MANSON'S
TROPICAL DISEASES

TWENTY-SECOND EDITION

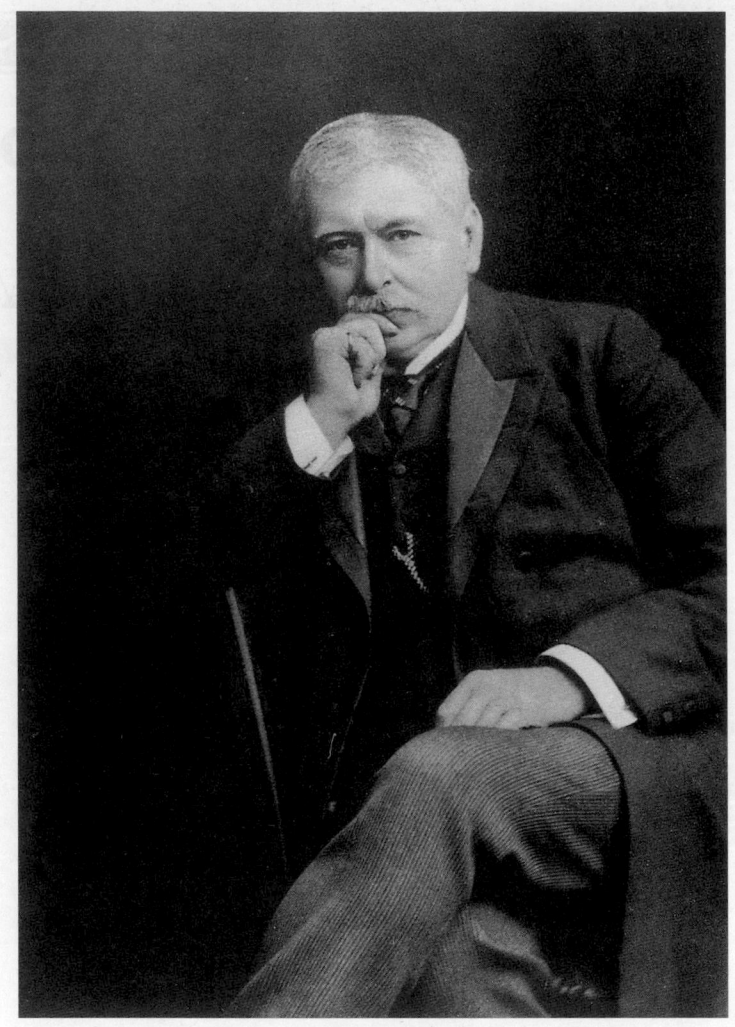

Sir Patrick Manson (1844–1922), GCMG, FRS

Commissioning Editor: Sue Hodgson
Development Editor: Louise Cook
Editorial Assistants: Rachael Harrison & Poppy Garraway
Project Managers: Glenys Norquay & Camilla Cudjoe
Design: Charles Gray
Illustration Manager: Merlyn Harvey
Illustrator: H. L. Studios
Marketing Managers (UK/USA): Clara Toombs/Courtney Ingram

MANSON'S

TROPICAL DISEASES

TWENTY-SECOND EDITION

Gordon C. Cook MD DSc FRCP(Lond) FRCP(Edin) FRACP FLS

Visiting Professor, Department of Medical Microbiology and Centre for Infectious Diseases, Royal Free and University College London Medical School, London, UK; President, The Royal Society of Tropical Medicine and Hygiene (1993–1995); Formerly Professor of Medicine, the Universities of Zambia, Riyadh (Saudi Arabia) and Papua New Guinea; Consultant Physician at University College Hospitals Trust, Hospital for Tropical Diseases, London; St Luke's Hospital for the Clergy and Senior Lecturer at the London School of Hygiene and Tropical Medicine, London, UK; President, The Fellowship of Postgraduate Medicine, London, UK 2000–2007; President, History of Medicine Section, Royal Society of Medicine, UK

Alimuddin I. Zumla BSc MBChB MSc PhD FRCP(Lond) FRCP(Edin)

Professor of Infectious Diseases and International Health, University College London, University College London Medical School; Director, Centre for Infectious Diseases and International Health, Windeyer Institute of Medical Sciences, University College London, London, UK; Honorary Consultant in Infectious Disease, University College London Hospitals NHS Trust and St. Luke's Hospital for Clergy, London UK; Honorary Professor, Liverpool School of Tropical Medicine, University of Liverpool, UK: Visiting Professor, Department of Medicine, University of Cape Town, South Africa; Honorary Professor, University of Zambia School of Medicine, Lusaka, Zambia; Formerly Associate Professor, Centre for Infectious Diseases, University of Texas Health Science Center at Houston, School of Medicine and Public Health, Houston, Texas, USA; Vice President, Royal Society of Tropical Medicine and Hygiene (2004–2006); Member of the Court of Governors, London School of Hygiene and Tropical Medicine, London, UK

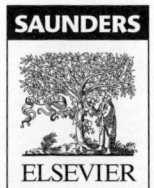

SAUNDERS

ELSEVIER

SAUNDERS
ELSEVIER

SAUNDERS an imprint of Elsevier Limited
© 2009, Elsevier Limited. All rights reserved.
© Dominic Kwiatkoski—Chapter 5 text; © David Yorston—Chapter 18 figures;
© David Warrell—Chapter 31 and 44 figures; © Suchitra Nimmannitya—Chapter 41 figures

First published 2009

First edition published in 1898
Twenty-first edition published 2003

The right of Gordon C. Cook and Alimuddin I. Zumla to be identified as authors of this work
has been asserted by them in accordance with the Copyright, Designs and Patents Act 1988.

Main Edition ISBN: *978-1-4160-4470-3*
International Edition ISBN: *978-1-4160-4471-0*

British Library Cataloguing in Publication Data
A catalogue record for this book is available from the British Library

Library of Congress Cataloging in Publication Data
A catalog record for this book is available from the Library of Congress

Notice
Medical knowledge is constantly changing. Standard safety precautions must be followed, but as
new research and clinical experience broaden our knowledge, changes in treatment and drug
therapy may become necessary or appropriate. Readers are advised to check the most current
product information provided by the manufacturer of each drug to be administered to verify the
recommended dose, the method and duration of administration, and contraindications. It is the
responsibility of the practitioner, relying on experience and knowledge of the patient, to determine
dosages and the best treatment for each individual patient. Neither the Publisher nor the author
assume any liability for any injury and/or damage to persons or property arising from this
publication.

The Publisher

ELSEVIER your source for books,
journals and multimedia
in the health sciences
www.elsevierhealth.com

Working together to grow
libraries in developing countries

www.elsevier.com | www.bookaid.org | www.sabre.org

ELSEVIER   BOOK AID   Sabre Foundation
            International

The
Publisher's
policy is to use
**paper manufactured
from sustainable forests**

Printed in China
Last digit is the print number: 9 8 7 6 5 4 3 2 1

Contents

Contents

Contents

Preface to the First Edition

A manual on the diseases of warm climates, of handy size, and yet giving adequate information, has long been a want; for the exigencies of travel and tropical life are, as a rule, incompatible with big volumes and large libraries. This is the reason for the present work.

While it is hoped that the book may prove of practical service, it makes no pretension to being anything more than an introduction to the important department of medicine of which it treats; in no sense is it put forward as a complete treatise, or as being in this respect comparable to the more elaborate works by Davidson, Schebe, Rho, Laveran, Corre, Roux, and other systematic writers in the same field. The author avails himself of this opportunity to acknowledge the valuable assistance he has received, in revising the text, from Dr. L. Westerna Sambon and Mr David Rees, MRCP LRCP lately Senior House Surgeon, Seamen's Hospital, Albert Docks, London. He would also acknowledge his great obligation to Mr Richard Muir, Pathological Laboratory, Edinburgh University, for his care and skill in preparing the illustrations.

Patrick Manson
April 1898

Preface to the Twenty-Second Edition

When Sir Patrick Manson GCMG, FRS (1844–1922) wrote his great text subtitled *'A manual of the diseases of warm climates'* in 1898, he could not have envisaged that a century and more later the work was to be in ever greater use by medical practitioners throughout the world. The textbook has in fact evolved and expanded to cover *all* of the diseases associated with tropical exposure, and not merely those about which something was known in the late nineteenth century, and about which the average medical practitioner in England and other temperate lands knew little.

The twenty-second edition of *Manson's Tropical Diseases* has in the main followed a pattern laid down in the twentieth edition (1996). The chapter headings are similar to those in the twenty-first edition, with the exception that, in order to keep the book to reasonable dimensions we have excluded the chapter on 'High Altitude problems'. The majority of the contributors to that edition have accepted our invitation to write again and update their chapters; however there are several new authors who share their experience and wisdom. We offer them a warm welcome and sincere thanks for their valuable input. There is a vast array of international talent included in this essentially British textbook which ranks as one of the oldest *clinical* treatises in the medical literature.

It is also our sad duty to record the sudden and tragic death of Professor CA Hart, one of our most prolific contributors, during the preparation of the present edition. We are indebted to Luis Cuevas for a tribute to Tony Hart, Professor of Microbiology at Liverpool University, who died in September 2007 aged 58 years.

We would again like to thank our Publishers for making our task relatively straightforward, especially our development editor Louise Cook, who has 'held the fort' throughout the publication of this edition. Finally we thank our respective wives Jane and Farzana for their continuing forbearance while we devoted countless hours to editorial tasks associated with this edition.

We trust that physicians, medical officers, postgraduate tropical medical students, infectious diseases physicians, parasitologists and other health personnel throughout the world will continue to delve into and benefit from what has rightly become widely known as the 'Bible' of tropical medicine. We commend the latest edition of this venerable work to all medical and paramedical health personnel throughout the world.

Gordon C Cook
Alimuddin I Zumla
2008

List of Contributors

Adewale O. Adebajo MBBS MSc FMCP FWACP FACP FRCP
Honorary Senior Lecturer and Associate Director
  of Teaching
Academic Rheumatology Group, Division of
Genomic Medicine
University of Sheffield Medical School
Sheffield, UK

Dwomoa Adu BCHIR MB MD FRCP
Consultant Physician and Nephrologist
Queen Elizabeth Medical Centre
Birmingham, UK

Yusuf Ahmed BM
Visiting Senior Lecturer
Department of Obstetrics and Gynaecology
School Of Medicine
University of Zambia
Lusaka, Zambia

Sandra Amor BSc PhD
Associate Professor
Department of Pathology – Neuropathology
VU Medical Center
Amsterdam, The Netherlands

Felix I. Anjorin MBBS FMCP FWACP
Professor of Medicine, Consultant Physician & Cardiologist,
  Vice-Chancellor and Provost
College of Medicine
Bingham University
Jos, Nigeria

Jeffrey K. Aronson MA MBChB DPhil FRCP FPharmacolS FFPM(Hon)
Reader in Clinical Pharmacology
University Department of Primary Health Care
University of Oxford
Oxford, UK

Masharip Atadzhanov MD PhD DSc FRCP
Professor of Neurology
Department of Internal Medicine
School of Medicine
University of Zambia
Lusaka, Zambia

Guy Baily MD FRCP
Consultant Physician
Department of Infection and Immunity
St Bartholomew's and The London NHS Trust
London, UK

John R. Baker BSc(Lond) PhD(Lond) DSc MA(Cantab) FiBol
Royal Society for Tropical Medicine and Hygiene
London, UK

Imelda Bates BSc MBBS MD MRCP MRCPath
Senior Lecturer in Tropical Haematology
Liverpool School of Tropical Medicine
Liverpool, UK

Raman Bedi BDS MSc DDS DSc FDSRCS FGDP FPHM DipHE
Professor
Global Child Health Dental Taskforce
King's College London
London, UK

Ronald H. Behrens MD BSc MBChB FRCP
Consultant in Travel Medicine
Hospital for Tropical Diseases
Mortimer Market Centre
London, UK

Solomon R. Benatar MBChB DSc(Med) FFA SA, FRCP(Lond)
FACP(Hon) FCP SA(Hon) FRS(SAfr)
Professor in Public Health Sciences
University of Toronto
Emeritus Professor of Medicine and Director
  Bioethics Centre
Faculty of Health Sciences
University of Cape Town
Cape, South Africa

Gerard C. Bodeker EdD MPsych
Adjunct Professor of Epidemiology
Columbia University;
Hon Senior Clinical Lecturer in Public Health
University of Oxford Medical School
London, UK

Bernard J. Brabin MB ChB MSc PhD FRCPC FRCPCH
Professor of Tropical Paediatrics
Child and Reproductive Health Group
Liverpool School of Tropical Medicine
Liverpool, UK

Rodney A. Bray BA PhD CBiol MIBiol FLS
Scientific Associate
Department of Zoology
Natural History Museum
Witham, Essex, UK

Simon Brooker DPhil
Reader in Tropical Epidemiology and Disease Control
Department of Infectious and Tropical Diseases
London School of Hygiene and Tropical Medicine
London, UK

Annette K. Broom BSC PhD
Senior Research Officer
Arbovirus Surveillance and Research Laboratory
Department of Microbiology
University of Western Australia
Nedlands, Western Australia, Australia

Reto Brun PhD
Research Group Leader
Parasite Chemotherapy
Swiss Tropical Institute
Basel, Switzerland

James E. G. Bunn MBBS MSc DCH MRCP DTM&H FRCPCH
Associate Professor
Community Health and Paediatrics
College of Medicine
Blantyre, Malawi

Donald A. P. Bundy PhD
Lead Specialist
School of Health and Nutrition
Human Development Division
The World Bank
Washington DC, USA

Christian Burri MSc PhD
Deputy Head of Department
Pharmaceutical Medicine Unit
Swiss Centre for International Health
Swiss Tropical Institute
Basel, Switzerland

Ana-Maria Cevallos PhD
Department of Gastroenterology
St Bartholomew's Hospital
London, UK

Richard E. Chaisson MD
Professor of Medicine, Epidemiology and International
Health
Centre for Tuberculosis Research
Johns Hopkins University School of Medicine
Baltimore, MD USA

Peter L. Chiodini BSc MBBS PhD MRCS FRCP FRCPath
FFTMRCPS(Glas)
Consultant Parasitologist
Department of Clinical Parasitology
Hospital for Tropical Diseases; and London School of
Hygiene and Tropical Medicine
London, UK

Sunil Chopra MD
Consultant Dermatologist
King George's Hospital, Ilford, Essex;
The London Dermatology Centre
London, UK

Timothy J. Coleman MB BS PhD
Director, Leptospira Reference Unit
Public Health Laboratory Service,
Health Protection Agency
Hereford, UK

Kenneth J. Collins MBBS MRCS BSc DPhil(Oxon) FRCP
Formerly Director of MRC, Thermoregulation Unit;
Honorary Senior Clinical Lecturer
University College and St Pancras Hospitals
London, UK

Gordon C. Cook MD DSc FRCP FRCPE FRACP FLS
Visiting Professor, Department of Medical Microbiology and
Centre for Infectious Diseases, Royal Free and University
College London Medical School, London, UK; President,
The Royal Society of Tropical Medicine and Hygiene (1993–
1995); Formerly Professor of Medicine, the Universities of
Zambia, Riyadh (Saudi Arabia) and Papua New Guinea;
Consultant Physician at University College Hospitals Trust,
Hospital for Tropical Diseases, London; St Luke's Hospital
for the Clergy and Senior Lecturer at the London School of
Hygiene and Tropical Medicine, London, UK; President, The
Fellowship of Postgraduate Medicine, London, UK 2000–
2007; President, History of Medicine Section, Royal Society
of Medicine, UK

John B. S. Coulter MD FRCP(I) FRCPCH
Honorary Clinical Lecturer
Liverpool School of Tropical Medicine
Liverpool, UK

George O. Cowan OBE FRCP
JCHMT
London, UK

Dorothy H. Crawford PhD MD DSc FRCPath
Professor of Medical Microbiology
Centre for Infectious Diseases
Edinburgh University Medical School
Edinburgh, UK

Julia A. Critchley MSc DPhil
Senior Lecturer
Institute of Health and Society
The Medical School
Newcastle University
Newcastle Upon Tyne, UK

Luis E. Cuevas MD DTCH MTropMed
Reader in Tropical Epidemiology
Liverpool School of Tropical Medicine
Liverpool, UK

Nigel A. Cunliffe BSc(Hons) MB ChB PhD MRCP DTM&H
Lecturer in Medical Microbiology
Department of Medical Microbiology and
    Genitourinary Medicine
The University of Liverpool
Liverpool, UK

David A. B. Dance MBChB MSc FRCPath
Regional Microbiologist
Health Protection Agency South West
Plymouth
Devon, UK

Andrew Davis MD FRCP(Edin) FFPHM DTM&H
Formerly Director, Parasitic Diseases Programme
World Health Organization
Geneva, Switzerland

P. Shanthamali de Silva MBBS DCH, MRCP(Paed) UK FRCP FSLCP
President
Sri Lanka College of Paediatricians
Colombo, Sri Lanka

Jean-Pierre Dedet MD MSc
Head, Laboratoire de Parasitologie-Mycologie
Centre Hospitalier Universitair, Montpellier;
Director, Centre National de Reference des Leishmania,
Montpellier;
Director, WHO Collaborating Centre on Leishmaniasis
Professor of Parasitology
Laboratoire de Parasitologie
Universite Montpellier 1
Montepellier, France

Mohammed R. Essop MBBCh MDCP FCP(SA) FACC FRCP(Lond)
Professor of Medicine and Cardiology
Baragwanath Hospital and University of the Witwatersrand
Chief-Division of Cardiology
Johannesburg, South Africa

Alice E. Eyers
c/o John E. Eyers

John E. Eyers BA MLS MIInfSc
Deputy Librarian
London School of Hygiene and Tropical Medicine
London, UK

Michael J. G. Farthing MD FRCP
Principal
St George's Hospital Medical School
University of London
London, UK

Alan F. Fleming MA MD FRCpath
Formerly Consultant Haemotologist
Somerset, UK

Neil French MBChB FRCP PhD
Reader in Infectious Diseases, Epidemiology
Karonga Prevention Study/London School of Hygiene and
    Tropical Medicine
Chilumba, Karonga District, Malawi

Göran Friman MD PhD
Professor
Department of Medical Sciences
Uppsala University Hospital
Uppsala, Sweden

Stephen H. Gillespie MD DSc FRCP FRCPath
Professor of Medical Microbiology
Department of Infection
Royal Free and University College Medical School
London, UK

Catherine Goodman PhD
Lecturer, Health Economics and Policy
Health Policy Unit
Department of Public Health and Policy
Kenya Medical Research Institute/Wellcome Trust Research
    Programme
Nairobi, Kenya

Stephen B. Gordon MA MD FRCP DTM&H
Senior Clinical Lecturer in Tropical Respiratory Medicine
Liverpool School of Tropical Medicine
Liverpool, UK

Bruno Gottstein PhD
Professor of Medical and Veterinary Parasitology
Institute of Parasitology
University of Bern
Bern, Switzerland

Stephen M. Graham MB BS FRACP DTCH
Associate Professor
Centre for International Child Health
University of Melbourne Department of Paediatrics
Royal Children's Hospital
Victoria, Australia

John M. Grange MSc MD
Visiting Professor
Centre for Infectious Diseases and International Heatlh
Royal Free and University College Medical School
London, UK

Goran Günther MD PhD
Section of Infectious Diseases
Department of Medical Sciences
Uppsala University Akademiska Sjukhuset
Uppsala, Sweden

Roy A. Hall PhD
Department of Microbiology and Parasitology
University of Queensland
Brisbane, Queensland, Australia

The late **C. Anthony Hart** MBBS BSc PhD FRCPCH PRCPath
Formerly Professor of Medical Microbiology
Department of Medical Microbiology
University of Liverpool Medical School
Liverpool, UK

Melissa Haswell-Elkins BA MSc PhD
Senior Lecturer Public Health (Mental Health)
North Queensland Health Equalities Promotion Unit
School of Medicine
University of Queensland
Queensland, Australia

Alan Haworth OBE FRCPsych DPM
Professor of Psychiatry
Department of Psychiatry
School of Medicine
University of Zambia
Lusaka, Zambia

Roderick J. Hay DM FRCP FRCPath
Professor of Dermatology
International Foundation for Dermatology
London, UK

Tran Tinh Hien MD
Vice Director
Wellcome Trust Clinical Research Unit
Hospital for Tropical Diseases
Ho Chi Minh City, Vietnam

Christopher J. Hoffman MD MPH
Fellow, Division of Infectious Diseases
John Hopkins School of Medicine
Baltimore, MD USA

Richard E. Holliman MD FRCPath DSc
Consultant and Reader in Clinical Microbiology
Department of Medical Microbiology
St George's Hospital and Medical School
London, UK

John E. Jellis FRCS(Eng & Edin) FCSECSA
Formerly Professor in Orthopaedic Surgery
University of Zambia
Consultant Orthopaedic Surgeon
Zambian-Italian
Orthopaedic Hospital
Lusaka, Zambia

Claire Jenkins BSc MSc PhD
Clinical Scientist
External Quality Assessment Department
Health Protection Agency
London, UK

Cheryl A. Johansen BSc MSc
Research Officer
Arbovirus Surveillance and Research Laboratory
Department of Microbiology
University of Western Australia
Nedlands, Western Australia, Australia

Sasithorn Kaewkes MD
Head
Department of Parasitology
Faculty of Medicine
Khon Khaen University
Khon Khaen, Thailand

Moses Kapembwa PhD MSc BSc MBChB FRCP(Lond) FRCP(Edin)
Consultant Physician and Senior Lecturer (Hon)
Department of Genitourinary and HIV Medicine
North West London Hospitals NHS Trust
Northwick Park and St Marks Hospitals
Middlesex, UK

Michael G. Kawooya MBChB MMed Radiology
Associate Professor of Radiology
Makerere University
Department of Radiology
Mulago Hospital
Kampala, Uganda

Paul Kelly MA MD FRCP
Reader in Tropical Gastroenterology
Department of Gastroenterology
St Bartholomew's and The London School of Medicine
London, UK

Mario A. Knight MD
c/o St Bartholomew's Hospital
London, UK

Dominic Kwiatkowski FRCP FRCPCH F Med Sci
MRC Clinical Research Professor
Wellcome Trust Centre for Human Genetics
Oxford, UK

Gary Maartens MBChB MMed FCP(SA) DTM&H
Professor of Clinical Pharmacology
Division of Clinical Pharmacology
University of Cape Town
Cape, South Africa

David C. W. Mabey DM FRCP
Professor, Clinical Research Unit
London School of Hygiene and Tropical Medicine
London, UK

John S. Mackenzie PhD
Emeritus Professor of Tropical Infectious Diseases
Australian Biosecurity CRC
Curtin University of Technology
Perth, Australia

Charles R. Madeley MB ChB MD FRCPath
Professor of Clinical Virology
University of Newcastle Upon Tyne
Newcastle-upon-Tyne, UK

M. Monir Madkour MD DM FRCP(Lond)
Consultant Physician
Department of Medicine
Riyadh Armed Forces Hospital
Riyadh, Saudi Arabia

D. D. Murray McGavin MD FRCS Ed, FRC Opth FRCP Ed
Honorary President
Icthes World Care
Glasgow, UK

Michael A. Miles MSc PhD DSc FRCPath
Professor of Medical Protozoology
Department of Infectious and Tropical Diseases
London School of Hygiene and Tropical Medicine
London, UK

Robert F. Miller MBBS, FRCP
Reader in Clinical Infection
Research Department of Infection and Population Health
University College London
London, UK

Alan E. Mills MA MB DCP DPath FRCPA FACTM FFPath RCPI
Pathologist
Dorevitch Pathology
Bendigo, Victoria, Australia

Anthony Moody MPhil MIBiol FIBMS
Formerly Head, BMS and Laboratory Manager
Department of Clinical Parasitology
University College Hospital
London, UK

Ayesha A. Motala MBChB MD FRCP
Professor of Medicine
Department of Endocrinology, Division of Internal Medicine
Nelson R. Mandela School of Medicine
University of KwaZulu-Natal
Durban, South Africa

Zeridah Muyinda MBChB MMed Radiology
Consultant Radiologist
Mulago Hospital
Makerere University
Kampala, Uganda

Peter Mwaba MMed
Research Fellow and Honorary Lecturer
Centre for Infectious Diseases, London;
Department of Medicine
University of Zambia School of Medicine
Lusaka, Zambia

Datshana P. Naidoo MD
Professor of Cardiology
Inkosi Albert Luthuli Central Hospital
Durban, South Africa

Osamu Nakagomi MD
Professor of Molecular Epidemiology
Department of Molecular Microbiology and Immunology
Graduate School of Biomedical Sciences
Nagasaki University
Nagasaki, Japan

Suchitra Nimmannitya MD MPH
Clinical Professor of Pediatrics, Senior Consultant
Queen Sirikit National Institute of Child Health
WHO/QSNICH Collaborative Centre for Case Management
of DF/DHF
Bangkok, Thailand

Stephen Owens MB ChB MTropPaed MRCPCH
Specialist Registrar in Paediatrics, Honorary Research Fellow
Child and Reproduction Health Group
Liverpool School of Tropical Medicine
Liverpool, UK

Shirley Owusu-Ofori CTM MB ChB BSc FGCP
Senior Specialist, Head of Transfusion Medicine Unit
Department of Medicine
Komfo Anokye Teaching Hospital
Kumasi, Ghana, West Africa

Joseph S. M. Peiris DPhil(Oxon) MBBS FRCPath FHKAM (Path)FRS
Chair Professor;
Honorary Consultant Microbiologist and Head of Division
   of Clinical Virology
Department of Microbiology
The University of Hong Kong
Queen Mary Hospital
Hong Kong, China

Fraser J. Pirie MBChB FCP(SA) MD(Natal)
Senior Lecturer
Department of Endocrinology
Division of Internal Medicine
Nelson R. Mandela School of Medicine
University of KwaZulu-Natal
Durban, South Africa

Francine Pratlong PhD
Curator of the International Cryobank of Leishmania
Centre National de Reference des Leishmania
Montpellier;
WHO Collaborating Centre on Leishmaniasis
Montpellier;
Laboratoire Parasitologie
Universite Montpellier
Montpellier, France

Jürg Reichen MD
Professor of Medicine
Department of Clinical Pharmacology
University of Berne
Berne, Switzerland

John Richens MA MBBS MSc FRCPE
Clinical Lecturer
Department of Sexually Transmitted Diseases
Division of Pathology and Infectious Diseases
Royal Free and University College Medical School
London, UK

Ivan M. Roitt DSc HonFRCP FRCPath FRS
Emeritus Professor of Immunology
Department of Immunology and Molecular Pathology
Royal Free and University College Medical School
Windeyer Institue of Medical Sciences
London, UK

Dirk Schoonbaert
Librarian
Institute of Tropical Medicine
Antwerpen, Belgium

Geoffrey M. Scott MD FRCP FRCPath DTM&H
Honorary Senior Lecturer
Department of Medicine;
Consultant Clinical Microbiologist
Department of Clinical Microbiology
University College London Hospitals
London, UK

Crispian Scully CBE MD PhD MDS MRCS FDSRCS FDSRCPS FFDRCSI
FRCPath FMedSci DSc
Professor of Special Care Dentistry
University College London;
Co-director, WHO Collaborating Centre
Eastman Dental Institute
London, UK

Paul Shears MD FRCPath
Consultant Medical Microbiologist
Royal Hallamshire Hospital
Sheffield Teaching Hospitals NHS Foundation Trust
Sheffield, UK

Nandini P. Shetty MSc MD FRCPath DipHIC
Consultant Microbiologist
Department of Clinical Microbiology
Health Protection Agency Collaborating Centre
University College Hospital London
London, UK

Prakash S. Shetty MD PhD FFPHM FRCP
Professor of Human Nutrition
Institute of Human Nutrition
Southampton General Hospital
University of Southampton
Southampton, UK

Paul E. Simonsen PhD
Senior Researcher
Danis Bilharziasis Laboratory - Centre for Health Research
and Development
University of Copenhagen
Charlottenlund, Denmark

Paiboon Sithithaworn MD
Department of Parasitology
Faculty of Medicine
Khon Kaen University
Khon Kaen, Thailand

Michael D. Smith BM MRCP FRCPath
Consultant Microbiologist
Department of Microbiology
Musgrove Park Hospital
Somerset, UK

David W. Smith BMeDSc MBBS FRCPA
Head of Department
Division of Microbiology and Infectious Diseases
PathWest Laboratory Medicine WA
Nedlands, WA, Australia

Eugene Sobngwi MD PhD
Senior Lecturer
Department of Epidemiology
Institute of Health and Society
Newcastle University
Newcastle-Upon-Tyne, UK

Tom Solomon DTMH FRCP PhD
Professor of Neurology, Medical Microbiology and Tropical
   Medicine
MRC Senior Clinical Fellow
Brain Infections Group
University of Liverpool
Liverpool, UK

Vaughan R. Southgate BSc PhD CBiol FIBiol FLS
Scientific Associate
Department of Zoology
The Natural History Museum
London, UK

Banchob Sripa PhD
Associate Professor of Pathology
Department of Pathology
Faculty of Medicine
Khon Kaen, Thailand

Robert Steffen MD
Director, WHO Collaborating Centre for Travellers'
   Health
Professor and Head
Division of Epidemiology and Prevention of
Communicable Diseases
Institute for Social and Preventative Medicine
University of Zurich
Zurich, Switzerland

John R. Sullivan MD
c/o Dr M Rinks
Dorevitch Pathology
Victoria, Australia

Gail Thomson MD
Specialist Registrar in Infectious Diseases
North Manchester General Hospital
Manchester, Greater Manchester, UK

Eric John Threlfall BSc PhD
Head of Antibiotic Resistance/Epidemiology Laboratory
Laboratory of Enteric Pathogens
Central Public Health Laboratory
London, UK

Raj C. Thuraisingham MD FRCP
Consultant Nephrologist
Department of Renal Medicine and Transplantation
Royal London Hospital
London, UK

Catherine L. Thwaites MD
Research Registrar
University of Oxford Wellcome Trust Clinical Research Unit
Ho Chi Minh City, Vietnam

Eli Tumba Tshibwabwa MD PhD
Associate Professor of Radiology
McMaster University Medical Centre
Department of Radiology
Ontario, Canada

Nigel Unwin DM FFPH FRCP
Professor of Epidemiology
Institute of Health and Society
The Medical School
Newcastle University
Newcastle upon Tyne, UK

Francisco Vega-López MD MSc PhD
Consultant Dermatologist and Honorary Senior Lecturer
University College London Hospitals NHS Trust
London School of Hygiene and Tropical Medicine
London, UK

Damian G. Walker BSc MSc PhD
Assistant Professor of Health Economics
Department of International Health
Johns Hopkins Bloomberg School of Public Health
Baltimore, MD USA

David C. Warhurst BSc PhD DSc FRCPath
Emeritus Professor of Protozoan Chemotherapy
Department of Infections and Tropical Diseases
London School of Hygiene and Tropical Medicine
London, UK

David A. Warrell MA DM DSc FRCP FRCPE FMedSci
Professor of Tropical Medicine and Infectious Diseases
Nuffield Department of Clinical Medicine
University of Oxford
Oxford, UK

Mary J. Warrell MB FRCPath MRCP
Honorary Senior Researcher
Centre for Clinical Vaccinology and Tropical Medicine
Churchill Hospital
Oxford, UK

Nicholas J. White OBE DSc MD FRCP FMedSci
Professor of Tropical Medicine
Mahidol University and Oxford University
Faculty of Tropical Medicine
Mahidol University
Bangkok, Thailand

Graham B. White MB ChB
Richmond
Surrey, UK

Hilary Williams MB ChB, BMedSci, MRCP
Clinical and Basic Virology Laboratory
School of Biomedical and Clinical Laboratory Services
University of Edinburgh
Edinburgh, UK

Stephen G. Withington MBChB FRACP
Consultant Physician
Department of Medicine
Ashburton Hospital
Ashburton, New Zealand

Sarah Wyllie PhD
Specialist Registrar
Department of Microbiology
Southampton General Hospital
Southampton, UK

Lam Mihn Yen MD
Director
Tetanus Unit
Hospital for Tropical Diseases
Ho Chi Minh City, Vietnam

David Yorston FRCOphth
Consultant Vitreo-Retinal Surgeon
Ophthalmic advisor to Christian Blind Mission
Tennent Institute
Gartnavel Hospital
Glasgow, UK

Arie J. Zuckerman MD DSc FRCP FRCPath FMedSci Dip Bact
Emeritus Professor of Medical Microbiology and
    Former Dean
Academic Centre for Travel Medicine and Vaccines
Royal Free and University College Medical School
London, UK

Jane N. Zuckerman MD FRCP(Ed) FRCPath FFPH
FFPM MRCGP FIBiol
Director, WHO Collaborating Centre for Reference,
    Research and Training in Travel Medicine
Senior Lecturer and Honorary Consultant
Academic Centre for Travel Medicine and Vaccines
Royal Free and University College Medical School
London, UK

Alimuddin I. Zumla BSc MBChB MSc PhD FRCP(Lon) FRCP(Edin)
Professor of Infectious Diseases and International Health,
University College London, University College London
Medical School; Director, Centre for Infectious Diseases and
International Health, Windeyer Institute of Medical Sci-
ences, University College London, London, UK; Honorary
Consultant in Infectious Disease, University College London
Hospitals NHS Trust and St Luke's Hospital for Clergy,
London UK; Honorary Professor, Liverpool School of Tropi-
cal Medicine, University of Liverpool, UK; Visiting Professor,
Department of Medicine, University of Cape Town, South
Africa; Honorary Professor, University of Zambia School of
Medicine, Lusaka, Zambia; Formerly Associate Professor,
Centre for Infectious Diseases, University of Texas Health
Science Center at Houston, School of Medicine and Public
Health, Houston, Texas, USA; Vice President, Royal Society
of Tropical Medicine and Hygiene (2004–2006); Member of
the Court of Governors, London School of Hygiene and
Tropical Medicine, London, UK

Charles Anthony Hart (1949–2007)

'Tony was the youngest professor to be appointed to this department and he also acted as Regional Microbiologist and Honorary Consultant. His prolific work focussed on infectious and tropical diseases and his papers had a great relevance for developing countries and for children in particular. He published more than 750 peer-reviewed papers and 12 textbooks, participated in numerous national and international committees and received many hundreds of lecture invitations. Despite this enormous workload his office was always open and visitors welcomed by a handshake, cup of tea and a nickname that made them feel at home. He travelled overseas many times to locations such as Brazil and South East Asia. Nothing could be better than a hard days work followed by a brainstorming session at the end of the day with a caipirinha or gin and tonic in hand. Colleagues anticipating his overseas arrival often asked what to do. The response: keep Tony busy, seek ideas for what studies to do, and avoid an idle day in the sun. If he was whistling at the end of the day it meant you had done well!

Tony's primary interest in paediatric infections led to ground-breaking work on meningitis, rotavirus diarrhoea and respiratory infections. He was always fascinated by differences between the profile of infection in developing countries and the UK, and how easily accepted dogmas could come crumbling down by competent research. He encouraged colleagues to undertake research and had the ability to identify promising research projects. Reports of pathogens were thus queuing on his desk, from first reports of Metapneumovirus and Bocavirus in Iran, Yemen, Brazil and Jordan, Cryptosporidium in Kenya, Malawi, Saudi Arabia, Brazil and Gaza, to clinical scores, quantitative PCR and pathogenesis of meningitis in Brazil and Ethiopia. The joint chapter on meningitis published in the present edition exemplifies his work. We have lost a great scientist and an excellent friend.'

Luis E. Cuevas
2008

Chapter 1

Gordon C. Cook

History of Tropical Medicine, and Medicine in the Tropics

European doctors practised in *tropical* countries as early as the seventeenth and eighteenth centuries in the English West Indies (the 'Sugar Islands'), India, the East Indies and later Africa, the western coast of which was widely termed the 'white man's grave'.[1-3] Many also produced monographs describing their experiences, with an outline of the disease pattern at these various locations. Many infections which now fall under the 'tropical' umbrella were widely distributed in northern Europe and northern America during the seventeenth to nineteenth centuries. For example, William Shakespeare (1564–1616) was well aware of malaria in England: 'he is so shak'd by the burning quotidian tertian that it is most lamentable to behold' (*Henry V*, II. i. 123). Thomas Sydenham (1624–1689) successfully used fever-tree bark (containing quinine) in the management of the 'intermittent fevers' during the seventeenth century.[4] Indigenous *Plasmodium vivax* infection remained a clinical problem in south-east England well into the twentieth century. Plague, typhoid, cholera, typhus and smallpox were major health hazards in Britain, London included, during the Victorian era.[5] John Bunyan (1628–1688) was well aware of the consumption (tuberculosis) – now such an important disease in 'tropical' countries – which so often 'took him down to the grave' (*The Life and Death of Mr Badman*).

What then is tropical medicine? Andrew Balfour (1873–1931)[2] summarized the position as he saw it, in his Presidential Address to the Royal Society of Tropical Medicine and Hygiene in 1925: 'there is in one sense no such thing as tropical medicine, and in any case many of the most erudite writings of Hippocrates are concerned with maladies which nowadays are chiefly encountered under tropical or subtropical conditions'. Some, including many historians, consider that 'tropical medicine' originated as a by-product of the British Empire and Raj.[6] The truth of the matter is that 'medicine in the tropics' was exploited by the Colonialists in order that the health of British personnel, both overseas and following return to the UK, could be improved (see below).[3] The specialty, in fact, as a formal discipline, had its origin(s) in a multidisciplinary background: major areas of progress during the nineteenth century were public health (and hygiene), travel and exploration, natural history, evolutionary theory, and a precise knowledge of the causation of disease (the 'germ theory').[3,7-9] The miasmatists and contagionists were previously at loggerheads. The development of clinical parasitology following the work of Manson, Ross and others (see below), and superimposed on this

complex backcloth, led to the inevitable genesis of 'tropical medicine' as a formal discipline.[3,9,10]

DEVELOPMENT OF TROPICAL MEDICINE AS A FORMAL DISCIPLINE

The Seamen's Hospital Society

In London, the Seamen's Hospital Society (SHS) (the 'foster mother of clinical tropical medicine') was formed in 1821, its predecessor being the Committee for Distressed (or destitute) Seamen, which was set up in the winter of 1817–1818; its raison d'être was to provide temporary relief to sick members of the mercantile marine then roaming in large number on London's docklands, streets.[1,3,11,12] The major objective was thus largely targeted at the management of illnesses (especially fevers and sexually transmitted diseases), many of which had been introduced into London from tropical and subtropical countries.[5] At a meeting held at the City of London Tavern on 8 March 1821 (William Wilberforce MP (1759–1833) was among those present), the committee resolved to establish a *permanent* floating hospital on the Thames for the exclusive use of sick and distressed seamen; the venture was to be supported by voluntary contributions. A series of hulks, HMS *Grampus* (lent by the Admiralty in 1821) (Figure 1.1), HMS *Dreadnought* (1831–1857) and HMS *Caledonia* (renamed *Dreadnought*) (1857–1870) were all anchored in Greenwich Reach and used successively; they had been 48, 98, and 120-gun vessels, respectively.[1,11,12] Although they served a valuable function, major practical problems arose: ventilation was poor, and nosocomial spread of disease occurred; lack of light was a major drawback during the winter months; and other problems (not least noise) associated with the situation in the midst of an extremely busy part of the River Thames proved tiresome.[12,13] In 1870, after protracted negotiations, the Commissioners of the Admiralty granted the SHS a 99-year lease of the Infirmary (and adjoining Somerset Ward) of the Royal Hospital, Greenwich, in lieu of the loan of the ship(s).[1,11,12] This move was made possible by a sharp decline in the number of pensioners residing in the hospital during the peaceful years following the battle of Waterloo (in 1815); the infirmary was therefore no longer required for them. In 1873, the hospital ceased being a permanent home for naval pensioners and

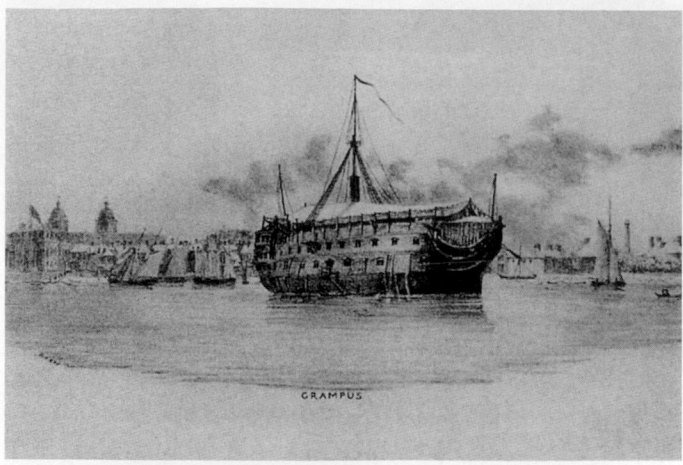

Figure 1.1 HMS *Grampus*. The first of three hospital-ships lent by the Admiralty to the Seamen's Hospital Society, anchored on Greenwich Reach. This disued 48-gun warship served in this capacity from October 1821 to October 1831.

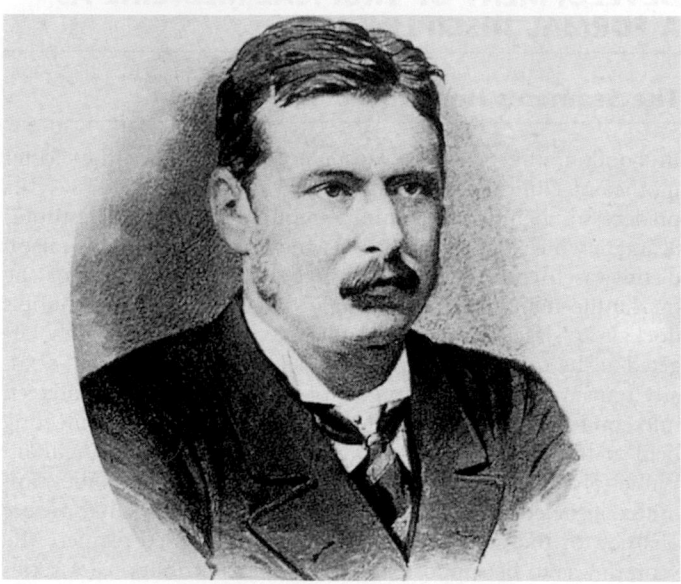

Figure 1.2 Dr (later Sir) Patrick Manson (1844–1922) aged 31 years. This photograph was probably taken while he was on leave in Britain from Amoy in 1875.

became the Royal Naval College (previously based at Portsmouth). The Royal Hospital[14] had been founded in 1694 by William III (1650–1702) and Mary as the naval equivalent of the Royal Hospital, Chelsea, founded by King Charles II, and is still in use for army pensioners today.

Emergence of the formal discipline in London

Following his return to London from Formosa and Amoy (where he had made his seminal discovery of man–mosquito transmission of the nematode *Filaria sanguinis hominis* (*Wuchereria bancrofti*), a causative agent of lymphatic filariasis) and Hong Kong, Patrick Manson (1844–1922)[3,8,15] (Figure 1.2) embarked on a

series of lectures devoted to 'tropical medicine' at several London medical schools.[1,3,16] The Rt Hon Joseph Chamberlain (1836–1914), Secretary of State for the Colonies, was immediately impressed at the possibility of sending Colonial medical staff on leave in Britain to these lectures, to give an update on the prevention and management of those diseases which seriously affected the 'servants of Empire'.[1,3] Regular trade, efficient administration and agricultural production were all seriously hampered by disease; Chamberlain's concept of 'constructive imperialism' could not be adequately developed in the presence of such a great deal of morbidity and mortality. Despite a great deal of opposition,[17] *clinical* tropical medicine emerged as both an important medical specialty and scientific discipline (the importance of parasites and their vectors in transmission of disease had only recently become clear – see above), Chamberlain considered that 'tropical medicine' was an essential component in the future development of British economic and social imperialism. It was, in fact, to become a 'colonial science'.[1,13] At the 1898 meeting of the British Medical Association held in Edinburgh, at which Ronald Ross's (1857–1932) work in Calcutta, India, on the role of the mosquito in *avian* malaria was announced (his initial demonstration at Secundarabad, India, of *Plasmodium* spp. development in the mosquito had been published in the *British Medical Journal* the previous year), a new section devoted to 'Tropical Medicine' was inaugurated.[10] There were several reasons why the discipline had not previously emerged. Many 'tropical diseases' had formerly existed in northern Europe (including England) and northern America. There was also widespread feeling that the high mortality rate affecting the white man in the tropics was inevitable, and that climate would prevent his living and working there successfully. The 'miasmatic theory' still held sway. Furthermore, there was an understandable pessimism regarding the possibility of significant environmental improvement in the foreseeable future, most British colonies being situated on unhealthy coastlines. Also, research had until then taken a very low priority for medical staff working in the tropics; their perceived task was solely to provide medical advice and care to the local British community.

The Manson–Chamberlain collaboration

In order to implement effective development of the 'new' discipline, Manson was appointed Medical Officer to the Colonial Office in 1897. Here, with Chamberlain's wholehearted support, he set about establishing a School of Tropical Medicine in London (LSTM).[1,3] A major problem relating to the venue of the proposed institution arose. Manson favoured the branch hospital of the Seamen's Hospital Society, situated near the Royal Albert Dock.[1,3,18] However, hostility to this suggestion arose from several quarters. The War Office favoured the Royal Victoria Hospital, Netley, which, situated on Southampton Water, had been founded in 1863;[1,3,19] it had been established principally for soldiers invalided from the Crimea and was then staffed by officers of the Royal Army Medical Corps. Manson considered this option unacceptable (he was already on the staff of the Albert Dock Hospital): the atmosphere and remote situation from London were, in his opinion, incompatible with the teaching of tropical medicine. The Royal College of Physicians was of the opinion that a new school was unnecessary. The senior medical staff of the Greenwich Hospital felt that removal of the 'tropical' cases to the Albert Dock Hospital (ADH) was a slight on their professional ability and was in any case undesirable because medical students from London's teaching hospitals were accustomed to visiting Greenwich for tuition in the diagnosis and management of these illnesses.[17] The end result was an outburst of acrimonious correspondence in the columns of the *Lancet*, the *British Medical Journal* and *The Times*, which later involved, among others, Sir William Broadbent, Sir William Church, Sir Jonathan Hutchinson and Sir Joseph Fayrer, the doyen of the Indian Medical Service. However, staunch determination from Manson and Herbert Read (Assistant Private Secretary to Chamberlain) to proceed with the project, strongly supported by Chamberlain himself, led to the rapid establishment of the proposed school at the ADH;[1,16,20] financial assistance to the tune of £3550 came from the Colonial Office. A subcommittee was set up to 'formulate a scheme for organisation and management of the LSTM in connection with the SHS'; the committee of management was to be composed of equal numbers of personnel from the SHS, the medical and surgical staff of the ADH, and teachers from the LSTM.

School and hospital in close proximity

The LSTM was officially opened on 2 October 1899.[1,3] The hospital (under SHS supervision) and teaching and research facilities at the LSTM were on the same site (Figure 1.3). With (Sir) Perceval Nairne (1841–1921) (Chairman of the SHS) presiding, the inaugural address – written by Manson – was read in his absence. He later declared: 'the school strikes, and strikes effectively, at the root of the principal difficulty of most of our Colonies-disease. It will cheapen government and make it more efficient. It will encourage and cheapen commercial enterprise. It will conciliate and foster the native'.[1,21] Meanwhile, a continuity funding was necessary, and several sources of income were exploited; two charity dinners, at which Chamberlain presided, were held at the Hotel Cecil in 1899 and 1905; they raised £12000 and £11000 respectively. At the former, Chamberlain declared:[1] 'The man who shall successfully grapple with this foe of humanity and find the cure for malaria, for the fever desolating our colonies . . . and shall make the tropics livable for white men . . . will do more for the world, more for the

British Empire, than the man who adds a new province to the wide Dominions of the Queen'. A 'Tropical Diseases Research Fund' was set up, and the Dean – (Sir) Francis Lovell (1844–1916) – raised funds on several overseas trips. In 1912, the school was enlarged and a new wing opened by Their Majesties King George V and Queen Mary. 'Tropical' cases were relatively few in the early days of the LSTM;[3,22] in fact, the ADH had been founded to care for seafarers and 'landsmen' in the London Docks – most of whom suffered from injuries.

In 1919, a decision was taken to relocate the school and hospital to central London; Endsleigh Palace Hotel, 25 Gordon Street, London WC1, was purchased (by the SHS with funding from the Red Cross) for £70000 and on 11 November, 1920 the Duke of York (later King George VI) (1895–1952) opened the joint LSTM and Hospital for Tropical Diseases (HTD) in this building.[1,13] The structure, which remains extant (and constitutes the student union of University College), provided five floors (at the top) for clinical tropical medicine, and four for the basic sciences; a radiology department was situated in the basement. Sir Philip Manson-Bahr (1881–1966)[12] considered the building 'dark, awkward and inconvenient, with multitudes of doors and narrow passages', but never before had there been 'more unanimity or good fellowship among the staff of the school and the hospital'. The Wellcome Tropical Museum was nearby and provided invaluable teaching resources.[1,13]

Between 1899 and 1929 the clinical specialty and the basic sciences were thus on the same site – first at the ADH[18] and later London WC1;[20] the close proximity was both valuable and productive, a great deal of teaching and clinical research being accomplished. For example, two research projects carried out by the clinical staff clinched the mosquito transmission of malaria saga in *Homo sapiens*. G. C. Low (1872–1952) (later in large part responsible for establishing the Royal Society of Tropical Medicine and Hygiene at Manson's House)[23,24] and three other investigators slept between dusk and dawn, for 3 months, in a mosquito-proof hut about 7 km from Rome, Italy (where *Plasmodium vivax* malaria was prevalent); by so doing they avoided a *P. vivax* infection.[1,3,8] Also, in 1900, three batches of mosquitoes infected with *P. vivax* were sent from Rome to London; Manson's elder surviving son – then a medical student at Guy's Hospital, and captain of rugby football – was exposed to them, and together with a technician, duly acquired a clinical attack of *P. vivax* infection, which responded to quinine.[1,3,7]

Foundation of the London School of Hygiene and Tropical Medicine: the close relationship between tropical physicians and basic scientific staff ends

In 1921, the Postgraduate Medical Committee recommended that an Institute of State Medicine Public Health be created in Bloomsbury, near the University of London; the Rockefeller Foundation was persuaded by Professor R. T. Leiper (1881–1969) to donate US$2 million to the Ministry of Health for the development of this facility.[1,13,20] On 18 July, 1929, the London School of Hygiene and Tropical Medicine (LSHTM) was officially opened at Keppel Street (Gower Street) by the Prince of Wales (later King Edward VIII) (1894–1972). Some years after this, the SHS ceased manag-

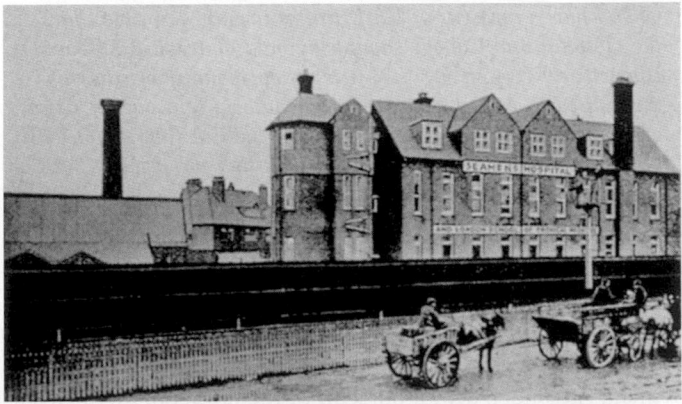

Figure 1.3 Newly opened London School of Tropical Medicine – situated on an adjoining site to the Seamen's Hospital Society's Branch (Albert Dock) Hospital – in October 1899.

ing the School, and *clinical* tropical medicine became detached from the basic sciences.

Clinical tropical medicine in London suffered a further temporary setback when the Ross Institute and Hospital for Tropical Diseases (Director: Sir Ronald Ross) was opened at Putney West Hill on 15 July, 1926.[1,13,25,26] It was, however, clear from the outset that there was insufficient clinical material in London to justify two hospitals devoted to the management of tropical disease; the project therefore had no chance of becoming viable from a clinical viewpoint. The institution ultimately became incorporated into the LSHTM, as the Ross Institute for Tropical Hygiene, with four beds at the HTD, in 1934; the Director had died 2 years previously.[3,26]

The itinerant saga of *clinical* tropical medicine in London continued unabated and the survival of Manson's original concept seemed at times in serious jeopardy – not least during World War II (1939–1945), when the specialty had to make do with a mere 10 beds – with no teaching facilities, at the *Dreadnought* (the SHS's land-based flagship) Hospital, Greenwich. For a brief period after the war, a nursing home in Devonshire Street, London W1, housed the discipline. In 1951, the HTD was transferred to St Pancras, NW1 and officially opened on 24 May (Empire Day) by the Duchess of Kent.[1,20] In late 1999, the latest (and possibly the final) move of the clinical discipline, to University College Hospital, took place;[20] regrettably, the facilities in that overcrowded setting were extremely limited.

Regarding the clinical discipline in London, Manson-Bahr[13] later concluded:

In recounting the chequered history of this institution, the Hospital for Tropical Diseases, a venture one would have thought essential to the greatest of all Empires, there runs the thread of insecurity . . . the hospital became the whipping boy of medical politics . . . The Board of the SHS was always a representative body of admirals whose interest lay in the sailor, but not in (clinical) tropical medicine.

The future of the clinical discipline in London remains anyone's guess![1,3,27]

DEVELOPMENT OF TROPICAL MEDICINE IN LIVERPOOL

This chapter has concentrated on the LSHTM because the principal catalyst for the 'formal discipline' – Manson (the 'Father of Tropical Medicine') established his school there. However, the Liverpool School of Tropical Medicine had opened about 6 months earlier.[1,3,28,29] Although the concept of a School of Tropical Medicine in Liverpool developed after that in London, the plan of action proceeded more rapidly, and the School was opened to students on 21 April, 1899. In many senses therefore, that one should be designated *the* Pioneer School of Tropical Medicine. The initial momentum had originated in a circular from Chamberlain to the General Medical Council and leading British medical schools (11 March, 1898), and a letter to the Governors of the Colonies (14 June, 1898). The timescale of the first appointments was impressive:[28,30] 20 January, 1899 – Dean appointed; 7 February – Demonstrator in tropical pathology (Dr H. E. Annett); 10 April – Lecturer in tropical medicine (Major Ronald Ross, IMS);

22 April – School officially opened by Lord Lister (1827–1912); May 1899 – teaching started. The Liverpool School was not a 'brainchild' of Manson/Chamberlain (unlike the LSTM), and it did not therefore receive Government support – a source of irritation (and perhaps even anger) at the time. It owed its inception to the initiative(s) of Mr (later Sir) Alfred Jones KCMG (1845–1909), a prominent Liverpool (an important seaport) figure, and an energetic leader in the development of Liverpool's overseas trade with the West African Colonies. He controlled the Elder Dempster shipping line, which traded with the Canary Islands and West Africa (and had a thriving business in bananas, groundnuts and oil nuts); local commerce had previously involved the 'triangular trade'. Together with several wealthy and generous Liverpool merchants, he also provided the financial backing for the School's foundation. The other major personality in the project was Dr (later Sir) Rubert Boyce, FRS (1863–1911) – the first Dean.

The project was encouraged by the Royal Society, whose Secretary wrote to the Principal of University College, Liverpool (18 November, 1898):[28,29]

I think the idea of starting something at Liverpool about Tropical Diseases in connection with the College, most admirable. The opportunities of studying Tropical Diseases are greater at Liverpool than anywhere else in England, excepting perhaps London. You have to arrange: 1. For teaching. 2. For investigation. No. 2 wants, I think, more support than No. 1. If you had a ward, say at the Southern Hospital, one of the physicians might take charge of it, and give lectures, clinical at the Hospital, and general say at the College – I suppose you might give him a title. For investigation you do not, I think, need a separate Laboratory at College, but a small Clinical Laboratory and the Hospital itself . . . The next point, I am in doubt about. I am inclined to think that the Pathology of Tropical Diseases should belong to the Professor of Pathology, who should, by virtue of this have some connection with the Tropical Diseases Ward in the Hospital, have access to the cases, . . . This system of a Pathologist working with the Physician or Surgeon in Clinical charge of the sick is being very largely worked with great success in America, and in this Tropical Disease seems to offer an opportunity for it. I have talked with Lord Lister (1827–1912) [President of the Royal Society], and he generally approves of what I have proposed, at least, thinks it most desirable that the Hospital and College should lay hold of Tropical Diseases. I myself feel very strong that it is an opportunity of study of these diseases. When the experts on Malaria sent out to Africa get to work on the West Coast, as they will in time do, it will be a great advantage to have an Institution for Tropical Diseases already in work at Liverpool. The experts abroad can work with the men at home.

At a meeting convened at the offices of Messrs Elder, Dempster and Co. on 23 November, 1898, the following were present:[28,29] Alfred L. Jones; William Adamson, President of the Royal Southern Hospital; R. T. Glazebrook, Principal of University College; William Alexander, Senior Surgeon of the Royal Southern Hospital; William Carter, Physician to the Royal Southern Hospital, Professor of Therapeutics, University College; and Boyce. The resulting minutes were as follows:

The following resolutions were unanimously passed: 1. That the gentlemen present form themselves into a Committee, with the approval of their various boards, for promoting the study of Tropical Diseases and to consider the best means of carrying out . . . Jones' intentions in the munificent offer he has made to further the above object. 2. That Mr Charles W. Jones (of Messrs Lamport and Holt) be asked to serve on this Committee. It was decided that the above resolutions should be printed, and that Jones would hand a copy to . . . Chamberlain . . . The Committee recommended that before the next meeting, the Professional Members should meet together to consider and suggest the best means for . . . carrying out these objects.

At a second meeting (12 December, 1898) a letter from Lord Ampthill (Colonial Office) to the Chairman (1 December) was read:[28]

I have shown your letter of the 28th ult. with regard to the School of Tropical Medicine [to] Chamberlain. He was much interested and very glad to hear of the important work you have thus commenced. You are no doubt aware of what . . . Chamberlain has been doing himself with regard to the establishment of a School of Tropical Medicine [in London] and he considers it a great advantage that Liverpool should be co-operating on similar lines. If it would interest you, I should be very glad to send you particulars of the Colonial Office scheme and information as to what has already been done, but I dare say you have learnt all that is essential from the newspapers.

In December 1898, the *Lancet*[30] reported:

. . . Chamberlain's scheme for the teaching of tropical diseases to colonial surgeons . . . has already borne practical fruit. Mr Alfred Jones [1845–1909] of Liverpool has offered £350 annually to establish and maintain a laboratory in Liverpool for the study of tropical diseases and the scheme will be carried out by a joint committee of the Royal Southern Hospital and of University College. A laboratory for immediate investigation will be built opposite the hospital, whilst prolonged research will be carried out in the pathological laboratory of University College, under the direction of Professor Boyce [1863–1911]. A large number of cases from the West Coast of Africa are taken into the wards of the Royal Southern Hospital, as Liverpool, being the centre of the African trade, is in constant communication with West Africa. We again have to congratulate Liverpool on the munificence of her citizens and would direct the attention of medical men about to practice in any capacity on the West Coast of Africa to the opportunity that is being afforded them for obtaining invaluable information.

In a letter (1 February 1899) from the Colonial Office,[28] read to a Committee meeting, it was stated that 'Chamberlain was very glad to learn that it had been decided to establish this School, but regretting that the Government could not grant any financial aid; however, in the selection of candidates for medical appointments in the Colonies, preference would be given to those who had received instruction in tropical medicine, such as that provided in the Liverpool School'. A further letter from Chamberlain (23 February) stated, however, that 'all doctors appointed to the Colonial Service must be attached to the ADH[3,18] for at least 2 months'. The Committee resolved to: (1) write to the Colonial Office and express regret that Chamberlain did not see his way to dispense with the latter condition in the case of students from the Liverpool School; and (2) approach the Colonial Office on the subject. On 20 March, Professor Boyce announced that Lord Lister (see above) had written stating that he intended to approach Chamberlain on behalf of the School, and it was therefore resolved to postpone further action in the matter pending receipt of information concerning the result of this interview. However, Government funding was never forthcoming and there can be no doubt that this led to a significant souring of relationships (some friendly rivalry still exists) between Liverpool and London.

Opening of the Liverpool school

In 1899, *The Lancet*[31] summarized the opening of the Liverpool School (Figure 1.4):

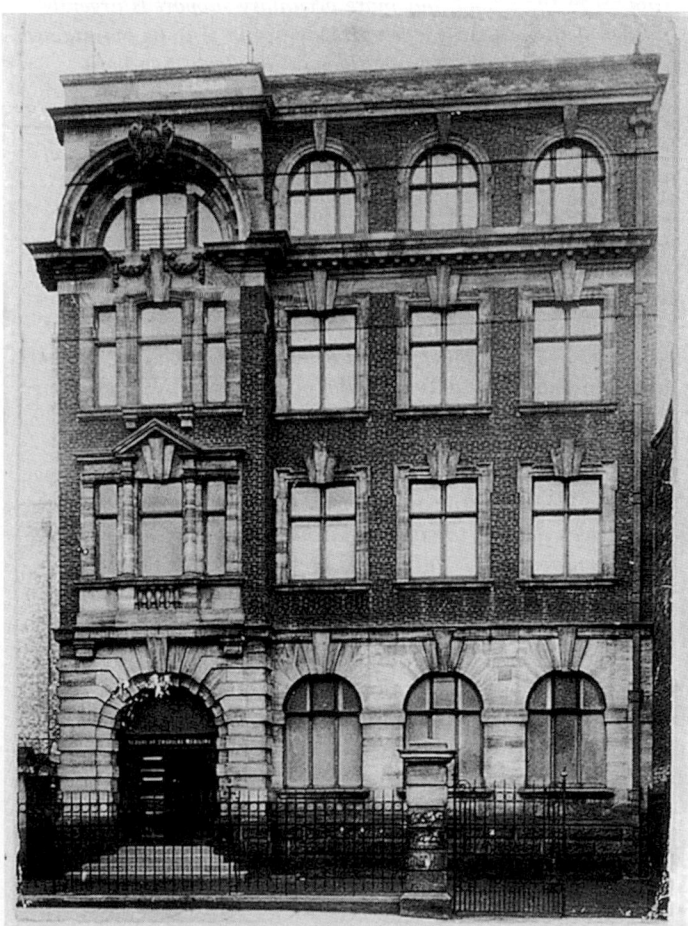

Figure 1.4 Liverpool School of Tropical Medicine; this building opened in 1920.

This School was inaugurated under fortunate auspices on April 22nd of this year by Lord Lister. At the annual dinner of the Royal Southern Hospital on Nov. 12th, 1898, Mr. Alfred L. Jones, a prominent Liverpool citizen and West Africa merchant, made an offer of £350 a year to start a school in Liverpool for the study of tropical diseases. The offer was made in the presence of Professor Rubert Boyce of University College, Liverpool, and Dr. William Alexander of the Royal Southern Hospital . . . The great interest subsequently taken in the project by Mr. Alfred L. Jones, aided by the indomitable energy of Professor Boyce, resulted in subscription and donations coming in from all quarters towards the expenses of the proposed school. To those two gentlemen, warmly supported by the committee and medical staff of the Royal Southern Hospital, is due the establishment of the Liverpool School of Tropical Diseases. The management of the school is in the hands of a strong committee, of which Mr. Alfred L. Jones is the chairman and Mr. William Adamson . . . the vice-chairman. The committee also consists of duly appointed representatives of University College, Liverpool, the Royal Southern Hospital, the Liverpool Chamber of Commerce, the Steamship Owners' Association, and the Shipowners' Association. A sum of over £1700 has already been promised, partly in annual subscriptions and partly in donations, in support of the school, but more pecuniary support is urgently needed if the practical work already begun is to be maintained at its excellent level. A large floor in the Royal Southern Hospital has been set apart for tropical cases. This floor includes a cheerful ward containing 12 beds, now fully occupied, also an extensive laboratory for the examination of blood, urine, faeces, etc., and furnished with the apparatus applicable to modern research. Professor Boyce superintends the pathological department of the school, with Dr. Annett as pathological demonstrator. The committee have been fortunate in securing the services of Major Ronald Ross, IMS [see above], as special lecturer [later professor] on tropical diseases . . . The number of malarial cases treated in Liverpool in 1898 amounted to 294. In the previous year . . . there were 242 cases of malaria, 14 of beri-beri, 30 of dysentery, and 39 of tropical anaemia. With the means of instruction in the varied forms of tropical diseases thus afforded there will be no need for Liverpool students to proceed to London [where there were fewer cases[22]] to obtain that which is ready to hand at their own doors. The authorities of the Liverpool School of Tropical Medicine have lost no time in getting to real work.

In June 1899, Ross (Figure 1.5) gave an inaugural lecture: he committed himself to the practical application of his malaria researches; extirpation of the mosquito, he envisaged, was the answer to the 'great malaria problem'. Ross had thus embarked on the 'sanitation' (or hygiene) tack, which was to dominate much of the Liverpool School's work for the forthcoming century.[3,29]

Subsequent developments in Liverpool

Shortly after its opening (in April 1899), the Liverpool School started on a series of 'expeditions': the first embarked for Sierra Leone in July, and 11 more had been carried out by the end of

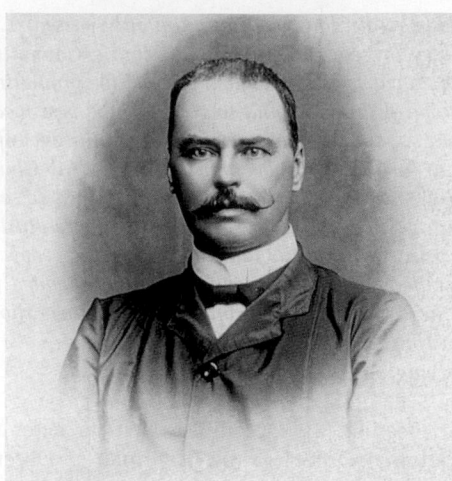

Figure 1.5 Major (later Sir) Ronald Ross (1857–1932).[35] The photograph was probably taken in the early twentieth century.

1903. Between its foundation and 1914, a total of 32 scientific expeditions to the tropics had taken place.[28,32] The *Annals of Tropical Medicine and Parasitology* was founded by the School's staff in 1907. The School was compelled, however, to survive by subscription; there was therefore no year-to-year stability.

At the outbreak of the Great War (1914–1918), teaching had been in full swing for 15 years;[33] two full courses were being given annually. An advanced practical course (of 1 month duration) was designed to meet the convenience of practitioners when at home on leave; those who attended this were excused the first month of the other course. Special courses on entomology designed for officers in the West African Medical Service and others were also given three times annually. Special research work was carried out at the School and the Runcorn Research Laboratories (about 16 miles from Liverpool).

Excellent historical accounts of the Liverpool School of Tropical Medicine are due to Miller[29] and Maegraith.[34] The School (unlike LSHTM) has established close collaborative links with some of the recently created Universities and Medical Schools of Africa, and other newly 'emergent' developing countries.

MEDICINE IN THE TROPICS AND TROPICAL MEDICINE

The practice of medicine in a tropical country differs in many ways from that in a temperate one – where the classical specialty (exemplified by the London and Liverpool Schools) has dominated the scenario. A major problem arises in the definition of 'tropical medicine'; this was accepted by Manson himself[3] in the preface to the first edition of this textbook in 1898:

The title I have elected to give to this work, TROPICAL DISEASES, is more convenient than accurate. If by 'tropical diseases' be meant diseases peculiar to, and confined to, the tropics, then half a dozen pages might have sufficed for their description . . . If . . . the expression 'tropical diseases' be held to include all diseases occurring in the tropics, then the work would require to cover almost the entire range of medicine . . . The tropical practitioner [he continued] enjoys opportunities for original research and discovery far superior in novelty and interest to those at the command of his fellow inquirer in the well-worked field of European and American research.

Figures 1.6 and 1.7 summarize some of the highlights in the development of these separate disciplines.[7]

In Britain (and other European countries) and northern America, infectious diseases dominated the medical scene until well into the twentieth century (Figure 1.6); however, following the introduction of improved sanitation/hygiene in Victorian England, their prevalence slowly declined,[1,3,35,36] the downward trend continued with the introduction of antibiotics in the 1940s and 1950s. Only recently has prevalence tended to increase – largely as a result of the HIV/AIDS pandemic. Tropical medicine, as an organized discipline, took off in the 1890s (see above) and reached a peak during the first half of the last century. Following World War II (1939–1945), or possibly before, a downward trend set in and as a result, this specialty continues to decline as a specific entity. The introduction of National Health Service 'reforms', following the Tomlinson report (published in 1992) and strategies of recent British governments, have rendered the future of this relatively small discipline extremely vulnerable. The major priority in Britain at present is to maintain a cadre of physicians well versed in the more 'exotic' infections encountered in the UK (e.g. trypanosomiasis, leishmaniasis and schistosomiasis), a requirement which also applies to other 'temperate' countries. More emphasis should also be given to 'travel medicine'.

In tropical countries situated in the tropics (Figure 1.7), the scenario is different.[7] Organized medical services began with the Indian Medical Service; this was followed by the Colonial Medical Service – with a far wider influence. Although Manson had started a Medical School in Hong Kong in 1887, the first School of Tropical Medicine in a tropical country was established by Sir Leonard Rogers (1868–1962) at Calcutta (now Kolkata) in 1920; this was a pioneering achievement.[3] When the former British Colonies acquired 'independence' in the 1950s and later, the 'wind of change' brought in its wake many newly created (indigenous) universities and medical schools, e.g. Makerere University College, Kampala; Ibadan University, Nigeria; and the University (and University Teaching Hospital), Lusaka; this led to much local teaching and research, and also simultaneously the introduction of local medical societies and examining boards.

These are changing times, and the future of the formal discipline specialty Tropical Medicine is at present uncertain. But that must on no account be confused with 'medicine in the tropics'.[3,37]

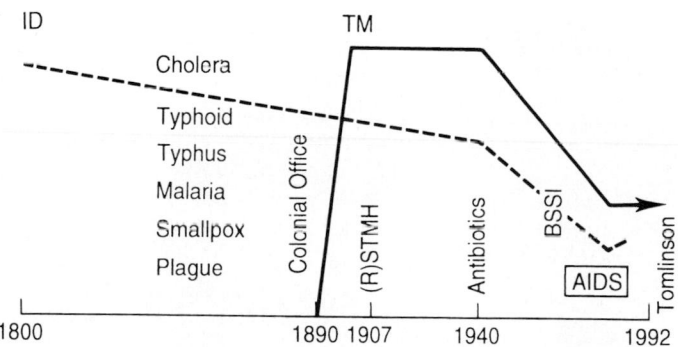

Figure 1.6 Approximate sequence of events in the foundation and development of the formal discipline of Tropical Medicine (TM). ID, infectious diseases; (R)STMH, (Royal) Society of Tropical Medicine and Hygiene; BSSI, British Society for the Study of Infection; AIDS, acquired immune deficiency syndrome; Tomlinson Report, published in 1992, which gave rise to sweeping changes in the British National Health Service.

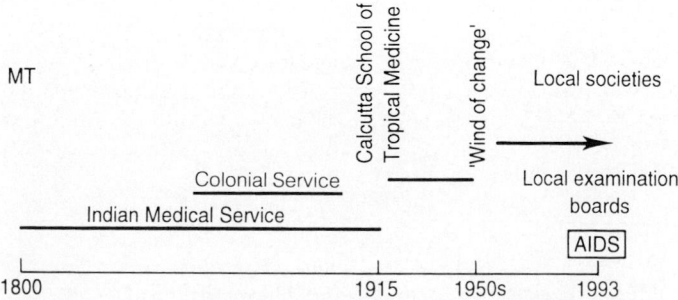

Figure 1.7 Approximate sequence of events in the progress of teaching/research in tropical (developing) countries. Medicine in the tropics (MT). AIDS, acquired immune deficiency syndrome.

REFERENCES

1. Cook GC. *From the Greenwich Hulks to Old St Pancreas: A History of Tropical Disease in London.* London: Athlone Press; 1992:338.
2. Balfour A. Some British and American pioneers in tropical medicine and hygiene. *Trans R Soc Trop Med Hyg* 1925; 19:189–231.
3. Cook GC. *Tropical Medicine: An Illustrated History of the Pioneers.* London: Academic Press; 2007:278.
4. Dewhurst K. *Dr Thomas Sydenham (1624–1689): His Life and Original Writings.* London: Wellcome Historical Medical Library; 1966:131–139.
5. Singer C, Underwood EA. *A Short History of Medicine.* 2nd edn. Oxford: Oxford University Press; 1962:221–223.
6. Arnold D. Introduction: diseases, medicine and empire. In: Arnold D, ed. *Imperial Medicine and Indigenous Societies.* Manchester: Manchester University Press; 1988:1–26.
7. Cook GC. Presidential Address. Evolution: the art of survival. *Trans R Soc Trop Med Hyg* 1994; 89:4–18.
8. Cook GC. Some early British contributions to tropical disease. *J Infect* 1993; 27:325–333.
9. Manson P. *Tropical diseases: A Manual of the Diseases of Warm Climates.* London: Cassell; 1898:624.
10. Ross R. *Memoirs: With a Full Account of the Great Malaria Problem and its Solution.* London: John Murray; 1923:547.
11. Cook GC. The Seamen's Hospital Society: a progenitor of the tropical institutions. *Postgrad Med J* 1999; 75:715–717.
12. Cook GC. *Disease in the Merchant Navy: A History of the Seamen's Hospital Society.* Oxford: Radcliffe; 2007:630.
13. Manson-Bahr P. *History of the School of Tropical Medicine in London: 1899–1949.* London: HK Lewis; 1956:328.
14. Cook GC. Changing role(s) for the Royal Hospital, Greenwich. *Hist Hosp* 2001; 22:35–46.

15. Manson-Bahr PH, Alcock A. *The Life and Work of Sir Patrick Manson*. London: Cassell; 1927:273.

16. Manson P. The necessity for special education in tropical medicine. *Lancet* 1897; ii:842–845.

17. Cook GC. Doctor Patrick Manson's leading opposition in the establishment of the London School of Tropical Medicine: Curnow, Anderson, and Turner. *J Med Biog* 1995; 3:170–177.

18. Cook GC, Webb AJ. The Albert Dock Hospital, London: the original site (in 1899) of Tropical Medicine as a new discipline. *Acta Tropica* 2001; 79:249–255.

19. Hoare P. *Spike Island: the Memory of a Military Hospital*. London: Fourth Estate; 2001:417.

20. May A. *London School of Hygiene and Tropical Medicine 1899–1999*. London: LSHTM; 1999:40.

21. Manson P. London School of Tropical Medicine: the need for special training in tropical disease. *J Trop Med* 1899; 2:57–62.

22. Cook GC. 'Tropical' cases admitted to the Albert Dock Hospital in the early years of the London School of Tropical Medicine. *Trans R Soc Trop Med Hyg* 1999; 93:675–677.

23. Low GC. The history of the foundation of the Society of Tropical Medicine and Hygiene. *Trans R Soc Trop Med Hyg* 1928; 22:197–202.

24. Cook GC. George Carmichael Low FRCP: Twelfth President of the Society and underrated pioneer of tropical medicine. *Trans R Soc Trop Med Hyg* 1993; 87:355–360.

25. Cook GC. Aldo Castellani FRCP (1877–1971) and the founding of the Ross Institute and Hospital for Tropical Diseases at Putney. *J Med Biog* 2000; 8:198–205.

26. Cook GC. A difficult metamorphosis: the incorporation of the Ross Institute and Hospital for Tropical Diseases into the London School of Hygiene and Tropical Medicine. *Med Hist* 2001; 45:483–506.

27. Cook GC. Future structure of clinical tropical medicine in the United Kingdom. *BMJ* 1982; 284:1460–1461.

28. Liverpool School of Tropical Medicine. *Historical Record 1898–1920*. Liverpool: University Press, 1920:103.

29. Miller PJ. *'Malaria, Liverpool': An Illustrated History of the Liverpool School of Tropical Medicine 1898–1998*. Liverpool: Liverpool School of Tropical Medicine 1898:78.

30. The study of tropical diseases in Liverpool. *Lancet* 1898; ii:1495.

31. The Liverpool School of Tropical Medicine. *Lancet* 1899; i: 1174–1176.

32. Worboys M. Manson, Ross and colonial medical policy: tropical medicine in London and Liverpool, 1899–1914. In: Macleod R, Lewis M, eds. *Disease, Medicine and Empire: Perspectives on Western Medicine and the Experience of European Expansion*. London: Routledge; 1988:21–37.

33. Liverpool School of Tropical Medicine. *BMJ* 1914; i:324.

34. Maegraith BG. History of the Liverpool School of Tropical Medicine. *Med Hist* 1972; 16:354–368.

35. Cook GC. Joseph William Bazalgette (1819–1891): a major figure in the health improvements of Victorian London. *J Med Biog* 1999; 7:17–24.

36. Cook GC. What can the Third World learn from the health improvements of Victorian Britain? *Postgrad Med J* 2005; 81:763–764.

37. Cook GC. Tropical medicine. *Lancet* 1997; 350:813.

Chapter 2 Nandini P. Shetty and Prakash S. Shetty

Primary Care and Disease Prevention and Control

INTRODUCTION

In 1978, the International Conference on Primary Health Care was held in Alma-Ata, USSR, and endorsed by the World Health Organization (WHO). This conference called for urgent and effective national and international action to develop and implement primary healthcare throughout the world, particularly in developing countries, in a spirit of technical cooperation and in keeping with a new international economic order. The Alma-Ata Declaration of 1978 states that the main social target should be the attainment by all peoples of the world, by the year 2000, of a level of health that will permit them to lead a socially and economically productive life.[1] However, the world almost 30 years on from the Alma-Ata Declaration is vastly different from that which saw the signing of the Declaration. Significant global changes – new epidemics, economic instability, continuing civil unrest and conflict, and triumph of the free market enterprise that has meant more pressure to produce profits – have all resulted in healthcare delivery systems across the world that are vastly different and hugely inequitable.[2]

DEFINITION OF PRIMARY HEALTHCARE

The Alma-Ata Declaration describes primary healthcare (PHC) as essential healthcare based on practical, scientific and socially acceptable methods and technology. It is made universally accessible to individuals and families in the community through their full participation and at a cost that the community and country can afford to maintain at every stage of their development in the spirit of self-reliance and self-determination. It is the first level of contact of individuals, the family and community with the national health system, bringing healthcare as close as possible to where people live and work, and constitutes the first element of a continuing healthcare process.[1]

THE KEY ELEMENTS OF PRIMARY HEALTHCARE

PHC addresses the main health problems in the community, providing promotive, preventive, curative and rehabilitative services accordingly. Key elements of the programme are:[1]

- Education concerning prevailing health problems and the methods of preventing and controlling them
- Promotion of food supply and proper nutrition
- An adequate supply of safe water and basic sanitation
- Maternal and child healthcare, including family planning
- Immunization against the major infectious diseases
- Prevention and control of locally endemic diseases
- Appropriate treatment of common diseases and injuries
- Provision of essential drugs.

Basic concepts drawn from the programme are summarized as follows:

- Primary healthcare should be shaped around the life patterns of the population
- It should both meet the needs of the local community and be an integral part of the national healthcare system
- Preventive, promotional and rehabilitative services for the individual, family and community need to be integrated
- The majority of health interventions should be undertaken as close to the community as possible by suitably trained workers
- The balance among these services should vary according to the community needs and may well change over time
- The local population should be involved in the formulation and implementation of healthcare activities
- Decisions about the community's needs and solutions to its problems should be based on a continuing dialogue between the people and the health professionals who serve them.

PRIMARY HEALTHCARE WORKERS

Based on experience of the success in Thailand, it was recognized that potential human resources exist in the community and are waiting to be mobilized. Two types of primary healthcare workers have thus been developed: village health communicators (VHCs) and village health volunteers (VHVs), who promote rural health and other development efforts through an organized community. The VHCs are responsible for a cluster of 8–15 households, the VHVs for the whole village. The functions of VHCs are to impart health education (prevention and promotion), and to disseminate and obtain health information from the villagers. The VHVs perform the same functions as VHCs, but also have the duty of caring for people who have had simple accidents or injuries and those with common diseases. Both VHCs and VHVs work on a voluntary basis. However, the government provides them with free medical services and a certificate when their training is completed. Other intangible incentives such as recognition from their peer group are also present. An informal 5-day training course for VHCs, covering the use of self-instruction modules, health problem identification, team working, etc. is organized by subdistrict health personnel. The 35 self-instruction modules for VHCs cover curative, preventive and promotive measures. The VHCs are expected to be able to disseminate such knowledge and gather information from villagers. VHVs obtain 17 additional modules on simple curative care and are trained for an additional 2 weeks.[3]

In India, multi-purpose health workers (MPWs) perform the role of village health workers. An evaluation of their role in a PHC in Kerala, India, revealed that MPWs apportion time to some national health programmes such as the malaria eradication programme and family welfare and immunization programmes to the detriment of others such as tuberculosis and acute respiratory infection. This demonstrated the need for continued training and evaluation of grass-root level workers to fulfil their multi-purpose role.[4]

The PHC programme in Thailand is often hailed as a success since it was responsible for solving many of the health problems of underserved people in rural areas. The concept of community participation and empowerment – consisting of the contribution of ideas, manpower, money and materials by the community – was fundamental and provided the key to success of the PHC programme. To educate the community to be self-reliant or self-supportive is another basic concept that the Thai PHC programme fostered. Their Ministry of Public Health was also a key player in that it recognized that strengthening of a health service delivery system and the development of a referral system were essential to support PHC activities.[5]

INTEGRATED MANAGEMENT OF THE SICK CHILD

While a great deal has been learned from disease-specific control programmes during the past 15 years, the challenge remained of how to combine the lessons learned into a single method for more efficient and effective management of childhood illness. WHO and UNICEF responded by jointly developing an approach referred to as integrated management of childhood illnesses (IMCI).[6]

The integrated management of the sick child initiative is seen as the intervention likely to have the greatest impact in reducing the global burden of disease. It is also among the most cost-effective health interventions in low- and middle-income countries. Inclusion of improved case management guidelines for children with symptomatic HIV infection and for better neonatal health have been included in IMCI from 2005.

Every year some 12 million children die before reaching their fifth birthday, many of them during their first year of life. Of these, 70% are killed due to one of five causes: diarrhoea, pneumonia, measles, malaria or malnutrition, and often in combination (Figure 2.1). Because their signs and symptoms may overlap, recognizing which of these conditions is present in a sick child can

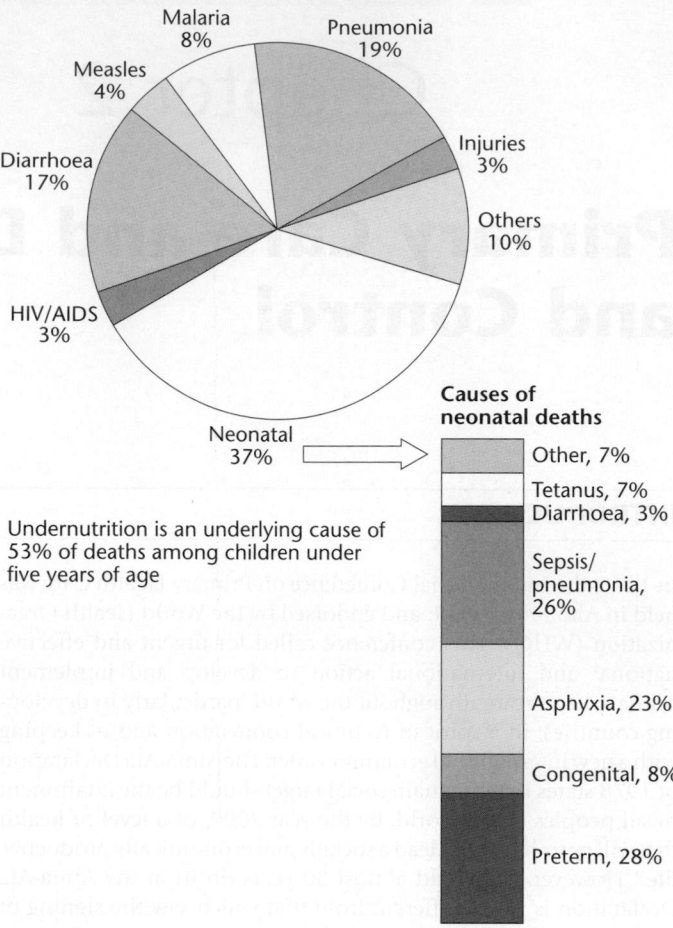

Figure 2.1 Major causes of death among children under 5 years of age and neonates, 2000–2003. (World Health Organization-UNICEF, Integrated Management of the Sick Child.)

be difficult and a single diagnosis is often inappropriate. Treatment of the sick child may also be complicated by the need to combine therapies for several conditions. The situation argues for child health programmes which address the sick child as a whole and not just single diseases.

Integrated management presents several key advantages. It leads to more accurate diagnoses in outpatient settings; ensures more appropriate and, where possible, combined treatment of major illnesses; and ensures and speeds up the referral of severely ill children. The approach gives due attention to prevention of childhood disease as well as its treatment, emphasizing immunization, vitamin A supplementation if needed, and improved infant feeding, including exclusive breast-feeding and appropriate complementary feeding. The role of the voluntary health worker or multi-purpose health worker is immediately evident in the IMCI programme.

Newly developed treatment guidelines for the sick child cover the most common potentially fatal conditions. The health worker is trained to assess every child for non-specific danger signs; for the four main symptoms of cough or difficult breathing, diarrhoea, fever and ear problems; for nutritional status; and for immunization status.

Case management process

1. The health worker assesses the child – asking questions, examining the child and checking immunization status.
2. The health worker then classifies the illness based on a colour-coded triage system, with which many health workers are already familiar through use of the WHO case management guidelines for diarrhoea and acute respiratory infections (ARI). The system classifies illnesses according to whether they require (a) urgent referral, (b) specific medical treatment and advice, or (c) simple advice on home management.
3. After classifying the illness, the health worker identifies specific treatments. If the child is being promptly referred, the health worker gives only urgent and appropriate treatment beforehand.
4. The health worker then provides practical instructions, such as how to administer oral drugs, increase fluids during diarrhoea and treat local infections at home. Mothers are advised on the signs which indicate the child should immediately be brought back to the clinic and when to return for follow-up.
5. For children under 2 years of age and those who are malnourished, the health worker assesses feeding, notes any feeding problems and provides counselling on feeding problems.

Training

Training health workers is a key activity in the long-term undertaking to improve the system for providing care to sick children. The WHO/UNICEF course Management of Childhood Illness trains health workers in first-level facilities (outpatient clinics and health centres), enabling them to effectively manage illnesses in an integrated fashion in sick children between the ages of 1 week and 5 years. The course also teaches them to communicate key health messages to mothers, helping them to understand how best to ensure the health of their children. The training course is based on the treatment guidelines and emphasizes hands-on practice. But course materials must be adapted to local situations so that, for example, local foods and drinks can be mentioned or locally appropriate drugs recommended.

Research

Research is an essential component of all programmes to reduce mortality and morbidity in children. WHO has drawn up a list of future research priorities related to integrated management of the sick child in order to improve the detection and treatment of the five major illnesses. Examples of areas where more information is needed are:

- Detection and management of anaemia and meningitis
- Management of malnutrition and feeding problems
- Management of severe disease in very young infants/neonates
- Management of children with symptomatic HIV infection
- Identification of high-risk children
- Adequacy of clinical management in first-level health facilities
- Reasons why families do not seek healthcare for sick children.

While much research is concerned with biomedical questions, there is also a need for further behavioural research on issues such as communicating with mothers and adaptation of advice on feeding to local conditions. In a cluster randomized evaluation of the integrated management of childhood illness (IMCI) strategy in Bangladesh, the mean index of correct treatment for sick children was 54 in IMCI facilities compared with nine in comparison facilities. Use of the IMCI facilities increased from 0.6 visits per child/year at baseline to 1.9 visits per child/year about 21 months after IMCI introduction. A total of 19% of sick children in the IMCI area were taken to a health worker compared with 9% in the non-IMCI area.[7]

The multi-country evaluation of integrated management of childhood illness (IMCI) effectiveness, cost and impact is a global evaluation to determine the impact of IMCI on health outcomes and its cost-effectiveness. Studies are under way in Bangladesh, Brazil, Peru, Uganda and the United Republic of Tanzania. The results indicate that in Tanzania children in IMCI districts received better care than children in comparison districts: their health problems were more thoroughly assessed, they were more likely to be diagnosed and treated correctly as determined through a gold-standard re-examination, and the caretakers of the children were more likely to receive appropriate counselling and reported higher levels of knowledge about how to care for their sick children. IMCI is therefore likely to lead to rapid gains in child survival, health and development if adequate coverage levels can be achieved and maintained.[8] Ethiopia contributed immensely to the development of IMCI and officially adopted it in 1997. Here it was found that the HIV/AIDS algorithm should be validated and included in the IMCI guidelines and essential IMCI drugs should be available to health facilities.[9]

The impact of PHC services on infant mortality assessed in the Gambia,[10] showed that PHC programmes had a significant impact on infant mortality, particularly when they were well supported and effectively mounted over a short time period. Significant impact of PHC on maternal and child mortality and morbidity could also be demonstrated in the Gomoa experience in rural Ghana.[11] In a landmark study from Maharashtra, India, health workers in communities were trained to use simple clinical criteria to identify neonates with potentially fatal sepsis and to identify the danger signs alerting mothers to seek care. Any one of the five maternally observed danger signs (reduced sucking, drowsy or unconscious, baby cold to touch, fast breathing and chest indrawing) gave 100% sensitivity and identified 23.9% neonates for seeking care.[12]

Shearley,[13] while commenting on the societal value of vaccination in developing countries, made the observation that immunization forms the basis of village operated PHC activity. Immunization programmes provide an opportunity for the provision of other primary care services, as it can be the only recurring activity in primary care that brings mother and child into contact with health services on a predictable and frequent basis. Immunization leads to a direct and measurable reduction of child mortality rates. This encourages smaller families and contributes to success of family planning programmes. Protecting the lives of children directly through immunization and other PHC activities is a major strategy towards improving the lives of women as it liberates their time, energy and resources. It empowers women to protect their own health and that of their children through their own actions. Therefore immunization services are best delivered along with other services needed by children in the first year of their life and by pregnant women – the persons who constitute the priority groups for PHC services in the developing world.

MATERNAL HEALTH

The global Safe Motherhood Initiative was launched in 1987 to improve maternal health and cut the number of maternal deaths in half by the year 2000.[14] New findings on maternal mortality by WHO, UNICEF and UNFPA (United Nations Population Fund) show that a woman living in sub-Saharan Africa has a 1 in 16 chance of dying in pregnancy or childbirth. This compares with a 1 in 2800 risk for a woman from a developed region. (Figure 2.2) Of the estimated 529 000 maternal deaths in 2000, 95% occurred in Africa and Asia, while only 4% (22 000) occurred in Latin America and the Caribbean, and less than 1% (2500) in the more developed regions of the world. Experience from successful maternal health programmes shows that much of this death and suffering could be avoided if all women had the assistance of a skilled health worker during pregnancy and delivery, and access to emergency medical care when complications arise.

Services for safe motherhood should be readily available through a network of linked community healthcare providers, clinics and hospitals. The integrated services that policy-makers from around the world have pledged to provide include:
- Community education on safe motherhood
- Prenatal care and counselling, including the promotion of maternal nutrition

- Skilled assistance during childbirth
- Care for obstetric complications, including emergencies
- Postpartum care
- Management of abortion complications, postabortion care and, where abortion is not against the law, safe services for the termination of pregnancy
- Family planning counselling, information and services
- Reproductive health education and services for adolescents.

Important lessons learned from the collaborative effort of several agencies highlight the following:

1. Empower women, ensure their choices. Gender inequalities and discrimination, especially in the developing world, limit women's choices and contribute directly to their ill-health and death (Figure 2.3). Legal reform and community mobilization can help women safeguard their reproductive health by enabling them to understand and articulate their health needs, and to seek services with confidence and without delay.

2. Every pregnancy faces risks (Figure 2.4). Every pregnant woman – even if she is well nourished and well educated – can develop sudden, life-threatening complications that require high-quality obstetric care. Attempts to predict these problems before they occur have not been successful, since most complications are unexpected and the majority of women with poor pregnancy outcomes do not fall into any high-risk categories. Therefore, maternal health programmes must aim to ensure that all women have access to essential services.

3. Ensure skilled attendance during childbirth. The single most effective way to reduce maternal death is to ensure that a health professional with the competence and skills to conduct a safe, normal delivery and manage complications is present during childbirth. Unfortunately, there is a chronic shortage of these professionals in poor and rural communities in the developing world. Research has shown that even trained traditional birth attendants (TBAs) have not significantly reduced a woman's risk of dying in childbirth, largely because they are unable to treat pregnancy complications. As an interim strategy for settings where TBAs attend a significant proportion of

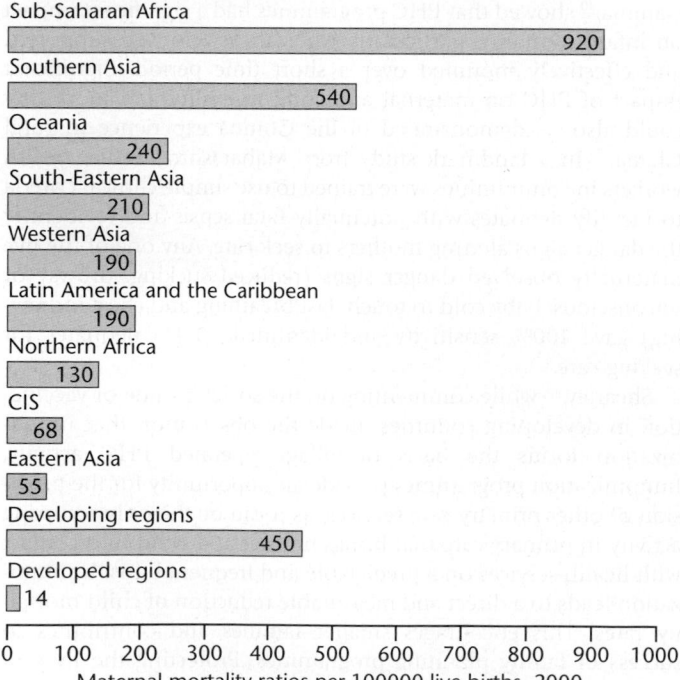

Figure 2.2 Maternal mortality in the developing countries. (United Nations. *The Millennium Development Goals 2005 Report*. New York: United Nations; 2005.)

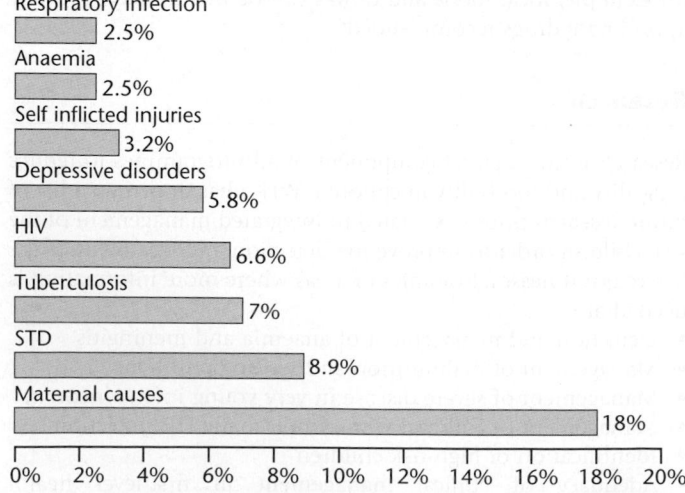

Figure 2.3 Leading causes of the burden of disease in women aged 15–44 in the developing world, 1990. (World Development Report 1993: Investing in Health. Washington, DC: World Bank; 1993.)

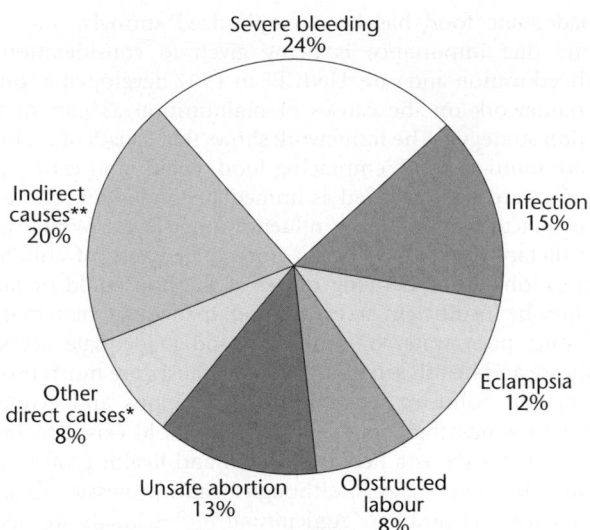

Figure 2.4 Causes of maternal deaths. *Other direct causes including, for example: ectopic pregnancy, embolism, anaesthesia related. **Indirect causes including, for example: anaemia, malaria, heart disease. ('Maternal Health Around the World' poster. World Health Organization and the World Bank 1997.)

deliveries, programme planners may want to provide TBAs with adequate training and support to help them refer complicated cases promptly and effectively. In all settings, however, skilled attendance at delivery should continue to be the long-term goal.

4. Improve access to high-quality maternal health services. A large number of women in developing countries do not have access to maternal health services. Many of them cannot get to, or afford, high-quality care. Cultural customs and beliefs can also prevent women from understanding the importance of health services, and from seeking them. In addition to legal reform and efforts to build support within communities, health systems must work to address a range of clinical, interpersonal and logistical problems that affect the quality, sensitivity and accessibility of the services they provide.

5. Address unwanted pregnancy and unsafe abortion. Unsafe abortion is the most neglected – and most easily preventable – cause of maternal death. These deaths can be significantly reduced by ensuring that safe motherhood programmes include client-centred family planning services to prevent unwanted pregnancy, contraceptive counselling for women who have had an induced abortion, the use of appropriate technologies for women who experience abortion complications and, where not against the law, safe services for pregnancy termination.

6. Measure progress. Female health workers in the Mwanza Region, Tanzania, distributed information and educated mothers regarding the use of a clean delivery kit for home births. Newborns whose mothers used the delivery kit were 13.1 times less likely to develop cord infection than infants whose mothers did not use the kit. Furthermore, women who used the kit for delivery were 3.2 times less likely to develop puerperal sepsis than women who did not use the kit.[15]

Dealing with HIV within the context of pregnancy must be an important focus of maternal and child health. UNFPA recognizes that an effective response requires a much more comprehensive, four-pronged approach:
- Prevent HIV infection among girls and women
- Prevent *unintended pregnancies* among women living with HIV
- Reduce *mother-to-child transmission* through antiretroviral drugs, safer deliveries and infant feeding counselling
- Provide care, treatment and support to women living with HIV and their families.[16]

MANAGEMENT OF SPECIFIC INFECTIOUS DISEASES

WHO has proposed a public-health approach to antiretroviral therapy (ART) to enable scaling-up access to treatment for HIV-positive people in developing countries, recognizing that the western model of specialist physician management and advanced laboratory monitoring is not feasible in resource-poor settings. Simplified tools and approaches to clinical decision-making, centred on the 'four Ss' – when to: start drug treatment; substitute for toxicity; switch after treatment failure; and stop – enable lower level healthcare workers to deliver care. To ensure access to ART in the poorest countries, the care and drugs should be given free at point of service delivery. Population-based surveillance for acquired and transmitted resistance is needed to address concerns that switching regimens on the basis of clinical criteria for failure alone could lead to widespread emergence of drug-resistant virus strains.[17]

Since 1990 the WHO Global Tuberculosis Programme has promoted the revision of national tuberculosis programmes to strengthen the focus on directly observed treatment, short course (DOTS). With direct observation of treatment, the patient does not bear the sole responsibility of adhering to treatment. Healthcare workers, public health officials, governments and communities must all share the responsibility and provide a range of support services patients need to continue and finish treatment. One of the aims of effective TB control is to organize TB services which are an integral part of PHC systems so that the patient has flexibility in where he or she receives treatment, for example in the home or at the workplace. Treatment observers can be anyone who is willing, trained, responsible, acceptable to the patient and accountable to the TB control services. The recording and reporting system is used to systematically evaluate patient progress and treatment outcome. The system consists of: a laboratory register that contains a log of all patients who have had a smear test done; patient treatment cards that detail the regular intake of medication and follow-up sputum examinations; the TB register, which lists patients starting treatment and monitors their individual and collective progress towards cure; and reporting from districts to the national level, which allows assessment of control efforts. Yet, DOTS is still not used widely. The consequences of not using DOTS more widely are alarming. TB cases and deaths will certainly continue, the global epidemic will remain uncontrolled, and harder-to-manage multidrug-resistant TB (MDR-TB) will be created. To address the problem of MDR-TB in areas where it has emerged, WHO has introduced the DOTS-Plus programme.[18]

The DOTS strategy has been successful in several centres in Asia and Africa. In Bangladesh,[19] success was attributed to decentralizing sputum smear microscopy and treatment delivery services to peripheral health facilities utilizing the existing PHC network. The large informal health workforce that exists in resource poor countries can be used to achieve public health goals. Involvement of village doctors in TB control has now become national policy in Bangladesh. Maintaining the quality of implementation, keeping it convenient and safeguarding confidentiality were important factors for its success. The success of DOTS in India has been documented from well designed community surveillance studies.[20] Involvement of private practitioners was suggested as a potential for spreading the DOTS strategy in the state of Kerala.[21] In Thailand DOTS was performed by health personnel, community members and supervised family members and contributed to effective and widespread implementation of the programme.[22] Community-based delivery systems for DOTS have been found to be successful in Ethiopia and other parts of sub-Saharan Africa. The community-based delivery systems used patients themselves in the form of 'TB Clubs'[23] or 'guardians' in the community,[24,25] thus effectively decentralizing the programme and empowering the community itself.

Utilizing PHC workers has been a successful strategy for case detection and control of leprosy.[26] Involvement of the community has been recognized as an important component for the control of visceral leishmaniasis in India.[27]

WATER SANITATION AND HEALTH

Deficiencies in water and sanitation contribute to the heavy disease burden imposed by diarrhoea, poliomyelitis, hepatitis, intestinal nematodes like hookworm and tropical diseases such as leishmaniasis. Food safety and hygiene are important factors in the prevalence of these illnesses. Few persons would dispute, however, that water and sanitation are important contributing factors. Furthermore, chemical contamination of drinking water is the main cause of illnesses such as arsenicosis and fluorosis. It has been suggested that local communities should be trained as guardians of sound water management practices, such as monitoring quality, protecting water sources from pollutants, and identifying and penalizing polluters. Consumers could even take the initiative, such as in many local communities, of mobilizing demand for proper sanitation and sewerage systems and implementing schemes.[28]

NUTRITION IN PRIMARY HEALTHCARE

Nutrition is an important element of PHC, and is a major determinant of the health of the community and for optimum growth and health of children. Nutrition and health are not synonymous, but without good nutrition health cannot be optimal. An essential prerequisite to prevent malnutrition or more appropriately undernutrition (since overnutrition and an unbalanced diet can also lead to poor health and disease) in a household or a community is to assure availability and access to adequate quantity, good quality and safe food to meet the nutrient needs of all people. However, the recognition that malnutrition is not just a problem

of inadequate food has been emphasized strongly, and more recently due importance is being given to considerations of health, education and care. UNICEF in 1997 developed a conceptual framework on the causes of malnutrition as part of their nutrition strategy.[29] The framework shows that causes of malnutrition are multi-sectoral, embracing food, health and caring practices. They are also classified as immediate, underlying and basic, whereby factors at one level influence other levels. While inadequate dietary intake may be an immediate cause of childhood malnutrition, the underlying causes at the household or family level may be insufficient access to food, inadequate maternal and child care, poor water or sanitation and inadequate access to healthcare and health services. The basic causes are much broader and include political, social, cultural, religious and economic systems in which the community or household exists. Malnutrition may manifest as a health problem and health professionals can provide some answers, although health professionals alone cannot solve the problem. Agricultural professionals are needed to ensure enough production of the right kinds of foods, while educators, both formal and non-formal, are required to assist people, particularly women, in achieving and ensuring good nutrition.

Breast-feeding

Promotion of exclusive breast-feeding at the primary healthcare level is crucial. This may include preparing the pregnant mother and helping her to decide to breast-feed the child. It also includes support in the postpartum period, through formal and informal activities, which may help women to have confidence in their ability to breast-feed and relieve doubts and anxieties they may have about it. Protection of breast-feeding should be aimed at guarding women who normally would successfully breast-feed against forces and situations that might cause them to alter this practice. Promotion of breast-feeding, which must be part of primary healthcare, includes motivating or re-educating mothers who might not be inclined to breast-feed, although promotion is difficult given changing work patterns of women in developing societies and changing demands on their time. The Baby Friendly Hospital Initiative (BFHI) launched in 1992 by UNICEF and WHO[29] to help protect, support and promote breast-feeding by addressing problems in hospitals may be less relevant for countries and communities where most babies are born outside hospital settings. However, there are lessons to be learned for application in PHC settings.

Complementary feeding

With a healthy mother providing adequate breast milk, breast-feeding alone should ensure good growth, nutrition and health of an infant up to 6 months of life. Continued breast-feeding with the addition of safe high-quality complementary foods into the second year of life provides the best nourishment and protects children from infections.[29] Thus at 6 months of age, complementary feeding should be introduced gradually while the infant continues to be breast-fed. The introduction of complementary feeds is a critical stage in a child's life. A child must have additional complementary feeds at 6 months of age since breast milk is no longer able to provide all the nutrients the child needs. Hence delaying the introduction of complementary feeds can cause a child's growth to falter. However, too early introduction can also increase the risk of malnutrition and infection in a child, particularly if the preparation and storage of food are not hygienic. From 6 to 18 months of age the child needs frequent feeding and will need meals that are dense in energy and nutrients and are also easily digestible. Foods the rest of the family normally eat will have to be adapted to suit the need of a growing child. Emphasis on hygiene in the preparation and storage of complementary feeds can never be considered excessive. The health worker at the PHC level can be an important player in educating the mother and other carers not only of the importance of good and nutritious complementary feeds, but also in promoting hygienic practices in the preparation, storage and handling of complementary feeds based on local foods for the child and in the imparting of knowledge of transmission of infectious agents.

Care

Of the three underlying causes of malnutrition, namely food, health and care, care is the one least investigated, least understood and least emphasized.[30] Adequate care is not only important for the child's survival but also for optimal physical and mental development. Care also contributes to the child's general well-being and happiness. Child care may be influenced by external factors such as war, conflict and civil unrest, by local factors such as equity and access to health services at the PHC level and availability of educational facilities, as well as factors within a family or household such as adequate housing, safe water, household hygiene and mother's knowledge and educational achievement. Care is manifested in the ways a child is fed, nurtured, taught and guided. It is the expression by individuals and families of the domestic and cultural values that guide them.[29] Nutritionally, care encompasses all measures and behaviours that transmit available food and health resources into good child growth and development. In most developing countries the mother is the care-giver for the infant and the very young child although in extended families older and young relatives (older siblings) often play an important role. Care-giving behaviour is often mistakenly assumed to be the exclusive domain of mothers; it should in fact be the responsibility of the entire family.

Care-giving behaviour that contributes to good nutrition and health varies enormously between societies and cultures. While the assumption that all societies value children and wish to see them grow in a healthy manner to become valuable assets of their society is very largely true, the assumption that societies have evolved with traditional or culturally determined caring practices, which are mostly good is often questioned. Identification of child-caring practices that are desirable should be the first step in any health promotion strategy that involves care. Protection of good practices that promote childcare from erosion or loss due to the developmental process is essential. Support is essential when good traditional practices of mothers or families are threatened or eroded by changes in society. A good example is the decline in breast-feeding that is seen in developing societies with urbanization. The PHC setting is obviously the focal point for integrating activities related to childcare in the community.

Promotion of growth monitoring

Growth monitoring was the first of UNICEF's GOBI (growth monitoring, oral rehydration, breast-feeding and immunization) strategy to improve child health and nutrition. Growth monitoring by itself does not improve health or promote adequate and appropriate growth in children. It ensures that children are growing well and in a healthy manner. It helps the early detection of the onset of malnutrition either because of inadequate and poor-quality food or because proper growth is affected adversely by other factors such as periodic episodes of infections. Hence the promotion of growth monitoring should form an important part of the PHC system. It should be closely integrated into primary healthcare activities and should not, as far as possible, be a separate programme. It should focus on maintaining and monitoring good and appropriate growth in infants and children in the community and help detect the early signs of growth faltering. It should not merely be used for following up and rehabilitating children who are recovering from malnutrition and whose growth is poor. Hence, it is important that growth-monitoring promotion when integrated into PHC activities should be aimed at all children in the community. In order to do that, it is essential that all children are entered into the growth-monitoring programme soon after birth, since all infants up to about 6 months who are exclusively breast-fed show satisfactory growth. Growth monitoring also derives other indirect benefits, since good physical growth is often related to other aspects of good child development and environments that promote good child development usually help promote optimum physical growth. The proper promotion of growth monitoring requires not only that the health worker at the PHC level is trained adequately in techniques used to measure and monitor growth in infants and children, but also has access to good, simple equipment for measuring length or height and weight, appropriate growth charts and record-keeping facilities. Above all, the health worker should have a good understanding of existing child-rearing practices and the cultural, social and dietary environment of the community. Growth-monitoring promotion is viewed as a strategy to empower mothers to maintain good nutritional status in their children and to prevent growth faltering or growth retardation. It is a preventive strategy designed to promote optimum growth and good health and not merely to help diagnose malnutrition and ill-health.

The promotion of good nutrition for health at the primary care level is an important role that can be played by the PHC-level health worker. Nutrition information and education are essential to improve nutrition knowledge for application during pregnancy to ensure the best possible birth outcome along with other aspects of antenatal care. This process of empowering communities with the requisite knowledge to promote the health and nutrition of their families should continue with the birth of the infant and the growth and development of the child. Special emphasis needs to be placed on promoting breast-feeding, the timely introduction of complementary feeding and the crucial role that growth monitoring plays in ensuring the optimum health of children. Increasing the awareness of food and nutrition and their important role in the good health of the entire household, good food hygiene practices and correction of false food beliefs and taboos is a role health workers at the PHC level can readily play. Providing

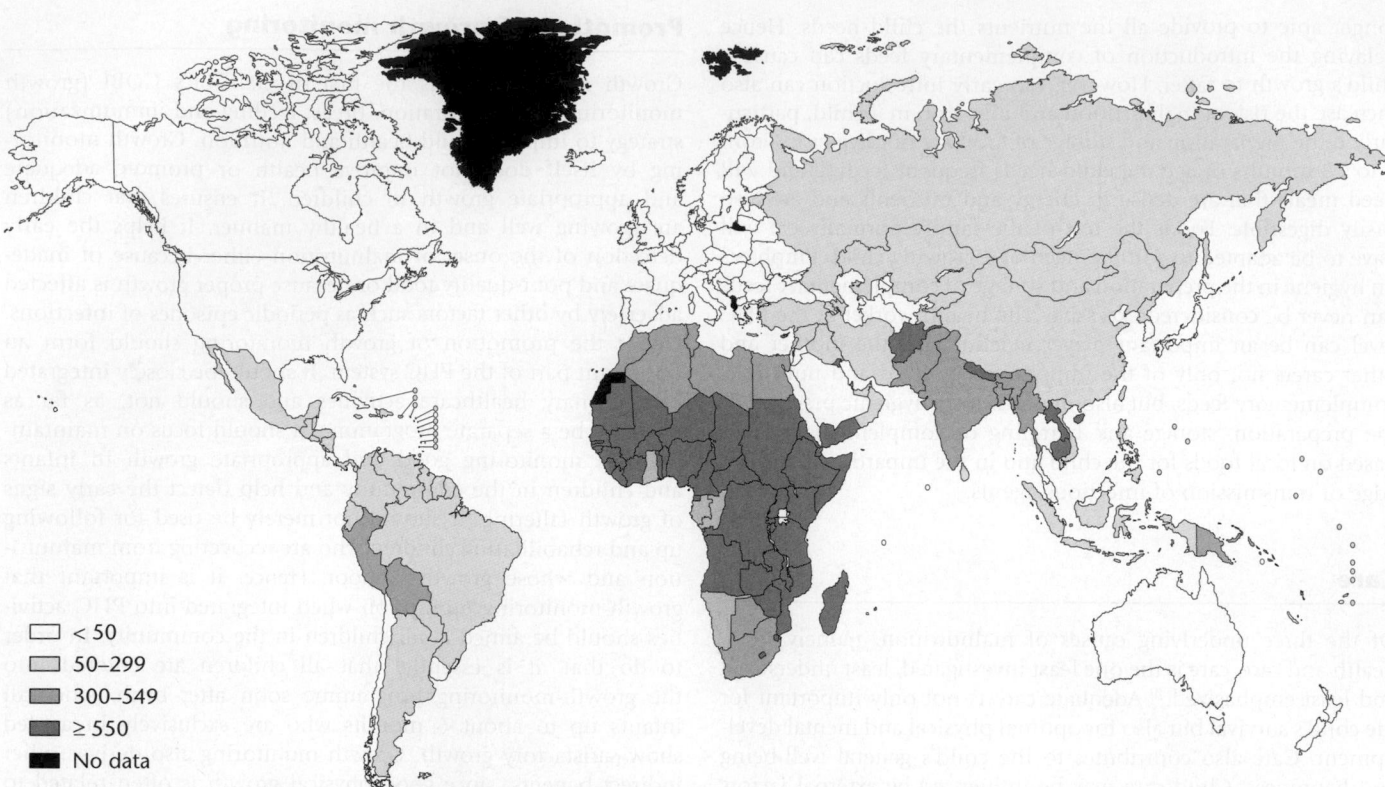

Figure 2.5 Maternal mortality per 100 000 live births in 2000. (The World Health Report 2005: *Make Every Mother and Child Count*. Geneva: WHO; 2005.)

adequate training in nutrition and the necessary resources along with support is crucial for the important role these workers at the community level can fulfil. Thailand has been a beacon to most countries in integrating nutritional activities into primary care and in empowering and involving the community in promoting the nutrition and health of its population. This is evidenced by the remarkable progress made by Thailand in reducing undernutrition of preschool children within a decade from the years 1982 to 1992.[31] It demonstrated how explicit support from the state along with the galvanization of grass-root involvement, based on a multi-sectoral and coordinated approach at the primary care level can have a dramatic impact on the health of the community.

CONCLUSION

In September 2000, at the United Nations Millennium Summit, 'leaders from every country agreed on a vision for the future – a world with less poverty, hunger and disease, greater survival prospects for mothers and their infants'.[32] This vision took the shape of eight Millennium Development Goals (MDGs), which range from halving extreme poverty to halting the spread of HIV/AIDS, reducing child mortality to providing universal primary education and improving maternal health (Figure 2.5) – all by the target date of 2015. These MDGs form a blueprint agreed to by all the world's countries and all the world's leading development institutions and have galvanized unprecedented efforts to meet the needs of the world's poorest.

The Millennium Development Goals (MDGs):
1. Eradicate extreme poverty and hunger
2. Achieve universal primary education
3. Promote gender equality and empower women
4. Reduce child mortality
5. Improve maternal health
6. Combat HIV and AIDS, malaria and other diseases
7. Ensure environmental sustainability
8. Develop a global partnership for development.

The 2005 UN World Summit in its report[32] showed that some progress had been made and, while the challenges the Goals represented were staggering, there were clear signs of hope. Thus, it would appear that through primary care we now have the opportunity, unprecedented in healthcare reform, to reduce maternal and child mortality and decrease the burden of deadly infectious disease and so meet the needs of the world's poorest.

REFERENCES

1. WHO. *Declaration of Alma-Ata*. International Conference on Primary Healthcare, Alma-Ata, 1978.
2. Chowdhury Z, Rowson M. The People's Health Assembly: Revitalising the promise of 'Health for All'. *BMJ* 2000; 321:1361–1362.
3. Nondasuta A, Ningsanon P, Chandavimol P, et al. Nutrition in primary healthcare. In: Andersen J, Valyasevi A, eds. *Effective Communications for Nutrition in Primary Healthcare*. Washington, DC: United Nations University Press; 1988:6.

4. Nair V, Thankappan K, Sarma P, et al. Changing roles of grass-root level health workers in Kerala, India. *Health Policy Plan* 2001; 16:171–179.

5. Nondasuta A. Primary healthcare and nutrition. In: Winichagoon P, Kachondham Y, Attig GA, et al, eds. *Integrating Food and Nutrition into Development*. Bangkok: UNICEF and Mahidol University, 1992:56–62.

6. WHO-UNICEF. *Integrated management of the sick child. Division of Child Health and Adolescent Development (CHD)*. 2005. Online. Available: http://www.who.int/child-adolescent-health/integr.htm 17 January 2007.

7. Arifeen SE, Blum LS, Hoque DME, et al. Integrated management of childhood illness (IMCI) in Bangladesh: early findings from a cluster-randomised study. *Lancet* 2004; 364:1595–1602.

8. Armstrong Schellenberg JR, Adam T, Mshinda H, et al. Effectiveness and cost of facility-based Integrated Management of Child Illness (IMCI) in Tanzania. *Lancet* 2004; 364:1583–1594.

9. Lulseged S. Integrated management of childhood illness: a review of the Ethiopian experience and prospects for child health. *Ethiop Med J* 2002; 40:187–201.

10. Hill AG, MacLeod WB, Joof D, et al. Decline of mortality in children in rural Gambia: the influence of village-level primary healthcare. *Trop Med Int Health* 2000; 5:107–118.

11. Afari EA, Nkrumah FK, Nakana T, et al. Impact of primary healthcare on child morbidity and mortality in rural Ghana: the Gomoa experience. *Cent Afr J Med* 1995; 41:148–153.

12. Bang A, Bang RA, Reddy MH, et al. Simple clinical criteria to identify sepsis or pneumonia in neonates in the community needing treatment or referral. *Pediatr Infect Dis J* 2005; 24:335–341.

13. Shearley A. The societal value of vaccination in developing countries. *Vaccine* 1999; 17(suppl 3):S109–S112.

14. Safe Motherhood Inter Agency Group. *What is safe motherhood?* 2002. Online. Available: http://www.safemotherhood.org/init_what_is.htm 18 Jan 2007.

15. Winani S, Wood S, Coffey P, et al. Use of a clean delivery kit and factors associated with cord infection and puerperal sepsis in Mwanza, Tanzania. *J Midwifery Womens Health* 2007; 52:37–43.

16. UNFPA, WHO. *Sexual and Reproductive Health of Women Living with HIV/AIDS*. 2006. Online. Available: http://www.unfpa.org/publications 17 Jan 2007.

17. Gilks CF, Crowley S, Ekpini R, et al. The WHO public-health approach to antiretroviral treatment against HIV in resource-limited settings. *Lancet* 2006; 368:505–510.

18. World Health Organization. *Stop TB Partnership Annual Report*. 2005. Online. Available: WHO/HTM/STB/2006.36.

19. Hamid Salim MA, Uplekar M, Daru P, et al. Turning liabilities into resources: informal village doctors and tuberculosis control in Bangladesh. *Bull World Health Organ* 2006; 84:427.

20. Subramani R, Santha T, Frieden TR, et al. Active community surveillance of the impact of different tuberculosis control measures, Tiruvallur, South India, 1968–2001. *Int J Epidemiol* 2007; 36(2):387–393.

21. Greaves F, Ouyang H, Pefole M, et al. Compliance with DOTS diagnosis and treatment recommendations by private practitioners in Kerala, India. *Int J Tuberc Lung Dis* 2007; 11:110–112.

22. Pungrassami P, Johnsen SP, Chongsuvivatwong V, et al. Practice of directly observed treatment (DOT) for tuberculosis in southern Thailand: comparison between different types of DOT observers. *Int J Tuberc Lung Dis* 2002; 6:389–395.

23. Getahun H, Maher D. Contribution of 'TB clubs' to tuberculosis control in a rural district in Ethiopia. *Int J Tuberc Lung Dis* 2000; 4:174–178.

24. Hadley M, Maher D. Community involvement in tuberculosis control: lessons from other healthcare programmes. *Int J Tuberc Lung Dis* 2000; 4:401–408.

25. Harries A, Kenyon T, Maher D, et al. 'Community TB care in Africa': a collaborative project coordinated by WHO. Report on a 'lessons learned' meeting in Harare, 27–29 December 2000. (WHO/CDS/TB/2001.291).

26. World Health Organization Regional Office for South-East Asia New Delhi. Global strategy for further reducing the leprosy burden and sustaining leprosy control activities 2006–2010. Operational guidelines. *Lepr Rev* 2006; 77:IX, X, 1–50.

27. Singh SP, Reddy DC, Mishra RN, et al. Knowledge, attitude, and practices related to Kala-azar in a rural area of Bihar state, India. *Am J Trop Med Hyg* 2006; 75:505–508.

28. World Health Organization. *Global Water Supply and Sanitation Assessment 2000 Report*. Online. Available: http://www.who.int/water_sanitation_health/Globassessment/GlasspdfTOC.htm 17 Jan 2007.

29. UNICEF. *State of the World's Children 1998*. New York: UNICEF; 1998.

30. Latham MC. *Human nutrition in the developing world*. FAO Food and Nutrition Series 29. Rome: Food and Agriculture Organisation; 1997.

31. SCN. *Ending malnutrition by 2020: An Agenda for Change in the Millennium*. Report of the Commission on the nutritional challenges of the 21st century. SCN; 2000.

32. United Nations. *The Millennium Development Goals Report 2006*. New York: UN; 2006.

Chapter 3 — Nandini P. Shetty and Prakash S. Shetty

Epidemiology of Disease in the Tropics

Ingenuity, knowledge, and organization alter but cannot cancel humanity's vulnerability to invasion by parasitic forms of life. Infectious disease which antedated the emergence of humankind will last as long as humanity itself, and will surely remain, as it has been hitherto, one of the fundamental parameters and determinants of human history. (William H. McNeill in Plagues and Peoples, *1976)*

INTRODUCTION

The study of epidemiology in the tropics has undergone major changes since its infancy when it was largely a documentation of epidemics. It has now evolved into a dynamic phenomenon involving the ecology of the infectious agent, the host, reservoirs and vectors as well as the complex mechanisms concerned in the spread of infection and the extent to which this spread occurs.[1] Similar concepts in the study of epidemiology apply to communicable as well as non-communicable diseases. The understanding of epidemiological principles has its origins in the study of the great epidemics. Arguably, the most powerful example of this is the study of that ancient scourge of mankind, the so-called black death or plague. A study of any of the plague epidemics throughout history has all the factors that govern current epidemiological analysis: infectious agent, host, vector, reservoir, complex population dynamics including migration, famine, fire and war; resulting in spread followed by quarantine and control.

The World Health Report 1996: 'Fighting disease, fostering development', states that infectious diseases are the world's leading cause of premature death.[2] Infectious diseases account for 45% of deaths in low-income countries (Figure 3.1) and up to 63% of deaths in children under 4 years of age worldwide. Africa and South-east Asia carry the highest mortality due to infectious diseases (Figure 3.2). In addition, new and emerging infections pose a rising global threat (Table 3.1).

THE SIX DEADLY KILLERS

No more than six deadly infectious diseases: pneumonia, tuberculosis, diarrhoeal diseases, malaria, measles and more recently, HIV/AIDS, account for half of all premature deaths, killing mostly children and young adults (Figure 3.3).

ACUTE RESPIRATORY INFECTIONS

Acute respiratory infections (ARIs) are the leading cause of death of infectious aetiology, killing more than 4 million people a year, 1.9 million of which constitute children under the age of five.[3]

Among the 42 countries of the world that carry 90% of the child mortality burden, 14–24% of the under-5 mortality is due to pneumonia and nearly 70% of this pneumonia mortality occurs in the Africa and South and South-east Asia regions. The majority of this burden is borne during early childhood, with the greatest risk from mortality occurring during the neonatal period. The global incidence of ARI in children is estimated to be 154 million cases per year.[3]

This range of infections, which includes pneumonia in its most serious form, accounts for more than 8% of the global burden of disease. Pneumonia often affects children with low birth weight or those whose immune systems are weakened by malnutrition or other diseases. Caused by different viruses or bacteria, ARI is closely associated with poverty, overcrowding and unsanitary household conditions. Several other factors seem to exacerbate the disease. Exposure to tobacco smoke increases the risk of contracting these infections, and many studies implicate both indoor and outdoor air pollution. Indoor air pollution has been the focus of particular concern: specifically, the soot and smoke associated with the burning of biomass fuels such as wood, coal, or dung. Many people in the developing world, mostly in rural areas, rely on biomass fuels for heating or cooking. A cause-and-effect relationship between indoor air pollution and ARI has been difficult to prove. Even so, the World Bank estimated in 1992 that switching to better fuels could halve the number of pneumonia deaths.[4] Approaches to the management of childhood pneumonia in the tropics are hampered by lack of diagnostic facilities to identify the aetiological agent. The WHO has devised a simple algorithm for use in field situations, by primary healthcare workers, using clinical criteria such as respiratory rate and indrawing of ribs to decide whether a child needs hospitalization. Proper implementation of this strategy has been shown to reduce the mortality from childhood pneumonias by 25–50%.[5] However, implementation of community ARI treatment programmes remains patchy and current rates of children with ARI being taken to a health provider are ~40% in Africa and South Asia. In nearly half of the 81 countries with available data, less than 50% of the children with ARI were taken to an appropriate healthcare provider.[5]

HIV/AIDS

The AIDS pandemic has emerged as the single most defining occurrence in the history of infectious diseases of the late twentieth and early twenty-first centuries. According to the AIDS epidemic update of December 2005 (UNAIDS and WHO),[6] the epidemiology of HIV in the tropics varies enormously from place to place (Figure 3.4). The Joint United Nations Program on HIV/AIDS (UNAIDS) estimated that by the end of 2005, there were about 40 million people living with HIV worldwide: 38 million were adults, including 17.5 million women, and 2.3 million children (under 15 years old). During 2005, there were 4.9 million new cases of HIV infection (4.2 million adults and 0.7 million

children), and 3.1 million AIDS-related deaths (2.6 million adults and 0.57 million children).[6]

Asia

Latest estimates show some 8.3 million people (2 million adult women) were living with HIV in 2005, including the 1.1 million people who became newly infected in the past year. AIDS claimed some 520 000 lives in 2005. These estimates are in line with known risk behaviour in this region, where men account for the majority of injecting drug users, and are responsible for sexual transmission of HIV, largely through commercial sex. Commercial sex accounts for a large part of the estimated 20% of HIV infections in China that are due to unprotected heterosexual contact. It also features in the transmission of the virus among men who have sex with men: a recent survey among male sex workers in the southern city of Shenzhen found that 5% of them were HIV-positive. However, it is the potential overlap between commercial sex and injecting drug use that is likely to become the main driver of China's epidemic.

Diverse epidemics are underway in India, where, in 2003, an estimated 5.1 million Indians were living with HIV. Although levels of HIV infection prevalence appear to have stabilized in some states (such as Tamil Nadu, Andhra Pradesh, Karnataka and Maharashtra), it is still increasing in at-risk population groups in several other states. As a result, overall HIV prevalence has continued to rise. A significant proportion of new infections is occurring in women who are married and who have been infected by husbands who (either currently or in the past) frequented sex workers. Commercial sex (along with injecting drug use, in the states of Nagaland and Tamil Nadu) serves as a major driver of the epidemics in most parts of India. HIV surveillance in 2003 found 14% of commercial sex workers in Karnataka (26% in the city of Mysore) and 19% in Andhra Pradesh were infected with HIV. The well-known achievements among sex workers of Kolkata's Sonagachi red-light area (in West Bengal, India) have shown that safe sex programmes that empower sex workers can curb the spread of HIV. Condom use in Sonagachi has risen as high as 85% and HIV prevalence among commercial sex workers declined to fewer than

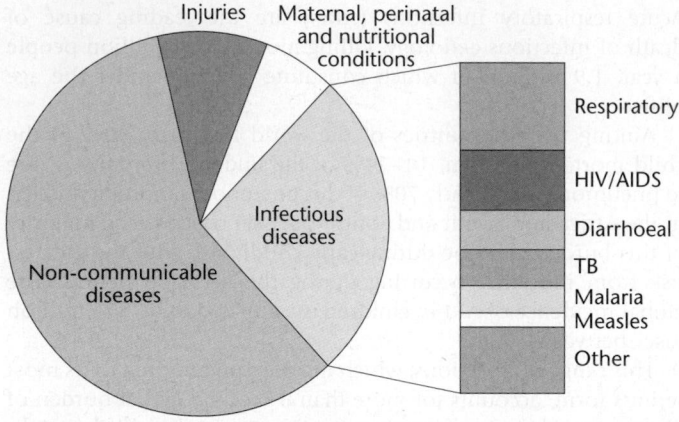

Figure 3.1 Main causes of death in low-income countries, 2002 (WHO 2003).

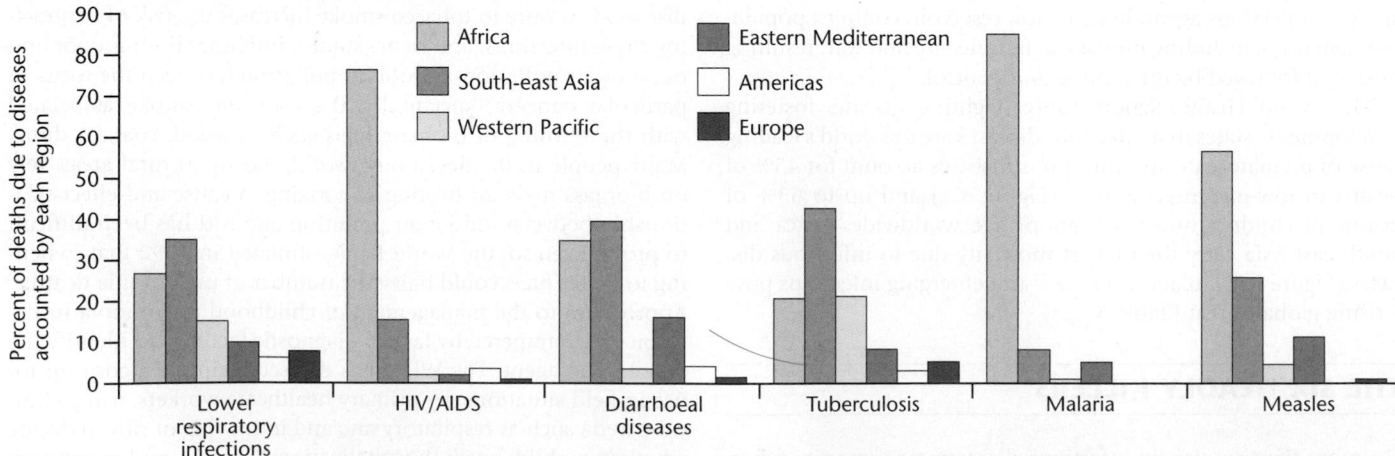

Figure 3.2 Global view of the mortality associated with infectious diseases, 2001 (WHO 2006).

Table 3.1 Examples of pathogenic microbes and the diseases they cause, identified since 1973

Year	Microbe	Type	Disease
1973	*Rotavirus*	Virus	Infantile diarrhoea
1977	*Ebola virus*	Virus	Acute haemorrhagic fever
1977	*Legionella*	*Bacterium pneumophila*	Legionnaires' disease
1980	Human T- lymphotrophic virus I (HTLV 1)	Virus	T cell lymphoma/leukaemia
1981	Toxin-producing *Staphylococcus aureus*	Bacterium	Toxic shock syndrome
1982	*Escherichia coli* O157:H7	Bacterium	Haemorrhagic colitis; haemolytic uraemic syndrome
1982	*Borrelia burgdorferi*	Bacterium	Lyme disease
1983	Human immunodeficiency virus (HIV)	Virus	Acquired immuno-deficiency syndrome (AIDS)
1983	*Helicobacter pylori*	Bacterium	Peptic ulcer disease
1989	Hepatitis C	Virus	Parentally transmitted non-A, non-B liver infection
1992	*Vibrio cholerae* O139	Bacterium	New strain associated with epidemic cholera
1993	Hantavirus	Virus	Adult respiratory distress syndrome
1994	*Cryptosporidium parvum*	Protozoa	Enteric disease
1995	*Ehrlichiosis*	Bacterium	Severe arthritis?
1996	nvCJD	Prion	New variant Creutzfeldt–Jakob disease
1997	HVN1	Virus	Influenza
1999	Nipah	Virus	Severe encephalitis
1999	West Nile	Virus	Severe encephalitis and multi-organ involvement
2002/3	SARS	Virus	Severe acute respiratory syndrome

World Health Organization: Report on infectious diseases; removing obstacles to healthy development, WHO 1999.

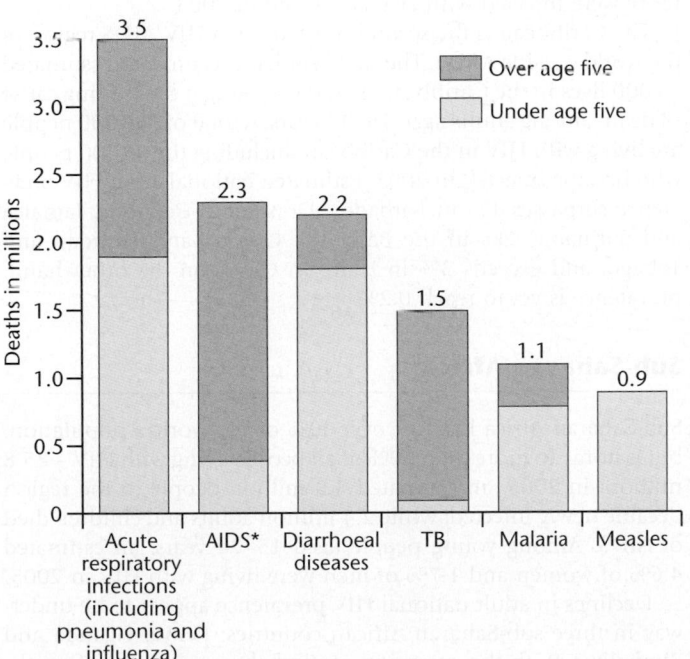

Figure 3.3 Leading infectious killers (millions of deaths, worldwide, all ages, 1998). HIV positive people who died with TB have been included in AIDS deaths (World Health Organization: Report on infectious diseases; removing obstacles to healthy development, WHO 1999).

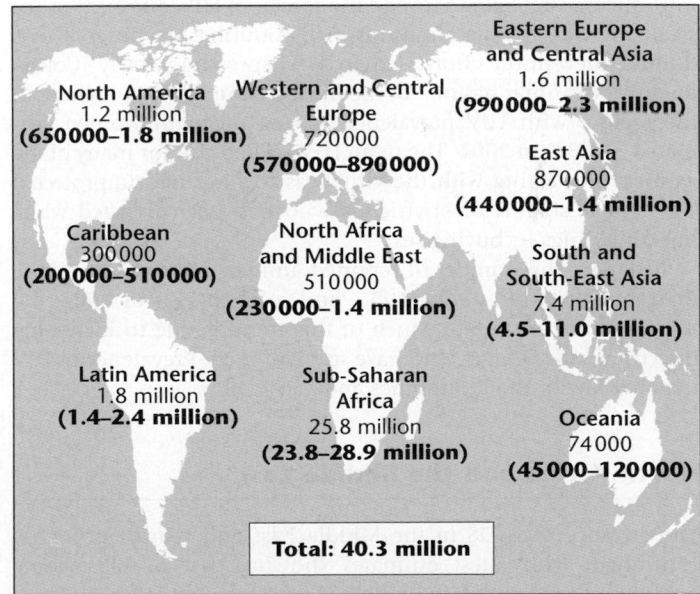

Figure 3.4 Adults and children estimated to be living with HIV in 2005 (WHO/UNAIDS December 2005).[6]

4% in 2004 (having exceeded 11% in 2001). In Mumbai, by contrast, available data suggest that sporadic and piecemeal efforts to promote condom use during commercial sex have not been as effective; there, HIV prevalence among female sex workers has not fallen below 52% since 2000.

The combination of high levels of risk behaviour and limited knowledge about AIDS among drug injectors and sex workers in Pakistan favours the rapid spread of HIV, and new data suggest that the country could be on the verge of serious HIV epidemics. Most countries in Asia still have the opportunity to prevent major epidemics. Bangladesh, where national adult HIV prevalence is well below 1%, began initiating HIV prevention programmes early in its epidemic.

Indonesia is on the brink of a rapidly worsening AIDS epidemic. With risk behaviour among injecting drug users common, a mainly drug-injection epidemic is already spreading into remote parts of this archipelago. In Malaysia, approximately 52 000 people were living with HIV in 2004, the vast majority of them young men (aged 20–29 years), of whom approximately 75% were injecting drug users. After peaking at 3% in 1997, national adult HIV prevalence in Cambodia fell by one-third, to 1.9% in 2003. The reasons for this are two-fold: increasing mortality and a decline in HIV incidence due to changes in risk behaviour. Thailand has been widely hailed as one of the success stories in the response to AIDS. By 2003, estimated national adult HIV prevalence had dropped to its lowest level ever, approximately 1.5%. However, Thailand's epidemic is far from over; infection levels in the most at-risk populations are much higher: just over 10% of brothel-based female sex workers were HIV-infected in 2003, as were 45% of injecting drug users who attended treatment clinics.

While Cambodia and Thailand in the 1990s were planning and introducing strategies to reverse the spread of HIV, another serious epidemic was gaining ground in neighbouring Myanmar. There, limited prevention efforts led to HIV spreading freely. Consequently, Myanmar has one of the most serious AIDS epidemics in the region, with HIV prevalence among pregnant women estimated at 1.8% in 2004. The main HIV-related risk for many of the women now living with the virus was to have had unprotected sex with husbands or boyfriends who had been infected while injecting drugs or buying sex.

In Japan, the number of reported annual HIV cases has more than doubled since 1994–1995, and reached 780 in 2004; the highest number to date. Much of this trend is due to increasing infections among men who have sex with men. Prevalence of HIV remains low in the Philippines and Lao PDR.

North Africa and the Middle East[6]

The advance of AIDS in the Middle East and North Africa has continued, with latest estimates showing that 67 000 people became infected with HIV in 2005. Approximately 510 000 people are living with HIV in this region. An estimated 58 000 adults and children died of AIDS-related conditions in 2005. Although HIV surveillance remains weak in this region, more comprehensive information is available in some countries (including Algeria, Libya, Morocco, Somalia and Sudan). Available evidence reveals trends of increasing HIV infections (especially in younger age groups) in such countries as Algeria, Libya, Morocco and Somalia.

The main mode of HIV transmission in this region is unprotected sexual contact, although injecting drug use is becoming an increasingly important factor (and is the predominant mode of infection in at least two countries: Iran and Libya). Infections as a result of contaminated blood products, blood transfusions or a lack of infection control measures in healthcare settings are generally on the decline.

By far the worst-affected country in this region is Sudan. In a country with a long history of civil conflict and forced displacement, internally displaced persons face higher rates of HIV infection. For instance, among displaced pregnant women seeking antenatal care in Khartoum in 2004, HIV prevalence of 1.6% was found compared with under 0.3% for other pregnant women.

Latin America and the Caribbean[6]

The epidemic in Latin America is a complex mosaic of transmission patterns in which HIV continues to spread through male-to-male sex, sex between men and women, and injecting drug use. The number of people living with HIV in Latin America has risen to an estimated 1.8 million. In 2005, approximately 66 000 people died of AIDS, and 200 000 were newly infected. Among young people 15–24 years of age, an estimated 0.4% of women and 0.6% of men were living with HIV in 2005. Primarily due to their large populations, the South American countries of Argentina, Brazil and Colombia are home to the biggest epidemics in this region. Brazil alone accounts for more than one third of the estimated 1.8 million people living with HIV in Latin America. The highest HIV prevalence, however, is found in the smaller countries of Belize, Guatemala and Honduras, where approximately 1% of adults or more were infected with HIV at the end of 2003.

The Caribbean is the second-most affected HIV/AIDS region in the world outside Africa. The AIDS epidemic claimed an estimated 24 000 lives in the Caribbean in 2005, making it the leading cause of death among adults aged 15–44 years. A total of 300 000 people are living with HIV in the Caribbean, including the 30 000 people who became infected in 2005. Estimated national adult HIV prevalence surpasses 1% in Barbados, Dominican Republic, Jamaica and Suriname, 2% in the Bahamas, Guyana and Trinidad and Tobago, and exceeds 3% in Haiti. In Cuba, on the other hand, prevalence is yet to reach 0.2%.

Sub-Saharan Africa[6]

Sub-Saharan Africa has just over 10% of the world's population, but is home to more than 60% of all people living with HIV – 25.8 million. In 2005, an estimated 3.2 million people in the region became newly infected, while 2.4 million adults and children died of AIDS. Among young people aged 15–24 years, an estimated 4.6% of women and 1.7% of men were living with HIV in 2005.

Declines in adult national HIV prevalence appear to be underway in three sub-Saharan African countries: Kenya, Uganda and Zimbabwe. With the exception of Zimbabwe, countries of southern Africa show little evidence of declining epidemics. HIV prevalence levels remain exceptionally high (except for Angola), and might not yet have reached their peak in several countries – as the expanding epidemics in Mozambique and Swaziland suggest. West and Central Africa also show no signs of changing HIV infection levels, except for urban parts of Burkina Faso (where prevalence appears to be declining).

The rights and status of women and young girls deserve special attention. Around the world – from south of the Sahara in Africa and Asia to Europe, Latin America and the Pacific – an increasing number of women are being infected with HIV. It is often women with little or no income who are most at risk. Widespread inequalities including political, social, cultural and human security factors also exacerbate the situation for women and girls. In several southern African countries, more than three quarters of all young people living with HIV are women, while in sub-Saharan Africa overall, young women between 15 and 24 years old are at least three times more likely to be HIV-positive than young men (Figure 3.5).[6] In many countries, marriage and women's own fidelity are not enough to protect them against HIV infection. Among women surveyed in Harare (Zimbabwe), Durban and Soweto (South Africa), 66% reported having one lifetime partner, 79% had abstained from sex at least until the age of 17 (roughly the average age of first sexual encounter in most countries in the world). Yet, 40% of the young women were HIV-positive. Many had been infected despite staying faithful to one partner.

DIARRHOEAL DISEASE

Diarrhoea remains one of the most common diseases afflicting children under 5 years of age and accounts for considerable mortality in childhood. Estimates from studies published between 1992 and 2000 show that there was a median of 3.2 episodes of diarrhoea per child-year in developing countries. This indicates little change from previously described incidences. Estimates of mortality revealed that 4.9 children per 1000/year in these countries died as a result of diarrhoeal illness in the first 5 years of life, a decline from the previous estimates of 5.6–3.6 per 1000/year. The decrease was most pronounced in children aged under one year. Despite improving trends in mortality rates, diarrhoea accounted for a median of 21% of all deaths of children aged under 5 years in developing countries, being responsible for 2.5 million deaths per year. There has not been a concurrent decrease in morbidity rates attributable to diarrhoea. As population growth is focused in the poorest areas, the total morbidity component of the disease burden is greater than previously.[7]

Diarrhoea remains a disease of poverty afflicting malnourished children in crowded and contaminated environments. Efforts to immunize children against measles, provide safe water and adequate sanitation facilities, and to encourage mothers to exclusively breast-feed infants through to 6 months of age can blunt an increase in diarrhoea morbidity and mortality. Preventive strategies to limit the transmission of diarrhoeal disease need to go hand in hand with national diarrhoea disease control programmes that concentrate on effective diarrhoea case management and the prevention of dehydration.[8] The factors contributing to childhood mortality and morbidity due to diarrhoea are described in Table 3.2.[8]

Studies in Asia and Africa have clearly shown that establishment of an oral rehydration therapy (ORT) unit with training of hospital staff can significantly reduce diarrhoea case fatality rates. For instance, at Mama Yemo Hospital in Kinshasa, Zaire, there was a 69% decline in diarrhoea deaths after creation of an ORT unit.[9] In May 2002, the World Health Organization and the United Nations Children's Fund recommended that the formulation of oral rehydration solution (ORS) for treatment of patients with diarrhoea be changed to one with a reduced osmolarity and that safety of the new formulation, particularly development of symptomatic hyponatremia, be monitored.[10] A total of 53 280 patients, including 22 536 children younger than 60 months, were monitored at the Dhaka and Matlab hospitals, Bangladesh. The risk of symptoms associated with hyponatraemia in patients

Table 3.2 Factors contributing to diarrhoea morbidity and mortality[8]

Biological factors	Socioenvironmental factors
Age of the child	Family income
Age of the caretaker	Education level of caretaker
Birth order of child	Water quality and/or quantity
Feeding mode	Sanitation facilities

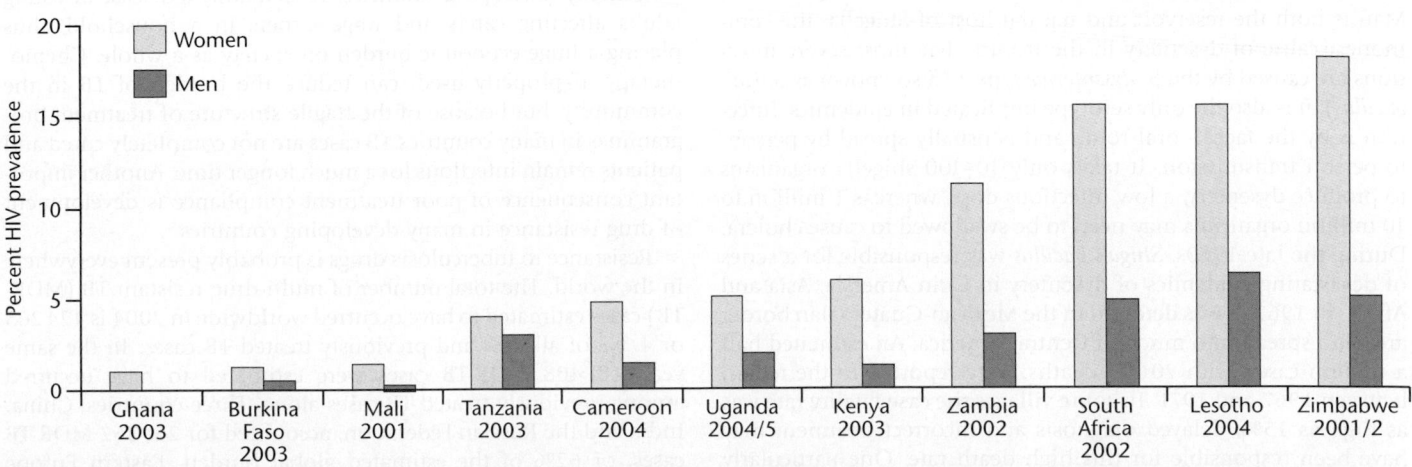

Figure 3.5 HIV prevalence among 15–24-year-old men and women in sub-Saharan Africa, 2001–2005. (WHO/UNAIDS December 2005.)

treated with the reduced osmolarity ORS was found to be minimal and did not increase with the change in formulation.[10]

Changing patterns in the epidemiology of diarrhoea have been noted in many studies. In Matlab, Bangladesh, acute watery diarrhoea accounted for 34% of diarrhoea deaths in under-fives, while the remaining 66% were related to dysentery or persistent diarrhoea and malnutrition. This pattern was age dependent, with acute watery deaths being more important in infancy, being associated with 40% of deaths, and less important in later childhood, being associated with 10% of deaths.[11]

Watery diarrhoea

Rotavirus is the most common cause of severe diarrhoeal disease in infants and young children all over the world, and an important public health problem, particularly in developing countries where 600 000 deaths each year are associated with this infection. More than 125 million cases of diarrhoea each year are attributed to rotavirus. In tropical developing countries, rotavirus disease occurs either throughout the year or in the cold dry season. Almost all children are already infected by the age of 3–5 years. Although the infection is usually mild, severe disease may rapidly result in life-threatening dehydration if not appropriately treated. Natural infection protects children against subsequent severe disease.

Globally, four serotypes are responsible for the majority of rotaviral disease, but additional serotypes are prevalent in some countries. The only control measure likely to have a significant impact on the incidence of severe disease is vaccination. Since the withdrawal from the market of the tetravalent rhesus–human reassortant vaccine (RotaShield, Wyeth Laboratories) because of an association with intussusception, ruling out such a risk has become critical for the licensure and universal use of any new rotavirus vaccine. Recent studies have shown that two oral doses of the live attenuated G1P[8] human rotavirus vaccine were highly efficacious in protecting infants against severe rotavirus gastroenteritis, significantly reduced the rate of severe gastroenteritis from any cause, and were not associated with the increased risk of intussusception linked with the previous vaccine.[12]

Dysentery

Man is both the reservoir and natural host of Shigella, the commonest cause of dysentery in the tropics. The most severe infections are caused by the S. dysenteriae type 1 (also known as Shiga's bacillus); it is also the only serotype implicated in epidemics. Infection is by the faecal- oral route and is usually spread by person-to-person transmission. It takes only 10–100 shigella organisms to produce dysentery, a low infectious dose, whereas 1 million to 10 million organisms may need to be swallowed to cause cholera. During the late 1960s, Shiga's bacillus was responsible for a series of devastating epidemics of dysentery in Latin America, Asia and Africa. In 1967, it was detected in the Mexican-Guatemalan border area and spread into much of Central America. An estimated half a million cases, with 20 000 deaths, were reported in the region between 1967 and 1971. In some villages the case fatality rate was as high as 15%; delayed diagnosis and incorrect treatment may have been responsible for this high death rate. One particularly disturbing feature was the resistance of the bacteria to the most commonly used antibacterial drugs: sulfonamides, tetracycline and chloramphenicol.[13]

Serious epidemics due to the multiple-drug resistant S. dysenteriae type 1 have occurred recently in Bangladesh, Somalia, South India, Burma, Sri Lanka, Nepal, Bhutan, Rwanda and Zaire. West Bengal in India has always been an endemic area for bacillary dysentery. Preventive measures include boiling or chlorination of drinking water, covering faeces with soil, protecting food from flies, avoiding eating exposed raw vegetables and cut fruits, and washing hands with soap and water before eating and after using the latrine. However, such measures are not easy to implement in most areas. Consequently epidemics take their own course and subside only gradually.[13]

TUBERCULOSIS

Tuberculosis (TB) is the leading cause of death associated with infectious diseases globally. The incidence of TB will continue to increase substantially worldwide because of the interaction between the TB and HIV epidemics. The 4.9 million new and relapse cases of TB (all forms)notified in 2004 represent 56% of the 9.2 million estimated new cases; the 2.5 million new smear-positive cases notified account for 64% of the 4.1 million estimated. The detection rate of new smear-positive cases from all sources slowly increased from 1995 to 2001, and then more quickly from 2002 to 2004. In 2006, there were 14.4 million prevalent cases (219/100 000 population), of which 6.1 million were smear-positive (95/100 000 population). Based on surveillance and survey data, we estimate that there were 9.2 million new cases of TB in 2006 (139 per 100 000 population), including 4.1 million (62 per 100 000 population) new smear-positive cases. Country-wide estimates of the incidence rate of TB in 2006 are shown in Figure 3.6. An estimated 1.7 million people (25/100 000 population) died from TB in 2006, including those co-infected with HIV (231 000). The African Region alone accounts for 85% of the estimated 709 000 cases of TB among HIV-positive people in the world, but for only 4% of those reported to have begun antiretroviral therapy (ART) in 2003. The region of the Americas (mainly Brazil), on the other hand, accounts for 2% of the estimated cases but for 96% of the 9388 people reported to have started on ART in 2006.[14]

In many developing countries, TB is mainly a disease of young adults affecting carers and wage-earners in a household, thus placing a huge economic burden on society as a whole. Chemotherapy, if properly used, can reduce the burden of TB in the community, but because of the fragile structure of treatment programmes in many countries TB cases are not completely cured and patients remain infectious for a much longer time. Another important consequence of poor treatment compliance is development of drug resistance in many developing countries.

Resistance to tuberculosis drugs is probably present everywhere in the world. The total number of multi-drug resistant TB (MDR-TB) cases estimated to have occurred worldwide in 2004 is 424 203 or 4.3% of all new and previously treated TB cases. In the same year, 181 408 MDR-TB cases were estimated to have occurred among previously treated TB cases alone. Three countries: China, India and the Russian Federation, accounted for 261 362 MDR-TB cases, or 62% of the estimated global burden. Eastern Europe reported the highest prevalence of MDR-TB among new cases, and

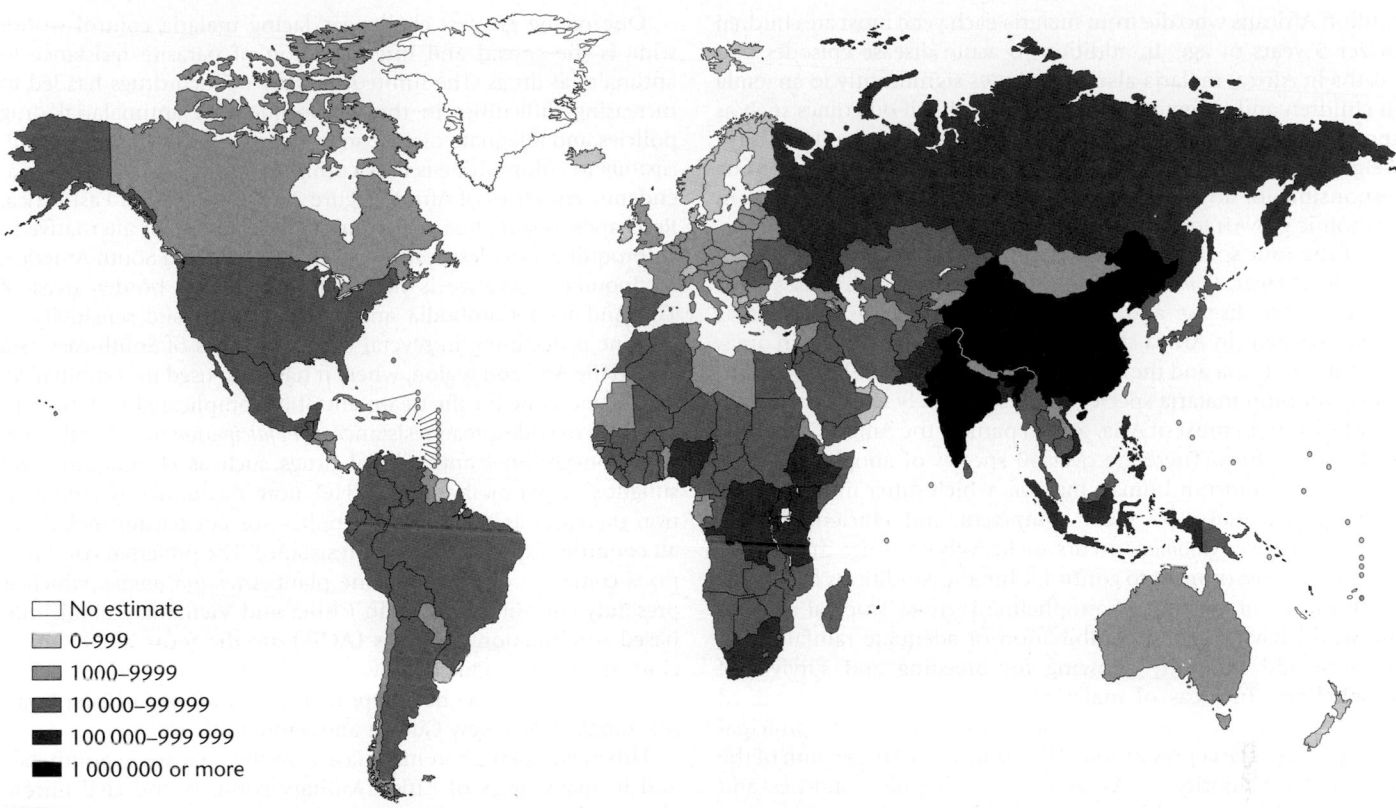

Figure 3.6 Estimated new TB cases (all forms) per 100 000 population. (WHO 2008[14].)

No estimate
0–999
1000–9999
10 000–99 999
100 000–999 999
1 000 000 or more

figures from former Kazakhstan and Israel both had an MDR prevalence rate of 14.2%. Other high prevalence areas include Uzbekistan (13.2%), Estonia (12.2%) and China's Liaoning Province (10.4%).[15]

Worldwide attention was focused on South Africa, when in October 2006 a research project publicized a deadly outbreak of XDR-TB in the small town of Tugela Ferry in KwaZulu-Natal. XDR-TB is the abbreviation for extensively drug-resistant tuberculosis (TB). This strain of *Mycobacterium tuberculosis* is resistant to first- and second-line drugs, and treatment options are seriously limited. Of 536 TB patients at the Church of Scotland Hospital, which serves a rural area with high HIV rates, some 221 were found to have multi-drug resistance and of these, 53 were diagnosed with XDR-TB. Some 52 of these patients died, most within 25 days of diagnosis. Of the 53 patients, 44 had been tested for HIV and all 44 were found to be HIV-positive. The patients were receiving antiretrovirals and responding well to HIV-related treatment, but they died of XDR-TB. Since the study, 10 more patients have been diagnosed with XDR-TB in KwaZulu-Natal. Only three of them are still alive (see: http://www.who.int/tb/xdr/xdr_jan.pdf).

Directly observed treatment, short course (DOTS), is the most effective strategy available for controlling the TB epidemic today. DOTS uses sound technology and packages it with good management practices for widespread use through the existing primary healthcare network. It has proven to be a successful, innovative approach to TB control in countries such as China, Bangladesh, Vietnam, Peru and countries of West Africa. However, new challenges to the implementation of DOTS include health sector reforms, the worsening HIV epidemic, and the emergence of drug-resistant strains of TB. The technical, logistical, operational and political aspects of DOTS work together to ensure its success and applicability in a wide variety of contexts.[14] Between 1995 and 2006, about 24 million patients were treated under the DOTS strategy. Worldwide, 183 countries were implementing the DOTS strategy by the end of 2004, and 83% of the world's population was living in regions where DOTS was in place. DOTS programs reported 2.4 million new TB cases through laboratory testing in 2006, a case detection rate of 61%, and the average success rate for DOTS treatment exceeded 85%. WHO aimed to achieve a 70% case detection rate of TB cases and cure 85% of those detected by 2005.[14]

A number of smaller countries appear to have declining TB incidence rates that are linked to high rates of case detection and cure; these include Cuba, Lebanon, the Maldives, Nicaragua, Oman and Uruguay.

MALARIA

Close to 100 countries or territories in the world are considered malarious, almost half of which are in Africa, south of the Sahara (Figure 3.4). As of 2004, 107 countries and territories have reported areas at risk of malaria transmission. The incidence of malaria worldwide is estimated to be 300–500 million clinical cases each year. Around 60% of the cases of clinical malaria and over 80% of the deaths occur in Africa south of the Sahara. Of the more than 1 million Africans who die from malaria each year, most are children under 5 years of age. In addition to acute disease episodes and deaths in Africa, malaria also contributes significantly to anaemia in children and pregnant women, adverse birth outcomes such as spontaneous abortion, stillbirth, premature delivery and low birth weight, and overall child mortality. The disease is estimated to be responsible for an estimated average annual reduction of 1.3% in economic growth for those countries with the highest burden.[16]

Of the four species of Plasmodium that infect humans: *P. falciparum*, *P. vivax*, *P. malariae* and *P. ovale*, *P. falciparum* causes most of the severe disease and deaths attributable to malaria and is most prevalent in Africa south of the Sahara and in certain areas of South-east Asia and the Western Pacific (Figure 3.7). The second most common malaria species, *P. vivax*, is rarely fatal and is commonly found in most of Asia, and in parts of the Americas, Europe and North Africa. There are over 40 species of anopheline mosquitoes that transmit human malaria, which differ in their transmission potential. The most competent and efficient malaria vector, *Anopheles gambiae*, occurs exclusively in Africa and is also one of the most difficult to control. Climatic conditions determine the presence or absence of anopheline vectors. Tropical areas of the world have the best combination of adequate rainfall, temperature and humidity allowing for breeding and survival of anophelines. In areas of malaria transmission where sustained vector control is required, insecticide treated nets are the principal strategy for malaria prevention. All countries in Africa south of the Sahara, the majority of Asian malaria-endemic countries and some American countries have adopted insecticide treated nets as a key malaria control strategy.[16]

One of the greatest challenges facing malaria control worldwide is the spread and intensification of parasite resistance to antimalarial drugs. The limited number of such drugs has led to increasing difficulties in the development of antimalarial drug policies and adequate disease management.[16] Resistance of *P. falciparum* to chloroquine is now common in practically all malaria-endemic countries of Africa (Figure 3.7), especially in East Africa. Resistance to sulfadoxine/pyrimethamine, the main alternative to chloroquine, is widespread in South-east Asia and South America. Mefloquine resistance is now common in the border areas of Thailand with Cambodia and Myanmar. Parasite sensitivity to quinine is declining in several other countries of South-east Asia and in the Amazon region, where it has been used in combination with tetracycline for the treatment of uncomplicated malaria.[16] In response to widespread resistance of *P. falciparum* to monotherapy with conventional antimalarial drugs such as chloroquine and sulfadoxine-pyrimethamine, WHO now recommends combination therapies as the treatment policy for falciparum malaria in all countries experiencing such resistance. The preferred combinations contain a derivative of the plant *Artemisia annua*, which is presently cultivated mainly in China and Vietnam. Artemisinin-based combination therapies (ACTs) are the most highly efficacious treatment regimens now available. Resistance of *P. vivax* to chloroquine has now been reported from Indonesia (Irian Jaya), Myanmar, Papua New Guinea and Vanuatu.[17]

Urban and periurban malaria are on the increase in South Asia and in many areas of Africa. Military conflicts and civil unrest, along with unfavourable ecological changes, have greatly contributed to malaria epidemics, as large numbers of unprotected, non-

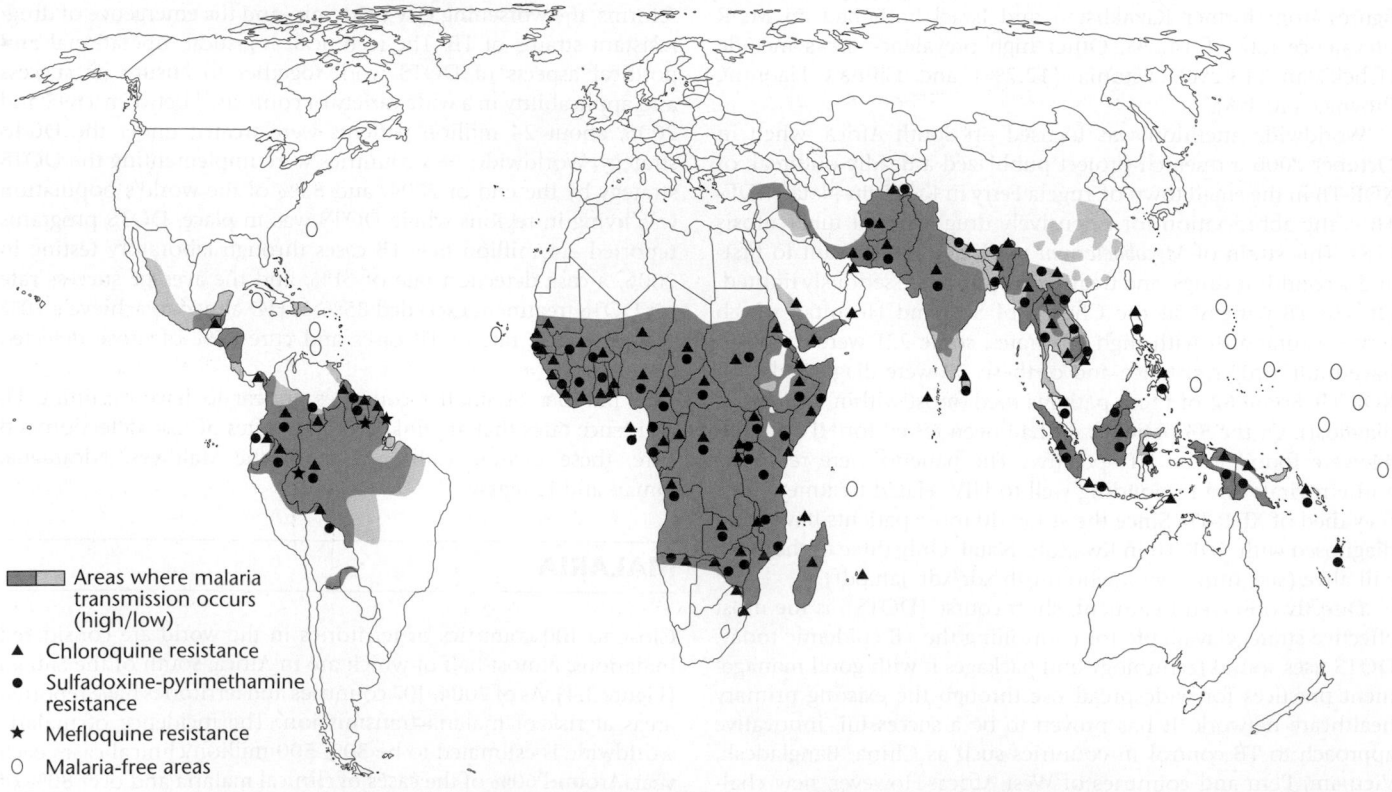

Areas where malaria transmission occurs (high/low)
▲ Chloroquine resistance
● Sulfadoxine-pyrimethamine resistance
★ Mefloquine resistance
○ Malaria-free areas

Figure 3.7 Drug resistance to *P. falciparum* from studies in sentinel sites, up to 2004. (World Malaria Report 2005, WHO 2005.)

immune and physically weakened refugees move into malarious areas. Such population movements contribute to new malaria outbreaks and make epidemic-prone situations more explosive.[16] Another disquieting factor is the re-emergence of malaria in areas where it had been eradicated (e.g. Democratic People's Republic of Korea, Republic of Korea and Tadjikistan), or its increase in countries where it was nearly eradicated (e.g. Azerbaijan, northern Iraq and Turkey). Current malaria epidemics in a majority of these countries are the result of a rapid deterioration of malaria prevention and control operations. Climatic changes have also been implicated in the re-emergence of malaria. In the past 5 years, the worldwide incidence of malaria has quadrupled, influenced by changes in both land development and regional climate. In Brazil, satellite images depict a 'fish bone' pattern where roads have opened the tropical forest to localized development. In these 'edge' areas malaria has resurged. Temperature changes have encouraged a redistribution of the disease; malaria is now found at higher elevations in central Africa and could threaten cities such as Nairobi, Kenya. This threat has been hypothesized to extend to temperate regions of the world that are now experiencing hotter summers year on year.[18]

VACCINE-PREVENTABLE INFECTIOUS DISEASES

Measles

Although substantial progress has been made in reducing measles deaths globally, in 2000 measles was estimated to be the fifth leading cause of mortality worldwide for children aged <5 years. Measles deaths occur disproportionately in Africa and South-east Asia. In 2000, the African Region of WHO, with 10% of the world's population, accounted for 41% of estimated measles cases and 58% of measles deaths; the South-east Asia region, with 25% of the world's population and 28% of measles cases, accounted for 26% of measles deaths. The burden of mortality in Africa reflects low routine vaccination coverage and high case-fatality ratios. In South-east Asia, where vaccination coverage is slightly below average worldwide levels, the large population amplifies the number of cases and deaths resulting from ongoing measles transmission.

The overwhelming majority of measles deaths in 2000 occurred in countries eligible to receive financial support from the Global Alliance for Vaccines and Immunization's Vaccine Fund (WHO, unpublished data 2003). The majority of measles deaths occur among young children living in poor countries with inadequate vaccination services. Like human immunodeficiency virus, malaria, and tuberculosis, measles can be considered a disease of poverty. However, unlike these diseases, measles can be prevented through vaccination.[19,20]

Hepatitis B

In much of the world, particularly sub-Saharan Africa, South-east Asia, China and the Pacific Basin, infection with hepatitis B virus (HBV) is very widespread. The carrier rate in some of these populations may be as high as 10–20%. In developing countries most hepatitis B transmission occurs during the perinatal period. Infection between children is another common route of infection; it is not uncommon to find up to 90% of 15-year-olds have serological evidence of infection with HBV. Intermediate levels of infection (2–7%) are seen in parts of the former Soviet Union, South Asia, Central America and the northern zones of South America. These high rates of infection lead to a high burden of disease, mainly from the clinical consequences of long-term carriage of the virus, which may include chronic hepatitis, cirrhosis and liver cancer. It has been estimated that HBV infection is the second most common cause of cancer deaths in the world (after tobacco consumption). In India hepatitis B is linked to 60% of cases of hepatocellular carcinoma and 80% of cases of cirrhosis of the liver.[21]

On the basis of disease burden and the availability of safe and effective vaccines, the WHO recommended that by the end of the twentieth century, hepatitis B vaccine be incorporated into routine infant and childhood immunization programmes for all countries. The efficacy of universal immunization has been shown in different countries, with striking reductions of the prevalence of HBV carriage in children. Most important, hepatitis B vaccination can protect children against hepatocellular carcinoma and fulminant hepatitis, as has been shown in Taiwan. Nevertheless, the implementation of worldwide vaccination against HBV requires greater effort to overcome the social and economic hurdles. Safe and effective antiviral treatments are available but are still far from ideal, a situation that, hopefully, will be improved soon. With hepatitis B immunization, the global control of HBV infection is possible by the end of the first half of twenty-first century.[22]

Neonatal tetanus

Tetanus is a vaccine-preventable disease that causes a total of 309 000 deaths annually. Of particular concern is maternal and neonatal tetanus (MNT), which can be prevented through immunization of the mother in pregnancy. In 2000, neonatal tetanus alone was responsible for an estimated 200 000 deaths. In addition, an estimated 15 000–30 000 non-immunized women worldwide die each year from maternal tetanus that results from postpartum, postabortal or postsurgical wound infection with *Clostridium tetani*.

While the focus is on 57 priority countries, 90% of the neonatal tetanus deaths occur in 27 countries. UNICEF spearheaded the effort to eliminate MNT by the year 2005, with the support of numerous partners. MNT elimination is defined as less than one case of neonatal tetanus per 1000 live births at district level. The main strategies consist of promotion of clean delivery practices, immunization of women with a tetanus toxoid (TT) containing vaccine, and surveillance. Maternal tetanus immunization is, in most developing countries, implemented as part of the routine immunization programme. However, large areas remain underserved, due to logistical, cultural, economical or other reasons. In order to achieve the target of MNT elimination by 2005, and to offer protection to women and children otherwise deprived from regular immunization services, countries are encouraged to adopt the high risk approach. This approach implies that, in addition to routine immunization of pregnant women, all women of child-bearing age living in high risk areas are targeted for immunization with three doses of a tetanus toxoid containing vaccine (TT or Td).[23]

By the end of 2007 11 countries have been validated as having achieved MNT elimination: Egypt, Eritrea, Malawi, Namibia, Nepal, Rwanda, South Africa, Togo, Viet Nam, Zambia and Zambabwe. In addition, 13 States and Union Territories in India were also validated as having eliminated MNT: Andhra Pradesh, Chandigarh, Goa, Haryana, Karnataka, Kerala, Lakshadweep, Maharashtra, Pondicherry, Punjab, Sikkim, Tamil Nadu & West Bengal. By the end of 2007, 47 countries remained that had not eliminated MNT.

Vaccination against a range of bacterial and viral diseases is an integral part of communicable disease control worldwide. Vaccination against a specific disease not only reduces the incidence of that disease, but it also reduces the social and economic burden of the disease on communities. Very high immunization coverage can lead to complete blocking of transmission for many vaccine-preventable diseases. The worldwide eradication of smallpox and the near-eradication of polio from many countries provide excellent examples of the role of immunization in disease control. Despite these advances many of the world's poorest countries do not have access to vaccines and these infections remain among the leading global causes of death.

NEGLECTED TROPICAL DISEASES

The Special Programme for Research and Training in Tropical Diseases (TDR) of the World Health Organization has designated several infectious diseases as 'neglected tropical diseases' (NTDs) that disproportionately afflict the poor and marginalized populations in the developing regions of *sub-Saharan Africa, Asia* and the *Americas*.[24] Infectious diseases are considered as 'neglected' or 'orphan' diseases when there is a lack of effective, affordable, or easy to use drug treatments. As most patients with such diseases live in developing countries and are too poor to pay for drugs, the pharmaceutical industry has traditionally ignored these diseases. NTDs cause an estimated 500 000 to 1 million deaths annually and cause a global *disease burden* equivalent to that of *HIV-AIDS*. WHO estimates that at least 1 billion people, i.e. one-sixth of the world's population suffers from one or more neglected tropical diseases, while other estimates suggest the number to be much higher. Some diseases affect individuals throughout their lives, causing a high degree of morbidity and physical disability and, in certain cases, gross disfigurement. Others are acute infections, with transient, severe and sometimes fatal outcomes. Patients can face social stigmatization and abuse, which only add to the already heavy health burden.

Neglected tropical diseases are contrasted with the 'big three' diseases (*HIV/AIDS, tuberculosis* and *malaria*) which receive much more attention and funding. The current neglected diseases portfolio includes parasitic diseases of protozoan origin like Kala-azar (*leishmaniasis*), *African sleeping sickness (African trypanosomiasis)* and *Chagas' disease* (American trypanosomiasis) as well as those caused by helminths such as *Schistosomiasis, lymphatic filariasis, Onchocerciasis* (river blindness) and *Dracunculiasis* (guinea worm). Infestations due to soil transmitted helminths such as *Ascariasis, Trichuriais* and *Hookworm* also belong to the latter category. Other neglected diseases include those of bacterial origin such as Leprosy, Buruli ulcer and Trachoma as well as those of viral origin like *dengue fever* which are vector-borne. Even cholera and yellow fever are considered by some as NTDs, while some include cysticercosis, hydatidosis and food-borne trematode infections. It is now believed that ramped up efforts against the 'big three', will yield far bigger dividends if they are coupled with concerted attack on NTDs[25]. Evidence now points to substantial geographical overlap between the neglected tropical diseases and the 'big three', suggesting that control of the neglected tropical diseases could become a powerful tool for effectively combating HIV/AIDS, tuberculosis, and malaria.[25]

EMERGING AND RESURGENT INFECTIOUS DISEASES

Since 1991, resurgent and emerging infectious disease outbreaks have occurred worldwide. In addition, many diseases widely believed to be under control, such as cholera, dengue and diphtheria, have re-emerged in many areas or spread to new regions or populations throughout the world (Figure 3.8).[26] A growing population and increasing urbanization contribute to emerging infectious disease problems. In many parts of the world, urban population growth has been accompanied by overcrowding, poor hygiene, inadequate sanitation and unclean drinking water. Urban development has also caused ecological damage. In these circumstances, certain disease-causing organisms and some of the vectors that transmit them have thrived, making it more likely that people will be infected with new or re-emerging pathogens. The existing public health infrastructure is already overtaxed and ill prepared to deal with new health threats. Breakdown of public health measures due to civil unrest, war and the movement of refugees has also contributed to the re-emergence of infectious diseases (Table 3.3).[26] International travel and commerce have made it possible for pathogens to be quickly transported from one side of the globe to the other (Figure 3.9).[26]

Examples of new and resurgent infections include Ebola, dengue fever, Rift Valley fever, diphtheria, cholera, Nipah virus infection, West Nile virus infection, severe acute respiratory syndrome (SARS) and avian influenza.

Ebola

In 1976 Ebola (named after the Ebola River in Zaire) first emerged in Sudan and the Democratic Republic of the Congo (formerly Zaire). Ebola virus occurs as four distinct subtypes: Zaïre, Sudan, Côte d'Ivoire and Reston. Three subtypes, occurring in the Democratic Republic of the Congo, Sudan and Côte d'Ivoire, have been identified as causing illness in humans. Ebola haemorrhagic fever (EHF) is a febrile haemorrhagic illness which causes death in 50–90% of all clinically ill cases. The natural reservoir of the Ebola virus is unknown despite extensive studies, but seems to reside in the rain forests on the African continent and in the Western Pacific.

Through June 1997, 1054 cases had been reported to the WHO, 754 of which proved fatal, mainly from Côte d'Ivoire, Democratic Republic of Congo, Gabon and Sudan. In October 2000, the first ever cases of Ebola were reported to the WHO from Uganda. By January 2001, there were 426 cases and 224 deaths in Uganda.

From October 2001 to December 2003, several EHF outbreaks of the Zaïre subtype, were reported in Gabon and the Republic of Congo with a total of 302 cases and 254 deaths.[27]

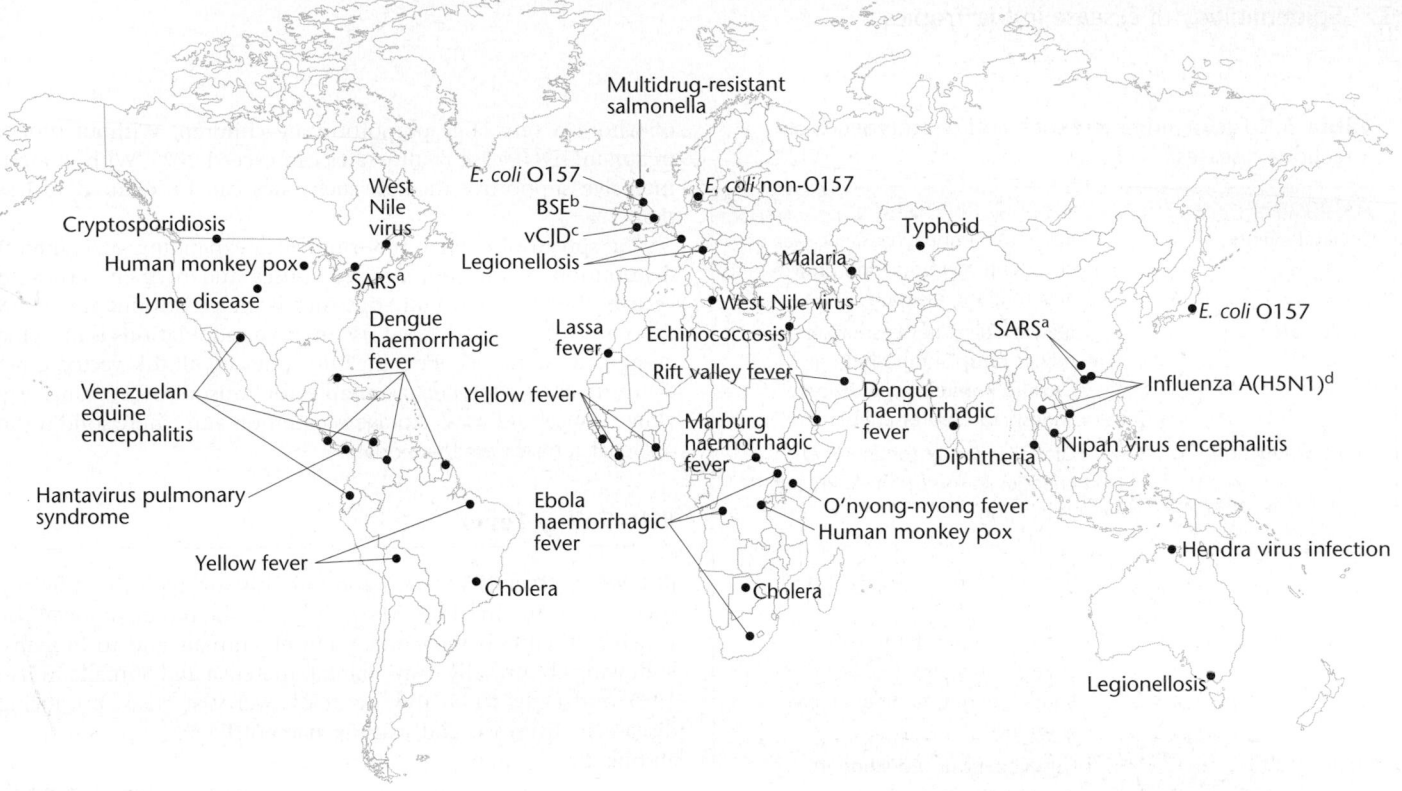

Figure 3.8   Selected emerging and re-emerging infectious diseases 1996–2004. [a]SARS, severe acute respiratory syndrome. [b]BSE, bovine spongiform encephalopathy; or mad cow disease. [c]vCJD, variant Creutzfeldt–Jakob disease. [d]Influenza A, (H5N1) or avian influenza (CDC and WHO 2006).

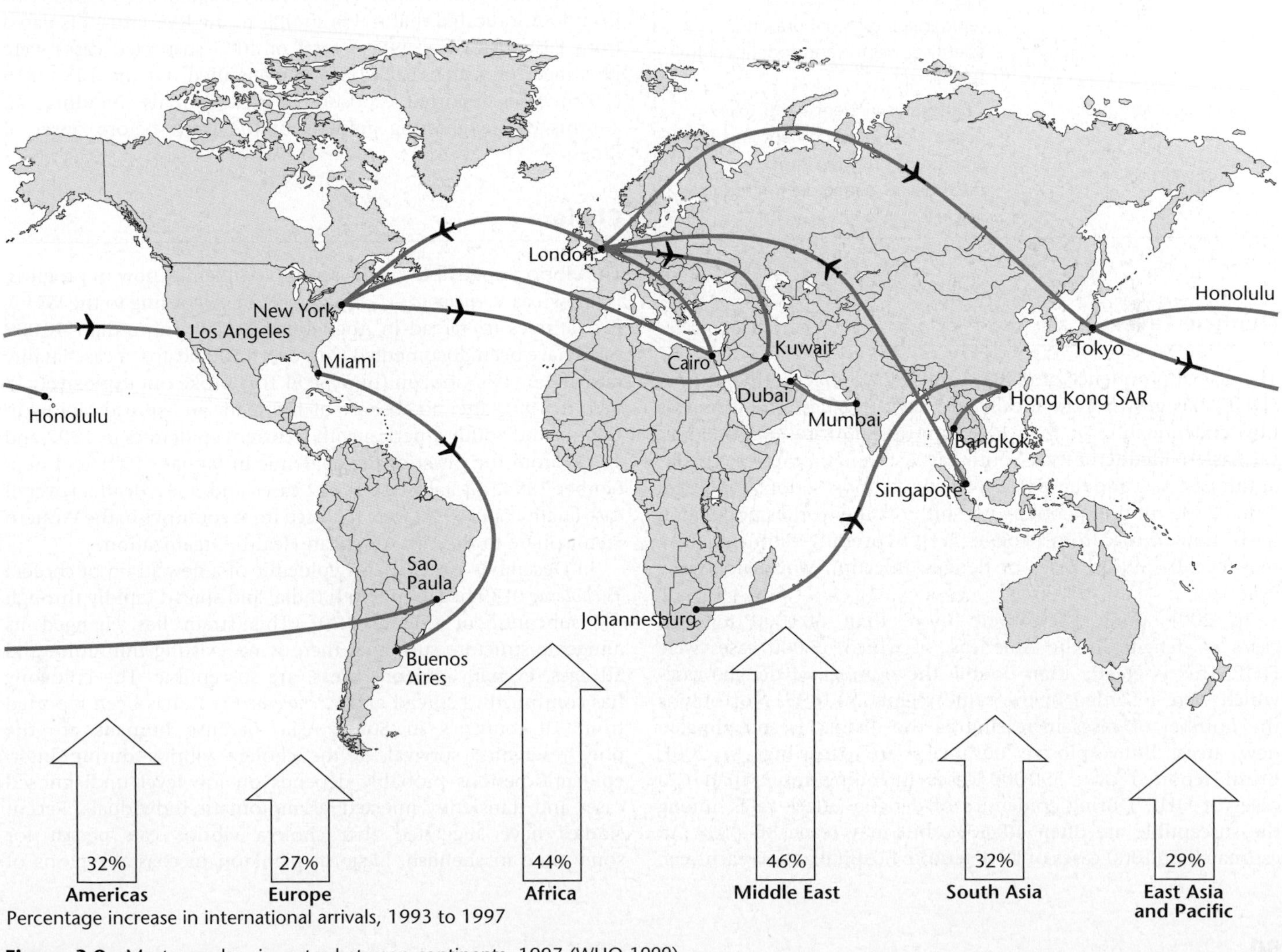

Percentage increase in international arrivals, 1993 to 1997

Americas	Europe	Africa	Middle East	South Asia	East Asia and Pacific
32%	27%	44%	46%	32%	29%

Figure 3.9   Most popular air routes between continents, 1997 (WHO 1999).

Table 3.3 Factors in emergence and re-emergence of infectious diseases[24]

Categories	Specific examples
Societal events	Economic impoverishment; war or civil conflict; population growth and migration; urban decay
Healthcare	New medical devices; organ or tissue transplantation; drugs causing immunosuppression; widespread use of antibiotics
Food production	Globalization of food supplies; changes in food processing and packaging
Human behaviour	Sexual behaviour; drug use; travel; diet; outdoor recreation; use of childcare facilities
Environmental changes	Deforestation/reforestation; changes in water ecosystems; flood/drought; famine; global warming
Public health	Curtailment or reduction in prevention programmes; infrastructure and communicable disease surveillance inadequate; lack of trained personnel (epidemiologists, laboratory scientists, vector and rodent control specialists)
Microbial adaptation	Changes in virulence and toxin production; development and change of drug resistance; microbes as co-factors in chronic diseases

Dengue fever

The global prevalence of dengue and dengue haemorrhagic fever (DHF) has grown dramatically in recent decades. The disease is now endemic in more than 100 countries in Africa, the Americas, the Eastern Mediterranean, South-east Asia and the Western Pacific. South-east Asia and the Western Pacific are most seriously affected. Some 2500 million people – two-fifths of the world's population – are now at risk from dengue. WHO currently estimates there may be 50 million cases of dengue infection worldwide every year.

In 2001 alone, there were more than 609 000 reported cases of dengue in the Americas, of which 15 000 cases were DHF. This is greater than double the number of dengue cases which were recorded in the same region in 1995. Not only is the number of cases increasing as the disease is spreading to new areas, but explosive outbreaks are occurring. In 2001, Brazil reported over 390 000 cases including more than 670 cases of DHF. During epidemics of dengue, attack rates among the susceptible are often 40–50%, but may reach 80–90%. An estimated 500 000 cases of DHF require hospitalization each year,

of whom a very large proportion are children. Without proper treatment, DHF case fatality rates can exceed 20%. With modern intensive supportive therapy, such rates can be reduced to less than 1%.

The spread of dengue is attributed to expanding geographical distribution of the four dengue viruses and of their mosquito vectors, the most important of which is the predominantly urban species *Aedes aegypti*. A rapid rise in urban populations is bringing ever greater numbers of people into contact with this vector, especially in areas that are favourable for mosquito breeding, e.g. where household water storage is common and where solid waste disposal services are inadequate.[28]

Rift Valley fever

Rift Valley fever (RVF) is a zoonotic disease typically affecting sheep and cattle in Africa. Mosquitoes are the principal means by which RVF virus is transmitted among animals and to humans. Following abnormally heavy rainfall in Kenya and Somalia in late 1997 and early 1998, RVF occurred over vast areas, producing disease in livestock and causing haemorrhagic fever and death among the human population. As of December 2006, WHO figures indicate that the outbreak continues to affect the north western provinces of Kenya. In September 2000 WHO documented the first ever RVF outbreak outside Africa, in Yemen and the Kingdom of Saudi Arabia (KSA). RNA sequencing of the virus from KSA indicated that it was similar to the RVF viruses isolated from East Africa in 1998. A total of 1087 suspected cases were identified, of which 121 (11%) persons died. Of the 1087, 815 (75%) cases reported exposure to sick animals, handling an abortus or slaughtering animals in the week before onset of illness.[29]

Cholera

The vibrio responsible for the seventh pandemic, now in progress, is known as *V. cholerae* O1, biotype El Tor. According to the WHO, it continues to spread in Angola and Sudan; more than 40 000 cases have been documented with over 1500 deaths: a case fatality rate of 3.5–4%. Cholera (biotype El Tor) broke out explosively in Peru in 1991, after an absence of 100 years, and spread rapidly in Central and South America, with recurrent epidemics in 1992 and 1993. From the onset of the epidemic in January 1991 to 1 September 1994, a total of 1 041 422 cases and 9642 deaths (overall case fatality rate 0.9%) were reported from countries in the Western Hemisphere to the Pan American Health Organization.

In December 1992, a large epidemic of a new strain of cholera *V. cholerae* 0139 began in South India, and spread rapidly through the subcontinent (Figure 3.10). This strain has changed its antigenic structure such that there is no existing immunity and all ages, even in endemic areas, are susceptible. The epidemic has continued to spread and *V. cholerae* O139 has been reported from 11 countries in South Asia. Because humans are the only reservoirs, survival of the cholera vibrios during inter-epidemic periods probably depends on low-level undiagnosed cases and transiently infected, asymptomatic individuals. Recent studies have suggested that cholera vibrios can persist for some time in shellfish, algae or plankton in coastal regions of

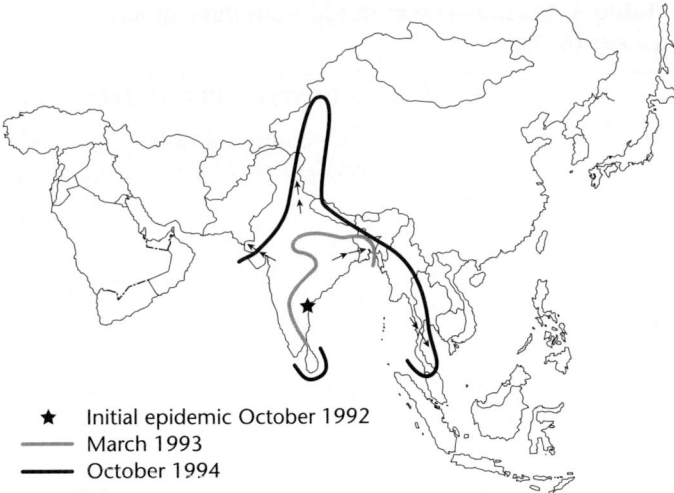

★   Initial epidemic October 1992
—   March 1993
—   October 1994

Figure 3.10 Spread of *Vibrio cholerae* O139-Asia, 1992–1994. (CDC MMWR Weekly March 1995.)

infected areas and it has been claimed that they can exist in a viable but non-culturable state.[30]

Nipah virus

In early 1999, health officials in Malaysia and Singapore investigated reports of febrile encephalitis and respiratory illnesses among workers who had been exposed to pigs. A previously unrecognized paramyxovirus (formerly known as Hendra-like virus), now called Nipah virus, was implicated by laboratory testing in many of these cases.

As of April 1999, 257 cases of febrile encephalitis were reported to the Malaysian Ministry of Health, including 100 deaths. Laboratory results from 65 patients who died suggested recent Nipah virus infection. The apparent source of infection among most human cases continues to be exposure to pigs. Human-to-human transmission of Nipah virus has not been documented. Outbreak control in Malaysia has focused on culling pigs; approximately 890 000 pigs have been killed. Other measures include a ban on transporting pigs within the country, education about contact with pigs, use of personal protective equipment among persons exposed to pigs, and a national surveillance and control system to detect and cull additional infected herds.[31] Nipah virus cases and deaths have also been reported from Bangladesh.

SARS

Severe acute respiratory syndrome (SARS) refers to an emerging infectious disease first recognized in late-2002, early-2003. The disease appeared initially as an outbreak of atypical pneumonia of unknown aetiology in November 2002 in Foshan, Guangdong Province in southern China. The disease soon spread to neighbouring cities, and escalated in February 2003 to involve Vietnam, Hong Kong, Canada and more than 30 countries subsequently, worldwide. The global outbreak ended in July 2003, with a total of 8098 probable cases and at least 774 deaths. After a period of

quiescence, a cluster of infection was detected again in December 2003 and January 2004 in Guangdong Province. Since then, no more human cases have been reported. SARS is due to infection with a newly identified coronavirus named as SARS-associated coronavirus (SARS-CoV).[32]

The source of infection is likely to be a direct cross-species transmission from an animal reservoir. This is supported by the fact that the early SARS cases in Guangdong Province had some history of exposure to live wild animals in markets serving the restaurant trade. Animal traders working with animals in these markets had higher seroprevalence for SARS coronavirus, though they did not report any illness compatible with SARS. More importantly, SARS-CoV-like virus detected from some animal species had more than a 99% homology with human SARS-CoV.[32]

The clinical course of SARS varies from a mild upper respiratory tract illness, usually seen in young children, to respiratory failure which occurred in around 20–25% of mainly adult patients. As the disease progresses, patients start to develop shortness of breath. From the second week onwards, patients progress to respiratory failure and acute respiratory distress syndrome, often requiring intensive care.[32]

Avian influenza virus in humans in Hong Kong

In May 1997, a 3-year-old boy in Hong Kong contracted an influenza-like illness, was treated with salicylates, and died 12 days later with complications consistent with Reye's syndrome. Laboratory diagnosis included the isolation in cell culture of a virus that was identified locally as influenza type A but could not be further characterized with reagents distributed for diagnosis of human influenza viruses. By August, further investigation with serological and molecular techniques in the Netherlands and in the USA had confirmed that the isolate was A/Hong Kong/156/97 (H5N1), which was very closely related to isolate A/Chicken/Hong Kong/258/97 (H5N1). The latter virus was considered representative of those responsible for severe outbreaks of disease on three rural chicken farms in Hong Kong during March 1997, during which several thousand chickens had died. Molecular analysis of the viral haemagglutinins showed a proteolytic cleavage site of the type found in highly pathogenic avian influenza viruses.

By late December, the total number of confirmed new human cases had climbed to 17, of which five were fatal; the case fatality rates were 18% in children and 57% in adults older than 17 years. Almost all laboratory evidence of infection was in patients who had been near live chickens (e.g. in marketplaces) in the days before onset of illness, which suggested direct transmission of virus from chicken to human rather than person-to-person spread. In December 1997, veterinary authorities began to slaughter all (1.6 million) chickens present in wholesale facilities or with vendors within Hong Kong, and importation of chickens from neighbouring areas was stopped.

Knowledge of how humans are infected, the real level of human-to-human transmission, the spectrum of disease presentation and the effectiveness of treatment remains scanty. Human-to human transmission is known to have occurred, but there is no evidence that transmission has become more efficient. All the human-to-human infections with H5N1 to date seem not to have transmitted on further. Therefore, although the case fatality rate for human

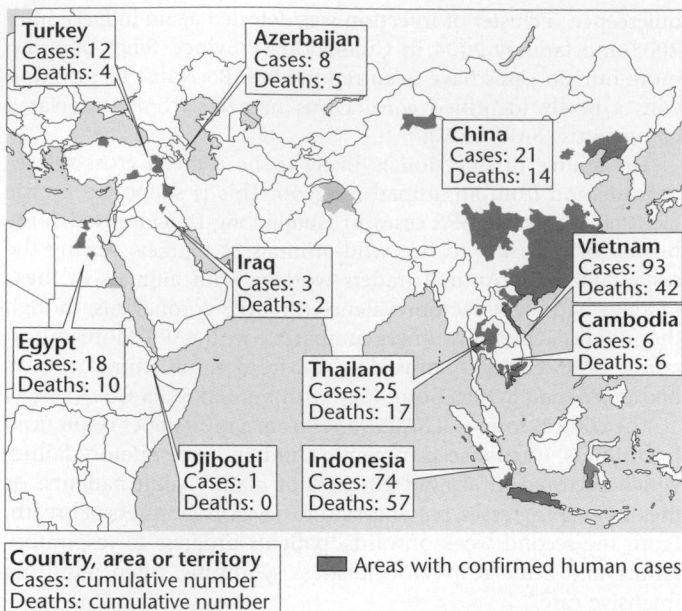

Figure 3.11 Confirmed human cases of H5N1 avian influenza since 2003 (status as of 27 December 2006; latest available update) (WHO 2006).

Table 3.4 Distribution of deaths from three groups of causes by region

Region	NUMBER OF DEATHS, ATTRIBUTED (%)		
	Infectious causes	Non-communicable causes	Injuries
Established market economies	6.2	87.6	6.2
Former socialist economies	3.6	86.8	9.6
China	15.1	73.4	11.5
Latin America	32.3	57.9	9.8
Middle Eastern crescent	46.2	44.8	8.9
India	43.3	50.2	6.5
Sub-Saharan Africa	68.2	23.9	7.9
Other Asia and islands	41.8	49.6	8.6
World	33.4	58.1	8.5

infection remains high (around 57% for cases reported to WHO), it seems that H5N1 avian viruses remain poorly adapted to humans.[33]

Global prevalence studies (Figure 3.11) indicate that Indonesia is currently the most active site of bird to human H5N1 transmission in the Asia Pacific region, and a large number of human cases have been detected here in 2005–06. China and Cambodia have also reported human cases in 2006. In south Asia (India and Pakistan), there have only been sporadic reports of infection in poultry to date. In Vietnam and Thailand there have been official reports of poultry outbreaks; these show a decline since 2006. Surveillance in Africa is especially weak, and there is evidence of widespread infection in domestic poultry in parts of north, west and central Africa. Prospects of control are bleak here because of weaknesses in veterinary services, and a number of competing animal and human health problems. The outbreaks in Egypt have been well described. These involved both commercial and backyard flocks, with considerable impact on economic life and food security. It is probable that large numbers of people in African countries are at risk of H5N1 infection. If that virus had pandemic potential then a pandemic arising from Africa must be considered a possibility.[33]

EMERGING NON-INFECTIOUS KILLERS IN THE TROPICS

Non-infectious diseases take an enormous toll on lives and health worldwide. Non-communicable diseases (NCDs) account for nearly 60% of deaths globally, mostly due to heart disease, stroke, cancer, diabetes and lung diseases. The rapid rise of NCDs represents one of the major health challenges to global development in the twenty-first century and threatens the economic and social development of nations as well as the lives and health of millions of their subjects. In 1998 alone, NCDs were estimated to have contributed to 31.7 million deaths globally and 43% of the global burden of disease.[34] Until recently, it was believed that NCDs were a minor or even non-existent problem in developing countries in the tropics. A recent analysis of mortality trends from NCDs suggests that large increases in NCDs have occurred in developing countries,[35] particularly those in rapid transition like China and India (Table 3.4). According to these estimates at least 40% of all deaths in the tropical developing countries are attributable to NCDs, while in industrialized countries NCDs account for 75% of all deaths. Low- and middle-income countries suffer the greatest impact of NCDs. The rapid increase in these diseases is seen disproportionately in poor and disadvantaged populations and is contributing to widening health gaps between and within countries. In 1998, of the total number of deaths attributable to NCDs 77% occurred in developing countries, and of the disease burden they represent 85% was borne by low- and middle-income countries.[34] It has now been projected that, by 2020, NCDs will account for almost three-quarters of all deaths worldwide, and that 71% of deaths due to ischaemic heart disease (IHD), 75% of deaths due to stroke, and 70% of deaths due to diabetes will occur in developing countries[36] and the number of people in the developing world with diabetes is expected to increase by more than 2.5-fold, from 84 million in 1995 to 228 million in 2025.[37] On a global basis, 60% of the burden of NCDs will occur in developing countries and the rate at which it is increasing annually is unprecedented. The public health and economic implications of this phenomenon are staggering, and are already becoming apparent.

It is important to recognize that these trends, indicative of an increase in NCDs, may be partly confounded by factors such as an increase in life expectancy, a progressive reduction in deaths due to communicable diseases in adulthood, and improvements in case detection and reporting in the tropics. However, increase in the incidence of these chronic degenerative diseases is real. The complex range of determinants (below) that interact to determine the nature and course of this epidemic[38] needs to be understood in order to adopt preventive strategies to help developing societies in the tropics to deal with this burgeoning problem.

The determinants of non-communicable diseases in developing societies are as follows:[1]

- Demographic changes in population
- Epidemiological transition
- Urbanization and internal migration
- Changes in dietary and food consumption patterns
- Lifestyle changes (changes in physical activity patterns, sociocultural milieu and stress as well as increased tobacco consumption)
- Adult-onset effects of low birth weight and the effects of early life programming
- Infections and their associations with chronic disease risk
- Effect of malnutrition and nutrient deficiencies
- Poverty, inequalities and social exclusion
- Deleterious effects of environmental degradation
- Impacts of globalization.

Four of the most prominent NCDs: cardiovascular disease, cancer, chronic obstructive pulmonary disease and diabetes, are linked to common preventable risk factors related to diet and lifestyle. These factors are tobacco use, unhealthy diet and lack of physical activity. Interventions to prevent these diseases should focus on controlling these risk factors in an integrated manner and at the family and community level since the causal risk factors are deeply entrenched in the social and cultural framework of society. Developing countries in the tropics have to recognize that the emerging accelerated epidemic of NCDs is a cause for concern and that it needs to be dealt with as a national priority. They have to learn from the experience of industrialized and affluent countries to tackle the emerging crisis of chronic diseases that they are likely to face in the near future. The emerging health burden of chronic disease affecting mainly the economically productive adult population will consume scarce resources. It is important, however, to realize that the poorer countries will be burdened even more in the long run, if attempts are not made to evolve and implement interventions to address these emerging health issues on an urgent basis. Ensuring that health policies are aimed at tackling the 'double burden' of the continued existence of the huge burden of infectious/communicable diseases alongside the emerging epidemic of non-communicable diseases in developing countries of the tropics becomes a priority.[39]

CONCLUSION

The world we live in is constantly changing. In the past 25 years, we have witnessed significant progress in sustainable and technological development. However, increases in mass population movements, continuing civil unrest and deforestation have helped carry diseases into areas where they have never been seen before. This has been aided by the massive growth in international travel. Effective medicines and control strategies are available to dra-

matically reduce the deaths and suffering caused by communicable and non-communicable diseases. Despite reduced global military spending many governments are failing to ensure that these strategies receive enough funding to succeed. WHO priorities for the control of infectious diseases in developing countries include childhood immunization, integrated management of childhood illnesses, use of the DOTS strategy to control TB, a package of interventions to control malaria, a package of interventions to prevent HIV/AIDS, access to essential drugs, and the overall strengthening of surveillance and health service delivery systems. Over 10% of all preventable ill-health today is due to poor environmental quality-conditions such as bad housing, overcrowding, indoor air pollution, poor sanitation and unsafe water. The challenge of disease in the tropics has continued into the new millennium – never before have we been so well equipped to deal with disease threats. It remains for humankind to summon the collective will to pursue these challenges and break the chain of infection and disease.

REFERENCES

1. Raska K. National and international surveillance of communicable diseases. *World Health Organ Chron* 1966; 20:315–321.
2. WHO. *World Health Report. Fighting Disease Fostering Development.* Geneva: World Health Organization; 1996.
3. WHO. *Acute Respiratory Infections.* Geneva: World Health Organization; 2002.
4. World Bank Group. *Indoor Air Pollution Energy and Health for the Poor.* Washington, DC: World Bank; 2000.
5. Rudan I, Tomaskovic L, Boschi-Pinto C, et al. Estimate of global incidence of clinical pneumonia in children under five years. *Bull WHO* 2004; 82:895–903.
6. WHO-UNAIDS. *AIDS Epidemic Updated.* Geneva: UNAIDS; 2005.
7. Kosek M, Bern C, Guerrant RL. The global burden of diarrhoeal disease, as estimated from studies published between 1992 and 2000. *Bull WHO* 2003; 81:197–204.
8. UNICEF Staff Working Papers. *Evaluation, Policy and Planning Series.* Number EVL-97-002. A global review of diarrhoeal disease control. New York. UNICEF; 1997.
9. Moore M, Davachi F, Bongo L, et al. New parameters for evaluating oral rehydration therapy: one year's experience in a major urban hospital in Zaire. *J Trop Pediatr* 1989; 35:179–184.
10. Alam NH, Yunus M, Faruque AS, et al. Symptomatic hyponatremia during treatment of dehydrating diarrheal disease with reduced osmolarity oral rehydration solution. *JAMA* 2006; 296:567–573.
11. Fauveau V, Yunus M, Zaman K, et al. Diarrhoea mortality in rural Bangladeshi children. *J Trop Pediatr* 1991; 37:31–36.
12. Ruiz-Palacios GM, Pérez-Schael I, Velázquez FR, et al. for the Human Rotavirus Vaccine Study Group. Safety and efficacy of an attenuated vaccine against severe rotavirus gastroenteritis. *N Engl J Med* 2006; 354:11–22.
13. WHO. *Guidelines for the Control of Epidemics due to Shigella dysenteriae 1.* Publication No. WHO/CDR/95.4. Epidemiology of dysentery caused by shigella. Geneva: World Health Organization; 1995.
14. WHO. *Global Tuberculosis Control*—Surveillance, Planning Financing, Geneva: World Health Organization; 2008.
15. Aziz MA, Wright A, Laszlo A, et al. WHO/International Union against Tuberculosis and Lung Disease Global Project on Anti-tuberculosis Drug Resistance Surveillance. Epidemiology of antituberculosis drug resistance (the Global Project on Anti-tuberculosis Drug Resistance Surveillance): an updated analysis. *Lancet* 2006; 368:2142–2154.
16. WHO. *WHO World Malaria Report.* Geneva: World Health Organization; 2005.
17. WHO Expert Committee on Malaria. *World Health Organ Tech Rep Ser* 2000; 892:i–v, 1–74.

18. Epstein PR. *Climate, ecology and human health*. Consequences 1997; 3:3–12. Online. Available: http://www.gcrio.org/CONSEQUENCES/vol3no2/climhealth.html 2 November 1997.

19. Lopez AD, Mathers CD, Ezzati M, eds. *Global Burden of Disease and Risk Factors*. Geneva: World Health Organization; 2006.

20. Morbidity and Mortality Weekly Report. Update: global measles control and mortality reduction – worldwide, 1991–2001. *MMWR* 2003; 52(20): 471–475.

21. WHO. *Towards the elimination of hepatitis B: a guide to the implementation of national immunization programs in the developing world*. The International Task Force on hepatitis B Immunization. Geneva: World Health Organization; 1991.

22. Kao JH, Chen DS. Global control of hepatitis B virus infection. *Lancet Infect Dis* 2002; 2:395–403.

23. Vandelaer J, Birmingham M, Gasse F, et al. Tetanus in developing countries: an update on the maternal and neonatal tetanus elimination. *Vaccine* 2003; 21:3442–3445.

24. WHO. *Control of neglected tropical diseases (NTD)*. Online. Available: http://www.who.int/neglected_diseases/en/ 16 February 2007.

25. Hotez PJ, Molyneux DH, Fenwick A, et al. Incorporating a rapid-impact package for neglected tropical diseases with programs for HIV/AIDS, tuberculosis, and malaria. *PLoS Med* 2006; 3(5):e102.

26. United States Government Accountability Office. *Emerging infectious diseases review of state and federal diseases surveillance*. September 2004. Online. Available: http://www.gao.gov/new.items/d04877.pdf

27. WHO. *WHO Fact Sheet: Ebola Haemorrhagic Fever*. Fact sheet No. 103. Geneva: World Health Organization; 2004.

28. National Institute of Health. *Dengue and Dengue haemorrhagic fever*. Report of the Public Health Laboratories Division. WHO Collaborating Centre for Research and Training in Viral Diagnostics National Institute of Health, Baltimore, USA: 2006. Online. Available: http://www.nih.org.pk/

29. WHO. *WHO Fact Sheet: Rift Valley Fever*. Fact sheet No. 207. Geneva: World Health Organization; 2000.

30. Morbidity and Mortality Weekly Report. Update: Vibrio cholerae O1-Western Hemisphere, 1991–1994, and V. cholerae O139-Asia, 1994. *MMWR* 1995; 44:215–219.

31. Morbidity and Mortality Weekly Report. Update: outbreak of Nipah virus: Malaysia and Singapore, 1999. *MMWR* 1999; 48:335–337.

32. Heymann DL. SARS and emerging infectious diseases: a challenge to place global solidarity above national sovereignty. *Ann Acad Med Singapore* 2006; 35:350–353.

33. Influenza team. European Centre for Disease Surveillance and Control, Stockholm, Sweden. World avian influenza update: H5N1 could become endemic in Africa. *Euro Surveill* 2006; 11(6). Online. Available: http://www.eurosurveillance.org/ew/2006/060622.asp#3.

34. WHO. *Global Strategy for the Prevention and Control of Non-Communicable Diseases*. Geneva: World Health Organization; 2000.

35. Murray CJL, Lopez AD. *Global Comparative Assessments in the Health Sector*. Geneva: World Health Organization; 1994.

36. WHO. *The World Health Report 1998. Life in the 21st Century: A vision for All*. Geneva: World Health Organization; 1998.

37. Aboderin I. *Life Course Perspectives on Coronary Heart Disease, Stroke and Diabetes: Key Issues and Implications for Policy and Research*. Geneva: World Health Organization; 2001: WHO/NMH/NPH/01.4.

38. Shetty PS. Diet and life-style and chronic non-communicable diseases: what determines the epidemic in developing societies? In: Krishnaswami K, ed. *Nutrition Research: Current Scenario and Future Trends*. New Delhi: Oxford and IBH Publishing; 2000:153–167.

39. Boutayeb A. The double burden of communicable and non-communicable diseases in developing countries. *Trans Roy Soc Trop Med Hyg* 2006; 100: 191–199.

Chapter 4   Gerard C. Bodeker

Traditional Medicine

WHY SHOULD TROPICAL MEDICINE PRACTITIONERS BE INFORMED ABOUT TRADITIONAL MEDICINE?

More than 80% of US medical schools now offer courses in complementary medicine and in Britain the General Medical Council requires medical schools to offer introductory courses on complementary medicine for medical students, in order to bridge the gap between patients and doctors in this field. In tropical countries, where a greater percentage of the population use traditional medicine than use conventional medicine, or than use complementary medicine in the industrialized countries, the need for information and understanding is greater.

There has been a historic mistrust between traditional health practitioners (THPs) and modern medical doctors. This has come in part from colonial policies which have attempted to suppress and replace traditional medicine. It also comes from the modern medical view that traditional medicine is at best of low therapeutic value and at worst dangerous. In reality, what appears to happen is that each side sees the other's worst cases and builds their impressions based on this sample. With the emergence of a global political consensus that traditional medicine in developing countries – and complementary medicine in industrialized countries – must take a role in comprehensive health sector development, an understanding of traditional medicine is necessary on the part of mainstream health personnel.

At the local level, there will be questions of traditional medicine's claims of efficacy, and concerns over whether particular traditional medicines are responsible for presenting renal or liver pathology. There will also be questions about interactive effects of traditional and conventional drugs. There may also be consideration of whether traditional means can be used in the management of common conditions such as wounds and tropical ulcers when conventional means are not available or have not worked.

This chapter attempts to provide an introduction to some of the above issues although, within the available space, clearly they will not be able to be addressed in their entirety or in depth. This will be up to the clinician, including by means of open enquiry with local THPs and through searches of relevant databases such as CABI, Medline, the British Library's AMED database, SOCIO-FILE and EMBASE.

BACKGROUND

The field of traditional medicine is as diverse as the societies in which it is found. *Materia medica* differ, and diagnosis, treatments and theories of disease also vary. In view of this immense diversity of traditional practice, it is clearly unrealistic to attempt to provide a comprehensive review of the various systems of traditional medicine found in tropical countries or to review their various clinical applications. What this chapter aims to do is to provide a framework for understanding what traditional medicine is, who uses it and why, and how it is moving towards being given a place in the formal healthcare systems of many countries. There is also a review of the use of traditional medicine in the management of common conditions: malaria, HIV/AIDS, wounds and eye disease. These have been selected for consideration as they are among the commonest reasons for people seeking treatment – from both modern and traditional health professionals. Other areas which have not been able to be included in this chapter, but which are of importance, include traditional birth practices, the very important mental health dimensions of traditional medicine, and the use of traditional anthelmintics and traditional orthopaedics. Each is a subject in itself and each has been the subject of review and policy consideration. Searches of the relevant databases will yield literature for those interested in further exploring these and related fields.

What is missing in the international literature is a body of sound clinical research. This is due to the low value ascribed to this sector by funders and health authorities, despite the fact that the majority of the public continue to use medical approaches about which little is known with respect to safety, efficacy, dosage or mechanisms of action. Clearly, the call for evidence must be matched by a commitment of resources to enable high-quality, sound research to be conducted. This is necessary to determine what constitutes best practice and safe practice as well as to open up the possibility of new discoveries for healthcare generally. These may be discoveries such as has been found for the evaluation of the traditional Chinese febrifuge, *Artemisia annua*, which has given rise to artemisinin and the class of antimalarial drugs derived from this compound[1] or that cited in the section on HIV/AIDS, where a Ugandan herbal preparation has been found to be more effective and considerably cheaper than the conventional treatment for herpes zoster. (For information on safety/toxicity issues, the reader is referred to Chapter 32).

While many of the studies presented in this chapter may need further replication, better trial design, etc. they do point to general trends in efficacy and safety as well as highlight the importance of further research and investment in the traditional healthcare sector.

TRADITIONAL HEALTH SYSTEMS

The World Health Organization estimates that the majority of the population of most non-industrial countries still relies on traditional forms of medicine for their everyday healthcare. In many countries, up to 80–90% of the population are in this category.

Traditions vary from region to region and even within a single country. Attempts to classify these traditions into meaningful systems and sets of practices have generally adopted a two-fold classification.

In Asia, traditional medical knowledge has often been classified into two broad groupings: codified and folk traditions.[2] The codified traditions of Asia typically have a written materia medica and clinical texts, a systematic theory of pathogenesis and treatments based on a formal diagnostic system, and a pharmacological tradition with precise standards of dosage and an awareness of toxicity and its management. These traditions include the Ayurvedic medical system of India and South Asia, traditional Chinese medicine and its related systems in Vietnam and Korea, Unani medicine, and the Graeco-Arabic tradition found in Pakistan, India and many other countries with Islamic traditions.

Folk traditions are generally seen as the collection of community knowledge about the use of plants in the management of common illness, non-pharmacological interventions such as massage, meditation, the use of steam and other physical means of effecting cure.

In studying Mayan medicine of Mexico, Berlin and Berlin have adopted Foster's[3] dual division of medical systems into naturalistic and personalistic frameworks. In the naturalistic system, a health condition is empirically determined. Diagnosis is based primarily on immediately apparent signs and symptoms. For a condition such as bloody diarrhoea, it is the norm for people to treat themselves with medicinal plants or to seek local expert advice in the use of plants as treatment. However, diagnosis of a personalistic condition is based on a retrospective analysis of possible causative factors, such as an encounter with ancestral spirits.

Berlin and Berlin[4] have noted in their study of Mayan traditional medicine that:

. . . such cases are first treated with plant medicinals, and later classed as personalistic in cases that are unresponsive to herbal remedies or that are either prolonged or progressively worsen. These patterns of diagnosis have been extensively described by virtually everyone who has studied the subject. Diagnosis and treatment frequently involve the intervention of healers with special powers, such as a pulser or diviner. While personalistic conditions may at times also be treated with herbal medications, Maya curers normally employ remedies that require ceremonial healing rituals and special prayers.

In the context of tropical medicine, it is sufficient to note that what may appear to the clinician as the practice of herbal medicine, with varying degrees of competence, is often grounded in theoretical assumptions, beliefs about disease and its origins, and what constitutes a real cure as opposed to simply the management of symptoms. An understanding of these perspectives is necessary to understand the beliefs and health practices of patients, many of whom will use both conventional and traditional medicine in the management of a condition.

What has become clear since the publication of the *World Health Organization Global Atlas on Traditional Complementary & Alternative Medicine,*[5] is that traditional medicine is widespread and is increasingly being given a place in formal healthcare in tropical and other countries.

Accordingly, this chapter will give an introduction to the prevailing views of what traditional medicine is, how widely it is used, by whom and for what, some examples of the use of traditional medicine for commonly occurring conditions in the tropics, and how the clinician may gain more information about traditional medicine.

DEFINITIONS AND CONCEPTUALIZATIONS OF TRADITIONAL MEDICINE

The following is a selection of definitions and characterizations of traditional medicine:

- Traditional medicine is widespread throughout the world. As its name implies, it is part of the tradition of each country and employs practices that are handed down from generation to generation of healer. Its acceptance by people receiving care is also inherited from generation to generation. Traditional medicine originated aeons before the modern medical era.[6]
- WHO definition of herbal medicines: Finished, labelled medicinal products that contain as active ingredients aerial or underground parts of plants, or other plant material, or combinations thereof, whether in the crude state or as plant preparations. Plant material includes juices, gums, fatty oils, essential oils, and any other substances of this nature. Herbal medicines may contain excipients in addition to the active ingredients. Medicines containing plant material combined with chemically defined active substances, including chemically defined, isolated constituents of plants, are not considered to be herbal medicines.[7]
- Traditional medicine is the totality of all knowledge and practices, whether explicable or not, used in diagnosing, preventing or eliminating a physical, mental or social disequilibrium and which rely exclusively on past experience and observation handed down verbally from generation to generation.[8]
- African Traditional Medicine: The sum total of all knowledge and practices, whether explicable or not, used in diagnosis, prevention and elimination of physical, mental, or societal imbalance, and relying exclusively on practical experience and observation handed down from generation to generation, whether verbally or in writing. Traditional medicine might also be considered to be the sum total of all practices, measures, ingredients and procedures of all kinds, whether material or not, which from time immemorial had enabled the African to guard against disease, to alleviate his suffering and to cure himself.[9]

The above definitions characterize traditional medicine as a collection of knowledge and skills. While these are aspects of the traditional systems that can be the subject of training, regulation and formalization, other aspects such as the traditional theory of physiological function and disease, and the role of spiritual practice and belief, are more elusive yet perhaps more fundamental to most traditional healthcare systems.

THEORETICAL FRAMEWORK

An essential feature of traditional health systems is that they are based in theories or cosmologies that take into account mental, social, spiritual, physical and ecological dimensions of health and well-being. A fundamental concept found in many systems is that of balance – the balance between mind and body, between different dimensions of individual bodily functioning and need, between individual and community, individual/community and environment, and individual and the universe. The breaking of this interconnectedness of life is a fundamental source of disease, which can progress to stages of illness and epidemic. Treatments, therefore, are designed not only to address the locus of the disease but also to restore a state of systemic balance to the individual and his or her inner and outer environment.

The World Health Organization has referred to the world's traditional health systems as holistic, i.e. 'that of viewing man in his totality within a wide ecological spectrum, and of emphasizing the view that ill health or disease is brought about by an imbalance, or disequilibrium, of man in his total ecological system and not only by the causative agent and pathogenic evolution'.[10]

Arthur Kleinman, of Harvard University's Center for Culture and Medicine, has noted that 'for members of non-Western societies, the body is an open system linking social relations, the self, a vital balance between interrelated elements in a holistic cosmos. Emotion and cognition are integrated into bodily processes. The body-self is not a secularized private domain of the individual person, but an organic part of a sacred, sociocentric world, a communication system involving exchanges with others (including the divine)'.[11]

The natural world is thus not only imbued with non-material attributes but also, in many traditions, is an expression of a more fundamental level of spiritual reality with which the individual is linked. Vitalistic traditions were present in the early days of Western medicine in ancient Greece. Aesculapian traditions drew on spiritual healing as a basis for complete recovery. Subsequently, the systematic, natural science approach of Hippocrates, while emphasizing the observable, acknowledged the value of the sacred in the healing process.

In Ayurvedic medicine, the classical healthcare system of India, consciousness is of primary significance and matter is deemed secondary. Accordingly, Ayurvedic medical treatment, when practised according to the high traditions of Ayurveda, will first address the spiritual and mental state of the individual – through meditation,[12] intellectual understanding of the problem, behavioural and lifestyle advice, etc. and then address the physical problem by means of diet, medicine and other therapeutic modalities.[13]

In the shamanic traditions of the Americas, spiritual healing is fundamental to the recovery process. Traditional health practices are part of a cultural identity that goes from the particular to the collective and vice versa. The forces which allow traditional health practices to function are based on spirituality, the wholeness of the person, the maintenance of balance and harmony with habitat and Nature. The practice strengthens and reinforces family and community connections. Therefore the traditional doctor re-establishes the patient's lost harmony'.[14]

UTILIZATION

The widespread demand for traditional medical services has been recognized as an enduring phenomenon. Earlier calls for traditional medicine to be replaced by modern medical services have now given way to recognition that some degree of formalization of these health services might offer the public increased standards of quality and safety.[5]

In many countries, life begins with the support of traditional medicine. An estimated 60–70% of births in developing countries still take place with the sole help of traditional birth attendants.[15]

Africa

There have been many general estimates of the extent of use of traditional medicine in Africa. The African regional report in the *WHO Global Atlas on Traditional, Complementary & Alternative Medicine* re-affirms a long-standing view that at least 80% of the population of Africa regularly use traditional medicine.[5]

However, some estimates of use are strikingly low. In a survey of perceived morbidity in a rural community in south western Ethiopia, 55.4% of those reporting illness took no action at all; 30.3% applied to health institutions; 9.2% reported self-care and only 5.2% visited a traditional healer.[16] By contrast, research done at Mogopane Hospital in north-eastern Transvaal, South Africa, showed that 9 out of 10 patients who come to the outpatients department first consult traditional healers.[17] Clearly, studies of community groups and of hospital populations address the needs and choices of different populations with different health profiles. In planning services, such differences need to be accounted for.

It is common in African healing traditions for illness to be understood as arising from psychological disturbances or disturbed relationships with either the living or the dead. Accordingly, traditional African medicine has strong psychosocial dimensions which have valuable potential for traditional and modern medical partnerships in addressing mental health concerns.[18,19]

Age and gender are factors in the utilization of traditional healthcare services. A study of visitors to traditional healers in central Sudan indicated that children under 10 years did not take part in visits. Most visitors were between 21 and 40 years (61%) and were women (62%). They were less educated compared with the general population in the area. The main reasons given for attending traditional healers were treatment (60%) and blessing (26%).[20]

In Mali, men are more likely to prefer traditional treatments for malaria than women,[21] and more boys than girls believed in herbal medicine in a survey in the Sudan.[22] It has been suggested that women are less likely to be treated at modern facilities, and are more likely to resort to traditional medicines.[23] Travel time can be a factor in the choice of traditional over modern medical services.

People with a serious health condition may seek traditional healthcare before accepting modern medical services. In Malawi, 37% of tuberculosis patients reported attending a traditional healer prior to attending the health service. By the time a final diagnosis of tuberculosis had been made, most patients had visited several different care providers: private practitioner (69 visits), village clinic (64) and traditional healer (40), and 32 patients reported taking some form of traditional remedy at home.[24]

Among comments made by traditional midwives in South Africa, in a study by Troskie,[8] was that 'the nearest hospital is 20 kilometres far'. By contrast, traditional healthcare services are readily available. Every village has a number of traditional healers and birth attendants, each with their own specializations.[25]

Similarly, in India, rural women in Gujarat were more likely to use services which were closer to home, other things being equal. The 'travel' variable (including time and travel costs) is a more important factor determining use of modern and traditional services among women in the study area than the actual direct costs of the service.[26]

In the case of malaria, selection of first-line treatment varies from area to area. Sometimes, herbal remedies are given at home as the first-line treatment,[27,28] especially in mild cases of malaria.[29,30] Sometimes, herbs are the second-line treatment when chemotherapy has failed.[31–33] Munguti[34] found that in a rural area of Kenya 7% used herbs as first choice of treatment, 17% as second choice and 14% as third choice.

There can be contrasting patterns of use across countries and regions. Whereas young children in the Sudan were found not to attend traditional healers, in Kenya 40% of sick children were taken to the mganga (traditional healer) and 55% to the clinic; 26% of the mothers said that both sources of treatment were consulted. There are usually differences between urban and rural populations in their use of traditional and modern medicine. While 95% of urban women who attended modern medical clinics in South Africa strongly advocated mixing traditional and Western antenatal care, only 63% of rural clinic attenders found this practice acceptable. All groups favoured Western over traditional care in cases of serious pregnancy complications.[35]

Asia

In India, it has been found that the influence of family structure is significant. The presence of the mother-in-law is associated with a greater use of traditional healers.[26]

Ethnic minorities in industrialized countries often continue to use the traditional medicine from their culture alongside, or even in place of, conventional medicine. This can apply even in settings where conventional healthcare is provided free of charge, but traditional healthcare services must be paid out of pocket, as in the case of Chinese communities in the UK.[36] As in developing countries, the affordability, availability and cultural familiarity of traditional medicine, together with family influence, contribute to the continued use of traditional medical providers and medicines in 'ethnic enclaves'.

In a study of health service utilization in four villages in India, the most common complaint by a majority of those surveyed was that 'medicines are never available' at the Primary Health Centre, followed by discourteous behaviour of the staff and health personnel, 'doctors never available', 'doctors demand money for better treatment', and so on. Almost one-quarter of the women initially tried homeopathic treatment, followed by 9% who administered Western medicine at home, while 2% opted for traditional home remedies for cure and treatment, before visiting and consulting a trained medical practitioner. Medical pluralism was found to be flourishing as people switched from one medical system to another depending on affordability and time.[37]

In Sri Lanka, two patterns of healthcare seeking which cut across modern and traditional medical systems have been identified. The first involved patients who searched for a medicine which could cure. The second pattern involved the search for a practitioner who had the power of the hand to cure one's illness.[38]

Medical pluralism is common worldwide and consumers practise integrated healthcare irrespective of whether or not it is present at the formal level. In Taiwan, 60% of the public have been found to be users of multiple healing systems, including modern Western medicine, Chinese medicine and religious healing.[39]

Indigenous communities

Native American communities incorporate traditional forms of treatment into the US Indian Health Service (IHS) alcohol rehabilitation programmes. In a study of 190 IHS contract programmes, it was found that 50% of these offered a traditional sweat lodge or encouraged its use. Treatment outcomes were found to be better for alcoholic patients when a sweat lodge was available. In addition, the presence of medicine men or healers, when used in combination with the sweat lodge, greatly improved the outcome.[40]

In the tropical regions of Australia, traditional Aboriginal medicine is widely practised.[41] In most regions of the Northern Territory, more than 22% of indigenous people had used bush medicine in the previous 6 months when surveyed.[41] A decrease in use of traditional medicine seems to be because Western medicine is easier to access, not because of a lack of faith in its efficacy.[41] Indigenous Australian medicine includes herbal preparations, diet, rest, massage, restricted diet and external remedies such as ochre, smoke, steam and heat.[41]

Traditional medicine and the formal health sector in Africa

Healers have for long been treated like trees on savanna farms – not formally cultivated, yet valued and used, particularly by women and children.[42]

There has been a long-reported willingness on the part of traditional healers in Africa to collaborate with the formal sector and to establish joint training. Burnett et al.[43] note that 37 of the 39 traditional healers (94%) and 14 of the 27 formal health workers (52%) interviewed in a Zambian study were keen to collaborate in training and patient care relating to HIV/AIDS.

However, this is not generally a reciprocal view. Although 1% of nurses in South Africa are reported to be traditional healers, rural nurses in Swaziland perceived themselves as being teachers to healers, but not learning from healers. They saw themselves as a source of referral for healers, but not the reverse.[44]

One view is that it may be more appropriate to work towards a system of cooperation between two independent systems, with each recognizing and respecting the character of the other.[42] This has been the policy in Botswana, where parallel development has been encouraged, since it is felt that one or other of the two systems might suffer in the process of integration.[43]

In South Africa, many traditional healers are members of well-organized national organizations that are seeking formal recognition from the government. In one instance of WHO-sponsored collaboration, it has been recognized that the rapid increase in TB caseload, especially in African countries heavily affected by the HIV epidemic, requires a search for effective ways to treat patients outside hospital. As a component of the WHO's Community Care for Tuberculosis in Africa Project, Wilkinson et al.[24] studied the potential role for collaboration between the health service and traditional healers, especially as tuberculosis treatment supervisors, and examined what precedent and potential exist for traditional healers to act in this role.

Before commencing collaborative effort in healthcare between modern and traditional sectors, a careful assessment of potential benefits and obstacles should be made. The medical services utilization patterns of the communities need to be ascertained and the specific role of traditional health practitioners considered. In such efforts the ideas of healers themselves about possible collaboration are crucial.[25]

Ghana passed the Traditional Medicine Practice Act 2000, Act 595, to establish a Council to regulate and control the practice of traditional medicine. The primary draft of this Act originated from the traditional healers themselves. The Act defines traditional medicine as 'practice based on beliefs and ideas recognized by the community to provide healthcare by using herbs and other naturally occurring substances', and herbal medicine as 'any finished labelled medicinal products that contain as active ingredients aerial or underground parts of plants or other plant materials or the combination of them whether in crude state or plant preparation'. It is arranged into four sections, namely the establishment and functions of a Traditional Medicine Practice Council; registration of practitioners; licensing of practices; and miscellaneous provisions.

Ghana's Ministry of Health has incorporated a Traditional Medicine Unit since 1991, and in 1999 this was upgraded to the status of a Directorate. The Ministry, in collaboration with the Ghana Federation of Traditional Medicine Practitioners Associations and other stakeholders, has now developed a 5-year strategic plan for traditional medicine which proposes, among other aspects, the need to develop comprehensive training in traditional medicine from basic and secondary to tertiary levels.

A 'Ghana Herbal Pharmacopoeia', containing scientific information on common medicinal plants, has been published. Efforts are being made to integrate traditional medicine into the official public health system, including dispensing certified and efficacious herbal medicines in hospitals and pharmacies.

In Nigeria, the National Agency for Food and Drug Administration and Control (NAFDAC) has taken steps to regulate and control traditional medicine products with a view to ensuring their safety, efficacy and quality. In consultation with traditional healers and researchers NAFDAC has developed guidelines on regulating herbal medicines. Recently, the government of Nigeria approved a national policy on a Traditional Medicine Code of Ethics. There is also legislation for national and state Traditional Medicine Boards to enhance the regulation of traditional medicine practice and promote cooperation and research in traditional medicine.[45]

PRIORITY DISEASE AREAS: HIV/AIDS AND MALARIA

Traditional medicine has a central role to play in combating new and re-emerging diseases. Global priority is currently placed on combating malaria and HIV/AIDS and new partnerships between the communities of traditional medicine, public health and health research are being formed. Two diseases are addressed below, but partnerships are being developed with other diseases such as tuberculosis and control of vector-borne diseases such as trypanosomiasis.

Partnership with the traditional sector in HIV/AIDS prevention and management

As the AIDS crisis leads an increasing number of countries to question their priorities in health expenditures, there is an emerging awareness that traditional health practitioners (THPs) can play an important role in delivering an AIDS prevention message. There is growing recognition that some THPs may be able to offer treatment for opportunistic infections (OIs). At the same time, there are concerns about unsafe practices and a growth in claims of traditional cures for AIDS. Partnerships between the modern and traditional health sectors are a cornerstone for building a comprehensive strategy to manage the AIDS crisis.[46]

Africa

In Uganda, where there is only one doctor for every 20 000 people, there is one traditional health practitioner per 200–400 people.[47] In such settings, partnerships may be the only way that effective healthcare coverage can be achieved in managing the twin epidemics of AIDS and malaria. Clearly, such partnerships not only make good public health sense but, based on a growing body of pharmacological evidence, may also yield important preventive and treatment modalities.

In light of the widespread availability of traditional healthcare services and the reliance of the population on these services, it is inevitable that people suffering from AIDS will turn to THPs for treatment. Collaborative AIDS programmes have been established in many African countries, including Malawi, Mozambique, Uganda, Senegal, South Africa, Swaziland, Zambia and Zimbabwe.

Information sharing and educational programmes in South Africa have resulted in THPs providing correct HIV/AIDS advice as well as demonstrations of condom use. One such programme trained 1510 THPs and it was calculated that during the first 10 months of the programme some 845 600 of their clients may have been reached with AIDS/STD prevention messages. In similar programmes in Mozambique, traditional healers learned that AIDS is transmitted by sexual contact, by blood and non-sterile razor blades used in traditional practice. In a follow-up evaluation, 81%

of those trained reported that they had promoted condom use with at least their STD patients.[48]

One of the challenges in such workshop situations is to move beyond 'training' to genuine information sharing. It has been noted that it is difficult to modify the manner in which health professionals teach about AIDS – a style that tends towards the didactic and use of scientific jargon. Removing communication barriers such as these is a necessary first step in ensuring that training is an effective tool in mobilizing traditional health practitioners as partners in AIDS control.

An important example of how this may be done was conducted in Brazil, where a face-to-face educational intervention by healers blended traditional healing – with its language, codes, symbols and images – with scientific medicine, and simultaneously addressed social injustices and discrimination. New information about HIV/AIDS transmission was conveyed using languages and concepts intimately familiar to traditional health practitioners. A controlled evaluation found significant increases in AIDS awareness, knowledge about risky HIV behaviour, information about correct condom use, and acceptance of lower-risk, alternative ritual blood practices among the 126 members of the trainee group compared with 100 untrained controls. There were significant decreases in prejudicial attitudes related to HIV transmission among the trainee group compared with controls.[49]

The Ugandan NGO, Traditional and Modern Health Practitioners Together Against AIDS (THETA), was established in 1992 to conduct research on potentially useful traditional medicines with HIV-related illness and to promote a mutually respectful collaboration between traditional and modern health workers in the fight against AIDS. THETA has conducted workshops to share knowledge on AIDS prevention and also treatment of opportunistic infections using local herbal remedies.

Traditional healers participating in clinical observational studies of their herbal medicines have subsequently sought training in prevention, education and counselling issues, as well as in basic clinical diagnostic skills. A 1998 UNAIDS-sponsored evaluation of THETA found that it had reached 125 THPs (44 women and 81 men) in five districts of Uganda. A total of 50 000 people were found to have benefited from the improved services offered by traditional health practitioners over a period of 2 years.[46]

In South Africa, a follow-up of educational workshops found that some THPs reported that local medical staff had begun referring HIV-positive and STD patients to them for condom demonstrations and HIV counselling. All THPs reported having given condom demonstrations not only to clients but also to any member of their communities with potential interest.

Giving a perspective on the benefits from investment in this involvement of local traditional health practitioners in AIDS prevention exercises, Edward C. Green, an organizer of the workshops, reported that: '630 second generation healers had been trained in 12 workshops held in diverse parts of South Africa. The total direct cost of training these 630 was about US$23.30 per healer, or US$5.90/day per healer. In addition to these 630 direct beneficiaries of training, up to 229 320 patients or clients of these healers may have benefited from AIDS education within 7 months of the first generation training (calculated as 26 weeks times an average of 14 patients a week per healer (see below) times 630 healers trained). Not all these healers specialize in STDs or AIDS, but most of them see a great number of at least STD patients.

Finally, an inestimable number of friends, family members, and others in the local community (local associations, sports teams, youth groups, etc.) benefited from informal AIDS education'.[47]

Research

Healthcare consumers and THPs want information on the safety and efficacy of local treatments, their effect on opportunistic infections, and how to test claims of cure in an efficient and cost-effective manner.[50]

There has been little official response from governments on this front. However, in one of the more forward-looking national programmes, the Uganda AIDS Commission and the Joint Clinical Research Centre in Kampala have worked with traditional healers in evaluating several traditional treatments used locally for OIs. The research has found traditional medicine to be 'better suited to the treatment of some AIDS symptoms such as herpes zoster (HZ), chronic diarrhoea, shingles and weight loss'. THETA has conducted controlled clinical trials on a Ugandan herbal treatment for HZ. Comparing subjects with herbal treatments with controls using aciclovir, the conventional treatment for HZ, both groups were found to experience similar rates of resolution of HZ attacks. The traditional medicine group had less super-infection and showed less keloid formation than did subjects on aciclovir. HZ pain resolved significantly faster in the herbal group. The investigators concluded that herbal treatment is an important local and affordable alternative in managing HZ in HIV-infected patients in Uganda.[46]

A study conducted by the Blair Research Institute Clinic in Harare, Zimbabwe, evaluated the impact of traditional medicine in persons with HIV infection and assessed their quality of life with respect to HIV disease progression. There were 105 HIV-infected persons in the study, at various stages of HIV infection, of whom 79% were on traditional herbal medicine and 21% were on conventional medical care (CMC). Using the WHO Quality of Life Scale, it was found that the proportions of scores on five domains measuring different aspects of quality of life for patients on traditional medicine were much lower than those on conventional therapy ($p < 0.0001$, for all variables). The research team concluded that the data supported the role of traditional medicine in improving the quality of life of HIV-1 infected patients, although its pharmacological basis is unknown.[51]

While clinical research has been slow to begin in the evaluation of traditional herbal treatments for HIV-related illness, there has been screening for antiviral effects of locally used plants since the early 1990s. A recent study reported promising antiviral effects from selected Ethiopian medicinal plants. Asres et al.[52] found that the highest selective inhibition of HIV-1 replication was found with the acetone fraction of *Combretum paniculatum Vent.*, and the methanol fraction of *Dodonaea angustifolia L.f.*[52] These showed selectivity indices (ratio of 50% cytotoxic concentration to 50% effective antiviral concentration) of 6.4 and 4.9, and afforded cell protection of viral-induced cytopathic effect of 100% and 99%, respectively, when compared with control samples. Asres et al. found that the greatest degree of antiviral activity against HIV-2 was achieved with the acetone extract of *C. paniculatum* (EC(50): 3 mg/mL), which also showed the highest selectivity index (32). The 50% cytotoxic concentration ranged from 0.5 mg/mL for the hexane extract of *D. angustifolia L.f.*, the most cytotoxic of the extracts tested, to >250 mg/mL for some extracts such as the methanol fraction of *Alcea rosea L.*, the least toxic tested. While there is the obvious potential for commercial development of fractions of these plants as pharmaceutical leads, there is growing recognition of the need to evaluate such plants clinically in order to determined the viability of affordable, locally available medicines for managing HIV-related illness.

Asia

While much of the international focus on AIDS in the developing world has been on Africa, there has been growing awareness of the rapid spread of the disease in Asia. Reflecting the concerns now beginning to be addressed in many African countries, India's national AIDS policy states: In a scenario where antiretroviral drugs are extremely expensive, there is a great need to look into the indigenous systems of medicine (ISM), like Ayurveda, Unani and Siddha. Some of the medicines in these systems have the potential of reducing the viral load in the body of the patient thus ensuring a healthier and longer life with the infection. The Government has sponsored research projects in ISM and is receiving encouraging response. It will pursue a policy of sponsoring research in ISM for development of drugs which can serve the purpose of antiretrovirals.

The policy statement cautions about false claims of cures among unscrupulous practitioners and makes the point that: 'Any medicine or system of treatment which cannot stand the test of scrutiny by the professional organizations like the Ayurveda Council cannot be accepted as a drug or a system of treatment in the country'. Clearly, drugs which are shown by rigorous research methods to have an effect can become part of a system of treatment in India.[53]

Traditional Chinese medicine is also being used in HIV management, not only in China but also in Africa and in other parts of Asia, where traditional Chinese medicines are exported. In one study, qian-kun-nin, a Chinese herbal formulation considered to have anti-infection, anti-tumour, antiretroviral and immunomodulatory properties, was evaluated for its anti-HIV effects.

Eight HIV-positive subjects were given oral qian-kun-nin capsules for 24 consecutive weeks in a single-blind design. Compared with baseline level, the plasma virus load decreased significantly at the end of week 12 ($p < 0.01$) and week 24 ($p < 0.01$), respectively. Four weeks after cessation of qian-kun-nin treatment, plasma virus load was still significantly lower compared with baseline ($p < 0.01$). Blood CD4 cell counts were increased significantly at the end of the 12th week compared with the baseline level ($p < 0.01$). No adverse effects were observed, and no significant side-effects were recorded in any subjects.[54]

This is one of many emerging studies that require adequate funding to ensure that the research methodology is sound. While these data appear to suggest that qian-kun-nin has therapeutic potential in the treatment of HIV-positive patients, the trial design and the sample size make it difficult to draw solid conclusions from the study. What this study does highlight is the potential for anti-HIV effects in traditional medicines and the need for standard operating procedures for the clinical evaluation of these medicines.

In Africa, Asia and elsewhere in the world, partnerships between modern and traditional health systems are being seen to be the clear way forward to build on existing community resources and to harness the potential therapeutic benefit of local and affordable treatments for HIV-related illness, as well as to screen out false claims and unsafe medicines and practices.[55,56]

Malaria

The emergence of multidrug-resistant strains of malaria which has accompanied each new class of antimalarial drugs may be viewed as one of most significant threats to the health of people in tropical countries. While there is widespread agreement that a fresh approach to the prevention and treatment of malaria is urgently needed, solutions have tended to focus on the development of new classes of drugs. More recently, there has been an emphasis on promoting combination therapy of existing drugs as a means of preventing resistance.

Historically, however, local communities in tropical regions have used local flora as a means of preventing and treating malaria.[57] It can be argued that these traditional medicines, based on the use of whole plants with multiple ingredients or of complex mixtures of plant materials, constitute combination therapies that may well combat the development of resistance to antimalarial therapy.

Resistance, synergism and traditional medicines

While combination therapy in malaria, cancer and AIDS is based on the principle of synergistic action among multiple drugs, little significance has as yet been given to the obvious point that all of the major antimalarials have been derived from plants and that combination existed in the traditional formulations before the process of extraction took place. For example, flavonoids in *Artemisia annua*, which are structurally unrelated to the antimalarial drug artemisinin, enhance the in vitro antiplasmodial activity of artemisinin.[57]

Elsewhere, synergism has been observed between the alkaloids of the antimalarial plant *Ancistrocladus peltatum*. A total alkaloid extract of this plant had far greater antiparasitic activity than any of the six alkaloids isolated subsequently. In studies on antimalarial plants from Madagascar, the alkaloids bisbenzylisoquinoline, novel pavine and benzyl tetrahydroisoquinolines, were all found to potentiate the antiparasitic activity of chloroquine in vitro and, in some cases, in vivo. Preparations of these plants are currently being tested as adjuvants to chloroquine therapy in Madagascar.[57] In Uganda, there are data from clinical case reports and a cohort study that a traditional Ugandan herbal remedy is effective against malaria.[33,58]

As with other conditions, people with malaria will often combine conventional drugs and traditional medicines, sometimes simultaneously or as first- or second-line treatments,[27,59-64] with herbalists reporting their view that this combination gives an additional therapeutic effect.[65] Perceived efficacy is an important reason for people using traditional antimalarial medicines. Affordability is another. However, when patients themselves were asked why they chose traditional medicine over conventional drugs, a study in Burkina Faso found that the cost of medicines accounted for only 50% of respondents. Lack of faith in doctors was the reason for the other 50% resorting to traditional medicine.[66] Elsewhere it has been reported that medical staff at Burkina Faso hospitals are less trusted as they are frequently young, do not speak the local languages, and are not courteous or welcoming to patients.[59]

Several cohort studies have been conducted to evaluate the outcomes of traditional herbal treatments used by herbalists in managing malaria. A few of these have shown complete parasite clearance by day 7.[67] Phetsouvanh's study[67] of the antimalarial effects of *Alocaci macrorhiza* root decoction showed 100% parasite clearance by day 7, without any recrudescence for the duration of follow-up (21 days), although this study has not been published or replicated. Makinde et al.[67] showed 100% parasite clearance in adults by a leaf extract of Morinda lucida. However, there was not full parasite clearance from infected children. Further clinical studies on the antimalarial effects of plants have been reviewed by Willcox and Bodeker.[67]

The research initiative for traditional antimalarial methods (RITAM)

To redress this situation, a partnership was established in December 1999 between the Global Initiative for Traditional Systems (GIFTS) of Health and the Tropical Disease Research Programme of WHO.[68] Through the Research Initiative for Traditional Antimalarial Methods (RITAM, http://mim.nih.gov/english/partnerships/ritam_repotr.pdf), individual scientists, traditional health practitioners and others have formed a partnership to investigate, evaluate and, where appropriate, develop traditional herbal medicines to combat malaria. Standard operating procedures have been developed for experimental, toxicological and clinical research on traditional antimalarials. A research network to evaluate the potential of classically prepared *Artemisia annua* has also been established by RITAM.[69]

WOUNDS

Dermatological problems are the third most common reason for people seeking medical care in developing countries.[70] Among the most common dermatological problems of non-industrialized countries are non-healing tropical ulcers, particularly among young men of working age.[71] Tropical or seasonal environments with occupational exposure to the damp are typical for tropical ulcer,[72] where malnutrition may also be a factor.

Many wounds are inadequately treated in these countries because of issues of treatment cost, storage, manufacture and supply.[73,74] Bacterial and viral contamination of wounds is usual and some form of antisepsis is helpful. Reliance on imported agents in health centres and from pharmacies is expensive and unsustainable and the widespread casual use of antibiotics should be discouraged. The use of hypochlorite, iodine or gentian violet in the tropics follows now-questionable conventional Western therapies.

This has led to calls for research and rationalization of wound treatment in this setting.[75] In non-industrial countries the majority of the population uses traditional healthcare, and commonly uses herbal treatment for wounds.[76–78] These treatments warrant investigation for this reason and because they may be more readily available and efficacious than the alternatives.[79]

There is growing evidence that a number of plant treatments are useful in a variety of dermatological conditions, including wounds.[70,80,81] *Centella asiatica* extract is one of the most widely studied plant-based wound treatments. It is used in Madagascar and several other tropical countries. In vivo laboratory studies have shown its topical application to significantly accelerate wound healing, and in vitro studies of treated granulating tissues have demonstrated a significant increase in fibroblast activity, total DNA and collagen content.[82,83]

Recent research on *Aloe barbadensis* has shown it to be a powerful wound-healing agent.[84] Extracts from *Aloe barbadensis,* or aloe vera as it is commonly known, have been found to penetrate tissue, have anaesthetic properties, have antibacterial, antifungal and antiviral properties, serve as an antiinflammatory agent, and dilate capillaries and increase blood flow.[85,86]

Research at the National Institute for Traditional Medicine in Hanoi has examined the mechanism by which *Cudrania cochinchinensis* (Moraceae), commonly used in Vietnam as a traditional wound-healing agent, produces a wound-healing effect. Tran et al.[87] examined its effect on fibroblast proliferation and the protection of both fibroblast and endothelial cells against oxidative damage. An ethyl acetate extract of the plant was found to protect fibroblasts and endothelial cells against hydrogen peroxide-induced damage. The research team has suggested that stimulation of fibroblast proliferation and protection of cells against destruction by mediators of inflammatory processes may be ways in which the polyphenolic substances from this plant contribute to wound healing.

Phan et al.[88] studied the wound-healing properties of Eupolin, a topical agent produced from the leaves of *Chromolaena odorata,* and which is used widely for the treatment of burns and soft tissue wounds in Vietnam. Eupolin was found to enhance haemostasis, stimulate granulation tissue and re-epithelialization, and inhibit collagen contraction. These results suggest a mechanism for clinical reports on the effectiveness of Eupolin in reducing wound contraction and scarring, which are critical complications in post-burn trauma. Other studies have found Eupolin to have antibacterial properties.[89]

Chen et al.[90] studied the effects of 'dragon's blood', sap from the bark of *Croton lechleri* used as a wound-healing agent in South America. The researchers found that *Croton lechleri* has no isolable 'wound-healing principle', but acts as a natural dressing which forms an occlusive layer with an antimicrobial environment and cell proliferative effects. This is due to the combined effects of several compounds. This synergistic effect was further investigated by Pieters et al.,[91] who compared the in vivo effects of dragon's blood on wound repair with a polyphenolic fraction of dragon's blood and with a solution of artificial polyphenols. Wound repair was defined as the percentage of the wound volume filled with new tissue. Pieters and colleagues found:

- 90% wound repair with traditionally prepared dragon's blood
- 50% with a polyphenolic fraction of dragon's blood
- 40% when a solution of artificial polyphenols was used.

This finding lends support to the traditional practice of the complex mixture of compounds found in the bark rather than an isolated 'active ingredient' approach to the development of an effective wound treatment typical of conventional natural products research.

OPHTHALMIC CONDITIONS

Traditional eye treatment (TET) has been the cause of much concern due to serious eye infections and injury associated with many traditional treatments. In addition to directly contributing to corneal disease, use of traditional medicine has been found often to delay the use of modern medical treatment for eye disease. Public health programmes have focused on training traditional practitioners to refer patients for eye treatment.[92]

Research in Tanzania found that of 26 corneal ulcers present in a sample of TET users, 58% ($n = 15$) had no other identified cause of ulceration apart from TET use. There was a trend to more central and dense corneal scarring in the TET users group (42% vs 23%, $p = 0.06$).[93]

Courtright and co-workers[94] have assessed the rates of corneal disease in a district in Malawi following an interactive training programme with traditional healers, based on a collaborative approach to eye care. It was found that among the 175 pre-intervention and 97 post-intervention patients, delay in presentation improved only slightly. However, blindness among patients using TEM decreased from 44% to 21% and bilateral corneal disease in patients using TEM decreased from 31% to 10%. Despite this success, the research team note that distance to a hospital continues to be a barrier to the use of modern medical approaches to eye care.

At the same time, clinical and experimental studies on selected Indian Ayurvedic herbal treatments show promise in the management of specific ocular diseases. In a multicentre RCT at the All India Institute of Medical Sciences, an Ayurvedic herbal eye drop formulation was significantly more effective in treating trachoma and chronic conjunctivitis than placebo. The eye drops produced no side-effects, unlike the saline placebo which produced a burning sensation. Research by the same group has found that an Ayurvedic herbal eye drop significantly improved dry eye syndrome and ocular asthenia.[95] Experimental research in India has demonstrated a protective effect of the Ayurvedic herbs *Momordica charantia* and *Eugenia jambolana* against the development of murine alloxan diabetic cataract.

Clearly, TETs are causing much eye damage through traditional practitioners' ignorance of the functioning of the eye as well as through the use of ineffective and unsafe ingredients. Re-training programmes show a willingness on their part to learn new skills. At the same time, Indian studies suggest that some of the herbal ingredients traditionally used may warrant controlled investigation for possible therapeutic value.

SAFETY

A primary concern regarding traditional and complementary therapies is 'Are they safe?' As noted above, traditional eye medicine has been found to have serious effects on eye health.

Recent studies in the UK have found that there has been adulteration with steroids of some traditional Chinese dermatological preparations. In an analysis of Chinese herbal creams prescribed for dermatological conditions, it was found that eight of eleven creams analysed contained steroids.[96]

One prominent example of dangerous plant-based medicines is plant species which contain pyrrolizidine alkaloids, widely known to produce adverse effects. In a number of countries, plants containing alkaloids are prohibited from use in herbal medicines intended for internal use. This is due to the hepatotoxic effect of these alkaloids. Following absorption from the gut, pyrrolizidine alkaloids are carried to the liver, where they are converted by microsomal mixed function oxygenation to highly reactive pyrrole esters, which are the primarily toxic metabolites. At high doses these compounds bind to liver cell proteins and other macromolecules and cause extensive periacinar hepatocellular necrosis and hepatic failure. With lower, repeated doses, the progressive damage to liver cells results in a gradual increase in connective tissue in the liver and cirrhosis develops.[97] Chapter 32 further elaborates the risks associated with ingestion of or contact with poisonous plants.

Safety must be the starting point for national drug development strategies for herbal medicines. WHO Guidelines on the Evaluation of Herbal Medicines consider that clinical evaluation is ethical where drugs have long been in traditional use and a range of models for safety testing now exist.[98]

Research should consider best evidence for safety, including evidence for adverse effects from treatments (including magnitude, percentage of people so affected, etc.), as well as from inappropriate applications of traditional therapies. Post-market surveillance studies can provide information on adverse effects of botanical herbal preparations. Pharmacognostic and pharmacological research can provide information on the quality, efficacy, safety or toxicity of botanical/herbal medicinal preparations.

It is also important to keep a balanced perspective on the issue of safety of herbal medicines, while recognizing the very real risks associated with a number of these and with the untrained use of plants as medicines. A basic question often asked in addressing safety in herbal medicines is 'Safe with respect to what?' Research has found that in the USA, 51% of FDA-approved drugs have serious adverse effects not detected prior to their approval. One and a half million people are sufficiently injured by prescription drugs annually that they require hospitalization.[99] Once in hospital, the problem may be compounded. The incidence of serious and fatal adverse drug reactions (ADRs) in US hospitals is now ranked as between the fourth and the sixth leading cause of death in the USA, after heart disease, cancer, pulmonary disease and accidents. The first study to evaluate the ADRs in a large population (8 208 960) of hospitalized US Medicare patients found that in a sample of 141 398 patients who experienced an ADR, death rates were 19.18% higher and length of hospital stay was 8.25% higher. Increased charges for patients with an ADR were: total Medicare 19.86% (US$339 496 598), drugs 9.15% (US$24 744 650) and laboratory charges 2.82% (US$6 221 512).[100]

Clearly, the safety of and risks associated with medical interventions is an issue across all categories of healthcare. A regulatory response is necessary on the part of governments.

In developing health systems for traditional medicine, safety and quality control of herbal medicines go hand in hand. A case in point is the development of new standards of safety and quality for herbal medicines produced in India, where regulations were introduced in 2000 to improve the standard and quality of Indian herbal medicines. Regulations established standard manufacturing practices and quality control, requirements for infrastructure and manpower, and for raw material authenticity and absence of contamination. The government also established 10 drug-testing laboratories for the Indian Systems of Medicine and upgraded existing ones to provide high-quality evidence to licensing authorities of the safety and quality of herbal medicines.

Other special considerations

Traditional orthopaedics

The World Health Report for 1999 attributes over 21 million disability-adjusted life years to the effects of musculoskeletal disease globally. A range of traditional approaches are used in managing musculoskeletal problems, with varying degrees of success and/or adverse outcomes. While space does not allow for these to be addressed here, traditional orthopaedic approaches are reviewed and discussed elsewhere.[97]

Refugee populations

Forced migration due to war or persecution of political dissidents can remove people from mainstream medical care and force an increased reliance on medical practices from their cultural traditions, even in the face of unfamiliar biodiversity. Many studies on psychosocial and primary health practices among refugees validate the effects of integrating traditional practices into refugee care. In one study of Burmese refugees at the Thai-Burma border, high traditional medicine use was found despite health official views that there was little or no traditional medicine use among these displaced groups. Drawing on local knowledge of the therapeutic potential of medicinal plants, self-help networks were established and served as a public health infrastructure in areas where no other medical services were available due to heavy conflict.[101]

FOOD AND MEDICINE

A final consideration in the understanding of traditional health systems is the relationship between food and medicine that exists in these traditions.

In many traditional societies, and also in urban communities where traditional medicine is used and traditional medical theory influences household cooking and self-medication practices, food is considered central to health and the management of disease. Typically, there is not a clear distinction made between food and medicine, as food is often viewed medicinally and many plants used for medicine may also be included in the diet according to seasonal changes and family requirements.

The Hausa of Nigeria use certain plants as both food and medicine, including plants identified as having antimalarial effects. Nina Etkin of the University of Hawaii has reported that the use of plants with antimalarial effects 'as both food and medicine exposes individuals to more pharmacologically remarkable constituents than does either category of use alone. Thus of the 54 most commonly used Hausa antimalarials, 82% also appeared in diet, and among those there was 89% concordance that the same plant structure (root, leaves, etc.) served as both antimalarial and food. Further, among those 39 plants, 67% were maximally available during the period of highest risk of malaria infection'.[102]

In Cameroon and the Central African Republic, the Aka and Baka Pygmies have a view of illness that includes both physical causes and a more fundamental view of equilibrium having been disturbed. Disequilibrium may pertain to the relationships between an individual and the worlds of which he or she is a part, including nature, society, the cosmos and the invisible. The Aka search for balance extends to food, where moderation in taste and quantity is preferred. Excess intake of food is considered to be life-threatening. The feeling of well-being associated with balance can only, in the Aka view, be obtained through a diet based around meat and honey. Meat is a sign of the hunter's prowess and is considered essential for health. Meat is obtained through hunting and skill in hunting requires clarity or peace of mind. Vital energy, intuition and keenness of eye are all attributes of the skilled hunter.[103]

The Masai of East Africa cook the bark of *Acacia goetzei* (Mimosaceae) and *Albizia anthelmintica* (Mimosaceae) with their traditional diet of boiled meat, milk and blood – sometimes described as 'the world's worst diet'. Research by Timothy Johns of McGill University has shown that combining the bark with the other foods results in cholesterol levels one-third that of the average American. Unique saponins in these plants are considered to be implicated in producing the cholesterol-lowering effects.[104]

The impact of traditional diet on health has been studied in Japan, where a high variety of foods, especially plant foods, is characteristic of a traditional Japanese diet. A Japanese survey of the diets of 200 elderly women revealed that they consumed a variety of over 100 biologically different foods per week. By contrast, in most Western countries the recommended minimum is only 30. The higher the variety, the less risk of many diseases, including cardiovascular disease, diabetes and many cancers. A high intake of soy products is also found in Japan: approximately 40 times more than the Western intake. Green tea, common in traditional Japanese diet, is rich in antioxidants (see, http://members.tripod.com).

Japanese who move overseas and adopt a Western-style diet have an increased risk of breast cancer, coronary heart disease and diabetes. Breast cancer is rare in Japan due to a low dietary fat intake, and a high intake of soy (with protective phyto-oestrogens), antioxidants and fibre. In addition, high food variety may be involved, as well as a possible genetic element. A low intake of meat is a major factor in the low bowel cancer rate in Japan. The traditional diet is based on the healthy combination of a high food variety, with minimal saturated fat, more fish, less meat, and especially more fruit, vegetables and grains.

In the context of tropical medicine, an understanding of traditional dietary practices can be helpful in the management and possibly the prevention of certain common conditions. It is an area worth enquiring into when taking a patient's history, as diet may include herbal ingredients that may influence the course of conventional treatment. More generally, the role of diet in the management of illness in the tropics is worthy of evaluation. While it will be complex to design dietary studies due to the multiple components in traditional diet, clinical and epidemiological research into the preventive and nutritional effects of traditional diet could examine their impact on the diseases which they have been used to combat in the tropics as well as on the emerging diseases of urban communities related to Western-style diet and lifestyle – particularly, diabetes, hypertension, stroke, heart disease and cancer.

CONCLUSION

Traditional medicine continues to exist in the tropics as a major source of healthcare for the majority of the population. National and international policies are calling for partnerships between conventional and traditional health practitioners in order to provide adequate healthcare coverage in the face of limited resources.

The tropical medicine practitioner may be faced with the negative effects of traditional medicine practice, such as renal and liver failure associated with improper use of traditional medicine; or, faced with unavailability of conventional medicines for common conditions, the tropical medicine practitioner might consider that partnerships with traditional practitioners in research-based practice are called for to evaluate possible traditional treatments for common conditions. In all cases, research ethics and medical ethics clearly take priority in evaluating and applying traditional treatments.

The move towards partnerships is clearly justified in the face of beneficial outcomes of such programmes in the fields of AIDS prevention and care and in reducing eye disease associated with traditional practices. Other research suggests that important discoveries may also result from such collaborative partnerships in a range of communicable diseases and common ailments, expanding the range of treatment options available for the management of disease in the tropics.

REFERENCES

1. Willcox M, Bodeker G. Malaria. In: Bodeker G, Burford G, eds. *Traditional, Complementary and Alternative Medicine: Policy & Public Health Perspectives.* London: Imperial College Press; 2007.
2. Shankar D. The spiritual dimensions of medicinal plants in the Vedic tradition of India. In: Posey D, ed. *Cultural and Spiritual Values in Biodiversity.* Nairobi: UN Environment Programme; 2000.
3. Foster G. Disease etiologies in non-western medical systems. *Am Anthropol* 1976; 78:773–782.
4. Berlin E, Berlin B. General overview of Maya ethnomedicine. In: Posey D, ed. *Cultural and Spiritual Values in Biodiversity.* Nairobi: UN Environment Programme; 2000.
5. Bodeker G, Ong C-K, Burford G, et al, eds. *World Health Organization Global Atlas on Traditional & Complementary Medicine*: World Health Organization, Geneva; 2005.
6. WHO. *SEARO*; 2000.
7. WHO. Guidelines for training traditional health practitioners in primary healthcare. Geneva: WHO Division of Strengthening of Health Services and Traditional Medicine, 1995 (unpublished).
8. Troskie TR. The importance of traditional midwives in the delivery of healthcare in the Republic of South Africa. *Curationis* 1997; 20(1):15–20.
9. WHO Regional Office for Africa. Report of a consultation on the coordination of activities relating to traditional medicine in the African region, Brazzaville, 2–6 July 1984. Brazzaville: WHO-AFRO (unpublished, ref. AFR/TRM/3).
10. WHO/UNICEF. *Primary Healthcare: A Joint Report.* Geneva: WHO; 1978.
11. Kleinman A. *The Illness Narratives.* New York: Basic Books; 1988; 12.
12. Herron RE, Hillis SL. The impact of the Transcendental Meditation program on government payments to physicians in Quebec: an update. *Am J Health Promotion* 2000; 14(5):284–291.
13. Sharma H, Clarke C. *Contemporary Ayurveda.* London: Churchill-Livingstone; 1998.
14. Alderete W, Guevara G. South and Central America regional workshop on traditional health systems: GIFTS of health. Conclusions and recommendations. *J Altern Complement Med* 1996; 2(3):398–401.
15. Stephens C. Training urban traditional birth attendants: balancing international policy and local reality. Preliminary evidence from the slums of India on the attitudes and practice of clients and practitioners. *Soc Sci Med* 1992; 35(6):811–817.
16. Shiferaw T. Illness burden and use of health services in a rural community, southwestern Ethiopia. *East Afr Med J* 1993; 70(11):717–720.
17. Oskowitz B. Bridging the communication gap between traditional healers and nurses. *Nursing RSA* 1991; 6(7):20–22.
18. Yen J, Wilbraham L. Discourses of culture and illness in South African mental healthcare and indigenous healing, Part II: African mentality. *Transcult Psychiatry* 2003; 40(4):562–584.
19. Ayonrinde O, Gureje O, Lawal R. Psychiatric research in Nigeria: bridging tradition and modernization. *Br J Psychiatry* 2004; 184:536–538.
20. Ahmed IM, Bremer JJ, Magzoub MM, et al. Characteristics of visitors to traditional healers in central Sudan. *Eastern Mediterranean Health J* 1999; 5(1):79–85.
21. Traore S, Coulibaly SO, Sidibe M. *Comportements et coûts liés au Paludisme chez les femmes des campements de pêcheurs dans la zone de Sélingué au Mali.* Bamako, Mali: Institut National de Recherche en Santé Publique, 1993. TDR/SER/PRS/12.
22. Elzubier AG, Ansari EHH, El Nour MH, et al. Knowledge and misconceptions about malaria among secondary school students and teachers in Kassala, Eastern Sudan. *J R Soc Health* 1997; 117(6):381–385.
23. Tanner M, Vlassoff C. Treatment-seeking behaviour for malaria: a typology based on endemicity and gender. *Soc Sci Med* 1998; 46(4–5):523–532.
24. Wilkinson D, Gcabashe L, Lurie M. Traditional healers as tuberculosis treatment supervisors: precedent and potential. *Int J Tuberc Lung Dis* 1999; 3(9):838–842.
25. Mbindyo P. Public-Private Partnerships: A Case Study from East Africa. In: Bodeker G, Burford G, eds. *Traditional, Complementary and Alternative Medicine: Policy & Public Health Perspectives.* London: Imperial College Press; 2007.
26. Vissandjee B, Barlow R, Fraser DW. Utilization of health services among rural women in Gujarat, India. *Public Health* 1997; 111(3):135–148.
27. Agyepong IA, Manderson L. The diagnosis and management of fever at household level in the Greater Accra Region, Ghana. *Acta Tropica* 1994; 58:317–330.
28. Ruebush TK, Kern MK, Campbell CC, et al. Self-treatment of malaria in rural areas of western Kenya. *Bull World Health Organ* 1995; 73:229–236.
29. Miguel CA, Manderson L, Lansang MA. Patterns of treatment for malaria in Tayabas, the Philippines: implications for control. *Trop Med Int Health* 1998; 3(5):413–421.
30. Miguel CA, Tallo VL, Manderson L, et al. Local knowledge and treatment of malaria in Agusan del Sur, the Philippines. *Soc Sci Med* 1999; 48:607–618.
31. Théra MA, Sissoko MS, Heuschkel C et al. Village level treatment of presumptive malaria: experiences with the training of mothers and traditional healers as resource persons in the Region of Mopti, Mali. In: *Clone, Cure and Control: Tropical Health for the 21st Century.* Second European Congress on Tropical Medicine, Liverpool. Poster P72; 1999:139.
32. Hausmann Muela S, Muela Ribera J, Tanner M. Fake malaria and hidden parasites – the ambiguity of malaria. *Anthropol Med* 1998; 5:43–61.
33. Bitahwa N, Tumwesigye O, Kabariime P, et al. Herbal treatment of malaria: four case reports from the Rukararwe Partnership Workshop for Rural Development (Uganda). *Trop Doct* 1997; (suppl 1):17–19.
34. Munguti KJ. Community perceptions and treatment seeking for malaria in Baringo District, Kenya: implications for disease control. *East African Med J* 1998; 75(12):687–691.
35. Varga CA, Veale DJH. Isihlambezo: utilization patterns and potential health effects of pregnancy-related traditional herbal medicine. *Soc Sci Med* 1997; 44(7):911–924.

36. Ong CK, Peterson S, Doll H, et al. *Do factors which influence preference for Traditional Chinese Medicine (TCM) in the Oxfordshire Chinese community affect access to GP care?* University of Oxford: Health Services Research Unit; 2001.

37. Bandyopadhyay M, MacPherson S. *Women and Health: Tradition and Culture in Rural India*. Brookfield: Ashgate; 1998.

38. Nichter M. Ethnomedicine: diverse trends, common linkages. Commentary. *Med Anthropol* 1991; 13:137–171.

39. Chi C. Integrating traditional medicine into modern healthcare systems: examining the role of Chinese medicine in Taiwan. *Soc Sci Med* 1994; 39(3):307–321.

40. Hall RL. Alcohol treatment in American Indian populations: an indigenous treatment modality compared with traditional approaches. *Ann NY Acad Sci* 1986; 472:168–178.

41. Maher P. A review of 'traditional' aboriginal health beliefs. *Aust J Rural Health* 1999; 7(4):229–236.

42. Last M, Chavanduka GL. *The Professionalisation of African Medicine*. Manchester: Manchester University Press; 1986.

43. Burnett A, Baggaley R, Ndovi-MacMillan M, et al. Caring for people with HIV in Zambia: are traditional healers and formal health workers willing to work together? *AIDS Care* 1999; 11(4):481–491.

44. Upvall MJ. Nursing perceptions of collaboration with indigenous healers in Swaziland. *Int J Nurs Stud* 1992; 29(1):27–36.

45. Osuide GE. Regulation of herbal medicines in Nigeria: the role of the National Agency for Food and Drug Administration and Control (NAFDAC). Paper presented at the International Conference on Ethnomedicine and Drug Discovery, Silver Spring, MD, 3–5 November 1999.

46. Bodeker G, Dvorak-Little M, Carter G, et al. HIV/AIDS: Traditional systems of healthcare in the management of a global epidemic. *J Altern Complem Med* 2006; 12(6):563–576.

47. Green EC. *AIDS and STDs in Africa: Bridging the Gap Between Traditional Healers and Modern Medicine*. Boulder: Westview Press; 1994. (South African edition published by University of Natal Press; 1994).

48. Green EC. The participation of African traditional healers in AIDS/STD prevention programmes. *Trop Doct* 1997; 27(suppl 1):56–59.

49. Nations MK, de Souza MA. Umbanda healers as effective AIDS educators: case-control study in Brazilian urban slums (favelas). *Trop Doct* 1997; 27(suppl 1):60–66.

50. Bodeker G, Kabatesi D, Homsy J, et al. A regional task force on traditional medicine and AIDS in East and Southern Africa. *Lancet* 2000; 355: 1284.

51. Sebit MB, Chandiwana SK, Latif AS, et al. Quality of life evaluation in patients with HIV-1 infection: the impact of traditional medicine in Zimbabwe. *Cent Afr J Med* 2000; 46(8):208–213.

52. Asres K, Bucar F, Kartnig T, et al. Antiviral activity against human immunodeficiency virus type 1 (HIV-1) and type 2 (HIV-2) of ethnobotanically selected Ethiopian medicinal plants. *Phytother Res* 2001; 15(1):62–69.

53. Bodeker G, Dvorak-Little M. AIDS control in India. A perspective from the traditional medicine sector. *J Altern Complement Med* 2006; 6:501–503.

54. Zhan L, Yue ST, Xue YX, et al. Effects of qian-kun-nin, a Chinese herbal medicine formulation, on HIV positive subjects: a pilot study. *Am J Chin Med* 2000; 28(3–4):305–312.

55. Liu J. An overview of clinical studies in complementary and alternative medicine in HIV infection and AIDS. In: Bodeker G, Burford G, eds. *Traditional, Complementary and Alternative Medicine: Policy & Public Health Perspectives*. London: Imperial College Press; 2007.

56. Chaudhury RR. A clinical protocol for the study of traditional medicine and human immunodeficiency virus-related illness. *Altern Complement Ther* 2001; 7(5):553–566.

57. Bodeker G. New research directions with antimalarial plants: An introduction. In: Willcox M, Bodeker G, Rasoanaivo P, eds. *Traditional Medicinal Plants and Malaria*. Boca Raton: CRC Press; 2004.

58. Willcox ML. A clinical trial of 'AM', a Ugandan herbal remedy for malaria. *J Public Health* Med 1999; 21(3):318–324.

59. Bugmann N. Le concept du paludisme, l'usage et l'efficacité in vivo de trois traitements traditionnels antipalustres dans la région de Dori, Burkina Faso. Inaugural doctoral dissertation, Faculty of Medicine, University of Basel; 2000.

60. Gessler MC, Msuya DE, Nkunya MH, et al. Traditional healers in Tanzania: sociocultural profile and three short portraits. *J Ethnopharmacol* 1995; 48(3):145–160.

61. Jayawardene R. Illness perception: social cost and coping strategies of malaria cases. *Soc Sci Med* 1993; 37:1169–1176.

62. Lipowsky R, Kroeger A, Vazquez ML. Sociomedical aspects of malaria control in Colombia. *Soc Sci Med* 1992; 34:625–637.

63. McCombie SC. Treatment seeking for malaria: a review of recent research. *Soc Sci Med* 1996; 43:933–945.

64. Pagnoni F, Convelbo N, Tiendrebeogo J, et al. A community-based programme to provide prompt and adequate treatment of presumptive malaria in children. *Trans R Soc Trop Med Hyg* 1997; 91:512–517.

65. Rasoanaivo P, Ratsimamanga-Urverg S, Milijaona R. In vitro and in vivo chloroquine-potentiating action of Strychnos myrtoides alkaloids against chloroquine-resistant strains of Plasmodium malaria. *Planta Medica* 1994; 60:13–16.

66. Abyan IM, Osman AA. *Social and behavioural factors affecting malaria in Somalia*. TDR/SER/PRS/11; 1993.

67. Willcox M, Bodeker G. Herbal remedies for malaria: an overview of clinical studies. In: Willcox M, Rasoanaivo P, Bodeker G, eds. *Traditional Medicine, Medicinal Plants and Malaria*. London: Harwood Press; 2004.

68. Bodeker G, Willcox M. New research initiative on plant-based antimalarials. *Lancet* 2000; 355:761.

69. Willcox M, Rasoanaivo P, Bodeker G, eds. *Traditional Medicine, Medicinal Plants and Malaria*. London: Harwood Press; 2004.

70. Burford G, Bodeker G, Ryan TJ. Skin and wound care: Traditional, complementary and alternative medicine in public health dermatology. In: Bodeker G, Burford G, eds. *Traditional, Complementary and Alternative Medicine: Policy & Public Health Perspectives*. London: Imperial College Press; 2007.

71. Ryan TJ. The epidemiology of leg ulcers. In: Westerhof W, ed. Leg Ulcers: Diagnosis and Treatment. Amsterdam: Elsevier Science; 1993.

72. Robinson DC, Adriaans B, Hay RJ, et al. The clinical and epidemiological features of the tropical ulcer (tropical phagedenic ulcer). Int J Dermatol 1988; 27:49–53.

73. Ryan TJ. Wound healing in the developing world. Dermatol Clin 1993; 11:791–799.

74. Zeina B, Zohra BI, al-Assad S. The effects of honey on Leishmania parasites: an in vitro study. Trop Doct 1997; 27(suppl 1):36–38.

75. Ryan TJ. International Foundation for Dermatology: solving the problems of skin disease in the developing world. Trop Doct 1992; 22(suppl 1): 42–43.

76. Vaqas B, Ryan TJ. Lymphoedema: pathophysiology and management in resource-poor settings – relevance for lymphatic filariasis control programmes. Filaria J 2003; 2:4.

77. Bodeker G, Hughes MA. Wound healing, traditional treatments and research policy. In: Etkin N, Prendergast H, Houghton P, eds. *Modern Medicine and Traditional Remedies*. London: Kew Press; 1998.

78. Bodeker G. Lessons on integration from the developing world's experience. *BMJ* 2001; 322:164–167.

79. Bodeker G, Ryan TJ, Ong C-K. Traditional approaches to wound healing. *Clin Dermatol* 1999; 17(1):93–98.

80. Bakhiet A, Adam S. Therapeutic utility, constituents and toxicity of some medicinal plants: a review. *Vet Hum Toxicol* 1995; 37(3):255–258.

81. Brantner A, Grein E. The antibacterial activity of plant extracts used externally in traditional medicine. *J Ethnopharmacol* 1994; 44(1):35–40.

82. Sasaki S, Shinkai H, Akashi Y, et al. Studies on the mechanism of action of asiaticoside (Madecassol) on experimental granulation tissue and cultured fibroblasts and its clinical application in systemic scleroderma. *Acta Dermato-Venerol* 1972; 52(2):141–150.

83. Suguna L, Sivakumar P, Chandrakasan G. Effects of Centella asiatica on dermal wound healing in rats. *Indian J Exp Biol* 1996; 34(12):1208–1211.

84. Heggers JP, Pelley RP, Robson MC. Beneficial effects of Aloe in wound healing. *Phytother Res* 1993; 7:S48–52.

85. Grindlay D, Reynolds T. The Aloe Vera phenomenon: a review of the properties and modern uses. *J Ethnopharmacol* 1986; 16:117–151.

86. Robson MC, Heggers JP, Hagstrom WJ. Myth, magic, witchcraft or fact? Aloe vera revisited. *JBCR* 1982; 3:157–163.

87. Tran VH, Hughes MA, Cherry GW. In vitro studies on the antioxidant and growth stimulatory activities of a polyphenolic extract from Cudrania cochinchinensis used in the treatment of wounds in Vietnam. *Wound Repair Regen* 1997; 5:159–167.

88. Phan TT, Hughes MA, Cherry GW, et al. An aqueous extract of the leaves of Chromolaena odorata (Eupolin) inhibits hydrated collagen lattice contraction by normal human dermal fibroblasts. *J Altern Complement Med* 1996; 2: 349–358.

89. Irobi ON. Activities of Chromolaena odorata (Compositae) cus faecallis. *J Ethnopharmacol* 1992; 37:81–83.

90. Chen ZP, Cai Y, Phillipson JD (1994). Studies on the antitumour, antibacterial and wound healing properties of dragon's blood. *Planta Med* 1994; 60:541–545.

91. Pieters L, de Bruyne T, van Poel B, et al. In vivo wound healing of Dragon's blood (Croton spp.), a traditional South American drug, and its constituents. *Phytomedicine* 1995; 2:17–22.

92. Poudyal AK, Jimba M, Poudyal BK, et al. Traditional healers' roles on eye care services in Nepal. *Br J Ophthalmol* 2005; 89(10):1250–1253.

93. Mselle J. Visual impact of using traditional medicine on the injured eye in Africa. *Acta Trop* 1998; 70(2):185–192.

94. Courtright P, Lewallen S, Kanjaloti S. Changing patterns of corneal disease and associated vision loss at a rural African hospital following a training programme for traditional healers. *Br J Ophthalmol* 1996; 80(8):694–697.

95. Biswas NR, Beri S, Das GK, et al. Comparative double blind multicentric randomised placebo controlled clinical trial of a herbal preparation of eye drops in some ocular ailments. *J Indian Med Assoc* 1996; 94(3):101–102.

96. Keane FM, Munn SE, du Vivier AWP, et al. Analysis of Chinese herbal creams prescribed for dermatological conditions. *BMJ* 1999; 318:563–564.

97. Burford G, Bodeker G, Ong C-K, et al. Musculoskeletal conditions. In: Bodeker G, Burford G, eds. *Traditional, Complementary and Alternative Medicine: Policy & Public Health Perspectives*. London: Imperial College Press; 2007.

98. Shia G, Noller B, Burford G. Safety: Issues and policy. In: Bodeker G, Burford G, eds. *Traditional, Complementary and Alternative Medicine: Policy & Public Health Perspectives*. London: Imperial College Press; 2007.

99. Barnes J. Pharmacovigilance of herbal medicines: A UK perspective. In: Bodeker G, Burford G, eds. *Traditional, Complementary and Alternative Medicine: Policy & Public Health Perspectives*. London: Imperial College Press; 2007.

100. Bond CA, Raehl CL. Adverse drug reactions in United States hospitals. *Pharmacotherapy* 2006; 26(5):601–608.

101. Bodeker G, Neumann C, Lall P, et al. Traditional Medicine Use & Health worker Training in a Refugee Setting at the Thai-Burma Border. *J Refugee Stud* 2005; 18, 1:76–99.

102. Etkin N. Antimalarial plants used by Hausa in northern Nigeria. *Trop Doct* 1997; 27(suppl 1):12–16.

103. Motte-Florac, Bahuchet S, Thomas JMC. The role of food in the therapeutics of the Central African Republic. In: Hladik CM, Hladik A, Linars OF, et al., eds. *Tropical Forests, People and Food: Biocultural Interactions and Applications to Development* Man and the Biosphere Series, Vol. 13. Paris: UNESCO and Parthenon Press; 1993.

104. Johns T, Mahunnah RL, Sanaya P et al. Saponins and phenolic content in plant dietary additives of a traditional subsistence community, the Batemi of Ngorongoro District, Tanzania. *J Ethnopharmacol* 1999; 66(1):1–10.

Chapter 5   Dominic Kwiatkowski

Genetics

INDIVIDUAL VARIATION

Apart from identical twins, no two human beings are exactly alike. A range of variation is found in almost every characteristic that it is possible to quantify, whether it is a simple physical attribute such as height, or something that is more complicated to measure, such as a hormone level. Sometimes there are striking differences between populations, for example in skin colour. But the phenomenon of human individuality goes much deeper than ethnic differences, and the vast majority of characteristics show significant variation within a single village or even within a single family. In this chapter, the characteristics that interest us are those that determine susceptibility to disease.

Since ancient times it has been debated whether nature or nurture is primarily responsible for individual variation – i.e. how much is due to genetics as opposed to environment. A substantial proportion of disease in the tropics is caused by environmental factors such as infectious agents or inadequate diet, so it might be thought that genetics would play a very small role, at least for the common ailments. Two lines of epidemiological evidence indicate that this view is incorrect. If a parent dies prematurely of infection, the children are more likely to die of infection, even if they are adopted in childhood and thus live in a different environment from the parent[1] And the risk of developing tuberculosis,[2] leprosy[3] or malaria[4] has been demonstrated to have a significant heritable component by comparing monozygous twins (who are genetically identical) with dizygous twins (who are genetically related but not identical). Such observations, together with a growing body of molecular data, have led to the view that genetic factors play a role in almost all human disease, even if the primary cause is environmental. For example, genetic variation may partly explain why one child develops fatal cerebral malaria, or kwashiorkor, while other children living in the same compound are equally exposed to malaria parasites and to poor diet but do not develop these severe clinical syndromes. A study in Kenyan children found that host genetic factors appeared to account for 25% of variation in risk of severe malaria, whereas household factors accounted for only 14%.[5] A huge amount of scientific effort is now being put into investigating the many different genetic factors that influence susceptibility to common diseases, in the hope that this will provide fundamental insights into molecular pathogenesis and ultimately lead to better ways of disease prevention.

Human disease genetics in the twentieth century was dominated by a set of rules deduced by Gregor Mendel in 1865. The observable characteristics that Mendel measured in his flowering peas, and that epidemiologists measure in human subjects, comprise the 'phenotype' of the individual. Mendelian rules apply when a specific genetic variant, for example a deletion or change in part of a DNA sequence, causes a predictable phenotypic change.[6] Humans generally have two copies of each gene, one from the mother and one from the father. A genetic effect is termed dominant if the phenotypic effect is observed in the heterozygote, i.e. when one copy of the gene is affected and the other copy is not. In contrast, a recessive effect is one where the affected phenotype is observed only in the homozygous state, i.e. when both copies of the gene are of the variant type. Here, the affected individual must receive the genetic variant from both parents, who may or may not be affected themselves. Genes on the X and Y chromosomes are a special case, as females carry two copies of the X chromosome while males carry one X plus one Y chromosome: thus, only one copy of a recessive X-linked genetic character is sufficient to cause the affected phenotype in a male. Based on these principles, clinical investigators have identified many major genetic diseases simply by analysing how the phenotype segregates in affected families. A classical example of a recessive effect is sickle cell disease, caused by a mutation that substitutes valine for glutamic acid in the sixth position of the β-globin chain. In homozygotes this causes anaemia and severe clinical complications resulting from major erythrocyte deformities at low oxygen saturations. Heterozygotes have a much milder phenotype and are normally asymptomatic. Thus, the typical patient with sickle cell disease is born to heterozygous parents, who each carry one copy of the affected gene but have no overt manifestations of the disease. Molecular geneticists have now identified over 7000 forms of DNA variation that act in a Mendelian fashion to alter human phenotype.[7] Mendelian genetic diseases are mostly at low prevalence in the general population, with the notable exception of erythrocyte defects such as sickle cell disease and thalassaemia.

The challenge for the twenty-first century is to unravel the genetic basis of common human diseases that do not show a Mendelian pattern of inheritance. These include major infectious diseases such as malaria, HIV/AIDS and tuberculosis, as well as non-infectious conditions such as hypertension, diabetes, dementia and the different cancers. The lack of Mendelian inheritance simply indicates that these conditions are not determined by a single major gene. Probably hundreds of different genes are involved, interacting with each other as well as with multiple environmental risk factors. Up till now such complexity has been impossible to dissect, but this field has recently been revolutionized by the sequencing of the human genome, and by novel technologies that will permit analysis of many thousands of genetic variants at the epidemiological level.

DIVERSITY OF THE HUMAN GENOME

A draft sequence of the human genome was published in early 2001[8,9] and the finished sequence was published in 2004.[10] The entire sequence can be browsed and interrogated in detail on websites such as Ensembl.[11] The total size of our genome is slightly over 3 billion base pairs but genes that encode protein account for only a small proportion of this. What the rest of our DNA does is open to question, but there is growing evidence that it may be extremely important for gene regulation.[12] Surprisingly, we are estimated to have slightly under 23 000 genes, which seems a remarkably small number given that the worm *C. elegans* has about 20 000 and the fruitfly about 14 000. This highlights the potential importance of gene regulation in determining uniquely human attributes. By the same token, a large part of human phenotypic diversity may stem from DNA polymorphisms that alter gene regulation rather than protein structure.

The term polymorphism is used to describe genetic variants that are found in a significant proportion (e.g. >1%) of the general population. The most common form of DNA variation, where one nucleotide is substituted for another, is called a single nucleotide polymorphism or SNP (pronounced 'snip'). The different forms of a polymorphism are called alleles: thus, a typical SNP has two alleles. Over 6 million common SNPs have so far been discovered and the total is likely to be in the order of 10 million. If we consider an average 10 kb region of the genome (i.e. one where the length of DNA sequence is 10 000 base pairs), there might typically be about 30 SNPs. If each SNP has two alleles, this amounts to over a billion (2^{30}) possible combinations, but in practice only a relatively small number of combinations are seen in any population. A particular combination of alleles that is seen in the population is known as a haplotype. One of the most important advances in human genetics in recent years has been the publication of a detailed haplotype map of the human genome, and in the later part of this chapter we will discuss why this is so important for investigation of the genetic basis of common diseases.[13,14] A second common form of variation involves repetition of a part of the sequence. In some cases the sequence that is repeated is very short (e.g. a two-base-pair repeat would be of the form . . . ATATATAT . . .) and variation occurs in the number of times it is repeated (e.g. 10 to 20): this is known as a microsatellite. In other cases the sequence that is repeated is much larger (e.g. >1 kb): this is known as copy number variation and it is emerging as a much more common form of human genome variation than was formerly thought.[15] A third common form of variation is insertion or deletion of a segment of DNA, known as an indel, which again may be just a few base pairs or a much larger segment. A fourth form of variation, which may be linked to all of the above, involves structural rearrangements of the genome.[16]

Despite the recent explosion in our knowledge of human genome variation it will be many years before we have a comprehensive catalogue of common genetic variants. In very crude terms, if two random chromosomes from a single population were compared, e.g. the maternal and paternal chromosomes contained in a single individual, it is likely that there would be over a million differences in the sequence. Remarkably, the level of nucleotide diversity within a single African village is not much less than the values observed when chromosomes are randomly sampled from around the world. This reinforces a point which population geneticists have known for some time, namely that the level of genetic differentiation between human populations is low, relative to the amount of genetic diversity that is typically present within a single population. Overall, nucleotide diversity within Africa tends to be greater than in other populations, consistent with the view that modern humans migrated out of Africa relatively recently in our evolutionary history.

SELECTIVE PRESSURE OF INFECTIOUS DISEASE ON THE HUMAN GENOME

At a global level, by far the most common group of known genetic disorders are those that involve the red blood cell. They include disorders of haemoglobin regulation (α- and β-thalassaemia due to mutations that suppress production of α- and β-globin, respectively); haemoglobin structure (sickle cell disease due to haemoglobin S, and other structural mutations of β-globin such as haemoglobin C and haemoglobin E), red cell enzymes (glucose-6-phosphate dehydrogenase deficiency due to *G6PD* mutations) and red cell ultrastructure (ovalocytosis due to mutations of the gene encoding band III protein). Although these genetic variants have different geographical distributions, they share one remarkable feature, namely that all are commonest in populations whose ancestors were highly exposed to malaria.[17] Over 50 years ago Haldane proposed an explanation, namely that these polymorphisms confer protection against malaria.[18]

There is now substantial evidence that this hypothesis is correct. The *HbS* allele, which encodes haemoglobin S, is a classical example of what Haldane termed balanced polymorphism, whereby heterozygotes are protected against malaria while the harmful genetic effects are restricted to homozygotes. African children who are heterozygous for *HbS* are 10 times less likely to develop life-threatening complications of *Plasmodium falciparum* infection than those who lack this allele[19] but they suffer none of the severe clinical problems seen in *HbS* homozygotes. Different degrees of protection against severe malaria have been documented for the *HbC* allele and for *G6PD* variants in African populations, and for band III polymorphisms in Papua New Guinea.[20-23] The frequency of α⁺-thalassaemia shows a close epidemiological relationship with malarial endemicity,[24] and it has been shown to protect against severe malaria,[25,26] but the story is complex, as it appears to be associated with increased malaria incidence in some settings[27] and there is evidence that the protective effect is lost in the presence of HbS.[28]

The potential value of population genetics in elucidating fundamental aspects of infectious disease is beautifully illustrated by the story of Duffy blood group antigen. West Africans lack Duffy antigen on their erythrocytes because of a SNP in the corresponding gene, and this makes them highly resistant to infection with *P. vivax*.[29,30] This discovery has yielded fundamental insights into the molecular mechanism by which malaria parasites invade human erythrocytes,[31] the type of information which could be invaluable in the development of an effective vaccine.

How has the selective pressure of infectious disease affected genetic diversity of the immune system? Certain HLA types appear to have risen to a high frequency in West Africa because of their protective effect against malaria,[19] but this is just the tip of the iceberg, and many similar examples for other infectious agents and for other immune genes undoubtedly remain to be discovered. Analysis of human genome sequence diversity may provide important clues to recent positive selection – e.g. when a new allele rapidly rises to high frequency in the population, it tends to carry surrounding alleles with it, resulting in extended haplotypes (a haplotype is a particular combination of alleles found in a localized region of the genome).[32] A survey of over 3 million SNPs in people of African, European and Asian ancestry found more than 300 regions of the genome that appeared to be under strong recent positive selection.[33] In some cases evolutionary selection appeared to involve multiple genes involved in a single biological process, including the *LARGE* and *DMD* genes which are both related to infection by the Lassa virus in West Africa.

GENETIC CONTRIBUTION TO COMMON DISEASES

There is now much information about those human diseases that are primarily caused by a major defect in a single gene.[7] They include a large number of fatal or highly debilitating diseases, such as muscular dystrophy, cystic fibrosis and Tay–Sachs disease, which are of huge consequence for the affected family, but fortunately they are relatively uncommon. From the perspective of the developing world, sickle cell disease and thalassaemia are of great importance but most other single gene disorders are not major public health priorities. The commonest infectious and non-infectious diseases of the developing world are influenced by many different environmental factors plus a genetic component which is largely unknown but undoubtedly complex. Here we will consider two different ways in which genetic factors may contribute to common disease of complex aetiology.

At one end of the spectrum, even if many environmental and genetic variables influence the disease process, there may exist certain families where the predominant factor is a single gene. For example, in a population with an extremely high prevalence of *P. vivax* infection, where a small minority of individuals are Duffy-negative, complete resistance to *P. vivax* is a rare phenomenon which segregates in certain families according to classical Mendelian rules. Another example is the group of genetic defects that result in primary immunodeficiencies.[34] In parts of the world with a high burden of infectious disease, it is extremely difficult for doctors and nurses to distinguish the child with congenital severe immunodeficiency from all the other infants and children who die of infectious causes. Thus, a clinical syndrome such as 'infant death due to disseminated staphylococcal infection' is a highly complex phenotype, of which a small subgroup may come from families afflicted with a major genetic defect. Table 5.1 gives some examples of the 100 or so major genetic defects of the immune system that have been identified, mostly due to a rare mutation of a single gene. Apart from the importance of this information for affected families, it has provided valuable insights into the molecular and cellular basis of host immunity against different microbial species.

At the other end of the spectrum are genetic variants with a much more modest effect on disease susceptibility. In recent years there has been an explosion of information about DNA polymorphisms that appear to increase or decrease the risk of common diseases by a factor of two or even less. Being only a small part of a complex picture, such genetic effects do not show Mendelian segregation within families, but they can be detected by large-scale epidemiological studies such as case–control analysis. Why are scientists concerned about such weak genetic effects? Even a modest genetic effect may be of considerable public health importance if it acts on an extremely common disease, and if many different genes each make a modest contribution, the overall genetic effect may be huge. And even modest association with specific genetic variants may be sufficient to gain novel insights into the molecular pathogenesis of common diseases – by provid-

Table 5.1 Severe immunodeficiency disorders with Mendelian inheritance

Example of genetic defect	System involved	Typical clinical syndrome
B cell cytoplasmic tyrosine kinase CD40 ligand	B lymphocyte	Recurrent bacterial infection due to defective antibody production
Interleukin-2 receptor γ chain Adenosine deaminase	T lymphocyte	Severe bacterial, viral and fungal infection due to defective humoral and cellular immunity
Cytochrome b558 Integrin β chain	Neutrophil	Severe bacterial infection due to defective phagocytosis
Interferon-γ receptor	Macrophage	Extreme susceptibility to infection with environmental mycobacteria
Terminal complement components	Complement	Recurrent *Neisseria* infection
Toll-like receptor 3	Innate sensing	Herpes simplex encephalitis[35]

Almost 100 severe deficiency disorders have been identified. Each is caused by a rare mutation of a single gene. Different mutations in the same gene may cause subtle variations in clinical phenotype. Mutations of different genes may lead to similar clinical syndromes if they disrupt a common immune pathway. For a more in-depth review of the problem see (34).

Table 5.2 Examples of genetic factors associated with risk of common infectious diseases

Infectious disease	Gene locus	Function	Selected references
HIV/AIDS	CCR5/CCR2	Chemokine receptor	36, 37
	HLA class I	Antigen presentation	38, 39
Meningococcal disease	C5 to C9	Terminal complement pathway	40, 41
	PAI-1	Inhibitor of fibrinolysis	42, 43
Tuberculosis	HLA-DR	Antigen presentation	44
	TIRAP	Toll-like signalling	45
Dengue	CD209	Attachment receptor	46
Norovirus	FUT2	ABO secretor status	47, 48
Malaria	HLA class I and II	Antigen presentation	19
	α- and β-globin	Haemoglobin structure and regulation	19, 25, 26, 28
	SLC4A1	Erythrocyte structure	21, 49
	G6PD	Cytosolic enzyme	20, 50
Leprosy	HLA class II	Antigen presentation	51
	PARK/PACRG	Molecular chaperone	52

Gene regions in which allelic variants have been associated with increased or decreased susceptibility to infectious disease. Often the variant allele is common in the population (e.g., above 10%) but the alteration in disease risk is relatively modest (e.g., two to fourfold). These examples probably represent a small minority of the total number of genetic factors involved. By dissecting the functional basis of such genetic associations, through detailed epidemiological and experimental analyses of the candidate gene regions in question, it may be possible to gain important insights into the molecular basis of immunity and pathogenesis. For detailed reviews of these and other examples see 17, 43, 78, 79.

ing categorical evidence about the host factors that are involved – that may point to new strategies for treating or preventing the disease. Table 5.2 lists some genetic polymorphisms that have been associated with susceptibility to common infectious diseases, and here we will discuss the possible significance of a few of these associations.

The great diversity of human leukocyte antigens (HLA), which act to present antigens for recognition by T lymphocytes, is postulated to have arisen as a host strategy to counter antigenic diversity in infectious organisms. Attempts to identify HLA types that confer resistance or susceptibility to specific pathogens have often been inconclusive or difficult to replicate, possibly reflecting geographical and temporal fluctuation in critical microbial antigens, but a few general themes have emerged. Several studies in Asian populations and elsewhere have identified HLA-DR2 as a risk factor for susceptibility to tuberculosis and leprosy.[44,51] HLA-DRB1*1302 has been associated with resistance to chronic hepatitis B infection in both African and European populations.[53,54] HLA-B*35 is associated with rapid progression of HIV-1 infection in Caucasian populations[38] and other associations have also been reported. HLA-B*5301 and HLA-DRB1*1302 show highly significant associations with protection from severe malaria in West Africa.[19]

The human chemokine receptors CCR5 and CXCR4 serve as co-receptors with CD4 for entry on HIV-1 into human cells. Homozygotes for a 32-base-pair deletion of the *CCR5* gene have a high level of resistance to AIDS infection[36] and rates of AIDS progression appear to be affected by other mutations in *CCR5*,[37] *CCR2*[55] and other genes thought to be involved in HIV entry (reviewed by O'Brien & Nelson[56]).

One approach to discovering human disease genes for complex diseases is to identify mouse strains that differ in disease suscep-tibility and then, by a process of cross-breeding and genetic mapping, to track down some of the genes responsible. For example, following a laborious and systematic effort to identify genetic locus for resistance to infection with mycobacteria, *Salmonella* and leishmania in inbred strains of mice, the gene responsible was eventually identified by positional cloning[57] and has subsequently been named *SLC11A1*. It is a divalent ion transporter located in the macrophage phagosomal membrane. Another example of the positional cloning approach is the murine tuberculosis susceptibility gene *SP110*, which appears to inhibit the multiplication of *M. tuberculosis* and switches a cell death pathway in infected macrophages from necrosis to apoptosis.[58] There is some evidence that polymorphisms in *SLC11A1* (also known as *NRAMP1*) and *SP110* are associated with human susceptibility to tuberculosis in West Africa.[59,60]

THE FUTURE OF GENETIC EPIDEMIOLOGY

The classical genetic approach used to study Mendelian disease, i.e. single gene defects with major clinical consequences, is known as linkage analysis. This has two essential components. First, it requires families with more than one case of the disease, ideally extensive pedigrees with several affected individuals. Second, it requires highly polymorphic genetic markers distributed throughout the genome, which are used to localize chromosomal regions that segregate with disease susceptibility within families. Of the thousands of major single gene defects that are now known, most have been discovered through this approach. These include severe defects of the immune system, some of which are given in the Table 5.1, and important diseases such as cystic fibrosis and muscular dystrophy.

In the decade or so before the human genome sequence was published, significant efforts were made to extend the principle of linkage analysis to common diseases that are clearly not single gene defects but are known to have a significant heritable component that is most likely to arise from multiple genetic factors, interacting with multiple environmental factors. One approach, known as affected sib-pair analysis, which studies large numbers of families with two or more affected siblings, has had a few major successes in discovering genes that affect risk of common diseases, notably the identification of *NOD2* as a susceptibility gene for Crohn's disease.[61,62] In infectious diseases, genetic linkage studies have identified susceptibility loci for schistosomiasis (in the chromosomal region 5q31–33 containing a high concentration of Th2 cytokines[63]), malaria (also on 5q31–33[64]), leprosy (on 10p13[65] and on 6q25[52]), tuberculosis (on 15q and Xq[59]), and hepatitis B (on 21q22 containing a cluster of class II cytokine receptor genes[66]). However, it remains a major undertaking to proceed from the discovery of an interesting chromosomal region by linkage analysis to identification of the genes responsible, and it is becoming increasingly clear that common diseases are typically determined by a large number of different genetic factors, each with modest effects, most of which would not be apparent using the genetic linkage approach unless the sample size was vast.

Investigation of the genetic basis of common diseases has been revolutionized by knowledge of the sequence of the human genome,[8–10] and by two major advances that this has led to. The first major advance is a rapidly growing body of information about common forms of genomic variation as outlined in the earlier part of this chapter, and particularly a haplotype map of the human genome.[13,14] The advantage of a haplotype map is that it allows researchers to identify common patterns of variation, and to select 'tagging' SNPs that are characteristic of the common variants. This allows a great deal of information about genetic variation across the whole genome to be gained by genotyping about half a million SNPs, which, though a large task, is vastly easier than having to type all 10 million or so common variants. The second major advance has been a series of radical innovations in high-throughput genotyping and sequencing technology which currently allow over half a million SNPs to be genotyped in thousands of individuals, and the race is on to devise a method of sequencing the whole human genome for US$1000 or less.

The first major application of these new technologies has been to develop statistically robust methods of genome-wide association analysis to discover novel genetic determinants of common diseases. Typically this is in the form of a case–control study, where the frequency of a particular genetic variant is measured in diseased individuals, and compared with controls recruited from exactly the same ethnic group. To understand why ethnic matching is so important, consider a mixed population within which a certain ethnic group is liable to develop a specific disease for entirely sociocultural reasons. In this situation, a random sample of disease cases will contain a higher proportion of this ethnic group than is found in the general population, and there is a danger that apparent 'genetic associations' may simply reflect ethnic differences rather than true disease susceptibility genes. Fortunately, methods are emerging to correct for this statistically, using genome-wide SNP data, and one way of definitively excluding artefacts is to supplement case–control approaches with intra-familial association studies, where the distribution of genotypes

among index cases is compared with that predicted from their parental genotypes using statistical techniques such as the transmission disequilibrium test.[67,68]

A critical requirement of genome-wide association studies is sample size, for several reasons. First, common diseases may have many different genetic influences that are individually of modest magnitude. Second, false-positive associations arise when hundreds of thousands of SNPs are tested, and large sample sizes are needed to differentiate these from true positives. Third, there are gene–gene and gene–environment interactions, with a vast number of combinatorial possibilities; any given combination of factors may be present in only a small proportion of individuals. This area of research increasingly relies on the formation of consortia to bring together large epidemiological sample sizes with state-of-the-art genome technologies and complex statistical analyses. A particularly successful example is the Wellcome Trust Case Control Consortium, which carried out genome-wide association analysis on a total of 17 000 individuals from the UK population, including 3000 controls and 2000 cases for each of seven common UK diseases.[69] This has led to important genetic discoveries across a range of conditions including cardiovascular disease[70], type 1 diabetes[71], type 2 diabetes[72], inflammatory bowel disease[73] and ankylosing spondylitis[74] and has catalysed studies on broader aspects of human variation including obesity[75] and height.[76]

A parallel initiative is the Malaria Genomic Epidemiology Network (MalariaGEN), a consortium of malaria researchers in 20 countries who have collectively collected DNA samples and detailed clinical data from thousands of individuals with severe malaria.[77] Previously this resource has been fragmented, with different groups pursuing relatively small studies on their own samples, and the goal of the MalariaGEN consortium is to join efforts to undertake a systematic and comprehensive search for the human genetic determinants of resistance to malaria.

Discovering a genetic association is not the end of the story. Every polymorphism shows a greater or lesser degree of association with neighbouring polymorphisms (a phenomenon known as linkage disequilibrium). So when we find a disease association with a polymorphism in gene X, the next step is to search for other polymorphisms in the region of X, and then to compare the strength of disease association with different combinations of linked polymorphisms (known as haplotypes), in order to dissect the causative polymorphism from linked markers that are functionally irrelevant. If gene X is just one of a large number of environmental and genetic factors that determine disease susceptibility, the process of fine-mapping may be extremely complex (e.g. it is much more difficult for diabetes than for cystic fibrosis) and this is the area where the most questions remain about the feasibility of the new genetic approach to the analysis of common human diseases.

HOW IS GENETICS GOING TO SHAPE MEDICAL PRACTICE?

What is the practical purpose of understanding the molecular genetic basis of susceptibility to infection? Efforts to develop vaccines and improved treatments for major diseases such as tuberculosis, HIV/AIDS and malaria are hindered by our poor understanding of the molecular and cellular mechanisms that determine clinical outcome. Genetic epidemiology may identify novel molecular mechanisms and improve understanding of critical events in the evolution of disease. For example, if an infectious disease is associated with high levels of factor X in the blood, it is often difficult to know whether this is of pathogenic importance or simply an epiphenomenon of the disease process. But if the production of factor X is known to be determined by a genetic polymorphism, and if this polymorphism is shown to predispose to the disease in question, then there is a much stronger case for factor X playing a causal role.

The human genome project has generated huge expectations but it will take decades for the full clinical implications to be revealed. For severe genetic disorders, detailed understanding of the molecular causes will improve diagnostic screening and genetic counselling, and will spawn novel therapeutic strategies including gene therapy. But for common human diseases, the long-term impact of genetic research will be at the level of the population rather than the individual patient. Genetic epidemiology provides a potentially powerful way of identifying the critical molecular events required for an infectious agent to invade the human host, and for the host to eradicate or succumb to the infection. This information is likely to revolutionize the process of drug discovery and vaccine development, a point that has already been taken on board by many of the major pharmaceutical agencies.

Humankind has evolved in a hostile microbial environment, and natural selection by infectious disease may be one of the major causes of human genetic diversity, particularly in the immune system. The high frequency of the sickle haemoglobin gene in West Africa, which has arisen because of its protective effect against malaria and despite the lethal nature of the homozygous state, gives some idea of the strength of genetic selection that may be involved. It is possible that some chronic non-infectious ailments such as atopy and autoimmune disease are a legacy of the evolutionary impact of infectious disease, where immune gene variants selected for protection against parasites and other infectious pathogens may have deleterious effects in an increasingly hygienic environment. The main reason for gaining a deeper understanding of the genetic factors that determine susceptibility to major infectious diseases is to learn about molecular mechanisms of disease and immunity that will inform efforts to prevent those diseases, but it may at the same time provide clues to the prevention of a much broader range of common diseases that afflict populations around the world.

REFERENCES

1. Sorensen TI, Nielsen GG, Andersen PK, et al. Genetic and environmental influences on premature death in adult adoptees. *N Engl J Med* 1988; 318:727–732.

2. Comstock GW. Tuberculosis in twins: a re-analysis of the Prophit survey. *Am Rev Respir Dis* 1978; 117:621–624.

3. Fine PE. Immunogenetics of susceptibility to leprosy, tuberculosis, and leishmaniasis: an epidemiological perspective. *Int J Lepr Other Mycobact Dis* 1981; 49:437–454.

4. Jepson AP, Banya WA, Sisay-Joof F, et al. Genetic regulation of fever in Plasmodium falciparum malaria in Gambian twin children. *J Infect Dis* 1995; 172:316–319.

5. Mackinnon MJ, Mwangi TW, Snow RW, et al. Heritability of malaria in Africa. *PLoS Med* 2005; 2:e340.

6. Strachan T, Read AP. *Human Molecular Genetics.* 3rd edn. New York: Garland Science; 2003.

7. http://www.ncbi.nlm.nih.gov/omim/. Online Mendelian Inheritance in Man, OMIM™.

8. Lander ES, Linton LM, Birren B, et al. Initial sequencing and analysis of the human genome. *Nature* 2001; 409:860–921.

9. Venter JC, Adams MD, Myers EW, et al. The sequence of the human genome. *Science* 2001; 291:1304–1351.

10. International Human Genome Sequencing Consortium. Finishing the euchromatic sequence of the human genome. *Nature* 2004; 431:931–945.

11. http://www.ensembl.org/. Ensembl Genome Browser.

12. Weinstock GM. ENCODE: more genomic empowerment. *Genome Res* 2007; 17:667–668.

13. International HapMap Consortium. A haplotype map of the human genome. *Nature* 2005; 437:1299–1320.

14. Frazer KA, Ballinger DG, Cox DR, et al. A second generation human haplotype map of over 3.1 million SNPs. *Nature* 2007; 449:851–861.

15. Redon R, Ishikawa S, Fitch KR, et al. Global variation in copy number in the human genome. *Nature* 2006; 444:444–454.

16. Conrad DF, Hurles ME. The population genetics of structural variation. *Nat Genet* 2007; 39(suppl):S30–S36.

17. Kwiatkowski DP. How malaria has affected the human genome and what human genetics can teach us about malaria. *Am J Hum Genet* 2005; 77: 171–190.

18. Haldane JBS. Disease and evolution. *Ricerca Sci* 1949; 19(suppl 1):3–10.

19. Hill AV, Allsopp CE, Kwiatkowski D, et al. Common west African HLA antigens are associated with protection from severe malaria. *Nature* 1991; 352:595–600.

20. Ruwende C, Khoo SC, Snow RW, et al. Natural selection of hemi- and heterozygotes for G6PD deficiency in Africa by resistance to severe malaria. *Nature* 1995; 376:246–249.

21. Genton B, al-Yaman F, Mgone CS, et al. Ovalocytosis and cerebral malaria. *Nature* 1995; 378:564–565.

22. Agarwal A, Guindo A, Cissoko Y, et al. Hemoglobin C associated with protection from severe malaria in the Dogon of Mali, a West African population with a low prevalence of hemoglobin S. *Blood* 2000; 96:2358–2363.

23. Modiano D, Luoni G, Sirima BS, et al. Haemoglobin C protects against clinical Plasmodium falciparum malaria. *Nature* 2001; 414:305–308.

24. Flint J, Hill AV, Bowden DK, et al. High frequencies of alpha-thalassaemia are the result of natural selection by malaria. *Nature* 1986; 321:744–750.

25. Allen SJ, O'Donnell A, Alexander ND, et al. alpha+-Thalassemia protects children against disease caused by other infections as well as malaria. *Proc Natl Acad Sci USA* 1997; 94:14736–14741.

26. Williams TN, Wambua S, Uyoga S, et al. Both heterozygous and homozygous alpha+ thalassemias protect against severe and fatal Plasmodium falciparum malaria on the coast of Kenya. *Blood* 2005; 106:368–371.

27. Williams TN, Maitland K, Bennett S, et al. High incidence of malaria in alpha-thalassaemic children. *Nature* 1996; 383:522–525.

28. Williams TN, Mwangi TW, Wambua S, et al. Negative epistasis between the malaria-protective effects of alpha+-thalassemia and the sickle cell trait. *Nat Genet* 2005; 37:1253–1257.

29. Miller LH, Mason SJ, Clyde DF, et al. The resistance factor to Plasmodium vivax in blacks: the Duffy-blood-group genotype, FyFy. *N Engl J Med* 1976; 295:302–304.

30. Tournamille C, Colin Y, Cartron JP, et al. Disruption of a GATA motif in the Duffy gene promoter abolishes erythroid gene expression in Duffy-negative individuals. *Nat Genet* 1995; 10:224–228.

31. Chitnis CE, Miller LH. Identification of the erythrocyte binding domains of Plasmodium vivax and Plasmodium knowlesi proteins involved in erythrocyte invasion. *J Exp Med* 1994; 180:497–506.

32. Sabeti PC, Schaffner SF, Fry B, et al. Positive natural selection in the human lineage. *Science* 2006; 312:1614–1620.

33. Sabeti PC, Varilly P, Fry B, et al. Genome-wide detection and characterization of positive selection in human populations. *Nature* 2007; 449:913–918.

34. Casanova JL, Abel L. Primary immunodeficiencies: a field in its infancy. *Science* 2007; 317:617–619.

35. Zhang SY, Jouanguy E, Ugolini S, et al. TLR3 deficiency in patients with herpes simplex encephalitis. *Science* 2007; 317:1522–1527.

36. Dean M, Carrington M, Winkler C, et al. Genetic restriction of HIV-1 infection and progression to AIDS by a deletion allele of the CKR5 structural gene. Hemophilia Growth and Development Study, Multicenter AIDS Cohort Study, Multicenter Hemophilia Cohort Study, San Francisco City Cohort, ALIVE Study. *Science* 1996; 273:1856–1862.

37. Martin MP, Dean M, Smith MW, et al. Genetic acceleration of AIDS progression by a promoter variant of CCR5. *Science* 1998; 282:1907–1911.

38. Carrington M, Nelson GW, Martin MP, et al. HLA and HIV-1: heterozygote advantage and B*35-Cw*04 disadvantage. *Science* 1999; 283:1748–1752.

39. Fellay J, Shianna KV, Ge D, et al. A whole-genome association study of major determinants for host control of HIV-1. *Science* 2007; 317:944–947.

40. Wurzner R, Orren A, Lachmann PJ. Inherited deficiencies of the terminal components of human complement. *Immunodefic Rev* 1992; 3:123–147.

41. Ellison RT 3rd, Kohler PF, Curd JG, et al. Prevalence of congenital or acquired complement deficiency in patients with sporadic meningococcal disease. *N Engl J Med* 1983; 308:913–916.

42. Westendorp RG, Hottenga JJ, Slagboom PE. Variation in plasminogen-activator-inhibitor-1 gene and risk of meningococcal septic shock. *Lancet* 1999; 354:561–563.

43. Hermans PW, Hibberd ML, Booy R, et al. 4G/5G promoter polymorphism in the plasminogen-activator-inhibitor-1 gene and outcome of meningococcal disease. Meningococcal Research Group. *Lancet* 1999; 354:556–560.

44. Singh SP, Mehra NK, Dingley HB, et al. Human leukocyte antigen (HLA)-linked control of susceptibility to pulmonary tuberculosis and association with HLA-DR types. *J Infect Dis* 1983; 148:676–681.

45. Khor CC, Chapman SJ, Vannberg FO, et al. A Mal functional variant is associated with protection against invasive pneumococcal disease, bacteremia, malaria and tuberculosis. *Nat Genet* 2007; 39:523–528.

46. Sakuntabhai A, Turbpaiboon C, Casademont I, et al. A variant in the CD209 promoter is associated with severity of dengue disease. *Nat Genet* 2005; 37:507–513.

47. Lindesmith L, Moe C, Marionneau S, et al. Human susceptibility and resistance to Norwalk virus infection. *Nat Med* 2003; 9:548–553.

48. Thorven M, Grahn A, Hedlund KO, et al. A homozygous nonsense mutation (428G->A) in the human secretor (FUT2) gene provides resistance to symptomatic norovirus (GGII) infections. *J Virol* 2005; 79:15351–15355.

49. Allen SJ, O'Donnell A, Alexander ND, et al. Prevention of cerebral malaria in children in Papua New Guinea by southeast Asian ovalocytosis band 3. *Am J Trop Med Hyg* 1999; 60:1056–1060.

50. Luzzatto L, Usanga FA, Reddy S. Glucose-6-phosphate dehydrogenase deficient red cells: resistance to infection by malarial parasites. *Science* 1969; 164:839–842.

51. Todd JR, West BC, McDonald JC. Human leukocyte antigen and leprosy: study in northern Louisiana and review. *Rev Infect Dis* 1990; 12:63–74.

52. Mira MT, Alcais A, Van Thuc N, et al. Chromosome 6q25 is linked to susceptibility to leprosy in a Vietnamese population. *Nat Genet* 2003; 33:412–415.

53. Thursz MR, Kwiatkowski D, Allsopp CE, et al. Association between an MHC class II allele and clearance of hepatitis B virus in the Gambia. *N Engl J Med* 1995; 332:1065–1069.

54. Hohler T, Gerken G, Notghi A, et al. HLA-DRB1*1301 and *1302 protect against chronic hepatitis B. *J Hepatol* 1997; 26:503–507.

55. Smith MW, Dean M, Carrington M, et al. Contrasting genetic influence of CCR2 and CCR5 variants on HIV-1 infection and disease progression. Hemophilia Growth and Development Study (HGDS), Multicenter AIDS Cohort Study (MACS), Multicenter Hemophilia Cohort Study (MHCS), San Francisco City Cohort (SFCC), ALIVE Study. *Science* 1997; 277:959–965.

56. O'Brien SJ, Nelson GW. Human genes that limit AIDS. *Nat Genet* 2004; 36:565–574.

57. Vidal SM, Malo D, Vogan K, et al. Natural resistance to infection with intracellular parasites: isolation of a candidate for Bcg. *Cell* 1993; 73:469–485.

58. Pan H, Yan BS, Rojas M, et al. Ipr1 gene mediates innate immunity to tuberculosis. *Nature* 2005; 434:767–772.

59. Bellamy R, Beyers N, McAdam KP, et al. Genetic susceptibility to tuberculosis in Africans: a genome-wide scan. *Proc Natl Acad Sci USA* 2000; 97:8005–8009.

60. Tosh K, Campbell SJ, Fielding K, et al. Variants in the SP110 gene are associated with genetic susceptibility to tuberculosis in West Africa. *Proc Natl Acad Sci USA* 2006; 103:10364–10368.

61. Hugot JP, Chamaillard M, Zouali H, et al. Association of NOD2 leucine-rich repeat variants with susceptibility to Crohn's disease. *Nature* 2001; 411:599–603.

62. Ogura Y, Bonen DK, Inohara N, et al. A frameshift mutation in NOD2 associated with susceptibility to Crohn's disease. *Nature* 2001; 411:603–606.

63. Marquet S, Abel L, Hillaire D, et al. Genetic localization of a locus controlling the intensity of infection by Schistosoma mansoni on chromosome 5q31–q33. *Nat Genet* 1996; 14.181–184.

64. Rihet P, Traore Y, Abel L, et al. Malaria in humans: Plasmodium falciparum blood infection levels are linked to chromosome 5q31–q33. *Am J Hum Genet* 1998; 63:498–505.

65. Siddiqui MR, Meisner S, Tosh K, et al. A major susceptibility locus for leprosy in India maps to chromosome 10p13. *Nat Genet* 2001; 27:439–441.

66. Frodsham AJ, Zhang L, Dumpis U, et al. Class II cytokine receptor gene cluster is a major locus for hepatitis B persistence. *Proc Natl Acad Sci USA* 2006; 103:9148–9153.

67. Spielman RS, McGinnis RE, Ewens WJ. Transmission test for linkage disequilibrium: the insulin gene region and insulin-dependent diabetes mellitus (IDDM). *Am J Hum Genet* 1993; 52:506–516.

68. Risch NJ. Searching for genetic determinants in the new millennium. *Nature* 2000; 405:847–856.

69. Wellcome Trust Case Control Consortium. Genome-wide association study of 14,000 cases of seven common diseases and 3,000 shared controls. *Nature* 2007; 447:661–678.

70. Samani NJ, Erdmann J, Hall AS, et al. Genomewide association analysis of coronary artery disease. *N Engl J Med* 2007; 357:443–453.

71. Todd JA, Walker NM, Cooper JD, et al. Robust associations of four new chromosome regions from genome-wide analyses of type 1 diabetes. *Nat Genet* 2007; 39:857–864.

72. Zeggini E, Weedon MN, Lindgren CM, et al. Replication of genome-wide association signals in UK samples reveals risk loci for type 2 diabetes. *Science* 2007; 316:1336–1341.

73. Parkes M, Barrett JC, Prescott NJ, et al. Sequence variants in the autophagy gene IRGM and multiple other replicating loci contribute to Crohn's disease susceptibility. *Nat Genet* 2007; 39:830–832.

74. Burton PR, Clayton DG, Cardon LR, et al. Association scan of 14,500 nonsynonymous SNPs in four diseases identifies autoimmunity variants. *Nat Genet* 2007; 39:1329–1337.

75. Frayling TM, Timpson NJ, Weedon MN, et al. A common variant in the FTO gene is associated with body mass index and predisposes to childhood and adult obesity. *Science* 2007; 316:889–894.

76. Weedon MN, Lettre G, Freathy RM, et al. A common variant of HMGA2 is associated with adult and childhood height in the general population. *Nat Genet* 2007; 39:1245–1250.

77. Malaria Genomic Epidemiology Network. Online: http://www.malariagen.net.

78. Emonts M, Hazelzet JA, de Groot R, et al. Host genetic determinants of Neisseria meningitidis infections. *Lancet Infect Dis* 2003; 3:565–577.

79. Hill AV. Aspects of genetic susceptibility to human infectious diseases. *Annu Rev Genet* 2006; 40:469–486.

Chapter 6

Ivan M. Roitt and Alimuddin I. Zumla

Immunological Aspects of Tropical Diseases

INTRODUCTION

The host is a continuous battleground between the immune system of the body[1] and invading antigens, whether they are microorganisms,[2] chemicals or cancer cells. At-risk patients are commonplace in the tropics because of malnutrition, HIV/AIDS, high parasite load, cancers, alcoholism, chronic renal and hepatic diseases, famine and poverty. While a vast amount of literature is accumulating on the subject of immune responses to pathogens,[3] the mechanisms underlying specific immunity to many microorganisms remain unknown.[4] Paradoxically, while the immune response has evolved to confer protection against invading antigens, much human pathology arises when the immune responses are evoked[5–8] (Tables 6.1, 6.2).

COMPONENTS OF THE IMMUNE SYSTEM

The human immune system, which has evolved to resist infection by microorganisms, has traditionally been classified into two parts:
1. The non-specific immune system consisting of:
   a. External barriers
   b. Innate immune system
2. The specific immune system, or the acquired immune response.

Immunology impinges on the practice of tropical medicine[4] in four main ways:
1. Protective immunity to particular tropical parasitic infections is frequently inadequate and sometimes non-existent; this

Table 6.1 Immunopathological consequences of tropical infections

Hypersensitivity type*		Mechanism involved	Examples
Type I	(allergic)	IgE	*Ascaris larvae* (lung)
		Mast cells, basophils	*Schistosomiasis* (swimmers' itch)
		IgE, mast cells	
	(anaphylactic)	IgG	Hydatid cyst leak/rupture
		Complement	
Type II (antibody-mediated)		Autoantibody	Malaria anaemia?
		Immune complexes	Goodpasture's syndrome
			Chagas' disease (*T. cruzi*)
			Streptococci (rheumatic heart disease, glomerulonephritis)
Type III (immune complex)		Complement	Malaria (kidney)
			Trypanosomiasis
			Schistosomiasis (Katayama fever)
			Streptococci
			Serum sickness
			Pulmonary eosinophilia
		Neutrophils	
Type IV (cell-mediated)		T cells	*Schistosomiasis* (egg granuloma)
		Cytokines	Tuberculosis
		Macrophages	Tuberculoid leprosy
			Lymphatic filariasis
			Lung flukes (*Paragonimiasis*)

* Gell and Coombs' classification.

Table 6.2 Immunopathology associated with acute bacterial infections

Bacteria	Toxins	Disease
Staphylococci	Enterotoxin A	Food poisoning
	Enterotoxin B	
	Enterotoxin C1–3	
	Enterotoxin D	
	Enterotoxin E	
	Toxic shock syndrome toxins	Toxic shock syndrome
	Exfoliating toxin A	Scaled-skin syndrome
	Exfoliating toxin B	
Group A streptococci	Pyrogenic exotoxin A	Streptococcal sore throat
	Pyrogenic exotoxin B	
	Pyrogenic exotoxin C	
	Pyrogenic exotoxin D	
	Erythrogenic exotoxin	Scarlet fever
	Haemolysis exotoxin	Erysipelas
Clostridium perfringens	Enterotoxin	Gas gangrene
Yersinia enterocolitica	Enterotoxin	Terminal ileitis
Mycoplasma arthritidis	Exotoxin	Arthritis
Gram-negative bacteria	(Endotoxin, LPS)	Gram-negative shock

affects both the normal course of the disease and the prospects for vaccination.

2. The prolonged ineffective immune responses can give rise to serious immunopathological consequences.
3. People afflicted with tropical infections often suffer a general immunodeficiency that weakens their response to normally mild infections.
4. The monitoring of immune responses, even when they are not protective, can often be of help in diagnosis and management.

Non-specific immunity: external barriers

External barriers (Figure 6.1) are normal mechanical and physiological properties of the host, which include:
- Skin (e.g. keratin, sebum, normal flora)
- Mucosal surfaces (e.g. intestinal, vaginal, cornea)
- Flushing mechanisms (e.g. urinating, ciliary movement)
- Enzymes (e.g. gut, tears)
- Normal microbial flora (e.g. commensals in skin, gut, vagina).

Skin

The skin is probably the most important physical barrier to invading microorganisms. The skin secretes sebum which inhibits growth of microorganisms. The skin's normal microflora compete with pathogenic organisms. This effect, called 'colonization inhibition', is also seen in the gut and pharynx. The physical barrier of the skin is usually only overcome when it is breached by scratches, wounds, bites, burns, trauma or injections.

Abrasions, ulcers, trauma

Breach in the continuity of the skin permits entry of skin pathogens such as *staphylococci*, *streptococci* or *leptospira*.

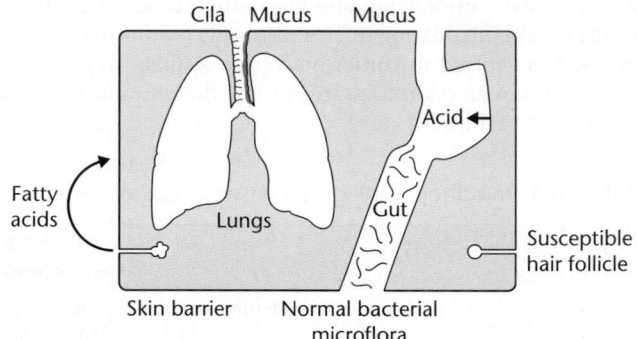

Figure 6.1   The first-lines of defence against infection: protection at the external body surfaces. (Redrawn with permission from Delves PJ, Martin SJ, Burton DR, Roitt IM. *Roitt's Essential Immunology*. 11th edn. Oxford: ©Blackwell; 2006.)

Insect bites

A number of infectious agents have used the vehicle of blood-sucking insects to get through the skin. Transmission by blood-sucking insects is a good example of how a resourceful parasite overcomes the external skin barrier and simultaneously solves the problem of spreading in a thinly populated country, but of course it also restricts the parasite to areas where the vector flourishes. They are further restricted to flourish in warmer parts of the world because they are not able to complete their life cycles in colder climates when their insect hosts assume the temperature of the environment. Nevertheless, only a tiny minority of potential parasites actually succeed in gaining a foothold in man. When they do, the responsibility for dislodging them passes to the adaptive immune system.

Active penetration by parasite larvae

Helminth parasites such as hookworm larvae and schistosome cercariae invade the human skin by use of proteolytic enzymes before gaining entry into the bloodstream.

Injections and razors

The use of contaminated needles and razors (traditional medicine cuts) breaches the skin and may enable bacteria and fungi to cause septicaemia. They may also transmit hepatitis viruses, HIV, malaria and trypanosomes.

Mucosal surfaces

Mucosal surfaces are not keratinized and thus are prone to invasion by bacteria and viruses. However, natural defences occur at mucosal surfaces[9] and these include:

- Ciliary movement to expel the debris
- Surface phagocytes
- Enzymes and surface antibody (secretory IgA)
- Mechanical washing by tears or urine
- Bacteriocins from normal flora.

There are a number of physico-chemical barriers which provide important mechanisms for limiting infectious agents. These include the tears from the eyes, lysozyme in saliva, ear wax and vaginal acidity. The mechanical barrier produced by the cilia and mucus of the respiratory tract traps 95% of inhaled organisms. The constant flow of bile in the biliary system as well as continuous production and flow of urine are other important mechanisms by which invading microorganisms may be kept at bay.

Commensal microbial flora

The role of the normal flora of the mouth, the vagina and the alimentary and urinary tracts deserves special mention. The human host provides a safe haven for these less harmful bacteria, which are then able to antagonize and prevent the flourishing of pathogenic bacteria. The facultative and obligate aerobes produce potent inhibitors of bacterial growth called bacteriocins, which act to inhibit the growth of competing organisms. In addition, many obligate anaerobes produce free fatty acids and alter the local redox potential, making the environment less supportive to other microorganisms. This delicate balance can be upset by disease or by the use of antibiotics. There is an increasing scientific and commercial interest in the use of beneficial microorganisms, or 'probiotics', for the prevention and treatment of disease. The microorganisms more frequently used as probiotic agents are lactic acid bacteria, such as *Lactobacillus rhamnosus* GG (LGG), which has been extensively studied in recent literature. Multiple mechanisms of action have been postulated, including lactose digestion, productive antimicrobial agents, competition for space or nutrients and immunomodulation. Studies of paediatric diarrhoea show substantial evidence of clinical benefits from probiotic therapy in patients with viral gastroenteritis, and data on LGG treatment for *Clostridium*

difficile diarrhoea appear promising. However, data to support use of probiotics for prevention of traveller's diarrhoea are more limited.[10]

Parasite evasion mechanisms for avoiding innate immunity

Complex multicellular microorganisms such as helminths have developed extensive strategies, not only for gaining access through direct intact skin, but also for migrating through subcutaneous tissues of the body until they reach their favorite habitats where they can thrive and multiply. In the tropics most infectious agents (apart from a few helminths such as cercariae of schistosomes and larvae of hookworm) use the faecal–oral route to overcome the external barriers. This route is more effective in tropical areas where clean water supplies are not highly organized and where sanitary facilities are often rudimentary. Clearly external barriers, while highly effective in preventing infections with harmless agents, are relatively ineffective against highly virulent organisms.

Non-specific immune system: innate immune responses

These can be divided into those that are mediated by:

- Phagocytic cells
- Natural killer (NK) cells
- Soluble factors
- Complement system.

Phagocytic cells

The cells of the innate immune system are collectively termed phagocytic cells because they are able to ingest simple unicellular organisms such as viruses, bacteria and rickettsiae and kill them by a variety of different mechanisms. These cells include (a) neutrophil leucocytes[11] and (b) monocytes/macrophages.[11,12] Phagocytosis of invading organisms occurs when phagocytic cells are attracted to sites of invasion/inflammation by soluble mediators. The efficiency of phagocytosis is enhanced when organisms are covered or 'opsonized' by complement or antibody, which provide receptors for the attachment for antibody. Organisms are phagocytosed and taken up into phagosomes which fuse with the lysosomes containing free radicals and lytic enzymes, resulting in killing (Figure 6.2).

The neutrophils are produced in large numbers (10^{11}/day) but circulate for only a few hours before passing through capillary walls into the extravascular space. Peripheral blood neutrophils are appropriately placed to prevent infections with circulating microorganisms, especially bacteria. Patients with deficiencies in neutrophil phagocyte function are prone to repeated pyogenic infections or develop chronic pyogenic granuloma.

Monocytes are larger phagocytic cells produced in the bone marrow. They circulate for hours to days in the peripheral blood, before differentiating into tissue macrophages.[12,13] They acquire specific characters depending on the tissue in which they reside, e.g. liver Kupffer cells, lung alveolar macrophages, synovial membrane A cells. Macrophages secrete lysozyme, neutral proteases, interleukin 1 (IL-1), tumour necrosis factor (TNF), superoxidases,

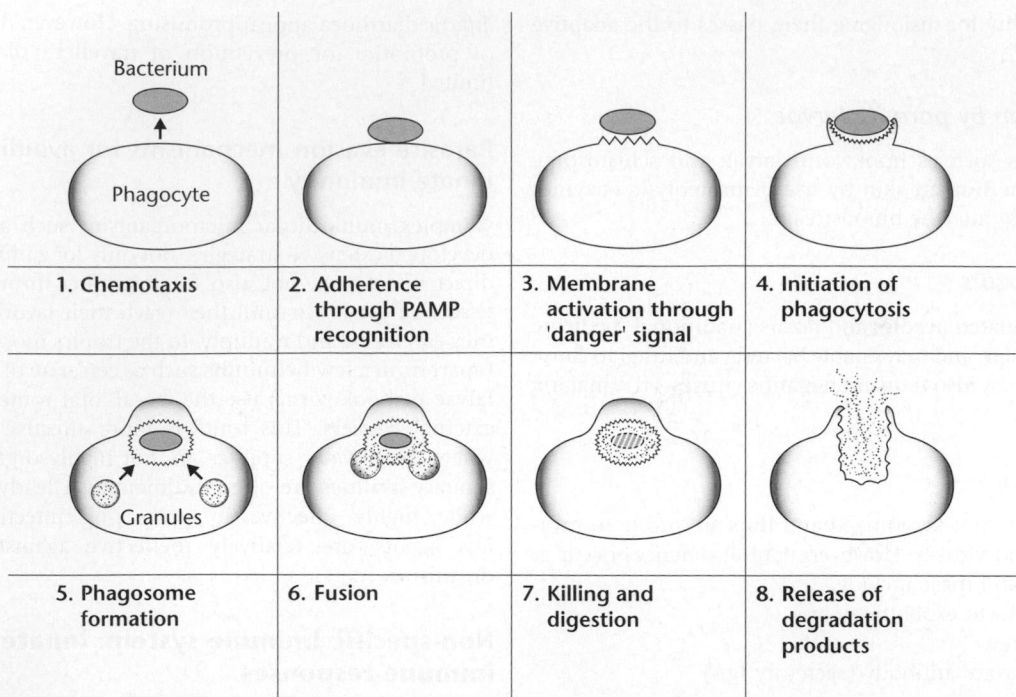

| 1. Chemotaxis | 2. Adherence through PAMP recognition | 3. Membrane activation through 'danger' signal | 4. Initiation of phagocytosis |

| 5. Phagosome formation | 6. Fusion | 7. Killing and digestion | 8. Release of degradation products |

Figure 6.2 Phagocytosis and killing of a bacterium. Stage 3/4, respiratory burst and activation of NADPH oxidase; stage 5, damage by reactive oxygen intermediates; stage 6/7, damage by peroxidase, cationic proteins, antibiotic peptide defensins, lysozyme and lactoferrin. (Redrawn with permission from Delves PJ, Martin SJ, Burton DR, Roitt IM. *Roitt's Essential Immunology*. 11th edn. Oxford: ©Blackwell; 2006.)

leukotrienes and complement components. They can ingest bacteria via the macrophage mannose receptor or the macrophage scavenger receptor. They are also capable of ingesting other microorganisms, opsonized by IgG and/or complement. They kill the ingested organisms by using oxygen-dependent mechanisms. Macrophages are also capable of processing antigens and presenting them to T cells as peptides bound to major histocompatibility complex (MHC) molecules. All three functions of macrophages, i.e. secretion, phagocytosis and antigen presentation, are enhanced when macrophages become 'activated' by exogenous stimuli, particularly the lipopolysaccharide (LPS) of invading microorganisms and interferon-α (IFNα) derived from virally infected cells.

Natural killer (NK) cells are large granular lymphocytes derived from the bone marrow that circulate in the blood.[14,15] They recognize and kill targets in the absence of antigenic stimulation and antibody. This killing is not MHC restricted. Many NK cells have surface Fc receptors through which they are able to mediate antibody-dependent cellular cytotoxicity (ADCC). NK cells seem to recognize virus-infected and tumour-derived cells, through targets that are carbohydrate, glycolipid or glycoprotein. The cytotoxicity of NK cells is also enhanced by IFN and IL-2. NK cells are not a homogeneous population, each one containing a combination of different inhibitory and activating receptors which promote killing.

Dendritic cells are specialized antigen-presenting cells (APCs) derived from the bone marrow.[16,17] They are distributed throughout the tissues and when activated by inflammatory stimuli take up and process antigen and migrate to the local lymph nodes where they present the antigen to naive T cells (Figure 6.3).

Dendritic cells express high levels of MHC class 1 and class 2 molecules and are highly susceptible to infection by human immunodeficiency virus (HIV) because they express CD4.

Evasion of killing by phagocytic cells by microorganisms

A number of both unicellular and multicellular microorganisms have developed evasion mechanisms to enable them to survive inside the normally destructive phagocytic cells (Table 6.3). For instance, *Haemophilus* bacteria are able to do so by developing an outer capsular coat. The special cell wall of *Mycobacteria* also renders them difficult to kill by phagocytic cells. The bacteria *Staphylococcus* are able to destroy phagocytes by producing toxins which reduce their number. The protozoan *Leishmania* and the bacteria *Listeria* and *Rickettsia* are able to prevent phagocytosis by escaping from the phagosome into the cytoplasm of the phagocytic cell. The protozoan Toxoplasma is able to prevent intracellular killing by preventing phagolysosome fusion. The bacteria *Legionella* demonstrates a similar ability. Some bacteria, namely *Legionella*, *Salmonella* and *Mycobacterium* spp, can survive and replicate within the phagolysosome in a location specifically designed to kill them by somehow remodelling the phagosome.

The ability of a wide variety of infectious microorganisms to survive and sometimes thrive in the intracellular environment in which they are meant to be killed is the mechanism by which many of them become chronic infections (Table 6.3). In this intracellular 'haven' they are able to escape other immune mechanisms which would lead to their destruction. Herpes simplex virus and the varicella zoster virus cause recurrent infections by

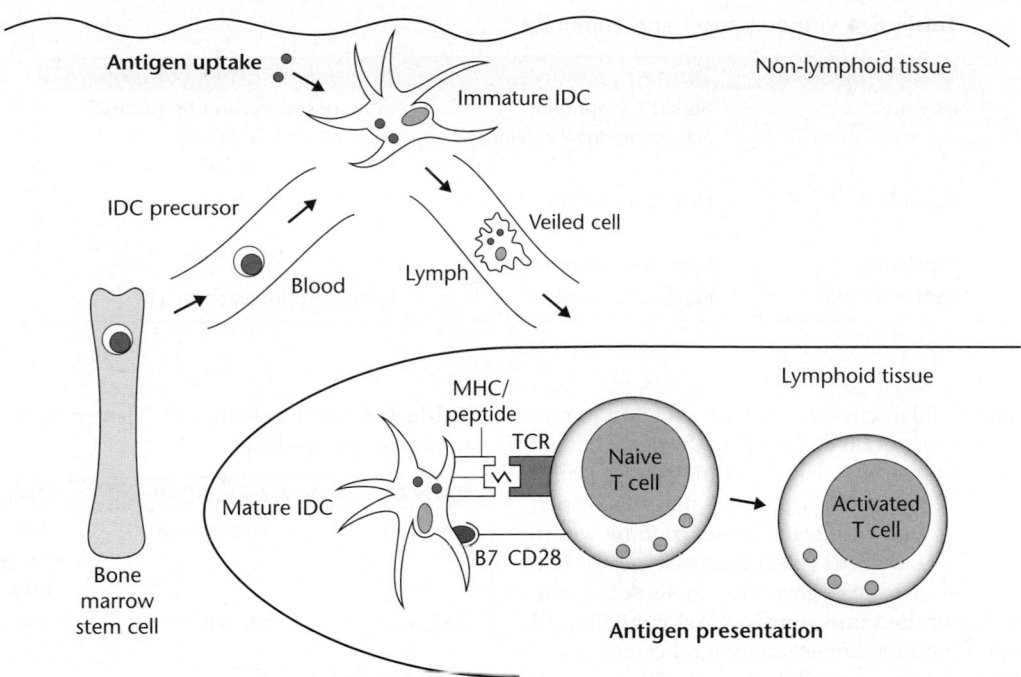

Figure 6.3 Migration and maturation of interdigitating dendritic cells (IDC). The precursors of these cells are derived from bone marrow stem cells. They travel via the blood to non-lymphoid tissues. These immature dendritic cells, e.g. Langerhans' cells in skin, are specialized for antigen uptake. Subsequently they travel via the afferent lymphatics as veiled cells to take up residence within secondary lymphoid tissues, where they express high levels of MHC class II and co-stimulatory molecules such as B7. These cells are highly specialized for the activation of naive T cells. The activated T cell may carry out its function in the lymph node, or after imprinting with relevant homing molecules, recirculate to the appropriate tissue. (Redrawn with permission from Delves PJ, Martin SJ, Burton DR, Roitt IM. *Roitt's Essential Immunology*. 11th edn. Oxford: ©Blackwell; 2006.)

Table 6.3 Some important persistent intracellular infections

Parasite persistence	Site of manifestation	Clinical
Herpes simplex virus	Dorsal root ganglia	Recurrent herpes simplex
Varicella zoster virus	Dorsal root ganglia	Recurrent shingles
Hepatitis B	Liver	Chronic hepatitis Carrier state Hepatoma
Epstein–Barr virus	B cells Nasal epithelium	Burkitt's lymphoma Nasopharyngeal cancer
Human immunodeficiency virus (HIV)	T cells Macrophages	AIDS
Mycobacterium tuberculosis	Macrophages	Reactivation
Salmonella typhi	Macrophages	Systemic spread Carrier state
Brucella	Macrophages	Chronic infection
Toxoplasma	Macrophages	Chronic infection or reactivation
Trypanosoma cruzi	Macrophages	Chronic infection
Leishmania spp.	Macrophages	Chronic infection
Plasmodium vivax	Hepatocytes	Recurrence

Table 6.4 Viruses, cancer and immunity

Virus implicated	Tumour	Immune or other component
EB virus	Burkitt's lymphoma	Immunosuppression by malaria?
	Nasopharyngeal carcinoma	High EB virus antibody
		Dietary carcinogens?
Hepatitis B	Hepatic carcinoma	Neonatal tolerance to virus?
		Aflatoxins
Papilloma	Cervical carcinoma	
KSAHV (HHV8)	Kaposi's sarcoma	Immunosuppression by HIV

persisting in the intracellular environment of the dorsal root ganglia. Persisting viruses may act as co-factors in the development of certain malignancies (Table 6.4). The Hepatitis B virus (HBV) is able to cause chronic hepatitis and hepatoma, not only by persisting in hepatocytes but also by integrating its genome within the host cells. The Epstein–Barr virus (EBV) is able to persist in B lymphocytes and in malarial areas gives rise to Burkitt's lymphoma. The persistence of the same virus in nasal epithelium is associated with the development of nasopharyngeal carcinoma. It is the ability of HIV to persist intracellularly in T cells 'amongst other cells' that leads to the development of the acquired immunodeficiency syndrome (AIDS).

Viruses are not alone in their ability to cause chronic infection by persisting in intracellular sites. Chronic infection with Brucella is possible because of the ability of this bacterium to survive in macrophages. Similarly, the reactivation of previously healed *Mycobacterium tuberculosis* infections is due to the ability of this organism to lie dormant within macrophages.[18] The ability of *Salmonella typhi* to persist in macrophages is partially responsible for the carrier state although the importance of the enterohepatic cycle via the biliary system should not be underestimated.

The protozoa *Leishmania* species[8] and *Trypanosoma cruzi* cause chronic infection by persisting within macrophages although this is a pretty precarious strategy. Under certain conditions, the infected macrophages become activated and become capable of killing these intracellular parasites. Not only have IFNa and IL-4 been demonstrated to be important for this activation process, but the macrophage divalent cation transporter, natural resistance-associated macrophage protein (NRAMP-1), has been demonstrated in mice to play an important role.[1] The ability of certain strains of the protozoan *Plasmodium* species, especially *Plasmodium vivax*, to remain dormant within infected hepatocytes, has been responsible for the recurrence of attacks of malaria in individuals many years after leaving malaria endemic areas.[19]

Soluble factors

Just as there are many different types of phagocytic cells making up the innate immune defences, numerous families of soluble factors (Table 6.5) are also involved in antimicrobial activity.[20,21]

Interferons

The interferons[22–24] (IFNα, β and γ), originally described through their antiviral effect, are now recognized to have antiproliferative and immunomodulatory roles. In response to viral infections

Table 6.5 Some activities of T lymphocytes that are mediated by cytokines

Cytokine	Target cell	Result
IFNγ, IL-4	Macrophage	Activation
		Parasite killing
		MHC class II increased
IFNγ, IL-2	NK cell	Activation
		Virus killing
IL-1 to -6	B cell	Antibody formation
IL-5	Eosinophil	Activation
		Worm killing
IL-2	CD4 T cell	Clonal T cell growth
	CD8 T cell	Clonal T cell activation

IFNα and IFNβ are released from a wide variety of virus-infected cells. They react with specific receptors on neighbouring uninfected cells, rendering them immune to virus infection. This binding induces the production of protein kinase and double-stranded RNA (dsRNA)-activated inhibitor of translation (DAI). In the presence of viral dsRNA, DAI inactivates the cellular protein (eIF-2a) required for translation of messenger RNA (mRNA) which inhibits protein synthesis and therefore viral replication.

IFNγ is a cytokine produced by T cells that activates both macrophages and natural killer cells. Although the IFNs are used in cancer therapy and in multiple sclerosis, it is their use as antiviral agents against chronic hepatitis B and chronic hepatitis C infections that is most relevant to tropical diseases.

Defensins and cathelicidins are two major families of antimicrobial peptides.[25] They are positively charged polar molecules which have a high affinity for negatively charged phospholipids in microbial cell membranes. They insert and disrupt the cell membrane, causing lysis of the microorganism. In response to microbial invasion, exposure to bacterial LPS and TNF, α-defensins are produced by neutrophils and intestinal Paneth cells. Under similar provocation β-defensins are produced by epithelial cells of the skin, pancreas, kidney and respiratory tract. In addition to their anti-membrane effects, both α- and β-defensins chemoattract memory T cells to sites of infection. β-Defensins also chemoattract immature dendritic cells which then develop and take up antigens and present them to T cell-dependent regions of local lymph nodes, initiating acquired immune responses.

Acute-phase proteins are an assorted group of plasma proteins which are synthesized by the liver in response to infection.[26] They are normally present at undetectable levels but rapidly increase, some by over 1000 times, during the process of acute inflammatory responses.[27] C-reactive protein (CRP), a-1 acid glycoprotein (AGP) and fibrinogen are amongst this group of proteins. Albumin is unusual in being a negative acute-phase protein; i.e. it is present in detectable amounts but the levels fall precipitously during infection with invading microorganisms. CRP is probably the most widely studied. It is so called because it binds to the C polysaccharide of *Streptococcus*, rendering the bacterium opsonized for phagocytosis and intracellular killing. AGP increases four-fold in malaria and has been demonstrated to inhibit invasion of red blood cells by *Plasmodium* species by up to 80%, probably by blocking the merozoite binding site.

The complement system is a complex system of serum proteins and serum enzymes working as an amplification cascade system which has important inflammatory and antimicrobial function.[28-30] There are three pathways of complement activation: the antibody-dependent classical pathway, the mannose-binding lectin pathway and the phylogenetically older antibody-independent alternative pathway, all of which generate enzymes (C3 convertases) capable of splitting the most abundant complement component, C3, into C3a and C3b fragments.

The net result of both mechanisms of activation is the deposition of C3b on microorganisms, opsonizing them for phagocytosis by neutrophils which are attracted to the site by chemotactic factors associated with C3a and the later fragment C5a, together with mast cells. Figure 6.4 shows the basis of these mechanisms which underline the defensive acute inflammatory response. Deposition of the C3b cleavage product C3d greatly enhances the uptake and presentation of microbial antigen by antigen-specific B cells and so potentiates the development of strong antibody responses. Finally, activation of the terminal components C5–9 is associated with the lysis of the cell walls of microorganisms.

Complement activation by the classical pathway is more highly effective than by the alternative pathway and genetic deficiencies of C3 are associated with severe bacterial infections. Deficiencies of the terminal components C5–9 are specifically associated with meningococcal septicaemia.

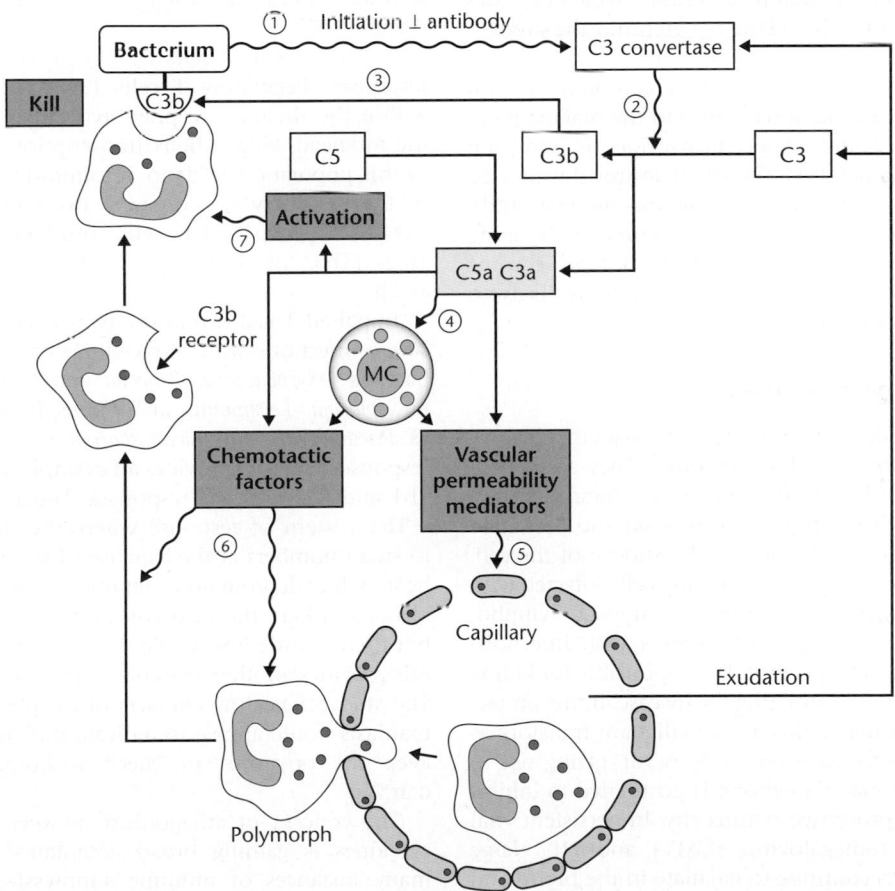

Figure 6.4 The defensive strategy of the acute inflammatory reaction initiated by bacterial activation of the complement system. Directions: (1) start with the activation of the *alternative pathway* C3 convertase through stabilization of the C3b Factor Bb complex by microbial polysaccharides or of the *classical pathway* C3 convertase through formation of the C142 complex by IgG or IgM opsonized microbes, (2) notice the generation of C3b, (3) which binds to the bacterium, C3a and C5a, (4) which recruit mast cell mediators, (5) follow their effect on capillary dilatation and exudation of plasma proteins and (6) their chemotactic attraction of neutrophils to the C3b-coated bacterium and triumph in (7) the adherence and final activation of neutrophils for the kill. (Redrawn with permission from Delves PJ, Martin SJ, Burton DR, Roitt IM. *Roitt's Essential Immunology*. 11th edn. Oxford: ©Blackwell; 2006.)

Specific acquired immune responses

The specific immune responses are mediated by T and B lymphocytes. These responses are generally more effective than innate immune responses and are much more antigen specific. Acquired immune responses also generate a large population of antigen-specific memory cells that mediate stronger and more rapid responses on re-exposure to the same infectious agent. These more rapid and exaggerated responses are always referred to as secondary immune responses, even after repeated exposure to the same antigen (i.e. not the primary immune response).

T lymphocytes are derived from the bone marrow but undergo maturation in the thymus gland. They bear a T cell receptor which can recognize a peptide bound to an MHC molecule on the surface of other cells (Figure 6.3).[20] Generally peptides derived from protein synthesized in the cytoplasm bind to MHC class I molecules (HLA A, B and C) and are usually recognized by CD8+ cytotoxic T lymphocytes (CTL). Peptides derived from extracellular proteins that are taken into APCs by endocytosis bind to MHC class II molecules (HLA DP, DQ and DR) and are usually recognized by CD4+ helper T lymphocytes (Th). The MHC molecules that an individual possesses, therefore, determine which peptides are efficiently presented to T cells and hence determine the strength of the acquired immune responses against a given infection. The MHC class I molecule (HLA-B53), which is common in West Africa, is associated with increased resistance to the malaria parasite, *Plasmodium*. HLA-B53 binds to specific peptides derived from malaria sporozoites and generates CTLs which destroy the infected hepatocytes and inhibit malaria infection within the liver. Individuals with the MHC class II molecule DR7 mount weak immune responses against HBV and are more likely to become chronic carriers, whereas those with the DR13 allele are more likely to eradicate HBV infection permanently.

Cell-mediated immune responses

Cell-mediated immunity describes immune responses that involve T lymphocytes without the need for antibody.[31] They are dependent on the recognition of antigens from intracellular parasites, otherwise hidden from view, which are processed and presented in combination with MHC molecules on the surface of the cell. CTLs reduce the severity of infections by killing cells infected with intracellular microorganisms. The abundant 'atypical lymphocytes' seen in the peripheral blood of patients with infectious mononucleosis represent EBV-specific CTLs responsible for killing the EBV-infected B cells and terminating the disease. If this protective cytotoxicity does not materialize then malignant transformation of the chronically infected B cells may occur, giving rise to Burkitt's lymphoma. The malaria parasite is postulated to inhibit the development of this protective cytotoxicity. In persistent viral infections with EBV, cytomegalovirus (CMV) and HIV, large numbers of memory CTLs continue to circulate in the blood and participate in the control of virus reactivation from latent infections.

CTLs have been implicated in leprosy, where they have been demonstrated in vitro to kill neuronal Schwann cells and liberate intracellular *Myobacterium leprae*, which can then be taken up by macrophages and killed. Similarly CTLs have been implicated in the killing of lymphocytes harbouring the protozoa *Theileria* (East Coast fever) in cattle. While the importance of CTLs in limiting episodes of infection is not in doubt, there is no established example of CTLs directly killing an infectious agent.

CD4+ helper T cells (Th) are classified as either Th0, Th1 or Th2, according to the pattern of soluble factors or cytokines they secrete. Most human Th cells are Th0, producing a broad range of cytokines, including IL-2, IFNγ, IL-4, IL-5, IL-6 and IL-10. Highly differentiated Th1 and Th2 cells secrete a narrow, non-overlapping range of cytokines which tend to have mutually antagonistic biological actions. For optimum control on intracellular infections the Th1 subset is required. They are generated during strong cell-mediated immune responses in response to IL-12 secreted by macrophages. Th1 cells secrete IL-2 and IFNg and induce delayed hypersensitivity skin reactions to antigens from the organism in question. In certain situations it is the Th2 subset which is preferentially stimulated, resulting in the secretion of IL-4 (induces IgE synthesis in B cells), IL-5 (activates eosinophils), IL-6 and IL-10 (inhibits Th1 cells). Th2 cell stimulation results in copious antibody production (which is usually of no benefit against intracellular parasites), while macrophage activation and intracellular parasite killing are reduced or absent (Figure 6.5).

Other classes of T cells are capable of downregulating immune responses. Regulatory T cells (Tregs) produced spontaneously within the thymus are phenotypically CD4+CD25+ and express the forkhead/winged helix transcription factor Foxp3; deficiency in this population leads to autoimmunity. Contact with antigen in the periphery can generate two other classes of Tregs, the CD4+CD25−Foxp3+ Trl cells producing IL-10 and induced Tregs (Th3) of phenotype CD4+CD25+Foxp3+ which produce TGFβ.

Impaired T cell immunity is associated with susceptibility to severe infections with intracellular organisms including viruses, bacteria (*Mycobacteria*, *Brucella* and *Salmonella typhi*), protozoa (*Toxoplasma*, *Leishmania* and *Plasmodium vivax*) and fungi such as *Pneumocystis* and *Cryptosporidium*. A study of the immune response in leprosy provides an example of the distinction between Th1 and Th2 immune responses. Tuberculoid leprosy represents a Th1 pattern of response where the microorganisms are kept to small numbers at the expense of serious tissue damage to the host, while lepromatous leprosy represents a Th2 pattern of response where the host tissues are teeming with mycobacteria but there is little host tissue destruction. The study of leishmaniasis provides another example of these two extremes of response. The study of healthy contacts of people with leprosy and leishmaniasis would appear to indicate sufficient immune response to keep the organism in check without causing severe tissue damage.

The concept of antagonism between the Th1 and Th2 cell cytokines is gaining broad acceptance and may account for many instances of immune suppression. The possibility that we may be able to switch an immune response from one spectrum to another is something that makes this hypothesis an attractive one. A number of academic units as well as pharmaceutical companies are trying to produce monoclonal antibodies and other immunological tools that will enable us to be able to modulate immune responses in whichever direction we choose.

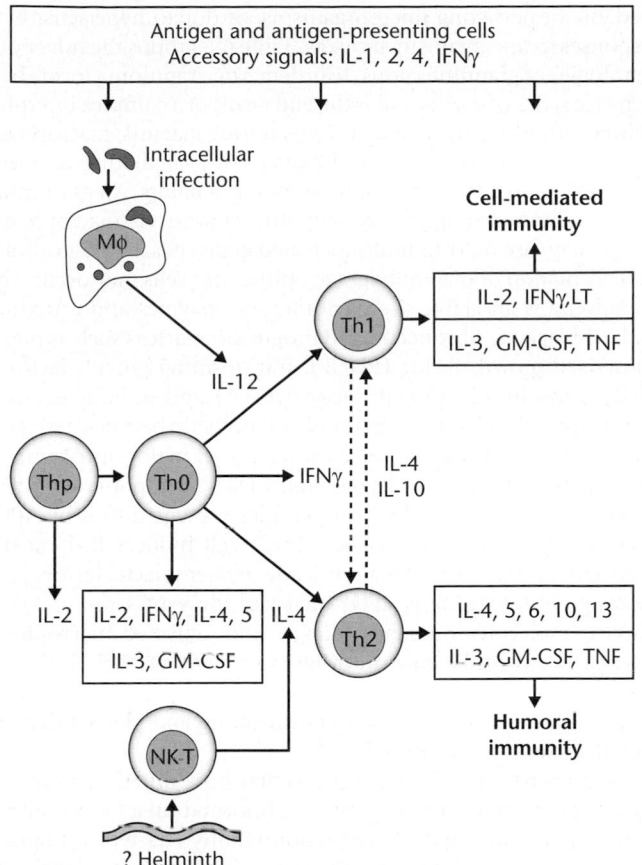

Figure 6.5 The generation of Th1 and Th2 CD4 subsets. Following initial stimulation of T cells, a range of cells producing a spectrum of cytokine patterns emerges. Depending on the nature of the pathogen and the response of cells of the innate immune system during the initial stages of infection, the resulting population can be biased towards two extremes. Th1-promoting pathogen products (such as LPS) engage Toll-like receptors (TLRs) on dendritic cells (DC) or macrophages and induce the secretion of Th1-polarizing cytokines such as IL-12 and IL-27. The latter cytokines promote the development of Th1 cells which produce the cytokines characteristic of *cell-mediated immunity*. IL-4 possibly produced by interaction of micro-organisms with the lectin-like NK1.1⁺ receptor on NK-T cells or through interaction of Th2-promoting pathogen products with TLRs on DCs, skews the development to the production of Th2 cells, whose cytokines assist the progression of B cells to antibody secretion and the provision of *humoral immunity*. Cytokines produced by polarized Th1 and Th2 subpopulations are mutually inhibitory. LT, lymphotoxin (TNFβ); Th0, early helper cell producing a spectrum of cytokines; IL, interleukin. (Redrawn with permission from Delves PJ, Martin SJ, Burton DR, Roitt IM. *Roitt's Essential Immunology*. 11th edn. Oxford: ©Blackwell; 2006.)

Humoral (antibody) responses

The bone marrow and spleen produce in the region of 10⁹ new B lymphocytes daily. These cells recognize antigens through their specific surface immunoglobulin (Ig or antibody) receptor, which is a product of the single light and heavy chain Ig genes which each B lymphocyte has been programmed to express. Sometimes when this surface immunoglobulin binds to the antigens (usually with repeating motifs such as polysaccharides) of invading micro-organisms, the B cell is induced to proliferate and change to plasma cells, producing specific antibody[21] to the antigen in question. The antigens that are capable of doing this directly are referred to as T cell-independent antigens and tend to give rise to the production of low-affinity pentavalent IgM antibodies which, however, have high 'functional affinity' (avidity) for the repeating groups on these polymeric antigens.

More commonly when antigens bind to the surface antibody of B cells, the complex becomes internalized inside the cell and antigenic peptides are presented to Th cells. This induces B cell proliferation and somatic mutation, resulting in the production of high-affinity IgG antibodies. This so-called 'isotype' class switching can also result in the production of other classes of immunoglobulin with different effector functions (i.e. IgA and IgE). Th cells also induce the differentiation of antigen-specific B cells into plasma cells and the production of memory B cells.

The different classes of immunoglobulin serve different functions. IgM circulates in the bloodstream and is responsible for immune surveillance in the vascular compartment. IgG provides defence against extracellular microorganisms in both intravascular and extravascular body fluids. IgA is usually secreted on to the mucosal surfaces of the respiratory, alimentary and genital tracts, where it is responsible for mucosal immunity. IgE is usually to be found in the tissues bound to mast cells, where it mediates immune responses against invading helminths, but is also intimately involved in allergic reactions.

The antiviral effect of antibody is easy to understand. In neutralization, the antibody binds to specific regions of the virion of the virus that is responsible for binding and penetration into cells. The virus is said to be neutralized as it can no longer gain entry into the cell and cause infection. Similarly, envelope viruses that have an LPS coat can be neutralized when antibody binds to their coat and induces antibody-dependent lysis of the viral envelope involving complement activation by the classic pathway. Also, viruses with attached antibody can be more readily destroyed by phagocytosis through binding the Fc receptor region of the antibody molecule. A word of caution here: one rather undesirable effect of antibody is, via binding to Fc receptors, the enhanced uptake into macrophages of organisms that thrive there, the most striking example of this being dengue virus.

The antibacterial affect of antibody includes the mechanism of opsonization and phagocytosis just described for viruses as well as the complement-dependent lysis of bacterial cell walls. Antibody can also have an antibacterial affect by neutralizing their extracellular toxins. Obviously, this mechanism is particularly important in limiting the clinical effects of the infections with bacteria whose clinical symptoms are caused mainly through the production of toxins, e.g. scarlet fever, diphtheria, tetanus and cholera.

In the past we have made use of the production of these antitoxin antibodies in animals to ameliorate clinical disease. Antitoxin antibodies have also been used to alleviate the symptoms of snake bites. Unfortunately antibodies produced in other animals are in themselves immunogenic to humans. Therapy with these agents is therefore limited as repeated exposure will either give rise to anaphylactic reactions in humans or to such rapid immune elimination of the antibodies as to render them non-effective. So far, attempts to generate human monoclonal antibodies that will have such an effect has met with very limited success. Attempts have therefore been made to 'humanize' monoclonal antibodies generated in laboratory animals by genetically engineering the antigen binding sites of murine monoclonal antibodies into human monoclonal immunoglobulin molecules. Interestingly, it is not in the field of tropical or infectious disease that these humanized antibodies are being commonly used, as these diseases caused by bacterial toxins have been very effectively controlled by vaccination programmes.

Antibody fragments such as scFv (VH/VL combination) or variable region domains (VH or VL) alone can be selected by antigen from engineered phage libraries. These can be used to block the adherence of microbes such as *Helicobacter pylori*, rotavirus and vaginal *Candida*[32] to specific receptors on the mucosal epithelium.

It is very rare for a parasite not to induce an antibody response. Even the higher eukaryotic organisms such as protozoa and helminths display large numbers of antigens foreign to humans, who as a general rule make antibody to most of them. Indeed, serum antibody is a most useful guide to infection, the general principle being that a predominance of IgM is a sign of recent infection. As mentioned earlier, antibody is only likely to provide effective defence when the parasite (or a parasite product such as a toxin) is in the extracellular compartment – blood, tissue spaces, secretions, etc. Even then, however, the existence of an antibody response does not ensure parasite disposal. The antibody may be of the wrong class or subclass (isotype) or of inadequate amount or affinity. Many of the effects of antibody rely on attachment of the antibody molecule not only to the antigen but also to phagocytes and/or complement, and here IgG is the most desirable isotype. Isotype switching and affinity maturation are both dependent on help from T cells, as is the development of memory. The involvement of T as well as B cells in antibody responses is therefore crucial, and protein antigen sequences from parasites are increasingly being analysed for antigenic portions, or 'epitopes' with the characteristic B cell or T cell recognition patterns; this is felt to be particularly important when identifying antigens for incorporation into vaccines (see below). Circulating antibody leads to the destruction of blood forms of *Trypanosoma brucei*, blocks invasion of erythrocytes by *Plasmodium merozoites* which it opsonizes for phagocytosis, and helps to limit the spread of *Trypanosoma cruzi* and *Leishmania* infections.

There tend to be vigorous Th2 responses to helminths generating copious IgE synthesis and chemoattraction of eosinophils through IL-5 production. Thus eosinophils binding to the larvae of *Schistosoma mansoni* or *Trichinella spiralis* coated with specific IgE or IgG bring about their killing through release of the crystalloid major basic protein and activation of oxygen-dependent microbicidal mechanisms. Th2 responses also facilitate the expulsion of intestinal nematodes by the mechanisms set out in Figure 6.6.

GRANULOMA FORMATION

Granulomas form as a consequence of the body's defence mechanism for walling off pathogens.[33] A granuloma can be defined as a focal, compact collection of inflammatory cells in which mononuclears predominate and are usually formed as a result of unde-

gradable or persisting microorganisms, or due to hypersensitivity responses to the organism antigens. Table 6.6 groups the infectious aetiologies of granulomatous disorders. The granuloma forms by a stepwise series of events and is the end result of a complex interplay between invading organism, prolonged antigenaemia, macrophage activity, T cell responses, B cell overactivity, circulating immune complexes and a vast array of biological mediators. Areas of inflammation of immunological reactivity attract monocyte-macrophages which may fuse to form multinucleated giant cells. Further cellular transformation of macrophages to epithelioid cells may occur. The granuloma is an active site of numerous enzymes and cytokines and, with ageing, fibronectin and progression factors such as platelet-derived growth factor (PDGF), transforming growth factor β (TGFβ), insulin-like growth factor (IGF-1) and tumour necrosis factor alpha (TNFα). There is a close relationship between activated macrophages bearing increased expression of major histocompatibility (MHC) Class II molecules and CD4+ T lymphocytes. These T helper cells recognize protein peptides presented to it by APCs bearing MHC class II molecules. The T cell induces IL-1 on the macrophage and thereafter a cavalcade of chemotactic factors promotes granulomagenesis. IFNγ increases the expression of MHC Class II molecules on macrophages, and activated macrophage receptors carry an Fc fraction of IgG to potentiate their ability to phagocytose. The end result is the epithelioid granuloma, which progresses under the impact of transforming and platelet-derived growth factor towards fibrosis.

Granulomas of various infections may have different immunoregulatory mechanisms governing their formation and resolution. Granulomas which synthesize predominantly Th2-type cytokines, such as those that form in response to parasite ova, make only small quantities of Th1-type cytokines chronically, whereas granulomas such as those of tuberculoid leprosy make large quantities of Th1-type cytokines and fewer of the Th2-type cytokines.

PARASITE EVASION OF HOST DEFENCE MECHANISMS

Infectious agents have developed a number of mechanisms for evading the body's immune system (Table 6.7). Many infectious microbes avoid antibody responses by adapting to an intracellular environment where it is impossible for them to come into contact with antibody. The helminth, *Schistosoma* species and the protozoan, *Trypanosoma cruzi*, have been demonstrated to cleave the Fc portion of antibody and evade antibody responses by this mechanism.

In malaria, where the *Plasmodium* undergoes a complicated life cycle within the infected host, different antigens are being produced at different stages and antibody responses are constantly having to adapt. Schistosoma represent another example of this 'stage-specific' immune response, because the adult worms seem to provoke very little immune response, while their eggs are highly immunological and induce immunopathology.[33]

It has often been proposed that parasites adapt to their host by mimicking their antigens. The acquisition of the ABO blood group antigen on the surface of mature Schistosoma may be one mechanism by which the mature worms evade antibody reactions. However, if this 'antigenic mimicry' is not fully effective, then the

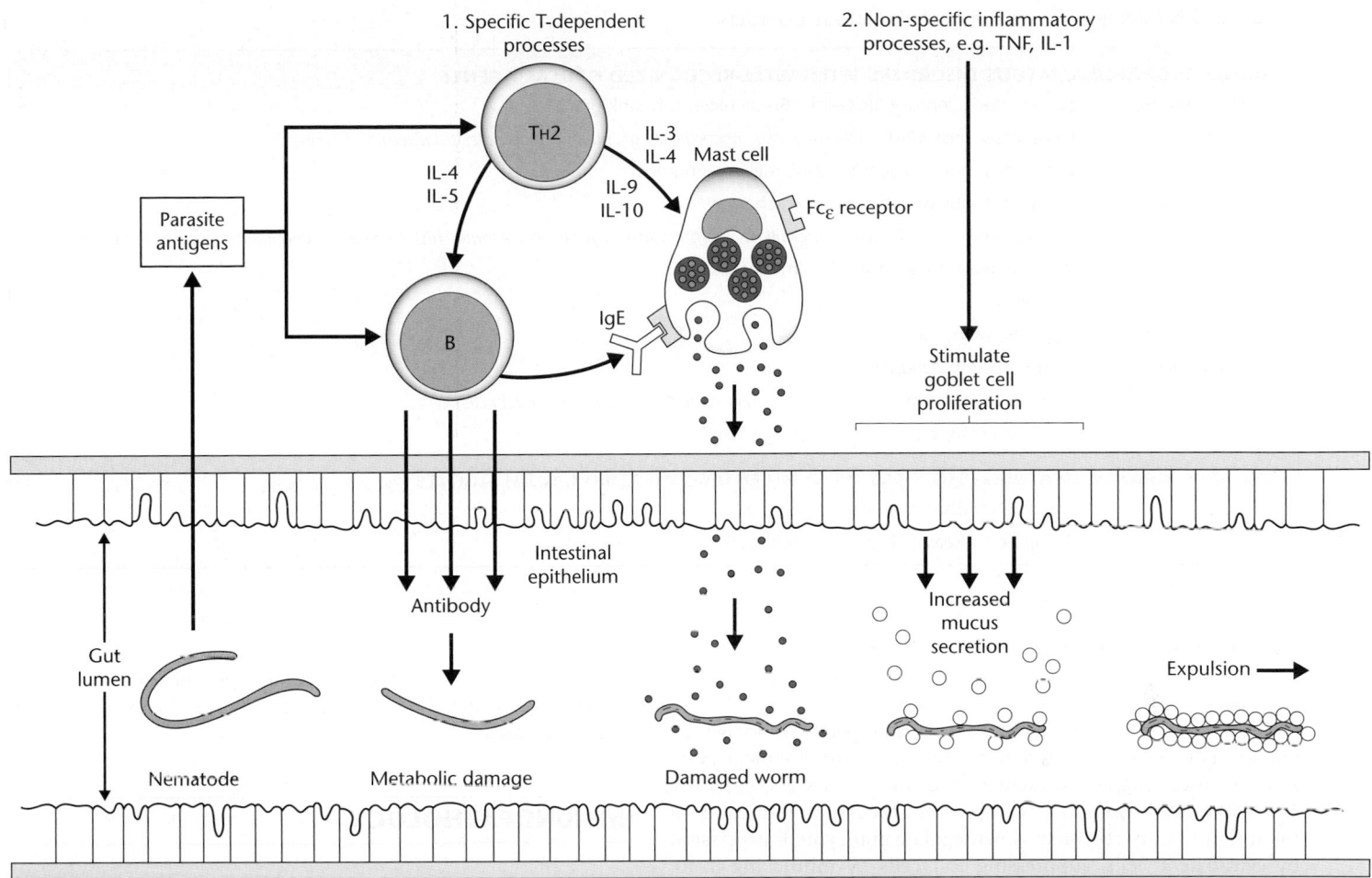

Figure 6.6 The expulsion of some intestinal nematodes occurs spontaneously a few weeks after primary infection. There seem to be two stages in the expulsion, which is achieved by a combination of T-dependent and T-independent mechanisms. (1) T cells (predominantly Th2 cells) respond to parasite antigens and induce (a) the production of antibody by B cells that have proliferated in response to IL-4 and IL-5, (b) the proliferation of mucosal mast cells, in response to IL-3, IL-4, IL-9 and IL-10, and (c) hyperplasia of mucus-secreting goblet cells in the intestinal epithelium. The worms are damaged by antibody together with products of IgE-sensitized mast cells which degranulate following contact with antigen, and so release histamine which increases the permeability of the intestinal epithelium. These processes are not sufficient to eliminate the worms. (2) Non-specific inflammatory molecules secreted by macrophages, including TNF and IL-1, contribute to goblet cell proliferation and cause increased secretion of mucus. The numbers of goblet cells in the jejunal epithelium and the secretion of mucus increase in proportion to the worm burden. The mucus coats the damaged worms and facilitates their expulsion from the body by increased gut motility induced by mast cell mediators, such as leukotriene-D_4, and diarrhoea resulting from inhibition of glucose-dependent sodium absorption by mast cell-derived histamine and PGE_2. The antigen-specific effector T cells are generated early in infection and the rate-limiting step is the onset of antibody damage. The relative importance of these various processes varies with the infecting nematode. (From Roitt I, Brostoff J, Male D. *Immunology*. 6th edn. London: ©Mosby International; 2001.)

development of antibodies to the infection may cross-react with autoantigens in the host and give rise to immunopathology. Such mechanisms may be responsible for the rheumatic carditis seen in Group A β-haemolytic streptococcal infections and the carditis and neuritis of Chagas' disease seen in *Trypanosoma cruzi* infections.

Infectious agents also evade antibody responses through the mechanism of 'antigenic drift' and 'antigenic shift'. Thus the influenza virus can escape neutralizing antibody by subtly changing its antigens, not only in going from patient to patient but also within the individual. 'Antigenic shift' is said to occur when a completely new haemagglutinin gene is incorporated into a new influenza strain and gives rise to the pandemic that occurs from time to time. Similar antigenic shift is seen in the envelope proteins of HIV and makes the epidemiological tracing of infections that much more difficult. The variation in the pilin genes of gonococci is a good example of antigenic variation in bacteria. In relapsing fever, the spirochaete *Borrelia hermsi* changes its surface major protein with each episode of fever. Similarly in African sleeping sickness, the protozoa *Trypanosoma brucei* constantly changes its variant antigenic type (VAT) and its variant specific glycoprotein (VSG) during the infection.[34] In this way the antibody response tends to be primarily of the IgM class, which has low affinity for the organism.

Table 6.6 Infectious causes of granulomatous disorders

GROUP 1: GRANULOMATOUS DISORDERS WITH WELL-RECOGNIZED CAUSAL AGENTS	
Mycobacteria	(tuberculosis, leprosy, BCGiosis, Buruli ulcer, fish tank granuloma)
Bacteria	(*brucellosis, melioidosis, actinomycosis, nocardiosis, granuloma inguinale, tularaemia, listeriosis*)
Viruses	(infectious mononucleosis, CMV, measles, mumps)
Chlamydia	(lymphogranuloma venereum, trachoma)
Fungi	(*cryptococcosis, candidiasis, aspergillosis, chromoblastomycosis, mycetoma, histoplasmosis, coccidioidomycosis, sporotrichosis*)
Protozoa	(leishmaniasis, toxoplasmosis, amoeboma)
Rickettsia	(Q fever)
Spirochaetes	(syphilis, yaws, pinta)
Nematodes	(*ascariasis, toxocariasis*)
Trematodes	(*schistosomiasis, paragonimiasis, fascioliasis, opisthorchiasis, clonorchiasis*)
Cestodes	(*echinococcosis, cryptococcosis, sparganosis*)
GROUP 2: GRANULOMATOUS DISORDERS WITH RECENTLY IDENTIFIED CAUSAL AGENTS	
Bacteria	(cat scratch disease: *Bartonella henselae*)
Actinomyces	(Whipple's disease: *Tropheryma whippelii*)

The protozoa *Entamoeba histolytica*, which causes amoebiasis, constantly sheds its surface antigen thereby evading antibody responses.

Virtually no biological process is safe from sabotage by viruses. For example, different viruses can subvert almost every step in processing and presentation of MHC class I to cytotoxic T cells; others can block complement-mediated induction of the inflammatory response, downregulate granzyme B expression by cytotoxic T cells, suppressing Th1 cells by mimicking IL-10, block apoptosis by producing a homologue of caspase 8 and so on.

Exposure to infective larvae of the filarial nematode *Onchocerca volvulus* (Ov) either results in patent infection (microfilaridermia) or it leads to a status called putative immunity, characterized by resistance to infection. Similar to other chronic helminth infections, there is T cell proliferative hyporesponsiveness to Ov antigen (OvAg) by peripheral blood mononuclear cells (PBMC) from individuals with patent infections, i.e. generalized onchocerciasis, compared to PBMC from putatively immune individuals. Recent studies argue against a general shift towards a Th2 response being the cause of hyporesponsiveness.[35]

CONCOMITANT INFECTIONS

Concomitant infections (existence of two or more parasites in one host) occur in nature and a number of interactions between protozoa and viruses; protozoa and bacteria; protozoa and other protozoa, protozoa and helminths; helminths and viruses; helminths and bacteria and helminths and other helminths have been described.[36] The interactions vary and the burden of one or both of the infectious agents may be increased; one or both may be suppressed, or one may be increased and the other suppressed. These interactions may be explained by the effects of parasites on the immune system, particularly parasite-induced immunosuppression, parasite-induced cytokine production and effects of cytokines controlling polarization to the Th1 or Th2 type T cell responses.

IMMUNOPATHOLOGY

Immune responses that do not achieve their purpose within a few weeks very often cause tissue damage to the host, and nowhere is this more true than with chronic tropical infections. All four types of hypersensitivity reaction are seen in chronic tropical infections (Table 6.1) and sometimes they are responsible for almost all the symptoms of infection. Schistosomiasis is an example where, judging by single-sex experiments in animals, the worms themselves are perfectly well tolerated but their eggs, deposited in the liver or bladder wall, induce T cell-mediated granulomas that can ultimately kill the patient. Hydatid disease is an infection in which the symptoms are due mainly to the large space-occupying cysts (essentially a host fibrotic response to the worms), with the added possibility, upon cyst rupture, of life-threatening anaphylaxis due to the encounter of massive amounts of worm antigen and IgE-loaded mast cells. In *Plasmodium falciparum* malaria there has always been debate as to the cause of the very diverse symptoms, and interest is currently being focused on the possibility that many of them may be secondary to the overproduction of cytokines, notably tumour necrosis factor (TNF). TNF has been found in the blood of severely ill malaria patients, and the levels correlate with the incidence of cerebral malaria and of hypoglycaemia. In animal models, evidence has also been obtained for a role of TNF in pulmonary oedema and anaemia. The roles of other cytokines such as IL-1, which resembles TNF in many of its actions, and of IFNg, also deserve investigation.

Table 6.7 Some parasite evasion mechanisms

Immune mechanism	Evasion strategy	Examples
Complement	Cell wall protected	*Salmonella* spp.
	Lytic complex expelled	*Leishmania* spp.
Phagocytosis	Capsule formation	*Haemophilus* spp.
	Phagolysosome blocked	Toxoplasmosis
	Oxygen radicals neutralized	Malaria
	Escape into cytoplasm	*Leishmania* spp.
	Difficult to kill	Mycobacteria
	Phagocytes destroyed	*Staphylococcus* spp. (toxins)
Antibody	Intracellular habitat	Mycobacteria
		Viruses
	Cyst formation	*Echinococcus granulosus*
		Paragonimus westermani
	Antigenic variation	
	by mutation	Influenza, poliovirus, HIV
	by recombination	Influenza
	by gene switching	Trypanosomes
		Borrelia spp.
		Brucella spp.
	Antibody binding factors	*Staphylococcus* protein A
	Antibody destroyed	Bacterial proteases
T cells	Inhibition of MHC expression	Herpesvirus
		Adenovirus
	Th2 stimulation	Leprosy
	Polyclonal activation	*Staphylococcus* spp. (enterotoxins)
T and B cells	Host antigen uptake	Schistosomiasis
	Tolerance	Congenital cytomegalovirus?
	Immunosuppression	Measles, HIV
		EB virus
		Trypanosomes
		Malaria
		Toxoplasmosis

BACTERIAL TOXINS AND THE IMMUNE SYSTEM

Acute bacterial infections can also cause immunopathology through the actions of their exo- and endotoxins.[5,37] It is thought that the activation of large numbers of T cells with a subsequent release of cytokines, especially TNF and IL-1, are responsible (Table 6.2). Bacterial endotoxin or LPS, a component of the cell wall of Gram-negative bacteria, comprises an outer polysaccharide and an inner lipid A moiety, and is responsible for the features of Gram-negative shock. When LPS is bound by the acute-phase protein, LPS-binding protein, it activates macrophages through a series of complex surface proteins comprising CD14, toll-like receptor and MD-2 to release TNF and IL-1. LPS can activate complement by the alternative pathway and is a powerful polyclonal B cell activator. The Jarisch–Herxheimer reaction is seen when human spirochaete infections are treated with antibiotics. The sudden killing of large numbers of spirochaetes produces severe hypotension as a result of the release of LPS from dead bacteria. The fact that this reaction can be attenuated by treatment with neutralizing antibody against TNF implicates this as the main cytokine involved in this reaction.

MALNUTRITION, IMMUNE RESPONSES AND INFECTION

A complex two-way interaction exists between infection and malnutrition[38] (Figure 6.7). There are two aspects: the effect of infection on metabolism and the nutritional state and the effect of

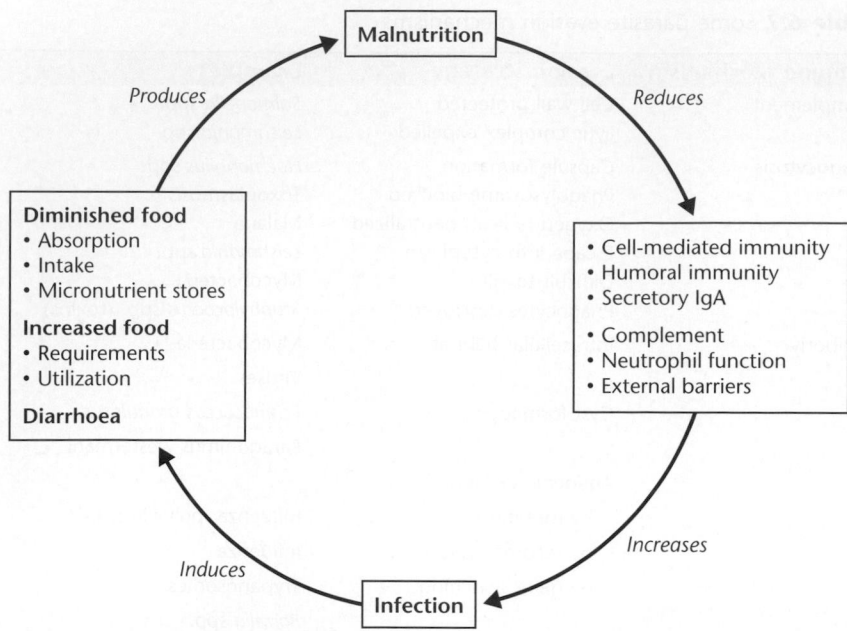

Figure 6.7 The malnutrition–infection cycle.

Table 6.8 Some immunodeficiency syndromes secondary to malnutrition

Deficiency components affected	Immune	Effect on disease
Calorie (marasmus)	Neutrophils Complement T cells	Susceptibility to bacterial and viral infections
Protein–calorie (kwashiorkor)	T cells Antibody Macrophages	Susceptibility to all infections
Iron	Neutrophils	Bacterial infections Malaria reduced?
Zinc, copper	T cells	Susceptibility to most infections
Selenium	T cells	Susceptibility to bacterial and viral infections
Vitamin A	T cells	Susceptibility to most infections

malnutrition on the susceptibility and severity of infections. Malnutrition causes depression of cell-mediated and humoral immune responses. The term 'malnutrition' usually refers to deficiency of macronutrients such as carbohydrate, protein and lipid, but may also be used for deficiencies of micronutrients such as vitamins, minerals and trace elements. Immunodeficiency syndromes secondary to malnutrition are shown in Table 6.8. Classically, patients who are calorie deficient (marasmus) are prone to viral, bacterial and tuberculosis infections, whereas those who suffer the more severe protein-calorie deficiency (kwashiorkor) are prone to all infections and have an impaired response to vaccination. Deficiency of zinc, copper and vitamin A also makes the host susceptible to infections, especially tuberculosis and fungal infection. While iron deficiency may seem to render people susceptible to bacterial infections,[39] it has been suggested that it can keep malarial infection at bay. It is not unusual for people who are having

their nutrition restored or who are receiving iron therapy for anaemia to experience a flare-up of malarial infection.

INFECTIONS CAUSING IMMUNODEFICIENCY

Infections which cause immunodeficiency are listed in Table 6.9. The much more serious course run by certain worldwide diseases in tropical countries, for example measles, meningococcal infection and gastroenteritis, is mainly due to the lowered immune status of the patients. Often it is not possible to pinpoint the reason for this, since inhabitants of the tropics are exposed to such a large number of different causes of immunodeficiency. The links between nutrition and immunity are much more complex than might be supposed. Many diseases are undoubtedly more severe in patients who are malnourished or underweight, measles being among the

Table 6.9 Some infections that cause immunodeficiency

Infection	Immune components affected	Effect on disease
HIV	CD4 T cells, macrophages	Opportunistic infections, e.g. *Pneumocystis carinii* *Toxoplasma gondii* *Mycobacterium tuberculosis*
Measles	T cells, neutrophils	Pneumonia, otitis media
Malaria	Antibody	? increased infections
	T cells	? Burkitt's lymphoma
Trypanosomiasis (African)	Antibody	Bacterial infection

most striking examples. Occasionally the opposite is true, as in the case of malaria, where iron deficiency inhibits the growth of the parasite and restoration of nutrition may induce a flare-up of the infection. A distinction is usually made between calorie deprivation and protein deprivation, the latter being generally more serious because both cell-mediated and antibody responses are impaired. There are also specific effects of deficiencies of iron, zinc, copper and vitamins on immune performance (Table 6.8).

Immunosuppression as a result of infection is extremely common, though it has usually proved very difficult to analyse the precise mechanisms involved, some of which have only been properly demonstrated in vitro. Thanks to the existence of animal models, malaria and African trypanosomiasis have been studied in particular detail, and the reality of the problem is well illustrated by the finding that treatment of even quite mild malaria improves the ability of patients to respond to unrelated vaccines (pneumococcal and meningococcal). Measles has long been known to suppress T cell responses and predispose to secondary infection, but all previous examples have been put in the shade by HIV, the most immunosuppressive and the most intensively studied parasite ever. Measles infection is undoubtedly more severe in the underweight or malnourished children in the tropics. Once they have caught the infection they are much more likely to develop pneumonia and otitis media.

AIDS AND TROPICAL INFECTIONS

The impact of AIDS in the tropics has, of course, been catastrophic (see Chapter 20). The original assumption that all the complications were due to a simple infection and destruction of CD4 T cells has turned out to be greatly oversimplified, and current research is also focused on the effects of HIV on macrophages, antigen-presenting cells, B cells and the cytokine network. It was a protozoan (or perhaps, according to recent data, fungal) infection, *Pneumocystis carinii*, that first drew attention, at the beginning of the 1980s, to the impending AIDS epidemic, and this strange

parasite remains a major cause of death in AIDS patients in the developed world, along with *Toxoplasma, Cryptococcus, Cryptosporidium* and other previously rare organisms. However, in tropical countries it is mycobacterial infections which have been most dramatically enhanced by AIDS, not only *Mycobacterium tuberculosis* but also the normally well-controlled *M. avium*, while some other parasites have been surprisingly unaffected. Malaria, for instance, shows virtually no change in either the density or the severity of infection, and nor, so far, do intestinal parasites such as *Entamoeba* or *Giardia*, or the major helminths.[8] Parasite immunologists are still digesting the implications of these unexpected findings, which seem to point to a particularly suppressive effect of HIV on those T cells that are concerned with parasites inhabiting macrophages, though Pneumocystis remains a puzzle because the parasite lives extracellularly in the lung alveoli. A sinister aspect of the relationship between HIV and *M. avium* is that each infection appears to enhance both the growth of the other within macrophages and the clinical progress of the disease, and it has been proposed that these effects are mediated by cytokines such as IL-1 and TNF. Infection with HIV makes people in tropical areas susceptible to a whole range of bacterial, viral and fungal infections. Mycobacterial infections, acute *bacterial sepsis, cryptococcal meningitis, Pneumocystis carinii* and *Cryptosporidium diarrhoea* are important opportunistic infections in AIDS patients worldwide.

IMMUNODEFICIENCY AND CANCER

Some of the best evidence for a role of the immune system in preventing malignancy comes from tropical conditions. In four tropical tumours a virus has been implicated, and in two, Burkitt's lymphoma and Kaposi's sarcoma, immunodeficiency appears to be a contributory factor (Table 6.4). Burkitt's lymphoma was recognized by Burkitt himself to have a very similar distribution to malaria in Africa and Papua New Guinea, and although the full aetiology is still not established, one plausible theory is that malaria suppresses the normal cytotoxic T cell response against the EB virus-infected B cells. The precise stage at which the well-known translocation of the c-myc proto-oncogene to one or other of the immunoglobulin gene loci occurs is not clear. Kaposi's sarcoma is found mainly in patients with T cell deficiencies, including AIDS. However, Kaposi's sarcoma is not particularly associated with malaria, nor is Burkitt's lymphoma with AIDS, which again emphasizes the range of different defects to which T cells are susceptible. Chronic infection with the human papilloma virus (HPV) can lead to cervical carcinoma, not only in the tropics but throughout the world.

IMMUNODIAGNOSIS

While the diagnosis of tropical infections is undoubtedly heavily reliant on clinical skills of history taking and physical examination, a number of laboratory tests are extremely helpful in confirming the diagnosis. However, as microbiological and pathological procedures are tedious, time consuming and relatively inefficient, several immunodiagnostic procedures[40] have found their way into general use. The four main immunodiagnostic tests for detection of antigen or antibody are:

1. ELISA test (enzyme-linked immunosorbent assay) and its development into multiplexing diagnostic microarrays where each spot in the array represents a unique 'micro-ELISA'. An alternative multiplexing technology involves the use of mixtures of beads, individually capable of binding a specific antigen or antibody, finally identified with a fluorescent readout in a flow cytometer.
2. Fluorescent antibody test using either the fluorescence microscope for tissue sections or flow cytofluorimetry for phenotyping individual cells.
3. Complement fixation test.
4. Agglutination test.

Neither of the latter two are currently being widely used.

Unfortunately, many of the early serological tests, although sensitive, lacked specificity and have been replaced by the detection of parasite antigens using monoclonal antibodies. The advent of the molecular biological tool of polymerase chain reaction, which allows the detection of small amounts of microbial DNA and RNA, has increased the sensitivity of immunodiagnosis. This tool has moved from the experimental to clinical laboratory, but is hampered by the problems of cross-contamination and false positive results, in addition to the enormous cost of performing the tests.

IS IMMUNITY EVER PROTECTIVE?

The combination of inappropriate immune responses with sophisticated parasite evasion ensures that virtually all protozoa and helminths can avoid elimination; the only case of 'proper' self-cure with resulting immunity, in the sense that we expect it with, for example, the childhood viruses (e.g. chickenpox, measles, mumps), is seen with Old World cutaneous leishmaniasis (oriental sore). However, it is nowadays accepted that the reduced parasite load with age in malaria and schistosomiasis is genuinely due to the development of a partial state of immunity, though the exact mechanisms in both cases are controversial. It should be remembered that there are also bacterial infections where immunity is precarious (e.g. tuberculosis) or non-existent (e.g. syphilis), and viral infections where it is ineffective in practice because of extensive antigenic variation (e.g. influenza, HIV).

IMMUNIZATION

A number of infectious diseases can now be controlled by immunization.[41] Generally speaking, immunization is likely to succeed in diseases in which good protective immunity follows natural infection. Sometimes immunization may result in better immunity than that seen after natural infection. In tetanus, the patient is only immune for about 3 or 4 months after recovery from infection. However, vaccination with three doses of tetanus toxoid induces a state of immunity that lasts between 5 and 10 years.

Table 6.10 shows the list of infections that are currently controlled by immunization programmes and is dominated by viruses and other simple organisms. Eradication of certain viral infections through vaccines (e.g. smallpox) has been a great success. Immunization may not always evoke a protective immune response. In dengue fever, an arthropod-borne virus infection, immunization

Table 6.10 WHO recommended vaccines

Vaccines against viruses	Vaccines against bacteria
Polio	Tetanus
Measles	Diphtheria
Hepatitis A – not for <12 years	Typhoid
Mumps	Meningococcal meningitis
Rubella	Tuberculosis (BCG)
Hepatitis B	Cholera
Rabies	
Japanese B encephalitis	
Influenza	

can give rise to more serious infection. Similarly in natural infections, previous infection to one strain of Dengue seems to give rise to a more exaggerated clinical course when one is exposed to another strain of Dengue, possibly due to Fc-mediated uptake of antibody-coated virus into productive macrophages, as mentioned earlier. Generally speaking, the longer the infection the more common is the likelihood of immunopathology.

The question is whether vaccines will ever succeed against infections that do not induce good immune responses. Opinion fluctuates on this point, but is at present guardedly optimistic. Great efforts are going into the production and testing of vaccines[42–47] against HIV/AIDS, malaria, schistosomiasis, leishmaniasis, tuberculosis and leprosy and at the research level filariasis and trypanosomiasis are targeted, though with less certain prospects. Unfortunately vaccine development programmes have only had limited success against more complicated multicellular organisms such as protozoa and helminths and against the more elusive HIV.

The advent of molecular and genetic techniques and availability of sophisticated methods for identifying and modifying genes which produce immunogenic proteins have revolutionized vaccine development. As more infectious agents become targets for immunization programmes, the spectrum of adverse events linked to vaccines has been widening.[43] Although some of these are tenuous, relatively little is known about the immunopathogenesis of even the best characterized vaccine-associated adverse events (VAAEs). The range of possible use of active immunization is rapidly expanding to include vaccines against infectious diseases that require cellular responses to provide protection (e.g. HIV infection, viral hepatitis B and C), and vaccines against non-infectious conditions (e.g. cancer, autoimmune disease). Less virulent pathogens (e.g. varicella, rotavirus in the developed world) are also beginning to be targeted, and vaccine use is being justified in terms of societal and parental 'costs' rather than in straightforward morbidity and mortality costs. In the developed world, the paediatric immunization schedule is becoming crowded, with pressure to administer increased numbers of antigens simultaneously in ever simpler forms (e.g. subcomponent, peptide and DNA vaccines). This trend, while attractive in many ways, brings hypothetical risks (e.g. genetic restriction, narrowed shield of protection and loss of randomness), which will need to be evaluated and monitored. The available epidemiological and laboratory tools to address issues outlined above are somewhat limited. As immunological and genetic tools improve, VAAEs will decrease and perhaps even avoid some of them.[43]

REFERENCES

1. Reynolds HY. Defense mechanisms against infections. *Current Opin Pulmon Med* 1999; 5:136–142.

2. Mims C, Dockrell HM, Goering RV, et al. *Medical Microbiology.* 3rd edn. London: Mosby; 2004.

3. Kotwal GJ. Microorganisms and their interaction with the immune system. *J Leucocyte Biology* 1997; 62:415–429.

4. Zumla A, James DG. Lung immunology in the tropics. In: Sharma OP, ed. *Lung Disease in the Tropics.* New York: Marcel Dekker; 1991:1–64.

5. Zumla A. T cells, superantigens and microbes. *Clin Infect Dis* 1992; 15(2): 313–320.

6. Penninger JM, Bachmaier K. Review of microbial infections and the immune response to cardiac antigens. *J Infect Dis* 2000; 181:S498–S504.

7. Ong RK, Doyle RL. Tropical pulmonary eosinophilia. *Chest* 1998; 113: 1673–1679.

8. Mosser DM, Brittingham A. Leishmania, macrophages and complement: a tale of subversion and exploitation. *Parasitology* 1997; 115:S9–S23.

9. Freihorst J, Ogra PL. Mucosal immunity to viral infections. *Ann Med* 2001; 33:172–177.

10. Alvarez-Olmos MI, Oberhelman RA. Probiotic agents and infectious diseases: a modern perspective on a traditional therapy. *Clin Infect Dis* 2001; 32: 1567–1576.

11. Burg ND, Pillinger MH. The neutrophil: function and regulation in innate and humoral immunity. *Clin Immunol* 2001; 99:7–17.

12. Paulnock DM, Collier SP. Analysis of macrophage activation in African Trypanosomiasis. *J Leuco Biol* 2001; 69(5):685–690.

13. Pieters J. Entry and survival of pathogenic mycobacteria in macrophages. *Microbes Infect* 2001; 3:249–255.

14. Brooks AG, Boyington JC, Sun PD. Natural killer cell recognition of HLA class I molecules. *Rev Immunogenet* 2000; 2:433–448.

15. Tefferi A, Morice WG, Leibson PJ. Natural killer cells and the syndrome of chronic natural killer cell lymphocytosis. *Leuk Lymphoma* 2001; 41:277–284.

16. Steinman RM. Dendritic cells and the control of immunity. *Mount Sinai J Med* 2001; 68(3):160–166.

17. Sousa CR. Dendritic cells as sensors of infection. *Immunity* 2001; 14:495–498.

18. Collins HL, Kaufmann SH. The many faces of host responses to tuberculosis. *Immunology* 2001; 103:1–9.

19. Plebanski M, Hill AV. The immunology of malarial infection. *Curr Opin Immunol* 2000; 12:437–441.

20. Matsukawa A, Hogaboam CM, Lukacs NW, et al. Chemokines and innate immunity. *Rev Immunogenet* 2000; 2:339–358.

21. Banyer JL, Hamilton NH, Ramshaw IA, et al. Cytokines in innate and adaptive immunity. *Rev Immunogenet* 2000; 2:359–373.

22. Le Page C, Genin P, Baines MG, et al. Interferon activation and innate immunity. *Rev Immunogenet* 2000; 2:374–386.

23. Levy DE, Garcia-Sastre A. The virus battles: IFN induction of the antiviral state and mechanisms of viral evasion. *Cytokine Growth Factor Rev* 2001; 12:143–156.

24. Shtrichman R, Samuel CE. The role of gamma interferon in antimicrobial immunity. *Curr Opin Microbiol* 2001; 4:251–259.

25. Yang D, Chertov O, Oppenheim JJ. Participation of mammalian defensins and cathelicidins in antimicrobial immunity: receptors and activities of human defensins and cathelicidin (LL-37). *J Leukoc Biol* 2001; 69:691–697.

26. Dhainaut JF, Marin N, Mignon A, et al. Hepatic response to sepsis: interaction between coagulation and inflammatory processes. *Crit Care Med* 2001; 29: S42–S47.

27. Thorn J. The inflammatory response in humans after inhalation of bacterial endotoxin: a review. *Inflamm Res* 2001; 50:254–261.

28. Walport MJ. Complement: Part I. *N Engl J Med* 2001; 344:1058–1066.

29. Walport MJ. Complement: Part II. *N Engl J Med* 2001; 344:1140–1144.

30. Jokiranta TS, Jokipii L, Meri S. Complement resistance to parasites. *Scand J Immunol* 1995; 42:9–20.

31. Johnson RM, Brown EJ. Cell-mediated immunity in host defense against infectious diseases. In: Mandell GL, Bennett JE, Dolin R, eds. *Principles and Practice of Infectious Diseases.* 5th edn. Edinburgh: Churchill Livingstone; 2000:31–155.

32. De Bernardis F, Liu H, O'Mahony R, et al. Human domain antibodies against virulence traits of *Candida albicans* inhibit fungus adherence to vaginal epithelium and protect against experimental vaginal candidiasis. *J Infect Dis* 2007; 195(1):149–157.

33. Zumla A, James DG. Granulomatous infections: an overview. In: James DG, Zumla A, eds. *Granulomatous Disorders.* Cambridge: Cambridge University Press; 2000:103–122.

34. Boros DL. The role of cytokines in the formation of the schistosome egg granuloma. *Immunobiology* 1994; 191:441–450.

35. Donelson JE, Hill KL, El-Sayed NM. Multiple mechanisms of immune evasion by African trypanosomiases. *Mol Biochem Parasitol* 1998; 91: 51–66.

36. Doetze A, Satoguina J, Burchard G, et al. Antigen-specific cellular hyporesponsiveness in a chronic human helminth infection is mediated by T(h)3/T(r)1-type cytokines IL-10 and transforming growth factor beta but not by T(h)1 to T(h)2 shift. *Int Immunol* 2000; 12:623–630.

37. Cox FE. Concomitant infections, parasites and immune responses. *Parasitology* 2001; 122:S23–S38.

38. Lencer WI. Microbes and microbial toxins: paradigms for microbial-mucosal interactions. *Am J Physiol Gastrointest Liver Physiol* 2001; 280(5): G781–G786.

39. Watzl B. Review of nutrition and immunity in man. *Am J Clin Nutr* 2001; 73:11–14.

40. Oppenheimer SJ. Iron and infection in the tropics: paediatric clinical correlates. *Ann Trop Paediatr* 1998; 18:S81–S87.

41. Harnett W, Bradley JE, Garate T. Molecular and immunodiagnosis of human filarial nematode infections. *Parasitology* 1998; 117:S59–S71.

42. Wenger J. Vaccines for the developing world: current status and future directions. *Vaccine* 2001; 19:1588–1591.

43. Minoprio P. Parasite polyclonal activators: new targets for vaccination approaches? *Int J Parasitol* 2001; 31:587–590.

44. Ward BJ. Vaccine adverse events in the new millenium: is there reason for concern? *Bull World Health Organ* 2000; 78:205–215.

45. Rowland-Jones S. Vaccines out of Africa. *Biologist* 2001; 48:64–66.

46. Tsuji M, Rodrigues EG, Nussenweig S. Progress towards a malaria vaccine: efficient induction of protective anti-malaria immunity. *Biol Chem* 2001; 382:553–570.

47. Moore JP, Parren PW, Burton DR. Genetic subtypes, humoral immunity and human immunodeficiency virus type 1 vaccine development. *J Virol* 2001; 75:5721–5729.

48. Cohen J. 'Breeding' antigens for new vaccines. *Science* 2001; 293:236–239.

Chapter 7

Damian G. Walker and Catherine Goodman

The Economics and Financing of Tropical and Infectious Disease Control

INTRODUCTION

The burden of tropical and infectious diseases on households is substantial, partly because a large proportion of health costs in low- and middle-income countries is met out-of-pocket. Consequently, households are pushed into poverty, or their poverty deepened.[1] The impact of HIV/AIDS in particular is dramatic, destroying family structures and long-established mechanisms of caring for the sick and sharing the financial burden of doing so. Many African countries are being fundamentally changed because of HIV/AIDS in ways that are only beginning to be understood. Similar changes could emerge in parts of South and East Asia without immediate action. With respect to malaria, Gallup and Sachs[2] found that, after taking into account initial poverty, economic policy, tropical location, and life expectancy, among other factors, countries with intensive malaria grew 1.3% less per person per year, and a 10% reduction in malaria was associated with 0.3% higher growth. Thus, while the impact of these diseases on GDP *per capita* has yet to be demonstrated conclusively, there is reason to believe that it is substantial.

This burden is not due to a lack of effective interventions. Indeed, the array of existing effective interventions is impressive. For example, while diarrhoea, pneumonia and malaria account for 40% of deaths among children in developing countries, there is at least one proven effective preventive intervention and at least one proven effective treatment intervention for each of these causes, each capable of being delivered in a low-income setting. For diarrhoea, there are no fewer than five proven preventive interventions and three proven treatment interventions. However, as Table 7.1 demonstrates, large numbers of people do not have access to prevention and treatment, and as a result die prematurely. And just as shortfalls in coverage vary across countries, so they vary within countries, with the poor and other deprived groups invariably lagging behind. For example, Victora et al.[3] found that the percentage of children in Cambodia who did not receive BCG, DPT, measles vaccines, vitamin A supplementation or safe water was 0.3%, but only 0.8% of children received all of the interventions. In the poorest wealth quintile, 31% of Cambodian children received no interventions and 17% only one intervention. To further compound the situation, even where services are obtained, the quality of provision is often low.

The under-use, and low quality of provision, of effective interventions helps to explain the current international focus on tackling these diseases, e.g. The Global Fund to Fight HIV/AIDS, Tuberculosis and Malaria, The GAVI Alliance, Stop TB, Roll Back Malaria and the US President's Emergency Plan for AIDS Relief (PEPFAR).

This chapter describes the armamentarium at the health economist's disposal in order to help guide policy-making to control tropical and infectious disease in the face of scarce resources. Specifically, we highlight three key areas: the demand for, and supply of, healthcare; the efficiency of healthcare; and the financing of healthcare.

THE DEMAND FOR, AND SUPPLY OF, HEALTHCARE

As described above, two key concerns in infectious and tropical disease control are the low coverage of effective interventions and the poor quality of service delivery. Economists use the tools of demand and supply analysis to address these issues by investigating how markets function for treatment and prevention services, and how they can be improved.

On the supply-side, the behaviour of providers is influenced by their knowledge, financial incentives, competition with other providers, perceptions of patients' attitudes, and any legal or regulatory sanctions for inappropriate behaviour. Treatment and prevention are delivered by a wide range of providers in the developing world. In the *public* sector, care is provided through a mix of hospitals and more peripheral health centres, clinics and dispensaries, which are generally staffed by nurses or similar cadres. Staff provide preventive services such as vaccines, growth monitoring and prevention of mother-to-child transmission (PMTCT) of HIV, and treatment for common illnesses such as malaria, tuberculosis, diarrhoea and respiratory infections. Increasingly they are also involved in the delivery of antiretrovirals (ARVs). There may also be outreach activities to remote areas, or community-based services delivered through local volunteers. For example, community-based volunteers in Uganda deliver a pre-packaged malaria treatment, and community members are widely used in the provision of directly observed therapy short-course (DOTS) for tuberculosis.

Table 7.1 Coverage levels in countries with a gross national income (GNI) per capita less than US$1200

Vaccination (polio, diphtheria, pertussis and tetanus)	75
Vaccination (measles)	68
Treatment of childhood illnesses (ARI)	59
Treatment of childhood illnesses (diarrhoea)	52
Insecticide-treated nets, residual indoor spraying	2
Treatment of clinical episodes of malaria	31
Short course TB treatment; smear + and − patients	44
HIV/AIDS interventions outside the health sector	10–20
Other HIV/AIDS preventive interventions	0–10
Palliative care for AIDS	6–10
Highly active antiretroviral therapy	<1

Source: Commission for Macroeconomics and Health (2001).

While public facilities often provide free or subsidized, and thus more affordable care, they often have weak management and poorly motivated and unproductive staff. High rates of absenteeism are common.[4] When staff are present they are often providing care of low clinical and consumer quality. This is partly because public sector providers generally have few incentives to increase coverage or quality as they are often remunerated purely by salary, and salary levels are often very low. As a result, informal payments are common. The potential to introduce performance or output-based payments to staff or facilities is increasingly being considered, though this brings its own challenges including accurate performance measurement, and the potential for fraud, demand inducement and neglect of quality.[5]

Private providers come in three broad guises:

- For-profit formal providers including registered self-employed doctors, clinics, hospitals, and diagnostic clinics, but also registered, organized, formally trained traditional healers
- Non-profit formal providers or non-governmental organizations (NGOs) who often operate primary healthcare facilities, but also district, and sometimes referral, hospitals. They often include organizations undertaking outreach activities, such as information, education, and communication programmes and social marketing
- For-profit informal providers include traditional healers, drug sellers, pharmacists (in offering healthcare, such as informal diagnosis and recommendations on medications to take), unqualified practitioners of allopathic medicine and traditional birth attendants.

The private for-profit sector plays a crucial role all over the world, accounting for a high proportion of treatment and preventive services. For example, around 60% of all malaria episodes in sub-Saharan Africa are initially treated by private providers, mainly through the purchase of drugs from retailers.[6] In India, more than 80% of children treated for diarrhea or ARI are seen by a private provider.[7] Preventive products such as insecticide-treated nets (ITNs) and condoms are available in some health facilities, but are primarily distributed through commercial retailers. Box 7.1 illustrates the range of private providers of TB and HIV/AIDS treatment in India, and recent government efforts to work with these groups.

Box 7.1 Supply of HIV/AIDS and TB treatment in India

In the city of Pune in the western Indian state of Maharashtra, 77% of private providers test for HIV, and 38% treat patients for HIV/AIDS.[8] However, there are major concerns over the quality of care among some private providers. For example, private providers predominantly use X-rays rather than sputum examination for the diagnosis of TB, and administer a variety of treatment regimens not conforming to national guidelines, some of which are inadequate and inappropriate. Routine HIV testing is undertaken without informed consent, and providers often fail to offer pre-test counselling to patients. ART therapy is still poorly understood and inappropriately prescribed. For both TB and HIV patients, private providers lack mechanisms to monitor treatment, ensure adherence and continuity of care.

While the government has tended to focus on the provision of DOTS for TB through public facilities, there have been recent attempts to involve the private sector through public-private partnerships in order to enhance access for patients. Key components of the public-private mix approach include diagnosis, treatment, supervision and monitoring of referred cases from private practitioners, improving the operation of private laboratories, registration of confirmed cases, and provision of DOTS by private providers. The approach is credited with increased acceptance of DOTS, creating a referral link between the public and private sectors, and enhanced training and information dissemination for private providers. However, challenges such as the difficulties in sustained monitoring of private providers, and the adversarial relationships between the public and private sectors highlight the need for strong commitment from both sectors at a national level.

In many developing countries, a substantial proportion of rural healthcare is provided by non-profit organizations. These providers are often perceived to deliver higher quality services, and to be more accessible and more efficient, though this depends on the performance of their own internal accountability structures. In many cases non-profit providers have proven more effective than public or for-profit providers in reaching stigmatized groups, e.g. those with sexually transmitted infections (STIs), including HIV/AIDS. However, while non-profit providers have many strengths, they also exhibit a number of weaknesses. In many countries, they are limited in terms of scale and coverage. Financial sustainability can be a particular problem for domestic organizations. Their need to cover costs (in the absence of public subsidy) can constrain the provision of services to poor people. Often they are not integrated or coordinated well with the public provider system, so duplication occurs and higher costs result.

Use of traditional practitioners is also widespread, although their significance varies considerably across geographical areas and medical condition. Two parallel explanatory models of disease may co-exist side by side, with both traditional and western medical providers consulted in turn.[9] In Malawi, families sought relief from AIDS symptoms by first using traditional remedies at home, followed by visiting traditional healers, only visiting a hospital after experiencing severe symptoms for anywhere from 6–12 months.[10] On the other hand, the reported use of traditional healers and medicines for uncomplicated malaria is low.[6] However, in various parts of Africa they are more commonly used for severe malaria, where symptoms such as convulsions may be perceived as supernatural in origin.[11]

When there is only one provider, e.g. a hospital, in a geographical area, it has the opportunity to control the price for services. A monopolistic for-profit provider will set prices in order to maximize profits. However, if a non-governmental organization is acting as the monopolist, it can choose to price discriminate and use its profits from some consumers to subsidize the purchase of a good or service by other consumers. A real-world example of such a market is the Aravind Eye Hospital system, which is the largest eye care provider in the world. It performs 220 000 eye operations per year, 80% of which are cataract surgeries. 47% of the patients pay nothing for surgery, 18% pay two-thirds of the cost and 35% pay well above the cost. This private-not-for-profit monopolistic model with price discrimination ensures greater access by the poor and hence reduces inequities. It does not mean that Aravind is a loss-maker either. With this model, they are able to be self-sustaining and profitable; for every dollar they spend, they make about US$1.60. Similar models are being piloted for typhoid vaccination in Vietnam by the Ministry of Health in collaboration with the International Vaccine Institute, in which a fee will be charged for the vaccine in private schools in order to cross-subsidize free provision in public schools. Of course, these models require individuals to demand the service or good.

Economists use the term *demand* to refer to the ability and willingness to pay for a product or service. The concept of demand therefore differs from 'medical need' or 'capacity to benefit,' and is useful in furthering our understanding of the factors influencing care seeking, utilization and adherence. These factors include prices of products and services, incomes, patient preferences and access to alternative providers. Demand is also influenced by the information that patients have at their disposal, including their knowledge of the price, quality and potential benefit of the alternatives available. The importance of these influences can be explored empirically in a number of ways, including cross sectional household surveys, before and after analyses (e.g. the introduction or removal of user fees), in-depth interviews and willingness-to-pay studies. Box 7.2 demonstrates the use of regression analysis of household survey data to assess the importance of a range of demand determinants.

Two of the most important influences on demand are the price of services and the income levels of households. A critical issue for policy-makers is the responsiveness of demand to price (the price elasticity of demand). A strong body of evidence indicates that introducing or increasing user fees has detrimental effects on the demand for services, particularly among the poorest groups.[14] Exemption policies are seldom sufficiently well managed to mitigate such negative impacts. Price can also be a barrier to prevention; mosquito nets are relatively expensive in the private sector, costing US$5–10 or more in many countries, and the average household will need to purchase more than one net to cover all beds/sleeping mats. In addition to the cost of drugs and services, ability to pay may also be influenced by credit availability, the acceptability of payment-in-kind, and the availability of loans or gifts, for example through savings schemes or from the extended family.[15]

The cost to households of obtaining services is not limited to the official prices charged. Unofficial payments or bribes are charged in many public facilities,[16] and care-seekers may incur

---

Box 7.2 The demand for malaria treatment and prevention in The Gambia

The Demand for Malaria Treatment and Prevention study assessed the importance of factors influencing demand for bed net ownership and malaria treatment seeking behaviour in The Gambia and Tanzania using household surveys and logit regression models.[12,13] Some of the key results for the Farafenni region of The Gambia are summarized below.

It was shown that older people were more likely to opt for self-care or no treatment. The longer the time spent ill or the more severe the fever then the more likely treatment was sought outside the home. Time of the year and availability of community infrastructure played a key role both in seeking malaria treatment and in choosing a healthcare provider. Poorer households were much more likely to visit another provider than incur the relatively higher cost of a hospital visit compared to wealthier households. The more a household spent on other forms of malaria prevention the less likely they were to own a bednet. The older the household head and the more education he or she had, the greater the likelihood of bed net ownership. Households where the head was a business person were also more likely to own a net. Lastly, households located in communities cut-off from main roads at certain times of the year due to flooding and other causes were less likely to own a net. The results imply that the demand for bed nets and malaria treatment can be significantly increased if certain aspects of public infrastructure are improved. They also inform price setting practices for subsidized bed nets. Finally, they show that greater attention needs to be paid to cultural or ethnic related reasons for bed net ownership and provider choice.

---

transport costs, and the time costs of travel and waiting, which can frequently take more than half a day. This represents an important cost, particularly during peak periods of economic activity such as harvest. Women are generally the primary caregivers, but often consult senior male household members before selecting providers. It may also take time for mothers to mobilize the money and approval necessary to take their children to a health facility, leading to dangerous delays in care seeking. Delays in diagnosing and/or treating an infectious disease can cause prolongation of the period of infectivity in the community, and may result in the disease state being more advanced at presentation, with consequent increases in acute morbidity, late sequelae and overall mortality.

High costs may lead patients to use alternative informal providers such as shops which are cheaper and more geographically accessible, but where quality of care may be lower. Another important reason for high use of shopkeepers is that they are more likely to sell an incomplete dose of drugs, which may be appreciated (although less effective) when cash is not available to buy a full treatment course.[17] Such under-dosing is widespread for TB, and other diseases such as malaria, diarrhoea and pneumonia.

Lack of information on the part of consumers severely limits the demand for preventive services. Individuals tend to underestimate their risk of HIV and other STIs.[18] In many places there is demand for untreated mosquito nets; demand for insecticide treatment is much lower, partly due to poor knowledge about its effectiveness.[19] Lack of knowledge about the benefits from intermittent preventive treatment in pregnancy similarly limits demand, as does concern amongst some pregnant women that drug use may pose health risks to the unborn child. However, patients may be willing to come forward for diagnosis and consultation if they are aware of the availability and effectiveness of treatment.

Information problems are crucial in explaining why the quality of treatment is so frequently poor. Patients often do not know what treatment they require, so they hand over responsibility for these choices to a provider as their 'agent.' However, agents' knowledge may also be imperfect; for example, many providers cannot accurately state antimalarial drug dosages. Limited information is likely to be most pronounced in shops and other commercial outlets where staff have minimal training, but is also surprisingly common in the more formal health sector. Where providers are more knowledgeable than patients they have the power to advise patients incorrectly and induce them to demand unnecessary treatment, termed supplier-induced demand. This is particularly likely where providers have financial incentives, for instance, to recommend unnecessary investigations, or report false-positive test results to induce drug purchase. This may be most common in the commercial sector, but also occurs in the public or NGO sector if certain behaviours generate extra money for the facility or individual. A study of prescribing practice in public facilities in Ghana found that introducing drug charges led to less rational drug prescription, with the proportion of patients treated for malaria receiving injections or three or more drugs rising from 56 to 89% following the policy change.[20]

People's perceptions of the technical quality of the service they receive also matters. They may, of course, not be the best judges of technical quality, but the fact is that perceptions of quality, based primarily on the more observable elements of provision, influence demand. In addition to the long waiting times mentioned above, there are frequent complaints that public facilities have rude and insensitive staff, lack diagnostic facilities, and suffer from poor infrastructure and drug shortages. Drug retailers may be perceived to have better stock availability, and more courteous staff. High use of traditional healers in some contexts has been attributed to the time taken over consultation and treatment and the greater communication between patient and provider. Most individuals with a STI seek care in the private sector in part because of the stigma attached to these infections and therefore the desire for confidentiality.[21]

Even in situations of perfect information, utilization of some health services will be sub-optimal if left to the private market because of the nature of their benefits.[19] Positive externalities are said to arise when a service provides benefits to the community above and beyond those enjoyed by the individual. There are numerous examples in the field of infectious disease. Rational drug use provides positive externalities to future patients in the form of a reduction in the rate of growth of drug resistance. Treatment for STIs benefits others through the reduction in disease transmission to future partners, and ITNs may have positive externalities if they reduce malaria transmission through the 'mass effect.'[22] Vaccination also provides benefits to others, particularly once levels of 'herd' immunity are reached. In making choices, individuals will not take into account these additional positive effects and therefore will consume less than the socially desirable quantity. In such cases, it may benefit society to provide incentives for people to consume enough of these services – immunizations,

for example – to ensure that society as a whole is protected. An innovation in Latin America is the use of conditional cash transfers, which provide direct cash payment contingent on households accessing preventive health services such as immunization. They thus represent a negative user fee.[14]

Although many health services exhibit externalities, a few have *public good* characteristics, meaning that they may not be provided by the market at all. With public goods no one can be excluded from consuming them once they are provided (they are non-excludable), and one person's consumption does not prevent anyone else's (they are non-rival). These attributes give rise to a paradox; although there is significant benefit to be gained from public goods by many people, there is no commercial incentive for producing them, since the benefit cannot be made conditional on payment. Examples in infectious disease control include provision of health education to the general population, epidemic surveillance, and indoor residual spraying against malaria because the main benefit is felt at the community level in terms of reduced vectorial capacity.

In recent years, the term Global Public Good (GPG) has been coined to refer to goods whose benefits cross borders and are global in scope.[23] For example, the eradication of infectious diseases such as smallpox or polio provides a benefit from which no country is excluded, and from which all countries will benefit without detriment to others. With *national* public goods, governments intervene either financially, through such mechanisms as taxation or licensing, or with direct provision. For *global* public goods this is harder to do, because no global government exists to ensure that they are produced and paid for.

The presence of externalities, public good characteristics, poor information, monopoly power and poverty are all potential justifications for government intervention in the financing and provision of health services. However, in many countries, particularly in sub-Saharan Africa, expenditure on health has been constrained by very limited government revenues and restrictive macroeconomic policies. It is therefore imperative to consider both the value for money of health sector interventions and the sources of finance, the topics addressed in the following two sections.

THE EFFICIENCY OF HEALTHCARE

The growth in the infectious disease burden in terms of new cases is much greater in many countries than the growth in the resources available for control. The desire to implement evidence-based policy decisions has arisen as limited healthcare budgets have emphasized the need to use resources effectively *and* efficiently. Consequently, economic evaluation has acquired greater prominence among decision-makers as there is a need to know which interventions represent 'value for money'.

Economic evaluation compares the costs *and* outcomes of *at least two* alternative programmes, one of which may be 'doing nothing', although most usually it is current practice (of course, in many settings, current practice may be 'doing nothing').[24] There exist several types of economic evaluation, which differ in the way that outcomes or consequences are measured.

In *cost-minimization analysis* (CMA) two or more interventions that have identical outcomes are assessed to see which provides the cheapest way of delivering the same outcome, e.g. assume two rotavirus vaccines have equivalent levels of effectiveness against severe gastroenteritis; this form of analysis would identify the least costly of the two vaccines. *Cost-effectiveness analysis* (CEA) measures the outcome of approaches in terms of 'natural units', e.g. if the outcome of interest were a reduction in childhood pneumonia, this form of analysis might compare vaccines against *Haemophilus influenzae* type b (Hib) and pneumococcal diseases in order to identify which averts a case of pneumonia more cheaply. *Cost-utility analysis* (CUA) uses measures of utility, which reflect people's preferences, in order to value outcomes. The outcomes are then expressed in terms of measures such as quality – (QALYs) or disability-adjusted life-years (DALYs), e.g. it might compare vaccines against rotavirus and Hib in terms of which averts a DALY more cheaply, but it also enables comparisons among different health sector interventions, e.g. those to control HIV/AIDS, TB and malaria. In practice, there has been a blurring of the distinctions between CEA and CUA, with the latter seen as an extension of the former. And finally, *cost-benefit analysis* (CBA), which expresses health outcomes in terms of monetary units; this form of analysis enables comparisons among interventions in the health sector, and other sectors, e.g. education, in order to identify which generates the greatest return on investment. The Copenhagen Consensus is a recent, and rare, example of an inter-sectoral priority-setting exercise (Box 7.3). The requirement of measuring outcomes in monetary units has limited the use of this type of analysis in health policy.

Economic evaluation attempts to identify ways in which scarce resources can be efficiently employed. However, efficiency has two meanings. First, there is allocative efficiency, which can be viewed as *doing the right things*, i.e. choosing the optimal mix of interventions for a given level of expenditure – optimal in the sense that they maximize health gain. In this definition of efficiency, different healthcare interventions with different objectives and outcomes are compared, e.g. malaria vs TB vs diarrhoeal disease control, or more generally, how should the Ministry of Health's budget be distributed between programmes? It thus follows that, while interventions may have different objectives and outcomes

of interest, these outcomes must be converted into commensurable units if the optimal mix is to be defined. Second, there is technical efficiency, which is a narrower definition as it concentrates on maximizing the achievement of a given objective within a given budget, i.e. *doing things right*. For example, an economic evaluation might compare the costs and effects of vaccination of children through fixed, outreach or mobile clinics in order to identify the most efficient means of vaccinating a child. While only CBA (and CUA within the health sector) can be used to assess allocative efficiency, all of the different types of economic evaluation can be used to assess technical efficiency.

The ceiling ratio represents a decision-maker's valuation of a unit of health gain. It is a particularly crucial element of CEA/CUA, as it is the relative value against which the value for money of an intervention is judged. If an intervention has a cost-effectiveness ratio below the ceiling ratio an intervention is deemed acceptable on grounds of cost-effectiveness. In economic evaluations of interventions to control tropical and infectious diseases in developing countries to date, many analysts have simply presented results without interpretation.[25] However, in 1996 in an effort to define research priorities,[26] interventions costing less than US$25 and US$150 per DALY averted were respectively cited as 'highly attractive' and 'attractive' uses of scare resources in low-income countries. For middle-income countries, these figures were US$100/DALY and US$500/DALY, respectively. More recently, based on the recommendation of the Commission on Macroeconomics and Health,[27] WHO classifies interventions as 'highly cost-effective' for a given country if results show that they avert a DALY for less than the per capita national gross domestic product.

The cost-effectiveness evidence-base for interventions to control tropical and infectious diseases is limited.[25,28] However, for some diseases, there are more cost-effectiveness data than for others. The following paragraphs summarize what is known regarding the relative cost-effectiveness of interventions to control HIV/AIDS, TB and malaria.

Many governments, particularly those in sub-Saharan Africa, face difficult choices in striking the right balance between prevention, treatment and care, all of which are necessary to deal comprehensively with the HIV/AIDS epidemic. Creese et al. (2002) illustrated that a strong economic case exists for prioritization of preventive interventions. For example, a case of HIV/AIDS can be prevented for US$11, and a DALY averted for US$1, by selective blood safety measures, and by targeted condom distribution with treatment of STIs. Single-dose nevirapine and short-course zidovudine for PMTCT, voluntary counselling and testing, cost under US$75 per DALY averted. Other interventions, such as formula feeding for infants, home care programmes, and ARV therapy for adults, cost several thousand dollars per infection prevented, or several hundreds of dollars per DALY averted. However, reductions in drug prices have raised the priority of treatment, though access to treatment remains restricted at present.

Borgdorff et al.[30] examined the impact and cost-effectiveness of TB control measures in developing countries. The authors found that treatment of smear-positive TB using the WHO DOTS strategy has by far the highest impact. While BCG immunization reduces childhood mortality, its impact on TB transmission is probably minimal. Under specific conditions, an additional impact on mortality and transmission can be expected through treatment of smear-negative cases, intensification of case-finding for smear-

---

Box 7.3 The Copenhagen consensus

The goal of the Copenhagen Consensus project was to use cost-benefit analysis to set priorities among a series of proposals for confronting ten great global challenges. These challenges, selected from a wider set of issues identified by the United Nations, were: civil conflicts; climate change; communicable diseases; education; financial stability; governance; hunger and malnutrition; migration; trade reform; and water and sanitation. A panel of economic experts was invited to consider these issues. The panel was asked to address the ten challenge areas and to answer the question, 'What would be the best ways of advancing global welfare, and particularly the welfare of developing countries, supposing that an additional $50 billion of resources were at governments' disposal?' Ten challenge papers, commissioned from acknowledged authorities in each area of policy, set out more than 30 proposals for the panel's consideration. The 2004 meeting found that combating HIV/AIDS had a very high rate of return and should be at the top of the world's priority list. About 28 million cases could be prevented by 2010. The cost would be US$27 billion, with benefits almost 40 times as high. (See www.copenhagenconsensus.com/ for further details.)

positive TB, and preventive therapy among individuals with dual TB-HIV infection. Of these interventions, DOTS is the most cost-effective at around US$5–40 per DALY averted. The cost for BCG immunization is likely to be under US$50 per DALY averted. Treatment of smear-negative patients has a cost per DALY averted of up to US$100 in low-income countries, and up to US$400 in middle-income settings. Other interventions, such as preventive therapy for HIV-positive individuals, appear to be less cost-effective.

In the field of malaria control, analysis by Goodman et al.[31] of the cost-effectiveness of malaria interventions showed that many interventions represent good value for money. For example, insecticide treatment of existing mosquito nets was estimated to cost US$4–10 per DALY averted, providing nets and retreatment US$19–85 per DALY averted, and intermittent presumptive treatment of pregnant women (IPTp) through existing antenatal services US$4–29 per DALY averted. However, most cost-effectiveness evidence is based on very specific delivery mechanisms. In the case of ITNs, for example, the above analysis was costed on the basis of providing free nets with regular retreatment by project staff. For IPTp, it was assumed that delivery would be through public sector static health facilities. Little systematic evidence has been collected about costs and health consequences of other delivery approaches, although one study showed that social marketing of ITNs can be at least as cost-effective (US$37–57 per DALY averted) as public sector delivery.[32] Costs of alternative delivery mechanisms will also vary across settings. For example, social marketing of ITNs costs US$3–5 per net in Tanzania, but up to US$10 in Mozambique.[19]

To date economic evaluations have not taken full account of the broader economic impacts of measures to control tropical and infectious diseases, particularly those targeted at infants and children. Examples of these broader economic impacts include[33]:

- the fact that healthy children are better able to attend school and to learn effectively while in class
- like school children, healthier workers have better attendance rates and are more energetic and mentally robust. Workers in healthy communities, moreover, need to take less time off to care for sick relatives
- healthier people expect to live longer, so they have a greater incentive to save for retirement. They are also able to work productively for longer, giving them more time to save. Workers and entrepreneurs therefore have a larger capital base to draw on for investment, leading to greater job creation and higher incomes.

These impacts stem from the fact that many interventions not only treat, or protect individuals against getting a disease *per se*, but also against the long-term effects of that disease on their physical, emotional and cognitive development. For example, by stunting physical growth, childhood diseases can curtail opportunities for carrying out manual labour during adulthood. In developing countries, where manual work is frequently the only option, physical handicaps are particularly damaging. Cognitive development may also be affected by tropical and infectious disease. For example, measles and malaria, among others, can cause brain damage or impair learning abilities, with severe impacts on a child's life prospects.

The importance of these effects is borne out by recent work demonstrating the link from improved health to economic growth.[27] This research has made clear the importance of health

interventions for achieving growth and suggests that economic evaluations, as currently conducted, are likely to underestimate the benefits of many interventions aimed at tropical and infectious diseases.

While the emphasis of this section has been on value for money, efficiency is only one of at least nine criteria relevant for priority-setting in health if the object is to decide how to spend public funds.[34] Other criteria include horizontal equity (equal treatment for people in equal circumstances); vertical equity (priority for people with worse problems); adequacy of demand; and public attitudes and wants. As we have seen already, two criteria – whether an intervention is a public good and whether it yields substantial externalities – are classic justifications for public intervention, because private markets could not supply them efficiently, just as in other sectors. Finally, cost matters by itself, as do the capacities of potential beneficiaries to pay for an intervention. The following section focuses on who pays, and how, for healthcare.

FINANCING HEALTHCARE

High-income countries spend about 100 times more on health per capita than low-income countries (US$3039 vs US$30).[35] Furthermore, the poorer the country the larger the amount of total health spending that is out-of-pocket; more than 60% of the meagre spending in low-income countries is from out-of-pocket payments by patients/households whereas the same statistic in high-income countries is 20%. Out-of-pocket payment for healthcare is the most inequitable type of financing because it hits the poor hardest and denies individuals financial protection from catastrophic illness, commonly classified as healthcare payments above 10% of household income.

User fees, one of the reasons for such high levels of out-of-pocket expenditure in developing countries, have been a contentious source of financing in low-income country settings.[36] In most cases they have occurred as a result of the scarcity of public financing, the prominence of the public system in the supply of essential healthcare, the government's inability to allocate adequate financing to its health system, the low salaries of health workers, the limited public control over pricing practices by public providers and the lack of key medical supplies such as drugs (discussed in the section on the supply of healthcare above). User fees are likely to remain in place until governments are ready and more able to mobilize greater funding for healthcare. Until that time, the global community should focus on helping countries design policies that can foster access by the poor to health-enhancing services and protect the poor and near-poor from catastrophic health spending.

Because tropical and infectious diseases often trigger catastrophic payments for healthcare,[1] low-income countries must improve *risk pooling* to improve financial protection. Risk pooling is the collection and management of financial resources so that large unpredictable individual financial risks become predictable and are distributed among all members of the pool. The challenge for low- and middle-income countries is to somehow direct the high levels of out-of-pocket spending into either public or private pooling arrangements, so that individuals will have real financial protection.

The most globally prominent and straightforward way to increase risk pooling in most developing countries is through

Ministries of Health acting as national health services. To exploit the potential strengths of national health service-style systems, it is important for developing countries to improve the capacity to raise revenue. Unfortunately, revenue collection in developing countries is the art of the possible, not the optimal.[35] Furthermore, as this chapter has already described, there are many problems with the public provision of healthcare in developing countries, which result in limited access to, and poor quality of, health services as well as limited financial protection against catastrophic health expenditures.

Social health insurance has the potential not only to improve risk pooling but also to bring additional funding into the health sector. Proponents of social health insurance argue that giving contributors a clear stake in the system, earmarking funds to protect health expenditures, and improving efficiency through competition on the purchasing side are sufficient justifications to pursue it. At issue are the pre-conditions for social health insurance: a growing economy and level of income capable of absorbing new contributions; a large payroll contribution base and thus a small informal sector; a concentrated beneficiary population; and good administrative and supervisory capacity. Such preconditions are absent in many developing countries. Voluntary health insurance can also increase risk pooling using private funding, but it accounts for less than 5% of private health spending in low-income countries,[35] and clearly fares poorly on equity grounds. In most middle- and high-income countries, it generally supplements other types of public insurance.

Community-based health insurance may provide some marginal benefits in increased risk pooling and resources, but alone is unlikely to significantly improve financial protection in low-income settings.[35] The schemes can be broadly defined as not-for-profit prepayment plans for healthcare that are controlled by a community that has voluntary membership. There is evidence that such schemes reduce out-of-pocket spending, but the protection provided by, and sustainability of, most community-based health insurance schemes are questionable. They are often unable to raise significant resources because of the limited income of the community, and the pool is often small, making it difficult to serve a broad risk-spreading and financial protection function. They are also placed at risk by the limited management skills available in the community, and they have limited impact on the delivery of healthcare, because few negotiate with providers on quality or price. They also cannot cover the poorer parts of the population; even small premiums may be out of reach for the poor. Therefore, community-based health insurance is not likely to be the 'magic bullet' for solving the bulk of health financing problems in low-income countries. It should be regarded more as a complement to, rather than a substitute for, other forms of strong government involvement in healthcare financing.

In 2000, 189 countries signed the United Nations Millennium Declaration. The document includes eight Millennium Development Goals (MDGs) with specific targets for poverty eradication and development that are to be achieved by 2015. Three of the eight MDGs are directly related to health, of which one is specifically related to infectious and tropical diseases: reducing child mortality (MDG4); improving maternal health (MDG5); and combating HIV/AIDS, malaria, and other diseases (MDG6). Health also underpins many of the other MDGs. Donor funding will be critical for most countries to meet the MDGs. Donors need

---

Box 7.4 Innovative financing mechanisms

AMCs offer a market-based financing mechanism to accelerate the development and availability of new vaccines. An AMC for vaccines is a financial commitment to subsidize the future purchase (up to a pre-agreed price) for a vaccine not yet available *if* an appropriate vaccine is developed and *if* it is demanded by developing countries. An AMC is not a purchase guarantee, as industry will only receive the subsidized price if the product meets targeted standards and countries demand the product. Thus the commitment itself has no cost unless and until an appropriate vaccine is developed. This means that an AMC for a malaria vaccine would not divert money from being invested in existing malaria control measures while the new vaccines were being developed. A pilot AMC has been designed for pneumococcal vaccines to demonstrate both the feasibility of the AMC mechanism and its impact on accelerating vaccine development, production scale-up and introduction. (See www.vaccineamc.org/ for further details.)

A second innovative financial instrument is the International Finance Facility (IFF). The IFF for Immunization (IFFIm) will provide proof of concept for this novel financing mechanism by raising up to US$4 billion for financing immunization programmes in low-income countries over the next 10 years. The IFFIm mechanism front-loads funding by using long-term government commitments as security for bonds issued in the capital markets. The proceeds from the bonds can be disbursed immediately to fund national immunization programmes or to guarantee the purchase of future vaccines, for example, through an AMC. If tied to the latter, the bond issuance would be timed to correspond with the procurement of the new product once it is on the market. (See www.iff-immunization.org/ for further details.)

---

to reduce the volatility, improve the predictability, and improve the longevity of aid. With that in mind, two recent, creative market-based mechanisms are currently being piloted: Advance Market Commitments (AMCs) and the International Financing Facility (IFF) (Box 7.4).

Much of the recent increase in development assistance for health has been directed to specific diseases and interventions (e.g. The Global Fund to Fight HIV/AIDS, Tuberculosis and Malaria and PEPFAR), and there is growing concern about the disease and intervention-specific focus of aid. Such a focus can be very effective in achieving rapid short-term health benefits in resource-scarce environments. However, as health systems develop, waste can result from separate delivery silos for different diseases. And given the severe human resources constraints in many African countries, aid programmes may compete with each other to hire away the few skilled professionals needed to run the public health system. Support to broad health systems development is vital to address this issue.

CONCLUSIONS

Tropical and infectious diseases continue to be the major cause of death and illness in poor countries. Effective, low cost methods for preventing tropical and infectious diseases exist – they are among the most cost-effective interventions possible. Furthermore, never before have such sizeable funds been made available to tackle infectious and tropical diseases. And yet, most developing countries are being severely challenged to provide essential services to their populations and to provide financial protection against infectious and tropical diseases.

Given the constrained resources of most countries heavily affected by infectious diseases, economic analyses provide a powerful tool to facilitate the prioritization of resources; it is important that the maximum possible benefit be gained from the scarce resources available. Moreover, the economic tools of demand and supply analysis, and application of economic principles to issues such as the role of government and financing of healthcare, can help countries improve the design and performance of their health system.

ACKNOWLEDGEMENTS

We thank Karina Kielmann (London School of Hygiene and Tropical Medicine) and Sheela Rangan (Maharashtra Association of Anthropological Sciences) for their assistance in preparing Box 7.1, and Virginia Wiseman (London School of Hygiene and Tropical Medicine) for her assistance in preparing Box 7.2. We are also grateful to Anne Mills (London School of Hygiene and Tropical Medicine) for her comments on an earlier draft.

REFERENCES

1. Russell S. The economic burden of illness for households in developing countries: a review of studies focusing on malaria, tuberculosis, and human immunodeficiency virus/acquired immunodeficiency syndrome. *Am J Trop Med Hyg* 2004; 71(suppl 2):147–155.

2. Gallup JL, Sachs JD. The economic burden of malaria. *Am J Trop Med Hyg* 2001; 64(suppl 1–2):85–96.

3. Victora CG, Fenn B, Bryce J, et al. Co-coverage of preventive interventions and implications for child-survival strategies: evidence from national surveys. *Lancet* 2005; 366(9495):1460–1466.

4. Chaudhury N, Hammer JS. Ghost doctors: absenteeism in rural Bangladeshi health facilities. *World Bank Econ Rev* 2004; 18(3):423–441.

5. Meessen B, Kashala J-PI, Musango L. Output-based payment to boost staff productivity in public health centres: contracting in Kabutare district, Rwanda. *Bull World Health Organ* 2007; 85:108–115.

6. McCombie SC. Treatment seeking for malaria: a review of recent research. *Soc Sci Med* 1996; 43(6):933–945.

7. Waters H, Hatt L, Peters D. Working with the private sector for child health. *Health Policy Plan* 2003; 18(2):127–137.

8. Sheikh K, Porter J, Kielmann K, et al. Public-private partnerships for equity of access to care for tuberculosis and HIV/AIDS: lessons from Pune, India. *Trans R Soc Trop Med Hyg* 2006; 100(4):312–320.

9. Hausmann Muela S, Muela Ribera J, Tanner M. Fake malaria and parasites – the ambiguity of malaria. *Anthropol Med* 1998; 5(1):43–61.

10. Hatchett LA, Kaponda CP, Chihana CN, et al. Health-seeking patterns for AIDS in Malawi. *AIDS Care* 2004; 16(7):827–833.

11. Ahorlu CK, Dunyo SK, Afari EA, et al. Malaria-related beliefs and behaviour in southern Ghana: implications for treatment, prevention and control. *Trop Med Int Health* 1997; 2(5):488–499.

12. Wiseman V, McElroy, Conteh L, et al. Household expenditure on mosquito control in The Gambia: patterns of expenditure and determinants of demand. *Trop Med Int Health* 2006; 11(4):419–431.

13. Wiseman V, Scott A, McElroy B, et al. Determinants of bed net use in The Gambia: implications for malaria control. *Am J Trop Med Hyg* 2007; 76: 830–836.

14. Palmer N, Mueller DH, Gilson L, et al. Health financing to promote access in low income settings – how much do we know? *Lancet* 2004; 364(9442): 1365–1370.

15. Hausmann Muela S, Mushi AK, Muela Ribera J. The paradox of the cost and affordability of traditional and government health services in Tanzania. *Health Pol Plann* 2000; 15(3):296–302.

16. McPake B, Asiimwe D, Mwesigye F, et al. Informal economic activities of public health workers in Uganda: implications for quality and accessibility of care. *Soc Sci Med* 1999; 49:849–865.

17. van der Geest S. Self-care and the informal sale of drugs in south Cameroon. *Soc Sci Med* 1987; 25(3):293–305.

18. Eaton L, Flisher AJ, Aaro LE. Unsafe sexual behaviour in South African youth. *Soc Sci Med* 2003; 56(1):149–165.

19. Hanson K. Public and private roles in malaria control: the contributions of economic analysis. *Am J Trop Med Hyg* 2004; 71(suppl 2):168–173.

20. Biritwum RB. The cost of sustaining Ghana's 'Cash and Carry' system of healthcare financing at a rural health centre. *West Afr J Med* 1994; 13(2): 124–127.

21. Brugha R. Antiretroviral treatment in developing countries: the peril of neglecting private providers. *BMJ* 2003; 326(7403):1382–1384.

22. Hawley WA, Phillips-Howard PA, ter Kuile FO, et al. Community-wide effects of permethrin-treated bed nets on child mortality and malaria morbidity in western Kenya. *Am J Trop Med Hyg* 2003; 68(suppl 4):121–127.

23. Smith R, Woodward D, Acharya A, et al. Communicable disease control: a 'Global Public Good' perspective. *Health Policy Plan* 2004; 19(5):271–278.

24. Drummond MF, Sculpher MJ, Torrance GW, et al. *Methods For Economic Evaluation of Healthcare Programmes.* Oxford: Oxford University Press; 2005.

25. Walker D, Fox-Rushby J. Economic evaluation of communicable disease interventions in developing countries: a critical review of the published literature. *Health Econ* 2000; 9(8):681–698.

26. WHO. *Investing in health research and development: report of the ad hoc committee on health research relating to future intervention options.* Geneva: World Health Organization; 1996.

27. Commission for Macroeconomics and Health. *Macroeconomics and health: investing in health for economic development.* Report of the Commission for Macroeconomics and Health. Geneva: WHO; 2001.

28. Jamison DT, Measham AR, Breman JB, et al. *Disease Control Priorities for Developing Countries.* Washington, DC: World Bank; 2006.

29. Creese A, Floyd K, Alban A, et al. Cost-effectiveness of HIV/AIDS interventions in Africa: a systematic review of the evidence. *Lancet* 2002; 359(9318): 1635–1643.

30. Borgdorff MW, Floyd K, Broekmans JF. Interventions to reduce tuberculosis mortality and transmission in low- and middle-income countries. *Bull World Health Organ* 2002; 80(3):217–227.

31. Goodman C, Coleman P, Mills A. Cost-effectiveness of malaria control in sub-Saharan Africa. *Lancet* 1999; 354:378–385.

32. Hanson K, Kikumbih N, Armstrong Schellenberg JAS, et al. Cost-effectiveness of social marketing of insecticide-treated nets for malaria control in the United Republic of Tanzania. *Bull World Health Organ* 2003; 81: 269–276.

33. Bloom DE, Canning D, Weston M. The value of vaccination. *World Econ* 2005; 6(3):15–39.

34. Musgrove P. Public spending on healthcare: how are different criteria related? *Health Pol* 1999; 47(3):207–223.

35. Gottret P, Schieber G. *Health Financing Revisited: A Practitioners Guide.* Washington, DC: World Bank; 2006.

36. James CD, Hanson K, McPake B, et al. To retain or remove user fees?: reflections on the current debate in low- and middle-income countries. *Appl Health Econ Health Pol* 2006; 5(3):137–153.

Chapter 8

Solomon R. Benatar

Ethics and Tropical Diseases: Some Global Considerations

The persistence of tropical diseases in an era that could have seen these largely eradicated is inextricably linked to poverty, inequality and global injustice. The root causes of such disruptive forces, and how they are perpetuated need to be recognized, studied and debated more constructively in order to make progress towards eradicating preventable diseases. Rather than focusing exclusively on such ethical considerations as what is right and wrong at the micro-level of the physician–patient relationship, ethical inquiry should be extended to include considerations of right and wrong behaviour within institutions and between nations – at which levels political decisions have a major impact on the health of whole populations. In a globalizing world the ethical imperatives that should be addressed include the need to relieve hunger, alleviate poverty and improve living conditions; reduce military expenditure; restructure third world debt; foster sustainable development; implement appropriate methods of taxing international financial transactions; and restructure international relations – all with a view to promoting a broader approach to moral behaviour that includes, but goes beyond, respecting human rights. New perspectives are also required on how to undertake clinical trials ethically in developing countries and on improving ethical relationships between researchers and participants. The impact of tropical diseases will only be reduced if all these issues are addressed in a wise, scholarly and morally imaginative manner.

INTRODUCTION

A proper understanding of the distribution and impact of infectious diseases on humankind in the broadest temporal and spatial contexts requires some knowledge of the trajectory of history over thousands of years. A less ambitious perspective on the forces promoting and sustaining tropical diseases would acknowledge the influence of imperialistic and colonial forces over the past 500 years. However, such historical considerations from the distant past tend to be eclipsed by more recent spectacular advances in science and technology. These advances and the extent to which they have facilitated control of infectious diseases in industrialized countries favour a narrow biomedical approach to health and disease focused on the prospects offered by modern vaccines and drugs. The World Health Organization's success in eradicating

smallpox provided hope that many other major infectious diseases that plagued humankind could be largely eliminated.

The persistence of many diseases, for example malaria and tuberculosis, the emergence of multi-drug resistance to both of these and the appearance of HIV (and other new infections, most notably SARS in recent years) illustrate the limitations of an approach to public health that does not embrace consideration of the social determinants of health. Infections have no respect for geographical boundaries, particularly in a globalizing world in which new ecological niches are being created and where speed of travel and transport allow enhanced transmission. This became particularly relevant with the outbreak of SARS and is further emphasized by the threat of an epidemic of avian flu. Control of infectious diseases thus poses not merely scientific challenges for individual nations but also global political and economic challenges that have wider ethical implications than previously considered.

In the previous edition of this text, a synoptic overview was provided of the powerful global forces that play a dominant role in perpetuating inequities that impair human flourishing and frustrate the control of infectious diseases. Some challenging ethical imperatives were identified and some potential solutions offered. Ethics is the branch of philosophy that rigorously evaluates and provides justification for what is right and wrong in human behaviour. Such considerations are usually focused within the context of one-to-one personal interactions. However, relationships also exist between individuals and institutions and between institutions and nations. My thesis is that massive differences in wealth, and how these have arisen and are perpetuated, lie at the heart of inequality and inequity in health between nations; and that the major ethical imperatives of our time are to narrow these gaps by considering the ethics of higher level relationships with a view to structuring more just societies in which premature death and unnecessary suffering from tropical diseases could be diminished.[1]

In this updated chapter some of some of the above-mentioned data will be even more synoptically covered and with exclusion of most of the original references to sources of data. Interested readers are referred back to the previous edition for such details. New sections in this chapter will focus on some considerations about the practice of tropical medicine and on ethical issues in relation to conducting research in developing countries.

A STARTING POINT: THE FACTS

The world today is in a tragic state (Box 8.1). Despite massive growth of the economy over the past 50 years, hundreds of millions of people live under conditions of 'absolute poverty' defined as 'a condition of life so limited by malnutrition, illiteracy, disease, squalid surroundings, high infant mortality, and low life expectancy as to be beneath any reasonable definition of human decency'.[2] Growing economic disparities are associated with growing inequalities in the burden of disease and premature death, and vast inequities in access to healthcare and medical research.[3]

MORAL JUSTIFICATION FOR CHANGE

These facts about the state of the world arouse moral indignation and must be addressed for several reasons. First, and foremost, is the ethical imperative to respect equally the dignity of all people. With the 60th anniversary of the Universal Declaration of Human Rights (UDHR) behind us, it is necessary to reflect on its content (and that of subsequent supportive covenants and declarations) and on the extent to which these aspirations have not been achieved. Moreover, concerns about human rights become magnified in an era in which there will be the potential to modify nature by applying genetic engineering techniques to all forms of life.[4,5]

Second, is the ethical requirement to promote the solidarity and social stability necessary for human flourishing in a complex world. The twentieth century was characterized by spectacular scientific and technological progress from which many have benefited greatly, but it was also characterized by ongoing wars since 1945, especially in the developing world. While wars have complex causes, they were certainly fuelled by the economic and ideological interests of the great powers during the Cold War, and continue under the influence of powerful global economic forces driving the extraction of human and material resources from poor regions to promote economic growth of the rich. Consequent hunger, miserable living conditions, lack of education, illiteracy and lack of control over personal destiny have bred anger, violence, crime, drug dealing and abuse of vulnerable humans – all of which reflect injustice and erode the fabric of society.[6-12] Third, is the ethical imperative to be aware of the adverse ecological effects of high and wasteful consumption patterns of modern life and to develop processes necessary to protect the environment for the well-being of future generations.[13]

CAUSES OF WIDENING DISPARITIES AND ONGOING POVERTY

Disparities in wealth and health are symptoms of an unjust world – a well known fact that is widely stated, but about which most privileged people have become complacent in pursuit of their own economic goals,[6,12,14] and in the deluded belief that we live in a just world.[15] Some believe that poverty is not the fault of wealthy countries, but rather the result of bad government elsewhere, and can be alleviated by market forces. Others believe either that the problems are of such great magnitude that there is little that can be done to ameliorate them, or that there is too much disagreement about values to focus on solutions. These views are all contestable and wealthy industrialized nations are deeply implicated in creating and sustaining poverty.[12,*]

The extent of injustice, the underlying causes of such injustice (described synoptically below) and potential solutions previously suggested[1] should be constructively addressed by scholars, politicians and policy-makers. Progress towards reducing inequalities and the burden of preventable diseases will be limited if these causes of injustice are ignored and a merely biomedical approach adopted to addressing inequalities in health. The World Health Organization's renewal strategy[16] indirectly acknowledges these issues but its approach is inadequate and a bolder thrust is required.

Globalization, economic exploitation and the debt problem

Globalization describes the development of a complex web of material, institutional and ideological forces that influence the

---

> **Box 8.1** Some facts about the world today
>
> ■ Gap between the richest 20% and poorest 20% of the world's population
>   – Widened from 9× at the beginning of the century to over 80× by 2000
> ■ Scale of absolute poverty has increased
>   – Number of extremely poor people more than doubled between 1975 and 1990
> ■ 2.8 billion (46% world population) live on <$2/day
> ■ 2.0 billion lack access to essential drugs
> ■ 2.8 billion lack access to sanitation
> ■ 2.0 billion do not have electricity
> ■ 1.2 billion lack access to safe water
> ■ 1.0 billion have no adequate shelter
> ■ 831 million are chronically undernourished
> ■ 18 million die prematurely every year from poverty related causes
> ■ 34 000 children die each day from hunger and preventable diseases
> ■ US$50 billion could prevent 50% premature deaths
>   – (0.2% combined GDP of affluent countries)
> ■ 90% of annual global expenditure on healthcare is spent on patients who bear less than 10% of the burden of disease expressed in disability adjusted life years (DALYs)
> ■ 90% of expenditure on health research is on those diseases accounting for 10% of the global burden of disease.

The facts and interpretations offered above are not intended to imply that the wealthy, productive and fortunate in the world should bear the whole burden of the blame for the complex series of historical developments that polarize the world. Political realities within developing countries, including corruption, ruthless dictatorships, ostentatious expenditure by elites and under-investment in education and health, have contributed greatly to the suffering of billions. However, it is vital for privileged people to have insight into the extent to which these deficiencies in many developing countries have been facilitated by the policies of wealthy nations in pursuit of their own interests. Powerful nations, intent on continuing to extract material resources (e.g. oil, diamonds, platinum) and human resources (recruitment of health professionals without any recompense), are often complicit in supporting despots and kleptocrats by legitimizing sale of their countries' assets to arm and enrich themselves.

balance of power, and effectively blur the boundaries between states. Globalization has been ostensibly spearheaded by a few hundred corporate giants, the development of earth-spanning technologies and products that can be produced anywhere and sold everywhere, and the spreading of credit through pervasively penetrating global channels of communication. However, globalization is both a more complex and ambiguous concept than this, going beyond economics to include social, cultural and ecological dimensions. Nor is it a new phenomenon, but rather the outcome of a long and interwoven economic and political history, involving a wide range of actors. Its effects are both beneficial and damaging – and as with the effects of population growth and global warming, adverse manifestations are now becoming starkly apparent.

Positive manifestations of progress associated with globalization include advances in science and technology; increased longevity; enhanced economic growth; greater freedom and prosperity for many; improvements in the speed and cost of communications and transport; and popularization of the concept of human rights. Negative effects of globalization include widening economic disparities between rich and poor (within and between nations), and increases in both absolute and relative poverty.[11,12] Economic disparities have become so marked and their adverse effects so apparent that a very significant degree of incompatibility has arisen between neo-liberal economic policies and the goals of democracy.[17,18]

The power of massive multinational corporations in a globalizing world has profound implications for the accumulation of capital and for the way in which resources are controlled. In 1970, 70% of all money that exchanged hands on a daily basis was payment for work, while speculative financial transactions accounted for 30%. By 1997 these proportions had changed to 5% and 95%, respectively. Such a striking shift in the distribution of money arguably reflects devaluation of the lives and work of most people in the world. The influence of the shift in the locus of economic power from the nation-state to global corporations thus alters the balance of power in the world, effectively blurring boundaries between states, and between foreign and domestic policies – in the process undermining small states' control over their own economies, and threatening their ability to provide for their citizens.

During the second half of the twentieth century, the evolution towards a globalized economy has perpetuated and aggravated centuries of exploitative processes that facilitate the enrichment of some people at the expense of others – within and between nations. Such exploitation (made possible by processes that devalue and dehumanize the 'other', relegating them to lower standards of life), overtly underpinned slavery, racism and industrial labour abuse. Over the past 50 years, covert erosion of the economies of many poor countries, under the impact of the neoliberal economic policies driving globalization, has obstructed real development and prevented the introduction of effective forms of modern medicine into many poor countries and the achievement of widespread access to even basic healthcare for billions of people.[19] Average national per capita GNP has risen to above US$30 000 in some countries and remained static or dropped to less than US$200 in others – and similar gaps can be observed within many societies.[20,21] The debt owed to rich countries by the poor amounted to US$2.2 trillion in 1997 – a debt developed and perpetuated through arms trading and ill conceived 'development projects' that did more harm than good and usually benefited developed nations more than those they were allegedly 'developing'. Such debt can never be repaid and perpetuates economic slavery and human misery in more covert guises.[8]

The adverse effects of globalization on health and health policy are evident in the policies of the World Bank and IMF, institutions that have held the balance of power for over 20 years in formulating global health policy. Liberalization of economies, reduced subsidies for basic foods, and shifts in agricultural policy that promote growing export crops to the detriment of home-grown food production, have resulted in devastating malnutrition and starvation that have caused billions to suffer, especially in Africa. Farming subsidies of US$350 billion per year in the USA and Europe coupled to trade protectionism cost developing countries US$50 billion per year in lost income.

It is an indictment of the IMF and World Bank's structural adjustment programmes that they imposed reduced government expenditure on healthcare, education and other social services and encouraged privatization, even within healthcare. Structural adjustment programmes, debt repayments, cuts in aid budgets (especially by the USA), discrimination against African trade, increasing malnutrition and the cold-war activities of the great powers have all played a significant part in sustaining high rates of infectious disease, destabilizing already dysfunctional health services and in fanning the AIDS pandemic.[21,22]

The debt of poor countries is maintained by liaisons between eager lenders, corrupt borrowers and linkages to arms trading. So from 1980–1994, more than 60% of economic aid was spent by developing countries on acquiring arms. The annual interest paid on debt by Africans far exceeds the US$21 billion per year of foreign aid to Africa, and there are many shortcomings in how international aid is applied – thus failing to achieve desired development goals. It is also noteworthy that development aid was progressively reduced over many years (although increased recently) but is now being directed more towards emergency humanitarian aid and the perceived security needs of wealthy nations, rather than towards sustainable development.[23,24]

Military expenditure

A concept of security that relies on force has resulted in industrialized countries spending vast sums of money on the military. In the 1990s, such expenditure averaged 5.3% of GNP (as contrasted with 0.3% on aid for developing countries). By deflecting resources away from true human development over many decades, such militarization and the associated militarism have compromised the health of individuals and nations directly and indirectly – killing, maiming, torture, refugeeism, destruction of livelihoods, starvation, rape, impoverishment of physical, social and mental health, environmental damage and social destabilization, most especially within developing countries where children too have become hardened warriors. Even though military expenditure fell during the 1990s it remained exorbitant and has increased since the onset of the Iraq war.[25,26]

SOCIAL INJUSTICE

Assuming that economic disparities and the causal processes behind these are a major global problem, the dilemma becomes one of addressing the question of economic or distributive justice.

This involves consideration of such overlapping notions as: rights, fairness (equity), equality and what may be deserved. Each of these are complex notions and they may be in conflict with each other. No attempt will be made here to review the many theories of justice that have been formulated as potentially coherent, comprehensive and plausible unifying solutions to such complex issues,[27] except to say that none have provided workable solutions. Some have proposed that theories of imperfect justice could be useful in making progress.[28]

While it is unrealistic to imagine that economic equality can be achieved globally, it is increasingly agreed that it is an ethical requirement that extreme poverty should be alleviated and prevented, and that social injustice be addressed within societies and across national boundaries. Some have suggested that the only way to achieve social justice is to abandon the capitalist system. Others have argued that this is both implausible and impossible, yet agree that major changes are required in the way in which economic systems operate.[10,11,14,18,28,29]

The absence of definitive answers to such complex questions should not engender paralysis. Moral solutions can be identified at the level of institutions and nations. For example in the context of the American healthcare system that is manifestly unjust, inefficient and extraordinarily expensive, a philosophically coherent and practically applicable outline has been provided for progress towards greater justice in healthcare.[30] If a powerful and wealthy country were to set such an example the global impact could be profound.

ETHICS AT THE LEVEL OF INTERNATIONAL RELATIONS

It is also necessary to move beyond considerations of justice only within nations and to attempt reducing injustice at a global level. Searching for and implementing solutions to the problems of poverty, inequality and inequity requires some understanding of how unethical relationships between nations have fostered global disparities and of seeking means of making such relationships more ethical in the future.[12,29,31,32]

INTERNATIONAL LAW AND HUMAN RIGHTS

Cutting across these complex political, social and economic developments there has been growing support for the concept of universal human rights and indeed the idea of Universal Human Rights is now becoming a new standard of civilization, superseding those standards of civilization that dominated over many centuries,[†] and since 1945 an extensive body of international human rights law has been developed.[33]

This new inclusive standard, adherence to which is required for full membership of international society, is now advocated to prevent the violation of human rights within states, and to allow intervention where required to protect the rights of the vulnerable and abused. The UDHR and international human rights law are considered to be capable of playing this role. Human rights consid-

†These range from common culture and language in Ancient Greece, through religion in the medieval era to the concept of the 'white man's civilization' during the age of empire, and the sovereignty of states.

erations have indeed become an everyday, (allegedly) non-partisan part of foreign policy and are of greatest concern in cases of shocking barbarism – for example in Rwanda and in Bosnia, but regrettably also in prisons in the highly industrialized and privileged world.[34,35]

Whether states can respond to moral issues remains contentious. On the one hand sceptics doubt that moral behaviour can be expected of states. On the other hand moralists insist on the highest standard of morality from states. Both extremes seem untenable and yet it seems reasonable to expect at least some degree of moral behaviour from states. Such expectations lie behind the UDHR, International Law and the rules of war. NATO attacks on Serbia (without United Nations approval), in response to the crisis in Kosovo, illustrate the potential for the use and abuse of power and the implications of actions seemingly based on 'humanitarian' concerns.[32,36]

The impact of globalization on human rights

Because the concept of rights was developed in an era in which national sovereignty was respected it becomes clear that another level of complexity is introduced when there is a need to implement human rights under conditions in which the power of states to deliver the rights expected by its citizens is being diluted by the adverse effect of globalizing forces on national economies. Even the extent to which states can control warfare is being diminished and independent warlords and militant groups are capable of waging uncontrollable conflict.[37] As all gradually become citizens of the world, as well as of states, so the ability to deliver on human rights requires both capacity and responsibility that extend beyond the state.[29,32]

WORLD VIEWS: UNDERSTANDING OTHER CULTURES

Optimism for the role of a universal concept of human rights within a state-centric system is not only threatened by globalizing forces. Donnelly, a champion of the human rights approach, has suggested that it can also reasonably be doubted whether universal human rights can constitute an effective international morality, given the degrees of ideological and political diversity that remain in the world. He expresses concern that even if the UDHR appears to be widely accepted it is not clear that its values have genuine significance for all.[33] It is thus necessary to acknowledge that there are many world views and that the West has not worked hard enough to understand the implications of these for making real progress towards a more peaceful world. Attempts by theologians to find the common ground on which all world religions can meet,[38] approaches to understanding how world views are constructed[39] and attention to human needs[40] offer at least some hope that there may be some potential for facilitating processes of peaceful interaction between diverse peoples.

REFLECTIONS ON SOME ETHICAL IMPERATIVES IN OUR MODERN WORLD

The major ethical imperatives of our time – and we should have no difficulty recognizing these unless we are morally blind – are to relieve hunger, alleviate profound poverty, sustainably improve the lives of those living under abominable conditions and to foster global peace and ecological security.[12,29,31] Several United Nations conferences – Rio 1992, Cairo 1994, Copenhagen and Beijing 1995 – and others testify to the growing acknowledgement of these ethical imperatives and the need to enable the processes by educating and empowering women and children. However, insufficient attention has been devoted to the ways in which resources can be generated to achieve these ambitious goals. Scholarly attention and political action directed at ethical and effective use of resources are central to the imperatives to be faced. Suggestions detailed in Chapter 8 in the previous edition include reduction of military expenditure, debt restructuring, implementation of appropriate international taxation, development of imaginative development programmes and new ways of viewing the world and international relations in an increasingly interdependent world.[1] New paradigms of thinking would embrace concern for population well-being as well as individual well-being; deeper insights into how complex systems function; and development of an ethic for institutions and international relations that recognizes the responsibility to balance individual goods and social goods, and not to harm weak and poor nations or groups of people through economic and other forms of exploitation that frustrate the achievement of human rights and well-being.[1,41]

SOME PRACTICAL AND ETHICAL CONSIDERATIONS FOR THE PRACTICE OF TROPICAL MEDICINE

Those who have trained under privileged conditions and then practice or undertake research in deprived contexts are generally ignorant about the local social, economic and political milieu that frames the context in which practice and research is being undertaken. In addition, they seldom have adequate insight into the mind-sets and belief systems of non-westernized peoples and they are insensitive to the differing perceptions of research and healthcare that may prevail in such contexts.[42] Their research generally does little to improve overall healthcare in the regions in which they work. For example the UK MRC has been doing research in the Gambia for over 50 years, yet this research has not been linked to making improvements in healthcare services in this region.[43] Privileged physicians need to better understand that their scientific world view, that allows them to see themselves as nobly advancing knowledge, is to some degree a reflection of their 'local' values. Impoverished research subjects who have benefited little from previous research may have different 'local' values within which a lower value is placed on research and healthcare professionals are seen primarily as providers of care.

The gap between these views could potentially be narrowed by seeking a middle ground through education of physicians and researchers about life in developing countries and about the perceptions of the medical care and research endeavours within specific local contexts. Acquiring such knowledge could facilitate linking to research medical care that would otherwise be unavailable in the research setting in developing countries. Negotiations to achieve these goals should be initiated by researchers and supported both by research ethics committees and by the development of partnerships as discussed below. By meeting the 'local' needs of

researchers, participants and the local healthcare system, the most admirable universal goal could be achieved – advancing knowledge for the purpose of improving health locally and globally.

In order to make the progress mentioned above new paradigms of thinking will be needed. First, we must acknowledge that research does not take place in a vacuum but rather in a world with wide disparities in which much research on vulnerable people has rarely been applied for their benefit. Second, researchers should increasingly view continuation of current patterns of exploitative research as ethically unacceptable. Third, the need to link moral progress to scientific progress should become a high priority. Progress could be made towards such goals by coupling research to improvements in health by linking research to development through partnerships and strategic alliances that could promote sustainability.[44–46]

CONTROVERSIES IN THE ETHICS OF CLINICAL TRIALS

Stimulated by the pharmaceutical industry's desire for new, marketable drugs, clinical research has become a burgeoning activity in recent years. More and more research is being undertaken in developing countries as large numbers of research subjects are needed and it is often easier and more economically favourable to recruit them in developing countries where costs are lower, ethics committees may be viewed as more lenient, and underprivileged subjects are eager to participate regardless of any benefits or the standard of care offered.

This raises serious ethical questions about the relevance and benefit of such research in the developing world. Recent controversies over proposed revisions to the Helsinki Declaration and to the Council for International Organizations of Medical Sciences (CIOMS) guidelines have stimulated renewed interest in the ethics of clinical research in developing countries. The contentiousness of the debate can be explained in part by different perceptions of social relations and of the relationship between research and healthcare. Researchers largely share a scientific world-view and have a primary, if not exclusive interest in advancing knowledge, often accompanied by an interest in financial and other personal and institutional benefits that flow from pharmaceutical companies in search of profit. Underprivileged and deprived research subjects within traditional cultures tend to share a non-scientific world-view, are less wedded to foreign imposition of market rules that do not seem to benefit them, and have a predominant interest in receiving care for their illnesses. Although these differences lie along a spectrum and many values may be shared, the extent of such differences is not trivial and they are of practical importance in developing ethical policies for research.

Despite seeming agreement on several issues, and widespread acceptance of the Declaration of Helsinki and the CIOMS guidelines for research ethics, some conclude that different viewpoints persist on fundamental issues and that it unlikely that current disagreements will be easily resolved.[47] We have argued that disagreements may in part be explained by differing perceptions of social relations and by failure to use moral reasoning to identify the rational middle ground between ethical universalism and moral relativism. We contend that progress can be made towards resolving contentious issues in international research ethics by acknowledging many areas of agreement, and developing a framework for understanding the different perspectives on life by researchers and vulnerable subjects that could facilitate rational responses to disagreements.[48] We reiterate here our summarized approach to resolving these disagreements by posing and answering a series of questions (Boxes 8.2–8.5).[48,49,††]

Attempts to resolve the vexed question of the 'standard of care' for research in developing countries by utilizing arguments totally within a single world-view are unlikely to convince those who have a different perspective on social relations and how these should influence social policy in research. An expanded concept of the standard of care is outlined in Box 8.5.

Box 8.2 What research should be undertaken in developing countries and how should priorities be decided?

- Clinical trials conducted by overseas sponsors in developing countries should be relevant to the health needs of the host country.
- For consideration of the host nation's health priorities host country researchers, research ethics committees and policy makers should be involved in the design, review and conduct of trials.
- They should pursue with overseas investigators, before a trial is approved by the host country research ethics committee, how study findings and other benefits that flow from the research will be incorporated into local healthcare systems.
- Through such advance collaboration host country researchers, subjects and health systems can all benefit in ways that significantly improve local research processes and build capacity for the public health sector.

Box 8.3 What sorts of study designs are acceptable? Can placebos be used and what comparative arms should be included?

- Conditions for use of placebos are described in the Declaration of Helsinki and the CIOMS guidelines but we have suggested that it is not always possible to decide whether it is ethical to use placebos in a particular research project simply by examining a few clauses in such guidelines as general principles, whether in law or ethics, are not self-interpreting.
- Moral reasoning requires consideration of context in the process of applying general, universally-applicable principles.
- Each study in which a placebo arm is anticipated should be considered on its merits, taking into account the research question posed, how this could best be answered, potential harms and benefits, ethical principles and relevant local circumstances.
- Where morally valid reasons can be mounted for placebo-controlled trials, and where such studies are designed specifically for the benefit of local populations rather than as surrogates for acquiring information for wealthy countries (e.g. studies of 'me too' drugs), the use of a placebo may be justified on rational grounds.
- Utilitarian calculations for the benefit of whole groups of people, even with their agreement, should almost never be used to justify a placebo arm when this may result in unnecessary suffering, avoidable injuries or death.
- These recommendations do not imply moral relativism, and the arguments for this have been explicated in greater detail elsewhere.[44,48]

Box 8.4 How do we avoid exploiting research subjects in developing countries?

Exploitation in the research context should be defined to include several acts or omissions:
- Taking advantage of power differentials to meet the researchers' goals through any means they choose, without first giving serious consideration to the harms that may be perceived by research participants or their communities.
- Using research subjects as a means to achieving only the ends of researchers, e.g. advancing knowledge and in many cases the commercial interests of Pharma, when the benefits of the research will not be relevant, affordable, or fairly available to research participants and their communities.
- Undertaking studies in which minimal benefits accrue to participants and large benefits, especially financial, may accrue in the long term to research sponsors, thus failing to ensure fair balance of benefits and burdens to sponsors/researchers and research participants over the longer term.
- Denying participants post-trial use of therapies identified as safe and beneficial in environments where such treatments would not otherwise be affordable and available to subjects in the public health sector.

To avoid exploitation:
- Priority should be given to trials that will provide useful knowledge for the host country.
- The balance of benefits and burdens should be fairly distributed.
- The benefits of research should be seen to flow into healthcare settings.
- While individual subjects' safety and benefits are always important, community and national health priorities must be identified and negotiated with relevant authorities, not just left to individual subjects, the IRB, or the local researcher.
- In no event should existing disparities be further entrenched by deflecting local human or material resources away from healthcare systems in host countries towards research that fails to advance subject, community or national health priorities.

---

††Material is used in this section from previous publications with permission from the journals.[48,49]

> **Box 8.5** What is the standard of care? How is this defined and how can it be justified?
>
> Attempts to resolve the vexed question of the 'standard of care' for research in developing countries by utilizing arguments totally within a single world-view are unlikely to convince those who have a different perspective on social relations and how these should influence social policy in research. An expanded concept of the standard of care is outlined.
>
> ■ A well-reasoned universal standard of care should be translatable into feasible local practices and a universally applicable ethical framework for a standard of care in research must acknowledge practical and morally relevant differences between countries.[44]
> ■ In order to apply universal principles to the context of a specific research project in a particular place, researchers should:
>   – Conduct research with the same respect for the dignity of all subjects wherever they are in the world and always treat them as ends in their own right and not use them merely to acquire knowledge that could benefit only others.
>   – Obtain authentic informed consent that reflects the realities of the economic, social, linguistic and cultural framework of research subjects and their communities.
>   – Provide care for other diseases concomitantly afflicting the subjects and for which treatment may not otherwise be available.
> ■ This alternative to providing the higher level of care that would be available in wealthy countries, but neither relevant nor affordable in local settings, would enhance community benefit from research and progressively ratchet up the standard of care in host countries.
> ■ The above require that researchers, research ethics committees and the community of subjects shape an acceptable standard of care for a particular study through a deliberative, respectful process of moral and scientific reasoning. In this way healthcare could be improved through successive research projects that would step up the standard of care in research towards a global universal level.[44–50]

Moral arguments have been advanced to justify this as opposed to a narrow standard of care (usually limited to which drug can be used in the control arm) that insists on worldwide uniformity.[44]

Simply put, the above position is based on the obligations to:

- Do no harm, do good and to be fair
- Respect practices within other cultures that pose no significant risk to health and safety, but reject those that infringe on universally agreed human rights
- Be sensitive to the adverse invasive social impact of their intrusion into lives and cultures in countries that they do not fully understand.

An improved standard of care that progressively approaches that of rich countries would enhance, not deter, successful achievement of research goals in developing countries.

When a broader standard of care in research is implemented in poor countries, this will highlight the existence of different standards of care in rich and poor countries. Some view the existence of different standards in the context of research as ethically impermissible. It is arguable that when an alternative, locally negotiated standard of care is applied in a poor country and the overall standard of care is ratcheted upwards through research, this represents progress towards better healthcare for vulnerable research participants and populations in poor countries. In research, as in healthcare generally, the perfect should not become the enemy of the realistically achievable. In light of the centuries of neglect and impoverishment of healthcare in poor countries, our inability to achieve immediate equity should not impede realistic, substantial research that could progressively improve healthcare more widely with time and effort. Some might characterize additional and enhanced care offered to poor, vulnerable research subjects as an ethically problematic means of inducement or even coercion. But inducements are only morally wrong if they result in participants taking risks with their health and lives.

Forming partnerships

Growing acknowledgement that much research in developed and developing countries has been exploitative has also led to greater emphasis on the need to focus on diseases of direct relevance to developing countries and to include scientists and others from developing countries in the design and planning of clinical trials.[44–46]

Prior evaluation by a local committee or governing body allows consideration of whether the study findings can, and will, be incorporated into the local healthcare system.

Care should be taken that the research will not inappropriately deflect local human or material resources away from the healthcare system in the host country towards the research project, thus more deeply entrenching existing disparities.

Since the goal of medical research is to improve healthcare for research subjects and their communities, as well as to advance scientific knowledge, closer links should be encouraged between overseas researchers, their sponsors, host country investigators, communities, and health authorities. To be effective, this collaboration must be authentic, not simply pro forma, and must be done in advance of submitting research protocols to the host country research ethics committee. These justifications and examples of how they have been applied in practice have been described in detail elsewhere.[44]

RESEARCH ETHICS COMMITTEES

The role of research committees is to evaluate research proposals with special attention to risk/benefit ratios, equity in distribution of benefits and burdens, potential conflicts of interest, the adequacy of information provided for subjects, and the protection of freedom of choice. Their second, equally important but less widely implemented role is to educate and assist faculty, researchers and other stakeholders in the community to understand and appreciate the ethics of research. A third, increasingly acknowledged but even less widely implemented, function is to monitor and audit research, and to provide accountability to the public.[42]

Given the growth of research in developing countries and the relative lack of training in research ethics the United States NIH's Fogarty International Center has in recent years sponsored capacity building programmes in international research ethics and bioethics in developing countries.[51] The contribution being made to educational and capacity-building endeavours by these programmes is of great importance in an era in which international collaborative research is expanding rapidly, and cross-cultural understanding is required. Research committees are being encouraged to proactively work to ensure benefits to participants, and the community.

BIOBANKS

Although personal information regarding genetic and other diseases has long been uncontroversially stored in databases, the storage of biological material for the purpose of future research has taken on new implications in the era of genetic biotechnology and computerization. Concerns include the use of such information to stigmatize and discriminate against individuals or groups; exploitation through commercialization of new information with limited if any benefits to those who provided the samples; emphasis on DNA sequences and neglect of social and environmental factors shaping health and disease. Reliance on adequate informed consent has been suggested as a means of overcoming such concerns. However, the difficulty in obtaining truly informed consent, especially from vulnerable subjects, undermines this as a protective measure. Some authors have suggested that other ethical principles can be invoked. For example, the duty to contribute to research by showing solidarity with fellow humans in order to facilitate scientific and medical advances. If it were possible to link the sharing of benefits from research with individuals and communities this would strengthen the validity of the principle of solidarity.[52] Give the extent to which vulnerable subjects in poor countries have not benefited proportionately from research involving them it is likely that controversies over biobanks will continue, although a single study in Uganda has shown that the majority were willing to participate in such research.[53]

CONCLUSIONS

Reducing the burden of tropical diseases and fostering greater human well-being on a global scale will require acknowledgement that unbridled materialism and wasteful consumerism are associated with impoverishment of the human spirit and threaten the lives of billions. Perpetual economic growth for some cannot continue at the expense of others without sacrificing our humanity. The forces that sustain poverty should be studied more seriously and constructively addressed. The poor are not poor because they are lazy, incompetent or corrupt. While poor countries must also accept some blame for their condition, the causes of poverty are much more complex. Powerful nations need to resolve to deal with the upstream causes of intolerable economic disparities in which they are deeply implicated through such processes as described above. Their wealth, their sense of entitlement and their moral insensitivity are as problematic as the existence of poverty.

Crucial to a new approach will be the recognition that it is not merely altruism that is called for but more importantly a long-term perspective on rational self-interest in an increasingly interdependent world. To achieve this will require a broader approach to morality that firmly embraces but also goes beyond the concept of human rights, and includes concern for human needs worldwide and for the environment on which all life is crucially dependent. Sustainable development and respect for human rights and

human dignity are in the interest of all worldwide. These can only be achieved through a combination of analytically incisive and honest thinking about global problems and the active promotion of solidarity devoid of economic, cultural, and ethical imperialism. It should also be acknowledged that all people and cultures have something to contribute to the development of a more just world. The goal of achieving a global mindset to which all can contribute is the challenge for the twenty-first century.[54] If this can be achieved the prospects of reducing suffering from tropical diseases will be greatly enhanced.

REFERENCES

1. Benatar SR. Ethics and tropical diseases: a global perspective. In: Cook G, Zumla A, eds. *Manson's Tropical Diseases.* 21st edn. Edinburgh: Elsevier Science; 2003:85–93.
2. United Nations Development Program. *Human Development Report.* New York: Oxford University Press; 1998.
3. Commission on Health Research for Development. *Health research: essential link to equity in development.* Oxford: Oxford University Press; 1990.
4. Benatar SR. Human rights in the biotechnology era: a story of two lives and two worlds. In: Bhatia GS, O'Neil JS, Gall GL, et al., eds. *Peace, Justice and Freedom.* Edmonton: University of Alberta Press; 1998:245–257.
5. Burley J, ed. *The Genetic Revolution and Human Rights.* Oxford: Oxford University Press; 1999.
6. Alexander T. *Unravelling Global Apartheid: An Overview of World Politics.* Cambridge: Polity Press; 1996.
7. Richmond AH. *Global Apartheid: Refugees, Racism and the New World Order.* Toronto: Oxford University Press; 1996.
8. Pettifor A. *Debt, The Most Potent Form of Slavery: A Discussion of The Role of Western Lending Policies in Supporting the Economies of Poor Countries.* London: Debt Crisis Network; 1996.
9. WHO. *Investing in Health, Research and Development. Report of the Ad-hoc Committee on Health's Research Relating to Future Intervention Options.* Geneva: World Health Organization; 1996.
10. Heilbroner R. *Twenty-first Century Capitalism.* London: WW Norton; 1993.
11. Falk R. *Predatory Globalisation: A Critique.* Cambridge: Polity Press; 1999.
12. Pogge T. *World Poverty and Human Rights.* Cambridge: Polity Press; 2002.
13. McMichael T. *Human Frontiers, Environments and Disease: Past Patterns, Uncertain Futures.* Cambridge: Cambridge University Press; 2001.
14. Galbraith JK. *The Culture of Contentment.* Boston: Houghton Mifflin; 1992.
15. Lerner M. *The Belief in a Just World: A Fundamental Delusion.* New York: Plenum Press; 1980.
16. WHO. *Renewing health for all strategy: elaboration of a policy for equity, solidarity and health.* Geneva: World Health Organization; 1995.
17. Ralph J. American democracy and democracy promotion. Review article. *Int Affairs* 2001; 77:129–140.
18. Gill S, Bakker I. New constitutionalism and the social reproduction of caring institutions. *Theoretical Medicine and Bioethics* 2006; 27(1):35–57.
19. Koivusalo M. The impact of economic globalization on health. *Theor Med Bioethics* 2006; 27(1):13–34.
20. Abbasi K. The World Bank and health. *BMJ* 1999; 318:1132–1135.
21. Global Health Watch. *Global Health Watch 2005–2006: An Alternative World Health Report.* London: Zed Books; 2005.
22. Nandy S, Scott R, Logie TE, et al. Realistic priorities for AIDS control. *Lancet* 2000; 356:1525–1526.
23. Lancaster C. *Transforming Foreign Aid: United States Assistance in the 21st Century.* Washington, DC: Institute for International Economics; 2000:108.
24. Woods N. The shifting politics of foreign aid. *Int Aff* 2005; 81:393–409.
25. Sivard RL. *World Military and Social Expenditure.* 16th edn. Washington, DC: World Priorities Press; 1996.

26. Mahmudi-Azer S. Arms trade and its impact on health. *Theoretical Medicine and Bioethics* 2006; 27(1):81–93.

27. Arthur J, Shaw WH. *Justice and Economic Distribution.* 2nd edn. Englewood Cliffs, NJ: Prentice-Hall, 1991.

28. Sreenivasan G. International justice and health: a proposal. *Ethics Int Aff* 2002; 16:81–90.

29. Caney S. *Justice Beyond Borders: A Global Political Theory.* Oxford: Oxford University Press; 2005.

30. Buchanan AE. Privatisation and just healthcare. *Bioethics* 1995; 9: 220–239.

31. Singer P. *One World: The Ethics of Globalization.* New Haven: Yale University Press; 2002.

32. Buchanan A. *Justice, Legitimacy, and Self-Determination: Moral Foundations for International Law.* Oxford: Oxford University Press; 2004.

33. Donnelly J. Human rights: a new standard of civilisation? *Int Relations* 1998; 74:1–24.

34. Amnesty International. *The United States of America: Rights for All.* London: Amnesty International; 1998.

35. Cassese A. *Inhuman States: Imprisonment, Torture and Detention in Europe Today.* Cambridge: Polity Press; 1996.

36. Brown C. *Understanding International Relations.* London: Macmillan; 1997.

37. Friman HR, Andreas P, eds. *The Illicit Global Economy and State Power.* Oxford: Rowman and Littlefield; 1999.

38. Kung H. *Global Responsibility: In Search of a New World Ethic.* New York: Continuum Press; 1993.

39. Smart N. *World Views Cross-Cultural Explorations of Human Beliefs.* 2nd edn. Englewood Cliffs: Prentice-Hall; 1995.

40. Doyal L, Gough I. *A Theory of Human Need.* London: Macmillan; 1991.

41. Challenges for global health in the 21st century: some upstream considerations. *Theor Med Bioeth* 2006; 27(1):3–114.

42. Benatar SR. Some reflections and recommendations on research ethics in developing countries. *Soc Sci Med* 2002; 54:1131–1141.

43. WHO. Country Health System Fact Sheet 2006: Gambia. Online. Available: http://www.afro.who.int/home/countries/fact_sheets/gambia.pdf possible to compare with http://www.afro.who.int/home/countries/fact_sheets/malawi.pdf 24 June 2008.

44. Shapiro K, Benatar SR. HIV prevention research and global inequality: towards improved standards of care. *J Med Ethics* 2005; 31:39–47.

45. Costello A, Zumla A. Moving to research partnerships in developing countries. *BMJ 2000*; 321:827–829.

46. Lo B, Bayer R. Establishing ethical trials for treatment and prevention of AIDS in developing countries. *BMJ* 2003; 327:337–339.

47. Macklin R. After Helsinki: unresolved issues in international research. *Kennedy Inst Ethics J* 2001; 11(1):17–36.

48. Benatar SR. Towards progress in resolving dilemmas in international research ethics. *J Law Med Ethics* 2004; 32(4):574–582.

49. Benatar SR, Fleischer TE. Ethical and policy implications of clinical drug trials in developing countries. *Harvard Health Policy Rev* 2005; 6(1): 97–105.

50. Benatar SR, Singer PA. A new look at international research ethics. *BMJ* 2000; 321:824–826.

51. Fogarty International Center. *International Research Ethics Education and Curriculum Development Award.* Online. Available: http://www.fic.nih.gov/programs/training_grants/bioethics/index.htm 20 Nov 2006.

52. Chadwick R, Berg K. Solidariy and Equity: new ethical frameworks for genetic databases. *Nat Rev Genet* 2001; 31(2):80321.

53. Wendler D, Pace C, Talisuna AO, et al. Research on stored biological samples: the views of Ugandans. *IRB: Ethics Hum Rights* 2005; 27(2): 1–5.

54. Benatar SR, Daar AS, Singer PA. Global health ethics: the rationale for mutual caring. *Int Aff* 2003; 79:107–138.

Chapter 9   Gary Maartens, Peter Mwaba and
Alimuddin I. Zumla

General Approach to the Patient

INTRODUCTION

The knowledge base of medicine in the tropics has grown rapidly[1,2] yet the fundamental practice of clinical medicine in the tropics remains more of an 'art' than a 'science'. The ability to establish a sympathetic rapport with the patient, understand the social, cultural and economic reasons underlying the patient's ill health, elicit the important parts of the history, identify the important physical signs and make sound judgements in the absence of sophisticated technological help, and maintain the highest ethical standards when dealing with patients from different ethnic and cultural backgrounds constitutes the 'art' of the practice of medicine in the tropics.

Despite the technological advances of the past two decades,[3] history taking and physical examination remain the mainstay of the practice of medicine.[4-6] Clinical acumen is of paramount importance in arriving at a correct diagnosis when medicine is practised in rural areas of the tropics or where laboratory back-up is scarce or unavailable. Even when modern technology is available, the medical practitioner can greatly enhance patient management by meticulous evaluation and by recognizing the multiple, often asymptomatic, pathologies that are a frequent feature of disease in the tropical context. Furthermore, non-infectious medical conditions are also common and may easily be overlooked (Figures 9.1–9.19).

The spectrum of diseases in tropical areas has changed considerably in the last two decades.[1] Rapid urbanization in the tropics has led to a rise in diseases associated with obesity, smoking and reduced physical activity: diabetes mellitus, hypertension and atheromatous cardiovascular diseases (see Chapters 12, 37 and 38).[7] At the same time, there have been successful campaigns that have reduced the incidence of many tropical diseases: examples include measles, polio, onchocerciasis, dracunculiasis, and leprosy. However, the rapid and devastating spread of the human immunodeficiency virus (HIV) epidemic has substantially changed the practice of medicine in the tropics and has added another complex dimension to the interpretation of symptoms and signs.[8,9] HIV/AIDS, because of its protean manifestations, should be at the back of every clinician's mind and included in the differential diagnosis of many clinical problems.

As the numbers of tourists from industrialized countries travelling to developing countries continue to increase, medical practitioners, particularly those in temperate countries, need to be mindful of the importance of taking an accurate travel history. This chapter attempts to cover 'a general approach' to the patient who lives in the tropics or acquired disease while visiting the tropics.

CLINICAL HISTORY

Most symptoms in tropical practice are system-specific. The physician's knowledge of clinical syndromes, disease epidemiology and geographical medicine will often lead to a specific diagnosis. There are several important aspects of the history to which particular attention should be given, irrespective of whether the patient lives in the tropics or is a returning traveller. A checklist for important components of the history is presented in Table 9.1.

Travel

A precise list of places visited in chronological order, together with the extent of rural travel and exposure to water (rivers, streams, lakes) and animals, must be obtained, as many diseases show a marked geographical variation in endemicity and prevalence. For instance, in the differential diagnosis of a feverish illness, bartonellosis would only be considered in visitors to, or residents of, Andean valleys in Peru, Ecuador or Colombia, whereas malaria and typhoid are so widespread as to necessitate consideration after any tropical or subtropical exposure. Some infections are common and widespread but are only acquired in certain well-defined circumstances or exposures. For example: (a) mosquitoes are widespread in the tropics and a range of infections can be transmitted by them including malaria (Chapter 73), arboviruses (Chapter 40) and filariasis (Chapter 84); (b) tick bites can transmit typhus, Colorado tick fever, Lyme disease and relapsing fever (see Chapter 49); (c) dog bites may be responsible for rabies (Chapter 44) or bacterial sepsis, sometimes with esoteric bacteria such as *Capnocytophaga canimorsus*; (d) schistosomiasis after contact with fresh water (see Chapter 82), (e) rickettsial diseases following the bite of specific arthropod vectors in restricted ecological niches, (f) variant Creutzfeldt–Jakob disease after contact with bovine spon-

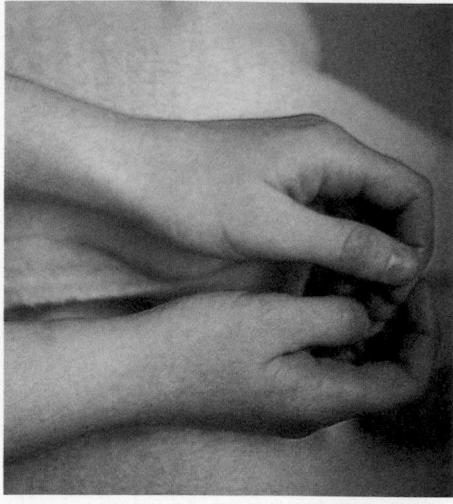

Figure 9.1 Transient swelling over the wrist in *Loa loa* infection.

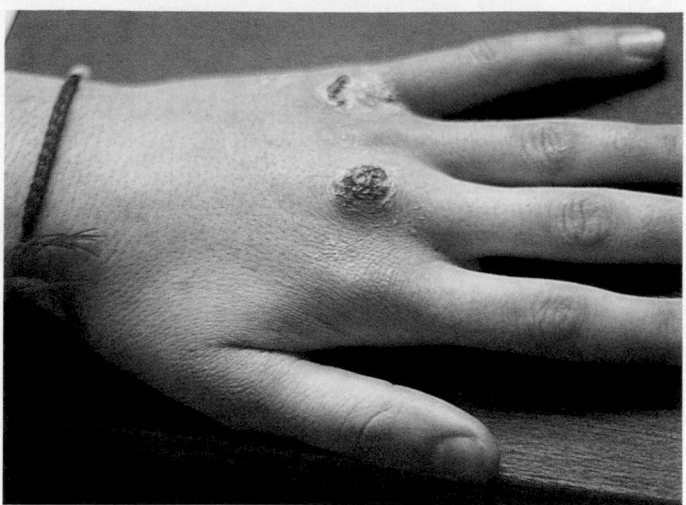

Figure 9.4 Crusted ulcers in *Staphylococcus* species: infected insect bites.

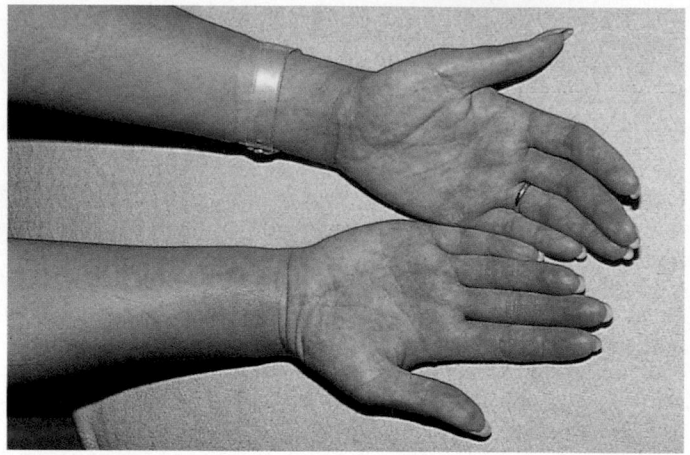

Figure 9.2 Transient swelling over the wrist in gnathostomiasis.

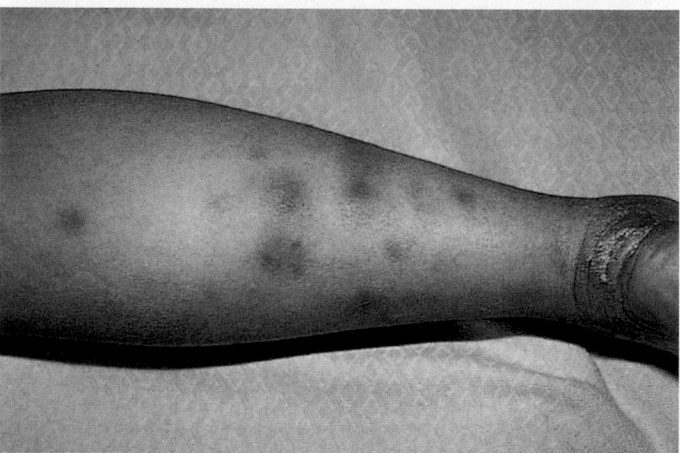

Figure 9.5 Painful nodules on the legs in erythema induratum (Bazin's disease) – related to tuberculosis.

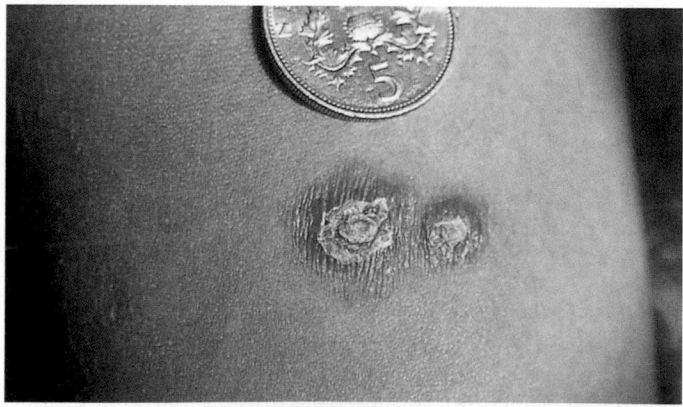

Figure 9.3 Crusted ulcers in cutaneous leishmaniasis.

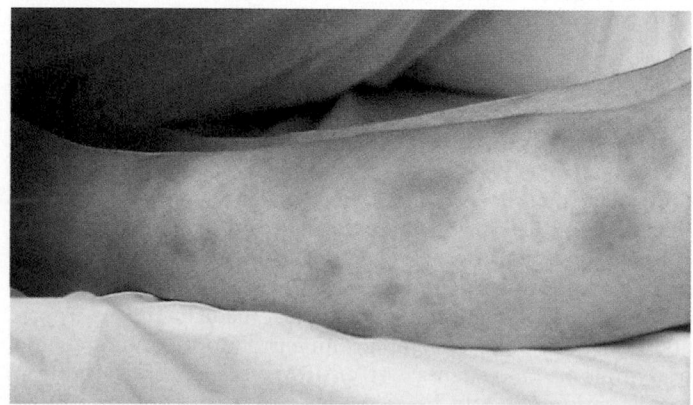

Figure 9.6 Painful nodules on the legs in erythema nodosum – related to tuberculosis.

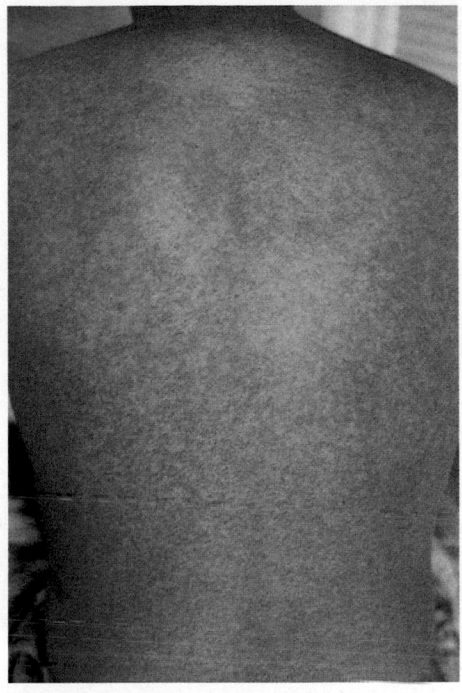

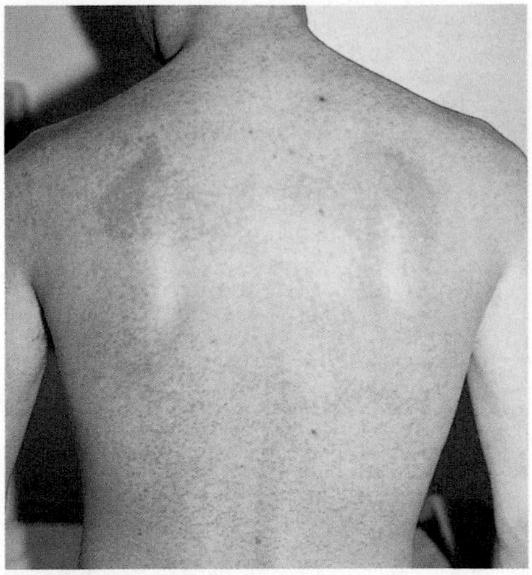

Figure 9.8 Non-confluent maculopapular rash due to rubella infection.

Figure 9.7 Non-confluent maculopapular rash due to Dengue fever.

Table 9.1 Checklist in history taking

Ethnic origin	
Occupation	e.g. farmer, fisherman, abattoir worker, cave explorer
Travel history	e.g. countries and places visited, contact with rivers, lakes, animals
Prophylaxis	e.g. immunizations, malaria prophylaxis, insect repellants, sunscreens
Treatment	e.g. blood transfusions, injections, traditional medicine, scarification, tattoos, splenectomy, gastrectomy
Drugs	e.g. antimalarials, antibiotics, antihypertensives, analgesics, hypoglycaemics, intravenous drug abuse, alcohol and other substance abuse, traditional medicines, over-the-counter medications
Diet	e.g. vegans, food fads, seafood, undercooked meat/fish/snails, traditional brews, safety of drinking water
Sex	e.g. sexual orientation, unprotected sex, multiple sexual partners, commercial sex
Allergies	e.g. seasonal, antibiotic, food, insect bite, plant
Bites	insect (e.g. mosquito, fleas, lice, tick, mite, tsetse fly, blackfly, horsefly), snake (see Chapter 31), carnivore (e.g. dog, cat, mongoose, jackal, leopard); arachnid (e.g. spider, scorpion, tarantula); monkey; human
Pets	birds (e.g. parakeets, budgies), dogs, cats
Family history	e.g. diabetes, sickle cell anaemia, tuberculosis, asthma, hypertension, epilepsy, partner with HIV/AIDS

giform encephalopathy-infected cattle products (although not yet a problem in tropical countries, a tropical student studying in Britain may have contracted it). It follows that the physician should be aware of the epidemiology of the disease(s) under consideration.

Ethnic origin, gender issues and cultural factors

There are marked ethnic differences in disease incidence. Some of these differences are due to genetic disorders. Familial Mediter-ranean fever may present with acute fever and pain in certain Middle Eastern races, whereas a similar presentation in a West African would bring sickle cell disease to mind. Other ethnic differences in incidence are related more to exposure to pathogens than to genetic predisposition – for instance, tuberculosis in the UK is more common in patients originating from the Indian subcontinent.

The presentation of disease is greatly influenced by cultural factors and gender issues.[10] Sensitivity to different cultures and the role of gender is of paramount importance for all clinicians in

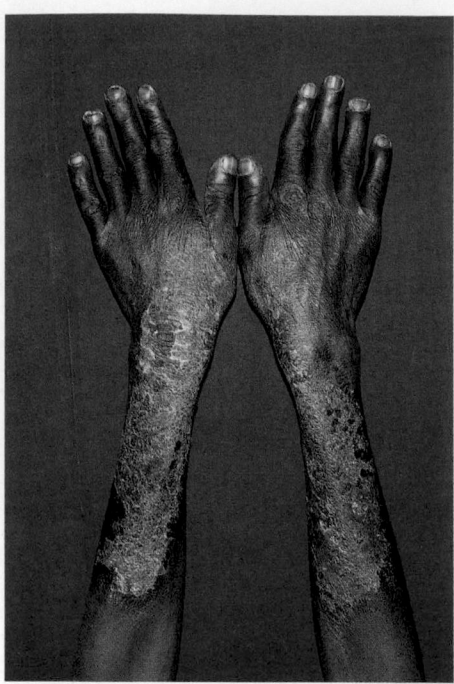

Figure 9.9 Skin rash (dermatitis) in pellagra.

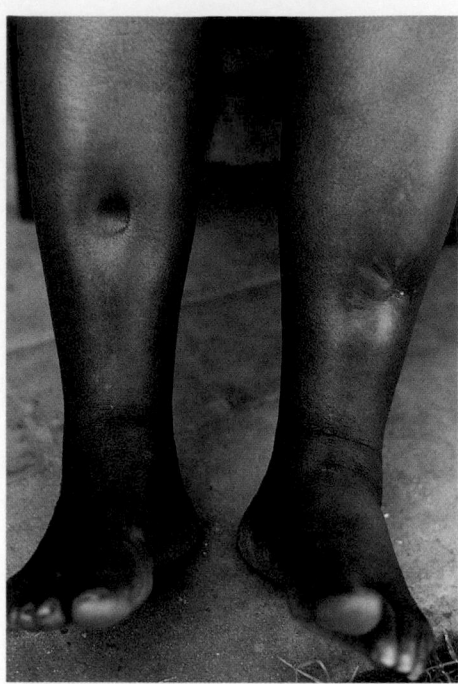

Figure 9.10 Pitting oedema in a patient with nephrotic syndrome.

tropical areas, especially when the clinician is from a different cultural background. In many cultures diseases are believed to result from bewitchment or disturbed ancestors. Although these beliefs contradict scientific understanding, they must be respected. It can be very difficult to distinguish appropriate but exaggerated religious experiences from psychiatric disease in certain ethnic groups and a great deal of reliance must be placed on the opinions of others from the same culture. Many patients will first consult a traditional healer. This, together with the fact that access to health-care facilities is often poor, frequently results in late presentation of disease. It is clearly desirable to speak and understand a patient's language when taking a history, but this is not always possible. Interpreters who have not undergone medical training may unintentionally change the patient's or clinician's intended meaning.

Diet

Malnutrition is common in tropical areas, particularly in children who may present with marasmus or kwashiorkor (see Chapter 23). 'Road to health' height and weight charts are essential tools in tropical paediatrics. Malnutrition becomes almost universal in extended droughts or when large groups of people are displaced by war or persecution. Vitamin deficiencies are frequently seen in areas where people depend on limited staple foods – beriberi is common in areas where rice is a staple food and pellagra where maize is a staple. Nutritional megaloblastic anaemia is common in pregnancy or lactation due to folate deficiency or in vegans due to vitamin B_{12} deficiency. Iron deficiency anaemia is very common in children and menstruating women due to a combination of poor diet and hookworm infestation. Abdominal pain in a Muslim patient during Ramadan may be caused by renal colic due to ureteric stones after self-imposed water deprivation during day-

light hours in a hot environment. Diseases due to dietary excess are becoming increasingly common in the tropics. Obesity occurs frequently with urbanization, resulting in increased frequency and severity of diabetes and hypertension. Dietary iron overload is common in central and southern Africa due to cooking and beer brewing in iron pots.

Ingestion of contaminated water or unwashed fruit and vegetables can lead to several infections such as amoebiasis, hepatitis A and E, leptospirosis, typhoid, cholera, salmonellosis and shigellosis. Unpasteurized milk and dairy products are responsible for the transmission of brucellosis, listeriosis, Q fever and tuberculosis. Undercooked meat may transmit a range of infections, including tapeworm, trichinosis, salmonellosis and toxoplasmosis. Fish or shellfish, particularly if uncooked, can transmit infections such as cholera, gastroenteritis (e.g. *Vibrio parahaemolyticus*), hepatitis A or parasites (e.g. anisakiasis, gnathostomiasis, diphyllobothriasis or paragonimiasis). Ciguatera poisoning is caused by the consumption of fish that have accumulated toxic dinoflagellates in certain tropical areas.

Sexual contacts

Sexually transmitted infections (STIs) are rampant worldwide (see Chapter 21). Several STIs occur much more frequently in the tropics, e.g. chancroid. Care and sensitivity are required in approaching a patient with STIs and patients must be encouraged to bring their partners for treatment. STIs frequently present with extragenital manifestations; hence, polyarthropathy, papular skin rash and fever may be the presenting features of gonococcaemia; likewise, an illness that includes a generalized rash and lymphadenopathy could be caused by secondary syphilis. HIV is endemic throughout the tropics, where it is mainly transmitted by hetero-

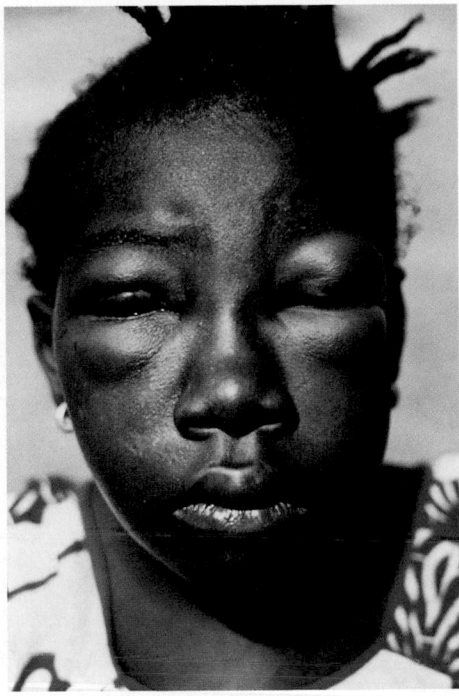

Figure 9.11 Bilateral facial oedema in nephrotic syndrome.

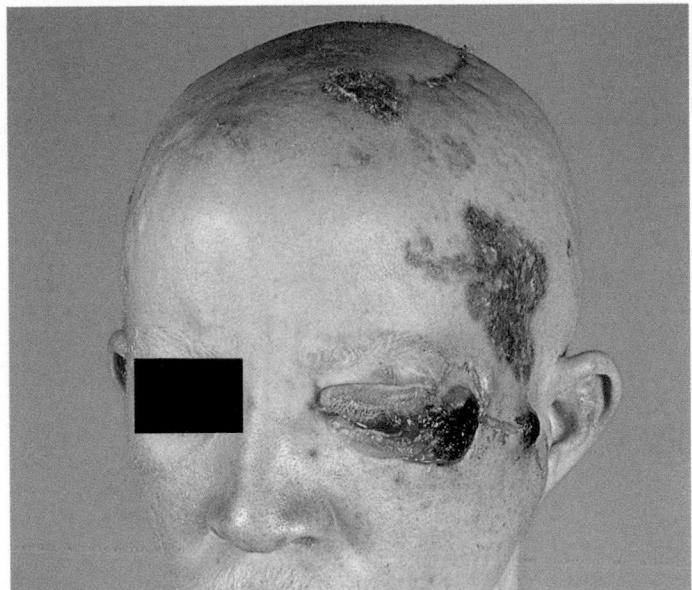

Figure 9.13 Squamous cell carcinoma in an African patient with albinism.

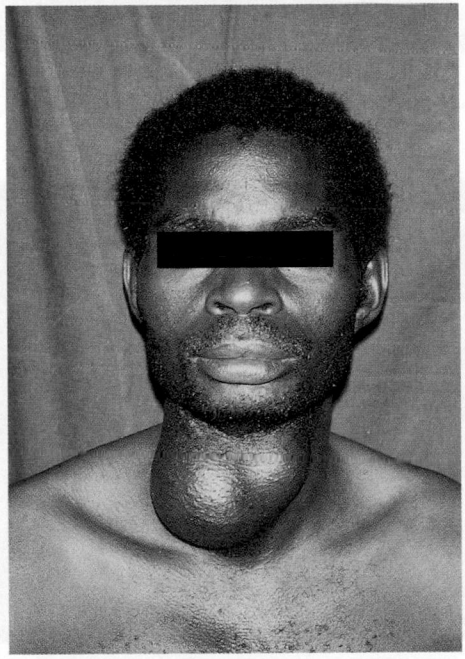

Figure 9.12 Endemic goitre.

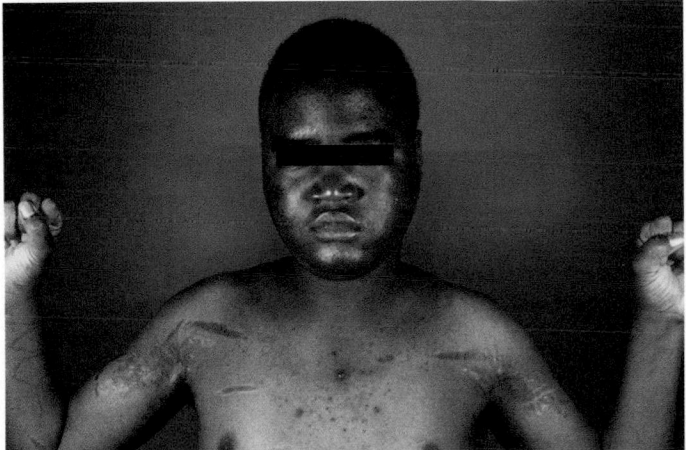

Figure 9.14 Cushingoid facies with cutaneous striae.

sexual coitus, and should be suspected as a cause or co-factor in virtually any febrile illness.

Vaccines, drugs and traditional medicines

A history of relevant vaccination should not be used as a reason to exclude any infection from the differential diagnosis, since vac-cination is never 100% effective and errors within the vaccine chain do occur. In the same way, the appropriate use of antima-larial prophylactic drugs does not eliminate all risk for this infec-tion but may decrease blood parasite counts to undetectable levels, thereby delaying diagnosis. Broad-spectrum antibiotics are freely available to the general public without prescription in many parts of the world and their prior use may prevent microbiological diagnosis in bacterial disease, as well as actually causing ill-health through side-effects, such as diarrhoea. Patients often consult tra-ditional medicine healers (see Chapter 4) and use herbal remedies but they may be reluctant to admit this. There are undoubtedly many effective traditional therapies. For example, the highly effica-cious artemesinin antimalarials are derived from the Chinese

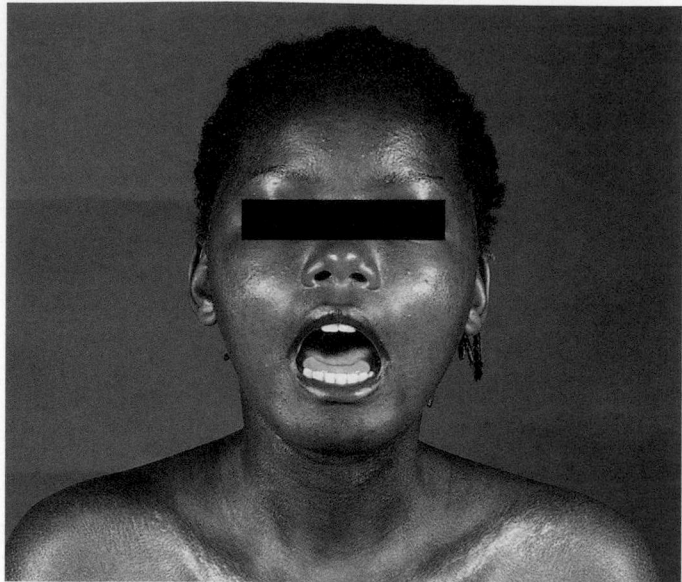

Figure 9.15 Systemic sclerosis restricting mouth opening.

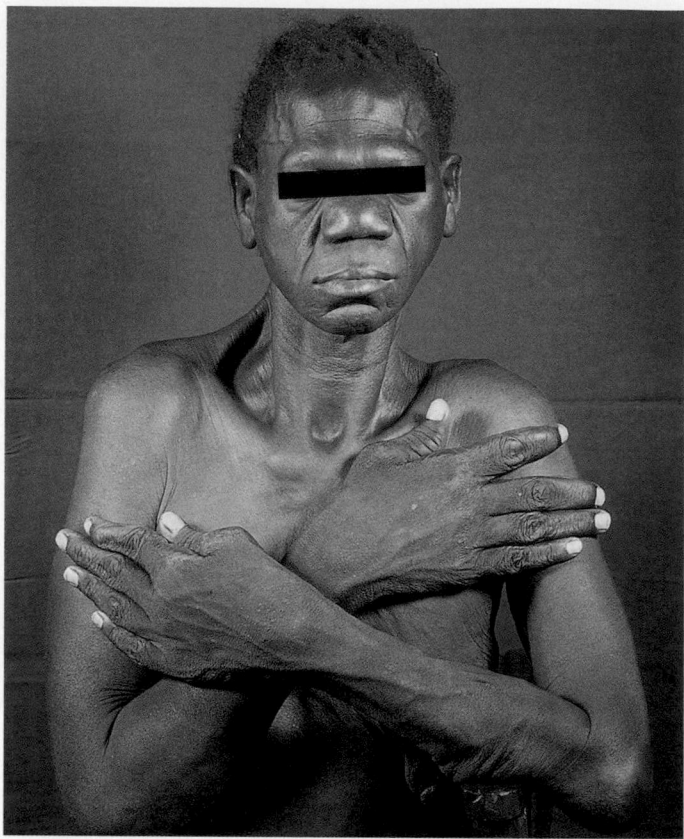

Figure 9.17 Acromegaly (large hands and prominent facial features).

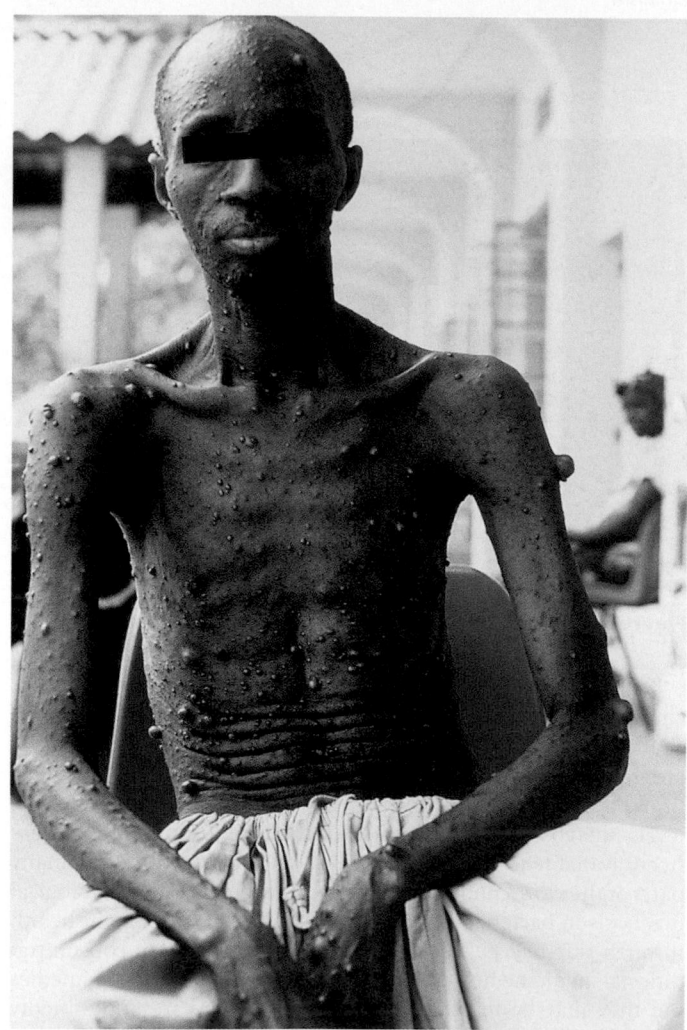

Figure 9.16 Multiple nodules of neurofibromatosis.

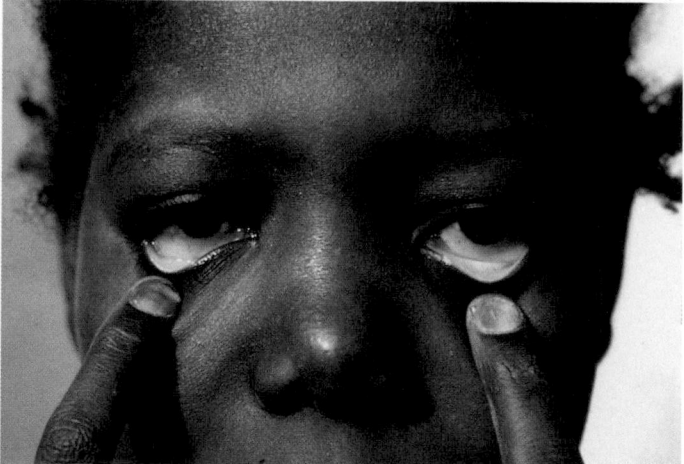

Figure 9.18 Pallor (anaemia) and koilonychia due to iron deficiency anaemia resulting from hookworm infestation.

herbal remedy qinghaosu. However, some herbal preparations can also cause ill-health, especially when impurities such as heavy metals are present, and severe symptoms may ensue. Acute toxicities which have been described in patients after consuming substances from traditional healers include psychosis, coma, renal failure, haemorrhagic gastroenteritis and fulminant hepatic

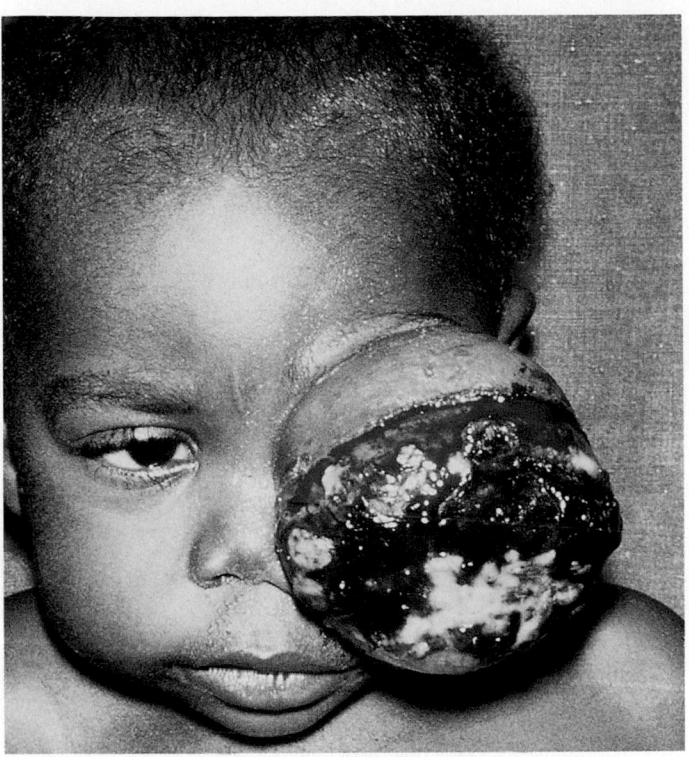

Figure 9.19 Advanced retinoblastoma in a Zambian child.

Table 9.2 Cryptic causes of weight loss

WEIGHT LOSS WITH ANOREXIA
Acquired immune deficiency syndrome
Extrapulmonary tuberculosis
Malignancy (hepatoma, lymphoma, cervical carcinoma, colon and others)
Amoebic liver abscess
Infective endocarditis
Visceral leishmaniasis
Brucellosis
Giardiasis
Hydatid disease
Schistosomiasis
Depression
WEIGHT LOSS WITHOUT ANOREXIA
Gut helminths
Diabetes mellitus
Thyrotoxicosis
Malabsorption
Drugs

failure. Chronic toxicities include hepatic fibrosis and hepatic veno-occlusive disease.

Weight loss, anorexia and malaise

These are relatively common presenting complaints and, for the most part, are readily attributable to associated disease; however, they may dominate the clinical presentation in situations where the aetiology is not obvious. Diseases to be considered in this circumstance are listed in Table 9.2.

Diarrhoea and vomiting

Diarrhoea is a frequent presenting complaint and in most patients will be caused by an acute gastrointestinal infection (Table 9.3). Gastrointestinal symptoms are frequent in patients with advanced HIV disease. Some extraintestinal diseases, such as Legionnaires' disease, malaria, measles, Addison's disease or diabetic ketoacidosis, can occasionally masquerade as gastroenteritis. Vomiting commonly accompanies diarrhoea and may predominate in viral gastrointestinal infections and toxin-associated food poisoning (*Staphylococcus aureus*, *Bacillus cereus*, ciguatera poisoning). Vomiting may also occur with a wide variety of non-gastrointestinal infections (severe malaria, meningitis and hepatitis).

GENERAL EXAMINATION

Multiple pathology is common within the context of tropical disease[11] and the clinician should not be surprised to find physical abnormalities additional to those expected from the primary com-

plaint (Figures 9.1–9.19). The general examination should include an assessment of nutritional status. Wasting or failure to thrive due to HIV/AIDS, the cachexia of chronic disease (especially tuberculosis), malnutrition or malabsorption, is a common finding. Anaemia, often on a nutritional basis, is common. Several vitamin deficiencies (pellagra, rickets and scurvy) produce characteristic features on general examination (described in Chapter 30). Angular stomatitis and glossitis may suggest associated vitamin B deficiencies. Clinical features of kwashiorkor include oedema, thin hypopigmented hair and dermatological lesions (described in Chapter 30).

Common causes of generalized oedema are the same clinical syndromes as those in industrialized countries (cardiac failure, glomerulonephritis, nephrotic syndrome and cirrhosis) but with a different aetiological spectrum (see Chapters 10, 12 and 15). Lymphoedema in the tropics may be due to filariasis (see Chapter 84) or Kaposi's sarcoma. Focal migratory oedema, typically on the limbs, occurs in loiasis (Calabar swellings) and gnathostomiasis. Unilateral orbital oedema (Romaña's sign) suggests acute Chagas' disease in endemic areas. Bilateral periorbital oedema is a feature of trichinosis but is more commonly found in renal disease and malnutrition.

Classic facies of selected diseases in the tropics include frontal bossing (associated with sickle cell anaemia or β-thalassaemia major), risus sardonicus (tetanus), leonine facies (lepromatous leprosy), lupus vulgaris (tuberculosis) and saddle nose (congenital syphilis).

Erythema nodosum has a wide differential diagnosis – in the tropics streptococcal infection, primary tuberculosis, leprosy, yersiniosis, lymphogranuloma venereum and the endemic mycoses should be considered.

Table 9.3 Common aetiologies of diarrhoea (and vomiting)

ACUTE WATERY DIARRHOEA (DURATION <2 WEEKS)	
Bacterial infections	*Vibrio cholerae*
	Salmonella spp.
	Campylobacter jejuni
	Escherichia coli (enterotoxigenic, enteropathogenic and enteroadherent)
	Shigella sonnei
	Yersinia enterocolitica
	Legionella pneumophila
Viral infections	HIV enteropathy
	Rotavirus and other enteric viruses
Protozoal infections	Malaria (*Plasmodium* spp.)
	Giardia lamblia
	Cryptosporidium parvum
	Microsporidia spp.
	Isospora belli
	Sarcocystis spp.
Toxin diarrhoea	*Clostridium perfringens* (toxin)
	Staphylococcus aureus (toxin)
	Bacillus cereus (stable toxin)
	Ciguatera fish poisoning

BLOODY DIARRHOEA	
	Shigella spp.
	Campylobacter jejuni
	Salmonella spp.
	Enteroinvasive and enterohaemorrhagic *E. coli*
	Clostridium perfringens (necrotizing enterocolitis, pigbel)

	Yersinia spp.
	Clostridium difficile (pseudomembranous colitis)
	Schistosoma spp. (intestinal schistosomiasis)
	Entamoeba histolytica (amoebiasis)
	Balantidium coli
	Inflammatory bowel disease (Crohn's disease or ulcerative colitis)

CHRONIC DIARRHOEA (DURATION >3 WEEKS)
Giardia lamblia
Entamoeba histolytica
Tropical enteropathy and tropical 'sprue'
HIV enteropathy
Ileocaecal tuberculosis
Shigella spp.
Enteroadherent *E. coli*
Strongyloides stercoralis
Trichuris trichiura
Capillaria philippinensis
Chronic pancreatitis
Schistosomiasis
Disaccharide intolerance
Lactose intolerance
Post-infective irritable bowel syndrome (IBS)
Inflammatory bowel disease (IBD)
Coeliac disease

Several features on general examination are highly suggestive of HIV/AIDS (see Chapter 20): generalized lymphadenopathy (see below), bilateral cystic parotidomegaly, oral hairy leucoplakia, oral candidiasis, zoster in patients younger than 50 years, papular pruritic eruption (associated marked postinflammatory hyperpigmentation is particularly common in Africa), hyperpigmantation of the nails (melanonychia), extensive seborrhoeic dermatitis, giant mucocutaneous herpes simplex virus ulcers and Kaposi's sarcoma.

Skin

The skin is frequently involved in systemic disease, e.g. petechiae in meningococcal sepsis, the hypopigmentation and flaking appearance of kwashiorkor and the photosensitive dermatitis of pellagra. Many problems in tropical disease practice may manifest themselves dermatologically and infections of the skin are especially common. It is often difficult to recognize many of the exanthemas on a dark-coloured skin. This subject is extensively dealt with in Chapter 19.

Fever

The symptom of fever should always be confirmed by measuring the temperature. Normal temperature is <37.2°C, but fever is generally diagnosed when it is 38°C or more. Most patients with significant fever will have an infection, but non-infectious diseases may also cause fever; this is particularly true of patients presenting with chronic fever (>2 weeks' duration). Absence of fever does not exclude severe infection, particularly in the elderly. Hypothermia may occur in severe sepsis. Many patients present with fever with no obvious focus of infection.

Fever patterns

The pattern of fever may be helpful in determining the underlying cause but the importance of fever patterns has been over-emphasized in earlier texts. The most characteristic pattern is periodic fever every second or third day in established tertian or quartan malaria, respectively (Figure 9.20). It is important to note that in

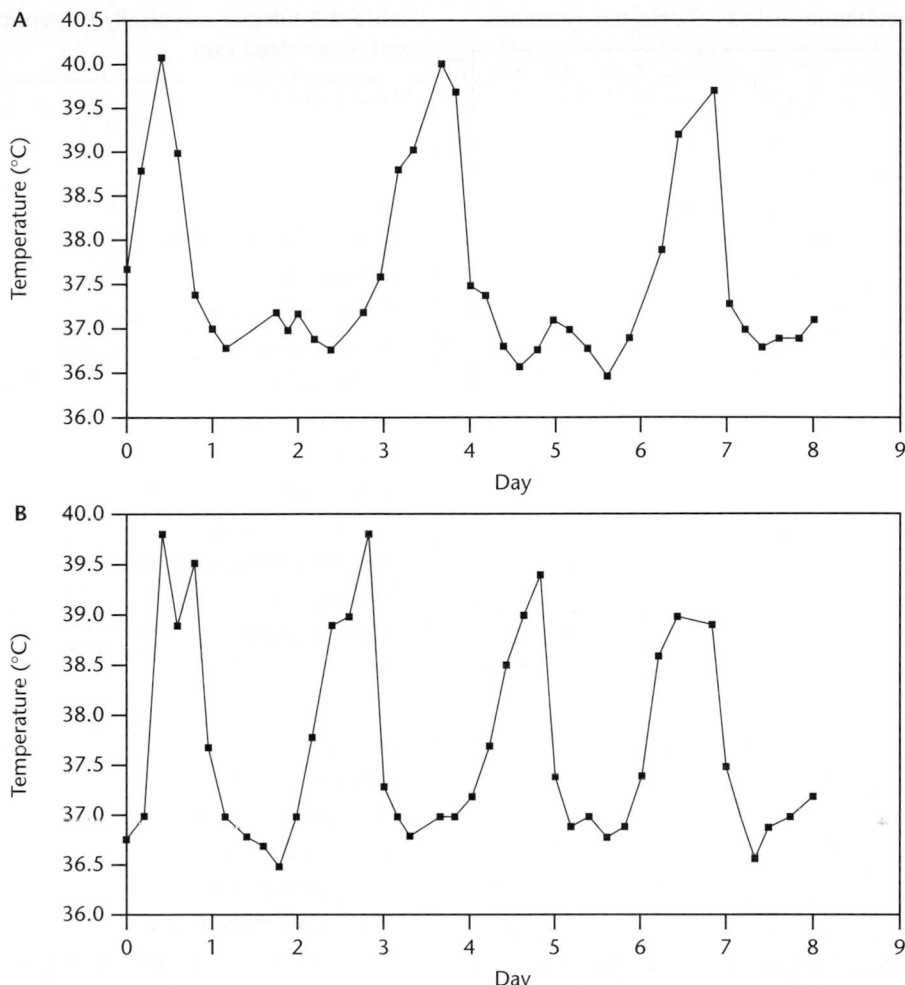

Figure 9.20 On rare occasions, a fever pattern can be so characteristic as to be virtually diagnostic as in (A) the quartan (2-day gap) fever of *Plasmodium malariae* infection, or (B) the tertian (1-day gap) fever of *Plasmodium vivax* infection.

malaria the tertian or quartan fever patterns are not present at the onset, and the tertian pattern is generally not present in non-immune patients with *Plasmodium falciparum* malaria. A biphasic or 'saddle-back' fever pattern with a short afebrile interval occurs in dengue and leptospirosis. Undulant fever that waxes and wanes over days may occur in brucellosis, visceral leishmaniasis and lymphoma (Pel–Ebstein fever). Fever that settles spontaneously with recurrences after intervals of a few days or weeks is characteristic of relapsing fever. Relative bradycardia (pulse rate increase less than the expected 15 bpm for each 1°C rise in temperature) is associated with several infections, particularly typhoid, yellow fever and Legionnaires' disease.

Incubation periods

Knowledge of the incubation period of infections can be very helpful in differential diagnosis if the exposure period is known. This applies particularly to travellers. Incubation periods are most useful in ruling out infections. Table 9.4 lists the average incubation periods of common tropical infections.

Evaluation of patients with acute fever

When evaluating patients with acute fever (<2 weeks) it is important to exclude infections which may require urgent intervention. These include malaria (especially falciparum malaria), bacteraemia (especially meningococcaemia), typhoid, rickettsioses and viral haemorrhagic fevers. The latter must be considered in any febrile patient with a bleeding tendency. The presence of rigors suggests bacteraemia, severe viral infections or malaria. The skin should be carefully examined for early petechial lesions suggesting meningococcaemia, rose spots of typhoid (difficult to see on dark skin), eschars suggesting rickettsiosis (these are usually found on the legs or the perineum), sparse papular or pustular lesions of disseminated gonococcal infection and stigmata of infective endocarditis. Features indicating severe sepsis include tachypnoea, confusion, hypotension and organ failure.

The extent of laboratory work-up of patients with acute fever in the tropics or the returning traveller from the tropics[12–14] will depend on the available facilities and how ill the patient is. Microscopic examination of thick and thin blood smears is the most

101

Table 9.4 Average incubation periods of selected infections

Short (<10 days)
Arboviruses
Bacillary dysentery
Rickettsial spotted fevers
Rickettsialpox
Scrub typhus
Relapsing fever
Plague
Intermediate (10–21 days)
Typhoid
Falciparum malaria
Leptospirosis
HIV
Brucellosis
Typhus (louse-borne)
Q fever
African trypanosomiasis
Acute Chagas' disease
Long (>21 days)
Viral hepatitis
Malaria (including *P. falciparum*)
Amoebic liver abscess
Visceral leishmaniasis

Table 9.5 Infections typically presenting with acute fever and generalized rash

Maculopapular
Measles
Rubella
Dengue
Rickettsial spotted fevers
Primary HIV
Louse-borne typhus
Scrub typhus
Chikungunya
O'nyong-nyong
Vesicular
Chickenpox
Disseminated zoster
Disseminated herpes simplex
Monkey pox
Rickettsia africae
Rickettsialpox
Erythroderma
Scarlet fever
Kawasaki's disease
Toxic shock syndrome
Haemorrhagic
Meningococcaemia
Viral haemorrhagic fevers
Disseminated intravascular coagulation
Louse-borne typhus (severe)
Rickettsial spotted fevers (severe)
Chickenpox (haemorrhagic)

important initial investigation and may identify malaria, Borrelia (relapsing fever) and African trypanosomiasis. However, it is important to recognize that the identification of malarial parasites in the indigenous population from a holoendemic area does not necessarily mean that malaria is the cause of fever as asymptomatic parasitaemia is common in this context. A complete blood count is often helpful. Significant anaemia suggests malaria, bartonellosis or acute haemolytic anaemia complicating sickle cell disease or glucose-6-phosphate dehydrogenase deficiency. Neutrophilia is present in many infections and is not of much diagnostic value. However, neutropenia suggests viral infections, typhoid or fulminant sepsis. Eosinophilia suggests acute parasite invasion (particularly acute schistosomiasis) or drug hypersensitivity reaction (see below). Thrombocytopenia is common in severe sepsis, viral infections and malaria. Urinalysis and chest radiography may indicate the source of infection. A blood culture should be done if there is no clear diagnosis. Liver function tests may suggest viral hepatitis, which typically presents with fever in the pre-icteric phase. Arterial blood gas analysis and renal function should be done in patients with features of severe sepsis.

Fever and generalized rash

Many infections present as an acute febrile illness with a generalized rash. The pattern of the rash is important in the differential diagnosis. The least specific pattern is maculopapular. Other patterns are diffuse erythroderma, vesicular and haemorrhagic lesions (petechiae, purpura or ecchymoses). Table 9.5 lists infections that typically present with these patterns. Drug hypersensitivity reactions and connective tissue diseases should also be considered.

Fever and jaundice

There are several pitfalls in managing the patient with jaundice.[6] The primary viral hepatitides (A–E) are febrile illnesses primarily in the prodromal, non-icteric phase. Fever normally subsides with the onset of jaundice but may persist for a few days after the development of jaundice. A patient who is febrile and jaundiced concurrently is more likely to be afflicted with another, usually more severe condition, such as *P. falciparum* malaria, typhoid or leptospirosis (Table 9.6). In view of the appreciable mortality of the latter conditions, their diagnosis should always be carefully considered.

Fever and eosinophilia

This is usually due to immature parasites that migrate through tissue. This clinical syndrome is generally called visceral larva

Table 9.6 Jaundice with concurrent fever

Hepatic
Severe *P. falciparum* malaria
Typhoid
Leptospirosis (Weil's disease)
Viral hepatitis A-E (fever usually settles before jaundice)
Septicaemia
Pneumococcal pneumonia
Relapsing fever
Yellow fever (and other viral haemorrhagic fevers)
Typhus
Alcoholic hepatitis
Post-hepatic
Ascending cholangitis (may complicate liver flukes or ascariasis)
Cholecystitis (bacterial, *Cryptosporidium parvum*), cytomegalovirus
Haemolytic
Malaria
Haemoglobinopathies (especially sickle cell disease)
Glucose-6-phosphate dehydrogenase deficiency (favism, drug-induced crisis)
Bartonella bacilliformis
Haemolytic–uraemic syndrome (*Shigella dysenteriae*, *E. coli*)

Table 9.7 Common causes of HIV-associated fever of unknown origin (FUO) in the tropics

Tuberculosis
Bacteraemia (*Salmonella* spp. and *S. pneumoniae*)
Pneumocystis jiroveci pneumonia
Community-acquired pneumonia
Cryptococcosis
Toxoplasmosis
Visceral leishmaniasis
Disseminated atypical mycobacteriosis
Disseminated endemic mycoses
Non-Hodgkin's lymphoma
Cytomegalovirus

Table 9.8 Important infectious causes of classical fever of unknown origin (FUO) in the tropics

Extrapulmonary tuberculosis
Typhoid fever
Amoebic liver abscess
Infective endocarditis
Pyogenic intra-abdominal abscesses
Brucellosis
Relapsing fever
Visceral leishmaniasis
Cryptococcosis
Strongyloides hyperinfection syndrome
Katayama fever
Visceral larva migrans
Q fever
Trypanosomiasis
Toxoplasmosis
Histoplasmosis
Coccidioidomycosis

migrans. It is commonly accompanied by pulmonary symptoms or infiltrates, as many parasites which present with fever and eosinophilia migrate through the lungs. Diagnosis of the specific parasite involved is difficult as the parasites have often not yet arrived at their final destination and laid eggs, which is the simplest definitive diagnostic test. Serological tests are available for some parasites, but are not always very specific. The commonest diseases presenting with fever and eosinophilia in the tropics are acute schistosomiasis (Katayama fever) and ascariasis. Other diseases include toxocariasis, hookworm, trichinosis, fascioliasis, gnathostomiasis and paragonimiasis. Hypersensitivity reactions to drugs should always be considered.

HIV-associated fever of unknown origin (FUO)

This has been defined as FUO in an HIV-infected person with no diagnosis after 3 days of inpatient investigation. HIV itself can cause a fever, but this is a diagnosis by exclusion as the vast majority of patients will have another treatable cause. Mycobacterial infections account for almost half of these. Table 9.7 lists the likely causes of FUO in the HIV-infected patient in the tropics. Bacteraemias are listed in the table, as blood culture results in resource-poor settings often take longer than 3 days.

Classical FUO

Classical FUO is chronic fever (>2 weeks) with no cause identified after initial investigations on two outpatient visits or three inpatient days.[13] In industrialized countries malignancies (particularly lym-phoproliferative disorders), infections and connective tissue disorders are collectively the cause in about three-quarters of cases of classical FUO, with malignancies being the commonest. In the tropics infectious causes are far more important and connective tissue diseases are relatively uncommon. Extrapulmonary tuberculosis is the commonest infectious cause. Table 9.8 lists some important infections presenting as classical FUO in the tropics.

Lymphadenopathy

Residents of the tropics are frequently exposed to infectious disease and palpable shotty lymph nodes are a common finding that does not necessarily indicate active pathology. Larger palpable inguinal nodes of no clinical significance are particularly common in people who walk barefoot. However, inguinal nodes should always be examined as several important diseases typically cause inguinal

Table 9.9 Diseases associated with lymphadenopathy

	Acute	Chronic
Generalized	Measles	HIV
	Dengue	Disseminated
	Primary HIV	tuberculosis
	Cytomegalovirus	Secondary syphilis
	Epstein-Barr virus	Brucellosis
	Rubella	Toxoplasmosis
	Scrub typhus	African trypanosomiasis
	Leptospirosis	Chagas' disease
	Leukaemia	Kala azar
		Leprosy
		Disseminated endemic
		mycoses
		Sarcoidosis
		Connective tissue
		diseases
Regional	Pyogenic adenitis[a]	Tuberculosis[a]
	Adenovirus	Lymphoma
	STD:	Metastatic carcinoma/
	Chancroid[a]	sarcoma
	Primary genital herpes	Non-tuberculous
	Primary syphilis	mycobacteria[a]
	Lymphogranuloma	Endemic mycoses
	venereum[a]	Chronic lymphatic
	Rickettsia:	filariasis
	R. conorii	Onchocerciasis
	R. africae	Loiasis
	R. akari	Cat scratch disease[a]
	Recurrent lymphatic	Melioidosis[a]
	filariasis	Kawasaki's disease
	Diphtheria	Kikuchi's disease[a]
	Bubonic plague[a]	
	Tularaemia[a]	
	Anthrax	

[a] Denotes that suppuration or caseation may occur.

lymphadenitis (many STIs, bubonic plague and lymphatic filariasis). Lymphadenopathy may be generalized or regional, acute or chronic, and accompanied by suppuration (with bubo formation) or caseation. Table 9.9 lists diseases in the tropics that may present with lymphadenopathy. The majority of diseases causing generalized lymphadenopathy also cause splenomegaly.

HIV-associated persistent generalized lymphadenopathy is very common in early disease, but in advanced disease, the nodes regress. Lymphadenopathy at this stage of the illness is usually due to opportunistic infections (overwhelmingly tuberculosis) or malignancies (Kaposi's sarcoma or lymphoma). Tuberculosis may present with generalized adenopathy, nodes matted together or with large asymmetrical nodes, which may be fluctuant if there is extensive caseation necrosis. Sinus formation is common; in the neck this may present with 'collar stud' abscesses.

Ulceroglandular syndromes present with a lesion at the site of inoculation (occasionally this may be the eye, producing the oculoglandular syndrome) associated with regional lymphadenitis. The classic example is tularaemia, but this pattern is also seen with anthrax, cat scratch disease (the site of inoculation is usually a

Table 9.10 Common causes of splenomegaly, hepatomegaly or hepatosplenomegaly

Malaria[a]
Typhoid
Brucellosis
Relapsing fever (louse and tick-borne)
Typhus
Visceral leishmaniasis[a]
Trypanosomiasis
Schistosomiasis (portal hypertension)
Haemoglobinopathies
HIV infection
Hepatitis B infection
Hydatid disease
Lymphoma[a]
Chronic myeloid leukaemia[a]
Myelofibrosis[a]
Leptospirosis
Bartonellosis

[a] May cause massive splenomegaly.

papule rather than an ulcer) and rickettsiae that are associated with an eschar.

Lymphangitis is inflamed subcutaneous lymphatic vessels. Acutely these are commonly associated with subcutaneous pyogenic infections or with recurrent attacks of lymphatic filariasis. Chronic nodular lymphangitis presents with granulomatous nodules along thickened lymphatic vessels. Sporotrichosis is the classic cause, but non-tuberculous mycobacteria (especially *Mycobacterium marinum*) and *Nocardia* species can also present in this way.

Glandular fever in the tropics is very uncommon as Epstein–Barr virus and cytomegalovirus are typically subclinical diseases of early childhood. Primary HIV infections should be considered in sexually active patients with a glandular fever-type illness. Features that strongly suggest this diagnosis are a maculopapular rash (without a history of prior aminopenicillin use) and small orogenital ulcers.

Splenomegaly

Splenomegaly and hepatomegaly or hepatosplenomegaly are common findings in patients living in the tropics.[15] A wide range of tropical infections and other systemic diseases can cause these signs (Table 9.10). The common causes of a very large spleen reaching the right iliac fossa are (a) tropical splenomegaly syndrome due to malaria, (b) visceral leishmaniasis, (c) portal hypertension (often due to schistosomiasis), (d) myelofibrosis and (e) lymphoma/chronic myeloid leukaemia.

CONCLUSION

History taking and physical examination remain the mainstay of the practice of medicine. Clinical acumen is of paramount importance in arriving at a correct diagnosis when medicine is practised in rural areas of the tropics or where laboratory back-up is scarce or unavailable. Medical practitioners in the tropics must take a practical and common-sense approach to the diagnosis and management of patients who present with infectious and non-infectious conditions. Where the diagnosis is uncertain the answer often lies in retaking a history and redoing the physical examination. In problematic cases, they should know where to seek assistance to obtain information on diseases specific to certain geographical areas (see Appendix V). Subsequent chapters in this book highlight the main symptoms and signs of infectious and non-infectious diseases relating to each system of the body.

REFERENCES

1. Gilles HM, Lucas AO. Tropical medicine: 100 years of progress. *Br Med Bull* 1998; 54:269–280.

2. Murray H, Pépin J, Nutman T, et al. Tropical medicine. *BMJ* 2000; 320: 490–494.

3. Weatherall D. The future role of molecular and cell biology in medical practice in the tropical countries. *Br Med Bull* 1998; 54: 489–501.

4. Cook GC. Dealing with disease related to tropical exposure. In: Toghill PJ, ed. *Examining Patients: An Introduction to Clinical Medicine.* 2nd edn. London: Edward Arnold; 1995:245–258.

5. Hoffman SH. Tropical medicine and the acute abdomen. *Emerg Med Clin North Am* 1989; 7:591–609.

6. Maher D, Harries A. Pitfalls in the diagnosis and management of the jaundiced patient in the tropics. *Trop Doctor* 1994; 24:128–130.

7. Holocombe C, Weedon R, Llwin M. The differential diagnosis and management of breast lumps in the tropics. *Trop Doctor* 1999; 29:42–46.

8. Karp CL, Neva FA. Tropical infectious diseases in human immunodeficiency virus-infected patients. *Clin Infect Dis* 1999; 28:947–965.

9. Polsky B, Kotler D, Steinhart C. HIV-associated wasting in the HAART era: guidelines for assessment, diagnosis, and treatment. *AIDS Patient Care STDS* 2001; 15:411–423.

10. Dias JC. Tropical diseases and the gender approach. *Bull Pan Am Health Organ* 1996; 30:242–260.

11. Peters W, Gilles HM. *Tropical Medicine and Parasitology.* 5th edn. Philadelphia: Mosby-Wolfe; 2000.

12. Suh KN, Kozarsky PE, Keystone JS. Evaluation of fever in the returned traveler. *Med Clin North Am* 1999; 83:997–1017.

13. Durack D, Street AC. Fever of unknown origin re-examined and redefined. *Curr Clin Top Infect Dis* 1991; 11:35–51.

14. Norman G, Joseph A, Theodore A, et al. Community-based teaching of tropical diseases: an experience with filariasis. *Trop Doctor* 1999; 29:86–89.

15. Onuigbo MA, Mbah AU. Tropical splenomegaly syndrome in Nigerian adults. *West Afr J Med* 1992; 11:72–78.

Chapter 10   Gordon C. Cook

Tropical Gastroenterological Problems

The portals of entry for organisms responsible for most infections which dominate medicine in tropical countries (as elsewhere) are the skin, and respiratory and intestinal tracts. A very high proportion of infections of warm climes originates from ingestion of contaminated water and foodstuffs; many resultant diseases therefore fall into the subspecialty tropical gastroenterology.[1-3]

Most gastroenterological emergencies which occur in a temperate climate also occur in tropical and subtropical countries. However, there are notable differences in prevalence.[4] Some are probably ethnically related (although elimination of environmental factors is often difficult), but the majority are superimposed upon an underlying communicable (infective) disease; important examples are ileal perforation or haemorrhage resulting from typhoid (enteric) fever, colonic perforation – and far less often haemorrhage – in amoebic colitis and shigellosis, and hepatic 'abscess' in invasive amoebiasis.[4]

MOUTH AND PHARYNX

The mouth and rectum are the most accessible parts of the gastrointestinal tract from a clinical viewpoint;[5] therefore, where endoscopic procedures are impossible (and that applies to many tropical and subtropical countries), as much information as possible should be derived from careful examination of these organs.

Viral, bacterial, mycotic and parasitic infections all give rise to oropharyngeal pathology, which is frequently most pronounced in the presence of associated malnutrition (especially in infants and children). Herpes simplex virus, Epstein–Barr virus (EBV) (see Chapter 43) and many enteroviruses can produce a stomatitis; oral ulceration is also a frequent manifestation of Behçet's syndrome-common in the Middle East and Japan. Lassa fever (see Chapter 42) and diphtheria (see Chapter 67) are frequently characterized by severe pharyngeal involvement, and in rabies (see Chapter 44) dysphagia caused by spasm of the pharyngeal muscles is an important feature of the disease. In addition to acute bacterial infections, tuberculosis, leprosy, syphilis and yaws all exert oral manifestations. Candidiasis (exceedingly common in the acquired immune deficiency syndrome, AIDS) (Chapter 20), histoplasmosis, South American blastomycosis and coccidioidomycosis can also produce buccal lesions. Acute pharyngitis caused by infection with young adult *Fasciola hepatica* (ingested in raw sheep

or goat liver – reported from the Middle East and India – and known locally as 'halzoun'; Chapter 83) is caused by pentastomids.[1] Therapeutic agents, such as sulfonamides (included in some antimalarial prophylactics, e.g. pyrimethamine + sulfamethoxazole, 'Fansidar') can give rise to the Stevens–Johnson syndrome, in which oral ulceration is common. Manifestations of specific malnutrition states (vitamin B and C deficits, and iron deficiency anaemia) are usually obvious, whereas in kwashiorkor, these are frequently combined with infective complications. Cancrum oris is a gangrenous condition involving the gums and cheeks and is associated with *Borrelia vincentii* and *Fusiformis fusiformis* infection; it is especially common in malnourished children,[1] especially in West Africa. Descriptions of the mouth, especially the tongue, in post-infective malabsorption (tropical sprue) (see below) were dominant in clinical accounts of this disease in the nineteenth century (i.e. before the advent of laboratory investigation).

Periodontal disease and dental caries are also a major problem in tropical countries.[1] Oral submucous fibrosis – a chronic disease of unknown aetiology – may affect any part of the oral cavity;[1] most reports are from the Indian subcontinent and Southeast Asia. Fibroelastosis of the submucous tissues, accompanied by epithelial atrophy, are important sequelae and are probably premalignant.

Of malignant disease(s), buccal carcinoma is pre-eminent;[5] Burkitt's lymphoma, ameloblastoma and nasopharyngeal carcinoma (Chapter 35) are other malignancies that have important geographical distributions in tropical countries.

Hypertrophy of the salivary glands is common in malnourished children; it can also be associated with *Ascaris lumbricoides* infection and chronic calcific pancreatitis (see below).[1] Tumours of the salivary glands are probably no more common than in temperate regions.

OESOPHAGUS

The most important disease to involve this organ is oesophageal carcinoma[6] (Figure 10.1) (Chapter 35); this malignancy possesses an enigmatic geographical distribution. It has a high prevalence in certain geographical locations:[1,6] central and east-Africa (western Kenya, Malawi and eastern Zambia have the highest rates), the southern Caspian littoral (especially north-eastern Iran) and

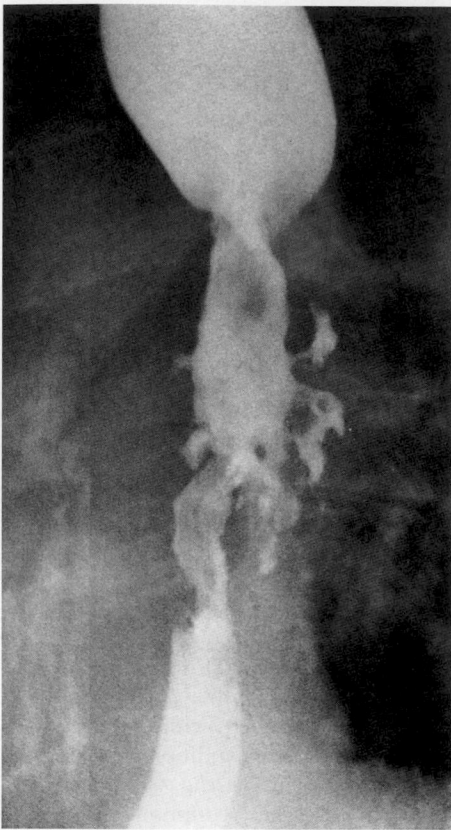

Figure 10.1 Barium swallow showing oesophageal carcinoma with gross mediastinal invasion.

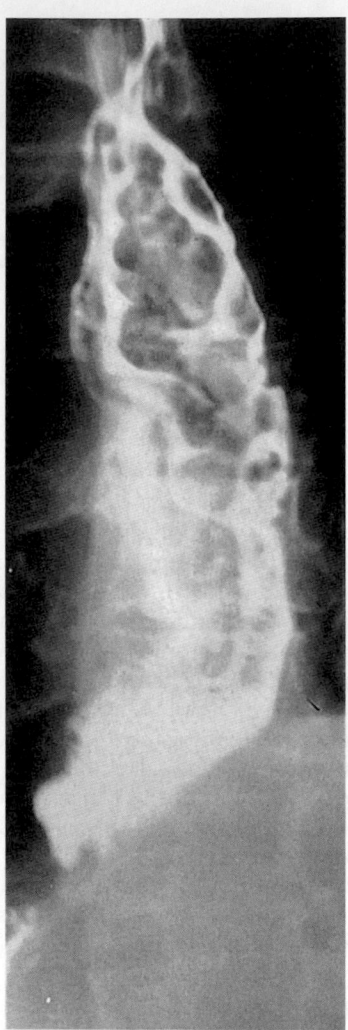

Figure 10.2 Advanced oesophageal varices in a Zambian woman with severe macronodular cirrhosis associated with HBV infection; barium swallow examination.

northern China (in and around the Taihang mountains). Various hypotheses have been advanced to explain the high incidence of this tumour in these areas (Chapter 35).[1,6]

Megaoesophagus, a feature of chronic *Trypanosoma cruzi* infection (Chagas' disease), is described in Chapter 76. Table 10.1 lists some major causes of dysphagia in a tropical environment.

Oesophageal varices (Figure 10.2) usually result from advanced macronodular cirrhosis (see below); however, hepatic schistosomiasis (caused by *Schistosoma mansoni, Schist. japonicum, Schist. intercalatum, Schist. matthei* and *Schist. mekongi*) are also important (Chapter 82). Portal vein obstruction (see below) is also common in some parts of Africa and Asia; this probably results in most cases (although more research is required) from umbilical sepsis in the neonatal period;[1] it is occasionally a sequel to hepatocellular carcinoma. A very high splenic blood flow associated with hyperreactive malarious splenomegaly (HMS; tropical splenomegaly syndrome) can also give rise to oesophageal varices (see below).[1] Where and when available, upper gastrointestinal endoscopic sclerotherapy is of enormous value in the management of oesophageal varices, but an ideal method of dealing with bleeding varices has yet to appear; in most tropical countries, older methods (see below) remain extant.

Oesophageal trauma is a major problem in several African countries; foreign bodies (e.g. kola nuts and fish bones) and corrosive agents – which give rise to strictures – are also relatively

Table 10.1 Some causes of dysphagia in tropical countries

Trauma	Gastritis
	Foreign bodies
	Corrosive agents
Infection	South American trypanosomiasis (Chagas' disease)
	Candidiasis (usually associated with AIDS)
	Rhizopus, Absidia (mucormycosis)
Neoplasia	Oesophageal carcinoma
Oesophageal	Macronodular cirrhosis (usually varices, postviral)
	Schistosomiasis
	Portal vein thrombosis
	Hyperreactive malarious splenomegaly
Others	Achalasia
	Peptic oesophagitis
	Hiatus hernia
Extrinsic pressure	Endemic goitre

common.[1] Achalasia, peptic oesophagitis and hiatus hernia are all encountered, but are not unduly common.

In HIV/AIDS infection, oesophageal candidiasis is a common manifestation; other systemic mycoses (Chapter 71) can also produce an oesophagitis.

Emergencies

The most common oesophageal lesions in tropical countries are varices (Table 10.1 summarizes the major causes) and carcinoma (see above);[4] resultant acute complications are upper gastrointestinal haemorrhage and obstruction, respectively. Hookworm and *Ascaris lumbricoides* infections (Chapter 85) should not be neglected in this context.[7] Of lesser importance, foreign bodies in the oesophagus (e.g. kola nuts) can cause dysphagia; corrosive lesions can result in stricture formation.[1]

Oesophageal varices

Reported prevalence of bleeding oesophageal varices in tropical countries is unreliable.[4] Transport facilities are usually exceedingly unsatisfactory; therefore, the majority of those afflicted die before reaching medical care. Also, high technology (e.g. endoscopic sclerotherapy) and blood transfusion are less often available; outcome following medical intervention is therefore frequently less satisfactory than in a Western country.[8] The cause of upper gastrointestinal bleeding in 131 successive patients admitted with haematemesis or melaena to a hospital at Harare, Zimbabwe, has been analysed;[9] in 36 (27%) admissions (mean age 42 years) oesophageal varices were responsible. In 21, conservative management was followed by cessation of bleeding; however, nine suffered continuous bleeding, and six re-bleeding; five patients died (four within 24 h of admission) from haemorrhagic shock. Vasopressin infusions were used in four with the addition of oesophageal tamponade in two.

The pathophysiological mechanisms underlying oesophageal bleeding have been addressed on numerous occasions.[10] Both erosive and eruptive bases seem the most likely explanations; in addition, pressure and variceal size are probably important. In Egypt, endoscopic biopsies obtained from intervariceal mucosa (within 5 cm of the cardia) in 20 individuals with, and 30 without, a history of variceal bleeding (most suffered from schistosomal liver disease) were examined histologically;[11] they showed dilated intraepithelial blood-filled channels within the squamous epithelium and lamina propria in all of the 'bleeders' and in 15 (50%) of the 'non-bleeders'. Furthermore, oesophagitis was more pronounced in the bleeders compared with the non-bleeders: 11 (55%) and 7 (23%), respectively.

The role of upper gastrointestinal endoscopy in a developing country has been studied in Kuwait;[12] 345 (4%) of 8680 patients examined successively using this technique had evidence of oesophageal varices, the usual cause being chronic schistosomal liver disease (usually in Egyptian labourers). By examining 718 successive patients who presented with upper gastrointestinal bleeding within 24 h of admission, the exact site of the haemorrhage was delineated in 651 (91%), and the responsible lesion detected in 685 (97%). At Ibadan, Nigeria, a recent study has indicated that endoscopy gives a superior result to radiology in the diagnosis of variceal disease, resulting in upper gastrointestinal

haemorrhage;[13] endoscopy was successful in 64 (85%), but a barium meal correctly located the source of bleeding in only 38 (51%) of 75 patients.

Three reports from New Delhi, India, focused on the role of endoscopic sclerotherapy in the management of bleeding oesophageal varices.[14-16] A total of 79 patients underwent treatment (with either absolute or 50% alcohol) every 3 weeks, for oesophageal varices; active bleeding was controlled in 14 of 15 (93%) and 5 of 13 (54%) using the two fluids, respectively ($p < 0.05$); the sole disadvantage of absolute alcohol was that it produced a higher incidence of retrosternal pain. In another study, using a similar regimen, 5% ethanolamine oleate was compared with absolute alcohol in 47 randomly allocated patients; the latter solution eradicated oesophageal varices earlier (12.9 vs 8.2 weeks, respectively) ($p < 0.001$); the mean number of injection courses and necessary amount of sclerosant were also lower in the alcohol-treated group ($p < 0.001$), but the frequency of re-bleeding did not differ significantly ($p > 0.05$). A total of 31 children with variceal bleeding caused by extrahepatic portal vein obstruction (19), non-cirrhotic portal fibrosis (5) or cirrhosis (7) were treated by sclerotherapy using absolute alcohol; arrest of acute bleeding was achieved in 10 by emergency sclerotherapy, and a 3-week schedule was able to achieve variceal obliteration in all of them. During a 23-month follow-up period, recurrent varices occurred in three (two with cirrhosis and one with non-cirrhotic portal fibrosis) patients; a re-bleed was successfully controlled with emergency sclerotherapy in five, and an oesophageal stricture in four of them (which was easily dilated) which were the only significant complications.

Although now rarely used in the Western world, oesophageal compression using a Sengstaken tube is often the only technique available. Intravenous pitressin is of limited value in acute bleeding. In long-term management, propranolol undoubtedly has a place in a developing country scenario.

In an attempt to provide clinical guidelines for the prediction of outcome of upper gastrointestinal bleeding in a developing country, Clamp et al.[8] carried out a multicentre study based on two centres, in Sikkim and China; in the former country, 60 (69%) of the patients put into the 'high-risk' group (by applying Bayes' theorem using a computer system) for re-bleeding experienced this event (27 (54%) died), whereas this complication occurred in only six (2%) in the 'low-risk' group; furthermore, a simplified scoring system (little computer technology was available at Sikkim) gave almost exactly the same predictive accuracy. The authors suggest that, by using one of these systems, patients in remote areas can be categorized in order that scarce resources (which are available there) can be put to the best use.

The optimal means of managing haemorrhage resulting from extrahepatic portal venous obstruction is summarized in the section on liver disease (see below).

Oesophageal carcinoma

Presence of histologically diagnosed chronic oesophagitis (using upper gastrointestinal endoscopy) has been shown to be common in a high-risk population (15–26 years) in China.[17] This lesion was significantly associated with: (1) consumption of 'burning hot' beverages; (2) a family history of oesophageal carcinoma (including second-degree relatives); (3) infrequent consumption of fresh fruit; and (4) infrequent consumption of dietary staples, other than maize. Associated factors which have been recorded in that population include: (1) positive cytological smears (568 individuals >30 years of 42 190 had a positive result); and (2) a high prevalence of pharyngeal carcinoma in free-range chickens, which lived off domestic scraps[18] in the local environment.

This tumour often presents late in its clinical course in the heavily affected areas; in fact, complete luminal obstruction (accompanied by inability to swallow saliva) is not uncommon at presentation. Passage of a Celestin latex rubber tube (a palliative technique) is often the only available procedure;[6] however, blockage is a frequent problem resulting largely from the bulky African (or other) diet. Chemotherapy and radiotherapy (when available) are of very limited value.

STOMACH AND DUODENUM

Peptic ulceration was at one time considered an unusual cause of abdominal pain in tropical countries; it was felt by many physicians to be a rare disease.[1] It is now clear, however, that this is not the case; many difficulties facing the clinical epidemiologist in a developing country are highlighted by studies of the geographical distribution of this disease. Because sophisticated methods of diagnosis, including barium meal and upper gastrointestinal endoscopy, have not until relatively recently been widely used in developing countries, diagnosis and attempts at establishing accurate prevalence rates have depended upon recording incidence rates of complications, especially pyloric stenosis; upper gastrointestinal haemorrhage seems an unusual presentation overall, but this probably results from the fact that such patients do not reach hospital before exsanguinations occur. Therefore, serious deficiencies exist in knowledge regarding the true prevalence of peptic ulceration, and it is currently impossible to draw accurate conclusions on regional and rural/urban patterns, and also on variations with time, i.e. during the course of 'westernization'.

As recently as the 1950s, duodenal ulcer (DU) was considered a rare disease in Africa;[1] this is not so, because satisfactory radiological, and more recently endoscopic, investigations have yielded accurate facts on true prevalence rate(s). Prevalence of DU in Africa has been reviewed using the available literature;[1,19] high-prevalence areas seem to exist in parts of West Africa, Rwanda, Burundi, eastern Zaire, western Tanzania, south-western Uganda and the Ethiopian highlands. In southern India[19] (and Fijians descended from this population[20]) and Papua New Guinea, the disease also seems relatively common. It has a marked male predominance; it is frequently post-bulbar, and presentation with pyloric obstruction is relatively usual. Genetic factors might be important;[19] the role of diet remains difficult to assess. Whether low rates of presentation resulting from haemorrhage and/or perforation accurately reflect incidence, or are biased by the inability to transport a sick patient to hospital, is also impossible to evaluate. In Lima, Peru there is evidence that the prevalence of peptic ulcer (and also gastric adenocarcinoma) has declined; between 1985 and 2002 a reduction from 3.15% to 5.05% was documented.[21] Evidence for a causative role for *Helicobacter pylori* in

chronic active gastritis, peptic ulceration and possibly gastric malignancy has escalated during the last decade;[19,22] however, Koch's postulates have not all been satisfied, and infection rate with this organism frequently approaches 100% at an early age in an affected population. In a study carried out in Belgium, South Africa, China and North America, a significantly higher rate was found in the presence of gastric carcinoma but not duodenal ulceration.[23]

Overall, gastric ulcer (GU) is uncommon in developing countries.[1] In a study carried out at Kumasi, Ghana, however, perforated duodenal ulcer was less common than perforated gastric ulcer; the latter was related to the widespread use of NSAIDs and herbal medicines.[24] An overall decline in ulcer mortality might be associated with a worldwide reduction in the occurrence of *H. pylori* infection.[25,26] When it occurs, it usually has a male predominance, is most common in the fifth and sixth decades, and afflicts predominantly the lower social strata. Pyloric obstruction is a common presentation, due frequently to late-stage disease at presentation. Management of a bleeding peptic ulcer has been reviewed.[1,4]

Gastritis, often resulting from alcohol and spicy foods, is a major cause of abdominal pain/discomfort[22] (Table 10.2). Infective causes (including tuberculosis) are overall rare, although occasionally encountered; infections which involve predominantly lower sections of the gastrointestinal tract (e.g. *Salmonella typhi* and *Shigella* spp.) occasionally produce significant gastric pathology. A heavy infection with hookworm and/or *Ascaris lumbricoides* can also account for epigastric discomfort (see below) and should be differentiated from peptic ulceration.

When H_2-receptor antagonists (e.g. cimetidine and ranitidine) are used in developing countries, a possibility exists that they will encourage proliferation of intestinal pathogen(s) – bacterial and parasitic – for the gastric acid defence mechanism is largely removed;[27] available data are, however, presently inadequate for assessing the practical importance of this. Several studies of gastric acid production indicate that mean acid production probably varies little in different ethnic groups. Hypochlorhydria is relatively common in the tropics;[1] whether it is the cause or consequence of intestinal infection (of bacterial, including *S. typhi*, and/or parasitic origin) remains far from clear.

Gastric carcinoma is overall an uncommon malignancy in tropical countries (Chapter 35). At Sura, Fiji, gastric ulcer and carcinoma have been shown to be more common in Fijians than Indians.

Emergencies

Many facts remain unclear regarding upper gastrointestinal haemorrhage in tropical countries. For example, DU is apparently common in descendants of southern Indians in Fiji (see above); however, haematemesis from a chronic DU is more common in Fijians.

Many data suggest that pyloric obstruction is the most common complication of DU in developing countries. A report from Zaria, northern Nigeria, indicates that at that location perforation is by no means uncommon;[28] between 1971 and 1983, 74 (24%) of 302 patients operated for DU, and 29 (58%) of 50 for GU, pre-

Table 10.2 Some causes of severe abdominal pain (without features of intestinal obstruction) in relation to tropical exposure

Site of pain	Cause
Epigastrium	Heavy nematode infection (e.g. *Ascaris lumbricoides*, hookworm) Mesenteric adenitis (helminthic eggs or tuberculosis) Acute pancreatitis (helminth related)
Generalized	Peritonitis Typhoid perforation Amoebic colitis with perforation (appendix, perforated peptic ulcer or diverticulitis) Abdominal tuberculosis Ruptured hydatid cyst Sickle cell crisis Recurrent familial polyserositis (familial Mediterranean fever) (Chapter 34) Hyperinfective syndrome caused by *Strongyloides stercoralis* *Angiostrongylus costaricensis*
Right upper quadrant	Helminthic infection involving biliary system
Left upper quadrant	Splenomegaly (e.g. hyperreactive malarious splenomegaly [HMS]) Splenic rupture Solitary splenic abscess
Right iliac fossa	Appendicitis *Anisakis* spp. infection Ileocaecal tuberculosis

sented with perforation; furthermore, there was a progressive increase in the years 1971–1974 to 1979–1983 of from 16% to 45%, respectively. A rare case report from India has recorded massive haematemesis and melaena from a cholecystoduodenal fistula secondary to DU in a 24-year-old man;[29] he was successfully managed surgically.

Ideally, management of the complications of gastritis and peptic ulceration is exactly the same as in a Western country. In a study carried out at Ankara, Turkey, age, delayed surgery, presence of shock, status of the anaesthetist, and 'definitive surgery' were significantly associated with a fatal outcome in patients undergoing emergence surgery for perforated peptic ulcer.[30]

Although usually associated with oesophageal varices, gastric varices also occur alone. In New Delhi, India, 48 (16%) out of 309 patients with portal hypertension were shown to have gastric varices;[31] in six (12%) there was no evidence of associated oesophageal varices. In 11 (28%) of 40 patients who completed endoscopic sclerotherapy for oesophageal varices, gastric varices disappeared concurrently with the former, or during the following 6 months. In the light of their experience, these authors considered that 'if they persist for 6 months after eradication of oesophageal varices, a combination of paravariceal and intravariceal sclerotherapy should be attempted for their obliteration'.

ABDOMINAL PAIN

Epigastric pain/discomfort is a common presenting symptom in medical practice in tropical countries (see above);[1,32] this frequently results from heavy small-intestinal helminthic infections, especially with *A. lumbricoides* and hookworm. Mesenteric adenitis as a sequel to the presence of helminthic ova, and tuberculosis, are further causes. Helminth-related acute pancreatitis is another possibility.

Table 10.2 summarizes some causes of severe generalized abdominal pain. This most commonly results from peritonitis, which has numerous aetiologies. Right upper quadrant pain is less likely to result from biliary tract disease than in a 'temperate' area of the world (see below); nevertheless, helminthic infections of the biliary system are occasionally encountered. Left upper quadrant pain can result from splenomegaly (following numerous 'tropical' infections; see below); an extreme example (HMS) occurs in most areas which are endemic for human *Plasmodium* spp. Ruptured spleen is a further cause of left hypochondrial pain; this event usually presents acutely. Solitary splenic abscess is by no means an uncommon event in West and Central Africa; the aetiology remains unclear.

Right iliac fossa pain is less likely to be caused by appendicitis (see below) than in most Western countries. However, an appendix-like syndrome has been recorded in *Yersinia* spp., and *Anisakis* spp. infections and ileocaecal tuberculosis (see below). *Enterobius vermicularis* is not infrequently detected in an appendicectomy specimen; whether there is a cause–effect relationship to acute appendicitis is frequently unclear. Less common parasites involving the appendix include *Taenia* species, *Trichuris trichiura* and *Angiostrongylus costaricensis* (see below). A peripheral blood eosinophilia is often (but by no means always) present when a helminthiasis is causatively related to appendicitis. Ileocaecal tuberculosis can account for chronic right iliac fossa pain; an ileocaecal mass is often palpable clinically (this can be confirmed by ultrasonography when this technique is available). A colonic amoeboma represents a possible source of diagnostic confusion.

SMALL INTESTINE

Tropical enteropathy, subclinical malabsorption and mechanism of diarrhoea

The small-intestinal mucosa of an individual living in a developing country possesses minor structural differences compared with that in one always resident in a temperate zone.[1,33,34] Changes are not related to the clinical syndrome: post-infective malabsorption (tropical sprue; see below). Although the cause of these changes is not entirely clear, they seem to result from repeated low-grade viral and bacterial infection(s). Similarly, marginal xylose and glucose malabsorption has been demonstrated in large numbers of people indigenous to tropical countries; these abnormalities are certainly greater in lower socioeconomic groups. Using a breath-hydrogen test, bacterial overgrowth in the small-intestine was demonstrated in 37.5% of children living in slum conditions compared with only 2.1% ($p < 0.001$) controls in urban Brazil.[35] Subclinical malabsorption exists in many people in developing countries;[1] xylose and B_{12} malabsorption have been demonstrated in 39% and 52%, respectively, of Peace Corps workers living under rural conditions in Pakistan. Apart from repeated small-intestinal infections, other factors are probably also important.[36] Xylose, glucose and folic acid absorption have been shown to be impaired in individuals with systemic bacterial infections, e.g. pulmonary tuberculosis and pneumococcal pneumonia. Dietary folate depletion also results in xylose malabsorption. Marginal malnutrition and pellagra have both been suggested as causing subclinical malabsorption, but evidence is contradictory.

The practical importance of subclinical malabsorption is unclear.[1,33,34] It seems likely that it significantly contributes to malnutrition in people in developing countries who subsist on a marginally adequate dietary intake consisting largely of carbohydrate. Before any rigid conclusions are drawn, however, it should be appreciated that the small intestine has a very substantial functional reserve, and that the role of the colon in absorption of carbohydrate (and other substances) (see above) remains unclear.

Diarrhoea resulting from small-intestinal disease consists of two main types;[1,33] (1) profuse watery (e.g. cholera), and (2) steatorrhoeic (exemplified by post-infective tropical malabsorption (tropical sprue)). Table 10.3 summarizes the most important causes; several of those responsible for the former type are infective, and then exert their pathogenic effect via an enterotoxin (either heat stable or heat labile); invasive disease involving the enterocyte is less important. The role of intestinal hormones – especially vasoactive intestinal peptide – in the production of watery diarrhoea has become clearer.[34] The pathogenesis of diarrhoea in AIDS has a multifactorial basis, and is often by no means clear;[37] some but not all cases are associated with an opportunistic infection(s), especially *Cryptosporidium parvum* (Chapter 79).[34] The bacteria *Escherichia coli*, fungi *Candida albicans* and Histoplasma capsulatum, and the astroviruses and caliciviruses are also relevant. Other opportunistic infections in this syndrome include cytomegalovirus, *Mycobacterium avium intracellulare*, *Salmonella* species, and the protozoa *Isospora belli*, *Cyclospora cayatenensis*, *Sarcocystis hominis* and *Microsporidium* species infections; in addition, Kaposi's sarcoma (Chapter 35) causes severe small-intestinal disease.

Many of the problems encountered in management, including chemoprophylaxis and chemotherapy, are exemplified by traveller's diarrhoea (see below).

Traveller's diarrhoea

The clinical syndrome traveller's diarrhoea (TD)[1,38–42] is arguably the world's most common disease entity; only rarely is it associated with mortality (usually in the presence of debility, or at the extremes of life), but the significant morbidity with which it is associated not infrequently interferes with a crowded schedule or a leisure or sporting activity. Numerous titles have been applied, including 'turista', 'Montezuma's revenge', 'Hong Kong dog' and 'Delhi belly'. One estimate is that 12 million individuals travel annually from an industrialized (Western) country

to one in the tropics or subtropics;[43] in this group incidence of TD varies from around 20–50%. There is a highly significant geographical variation in prevalence; high-risk areas include North Africa, sub-Saharan Africa, the Indian subcontinent, Southeast Asia, South America, Mexico and the Middle East; intermediate ones include the north Mediterranean, Canary Islands and the Caribbean islands; low-risk ones include North America, Western Europe and Australia. In a retrospective study carried out in Switzerland, a large group of travellers were asked to complete a questionnaire after travelling abroad; incidence of the disease varied greatly, the highest figure (50%) being associated with travel to Tunisia. (No detailed study exists of TD acquired in a European country.[44])

Table 10.3 Small-intestinal diarrhoea

Watery diarrhoea (large volume, fluid stool(s)):

Traveller's diarrhoea (TD) (turista)

Vibrio cholerae (and other vibrios)

Escherichia coli (enterotoxigenic)

Salmonella spp.

Campylobacter jejuni

Rotavirus (and other enteric viruses)

Cryptosporidium spp.

(Food poisoning – *Staphylococcus*, *Clostridium perfringens*)

Hypolactasia: Primary – genetically determined
                          Secondary – resulting from enterocyte damage

Steatorrhoeic diarrhoea (malabsorption) (characteristically large pale, fatty, offensive stools; microscopy often shows fat globules in faecal smear):

Post-infective tropical malabsorption ('tropical sprue')

Intestinal parasites

  Giardia lamblia

  Strongyloides stercoralis

  Capillaria philippinensis

  Coccidia: *Cryptosporidium parvum*

         Isospora belli

         Sarcocystis hominis

         Microsporidium spp.

         Cyclospora cayetanensis

HIV enteropathy

Trauma – short bowel syndrome (e.g. recovered pigbel disease)

Lymphoma – Burkitt's, Mediterranean lymphomas

Ileocaecal tuberculosis

Chronic calcific pancreatitis

Acute and chronic liver disease

(Gluten-induced enteropathy (coeliac disease) seems to be uncommon or even rare in most tropical populations. Occasionally it can become clinically obvious in visitors from Western countries to the tropics)

The disease tends to become less common with advancing years; it is unclear whether this is due to the fact that older travellers (≥60 years) have a more discerning lifestyle, or whether relative immunity increases with advancing age.[38] Individuals resident for substantial periods in areas where TD is common seem to experience it less frequently than those not previously exposed.[38,39]

Clinical features

TD is contracted by ingestion of contaminated water/food; it is characterized by acute-onset watery diarrhoea (usually of small-intestinal origin);[38–42] when colorectal involvement exists, diarrhoea is often bloody (see below). Abdominal colic, nausea and vomiting may be present; fever is unusual, being recorded in 1–10% of infected individuals. Prostration and resultant dehydration (with electrolyte imbalance) cause major problems in a severe case. Rarely, symptoms become chronic, and it seems likely that a small proportion of cases of TD proceeds to post-infective malabsorption (see below).[33] Unfortunately, for the investigator, by the time disease has become clinically overt, the initiating infection(s) has invariably been cleared. Chronic diarrhoea of lesser severity is a relatively common problem following recovery from acute disease; this can usually be attributed to (1) tropical enteropathy (in which there is major derangement of enterocyte structure and function) (see above) or (2) the irritable bowel syndrome (see below).

On clinical grounds, an important differential diagnosis is inflammatory bowel disease presenting for the first time during, or immediately after, tropical exposure.[45,46] In a retrospective review of UK residents presenting at the Hospital for Tropical Diseases, London, with acute onset/bloody diarrhoea, the majority had inflammatory bowel disease (usually ulcerative colitis); it was numerically more important than shigellosis and amoebic colitis.[45]

Acute disease pursues an especially virulent course in certain high-risk groups,[38,39] e.g. those suffering from achlorhydria (*Salmonella* species and *Vibrio* species infections are known to be significantly more common in this group), known inflammatory bowel disease (see below), previous gastrointestinal tract surgery, a malignancy involving the gastrointestinal tract, and acquired or congenital immunodeficiency (including immunosuppressive therapy and HIV/AIDS). In addition, individuals on diuretic therapy (in whom maintenance of electrolyte balance is precarious) and others at the extremes of life also fall within the high-risk group. It is important to recognize these factors when advising chemoprophylaxis (see below).

Aetiology

In 1970, Rowe et al.[47] recorded results of a study involving British soldiers newly arrived in Aden; in 19 (54.3%) of 33 cases in which a recognized pathogen was not apparent, a 'new' serotype of *Escherichia coli* was isolated in the acute phase of TD; in a further 14 (40%), several different *E. coli* serotypes were also isolated. (B. H. Keane had suggested in the 1950s (on circumstantial evidence) that bacterial pathogens were implicated.[33,34]) Sack[48] recorded the identity of *E. coli* serotypes isolated from US Peace Corps volunteers serving in various countries: Kenya 06:

H16, 06H⁻, 027:H7, 0159:H4 and 0159:H34; Morocco 06:H16, 0128:H12, 027:H20 and 0169:H⁻; Honduras 08:H9, 015:H49, 015:H⁻ and 027:H20. Therefore, many common strains of enterotoxigenic *E. coli* (ETEC) are relevant. Many other microorganisms are also involved. *Salmonella* species, *Shigella* species, *Campylobacter jejuni*, enteroadherent *E. coli* (EAEC) and *Vibrio* spp. (see Chapter 51); rotavirus and norovirus (Chapter 45), and *Giardia lamblia*, *Coccidia* species (including *Cryptosporidium* species, *I. belli* and *Blastocystis hominis*) and *Entamoeba histolytica* (Chapter 79). Other bacteria which have been implicated include *Aeromonas hydrophila*, *Plesiomonas shigelloides* and *Yersinia enterocolitica*. The causative agent(s) vary significantly in different locations, e.g. in an affected individual in Asia, Central America or Africa the likely organism is different on statistical grounds, although not relevant to a specific case. Furthermore, more than one organism is frequently present; in a study involving US Peace Corps workers in Thailand, 33% were infected by two to four different pathogens.[38] Although protozoan parasites are usually incorporated in the list of aetiological agents, the incubation period is usually somewhat longer than is usual in TD; this applies especially to *G. lamblia*. When the colorectum is predominantly involved, *Shigella* species, enteroinvasive *E. coli* (EIEC), enterohaemorrhagic *E. coli* (EHEC) and *Ent. histolytica* may be responsible. Rarely, herpes simplex virus and *Chlamydia trachomatis* have been implicated. New pathogens will doubtless emerge in future years.

Pathophysiology

The pathophysiology varies and depends on the site within the gastrointestinal tract to be involved.[1,38–41] Whereas in the small intestine toxigenic diarrhoeas predominate (see above), in the colorectum (see below) invasive disease is more common.

ETEC are characterized by both toxin production and mucosal adherence (via specific fimbriae); the latter property is required for disease production, for toxin-producing non-adherent mutants do not cause disease. Enteropathogenic *E. coli* (EPEC) (probably not a major cause of TD) adhere to intestinal mucosal cells and although they do not invade, destroy microvilli. EAEC (detected in up to 15% of patients suffering from TD) do not belong to classical serotypes of EPEC, but adhere to Hep-2 cells in culture; they neither produce a toxin nor invade.[49] EIEC behave similarly to *Shigella* species and account for up to 5% of cases; the main site of action is the colorectum, and the major clinical manifestation is therefore dysentery resulting from epithelial cell invasion and intracellular multiplication; there is resultant mucosal inflammation and ulceration.[49] EHEC (an uncommon cause of TD) produces disease via verotoxin production.

Prophylaxis

Travellers should take maximal care to avoid water/food likely to be contaminated; common sense is of paramount importance! Use of prophylactic agents is controversial. Many chemoprophylactics have been used: doxycycline, co-trimoxazole, trimethoprim, mecillinam, bicozamycin and the fluroquinolone compounds (norfloxacin and ciprofloxacin). High protection rates (≥90%) have been claimed for co-trimoxazole and the fluoroquinolones; for trimethoprim a rate of around 50% has been recorded. Most cases of TD therefore possess a bacterial aetiology. The major problem with antibiotic chemoprophylaxis, however, is the risk of significant side-effects, dominated by dermatological reactions (including Stevens–Johnson syndrome) and pseudomembranous colitis (see below); using co-trimoxazole, a rate of up to 20% of significant skin reactions, necessitating discontinuation of prophylaxis, has been recorded. Also, the acquisition of resistant faecal *E. coli* during chemoprophylaxis has been recorded in several studies; an increase from 21% to 100% has been recorded using doxycycline in Kenya, and one of 3% to 100% with co-trimoxazole in Mexico. When chemoprophylaxis is used, either norfloxacin or ciprofloxacin seems to be the most appropriate, although strains of *Campylobacter jejuni* rapidly acquire resistance.[44] In a recent study in Egypt, two of 105 individuals on norfloxacin developed TD, compared with 30 (26%) of 117 given a placebo.[49] (Ciprofloxacin should be avoided in children because of experimental evidence indicating cartilaginous damage in young experimental animals; there is no evidence in *Homo sapiens*.)

Should chemoprophylaxis be recommended widely in this essentially benign clinical syndrome? In addition to the objections so far outlined (see above), there is a possibility of inducing a false sense of security, resulting in increased exposure to other infections, e.g. viral hepatitis.[49] The following groups should be seriously considered for chemoprophylaxis (for <3 weeks):

- Travellers with a bad 'history' of TD[38–41]
- Those in whom hypochlorhydria is proven (or a possibility)
- Individuals suffering from inflammatory bowel disease
- HIV-infected patients
- Those in whom electrolyte balance is precarious (e.g. those receiving diuretic therapy) and others with chronic renal failure
- The 'elderly' (not easily defined)
- A nebulous group in whom TD is professionally embarrassing (e.g. members of the armed services, airline pilots, athletes, politicians, businessmen and other professionals on tight schedules, etc.).

The role of prophylactic antiperistaltic agents is likewise controversial: action is unphysiological. It has been suggested that they can mask a more serious infection, e.g. *S. typhi*, although in this disease diarrhoea is an unusual presenting symptom (Chapter 52). By delaying excretion of pathogen(s) it is also possible that clinical disease is prolonged. In children, paralytic ileus is a major complication and has occasionally precipitated mortality.[50]

Bismuth subsalicylate has a role in prophylaxis; the bismuth moiety possesses antimicrobial activity and salicylate antisecretory properties.[39] Early studies in Mexico by DuPont et al.[51] showed that, given as a suspension (the sheer bulk required precluded its use by travellers), this agent significantly reduced TD; the same group, also working in Mexico, has demonstrated that, when given in tablet form (2 tablets 4 × daily for 3 weeks, i.e. 2.1 g daily), a 65% protection rate can be achieved;[51] at half that dose, efficacy was greatly reduced. The number(s) of pathogen-positive TD cases in a group of treated patients was seven of 29, compared with 35 of 59 in a placebo group; ETEC was present in 3 and 22, respectively, and *Shigella* species in two and eight, respectively.[51]

A B-subunit/whole-cell (BS-WC) cholera vaccine has been shown to produce relative protection.[52] In a study involving Finnish tourists to Morocco, BS-WC induced 52% protection

against diarrhoea caused by ETEC, 65% with mixed infection, 71% when ETEC was present with another pathogen, and 82% when ETEC and *S. enterica* were present concurrently. (Sack[48] has concluded that 'any advances in prevention and treatment of diarrhoea in travellers will be directly applicable to the worldwide problem of diarrhoea in children, which is far more important on a global scale'. This statement does not apply to this BS-WC vaccine, because protection only lasts for about 3 months.) A further approach under consideration consists of oral administration of colostrum-derived antibodies against ETEC.[39]

A recent experimental investigation indicates that lactobacilli, which have the ability to adhere to the intestinal mucosa, can prevent *E. coli* colonization. In a limited clinical study, *Lactobacillus GG* reduced prevalence of TD by up to 40%.[39]

Management

Treatment (as in cholera, see below) devolves around oral rehydration (see below); all travellers should carry suitable preparations.[1,41,53] When properly constituted, Dioralyte (Rhône-Poulenc Rorer) solution contains glucose 90, Na^+ 60, K^+ 25, Cl^- 45 and citrate 20 mmol/L. Corresponding concentrations for another proprietary preparation, Rapolyte (Janssen), are 111, 60, 20, 50 and 10 mmol/L. WHO/UNICEF rehydration fluid contains glucose 111, Na^+ 90, K^+ 20, Cl^- 80 and citrate 10 mmol/L. In a mild case adequate rehydration can usually be achieved using ordinary mineral water.

The role of chemotherapy in established TD remains controversial. Early work carried out by DuPont et al.[38] in Mexico showed that both co-trimoxazole and trimethoprim reduced the length of symptoms. Recent trials, using antibiotics which have been given for chemoprophylaxis (see above), have also indicated that the length of symptoms can be shortened; in Mexico, ofloxacin (600 mg daily for 3 days) produced cure in 77 (95%) of 81, compared with 56 (71%) patients who received placebo ($p = 0.0001$).[54] In a study carried out in Thailand where the causative organism is usually *Campylobacter jejuni*, cure rate at 72 h was highest with single-dose azithromycin (96%), compared with lower rates with 3-day azithromycin and levofloxacin.[55] Short-course chemotherapy can only be justified in a severe case; this applies at the extremes of life and in high-risk groups (see above), especially HIV-infected individuals.[56]

Cholera

Cholera (see also Chapter 51) represents the archetypal disease in the context of small-intestinal secretory (watery) diarrhoea.[34,36,57]

The causative organism, *Vibrio cholerae*, is not invasive and exerts its effect by means of an enterotoxin.[58] If untreated, the disease has a 20–80% mortality; with modern oral rehydration regimens that figure should be <1%. Death results from dehydration, vascular collapse and renal failure.

Historically, cholera was not confined to tropical countries and involved many temperate areas, including much of northern Europe. An epidemic in 1854 in London was traced to contaminated water supplied from the Broad Street pump in Soho. According to legend, when the handle of the pump was tied down by Dr John Snow, the London anaesthetist, a rapid decline in the incidence of new cases was recorded.[59]

Epidemiology

Cholera is endemic in India, Pakistan, Bangladesh, Afghanistan and many other countries of South-east Asia. Nosocomial transmission is reported. In recent years, epidemics have occurred in the Middle East, South America and Africa;[58] most have been localized. Cholera is endemic along the Gulf Coast of the USA. The disease is closely associated with poverty, overcrowding and low socioeconomic status.

In former times cholera was spread by population movements such as the annual 'hajj' to Mecca; outbreaks involving air travellers have been recorded. Overall, however, the disease is rare in British travellers.[60] It tends to affect young people more often than the elderly.

Aetiology and pathogenesis

There is probably a genetic predisposition: blood group O is associated with a higher infection rate than group A.[34]

Classical cholera is caused by V. cholerae, and is now localized to the Indian subcontinent, particularly the deltas of the Ganges and Brahmaputra rivers. Elsewhere, the El Tor biotype, which originated in Indonesia around 1960, and the O139 strain have been responsible for most epidemics. Vibrio species are curved, Gram-negative, flagellated rods approximately 2 mm in length. Each biotype of cholera contains three serotypes: Inaba, Ogawa and Hikojima. For details of the organism and its pathophysiological effects, see Chapter 51.

Pathology

Histologically, the small-intestinal mucosa is intact. Light and electron microscopical appearances are normal. Following circulatory collapse following gross dehydration, renal tubular necrosis can be demonstrated.

Clinical features

There are no prodromal symptoms. The incubation period varies from a few hours to 5 days. The disease is similar whichever biotype is involved, but there is a wide spectrum of severity. When the El Tor biotype is responsible, a higher proportion of patients are asymptomatic. Onset is sudden, and mild diarrhoea rapidly gives way to the passage of a large volume of opalescent fluid – the classic 'rice-water' stools. Up to 30 L of fluid, containing a high concentration of Vibrio spp. organisms, may be passed in 24 h.[57] Vomiting of fluid of a similar composition is a later feature. Thirst, muscle cramps, hoarseness and anuria follow.

Clinical signs of severe dehydration may be present by 24 h after onset in an untreated case. The body temperature is normal or mildly elevated. Circulatory failure and acute renal failure follow. Confusion, disorientation and hypoglycaemic convulsions may occur. Mortality rate is directly related to the degree of dehydration. Relative immunity is short lived. A carrier state, which lasts a few weeks, may occur, and gallbladder foci have been identified.

Investigations

Vibrio spp. organisms are easily identified in a faecal specimen; material should be transported to the laboratory in alkaline peptone water (pH 9.0). A rapid diagnostic technique for field use has been described. For accurate serological identification of V. cholerae, rigid criteria are necessary. With classic cholera, organisms are present during the incubation period and up to 5 days after an attack; in the El Tor variety, Vibrio spp. can persist for weeks or months.

Faecal samples are isotonic, with a protein concentration of approximately 10 g/L; pH is about 7.5; typical electrolyte concentrations are: sodium 139 mmol/L, potassium 23 mmol/L, chloride 106 mmol/L and bicarbonate 48 mmol/L. Specimens contain a high concentration of IgA. Serum IgA and IgM are elevated, the former most markedly in patients with an El Tor infection. In vitro animal studies, indicate that cholera toxin enhances IgA secretion from crypt epithelium to ileal lumen.[56]

Serum electrolyte, urea and creatinine concentrations vary with the stage and severity of the disease. Excessive potassium loss exacerbates metabolic acidosis. Urine is concentrated; its composition depends on the severity of the disease.

Differential diagnosis

Diagnosis is usually straightforward; however, all other causes of small-intestinal diarrhoea (with and without vomiting) of acute onset (see below) should be considered. These include traveller's diarrhoea, E. coli, Staphylococcus species, Clostridium perfringens, Cl. botulinum, Campylobacter jejuni and viral causes (e.g. rotavirus, norovirus). Salmonella and Shigella spp. should also be considered. Vibrio parahaemolyticus (conveyed by infected raw seafood) and other non-cholera Vibrio species can produce a similar disease. Very occasionally, Plasmodium falciparum malaria presents with severe watery diarrhoea, especially in infants and children. Food poisoning, caused by toxic agents, should be added to the list of differential diagnoses.

Prevention

Basic sanitation and public health procedures should be improved.[61] Sterility of water supplies is of paramount importance. Contacts of proven cases should be vaccinated; all faeces and bed linen should be destroyed. Vaccination with inactivated (dead) Vibrio species organisms gives only limited protection;[62] 0.5 mL and 1.0 mL vaccine should be given at an interval of 1 week, and a 0.5 mL booster every 6 months.

The 26th Assembly of the WHO recommended, in 1973, that cholera vaccination should not be compulsory, due to its limited public health value. Despite this, a few countries continue to demand vaccination before entry. Important progress is being made towards an effective oral bivalent cholera–typhoid vaccine.[63]

Management

Rehydration regimens

Treatment was revolutionized by the introduction of oral rehydration regimens.[64–66] The enterocyte sodium-glucose carrier system is not affected by cyclic AMP, and thus glucose (and glycine)-stimulated membrane transport takes place normally.

It is impossible to overload the circulation by the oral route in a previously fit person. Quantity of ingested fluid should be regulated by faecal loss, best measured 2-hourly. Rehydration should be accomplished within 48 h. In an unsophisticated situation, sucrose is often more easily obtainable than glucose; results are usually good, although if severe mucosal damage pre-exists, sucrase concentration is lowered and satisfactory rehydration is less readily achieved. Cereal-based electrolyte solutions have also given satisfactory results.[66]

In a severe case, intravenous fluids may be necessary for initial rehydration.[65] A widely-used formula consists of; sodium chloride 5.0 g, sodium bicarbonate 4.0 g, potassium chloride 1.0 g, made up to 1 L. Severity of dehydration should be assessed on clinical grounds; in a case of average severity, 5 L should be given (the first litre within 10 min) to a 50 kg subject.

Drug treatment

Analgesics may be necessary for severe muscle cramps. Intravenous calcium gluconate is of value for tetany.

Tetracycline hydrochloride, 1 g/day for 5 days, shortens duration of diarrhoea and clears the luminal content of *Vibrio* spp. organisms in the case of the El Tor biotype.[66] A single dose (1 g or 2 g) has also been shown to be effective in *V. cholerae* infection, but is associated with asymptomatic bacteriological relapse.[67,68] Tetracycline should be started several hours after rehydration therapy has begun. Single-dose doxycycline (300 mg) is probably as effective as tetracycline.[69] There is clear evidence that in epidemics the El Tor biotype rapidly develops resistance not only to tetracycline, but also to several other antibiotics (including trimethoprim plus sulfamethoxazole), and is therefore of very limited value. Recently, *Vibrio cholerae* 01 biotype El Tor strains have proved resistant to furazolidone and co-trimoxazole.[70]

Prognosis

If cholera is adequately treated, there should be zero mortality, and complete recovery. A suggestion has been made that individuals who have suffered from cholera might be predisposed to α-chain disease (see below).

Malabsorption in the tropics

Apart from infective causes, primary hypolactasia (lactase deficiency)[1,71] accounts for watery small-intestinal diarrhoea in some people indigenous to tropical countries. A low concentration of this enzyme in the enterocyte brush border is normal for adult *Homo sapiens* (as for other species within the mammalian kingdom); the enzyme is under genetic control. In a minority of the world's population, i.e. northern Europeans, Africans with an Hamitic ancestry, certain Middle Eastern populations (e.g. Saudi Arabians) and others in northern parts of the Indian subcontinent, a high concentration continues into adult life. Secondary hypolactasia results from brush border damage;[1,71] concentration of all disaccharidases (and other digestive enzymes) is reduced, and slow recovery occurs after the initiating insult has disappeared. Thus, whenever there is enterocyte destruction (this includes post-infective malabsorption, see below) hypolactasia develops.

Following ingestion of milk or another milk produce, in which lactose is incompletely hydrolysed, osmotic diarrhoea results; this is accompanied by abdominal colic, distension and flatulence ('lactose intolerance'). In a study carried out at Penang, Malaysia, hypolactasia was demonstrated in all ethic groups, and although there was no clear association with gastrointestinal symptoms, the authors recommend a low lactose diet in all Asian countries.[72] Yoghurt contains adequate bacterial lactase to hydrolyse the lactose component and is usually well tolerated. Lactic acid production (derived from hydrolysis of lactose by colonic bacteria) produces irritative diarrhoea, which contributes to the symptoms. The precise role of the colon in adaptation remains unclear; carbohydrate, in the form of free fatty acid(s) (and also nitrogen and electrolytes), can be absorbed from this organ. Investigation of hypolactasia most often utilizes the breath hydrogen test; lactose 'tolerance' test and lactase assay in a jejunal biopsy specimen are alternatives. In management, milk and all lactose-containing dairy products should be eliminated from the diet;[1,71] individuals in countries with a high prevalence of primary hypolactasia can regulate bowel function by varying lactose ingestion.

Post-infective malabsorption (PIM) (tropical sprue)

Relatively little is known about the prevalence and severity of malabsorption in acute infective conditions of the small intestine (viral, bacterial and parasitic) and the duration for which it can continue after the specific organism(s) has been eliminated.[73]

In some cases, malabsorption persists in the presence of mixed luminal flora, and a single infective agent cannot be detected. In others the recognizable initiating infective cause (or causes) may continue, culminating in a chronic form; a more precise term is therefore 'postacute infective' malabsorption. As with all infective diseases, the clinical spectrum of disease varies from subclinical to gross pathology (malabsorption). PIM is of particular clinical significance in tropical countries, where small (and large) intestinal infections are exceedingly common.

PIM related to tropical exposure has been reviewed by Cook,[1,33,74] Tomkins,[75] Baker[76] and Mathan.[77]

History and definition

Confusion has existed between PIM and tropical sprue; however, in tropical and subtropical countries, these entities are synonymous, and the difficulty is primarily one of semantics.[1,33] Patrick Manson first coined the term tropical sprue (derived from a word used by Dutch workers in the East Indies) in 1880.[78] The term was rapidly applied to all cases of malabsorption in tropical countries, undoubtedly including some resulting from tuberculosis and various parasitoses (both protozoan and helminthic). Historically, chronic diarrhoea accompanied by wasting was recognized in India before 600 BC; although the Englishman William Hillary is often credited with the first precise description of tropical sprue at Barbados,[79] it now seems likely that he described either epidemic *G. lamblia* infection, or possibly strongyloidiasis. The clinical syndrome was well known to British physicians in India during the eighteenth and nineteenth centuries; most descriptions were made in British expatriate populations. It was in the early 1960s that reports of a high prevalence of epidemic PIM in indigenous Indians became available.[1,76,77] Despite early suggestions that chronic tropical diarrhoea had an insidious onset, it is clear (after careful assessment) that the vast majority of cases always presented acutely. Confusion has been compounded further when acute epidemic cases of small-intestinal infection, associated with gross dehydration (in addition to xylose and fat malabsorption) and acute mortality, have been designated tropical sprue, as in numerous reports from southern India.[77] It is essential to include a time factor in the definition of this clinical syndrome, e.g. chronic diarrhoea and malabsorption, with weight loss, of at least 3–4 months duration. The term tropical sprue (if used at all) would be better reserved for a condition where malabsorption of nutrients is quantitatively more important than that of water and electrolytes. Although the aetiology of PIM is not yet completely clear (see below), in most cases it undoubtedly follows an acute small-intestinal insult by either a bacterial, viral or parasitic (or mixed) infection.

Overall, evidence for PIM following a small-intestinal insult is most complete for bacterial and parasitic infections; those of viral origin might, however, be more important numerically. Lack of precise data can be largely attributed to the fact that virology remains a relatively neglected discipline in most developing countries, where infections of all types are far more common than in the Western world.

The effect of malabsorption on overall nutritional status is largely unknown (see above); children are especially at risk. The magnitude of energy loss is unclear; a deficit of 10% of dietary energy (one estimate) is substantial in tropical populations subsisting on a 'marginal' diet. The importance of anorexia in exacerbating associated malnutrition is also underexplored.

Geographical distribution

Figure 10.3 summarizes the geographical localities where PIM has been reported either commonly or less frequently;[33,34] the map does not include areas where sporadic cases have been rarely recorded. Although the disease is common (and endemic) in Asia and the northern part of South America, it is a very unusual condition in tropical Africa. It remains a problem in travellers to many tropical locations.[80–82] Until recently, it was a common entity in overland travellers from the UK to Asia; the fact that it is now rarely seen is probably associated with early antibiotic administration. In the Middle East and Mediterranean littoral PIM is unusual, but undoubtedly occurs.[74]

Aetiology

There can now be no reasonable doubt that PIM has an infective basis (see above): it is (1) more common in geographical areas where enteric infection abounds; (2) epidemic in certain areas, including southern India; (3) the small-intestinal lumen is colonized by aerobic enterobacteria; and (4) recovery usually occurs rapidly (and dramatically) following initiation of broad-spectrum antibiotic treatment. Despite this, however, Mathan[77] is of the opinion that in southern India the primary lesion is enterocyte damage resulting from a 'persistent' lesion of the stem cell compartment on a 'background of tropical enteropathy'. He further considers that 'an immunity-conferring agent may be responsible for the initiating damage'. The widely used definition for this clinical syndrome in southern India, 'intestinal malabsorption of at lease two nutrients and the exclusion of diseases that give rise to secondary malabsorption in a tropical environment', is inadequate; it does not exclude tropical enteropathy (see above), nor does it introduce a time (chronicity) factor.

Genetic predisposition

All infective diseases, without exception, have a genetic background. In a limited study at Puerto Rico, 25 of 27 patients with PIM (not well defined) had at least one antigen of the HLA-Aw19 series;[83] the strongest associated link was with Aw31. In India, a high frequency of HLA-B8 was documented;[84] HLA-A1, A28 and Bw35 were significantly decreased in the affected group. More data are undoubtedly required on genetic markers in PIM.

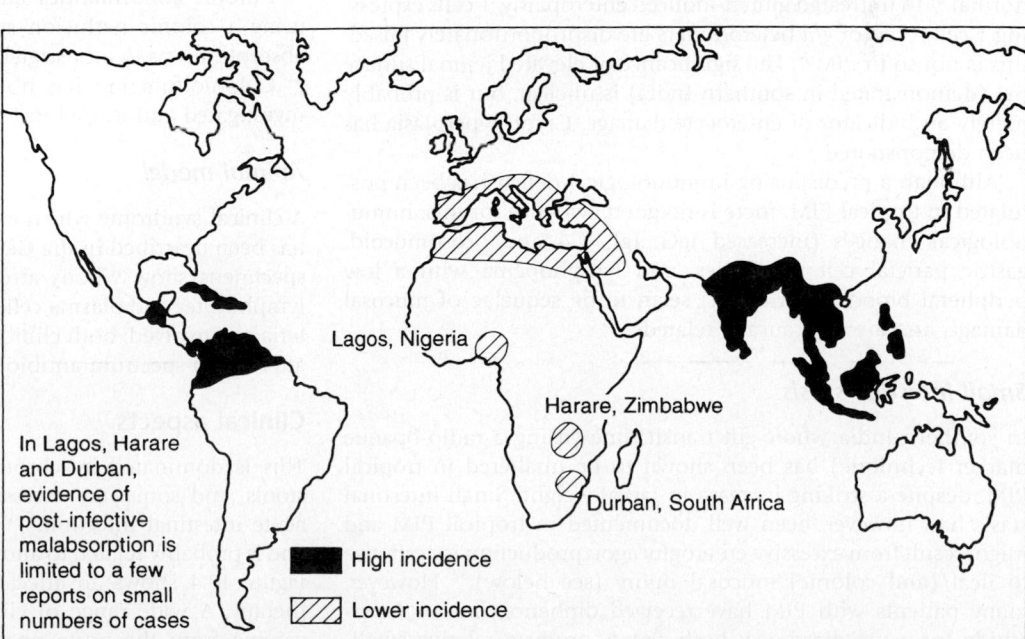

In Lagos, Harare and Durban, evidence of post-infective malabsorption is limited to a few reports on small numbers of cases

Lagos, Nigeria

Harare, Zimbabwe

Durban, South Africa

■ High incidence

▧ Lower incidence

Figure 10.3 World map showing areas where post-infective tropical malabsorption is a significant problem.

Infection

In severe PIM (in the absence of parasites) bacterial colonization has been demonstrated both within the jejunal lumen and in biopsy specimens. The importance of adhesive properties of bacteria in pathogenesis is unclear; many bacteria, including *E. coli*, *S. typhimurium* and *V. cholerae*, possess such properties, mediated by a transmissible plasmid. In tropical PIM, several groups have demonstrated a higher concentration of aerobic enterobacteria in relation to the enterocyte compared with luminal fluid. (In the normal individual, anaerobes outnumber aerobes by about 1000-fold.) It seems likely that a variety of toxins released by these enterobacteria induce net water secretion and malabsorption. In the blind-loop syndrome, enterobacteria (which are invariably obligate anaerobes) do not produce toxins. Several months after tropical exposure the upper small-intestinal intraluminal bacterial flora (mucosal biopsy or luminal fluid) remains abnormal;[85] seven of 11 patients studied had enterobacteria in numbers ranging from 10^3 to 10^8/g or mL. The most common organisms were *Klebsiella pneumoniae*, *Enterobacter cloacae* and *E. coli*; *Citrobacter feundii*, *Serratia marcescens* and *Pseudomonas* spp. have also been detected. It seems highly likely, therefore, that these organisms were present since the onset of disease.[86] In southern India, a viral aetiology has been sought, but there is little evidence for this. The origin of continuing overgrowth has not been adequately studied in tropical PIM; in patients in England with small-intestinal bacterial overgrowth, faecal flora account for most of the organisms, but salivary flora are probably important in some cases.

Jejunal morphology

Morphological changes are non-specific and range in severity.[74] Blunting of villi ('partial villous atrophy') with increased lymphocyte and plasma cell infiltration (not a feature of tropical enteropathy) are present to a variable degree; a 'flat' mucosa is exceedingly unusual. Although the number of plasma cells is increased, distribution of IgA-, IgM- and IgG-containing cells is normal.[87] In untreated gluten-induced enteropathy, T cells expressing T cell receptor g/d heterodimers are disproportionately raised; this is not so in PIM.[87] The significance of elevated jejunal surface pH (demonstrated in southern India) is unclear, but is probably merely an indicator of enterocyte damage. Crypt hyperplasia has been demonstrated.

Although a predisposing immunological deficit has been postulated in tropical PIM, there is no good evidence for this; immunological changes (increased IgG, IgE, C4 and orosomucoid, gastric parietal cell antibodies, and lymphopenia with a low peripheral blood T cell count) seem to be sequelae of mucosal damage, and are not causally related.

Small-intestine stasis

In southern India whole-gut transit time (using a radio-opaque marker technique) has been shown to be unaltered in tropical PIM, despite a striking increase in faecal weight. Small-intestinal stasis has, however, been well documented in tropical PIM and might result from excessive enteroglucagon production in response to ileal (and colonic) mucosal injury (see below).[88] However, many patients with PIM have received diphenoxylate or loperamide for acute diarrhoea; both agents produce relative small-intestinal stasis. Both of these agents interfere with peristalsis and prevent prostaglandin-induced diarrhoea; inhibition of small-intestinal secretion also occurs. Such stasis is of particular interest because peristalsis is usually increased in the presence of intraluminal bacteria.

Gut hormones

Gut hormones have been studied in tropical PIM in the fasting state and following a standard meal.[88] Fasting and postprandial plasma enteroglucagon concentrations (produced by cells in the distal ileum and colon) and motilin were markedly elevated; furthermore, the elevated enteroglucagon concentration is significantly correlated with a reduction in small-intestinal transit (using the H_2 breath test). Both enteroglucagon and motilin concentrations fall after treatment. Concentration of another gut hormone, plasma peptide YY (also produced by endocrine cells in the ileum and colon and known to delay gastric emptying and small-intestinal transit, and to reduce gastric and pancreatic secretion) has been shown to be grossly elevated in PIM;[89] it seems possible that this results from a change in peptide YY secretion, resulting from malabsorption, and is a compensatory mechanism in diarrhoea. Patients with PIM also have a reduced post-prandial rise in gastric-inhibiting polypeptide; gastrin and pancreatic polypeptide are normal.

Role of the colon

The colonic mucosa, in addition to that of the small intestine, is abnormal in tropical PIM ('tropical colonopathy').[90] Few causes of diarrhoea are strictly confined to one or other of these organs; for example, *shigellosis* frequently involves the small intestine, and *salmonellosis* and *Campylobacter jejuni* infection of the colon.

The normal colon is able to absorb 4–7 L of water/24 h,[91] together with 100–160 mmol carbohydrate (as volatile fatty acid(s)). Failure of the diseased colon to 'salvage' the increased ileal effluent must increase the intensity of diarrhoea.

Colonic abnormalities have been reported in tropical sprue; using a colonic perfusion system, impaired water and sodium absorption was demonstrated.[92]

Colonic function has not been investigated in tropical PIM investigated and treated in London.

Animal model

A clinical syndrome which exhibits very close similarities to PIM has been described in the German shepherd dog.[93] Jejunal biopsy specimens show villous atrophy with a variable infiltration of lymphocytes and plasma cells in the lamina propria. Aerobic bacteria are involved; both clinical and laboratory recovery take place after broad-spectrum antibiotic therapy.

Clinical aspects

This is dominated by chronic diarrhoea with large, pale, fatty stools, and sometime excessive flatulence, usually following an acute intestinal infection.[1,33,34,74] Weight loss is sometimes gross and is probably related to anorexia as much as to intestinal disease. Figure 10.4 shows an affected patient before and after chemotherapy. A wide range of clinical presentations exists, however, varying from the acute onset type (not strictly postinfective),

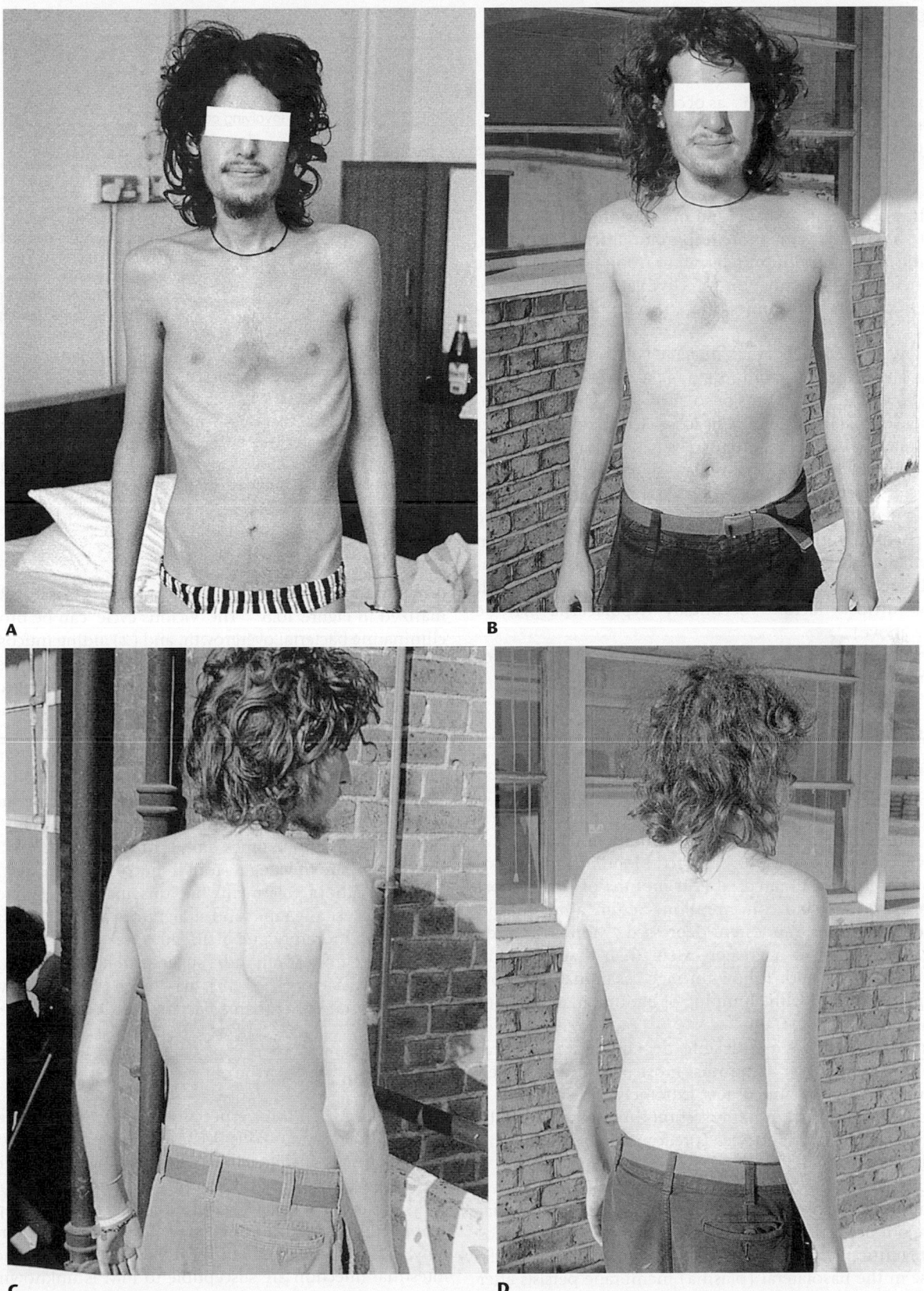

Figure 10.4 (A and C) A 19-year-old Englishman presented in London with post-infective tropical malabsorption (tropical sprue). Acute diarrhoea started soon after his arrival in Nepal and he lost approximately 12 kg in weight during the subsequent 2 months. The total urinary xylose excretion after a 25 g oral load was 2.5 mmol/5 h (normal range 8.0–16.0 mmol/5 h); the 24-h faecal fat was 83 mmol (normal range 11–18 mmol); the Schilling test result was 0.16% urinary excretion at 24 h (normal >10%) and the 8-h serum concentration was 0% (normal >0.6%) of the loading dose. Jejunal biopsy histology showed marked villous blunting with increased lymphocytes in the lamina propria. Parasites were not found in several faecal samples. Serum albumin 36 g/L; haemoglobin 13.2 g/dL; mean corpuscular volume 102.9; red blood cell folate 113 ng/L (normal >150 ng/L); serum vitamin B_{12} 322 pg/L (normal >150 pg/L). He responded rapidly to treatment with oral tetracycline and folic acid. (B and D) The same man 4 weeks after initiation of treatment when all investigations were normal.

described by Baker[76] and Mathan[77] as occurring in epidemics (with vomiting and pyrexia in up to 50%) at Vellore, India, to a far more chronic entity. Other clinical features, such as glossitis (aphthous ulceration was common in nineteenth-century reports), megaloblastic anaemia, fluid retention, depression, apathy, amenorrhoea and infertility, occur only after several months duration.

Table 10.3 summarizes the more important differential diagnoses of chronic malabsorption in relation to tropical exposure (see below).[80] There are also many non-infective causes of malabsorption in the tropics and subtropics; these should be excluded systematically.[94]

During, and immediately after, an acute small-intestinal infection, xylose, glucose, fat, B_{12} and folate malabsorption frequently occur (see above). After 4 months or so, moderate/severe morphological change occurs in the jejunal mucosa; serum folate and later B_{12} concentrations decline – often to very low concentrations. Hypoalbuminaemia and oedema are late signs.

Gastric acid secretion is often depressed, but whether this precedes, or is a sequel to, the initiating infection is unknown. The role of hypochlorhydria in the production of small-intestinal infection remains unclear. In a small proportion of cases in southern India, B_{12} absorption either improved or became normal with addition of intrinsic factor.[90] Secondary hypolactasia may be present (see above).[71]

There is no good evidence that PIM predisposes to any gastrointestinal malignancy.

Investigations

Investigations should include urinary D-xylose excretion, 72-h faecal fat estimation, a Schilling test and jejunal biopsy; faecal parasites should be excluded (1-h blood xylose concentration is in practice probably superior to a 5-h urinary collection in a tropical environment[95]): serum B_{12} and red blood cell folate concentrations should be estimated; after 4 months of illness most patients have a low folate concentration. Serum albumin and globulin concentrations are often depressed. Monosaccharide absorption is impaired to a greater extent than that of amino acids.[74] Barium meal and follow-through examination show dilated loops of jejunum with clumping of barium, in addition to reduced transit rate.

Jejunal mucosal changes are variable, depending on the duration of the disease. By 3 or 4 months, most biopsies are ridged and/or convoluted; a flat mucosa is extremely unusual and, if present, gluten-induced enteropathy[94] should be suspected. Submucosal invasion with lymphocytes (predominantly T cells) and plasma cells is usual.

Ultrastructural changes in jejunal biopsy specimens have been studied;[96] although lysosomes, peroxisomes and mitochondrial enzymes are not depressed, the organelles are more fragile. Endoplasmic reticulum is unchanged. A significant reduction in 5-nucleotidase in the basolateral (plasma) membrane persists after recovery. The latter finding might reflect an underlying abnormality in the enterocyte of individuals susceptible to PIM.

Intestinal permeability has also been investigated;[36,97] abnormalities in urinary excretion of lactulose and rhamnose following an oral load are similar to results obtained in gluten-induced enteropathy.

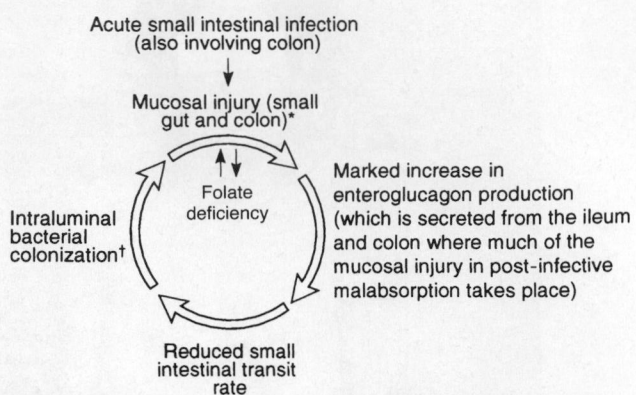

Figure 10.5 Hypothetical scheme to illustrate the pathogenesis of post-infective malabsorption. The open arrows indicate the vicious cycle which, once set in motion, is only broken by elimination of the abnormal intraluminal flora (†), and hastening of enterocyte recovery (*).

Aetiology and treatment

A hypothesis to account for the aetiology of tropical PIM is summarized in Figure 10.5.[98] The 'vicious cycle' can be broken by (1) eliminating bacterial overgrowth, and (2) aiding mucosal recovery (with folic acid supplements). While this hypothesis has been challenged,[99] a satisfactory alternative has not been produced. An adequate diet should be combined with tetracycline (250 mg three times a day for at least 2 weeks) and folic acid (5 mg three times a day for 1 month). Evidence of susceptibility of the responsible flora to antibiotics other than tetracycline is limited. Symptomatic treatment may be necessary in the acute stage of the disease; codeine phosphate (30 mg three times a day), diphenoxylate (2.5–5 mg four times daily), or loperamide (5–10 mg four times daily) are of value if stool frequency is excessive. Mild cases respond without treatment, but this may take several months. Recovery is usually rapid and straightforward;[1,74,98] in the pre-antibiotic era a mortality rate of 10–20% was usual.

Evidence from south India suggests that response to antibiotics is less satisfactory;[76,77] this has been used as evidence to support a viral rather than a bacterial aetiology being causative in that locality.

Conclusion

The aetiology of PIM – especially that presenting in association with tropical exposure – is becoming clearer.[99] It is probable that several primary insults to the enterocyte (of an infective nature) are involved. Whereas PIM resulting from most viral, bacterial and parasitic causes is usually self-limiting, this does not apply to the 'tropical sprue' syndrome, when well established. The reason why only a minority of affected individuals who suffer an acute small-intestinal infection are susceptible to PIM is unknown; a genetic (or ethnic) basis for susceptibility seems likely.

Other causes of malabsorption in the tropics

Table 10.3 summarizes some of these. The role of parasitic infection has been highlighted by AIDS, in which prolonged diarrhoea accompanied by malabsorption and weight loss can be very troublesome.[37] Incontrovertible evidence exists that HIV itself causes chronic enteropathy with villous blunting; crypt hypoplasia results from a direct effect of the viruses on cell replication, or by an unknown immunological reaction. This is a very common cause of persisting malabsorption in Africa. In this context, *Cryptosporidium parvum* and *Isospora belli* have recently come to the fore and it is now also clear that these organisms can produce a self-limiting illness simulating TD in immunocompetent adults and children (see below). *G. lamblia* (see below) is undoubtedly the most common cause of parasitic malabsorption.[74,100,101] *Strongyloides stercoralis* (see below), which is widespread in tropical countries, was until very recently still present in approximately 15–30% of former prisoners of war in South-east Asia during World War II; it is an underdiagnosed cause.[1,102]

Of all causes of malabsorption related to tropical exposure, intestinal tuberculosis – usually involving the ileocaecal region – is probably that with the lowest index of suspicion among medical personnel.[74,103] Abdominal tuberculosis can assume several clinical forms: apart from the hypertrophic ileocaecal form, glandular (involving the mesenteric glands), peritoneal (sometimes with ascites) and hepatic involvement (with granulomatous disease) are relatively common. With the first of these presentations, weight loss and diarrhoea are often accompanied by a low-grade febrile illness; in severe cases stools are large, pale and bulky. Examination reveals an ileocaecal mass in 35–50% of cases,[103] and occasionally enlargement of one or more lymph glands; however, there is often no clinical abnormality. Late presentation can be as adult kwashiorkor. Anaemia and hypoalbuminaemia are common.[103] Chest radiography is usually normal. Absorption tests are frequently abnormal; fat and B$_{12}$ absorption are affected most severely. A protein-losing enteropathy may be present. Pathologically, the disease results either from miliary dissemination, or follows ileal ulceration. Malabsorption is caused by chronic bile salt loss; unabsorbed bile salts (normally re-absorbed in the terminal ileum) in turn interfere with colonic absorption. Barium meal and follow-through examination show ileal strictures,[103] frequently multiple, in a high percentage of cases; the ascending colon may also be shortened. The major differential is Crohn's disease, which is statistically much less common in people indigenous to the tropics. *Yersinia* infection should also be considered. Chest radiography is usually normal. The tuberculin test is positive in 70–90% of cases.[103] A needle liver biopsy specimen occasionally shows hepatic granulomas with caseation. Diagnostic laparotomy or peritoneoscopy (and peritoneal biopsy) is sometimes necessary in order to obtain a tissue diagnosis.[103] Treatment is with an antituberculosis regimen (Chapter 56). Resection of stricture(s) and occasionally hemicolectomy are sometimes necessary; chemotherapy should be initiated before surgical intervention.

A further cause of malabsorption in a tropical environment consists of the Mediterranean (α-chain) lymphoma,[104,105] which occurs sporadically in many parts of the tropics. If started early, tetracycline usually produces a good result, but not always so.

Although it seems overall uncommon in most indigenous populations in tropical countries recent reports of coeliac disease have been made from India[106] and Turkey[107] and some evidence exists that it might be increasing in prevalence.[108]

Other small-intestinal infections

Viral infections

Significant intestinal protein loss (mean 1.7 g daily) and xylose malabsorption have been demonstrated in northern Nigerian children with measles (see Chapter 47); approximately 25% also had lactose malabsorption.[109] Other infections in children caused by enteroviruses and herpes simplex viruses are also associated with diarrhoea and weight loss; malnutrition may result; the mechanism(s) (involving enterocyte damage) is probably similar to that in measles.

Volunteers infected with enteric viruses develop small-intestinal morphological lesions which are not always associated with symptoms.

Jejunal mucosal changes giving rise to severe malabsorption have been well documented in viral hepatitis;[110] these may persist for a considerable time after resolution of the hepatic abnormalities. The norovirus (a 27 nm piconavirus) can also produce mucosal damage and malabsorption.[111] Rotavirus infections give rise to morphological abnormalities and (especially in children) malabsorption.[112,113]

These viral infections are invasive, and the resulting diarrhoea and malabsorption are caused by enterocyte destruction. Malabsorption usually occurs after the virus has been shed into the intestinal lumen; the villi contain immature crypt-type enterocytes. In coronavirus infection(s) in piglets, which resemble human rotavirus infections, glucose absorption is significantly impaired.[114] This has practical importance in management because sodium and water secretion cannot be reversed by glucose; oral rehydration fluids, commonly used in small-intestinal (including travellers') diarrhoea (see above), contain a high glucose concentration which overwhelms the limited absorptive capacity.

Baker[76] and Mathan[77] have suggested that coronavirus infections are responsible for at least some cases of 'tropical sprue' in southern India (see above); this might be the case, but asymptomatic individuals often excrete these viruses and this does not therefore indicate a cause-effect relationship. Also at *Vellore*, a search for evidence of *Berne* virus infection in 'epidemic tropical sprue' proved negative.[115]

Bacterial infections

Moderate to severe malabsorption is commonplace during acute intestinal infections of bacterial origin; subnormal absorptive capacity persists for variable periods after termination of the diarrhoea and apparent clinical recovery. In a study in Bangladesh, approximately 70% of patients had evidence of xylose malabsorption 1 week after the diarrhoea had ceased; this was less common after cholera than *Shigella* species, *Salmonella* species and/or *Staphylococcus* species infections; xylose and B$_{12}$ malabsorption persisted for up to 378 and 196 days, respectively, after the diarrhoea had cleared.

Although many different infective insults to the enterocyte are probably important in PIM (see above), evidence for bacteria being responsible currently has more solid support than that involving other agents.

Escherichia coli

These organisms (with varying modes of pathogenicity) produce a spectrum of disease from TD to malabsorption by enterotoxin production and mucosal invasion-similar to that caused by Shigella species (Chapter 51). They are frequently food- or water-borne, and may cause outbreaks of gastroenteritis. Heat-labile enterotoxins exert an effect by activating adenylcyclase by a mechanism(s) similar to *V. cholerae*. Both heat-labile and heat-stable enterotoxins are probably important in TD (see above). A large pool of resistant *E. coli* (often showing resistance to multiple antimicrobials) now exists in the community. Enterotoxin production by *E. coli* may be transferred simultaneously with antibiotic resistance (Chapter 53); in a study, 72% and 44% of ETEC isolated in South-east Asia were resistant to one or more, and four or more antibiotics, respectively.[116] Enterocyte adhesiveness of *E. coli* is also a property of some strains and that might be important in continuing colonization and subsequent malabsorption. The relationship between adherence and verotoxin production remains unclear.[106] Attachment of microorganisms to the enterocyte prevents clearance by peristaltic activity; such mucosal receptors may be determined genetically.[117] Ultrastructural studies have shown *E. coli* adherent to mucosal cells, with flattering of the microvilli, loss of the cellular terminal web and cupping of the plasma membrane around individual bacteria; intracellular damage was marked in the most heavily colonized cells. Histological improvement was demonstrated following clearing of *E. coli* with neomycin and nutritional support. This mechanism can lead to protracted diarrhoea in infants. In most cases, resultant malabsorption is short lived.

Salmonellosis

Malabsorption occasionally follows infection with *Salmonella* species (Chapter 52),[118] but the frequency is unknown.

Campylobacter jejuni

Although unusual, dysenteric disease (bloody diarrhoea) has for long been known to predispose to tropical PIM;[74] in addition to shigellosis it is clear that some cases are caused by *E. coli* (see above) and others by *Campylobacter jejuni* (Chapter 51).

Although most cases of *Campylobacter jejuni* infection are acute, present with gastroenteritis and are self-limiting, initial symptoms can be prolonged.[119] The disease is a zoonosis; poultry are frequently contaminated. Many outbreaks have been traced to infected cow's milk. Dogs also constitute a reservoir of infection. Although the infection is self-limiting, erythromycin probably hastens recovery when given early in a severe case. The carrier state is common.

Enteritis necroticans (pigbel disease)

Although described in Germany at the end of World War II (1939–1945), and named Darmbrand,[4,34] this acute infection (Figure 10.6), which is more common in children than adults, occurs in several tropical countries, notably the highlands of Papua New Guinea (where it is endemic),[120] Thailand and Uganda. Recently, enteritis necroticans has been recorded in Khmer children at an evacuation site on the Thai-Kampuchean border of Thailand; in the former report 36 (58%) out of 62 affected children (10 months to 10 (mean 4) years) died.[4] It seems likely that a disease termed 'necrotizing jejunitis' in rural areas of Bihar, India – which also affects children – represents the same entity; this condition ('segmental necrotizing enteritis') has also been recorded in Jaipur, India, and in Sri Lanka.[4] Scanty reports of a similar condition have also been made from northern Europe, which suggests that the disease exists worldwide, but only reaches epidemic proportions when suitable conditions exist, most importantly for the β-toxin of *Clostridium perfringens* type C (ingested in contaminated foodstuffs) to take its toll. Murrell[121] has suggested (in the light of historical evidence) that the disease was widespread in medieval Europe when 'human habitats, food hygiene, protein deficiency and periodic meat feasting formed the basics of village life as they do in many Third World cultures today'. Enteritis necroticans is now known to be caused by the ingestion (often at pig feasts or 'mumus') of food contaminated by *Cl. perfringens* type C.[120] The pathophysiology of the disease is complex, but the presence of a low concentration of trypsin (resulting from

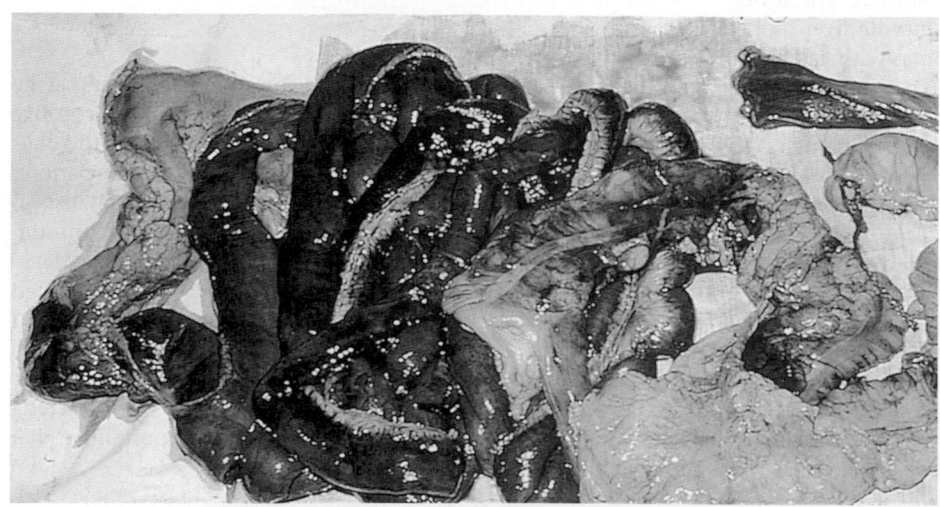

Figure 10.6 Gangrenous small intestine at post-mortem in a Papua New Guinean child who had died from necrotizing enteritis (pigbel disease).

trypsin inhibitors in foodstuffs and chronic protein-energy malnutrition) allows the β-toxin of *Cl. perfringens* to survive and produce mucosal injury.[34] It is sometimes associated with persisting structural changes in the small intestine; malabsorption may be a sequel.

Fluid and electrolyte replacement are essential (see below). Tetracycline or chloramphenicol, and type C gas gangrene antisera are of value; laparotomy is often indicated. In Papua New Guinea, immunization against *Cl. perfringens* type C has given good results;[34] in a controlled trial, marked reduction in incidence and mortality was demonstrated in the treatment group. A management strategy has been outlined.[120]

Parasitic infections

A study carried out in Sierra Leone has indicated that both protozoan and helminthic infections are particularly common in displacement camps.[122]

Giardiasis

The spectrum of disease caused by this flagellated protozoan is broad.[1,74,100,101] Symptoms vary from subclinical cases to those with severe malabsorption and malnutrition. The reason why some individuals are prone to symptomatic giardiasis is not clear; size of infecting dose, strain variability, genetic predisposition, acquired immunity factors, achlorhydria, a local secretory IgA deficiency and the presence of blood group A phenotype have all been considered. An increase in IgE and IgD cell numbers has been reported in the jejunal mucosa of 20 affected patients;[123] the former reversed after treatment, when an increase in IgA cell numbers was also recorded. Genetic characterization has recently been reported from Ethiopia.[124] The actual mechanism by which the trophozoites cause an absorptive defect is also unclear. Mucosal injury, with or without invasion, bacterial overgrowth in association with parasitization, and bile salt deconjugation by bacteria and/or parasites have all been considered. The extent of jejunal morphological abnormality varies widely.

Clinical presentation is usually between 1 and 3 weeks after infection; contaminated water and, less commonly, food are the usual sources of infection. Infection occurs both endemically and epidemically. The disease can probably be contracted from domestic animals.[125] It is more common in male homosexuals, but is not an opportunistic infection in AIDS sufferers. Diarrhoea of acute onset, flatus and weight loss may all be present; the stools have the characteristics of malabsorption. The disease is clinically indistinguishable from PIM; investigations also give similar results. A full-blown case has all of the clinical and laboratory features of the classical (historical) reports of 'tropical sprue' (see above). Cysts may be found in a faecal specimen; trophozoites can be detected in either a jejunal biopsy or jejunal fluid, or with the string test ('Enterotest'). If mucosal changes and malabsorption exist, circulating antibodies to *G. lamblia* cysts can often be detected.

Treatment is with metronizadole (2 g on three consecutive days); alcohol should be avoided during the treatment period. A single dose of tinidazole (2 g orally) has been used with success. Two 5-nitroimidazoles – ornidazole and tinidazole (as a single 1.5 g dose) – have been compared;[126] recurrence of infection during the subsequent 2 months was similar in each case (about 10%). Nimorazole has also been used. An alternative is mepacrine (100 mg three times daily for 10 days), which is less often used.

Cryptosporidium parvum

The importance of farms as a source of infection has been emphasized in a study from Zambia.[127] Importance of domestic pets as a source of infection has also recently been emphasized in a study carried out in Peru.[128] Like *G. lamblia*, this organism produces a broad spectrum of disease; prolonged infection usually, but not always, occurs in the immunosuppressed (including AIDS) sufferer where the organism is opportunistic. Diagnosis is similar to that for *G. lamblia* infection; oocysts are usually detectable in a faecal sample. Treatment (rarely indicated in the immunointact) is with spiramycin, but is usually ineffective in the immunosuppressed; although at least 70 other compounds have been tested, none, including spiramycin, has proven efficiency in vitro.

Other parasites

The vast majority of small-intestinal parasitic infections do not result in signs/symptoms unless present at a high concentration.[32] In a heavy infection, hookworm is responsible for hypochromic anaemia; *A. lumbricoides* rarely accounts for obstruction in the small intestine and biliary and pancreatic ducts (Chapter 85). The major clinical sequel of tapeworm infection is neurocysticercosis (*Taenia solium*) (Chapter 87) – a complication unrelated to the intestinal tract.

Although *A. lumbricoides*, *Ancylostoma duodenale* and *Necator americanus* have at various times been implicated in malabsorption, there is no clear evidence except in rare or anecdotal case reports.[129] *Diphyllobothrium latum* infections are occasionally associated with a low serum B_{12} concentration; however, this is caused by B_{12} uptake within the small-intestinal lumen, and is not an example of true malabsorption.

Clear evidence exists that *Strongyloides stercoralis* is causally related to malabsorption.[1,34,74,102] This helminth can survive in the human host for several decades; some 10–20% of ex-prisoners of war in South-east Asia during World War II (1939–1945) remained infected until recently. Onset of diarrhoea is less acute than with *G. lamblia*. Larvae can be demonstrated by the 'Enterotest', and less often by jejunal biopsy. Ova and larvae can occasionally be detected in faecal specimens. Eosinophilia may be gross; however, it is often absent. The immunofluorescent antibody test (IFAT) is positive in approximately 70% of cases; however, cross-reaction with filaria is common. The enzyme-linked immunosorbent assay (ELISA) test, when available, is more specific. A negative serological result is common in the immunosuppressed patient. Treatment is with thiabendazole (1.5 g twice daily on three successive days); repeated courses may be required. Albendazole (400 mg daily for 3 days) seems less effective. In animal experiments, cambendazole has given encouraging results; this has also been the case in limited clinical studies, but the compound has not been officially released for human use. Other *Strongyloides* species are important, especially in children. *Stongyloides fülleborni* has been implicated in the pathogenesis of severe PIM (see above) in Zambia and Papua New Guinea, where a significant mortality rate has been recorded.[74]

In the northern Philippines and Thailand, *Capillaria philippinensis* has been causally associated with PIM.[1] It can occur in epidemics. Diarrhoea of acute onset is followed by malabsorption and, if untreated, infection carries a substantial mortality rate. Protein-losing enteropathy may also be present. Treatment with one of the benzimidazole compounds has given good results.

The protozoa *Isospora belli* and *Sarcocystis hominis* (usually conveyed by undercooked pork and beef)[130] also cause malabsorption. These organisms replicate within the enterocyte. *I. belli*, like *Crytosporidium parvum*, causes a spectrum of disease, from TD to PIM, and is more common in the immunosuppressed individual. Pyrimethamine + sulfadiazine, and co-trimoxazole + nitrofurantoin, have been used with some success. Other protozoan parasites, such as *P. falciparum* (in an acute infection) and visceral leishmaniasis (kala azar), can also produce significant malabsorption. Other protozoa which have assumed practical importance in the wake of the HIV/AIDS pandemic are *Cyclospora cayetanensis*,[131-133] *microsporidiosis*,[134,135] and *Blastocystis hominis*.[136] All can be implicated in a wide range of small-intestinal problems ranging from traveller's diarrhoea to malabsorption.

Emergencies

Severe dehydration consequent upon secretory watery diarrhoea accounts for enormous amounts of acute morbidity throughout the tropics; this applies especially to infants and children. Intravenous replacement therapy has been in use for more than 150 years; Dr Robert Lewins MD FRCP, of Leith, recorded that he had witnessed Dr Thomas Latta inject saline intravenously into a patient suffering from cholera (see above) in 1832,[65] and George Leith Roupell,[137] a physician at St Bartholomew's Hospital, London, seems to have been an early user of this technique. It is unlikely, however, that these were the first attempts at intravenous rehydration (in fact, Sir Christopher Wren, better known for his architectural achievements, had used the technique experimentally in 1657). Nearly three-quarters of a century passed before Sir Leonard Rogers, working at Calcutta, demonstrated a reduction in the mortality rate in cholera patients from 70% to 20% by use of this technique. Introduction of oral rehydration regimens had to wait much later, in fact until the latter half of the twentieth century. Introduction of this form of management, which followed upon important basic applied physiological observations, was, in a world context, one of the most important medical advances during the twentieth century.[1] In many acute medical conditions, gastric emptying is delayed; however, this is not the case in cholera (and presumably other acute small-intestinal infections) and does not constitute a barrier to oral rehydration, even when fluid and electrolyte loss (in the stool) is severe.[138] Oral rehydration therapy remains grossly underused,[139] however, and infants and children in developing countries with acute gastroenteritis continue to die unnecessarily because this simple technique is not readily applied. The authors of this latter article have concluded: 'the impediment to its wide acceptance may be that it is counterintuitive for a simpler and much less expensive treatment

to be an improvement over an effective but more complicated technology'!

Enteritis necroticans (pigbel disease)

This acute small-intestinal emergency (see above), which usually affects infants and children (see above) is characterized by gangrenous changes in the small-intestinal wall (in patchy distribution); the jejunum is most markedly affected, but the ileum is also involved. Presentation is usually as an acute abdominal (surgical) emergency, with abdominal pain, fever and bloody diarrhoea (see above). A chronic stage of the disease may ensue in which there is narrowing of the small-intestinal lumen (in one or more places) by a fibrotic stenosis or adhesion; clinical presentation is with subacute obstruction, often accompanied by malabsorption and malnutrition. Fluid and electrolyte replacement are vitally important in management; gastric suction is also required. Penicillin or another antibiotic should be given (see above). Laparotomy is frequently indicated to confirm the diagnosis and to resect the necrotized, haemorrhagic, segment(s) of small intestine. Fortunately, active immunization against the β-toxin has proved effective prophylaxis in Papua New Guinea; hospital admissions for pigbel in one area of the country fell to less than one-fifth of the previous figure ($p < 0.001$) when a vaccination programme was introduced.[140] Morbidity due to this acute abdominal emergency (with a very high mortality rate) should eventually fall in the seriously affected countries.

Paralytic ileus and acute obstruction

In Pakistan, paralytic ileus has been recorded as a late complication of acute diarrhoeal disease in infants;[141] despite rehydration and total parenteral nutrition, the mortality rate was 25%. When compared with others who did not develop ileus (following acute diarrhoeal disease), these infants were shown to have had significantly more antimotility agents preceding the ileus; furthermore, many had a depressed serum potassium concentration. The potential dangers associated with antiperistaltic agents, especially in infancy and childhood, are thus re-emphasized.

Acute intestinal obstruction constitutes a common surgical emergency in both children and adults in many parts of the tropics, including Africa. Strangulated hernia (usually of inguinal origin) is usually the most common cause; volvulus and intussusception are relatively common in tropical Africa; tuberculosis is a further cause due either to stenosis or to pressure on the third part of the duodenum or jejunum. A heavy *A. lumbricoides* infection (especially in children) can also produce small-intestinal obstruction;[142] when diagnosed clinically, laparotomy can usually be avoided. Management consists of intravenous hydration, nasogastric suction and appropriate anthelmintic chemotherapy. Strangulated hernia, volvulus and intussusception nearly always require laparotomy.[142] In a report from southern India, 904 children presented with intestinal obstruction;[143] the most common causes in order of frequency were necrotizing enteritis (see above), acute intussusception, band obstruction, subacute obstruction, and remnants of the vitello-intestinal duct. Rare causes of small-intestinal obstruction include: Burkitt's lymphoma, Mediterranean lymphoma (α-chain disease) (see above) and intestinal schistosomiasis. Small-intestinal trauma – caused by a road accident or knife, arrow or gunshot wound – is also important in a tropical context.

Typhoid (enteric) fever

In most areas within the developing world, typhoid (see also Chapters 52 and 53) (and to a lesser extent tuberculosis) accounts for much small-intestinal disease encountered in surgical practice;[144] perforation, obstruction and less often haemorrhage constitute acute surgical emergencies. This seems especially important in West Africa. S. typhi infection is also an increasing problem in travellers from industrialized countries to the tropics;[145] in the USA, 2666 cases (fatality rate 1–3%) of acute enteric fever were officially notified between 1975 and 1984; 62% of them were imported, the majority of infections having originated in either Mexico or India. Statistically, surgical complications are unusual; thus in a series of 82 culture-positive cases in The Gambia there were no surgical complications;[146] this was also the case in a series of 192 cases of enteric fever – most caused by S. typhi – in Thailand.[147] Despite its relative rarity, however, (perhaps 2–4% of cases worldwide), typhoid perforation is an extremely serious event, accounting for 20–60% of deaths in this disease (a statistic which is increased by late presentation, female sex, age ≥40 years and the presence of multiple perforations). Late perforation is often indistinguishable from a perforated appendix, amoebic liver abscess, tuberculous peritonitis, an infected ruptured ectopic pregnancy or intestinal strangulation. The optimal form of management seems to be surgical, provided the patient is not too shocked to endure such a procedure (a prolonged period of pre-operative resuscitation is often required). There is as yet no general agreement, however, regarding the ideal type of operative intervention;[148] simple closure, ulcer excision and closure, wedge excision and closure, ileal resection and anastomosis, resection and transverse ileotransverse colostomy, and right hemicolectomy have all found favour. When the perforation is single, simple closure (with or without excision) is the procedure of choice; an area(s) of impending perforation should not be oversewn; closure should always be in two layers: an inner one of chromic catgut and an outer of silk. When there are three or more perforations, bowel resection is probably advisable. Peritoneal lavage with a copious amount of washing with normal saline should be carried out. The incidence of postoperative complications is high, and includes peripheral vascular failure, respiratory infections, anaemia, sepsis, abscess formation, burst abdomen and intestinal obstruction.[148] Re-perforation or a new perforation is possible. In a series of 108 consecutive cases of perforated typhoid enteritis managed in western Nigeria, 100 (93%) underwent 'debridement of the perforation and two-layer bowel closure';[149] 35 patients died, usually from overwhelming sepsis. In addition to specific chemotherapy, although chloramphenicol (1 g four times daily in an average adult, reduced to 1 g twice daily when body temperature is normal) remains the agent of choice, increasing numbers of reports of multiple-antibiotic-resistant strains of S. typhi are being reported (especially from India), metronidazole, and possibly corticosteroids, seem to improve the prognosis. Alternative chemotherapeutic agents include amoxicillin, co-tri-moxazole, trimethoprim and ciprofloxacin; the last agent is indicated when there are serious doubts about sensitivity to the other compounds, as is frequently the case when infection has resulted in Asia. Despite these advances therefore, ileal perforation in enteric fever remains a potentially lethal complication, especially in children.[150]

Haemorrhage is rarely life-threatening, although recorded;[151] whereas the majority of cases can be treated conservatively (blood transfusion when indicated), when selective angiography, fibreoptic endoscopy and high-resolution radionuclide imaging are available, localization of the bleeding site can be delineated and appropriate surgery instituted.

Emergencies associated with helminthiases

Abdominal discomfort (and pain) are common sequelae to heavy small-intestinal nematode infections (see above), especially ancylostomiasis and A. lumbricoides (see above), but serious acute complications (see above) are fortunately rare.[152] Anisakiasis, for example – usually acquired from ingestion of undercooked or raw infected fish (sushi and sashimi) – can present with an acute appendicitis-like illness.[153-155] Invasive disease caused by this organism is usually localized to the ileocaecal region; there is no satisfactory parasitological or serological test, and chemotherapy is not effective. A diagnostic laparotomy is often necessary.

Eosinophilic enteritis is an entity of multiple aetiology.[156] A report from Townsville, Australia, suggested that Ancylostoma caninum (the dog hookworm) was responsible for an epidemic (93 cases) encountered there;[157] nine were subjected to diagnostic laparotomy: eosinophilic infiltration involving a segment of ileum with indurated thickening of the distal small intestine and proximal dilatation was the usual underlying pathology. A rare case of acute mesenteric ischaemia (accompanied by segmental small-intestinal infarction and gangrene) caused by Schist. mansoni has been reported from Baghdad, Iraq.[158] The small intestine can also be involved in Schist. japonicum infection; intestinal obstruction resulting from mesenteric ischaemia, an intussuscepting polypoid mass or fibrotic stenosis are possible sequelae. Intestinal perforation resulting from infection with the acanthocephalan helminth Macracanthorhynchus hirudinaceus, a natural intestinal parasite of the pig, has been described in Bangkok, Thailand[159] (eight other cases are on record); this infection has also been reported from several other parts of the world, including China and southern Europe. Fatal gastrointestinal haemorrhage (associated with fluctuating jaundice, a tender liver, palpable gallbladder and an eosinophilia) has been attributed to Fasciola hepatica (liver fluke) infection in Harare, Zimbabwe;[160] the site of bleeding was probably the biliary tree.

COLORECTUM

Most cases of colorectal disease occurring in a tropical environment have an infective basis (Table 10.4); they are dominated by bacterial (Shigella species[161] (Chapter 51) (Figure 10.7), Campylobacter jejuni and invasive E. coli) and protozoan (Ent. histolytica (Chapter 79) and Balantidium coli) infections. Amoebic colitis[162] and shigellosis present classically with bloody diarrhoea; this should be

Table 10.4 Colorectal diarrhoea[a]

Bacterial infection
  Shigellosis
  Campylobacter jejuni
  Escherichia coli (enteroinvasive)
Protozoan infection
  Entamoeba histolytica
  Balantidium coli
Schistosomiasis (usually *Schistosoma mansoni* and *Schist. japonicum*)
Unusual causes
  Non-specific ulcerative colitis – inflammatory bowel disease[b]
  Crohn's disease[b]
  Appendicitis
  Diverticulitis
  Haemorrhoids
  Colonic carcinoma
  Irritable bowel syndrome

[a]Characteristically, numerous small stools containing mucus, pus and blood; microscopy shows pus cells and/or red blood cells in a faecal smear.
[b]Although these diseases are uncommon, or even rare, in most tropical populations, they can become clinically overt for the first time in visitors from Western countries to the tropics.

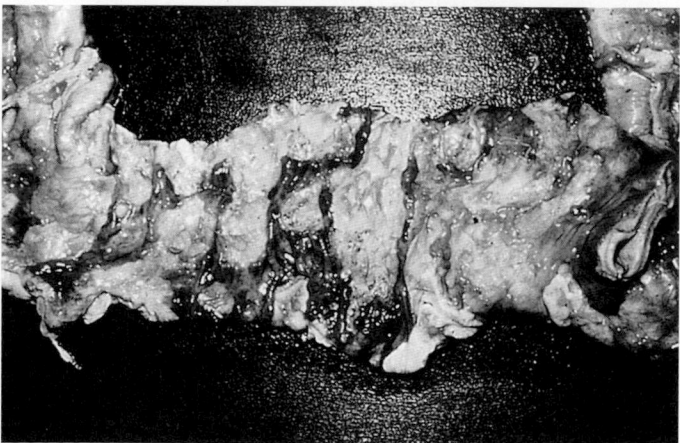

Figure 10.7 Severe amoebic colitis: operative specimen obtained from an Australian nurse misdiagnosed as having non-specific ulcerative colitis (inflammatory bowel disease) while working in Papua New Guinea.

differentiated from carcinoma, necrotizing colitis, antibiotic-associated colitis and inflammatory bowel disease (which is overall not very common in tropical countries). Whether or not amoebic colitis can proceed to inflammatory bowel disease is debatable; however, misdiagnosis of amoebic colitis as inflammatory bowel disease (with subsequent corticosteroid therapy) can result in fatality. In AIDS, cytomegalovirus colitis is common; *Cryptosporidium* is usually a small-intestinal parasite, but colonic involvement can also occur. In addition, megacolon resulting

from South American trypanosomiasis (Chagas' disease) (Chapter 76) is another cause of colonic pathology. Of diseases localized to the anal region, lymphogranuloma is perhaps the most important although bacterial (including donovanosis, syphilis and gonorrhoea (Chapter 21)) and parasitic (including *Ent. histolytica*, *Schistosoma* species and *Enterobius vermicularis*) infections constitute differential diagnoses.

Overall, diseases of the colorectum are far less common in indigenous people in developing countries compared with individuals in industrialized ones;[1,163] colonic carcinoma seems, for example, to be an unusual lesion in rural communities. Good evidence now exists that frequency of these diseases is increasing as urbanization advances, in Africa especially. Hypotheses to account for these differences include high dietary fibre consumption in most tropical countries; however, such associations rarely have a proven cause–effect relationship.

Many data have been collected on colonic function in indigenous inhabitants of developing countries;[1] it seems likely that mean 24-h faecal weight and volume is higher in Africa, and constipation unusual. Overall, intestinal transit rate also seems more rapid. Limited evidence indicates that colorectal histology is mildly different in indigenous people in developing countries, and is comparable to tropical enteropathy (see above). In PIM in India (see above) in vivo colonic functional abnormalities have been demonstrated. Whether colonic pathology is important in a nutritional context remains difficult to evaluate (see above): evidence now exists that this organ is important in the absorption of nitrogen and free (volatile) fatty acids.

Inflammatory bowel disease (non-specific ulcerative colitis and Crohn's disease)[164] is probably less common overall in indigenous people in developing countries compared with the UK and other Western countries.[165,166] However, a recent study from Lebanon demonstrated a high prevalence of the disease there.[167] The aetiology of this disease is unknown, although an infective basis has frequently been suggested; satisfactory evidence for a viral or bacterial (possibly mycobacterial) origin is at present lacking. A handful of reports of ulcerative colitis have been made from African countries, and a few more from Asia.[164] In individuals in the UK with an ancestry in the Caribbean or Indian subcontinent this disease clearly exists but is unusual. Such differences also apply to Crohn's disease, although this disease also is well recognized in Caribbean people in the UK. Although Crohn's disease behaves very much like intestinal tuberculosis in clinical practice, response to antituberculous therapy is disappointing. When inflammatory bowel disease occurs, it seems to behave similarly to that in the indigenous population of the UK. It is a common cause of bloody diarrhoea in travellers who have returned to temperate from tropical countries (Figure 10.8).[39-41] Similarly, appendicitis, diverticular disease and haemorrhoids are overall less common in a developing country population, where a high-fibre intake has been implicated in their prevention; a causative association has not, however, been proved.

Although irritable bowel (IBD) syndrome (spastic colon)[168] is extremely common in UK residents (and others) following an intestinal infection acquired in a tropical country, it seems to be far less significant in indigenous peoples in Africa[169] and Asia. Whether this constitutes a genuine difference is unclear because so many of the latter have more severe symptoms of different origin(s), which might mask symptoms resulting from IBD. This

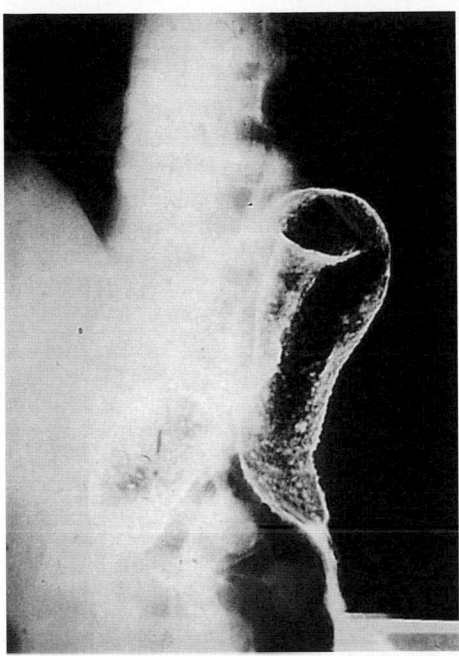

Figure 10.8 Barium enema in a 35-year-old English woman who experienced bloody diarrhoea during a visit to Africa; she had not previously had significant gastrointestinal problems. Colonic biopsy specimen obtained at colonoscopy confirmed inflammatory bowel disease.

syndrome does not constitute a single entity;[170,171] although some cases respond to mebeverine or peppermint oil, many do not. There is no doubt that recognition of the syndrome in developing countries leaves much to be desired.[172] More studies are required.

Enterobius vermicularis infection (Chapter 85) is arguably the most common gastrointestinal infection in the world;[173] it exists in both tropical and temperate areas.

Colonoscopy is an endoscopic technique which is now available in some, but by no means all, developing countries; frequently, it is available only at the teaching hospital and/or other (tertiary referral) centre(s).

Emergencies

Invasive amoebic colitis

Perforation, although a rare event, can complicate this disease, with the production of amoebic peritonitis;[1] there may be diffusion of *Ent. histolytica* from a 'blotting-paper'-like colon, and perforation (especially in the rectosigmoid or caecal regions or to the retroperitoneal tissues) or leakage into a confined space (resulting in a pericolic abscess or internal intestinal fistula). Management consists of gastric suction and intravenous fluid replacement; metronizadole, 500 mg 8-hourly (preferably by the intravenous route), and a broad-spectrum antibiotic should immediately be given. The colon is extremely fragile; laparotomy is usually best avoided;[174] overall, mortality is of the order of 50% and after surgery close on 100%. Two reports have recorded results of surgical intervention in 15 patients with fulminant amoebic colitis.[175,176] In the first, five out of six patients (four had a subtotal colectomy

with ileostomy, and two a right hemicolectomy and ileostomy) subsequently died (none was diagnosed either preoperatively or during surgery); in the second, three out of nine died, all of whom had exteriorization of the cut ends of the bowel following resection of the necrotic segment (four of those who died had end-to-end anastomoses, and two peritoneal drainage).

Shigellosis

A recent study in China has drawn attention to a significant climatic factor in prevalence.[177] Although perforation is less common in shigellosis compared with amoebic colitis, haemorrhage is well documented. The most recent pandemic of this disease in the Western Hemisphere began in Guatemala in 1969 and ended in 1973. It spread rapidly to Nicaragua, Belize, Honduras, Costa Rica, Panama and Mexico; with an estimated 500 000 affected, of whom 20 000 died.[178]

Appendicitis

Overall, this entity is less common in developing compared with 'westernized' countries. Nevertheless it certainly exists, and a predominance of appendicectomies in women has been recorded.[179] Confusion with an acute gynaecological condition is a real problem and more widespread use of ultrasound and laparoscopy might be the solution.[180] In Calabar, Nigeria, 603 consecutive cases were investigated prospectively during a 5-year period;[181] there were no major differences from this disease in industrialized countries, and it constituted the second most common abdominal emergency during the study period, being less common than acute intestinal obstruction. Many causative agents have been implicated; in a retrospective review of 2921 appendicectomies carried out at Allahabad, India, during a 25-year period, 153 produced histological evidence of a specific infection:[182] tuberculosis (70), *Ent. histolytica* (17), *A. lumbricoides* (13), *A. lumbricoides* and *Trichuris trichiura* (2), *Enterobius vermicularis* (41), and *Taenia* species (2). This acute disease should be differentiated from pelvic inflammatory disease, typhoid enteritis, ruptured ectopic pregnancy, psoas abscess, acute amoebic colitis, and *Schist. mansoni* colitis.[183] Although the vast majority of cases of appendicitis in developing countries result from a bacterial cause, helminths, including *Schist. mansoni*, *Strongyloides stercoralis*, *Trichuris trichiura* and *E. vermicularis* have also been implicated.[1,184]

Volvulus of the colon

This is a disease with clear geographical differences; it is common in much of Central and East Africa, India and South America;[1] numerous reports have been made from Uganda and Zimbabwe. Although genetic factors have been suggested for these high rates; a high-fibre diet, common in most of Africa, has also been implicated. The major complication is strangulation, and gangrene of a colonic segment; this should be differentiated from primary volvulus of the small intestine, compound volvulus (usually ileosigmoid) and internal herniae. Distension can be relieved with a flatus tube; at laparotomy the nature of the operation, and extent of resection, depends on the length of gangrenous colon. With simple volvulus, mortality rate should be low. Zimmerman et al.[185] have emphasized the value of emergency colonoscopy in the diagnosis of colonic volvulus; when the mucosa is ischaemic or necrotic, emergency laparotomy is indicated, but when appearances are normal, relief of flatus (with a flatus tube passed per rectum) together with medical management followed by elective surgery (resection and anastomosis) 10 days later is recommended.

Colonic intussusception

The common variety, especially in West Africa, is the caecocolic one; although children may be afflicted, the vast majority are in adults.[1] The condition has also been reported to be by no means uncommon in Ethiopian adults.[186] Aetiology, as with that of volvulus, is conjectural; while an intestinal polyp or amoeboma accounts for some, there is no obvious clue in most cases. Gangrene is about three times more common with the ileoileal and ileocaecal varieties compared with the caecocolic type.

Acute colonic dilatation

Several gastrointestinal infections can cause toxic megacolon. These include: *Salmonella species*, *Campylobacter* species and *Y. enterocolitica* infection; however, there has been a growing recognition of *Shigella* species in this potentially lethal condition.[187] Correct diagnosis is essential; an unnecessary laparotomy can thus usually be avoided. If the condition is misdiagnosed as ulcerative colitis, and corticosteroids administered, potentially fatal consequences can ensue. Diagnostically, the causative organism can usually be identified in a faecal sample. Choice of an appropriate antibiotic is often difficult; in *Shigella* species infection, a fluoroquinolone, e.g. ciprofloxacin (200 mg intravenously 12-hourly for 10 days), seems most appropriate. Toxic dilatation of the colon has also been reported, albeit rarely, in *Ent. histolytica* infection;[188] these authors recorded a single case (in which total colectomy, and administration of metronidazole and emetine, was followed by recovery); they were able to detect seven cases in the world literature.

Other colorectal lesions

Anorectal infections in relation to tropical exposure have been reviewed.[189] Trauma to the colon, often resulting from road accidence, constitutes a medical emergency in most tropical countries.[1] Necrotizing colitis (the pathology is similar to that of enteritis necroticans; see above) is rarely encountered. Colonic obstruction is rarely caused by carcinoma (a rare tumour in the rural tropics[190]) but is recorded following introduction of a foreign body per rectum. Colorectal tuberculosis is an unusual cause of stricture formation, which occasionally requires surgical intervention.[191]

While the true prevalence of *Clostridium difficile* infection in developing countries is considered to be low, many more studies are required.[192]

LIVER AND BILIARY SYSTEM

Liver histology in an individual indigenous to a tropical country differs from that in one who has spent his/her life in a temperate region of the world.[1] This organ is subjected to numerous systemic infections – viral, bacterial and parasitic – and it lies at the distal end of the portal circulation; it is therefore bathed with portal blood containing viruses, bacteria, parasites, ova, products of digestion and other antigens. Thus, Kupffer cell hyperplasia and periportal infiltration (with lymphocytes, plasma cells and eosinophils) are more common, and stellate fibrosis occurs more frequently. Also, nuclear pleomorphism in hepatocytes and sinusoidal lymphocytes are frequently prominent; these appearances are unusual in biopsies obtained in a temperate country. Malaria and schistosomal pigment are often also present. Granulomas are common (Figure 10.9) and a large number of differential diagnoses exist; Table 10.5 lists some of them.

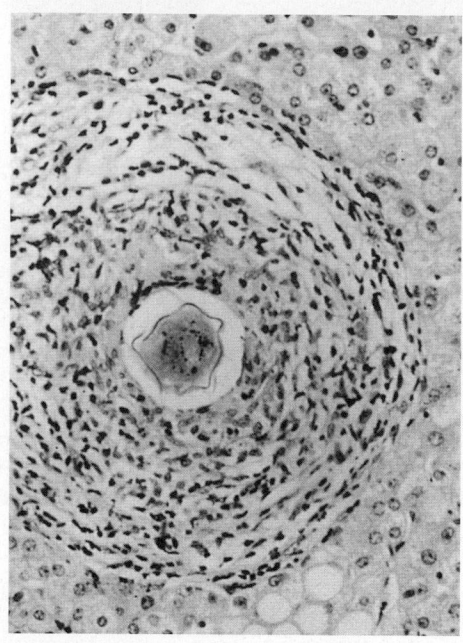

Figure 10.9 Liver biopsy specimen from a 30-year-old Zambian woman. A degenerating *Schistosoma mansoni* egg is surrounded by a well-formed granuloma.

Table 10.5 Some causes of hepatic granulomas in tropical countries

Infection	Viral cytomegalovirus, Epstein–Barr virus
Bacterial	Tuberculosis and atypical mycobacteria, leprosy, syphilis, Q fever, brucellosis
Parasitic	Schistosomiasis, ascariasis, strongyloidiasis, toxocariasis, filariasis, enterobiasis, visceral leishmaniasis
Fungi	Histoplasmosis, coccidioidomycosis, aspergillosis, actinomycosis, candidiasis
Neoplasms	Lymphomas – especially intra-abdominal Hodgkin's disease
Others	(sarcoidosis) therapeutic agents – especially sulfonamides

Table 10.6 Some causes of jaundice in the tropics

Jaundice of acute bacterial infection: pneumococcal lobar pneumonia, pyomyositis	
Viruses	Hepatitis (A–F)
	Yellow fever
	Epstein–Barr virus
	Cytomegalovirus
	Marburg and Ebola diseases
	Lassa fever
Bacteria	Leptospirosis
	Typhoid fever
	Syphilis
	Gonococcal disease
	Bartonellosis
Parasites	Malaria (acute *Plasmodium falciparum* and *P. vivax*)
	Schistosomiasis
	Amoebiasis (rarely)
	Toxoplasmosis
	Trichinellosis
	Fascioliasis
	Clonorchiasis ⎫
	Opisthorchiasis ⎬ predominantly large-duct
	Ascariasis ⎭ obstructive jaundice
	Hydatidosis (rarely)
Genetic	Sickle cell disease
	Glucose-6-phosphate dehydrogenase deficiency
	Dubin–Johnson syndrome

intracellulare, atypical mycobacteria, *Cryptosporidium parvum*, *Pneumocystis carinii*, *Cryptococcus* species and/or Kaposi's sarcoma. Cholestatic features are common. The co-existence of HIV and HBV should not be underestimated.[202]

In addition to septicaemia, several other infections can produce jaundice;[1,203,204] leptospirosis is frequently accompanied by renal involvement, while overt jaundice in typhoid fever 'hepatitis' is unusual.[205,206] Melioidosis, plague, tularaemia and relapsing fever can also produce hepatitis. Of parasitic causes, acute *P. falciparum* infection is probably the most important. In acute (Katayama syndrome) and severe chronic schistosomiasis jaundice may be present, but is rare in invasive hepatic amoebiasis. Most parasitic infections, including African trypanosomiasis (Chapter 75) and visceral leishmaniasis (Chapter 77), can produce significant hepatitis and deranged hepatocellular function – often in the absence of clinical jaundice.

Several parasites produce large duct biliary obstruction; for practical purposes, *A. lumbricoides* is the most important to recognize and treat urgently.[207]

Sickle cell disease and haemoglobinopathies (Chapter 13) are important causes of haemolytic jaundice; they possess a genetic basis. Jaundice in the presence of G6PD deficiency is frequently precipitated (or worsened) by therapeutic agents and/or toxins. In some parts of the tropics, especially Indonesia and Papua New Guinea, the Dubin-Johnson syndrome seems unusually common.

Chronic liver disease

Most cases of chronic active hepatitis in tropical countries result from HBV and HCV infections;[208] corticosteroids should not be administered for they exacerbate hepatocyte viral infection; interferon-γ and adenine arabinoside have given encouraging results, but ethnic factors are probably important. There is no reliable evidence that either malnutrition (including kwashiorkor) or *Plasmodium* species infection are aetiologically important, although such beliefs linger.[1]

In tropical countries most cases of macronodular cirrhosis result from viral hepatitis, most commonly HBV, and to a lesser extent HCV hepatitis.[201] The sequence of events is: acute hepatitis → chronic active hepatitis → macronodular cirrhosis → and, ultimately, hepatocellular carcinoma[209–212] (hepatoma) (acute viral hepatitis is covered in Chapter 39 and hepatoma in Chapter 35). HBV and HCV are undoubtedly the most important aetiological factors in hepatoma, but the role of aflatoxin[1] should not be totally disregarded. The true prevalence of autoimmune hepatitis, which has been studied in Brazil, is unknown.[213]

An important and probably underrated cause of chronic liver disease in a tropical context is schistosomiasis (Chapter 82).[214,215] Although hepatocellular function is preserved until late in the disease, portal hypertension and its various complications (see below) are as important as in the various forms of cirrhosis.

Clinically, cutaneous stigmata of chronic hepatocellular disease are difficult to detect in brown or black skins;[1] similarly, other cutaneous stigmata of chronic liver disease may be absent. Diagnosis is often first suspected by abnormal liver function tests; a needle liver biopsy specimen is usually diagnostic. Peritoneoscopy is relatively simple and underused in developing countries; refined

Acute liver infections

Jaundice in a tropical context (Table 10.6) is most commonly a result of viral hepatitis (types A,[193,194] B (sometimes a combined infection with D), C,[195] E[196–200] and F) (Chapter 39), but other causes should also be considered; Table 10.6 summarizes some of them. An important cause is the jaundice of acute bacterial infection – most commonly caused by pneumococcal lobar pneumonia or pyomyositis.[1] The mechanism of this form of jaundice is complex and consists of hepatocellular, cholestatic and haemolytic elements; the importance of the latter depends on the underlying prevalence of glucose-6-phosphate dehydrogenase (G6PD) deficiency in the population under consideration (Chapter 13). It is important to differentiate this form of jaundice from viral hepatitis, otherwise the appropriate antibiotic will not be administered for an underlying bacterial infection. In addition to yellow fever, several other viruses are implicated;[195] dengue fever, Kyasanur Forest disease, herpes simplex and Coxsackie virus should also be considered.

In AIDS, the liver is affected by many opportunistic organisms. These include viruses; hepatitis B (HBV) and C (HCV)[201] infections can be especially virulent. A liver biopsy specimen may also yield evidence of cytomegalovirus, *Mycobacterium tuberculosis*, *M. avium*

diagnostic techniques are rarely available. No treatment is of any avail in established cirrhosis, but some of the chromolytics in chronic schistosomal disease of the liver are reversible after treatment (Chapter 82). Major complications (see below) resulting from portal hypertension are: (1) haemorrhage, from oesophageal varices (see below); (2) fluid retention, including ascites; and (3) hepatic encephalopathy. Fluid retention is a major long-term problem, largely the result of a very low serum albumin concentration. This complication is often difficult to manage, largely because salt restriction is virtually impossible to impose in a tropical setting; diuretics, e.g. furosemide (Lasix) (40–120 mg daily) and spironolactone (Aldactone) (100 mg daily), usually achieve success. Paracentesis abdominis should rarely be undertaken; this procedure depletes albumin stores further, and electrolyte balance can be seriously disturbed; tapping ascitic fluid should be reserved for: (1) diagnostic purposes, to understand whether a bacterial infection, tuberculous peritonitis or hepatocellular carcinoma is present concurrently; and (2) management of tense ascites, accompanied by respiratory embarrassment. Hepatic encephalopathy is managed by accepted methods: oral neomycin (6 g daily) and/or lactulose (20–35 g three times daily); in the presence of hypolactasia, lactose can be substituted for lactulose.

Other forms of chronic liver disease (with subsequent decompensation) (see below) include those resulting from excessive alcohol ingestion, Indian childhood cirrhosis, haemosiderosis and veno-occlusive disease. Wilson's disease (hepatolenticular degeneration) and other genetically determined forms of cirrhosis are of limited importance numerically in the tropics, although they too should enter the list of differential diagnoses.

Alcoholic liver disease

Alcohol-related disease (including cirrhosis) is common in both indigenous and expatriate populations in tropical countries.[1,216] Genetic factors are undoubtedly involved; HBsAg carriers are especially vulnerable. The liver in chronic alcoholic disease is classically micronodular, but not always so; liver biopsy histology sometimes shows characteristic Mallory's hyaline deposits, and haemosiderin may be present in excess. There are no major differences from the disease in temperate climates. The quantity of daily alcohol required to produce this disease is not known with accuracy, and estimates differ widely; an individual variation exists, and women seem to tolerate chronic alcohol ingestion less well than men. Acute alcoholic hepatitis is underdiagnosed and possesses a high mortality rate; the role of corticosteroids continues to be disputed;[1,216] any beneficial effect is at best marginal and administration should probably be confined to severe and advanced cases.

Indian childhood cirrhosis

Indian childhood cirrhosis[217] is largely confined to India (especially south India, Calcutta and the Punjab) and surrounding countries; it is frequently familial. Diagnosis is usually made between 1.5 and 3 years of age; members of the upper strata of Hindu society are often affected. The disease may pursue fulminant, acute or subacute courses, and carries a high mortality

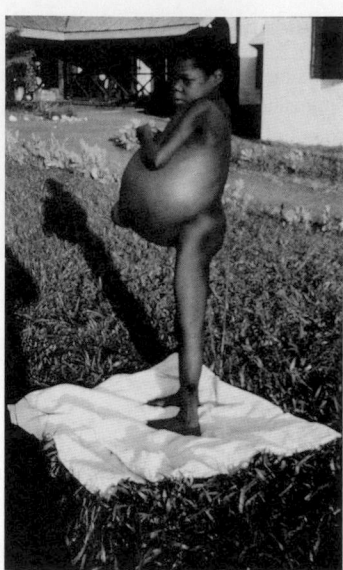

Figure 10.10 Indian child suffering from decompensated chronic liver disease – Indian childhood cirrhosis.

rate. The clinical course therefore varies widely and is comparable to viral hepatitis (see above), with acute fulminant hepatitis at one extreme of the spectrum and cirrhosis (with one or all of its classic complications) (Figure 10.10) at the other. Histologically, there is usually progressive fibrosis, with absence of regeneration; macronodular and micronodular cirrhosis result. Hepatocellular carcinoma is an uncommon complication. The disease is associated with a high copper intake; epidemiological evidence suggests that early weaning followed by milk-feeding from copper vessels imparts an excessive copper intake.[218] However, the possibility of an inherited defect resulting in excess copper absorption and/or metabolism has not been eliminated. There is no adequate treatment; in prevention, non-human milk for infant and childhood consumption should not be stored in copper-containing vessels.

Haemosiderosis

Haemosiderosis (African or Bantu siderosis) is a disease of southern, and to a lesser extent other parts of (tropical) East and West Africa.[219,220] Whether it can proceed to clear-cut cirrhosis is arguable; heavy alcohol intake is commonplace in many geographical areas where the disease is common; it is frequently impossible to exclude this as an aetiological factor (as with haemochromatosis). Iron-containing pots for cooking are commonly used in most areas, such as Zimbabwe, where haemosiderosis is common, but other factors also seem relevant. Also, chronic pancreatitis is relatively common in these areas; evidence exists that an excess of iron (and fat) is common.

Veno-occlusive disease

Although first described in Jamaica, distribution of veno-occlusive disease is now known to be much wider.[224] Bush-teas, which contain pyrrolizidine alkaloids (*Heliotropium, Crotalaria* and *Senecio*) are important aetiologically. Veno-occlusive disease occurs in many localized areas of the tropics, and is certainly not confined to the Caribbean.

Other chronic liver diseases

The liver is involved in most chronic infective diseases; tuberculosis, leprosy, syphilis, actinomycosis, visceral leishmaniasis and African histoplasmosis are examples. It is, however, unusual for decompensation (and liver failure) to result. Major space-occupying lesions involving the liver are amoebic abscess (see below), pyogenic abscess and hydatid disease; tuberculomas, cysticercosis and melioidosis are of lesser importance. Of non-infective diseases, sickle cell disease, β-thalassaemia, haemoglobin-H disease, porphyria and α_1-antitrypsin deficiency produce significant hepatic pathology. A change in disease profile of the Budd-Chiari Syndrome has been recorded over the past three decades in India.[222]

Portal hypertension

Portal hypertension[1,223] is a sequel to any form of chronic liver disease; Table 10.7 summarizes some causes in a tropical country. Cirrhosis and schistosomal liver disease (Chapter 82) are numerically very important; however, in the latter entity hepatocellular function is preserved to a greater extent, and for longer in the course of disease than in cirrhosis; therefore, fluid retention and more importantly encephalopathy are less common. A form of non-cirrhotic chronic liver disease, sometimes associated with portal hypertension, exists in India; despite various suggestions (including arsenic poisoning), the aetiology remains unclear. Of pre-hepatic causes, HMS (see Table 10.7) is the most common; portal hypertension results from an increased splenic blood flow. Portal/splenic vein obstructions, probably resulting from neonatal umbilical sepsis, are important causes throughout tropical countries, and are undoubtedly underdiagnosed;[223] hepatocellular function is usually intact. Posthepatic causes of portal hypertension include (Table 10.7) cardiac failure (usually resulting from chronic rheumatic cardiac disease), right-sided endomyocardial fibrosis (Chapter 12) and constrictive pericarditis, usually but not always resulting from tuberculosis. Other causes of portal hypertension are hepatocellular carcinoma (see above) and various dehydrating diseases, including dysentery and cholera. Splenomegaly is present whatever the cause of portal hypertension (which should be distinguished from other causes of enlargement of this organ in a tropical country). Barium swallow or upper gastrointestinal endoscopy usually confirms the presence of oesophageal varices. When available, ultrasonography is valuable in assessing portal vein patency.

Biliary tract disease

In tropical countries biliary pathology is largely attributable to parasites,[1,207,224] ascariasis (Chapter 85), clonorchiasis and opisthorchiasis (Chapter 83); pigment stones (often intrahepatic) occasionally complicate sickle cell disease. *A. lumbricoides* infection (Chapter 85) is an underdiagnosed cause of large-duct obstruction. It should always be considered in this clinical situation, for it may be confused with pancreatic carcinoma. Endoscopy, if available, is of value; medical treatment is usually successful. Clonorchiasis and opisthorchiasis (Chapter 83), acquired from ingestion of raw fresh-water fish, may result in cholangiohepatitis and biliary obstruction; cholangiocarcinoma is a late complication of both infections. *F. hepatica* infection (Chapter 83) can give rise to tender hepatomegaly accompanied by jaundice; difficulty in diagnosis from viral hepatitis may be a problem; an eosinophilia is, however, common with this and all biliary trematode infections. Praziquantel is of no value in treatment; triclabendazole has now replaced it.[225-227] Overall, cholesterol stones (and associated secondary infection) are uncommon in rural populations, especially in Africa. Gallbladder infection by *S. typhi* can result in the typhoid carrier state (Chapter 52); the focus of infection is usually intrahepatic. Gallbladder carcinoma is unusual.

Table 10.7 Causes of portal hypertension and oesophageal (and gastric) varices, showing those which are more common in developing countries

Level of obstruction	Cause
Pre-hepatic	Hyper-reactive malarious splenomegaly (HMS) (increased portal blood flow)[a]
	Portal vein occlusion[a]
	Splenic vein occlusion
Hepatic macronodular cirrhosis[a]	Hepatosplenic schistosomiasis[a]
	Veno-occlusive disease[a]
	Congenital hepatic fibrosis
Post-hepatic	Cardiac failure (secondary to chronic rheumatic disease)[a]
	Endomyocardial fibrosis[a]
	Constructive pericarditis[a]
	Inferior vena caval obstruction
	Hepatic vein thrombosis (Budd–Chiari syndrome)

[a]More common in a developing than a developed country.

Emergencies

Acute hepatocellular failure

Acute liver failure (acute hepatic necrosis) is a major clinical problem in all developing countries (see above);[4,228] various hepatitis viruses (most commonly B, C, D and E, and to lesser extent A) are all involved (see above), but some cases are caused by other viruses, bacteria or toxins. Although acute hepatocellular failure has been recorded in severe acute *P. falciparum* infection, this is of very limited clinical importance; it occurs as a terminal event but is of far lesser importance than other major organ failure.[229]

The role of several viruses involved in the production of acute liver injury has been summarized.[201] Several reports highlight the aetiological basis of hepatitis in tropical countries; in Egypt, HBV and hepatitis A virus (HAV) accounted for 47% and 0.7% of cases of acute hepatitis (there was serological evidence of both viral

131

infections in a further 1.4%), whereas 14.2% of cases were HBsAg carriers, 31% 'non-A, non-B' hepatitis and 6% were drug-induced.[230] In other locations, however, hepatitis D virus (HDV) is important, especially in southern America, South-east Asia (and probably India) and northern Africa. Thus in Thailand, HDV is frequently present in drug abusers; it is also endemic in Chandigarh, India,[231] and has been described in an epidemic of acute hepatitis in the Himalayan foothills in south Kashmir.[232] In India and South-east Asia, hepatitis E virus (HEV) (see above) is responsible for most cases of the entity previously termed 'non-A, non-B' hepatitis; a similar situation probably pertains in Africa and South America. This virus is transmitted by the faecal–oral route and is transmitted in contaminated drinking water; the major importance of this infection is that it produces a high incidence of hepatocellular failure in pregnant women. HCV also causes severe disease – including acute hepatic failure – similar to that produced by HBV (Chapter 39).

Differential diagnosis

Many other viruses present in tropical and subtropical regions may also produce acute hepatic necrosis; these include herpes simplex type 1, herpes virus 6,[233] Epstein–Barr virus, cytomegalovirus, yellow fever[234] and the haemorrhagic fever viruses, which include the Lassa fever virus, the Marburg virus, Ebola virus and Rift Valley fever virus (see above).[235,236] Of bacterial causes of hepatitis, enteric fever is common, but rarely (if ever) proceeds to hepatocellular necrosis (see above). The jaundice of systemic bacterial infection[1] often follows pyomyositis, especially in Africa. *P. falciparum* malaria causes deranged liver function tests resulting from centrilobular necrosis (see above). Hepatotoxicity resulting from herbal remedies is not confined to tropical countries.[237] Alcoholic hepatitis is a significant clinical problem in both indigenous and expatriate populations.

Management

Tandon et al.[238] have outlined their experience of acute hepatic failure (resulting from viral hepatitis) in 145 (>12 years old) patients managed by them using a 'simple supportive therapeutic regimen' during a 5.5-year period at New Delhi, India. Criteria for inclusion were:
- Development of hepatic encephalopathy within 4 weeks of onset of symptoms and signs of acute hepatitis; and
- Absence of evidence of pre-existent liver disease.

There were 65 men and 80 women; 46 of them were pregnant and presumably infected by HEV.

They used a simple intensive support mechanism; this consisted of:
1. Isolation in an intensive care room.
2. Attention to general hygiene and care of a comatose patient.
3. Intravenous fluid to provide 1000–1500 calories daily using 10% dextrose, supplemented if necessary, by 20% dextrose.
4. Nasogastric tube for aspiration of gastric contents and instillation of drugs.
5. Gut sterilization by ampicillin (1.5 g 6-hourly via nasogastric tube); colonic washes twice daily.
6. Liquid antacids (30 mL 2-hourly).

7. 'Lactisyn' (1 ampoule = Lactobacillus lactus 490 million, L. acidophilus 490 million, Streptococcus lactus 10 million) three times daily.
8. Condom or catheter drainage of the urinary bladder.
9. Maintenance of electrolyte and fluid balance by intravenous supplementation.

Complications were managed as follows:
- Infection (diagnosis was based on clinical findings, leukocyte count $>15 \times 10^9$/L, and/or chest radiograph abnormality): gentamicin 3.5 mg/kg body weight (as three divided doses), and/or cephalexin (2 g daily as four divided doses)
- Cerebral oedema (criteria for diagnosis were: focal or generalized seizures, abnormal reactive or unequal pupils, decerebrate posture of the body after minor stimuli, and/or sudden deterioration of vital signs): intravenous mannitol (200 mL administered during 30 min and repeated three or four times per 24 h).
- Gastrointestinal bleeding (diagnosed by aspiration of fresh or altered blood via nasogastric tube): liquid antacid (30–45 mL every 2 h), gastric lavage (with 100 mL cold saline containing 8 mg noradrenaline every 30 min) and occasionally cimetidine. (When the prothrombin time was >7 s compared with a control, fresh frozen plasma was administered.)
- Renal failure (the criterion used was: oliguria (urine output <400 mg/24 h, and rising blood urea) despite adequate hydration): diuretics (judiciously used).

Overall, 42 (28.9%) survived; of those ≤40 years old, 41 (33%) recovered, compared with only one (4.8%) of those ≥40 years; survival was not affected by pregnancy. Indicators of poor prognosis were: grade IV coma, presence of HBsAg, serum bilirubin concentration >20 mg/100 mL and sodium <119 mmol/L. In fatal cases the immediate complications resulting in death were cerebral oedema (65), bleeding (31), renal failure (11) and infection (8). The authors concluded that these results were comparable with results from centres using a variety of complex therapeutic regimens (e.g. exchange blood transfusion, charcoal perfusion and haemodialysis).

Chronic hepatocellular failure and hepatoma

Cirrhosis, generally resulting from one of the hepatitis viruses (see above), is a very common problem throughout tropical and subtropical countries. A study carried out at New Delhi, India, has addressed the problem of survival in young (<35 years old) and older patients with cirrhosis;[239] numbers in the two groups were 63 and 106, respectively. Aetiology of cirrhosis in the young and adult groups was: HBV-related (32 and 51), alcohol-related (10 and 28), while 19 and 21, respectively, were labelled 'cryptogenic'; in the former group, one had Wilson's disease and another α_1-antitrypsin deficiency. During the surveillance period 27 and 47 deaths occurred: 40% and 64% from hepatic failure, and 52% and 26% from variceal bleeding. The 5-year survival (62% and 56%) and probability of survival within a similar grade of liver disease (Child's classification) were comparable. As anticipated, probability of survival was significantly higher in grade A and lowest in C. Aetiology of cirrhosis did not significantly influence prognosis in this study.

Hepatocellular carcinoma usually presents as a rapidly progressive malignancy; however, an acute or chronic presentation can occur due to internal necrosis and haemorrhage.[142] Such a lesion can in fact rupture into the peritoneal cavity, posing problems in differential diagnosis.

In a patient with actively bleeding oesophageal varices, differentiation of the aetiology of underlying liver disease (from postviral (or another aetiology) cirrhosis and chronic schistosomal disease) is usually impossible on clinical grounds alone. In a study carried out at Cairo, Egypt, liver ultrasonography was undertaken in 50 patients who were undergoing an operation for bleeding oesophageal varices;[240] ultrasonographic diagnosis was compared with a surgically obtained wedge biopsy specimen. The authors concluded that ultrasonography gave the more accurate diagnosis; the findings in schistosomal periportal (pipe-stem) fibrosis were characteristic and were not mimicked by other liver diseases (including cirrhosis); ultrasonography agreed with the histological diagnosis in 44 cases.

Role of ultrasonography in management

The overall value of ultrasonographic scanning and scintigraphy in the diagnosis of chronic liver disease in developing countries has been addressed.[241] Needle biopsy is frequently necessary to diagnose diffuse disease, but a high degree of specificity can be anticipated with a space-occupying lesion.[155] A further problem surrounding ultrasonography has been highlighted:[241] in Africa and other developing countries, focal lesions 'often present so late that lesions revealed by ultrasound are huge and bizarre', and the inexperienced radiologist may therefore be baffled.

Portal hypertension and its complications

The major causes of portal hypertension (and oesophageal varices) are summarized in Table 10.7. Some geographical variations have been reviewed.[1,9] While in many parts of the world cirrhosis is the most common cause, in India non-cirrhotic portal fibrosis is relatively common.[9] Indian childhood cirrhosis (see above) also accounts for cases in the younger age group(s). Extrahepatic portal vein obstruction is common in some countries (including India);[223,242] however, in Egypt, Africa, the Middle East, South America and China, *Schist. mansoni* and *Schist. japonicum*, respectively, are frequently responsible. In Jamaica, South Africa, central Asia and the south-western USA, epidemic veno-occlusive disease (see above) (caused by *Heliotropium*, *Crotalaria*, *Senecio* and other alkaloids; see above) is important.

Pitressin (vasopressin) forms the basis of management of variceal haemorrhage; if and where available, upper gastrointestinal endoscopic sclerotherapy is of value, but this technique usually has to be repeated at 6-monthly intervals. The Sengstaken tube (for variceal compression) still has a place in developing countries. Haemorrhage is not a major presenting feature at most tropical hospitals (see above).

Bleeding varices resulting from extrahepatic portal obstruction

The cause of portal vein thrombosis in developing countries remains unclear; it is, however, a relatively common condition, and neonatal umbilical sepsis is usually cited as the likely aetiological factor.[1] During an 8.5-year period, 136 patients with extrahepatic portal hypertension were treated surgically at New Delhi, India;[242] in 22 it was carried out as an emergency (for variceal bleeding), and in 114 as an elective procedure (in 104 for a past haematemesis and in 10 for massive splenomegaly). The emergency strategy consisted of: splenectomy and splenorenal shunt (14), transoesophageal variceal ligation (4), splenectomy and gastro-oesophageal devascularization (3) and mesocaval shunt (1). Elective procedures were: splenectomy and splenorenal shunt (94), mesocaval shunt (8) and splenectomy and gastro-oesophageal devascularization (12). Operative mortality was 2 (9%) and 1 (1%), respectively; none of the survivors developed encephalopathy or postsplenectomy sepsis. One hundred and seventeen (86%) were followed up for 2–10 years; 17 had a further haematemesis, but 90% and 75% were alive at 5 and 10 years, respectively. Patients experiencing haematemesis are often far from medical facilities in a developing country; the authors therefore considered that in this setting operative intervention was more satisfactory than endoscopic sclerotherapy or management with propranolol (variceal compression was not considered).

Space-occupying hepatic lesions

Invasive hepatic amoebiasis

Amoebic liver abscess is a cause of right upper quadrant pain (and hepatomegaly); this is usually accompanied by fever, and not infrequently right shoulder-tip pain. Travellers to infected areas as well as the indigenous population(s) of the tropics may be affected.[1,243] Pathogenesis is dependent on an oral infection with a potentially invasive strain (zymodeme) of *Ent. histolytica*.[244] The mode of evolution remains unclear.[245] Diagnosis is based on an appropriate serological technique (IFAT, cellulose acetate or countercurrent immunoelectrophoresis) and hepatic ultrasonography or computed tomography.

Clinical characteristics in a group of 52 patients suffering from amoebic liver abscesses have been recorded at Cairo, Egypt;[246] while 22 (42%) presented with an acute illness (see above), 30 (58%) had a more chronic illness with dull aching in the right hypochondria, weight loss, fatigue, moderate to low-grade pyrexia and anaemia. A right-sided pleural effusion, emphysema, ascites and jaundice were present in three (6%), four (8%), seven (13%) and seven (13%), respectively. Forty-two (81%) abscesses were solitary and in the right lobe; 29 (43%) were initially solid or heterogeneous. Response to metronidazole (750 mg three times daily for 10 days) was described as good in 50; in four aspiration was carried out on account of the large abscess size.

Whether needle aspiration of an amoebic abscess (in addition to satisfactory chemotherapy) is indicated remains controversial. A prospective, randomized controlled study carried out at New Delhi, India, has addressed this issue;[247] in 17 of 37 patients (all received appropriate chemotherapy, 2–4 g metronizadole for 10 days) who completed the study, aspiration was carried out on the day of hospital admission; clinical improvement (and cure) was similar to that in 20 controls. 'Abscess' diameter was slightly lower in those who underwent aspiration (54 vs 72 mm). However, at Benin, Nigeria, needle aspiration was considered to 'enhance clinical recovery';[248] in a non-randomized trial, 19 patients were managed by needle aspiration in addition to chemotherapy, and 17 were given chemotherapy (metronidazole, diloxanide and chloroquine) alone; 18 and 10, respectively, experienced complete resolution (as shown by ultrasonography) after 21 days ($p < 0.021$), and clinical response was also considered more rapid ($p < 0.01$), especially when the abscess was >6 cm in diameter. Delay in ultrasonographic 'recovery' is not important, there being good evidence that a residual abnormality after a year or more is compatible with complete, uncomplicated resolution.

Although no in vitro evidence of *Ent. histolytica* resistance to the 5-nitroimidazole compounds exists, reports continue to be made from India of drug-resistant cases. The main problem with such reports is that, in few (if any) has diloxanide furoate (500 mg three times daily for 10 days) been administered; this is essential for a definitive cure because it is a far superior luminal amoebicide compared with the 5-nitroimidazole compounds – and therefore kills the cysts (which could belong to invasive zymodemes). In a prospective randomized study of 50 such 'resistant' cases at New Delhi, four management regimens were used:[249] (1) a repeat course of conservative therapy (with 1.25 mg/kg dehydroemetine given intramuscularly daily for 10 days); (2) needle aspiration (under ultrasonographic guidance); (3) percutaneous catheter drainage (under ultrasonographic guidance); and (4) open surgical drainage with catheter insertion. The authors concluded that 'the most impressive results' were obtained with regimen 3.

To summarize, in the uncomplicated case, needle aspiration (under cover of a 5-nitroimidazole compound) is indicated when: (1) the abscess(es) cavity is large and the patient seriously ill; and (2) the site of the lesion is such that perforation into a nearby viscus (most importantly the pericardium) seems probable. All cases of invasive amoebiasis should receive a course of the luminal amoebicide, diloxanide furoate (500 mg three times daily for 10 days) after metronidazole (800 mg three times daily for 10 days) or tinidazole (2 g daily for 3 days). If this regimen is omitted, *Ent. histolytica* cysts remain in the colonic lumen and, in the event of their being of a pathogenic zymodeme, further tissue invasion (including liver abscess) might occur.

Spontaneous perforation of an amoebic liver abscess is a serious complication which is associated with high morbidity and mortality rates;[243] this applies especially when perforation takes place into the pericardial cavity. Successful percutaneous drainage (for 7–34 days) of a perforated abscess in five 'severely ill' patients (with a total of 11 lesions) under metronidazole cover has been recorded;[250] there were resultant abscesses in the subhepatic space, pelvis, chest, right and left paracolic gutters, lesser sac, retroperitoneum and flank, and associated fistulas were demonstrated with the bile duct, duodenum and the colon; all healed completely. No patient required a laparotomy. These authors recommend wider use of catheter drainage for this serious complication of hepatic amoebiasis.

Pyogenic liver abscess

Although in a tropical context it is far less common than invasive amoebiasis (see above), pyogenic abscess is a serious disease with high morbidity and mortality, even when managed in experienced hands.[1] In most cases, a primary intra-abdominal focus of infection can be detected. Differentiation from invasive hepatic amoebiasis is usually straightforward, the patient being more severely and acutely ill; jaundice, septicaemia and renal impairment are common accompaniments. Ultrasonography is usually diagnostic. In Kuala Lumpur, 25 pyogenic abscesses were encountered between 1970 and 1985;[251] during the same period, there were 90 amoebic and one tuberculous abscesses, while in 89 others the cause of the abscess was not discovered. At Kingston, Jamaica, fever and abdominal pain were present in 21 (80%) out of 24 cases of pyogenic abscess encountered between 1977 and 1986;[252] the most common signs were right upper quadrant tenderness and hepatomegaly; leukocytosis, elevated alkaline phosphatase and hypoalbuminaemia were common. Reports from London[253] and California[254] have given encouraging reports of management by needle aspiration under antibiotic (usually gentamicin and metronidazole or clindamycin) cover. Another study has also recorded satisfactory results in 18 of 21 patients using this form of percutaneous drainage. Other authors have intimated, however, that this form of management should be reserved for selected patients.[255] A report from Riyadh, Saudi Arabia, has provided results which were less encouraging. In Jamaica surgical drainage using a guided percutaneous technique gave comparable results.[256] Taking all reports into account, it seems wise to perform a laparotomy and to institute surgical drainage as soon as possible after diagnosis. Using ultrasonographic control, a pyogenic abscess can be seen to 'resolve' significantly more rapidly than an amoebic abscess. It should be appreciated, however, that this disease carries a significant mortality rate; between 1975 and 1986, these authors treated 109 children with pyogenic liver abscess; the mortality rate was 15%.[257] There is limited (suggestive) evidence that the overall prognosis is improving.

Hydatid disease and schistosomiasis involving the liver

Only rarely, usually following trauma, does hydatidosis[207,258,259] present as an abdominal emergency. Perforation into the peritoneal cavity may produce an anaphylactoid reaction with hypotension, and/or seeding of daughter hydatid cysts within the peritoneal cavity. A relatively high prevalence of alveolar echinococcosis has been recorded in China.[260] Secondary bacterial infection is an unusual event. Chemotherapy is with albendazole and/or praziquantel (Chapter 86).

Hepatic schistosomiasis[261] is complicated by portal hypertension and oesophageal varices in an advanced case; however, hepatocellular function is maintained late into the course of disease and hepatic encephalopathy and ascites occur as advanced (usually terminal) signs. Praziquantel is the chemotherapeutic agent of choice; evidence of reversal of fibrotic changes is now available.

PANCREAS

The two major diseases involving this organ encountered in tropical countries, and which differ from those in temperate ones, are (1) 'J-type' diabetes, first reported in Jamaica (Chapter 36) and (2) chronic calcific pancreatitis.

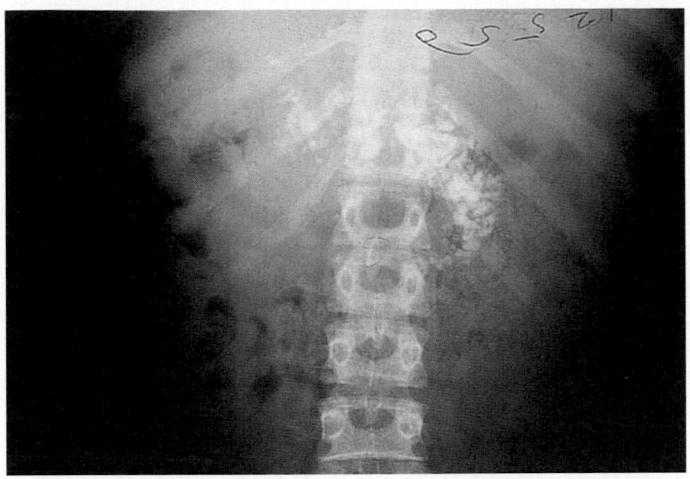

Figure 10.11 Abdominal radiograph showing calcified pancreas in the chronic calcific pancreatitis syndrome. There was no history of alcohol excess or infant malnutrition; aetiology was therefore undetermined.

Diabetes, which is *not* associated with pancreatic calcification in young people, is encountered throughout tropical countries; those affected are usually thin, and require high doses of insulin; however, they do not rapidly develop ketosis when insulin is discontinued. J-type diabetes might have a viral aetiology, a Coxsackie virus being involved; a raised incidence of antibody to Coxsackie B$_4$ has been demonstrated in affected patients in India. A suggestion has been made that these patients, especially those in Africa, are less susceptible to chronic diabetic complications than Europeans; this now seems unlikely.

A popular Indian and Chinese vegetable, karela (*Momordica charantia*) possesses hypoglycaemic properties; these are enhanced by chlorpropamide, a fact that should be taken into account in the management of diabetes in a number of Asian countries.

A syndrome consisting of pancreatic calcification associated with both exocrine and endocrine impairment is common in many tropical countries (Figure 10.11);[1,262,263] most observations have been made in Africa (East and West), southern India and Indonesia. The aetiology of *chronic calcific pancreatitis* remains unknown. Pancreatic disruption in childhood kwashiorkor can be severe and might be relevant. Cassava (*Manihot esculenta*) has also been implicated. Long-standing pancreatic damage can also follow viral hepatitis. A further hypothesis is that pancreatic ducts blocked by secretions and inspissated mucous plugs later calcify; this might be more common after starvation, gastroenteritis and dehydration. Presentation is with weight loss and malabsorption (in some parts of Africa, this is the most common cause of overt malabsorption); diabetes mellitus and pancreatic pain are important features. Management consists of providing pancreatic supplements (e.g. pancreatin BP, 6 g orally with meals) together with diabetic control.[1] Pain is often difficult to manage and may be so severe that suicide is a sequel.

The pancreas can also be involved in many infections including *Schist. mansoni* and *Schist. japonicum*, trichinellosis, cysticercosis and hydatid disease.

Pancreatic duct obstruction, complicated by acute pancreatitis, is most commonly a sequel to *A. lumbricoides* infection (see below); tapeworms are rarely implicated. Clonorchiasis and opisthorchiasis may involve the pancreatic duct system.

Emergencies: pancreas, and biliary system

One of the most widely distributed nematodes in tropical and subtropical countries is *A. lumbricoides*. By entering the biliary system (from the duodenum) this parasite can cause several acute medical and surgical conditions. Reporting from Kashmir, India, Khuroo et al.[264] collected 500 cases in which *A. lumbricoides* involved the liver, biliary tract and pancreas; biliary ascariasis was present in 171 cases, and in 140 there was hepatic, in eight gallbladder and in seven pancreatic involvement. These authors recognized five clinical presentations: acute cholecystitis (64), acute cholangitis (121), biliary colic (280), acute pancreatitis (31) and hepatic abscess (4). Twenty-seven had a pyogenic cholangitis, which was treated by decompression and drainage, surgically in two and endoscopically in 25; removal of adult worms from the ampullary orifice (with extraction per os) led to rapid relief of biliary colic in 214, and acute pancreatitis in 16; four patients died, from acute pancreatitis (2), pyogenic cholangitis (1) and hepatic abscess (1). Worms persisted at 3 weeks in the biliary tree in 12 patients; dead worms were removed either by surgery (5) or by using an endoscopic basket (7). *A. lumbricoides* moved out of the ductal system in 211 cases. The patients were followed-up for a mean of 48 months; 76 became re-infected and had re-invasion of the biliary tree; in seven cases intrahepatic duct and bile duct calculi (superimposed on dead worms) were present.

In South-east Asia, the two most common biliary parasites are *Clonorchis sinensis* and *Opisthorchis* spp. Although these cause chronic problems, notably secondary bacterial cholangitis[142] and adenocarcinoma of the biliary system, an acute presentation[1] is unusual.

In most indigenous people of developing countries, gallstones are unusual; when they occur they are usually of the pigment variety, and often associated with haemolysis. A report from Saudi Arabia, where the average lifestyle has rapidly become westernized (with striking changes in diet) over the last few decades, indicates that cholecystectomy for cholelithiasis is now one of the most common major abdominal operations to be carried out;[265] between 1977 and 1986, for example, 2854 individuals (most of them young Saudis) underwent this operation at 14 hospitals in the Eastern Province of the country.

Acute pancreatitis is uncommon overall in developing countries, although severe abdominal pain caused by chronic calcific pancreatitis[1] can give rise to problems in differential diagnosis. The pain may be severe. Biliary involvement by *A. lumbricoides* can result in acute pancreatitis.[1,142] Other helminths, including *Clonorchis sinensis*, *Opisthorchis* and *Anisakis* species have also been associated with this condition.

Table 10.8 Some causes of splenomegaly in the tropics

Infections	
Viral	Epstein–Barr virus, cytomegalovirus, viral hepatitis and other virus diseases
Bacterial	typhoid fever, brucellosis, tuberculosis
Parasitic	malaria (especially hyper-reactive malarious splenomegaly (HMS)), schistosomiasis, visceral leishmaniasis, African trypanosomiasis

Portal hypertension
Haemopoietic diseases
Sickle cell disease, thalassaemia
Reticuloendothelial diseases
Burkitt's lymphoma, leukaemia, reticuloses
Cystic lesions
Hydatid disease
Abscess
Amoebic; unknown aetiology
Spontaneous haemorrhage and rupture
Metabolic
Amyloidosis

SPLEEN

Table 10.8 summarizes some causes of splenomegaly in the tropics.[1] Most of these receive attention in other chapters. The most extreme form of splenomegaly (HMS) (Figure 10.12) is covered in Chapters 13 and 72; those caused by various viral, bacterial and parasitic infections are dealt with under these respective headings.

The spleen is an extremely important line of defence against many infections, especially pneumococcal and *Plasmodium* species infections. Splenectomized individuals in tropical countries should receive pneumococcal vaccine; prudent advice regarding malaria prophylaxis is mandatory.

Splenic abscess is a well-documented tropical disease.[1] Aetiology is usually unknown; underlying viral and parasitic diseases have been suggested, but not proved. A connection with carriage of the sickle cell gene has also been suggested, but this has also not been proved. Most reports have been made in West Africa and Zimbabwe. In most, the aetiology is unknown, but some undoubtedly result from a *S. typhi* infection. The clinical history is usually one of 2–3 weeks duration, and consists of pain/swelling in the left hypochondrium, associated with pyrexia. The splenic swelling is tender, often exquisitely so, and fluctuant. A radiograph may show gas within the abscess. Untreated, the abscess can rupture into the peritoneal cavity; splenectomy therefore has an important role in management. Should the condition become chronic – an unusual event – splenectomy is also the correct course of management.

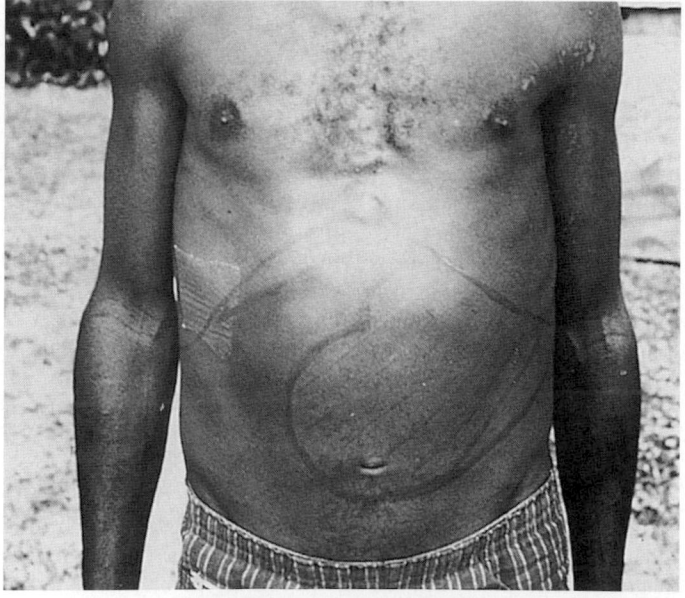

A

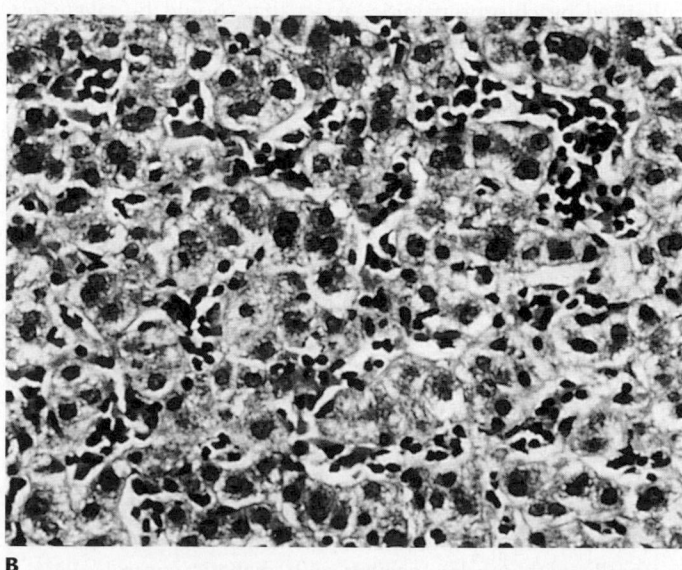

B

Figure 10.12 Papua New Guinea man suffering from hyperreactive malarious splenomegaly (HMS); all of the features of this syndrome were present. (B) Liver biopsy specimen showing severe sinusoidal lymphocytosis, a component of the syndrome.

REFERENCES

1. Cook GC. *Tropical Gastroenterology.* Oxford: Oxford University Press; 1980:484.

2. Cook GC, ed. *Gastroenterological Problems from the Tropics.* London: BMJ Publishing; 1995:146.

3. Cook GC, ed. *Travel-Associated Disease.* London: Royal College of Physicians 1995:179.

4. Cook GC. Gastroenterological emergencies in the tropics. *Baillière's Clin Gastroenterol* 1991; 5:861–886.

5. Ferguson R. Diseases of the mouth. In: Misiewicz JJ, Pounder RE, Venables CW, eds. Diseases of the Gut and Pancreas. 2nd edn. Oxford: Blackwell; 1994:93–101.

6. Watson A. Carcinoma of the oesophagus. In: Misiewicz JJ, Pounder RE, Venables CW, eds. Diseases of the Gut and Pancreas. 2nd edn. Oxford: Blackwell; 1994:159–172.

7. Sharma BC, Bhasin DK, Bhatti HS, et al. Gastrointestinal bleeding due to worm infestation, with negative upper gastrointestinal endoscopy findings: impact of enteroscopy. *Endoscopy* 2000; 32:314–316.

8. Clamp SE, Morgan AG, Kotwal MR, et al. Use of a multinational survey to provide clinical guidelines for upper gastrointestinal bleeding in developing countries. *Scand J Gastroenterol* 1988; 23(suppl 144):63–66.

9. Kiire CF, Kitai I, Sigola L, et al. Upper gastrointestinal bleeding in an African setting. *J R Coll Physicians Lond* 1987; 21:107–110.

10. Okumura H, Aramaki T, Katsuta Y. Pathophysiology and epidemiology of portal hypertension. *Drugs* 1989; 37(suppl 2):2–12.

11. El-Zayadi A, Montasser MF, Girgis F, et al. Histological changes of the esophageal mucus in bleeding versus non-bleeding varices. *Endoscopy* 1989; 21:205–207.

12. Nakib BAI, Radhakrishnan S, Liddawi HAI, et al. The role of gastrointestinal endoscopy in a developing country. *Endoscopy* 1986; 18:37–39.

13. Atoba MA, Ayoola EA, Olubuyide IO. Radiological and endoscopic correlation in upper gastrointestinal haemorrhage and malignancy. *Scand J Gastroenterol* 1986; 21(suppl 124):149–151.

14. Sarin SK, Nanda R, Sachdev G. Relative efficacy and safety of absolute alcohol and 50% alcohol as variceal sclerosants. *Gastrointest Endosc* 1987; 33:362–365.

15. Sarin SK, Mishra SP, Sachdev GK, et al. Ethanolamine oleate versus absolute alcohol as a variceal sclerosant: a prospective, randomised, controlled trial. *Am J Gastroenterol* 1988; 83:526–530.

16. Sarin SK, Misra SP, Singal AK, et al. Endoscopic sclerotherapy for varices in children. *J Pediatr Gastroenterol Nutr* 1988; 7:662–666.

17. Wahrendorf J, Chang-Claude J, Liang QS, et al. Precursor lesions of oesophageal cancer in young people in a high-risk population in China. *Lancet* 1989; ii:1239–1241.

18. Clarke CA, Bodmer WF. Oesophageal cancer in China. *Lancet* 1989; ii:1525.

19. Langman MJS. Aetiologies of peptic ulcer. In: Misiewicz JJ, Pounder RE, Venables CW, eds. Diseases of the Gut and Pancreas. 2nd edn. Oxford: Blackwell; 1994:249–259.

20. Scobie BA, Beg F, Oldmeadows M. Peptic diseases compared endoscopically in indigenous Fijians and Indians. *N Z Med J* 1987; 100:683–684.

21. Ramirez-Ramos A, Watanabe-Yamamoto J, Takano-Morón J, et al. Decrease in prevalence of peptic ulcer and gastric adenocarcinoma at the Policlinico Peruano Japones, Lima, Peru, between the years 1985 and 2002. Analysis of 31,446 patients. *Acta Gastroent Latinoam* 2006; 36:139–46.

22. Mattar R, Marques SB, Monteiro Mdo S, et al. *Helicobacter pylori cag* pathogenicity island genes: clinical relevance for peptic ulcer disease development in Brazil. *J Med Microbiol* 2007; 56:9–14.

23. Argent RH, Burette A, Miendje Deyi VY, et al. The presence of *dupA* in *Helicobacter pylori* is not significantly associated with duodenal ulceration in Belgium, South Africa, China, or North America. *Clin Infect Dis* 2007; 45:1204–1206.

24. Ohene-Yeboah M, Togbe B. Perforated gastric and duodenal ulcers in an urban African population. *West Afr J Med* 2006; 25:205–211.

25. Tytgat GNJ. Gastritis. In: Misiewicz JJ, Pounder RE, Venables CW, eds. Diseases of the Gut and Pancreas. 2nd edn. Oxford: Blackwell; 1994:221–235.

26. Sonnenberg A. Time trends of ulcer mortality in non-European countries. *Am J Gastroenterol* 2007; 102:1101–1107.

27. Cook GC. Hypochlorhydria and vulnerability to intestinal infection. *Eur J Gastroenterol Hepatol* 1994; 6:693–695.

28. Craven JL. Carcinoma of the stomach. In: Misiewicz JJ, Pounder RE, Venables CW, eds. Diseases of the Gut and Pancreas. 2nd edn. Oxford: Blackwell; 1994:335–352.

29. Kochhar R, Krishna PR, Gupta NM, et al. Massive gastrointestinal bleeding due to cholecystoduodenal fistula. *Acta Chir Scand* 1988; 154:471–472.

30. Kocer B, Surmeli S, Solak C, et al. Factors affecting mortality and morbidity in patients with peptic ulcer perforation. *J Gastroent Hepatol* 2007; 22:565–570.

31. Sarin SK, Sachdev G, Nanda R, et al. Endoscopic sclerotherapy in the treatment of gastric varices. *Br J Surg* 1988; 75:747–750.

32. Jernigan J, Guerrant RL, Pearson RD. Parasitic infections of the small intestine. *Gut* 1994; 35:289–293.

33. Cook GC. The small intestine and its role in chronic diarrheal disease in the tropics. In: Gracey M, ed. *Diarrhea.* Boca Raton: CRC Press; 1991:127–162.

34. Cook GC. Tropical disease and the small intestine. In: Misiewicz JJ, Pounder RE, Venables CW, eds. Diseases of the Gut and Pancreas. 2nd edn. Oxford: Blackwell; 1994:597–615.

35. dos Reis JC, de Morais MB, Oliva CA, et al. Breath hydrogen test in the diagnosis of environmental enteropathy In children living in an urban slum. *Dig Dis Sci* 2007; 52:1253–1258.

36. Menzies IS, Zuckerman MJ, Nukajam WS, et al. Geography of intestinal permeability and absorption. *Gut* 1999; 44:483–489.

37. Ramakrishna BS. Prevalence of intestinal pathogens in HIV patients with diarrhea: implications for treatment. *Indian J Pediatr* 1999; 66:85–91.

38. DuPont HL. Travelers' diarrhea. In: Gracey M, ed. *Diarrhea.* Boca Raton: CRC Press; 1991:115–126.

39. Gorbach SL. Travelers' diarrhea. In: Gorbach SL, Barlett JG, Blacklow NR, eds. *Infectious Diseases.* Philadelphia: W B Saunders; 1992:622–628.

40. Okhuysen PC, Ericsson CD. Travelers' diarrhea. *Curr Opin Gastroenterol* 1992; 8:110–114.

41. Farthing MJG. Travellers' diarrhoea. *Gut* 1994; 35:1–4.

42. Ansdell VE, Ericsson CD. Prevention and empiric treatment of traveler's diarrhea. *Med Clin North Am* 1999; vi: 83:945–973.

43. Black RE. Epidemiology of travelers' diarrhea and relative importance of various pathogens. *Rev Infect Dis* 1990; 12(suppl 1):S73–S79.

44. Ljungh AH. Travellers' diarrhoea and the European tourist. *Eur J Gastroenterol Hepatol* 1992; 4:764–770.

45. Harries AD, Myers B, Cook GC. Inflammatory bowel disease: a common cause of bloody diarrhoea in visitors to the tropics. *BMJ* 1985; 291:1686–1687.

46. Schumacher G, Kollberg B, Ljungh A. Inflammatory bowel disease presenting as travellers' diarrhoea. *Lancet* 1993; 341:241–242.

47. Rowe B, Taylor J, Bettelheim KA. An investigation of travellers' diarrhoea. *Lancet* 1970; i:1–4.

48. Sack RB. Travelers' diarrhea: microbiologic bases for prevention and treatment. *Rev Infect Dis* 1990; 12(suppl 1):S59–S63.

49. Tellier R, Keystone JS. Prevention of travelers' diarrhoea. *Infect Dis Clin North Am* 1992; 6:333–354.

50. Bhutta TI, Tahir KI. Loperamide poisoning in children. *Lancet* 1990; 353:363.

51. DuPont HL, Ericsson CD, Johnson PC, et al. Use of bismuth subsalicylate for the prevention of travelers' diarrhea. *Rev Infect Dis* 1990; 12(suppl 1):S65–S67.

52. Peltola H, Siitonen A, Kyronseppa H, et al. Prevention of travellers' diarrhoea by oral B-subunit/whole cell cholera vaccine. *Lancet* 1991; 338:1285–1289.

53. CHOICE Study Group. Multicenter, randomised, double-blind clinical trial to evaluate the efficacy and safety of a reduced osmolarity oral rehydration salts solution in children with acute watery diarrhea. *Pediatrics* 2001; 107:613–618.

54. DuPont HL, Ericsson CD, Matthewson JJ, et al. Five versus three days of ofloxacin therapy for travelers' diarrhea: a placebo-controlled study. *Antimicrob Agents Chemother* 1992; 36:87–91.

55. Tribble DR, Sanders JW, Pang LW, et al. Traveler's diarrhea in Thailand: randomized, double-blind trial comparing single-dose and 3-day azithromycin- based regimens with a 3- day levofloxacin regimen. *Clin Infect Dis* 2007; 44:338–346.

56. Hamilton SK, Keren DF, Boitnott JK, et al. Enhancement of cholera toxin of IgA secretion from intestinal crypt epithelium. *Gut* 1980; 21:365–369.

57. Phillips SF. Asiatic cholera: nature's experiment? *Gastroenterology* 1986; 91:1304–1307.

58. Nalin DR. Cholera and severe toxigenic diarrhoeas. *Gut* 1994; 35:145–149.

59. Cook GC. The Asiatic cholera: an historical determinant of human genomic and social structure. In: Drasar BS, Forrest BD, eds. *Cholera and the ecology of vibrio cholerae.* London: Chapman & Hall; 1996.

60. Steffen R. Epidemiologic studies of travelers' diarrhea, severe gastrointestinal infections, and cholera. *Rev Infect Dis* 1986; 8:S122–S130.

61. Cook GC. Preventive strategies for the avoidance of infectious diarrhoea. In: Gracey M, Bouchier IAD, eds. *Infectious diarrhoea.* Vol. 7(2). London: Baillière Tindall; 1993:519–545.

62. Levine MM. Modern vaccines: enteric infections. *Lancet* 1990; 335:958–961.

63. Kaper JB. Vibrio cholerae vaccines. *Rev Infect Dis* 1989; 11:S568–S573.

64. Avery ME, Snyder JC. Oral therapy for acute diarrhea: the underused single solution. *N Engl J Med* 1990; 323:891–894.

65. Cosnett JE. The origins of intravenous fluid therapy. *Lancet* 1989; ii:768–771.

66. Cook GC. Management of cholera: the vital role of rehydration. In: Drasar BS, Forrest BD, eds. *Cholera and the ecology of vibrio cholerae.* London: Chapman & Hall; 1996.

67. Islam MR. Single-dose tetracycline in cholera. *Gut* 1987; 28:1029–1032.

68. Rabbani GH, Islam MR, Butler T, et al. Single-dose treatment of cholera and furazolidone or tetracycline in a double-blind randomised trial. *Antimicrob Agents Chemother* 1989; 33:1447–1450.

69. Alam AN, Alam NH, Ahmed T, et al. Randomized double blind trial of single dose doxycycline for treating cholera in adults. *BMJ* 1990; 300: 1619–1621.

70. Sengupta PG, Niyogi SK, Bhattacharya SK. An outbreak of El Tor cholera in Aizwal town of Mizoram, India. *J Commun Dis* 2000; 32:207–211.

71. Cook GC. Hypolactasia: geographical distribution, diagnosis, and practical significance. In: Chandra RK, ed. *Critical Reviews in Tropical Medicine.* Vol. 2. New York: Plenum Press; 1984:117–139.

72. Asmawi MZ, Seppo L, Vapaatalo H, et al. Hypolactasia & lactose intolerance among three ethnic groups in Malaysia. *Indian J Med Res* 2006; 124:697–704.

73. Lim ML, Wallace MR. Infectious diarrhea in history. *Infect Dis Clin North Am* 2004;18:261–274.

74. Cook GC. Persisting diarrhoea and malabsorption. *Gut* 1994; 35:582–586.

75. Tomkins A. Tropical malabsorption: recent concepts in pathogenesis and nutritional significance. *Clin Sci* 1981; 60:131–137.

76. Baker SJ. Idiopathic small intestinal disease in the tropics. In: Chandra RK, ed. *Critical Reviews in Tropical Medicine.* Vol. 1. New York: Plenum Press; 1982:197–245.

77. Mathan VI. Tropical sprue in southern India. *Trans R Soc Trop Med Hyg* 1988; 82:10–14.

78. Manson P. Notes on sprue. *Medical Reports for the half year ended 31 March 1880,* 19th issue. Imperial Maritime Customs 11, spec. ser. 2. Shanghai: Statistical Department of the Inspectorate General; 1880:33–37.

79. Hillary W. Of chronical diseases. *Observations on the Changes of the Air and the Concomitant Epidemical Diseases, in the Island of Barbados,* 2nd edn. Hawes, Clarke, Collins; 1799:276–297.

80. Taylor DN, Connor BA, Shlim DR. Chronic diarrhea in the returned traveler. *Med Clin North Am* 1999; vii(83):1033–1052.

81. Gerson CD. The small intestine. *Mt Sinai J Med* 2000; 67:241–244.

82. Peetermans WE, Vonck A. Tropical sprue after travel to Tanzania. *J Travel Med* 2000; 7:33–34.

83. Menendez-Corrada R, Netthleship E, Santiago-Delpin EA. HLA and tropical sprue. *Lancet* 1986; ii:1183–1185.

84. Naik S. HLA and gastrointestinal disorders. *Indian J Gastroenterol* 1986; 5:121–124.

85. Klipstein F, Engert RF, B Short HB. Enterotoxigenicity of colonising coliform bacteria in tropical sprue and blind-loop syndrome. *Lancet* 1978; ii:342–344.

86. Tomkins AM, Wright SG, Drasar BS. Bacterial colonization of the upper intestine in mild tropical malabsorption. *Trans R Soc Trop Med Hyg* 1980; 74:752–755.

87. Spencer J, Isaacson PG, Diss TC, et al. Expression of disulfide-linked and non-disulfide-linked forms of the T cell receptor g/d heterodimer in human intestinal intraepithelial lymphocytes. *Eur J Immunol* 1989; 14:1335–1338.

88. Besterman HS, Cook GC, Sarson DL, et al. Gut hormones in tropical malabsorption. *BMJ* 1979; ii:1252–1255.

89. Adrian TE, Savage AP, Bacarese-Hamilton AJ, et al. Peptide YY abnormalities in gastrointestinal disease. *Gastroenterology* 1986; 90:379–384.

90. Mathan VI. Tropical sprue in southern India. *Trans R Soc Trop Med Hyg* 1988; 82:10–14.

91. Read NW. Diarrhoea: the failure of colonic salvage. *Lancet* 1982; 11:481–483.

92. Ramakrishna BS, Mathan VI. Role of bacterial toxins, bile acids, and free fatty acids in colonic water malabsorption in tropical sprue. *Dig Dis Sci* 1987; 32:500–505.

93. Batt RM, McLean L. Comparison of the biochemical changes in the jejunal mucosa of dogs with aerobic and anaerobic bacterial overgrowth. *Gastroenterology* 1987; 93:986–993.

94. Catassi C, Ratsch IM, Gandolfi L, et al. Why is coeliac disease endemic in the people of the Sahara? *Lancet* 1999; 354:647–648.

95. Gupta B, Narru N, Dhar KL. Evaluation of surface area corrected peak blood xylose as a screening test of intestinal malabsorption in the tropics. *Indian J Gastroenterol* 1987; 6:89–91.

96. Peters TJ, Jones PE, Wells G, et al. Sequential enzyme and subcellular fractionation studies on jejunal biopsy specimens from patients with post-infective tropical malabsorption. *Clin Sci Mol Med* 1979; 56:479–486.

97. Cook GC, Menzies IS. Intestinal absorption and unmediated permeation of sugars in post-infective tropical malabsorption (tropical sprue). *Digestion* 1986; 33:109–116.

98. Cook GC. Aetiology and pathogenesis of post-infective tropical malabsorption (tropical sprue). *Lancet* 1984; i:721–723.

99. Glynn J. Tropical sprue: its aetiology and pathogenesis. *J R Soc Med* 1988; 79:599–606.

100. Jelinek T, Loscher T. Epidemiology of giardiasis in German travellers. *J Travel Med* 2000; 7:70–73.

101. Yong TS, Park SJ, Hwang UW, et al. Genotyping of Giardia lamblia isolates from humans in China and Korea using ribosomal DNA sequences. *J Parasitol* 2000; 86:887–891.

102. Grove DI. Strongyloidiasis: a conundrum for gastroenterologists. *Gut* 1994; 35:437–440.

103. Tandon RK. Abdominal tuberculosis. In: Bouchier IAD, Allan RN, Hodgson HJF et al., eds. *Gastroenterology: Clinical Science and Practice.* 2nd edn. London: W B Saunders; 1993:1459–1468.

104. Rambaud J-C, Ruskoné-Fourmestraux A. Small intestinal lymphomas: immunoproliferative small intestinal disease, a-chain disease and Mediterranean lymphomas. In: Bouchier IAD, Allan RN, Hodgson HJF et al., eds. *Gastroenterology: Clinical Science and Practice.* 2nd edn. London: W B Saunders; 1993:636–643.

105. Ghoshal UC, Chetri K, Banerjee PK, et al. Is immunoproliferative small intestinal disease uncommon in India? *Trop Gastroenterol* 2001; 22:14–17.

106. Rana SV, Thapa BR, Pal R. Comparison of D-xylose hydrogen breath test with urinary D-xylose test in Indian children with celiac disease. *Dig Dis Sci* 2007; 52:681–684.

107. Arikan C, Zihni C, Cakir M, et al. Morphometric analysis of small-bowel mucosa in Turkish children with celiac disease and relationship with the clinical presentation and laboratory findings. *Dig Dis Sci* 2007; 52:2133–2139.

108. Cataldo F, Montalto G. Celiac disease in the developing countries: a new and challenging public health problem. *World J Gastroent* 2007; 13:2153–2159.

109. Dossetor JFB, White HC. Protein-losing enteropathy and malabsorption in acute measles enteritis. *BMJ* 1975; 2:592–593.

110. Conrad ME, Schwartz FD, Young AA. Infectious hepatitis: a generalised disease. *Am J Med* 1964; 37:789–801.

111. Schreiber DS, Blacklow NR, Trier JS. The intestinal lesion of the proximal small intestine in acute infectious nonbacterial gastroenteritis. *N Engl J Med* 1973; 288:1318–1323.

112. McCormack JG. Clinical features of rotavirus gastroenteritis. *J Infect* 1982; 4:167–174.

113. Pun SB, Nakagomi T, Sherchand JB et al. Detection of G12 human rotaviruses in Nepal. *Emerg Infect Dis* 2007; 13:482–484.

114. Telch J, Shephard RW, Butler DG, et al. Intestinal glucose transport in acute viral enteritis in piglets. *Clin Sci* 1981; 61:29–34.

115. Brown DWG, Selvakumar R, Daniel DJ, et al. Prevalence of neutralising antibodies to Berne virus in animals and humans in Vellore, South India. *Arch Virol* 1988; 98:267–269.

116. Lindenbaum J. Malabsorption during and after recovery from acute intestinal infection. *BMJ* 1965; ii:326–329.

117. Editorial. Mechanisms in enteropathogenic *Escherichia coli* diarrhoea. *Lancet* 1983; i:1254–1256.

118. Mandal BK. Salmonella typhi and other salmonellas. *Gut* 1994; 35:726–728.

119. Editorial. Campylobacter enteritis. *Lancet* 1982; ii:1437–1438.

120. Murrell TGC, Walker PD. The pigbel story of Papua New Guinea. *Trans R Soc Trop Med Hyg* 1991; 85:119–122.

121. Murrell TGC. Pigbel disease in Papua New Guinea: an ancient disease rediscovered. *Int J Epidemiol* 1983; 12:211–214.

122. Gbakima AA, Konteh R, Kallon M, et al. Intestinal protozoa and intestinal helminthic infections in displacement camps in Sierra Leone. *Afr J Med Sci* 2007; 36:1–9.

123. Gillon J, Andre C, Descos L, et al. Changes in mucosal immunoglobulin-containing cells in patients with giardiasis before and after treatment. *J Infect* 1982; 5:67–72.

124. Gelanew T, Lalle M, Hailu A, et al. Molecular characterization of human isolates of Giardia duodenalis from Ethiopia. *Acta Trop* 2007; 102:92–99.

125. Farthing MJG. Giardia lamblia. In: Farthing MJG, Keusch GT, eds. *Enteric Infection: Mechanisms, Manifestations and Management*. London: Chapman & Hall; 1988:397–413.

126. Jokipii L, Jokipii AMM. Treatment of giardiasis: comparative evaluation of ornidazole and tinidazole as a single oral dose. *Gastroenterology* 1982; 83:399–404.

127. Siwila J, Phiri IG, Vercruysse J, et al. Asymptomatic cryptosporidiosis in Zambian dairy farm workers and their household members. *Trans R Soc trop Med Hyg* 2007; 101:733–734.

128. Xiao L, Cama A, Cabrera L, et al. Possible transmission of Cryptosporidium canis among children and a dog in a household. *J Clin Microbiol* 2007; 45:2014–2016.

129. Crosby WH. The deadly hookworm: why did the Puerto-Ricans die? *Arch Intern Med* 1987; 147:577–578.

130. Bunyaratvej S, Bunyawongwiroj P, Nitiyanant P. Human intestinal sarcosporidiosis: report of six cases. *Am J Trop Med Hyg* 1982; 31:36–41.

131. Eberhard ML, Nace EK, Freeman AR, et al. Cyclospora cayetanensis infections in Haiti: a common occurrence in the absence of watery diarrhea. *Am J Trop Med Hyg* 1999; 60:584–586.

132. Green ST, McKendrick MW, Mohsen AH, et al. Two simultaneous cases of Cyclospora cayatensis enteritis returning from the Dominican Republic. *J Travel Med* 2000; 7:41–42.

133. Verdier RI, Fitzgerald DW, Johnson WD, et al. Trimethoprim-sulfamethoxazole compared with ciprofloxacin for treatment and prophylaxis of Isospora belli and Cyclospora cayetanensis infection in HIV-infected patients: a randomised, controlled trial. *Ann Intern Med* 2000; 132:885–888.

134. Lopez-Velez R, Turrientes MC, Garron C, et al. Microsporidiosis in travellers with diarrhea from the tropics. *J Travel Med* 1999; 6:223–227.

135. Bicart-See A, Massip P, Linas MD, et al. Successful treatment with nitazoxanide of Enterocytozoon bieneusi microsporidiosis in a patient with AIDS. *Antimicrob Agents Chemother* 2000; 44:167–168.

136. Vdovenko AA. Blastocystis hominis: origin and significance of vacuolar and granular forms. *Parasitol Res* 2000; 86:8–10.

137. Cook GC. George Leith Roupell FRS (1797–1854): significant contributions to the early nineteenth-century understanding of cholera and typhus. *J Med Biog* 2000; 8:1–7.

138. Collins BJ, van Loon FPL, Molla A, et al. Gastric emptying or oral rehydration solutions in acute cholera. *J Trop Med Hyg* 1989; 92:290–294.

139. Avery ME, Snyder JD. Oral therapy for acute diarrhea: the underused simple solution. *N Engl J Med* 1990; 323:891–894.

140. Lawrence GW, Lehmann D, Anian G, et al. Impact of active immunisation against enteritis necroticans in Papua New Guinea. *Lancet* 1990; 336:1165–1167.

141. Murtaza A, Khan SR, Butt KS, et al. Paralytic ileus, a serious complication in acute diarrhoeal disease among infants in developing countries. *Acta Paediatr Scand* 1989; 78:701–705.

142. Hoffman SH. Tropical medicine and the acute abdomen. *Emerg Med Clin North Am* 1989; 7:591–609.

143. Gopi VK, Joseph TP, Varma KK. Acute intestinal obstruction. *Indian Pediatr* 1989; 26:525–530.

144. Archampong EQ. Tropical diseases of the small bowel. *World J Surg* 1985; 9:887–896.

145. Ryan CA, Hargrett-Bean NT, Blake PA. Salmonella typhi infections in the United States, 1975–1984: increasing role of foreign travel. *Rev Infect Dis* 1989; 11:1–8.

146. Weeramanthri TS, Corrah PT, Mabey DCW, et al. Clinical experience with enteric fever in The Gambia, West Africa 1981–1986. *J Trop Med Hyg* 1989; 92:272–275.

147. Thisyakorn U, Mansuwan P, Taylor DN. Typhoid and paratyphoid fever in 192 hospitalized children in Thailand. *Am J Dis Child* 1987; 141:862–865.

148. Gibney EJ. Typhoid perforation. *Br J Surg* 1989; 76:887–889.

149. Meier DE, Imediegwu OO, Tarpley JL. Perforated typhoid enteritis: operative experience with 108 cases. *Am J Surg* 1989; 157:423–427.

150. Ameh EA. Typhoid ileal perforation in children: a scourge in developing countries. *Ann Trop Paediatr* 1999; 19:267–272.

151. Rubin CME, Fairhurst JJ. Life-threatening haemorrhage from typhoid fever. *Br J Radiol* 1988; 61:415–416.

152. Raj SM, Sivakumaran S, Vijayakumari S. Morbidity due to intestinal helminthiasis. *Lancet* 1990; 336:811–812.

153. Nuchjangreed C, Hamzah Z, Suntornthiticharoen P, et al. Anisakids in marine fish from the coast of Chon Buri Province, Thailand. *Southeast Asian J Trop Med Publ Hlth* 2006; 37(suppl 3):35–39.

154. Umehara A, Kawakami Y, Araki J, et al. Molecular identification of the etiological agent of the human anisakiasis in Japan. *Parasit Int* 2007; 56:211–215.

155. Cook GC. *Parasitic Disease in Clinical Practice*. London: Springer; 1990:272.

156. Hepburn NC. Aetiology of eosinophilic enteritis. *Lancet* 1990; 336:571.

157. Prociv P, Croese J. Human eosinophilic enteritis caused by dog hookworm Ancylostoma caninum. *Lancet* 1990; 335:1299–1302.

158. Anayi S, Al-Nasiri N. Acute mesenteric ischaemia caused by Schistosoma mansoni infection. *BMJ* 1987; 294:1197.

159. Radomyos P, Chobchuanchom A, Tungtrongchitr A. Intestinal perforation due to Macracanthorhynchus hirudinaceus infection in Thailand. *Trop Med Parasitol* 1989; 40:476–477.

160. Bannerman C, Manzur AY. Fluctuating jaundice and intestinal bleeding in a 6-year-old girl with fascioliasis. *Trop Geogr Med* 1986; 38:429–431.

161. Acheson DWK, Keusch GT. The shigella paradigm and colitis due to enterohaemorrhagic Escherichia coli. *Gut* 1994; 35:872–874.

162. Ravdin JI. Diagnosis of invasive amoebiasis: time to end the morphology era. *Gut* 1994; 35:1018–1021.

163. Fielding L, Padmanabhan A. Clinical features of colorectal cancer. In: Misiewicz JJ, Pounder RE, Venables CW, eds. *Diseases of the Gut and Pancreas*. 2nd edn. Oxford: Blackwell; 1994:877–892.

164. Misiewicz JJ, Pounder RE, Venables CW, eds. *Diseases of the Gut and Pancreas*. 2nd edn. Oxford: Blackwell; 1994:675–804.

165. Jiang L, Xia B, Li J, et al. Risk factors for ulcerative colitis in a Chinese population: an age-matched and sex-matched case-control study. *J Clin Gastroenterol* 2007; 41:280–284.

166. Wang YF, Zhang H, Ouyang Q. Clinical manifestations of inflammatory bowel disease: East and West differences: *J Dig Dis* 2007; 8:121–127.

167. Abdul-Baki H, ElHajj I, El-Zahabi LM, et al. Clinical epidemiology of inflammatory bowel disease in Lebanon. *Inflamm Bowel Dis* 2007; 13: 475–480.

168. Holdsworth CD. Irritable bowel syndrome. In: Misiewicz JJ, Pounder RE, Venables CW, eds. *Diseases of the Gut and Pancreas*. 2nd edn. Oxford: Blackwell; 1994:921–930.

169. Ladep NG, Okeke EN, Samaila AA, et al. Irritable bowel syndrome among patients attending General Outpatients' clinics in Jos, Nigeria. *Eur J Gastroenterol Hepatol* 2007; 19:795–799.

170. Uz E, Türkay C, Aytac S, et al. Risk factors for irritable bowel syndrome in Turkish population: role of food allergy. *J Clin Gastroenterol* 2007; 41: 380–838.

171. Soyturk M, Akpinar H, Gurler O, et al. Irritable bowel syndrome in persons who acquired trichinellosis. *Am J Gastroenterol* 2007; 102:1064–1069.

172. Chang FY, Lu C L. Irritable bowel syndrome in the 21st century: perspectives from Asia or South-east Asia. *J Gastroenterol Hepatol* 2007; 22:4–12.

173. Cook GC. Enterobius vermicularis infection. *Gut* 1994; 35:1159–1162.

174. Ravdin JI. Intentional disease caused by Entamoeba histolytica. In: Ravdin JI, ed. *Amebiasis: Human Infection by Entamoeba histolytica*. New York: Churchill Livingstone; 1988:495–510.

175. Ellyson JH, Bezmalinovic Z, Parks SN, et al. Necrotizing amebic colitis: a frequently fatal complication. *Am J Surg* 1986; 152:21–26.

176. Shukla VK, Roy SK, Vaidya MP, et al. Fulminant amebic colitis. *Dis Colon Rectum* 1986; 29:398–401.

177. Zhang Y, Bi P, Hiller JE, et al. Climate variations and bacillary dysentery in northern and southern cities of China. *J Infect* 2007; 55:194–200.

178. Parsonnet J, Greene KD, Gerber AR, et al. Shigella dysenteriae type 1 infections in US travellers to Mexico. *Lancet* 1989; ii:543–545.

179. Lanenscheidt P, Lang C, Puschel W, et al. High rates of appendicectomy in a developing country: an attempt to contribute to a more rational use of surgical resources. *Eur J Surg* 1999; 165:248–252.

180. Ameh EA. Appendicitis versus genital disease in young women in tropical Africa. *Trop Doct* 2000; 30:103–104.

181. Out AA. Tropical surgical emergencies: acute appendicitis. *Trop Geogr Med* 1989; 41:118–122.

182. Gupta SC, Gupta AK, Keswani NK, et al. Pathology of tropical appendicitis. *J Clin Pathol* 1989; 42:1169–1172.

183. Badmos KB, Komolafe AO, Rotimi O. Schistomiasis presenting as acute appendicitis. *East Afr Med J* 2006; 83:528–532.

184. Ramezani MA, Dehghani MR. Relationship between Enterobius vermicularis and the incidence of acute appendicitis. *Southeast Asian J Trop Med Publ Hlth* 2007; 38:20–23.

185. Zimmerman J-M, de Graeve B, Coblence J-F, et al. Attitude thèrapeutique actuelle devant le volvulus du colon pelvien en milieu tropical. *Méd Trop* 1989; 49:371–374.

186. Kotisso B, Bekele A. Intussusception in adolescents and adults: a report on cases from Addis Abaka, Ethiopia, during a three-year period. *Ethiop Med J* 2007; 45:187–194.

187. Wilson APR, Ridgway GL, Sarner M, et al. Toxic dilatation of the colon in shigellosis. *BMJ* 1990; 301:1325–1326.

188. Gradon JD, Lutwick LI. Toxic dilation and amebiasis. *Am J Gastroenterol* 1988; 83:206–207.

189. Cook GC. Anorectal infections in relation to tropical exposure. In: Demling L, Frühmorgan P, eds. *Non-neoplastic Diseases of the Anorecturm*. Dordrecht: Kluwer; 1992:187–226.

190. Segal I, Edwards CA, Walker AR. Continuing low colon cancer incidence in African populations. *Am J Gastroenterol* 2000; 95:859–860.

191. Misra SP, Misra V, Dwivedi M, et al. Colonic tuberculosis: clinical features, endoscopic appearance and management. *J Gastroenterol Hepatol* 1999; 14:723–729.

192. Koh TH, Tan AL, Tan ML, et al. Epidemiology of Clostridium difficile infection in a large teaching hospital in Singapore. *Pathology* 2007; 39:438–442.

193. Kunasol P, Cooksley G, Chan VF, et al. Hepatitis A virus: declining seroprevalence in children and adolescents in Southeast Asia. *Southeast Asian J Trop Med Publ Hlth* 1998; 29:255–262.

194. Shah U, Habib Z, Kleinman RE. Liver failure attributable to hepatitis A virus infection in a developing country. *Pediatrics* 2000; 105:436–438.

195. Anonymous. Hepatitis C: global prevalence (update). *Wkly Epidemiol Rec* 1999; 74(10 December):425–427.

196. Coursaget P, Buisson Y, N'Gawara MN, et al. Role of hepatitis E virus in sporadic cases of acute and fulminant hepatitis in an endemic area. *Am J Trop Med Hyg* 1998; 58:330–334.

197. Labrique AB, Thomas DL, Stoszek SK, et al. Hepatitis E: an emerging infectious disease. *Epidemiol Rev* 1999; 21:162–179.

198. Potasman I, Koren L, Peterman M, et al. Lack of hepatitis E infection among backpackers to tropical countries. *J Travel Med* 2000; 7:208–210.

199. Tarrago D, Lopez-Velez R, Turrientes C, et al. Prevalence of hepatitis E antibodies in immigrants from developing countries. *Eur J Clin Microbiol Infect Dis* 2000; 19:309–311.

200. Bircher J, Benhamou J-P, McIntyre N, et al., eds. In: *Oxford Textbook of Clinical Hepatology*. 2nd edn. Vol. 2. Oxford: Oxford University Press; 1999:825–985.

201. Summerfield JA. Virus hepatitis update. *J R Coll Physicians Lond* 2000; 34: 381–385.

202. Hoffmann CJ, Thio CL. Clinical implications of HIV and hepatitis B co-infection in Asia and Africa. *Lancet Infect Dis* 2007; 7:402–409.

203. Acharya SK, Madan K, Dattagupta S, et al. Viral hepatitis in India. *Natl Med J India* 2006; 19:203–217.

204. Mukhopadhya A. HCV: the Indian scenario. *Trop Gastroenterol* 2006; 27:105–110.

205. Pramoolsinsap C, Viranuvatti V. Salmonella hepatitis. *J Gastroenterol Hepatol* 1998; 13:745–750.

206. Shetty AK, Mital SR, Bahrainwala AH, et al. Typhoid hepatitis in children. *J Trop Pediatr* 1999; 45:287–290.

207. Da Dilva LC, Chieffi PP, Carrilho FJ. Protozoal and helminthic diseases of the liver. In: Prieto J, Rodes J, Shafritz DA, eds. *Hepatobiliary Disease*. Berlin: Springer; 1992:631–664.

208. Bircher J, Benhamou J-P, McIntyre N, et al., eds. Cirrhosis. In: *Oxford Textbook of Clinical Hepatology*. 2nd edn. Vol. 1. Oxford: Oxford University Press; 1999:605–641.

209. Okuda K, Okuda H. Primary liver cell carcinoma. In: Bircher J, Benhamou J-P, McIntyre N, et al., eds *Oxford Textbook of Clinical Hepatology*. 2nd edn. Vol. 2. Oxford: Oxford University Press; 1999:1491–1530.

210. Bosch FX, Ribes J, Borras J. Epidemiology of primary liver cancer. *Semin Liver Dis* 1999; 19:271–285.

211. Haworth EA, Soni-Raleigh V, Balarajan R. Cirrhosis and primary liver cancer amongst first generation migrants in England and Wales. *Ethn Health* 1999; 4:93–99.

212. Wild CP, Hall AJ. Primary prevention of hepatocellular carcinoma in developing countries. *Mutat Res* 2000; 462:381–393.

213. Goldberg AC, Bittencourt PL, Oliveira LC, et al. Autoimmune hepatitis in Brazil: an overview. *Scand J Immunol* 2007; 66:208–216.

214. Pan KT, Hung CF, Tseng JH, et al. Hepatic calcification by sequelae of chronic schistosomiasis japonica: report of four cases. *Changgeng Yi Xue Za Zhi* 1999; 22:265–270.

215. El-Hawey AM, Amr MM, Abdel-Rahman AH, et al. The epidemiology of schistosomiasis in Egypt: Gharbia Governorate. *Am J Trop Med Hyg* 2000; 62(suppl 2):42–48.

216. Bircher J, Benhamou J-P, McIntyre N, et al., eds. Alcoholic liver disease. In: *Oxford Textbook of Clinical Hepatology*. 2nd edn. Vol. 2. Oxford: Oxford University Press; 1999:1155–1247.

217. Mowat AP. Paediatric liver disease. In: Bircher J, Benhamou J-P, McIntyre N, et al., eds. *Oxford Textbook of Clinical Hepatology*. 2nd edn. Vol. 2. Oxford: Oxford University Press; 1999:1875–1889.

218. Scheinberg IH, Sternlieb I. Is non-Indian childhood cirrhosis caused by excess dietary copper? *Lancet* 1994; 344:1002–1004.

219. Brissot P, Deugnier Y. Genetic haemochromatosis. In: McIntyre N, Benhamou J-P, Bircher J, et al., eds. *Oxford Textbook of Hepatology*. Oxford: Oxford University Press; 1991:948–958.

220. Kew MC, Asare GA. Dietary iron overload in the African and hepatocellular carcinoma. *Liver Int* 2007; 27:735–741.

221. Valla D, Benhamou J-P. Vascular abnormalities. In: Bircher J, Benhamou J-P, McIntyre N, et al., eds. *Oxford Textbook of Clinical Hepatology*. 2nd edn. Vol. 2. Oxford: Oxford University Press; 1999:1457–1479.

222. Eapen CE, Mammen T, Moses V, et al. Changing profile of Budd Chiari Syndrome in India. *Indian J Gastroenterol* 2007;26:77–81.

223. Arora NK, Lodha R, Gulati S, et al. Portal hypertension in north Indian children. *Indian J Pediatr* 1998; 65:585–591.

224. Osman M, Lausten SB, El-Sefi T, et al. Biliary parasites. *Dig Surg* 1998; 15:287–296.

225. Richter J, Freise S, Mull R, et al. Fascioliasis: sonographic abnormalities of the biliary tract and evolution after treatment with triclabendazole. *Trop Med Int Health* 1999; 4:774–781.

226. El-Morshedy H, Farghaly A, Sharaf S, et al. Triclabendazole in the treatment of human fascioliasis: a community-based study. *East Mediterr Health J* 2000; 5:888–894.

227. Millan JC, Mull R, Freise S, et al. The efficacy and tolerability of triclabendazole in Cuban patients with latent and chronic Fasciola hepatica infection. *Am J Trop Med Hyg* 2000; 63:264–269.

228. Khan SA, Shah N, Williams R, et al. Acute liver failure: a review. *Clin Liver Dis* 2006; 10:239–258.

229. Cook GC. Hepatic structure and function in experimental and human malaria. In: Bianchi L, Gerok W, Maier K-P, Dienhardt F, eds. *Infectious Diseases of the Liver (Falk Symposium 54)*. Dordrecht: Kluwer; 1990:191–213.

230. Zakaria S, Goldsmith RS, Kamel MA, et al. The etiology of acute hepatitis in adults in Egypt. *Trop Geogr Med* 1988; 40:285–292.

231. Pal SR, Prasad SR. Delta virus infections in and around Chandigarh, Northern India: evidence for endemicity. *Trop Geogr Med* 1987; 39:123–125.

232. Khuroo MS, Zargar SA, Mahajan R, et al. An epidemic of hepatitis D in the foothills of the Himalayas in South Kashmir. *J Hepatol* 1988; 7:151–156.

233. Asano Y, Yoshikawa T, Suga S, et al. Fatal fulminant hepatitis in an infant with human herpesvirus-6 infection. *Lancet* 1990; 335:862–863.

234. Boulos M, Segurado AAC, Shiroma M. Severe yellow fever with a 23-day survival. *Trop Geogr Med* 1988; 40:356–358.

235. Holmes GP, McCormick JB, Trock SC, et al. Lassa fever in the United States: investigation of a case and new guidelines for management. *N Engl J Med* 1990; 323:1120–1123.

236. Lucia HL, Coppenhaver DH, Harrison RL, et al. The effect of an arenavirus infection on liver morphology and function. *Am J Trop Med Hyg* 1990; 43:93–98.

237. MacGregor FB, Abernethy VE, Dahabra S, et al. Hepatoxicity of herbal remedies. *BMJ* 1989; 299:1156–1157.

238. Tandon BN, Joshi YK, Tandon M. Acute liver failure: experience with 145 patients. *J Clin Gastroenterol* 1986; 8:664–668.

239. Sarin SK, Chari S, Sundaram KR, et al. Young v adult cirrhotics: a prospective, comparative analysis of the clinical profile, natural course and survival. *Gut* 1988; 29:101–107.

240. Abdel-Wahab MF, Esmat G, Milad M, et al. Characteristic sonographic pattern of schistosomal hepatic fibrosis. *Am J Trop Med Hyg* 1989; 40:72–76.

241. Editorial. Clinical ultrasound in developing countries. *Lancet* 1990; 336:1225–1226.

242. Pande GK, Reddy VM, Kar P, et al. Operations for portal hypertension due to extrahepatic obstruction: results and 10 year follow-up. *BMJ* 1987; 295:1115–1117.

243. Reed SL, Braude AI. Extraintestinal disease: clinical syndromes, diagnostic profile, and therapy. In: Ravdin JI, ed. *Amebiasis: Human Infection by Entamoeba histolytica*. New York: Churchill Livingstone; 1988:511–532.

244. Sargeaunt PG. Zymodemes of Entamoeba histolytica. In: Ravdin JI, ed. *Amebiasis: Human Infection by Entamoeba histolytica*. New York: Churchill Livingstone; 1988:370–387.

245. Robinson SP, Remedios D, Davidson RN. Do amoebic liver abscesses start as large lesions? Case report of an evolving amoebic liver abscess. *J Infect* 1998; 36:338–340.

246. Ahmed L, Rooby AEI, Kassem MI, et al. Ultrasonography in the diagnosis and management of 52 patients with amebic liver abscess in Cairo. *Rev Infect Dis* 1990; 12:330–337.

247. Sharma MP, Rai RR, Acharya SK, et al. Needle aspiration of amoebic liver abscess. *BMJ* 1989; 299:1308–1309.

248. Freeman O, Akamaguna A, Jarikre LN. Amoebic liver abscess: the effect of aspiration on the resolution or healing time. *Ann Trop Med Parasitol* 1990; 84:281–287.

249. Singh JP, Kashyap A. A comparative evaluation of percutaneous catheter drainage for resistant amebic liver abscesses. *Am J Surg* 1989; 158:58–62.

250. Ken JG, van Sonnenberg E, Casola G, et al. Perforated amebic liver abscesses: successful percutaneous treatment. *Radiology* 1989; 170:195–197.

251. Goh KL, Wong NW, Paramsothy M, et al. Liver abscess in the tropics: experience in the University Hospital, Kuala Lumpur. *Postgrad Med J* 1987; 63:551–554.

252. Bansal AS, Prabhakar P. Clinical aspects of pyogenic liver abscess: the University Hospital of the West Indies experience. *J Trop Med Hyg* 1988; 91:87–93.

253. Berger LA, Osborne DR. Treatment of pyogenic liver abscesses by percutaneous needle aspiration. *Lancet* 1982; i:132–134.

254. Herbert DA, Fogel DA, Rothman J, et al. Pyogenic liver abscesses: successful non-surgical therapy. *Lancet* 1982; i:134–136.

255. Bowers ED, Robison DJ, Doberneck RC. Pyogenic liver abscess. *World J Surg* 1990; 14:128–132.

256. McCorkell SJ, Niles NL. Pyogenic liver abscesses: another look at medical management. *Lancet* 1985; i:803–806.

257. Pineiro-Carrero VM, Andres JM. Morbidity and mortality in children with pyogenic liver abscess. *Am J Dis Child* 1989; 143:1424–1427.

258. Shaw JM, Bornman PC, Krige JE. Hydatid disease of the liver. *S Afr J Surg* 2006; 44:70–72, 74–77.

259. Franchi C, Di Vico B, Teggi A. Long-term evaluation of patients with hydatidosis treated with benzimidazole carbamates. *Clin Infect Dis* 1999; 29:304–309.

260. Craig PS, The Echinococcus working group in China. Epidemiology of human alveolar echinococcosis in China. *Parasit Int* 2006; 55:S221–S225.

261. Strickland GT. Gastrointestinal manifestations of schistosomiasis. *Gut* 1994; 35:1334–1337.

262. Castillo CF del, Richter JM, Warshaw AL. Chronic pancreatitis. In: Bouchier IAD, Allan RN, Hodgson HJF, et al., eds. *Gastroenterology: Clinical Science and Practice*. 2nd edn. London: WB Saunders; 1993:1615–1634.

263. Chattopadhyay PS, Chattopadhyay R, Goswami R, et al. Observations on hepatic structure and function in fibro-calculous pancreatic diabetes (FCPD) vis-à-vis other diabetic subtypes. *Indian J Pathol Microbiol* 1998; 41:141–146.

264. Khuroo MS, Zarger SA, Mahajan R. Hepatobiliary and pancreatic ascariasis in India. *Lancet* 1990; 335:1503–1506.

265. Tamimi TM, Wosornu L, Al-Khozaim A, et al. Increased cholecystectomy rates in Saudi Arabia. *Lancet* 1990; 336:1235–1237.

REFERENCES

Chapter 11 — Stephen M. Graham and Stephen B. Gordon

Respiratory Problems in the Tropics

INTRODUCTION

In an average tropical hospital, 20–50% of out-patients have come with respiratory complaints, and 20–30% of hospital medical admissions are for disorders predominantly affecting the lungs. The incidence is highest in infants and young children, especially for those living in urban areas. It is estimated that acute respiratory infection (ARI) is responsible for one-third of deaths of children under 5 years of age globally and the majority of these deaths occur in children from tropical countries. The major burden of adult disease has traditionally been due to pneumonia (Chapter 54) and tuberculosis (TB: Chapter 56) but the incidence of chronic obstructive pulmonary disease is rising globally due to the increasing use of tobacco and continuing use of biomass fuel. Occupational lung disease and asthma are problems of polluted and urban environments and the pulmonary complications of HIV infection include empyema and pulmonary hypertension as well as opportunistic infections.

CLINICAL ASSESSMENT IN CHILDREN

History

Most of the morbidity and mortality due to ARI in children occurs in infants and young children. This influences clinical approach as there is less detail of symptoms than for older children and adults, and abnormalities of auscultation or percussion may be absent or hard to define in small chests. The child usually presents with cough and/or difficulty breathing. Factors that increase the incidence and severity of childhood pneumonia include young age, low birth weight, malnutrition, exposure to indoor smoke and underlying disease such as HIV infection, cardiac abnormalities or cerebral palsy. Poor immunization coverage for measles and whooping cough may be a factor in some regions.

Examination

A raised respiratory rate is consistently the most reliable clinical sign for lower respiratory tract infection. There is some clinical overlap with the presentation of other common childhood illnesses such as malaria or septicaemia. More severe pneumonia is indicated by chest indrawing, difficulty with feeding in infants or cyanosis. School-aged children often present with acute lobar pneumonia and initially cough may not be a prominent symptom. They may complain of pleuritic chest pain and sometimes present with acute abdominal pain or with headache and neck pain, depending on the site of lobar involvement. The presence of stridor suggests large airway obstruction (e.g. croup), while wheeze indicates small airway obstruction (e.g. bronchiolitis in the infant or asthma in the toddler or older child).

In children with persistent cough or wheeze not responding to standard treatment consider pulmonary TB (PTB), foreign body, HIV-related lung disease or cardiac failure. A review of the growth chart is often helpful. Mild asthma or recurrent viral respiratory infection causing persistent symptoms usually occurs in thriving well-nourished children while TB is marked by significant failure to thrive or weight loss. A history of TB contact (or of household contacts with chronic cough), particularly close contact with sputum smear-positive PTB, is important. In HIV endemic regions, consider *Pneumocystis jiroveci* pneumonia (PcP) in an infant with severe pneumonia not responding to standard antibiotic treatment. PcP is usually the first presentation of HIV-related disease. Lymphocytic interstitial pneumonitis (LIP) is an HIV-related lung disease that usually presents in older children and is often misdiagnosed as PTB. Look for features suggestive of HIV infection such as generalized lymphadenopathy, extensive oral candidiasis, parotid swelling, digital clubbing or typical skin rashes. A history of a choking episode in a child with persistent wheeze suggests foreign body aspiration. Children with congenital or acquired heart disease often present with recurrent or persistent respiratory symptoms.

CLINICAL ASSESSMENT IN ADULTS

History

The most common respiratory symptoms are cough and dyspnoea. Carefully determine the duration of cough and degree of dyspnoea. In a patient with cough, ask for associated symptoms such as fever, chest pain, haemoptysis, night sweats and weight loss. Ask about previous anti-TB therapy, the basis for the diagnosis of PTB and successful completion of treatment. In a patient with dyspnoea, determine the speed of onset and a careful smoking and occupational history. In a patient with a short history of dyspnoea, consider pneumothorax or an inhaled foreign body; in all patients with cough, fever and dyspnoea, consider the possibility of HIV infection. HIV infection is suggested by chronic ill-health of either the patient or their partner, and is common in migrant workers and truck drivers.

In your differential diagnosis, remember that cardiac disease can present with dyspnoea. Mitral valve disease and pericardial tamponade (often due to TB) are much more common in developing than in industrial countries and cardiomyopathy is not uncommon.

Examination

Always start by assessing a patient with respiratory symptoms from the end of the bed in order to observe the severity of respiratory distress, as well as the symmetry of chest movement. Many patients have advanced disease by the time they reach medical attention, and have florid signs rarely seen in developed countries. Abnormalities of chest movement or shape and mediastinal (tracheal) shift may indicate contraction from chronic fibrosis within the chest. Hydropneumothorax or pyopneumothorax can be identified clinically by the succussion splash and shifting dullness (percussion over the 5th intercostal space anteriorly is dull with the patient erect, and hollow when supine). Amphoric breathing and post-tussive crackles may be heard over a large pulmonary cavity. Look for features suggestive of chronic lung disease such as a barrel-shaped chest or finger clubbing. Marked wasting, generalized lymphadenopathy and enlarged non-tender parotid glands are consistent with HIV infection but may also occur with disseminated TB or malignancy. Severe fungal infections such as histoplasmosis, cryptococcosis or paracoccidioidomycosis can also present as pneumonia in an emaciated patient and occur more commonly, but not exclusively, in HIV-infected individuals (see Chapter 20). Palpable lymph nodes may provide a source of diagnostic material and should be sought routinely.

Finally, look carefully for evidence of cardiac or abdominal abnormalities. Pericardial constriction or effusion may mimic or complicate pulmonary disease such as TB. Right ventricular hypertrophy with cor pulmonale may develop secondary to chronic pulmonary disease, e.g. pulmonary schistosomiasis or chronic pulmonary histoplasmosis.

PULMONARY INVESTIGATIONS IN CHILDREN AND ADULTS

The diagnosis of bacterial pneumonia is clinical. Blood culture is often not available, has a low sensitivity (<30%) and a decision to treat with antibiotics must be made before the result is available. Transthoracic needle aspiration of consolidated lung has a higher yield and has been an important research technique for studies of aetiology, particularly in children, that guide standard management policy, but usually is not practical for routine clinical management.

Sputum smear microscopy for acid-fast bacilli is the initial investigation of choice for PTB diagnosis. Appropriate patient selection, proper sputum collection and optimal specimen pro-

cessing are all important.[1] HIV-infected patients have increased susceptibility to TB (both reactivation and new infections) but PTB is more likely to be sputum-negative in HIV-infected patients than in other people due to the decreased immune response and hence decreased cavitation seen in the HIV-infected group. Children of <8 years of age are usually unable to expectorate sputum and so the diagnosis of PTB can be particularly difficult. Improved samples can be obtained in adults by initiating a deep cough using physiotherapy or nebulized hypertonic saline to induce sputum production. These techniques are also showing promise for infants and young children.[2]

Good sputum samples may yield other information, depending on available microbiology services. Bacterial culture is of very limited value because of the plentiful commensal flora in the pharynx but culture for tubercle bacilli yields a delayed diagnosis in some smear-negative subjects. Nocardiosis is difficult to distinguish clinically and radiologically from PTB but *Nocardia asteroides* is identifiable by Gram stain or culture of the sputum. Other organisms that are identifiable from sputum include *Burkholderia pseudomallei* (causing melioidosis), *Pneumocystis jiroveci*, *Histoplasma capsulatum*, *Cryptococcus* spp. and *Paracoccidioides brasiliensis*. Sputum microscopy may occasionally reveal larval helminths, *Strongyloides*, *Paragonimus ova*, hydatid scolices or fungal hyphae (aspergilloma).

Bedside lung function testing is unusual in many parts of the tropics and under-used elsewhere. A peak flowmeter provides an index of airways obstruction, both for diagnosis and for observing changes and response to treatment. Duration and force of blowing a full breath out can yield similar information (duration >4 s indicating severe obstruction). Pulse oximetry is a useful method for determining severity of hypoxia and response to oxygen therapy.

Chest radiographs are important but expensive. They should be used with discretion and not simply to prove what is clearly deducible from clinical features, as in lobar pneumonia, massive pleural effusion or sputum smear-positive PTB. It is better to reserve radiography for circumstances such as the management of pneumothorax or the investigation of unresolving pneumonia. HIV infection has affected the specificity and sensitivity of chest X-ray abnormalities for patients with PTB. The appearance may be atypical, e.g. lower zone infiltrates, or even normal, especially in the severely immunocompromised patient (see Chapters 20 and 57).

Lymph node aspiration and biopsy can provide useful diagnostic information, particularly if TB or disseminated malignancy is suspected. If a large effusion is present, a pleural tap is often helpful to differentiate causes such as TB (straw-coloured fluid, by far the most common cause of effusion in TB endemic areas), empyema (thick purulent fluid) or pulmonary Kaposi's sarcoma (bloody tap in the presence of palatal KS). Pleural biopsy, using an Abrams' needle and taking two or three specimens in different directions at the same site, may assist with histological diagnosis. HIV serology is now widely available but remember caution must be used in order not to miss multiple diagnoses in HIV-infected patients.

If available, fibreoptic bronchoscopy may provide useful additional diagnostic information: by identifying causes of local bronchial obstruction (e.g. foreign bodies, tumours) or obtaining secretions and specimens by bronchoalveolar lavage and transbronchial biopsy. As for sputum sampling, the value of fibreoptic bronchoscopy is limited by the quality of laboratory facilities that can be applied to fluid or tissues obtained. It is rarely indicated in young children except for foreign body removal.

ACUTE RESPIRATORY INFECTION IN CHILDREN

The urban child suffers an average of five to eight episodes of ARI per year and the rural child three to four episodes per year, whether in the tropics or non-tropics. The majority are mild upper respiratory tract infections due to viruses. The important difference in epidemiology between the regions is that acute lower respiratory tract infection (pneumonia) is more common, more frequently due to bacteria, more severe and much more likely to be lethal in the tropics. Although respiratory diseases are seasonal, especially in temperate regions, the contrast in severity is a reflection of socioeconomic differences rather than differences in climate.

Simple clinical criteria, such as breathing rate and the presence of subcostal indrawing are very useful in determining severity of ARI. Bacteria are responsible for up to 60% of severe pneumonia cases and for the majority of pneumonia-related deaths. The most common bacteria in children >2 months of age are *Streptococcus pneumoniae* and *Haemophilus influenzae*. These facts provided the foundation for the case management approach that aimed to reduce pneumonia deaths by identification and appropriate antibiotic (and supportive, i.e. oxygen/feeding) management of children with severe pneumonia and to reduce unnecessary use of antibiotics in children with mild ARI.[1]

There is increasing resistance of pneumococcus and *Haemophilus* to co-trimoxazole, penicillin and chloramphenicol, common first-line antibiotics for children with suspected acute bacterial pneumonia in low-income countries. As the bacteria are rarely isolated in cases of pneumonia, useful information of the pattern of resistance in the community can be obtained from nasopharyngeal sampling of healthy young children or by reviewing the pattern of resistance among isolates from children with bacterial meningitis. However, unlike for meningitis, in vitro resistance may not necessarily affect treatment response for pneumococcal pneumonia.

Pneumonia is due to a wider range of bacteria in neonates, malnourished children and HIV-infected children, and they are at greater risk of death. *Staphylococcus aureus* and Gram-negatives, such as *Klebsiella*, *Escherichia coli* or *Salmonella* are also important in these children. Staphylococcal pneumonia with pneumatoceles seems to be less common than it was and this may in part be due to less frequent and less severe measles in many countries. Non-typhoidal *Salmonella* is a common isolate from young children presenting with pneumonia in tropical Africa.[3]

WHO recommendations for first-line treatment for acute childhood pneumonia in tropical countries are aimed at reducing deaths due to bacterial pneumonia and are currently under review. A recent meta-analysis concluded that amoxicillin is superior to co-trimoxazole for the outpatient treatment of non-severe pneumonia and that penicillin and gentamicin is superior to chloramphenicol alone for hospitalized children with severe pneumonia.[4]

Of the responsible viruses causing pneumonia, respiratory syncytial virus (RSV), the influenza and parainfluenza viruses, human metapneumovirus and measles are numerically most important. Bronchiolitis and croup occur but are less seasonal and less common than in cooler climates. Again, nutritional state affects presentation and outcome. RSV is the commonest viral cause of childhood pneumonia in tropical countries. The typical clinical picture of RSV bronchiolitis in infants is recognized, but in malnourished and HIV-infected children wheeze is unusual and secondary bacterial infection more common. Common and often fatal complications of measles were severe laryngotracheitis and/or pneumonia. However, measles is now less common owing to effective immunization and vitamin A supplementation and treatment has further reduced the frequency of such complications in children with measles.

Mycoplasma pneumoniae and *Chlamydia pneumoniae* cause atypical pneumonia, particularly in school-aged children, usually not severe, and characterized by a protracted course over a few weeks and fine crackles on auscultation. Their relative importance in the tropics is not clear. Treatment of choice is erythromycin. *Chlamydia trachomatis* causes pneumonia in up to 20% of infants born to infected women and presents between 1 and 3 months of age. There is often a history of neonatal conjunctivitis. Finally, remember that TB does present as acute pneumonia, particularly in infants. The contact will usually be the mother.

Immunization against measles and pertussis, breast-feeding and improved socioeconomic circumstances can reduce the incidence and mortality of childhood ARI. The successful development of effective conjugate vaccines against invasive pneumococcus and *Haemophilus influenzae* type b (Hib) means that there is great potential for prevention of severe bacterial pneumonia in the tropics. Following efficacy studies, the Hib vaccine has already been added to routine immunization in a number of low-resource countries with great effect in reducing the burden of Hib meningitis and pneumonia.[5] More recent field trials of a 9-valent pneumococcal conjugate vaccine in South Africa and The Gambia showed similar efficacy against invasive pneumococcal disease due to vaccine serotypes resulting in significant improvements in child survival and making a very strong case for routine implementation of bacterial conjugate vaccines in developing countries.[6]

ACUTE RESPIRATORY INFECTION IN ADULTS

Acute pneumonia is common in adults in tropical countries and as in developed countries, the most common cause is *Streptococcus pneumoniae*. The higher incidence of pneumonia in tropical countries is primarily due to immunocompromise due to HIV infection but is also due to increased carriage of pneumococci by children and adults, large family size, crowding in small houses, exposure to domestic and tobacco smoke and the impaired immunity due to poor diet and parasitic diseases. Individuals with increased susceptibility to pneumonia include those with reduced splenic function (sickle cell disease, postsplenectomy), pregnant women, patients with diabetes mellitus and those with excess alcohol intake. Bacterial pneumonia may be preceded by a viral infection such as influenza that damages mucosal defence mechanisms.

The symptoms and signs of lobar pneumonia may be confusing. In early pneumonia, the diagnosis may have to be made in a patient with symptoms, fever and shallow tachypnoea in the absence of any auscultatory signs. The patient will often point to the place where pain occurs when asked to cough. When pleurisy is diaphragmatic, the patient may present with suspected abdominal disease. In some populations a considerable proportion of patients with lobar pneumonia develop jaundice.

The aetiological cause of pneumonia cannot usually be determined at the bedside but a clinical assessment of severity is more important as it can be used to guide management. In particular, young patients with uncomplicated lobar pneumonia can be managed at home with oral therapy. Patients with indicators of severity (age, co-existing disease, multi-lobar disease, shock, hypoxia) should be managed in hospital with broad-spectrum antibiotic cover to include likely (*Streptococcus pneumoniae*, *Haemophilus influenzae*) and atypical organisms.

Mycoplasma pneumoniae, *Chlamydia pneumoniae* and *Legionella pneumophila* also cause pneumonia in adults but are rare in Africa. In South-east Asia and northern Australia, melioidosis should be considered as a possible cause of both acute and of unresolving pneumonia, especially in the debilitated or immunocompromised. Appropriate media are needed to culture the organism *Burkholderia pseudomallei*. Paracoccidioidomycosis is common in Latin America and may present with pulmonary disease. Histoplasmosis and blastomycosis are also endemic in the Americas. It is important to remember that PTB may present with a clinical syndrome indistinguishable from acute bacterial pneumonia. William Osler recognized this when working in Boston in 1900, and PTB was the second most common cause of pneumonia described in Kenyan adults in 2000.[7]

PULMONARY TUBERCULOSIS IN CHILDREN AND ADULTS

Mycobacterium tuberculosis is now the second leading cause of death due to infectious disease in the world after HIV infection. The epidemiology and clinical management of TB in children and adults are covered in detail in Chapter 56. The differential diagnoses of PTB include a range of fungal diseases, parasitic diseases and non-infectious granulomatous disorders (Table 11.1).

HIV INFECTION AND PULMONARY PRESENTATIONS IN CHILDREN AND ADULTS

HIV infection is common in many regions of the tropics, particularly in sub-Saharan Africa. This subject is dealt with in detail in Chapter 20. The peak prevalence is among young adults and mother-to-child transmission is common. Respiratory disease, acute or chronic, is the commonest cause of morbidity and mortality in HIV-infected adults and children. Pulmonary symptoms are often the first clinical manifestation of the disease, but clinical evidence of underlying immunosuppression should be sought.

There are important differences in the pattern of HIV-related pneumonia between adults and children within the tropics, and in comparison to non-tropical regions (Table 11.2).[8,9] The incidence of bacterial pneumonia is greatly increased in both HIV-infected children and adults, but is highest in children.[10] The range of causative organisms is similar to that which occurs in HIV-uninfected children of similar nutritional status. Although HIV-

Table 11.1 Differential diagnoses of pulmonary tuberculosis

Fungal disease	PCP
	Cryptococcosis
	Aspergillosis
	Histoplasmosis
	Candidiasis
	Paracoccidioidomycosis[a]
	Coccidioidomycosis[a]
	Penicilliosis[b]
Bacterial disease	Nocardiosis
	Melioidosis[b]
	Lung abscess
	Brucellosis
	Actinomycosis
Parasitic disease	Paragonimiasis
	Amoebiasis
	Echinococcosis
	Strongyloidiasis
Non-infectious	Sarcoidosis
	Emphysema
	Cardiac disease
	Neoplasm

[a]In Central and South America.
[b]In South-east Asia.

Table 11.2 Causes of HIV-related lung disease in low-income tropical regions

Age group	Most common	Less common
Infants	Bacterial pneumonia	Viral pneumonia (e.g. CMV)
	PCP	Tuberculosis
Children	Bacterial pneumonia	Viral pneumonia (e.g. measles)
	LIP	Pulmonary Kaposi's sarcoma
	Tuberculosis	Nocardiosis
		Candidiasis
Adults	Bacterial pneumonia	PCP
	Tuberculosis	Cryptococcosis
		Nocardiosis
		Pulmonary Kaposi's sarcoma
		Penicilliosis[a]
		Melioidosis[a]
		Paracoccidioidomycosis[b]
		Histoplasmosis[b]

[a]In South-east Asia.
[b]In Central and South America.

infected children are more susceptible to PTB, the actual incidence of PTB is low. A common cause of chronic lung disease in HIV-infected children, which is often misdiagnosed as PTB or miliary TB, is LIP.[9] LIP is an HIV-related disease that usually occurs in children. Common clinical markers include marked generalized lymphadenopathy, finger clubbing, enlarged parotid glands and massive hepatomegaly. The typical radiographic abnormalities are diffuse reticulonodular infiltration with bilateral hilar lymphadenopathy, which contrasts with the focal and often unilateral abnormalities of PTB. Bronchiectasis presents with a chronic cough productive of copious purulent and sometimes blood-stained sputum, finger clubbing and halitosis. Bronchiectasis may complicate LIP or PTB.

PTB and bacterial pneumonia are the major causes of respiratory morbidity in HIV-infected adults living in the poorer regions of the tropics. The clinical features of bacterial pneumonia are similar to those in HIV-seronegative patients, although bacteraemia is more common.[7] The HIV pandemic has had a profound effect on the epidemiology, clinical presentations, diagnosis, drug treatment and treatment response in TB. In many HIV-infected adults, the clinical presentation is atypical (e.g. diffuse, miliary or basal in its distribution) due to the impaired Th1 type immunity in HIV-infected adults that prevents formation of the usual granulomatous inflammation followed by cavitation. Drug reactions are more common among patients with HIV-related disease and there is a high mortality in early treatment. The introduction of appropriate antiretroviral therapy during TB treatment makes management of HIV/TB more difficult than TB alone. Case holding is difficult in chronically ill patients and cure rates are lower in HIV-infected patients than in individuals without HIV.

Less common diseases in HIV-infected adults living in tropical Africa include cryptococcosis, pulmonary Kaposi's sarcoma and PcP.[8] The clinical presentation of pneumonitis caused by *Pneumocystis jiroveci* is described in Chapter 72. This is a common cause of severe pneumonia in HIV-infected African infants but is rare beyond 6 months of age.[9] In comparison to bacterial pneumonia, PcP is characterized by a low-grade or absent fever, a clear chest with good air entry or diffuse rather than focal abnormalities, severe and persistent hypoxia, and a poor clinical response to usual broad-spectrum antibiotics (e.g. chloramphenicol) and to oxygen. Hyperinflation and diffuse interstitial infiltration are the usual radiographic abnormalities. PcP is usually fatal even when treated with high-dose co-trimoxazole, prednisolone and oxygen. Co-trimoxazole prophylaxis is very effective in preventing PcP in HIV-infected infants and is recommended by WHO for all HIV-exposed infants until HIV infection can be excluded. Co-trimoxazole prophylaxis is also effective in improving survival for HIV-infected adults and children and in some studies, improved outcome has been to reduction in non-PcP pneumonia.[11]

HIV-related infections in other tropical regions include paracoccidioidomycosis in tropical America and penicilliosis due to *Penicillium marneffei* in South-east Asia.[12,13] Although a variety of parasites causes lung problems in the tropics (see below), these infections do not appear to be increased in frequency or altered in their clinical manifestations by concomitant HIV infection or AIDS.

ASTHMA AND ALLERGY IN CHILDREN AND ADULTS

Asthma is less common in the tropics than in some temperate regions and there are differences in the pattern of presentation.[14] However, the prevalence of asthma in tropical countries is increasing, particularly in urban communities. Many asthmatics first develop symptoms in adult life and there is less likely to be a history of other atopic conditions. The low but increasing incidence of atopic disease and asthma in tropical countries is an area of current research interest with the hope that it may provide important information as to why such diseases have become so common in more affluent countries. Nutrition is likely to be one factor: asthma is extremely rare in malnourished children. Relationship to infections more prevalent in the tropics such as the higher burden of parasitic disease may also be important.

Patients with asthma should be assessed for possible precipitating factors including seasonal allergy, nocturnal and exertional exacerbation, dust including house-dust, farm and industrial dusts, fumes including perfumes, drugs (e.g. salicylates and beta blockers), cigarette smoking and animals. Measurements of peak expiratory flow rate and a sleep diary can help to monitor health status and response to treatment.

Treatment should be appropriate to the frequency and severity of attacks but often the range of therapeutic options available is limited. Oral salbutamol or aminophylline are perhaps the most widely available but have limited efficacy. Inhaled β2-agonists such as salbutamol or terbutaline are very useful in symptom relief particularly if patients are taught to use the inhaler effectively either by direct delivery or via a spacer. The mainstay of asthma management is inhaled corticosteroid therapy which is stepped up and down in response to symptom control and peak expiratory flow rate. Combination therapy with long acting inhaled β-agonists and steroid preparations is highly effective. Cromoglycate may be assessed for prophylactic efficacy over a period of weeks for those suffering frequent attacks of exercise-induced asthma – it is particularly useful in children. The availability of effective asthma therapy in developing countries is still poor and is being addressed by global initiatives including GINA and the WHO asthma treatment initiative.

Severe episodes of asthma can be treated with oxygen, nebulized β2-agonists and short courses of oral corticosteroids. Subcutaneous adrenaline can be very useful for the life-threatening episode especially as it is usually available.

BIOMASS FUEL USE AND RESPIRATORY HEALTH

Biomass fuel (burned organic products such as wood, charcoal or animal dung) are used by 2 billion people daily for cooking and heating. This form of energy produces particulate smoke which is often poorly vented resulting in very high exposures to smoke, particularly among women and young children. Biomass fuel smoke increases susceptibility to acute and chronic pulmonary infection in children and is associated with chronic obstructive pulmonary disease (COPD) and lung cancer in adults.[15] The impact of indoor smoke on the incidence of respiratory disease in developing countries is likely to be enormous but has been poorly documented.[16] Indoor air pollution is also associated with increased rate of disease and increased mortality due to TB.[17]

Many new forms of environmentally sensitive cooking stoves have been designed in the last 50 years (http://stoves.bioenergylists.org/), primarily with the aim of reducing deforestation and consumption of fossil fuel. It is likely that these improved stoves will also have a beneficial health effect but health impact assessments have only been described in a few studies to date.[18,19]

TOBACCO AND HEALTH

Many developing countries have a tobacco industry that was created hoping to create revenue, employment and trade but it is now realized that the economic cost of this industry exceeds its benefit. In particular, poor agricultural practice leads to loss of soil fertility, pesticide toxicity and green tobacco leaf related illnesses are a major problem in the workforce and curing the leaf requires large amounts of firewood, making this process a major cause of deforestation. Furthermore, the processed end-product is expensive and tobacco companies curtailed by strict advertising regulations and costly litigation in rich countries are now targeting middle- and low-income countries as their future market. Particularly alarming are figures from secondary schools: 30–40% of pupils in some areas have been found to be regular smokers.[20]

Smoking-related diseases have increased in tandem. Emphysema and lung cancers are becoming more common in China, Nigeria, India and Malaysia. Because of the delayed effects of smoking, a great increase of these and other smoking-related diseases can be expected within the coming decade in tropical countries. COPD is still primarily related to the use of biomass fuel (see below) in many developing countries but tobacco smoking related COPD will increase dramatically as tobacco consumption increases.

OCCUPATIONAL LUNG DISEASES

Respiratory disease often relates to occupation. In particular, mining dusts may cause pulmonary fibrosis, a wide variety of aerosolized compounds cause asthma and rare infections are common in exposed professional groups.

Work in mines, even in the distant past, may have been responsible for fibrotic lung disease (e.g. silicosis, asbestosis or berylliosis) or anthracosis and is associated with an increased risk of lung cancer. Retired miners are often debilitated if they have worked in poorly regulated conditions and the pulmonary damage sustained is increased by concomitant cigarette smoking. Exposure to asbestos and industrial air pollutants (e.g. diesel fumes, acid fumes such as SO_2 and NO_2) is associated with mining and other heavy industry.

Several hundred causes of occupational asthma have now been described including both high molecular weight compounds (flour, seafood proteins, starch) and low molecular weight compounds (glutaraldehyde, isocyanates). It is important to enquire about both current and past place and conditions of work, with particular emphasis on the relation of symptoms to the time of work. The 'healthy worker effect' where affected workers leave the workplace can result in poor association between current exposure and symptoms in exposed workforces.

Infectious occupational lung disease is common. Most cases of melioidosis in South-east Asia occur in rice farmers. A patient who works with animals or birds may be exposed to zoonotic diseases that sometimes have a pulmonary component: histoplasmosis, brucellosis, tularaemia, Q-fever, leptospirosis or psittacosis. In areas where paragonimiasis and gnathostomiasis occur, enquire about eating raw or undercooked fish; where schistosomiasis is prevalent consider the likelihood of environmental contact (e.g. fishermen and bus washers in Lake Victoria).

PULMONARY PROBLEMS IN PARASITIC DISEASES AND TROPICAL PULMONARY EOSINOPHILIA

Parasitic infection often involves the lung. In Paragonimiasis, the lung is the predominant organ involved (see Chapter 83). Paragonimiasis may present with cough, haemoptysis and cavitating lung disease. It is often mistaken for PTB and must be considered in areas where raw fish is eaten.

More usually, however, parasitic disease is systemic, with lung symptoms presenting with other features. Hydatid cysts (see Chapter 86) may produce a variety of lung problems as a result of mechanical compression of intrathoracic structures. In schistosomiasis, especially where portal hypertension has led to venous shunts bypassing the liver, eggs may be deposited in pulmonary capillaries and arterioles, eliciting a granulomatous reaction resulting either in pulmonary hypertension or the accumulation of large masses of granulation tissue (see Chapter 82). In a number of helminth infections (hookworm, Ascaris, Strongyloides, schistosomiasis) a larval stage of the parasite migrates through the lungs, when it may cause cough, fever, dyspnoea and sometimes wheeze or haemoptysis (see Chapter 85). The severity of the illness probably depends on how many larvae are migrating at one time; the classical self-experiment of Koino illustrated this. He swallowed 2000 viable Ascaris eggs, and within a week suffered a severe illness with high fever, dyspnoea, cyanosis, severe cough and frothy, blood-stained sputum lasting for 7 days. There was eosinophilia, and many Ascaris larvae were recovered from his sputum. It would be unusual for such a large number of eggs to be ingested simultaneously in natural circumstances.

Malaria may be complicated by pulmonary problems; cough is not uncommonly a symptom, even in moderately severe malaria, and in severe *Plasmodium falciparum* malaria pulmonary problems have been reported in 5–15% of cases. Although pulmonary oedema due to therapeutic fluid overload, or bronchopneumonia complicating deep coma, may occur, a more specific malarial lesion indistinguishable from adult respiratory distress syndrome has been recognized in which there is septal oedema, endothelial cell swelling and hyaline membrane formation within the alveoli (see Chapter 73). In children in endemic areas, anaemia and acidosis with resultant tachypnoea are common in severe malaria, but respiratory distress syndrome is rare.

TROPICAL PULMONARY EOSINOPHILIA

In areas where *Wuchereria bancrofti* and *Brugia malayi* are common, patients with cough or wheeze may have tropical pulmonary eosinophilia, in which marked eosinophilia (eosinophil count often >3000 per mm^3) and lung shadows on radiography are supported by a positive filarial antibody test. The condition improves rapidly with antifilarial treatment (see Chapter 83).[21,22] Filariasis is most common in Southern and Eastern Asia, the Pacific and Brazil. The condition is uncommon in Africa, but a similar combination of cough, wheeze and eosinophilia may occur due to the migrating larval stages of *Ascaris*, hookworm, schistosomiasis or *Strongyloides* infection (see Chapter 84).[23]

PLEURAL DISEASES – PNEUMOTHORAX, EFFUSION AND EMPYEMA

Pneumothorax

Primary pneumothorax (air in the pleural space) occurs in the absence of any previous lung pathology and has a good prognosis; secondary pneumothorax occurs on a background of damaged lung (e.g. chronic obstructive pulmonary disease; PcP) and the prognosis is often poor. The immediate management of pneumothorax depends on the size and complications of the pneumothorax. Small primary pneumothoraces can be managed conservatively or with simple aspiration. Large or tension pneumothoraces require urgent aspiration and if this is unsuccessful, a drain must be used. Secondary pneumothoraces are often very slow to respond and may required prolonged drainage for up to several weeks. Prolonged drainage carries a high risk of secondary infection.

Effusion

Pleural effusion (fluid in the pleural space) is most commonly caused by TB in endemic areas. Parapneumonic effusion and malignant effusion (often blood stained) are the important differential. The cause of the effusion must be diagnosed and treatment designed to relieve symptoms while treating the underlying cause. Asymptomatic effusion due to tuberculosis need not be drained.

Empyema

Empyema (infection in the pleural space) is a common complication of pleural effusion and can occur as a primary presentation of TB. Empyema must always be removed either by repeated aspiration, drainage or surgery. Full recovery requires prolonged (6 weeks or more), appropriate antibiotic therapy. Intercostal drainage of empyema can result in super-infection; mixed pleural infections in AIDS patients are difficult to cure and sometimes permanent drainage or fistula is the best that can be achieved.

VASCULAR DISEASES – PULMONARY EMBOLISM AND PULMONARY ARTERIAL HYPERTENSION

Thromboembolic pulmonary embolism

Thromboembolic pulmonary embolism is a potentially life-threatening complication of immobilization and dehydration that can be prevented by anticoagulant prophylaxis. Large thrombi form in deep veins, typically of the pelvis and legs, and embolize to the pulmonary circulation. Large pulmonary emboli present with sudden cardiac collapse and death, and smaller emboli may present with dyspnoea and chest pain. Patients have few signs or present with tachycardia, prominent pulmonary heart sounds or abnormal ECG features. Due to resource constraints, many immobilized in-patients in tropical hospitals do not receive prophylactic heparin or low molecular weight heparin and so thromboembolism is common. This is a particular problem in obstetrics, orthopaedics and among medical patients recovering from dehydrating conditions such as diabetic ketoacidosis.

Pulmonary arterial hypertension

Pulmonary arterial hypertension can be primary or secondary. The most common causes of secondary pulmonary arterial hypertension in tropical hospitals are as a complication of pulmonary thromboemboli and HIV infection. Patients present with shortness of breath and signs of right heart failure but definitive diagnosis and treatment are difficult. Treatment with high dose calcium channel blockers (e.g. amlodipine) or sildenafil (Viagra) may be of benefit.

SARCOIDOSIS

In many tropical countries, sarcoidosis has never been identified. However, in temperate countries, Africans, West Indians and Asians have a much higher incidence of sarcoidosis than do Caucasians living in the same vicinity. Caucasians are also found to have less severe disease, with fewer systemic manifestations, than the other ethnic groups. There is now evidence that sarcoidosis has been under-reported from tropical countries and is often misdiagnosed as TB.[24] The possibility of sarcoidosis should be considered in patients with unresolving lung disease, especially if there are accompanying extrathoracic features such as iridocyclitis, lymphadenopathy, central nervous system complications or hypercalcaemia.

REFERENCES

1. Rasmussen Z, Pio A, Enarson P. Case management of childhood pneumonia in developing countries: recent relevant research and current initiatives. *Int J Tuberc Lung Dis* 2000; 4:807–826.
2. Zar HJ, Hanslo D, Apolles P, et al. Induced sputum versus gastric lavage for microbiological confirmation of pulmonary tuberculosis in infants and young children: a prospective study. *Lancet* 2005; 365:130–134.
3. Berkley JA, Maitland K, Mwangi I, et al. Use of clinical syndromes to target antibiotic prescribing in seriously ill children in malaria endemic area: observational study. *Brit Med J* 2005; 330:995–960.
4. Kabra SK, Lodha R, Pandey RM. Antibiotics for community acquired pneumonia in children. *Cochrane Database Syst Rev* 2006; 3:CD004874.
5. Adegbola RA, Secka O, Lahai G, et al. Elimination of *Haemophilus influenzae* type b (Hib) disease from The Gambia after the introduction of routine immunization with a Hib conjugate vaccine: a prospective study. *Lancet* 2005; 366:144–150.
6. Levine OS, O'Brien KL, Knoll M, et al. Pneumococcal vaccination in developing countries. *Lancet* 2006; 367:1880–1882.

7. Scott JA, Hall AJ, Muyodi C et al. Aetiology, outcome and risk factors for mortality among adults with acute pneumonia in Kenya. *Lancet* 2000; 355:1225–1230.

8. Daley CL. Pulmonary infections in the tropics: impact of HIV infection. *Thorax* 1994; 49:370–378.

9. Graham SM. Non-tuberculosis opportunistic infections and other lung diseases in HIV-infected infants and children. *Int J Tuberc Lung Dis* 2005; 9:592–602.

10. Madhi SA, Petersen K, Madhi A, et al. Increased disease burden and antibiotic resistance of bacteria causing severe community-acquired lower respiratory tract infections in human immunodeficiency type 1-infected children. *Clin Infect Dis* 2000; 31:170–176.

11. Guidelines on co-trimoxazole prophylaxis for HIV-related infections among children, adolescents and adults in resource-limited settings. World Health Organization 2006.

12. Sirisanthana T, Supparatpinyo K. Epidemiology and management of penicilliosis in human immunodeficiency virus-infected patients. *Int J Infect Dis* 1998; 3:48–53.

13. Saubolle MA. Fungal pneumonias. *Semin Respir Infect* 2000; 15:162–177.

14. Beasley R, Crane J, Lai CK, et al. Prevalence and etiology of asthma. *J Allergy Clin Immunol* 2000; 105:S466–S472.

15. Ezzati M, Kammen D. Indoor air pollution from biomass combustion and acute respiratory infections in Kenya: an exposure-response study. *Lancet* 2001; 358:619–624.

16. Bruce N, Perez-Padilla R, Albalak R. Indoor air pollution in developing countries: a major environmental and public health challenge. *Bull World Health Org* 2000; 78:1078–1092.

17. Smith KR. Inaugural article: national burden of disease in India from indoor air pollution. *Proc Natl Acad Sci* USA 2000; 97:13286–13293.

18. Perez-Padilla R, Regalado J, Vedal S, et al. Exposure to biomass smoke and chronic airway disease in Mexican women. A case-control study. *Am J Respir Crit Care Med* 1996 ; 154:701–706.

19. Diaz E, Bruce N, Pope D, et al. Lung function and symptoms among indigenous Mayan women exposed to high levels of indoor air pollution. *Int J Tuberc Lung Dis* 2007; 11:1372–1379.

20. Warren CW, Riley L, Asma S et al. Tobacco use by youth: a surveillance report from the Global Youth Tobacco Survey project. *Bull World Health Org* 2000; 78:868–876.

21. Ong RK, Doyle RL. Tropical pulmonary eosinophilia. *Chest* 1998; 113:1673–1679.

22. Cooray JH, Ismail MM. Re-examination of the diagnostic criteria of tropical pulmonary eosinophilia. *Respir Med* 1999; 93:655–659.

23. Sarinas PS, Chitkara RK. Ascariasis and hookworm. *Semin Respir Infect* 1997; 12:130–137.

24. Jindal SK, Gupta D, Aggarwal AN. Sarcoidosis in developing countries. *Curr Opin Pulm Med* 2000; 6:448–454.

Chapter 12 Felix I. Anjorin

Cardiovascular Disease in the Tropics

Cardiovascular disease is changing continuously in the tropics,[1-4] and so the pattern of disease described in any country describes point prevalence. Cardiovascular disease burden is increasing in Africa, constituting a public health problem throughout the region.[5] In Abidjan and Accra[6] coronary arterial disease now accounts for about 10% of cardiovascular cases, but this is not seen in rural people,[7] and the predictions of the World Health Report of 1993 were made without reliable data. HIV infection now dominates clinical practice in many countries[8] and is responsible for the rise of cases of tuberculous pericarditis.

Some cardiac diseases depend on the local environment and/or its microbes[9]: Chagas' disease in Latin America, schistosomal cor pulmonale in Egypt, Sudan and Brazil,[10] and cor pulmonale in parts of India and Papua New Guinea. The chief diseases are still rheumatic heart disease, dilated cardiomyopathy, hypertension, cardiomyopathy and pericardial tuberculosis associated with HIV, and, with urbanization, coronary arterial disease.

RHEUMATIC HEART DISEASE

This important disease accounts for 12–30% of cardiovascular admissions. It prevails among the poorly housed and is an indicator of their plight.[11-14] Rheumatic fever in poor communities in the tropics differs from the formerly familiar pattern in the industrialized countries:[15] it affects young children;[16] it has different clinical features;[17,18] it affects the heart more commonly both in the first attack and in recurrences; and, on account of weak health services, its secondary prevention is very difficult indeed,[19] and comprehensive programmes are needed to control it.[20] Some come to medical attention for the first time in their thirties and forties, sometimes after giving birth to four children!

Epidemiology

Risk factors are poverty and overcrowded housing in the drier areas of the tropics. This is presumably due to easier transmission and/or acquisition of *Streptococcus pyogenes* in a hot dry climate. WHO has used, as a baseline for further studies,[21] a mean prevalence of 10/1000 for established rheumatic heart disease and an incidence of rheumatic fever of 100/100 000, but methods of study vary greatly.

Criteria for diagnosis

The Duckett Jones criteria have been successively modified because chorea, subcutaneous nodules and erythema marginatum are rare in the tropics: carditis is allowed as the only major manifestation,[22] and arthralgia instead of arthritis. Rheumatic fever[21] follows infection with *Strep. pyogenes*. For every 100 cases of sore throat, 20 are caused by *Strep. pyogenes*. For every 100 of those caused by *Strep. pyogenes*, 20 are symptomatic with fever and cervical lymph nodes. Out of the 20 symptomatic cases, two of rheumatic fever may develop, whereas only one case may develop in the 80 without symptoms, except during an epidemic, when the numbers are increased five times.

Clinical features

Echocardiography is important for confirming a diagnosis and for following the evolution of the disease.[23]

Rheumatic fever

Carditis in a child may present as a low grade fever and a tachycardia and nothing else. Dissociation between the height of the temperature and the tachycardia, and a cardiac murmur – systolic or diastolic – at the apex of the heart may help in diagnosis.

Rheumatic heart disease

Established disease affects (1) the mitral valve alone, which leads to mitral incompetence, the most common lesion; next, mitral stenosis or mixed stenosis and incompetence (2); both mitral and aortic valves; and (3) least commonly, the aortic valve alone (Figure 12.1).

Streptococcal sore throat

A clinical episode may precede some cases of acute rheumatic fever, and it must be recognized in the community if primary prevention is to have any hope of success. The distinction between a streptococcal and a viral infection may be difficult (Table 12.1).

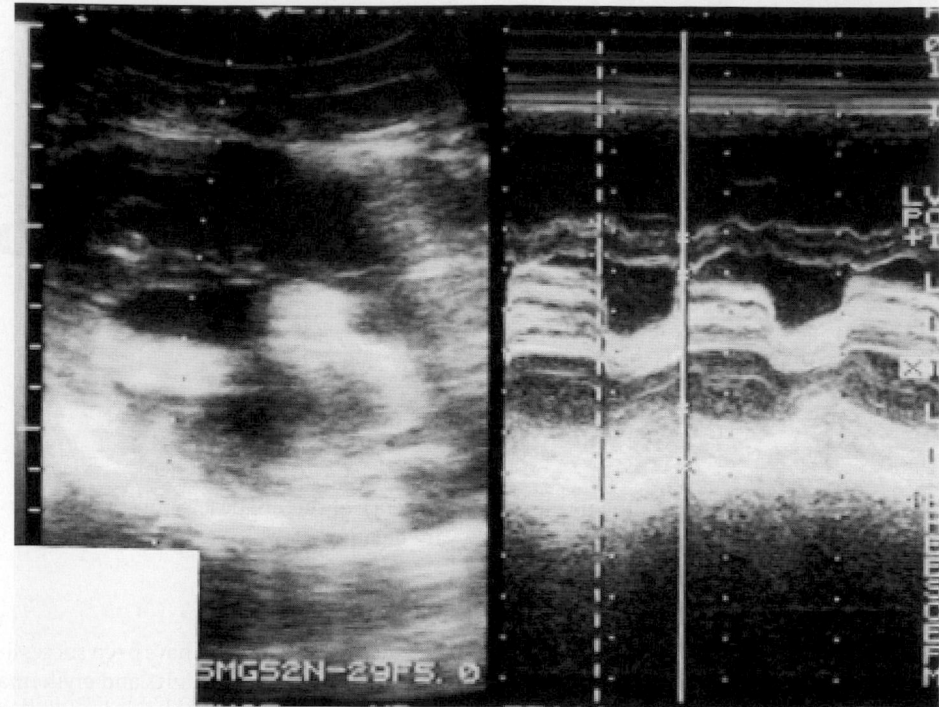

Figure 12.1 Echocardiogram of a 39-year-old Nigerian man showing mitral valve (MV) stenosis with dense calcification. He subsequently underwent a successful mitral valve replacement.

Table 12.1 Comparison of streptococcal and viral sore throat

Feature	Streptococcal	Viral
Onset	Abrupt	Gradual
Throat	Painful	Uncomfortable
Cervical nodes	Enlarged, tender	Not enlarged
Eyes and nose	Not affected	Watery eyes, runny nose
Throat/tonsils	Red, swollen, exudate	Red, vesicles, ulcers

Prevention

The fundamental aims are as follows:
1. *Environment:* to improve homes and housing, food and health-care.
2. *Primary prevention:* to detect and treat symptomatic *Strep. pyogenes* sore throat – with either benzathine penicillin 1.2 megaunits, penicillin V for 10 days, or benzyl penicillin.
3. *Secondary prophylaxis:* to prevent streptococcal infection, with benzathine penicillin every 3 weeks, in those with known rheumatic heart disease,[20] through dedicated community nurses.

Management

Acute rheumatic fever

Eradicate *Strep. pyogenes* with benzyl penicillin and establish maintenance prophylaxis with benzathine penicillin. Manage cardiac failure with bed-rest for acute carditis and give aspirin or cortico-

steroids, for as long as there is evidence of carditis, provided there is no evidence of cardiac failure.[10]

Chronic rheumatic heart disease

Maintain penicillin prophylaxis to prevent recurrences (and infective endocarditis), and give standard treatment for valvular disease, disorders of rhythm or cardiac failure.

DILATED CARDIOMYOPATHY

In some tropical countries, patients who have a dilated heart, without any identifiable cause, account for about 20% of cardiovascular cases.[24]

Pathogenesis

There are many possible factors and this is, at best, a syndrome. Men are affected more than women, predominantly in the age group 40–49 years.

Poverty and social class

The condition is much more common in patients of low social class in West Africa than is found with other types of heart disease.[25]

Anaemia

While severe anaemia may be associated with cardiac failure it does not appear to be a causal factor in dilated cardiomyopathy in the tropics.

Toxins

These are often suggested but rarely incriminated.

Alcohol

Alcohol, often a strong traditional brew, is an important cause of dilated cardiomyopathy in many areas of the tropics.

Nutrition and micronutrients

There is no evidence for a direct nutritional cause of dilated cardiomyopathy in the tropics, except the rare cases of beriberi, and micronutrient deficiency (e.g. selenium) has not yet been proved. The wasting associated with HIV infection is associated with a loss of left ventricular mass and of diastolic function.[26]

Myocarditis

A previous viral myocarditis may prove to be more significant than is currently appreciated.

Hypertension

There is evidence that some patients may be former hypertensives: the age groups of those with hypertensive cardiac failure and dilated cardiomyopathy are similar; the aortic arch diameter in all cases of dilated cardiomyopathy is intermediate between that of hypertensive and normal individuals; in some cases the blood pressure rises to abnormal levels as cardiac failure responds to treatment; and in East Africa formerly-proved hypertensives presented years later with dilated cardiomyopathy but with normal blood pressures.

Clinical features

Most patients have symptoms of pulmonary and/or systemic oedema for up to 2 years and thus often present with pulmonary oedema or dependent oedema, ascites and a large liver, a large left ventricle and signs of atrioventricular valvular incompetence. Some patients present with systemic embolization, for example a 'cerebrovascular accident', from an intracavitary left ventricular thrombus.

Diagnosis

In a man with normal arterial pressure and no evidence of valvular disease the diagnosis is not difficult, but if there is raised arterial pressure, retinal arterial changes and a left ventricle which is thickened but dilated, the distinction from hypertensive cardiac failure may be difficult. Similarly, mitral incompetence in a younger patient may indicate rheumatic heart disease or even endomyocardial fibrosis, but the mitral valvular incompetence in cardiomyopathy may be reversed by treatment of the cardiac failure.

Management and prognosis

Management depends on the resources and drugs available. In district hospitals, diuretics, with digoxin when there is an atrial arrhythmia, are essential. Other forms of treatment with ACE inhibitors and angiotensin receptor blockers are available at specialist hospitals. The prognosis[27] depends on the function of the left ventricle:[19] those who do worst have a high left ventricular end-diastolic pressure, end-systolic volume and end-diastolic volume with a reduced ejection fraction. If alcohol is incriminated as a causative factor then somehow the patient has to stop drinking it.

PERIPARTUM CARDIAC FAILURE (PPCF)

The definition of PPCF varies but only in the time interval related to delivery. In Nigeria, the following definition has been used: 'cardiac failure, with symptoms beginning in pregnancy or up to 6 months postpartum – of up to 6 months duration, with no history of cardiac failure other than PPCF itself, and with no discernible cause for cardiac failure other than anaemia or hypertension, presumed to be acute'.[28]

Distribution

The syndrome has been reported from tropical Latin America,[29] the Caribbean, East, West[28,30–32] and South Africa,[33] India, China and Korea. Occasional cases are also seen in temperate countries and some important series of cases have been reported in the USA,[34] almost exclusively among black women.

Factors in the pathogenesis

This syndrome may conceal a number of conditions: some cases resemble dilated cardiomyopathy and therefore its possible causes have to be considered in PPCF.

Race

The largest reported series have been in West Africans and black Americans. The syndrome is apparently also common in Korea, and cases are reported in all races.

Parity

PPCF is more common in multiparous women, and this appears to be independent of age, although increasing age is itself a risk factor.

Twin births

Data are few but the risk has been reported to be two-fold in a twin pregnancy.

Blood pressure

The question therefore arises as to whether PPCF patients are a potentially hypertensive cohort and whether PPCF is a form of hypertensive heart failure, as suggested in southern Nigeria, or can the hypertension in some cases be explained by some other mechanism? There is persuasive evidence from northern Nigeria that this is indeed the case in some patients. Some women develop hypertension soon after treatment for their cardiac failure and, although the numbers were small, more Nigerian PPCF women had hypertensive immediate family members than controls. Similarly, a highly significant number took extra salt compared with controls and so there may be a genetically determined disorder of salt taste resulting in excess salt intake. The group probably represents a salt-sensitive subset with resultant actual or potential hypertension, masquerading as PPCF but revealed as hypertension later in life.

Infection

There is a rapidly advancing myocarditis, possibly viral, in some non tropical cases, confirmed by endomyocardial biopsy in over 50% of such cases, but its mechanism is not known.[31,35]

The northern Nigerian PPCF syndrome

Cultural practices

After delivery, the Hausa women around Zaria traditionally take *kanwa*, a rock salt rich in sodium and potassium, in order to promote the flow of breast milk. They also lie on a heated bed for at least 40 days postpartum and take 'hot baths' twice daily to prevent themselves from becoming diseased from cold.

Seasonal variation

The peak of admissions follows about 2 months after the hottest humid season.

The Nigerian syndrome – a possible mechanism

The factors are postpartum state, hot season and hot beds and baths, and ingestion of sodium-rich rock salt. The heat causes vasodilatation so that the cardiac output rises in order to maintain flow and arterial pressure, but the excessive sodium load demands a high renal arterial pressure for its excretion. This can only be at best partially achieved by a further rise of cardiac output and blood pressure.[32] Oedema therefore develops and the cycle is set for it to increase daily. The syndrome is thus established with a high output state and vasodilatation, oedema, and systemic and pulmonary venous congestion. Physiologically, it is not true cardiac failure because the stroke volume can rise in response to a rise in filling pressure. This group responds rapidly with a massive diuresis, but it does not include a smaller number whose heart is dilated and who do not respond with a diuresis.

Clinical picture

Symptoms of pulmonary and/or systemic venous congestion develop, often with massive swelling of body and face. The blood pressure is often raised when the patient is first seen, but falls within a few days during diuretic treatment. Systemic and pulmonary emboli are seen when the heart is very large. Imaging shows a dilated heart, pulmonary venous congestion and oedema.

Disordered physiology

There is no homogeneous pattern of cardiac function. Most Brazilian patients showed a raised ventricular filling pressure with low cardiac output but a subset, similar to the Nigerian group, had high output 'failure'.[29] Volume overload was thought to be respon-

sible: this hypervolaemia, when cured by diuretics, can leave a normal heart.[36] Some cases, however, have irreversible cardiac damage.

Evolution and treatment

The prognosis of this syndrome varies with its pathogenesis, from the rapidly progressive myocarditis for which cardiac transplantation may be needed, to a syndrome of oedema and uncomplicated cardiomegaly which resolves very quickly with treatment by diuretics. Bad signs are an arrhythmia, persistent hypertension, cardiomegaly, or systemic or pulmonary emboli.[37] There is no reason to take the baby off the breast, and as soon as the mother has had a major diuresis she can be treated at home.

Subsequent pregnancies

The syndrome may recur,[9,37] but if the heart returns to normal after the first episode,[25] there is no reason to advise against subsequent pregnancy.

HYPERTENSION AND HYPERTENSIVE HEART DISEASE

Most people in the tropics with high blood pressure (defined by the WHO criteria) do not know that they are hypertensive, and even if they were aware and sought treatment, in many countries the public budget can not possibly stretch to supply the ideal combination of antihypertension drugs.

Blood pressure in rural and urban societies

Rural societies in the tropics have a very low prevalence of hypertension and only a modest rise in blood pressure throughout adult life. In urban settings the prevalence is high and rises with advancing age.[38,39] Rural–urban migration is associated with increase in the prevalence of hypertension; increase in body mass index and waist–hip ratio are also associated with increased prevalence. So also is high sodium intake,[40] often coupled with low potassium intake.[41–44] Some individuals who traditionally take a low salt diet have been found to be sensitive to an increase in salt intake with attendant development of hypertension.[45]

Race

Different origins apparently govern both the prevalence and pattern of hypertension.[41,42] In any society, those of black African origin are most susceptible and, as discussed below, they are vulnerable to stroke; low renin hypertension is also more common.

Sequelae of hypertension

Stroke is a common complication of hypertension, especially in previously undiagnosed patients or in those who default from treatment.[46] In one study, over 27 years, stroke mortality was 11.4% in hypertensives but only 1.8% in normotensives. Adequate control of hypertension considerably reduces the risk of stroke but does not completely eliminate it. Control of diabetes mellitus, dyslipidaemias, regular, judicious physical exercise and avoidance/cessation of smoking are all also important in stroke prevention.

Hypertensive cardiac disease and failure[47] has already been discussed in relation to dilated cardiomyopathy. In some cases of hypertensive heart disease, left ventricular hypertrophy is asymmetrical. It accounts for 20–35% of cases of cardiovascular admissions in many tropical countries.

Malignant hypertension is well recognized and renal failure with severe hypertension is also often seen, but without a definite diagnosis of the underlying renal disease. The cause for this remains conjectural.[48] Retinopathy occurs in hypertension, as it does in northern countries.

Coronary arterial events are much more common in Asian hypertensives than among those of black African origin.

The problem of management

As life expectancy increases, there are inevitably more untreated and later disabled victims of hypertension. Severe hypertension may be detected if there is an efficient primary healthcare service, but few tropical countries can afford to treat hypertension in all those who need drugs. This problem is compounded because angiotensin-converting enzyme (ACE) inhibitors are less efficacious in black people than they are in white people.

For the individual who needs drugs it is essential both to establish that drug supply can be sustained indefinitely and to ensure that treatment will be followed.[49] The drug regimen will depend on national drug policy, the essential drug list, and thus what drugs are available at each level of healthcare. Follow-up with good records can be handled by a well-trained medical assistant or nurse, who has defined criteria for referral if there is an unexpected change.

ENDOMYOCARDIAL FIBROSIS

EMF has distinctive clinical and pathological features[50,51] and a novel pathogenesis,[52] but even in specialist centres in endemic areas it comprises only about 1–5% of cases. Nevertheless, in some parts of the hot and humid tropics, e.g. Kerala, Malaysia, West and Central Africa and Brazil,[53] EMF is seen much more commonly than in other areas.

What is EMF?

Endocardial thickening of the ventricle leads to cardiac constriction or restriction and atrioventricular valvular incompetence, leading to regurgitation.[50,51,53,54] In the left ventricle, dense fibrous tissue at the apex spreads around the cavity of the ventricle or may first appear around the papillary muscle of the posterior cusp of the mitral valve. This muscle is anchored so that the valve becomes incompetent. The right ventricular cavity is obliterated from below by the advancing fibrosis of layered mural thrombi. In late cases the papillary muscles are lost in a bed of fibrous tissue, the tricuspid valve becomes functionless and the right atrium becomes aneurysmal. The left, right, or both ventricles can be affected. Chronic pericardial effusion can complicate right ventricular EMF; a pleural effusion is more common with left or bi-ventricular disease.

The anatomical changes explain physiological dysfunction and the physical signs in established disease. Dense avascular fibrous tissue, often sharply defined from or 'dipping into' the myocardium, is characteristic of established disease. In acute disease, however, the pericardium, myocardium and endocardium show active inflammation with lymphocytes, eosinophils which may be degranulated,[52] and many small blood vessels packed with cells. In addition, irregularly scattered throughout the myocardium, and often unrelated to overlying endocardial change, there are foci where myocardial fibres are disappearing and fibroblasts are evident.

Pathogenesis

The term eosinophilic endomyocardial disease has been suggested to replace endomyocardial fibrosis because the cardiac changes are explained in terms of the eosinophil and its constituents.[55] Thus EMF has changes similar to those found in the heart in patients with hypereosinophilic syndromes.[56] The critical questions are: what is the trigger for an eosinophilia in EMF,[18] and is it found consistently? Eosinophilia is not consistent, but that could be because the disease is often not present until its pathogenetic process is burnt out. Early reports from West Africa linked filariasis with EMF, and particularly *Loa loa*, or any other helminth which provokes an eosinophilia.[56] A clear initial illness[54,57] has been described, when there may be a significant eosinophilia.

The suggested sequence is as follows: a trigger to eosinophilia (helminthic or other infection) leads to hypereosinophilia and liberation of eosinophilic major basic proteins and cationic protein which are toxic to a wide range of cells, including endocardial and myocardial cells. The damaged endocardium serves as a focus for mural thrombi, which are themselves promoted by the release of platelet activation factor(s) from the eosinophils. Further mural thrombi are then laid down at the original and adjacent sites, and a fibrotic mass, sometimes calcified,[58] results. This is a logical and clear sequence following hypereosinophilia but the difficulty lies in reconciling it with all the data, particularly from Uganda, where for example the prevalence of EMF differed between immigrant Rwanda and native Baganda, in a ratio of about 4–5 : 1, whereas rheumatic heart disease was just the reverse.[59] Similarly, in kindred with the tropical splenomegaly syndrome, EMF was apparently more prevalent.[60] Causes of eosinophilia are abundant in the tropics but EMF is not. Additionally, it appears to be much less prevalent in dry grassland areas – but why? On the whole, available evidence suggests that hypereosinophilia in a hot and humid environment promotes features leading to the development of endomyocardial fibrosis. The role of trace elements is not yet established.[61]

Clinical features

These depend on the stage of the disease and the anatomical distortion of the affected ventricle(s), together with the resultant effects on cardiac function.

Initial illness

Some patients have a febrile illness with facial swelling, and symptoms of pulmonary venous congestion. This can be fatal within months, but little is known about this phase of the disease.[57]

Left ventricular disease

The ventricle is not enlarged and there are inevitably, in almost every case, signs of mitral valvular incompetence with a loud pulmonary closure sound, and progressive pulmonary hypertension. A third heart sound is usually early and crisp, and is dominant when the physiological pattern is a restricted ventricle.

Right ventricular disease

The classical picture, described from Ibadan,[54] is of a young patient, often with delayed puberty, slight exophthalmos, central cyanosis, no peripheral oedema and massive ascites. Many cases of established right ventricular EMF are at first missed because the ascites is so dominant and the jugular pressure so high that it is missed clinically. The jugular systolic wave, secondary to tricuspid regurgitation, may even move the ear lobe. The arterial pulse has a small pulse pressure and atrial fibrillation is common. The heart may be impalpable either because there is a large pericardial effusion or because it is rotated by the massive right atrium, which lies under the sternum, so that the left ventricle lies more posteriorly. There may be no murmur at the defunct tricuspid valve but only an abrupt third heart sound.

Investigations

The stage and site of disease determine findings on the chest radiograph; these vary from a massive cardiac shadow (aneurysmal right atrium or pericardial effusion) (Figure 12.2) to an almost normal heart with perhaps a prominent pulmonary artery. Echocardiography[62] is valuable, as it shows distinctive patterns.

Management

Established disease

Cardiac surgery[27] is economically adventurous, but it is clinically logical in deforming inactive disease.

The acute illness

Treatment aims to maintain cardiac function and possibly suppress the eosinophilia with corticosteroids.

PERICARDIAL DISEASE

In the tropics, the two important forms of pericarditis are both secondary to a major infection: (1) acute pyogenic pericarditis; and (2) tuberculous pericarditis, which has been catapulted into prominence by HIV. Rarely, pericarditis complicates amoebic liver abscess.

Pyogenic pericarditis

The pericardium is affected in a bacteraemia associated with a pyogenic infection, for example pyomyositis, lobar pneumonia or pelvic infection, when local and systemic signs are dominant and pericarditis may not be recognized until it causes circulatory effects.

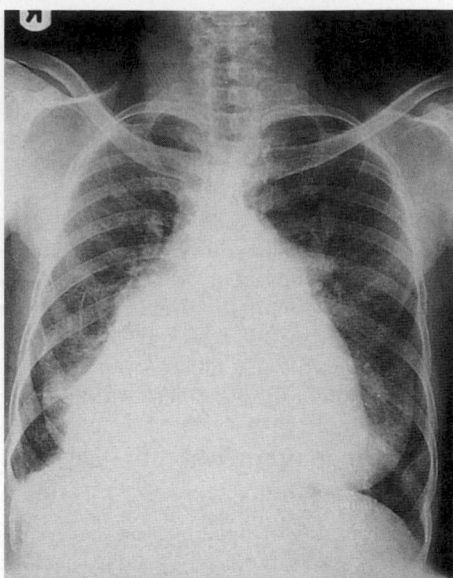

Figure 12.2 Biventricular endomyocardial fibrosis: the cardiac shadow is totally distorted with the enlarged right atrium prominent.

Clinical features

These depend on whether or not there is a pericardial effusion and the speed at which this has formed. If the fluid forms quickly, the parietal pericardium cannot stretch adequately to accommodate it and symptoms and signs of cardiac tamponade develop. The heart is compressed and the signs therefore depend on obstruction to venous inflow and a subsequent fall in stroke output, cardiac tamponade. There may be evidence of pericarditis – a pericardial rub or signs of fluid, dullness to percussion at the right border of the sternum, an impalpable cardiac impulse and very quiet heart sounds.

Management

In an uncomplicated effusion, in a district hospital without echocardiography, a chest radiograph may reveal a large cardiac shadow but this may be difficult to interpret if there is lobar pneumonia or a pleural effusion (Figure 12.3). Purulent pericardial fluid confirms the diagnosis; it should be aspirated totally by the epigastric approach, with the patient sitting up in bed. Use a 50 mL or 20 mL syringe with a long needle fitted with a two-way tap so that fluid can easily be expelled. Aspirate daily, but be prepared to transfer the patient to a cardiac surgical unit if there are persistent signs of fluid or cardiac compression. Early diagnosis with aspiration and instillation of the appropriate antibiotic into the pericardial sac may prevent this.

In pericardial effusion with cardiac tamponade the fluid must be aspirated immediately and completely.

Tuberculous pericarditis

This is now a major problem in patients with HIV infection. Before the HIV epidemic an unusually high prevalence was described

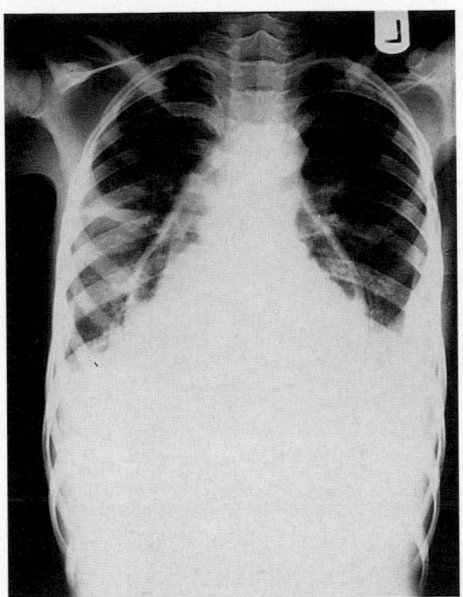

Figure 12.3 Pyogenic pericarditis. Note the thickness of pericardium and the associated pleural effusion and pulmonary changes.

in Transkei.[22] *Mycobacterium tuberculosis* reaches the pericardium from adjacent lymph nodes or possibly pleura.

Clinical picture

This depends on the stage of the disease. Many patients present late and are thought to have liver disease because they are wasted and have tense ascites, or because the jugular venous pressure is not examined, or is very high. Those who have HIV/AIDS often show evidence of early pericardial infection, with a pericardial rub and some precordial pain.[8] Most patients have a pericardial effusion which may be large or small, with underlying pericardial fibrosis. This is constrictive pericarditis with its distinctive signs: a small arterial pulse pressure, sometimes with pulsus paradoxus, and a venous pulse which has a high pressure and can be seen to fall sharply immediately after carotid pulsation (*y* descent): the heart may be impalpable and, when constriction is established, a third heart sound is audible.

Diagnosis

In patients with HIV/AIDS, signs of pericarditis must be assumed to be caused by tuberculosis. Aspiration of pericardial fluid is helpful: the fluid has a high protein content around 40 g/L and in about 80% of cases it is bloodstained; the cells are lymphocytes. There is no characteristic chest radiograph: this depends on the volume of pericardial fluid, the presence of a pleural effusion, and whether the pericardium has calcified or not (Figure 12.4).

Treatment

Give antituberculosis drugs with corticosteroids. Strang et al. showed that steroids prevent constriction.[63,64] The currently recommended initial dose is prednisolone 2 mg/kg. The course of steroids is 11 weeks. This makes patients rapidly better, constriction is prevented, and pericardial fluid disappears.

Other infections

Viruses

There is nothing distinctive about viral pericarditis in the tropics.

Meningococcus

Signs of pericarditis may be detected in patients with meningococcal disease who have bacteraemia and antigenaemia. Immune complexes are formed and are deposited on the pericardium. The pericarditis is transient and the prognosis is dominated by the severity of infection.

Parasites

Rarely trophozoites of *Entamoeba histolytica* reach the pericardium from an adjacent liver abscess. The prognosis is bad. Pericardial tamponade demands urgent aspiration. Metronidazole and chloroquine orally, and metronidazole injected into the pericardial sac, have been advocated for treatment.

ARTERIAL DISEASE

Aorta and large arteries

Idiopathic 'tropical' aortitis is more common in the tropics, particularly in Asian countries: Malaysia, Thailand, Singapore, Korea, China and India,[65] where some cases are named Takayasu's disease. It has been described in many African countries, with notable studies in South Africa.[66] Whether the disease in Asia is the same as that seen in African countries, is not known. The questions are: what are the triggers for the disease?

The clinical features are determined by the pathological/anatomical damage to the aorta and its large branches, so that regional ischaemia in a tissue or organ is the most common clinical presentation. Imaging shows aneurysmally dilated or stenosed segments of aorta with an irregular lumen so that the orifices of any of its branches may be occluded.

The disease affects the abdominal aorta in over 90% of cases, the subclavian arteries in over 60%, and renal arteries in over 80%.

Pathogenesis

The cause of the arteritis is not known. There is a systemic inflammatory phase in some patients, and the morphological changes are those of a giant-cell arteritis. Therefore, while an immune mechanism has been suggested (an associated glomerulonephritis in some patients may be suggestive evidence), there are no consistent markers of an immune reaction. HLA-B5 has been linked to both Takayasu's disease and HLA-DRB1 in Buerger's disease.

Clinical features

The symptoms depend on the artery affected. Most patients are young adults; in some series women predominate. About one-third have hypertension, and another third have visual symptoms.

157

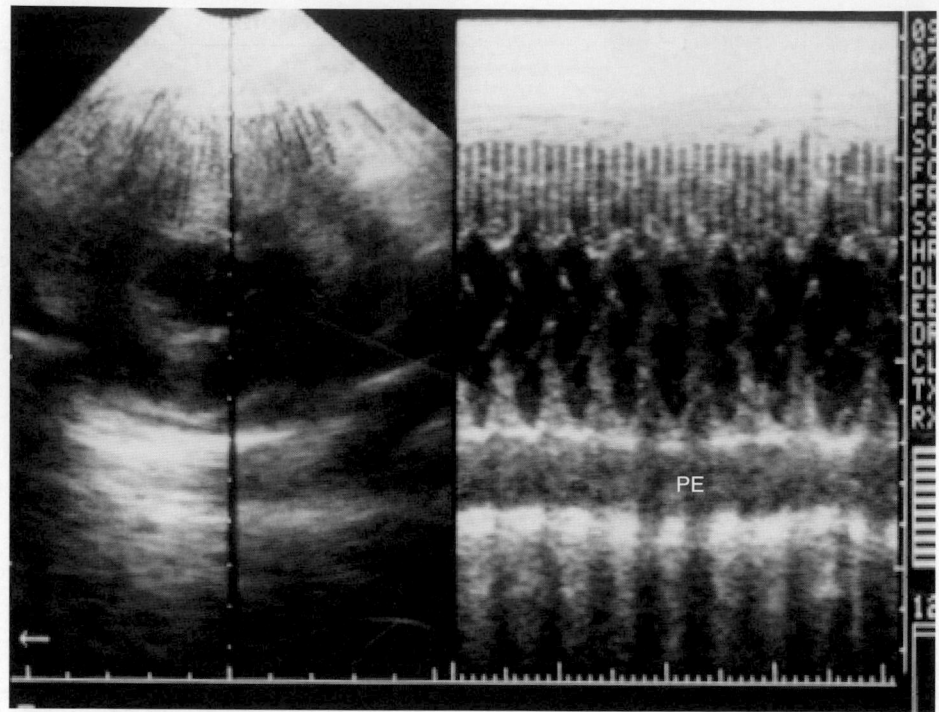

Figure 12.4 Echocardiogram of a 37-year-old Nigerian woman showing a large pericardial effusion (PE) due to tuberculous pericarditis. She had an effusive, constrictive pericarditis; there was a good response to antituberculosis therapy and pericardiectomy.

Physical signs depend on the vessel affected; for example, a renal arterial bruit.

Management

The arteritis is widespread and treatment is unlikely to help, but in advanced hospitals angioplasty or an arterial bypass can be advised for limited disease; for example, renal arterial disease with severe hypertension.

Coronary arterial disease

The remarkable differences in the prevalence of coronary artery diseases between different countries in the tropics have led to many comparative studies. Similarly, the pattern of disease is changing as countries become industrialized and where habits and diet are changing.[5]

Clinically, coronary arterial disease causes the same symptoms, whether in tropical or temperate countries. Cardiac pain on effort, however, in a patient who is at low risk – a young adult from a rural African community – may cause a problem with diagnosis. Severe anaemia from untreated heavy hookworm infection can lead to a qualitative defect in coronary arterial flow in spite of a greatly increased cardiac output. In a patient who is not anaemic the orifices of the coronary arteries or their lumens may be occluded (e.g. by sickled erythrocytes in homozygous HbSS disease) or stenosed. Tropical or syphilitic aortitis may involve the orifice(s); the lumen may be occluded by emboli in rheumatic cardiac disease or dilated cardiomyopathy with a left ventricular mural or cavitary thrombus. A rare curiosity which may distort a coronary artery is annular subvalvular aneurysm of the left ventricle.[67] Described in a number of tropical countries, a pouch forms and enlarges so that it may stretch the circumflex branch of the left coronary artery, appear as a rounded shadow on the left ventricle in a chest radiograph, or grow into the septum. Mural thrombi form and may partially fill the aneurysm and lead to systemic emboli.

Left ventricular cavitary thrombus

Originally described at autopsy in Senegal in patients with dilated cardiomyopathy, these thrombi are now being detected by echocardiography in similar cases in West Africa and in patients with peripartum cardiac failure. In some, thrombolytic therapy has been remarkably effective.[68]

REFERENCES

1. Astagneau P, Lang T, Delarocque E, et al. Arterial hypertension in urban Africa: An epidemiological study on a representative sample of Dakar inhabitants in Senegal. *J Hypertens* 1992; 10:1095–1101.
2. Hakim JG, Manyemba J. Cardiac disease distribution among patients referred for echocardiography in Harare, Zimbabwe. *Cent Afr J Med* 1998; 44:140–144.
3. Lodenyo HA, McLigeyo SO, Ogola EN. Cardiovascular disease in elderly in-patients at the Kenyatta National Hospital, Nairobi, Kenya. *E Afr Med J* 1997; 74:647–651.
4. Stephen SJ. Changing patterns of mitral stenosis in childhood and pregnancy in Sri Lanka. *J Am Coll Cardiol* 1992; 19:1276–1284.

5. WHO Regional Director. Cardiovascular disease in the African region: current situation and perspectives. *WHO Executive summary of Regional Committee for Africa.* AFR/RC55/12. 2005.

6. Amoah GB, Kallen C. Aetiology of heart failure as seen from a national cardiac referral centre in Africa. *Cardiology* 2000; 93:11–18.

7. Swai AB, McLarty DG, Kitange HM, et al. Low prevalence of risk factors for coronary heart disease in rural Tanzania. *Int J Epidemiol* 1993; 22: 651–659.

8. Silva-Cardoso J, Moura B, Martins L, et al. Pericardial involvement in human immunodeficiency virus infection. *Chest* 1999; 18:415–422.

9. Adoh A, Kouassi-Yapo F, N'Dori R, et al. Etiologie des arteriopathies des membres inferieurs chez les Noirs Africains à Abidjan. *Cardiol Trop* 1991; 17:59–65.

10. Barbosa MM, Lamounier JA, Oliveira EC, et al. Pulmonary hypertension in Schistosomiasis mansoni. *Trans R Soc Trop Med Hyg* 1996; 90: 663–665.

11. Carapetris JR, Wolf DR, Currie BJ. Acute rheumatic fever and rheumatic heart disease in Top End of Australia's Northern Territory. *Med J Aust* 1996; 164:146–149.

12. Ibrahim Khalil S, Elhaq M, Ali E, et al. An epidemiological survey of rheumatic fever and rheumatic heart disease in Sahafa Town, Sudan. *J Epidemiol Community Health* 1992; 46:477–479.

13. Ilyas M, Peracha MA, Ahmed R, et al. Prevalence and pattern of rheumatic heart disease in the frontier province of Pakistan. *JPMA* 1997; 29:165–198.

14. Quinn RW. Comprehensive review of morbidity and mortality trends for rheumatic fever, streptococcal disease, and scarlet fever: the decline of rheumatic fever. *Rev Infect Dis* 1989; 11:928–953.

15. Majeed HA, Batnager S, Yousof AM, et al. Acute rheumatic fever and the evolution of rheumatic heart disease: a prospective 12 year follow-up report. *J Clin Epidemiol* 1992; 45:871–875.

16. Chauvet J, Kakou Guikahue M, Aka F, et al. La gravite des cardites rheumatismales à Abidjan. A propos de 52 cas à Abidjan chez les enfants de moins de 15 ans. *Cardiol Trop* 1989; 15:77–81.

17. Serme D. Etude epidemiologique, clinique et evolutive de valvulopathies rheumatismales observees a Ouagadougou. *Cardiol Trop* 1992; 18:93–99.

18. Rutakinggirwa M, Ziegler JL, Newton R, et al. Poverty and eosinophilia are risk factors for endomyocardial fibrosis in Uganda. *Trop Med Int Health* 1999; 4:229–235.

19. Edington ME, Gear JSS. Rheumatic heart disease in Soweto: a programme for secondary prevention. *S Afr Med J* 1982; 62:523–525.

20. Bach JF, Chalons S, Forier E, et al. 10-year educational programme aimed at rheumatic fever in two French Caribbean islands. *Lancet* 1996; 347:644–648.

21. Stollerman GH. Rheumatic fever. *Lancet* 1997; 349:935–942.

22. Strang JIG. Tuberculous pericarditis in Transkei. *Clin Cardiol* 1984; 7: 667–670.

23. Sagie A, Frietas N, Padial LR, et al. Doppler echocardiographic assessment of long term progression of mitral stenosis in 103 patients: valve area and right heart disease. *J Am Coll Cardiol* 1996; 28:472–479.

24. Malu K, Ticolat R, Renambot I, et al. Enquête épidémiologique sur les myocardopathies chroniques dilatées apparemment primitives: 69 cas. *Cardiol Trop* 1991; 17:127–132.

25. Sutton M St J, Cole P, Plappert M. Effects of subsequent pregnancy on left ventricular function in peripartum cardiomyopathy. *Am Heart J* 1991; 121:1776–1778.

26. Matinez-Garcia T, Sobrino JM, Pujol E, et al. Ventricular mass and diastolic function in patients infected by the human immunodeficiency virus. *Heart* 2000; 84:620–624.

27. Moraes F, Lapa C, Hazin S, et al. Surgery for endomyocardial fibrosis revisited. *Eur J Cardiothorac Surg* 1999; 15:309–312.

28. Davidson NM, Parry EH. Peri-partum cardiac failure. *Q J Med* 1978; 47: 431–461.

29. Marin-Neto JA, Maciel BC, Teran Urbenetz LL, et al. High output failure in patients with peripartum cardiomyopathy: a comparative study with dilated cardiomyopathy. *Am Heart J* 1991; 121:134–140.

30. Cenac A, Djibo A. Postpartum cardiac failure in Sudanese-Sahelian Africa: clinical prevalence in Western Niger. *Am J Trop Med Hyg* 1998; 58:319–323.

31. Sanderson JE, Olsenb EGJ, Gatei D. Peripartum heart disease: an endomyocardial biopsy study. *Br Heart J* 1986; 56:285–291.

32. Sanderson JE, Adesanya CO, Anjorin FI, et al. Postpartum cardiac failure – heart failure due to volume overload? *Am Heart J* 1979; 97: 613–621.

33. Desai D, Moodley J, Naidoo D. Peripartum cardiomyopathy: experiences at King Edward VIII Hospital, Durban, South Africa and a review of the literature. *Trop Doct* 1995; 25:118–123.

34. Homans DC. Current concepts: peripartum cardiomyopathy. *N Engl J Med* 1985; 312:1432–1437.

35. Midel MG, De Ment SH, Feldman AM, et al. Peripartum myocarditis and cardiomyopathy. *Circulation* 1990; 81:922–926.

36. Albanese Filho FM, da Silva TT. Natural course of subsequent pregnancy after peripartum cardiomyopathy. *Arq Bras Cardiol* 1999; 73:47–57.

37. Ford L, Abdullahi A, Anjorin FI, et al. The outcome of peripartum cardiac failure in Zaria, Nigeria. *Q J Med* 1998; 91:93–103.

38. Edwards R, Unwin N, Mugusi F, et al. Hypertension prevalence and care in an urban and rural area of Tanzania. *J Hypertens* 2000; 18:145–152.

39. Poulter NR, Khaw KT, Hopwood BEC, et al. The Kenya Luo migration study: observations of initiation of a rise in blood pressure. *BMJ* 1990; 309:967–972.

40. Olubodun JO, Akingbade OA, Abiola OO. Salt intake and blood pressure in Nigeria hypertensive patients. *Int J Cardiol* 1997; 59:185–188.

41. Cooper RS, Rotimi CN, Atman SL, et al. The prevalence of hypertension in seven populations of West African origin. *Am J Public Health* 1997; 87: 160–168.

42. Cooper RS, Rotimi CN, Kaufman JS, et al. Hypertension treatment and control in sub-Saharan Africa: the epidemiological basis for policy. *BMJ* 1998; 316:614–617.

43. James SA, de Almeida-Filho N, Kaufman JS. Hypertension in Brazil: a review of the epidemiological evidence. *Ethn Dis* 1991; 1:91–98.

44. Kaufman JS, Rotimi CN, Brieger WR, et al. The mortality risk associated with hypertension: preliminary results of a prospective study in rural Nigeria. *J Hum Hypertens* 1996; 10:461–464.

45. Mtabaji JP, Nara Y, Yamori Y. The cardiac study in Tanzania: salt intake in the causation and treatment of hypertension. *J Hum Hypertens* 1990; 4:80–81.

46. Walker RW, Mclarty DG, Kitange HM, et al. Stroke mortality in urban and rural Tanzania. *Lancet* 2000; 355:1684–1687.

47. Falase AO, Ayeni O, Sekoni GA, et al. Heart failure in Nigerian hypertensives. *Afr J Med Sci* 1983; 12:7–15.

48. Plange-Rhule J, Philips R, Achampong J, et al. Hypertension and renal failure in Kumasi, Ghana. *J Hum Hypertens* 1999; 13:37–40.

49. Maro EE, Lwakatare J. Medication compliance among Tanzanian Hypertensives. *E Afr Med J* 1997; 74:539–542.

50. Connor DH, Somers K, Hutt MSR, et al. Endomyocardial fibrosis in Uganda (Davies' disease). *Am Heart J* 1968; 75:107–124.

51. Connor DH, Somers K, Hutt MSR, et al. Endomyocardial fibrosis in Uganda (Davies' disease). *Am Heart J* 1967; 74:687–700.

52. Po-chun Tai, Spry CJF, Olsen EGJ, et al. Deposits of eosinophil granule proteins in cardiac tissues of patients with endomyocardial fibrosis. *Lancet* 1987; i:643–647.

53. Guimaraes AC, Esteves JP, Filho AS, et al. Clinical aspects of endomyocardial fibrosis in Bahia, Brazil. *Am Heart J* 1971; 81:7–19.

54. Parry E, Abrahams DG. The natural history of endomyocardial fibrosis. *Q J Med* 1965; 34:383–408.

55. Spry CJF. Eosinophil in eosinophilic endomyocardial disease. *Postgrad Med J* 1987; 62:609–613.

56. Andy JJ, Ogunowo PO, Akpan NA, et al. Helminth associated hypereosinophilia and tropical endomyocardial fibrosis (EMF) in Nigeria. *Acta Trop* 1998; 69:127–140.

57. Andy JJ, Bishara FF. Observations on clinical features of early disease of African endomyocardial fibrosis. *Cardiol Trop* 1982; 8:23–33.

58. Canesin MF, Gama RF, Smith DL, et al. Endomyocardial fibrosis associated with massive calcification of the left ventricle. *Arq Bras Cardiol* 1999; 73: 499–506.

59. Shaper AG, Coles RM. The tribal distribution of endomyocardial fibrosis in Uganda. *Br Heart J* 1965; 27:121–127.

60. Patel AK, Zeigler JL, D'Arbela PG, et al. Familial cases of endomyocardial fibrosis in Uganda. *BMJ* 1971; 4:331–334.

61. Kartha CC, Eapen JT, Radhakumary C, et al. Pattern of cardiac fibrosis in rabbits periodically fed a magnesium-restricted diet and administered rare earth chloride through drinking water. *Biol Trace Elem Res* 1998; 63: 19–30.

62. Berenzstein C, Pineiro D, Marcotegui M, et al. Usefulness of echocardiography and Doppler echocardiography in endomyocardial fibrosis. *J Am Soc Echocardiogr* 2000; 13:385–392.

63. Strang JIG, Gibson DG, Nunn AJ, et al. Controlled trial of prednisolone as adjuvant in treatment of tuberculous constrictive pericarditis in Transkei. *Lancet* 1987; i:1418–1422.

64. Strang JI G, Gibson DG, Mitchison DA, et al. Controlled clinical trial of complete open surgical drainage and of prednisolone in treatment of tuberculous pericardial effusion in Transkei. *Lancet* 1988; ii:759–764.

65. Chugh KS, Jain S, Sakhuja V, et al. Renovascular hypertension due to Takayasu's arteritis among Indian patients. *Q J Med* 1992; 85:833–843.

66. Isaacson CA. An idiopathic aortitis in young Africans. *J Pathol Bacteriol* 1961; 81:69–79.

67. Abrahams DG, Barton J, Cockshott WP, et al. Annular subvalvular left ventricular aneurysms. *QJ Med* 1962; 31:345–360.

68. Muoghalu K, Menta M, Okeahialam BN, et al. Lysis of left ventricular thrombus with urokinase in a patient with alcohol heart disease. *West Afr J Med* 1998; 17(1):47–49.

Chapter 13   Alan F. Fleming and P. Shanthamali de Silva

Haematological Diseases in the Tropics

REFERENCE RANGES

The normal values of red cell counts and indices, white cell counts, platelet counts and activities of haemostatic mechanisms vary with age, sex and pregnancy state.[1,2] There are also genetic and common environmental factors which can affect the reference ranges in certain populations.[3] It is especially important that the difference in reference ranges in all stages of life be appreciated by health workers in tropical countries, where up to half the population are aged under 15 years and women experience numerous and often complicated pregnancies.

Red cell values

Age

Full-term infants

Red cell values of the fetus are almost unchanged during the last trimester of pregnancy. The full-term infant is born with a high haemoglobin (Hb) concentration, red blood cell (RBC) count and mean cell volume (MCV) (Table 13.1). A rapid rate of red cell production and low splenic function are shown by the presence of nucleated RBCs, occasional Howell–Jolly bodies (red cell nuclear fragments), polychromasia, a high reticulocyte count (mean 150×10^9/L) and target cells in the peripheral blood. In the first few hours of life, the Hb concentration of capillary blood is on average 35 g/L higher than in venous blood, due to haemoconcentration. If the blood from the placenta is allowed to transfuse into the infant, the Hb rises about 10–20 g/L.

The blood volume ranges from 50 to 100 mL (mean 85 mL)/kg body weight.

During the first few weeks of life, the ability of the blood to deliver oxygen is in excess of what is required, so that erythropoietin secretion is low and the bone marrow is relatively hypoplastic. Red cell survival is short: 80–100 days compared with 90–150 (mean 120) days in adults. Plasma volume increases as the infant grows. As a consequence, the Hb, packed cell volume (PCV) and RBC count decline, to reach a nadir between 8 and 12 weeks of life. The large fetal red cells are replaced, and the MCV declines (Table 13.1). Fetal haemoglobin (HbF) is replaced by adult haemoglobin (HbA) (Table 13.2).[4]

Premature infants

Infants born prematurely during the third trimester have red cell values initially the same as those of full-term infants. However, their basal metabolic rates, oxygen consumption, erythropoietin secretion, red cell production and red cell survival (60–80 days) are all lower. After birth, red cell values fall faster and to lower levels than in mature infants: at around 8 weeks of life the most premature but otherwise normal and well-nourished infant can have an Hb as low as 70 g/L (Table 13.3).[2]

Childhood

After the third month of life, oxygen needs exceed oxygen delivery and provide the necessary stimulus to erythropoietin secretion and red cell production: the Hb, PCV and RBC count rise steadily until puberty (Table 13.1).

Sex

The Hb continues to rise in boys but levels off in girls at puberty, so that men have on average Hb 15 g/L higher than non-pregnant women (Table 13.1). Red cell volumes are 30 ± 5 mL/kg in men and 25 ± 5 mL/kg in women; plasma volume (45 ± 5 mL/kg) and total blood volume (70 ± 10 mL/kg) are the same in both sexes. Testosterone is the stimulus to additional erythropoiesis in men, whereas oestrogen depresses erythropoiesis.

Pregnancy

From the 12th week of gestation there is an increase of erythropoietin secretion, erythroid hyperplasia, reticulocytosis (2–6%) and an increase of the total red cell volume by 400–450 mL in normal and iron-sufficient pregnant women. The plasma volume increases also, by about 1250 mL in primigravidae and 1500 mL in multigravidae. As the increase in plasma volume is greater than that of the red cell volume, there is haemodilution (Figure 13.1B, C): Hb 110 g/L and PCV 0.31 are the accepted lower limits of normal. There is a mild macrocytosis (increase of MCV) during pregnancy.[5]

Genetic and environmental differences

When large series of persons of European descent (whites) and of sub-Saharan African descent (blacks) have been matched for age,

Table 13.1 Red blood cell values at various ages

	Hb (g/L)	PCV (L/L)	RBC (×10¹²/L)	MCV (fL)	MCH (pg)	MCHC (g/L)
Birth (cord blood)	165 ± 30	0.54 ± 0.10	6.0 ± 1.0	120 (mean)	–	300 ± 27
3 months	115 ± 20	0.38 ± 0.04	4.0 ± 0.8	95 (mean)	29 ± 5	325 ± 25
1 year	120 ± 15	–	4.4 ± 0.08	78 ± 8	27 ± 4	325 ± 25
3–6 years	130 ± 10	0.40 ± 0.04	4.8 ± 0.7	84 ± 8	27 ± 3	325 ± 25
10–12 years	130 ± 15	0.41 ± 0.04	4.7 ± 0.7	84 ± 7	27 ± 3	325 ± 25
Men	155 ± 25	0.47 ± 0.07	5.5 ± 1.0	86 ± 10	29.5 ± 2.5	325 ± 25
Women	140 ± 25	0.42 ± 0.05	4.8 ± 1.0	86 ± 10	29.5 ± 2.5	325 ± 25

Table 13.2 Proportion of haemoglobin F found at various ages

Age	HbF (%)
Birth	70–90
1 month	50–75
2 months	25–60
3 months	10–35
4 months	5–20
6 months	<8
9 months	<5
1 year	<2
Adults	<0.4

Table 13.3 Haemoglobin (g/L) observed in iron-sufficient pre-term infants

Age	BIRTH WEIGHT (G)	
	1000–1500	1501–2000
2 weeks	163 (117–184)	148 (188–196)
1 month	109 (87–152)	115 (82–150)
2 months	88 (71–115)	94 (80–114)
3 months	98 (89–112)	102 (93–118)
4 months	113 (91–131)	113 (91–131)
5 months	116 (102–143)	118 (104–130)
6 months	120 (94–138)	118 (107–126)

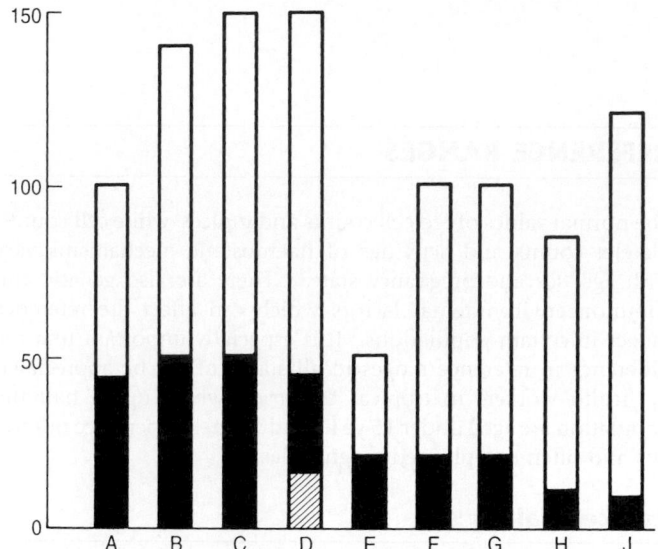

Figure 13.1 Blood volume changes in health and disease. (A) Normal (non-pregnant) adult. (B) Normal single pregnancy. (C) Normal twin pregnancy. (D) Hypersplenism, not anaemic. (E) Acute haemorrhage. (F) Acute haemorrhage, 48 h later. (G) Moderate anaemia. (H) Severe anaemia. (J) Severe anaemia with circulatory congestion. Note that two or more of these conditions may be present in the same patient; in particular E–J are variations on A (non-pregnant), but could be shown again as variants on B (pregnant), C (multiple pregnancy) or D (hypersplenism). Solid bars, red cells; hatched bar, red cells sequestered in the spleen; white bars, plasma. (Reproduced with permission of the publisher, from Fleming AF. In: Parry EHO, ed. *Principles of Medicine of Africa*, 2nd edn. Oxford: Oxford University Press; 1984:706).

sex, pregnant state and socioeconomic status, it has been found that at all ages and in both sexes blacks have on average Hb 5–10 g/L lower than whites, and that this difference is independent of environment. A high frequency of a^+ thalassaemia, up to 50% of some black populations, explains this small genetically determined difference.

Of much greater importance are environmental factors, including malaria, other intercurrent infections and malnutrition, especially deficiencies of iron and folic acid. Apparently healthy members of communities living in the tropics frequently show an average Hb 20 g/L lower at all ages and in both sexes than the internationally accepted reference means. The control of malaria, improvements in hygiene and nutrition, and rises in social class are all associated with the range of Hb concentrations increasing towards the standard ranges.[3]

Altitude

For every 1000 m above sea level, the Hb increases on average by 2.5 g/L, due to low oxygen tension stimulating erythropoietin production.

Miscellaneous factors

The Hb rises slightly with muscular exercise and in assuming the upright posture. It is somewhat higher in the morning than the evening. It is lower in athletes in training, and is raised in tobacco-smokers.

White cell count

Neutrophils

Age

There is a transiently high total white blood cell (WBC) count and a neutrophil leukocytosis at and following birth, peaking at about 12 h of life (Table 13.4), with a high number of non-segmented neutrophils (up to 1.8×10^9/L). The number of neutrophils declines and is exceeded by the lymphocyte count after 2 weeks. From 2 years, the number of circulating neutrophils increases with age until adult life, when they contribute 40–75% of the total count of $4.0–11.0 \times 10^9$/L in Caucasian adults.[2]

Sex

Women during their reproductive period of life have slightly higher WBC and neutrophil counts (average difference 0.66×10^9/L) than men, and oral contraceptives increase counts further: there are two peaks of neutrophil leukocytosis coinciding with peaks of oestrogen secretion and a fall following menstruation. Postmenopausal women have counts slightly lower than men.

Pregnancy

The WBC and neutrophil counts rise to a plateau by the second trimester (WBC mean 9.0×10^9/L, range $5.0–16.0 \times 10^9$/L; neutrophils mean 7.0×10^9/L, range $2.5–14.0 \times 10^9$/L) (Figure 13.2).[5] There is a sharp peak of neutrophil leukocytosis during obstetric delivery, when the total WBC count may reach 40×10^9/L in an uninfected patient. Neutrophil and total WBC counts fall to non-pregnant levels by the 6th day postpartum. The circulating neutrophils in pregnant women are relatively young, with a shift to the left (<3% metamyelocytes and myelocytes), raised activity of

neutrophil alkaline phosphatase and other enzymes and enhanced bactericidal function.

Genetic and environmental factors

A relative and absolute neutropenia has been described in children over 6 months and adults who are black Africans or of black African descent in the Americas and Europe (Table 13.5),[3] and in Palestinians, Yemeni Jews and Saudi Arabians. The total body neutrophils have been found to be the same in adults of West Indian origin living in the UK as in the white Britons, but the West Indians have a greater number of neutrophils in the bone marrow storage pool, while Europeans have more in circulation; provocation of a neutrophil response, either experimentally or by natural infection, leads to rises to the same level in both races. There is probably a genetic factor underlying this ethnic neutropenia, but environmental factors may also play a role, for example those causing splenomegaly and hypersplenism. The neutrophil count rises with higher socioeconomic status in Africans, and declines in Europeans living in West Africa.

The WBC and neutrophil counts rise during pregnancy in African women, but remain about 3.0×10^9/L lower than in pregnant Caucasians (Figure 13.2).

Miscellaneous factors

Counts are higher in the afternoon than in the morning, by about 0.5×10^9/L. Exercise mobilizes the cells marginated on the endothelium, and so raises the number of circulating cells, even up to a WBC count of 30×10^9/L with the most strenuous exertion. Emotional stress can raise counts transiently. Tobacco-smokers have persistently higher neutrophil counts.

Acute reactive neutrophil leukocytosis is seen most commonly in response to pyogenic infections (Table 13.6): immature neutrophils (metamyelocytes) are released from the bone marrow; there is an excess of deeply purple-staining primary cytoplasmic

Table 13.4 Normal leukocyte counts

Age	TOTAL LEUKOCYTES		NEUTROPHILS			LYMPHOCYTES			MONOCYTES		EOSINOPHILS	
	Mean	Range	Mean	Range	(%)	Mean	Range	(%)	Mean	(%)	Mean	(%)
Birth	18.1	(9.0–30.0)	11.0	(6.0–26.0)	61	5.5	(2.0–11.0)	31	1.1	6	0.4	2
12 h	22.8	(13.0–38.0)	15.5	(6.0–28.0)	68	5.5	(2.0–11.0)	24	1.2	5	0.5	2
24 h	18.9	(9.4–34.0)	11.5	(5.0–21.0)	61	5.8	(2.0–11.5)	31	1.1	6	0.5	2
1 week	12.2	(5.0–21.0)	5.5	(1.5–10.0)	45	5.0	(2.0–17.0)	41	1.1	9	0.5	4
2 weeks	11.4	(5.0–20.0)	4.5	(1.0–9.5)	40	5.5	(2.0–17.0)	48	1.0	9	0.4	3
1 month	10.8	(5.0–19.5)	3.8	(1.0–9.0)	35	6.0	(2.0–16.5)	56	0.7	7	0.3	3
6 months	11.9	(6.0–17.5)	3.8	(1.0–8.5)	32	7.3	(4.0–13.5)	61	0.6	5	0.3	3
1 year	11.4	(6.0–17.5)	3.5	(1.5–8.5)	31	7.0	(4.0–10.5)	61	0.6	5	0.3	3
2 years	10.6	(6.0–17.0)	3.5	(1.5–8.5)	33	6.3	(3.0–9.5)	59	0.5	5	0.3	3
4 years	9.1	(5.5–15.5)	3.8	(1.5–8.5)	42	4.5	(2.0–8.0)	50	0.5	5	0.3	3
6 years	8.5	(5.0–14.5)	4.3	(1.5–8.0)	51	3.5	(1.5–7.0)	42	0.4	5	0.2	3
8 years	8.3	(4.5–13.5)	4.4	(1.5–8.0)	53	3.3	(1.5–6.8)	39	0.4	4	0.2	2
10 years	8.1	(4.5–13.5)	4.4	(1.8–8.0)	54	3.1	(1.5–6.5)	38	0.4	4	0.2	2
16 years	7.8	(4.5–13.0)	4.4	(1.8–8.0)	57	2.8	(1.2–5.2)	35	0.4	5	0.2	3
21 years	7.4	(4.5–11.0)	4.4	(1.8–7.7)	59	2.5	(1.0–4.8)	34	0.3	4	0.2	3

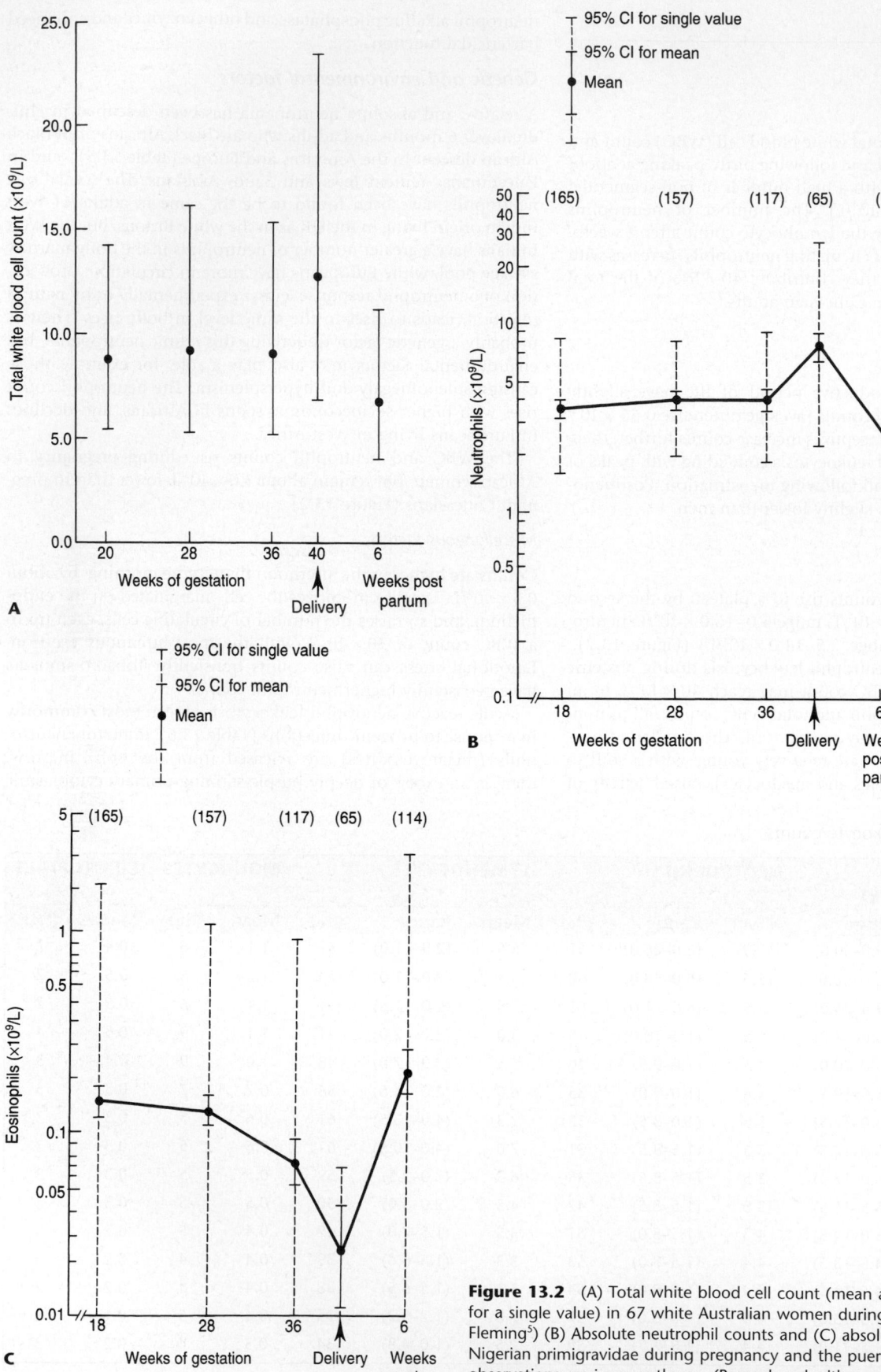

Figure 13.2 (A) Total white blood cell count (mean and 95% confidence limits for a single value) in 67 white Australian women during pregnancy. (From Fleming[5]) (B) Absolute neutrophil counts and (C) absolute eosinophil counts in Nigerian primigravidae during pregnancy and the puerperium: numbers of observations are in parentheses. (Reproduced with permission from Fleming AF, Akintunde EA, Harrison KA, Dunn D. *E Afr Med J* 1985; 62:175–184.)

Table 13.5 Leukocyte counts in 123 non-elite male Nigerian blood donors in Zaria

	Mean	Range	(%)
Total white cells	5.1	2.6–10.2	–
Neutrophils	2.8	1.1–7.1	30–85
Eosinophils	0.11	0–2.0	1–30
Basophils	0.002	0–0.02	0–1
Lymphocytes	2.1	0.7–3.1	15–60
Monocytes	0.13	0–1.3	0–8

Table 13.6 Some causes of reactive leukocytosis

Leukocytosis	Causes
Neutrophilia	Acute viral infections (e.g. poliomyelitis)
	Acute bacterial infections (e.g. staphylococcal)
	Tissue damage
	Haemorrhage
	Malignancies
	Stress states
	Diabetic ketoacidosis
	Miscellaneous (drugs, corticosteroids, chemicals, renal failure, collagen diseases)
	Pregnancy and delivery
Eosinophilia	Helminthic infections of tissues
	Löffler's syndrome (larval migration of nematodes)
	Convalescence from viral or other infections
	Malignancies
	Cytotoxic therapy
	Allergic disorders
	Miscellaneous (post splenectomy, familial, lead ingestion, polyarteritis nodosa, pulmonary aspergillosis, rheumatoid arthritis)
Basophilia	Miscellaneous (hypersensitivity, myxoedema, iron deficiency, chronic haemolysis)
Lymphocytosis	Childhood infections generally
	Protozoan infections (malaria, toxoplasmosis)
	Viral infections
Monocytosis	Protozoan infections (malaria)
	Rickettsial infections
	Subacute/chronic bacterial infections (tuberculosis, brucellosis, subacute bacterial endocarditis)

granules ('toxic granulation'); occasionally oval blue-staining Döhle bodies, which are RNA, are present in the cytoplasm. Neutrophil damage shows as ragged and vacuolated cytoplasm and pyknotic nuclei. With severe infections there can be a leukaemoid reaction, when the total count is above $80 \times 10^9/L$ with a shift to the left as far as promyelocytes and blast cells.

Eosinophils and basophils

The eosinophil count is high at birth and declines slowly throughout childhood to less than $0.4 \times 10^9/L$ in adult life (see Table 13.4).[2] There is a diurnal variation, more considerable than that of neutrophils. The eosinophil count is lower during pregnancy; the stress of obstetric delivery causes the eosinophils to vanish from the peripheral blood almost entirely, even if there was an initially high count (Figure 13.2). Symptom-free individuals living in the tropics often have high eosinophil counts due to subclinical infections by helminths (see Table 13.5); counts are higher in rural and non-elite groups than in urban and elite groups. In the tropics eosinophilia is more likely to be a response to helminthic infection than to be an indication of allergy (Table 13.6).

The basophil count is normally low (see Table 13.4); accurate electronic counting demonstrates diminished counts during stress, pregnancy, acute infections and the administration of corticosteroids. A raised count is always suggestive of leukaemia or a myeloproliferative disorder, but may be seen in some allergic conditions (Table 13.6).

Lymphocytes

The lymphocyte count is normally high in the first year of life and then declines to adult levels (see Table 13.4). There are no reported differences between adult males and non-pregnant females, but the total lymphocyte count declines slightly during pregnancy; of more importance is a functional reduction of T cell-mediated immunity during pregnancy.

A proliferation of B cell lymphocytes is commonly seen in the tropics in response to malaria and other intercurrent infections, especially in childhood in rural and non-elite groups (Table 13.6). An absolute lymphocytosis with numerous activated lymphocytes (plasmacytoid cells) is frequently seen in children in the tropics. Atypical lymphocytes with slate-grey or blue cytoplasm are suggestive of viral infections. African adults have a relative lymphocytosis, due to neutropenia, and often an absolute lymphocytosis (see Table 13.5). Of peripheral blood lymphocytes of adults in the industrialized countries, approximately 80% are T cells, 10–15% B cells and 5–10% null cells; rural Nigerians have been reported to have higher proportions of B cells (about 30%), whereas elite Nigerians and Europeans had similar distribution of lymphocyte subsets.

Monocytes

The monocyte count is highest during the first 2 weeks of life (see Table 13.4); there is no other significant physiological change, except a fall during obstetric delivery. In the tropics counts may be raised in association with subclinical protozoan or other infections or lowered in subjects with splenomegaly (see Tables 13.5 and 13.6).

Haemostasis

Age

Platelet counts (normal $150–400 \times 10^9/L$) and function do not vary with age to any clinically significant degree.

Vitamin K is a fat-soluble vitamin, widely distributed in both vegetable and animal foods as well as being absorbed from that produced by the microbiological flora of the normal gut. Vitamin

K levels of infants, especially premature infants, are critically low in the first 3 days of life because of a slow rate of transport across the placenta, low hepatic stores, the absence of an intestinal bacterial flora, and low concentrations in colostrum and breast milk. In addition, the immature liver has limited capacity for the synthesis of clotting factors. Vitamin K is essential for the synthesis by the liver of clotting factors (II, VII, IX and X) and protein C and protein S; these have low activity in umbilical cord blood, especially in preterm infants, so that the prothrombin time (PT) and partial thromboplastin time (PTT) are prolonged (Table 13.7).[2] Vitamin K-producing bacteria colonize the bowel and the deficiency is usually rectified by 72–120 h. However, a few infants, especially the pre-term, progress to haemorrhagic disease of the newborn. Fibrinolytic activity is essentially functional in infants.

Sex

Platelet counts are higher in women than men by about 20%, and fall following menstruation.[1]

Pregnancy

Plasma volume expansion causes the platelet count to fall about 20% during pregnancy, but function remains unchanged. The activity of the extrinsic pathway is enhanced during pregnancy, with high levels of factors VII, X and fibrinogen. On the intrinsic pathway, activity of factors XII, IX and VIII are also moderately raised, but factor XI decreases. A decline of antithrombin III (AT III) adds to hypercoagulability in pregnancy, so that the thromboplastin generation time and PT are accelerated. This potential hypercoagulability is balanced by lower levels of factor XIII. Plasminogen levels are increased parallel to the rise of fibrinogen, while antiplasmin activity is unchanged. This potential for fibrinolysis is suppressed normally by the placenta producing inhibitors to plasminogen activator synthesis and release by endothelium. Fibrin/fibrinogen degradation products (FDPs) are present in plasma in low concentrations in the third trimester only.

During obstetric delivery and following separation of the placenta there is activation and consumption of platelets and coagulation factors; the fibrinolytic pathway is activated, with a transient appearance of FDPs reaching a maximum in the first 4 h post

partum. There is a return of all haemostatic factors to non-pregnant levels by the end of the second week of the puerperium.

Genetic and environmental differences

The platelet counts in the African newborns up to around 6 months of age do not differ significantly from those of European newborns and adults. Older children and adults throughout tropical Africa have a moderate thrombocytopenia, for example $70–370 \times 10^9/L$ in symptom-free adult male Nigerians. This is probably the result of increased pooling of platelets in subclinically enlarged spleens.[1,3]

Platelets from non-elite Nigerians have been shown to be relatively resistant to aggregation by ADP, thrombin and ristocetin: aggregation can be induced either by increasing concentrations of the agonists or by resuspending the platelets in European plasma, suggesting that there are inhibitory plasma factors; these could be merely high levels of macroglobulins in response to intercurrent infections. The bleeding time and clot retraction are within standard reference ranges and there is no tendency to purpura, but the inhibition of platelet adhesion and aggregation could contribute to the low incidence of atheroma and thrombosis.[6]

Factor VIII coagulant activity of Africans is commonly greater than 150% of the activity of pooled European plasma. Levels in plasma of fibrinogen, plasminogen activators and spontaneous fibrinolysis are high in Africans and Papua New Guineans who perform heavy manual work, but levels fall with rising economic status and a more sedentary life. In Kenya and Papua New Guinea the frequency distribution of PT was shown to be skewed to the right; that is, there was a subpopulation with prolonged times; subclinical hepatic disease is a probable cause, and this is likely to apply to other tropical populations.

ANAEMIA

Definition

Anaemia is defined as a condition in which the Hb concentration in peripheral blood is lower than normal for age, sex and pregnancy state of the subject (Table 13.8).[7] The Hb is usually directly related to the total red cell volume, but there are exceptional circumstances: (1) during the first hours of life, when there is haemoconcentration in the capillaries, capillary blood samples

Table 13.7 Haemostatic measurements in the newborn and adults

	Pre-term infants	Full-term infants	Children over 2 months and adults
Platelets ×10⁹/L	150–400	150–400	150–400
Prothrombin time (s)	13–18	12–16	11–14
Partial thromboplastin time (s)	35–50	30–45	23–35
Fibrinogen (g/L)	2–4	2–4	2–4
FDP (mg/L)	<10	<10	<10

Table 13.8 Haemoglobin concentrations below which anaemia is likely to be present in populations living at sea level

	Hb (g/L)
Newborn infants	140
6 months–6 years	110
6–14 years	120
Adult males	130
Adult females (non-pregnant)	120
Adult females (pregnant)	110

will underestimate anaemia, especially in premature, acidotic, hypotensive or hypovolaemic infants; (2) immediately following acute haemorrhage, the Hb remains unchanged until there has been compensatory expansion of the plasma volume over the following 48 h (see Figure 13.1E, F); (3) with splenomegaly there is both an expansion of plasma volume and sequestration of red cells, so that patients with massive splenomegaly may have a Hb of 80 g/L, for example, while the total red cell mass is normal (see Figure 13.1D).

Aetiology

Anaemia results from three basic mechanisms: (1) blood loss (haemorrhage); (2) decreased production of red cells; and (3) increased destruction of red cells (haemolysis) (Table 13.9). Only those causes which are of major public health importance in the tropics will be discussed. These include: (a) infections such as malaria, the human immunodeficiency viruses (HIV-1 and HIV-2), tuberculosis, hookworm and schistosomiasis; (b) nutritional deficiencies of iron and folate; and (c) inherited disorders of red cells, including the thalassaemias, sickle cell disease, glucose 6 phosphate dehydrogenase (G6PD) deficiency and ovalocytosis.

Epidemiology

Anaemia is the most common manifestation of disease observed in the tropics (Table 13.10).[8] Prevalence and morbidity are greatest in preschool children and pregnant women, in whom it is usual to find about half to be anaemic in rural and impoverished communities. The most common causes in preschool children are iron deficiency, malaria, thalassaemias (in Asia) and sickle cell disease (in Africa). The conditions leading most frequently to an anaemia in pregnancy are iron and folate deficiencies, malaria, thalassaemia minor (in Asia) and milder forms of sickle cell disease (in Africa). Although anaemia is less common and usually less severe in school children, men and non-pregnant women, it is still a major health problem in these groups: in them, anaemia is often secondary to tuberculosis or other chronic infections. HIV infection is now an extremely common cause of anaemia in men and women in the sexually active age range, but also in children: it is now the commonest cause of anaemia in adults requiring admission to hospital in sub-Saharan Africa.

Pathophysiology

Anaemia reduces the oxygen-carrying capacity of the blood. The body compensates for this by: (a) increasing the release of oxygen from Hb to the tissues; (b) increasing cardiac output; (c) enhancing blood flow to vital tissues with high oxygen requirements, while reducing flow to other organs; and (d) increasing respiration. The severity of anaemia is best considered as passing through three stages: (1) compensated, (2) decompensated and (3) life-threatening anaemia. The severity of anaemia does not depend on the Hb concentration alone, so that cut-off points of Hb 70 g/L and 30 g/L for when decompensation and cardiac failure respectively are likely must be taken as very approximate. Older patients are more likely to progress to decompensation or heart failure than the young; infants and young children are able to tolerate

Table 13.9 Aetiology of anaemia

1. BLOOD LOSS	
(a) Acute	(b) Chronic (e.g. hookworm) leading to iron deficiency

2. DECREASED RED CELL PRODUCTION	
(a) Nutritional deficiencies	(b) Depressed bone marrow function
Iron	Secondary anaemias
Folate	HIV/AIDS
Vitamin B$_{12}$	tuberculosis
Various	other chronic infections
protein–energy	chronic hepatic disease
vitamin A	chronic renal disease
vitamin C	carcinomatosis
vitamin E, riboflavin	Aplastic anaemia
pyridoxine, Cu	drugs and chemicals
	infiltration
	idiopathic
	irradiation
	congenital
Thalassaemias	
α thalassaemias	
β thalassaemias	

3. INCREASED RED CELL DESTRUCTION	
(a) Abnormalities of red cells	(b) Abnormal haemolysis
Haemoglobin	Immune haemolysis
sickle-cell disease	autoimmune
Enzymes	fetomaternal incompatibility
G6PD deficiency	incompatible blood transfusion
Membrane	Non-immune haemolysis infections (e.g. malaria)
elliptocytosis	hypersplenism
ovalocytosis	drugs and chemicals
spherocytosis	venoms
	burns
	mechanical

extremely low Hb concentrations with few complaints. Patients who develop an anaemia acutely have less time to compensate than patients with chronic anaemias such as sickle cell disease or aplastic anaemia. Patients who are hypervolaemic as a result of pregnancy (see Figure 13.1B), especially multiple pregnancy (see 13.1C), or of splenomegaly (see Figure 13.1D) are more liable to progress as far as congestive cardiac failure, as are patients with underlying cardiac, vascular or respiratory diseases. In contrast, patients with low levels of activity, including the bedridden, are less likely to become decompensated.

Table 13.10 Estimated prevalence of anaemia by geographical region and age/sex category, around 1980 (population data in millions)

Region	CHILDREN (0–4 YEARS)			CHILDREN (5–12 YEARS)			MEN (15–59 YEARS)			WOMEN (15–49 YEARS) PREGNANT			WOMEN (15–49 YEARS) ALL		
	Total	ANAEMIC		Total	ANAEMIC		Total	ANAEMIC		Total	ANAEMIC		Total	ANAEMIC	
	(n)	(%)	n	(n)	(%)	n	(n)	(%)	n	(n)	(%)	n	(n)	(%)	n
Africa	85.7	56	48.0	96.6	49	47.3	116.8	20	23.4	17.9	63	11.3	106.4	44	46.8
Northern America	19.6	8	1.6	27.5	13	3.6	76.3	4	3.1	3.4	–	–	64.2	8	5.1
Latin America	52.9	26	13.7	69.8	26	18.1	98.1	13	12.8	9.9	30	3.0	86.5	17	14.7
East Africa	16.1	20	3.2	25.4	22	5.6	55.8	11	6.1	2.7	20	0.5	46.9	18	8.4
South Asia	212.0	56	118.7	278.4	50	139.2	386.3	32	123.6	41.7	65	27.1	329.4	58	191.0
Europe	33.4	14	4.7	55.0	5	3.0	147.2	2	3.0	5.7	14	0.8	117.5	12	14.1
Oceania	2.3	18	0.4	3.6	15	0.5	6.9	7	0.5	0.4	25	0.1	5.5	19	0.1
Former Soviet Union	23.1	–	–	31.1	–	–	80.3	–	–	4.0	–	–	68.7	–	–
World[a]	445.1	43	193.5	587.6	37	217.4	967.7	18	174.2	85.8	51	43.9	825.0	35	288.4
Developed regions	86.1	12	10.3	130.7	7	9.1	346.5	3	12.0	14.8	14	2.0	285.5	11	32.7
Developing regions[a]	395.0	51	183.2	456.8	46	208.3	621.2	26	162.2	71.0	59	41.9	539.5	47	255.7

[a]Excluding China.

Compensated anaemia

The major compensatory mechanism in mild to moderate anaemia is the increase of 2,3-diphosphoglycerate (2,3-DPG) concentration in red cells: this binds to deoxyhaemoglobin, shifts the oxygen dissociation curve of Hb to the right (decreased oxygen affinity) and increases oxygen release to tissue by up to 40%.[9] Cardiac output is raised by an increase in stroke volume at rest: on exertion there is both an exaggerated tachycardia and further rise in stroke volume. Vasodilatation enhances the blood flow to the myocardium, skeletal muscle and brain, while there is vasoconstriction in the skin and kidneys. The plasma volume expands, but the total blood volume remains normal (see Figure 13.1G).

Patients complain of breathlessness on exertion only, and there are no physical signs except pallor, unless there are symptoms and signs from the underlying cause of the anaemia.

Work capacity

Maximal work capacity, as measured by the Harvard Step Test (HST), correlates directly with Hb at all levels, and is reduced by even mild anaemia: the average HST of Guatemalan labourers was 65 at Hb 130–150 g/L and 30 at Hb 70–90 g/L.[10]

Productivity and earnings of anaemic male manual workers are seriously reduced.[11,12] The earnings of anaemic women performing less strenuous factory work are also reduced.[13] Anaemia in either parent has an adverse effect on the family through low food production, low income and poor care for children; village life suffers from there being less ground under cultivation, and the national economy declines from overall low productivity.

The incidence of low birth weight and perinatal mortality rises rapidly when the maternal haematocrit (Hct) falls below 0.30.[14]

In childhood, anaemia is associated with slow growth, delayed development and poor cognitive abilities.

Decompensated anaemia

When the Hb falls below about 70 g/L, the major mechanism for improving oxygen delivery is an increase in cardiac output.[9] Both stroke volume and the heart rate are raised at rest. The work of the ventricles is reduced by the low viscosity of anaemic blood and by peripheral vasodilatation; the circulation time is short. The blood volume is reduced in about 25% of patients (see Figure 13.1H).

Patients are breathless even at rest. There is tachycardia, arterial and capillary pulsation, a wide pulse pressure and haemic ejection systolic murmurs. It is common experience that patients who are subsistence farmers, or others wholly dependent on their own manual labour, do not seek treatment until they have reached this stage of anaemia.

Life-threatening anaemia

Hypoxia and acidosis

If anaemia progresses in children with malaria until Hb falls to <50 g/L, respiratory distress develops, showing as tachypnea and at least one of the signs of nasal flaring, indrawing of the chest wall or diaphragm, grunting or deep breathing. The children are hypovolaemic (Figure. 13.1H) and acidotic with lactic acidaemia.[15] Without appropriate treatment, mortality is high.

Anaemic heart failure

If anaemia progresses (Hb <30 g/L approximately), the oxygen supply to the myocardium is insufficient, no further increase of cardiac output is possible, and high-output cardiac failure develops. The plasma volume expands (see Figure 13.1J): patients who are already hypervolaemic from pregnancy or splenomegaly are most liable to develop anaemic heart failure.

Patients are severely breathless and may complain of angina, night cramps or claudication. There is cardiomegaly, engorgement of jugular veins, pulmonary oedema, hepatomegaly, peripheral oedema and sometimes ascites. Without appropriate treatment there is a high morbidity rate. Maternal deaths rise sharply when the Hct is below 0.20 at the time of delivery: up to 20% of maternal deaths in Africa and India used to be due to anaemic heart failure, and this may still be true where obstetric and blood transfusion services have not developed.[16]

Management

The first principle of management is the diagnosis and treatment of the cause of the anaemia. The transfusion of concentrated red cells is required by anaemic patients in three circumstances only: (1) a patient is in danger of dying of anaemic heart failure or hypoxia before specific medication can raise the Hb; (2) a patient is about to experience stress, such as emergency major surgery, obstetric delivery or cytotoxic therapy; and (3) the anaemia is incurable, for example thalassaemia or aplastic anaemia, as will be discussed under these conditions. Children with severe malarial anaemia are hypovolaemic, not hypervolaemic, and should be transfused whole blood, not concentrated red cells, when the Hb is <50 g/L and there is respiratory distress or when the Hb is <40 g/L with or without respiratory distress. (Management of severe malaria is discussed in Chapter 73.) The inappropriate use of blood transfusion is not to be condoned, especially since the advent of HIV and the acquired immunodeficiency syndrome (AIDS).[17]

Haemolytic anaemias

This is a group of anaemias in which there is an increase of red cell turnover due to a shortening of the red cell lifespan from the normal range of 90–150 (mean 120) days. Haemolysis may be the consequence of an abnormal haemolytic process, or of abnormalities (usually congenital) of the red cells (see Table 13.9). Clinical and laboratory features common to all haemolytic anaemias are due to the increased breakdown of haemoglobin and the compensatory mechanisms of increased red cell production (Table 13.11). Haemolysis may be extravascular, that is, within the reticuloendothelial system (RES), when the breakdown products of haemoglobin follow the normal metabolic pathways of bilirubin. Lysis of red cells within the circulation results in the release of haemoglobin into plasma, the saturation and removal of haemoglobin- and haem-binding proteins (haptoglobins and haemopexin), and the presence of haemoglobin and its degradation products in the plasma and urine. Chronic haemolysis can lead to the formation of pigment stones in the gallbladder.

The bone marrow is capable of increasing red cell production around eight times the normal rate. Compensatory erythroid hyperplasia may be sufficient to maintain a normal or near-normal Hb, but is insufficient when rates of haemolysis are most rapid. Often the haemolytic process is accompanied not by erythroid hyperplasia, but by depression of marrow activity, either as part of the pathology of the disease (e.g. malaria) or due to complicating infections, such as parvovirus B19, which precipitates the so-called aplastic crises of sickle cell disease. A rapid rate of red cell production leads to high demands for folic acid, and long-standing haemolytic anaemias are frequently complicated by

Table 13.11 Features of the haemolytic anaemias

FEATURES OF EXTRAVASCULAR AND INTRAVASCULAR HAEMOLYSIS
Jaundice
Hyperbilirubinaemia (unconjugated)
Increased urinary urobilinogen
Increased faecal urobilinogen (stercobilinogen)
FEATURES OF INTRAVASCULAR HAEMOLYSIS
Reduced/absent haptoglobins
Reduced haemopexin
Haem/methaemoglobinaemia
Methaemalbumin (positive Schumm's test)
Haem/methaemoglobinuria
Haemosiderinuria
FEATURES OF INCREASED RBC PRODUCTION
Polychromasia
Reticulocytosis
Bone marrow erythroid hyperplasia

folate deficiency and megaloblastic erythropoiesis, followed by more profound anaemia. Chronic erythroid hyperplasia, as in sickle cell disease and the thalassaemias, results in expansion of the bone marrow cavity, seen clinically as bossing of the vault of the skull and projection of the maxilla (gnathopathy), and on radiography of the skull as the hair-on-end appearance (see Figure 13.10).

Splenomegaly and hypersplenism

Palpable enlargement of the spleen is a common clinical finding in the tropics, especially where malaria is endemic (Table 13.12). In many instances splenomegaly is accompanied by the syndrome of hypersplenism, when there is pancytopenia, the severity of which is usually related to the size of the spleen. The anaemia is due to: (1) increased red cell pooling in the spleen, (2) shortened red cell lifespan with increased destruction of the spleen, and (3) haemodilution from an increased plasma volume (see Figure 13.1D). The mechanisms of granulocytopenia and thrombocytopenia are similar: an eosinophilic response to helminthic infection may not be apparent in the peripheral blood because the eosinophils are held in the spleen, but it will be obvious in the bone marrow. The anaemia is usually normocytic and normochromic, there is a reticulocytosis and the bone marrow shows hyperplasia.

Malaria

The features of malaria are described in detail in Chapter 73; here are discussed only the haematological consequences, which include anaemia, changes in the white cells and disorders of haemostasis.[18,19] Of the different species of parasite, *Plasmodium falciparum* is the most common and has the most profound haematological consequences; this species of malaria is implied except where stated otherwise.

Table 13.12 Some causes of splenomegaly (see also Chapter 10)

GENERALLY SLIGHT (<5 CM BELOW THE COSTAL MARGIN)	
Acute infections	malaria, septicaemias, viraemias, hepatitis, trypanosomiasis, brucellosis, toxoplasmosis, typhus
Subacute, chronic infections	tuberculosis, brucellosis[a], syphilis, hydatid, meningococcal septicaemia, histoplasmosis, bacterial endocarditis
Miscellaneous	megaloblastic anaemia, iron deficiency anaemia, immune thrombocytopenia, rheumatoid arthritis[a], hyperthyroidism, myeloma, disseminated lupus erythematosus, sarcoidosis[a], amyloidosis
GENERALLY MODERATE (5–10 CM BELOW THE COSTAL MARGIN)	
Chronic haemolysis	recurrent malaria[a], haemoglobinopathies, spherocytosis
Portal hypertension[a]	hepatic cirrhosis
Haematological malignancies	chronic lymphocytic leukaemia[a], lymphomas[a], acute leukaemias, polycythaemia vera
USUALLY GROSS (>10 CM BELOW THE COSTAL MARGIN)	
Hyperreactive malarial splenomegaly (HMS)[a]	
Schistosomiasis[a]	
Kala-azar[a]	
Thalassaemia major[a]	
Haematological malignancies	chronic granulocytic leukaemia, myelofibrosis[a]
Miscellaneous	splenic cysts and tumours, lipid storage diseases

[a]These conditions are commonly associated with hypersplenism.

Malarial anaemia

Where malaria is endemic, for example in tropical Africa, the severity and pathology (including anaemia) progress through three phases as individuals acquire partial immune protection: (1) acute malaria in non-immune children after about 6 months of age when maternally derived immunity is lost; (2) recurrent malaria in children less than about 5 years of age; and (3) recurrent mild parasitaemia in partially immune older children and adults. Malaria in non-immune adults, such as expatriate visitors to endemic areas or inhabitants of countries where malaria is unstable, have haematological complications of acute or recurrent malaria essentially similar to those of children in the endemic areas.

Acute malaria

In non-immune individuals, there is usually no anaemia within 24–48 h of the onset of fever, but there is then a rapid fall of the Hb and Hct over 4–5 days, with the degree of anaemia corresponding approximately to the intensity of parasitaemia. The anaemia is normochromic and normocytic. The reticulocyte count is low at this stage, although the bone marrow shows erythroid hyperplasia with minimal dyserythropoietic changes. The total plasma bilirubin and unconjugated fraction are raised: increased conjugated bilirubin indicates complicating hepatic dysfunction. Haptoglobins are reduced or absent (see Table 13.11).

A major mechanism of haemolysis is rupture of red cells at the time of release of merozoites, but anaemia is often more severe and more persistent than can be accounted for directly by parasitaemia. The Hb may continue to fall for between 7 and 21 days following clearing of the parasites, due apparently to both continued haemolysis and delayed release of red cells from the marrow. Survival of both autologous non-parasitized red cells and donated red cells is shortened. There is phagocytosis of the parasitized and unparasitized red cells, seen easily in the bone marrow. The direct Coombs' test (DCT) is frequently positive, associated with adsorption by red cells of immunoglobulin (Ig) G and the C3 component of complement; however, auto-immune haemolysis is not an important mechanism, although IgG-coated red cells are more rapidly removed by the RES than uncoated cells. Haemolysis of unparasitized red cells appears, therefore, to be due to a non-specific activation of the RES, hypersplenism and Fc receptor-mediated uptake.

Malaria is immunosuppressive and is frequently complicated by secondary infections, such as bronchopneumonia, urinary tract infections and Gram-negative septicaemias; anaemia is generally more profound when there is secondary infection, especially with non-typhoid *Salmonella* septicaemia. It has been suggested that profound anaemia in some children may be the result of concurrent infection by parvovirus B19, which infects early red cell precursors preferentially and causes a transient red cell hypoplasia.

During acute malaria there is immobilization of iron in the macrophages, and low serum iron concentrations: serum ferritin is massively increased, being an acute reactive protein. Red cell folate levels are raised above normal through mechanisms which are uncertain, but possibly due to synthesis of folate by the parasites themselves.

Following clearance of the parasitaemia and during recovery, the peripheral blood shows a reticulocytosis, anisocytosis, macrocytosis and polychromasia (see Table 13.11).

Recurrent malaria

Children living where malaria is endemic suffer from recurrent attacks: they complain of intermittent fever and general ill health, and on examination often have moderate splenomegaly. They have a chronic normocytic, normochromic anaemia with a low reticulocyte count; anaemia may be profound during acute exacerbations but there is only a scanty parasitaemia, although gametocytes and malarial pigment may be seen in the monocytes. The anaemia is a result of both hypersplenism and severe dyserythropoietic disturbance of the bone marrow (Figure 13.3). The mechanism of dyserythropoiesis is uncertain, but it could be secondary to hypoxia from the packing of bone marrow sinusoids with parasitized red cells, or be mediated by an imbalance of cytokines.

Serum tumour necrosis factor (TNF) and interferon γ (IFNγ) are raised in acute malaria: they play an essential role in the

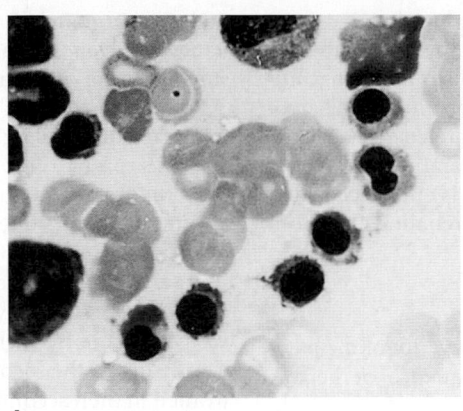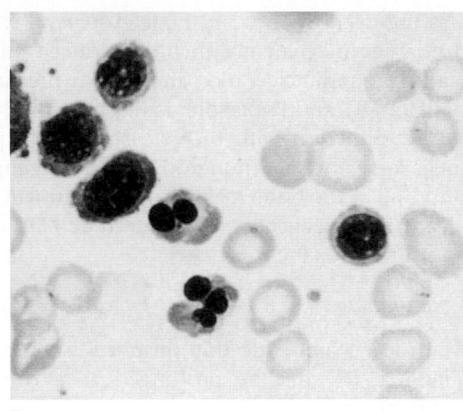

Figure 13.3 (A) and (B)
Dyserythropoiesis: a term used to describe specific morphological changes in bone marrow which usually denotes ineffective erythropoiesis. These changes include cytoplasmic vacuolation, basophilic stippling, intracytoplasmic bridges, nuclear fragmentation (karyorrhexis), incomplete and unequal nuclear division and multinuclearity.

A   **B**

control of parasitaemia and in inflammatory reactions. Interleukin 10 (IL-10) is also raised, and modulates the inflammatory responses. Low IL-10 concentrations have been found in African children with severe malaria, and it has been suggested that a failure of IL-10 may allow the uncontrolled actions of TNF in promoting dyserythropoiesis and erythrophagocytosis.

Disturbed marrow function is reversed by successful antimalarial treatment, which is followed by a brisk reticulocytosis and rise in Hb.

Haemoglobinuria and blackwater fever

The majority of patients presenting with haemoglobinuria seen today are G6PD deficient and have been treated with oxidant drugs (see below). However, some are G6PD normal and the trigger to severe intravascular haemolysis cannot be found. In the past patients were not infrequently seen with blackwater fever. Typically such a patient was a non-immune adult expatriate who had been taking quinine irregularly as prophylaxis. The patient complained of loin pain, vomiting and diarrhoea; initially there was polyuria, but later oliguria with dark-brown or black urine. There was tender hepatosplenomegaly, jaundice and profound anaemia; malarial parasites were scanty or even absent. There was massive haemoglobinuria and all other features of intravascular haemolysis (see Table 13.11). The mechanism was probably quinine-induced immune haemolysis. Blackwater fever is increasing in incidence as quinine comes back into use, and may be triggered also by mefloquine, artemisinin and halofantrine.

Malaria in the partially immune

Where malaria is endemic, older children and adults experience recurrent malarial parasitaemia contained by acquired immunity, with moderate haemolysis and compensatory erythroid hyperplasia. This contributes largely to the mean Hb being about 20 g/L lower than accepted reference figures in both sexes in many communities.[3] There is moderate anisocytosis, macrocytosis and polychromasia. The balance between haemolysis and erythroid hyperplasia is disturbed during pregnancy (see below), after splenectomy and immune anergy, for example from malignant disease, and with hyperreactive malarial splenomegaly (HMS) (see below).

HIV infection is associated with increased parasite densities and incidence of clinical malaria, which has significance particularly during pregnancy (see below).[20]

Leukocytes in malaria

Lymphocytes

From about the 3rd day of fever onwards, there are, in the peripheral blood, numerous transformed lymphocytes or plasmacytoid cells with dark blue cytoplasm and large nuclei with nucleoli. These are activated B cells. Sometimes in African children a leukaemoid reaction is seen, difficult to distinguish on simple blood film examination from acute lymphoblastic leukaemia.[21]

Neutrophils

Many patients with acute malaria show a neutropenia due to margination to the endothelial surface of neutrophils in the circulation. During recovery from uncomplicated malaria there is often a leukocytosis with a shift to the left, toxic granulation, vacuolation and ragged cytoplasm. A neutrophil leukocytosis is seen often in reaction to secondary infections, and carries a poor prognosis.[18] Rarely, there is a myeloid leukaemoid reaction, with an extremely high neutrophil count and shift to the left as far as myelocytes or promyelocytes and blast cells.[21]

Eosinophils

The eosinophil count is low during acute malaria, even if the initial count is high in response to helminthic infections. During recovery, there may be an eosinophilia.[21]

Monocytes

The monocyte count is raised; the cells are frequently vacuolated, and erythrophagocytosis and malarial pigment may be seen. The examination of monocytes in a thin blood film is most valuable in diagnosis as malarial pigment persists for several days after the clearance of parasitaemia; pigment remains in bone marrow macrophages for up to 20 weeks after infection.

Disorders of haemostasis in malaria

Platelets

The platelet count is reduced regularly in acute malaria; for example, in 105 Nigerian children with malaria, the mean platelet count was 132×10^9/L, as compared with 234×10^9/L in the same subjects 12 days later after receiving treatment with chloroquine. However, severe thrombocytopenia ($<50 \times 10^9$/L) was observed in only 5%. Platelet survival is reduced to 2–4 days; probable mechanisms include reduced membrane sialic acid leading to rapid clearance, an immune mechanism involving antiplatelet IgG and hypersplenism. There may be some megakaryocyte dysfunction with the release of giant platelets, but usually megakaryocytes are numerous, normal in appearance and actively budding in the bone marrow. Platelet function is enhanced generally, including aggregation induced by ADP, adrenaline, thrombin and thromboxane A_2 (TXA_2).[18,22]

Coagulation

AT III levels are reduced in proportion to the severity of the parasitaemia. PT may be prolonged as a consequence of hepatic dysfunction.

In a small proportion, for example <10% of Thai adults, acute malaria may be complicated by disseminated intravascular coagulation (DIC). The process is triggered by the release of thromboplastin during massive haemolysis, toxic destruction of endothelium and the activation of complement. DIC is reversed usually following active antimalarial therapy: patients may require transfusion with fresh whole blood, or even exchange transfusion; the use of heparin is controversial.[18,21]

Management of severe malarial anaemia

The management of acute malaria and its complications is discussed in Chapter 73. Malarial anaemia generally responds to antimalarial therapy, but is a major cause of morbidity and of mortality. In different series, between 10% and 16% of all deaths in childhood in Africa have been attributed to malarial anaemia, but these are certain to be underestimates.

In the past, there has been far too great a willingness to treat malarial anaemia by blood transfusion. With the advent of HIV in Africa, many thousands of children have been treated successfully for anaemia, but at the cost of developing AIDS later. Even where blood donations are screened for anti-HIV, donors may be in the window between infection and seroconversion, so that more stringent criteria for transfusion must be applied, which will prevent mortality from anaemia but minimize the transmission of HIV.[15,19]

1. Hb >50 g/L with or without respiratory distress: intravenous normal saline in aliquots of 10 mL/kg.
2. Hb 40–50 g/L without respiratory distress: intravenous saline as above, with careful monitoring and reviewing over 48 h.
3. Hb <50 g/L with respiratory distress or impaired consciousness: transfusion of whole blood 20 mL/kg, without a diuretic; with mild distress (nasal flaring) transfuse over 4–6 h; with severe distress, transfuse 10 mL/kg over 1 h and the remaining 10 mL/kg over the next 2–4 h.
4. Hb <40 g/L with or without respiratory distress: transfuse as in (3).

Malaria in pregnancy

There is a reduction in resistance to malaria during pregnancy.[23] The mechanisms of increased susceptibility may include (1) a physiological suppression of cell-mediated immunity, (2) high serum cortisol and oestrogen concentrations, (3) cytoadherence of parasites in the placenta,[24] leading to intense infection within the placenta and extensive placental damage, and (4) a higher risk of mosquito bites during pregnancy.[25] Humoral immunity to malaria is unaltered. The presentation of malaria during pregnancy varies enormously according to the woman's previous exposure and level of acquired immunity to malaria.[25,26]

Women with no or low levels of acquired immunity to malaria, if infected during pregnancy, suffer from severe malaria, frequently complicated by cerebral malaria, renal failure, blackwater fever, profound anaemia and DIC. Women of all ages and parities are affected equally. Maternal and fetal morbidity and mortality are heavy.

In women who live where malaria is stable (hyper- or holoendemic), and who have acquired high levels of immunity to *P. falciparum*, the frequency and density of parasitaemia rise to plateaux early in the second trimester, especially in primigravidae, or women in their second pregnancies to a lesser extent. The densities of parasitaemias do not reach levels seen in early childhood, and the women are generally asymptomatic or have mild symptoms only. However, there is haemolysis and anaemia, seen most commonly in the mid-second trimester and in primigravidae. Compensatory erythroid hyperplasia leads to high demands for folate, demands which are already increased because of pregnancy. The haemolytic process is often complicated by megaloblastic erythropoiesis, and profound anaemia follows.

The frequency of palpable splenomegaly increases during pregnancy in all gravida classes, and a peak spleen rate about double that of non-pregnant women can be reached at around 16 weeks' gestation. Even higher spleen rates (e.g. 70% in Nigeria) are seen in anaemic pregnant women; in Nigeria about 25% of severe anaemias in pregnancy were complicated by HMS (see below) and hypersplenism. About 5% of women in the same series had a severe haemolytic process, which was not controlled by antimalarials but responded to prednisolone and was presumed to be due to an immune process triggered by malaria.[26,27]

The presentation of malaria in pregnancy is intermediate between the two patterns where malaria is unstable (mesoendemic), as for example in Thailand and Zambia.

Patterns of resistance to malaria during pregnancy are further complicated by co-infection with HIV; in Malawi, for example, women attending antenatal clinic for the first time during their present pregnancy were found to be around 30% HIV-infected and more than 40% with malarial parasitaemia. HIV positivity in pregnancy was associated with increased prevalence and density of *P. falciparum* parasitaemia and placental infection, increased incidence of clinical malaria and decreased effectiveness of prophylactic antimalarials, in women of all parities.[28]

The peripheral blood picture of malarial plus folate deficiency anaemia in pregnancy is characterized by great anisocytosis, macrocytosis and polychromasia with or without nucleated red cells, but no poikilocytosis; there is a reticulocytosis; malarial parasites are usually absent or scanty. The white cell count is variable and there may be a myeloid leukaemoid reaction; the expected hypersegmentation of folate deficiency is often masked by a shift to the left. The bone marrow shows megaloblastic changes which may be gross; malarial pigment is present in the macrophages; iron stores tend to be increased unless there is concurrent iron deficiency. Maternal and fetal morbidity and mortality are extremely high (see Anaemia: pathophysiology).

Blood transfusion is indicated only if the patient is in incipient or established cardiac failure, or if the patient is approaching delivery with an Hb <70 g/L.[17] Anaemia responds rapidly in most patients following antimalarial therapy and folic acid; the haematocrit tends not to rise, but remains steady in patients with HMS;[26] in the few patients with immune haemolysis the haematocrit rises rapidly following treatment with prednisolone 60 mg/day for 1 week, 45 mg/day for 1 week and 30 mg/day maintenance in three divided doses, up to about 36 weeks' gestation.[27]

Malaria and anaemia can be effectively prevented by the administration of prophylactic antimalarials and folic acid supplements to pregnant women.[26] There are, however, great problems in the delivery of effective regimens to more than the few who attend antenatal clinics regularly: malaria chemoprophylaxis (Maloprim) has been given by traditional birth attendants in The Gambia, with beneficial effects on parasite rates, the haematocrit and birthweight, especially in primigravidae and also grandes multigravidae.[29]

Administration of sulfadoxine/pyrimethamine (Fansidar®) in two or more intermittent doses from first attendance to the third trimester has the advantages of practicality and cost-effectiveness, and results in higher maternal Hb, decreased placental malaria and decreased low birth weight. This strategy should be applicable in remote communities.[30]

The efficacy of insecticide-impregnated bed nets (IIBN) (see Chapter 73) during pregnancy, alone or in combination with prophylactics, in the reduction of malaria and its consequences for mothers and infants, needs research in the field, as reports so far are contradictory.

The prevention of malaria in pregnancy in endemic areas has focused on first (or second) pregnancies as being the worst affected. With the advent of HIV, however, more attention should be given to multigravidae as well, because HIV infection decreases the ability to control malaria in women of all parities, and it is possible that malaria infection may also increase vertical transmission of HIV.[31]

Hyperreactive malarious splenomegaly

In malarious areas a varying proportion of children (and non-immune adult visitors) have splenomegaly associated with intermittent parasitaemia, and regressing with the gradual acquisition of relative immunity. In some, however, the spleen does not regress but enlarges progressively with increasing age. This condition is known as hyperreactive malarious splenomegaly (HMS) (see also Chapter 73), and was previously called the tropical splenomegaly syndrome (TSS). Its defining features are: (1) residence in a malarious area; (2) chronic splenomegaly, often massive; (3) serum IgM elevated to more than 2 standard deviations above the local reference mean; (4) high malarial antibody titres; (5) hepatic sinusoidal lymphocytosis; and (6) clinical and immunological response to long-term antimalarial prophylaxis.[32,33]

Pathophysiology

Central to the pathophysiology of HMS is the overproduction of IgM in response to recurrent infection by *P. falciparum*, *P. malariae* or *P. vivax*. There is familial and ethnic clustering suggesting a genetic basis. It is seen most often in groups who have migrated relatively recently to endemic malarial areas, and so are likely to lack genetic polymorphisms which confer partial protection against malaria. Such polymorphisms could include HLA-linked genetically controlled processing of malarial antigens and antibody production.[34,35] During acute malaria, there is transient production of IgM lymphocytotoxic antibodies which are specific for activated suppressor T lymphocytes (CD8+), which normally downregulate synthesis of IgM by B cells. It has been shown in Indonesian patients with HMS that these lymphocytotoxic antibodies persist, with consequent imbalance between helper T cells (CD4+) which are normal, and suppressor T cells which are greatly reduced, so that there is a lack of inhibition of B cell activity.[36] Recurrent antigenic and mitogenic stimuli from malaria to the B cells result in gross overproduction of polyclonal IgM, of which only a small part has antimalarial specificity. The IgM forms aggregates (cryoglobulins) and immune complexes. These are phagocytosed by the RES, including the macrophages of the liver (Kupffer cells), spleen and bone marrow, stimulating macrophage hyperplasia and T cell proliferation, seen as hepatic sinusoidal infiltration and the lymphocytosis of spleen and bone marrow. Overproduction of IgM and its complexes precedes and is the stimulus to progressive and eventual massive splenomegaly and hepatomegaly. Pancytopenia of variable severity results from hypersplenism. The apparent anaemia is caused mainly by the expansion of plasma volume (up to 130 mL/kg) and sequestration of up to one-third of the total red cells in the spleen (see Figure 13.1D). There is haemolysis of cells pooled in the spleen, and erythrophagocytosis mediated by the adsorption of immune complexes; haemolytic crises are associated with pregnancy and infection. Patients are liable to frequent and prolonged infections related to neutropenia and disturbed immune function.[37,38]

Distribution and clinical presentation

HMS has been described in Africa (Nigeria, Uganda, Kenya and Zambia), western Asia (Aden), the Indian subcontinent (Bengal, Sri Lanka), South-east Asia (Vietnam, Thailand, Indonesia), Oceania (Papua New Guinea) and South America (Amazon basin). High incidences are reported in the Fulani in northern Nigeria, Rwandan immigrants in Uganda, the Angas of Upper Watut Valley and the related Menya of Tauri Valley (Papua New Guinea), and the Yanomani in Venezuela. Prevalence rates of over 50% have been reported only in the Papua New Guinea groups and the Indonesians of the island of Flores.[32-38]

Presentation is usually in young to middle-aged adults, but can occur as early as 8 years of age and in old age. In some series women have outnumbered men, but in others there is an equal sex incidence. Patients complain most commonly of abdominal swelling and a dragging feeling or pain from the enlarged spleen. The spleen may be huge, reaching to the left iliac fossa and across the midline. There is usually hepatomegaly. Lymphadenopathy is not a feature.[33,36]

Haematology

The anaemia is generally moderate, but may be severe during pregnancy or following acute infections; it is normocytic, but there may be macrocytosis and polychromasia with a reticulocytosis. The total WBC is generally low, with granulocytopenia. However, in West Africa in about 10% of patients, there is a lymphocytosis which may mimic chronic lymphocytic leukaemia (CLL). There is a mild thrombocytopenia, but not usually sufficient to lead to haemorrhage. Malarial parasites are absent as a rule. Sickle cell trait confers significant but partial protection against the development of HMS.

The bone marrow shows hyperactivity of erythroid, granulocyte and megakaryocyte lines. Megaloblastic changes are rare. An excess of normal lymphocytes is observed in West African patients. The frequency of depleted iron stores is not different from that of the population. Malaria pigment is not seen.[33,37]

Diagnosis

The defining feature is excessively high serum IgM. When there is a leukaemoid reaction, HMS may be distinguished from CLL by (1) the absence of lymphadenopathy, (2) the high serum IgM, whereas levels are lower than normal in CLL except when there is a monoclonal paraprotein, (3) normal lymphocyte transformation with phytohaemagglutinin (PHA), whereas transformation is reduced in CLL, (4) polyclonal lymphoproliferation and polyclonal Ig heavy chain gene rearrangement, as compared with monoclonal proliferation in CLL.[32,33,37,39]

Prognosis

The condition appears benign in most patients when seen first, but there is a high mortality without treatment; for example 46% over 15 years rising to nearly 90% in those with gross splenomegaly in the Upper Watut Valley. Death is usually from acute bacterial or other overwhelming infections.[38]

Some patients show a haematological and immune status suggestive of transition to a clonal lymphoproliferation, sometimes called 'African CLL' or 'tropical splenic lymphoma' (see 'Chronic lymphocytic leukaemia'). It is probable that the polyclonal expansion of B lymphocytes provides targets for somatic mutation, followed by selection of a single clone. A previous suggestion that 'African CLL' was splenic lymphoma with villous lymphocytes (SLVL) has not been supported as the cells have an origin from naive B cells:[40] surface markers of cells from a small series of Zambian patients are consistent with B cell prolymphocytic leukaemia.[41] Multicentre studies into the nature of HMS and its transition to malignancy are much needed.

Management

The treatment of choice is the administration of antimalarial chemoprophylaxis for life. The choice of prophylactic depends on the local pattern of sensitivity of the malarial parasites: proguanil has been the most effective agent in tropical Africa. After about 3 months of treatment, there is a steady decrease in splenomegaly over many months and a return of all immunological and haematological parameters to normal. Failure of treatment suggests non-compliance, ineffectiveness of the prescribed antimalarial prophylactic, malignant transformation or incorrect diagnosis. Non-compliance leads to relapse, morbidity and increased mortality.

There is no place for splenectomy, despite the immediate improvement it causes, because of high operative and later mortality, the transfer of disease from splenomegaly to hepatomegaly, and the need in any case for lifelong antimalarial prophylaxis to prevent acute malaria.[33,37]

Other protozoa

Visceral leishmaniasis

Infection by *Leishmania donovani* (see also Chapter 77) is followed by hyperplasia of macrophages and lymphocytes, massive production of IgG and progressive hepatosplenomegaly (kala-azar). The size of the spleen is related directly to the duration of infection and to the severity of pancytopenia.[21,42] Anaemia is due primarily to hypersplenism (expansion of plasma volume, haemodilution, splenic sequestration and haemolysis) (see Figure 13.1D). There are plasma cold anti-I agglutinins, the adsorption of IgG by red cells and the fixation of complement, but no convincing evidence that autoimmune haemolysis contributes to the severity of anaemia in kala-azar.[43] Dyserythropoiesis and ineffective erythropoiesis have a role in the causation of anaemia in at least some patients.[44] In India about half of patients are reported to have moderate to severe megaloblastosis, due to folate deficiency secondary to increased demands from haemolysis.[45] Pancytopenia is particularly severe in subjects who are also infected by HIV.

In the early stages there may be leukocytosis with a shift to the left, but neutropenia becomes increasingly severe with advancing disease. Neutrophil function has been reported to be normal by some, but Italian workers have reported reduced phagocytic and bactericidal activity.[46] Neutropenia may become profound: children in particular are liable to secondary bacterial infections, or the development of cancrum oris. The eosinophil count is reduced; lymphocyte and monocyte counts are raised and occasionally there may be leukaemoid reactions.[21]

Platelets are sequestered in the spleen and platelet survival is short: thrombocytopenia may be sufficiently severe to cause mucosal bleeding but cutaneous purpura is unusual. Hepatic dysfunction can lead to hypoprothrombinaemia with prolonged coagulation time and PT. There is increased fibrinolytic activity and reduced fibrinogen concentration in some patients with advanced disease.[21] Immune complex-mediated vasculitis and DIC have been reported from Sudan.[47]

The bone marrow is usually hyperplastic and often megaloblastic, with increased erythroid, granulocytic and megakaryocytic activity; lymphocytes and plasma cells are numerous, as are macrophages, many of which contain Leishman–Donovan bodies. In long-standing chronic kala-azar there may be bone marrow hypoplasia and fibrosis; gelatinous transformation of bone marrow has been described in one patient.[48] Pure red cell aplasia has been reported, which could have been due to coincidental infection by parvovirus B19.[49]

Successful treatment of leishmaniasis is followed by regression of the spleen and a return to haematological normality over 9 months following cure. The Hb response may be delayed due to the anaemia of chronic disorder (see below).[50,51]

Trypanosomiasis

African trypanosomiasis (see also Chapters 75 and 76) is accompanied by a haemolytic anaemia, which is usually moderate but may be severe.[21] Haemolysis has several mechanisms: (1) trypanosomes release haemolysins, which enable the parasites to utilize haem and other nutrients from the red cells; (2) there is adsorption of IgM immune complexes on to red cells with fixation of complement, and the sensitized red cells are phagocytosed throughout the RES; and (3) there is hypersplenism. There is a moderate leukocytosis, with raised lymphocyte and monocyte counts, but a neutropenia from hypersplenism. Thrombocytopenia is usual during acute infections, and may be profound due to hypersplenism. With *Trypanosoma brucei rhodesiense* infections there is, in addition, platelet aggregation and destruction, and in some patients DIC.

In infections with *T. cruzi* (American trypanosomiasis, Chagas' disease) there may be a normocytic anaemia, leukocytosis, lymphocytosis and hypoprothrombinaemia.

Toxoplasmosis

There is a high rate of transmission of *Toxoplasma gondii* in childhood in the developing countries, causing only mild disease generally; some patients may have a persistent lymphocytosis with atypical mononuclear cells like glandular fever cells and a thrombocytopenia.[21] Congenital toxoplasmosis is rare as women are almost invariably immune. Severe and congenital toxoplasmosis may be seen more commonly as a result of the AIDS pandemic.

Amoebiasis

Patients with chronic disease have a hypochromic microcytic anaemia as a result of either chronic blood loss and iron deficiency, and/or the anaemia of chronic disorders. Neutrophil leukocytosis, sometimes amounting to a leukaemoid reaction, is associated with perforation of the bowel, peritonitis, secondary bacterial infections and amoebic liver abscesses. Hepatic disease results in prolonged PT and excessively high serum vitamin B_{12} levels.

Giardiasis

Acute diarrhoea due to *Giardia lamblia* causes a malabsorption of folate, whereas about half of the patients with chronic infections have impaired absorption of vitamin B_{12} which is multifactorial, including damage to ileal receptors, utilization of the vitamin by the parasite, and bacterial overgrowth of the bowel.[21]

Haemoglobinopathies

The inherited disorders of haemoglobin synthesis, the haemoglobinopathies, form by far the largest group of single-gene disorders in the world population, and also the largest group of genetically determined anaemias. There are hundreds of millions of carriers, and each year 200 000–300 000 severely affected homozygotes or compound heterozygotes are born.[52,53]

In many of the developing countries, where there is still a very high mortality from infection and malnutrition in the first years of life, these conditions are not yet recognized as important public health problems. However, once economic conditions improve and the infant death rates fall, the genetic disorders of haemoglobin will start to place a major burden on the health services. They occur most frequently in Asia, Africa and the Mediterranean region and in the immigrant population from these areas, but can be encountered in every ethnic group.

Normal human haemoglobins

The oxygen-carrying pigment in the RBC of vertebrates is haemoglobin, a globular protein molecule (molecular weight 64 450), made up of four subunits (Figure 13.4). Each subunit contains a haem moiety (iron-containing porphyrin) conjugated to a polypeptide (globin) chain. The four polypeptide chains consist of two identical pairs each of over 140 amino acids. One pair belong to the α family (α or ζ chains) and other to the β family (β, γ, δ or

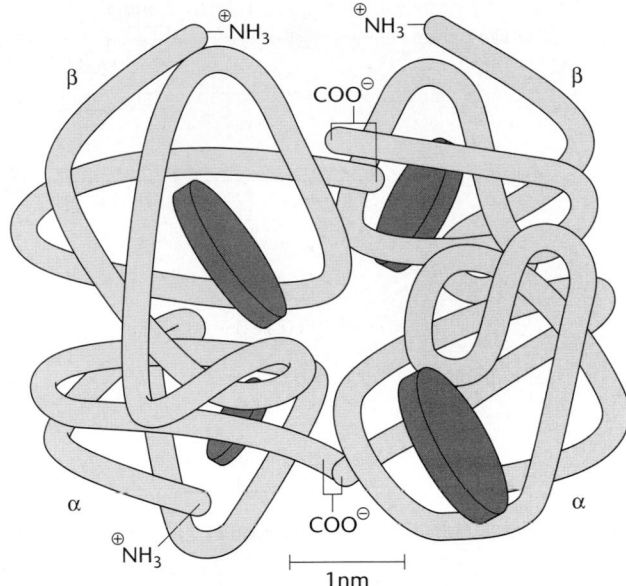

Figure 13.4 The structure of haemoglobin. Diagrammatic representation of adult haemoglobin (HbA) showing four subunits. There are two α and two β polypeptide chains, each containing a haem moiety, represented by disks.

ε chains). The productions of the α and β families are controlled by gene clusters on chromosome 16 and chromosome 11, respectively (Figure 13.5).

The embryonic haemoglobins consist of Hb Gower 1 ($\zeta_2\varepsilon_2$), Hb Portland ($\zeta_2\gamma_2$) and Hb Gower 2 ($\alpha_2\varepsilon_2$). They are produced in the yolk sac before the tenth week of embryonic–fetal life. Fetal haemoglobin (HbF) is $\alpha_2\gamma_2$: it has a higher oxygen affinity than the adult haemoglobin and hence allows efficient extraction of oxygen from the maternal circulation. It is produced by the liver and spleen from about the 10th week of fetal life and declines from about the 30th week to reach the adult level by 1–2 years of age (see Table 13.2). In certain pathological conditions, the embryonic and fetal globin chain synthesis persists to a later period.

In the adult, two types of haemoglobin are present – HbA and HbA_2 – constituting 95% and 1–3% respectively. HbA is composed of two α and two β chains ($\alpha_2\beta_2$), and HbA_2 of two a and two γ chains ($\alpha_2\gamma_2$). The α chain consists of 141 amino acid residues, and the β chain contains 146 amino acid residues. The γ chain also has 146 amino acids but 10 individual residues differ from those in the β chains. HbA is detectable at the eleventh week of fetal life. By the 18th week of gestation, it comprises approximately 8%. It replaces HbF during late gestation and infancy, reaching adult levels by 6 months of age. HbA_2 begins to appear at birth and increases over the 2 years of life. Because it is present in such low concentrations, it is of no practical use as an oxygen carrier. However, it is a useful diagnostic tool for evaluating patients with certain types of thalassaemia.

Inherited disorders of haemoglobin synthesis

The mutations leading to abnormalities of haemoglobin synthesis may result from either a deletion of a gene or part of the gene, as

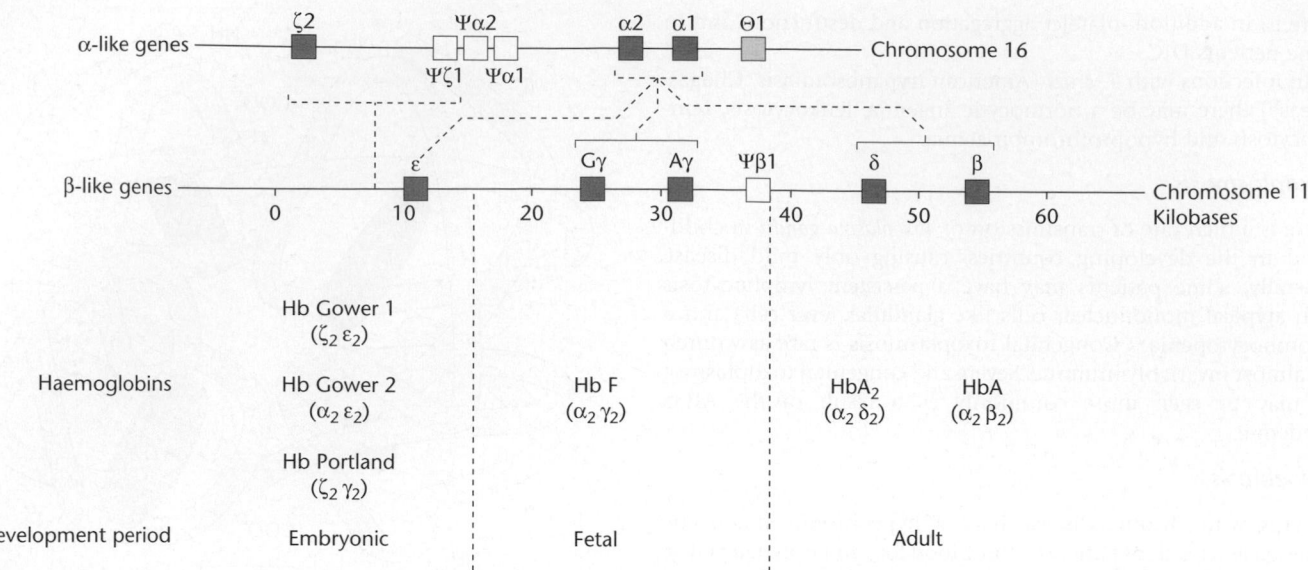

Figure 13.5 Chromosomal organization of the globin genes and their expression during development. The solid boxes indicate functional globin genes, whereas the open boxes indicate pseudo-genes. The scale of the depicted chromosomal segment is in kilobases of DNA (Kb). The switch from the embryonic to fetal haemoglobin occurs between 6 and 10 weeks' gestation, and the switch from the fetal to adult haemoglobin occurs at about the time of birth. (Reproduced with the permission of the publishers, from Nathan DG, Oski FA, eds. *Hematology of Infancy and Childhood,* 4th edn. Philadelphia: WB Saunders; 1993.)

seen in most α thalassaemias, or may result in a single base change (point mutation), as seen in most β thalassaemias. In point mutations there is a deletion, substitution or insertion of one or two bases in the nucleotide strand of the gene. The haemoglobinopathies are inherited in a single Mendelian codominant fashion: the carriers are relatively symptom free and the homozygotes manifest the disease.

The main genetic disorders of haemoglobin productions are due to: (1) either a complete absence or reduced production of α or β polypeptides chains, the thalassaemias, or (2) a structural defect of the polypeptide chains, the haemoglobin variants, leading to instability of the molecule or abnormal oxygen transport. In addition, there is a harmless group of mutations which interfere with the normal switching of fetal to adult haemoglobin production, called hereditary persistence of fetal haemoglobin (HPFH).

The common thalassaemias are the β thalassaemias, when there is a defective rate of synthesis of β chains, and the α thalassaemias, when there is defective synthesis of α chains. Of the structural defects, variants of the β chain are the most common and clinically important: they include HbS, HbC, HbD, HbE and HbO, which occur in certain populations at polymorphic frequencies. These populations all live in regions where *P. falciparum* malaria is or was endemic or are migrant populations from these areas. On geographical evidence, and in some instances demographic and parasitological evidence as well, it is thought that heterozygous inheritance of these abnormalities of haemoglobin synthesis renders the red cell less favourable than normal for the development of malarial parasites. Carriers enjoy, therefore, some protection against severe malaria, and hence survival and genetic advantages, which balance in the population the genetic disadvantages arising from the ill health and early deaths in the homozygotes.[35,52,53]

Thalassaemia syndromes

The thalassaemias are a heterogeneous group of disorders of haemoglobin synthesis, all of which result from an absent or a reduced rate of production of one or more of the globin chains. They are divided into α, β, δβ or γδβ thalassaemias according to which globin is deficient. When globin chains are not synthesized at all, they are designated as α^0 or β^0 thalassaemias, and when globin chains are produced at a reduced rate, α^+ or β^+ thalassaemias. δβ and γδβ thalassaemias are always characterized by absence of chain synthesis: thus they are $(\delta\beta)^0$ and $(\gamma\delta\beta)^0$ thalassaemias.

Because thalassaemias occur in populations in which structural haemoglobin variants are also common, it is not unusual for an individual to receive a thalassaemia gene from one parent and a gene for a structural variant from the other. Furthermore, both α and β thalassaemia occur commonly in some countries, and hence individuals may receive genes for both types. These different interactions produce an extremely complex and clinically diverse series of genetic disorders, which range in severity from death in utero to extremely mild, symptomless hypochromic anaemia.

Clinically thalassaemias are classified according to their severity into major, intermedia and minor forms. Thalassaemia major is a severe transfusion-dependent disorder. Thalassaemias intermedia are characterized by anaemia and splenomegaly but not so severe as to require regular blood transfusions. Thalassaemia minor is a symptomless carrier state.

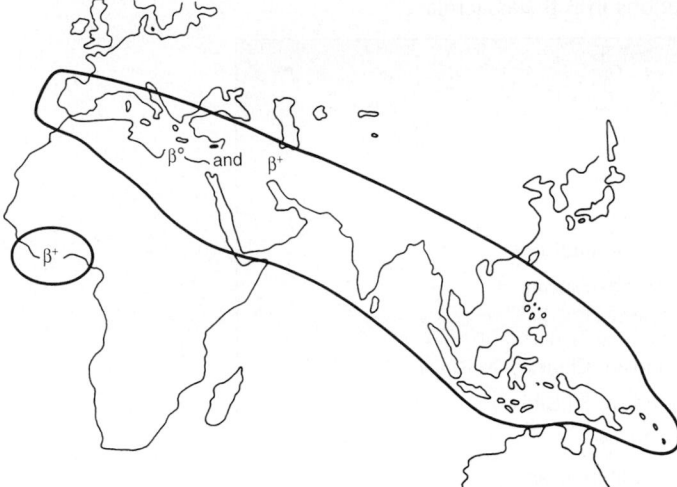

Figure 13.6 Areas of the Old World where β thalassaemias reach polymorphic frequencies. (Reproduced with permission of the publishers, from Fleming AF. In: Strickland GT, ed. *Hunter's Tropical Medicine*, 7th edn. Philadelphia: WB Saunders; 1991:36–64.)

The β thalassaemias

The β thalassaemias are the most important types of thalassaemia because they are so common and produce severe anaemia in their homozygous and compound heterozygous states. They occur commonly in a broad belt ranging from the Mediterranean and parts of North and West Africa through the Middle East and the Indian subcontinent to South-east Asia (Figure 13.6). The disease is particularly common in South-east Asia, where it occurs in a line starting in southern China and stretching down through Thailand, the Malay Peninsula and Indonesia to the Pacific islands.

The carrier frequency for various forms of the disease ranges between 2% and 30%. About 3% of the world's population, or over 150 million individuals, mostly in Asia, are carriers. Over 50 000 infants are born annually with β thalassaemias major. In many of these regions β thalassaemia is a major public health problem and a drain on medical resources.

Molecular pathology

The molecular lesions responsible for the defective synthesis of the β chains are extremely heterogeneous: nearly 200 different mutations, mostly point mutations, can produce the clinical phenotype of β thalassaemia but only about 20 alleles account for 90% of all β thalassaemia genes (Table 13.13).[35,52–54]

Pathophysiology

The basic molecular defect in β thalassaemia results in absent or reduced β chain production: α chain synthesis proceeds at the normal rate and hence there is an excess of α chains (Figure 13.7). In the absence of their partner β chains, α chains are unstable and precipitate in the red cell precursors, giving rise to large intracellular inclusions, demonstrable on methyl violet staining of the peripheral blood of splenectomized patients. In non-splenectomized individuals, the inclusions are difficult to demonstrate as they are removed during passage of RBC through the splenic sinusoids, generating fragments and teardrops. The inclusions have several detrimental effects on red cells. They interfere with the division of RBC precursors causing ineffective erythropoiesis: they damage the cell membrane and contribute to the intramedullary death of red cells; and they disturb red cell deformability, interfering with the egress of cells from the bone marrow spaces. Red cells which do mature and enter the circulation contain α chain inclusions, which interfere with their passage through the microcirculation particularly in the spleen, leading to their premature destruction. Thus the anaemia of β thalassaemia results from both ineffective erythropoiesis and a shortened red cell survival.

The anaemia is a stimulus for erythropoietin production, which causes a massive expansion of the bone marrow and leads to serious deformities of the skull and long bones. Because the spleen is constantly bombarded with abnormal red cells, it hypertrophies and the resulting splenomegaly gives rise to a massive increase of the plasma volume, which exacerbates an already severe degree of anaemia.

Normally HbF production decreases to a low level over the first 6 months of postuterine life. However, some adult red cells precursors retain the ability to produce a small number of γ chains. Because the latter can combine with excess α chains to form HbF, cells which make relatively more γ chains in the bone marrow of β thalassaemia are partially protected against the deleterious effects of α chain precipitation. Hence the red cell precursors which produce HbF are selected in the marrow, and there are relatively large amounts of HbF in the peripheral blood RBC. Because δ chain synthesis is unaffected the disorder is characterized by increased HbA$_2$ production.

β Thalassaemia major

Clinical features

Patients with most severe forms of β thalassaemia present within the first year of life with a failure to thrive, poor feeding, intermittent fever and intercurrent infections. At this stage the affected infant is pale with splenomegaly. There are no other specific clinical signs and the diagnosis depends on the haematology.

If the anaemia is not corrected the child will die of complications due to anaemia by the age of 5 years (Figure 13.8). If the anaemia is corrected with blood transfusions the erythropoietic drive is shut off, growth and development are normal and bone deformities do not occur. However, each unit of blood contains 200 mg of iron; with regular transfusions there is a steady accumulation of iron in the liver, endocrine glands and myocardium. Thus, although well-transfused thalassaemic children grow and develop normally until puberty, they die of iron overload unless steps are taken to remove iron.

The clinical picture in children who are inadequately transfused is of growth retardation, progressive splenomegaly and hypersplenism, which causes a worsening of the anaemia, sometimes associated with thrombocytopenia and a bleeding tendency (Figures 13.7, 13.9). Because of the bone marrow expansion, there are deformities of the skull, marked bossing and overgrowth of the zygomata, giving rise to the classical facies of β thalassaemia (Figure 13.10). Expansion of medullary cavities by bone marrow and thinning of cortical bone in bones of arms, hands,

Table 13.13 Some examples of point mutations in β thalassaemia

Mutant class	Genotype	Origin
I. NON-FUNCTIONAL mRNA		
(a) Nonsense mutants		
Codon 17 (A–T)	β⁰	Chinese
Codon 15 (G–A)	β⁰	Indian
Codon 37 (G–A)	β⁰	Saudi Arabian
Codon 39 (C–T)	β⁰	Mediterranean
(b) Frameshift mutants		
Codon 41/42	β⁰	Indian, Chinese, Sri Lanka
Codon 8/9	β⁰	Indian, Sri Lanka
Codons 71/72	β⁰	Chinese
Codon 6	β⁰	Mediterranean
II. RNA PROCESSING MUTATIONS		
(a) Splice junction alteration		
IVS1–1 (G–A)	β⁺	Mediterranean
IVS1–1 (G–T)	β⁰	Indian, Chinese
IVS1–5 (G–C)	β⁺	Indians, Sri Lanka, Chinese, Mediterranean
IVS2–1 (G–A)	β⁰	American black, Mediterranean
(b) Creation of new splice signals in IVS		
IVS1–110 (G–A)	β⁺	Mediterranean
IVS2–654 (C–T)	β⁰	Chinese
(c) Coding region substitution after the RNA processing		
Codon 26 (G–A)	HbE	SE Asian, Sri Lanka
Codon 24 (T–A)	β⁺	American black
III. TRANSCRIPTIONAL MUTATIONS		
–88 C–T	β⁺	Indian
–31 A–G	β⁺	Japanese
–28 A–G	β⁺	Chinese
IV. RNA CLEAVAGE = POLYADENYLATION MUTANTS		
AATAAA-AACAAA	β⁺	American black
V. CAP SITE MUTATIONS		
+1 A–C	β⁺	Indian
VI. UNSTABLE GLOBINS DUE TO MISSENSE MUTATIONS		
Codon 112	β⁺	European
Codon 10	β⁺	Japanese

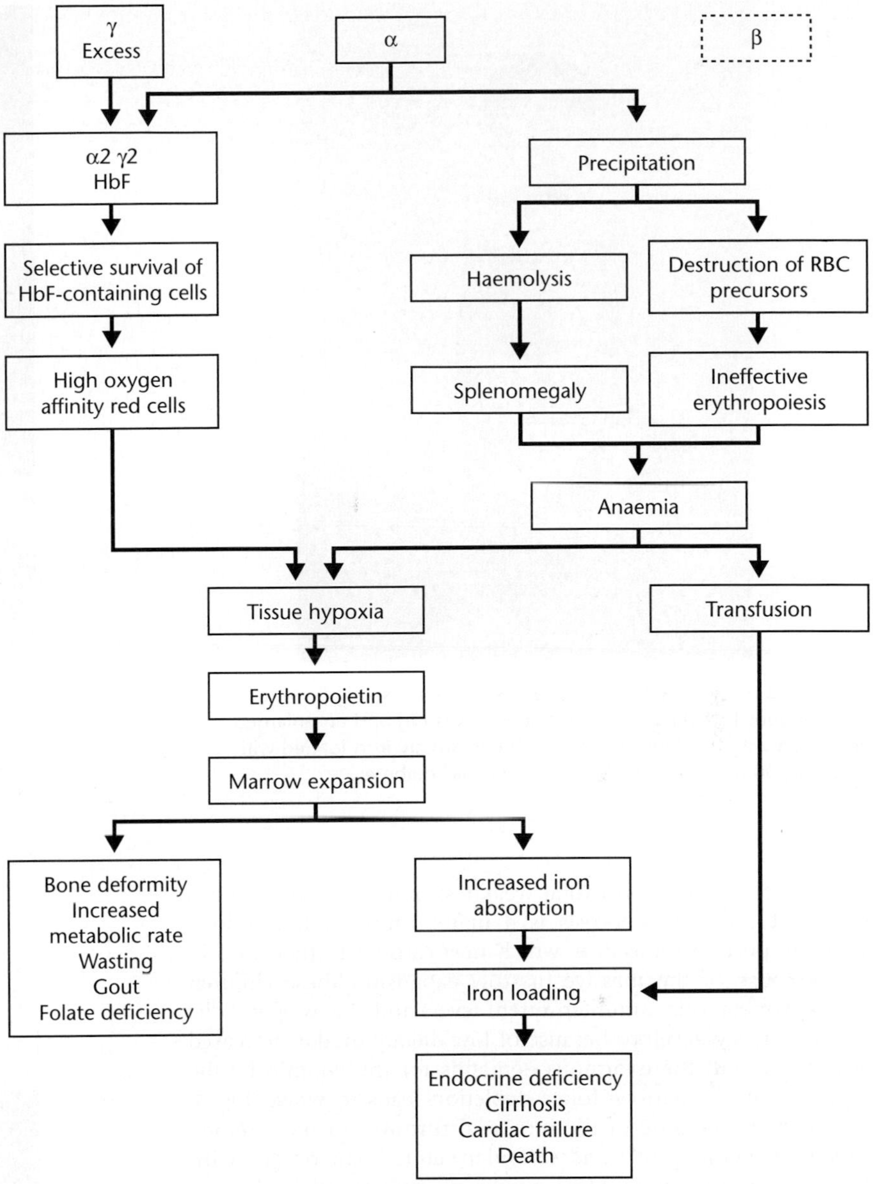

γ
Excess
α
β
α2 γ2
HbF
Precipitation
Selective survival of
HbF-containing cells
Haemolysis
Destruction of RBC
precursors
High oxygen
affinity red cells
Splenomegaly
Ineffective
erythropoiesis
Anaemia
Tissue hypoxia
Transfusion
Erythropoietin
Marrow expansion
Bone deformity
Increased
metabolic rate
Wasting
Gout
Folate deficiency
Increased iron
absorption
Iron loading
Endocrine deficiency
Cirrhosis
Cardiac failure
Death

Figure 13.7 The pathophysiology of β thalassaemia.

100
80
60
40
20
0
Survival (%)
0
5
10
15
20
25
30
Age (years)
Transfusion + Desferal
Transfusion only
No treatment

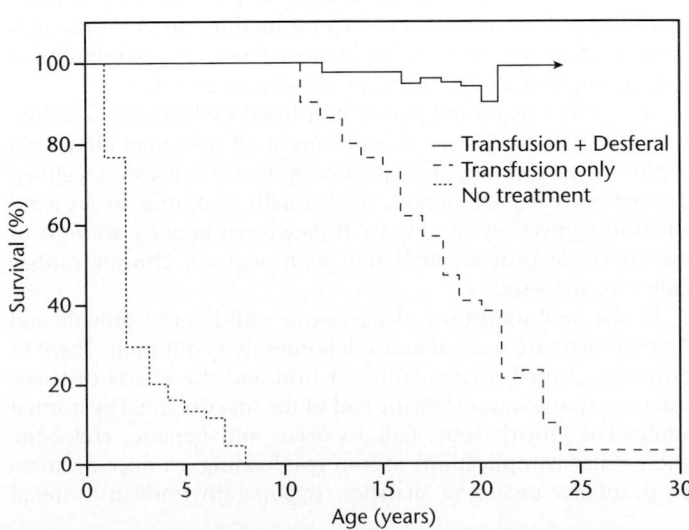

Figure 13.8 The prognosis of patients with β thalassaemia major.

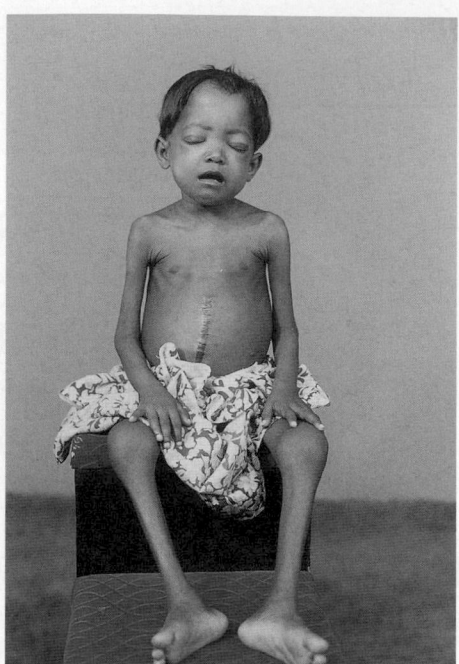

Figure 13.9 Typical features of a poorly transfused child with homozygous β thalassaemia, with severe wasting and an enlarged abdomen with a splenectomy scar. She is grossly iron loaded with a liver iron 30 mg/dry weight of liver, and has diabetes.

legs and feet lead to structural weakness and recurrent fractures (Figure 13.11). Osteoporosis is a major cause of morbidity.[55] They are prone to infection, which may cause a further drop in Hb. Because of the massive marrow expansion these children are hypermetabolic, run intermittent fevers and lose weight. Folic acid deficiency develops because of low dietary intake, decreased absorption and the enormous demands for the vitamin by the expanded bone marrow: folate depletion leads to worsening of the anaemia. Because of the increased turnover of red cell precursors, hyperuricaemia and secondary gout occur occasionally. If these unfortunate children survive to puberty, they develop in addition the complications of iron loading: some of the iron accumulation results from an increased rate of gastrointestinal iron absorption as well as from transfused blood.

The prognosis for the poorly transfused thalassaemic children is bad. If they receive no transfusions at all they may die within the first 2 years; if they are kept alive by a low transfusion regimen throughout early childhood, they usually succumb to an overwhelming infection by 10 years. If they reach puberty, they die of the effects of iron accumulation with acute or chronic cardiac failure or diabetes.

In the well-transfused thalassaemic child, early growth and development are normal and splenomegaly is minimal. There is, however, gradual accumulation of iron and the effects of tissue siderosis start to appear by the end of the first decade. The normal adolescent growth spurt fails to occur and hepatic, endocrine and cardiac complications of iron overloading produce a variety of problems including diabetes, hypoparathyroidism, adrenal

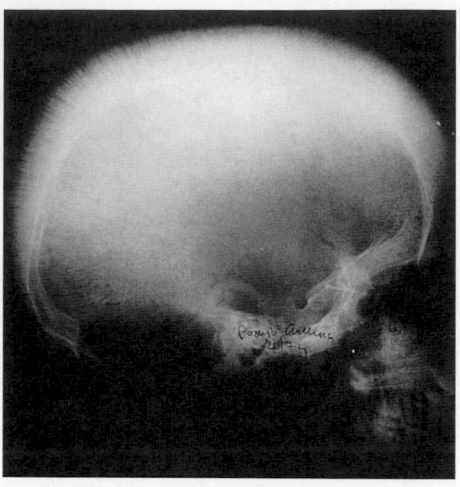

A

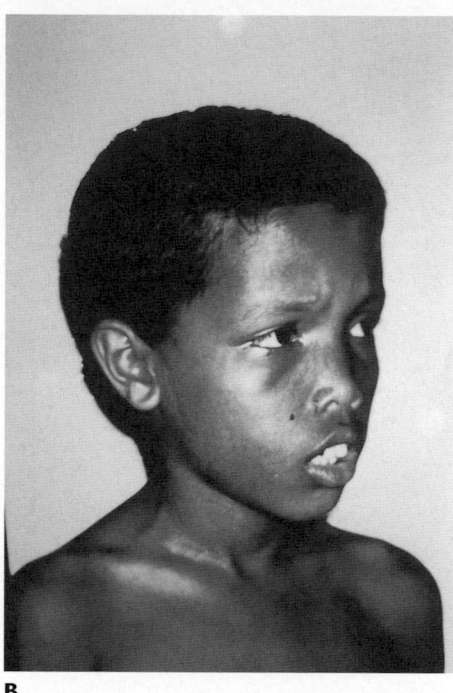

B

Figure 13.10 (A) Skull radiograph in β thalassaemia major, showing hair-on-end appearance which is the result of massive expansion of the bone marrow cavity. (B) Thalassaemia facies (with permission of the patient).

insufficiency and progressive liver failure. Secondary sexual development is delayed, or does not occur at all. The short stature and lack of sexual development may lead to serious psychological problems. By far the commonest cause of death, which usually occurs towards the end of the second or early in the third decade, is progressive cardiac damage. Patients die ultimately either from protracted cardiac failure or suddenly from an acute arrhythmia. The use of intensive chelation may prevent or delay this distressing termination (Figure 13.8).

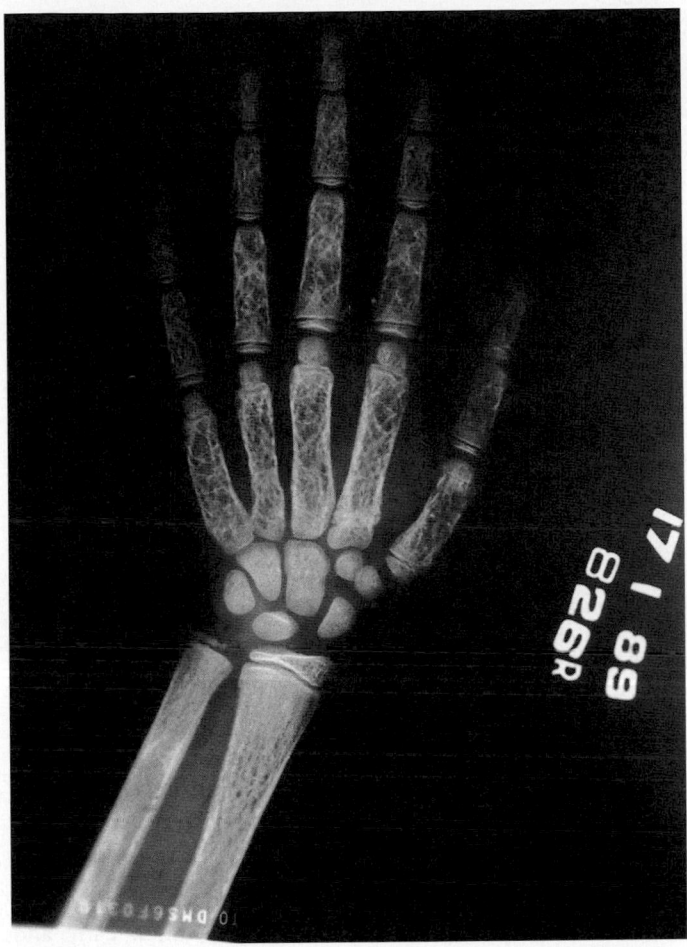

Figure 13.11 X-ray of the hand of a homozygous β thalassaemia patient showing the lace-like appearance, and the thinning of cortical bone.

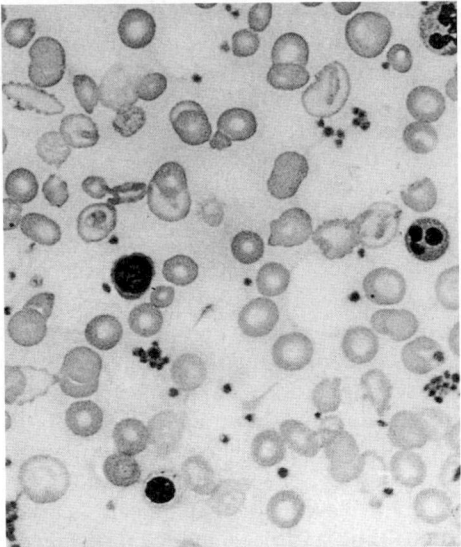

Figure 13.12 Peripheral blood film in β thalassaemia major, showing gross hypochromia, numerous target cells and nucleated red cells.

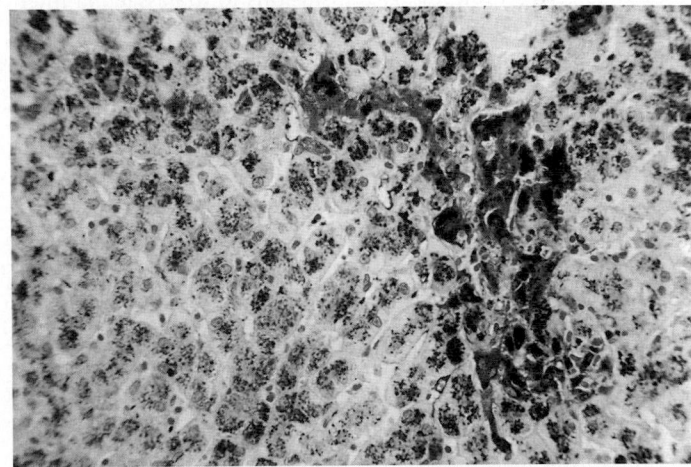

Figure 13.13 Histological appearance of the liver in homozygous β thalassaemia showing gross iron deposition.

Haematological changes

There is always a severe anaemia and the Hb value on presentation ranges from 20 to 80 g/L. The mean cell Hb (MCH) and the MCV are reduced (MCH 12–18 pg; MCV 50–60 fL). RBC show variation in size (anisocytosis) with both microcytes and macrocytes; variations in shape (poikilocytosis) with target cells, teardrops, microspherocytes and fragmented cells (schistocytes); hypochromia; blue-stained red cells (polychromasia), stippling (punctate basophilia) and nucleated RBC (Figure 13.12). In the post-splenectomy film many of the nucleated and mature red cells show ragged inclusions after incubation of blood with methyl violet. The reticulocyte count is slightly elevated. The white cells and platelets are normal, unless there is hypersplenism when they are reduced, or the white cells are raised during infection. Bone marrow shows marked erythroid hyperplasia with a myeloid/erythroid (M/E) ratio of unity or less. Many red cell precursors show ragged inclusions after incubation of the marrow with methyl violet. Serum bilirubin is raised and haptoglobins are absent. Red cell survival is shortened. The serum iron rises progressively and the iron binding capacity is saturated. Plasma ferritin is high and the liver biopsy shows a marked increase in iron in both RES and parenchymal cells (Figure 13.13).

Haemoglobin changes

HbF level is always elevated. In β^0 thalassaemia there is no HbA and the haemoglobin consists of HbF and HbA_2 only. In β^+ thalassaemia some HbA is present, and the level of HbF ranges from 30% to 90% of the total; the HbA_2 level is usually normal.

Management

The management of β thalassaemia major needs a multidisciplinary team, which should include (1) dedicated physicians who give continuity of care, (2) dedicated nurses to allow the critically important relationship to develop with each patient,

(3) other specialists such as cardiologists, endocrinologists, ophthalmologists, orthopaedic surgeons, general surgeons, hepatologists, neurologists, obstetricians and psychologists and (4) social workers.

The principles of management are (1) a regular blood transfusion regimen, (2) the administration of chelating agents to reduce iron overload, (3) splenectomy when hypersplenism develops, (4) folic acid supplementations, 1 mg per day, (5) psychological and financial support, (6) bone marrow transplantation and (7) genetic counselling.

Blood transfusion

The decision to initiate regular transfusions in patients with β thalassaemia may be difficult and should be based on the presence and severity of symptoms and signs of anaemia, including failure of growth and development. Even when the Hb is 70 g/L, if the child has no symptoms of anaemia and is thriving the patient need not be transfused.

It is important to have an accurate diagnosis prior to starting treatment. The clinical and haematological diagnosis should be confirmed by DNA studies whenever possible. This is mainly to distinguish β thalassaemia major from thalassaemia intermedia and to permit prenatal diagnosis in subsequent pregnancies. Countries where facilities for DNA studies are not available embark on regular blood transfusion to all the phenotypical thalassaemics, thus giving unnecessary transfusions to thalassaemia intermedia patients and increasing the financial burden to the country unnecessarily.

The current recommendation for thalassaemia major is to maintain a pre-transfusion Hb concentration at 95–100 g/L. This prevents chronic hypoxaemia, reduces compensatory marrow hyperplasia, promotes normal physical activity and growth, prevents bone changes, hypersplenism and hypervolaemia, and reduces gastrointestinal iron absorption. The post-transfusion Hb should not rise above 155 g/L, as higher Hb levels raise blood viscosity, reduce tissue oxygenation and increase the risk of thrombosis, especially in the presence of other risk factors such as infections, metabolic acidosis, diabetes, or high platelet count following splenectomy. Higher Hb levels also increase blood consumption and accelerate iron overload. This regimen requires blood to be given at 4- to 6-weekly intervals throughout the patient's life.

Unless one gives good-quality and safe blood, patients are exposed to risks of: (1) alloimmunization against donor red cell, platelet and white cell antigens, (2) allergic reactions to plasma and (3) transmission of infections. The aim is to give red cells with the smallest possible amount of white blood cells or plasma. Antibody reactions manifest as fever during or 8 h after transfusions without any other apparent cause. Allergic reactions to plasma show as urticaria during the transfusion. Leukocytes can also transmit leukocyte-borne viruses, including cytomegalovirus (CMV), Epstein–Barr virus (EBV), hepatitis B and C viruses (HBV, HCV) and human T-lymphotropic virus type 1 (HTLV-1). Leukocytes induce graft-versus-host disease and may be immunosuppressive. Therefore, it is best to give packed red cells via leukodepleting filters as this removes 99.9% of the white cells and platelets. An Italian and a Greek study showed that by using filters there was a 90% reduction of febrile illness in thalassaemias. Transmission of HBV, HCV, HIV, HTLV-1, syphilis and malaria are reduced to a minimum through donor selection, donor screening and immunization of the patient against HBV.

The volume of blood to transfuse is calculated according to the patient's weight, Hct of the available blood preparation and the patient's pre-transfusion Hb level. The rate at which blood can be transfused without overloading the circulation depends on the patient's Hb level and cardiovascular status. If there is no cardiac problem, it is acceptable to give 5–7 mL of packed red cells/kg body weight per hour. If cardiac failure is present it is advisable to give 2 mL/kg per hour. Hypertension, convulsions and cerebral haemorrhage have been observed in patients whose Hb is raised rapidly, especially when they were maintained at a very low Hb level.

It is important to evaluate the annual mean Hb level and the annual red cell consumption. The usual red cell consumption for splenectomized patients with a mean Hb of 120 g/L ranges from 100 to 200 mL/kg per year. An unsplenectomized patient may consume 130–240 mL/kg per year. If the consumption of red cells is higher than this, the cause should be identified and corrected. The main causes of increased blood consumption are hypersplenism, red cell incompatibility and poor quality of transfused blood.

Chelation therapy

Regular chelation with desferrioxamine has proved remarkably effective in reducing the iron burden of transfused patients.[54] Cardiac disease is delayed or prevented and life expectancy is significantly extended, but endocrinopathy may develop and persist (Figure 13.8). Unfortunately, effective use of the drug requires devotion to a mechanical pump that slowly infuses the medication into a subcutaneous site (Figure 13.14). Nearly normal concentration of hepatic iron can be maintained with modern regimens of desferrioxamine, and the progression of hepatic fibrosis to cirrhosis can be arrested. There are relatively low prevalences of thyroid, parathyroid and adrenal abnormalities. Early and intensive desferrioxamine therapy increases the incidence of normal sexual maturation, but it apparently does not reverse established abnormalities. Desferrioxamine prevents diabetes mellitus, but does not reverse this complication.

A balance between the effectiveness of desferrioxamine and its toxicity (the later observed primarily in the presence of relatively low body iron burden) can be maintained through regular determination of body iron burden. The serum ferritin concentration, measured 6-monthly, is commonly used to assess the effectiveness of treatment, but this test may lead to errors in the management; many factors influence ferritin levels, such as presence of inflammatory disease, liver disease or vitamin C deficiency. By contrast, the annual or biannual measurement of hepatic stores, whose concentrations are highly correlated with total body iron stores, provides the best quantitative, specific and sensitive method of evaluating iron burden in patients with thalassaemia. Determination of hepatic iron concentration in liver biopsy specimens obtained with ultrasonographic guidance is safe and permits rational adjustments in iron chelating therapy (Figure 13.13).

Chelation therapy should be started as soon as transfusions have deposited enough iron to protect against desferrioxamine toxicity. The current recommendation is to start therapy when serum transferrin is completely saturated, which happens usually after 10–20 transfusions, or when the ferritin level rises above 1000 ng/mL, or at least by the age of 3 years. Administration recommended is by slow subcutaneous infusion via a thin needle

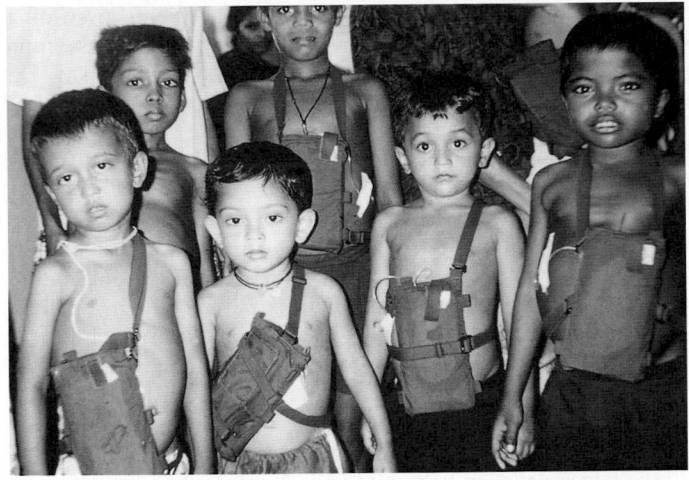

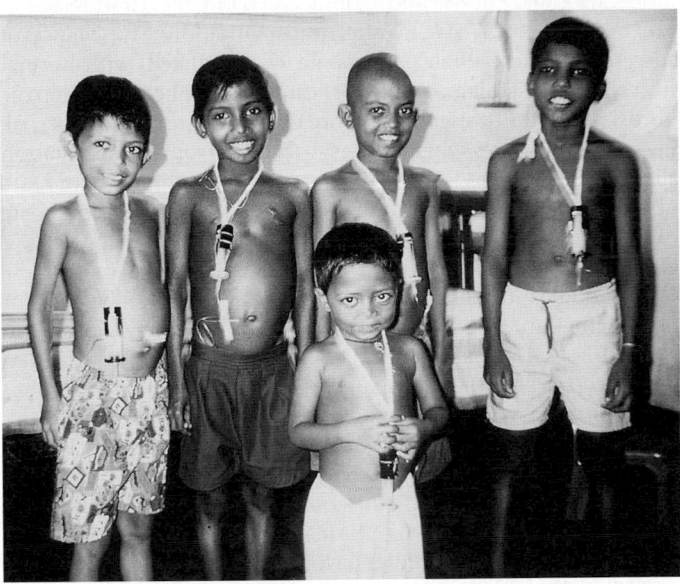

Figure 13.14 (A) A group of thalassaemic patients using infusion pumps (cost US$260 per pump). (B) Using hand-made pumps (cost: 'quarter of a dollar').

inserted subcutaneously, over 8–12 h using an infusion pump, given five to seven times per week at a mean daily dose of 20–50 mg/kg body weight. The dose is adjusted according to hepatic iron value or serum ferritin levels. If the patient's serum ferritin is <2000 ng/mL about 25 mg/kg per day is required; if the ferritin level is 2000–3000 ng/mL about 35 mg/kg per day is required; patients with a higher serum level require up to 55 mg/kg per day.

Continuous infusion of desferrioxamine is more beneficial than periodic infusions, because of the constant removal of toxic free iron which returns to the pretreatment levels within minutes of stopping a continuous intravenous infusion. When intensive chelation is needed an implanted intravenous delivery system (portacath) can be used. Patients who have cardiac problems

secondary to iron overload will benefit with continuous intravenous desferrioxamine as this removes large quantities of iron. It can reverse deteriorating cardiac function by removing the toxic non-transferrin bound iron. The recommended dose is 50–70 mg/kg per day for 5–6 days. Individuals with refractory congestive cardiac failure or hypotension due to cardiac disease are poor candidates for intravenous desferrioxamine.

It is best to avoid desferrioxamine during pregnancy. Treatment can be resumed at full dosage during lactation, as the drug is not absorbed orally.

Desferrioxamine treatment is burdensome and can be painful, and non-compliance is an important and common problem. Compliance requires a constant and secure relationship between doctor, patient and parents, and regular discussion of its importance.

Complications of desferrioxamine administration

Infection with Yersinia enterocolitis is the most important acute risk associated with desferrioxamine treatment. Treatment should be discontinued temporarily in any patient with an acute febrile illness, especially if any or all of the following symptoms are present: sore throat, high fever, acute abdominal pain or severe diarrhoea.

Rashes of more or less intense hyperaemia are common. They may be due to the injection of a concentrated solution of desferrioxamine (usually 500 mg in 5 mL of distilled water for injection). It is better to dilute the preparation further. If the rash persists, adding hydrocortisone to the infusion should be tried. Severe allergic reactions to desferrioxamine are rare.

Desferrioxamine overdose is seen if it is administered in high doses to patients who are not heavily iron loaded. The complications are toxic effects on the eye, including night blindness, reduction in visual fields and reduction of visual acuity. These usually regress when treatment is stopped. High tone deafness is seen particularly in the young; this is usually not reversible. Patients should be questioned frequently regarding the symptoms and formal audiometry and ophthalmological examination should be performed regularly. There may be retardation of growth, with skeletal changes such as short trunk, genu valgum and short stature, which can be reversible with dose reduction.

Other ways to reduce the iron overload

The oral iron chelating drug deferiprone is effective in removing iron, at least in the short term.[56] Long-term studies have suggested that hepatic iron may stabilize at or rise to concentrations associated with hepatic fibrosis, an increased risk of cardiac disease and early death in approximately half of patients. Previously recognized adverse effects of deferiprone include embryo toxicity, teratogenicity, neutropenia and agranulocytosis.

The results of long-term follow-up of the effectiveness of other modes of administration of desferrioxamine are awaited. These include desferrioxamine attached to high-molecular starch, or given in a lipid vehicle permitting slow release.

Role of vitamin C

Iron-loaded patients usually become vitamin C deficient, probably because iron oxidizes the vitamin. When this is the case, administration of vitamin C increases the availability of iron and so increases its toxicity if large doses are taken without simultaneous desferrioxamine infusion. Vitamin C supplements should be started only if the patient is receiving desferrioxamine regularly. The minimum effective dose is 5 mg/kg (50 mg for children under

10 years and 100 mg for children over 10 years) and should be given after starting the desferrioxamine.

Splenectomy

Massive splenomegaly with hypersplenism that causes leucopenia, thrombocytopenia and an increasing transfusion requirement is frequent at a relatively early age in patients on moderate transfusion regimens. Early splenectomy is required. The benefits of splenectomy on iron balance occur if the transfusion requirements exceed 200–250 mL/kg per year of packed red cells when the minimum Hb is maintained at 100 g/L; a spleen which is very large, in the absence of overt hypersplenism, accounts for a relatively large portion of the total blood volume, and its removal often leads to a marked reduction in blood requirement. The surgical risks in experienced hands are minimal. Removal of the spleen may blunt the primary immune response to encapsulated organisms *Diplococcus pneumoniae*, *Haemophilus influenzae* or *Neisseria meningitidis*, and therefore delay of splenectomy until after 4 or 5 years of age is most desirable, so that the child has an opportunity to develop some resistance to these organisms. It advisable to immunize patients with the appropriate vaccines against these organisms about 2 weeks prior to surgery, and to prescribe long-term prophylactic oral penicillin to prevent colonization by strains of pneumococcus not covered by the vaccine, especially in young children. Any illness accompanied by high fever of uncertain aetiology should be treated aggressively with parenteral antibiotics, usually an ampicillin derivative such as amoxicillin, until culture results become known. Splenectomized patients are also more susceptible to malaria, and should receive lifelong prophylaxis when living in endemic regions.

Splenectomy usually results in a transitory or persistent thrombocytosis. As a rule this carries no risk for patients, possibly because it is balanced by a simultaneous reduction in platelet aggregation, but studies in Thailand claim that splenectomized patients have evidence of pulmonary vascular disease due to thrombocytosis. Low-dose prophylactic aspirin may be considered for patients whose platelet count exceeds 800×10^9/L.

Psychological support

The inherited nature of the disease, its appearance during the first year of life, the possibility of physical deformity and the need for continuous punishing treatment have important implications for the child's emotional development and relationships with the rest of the family. An appropriately constituted therapeutic team can help patients to cope successfully with the psychological consequences of their illness, to integrate themselves into society and to see themselves as essentially normal people.

All members of the management team, especially nursing staff, should remain the same for as long as possible and should have a thalassaemia-oriented training. The team should reserve time and space for meeting with both patients and parents before, during or after the visit to the treatment centre. Patients should be helped to understand and accept their illness, so that they can also accept the necessary treatment.

Integration into school constitutes a critical step in psychological development. The ultimate goal is the development into an adult who can actively participate in society. In general, school staff should be advised to avoid limiting the patient's activity or allowing special privileges (unless they are medically indicated)

which could lead to continued dependency. Patients' overriding right not to inform teachers or peers that they have thalassaemia should always be respected.

Patients' and parents' associations help families to feel less isolated, and offer them the help and comfort of others in the same situation. Participation helps patients and families to comply with the treatment regimen.

Bone marrow transplant

Over 1000 patients have received bone marrow transplants in several highly experienced centres.[52–54] The donor should be an HLA-matched sibling, or occasionally a parent. When a patient has an HLA-compatible donor, if transplantation is chosen it should be done as soon as possible. Transplantation from an unrelated donor carries a substantially increased risk, and should be considered only in exceptional circumstances. Graft-versus-host disease (GVHD) is less common in children than in adults: in the largest series in Italy mild GVHD occurred in 10% of cases, moderate GVHD in 8% and serious GVHD in 2%. Graft rejection can occur up to 3–5 years after transplantation. The chance of success is highest when patients are well chelated, with normal liver size and histology, and free of cardiac complications. Hepatic fibrosis and the presence of iron overload are important risk factors. In countries where it is available, marrow transplantation should be considered for all patients with a suitable donor (30–40% of patients in most populations) and who have a low score of these risk factors.

Cord blood transplantation

Cord blood contains haemopoietic stem cells that can be used for transplantation. Preliminary experience is encouraging and all new siblings of thalassaemic patients should have cord blood preserved for possible future use.

Augmentation of fetal haemoglobin synthesis

Several trials have attempted to augment the synthesis of HbF in an effort to ameliorate the severity of thalassaemia.[52–54] Therapy with hydroxyurea, butyric acid compounds and these agents in combination has reduced or eliminated transfusion requirements in some patients. Other studies have reported only a small increase in HbF and total Hb concentrations during the administration of oral hydroxyurea and intravenous or oral butyrates. Erythropoietin has not been proved useful in thalassaemia, either alone or in combination with hydroxyurea. Therapies to increase the synthesis of HbF in β thalassaemia have, with few exceptions, proved disappointing to date.

Gene therapy

Permanent correction of genetic deficit of the haemopoietic system requires the transfer of genes into stem cells, with long-term, high-level and lineage-specific expression of these cells after autologous transplantation. Over the last decade, there has been progress in the development of transduction methods and vectors, but many problems remain.[54]

Thalassaemia Intermedia

The term thalassaemia intermedia is used to describe patients with clinical thalassaemia which, although not transfusion dependent, is associated with a much more severe degree of anaemia than that found in heterozygous carriers for α and β thalassaemia. This clinical course is seen in β+ thalassaemia homozygotes with mild decrease in the β globin expression (e.g. in West Africa and Afro-Americans), HbC β⁰ thalassaemia and various δβ thalassaemias. It is also seen in homozygous thalassaemia patients who have inherited an α thalassaemia determinant, thereby reducing the overall degree of globin chain imbalance. Co-inheritance of a triplicated α globin locus with heterozygous β thalassaemia also causes thalassaemia intermedia phenotype (Table 13.14).

The clinical features of the intermedia forms are extremely variable. At one end of the spectrum are individuals who are virtually symptom free except for moderate anaemia. At the other end, there are patients who have Hb in the range 50–70 g/L, who develop marked splenomegaly, severe skeletal deformities due to expansion of bone marrow and, as they get older, become heavily iron loaded because of increased intestinal absorption of iron. Recurrent leg ulcers, folate deficiency, symptoms due to extramedullary haemopoietic tumour masses in the chest and skull, gallstones and a marked proneness to infection are particularly characteristic of this group of thalassaemics. Many of them are identified with anaemia later in life than is usual for homozygous α thalassaemia.

β Thalassaemia minor

Heterozygous inheritance of either β⁰ or β⁺ thalassaemia genes results in β thalassaemia minor; there are over 150 million such carriers alive today.

Clinical

The condition is asymptomatic. A small proportion of subjects have just palpable splenomegaly. The moderate but persistent anaemia during pregnancy causes fetal hypoxia, compensatory placental hypertrophy, mild intrauterine growth retardation, low urinary oestradiol excretion, an increased frequency of fetal distress during delivery and a high frequency, about 12%, of Apgar scores of 3 or less at 1 min, but no significant increase of perinatal mortality.[57]

Haematology

The Hb is in the range 90–110 g/L, and during pregnancy about 20 g/L lower; the MCV and MCH are low, especially with β⁰ thalassaemia (Table 13.15), and the blood film shows moderate anisocytosis, microcytosis and hypochromia with occasional target cells and a few cells with punctate basophilia; the red cell changes are greater than expected for the mild degree of anaemia. There is mild to moderate erythroid hyperplasia in the bone marrow; there is no tendency to iron overload unless the patient has received inappropriate parenteral iron therapy, and the prevalence of iron deficiency is the same as that of the general population.

The diagnosis is made by observing that the HbA_2 is raised to 4–6%; the HbF is also raised to about 3% in approximately half of the subjects. Osmotic fragility is reduced.

Management

It is important for the diagnosis to be made so as to avoid unnecessary treatment of the hypochromic anaemia with iron. Subjects should be reassured as to the benign nature of the condition and be offered genetic counselling (see below).

Malaria

J. B. S. Haldane was the first to hypothesize that the geographical coincidence of malaria and β thalassaemia could be due to the heterozygotes being at genetic advantage through a partial protection against *P. falciparum*. A relative resistance to malaria was confirmed in Liberian children with thalassaemia minor.[58] Suggested mechanisms of limiting parasitaemia have included: (1) a slower than normal decline of HbF in the first 2 years of life;[59] (2) a greater rigidity of red cell membranes resisting parasite invasion; (3) modified expression of parasite-induced neoantigens on red cell surfaces enhancing the development of protective cell mediated immunity;[60] and (4) high oxidant stress in thalassaemic cells inhibiting parasite growth.[61]

β Thalassaemia in association with Hb variants

In many populations, because there is a high incidence of both β thalassaemia and Hb variants, it is quite common for an individual to inherit a β thalassaemia gene from one parent and a gene for structural Hb variant from the other, e.g. HbS β thalassaemia

Table 13.14 Molecular basis of thalassaemia intermedia

HOMOZYGOUS β THALASSAEMIA
Mild β⁺ point mutation
Co-inheritance α⁺ thalassaemia
Enhanced production of HbF
δβ THALASSAEMIA
Homozygous δβ thalassaemia
HETEROZYGOUS β THALASSAEMIA
Co-inheritance of triplicated α globin loci (ααα)

Table 13.15 Red cell indices in iron deficiency and in thalassaemia compared with normal individuals

Red blood cell indices	Normal range	Iron deficiency	Typical α or β thalassaemia trait
Red blood cell count (×10¹²/L)	4–5	<4	6.32
Mean corpuscular volume (MCV) (fL)	75–99	<76	63
Mean cellular haemoglobin (MCH) (pg)	27–31	27.5	20.3
Mean corpuscular haemoglobin concentration (MCHC) (g/dL)	32–36	30	32.2

(discussed under 'Sickle cell disease'), HbC β thalassaemia, HbE β thalassaemia and HbD β thalassaemia.

Haemoglobin C thalassaemia

This disorder is restricted to West African, some North African, southern Mediterranean and American populations. HbC β+ thalassaemia in West Africans is characterized by a mild haemolytic anaemia associated with splenomegaly: the peripheral blood film shows numerous target cells and thalassaemic red cell changes with a moderately elevated reticulocyte count. Hb electrophoresis shows a preponderance of HbC, some HbA and HbF. HbC β0 thalassaemia, in Mediterranean people and Americans, is somewhat more severe clinically, resembling thalassaemia intermedia: there is only HbC and HbF. (HbA2 cannot be separated from HbC.) Diagnosis is confirmed by checking the parents.

Haemoglobin E thalassaemia

This is the commonest severe form of thalassaemia in South-east Asia and eastern India. HbE is inefficiently synthesized, and hence when an HbE gene is inherited together with a β0 thalassaemia determinant, there is a marked deficiency of β chain production. The resulting clinical picture can closely resemble homozygous β0 thalassaemia, and is seen commonly in South-east Asia.[62]

In contrast, in Sri Lanka, where HbE thalassaemia constitutes 40% of all thalassaemias, the clinical picture varies from an almost normal to a mild anaemia to a severe anaemia.[63] The majority in Sri Lanka have a mild anaemia with splenomegaly: they grow and develop normally with few complications, and there are many recorded cases of pregnancy in women with this disorder. They usually have an average Hb of 60–70 g/L, are rarely symptomatic because the Hb O_2 dissociation curve is shifted to the right and more oxygen is released to tissues than from HbF in β thalassaemia major, and may not be transfusion dependent. They are liable to become more anaemic and may require transfusions during an infection, to which these patients are more prone. These patients continue to become iron overloaded in spite of not receiving blood transfusions, probably due to increased gastrointestinal absorption of iron.

The diagnosis of HbE β thalassaemia is confirmed by finding only HbE and HbF on electrophoresis, and by demonstrating the HbE trait in one parent and β thalassaemia trait in the other parent.

The δβ thalassaemias

The disorders due to reduced β and δ chain synthesis are much less common than those due to defective β chain production alone. They result from deletions of the β and δ globin genes or may be due to unequal crossing over between the δ and β globin gene loci with the production of δβ fusion genes. The latter produce δβ fusion chains which combine with a chain to form haemoglobin variants called Lepore haemoglobins.

Clinical features

The δβ thalassaemias have been reported in many populations although there are no high-frequency areas. In the homozygous state there is a mild degree of anaemia with Hb values of 80–100 g/L. There is often a moderate degree of splenomegaly, but these patients are usually symptomless except during periods of stress, such as infections or pregnancy. Haemoglobin analysis shows 100% HbF in homozygotes; heterozygous carriers have a thalassaemic blood picture, elevated levels of HbF of 5–20% and normal levels of HbA2.

The homozygous state for Hb Lepore is characterized by a clinical picture which is usually similar to that of homozygous β thalassaemia, although in some cases it might be milder and not transfusion dependent. The clinical and haematological findings are similar to those of β thalassaemia. The haemoglobin consists of HbF and Hb Lepore only.

Hereditary persistence of fetal haemoglobin (HPFH)

HPFH results from a combined deletion of the δ and β chains, but the deficit of β globin chains is compensated for by a high rate of synthesis of γ chains. Heterozygotes have no clinical or haematological abnormalities except that they have HbF 20–30%; acid elution and staining for HbF on a peripheral blood film shows that HbF is homogeneously distributed in all red cells, so distinguishing this from other conditions such as β+ thalassaemia, where HbF is distributed unevenly in the erythrocytes. The homozygotes are entirely asymptomatic, but have a thalassaemic-like appearance in the red cells and 100% HbF.

γδβ thalassaemia

This rare thalassaemia results from long deletion of β globin gene clusters which, as well as removing the entire β gene, removes the γ and δ genes. There is no output of globin from this gene cluster at all. The homozygous state leads to an absence of HbF and is not compatible with fetal survival; heterozygotes have severe haemolytic disease of the newborn with anaemia and jaundice. If they survive the neonatal period, they grow and develop normally; in adult life they have a haematological picture resembling heterozygous β thalassaemia.

The α thalassaemias

Although the α thalassaemias are commoner than the β thalassaemias they pose less of a public health problem, because the severe homozygous forms cause death in utero or in the neonatal period and the milder forms do not produce major disability.

The α thalassaemias occur widely throughout the Mediterranean region, sub-Saharan Africa, the Middle East, isolated parts of the Indian subcontinent, and throughout South-east Asia in a line stretching from south China through Thailand, Malaysia and Indonesia (Figure 13.15).

Definition and inheritance

Genetic disease of α chain synthesis results in defective HbF and HbA production, as both contain α chains. In the fetus the deficiency of α chains leads to the production of excess γ chains, which form γ_4 tetramers or Hb Bart's. In the adult a deficiency of α chains leads to an excess of β chains which forms β_4 tetramers or HbH. Hb Bart's and HbH are the hallmarks of α thalassaemia, but the carrier states of different forms of α thalassaemia are difficult to diagnose as only trace amounts of these haemoglobins are produced.

Genetically determined reductions of α globin synthesis are most often the outcomes of a variety of deletions from α globin clusters on chromosome 16 (Figure 13.5).[52,53,64] There are two α genes (α_2 and α_1) responsible for the production of α globin chain in the chromosome. Thus there are four genes in a human diploid cell, two coming from each parent, represented as αα/αα. Deletion of one of the two α globulin genes is denoted as (−α) and this results in α+ thalassaemia, with partial suppression of the α globin

Table 13.16 The α thalassaemia syndromes

Genotype (normal αα/αα, ββ)	Globin genes affected by mutations	Syndrome	Clinical features	Haemoglobin pattern
α–/αα. ββ	1 (α_2)	Silent carrier	No anaemia Normal red cell	Hb Bart's 1–2% at birth HbCS 1–2% Remainder HbA
– –/αα. ββ or α–/α–. ββ	2 ($\alpha_2\ \alpha_1$) or 2 (α_2)	Thalassaemia trait	Mild anaemia Hypochromic microcytic red cells	Hb Barts 5–10% HbCS 1–2% Remainder HbA
– –/–α. ββ	3 (α genes)	HbH disease	Moderate anaemia Hypochromic microcytic, fragmented red cells May demonstrate inclusion bodies	Hb Bart's 5–30% HbCS 1–2% Remainder HbA
– –/– –. ββ	4 (α genes)	Hydrops fetalis	Severe anaemia Death in utero	Mainly Hb Bart's (γ_4)

synthesis: this is caused by unequal cross-over events, generating at the same time a triple α gene (ααα), which can be observed in the normal population. Deletions of both genes, denoted as (– –), result in α^0 thalassaemia with total absence of α globin synthesis. A further refinement of this nomenclature includes the designation of specific mutations; (– –^{SEA}) signifies the α^0 deletion mutation that is confined to South-East Asia, while (–$\alpha^{3.7}$) symbolizes the α^+ rightward gene deletion common in Africa.

A few α^+ thalassaemias are due to point mutations, giving rise to more severe reduction of α globulin synthesis than due to the single gene deletions. These are designated by the superscript T ($\alpha\alpha^T$). The most important non-deletional α thalassaemia gene is a termination codon mutation on α_2 globin gene, designated as ($\alpha^{CS}\alpha$), leading to the production of an elongated α chain which combines with β chains to form Hb Constant Spring: the abnormal mRNA is unstable so that only low levels of Hb Constant Spring are synthesized and the phenotype is a moderately severe α thalassaemia.

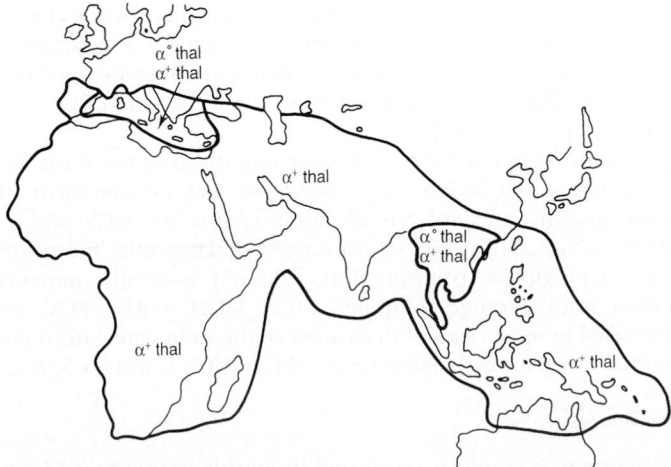

Figure 13.15 Areas of the Old World where α thalassaemias reach polymorphic frequency.

Genetics of α thalassaemia

Three genotypes are associated with clinically asymptomatic states: (1) heterozygous α^+ thalassaemia (–α/αα); (2) homozygous α^+ thalassaemia (–α/–α); and (3) heterozygous α^0 thalassaemia (– –/αα) (Table 13.16).

Doubly heterozygous α^0 thalassaemia/α^+ thalassaemia (– –/–α) leaves only one active α globulin gene. Both Hb Bart's and HbH have high oxygen affinity, resulting in tissue hypoxia; in addition, HbH is unstable and is precipitated as intracellular inclusion bodies, causing haemolysis and the clinical condition of HbH disease.

Homozygous α^0 thalassaemia (– –/– –) allows for only Hb Bart's to be formed in fetal life; because of its high oxygen affinity, infants are hypoxic and hydropic, inevitably dying in utero or shortly after delivery.

Geographical distribution

The α^0 thalassaemia gene frequencies are highest in South-east Asia and China (Figure 13.15);[64] in Thailand, for example, gene frequency for α^0 thalassaemia is 0.025, for α^+ thalassaemia 0.10–0.15, and for Hb Constant Spring 0.05–0.15. In consequence, Hb Bart's hydrops fetalis affecting 25 000 infants each year, and HbH disease affecting about 68 000 infants each year, are major health problems.

Both α^+ thalassaemia and α^0 thalassaemia deletions are seen at low frequencies in the Mediterranean region, so that HbH disease and hydrops fetalis can occur: in addition, HbH disease arises rarely from non-deletional mutations. The α^+ thalassaemias are common in Saudi Arabia (frequency 0.37), as is a severe non-deletional form of α thalassaemia resulting in HbH disease.

On the Indian subcontinent α^+ thalassaemia gene frequencies are extremely high (above 0.70) in tribal or scheduled groups and in the Tharu of Nepal. In Sri Lanka 15.5% of the population are heterozygous for α^+ thalassaemia and about 3% of the population were heterozygous for the triplicated α-globin gene arrangement (ααα).[63] Similarly the α^+ thalassaemia gene frequency reaches up to 0.70 on coastal areas of Papua New Guinea. α^+ Thalassaemia gene frequencies are in the range 0.10–0.27 throughout sub-Saharan Africa.[65] However, α^0 thalassaemia is not present in these populations and there is no disease.

Pathophysiology

The pathophysiology of α thalassaemia is different from that of β thalassaemia. Hb Bart's and HbH respectively do not precipitate in the marrow and hence there is less intramedullary destruction of red cell precursors, and erythropoiesis is more effective than in β thalassaemia. However, HbH is unstable and precipitates in red cells as they age. The resulting inclusion bodies are trapped in the spleen and other parts of the microcirculation, leading to shortened red cell survival. Furthermore, both Hb Bart's and HbH have a very high oxygen affinity. Thus the pathology of severe forms of α thalassaemia is based on defective haemoglobin production, the synthesis of homotetramers which are physiologically useless, and the haemolytic component due to their precipitation in older red cells.

Haemoglobin Bart's hydrops syndrome

The homozygous state for α^0 thalassaemia $(- -/- -)$ is a common cause of fetal loss throughout South-east Asia, Greece and Cyprus. Affected infants do not produce HbF or HbA. The infants are usually stillborn between 28 and 40 weeks or die within a few hours after delivery.[52,53] They have the typical features of hydrops fetalis with gross pallor, generalized oedema and massive hepatosplenomegaly. There is a very large friable placenta. All these findings are due to severe intrauterine anaemia. The Hb values are in the 60–80 g/L range, and there are gross thalassaemic changes of the peripheral blood film with many nucleated red cells. The haemoglobin consists of approximately 80% Hb Bart's and 20% of embryonic Hb Portland $(\zeta^2\gamma^2)$. It is believed that these infants survive to term because they continue to produce embryonic haemoglobin which transports oxygen functionally.

The syndrome is characterized also by a high incidence of toxaemia of pregnancy and considerable obstetric difficulties due to the presence of the large, friable placenta. Both parents have minor thalassaemic red cell changes with normal HbA$_2$ values, which is a characteristic finding of the heterozygous state of α^0 thalassaemia.

Haemoglobin H disease

HbH disease usually results from the inheritance of doubly heterozygous α^0 thalassaemia/α^+ thalassaemia $(- -/-\alpha)$, or from the inheritance of α^0 thalassaemia and Hb Constant Spring $(- -/\alpha^{cs}\alpha)$, or from the homozygous state for severe non-deletion form of α thalassaemia particularly common in Saudi Arabia.[52,53]

There is a variable degree of anaemia and splenomegaly, but it is most unusual to see severe thalassaemic bone changes or growth retardation. Affected patients survive into adult life as they have sufficient HbA, but their course may be interspersed with severe episodes of haemolysis associated with infection, or worsening of the anaemia due to progressive hypersplenism. In addition, oxidant drugs such as sulphonamides, or pregnancy, may increase the rate of precipitation of HbH and exacerbate the anaemia. Iron overload is uncommon.

The Hb values range from 70 to 100 g/L and the blood film shows typical thalassaemic changes. There is moderate reticulocytosis, and on incubating the red cell with brilliant cresyl blue numerous inclusion bodies are generated by precipitation of the HbH under the redox action of the dye. Haemoglobin analysis reveals from 5% to 40% HbH, together with HbA and normal or reduced level of HbA$_2$.

Consistent with the mild nature of the disease, treatment is primarily supportive.

Asymptomatic α thalassaemia

The silent carrier state $(-\alpha/\alpha\alpha)$ is due to the presence of a mutation affecting the deletion of a single α globin gene. α Thalassaemia trait is commonly associated with two genotypes: $(- -/\alpha\alpha)$ and $(-\alpha/-\alpha)$. Point mutation affecting the α_2 gene $(\alpha^T\alpha/\alpha\alpha)$ may also lead to α thalassaemia trait. Subjects develop mild hypochromic, microcytic anaemia. At birth, Hb Bart's contributes about 2.5% of the total Hb in heterozygous α^0 thalassaemia $(- -/\alpha\alpha)$ and homozygous α^+ thalassaemia $(-\alpha/-\alpha)$, and may be seen in trace amounts in about 10% of heterozygous α^+ thalassaemia $(-\alpha/\alpha\alpha)$. HbH is not detected.

α^+ Thalassaemia is of some importance in Africa as, besides causing a slight anaemia, it ameliorates the severity of sickle cell disease as well as the anaemia of homozygous β^+ thalassaemia, and is associated with a lower proportion of HbS in sickle cell trait.

Malaria

The strongest evidence that α^+ thalassaemia has been selected for by malaria is epidemiological: for example, gene frequency is closely and positively correlated with endemicity of malaria in Papua New Guinea and in island Melanesia.[66] As the disadvantage of α^+ thalassaemia, or even α^0 thalassaemia, is not great, only mild selective pressure would be required to achieve polymorphism. In fact, no increased fitness or control of parasitaemia has been demonstrated in heterozygotes. However, in α^+ thalassaemia increased amounts of malaria-induced neoantigens are displayed on red cell surfaces, and rapid immune clearance of parasitized cells is one probable mechanism of advantage.[60] Also, an increased incidence of mild *P. falciparum* malaria has been described in children with α thalassaemia, stimulating high levels of immunity.[66]

Screening for thalassaemia syndromes

Thalassaemia syndromes may be easily recognized from clinical presentation of anaemia, growth retardation, jaundice and splenomegaly, and changes in the red cell morphology. However, carrier detection including genotype determination requires certain laboratory investigations.[67]

Usually, Hb levels of 100 g/L and below are considered as indications for the screening of thalassaemia for subjects without iron deficiency. However, the Hb level may be normal in the carrier or heterozygous states. In all cases, iron deficiency must be ruled out before the diagnosis is made since its interference can cause misdiagnosis (Table 13.15).

Routine haemoglobinopathy screening includes the measurement of red cell indices, electrophoresis and measurement of haemoglobins, and analysis of globin chains. An MCV <80 fL, MCH <27 pg and/or Hct <36% suggest thalassaemia: the mean cell haemoglobin concentration (MCHC) generally remains within normal range. Although MCV, MCH and/or PCV are decreased in most cases of thalassaemia, the values are within the normal range for α thalassaemias, HbE and Hb Constant Spring.

Prevention

Thalassaemias produce severe public health problems and are serious drains on medical resources in many populations. Since there is no definitive treatment and supportive treatment is extremely expensive, most countries in which the disease is common are putting a major effort into prevention.

There are two major approaches to the prevention of thalassaemia. Since the carrier states for β thalassaemia can be recognized easily, it is possible to screen populations and offer genetic counselling about the choice of marriage partners. If a β thalassaemic heterozygote marries another carrier, one in four (on average) of their children will have the severe transfusion-dependent homozygous disorder. It is well to remember that this risk applies to each pregnancy. Large-scale programmes of this type have had variable outcomes.

Most countries are developing screening programmes at antenatal clinics. When heterozygous carrier mothers are found their husbands are tested, and if they are also carriers the couple is offered the possibility of prenatal diagnosis and termination of pregnancies carrying fetuses with severe forms of thalassaemia.

In view of the considerable burden of the disease, most parents of children with thalassaemia major find the 25% risk of recurrence to be unacceptable. They prefer to have prenatal diagnosis of the disease in the next pregnancy. It has been observed that where the prenatal diagnosis is not available, most of the couples at risk restrict family size subsequent to the birth of an affected child.

Prenatal diagnosis

Prenatal diagnosis is by DNA studies on chorionic villus sampling at 9–12 weeks of gestation or by testing the fetal blood obtained at 18–20 weeks of gestation. The preferred method is through DNA studies: the diagnosis is highly accurate, and in the event of an affected fetus preventive abortion can be undertaken early and easily.[68]

Chorionic villus sampling can be done as an out-patient investigation either transcervically or transabdominally with ultrasound guidance. There is a 2–4% risk of a miscarriage. There is always a 1–2% chance of error of DNA diagnosis because of mixing with some maternal cells; therefore collection, cleaning and selection of villi is critically important. Prenatal diagnosis of thalassaemia is now well established in many countries, and in Sardinia, Greece and Cyprus has already reduced by up to 97% the number of new cases of thalassaemia major in the community.[68]

The control of thalassaemia in the community

In developing countries optimal management of all patients having β thalassaemia is extremely difficult, if not impossible, to provide. This is not to deny that there are many individual success stories where affected children have received the optimal management, have excellent growth, and can even go on to marry and have children. However, the availability of blood for transfusion is always limited, while desferrioxamine and pumps for infusing are expensive and unaffordable by the vast majority.

Strategy for control involves: (1) educating the community to the problem, and making people aware of the burden of the disease and the desirability of control; (2) screening the community to identify carriers of β thalassaemia genes, and to recognize couples at risk of having homozygous children. Carrier screening can be done at various times, such as at birth, in school, in college, before marriage, just after marriage or during pregnancy. Many scientists have suggested that carrier screening be done at high school or college, so that counselling may prevent marriage between carriers. In most Asian countries this strategy is not satisfactory and it would be better to permit free choice of partner,

and then to screen the couple. If they are carriers, they can be counselled appropriately.

It is essential for success that all the components of the programme (health education, carrier screening and prenatal diagnosis) be in place for proper implementation. Such a community programme requires two other essential ingredients: a strong political will and active participation by the community and by parents and children with thalassaemia. People for their part must be motivated enough to accept a screening and control programme. Health education to all sections of the population – politicians, bureaucrats, professionals and the community as a whole – is the key to success.

Sickle cell disease

A point mutation replaces glutamic acid with valine at position 6 on the β globin. The combination of normal α chains with the abnormal βˢ chains forms sickle haemoglobin (HbS).[53,69-71] Sickle cell disease is defined as the condition resulting from the inheritance of two abnormal allelomorphic genes controlling β globin formation, of which at least one is the βˢ gene. Sickle cell disease includes the most common type, homozygous HbSS (referred to as sickle cell anaemia), and the compound heterozygous conditions of HbS β thalassaemias, HbSC, HbSD, HbSO^Arab and others. Sickle cell trait (HbAS) is the condition arising from the inheritance of one normal β globin gene and one βˢ gene.

There were about 78 million carriers of sickle cell trait in the world in 1992; of these, 65 million were in Africa south of the Sahara and north of the Zambesi River and Kalahari Desert. In tropical Africa βˢ gene frequencies reach to over 0.15; that is, >30% of the adult population have HbAS (Figure 13.16).[72] The βˢ gene is found at polymorphic frequencies also in the tribal (scheduled) groups of India, in the Arabian peninsula and the Mediterranean region. High gene frequencies are encountered also in populations derived from the slave trade or voluntary emigration from Africa and the Mediterranean, such as in the Americas, the UK, other northern European countries and Australia.

DNA analysis of the β globin gene cluster has shown that the βˢ gene is linked to various β chain haplotypes, each with a distinct

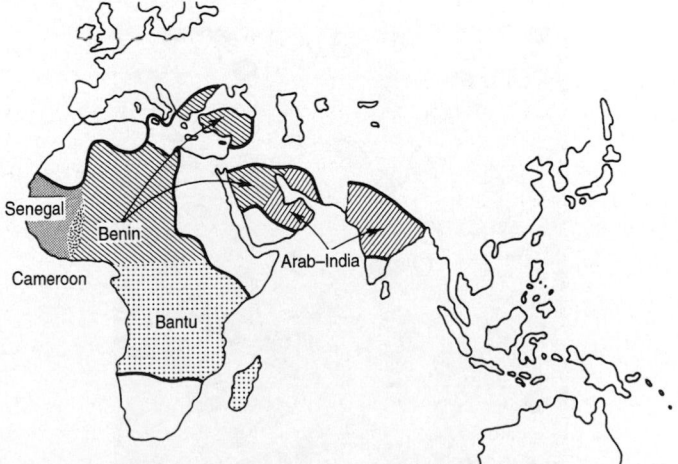

Figure 13.16 Areas of the Old World where haemoglobin S gene frequency is >0.02, and distribution of βˢ haplotypes. Heavy arrows indicate probable spread of the Benin haplotype to the Mediterranean and western Asia.

geographical distribution (Figure 13.16). This implies that the sickle mutation arose independently at different times, linked to the different haplotypes. The Arab–India haplotype is found throughout the Indian tribal groups and in eastern Saudi Arabia. The Senegal haplotype is confined to the western seaboard of West Africa. The Benin haplotype is common in central West Africa, and would seem to have spread through the trans-Saharan slave trade to North Africa, the Mediterranean region and western Arabia. The Bantu haplotype (previously called Central African Republic or CAR haplotype) is found uniformly throughout the Bantu speakers of central and southern Africa. The fourth African β^S mutation, linked to the Cameroon haplotype, is restricted to the Eton ethnic group of central Cameroon.[72] These distributions are of interest not only in our understanding of selective pressures and human evolution, but also because clinical expression is modified by haplotype linkages.

Each year about 156 000 infants are born with sickle cell disease, of whom 130 000 are in Africa and 33 000 in Nigeria alone. Most have sickle cell anaemia (HbSS); HbSC is also common in central West Africa (Burkina Faso, Ghana, Benin and south-western Nigeria); HbS β^+ thalassaemia is seen in West Africa, especially Liberia; HbS β^0 thalassaemia occurs in North Africa, the Mediterranean and mixed populations of the Americas; HbSD is seen most in the Punjab (see Figures 13.6, 13.16 and 13.18).

Pathophysiology

Valine is a hydrophobic amino acid, whereas glutamic acid is hydrophilic: as position 6 of the β globin is externally situated, the solubility of the HbS molecule is much reduced compared to HbA, especially in the deoxygenated state. Deoxy-HbS polymerizes the contact points between molecules involving the $\beta6$ valines. The polymers form long chains of haemoglobin molecules; in cross-section, each chain consists of 14 molecules. The polymers align in parallel, and this is the probable mechanism for the distortion of red cells into the characteristic sickle cell shape (Figure 13.17), as the polymers lie parallel to the long axis of the sickled cells. With alternating deoxygenation and oxygenation, the red cell sickles and unsickles, but eventually ill-defined losses and changes of membrane lipids and proteins lead to the membrane becoming

rigid in the sickle form. The red cell is then an irreversible sickled cell, although within the membrane the haemoglobin is still capable of degelling on oxygenation. Failure of transmembrane ion exchange mechanisms leads to the loss of K^+ and water from the cell, while intracellular concentrations of Na^+ and Ca^{2+} rise.

Sickled cells are fragile and are phagocytosed by cells of the RES, so that there is both intravascular and extravascular haemolysis. Sickled cells adhere to each other and to the endothelium, so causing blockage of small blood vessels, infarction and death of tissues. Important secondary effects include an increased susceptibility to infection, which has several mechanisms: (1) mucosal and skin integrity may be breached following infarction; (2) haemoglobinaemia activates and consumes complement, so that there is a chronic defect of the alternative pathway of activation and diminished opsonization and phagocytosis of, for example, pneumococci; (3) recurrent infarction in the spleen leads to destruction of the organ (autosplenectomy) and functional hyposplenism; and (4) post-infarctive tissue necrosis provides a microenvironment favouring bacterial growth, and precedes the development of osteomyelitis and pyelonephritis. Recurrent infections and chronic ill health are associated with retardation of growth and development: chronic haemolysis creates high demands for folate, and deficiency contributes to the impaired growth and development besides leading to anaemic crisis.

Disease is worst in HbSS and HbS β^0 thalassaemia, and is in diminishing order of severity in HbSC, HbSD, HbSO^{Arab} and HbSβ^+ thalassaemia. Sickle cell trait (HbAS) and HbS/HPFH are essentially without clinical abnormality except when under extreme stress.

Clinical presentation

Infants with HbSS have complications only rarely in the early months of life, while HbF concentrations remain high. The disease is manifest clinically from the 3rd month onwards: the earliest presentation is frequently the 'hand-foot' syndrome of painful swelling of the dorsum of the hands or feet, often symmetrical, resulting from infarctions into the small bones. Due to parents coming late for advice and limited diagnostic skills at the first levels of care, the diagnosis is commonly delayed in tropical Africa (where about five out of six patients are born with sickle cell anaemia) with consequent morbidity and mortality, which could have been prevented.[73] The diagnosis is made in the 1st year of life in only about 10% of Nigerian children with sickle cell anaemia receiving hospital care. The most common age is 1–3 years, but up to 20% of patients are over 10 years at the time of diagnosis.

Patients suffer from chronic ill health interspersed with acute anaemic, infarctive and infective crises.

The steady state

Height and weight are below average for age throughout childhood. There is little body fat. The limbs are long and thin, and much of the loss of height is in the spinal column; there is an exaggerated lumbar lordosis and the chest is often barrel shaped due to an increase in the anteroposterior distance. The bones of the vault of the skull and the face show bossing similar to that of β thalassaemia major (see Figure 13.10A): rounding of the forehead causes exaggeration of the supraorbital sulcus; the bridge of the nose appears sunken because of expansion of the bones around it; expansion of the maxilla causes the upper teeth to protrude. Bossing is much more pronounced in African than

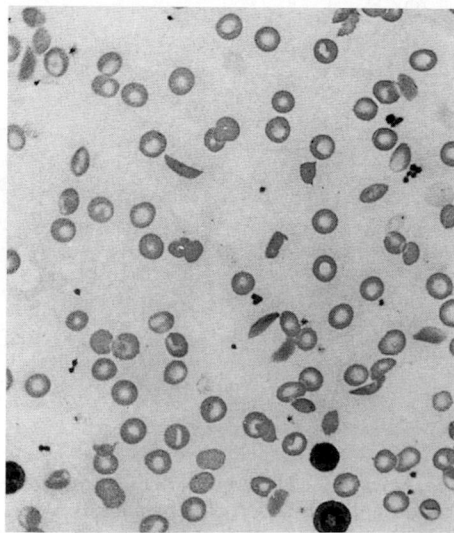

Figure 13.17 Peripheral blood film in sickle cell anaemia.

American patients; it is largely reversible with long-term antimalarial prophylactics, which suggests that malarial haemolysis is a contributory factor.

There is pallor and usually clinically obvious jaundice. The liver is invariably enlarged. Gallstones can be demonstrated in about 10% of African and 30% of American adult patients, but only rarely do they cause symptoms. The spleen is large in early childhood, but shrinks due to infarction, and is palpable in about 7% of patients only after puberty. In only the occasional patient is there hypersplenism. Moderate chronic cervical adenopathy is usual.

The heart is enlarged: the apex beat is displaced laterally and may be visible. The pulse rate is normal at rest but is rapid after minimal exertion or with apprehension and excitement. Midsystolic murmurs are heard in most patients, and third heart sounds are common. Patients complain of polydipsia and polyuria, related to renal medullary infarction and loss of ability to concentrate urine; enuresis in childhood and nocturia are usual.

Most patients are remarkably well adapted psychologically, and perform their schooling well, although achievement may be poor from loss of time through ill health.

After the age of about 11 years skeletal maturation is delayed. Fusion of the epiphyses is late, and growth may continue for longer than normal, so that post-pubertal HbSS subjects catch up on growth and a few even go on to reach well above average height (e.g. 190 cm). Puberty is delayed, and menarche occurs in girls on average 1 year later than in the normal population. Post-adolescent patients, girls in particular, persist in a non-adult lifestyle, so that first sexual experience and marriage are often at a relatively late age; many men are impotent following priapism (see below). Rarely, growth and development are so retarded that the patient has the appearance of a pituitary dwarf.

Haematology in the steady state

The Hb is generally in the range 60–100 g/L; patients are not in distress, even with levels constantly lower than this range, as they are compensated by high levels of erythrocyte 2,3-DPG and efficient oxygen delivery to the tissues. The red cells show great anisocytosis, macrocytosis with microcytosis, sickle cell forms, target cells, poikilocytes, polychromasia and a variable number of nucleated red cells (Figure 13.17); with hyposplenism the red cell appearance is more abnormal, and punctate basophilia and Howell–Jolly bodies may be seen. The reticulocyte count is raised up to 20%. The total white cell count is generally raised, showing a neutrophil leukocytosis with a shift to the left and toxic granulation, or a lymphocytosis with activated forms, even in the absence of obvious infection. The platelet count is high, especially when there has been autosplenectomy and following an infarctive crisis.

Haemoglobin electrophoresis shows the major fraction in the position of HbS, with a variable proportion of HbF and normal HbA_2. That the major haemoglobin is HbS can be confirmed by the solubility test.[1,67]

The biochemical features of both intravascular and extravascular haemolysis are present (see Table 13.11); conjugated bilirubin is usually raised due to liver dysfunction.

Anaemic crises

Catastrophic declines of Hb are the result of (1) malaria, (2) acute splenic sequestration, (3) folate deficiency and (4) aplastic crises.[73]

Acute *P. falciparum* malaria in subjects with sickle cell disease causes a severe haemolytic crisis and profound anaemia, often leading to anaemic cardiac failure, which used to be the most common observed cause of death in Africa. The most severe anaemias in acute illness are still associated with malaria, even in patients who are supposedly receiving prophylactics.

A sequestration crisis is characterized by an acutely enlarging spleen and a precipitate fall of Hb by more than 20 g/L, with a high reticulocyte count. It is most frequent in the second 6 months of life but can occur at older ages, even adulthood, in subjects who retain their spleens. Anaemic cardiac failure can develop, and it is the single most common cause of death in early life in non-malarial areas, such as the West Indies.[69]

More than 10% of untreated African patients have megaloblastic erythropoiesis from folic acid deficiency when seen first. Megaloblastosis is almost inevitable during pregnancy unless prevented. Life-threatening anaemia develops rapidly.

During almost any acute infection erythropoiesis is depressed, and as patients with sickle cell anaemia are dependent on abnormally high rates of erythropoiesis the Hb drops rapidly. Of greater severity is infection by parvovirus B19 (see below). 'Aplastic' crises occur in clusters in patients with sickle cell anaemia, associated with epidemic transmission of parvovirus B19 and outbreaks of erythema infectiosum in the population of normal children.

Infarctive crises

Sickling can lead to infarction in almost any organ or tissue in the body. The common sites of infarction crises are the bones, chest and abdomen.[53,69,70,73]

Up to 90% of African children seen with sickle cell anaemia between 6 months and 2 years of age have the hand–foot syndrome. If the swelling is hot, red and fluctuant, a superimposed osteomyelitis must be suspected. After about 2 years of age the sites of bone pain crises shift to the long bones. Pain is frequently localized around the joints, may be in multiple sites, be symmetrical in its distribution, and move from site to site. Onset is sudden; severity is variable, but often intense; duration is also variable, but usually there is spontaneous resolution within 5 days. Often there are no physical signs except warmth and tenderness over the affected bone, and the unwary physician is liable to underestimate the severity of the pain and overestimate the patient's reaction. Malaria, other infections, cold or damp (in the rainy season) are recognized precipitating factors, but often crises start for no apparent reason. Necrosis can lead rarely to emboli of bone marrow fat or bone to the lungs, brain, kidneys or other tissues.

Acute severe pain in the chest can be due to (1) lower respiratory tract infection, (2) bone marrow fat embolism, (3) pulmonary infarction, (4) acute pulmonary sequestration and (5) bone pain crisis in the thoracic cage.[71,74] The first four conditions are serious and often difficult to distinguish clinically or radiologically; as one may precede and precipitate the others, the phrase 'acute chest syndrome' is used. Lobar pneumonia and infection by the pneumococcus are more likely in early childhood, and infarction to be the primary pathology in adults.

Patients commonly complain of recurrent mild abdominal pain, but this may be severe and require admission to hospital. Pain is usually localized centrally or in the epigastrium. The patient may be vomiting. There is a history of constipation; bowel sounds are reduced and fluid levels can be seen radiologically.

Aetiology is obscure, but is thought to be due to mesenteric infarcts. The condition resolves spontaneously, usually within 5 days. Other abdominal painful crises related to sickle cell disease are splenic infarction, infarction in lumbar vertebrae, duodenal ulceration, acute cholecystitis, obstruction of cystic or bile ducts and pancreatitis. Patients may also present with abdominal crises unrelated to sickle cell disease, for example acute appendicitis.

Sickling in cerebral vessels can cause obstruction, infarction and haemorrhage. The immediate consequences of stroke include convulsions, coma, paralyses of varying extent and depth, or death. The late sequelae are contractions of limbs if no physiotherapy is available, faecal and urinary incontinence, speech defects and serious impairment of intellectual function. Two-thirds of untreated children have recurrent clinical strokes.[75]

Older patients can complain of blurred vision: examination reveals tortuous retinal vessels, proliferation of the retinal vessels, intraocular haemorrhages and sometimes retinal detachment. Pathology can develop until there is severe or total loss of vision.

Leg ulceration is a most common complication in the West Indies and North America, starting most often between 10 and 20 years of age. For reasons which remain obscure, ulcers are uncommon (<10%) in Africa even in those above 12 years of age; males are affected six times more often than females. The ulcers are usually on the lower third of the leg above the medial or lateral malleoli. They start as infarcts into the skin which show as small blisters; these develop into necrotic sloughs after 2 weeks and ulcers in about 3 weeks. Small ulcers may heal or may spread to up to 10 cm in diameter, causing serious incapacity.

Infarction in the renal pelvis leads to papillary necrosis, often complicated by haematuria and bacteriuria. Priapism is seen in adolescent or young adult males, but can occur in childhood; severity can vary from mild and transient, to moderate which resolves with 24 h, to when the penis is hot and exquisitely tender, with pain referred to the perineum and lower abdomen. Untreated, severe priapism subsides over about 2 weeks but leads to fibrosis of the corpora cavernosa and permanent impotence.

Bacterial infections

The pneumococcus (*Streptococcus pneumoniae*) is the most common infectious cause of death in non-malarial areas; its frequency in Africa has been underestimated, and it is probably second only to malaria as a cause of morbidity and mortality.[73] Pneumococcal pneumonia, septicaemia and meningitis are seen in children between 5 months and 5 years old, and most frequently under the age of 2 years; the children have high fevers (>39.5°C) and are liable to convulsions, coma, shock and the Waterhouse–Friderichsen syndrome. Without appropriate treatment mortality is >50%.

Other organisms commonly associated with acute upper or lower respiratory tract infections and bacteraemia are *Haemophilus influenzae*, staphylococci, streptococci and various Gram-negative bacilli. Bone infarction is complicated by acute osteomyelitis in less than 10% of all patients; invading organisms in Africa are *Salmonella* (usually *S. typhi*) in about half, other coliforms in less than half and *Staph. pyogenes* in about one-fifth.

Chronic degenerative disease

As more patients live into adult life, chronic and irreversible degenerative changes after the age of 20 years are becoming increasingly important. Irreversible organ damage leading to death includes hepatic failure, renal failure, stroke and pulmonary fibro-sis, pulmonary hypertension and respiratory failure.[69–71] Major debilitation is the result of (1) avascular necrosis of bones, which can lead to loss of mobility when affecting the head of the femur or vertebral bodies, (2) retinopathy with loss of vision and (3) leg ulcers. Men over 25 years commonly present with duodenal ulcers (over 30% in Jamaica), which have complicated clinical courses, including pyloric stenosis.[69] There can be a progressive bone marrow failure after the age of 40.[76]

Pregnancy

African women with sickle cell anaemia invariably become severely depleted of folic acid by mid-pregnancy if they are without medical supervision. About one-quarter may experience sequestration crises. Shortly before and shortly after delivery they are liable to severe bone pain crises, which may be complicated by marrow and bone embolus and systolic hypertension with albuminuria ('pseudotoxaemia'). They have high frequencies of urinary tract and other infections.

Obstetric delivery is often complicated by pelvic disproportion, the result of impaired growth during childhood. In Nigeria, about half are delivered by caesarean section. During the puerperium they are liable to infection, especially wound sepsis.

Maternal mortality rates depend largely on the obstetric care available: in early series it was about 33%, but this has been reduced to nearly zero in the USA. In Nigeria mortality remains around 12%.

There is fetal growth retardation, and one-third of infants are of low birth weight. Perinatal mortality can be as high as 33% but can be reduced to around 10% with good antenatal care and careful supervision of delivery and the puerperium.[77]

Prognosis

The pattern and severity of disease are governed by both environmental and genetic factors.[73] In Africa, the environmental factors are of far greater importance in determining prognosis; in the USA, the impact of the environment is largely controlled and the severity of disease depends more on the inherited factors.

In Jamaica, where there has been a long-running intensive, nationwide and successful programme of sickle cell care, calculated mean survival for men is 53 years and for women 58.5 years.[78] In contrast in rural tropical Africa, when there was inadequate nutrition, poor hygiene, no avoidance of mosquitoes and no practice of modern medicine, <2% of infants born with sickle cell anaemia survived beyond 4 years.[79] The family are all-important: when they are caring, intelligent, educated and wealthy, children with HbSS do much better, even without regular medical care. The principal role of the medical profession is to support the family in the maintenance of the good health of family members with sickle cell disease (see below). Since the 1960s, the provision of care has spread and improved throughout much of tropical Africa, so that it is now not unusual to see African patients with HbSS entering professional life (e.g. law, medicine, nursing) and achieving parenthood.

The expression of sickle cell disease is modified by a range of other mutations on the β globin gene cluster, the so-called β globin haplotypes (Figure 13.16).[72] The Arab–India and the Senegal haplotypes are linked to determinants of high levels of persisting HbF (means 20% and 12%, respectively) in subjects with HbSS. The Benin and Bantu haplotypes are associated with lower levels of HbF (means 8%), but for reasons which are not yet understood disease is more severe with the Bantu than the Benin haplotype. Sickle cell anaemia with high levels of HbF, linked to Arab–India and Senegal haplotypes, is associated with a more normal body build, more subcutaneous fat, less dactylitis, less acute chest pain, less splenic atrophy and less major organ failure in adult life; Hb concentrations are higher, red cell survival is longer, there are fewer sickled cells, and reticulocyte and platelet counts are lower.

Coincidental inheritance of homozygous α^+ thalassaemia $(-\alpha/-\alpha)$ with HbSS results in less anaemia, less haemolysis, lower MCH and MCV, fewer sickled cells and lower reticulocyte counts. Values with heterozygous α^+ thalassaemia are intermediate between those with $-\alpha/-\alpha$ and $\alpha\alpha/\alpha\alpha$. α Gene deletions do not seem to have much influence on the severity of acute complications of sickle cell disease but do decrease the risks of chronic organ damage in adults.

Maintenance of health

Wherever the β^S gene has high frequency, priority should be given to a system for maintaining patients in a steady state of good health through early diagnosis, supportive care at sickle cell clinics and obstetric units, easy access to appropriate care in crises, and education of the public, patients and health professionals (Table 13.17).[73]

To facilitate early diagnosis all pregnant women should be screened by Serjeants' HbS solubility test, with confirmation of positive results by haemoglobin electrophoresis; screening of fathers would identify couples at risk of having affected infants

but it is more practical if a woman has HbS to test the newborn infant by electrophoresis (on citrate agar at pH 6–6.5). Other children at risk and to be screened are all with severe anaemia and the ill siblings of known patients with sickle cell disease. Serjeants' HbS solubility test is preferable by far to the sickling test as it distinguishes heterozygotes from homozygotes and is simpler to perform; it is the test of choice in the primary healthcare setting. Haemoglobin electrophoresis should be set up in all hospitals of around 100 beds or more in tropical Africa and should be available for all clinicians.

Once diagnosed, sickle cell disease should be explained in detail to parents, guardians and patients in a language and phraseology they can understand. Their knowledge and comprehension must be reinforced with the aid of pamphlets and further discussions. The first essential intervention is the prevention of malaria: patients should receive a curative course of antimalarials at first attendance or following any break in attendance at the sickle cell clinic; they must be kept free from malaria through regular antimalarial prophylaxis, the choice of prophylactic depending on the prevailing pattern of resistance in *P. falciparum* strains and national policies. A regimen of once-daily folic acid supplement and once-daily proguanil is easy to remember and comply with. Prophylactic oral penicillin V potassium 125 mg twice daily up to the age of 5 years (or to adolescence) has substantially reduced the morbidity and mortality associated with pneumococcal septicaemia in the USA and the UK.[80] Controlled trials are needed in Africa but present problems of cost and logistics. Widespread immunization against the pneumococcus is not an option for reasons of cost, difficulties of the cold chain and the inadequate response of

Table 13.17 Maintenance of health in sickle cell disease.

Early diagnosis	Laboratory techniques	HbS solubility
		Hb electrophoresis
	Screening	pregnant women
		newborn of mothers with S gene
		anaemic children
		siblings of patients
	Clinical awareness	
Education	Parents and patients	
	Health professionals	
	General public	
Sickle cell clinics	Prevent infection	prophylactic antimalarials
		immunization
		prophylactic penicillin
	Nutrition	folic acid supplements
		general nutritional advice
	Advice	avoid cold, fatigue, dehydration, excessive alcohol
		no useless treatment
		attend clinic regularly
		report when ill
		report when pregnant
Induction of fetal haemoglobin	Hydroxyurea	
Hospital	Prompt treatment of crises	
Obstetrics	Supervision of pregnancy, delivery, puerperium	
	Family limitation to ≤3 viable children	

children under 3 years. On the other hand it is important for children with sickle cell disease to receive the expanded programme of immunization against other common infections.[73]

The coincidence of the area of Africa where the β^S gene has high frequency and where HIV is now epidemic makes it more important than ever that the health of patients with sickle cell disease be maintained so as to avoid situations where it is necessary to transfuse blood. Where there are no programmes of healthcare for sickle cell disease sufferers, but merely treatment of crises, which often involves transfusions of blood (appropriate and inappropriate), 20% or more of patients with sickle cell disease have been infected with HIV. In Africa 130 000 infants are born each year with sickle cell disease, and only 400 with haemophilia, who are at risk of infection by HIV through blood and blood products.[73]

Induction of fetal haemoglobin

Various agents have been tried for their efficacy in raising the concentration of HbF in patients with sickle cell disease. The oral cytotoxic agent hydroxyurea is the only one to date which has an established place in the management of sickle cell disease.[80]

Treatment with hydroxyurea for 2 years: (1) increases the concentration of HbF up to 15–20% of the total haemoglobin; (2) decreases the number of granulocytes and monocytes, and hence the release of oxidative radicals; and (3) reduces the adherence of sickled cells to the endothelium. Clinically, hydroxyurea reduces the frequency of painful crises, of acute chest syndrome, of hospitalization and of the need for blood transfusion.

Treatment is started with hydroxyurea 500 mg per day (10–15 mg/kg body weight). If this is tolerated, the dosage is increased to 1000 mg per day after 6–8 weeks; the dose can be increased further to 2000 mg (20–30 mg/kg body weight). The full blood count HbF renal function and hepatic function need to be monitored.

Short-term toxicity is minimal, but the long-term effects of hydroxyurea are not known, and it may be mutagenic. In Africa, hydroxyurea is available at present only to those who are able to purchase it.

Management of the patient in crisis

Prompt treatment is essential and arrangements should be made for patients in crisis to be able to report and receive attention without having to compete with the mass of sick people seen in the outpatient clinics of equatorial Africa. Regardless of the nature of the crisis it should be assumed that the patient has malaria, and treatment started without waiting for the results from a thick blood film. Antimalarial prophylaxis and supplementary folic acid should continue.

Anaemic crises

In the great majority of patients the haematocrit will cease to fall and will rise rapidly following treatment with antimalarials, folic acid and antibiotics if indicated. Blood transfusion is necessary only if: (1) there is respiratory distress, or incipient or established heart failure, (2) there is a sequestration crisis, with Hb <60 g/L and falling rapidly, (3) obstetric delivery is imminent, with Hb <80 g/L, or (4) there are coincidental indications, such as haemorrhage or emergency surgery.[17,73]

Infarctive crises

Management is based on three principles: (1) the control of pain, (2) the restoration and maintenance of hydration and acid-base balance and (3) the treatment of infection.[53,69,73,80]

The physician should assess the severity of pain and prescribe appropriate analgesics to be given at determined dosage and intervals; the physician must reassess pain at regular intervals and be prepared to increase or decrease the analgesics. Analgesic dosage should never be left to the judgement of different ward staff and the persuasive powers of the patients. Mild pain can be controlled with paracetamol, moderately severe pain with dihydrocodeine tartrate (DF118) and severe pain with opiates, such as diamorphine 10 mg at once, followed by an infusion, assessed by body size and the patient's response.[80]

Hydration is maintained by encouraging the mildly affected patient to drink; a more severely ill patient may be treated with nasogastric fluids if bowel sounds can be heard, or by intravenous fluids.

Acute infections

Antibiotics should be withheld unless there are clear indications for their use. If there are indications, antibiotics should be given promptly and in adequate dosage. Treatment must be started before results of bacteriological investigations are completed when there is (1) fever of >39°C, unless due to malaria, (2) the acute pulmonary syndrome, or (3) suspected meningitis. Initial treatment could be with cefuroxime sodium 150 mg/kg per 24 h, or alternatively ampicillin or penicillin plus chloramphenicol. Treatment of acute osteomyelitis can commence with chloramphenicol and cloxacillin.[73]

Cerebrovascular accidents

Patients should be rehydrated immediately. Some physicians advocate exchange blood transfusion but it is not possible to give general advice on this question.[75,80] Patients should be managed individually, taking into consideration the safety of blood transfusion in the locality. Repeated transfusions, aimed at reducing HbS concentrations to <30%, largely prevent recurrent strokes, but such a regimen can only be embarked upon if there is an assured supply of safe blood.

Priapism

Treatment is aimed at relieving pain and preventing fibrosis of the corpora cavernosa. Mild or 'stuttering' priapism can be relieved by micturition, walking around, avoiding sexual arousal and bathing in cold water. Moderately severe priapism will respond, usually within 24 h, to bed-rest, sedation, analgesics, intravenous hydration, and cyproterone or stilboestrol. Initial therapy of severe priapism should include opiate analgesics and rehydration; under general or spinal anaesthetic, a wide-bore needle is inserted into the lateral side of the base of the penis and the viscous blood aspirated; this is followed by repeated irrigation with adrenaline $1:10^6$ in saline and aspiration until fresh blood only is obtained.

Leg ulceration

Small and clean ulcers are treated successfully with daily antiseptic washing and dressing. Large ulcers will heal slowly with (1) prolonged bed-rest with the affected leg raised, (2) appropriate antibiotic therapy, (3) hydrogen peroxide lotion or surgical debridement to remove the slough, and (4) antitetanus prophylaxis. Larger ulcers or those which fail to heal require skin grafts. Once healed, the legs should be protected by crepe or elastic stockings.[70]

Management during pregnancy

Health must be maintained through careful antenatal supervision and the insistence on prophylactic antimalarials and supplementary folic acid.[17] Prophylactic red cell transfusion has been advocated, but benefits are slight, if any, and are certainly outweighed by the risk of complications from transfusion in the tropics. Transfusion of red cells is indicated if a patient approaches obstetric delivery with Hb <80 g/L.[17] Patients should be assessed as to the danger of pelvic disproportion, and elective Caesarean delivery planned if necessary.

Prevention of sickle cell disease

Strategies for prevention of sickle cell disease include (1) screening to recognize couples at risk, (2) genetic counselling, and (3) prenatal diagnosis followed by termination of homozygous or doubly heterozygous fetuses. Postmarital screening and counselling are widely available for African couples who have had affected children already: in Nigeria in particular, there have been attempts to educate the population and to make premarital counselling available.[81]

Prenatal diagnosis is technically possible and is becoming relatively inexpensive to apply in a few centres.[53] National programmes in Africa suffer restraints of low priority from government, lack of knowledge in the whole community, lack of trained staff, lack of facilities and the illegality or ethical non-acceptance of termination of pregnancy.

Haemoglobin SC disease

The compound heterozygous inheritance of HbS and HbC occurs often in West Africa and in populations derived from West Africa (see Figures 13.16 and 13.18). The pathophysiology and clinical features are similar to those of HbSS, but the severity is much less, and some patients are nearly asymptomatic.[69] Age at presentation is generally later. Because many girls survive childhood, HbSC is the most common form of sickle cell disease to present with complications during pregnancy in West Africa.[77] Eye disease is more frequent, related to the higher Hb concentration. Because the spleen is not destroyed, acute sequestration crises and splenic

infarcts during flight, including in pressurized aircraft, occur during adult life.

The Hb concentration is intermediate between that of HbSS and normals. The MCV is lower than in HbSS; reticulocyte counts are moderately raised. The red cell appearance is of anisocytosis, some macrocytes, some microspherocytes, numerous target cells, occasional sickle cell forms but with rounded ends, and occasional intraerythrocytic crystals of precipitated HbC (Figure 13.19). Electrophoresis shows two major fractions in the position of HbS and HbC.

The condition of combined inheritance of HbSS plus the α globin variant HbG^Philadelphia is commonly mistaken for HbSC in West Africa. On electrophoresis the subject with HbSS + G shows HbS and the hybrid HbS/G, which moves into the position of HbC; HbS solubility easily differentiates between the two, showing the heterozygous pattern (half precipitated) with HbSC and the homozygous pattern (all haemoglobin precipitated) with HbSS + G.

Haemoglobin S β⁰ thalassaemia

The inheritance of both HbS and β⁰ thalassaemia occurs most often in North Africa, Sicily and in the mixed population of the Americas (see Figures 13.6 and 13.16).[69,70,72]

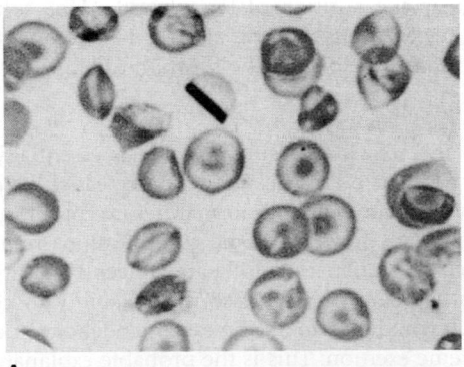

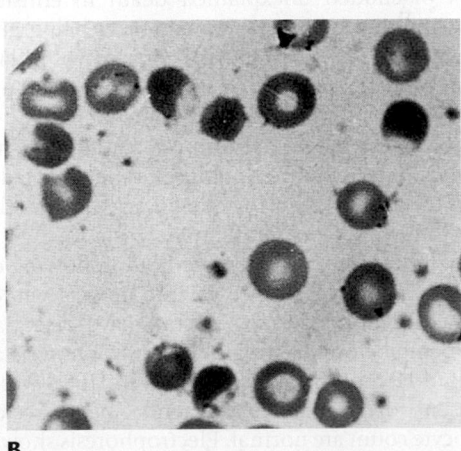

Figure 13.19 Peripheral blood films. (A) Haemoglobin C disease: there are numerous target cells and one red cell shows intracellular crystal formation. (B) G6PD deficiency: red cells showing oxidative damage. The haemoglobin seems to be separated from the membrane of the cells in certain areas ('blister' cells) and 'bite' cells where the Heinz bodies have been removed in the spleen; the rest of the cell looks dense. These changes occur only during a haemolytic episode.

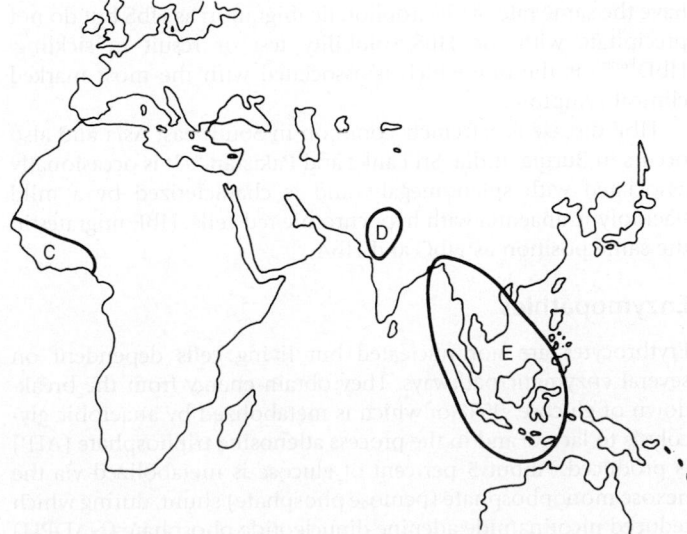

Figure 13.18 Areas of the Old World where haemoglobins C, D (Punjab or Los Angeles) and E reach polymorphic frequencies. (Reproduced with permission of the publishers, from Fleming AF. In: Strickland GT, ed. *Hunter's Tropical Medicine*, 7th edn. Philadelphia: W B Saunders; 1991:36–64.)

The clinical course is very similar to that of HbSS. Haematologically the two conditions are difficult to distinguish: the peripheral blood pictures are similar, the MCV and MCH are lower in HbS β^0 thalassaemia; HbS is the only major fraction and the HbF is raised in both conditions, but HbA$_2$ is raised only in HbS β^0 thalassaemia. The diagnosis is made with certainty when one parent carries the β^S gene and the other has β^0 thalassaemia trait.

Haemoglobin S β^+ thalassaemia

This doubly heterozygous condition is most common in Liberia and other parts of West Africa (see Figures 13.6 and 13.16). The clinical course is mild. Anaemia is often slight, and irreversibly sickled cells are seen rarely in the blood. Haemoglobin electrophoresis shows HbA 5–30%, and HbS >50%. It is important not to mistake HbS β^+ thalassaemia for HbAS, in which the HbS is always <50%.

Haemoglobin S D^{Punjab}

There are several HbDs, but only HbD^{Punjab} interacts with HbS, leading to a disease similar to HbSS, and is seen amongst Sikhs and mixed populations (see Figures 13.16 and 13.18).[69,70] There is moderately severe haemolytic anaemia; the peripheral blood picture resembles HbSS; electrophoresis at alkaline pH shows a single band in the position of HbS, but the HbS solubility test yields the heterozygous pattern, and electrophoresis on agar gel separates HbS from HbD (in the position of HbA).

Sickle cell trait

The inheritance of HbAS results in what is essentially a benign condition, which is not associated with decreased life expectancy or with any haematological abnormalities except for the presence of HbS. There are, however, some complications resulting from microinfarcts in the renal medulla and spleen.[53,69,70]

There is a progressive decrease in the ability to concentrate urine, which could lead to an increased tendency to dehydration during extreme exertion. This is the probable explanation for the relative risk of sudden unexplained death in enlisted recruits during basic training in the US Armed Forces being 28–40 times higher among those with HbAS as compared with black recruits or recruits of all races; the relative risk increases with age.[82] These sudden deaths are rare, however, as there were only 12 deaths among 38 600 HbAS individuals in over 2 million recruits. Other renal complications include a doubling of the expected frequency of significant bacteriuria during pregnancy, and rarely painless haematuria following renal papillary necrosis.

Incidents are reported of splenic infarcts following exertion at high altitudes. Earlier reports of splenic infarcts while flying at high altitudes in unpressurized aircraft have been largely discounted as being before haemoglobin electrophoresis and differentiation from HbS β^+ thalassaemia or even HbSC was possible.

In the absence of other causes of anaemia, the Hb, red cell indices and reticulocyte count are normal. Electrophoresis shows HbA and HbS: the proportion that is HbS has a trimodal distribution associated with the coincidental inheritance of α-thalassaemia genes; HbS is 34–38% with $\alpha\alpha/\alpha\alpha$, 28–34% with $-\alpha/\alpha\alpha$ and 20–28% with $-\alpha/-\alpha$. HbS above 45% is suggestive of HbS β^+ thalassaemia.

A partial protection against *P. falciparum* malaria has been more clearly demonstrated to be associated with sickle cell trait than it has with any other inherited abnormality of the red cells.[35,72]

In the non-immune, parasite densities, the frequency of severe malaria (e.g. cerebral malaria or malarial anaemia) and the frequency of death from severe malaria are all lower, and survival rates in childhood are higher. In areas of low endemicity female fertility is higher. In areas of stable malaria HbAS gives partial protection against HMS and severe anaemia associated with HMS during pregnancy.[26,33] There appear to be several mechanisms by which the density of parasitaemias is controlled:[35,72] (1) there is an increase of sickling of parasitized red cells, with subsequent removal of the parasitized and sickled cells by the spleen, so limiting the number of early parasite forms; (2) the intraerythrocyte growth during schizogony is inhibited by HbS gelling during the last 12 h of the cycle spent in relatively hypoxic deep tissues; (3) enhancement of cell-mediated immune responses against *P. falciparum* antigens has been described, possibly related to a modified expression of parasite antigens.[83]

Other haemoglobinopathies associated with haemolytic anaemia

The other common haemolytic haemoglobin disorders are Hbs C, D and E diseases (see Figure 13.18).[53]

HbC disease occurs commonly in West Africa, the carrier rate being highest in northern Ghana, with an incidence of 16–28%. The homozygous disorder is characterized by a mild haemolytic anaemia and splenomegaly. It can be recognized by examination of a blood film which shows up to 100% target cell formation with intracellular crystals (Figure 13.19A). Mild microcytosis is a common but not universal feature of HbC trait and disease. Folic acid deficiency and megaloblastic erythropoiesis frequently complicate the course of pregnancy. The diagnosis can be confirmed by haemoglobin electrophoresis.

HbD disease has been found in several racial groups. The clinical picture is that of a moderately severe haemolytic anaemia with splenomegaly. The blood film usually shows moderate numbers of target cells. There are several different types of HbD, all of which have the same rate of electrophoretic migration as HbS but do not precipitate with the HbS solubility test or result in sickling. HbD^{Punjab} is the one which is associated with the most marked clinical symptoms.

HbE disease is extremely common in South-east Asia and also occurs in Burma, India, Sri Lanka and Pakistan.[62] It is occasionally associated with splenomegaly, and is characterized by a mild haemolytic anaemia with hypochromic red cells. HbE migrates in the same position as HbC and HbA$_2$.

Enzymopathies

Erythrocytes are non-nucleated but living cells dependent on several enzymatic pathways. They obtain energy from the breakdown of glucose, 95% of which is metabolized by anaerobic glycolysis to lactate and in the process adenosine triphosphate (ATP) is produced. About 5 per cent of glucose is metabolized via the hexose monophosphate (pentose phosphate) shunt, during which reduced nicotinamide adenine dinucleotide phosphate (NADPH) is produced. There are many enzymopathies or inherited defects of enzymes affecting the red cells, for example pyruvate kinase deficiency, but of these only deficiencies of G6PD, the first and rate-limiting enzyme of the hexose monophosphate shunt, reach polymorphic frequencies in different populations.[84,85]

G6PD deficiency

Role of the enzyme

G6PD is vital to and occurs in all cells, but in the red cell this enzyme with the hexose monophosphate pathway is the only source of NADPH. Reduced glutathione (GSH) is synthesized at high concentration in red cells, and has the function of restoring oxidized SH groups and reducing superoxides and peroxides (through the actions of superoxide dismutase and glutathione peroxidase), but is itself oxidized to GSSG. NADPH is essential for the regeneration of GSH (with the enzyme glutathione reductase). G6PD deficiency and a reduction of synthesis of NADPH expose the red cell to oxidation of haemoglobin with the intracellular precipitation of globin as Heinz bodies, of several enzymes and of lipids and proteins of the membrane, with consequent haemolysis.

G6PD variants

Over 400 allelic variants of G6PD have been differentiated by electrophoretic mobility, kinetic properties and spectrophotometric assay of enzymatic activity. They have been classified according to their enzymatic activity and clinical manifestations (Table 13.18). Variants of class I, causing chronic non-spherocytic haemolytic anaemias, occur sporadically in all populations. Variants of class II (e.g. Gd^{Mediterranean}) and of class III (e.g. GdA$^-$) are associated with intermittent haemolytic crises triggered by oxidant stresses: all variants of major public health importance are in these two groups. Class IV includes GdB, the most common enzyme and referred to as the normal: other variants with normal activity achieve polymorphic frequency, for example GdA in Africa.

The gene controlling G6PD structure is carried on the X chromosome. Males who inherit an abnormal gene ($^-$XY) will have the variant enzyme in all their erythrocytes, as will homozygous females ($^-$X$^-$X). Heterozygous females ($^-$XX) will have on average half of their red cells containing normal enzyme and half containing variant enzyme, due to the random suppression of one X chromosome in all female somatic cells. Clinically significant enzyme deficiency will be seen most often in hemizygous males; homozygous females contribute about 10% of those genetically deficient, and about 10% of female heterozygotes are also effectively deficient due to unequal inactivation of their X chromosomes. Frequency in populations is usually expressed as a percentage of males who are hemizygotes.

World distribution

About 400 million of the world's population carry one or two genes for G6PD deficiency: the highest frequencies are in sub-Saharan Africa (e.g. 32% of males among the Luo on the shores of Lake Victoria), Saudi Arabia and South-east Asia (Figure 13.20). There are populations, for example Sardinians and Kurdish Jews, in which the frequency of G6PD deficiency in males exceeds 50%. The Old World can be divided into three zones according to which G6PD variants achieve polymorphic frequency. In zone I, covering the Mediterranean, North Africa, western Asia and the Indian subcontinent, the severely deficient (class II) Gd^{Mediterranean} is prevalent. In zone II, covering South-east Asia, China, Korea and Oceania, two class II variants (Gd^{Mediterranean} and Gd^{Union}) and two moderately severely deficient (class III) variants (Gd^{Mahidol} and Gd^{Canton}) are common: Asia is remarkable for the number of variants, for example in the population of Taiwan there are at least nine different deficient enzymes, of which Gd$^{Taiwan-Hakka}$ is the most prevalent.[86] In the third zone, sub-Saharan Africa, the class III enzyme GdA$^-$ is frequent, the class II Gd^{Mali} achieves local polymorphic frequency, and up to 40% carry the GdA variant with normal activity. G6PD deficiency is not found in the indigenous populations of America or Australia, but deficient variants occur commonly in the descendants of African, Mediterranean and Asian immigrants.

About 4.5 million infants born each year are at risk for the complications of G6PD deficiency.

Clinical manifestations

Episodes of haemolysis and jaundice occur in four situations: (1) the neonatal period, (2) severe viral and bacterial infections, (3) following ingestion of certain foods and (4) following exposure to various drugs and chemicals (Table 13.19). These intermittent episodes tend to be more severe with class II (e.g. Gd^{Mediterranean}) than class III (e.g. GdA$^-$) variants.

Neonatal jaundice

Newborn infants are frequently jaundiced (defined as serum bilirubin >250 mmol/L (15 mg/dL) on about the 4th day of life in all parts of the world where G6PD deficiency is common (see Figure 13.20), and neonatal jaundice is recognized as a major public health problem in Greece, Saudi Arabia, tropical Africa, the Caribbean, South-east Asia and China, although incidence figures are not often available; in Hong Kong 12% and Singapore 10% of newborns were jaundiced before the introduction of successful control programmes.[87] Jaundice is often multifactorial: common causes include sepsis, prematurity, G6PD deficiency, fetomaternal ABO incompatibility, and haematomas from birth trauma. G6PD deficiency contributes in 30–80% of patients. Globally, infant mortality due to jaundice associated with G6PD deficiency is 0.7–1.6 per 1000 births, with an equal number suffering lifelong morbidity.

Identified variables which potentiate jaundice due to G6PD deficiency are: (1) the severity of the enzyme deficiency (e.g. Mediterranean vs African variants) and lower levels of G6PD in the liver; (2) prematurity; (3) genetically determined slower maturity of the liver in Asians; (4) infections, such as umbilical sepsis, septicaemia and pneumonia; (5) exposure of either the mother or

Table 13.18 Classification of variants of G6PD

Class	G6PD activity	Haematological manifestations	Polymorphic variants
I	Nearly absent	Congenital non-spherocytic haemolytic anaemia	–
II	Severe <10%	Intermittent haemolysis	Mediterranean, Mali, Union
III	Moderate 10–60%	Less severe intermittent haemolysis	A$^-$, Canton, Mahidol
IV	Normal 60–100%	None	B, A, Gambia
V	Increased >150%	None	

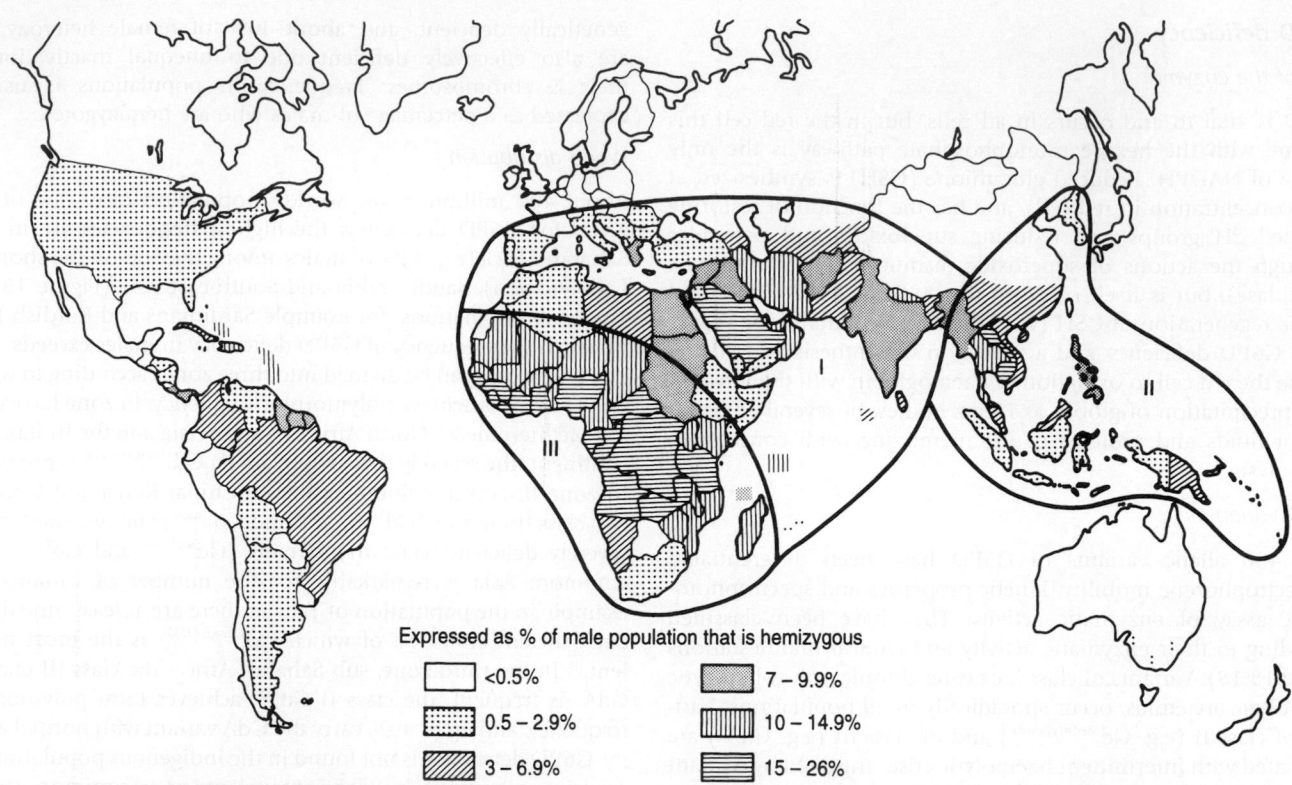

Expressed as % of male population that is hemizygous

<0.5%	7 – 9.9%
0.5 – 2.9%	10 – 14.9%
3 – 6.9%	15 – 26%

Figure 13.20 World distribution of G6PD deficiency. Superimposed are three zones where different G6PD variants reach polymorphic frequencies: Zone I, Gd^Mediterranean; zone II, Gd^Mediterranean, Gd^Canton, Gd^Union, Gd^Mahidol; Zone III, Gd A-. (Reproduced with permission of the World Health Organization from WHO Working Group 84.)

the infant to oxidant drugs (Table 13.19), e.g. mothballs (in the preservation of towelling saved from an older infant), herbal medicines (e.g. Chinese hung lian), 'mentholated' powders applied to the umbilical cord, vitamin K analogues, sulphonamides and nitrofurantoins; and (6) breast-feeding, which, however, should not be discouraged unless there are exceptional circumstances. Jaundice results from both haemolysis and poor hepatic function. Anaemia is generally moderate (e.g. Hb 130 g/L), with red cell anisocytosis, spherocytosis, polychromasia and numerous nucleated cells. Total unconjugated bilirubin levels are raised, and when above 300 mmol/L there is the danger of kernicterus and severe permanent brain damage.

While the serum bilirubin is in the range of 250–300 mmol/L in mature and otherwise healthy infants, treatment should be with phototherapy. In the absence of designed equipment, sufficient irradiance can be obtained from a unit of at least seven 20-watt fluorescent tubes placed 40 cm above the naked infant, whose eyes are shielded.[85] Alternatively, exposure to the morning sunlight, with cooling of the body and shielding of the eyes, is effective. When the unconjugated bilirubin rises above 300 mmol/L, treatment is by exchange blood transfusion with blood from G6PD normal donors compatible with both mother and infant, at a volume twice that of the infant's blood volume (i.e. 2 × 85 mL/kg body weight), in 20 mL aliquots over 2 h. Phototherapy and exchange transfusion are indicated at lower bilirubin levels in low-weight and ill infants.[85–88]

Neonatal jaundice has been controlled and kernicterus virtually abolished in Singapore by a highly successful national campaign in which (1) G6PD activity is screened in cord blood of all infants; (2) all those deficient are observed in hospital for 2 weeks, and treated promptly if jaundice develops; (3) both the general public and health professionals are informed and educated; (4) letters are given to parents with G6PD deficiency addressed to the obstetrician who delivers the next baby; and (5) G6PD-deficient infants are issued with cards warning against potentially haemolysing drugs.[87] Other measures preventing neonatal jaundice include: (1) adequate prenatal care, so avoiding many premature deliveries; (2) non-traumatic delivery, so avoiding extensive haematomas; and (3) hygiene in the puerperium, so avoiding sepsis.

Infection-induced jaundice

Viral infections, including hepatitis, infections of the respiratory and gastrointestinal tracts, and bacterial infections, including lobar pneumonia, typhoid, paratyphoid and septicaemia, may cause severe jaundice in G6PD-deficient subjects.[85] Possible mechanisms are the generation of H_2O_2 by activated neutrophils and macrophages triggering haemolysis of G6PD-deficient cells, and liver dysfunction leading to hepatocellular jaundice. Anaemia will be more severe as a result of suppression of erythropoiesis by infection. The course may be complicated in adults, but only rarely in children, by renal failure, which can be the result of pre-existing renal disease, nephrotoxic drugs, urinary tract infection, hepatic virus infection, renal ischaemia and tubular obstruction by haemoglobin. The administration of oxidant drugs may lead to further intravascular haemolysis and life-threatening renal failure.

Table 13.19 Drugs and other agents commonly associated with oxidative damage to red cells

DRUGS AND CHEMICALS WHICH CAUSE OXIDATIVE DAMAGE TO RED CELLS IN NORMAL SUBJECTS AND MORE SEVERE HAEMOLYSIS IN G6PD-DEFICIENT SUBJECTS
Phenylhydrazine
Dapsone and other sulfones
Naphthalene (moth balls)
Phenacetin and acetanilide (in large doses only)
Sulfasalazine (Salazopyrin)

DRUGS AND CHEMICALS WHICH ARE SHOWN TO CAUSE HAEMOLYSIS IN G6PD-DEFICIENT SUBJECTS
Acetanilide and phenacetin (therapeutic doses)
Henna dye
Methylene blue
Nalidixic acid
Niridazole (Ambilhar)
Nitrofurantoins
Orange RN (red suya food colouring)
Pamaquine
Primaquine
Pentaquine
Sulfonamides: sulfacetamide sulfamethoxale/co-trimoxazole sulfanilamide sulfapyridine
Thiazosulfone
Toluidine blue
Trinitrotoluene (TNT)
Vicia faba (broad beans)

DRUGS AND CHEMICALS THAT MAY CAUSE HAEMOLYSIS IN SOME TYPES OF G6PD-DEFICENT SUBJECT BUT NOT SHOWN TO BE HAEMOLYTIC IN GDA⁻ TYPE
Aspirin (in large doses)
Chloroquine
Quinine
Quinidine
Vitamin K analogues
Chloramphenicol
Dimercaprol (BAL)

Management is supportive: the treatment of the primary infection, the avoidance of oxidative drugs (Table 13.19) and a regimen for renal failure.

Food-induced haemolysis

Favism is a condition of severe intravascular haemolysis precipitated by eating fava beans (Vicia faba) or inhalation of the pollen; it occurs commonly in G6PD-deficient inhabitants of the Mediterranean area, North Africa and western and eastern Asia. It had

been thought to be associated only with class II variants (e.g. Gd^{Mediterranean}), but has been described with other variants including GdA⁻.[89] Favism occurs with the ingestion of fresh, dried or frozen beans, but fresh young beans in the spring are the most potent. Haemolysis in breast-fed infants may follow when mothers eat fava beans. Which ingredients trigger haemolysis is not proven.

Favism affects children under 5 years most commonly. Its pathogenesis is uncertain, as some G6PD subjects are spared altogether, while others have attacks for the first time after eating beans for years without trouble. There is intravascular haemolysis of sudden onset 24–48 h after ingestion of beans: patients show pallor and haemoglobinuria; jaundice is less pronounced than with the haemolysis triggered by infections or drugs. Anaemia may be profound and renal failure can develop.

There is no specific treatment: transfusion of G6PD normal blood may be required if there is incipient or established cardiac failure.

Haemolytic episodes are best prevented by screening of G6PD deficiency in populations with high frequency, education and avoiding eating beans.

Milder acute haemolytic episodes have followed eating red suya, a peppered kebab-like roasted meat, in Nigeria; the offending substance was Orange RN (monosodium salt of 1-phenylazo-2-naphthol-6-sulfonic acid) used as colouring. It can be predicted that other foods could have the same effect in developing countries where there is inadequate control of additives.[90]

Drug-induced haemolysis

Ingestion of a wide variety of drugs and chemicals induces haemolysis in G6PD-deficient subjects (Table 13.19). The range of precipitating substances and the severity of the crises are greater with class II (e.g. Gd^{Mediterranean}) than class III (e.g. GdA⁻) variants. There is also considerable intrapatient variability of severity between subjects with the same G6PD variant and drug exposure.[84,85,88]

Starting from between a few hours and 3 days after exposure, there may be only transient mild anaemia, or in some there is a rapidly progressive severe anaemia reaching a nadir at 7–8 days. Patients can complain of loin and abdominal pain; there is jaundice, haemoglobinuria and transient splenomegaly. Recovery is marked by a reticulocytosis and a rise of haemoglobin after 8–9 days.

Continued exposure to the drug can lead to fatal anaemia or renal failure in the case of class II variants. However, in the milder haemolysis of GdA⁻ it is sometimes possible to continue with essential therapy, for example dapsone in the treatment of leprosy; patients have a transient haemolytic anaemia, followed by a state of compensated haemolysis.

Treatment is supportive and by withdrawal of the offending agent. Further attacks can be prevented by giving the patient a list of drugs to be avoided. Community strategies include screening and education.

Diagnosis

Haematology

During the steady state, subjects with the common forms of G6PD deficiency have a very mild chronic haemolysis, with a red cell lifespan of around 100 days. With Gd^{Mediterranean} the mean Hb in males is slightly decreased (141 vs 157 g/L in controls in one series). Red cell indices and appearance on blood film are normal, but there is a slight reticulocytosis (±1.5%).

During a haemolytic crisis there are all the features of intravascular haemolysis (see Table 13.11) and a characteristic peripheral blood film appearance (see Figure 13.19B): supravital staining shows the presence of Heinz bodies.

G6PD screening and identification

There are several screening tests available that depend on NADPH production and its detection by direct fluorescence or by reduction of a coloured dye (e.g. methylene blue) to its colourless form.[85] These are simple, inexpensive and sensitive for the detection of hemizygous males and homozygous females when in the steady state. However, immediately following haemolytic crises, when there is a high population of young red cells, G6PD activity of whole blood may be normal, especially with class III (e.g. GdA⁻) variants; in this situation blood should be centrifuged and the older cells at the bottom of the column tested, or the test delayed for about 6 weeks.

G6PD activity can be measured quantitatively by the spectrophotometric assay of NADPH formation by red cells: this requires a basic biochemistry laboratory. Male hemizygotes, female homozygotes and more than 80% of female heterozygotes can be identified.

The different G6PD variants are identified by several techniques, including electrophoresis and enzyme kinetic studies: these investigations are performed in reference or research laboratories only.

G6PD and malaria

Evidence that G6PD deficiency may confer advantage is derived from geography, parasitology of patients and in vitro cultures of *P. falciparum*.[84,85] Globally, G6PD deficiency reaches polymorphic frequency only where *P. falciparum* is or was endemic (see Figure 13.20), suggesting that in these areas deficient subjects have a genetic advantage; this view is supported by micromapping, for example in Sardinia where deficient gene frequency declines with increasing altitude and decreasing transmission of malaria. In a clinical study, female Nigerian children with GdB/GdA⁻ had significantly lower *P. falciparum* densities than normal children with malaria; furthermore, GdB (normal) red cells were much more often parasitized than GdA⁻ (deficient) red cells in the same individual.[85] It had been thought that limitation of malaria was confined to female heterozygotes only and was not enjoyed by male hemizyotes, but large case-control studies of children in West and East Africa have shown that both female heterozygotes and male hemizygotes had significant protection against severe malaria (about 46% and 58%, respectively), but protection against mild malaria was statistically significant only in female heterozygotes.[91] In vitro cultures of *P. falciparum* have demonstrated that parasite growth is impaired in G6PD-deficient compared with normal red cells, but in some studies additional oxidative stress was needed before the difference became apparent. Oxidant radicals in parasitized red cells could lead to both impaired parasite development and to damage to the red cell membrane with early phagocytosis.[92]

Membrane defects

The red cell membrane is supported by a protein skeleton consisting of a lattice of hexagons, the sides of which are spectrin tetra-

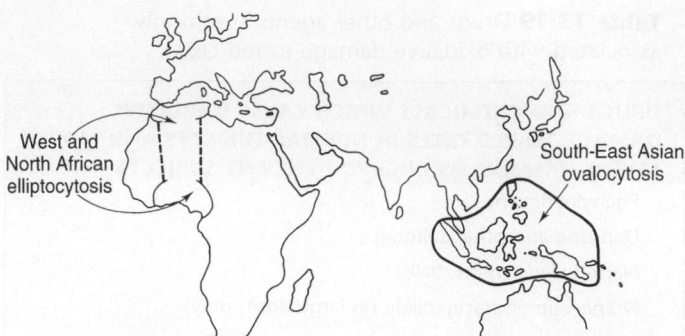

Figure 13.21 Areas of the Old World where ovalocytosis and elliptocytosis achieve (or approach) a polymorphic frequency.

mers: these are linked at the corners of the hexagons by actin, tropomyosin and protein 4.1, and attached to the lipid bilayer by ankyrin and protein band 3 (the major transmembrane protein and anion transporter), as well as by glycoproteins such as glycophorin C. Inherited variants of either the integral or skeletal proteins of the red cell membrane may be manifest as abnormalities of shape, such as hereditary spherocytosis, elliptocytosis and ovalocytosis.[93] Membrane defects occur sporadically in all populations, hereditary spherocytosis being the most studied; only ovalocytosis in South-east Asia and Oceania achieves polymorphic frequency, but elliptocytosis is approaching polymorphic frequency in West and North Africa (see Figure 13.21).

South-east Asian ovalocytosis

The molecular basis of South-east Asian ovalocytosis (SAO) is a deletion of 27 nucleotides, resulting in the deletion of nine amino acids from band 3: the abnormal SAO band 3 has a higher than normal affinity for ankyrin, resulting in increased membrane rigidity and the oval shape (Figure 13.22A).[93,94] Inheritance is autosomal and dominant. Homozygotes have not been observed and this condition is probably lethal.

Ovalocytosis is seen at high frequency in populations of Malaysia, Indonesia, the Philippines, Papua New Guinea and the Solomon Islands, and possibly in Micronesian populations further out into the Pacific (see Figure 13.21). The distribution is extremely uneven within this area, but reaches up to 50% in Sulawesi (Celebes) and 27% in coastal Papua New Guinea.

A high proportion of red cells are ovalocytes (with a long axis less than twice the transverse axis), stomatocytes and knizocytes (with duplicated central pallor) (Figure 13.22A). Osmotic fragility is reduced. In otherwise healthy children, SAO is not associated with haemolysis or anaemia.

It had been reported earlier that in vivo both *P. falciparum* and *P. vivax* parasite rates were significantly lower in subjects with ovalocytes than in those with normal red cells, and that in vitro there was reduced parasite invasion of the rigid membranes of ovalocytes. More recently, however, when the diagnosis was made by detection of the SAO band 3 and not by subjective microscopy, similar rates of densities of both *P. falciparum* and *P. vivax* parasitaemias have been observed in community controls with and without SAO. Malarial anaemia was exacerbated by ovalocytosis, the median Hb being 12 g/L lower during acute malaria in

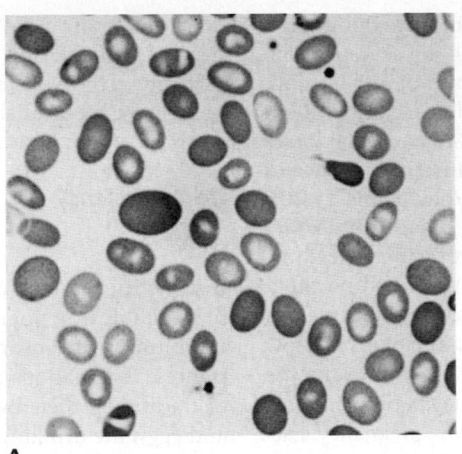
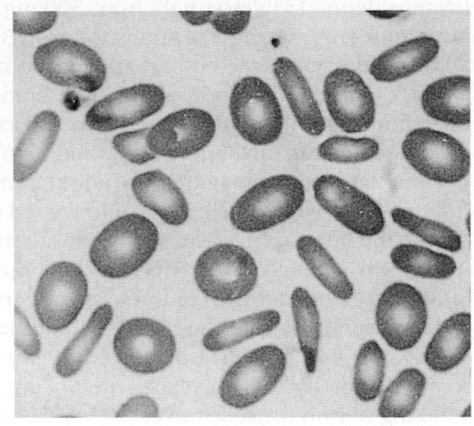

Figure 13.22 Peripheral blood films. (A) South-east Asian ovalocytosis. A high proportion of cells have a long axis which is less than twice the transverse axis (ovalocytosis). Some have two areas of central pallor (knizocytes), e.g. on the horizontal midline, towards the right edge. Some have mouth-like slits of pallor (stomatocytes), e.g. near the lower edge towards the left. (Reproduced with permission of the author and publisher, from Dacie JV. *The Haemolytic Anaemias* 1, 3rd edn. Edinburgh: Churchill Livingstone; 1985.) (B) Elliptocytosis. The long axis is more than twice the transverse axis.

A　　　　　**B**

subjects with SAO than in controls. On the other hand, SAO prevented cerebral malaria, being observed in none of 68 children with cerebral malaria and in six (8.8%) of 68 matched controls in Papua New Guinea.[95] The mechanism of protection is likely to be related to differences of adherence of parasitized RBC to endothelium.

Elliptocytosis in West and North Africa

There are many mutations which result in elliptocytosis, and several have been described in West and North Africa.[94] Two variants of spectrin (Spa$^{I/65}$, Spa$^{I/46-50a}$) are at least approaching polymorphic frequency. Spectrin aI/65 is the more common, but both are found throughout West Africa, the Maghreb (Tunisia, Algeria and Morocco), southern Italy and the Americas;[96] Tuaregs who inhabit the Sahara between West and North Africa have elliptocytosis, but this has not been characterized (see Figure 13.22). Up to 2–3% of both northern and southern Nigerians have an uncharacterized elliptocytosis. Inheritance is dominant. The condition is usually symptomless, but there may be mild haemolysis, especially in homozygotes with the spectrin aI/65 variant. Red cells have a long axis more than twice the transverse axis (Figure 13.22B). There can be periodic episodes of slight jaundice and moderate splenomegaly following intercurrent infections; children with elliptocytosis and malaria sometimes develop profound anaemia (personal observations). Some elliptocyte variants in vitro are resistant to invasion by *P. falciparum*,[97] but there is no evidence at present as to whether there is selection for elliptocytosis in West Africa.

Nutritional anaemias

Iron

Iron is essential for the formation of haemoglobin, myoglobin and various enzymes. Its deficiency is the most common of all nutritional disorders: about 1000 million individuals suffer from anaemia due to iron deficiency (see Table 13.10), while an even larger number have iron depletion which has not reached the stage of anaemia.[98,99]

Dietary iron and absorption

In early postnatal life iron is derived normally from breast milk, which contains 0.3–0.5 mg/L in a readily available form (50% absorbed). Iron in all other foods is in three forms: (1) haem iron, (2) non-haem iron and (3) contamination iron.

Haem iron is a constituent of haemoglobin and myoglobin in meat, poultry, fish and blood products; it is readily absorbed (20–30%) by the duodenal mucosal cells and utilized.

Non-haem iron is found in varying concentrations in all foods of plant origin, including cereals, tubers, vegetables and pulses. It is poorly absorbed (<5%) from common staples such as rice, maize, wheat, sorghum and millet when eaten alone. Absorption is inhibited by many vegetable ligands, including phytates in cereals, polyphenols in nuts and legumes, tannin in tea and soy protein, and by fibre; other inhibitors are egg phosphoproteins, and in those with pica, ash and clay. Absorption may be enhanced to up to 20% by consumption during the same meal of (1) fresh fruits and vegetables rich in ascorbic acid (e.g. guava, citrus, pineapple, mango, green or red peppers, cauliflower, some green leaves, potato, sweet potato, tomato and turnip), (2) amino acids from meat, poultry, fish and other seafoods, and (3) acids (e.g. lactic, citric).

Contamination iron is from two sources: dirt and iron cooking vessels. An adult male can take in 40–500 mg of contaminating iron on rice, sorghum or tef (*Eragrostis abyssinica*, a staple of the Ethiopian highlands) from the dirt picked up during threshing on earth floors and the dust of the marketplace; little of this is absorbable. Cooking food in iron pots may increase the iron content several-fold, especially with soups containing acid-rich vegetables which are simmered for a long time. Beer brewed in iron pots is rich in available iron, and nutritional iron overload can follow after years of steady consumption (see below).

Absorption is by duodenal mucosal cells and is regulated by the iron status of the individual, being more efficient in the iron depleted than in the iron replete.

Iron balance

The iron in the body is in four compartments: (1) haemoglobin iron 1.5–3.0 g, (2) storage iron 1.0–1.5 g as ferritin and haemosiderin, (3) 'essential' iron 300 mg in myoglobin and numerous enzymes, and (4) transport iron 3–4 mg as transferrin, all quantities relating to adult males. The turnover of iron is rapid, about 23 mg entering and leaving the haemoglobin compartment of an adult each day, but iron is highly conserved and basal losses by desquamation in faeces, urine and skin for adult men and postmenopausal women are only about 1 mg/day (Table 13.20). Infants have low requirements while the red cell mass diminishes during the first 4–6 months, and these are met by breast-feeding. Iron needs are high relative to body size during growth in older infancy, childhood and the adolescent growth spurt. Menstruation approximately doubles the basal demand. Requirements are low during the first trimester of pregnancy but rise rapidly in the second trimester, to reach around 6–7 mg/day; approximately 1000 mg of iron is needed over the whole of one pregnancy. Lactating women secrete about 0.3 mg of iron per day in breast milk, but while they have amenorrhoea daily requirements are relatively low.

Diets with high contents of bioavailable iron are eaten by most populations in industrialized countries, and also, until recently, surviving communities of hunter-gatherers, pastoralists who eat meat and blood (e.g. Masai in Kenya) and some groups with high ascorbic acid intake (e.g. Yoruba in Nigeria); physiological demands for iron are usually met, except during pregnancy when negative balance and some depletion of stores is inevitable. The majority of the world's population eat food with intermediate, low or very low bio-available iron, from which it is impossible to meet the basic physiological requirements for iron (Table 13.20).[99]

Iron deficiency

Aetiology

Iron deficiency is commonly the result of inadequate intake of bioavailable iron not meeting physiological requirements. Ligands inhibiting iron absorption can be increased in special circumstances: food taboos applied during pregnancy; the replacement of traditional diets by convenience foods including wheat-bread and eggs; the drinking of tea (or coffee to a lesser extent) with the meal. Premature infants are a special case of nutritional deficiency as the transplacental transport of iron to the infant takes place almost wholly in the last 4 weeks' gestation.

Those with the greatest physiological demands for iron are at the highest risk of deficiency; these are preschool children, adolescents during the growth spurt, and especially menstruating girls, and pregnant women. Women who have many pregnancies, closely spaced, are especially liable to deficiency.

Table 13.20 FAO/WHO recommended iron intakes (mg/day) to cover requirements of 97.5% individuals in each age/sex group for diets with different bioavailabilities.[98]

Age/sex group	Absorbed iron required	BIOAVAILABILITY OF DIETARY IRON (% OF IRON ABSORBED)			
		Very low[a] (<5%)	Low[b] (5–10%)	Intermediate[c] (11–18%)	High[d] (>19%)
Children, both sexes					
0–4 months	0.5	[e]	[e]	[e]	[e]
4–12 months	0.96	24	13	6	4
13–24 months	0.61	15	8	4	3
2–5 years	0.70	17	9	5	3
6–11 years	1.17	29	16	8	5
Adolescents					
12–16 years (girls)	2.02	50	27	13	9
12–16 years (boys)	1.82	45	24	12	8
Adults					
Men	1.14	28	15	8	5
Women					
Menstruating	2.38	59	32	16	11
Pregnant					
1st trimester	0.8	–	–	–	–
3rd trimester	6.3	[f]	[f]	[f]	–
Lactating	1.31	33	17	9	6
Postmenopausal	0.96	24	13	6	4

[a]*Very low bioavailability*. Diet composed almost entirely of cereals (e.g. in India).
[b]*Low bioavailability*. Monotonous diet based on cereals, roots and tubers, with a preponderance of foods which inhibit iron absorption (maize, rice, beans, wheat, sorghum) and with negligible quantities of meat, fish or ascorbic acid.
[c]*Intermediate bioavailability diet*. Similar to above, but including some foods of animal origin and/or ascorbic acid.
[d]*High bioavailability*. A diversified diet containing generous quantities of meat, poultry, fish or foods rich in ascorbic acid: typical of most populations in industrialized countries. The regular consumption with meals of inhibitors of absorption (e.g. tea or coffee) can reduce bioavailability to the intermediate level.
[e]Iron from breast milk is sufficient for about the first 6 months.
[f]Supplementation essential.

As normal red cells contain iron as haemoglobin 1 mg per 1 mL, chronic blood loss can lead easily to negative balance and depletion of iron stores. Common causes in the tropics are infection by hookworm, Schistosoma species and whipworm (*Trichuris trichiura*).[98–100] Many conditions leading to chronic haemorrhage (e.g. menorrhagia, aspirin ingestion, peptic ulcers, carcinomas) occur in tropical as well as in non-tropical environments.

Hookworm

Infections with *Ancylostoma duodenale* and *Necator americanus* are widespread, and approximately 1200 million individuals, almost a quarter of the world's population, are infected (see Chapter 85).[100] Prevalence of 80–90% in the population in the moist tropics is not unusual.

The adult worms ingest, detach and digest the host's intestinal mucosa, causing bleeding. The daily loss of iron has been calculated as 1.2 mg and 0.8 mg per 1000 ova/g of faeces for *A. duodenale* and *N. americanus*, respectively, but as both species are now found more or less worldwide and mixed infections are common, the daily loss of iron of 1 mg per 1000 ova/g of faeces regardless of species is a good working figure.[99,100]

Depletion of iron stores depends on (1) the daily absorption of iron, (2) the size of the body's iron stores and (3) the intensity of the hookworm infection. Subjects with diets poor in bioavailable iron and with low or no stores need only light infections to deplete them of iron; in contrast, adults in West Africa on traditional diets had a threshold of at least 20 000 ova/g of faeces, equivalent to an iron loss of 20 mg/day, above which they went into negative balance. Women have lower thresholds than men. Children expose their whole body surfaces to infection when playing on the ground, and have heavy hookworm loads in relation to their body weights; the resultant subacute hookworm anaemia has an element of acute haemorrhage in its aetiology.

Acute hookworm anaemia is rare but follows extremely heavy infections, usually in infants but sometimes in older children or even adults. *A. duodenale* is able to cross the placenta and infect the infant in utero. Anaemia is from acute blood loss, shows a normochromic picture and may be severe and life-threatening.[21,100]

Schistosomiasis

About 200 million people are infected by *Schistosoma*, and transmission is increasing with the spread of irrigation (see Chapter 82).

The haematuria from *S. haematobium* is short lived but can give rise to a loss of 30–40 mg of iron per day and contribute significantly to iron deficiency, especially in adolescent boys, for example in Somalia and coastal East Africa.

The mechanisms of anaemia caused by *S. mansoni* and *S. japonicum* infections are complex. Ulcers and polyps in the colon bleed and can result in a chronic loss of iron of 7–8 mg/day. Infection of the liver is followed by hepatic fibrosis and the anaemia of chronic disorders; portal hypertension leads to splenomegaly and the pancytopenia of hypersplenism; oesophageal varices may bleed acutely or intermittently, leading to iron loss.[21,100]

Trichuriasis

T. trichiura is one of the most prevalent helminths in the world, infecting about 1000 million people (see Chapter 85).[100] Blood is lost from the inflamed colonic mucosa. Heavy infections in excess of 800 worms (16 000 ova/g of faeces) result in a blood loss of 4 mL, or iron loss of 1.5 mg/day. Trichuriasis can contribute to

iron deficiency, or be a major cause in children, as has been reported from Central America and Malaysia.[100]

Stages of iron deficiency

Iron deficiency passes through three stages. In the first stage, iron depletion, iron stores are reduced, but haemopoiesis remains unaffected: plasma ferritin is below normal and staining for iron in a bone marrow aspirate shows scanty (1+) or zero iron in the macrophages of a cellular fragment; plasma iron is low normal, plasma transferrin raised and its percentage saturation reduced within the normal range. In the second stage, iron-deficient erythropoiesis, iron stores have been exhausted: plasma ferritin is reduced further, iron is absent from the bone marrow and there are no sideroblasts; plasma iron and transferrin saturation are below normal and red cell protoporphyrin is raised; the Hb is likely to be within the normal range or there may be a slight normochromic anaemia. With further depletion, iron is not available for haemoglobin synthesis, and iron deficiency anaemia develops.

Iron deficiency anaemia

Clinical

Patients present with symptoms and signs of anaemia from any cause; in addition they may show angular stomatitis, koilonychia and loss of melanin skin pigmentation.

Iron is essential for many metabolic processes, and its deficiency even without anaemia has adverse effects on development during childhood, the outcome of pregnancy and work capacity. In practice it is not feasible to distinguish the results of iron deficiency per se from those of anaemia. The consequences of iron deficiency, and especially iron deficiency anaemia are: in infants, children and adolescents, impaired motor development, coordination, language development and scholastic achievement, psychological and behavioural effects (inattention, fatigue, insecurity, etc.) and decreased physical activity;[101] in adults of both sexes, decreased physical work, earning capacity and resistance to fatigue; in pregnant women, increased maternal and infant morbidity and mortality, placental hypertrophy premature delivery, and risk of low birthweight.[98,99,102,103] There is no convincing evidence that iron deficiency either enhances or significantly impairs resistance to infections, although there is some reduction of cellular immune responses.[99]

Haematology

Anaemia varies from mild to profound. The MCV, MCH and MCHC are all reduced; the peripheral blood film shows microcytic hypochromic red cells and sometimes numerous target cells (Figure 13.23). In the bone marrow aspirate there are micronormoblastic red cell precursors and the total absence of storage iron. Plasma, for example in a microhaematocrit tube, is nearly colourless and water clear.

There are three considerations in confirming the diagnosis of iron deficiency anaemia: (1) limited laboratory facilities, (2) biochemical measurements of iron status giving misleading results in patients with multiple pathology and (3) differentiation from the microcytic hypochromic anaemias of chronic disorders and β thalassaemia minor.

Within a limited laboratory, the diagnosis of iron deficiency anaemia can be usually made with certainty from the blood film appearance, colourless plasma and the absence of iron in the bone marrow. However, iron is immobilized in the RES in the anaemia

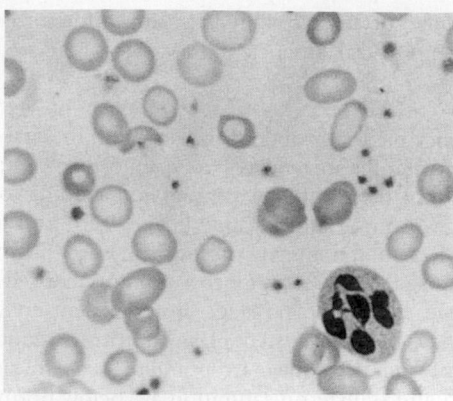

Figure 13.23 Peripheral blood film. Iron deficiency anaemia: there is variation in size of the red cells (anisocytosis) with many small cells (microcytosis), variation of shape (poikilocytosis) and hypersegmented neutrophil, suggestive but not diagnostic of folate or vitamin B_{12} deficiency; there are numerous platelets (thrombocytosis) which are likely to be a response to chronic haemorrhage.

of chronic disorders, megaloblastic anaemia and protein-energy malnutrition (PEM); although iron is seen in the bone marrow and iron deficiency is not limiting erythropoiesis at the time, treatment of the primary condition can lead to the mobilization of all iron and the uncovering of iron deficiency.

Ferritin is an acute reactive protein and plasma ferritin levels are generally raised in rural populations in the tropics, and although levels correlate with the body iron stores, higher cut-off points have to be applied. Malaria, other recurrent infection and chronic hepatic disease can be accompanied by abnormally high plasma ferritins even in the face of severe iron deficiency, making the measurement of plasma ferritin of limited diagnostic value, especially in children.

In iron deficiency, the plasma iron is low and the plasma transferrin is raised, so that transferrin saturation is <16% in adults, <14% in children and <12% in infants. In contrast, in anaemia of chronic disorders and PEM, both plasma iron and plasma ferritin are reduced, and although the saturation of transferrin is decreased it remains >15%.

In β thalassaemia minor the red cell count is higher (>5.0 × 10^{12}/ L), there is less anisocytosis (normal RBC distribution width (RDW)), greater microcytosis and less hypochromia than with iron deficiency (Table 13.15). From these characteristics are derived several formulae to differentiate the two conditions; for example, the ratio MCV:RBC is >14 in iron deficiency and <14 in thalassaemia.

Management

Oral treatment
Tablets of ferrous salts (e.g. exsiccated ferrous sulfate 200 mg, containing 60 mg of elemental iron) taken orally are the cheapest effective treatment.[98,104] For adults and adolescents, the recommended dosage is 60 mg of elemental iron per day for mild anaemia and 120 mg (plus folic acid 400 mg) per day for moderate or severe anaemia. Absorption is best if the tablets are taken on an empty stomach. Treatment should continue until the Hb has reached normal limits and ceased to rise, and then for at least another 4–6 weeks in order to build up body stores.

Pregnant women should receive a combination tablet containing 400 mg of folic acid and 60 mg of iron twice a day; suitable tablets are supplied by UNICEF for US$1 per 1000 tablets.

Infants and children may be treated with liquid preparations in divided doses to provide 5 mg of iron per kilogram body weight (plus folic acid 100–400 mg) per day.

Oral iron can cause upper gastrointestinal side effects (epigastric discomfort, nausea and vomiting), or lower gastrointestinal side effects (diarrhoea or constipation). The frequency of adverse reactions is related directly to the dosage of iron and not to the ferrous compound prescribed. Oral treatment must continue if possible: dosage should be reduced and then stepped up again slowly within the patient's tolerance, or the tablets taken with meals (although this reduces absorption), or the formulation changed to a better tolerated but much more expensive slow-release preparation.

Where folate intake is poor, deficiency may develop during the response to iron therapy: folic acid 5 mg/day for 3 weeks should be given.

Parenteral treatment
A parenteral route is justified when (1) oral treatment has not been tolerated, (2) there is persistent non-compliance, (3) it is nearly impossible for a patient to comply because of the severity of the iron deficiency and the length of time required for oral therapy, and (4) an advanced period of gestation does not allow for full oral treatment before obstetric delivery. The extra cost of parenteral preparations is offset by savings on hospital bed occupancy and staff time, and by the rapid return of the patient to productive life.[100]

Complementary parasite treatment
Where hookworm is endemic (prevalence >20%), those above 2 years of age should receive albendazole 400 mg in a single dose as the simplest to administer effective anthelmintic; treatment should be withheld during the first trimester of pregnancy. Where urinary schistosomiasis is endemic, any person over 5 years of age who has visible haematuria should be treated with oral praziquantel 50 mg/kg body weight in a single dose. Recovery may be delayed by coincidental malaria: children under 5 years of age in malaria endemic areas should receive curative antimalarial therapy followed by prophylaxis for 3 weeks, appropriate to the area.[104]

Prevention

There are four strategies for the prevention of iron deficiency: (1) iron supplementation; (2) fortification of a staple food with iron; (3) measures to increase dietary intake of bioavailable iron; and (4) the control of hookworm and other helminthic infections.[98,100]

Supplementation
Supplementation with medicinal iron has the advantages of having immediate impact and of being targeted on specific groups which are known to be liable to deficiency, including pregnant women, premature infants, preschool children and adolescent girls.[104]

Iron supplementation for pregnant women should be given the highest priority in all national programmes of prenatal care delivery.[26,98,102] A successful programme must involve policy makers, planners, managers, educators, workers, midwives, obstetricians, the pregnant women themselves and their families, in order to ensure the utilization of antenatal services, the provision of medication and compliance by pregnant women; administration of iron supplements by traditional birth attendants reduced the prevalence of iron deficiency and anaemia and increased the mean birth weight, without enhancing peripheral blood or placental malaria, in The Gambia.[105] Pregnant women with sickle cell trait and their infants may not benefit from iron supplementation, through mechanisms which are not understood.[106] Recommended supplementation is the UNICEF combined tablet of elemental iron 60 mg (as ferrous sulfate) and folic acid 400 mg, taken twice daily without food throughout the second half of pregnancy; if compliance is poor or if there are unacceptable side-effects, the two tablets can be taken together, or taken with meals or reduced to 1/day. Where malaria is endemic, antimalarial prophylaxis should start from the time of first antenatal attendance. Where women are exposed to heavy hookworm infestations, albendazole 400 mg should be given orally on first attendance after the first trimester. Vitamin A (2.4 mg retinol/day) supplements dramatically enhanced the efficacy of iron in the prevention of anaemia in pregnancy in Indonesia.[100]

Breast-feeding for 6 months or more protects full-term infants; breast-fed pre-term infants require iron supplements by no later than 2 months of age. Recommended dosage is 2 mg/kg body weight, up to a maximum of 15 mg/day until iron-fortified cereal foods can be introduced. Parents must be warned about the toxicity of iron overdosage. Bottle-fed infants should receive formulae containing iron 12 mg/L and vitamin E 10 IU/L;[2] unfortified brands are still being sold by the unscrupulous in developing countries. Children aged 6–24 months of age can be given supplements of 12.5 mg iron plus 50 mg folic acid daily.[104] It is the consensus that this does not increase significantly the risk of malaria.[107]

Food fortification

The fortification with iron of widely consumed and centrally processed staple foods is the main strategy for anaemia control in many countries.[11,99] Vehicles for fortification have included acidified milk formulae and biscuits (with added bovine haemoglobin) in Chile, sugar in Guatemala, salt in India and fish sauce in Thailand. Fortification has been followed by a slow but steady decrease of prevalence of anaemia at low cost. Fortification programmes require industrial infrastructure and organized marketing which do not exist in many countries, particularly in Africa.

Dietary modification

In the long term, the ideal is for people to eat food from which they can absorb sufficient iron for normal physiological requirements.[98] Improved iron status can be achieved by increasing enhancers of iron absorption (e.g. ascorbic acid and animal protein), decreasing inhibitors (e.g. tannin and phytic acid), or by increasing total food intake so that energy needs are met fully and total iron intake improved by up to 30%. Ethiopian children fed on food cooked in iron pots had lower rates of anaemia and improved growth compared with children whose food was cooked in aluminium pots: provision of iron pots may be a cheap and effective way of preventing iron deficiency anaemia.[108]

Even when the value of ascorbic acid-rich foods is understood, there are restraints of cost if purchased, and of limited water supply and expense of fencing if grown in home gardens. As ascorbic acid is destroyed by heat, encouragement should be given to eating food raw or cooked only lightly and not reheated. Germination, malting and fermentation of grains both increase ascorbic acid and decrease tannin and phytates. Attempts to increase intake of animal protein are restrained by high costs and by religious objections, for example Hinduism.

Control of helminthic infections

It has been shown, for example in Korea, that transmission of hookworm can be reduced highly effectively and cheaply by simple sanitary measures, such as pit latrines, wearing plastic sandals and abandoning human faeces as fertilizer[99] (see also Chapter 85 and Appendix II).

Iron overload

There are many congenital and acquired conditions leading to systemic iron overload, including hereditary haemochromatosis and thalassaemia.[109] In sub-Saharan Africa, dietary iron overload is associated with drinking regularly for many years beers brewed from sorghum, millet and maize (Chapter 10). The beers are fermented in iron pots or, in more recent times, steel (oil) barrels, and contain absorbable iron at a concentration of up to 80 mg/L; as acid and alcohol stimulate gastric acid secretion, absorption is enhanced further.[110] Men especially commonly drink several litres at weekends.

Dietary iron overload, as defined as hepatic iron >360 mmol/g dry weight (normal <17 mmol/g), was present in 26% of male and 8% of female black South Africans over 40 years of age in necropsies at Baragwanath Hospital, Soweto, in 1959–1960. The 'liberalization' of the drinking laws, allowing black South Africans to drink bottled beer, was followed by a substantial decline in prevalence of the condition. However, dietary iron overload remains common in rural areas of much of southern Africa; e.g. 21% of Zimbabwean men aged 45 years or more had high serum ferritins and transferrin saturation >70% in 1986, and the condition is reported in several countries of East and West Africa. It seems probable that a high dietary intake is not the only factor but that it is interacting with an inborn error of metabolism in the causation of iron overload in Africa.[111]

Once the hepatic iron is above 360 mmol/g dry weight, portal fibrosis and cirrhosis develop. Other complications include pancreatic fibrosis and diabetes mellitus, cardiac fibrosis and heart failure, chronic scurvy and osteoporosis. Patients have a history of beer consumption over years, hepatomegaly with or without ascites and hyperpigmentation. The diagnosis is confirmed by finding excessively high serum iron, transferrin saturation and ferritin, and excessive iron in a liver biopsy. Benefit is described from repeated venesections; chelating agents have had no extensive trials.

Folic acid

Normal metabolism

The vitamin folic acid is not found naturally in the form of the core molecule pteroylglutamic acid (PGA), but as active folates, which are reduced, conjugated and condensed forms of PGA.[112] The enzyme dihydrofolate reductase, found in mammalian liver cells, reduces PGA to dihydro- and tetrahydrofolates. Folates are transported and absorbed as monoglutamates, but intracellularly are often conjugated to form polyglutamates. Folates are metabolically active when condensed with one-carbon radicals (e.g. methyl, methenyl, methylene, formyl); folates function as cofactors for the transfer of these one-carbon radicals in the synthesis of purines and pyrimidines (and hence nucleic acids) and in amino acid interconversions (e.g. histidine/glutamic acid, homocysteine/methionine and glycine/serine). Folate is essential for the conversion of uridine to thymidine required for DNA synthesis; therefore, folate is necessary for normal cell division, and tissues with rapid rates of cell division, for example bone marrow and gastrointestinal mucosa, have the highest requirements.

Folates are found in a wide variety of both animal and vegetable foods. Good sources include liver, green vegetables, tubers (e.g. yams, sweet potatoes), bananas and plantains, mangoes, fresh green and red peppers, locust beans, eggs, cheese and yeast products (e.g. bread and beer). Red meat and poultry are moderately good sources. Poor sources are grains (e.g. rice, maize, sorghum, millet), roots (e.g. cassava), non-green vegetables and distilled alcohols. Folates are heat labile and water soluble, so that prolonged cooking, reheating or boiling in large volumes of water greatly reduces the available folate.

Polyglutamates are deconjugated and folates are absorbed actively as monoglutamates in the upper jejunum. Serum transport is as N-5-methyltetra-hydrofolate. Storage is mainly in the liver, and is normally sufficient to meet requirements for about 3 months only. Folate is excreted in bile, but most of this is reabsorbed. There is a small loss in urine; faeces are rich in folate, but this is derived from bacterial synthesis in the colon and is extraneous to the body's metabolism. Folate is consumed in intermediary metabolism: requirements are highest during growth, pregnancy and lactation (Table 13.21).

Folate deficiency

Aetiology

Despite folates being found in a wide range of commonly eaten foods, dietary deficiency is common, often related to food shortages, destruction by cooking or eating of inappropriate foods (Table 13.22).[112,113] In some communities of subsistence farmers, folate deficiency is seen most frequently at the end of the dry season and in the early rainy season before the new harvest. Sometimes all the folate-rich foods are cooked in a soup or relish added to the bulky staple; this may be cooked for several hours and reheated many times before being finished, so destroying most of the folate. Individuals with highest requirements, especially pregnant women and premature infants, are the most likely to be severely deficient.[26]

Malabsorption of folate results from tropical sprue and from acute or chronic intestinal infections (e.g. giardiasis), and may also complicate systemic infections, including acute pneumonias, tuberculosis and malaria.

Haemolysis leads to erythroid hyperplasia and high demands for folate: patients with severe chronic haemolytic anaemias (e.g. sickle cell disease, thalassaemia major, spherocytosis) are almost inevitably seriously deficient if untreated. Recurrent malaria in childhood leads to dyserythropoiesis but not folate deficiency; in contrast, the main pathology of malaria in partially immune pregnant women is haemolysis and an anaemia which is normocytic at first but can progress to a profound folate deficiency megaloblastic anaemia.[26]

Dihydrofolate reductase is inactive at $39°C$: high or prolonged pyrexia can lead to acute megaloblastic arrest of erythropoiesis due to this block in folate metabolism. The 2,4-diaminopyrimidines (pyrimethamine and trimethoprim) are analogues of PGA and competitive inhibitors of dihydrofolate reductase. Their affinities for the enzymes of protozoa or bacteria are high and for the enzymes of mammals low, but overdosage can lead to severe disturbance of folate metabolism and megaloblastic anaemia. This has occurred in epidemics in China following the addition of pyrimethamine to table salt. Infants are liable to be overdosed, and individuals may overtreat themselves with antimalarial prophylactics (e.g. pyrimethamine daily instead of weekly), or with therapies containing pyrimethamine (e.g. Fansidar), or with simultaneous antimalarials and co-trimoxazole in high dose.

Aetiology is often multiple. In infancy and childhood, folate deficiency commonly complicates prematurity, feeding with boiled cows' milk or with goats' milk (which contains only folate unavailable for man), poor weaning foods, diarrhoea, repeated systemic infections, and haemoglobinopathies;[112] in West Africa, for example, about one-third of children with either PEM or moderate to severe anaemia are folate deficient. Factors leading to folate deficiency during pregnancy are commonly low intake, high demands from pregnancy, especially multiple pregnancy, malarial haemolysis, especially in primigravidae, pyrexia and haemoglobinopathies; folate deficiency is a major aetiological factor in severe anaemias in pregnancy in around three-quarters of West African patients and two-thirds of Indian patients.[11,26] In southern Africa women present commonly about 6 months postpartum with megaloblastic anaemia due to a low intake of folate from a maize-based diet not meeting the high demands of repeated pregnancies and prolonged lactation.[113]

Clinical

Patients with folate deficiency present with the symptoms and signs of anaemia. They have an increased susceptibility to infection related to neutropenia and immune deficiency. Rarely, there is a history of purpura or menorrhagia associated with thrombocytopenia. Mild splenomegaly is not unusual. Patients may have depression of mood and mental alertness, but not the major neurological signs of vitamin B_{12} deficiency. Long-standing folate deficiency can cause hyperpigmentation of the skin, but this is not so obvious as with vitamin B_{12} deficiency. Changes in the intestinal tract are glossitis, angular cheilosis, mild malabsorption and

Table 13.21 Daily dietary requirements[7] for folates and vitamin B_{12}

Nutrient	Group	Daily dietary requirement (μg)
Folate	0–6 months	40–50
	7–12 months	120
	1–12 years	200
	≥13 years	400
	Pregnant women	800
	Lactating women	600
Vitamin B_{12}	0–12 months	0.3
	1–3 years	0.9
	4–9 years	1.5
	≥10 years	2.0
	Pregnant women	3.0
	Lactating women	2.5

Table 13.22 Some causes of folate and vitamin B$_{12}$ deficiencies

	Folate	Vitamin B$_{12}$
Inadequate intake	Boiling of bottle-feeds	Breast-feeding by B$_{12}$-deficient women
	Goats' milk feeding of infants	
	Inappropriate weaning foods	Veganism
	Anorexia (recurrent infection, old age)	
	Seasonal shortage (end of dry season)	
	Prolonged cooking/re-heating	
	Prolonged storage of food	
	Famine	
	Taboos and food fads	
	Alcoholism	
Malabsorption	Diarrhoea in infancy	Pernicious anaemia
	Acute enteric infections	Gastrectomy
	Giardia lamblia	Chronic *Giardia lamblia*
	Ileocaecal tuberculosis	*Diphyllobothrium latum*
	Systemic infections (pneumonia, tuberculosis)	Stagnant loop syndrome
	Coeliac disease	Tropical sprue (chronic) (Chapter 10)
	Tropical sprue (acute)	Crohn's disease
	Crohn's disease	
High physiological demands	Growth (prematurity, infancy, adolescence)	
	Pregnancy	Pregnancy
	Lactation	
Pathologically high demands	Haemolysis (sickle cell, thalassaemia, etc.; recurrent malaria)	
	Malignant disease (Burkitt's, choriocarcinoma)	
Disturbed metabolism	Pyrexia	Nitrous oxide
	Overdosage of antagonists (pyrimethamine, trimethoprim)	Chronic cyanide intoxication (cassava)

delayed regeneration of liver cells. Chronic deficiency causes sterility in both sexes and retarded growth and development in childhood, for example in patients with sickle cell disease. Folate deficiency in early pregnancy has an association with neural tube defects in the infants, and in later pregnancy with fetal growth retardation, premature delivery and low birth weight.[114]

Haematology

Anaemia varies in severity but may be profound. The MCV and MCH are raised, but the MCHC is normal. Macrocytosis may be masked if there is a coincidental cause for microcytosis, such as iron deficiency or thalassaemia trait. The reticulocyte count is high if the underlying cause is haemolysis, but otherwise is normal or low. The red cells show anisocytosis and macrocytosis; there is a tendency to oval forms, but poikilocytosis is unusual unless the anaemia is long-standing; cells are normochromic; there is polychromasia, punctate basophilia occasionally, nucleated cells (which may be obvious megaloblasts) and Howell–Jolly bodies (Figure 13.24A). Macrocytosis and raised MCV may not be apparent in patients who have concomitant iron deficiency or α thalassaemia. The total WBC and neutrophil counts are usually low, with hypersegmented neutrophils in the peripheral blood (Figure 13.24B); however, with complicating infections, as are common in the tropics, there may be leukaemoid reactions, with excessively high total WBC and neutrophil counts, showing a shift to the left as far as the

promyelocytes or even blasts, and numerous giant metamyelocytes. The platelet count is moderately reduced commonly, but sometimes severely. Bone marrow aspirates reveal megaloblastic haemopoiesis (Figure 13.25); iron stores tend to be raised due to immobilization, but in patients with dual deficiencies megaloblastic changes can be masked and iron absent from the marrow. Serum lactate dehydrogenase levels are extremely high; serum bilirubin is moderately raised.

With many patients, for example pregnant women or patients with sickle cell disease, it is obvious that megaloblastic erythropoiesis is the result of folate deficiency, but with others it is necessary to distinguish folate from vitamin B$_{12}$ deficiency by assaying serum folate, red cell folate and serum vitamin B$_{12}$ levels. If assays are not available, the two deficiencies can be distinguished by a therapeutic trial of physiological doses of folic acid 50 mg/day: if there is no reticulocyte or haemoglobin response within 1 week, vitamin B$_{12}$ 1 mg/day intramuscularly is tried; coincidental infections suppress haematological responses, making results difficult to interpret.

Management

Folic acid 5 mg/day is followed by a reticulocyte response after about 5 days, and the slow restoration of normal haematology; treatment for 3 weeks is sufficient to replace the body stores but should be continued if there are ongoing high demands or malabsorption. This dosage is in excess of requirements and there is

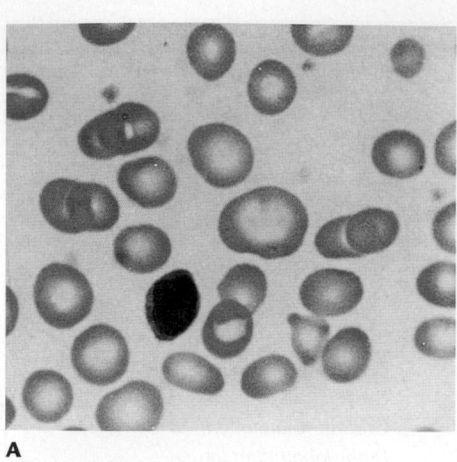
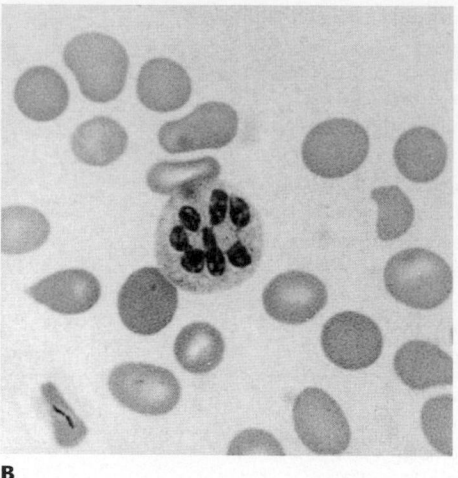

A

B

Figure 13.24 Peripheral blood films. (A) Macrocytic megaloblastic anaemia. Red cells show variation of size (anisocytosis) and large cells (macrocytes), some of which are oval. (B) Hypersegmented neutrophil of a patient with dietary vitamin B_{12} deficiency.

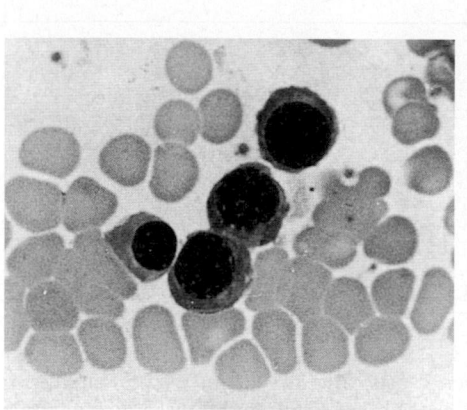
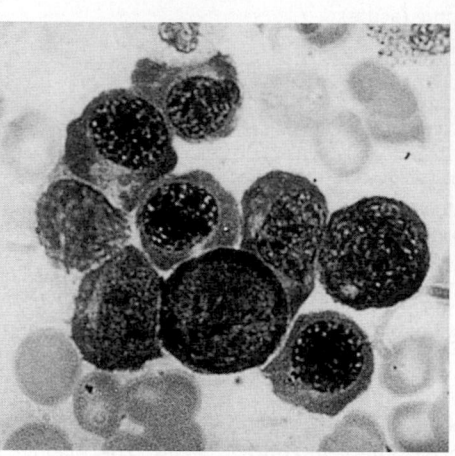
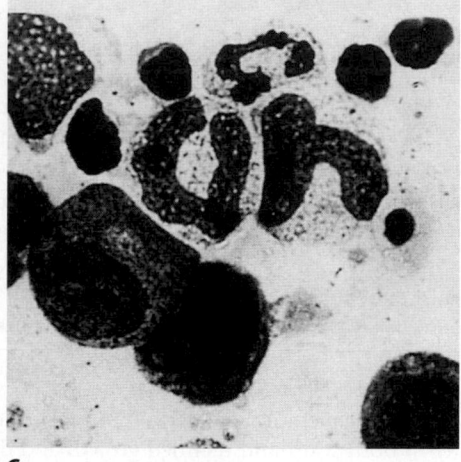

A

B

C

Figure 13.25 Bone marrow. (A) Normoblastic erythroid hyperplasia from a patient with haemolytic anaemia, to show the normal stages of maturation of erythroblasts. (B) Megaloblastic bone marrow: the erythroblasts are large; the nuclei are grainy (deficient in chromatin); the nuclei remain immature whereas the cytoplasm continues to develop (nuclear-cytoplasmic dissociation); there are bizarre-shaped nuclei and Howell–Jolly bodies; there is a high proportion of early forms which do not develop to late forms, but suffer intramedullary destruction. (C) Giant metamyelocytes: these are about twice the size of normal metamyelocytes and characteristic of megaloblastic bone marrows, but may be seen also following cytotoxic therapy.

never any need to increase to 15 mg/day; parenteral treatment is indicated only rarely with severe malabsorption, and the reduced form folinic acid is needed only to counteract dihydrofolate reductase inhibitors.

Patients with a megaloblastic anaemia can be treated initially with both folic acid and vitamin B_{12} while awaiting the results of vitamin assays, provided all blood and marrow samples have been collected for necessary investigations.

Prevention

The same three strategies of supplementation, fortification of food and dietary modification apply as in the prevention of iron deficiency.

Premature infants should be given supplements of 50 mg/day. Infants with diarrhoea should receive 50 mg in addition. Defi-

ciency in pregnancy is prevented with the combined iron (60 mg) and folic acid (400 mg) tablets twice a day. Preconceptional supplements of folic acid are required to prevent recurrence of neural tube defects.[114] Patients with chronic haemolytic anaemias (e.g. thalassaemia, sickle cell disease, congenital spherocytosis) are generally given folic acid 5 mg/day, this large dose being the pharmaceutical preparation usually available.

For populations with high frequencies of nutritional deficiency there is a strong case for the fortification of the staple with folic acid, for example maize flour in southern Africa; however, this has not yet been enforced.[113]

The natural folate content of food can be enhanced by cultivating and eating folate-rich vegetables, which are generally those which are also rich in ascorbic acid (see 'Prevention of iron deficiency'). Encouragement should also be given to eating raw or only lightly cooked vegetables and fruit.

Vitamin B$_{12}$

The natural forms of vitamin B$_{12}$ in mammals are: (1) deoxyadeno-sylcobalamin, which accounts for about 80% of intracellular vitamin B$_{12}$; (2) methylcobalamin, which is the main form in plasma; and (3) hydroxocobalamin, which occurs in small quantities both intracellularly and extracellularly.[112] Cyanocobalamin occurs naturally in trace amounts only, but is stable and so finds diagnostic and therapeutic applications. There are only three biochemical reactions known to involve vitamin B$_{12}$ in man: (1) the isomerization of methylmalonyl CoA to succinyl CoA; (2) the isomerization of α-leucine to β-leucine; (3) the methylation of homocysteine to methionine, a reaction which results in conversion of methyltetrahydrofolate to tetrahydrofolate. Vitamin B$_{12}$ is vital for normal folate metabolism and for the myelination of nerve fibres.

Vitamin B$_{12}$ is synthesized by microorganisms and is available to man in animal foods, especially liver, and animal products, including milk and its derivatives and eggs. Vitamin B$_{12}$ is not found in vegetables: it is available, however, from faecally contaminated water, and this source is important in the poorest vegetarian societies.[115] Requirements are extremely low, and are met by very small intakes of animal food (Table 13.21).

Vitamin B$_{12}$ is released from food in the stomach, and then bound to intrinsic factor (IF), a glycoprotein secreted by parietal cells. The IF-B$_{12}$ complex is adsorbed by means of a specific receptor on to the mucosal cells of the terminal ileum; the vitamin B$_{12}$ is absorbed and transported to the liver by the plasma protein transcobalamin II (TC-II). Storage, mainly in the liver, amounts to 3–5 mg and is sufficient to meet requirements for 3–4 years. There is an enterohepatic circulation: there is a minimal loss in urine; faeces are rich in vitamin B$_{12}$, but this is synthesized by colonic bacteria and not absorbed.

Serum vitamin B$_{12}$ is bound about 80% to TC-I, derived from neutrophils; the function of this fraction is not understood. TC-II, derived from macrophages and hepatocytes, carries metabolically available vitamin B$_{12}$ between tissues. The reference range of serum vitamin B$_{12}$ is usually given as 150–900 ng/L, but higher levels (160–2250 ng/L) are normal in blacks, who have a genetically determined higher TC-II binding capacity.[116] High serum vitamin B$_{12}$ is associated also with PEM, hepatic disease and granulocytic proliferations.

Vitamin B$_{12}$ deficiency

Aetiology

Vitamin B$_{12}$ deficiency can be the result of (1) inadequate intake, (2) malabsorption due to a failure of IF secretion by gastric parietal cells, (3) disease of the ileum, (4) competition by the fish tapeworm, Diphyllobothrium latum, and (5) disturbed metabolism (Table 13.22).[112,115] Demands are raised during pregnancy and lactation (Table 13.21), but this precipitates overt deficiency only in those whose status was marginal before pregnancy.

Dietary inadequacy

The requirements for vitamin B$_{12}$ are so low that nutritional deficiency is rare. It is seen most commonly in infants born to and breast-fed by women who are vitamin B$_{12}$ deficient; the disorder occurs predominantly in Indians whose mothers have tropical sprue and/or inadequate nutrition, but can result from maternal pernicious anaemia.[115]

Strictly vegan diets, which exclude all animal products such as milk and eggs, contain inadequate vitamin B$_{12}$ and deficiency occurs in some impoverished Indian Hindu populations and other vegans such as Rastafarians. Indian immigrants in the UK seem to be at an increased risk of deficiency, possibly because there is less bacterial contamination of water and food. Severe vitamin B$_{12}$ deficiency has been described in long-term prisoners of oppressive governments.

Malabsorption

Classical Addisonian pernicious anaemia (PA) is an autoimmune disease characterized by antiparietal cell and/or anti-IF antibodies, and a failure of IF secretion. It has the highest incidence in populations of northern European descent, but it is being diagnosed with increasing frequency in Arabs, Asians and blacks.[116,117] Undefined environmental factors appear to protect against the development of PA in tropical Africa, as it is rare in Zambia (personal observations) and Nigeria.[118] In contrast, PA accounts for about half of all megaloblastic anaemias in Soweto, South Africa,[113,116] and for 86% of megaloblastic anaemias not occurring in pregnancy in Zimbabwe.[119]

Sprue is the most common cause of malabsorption, probably as a result of interfering with adsorption of IF-B$_{12}$ by ileal mucosal cells. Subnormal serum vitamin B$_{12}$ is reported in up to 40% of people with AIDS; this may not be a true deficiency but the result of neutropenia and low synthesis of TC-I.[120] The fish tapeworm is a rare cause of deficiency, even where the infestation is common.

Disturbed metabolism

Cassava flour is an important staple in sub-Saharan Africa, especially in Mozambique, Tanzania and the Democratic Republic of Congo, and in Indonesia and Brazil.[121] The peel of the roots of cassava contains linamarin, a cyanogenic glycoside from which is released hydrocyanic acid. Cassava is usually prepared by peeling, washing and drying in the sun; this destroys the source of cyanide through fermentation. Chronic cyanide intoxication can follow drought, for example in Mozambique, when the linamarin content is excessively high, or from imperfect preparation, for example in refugees during the Nigerian civil war. Patients suffer from chronic cyanide intoxication, leading to tropical amblyopia. Urinary thiocyanate excretion is high, serum cyanocobalamin is raised but total serum vitamin B$_{12}$ is low. The neurological complications have been linked to disturbed metabolism of vitamin B$_{12}$, but megaloblastic anaemia has not been reported. Tobacco amblyopia has a similar pathogenesis.

Exposure to nitrous oxide for 5–6 days or recurrent exposure induces megaloblastic anaemia through the oxidation of cobalamins to inactive forms.

Clinical

Vitamin B$_{12}$ deficiency has the same haematological and systemic consequences as folate deficiency. In addition, the course can be complicated by peripheral neuropathy, optic atrophy, psychiatric disturbances and subacute combined degeneration of the cord, characterized by demyelination in the lateral and posterior columns. A common clinical finding is melanin hyperpigmentation, especially of palms, soles and across the small joints of the hands and feet.[115] PA is seen at a younger age in blacks and Arabs, and the rate of progression of the disease may be more rapid than in other ethnic groups.[116,117]

Neonatal deficiency, as seen in Indian infants, shows as a failure of normal development, involuntary movements, loss of muscle tone, pallor and hyperpigmentation of skin and mucous membranes; untreated the condition can progress to coma and death.[115]

Haematology

The peripheral blood and bone marrow findings are identical to those of folate deficiency, except that as vitamin B_{12} deficiency is likely to be more long standing, there tends to be more poikilocytosis and thrombocytopenia. Diagnosis is confirmed by the serum vitamin B_{12} level being well below the reference range. Measurement of vitamin B_{12} absorption, without and with IF (the Schilling test), is cumbersome, expensive, involves radioactivity and is generally not available in developing countries. Both blacks and Arabs with PA have high frequencies of anti-IF antibodies.[116,117] A diagnosis of PA is established without resorting to the Schilling test, in a patient with megaloblastic anaemia, low serum vitamin B_{12} and anti-IF antibodies, a test shown to have high sensitivity in black South Africans.[122]

Management

Normal stores are restored with hydroxocobalamin 1000 mg intramuscularly, six times over 1–2 weeks; thereafter, 1000 mg is given every 3 months to all patients with permanent malabsorption. Vegans may be treated orally, or be encouraged to eat some vitamin B_{12}-containing food. Infants should receive 0.1 mg per day orally, and deficient mothers treated at the same time.

Cyanocobalamin is still used in some developing countries but is not as satisfactory because maintenance doses have to be given monthly, and it is useless in the treatment of cyanide intoxication.

Other deficiencies

Vitamin A deficiency

About 250 million children worldwide are at risk of vitamin A deficiency. Vitamin A deficiency has distinct haematological actions: (1) there is immobilization of iron in the reticuloendothelial system; (2) there is increased susceptibility to infection, and hence anaemia and further immobilization of iron. Vitamin A may also have a role in red cell differentiation. Simultaneous supplementation with iron and with vitamin A results in greater haemopoietic benefit than supplementation with iron alone to children, pregnant women and non-pregnant adults.

Vitamin A deficiency in children should be improved by (1) breast-feeding, (2) dietary improvements, (3) food fortification, (4) supplementation to the child, and (5) supplementation to the mother. It is recommended that children at risk of vitamin A deficiency should receive vitamin A 100 000 IU at 9 months at the time of measles vaccination, and 200 000 IU between 15 and 21 months. Women should receive 10 000 IU daily or 25 000 IU weekly while pregnant, and 200 000 IU once after delivery.[123]

Riboflavin deficiency

Low dietary intake and overcooking are the usual causes of deficiency of riboflavin: high prevalences of deficiency have been reported amongst children and pregnant or lactating women in West Africa. Riboflavin deficiency is associated with erythroid hypoplasia and immobilization of iron.[124] Supplementation with riboflavin has enhanced the response to supplementation with iron in children, women who are pregnant or lactating, and men with anaemia in West Africa.[125,126]

Protein-energy malnutrition

PEM is a serious cause of disease, but not of anaemia. Anaemia is usually moderate (Hb 80–90 g/L), normocytic and normochromic, although the MCV may be slightly elevated.[124] The reticulocyte count is low and the marrow shows a normoblastic erythroid hypoplasia. Erythropoietin levels are increased appropriately for the degree of anaemia but there is an impaired response by erythroid precursors. Red cell survival may be moderately shortened, especially in kwashiorkor. Anaemia is more severe when there is concomitant infection related to impaired cell-mediated immunity, and deficiencies of iron and folate, as occur commonly.

Vitamin C deficiency

Severe scurvy is associated with normochromic normocytic anaemia.[124] Vitamin C-deficient diets are certainly deficient in folate and bioavailable iron as well, and anaemia of multiple deficiencies is usual.

Vitamin E deficiency

Premature infants bottle-fed with milk rich in polyunsaturated fatty acids, deficient in vitamin E and supplemented with iron, develop a haemolytic anaemia due to oxidation of the red cell membrane.

Pyridoxine deficiency

Naturally occurring pyridoxine deficiency is rare, but administration of pyridoxine antagonists, such as cycloserine and pyrazinamide, causes a failure of incorporation of iron into haemoglobin and sideroblastic anaemia.[127]

Copper deficiency

Premature infants and infants or children with severe chronic diarrhoea and malnutrition may become deficient of copper.[124] There is anaemia and severe neutropenia. The marrow shows vacuolated erythroid cells, megaloblasts and ringed sideroblasts; myeloid cells are also vacuolated and have an arrest of maturation at the myelocyte stage.

Anaemia due to marrow depression

Acute infections

Any acute infection may result in a temporary depression of erythropoiesis, which generally goes unnoticed. Significant anaemia results if the patient is dependent on a rapid rate of erythropoiesis (e.g. sickle cell disease), or if the infection causes haemolysis as well; mechanisms of haemolysis may be: (1) specific to the infection (e.g. malaria, the lecithinases of Clostridium); (2) DIC and microangiopathic haemolysis following septicaemias or viraemias; (3) immune, for example complicating infection by *Mycoplasma pneumoniae*; or (4) idiosyncrasies of the patient, for example G6PD deficiency.

Anaemia of chronic disorders

With chronic infections, and also malignant disease and some collagen diseases (e.g. rheumatoid arthritis), anaemia can progress over weeks to reach a constant state known as the anaemia of chronic disorders. There are at least four mechanisms: (1) there are factors which depress erythropoiesis and reduce the sensitivity to erythropoietin; (2) there is a depression of production of erythropoietin; (3) there is moderate reduction of red cell lifespan; (4) iron is sequestered into the RES; possibly this is mediated at sites of inflammation through the release from granulocytes of lactoferrin, a protein with a high affinity for iron and for which there is a specific receptor on macrophages.

The anaemia is usually moderate (Hb >80 g/L, Hct >0.30) and normocytic, but may progress to being hypochromic and rarely microcytic. The plasma iron is reduced (<12 mmol/L), plasma transferrin is low (unlike iron deficiency) and the saturation of transferrin is low (15–25%) but generally higher than in iron deficiency; serum ferritin is raised (>200 mg/L) (unlike iron deficiency). In the bone marrow, iron is seen in increased quantities in the macrophages (unlike iron deficiency), but the number of siderocytic granules in normoblasts (sideroblasts) is low; erythropoiesis is normoblastic with occasional mild dyserythropoietic changes; there tends to be granulocytic hyperplasia and often an obvious increase in the number of plasma cells.

The haematological complications of three infections – tuberculosis, HIV and parvovirus B19 – need to be discussed in detail because they show certain features and because of their public health importance. The anaemias of protozoal and helminthic infections have already been discussed.

Tuberculosis

Approximately one-third of the world's population is infected by *Mycobacterium tuberculosis* (see also Chapter 56). It is estimated that 8 million develop tuberculosis each year, of whom more than 4.5 million are in Asia, including China; 2.6–2.9 million die each year. The highest incidence (220/100 000 per year) was in sub-Saharan Africa, and this has now risen further to about 400/100 000 per year, due to the pandemic of HIV. It is predicted that during the next decade the incidence of tuberculosis will continue to rise in Africa, and as it seems inevitable that the incidence of HIV infections in Asia will overtake that of Africa, the impact of AIDS on tuberculosis in Asia will be catastrophic.

Tuberculosis is one of the most common causes of anaemia in adult males and non-pregnant females in the developing world, probably the most common cause amongst adults requiring hospital care, and in some communities, for example in southern Africa, the most common underlying disease leading to the need to administer blood transfusions in the management of anaemia.[127]

The major mechanism is the anaemia of chronic disorders: anaemia is more common and tends to be more severe in patients with extrapulmonary and disseminated disease. Patients, especially vegetarians, are frequently undernourished, with specific deficiencies of vitamin B_{12}, folate, iron and protein, both as predisposing factors through impairment of cell-mediated immunity and as complications of tuberculosis through anorexia and malabsorption, especially with abdominal tuberculosis. Metastatic fibrocaseous granulomas in the bone marrow give rise to a leukoerythroblastic picture and severe anaemia.

Abnormalities of the white cells are most pronounced with disseminated non-reactive miliary tuberculosis. These include: a neutrophil leukocytosis with a shift to the left and toxic granulation, and this may amount to a leukaemoid reaction; eosinophilic reactions, which are likely to reflect coincidental helminthic infections; increased basophils, which are suggestive of an underlying myeloproliferative disease; monocytosis and lymphocytosis. Many patients have reactive thrombocytosis, sometimes exceeding 1000×10^9/L. Other patients have neutropenia, lymphopenia or thrombocytopenia due to inhibition of production related to tuberculosis, hypersplenism of tuberculous splenomegaly, or HIV infection.

The bone marrow is commonly normoblastic but may show micronormoblastic, dyserythropoietic or megaloblastic features; granulocytic and megakaryocytic hyperplasia and plasma cell excess are usual; there is an excess of iron in the macrophages unless the patient is iron deficient. Some patients may show hypoplasia of one or more cell lines, associated with severe anaemia, neutropenia and thrombocytopenia.

The various therapeutic agents used in the management of tuberculosis can lead to haematological complications. These include: (1) the sideroblastic anaemia of pyridoxine inhibitors (isoniazid, pyrazinamide, cycloserine); (2) hypoplasia or aplasia of one or more of the cell lines; (3) disturbances of folate or vitamin B_{12} metabolism; and (4) immune haemolysis.[127]

Immune deficiency states predispose to the reactivation of latent tuberculosis. For many years it has been known that tuberculosis is associated with lymphomas, leukaemias (especially chronic myeloid leukaemia), the myeloproliferative diseases and aplastic anaemia. Currently in Africa, one-third of patients presenting with AIDS have active tuberculosis; where the HIV epidemic is mature, up to 60% of all patients newly diagnosed as having pulmonary tuberculosis and a higher proportion with extrapulmonary tuberculosis are anti-HIV seropositive.

Human immunodeficiency virus (HIV)

The pattern of disorders of the blood, and the practice of haematology as with other disciplines in medicine, has been changed profoundly in sub-Saharan Africa by the epidemic of HIV (see also Chapter 20). AIDS is now the commonest cause of anaemia, leucopenia and thrombocytopenia encountered both in patients and in the community.[128]

There is often an infectious mononucleosis-like illness 6–8 weeks following infection by HIV, at the time of acute viraemia and seroconversion: the peripheral blood shows initially lymphopenia, but after a few days there is a lymphocytosis with atypical mononuclear cells (virocytes); moderate neutropenia, thrombocytopenia or anaemia can occur, but resolve over 2 weeks.[129]

During the asymptomatic period of HIV infection, which lasts on average 8–10 years, the only haematological abnormalities, which are commonly detected are thrombocytopenia in up to 12% of subjects due to immune destruction and significant neutropenia in 5–10%.[129]

Patients who have progressed to AIDS commonly have an absolute lymphopenia; atypical lymphocytes and lymphocytes with lobulated nuclei are usual. Around half of patients have a neutropenia from marrow dysfunction. There are two patterns seen: some neutrophils show the hypogranularity and non-segmented forms typical of myelodysplasia; some neutrophils have toxic granulation, a shift to the left (sometimes with the presence of myelocytes, promyelocytes or blasts) and vacuolated and ragged cytoplasm in response to intercurrent infection.[129]

Anaemia becomes increasingly common (up to 95%) and more severe (Hb <50 g/L in terminal stages) with the progression of AIDS. Anaemia is not uncommonly the first presentation of AIDS in Africa. The anaemia is normochromic and normocytic, but anisocytosis and macrocytosis are not infrequent. The main mechanism of anaemia is probably infection by HIV of bone marrow stromal cells, disturbed production of haemopoietic growth factors and hence dyserythropoiesis. Other mechanisms include (1) the anaemia of chronic disorders secondary to opportunistic infections or activation of latent infection such as tuberculosis, (2) chronic parvovirus B19 infection (see below), (3) folate deficiency from inadequate intake, malabsorption and self-medication with overdosage of trimethoprim (in co-trimoxazole) or pyrimethamine (in Maloprim® and Fansidar®) (Table 13.22), (4) vitamin A deficiency, (5) microangiopathic haemolysis associated with DIC or a thrombotic thrombocytopenic purpura (TTP)-like syndrome, and (6) autoimmune haemolysis, which is rare although the DCT is commonly positive. Serum vitamin B_{12} is low in up to 40% of people with AIDS, but this is thought not to reflect a true deficiency (see above).[120,129]

Up to 70% of people with AIDS develop thrombocytopenia as a consequence of immune destruction, low production and, in some, hypersplenism. Spontaneous haemorrhage or purpura is uncommon, but there can be excessive bleeding following trauma and surgery. Severe thrombocytopenia is seen when the rare TTP-like syndrome develops.[129]

In early stages of HIV/AIDS, the bone marrow is hypercellular but there is a decline of cellularity as disease progresses, and hypocellularity is usual in the late stages. Red cell and granulocyte precursors and megakaryocytes are increasingly dysplastic with severity of AIDS. Macrophage numbers are commonly raised; haemophagocytosis is often present. There is frequently a markedly increased number of plasma cells: this may lead to a mistaken diagnosis of myeloma, especially if there is also hypergammaglobulinaemia. There may be heavy deposits of iron in macrophages as a result of immobilization of iron with infections and of high intake, for example from traditional beers. Tuberculosis of the marrow was diagnosed in about a half of South Africans with AIDS, either by culture or the presence of granulomas.[130] The bone marrow may be infiltrated by AIDS-related Burkitt's lymphoma.[131]

Patients with AIDS and haematological cytopenias should receive supportive management with red cell and platelet transfusions when required, treatment of opportunistic infections, and antiretrovirals if these are available.

Treatment with nucleoside reverse transcriptase inhibitors, for example zidovudine or stavudine, causes dose-related macrocytosis, megaloblastosis and pancytopenia, limiting their usefulness in the already anaemic patient. Overdosage of trimethoprim-containing therapies can precipitate profound megaloblastosis and pancytopenia. Dapsone, in the management of pneumocystis, may precipitate haemolysis in G6PD-deficient or, more rarely, G6PD-normal subjects.[129]

AIDS-related lymphomas

The increased risk of developing lymphomas is well documented in the industrialized countries.[129,131] Non-Hodgkin's lymphomas (NHL) are 60–200 times more common in HIV-positive patients than in the general population. The incidence of Hodgkin's disease (HD) is increased by eight times.

AIDS-related NHL has been observed in Africans, but relatively infrequently. Possible reasons for the low frequency in sub-Saharan Africa are: (1) lack of diagnostic facilities, (2) a high death rate from infection early in the course of AIDS, (3) the absence of antiretroviral therapy which prolongs life until lymphomas develop, and (4) genetic factors. The chemokine stromal cell-derived factor 1 (SDF-1) is polymorphic: 37% of Caucasians and only 11% of Afro-Americans carry the 3^1A variant; the risk of AIDS-related lymphoma is doubled in heterozygotes for SDF1–3^1A and quadrupled in homozygotes.[131]

Over 90% of AIDS-related lymphomas are high-grade B cell tumours. About two-thirds are diffuse large cell lymphomas, and about one-third are Burkitt's lymphomas. In these tumours there are two recognized factors associated with tumorigenesis: (1) reactivation of latent EBV, contributing to 70% of diffuse large lymphomas and 30% of Burkitt's lymphomas, and (2) HIV-induced production of cytokines that cause B cell stimulation, proliferation and activation. Causative factors in other rarer AIDS-related lymphomas are (1) the human herpes virus 8 (HHV8, also known as the Kaposi's sarcoma-associated virus) plus EBV in body cavity lymphoma (also called primary effusion lymphoma), (2) HHV8 and sometimes co-infection with EBV in multicentric Castleman's disease, (3) HIV acting as an oncogenic virus in peripheral T cell lymphoma, and (4) EBV in HD.

Prognosis remains poor for all persons with AIDS-related lymphomas, despite management which involves cytotoxic and antiretroviral therapy, and the treatment of opportunistic infections.[131]

Parvovirus B19

Parvovirus B19 is a single-stranded DNA virus which is common and distributed worldwide.[132] Transmission is by respiratory droplets, but also transplacentally and by exchange of blood. In tropical countries children are usually infected in the first 2 years of life, and protective antibodies are present in about 90% of adults. Between 7 and 10 days after infection there is a transient viraemia for not more than 2 weeks; this may be symptomless in up to 30%, or be accompanied by flu-like symptoms, or cause self-limiting erythema infectiosum (fifth disease) after 1 week, or in adults arthritis or arthralgia; vascular purpura is a rare complication.

The virus has a tropism for early erythroid cells: during viraemia there is an absence of reticulocytes, a great reduction of erythroid progenitors and the presence of giant pronormoblasts in the bone marrow. In subjects with previously normal erythropoiesis and normal immunocompetence there is only a transient depression of erythropoiesis coinciding with the viraemia, but this is tolerated and usually unnoticed. There are three situations in which parvovirus B19 has serious consequences: pregnancy, haemolytic anaemias and immune deficiency.

When parvovirus B19 infection is acquired for the first time during the first half of pregnancy, there is transplacental transmission which can cause spontaneous abortion or hydrops fetalis or congenital anaemia, increasing by 20 times the risk of fetal wastage.

Patients with a short red cell life are dependent on a compensatory rapid rate of erythropoiesis and suffer from 'aplastic crises' when infected by parvovirus B19; morbidity and mortality rates are high. This was described first with sickle cell disease but has been observed with thalassaemia, spherocytosis, enzymopathies and acquired haemolytic anaemias.[69] It has been suggested that concomitant infection with parvovirus B19 could be a cause of severe anaemia and death in children with malaria.[133]

Parvovirus B19 viraemia can persist in patients who are immunocompromised, including those with leukaemias, lymphomas and HIV disease. There is severe chronic anaemia due to erythroid hypoplasia; occasionally there is also neutropenia and thrombocytopenia. It is certain that parvovirus B19 infections are occurring frequently in infants and young children already infected transplacentally with HIV, and it is probable that this is a common cause of profound anaemia in Africa and elsewhere.

During epidemics of parvovirus B19, susceptible subjects, such as patients with sickle cell disease and non-immune pregnant women, can be protected with intravenous normal immunoglobulin. Immunoglobulin therapy is curative of persistent viraemia and chronic anaemia in immunocompromised patients, but failures have been reported with AIDS. Vaccines are being developed.

Aplastic anaemia

Aplastic anaemia is a rare condition. The annual incidence is $2-3/10^6$ in the Western world, with peaks at 10–24 years and in old age, and a male predominance. High annual incidence is observed in Thailand, up to 5.0×10^6 in the north of the country; there is a male predominance, a peak incidence in young adults (15–24 years) and an association with low socioeconomic status.[134] This high incidence is probably to be found also in Japan and other Far Eastern countries, for unknown reasons. No cause is found in the majority of patients, but in some exposure to antibiotics (e.g. chloramphenicol), non-steroidal antiinflammatory drugs (e.g. indomethacin, butazones), paint, benzene and irradiation have proven aetiological associations. The easy availability of potent pharmaceuticals without prescription, and the constant exposure to benzene of unofficial vendors of petrol and sweatshop factory workers are serious, if unmeasured, risk factors in developing countries.[135] The role of hepatitis and other viruses remains unclear.

Alcoholism

Excessive consumption of alcohol is a large and growing social and health problem in tropical communities whose traditional ways of life have been disrupted. The haematological consequences are anaemia, macrocytosis, vacuolation of the normoblasts and excess sideroblasts, as a direct result of the toxicity of alcohol on early red cell precursors (CFU-E and BFU-E). Thrombocytopenia is common, but leucopenia is unusual. Other results of alcoholism include malnutrition leading to folate deficiency and megaloblastic anaemia, and haemosiderosis (see 'Iron overload').

Hepatic failure can be complicated by hypoprothrombinaemia (see below).

DISORDERS OF WHITE CELLS

The peripheral blood white cell counts of healthy individuals (see Tables 13.4, 13.5 and Figure 13.2) and the causes of reactive leukocytosis (see Table 13.6) have been discussed under 'Reference ranges'.

Leucopenia

The number of circulating WBCs may be abnormally low as a result of failure of production, inhibition of release, increased margination in the circulation, pooling in an enlarged spleen or excessive consumption, and there is often a combination of these factors in one patient. Both neutropenia and lymphopenia are common in the tropics, usually as the direct or indirect result of infections (Table 13.23).

Lymphomas and paraproteinaemias

Only the epidemiological and possible aetiological factors in the tropics will be discussed; lymphomas are described in detail in Chapter 35 and in standard texts.

Table 13.23 Some causes of leucopenia in the tropics

NEUTROPENIA: <2.0 × 10⁹/L
AIDS
Viral infections in early stages
Acute malaria
Typhoid
Brucellosis
Overwhelming bacterial infections
Megaloblastosis
Hypersplenism
Bone marrow infiltration (e.g. leukaemia)
Exposure to chemicals (e.g. benzene)
Idiosyncratic reactions to drugs and herbal remedies
Acute leukaemias
Aplastic anaemia
Felty's syndrome
Miscellaneous (racial, familial, cyclic, chronic, idiopathic)
LYMPHOPENIA: <1.5 × 10⁹/L
AIDS
Viral infections in prodromal stages
Corticosteroids
Lymphoma
Acute leukaemias

Burkitt's lymphoma

The highest age-specific incidence of cancers (all types) in childhood has been reported from tropical Africa; there is a peak of incidence between the ages of 5 and 9 years, more marked in boys than girls and predominantly due to Burkitt's lymphoma (BL) (Figure 13.26) (see also Chapter 43).[136] There are three epidemiological patterns: (1) BL is endemic in tropical Africa and Papua New Guinea, where annual incidence is 8–12/100 000, with a peak at 4–9 years of age; (2) intermediate incidence of 1–2/100 000/year is found in North Africa, western Asia and South America; (3) BL occurs sporadically, <0.1/100 000/year, in the Western world.[137]

The causation of endemic BL may be summarized as follows: the majority of children in developing countries are infected by the EBV before the age of 1 year; infection by EBV immortalizes B cells, resulting in their proliferation; where *P. falciparum* is endemic,

recurrent infections suppress T cell regulation of B cell proliferation, and also stimulate antigenically and mitogenically further B cell proliferation; somatic mutations are more probable the larger is the polyclonal pool of proliferating B cells; one such mutation is a translocation involving chromosome 8 at the site of the *c-myc* proto-oncogene, with its juxtaposition to an immunoglobulin heavy chain gene sequence on chromosome 14; BL is the result of the monoclonal proliferation of cells with t8:14 in 85% of cases, or in the minority of cases the juxtaposition of the chromosome 8 *c-myc* to immunoglobulin κ or λ light chain sequences on chromosomes 2 and 22, respectively. In areas of intermediate endemicity there are high rates of EBV transmission in early childhood, but no or low malaria transmission. Less than 20% of sporadic cases of BL are associated with EBV. BL also results as a complication of AIDS (see above).

Hodgkin's disease

There are four histological types of Hodgkin's disease (HD): nodular sclerosing (NS), mixed cellularity (MC), lymphocyte depleted (LD) and lymphocyte predominant (LP). The last form, LP, may be a distinct and separate entity. HD is not common, having a crude annual incidence of 2.4–3.0/100 000 in North America and Western Europe; overall, the male:female ratio is 1:1.5. There are four epidemiological patterns. Pattern I: there are high incidences (or relative frequencies) of HD in childhood in Central and South America, North Africa, western Asia and sub-Saharan Africa; there is a predominance of MC and LD, which carry poor prognoses.[138] Pattern III: in developed countries, there is a peak of incidence in young adults (20–34 years), in whom NS is the predominant type; a second peak of HD in middle age has been described in the past, but this may have been due to overdiagnosis. Pattern II: this is intermediate between patterns I and III, and is found in rural areas of developed countries, including Eastern Europe and southern USA. Pattern IV: HD has a low incidence in eastern Asia.[139]

EBV genomes are expressed by the malignant Reed-Sternberg cells from a high proportion (50–70%) of HD patients aged under 15 or over 50 years, and it is most probable that EBV plays an aetiological role in these patients. In contrast, EBV genome positivity is rare in patients aged 15–34 years and with NS, suggesting a different aetiology.[139] HIV-infected persons appear to be at greater risk of developing HD (see above).

Non-Hodgkin's, non-Burkitt's lymphomas

The remaining lymphomas, excluding BL and HD, are a heterogeneous group of tumours of B cell and T cell origin, the classification of which is complex and not wholly agreed. The combined incidence of all non-Hodgkin's lymphomas (NHLs) generally exceeds the incidence of HD, for example 4.9/100 000 per year for males and 4.1/100 000 per year for females in England and Wales; incidence rises with age to peak at 55–74 years.

In developed countries, follicle centre cell lymphomas with follicular pattern are the most common NHL, with increasing incidence with age. About 75% have a translocation of chromosomes 14 and 18, juxtaposing the immunoglobulin heavy chain locus and the bcl-2 putative proto-oncogene. In contrast, these low or intermediate grade tumours are relatively rare in developing

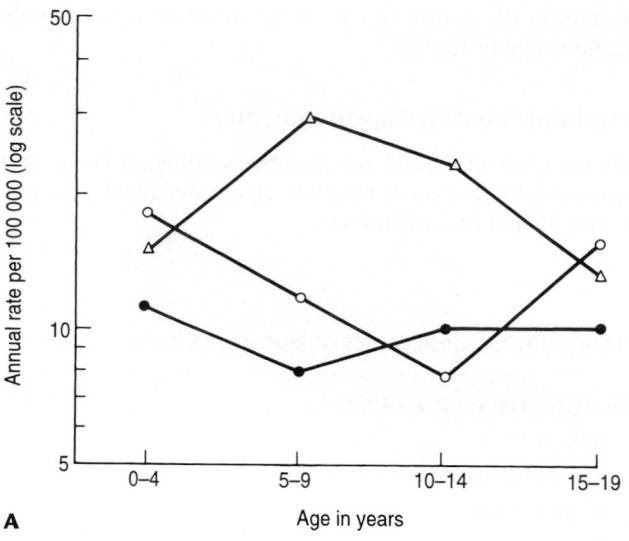

A

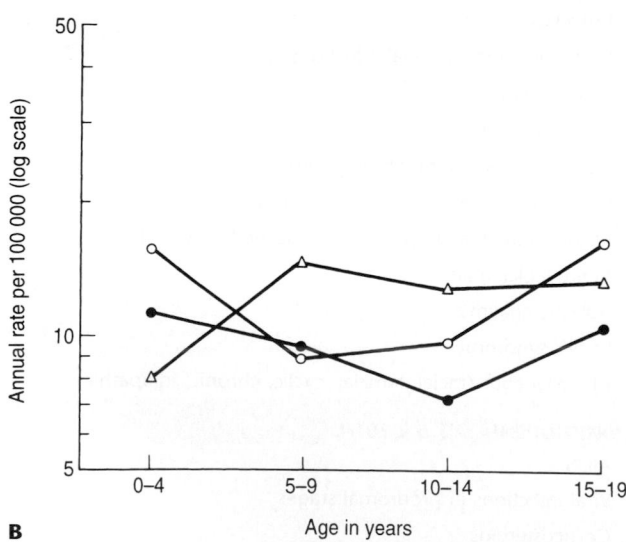

B

Figure 13.26 Age-specific incidence of childhood cancer (all types) in (A) males and (B) females in US whites (○) and blacks (●) (Michigan) and Nigerians (△) (Ibadan).[136]

countries.[137] High-grade NHLs have higher frequencies in Asia and Africa: a strong association has been reported in Africa between frequency of high-grade NHLs and malarial endemicity, but as high incidence persists into the second generation of immigrants in Israel, there may be some inherited susceptibility.[140–142]

Immunoproliferative small intestinal disease

This is a condition which occurs at high incidence in children and young adults in North Africa, western Asia, eastern Asia and sub-Saharan Africa. Sporadic cases have been reported in South, Central and North America, and Europe.[137,143] It is associated with low socioeconomic status and recurrent or chronic enteric infections. Prolonged antigenic stimulation of intestinal lymphoid tissues and a genetic predisposition are proposed mechanisms. In its premalignant phase, there is steatorrhoea, malabsorption and weight loss; histologically there is a lymphoproliferation and plasma cell infiltration of the small bowel mucosa and mesenteric lymph glands. The proliferating cells are IgA-producing B cells, which synthesize defective immunoglobulin α heavy chains (α heavy chain disease). The condition responds at this stage to ampicillin, metronidazole and anthelmintic agents, followed by long-term tetracycline. Untreated, the condition may progress to a high-grade malignant lymphoma of large cell immunoblastic plasmacytoid type (sometimes called 'Mediterranean lymphoma'). The annual incidence of intestinal lymphoma used to be as high as $4.8/10^6$ in Israel, but this has now dropped; the male to female ratio is around 2:1. The anaemia of chronic disorders is usual and is complicated in about 40% of patients by malabsorption of iron, folate or vitamin B_{12}. The lymphoma responds to combination chemotherapy, e.g. cyclophosphamide, Adriamycin, vincristine and prednisolone (CHOP).

Adult T cell leukaemia/lymphoma

Epidemiology

The human T cell lymphotropic virus type 1 (HTLV-1) is a type C retrovirus which is causative of adult T cell leukaemia/lymphoma (ATL) and tropical spastic paraparesis/HTLV-1-associated myelopathy (TSP/HAM) in a small number of infected individuals.[144,145] HTLV-1 is transmitted by sexual intercourse, through breast-feeding and by the exchange of blood. Male to female transmission is more efficient than female to male, and is enhanced by other concomitant sexually transmitted diseases: female prostitutes have higher seroprevalence than the general population. Unidentified receptors for HTLV-1 are on surfaces of CD4 +ve T cells, CD8 +ve T cells and monocyte-derived cells. After invasion of cells and transcription, proviral DNA is integrated into the DNA of host cells.

HTLV-1 is endemic in geographical clusters in Asia, Africa, the Americas, Australasia and Oceania. Seroprevalence is high (up to 30%) in south-west Japan, especially on Kyusha and Shikoku islands. HTLV-1-associated ATL is encountered sporadically in other parts of Japan and on Taiwan, and only occasionally in other Asian countries.[141] The largest pool of the virus is in sub-Saharan Africa, where there are probably about 10 million infected subjects. The highest rates of seropositivity are in the rainforests of west Central Africa: up to 15% has been reported in the Equateur region of the Democratic Republic of Congo, and 10% in Gabon and southern Cameroon; prevalence declines northwards into the savannah and Sahel. In West Africa seroprevalence is 3–6% in the savannah of

Nigeria and Benin; rates are lower (1–2%) in coastal areas and further west as far as Senegal. HTLV-1 has low endemicity (about 1%) in populations of East and Central Africa, except in the Seychelles, where overall frequency is 6.2%. There is a geographical cluster in northern Kwazulu (3.5%), northern Transkei and Free State of South Africa. The virus is also endemic in populations of African descent in the Caribbean, Central America, southern USA and Britain (e.g. 3–6% among Jamaican adults). Clusters have been reported among Iranian Jews, Iraqis, Georgians of the Caucasus, Australian Aborigines and the inhabitants of Papua New Guinea and the Solomon Islands. Seroprevalence rises slowly with age, compatible with the slow rate of transmission in endemic areas.[146]

HTLV-1 is spreading epidemically amongst intravenous drug users and male homosexuals in North and South America and Western Europe.

The structurally similar HTLV-2 is endemic among groups of the aboriginal population of Central America, and is being spread epidemically amongst blood transfusion recipients and intravenous drug users in the USA and Italy. Associations with disease, such as hairy cell leukaemia, cutaneous T cell lymphoma, chronic neurodegenerative disease or the chronic fatigue syndrome, remain indefinite.

Pathogenesis

HTLV-1 (and HTLV-2) induces a latent infection in a small subset of cells predominantly CD4 +ve T cells. HTLV-1 does not possess oncogenes, but the regulatory gene tax has oncogenic potentials through inducing expression of both IL2 and IL2 receptor. The lifetime risk of developing ATL is about 5% in subjects infected by HTLV-1 before 20 years of age. The incubation period is decades: the mean age of onset is 40–45 years, but it can be seen rarely in adolescence; women are affected more often than men in Africa and the Americas. In contrast, in Japan the mean age at diagnosis is nearly 60 years, and men are affected more often than women. It is possible that HIV accelerates progression to ATL.

T cell function is defective; Strongyloides stercoralis hyperinfection and other opportunistic infections are associated with HTLV-1 infection at any stage. The pathogenesis of TSP/HAM is discussed in Chapter 16.

Clinical

Five clinical phases are recognized: (1) asymptomatic, (2) acute ATL, (3) chronic ATL, (4) smouldering ATL, and (5) lymphoma type. Some asymptomatic patients show a preleukaemic condition, diagnosed from the incidental observation of lymphocytosis, with abnormal cells characterized by pleomorphism, multilobed nuclei ('flower' or 'clover-leaf' cells), or cytoplasmic vacuoles; pre-ATL is transient in about half of patients, but may persist and progress to ATL.

About half of African and Caribbean patients have acute ATL. Predominant clinical findings are lymphadenopathy, hepatosplenomegaly and skin lesions, which include papules, nodules, plaques, tumours and ulcers.

Histology of the lymph nodes and of skin lesions is of a high-grade NHL. The cells originate usually from helper T cells (CD4 +ve, CD8 −ve) with functional suppressor activity. Radiology shows pulmonary infiltration and osteolytic lesions which are associated with hypercalcaemia. Anaemia and thrombocytopenia are rare. The WBC count is raised, $30-130 \times 10^9$/L, with a predominance of the characteristic abnormal lymphocytes; the bone marrow shows infiltration, but less than would be expected from the leukaemic blood picture. The disease is generally resistant to aggressive cytotoxic therapy, and patients die within 12 months of diagnosis. The most effective treatment is IFNα in combination with zidovudine, but relapses are frequent.[144] Patients should receive anthelmintic, antifungal, antibacterial, antimalarial and antiviral treatment and prevention, as indicated clinically or by assessment of risk.

Chronic ATL, seen in about one-fifth of African and Caribbean patients, is associated with skin lesions, mild lymphocytosis only, and a prolonged course. Smouldering ATL, seen in about 5% of patients, shows as skin rashes and a low count of ATL cells, and remains stable for many years. The lymphoma type, seen in about one-fifth of patients, is clinically like NHL, without the leukaemic manifestations; prognosis is poor.

ATL (and TSP/HAM) develops amongst individuals wherever HTLV-1 is endemic: the low reported frequency, for example in tropical Africa, reflects a low rate of diagnosis.

Myeloma in black Africans

The age-adjusted incidence rates of myeloma have been reported to be 9.9/100 000 in blacks and 4.3/100 000 in whites in the USA. Similar high incidence is observed in black South Africans, and the diagnosis is made at high frequencies in the Caribbean and tropical Africa.[147,148] The high incidence in black Africans and those of black African descent may be genetically determined. The disease is seen in sub-Saharan Africa not infrequently in patients of 30-39 years of age, and around 65% of patients are 40-60 years old. Plasmacytomas are not uncommon.

Leukaemias

The crude incidence of all leukaemias is probably very much the same in tropical and non-tropical regions, but there are distinct differences in the age and gender distribution of the four main types: (1) acute lymphoblastic leukaemia (ALL), (2) acute myeloblastic leukaemia (AML), (3) chronic myeloid leukaemia (CML), and (4) chronic lymphocytic leukaemia (CLL). There are only a few clinical and haematological manifestations and diagnostic problems peculiar to the tropics, but there are severe limitations to their management, especially of the acute leukaemias, in the developing countries.

Acute lymphoblastic leukaemias

Immunophenotypic markers distinguish ALL according to the cells of origin of the blast cells, as precursor B-ALL (including null-ALL, common ALL (c-ALL) and pre-B-ALL), B-ALL and T-ALL. There are three epidemiological patterns of childhood ALL.[149] Pattern I: in countries with the poorest economic development, for example much of tropical Africa and Asia, the incidence of diagnosed ALL is low (<0.1/100 000 per year). Pattern II: in countries of intermediate economic development and where there has been the establishment of some haematological services, for example North Africa, Nigeria, Kenya and southern Africa, ALL remains uncommon (<1/100 000 per year), cALL is rare but there is a peak of T-ALL at 5-14 years of age. Pattern III: in the developed or Western countries, the incidence of ALL is 2-3/100 000 per year,

with a marked peak of cALL at 2-4 years of age. ALL of all types is seen at low incidence in adults at all ages. The male to female ratio is generally 2:1. Pattern I is largely the result of the lack of medical facilities and diagnostic abilities. The rarity of cALL in pattern II is true; T-ALL has only a relatively high incidence, due to the absence of cALL, not an absolutely high incidence. It is unlikely that the deficit of cALL in developing countries compared with industrialized countries is genetically determined, as the peak of cALL in childhood is now emerging in Arabia, South-east Asia, Afro-Americans, black South Africans and Zimbabweans.[150-152] It is postulated that cALL is the rare consequence of an unidentified virus, or other agent, of high infectivity but low pathogenicity. The risk of cALL is increased in the industrialized countries as a consequence of delayed exposure to the infection, associated with reduced infection rates in childhood, deficit of social contacts in infancy and possibly the absence of prolonged breast-feeding.[153,154] Small epidemics of cALL in childhood follow mixing of populations, which exposes a non-immune, often remote, population to infection introduced by another population, often urban, carrying the infection.[155] The factors increasing the risk of cALL in childhood may be becoming prevalent in South Africa and Zimbabwe, but not yet in Zambia, where cALL is still rare.[41] The children of immigrants (e.g. Asians and West Indians in the UK) have patterns of incidence similar to the population of their country of residence, illustrating the importance of the environment.

Clinical

The symptoms and signs of ALL are those arising from malignant infiltration (lymphadenopathy, hepatosplenomegaly, bone pain), anaemia, haemorrhage or thrombosis, and infections from immune depression. Being uncommon in the developed countries, these symptoms and signs arouse the suspicion of leukaemia, but in the tropical world the diagnosis may be overlooked in the mass of children with anaemia, infection and hepatosplenomegaly.

Diagnosis

The total WBC count is raised in around two-thirds, but may be normal or low in one-third of patients. The leukaemic blast cells can be mistaken for activated or transformed lymphocytes in response to malaria, viral or other infections, and the diagnosis missed in the laboratory. The bone marrow is infiltrated with blasts. ALL is classified according to the French-American-British (FAB) criteria by the light microscopic appearance of the blasts: L1, the blasts are uniformly small and have little or no cytoplasm; L2, the blasts are pleomorphic with more abundant, agranular cytoplasm; L3, the blasts have dark-blue staining cytoplasm with vacuoles in both cytoplasm and nucleus. L3 often corresponds to B-ALL or the leukaemic presentation of BL.

Management and prognosis

Supportive treatment includes red cell transfusion for anaemia, platelet transfusion for haemorrhage from thrombocytopenia, antibiotics for infection, allopurinol for hyperuricacidaemia, and antimalarial therapy and prophylaxis. Specific treatment is with complex regimens of cytotoxic agents and radiotherapy of the central nervous system: it is highly effective, especially for cALL in childhood, but cannot be undertaken except in specialized units. Regrettably, patients in most of the developing world have not benefited from the strides made in leukaemia management during the last 30 years, because of both social and biological handicaps. Patients, or parents, are not able to comply with therapeutic regimens because of their complexity, cost, distances of travel, lack of comprehension or distrust of modern medicine. Supplies of cytotoxic drugs are uncertain and radiotherapy usually wholly unavailable. Patients often show indicators of poor prognosis, including late presentation, poor nutrition, high leukocyte counts, severe thrombocytopenia, L2 blasts, T cell markers and mediastinal masses.

Acute myeloblastic leukaemias

AML is classified by FAB criteria as: M0 and M1, with malignant blast cells that have few or no granules; M2, with blasts that have granules and Auer rods; M3, promyelocytic leukaemia, of hyper- or hypogranular variants; M4, myelomonocytic leukaemia; M5, monocytic leukaemia; M6, erythroleukaemia; and M7, megakaryocytic leukaemia, the last two being rarities.

AML is diagnosed at equal frequency as ALL in childhood in tropical Africa, whereas in the Western world there are four cases of ALL to one of AML; this is due in part to the low incidence of cALL in Africa, but there is also a high frequency of AML in boys (male to female ratio as high as 3.8 : 1), associated with low socioeconomic status.[41,149] AML in adults has about equal gender frequency and no association with economic status. Recognized risk factors in adults include cigarette smoking, which may account for up to 20% of AML in some communities;[156] a rising incidence of AML will be one part of the large increases of cancer, mostly tobacco related, predicted for developing countries during the next few decades. Exposure to chemicals and toxic or radioactive waste at work and in the environment is increasing and is uncontrolled in the Third World; factors related causatively to AML include benzene, to which are exposed informal petrol vendors and workers in the rubber, shoe, petroleum, leather, printing and chemical industries, asbestos, chemical fertilizers, pesticides and irradiation.[135,155] As alkylating agents (e.g. cyclophosphamide) are associated causatively with AML and as they are used in the treatment of BL, NHL, HD, myeloma and CLL, all of which occur in the young or relatively young in the tropics, it may be anticipated that AML will be observed at higher than expected incidence in patients who have received cytotoxic therapy.[149] The myelodysplastic syndromes are not diagnosed often in tropical countries, but are significant causes of anaemia, have the same environmental risk factors as AML (tobacco, benzene, myelotoxic agents) and are preleukaemic conditions.[135,153,156,157]

Clinical

AML is indistinguishable from ALL clinically, except that in tropical Africa between 10% and 25% of all patients and about one-third of boys may present with a chloroma.[149] Chloromas are solid tumours usually arising in the orbit but occurring at other sites: the freshly cut surface is characteristically green (hence the name); histologically the tumour is a myeloblastic deposit.[41]

Diagnosis

Monocytic and myelomonocytic leukaemoid reactions from tuberculosis may be mistaken sometimes for M4 and M5 AML.[127] L2 ALL and M1 AML are differentiated by the myeloperoxidase and Sudan black reactions, which are positive with AML. The nonspecific esterase reaction is strongly positive with M5 and positive with M4 AML.

Management and prognosis

Supportive treatment should be given as with ALL (see above). Survival without specific treatment is about 2 months. Cytotoxic therapy should be undertaken in specialist centres only: conventional chemotherapy allows for a median survival of about 9 months. Marrow ablation followed by bone marrow transplant carries much better prognosis and the possibility of cure, but needs sophisticated and expensive facilities.

In promyelocytic leukaemia (M3) there is a specific translocation which fuses the retinoic acid receptor α gene on chromosome 17 to a locus, PML on chromosome 15. All-trans-retinoic therapy has been followed by differentiation of M3 blasts down the neutrophil pathway, a treatment which it is possible to administer and control with limited resources.

Chronic myeloid leukaemia

Over 90% of CMLs have cells with the Philadelphia (Ph[1]) chromosome, which is a chromosome 22 that has lost much of its long arm in reciprocal translocation with chromosome 9. The translocation juxtaposes the Abelson proto-oncogene (Abl) from the long arm of chromosome 9 with a breakpoint cluster region (bcr) on chromosome 22. Bcr/Abl may be detected by polymerase chain reaction in many patients in whom the Ph[1] chromosome cannot be demonstrated. The combination produces a chimeric mRNA, which translates a protein with tyrosine kinase activity able to confer independence from control by growth factors on several cell lines.

Annual incidence is about 1/100 000 throughout the world, with a slightly higher rate in male blacks; males are affected more often than females. Age-specific incidence rises progressively with age from childhood; frequency peaks in the industrialized countries in the fifth decade, but in the developing countries with younger populations more patients are seen under 40 years than over. CML is the third leukaemia of childhood, and in Africa between 10% and 20% of cases occur in patients below the age of 15 years.[41,149] Environmental factors associated with CML are excessive exposure to ionizing irradiation and benzene.[149]

Clinical

Patients complain most often of abdominal discomfort from gross hepatosplenomegaly. They may be emaciated, have generalized lymphadenopathy, and be anaemic. African patients have on average larger spleens and more severe anaemia than European patients.

Diagnosis

The WBC count is raised up to 500×10^9/L; all stages of granulocyte development are present in increasing proportions from blasts to mature granulocytes, with neutrophils predominating usually, but eosinophils and basophils are also present. Tuberculosis, meningococcal meningitis, septicaemia, megaloblastosis in pregnancy, eclampsia, acute liver necrosis, amoebic liver abscess, burns, mercury poisoning from skin-lightening ointments, and severe haemorrhages may give leukaemoid reactions resembling CML. CML and leukaemoid reactions can be distinguished by: (1) a gap in the progression of granulocyte development in CML, e.g. relatively few metamyelocytes; (2) a high basophil count in CML; (3) toxic granulation and other reactive features in leukaemoid reactions; and (4) the neutrophil leukocyte alkaline phosphatase reaction, which is strongly positive with leukaemoid reactions and negative with CML.

Management and prognosis

Supportive therapy should include initial antimalarial treatment and prophylaxis for life in endemic regions, and allopurinol. There are five therapeutic options. (1) Oral busulfan reduces the WBC and splenomegaly, improves the quality of life, but does not prolong survival. Median survival is 40–47 months from diagnosis, with the most usual cause of death being transformation of CML to AML or ALL. Busulfan is wholly superseded in the developed countries, but it still has a place in the tropics as it is inexpensive and the control of WBC is easy, so allowing patients to travel long distances to their homes and to have long intervals between blood counts and reassessment. (2) Oral hydroxyurea reduces the WBC more rapidly and may prolong life slightly, but it is more difficult to control myelotoxicity; it is to be preferred to chlorambucil when the patient has easy access to the hospital and laboratory monitoring. (3) Subcutaneous IFNα, in combination with hydroxyurea or cytosine arabinoside, has resulted in definite prolongation of life, and rarely in the elimination of detectable bcr/abl. This represents an advance in the management of CML, but IFNα is too expensive for use in most developing countries. (4) Imatinib is a recently synthesized inhibitor of the bcr/abl tyrosine kinase.[158] Oral administration is impressively effective against CML, including blastic crisis, and also bcr/abl-positive ALL. It is well tolerated. It promises to be an agent which could be administered with a minimum of laboratory monitoring, as in the developing world. The cost is very high. (5) Bone marrow transplant, which if successful is curative.

Chronic lymphocytic leukaemia

In 90–95% of CLLs the cells are of mature B cell origin; other variants are hairy cell leukaemias (5–10%) usually of B cell origin, T-CLL (about 1%) and B- or T-prolymphocytic leukaemias (<1%). Age-adjusted incidence rates differ more than 10-fold among populations, showing greater variation than any other major leukaemia type. There are three main epidemiological patterns.

Pattern I: the highest age-adjusted rates (>3/100 000 per year for males) are in Canada and Scandinavia; the rest of the Western world has intermediate rates (>2/100 000 per year for males); lower rates (about 1/100 000 per year for males) are found in Central and South America. CLL is rare under 40 years of age, and thereafter incidence rises rapidly with age. The male to female ratio is about 2:1.

Pattern II: in tropical Africa, CLL occurs from the age of about 17 years, with equal numbers of men and women affected.[149,159] There is a bimodal distribution. About half the patients are aged <45 years; in these younger adults CLL is associated with low socioeconomic status and rural habitation; females predominate by about 2:1 in most West African series, but not in some East and Central African series; frequency rises with age in females to peak at the end of reproductive life. Over the age of 45 years the male to female ratio is 2:1, as in pattern I.

It is hypothesized that the probability of somatic mutation in B cells is increased in an enlarged pool of proliferating B cells resulting from recurrent malaria and other infections; probability is greatest in individuals of low socioeconomic status and high rates of exposure to infection, and in women whose cell-mediated immunity has been depressed repeatedly during pregnancies; the probability is further enhanced in individuals with HMS (see above). A second genetic event could follow infection by a virus, whose transmission is more likely in poor communities and whose proliferation may be more rapid with depression of immunity by malaria and pregnancy; HTLV-1, EBV, HCV and HHV8 have been excluded as likely causative agents.[159,160] The condition is referred to variously as 'tropical splenic lymphoma' or 'African CLL'. Analysis of V_H genes showed that the cells have an origin from naive B cells which have not undergone somatic mutation in the germinal centres; this is not consistent with the lymphoma/leukaemia being splenic lymphoma with villous lymphocytes as had been suggested.[161] Immunophenotyping of cells in Zambian patients was consistent with B cell prolymphocytic leukaemia.[41]

Pattern III: CLL is rare throughout the Indian subcontinent, South-east Asia and the Far East. Genetic factors are important determinants, as Asian immigrants to Hawaii, North America and Europe have continued low incidence.

Clinical

Onset is insidious. Patients present with hepatosplenomegaly and lymphadenopathy. Spleens tend to be larger where malaria is endemic and may reach across to the right iliac fossa.

Diagnosis

The WBC count is commonly $>40 \times 10^9/L$, with the majority of cells mature lymphocytes. Following acute malaria, cells are marginated and the count in the peripheral blood falls temporarily. It is common to see two populations of lymphocytes in the blood: one representing the malignant clone, the other reactive to recurrent malaria or other infections. The bone marrow is infiltrated with the malignant clone only.

The only condition which can give a CLL leukaemoid reaction is HMS (see above); the differentiation of the two conditions has been discussed.

Management and prognosis

Initial curative antimalarial therapy followed by long-term prophylaxis, for example with proguanil, is followed by a partial reduction of spleen size and peripheral lymphocyte count, supporting the view that patients with CLL have a loss of acquired immunity to malaria. In mild disease this may be the only necessary treatment. Most patients will require reduction of tumour mass by chlorambucil or chlorambucil plus prednisolone, following standard regimens. Response can be monitored and treatment controlled wherever there is a minimum of laboratory support. Median survival is about 8 years, but is dependent on the stage of disease, and is certainly shorter in tropical countries. Infections are often the terminal events.

Haemato-oncology services

Most patients with leukaemias in tropical countries have not benefited from the great advances in management which have occurred in the past 30 years. Diagnostic facilities are often not developed; supplies of cytotoxic agents are insufficient for the protocols which are now standard; radiotherapy units are few, and liable to break down; staff in all disciplines have not received appropriate training. Sustainable haemato-oncology services can be established through the twinning of centres in the developing world with centres in the industrialized countries, as shown by the successful Italian-Swiss cooperative with Nicaragua in the La Mascota Programme.[162] The developing country benefits from (1) rational treatment of patients, (2) training of different cadres in oncology practice, and (3) training in research methods. The centre in the developed country gains advantage from (1) the experience in the range of malignant disease seen in the tropics, (2) research opportunities, (3) the intellectual stimuli derived from living in a different community and environment and (4) a sense of fulfilment.[41]

DISORDERS OF HAEMOSTASIS

Abnormal bleeding can arise from disorders of: (1) the initiation of haemostasis, involving the vascular endothelium and platelets, and manifest as purpura and haemorrhage from or into superficial surfaces; and (2) the consolidation of haemostasis, involving the coagulation and fibrinolytic pathways, and showing clinically as uncontrolled haemorrhages from or into deeper tissues. The pathogenesis of haemorrhage is often multiple; for example, a viraemia can cause damage to both endothelium and platelets, and this can lead to the consumption of platelets and coagulation factors, and the activation of fibrinolysis.

Purpuras

Disorders of the initiation of haemostasis result from (1) abnormalities of the endothelium, (2) abnormalities of platelet function or (3) thrombocytopenia.

Vascular purpuras

Damage to endothelium is a common cause of purpura and haemorrhage in the tropics (Table 13.24). Infections are important, leading to haemorrhage through either direct toxicity to the endothelium (the haemorrhagic fevers), or to an immune damage during convalescence from several of the common childhood diseases, or to late immune damage as in Henoch–Schönlein purpura. The viral haemorrhagic fevers include dengue, yellow fever, Lassa fever, Rift Valley, Argentinian, Bolivian, Venezuelan, Crimea–Congo, Omsk, Kyasanur Forest, Korean, Marburg and Ebola haemorrhagic fevers. In immunocompromised individuals, herpes viruses (simplex and varicella) and arboviruses (O'nyong-nyong,

African chikungunya) can cause haemorrhages which are sometimes fatal. Dengue is the most common of the haemorrhagic fevers, being hyperendemic in South-east Asia and spreading epidemically, especially to the Americas and China: the annual incidence in Thailand was 345/100 000 in 1987.

Defective platelet function

Purpura resulting from disordered platelet function (thrombopathy) can complicate the course of some of the haemorrhagic fevers (Lassa, dengue, Marburg, Ebola), alcoholism, hepatic cirrhosis, uraemia, paraproteinaemias, leukaemias and myeloproliferative disorders, or can result from ingestion of non-steroidal antiinflammatory agents (aspirin, indometacin) and other drugs. The bleeding tendency of patients with uraemia can be corrected temporarily by cryoprecipitate (see under 'Haemophilia').

Thrombocytopenia

An abnormally low platelet count may result from defective production, destruction or consumption in the peripheral blood, splenic pooling, or a combination of these mechanisms. Many of the common causes in the tropics have been discussed already (viral, bacterial and protozoal infections, AIDS, hypersplenism, megaloblastosis, alcoholism, overdosage with pyrimethamine and trimethoprim, benzene exposure) (Table 13.25). Other conditions, such as idiopathic thrombocytopenic purpura (ITP), have no epidemiological or clinical features peculiar to the tropics, except that patients tend to have splenomegaly and anaemia.[22]

Onyalai

The word onyalai means blood blister in the language of the Kimbundu in western Angola.[163] It is an acquired immune thrombocytopenia which differs epidemiologically, immunologically and clinically from ITP.

Epidemiology

Onyalai has been described only in Africa south of the equator. The geographical area of distribution has shrunk over the last 60 years, due partly to the discontinuation of the habit of calling any thrombocytopenia an African onyalai, and probably because changing lifestyles have removed unknown aetiological factors. Onyalai is encountered commonly in Kavango and Ovambo territories of northern Namibia and in neighbouring southern

Table 13.24 Some causes of haemorrhage due to vascular endothelial disorders in the tropics

Infections	direct toxicity:	viraemias (dengue, yellow fever, Lassa fever, other haemorrhagic fevers)
		bacteria (typhoid, Gram-negative septicaemia, meningococcal septicaemia)
	early immune damage:	measles, scarlet fever, chickenpox, rubella, tuberculosis
	late immune damage:	Henoch–Schönlein purpura, purpura fulminans
Drugs	idiosyncratic reactions:	streptomycin, isoniazid, penicillin, sulphonamides, aspirin, quinine, etc.
Uraemia		
Scurvy		
Dysproteinaemias (e.g. myeloma)		
Fat embolism (e.g. marrow embolism in sickle cell disease)		
Congenital (Ehlers–Danlos, Osler–Rendu–Weber, etc.)		
Miscellaneous (purpura simplex, senile purpura, factitious bleeding)		

Table 13.25 Some causes of thrombocytopenia in the tropics

PRIMARILY LOW PRODUCTION	
Infections (e.g. typhoid, brucellosis)	
Megaloblastic anaemia	
Alcoholism	
Marrow infiltration (e.g. leukaemia)	
Aplastic anaemia	
Drugs and chemicals	cytoxic drugs
	overdosage (e.g. pyrimethamine, trimethoprim)
	idiosyncratic reactions
	occupational exposure (e.g. benzene)
Miscellaneous (cyclic, congenital)	
PRIMARY INCREASED CONSUMPTION OR DESTRUCTION	
Infections (e.g. acute malaria, trypanosomiasis, dengue)	
Hypersplenism (see Table 13.12)	
Chronic hepatic disease	
Disseminated intravascular coagulation (see Table 13.26)	
Immune	idiopathic thrombocytopenia (ITP)
	acute viral infections
	drugs (e.g. quinine, penicillin)
	AIDS
	onyalai
	other autoimmune diseases
	lymphomas, CLL

Angola. Onyalai accounts for over 1% of all hospital admissions in Kavango, where the minimum annual incidence has been calculated to be 151/100 000. There is no significant seasonal variation of frequency. Over half of all patients are aged under 20 years, which may not differ from the age structure of the whole population. The male to female ratio is 1 : 1.5.

Aetiology is linked clearly to some factor(s) in rural life in the Okavango valley, where millet is the main staple, and mycotoxins from fungal contamination of grain are suspected. Recently, auto-antibodies to glycoprotein (GP) IIb/IIIa of platelets have been demonstrated in 12 out of 14 patients with onyalai; both IgG and IgM antibodies were present. In contrast, anti-GPIIb/IIIa is found in only about one-third of patients with ITP, and it is mainly IgG.[163]

Clinical

The clinical hallmark is the acute appearance of haemorrhagic bullae in the mucous membranes of the mouth, tongue and palate, and less frequently on the skin, including the soles of the feet. Epistaxis is often present and may be severe. Blood loss can lead to haemorrhagic shock. The median duration of haemorrhage is about 8 days, but the condition may persist for months and tends to recur.

Haematology

Patients have profound thrombocytopenia, and many are anaemic from blood loss. The bone marrow shows hyperplasia of the erythron and megakaryocytes. Platelets are morphologically normal.

Management and prognosis

Mortality in the acute phase used to be about 10%: patients dying of haemorrhagic shock or from cerebral haemorrhage. Treatment with transfusions of whole blood for haemorrhagic shock and of platelets, and supportive measures including oral hygiene, has reduced mortality to <3%. Prednisolone is not effective. Splenectomy is indicated for otherwise uncontrollable bleeding, and is followed by a return to normal platelet counts, but the condition has recurred fatally in some splenectomized patients. Intravenous immunoglobulin has been effective in four patients, but the cost is prohibitive. Vincristine may benefit some patients.

Coagulation disorders

The disorders of blood coagulation may be acquired or congenital. The acquired disorders occur more commonly in clinical practice, but have not attracted the intense medicoscientific interest given to the congenital diseases such as haemophilia.[164]

Acquired coagulopathies

Hypoprothrombinaemias

Vitamin K deficiency

Haemorrhagic disease of the newborn
The newborn, especially the premature, have normally low levels of vitamin K and somewhat prolonged PTs (see 'Reference ranges' and Table 13.7).[165] Classical haemorrhagic disease of the newborn (HDN) is the result of vitamin K deficiency: premature infants and infants of mothers receiving antituberculous therapy, anticonvulsants or warfarin are at increased risk; bleeding is usually into skin, mucosal surfaces, the gastrointestinal tract, or from the umbilical stump or from circumcision. Infants may present between 1 and 3 months with intracranial haemorrhage of late HDN due to vitamin K deficiency: they are exclusively breast-fed and may have received antibiotics.

The incidence of HDN is not known, but is obviously high where premature infants are breast-fed exclusively; late HDN has been estimated to occur in 3/1000 Thai infants. The diagnosis is confirmed by a prolonged PT. HDN is prevented by prophylactic vitamin K, 1 mg intramuscularly on the first day of life; in treatment, vitamin K should be given intravenously.

Malabsorption
Patients with biliary obstruction or small bowel disease become deficient of the fat-soluble vitamin. Gut sterilization by antibiotics can contribute to but does not cause deficiency alone. Diagnosis is based on a prolonged PT, which reverts rapidly to normal following vitamin K, 10 mg intravenously; the response will be partial only if there is liver disease.

Vitamin K antagonism
Warfarin is a competitive inhibitor of vitamin K. Haemorrhage follows inadvertent overdosage, self-administration by the psychiatrically disturbed, the simultaneous administration of medications which potentiate warfarin (e.g. co-trimoxazole, chloramphenicol), or the eating by children of warfarin laid out as rat poison. Patients remain anticoagulated for several days after warfarin has been stopped, so that severe overdosage or poisoning has to be reversed by intravenous vitamin K.

Hepatic disease

Bleeding in liver disease is multifactorial. During acute infectious hepatitis, a mild disorder of haemostasis, consisting of reduced levels of V, VII and X and a prolonged PT, is not unusual. In association with liver failure, there is severe factor deficiency, afibrinogenaemia and DIC (see below). Patients with chronic hepatic disease or cirrhosis show impairment of synthesis of all vitamin K-dependent factors and fibrinogen and reduced platelet function; some patients show a reduced clearance of FDPs, which contributes to chronic DIC.

The PT is prolonged and vitamin K has little or no effect. If the PT is four times the normal or more, it is hazardous to perform a percutaneous liver biopsy. Bleeding with liver disease should be treated by transfusion of cryosupernate (residual plasma following removal of cryoprecipitate), or fresh frozen plasma or factor concentrates (if available).[17]

Disseminated intravascular coagulation

The widespread or uncontrolled deposition of fibrin in the circulation may be triggered by a large range of conditions (Table 13.26).[164,166] Pathogenesis starts with (1) damage to the endothelium, often from infectious causes in the tropics or (2) the release of tissue factor from traumatized tissues with the activation of platelets and coagulation or (3) the injection of procoagulants of various snake venoms (Table 13.27) or contact by South American rubber-tappers with caterpillars of the moths *Lonomia achelous* and *L. obliqua*, which feed on the leaves of rubber trees. During pregnancy there is normally a potential hypercoagulable and hyperfibrinolytic state (see 'Reference ranges') and a wide range of obstetric disorders can trigger severe DIC (see Table 13.26).

The dominant feature of acute DIC is haemorrhage, which is multifactorial (Figure 13.27): there is endothelial damage, and consumption of platelets, coagulation factors and fibrinogen, rendering the blood incoagulable; plasmin is activated, both fibrin and fibrinogen are degraded, and FDPs are released into the circulation; FDPs have antithrombin activity and are incorporated into clot, rendering it friable. In subacute and chronic DIC red cells are ruptured by being forced through fibrin networks in small blood vessels, resulting in microangiopathic haemolytic anaemia. The obstruction of small blood vessels can cause ischaemia, tissue necrosis and renal failure; pituitary and suprarenal failure are rarer complications.

Clinical

Patients have the clinical features of their primary condition. DIC can range from a minor derangement of coagulation without bleeding to a severe haemorrhagic state. It is a dynamic condition which can progress rapidly, so that attention must be paid to minor abnormalities of clotting tests. The most usual presentation

Table 13.26 Main causes of DIC encountered in clinical practice in the tropics

Acute	Subacute	Chronic
INFECTIONS	**OBSTETRIC**	**METABOLIC**
Viraemias	Pre-eclampsia/eclampsia	Liver disease
Septicaemias (Gram-negative, typhoid, meningococcal)	Retention of dead fetus	Renal disease
Protozoan (African trypanosomiasis)	Hydatidiform mole	
OBSTETRIC DISORDERS	**MALIGNANCY**	**MALIGNANCY**
Septic abortions	Acute leukaemias (M3)	Prostatic carcinoma
Abruptio placentae	**OTHERS**	**OTHERS**
Ruptured uterus	Purpura fulminans	Purpura fulminans
Amniotic fluid embolus		
SHOCK		
Accidental trauma (birth trauma or anoxia, head injuries, thoracic, fractured femur)		
Surgical trauma (thoracic)		
Burns		
Heat stroke		
ENVENOMATION		
Snake bites (see Table 13.27)		
Lonomia achelous caterpillars		
OTHERS		
Acute hepatic necrosis		
Cytotoxic therapy		
Incompatible blood transfusion		

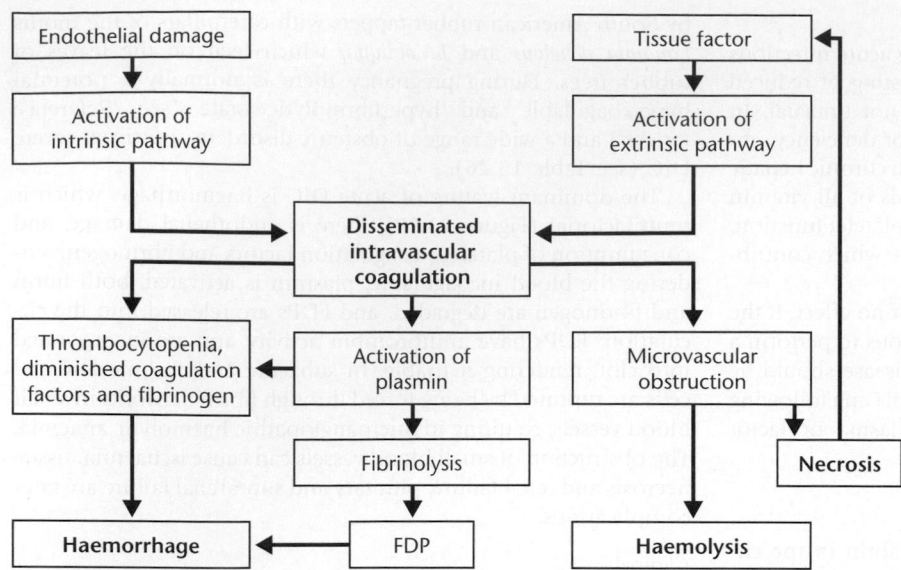

Figure 13.27 The pathogenesis of disseminated intravascular coagulation (DIC). (Reproduced with permission of the publishers, from Fleming AF. In: Parry EHO, ed. *Principles of Medicine in Africa,* 2nd edn. Oxford University Press; 1984:733.)

is bleeding from mucous membranes, skin, venepuncture sites or from the uterus.

Diagnosis

The platelet count is reduced, kaolin-cephalin clotting time (KCCT), PT and thrombin times are prolonged, and the plasma FDPs are raised. In severe DIC the simple clotting time is prolonged or the blood may be incoagulable or nearly so, allowing for confirmation of the diagnosis in the absence of other laboratory tests. Microangiopathic haemolytic anaemia shows the features of intravascular haemolysis (see Table 13.11); in the peripheral blood there are many small fragmented red cells with bizarre shapes (schizocytes).

Subacute or chronic DIC is confirmed when there are thrombocytopenia, raised plasma FDPs, moderate decreases in coagulation factors and evidence of microangiopathic haemolysis.

Management

The first principle is to treat the primary cause. If the underlying disease responds rapidly (e.g. meningococcal septicaemia to antibiotics, snake envenomation to specific antivenom, or abruptio placentae to the completion of obstetric delivery), DIC will correct spontaneously in most instances.

Second, the blood volume must be restored and maintained with the transfusion of whole blood (or if not available, concentrated red cells plus saline, or saline and colloids).

Third, if haemorrhage cannot be controlled, platelets, fresh frozen plasma and cryoprecipitate may have to be transfused to restore the missing factors.[17]

Fourth, in subacute or chronic conditions in which the primary cause cannot be cured, the patient may be heparinized, with the aim of keeping the clotting time just above 15 min, in order to break the chain of pathogenesis.

Snake envenomation

Snake bites (see also Chapter 31) are of major public health importance in many communities as causes of haemorrhage,

other morbidity and mortality, but are largely neglected in health-care planning (Table 13.27).[164] Those at highest risk of envenomation include: (1) farmers working in paddy fields, or at the beginning of the rains in dryer climates, when small rodents and reptiles attract the snakes to the fields at the same time as farmers are digging; (2) nomadic herdsmen; (3) hunter-gatherers; (4) workers on development sites. Epidemics of snake bites follow floods, when human and snake populations are concentrated together. Snake venoms contain up to about 20 components with a wide range of toxicity (see Chapter 31); only snake venoms causing haemorrhage through procoagulant activities are briefly discussed here (Figure 13.28).

Africa

Echis ocellatus

The carpet or saw-scale viper is probably the most dangerous snake in the world, and is found throughout Africa north of the equator, as well as in the Middle East, the Indian subcontinent and South-east Asia. The snake is particularly prevalent in West Africa, where in rural areas during the early rains up to one-third of adult male hospital beds may be occupied by envenomed farmers. The annual incidence in the Bambur area of the Benue valley, Nigeria, has been estimated to be 600/100 000; mortality is 10–20% in those who attend hospital but do not receive appropriate attention; this has been projected to an estimated 23 000 deaths annually in West Africa.

The venom contains an activator of thrombin (Figure 13.28), causing consumption of coagulation factors, but not usually of platelets, and high levels of FDPs. The blood is incoagulable, which is diagnostic of severe *E. ocellatus* envenomation where this is common. Death follows intracranial haemorrhage after 1 or 2 days, or haemorrhagic shock and renal failure after 1 week.

Therapy is with an antivenom, which must be known to be effective in the locality because antigenic specificity of venoms varies, for example between East and West Africa. Both Pasteur Paris Echis and South African Institute for Medical Research (SAIMR) antivenoms are reliable in West Africa.

Table 13.27 Species of snake commonly responsible for morbidity or death from haemorrhage (see also Chapter 32)

Area	Latin name	Vernacular names
AFRICA		
	Echis ocellatus[c]	Carpet or saw-scale viper
	Bitis arietans	Puff adder
	Naja nigricollis	Spitting cobra
	Dispholidus typus	Boomslang
ASIA		
Middle East; South-east	*E. ocellatus*[c]	Carpet or saw-scale viper
	Daboia russelii[a]	Russell's viper
	E. carinatus	Carpet or saw-scale viper
	Calloselasma rhodostoma[b]	Malayan pit viper
	Trimeresurus species	Green pit viper
AUSTRALIA		
	Notechis scutatus	Tiger snake
	Oxyuranus scutellatus	Taipan
	Pseudonaja textilis	Eastern brown snake
AMERICA		
North	*Crotalus adamanteus*	Eastern diamond-backed rattlesnake
	C. atrox	Western diamond-backed rattlesnake
Central	*C. durissus durissus*	Central American rattlesnake
	Bothrops asper	Terciopelo, caissaca
South	*B. atrox*	Fer-de-lance, barba amirilla
	B. jararaca	Jararaca
	C. durissus terrificus	South American rattlesnake

[a]Formerly *Vipera russellii*.
[b]Formerly *Agkistrodon rhodostoma*.
[c]Formerly *Echis carinatus*.

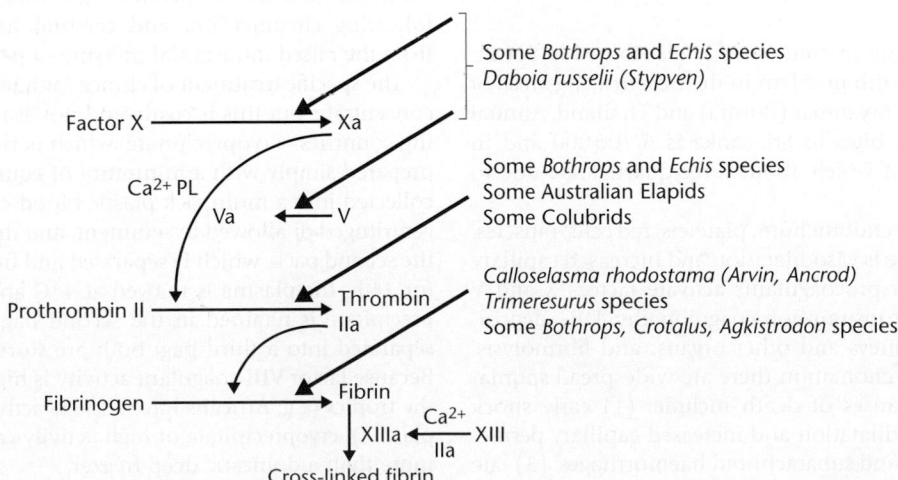

Figure 13.28   Sites of action of some snake procoagulants. (Reproduced with the kind permission of D A Warrell.)

Naja nigricollis

The spitting cobra is common throughout sub-Saharan Africa, except in the central African forest and the temperate south. Besides spitting, the snakes bite, and about one-fifth of systematically envenomed victims have spontaneous haemorrhages, which may be fatal.

Procoagulant activity has been shown in vitro, but is probably not important. FDPs can be raised from about the fifth day, associated with tissue necrosis, but DIC is not a serious feature. One specific action is the destruction of platelet actin and a failure of clot retraction. In the clotting time test, clot forms normally (unlike with *E. carinatus*), but fails to retract on standing.

Polyvalent antivenoms are not effective.

Bitis arietans

The puff adder is found throughout sub-Saharan Africa except in dense forest, and occurs also up the west Atlantic seaboard to Morocco and in western Arabia. The main effects of envenomation are cytotoxic on the heart, the automatic nervous system and the kidney. Some patients have spontaneous haemorrhages, usually of gums and nose, as a result of endothelial damage, consumption of platelets and thrombocytopenia; DIC is not usual, but may occur and be complicated by microangiopathic haemolytic anaemia.

Bites by the Gaboon viper (*B. gabonica*) found throughout sub-Saharan Africa, and by the rhinoceros-horned viper (*B. nasicornis*) found in a belt between West Africa and western Kenya, have similar effects.

Treatment includes specific polyvalent antivenom.

Dispholidus typus

The green African tree-snake or boomslang is widespread in wooded areas of sub-Saharan Africa, except in the dense central African forest. It is not aggressive and is inefficient in envenomation as it is back-fanged. Only those who handle snakes are liable to be bitten. Envenomation is followed after 1–2 days by spontaneous haemorrhage, due to the activation of factors II, X and XIII leading to DIC. The course may be complicated by microangiopathic haemolysis and renal failure. Mortality without treatment is high, but antivenoms are effective.

Asia

Daboia russelii

Russell's viper is widely but discontinuously distributed in South-east Asia; it is a major health problem in the rice-growing areas of the Indian subcontinent, Myanmar (Burma) and Thailand. Annual incidence of fatal snake bites in Sri Lanka is 6/100 000 and in Myanmar 3.3/100 000, of which about three-quarters are due to *D. russelii*.

Venom is cytotoxic for endothelium, platelets, red cells, muscles, nerve cells and liver; there is vasodilatation and increased capillary permeability. Two major procoagulants activate factors X and V (Figure 13.28), causing consumption coagulopathy, DIC, deposition of fibrin in the kidneys and other organs, and fibrinolysis. With severe systemic envenomation there are widespread spontaneous haemorrhages. Causes of death include: (1) early shock from haemorrhage, vasodilatation and increased capillary permeability; (2) intracerebral and subarachnoid haemorrhages; (3) late shock from massive gastrointestinal bleeding; (4) late shock from pituitary-adrenal insufficiency following haemorrhage or infarction; and (5) acute renal failure. Blood is usually incoagulable, FDPs are high and there is often thrombocytopenia.

Antivenom restores haemostasis but does not prevent the complications of renal failure.

Asian pit vipers

Calloselasma rhodostoma, the Malayan pit viper, is the second most important cause of envenomation in South-east Asia. There is more local swelling, pain, lymphadenopathy and tissue necrosis than with *D. russelii* bites. The proteolytic enzyme 'arvin' or 'ancrod' cleaves fibrinogen (Figure 13.28), defibrinating the victim in about half an hour: platelets are damaged, fibrinolysis is activated and the FDPs raised. Haemorrhage may be local, spread up the bitten limb or become generalized.

Many species of *Trimeresurus*, the green pit vipers, bite frequently but with less serious effects than with the Malayan pit viper.

Central and South America

About 200 deaths in Brazil and 100 in Venezuela each year are due to bites by *Crotalus* species (rattlesnakes) and *Bothrops* species (Table 13.27). Envenomation causes (1) extensive tissue necrosis, (2) defibrination from cleavage of fibrinopeptide A from fibrinogen (Figure 13.28), (3) intravascular haemolysis, (4) renal failure, and (5) neurotoxicity.

Antivenom should be administered in all cases of rattlesnake bite, even before there is evidence of systemic envenomation.

Congenital disorders

The prevalence of haemophilia A (congenital deficiency of factor VIII) is about 10/100 000, that of von Willebrand's disease (congenital deficiency or abnormality of factor VIII-related antigen) is >10/100 000, and that of haemophilia B (congenital deficiency of factor IX) is about 0.1/100 000 population.[164] All other congenital disorders of coagulation are rarities. Except in consanguineous communities, there is probably little true variation of incidence between populations in the world, although the rate of diagnosis may be low in developing countries due to early death, low clinical suspicion and lack of laboratory facilities.[167]

The clinical presentation of these disorders is much the same in the tropics as in the temperate zones. Boys present not infrequently following circumcision, and cerebral haemorrhages can result from the raised intracranial pressure of persistent coughing.

The specific treatment of choice for haemophilia A is factor VIII concentrate, but this is costly and not available in many developing countries. Cryoprecipitate, which is rich in factor VIII, can be prepared simply with a minimum of equipment. Donor blood is collected into a multipack plastic blood collection set: the unit is centrifuged or allowed to sediment, and the plasma separated into the second pack, which is separated and frozen at −20°C or colder for 24 h; the plasma is thawed at 4°C and centrifuged; the cryoprecipitate is retained in the second bag and the cryosupernate separated into a third bag; both are stored at −20°C until used. Because factor VIII coagulant activity is high in normal subjects in the tropics (e.g. Africans have >150% activity of pooled European plasma), cryoprecipitate of high activity can be produced with no more than a domestic deep-freezer.

During the first half of the 1980s a large number of haemophiliacs treated with factor VIII concentrates were infected with HIV through this product. Patients escaped infection when they were treated only with locally produced cryoprecipitate from donors in communities which were not yet infected by HIV, for example in Nigeria. The present situation (2002) is that factor VIII concentrates are non-infective if the virus is correctly inactivated, whereas cryoprecipitate is potentially infective. In the future, many haemophiliacs in tropical Africa, America and Asia are liable to be infected through contaminated cryoprecipitate, unless virus-inactivated concentrates or the more expensive recombinant factors VIII and IX are made available.

Haemophilia B is best treated with virus-inactivated factor IX concentrate; cryosupernate and fresh frozen plasma can be given in the absence of the concentrate, but are potentially infectious for HIV.

Wherever possible, von Willebrand's disease should be managed with desmopressin, but cryoprecipitate may be necessary.

All blood products which are not heat inactivated are potentially infectious for HIV, HBV (if donors are not screened for HBsAg), HCV and other micro-organisms. Blood and blood products should be used appropriately: that is, only when there are definite indications for which the advantages are judged to outweigh the risks of infection.[17]

Haemophilia care in developing countries

Only about 25% of people with haemophilia in the world are receiving adequate comprehensive care. National programmes for haemophilia care can be launched and be successful, with the guidance and support of the World Federation of Hemophilia (Contact: Executive Director, WFH Secretariat, 1310 Greene Avenue, Suite 500, Montreal, Quebec, Canada H3Z 2BZ. Tel: 1-514-933-7944; Fax: 1-514-933-8916; e-mail: wfh@wfh.org).[168]

Components of a national programme of comprehensive care include (1) the establishment of centres for care, (2) the training of care providers, (3) diagnosis and registration of people with haemophilia, (4) the education of patients and their families, (5) education of the whole community, (6) the provision of safe and effective therapeutic products, and (7) the prevention of haemophilia through counselling and antenatal diagnosis.

REFERENCES

1. Lewis SM, Bain B, Bates I. Dacie, Lewis's *Practical Haematology*, 9th edn. Edinburgh: Churchill Livingstone; 2001.

2. Lubin BH. Reference values in infancy and childhood. In: Nathan DG, Oski FA, eds. *Hematology of Infancy and Childhood*, 4th edn. Philadelphia: W B Saunders; 1993:Appendix i–xx.

3. Gilles HM. Normal haematological values in tropical areas. *Clin Haematol* 1981; 10:697–706.

4. Huehns ER. The structure and function of haemoglobin: clinical disorders due to abnormal haemoglobin structure. In: Hardisty RM, Weatherall DJ, eds. *Blood and its Disorders*. Oxford: Blackwell; 1974:526–629.

5. Fleming AF. Haematological changes in pregnancy. *Clin Obstet Gynecol* 1975; 2:269–283.

6. Dupuy E, Fleming AF, Caen JP. Platelet function, factor VIII, fibrinogen, and fibrinolysis in Nigerians and Europeans, in relation to atheroma and thrombosis. *J Clin Pathol* 1978; 31:1094–1101.

7. World Health Organization. Nutritional anaemias. *WHO Tech Rep Ser* 1972; 503.

8. DeMaeyer E, Adiels-Tegman M. The prevalence of anaemia in the world. *World Health Stat Q* 1985; 38:302–316.

9. Bellingham AJ. The red cell in adaption to anaemic hypoxia. *Clin Haematol* 1974; 3:577–594.

10. Viteri FE, Torún B. Anaemia and physical work capacity. *Clin Haematol* 1974; 3:609–626.

11. Baker SJ, DeMaeyer EM. Nutritional anemia: its understanding and control with special reference to the work of the World Health Organization. *Am J Clin Nutr* 1979; 32:368–417.

12. Wolgemuth JC, Latham MC, Hall A, et al. Worker productivity and nutritional status of Kenyan road construction laborers. *Am J Clin Nutr* 1982; 36:68–78.

13. Florencio CA. Effects of iron and ascorbic acid supplementation on hemoglobin level and work efficiency of anemic women. *J Occup Med* 1981; 23:699–704.

14. Harrison KA, Lister UG, Rossiter DE, et al. Perinatal mortality. *Br J Obstet Gynaecol* 1985; 92(suppl 5):86–99.

15. English M. Life-threatening severe malarial anaemia. *Trans R Soc Trop Med Hyg* 2000; 94:585–588.

16. Harrison KA, Rossiter CE. Maternal mortality. *Br J Obstet Gynaecol* 1985; 92(suppl 5):100–115.

17. World Health Organization, Global Programme on AIDS, Global Blood Safety Initiative. *Guidelines for the Appropriate Use of Blood*. WHO/GPA/Int/89; 18. Geneva: WHO; 1989.

18. World Health Organization. Severe falciparum malaria. *Trans R Soc Trop Med Hyg* 2000; 94(suppl 1).

19. Mendendez C, Fleming AF, Alonso P. Malaria-related anaemia. *Parasitol Today* 2000; 16:469–476.

20. French N, Gilks CF. HIV and malaria, do they interact? *Trans R Soc Trop Med Hyg* 2000; 94:233–237.

21. Fleming AF. Haematological manifestations of malaria and other parasitic diseases. *Clin Haematol* 1981; 10:983–1011.

22. Essien EM. Platelets and platelet disorders in Africa. *Baillière's Clin Haematol* 1992; 5:441–456.

23. Menendez C. Malaria during pregnancy: a priority area of malaria research and control. *Parasitol Today* 1995; 11:178–183.

24. Wahlgren M, Spillman D. Sticky sugars attract malaria to the fetus. *Nature Med* 2000; 6:25–26.

25. Lindsay S, Ansell J, Selman C, et al. Effect of pregnancy on exposure to malaria mosquitoes. *Lancet* 2000; 355:1972.

26. Fleming AF. Tropical obstetrics and gynaecology. 1. Anaemia in pregnancy in tropical Africa. *Trans R Soc Trop Med Hyg* 1989; 83:441–448.

27. Fleming AF, Allan NC. Severe haemolytic anaemia in pregnancy in Nigerians treated with prednisolone. *BMJ* 1969; iv:461–466.

28. Steketee RW, Wirima JJ, Bloland PB, et al. Impairment of a pregnant woman's acquired ability to limit Plasmodium falciparum by infection with human immunodeficiency virus type-1. *Am J Trop Med Parasitol* 1996: 55(suppl 1):42–49.

29. Greenwood BM, Greenwood AM, Snow RW, et al. The effects of malaria chemoprophylaxis given by traditional birth attendants on the course and outcome of pregnancy. *Trans R Soc Trop Med Hyg* 1989; 83:589–594.

30. Rogerson SJ, Chaluluka E, Kanjala M, et al. Intermittent sulfadoxine-pyrimethamine in pregnancy: effectiveness against malaria morbidity in Blantyre, Malawi, in 1977–99. *Trans R Soc Trop Med Hyg* 2000; 94:549–553.

31. Fleming AF, MacIntyre JA, Johnstone FD. HIV infection and AIDS in pregnancy. In: Lawson JB, Harrison KA, Bergström S, eds. *Maternity Care in the Developing Countries*. London: Royal College of Obstetricians and Gynaecologists; 2001:337–359.

32. Bryceson A, Fakunle YM, Fleming AF, et al. Malaria and splenomegaly. *Trans R Soc Trop Med Hyg* 1983; 77:879.

33. Bryceson ADM, Fleming AF, Edington GM. Splenomegaly in northern Nigeria. *Acta Trop* 1976; 33:185–214.

34. Crane G. The genetic basic of hyperreactive malarial splenomegaly. *Papua New Guinea Med J* 1989; 32:269–276.

35. Hill AVS. Malaria resistance genes: a natural selection. *Trans R Soc Trop Med Hyg* 1992; 86:225–226, 232.

36. Piessens WF, Hoffman SL, Wadee AA, et al. Antibody-mediated killing of suppressor T lymphocytes as a possible cause of macroglobulinemia in the tropical splenomegaly syndrome. *J Clin Invest* 1985; 75:1821–1827.

37. Fakunle YM. Tropical splenomegly. Part 1: tropical Africa. *Clin Haematol* 1981; 10:963–973.

38. Crane GG. Hyperreactive malarious splenomegaly (tropical splenomegaly syndrome). *Parasitol Today* 1986; 2:4–9.

39. Jimmy EO, Bedu-Addo G, Bates I, et al. Immunoglobulin gene polymerase chain reaction to distinguish hyperreactive malarial splenomegaly from 'African' chronic lymphocytic leukaemia and splenic lymphoma. *Trans R Soc Trop Med Hyg* 1996; 90:37–39.

40. Zhu A, Thompsett AR, Bedu-Addo G, et al. V$_H$ genes sequences from a novel tropical splenic lymphoma reveal a naïve B cell as the cell of origin. *Br J Haematol* 1999; 107:114–120.

41. Fleming AF, Terunuma H, Tembo C, et al. Leukaemias in Zambia. *Leukemia* 1999; 13:1292–1293.

42. Cartwright GE, Chung H-L, Chang A. Studies on the pancytopenia of kala-azar. *Blood* 1948; 3:249–275.

43. Kager PA, van der Plas-van Dalen C, Rees PH, et al. Red cell, white cell and platelet autoantibodies in visceral leishmaniasis. *Trop Geogr Med* 1984; 36:143–150.

44. Wickramasinghe SN, AbdallaS H, Kasili EG. Ultrastructure of bone marrow in patients with visceral leishmaniasis. *J Clin Pathol* 1987; 40:267–275.

45. Marwaha N, Sarode R, Gupta RK, et al. Clinico-hematological characteristics in patients with kala azar. *Trop Geogr Med* 1991; 43:357–362.

46. Lazzarin A, Esposito R, Almaviva M. Modifications of leucocyte function in visceral leishmaniasis. *Boll Ist Sieroter Milan* 1981; 60:222–224.

47. El-Hassan AM, Ahmed MAM, Rahim AA, et al. Visceral leishmaniasis in the Sudan: clinical and hematological features. *Ann Saudi Med* 1990; 10:51–56.

48. Varma N, Bhoria U, Bambery P, et al. Gelatinous transformation of the bone marrow and Leishmania donovani infection. *J Trop Med Hyg* 1991; 94:310–312.

49. Solano C, Gomez-Reino F, Fernandez-Rañada JM. Pure red cell aplasia in kala azar. *Acta Haematol* 1984; 72:205–207.

50. Kager PA, Rees PH. Haematological investigations in visceral leishmaniasis. *Trop Geogr Med* 1986; 38:371–379.

51. Pippard MJ, Moir D, Weatherall DJ. Mechanism of anaemia in resistant visceral leishmaniasis. *Ann Trop Med Parasitol* 1986; 80:317–323.

52. Weatherall DJ, Clegg JB. *The Thalassaemia Syndromes*, 4th edn. Oxford: Blackwell Science; 2000.

53. Steinberg MH, Forget BG, Higgs DR, et al. *Disorders of Hemoglobin*. Cambridge: Cambridge University Press; 2001.

54. Olivieri NF. The β-thalassaemias. *N Engl J Med* 1999; 341:99–109.

55. Wonke B. Bone disease in β-thalassaemia major. *Br J Haematol* 1998; 103:897–901.

56. Pippard MJ, Weatherall DJ. Oral iron chelation therapy for thalassaemia: an uncertain scene. *Br J Haematol* 2000; 111:2–5.

57. Fleming AF. Maternal anemia and fetal outcome in pregnancies complicated by thalassemia minor and 'stomatocytosis'. *Am J Obstet Gynecol* 1973; 116:309–319.

58. Willcox M, Björkman A, Brohult J. Falciparum malaria and β-thalassaemia trait in northern Liberia. *Ann Trop Med Parasitol* 1983; 77:335–347.

59. Metaxotou-Mavromati AD, Antonopoulou HK, Laskari SS et al. Developmental changes in hemoglobin F levels during the first two years of life in normal and heterozygous β-thalassemia infants. *Pediatrics* 1982; 69:734–738.

60. Luzzi GA, Merry AH, Newbold CI, et al. Surface antigen expression of Plasmodium falciparum-infected erythrocytes is modified in alpha- and beta-thalassemia. *J Exp Med* 1991; 173:785–791.

61. Senok AC, Nelson EAS, Li K, et al. Thalassaemia trait, red blood cell age and oxidant stress: effects on Plasmodium falciparum growth and sensitivity to artemisinin. *Trans R Soc Trop Med Hyg* 1997; 91:585–589.

62. Fucharoen S, Winichagoon P. Clinical and hematologic aspects of hemoglobin E β-thalassemia. *Current Opinions Hematol* 2000; 7:106–112.

63. de Silva S, Fisher CA, Premawardhena A, et al. Thalassaemia in Sri Lanka: implications for the future health burden of Asian populations. *Lancet* 2000; 355:786–791.

64. Chen FE, Ooi C, Ha SY et al. Genetic and clinical features of hemoglobin H disease in Chinese patients. *N Engl J Med* 2000; 343:544–550.

65. Muklwala EC, Banda J, Siziya S, et al. Alpha thalassaemia in Zambian newborn. *Clin Lab Haematol* 1989; 11:1–6.

66. Williams TN, Maitland K, Bennett S, et al. High incidence of malaria in α-thalassaemic children. *Nature* 1996; 383:522–525.

67. Bain BJ. *Haemoglobinopathy Diagnosis*. Oxford: Blackwell Science; 2001.

68. Modell B, Bulyzhenkov V. Distribution and control of some genetic disorders. *World Health Stat Q* 1988; 41:209–218.

69. Serjeant GR, Serjeant BE. *Sickle Cell Disease*, 3rd edn. Oxford: Oxford University Press; 2001.

70. Platt OS, Dover GJ. Sickle cell disease. In: Nathan DG, Oski FA, eds. *Hematology of Infancy and Childhood*, 4th edn. Philadelphia: W B Saunders; 1993:732–782.

71. Serjeant GR. The emerging understanding of sickle cell disease. *Br J Haematol* 2001; 112:3–18.

72. Nagel RL, Fleming AF. Genetic epidemiology of the β^s gene. *Baillière's Clin Haematol* 1992; 5:331–365.

73. Fleming AF. The presentation, management and prevention of crisis in sickle cell disease in Africa. *Blood Rev* 1989; 3:18–28.

74. Vichinsky EP, Neumayr LD, Earles AN, et al. Causes and outcomes of the acute chest syndrome in sickle cell disease. *N Engl J Med* 2000; 342:1855–1865.

75. Powars DR. Management of cerebral vasculopathy in children with sickle cell disease. *Br J Haematol* 2000; 108:666–678.

76. Morris J, Dunn D, Beckford M, et al. The haematology of homozygous sickle cell disease after the age of 40 years. *Br J Haematol* 1991; 77:382–385.

77. Harrison KA. Haemoglobinopathies in pregnancy. In: Lawson JB, Harrison KA, Bergström S, eds. *Maternity Care in Developing Countries*. London: Royal College of Obstetricians and Gynaecology; 2001:129–145.

78. Wierenga KJJ, Hambleton IR, Lewis NA. Survival estimates for patients with homozygous sickle-cell disease in Jamaica: a clinic-based population study. *Lancet* 2001; 357:680–683.

79. Molineaux L, Fleming AF, Cornille-Brøgger R, et al. Abnormal haemoglobins in the sudan savanna of Nigeria. III. Malaria, immunoglobulins and antimalarial antibodies in sickle cell disease. *Ann Trop Med Parasitol* 1979; 73:301–310.

80. Steinberg MH. Management of sickle cell disease. *N Engl J Med* 1999; 340:1021–1030.

81. Akinyanju OO, Anionwu EN. Training of counsellors in sickle-cell disorders in Africa. *Lancet* 1989; i:653–654.

82. Kark JA, Posey DM, Schumacher HR, et al. Sickle-cell trait as a risk factor for sudden death in physical training. *N Engl J Med* 1987; 317:781–787.

83. Abu-Zeid YA, Abdulhadi NH, Theander TG, et al. Seasonal changes in cell mediated immune responses to soluble Plasmodium falciparum antigens in children with haemoglobin AA and haemoglobin AS. *Trans R Soc Trop Med Hyg* 1992; 86:20–22.

84. WHO Working Group. Glucose-6-phosphate dehydrogenase deficiency. *Bull World Health Organ* 1989; 67:601–611.

85. Luzzatto L. G6PD deficiency and hemolytic anemia. In: Nathan DG, Oski FA (eds) *Hematology of Infancy and Childhood,* 4th edn. Philadelphia: W B Saunders; 1993:674–695.

86. Huang C-S, Hung K-L, Huang M-J, et al. Neonatal jaundice and molecular mutations in glucose-6-phosphate dehydrogenase deficient newborn infants. *Am J Hematol* 1996; 51:19–25.

87. Ho NK. Neonatal jaundice in Asia. *Baillière's Clin Haematol* 1992; 5:131–142.

88. Chan MCK. Glucose-6-phosphate dehydrogenase (G6PD) deficiency. *Postgrad Doct Middle East* 1992; 15:10–15.

89. Galiano S, Gaetani GF, Barabino A, et al. Favism in the African type of glucose-6-phosphate dehydrogenase deficiency (A⁻). *BMJ* 1990; 300:236.

90. Williams CKO, Osotimehim BO, Ogunmola GB, et al. Haemolytic anaemia associated with Nigerian barbecued meat (red suya). *Afr J Med Sci* 1988; 17:71–75.

91. Ruwende C, Hill A. Glucose-6-phosphate dehydrogenase deficiency and malaria. *J Mol Med* 1998; 76:581–588.

92. Cappadora M, Giribaldi G, O'Brien E, et al. Early phagocytosis of glucose-6-phosphate dehydrogenase (G6PD)-deficient erythrocytes parasitized by Plasmodium falciparum may explain malaria protection in G6PD deficiency. *Blood* 1998; 92:2527–2534.

93. Tse WT, Lux SE. Red blood cell membrane disorders. *Br J Haematol* 1999; 104:2–13.

94. Nurse GT, Coetzer TL, Palek J. The elliptocytoses, ovalocytosis and related disorders. *Baillière's Clin Haematol* 1992; 5:187–207.

95. Allen SJ, O'Donnell A, Alexander NDE, et al. Prevention of cerebral malaria in children in Papua New Guinea by Southeast Asian ovalocytosis band 3. *Am J Trop Med Hyg* 1999; 60:1056–1060.

96. Glele-Kakai C, Garbarz M, Lecomte M-C, et al. Epidemiological studies of spectrin mutations related to hereditary elliptocytosis and spectrin polymorphisms in Benin. *Br J Haematol* 1996; 95:57–66.

97. Chishti AH, Palek J, Fisher D et al. Reduced invasion and growth of Plasmodium falciparum into elliptocytic red blood cells with a combined deficiency of protein 4.1, glycophorin C, and p 55. *Blood* 1996; 87:3462–3469.

98. DeMaeyer EM, Dallman P, Gurney JM, et al. *Preventing and Controlling Iron Deficiency Anaemia through Primary Healthcare*. Geneva: WHO; 1989.

99. Fleming AF. Iron deficiency in the tropics. *Clin Haematol* 1982; 11:365–388.

100. *Report of the WHO Informal Consultation on Hookworm Infection and Anaemia in Girls and Women*, WHO/CTD/SIP/96.1. Geneva: WHO; 1996.

101. Bruner AB, Joffe A, Duggan AK, et al. Randomised study of cognitive effects of iron supplementation in non-anaemic iron-deficient adolescent girls. *Lancet* 1996; 348:992–996.

102. Allen LH. Anemia and iron deficiency: effects on pregnancy outcome. *Am J Clin Nutr* 2000; 71(suppl):1280S–1284S.

103. Hindmarsh PC, Geary MPP, Rodeck CH, et al. Effect of maternal iron stores on placental weight and structure. *Lancet* 2000; 356:719–723.

104. Stoltzfus RJ, Dreyfuss ML. *Guidelines for the Use of Iron Supplements to Prevent and Treat Iron Deficiency Anemia*, INACG/WHO/UNICEF Washington: ILSA Press; 1998.

105. Menendez C, Todd J, Alonso PL, et al. The effect of iron supplementation during pregnancy, given by traditional birth attendants, on the prevalence of anaemia and malaria. *Trans R Soc Trop Med Hyg* 1994; 88:590–593.

106. Menendez C, Todd J, Alonso PL, et al. The response to iron supplementation of pregnant women with the haemoglobin genotype AA or AS. *Trans R Soc Trop Med Hyg* 1995; 89:289–292.

107. INACG. *Safety of Iron Supplementation Programs in Malaria-Endemic Regions*. Washington: INACG; 1999.

108. Adish AA, Esrey SA, Gyorkos TW, et al. Effect of consumption of food cooked in iron pots on iron status and growth of children: a randomized trial. *Lancet* 1999; 353:712–716.

109. Gordeuk V. Hereditary and nutritional iron overload. *Baillière's Clin Haematol* 1992; 5:169–186.

110. Saungweme T, Khumalo H, Mvundura E, et al. Iron and alcohol content of traditional beers in rural Zimbabwe. *Centr Afr J Med* 1999; 45:136–140.

111. Moyo VM, Mandishona E, Hasstedt SJ, et al. Evidence of genetic transmission in African iron overload. *Blood* 1998; 91:1076–1082.

112. Cooper BA, Rosenblatt DS, Whitehead VM. Megaloblastic anemia. In: Nathan DG, Oski FA, eds. *Hematology of Infancy and Childhood*, 4th edn. Philadelphia: W B Saunders; 1993:354–390.

113. Ingram CF, Fleming AF, Patel M, et al. Pregnancy- and lactation-related folate deficiency in South Africa: a case for folate food fortification. *S Afr Med J* 1999; 89:1279–1284.

114. Scholl TO, Johnson WG. Folic acid: influence on the outcome of pregnancy. *Am J Clin Nutr* 2000; 71(suppl):1295S–1303S.

115. Baker SJ. Nutritional anaemias. Part 2: Tropical Asia. *Clin Haematol* 1981; 10:843–871.

116. Carmel R. Ethnic and racial factors in cobalamin metabolism and its disorders. *Semin Hematol* 1999; 36:88–100.

117. Harakati MSE. Pernicious anaemia in Arabs. *Blood Cells Mol Dis* 1996; 22:98–103.

118. Akinyanju OO, Okany CC. Pernicious anaemia in Africans. *Clin Lab Haematol* 1992; 14:33–40.

119. Savage D, Gangaidzo I, Lindenbaum J, et al. Vitamin B$_{12}$ deficiency is the primary cause of megaloblastic anaemia in Zimbabwe. *Br J Haematol* 1994; 86:844–850.

120. Remacha AF, Cadafalch J. Cobalamin deficiency in patients infected with the human immunodeficiency virus. *Semin Hematol* 1999; 36:75–87.

121. Cardosa AP, Ernesto M, Cliff J, et al. Cyanogenic potential of cassava flour: field trial in Mozambique of a simple kit. *Int J Food Sci Nutr* 1998; 49:93–99.

122. Ingram CF, Fleming AF, Patel M, et al. The value of the intrinsic factor antibody test in diagnosing pernicious anaemia. *Cent Afr J Med* 1999; 44:178–181.

123. WHO/UNICEF/IVACG/HKI. *Vitamin A Supplements: A Guide to their Use in the Treatment and Prevention of Vitamin A Deficiency*, 3rd edn. Geneva: World Health Organization; 2001.

124. Wickramasinghe SN. Nutritional anaemias. *Clin Lab Haematol* 1988; 10:117–134.

125. Powers HJ, Bates CJ, Prentice AM, et al. The relative effectiveness of iron with riboflavin in correcting a microcytic anaemia in men and children in rural Gambia. *Hum Nutr Clin Nutr* 1983; 37C:413–425.

126. Power HJ, Bayes CJ, Lamb WH. Haematological response to supplements of iron and riboflavin to pregnant and lactating women in rural Gambia. *Hum Nutr Clin Nutr* 1984; 39C:117–129.

127. Knox-Macaulay HHM. Tuberculosis and the haemopoietic system. *Baillière's Clin Haematol* 1992; 5:101–129.

128. Malyangu E, Abayomi EA, Adewuyi J, et al. AIDS is now the commonest clinical condition associated with multilineage blood cytopenia in a central referral hospital in Zimbabwe. *Cent Afr J Med* 2000; 46:59–61.

129. Bain BJ. The haematological features of HIV infection. *Br J Haematol* 1997; 99:1–8.

130. Karstaedt AD, Pantanowitz L, Gavalakis C, et al. Bone marrow morphology in human immunodeficiency virus-infected South Africans with and without tuberculosis. *Br J Haematol* 2001; 112:824–827.

131. Bower M. Acquired immunodeficiency syndrome-related systemic non-Hodgkin's lymphoma. *Br J Haematol* 2001; 112:863–873.

132. Alter BP, Young NS. The bone marrow failure syndromes. In: Nathan DG, Oski FA, eds. *Hematology of Infancy and Childhood*, 4th edn. Philadelphia: W B Saunders; 1993:216–316.

133. Yeats J, Daley H, Hardie D. Parvovirus B19 infection does not contribute significantly to severe anaemia in children with malaria in Malawi. *Eur J Haematol* 1999; 63:276–277.

134. Issaragrisil S, Leaverton PE, Chansung K, et al. Regional patterns in the incidence of aplastic anemia in Thailand. *Am J Hematol* 1999; 61:164–168.

135. Niazi GA, Fleming AF, Siziya S. Blood dyscrasia in unofficial vendors of petrol and heavy oil and motor mechanics in Nigeria. *Trop Doct* 1989; 19:55–58.

136. Waterhouse J, Muir C, Correa P, et al. *Cancer Incidence in Five Continents*, 3. Lyon: International Agency for Research on Cancer; 1976.

137. Ramot B, Rechavi G. Non-Hodgkin's lymphomas and paraproteinaemias. *Baillière's Clin Haematol* 1992; 5:81–99.

138. Glaser SL. Hodgkin's disease in black populations: a review of the epidemiologic literature. *Semin Hematol* 1990; 17:643–659.

139. Jarrett RF. Hodgkin's disease. *Baillière's Clin Haematol* 1992; 5:57–79.

140. Schmauz R, Mugerwa JW, Wright DH. The distribution of non-Burkitt, non-Hodgkin's lymphomas in Uganda in relation to malarial endemicity. *Int J Cancer* 1990; 45:650–653.

141. Shih L-Y, Liang D-C. Non-Hodgkins lymphomas in Asia. *Hematol Oncol Clin North Am* 1991; 5:983–1001.

142. Iscovich J, Parkin DM. Risk of cancer in migrants and their descendants in Israel: I. Leukaemias and lymphomas. *Int J Cancer* 1997; 70:649–653.

143. Foerster J. Heavy chain disease. In: Nathan DG, Oski FA, eds. *Hematology in Infancy and Childhood*, 4th edn. Philadelphia: W B Saunders, 1993:2693–2704.

144. Pawson R, Mufti GJ, Pagliuca A. Management of adult T-cell leukaemia/lymphoma. *Br J Haematol* 1998; 100:453–458.

145. Manns A, Hisada M, La Grenade L. Human T-lymphotropic virus type 1 infection. *Lancet* 1999; 353:1951–1958.

146. Weber T, Hunsmann G, Stevens W, et al. Human retroviruses. *Baillière's Clin Haematol* 1992; 5:273–314.

147. Blattner WA, Jacobson RJ, Shulman G. Multiple myeloma in South African Blacks. *Lancet* 1979; i:928–929.

148. Mukiibi JM, Mkwananzi JB. Multiple myeloma in Zimbabweans. *East Afr Med J* 1987; 64:471–481.

149. Fleming AF. Leukaemias in Africa. *Leukemia* 1993; 7(suppl):S138–S141.

150. Greaves MF, Colman SM, Beard MEJ et al. Geographical distribution of acute lymphoblastic leukaemia subtypes: second report of the Collaborative Group study. *Leukemia* 1993; 7:27–34.

151. Fleming AF, Glencross DK, Adam F, et al. Acute lymphoblastic leukaemia in Johannesburg: distribution of phenotypes by race, age and sex. *24th Congress of the International Society of Haematology*, London; 1992:Abstract 144:382.

152. Paul B, Mukiibi JM, Mandisodsa A, et al. A three-year prospective study of 137 cases of acute leukaemia in Zimbabwe. *Cent Afr J Med* 1992; 38: 95–99.

153. Greaves MF. Aetiology of acute leukaemia. *Lancet* 1997; 349:344–349.

154. Greaves M. Childhood leukaemia. *Br Med J* 2002; 324:283–287.

155. Kinlen LJ, Balkwill A. Infective cause of childhood leukaemia and wartime population mixing in Orkney and Shetland, UK. *Lancet* 2001; 357:858.

156. Pasqualetti P, Festuccia V, Acitelli P, et al. Tobacco smoking and risk of haematological malignancies in adults: a case-control study. *Br J Haematol* 1997; 97:659–662.

157. Mukiibi JM, Paul B. Myelodysplastic syndromes (MDS) in Central Africans. *Trop Geog Med* 1994; 46:17–19.

158. Goldman JM, Melo JV. Targeting the BCR-ABL tyrosine kinase in chronic myeloid leukemia. *N Engl J Med* 2001; 344:1084–1086.

159. Fleming AF. Chronic lymphocytic leukaemia in tropical Africa: a review. *Leuk Lymphoma* 1990; 1:169–173.

160. Bates I, Bedu-Addo G, Jarrett RF, et al. B-lymphotropic viruses in a novel tropical splenic lymphoma. *Br J Haematol* 2001; 112:161–166.

161. Zhu D, Thompsett AR, Bedu-Addo G, et al. V_H gene sequences from a novel tropical splenic lymphoma reveal a naïve B cell as the cell of origin. *Br J Haematol* 1999; 107:114–120.

162. Masera G, Baez F, Biondi A, et al. North-South twinning in paediatric haemato-oncology. The La Mascota programme, Nicaragua. *Lancet* 1998; 352:1923–1926.

163. Hesseling PB. Onyalai. *Baillière's Clin Haematol* 1992; 5:457–473.

164. Nathwani AC, Tuddenham EGD. Epidemiology of coagulation disorders. *Baillière's Clin Haematol* 1992; 5:383–439.

165. Zipursky A. Prevention of vitamin K deficiency bleeding in newborns. *Br J Haematol* 1999; 104:430–437.

166. Levi M, ten Cate H. Disseminated intravascular coagulation. *N Engl J Med* 1999; 341:586–592.

167. Adewuyi JO, Coutts AM, Levy L, et al. Haemophilia care in Zimbabwe. *Cent Afr J Med* 1996; 42:153–156.

168. World Health Organization. *Control of Haemophilia:Haemophilia Care in Developing Countries. Report of a Joint WHO/World Federation of Haemophilia Meeting*, WHO/HGN/WFH/WG/98.3 Geneva: WHO; 1998.

Chapter 14

Imelda Bates and Shirley Owusu-Ofori

Blood Transfusion

Only 39% of the global blood supply is donated in the poorest countries where 82% of the world's population lives.[1]

Blood transfusion is a vital component of every country's health service (Table 14.1). It can be a life-saving intervention for severe, acute anaemia, but mistakes in the transfusion process can be life-threatening, either immediately or years later through transmission of infectious agents. It is imperative that clinicians have a good understanding of how blood is acquired and prepared for transfusion, and when it should be used, and that governments put in place quality assurance mechanisms to guarantee that blood for transfusion is safe.

BLOOD TRANSFUSION SERVICE AT THE NATIONAL LEVEL

Transfusion medicine is critical to the success of most clinical specialties and should be incorporated into all national health plans and budgets. Only 16% of member states meet all the World Health Organization's (WHO) recommendations for a national quality blood transfusion system.[1] At the national level the transfusion service should have a director, an advisory committee and clear transfusion policies and strategies (Table 14.2). Blood collection, testing and distribution need to be standardized. Although centralization of these services may offer the best guarantee of quality, it is often not practical in countries with poorly developed communications and transport infrastructure. In such countries, each hospital organizes its own blood transfusion service and it is then difficult to ensure national standardization and quality. Hospital-based transfusion services place an enormous burden on laboratory resources and on the families of patients because they are responsible for finding suitable blood donors. In a typical district hospital in Malawi, the overall cost of the transfusion service, including consumables, proportional amounts for capital equipment, staff time and overheads, was 53% of total laboratory costs and each unit of whole blood cost the laboratory approximately £10 to collect and process.[2]

In wealthy countries with nationally or regionally centralized transfusion services, blood donor recruitment, and screening and processing of donated blood, are carried out in purpose-built centres which are separate from the hospitals where the blood is transfused. These centres operate to good manufacturing standards similar to those laid down for the pharmaceutical industry. After donation and exclusion of potentially infected units, the blood is separated into components and filtered to remove white cells. Computerization enables individual components to be barcoded so they can be tracked back to the original donor. Hospitals are proficient at predicting how much blood they will require and they receive regular consignments through a well-established delivery network. The efficiency of the system means that one donor centre may provide blood to many hospitals and cover a population of several million. This process is expensive and one unit of blood currently costs over £100.[3]

Separation of whole blood into components

In wealthy countries it is standard practice to optimize the use of each donation of blood by separating it into individual components. These components, which may include plasma, platelets and cryoprecipitate, are prepared by centrifugation using a closed, sterile system. Each component has different storage requirements. Plasma and cryoprecipitate are kept frozen, red cells are stored at 1–5°C, and platelets at 18–22°C with constant agitation. Separation of blood, even into simple components such as cells and plasma, requires equipment and expertise, so in the poorest countries blood components may only be accessible to those living close to a central hospital with blood separation facilities.

Ensuring safety of blood for transfusion

An unsafe blood supply is costly in both human and economic terms. Transfusion of infected blood causes morbidity and mortality in the recipients, and has an economic and emotional impact on their families and communities. Those who become infected through blood transfusion are infectious to others and contribute to the spread of disease throughout the wider population. This increases the burden on health services and reduces productive labour.

Selecting low-risk blood donors

Strategies for recruiting blood donors have to balance supply with demand, and yet ensure that the blood is as safe as possible. In general, the safest sources of blood are altruistic voluntary unpaid donors who should be anonymous to the recipient. Only 32% of WHO member states report having at least 90% of their blood supply from voluntary donors, and developing countries have not shown any improvement in recruitment of voluntary donors for several years.[1]

In countries without a national transfusion service, each hospital is responsible for finding its own donors and processing blood for transfusion. Recruiting voluntary donors from the community is expensive and logistically complicated, requiring resources such as a local education programme, dedicated venesection team, vehicles and cold storage. Paid donors or 'loan' systems, where family members are responsible for providing blood for their relatives in the hospital, are therefore widespread in poorer countries. Cultural taboos and misinformation about donating blood (e.g. 'men will become impotent if they donate blood'; 'HIV can be caught from the blood bag needle') mean that relatives may be reluctant to donate. Families are open to exploitation by 'professional donors' who charge a fee to donate in place of a family member. By the time a donor has been found, screened and venesected, and the blood is transfused into the patient, several hours or even days can elapse, especially if blood of a rare group is required. Because patients in poorer countries often present late in the course of their disease, severely anaemic patients may die in hospital without ever receiving a blood transfusion. It is unfortunate that in many countries where the majority of transfusions are performed as an emergency and where it is imperative to have a well-stocked blood bank, the 'loan' system, with its inherent delays, predominates.

Potential 'high-risk' donors, such as commercial sex workers or those having frequent contact with these individuals, intravenous drug abusers, or persons with itinerant or fluctuating activities such as traders, drivers and military personnel, should be permanently deferred from the donor pool.[4] Even in areas where HIV infection rates in the general population are high, donor deferral can be effective in excluding HIV-infected donors.[5] The whole donation process, including tests for HIV and other infections, should be explained to the donor before blood is collected and donors should have the option of knowing the results and receiving counselling. It is imperative that complete confidentiality is maintained throughout all procedures.

Screening for transfusion-transmitted infections

Infections with organisms that are common in tropical countries, such as HIV-1 and -2, hepatitis A, B, C and D, cytomegalovirus, syphilis, lyme borreliosis, malaria, babesiosis, American trypanosomiasis (Chagas' disease) and toxoplasmosis, can all be acquired through blood transfusions. There have also been recent reports of transmission of variant Creutzfeldt–Jakob disease through blood transfusion and there is a theoretical risk of acquiring severe acute respiratory syndrome (SARS) through transfusion of labile blood products.[6,7] WHO recommends that all donated blood should be screened for HIV, hepatitis B and syphilis and, where feasible and appropriate, for hepatitis C, malaria and Chagas' disease.

Between 5% and 10% of HIV infections worldwide are thought to have been transmitted through the transfusion of infected blood and blood products. HIV testing of blood donors needs to be highly sensitive, and blood which tests positive should be rejected. Before informing the donor of the outcome, all positive results should be confirmed using a test with a high degree of specificity. Where blood donation is organized locally, the confirmatory test is often performed at a central laboratory, so there may be delay in informing the donor of the result.

Malaria can be transmitted by transfusion and has an incubation period of between 7 and 50 days, depending on the species. In areas of low or no malaria transmission, screening for the parasite is important, as recipients are likely to have no immunity. In countries with high malaria transmission, exclusion of parasitaemic donors could result in deferral rates exceeding 30% and consequently would have a major impact on blood supply.[8] It is unclear whether malaria screening is necessary in regions where

Table 14.1 Global facts about blood transfusion

80% of the world's population has access to 20% of the world's safe blood supply
Transfusion or injection of unsafe blood accounts for 8–16 million hepatitis B virus infections, 2.3–4.7 million hepatitis C virus infections, and 80 000–160 000 HIV infections each year
25% of maternal deaths from pregnancy-related causes are linked with blood loss

Table 14.2 Elements and national strategies for blood safety[1]

Essential element	Supporting strategy
Well-organized, nationally coordinated blood transfusion service	Government commitment; specific, adequate budget; implementation of national blood policy and plan; legislative and regulatory framework
Quality systems covering all aspects of activities	Organizational management; quality standards; documentation systems; staff training; quality assessments
Blood collection only from voluntary, non-remunerated donors	Effective donor recruitment programmes; stringent donor selection criteria; donor care programme
Quality assured testing of all donated blood	Testing for transfusion-transmissible infections; accurate blood group serology and compatibility testing procedures
Reduction in unnecessary use of blood	Use of appropriate component therapy; safe administration of blood and blood products

the disease is common, particularly because most of the blood is given to hospitalized children with malaria who are likely to be receiving antimalarial drugs, or adults who are clinically immune. Further research to assess the risks and benefits of screening blood for malaria is needed, particularly in relation to pregnant women and patients with HIV infection.

Screening for hepatitis B surface antigen should be carried out on all donated blood, as hepatitis B-infected blood is almost 100% infectious. Fresh blood is potentially infectious for syphilis, but storage at 4°C can inactivate *Treponema pallidum*. Globally, the prevalence of hepatitis C, HTLV-1 and -2 and Chagas' disease is variable and the decision to introduce donor screening for these infections will be based on local assessments of the risks, benefits, feasibility and costs. Blood should not be separated into components if the residual risk of infection is high, as this will increase the number of potentially infected recipients. In some wealthy countries nucleic acid amplification techniques (NAT) have been introduced to improve the safety of blood. Although NAT may not be cost-effective where infection prevalence is low, it has reduced the residual risk for HIV, hepatitis C virus (HCV) and hepatitis B virus (HBV) infection in Germany to 1 in 5 540 000, 1 in 4 400 000 and 1 in 620 000, respectively.[9]

Blood is usually taken from donors and stored in a blood bank until screening tests for infections have been completed. This system has several drawbacks: potentially infected blood may be mixed up with units that have already been screened, and the whole process of venesection with wastage of blood collection bags is costly. Pre-donation screening, by which potential donors are tested for HIV, hepatitis B and possibly hepatitis C at the site of donation before being venesected, may be a more cost-effective way of ensuring safe blood.[10]

CLINICAL USE OF BLOOD

Reasons for transfusion in poorer countries

In wealthy countries the majority of transfusions are planned and carried out electively. By contrast, in poorer countries, and particularly those where the malaria transmission rate is high, most transfusions are given for life-threatening emergencies. In these countries 50–80% of transfusions are administered to children, predominantly for malaria-related anaemia. Transfusion can significantly reduce the mortality of children with severe anaemia but it may not have any benefit unless it is given within the first 2 days of hospital admission.[11] In areas of high HIV prevalence, young children have a relatively low risk of being infected with HIV and potentially have a long life expectancy. However, this is the age group that is predominantly affected by severe malaria-related anaemia and so they are particularly at risk of transfusion-acquired HIV infection.[12] Pregnant women are the second most common recipients of blood, particularly for haemorrhagic emergencies.[13] Other specialities which are significant users of blood are surgery, trauma and general medicine.

Avoiding unnecessary transfusions

Whether a patient needs a blood transfusion or not is ultimately a clinical decision. Emergency transfusions can be life-saving for patients in whom the anaemia has developed too quickly to allow physiological compensation. Examples of such emergencies include severe malaria-related anaemia in children, and sudden, severe obstetric bleeding. In contrast, if the anaemia has developed slowly, for example due to hookworm infestation or nutritional deficiency, patients can generally be managed conservatively by treating the cause of the anaemia and prescribing haematinic replacements. These should be continued for at least 3 months after the haemoglobin has returned to normal, so that body stores can be replenished.

Guidelines for transfusion practice

It is possible to avoid unnecessary transfusions through the use of clinical transfusion guidelines, and most institutions or organizations have developed guidelines to help clinicians make rational decisions about the use of blood transfusions (Table 14.3).[14] Strict enforcement of a transfusion protocol in a Malawian hospital reduced the number of transfusions by 75% without any adverse effect on the mortality rate.[15] While the details may vary, the principles underlying most transfusion guidelines are similar and combine a clinical assessment of whether the patient is developing complications of inadequate oxygenation, with measurement of their haemoglobin. The haemoglobin level is used as a surrogate measure for intracellular oxygen concentration. Increasingly, transfusion guidelines are making use of evidence which shows that adequate oxygen delivery to the tissues can be achieved at haemoglobin levels that are significantly lower than the normal range.[16]

Table 14.3 Prescribing blood: a checklist for clinicians[14]

Always ask yourself the following questions before prescribing blood or blood products for a patient:
1. What improvement in the patient's clinical condition am I aiming to achieve?
2. Can I minimize blood loss to reduce this patient's need for transfusion?
3. Are there any other treatments I should give before making the decision to transfuse, such as intravenous replacement fluids or oxygen?
4. What are the specific clinical or laboratory indications for transfusion in this patient?
5. What are the risks of transmitting HIV, hepatitis, syphilis or other infectious agents through the blood products that are available for this patient?
6. Do the benefits of transfusion outweigh the risks for this particular patient?
7. What other options are there if no blood is available in time?
8. Will a trained person monitor this patient and respond immediately if any acute transfusion reactions occur?
9. Have I recorded my decision and reasons for transfusion on the patient's chart and the blood request form?
Finally, if in doubt, ask yourself the following question:
If this blood were for myself or my child, would I accept the transfusion under these circumstances?

It is easier to develop guidelines than to ensure that they are used in routine practice. Implementation of transfusion guidelines is particularly difficult if clinicians do not have confidence in the quality of haemoglobin measurements. It has been shown that when doubtful of the quality of haemoglobin result, clinicians rely entirely on clinical judgement to guide transfusion practice. This may lead to significant numbers of inappropriate transfusions.[17] In a typical district hospital in Africa, the cost of providing a unit of blood through the family 'loan' system is approximately 30 times the cost of a quality-assured haemoglobin test. A lack of investment in assuring the quality of a basic but critical test such as haemoglobin measurement can result in a significant waste of resources downstream in the transfusion process, with the additional unnecessary exposure of recipients to the risk of transfusion-related infections.

Haemoglobin thresholds for transfusion

In resource-poor countries, the recommended haemoglobin threshold for transfusions is often well below that which would be accepted in more wealthy countries. For example, American anaesthetists suggest that transfusions are almost always indicated when the haemoglobin level is less than 6 g/dL,[18] whereas in Malawi transfusions are recommended for children with haemoglobin levels less than 4 g/dL, provided there are no other clinical complications.[19] Complications such as cardiac failure or infection may necessitate transfusion at a higher haemoglobin level. Transfusion should be combined with adequate iron and folate replacements and treatment of any underlying conditions that contribute to anaemia, so that a normal haemoglobin count can be achieved during the weeks following transfusion.

Any transfusion service must be able to guarantee the quality of haemoglobin results. These results are crucial in donor selection and are also used to guide the decision to transfuse patients. Although it is the most commonly performed test, accurate haemoglobin estimation is difficult to achieve in laboratories without automated blood analysers.[20] The reference technique for haemoglobin measurement is the haemiglobincyanide method. Not only does this method need a constant electricity source for the spectrophotometer, but also technicians need arithmetic expertise to calibrate the equipment and automatic pipettes for accurate measurements. In under-resourced countries, district hospitals may use simpler, cheaper and less accurate methods of haemoglobin measurement, many of which are based on visual colour comparisons. While a few individual laboratories in resource-poor countries may be registered with an external system to monitor the quality of laboratory tests, almost no country has a nationwide programme. This means that for many laboratories and their users, the quality of tests, including haemoglobin and those used for screening and determining blood groups, is unknown.

COMPLICATIONS OF BLOOD TRANSFUSION

Complications can occur immediately during transfusion, within a few hours of its completion, or be delayed for many years, as in the case of viral infections. See Table 14.4.

Table 14.4 Complications of blood transfusion

- Febrile non-haemolytic transfusion reactions. Haemolytic reactions include chills, headache, backache, dyspnoea, cyanosis, chest pain, tachycardia and hypotension
- Risk of severe bacterial infection and sepsis
- Transmission of viral infection (hepatitis B, HIV or hepatitis C)
- Transmission of blood-borne trypanosomes, filaria, malaria, etc.
- Cardiac failure
- Air embolism
- Transfusion-associated acute lung injury (TRALI) – a syndrome of acute respiratory distress, often associated with fever, non-cardiogenic pulmonary oedema, and hypotension, which may occur as often as 1 in 2000 transfusions
- Other risks: volume overload, iron overload (with multiple red blood cell transfusions), transfusion-associated graft-versus-host disease, anaphylactic reactions (in people with IgA deficiency), and acute haemolytic reactions (most commonly due to the administration of mismatched blood types)

Acute and delayed haemolysis due to red cell incompatibility

Transfusion of blood into a recipient who possesses antibodies to the donor's red cells can cause an acute, and occasionally fatal, intravascular haemolysis. This could occur, for example, if group A cells are transfused into a group O recipient who has naturally occurring antibodies to group A cells. The profound haemolysis induces renal vasoconstriction and acute tubular necrosis. Treatment involves stopping the transfusion, cardiorespiratory support and inducing a brisk diuresis. In addition to abnormalities indicating renal failure, laboratory findings include haemoglobinuria and haemoglobinaemia. Proof of the diagnosis involves rechecking the whole transfusion process including all documentation stages, regrouping the donor and the recipient, and screening for antibodies on red cells with a direct antiglobulin test. These tests are usually available in any hospital laboratory capable of providing a transfusion service. Delayed haemolysis has a similar physiological basis to acute intravascular haemolysis but tends to be less severe. The antibody–antigen reaction develops 7–10 days after the transfusion and it is less likely than acute haemolysis to present as a clinical emergency.

Bacterial contamination

Bacteria can enter the blood bag during venesection or if the bag is perforated at a later stage, perhaps to reduce the volume for a paediatric recipient or during component preparation. Gram-negative bacteria, including *Pseudomonas* and *Yersinia*, grow optimally at refrigerator temperatures and infected blood may not necessarily appear abnormal. Reactions following infusion of infected blood are often due to endotoxins and may occur several hours after the transfusion has finished. Although these reactions are rare, they can be severe and fatal. If bacterial contamination is suspected, the transfusion should be stopped and samples from the patient and the blood bag sent to the laboratory for culture. Cardiorespiratory support may be needed and broad-spectrum antibiotics should be started immediately and continued until culture results are available.

Non-haemolytic febrile reactions

These are episodes of fever (i.e. ≥1°C rise in temperature) and chills for which no other cause can be found. They are due to the recipient's antibodies reacting against antigens present on the donor's white cells or platelets. These reactions are most common in patients who have received multiple transfusions in the past and have therefore been exposed to a broad range of antigens. Mild febrile reactions usually respond to simple antipyretics such as paracetamol. More severe reactions may be the first indication of a haemolytic transfusion reaction or bacterial contamination and should be investigated and managed accordingly.

Allergic reactions

These are due to infusion of plasma proteins and manifestations include erythema, rash, pruritus, bronchospasm and anaphylaxis. The transfusion should be stopped and the patient treated with antihistamines. If the reaction is mild and the symptoms and signs completely disappear, the transfusion can be restarted. If this type of mild reaction occurs repeatedly with more than one unit of blood, the red cells can be washed before transfusion. This should only be done if absolutely necessary, as it carries the risk of introducing potentially fatal bacterial infection. Severe allergic reactions with evidence of systemic toxicity should be managed as acute anaphylaxis.

Circulatory overload

Blood should always be transfused slowly, to avoid overloading the circulation, unless the patient is actively and severely bleeding. Overload may be a particular problem when paediatric blood bags are not available, as children may be over-transfused due to miscalculation of the required volume, lack of accurate infusion devices or inadvertent administration of an adult-sized unit of blood.

Transfusion-transmitted infections (see above)

In tropical practice, blood transmission of hepatitis B, HIV-1 and -2, and, in some areas, American trypanosomiasis (Chagas' disease) is of particular concern. In general, transfusions are not the major route of transmission of these infections and they may not cause clinical problems until many months or years after the transfusion.

Haemosiderosis

Four units of blood contain the equivalent of the amount of iron stored in the bone marrow (approximately 1 g). Repeated transfusions for chronic haemolytic anaemia, as in thalassaemia major and sickle cell disease, lead to iron deposition in parenchymal cells. Eventually, failure of the heart, liver and other organs supersedes. Adequate doses of iron chelators, such as injectable desferrioxamine or the newer oral chelator, deferiprone, are able to maintain acceptable iron balance in patients with chronic anaemia receiving regular transfusions.

Hypothermia

It is not usually necessary to warm blood unless rapid transfusion of large quantities is needed. This may lower the temperature of the sino-atrial node to below 30°C, at which point ventricular fibrillation can occur. If blood needs to be warmed, an electric blood warmer specifically designed for the purpose should be used. This keeps the temperature below 38°C, thereby avoiding the haemolysis associated with overheating blood.

Graft-versus-host disease

Graft-versus-host disease occurs when donor lymphocytes engraft in an immune-suppressed recipient. The lymphocytes recognize the recipient's bone marrow as foreign and induce aplasia. Graft-versus-host disease is almost universally fatal and can be prevented by irradiating the donor blood, which inactivates the donor lymphocytes.

REDUCING THE USE OF BLOOD TRANSFUSIONS

Minimizing surgical blood loss

Where blood is in short supply, it is particularly important to ensure that the best anaesthetic and surgical techniques are used, to minimize blood loss during surgery. Drugs which improve haemostasis or reduce fibrinolysis, such as aprotinin and cyklokapron, and fibrin sealants, can be effective in reducing perioperative blood loss and hence the need for blood transfusion. Cost is a major limiting factor to the use of these therapies in poorer countries, and surgical blood loss is generally not a major contributor to the overall transfusion needs.

Preoperative autologous blood deposit

Patients undergoing planned surgery who are likely to require a blood transfusion can have units of their own blood removed and stored prior to surgery for use by themselves only, if significant intraoperative blood loss is anticipated. Preoperative autologous donation can reduce the need for allogeneic transfusions by 46–74%[21] but it requires careful organization: the surgeon needs to predict how much blood will be required, the patient has to be fit enough to withstand removal of one or more units of blood over the weeks preceding the surgery (preoperative haemoglobin will drop by about 1 g/dL), and the surgery must take place within the shelf-life of the blood. As the blood has to be stored in the blood bank there is still a risk that the patient may receive blood which is not his or her own or that the blood may become infected with bacteria during the process.

Intraoperative blood salvage

This involves collecting blood lost during the operation and reinfusing it into the patient either during or after surgery. Although this technique is practical and safe, and reduces the need for donor blood by 27–53%,[21] it requires specialized equipment and training and may be more expensive than routinely donated blood.[22]

Other methods

Normal saline or intravenous replacement fluids can be used judiciously in acute blood loss, and in certain circumstances may be as effective as whole blood, red cells or plasma. Erythropoietin, which stimulates endogenous red cell production, has well-established uses in chronic anaemias such as those due to renal failure, cancer and HIV infection. Its delayed action makes it unsuitable for use in acute anaemias, the major reason for transfusions in poorer countries. The development of synthetic oxygen carriers, generally perfluorocarbons, has been fraught with problems and they are not routinely available.[23]

In under-resourced countries, especially those with a heavy burden of malaria, the most effective way to avoid the need for transfusions is to reduce the prevalence of anaemia in the community. More studies on the ability and cost of combined interventions such as the provision of bed nets, nutritional supplements and anthelmintic drugs to children to prevent anaemia and reduce transfusion requirements are needed. When resources are very limited, governments may need to make some difficult decisions in order to achieve an equitable balance between investing in a transfusion service and public health measures to reduce anaemia.

REFERENCES

1. World Health Organization. *Global database on blood safety 2001–2002*. WHO/EHT/04.09. 2004. Online. Available: http://www.who.int/bloodsafety/GDBS_Report_200-2002.pdf.
2. Medina Lara A, Kandulu J, Chisuwo L, et al. Laboratory costs of a hospital-based blood transfusion service in Malawi. *J Clin Pathol* 2007; 60:1117–1120.
3. Provan D. Better blood transfusion. *BMJ* 1999; 381:1435–1436.
4. Gerard C, Sondag-Thull D, Watson-Williams EJ, et al. *Safe Blood in Developing Countries*. Brussels: European Commission; 1995:48.
5. Schutz R, Savarit D, Kadjo J-C, et al. Excluding blood donors at high risk of HIV infection in a West African city. *BMJ* 1993; 307:1517–1519.
6. Llewelyn C, Hewitt P, Knight R, et al. Possible transmission of variant Creutzfeldt-Jakob disease by blood transfusion. *Lancet* 2004; 363:417–421.
7. World Health Organization. *WHO recommendations on SARS and blood safety*. 15 May 2003. Online. Available: http://www.who.int/csr/sars/guidelines/bloodsafety/en/.
8. Kinde-Gazard D, Oke J, Gnahoui I, et al. The risk of malaria transmission by blood transfusion at Cotonou, Benin. *Sante* 2000; 10:389–392.
9. Offergeld R, Faensen D, Ritter S, et al. Human immunodeficiency virus, hepatitis C and hepatitis B infections among blood donors in Germany 2000–2002: risk of virus transmission and the impact of nucleic acid amplification testing. *Euro Surveill* 2005; 10:8–11.
10. Owusu-Ofori S, Temple J, Sarkodie F, et al. Predonation screening of blood donors with rapid tests: implementation and efficacy of a novel approach to blood safety in resource-poor settings. *Transfusion* 2005; 45:133–140.
11. Lackritz E, Campbell C, Ruebush T, et al. Effect of blood transfusion on survival among children in a Kenyan hospital. *Lancet* 1992; 340:524–528.
12. Shaffer N, Hedberg K, Davachi F, et al. Trends and risk factors of HIV-1 seropositivity among outpatient children, Kinshasa, Zaire. *AIDS* 1990; 4:1231–1236.
13. Zucker J, Lackritz T, Ruebush T, et al. Anaemia, blood transfusion practices, HIV and mortality among women of reproductive age in western Kenya. *Trans R Soc Trop Med Hyg* 1994; 88:173–176.
14. World Health Organization. *Blood safety . . . for too few*. Press release WHO/25. 7 April 2000. WHD/3 Information sheet for clinicians. Online. Available: www.who.int/inf-pr-2000/en/pr2000-25.html.
15. Craighead I, Knowles J. Prevention of transfusion-associated HIV transmissions with the use of a transfusion protocol for under 5s. *Trop Doc* 1993; 23:59–61.
16. Leung J, Weiskopf R, Feiner J, et al. Electrocardiographic ST-segment changes during acute, severe isovolemic hemodilution in humans. *Anesthesiology* 2000; 93:1004–1010.
17. Bates I, Mundy C, Pendame R, et al. Use of clinical judgement to guide administration of blood transfusions in Malawi. *Trans R Soc Trop Med Hyg* 2001; 95:510–512.
18. American Society of Anesthesiologists Task Force. Practice guidelines for blood component therapy. *Anesthesiology* 1996; 84:732–747.
19. Ministry of Health and Population, Malawi. AIDS control programme. Recommended guidelines for the practice of safe blood transfusion in Malawi, 1997.
20. Lara A, Mundy C, Kandulu J, et al. Evaluation and costs of different haemoglobin methods for use in district hospitals in Malawi. *J Clin Pathol* 2005; 58:56–60.
21. Carless P, Moxey A, O'Connell D, et al. Autologous transfusion techniques: a systematic review of their efficacy. *Transfus Med* 2004; 14:123–144.
22. McMillan D, Dando H, Potger K, et al. Intra-operative autologous blood management. *Transfus Apher Sci* 2002; 27:73–81.
23. Spahn D, Kocian R. Artificial O2 carriers: status in 2005. *Curr Pharm Des* 2005; 11:4009–4114.

Chapter 15

Raj C. Thuraisingham and Dwomoa Adu

Renal Disease in the Tropics

There are variations in the causes of renal diseases in different parts of the world and this is most marked between temperate and tropical regions. Even within tropical regions differences are seen in the pattern of renal diseases. The main factor that differentiates renal disease in the tropics from that in temperate regions of the world is the much higher frequency with an infectious aetiology. Much renal disease in the tropics is, however, idiopathic and similar to renal disease found elsewhere in the world. Whether caused by infections or not, the principles underlying the understanding of renal disease are the same in all parts of the world.

ASSESSMENT OF KIDNEY DISEASE

Abnormalities in the kidneys are assessed by estimating GFR using serum creatinine levels and determining the presence of blood or protein in urine. This is complemented by imaging techniques and in particular ultrasound. The glomerular filtration rate (GFR) is generally considered the best measure of renal function. Inulin satisfies all the criteria for an ideal filtration marker and is the 'gold standard' for the measurement of GFR. But this remains a research tool.[1] The normal GFR is approximately 130 mL/min per 1.73 m^2 in young males and 120 mL/min per 1.73 m^2 in young females and these values decline with age.

SERUM CREATININE CONCENTRATION

Serum creatinine determination is widely used; however, its concentration is insensitive to detection of mild to moderate reductions in GFR due to the non-linear relation between concentration of creatinine in the blood and GFR. This means that GFR must decline to approximately half the normal level before the serum creatinine concentration rises above the upper limit of normal. Correspondingly many patients with chronic kidney disease (CKD) maintain serum creatinine levels in the normal range despite having significantly impaired renal function. Serum creatinine levels are dependent on dietary protein intake, total muscle mass, and the use of medications such as cimetidine and trimethoprim which interfere with renal creatinine handling. Additionally, several substances can interfere with the laboratory measurement of creatinine. Glucose, uric acid, ketones, plasma proteins and cephalosporins may lead to falsely high creatinine values when the Jaffe reaction method is used. The effect of non-creatinine chromogens in serum is markedly reduced in the kinetic rate Jaffe reaction, which is implemented in many autoanalyzers.

CYSTATIN C

Cystatin C, a non-glycosylated basic protein with a low molecular mass (13 kD) that is freely filtered by the glomerulus, is currently under investigation as a replacement for serum creatinine in estimating the GFR.[1]

GFR ESTIMATION USING PREDICTION EQUATIONS

In an attempt to overcome the drawbacks using serum creatinine alone, several equations have been developed to estimate GFR.[1] The most widely used equations for estimating GFR are the Cockcroft and Gault proposed equation and the Modification of Diet in Renal Disease (MDRD) equation. The Cockcroft–Gault (CG) formula is an estimate of creatinine clearance originally developed in a population of 236 Canadian patients, 209 of whom were male, and has been tested widely in its prediction of GFR. The MDRD equation was developed on a large ($n = 1785$) database containing persons with various kidney diseases. These patients had been enrolled in the Modification of Diet in Renal Diseases Study and had serum creatinine as well as isotopic GFRs measured. The equation was subsequently tested on a validation database containing more than 500 additional patients.[2] The MDRD equation has been widely validated in several other groups including African-Americans with hypertension (Table 15.1).[3]

The equation is not valid in children. Most guidelines advocate the use of the MDRD equation to predict glomerular filtration rate in clinical practice. This is because the equation detects impaired kidney function more accurately than using serum creatinine concentration alone, and it also serves as a monitoring tool for patients with known renal disease.

Table 15.1 MDRD equation for GFR

GFR = 186 × (Creatinine/88.4)$^{-1.154}$ × age$^{-0.203}$
Women = Multiply × 0.742
Black = Multiply × 1.210
Creatinine μmol/L

MDRD, Modification of Diet in Renal Disease; GFR, glomerular filtration rate. Calculator on: http://www.renal.org/eGFRcalc/GFR.pl

PROTEINURIA

Proteinuria[4] is a marker of renal damage. Physiologically, the glomerular basement membrane provides both a mechanical and a charge barrier to the passage of plasma proteins into the glomerular filtrate. Nevertheless, some plasma proteins cross this barrier in the concentrations that are related to the protein's size, charge, deformability and concentration in the plasma. Under normal circumstances, the mechanical barrier to filtration excludes large molecules like globulins from entering the glomerular filtrate; only low molecular weight proteins, such as peptide hormones, insulin, and derivatives of immunoproteins cross the glomerular basement membrane. Normal persons usually excrete very small amounts of protein in the urine. Increased excretion of protein is therefore a sensitive marker for chronic kidney disease due to diabetes, glomerular disease and hypertension. Proteinuria is not only a marker of kidney damage but also a strong predictor of clinical progression of kidney disease[5] and can be of considerable value in assessing the effectiveness of therapy and the progression of the disease.[6]

The assessment of proteinuria in clinical practice is generally carried out using dipstick methods and/or quantification of proteinuria. The quantitative methods widely used are the untimed (spot) urine and the timed (overnight or 24 h) urine specimen. The standard commercial dipsticks measure total protein or albumin, they are simple to use, and provide high specificity. This is advantageous for clinicians because only a few false-positive results are identified. The standard urine dipstick is insensitive for low concentrations of albumin that may occur in patients with microalbuminuria. In addition, the standard dipstick is also insensitive to positively charged serum proteins, such as immunoglobulin light chains. Quantification of proteinuria based on the timed urine collection over 24 h is a definitive measure of protein or albumin excretion. However, the 24 h urine collection is time consuming, subject to collection error and requires good compliance. In recent years, the ratio of protein or albumin to creatinine ratio in an untimed ('spot') urine specimen has replaced protein excretion in a 24-h collection as the preferred method for measuring proteinuria.[7] These ratios correct for variations in urinary concentration due to hydration and provide a more convenient method of assessing protein and albumin excretion than that involved with timed urine collections. Single void urine samples have been evaluated as a semi-quantitative estimate of proteinuria. Many studies have found that values for urine protein/creatinine ratios measured in random urine samples correlate well with measurements of protein excretion in 24-h urine collections from the same patients. While some authors may have a preference for early morning or random samples obtained during the daytime most guidelines recommend the use of a first morning urine sample but when not available, a random urine sample to estimate protein creatinine ratio is acceptable.

GLOMERULONEPHRITIS

Glomerulonephritis is more common in the tropics than in temperate countries. It has been calculated that the incidence of nephrotic syndrome is 60–100 times higher in some tropical countries than in the USA and UK.[8] In tropical areas, infections are a major cause of both acute and chronic glomerulonephritis. In most instances, infection-induced acute glomerulonephritis resolves when the infection is cured, although glomerulonephritis resulting from chronic infection (e.g. malaria and schistosomiasis) is not reversed following measures that eradicate the infection.

Pathogenesis of infection-associated glomerulonephritis

The classical studies of Dixon et al.[9] established that glomerulonephritis could be induced in experimental animals following immunization with antigen. The development of glomerulonephritis coincided with the rise in specific antibody titres and the development of circulating immune complexes. Renal tissue studied by immunofluorescence showed glomerular mesangial or capillary wall deposits of immunoglobulin (Ig), complement and antigen. These studies provided the theoretical basis for the concept of immune complex-mediated glomerulonephritis. Subsequent studies, however, showed that it was difficult to induce a glomerulonephritis by the injection of preformed antigen-antibody complexes in 'naive' animals. It therefore seems unlikely that circulating immune complexes are important in the pathogenesis of glomerulonephritis. Other factors are likely to be responsible for the development of nephritis.[10] Cationic antigen or antibody is more likely to bind to the anionic surface of glomerular basement membrane and induce a glomerulonephritis. In situ antigen-antibody complexes formed following prior fixation of antigen or antibody to glomerular structures have been shown experimentally to lead to the development of a glomerulonephritis. Finally, some antibodies formed in response to non-renal antigens have been shown to bind to glomerular structures. Only a minority of individuals with a given infection develop a glomerulonephritis, demonstrating the importance of host factors in pathogenesis. Often with a single infecting organism, a variety of glomerulonephritides is seen in different individuals (Table 15.2).

Classification

The most helpful classification is one based on aetiology and histology. The histological changes may be of unknown aetiology (idiopathic), or secondary to well-defined aetiological factors. The types and clinical features of idiopathic glomerulonephritis have been reviewed elsewhere.[11]

Table 15.2 Infection-associated glomerulonephritis

Glomerulonephritis	Infection
Membranous nephropathy	Hepatitis B
	Schistosoma mansoni
	Leprosy
	Loa loa
	Syphilis
Mesangiocapillary glomerulonephritis	*Schistosoma mansoni*
	Leprosy
	Loa loa
	Onchocerciasis
	Tuberculosis
	Candidiasis
Focal segmental glomerulosclerosis	HIV
	Schistosoma mansoni
Proliferative glomerulonephritis	*Streptococcus* spp.
	Staphylococcus spp.
	Schistosoma mansoni
	Leprosy
	Wuchereria bancrofti
	Onchocerciasis
	Syphilis
Amyloid	Leprosy
	Schistosoma mansoni

Table 15.3 Clinical presentation of glomerulonephritis

Persistent microscopic haematuria
Persistent proteinuria
Nephrotic syndrome
Acute nephrotic syndrome
Acute renal failure
Chronic renal failure

Clinical presentation

The ways in which glomerulonephritis may present are fairly limited and are summarized in Table 15.3. Patients with glomerulonephritis can present with asymptomatic proteinuria and/or haematuria, with proteinuria that is heavy enough to cause a nephrotic syndrome, with an acute nephritic syndrome, which may be severe enough to cause acute renal failure (ARF), or with chronic renal failure.

Diagnosis

Definitive diagnosis of most forms of glomerulonephritis is dependent on a renal biopsy with careful interpretation of the renal histology in the light of clinical, biochemical and immunological features of the disorder.

Overview of management of glomerulonephritis

Conservative management of the nephrotic syndrome is with salt restriction, careful use of diuretics and of angiotensin converting enzyme inhibitors (ACEI) or angiotensin receptor blockers. There is now good evidence that a reduction in blood pressure and in urine protein retards the rate at which renal function deteriorates. ACE inhibition is more effective than other hypotensive drugs in reducing proteinuria and the rate of decline in renal function in patients with a glomerulonephritis and proteinuria.[12-14] There have been real improvements in the long-term prognosis of patients with a glomerulonephritis although the evidence base in terms of randomized controlled trials of therapy is small. The trials that have been done are few and often the numbers of patients in each trial are small. The treatment of glomerulonephritis is often with steroids and immunosuppressants and these drugs have major toxicities which need to be offset against any benefit. The aims of treatment of glomerulonephritis are the induction of remission, the maintenance of remission and the prevention of progression of glomerular injury. Choice of treatment is based on the clinical syndrome as well as on the acuteness and hence potential reversibility of the glomerular lesion and the extent of scarring, which is irreversible.

Pattern of glomerular disease in the tropics

This has been reviewed by Jha and Chugh.[15] In most tropical countries primary glomerular diseases are more common than secondary glomerular disease. In Jamaica, however, 54% of patients with a nephrotic syndrome have secondary glomerular disease, usually lupus nephritis.[16] In Zimbabwe, 80% of children with a nephrotic syndrome have hepatitis B or streptococcal infection,[17,18] although in a later study these aetiologies were uncommon.[19] This emphasizes the point that the aetio-pathogenesis of glomerulonephritis in tropical countries does seem to be changing. Over the last two decades there have been only infrequent reports of quartan malarial nephropathy, which had been a common cause of the nephrotic syndrome in children in Nigeria and Uganda.[20] In Ghana, Kenya, the Indian subcontinent and South-east Asia, however, 70–90% of adults and also children with a nephrotic syndrome have a primary glomerular disease.[21-27] Indeed there is now increasing evidence that idiopathic glomerulonephritis is common in tropical countries, making the diagnosis and treatment of these disorders important. The wide range of causes of the nephrotic syndrome in children in the tropics means that renal histology is usually required to determine whether treatment with steroids or immunosuppressants is appropriate. This is a particular problem as the facilities for renal biopsy are rarely available.

Idiopathic glomerulonephritis

Minimal change nephropathy

In this condition, the glomeruli are normal on light microscopy and there are no glomerular deposits of immunoglobulin and complement. This is uncommon in tropical Africa, where it is found in between 4% and 46% of cases.[17,20,25,26,28,29] In India, 32%

of children with a nephrotic syndrome have minimal change nephropathy.[30]

Management[31-33]

Children

Steroids

Meta-analysis showed that treatment with prednisolone for three months or more during the first episode of a nephrotic syndrome in children significantly reduced the risk of relapse at 12–24 months as compared with treatment for 2 months (RR 0.70; 95% CI 0.58–0.84). It is therefore recommended that children receive at least 6 weeks of treatment with daily oral prednisolone 60 mg/m^2 followed by 6 weeks of alternate day prednisolone 40 mg/m^2.

Treatment of frequent relapsers

Approximately 30–50% of children with steroid sensitive nephrotic syndrome have frequent relapses. An eight week course of cyclophosphamide (2–3 mg/kg per day) or chlorambucil (0.2 mg/kg per day) significantly reduced the risk of further relapse as compared with prednisolone alone, RR 0.44, 95% CI 0.26–0.73 and RR 0.13; 95% CI 0.03–0.57, respectively. Approximately 50% of treated children are in remission at 2 years and 40% at 5 years. Cyclophosphamide has been carefully evaluated in these children and is the drug of choice. Ciclosporin (6 mg/kg per day) was as effective as cyclophosphamide or chlorambucil but the effect was maintained only during treatment. Levamisole has also been used and is more effective in reducing relapses than prednisolone alone (RR 0.60; 95% CI 0.45–0.79) but again the effect was only restricted to the period of treatment. Levamisole can cause a reversible neutropenia.

Steroid resistant nephrotic syndrome in children

In children presenting with a first episode of nephrotic syndrome about 90% go into remission with steroid treatment. Steroid resistant children will, if biopsied, have minimal change nephrotic syndrome, mesangioproliferative glomerulonephritis or focal segmental glomerulosclerosis. In these patients ciclosporin is more effective in inducing complete remission than placebo or no treatment (RR for persisting nephrotic syndrome 0.64; 95% CI 0.47–0.88). The long-term prognosis for renal function in minimal change nephropathy is excellent.

Adults

Minimal-change nephropathy in adults

About 20% of adults with a nephrotic syndrome have minimal-change nephropathy. The mean age of onset is 40 years but the condition can occur at any age. The histology is identical to that found in children, with the exception of a higher incidence of globally sclerosed glomeruli that are a feature of ageing.

Clinical presentation

As in children, the clinical presentation is with a nephrotic syndrome, although this is not generally as severe. Profound hypoalbuminaemia (serum albumin level under 10 g/L) is rare in adults. The disease is slightly more common in men than in women, with a male to female ratio of 1.3 : 1. More adults than children are hypertensive (30%), have microscopic haematuria (28%), and have renal impairment at diagnosis (60%). These abnormalities are more severe in patients aged over 60 years who are also at particular risk of developing acute renal failure.

Diagnosis

A renal biopsy is essential to make the diagnosis in adults with a nephrotic syndrome.

Treatment of minimal-change nephropathy in adults

Treatment is with prednisolone at an initial dose of 60 mg/day: response occurs slightly less often than in children and also more slowly. Response to steroid treatment takes longer and is also less complete in adults at 75% at 6 months. Up to 60% of patients who go into a remission have a relapse and 39% have frequent relapses. In frequent relapsers treatment with cyclophosphamide induces a sustained remission of 60% over a five year period. Ciclosporin is also of benefit in frequent relapsers but most patients relapse when this is discontinued. Patients who are steroid-responsive or multiple relapsers are more likely to respond with complete or partial remissions (70–80%) than patients who are resistant to steroids (40–50%). Ciclosporin should be considered in those patients who develop steroid toxicity because they have multiple relapses or who are steroid-dependent. However, relapses appear to recur with the same frequency after ciclosporin A has been discontinued as before, and for that reason it is still advisable to use cyclophosphamide as the first-choice treatment in patients with a multiple relapsing or steroid-dependent minimal-change nephropathy in the hope of inducing a sustained remission. Ciclosporin A appears to be effective at blood levels of between 100 and 200 ng/mL, and at these levels significant short-term nephrotoxicity and hypertension are uncommon. In this author's view, ciclosporin A can best be viewed as a steroid-sparing agent in patients with minimal-change nephropathy.

New treatments

More recently, mycophenolate mofetil and also tacrolimus have been reported in uncontrolled trials to be effective in inducing and maintaining remission in patients with steroid resistant or relapsing minimal-change disease and in focal segmental glomerulosclerosis.

Long-term outcome

Some 6% of adult patients are still nephrotic after a mean follow-up of 7.5 years. The survival in patients over 60 years of age has been reported to be 50% at 10 years, and in those aged 15–59, it was 90%.

Focal segmental glomerulosclerosis

This is particularly common in Ghana,[26] Senegal,[34] Zaire[24,35] and South Africa.[29] Renal biopsies from the patients described in Senegal had an unusual fibrillary splitting of glomerular capillary walls with interposition of basement membrane-like material. Immunohistochemistry reveals deposits of IgM and C3 in sclerosed areas.

Focal segmental glomerulosclerosis

Focal segmental glomerulosclerosis (FSGS) was first described by Rich in 1957 at autopsy in children who died from a nephrotic syndrome. Fewer terms have generated more disagreement amongst pathologists and nephrologists: it is not a disease entity but a histological lesion that is often of unknown aetiology.

Secondary FSGS

Segmental scarring of glomeruli is the end product of a variety of pathological processes. These include, for example, sickle cell anaemia, reduced renal mass, HIV infection, inherited mutations of podocyte related genes and immune complex nephritis. Some of these causes lead to well defined glomerular lesions, e.g. collapsing glomerulopathy in HIV-associated nephropathy and prominent hilar segmental lesions in reduced renal mass. Mutations in genes encoding slit diaphragm proteins are found in up to 20–30% of children with steroid resistant nephrotic syndrome but not in patients with steroid sensitive nephrotic syndrome and are uncommon in adults. Importantly, patients with a genetic cause for their nephrotic syndrome show no response to steroids or immunosuppressants and these should not be used.

Pathology

The histological lesions of FSGS comprise segmental areas of glomerular sclerosis with hyalinization of glomerular capillaries, the segmental areas usually being adherent to Bowman's capsule.[36] In childhood FSGS, these lesions predominantly affect juxtamedullary glomeruli. One suggested classification is the Columbia FSGS classification.[37] Several variants have been described based on the site of the segmental sclerosing lesion (perihilar variant and glomerular tip lesion), the presence of glomerular collapse (collapsing variant) and endocapillary cellularity with visceral epithelial cell hyperplasia (cellular variant). Having excluded these variants, this leaves FSGS (not otherwise specified). This latter lesion is equivalent to classical nephrotic associated FSGS. Typically, the areas of segmental sclerosis are randomly distributed within the glomerular tuft with a predilection for the hilar regions (Figure 15.1). Focal areas of tubular atrophy and interstitial nephritis are prominent. On immunofluorescent microscopy, deposits of IgM and C3 may be seen in the sclerotic areas. Electron microscopy shows diffuse foot-process effacement in apparently unaffected glomeruli.

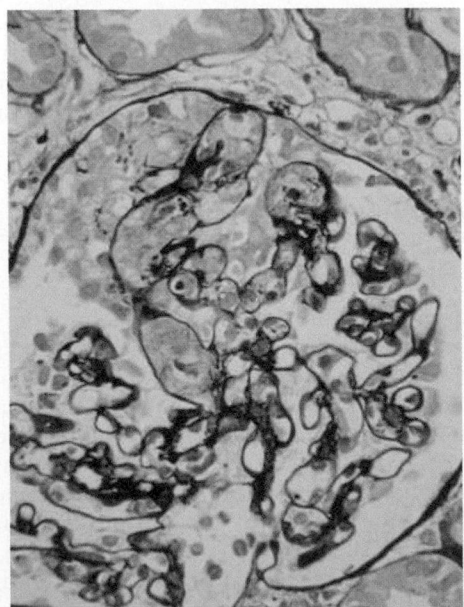

Figure 15.1 Early focal segmental sclerosing glomerular disease. (Courtesy of Professor A. J. Howie.)

Management

Steroids

There have been no randomized controlled trials of steroid therapy in FSGS. Cohort studies report that 40–60% of patients treated with a 6-month course of prednisolone go into complete or partial remission.[38] Complete as well as partial remissions are associated with a significant reduction in the risk of developing end-stage renal failure as compared with no remission. Adult patients who achieve a complete remission have a 5-year survival off dialysis of 94% as compared with 53% of those who do not achieve remission. Children who achieve a complete remission have a 100% renal survival as compared with 92% with a partial remission and 47% with no remission. Relapses are, however, common and found in 40–56% of patients. All patients with idiopathic FSGS and a nephrotic syndrome should be treated with prednisolone for 6 months. Children are treated with prednisolone at an initial dose of 60 mg/m² per day and adults with a dose of 60 mg/day with tapering of the steroid dose.

Ciclosporin

Patients whose nephrotic syndrome is resistant to 6 months treatment with prednisolone should receive ciclosporin for 26–52 weeks.[39] A meta-analysis of three studies in patients with FSGS who were resistant to an 8-week course of prednisolone indicates that ciclosporin was more effective than prednisolone or placebo in inducing remission (RR for persisting nephrotic syndrome 0.34; 95% CI: 0.18–0.69) and in preventing end-stage renal failure (RR 0.45; 95% CI: 0.21–0.97).[40]

Other immunosuppressants

There is no evidence that cyclophosphamide or chlorambucil are of benefit in the treatment of FSGS.

ACE inhibition/ARB

Children

Angiotensin converting enzyme inhibitors have been shown to be of benefit in reducing proteinuria in patients with a steroid resistant nephrotic syndrome.[41]

Prognosis

There is no difference in prognosis between adults and children. Adverse prognostic factors include tubulointerstitial fibrosis, renal impairment and a failure of remission with treatment.

Membranous nephropathy

This is common in children in Zimbabwe,[17] Namibia[42] and South Africa,[43,44] and also in adults in Sudan[28,45] and Pakistan.[45] In both Africa and Asia it is frequently a complication of hepatitis B infection. The glomerular basement membranes are uniformly thickened in membranous nephropathy, with regular spikes on the epithelial side when stained with periodic acid-methenamine silver. Immunohistology shows uniform granular deposition of IgG and complement on the epithelial side of glomerular basement membranes.

Renal vein thrombosis in membranous nephropathy[46]

Patients with membranous nephropathy appear to be at particular risk of developing renal vein thrombosis, although this is not as high as originally suggested. Most such patients are asymptomatic, but they may present with pulmonary emboli. Detection is by Doppler ultrasound of the renal veins, computed tomography (CT) or magnetic resonance (MRI) imaging. In practice, a renal vein thrombosis should be looked for if there is a sudden deterioration of renal function in a patient with membranous nephropathy. It is now known that renal vein thrombosis is a consequence of the hypercoagulable state of the nephrotic syndrome and is not a cause of membranous nephropathy.

Management

About 70% of patients with membranous nephropathy and a nephrotic syndrome survive free of end-stage renal failure at 10 years.[47] Therefore any therapy that benefits the 30% of patients who develop renal failure exposes the other 70% to unnecessary toxicity. The twin aims of treating membranous nephropathy are first to induce a remission of the nephrotic syndrome and second to prevent the development of end-stage renal failure. Despite several careful studies using steroids and immunosuppressants, there is still no agreement that these aims can be achieved.

Meta-analysis of the treatment of membranous nephropathy[48]

There have been several meta-analyses on the treatment of idiopathic membranous nephropathy. These show that steroids alone are of no benefit in inducing remission or preventing end-stage renal failure. Treatment with cyclophosphamide or chlorambucil together with prednisolone leads to more complete remissions (RR 2.37; 95% CI 1.32–4.25) and more partial remissions (RR 1.22; 95% CI 0.63–2.35) than prednisolone alone. No beneficial effect was seen on end-stage renal failure (RR 0.56; 95% CI 0.18–1.68). In this meta-analysis ciclosporin as compared with prednisolone or no treatment did not appear to be associated with any important clinical benefit. Our own analysis indicates that ciclosporin as compared with prednisolone or placebo increases the likelihood of remission but does not reduce the risk of developing end-stage renal failure. Between 40 and 60% of patients with a membranous nephropathy and a nephrotic syndrome go into spontaneous remission. Our current strategy is to wait for 12–18 months and then only treat those patients who are still nephrotic with ciclosporin or with prednisolone and cyclophosphamide. An ongoing MRC randomized controlled trial is testing the efficacy of this approach.

Mesangiocapillary (membranoproliferative) glomerulonephritis

This has been described in Indonesia,[49] India,[30] Ghana,[22] Nigeria[50,51] and South Africa[52] and may be idiopathic but is also commonly seen in post-infectious glomerulonephritis.[53] Most cases of mesangiocapillary glomerulonephritis (MCGN) in the tropics are of the Type I (subendothelial) variety. Here immunohistology reveals subendothelial deposits of IgG and less frequently of IgM and IgA

and C3. In Type II MCGN (dense-deposit disease), basement membrane and mesangial deposits of C3 are found.

Management

Randomized controlled trials of steroids in MCGN showed no benefit. At time of writing, treatment with angiotensin blockade and diuretics is recommended.

IgA nephropathy

This is common in Singapore, Malaysia, Hong Kong and Taiwan; in Singapore 75% of patients with more than 1 g of proteinuria per 24 h have IgA nephropathy.[54] IgA nephropathy is, however, uncommon in blacks in Africa,[55] although it has been recently reported in patients with HIV infection. Renal histology is characterized by the presence of mesangial proliferation and diffuse mesangial deposits of IgA and C3.

Management

Between 20% and 30% of patients with IgA nephropathy will develop end-stage renal failure by 20 years. Adverse prognostic features for renal function include proteinuria in excess of 1.0 g/24 h, renal impairment at the time of diagnosis and possibly hypertension. The options for treatment of patients with IgA nephropathy, and proteinuria >1.0 g/24 h and serum creatinine <250 mmol/L are (a) supportive treatment only with ACE inhibitors, (b) prednisolone (methylprednisolone 1 g i.v. daily for 3 days at 0, 2 and 4 months and oral prednisolone 0.5 mg/kg on alternate days for 6 months, or (c) fish-oil (MaxEPA) 6 g twice daily for 2 years. Further randomized clinical trials are necessary to establish the effectiveness of these treatments.

Mesangial IgM proliferative glomerulonephritis

Mesangial IgM proliferative glomerulonephritis is a major cause of the nephrotic syndrome in Thailand and other parts of South-east Asia[56] and in parts of Africa.[19] This type of glomerulonephritis can also present with asymptomatic proteinuria and haematuria.

Secondary glomerulonephritis

Systemic lupus erythematosus

Lupus nephritis is common in Malaysia and Singapore and other parts of South-east Asia, and in these areas is found mostly in people of Chinese origin.[57] Lupus nephritis is also common in Jamaica[16] and also in black Americans but is relatively uncommon in blacks in Africa.[22,58] Clinically apparent nephritis develops in about 40–75% of patients with systemic lupus erythematosus. The renal manifestations of lupus nephritis are heterogeneous both in clinical presentation and in histology. Patients with minimal changes or mesangial glomerulonephritis usually have an inherently low rate of progressive renal failure. Patients with membranous nephropathy have an intermediate prognosis for renal function. In contrast, patients with focal or diffuse proliferative glomerulonephritis have a high risk of progressive renal failure.

Management

Lupus mesangial proliferative glomerulonephritis

In the absence of controlled trials to guide treatment, it is reasonable to treat such patients with corticosteroids in the hope that this will prevent progression to a more severe glomerulonephritis, although that is not certain.

Lupus membranous nephropathy

Here again, there are no controlled trials of treatment and thus there is no consensus on treatment. Patients with pure lupus membranous nephropathy will respond to treatment with prednisolone only and azathioprine or mycophenolate mofetil may be used as a steroid sparing agent in these patients. Patients with lupus membranous nephropathy and proliferative glomerulonephritis lesions are at high risk of developing progressive renal failure and should be treated as for patients with a proliferative lupus nephritis.

Focal and diffuse lupus proliferative glomerulonephritis

Cyclophosphamide for remission induction

The careful randomized controlled studies from the NIH made intravenous cyclophosphamide and oral prednisolone the accepted method for the management of severe lupus nephritis (WHO Classes III and IV).[59] A recent study[60] showed that a shorter 12-week course of i.v. cyclophosphamide every two weeks at a dose of 500 mg followed by azathioprine was as effective as an abbreviated NIH regime (6 monthly pulses of 0.5 g/m^2) followed by 2 quarterly pulses. In a recent meta-analysis of randomized controlled studies,[61] when compared with prednisolone, cyclophosphamide and prednisolone reduced the risk of doubling of the serum creatinine (RR 0.59; 95%CI 0.4–0.88) while azathioprine did not (RR 0.98; 95% CI 0.36–2.68). However, azathioprine reduced the risk of death (RR 0.60; 95% CI 0.36–0.99), while cyclophosphamide did not (RR 0.95; 95%CI 0.53–1.82). Lupus affects predominantly women of childbearing age and the documented gonadotoxicity of cyclophosphamide (RR 2.18 95%CI: 1.10–4.34) makes it an inherently unattractive agent for therapy and one that could only be justified by its effectiveness in reducing the risk of renal failure. The search for more effective and less toxic treatments for remission induction led to studies of mycophenolate mofetil. Mycophenolate mofetil (MMF) is a powerful immunosuppressant that is licensed for renal transplantation. Pilot studies suggested that it might be effective together with steroids in the induction treatment of lupus nephritis and this has now been tested by randomized controlled trials.[62,63] These indicate that mycophenolate mofetil is probably as effective as and less toxic than cyclophosphamide in patients with new onset mild to moderate lupus nephritis. MMF may also have a role as remission maintenance therapy in lupus nephritis.

Crescentic glomerulonephritis

Most renal biopsy series from the tropics report that between 4% and 7% of patients have a crescentic glomerulonephritis with extracapillary proliferation. This is seen in a wide variety of disorders, including post-streptococcal glomerulonephritis, hepatitis B and C-associated glomerulonephritis, microscopic polyarteritis (polyangiitis), Wegener's granulomatosis and lupus nephritis. The importance of crescentic glomerulonephritis is that it is usually associated with a rapid decline in renal function. Treatment is usually with prednisolone and cyclophosphamide.

Infection-associated glomerulonephritis

Acute endocapillary proliferative glomerulonephritis

The most common cause of acute proliferative glomerulonephritis (APGN) is an infection with group A streptococci. This is common in Africa,[17] the Caribbean countries[64] and in India.[65] A similar type of glomerulonephritis has been reported with other bacteria in patients with infective endocarditis, shunt nephritis and visceral abscesses. APGN commonly develops 1–2 weeks after a streptococcal pharyngitis and 3–6 weeks after a skin infection (impetigo). With both sites of infection the risk of an ensuing glomerulonephritis is higher in children aged between 2 and 12 years. APGN has become quite rare in Western countries but epidemic outbreaks following skin infections with streptococci still occur in tropical countries.[66]

Pathogenesis[67]

Only certain M types (cell wall protein antigens) of Lancefield group A streptococcal infections are followed by the development of glomerulonephritis. This is an immune-mediated nephritis and would by convention be termed an immune complex nephritis. The frequent observation of hypocomplementaemia fits in with antigen-antibody-mediated nephritis. The candidate 'nephritogenic' antigen is as yet not known. Some studies have suggested that this is a soluble water-extractable antigen called 'endostreptosin'. Other studies have suggested that M proteins or M-associated proteins may be pathogenic antigens, and in yet others a cationic streptococcal proteinase has been suggested. The sera of patients with post-streptococcal glomerulonephritis also contain rheumatoid factors and antinuclear antibodies and the role of these autoantibodies in the pathogenesis of the nephritis is unclear.

Pathology

This is the classical endocapillary proliferative glomerulonephritis. There is increased hypercellularity of glomeruli from mesangial proliferation and an influx of polymorphonuclear leucocytes, monocytes and T lymphocytes (Figure 15.2). Subepithelial humps on electron microscopy are characteristic of this disorder. Extracapillary proliferation (crescents) is infrequent. Renal biopsies show deposits of C3, IgG and sometimes IgM in the glomerular mesangium and also large subepithelial deposits (humps) on immunofluorescence and electron microscopy.

Serology

Antibodies to various streptococcal antigens form the basis of diagnosis in culture-negative cases: after pharyngitis 95% of children will have an antibody response to streptolysin O, deoxyribonuclease, deoxyribonuclease B, hyaluronidase and streptokinase. After pyoderma antibody responses to deoxyribonuclease B are found, while responses to streptolysin O are infrequent.

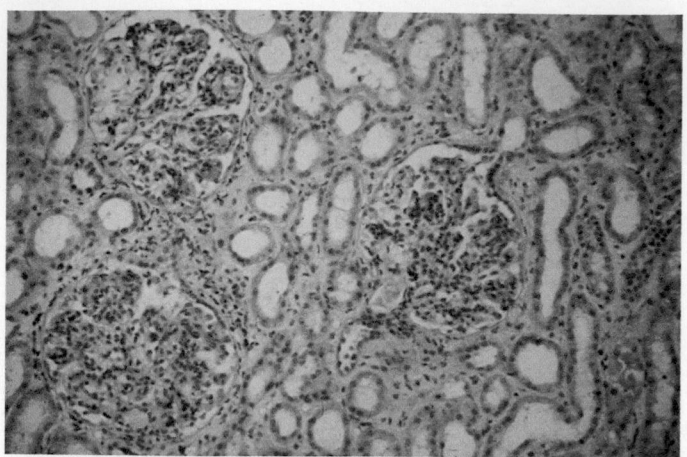

Figure 15.2 Acute post-infective glomerulonephritis. Solid looking glomeruli filled with neutrophil polymorphs. (Courtesy of Professor A. J. Howie.)

Clinical

The clinical presentation ranges from asymptomatic haematuria and proteinuria, through an acute nephritic syndrome, at times accompanied by a nephrotic syndrome, and rarely a rapidly progressive glomerulonephritis. The patient with an acute nephritic syndrome presents with oliguria, reddish-brown urine due to haematuria, proteinuria, a puffy face and ankle oedema, and this is often accompanied by hypertension. Hypertension and cardiac failure are usually due to salt and water overload. Headache, vomiting and fits may complicate the rise in blood pressure. A full-blown nephrotic syndrome is infrequent and acute renal failure from extracapillary glomerulonephritis is rare, being found in less than 2% of affected children.

Management

All patients should be given a 10-day course of penicillin or erythromycin to eradicate the organism and prevent secondary spread, although this treatment has no effect on the outcome of the renal illness. The management of the acute nephritic illness is based on conventional treatment, with meticulous attention to fluid balance, together with diuretics and hypotensive drug therapy as necessary. Rarely there may be the development of a crescentic glomerulonephritis and if renal failure is severe then treatment with prednisolone and cyclophosphamide should be considered.

Outcome

The long-term prognosis of post-streptococcal glomerulonephritis is good and there are few reports of end-stage chronic renal failure as a long-term sequel. Long-term prospective studies of epidemic post-streptococcal glomerulonephritis following skin infection showed little evidence of progressive chronic renal failure or hypertension. Other studies of sporadic post-pharyngitic glomerulonephritis, however, showed that up to 50% of patients have some evidence of chronic renal damage.[20]

Eosinophilic proliferative glomerulonephritis in Uganda

An eosinophilic diffuse proliferative glomerulonephritis was reported by Walker et al.[68] from Uganda, in children with proteinuria. Immunostaining showed granular deposits of C3 and IgG and electron microscopy revealed subepithelial and intramembranous dense deposits. The eosinophilia raised the possibility of a parasitic contribution to the cause of the glomerulonephritis. There was no clear association with streptococcal infection or evidence of malaria or HIV infection in the whole series.

Hepatitis B infection and renal disease

The renal complications of hepatitis B infection are found mainly in individuals who are chronically infected. The observation by immunological techniques of hepatitis B antigen or its antibody in glomeruli strongly suggests that the renal injury is immune mediated, although the precise mechanisms are unknown. The major renal lesions of hepatitis B infection are membranous nephropathy, which is more common in children, and less commonly a mesangiocapillary glomerulonephritis, IgA nephropathy (more common in adults) and polyarteritis.[69,70]

Hepatitis B-associated membranous nephropathy

This is seen particularly in children who are chronic carriers of hepatitis B virus. The frequency of hepatitis B as a cause of membranous nephropathy parallels the general carrier rate of this virus in the population. Between 60% and 100% of children with membranous nephropathy in Japan, Hong Kong, South Africa and Zimbabwe have HBsAg,[5,7,16,21,22,32,43,44,53,70] and by contrast this is infrequent in the USA and the UK. In children the age of onset is between 2 and 12 years, and over 80% of affected children are male. The clinical presentation is usually with a nephrotic syndrome. Most affected children have no clinical evidence of liver disease; this is more common in adults.

Serology

Sera from almost all patients with hepatitis B-associated membranous nephropathy show evidence of infection in the form of HBsAg, HBc antibodies, HBeAg, and HBe antibodies.

Pathology

The histological lesion of hepatitis B-associated membranous nephropathy differs from the idiopathic variety in that in addition to subepithelial immune deposits there are often subendothelial and mesangial deposits of immunoglobulin. (Figure 15.3A,B). Glomerular capillary deposits of the hepatitis B antigens HBsAg, HBcAg and HBeAg have been demonstrated in renal biopsies.

Management and outcome

There is no evidence that corticosteroids are beneficial and indeed their use and withdrawal may lead to rebound hepatitis. The antiviral agents interferon α and lamivudine may be of benefit in this dis-

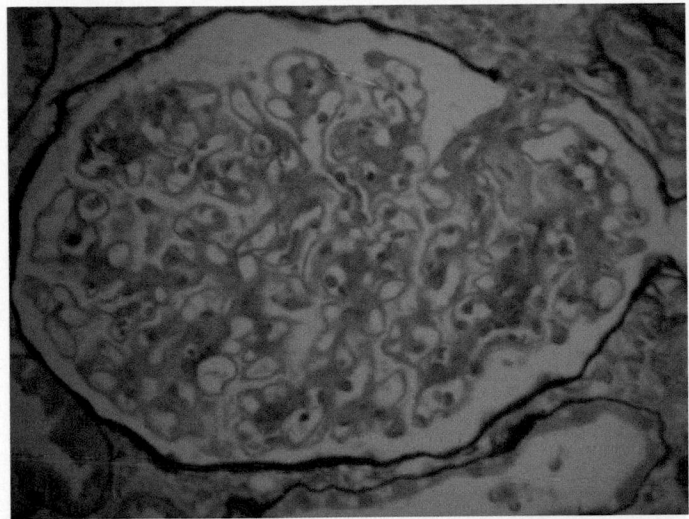

A

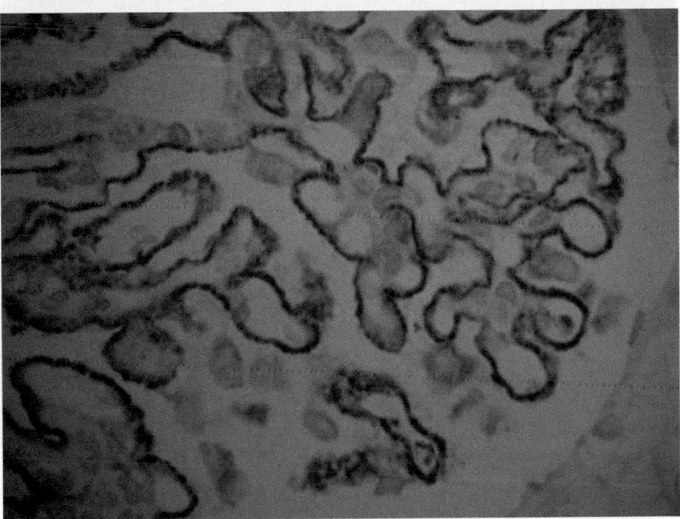

B

Figure 15.3 (A) Glomerulus showing thickening of the basement membrane in hepatitis B-associated membranous nephropathy (Courtesy of Professor A. J. Howie.); (B) Immunoperoxidase staining showing sub-epithelial deposits of IgG in hepatitis B-associated membranous nephropathy. (Courtesy of Professor A. J. Howie.)

order but there are no controlled trials of treatment. In a recent study, Tang et al.[71] treated 10 patients with hepatitis B-associated membranous nephropathy with lamivudine. As compared with historical controls, lamivudine increased the proportion of patients going into complete remission from 25% to 60% and reduced renal failure from 60% to nil (0). There was a need for long-term treatment as cessation of this at 2 years led to a relapse of the nephrotic syndrome. The prognosis in children is good, with reported spontaneous remissions of the nephrotic syndrome in up to two-thirds of cases. Approximately 5% of children progress to end-stage renal failure, while adults fare worse with 10% developing renal failure. Vaccination of all neonates has been shown to reduce the rate of hepatitis B carriage and hepatitis B-associated glomerulonephritis.

Hepatitis B-associated polyarteritis nodosa

HBsAg has been reported in 10–40% of patients in the USA, 18–50% of patients in France and 4–8% of patients in the UK who have classical polyarteritis. This association is uncommon in tropical countries.

Hepatitis C-associated nephropathy

Hepatitis C virus infection is found in less than 0.6% of the population of North America and Northern Europe but is more common in southern Europe and Africa and has a high prevalence in haemophiliacs and intravenous drug abusers. Hepatitis C infection may lead to chronic active hepatitis and cirrhosis. Hepatitis C infection is the main cause of mixed essential cryoglobulinaemia. The clinical presentation is with a fever, purpuric rash, arthralgia and peripheral neuropathy. The renal presentation is with proteinuria or a nephrotic syndrome often accompanied by mild to moderate renal impairment.[72-74]

Pathology

The renal lesion in cryoglobulinaemic glomerulonephritis is a type of membranoproliferative glomerulonephritis characterized by intraluminal and subendothelial deposits but other types of glomerulonephritis, e.g. a mesangioproliferative glomerulonephritis, have been reported and rarely there is a renal arteritis. Immunofluorescent microscopy shows subendothelial as well as mesangial and capillary wall deposits of IgM, IgG and C3. On electron microscopy these deposits may show the characteristics of cryoglobulins.

Management

Treatment with interferon α improves proteinuria and possibly renal function in patients with hepatitis C-associated mesangiocapillary glomerulonephritis although renal disease and viraemia mostly relapse after cessation of therapy. There is some evidence that the addition of ribavirin to interferon α confers additional benefit.[75] Treatment of acute cryoglobulinaemic glomerulonephritis and vasculitis has usually been with prednisolone and cyclophosphamide. Interpretation of these studies of treatment is complicated by the lack of controlled studies and also by the fact that many of these studies were performed prior to the recognition of the role of HCV infection in the pathogenesis of mixed cryoglobulinaemia. Plasma exchange reduces cryoglobulin and immune complex levels and has been reported to lead to an improvement of renal function. However, the effects are usually temporary, since depletion of cryoglobulins leads to rapid rebound immunoglobulin synthesis.

Human immunodeficiency virus-associated glomerulonephritis[76,77]

Renal complications of HIV could become a large burden on the healthcare systems in Africa as 3–12% of Black Africans with HIV are likely to develop chronic kidney disease. A variety of renal disorders occur in patients with HIV infection. Acute deterioration of renal function may develop as a result of volume depletion from renal salt wasting or from diarrhoea and vomiting. In addition, some of the antiviral drugs used in therapy are potentially nephrotoxic, as are some of the drugs used to treat opportunistic infections. In addition, there may be renal disease from coexistent hepatitis B or C infection, post-infectious glomerulonephritis or an IgA nephropathy. A major clinical problem in these patients is the development of proteinuria, a nephrotic syndrome and renal impairment.[78–80] In Africa, in addition to HIVAN (HIV-associated nephropathy), a collapsing variant of focal and segmental glomerulosclerosis, other lesions are commonly found.[79] In a recent study from South Africa HIVAN was found in only 27% of cases.[80] An immune complex deposition disease (HIVICK) with a characteristic 'ball in cup' appearance was found in 21% of cases and other glomerular lesions such as membranous nephropathy and IgA nephropathy were also frequently seen.[80]

Clinical presentation

The clinical presentation of HIVAN and HIVICK is usually with a nephrotic syndrome and renal impairment. Hypertension is uncommon and ultrasound examination shows large echogenic kidneys. Without antiretrovirals, these lesions carry a poor prognosis with at least a 50% mortality within 2 years and it is now clear that antiretrovirals markedly improve the prognosis.

Pathology

Collapsing glomerulopathy was initially described in patients with HIV-associated nephropathy (HIVAN), where it was associated with a severe nephrotic syndrome and rapid progression to end-stage renal failure. There are now two characteristic histological lesions in HIV. The first, HIVAN, is a type of focal segmental sclerosing glomerulonephritis characterized by segmental or global collapse of glomerular capillaries with basement membrane wrinkling and crowding of glomerular epithelial cells (Figure 15.4A).[78] There is often a marked interstitial infiltrate of lymphocytes and plasma cells and dilated tubules with casts (Figure 15.4B). In addition there are endothelial tubuloreticular inclusions. On immunofluorescent microscopy mesangial and capillary wall deposits of IgM and C3 are seen. Collapsing glomerulopathy may also be seen in patients without HIV infection and may be idiopathic or associated with parvovirus B19 infection. The second lesion, HIVICK, results in mesangial proliferation and immune complex deposition. Large subepithelial deposits are present, often with a mesangial reaction, giving a 'ball in cup' appearance. IgA, IgM and IgG may be present along with C3 and in some cases the immunohistochemical appearances may be similar to those seen in lupus.[80]

Management

There is increasing evidence to suggest that treatment with highly active antiretroviral drugs improves both the renal and overall prognosis of affected patients.[77,81] As with other proteinuric renal diseases there is evidence that treatment with ACEI may be of long-term benefit. Patients with HIV infection and end-stage renal failure have been treated with chronic haemodialysis with benefit. Haemodialysis is safe in patients with HIV-associated renal failure and in those patients with undetectable viral loads and preserved

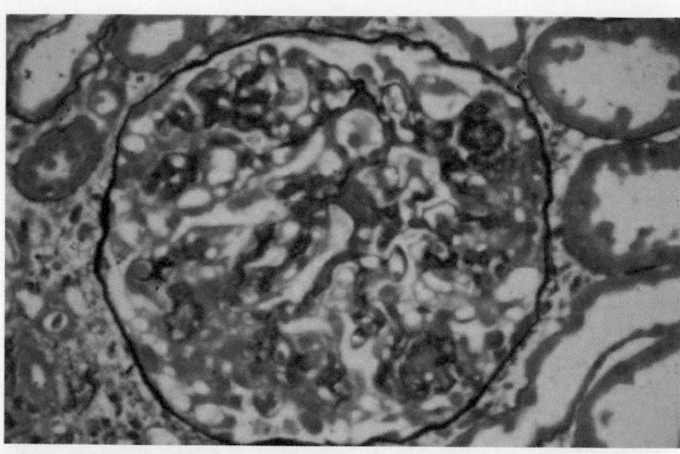

A

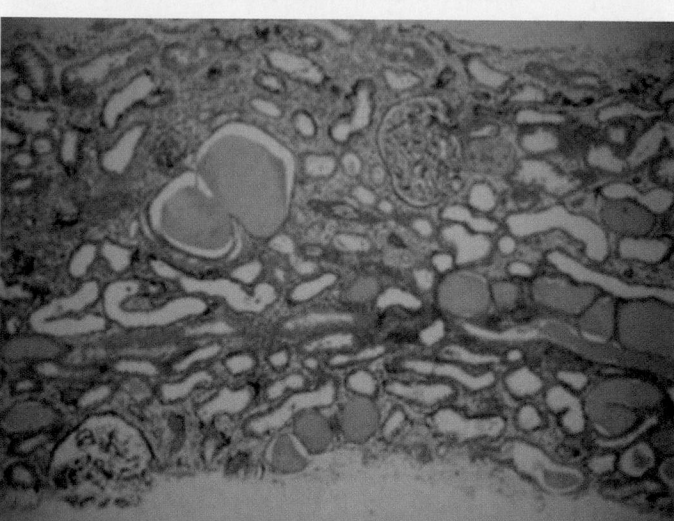

B

Figure 15.4 (A) HIV-associated nephropathy: glomeruli have changes of collapsing glomerulopathy (Courtesy of Professor A. J. Howie.); (B) Renal cortex in HIV nephropathy. Tubules are dilated and contain casts. (Courtesy of Professor A. J. Howie.)

CD4 counts transplantation can also be considered if the patient is stable on antiretrovirals.

Highly active antiretroviral drugs and nephrotoxicity[82,83]

Some of the antiretroviral drugs used in the treatment of HIV are nephrotoxic and these effects are summarized in Table 15.4.

Schistosomiasis

Schistosomiasis (see also Chapter 82) is widespread in the tropics. *Schistosoma haematobium* affects the urinary tract, and *S. mansoni* and *S. japonicum* the intestine(s) and liver. Significant glomerular disease has been mostly in patients with *S. mansoni* infection and hepatosplenic disease[84–86] but also rarely in patients with hepatointestinal disease.[87] Overall, just under 5% of patients with *S. mansoni* infection have hepatosplenic disease, and of these about 10–15% develop glomerular lesions over a period of up to 10

Table 15.4 Nephrotoxicity of highly active antiretroviral drugs

Antiretroviral class	Name	Renal abnormalities	Histology
Protease inhibitors	Indinavir	Renal calculi, crystalluria, ARF, CRF	Tubulointerstitial nephritis with crystals
	Nelfinavir	Renal colic	
	Ritonavir	ARF	
Nucleoside reverse transcriptase inhibitors	Abacavir	ARF	Interstitial nephritis
	Didanosine	Proximal tubular dysfunction	
	Lamivudine	Proximal tubular dysfunction	
	Stavudine	Proximal tubular dysfunction	
Nucleotide reverse transcriptase inhibitors	Tenofovir	Proximal tubular dysfunction, ARF Nephrogenic diabetes insipidus, Nephrotic syndrome	
HIV-1 fusion inhibitor	Enfuvirtide	Glomerulonephritis	Membranoproliferative nephritis

years. The clinical presentation is with proteinuria or nephrotic syndrome. In Egypt there is evidence that schistosomal glomerulonephritis is more common in individuals with concomitant chronic infections with Salmonella species.[88,89]

Pathology

A mesangial proliferative glomerulonephritis is seen in mild or early cases and the most common histological change in advanced cases is a mesangiocapillary (membranoproliferative) glomerulonephritis, seen in about 50% of patients. The next most frequently seen histological lesion is a focal segmental glomerulosclerosis. There are also infrequent reports of a membranous nephropathy and a proliferative glomerulonephritis. Immunofluorescent microscopy of renal biopsies shows granular deposits, predominantly of IgM but also of IgG, IgA, IgE and C3 in the mesangium and the subepithelial and subendothelial sites. Co-existing infection with hepatitis B and hepatitis C should be excluded in patients with S. mansoni infection and glomerulonephritis.[90] Renal amyloidosis has been described in patients with S. mansoni infection in Sudan and in Egypt[91,92] but not in Brazil.[93]

Management

Treatment of schistosomal glomerulonephritis with antischistosomal drugs, prednisolone and cyclophosphamide has been of no benefit and progression to renal failure is usual.

Leprosy

The major renal lesions found in leprosy (see also Chapter 58) are amyloidosis and glomerulonephritis, although chronic interstitial nephritis has also been described.

Amyloidosis

Renal amyloid is a complication of long-standing leprosy and has been most often described in patients with lepromatous leprosy and rarely in patients with tuberculoid leprosy.[94,95] In earlier autopsy studies, renal amyloid was described in up to 30% of cases in North and South America, but is relatively uncommon (<10% of cases) in India, Papua New Guinea and Africa. The amyloid

fibrils in leprosy are of the AA variety, which is derived from the acute-phase reactant serum amyloid A (SAA). Serum levels of SAA rise in patients with erythema nodosum leprosum (ENL) reactions and there are suggestions that amyloidosis is more common in patients with recurrent ENL.[94] The clinical presentation is with proteinuria, microscopic haematuria and the nephrotic syndrome, and progression to renal failure is common.

Glomerulonephritis

Glomerulonephritis is found in up to 10% of patients with leprosy at autopsy. It tends to be more common in patients with lepromatous than with tuberculoid leprosy, and the onset of glomerulonephritis may coincide with an episode of ENL. The most common glomerular lesions are a mesangial proliferative glomerulonephritis and a focal or diffuse proliferative glomerulonephritis. Rarely a membranous nephropathy or mesangiocapillary glomerulonephritis is seen. Immunofluorescent microscopy shows granular glomerular deposits of IgG, IgM and C3 in the mesangium or on capillary walls.[95,96] The renal disease progresses to renal failure and it is unclear whether treatment for leprosy influences progression.

Filariasis

There are several reports of an association between filariasis and glomerulonephritis from India and Cameroon.[97,98] The clinical presentation is usually with nephrotic syndrome and rarely with an acute nephritic syndrome. Patients with Wuchereria bancrofti infection may develop a mesangial proliferative or a diffuse proliferative glomerulonephritis.[98] In patients with Loa loa infections a membranous and a mesangiocapillary glomerulonephritis have been reported. Onchocerciasis infections have been reported to be associated with a nephrotic syndrome due to minimal-change nephropathy, mesangial proliferative glomerulonephritis or a mesangiocapillary glomerulonephritis.[98]

Pathology

On immunofluorescent microscopy glomerular deposits of IgG, IgM and C3 are seen in the mesangium and capillary walls, and in one study onchocercal antigens were identified on glomerular capillaries.

Management

Treatment with diethylcarbamazine probably hastens recovery in those patients with an acute nephritic presentation but has no effect in patients presenting with nephrotic syndrome.

Malaria

Malaria (see also Chapter 73) is widespread in the tropics and is a major cause of death. In the 1930s in British Guyana, Giglioli established the long-suspected association between *Plasmodium malariae* infection and a nephrotic syndrome. Proteinuria, nephritis and deaths from nephritis were common in British Guyana. Patients with nephrotic syndrome in this area had a higher incidence of *P. malariae* parasitaemia than unaffected individuals, who more often had *P. vivax* and *P. falciparum* infection. In 1962, Giglioli[99,100] summarized his observations that following eradication of malaria from British Guyana there was a reduction in the incidence of proteinuria and nephritis and deaths from malaria.

Quartan malarial nephropathy

The association between *P. malariae* infection and glomerulonephritis was confirmed by clinicopathological studies from Nigeria and Uganda in children with nephrotic syndrome. These children mostly had an incidence of *P. malariae* parasitaemia (up to 88% of children) that was significantly higher than in healthy controls (20%).[8,101,102] There have, however, been few recent reports of quartan malarial nephropathy from tropical Africa.

Sickle cell disease[103]

Patients with sickle cell disease often have an impaired ability to concentrate and acidify urine and to excrete a potassium load but these changes are minor and usually of no clinical significance. Glomerular filtration rate (GFR) and effective renal plasma flow are increased in children with sickle disease and it is suggested that the increased GFR may lead to glomerular damage in later life.

Haematuria

Microscopic haematuria is common in patients with both sickle cell disease and trait, and less commonly macroscopic haematuria, that may be persistent, is seen. The management is with conservative measures only. It is worthwhile screening for other causes of haematuria in these patients, e.g. schistosomiasis.

Renal papillary necrosis

This is found in both sickle cell disease and sickle cell trait. The clinical presentation is with haematuria that on occasion may be complicated by clot colic. Diagnosis is confirmed by intravenous pyelography, showing changes ranging from clubbing of calyces to a ring sign in which an often calcified, partly attached papilla is surrounded by a ring of contrast.

Glomerulonephritis

Focal segmental glomerulosclerosis[104]

This is the most frequently described lesion. It is found in older patients, usually aged over 30 years. The incidence of this lesion is unclear. Histologically the glomeruli are larger than normal and show segmental areas of glomerular sclerosis. Because the GFR is raised in early life in patients with sickle cell disease, it has been suggested that the segmental sclerosis is a consequence of hyperfiltration and intraglomerular hypertension. The clinical presentation is with proteinuria and the clinical course is with progressive renal impairment. The proteinuria reduces with treatment with angiotensin converting inhibitors and it is possible that these agents, by reducing intraglomerular pressures, might reduce the rate at which renal function declines.

Mesangiocapillary glomerulonephritis[105,106]

The second most commonly described lesion in patients with sickle cell anaemia and proteinuria is a mesangiocapillary glomerulonephritis. The pathogenesis of this is unclear and suggestions that it is caused by the glomerular deposition of renal tubular epithelial cell antibodies and antigen await confirmation.

Acute proliferative glomerulonephritis[107]

An increased predisposition to post-streptococcal glomerulonephritis from infected leg ulcers has also been reported in older patients with sickle cell anaemia.

End-stage renal failure in sickle cell anaemia

Both continuous ambulatory peritoneal dialysis and haemodialysis have been successfully used in these patients. Anaemia is a major problem and can be helped by the cautious use of erythropoietin. It is necessary to perform exchange transfusion with AA blood prior to transplantation to prevent sickling of the renal graft.

ACUTE RENAL FAILURE[108–111]

Acute renal failure complicates a wide variety of diseases. The abrupt cessation of renal function leads to uraemia, with abnormalities of fluid and electrolyte balance. The persistently high mortality in these patients leaves no room for complacency in management. Patients with acute renal failure do not necessarily present in neat diagnostic categories but more often as unexplained acute uraemic emergencies. Investigation, diagnosis and initial management must often be compressed into a few hours. The priorities in this early phase are to manage acute uraemia and electrolyte abnormalities, in particular hyperkalaemia, to establish the reversibility of the renal failure and to define its cause.

Causes of acute uraemia

The main cause of acute renal failure in the tropics is acute tubular necrosis, often as a result of infection, with glomerulonephritis presenting less commonly. Of all cases of acute renal failure in the tropics, 60% have a medical cause, 25% a surgical cause and 15%

an obstetric cause.[109,112,113] In the more developed areas the pattern is akin to that found in the West, where medical and surgical causes predominate and obstetric cases are rare.[109] The differences in aetiology are largely dependent on socioeconomic factors and the availability of therapeutic pregnancy termination services. The classification of the causes of acute renal failure into pre-renal, intrinsic and post-renal categories remains clinically useful in that it allows a structured approach to diagnosis and management. In an Egyptian series, 38% had pre-renal, 24% post-renal and the rest intrinsic renal disease as a cause of their acute renal failure.[114] The major causes of acute renal failure are summarized in Table 15.5. This list is not exhaustive and is meant to emphasize the importance of seeking an aetiology in a patient with unexplained acute renal failure.

Clinical syndromes

Acute tubular necrosis

A variety of infections and hypovolaemia may lead to renal ischaemia with renal vasoconstriction and tubular cell damage with a reduction in GFR. In addition there may be tubular obstruction and back-leakage of filtrate. A similar outcome may be the result

Table 15.5 Causes of acute renal failure

PRE-RENAL
Renal hypoperfusion (leading to acute tubular necrosis)
Hypovolaemia
Septicaemia
Obstetric accidents
Massive intravascular haemolysis
Rhabdomyolysis
RENAL
Acute tubular necrosis
Acute interstitial nephritis
Diffuse extracapillary glomerulonephritis
Acute pyelonephritis
Nephrotoxins
Haemolytic–uraemic syndrome
POST-RENAL
Obstructive uropathy
Renal tubule blockage
Myeloma (light chains)
Uric acid, sulfadiazine
Bilateral urinary tract blockage
Calculi
Schistosoma haematobium
Urethral stricture
Prostatic hypertrophy
Pelvic malignancy
Posterior urethral valves

of nephrotoxic drugs, such as aminoglycosides, and also traditional herbal remedies. There has been considerable research into the mediators involved in this injurious process. Nitric oxide, oxygen radicals, endothelin and free iron have all been implicated. To date there have been few convincing data to suggest that manipulation of these systems improves outcome, although some studies do suggest beneficial outcomes with N-acetylcysteine in preventing acute tubular necrosis secondary to radio contrast-induced acute renal failure.

The clinical consequence of acute tubular necrosis is uraemia, which is usually associated with oliguria, although some patients may be non-oliguric, producing urine volumes of 1–2 L or higher. In the vast majority of cases acute tubular necrosis is self-limiting and with spontaneous recovery occurring between 10 days and 6 weeks, provided the initial insult is treated. When the initial insult is very severe, cortical necrosis may occur, leading to irreversible renal failure.

Renal parenchymal causes

Acute glomerulonephritis, especially when accompanied by extracapillary proliferation (crescent formation), may lead to acute renal failure. Acute interstitial nephritis is seen in leptospirosis and may also be a complication of drugs such as the penicillins, sulfonamides, thiazide diuretics and frusemide as well as non-steroidal antiinflammatory drugs.

Obstructive uropathy

Obstruction to the urinary tract is important because it is a common and potentially reversible cause of acute renal failure. The most common site of obstruction is at the bladder outlet due to prostatic hypertrophy or cancer, and urethral stricture. Urethral stricture is particularly common in tropical Africa. Pelvic tumours in women (cervical and disseminated ovarian tumours), and in both sexes bladder cancer and less commonly retroperitoneal fibrosis or malignancy, may also obstruct the urinary tract. Obstruction at the level of the ureters or higher must be bilateral, unless there is a solitary functioning kidney, to cause acute renal failure. This is usually due to renal calculi or schistosomal-induced ureteric stenosis.[115,116] Renal tubules may become blocked by uric acid crystals, particularly in patients with hyperuricaemia following chemotherapy for lymphoma, leukaemia or myeloma. Prophylactic treatment with allopurinol, hydration and alkalinization of urine in these patients now make this an infrequent cause of acute renal failure. Other causes of renal tubular obstruction include sulfadiazine therapy, antiretrovirals (outlined above) and high-dose methotrexate treatment.

Causes of acute renal failure in the tropics

Acute renal failure in pregnancy

Acute renal failure from obstetric causes is common in the tropics. In the West, 3% of all causes of acute renal failure have an obstetric aetiology, whereas this figure is much higher in the tropics: 25% in Ghana[112] and 9–15 % in India.[113,117] The actual cause varies according to the different stages of pregnancy. In the first trimester, septic abortions account for the vast majority of cases. This is common because of the lack of legal abortion services in many tropical countries, resulting in a high prevalence of 'back street' abortions. In the third trimester the causes include pre-eclampsia and eclampsia, HELLP syndrome, puerperal sepsis, haemorrhage and abruption placentae. The most common histological lesion found is acute tubular necrosis, although cortical necrosis is found more frequently in the tropics. The striking decline in the incidence of acute renal failure during pregnancy in some developing countries can be attributed to improved obstetric care and also to liberalization of abortion laws.[118]

Massive intravascular haemolysis

Glucose-6-phosphate dehydrogenase deficiency

Glucose-6-phosphate dehydrogenase (G6PD) deficiency is a red cell abnormality which is inherited as a sex-linked gene of partial dominance. The gene abnormality is widespread in tropical Africa, India and South-east Asia and world wide affects more than 400 million people. The product of the G6PD reaction is NADPH, which is essential for the function of enzymes that protect against oxidants (catalase and glutathione peroxidase). Hence in G6PD deficiency, erythrocytes are susceptible to the effects of oxidant stress. The major clinical consequence of this is haemolysis due to infections and drugs. Acute renal failure has been reported in G6PD-deficient individuals following haemolysis due to drugs[119,120] and infections such as typhoid fever, malaria and hepatitis.[121,122]

Malaria

Acute renal failure is a well-recognized complication of malarial infection by *Plasmodium falciparum*.[123,124] The prevalence of acute renal failure is of the order of 1% but in cases of severe infection can be much higher.[124–126] The major causes of acute renal failure are volume depletion, severe parasitaemia and blackwater fever from massive intravascular haemolysis.[127–129] The latter may be a consequence of severe infection alone, but is often triggered by drugs such as quinine, or caused by G6PD deficiency. The acute renal failure seen in *P. falciparum* infection usually occurs 4–7 days after the onset of fever. It can be of the oliguric or non-oliguric type and most patients are hypercatabolic. Cholestatic jaundice is often seen and there have been reports of disseminated intravascular coagulation. Jaundice, oliguria, hypotension and multiple organ failure signify a poor prognosis.

The mechanism of acute renal failure involves erythrocytes containing *P. falciparum* becoming adherent to capillaries and venules and being sequestered in organs such as the kidney, causing alterations in the microcirculation. The infected red cells also display reduced deformability, which results in predominantly extravascular haemolysis. The combination of these two phenomena causes renal vasoconstriction, renal tubular toxicity and activation of intravascular coagulation.[130] Activation of cytokines also contributes to the increased adhesion and alteration of the renal microcirculation.

The histological changes are those of acute tubular necrosis, more marked in the distal tubule, and there may be casts of haemoglobin and malarial pigment. Quinine was the drug of choice in the treatment of severe *P. falciparum* malaria; however, a recent study has shown Artemisinin compounds to be safer and perhaps more effective.[131] The renal failure should be treated along standard lines with either peritoneal dialysis or haemodialysis, although continu-

ous haemofiltration is probably more effective than peritoneal dialysis. Of those patients who develop acute renal failure, 60% will require dialysis but the overall mortality is less than 10%.

Diarrhoeal diseases

The acute renal failure that occurs with diarrhoeal disease is usually due to volume depletion. This is common in tropical countries.[109–111]

Typhoid fever

Renal complications occur in around 10% of cases of typhoid fever. Acute renal failure may be caused by massive intravascular haemolysis and this is particularly common in patients with G6PD deficiency.[121,122] There have been reports of haemolytic–uraemic syndrome in association with *Salmonella* species infections,[132] and also of a transient mesangial proliferative glomerulonephritis.

Shigella *species*

Shigella dysentery may also lead to childhood acute renal failure in the tropics.[133] In severe *Shigella* species infection, volume depletion and toxaemia can lead to acute renal failure from acute tubular necrosis. Acute renal failure may also occur from a haemolytic–uraemic syndrome during the diarrhoeal phase of the illness.[134] The mortality from this condition is high at 70%, with 14% of the survivors going on to develop chronic renal impairment as a result of chronic interstitial nephritis and cortical necrosis.[135] There are some promising developments, however, with the development of neutralizing antibodies to the A subunit of the Shiga toxin molecule that have shown promise in animal studies.[136]

Cholera[137]

The WHO received reports of over 131 943 cases of cholera worldwide in 2005, of which there were over 2200 deaths. Though this represents a significant fall since 1999 (250 000 cases and 2200 deaths) this was an increase from the figure in 2004. The vast majority of deaths are due to renal failure secondary to volume depletion as a result of the profuse diarrhoea. Given the degree of diarrhoea in cholera, hypokalaemia is frequently present, and in addition to acute tubular necrosis there may also be evidence of vacuolation of the proximal tubular epithelium. These complications can usually be prevented by adequate fluid replacement in most cases, using oral rehydration solutions. An oral cholera vaccine is now available but its use in preventing and treating outbreaks is yet to be fully evaluated.

Leptospirosis[138,139]

Leptospirosis is contracted following exposure to contaminated water, either in rivers or sewage. The clinical presentation is with myalgia, pyrexia, conjunctival congestion, headache and jaundice. There may be a bleeding diathesis with gastrointestinal and pulmonary haemorrhage. Acute renal failure occurs during the acute leptospiraemia stage and is usually accompanied by jaundice (Weil's syndrome). All patients with leptospirosis will have a tubulointerstitial infiltrate if biopsied, but approximately 50% of patients go on to develop acute renal failure, the major histological lesion being tubulointerstitial nephritis with acute tubular necrosis. Minor glomerular mesangial proliferation may be seen. Characteristic features of the acute renal failure are that it is hypercatabolic and that hyperuricaemia, hyperkalaemia and the rise in blood urea are disproportionate to the serum creatinine. Dark-field microscopy of urine may reveal leptospires and they may also be grown from blood culture specimens. The diagnosis may also be established by serological tests. Treatment of leptospirosis when there is renal failure is with penicillin or erythromycin although data suggest that cephalosporins can also be used and indeed the treatment failure rate may be lower with these drugs. The use of penicillin may be complicated by a Jarisch–Herxheimer reaction and in certain studies has been ineffective in preventing the need for dialysis.[140] Patients with severe renal failure require treatment with haemodialysis or peritoneal dialysis.

Post-streptococcal glomerulonephritis

Beta haemolytic streptococcal infections of the throat or skin can be complicated by an endocapillary proliferative glomerulonephritis. In Ethiopia, 5% of children with these infections developed renal complications.[141] There is evidence that the incidence is decreasing in some tropical countries; however, it still accounts for up to 13% of all paediatric acute renal failure cases.[142] This disease is discussed in more detail above.

Heatstroke

Heatstroke[143] occurs in hot climates, usually in association with exertion and poor fluid input, and can lead to acute renal failure. The mechanism of the renal failure is rhabdomyolysis and disseminated intravascular coagulation. Fulminant hepatic failure may also occur, contributing to the coagulopathy and renal failure. Investigations reveal evidence of haemoconcentration with a raised creatinine kinase, hyperuricaemia, myoglobinuria, hyperkalaemia, hypocalcaemia, proteinuria and often microscopic haematuria. Renal failure is treated along standard lines.

Melioidosis

This infection is caused by *Burkholderia pseudomallei*, an organism found in soil and water, and the infection is endemic in South-east Asia, Central and South America and the West Indies.[144] Patients with diabetes mellitus and tuberculosis have an increased susceptibility to this infection. There is a marked seasonal variation in this disease, with the majority of cases occurring in the rainy season. In northern Thailand it accounts for 20% of all community-acquired septicaemias. Patients can present with a localized form of the illness with discrete foci of infection or they can present with septicaemia without any obvious site of infection. Acute renal failure is more common in patients with septicaemia (60%) than in those with the localized form of the infection (35%). In the septicaemic form the presentation is usually one with a short history of a high temperature with diarrhoea, shock and a metabolic acidosis. There is usually radiological evidence of pneumonia, although there may be no symptoms or signs to support this. Microabscesses are sometimes seen in the skin. Other features include hypoglycaemia, hyponatraemia and a low white cell count. In patients with acute renal failure the mortality is high. The renal lesion is most often acute tubular necrosis but an inter-stitial nephritis and renal microabscesses have been seen. Treatment is with ceftazidime or a combination of ceftazidime and trimethoprim-sulfamethoxazole. Imipenem can also be used but this is not as readily available. The organism is resistant to gentamicin and penicillin.

Snake bite

Snake bites (see also Chapter 31) are a relatively common event in the tropics. In Papua New Guinea, snake bite victims account for 60% of all ventilator bed-days in intensive care units.[145] Acute renal failure is a well-recognized complication of snake bite. In a series from Chandrigah in India, out of 1862 patients with snake bites 3% developed acute renal failure.[146] Acute renal failure has been reported in patients bitten by snakes of the viper, colubrid and sea snake class. Following the bite of a Russell's viper, between 3% and 30% of patients go on to develop renal failure; the figure following rattlesnake envenomation is around 15%. The risk of developing acute renal failure depends on the venom dose and the time between the bite and the administration of antivenom. Gastrointestinal bleeding and also bleeding into the muscle, viscera and subarachnoid space may develop. Acute renal failure develops within hours to 3 days after envenomation. The mechanism for the acute renal failure differs among the various snake families. Vipers cause intravascular haemolysis and disseminated intravascular coagulation but there is also evidence for direct nephrotoxicity. The mechanism whereby sea snake bites cause acute renal failure is rhabdomyolysis and myoglobinuria. The most common renal histological change seen is acute tubular necrosis, but cortical necrosis may be seen in up to 3% of cases. Other renal lesions reported include proliferative glomerulonephritis (occasionally with crescents), arteritis and renal infarcts. The main aim of treatment is adequate volume replacement and the administration of as specific an antivenom as is available as soon as possible. Treatment of renal failure is along standard lines.

Nephrotoxins

A wide variety of plants used as herbal remedies in the tropics have been reported to be nephrotoxic[56] (see also Chapter 32).[147] Renal failure has also been reported following multiple bee and wasp stings, spider bite and scorpion sting. In addition to direct nephrotoxicity the causes of acute renal failure include haemolysis and disseminated intravascular coagulation. Other causes of nephrotoxic acute renal failure include paraquat and copper sulphate poisoning. More recently, ingestion of the hair dye paraphenylene diamine has been reported to cause acute renal failure in North Africa and in India.[148] This is associated with neck and upper respiratory oedema, rhabdomyolysis and respiratory failure.

Haemolytic–uraemic syndrome

This is a syndrome of thrombocytopenia, microangiopathic haemolytic anaemia with fragmented red blood cells and acute renal failure. The main cause of epidemic diarrhoea-associated haemolytic–uraemic syndrome (HUS) is Shiga toxin-producing *Escherichia coli* (STEC), although HUS can occur as part of many other disease processes including HIV infection. Mortality from this condition can be as high as 40% in some countries. The clinical syndromes of STEC infections include mild diarrhoea, haemorrhagic colitis and HUS in 7–24% of patients. Sporadic cases of HUS also occur and this is more common in adults. In the Indian subcontinent HUS may complicate *Shigella dysenteriae* type I infection.[133] Rare infective causes of HUS include neur-aminidase-producing pneumococci and also *Salmonella typhi* infection.[132] Most cases of endemic HUS occur in infants and young children. There is usually a prodromal bloody diarrhoeal illness followed by renal failure and bleeding from the gut. Hypertension is common and focal neurological abnormalities such as fits and strokes may develop.

The pathological lesion is believed to be caused by the transport of Shiga toxin by neutrophils to the kidney.[149] This binds to receptors on glomerular endothelial and tubular epithelial cells, whereby the toxin is internalized via receptor mediated endocytosis. This process leads to endothelial swelling and detachment and secondary activation of platelets and the coagulation cascade. The end result of this process is the characteristic microangiopathic haemolytic anaemia. Histological abnormalities on renal biopsy include glomerular changes, such as endothelial swelling, proliferation and capillary loop thrombosis. Afferent glomerular arterioles may show fibrin deposition and may be thrombosed. The use of antibiotics in preventing patients with *E. coli* infection from developing HUS, however, is more controversial, with some studies showing benefit and others a detrimental effect.[150]

Investigations in acute renal failure

These are aimed at establishing the presence and severity of acute renal failure and its aetiology, together with the history and physical examination; it is then possible to plan rational management for these patients.

Urine

Microscopic haematuria with red cell casts in the presence of proteinuria points strongly to a glomerulonephritis, while eosinophiluria suggests a drug-induced acute interstitial nephritis. The presence of urinary myoglobin is diagnostic of rhabdomyolysis.

Haematology

In acute renal failure an elevated neutrophil count usually suggests underlying sepsis. In STEC or Shigella-associated HUS the neutrophil count also correlates with disease severity. Anaemia with thrombocytopenia and fragmented red cells in the presence of normal clotting indices is also indicative of HUS, whereas the presence of a coagulopathy and raised serum levels of fibrinogen degradation products suggests disseminated intravascular coagulation. In severe drug-induced interstitial nephritis there may be an increase in the circulating peripheral blood eosinophil count. Blood should also be examined for the presence of malarial parasites.

Chemistry

An elevation of blood urea and creatinine will be found in acute renal failure. An inappropriately elevated urea compared with creatinine, however, may suggest volume depletion and a pre-renal aetiology. Gastrointestinal haemorrhage in the presence of acute renal failure will also produce a similar picture. If rhabdomyolysis is suspected the blood creatinine phosphokinase concentrations should also be measured as these are grossly elevated in this condition.

Radiological investigations

A chest radiograph should be performed in all patients with acute renal failure and a plain abdominal radiograph may reveal renal or ureteric calculi. An ultrasound examination of the kidneys helps to exclude obstruction and determine renal size. In patients with an obstructive uropathy, percutaneous antegrade pyelography allows visualization of the pelvis and ureter, defines the site of obstruction and allows both drainage and decompression, allowing recovery of renal function. If access to the renal pelvis is not achieved the site of the obstruction may be determined using retrograde pyelography. Computed tomography is another useful tool for defining the nature and the level of obstruction in obstructive nephropathy. Radionuclide scanning with DTPA or DMSA demonstrates renal perfusion.

Renal biopsy

Renal histology is useful in all patients with unexplained acute renal failure and normal-sized unobstructed kidneys, especially if they have features suggestive of glomerulonephritis or other systemic diseases.

Management

Prevention of acute tubular necrosis

Many patients develop acute tubular necrosis after a severe infection. It is likely that many of these cases can be prevented by paying careful attention to fluid balance and avoiding nephrotoxic drugs. In this early phase acute renal failure may be potentially reversible. Oliguria, with a low urinary Na^+ (<10 mmol/L), a low fractional excretion of Na^+ and urine that is more concentrated than plasma, is indicative of incipient or pre-renal acute renal failure. The ability of these urinary indices to differentiate reversible from established renal failure is imprecise and is invalidated by loop diuretics. We and others find them of little value in practice. In patients with oliguria the first step is to correct hypovolaemia and a low cardiac output. The use of central venous pressure monitoring may be helpful in difficult cases. A potential pitfall is that if the patient remains oliguric pulmonary oedema may be precipitated. Low-dose dopamine does not improve the outcome of patients with acute renal failure and may adversely affect outcome. Frusemide may make fluid overload easier to manage and avoid the need for dialysis but some studies suggest a poorer outcome for patients treated in this way.

Fluid balance

A daily weight chart is valuable in assessing the fluid balance of patients with acute renal failure. Volume depletion is usually present if the jugular venous pressure is not visible; there is a resting tachycardia and a postural drop in blood pressure. Skin turgor is more difficult to interpret as it depends on other factors such as age. The amount of fluids given to a patient in acute renal failure is based on: (1) measured fluid losses; (2) insensible losses minus metabolically produced water (about 600 mL/day in an adult); and (3) fluid removed by dialysis. Crystalloids such as either normal saline or isotonic sodium bicarbonate should be used unless there has been blood loss, in which case blood transfusions are required.

Hyperkalaemia and acidosis

Serum potassium can rise rapidly in patients who are hypercatabolic or acidotic or who have rhabdomyolysis. Hyperkalaemia is cardiotoxic and the electrocardiographic features include tall peaked T waves, prolongation of the PR interval, broadening of the QRS complex, which merges into the T wave, and ventricular arrhythmias with cardiac arrest. The serum potassium must be measured daily in patients with acute renal failure and more frequently in patients who are hypercatabolic. With milder degrees of hyperkalaemia (K^+ <6.0 mmol/L) cation exchange resins may be used to increase faecal potassium excretion, although these can lead to severe constipation and should be administered with laxatives. Serum potassium levels higher than 6.0 mmol/L are an indication for urgent dialysis. Intravenous glucose and soluble insulin are often helpful in reducing serum potassium pending dialysis. Most patients with acute renal failure have a metabolic acidosis and this can be severe in patients who are hypercatabolic. Intravenous isotonic sodium bicarbonate is useful in that it can be administered peripherally, corrects the acidosis and by doing so also lowers serum potassium. It should only be used in patients who are volume depleted and should not be used in the presence of hypocalcaemia as it will lower ionized calcium and provoke tetany and convulsions.

Dialysis

There are now a variety of techniques for treating uraemia and removing fluid from patients with acute renal failure. These include haemodialysis, peritoneal dialysis, haemofiltration, continuous arteriovenous haemofiltration, and continuous venovenous haemodialysis (CVVHD).

Peritoneal dialysis

This has the advantage of being widely available, easy to set up and easy to run. The advent of percutaneous peritoneal dialysis catheter insertion techniques has made this procedure safer. It is effective in patients with milder degrees of renal failure who are not hypercatabolic. It has the advantage of not needing specialized equipment, avoids anticoagulation and is carried out at the bedside. Because it is a continuous process it is suitable for patients who are cardiovascularly unstable. The main complication of peritoneal dialysis is peritonitis.

Haemodialysis

Haemodialysis is now the mainstay of treatment for acute renal failure in the non-ITU setting. Access to the circulation is achieved by means of temporary or semi-permanent central venous catheters. Ideally these should be placed in the internal jugular vein. The femoral vein can be used if the patient is unable to lie flat but this route is prone to infective complications. Tunnelled semi-permanent venous catheters should be employed if prolonged dialysis is likely to be required.

Patients are usually dialysed for between 3 and 4 h either daily or every other day. This is an extremely efficient form of treatment as it has the ability to clear large quantities of catabolic products and fluid over a relatively short period of time. Its intermittent nature also means that patients do not require the continuous anticoagulation needed for the other forms of haemodialysis (discussed below). The disadvantages of intermittent haemodialysis are that patients who are hypotensive or cardiovascularly unstable are often not able to tolerate the procedure.

In the unstable patient continuous forms of dialysis are better tolerated. Peritoneal dialysis has been discussed above. Continuous forms of haemodialysis are also available but require intensive care. The standard mode of continuous haemodialysis is continuous veno-veno haemofiltration with fluid replacement. A dual-lumen venous catheter is required and blood is pumped through an artificial kidney. It requires continuous anticoagulation. Fluid removal takes place constantly, making this suitable treatment for unstable patients.

Nutrition

Patients with acute renal failure should be given adequate nutrition in an attempt to minimize muscle catabolism and reduce malnutrition with the added risks of delayed wound healing and impaired resistance to infection.

Sepsis

Sepsis is important both as a cause and as a complication: most studies show that sepsis is still a major cause of death in patients with acute renal failure. The major sites of sepsis are intra-abdominal and pulmonary, and septicaemia is a frequent complication. Antibiotic doses may need to be adjusted as many are cleared by the kidney. More importantly, if drugs such as gentamicin and vancomycin are required, strict monitoring of trough levels is required almost on a daily basis.

Drugs

Many drugs used in patients with acute renal failure are excreted by the kidneys and, unless their dose is modified, will accumulate with potentially toxic effects. It is therefore essential to know the precise pharmacokinetics of any drug before it is given to a patient with acute renal failure. Detailed guidelines of drug treatment in these patients are available.

CHRONIC RENAL FAILURE

Definition

Chronic renal failure results from the progressive and irreversible loss of kidney function. When the GFR is <10 mL/min then uraemic symptoms develop and dialysis and/or transplantation is required for survival. It may be staged based on the level of GFR as shown in Table 15.6. Chronic Kidney Disease (CKD) is common in the tropics but there are very few data on the prevalence of this condition.

Table 15.6 KDOQI stages of chronic kidney disease

Stage	Description	GFR (mL/min per 1.73 m²)
1	Kidney damage with normal or increased GFR	>90
2	Kidney damage with mild decrease in GFR	60–89
3	Moderate decrease in GFR	30–59
4	Severe decrease in GFR	15–29
5	Kidney failure (ESRD)	<15 or dialysis

The stages of chronic kidney disease are set out above. Stage 1 refers to patients with known proteinuria or haematuria or structural abnormalities, e.g. polycystic kidneys.
KDOQI, Clinical Practice Guidelines and Clinical Practice Recommendations for Diabetes and Chronic Kidney Disease.

Table 15.7 Causes of chronic renal failure in the tropics

Cause	Africa	India	Malaysia
Hypertensive renal disease (nephrosclerosis)	32–49	5–23	?
Glomerulonephritis	25–62	35–65	30
Pyelonephritis	2–29	7–18	2
Diabetic nephropathy	3–9	7–23	9
Obstructive uropathy	?	3–14	6
Renal calculi	12	7	?
Tuberculosis	?	1–5	?
Polycystic kidney disease	?	1–6	0.5

Aetiology

There are many causes of chronic renal failure in the tropics and these are summarized in Table 15.7. In tropical countries, glomerulonephritis, hypertension and diabetic nephropathy are major causes of chronic renal failure, as are nephrolithiasis and obstructive uropathy.[151–157]

Diabetic nephropathy

The number of patients with type 2 diabetes is growing rapidly and the prevalence of diabetes in the general population of some tropical countries is high, with up to 23% of those between 30 and 64 years being affected. This appears to be, in part at least, a problem related to urbanization. Diabetic nephropathy has been reported in tropical Africa, the Caribbean, the Indian subcontinent and Southeast Asia. In most areas the prevalence of diabetic nephropathy in patients with diabetes mellitus varies between 10% and 20%. The progressive nature of diabetic nephropathy makes this likely to be a major cause of end-stage renal failure in these areas.

Hypertension

Hypertension is a major cause of chronic kidney disease and an important determinant of progression regardless of the cause of renal disease. Worldwide, hypertension is common[158] and this is a major cause of chronic renal failure in tropical countries.[151,153–155]

Prevalence of CKD

Population studies on the prevalence of CKD that estimate GFR using prediction equations in relation to the general population show that CKD is common. In studies from the USA and Europe the prevalence of chronic kidney disease is around 10%[159,160] and it is likely that the prevalence of CKD in the tropics is at least as high as this. In the tropics the prevalence of patients receiving dialysis is largely governed by socioeconomic forces. In Singapore approximately 500 per million population are on dialysis, whereas dialysis prevalence rates are lower in countries such as Eygpt (264 per million population), the Philippines (40 per million population), and Pakistan (15 per million population).[98] There is little dialysis availability in many tropical countries and in low income societies, patients with end-stage renal failure die as dialysis is unavailable or unaffordable.

Pathophysiology

When a critical proportion of functioning nephrons is lost, glomerular hypertrophy is accompanied by glomerular hyperperfusion, hyperfiltration and hypertension and these in turn lead to progressive glomerular sclerosis, tubulointerstitial atrophy and scarring.[161] In rats, reduction of intraglomerular pressures, either by a low protein diet or by an angiotensin-converting enzyme inhibitor (ACEI) (which reduces intraglomerular pressures by afferent arteriolar vasodilatation), slowed down the rate at which renal failure progressed. A common consequence of hyperfiltration injury is proteinuria, which is associated with the development of tubulointerstitial injury. Patients with proteinuria are more likely to progress to end-stage renal failure independent of initial diagnosis.[162]

Early detection and management

Recent guidelines and public health campaigns have focused on early detection and treatment of CKD as treatments that are initiated early in the disease course will slow the progression of kidney disease and delay the onset of kidney failure. In developing countries without the resources or infrastructure to provide for universal renal replacement treatment this is an important strategy. Detection of CKD is generally based on renal function and proteinuria. Serum creatinine levels and glomerular filtration rate (GFR) are used as markers for renal function. Due to the difficulties of measuring GFR using radioisotopic techniques, derived prediction equations, in particular the MDRD equation, are used to estimate renal function. As described in the introduction, proteinuria is a marker of renal damage and also a strong predictor of clinical progression of kidney disease.

There are certain basic principles that can be applied to all patients to retard the rate of progression of chronic renal failure. Specific treatment for CKD should depend on the cause of kidney disease and a thorough search for reversible causes, e.g. obstruction to the renal tract. Nephrotoxic drugs such as non-steroidal antiinflammatory drugs should be discontinued. There is now compelling evidence that inhibiting the effects of angiotensin using angiotensin-converting enzyme (ACE) or angiotensin-II- receptor blockers slows the progression of diabetic as well as non-diabetic CKD.[12,163–168] Caution, however, needs to be exercised in patients with both large and small vessel renal disease as in this setting these drugs may cause an acute but usually reversible deterioration in renal function. Because of this, high-risk patients require close monitoring of renal function after the initiation of therapy. Good blood pressure control also reduces the rate at which renal failure progresses.[169] The blood pressure target aimed for is 130/80 or 125/75 mmHg in patients with proteinuria (Table 15.8). A low salt intake reduces blood pressure and probably slows progression of renal failure.[170] In patients with diabetes good glycaemic control has been shown to slow down the progression of renal failure.[171,172] A low-protein diet reduces the progression of renal damage in rats and possibly in humans. We advise against excessive protein intake in patients with renal impairment.

Table 15.8 Management of chronic kidney disease

1.	Maintain blood pressure <130/80 mmHg and 125/75 mmHg for patients with significant proteinuria
2.	ACE inhibitors (ACEI) and Angiotensin II receptor blockers (ARBS)are effective in slowing progression of renal failure and should be used when there is proteinuria
3.	Check creatinine and potassium 2 weeks after starting an ACE Inhibitor or Angiotensin II receptor blocker and after any increase in dose. There is usually a slight decline in GFR. Discontinue drugs only if GFR drops by more than 20 mL/min and exclude renal artery stenosis
4.	In patients with impairment of renal function who are on ACEI or ARBS do not use potassium sparing diuretics (spironolactone/amiloride) or NSAIDs because of the risk of hyperkalaemia
5.	Treat hyperkalaemia (K+ 5.5–6.0) with frusemide and recheck in 2 weeks. Discontinue angiotensin blockade if K+ still ≥6.0 mmol/L
6.	Discontinue non-steroidal antiinflammatory drugs in patients with renal impairment
7.	Annual mortality from cardiovascular disease is 10–100 times higher with kidney failure so monitor and treat risk factors
8.	Patients with type 2 diabetes mellitus and microalbuminuria or proteinuria should be managed according to current guidelines (National Institute for Clinical Excellence 2002). Pending publication of NICE guidelines, patients with type 1 diabetes mellitus and microalbuminuria or proteinuria should be managed according to SIGN guidelines
9.	Arrange urgent ultrasound of kidneys and bladder in patients with urological symptoms

The maintenance of GFR in advanced renal failure is critically dependent on salt and water balance. Salt and water overload leads to heart failure, a reduction in cardiac output and worsening of renal function. Salt and water depletion leads to volume depletion, a reduction in cardiac output and a reduction in GFR. Each patient must have careful regular assessments of their fluid status and salt and water intake and this is then optimized, if necessary, using diuretics. Once the GFR falls below 20 mL/min plasma potassium tends to rise, justifying a reduction in dietary potassium intake. Expert dietetic help adjusted to the local foods is invaluable in the management of these patients.

Consequences of CKD

Hyperkalaemia and acidosis

These are not marked until the GFR falls below 20 mL/min. Exceptions to this are patients with tubulointerstitial disorders.

Salt and water handling

In most patients, salt and water balance is maintained until the GFR falls below 15% of normal, although in diabetes this may occur earlier. Nevertheless some individuals with tubulointerstitial disease are salt and water losers and tend to dehydration at a higher GFR. Others with glomerular disease and hypertension, especially with hypertensive heart disease, may retain salt and water and develop heart failure.

Bone[173]

Increased blood levels of parathormone are found in very early renal failure when GFR falls below 50–60 mL/min. This is due to inappropriately low levels of 1,25-dihydroxycholecalciferol, hyperphosphataemia and consequent hypocalcaemia. With advanced renal failure there is impaired renal synthesis of 1,25-cholecalciferol from its precursor 25-cholecalciferol. A reduction in intestinal absorption of calcium and also hyperphosphataemia increase the tendency to hypocalcaemia. This stimulates parathyroid glands to hyperplasia and in severe cases to adenoma formation. The consequence of this is renal osteodystrophy. Vitamin D deficiency leads to osteomalacia, and hyperparathyroidism to the development of bone erosions and osteitis fibrosa.

Renal osteodystrophy is becoming more of a problem as more patients are now receiving maintenance dialysis. Key principles in management include control of hyperphosphataemia with phosphate binders which bind ingested phosphate and the use of 1a-hydroxycholecalciferol or 1,25-dihydroxycholecalciferol in patients who are (1) hypocalcaemic, (2) have a raised alkaline phosphatase, and/or (3) have a raised parathormone. Available phosphate binders include calcium carbonate, calcium acetate and sevelamer. The dose of calcium carbonate must be adjusted to avoid hypercalcaemia and subsequent vascular and soft tissue calcification.

Anaemia[174,175]

Haemoglobin concentrations tend to be maintained until the GFR falls below 30 mL/min. At this time anaemia ensues. There are several reasons for the anaemia of chronic renal failure. Perhaps the most important is the failing kidney's inability to produce sufficient quantities of erythropoietin, the hormone that drives the bone marrow to produce red blood cells. Other factors, such as reduced red cell survival are also important. In addition, the uraemic environment renders the bone marrow relatively resistant to the action of erythropoietin, especially if inflammation and infection are present. Recombinant human erythropoietin is now readily available but at considerable cost. Careful monitoring of anaemia is also required so that treatment can begin early. The use of subcutaneous recombinant human erythropoietin on a regular basis can be initiated in order to achieve a haemoglobin level of 11 g/L. Normalization of haemoglobin should be avoided as this increases mortality. Adequate utilizable iron is required to minimize erythropoietin dosage and many centres in the West now administer regular intravenous iron to dialysis patients.

Aluminium intoxication

This arises from dialysis against fluid containing aluminium and to a lesser extent absorption of aluminium-containing phosphate binders. The bony consequence is osteomalacia. Aluminium intoxication can also cause an encephalopathy. This is now less of a problem as pure aluminium free dialysate is routinely used and aluminium-containing phosphate binders are now not routinely used.

Dialysis and transplantation

Once the GFR falls below 10 mL/min, renal replacement with either dialysis or a renal transplant is necessary if life is to be maintained. The costs of dialysis – both continuous ambulatory dialysis and haemodialysis – are substantial, but increasingly tropical countries are providing chronic dialysis facilities. In the more developed tropical countries the level of dialysis provision approaches that of the West. Singapore, for instance, has 500 dialysis patients per million population and neighbouring Malaysia has 253 dialysis per million population; however, other countries lag far behind, with figures of between 15 and 40 per million population (Pakistan and Philippines). Renal transplantation once set up is less costly in the long term.

Haemodialysis

This is the most popular method for the delivering of long-term dialysis worldwide. In the USA, nearly 90% of all patients on dialysis receive haemodialysis. In the UK the proportion receiving haemodialysis is somewhat lower at 60%. In tropical countries the majority of chronic dialysis programmes have more patients on haemodialysis. This method of dialysis delivery has the advantage of being able to treat a large number of patients and is fast and efficient. Technique survival is only limited by vascular access. It is, however, limited by staff, space and availability of machines. Also patients have to travel to centres to have this treatment as very few tropical countries have home haemodialysis programmes.

Peritoneal dialysis

Several techniques are now on offer: continuous ambulatory peritoneal dialysis (CAPD), automated peritoneal dialysis (APD) and intermittent peritoneal dialysis (IPD). Both CAPD and APD are

domiciliary treatments and hence are less dependent on staff or space. Patients living far from dialysis centres may benefit from these modalities although provision and delivery of dialysate may prove difficult. Unfortunately, most commercially produced dialysates are expensive and hence render this treatment no cheaper than haemodialysis. Because of membrane failure median technique survival for CAPD is 7–8 years.

Transplantation

This form of renal replacement therapy provides patients with the best long-term outlook, with living donation providing the best graft survival figures. Many tropical countries have established live donor programmes but cadaveric programmes are also being established in some. The previous practice of 'organ trade' is now illegal in countries such as India following the passage of Act 42. The Transplantation of Human Organs Act. Transplantation provides patients with a near-normal lifestyle, most of the complications occurring as a result of side-effects of the immunosuppressive therapy. The mainstay of immunosuppression is steroids, azathioprine, mycophenolate mofetil and calcineurin inhibition with ciclosporin and tacrolimus. The patent on ciclosporin has recently expired, resulting in numerous cheaper generic forms. This will hopefully afford greater access to this drug. This is especially important when graft failure secondary to poor compliance, for economic reasons, is common.

OBSTRUCTIVE UROPATHY

Renal tuberculosis[176]

Tuberculosis can affect the urinary tract in many ways. Most commonly there is parenchymal renal involvement with ureteric and bladder involvement. Parenchymal renal involvement often leads to cavitation, seen on intravenous urography as papillary ulceration or cavities in the parenchyma, and these may communicate with the pelvicaliceal system. Advanced parenchymal lesions lead to a non-functioning kidney – so-called autonephrectomy. On plain abdominal radiographs renal calcification is often a clue to the diagnosis of tuberculosis. Bladder involvement leads to ulceration and there may be inflammation of the ureters. In advanced disease, the bladder becomes obstructed and fibrosed and this, together with ureteric stricture or incompetence of the vesicoureteric junction, can lead to an obstructive uropathy. Extrarenal tuberculosis may lead to the late development of glomerular amyloid. The clinical presentation is that of renal amyloid from any other cause. Rarely tuberculosis has been associated with the development of a mesangiocapillary glomerulonephritis.

Renal calculi[177]

Renal and ureteric calculi tend to be uncommon in blacks in tropical Africa but are common in the Middle East, the Indian subcontinent and the rest of Asia. The overall probability of forming stones ranges from 1–5% in Asia to 20% in Saudi Arabia compared with 5–9% in Europe and 13% in North America. The Indian population of Fiji is noted for their high incidence of renal calculi, unlike their native Fijian counterparts.

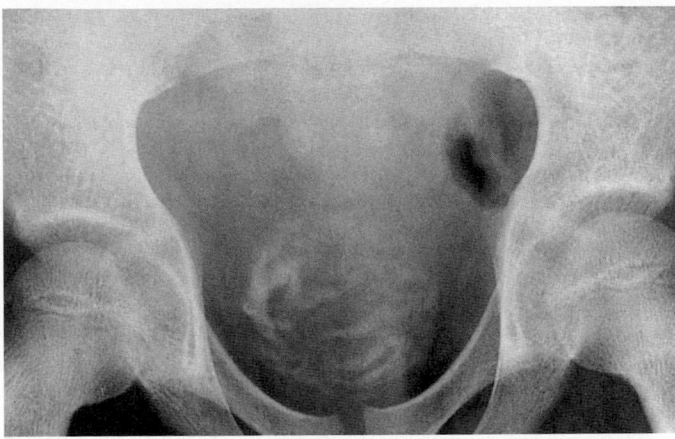

Figure 15.5 Bladder wall calcification in schistosomiasis. (Courtesy of Judy Webb, St Bartholomew's Hospital.)

In areas with a high incidence of schistosomiasis, bladder stones may be common. It is suggested that a high temperature, inadequate fluid intake and low urine volume predispose to stone formation in some areas. Bladder stones are common in Central Africa and parts of South-east Asia.

Schistosoma haematobium

S. haematobium[86,178,179] infections are widespread in the tropics. *Schistosoma*-mediated inflammation of the bladder and ureters can lead to fibrosis and to obstructive uropathy. The bladder and the juxtavesical ureter are initially involved by granuloma formation. Ureteric involvement leads to ureteric dilatation, stricture and vesicoureteric reflux. Functionally these abnormalities may lead to renal failure. Diagnosis is by examining the urine for *S. haematobium* ova. A calcified bladder or ureters may be seen on abdominal radiographs (Figure 15.5). Intravenous urography shows a variety of changes including segmental dilatation of the ureter, ureteric stenosis and dilatation of the upper tracts. More recently, the ultrasonographic features have been described and this technique is gaining popularity. Treatment with praziquantel results in high cure rates and when used community-wide in endemic areas has been shown to reduce the prevalence of urinary tract abnormalities. There is good evidence of an association between *S. haematobium* infection and the subsequent development of bladder cancer. The majority of these tumours are squamous cell carcinomas.

REFERENCES

1. Stevens LA, Coresh J, Greene T, et al. Assessing kidney function – measured and estimated glomerular filtration rate. *N Engl J Med* 2006; 354(23): 2473–2483.
2. Levey AS, Coresh J, Greene T, et al. Using standardized serum creatinine values in the modification of diet in renal disease study equation for estimating glomerular filtration rate. *Ann Intern Med* 2006; 145(4):247–254.
3. Lewis J, Agodoa L, Cheek D, et al. Comparison of cross-sectional renal function measurements in African Americans with hypertensive nephrosclerosis and of primary formulas to estimate glomerular filtration rate. *Am J Kidney Dis* 2001; 38(4):744–753.
4. KDOQI. KDOQI Clinical Practice Guidelines and Clinical Practice Recommendations for Diabetes and Chronic Kidney Disease. *Am J Kidney Dis* 2007; 49(2, suppl 2):S12–S154.
5. Keane WF. Proteinuria: its clinical importance and role in progressive renal disease. *Am J Kidney Dis* 2000; 35(4, suppl 1):S97–S105.
6. Jafar TH, Stark PC, Schmid CH, et al. Proteinuria as a modifiable risk factor for the progression of non-diabetic renal disease. *Kidney Int* 2001; 60(3):1131–1140.
7. Ginsberg JM, Chang BS, Matarese RA, et al. Use of single voided urine samples to estimate quantitative proteinuria. *N Engl J Med* 1983; 309(25):1543–1546.
8. Kibukamusoke JW, Hutt MS, Wilks NE. The nephrotic syndrome in Uganda and its association with quartan malaria. *Q J Med* 1967; 36(143):393–408.
9. Dixon FJ, Vazquez JJ, Weigle WO, et al. Pathogenesis of serum sickness. *AMA Arch Pathol* 1958; 65(1):18–28.
10. Feehally J, Floege J, Savill J, et al. Glomerular injury and glomerular response. In: Davison AM, Cameron JS, Grunfeld JP, et al., eds. *Oxford Textbook of Clinical Nephrology*. 3rd edn. Oxford: New York: Oxford University Press, 2005:363–387.
11. Adu D. Minimal-change nephropathy, focal segmental glomerulosclerosis, and membranous nephropathy. In: Warrell D, Cox TM, Firth JD, Benz JE, eds. *Oxford Texbook of Medicine*. Oxford: Oxford University Press; 2004.
12. Ruggenenti P, Perna A, Benini R, et al. In chronic nephropathies prolonged ACE inhibition can induce remission. dynamics of time-dependent changes in GFR. Investigators of the GISEN Group. Gruppo Italiano Studi Epidemiologici in Nefrologia. *J Am Soc Nephrol* 1999; 10(5):997–1006.
13. Ruggenenti P, Schieppati A, Remuzzi G. Progression, remission, regression of chronic renal diseases. *Lancet* 2001; 357(9268):1601–1608.
14. Chiurchiu C, Remuzzi G, Ruggenenti P. Angiotensin-converting enzyme inhibition and renal protection in nondiabetic patients: the data of the meta-analyses. *J Am Soc Nephrol* 2005; 16(suppl 1):S58–S63.
15. Jha V, Chugh KS. Glomerular disease in the tropics. In: Davison AM, Cameron JS, Grünfeld J-P, et al., eds. *Oxford Textbook of Clinical Nephrology*. 3rd ed. Oxford: Oxford University Press; 2005:639–655.
16. Morgan AG, Shah DJ, Williams W, et al. Proteinuria and glomerular disease in Jamaica. *Clin Nephrol* 1984; 21(4):205–209.
17. Seggie J, Davies PG, Ninin D, et al. Patterns of glomerulonephritis in Zimbabwe: survey of disease characterised by nephrotic proteinuria. *Q J Med* 1984; 53(209):109–118.
18. Seggie J, Nathoo K, Davies PG. Association of hepatitis B (HBs) antigenaemia and membranous glomerulonephritis in Zimbabwean children. *Nephron* 1984; 38(2):115–119.
19. Borok MZ, Nathoo KJ, Gabriel R, et al. Clinicopathological features of Zimbabwean patients with sustained proteinuria. *Cent Afr J Med* 1997; 43(6):152–158.
20. Seggie J, Adu D. Nephrotic syndrome in the tropics. In: Cameron JS, Glassock RJ, eds. *The Neprotic Syndrome*. New York: Marcel Dekker, 1988:653–695.
21. Morel-Maroger L, Saimot AG, Sloper JC, et al. 'Topical nephropathy' and 'tropical extramembranous glomerulonephritis' of unknown aetiology in Senegal. *BMJ* 1975; 1(5957):541–546.
22. Adu D, Anim-Addo Y, Foli AK, et al. The nephrotic syndrome in Ghana: clinical and pathological aspects. *Q J Med* 1981; 50(199):297–306.
23. Chugh KS, Sakhuja V. Renal disease in Northern India. In: Kibukamusoke JW, ed. *Tropical Nephrology*. Canberra: Citforge; 1984:428–440.
24. Pakasa M, Mangani N, Dikassa L. Focal and segmental glomerulosclerosis in nephrotic syndrome: a new profile of adult nephrotic syndrome in Zaire. *Mod Pathol* 1993; 6(2):125–128.
25. McLigeyo SO. Glomerular diseases in Kenya – another look at diseases characterised by nephrotic proteinuria. *Afr J Health Sci* 1994; 1(4):185–190.
26. Doe JY, Funk M, Mengel M, et al. Nephrotic syndrome in African children: lack of evidence for 'tropical nephrotic syndrome'? *Nephrol Dial Transplant* 2006; 21(3):672–676.
27. Mathieson PW. Glomerulonephritis in the tropics: who are the culprits? *Ethn Dis* 2006; 16(2, suppl 2):52–55.

28. Musa AR, Veress B, Kordofani AM, et al. Pattern of the nephrotic syndrome in the Sudan. *Ann Trop Med Parasitol* 1980; 74(1):37–44.

29. Bhimma R, Coovadia HM, Adhikari M. Nephrotic syndrome in South African children: changing perspectives over 20 years. *Pediatr Nephrol* 1997; 11(4):429–434.

30. Kumar J, Gulati S, Sharma AP, et al. Histopathological spectrum of childhood nephrotic syndrome in Indian children. *Pediatr Nephrol* 2003; 18(7):657–660.

31. Hodson EM, Knight JF, Willis NS, et al. Corticosteroid therapy for nephrotic syndrome in children. *Cochrane Database Syst Rev* 2005(1):CD001533.

32. Durkan A, Hodson EM, Willis NS, et al. Non-corticosteroid treatment for nephrotic syndrome in children. *Cochrane Database Syst Rev* 2005(2): CD002290.

33. Hodson EM, Habashy D, Craig JC. Interventions for idiopathic steroid-resistant nephrotic syndrome in children. *Cochrane Database Syst Rev* 2006(2): CD003594.

34. Diouf B, Ka E F, Niang A, et al. Analysis of 115 kidney biopsies performed in Dakar (Senegal). *Dakar Med* 2001; 46(1):51–53.

35. Pakasa NM, Sumaili EK. The nephrotic syndrome in the Democratic Republic of Congo. *N Engl J Med* 2006; 354(10):1085–1086.

36. Howie AJ, Pankhurst T, Sarioglu S, et al. Evolution of nephrotic-associated focal segmental glomerulosclerosis and relation to the glomerular tip lesion. *Kidney Int* 2005; 67(3):987–1001.

37. D'Agati VD, Fogo AB, Bruijn JA, et al. Pathologic classification of focal segmental glomerulosclerosis: a working proposal. *Am J Kidney Dis* 2004; 43(2):368–382.

38. Korbet S, Schwartz M, Lewis E. Primary focal segmental glomerulosclerosis: Clinical course and response to therapy. *Am J Kidney Dis* 1994; 23:773–783.

39. Cattran DC, Appel GB, Hebert LA, et al. A randomized trial of cyclosporine in patients with steroid-resistant focal segmental glomerulosclerosis. North America Nephrotic Syndrome Study Group. *Kidney Int* 1999; 56(6): 2220–2226.

40. Adu D. Meta-analysis of cyclosporin treatment of FSGS. *unpublished* 2006.

41. Bagga A, Mudigoudar BD, Hari P, et al. Enalapril dosage in steroid-resistant nephrotic syndrome. *Pediatr Nephrol* 2004; 19(1):45–50.

42. van Buuren AJ, Bates WD, Muller N. Nephrotic syndrome in Namibian children. *S Afr Med J* 1999; 89(10):1088–1091.

43. Bhimma R, Coovadia HM, Adhikari M. Hepatitis B virus-associated nephropathy in black South African children. *Pediatr Nephrol* 1998; 12(6):479–484.

44. Gilbert RD, Wiggelinkhuizen J. The clinical course of hepatitis B virus-associated nephropathy. *Pediatr Nephrol* 1994; 8(1):11–14.

45. Sadiq S, Jafarey NA, Naqvi SA. An analysis of percutaneous renal biopsies in fifty cases of nephrotic syndrome. *J Pak Med Assoc* 1978; 28(9):121–124.

46. Llach F. Thromboembolic complications in nephrotic syndrome. Coagulation abnormalities, renal vein thrombosis, and other conditions. *Postgrad Med* 1984; 76(6):111–114, 116–118, 121–123.

47. Schieppati A, Mosconi L, Perna A, et al. Prognosis of untreated patients with idiopathic membranous nephropathy. *N Engl J Med* 1993; 329(2):85–89.

48. Schieppati A, Perna A, Zamora J, et al. Immunosuppressive treatment for idiopathic membranous nephropathy in adults with nephrotic syndrome. *Cochrane Database Syst Rev* 2004(4):CD004293.

49. Sidabutar RP, Lumenta NA. The patterns of glomerulonephritis in 'Tjikini' Hospital Jakarta. *Ann Acad Med Singapore* 1982; 11(1):42–45.

50. Abdurrahman MB, Babaoye FA, Aikhionbare HA. Childhood renal disorders in Nigeria. *Pediatr Nephrol* 1990; 4(1):88–93.

51. Asinobi AO, Gbadegesin RA, Adeyemo AA, et al. The predominance of membranoproliferative glomerulonephritis in childhood nephrotic syndrome in Ibadan, Nigeria. *West Afr J Med* 1999; 18(3):203–206.

52. Madala ND, Naicker S, Singh B, et al. The pathogenesis of membranoproliferative glomerulonephritis in KwaZulu-Natal, South Africa is unrelated to hepatitis C virus infection. *Clin Nephrol* 2003; 60(2):69–73.

53. Chugh KS, Sakuja V. Glomerular disease in the tropics. In: Warrell DA, Cox TM, Firth JD, et al., eds. *Oxford Textbook of Medicine.* 4th edn. Oxford: Oxford University Press; 2004.

54. Levy M, Berger J. Worldwide perspective of IgA nephropathy. *Am J Kidney Dis* 1988; 12(5):340–347.

55. Swanepoel CR, Madaus S, Cassidy MJ, et al. IgA nephropathy – Groote Schuur Hospital experience. *Nephron* 1989; 53(1):61–64.

56. Sitprija V. The kidney in acute tropical disease. In: Kibukamusoke JW, ed. *Tropical Nephrology.* Canberra: Citforge; 1984:148–169.

57. Prathap K, Looi LM. Morphological patterns of glomerular disease in renal biopsies from 1000 Malaysian patients. *Ann Acad Med Singapore* 1982; 11(1):52–56.

58. Seedat YK, Parag KB, Ramsaroop R. Systemic lupus erythematosus and renal involvement. A South African experience. *Nephron* 1994; 66(4):426–430.

59. Austin HA 3rd, Klippel JH, Balow JE, et al. Therapy of lupus nephritis. Controlled trial of prednisone and cytotoxic drugs. *N Engl J Med.* 1986; 314(10):614–619.

60. Houssiau FA, Vasconcelos C, D'Cruz D, et al. Immunosuppressive therapy in lupus nephritis: the Euro-Lupus Nephritis Trial, a randomized trial of low-dose versus high-dose intravenous cyclophosphamide. *Arthritis Rheum* 2002; 46(8):2121–2131.

61. Flanc RS, Roberts MA, Strippoli GF, et al. Treatment of diffuse proliferative lupus nephritis: a meta-analysis of randomized controlled trials. *Am J Kidney Dis* 2004; 43(2):197–208.

62. Chan TM, Li F K, Tang CS, et al. Efficacy of mycophenolate mofetil in patients with diffuse proliferative lupus nephritis. Hong Kong-Guangzhou Nephrology Study Group. *N Engl J Med* 2000; 343(16):1156–1162.

63. Ginzler EM, Dooley MA, Aranow C, et al. Mycophenolate mofetil or intravenous cyclophosphamide for lupus nephritis. *N Eng J Med* 2005; 353(21):2219–2228.

64. Poon-King T, Svartman M, Mohammed I, et al. Epidemic acute nephritis with reappearance of M-type 55 streptococci in Trinidad. *Lancet* 1973; 1(7801):475–479.

65. Rajajee S. Post-streptococcal acute glomerulonephritis: a clinical, bacteriological and serological study. *Indian J Pediatr* 1990; 57(6):775–780.

66. Parra G, Rodriguez-Iturbe B, Batsford S, et al. Antibody to streptococcal zymogen in the serum of patients with acute glomerulonephritis: a multicentric study. *Kidney Int* 1998; 54(2):509–517.

67. Rodriguez-Iturbe B, Batsford S. Pathogenesis of poststreptococcal glomerulonephritis a century after Clemens von Pirquet. *Kidney Int* 2007; 71(11):1094–1104.

68. Walker A, Ellis J, Irama M, et al. Eosinophilic glomerulonephritis in children in Southwestern Uganda. *Kidney Int* 2007; 71(6):569–573.

69. Johnson RJ, Couser WG. Hepatitis B infection and renal disease: clinical, immunopathogenetic and therapeutic considerations. *Kidney Int* 1990; 37(2):663–676.

70. Lai KN, Lai FM, Chan KW, et al. The clinico-pathologic features of hepatitis B virus-associated glomerulonephritis. *Q J Med* 1987; 63(240):323–333.

71. Tang S, Lai FM, Lui YH, et al. Lamivudine in hepatitis B-associated membranous nephropathy. *Kidney Int* 2005; 68(4):1750–1758.

72. D'Amico G, Fornasieri A. Cryoglobulinemic glomerulonephritis: a membranoproliferative glomerulonephritis induced by hepatitis C virus. *Am J Kidney Dis* 1995; 25(3):361–369.

73. D'Amico G. Renal involvement in hepatitis C infection: cryoglobulinemic glomerulonephritis. *Kidney Int* 1998; 54(2):650–671.

74. Sabry AA, Sobh MA, Irving WL, et al. A comprehensive study of the association between hepatitis C virus and glomerulopathy. *Nephrol Dial Transplant* 2002; 17(2):239–245.

75. Sabry AA, Sobh MA, Sheaashaa HA, et al. Effect of combination therapy (ribavirin and interferon) in HCV-related glomerulopathy. *Nephrol Dial Transplant* 2002; 17(11):1924–1930.

76. Bourgoignie JJ. Renal complications of human immunodeficiency virus type 1. *Kidney Int* 1990; 37(6):1571–1584.

77. Khan S, Haragsim L, Laszik ZG. HIV-associated nephropathy. *Adv Chronic Kidney Dis* 2006; 13(3):307–313.

78. Klotman PE. HIV-associated nephropathy. *Kidney Int* 1999; 56(3): 1161–1176.

79. Han TM, Naicker S, Ramdial PK, et al. A cross-sectional study of HIV-seropositive patients with varying degrees of proteinuria in South Africa. *Kidney Int* 2006; 69(12):2243–2250.

80. Gerntholtz TE, Goetsch SJ, Katz I. HIV-related nephropathy: a South African perspective. *Kidney Int* 2006; 69(10):1885–1891.

81. Szczech LA, Gupta SK, Habash R, et al. The clinical epidemiology and course of the spectrum of renal diseases associated with HIV infection. *Kidney Int* 2004; 66(3):1145–1152.

82. Wyatt CM, Klotman PE. Antiretroviral therapy and the kidney: balancing benefit and risk in patients with HIV infection. *Expert Opin Drug Saf* 2006; 5(2):275–287.

83. Valle R, Haragsim L. Nephrotoxicity as a complication of antiretroviral therapy. *Adv Chronic Kidney Dis* 2006; 13(3):314–319.

84. Andrade ZA, Rocha H. Schistosomal glomerulopathy. *Kidney Int* 1979; 16(1):23–29.

85. Nussenzveig I, De Brito T, Carneiro CR, et al. Human Schistosoma mansoni-associated glomerulopathy in Brazil. *Nephrol Dial Transplant* 2002; 17(1):4–7.

86. Barsoum RS. Schistosomiasis and the kidney. *Semin Nephrol* 2003; 23(1):34–41.

87. Abensur H, Nussenzveig I, Saldanha LB, et al. Nephrotic syndrome associated with hepatointestinal schistosomiasis. *Rev Inst Med Trop Sao Paulo* 1992; 34(4):273–276.

88. Bassily S, Farid Z, Barsoum RS, et al. Renal biopsy in Schistosoma-Salmonella associated nephrotic syndrome. *J Trop Med Hyg* 1976; 79(11):256–258.

89. Barsoum RS, Bassily S, Baligh OK, et al. Renal disease in hepatosplenic schistosomiasis: a clinicopathological study. *Trans R Soc Trop Med Hyg* 1977; 71(5):387–391.

90. Barsoum R. The changing face of schistosomal glomerulopathy. *Kidney Int* 2004; 66(6):2472–2484.

91. Omer HO, Abdel Wahab SM. Secondary amyloidosis due to Schistosoma mansoni infection. *BMJ* 1976; 1(6006):375–377.

92. Barsoum RS, Bassily S, Soliman M, et al. Amyloidosis in hepatosplenic schistosomiasis. *Trans R Soc Trop Med Hyg* 1978; 72(2):215–216.

93. Andrade ZA, Van Marck E. Schistosomal glomerular disease (a review). *Mem Inst Oswaldo Cruz* 1984; 79(4):499–506.

94. McAdam KP, Anders RF, Smith SR, et al. Association of amyloidosis with erythema nodosum leprosum reactions and recurrent neutrophil leucocytosis in leprosy. *Lancet* 1975; 2(7935):572–573.

95. Chugh KS, Damle PB, Kaur S, et al. Renal lesions in leprosy amongst north Indian patients. *Postgrad Med J* 1983; 59(697):707–711.

96. Johny KV, Karat AB, Rao PS, et al. Glomerulonephritis in leprosy – a percutaneous renal biopsy study. *Lepr Rev* 1975; 46(1):29–37.

97. Chugh KS, Singhal PC, Tewari SC, et al. Acute glomerulonephritis associated with filariasis. *Am J Trop Med Hyg* 1978; 27(3):630–631.

98. Ngu JL, Chatelanat F, Leke R, et al. Nephropathy in Cameroon: evidence for filarial derived immune-complex pathogenesis in some cases. *Clin Nephrol* 1985; 24(3):128–134.

99. Giglioli G. Malaria and renal disease, with special reference to British Guiana. II. The effect of malaria eradication on the incidence of renal disease in British Guiana. *Ann Trop Med Parasitol* 1962; 56:225–241.

100. Giglioli G. Changes in the pattern of mortality following the eradication of hyperendemic malaria from a highly susceptible community. *Bull World Health Organ* 1972; 46(2):181–202.

101. Hendrickse RG, Adeniyi A, Edington GM, et al. Quartan malarial nephrotic syndrome. Collaborative clinicopathological study in Nigerian children. *Lancet* 1972; 1(7761):1143–1149.

102. Adeniyi A, Hendrickse RG, Houba V. Selectivity of proteinuria and response to prednisolone or immunosuppressive drugs in children with malarial nephrosis. *Lancet* 1970; 1(7648):644–648.

103. Caruana R. The patient with sickle-cell disease. In: Davison AM, Cameron JS, Grunfeld JP, et al., eds. *Oxford Textbook of Nephrology*. Oxford: Oxford University Press, 2005:879–900.

104. Falk RJ, Scheinman J, Phillips G, et al. Prevalence and pathologic features of sickle cell nephropathy and response to inhibition of angiotensin-converting enzyme. *N Engl J Med* 1992; 326(14):910–915.

105. Iskandar SS, Morgann RG, Browning MC, et al. Membranoproliferative glomerulonephritis associated with sickle cell disease in two siblings. *Clin Nephrol* 1991; 35(2):47–51.

106. Okoro BA, Okafor HU. Nephrotic syndrome in Nigerian children with homozygous sickle cell disease. *East Afr Med J* 1997; 74(12):819–821.

107. Nicholson GD. Post-streptococcal glomerulonephritis in adult Jamaicans with and without sickle cell anaemia. *West Indian Med J* 1977; 26(2):78–84.

108. Adu D. Acute renal failure in the tropics. In: Kibukamusoke JW, ed. *Tropical Nephrology*. Canberra: Citforge; 1984:199–215.

109. Anandh U, Renuka S, Somiah S, et al. Acute renal failure in the tropics: emerging trends from a tertiary care hospital in South India. *Clin Nephrol* 2003; 59(5):341–344.

110. Agarwal I, Kirubakaran C, Markandeyulu V. Clinical profile and outcome of acute renal failure in South Indian children. *J Indian Med Assoc* 2004; 102(7):353–354, 356.

111. Olowu WA, Adelusola KA. Pediatric acute renal failure in southwestern Nigeria. *Kidney Int* 2004; 66(4):1541–1548.

112. Adu D, Anim-Addo Y, Foli AK, et al. Acute renal failure in tropical Africa. *BMJ* 1976; 1(6014):890–892.

113. Jayakumar M, Prabahar MR, Fernando EM, et al. Epidemiologic trend changes in acute renal failure – a tertiary center experience from South India. *Ren Fail* 2006; 28(5):405–410.

114. Essamie MA, Soliman A, Fayad TM, et al. Serious renal disease in Egypt. *Int J Artif Organs* 1995; 18(5):254–260.

115. Strickland GT, Abdel-Wahab MF. Abdominal ultrasonography for assessing morbidity from schistosomiasis. 1. Community studies. *Trans R Soc Trop Med Hyg* 1993; 87(2):132–134.

116. El-Khoby T, Galal N, Fenwick A, et al. The epidemiology of schistosomiasis in Egypt: summary findings in nine governorates. *Am J Trop Med Hyg* 2000; 62(2 suppl):88–99.

117. Chugh KS, Singhal PC, Sharma BK, et al. Acute renal failure of obstetric origin. *Obstet Gynecol* 1976; 48(6):642–646.

118. Utas C, Yalcindag C, Taskapan H, et al. Acute renal failure in Central Anatolia. *Nephrol Dial Transplant* 2000; 15(2):152–155.

119. Owusu SK, Addy JH, Foli AK, et al. Acute reversible renal failure associated with glucose-6-phosphate-dehydrogenase deficiency. *Lancet* 1972; 1(7763):1255–1257.

120. Chugh KS, Singhal PC, Sharma BK, et al. Acute renal failure due to intravascular hemolysis in the North Indian patients. *Am J Med Sci* 1977; 274(2):139–146.

121. Lwanga D, Wing AJ. Renal complications associated with typhoid fever. *East Afr Med J* 1970; 47(3):146–152.

122. Adu D, Anim-Addo Y, Foli AK, et al. Acute renal failure and typhoid fever. *Ghana Med J* 1975; 14(3):172–174.

123. Boonpucknavig V, Sitprija V. Renal disease in acute Plasmodium falciparum infection in man. *Kidney Int* 1979; 16(1):44–52.

124. Habte B. Acute renal failure due to falciparum malaria. *Ren Fail* 1990; 12(1):15–19.

125. Krishnan A, Karnad DR. Severe falciparum malaria: an important cause of multiple organ failure in Indian intensive care unit patients. *Crit Care Med* 2003; 31(9):2278–2284.

126. Naqvi R, Ahmad E, Akhtar F, et al. Outcome in severe acute renal failure associated with malaria. *Nephrol Dial Transplant* 2003; 18(9):1820–1823.

127. Dukes DC, Sealey BJ, Forbes JI. Oliguric renal failure in blackwater fever. *Am J Med* 1968; 45(6):899–903.

128. Canfield CJ, Miller LH, Bartelloni PJ, et al. Acute renal failure in Plasmodium falciparum malaria. Treatment of peritoneal dialysis. *Arch Intern Med* 1968; 122(3):199–203.

129. Mate-Kole MO, Yeboah ED, Affram RK, et al. Blackwater fever and acute renal failure in expatriates in Africa. *Ren Fail* 1996; 18(3):525–531.

130. Eiam-Ong S, Sitprija V. Falciparum malaria and the kidney: a model of inflammation. *Am J Kidney Dis* 1998; 32(3):361–375.

131. Dondorp A, Nosten F, Stepniewska K, et al. Artesunate versus quinine for treatment of severe falciparum malaria: a randomised trial. *Lancet* 2005; 366(9487):717–725.

132. Baker NM, Mills AE, Rachman I, et al. Haemolytic-uraemic syndrome in typhoid fever. *BMJ* 1974; 2(5910):84–87.

133. Raghupathy P, Date A, Shastry JC, et al. Haemolytic-uraemic syndrome complicating shiga dysentery in south Indian children. *BMJ* 1978; 1(6126):1518–1521.

134. Bhuyan UN, Srivastava RN, Choudhry VP. Pathology of acute renal failure and haemolytic uraemic syndrome in acute dysentery in children. *Indian J Med Res* 1985; 81:402–408.

135. Srivastava RN, Moudgil A, Bagga A, et al. Hemolytic uremic syndrome in children in northern India. *Pediatr Nephrol* 1991; 5(3):284–288.

136. Tzipori S, Sheoran A, Akiyoshi D, et al. Antibody therapy in the management of shiga toxin-induced hemolytic uremic syndrome. *Clin Microbiol Rev* 2004; 17(4):926–941, table of contents.

137. Benyajati C, Keoplug M, Beisel WR, et al. Acute renal failure in Asiatic cholera: clinicopathologic correlations with acute tubular necrosis and hypokalemic nephropathy. *Ann Intern Med* 1960; 52:960–975.

138. Visith S, Kearkiat P. Nephropathy in leptospirosis. *J Postgrad Med* 2005; 51(3):184–188.

139. Covic A, Goldsmith DJ, Gusbeth-Tatomir P, et al. A retrospective 5-year study in Moldova of acute renal failure due to leptospirosis: 58 cases and a review of the literature. *Nephrol Dial Transplant* 2003; 18(6):1128–1134.

140. Daher EF, Nogueira CB. Evaluation of penicillin therapy in patients with leptospirosis and acute renal failure. *Rev Inst Med Trop Sao Paulo* 2000; 42(6):327–332.

141. Tewodros W, Muhe L, Daniel E, et al. A one-year study of streptococcal infections and their complications among Ethiopian children. *Epidemiol Infect* 1992; 109(2):211–225.

142. Srivastava RN, Bagga A, Moudgil A. Acute renal failure in north Indian children. *Indian J Med Res* 1990; 92:404–408.

143. Shibolet S, Coll R, Gilat T, et al. Heatstroke: its clinical picture and mechanism in 36 cases. *Q J Med* 1967; 36(144):525–548.

144. Susaengrat W, Dhiensiri T, Sinavatana P, et al. Renal failure in melioidosis. *Nephron* 1987; 46(2):167–169.

145. McGain F, Limbo A, Williams DJ, et al. Snakebite mortality at Port Moresby General Hospital, Papua New Guinea, 1992–2001. *Med J Aust* 2004; 181 (11–12):687–691.

146. Chugh KS, Pal Y, Chakravarty RN, et al. Acute renal failure following poisonous snakebite. *Am J Kidney Dis* 1984; 4(1):30–38.

147. Luyckx VA, Steenkamp V, Stewart MJ. Acute renal failure associated with the use of traditional folk remedies in South Africa. *Ren Fail* 2005; 27(1): 35–43.

148. Kallel H, Chelly H, Dammak H, et al. Clinical manifestations of systemic paraphenylene diamine intoxication. *J Nephrol* 2005; 18(3):308–311.

149. Te Loo DM, van Hinsbergh VW, van den Heuvel LP, et al. Detection of verocytotoxin bound to circulating polymorphonuclear leukocytes of patients with hemolytic uremic syndrome. *J Am Soc Nephrol* 2001; 12(4):800–806.

150. Wong CS, Jelacic S, Habeeb RL, et al. The risk of the hemolytic-uremic syndrome after antibiotic treatment of Escherichia coli O157:H7 infections. *N Engl J Med* 2000; 342(26):1930–1936.

151. Matekole M, Affram K, Lee SJ, et al. Hypertension and end-stage renal failure in tropical Africa. *J Hum Hypertens* 1993; 7(5):443–446.

152. Diouf B, Ka EF, Niang A, et al. Etiologies of chronic renal insufficiency in an adult internal medicine service in Dakar. *Dakar Med* 2000; 45(1):62–65.

153. Naicker S. End-stage renal disease in sub-Saharan and South Africa. *Kidney Int Suppl* 2003; (83):S119–S122.

154. Sakhuja V, Sud K. End-stage renal disease in India and Pakistan: burden of disease and management issues. *Kidney Int Suppl* 2003; (83):S115–S118.

155. Barsoum RS. End-stage renal disease in North Africa. *Kidney Int Suppl* 2003; (83):S111–S114.

156. Sitprija V. Nephrology in South East Asia: fact and concept. *Kidney Int Suppl* 2003; (83):S128–S130.

157. Santa Cruz F, Cabrera W, Barreto S, et al. Kidney disease in Paraguay. *Kidney Int Suppl* 2005; (97): S120–S125.

158. Cooper RS, Wolf-Maier K, Luke A, et al. An international comparative study of blood pressure in populations of European vs. African descent. *BMC Med* 2005; 3:2.

159. Clase CM, Garg AX, Kiberd BA. Prevalence of low glomerular filtration rate in nondiabetic Americans: Third National Health and Nutrition Examination Survey (NHANES III). *J Am Soc Nephrol* 2002; 13(5):1338–1349.

160. Hillege HL, Janssen WM, Bak AA, et al. Microalbuminuria is common, also in a nondiabetic, nonhypertensive population, and an independent indicator of cardiovascular risk factors and cardiovascular morbidity. *J Intern Med* 2001; 249(6):519–526.

161. Remuzzi G, Bertani T. Pathophysiology of progressive nephropathies. *N Engl J Med* 1998; 339(20):1448–1456.

162. Ruggenenti P, Perna A, Mosconi L, et al. Proteinuria predicts end-stage renal failure in non-diabetic chronic nephropathies. The 'Gruppo Italiano di Studi Epidemiologici in Nefrologia' (GISEN). *Kidney Int Suppl* 1997; 63:S54–S57.

163. Lewis EJ, Hunsicker LG, Bain RP, et al. The effect of angiotensin-converting-enzyme inhibition on diabetic nephropathy. The Collaborative Study Group. *N Engl J Med* 1993; 329(20):1456–1462.

164. GISEN. Randomised placebo-controlled trial of effect of ramipril on decline in glomerular filtration rate and risk of terminal renal failure in proteinuric, non-diabetic nephropathy. The GISEN Group (Gruppo Italiano di Studi Epidemiologici in Nefrologia). *Lancet* 1997; 349(9069):1857–1863.

165. Lewis EJ, Hunsicker LG, Clarke WR, et al. Renoprotective effect of the angiotensin-receptor antagonist irbesartan in patients with nephropathy due to type 2 diabetes. *N Engl J Med* 2001; 345(12):851–860.

166. Brenner BM, Cooper ME, de Zeeuw D, et al. Effects of losartan on renal and cardiovascular outcomes in patients with type 2 diabetes and nephropathy. *N Engl J Med* 2001; 345(12):861–869.

167. Ruggenenti P, Perna A, Loriga G, et al. Blood-pressure control for renoprotection in patients with non-diabetic chronic renal disease (REIN-2): multicentre, randomised controlled trial. *Lancet* 2005; 365(9463):939–946.

168. Hou FF, Zhang X, Zhang GH, et al. Efficacy and safety of benazepril for advanced chronic renal insufficiency. *N Engl J Med* 2006; 354(2):131–140.

169. Klahr S, Levey AS, Beck GJ, et al. The effects of dietary protein restriction and blood-pressure control on the progression of chronic renal disease. Modification of Diet in Renal Disease Study Group. *N Engl J Med* 1994; 330(13):877–884.

170. Jones-Burton C, Mishra SI, Fink JC, et al. An in-depth review of the evidence linking dietary salt intake and progression of chronic kidney disease. *Am J Nephrol* 2006; 26(3):268–275.

171. DCCT. The absence of a glycemic threshold for the development of long-term complications: the perspective of the Diabetes Control and Complications Trial. *Diabetes* 1996; 45(10):1289–1298.

172. Stratton IM, Adler AI, Neil HA, et al. Association of glycaemia with macrovascular and microvascular complications of type 2 diabetes (UKPDS 35): prospective observational study. *BMJ* 2000; 321(7258):405–412.

173. KDOQI. KDOQI clinical practice guidelines for bone metabolism and disease in chronic kidney disease. *Am J Kidney Dis* 2003; 42(4, suppl 3):S1–201.

174. KDOQI. KDOQI clinical practice guidelines and clinical practice recommendations for anemia in chronic kidney disease. *Am J Kidney Dis* 2006; 47(5, suppl 3):S11–145.

175. Macdougall IC. Recent advances in erythropoietic agents in renal anemia. *Semin Nephrol* 2006; 26(4):313–318.

176. Eastwood JB, Corbishley CM, Grange JM. Tuberculosis and the kidney. *J Am Soc Nephrol* 2001; 12(6):1307–1314.

177. Robertson W. *Urolithiasis: Epidemiology and Pathogenesis.* In: Hussain I, ed. Edinburgh: Churchill Livingstone; 1984:143–164.

178. Kardorff R, Traore M, Doehring-Schwerdtfeger E, et al. Ultrasonography of ureteric abnormalities induced by Schistosoma haematobium infection before and after praziquantel treatment. *Br J Urol* 1994; 74(6):703–709.

179. Vester U, Kardorff R, Traore M, et al. Urinary tract morbidity due to Schistosoma haematobium infection in Mali. *Kidney Int* 1997; 52(2):478–481.

Chapter 16

Masharip Atadzhanov

Tropical Neurology

INTRODUCTION

Applying equally to other chapters in this book is the problem of a comprehensive yet pragmatic definition of tropical medicine – for which there appears to be no simple resolution. Even the nineteenth-century rubric – those diseases which prevail between the tropics of Cancer and Capricorn – was unsatisfactory because illnesses such as cholera, typhoid, typhus and malaria occurred widely in Europe until the beginning of the twentieth century. Now, when speed and facility of travel can dramatically influence presentation of disease, definitions must be appropriately elastic. No doubt controversy will continue concerning a more suitable, precise and contemporary name for this specialty. Maurice King's term 'the medicine of poverty' is probably as succinct as can be presently contrived – to embrace afflictions arising from primitive social conditions, malnutrition, high population growth, ignorance of 'overly traditional societies', high infant mortality rates and low life expectation, all fundamentally determined by major factors beyond the powers of physicians; only the economist, engineer, agriculturalist and those who can alter the distribution of global wealth can make a significant impact.

Tropical neurology encompasses a wide range of infectious and non-infectious clinical presentations. It is not limited to bizarre manifestations of viral, bacterial and parasitic infections, but also reflects the expression of many non-infectious diseases in a particular environment where malnutrition, trauma, perinatal injury, cerebrovascular, degenerative, and genetic diseases tend to show patterns of twentieth-century Western proportions; 'younger' societies may show different disease distributions. These are among the many factors that must be taken into consideration when assessing and comparing epidemiological surveys. Consider, for example, epilepsy: this is a major neurological disorder in the tropics and has important medical and social implications (Table 16.1).[1] Attempts to determine accurately the magnitude of the problem have encountered considerable difficulties, including differences in definition and methods of case detection. It is therefore difficult to determine what significance should be attributed to the reported relatively low prevalence in India and the fact that certain regions of Africa and Latin America have a very high prevalence, sometimes as much as 10 times the average for industrialized countries. It would appear that rural prevalence is lower than in urban areas, partial seizures more common than primary generalized ones and mortality rates for epilepsy appear to be higher in tropical countries in comparison to those in industrialized areas. Known aetiological factors present a bewildering spectrum.[2] Cysticercosis accounts for about half the cases of epilepsy of late onset in several countries. Other parasitic infections known to cause epilepsy include schistosomiasis, paragonimiasis, sparganosis, hydatid disease, toxoplasmosis, trypanosomiasis, cerebral malaria, cerebral amoebiasis and *Gnathostoma spinigerum*. Tuberculous, pyogenic, viral and fungal infections can also cause epilepsy as a late sequel as well as being a feature of the acute illness. Poor antenatal and perinatal care resulting in perinatal brain damage probably contributes to a higher prevalence. Despite these problems there have been impressive attempts to sharpen the epidemiological profile of epilepsy. Thus a recent survey[3] of a rural area in South Tanzania showed the active epilepsy prevalence in a rural African population. The study confirmed a pattern toward higher prevalence of epilepsy in tropical countries compared to Western countries. The authors observed a higher prevalence of epilepsy in children and adolescents, followed by a steady decline with increasing age. The epidemic of human immunodeficiency virus (HIV) has had significant effect on the epidemiology, clinical and pathological presentation of epilepsy. New-onset seizures are frequent manifestations of the central nervous system (CNS) disorders in patients infected with HIV.[4] In some patients the HIV infection itself may be the cause of the seizure.[5]

On September 2005 the world's population reached an estimated 6.5 billion[6] and by the year 2050 is likely to be 9.3 billion. 'The growth of the earth's population has been like a long thin powder fuse that burns slowly and haltingly until it finally reaches the charge and explodes' (Kingsley Davis). To this potential explosion must be added the impact of global environmental change[7] on disease patterns.[8] Thus the effects of global warming on the distribution of parasitic and other infectious diseases – disequilibrium in physical and biological ecosystems – and the potential impact of climate changes on world food supply indicate that the developing countries are likely to bear the brunt of the problem. The disparity between developed and developing countries may become even more conspicuous. Famine is as old as humanity and 'tropical diseases' and their neurological complications are likely to increase. The past three decades

Table 16.1 Causes of fits/convulsions

Infections
Meningitis
Encephalitis
HIV/AIDS
Cerebral malaria
Tuberculous meningitis/tuberculoma
Neurocysticerosis
Schistosomiasis
Cerebral hydatid diseases
Paragonimiasis
Cerebral toxoplasmosis
Cerebral amoebiasis
Tetanus (pseudoepilepsy)
Alcohol
Trauma (cerebral concussion, contusion, laceration, extradural or intracerebral haemorrhage)
Cerebrovascular accident (thrombosis, haemorrhage, embolism)
Aneurysm
Metabolic (hypoglycaemia, hyperglycaemia, insulinoma, uraemia)
Drugs (opiates, overdose)
Space-occupying lesions (primary and secondary tumours, cysts, abscesses, tuberculoma, hydatid)
Hydrocephalus

have seen the rapid spread of the HIV epidemic throughout the tropics and neurological manifestations of infection with HIV are common.

NUTRITIONAL AND TOXIC FACTORS

The clinical features of the major classical nutritional disorders of the central and peripheral nervous systems are well known, as is the importance of the vitamin B complex for the development and functioning of the nervous system. Thus beriberi ('I can't, I can't', depicting profound weakness), usually due to the discarded germinal layer of polished rice, presents clinically in the wet or dry form: the salient neurological features are painful polyneuropathy with tender calves and sensitive soles. Pellagra, due to a similar dietary deficiency mainly involving the nicotinic acid obtained in white maize, presents clinically – often in endemic spring attacks – with diarrhoea, a light-sensitive erythematous rash progressing to thickening and atrophy with glossitis, diplopia, dysarthria, myelopathy and neuropathy with psychological and behavioural changes. Wernicke's encephalopathy may be acute or insidious, with vomiting, nystagmus, diplopia, confusion, ophthalmoplegia, retinal haemorrhages, polyneuropathy, and a dramatic Korsakoff's syndrome with amnesia and confabulation. Alcoholism is the most frequent predisposing factor for Wernicke's encephalopathy. High levels of alcohol consumption and abuse were found in some tropical countries.[9] The effects of excessive alcohol consumption, and its relationship to current neurological practice, are

a potentially important area of future research in these countries. It will be appreciated that even in communities known to be thiamine deficient from the consumption of processed rice, or in maize-eating populations known to be vulnerable to pellagra from niacin deficiency, it is common to see the consequences of the lack of thiamine, pyridoxine and niacin and perhaps also pantothenic acid in combination, necessitating appropriate blunderbuss therapy. The manner in which thiamine depletion produces neurological disorders is unknown.

It will also be appreciated that there are numerous local and usually well-recognized (yet to appear in classical textbooks) nutritional syndromes. For example, among certain hill tribes in north-east Burma it is traditional for women to consume only polished rice while pregnant; their infants may develop an unusual pattern of beriberi with congestive heart failure, hepatosplenomegaly and aphonia due to bilateral recurrent laryngeal nerve lesions which respond promptly to parenteral pyridoxine. Strachan's syndrome (visual failure, painful neuropathy and oral, perianal and scrotal dermatitis and ulceration) has been described in several parts of the world and is another probable consequence of multiple nutritional deficiencies including riboflavin, thiamine, niacin and pyridoxine. The painful burning feet described in prisoner-of-war camps was probably another example of multiple nutritional deficiency.

Clinically and epidemiologically it is often difficult to separate the consequences of nutritional deficiency from environmental toxins because they tend to occur in similar settings and the manifestations may be indistinguishable. The problem is further compounded by increasing quantities of chemicals, often indiscriminately used in industry and agriculture as well as medicine. Toxic pesticides merit particular attention and many of the hazards arise from the lack of precautions and facilities for handling and storing these neurotoxic products safely.

The peripheral nervous system is commonly affected and has been frequently studied because it is easier to recognize clinically and to investigate electrodiagnostically and by nerve biopsy. While the pathophysiology may vary according to the putative toxin, distal axonal degeneration – so-called 'dying back' phenomenon[10] – is the most common mechanism; initially, longer or larger nerve fibres are involved, then degeneration begins in the distal regions of the nerve fibres, progressing proximally with time. However, mechanisms are probably more complex: experimental evidence suggests that many toxic agents act at the level of the axon rather than the cell body,[11] impairing axonal transport; others may disturb anabolic mechanisms in the region of the neuronal perikaryon. Whatever the precise mechanism, clinical features are similar. Early symptoms are usually sensory with paraesthesiae, suprasensitivity, hyperalgesia and pain, followed later by peripheral weakness and wasting. Impairment of tendon reflexes occurs early and all sensory modalities may be variably affected. Some have associated myelopathic disturbances with spasticity and extensor plantar responses. Involvement of the autonomic nervous system with defective sweating and vasomotor disturbances commonly occurs.

The list of known aetiological agents is legion (Table 16.2). Heavy metals such as arsenic, lead and thallium are often found in traditional folklore medications.[12] For example, arsenical polyneuropathy (acute, or more commonly chronic) occurs very widely. Acute symptoms may include vomiting, diarrhoea, burning

Table 16.2 Causes of neuropathy/weakness

INFECTIONS
Leprosy
HIV
Spinal schistosomiasis
Spinal tuberculosis
Spinal brucellosis
Tropical spastic paraparesis (HTLV-1)
Postinfectious ascending neuropathy (Guillain-Barré syndrome)
Diphtheria
Botulism
METABOLIC
Diabetes mellitus
Uraemia
Amyloidosis
Porphyria
TOXINS/METALS
Ciguatera fish
Snake (see Chapter 31)
Cassava (cyanide)
Lathyrism and cycad poisoning (plant toxins)
Heavy metals (lead, arsenic, thallium)
NUTRITIONAL DEFICIENCIES
Vitamin B complex
Vitamin B_{12} deficiency (subacute combined degeneration of spinal cord)
Thiamine (beriberi, alcoholism)
Nicotinic acid (pellagra)
Pyridoxine deficiency
DRUGS/CHEMICALS
Isoniazid, nitrofurantoin, vincristine, chloroquine
MECHANICAL
Trauma, compression, stretching
MISCELLANEOUS
Sarcoidosis
Rheumatoid arthritis
Malignancy
Hereditary neuropathies

discomfort in the eyes, excessive tears, photophobia, congestion and facial swelling, followed by a predominantly sensory neuropathy. Mees' lines (transverse white bands across the fingernails) frequently occur, as does increased pigmentation of the extremities with patches of depigmentation, hyperkeratosis and desquamation of palms and soles. Here the diagnosis may be confirmed, if facilities permit, by demonstrating high concentrations of arsenic in scalp hairs and nail clippings. Illicit liquor,

crude abortifacients and well water deliberately contaminated by an enemy have all been reported.[13] It will also be recalled that certain ocean fish and marine crustacea, such as the pomfret, plaice, halua and hilsa, may contain relatively high concentrations of arsenic. Another source of arsenical poisoning is said to be contaminated opium. The mechanism is thought to be direct reaction of arsenical compounds with the sulfhydryl group of proteins; electrophysiologically the signs of distal axonal degeneration and nerve biopsies show loss of myelinated fibres and degeneration of myelin into rows of myelin ovoids;[14] segmental demyelination and inflammatory changes do not occur. In the acute stages dimercaprol and/or penicillamine must be given early; when there is a delay, response may be poor.

Lead may cause a peripheral neuropathy in adults and an encephalopathy in children. Lead neuropathy tends to be predominantly motor, more evident in the upper limbs where the extensors of the wrists and fingers are affected early and asymmetrically, tending to affect the dominant hand.[15] Proximal involvement is slow and occurs later, and sensory disturbances are minimal or absent. Associated abdominal colic and the characteristic anaemia with punctate basophilia, when present, may suggest the diagnosis. Potential sources include reconditioning of car batteries and burning lead-containing batteries for cooking, illicit liquor distillation by means of lead pipes or radiators, and contaminated water.

Thallium may induce both neuropathy and encephalopathy. The acute painful neuropathy may be associated with gastrointestinal symptoms – non specific signs – but the occurrence of alopecia within 3 weeks should suggest the diagnosis.[16] Potassium ferrocyanide, given orally, is the present treatment of choice.

Of the many conventional medications that may provoke peripheral neuropathy brief mention will be made of those drugs widely used in the treatment of tropical bacterial and parasitic infections. Peripheral neuropathy, particularly in those genetically disposed to slow acetylation of isoniazid for the treatment of tuberculosis, is well known, as is the similar hazard of ethionamide, from sulfonamides widely used in bacillary dysentery and urinary tract infections; similarly the optic neuritis related to ethambutol. Chloroquine, a standard antimalarial agent, may produce a neuromyopathy after prolonged use, with muscle fibres showing vacuolation and peripheral nerves showing involvement of terminal axons with Schwann cell defects.[17] Clioquinol – previously widely used in the symptomatic treatment of diarrhoea and intestinal amoebiasis – is now known to be the causative agent of subacute myelo-optic neuropathy;[18] unfortunately clioquinol continues to be prescribed in certain countries and the complication is still sporadically encountered. The aromatic diamidines used in the treatment of leishmaniasis and trypanosomiasis have been associated with an odd, uncommon focal disturbance of sensory function of the trigeminal nerve.

Industrial chemicals of known potential neurotoxicity rarely cause hazards in developed societies; it is where appropriate safety measures and conditions are not practised that outbreaks continue to occur. Accidental contamination of food, particularly edible oils, may produce not only classical peripheral mixed neuropathy, but also signs of cord involvement. Unfortunately, the damage is permanent and there is no curative or generally available protective agent. In unprotected environments, carbon disulfide and acrylamide may produce similar hazards. Insecticides widely dispensed in tropical countries are a common cause. The most common culprit is the group of organophosphorus insecticides;[19] the defect is believed to be mainly at the postsynaptic border of the neuromuscular junction. Clinically the onset may be acute or delayed.

Particularly well documented in recent years are the toxic effects of the root crop cassava, a major crop sustaining millions of people in Africa.[20] Flour made from cassava roots may contain a high concentration of linamarin, a cyanogenic glycoside, resulting in chronic cyanide intoxication and clinically 'tropical ataxic neuropathy'. The clinical features in addition to painful neuropathy and ataxia may include blurred vision and impaired hearing of cochlear type; occasionally upper motor neurone lesions are seen. This pattern of illness is usually slowly progressive.

Konzo is a clinically distinct pattern of the abrupt onset of non-progressive spastic paraparesis caused by long-term intake of cassava.[21] It has been reported that linamarin is enzymatically converted to cyanide by bacteria in the intestine, and this is absorbed into the blood and then damages neural cells. However, a recent study[22] was able to confirm that linamarin can directly damage neural culture pheochromocytoma cells. Additional 10 µM-cytochalasin B, an inhibitor of a glucose transporter, prevented cell death. These results suggest that linamarin competes with cytochalasin B and glucose for binding to a glucose transporter and enters into cells via glucose transporter.

Lathyrism and cycad poisoning are two other well-known examples of neurotoxic plant poisons affecting the CNS. Lathyrism, endemic in parts of India, Bangladesh and Ethiopia, is caused by excessive consumption of peas of the lathyrus family (chickpeas). It presents as a slowly progressive spastic paraparesis: neuropathological studies have shown selective atrophy of the pyramidal, spinocerebellar and dorsal columns of the spinal cord. The neurotoxin is an amino acid b-N-oxalylamino-L-alanine, which is thought to act by excessive and prolonged exhaustion stimulation – a so-called excitatory amino acid. Once damage has occurred there is no effective treatment. In a similar manner excessive consumption of the seed of the false-sago palm – either as a foodstuff or as a medicinal component – may have an excitatory neurotoxic effect and may be one of the constellation of factors responsible for the occurrence of amyotrophic lateral sclerosis and Parkinsonism-dementia complex in the Pacific Mariana Islands.[23]

Rarer plant toxins include that of *Gloriosa superba* (glory lily):[24] accidental ingestion may cause alopecia, aplastic anaemia and polyneuropathy due to colchicine, which impairs exoplasmic transport in peripheral nerves and also damages skeletal muscle. Podophyllin (from the dried rhizome and root of the mandrake) also has neurotoxic properties. A report from Hong Kong[25] described encephalopathy and sensorimotor polyneuropathy and autonomic changes after ingestion of a broth containing herbal *guijiu*. Another poisonous shrub of the buckthorn family (*Karwinskia humboldtiana*), which grows freely in Mexico and Texas, may cause a progressive polyneuropathy, terminating in respiratory and bulbar paralysis.[26]

All these essentially irreversible and disabling toxic disturbances of the central, autonomic and peripheral nervous systems are preventable and presumably will continue to be observed and reported in the developing world until nutritional, economic and educational disparities are resolved.

CNS INFECTIONS

The variety of infectious agents which can damage the nervous system is vast and their clinical manifestations are protean. Table 16.3 lists those which cause meningitis and encephalitis, and Table 16.4 lists infectious and non-infectious causes of decreased consciousness and confusion. Symptoms related to CNS infections are (a) headache, (b) fever, (c) irritability, (d) confusion, (e) photophobia, (f) vomiting, (g) deteriorating consciousness levels and (h) fits; in addition, children may have listlessness and failure to feed.

In addition to the general predisposing factors mentioned above – poverty, ignorance, deprivation, inadequate education – is the prevalence and persistence of insect and other vectors which

Table 16.3 Causes of meningitis and encephalitis

MENINGITIS
Bacterial
Neisseria meningitidis
Streptococcus pneumoniae
Haemophilus influenzae
Mycobacterium tuberculosis
Listeria monocytogenes
Escherichia coli
Brucella spp.
Viral
Enterovirus (polio, echo, Coxsackie)
Mumps virus
HIV (also *Cryptococcus neoformans* in AIDS)
Protozoal
Amoebae (*Naegleria fowleri*, Acanthamoebae)
Helminths
Strongyloides stercoralis (hyperinfection syndrome)
Angiostrongylus cantonensis
Gnathostoma spp.
ENCEPHALITIS
Acute
Arboviruses
Herpes simplex
Measles
Chickenpox
Yellow fever
Rabies
Trichinella spiralis
Subacute/chronic
African trypanosomiasis
AIDS (cryptococcal, toxoplasmosis)
Rickettsia spp.
Kuru

Table 16.4 Confusion/decreased consciousness level

Infective	Non-infective
Meningitis	Drugs/alcohol/herbal
Encephalitis	medicines
Cerebral malaria	Dehydration
AIDS (e.g. HIV encephalopathy)	Liver failure (acute
Viral haemorrhagic fevers, e.g.	fulminant hepatitis)
dengue	Hypoglycaemia (e.g. in
Legionnaires' disease	malaria)
Leptospirosis	Hypertensive stroke
Typhus	Head injury
Relapsing fever	Renal failure
Septicaemia	Psychiatric illness
Rabies	(hysterical conversion)
Neurocysticercosis	

thrive in humid climates and which survive throughout the seasons. In a limited review it is possible to indicate only certain salient clinical features of some of these numerous disorders, which will be discussed under conventional categories.

Viruses

The acute exanthemas of childhood – measles, mumps and chickenpox – are still major killers, especially when epidemics occur in the presence of severe malnutrition (see also Chapters 20, 23, 47 and 48). The clinical scene and the therapeutic possibilities have changed considerably in recent years. Thus acute poliomyelitis (see below) is now rarely seen – an impressive example of the power of truly effective preventive medicine. Similarly, subacute sclerosing panencephalitis (SSPE) is disappearing in many parts of the world where measles vaccination is available, but is still relatively common and fatal in many parts of the Middle East, Far East, India, Africa and South America; racial and ethnic factors have been implicated. Recently started studies genetic evolution of mutated measles virus called SSPE virus isolated from brain tissues of a patient.[27,28] The introduction of therapy with intraventricular interferon alpha and its later association with ribavirin aroused new expectations.[29]

Acute viral encephalitis

Acute viral encephalitis, due to direct invasion of the brain parenchyma, is indistinguishable clinically from the postinfectious encephalitides where perivenous demyelination is probably triggered by allergic or immune reactions caused by a latent viral infection. Globally, viruses are by far the most common cause of encephalitis. The arboviruses cause epidemic encephalitides in many parts of the world. The majority is perpetuated by zoonoses, often inconspicuous infections obtained from birds and smaller vertebrates; transmission is by an arthropod vector such as a mosquito or tick. After replication and viraemia, encephalitis of unpredictable gravity develops. Many patients recover spontaneously after a mild attack; others may deteriorate and die within days or weeks. The clinical features are common to all: prodromal myalgia, fever and malaise, then headache, mental changes, drowsiness, with or without signs of meningeal irritation; focal neurological

abnormalities such as disturbances of behaviour, mood, disorientation, deterioration of speech, level of consciousness, fits (focal or generalized), raised intracranial pressure and a deepening coma. Even when sophisticated diagnostic neuroimaging techniques such as computed tomography (CT) or magnetic resonance imaging (MRI) are available, there may be no specific features and the EEG and cerebrospinal fluid (CSF) may not be diagnostically helpful. The demonstration of sequential changes in antibody titre in samples of serum or CSF may be the only means of establishing the true agent in sporadic cases and usually the illness has taken its course by the time the agent is confirmed.

Eastern equine encephalitis

Eastern equine encephalitis – mainly on the Atlantic and Gulf coasts of America – tends to occur in summer and autumn and the mortality may be as high as 70%;[30] Western equine encephalitis, which despite its name occurs throughout the USA and eastern South America, tends to be less severe.

Japanese encephalitis (JE) is a mosquito-borne arboviral infection which still claims many lives in South-east Asia. The virus is antigenically related to the flaviviruses of St Louis encephalitis and Murray Valley encephalitis and to the West Nile virus. The illness is usually severe, and fatal in about 25% of cases, with neuropsychiatric sequelae in a further 30%. It mainly affects the young, but a shift now to the elderly may be due to early immunization. CT and MRI show thalamic involvement (Figure 16.1). Recently it was shown that a single dose of SA 14-14-2 vaccine was 98.5% effective 12–15 months after vaccination.[31] Sporadic and epidemic attacks of encephalitis continue to be reported from different parts of the world and often the reasons for these fluctuations remain obscure. For example, Rift Valley fever (RVF) caused two simultaneous outbreaks in Yemen and Saudi Arabia in 2000, 2001. Clinical features included fever, nausea, vomiting, abdominal pain, diarrhoea, jaundice, encephalitis, haemorrhagic manifestations, symptoms of renal failure, retinitis and uveitis. Haemorrhagic fever, encephalitis and jaundice were independently associated with a high mortality rate.[32] In spite of the danger of the virus, neither veterinary nor human vaccines are available, although a RVF virus reverse genetics system is developing.

Poliomyelitis

The progress of the Polio Eradication Programme has encountered a number of hurdles in the past 2 years as the virus has spread from northern Nigeria across much of central Africa and into the Middle East and as far as Indonesia.[33] An outbreak of polio in the northern Indian states, which started in 2005, quadrupled in 2006. Moreover, by mid-September 2006, cases of polio were confirmed in Angola, Bangladesh, Congo, Nigeria, and Nepal.

Cases of vaccine-associated paralytic polio led to a switch from the oral polio vaccine (OPV) to inactivated vaccine (IPV) in Canada, USA, most European countries and New Zealand. However, Huang and colleagues[34] recommend doing studies on vaccine virus persistence in tropical, developing countries where transmission of OPV viruses is likely to be more intense. They conclude that the findings of such studies are vital to formulate polio immunization policies in the post-certification era.

Wild poliovirus-causing disease is still a problem in small pockets of individuals in Western Europe who, for religious

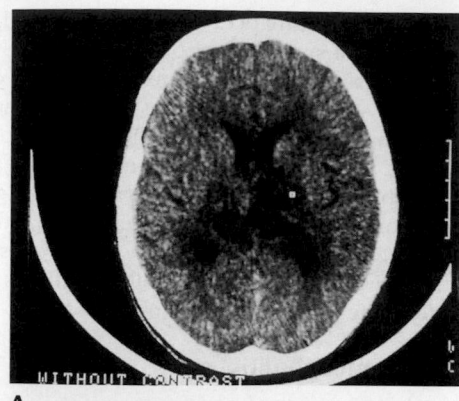

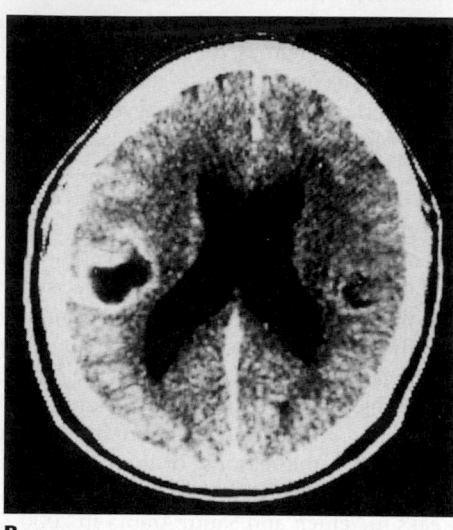

Figure 16.1 Japanese encephalitis. Brain scan (A) before and (B) after contrast showing thalamic lesions. (Courtesy of M. Gourie-Devi, National Institute of Mental Health and Neurosciences, Bangalore, India.)

reasons, refuse vaccination, as exemplified by the 1992 outbreak in Holland. Apparent outbreaks are still reported worldwide.[35,36]

Dengue

Dengue, especially the haemorrhagic variety, still causes considerable morbidity and fatality in South-east Asia, and yellow fever similarly in Africa and South America. Dengue virus is a flavivirus transmitted by the bite of the mosquito. Three distinct neurological syndromes have been reported during dengue infection: (1) Acute non-specific neurological symptoms (headache, retrobulbar pain, mood change, etc.). (2) Acute encephalitic or focal neurological symptoms (spastic paraparesis, seizures, mono-or polyneuropathy, etc.). (3) Post-infectious neurological complications (transverse myelitis, mononeuropathies).[37]

Lassa fever

Lassa fever, an acute haemorrhagic febrile illness occurring in West Africa, carries a fatality of up to 20%. It is caused by an arenavirus spread by a rodent (*Mastomys natalensis*) and causes a wide spec-

trum of clinical disease, from asymptomatic or trivial malaise to fatal illness, and is often associated with neurological manifestations during the acute disease or in early convalescence. Delirium, convulsions and coma occur in critically ill patients; deafness may occur towards the end of an acute illness and is believed to be the result of cochlear nerve damage. The importance of metabolic encephalopathy, severe tremor, self-limiting encephalitis, late ataxia and subacute or chronic neuropsychiatric sequelae has been emphasized.[38]

Rabies

Rabies is an acute, progressive, fatal encephalitis caused by viruses in the family Rhabdoviridae, genus *Lyssavirus*. Rabies is transmitted usually by saliva from infected bites of dogs, foxes, bats and others.[39] It remains a public-health threat in many parts of the world. After its onset, the disease presents as encephalitis (in 80%) with hydrophobia or a paralytic syndrome (in 20%), the outcome of which is always fatal and causes 30 000–70 000 deaths yearly, worldwide.[40] Whereas vaccines derived from cell cultures are now much safer and more effective than animal-derived preparations, effective and less expensive reduced dose post-exposure vaccination regimens have helped eliminate nerve tissue vaccines in Thailand, Philippines and Sri Lanka. India and Pakistan, the major users of dangerous nerve tissue-derived Semple type vaccine, are now considering following suit.[41] A cost analysis study of the system of oral vaccination implemented in France demonstrated that it is beneficial compared to the traditional expenses of rabies control. However, if dog and other animals rabies control is possible by vaccination and population control, if oral vaccination demonstrated its potential to eliminate rabies from terrestrial wildlife reservoir, it is unrealistic today to clear lyssaviruses from bats, while bat rabies is a growing concern for both public and animal health.[42] Srinivasan et al. recently reported on the transmission of 'bat' rabies virus from an organ donor to transplant recipients.[43]

HIV

About 65 million people globally are living with HIV/AIDS. The UN announced that almost 5 million people in the world were newly infected by HIV in 2005. A total of 25–28 million people with HIV live in sub-Saharan Africa and it is changing the face of tropical medicine. One-third of HIV-infected patients have at least one neurological complication. It is well known that all parts of the CNS, peripheral nerves and roots and muscles may be involved in the course of HIV infection.[44] However, HIV can have an impact on the nervous system in many ways, due to HIV itself, secondary viral infection, non-viral infection, neoplasms, cerebrovascular disease and complications related to antiretroviral treatment. It is not easy to create a simplified classification system of all neurological complications of HIV infection. One of the most useful classified complication systems is according to the degree of advancement of HIV disease: early, moderately advanced and advanced.[45] The introduction of highly actively antiretroviral therapy (HAART) has had a significant impact on epidemiology and the neurological manifestations of HIV infection and poses new challenges in diagnosis and treatment. HAART can stop or reduce the process of destruction of the immune system induced by the virus, but cannot protect the brain from HIV. Preliminary data indicate that the brain may serve as a long-term reservoir for the virus, and neuroinflammatory and neurodegenerative changes may continue despite HAART.[46] Lawn et al. recently described immune reconstitution inflammatory syndrome (IRIS) which results from the rapid restoration of immune function.[47] IRIS is an increasingly recognized complication of the initial weeks of HAART. HAART has also changed the incidence rates of neurological diseases and disorders; becoming mild, readily treatable or reversible or becoming less common. In our experience neurological manifestations of HIV/AIDS at the University Teaching Hospital (Lusaka) have changed in pattern and incidence during the last 6 years. In particular, the incidence of cryptococcal meningitis and cerebral toxoplasmosis decreased, whereas the incidence of primary CNS lymphoma (Figure 16.2) and stroke (Figure 16.3) has increased.

Human T lymphotropic virus

The human T lymphotropic virus (HTLV)-1 was discovered in the USA, and published in 1980, followed closely by the discovery of HTLV-2. HTLV-1 is a human retrovirus and its dominant modes of transmission are blood-borne, sexual and mother-to-child. The geographical distribution of the virus shows Japan, Africa, the Caribbean Islands and South America emerging as the areas of highest prevalence.[48] HTLV-1-associated myelopathy appears to correspond to human migrations that preceded recent European expansion. This suggests an ancient source. There are 3 types of HTLV-1 viruses based on envelope sequencing: 'cosmopolitan', 'central African' and 'Australo-melanesian'.[49]

Only a small proportion of the individuals carrying the virus show signs of HTLV-1-associated myelopathy. HTLV-1 is the aetiological agent for HTLV-1-associated myelopathy/tropical spastic paraparesis (HAM/TSP) and adult T cell leukaemia/lymphoma (ATL). HAM/TSP appears in children and adults, but more often age of onset is between 30 and 60, and is characterized by slowly progressive spastic paraparesis with urinary disturbance.[50] HAM/TSP is associated with high levels of Th1 cytokines, interferon-γ and tumour necrosis factor.[51] Many conditions have been recognized as being closely associated with HTLV-1: uveitis, dermatitis, polymyositis, intestinal pneumonitis and autoimmune disorders. In the past two decades much initiative has gone into the development of experimental vaccination and therapeutic strategies to combat HTLV-1 infection.[52]

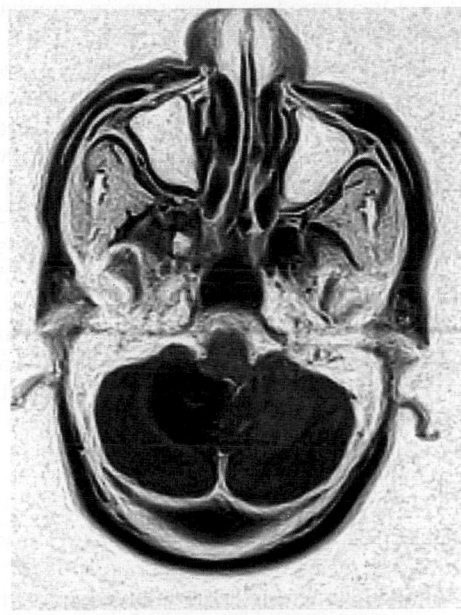

A

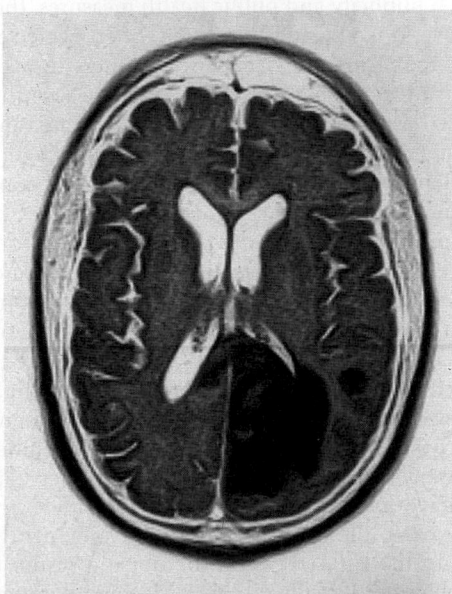

B

Figure 16.2 MRI of the brain showing primary multifocal right cerebellar (A) and left occipital part of the ventriculus (B) lymphoma in a Zambian patient with AIDS.

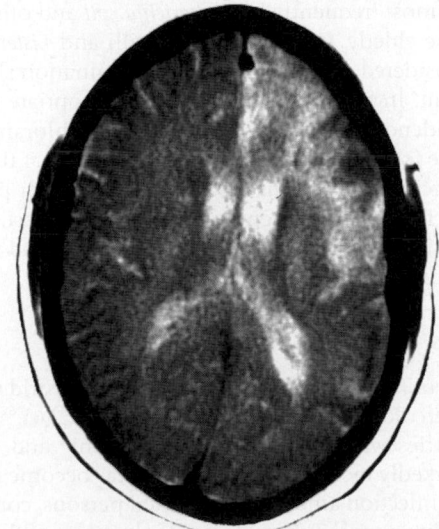

Figure 16.3 CT image shows a left middle cerebral artery infarction in a 28-year-old HIV patient.

Rickettsia

This group of illnesses,[53] which usually present as acute meningo-encephalitis, are transmitted to man via the bites of ticks or mites and occur throughout the world, except in Antarctica (see also Chapter 49). Mediterranean spotted fever (*Rickettsia conorii*) in Africa, Asia and the Mediterranean basin;[54] scrub typhus (*R. tsutsugamushi*) in Asia and the Pacific; typhus (*R. prowazekii*) and Q fever (*Coxiella burnetii*) are ubiquitous. Whereas the incubation period and clinical features vary between organisms, all patients manifest high fever, rash and headache, with meningoencephalitis developing during the second week of the illness.[55] Non-focal neurological features include headache, neck stiffness and photophobia, confusion, impairment of consciousness and fits. When present, the distinctive eschar at the site of the bite may suggest the diagnosis. CSF examination is rarely helpful and treatment should be started on clinical suspicion. The response to tetracycline or chloramphenicol is usually gratifying.

Bacterial infections

The organisms that produce bacterial infections (see also Chapters 54–71) of the nervous system in tropical regions are similar to those existing in the rest of the world. Despite the diagnosis of acute bacterial meningitis, which is an important cause of morbidity and mortality both in children and adults, there remains difficulty in tropical countries due to inadequate laboratory facilities.[56] Timely detection of meningitis epidemics in the tropics is still a serious problem, which became obvious in 1996 when the worst recorded meningococcal epidemics in history occurred in Africa.[57] In view of field experience and new evidence in 2000, WHO revised its guidelines for detecting meningococcal meningitis epidemics in highly endemic countries of Africa.[58] Outbreaks of meningococcal meningitis (meningitis caused by *Neisseria meningitidis*) remain a major public health problem in the African 'meningitis belt'.[59] Neonatal meningitis may be caused by almost any organism but most frequently by *Escherichia coli* and other enteric bacilli.[60] In the elderly, Gram-negative bacilli and *Listeria* species should be considered. Confirmatory CSF examination should not delay treatment. In the search for an early appropriate antibiotic in a high-incidence part of Africa, long-acting chloramphenicol injections were found to be as effective as ampicillin 4 times a day for 8 days. Vaccination remains the only real hope for preventing epidemics of meningitis. Recently, data on the effectiveness of conjugate vaccine for *Haemophilus influenzae* type b and meningococcus infection have been confirmed.[61]

Tuberculosis

The HIV epidemic has had a major impact on the world wide incidence of tuberculosis (see also Chapter 20 and 56).[62] In some tropical countries where tuberculosis is endemic and HIV incidence has markedly increased, tuberculosis has become the major opportunistic infection among HIV-infected persons, contributing to high mortality rates.[63] Tuberculosis involvement of the nervous system remains common, and despite the now worldwide availability of effective antituberculous therapy, the classical syndromes – spinal cord compression from tuberculous osteitis, tuberculous meningitis and intracranial tuberculomas – continue to cause significant morbidity and mortality.[64] As far as tuberculous osteitis is concerned it is important to appreciate that this may occur at any spinal level and is not restricted to the dorsal vertebrae; whereas in the early stages of the granulomatous process involving adjacent vertebrae and the intervening disc the cord is usually compressed anteriorly, this is not invariably so. There may be one or more posterior compressive lesions arising from tuberculous osteitis in the laminae and pedicles, and epidural tuberculomas can easily be confused with epidural tumours and other focal pathologies.

Intracranial tuberculoma – single or multiple – remains the most common cause of a space-occupying lesion in many parts of the world. CT facilities are now more widespread and the most common finding is a hypodense lesion on an unenhanced scan with a ring or disc-like enhancement with contrast and surrounding hypodensity. Where tuberculosis is common, physicians frequently promptly embark on a course of antituberculous therapy without histological verification. After 3 months of treatment, a repeat brain scan should show clearing of the lesion. While there are regional differences in the optimal combination of antituberculous drugs, chemotherapy is usually given for 6–12 months, depending upon the severity of the disease and response to treatment; corticosteroids are not given routinely, but dexamethasone in high doses during the acute phase of raised pressure may be helpful in reducing cerebral oedema. Obstructive hydrocephalus may develop at any stage of the illness, sometimes acutely; it is the most likely explanation for sudden neurological deterioration and should be treated promptly by surgical drainage.

Leprosy

Leprosy remains by far the most common cause of chronic mononeuritis multiplex in the world (see also Chapter 58).[65] The WHO currently estimates that there are 5.5 million patients with leprosy worldwide; a fall of about 50% since the 1980s. Nevertheless, despite much publicity and public health measures, the disease is frequently overlooked or misdiagnosed, often neglected and still generally feared. Thus the extent of the illness in a community may be difficult to estimate, but all reasonable attempts to do so indicate that, despite the availability of effective treatments, prevalence throughout the world is essentially unaltered. It remains true[66] that: 'leprosy should be considered whenever confronted by a chronic and symptomless skin rash that does not correspond with a common dermatosis or which does not respond to standard treatment for similar lesions. Leprosy should be considered in all cases of transient, recurrent or persistent numbness of paraesthesiae especially when this is localized to a more or less well-defined area of skin'. Hypopigmentation, with impaired sensitivity to light touch and pinprick, and particularly focal impairment or absence of sweating, should strongly suggest the diagnosis and a careful search should be made for thickening of peripheral nerves. Most commonly palpable are the great auricular nerve in the neck, the ulnar nerve just above the medial epicondyle, the median nerve at the wrist, the lateral popliteal nerve below the head of the fibula and the sural nerve on the dorsum of the foot. Early thickening may be difficult to clinch. Trained paramedical staff often become expert in detecting and confirming the presence of leprosy in suspects. Even those with advanced disease, severe neuropathy, deformity and incapacity may be helped by skilled reconstructive surgery.

Brucellosis

Brucellosis occurs in many tropical and subtropical areas and the nervous system may be affected in up to 5% of patients in a variety of ways (see also chapter 59).[67] It can cause an acute meningoencephalitis with papilloedema, convulsions and coma. Spinal presentation is with spastic or flaccid paraparesis due to cord compression or myeloradiculopathy, and central involvement with hemiparesis and ataxia. Diagnosis depends on blood or CSF culture of brucella, or more commonly on enzyme-linked immunosorbent assay (ELISA) of the blood and CSF.[68] Treatment with rifampicin, tetracycline and streptomycin should be for 3 months in those presenting with the subacute or chronic forms.

Spirochaetes

Neurosyphilis is again on the march and is increasingly occurring in the wake of HIV infection (see also Chapters 68, 69 and 70). The old clinical adage remains true: 'to know all the manifestations of syphilis is to know the whole of medicine' – but even here there are new twists to perplex even experienced physicians. When a young and apparently otherwise healthy male presents with acute onset of unilateral neural deafness, who would immediately suspect secondary syphilis? Other frequently occurring spirochaetal infections affecting the nervous system include borreliosis or relapsing fever (*Borrelia recurrentis*, louse borne; *B. duttonii*, tickborne), usually presenting as a febrile meningoencephalitis. Leptospirosis may affect any part of the nervous system, including an acute neuropathy.[69] Lyme disease (*B. burgdorferi*) is spread to man by infected ticks. While there is very extensive literature[70] on its diverse neurological and systemic manifestations – now recognized as the leading vector-borne disease in the USA – this malady occurs mainly in temperate climates. The neural manifestations span from meningitis, encephalitis, focal cranial neuropathies, radiculitis neuropathy, encephalopathy and post-borreliosis syndromes.

Protozoa

Cerebral malaria

The problems of malaria are considered in detail elsewhere in this book (see Chapters 14, 20 and 73). From the neurological aspect, cerebral malaria is a major life-threatening complication of *Plasmodium falciparum* in humans. *P. falciparum* is the predominant species in tropical countries and over 80% of these cases occur in Africa.[71] Despite over 100 years of research, mortality remains high.[72] It is characterized by a marked elevation in body temperature, disturbances of consciousness and coma along with convulsions, acute delirium and symmetrical motor signs. Children, pregnant women and non-immune adults are more susceptible to cerebral malaria.[73] Cerebral malaria-associated neurological sequelae and systemic complications, such as hypoglycaemia, hypovolaemia, hyperpyrexia, renal failure, bleeding disorders, anaemia, lactic acidosis and respiratory distress, may contribute to the pathogenesis of coma, and are responsible for high mortality.[74] The mechanisms underlying the fatal cerebral complications of *P. falciparum* are still not fully understood. That humans in endemic areas become immune to malaria led to the idea of protective vaccines. However, natural immunity to malaria is relatively inefficient.[75] The annual mortality attributed to malaria is increasing due primarily to widespread resistance to currently used drugs. Despite introducing new antimalarial drugs to clinical practice an effective and practical vaccine is still urgently required.[76] The complete genome sequence of *P. falciparum* has been determined, which has brought new approaches to the treatment and control of this disease.[77] The management of post-cerebral malaria syndromes (mental and physical retardation in young children, seizures, cranial neuropathies, encephalopathy, tremor and cerebellar dysfunction, sensory and motor deficit and cerebrovascular disorders) remains a challenge for neurologists in the tropics.

Trypanosomiasis

Two major diseases have been identified: human African trypanosomiasis (HAT), known as sleeping sickness and American trypanosomiasis, known as Chagas' disease. HAT produces progressive CNS damage, which if untreated results in death. Involvement occurs within a few weeks in the case of *Trypanosoma rhodesiense*, but usually takes much longer in the case of *T. gambiense*, i.e. months or even years. Brain involvement is caused mainly by cytokines (interferon-γ, tumour necrosis factor-α, and IL-10), nitric oxide and endothelial cell apoptosis.[78] The treatment for the early stage of HAT involves the drugs pentamidine and suramin. In the second stage of the disease, during which the trypanosomes reside in the cerebrospinal fluid, treatment is dependent exclusively on the arsenical compound melarsoprol, which crosses the blood–brain barrier. However, the drug is followed by a severe post-treatment reactive encephalopathy in 10% of cases, of which half die.[79] There is no current consensus on the diagnostic criteria for CNS involvement and the specific indications for melarsoprol therapy also differ. The problems of early diagnosis and introduction of cheap, safe and effective therapy before irreversible cerebral damage occurs are immense; meanwhile the prognosis for established sleeping sickness must remain grim.

Chagas' disease (CD) exists only on the American continent. It is caused by a parasite, *Trypanosoma cruzi*, transmitted to humans by blood-sucking triatomine bugs and by blood transfusion. Chagas' disease has two successive phases, acute and chronic. The acute phase lasts 6–8 weeks. Thanks to Chagas' disease control, acute cases are now disappearing and the incidence of new infections by *T. cruzi* in the whole continent has decreased by 70%.[80] CD is a major cause of cardiomyopathy and irreversible damage to the heart can develop 10–20 years after chagasic infection. American trypanosomiasis caused by *T. cruzi* can involve the nervous system in the acute stage with trypanosomes in the CSF. CD is recognized as a risk factor for stroke, independent of systolic dysfunction or presence of cardiac arrhythmias.[81] In its chronic stage, enlargement of hollow organs is the diagnostic hallmark. CD can reactivate in patients with HIV/AIDS and present as a brain mass lesion or an acute meningoencephalitis.[82] However, a cerebral tumour-like lesion is a more common manifestation of CD reactivation in AIDS patients.

Amoebiasis

Infection of the CNS by amoebae is an unusual event (see chapters 79 and 80). *Entamoeba histolytica* is an intestinal parasite and the causative agent of amoebiasis, which is a significant source of morbidity and mortality in developing countries.[83] E. histolytica can cause single or multiple cerebral abscesses which are noted on CT and may be clinically silent. Indirect haemagglutination antibody assay can be used for the diagnosis. Early treatment with metronidazole followed by rifampicin and tetracycline may improve both symptoms and radiographic images. Persons with HIV/AIDS are at significantly higher risk of E. histolytica infection.[84]

Three free-living amoebas: Naegleria fowleri, Acanthamoeba species and Balamuthia mandrillaris are recognized as causal agents for primary amoebic meningoencephalitis (PAM) (N. fowleri) and granulomatous amoebic encephalitis (GAE) (Acanthamoeba and Balamuthia). These amoebas are found in soil, water and air samples from all over the world. N. fowleri is a thermophilic amoeba that grows well in tropical and subtropical climates. PAM is characterized by an acute fulminant meningoencephalitis leading to death 3–7 days after exposure. GAE is usually seen in debilitated, malnourished individuals and in patients with AIDS. Clinical manifestations include headache, low fewer, seizures, hemiparesis and coma leading to death. A CT scan is non-specific. Clinical course is insidious and may mimic bacterial meningitis or tuberculous meningitis. Immunofluorescence antibody staining can be successful when used in patients whose clinical, laboratory and radiological findings suggest amoebic encephalitis.[85]

A sequential regime of anti-amoebic drugs, such as azithromycin, pentamidine, itraconazole, and flucystone is recommended. A recently recognized new human pathogen of Sappinia diploidea may lead to the diagnosis of S. diploidea encephalitis.[86]

Helminths

The diversity and complexity of the life cycles of the numerous parasites that may affect the nervous system are considered elsewhere in this book (see Chapters 82–87). Here, brief consideration will be given only to the salient clinical features.

Cysticercosis

This is an infection caused by Taenia solium larvae (cysticerci), the most common parasite to invade the CNS. When the cysticercus is lodged in the CNS, the disease is known as neurocysticercosis (NC). Neurocysticercosis is the most frequent and most widely disseminated neuroparasitosis. It is endemic in many parts of the world, particularly in Latin America, Africa and Asia.[87] Although neurocysticercosis is potentially eradicable, it remains neglected in most endemic countries and the infection has not been eliminated from any region by a specific programme and no national control programmes are yet in place.[88] Owing to massive emigration from endemic areas, frequency of NC has increased in developed countries.[89] Many people are exposed to cysticercosis but few become infected and human NC develops due to interaction of genetic and environmental factors. No familial aggregation was detected in studied cases of NC;[90] however, genetic heterogeneity of T. solium is significant for epidemiology and transmission of the disease.

The life cycle of T. solium involves pigs and humans. NC develops when humans become the intermediate host. In about 95%, this infection occurs when the individual ingests undercooked food or water that is contaminated with T. solium ova. Beginning weeks after ova ingestion, the larva creates a small oedematous lesion in the brain. Several weeks later, the larva develops into a cyst with a protoscolex surrounded by a bladder wall. The living cyst evokes only a minimal surrounding inflammation and remains viable from 2 to more than 10 years, before the osmotic barrier of the cyst wall breaks down. When the cyst wall begins to leak C. cellulosae antigens, an intense inflammatory reaction develops in the adjusted brain. The immune response is both humoral and cell-mediated. The CSF is characterized by increased levels of IgG subclasses, IL6/IL5/IL10, proteins and eosinophilis.[91]

In NC cysts develop in the brain parenchyma, meninges or ventricular spaces. The clinical features of NC depend on the number, type, size, localization and stage of development of cysticerci, as well as on the host immune response against the parasite. Cysticerci do not produce clinical symptoms until the cysts begin to degenerate (between 2 to 10 years).[92] Patients with 1–22 cysts may never develop clinical symptoms. Seizures are the most common symptom, occurring in 70–90% of patients, while NC is considered one of the main causes of late-onset epilepsy in endemic areas. When cysticerci lodge within the ventricular system, acute intracranial hypertension secondary to hydrocephalus may develop. Cysts in the subarachnoid space may grow to large sizes (giant cysts) causing intracranial hypertension with hemiparesis, partial seizures or other focal neurological signs. Racemose cysts in the basal cisterns can cause an intense inflammatory reaction at the base of the brain. Approximately 60% of the cases develop obstructive hydrocephalus. Some cases develop chronic cysticercotic meningitis, with headache and stiff neck. Ventricular and basal cisternal locations are considered to be malignant forms of NC.[93] About 1.5–3% of all cases develop spinal NC. Recent studies document significant age-related radiological, clinical and inflammatory differences in Mexican NC patients.[94]

Because the clinical presentation of NC is non-specific, diagnosis has been difficult. The diagnosis of NC should be considered in young adults from countries endemic for cysticercosis who present with the new onset of focal or generalized seizures, obstructive hydrocephalus, unexplained strokes, headache and stiff neck or unexplained cerebral cystic mass. CT and MRI have greatly facilitated diagnosis (Figure 16.4). The cystic lesions may be seen to contain more dense nodules, corresponding to the scolex; calcifications where cysts have died and cysts on nodules may enhance with contrast material as the cysticerci degenerate. However, there may be no radiological evidence of parasitic lesions and a negative scan does not eliminate the diagnosis if other clinical evidence is persuasive.

Serological tests for cysticercosis are improving. A monoclonal antibody-based antigen detection enzyme-linked immunosorbent assay has been developed. The test is sensitive (85%) for detection of cysticercus antigen in CSF. Recently it has been demonstrated that the PCR diagnosis of T solium DNA in the CSF may be a strong support for the diagnosis of neurocysticercosis.[95]

It is clear that cysticercosis cannot be regarded as a single disorder; treatment needs to be modified based on the location and number of cysticerci and the host response. The management of NC can be medical (anthelmintic drugs and corticosteroids) or surgical (removal of the cyst or replacement of CSF shunt). Optimal management depends on the location and the stage of the cysts.[92] Albendazole and praziquantel are effective drugs for the treatment of NC. However, there is controversy about their role in several forms of the disease. There is a strong consensus between

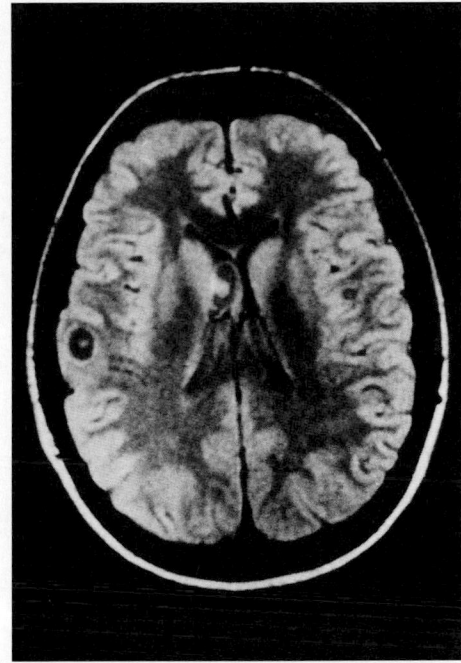

A

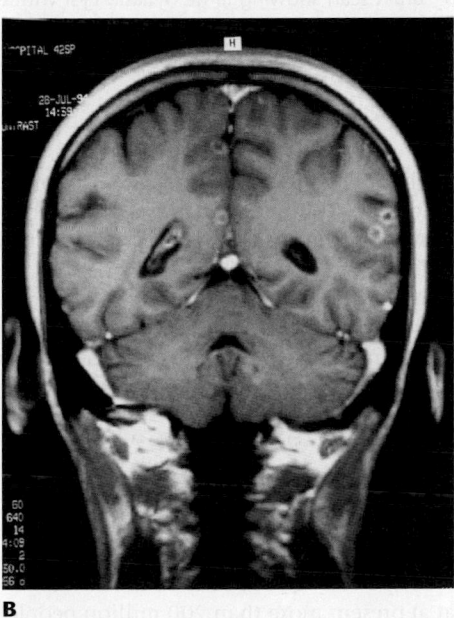

B

Figure 16.4 Neurocysticercosis. (A) Cysts in different stages of maturation. (B) Two cysts containing scolices.

experts that there is no role for antiparasitic drugs in patients with only calcified lesions. Studies suggest that patients with single enhancing lesions will do well regardless of antiparasitic therapy. Antiparasitic drugs are contraindicated in patients with cerebral oedema (cysticercal encephalitis) and most experts strongly recommend antiparasitic therapy in patients with multiple sub-arachnoid *cysticerci* or giant *cysticerci*. In patients with ventricular *cysticerci*, endoscopic removal is the preferred therapy but place-ment of a ventricular shunt followed by antiparasitic therapy is an acceptable alternative.[96] Standard treatment for localization-

related epilepsy is effective for seizures caused by cysticercosis. In general, seizures are easily controlled in NC: corticosteroid admin-istration along with the anthelmintic drug is often shown to min-imize transient worsening of the clinical symptoms that may occur early in the treatment. There are currently many differing opinions regarding the treatment of patients with NC and therapy of infected individuals must be individualized.

Filariasis

Human filariasis may be due to *Loa loa*, *Dracunculus medinensis* or *Onchocerca volvulus*. Loiasis can cause meningoencephalitis with microfilariae in the CSF. Severe adverse events following ivermec-tin treatment may occur in people harbouring high *Loa loa*, especially Loa encephalopathy.[97] Pion et al. recently developed a semi-empirical model to predict the prevalence of heavy *L. loa* loads in a community, given its overall microfilariae prevalence.[98]

W. bancrofti can cause Guillain–Barré syndrome. Three cases have been reported, in which microfilariae were identified in the cyst fluid of tumours of the brain.[99]

Onchocerciasis

Onchocerciasis (river blindness) is a filarial infection which causes blindness and debilitating skin lesions. The disease occurs in 37 countries, of which 30 are found in Africa (the most affected in terms of distribution and the severity of the clinical manifestations of the disease), six in the Americas and one in the Arabian Penin-sula.[100] It has been reported that the reduction in prevalence and intensity of *Onchocerca volvulus* infection differs between ethnic groups and communities. Recent studies found significant expres-sion of prostaglandin E(2) in *O. volvulus*-infected patients which was independent of antifilarial and antiendobacterial treatment.[101] In rural areas of central Cameroon and West Uganda, it was found that epilepsy was closely linked to onchocerciasis.[102] A higher incidence of epilepsy in zones of high endemicity of oncho-cerciasis may be due to various risk factors including genetic factors and low socioeconomic status. The possibility of a relationship between epilepsy and onchocerciasis might explain the presence of *O. volvulus* in the CNS and immunological mechanisms involv-ing cross-reactive immunization or cytokine production during infection. In many areas of Africa, where human onchocerciasis is endemic, there are now programmes for mass treatment with iver-mectin. However, ivermectin is a microfilaricide and does not kill the adult worms. Since it does not cross the blood–brain barrier, the drug is unlikely to have direct pro- or anti-convulsive activity. Distribution of the drug will be needed for at least 25 years and latest estimates indicate that 90 million people will need annual treatment if onchocerciasis is to be eliminated.[103]

Nematode infections

The gender *Gnathostoma* includes many species, the most frequent being *Gnathostoma spinigerum*. Human gnathostomiasis is endemic in some countries of South-east Asia, and Latin America. Since the beginning of the 1980s, there has been an increasing number of cases of gnathostomiasis described in Western countries in travel-lers returning from endemic countries.[104] The disease develops due to the consumption of raw or insufficiently cooked meat or fish.

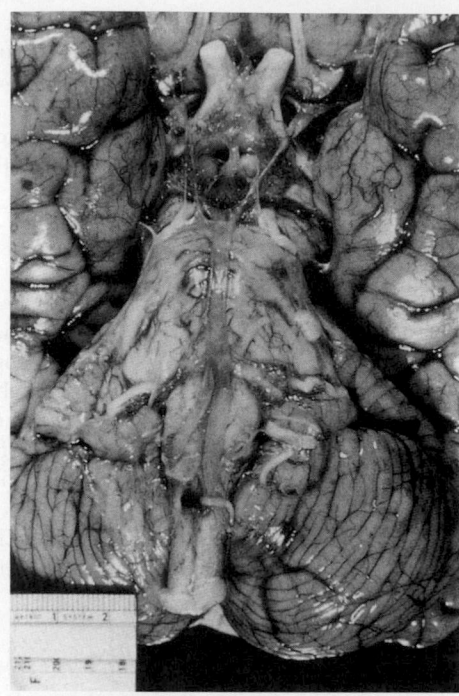

Figure 16.5 Gnathostomiasis. On the ventral surface of the lower medulla the nematodes can be seen emerging from a cavity (seen at autopsy). (Courtesy of Athasit Vejjajiva, Department of Neurology, Ramathibodi Hospital, Thailand.)

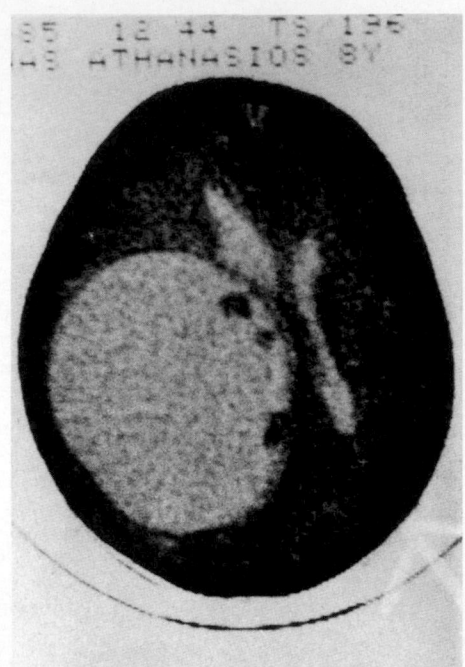

Figure 16.6 Brain scan showing large hydatid cyst with daughter cysts.

Gnathostomiasis is a cause of cutaneous and/or visceral larva migrans syndrome. The commonest neurological manifestations include encephalitis, myelitis, radiculomyelitis, radiculitis and subarachnoid haemorrhage.[105] The main laboratory finding is eosinophilia in blood and CSF. Some patients present with a curious and fatal multifocal neurological illness (Figure 16.5). It was recently reported that recognition of 21 kDa antigen in *G. spinigerum* advanced third-stage larvae crude extracts is the most specific diagnostic marker for human gnathostomiasis, with 100% sensitivity and specificity.[106] *Angiostrongylus cantonensis* (rat lungworm) similarly affects those in South-east Asia who consume poorly cooked snails, prawns and crabs. Neurological complications include meningitis, papilloedema and extraocular palsies with an eosinophilic CSF pleocytosis. Brain abscesses may occur and CT shows well-circumscribed enhancing lesions. Both these nematodes are treated with albendazole with steroid cover.

Strongyloides stercoralis is another nematode which affects the nervous system with an eosinophilic meningitis. HIV and tropical infections affect each other mutually. At present, there is a concept that strongyloides dissemination in endemic countries may be as a manifestation of HIV-associated immune reconstitution disease.[107]

Hydatid disease

Cerebral hydatid disease is very rare and usually secondary. The vast majority of patients affected are children. A cerebral hydatid cyst is always solitary unless the primary site is the brain; CT and MRI (Figure 16.6) may reveal diagnostic daughter cysts. Headache, vomiting and seizures are predominant symptoms in children, whereas focal neurological deficits are most common in adults. Intracranial hydatid cysts should always be surgically removed without rupture; the outcome remains excellent in these cases. Treatment with albendazole is beneficial both pre- and postoperatively. A spinal hydatid disease is a rarity. In spinal hydatidosis, the cysts are usually multiple and extradural, and paraplegia may result.[108] In endemic areas, the clinician should include spinal hydatid disease as part of the differential list for paraplegia and consider performing neuroimaging.

Schistosomiasis

The longest-known parasite of man: the earliest case known to have occurred was 5000 years ago in an Egyptian adolescent from the pre-dynastic period. It continues to afflict mankind and it is believed that at present more than 200 million people worldwide are affected. Of the Schistosoma species, *S. mansoni*, *S. hematobium* and *S. japonicum* are the most important to man and the most widely distributed. Schistosomiasis is endemic in parts of South America, sub-Saharan Africa, the Middle East, and some Caribbean islands.[109] Disorders of the liver and gastrointestinal tract are the most common clinical manifestations. The involvement of the CNS by the infection may or may not determine clinical manifestations. Neuroschistosomiasis (NS) develops through eggs or by anomalous migration of the parasite. More common neurological manifestations of spinal NS are transverse myelitis and myeloradiculopathy. Cerebral NS usually manifests with symptoms of increased intracranial pressure associated with focal neurological signs. Betting et al. described NS manifested by partial epileptic seizures caused by a granulomatous lesion due to

S. mansoni.[110] Antischistosomal drugs, corticosteroids and surgery are the resources for treating NC. The diagnosis of cerebral NS is established by biopsy of the nervous tissue and spinal NS is usually diagnosed according to a clinical criterion. The microscopic examination of excreta remains the gold standard for the diagnosis of schistosomiasis. Eosinophilia in the CSF and the CT and MRI findings (Figure 16.7) may clinch the diagnosis of NC. Praziquantel (PZQ) is active against all schistosome species. However, the drug has little or no effect on eggs and immature worms. Moreover, decreased susceptibility to PZQ has been observed in several countries and the prospects for developing an effective vaccine are encouraging.[111] Studies published over the past decade led to the hypothesis that helminth infections such as schistosomiasis may exacerbate HIV-1 transmission or progression.[112]

Trichinosis

This parasitic disease, which develops after ingestion of under-cooked meat contaminated with larvae of *Trichinella spiralis*, occurs both in tropical and temperate climates, and apparent outbreaks are still reported worldwide.[113] The acute illness, with fever, headaches, myalgia, weakness and malaise, arthralgia, periorbital oedema, nausea and diarrhoea with a marked blood eosinophilia, increased serum muscle enzymes and specific antibodies, is well known. Turk et al.[113] reported a benign course and a milder clinical picture of trichinellosis in children than adults. Neurological manifestations occurred in 10–15% of the diseased. There could be a serious diagnostic problem in the absence of corresponding epidemiological data and typical symptoms and signs of the disease. Neurotrichinosis may manifest with clinical symptoms of meningitis, encephalitis, polyradiculoneuritis, myasthaenia gravis and diseases of the connective tissue involving the nervous system. Brain lesions in trichinosis have been defined on CT and MRI as multifocal small lesions located in the cerebral cortex and white matter.[114] Early diagnosis and prompt treatment with anthelmintic therapy such as mebendazole with corticosteroids is mandatory.

Paragonimiasis

Paragonimiasis is a typical food-borne parasitic disease that is common in South-east Asia, the Far East, Latin American and Africa. Recently, however, this disease has been seen in many parts of the world, largely due to increases in the numbers of immigrants and overseas travellers.[115] *Paragonimiasis westermani* is a typical digenetic parasite. Cerebral paragonimiasis (CP) is not rare, but pleuropulmonary manifestations are the most prevalent. CP cases are more frequent in the Far East, especially Korea. It presents as an intracranial space-occupying lesion. Brain MRI shows a single or multiple conglomerated lesions.[116] The parasite is transmitted to man through ingestion of crab and crayfish; the metacercariae travel to the lungs and mature. The adult can live in the lung for several years and is usually asymptomatic. Neurological presentation is due to cerebral involvement as a result of the development of cysts in ectopic sites; various intracranial sites can be affected. The diagnosis is based on the identification of parasite eggs in sputum, faeces and pleural fluid and on ELISA serology. Studies suggest that Triclabendazole is the most effective and best tolerated drug for the treatment of food-borne trematode infections.

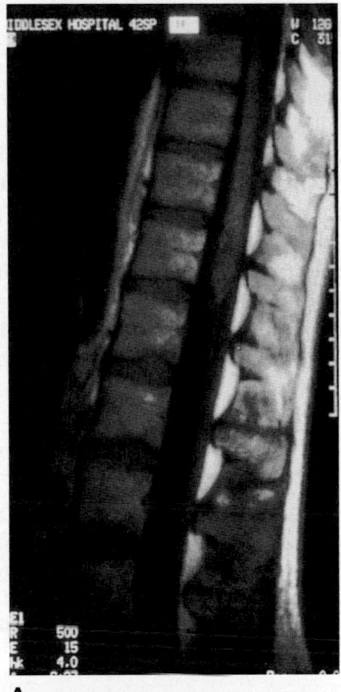

A

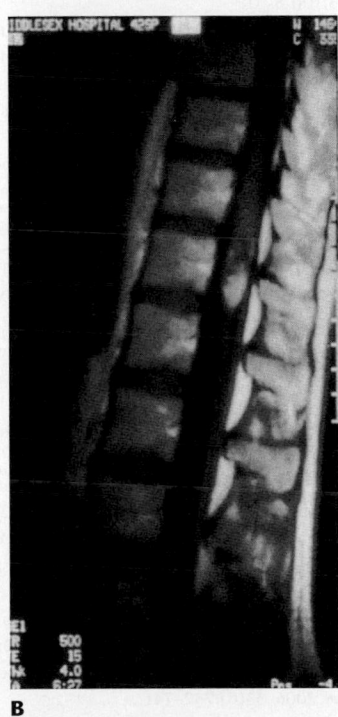

B

Figure 16.7 Schistosomiasis of the lower spinal cord and conus. (A) Before contrast. (B) After contrast with an irregular area of altered signal in surrounding oedema.

CONCLUSION

This chapter has briefly described an exceedingly diverse and fascinating group of illnesses which affect the CNS in tropical patients. While the extent and somewhat idiosyncratic depth of this coverage will not be beyond the criticism of the specialist, there is sufficient detail for clinical neurologists to be aware of CNS diseases that may affect many patients throughout the tropics and subtropics. Neurological manifestations are early and common in HIV-positive patients and early counselling and testing should be offered to the patient. For more specialist discussion of the subject, the reader is referred to a recently published book, *Tropical Neurology*.[117]

REFERENCES

1. Bittencourt PRM, Adamolekum B, Bharucha N, et al. ILAE Commission Report. Epilepsy in the tropics: I and II. *Epilepsia* 1996; 37(11):1121–1137.
2. Preux PM, Druet-Cabanac M. Epidemiology and aetiology of epilepsy in sub-Saharan Africa. *Lancet Neurol* 2005; 4:21–31.
3. Dent W, Helbok R, Matuja WB et al. Prevalence of active epilepsy in a rural area in South Tanzania: a door-to-door survey. *Epilepsia* 2005; 46(12):1963–1969.
4. Bhigjee AI. Seizures in HIV/AIDS: a southern African perspective. *Acta Neurol Scand Suppl* 2005; 181:8–11.
5. Mullin P, Green G, Bakshi R. Special population: the management of seizures in HIV-positive patients. *Curr Neurol Neurosci Rep* 2004; 4(4):308–314.
6. World Population Prospects. The 2005 Revision. Online. Available: http://www.un.org/esa/population/publications/pop_challenges/pressrelease_english.pdf
7. Hampton T. Researchers study health effects of environmental change. *JAMA* 2006; 296(8):913–920.
8. Epstein PR. Climate change and human health. *N Engl J Med* 2005; 353(14):1433–1436.
9. Neufeld KJ, Peters DH, Rani M, et al. Regular use of alcohol and tobacco in India and its association with age, gender, and poverty. *Drug Alcohol Depend* 2005; 77(3):283–291.
10. Cavanagh JB. The 'dying back' process: a common denominator in many naturally occurring and toxic neuropathies. *Arch Pathol Lab Med* 1979; 103:659–664.
11. Pratt RW, Weimer LH. Medication and toxin-induced peripheral neuropathy. *Semin Neurol* 2005; 25(2):204–216.
12. Ibrahim D, Floberg B, Wolf A, et al. Heavy metal poisoning: clinical presentations and pathophysiology. *Clin Lab Med* 2006; 26(1):67–97.
13. Mukherjee SC, Rahman MM, Chowdhury UK, et al. Neuropathy in arsenic toxicity from ground-water arsenic contamination in West Bengal, India. *J Environ Sci Health* 2003; 38(1):165–183.
14. Goebel HH, Schmidt PF, Bohl J, et al. Polyneuropathy due to acute arsenic intoxication: biopsy studies. *J Neropathol Exp Neurol* 1990; 49(2):137–149.
15. Thomson RM, Parry GJ. Neuropathies associated with excessive exposure to lead. *Muscle Nerve* 2006; 33(6):732–741.
16. Kuo HC, Huang CC, Tsai YT, et al. Acute painful neuropathy in thallium poisoning. *Neurology* 2005; 65(2):302–304.
17. Becerra-Cunat JL, Coll-Canti J, Gelpi-Mantius E, et al. Chloroquine-induced myopathy and neuropathy. *Rev Neurol* 2003; 36(6):523–526.
18. Konagaya M, Matsumoto A, Takase S, et al. Clinical analysis of longstanding subacute myelo-optico-neuropathy: sequelae of clioquinol at 32 years after its ban. *J Neurol Sci* 2004; 218(1–2):85–90.
19. Eddleston M, Eyer P, Worek F, et al. Differences between organophosphorus insecticides in human self-poisoning: a prospective cohort study. *Lancet* 2005; 366(9495):1452–1459.
20. Oluwole OS, Onabolu AO, Cotgreave IA, et al. Incidence of endemic ataxic polyneuropathy and its relation to exposure to cyanide in a Nigerian community. *J Neurol Neurosurg Psychiatry* 2003; 74(10):1417–1422.
21. Kaiser P. Endemic spastic paraparesis (konzo). *Nervenarzt* 2002; 73(10):946–951.
22. Sreeja VG, Nagahara, Li Q, et al. New aspects in pathogenesis of konzo: neural cell damage directly caused by linamarin contained in cassava (Manihot esculenta Crantz). *Br J Nutr* 2003; 90(2):467–472.
23. Spencer PS, Palmer VS, Ludolph AC. On the decline and etiology of high incidence motor system disease in West Papua (southwest New Guinea). *Mov Disord* 2005; 20(suppl 12):119–126.
24. Angunawela RM, Fernando HA. Acute ascending polyneuropathy and dermatitis following poisoning by tubers of Gloriosa superba. *Ceylon Med J* 1971; 16:233–235.
25. Ng T HK, Chan YW, Yu Y L, et al. Encephalopathy and neuropathy following ingestion of a Chinese herbal broth containing podophyllin. *J Neurol Sci* 1991; 101:107–113.
26. Martinez HR, Bermudez MV, Rangel-Guerra RA, et al. Clinical diagnosis in Karwinskia humboldtiana polyneuropathy. *J Neurol Sci* 1998; 154(1):49–54.
27. Hotta H, Nihel K, Abe Y, et al. Full-length sequence analysis of subacute sclerosing panencephalitis (SSPE) virus, a mutant of measles virus. *Microbiol Immunol* 2006; 50(7):525–534.
28. Kuhne M, Brown DW, Jin L. Genetic variability of measles virus in acute and persistent infections. *Infect Genet Evol* 2006; 6(4):260–276.
29. del Toro-Riera M, Macaya-Ruiz A, Raspall-Chaure M, et al. Subacute sclerosing panencephalitis: combined treatment with interferon alfa and intraventricular ribavirin. *Rev Neurol* 2006; 42(5):277–281.
30. Deresiewicz RL, Thaler SJ, Hsu L, et al. Clinical and neuroradiographic manifestations of eastern equine encephalitis. *N Engl J Med* 1997; 336(26):1867–1874.
31. Ohrr H, Tandan JB, Sohn YM, et al. Effect of single dose of SA 14–14–2 vaccine 1 year after immunisation in Nepalese children with Japanese encephalitis. *Lancet* 2005; 366:1375–1378.
32. Madani TA, Al-Mazrou YY, Al-Jeffri MH, et al. Rift Valley fever epidemic in Saudi Arabia: epidemiological, clinical, and laboratory characteristics. *Clin Infect Dis* 2003; 37(8):1084–1092.
33. Katz SL. Polio-new challenges in 2006. *J Clin Virol* 2006; 36(3):163–165.
34. Huang QS, Greening G, Baker MG, et al. Persistence of oral polio vaccine virus after its removal from the immunisation schedule in New Zealand. *Lancet* 2005; 366:394–396.
35. Liang X, Zhang Y, Xu W, et al. An outbreak of poliomyelitis caused by type 1 vaccine-derived poliovirus in China. *J Infect Dis* 2006; 194(5):545–551.
36. Sidley P. Seven die in polio outbreak in Namibia. *BMJ* 2006; 332(7555):1408.
37. Han MH, Walker M, Zunt JR. Neurological infections in the returning international traveler. In: *Infectious Disease*. American Academy Neurology CONTINUUM 2006; 12(2):133–158.
38. Richmond JK, Baglole DJ. Lassa fever: epidemiology, clinical features, and social consequences. *BMJ* 2003; 327(7426):1271–1275.
39. Rupprecht CE, Hanlon CA, Slate D. Oral vaccination of wildlife against rabies: opportunities and challenges in prevention and control. *Dev Biol (Basel)* 2004; 119:173–184.
40. Warrel MJ, Warrel DA. Rabies and other Lyssavirus diseases. *Lancet* 2004; 363(9413):959–969.
41. Wilde H, Khawplod P, Khamoltham T, et al. Rabies control in South and Southeast Asia. *Vaccine* 2005; 23(17–18):2284–2289.
42. Tordo N, Bahloul C, Jacob Y, et al. Rabies: epidemiological tendencies and control tools. *Dev Biol (Basel)* 2006; 125:3–13.
43. Srinivasan A, Burton EC, Kuehnert MJ, et al. Transmission of rabies virus from an organ donor to four transplant recipients. *N Engl J Med* 2005; 352(11):1103–1111.
44. McArthur JC, Brew BJ, Nath A. Neurological complications of HIV infection. *Lancet Neurol* 2005; 4:543–555.

45. Brew BJ. *HIV Neurology*. Oxford: Oxford University Press; 2001.

46. Nath A, Sacktor N. Influence of highly active antiretroviral therapy on persistence of HIV in the central nervous system. *Curr Opin Neurol* 2006; 19(4):358–361.

47. Lawn SD, Bekker LG, Miller RF. Immune reconstitution disease associated with mycobacterial infections in HIV infected individuals receiving antiretrovirals. *Lancet Infect Dis* 2005; 5:361–373.

48. Proietti FA, Carneiro-Proietti AB, Catalan-Soares BC, et al. Global epidemiology of HTLV-1 infection and associated diseases. *Oncogene* 2005; 24(39):6058–6068.

49. Oger J. HTLV-1 associated myelopathy. *Medlink Neurology* 2006.

50. Grindstaff P, Gruener G. The peripheral nervous system complications of HTLV-1 myelopathy (HAM/TSP) syndromes. *Semin Neurol* 2005; 25(3):315–327.

51. Guerreiro JB, Santos SB, Morgan DJ, et al. Levels of serum chemokines discriminate clinical myelopathy associated with HAM/STP disease from HTLV-1 carrier state. *Clin Exp Immunol* 2006; 145(2):296–301.

52. Kynch MP, Kaumaya PT. Advances in HTLV-1 peptide vaccines and therapeutics. *Curr Protein Pept Sci* 2006; 7(2):137–145.

53. Bassetti S. Rickettsioses of the spotted fever-group. *Internist (Berl)* 2004; 45(6):669–676.

54. Parker NR, Barralet JH, Bell AM. Q fever. *Lancet* 2006; 367:679–688.

55. Amaro M, Bacellar F, Franca A. Report of eight cases of fatal and severe Mediterranean spotted fever in Portugal. *Ann NY Acad Sci* 2003; 990:331–343.

56. Wiersinga WJ, van Dellen QM, Spanjaad L, et al. High mortality among patients with bacterial meningitis in a rural hospital in Tanzania. *Ann Trop Med Parasitol* 2004; 98(3):271–278.

57. Lewis R, Nathan N, Diarra L, et al. Timely detection of meningococcal meningitis epidemics in Africa. *Lancet* 2001; 358:287–293.

58. WHO. Detecting meningococcal meningitis epidemics in highly-endemic African countries. *Wkly Epidemiol Res* 2000; 75:306–309.

59. Mueller JE, Borrow R, Gessner BD. Meningococcal serogroup W135 in the African meningitis belt: epidemiology, immunity and vaccines. *Expert Rev Vaccines* 2006; 5(3):319–336.

60. Laving AM, Musoke RN, Wasunna AO, et al. Neonatal bacterial meningitis at the newborn unit of Kenyatta National Hospital. *East Afr Med J* 2003; 80(9):456–462.

61. Adegbola RA, Secka O, Lahai G, et al. Elimination of Haemophilus influenzae type b (HIB) disease from the Gambia after the introduction of routine immunisation with a HIB conjugate vaccine: a prospective study. *Lancet* 2005; 366:144–150.

62. Onyebjoh P, Zumla A, Ribeiro I, et al. Treatment of tuberculosis: present status and future prospects. *Bull World Health Organ* 2005; 83(11):857–865.

63. Charles M, Pape JW. Tuberculosis and HIV: Implications in the developing world. *Curr/AIDS Rep* 2006; 3(3):139–144.

64. Thwaites GE, Tran TH. Tuberculous meningitis: many questions, too few answers. *Lancet Neurol* 2005; 4(3):160–170.

65. Ooi WW, Srinivasan J. Leprosy and the peripheral nervous system: basic and clinical aspects. *Muscle Nerve* 2004; 30(4):393–409.

66. WHO regional strategy for sustaining leprosy services and future reducing the burden of leprosy, 2006–2010. *Indian J Lepr* 2006; 78(1):33–47.

67. Pappas G, Papadimitrou P, Akritidis N, et al. The new global map of human brucellosis. *Lancet Infect Dis* 2006; 6(2):91–99.

68. Al Dahouk S, Tomaso H, Nockler K, et al. Laboratory-based diagnosis of brucellosis – a review of the literature. Part II: serological tests for brucellosis. *Clin Lab* 2003; 49(11–12):577–589.

69. Panicker JN, Mammachan R, Jayakumar RV. Primary neuroleptospirosis. *Postgrad Med J* 2001; 77(911):589–590.

70. Halperin JJ. Central nervous system Lyme disease. *Curr Neurol Neurosci* 2005; 5(6):446–462.

71. Solomon T, Wondscrichanalai C, Hemachudha T. Malaria. *Medlink Neurology* 2006.

72. Idro R, Aketch S, Gwer S, et al. Research priorities in the management of severe Plasmodium falciparum malaria in children. *Ann Trop Med Parasitol* 2006; 100(2):95–108.

73. Duffy PE, Fried M. Malaria in the pregnant woman. *Curr Top Microbiol Immunol* 2005; 295:169–200.

74. Idro R, Jenkins NE, Newton CR. Pathogenesis, clinical features, and neurological outcome of cerebral malaria. *Lancet Neurol* 2005; 4(12):827–840.

75. Marsh K, Kinyanjui S. Immune effector mechanisms in malaria. *Parasite Immunol* 2006; 28(1–2):51–60.

76. Walther M. Advances in vaccine development against the preerythrocytic stage of Plasmodium falciparum malaria. *Expert Rev Vaccines* 2006; 5(1):81–93.

77. Montgomery J, Milner DA Jr, Tse MT, et al. Genetic analysis of circulating and sequestered populations of plasmodium falciparum in fatal pediatric malaria. *J Infect Dis* 2006; 194(1):115–122.

78. Bisser S, Ouwe-Missi-Oukem-Boyer ON, Toure FS, et al. Harboring in the brain: A focus on immune evasion mechanisms in malaria and human African trypanosomiasis. *Int J Parasitol* 2006; 36(5):529–540.

79. Kennedy PG. Diagnostic and neuropathogenesis issues in human African trypanosomiasis. *Int J Parasitol* 2006; 36(5):505–512.

80. Moncayo A. Chagas disease. Current epidemiological trends in the Southern Cone countries. *Mem Inst Oswaldo Cruz* 2003; 98(5):577–591.

81. Oliveira-Filho J, Viana LC, Vieira-de-Melo RM, et al. Chagas disease is an independent risk factor for stroke: baseline characteristics of a Chagas Disease cohort. *Stroke* 2005; 36(9):2015–2017.

82. Lambert N, Mehta B, Walters R, et al. Chagasic encephalitis as the initial manifestation of AIDS. *Ann Intern Med* 2006; 144(12):941–943.

83. Lottus B, Anderson I, Davies R, et al. The genome of the parasite Entamoeba histolytica. *Nature* 2005; 433(7028):865–868.

84. Tsai JJ, Sun HY, Ke L Y, et al. Higher seroprevalence of Entamoeba histolytica infection in associated with HIV-1 infection in Taiwan. *Am J Trop Med Hyg* 2006; 74(6):1016–1019.

85. Schuster FL, Honarmand S, Visvesvara GS, et al. Detection of antibodies against free-living amoebae Balamuthia mandrillaris and Acanthamoeba species in a population of patients with encephalitis. *Clin Infect Dis* 2006; 42(9):1260–1265.

86. Gelman BB, Popov V, Chaljub G, et al. Neuropathological and ultrastructural features of amebic encephalitis caused by Sappinia diploidea. *J Neuropathol Exp Neurol* 2003; 62(10):990–998.

87. Garcia HH, Del Brutto OH. Neurocysticercosis: updated concepts about an old disease. *Lancet Neurol* 2005; 4:653–661.

88. Willingham AL 3rd, Engels D. Control of Taenia solium cysticercosis/taeniasis. *Adv Parasitol* 2006; 61:509–566.

89. Alarcon F. Neurocysticercosis: its aetiopathogenesis, clinical manifestations, diagnosis and treatment. *Rev Neurol* 2006; 43(suppl 1):S93–S100.

90. Fleury A, Morales J, Bobes RJ, et al. An epidemiological study of familial neurocysticercosis in an endemic Mexican community. *Trans R Soc Trop Med Hyg* 2006; 100(6):551–558.

91. Chavarria A, Fleury A, Garcia E, et al. Relationship between the clinical heterogeneity of neurocysticercosis and the immune-inflammatory profiles. *Clin Immunol* 2005; 116(3):271–278.

92. Davis LE. Neurocysticercosis. *Medlink Neurology* 2006.

93. Takayanagui OM, Odashimba NS. Clinical aspects of neurocysticercosis. *Parasitol Int* 2006; 55(suppl):S111–S115.

94. Saenz B, Ruiz-Garcia M, Jimenez E, et al. Neurocysticercosis: Clinical, radiologic, and inflammatory differences between children and adults. *Pediatr Infect Dis J* 2006; 25(9):801–803.

95. Almedia CR, Ojopi EP, Nunes CM, et al. Taenia solium DNA is present in the cerebrospinal fluid of neurocysticercosis patients and can be used for diagnosis. *Eur Arch Psychiatry Clin Neurosci* 2006; 256(5):307–310.

96. Riley T, White AC Jr. Management of neurocysticercosis. *CNS Drugs* 2003; 17(8):577–591.

97. Pion DS, Gardon J, Kamgno J, et al. Structure of the microfilarial reservoir of Loa loa in the human host and its implications of monitoring the treatment with ivermectin carried out in Africa. *Parasitology* 2004; 129(Pt 5):613–626.

98. Pion SD, Filipe JA, Kamgno J, et al. Microfilarial distribution of Loa loa in the human host: population dynamics and epidemiological implications. *Parasitology* 2006; 133(Pt 1):101–109.

99. Aron M, Kapila K, Sarkar C, et al. Microfiliariae of Wuchereria bancrofti in cyst fluid of tumours of the brain: a report of three cases. *Diagn Cytopathol* 2002; 26(3):158–162.

100. Boatin BA, Richards FO Jr. Control of onchocerciasis. *Adv Parasitol* 2006; 61:349–394.

101. Brattig NW, Schwohl A Rickert R, et al. The filarial parasite Onchocerca volvulus generates the lipid mediator prostaglandin E(2). *Microbes Infect* 2006; 8(3):873–879.

102. Kaiser C, Asaba G, Kasoro S, et al. Mortality from epilepsy in an onchocerciasis-endemic area in West Uganda. *Trans R Soc Trop Med Hyg* 2007; 101(1):48–55.

103. Hopkins AD. Ivermectin and onchocerciasis: is it all solved? *Eye* 2005; 19(10):1057–1066.

104. Clement-Rigolet MC, Danis M, Caumes E. Gnathostomiasis, an exotic disease increasingly imported into Western countries. *Presse Med* 2004; 33(21): 1527–1532.

105. Schmutzhard E, Boongird P, Vejjajiva A. Eosinophilic meningitis and radiculomyelitis in Thailand caused by CNS invasion of Gnasthostoma spinigerum and Angiostrongylus cantonensis. *J Neurol Neurosurg Psychiatry* 1988; 51:80–87.

106. Anantaphruti MT, Nuamtanong S, Dekimoyo P. Diagnostic values of IgG4 in human gnathostomiasis. *Trop Med Int Health* 2005; 10(10):1013–1021.

107. Lawn SD, Wilkinson RJ. Immune reconstiution disease associated with parasitic infections following antiretroviral treatment. *Parasite Immunol* 2006; 28(11):625–633.

108. Rumana M, Mahadevan A, Nayl Khurshid M, et al. Cestode parasitic infestation: intracranial and spinal hydatid disease – a clinico-pathological study of 29 cases from South India. *Clin Neuropathol* 2006; 25(2):98–104.

109. Gryceels B, Palman K, Clerinx J, et al. Human schistosomiasis. *Lancet* 2006; 368:1106–1118.

110. Betting LE, Pirani C Jr, de Souza Queiroz L, et al. Seizures and cerebral schistosomiasis. *Arch Neurol* 2005; 62(6):1008–1110.

111. McManus DP. Prospects for development of a transmission blocking vaccine against Schistosoma japonicum. *Parasite Immunol* 2005; 27(7–8):297–308.

112. Secor WE. Interactions between schistosomiasis and infection with HIV-1. *Parasite Immunol* 2006; 28(11):597–603.

113. Turk M, Kaptan F, Turker N, et al. Clinical and laboratory aspects of a trichinellosis outbreak in Izmir, Turkey. *Parasite* 2006; 13(1): 65–70.

114. Gelal F, Kumral E, Vidini BD, et al. Diffusion-weighted and conventional MRI imaging in neurotrichinosis. *Acta Radiol* 2005; 46(2):196–199.

115. Jeon K, Koh WJ, Kim H, et al. Clinical features of recently diagnosed pulmonary paragonimiasis in Korea. *Chest* 2005; 128(3): 1423–1430.

116. Zhang JS, Huan Y, Sun LJ, et al. MRI features of pediatric cerebral paragonimiasis in the active stage. *J Magn Reson Imaging* 2006; 23(4): 569–573.

117. Misra UK, Kalita J (eds). *Tropical Neurology*. Georgetown: Landes Bioscience; 2003.

Chapter 17   Alan Haworth

Psychiatry

Psychiatric disorders account for more morbidity than is often recognized. The World Health Organization's 1999 World Health Report states that neuropsychiatric conditions make up an estimated 11.5% of the global burden of disease and on average these conditions account for 28% of total years lived with disability. A large proportion of the burden is attributable to major depression. Five of the ten leading causes of disability worldwide are mental disorders and suicide is the tenth leading cause of death in the world. Natural disasters with their psychosocial consequences tend to occur with more frequency in tropical countries. Malnutrition and its consequences affect both prenatal and postnatal growth in the child. Malnutrition and other physical stresses such as chronic anaemia, parasitic infections and the burden, for example, of trying to grow one's own food in drought conditions make their contribution to the occurrence of psychiatric morbidity generally. There are higher levels of head trauma resulting in long-term sequelae and of intracranial infections and especially in some countries of human immunodeficiency virus and associated opportunistic infections. In the past, a simple dichotomy between urban and rural was described, although there is no clear definition applicable worldwide of the term 'urban'. In many countries there is a lower limit of 20000 and many tropical countries also have very large cities. Much emphasis was in the past put on the many stresses of living in an urban environment with somewhat simplistic conceptualizations of rural serenity but more recent studies show that the main social determinant of psychiatric disorder remains poverty and its concomitants. Many of the migrants to vibrant urban centres move there because of the poverty and other stresses of rural life.[1]

Systematic psychiatry is covered in the standard textbooks on the subject. The aim of this chapter is to consider those aspects which are particularly relevant to practitioners who have to deal with psychiatric problems in the tropics but who have not had special training in the subject. Although psychiatrists working in the tropics are scarce (about 1/million population in most of sub-Saharan Africa, for example), some countries also employ professional psychiatric nurses or medical auxiliaries with experience in the field who can be called upon to assist and advise in the management of the mentally ill.[2] It should be stressed, however, that most mentally disturbed patients can be managed by the general medical officer in the wards of a district hospital or in the community. Most medical schools now give more time to psychiatry than in the past and doctors are better equipped to recognize psychiatric disorders. But most courses and many major general textbooks of psychiatry do not give sufficient attention to the 'cultural' element, which is so important in psychiatric practice. We use the word 'culture' in a very broad sense as referring to any socially determined influence impinging upon a person's lifestyle, means of coping with problems and conceptualization of illnesses. Table 17.1 lists some polar attributes of traditional and modern societies. These attributes vary in the extent of their application to any particular society, and not all would apply in any particular location. The concept of cultural sensitivity concerns the differences, of which any doctor should be aware, between his own cultural background, including his values and attitudes, and those of any patient coming from a different background, even in his own country. While practitioners who are foreign to a particular culture should not be expected to 'master' the culture (one can speak of culture as well as language-learning), they should make themselves skilled in working with local staff who can evaluate puzzling symptoms and signs. Knowledge of a language must include an appreciation of idiom and of the emotional loading attached to particular words in different contexts. In multi-ethnic societies no single practitioner will be able to communicate directly with all patients in their own vernaculars and the rapid changes in usage of a dominant rural language adopted as a local lingua franca, for example, in a capital city must be appreciated. Hence the skilful use of interpreters becomes essential in practice, caution being employed in their selection, however.[3]

Alternative and complementary healing practices

Traditional healers are an important aspect of life in most tropical areas. The term 'traditional healer' is misleading, however, and it tends to lump all non-Western-trained healers together. Much depends on the part of the world – India has its great tradition of Ayurvedic practice, for example. A comprehensive classification is impossible in a chapter of this length. The term 'alternative medicine' has come into more general usage and its techniques, successes and failures are being scrutinized more closely; traditional healing should be looked upon as part of alternative medicine. If many patients consult local healers, it is wise to learn something of their techniques and ways of interpreting illness. Some healers

Table 17.1 Polar attributes of traditional and modern societies

Traditional society	Modern society
Group oriented	Individual oriented
Extended family	Nuclear family
Income-producing linked to kinship ties	Income-producing independent of kinship ties
Economic functions non-specialized	Economic functions specialized
High mortality, high fertility	Low mortality, low fertility
Status determined by age and position in family	Status achieved by own efforts
Relationships between kin obligatory	Relationships between kin permissive
Relationships determined by role and position in family	Relationships determined by individual choice
Arranged marriages	Choice of marital partner
Individuals can be replaced by others filling same roles	Individuals unique and irreplaceable
Extensive classification terminology for distant relatives	Restricted classification terminology for close relatives only
Behaviour to specific kin prescribed	Great variation in kin behaviour
Emotional relationships stereotyped	Emotional relationships differentiated

use trance states (spirit possession, sometimes called shamanistic healing) or other means of divination. Spiritual healing also includes activities taking place within a formal religious context – for instance, casting out of demons. It should not be assumed that the traditional healer can always communicate better with patients or their families than orthodox medical workers, especially in an urban setting where they might accept patients from any ethnic group. Because a healer may often look to interpersonal conflict and jealousy as the cause of illness, some individual may be blamed, resulting in family or other social disruption. While a patient's belief in having been bewitched or affected by a magical charm may be understandable in terms of 'culture', it may equally well be a symptom which needs assessment within the total clinical context. The type of healer available for consultation, be he traditional or religious, is also part of the individual's culture. Some traditional healers are men and women of experience and wisdom and some know of herbs that seem to have potent neuroleptic or tranquillizing effects. It is wise to ask a patient if they have consulted a healer, or are currently receiving treatment or are intending to do so. Some of the constituents of herbs given by traditional healers may interact with prescribed medications or have other toxic effects[4] but it appears that the majority probably have only a placebo effect.[5] Should the doctor encourage or allow his patients to consult traditional healers? Clinical judgement must determine the response. One cannot prevent a patient seeking alternative help but should at least warn where this is seen as inappropriate or dangerous. Patients with organic disorders and those with psychotic symptoms and the severely depressed should be advised not to seek such help. Many healers tend to avoid looking after such patients.

Terminology and classification

There are currently two main systems of classification used in psychiatry. Although the 4th edition of the American Psychiatric Association's Diagnostic and Statistical Manual[6] (DSM-IV) is comprehensive and detailed in its definitions the International Classification of Diseases, 10th edition[7] (ICD-10), has the advan-

tage of being truly international and of being concise in its definitions while being very largely consistent with the larger American volume. All references to diagnostic categories in this chapter will be to ICD-10. Modern classifications have all but abandoned certain well-known but ill-defined terms. To merely diagnose 'psychosis' can be dangerous since typical symptoms occur in conditions having very different aetiologies and requiring very different management. The term 'neurosis' is not used in ICD-10 and the word 'neurotic' is found only in the title of a chapter. As an adjective, the word tends sometimes to carry a pejorative connotation and implies some form of innate weakness of character or inability to cope. It should never be used in this sense. The word 'hysteria' has also been abandoned since it had become ambiguous in its meaning and 'puerperal psychosis' is also redundant since a diagnosis should almost always be possible under some other heading. There are in addition a number of culture-bound symptoms or symptom complexes which have been described in the past. Such terms should now be looked upon as essentially obsolete. Making a more specific diagnosis enables all factors to be taken into account (as with many psychiatric conditions, the aetiology may be multiple) and should lead to more focused management. However the use of local terminology in describing an illness can be justified when it improves communication in increasing understanding of underlying social processes.

ORGANIC, INCLUDING SYMPTOMATIC MENTAL DISORDERS

Acute organic states

Although brief episodes of apparent clouding of consciousness may occur in psychoses such as schizophrenia or during an acute polymorphic psychiatric disorder (sometimes called a brief psychotic episode), it is best to assume that all such states are caused by organic dysfunction. It is wise to avoid the term 'confusional state', often used for acute organic states, since the expression is also generally used to refer to muddled thinking, which is found in other psychiatric disorders. Delirium may occur as a result of primary cerebral disorders or of systemic disease.

Common systemic conditions causing delirium in the tropics include:

- Heat: high fever, heat stroke, heat exhaustion
- Dehydration, electrolyte imbalance
- Infections, especially malaria, pneumonia, septicaemia, typhoid, typhus, urinary tract infection
- Poisons including carbon monoxide
- Vitamin deficiency, thiamine, niacine, B_{12}, folate
- Alcohol, drug intoxication or withdrawal
- Prescribed drugs, herbal remedies
- Endocrine and metabolic disorders, hypoglycaemia.

Disorders primarily affecting the central nervous system and causing delirium include:

- Infection: meningitis, encephalitis, brain abscess, tuberculoma, cerebral schistosomiasis, cysticercosis, hydatid disease, paragonimiasis
- Epilepsy and postepileptic states
- Head injury and its sequelae including cerebral haemorrhage, subdural haematoma
- Intracranial space-occupying lesions
- Raised intracranial pressure.

Since delirium refers to a constellation of psychiatric symptoms occurring in individuals suffering from some other underlying illness, the nature of this illness may also determine the presentation and may be a main feature; or the illness may present as a delirium and steps have to be taken to determine its cause. The main feature – impairment of consciousness – may be very mild and may vary, both according to the time of day (usually worse at night) and from moment to moment. It is characterized by disorientation in time and place and by an inability to recognize familiar people. There are typically visual hallucinations and possibly illusions or other disturbances of perception; the mood is often anxious, irritable or simply one of perplexity but often very labile; thinking is slow and muddled and there may be some paranoid ideation and such a degree of suspiciousness that it is difficult to nurse the patient. The patient can give little information about himself and registration of new memories is impaired.

The treatment of any delirious episode needs to be both general and specific. The general treatment, as well as focusing upon the underlying cause, must include adequate nursing and this is best complemented by the presence of family members. Nursing should be done in an environment where the patient is neither under- nor over-stimulated and is rapidly able to recognize those who are caring for him. Drug treatment should not sedate during the day and should assist sleep at night. While chlordiazepoxide is often the drug of choice in delirium tremens it may sometimes prove to be too sedative with other types of delirium (e.g. in an individual recovering from unconsciousness due to head injury) and in this case a neuroleptic such as haloperidol may be preferred during the day. Since alcohol withdrawal and vitamin deficiency states so often co-exist and may also be factors in a person who has been concussed after a road traffic accident, it is wise to give the full spectrum of B vitamins to all delirious patients. Delirium tremens should be treated, if severe, as a medical emergency. There may be severe dehydration and disturbance of electrolyte balance, seizures may occur and there may be hepatic pathology and a

cardiomyopathy. Infusing glucose without ensuring an adequate supply of thiamine can precipitate Wernicke's encephalopathy. Other specific treatments will depend on the cause of the delirium.

Chronic organic mental disorders and dementia (chronic brain syndrome)

Dementia is a syndrome due to disease of the brain, usually of a chronic or progressive nature, in which there is a disturbance of multiple functions including memory, thinking, orientation, comprehension, calculation, learning capacity, language and judgement. Consciousness is not clouded although episodes of clouding may occur during the course of a dementing process. Although there is no specific therapy for some forms of dementia it is important to be able to recognize those cases in which effective treatment can be given. Because some of the main causes of dementia arise from degenerative conditions (such as Alzheimer's disease, Huntington's chorea and cerebrovascular disease), they are more commonly seen in older patients and thus are less common in those countries with a lower life expectancy. As the population structure changes, so does the spectrum of diseases. It is likely that Alzheimer's dementia will become more common, although in some countries HIV infection has taken over as one of the commonest causes of a dementing process. Especially in younger persons, however, treatable forms of dementia may occur, such as that due to chronic subdural haematoma or prolonged lack of vitamin B_{12}. The dementia of HIV infection (typically subcortical) tends to occur late in the disease when the patient is seriously ill from other manifestations of AIDS. Few tropical countries have been able to provide sufficient drugs for the many needing antiretroviral (ARV) therapy; ARVs diminish the development of an AIDS encephalopathy but do not necessarily prevent it . Other opportunistic infections such as toxoplasmosis, tuberculous meningitis or cytomegalovirus may also lead to a dementing process and should also be kept in mind, especially with a view to possible treatment. In case one of these is found without any prior suspicion of HIV infection, the question of counselling and testing becomes part of the overall management. Depression may be mistaken for dementia, especially when older patients are admitted to the foreign environment of a hospital and their natural perplexity (perhaps confounded by inability to communicate well in the local lingua franca) gives a false impression of intellectual deterioration.

Mental and behavioural disorders due to psychoactive substance use

Alcohol remains the main substance of abuse in most countries. Since the consumption of alcohol is linked to so many forms of morbidity, it is advisable for practitioners in any tropical country to make themselves acquainted with the terminology related to consumption of local beverages (including usual alcohol content) and the consumption style of the population. Alcoholic beverages may be very cheap, especially grain-based opaque beers, whether commercial or home-brewed, which are drunk without previous filtration. While a country may have laws concerning the production and distribution of alcoholic beverages, these laws may often not be enforced and in remote rural areas their enforcement is in any case largely impractical. The definition of an illicit beverage is usually determined locally but the fact of being illicit seldom deters either producers or drinkers. More importantly, there is no formal quality control over such products and potency-enhancing contaminants may be added. Illicitly distilled beverages often contain about 20–30% or more alcohol by volume. When a spirit has been made, the most common and dangerous contaminant is methyl alcohol, which can lead to sudden death or bilateral optic neuritis and blindness. The drinking style of the population may be very heterogeneous in that different age and income bands may have different patterns, while there may be a sharp differentiation between the sexes. Consumption patterns are often related to cost as well as to availability. Many drinkers do not realize how much harm alcohol can do to the body but its social disruptiveness can often be mitigated by established customs in drinking.[8]

The concept of the alcohol dependence syndrome is now well established, but the common style of drinking may not usually lead to this particular complication. For a person to become dependent, it is usually necessary for there to be a high intake of alcohol on a daily basis over a long period. The main features of alcohol dependence include a strong desire or compulsion to take alcohol, difficulties in controlling drinking behaviour in terms of its onset, termination or levels of use; a physiological withdrawal state; evidence of tolerance; neglect of alternative pleasures or interests; and persisting with drinking despite clear evidence of overtly harmful consequences. Disorders related to thiamine deficiency (Wernicke's encephalopathy and Korsakov psychosis) may occur less commonly than, for example, pellagra. In some countries pellagra is seen when a heavy-drinking man is deprived for a time of the food provided by his wife and he turns to a diet of bread and an illicit spirit. There is often a mixed vitamin deficiency state, with either niacin or thiamine deficiency the more prominent. Although the features of Wernicke's encephalopathy are well known, those of niacin deficiency are not. The medical student's triad of three Ds is incorrect. There is no dementia but an acute or subacute organic state. While the skin changes may be typical, there may be no history of gastrointestinal symptoms. The clouding of consciousness is usually very labile and within a matter of a minute or so a patient may be able to give some personal details and then become inaccessible. Neurological signs are commonly present, with a marked snout reflex and increased deep-tendon reflexes but with (usually) down-going plantar reflexes. There may be features of a peripheral neuropathy from thiamine deficiency. It is common for health workers to successfully treat the pellagra while ignoring the underlying cause. Following up the patient and helping him with his drinking problem is an example of how prevention should be incorporated into all health programmes and practice.

Cannabis is often implicated as a cause of acute mental disorder in countries where it is grown and used. The plant Cannabis sativa (Indian hemp) is easily grown in the tropics and is widely available. Besides the well-known synonyms for cannabis products there is a constantly changing list of new names invented by current users in any locality. The main active ingredient is tetrahydrocannabinol; it enters the body usually by being smoked or sometimes by being eaten, and induces in most people a pleasant, dreamy state of altered perception. However, some people experience a panic attack or feel depressed. An acute psychotic state may be induced by heavy intoxication but it is generally agreed that

there is no cannabis psychosis as such. It seems likely, however, that cannabis use may be a factor in the development of schizophrenia in especially vulnerable persons. In countries where there is widespread use of cannabis, mental illness is often attributed to its use in a very uncritical way. Careful history taking will more often reveal that there is no association. Longer-term psychological effects include interference with memory and learning. Psychological dependence may occur in regular users. The concept of a cannabis amotivational syndrome has not been confirmed. Cannabis slows down reaction time and hence when combined with alcohol can be a factor in traffic or other accidents. Cannabis use is not especially associated with violence but this may occur when it is used at the same time as alcohol. There are no pharmacological effects producing fatal consequences.[9]

Alcohol and cannabis are widely available and relatively inexpensive. Many other drugs are much more expensive – but the scene is a constantly changing one. In countries swept by war, other drugs may be introduced (amphetamines for example) or tablets like diazepam looted from stores may be widely distributed. The taking of a drug like diazepam or an amphetamine may become fashionable in any country and particularly in schools and colleges. The drug 'ecstasy' is making its way round the world and other 'designer' drugs may well become widely available, especially in large cities. 'Street children' are especially prone to use volatile substances. Doctors should be aware of the effects of these drugs and be prepared to advise the authorities as well as treat individuals.

PSYCHOTIC STATES

Schizophrenia

The most characteristic symptoms of schizophrenia are remarkably consistent all over the world, whatever the culture. ICD-10 states that although there are no strictly pathognomonic symptoms of schizophrenia, the following often occur together: thought echo, thought insertion or withdrawal, and thought broadcasting; delusions of control, influence or passivity clearly referred to body movement, specific thoughts action or sensations; hallucinatory voices, commenting on the patient's actions, discussing the patient among themselves, or other types of voice coming from some part of the body; persistent culturally inappropriate or impossible delusions; breaks or interpolations in the train of thought, and incoherent or irrelevant speech or neologisms. Catatonic behaviour with excitement, posturing, waxy flexibility, negativism, mutism or stupor is uncommon.

Negative symptoms may also be present, including marked apathy, paucity of speech, blunting or incongruity of emotional responses. They usually result in withdrawal and lowering of social performance, with a significant change in the overall quality of personal behaviour, manifest in loss of interest, aimlessness, idleness and a self-absorbed attitude. Paranoid schizophrenia is the commonest type in most parts of the world but many patients present with an undifferentiated form. A dilemma presents itself with regard to diagnosis. On the one hand, making an early diagnosis and instituting treatment early improves the prognosis but, on the other hand, one should not be too hasty in attaching this diagnosis to an individual. However, if the symptoms are quite typical and there is no question of prior drug use or any other organic factor, a provisional diagnosis should be made and treatment instituted. Schizophrenia can run a variety of different courses. Very roughly, it may be said that in one-quarter of patients the symptoms continue unremittingly. In one-third the symptoms remit after an initial episode but, following this, the condition may relapse periodically though most can manage a reasonably normal social life. In the remainder, the patients recover and remain well. Favourable prognostic factors include a negative family history, good premorbid personality, an acute onset with early treatment and a good response to treatment. Although prognosis in the tropics is said to be better, it is possible that some patients with acute transient psychotic episodes, as described below, may be mis-diagnosed as schizophrenia. As much more is learnt about the underlying neurological mechanisms involved it is apparent that many neurotransmitters and neuropeptides have a role to play. Any drugs which are prescribed will inevitably have some unwanted effects and some may be dangerous. The patient's tolerance for these unwanted effects will be an important factor in adherence, as will the cost of treatment. More previously expensive later generation drugs such as risperidone and olanzapine are becoming available at an affordable price and these should be used for preference although there is as yet little evidence that they are more effective therapeutically.[10] Otherwise the older neuroleptics such as chlorpromazine, trifluoperazine and haloperidol should be used, keeping in mind the possible need for an antiparkinsonian drug such as trihexyphenidyl (benzhexol). For many patients the drug of choice will be a depot preparation, such as fluphenazine decanoate. An injection may need to be given only once per month and sometimes even less frequently. This drug requires an antiparkinsonian. Specialist advice should be sought regarding cessation of therapy and, with prolonged therapy, a watch needs to be made for the symptoms of tardive dyskinesia. Attending to psychosocial factors is important in helping the schizophrenic patient. Counselling for the family is especially important; for instance, many patients cannot tolerate highly emotional situations and are unwilling to be pushed into strong social interaction. The patient and his family must understand why the drugs are being given and know the difference between those given for the illness and those given to prevent unwanted effects.

Acute transient psychotic episodes

The concept of the parasuicidal 'cry for help' has proved to be very useful in some cultures but it needs some modification where a strong sense of group membership rather than self-identity is fostered (Table 17.1). Instead of violence directed against the self, it is directed towards the family and community. A young woman, quite often in the evening, begins to sing and dance and may exhibit destructive or other exhibitionistic behaviour. This behaviour may continue for many hours and even for 2 or 3 days; the patient may be taken to a traditional healer or church leaders. Admission or detention of such patients is usually desirable, not only because their behaviour is unacceptable at home but also because observation of the clinical course over the next few hours and days will provide essential information for future management. Such episodes are often incorrectly diagnosed as mania but

the typical elevation of affect, pressure of speech and flight of ideas are not seen. If sedation is required either a benzodiazepine or a neuroleptic may be used. The length of treatment is likely to be short. Once the patient is able to communicate, the psychological and social causes need to be explored. Not infrequently, symptoms of depression will be found to be present or there may be some history of an acute traumatic episode or of conflict within the family. This is the point at which familiarity with the patient's culture is especially important.

It is commonly assumed that violence is common in psychiatric patients but this is wrong. It may be precipitated because people are fearful and attempt to restrain an already fearful patient, perhaps perplexed by what is happening to him; if the police are involved this may only make the situation worse. A struggling, seemingly violent patient can often be left in the capable hands of an experienced nurse who is ready to listen and reassure. Where a patient is manifestly violent and no communication can be established, sufficient staff members experienced in working together should hold the patient so that intramuscular chlorpromazine or haloperidol may be administered. It should be kept in mind that chlorpromazine tends to cause local tissue necrosis. Overactive or violent patients may benefit from a cocktail of haloperidol and diazepam (given alternately) at three-hour intervals and withdrawn slowly over a period of 24–36 h.

Bipolar affective disorders

Mania is one pole of the affective disorder spectrum and its main feature is elevation of mood, often amounting to elation, although irritability may sometimes be present. There is reduced sleep – which others complain about, not the patient, and there is increased appetite. Behaviour is often socially inappropriate. On examination, there are expansive ideas or actual grandiose delusions, pressure of speech with flight of ideas is present and hallucinations may occur. Insight is impaired and may not be fully recovered, even by a compliant patient receiving a mood-stabilizing drug. There will often be a family history of similar episodes, or of depression and suicide, and the patient may have suffered from a previous episode or episodes, either of mania or depression. A first episode should be differentiated from schizophrenia or an acute transient psychotic episode, since long-term management differs in the three conditions. Even without treatment manic episodes are self-limiting after a few weeks or months, and the patients are able to live normal sociable lives between the episodes. Haloperidol is the drug of choice in the acute phase. There is usually no need to guard against a recurrence after a first episode of mania, but if two or more recur at relatively short intervals continuing medication with a 'mood stabilizer' will be advisable. While lithium may be best, its use requires experience and adequate blood lithium levels monitoring facilities. Carbamazepine and sodium valproate can also be used as mood stabilizers and besides being more readily available many families may be willing to take the burden of their cost rather than cope with further manic episodes. As with schizophrenia, careful counselling of the patient is required regarding continuing medication; one of the early signs of relapse is increasing reluctance to take the medication by a patient who increasingly doubts whether he has ever been ill.

DEPRESSION

There have been numerous attempts at the classification of depressive disorders. The niceties of classification in practice are less important than the ability to recognize depression in its milder as well as more extreme forms and the ability to offer appropriate therapy. While depression may form one pole of bipolar affective disorder, it may also be found as a component of many other disorders, including schizophrenia and dementia. Depression can have many causes and several may be operating at the same time – for example, in a woman who is at the menopause, is taking antihypertensive drugs, is just recovering from an attack of influenza and has a daughter with an unwanted pregnancy. While there may be multiple aetiologies, it can be taken that there is a final common pathway influencing many symptoms involving monoamine neurotransmitters.

Depression is characterized by depressed mood or sadness, loss of interest and enjoyment, reduced energy, increased fatiguability and diminished activity. Some of the following may also be present: reduced concentration and attention, reduced self-esteem and self-confidence, ideas of guilt and unworthiness, bleak and pessimistic views of the future, ideas or acts of self-harm or suicide, disturbed sleep, diminished appetite (including desire for sex). Some patients may feel worse at the end of the day and have difficulty getting off to sleep. Others feel worse on waking, sometimes linked with early-morning waking. Depression is often a hidden and unmentioned cause of distress and disability, particularly in housewives. Although depression in the tropics is similar to that seen elsewhere, cultural factors seem to be especially important in its expression; for example, somatic symptoms (such as burning sensations on the top of the head, may be more prominent. It has been noted that there is no exact translation for the word 'depression' into many African languages. Once the condition is suspected the presence of both typical psychological and vegetative symptoms of depression will rapidly confirm the diagnosis. Often a single question about 'thinking too much' will give an initial clue.

Both drugs and psychosocial therapy may be beneficial. As with the older neuroleptics, the older tricyclic antidepressants are much less well tolerated than newer products such as the selective serotonin re-uptake inhibitors. The antimuscarinic side-effects of the older tricyclics discourage many patients from continuing with an adequate dose – and too low a dose is one of the commoner causes for failure to respond to treatment. The newer drugs are better tolerated but more expensive. When only the older tricyclics, such as amitriptyline, are available, it is best to start with a relatively small dose and work up to the dose required while explaining and offering reassurance about the side-effects. The drug can be given in a single dose before going to bed and there is the double advantage of better sleep and less experience of side-effects. Patients should always be informed that there will be a delay of up to 2 weeks in feeling the full antidepressant effect. Great care must be taken with potentially suicidal patients when a tricyclic antidepressant and especially amitriptyline (because of its cardio-toxicity) is prescribed – some other person should always have charge of the drug which is given to the patient as required.

Suicide

When an individual talks of or threatens suicide the risk must be assessed. Recognizing suicidal intent can be life-saving, since suicide is mostly preventable when its possibility is kept in mind. It is not always possible after a 'failed attempt' to determine whether an individual really wished to die or not but there are indicators of possible future intent. The patient who is depressed should always be asked about suicidal ideation or plans. There is never any risk in doing so. These days, with the wide availability of pharmaceutical and poisonous domestic products, carrying out a suicidal act is far easier than in the past, when resort might have been had to hanging, drowning or self-immolation. Indicators of risk include: if an individual talks of committing suicide or killing themselves, has made definite plans including writing a note, putting affairs in order, accumulating tablets (e.g. of an antidepressant); the presence of a psychiatric disorder such as schizophrenia but especially severe depression; alcohol or drug dependence; being older, especially if suffering from any chronic illness or disability; and being socially isolated. Those who are more likely to carry out a 'parasuicidal act' are usually younger, female, less commonly suffer from a psychiatric disorder, have usually acted on impulse and used a less dangerous method.

Anxiety and stress-related disorders

In ICD-10 several groups of anxiety disorders are listed including phobic states, obsessive compulsive disorder, panic and generalized anxiety disorder, reactions to severe stress and adjustment disorder and dissociative (conversion) disorders. The term phobia refers to anxiety occurring in relation to specific situations. Since phobic states and obsessive compulsive disorders appear to be uncommon in tropical countries, and their management requires specialist training, they are not dealt with further. Panic attacks are brief episodes of severe anxiety, not associated with any precipitant, when the patient suddenly experiences autonomic symptoms accompanied by a fear of being about to die or lose control or become mad. They are often associated with hyperventilation with its typical symptoms of dyspnoea, hyperpnoea, chest pain, dizziness, weakness, paraesthesia and carpopedal spasm. A combination of explanation and reassurance with pharmacotherapy may be necessary. A selective serotonin re-uptake inhibitor or a tricyclic antidepressant such as imipramine may be effective in suppressing attacks. Generalized anxiety disorder manifests with persistent autonomic symptoms as well as somatic complaints such as abdominal discomfort and constriction of the chest, and accompanied by vague fears, irritability and poor concentration. Sometimes there is a more specific complaint such as tension headache (which must be distinguished from migraine). Generalized anxiety may occur with depression and often in clinical practice it is unnecessary to distinguish between the two; the designation 'common mental disorders' has been found useful for this group of disorders.[11] In all patients with a provisional diagnosis of anxiety or depression, a thorough physical examination is an important procedure, which can be reassuringly therapeutic. Anxiolytic drugs such as the benzodiazepines are only suitable for the relief of acute anxiety in the short term. Since many patients also have depressive symptoms, an antidepressant may prove helpful. Symptomatic treatment will not remove the need for intervention at the social level and counselling, but can be an important component of treatment.[12] Although it is often stated that the traditional healer can be especially helpful it will often be found that the patient has already visited several, with little practical help having been obtained.

Reference has been made to the strong pressure to conform in traditional society. In the modern world, there is also strong pressure from parents for their children to fulfil frustrated parental ambitions and many children are ambitious to go far in their schooling. This led in Nigeria to the naming of a syndrome which still merits attention, if not the special name (brain fag syndrome).[13] The symptoms (complained of more often by boys) may be attributed diagnostically to a mild anxiety/depressive disorder with marked somatization and they include difficulty in concentrating or retaining what has been read and blurred vision. Relating mainly to problems of study, symptoms tend to increase as examination time approaches. Medical intervention is rarely necessary and much distress can be prevented if the school can appoint a trained counsellor, able to give guidance on good study habits and deal with the problems of adolescence and of boarding school life, as well as giving guidance to parents.

Dissociative (conversion) disorders

The term 'hysteria' is no longer used. It formerly had many meanings attached to it, often with a pejorative connotation, especially when referring to personality (the designation is now 'histrionic') or to a constellation of physical complaints having no organic cause. The mechanism of dissociation implies a loss of conscious (and therefore voluntary) control over the integration of memories, current experiences and current behaviour, which results in psychological or apparent neurological dysfunction – the latter being designated 'conversion'. It is assumed that psychological discomfort has been converted to physical symptoms, thus allowing relief of distress and secondary gain.[14] Of psychological symptoms, dissociative amnesia and fugue states are most often seen and of conversion disorders, aphonia and paralysis, e.g. of a limb or even a particular movement. More dramatic manifestations are rare. The mechanism of dissociation is sometimes encountered in states of (spirit) possession, which often serve a useful function in allowing expression of psychosocial problems in socially acceptable ways; such states are not considered to be pathological.

Epidemic hysteria

One type of disorder which a doctor may be called upon to deal with can still conveniently be called 'epidemic hysteria'. Reports are regularly made of tens or even scores of school children being inflicted with a disease causing bizarre symptoms and defying immediate diagnosis in terms of any infectious agent, although the rapidity of spread of the symptoms suggests an 'epidemic'. Usually there is some cause of common distress or concern in the establishment, e.g. regarding the quality of food, or dislike for a particular staff member. A prominent figure (such as a head girl) may provide an example of easily imitated symptoms. Rapid iso-

lation of the afflicted and an understanding that perpetuation of the symptoms will result in leaving school quickly cure the epidemic.

Stress-related disorders

Natural and man-made disasters (including war and civil conflict) are common causes of stress to large numbers of people, including refugees, and many individuals are also subject to overwhelming stress in their personal lives, for example because of a serious traffic accident, involvement in a fire or being assaulted. Post-traumatic stress disorder is a reaction that can affect anyone, and not only the especially vulnerable. It often appears after a delay of some days or weeks and then persists with anxiety, insomnia and nightmares. Although there is difficulty in remembering details of the traumatic event, patients are troubled by intrusive and unwanted memories of what happened and try to avoid reminders of the event. There are also complaints of irritability, poor concentration and in some cases a feeling of detachment and of an inability to feel emotion. Early treatment is likely to be most effective and should be aimed first at reducing severe anxiety and restoring sleep by use of appropriate drugs over a short period while increasingly enabling individuals to recall their experiences and express their emotions in a supportive relationship. Planners need to pay attention to training of workers with the necessary counselling skills in disaster-prone areas. It is probable that the spread of HIV infection has drawn attention to gender-based violence and especially to sexual assault, including widespread child physical and sexual abuse. The health worker must be alert to the possibility of injuries having been inflicted in an abusive situation. Changes in a child's behaviour may be reported including: social isolation, sleep disturbances (nightmares, irrational fears, bed wetting, fear of sleeping alone), reluctance or refusal to participate in physical activities or to change clothes for activities, drug, alcohol, or solvent abuse, display of sexual knowledge beyond the child's years, unusual interest in the genitals of adults, children, or animals, lack of trust in adults or over-familiarity with adults, fear of a particular individual, sexual promiscuity. In areas with limited resources, new techniques of using 'group cognitive behaviour therapy' have recently been shown to be feasable.[15]

REFERENCES

1. Satterthwaite D. Will most people live in cities? *BMJ* 2000; 321:1143–1145.
2. Murthy RS. Reaching the unreached. *Lancet Perspect* 2000; 356:s39.
3. Swartz L. *Culture and Mental health: A South African View.* Cape Town: Oxford University Press; 1998, Ch. 2.
4. Escher M, Desmeules J, Giatra E, et al. Drug points: hepatitis associated with Kava herbal remedy for anxiety. *BMJ* 2001; 322:139.
5. Ernst E. The role of complementary and alternative medicine. *BMJ* 2000; 321:1133–1135.
6. American Psychiatric Association. *Diagnostic and Statistical Manual of Mental Disorder.* 4th edn. Washington, DC: American Psychiatric Association; 1994.
7. WHO. *ICD-10 Classification of Mental and Behavioural Disorders.* Geneva: World Health Organization; 1992.
8. Haworth A, Simpson R. Introduction. In: Haworth A, Simpson, eds. *R Moonshine Markets.* New York: Brunner-Routledge; 2004:1–90.

9. WHO. *Cannabis: A Health Perspective and Research Agenda.* Geneva: World Health Organization; 1997.

10. Byrne P. Managing the acute psychotic episode. *BMJ* 2007; 334:686–695.

11. Goldberg D, Huxley P. *Common Mental Disorders.* London: Routledge; 1992.

12. Patel V, Todd C, Winston M, et al. Outcome of common mental disorders in Harare, Zimbabwe. *Br J Psychiatry* 1998; 172:53–57.

13. Prince R. Concept of culture bound syndromes: anorexia and brain fag. *Soc Sci Med* 1985; 21:197–203.

14. Kendell RE. Hysteria, somatisation and the sick role. *Med Int* 1991; 95:3944–3947.

15. Bolton P, Bass J, Neugerbauer R, et al. Group interpersonal psychotherapy for depression in rural Uganda. *JAMA* 2003; 289:3117–3124.

Chapter 18   David H. Yorston and D. D. Murray McGavin

Ophthalmology in the Tropics and Subtropics

WORLD BLINDNESS

The World Health Organization (WHO) Programme for the Prevention of Blindness and Deafness estimates that the number of people blind in the world is now around 37 million.[1] The figure does not take into account the many millions who have only partial sight, an estimated further 124 million.[1] Over 90% of blind people live in the developing world and at least 70% of blindness could be 'avoided', that is, either prevented or cured.

WHO categories of visual impairment

At one time there were over 70 different definitions of blindness among United Nations member states. The WHO has now defined five categories of visual impairment (Table 18.1).

Blindness is defined as a best-corrected binocular visual acuity of less than 3/60 (less than counting fingers at 3 m) or where the central visual field is less than 10° around fixation in the better eye. Agreed definitions allow comparisons between countries and regions, and between the main causes of blindness affecting different populations, which is essential for planning effective eye care services.

Patterns of blindness

The prevalence of blindness around the world is influenced by a number of factors, including age, gender, ethnic origin, environment and socioeconomic factors.

Age

Life expectancy is increasing in developing countries, and with the increase in numbers of old people there is a corresponding increase of those who are blind. The WHO estimates that 82% of global blindness is found in people aged over 50, although in most countries less than 20% of the population belong to this age group.[1] In all countries, increased longevity has resulted in more older people with chronic blinding diseases. There is, however, a contrast in the common causes of blindness between the developed and the developing world (Table 18.2).[1]

Gender

Blinding eye disease throughout the world shows some differences between males and females (Table 18.3).[2] Some of the variation is due to differing access to eye services. Trachoma trichiasis is four to five times more common among women compared with men, due to the recurrent cycle of reinfection affecting children and mothers (Figure 18.1).[3] Onchocerciasis (river blindness), as a blinding disease, is more common in men, who are more exposed to the bites of the black biting fly.

Angle closure glaucoma in Inuit women is found three to four times more often when compared with Inuit men. Conversely, open angle glaucoma among Africans may be more common in men than women.

Climatic keratopathy, due to exposure to direct or reflected ultraviolet light, is more common among men than women. This relates to the exposure to sunlight of men working out of doors, and is common in desert areas.

Ethnic origin

Glaucoma, in its two primary forms, shows considerable variation among broad ethnic regions around the world.[4] Primary angle closure glaucoma is more common among the Inuit and Chinese. In contrast, primary open angle glaucoma is more common in people of African origin, often presenting in younger patients as compared with Caucasian races.

Environmental factors

Many environmental factors affect the prevalence of blindness in communities. Trachoma is found in communities with poor sanitation and inadequate water supplies.[5] Acute dehydration, which may be due to acute diarrhoeal disease, is a risk factor for the later onset of cataract.[6]

A village situated close to a river with turbulent, frothy water is more likely to have blinding eye disease due to onchocerciasis. The Simulium fly, which carries the microfilariae of the worm *Onchocerca volvulus*, breeds at the margins of these rivers – hence the name river blindness.

Poor environmental sources of fruits and vegetables, or lack of basic health education where these vitamin A-rich foods may be

Table 18.1 Categories of visual impairment*

Categories*	VISUAL ACUITY† WITH BEST POSSIBLE CORRECTION	
	Maximum less than:	Minimum equal to; or better than:
1 Visual impairment	6/18 20/70 3/10 (0.3)	6/60 20/200 1/10 (0.1)
2 Severe visual impairment	6/60 20/200 1/10 (0.1)	3/60 (finger counting at 3 m) 20/400 1/20 (0.05)
3 Blindness	3/60 (finger counting at 3 m) 20/400 1/20 (0.05)	1/60 (finger counting at 1 m) 5/300 (20/1200) 1/50 (0.02)
4 Blindness	1/60 (finger counting at 1 m) 5/300 (20/1200) 1/50 (0.02)	Light perception
5 Blindness	No light perception	

*If the extent of the visual field is taken into account, patients with a visual field radius no greater than 10° but greater than 5° around central fixation should be placed in category 3. Patients with a field no greater than 5° around central fixation should be placed in category 4, even if the central acuity is not impaired.
†For the first four categories of visual impairment, the different figures in each box of the visual acuity columns represent the same level of acuity expressed according to different notations. The first line gives the notation used with the Snellen 6-metre scale (and, where applicable, the corresponding ability to count extended fingers at a set distance); the second line gives the equivalent notation used with the 20-foot scale; the third gives the decimal notation.
Adapted from the International Classification of Diseases, ninth (1975) revision.

Table 18.2 Major causes of blindness

	United Kingdom	Tanzania
Children (0–15 years)	Genetic diseases	Vitamin A deficiency (measles)
	Retrolental fibroplasia	Congenital cataract
	Congenital anomalies	Ophthalmia neonatorum
Adults (45 years +)	Age-related macular degeneration	Cataract
	Chronic glaucoma	Chronic glaucoma
	Diabetic retinopathy	Corneal scar

Table 18.3 Blindness and gender

More common in women	More common in men
Trachoma	Onchocerciasis
Acute glaucoma	Chronic glaucoma
Cataract	Climatic keratopathy
Diabetic retinopathy	

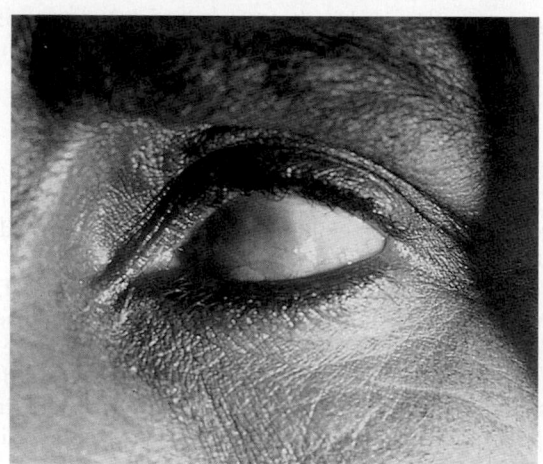

Figure 18.1 A blind eye due to trachoma in a 44-year-old woman. (Courtesy of John D. C. Anderson.)

available, place children, particularly between the ages of 1 and 6 years, at risk of xerophthalmia.

Socioeconomic factors

Prevalence rates of blindness in the developing countries of the world are higher when compared with those in the developed world. Estimates of the number of blind people in different regions of the world (see below) reflect population densities as well as available eye care services.

In richer countries, better perinatal care allows infants to survive, but with occasional eye abnormalities such as genetic defects and retinopathy of prematurity. In countries where obstetric and neonatal care is less advanced, premature babies do not survive.

Low literacy rates and poverty are linked to a greater risk of blindness.[7]

Common causes of worldwide blindness

We have briefly discussed the definition of blindness and some significant factors which influence blindness in the world. Table 18.4 gives estimates of world blindness from the WHO.[1]

Table 18.4 Major causes of blindness worldwide: estimates in millions

Cause of blindness	No. blind (millions)	%
Cataract	17.5	47.8
Glaucoma	4.5	12.3
Age-related macular degeneration	3.2	8.7
Corneal opacity	1.9	5.1
Diabetic retinopathy	1.8	4.8
Childhood blindness	1.4	3.9
Trachoma	1.3	3.6
Onchocerciasis	0.3	0.8
Others	4.8	13.0
Total	36.7	

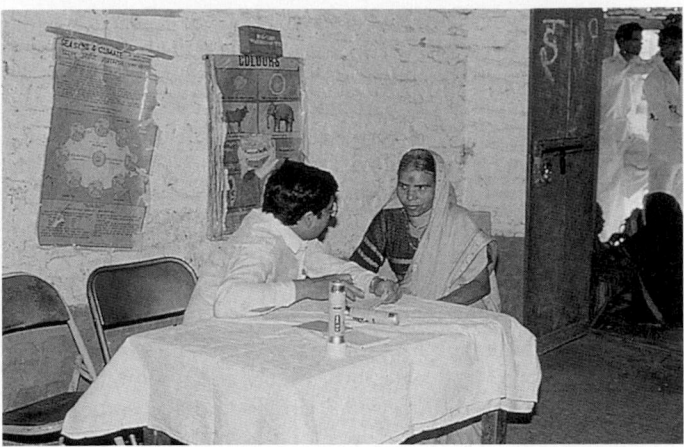

Figure 18.2 A screening/diagnostic eye camp in a school near Pune, India. (Courtesy of Murray McGavin.)

Eye care services

There is a huge disparity in the provision of eye care services between the developed and the developing world. In Europe and North America, there is one ophthalmologist for populations ranging from 20 000 up to 100 000. In sub-Saharan Africa, on average, there is one ophthalmologist for 1 million people.[8]

A universal feature of eye care services throughout the world is the 'urbanization' of ophthalmologists – drawn to major cities by the attractions of lifestyle and financial reward. Even where there are adequate numbers of ophthalmologists, this skewed distribution means that rural areas consistently suffer from inadequate eye care facilities and expertise. Some of those who have specialized in ophthalmology do contribute generously, giving their time and resources to visit distant and impoverished communities.

If we consider that over 90% of the world's blindness is in developing countries and that 70% of this blindness could be either prevented or cured, then the message of need and responsibility is clear.

To meet the needs of the huge numbers of cataract blind patients in Africa, surgeons are being trained who may not be medically qualified. Ophthalmic medical assistants (ophthalmic clinical officers) who have an interest and aptitude, possessing the hand and coordination skills required for eye surgery, make excellent surgeons.[8,9] Good hands and surgical skills are not confined only to those who are medically trained!

The most effective organization of eye care services, in developing countries, is a structure of primary healthcare workers, trained in the recognition of eye disease, who provide basic treatment and advice for patients and recognize those who should be referred to secondary eye care units. Secondary eye care facilities provide routine eye surgery, but have the option of referring patients to tertiary eye care centres, where more specialist services and technologies are concentrated.

At all levels of expertise and experience, ongoing training must be given high priority. Training materials such as textbooks, manuals, videos, CD ROMs, teaching slide sets and posters are widely available. These eye healthcare workers can in turn develop their own programmes to provide health education for the general public.

Eye camps

Where there are no established eye care facilities, eye services may be provided by eye camps (Figure 18.2). These ophthalmic outreach programmes may be described in two broad categories:

- Screening/diagnostic eye camps with referral to the base hospital
- Traditional surgical eye camps.

Although eye camps can deliver services to populations who would otherwise have no access to eye services, the results of surgery are worse in eye camps than in static units.[10,11] The provision of free surgery may undermine local attempts to achieve sustainable cost-recovery. It is now recommended that eye camps should be used primarily for screening/diagnosis rather than surgery.

EXAMINATION OF THE EYES

One of the advantages of ophthalmology is the opportunity to visualize eye abnormalities of both the anterior and posterior segments of the eye. With a focal light and magnification, the anterior eye can be examined, and, with an ophthalmoscope, the vitreous, optic nerve, retina and blood vessels can be seen.

Basic equipment and diagnostic materials

For effective examination of the eyes, only a few basic items are required:

- Test chart, e.g. Snellen's E chart
- Pin-hole disc to screen for refractive errors
- Hand torch (flashlight)
- Magnifying lens or loupe-uniocular or binocular
- Direct ophthalmoscope
- Lid speculum or retractor(s) (suitably shaped paper-clips may be used)

- Schiotz tonometer
- Eye drops: local anaesthetic drops, e.g. amethocaine 1%, benoxinate 0.4%; short-acting mydriatics (to dilate the pupil), e.g. tropicamide 1%, cyclopentolate 1%; fluorescein dye, e.g. minims (very small, disposable); paper strips. (Do not use fluorescein eye drops from bottles as pathogenic organisms may contaminate these bottles.)

Other equipment and medicines for treatment of eye patients

A few basic requirements for the removal of conjunctival or corneal foreign bodies, corneal abrasions, eyelid and periorbital lacerations, and infection of the eyelids, conjunctiva and cornea are as follows:

- Sterile hypodermic needles
- Fine suture material, needle-holding forceps, plain forceps
- Cotton-wool 'buds'
- Eye pads, adhesive tape, bandages
- Scissors
- Antibiotic eye drops and ointments, e.g. tetracycline 1% eye ointment, chloramphenicol 0.5% eye drops; vitamin A capsules (200 000 IU).

Clinical examination of the eyes

This chapter on eye diseases in the tropics and subtropics cannot describe the methods of examination in detail, which are best taught by demonstration. However, a systematic approach to examination should always be followed.

1. History of the complaint

Symptoms should be elicited and described. What is the nature of the complaint? How long has the condition been present? Is vision affected? Is there pain, irritation, itching or discharge? What is the nature of the discomfort? Is the condition improving or worsening? Is there a family history of a similar complaint?

2. Measurement of visual acuity

Visual acuity should be assessed both for distance and near. Distance visual acuity should be recorded for each eye separately at a distance of 6 m (Figure 18.3). If spectacles are worn, visual acuity should be recorded with the spectacles. If vision is reduced and there is no clear evidence of any eye disease, the pin-hole disc should be used. An improvement in vision in one or both eyes using the pin-hole indicates a likely refractive error – spectacles should improve vision.

3. Observe the general health of the patient

Note any obvious signs of systemic disease, e.g. malnutrition, Hansen's disease, rheumatoid arthritis.

4. Examine the periorbital region of each eye

Is there swelling or inflammation – for example in the region of the lacrimal sac? Are the eyelids in the normal position, or are they everted (ectropion) or inverted (entropion)?

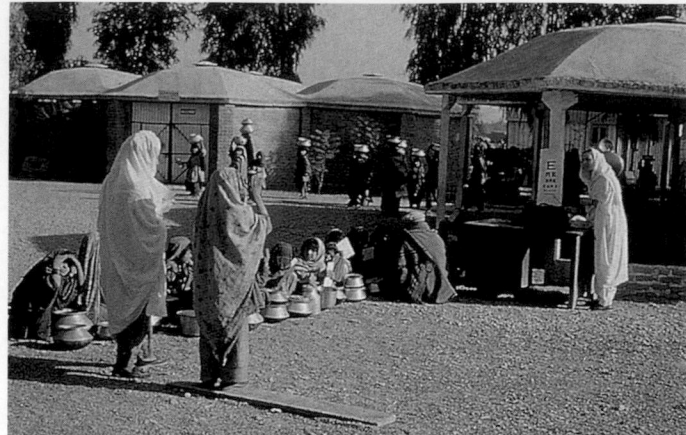

Figure 18.3 Testing the distance visual acuity of Afghan refugee children in Pakistan. (Courtesy of Murray McGavin.)

5. Examine both eyes together

Is there any squint (strabismus)? Is there evidence of proptosis of either eye?

6. Examine the anterior segment

Use a torch and a magnifier to examine the anterior segment systematically – the conjunctiva (bulbar and tarsal), cornea, anterior chamber, iris and pupil. Evert the upper lid to examine the tarsal conjunctiva.

7. Examine the posterior segment

Using the ophthalmoscope, examine the vitreous and the retina, optic nerve and retinal blood vessels.

8. Examine the intraocular pressure

A very crude estimate of the intraocular pressure can be obtained by gently palpating the eyeball through the upper eyelid, using the two index fingers, with alternating compression. This will indicate only a very hard eye with increased intraocular pressure, or a very soft eye. Much more accurate readings may be obtained using a tonometer. Extreme care should be observed in manipulation should there be an eye injury, particularly if perforation is a possibility.

These simple procedures can be carried out very quickly by a primary healthcare worker trained to examine the eyes.

VISION 2020: THE RIGHT TO SIGHT

The Global Initiative for the Prevention of Blindness – VISION 2020: The Right to Sight – was officially endorsed by Gro Harlem Brundtland MD MPH, Director-General, WHO, on 18 February 1999.[12]

Recognizing that 100 million people will needlessly go blind by the year 2020 without joint global action, VISION 2020's mission is 'to eliminate the main causes of blindness in order to give all people of the world, particularly the millions of needlessly blind, the right to sight'.

This global partnership involves the WHO and the Task Force of the International Agency for the Prevention of Blindness and incorporates the leading international non-governmental development organizations.

VISION 2020 focuses on three areas requiring action:
- Disease control
- Human resource development
- Infrastructure development and appropriate technology.

Disease control

The priorities are those conditions which are easily treatable or preventable, and are major causes of blindness and visual impairment. They include:
- Cataract
- Trachoma
- Childhood blindness
- Onchocerciasis
- Refractive errors and low vision.

Human resource development

More ophthalmologists will be trained, to achieve the following targets by 2020: in Africa, one ophthalmologist for 250 000 people; in Asia, from one ophthalmologist for 200 000 today to one per 50 000. Of equal importance is the training of ophthalmic medical assistants and ophthalmic nurses, to reach a ratio of one per 100 000 in Africa and one per 50 000 in Asia by 2020. Basic eye care must be taught in all medical schools worldwide by 2020. Other specialist personnel requiring training include refractionists, managers and equipment technicians.

Infrastructure and appropriate technology

Standard lists of equipment and consumable materials that are affordable and effective have reduced the cost of eye care and increased access.[13] Local production of instruments and consumables for ophthalmic surgery and basic eye examination, spectacles and other optical devices, and eye drops has been encouraged. The price of a standard rigid intraocular lens has dropped from approx US$200 in 1990 to about US$2 today.

BLINDING DISEASES IN ADULTS

Cataract

Cataract is found worldwide and is the most common cause of blindness (Figure 18.4). About 17.5 million people are blind due to cataract. Many millions more have visual impairment due to cataract. Most of the backlog of blind people requiring surgery is in Asia (70%), followed by Africa (20%).

The number of cataract blind people is increasing worldwide because of:
- Population growth
- Increasing longevity.

The world population over 60 years old will double during the next 20 years to around 800 million by 2020, with a corresponding increase in patients who are blind because of cataract.

The only treatment for cataract is surgical removal of the lens of the eye, usually with insertion of an intraocular lens implant.

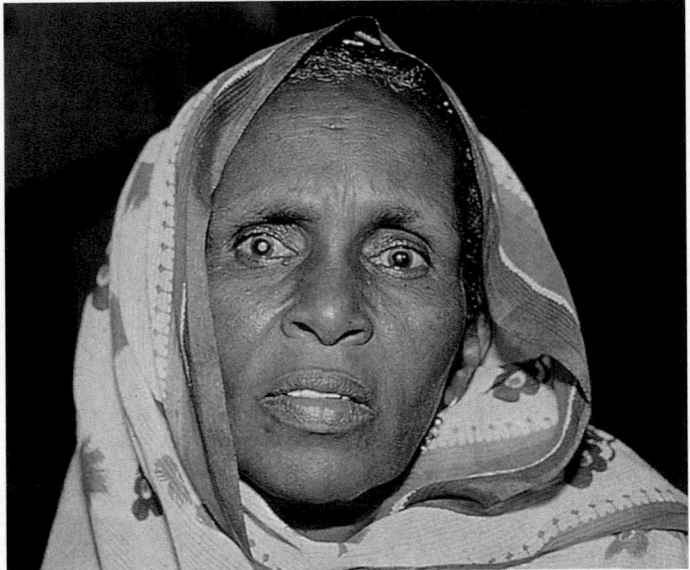

Figure 18.4 Bilateral cataract in a Somali woman. (Courtesy of Murray McGavin.)

Aetiology

Nutrition

A number of nutrients have been cited as playing a role in the development of cataract, based on animal and in vitro studies. These include: riboflavin, total protein, amino acids (especially tryptophan), vitamin C, vitamin E, selenium, calcium and zinc. The question of whether malnutrition predisposes to the development of cataract is difficult to elucidate. Researchers in Punjab associated a higher prevalence of cataract with inadequate diet of proteins, including beans, lentils, milk, eggs and curd. In this study, short height and low weight were also linked with a greater risk of cataract.[14]

The converse of this and other studies is the question of whether the regular taking of multivitamins provides protection against the development of cataract. A recent randomized trial in the USA found that vitamin supplements did not prevent progression of lens opacities.[15]

Diarrhoea/dehydrational crises

There is some evidence that episodes of acute dehydration, such as severe diarrhoea or heatstroke, increase the risk of cataract, at least in some localities. One of the authors was advised by a former professor of ophthalmology in Calcutta, India, that he recalled the 'acute' onset of cataract during epidemics of cholera. A history of severe diarrhoeal disease, sufficient to confine a patient to bed or mattress for 3 days, greatly increases the risk of the onset of cataract.[6] However, not all studies implicate acute dehydration so dramatically.[16]

Sunlight

There is some evidence for an association between exposure to sunlight and the development of cortical lens opacities. It is very difficult to estimate lifetime exposure to ultraviolet light, which limits the reliability of these studies. A cross-sectional survey of 838 watermen in Chesapeake Bay area of the USA reported that lifetime sunlight exposure was associated with cortical but not nuclear cataracts. Only ultraviolet B light (295–320 nm) was associated with a weak increased risk of cortical cataract formation.

A further 168 patients who required surgery for posterior subcapsular cataracts during 12 months in Maryland were compared with controls without posterior subcapsular cataracts selected from the same area and matched for age, sex and referral patterns. An association which was statistically significant was found between ultraviolet B and posterior subcapsular cataracts.

Smoking

A number of reports indicate an association between smoking and increased risk of nuclear cataracts and possibly posterior subcapsular cataracts.[17,18] It is possible that smokers can reduce the risk by stopping the habit.

Diabetes

Diabetes is known to increase the risk of cataract. Conversely, tight blood sugar control reduces the risk of cataract surgery.[19]

Genetics

Twin studies have suggested that genetic factors are important in cataract formation.[20]

Primary prevention

It is difficult or impossible to modify most of the risk factors associated with cataract, apart from smoking. At present it is unlikely that the incidence of cataract can be significantly reduced by public health measures.

Surgery

Barriers to cataract surgery

It has been shown that many patients remain cataract blind even if cataract surgery is available.[21] There is increasing recognition that a number of factors provide barriers to effective cataract surgery. These include:
- Cost of surgery[22]
- Distance to the hospital
- Cultural and social barriers
- Knowledge of services
- Trust in the outcome of surgery
- Lack of eye surgeons, particularly in Africa.

These issues must be addressed to achieve effective cataract surgical services.[23]

Cataract surgical rate

In order to eliminate cataract blindness it is necessary to operate on at least the total number of eyes that become blind or visually impaired every year. The cataract surgical rate (CSR) is the number of cataract operations performed per year, per million population. In the industrialized countries of the world, the CSR is usually between 4000 and 6000. India has significantly increased its CSR in the last 10 years, from less than 1500 to over 4000 today. However, in most of Africa, the CSR remains below 1000.

Cataract surgical coverage

Cataract surgical coverage (CSC) provides important information on the impact of cataract intervention programmes. CSC may be measured for both 'persons' and/or 'eyes'. CSC indicates the extent to which services have covered the needs in communities/populations. It is estimated by taking a random sample of the population, and identifying all those who either have visually significant cataract, or have had cataract surgery. For example, CSC (eyes) can be calculated by the following equation:

$$\text{Cataract surgical coverage} = \text{No. of operated eyes} / (\text{No. of operated eyes} + \text{Eyes with operable cataract})$$

The CSC (eyes) and the CSC (persons) are given as a percentage, where the percentage finding for eyes will be lower than that found for persons. By examining postoperative eyes, visual outcome and causes of poor outcome can also be determined.[10,24]

Surgical technique

Currently, the most popular method for cataract operation in the developing world is extracapsular cataract extraction with an intraocular lens implant (ECCE + IOL) (Figure 18.5).

Extracapsular cataract extraction (ECCE) leaves the posterior capsule of the lens intact, removing the nucleus and cortex of the lens. A posterior chamber intraocular lens (IOL) implant is then placed within the capsular bag. Optically, this is the best method, and restores normal vision with little distortion or magnification.

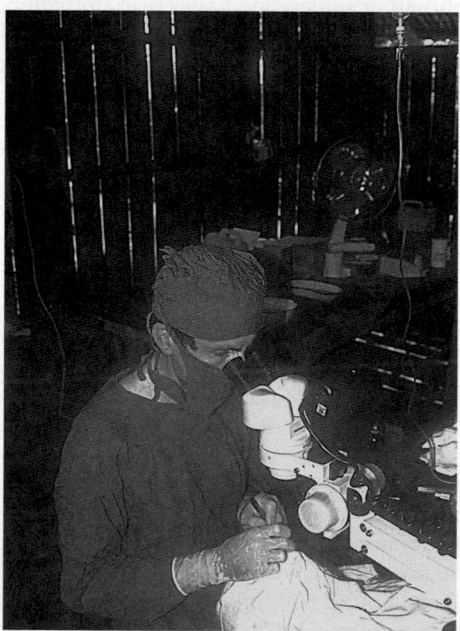

Figure 18.5 Extracapsular cataract surgery using a portable microscope in a refugee camp. (Courtesy of David Yorston.)

Better optical correction leads to better surgical outcomes, which permit earlier intervention.[10,24,25]

In recent years, the unit cost of high-quality IOLs has fallen to less than US$5. The disadvantages of ECCE + IOL include the need for an operating microscope, and the retention of the posterior capsule, which may opacify, causing loss of vision years after the cataract surgery.

Small-incision ECCE + IOL involves removal of the cataract through a self-sealing tunnel incision at the limbus. No sutures are required, and the procedure causes less astigmatism than a standard ECCE + IOL.[26,27] The surgery is very cost-effective.[28]

In developed countries, and in some middle-income countries, phacoemulsification is the technique of choice. Ultrasound energy is used to fragment and emulsify the cataract so that it can be removed through a 3 mm incision. A foldable IOL is then inserted. This technique is superior to ECCE, but much more costly and dependent on complex and fragile technology.[29]

Postoperative care

Community-based studies show that visual outcomes are frequently poor.[10,30,31] Outcomes may be improved by monitoring the results of surgery.[9,32] Postoperative refraction and provision of glasses will reduce poor outcomes due to uncorrected refractive error.

The Glaucomas

Glaucoma is not a single disease entity and, therefore, the group of conditions with different mechanisms involved is best described as 'the glaucomas'. The abnormal mechanisms involved may be the result of raised intraocular pressure which leads to optic nerve atrophy and corresponding visual field defects.

Glaucoma presents in two primary forms:
- Primary open angle glaucoma
- Primary angle closure glaucoma.

A congenital form of glaucoma may also occur (buphthalmos).

There are a number of secondary forms of glaucoma. Examples are:
- Glaucoma due to iridocyclitis
- Glaucoma following trauma
- Lens-induced glaucoma
- Neovascular glaucoma
- Steroid-induced glaucoma
- Epidemic dropsy.

Epidemiology of the primary glaucomas

Glaucoma is found throughout the world. It is a blinding disease, with 4.5 million blind worldwide. By 2010 there will be 44.7 million with open angle glaucoma and 15.7 million with angle closure glaucoma.[4]

Open angle glaucoma has a higher prevalence among people of African origin, in whom it occurs at a younger age, with a correspondingly serious prognosis if treatment is unavailable. The prevalence of open angle glaucoma among black Americans is 8–10 times higher than their white American compatriots.

Very late diagnosis of open angle glaucoma is the norm in most of the developing countries of the world. In one country in Central Asia, nearly 50% of patients diagnosed with glaucoma during one calendar year, were already completely blind in one eye, with vision at no light perception or only slightly better, and in the second eye the vision was commonly reduced to counting fingers.

Angle closure glaucoma is most prevalent in Asia, e.g. China, Myanmar and Singapore. It is also common among the Inuit.

It should be noted, however, that these separately described primary forms of glaucoma may occur among all races and there may be great variety in presentation.

Anatomy and physiology of aqueous fluid circulation

Aqueous fluid is produced by the ciliary body. It circulates around the lens and passes through the pupil, with most of the fluid draining through the trabecular meshwork at the angle of the anterior chamber. Any form of obstruction, whether due to the root of the iris, blood, inflammatory cells, pigment, etc., can reduce the drainage of aqueous from the eye, leading to raised intraocular pressure.

Open angle glaucoma

Known risk factors for open angle glaucoma include increasing age, ethnicity (see above), myopia, family history, evidence of vascular spasm elsewhere (e.g. Raynaud's syndrome, migraine) and possibly diabetes and hypertension (in older age).

The onset of open angle glaucoma is asymptomatic, and many patients are undiagnosed. The anterior segments appear normal. The anterior chamber is deep, and the angles are open. The intraocular pressure may be raised, but in many patients the pressure is normal. Equally, raised intraocular pressure alone does not mean that the patient has glaucoma. Glaucoma with visual field loss may be associated with normal pressure (normal tension glaucoma); and moderately raised pressures can occur in eyes that do not have field loss (ocular hypertension). Visual acuity is only affected very late in the disease when most of the visual field has been lost. Primary open angle glaucoma (POAG) is typically a bilateral condition, although it is often asymmetrical.

Examination of the optic nerve head is essential in the diagnosis of glaucoma. An abnormally cupped optic nerve head is highly suggestive of open angle glaucoma (Figure 18.6). Borderline cupping of the optic disc, when the cup : disc ratio may be between 0.5 and 0.7, requires further investigation, with examination of central visual fields. The finding of typical 'glaucomatous' visual field defects will often confirm the diagnosis. In the developing world the diagnosis is usually obvious as patients present late with advanced disease.

Management

The treatment of open angle glaucoma is to lower the intraocular pressure,[33] either by medication or by surgery. In developing countries, the approach should generally be surgical. Patients may use the antiglaucoma eye drops irregularly and may not replace them when finished. Eye drops must be instilled for the lifetime of the patient, and are costly.

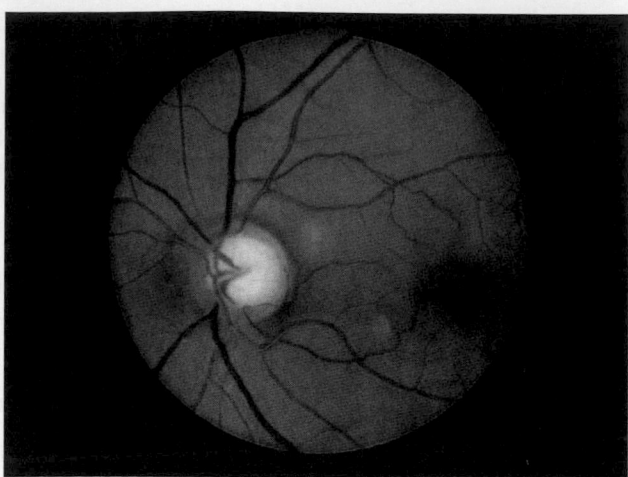

Figure 18.6 Cupping of the optic nerve head. (Courtesy of Gordon Johnson.)

If medical therapy is given, the following eye drops may be used:

- Beta-blocker, e.g. timolol 0.25% or 0.5%, (alternatives: levobunolol, carteolol or metipranolol)
- Prostaglandin analogue, e.g. latanoprost, travoprost or bimatoprost
- Topical carbonic anhydrase inhibitor, e.g. dorzolamide or brinzolamide
- Alpha-agonist, e.g. brimonidine.

Other topical medications such as pilocarpine or epinephrine may be used, but have more side-effects.

Topical treatment with eye drops may be supplemented with oral acetazolamide 250 mg, two to four times daily. However, acetazolamide should only be used as a short-term measure; if required for a longer period of time, the patient should also be given a potassium supplement. Side-effects of acetazolamide include paraesthesiae, gastrointestinal disturbance and kidney stones.

The most effective operation for open angle glaucoma is trabeculectomy. This procedure allows the aqueous fluid to drain into the subconjunctival space. African patients may have an inflammatory postoperative response with consequent scarring and blockage of the filtering site. This can be dealt with by using anti-metabolites (e.g. mitomycin C or 5-fluorouracil) at the time of surgery. Beta-irradiation improves the effectiveness of trabeculectomy in African eyes, but increases the risk of cataract.[34]

Angle closure glaucoma

Angle closure glaucoma occurs following occlusion of the angle by the iris in eyes with a shallow anterior chamber. It may be acute or chronic. Acute angle closure glaucoma is an ophthalmic emergency – delay will result in permanent loss of vision. Furthermore, without treatment, the second eye has a greater than 50% chance of developing angle closure glaucoma within 5 years.

Clinical presentation

In acute glaucoma the patient is distressed with severe pain and headache. Visual acuity is usually considerably reduced. The affected eye is red. The cornea is hazy due to oedema. The anterior chamber is shallow or flat, with the iris apposed to the peripheral cornea. The pupil is semi-dilated and unresponsive to light. The intraocular pressure is likely to be very high, over 40 mmHg. Using two index fingers and gently palpating the affected eye through the upper eyelid, will demonstrate the eye is hard compared to the other eye.

The other eye appears normal. Close examination is likely to reveal a shallow anterior chamber, which can be detected by shining a light from the side of the eye across the anterior segment.

Chronic angle closure presents in the same way as open angle glaucoma. It is asymptomatic and painless. Visual acuity is lost only after the optic nerve has been severely damaged. Chronic angle closure is the most common presentation in Asia.[35]

Predisposing factors for angle closure glaucoma include 'crowding' of the anterior segment of the eye – a smaller corneal diameter, an enlarged lens and a shorter axial length of the eye.

Risk factors for angle closure glaucoma are increasing age, gender (women are affected more often), ethnic origin (see earlier), refractive error (hypermetropia) and side-effects of drugs (e.g. mydriatics).

Management

In acute angle closure, treatment must be immediate. Acetazolamide 250 mg, four times daily, should be taken orally if possible. If the patient is vomiting, the drug may be given by slow intravenous infusion. This systemic treatment is supplemented with gutt. timolol 0.5% and gutt. apraclonidine. Pilocarpine should be given when the intraocular pressure has started to come down.

The definitive treatment for angle closure is iridectomy, which can be performed with a laser or surgically. This procedure creates another opening through which aqueous fluid can pass and deepens the anterior chamber of the eye. The second eye should have surgery as a prophylactic measure, as it is at high risk of developing angle closure.

Chronic angle closure glaucoma is usually treated in the same way as open angle glaucoma, by trabeculectomy or topical medication. If iridectomy is performed early, before the intraocular pressure rises, it may reduce the risk of developing chronic angle closure.

Central visual fields and medical treatment of glaucoma

If medical therapy is used, the central visual fields should be recorded at regular intervals, often every 6–12 months. Regular attendance at the glaucoma clinic must continue for the patient's lifetime.

Secondary glaucomas

Glaucoma may occur as a consequence of other eye diseases. These include the following.

Iridocyclitis

Iridocyclitis can be a complication of a number of systemic disorders, including leprosy, tuberculosis, syphilis, onchocerciasis and many others, but in most cases no underlying systemic condition is identified. Inflammation of the iris allows cells and protein to enter the aqueous. Using a focal light and magnification, a 'flare' may be seen in the anterior chamber – like a shaft of sunlight streaming into a room full of dust. The presence of cells and protein in the aqueous may lead to increased intraocular pressure. Because the iris is inflamed, adhesions may form between the pupil margin and the anterior lens surface (posterior synechiae) and/or in the angle of the anterior chamber (peripheral anterior synechiae). The pupil will dilate irregularly if posterior synechiae are present. Occasionally, the adhesions may involve the entire pupil margin. The iris bows forward as aqueous fluid cannot pass through the pupil, leading to closure of the drainage angle and acute glaucoma. This may be prevented by dilating the pupil. If the pupil is already completely adherent, a peripheral iridectomy will allow aqueous to enter the anterior chamber, and reopen the angle.

Haemorrhage into the anterior chamber (hyphaema)

Erythrocytes may block the trabecular meshwork, leading to a raised intraocular pressure. If the haemorrhage has been the result of a severe blunt injury, with damage to the angle of the anterior chamber, later healing with fibrosis may cause a severe type of secondary raised intraocular pressure (post-traumatic angle recession). If the hyphaema fills the anterior chamber, it should be removed.

Lens-induced glaucoma

In phacomorphic glaucoma, a mature cataract becomes swollen (intumescent) which pushes the iris forward and closes the angle (Figure 18.7). In phacolytic glaucoma, lens proteins may leak through the capsule of a hypermature lens. Macrophages, attempting to remove this abnormal material, and the lens matter itself, block the trabecular meshwork. Urgent cataract surgery is required to control the intraocular pressure in both cases.

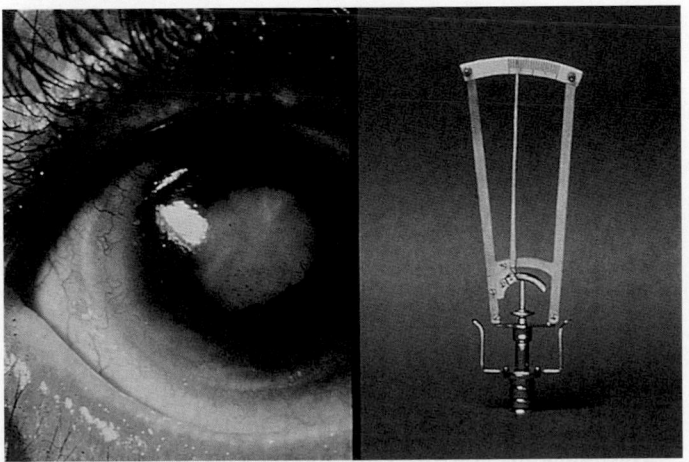

Figure 18.7 Secondary glaucoma caused by an intumescent cataract. A Schiotz tonometer is shown on the right. (Courtesy of John D. C. Anderson and David's Studio.)

Neovascular glaucoma (rubeotic glaucoma)

Severe ischaemia of the retina, most often due to central retinal vein occlusion or diabetic retinopathy, leads to the formation of new vessels. If these new vessels grow in the angle of the anterior chamber, they lead to peripheral anterior synechiae, and complete closure of the angle. Early and aggressive pan-retinal laser treatment may reverse the neovascularization, but treatment of established rubeotic glaucoma is very difficult.

Corticosteroid-induced glaucoma

The use of topical corticosteroids can result in a rise of intraocular pressure in some patients. Usually, the raised intraocular pressure falls when the steroids are stopped.

Epidemic dropsy

This acute toxic disease is caused by the ingestion of Argemone mexicana oil, an adulterant of cooking oils. It has been reported in India, Mauritius, Fiji, Bangladesh and southern Africa. Rash, oedema of the lower limbs, and gastrointestinal and cardiovascular disturbances may be accompanied by a secondary form of glaucoma and retinal vascular abnormalities.

Congenital glaucoma (buphthalmos)

Congenital glaucoma is rare but occurs throughout the world. The trabecular meshwork does not develop normally, leading to a reduction in aqueous fluid outflow. The intraocular pressure rises and in these small children, who have an elastic sclera, the eyeball enlarges. The optic disc may be cupped. Other clinical features include photosensitivity and corneal oedema.

If the condition is unilateral, the diagnosis is easy. However, bilateral buphthalmos may not be so immediately obvious. Management is surgical. Because of the rarity of the condition, children should be treated by a surgeon with specialist training in paediatric ophthalmology.

Trachoma

Trachoma is one of the major blinding diseases of the world. It is the most common infectious cause of blindness. Active trachoma is believed to affect over 100 million people. About 3.6 million are blind or at risk of blindness as a consequence of trachoma.[1] This eye disease is a serious public health problem in many parts of Africa, the Middle East and Asia. However, the prevalence is declining in many communities.[36]

Trachoma is a recurrent, chronic eye infection. The infecting organism is Chlamydia trachomatis – one of a group of organisms which share characteristics of both viruses and bacteria. Like bacteria, they contain both RNA and DNA, and are sensitive to some antibiotics. Like viruses, they are obligate intracellular parasites. Serotypes A, B, Ba and C cause the eye infection. Serotypes D–K mainly cause urogenital infection, which can also involve the eyes.

Eye infection begins in early childhood. Recurrent episodes of inflammation, together with secondary bacterial infection, may

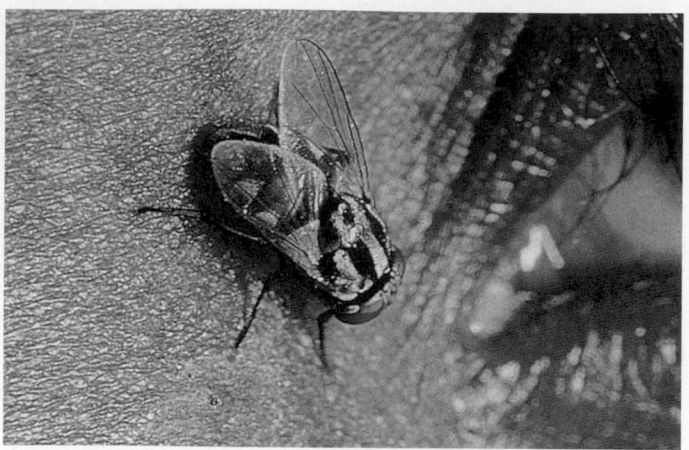

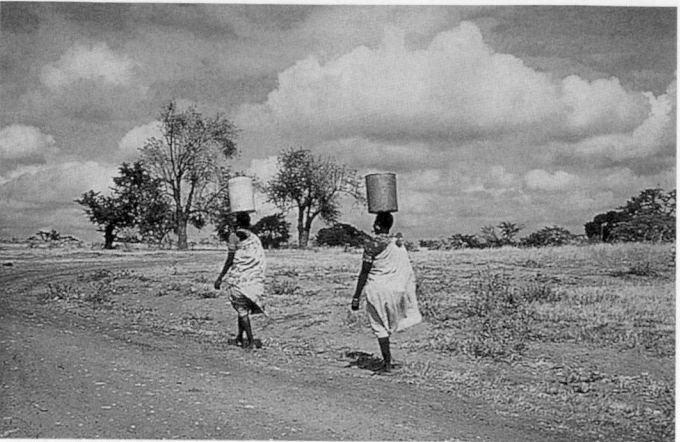

Figure 18.8 An eye-seeking fly which carries the organism *Chlamydia trachomatis*. (Courtesy of John D. C. Anderson.)

Figure 18.9 Collecting water – at a distance. (Courtesy of Erika Sutter.)

lead to scarring of the tarsal conjunctiva. Typically, the upper eyelid turns inwards (entropion), and distortion of the eyelashes occurs. These rub on the eyeball (trichiasis), leading to disturbance of the corneal surface, inflammation, corneal scarring and blindness.

Risk factors

Communities with a high prevalence of trachoma typically have a dry and dusty environment, a poor water supply, inadequate sanitation, overcrowding in the homes, and a large fly population.

Flies carry the organism[37] from child to child (Figure 18.8). They are attracted by discharging eyes and noses. Dirty, unwashed faces create an environment which predisposes to trachoma.

Exposed faeces will also attract flies. Well-designed ventilated pit latrines, which are properly used, will reduce the prevalence of trachoma within a community.[38]

An inadequate water supply is another risk factor for trachoma. There is a correlation between the distance travelled to collect water and the prevalence of trachoma within a community (Figure 18.9).

Poor education, especially of mothers, is yet another risk factor for trachoma. Health education emphasizing facial cleanliness reduces the transmission of trachoma.[39]

One can summarize the risk factors for trachoma by the six Ds:
- Dry
- Dusty
- Dirty
- Dung
- Discharge
- Density (overcrowding in the home).

The modes of transmission are summarized by the three Fs:
- Flies
- Fingers
- Fomites (contaminated material or objects such as clothing or towels).

Clinical examination

The eye should be examined with at least ×2.5 magnification and a good light.
1. Look for evidence of any discharge, and to see if any eyelashes are touching the cornea.
2. It should be noted if any eyelashes have been removed (epilation).
3. The cornea is examined for evidence of inflammation and/or corneal opacity.
4. Evert the upper lid by asking the patient to look down, but keep the eyes open. The eyelashes are gently grasped between finger and thumb, while the other hand places a glass rod or similar object on the skin at the upper border of the upper lid tarsal plate. The eyelid is rotated against the slim rod and everts, revealing the upper tarsal conjunctiva.
5. The tarsal conjunctiva is examined for evidence of follicles, intense inflammation or conjunctival scarring.

Simple grading system

A simplified grading classification for trachoma looks for five selected signs (Figures 18.10–18.15):[40]
- **Trachomatous inflammation – follicular (TF)**: the presence of five or more follicles in the upper tarsal conjunctiva. Follicles are accumulations of lymphoid cells. They look like small lumps, yellowish or white and paler than the rest of the conjunctiva. They should be at least 0.5 mm in diameter and situated on the flat surface of the tarsal conjunctiva.
- **Trachomatous inflammation – intense (TI)**: pronounced inflammatory thickening of the upper tarsal conjunctiva that obscures more than half of the deep tarsal vessels. In severe inflammation, the tarsal conjunctiva will appear red, rough and thickened. There is diffuse inflammatory infiltration, oedema and vascular papillary hypertrophy. This is the most infective stage of trachoma.
- **Trachomatous scarring (TS)**: the presence of scarring in the tarsal conjunctiva. White lines in the tarsal conjunctiva show early signs of the scarring stage of trachoma. The scarring may also appear as bands or sheets.

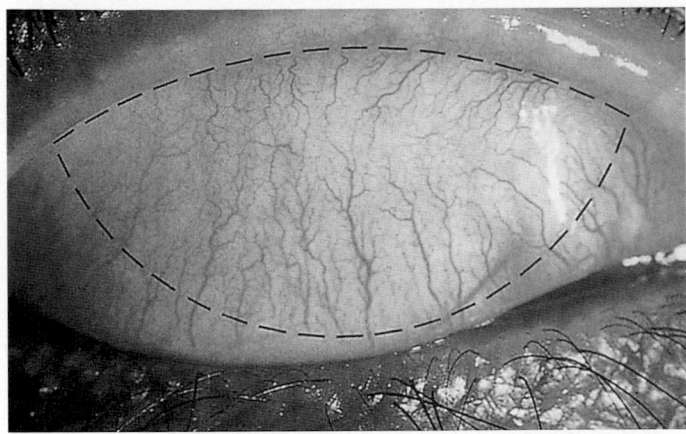

Figure 18.10 Normal upper eyelid. The area to be examined for inflammatory changes is outlined. (Courtesy of the *Journal of Community Eye Health*, International Centre for Eye Health, London.)

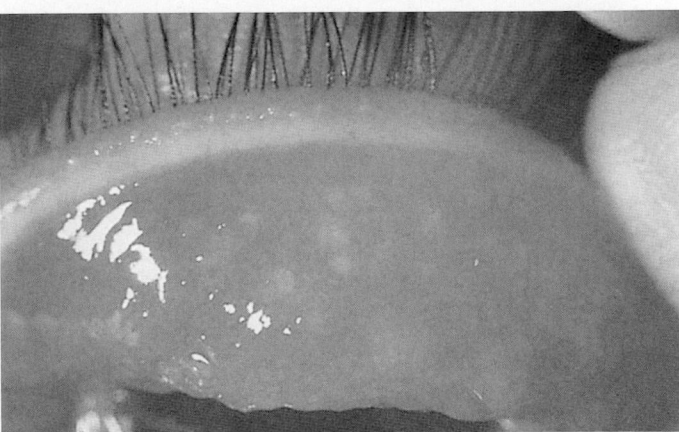

Figure 18.12 Trachomatous inflammation – intense (TI): marked inflammatory thickening of the upper tarsal conjunctiva; this obscures more than half the normal deep tarsal vessels. (Courtesy of Allen Foster and the *Journal of Community Eye Health*, International Centre for Eye Health, London.)

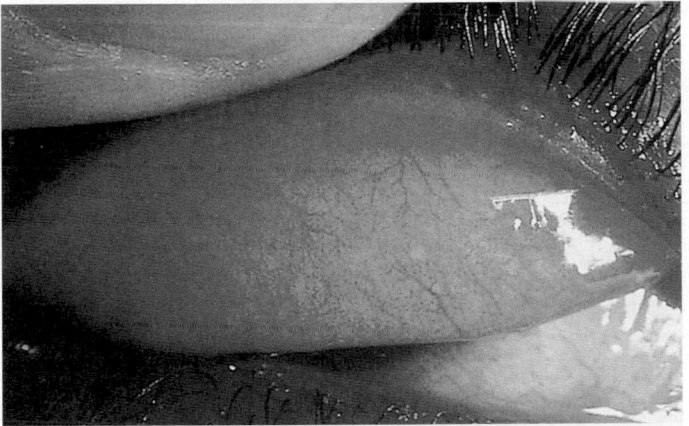

Figure 18.11 Trachomatous inflammation – follicular (TF): the presence of five or more follicles (each of which must be >0.5 mm diameter) on the flat surface of the upper tarsal conjunctiva. (Courtesy of John D. C. Anderson and the *Journal of Community Eye Health*, International Centre for Eye Health, London.)

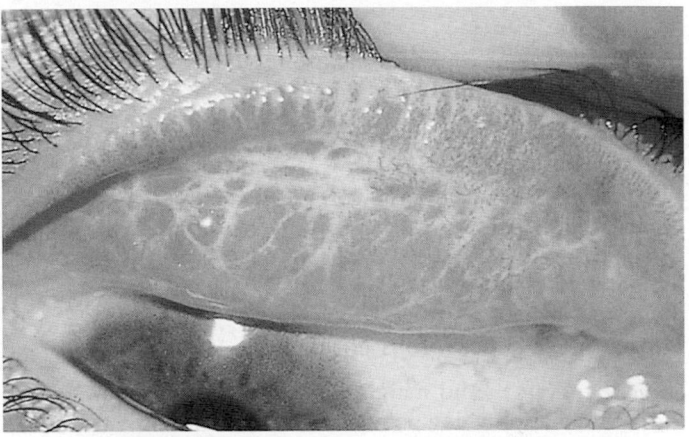

Figure 18.13 Trachomatous scarring (TS): involving the tarsal conjunctiva. (Courtesy of Hugh Taylor and the *Journal of Community Eye Health*, International Centre for Eye Health, London.)

- **Trachomatous trichiasis (TT):** at least one eyelash rubbing on the eyeball. Evidence of removal of eyelashes (epilation) should also be included in this category.
- **Corneal opacity (CO):** visible corneal opacity obscuring at least part of the pupil. This leads to visual impairment.

Trachoma control and the SAFE strategy

A new strategy, with the acronym SAFE, provides an appropriate and focused approach in control measures which involve tertiary prevention (surgery), secondary prevention (antibiotic treatment) and primary prevention (facial hygiene and environmental change).[41] These three elements are contained within the SAFE strategy:

- Surgery to prevent blindness in those who have trichiasis/ entropion

- Antibiotics (tetracycline eye ointment or azithromycin orally)
- Facial hygiene
- Environmental change.

Management

Medical treatment

Both tetracyclines and macrolides are effective against trachoma in its acute stages (TF and TI).[42] Topical tetracycline 1% ointment may be given twice daily for 6 weeks. In practice, compliance with this regimen is poor. A single dose of oral azithromycin is as effective as treatment with topical tetracycline,[43] and more convenient. Mass treatment of endemic communities may interrupt the transmission of infection, but at present it is not known how frequently treatment must be repeated, nor which populations require mass

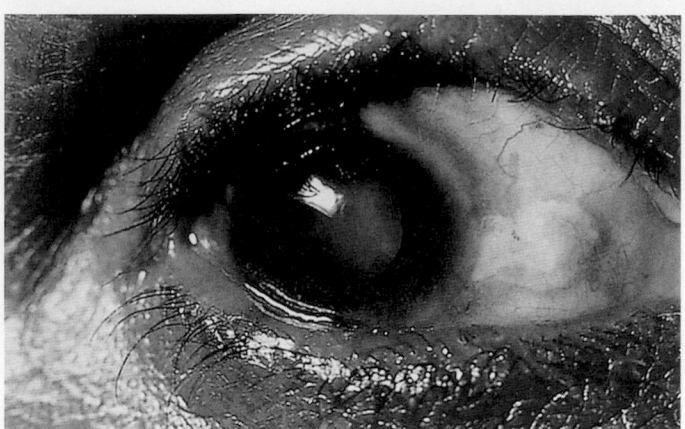

Figure 18.14 Trachomatous trichiasis (TT): evidence of one or more eyelashes rubbing on the eyeball. If one or a number of eyelashes have recently been removed, this should be graded trachomatous trichiasis. (Courtesy of John D. C. Anderson and the *Journal of Community Eye Health*, International Centre for Eye Health, London.)

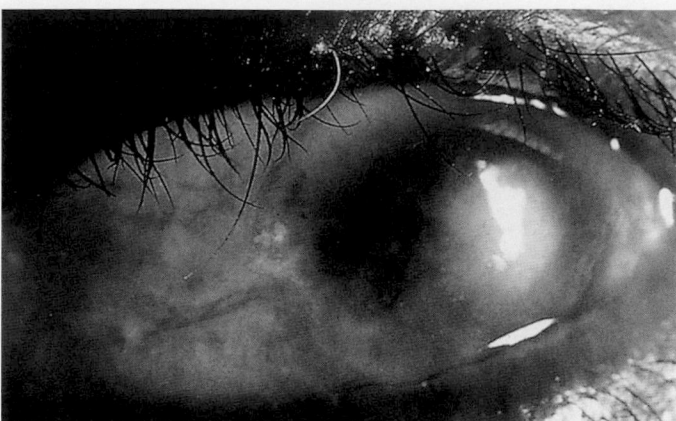

Figure 18.15 Corneal opacity (CO): corneal scarring due to trachoma where the scarring is central and sufficiently dense to obscure part of the pupil. (Courtesy of John D. C. Anderson and the *Journal of Community Eye Health*, International Centre for Eye Health, London.)

treatment. In some countries, azithromycin has been donated for use in trachoma control programmes.

Trichiasis and epilation

When an eyelash touches the cornea, causing extreme irritation, many patients remove it using forceps. Unfortunately, eyelashes will grow again in 4–6 weeks; however, epilation does provide temporary symptomatic relief.

Surgery for trachomatous entropion

Surgery to evert the lid margin and rotate the lashes away from the cornea may provide a permanent cure for trichiasis, and reduce the risk of visual loss. Several procedures have been described,[44] but there is a significant risk of recurrence following any operation. Uptake of trichiasis surgery is poor, and most patients never have an operation. Access to surgery may be improved by using ophthalmic assistants to perform the surgery in the patient's own village.

Surgery after corneal opacity

The outcome of corneal transplantation is usually poor, as there is an associate ocular surface disorder, with an unstable tear film, and possible corneal epithelial stem cell deficiency.

Prevention

Systemic treatment with azithromycin, if delivered to an entire community, may eliminate transmission of trachoma; however, reinfection is likely. Without additional preventive measures, antibiotic treatment will not have a permanent effect.

Communities must be educated in the prevention of trachoma. The following advice should be given:
- Secure a suitable water supply.
- Keep children's faces clean.
- Build and use well-designed ventilated pit latrines.

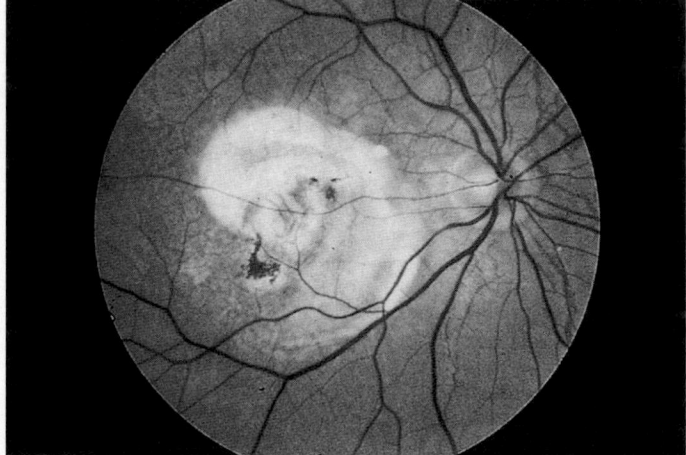

Figure 18.16 Age-related macular degeneration. (Courtesy of David Yorston.)

- Rubbish lying in the open should be burned or buried.
- Animals, especially cattle, should be housed some distance from the family home.

In many countries of the world, blinding trachoma has been eradicated due to improved environmental and socioeconomic conditions.[36] However, foci of severe disease remain, particularly in the most marginalized and disadvantaged groups. Trachoma will only be eradicated when we improve the quality of life of these communities.

Age-related macular degeneration

Age-related macular degeneration (AMD) is the most common cause of blindness in the industrialized world (Figure 18.16), where it accounts for about 50% of blindness. It is rare in people under 70 years old. As more people survive into old age, AMD prevalence is increasing.

Aetiology

There is a strong association between a single nucleotide polymorphism in complement factor H and AMD, possibly accounting for up to 50% of cases.[45] Smoking is another important risk factor that may be responsible for one-third of AMD.

Clinical appearance and treatment

AMD is a degenerative disorder of the central retina. The initial symptoms include distortion and loss of reading vision. In the early stages there are changes in the retinal pigment epithelium. This may lead to a slowly progressive atrophy of the photoreceptors (atrophic or dry AMD), or to choroidal neovascularization, leading to subretinal haemorrhage and scarring (CNV or exudative AMD). Choroidal neovascularization can be treated with intraocular injections of anti-VEGF drugs. These inhibit the formation of new blood vessels, and are effective, but must be given every month. They are also very expensive. Without treatment, central vision is lost. However, peripheral navigational vision remains intact.

Prevention

The most important measure is to stop smoking. Dietary supplements with high doses of antioxidant vitamins and zinc reduce the risk of progression in patients with early AMD in both eyes, or advanced AMD in one eye.[46]

Diabetes mellitus

The number of adults with diabetes is projected to rise from 135 million in 1995 to 300 million in 2025. Most of this increase will occur in developing countries. Certain ethnic groups have a very high prevalence of diabetes. In the USA, the prevalence of diabetes is highest among native Americans, followed by African-Americans and Hispanics.

Earlier estimates by the WHO indicate that about 1.8 million people are blind due to diabetic retinopathy, and it is still the leading cause of blindness in people under 65 in rich countries.

Diabetic retinopathy

Twenty years after the onset of diabetes, nearly all patients with type I diabetes (insulin-dependent) and more than 60% of those with type II diabetes (non-insulin-dependent) will have retinopathy.

Retinal changes which cause visual loss are:
- Oedema or ischaemia of the macula
- Proliferative diabetic retinopathy, leading to vitreous haemorrhage, traction retinal detachment or rubeotic glaucoma.

Diabetic retinopathy was classified by the Early Treatment of Diabetic Retinopathy Study (ETDRS). The detailed classification uses standard photographs, but this is beyond the scope of this chapter. However, a brief description of the classification is given below.

Non-proliferative retinopathy

1. Mild non-proliferative retinopathy: at least one microaneurysm and also dot, blot or flame-shaped haemorrhages in all four fundus quadrants.

2. Moderate non-proliferative retinopathy: intraretinal microaneurysms and dot and blot haemorrhages in one to three quadrants. Cotton-wool spots and venous calibre changes, including venous beading, may be seen.

3. Severe non-proliferative retinopathy: at least one of the following should be present:
   - Haemorrhages and microaneurysms in all four quadrants of the fundus
   - Venous beading in at least two quadrants
   - Intraretinal microvascular abnormalities in at least one quadrant.

Proliferative diabetic retinopathy

New vessels grow from the retina along the posterior surface of the vitreous, in fibrovascular bands and sheets (Figure 18.17). These may bleed, causing vitreous haemorrhage, or contract, leading to traction retinal detachment. Treatment of proliferative retinopathy is urgent.

Diabetic maculopathy

This is the most common cause of visual loss in diabetes mellitus. Retinal oedema or exudates within 1 mm of the fovea threaten central vision and require laser treatment (Figure 18.18). Macular ischaemia is harder to recognize clinically. The visual acuity is reduced and there is no macular oedema or exudate, but there is moderate/severe non-proliferative or proliferative retinopathy.

Treatment of diabetic retinopathy

Intensive control of blood sugar (in type I and type II diabetes) and tight control of blood pressure (in type II diabetes) delay the onset of retinopathy and slow the progression of the disease.[47]

Photocoagulation

Pan-retinal laser photocoagulation destroys the peripheral retina, reducing the stimulus to new vessel formation. Laser treatment of

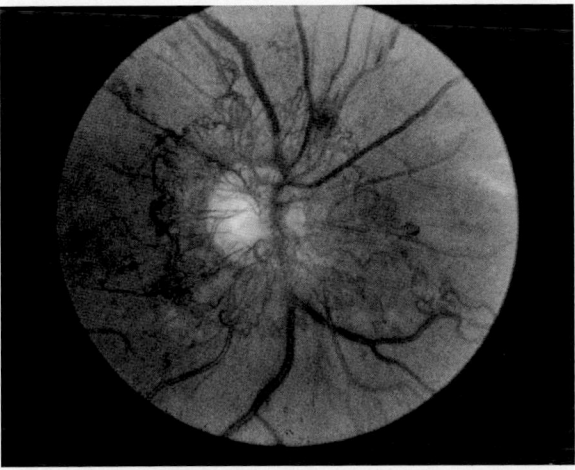

Figure 18.17 Proliferative diabetic retinopathy. (Courtesy of Gordon Johnson.)

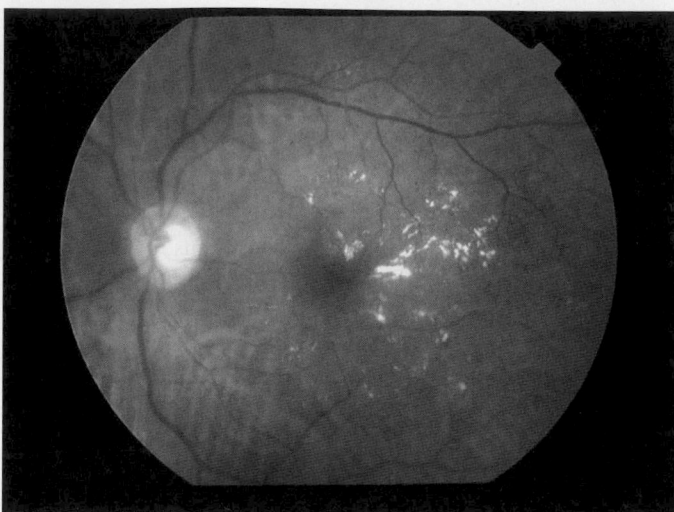

Figure 18.18 Diabetic maculopathy. Hard exudates close to the fovea. (Courtesy of David Yorston.)

macular oedema is less reliable, but still halves the risk of moderate visual loss.[48] Both forms of photocoagulation are most effective if delivered early, before there is a decrease in visual acuity.

Pars plana vitrectomy

Vitrectomy is indicated for persistent vitreous haemorrhage, or if the macula is detached or threatened by traction detachment. Endolaser photocoagulation is given at the same time. Relatively few eye clinics in developing countries have the expertise and equipment to perform this complex surgery.

Screening for diabetic retinopathy

Because laser treatment is most effective before vision is lost, retinopathy must be detected by screening. Everyone who cares for diabetics should be able to detect retinopathy with an ophthalmoscope.

Screening guidelines:
- Type I/juvenile-onset diabetes: dilated examination of the retina every year beginning after puberty and 5 years after diagnosis
- Type II/maturity-onset diabetes: dilated examination of the retina every year once diabetes is diagnosed.

Examinations should be more frequent if severe retinopathy is detected.

Onchocerciasis

Onchocerciasis is a parasitic disease caused by the filarial worm *Onchocerca volvulus*. The worm is transmitted by a vector, one of several species of the Simulium blackfly. The fly breeds in rivers, with a preference for turbulent and highly oxygenated waters. Both the skin and the eyes are affected by the condition, commonly known as 'river blindness'.

Epidemiology

The WHO Expert Committee has estimated that the number of people infected by *O. volvulus* is approximately 18 million, of whom 270 000 are blind. Once blind, affected individuals have a life expectancy only one-third that of the sighted. The disease is associated with poor school performance and a higher drop-out rate among infected children.

Of the 37 countries where the disease is endemic, 30 are in sub-Saharan Africa and 6 are in the Americas. Over 17 million of those infected with *O. volvulus* live in West and Central Africa. There are foci of infection in Yemen, and in Central America and northern countries of South America.

The social and economic consequences of this disease are huge. The prevalence of blindness in West African villages near fast-flowing rivers may reach 15%, leading to depopulation, and migration away from fertile land to areas with less risk of blindness.

The eye disease typically affects a relatively young man, 30–40 years old, who has lived and worked near to a fast-flowing river in West or Central Africa. During childhood and early adult life he will have been bitten many times by the Simulium fly and has been repeatedly infected with the larvae of *O. volvulus*. The eye problems are insidious, beginning with chronic inflammation that leads to scarring in both the anterior and posterior segments. Visual field is gradually lost in each eye, and vision is severely reduced, leading to blindness.

The vector: the Simulium fly

The disease is spread from person to person by the blackfly of the genus *Simulium*. The female Simulium lays her eggs on rocks and vegetation, where rivers are fast flowing and 'white' through turbulence, because the eggs and larvae of the fly need highly oxygenated water for their development.

The female fly can travel up to 80 km in one day, but she is more likely to fly 5–10 km on either side of a river. During the rainy season the flies may travel to new breeding sites, but in the dry season they are restricted to permanent rivers.

The female fly requires a blood meal to ensure development of her eggs, and she prefers to feed on human blood at dawn or dusk.

Life cycle of *O. volvulus*

When a person is already infected by *O. volvulus* and is bitten by the Simulium fly, the small embryo worms (microfilariae) present in the skin of the infected person enter the body of the fly. There they pass through the gut wall and enter the thoracic muscles, After about 7 days, the larvae move to the head of the fly, ready to be transmitted to the next human host when the fly requires another blood meal.

They will take 1–3 years to develop into adult worms. One female worm can produce 0.5–1 million microfilariae in 1 year. The cycle of transmission from person to person continues.

Clinical presentation

Skin complications

Itching is one of the first symptoms of onchocerciasis, and this can be very severe, disturbing sleep. There is a rash which may occur on most parts of the body but often affects the buttocks. Obvious scratch marks may indicate the severity of the itching.

Repeated episodes of dermatitis associated with the death of microfilariae lead to depigmentation, described as 'leopard skin'. There is subcutaneous fibrosis, skin atrophy and pigmentary changes. The skin may look and feel like the skin of a very old person. This has been described as 'lizard skin'.

Lymphoedema results in chronic thickened skin. Lymph node enlargement in the inguinal areas can lead to folds of skin known as the 'hanging groin' of onchocerciasis.

Subcutaneous nodules are found in different parts of the body, often over bony prominences. They are firm, discrete and painless. A nodule is formed by a fibrous reaction around coiled adult worms. Surgical removal of nodules (nodulectomy) may be considered, particularly where nodules are situated in the region of the head or shoulders.

Eye complications

Most of the symptoms and signs of onchocerciasis, including those affecting the eyes, are caused by the microfilariae of *O. volvulus*. Typically, both eyes will be involved. As with the skin changes, it is the dead microfilariae which cause most inflammatory reaction within the eye. Live microfilariae may be seen in the anterior chamber with a slit lamp microscope.

Eye inflammation can affect both the anterior and posterior eye.

- 'Snowflake' keratitis – White-grey spots may be seen in the superficial cornea, indicating a reaction to dead microfilariae within the cornea. The eye may be inflamed and photophobic. Topical corticosteroids may be used, but should only be prescribed by an eye specialist as they may cause glaucoma and corneal ulceration.
- Sclerosing keratitis – Sclerosing keratitis is a common feature of onchocerciasis which can cause blindness (Figure 18.19). Typically, it begins at the nasal and temporal aspects of the cornea, and the opacity then extends throughout the lower part of the cornea. Advanced sclerosing keratitis can result in complete corneal opacification. There is no specific treatment.
- Iridocyclitis – Inflammation of the iris (iritis) and of the ciliary body (cyclitis) can contribute to reduced vision. The pupil may be dragged inferiorly, like an inverted tear drop, due to inflam-

mation caused by accumulated dead microfilariae. Iridocyclitis should be treated with topical atropine sulphate 1% eye drops and antiinflammatory agents. Iritis may lead to cataract, which may require surgery, when the eye is quiet and there is no active inflammation.

- Optic neuritis and chorioretinitis – In the posterior segment, onchocerciasis causes optic nerve atrophy and chorioretinal atrophy. In severe optic atrophy, the optic disc is white, whereas the normal optic disc is a faint pink colour. Areas of the retina may be pale, with scattered clumps of pigmentation (Figure 18.20). There is no treatment for these conditions, which are the leading causes of blindness in onchocerciasis.

Diagnosis

The clinical signs are often sufficient to make a diagnosis: onchodermatitis, signs of scratching, depigmentation of the skin, 'lizard' skin and subcutaneous nodules. Characteristic eye changes and microfilariae in the anterior chamber will confirm the diagnosis.

The skin snip

A small piece of skin may be removed, often from the iliac crest or the shoulder, using a sterile needle and blade, or a purpose-designed skin punch. The fragment of skin is placed on a microscope slide and a drop of saline is added. After at least 30 minutes, and preferably even later, the slide is examined microscopically. Mobile microfilariae can be seen moving in the fluid when using ×40 magnification. Skin snips are used less frequently today, as treatment is largely based on community prevalence rather than individual diagnosis.

Control

Vector control

Vector control uses larvicides to kill the Simulium larvae. This has been most effectively carried out by the Onchocerciasis Control Project (OCP) in 11 countries of West Africa. Unfortunately, vector control is very expensive, as selective larvicides must be delivered to all breeding sites, including the most remote and inaccessible.

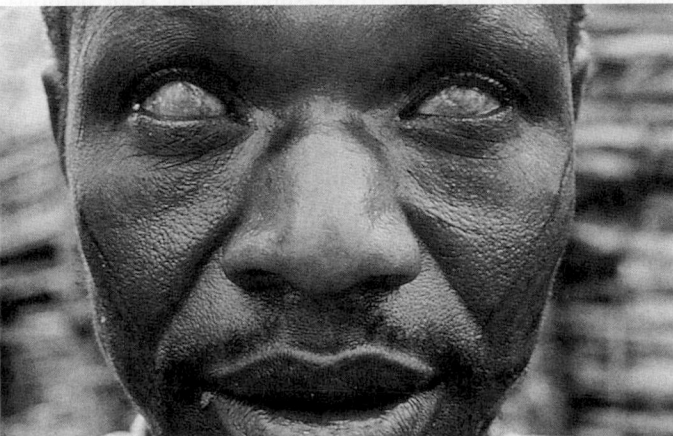

Figure 18.19 Sclerosing keratitis in onchocerciasis. (Courtesy of Pak Sang Lee.)

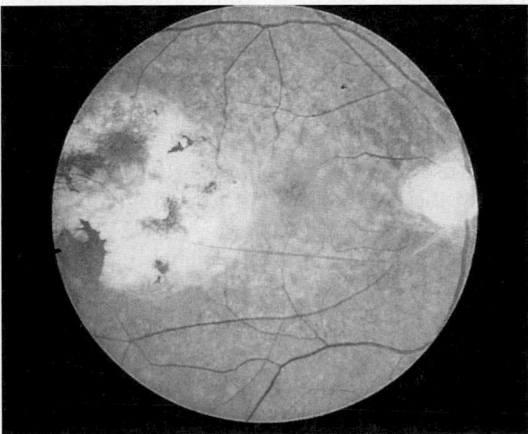

Figure 18.20 Chorioretinal atrophy and optic nerve atrophy after onchocerciasis. (Courtesy of Ian Murdoch.)

Nodulectomy

Removing the adult worms within the fibrous nodule which forms the subcutaneous lump may reduce the number of microfilariae. However, not all adult worms are in superficial nodules, so it is unlikely that nodulectomy can effect a complete cure.

Macrofilaricides

In the past, suramin has been used, given in weekly intravenous injections. However, suramin is toxic and can cause serious systemic and ocular reactions. It is not routinely recommended.

Diethylcarbamazine

Diethylcarbamazine (DEC) was the mainstay of treatment for many years. However, the sudden death of millions of microfilariae caused by diethylcarbamazine leads to a severe systemic reaction with intense itching, a skin rash, fever, headache and joint pains. This is known as the Mazzotti reaction, and it causes further ocular inflammation and loss of sight.

Ivermectin (Mectizan®)

Ivermectin kills the microfilariae but usually causes only mild reactions, and, unlike diethylcarbamazine, it does not cause additional ocular inflammation. In 2005, over 250 million tablets were distributed.

Ivermectin has the following advantages:

- It kills microfilariae.
- It reduces the risk of blindness due to optic atrophy by 50%.
- The production of microfilariae by the adult female worm is inhibited for some months.
- A single dose every 6–12 months eliminates microfilariae.
- It is sufficiently safe for mass distribution to entire communities.
- The oral route provides easy delivery of the drug.

A beneficial side-effect is the elimination of other parasites, including hookworm and scabies. Ivermectin has been donated free of charge by Merck & Co.

Because ivermectin is safe, effective and free, treatment is aimed at the whole community, in order to reduce the prevalence of the infection, rather than targeting symptomatic individuals. Rapid epidemiological mapping techniques identify the communities at greatest risk. The usual strategy is community-directed treatment with ivermectin (CDTI). This involves the affected communities in the planning, implementation and monitoring of treatment activities. Local people are trained to distribute the ivermectin, and to monitor its use. CDTI is the approved strategy used throughout Africa by both the OCP and the African Programme for Onchocerciasis Control (APOC).[49]

Ivermectin, 150 mg per kg by weight, is given every 6–12 months by mouth. A simplified dosage schedule uses patient height as a proxy for weight. It should not be given to the following groups of patients:

- Children under 5 years old or weighing less than 15 kg or less than 90 cm in height.
- Pregnant women
- Women breast-feeding a child under 1 week old
- Severely ill patients.

Table 18.5 Adverse reactions to ivermectin (Mectizan®) therapy

Mild	Severe
Pruritus	Hypotension
Fever	Asthma attacks (in known patients)
Rash	Bullous skin lesions (after 1–2 weeks)
Headache	
Oedema	
Lymphadenopathy	
Myalgia	
Generalized body aches	

Although ivermectin is generally safe, there have been neurological reactions, some fatal, in patients who have a severe infection with *Loa loa* (>30 000 mf/mL). Ivermectin should be used with great caution where loiasis is endemic.

Side-effects of ivermectin include mild itching, fever, rash, headache, oedema, lymphadenopathy, myalgia and generalized body aches (Table 18.5). More severe reactions, which are rare, include hypotension, asthma attacks in known asthmatics, and bullous skin lesions after 1–2 weeks. Most reactions occur within 2 or 3 days of the first dose. Aspirin or an antihistamine may be given.

There has been a significant expansion of onchocerciasis control activities due to the combined efforts of WHO, the World Bank, the pharmaceutical industry, and non-governmental development organizations. Three regional programmes have been established, one in Central and Latin America, and two in Africa, the OCP and the APOC. Millions of people are being treated annually. However, external funding for the APOC may not continue beyond 2010, and its future is uncertain.

Toxins and the optic nerve

In patients with nutritional deficiency, particularly of the vitamin B complex, the optic nerve is susceptible to toxic damage.

Tobacco smoking, combined with excess alcohol consumption and relatively poor nutrition, can result in a toxic optic neuropathy. Methanol is sometimes drunk with disastrous effects, including optic neuropathy and subsequent blindness. Methanol poisoning can be treated with fomepizole.[50]

Inadequately prepared cassava can cause optic neuropathy and peripheral nerve abnormalities due to cyanide toxicity. Cyanide is found particularly in the skin of the tubers. Water used for soaking cassava must be discarded, together with any fermenting cassava.

Drugs which may cause a toxic optic neuropathy include ethambutol, quinine and isoniazid.

An epidemic of bilateral optic neuropathy has affected people aged between 10 and 40 years in Dar es Salaam, Tanzania. The condition has an acute onset with accompanying impairment of colour vision and temporal pallor of the optic discs. There may be associated peripheral neuropathy and sensorineural hearing loss.[51]

The pigment beneath the macula was dispersed and clumped, sometimes forming a small ring. The cause is currently unknown, although the history and clinical appearance suggest a toxic agent.

An epidemic of neuropathy occurred in Cuba during 1992–1994. More than 50 000 cases were reported. Most patients were middle-aged and males were slightly more often affected (3:2). Painful paraesthesiae, mainly in the legs, with ataxia were reported. The number of patients with optic nerve involvement is uncertain, but some estimates suggested nearly 50% of cases. The aetiology is obscure but may include poor nutrition, toxins such as tobacco or alcohol, or a virus. Patients did seem to benefit by receiving B complex vitamins and the number of new cases declined dramatically.

BLINDING DISEASES IN CHILDREN

Although the exact number of blind children in the world is not known, it is estimated that the figure is approximately 1.4 million.[52] Approximately 75% of these children live in Africa and Asia. Up to 60% die within 1–2 years of becoming blind. Children have a much lower prevalence of blindness than adults, and there are few surveys large enough to estimate the prevalence of childhood blindness with any precision. However, there is a close correlation with childhood mortality.

Major causes and strategies for prevention

The major causes of blindness vary from region to region (Table 18.6), and accurate data are difficult to obtain. In industrialized countries, blind registers are one source, although these records may be incomplete. Indications of the common causes of blindness in children can be obtained from schools for the blind, although this information is likely to be biased as it only includes children who are in education.

A form developed by the International Centre for Eye Health, London, and the WHO provides a classification of blindness in children, with coding instructions, definitions, description of methods and guidelines.

Vitamin A deficiency disorders (VADD) and the eye

Vitamin A deficiency is an example of a condition with a simple remedy, which, however, blinds thousands of children.

The impact of subclinical vitamin A deficiency on the health of the young child is well known. Morbidity and mortality, immune status, growth and haemopoiesis can be significantly affected.

Table 18.6 Leading causes of childhood blindness

Poor countries	Middle-income countries	Rich countries
Corneal scar	Retinopathy of prematurity	CNS disorders
Cataract	Inherited retinal disease	Inherited retinal disease
Retinal disorders	Cataract	Retinopathy of prematurity

Magnitude of VADD worldwide and blindness

Vitamin A deficiency affecting the eye, also known as xerophthalmia ('dry eye'), is a common cause of blindness in children in very poor countries. In many cases, this acute nutritional deficiency is associated with measles.

The magnitude of VADD worldwide is indicated in Table 18.7.

Malnourished children are found in many countries of Asia and Africa, as well as in some areas of the Americas. There are encouraging signs that countries with a history of widespread VADD have shown distinct improvement in vitamin A status in recent years, particularly India, Indonesia and Bangladesh.

Vitamin A (retinol)

Deficiency results in an impaired immune response with decreased resistance to infection. Squamous metaplasia of epithelial surfaces allows, for example, a greater susceptibility to lung infection.

Stores of vitamin A are found in the liver, where 90% of the body's vitamin A is retained. Vitamin A deficiency is typically associated with other nutritional deficits, which make the young patient vulnerable to systemic disease.

Measles infection is particularly important in vitamin A deficiency. The measles virus affects all epithelial surfaces. Following an acute infection with measles, the body stores of vitamin A are quickly exhausted and corneal necrosis (keratomalacia) may occur.

In older children and adults who have chronic vitamin A deficiency, a history of night blindness is common. Vitamin A is required for the photosensitive pigment of the rods of the retina.

Eye changes in vitamin A deficiency

The following are the eye symptoms and signs of xerophthalmia (Figure 18.21 and Table 18.8):
1. Night blindness (XN). Vitamin A is an essential part of rhodopsin – without vitamin A, rod photoreceptor function is seriously impaired, leading to night blindness.
2. Conjunctival xerosis (X1A). The conjunctiva appears dry and wrinkled. This dry appearance provides the term xerophthalmia, which is commonly used to describe the condition of vitamin A deficiency affecting the eye.
3. Bitot's spots (X1B). Bitot's spots are foamy triangular patches, usually found on the temporal bulbar conjunctiva. They are

Table 18.7 Magnitude of VADD worldwide

- Approximately 300 000 preschool-age children are blind from xerophthalmia and up to 60% of these die within 1 year
- About 3 million children are blind worldwide
- Approximately 3 million children have clinical xerophthalmia which includes night blindness and Bitot's spots
- In the region of 250 million preschool-age children are subclinically vitamin A deficient, with the corresponding consequences of morbidity and mortality
- Around 500 000 women die in childbirth annually and an unknown percentage of these die because of impaired vitamin A status

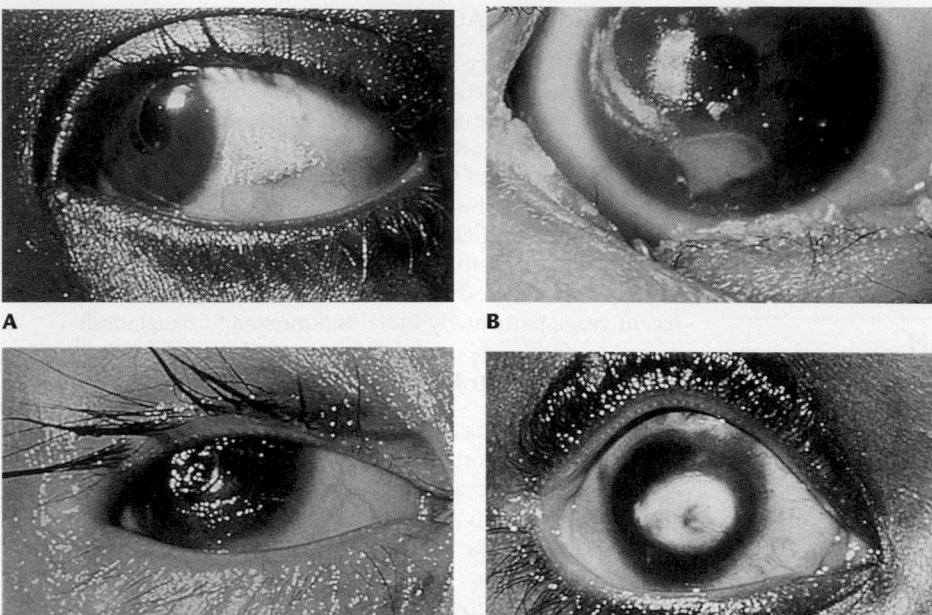

Figure 18.21 (**A**) Bitot's spot; (**B**) corneal xerosis with early ulceration; (**C**) corneal ulceration/keratomalacia; (**D**) corneal scarring. (Courtesy of: (**A**) Simon Franken; (**B**) Allen Foster; (**C**) Donald McLaren; (**D**) Gordon Johnson.)

Table 18.8 Eye changes and vitamin A status

Eye lesion	Vitamin A status*	Comments
Night blindness (XN)	Mild–moderate decrease (over 1 per 100)	Sensitive sign of low body vitamin A stores; still associated with increased illness and mortality
		Prevalence often increases into early school-age years
		Boys may be more affected than girls
		Cause is chemical deficiency in retina
Conjunctival xerosis (X1A)	Mild–moderate decrease (not used in WHO classification)	Dryness of conjunctiva due to decrease in goblet cells and epithelial change
		Difficult to diagnose reliably by clinical examination
Bitot's spots (X1B)	Mild–moderate decrease (over 5 per 1000)	White 'foamy' or 'cheese-like' spots on the conjunctiva: usually bilateral and temporal
		Caused by change in squamous epithelium with underlying xerosis
		In older children may not disappear with vitamin A treatment
Active corneal changes (X2/X3)	Severe decrease (over 1 per 10 000)	Danger signs of permanent loss of sight
		Cornea may 'melt' (keratomalacia) in a few hours
		Most common at age 2–4 years
		No sex differences
Corneal scars (XS)	Depends on examination timing (over 5 per 10 000)	End-stage of malnutrition eye damage
		Scarring (leukoma) often allows some residual vision
		Blinded eyes may be protuberant (anterior staphyloma) or shrunken (phthisis)

*Public Health problem criteria as defined by the WHO in children aged between 6 months and 6 years.
Source: WHO Programme for Prevention of Blindness.

an unreliable sign of vitamin A deficiency, as they may persist long after the vitamin A levels have been restored, and they can occur in other conditions (e.g. with contact lens wear).

4. Corneal xerosis (X2). The cornea appears dry and dull, indicating changes in the corneal epithelium due to vitamin A deficiency.
5. Corneal ulceration with xerosis (X3A). The damaged epithelium breaks down, leading to a corneal ulcer which may progress to involve the deeper layers of the cornea. A central corneal ulcer will profoundly affect vision.
6. Corneal ulceration/keratomalacia (X3B). The cornea may melt dramatically (keratomalacia), with an acute onset, sometimes over a few hours. Young children, aged 1–3 years, are particularly at risk. Sadly, keratomalacia is often bilateral, and usually leads to irreversible blindness.
7. Corneal scarring (XS). The healed state following severe vitamin A deficiency, with corneal ulceration and keratomalacia, can result in marked corneal scarring which will often affect both eyes. Vision is greatly reduced. Many children who have severe vitamin A deficiency will die because they are particularly susceptible to intercurrent infections, such as respiratory infections and diarrhoea. For those who survive, both their eyes, and their lives, will be scarred.

If a child has vitamin A deficiency, others in the same family and community are also at high risk.

Treatment of vitamin A deficiency

The recommended treatment of vitamin A deficiency affecting all age groups except women of reproductive age is given in Table 18.9.

If there is vomiting, an intramuscular injection of 100 000 IU of water-soluble vitamin A (not an oil-based preparation) may be used instead of the first oral dose.

When vitamin A treatment is started, a topical antibiotic (e.g. chloramphenicol 1%) is also given four times daily, to prevent bacterial infection, and the patient should be referred immediately to an eye specialist.

Table 18.9 Treatment schedule for xerophthalmia for all age groups except women of reproductive age*

Timing	Vitamin A dosage[†]
Immediately on diagnosis:	
• <6 months of age	50 000 IU
• 6–12 months of age	100 000 IU
• >12 months of age	200 000 IU
Next day	Same age-specific dose[‡]
At least 2 weeks later	Same age-specific dose[§]

*Caution: women of reproductive age with night blindness or Bitot's spots should receive daily doses ≤25 000 IU. However, all women of child-bearing age, whether or not pregnant, who exhibit severe signs of active xerophthalmia (i.e. acute corneal lesions) should be treated as above.
[†]For oral administration, preferably in an oil-based preparation.
[‡]The mother or other responsible person can administer the next-day dose at home.
[§]To be administered at a subsequent health service contact with the individual.

Prevention of xerophthalmia

A high-dose schedule for prevention of vitamin A deficiency is given in Table 18.10.

High doses of vitamin A are contraindicated in pregnancy, as there have been concerns about the effects of vitamin A on the unborn child.

Breast milk contains vitamin A, and this provides an adequate supply for the newborn child.

Communities which have endemic vitamin A deficiency should receive nutritional education as well as vitamin A supplements. Vitamin A-rich foods are often available, but for cultural or other reasons are not consumed by children (Figure 18.22).

The following should be emphasized:

• Encourage breast-feeding.
• Supplement the feeding of infants by 6 months with fruits such as mango or papaya. Children aged 1 year or older can be given dark-green leafy vegetables, which are rich in vitamin A. Health workers, and parents, should know which local foods have a high content of vitamin A. Examples are spinach, carrots, sweet potatoes, papaya, mango, eggs and green leafy vegetables. Red palm oil, which is widely used in West and Central Africa, has a very high content of vitamin A.
• Families should be encouraged to plant appropriate crops, whether in small gardens or in larger plantations.

Interventions by the health authorities

• Foods which are widely used – for example, sugar, flour or milk – may be fortified with vitamin A.
• Vitamin A supplementation may be combined with immunization.
• Public awareness of vitamin A deficiency should be increased by health education at mother and child health clinics and in schools.

Table 18.10 High-dose universal-distribution schedule for prevention of vitamin A deficiency

Age	Vitamin A dosage
Infants <6 months of age*	
• Non-breast-fed infants	50 000 IU orally
• Breast-fed infants whose mothers have not received supplemental vitamin A	50 000 IU orally
Infants 6–12 months of age	100 000 IU orally, every 4–6 months[*]
Children >12 months of age	200 000 IU orally, every 4–6 months[†]
Mothers	200 000 IU orally, within 8 weeks of delivery

*Programmes should ensure that infants <6 months of age do not receive the larger dose intended for mothers. It may therefore be preferable to dose infants with a liquid dispenser to avoid possible confusion between capsules of different dosages.
[†]Evidence suggests vitamin A reserves in deficient individuals can fall below optimal levels 3–6 months following a high dose: however, dosing at 4–6-month intervals should be sufficient to prevent serious consequences of vitamin A deficiency.

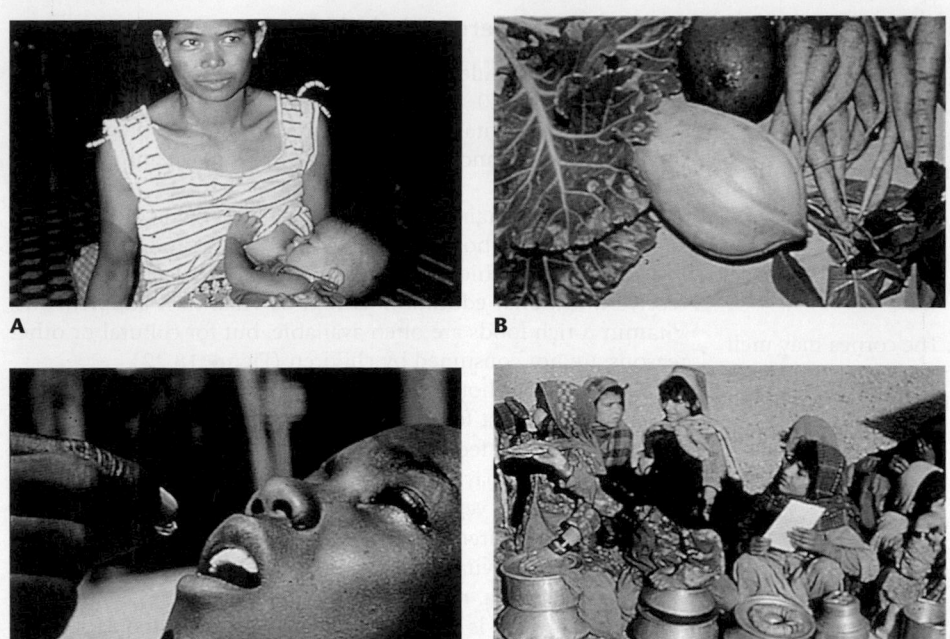

Figure 18.22 (**A**) Breast-feeding; (**B**) vitamin A-rich fruit and vegetables; (**C**) vitamin A capsule; (**D**) milk fortified with vitamin A. (Courtesy of: (**A, B, D**) Murray McGavin; (**C**) Christoffel Blindenmission.)

Measles and the eye

Measles is a serious infection, especially in the developing world. Up to 1 million children die from measles annually. Measles infection has been associated with the onset of eye problems in children who present with corneal scarring.[53]

Clinical presentation

Measles virus causes conjunctivitis, so children with measles will often have photosensitivity (sensitivity to light), watering and red eyes. There may be evidence of a punctate keratitis. However, measles conjunctivitis is self-limiting and it is the complications of measles which can cause blindness.

In a child with low reserves of vitamin A (mostly in the liver), acute vitamin A deficiency can result in corneal ulceration and keratomalacia (X3B).

The immune response may be depressed by measles infection, which may lead to severe herpes simplex keratitis.

A seriously ill child may be listless and fail to close the eyelids adequately. Corneal drying due to exposure can result in corneal ulceration. Antibiotic eye ointment should be used at least four times daily during the illness.

The use of traditional eye medicines may complicate the clinical picture. Often the mother will be reluctant to admit to attending a traditional healer.

Treatment of measles and its eye complications

Vitamin A 200 000 IU orally should be given at least once. If there is a known risk of vitamin A deficiency in the community or if there are any symptoms or signs of vitamin A deficiency affecting the eyes of the child, the full regimen of three doses of vitamin A should be prescribed.

A topical antibiotic should be given to each eye at least four times each day.

Supportive treatment should be given as appropriate, for example for gastroenteritis or respiratory infection.

Prevention

A programme of immunization should be instituted as soon as possible for the community or communities at risk. The WHO Expanded Programme on Immunization is promoting increased coverage of immunization around the world. Improved measles immunization is associated with a reduction in severe vitamin A deficiency.[54]

Newborn conjunctivitis (ophthalmia neonatorum)

By definition, newborn conjunctivitis occurs in a child within the first 28 days of life. Infection occurs during the birth of the child. It presents as a severe conjunctivitis, with purulent discharge. There is a danger of corneal ulcer and perforation.

Two organisms commonly cause newborn conjunctivitis: *Neisseria gonorrhoea* and *Chlamydia trachomatis*. Between 25% and 50% of infants exposed to *N. gonorrhoea* or *C. trachomatis* during birth develop the corresponding eye infection, if no eye prophylaxis is given.

The WHO has estimated a yearly adult incidence of 62 million cases of gonorrhoea and 89 million of genital chlamydial infection. The prevalence of gonorrhoea among antenatal attenders in African countries is disturbingly high, at between 4% and 15%. However, the global incidence of newborn conjunctivitis is not known.

Newborn conjunctivitis due to *N. gonorrhoea* typically has a dramatic onset with bilateral purulent conjunctivitis and profuse

Table 18.11 Management of newborn conjunctivitis

GONOCOCCAL

A. Admission to hospital
    Penicillin i.m. or i.v.
    Topical antimicrobial therapy, e.g. tetracycline 1%
    ointment, intensively at first (hourly) then reducing to three
    times a day for 14 days

B. *If PPNG* prevalence more than 1%*
    Single i.m. injection of cefotaxime 100 mg/kg or kanamycin
    25 mg/kg plus tetracycline 1% ointment or erythromycin
    0.5% ointment as indicated in (A)

Chlamydial: systemic treatment
Erythromycin estolate orally (syrup) 5 mg/kg per day for 14 days

Non-gonococcal, non-chlamydial
Tetracycline 1% ointment or erythromycin 0.5% ointment four
times a day for 14 days

Treatment of Parents

Table 18.12 Prevention of newborn conjunctivitis

Detection and treatment of infected pregnant women
Screening of all pregnant women is difficult in most countries
and expensive
May be possible to screen high-risk groups

Eye prophylaxis in the neonate at birth
Mechanical cleaning of the eyelids immediately at birth, plus
povidone iodine 2.5%, tetracycline 1% ointment or silver nitrate
1% drops

Treatment of the neonate as an index case
Only applicable where:
• prevalence of gonococcal infection low
• main sexually transmitted disease causing newborn
  conjunctivitis is *Chlamydia trachomatis*
• all infected infants can be detected and treated
• facilities exist for diagnosis of *C. trachomatis*

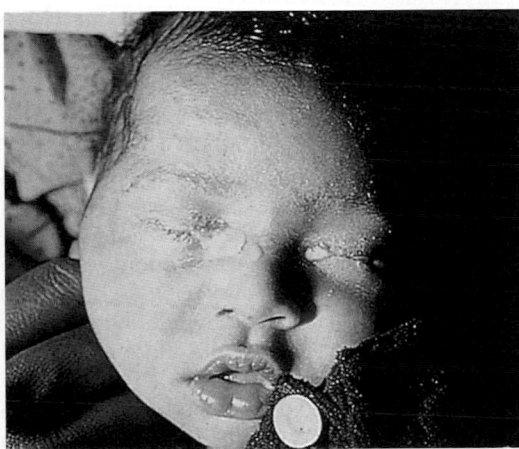

Figure 18.23 Newborn conjunctivitis due to *Neisseria gonorrhoeae*. (Courtesy of John D. C. Anderson.)

discharge of pus, associated with tense and swollen eyelids (Figure 18.23). The condition usually presents within the first few days of birth. This is an emergency and treatment must be started immediately with hourly topical antibiotic drops (e.g. ofloxacin or gentamicin), intensive cleaning of the eyes, and systemic antigonococcal treatment.

Newborn conjunctivitis due to *C. trachomatis* has similar clinical features, but does not lead to corneal ulceration. It may present later than gonococcal infection. Treatment for newborn conjunctivitis due to *C. trachomatis* is systemic erythromycin or azithromycin.

Treatment for these conditions should include systemic antimicrobial therapy because the infection is not confined to the eyes alone. Systemic treatment must also be given to both parents, who may be at high risk of other sexually transmitted diseases (Table 18.11).

Other bacteria which may cause newborn conjunctivitis include *Haemophilus*, *Streptococcus pneumoniae*, *Staphylococcus* and *Pseudomonas*.

To prevent newborn conjunctivitis, the eyelids should be carefully cleaned with sterile saline as soon as the child is born, and prophylactic treatment instilled (Table 18.12). Povidone iodine, 2.5% solution, is more effective than either silver nitrate drops or erythromycin ointment, and considerably cheaper than both.[55] As it is self-sterilizing, it may be used safely by traditional birth attendants as well as hospital midwives.

Retinitis pigmentosa

The hereditary dystrophies of the retina can be sporadic, recessive, dominant or X-linked. They are characterized by progressive loss of photoreceptor and retinal pigment epithelium function.

Symptoms include night blindness (nyctalopia) and gradual loss of peripheral vision. Dark adaptation is affected, a ring scotoma or severe constriction of the visual fields may be found, and characteristic 'bone corpuscle' pigment is seen in the peripheral retina. The blood vessels become attenuated and the optic disc is pale. The condition may be associated with other disorders or syndromes. It may also present with atypical forms.

The visual prognosis is variable. Dominantly inherited forms generally preserve central vision into the sixth or seventh decade. Recessive and X-linked forms are much more severe.

There is no specific treatment. Close intermarriage (consanguinity) in many countries increases the risk of this disorder, and genetic counselling should be offered to affected families.

Sickle cell disease

Ocular manifestation of sickle cell anaemia include conjunctival vascular abnormalities, focal iris ischaemia, peripheral retinal vascular disturbance with new blood vessel formation, haemorrhages, fibrosis and sometimes a detached retina. These lesions are due to focal ischaemia caused by sickling. The most severe eye disease is found not in homozygous patients with haemoglobin SS, but in heterozygotes with haemoglobin SC.

Laser photocoagulation should be used to treat peripheral ischaemic retina causing neovascularization. Late-stage disease with vitreous haemorrhage may require surgical removal of the vitreous (vitrectomy). Retinal detachment surgery may also be necessary.

Congenital cataract

In adults, cataract does not require urgent treatment, as the prognosis remains good even if the cataract has been present for years. In children under the age of 5, cataract leads to amblyopia (lazy eye). If surgery is delayed, the amblyopia may be irreversible, and the vision will not recover despite successful surgery.[56]

Congenital cataract may be the result of maternal infection with rubella during the early months of pregnancy. The most common cause is rubella; but chickenpox, cytomegalovirus and toxoplasmosis have also been implicated. Congenital cataract may be dominantly inherited and affect entire families. Down's syndrome, and other chromosomal abnormalities, are associated with congenital cataract.

Other causes of cataract include metabolic disorders with abnormal biochemical functions, for example, galactosaemia. However, in most cases no cause is found, and exhaustive investigations are unnecessary.

Congenital rubella syndrome may be prevented by immunization. If only a small proportion of the community is immunized, however, this may reduce the risk of infection in childhood, leading to more infections in early adulthood and an increase in congenital rubella syndrome.

A child with bilateral cataract (Figure 18.24) should be referred as soon as the diagnosis is made. Surgery should be carried out in a specialist children's eye centre, which has the necessary equipment and expertise.[57]

In most developing countries, the child who has had surgery for bilateral congenital cataract will be provided with aphakic spectacles or an intraocular lens. Refraction should be carried out

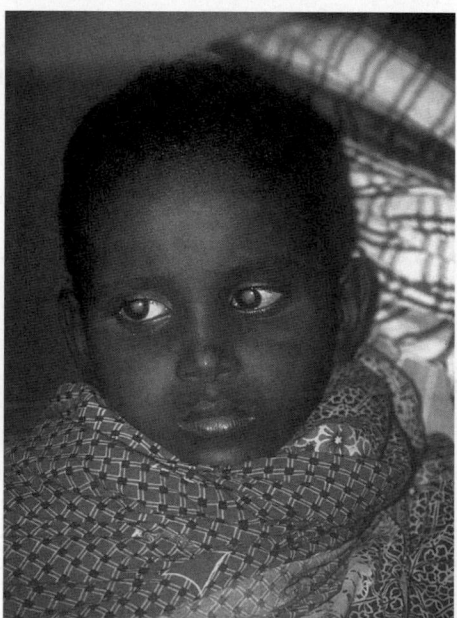

Figure 18.24 Bilateral congenital cataract. (Courtesy of David Yorston.)

every 6 months as the child's eye is growing rapidly. Despite surgery and adequate refractive correction, the child often has residual mild visual impairment, and will require additional support for schooling. Low-vision services are an integral part of the management of childhood cataract.

Unilateral congenital cataract causes profound amblyopia, and surgery is not justified. An exception is traumatic cataract, in which prompt surgery with an intraocular lens can have good results.[58]

Congenital glaucoma (buphthalmos)

Glaucoma in childhood may be present at birth or can develop during the first few years of life. In a young child the sclera is more elastic, and increased intraocular pressure stretches and enlarges the eye. For this reason the description of buphthalmos, or 'ox eye', is used. Congenital glaucoma may be unilateral or bilateral. The unilateral enlarged eye is usually more quickly recognized.

The condition causes discomfort, with photophobia, and inflammation. On examination the cornea is enlarged (>11 mm diameter) and may be hazy.

Treatment requires surgery to allow the aqueous fluid to drain out of the eye. Unfortunately, the prognosis for vision is frequently poor, as the diagnosis is often delayed.

Retinopathy of prematurity

Retinopathy of prematurity (RoP) is a leading cause of childhood blindness throughout the world apart from sub-Saharan Africa. Better neonatal care has increased the survival of premature babies who are at risk of this condition. In rich countries, blinding RoP is rare in babies with a birth weight over 1000 g or a gestational age greater than 28/40. However, in middle-income countries of Asia and Latin America, heavier and more mature babies are at risk.[59]

RoP is a proliferative retinopathy in babies with immature retinal blood vessels. Spasm of the retinal vessels is followed by dilated vessels, new vessel formation, vitreous haemorrhage, vitreoretinal traction, and retinal detachment.

Early detection, by screening all babies at risk, followed by prompt photocoagulation or cryotherapy of ischaemic retina has been shown to reduce the risk of blindness, and is one of the most cost-effective interventions in medicine. All premature babies at risk of RoP should be examined by an ophthalmologist with experience of the condition. Local guidelines must be developed to identify babies at risk. In middle-income countries, examining all babies weighing under 1750 g may be a reasonable strategy.

Retinoblastoma

This malignant tumour of children arises because of mutations in the *RB1* tumour-suppressing genes situated on the long arm of chromosome 13. Two-thirds of children with retinoblastoma develop the tumour because of random somatic mutations. These children present with a single tumour, typically at a relatively older age than other children with retinoblastoma. If they survive, these children do not pass on a genetic defect to their offspring.

The remaining one-third of children who develop retinoblastoma have a mutation in the *RB1* gene in every cell in the body.

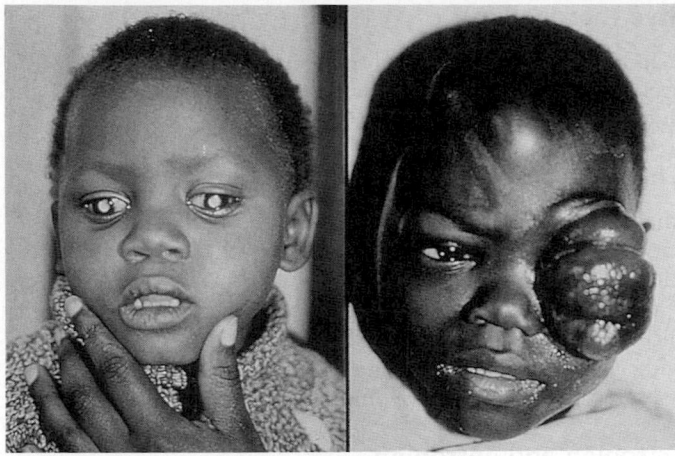

Figure 18.25 Bilateral retinoblastoma (left). Advanced retinoblastoma (right). (Courtesy of Volker Klauss.)

Either the defect is inherited or the mutation occurs at the time of conception. A sporadic mutation will then occur affecting the second *RB1* gene, often in more than one retinal cell. This causes multifocal, bilateral tumours, which occur at a younger age. These children are also at risk of other tumours if they survive the retinoblastoma.

Retinoblastoma may present with a white pupil, but many children in developing countries present late, with advanced fungating tumour, commonly extraocular and often extraorbital (Figure 18.25). The tumour extends along the optic nerve to the brain. In the later stages, metastases occur to other parts of the body. Other complaints which may lead to a discovery of retinoblastoma include a squint, glaucoma, visual loss, a painful red eye and proptosis. The tumour may present at any time during the first 5 years of life.

Following the discovery of a single tumour, both eyes must be examined carefully. Examinations must continue regularly, every 3–6 months, until at least the age of 5 years.

Adults who have had multiple retinoblastomas, and survived, must be advised that there is a 50% chance of their children being affected.

The differential diagnosis of this tumour (when still intraocular) includes infections such as toxocariasis and toxoplasmosis, vascular disorders such as retinopathy of prematurity and Coat's disease, and many other conditions. Investigations should include ultrasonography or computed tomography, if available.

Management

Effective treatment of retinoblastoma is largely dependent on early recognition of the tumour while it is still contained within the eye. The patient must be referred immediately to the specialist. In developing countries, most eyes will require enucleation, removing as much of the attached optic nerve as possible. Some specialist centres will be able to provide chemotherapy for these children, which is very effective. For smaller intraocular tumours, cryotherapy can be applied directly to the tumour. Radioactive plaques sutured to the sclera adjacent to the tumour may also be used.

HARMFUL TRADITIONAL EYE MEDICINES

Many patients will go to the local traditional healer before considering attendance at a health centre or eye clinic. It should be recognized that traditional healing can provide benefit to patients. However, some applications to the eyes used by these local healers can cause severe adverse reactions.

The clinical features of the original condition may be confused by the application of harmful eye medicines into an eye that is already abnormal. The patient, or the parent who has brought a child, may be very reluctant to admit that traditional eye medicine has been used.

A variety of harmful medications may be used: the juice of squeezed plant leaves, lime juice, kerosene, toothpaste and urine (either animal or human). A chemical or caustic keratoconjunctivitis may occur, or infection, such as with *N. gonorrhoea* from human urine. Infectious keratitis is common after the use of traditional eye medicines.[60] Topical therapy with an antibiotic every 2 to 6 hours, and a cycloplegic such as atropine sulphate once daily, should be used. The underlying eye disease should be treated as usual.

Programmes to develop a constructive approach of dialogue and cooperation with traditional healers have been developed in Zimbabwe, Malawi and Nepal, where it has been demonstrated that traditional healers can have a role in the prevention of blindness. These programmes have encouraged the following:

- Change specific practices that may be harmful and encourage those that are not harmful
- Improve the ability of healers to recognize and refer patients with cataract
- Build upon existing respect given to healers by the community
- Develop programmes in collaboration with healers, using their pre-existing knowledge and skills
- Maintain interaction between healers and eye care providers, establishing collaborative activities.

Couching

Couching is a traditional procedure for the treatment of cataract in parts of the developing world, in which the opaque lens is displaced from the visual axis. The procedure often leads to blinding complications.

Two methods of couching are reported:
1. 'Sharp' method: the eye is perforated and the lens is pushed backwards by a sharp instrument, for example a long thorn.
2. 'Blunt' method: the lens is pushed into the vitreous by massage or by blunt injury. In this method the eye is not perforated and it has been assumed to be safer.

The following example of a blunt method comes from Sudan. The coucher places the spent cartridge of a bullet filled with sand or gravel against the patient's closed eye. The end of the cartridge is struck sharply and the 'bolus' of sand or gravel hits the eye. This is repeated until the patient describes better vision because the cataractous lens is dislocated into the vitreous. There was no mention of the other injuries which may have occurred due to blunt trauma!

REFRACTIVE ERRORS

It is beyond the scope of this chapter to discuss refractive errors in detail. However, the recognition of refractive needs and the provision of spectacles are vital to most populations. Refractive error can affect the performance of a child in school. Programmes to detect refractive error in schoolchildren have been implemented in India. A pin-hole disc can indicate if poor vision is due to a refractive error. People aged 40 or more need presbyopic glasses – for reading, for sewing, or for picking stones out of rice! Aphakic spectacle corrections are required for aphakic patients.

It is estimated that 2.3 billion people worldwide have refractive errors. The vast majority of these could have their sight improved by spectacles, but only 1.8 billion people have access to eye examinations and affordable glasses. Therefore, around 500 million people, mostly in developing countries, have uncorrected refractive errors.

Vision 2020 includes refractive errors and low vision. The Vision 2020 strategy seeks to develop the following:

- Create awareness and demand for refractive services through community-based services/primary eye care and school screening
- Develop accessible refractive services for individuals identified with significant refractive errors, which will require training in refraction and dispensing
- Ensure that affordable spectacles are made available to individuals with significant refractive errors
- Develop and make available low-vision services and optical devices for all those in need, including children in blind schools and integrated education.

ACUTE RED EYE

The differential diagnosis of the acute painful red eye includes inflammations of the eyelids, conjunctivitis, uveitis, corneal ulcers, trauma and acute glaucoma. Conjunctivitis is the most common condition, and rarely causes loss of vision. As a rule, unilateral red eye is less likely to be conjunctivitis, and is more likely to cause blindness in the affected eye.

Disorders of the eyelids

Blepharitis

Blepharitis is common and usually chronic. Seborrhoeic blepharitis presents with redness of the lid margins with crusts on and at the base of eyelashes. Meibomitis is caused by blockage and inflammation of the meibomian glands in the tarsal plate. *Staphylococcus aureus* may be involved. Treatment of this chronic condition can be difficult and the inflammation will often recur. The eyelids should be massaged daily with hot compresses. If there is a severe blepharitis, systemic tetracycline 250 mg orally, four times daily for 1 week and then twice daily, for 6–12 weeks, may be used.

Inflammation of the eyelid skin or margins may be due to a virus such as papillomavirus, herpes simplex, herpes zoster or molluscum contagiosum.

Stye (hordeolum)

A localized staphylococcal abscess may form at the base of an eyelash. Epilation of the eyelash may speed resolution of the infection.

Chalazion (meibomian cyst)

The meibomian glands, which are situated in the tarsal plates of each eyelid, open along the lid margins. Ducts may become blocked, resulting in a retention cyst with ensuing inflammatory reaction. If present for more than 3 months, the cyst may require incision. Following local anaesthetic injection, the eyelid is everted with a chalazion clamp, and the cyst is incised vertically and curetted. A topical antibiotic eye ointment is given for 1 week.

Ectropion and entropion

Abnormal positions of the eyelids, such as an eyelid which turns out (ectropion) or turns in (entropion), may cause discomfort and inflammation.

Ectropion, which usually involves the lower eyelid, results in exposure of the tarsal conjunctiva. Ectropion can follow facial nerve paralysis. Injury or infection with associated scarring can cause a cicatricial ectropion.

Entropion can commonly affect both upper and lower eyelids. The scarring of trachoma is often associated with upper eyelid entropion. In older age, the lower eyelid may turn in, causing irritation due to eyelashes rubbing on the cornea.

Eyelid tumours

Both basal cell carcinoma and squamous cell carcinoma may cause nodular or ulcerating lesions on the eyelids. These occur in fair-skinned people who have prolonged or intense exposure to sunlight.

Other eyelid inflammations

Inflammation and scarring of the eyelids may be caused by conditions such as anthrax, actinomycosis, Leishmaniasis and yaws.

Orbital cellulitis

Infection within the orbital cavity leads to swelling of the eyelids, and proptosis. Eye movements are reduced. The patient usually has a fever and is unwell. Complications of orbital cellulitis include meningitis, cerebral abscess, and cavernous sinus thrombosis. Patients should be admitted and treated with high-dose intravenous antibiotics.

Dacrocystitis

Blockage of the nasolacrimal duct prevents drainage of the lacrimal sac, which may lead to infection causing a painful swelling at the side of the nose below the medial canthus of the eye. This can present as an acutely inflamed abscess or as a chronic watery and discharging eye.

The infection will recur unless the lacrimal sac is emptied by re-establishing drainage to the nose. This can be accomplished by dacryocystorhinostomy.

Inflammation of the conjunctiva

Infectious conjunctivitis

Both bacteria and viruses may cause suppurative conjunctivitis, characterized by foreign body sensation, conjunctival injection and a purulent discharge.

Most bacterial conjunctivitis is self-limiting and does not affect vision. Gonococcal conjunctivitis may affect adults, particularly young men who may inadvertently transfer genital gonorrhoea to their conjunctiva. This causes a very severe conjunctivitis, with a profuse purulent discharge, and may lead to corneal ulcers and perforation.

Viral conjunctivitis may be associated with transient corneal opacities, which can affect the vision. It is also associated with subconjunctival haemorrhages, which look dramatic but are harmless. Viral conjunctivitis is highly infectious and tends to occur in epidemics.

Allergic conjunctivitis

Allergic conjunctivitis is characterized by a slightly red eye, itching, and a watery or mucous discharge. This may be associated with other atopic conditions such as hay fever, eczema or asthma.

Vernal keratoconjunctivitis

This disorder, which mostly affects children and teenagers, is common in the more temperate parts of the tropics (e.g. highlands of East Africa). The precise aetiology remains obscure but IgE and cell-mediated immune mechanisms play an important role. It affects the upper tarsal conjunctiva and the bulbar conjunctiva at the corneoscleral junction. The eyes are red, irritable, and discharge mucus. Severe itching is typical. Papillae may be large and often have an appearance like 'cobblestones'.

The most effective treatment of vernal keratoconjunctivitis is topical corticosteroids; however, these should only be used under strict specialist ophthalmic supervision. Topical corticosteroids can have blinding side-effects, such as steroid-induced glaucoma. They also cause local immunosuppression, which may be catastrophic if a red eye is caused by infection, e.g. herpes simplex. Although the symptoms of vernal catarrh are troublesome and irritating, they are self-limiting, as the condition goes into remission as the patient enters adulthood, and it very rarely affects the sight. Topical steroids relieve the symptoms, but prolonged treatment may cause blindness.

Alternative treatments for vernal conjunctivitis include topical or systemic antihistamines. Mast cell stabilizers, such as sodium cromoglicate 2% (Opticrom®, Aarane®, Intal®) or nedocromil 2% may alleviate symptoms if used continuously over several weeks. Symptomatic relief may be obtained with cold compresses and artificial tears to irrigate the conjunctiva.

Subconjunctival haemorrhage

Subconjunctival haemorrhage usually occurs spontaneously and is evident as a dramatic red area over the white sclera. This will resolve in 2–3 weeks. Unless the patient has similar haemorrhages

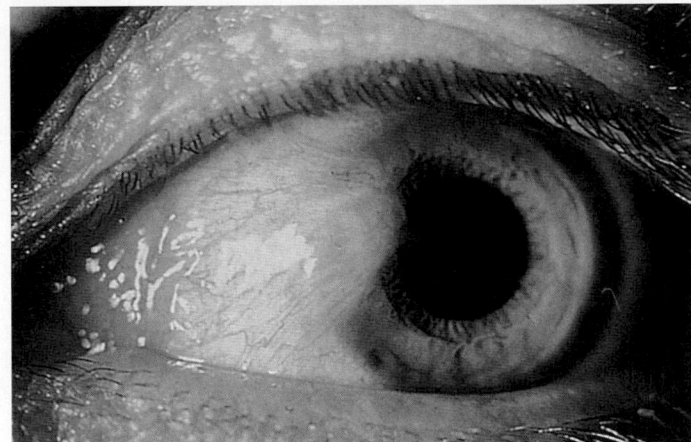

Figure 18.26 Nasal pterygium. (Courtesy of Murray McGavin.)

elsewhere, it is likely to be an isolated episode of no consequence. Occasionally it may be a manifestation of a bleeding disorder.

Pinguecula

The accumulation of yellow-white fatty deposits at the nasal or temporal conjunctival limbus is a common finding in middle or older age. Occasionally the pinguecula may become inflamed, when a topical antiinflammatory agent may be used. The best form of treatment is to leave them alone.

Pterygium

A pterygium is a 'wing' of conjunctival and fibrovascular tissue which grows across the cornea from either the temporal or the nasal side (Figure 18.26). Although poorly understood, it is associated with exposure to sunlight and dust. Most pterygia cause few problems, and do not encroach on the visual axis. If they are excised, they are likely to recur, and behave much more aggressively. If surgery is required, a conjunctival autograft should be used to reduce the risk of recurrence.

Phlyctenulosis

A phlycten appears most commonly at or near to the limbus and is evidence of a hypersensitivity reaction to staphylococci or other bacterial allergens. A phlycten is a microabscess which appears as a raised, pale nodule. It responds quickly to topical corticosteroids. Again, the diagnosis should be certain and any use of topical corticosteroids should be carefully monitored. Any patient with a phlycten should be examined for possible systemic disease, particularly tuberculosis.

Keratoconjunctivitis sicca (dry eye)

Keratoconjunctivitis sicca (KCS) is a common condition where dryness of the eyes causes symptoms of irritation, with grittiness and burning. It is more common in patients over 50 years of age. There is a recognized association with rheumatoid arthritis (Sjögren's syndrome: KCS, dry mouth and rheumatoid arthritis).

Dry eyes can follow trachoma, in which the lacrimal gland ducts, and conjunctival goblet cells, are damaged.

A Schirmer's test uses strips of filter paper which are hooked over the lower eyelid and the length of wetting of the strip is measured after 5 minutes. However, this test is unreliable. A drop of Rose Bengal 1% eye drops will reveal punctate staining of the cornea and conjunctiva and filaments of epithelium on the cornea (filamentary keratitis). In a dry eye, Rose Bengal will cause considerable discomfort.

Treatment is with artificial tear preparations such as hypromellose 0.3% eye drops.

In extreme cases of dry eyes, temporary occlusion of the lacrimal canaliculi (using plugs) or permanent occlusion (using cautery) can be very effective. However, permanent occlusion should only be done in patients who have severe symptoms, and are willing to accept a possible watering eye.

Trachoma

See pp. 291–294.

Suppurative keratitis

Suppurative corneal ulceration, due to either bacteria or fungi, is a common problem (Figure 18.27).[61] Central ulceration involving the stroma will leave a corneal scar when it heals. The treatment of this condition can be further complicated by lack of antibiotics and antifungal agents.

Epithelial ulceration, without stromal involvement, will heal without scarring. However, breached epithelium permits the entry of microorganisms, which leads to destruction of the stroma and scarring. If the infection penetrates the eye, it can result in endophthalmitis and phthisis.

Many organisms cause suppurative keratitis. The most frequent causes of bacterial keratitis are *Streptococcus pneumoniae*, *Pseudomonas* and *Staphylococcus aureus*. The most common fungi are *Aspergillus*, *Fusarium* and *Candida albicans*. Fungal keratitis is more frequent in humid tropical areas such as coastal West Africa and South-East Asia. Agricultural accidents and injuries with vegetable matter predispose to fungal infection.

Clinical appearance

The eye will be red, painful and photophobic, with profuse lacrimation. A corneal opacity, which stains with fluorescein, is visible. A hypopyon, which appears as a white fluid level in the anterior chamber, is the characteristic feature of suppurative keratitis.

It is not easy to determine whether a corneal ulcer is due to bacterial or fungal infection on clinical grounds alone. However, serrated margins, a raised slough, and coloured infiltrate suggest infection due to a fungus.[62]

Laboratory diagnosis

Gram staining and microscope examination are possible within half an hour. The procedure for obtaining and examining material from a corneal scrape is shown in Table 18.13. This may demonstrate the presence of bacteria or fungi. Bacteria will be identified as Gram-positive or Gram-negative, and as rods or cocci. The examination and interpretation of corneal scrapes requires skill and experience, and it is often impossible to detect any organism.

Management

The treatment of suppurative keratitis is urgent. Initial treatment may be guided by Gram stain results, and knowledge of the locally common causes of infectious keratitis. For example, fungal keratitis is common in South India, so an antifungal should be given when the organism is unknown. Treatment can be modified if culture and sensitivity results become available later.

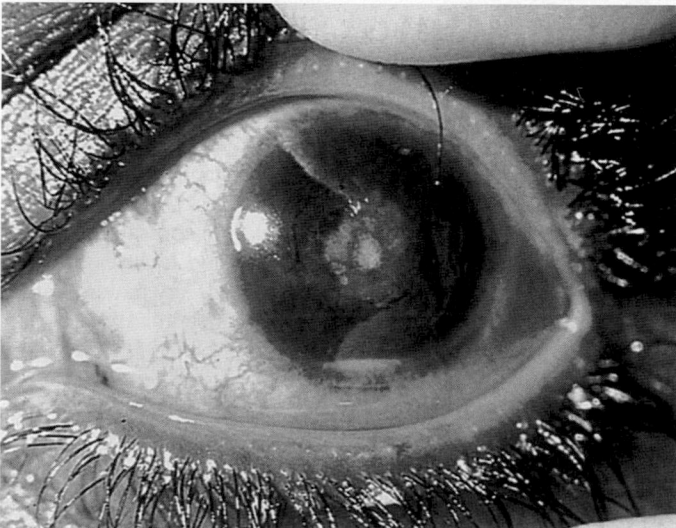

Figure 18.27 Corneal ulceration with hypopyon formation. (Courtesy of Allen Foster.)

Table 18.13 Materials and procedure for a corneal scrape

Material
Topical anaesthetic (ideally preservative-free if culture is to be performed)
Scalpel blades, needles or platinum spatula
Alcohol or gas burner
Matches or lighter
Clean glass microscope slides (labelled)
Wax or diamond marker
Culture media (labelled)

Procedure
Put nothing in the eye except anaesthetic until the specimen is taken
Explain the procedure to the patient
Children require sedation
Apply topical anaesthetic if required
Use sterile, cooled blade or needle to sample representative areas of ulcer (a spirit lamp may be used for sterilization)
Avoid touching lids and lashes
Use each scrape to prepare one smear or culture
Spread material thinly on to microscope slides
Re-sterilize and cool instrument between scrapes
Fix slides for microscopy with gentle heat (or alcohol)
Label slides and cultures with name and date

Table 18.14 Topical treatment of suppurative keratitis according to results of Gram stain

	Ideal circumstances	Practical alternatives
Gram-positive cocci	Cefuroxime 50 mg/mL or fluoroquinolone	Gentamicin 8 mg/mL
Gram-negative rods	Fluoroquinolone or gentamicin 8 mg/mL	
Fungal elements	Econazole 1% or natamycin 5%	
Unknown organism	Fluoroquinolone + antifungal if indicated	Gentamicin 8 mg/mL

All antibiotics should be given hourly for 48 hours and then reduced to every 6 hours.

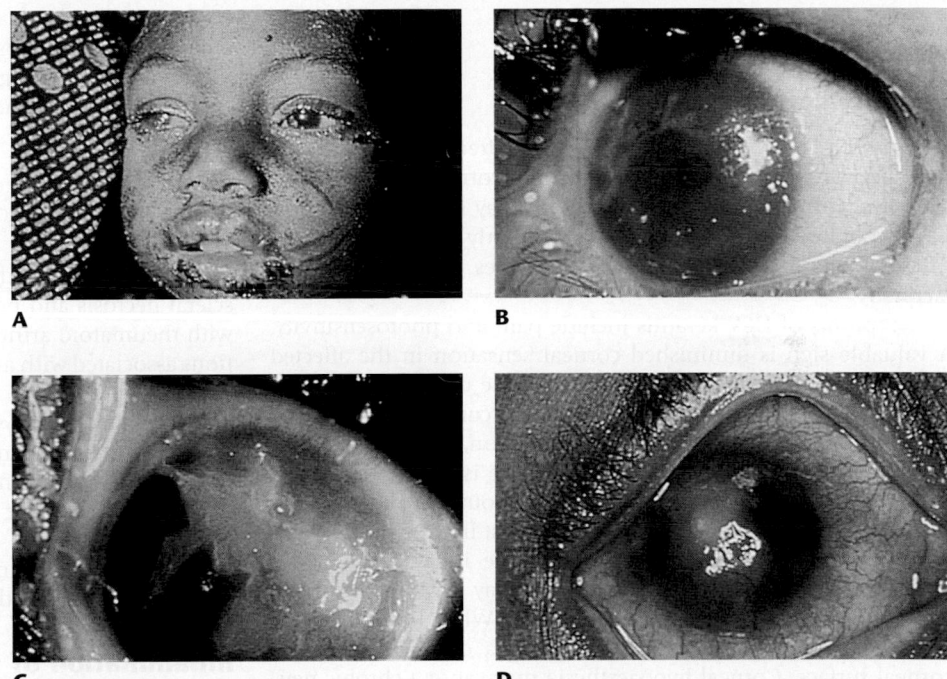

Figure 18.28 Herpes simplex keratitis. (Courtesy of: (**A**, **C**) John Sandford-Smith; (**B**) Allen Foster; (**D**) David Yorston.)

Different regimens of treatment are given in Table 18.14.

Fluoroquinolones, such as ciprofloxacin or ofloxacin, have good activity against all Gram-negative organisms, including *Pseudomonas*. They are also effective against many Gram-positive species and are recommended as monotherapy.

Natamycin or an imidazole, such as econazole, are the antifungals of choice. Natamycin has limited corneal penetration, but has been shown to be effective in randomized clinical trials.

Any eye with corneal ulceration should also be given a cycloplegic, such as atropine sulphate 1%, used at least once daily.

Any bacterial ulcer will be sterilized within 48 hours of intensive treatment, but healing may take much longer. Bacterial ulcers should be healed in 10–14 days, and fungal ulcers within 21–28 days. If the ulcer does not heal, a central tarsorrhaphy should be performed. If perforation is imminent, a conjunctival flap can save the eye.

Herpes simplex keratitis

The herpes simplex virus (HSV) is distributed worldwide and can have severe effects on the eye. Most individuals will have experienced a 'cold sore' on the face, but a similar lesion on the cornea is much more significant. Combined with the inappropriate use of topical corticosteroids (which are contraindicated in this infection unless used by an eye specialist), the results can be disastrous for the eye. Most HSV keratitis is caused by type I infection, although occasionally type II infections occur, particularly in the newborn – when infection occurs in the mother's birth canal.

The virus can remain latent within the nervous system, particularly the ganglion of the 5th cranial nerve. HSV infection is more severe in immunocompromised individuals and may, for example, complicate the picture of measles keratitis and malnutrition.

In one study in Tanzania, HSV was responsible for 36% of corneal ulcers found in children (1981–1985).[53]

Although HSV keratitis may be immediately obvious if there is a classical dendritic ulcer, the infection often has an atypical appearance in developing countries.[63] The ulcer may be larger and geographic or amoeboid in appearance (Figure 18.28). These presentations may relate to reduced host immune response, delay before treatment is sought, or to the effect of inaccurate diagnosis and inappropriate treatment, particularly with corticosteroids or traditional eye medicines.

Table 18.15 Distinguishing signs of herpetic corneal ulcers

Typical, narrow branching dendritic ulcer
Large, irregular geographic ulcer
Intense corneal vascularization
Dense stromal infiltrate
Stromal necrosis and/or facetting
Reduced corneal sensation
Scarring/facetting/vascularization from previous attacks
Central corneal oedema, with keratitic precipitates (disciform)

Eye complications

Herpes simplex ulceration of the cornea is often recurrent. Should the infection and inflammation affect the corneal stroma, it will lead to scarring and opacity. Recurrence may be stimulated by a number of factors, including fever (particularly malaria), exposure to ultraviolet light, minor trauma, measles and psychological factors.

Symptoms of HSV keratitis include pain and photosensitivity. A valuable sign is diminished corneal sensation in the affected eye. This can be tested with a wisp of sterile cotton wool. Other signs (Table 18.15) include lacrimation, circumcorneal injection and photophobia. In the classic presentation, the ulcer forms a branching dendritic figure. This appearance is clearly delineated by fluorescein dye. The same dye will also outline a larger ulcer, such as the geographic ulcer. An intense host immune reaction to the virus in the cornea can lead to severe inflammation, and destruction of the stroma. Blood vessels may invade the cornea, particularly with ulcers close to the limbus. When healing occurs, a scar remains and loss of corneal stroma causes an irregular corneal surface. Corneal hypoaesthesia may cause a chronic neurotrophic ulcer. Deep inflammation of the cornea due to HSV infection provides a complicated problem in treatment. A uveitis may develop and sometimes the evidence of previous corneal epithelial infection can only be found with careful examination under magnification.

Management

Previously, treatment of superficial HSV keratitis affecting only the corneal epithelium was mechanical removal of the infected cells of the epithelium.

Other forms of treatment are now more commonly used. These include aciclovir 3% eye ointment, which should be given five times daily, or trifluorothymidine 1% solution, five times daily. Aciclovir is also available for systemic treatment, either orally or intravenously. Cycloplegic eye drops should be given while the eye is painful.

Topical corticosteroids may be required when there is an immune response resulting in a deep stromal keratitis. The weakest effective dose of steroid should be used, and must be given with an antiviral agent.

Eye health workers should refer any patient with geographic or stromal HSV keratitis to an ophthalmologist, after beginning treatment with a topical antiviral agent, if this is available.

An unhealed HSV ulcer may require a conjunctival flap or a tarsorrhaphy to effect healing. (A tarsorrhaphy is a surgical procedure, in this situation usually temporary, in which the eyelids are partially sutured together.) Corneal scarring may require a corneal transplant, which has a poor prognosis in HSV keratitis, as the infection recurs in the graft, and may provoke graft rejection.

Inflammation of the episclera and sclera

Episcleritis

Episcleritis is a self-limiting condition, characterized by localized conjunctival and subconjunctival hyperaemia. It has been associated with herpes zoster ophthalmicus, gout and rheumatoid arthritis and is a recognized complication of leprosy, but in most cases no cause is found. Topical corticosteroids can be used when required.

Scleritis

Inflammation of the sclera is more serious than episcleritis. It causes severe pain and redness. Occasionally, scleritis may lead to scleral necrosis and perforation. It is most commonly associated with rheumatoid arthritis and systemic vasculitis. Infective conditions associated with a scleritis are leprosy, tuberculosis and herpes zoster ophthalmicus.

Scleritis requires systemic treatment, either with non-steroidal antiinflammatory agents or systemic corticosteroids. Other immunosuppressive agents may also be used. Subconjunctival injections of corticosteroids are contraindicated as they may cause focal scleral necrosis.

When the scleral inflammation has settled, the area of sclera may be thin and faintly translucent.

Inflammation of the anterior uvea (anterior uveitis, iridocyclitis)

Inflammation of the iris (iritis) and of the ciliary body (cyclitis) may be described as iridocyclitis or anterior uveitis.

Iridocyclitis presents typically with pain, redness and photophobia. The condition may be unilateral or bilateral. Examination with magnification will reveal a haziness of the aqueous fluid in the anterior chamber of the eye due to the presence of circulating proteins and inflammatory cells. Deposits of cells may be found on the inferior endothelium of the cornea (keratic precipitates). If there is very severe inflammation, the white cells may form a fluid level in the inferior anterior chamber (hypopyon). Inflammation of the iris and its pupil margin may result in adhesion of the pupil to the anterior lens surface (posterior synechiae). Synechiae may also occur at the base of the iris, across the angle of the anterior chamber to the cornea (anterior synechiae). Both posterior and anterior synechiae can lead to secondary glaucoma and, in some instances, secondary cataract formation.

The causes of iridocyclitis are many, but in most cases no cause will be identified. Systemic diseases which present with a classical granulomatous type of iridocyclitis with large keratic precipitates include sarcoidosis and tuberculosis.

Injury to an eye can occasionally result in a 'sympathetic' inflammation of the undamaged eye. This may occur weeks, months or even years after the original injury. Topical and systemic corticosteroid therapy is required.

There are a variety of factors influencing the onset of iridocyclitis which may relate to genetic characteristics. For example, the HLA-B27 antigen is often associated with ankylosing spondylitis and uveitis. Males are more likely to develop ankylosing spondylitis or Reiter's syndrome. Reiter's syndrome is recognized by non-specific urethritis, polyarthritis and iridocyclitis. Certain racial factors influence uveitis in conditions such as Behçet's syndrome, which is more common in eastern Mediterranean people and the Japanese. Behçet's syndrome typically presents with recurrent ulcers of the mouth and genitalia associated with a severe uveitis. Sarcoidosis is more common in African-Americans than in Caucasians in North America.

Acute angle closure glaucoma

See pp. 290.

Inflammation of the eyeball

Endophthalmitis

Infection can develop inside the eye, for example when a bacterial or fungal corneal ulcer perforates, or following a penetrating injury or intraocular surgery. This causes a severe intraocular inflammatory reaction which may destroy the eye. There is fibrin in the anterior chamber, and a hypopyon may be visible. Vigorous treatment is required with systemic and intravitreal antibiotics. If the organism is unknown, intravitreal amikacin and vancomycin are given.

Staphyloma

A staphyloma occurs when there is thinning and ectasia of the corneoscleral coat of the eye, leading to protrusion of uveal tissue with a thin covering of cornea or sclera. The eye is usually severely inflamed initially, leading to a weakened cornea or sclera. This appearance may follow vitamin A deficiency (Figure 18.29), necrotizing scleritis, or corneal ulceration.

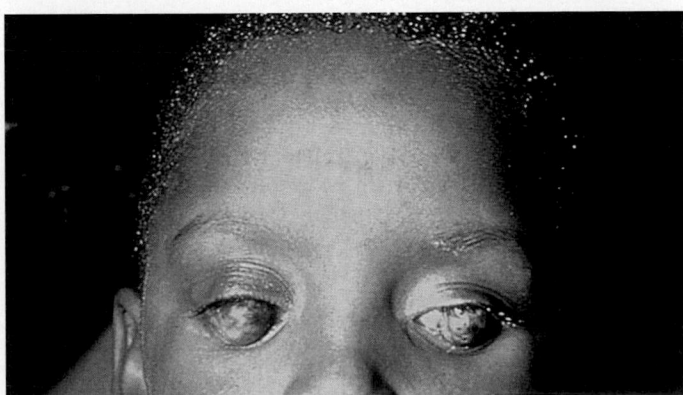

Figure 18.29 Gross staphyloma after measles and vitamin A deficiency. A blind unsightly eye will usually be enucleated. (Courtesy of Simon Franken.)

Phthisis bulbi

Severe inflammation, such as endophthalmitis, or injury may damage the ciliary body, and reduce aqueous production. This leads to low intraocular pressure (hypotony), and the eye becomes shrunken. If the patient is not complaining, no treatment is necessary. However, the appearance can be greatly improved by inserting an artificial eye either on top of the phthisical eye or following surgical removal of the eye.

Eye injuries

Trauma is a common cause of uniocular red eye and sometimes blindness. Injuries to the eye are classified as 'closed globe', which includes contusions and partial depth lacerations, and 'open globe', which includes globe ruptures, penetrating injuries and intraocular foreign body.

Corneal abrasion

Although this is a superficial injury involving only the corneal epithelium, it causes acute pain, lacrimation and photophobia.

Management

Instil topical antibiotics for 5 days. Give a cycloplegic, e.g. cyclopentolate 1%, once. If vegetable matter caused the injury, it may be complicated by fungal infection.

Superficial retained foreign body

These are often metallic but may also be stone, wood or an eyelash. The foreign body may lie on the upper tarsal conjunctiva, where it will be revealed by everting the eyelid.

Management

Instil local anaesthetic drops. Remove the foreign body with a cotton-wool bud or a sterile hypodermic needle. If the foreign body is ferrous, there may be some surrounding rust. Do not attempt to remove this without a microscope, as the cornea is only about 0.5 mm thick. Give topical antibiotics for 5 days, and a single dose of a cycloplegic.

Penetrating injuries

A penetrating injury may be due to any sharp object, such as a thorn, which penetrates the eye.

The evidence of injury is not always obvious. In some instances, only careful examination will reveal the track of a retained intraocular foreign body. There is no substitute for careful examination of the injured eye, using magnification. A retained foreign body which is radio-opaque will be seen on X-ray.

Management

As soon as a penetrating injury is recognized, the patient should be given antibiotic cover, both topically and systemically, and referred immediately to the eye specialist for surgical repair. Further examination is unnecessary, and may even harm the eye. The damaged eye should be protected with a shield.

Blunt injury

A blunt, or non-penetrating, injury may be caused by large slow-moving objects such as a stone or a fist.

Following a blunt injury, examine the eye systematically from the front to the back, beginning with the periorbital region and eyelids. Fractures may involve the orbital margin or the bony floor of the orbit (a blow-out fracture), which leads to adherence of the inferior rectus muscle. Bruising may occur affecting the eyelids, making it difficult to open the eye. There may be bleeding into the anterior chamber of the eye (hyphaema); if the hyphaema occupies more than 50% of the anterior chamber, there is a high risk of secondary glaucoma. Intraocular tissues such as the root of the iris may be torn (iridodialysis). The lens may be dislocated. Bleeding in the posterior segment of the eye may result in vitreous haemorrhage. Retinal oedema and haemorrhages may be apparent on ophthalmoscopy.

Management

In most instances the correct treatment of a blunt injury is observation until the condition resolves. Should there be a large hyphaema, the intraocular pressure must be monitored carefully. A hyphaema with a high pressure forces blood into the corneal stroma, leading to corneal blood staining. Raised intraocular pressure should be treated intensively, and, if medical treatment is insufficient, the patient should be referred urgently for surgical removal of the hyphaema.

It is advisable to give a topical antibiotic and cycloplegic eye drops. A topical steroid may be given. Any moderate intraocular pressure rise can be controlled by oral acetazolamide.

Chemical burns of the eye

Chemical injury may be caused by acid or alkali. Alkali burns are generally more serious.

Management

When a chemical injury has occurred, immediately irrigate the eye with water. Keep washing for 15–20 minutes, until all traces of the chemical have been washed out. Remember to irrigate under the eyelids as well. Any fragments of cement or solid material may be picked off with forceps. Antibiotic and steroid drops should be applied hourly for 2 days, and then reduced in frequency. Eyelids should be kept mobile with deliberate movement of the lids a number of times each day. Severe alkali burns should be urgently referred to the eye specialist, but most acid burns will heal within a few days.

Snake venom conjunctivitis

In regions of the world where the spitting cobra is found, snake venom can cause a conjunctivitis. Severe damage is rare, and is more likely to be caused by frantic attempts to remove the venom than by the toxin itself.

Solar burn (eclipse retinopathy)

Our natural precaution is to avoid the direct glare of the sun's rays, but in certain situations this does not happen. An eclipse of the

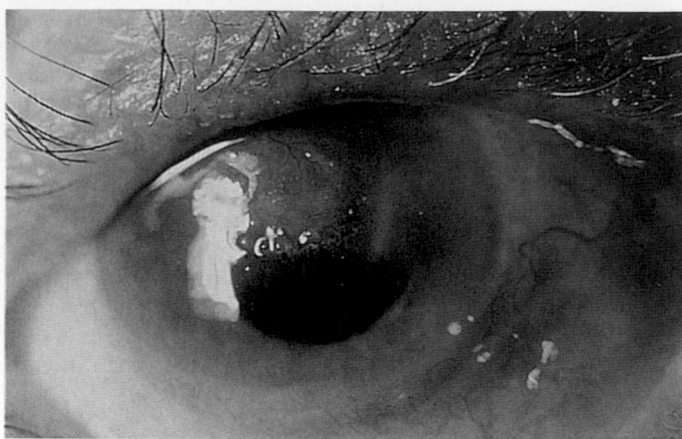

Figure 18.30 Climatic droplet keratopathy. (Courtesy of Gordon Johnson.)

sun should only be viewed with adequate filters, otherwise a macular burn will follow because sunlight will focus on the retina. This leads to a permanent central scotoma.

Caterpillar hair conjunctivitis (ophthalmia nodosum)

Caterpillar hairs in the conjunctiva provoke an unusual foreign body reaction known as ophthalmia nodosum. A granuloma forms around each caterpillar hair. Treatment requires removal of the hair, or deeper invasion may occur.

Landmine injuries

Antipersonnel landmines (APLs) inflict horrific injuries and often kill or maim civilians who have little or no part in any conflict. The problem is particularly serious in Afghanistan, Angola, Cambodia, Mozambique, Iraq and Somalia, but it is also present in more than 50 other countries. One estimate gives a figure of more than 100 million mines laid worldwide. Ophthalmic injuries typically occur when children play with ordnance, which then explodes in their faces.

Climatic droplet keratopathy

Climatic droplet keratopathy is a degenerative condition in which translucent droplets accumulate in the superficial stroma of the lower part of the cornea (Figure 18.30). It is caused by a high level of exposure to reflected ultraviolet light.

Treatment can involve sector iridectomy, debridement (scraping) of the central cornea, lamellar or penetrating keratoplasty and, more recently, ablation by excimer laser.

VIRAL INFECTIONS AND THE EYE

Measles

Measles and the eye, and its association with vitamin A deficiency disorders, are discussed on p. 302.

Rubella

The disease is frequently subclinical and is most often diagnosed when it appears in epidemics. The disease presents with an erythematous maculopapular rash on the face, trunk and extremities. The infection is self-limiting and harmless in children and males. However, maternal infection during the first trimester of pregnancy has an 80% chance of affecting the unborn child. The congenital rubella syndrome ranges from minimal to severe effects. Apart from eye complications, the child may be deaf or mentally retarded and there may be cardiovascular abnormalities. There is intrauterine growth retardation, and the most severe cases may cause spontaneous abortion or stillbirth.

Eye complications

Cataract may occur in around half of all children affected by rubella in utero. The virus may remain in the lens for some years after birth, and surgical removal of the cataract causes uveitis. Other eye defects include congenital glaucoma (buphthalmos), rubella retinopathy, which can have a 'salt and pepper' appearance, optic atrophy, squint, nystagmus and microphthalmos. Congenital cataract due to rubella has a poor prognosis.

Management

The treatment of rubella is preventive. Young females should be immunized; immunization may be carried out at 1 year of age or before puberty. This provides lasting immunity. However, immunization programmes must achieve at least 80% coverage of the population. Partial coverage may reduce the incidence of the disease in childhood, leading to a greater number of women reaching child-bearing age with no immunity.

Chickenpox (varicella)

This common virus infection of childhood is caused by the herpes zoster virus. The illness is characterized by fever, malaise and rash, which appears 12–16 days after infection has occurred. The rash is erythematous with vesicles occurring in groups which are widespread over the body surface. It may, however, occur at any age and can be a serious disease in adults. The patient has immunity to varicella following infection.

Eye complications

Vesicles may occur on the eyelids, conjunctiva and at the corneoscleral margin(s). Superficial punctate keratitis, deeper inflammation of the corneal stroma (interstitial keratitis) and iridocyclitis have been described. Occasionally, extraocular muscle involvement, pupil abnormalities and optic neuritis have occurred.

Management

Antibiotic ointment can prevent secondary bacterial infection of skin lesions. Any systemic complication, such as a pneumonia, will require suitable antibiotic cover for secondary bacterial infection.

Herpes zoster ophthalmicus

The herpes zoster virus lies dormant in sensory nerve ganglia after a previous infection with chickenpox (varicella). A variety of stimuli may precipitate herpes zoster (shingles). Herpes zoster most commonly affects older people and immunocompromised individuals. In Africa the development of shingles is often the first evidence of infection with the HIV/AIDS virus. Most often shingles affects the trunk, but herpes zoster ophthalmicus, affecting the periorbital region and eye, occurs in less than 10% of patients who develop shingles. In these patients the ophthalmic division of the 5th cranial nerve is affected. A distressing characteristic of the infection is post-herpetic neuralgia, which can persist for a year or more.

Eye complications

The clinical features of herpes zoster ophthalmicus include a red vesicular rash, which develops crusts and later resolves with multiple tiny scars. The rash is typically unilateral, respecting the midline of the forehead. In severe cases the rash may cause scarring, with cicatricial ectropion and exposure.

Eye involvement occurs in around 50% of patients and can be expected if the nasociliary branch of the ophthalmic division of the 5th nerve is affected, with vesicles on the side of the nose. There may be conjunctivitis, episcleritis, scleritis, keratitis and loss of corneal sensation (neuroparalytic keratitis), anterior uveitis, secondary glaucoma, extraocular nerve and muscle involvement, and optic neuritis. The virus can also infect the retina, causing acute retinal necrosis. Herpes zoster keratitis may take a variety of forms, including punctate epithelial erosions, filamentary keratitis and disciform keratitis. In patients with HIV/AIDS, the disease is particularly severe, and over 50% of eyes become blind.[64]

Management

The patient requires rest, adequate fluids and analgesia to allow relief of the often severe pain. Antiviral drugs should be given systemically, especially if a patient is immunocompromised. Alternatives include aciclovir, valaciclovir or famciclovir. A topical cycloplegic, such as atropine sulphate 1% eye drops, should be given. A topical corticosteroid may also be given if there is keratitis or anterior uveitis, but this should be under supervision of an eye specialist.

Corneal anaesthesia should be treated with a tarsorrhaphy. Acute retinal necrosis will require intravenous antivirals, and should be referred to a retinal specialist as these eyes often develop retinal detachment.

Cytomegalovirus

In recent years, infection with this virus has been particularly associated with the HIV/AIDS epidemic. Thus, it is a relatively common infection in the immunocompromised host. 'HIV/AIDS and the eye' is discussed further below.

Eye complications

Eye changes associated with the infection include anterior uveitis, retinitis with widespread necrosis, haemorrhages and sometimes

313

retinal detachment. The optic nerve may be involved, with progressive optic atrophy.

Infection affecting a woman who is pregnant can result in fetal abnormalities. These include low birth weight, purpura, deafness, mental retardation, pneumonitis, and an enlarged liver and spleen. Ocular abnormalities include cataract, uveitis, optic nerve atrophy, chorioretinitis and microphthalmos.

Epstein-Barr virus and Burkitt's lymphoma

The Epstein-Barr virus may cause a mild keratitis. It has been implicated in lymphoma, although no conclusive proof is available. The tumour is endemic in sub-Saharan Africa, but occurs sporadically elsewhere, particularly in immunosuppressed patients.

Most commonly found in children under 10 years old, the maxillary region and orbit are often involved. The abdomen and the central nervous system may also be affected. A cranial nerve palsy can occur. Periorbital infiltration may lead to proptosis, limitation of eye movements and exposure.

Treatment is by surgery, radiotherapy and chemotherapy (see Chapters 35 and 43).

Mumps

An acute fever with parotitis is the typical presentation, sometimes involving other organs, causing orchitis, oophoritis and pancreatitis. Following infection, the patient has long-term immunity.

Eye complications are uncommon but include dacryoadenitis, conjunctivitis, keratitis, iridocyclitis, scleritis, retinitis and optic neuritis. Treatment is supportive with analgesics and appropriate treatment of any eye complications.

Molluscum contagiosum

Molluscum contagiosum is caused by a DNA virus which usually infects children. Infection in adults, especially in Africa, may be a sentinel lesion for HIV infection. A small papule with a central umbilicus is typical. The lesion may be isolated or in clusters. Lesions on the eyelid may cause a follicular conjunctivitis or sometimes a keratitis. Curetting of the lesions, under local anaesthesia, with the application of chemical cautery using iodine or carbolic acid is usually successful.

HIV/AIDS and the eye

HIV infection is most often a sexually transmitted disease caused by the human immunodeficiency virus. It can also be transmitted by transfusion of infected blood and by contaminated needles.

HIV infection in industrialized countries occurs particularly in homosexual populations and among intravenous drug users. In Africa it is transmitted mainly by heterosexual activity. Seropositivity is significantly linked with a history of sexually transmitted disease, genital ulcer disease, contact with prostitutes and lack of male circumcision. Age-specific peaks of HIV infection are found among children under the age of 5 and among young adults.

Epidemiology of HIV/AIDS

HIV/AIDS emerged in the late 1970s and spread in America, Europe and Australia, mainly among homosexual and bisexual man and intravenous drug users. At the same time, an epidemic occurred in East and Central Africa and in the Caribbean, but in these regions the infections have been mainly among heterosexual men and women with multiple sexual partners. It is estimated that in 2006 there were approximately 40 million people living with HIV. Twenty-five million of them live in sub-Saharan Africa. Over four million new infections occurred in 2006, of which nearly 75% were in sub-Saharan Africa.

Modes of transmission

HIV has been isolated from most body fluids. Semen, vaginal secretions and blood are the most important in transmission of the disease.

HIV has also been found in the tears, conjunctiva, cornea, aqueous humour and the vascular endothelium of the retinal vessels. These findings may be important in relation to potential transmission of the infection, for example when examining patients with an applanation tonometer. However, there is no report of transmission occurring through tears. Isopropyl alcohol swabbing of the tonometer tip is an adequate means of sterilization. The possible transmission of HIV by corneal transplantation is an obvious concern.

Herpes zoster ophthalmicus

Herpes zoster ophthalmicus is a marker for HIV infection in Africa.[64] The course of this disease is more severe in HIV-positive patients, with more subjective discomfort. It also occurs in a younger age group. Intravenous or oral antiviral drugs, such as aciclovir, valciclovir and famciclovir, are the preferred treatments. Acute retinal necrosis may occur in association with herpes zoster, and in HIV/AIDS patients is typically florid, causing rapidly progressive outer retinal necrosis (PORN), with large areas of pale, necrotic retina and eventual retinal detachment. Treatment is with high doses of aciclovir or foscarnet intravenously, but the prognosis is very poor.

Molluscum contagiosum and papillomata

The eyelids may have multiple warts or the umbilicated papules of molluscum contagiosum, both suggestive of HIV/AIDS infection.

HIV-related retinopathy

The most common ocular manifestation of HIV-infected patients is abnormalities of the small vessels of the retina. These can be found in around one-third of AIDS patients, and are associated with a high viral load. These lesions consist of small nerve fibre layer infarcts ('cotton-wool' spots), microaneurysms and telangiectasia. HIV retinopathy does not cause visual loss.

AIDS and cytomegalovirus (CMV) retinitis

In HIV patients with severe immunosupression (CD4 count less than $50/mm^3$), reactivation of earlier infection with CMV may

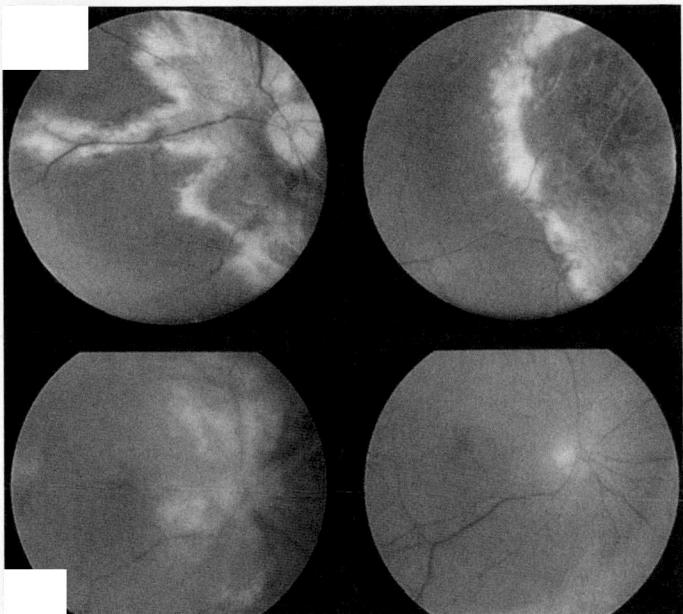

Figure 18.31 AIDS and cytomegalovirus (CMV) retinitis. (Courtesy of Philippe Kestelyn.)

cause gastrointestinal disease, pneumonitis, encephalitis and retinitis. CMV retinitis affects up to 30% of AIDS patients in the industrialized world, while in developing countries the prevalence seems to be much lower. AIDS patients in developing countries will often die from other diseases, such as tuberculosis, before they develop CMV retinitis.[65]

The classical appearance of CMV retinitis is that of a haemorrhagic retinal necrosis – sometimes described as tomato ketchup on cottage cheese, with extension of the lesions along the vascular arcades (Figure 18.31). There is surprisingly little vitritis or inflammation, as the patient is unable to mount an immune response. The disease is bilateral in about 50% of patients. It is slowly progressive, and, if no treatment is provided, the whole retina may be destroyed within 6 months.

The optimum treatment of CMV retinitis is daily intravenous ganciclovir or foscarnet. Ganciclovir suppresses the bone marrow, while foscarnet is nephrotoxic. An alternative drug to ganciclovir and foscarnet is cidofavir, which does have the advantage of once-weekly treatment, but causes severe uveitis. These drugs are very expensive and daily intravenous injections are inconvenient. An option is to use weekly intravitreal injections of 2 mg of ganciclovir. These stabilize the disease, and maintain the vision, provided central vision has not already been affected.[66]

The use of HAART (highly active antiretroviral therapy) leads to an improvement in the patient's immune system. Paradoxically, this can lead to a worsening of vision, as the cytomegalovirus provokes an immune response that may cause uveitis and macular oedema.

HIV/AIDS and syphilis

All patients with syphilis should be tested for HIV and vice versa. Ocular manifestations of syphilis and HIV-seropositive patients include uveitis, retinal vasculitis and optic nerve disease.

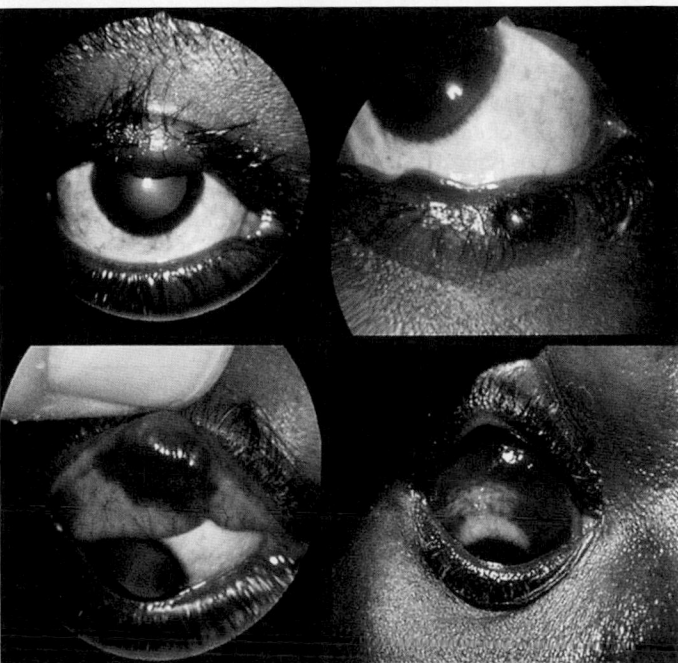

Figure 18.32 HIV/AIDS and tumours: Kaposi's sarcoma. (Courtesy of Philippe Kestelyn.)

The recommended treatment for ocular syphilis in HIV-seropositive patients is 12–24 million units of aqueous crystalline penicillin G intravenously per day for 10–14 days.

HIV/AIDS and tuberculosis

Because of the profound depression of cell-mediated immunity in HIV/AIDS patients, there is rapid dissemination of the infection to multiple organs (miliary disease). The alarming rise in the prevalence of tuberculosis parallels the spread of the HIV pandemic. In developing countries, 30–50% of adults have latent tuberculosis that may be reactivated in the presence of HIV infection. In patients with profound immunosupression, the presentation may be atypical, with extrapulmonary involvement and a negative tuberculin test. In patients with HIV/AIDS, massive choroidal invasion may lead to secondary retinal necrosis and blindness. Most patients die within a few months.

The treatment of tuberculosis is the same as in patients who are not HIV infected.

HIV/AIDS and tumours

Squamous cell caricinomas of the conjunctiva have been reported with greater frequency in HIV-infected individuals.

Kaposi's sarcoma is a malignant vascular tumour which occurs in 15–24% of patients with AIDS in the developing world. This tumour can present on the skin or mucous membranes. It may develop on the eyelid skin, on the eyelid margins, on the conjunctiva and, rarely, within the orbit. The clinical presentation of the tumour appears as a deep purple-red nodule (Figure 18.32). Typically, multifocal skin lesions appear which later ulcerate. They are usually slow-growing and rarely invasive. The tumours can be excised or given focal radiation therapy.

Squamous cell carcinomas have been reported with greater frequency in HIV-infected individuals. It may be that the oncogenic potential of the human papillomavirus acts as a co-factor.[67] The presence of a greyish-white keratinized mass surrounded by a blood supply of engorged conjunctival vessels, sometimes with pigmentation, is typical of the tumour. The tumour is often aggressive. Prompt and complete surgical excision is required. Topical treatment with mitomycin C or 5-fluorouracil may also be effective.[68]

CHLAMYDIAL AND RICKETTSIAL INFECTIONS AND THE EYE

Trachoma

Infection with *Chlamydia trachomatis* is described on pp. 291–294.

Lymphogranuloma venereum

Lymphogranuloma venereum is caused by an organism of the *Chlamydia* (or *Bedsonia*) group of infective agents. It is transmitted by sexual contact. The organism is widespread geographically.

The initial lesion, the primary sore, is usually in the genital region, and within days there follows a regional lymphadenitis, with fever, headache and malaise.

Eye complications

Eye changes include a follicular conjunctivitis with pre-auricular lymphadenopathy. These are the clinical features of Parinaud's oculoglandular syndrome. A keratitis may be associated with corneal infiltration and new vessel formation. Iridocyclitis has been described. Posterior eye changes include dilatation of the retinal veins, retinal haemorrhages and optic disc oedema.

Management

Tetracyclines are the drugs of choice. The treatment of lymphogranuloma venereum is described in Chapter 21.

Typhus

Typhus fever may be louse-borne, where the infecting organism is *Rickettsia prowazeki*, or tick-, mite- or flea-borne.

Eye complications

Eye complications associated with typhus fever include conjunctivitis, iridocyclitis, retinal haemorrhages and optic nerve oedema, which may lead to optic atrophy.

Management

See Chapter 49.

Rocky Mountain spotted fever

This rickettsial disease is caused by *R. rickettsii* and is found in the Western Hemisphere. The vector is the tick – carried by wild rodents and dogs.

A conjunctivitis with photosensitivity and petechial haemorrhages of the bulbar and tarsal conjunctivae are described.

Treatment is with doxycycline.

Cat-scratch disease

This is caused by the rickettsial organisms of the genus *Bartonella*. Patients develop a regional lymphadenopathy.

Eye complications

Uveitis has been reported. *Bartonella* is a well-recognized cause of neuroretinitis, in which the optic disc is swollen, and macular oedema leads to the deposition of exudates in a characteristic star-shaped pattern.

Bartonella is sensitive to tetracyclines and to macrolides such as erythromycin and azithromycin.

SYSTEMIC BACTERIAL INFECTIONS AND THE EYE

Leprosy and the eye

Epidemiology

At the beginning of 2000, 640 000 leprosy patients were being treated for active disease with multi-drug therapy (MDT) worldwide. Around 680 000 newly detected patients were registered in 1999. More than 10 million previous leprosy patients had been released from treatment (RFT). It is estimated that around 100 000 leprosy patients are blind due to the disease. However many thousands more are blind due to non-leprosy-associated eye disease.

Clinical presentation

Leprosy is a chronic bacterial disease caused by *Mycobacterium leprae*, which is an acid-fast bacillus of low-grade infectivity, and a preference for cooler temperatures. Thus, the slightly cooler anterior segment of the eye is particularly affected.

The clinical picture of leprosy is determined by the immune response of the individual.

If the cellular immune response is strong, the corresponding bacterial count will be low, and so-called paucibacillary (PB) leprosy will develop.

If the cellular immune response is weak, the corresponding bacterial count will be high, and so-called multibacillary (MB) leprosy will develop (more than five skin lesions).

MB leprosy patients may spread the disease. PB leprosy patients do not spread the disease.

The type of leprosy is important for both the treatment regimens and the type of systemic complications which may occur.

Two mechanisms are responsible for nerve damage and various disabilities in leprosy. These are described as type I and type II reactions.

Type I reaction (reversal reaction)

A type I reaction occurs as a result of a sudden increase in cellular immunity (paucibacillary leprosy patients) (Table 18.16).

Table 18.16 Eye complications in leprosy, related to classification*

Cause of complications	Complications	Paucibacillary	Multibacillary
Type I reaction	Lagophthalmos	+	+
	Corneal hypoaesthesia	+	+
Type II reaction	Acute iritis	−	+
	Scleritis	−	+
	Chronic iritis	−	+
Bacilli in high numbers	Madarosis	−	+
	Blepharochalasis	−	+
	Blocked lacrimal sac	−	+
	Limbal leproma	−	+
	Leprous keratitis	−	+
	Iris pearls	−	+
	Neuroparalytic iritis	−	+
	Iris atrophy	−	+

*Exceptions may occur due to variations in the grading of patients.

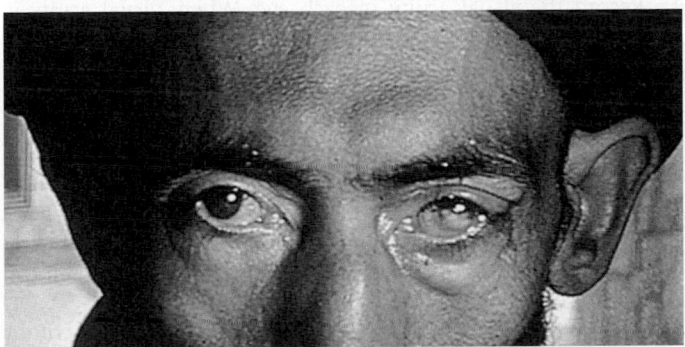

Figure 18.33 Bilateral facial paralysis due to leprosy. Temporal tarsorrhaphies have been carried out, but the left eye has severe corneal ulceration. (Courtesy of John D. C. Anderson.)

Acute inflammation in the skin lesions and the peripheral nerves can cause both motor and sensory deficits. Involvement of the 5th and 7th cranial nerves leads to corneal hypoaesthesia (5th nerve) and lagophthalmos (7th nerve). The facial skin patch may be red and raised (in reaction) – or hypopigmented.

Damage to the 7th cranial nerve leads to paresis of the orbicularis oculi and lagophthalmos. The patient is unable to close the eyes. This can be detected with both gentle and attempted forced closure of the lids. Lagophthalmos is a common eye complication of leprosy and may be associated with all forms of the disease (Figure 18.33). However, lagophthalmos and corneal hypoaesthesia are the expected complications found in association with a type I reaction.

Involvement of the 5th cranial nerve causes corneal hypoaesthesia which may occur in association with lagophthalmos. The combination of inadequate lid closure and corneal insensitivity poses a grave risk to the eye through exposure and the effects of minor trauma.

The management of eye complications associated with a type I reaction is recorded in Table 18.17.

Table 18.17 Treatment of lagophthalmos

Duration	Treatment
<6 months	Prednisolone (30 mg/day), decreasing over 6 months
	Blinking exercises
	Protective spectacles
>6 months No exposure keratitis Normal corneal sensation With exposure keratitis/ectropion and/or corneal sensation reduced	Eye health education
	Protective spectacles and other protective measures
	'Think-blink habit'
	Permanent tarsorrhaphy
	Ectropion surgical correction

Type II reaction (erythema nodosum leprosum: ENL)

ENL reactions occur only in multibacillary leprosy patients and are caused by antigen–antibody interaction leading to immune complex deposition.[24]

The typical clinical presentation is fever, subcutaneous nodules, swelling of nerves and inflammatory foci. A type II reaction affecting the eye can cause acute iridocyclitis, episcleritis and scleritis. Massive infiltration with *M. leprae* can cause secondary atrophy of the involved tissues, leading to madarosis, collapse of the nose and thin earlobes.

Eye complications associated with a type II reaction

- Acute iridocyclitis – Treatment of acute iridocyclitis is the same regardless of the cause. Atropine sulphate 1% eye drops and corticosteroid eye drops should be given. Systemic corticosteroids are not required.
- Episcleritis and scleritis – An episcleritis will respond quickly to topical corticosteroids. The deeper inflammation of scleritis, particularly severe bilateral scleritis, is a well-recognized complication of severe type II reactions. Topical treatment should be given as described above, with atropine sulphate 1% and

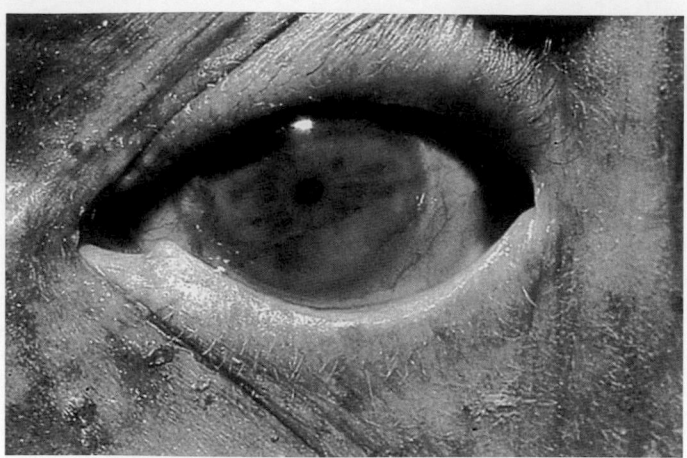

Figure 18.34 Chronic iridocyclitis in leprosy. (Courtesy of Hans Limburg.)

corticosteroids, but short courses of systemic corticosteroids – together with clofazimine – will be required. There is a risk of scleral staphyloma (bulging of the inflamed sclera with adherent choroid and ciliary body), associated with scleral thinning.

- Chronic iridocyclitis – This chronic inflammation presents with slight haziness in the anterior chamber due to cells and protein in the aqueous fluid (Figure 18.34). Although posterior synechiae are uncommon, the pupils may become small (miosis) and fixed. Keratic precipitates (foci of cells adherent to the back of the cornea) may be found on the corneal endothelium. When treating chronic iridocyclitis, keep the pupil as dilated and active as possible, using phenylephrine 2.5–5% eye drops.

There are other features which do not affect vision but can confirm the diagnosis of leprosy with eye complications.

- Madarosis – There is loss of the eyebrows which may be associated with loss of eyelashes. A hair-bearing skin graft may be used to provide a 'new' eyebrow. Alternatively, a dark pencil may be used.
- Blepharochalasis – Excessive folds of the skin of the upper eyelid can occur after swelling due to inflammation has resolved. The treatment is surgical.
- Lacrimal duct obstruction – This results in excessive watering of the affected eye (epiphora) and may occur following inflammation of the nasal mucosa and sometimes collapse of the nasal cartilage. Surgery to bypass the obstruction (dacrocysto-rhinostomy) may be indicated.
- Limbal leproma – A painless pinkish or yellowish nodule may present at the corneoscleral margin (limbus). This should resolve slowly with supervised multiple drug treatment.
- Leprous keratitis – Chalky corneal deposits may occur, often in both eyes at the upper temporal quadrant of the cornea. These usually do not affect visual acuity and are evidence of corneal invasion by *M. leprae.*
- Iris atrophy – In long-standing multibacillary leprosy, the iris stroma and pupil dilator muscle may become thin and atrophic, leading to a fixed miotic pupil. Irregular atrophy of the iris may result in pupil distortion.
- Iris pearls – Small white nodules may appear on the surface of the iris. These are pathognomonic for leprosy and are formed by calcified foci of dead leprosy bacilli.

Age-related cataract in leprosy patients

Management of cataract in leprosy patients can be complicated by intraocular inflammation and small rigid pupils. Surgery should be delayed until the patient has had 6 months of systemic anti-leprosy treatment, without any recognized reaction. Intraocular lenses may be used provided there is no active inflammation.

Raised intraocular pressure may occur in association with iridocyclitis. However, the intraocular pressure is often slightly lower than average (ocular hypotension) owing to atrophy of the ciliary body.

Summary: examination of the eyes in leprosy and eye health education

In examining the patient with leprosy, take particular note of the following:[69]
- Visual acuity of each eye
- Lagophthalmos and corneal sensation
- Red eye
- Facial skin patch
- Cataract.
1. Record the visual acuity in each eye. Where visual acuity is reduced below 6/12 in either eye, refer to the eye specialist.
2. Note if the patient blinks regularly. Ask the patient to close the eyes gently. If necessary, ask the patient to close the eyelids forcibly. If there is evidence of a lid-gap >5 mm, the patient should be referred for surgery.
3. The patient with lagophthalmos or corneal hypoaesthesia should be taught to think-blink – many times each day. This patient requires referral to the eye surgeon.
4. Note any redness of either eye. Any patient who has a red eye should be referred to the eye specialist.
5. Test the corneal sensation with a fine tip of 'rolled' cotton wool.
6. Examine, with magnification, the anterior chamber for evidence of iridocyclitis.
7. Note any evidence of cataract.
8. Dilate the pupil with cyclopentolate 1% eye drops. Posterior synechiae or a miotic pupil suggests current or previous iridocyclitis.
9. Confirm that each patient is on the correct systemic treatment for their leprosy.

The success of leprosy control has resulted in the closure of some specialized leprosy programmes and leprosy workers moving to other employment. In India, Tamil Nadu was the first state to integrate leprosy control fully into the general health services. Other states and countries are following this example. This poses a risk that new cases will be missed and disabilities in leprosy patients will not receive adequate care. This means that the guidelines and responsibilities of general health workers must be clarified and appropriate training provided.

Close collaboration between former leprosy control and prevention of blindness programmes will be required, at national, regional and local levels.

Tuberculosis

Tuberculosis is widespread and the prevalence is increasing. The WHO estimates that there are over 7 million new cases each year, with nearly 3 million deaths. In countries where HIV/AIDS is endemic, tuberculosis is spreading rapidly.

Eye complications

The disease may affect all systems of the body, including the eyes. Infection of the skin (lupus vulgaris) can result in eyelid scarring and secondary corneal involvement due to exposure. Phlyctenular keratoconjunctivitis is due to a hypersensitivity reaction to the tuberculoprotein, presenting as small yellow/pink nodules, often on the corneoscleral margin. This nodule is a microabscess, and any patient presenting with this allergic response should be examined for tuberculosis. Scleritis may be either anterior or posterior. Posterior scleritis may be associated with marked thickening of the sclera due to granuloma formation.

A granulomatous anterior uveitis (iridocyclitis) with large keratic precipitates (described as 'mutton fat') may occur. Examination with magnification may reveal small white nodules at the pupil margin (Koeppe nodules). Miliary choroidal tubercles can be present as part of widespread disease. Both optic neuritis and optic atrophy are described.

Management

The systemic treatment of tuberculosis with isoniazid, together with rifampicin or ethambutol and other medications, in a variety of regimens, is described in Chapter 56.

A phlycten responds quickly to topical corticosteroid therapy.

Retinal vasculitis

In developing countries, retinal vasculitis is often associated with systemic tuberculosis. However, association with other systemic diseases (e.g. sarcoidosis, Behçet's disease, systemic lupus erythematosus and multiple sclerosis) is well recognized. The vascular disturbance may vary from mild vascular sheathing in the retinal periphery, to new vessel formation, traction retinal detachment and bilateral vitreous haemorrhages. Eales' disease is a form of retinal vasculitis affecting mostly the retinal veins, and occurring in young men. It is particularly common in South Asia. Other causes of retinal neovascularization and vitreous haemorrhage must be excluded.

Brucellosis (undulant fever; Mediterranean fever)

Brucellosis is caused by infection with organisms which are Gram-negative bacilli: *Brucella abortus*, *B. melitensis* or *B. suis*. The disease is widespread throughout the world.

Eye complications

These include a chronic granulomatous uveitis which may involve the posterior segment. Keratitis may occur with epithelial opacities. An optic neuritis is rare. Extraocular muscle abnormalities can appear, as a result of either local inflammation or 6th cranial nerve paralysis due to a basal meningoencephalitis.

Management

Treatment of the eye disease is that given for an anterior uveitis, with topical mydriasis/cycloplegia, using eye drops such as atropine sulphate 1%, and topical corticosteroids.

Treatment of the systemic disease is described in Chapter 59.

Tularaemia

Tularaemia is caused by a small Gram-negative bacillus, *Francisella tularensis* (*Pasteurella tularensis*). The human infection is found in Europe, Japan and North America.

The systemic disease and its transmission from animals such as rabbits and other rodents are described in Chapter 62.

Eye complications

Ocular infection with tularaemia causes a severe conjunctivitis. After an incubation period of up to 2 weeks, the eye becomes itchy and photosensitive. The conjunctiva is red and oedematous, with granulomas, and the regional lymph nodes become enlarged. This clinical picture is known as Parinaud's oculoglandular syndrome.

Treatment

Details of systemic treatment are given in Chapter 65.

Meningococcal meningitis

Epidemics of meningococcal meningitis (cerebrospinal meningitis) occur in tropical countries, although the disease is found worldwide. The organism is the Gram-negative *N. meningitidis*, which typically is seen on microscopy as pairs of cocci or as a single coccus.

Eye complications

Extraocular muscle imbalance can occur due to involvement of the cranial nerves, in particular, the 6th nerve, although a partial 3rd nerve paralysis is not uncommon. Encephalitis with optic neuritis may result in post-neuritic atrophy.

Conjunctivitis and anterior uveitis can occur due to meningococcaemia. Petechial haemorrhages may be visible in the conjunctiva and are a valuable aid to diagnosis.

The pupils react in a variety of ways according to the particular site of inflammation intracranially. In the early stages there may be miosis, but mydriasis will occur with the onset of coma.

Involvement of the visual cortex can result in loss of vision with entirely normal ocular features and reactions.

Management

The treatment of the systemic disease with penicillin or chloramphenicol is described in Chapter 55.

Local inflammation involving the eye or eyes should be treated appropriately.

Diphtheria

Diphtheria is caused by infection with a Gram-positive bacillus, *Corynebacterium diphtheriae*.

The disease is a public health problem in some developing countries, for example Sudan and India. Due to immunization, there has been a worldwide reduction in incidence.

Eye complications

Infection of the conjunctiva causes a membranous conjunctivitis with eyelid oedema, discharge and local lymph node enlargement. Corneal ulceration can occur. The classical sign of infection with the bacillus is a grey membrane which forms where infection has occurred. On removal of the membrane, the surface uncovered is raw with petechial haemorrhages.

The exotoxins formed by the organisms are particularly damaging to the heart, kidneys and central nervous system. Cranial nerve paralysis can occur, affecting the extraocular muscles, particularly the 6th cranial nerve, but with the 4th and 3rd nerves sometimes also affected.

Membranous conjunctivitis may be caused by other infections, such as *Streptococcus*, *Pneumococcus* or adenovirus.

Management

Diphtheria antitoxin should be given as well as antibiotics. Treatment of the disease is given in Chapter 67.

Anthrax

Cutaneous anthrax can involve the eyelids and periorbital regions. Infection is by direct contact with contaminated skins and other animal products, most often among those who work with live or dead animals. The organism may also be transmitted by insects. A red papule forms at the site of inoculation with the organism, *Bacillus anthracis*. The area becomes black (eschar) and gangrenous. The woman from Central Asia shown in Figure 18.35 said

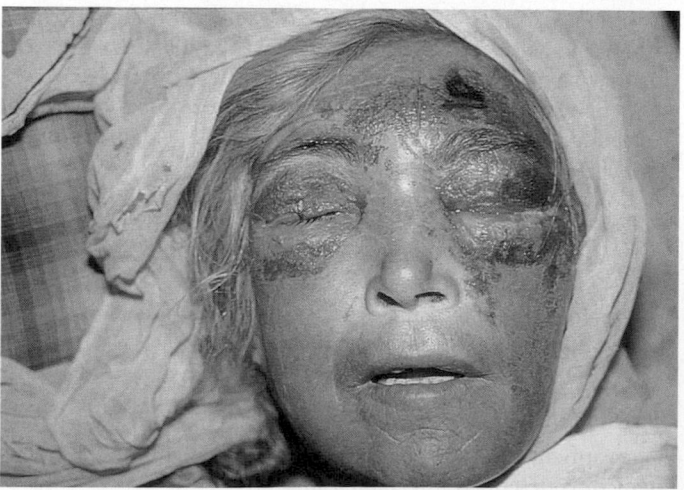

Figure 18.35 Anthrax in Central Asia. Notice the black eschar on the forehead. (Courtesy of Murray McGavin.)

that an insect had bitten her forehead, and a dark eschar can be seen at the site. Typically, the patient is very ill.

Eye complications

Eschar formation affecting the eyelids can progress to severe scarring, resulting in dramatic cicatricial ectropion – the eyelid can turn inside out. Exposure keratitis may cause corneal scarring and blindness.[70]

Management

Systemic treatment with the penicillins is described in Chapter 63.

Correction of the ectropion requires division of the scar tissue, and a full-thickness skin graft – to allow the eyelid to resume its original position.

Cholera

Cholera is a gastrointestinal disease caused by the bacillus *Vibrio cholerae*. The disease is widespread in tropical countries. Profuse watery diarrhoea and vomiting result in acute dehydration. The disease is described in Chapters 10 and 51.

Eye complications

The severely dehydrated patient will present with 'sunken' eyes. In a severely ill patient the eyelids may be left open, leading to exposure keratoconjunctivitis and corneal ulceration. There may be an increased risk of cataract due to acute systemic dehydration, and acute onset of cataract, which has been described during cholera epidemics in India.

Management

Treatment details are given in Chapters 10 and 51.

Typhoid fever

Infection with *Salmonella typhi* causes fever, abdominal pain and prostration. The bacilli may be harboured by a carrier of the infection, and the organism is also found in water, milk, ice-cream and other foodstuffs.

Eye complications

Rose spots may be found on the conjunctiva of patients with typhoid. They are found in association with similar rose spots on the trunk and limbs. During epidemics, cataract may form, possibly related in part to associated dehydration. Involvement of the nervous system may result in a variety of complications, including extraocular muscle involvement and pupillary abnormalities.

Management

For a full description of treatment options in typhoid fever, see Chapter 52.

SPIROCHAETAL DISEASES AND THE EYE

Syphilis

Syphilis is caused by the spirochaete *Treponema pallidum*, which may be transmitted by venereal contact or across the placenta to the unborn child. An annual incidence of 12 million with a world-wide prevalence of 28 million is reported by the WHO.

Congenital syphilis

The ocular manifestations of congenital syphilis include inflamed eyelids, dacryocystitis, conjunctivitis, extraocular muscle paresis, interstitial keratitis, iridocyclitis, pupil abnormalities (an Argyll Robertson pupil may be seen occasionally), chorioretinitis with the classical appearance of pigment granules and yellow/red spots (the 'salt and pepper' fundus), and optic neuritis and optic atrophy. Typically, congenital syphilis becomes latent and then reactivates, often during the teenage years, and may reappear as an interstitial keratitis. The patient complains of severe discomfort with photosensitivity and a red eye. The affected area of the cornea may attract new blood vessels and the oedematous and inflamed area appears pink, which has been described as a 'salmon patch'. The keratitis can lead to corneal scarring. The empty blood vessels in the cornea are described as 'ghost vessels'. Associated inflammation can include an iridocyclitis.

Adult acquired syphilis

Eye changes are associated with the secondary stage of syphilis, and can include iridocyclitis, retinal vasculitis and optic neuritis. Inflammation of the iris (iritis) may be obviously hyperaemic (roseolae). Tertiary syphilis may ensue after a variable period of time and can have similar clinical features. Also, the classical Argyll Robertson pupil may occur, with small irregular pupils which do not react to either direct or consensual light stimulation but will constrict on accommodation. Optic atrophy may be found.

Management

Treatment of the inflammatory disease of the anterior eye will require mydriasis and cycloplegia using eye drops such as atropine sulphate 1%, together with topical corticosteroids.

A description of the general treatment of syphilis, using penicillin, is given in Chapter 21.

Leptospirosis

Leptospirosis is caused by spirochaetes of the genus *Leptospira*. Man is infected by contact with a variety of domestic and wild animals, mostly due to contact with urine-contaminated water and soil. After an incubation period of 8–12 days, the patient develops fever and chills with general malaise and photosensitivity.

Eye complications

The conjunctival vessels may be dilated and there may be subconjunctival haemorrhages. An iridocyclitis can occur, although the onset of the intraocular inflammation may be weeks or some months after the initial infective phase has passed.

See Chapter 70 for details of appropriate treatment. Antibiotics in high doses are indicated.

Relapsing fever

Relapsing fever is caused by the spirochaetes *Borrelia recurrentis* and *Borrelia duttonii*, which may be louse-borne or tick-borne, respectively. The patient has a recurring fever with severe headache, photosensitivity, muscle and joint pains, upper respiratory tract inflammation, nausea and vomiting. A rash is common.

Eye complications

Eye complications of louse-borne relapsing fever include anterior uveitis, which may be acute or chronic in character. Haemorrhages and exudates of the retina have been described. A meningitis may result in ptosis and extraocular muscle abnormalities due to cranial nerve paralysis.

Management

A full description of the systemic disease, diagnostic tests and treatment is given in Chapter 69.

Lyme disease

This infection is caused by *Borrelia burgdorferi*, and is spread by the bite of an infected tick. The best-known systemic manifestation is erythema migrans; however, the infection can cause arthritis, neurological and cardiac problems as well as skin lesions.

Eye complications

Uveitis, optic neuritis, and cranial nerve palsies have all been described.

Yaws

Yaws is caused by the spirochaete *Treponema pertenue*, which is found in many geographical locations, including Asia, Africa, South America and the Caribbean. An ulcerating papilloma forms the primary lesion.

During later stages, the characteristic lesion is an ulcerating granuloma (gumma) which heals with scarring. This lesion can destroy tissue around the nose or orbit.

Eye complications

Periorbital gumma may cause severe scarring and deformity of the eyelids, with cicatricial ectropion, and possibly exposure.

FUNGAL INFECTIONS AND THE EYE

Over 100 fungal species, whether filamentous fungi, yeasts or dimorphic organisms, have been associated with eye infections. Difficulties in management of the oculomycoses relate to problems in diagnosis and inadequate antifungal agents. Suppurative keratitis may be due to bacteria or fungi but this cannot be firmly decided on clinical grounds alone. Gram staining is the simplest method of distinguishing bacterial and fungal infection.

Fungi causing eye infections are most commonly filamentous fungi and yeasts.

Filamentous fungi are multicellular organisms with projections known as hyphae. Hyphae may have divisions or be non-septate. Septate filamentous fungi include the most common causes of fungal eye infections: *Fusarium* and *Aspergillus*. Non-septate filamentous fungi, for example *Rhizopus* and *Phycomycetes*, less commonly involve the eye.

Candida albicans and *Cryptococcus neoformans* are species of yeasts that may be involved in eye infections. They are unicellular organisms that reproduce by budding.

Dimorphic fungi such as *Blastomyces dermatitidis* may be responsible for ocular and orbital disease following blood and lymphatic spread.

Oculomycoses are found worldwide but particularly in hot and humid climates. The geographical pattern of these infections is gradually emerging as the literature on mycotic infections of the eye increases. In some parts of the tropics, between a third and a half of adult corneal ulcers are caused by fungi.[71]

The most significant anatomical site of fungal eye infections is the cornea, where suppurative keratitis, ulceration, hypopyon formation and possible corneal perforation mean that early diagnosis and prompt treatment are vital.

A fungal corneal ulcer is suggested by a raised slough, with serrated margins, and a coloured infiltrate, particularly if the ulcer fails to respond to antibiotic treatment.[62] However, these signs are not consistently present.

Fungi are associated with vegetable matter, so abrasions of the cornea with twigs, thorns and husks must raise suspicion of a possible fungal infection.

Fungi may also involve the lacrimal canaliculi.

Aspergillosis

The genus *Aspergillus* contains over 300 identified species and is common in warm and humid climates. The nose and paranasal sinuses are often infected, which can lead on to ocular involvement with extraocular muscle palsies. Intracerebral abscess formation can cause eye complications due to a space-occupying lesion.

Fusariosis

Fusarium spp. may cause a suppurative keratitis. As with any suppurative keratitis, corneal scarring is likely when the area of infection and inflammation heals. At a later time, corneal grafting may be indicated.

Candidiasis (moniliasis)

Candida albicans is an organism commonly found in the mouth, throat and vulva.

The fungus may affect the eyelids, lacrimal system, conjunctiva and cornea. Often, infection will follow injury to the eye, whether accidental or (sometimes) surgical. *Candida* endophthalmitis is

associated with intravenous drug abuse or long-term intravenous catheters. There are characteristic spherical 'puff balls' in the vitreous. A vitrectomy is required to clear the visual axis and to provide specimens for diagnosis.

Cryptococcosis

Cryptococcus neoformans is a yeast-like fungus which may have systemic effects involving the skin, lungs and meninges. It may cause a suppurative keratitis. Endogenous spread through the bloodstream results in infective uveitis. Infection of the meninges may cause raised intracranial pressure with papilloedema and subsequent optic atrophy. Cranial nerve abnormalities also occur.

Blastomycosis

Blastomyces dermatitidis is found in the Americas and Africa and affects the skin, lungs and various other organs. The infection is characterized by suppurative granulomas which may be found in the mouth, nose and also sometimes involving the eyelids. The orbit, lacrimal canaliculi, conjunctiva and cornea may be affected.

Coccidioidomycosis

Infection with *Coccidioides immitis* usually begins with inhalation of the organism, causing a pneumonitis. The disease may also involve skin, subcutaneous tissues, bone and meninges. Eye involvement can include a hypersensitivity response, manifest as a phlyctenular conjunctivitis. The eyelids may be affected, and intraocular involvement has been recorded, causing a posterior uveitis.

Histoplasmosis

Infection by the fungus *Histoplasma capsulatum* is widespread. The organism is found in the soil and is inhaled. The eye changes associated with this infection are described as 'presumed ocular histoplasmosis syndrome' (POHS), and based on evidence of infection elsewhere, but no organism has been isolated from the eye. It is presumed that histoplasmosis has a predilection for the posterior uvea and the characteristic lesions are multifocal areas of choroidal atrophy. If one of these lesions is close to the fovea, it may be associated with a choroidal neovascular membrane, which often leads to subretinal scarring and loss of central vision. The membrane can be treated with photodynamic therapy, intravitreal injections of VEGF antagonists, or it may be surgically removed.

Treatment of fungal infections

If possible, immediate empirical antifungal treatment should be avoided until a Gram stain of a corneal scrape is available. If fungal keratitis is suspected when there has been no response to antibiotics after 48 hours, an antifungal agent should be used.

Natamycin 5% eye drops are most effective against filamentous fungi, including *Aspergillus* and *Fusarium*.[72] Dosage is one drop half-hourly, then six to eight times per day after 3–4 days.

Amphotericin B is most effective against yeasts, particularly *Candida* and *Cryptococcus*. It may be given intravenously and topically.

Flucytosine 1% is effective against yeasts, including *Candida* and *Cryptococcus*, although some strains are resistant. It must therefore be given with an imidazole. It may be given in oral form and topically.

The imidazoles have a broad spectrum of antifungal activity. All are used topically. Clotrimazole 1%, miconazole 1%, ketoconazole 2% and econazole 1% have all been used in treatment of fungal keratitis.

Antifungal treatment has to be continued for at least 3 weeks, and about two-thirds of fungal ulcers will heal within 1 month. Bacterial ulcers respond more rapidly.

Systemic antifungal treatment will be necessary in endogenous infections, such as with *Candida*, where flucytosine orally 200 mg/kg per day or ketoconazole orally 200 mg once per day for 2 weeks may be given. Alternatively, amphotericin B can be administered intravenously over several days.

DISEASES CAUSED BY PROTOZOA

Toxoplasmosis

Toxoplasmosis is caused by *Toxoplasma gondii*. The distribution of toxoplasmosis is worldwide, although there is some geographical variation related to the dietary habits of populations, particularly consumption of undercooked or raw meat, and the presence of cats, which are recognized hosts of the organism.

Eye complications

Retinochoroiditis is the common ocular manifestation of the disease. It is most often seen while quiescent, as a pigmented scar affecting the posterior segment of the eye (Figure 18.36).

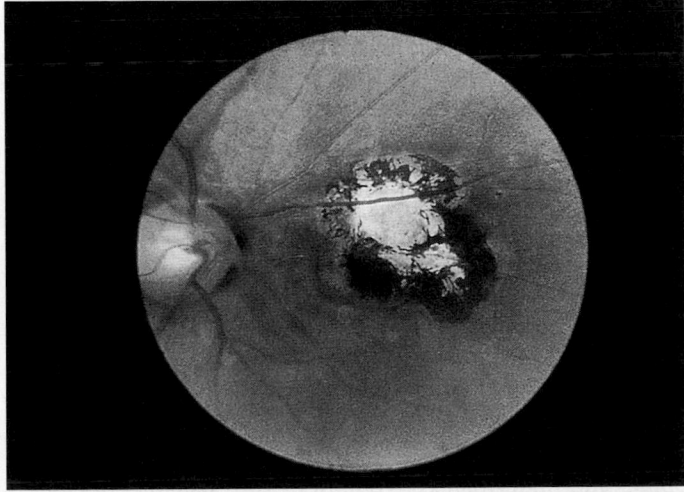

Figure 18.36 Old toxoplasmic retinochoroidal atrophy. (Courtesy of Gordon Johnson.)

If the scar involves the macula, the patient may complain of poor vision. However, the typical scarring is also found during routine eye examinations in asymptomatic teenage or adult patients.

The acute infection is characterized by focal, necrotizing retinitis, often arising at the border of a previously healed scar. The patient may complain of blurred vision, and floaters. In the acute phase, the foci of inflammation are 'fluffy' white with hazy margins. The vitreous is hazy due to vitritis, and there is an anterior uveitis. Cystoid macular oedema can develop. In patients with HIV/AIDS, the disease is multifocal and more aggressive.

Treatment

Anterior uveitis may be treated with mydriatics and topical steroids. Because of potential bone marrow toxicity, systemic treatment should only be given if the infection is close to the macula or optic nerve, and there is a reasonable prospect of preserving vision. A full description of systemic treatment is given in Chapter 78.

Leishmaniasis

Leishmaniasis is a protozoan disease caused by parasites of the genus *Leishmania*. The insect vector which transmits the parasite is the sandfly. It is found in many developing countries, with up to 2.5 million cases of 'visceral' disease and 9.5 million of the cutaneous form estimated.

Eye complications (visceral leishmaniasis)

The visceral form of leishmaniasis is known as kala-azar and eye disease is uncommon with this condition. Retinal haemorrhages have been described, typically bilateral and multiple in distribution. Iridocyclitis has been reported, with occasional descriptions of keratitis.

Eye complications (cutaneous leishmaniasis)

Cutaneous leishmaniasis has been described as tropical sore (oriental sore), mucocutaneous leishmaniasis (espundia) and disseminated anergic cutaneous leishmaniasis.

Eye changes commonly affect the eyelids, with occasional involvement of the lacrimal ducts or conjunctiva. The cutaneous lesion has a variety of appearances, with ulcer formation after the initial appearance of nodules or papules, often situated on the face, sometimes affecting the eyelids. Skin involvement leaves a characteristic scar.

Treatment

Details of treatment regimens are given in Chapter 77.

Amoebiasis

Amoebiasis is an intestinal protozoal disease due to the organism *Entamoeba histolytica*.

The disease is found worldwide, with possibly 500 million infected and an incidence of 48 million new cases each year. It is found in deprived communities, being associated with poverty and inadequate sanitation. It is a major health problem in parts of Africa, Asia and Latin America, where highly virulent strains may exist. Around 70 000 deaths probably occur each year.

Eye complications

In many populations where infection with *Entamoeba histolytica* is endemic, or even epidemic, it is difficult to determine whether eye changes are specifically associated with the systemic infection. A relatively uncommon but well-recognized complication of amoebiasis is a cerebral focus of infection, and reports of improvement in eye lesions, for example keratitis, associated with systemic treatment of amoebiasis do suggest an occasional association. Cysts close to the macula with associated small retinal haemorrhages and disturbance of the retinal pigment epithelium have been described.

Management

A description of systemic treatment is given in Chapter 79.

African trypanosomiasis

Trypanosomiasis in Africa is caused by *Trypanosoma brucei gambiense* and *T. b. rhodesiense*, which are transmitted by the tsetse fly of the genus *Glossina*.

The disease, commonly known as 'sleeping sickness', is found in Africa, between latitudes 15°N and 15°S. It is estimated that 400 000 people have active disease.

Eye complications

A variety of clinical eye abnormalities have been reported. Eyelid oedema with conjunctival redness and photosensitivity may occur. Interstitial keratitis and iridocyclitis are reported. In the severe form of the disease, with the onset of meningoencephalopathy, there may be widespread neurological changes, ptosis, extraocular muscle involvement, optic neuritis and papilloedema.

Management

A description of the treatment of African trypanosomiasis is given in Chapter 75.

American trypanosomiasis

Also known as Chagas' disease, American trypanosomiasis is caused by a protozoan parasite, *T. cruzi*.

The disease is found in Central and South America, extending from Mexico to Argentina.

Eye complications

Characteristic evidence of Chagas' disease is unilateral oedema of the eyelids (Romana's sign), which typically occurs when the inoculation site is close to the eye. The lacrimal gland can be involved in the inflammation.

Management

Please see Chapter 76 for details.

Malaria

Malaria is caused by infection with one of the four *Plasmodium* spp. – *P. falciparum. P. vivax, P. ovale* and *P. malariae*. Most eye complications are associated with *P. falciparum*, which causes the most severe disease.

Eye complications

Retinal signs are particularly common in cerebral malaria, where they are of diagnostic importance.[73] The retinal signs reflect the changes taking place in the cerebral circulation. The retinal findings include haemorrhages, oedema and papilloedema. White centred retinal haemorrhages may be associated with higher mortality.

In severe cerebral malaria there may be extraocular muscle pareses, optic neuritis and cortical blindness due to brain damage.

A rare complication associated with the treatment of malaria is chloroquine retinopathy. Chloroquine can damage the central retina, disturbing the retinal pigment epithelium around the macula and producing a 'bull's eye' maculopathy. The disturbed retinal pigment epithelium forms a ring or oval which provides the reason for the descriptive term. Chloroquine may be given at a dose of 6.5 mg/kg/day for some years with negligible risk of toxicity.

Management

The treatment of malaria is described in Chapter 73.

Pneumocystosis

Pneumocystis causes pneumonia in immunosuppressed individuals, particularly in HIV/AIDS.

Eye complications

Pneumocystis choroiditis is characterized by pale subretinal infiltrates that may be associated with exudative retinal detachments. These appearances are non-specific, and the diagnosis may be made postmortem. The condition responds to treatment with co-trimoxazole or atovaquone.

DISEASES CAUSED BY NEMATODES

Onchocerciasis

Onchocerciasis and its effects are discussed elsewhere in this chapter.

Toxocariasis

Toxocariasis is caused by *Toxocara canis*; it results from contact with the host, especially puppies. Toxocariasis is found in both developing and industrialized countries. The systemic disease is described as visceral larva migrans, which is further discussed in Chapter 85.

Eye complications

Ocular toxocariasis may present as a squint or a white pupil (leucocoria). The typical abnormality is an isolated granuloma at the posterior pole, although the lesion may occur peripherally and more than one focus may be evident. Granulomatous inflammation may lead to other clinical features, including severe uveitis, chronic endophthalmitis, detached retina and optic neuritis. In the 'quiet state' the retina and choroid may show atrophic scarring.

It is important to differentiate ocular toxocariasis from the malignant intraocular tumour of childhood, retinoblastoma. Both these conditions may present with leucocoria.

Management

Most eye lesions are quiescent and no therapy is indicated. Inflammation should be treated appropriately. If severe uveitis is present, systemic or periocular corticosteroids may also be required. Intraocular inflammation can result in endophthalmitis, membrane formation and traction retinal detachment. Expert surgical intervention can involve vitrectomy, division of membranes and retinal detachment surgery.

Treatment details are also described in Chapter 85.

Loiasis

Loiasis is found in West and Central Africa and is caused by the filarial helminth *Loa loa*. The insect vector of the worm is the fly of the genus *Chrysops*.

Eye complications

The most typical ophthalmic presentation of loiasis is a subconjunctival worm. There may be conjunctival redness and some discomfort. The more dramatic presentation shows considerable swelling due to oedema of the eyelids (Calabar swelling), caused by the presence of the worm subcutaneously. Usually this swelling will settle in a few days.

Other eye features described include worms in the anterior chamber, uveitis and retinopathy. Loiasis complicates the treatment of onchocerciasis, as treatment of a mixed infection with ivermectin can be associated with severe neurological adverse effects.

Management

The regimen of treatment is described in Chapter 74.

The removal of a subconjunctival worm requires topical anaesthesia. A suture is passed under the worm and tied tightly and the worm is dissected out. Alternatively, cryotherapy may immobilize the worm before surgical removal. The worms can move with surprising agility!

Thelaziasis

The oriental eye worm, *Thelazia callipaeda*, has principally been reported in patients from Japan and other countries in the Far East.

Eye complications

Typically, the patient complains of irritation and watering with a congested eye, often associated with pain. The worm may be seen within the conjunctival sac.

Management

Any worm present on the surface of the eye can be removed after the application of a local anaesthetic.

Bancroftian and Brugian filariasis

Filariasis caused by *Wuchereria bancrofti* has a widespread distribution in Africa, Asia and Latin America, with 119 million infected (WHO). *Brugia malayi* occurs principally in South-East Asia, while *Brugia timori* is found in Indonesia. These lymphatic filariases have a wide variety of clinical presentations. Transmission is by mosquitoes.

Eye complications

Adult worms have been isolated in the conjunctiva, with associated pain and redness. A subretinal adult worm has been found and larvae can infiltrate the anterior chamber, iris, lens capsule, retina and choroid. Worms have been found in the eyelid and also the lacrimal gland.

Management

An adult worm may be removed from beneath the conjunctiva after the application of topical anaesthetic to the bulbar conjunctiva.

The preferred treatment is described in Chapter 84.

Dracunculiasis

Dracunculiasis due to the guinea worm, *Dracunculus medinensis*, is widely distributed, mainly in sub-Saharan Africa but also in southern Asia. It is estimated by the WHO that the number of people infected is now around 70 000.[2] Few die of the disease. Water which is contaminated with the small crustacean *Cyclops* is ingested and the patient becomes infected. After an incubation period of up to 1 year, a worm emerges through the skin. This may involve the orbit. Emergence of the worm is associated with swelling, pain and fever.

Management

A description of treatment is given in Chapter 84.

Trichinosis

Trichinosis is caused by infection with the larvae of *Trichinella spiralis*.

Trichinosis is commonly the result of eating uncooked meat, most often pork. Many other animals are also infected, including dogs, rodents, bears and jackals. The disease is found worldwide, including both Europe and America, where raw meat may be eaten.

Eye complications

The most common ophthalmic presentation is bilateral eyelid oedema. This may follow invasion of the extraocular muscles by the organism, and pain on eye movement can be a feature. There may be associated oedema of the conjunctiva (chemosis).

Photosensitivity and blurring of vision can occur. Small haemorrhages may occur. These may present subconjunctivally and also within the eye, for example as a retinal haemorrhage. There may be an optic neuritis and optic nerve oedema.

Management

Treatment of the eyes is with a cycloplegic, such as atropine sulphate 1%, and topical corticosteroids. Swelling may be reduced with the application of cold compresses.

The systemic treatment of trichinosis with thiabendazole is described in Chapter 85.

Gnathostomiasis

Most reports of gnathostomiasis have come from Asia, but the disease has also been reported in Mexico.

Infection is caused by eating uncooked fish, chicken or pork.

The human disease has been mainly due to infection with *Gnathostoma spinigerum*, the inflammatory consequences being caused by the larvae, with hypersensitivity reactions within the tissues.

Eye complications

The eyelids, the anterior surface of the eye, and intraocular tissues may be involved, and there may be an orbital cellulitis. Uveitis, worms in the anterior or posterior chambers, cataract and secondary glaucoma are described. The worm may cause retinal disturbance and inflammatory changes can occur along the track made by the moving worm.

Management

The only form of treatment is the removal of the worm after anaesthesia. It has been suggested that cryotherapy could be used to immobilize the worm before surgery.

Diffuse unilateral subacute neuroretinitis

Diffuse unilateral subacute neuroretinitis (DUSN) was first described in the USA in the late 1970s; however, it is also found in Latin America, Asia and Africa.[74] It presents with loss of vision

Table 18.18 Essential eye drugs*[13]

Topical antimicrobial agents	Antibiotic[†]	0.5% Chloramphenicol eye drops
	Antiherpetic[†]	0.1% Idoxuridine eye drops
	Pan antiinfective[†]	5% Povidone-iodine
		1% Tetracycline eye ointment (enriched with polymyxin B)
		This last, being an ointment, has to be purchased in bulk
Local anaesthetic	Topical[†]	0.5% Amethocaine hydrochloride eye drops
Mydriatic	Diagnostic[†]	1% Cyclopentolate hydrochloride
	Therapeutic[†]	1% Atropine sulphate
Topical steroids	Weak[†]	0.1% Prednisolone
	Normal[†]	0.5% Prednisolone
	Strong[†]	1.0% Prednisolone
Corneal stain		Fluorescein paper strips
Subconjunctival drugs	Antibiotic	Gentamicin 40 mg/mL
	Steroid	Hydrocortisone succinate 100 mg ampoule
		Methylprednisolone 40 mg/mL (Depo-prep)
	Mydriatics	Atropine sulphate 1 mg/mL
		Adrenaline hydrochloride 1/1000
Oral agents		Tab. Acetazolamide 250 mg
		Tab. Prednisolone 5 mg
		Tab./Amp. Vitamin A 200 000 IU
		Tab. Ivermectin (in areas where onchocerciasis occurs)

*Many of these can be locally made and are already in use by some National Prevention of Blindness programmes.
[†]These drops can be locally prepared from raw materials.

in the affected eye, which may be accompanied by subretinal infiltrates, inflammation and vitritis. Later there is optic atrophy and diffuse subretinal pigmentary changes, with attenuation of the retinal vessels. A motile subretinal worm may be seen. Attempts have been made to remove the worm surgically, but the preferred treatment is to kill it with laser photocoagulation. Drugs such as thiabendazole are ineffective.

DISEASES CAUSED BY CESTODES

Cysticercosis

Cysticercosis is associated with the encysted form of the larvae of the tapeworm *Taenia solium*, and occasionally *T. saginata*. Faecal contamination of food and water is the most common cause of the acquired form of the disease, although the consumption of raw pork or beef means that the infection is widespread throughout the world.

T. solium cysticerci have been found in many tissues, including brain, spinal cord, muscles, lungs, subcutaneous tissues and eyes.

Eye complications

Ophthalmic cysticercosis is commonly intraocular and usually affects the posterior segment, either subretinally or within the vitreous. *T. solium* cysticerci may also occur in the anterior chamber and other eye tissues. The typical form of the intraocular cyst may show movement and the protoscolex may move 'in or out' of the cyst.

Symptoms and signs include pain, double vision, blurring of vision and sometimes flashes of light.

Management

The systemic treatment of cysticercosis with praziquantel is described in Chapter 87. Corticosteroids may be used in association with praziquantel. The intraocular cyst should be surgically removed if possible.

Echinococcosis

Also described as hydatid disease, this infection is most often due to the larvae of the tapeworm *Echinococcus granulosus*. The disease is widespread and other species are found in particular geographical locations. Most cysts are found in the liver and lungs.

Eye complications

Typically, echinococcosis causes a space-occupying lesion within the bony orbit. The most common sign is proptosis. There may be associated conjunctival chemosis, congestion and exposure keratitis. However, cysts may also be found within the eye.

Management

Treatment of the orbital cyst is by surgical removal.

The treatment of the systemic disease is described in Chapter 86.

Sparganosis

Sparganosis, due to infection with larvae of the cestode of the genus *Spirometra*, is found worldwide, but particularly in the Far East.

Humans can develop sparganosis by drinking contaminated water or eating infected snakes, birds or mammals. The flesh of an infected frog may be placed on ulcers, and eye problems are usually caused by direct contact. For example, in China, raw flesh may be applied to the eyes of patients who have fever.

Eye complications

The application of the flesh of a frog to inflamed or painful eyes can result in infection with the parasite, and eyelid oedema, watering and extreme irritation may develop. A worm may be found subconjunctivally and retrobulbar invasion can occur. The larva has been identified in the anterior chamber of the eye.

Management

The worm or nodule should be removed surgically.

DISEASES CAUSED BY TREMATODES

Paragonomiasis

A number of lung flukes of the genus *Paragonimus* have been implicated in this infection, which is particularly prevalent in the Far East but is also found in Africa and Latin America. The organism is carried by many animals, and human infection may follow the consumption of uncooked meats, including crab and other crustaceans.

Eye complications

Typically, the onset of eye inflammation is characterized by severe pain which is intermittent in nature. There is a uveitis leading to considerable intraocular inflammation. The immature worm may cause anterior segment inflammation with hypopyon formation. There may be vitreous and retinal haemorrhages.

Management

In ocular paragonomiasis, the helminth should be removed surgically.

Treatment of the systemic disease is described in Chapter 83.

Schistosomiasis

Schistosomiasis (bilharzia) probably affects around 200 million people, with as many as 600 million at risk and 20000 deaths each year. This infection is caused by *Schistosoma japonicum*, *S. mansoni* and *S. haematobium*. Dams and irrigation canals have increased the prevalence because these waters contain the snail which is the intermediate host for the worm.

Eye complications

Egg granulomas are found on the conjunctiva but also in the choroid and in the lacrimal gland. The most frequent infecting agent is *S. haematobium*.

An *S. mansoni* adult has been found in the anterior chamber of an eye.

There are records of uveitis and retinal haemorrhages that have been observed in patients with schistosomiasis.

Management

Systemic treatment regimens are given in Chapter 82.

DISEASE CAUSED BY ARTHROPODS

Myiasis

The larvae (maggots) of certain flies may cause ocular myiasis. These infestations are found in the Mediterranean region, Central America and Africa, but also in temperate regions. Orbital involvement has been reported in many countries around the world.

Eye complications

External ocular myiasis can affect the eyelids, nasolacrimal ducts, lacrimal sac and conjunctiva. There is acute redness with irritation and discharge. This extremely unpleasant infection requires surgical removal of the larvae.

Internal ocular myiasis may result in uveitis, which can be severe. Usually the inflammation is due to a single larva and the prognosis is relatively good.

Orbital myiasis is often found in patients with poor personal hygiene; maggots invade the periorbital regions.

Management

External ocular myiasis requires the careful removal of the larvae after applying local anaesthetic eye drops.

Internal ocular myiasis requires treatment of any inflammation with topical therapy, including corticosteroids. Occasionally it may be necessary to remove the larvae surgically.

Orbital myiasis requires removal of the maggots with the application of antiseptic solutions and the likely need of systemic antibiotics to deal with secondary bacterial infection.

Nairobi eye

The blister beetle – a red and black beetle of the genus *Paederus* – can occur in large numbers in Kenya and Tanzania.[75] Contact with the beetle leads to dermatitis with vesicle formation. Indirect contact with the eye causes an intense periorbital dermatitis and keratoconjunctivitis. Although the appearance is dramatic, the condition is self-limiting and resolves over a few days.

ESSENTIAL EYE DRUGS

Table 18.18 gives details of medications routinely used in ophthalmic practice. Many of these drugs can be locally manufactured from ready-prepared materials.[76]

GLOSSARY

Abrasion: injury to the cells lining the surface of the anterior eye, often describing superficial injury of the corneal epithelium.

Amblyopia: also described as a 'lazy' eye; the result of inadequate stimulus to the retina in the child, often in an eye that squints.

Anterior uveitis: inflammation of the anterior uveal tract.

Aphakia: an eye in which the lens has been removed.

Band keratopathy: deposition of calcium between the epithelium and Bowman's membrane across the middle and lower part of the cornea.

Bitot's spot: an often triangular foam-like plaque on the bulbar conjunctiva associated with vitamin A deficiency.

Blepharitis: inflammation of the eyelids.

Blepharospasm: tonic contraction of the eyelids.

Bowman's membrane: the interface between the corneal epithelium and the corneal stroma.

Buphthalmos: congenital glaucoma ('ox eye').

Cataract: opacity in the lens of the eye.

Chalazion: a cyst in the region of the meibomian glands of the eyelid.

Chemosis: oedema of the conjunctiva.

***Chlamydia*:** the genus of microorganisms that includes those causing trachoma.

Choroiditis: inflammation of the choroid.

Chorioretinitis: inflammation of the choroid and retina.

Climatic keratopathy (solar keratopathy, Labrador keratopathy): corneal changes and opacities caused by excessive exposure to ultraviolet light.

Cobblestones: a descriptive term used for the papillae of the tarsal conjunctiva found in vernal (spring) catarrh.

Conjunctivitis: inflammation of the conjunctiva.

Corneal anaesthesia: loss of corneal sensitivity.

Corneal grafting: the surgical technique used to replace a centrally scarred cornea with a donor graft.

Corneal stroma: the main thickness of the cornea (9/10) between Bowman's and Descemet's membranes.

Cryotherapy: treatment by freezing.

Cycloplegia: paralysis of the ciliary muscle of the eye.

Dacryocystectomy: surgical removal of the lacrimal sac.

Dacryocystitis: inflammation of the lacrimal sac.

Dacryocystorhinostomy (DCR): surgery to create a new opening from the lacrimal sac into the nose to allow tears to drain into the nose.

Dendritic ulcer: the typical appearance of a primary corneal ulcer caused by the herpes simplex virus.

Descemet's membrane: the membrane in the cornea between the stroma and the corneal endothelium.

Ectasia: outward bulge of thinned tissue.

Ectropion: outward turning of the eyelid.

Endophthalmitis: extensive inflammation inside the eye.

Entropion: inward turning of the eyelid.

Enucleation: removal of the eyeball, most often as a surgical procedure.

Epilation: removal of an eyelash.

Epiphora: overflow of tears.

Episcleritis: inflammation of the episclera.

Evert: turning inside out; for example, turning the upper eyelid to examine the tarsal conjunctiva.

Evisceration: removal of the contents of the eye by curettage, leaving the sclera, optic nerve and extraocular muscles.

Extraocular: outside the eye.

Facial nerve palsy: paralysis of the facial (7th cranial) nerve.

Filtration angle: the region between the base of the iris and the cornea where aqueous fluid drains through the trabecular meshwork.

Fluorescein: a dye used topically on the surface of the eye to stain an area of corneal ulceration. The dye is also used by injection to view vascular and other abnormalities of the retina and choroid (fluorescein angiography).

Follicles: small yellow/white lumps on the conjunctiva which vary from 0.2 to 2 mm in diameter. Histologically they consist of lymphoid tissue.

Foreign body: usually a tiny fragment causing eye injury; it may be metal, dust, wood, stone, etc.

Gonioscopy: examination of the filtration angle of the anterior chamber of the eye with a contact lens (gonioscope).

Goniotomy: a surgical procedure with a goniotomy knife used in congenital glaucoma.

Gram stain: a stain used to identify organisms, both bacteria and fungi, microscopically.

Halo: a diffuse circle of rainbow-like colours around a light when corneal oedema is present.

Hypermetropia: long sight.

Hyphaema: blood in the anterior chamber of the eye.

Hypopyon: pus in the anterior chamber of the eye.

Hypotony: low intraocular pressure.

Intumescent: swollen; often used to describe an enlarged hypermature cataractous lens.

Iridocyclitis: inflammation of the iris and the ciliary body.

Keratic precipitates (KP): clumps of cells and/or pigment on the corneal endothelium due to inflammation of the iris and possibly ciliary body.

Keratitis: inflammation of the cornea.

Keratoconjunctivitis: inflammation of the cornea and the conjunctiva.

Keratoconjunctivitis sicca: dry eyes due to a reduced and abnormal precorneal tear film.

Keratomalacia: destructive melting of the cornea associated with vitamin A deficiency.

Keratomycosis: fungal infection of the cornea.

Lacrimation: secretion and flow of tears.

Lagophthalmos: inability to close the eyelids; may be associated with facial nerve paralysis, e.g. in leprosy.

Laser iridotomy: the creation of a hole in the iris using the laser.

Lens-induced uveitis: inflammation of the uvea due to leakage of protein through the lens capsule.

Leucoma: a white scar of the cornea.

Madarosis: loss of eyebrow hair and/or eyelashes.

Mazzotti reaction: systemic reaction following the use of diethylcarbamazine and suramin for onchocerciasis.

Miosis: constriction of the pupil.

Molluscum contagiosum: a virus-induced small papilloma.

Mydriasis: dilatation of the pupil.

Myopia: short sight.

Night blindness: poor vision at night.

Nodulectomy: surgical removal of nodules (onchocercomas) in onchocerciasis.

Onchocercomas: nodules formed by the encapsulated mass of adult worms in onchocerciasis.

Ophthalmia neonatorum: infection of a newborn child's eyes within 28 days of birth.

Optical iridectomy: surgical enlargement of the pupil to improve vision.

Optic neuritis: inflammation of the optic nerve.

Orbit: the bony skeleton (part of the skull) which contains the eye and extraocular muscles, nerves, blood vessels and fat.

Pannus: a superficial fibrovascular membrane of the upper cornea, associated with trachoma.

Panretinal photocoagulation: multiple small burns of the retina with the laser photocoagulator; commonly used for proliferative diabetic retinopathy.

Papilloedema: oedema of the optic nerve head.

Peripheral anterior synechiae (PAS): inflammatory adhesions in the angle of the anterior chamber of the eye.

Peripheral iridectomy: the surgical removal of a small piece of peripheral iris.

Phacolytic glaucoma: raised intraocular pressure due to macrophages and lens protein blocking the filtration angle, often associated with hypermature cataract.

Phlycten: a microabscess, usually at the corneoscleral margin, often associated with an allergic reaction to the tubercle bacillus.

Photophobia: fear (dislike) of light.

Phthisis bulbi: shrunken eye.

Pinguecula: fatty deposit on the bulbar conjunctiva.

Pin-hole disc: a tiny aperture or multiple apertures in a card or plastic disc; used to assess visual acuity.

Posterior synechiae: inflammatory adhesions between the pupil margin and the anterior surface of the lens.

Proptosis: forward displacement of the eye.

Pseudoexfoliation: the accumulation of white particles within the anterior segment of the eye, collecting on the anterior lens capsule, pupillary margin, ciliary body and zonule.

Pterygium: fleshy growth which grows across the cornea from the conjunctiva and subconjunctiva.

Ptosis: drooping of the eyelid.

Refractive error: a variation from the accepted normal optics of an eye, usually corrected by suitable spectacles.

Retinoblastoma: a malignant tumour of the retina found in young children.

Rhodopsin (visual purple): a substance required by the rods of the retina to allow some vision at night.

Schiotz tonometer: an instrument designed to measure intraocular pressure.

Scleritis: inflammation of the sclera.

Sclerosing keratitis: scarring of the peripheral cornea in association with inflammation.

Snellen 'E' chart: a standard chart to measure visual acuity.

Staphyloma: outward bulge of the cornea or the sclera with the uvea adherent behind.

Stye: infection at or near an eyelash follicle.

Subconjunctival haemorrhage: bleeding under the conjunctiva.

Subluxated: partial dislocation, usually describing a lens which is out of position.

Tarsal conjunctiva: conjunctiva lining the inner surface of the eyelids.

Tarsorrhaphy: stitching together of the eyelids, usually partial and often a temporary measure.

Trabecular meshwork: a connective tissue network in the angle of the anterior chamber through which the aqueous fluid drains out of the eye.

Trabeculectomy: a surgical filtering procedure, usually for open angle glaucoma.

Trabeculotomy: a surgical procedure for congenital glaucoma.

Trachoma: eye infection caused by the microorganism *Chlamydia trachomatis.*

Traditional eye medicines (TEM): medicines used by traditional healers in developing countries.

Trichiasis: eyelashes turning inwards and scratching the external surface of the eyeball.

Vernal catarrh (spring catarrh): a type of allergic conjunctivitis.

Visual acuity: the measurement of vision.

Xerophthalmia: 'dry eye'; used to describe the eye changes associated with vitamin A deficiency.

Xerosis: dryness of the surface of the eye, often associated with vitamin A deficiency.

ACKNOWLEDGEMENTS

An authoritative source on parasites and the eye, *Ophthalmic Parasitology*, by B. H. Kean, Tsieh Sun and Robert M. Ellsworth (Igaku-Shoin), is the standard text in the field to which constant referral for that section of the chapter.

REFERENCES

1. Resnikoff S, Pascolini D, Etya'ale D, et al. Global data on visual impairment in the year 2002. *Bull World Health Organ* 2004; 82:844–851.
2. Abou-Gareeb I, Lewallen S, Bassett K, et al. Gender and blindness: a meta-analysis of population-based prevalence surveys. *Ophthalmic Epidemiol* 2001; 8:39–56.
3. Turner VM, West SK, Munoz B, et al. Risk factors for trichiasis in women in Kongwa, Tanzania: a case-control study. *Int J Epidemiol* 1993; 22:341–347.
4. Quigley HA, Broman AT. The number of people with glaucoma worldwide in 2010 and 2020. *Br J Ophthalmol* 2006; 90:262–267.
5. Pruss A, Mariotti SP. Preventing trachoma through environmental sanitation: a review of the evidence base. *Bull World Health Organ* 2000; 78:258–266.
6. Minassian DC, Mehra V, Verrey JD. Dehydrational crises: a major risk factor in blinding cataract. *Br J Ophthalmol* 1989; 73:100–115.
7. Dandona L, Dandona R, Srinivas M, et al. Blindness in the Indian State of Andhra Pradesh. *Invest Ophthalmol Vis Sci* 2001; 42:908–916.
8. Foster A. Who will operate on Africa's 3 million curably blind people? *Lancet* 1991; 337:1267–1269.
9. Yorston D, Gichuhi S, Wood M, et al. Does prospective monitoring improve cataract surgery outcomes in Africa? *Br J Ophthalmol* 2002; 86:543–547.
10. Mathenge W, Kuper H, Limburg H, et al. Rapid assessment of avoidable blindness in Nakuru district, Kenya. *Ophthalmology* 2007; 114:599–605.
11. Singh AJ, Garner P, Floyd K. Cost-effectiveness of public-funded options for cataract surgery in Mysore, India. *Lancet* 2000; 355:180–184.
12. World Health Organization. *Global initiative for the elimination of avoidable blindness.* WHO/PBL/97.61Rev2. Geneva: WHO; 2000.
13. International Centre for Eye Health. *Standard list for a VISION 2020 eye care service unit 2006/07.* 2006. Online. Available: http://www.iceh.org.uk/files/standardlist06.pdf. Accessed July 2008.
14. Chatterjee A, Milton RC, Thyle S. Prevalence and aetiology of cataract in Punjab. *Br J Ophthalmol* 1982; 66:35–42.
15. Age-Related Eye Disease Study Research Group. A randomized, placebo-controlled, clinical trial of high-dose supplementation with vitamins C and E and beta carotene for age-related cataract and vision loss: AREDS report no. 9. *Arch Ophthalmol* 2001; 119:1439–1452.
16. Bhatnagar R, West KP Jr, Vitale S, et al. Risk of cataract and history of severe diarrheal disease in southern India. *Arch Ophthalmol* 1991; 109:696–699.
17. Klein BE, Klein R, Lee KE, et al. Socioeconomic and lifestyle factors and the 10-year incidence of age-related cataracts. *Am J Ophthalmol* 2003; 136:506–512.
18. Krishnaiah S, Vilas K, Shamanna BR, et al. Smoking and its association with cataract: results of the Andhra Pradesh eye disease study from India. *Invest Ophthalmol Vis Sci* 2005; 46:58–65.
19. UKPDS. Intensive blood-glucose control with sulphonylureas or insulin compared with conventional treatment and risk of complications in patients with type 2 diabetes (UKPDS 33). UK Prospective Diabetes Study (UKPDS) Group. *Lancet* 1998; 352:837–853.

20. Hammond CJ, Snieder H, Spector TD, et al. Genetic and environmental factors in age-related nuclear cataracts in monozygotic and dizygotic twins. *N Engl J Med* 2000; 342:1786–1790.

21. Yorston D. High-volume surgery in developing countries. *Eye* 2005; 19:1083–1089.

22. Lewallen S, Geneau R, Mahande M, et al. Willingness to pay for cataract surgery in two regions of Tanzania. *Br J Ophthalmol* 2006; 90:11–13.

23. Lewallen S, Roberts H, Hall A, et al. Increasing cataract surgery to meet VISION 2020 targets; experience from two rural programmes in east Africa. *Br J Ophthalmol* 2005; 89:1237–1240.

24. Duerksen R, Limburg H, Carron JE, et al. Cataract blindness in Paraguay – results of a national survey. *Ophthalmic Epidemiol* 2003; 10:349–357.

25. Yorston D. Are intraocular lenses the solution to cataract blindness in Africa? *Br J Ophthalmol* 1998; 82:469–471.

26. Gogate PM, Deshpande M, Wormald RP, et al. Extracapsular cataract surgery compared with manual small incision cataract surgery in community eye care setting in western India: a randomised controlled trial. *Br J Ophthalmol* 2003; 87:667–672.

27. Hennig A, Kumar J, Yorston D, et al. Sutureless cataract surgery with nucleus extraction: outcome of a prospective study in Nepal. *Br J Ophthalmol* 2003; 87:266–270.

28. Gogate PM, Deshpande M, Wormald RP. Is manual small incision cataract surgery affordable in the developing countries? A cost comparison with extracapsular cataract extraction. *Br J Ophthalmol* 2003; 87:843–846.

29. Gogate PM, Kulkarni SR, Krishnaiah S, et al. Safety and efficacy of phacoemulsification compared with manual small-incision cataract surgery by a randomized controlled clinical trial: six-week results. *Ophthalmology* 2005; 112:869–874.

30. Dandona L, Dandona R, Naduvilath TJ, et al. Population-based assessment of the outcome of cataract surgery in an urban population in southern India. *Am J Ophthalmol* 1999; 127:650–658.

31. Bourne RR, Dineen BP, Jadoon Z, et al. Outcomes of cataract surgery in Pakistan: results from The Pakistan National Blindness and Visual Impairment Survey. *Br J Ophthalmol* 2007; 91:420–426.

32. Limburg H, Foster A, Gilbert C, et al. Routine monitoring of visual outcome of cataract surgery. Part 2: Results from eight study centres. *Br J Ophthalmol* 2005; 89:50–52.

33. Heijl A, Leske MC, Bengtsson B, et al. Reduction of intraocular pressure and glaucoma progression: results from the Early Manifest Glaucoma Trial. *Arch Ophthalmol* 2002; 120:1268–1279.

34. Kirwan JF, Cousens S, Venter L, et al. Effect of beta radiation on success of glaucoma drainage surgery in South Africa: randomised controlled trial. *BMJ* 2006; 333:942.

35. Foster PJ. The epidemiology of primary angle closure and associated glaucomatous optic neuropathy. *Semin Ophthalmol* 2002; 17:50–58.

36. Dolin PJ, Faal H, Johnson GJ, et al. Reduction of trachoma in a sub-Saharan village in absence of a disease control programme. *Lancet* 1997; 349:1511–1512.

37. Miller K, Pakpour N, Yi E, et al. Pesky trachoma suspect finally caught. *Br J Ophthalmol* 2004; 88:750–751.

38. Emerson PM, Lindsay SW, Alexander N, et al. Role of flies and provision of latrines in trachoma control: cluster-randomised controlled trial. *Lancet* 2004; 363:1093–1098.

39. West S, Munoz B, Lynch M, et al. Impact of face-washing on trachoma in Kongwa, Tanzania. *Lancet* 1995; 345:155–158.

40. Thylefors B, Dawson CR, Jones BR, et al. A simple system for the assessment of trachoma and its complications. *Bull World Health Organ* 1987; 65:477–483.

41. Bailey R, Lietman T. The SAFE strategy for the elimination of trachoma by 2020: will it work? *Bull World Health Organ* 2001; 79:233–236.

42. Mabey D, Fraser-Hurt N, Powell C. Antibiotics for trachoma. *Cochrane Database Syst Rev* 2005; (2):CD001860.

43. Bowman RJ, Sillah A, Van Dehn C, et al. Operational comparison of single-dose azithromycin and topical tetracycline for trachoma. *Invest Ophthalmol Vis Sci* 2000; 41:4074–4079.

44. Yorston D, Mabey D, Hatt S, et al. Interventions for trachoma trichiasis. *Cochrane Database Syst Rev* 2006; (3):CD004008.

45. Klein RJ, Zeiss C, Chew EY, et al. Complement factor H polymorphism in age-related macular degeneration. *Science* 2005; 308:385–389.

46. Age-Related Eye Disease Study Research Group. A randomized, placebo-controlled, clinical trial of high-dose supplementation with vitamins C and E, beta carotene, and zinc for age-related macular degeneration and vision loss: AREDS report no. 8. *Arch Ophthalmol* 2001; 119:1417–1436.

47. UK Prospective Diabetes Study Group. Tight blood pressure control and risk of macrovascular and microvascular complications in type 2 diabetes: UKPDS 38. *BMJ* 1998; 317:703–713.

48. Early Treatment Diabetic Retinopathy Study Research Group. Early photocoagulation for diabetic retinopathy. ETDRS report number 9. *Ophthalmology* 1991; 98:766–785.

49. Hopkins AD. Ivermectin and onchocerciasis: is it all solved? *Eye* 2005; 19:1057–1066.

50. Brent J, McMartin K, Phillips S, et al. Fomepizole for the treatment of methanol poisoning. *N Engl J Med* 2001; 344:424–429.

51. Bourne RR, Dolin PJ, Mtanda AT, et al. Epidemic optic neuropathy in primary school children in Dar es Salaam, Tanzania. *Br J Ophthalmol* 1998; 82:232–234.

52. Gilbert C, Foster A. Childhood blindness in the context of VISION 2020 – the right to sight. *Bull World Health Organ* 2001; 79:227–232.

53. Foster A, Sommer A. Corneal ulceration, measles, and childhood blindness in Tanzania. *Br J Ophthalmol* 1987; 71:331–343.

54. Foster A, Yorston D. Corneal ulceration in Tanzanian children: relationship between measles and vitamin A deficiency. *Trans R Soc Trop Med Hyg* 1992; 86:454–455.

55. Isenberg SJ, Apt L, Wood M. A controlled trial of povidone-iodine as prophylaxis against ophthalmia neonatorum. *N Engl J Med* 1995; 332:562–566.

56. Yorston D, Foster A, Wood M. Results of cataract surgery in young children in east Africa. *Br J Ophthalmol* 2001; 85:267–271.

57. World Health Organization. *Preventing blindness in children. Report of a WHO/IAPB scientific meeting.* WHO/PBL/00.77. Geneva: WHO; 2000.

58. Gradin D, Yorston D. Intraocular lens implantation for traumatic cataract in children in East Africa. *J Cataract Refract Surg* 2001; 27:2017–2025.

59. Gilbert C, Fielder A, Gordillo L, et al. Characteristics of infants with severe retinopathy of prematurity in countries with low, moderate, and high levels of development: implications for screening programs. *Pediatrics* 2005; 115:e518–e525.

60. Yorston D, Foster A. Traditional eye medicines and corneal ulceration in Tanzania. *J Trop Med Hyg* 1994; 97:211–214.

61. Whitcher JP, Srinivasan M. Corneal ulceration in the developing world – a silent epidemic. *Br J Ophthalmol* 1997; 81:622–623.

62. Thomas PA, Leck AK, Myatt M. Characteristic clinical features as an aid to the diagnosis of suppurative keratitis caused by filamentous fungi. *Br J Ophthalmol* 2005; 89:1554–1558.

63. Yorston D, Foster A. Herpetic keratitis in Tanzania: association with malaria. *Br J Ophthalmol* 1992; 76:582–585.

64. Lewallen S. Herpes zoster ophthalmicus in Malawi. *Ophthalmology* 1994; 101:1801–1804.

65. Lewallen S, Kumwenda J, Maher D, et al. Retinal findings in Malawian patients with AIDS. *Br J Ophthalmol* 1994; 78:757–759.

66. Visser L. Managing CMV retinitis in the developing world. *J Comm Eye Health* 2003; 16:38–39.

67. Waddell KM, Lewallen S, Lucas SB, et al. Carcinoma of the conjunctiva and HIV infection in Uganda and Malawi. *Br J Ophthalmol* 1996; 80:503–508.

68. Shields CL, Naseripour M, Shields JA. Topical mitomycin C for extensive, recurrent conjunctival-corneal squamous cell carcinoma. *Am J Ophthalmol* 2002; 133:601–606.

69. Courtright P. Recommendations of international workshop on practical eye care guidelines for leprosy patients. *J Comm Eye Health* 2001; 14:26.

70. Yorston D, Foster A. Cutaneous anthrax leading to corneal scarring from cicatricial ectropion. *Br J Ophthalmol* 1989; 73:809–811.

71. Leck AK, Thomas PA, Hagan M, et al. Aetiology of suppurative corneal ulcers in Ghana and south India, and epidemiology of fungal keratitis. *Br J Ophthalmol* 2002; 86:1211–1215.

72. Kalavathy CM, Parmar P, Kaliamurthy J, et al. Comparison of topical itraconazole 1% with topical natamycin 5% for the treatment of filamentous fungal keratitis. *Cornea* 2005; 24:449–452.

73. Lewallen S, Harding SP, Ajewole J, et al. A review of the spectrum of clinical ocular fundus findings in *P. falciparum* malaria in African children with a proposed classification and grading system. *Trans R Soc Trop Med Hyg* 1999; 93:619–622.

74. Cortez R, Denny JP, Muci-Mendoza R, et al. Diffuse unilateral subacute neuroretinitis in Venezuela. *Ophthalmology* 2005; 112:2110–2114.

75. Poole TR. Blister beetle periorbital dermatitis and keratoconjunctivitis in Tanzania. *Eye* 1998; 12:883–885.

76. World Health Organization. *The local small-scale preparation of eye drops. Eye drop update 2002.* WHO/PBL/01.83. Geneva: WHO/CBM; 2002.

FURTHER READING

Eye Disease in Hot Climates, by Dr John Sandford-Smith, is an excellent short textbook of ophthalmology that is particularly relevant to the developing world.

The *Journal of Community Eye Health* is freely accessible on the internet at *www.cehjournal.org*, and it contains a wealth of useful articles. The paper edition is sent free of charge to health workers in developing countries.

Chapter 19   Sunil Chopra, Mario A. Knight and
                       Francisco Vega-Lopez

Dermatological Problems

INTRODUCTION

Skin diseases are highly prevalent in the general population and represent one of the main causes of consultation for the general practitioner and other members of the health team. The skin also manifests as a sign of cryptic systemic diseases. In tropical regions of the world a high prevalence of skin diseases is in sharp contrast with the paucity or absence of specialist dermatologist services.

Poverty and disability are two main characteristics of the individual patient and the community affected by skin disease in the tropics. A number of quantitative and qualitative epidemiological studies as well as individual observations by clinicians support the aetiological role of poverty in skin conditions such as fungal diseases, leprosy, scabies and impetigo. The vicious circle is closed as chronic or recurrent skin disease results in further disability and loss of economic activity. Clear examples of this complex problem are overtly manifest in those individuals suffering from superficial pyogenic infections, cutaneous leishmaniasis, leprosy, scabies and fungal diseases, among others.

Skin infections and tropical diseases may present as a primary condition or as a secondary manifestation of illness elsewhere in the body. Madura foot, cutaneous larva migrans and localized cutaneous simple leishmaniasis are examples of the former, whereas the latter can be exemplified by systemic conditions such as leprosy, disseminated leishmaniasis secondary to kala-azar, and coccidioidomycosis. The clinical approach to a patient with skin tropical disease involves a thorough exercise in history-taking that leads to establishing a morphological and topographical diagnosis. The identification of primary and secondary elementary skin lesions as well as the anatomical region affected score high in terms of diagnostic sensitivity and specificity. Table 19.1 shows examples of lesions and symptoms that suggest or establish a particular diagnosis in clinical practice.

The dermatological history must include detailed information on previous skin disease, travel history, activities while travelling, occupation, drugs, duration of signs and symptoms, evolution of clinical signs, symptoms in relatives or household contacts, wild or domestic animal contacts, and a fast practical assessment of the patient's immune status. The identification of extracutaneous signs such as fever, enlarged lymph nodes, hepatosplenomegaly and general malaise indicates systemic illness and these findings should prompt immediate action for further investigations or an appropriate referral. Particular epidemiological settings in the tropics determine exposure and attack rates from specific diseases and, hence, an in-depth understanding of the global geographical pathology and living conditions of the overseas population is required in the practice of tropical dermatology.

SKIN DISEASES CAUSED BY BACTERIA

Pyogenic infections

Aetiology and pathogenesis

Common skin bacterial infections in the tropics are caused by *Staphylococcus* and *Streptococcus* spp. These infectious agents are ubiquitous in both urban and rural environments and are capable of causing disease in all age groups. Healthy and immunocompromised hosts develop pyogenic infections of the skin following direct inoculation of bacteria. Less often, haematogenous dissemination and even a septicaemic state may develop as a result of a minor skin injury. The port of entry for these pathogenic organisms is often unnoticed by both the patient and doctor, but minor injuries, insect bites, friction blisters or superficial fungal infection are the commonest found in clinical practice. Other clinical circumstances such as burns, use of indwelling catheters in children and minor surgical procedures also play a role as risk factors for these infections.

Pyogenic bacteria cause damage in the infected tissue by the pathogenic action of proteases, haemolysins, lipoteichoic acid and coagulases. Erythrogenic toxins are responsible for the erythema commonly observed in infections by *Streptococcus* spp.[1]

Clinical findings and diagnosis

The clinical spectrum of skin pyogenic infections includes folliculitis, furuncle and carbuncle formation on areas with hair follicles. Plaques of impetigo (Figure 19.1) and infiltrated thickened dermis commonly affect the lower limbs (Figure 19.2) and are respectively caused by *Staphylococcus* and *Streptococcus* spp. Abscess formation, cellulitis and necrotic ulceration represent the more severe end of the spectrum.

Table 19.1 Skin lesions and symptoms suggesting a variety of diagnoses

Clinical features	Working diagnosis
Itchy papules in clusters	Arthropod bites
Asymptomatic palmoplantar papules	Syphilis
Single ulcerated nodule on exposed skin	Cutaneous leishmaniasis
Asymptomatic chronic verrucous plaque	Tuberculosis or chromoblastomycosis
Dysautonomic changes and ulceration	Leprosy
Hyper/hypopigmented patch/plaques with atrophy and ulceration	Leprosy
Erythematous or hypopigmented plaques or nodules with peripheral neuropathy	Leprosy
Excoriated papules and burrows	Scabies
Ulcerated nodule and lymphangitis	Sporotrichosis or cutaneous leishmaniasis
Chronic scarring and sinus tracts	Mycetoma
Itchy serpiginous track	Cutaneous larva migrans
Haemorrhagic eschar, rash and fever	Tick typhus, Lyme disease
Pruritic lichenification, nodules and dyschromic changes	Onchocerciasis
Recurrent swellings	*Loa loa* or gnathostomiasis
Patchy alopecia and boggy inflammation	Scalp ringworm
Acute urticaria, fever and abdominal pain	Acute schistosomiasis (Katayama fever)
Painful, pruritic, plantar blisters	Acute tinea pedis or acute eczema
Furunculoid painful lesions	Myasis
Erythema, or urticaria, or exfoliative skin lesions with/without mucosal involvement	Drug reactions

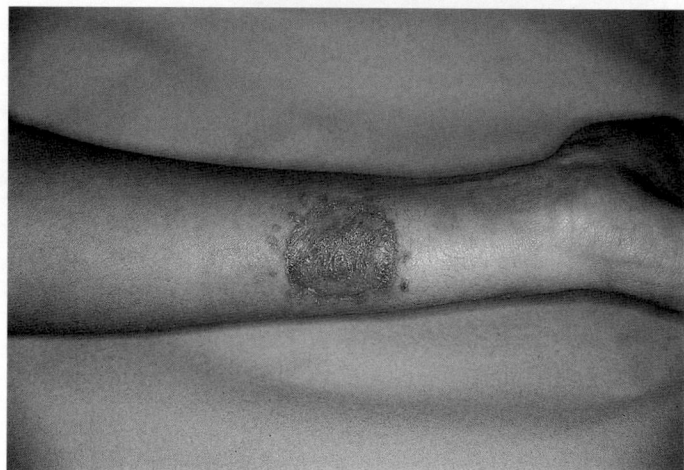

Figure 19.1 Erythematous plaque of superficial impetigo with satellite lesions.

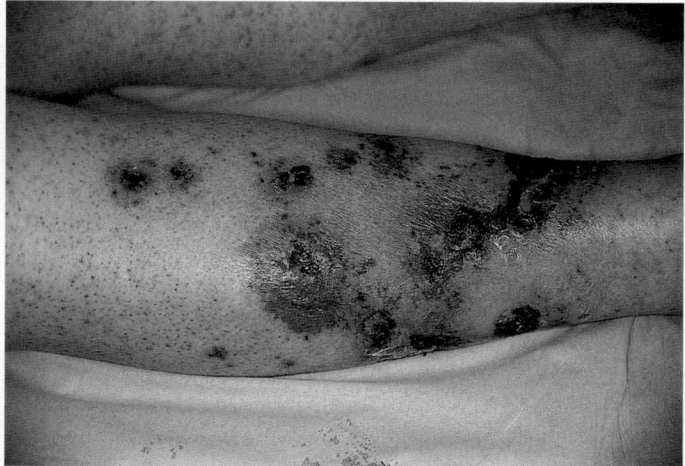

Figure 19.2 Pyogenic superficial lesions with purpuric plaques of cellulitis and proximal dissemination.

By far, the perimalleolar regions are more commonly affected than other areas of the lower limb as they are exposed to mechanical trauma; however, other common pyogenic infections may present on the upper limbs, face (Figure 19.3) and trunk. Common clinical signs of pyogenic infections include a variety of manifestations such as erythema, inflammation, pus discharge, abscess formation, ulceration, blistering, necrotizing lesions and gangrene. Severe scarring may result from pyogenic ulcers caused by friction injury or else in cases of ecthyma (Figure 19.4).

Most pyogenic skin infections are painful and the diagnosis is based on the clinical history and findings. Bacteriological investigations and sensitivity profile to antibiotics must be carried out if available. Disseminated, chronic or severe infections require an immediate referral to a dermatologist or to an infectious disease specialist. Uncommon cases of streptococcal infection of the throat may express clinically with a sudden eruption of guttate psoriasis as a result of bacterial superantigen stimulation.

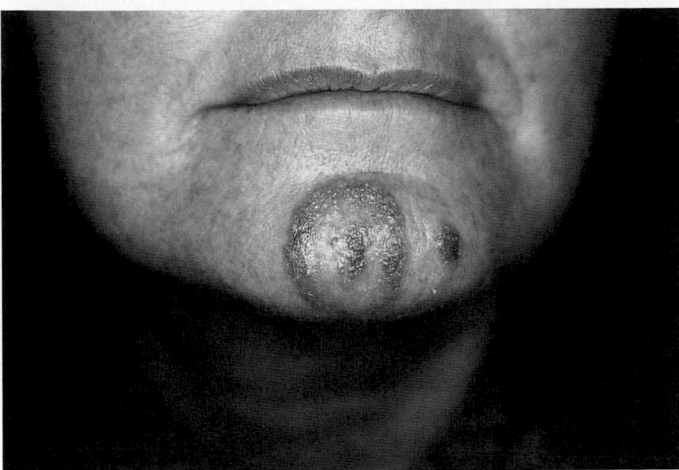

Figure 19.3 Circular plaque of staphylococcal pustular impetigo on the chin, with satellite lesions.

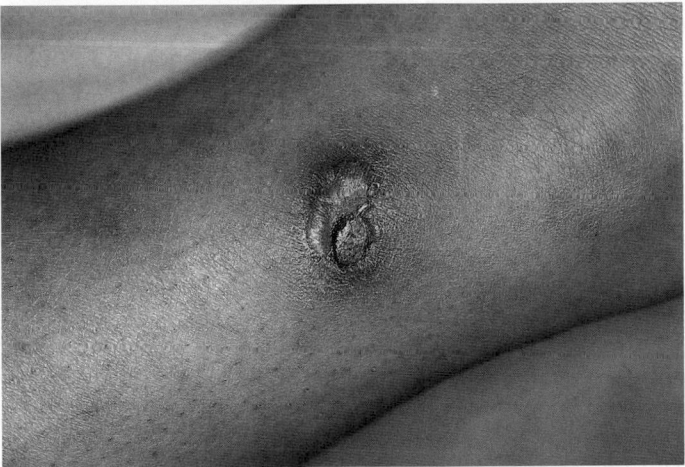

Figure 19.4 Localized ecthyma with surrounding cellulitis on the lower limb.

Management

Mild infections are successfully treated with bathing or soaking of the affected skin in potassium permanganate solution (1 : 10 000 dilution in water) for 20 minutes daily. Other mild superficial infections such as isolated plaques of impetigo or impetiginized eczema respond well to antiseptic or antimicrobial creams and ointments containing cetrimide, chlorhexidine, fucidic acid or mupirocin. Acute or chronic eczema requires treatment with potent topical steroids in order to eliminate risk factors for infection. Infections with multiple lesions or those involving larger areas of the skin require a complete course of systemic β-lactam or macrolide antibiotics in addition to the above topical treatments. Recurrent episodes of cellulitis require longer courses of these antibiotics, and hospitalization followed by surgical debridement is mandatory in necrotic lesions, gangrenous plaques and deeper infections with severe fasciitis. Superficial infections of the foot skin complicated by deeper involvement with necrosis of soft tissues carry a high mortality rate up to 25%.[2] Necrotizing soft tissue infections (NSTIs) are highly lethal and pose one of the few dermatological emergencies, with early diagnosis being crucial. Although the optimum treatment is surgical debridement combined with antimicrobial therapy, there are novel therapeutic measures that are currently being trialled with much success, including hyperbaric oxygen and intravenous immunoglobulin.[3]

Treponemal infections

These spirochaetal infections mainly consist of endemic syphilis, yaws and pinta.

Syphilis

Primary syphilis

This is characterized by the appearance of a painless papule (chancre) at the point of infection, usually the genital or oral mucosa.

Secondary syphilis

If the primary form is untreated, this may result in the secondary form from 20 to 60 days after infection, resulting in a maculopapular rash which is red to reddish brown in colour with common palmoplantar involvement. There may be a scarring alopecia, ulceration of mucous membranes and characteristic **condylomata lata** in the flexures. Condylomata lata are whitish grey and, due to their presence in flexures, tend to be moist. Systemic symptoms include fever, lethargy, myalgia and arthralgia.

Tertiary syphilis

This may develop approximately 3–5 years after infection. Tuberous syphilids with grouped red-brown papules occur on the skin. Such lesions develop with central regression and atrophy. Associated peripheral progression results in a serpiginous morphology. Gummata may be localized on the forehead, scalp, lips, tongue, genitals (Figure 19.5) or any part of the body. Morphologically, the gummata are various shades of red and may ulcerate and heal with extensive scarring.

Treatment

The treatment of choice is penicillin, but allergic individuals respond to erythromycin or tetracyclines.[4]

Yaws

This is a condition that tends to begin in childhood and is associated with overcrowding, as the main vector of transmission is skin-to-skin contact. Propagation of the causative organism *Treponema pertenue* is dependent on a hot humid climate and is seen in Africa, South-east Asia and parts of South America. The clinical presentation is divided into four stages: primary, secondary, latent and tertiary. The primary stage is characterized by a single papule, which enlarges to become a papilloma at the site of inoculation. The average incubation period is 20 days, during which the epidermis and cutaneous lymphatics are infected, leading to blood-borne infection. Deceptively, this papilloma resolves spontaneously, only for the same papillomas to appear

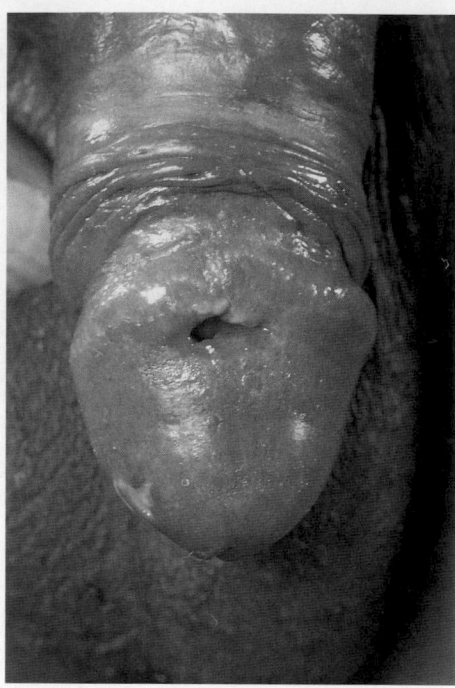

Figure 19.5 Asymptomatic exudative gummata of the penis in syphilis.

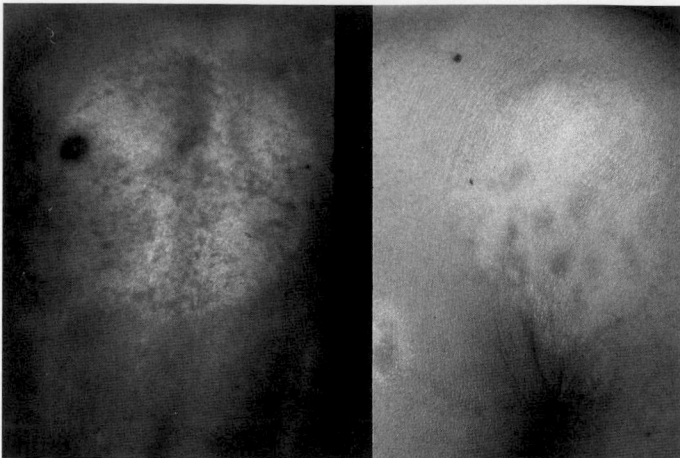

Figure 19.6 Circumscribed patches of hypopigmented truncal skin in 'mal del pinto'.

6 months later in a disseminated distribution in the secondary phase. These secondary stage papillomas tend to heal spontaneously, leading to an asymptomatic latent phase with sporadic appearance of papillomatous skin lesions which also spontaneously heal. Both secondary and latent phases may be associated with characteristic palmoplantar hyperkeratosis which makes it painful for the patient to walk and hence the associated 'crab gait'. The tertiary stage may occur in up to 10% of patients, with scarring of the skin manifesting in:

- juxta-articular nodules, which are hard nodules around joints, mainly on the extensor side of elbows and wrists and also on hips, ankles and sacrum
- the appearance of gummata on the nose, palate and upper lip, causing soft tissue destruction that results in scarred areas called gangosa.

There can also be inflammation of the bones of the nose and upper jaw, leading to destruction of bone and cartilage that results in scarred mutilated areas called goundou.[5]

Treatment

The prognosis of primary and secondary yaws is excellent, with a single dose of penicillin causing healing of cutaneous lesions within weeks. Alternative antibiotics are tetracyclines and erythromycin. Unfortunately, once the scarring lesions of tertiary yaws have been established these remain permanent.

Pinta

This is endemic and caused by *Treponema carateum*. It is characterized by chronic skin lesions only, with no systemic involvement, and occurs mainly in young adults. There are four stages: primary, secondary, latent and tertiary. Three weeks after inoculation, a papule or verrucous plaque appears on the periphery of the limbs, which enlarges and becomes gradually hyperkeratotic. Secondary pinta is said to occur 9 months later, when there is dissemination of such lesions throughout the skin. Years later, the tertiary form may develop, with hypo- and hyperpigmented scarred areas throughout the skin (Figure 19.6).

Treponemal organisms can be found in the early dyschromic lesions and cross-reactive positive serology is very helpful in establishing the diagnosis. Benzylpenicillin is the treatment of choice, with tetracyclines and erythromycin being useful alternatives.[6]

Mycobacterial infections

The main disease-causing mycobacteria are *M. tuberculosis* and *M. leprae*. However, there are several other relevant mycobacteria that cause skin disease:

- *M. marinum*
- *M. ulcerans*
- *M. chelonae* and *M. abscessus*.

Clinical findings and diagnosis

M. marinum

The fish tank granuloma more commonly affects the fingers or hand dorsum, but it has also been described on the foot and other anatomical sites. *M. marinum* frequently infects freshwater fish and, hence, individuals handling fish tanks represent the main population at risk.[7] The disease manifests as a localized progressing swelling with variable pain, and the appearance, within a few weeks, of nodular or verrucous skin lesions on the affected area (Figure 19.7). These lesions can show ulceration and bleeding from the disease process itself but also from mechanical trauma. The nodular lesions, measuring a few millimetres up to 2 or 3 cm, may resolve spontaneously after a few months, but they can also disseminate proximally by haematogenous or lymphatic spread. The dorsal aspects of the hand, foot and the malleolar regions are exposed to trauma and therefore direct inoculation commonly

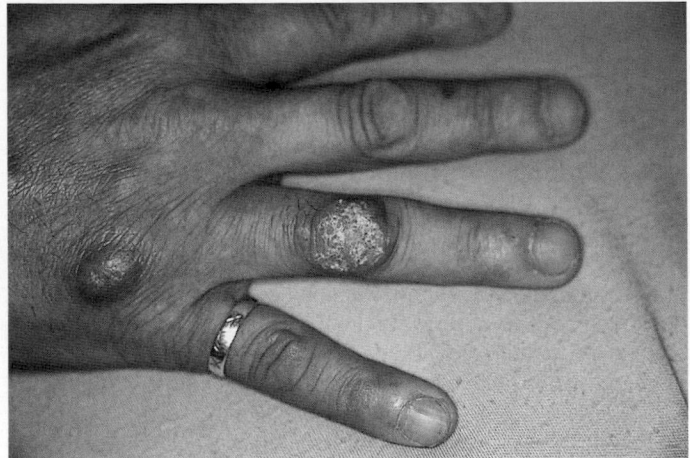

Figure 19.7 Nodular verrucous violaceous lesions with proximal dissemination caused by *Mycobacterium marinum*.

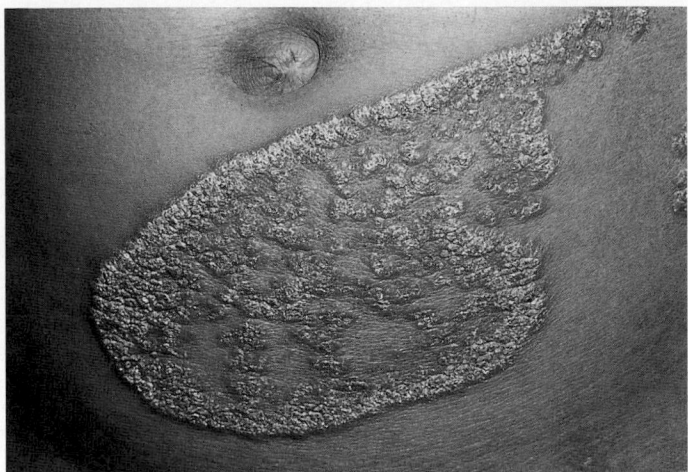

Figure 19.8 Circumscribed large verrucous plaque with erythematous islets in chronic tuberculosis verrucosa cutis. (Courtesy of Professor Amado Saúl, Mexico.)

takes place on these regions. Once the condition is suspected, microbiological and histopathological investigations represent the most sensitive tests to confirm the clinical diagnosis.

M. ulcerans

This causes the Buruli ulcer which affects mainly young individuals in rural Africa and particularly in West Africa, where an increase in incidence has been reported.[8] More than two-thirds of the total of cases present in children below age 15. The initial lesions present as papules or small nodules that slowly increase in size to the point of causing an area of inflammation and subsequent ulceration of the skin. The ulcer characteristically presents with undermined edges and manifests as active indolent phagedenism often involving large areas of the affected limb. A single ulcer or else smaller coalescing ulcers present more frequently on the lower leg above the ankles but other regions of the foot can be involved as well. Oedematous forms may progress rapidly and cause a panniculitis with destruction of underlying tissues such as fascia and bone. In cases where a large ulceration is followed by healing, contractures of the affected limb result from scarring.[9] Severe scarring and contractures have been identified as a high morbidity factor for disability and a significant percentage of them require amputation of the deformed limb.[10]

M. chelonae and M. abscessus

These can cause local cutaneous disease after trauma. Disseminated skin and soft tissue lesions only occur if the patient is immunocompromised.

Iatrogenic infections due to *M. chelonae* are well documented, with the source of contamination commonly tap-water and contaminated medical instruments. Lesions can be varied, with ulcerative lesions, subcutaneous nodules and fistula formation.

Tuberculosis of the skin

Aetiology

Tuberculosis of the skin is caused by *M. tuberculosis*. Those infected usually come into contact with the bacteria during childhood,

transmission occurs between susceptible individuals, and those who become infected have usually been in direct contact with people who are bacteriologically positive.

Primary tuberculosis

This form of tuberculosis is found in patients who are non-primarily infected. The initial infection can take place as a result of the bacteria coming into contact with a patient's skin but this is unusual.

This form of the disease manifests itself 3 to 4 weeks after infection, appearing as a papule, becoming a plaque (Figure 19.8), or in a nodular inflammatory form which evolves into an ulceration.

The tuberculin test starts negative; however, as the development of the disease progresses, the test will eventually become positive.[11]

Secondary tuberculosis

This form of tuberculosis occurs in patients previously infected. The patient will have given a positive result to a tuberculin test and will also have a sufficient level of immunity.

Types of skin tuberculosis

Lupus vulgaris

Indolent, erythematous nodules form plaques that may be scaly, ulcerated or crusted. It is most commonly found on the face, nose and ears, but may occur anywhere on the body. It is common to find the development of squamous cell carcinoma on the surface of the lesion; this will invariably be in a chronic form.

The diagnosis is made by undertaking a clinical examination, biopsy or culture.

The tuberculin test is strongly positive.

Scrofuloderma

This is the most common form of skin tuberculosis. The infection is localized to chains of lymph nodes (usually on the neck and chest) with sinuses draining onto the surface of the skin.

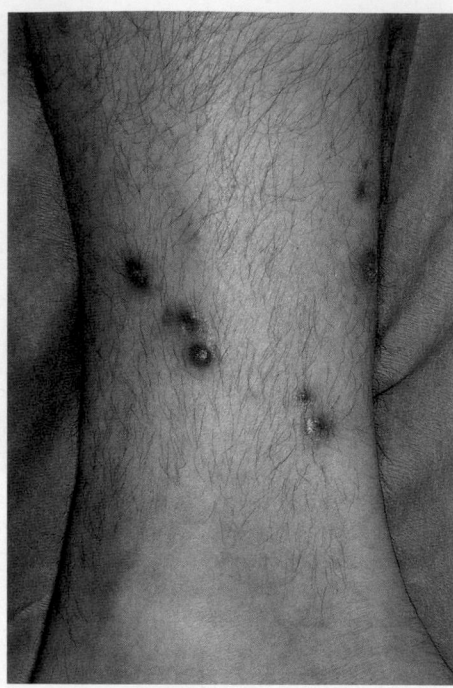

Figure 19.9 Erythematous papules, nodules, and scarring caused by MAIS complex infection in a patient with AIDS.

The diagnosis is made by clinical examination, biopsy, a positive tuberculin test and culture.

Acute haematogenous miliary tuberculosis

This form of tuberculosis is very rare. It normally occurs in children on account of the haematogenous dissemination. It is also seen in immunocompromised patients, presenting as multiple papules, plaques or nodules (Figure 19.9). The presence of these severe symptoms can be a basis upon which a diagnosis can be made.

Orificial tuberculosis

This is a rare form of tuberculosis of the mucous and periorificial skin as a result of self-infection; this takes place in patients with progressive visceral tuberculosis. This usually occurs in patients with advanced tuberculosis. The tuberculin test will give a positive result.

Patients with tuberculosis of the lungs will also have lesions in their mouth and on their lips.

Patients with intestinal tuberculosis will have lesions in the anus and patients with urogenital tuberculosis will have lesions in the genital areas.

It is easier to diagnose this form of the disease if the doctor is aware that the patient has visceral tuberculosis. The diagnosis is arrived at after undertaking the standard clinical tests.

The clinical appearance of the lesions is dependent on the route of entry of the organism and the state of immunity of the patient. A hypersensitivity state may occur in patients with good immunity. Erythema induratum, lichen scrofulosorum and papulonecrotic tuberculid are the skin manifestations.

Papulonecrotic tuberculid

This hypersensitivity reaction presents as crops of indolent papules with central pustules, which develop necrotic centres and finally atrophic scars. Lesions are found characteristically in acral areas such as the elbows, knees and ears.

The diagnosis is confirmed by a positive tuberculin test and biopsy.

Erythema induratum

This form may resemble erythema nodosum, but in contrast tends to be seen on the calves rather than the shins. The lesions are tender red nodules that break down and ulcerate, discharging onto the surface of the skin and healing with atrophic scars.

The diagnosis is confirmed with a biopsy, a positive tuberculin test and culture.

Lichen scrofulosorum

This is a rare form, occurring in children and teenagers with organic tuberculosis, primary tuberculosis or tuberculosis after vaccination.[12]

This form normally appears in the lateral part of the chest in the form of erythematous plaques, and sometimes can be followed by peeling.

Treatment

All forms of skin tuberculosis respond to standard antituberculosis regimens (see Chapter 56).

Leprosy

Leprosy is a disease with chronic development, caused by *M. leprae* (see Chapter 58). The bacterium is transmitted from individual to individual; for example, the bacillus can be easily dispersed by individuals when they exhale.

Leprosy is endemic in many areas of the globe. The disease results in sufferers having either mild or severe dermatological and neurological lesions. The lesions may, if the patient is not treated, result in the patient suffering from severe deformity and becoming incapacitated (Figure 19.10). Infection is likely to result in patients being both stigmatized and ostracized.

Aetiology

M. leprae is a Gram-positive, alcohol–acid-resistant bacillus. Analysis using the Ziehl–Neelsen staining method will show that the bacilli are arranged in globi, and this is the only bacterium that displays this kind of characteristic.

Transmission and evolution

M. leprae can be spread by non-infected individuals coming into contact with either nasal or throat mucus from an infected person. In most cases, the bacteria will have entered the body as a result of coming into contact with an area of skin that has become damaged.

The Hansen bacillus is a germ that is highly infectious and has a low pathogenicity and as a result this can give rise to serious concern among healthcare professionals that a large percentage of a defined population might become infected in endemic areas. Widespread infection is likely to commence very quickly after the

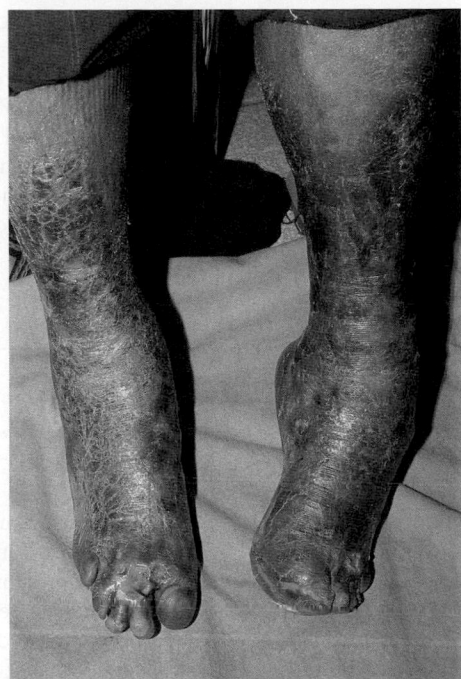

Figure 19.10 Pigmentary atrophic changes of the skin and mutilation in severe bilateral leprosy neuropathy.

bacillus has initially been detected. However, while it is of concern that a large percentage of a defined population might become infected, it is of equal concern that only a small number of those infected will show any immediate signs of sickness as a result of the infection. The reason for the latter is due to the fact that the incubation period varies from 2 to 5 years.

Research has shown that the majority of the population in those geographical areas where the disease is prevalent are in fact resistant to infection by *M. leprae*. Individuals can easily be tested for resistance by implementation of a programme to undertake testing of individuals using the Mitsuda test.[13] The test will show the level of resistance that the patient has to the disease. In essence, the test is carried out by giving the patient an intradermic injection of dead bacillus.

A positive Mitsuda reaction to the test is an indication that the patient has developed immunity to the disease. This is likely to be as a result of cellular maturation after being stimulated by *M. leprae*. The same result can also be ascertained by the use of other bacteria. It is possible that people in endemic countries can also have a positive result to the Mitsuda test.

Classification

The World Health Organization (WHO) classification, for purposes of treatment, divides leprosy into two groups:
- Paucibacillary cases – negative bacilloscopy. This group includes indeterminate leprosy and tuberculoid leprosy.
- Multibacillary cases – positive bacilloscopy. This group includes borderline leprosies and lepromatous leprosy.

WHO has adopted certain policies and developed protocols to be followed when administering multi-drug therapy to infected patients. Countries in which the disease is endemic are strongly advised to adopt those policies and protocols, details of which can be found on the WHO website.

Clinical manifestations

Neurological lesions

M. leprae has a specific tropism in the manner in which it affects the peripheral nervous system of those infected by the disease. It will be obvious that the peripheral nervous system has been compromised in all forms of the disease. The disease is initially diagnosed as a result of the patient experiencing sensitivity disorders.

As a result of the effect of the bacteria on the peripheral nervous system the patient will firstly lose the ability to detect heat, cold or a change in temperature. This will be followed by the patient losing the ability to feel pain and finally the patient will lose the ability to experience the usual sensations associated with touching.[14]

After the damage to the nerve branches there will be an immediate increase in the damage to the secondary branches and the peripheral nerves: palpably enlarged cutaneous nerve, great auricular nerve in the neck, the superficial branch of the radial nerve at the wrist, the ulnar nerve at the elbow, the lateral popliteal nerve at the knee, and the sural nerve on the lower leg.

When the nerve is percussed and the patient gets the sensation of shock, the condition is known as 'Tinel's sign'. It is possible that a patient may experience neurological disorders before any signs of there being any damage to the patient's skin, which can be a factor in causing late detection of the disease, especially when those who treat the disease have a lack of practical experience in recognizing its symptoms.

Skin damage

Indeterminate leprosy

Indeterminate leprosy is the first manifestation of the disease in a patient. It is characterized by macular or circumscribed areas with sensitivity disorders, sweat disorders and vasomotory disorders.

A patient may also suffer partial or total alopecia. Normally the macules are hypochromic or erythematous. Indeterminate leprosy has fewer than five lesions and no bacilli on smear testing.

Tuberculoid leprosy

This type of leprosy is characterized by macules or plaques with raised borders. Generally the disease in this form will appear as a single individual lesion; however, it is possible for the disease to manifest itself by the appearance of a number of lesions asymmetrically distributed over the patient's body. Negative bacilloscopy will be seen and also give rise to an extremely positive result to a Mitsuda test.

Borderline leprosy

See Chapter 58

Lepromatous leprosy

This form of the disease is characterized by a polymorphism of lesions; the skin and the nervous system are both severely affected by multiple lesions which are bilateral and symmetrically distributed.

Nerve damage occurs late in the progression of the disease and the skin lesions result in the patient suffering from a total loss of sensitivity. The effects of the disease result in the patient suffering from epistaxis and nasal obstruction.

The patient may develop leonine facies, hair loss from the eyebrows and eyelashes, misshapen nose, thickened deformed earlobes, ichthyosis of the calves, glove and stocking anaesthesia with skin ulcers, and deformity of fingers and toes.

Reactions in leprosy

There are two distinct types of reaction that a patient will have after becoming infected with M. leprae.

They have been classified as type 1 and type 2 symptoms. Type 1 appears in patients who have some level of cellular immunity such as in tuberculoid and borderline leprosy. These lesions become both more erythematous and oedematous. New acute lesions may appear with the same characteristics in other parts of the body. This reaction may appear before or after the course of treatment has been completed.

Type 2 is known as leprosy nodosum erythema, and can appear before the course of treatment has been completed; however, it is more common for this type of the disease to appear during the course of treatment.

The characteristics of type 2 leprosy are fever, sickness, neck pain, lymphadenomegaly, plaques, erythema nodosum, arthropathy, orqui-epididymitis and painful hepatosplenomegaly.

Diagnosis

There is a range of tests that a clinician can undertake in order to assist in the diagnosis of leprosy. These include: skin sensitivity testing, histamine test, pilocarpine test, Mitsuda test, bacilloscopy, biopsy, PCR and serology.

PCR helps to detect M. leprae before there are any visible symptoms present in the patient, making it extremely useful to detect minimum quantities of M. leprae.[15]

Treatment

WHO recommends the following multi-drug therapy regimens for adults:

- Paucibacillary leprosy: give at least 6 months of treatment within a 9-month period; treat with rifampicin 600 mg once a month (supervised) and dapsone 100 mg daily.
- Multibacillary leprosy: give at least 12 months of treatment within a period of 18 months; treat with rifampicin 600 mg once a month (supervised), clofazimine 300 mg once a month (supervised) and 50 mg daily, and dapsone 100 mg daily.

Management of mycobacterial infections

All mycobacterial diseases require highly specialized diagnostic investigations that in many cases can only be carried out in a tertiary hospital setting. Most mycobacterial diseases affecting the skin represent public health priorities not only for the endemic countries where they occur, but also at an international level as established by the WHO. Following the diagnosis of individual cases a long-term multi-drug therapeutic regimen can be prescribed only by specialized physicians. Mycobacteria are known to develop resistance to antibiotics and it is imperative that all cases are treated with combinations of at least two drugs. The main drugs with antimycobacterial activity are rifampicin, ethambutol,

pirazinamide, clofazimine, sulfone, isoniazid, macrolide antibiotics, tetracyclines and quinolones. Established combinations for particular infections are routinely administered according to international and local guidelines. The management of all mycobacterial diseases must consider not only the medical treatment but also a full range of educational initiatives aimed at the patient, the community and health personnel. Early lesions of fish tank granuloma, skin tuberculosis and particularly those caused by Buruli ulcer require surgical excision.

Bacterial mycetoma

Aetiology and pathogenesis

Nocardia, *Actinomadura* and *Streptomyces* spp. are the common aetiological agents of 'Madura foot' or actinomycetoma. This form of mycetoma occurs in tropical countries and the main case series have been reported from Sudan, Senegal, Nigeria, Saudi Arabia, India and Mexico. The infection is acquired by direct inoculation of bacteria into the skin and does not seem to represent a risk for travellers. Young male individuals living in endemic regions and dedicated to agricultural activities have been reported with the highest incidence of actinomycetoma. Bacteria causing actinomycetoma have a thick wall surrounding the cytoplasmic membrane which is rich in lipid and carbohydrate compounds.[16] Some of these compounds such as lipoarabinomannan and mycolic acids have been identified as virulence factors. These bacteria are capable of blocking the adequate killing mechanisms by the cells of the infected host; however, it is considered that they have a low pathogenic potential and most of them live as saprophytes in the soil.

Clinical findings and diagnosis

The clinical disease is characterized by a chronic course with inflammation, formation of sinus tracts discharging 'grains' and progressive deformity of the affected foot. Healing of discharging sinus tracts throughout years determines scarring with atrophic skin plaques and secondary pigmentary changes. Asymptomatic nodular or verrucous lesions can also be found and in a few cases a variable range of symptoms is present. These include pain that often results from superimposed pyogenic infection, acute inflammation and bone involvement. The chronic infection with deformity of the foot determines periosteal involvement and subsequently osteomyelitis. Variable but often severe degrees of disability complete the chronic course of actinomycetoma (Figure 19.11). The clinical picture manifested on one foot is highly suggestive of the diagnosis. The main differential diagnosis includes mycetoma caused by fungi (see 'Eumycetoma' below) but other forms of 'cold abscess' formation, histoplasmosis, chromoblastomycosis, cutaneous tuberculosis and sarcoidosis are the other main conditions to consider. Direct microscopy to disclose the 'grains' discharged from sinus tracts confirms the diagnosis and the culture of this material also provides a definite diagnosis of actinomycetoma.

Management

The current treatment of actinomycetoma is trimethoprim–sulfamethoxazole 7.5–40 mg/kg daily in three oral doses for

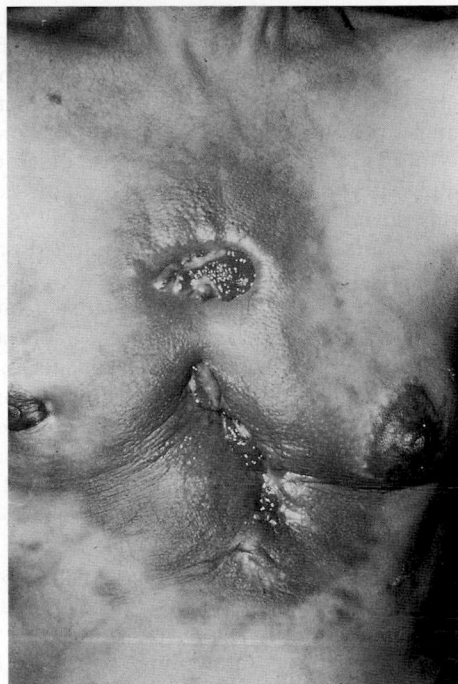

Figure 19.11 Sinus tract formation and severe scarring in chest actinomycetoma. (Courtesy of Dr Ruben López, Mexico.)

several months or years. In certain anatomical sites, extensive lesions, or cases resistant to this therapy, amikacin 15 mg/kg intramuscularly daily should be added.[17] However, treatment with co-amoxiclav represents an alternative or rescue treatment for cases that have previously failed standard therapies.[18] The treatment for mycetoma has to be administered for several months and the therapeutic response is variable. Early cases with small single lesions can be cured by surgical excision. In contrast, advanced cases with periosteal involvement and those with osteomyelitis do not respond to medical treatment and radical surgery of the foot represents the only therapeutic option.

Other bacterial infections

Tropical sea-borne infections by halophilic *Vibrio vulnificus* can produce localized or systemic disease manifested by acute and painful erythema, purpura, oedema and necrosis, particularly affecting the lower limbs. Cases of returning travellers presenting in inland metropolitan areas can be very difficult to diagnose and these patients carry a high mortality risk. Fatal septicaemia manifests with coalescing purpuric patches on one or both lower limbs that subsequently spread to the periumbilical region. The infection is acquired by direct traumatic inoculation in estuaries and seawater, or by ingestion of raw seafood, particularly oysters. Male individuals with a history of liver disease and iron overload states are the group at highest risk for this infection.[19] Severe cases require immediate referral to a specialist hospital physician as

intravenous antibiotics and early surgical debridement represent the treatment of choice.

Exfoliation of the face, truncal and palmoplantar skin is part of the complex and severe picture in cosmopolitan cases with staphylococcal scalded skin syndrome (SSSS),[20] whereas necrotic ulceration on a limb can result from tropical cutaneous diphtheria caused by *Corynebacterium diphtheriae*.[21] Cutaneous diphtheria commonly manifests as a non-healing single ulcerated lesion on the toe or toe cleft lasting between 4 and 12 weeks.

SKIN DISEASES CAUSED BY PARASITES, ECTOPARASITES AND BITES

Cutaneous larva migrans

Aetiology and pathogenesis

This dermatosis results from the accidental penetration of the human skin by parasitic larvae from domestic canine, bovine and feline hosts. Animals pass ova of these helminths with the stools and larval stages develop in the soil or beach sand. A close contact with human skin allows the infective larvae to burrow into the epidermis and cause clinical disease. The main aetiological agents are *Ancylostoma braziliense*, *A. caninum*, *A. ceylanicum* and *Uncinaria stenocephala* but other species affecting ruminants and pigs can also cause human disease. Following penetration into the skin, the larvae are incapable of crossing the human epidermodermal barrier and stay in the epidermis, creeping across spongiotic vesicles until they die a few days or weeks later. Multiple infections can, however, last for several months. Cases of systemic invasion with a Loeffler's syndrome have been exceptionally described.

Clinical findings and diagnosis

The plantar regions of one or both feet represent the main anatomical site affected by cutaneous larva migrans (Figure 19.12), but any part of the body in contact with infested soil or sand can be involved. Individuals of all age groups and both sexes can be affected and the disease is a common problem for tourists on beach holidays where they walk on bare feet or lie naked on the infested sand. A report of 44 cases presenting in returning travellers attending our specialized clinic in London revealed that 70% of the lesions were located on one foot, but the buttocks were also commonly affected.[22] The initial lesion is a pruriginous papule at the site of penetration that appears within a day following the infestation. An erythematous, raised larval track measuring 1–3 mm in width and height starts progressing in a curved or looped fashion. New segments of larval track reveal that the organism can advance at a speed of 2–5 cm daily. Commonly, the larval track measures between a few millimetres up to several centimetres in the region adjacent to the penetration site, but uncommon cases may present long larval tracks surrounding large areas of the foot with a well-defined perimalleolar distribution. Localized clinical pictures on the toes may present with only papular lesions but other presentations include eczematous plaques, blisters and urticarial wheals. Secondary complications to the presence of

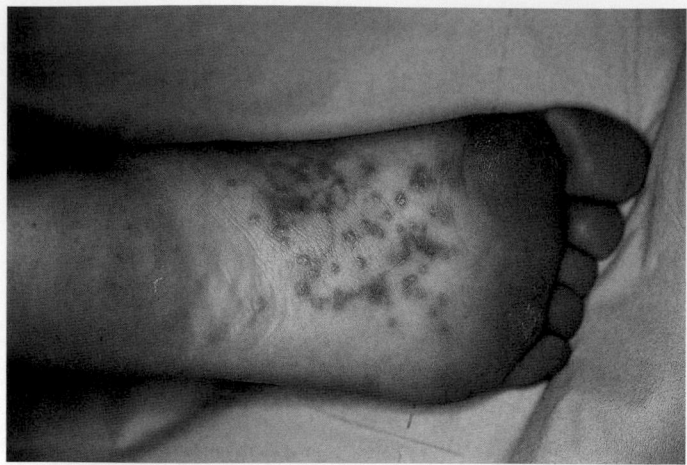

Figure 19.12 Erythematous larval track and papulovesicular eruption in unilateral cutaneous larva migrans of the plantar region.

the parasite in the epidermis include an inflammatory reaction, eczematization, impetiginized tracks or papules and even deeper pyogenic infections. Variable in severity, but most commonly, intense pruritus and burning sensation are the main symptoms.

The diagnosis is based on the clinical history and physical findings on the affected skin. The histopathological investigation has little if any value in the diagnosis of cutaneous larva migrans. The study of 332 cases in central Mexico throughout 10 years in the 1980s (Orozco, personal communication, 1993) revealed that haematoxylin–eosin (H&E) preparations of affected skin show a spongiotic acute or subacute dermatitis with a variable presence of larval structures. A mild perivascular lymphocytic infiltrate was frequently observed in the dermis, and a low proportion of cases may develop peripheral eosinophilia, but this is not a constant finding.

Management

Thiabendazole is currently considered the agent of choice: oral thiabendazole, 500 mg four times daily for 5 days, has been shown to be effective.[23]

Topical thiabendazole application is used for early localized lesions. Liquid nitrogen cryotherapy can be used on the end of the larval burrow.

Leishmaniasis

See Chapter 77.

Introduction

Aetiology and pathogenesis

Leishmania spp. parasites are protozoan organisms transmitted to humans and other vertebrates by the bite of female sandflies of the genera Phlebotomus or Lutzomya. Most *Leishmania* spp. can cause skin or mucocutaneous disease, but a few of them affect internal organs as well. It is estimated that 12 million individuals are infected by *Leishmania* in 88 countries and 1.5 million new

cases of cutaneous leishmaniasis occur every year (WHO 2006). The main endemic foci are found in Asia, the Middle East, India, Northern Africa, Southern Europe, Mediterranean basin and Latin America. A hot and humid environment such as that found in rainforest jungles provides adequate habitat for the animal reservoirs and vectors in Latin America. In contrast, desert conditions favour breeding sites for the vectors in the Middle Eastern and North African endemic regions.[24]

Following the bite from a *Leishmania*-infected sandfly the human skin can heal spontaneously or else develop localized or disseminated disease. Sandfly and *Leishmania* spp. causing skin disease in humans have been classified in geographical terms as Old World and New World cutaneous leishmaniasis. Both can affect one area of exposed thin skin, but multiple infective bites or disseminated forms may present with lesions on several anatomical regions. Common inoculation sites include facial bone prominent regions, external aspects of the wrists and malleolar regions. The bite of the sandfly commonly targets exposed areas such as the external ankles during sleep or else medial regions of the foot when the host is at rest. *Leishmania* parasites can resist phagocytosis and damage by complement proteins from the host by the action of lipophosphoglycan and glycoprotein antigens. Following phagocytosis, the intracellular forms of *Leishmania* parasites induce a delayed-type hypersensitive granulomatous reaction which adds to the tissue damage.[25]

Clinical findings and diagnosis

The bite of a sandfly may induce an inflammatory papular or nodular lesion that slowly progresses for several weeks. The incubation period can be as short as 15 days but commonly it is estimated at around 4–6 weeks. Certain forms may take longer to develop clinically. A non-healing papule with surrounding erythema and pain may also indicate superimposed bacterial infection that subsequently develops ulceration. On average 6–8 weeks after the sandfly bite a violaceous nodule starts enlargement and ulceration. The ulcer is partially or completely covered by a thick crust that following curettage reveals a haemorrhagic and vegetating bed. Cutaneous leishmaniasis can be clinically manifest as nodules covered with crust, ulceration with a raised inflamed solid border, tissue necrosis and lymphangitic forms. Advanced late forms present with scarring, skin atrophy and pigmentary changes. A particular localized form caused by *L. mexicana* or *L. braziliensis* is called 'chiclero ulcer' (Figure 19.13) and affects the helix of one ear; however, *L. braziliensis* more commonly manifests as a single destructive violaceous ulceration of the skin (Figure 19.14).

Other regions of the body surface may be affected by pigmented and hyperkeratotic lesions in patches and plaques in the clinical form named post-kala-azar dermal leishmaniasis (PKDL). This clinical form presents after an episode of visceral leishmaniasis by *L. donovani* in cases originating from India and Africa. Other common and characteristic clinical pictures include dry, single oriental sore by *L. tropica* (Figure 19.15), wet destructive single ulcer by *L. major*, diffuse anergic cases by *L. aethiopica* or *L. mexicana*, and cases of mucocutaneous leishmaniasis by *L. braziliensis* or *L. mexicana*.

The clinical picture of cutaneous leishmaniasis and the history of exposure in an endemic region of the world strongly suggest the diagnosis and the species involved. Complementary tests

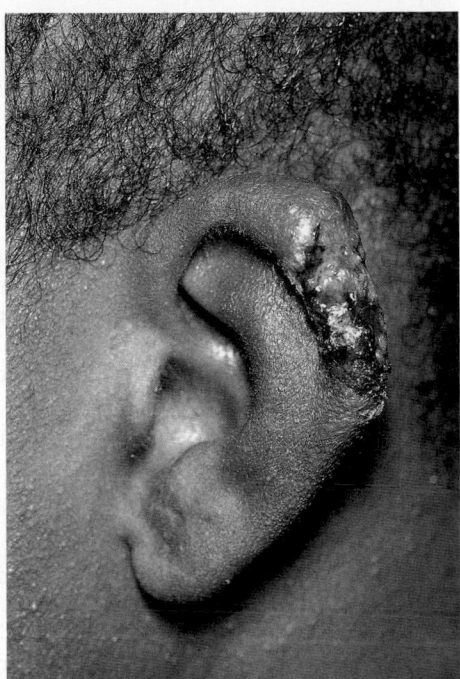

Figure 19.13 Chiclero ulcer in American cutaneous leishmaniasis caused by *Leishmania braziliensis*.

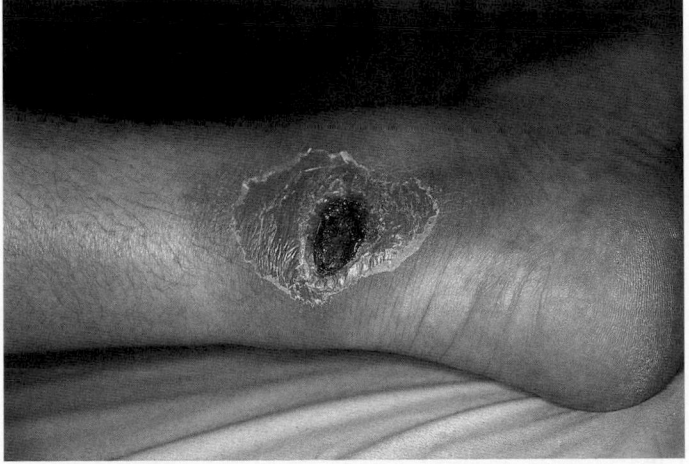

Figure 19.14 Erythemato-violaceous nodular ulceration with surrounding cellulitis caused by *Leishmania braziliensis*.

include histology of lesional skin, slit skin smears stained with Giemsa for direct microscopy, tissue samples for culture in NNN medium, and genetic analysis by PCR techniques. In our experience at the Hospital for Tropical Diseases we have found that in the context of a positive history of exposure and a typical clinical picture, the sensitivity for the histopathological diagnosis with dermal granulomata is 100%.

Management

Antimonials such as *meglumine antimoniate* and *sodium stibogluconate* are the conventional forms of treatment. In India, resistance

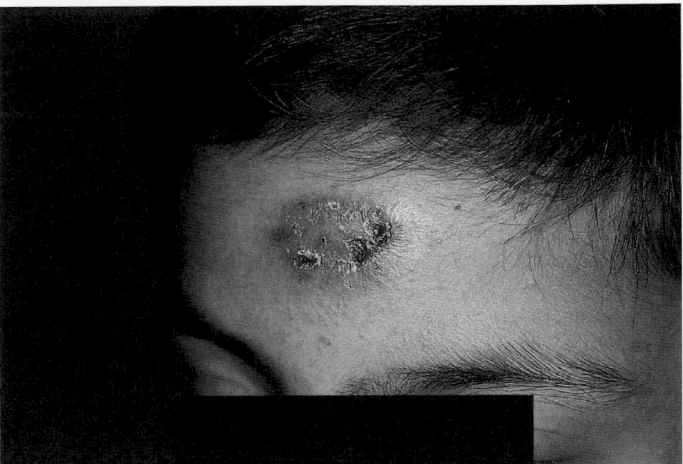

Figure 19.15 Single scarring erythematous sore with crusting in Old World leishmaniasis caused by *Leishmania tropica*.

has now become common,[26,27] and the treatment of choice for Indian-acquired visceral leishmaniasis is now *Ambisome*®,[28] *Abelcet*®, *Amphocil*®,[29] which are various forms of *amphotericin B*.[30]

The first oral treatment for this condition was *miltefosine* (Impavido®). Miltefosine had a 95% cure rate in phase III clinical trials; Ethiopian studies showed that it was also effective in Africa. In immunosuppressed HIV-positive patients who are coinfected with leishmaniasis, it has been shown that, even in resistant cases, two-thirds of the people responded to this new treatment in clinical trials. Miltefosine was approved by the Indian regulatory authorities in 2002 and in Germany in 2004. Its usage is now registered in many countries. The drug is generally better tolerated than other drugs. The main side-effect is gastrointestinal disturbance in the first or second day of treatment (a course of treatment is 28 days) which does not affect the efficacy. Because it is available as an oral formulation, the expense and inconvenience of hospitalization is avoided, which makes it a drug of choice.

The *Institute for OneWorld Health*, a non-profit organization, has developed the drug *paromomycin*, which is claimed to be effective and cheap.

Onchocerciasis

Aetiology and pathogenesis

This filarial disease is acquired through the inoculation into the skin of *Onchocerca volvulus* by black flies of the genus *Simulium*. This infection, also named 'river blindness' and 'Robles disease', is highly prevalent in Africa within latitudes 15°N and 15°S, and affects tropical countries in Central and South America. Fast-flowing brooks and small rivers provide breeding sites for the black fly vectors and only the female individuals are haematophagous. They can bite potential hosts throughout the day and principally those pursuing outdoor activities. Holiday-makers as well as those travelling for professional reasons have a risk of acquiring this parasitic disease, but it is the local population that suffers the highest toll from both clinical disease and subsequent disability.

Following an incubation period of approximately 1 year, the adult worms live freely in the skin or within fibrotic nodules or

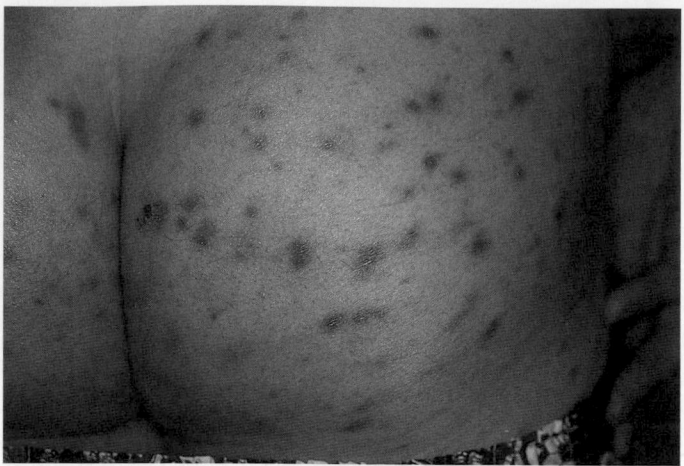

Figure 19.16 Pruritic papules and nodules on the buttocks in a patient with eosinophilia caused by onchocerciasis.

cysts named onchocercomata. The female adult worm releases microfilariae into the dermis and they are disseminated by the lymphatic system. Adult worms may live and reproduce for up to 15 years in the human host.

Clinical findings and diagnosis

The main clinical manifestations include pruritus and skin lesions with lichenified plaques, papular or prurigo eruptions, nodules, atrophic changes and pigmentary abnormalities. Early symptoms include fever, arthralgia and transient urticaria affecting the face and trunk. Pruritus and scratching lead to eczematization revealed as patches of lichenified and excoriated skin on the trunk and lower limbs. The buttocks are commonly involved (Figure 19.16) and oedematous plaques are characteristic in Latin American cases, locally named 'mal morado'. Late skin lesions show atrophy with hyper- and hypopigmented patches giving the appearance of 'leopard skin' described in African cases. The presence of filariae in the ocular anterior chamber causes acute symptoms and late ocular lesions lead to blindness.

The parasitological diagnosis includes the identification of microfilariae in samples taken from skin snips from the back, hips and thighs, specimens for histopathological investigation and serology. Most patients develop peripheral hypereosinophilia.

Management facets

The treatment of choice for onchocerciasis is a single dose of oral ivermectin every 6 months. However, this treatment does not cure the disease as ivermectin is a microfilaricide and does not kill adult worms. However, it significantly reduces the microfilarial load, which affects several aspects of the disease, especially reducing transmission and the prevalence of onchodermatitis and blindness. Recent research has shown that the combination of doxycycline plus ivermectin may be more effective as a long-term treatment.[31] The surgical excision of nodules is indicated and all patients require specialized attention in tertiary medical centres, including a comprehensive ophthalmological assessment. An active programme of mass therapy for individuals living in endemic regions of the world has been in place for more than a decade and other control strategies include the rotational spraying of breeding sites with insecticides.

Gnathostomiasis

Aetiology and pathogenesis

Several *Gnathostoma* spp. live as adult worms in the intestine of domestic cats, and humans can acquire the disease by eating contaminated fish that have ingested small crustaceans acting as intermediary hosts in this condition. The larval stages do not reach maturation in the human body; however, they are capable of causing disease in several internal organs as well as in the skin. The disease is prevalent in South-east Asia, China, Japan, Indonesia, Australia and Mexico.

Clinical findings and diagnosis

Episodes of migrating intermittent subcutaneous oedema with pruritus constitute the main clinical picture and cases can adopt a chronic protracted course for years. The trunk and proximal limbs are commonly affected. The episodes of oedema can be quite inflammatory and painful and the larvae can erupt out from the affected skin. Peripheral eosinophilia and positive serology support the clinical diagnosis.

Management

The surgical extraction of the larva from the skin results in cure.[32]

Tungiasis

Aetiology and pathogenesis

Tungiasis is a localized skin disease commonly affecting one foot and caused by the burrowing flea *Tunga penetrans*. This is also known as chigoe infestation, jigger, sandflea, chigoe and puce chique (Fr). It has been reported that this flea originated in Central and South America[33] and was subsequently distributed in Africa, Madagascar, India and Pakistan. It is a very small organism, measuring approximately 1 mm in length, and lives in the soil near pigsties and cattle sheds. Fecundated females require blood and their head and mouthparts penetrate the epidermis to reach the blood from the superficial dermis. After nourishment through several days, eggs are laid to the exterior and the flea dies.

Clinical findings and diagnosis

These fleas commonly affect one foot, penetrating the soft skin on the toe-web spaces, but other areas of toes and plantar aspects on the foot can be affected.[34] The initial burrow and the flea body can be evident in early lesions, but within 3–4 weeks a crateriform single nodule develops with a central haemorrhagic punctum (Figure 19.17). Superimposed bacterial infections may be responsible for impetigo, ecthyma, cellulitis and gangrenous lesions.

The diagnosis is clinical, but skin specimens for direct microscopy and histopathology with H&E stain reveal structures of the flea and eggs.

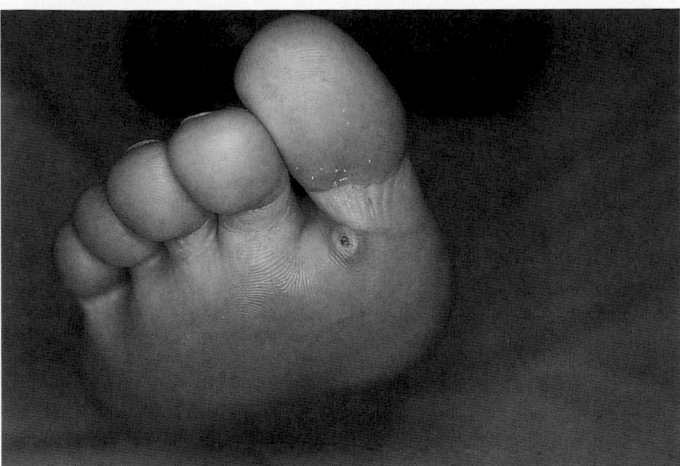

Figure 19.17 Single nodular lesion with central haemorrhage caused by *Tunga penetrans* acquired in Tanzania.

Management

Curettage, cryotherapy, surgical excision, or else careful removal of the flea and eggs are the curative choices. Medical management in the form of drugs such as ivermectin has proved unsuccessful.[35] Early treatment and avoidance of secondary infection are of the utmost importance in all infested hosts, and particularly in individuals with diabetes mellitus, leprosy or other debilitating conditions of the feet. A haemorrhagic nodule by *Tunga penetrans* may pose a diagnostic difficulty with an inflamed common wart or a malignant melanoma, but the short duration of the lesion and the history of exposure indicate the acute nature of this parasitic disease.

Myiasis

Aetiology and pathogenesis

Several dipteran species in larval stages (maggots) are capable of colonizing the human skin. The infestation mechanism involves direct deposition of eggs, contamination by soil or dirty clothes, other insects acting as vectors, or else actual penetration of larvae into the skin. Drying clothes on a line can be a common target where eggs become attached and subsequently reach contact with human skin. Species of *Dermatobia* and *Cordylobia* are the commonest found in the tropics, respectively in the Americas and Africa, whereas European cases originate from *Hypoderma* spp.[36] A local inflammatory reaction to the larvae with secondary infection is responsible for the signs and symptoms of disease.

Clinical findings and diagnosis

Elderly and debilitated individuals of both sexes with exposed chronic wounds or ulcers are at a higher risk of suffering from this infestation; however, most affected hosts are in good general health. Furunculoid and subcutaneous forms may affect any part of the body, but in children the scalp is a commonly affected site. Chronic ulcers of the lower legs and feet represent a predisposing factor and myiasis can complicate severe infections by bacteria or fungi. Larvae feed on tissue debris and may not cause discomfort or symptoms at all; however, cases with secondary local or systemic pyogenic infections can result from myiasis. Cases are observed throughout the year in tropical regions where the standards of hygiene, nutrition and general health are poor. The diagnosis is based on clinical suspicion and physical findings.

Management

The treatment of choice is the mechanical removal or surgical excision of the larvae.[37] Single furunculoid lesions can be covered by thick Vaseline® or paste to suffocate the larvae, which, following death, can subsequently be extracted. Superficial infestations respond to repeated topical soaks or baths in potassium permanganate at a 1:10000 dilution in water carried out for a few days. Cases with secondary pyogenic infection require a full course of β-lactam or macrolide antibiotics. Recent research has shown that it is possible to perform chemotherapy of myiasis with the antibiotic ivermectin.[38]

Scabies

Aetiology and pathogenesis

Scabies is a cosmopolitan problem but individuals in poor tropical countries with low standards of hygiene and particularly overcrowding suffer from cyclical outbreaks of severe and chronic forms.[39] This infestation is acquired by personal direct skin contact. The human scabies mite *Sarcoptes scabiei* commonly affects the skin of both feet of infants and children. Adults rarely manifest scabies on the lower limbs below the knees (Hebra lines), but exceptional cases of crusted scabies may present with lesions on both feet. The scabies mite burrows a tunnel of up to 4 mm into the superficial layer of the epidermis, where eggs are laid. The eggs hatch and reach the stage of nymph and subsequently become an adult male or female mite. Female individuals live up to 6 weeks and lay up to 50 eggs. A new generation of fecundated females penetrates the skin in adjacent regions to the nesting burrow, but the mite infestation can also be perpetuated by clothes or by reinfestation from another host in the household.

Clinical findings and diagnosis

Papules, with or without excoriation, and S-shaped burrows are the elementary classical lesions of scabies. Infants and young children present with papular, vesicular and/or nodular lesions on both plantar regions, but other parts of the feet can be affected. In contrast, adults present with bilateral lesions on fingers, finger web spaces, anterior wrists, upper limbs, anterior axillary lines, periumbilical region, external genitalia and buttocks.[40] A high proportion of males suffer involvement on prepuce and scrotum (Figure 19.18). Patients of all age groups suffering from chronic crusted scabies may present with eczematization, impetiginized plaques and hyperkeratosis masking the typical clinical signs of this infestation. Large crusts (Figure 19.19) covering inflammatory papular lesions contain a high number of parasites and a careful examination is required to prevent health personnel from acquiring the infestation.

The clinical findings and intense pruritus support the diagnosis. Confirmation is obtained by direct microscopy of skin scrapings

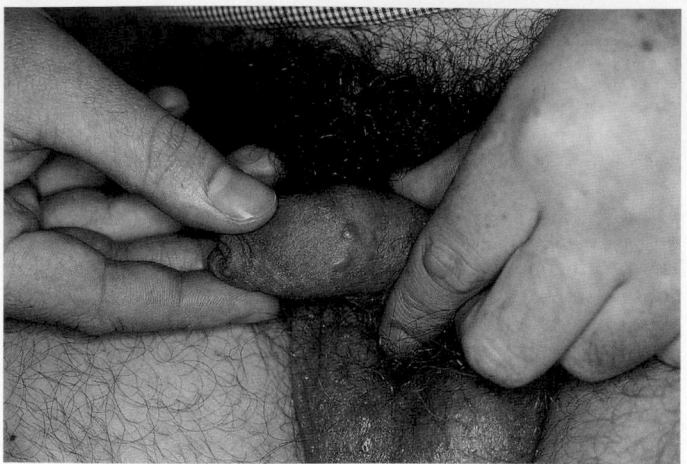

Figure 19.18 Pruritic erythematous papules of scabies on the prepuce and scrotum.

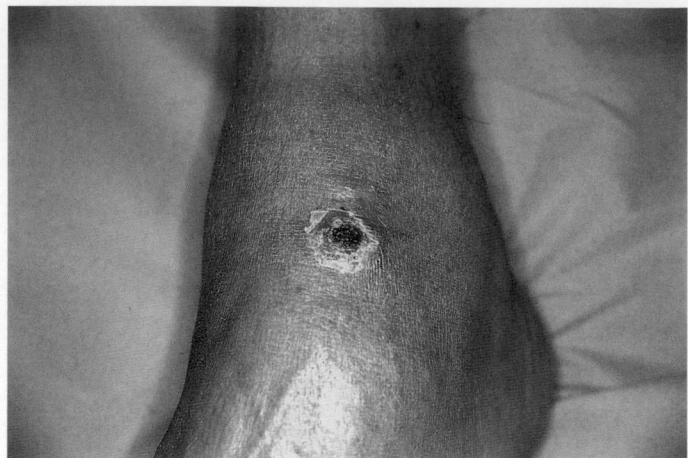

Figure 19.20 Small erythematous patch surrounding a haemorrhagic ulceration characteristic of an eschar produced by tick bite.

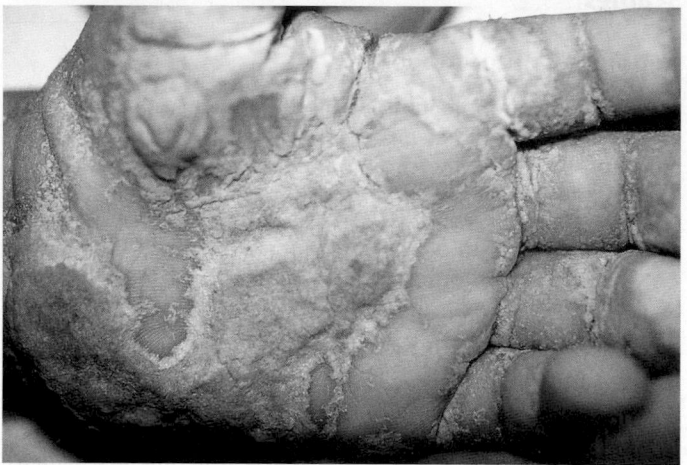

Figure 19.19 Disseminated crusted scabies in an immunodeficient child. (Courtesy of Dr Edmundo Velázquez, Mexico.)

from a burrow revealing the structures or faecal pellets of the mite. This test is carried out on a glass slide under low power and has a low sensitivity if carried out by non-experienced hands (potassium hydroxide should not be used since it can dissolve mite pellets). However, in vivo standard dermascopic mite identification with a handheld dermascope can also be used as a useful tool for diagnosing scabies, with high sensitivity. It greatly enhances clinical skills for making treatment decisions, reducing the number of cases of scabies left untreated.[41]

Management

Topical permethrin appears to be the most effective treatment for scabies. Ivermectin appears to be an effective oral treatment.[42] The patient should apply permethrin cream from head to toe before washing off after 12 hours. A second application 7 days after the original treatment must be prescribed and all the affected members of a household or community require treatment at the same time to prevent cyclical reinfestations. Recently, oral ivermectin is being

increasingly used as a first-line treatment.[43] Severe outbreaks require a second dose of ivermectin at a 2-week interval (150–200 µg/kg body weight). Other therapeutic measures are directed to control the symptoms, inflammation and secondary bacterial infection. Clothes and bed linen require washing at high temperature to kill all young fecundated females; however, a number of authors have demonstrated that this is not necessary, as the mites die from dehydration normally within 48 hours after losing a niche on human skin. In the right epidemiological context, scabies may represent a venereal disease. Pruritus may last for several weeks after cure and may be partially alleviated with an oral antihistamine.

Ticks

Aetiology and pathogenesis

Ticks are cosmopolitan ectoparasites capable of transmitting severe viral, rickettsial, bacterial and parasitic diseases. The transmission of infectious agents takes place at the time of taking a blood meal from a human host that becomes infested accidentally. Soft ticks of the Argasidae family are more prevalent in the tropics and subtropical regions of the world and transmit agents of tick-borne relapsing fever. The main genera of hard ticks are *Ixodes*, *Dermacentor*, *Haemaphysalis* and *Amblyomma* and these can transmit arboviral, bacterial and rickettsial diseases.

Clinical findings and diagnosis

The bite of a tick is painful and the patient is aware of this episode. The bite produces a local inflammatory reaction suggesting initially an ordinary papular insect bite that subsequently causes localized superficial vascular damage with necrosis. The characteristic clinical picture manifested as an eschar can be easily recognized on careful physical examination (Figure 19.20). This area of circular scaling of the skin surrounding the original haemorrhagic bite can be seen after 7–10 days. Residual chronic lesions may leave hyperpigmented patches with a central induration.

Management

Careful removal of the tick can be carried out by grabbing the tick as close to the skin as possible with a very fine forceps and pulling it firmly out from the skin. The bite site should then be thoroughly disinfected with a skin antiseptic solution. Squeezing of the tick during removal should be avoided as this may inject infectious material into the skin. Use of chloroform, petroleum and other organic solvents to suffocate ticks should be avoided.[44]

A careful follow-up and self-surveillance are indicated, as systemic illness may start a few days or weeks following the tick bite. Symptoms such as a fever, skin rash, lymph node enlargement, fatigue and night sweats indicate systemic disease and the patient requires referral to a hospital physician or to a specialist in tropical or travel medicine.

Fleas

Aetiology and pathogenesis

The common human flea *Pulex irritans* is cosmopolitan but a number of other species show preference for tropical climates. Such is the case of the tropical rat flea *Xenopsylla cheopis*. Fleas bite humans in order to obtain a blood meal and in doing so produce a localized inflammatory reaction.[45] History of exposure can reveal an individual host or family members recently moving house or acquiring a second-hand piece of wooden furniture where fleas can live for months without taking blood meals.

Clinical findings and diagnosis

A clinical picture of prurigo with papules, vesicles or small nodules on both feet and lower legs is characteristic and the lesions are often found in clusters (Figure 19.21). The papular discrete lesions

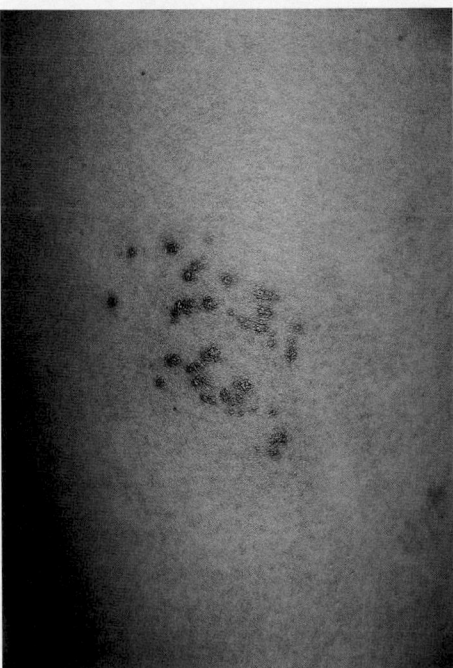

Figure 19.21 Cluster of pruritic erythematous papules on a thigh caused by *Pulex irritans*.

may reveal a central haemorrhagic punctum and the lesions in clusters often show a remarkable asymmetry. Modification of the initial pruriginous lesions may result from intense scratching and superimposed secondary bacterial infection.

Management

Fumigation can be successfully achieved by using common insecticide products approved for domestic use. Severe reactions of prurigo require a topical steroid cream and impetiginized cases topical or systemic antibiotics. Antihistamine lotions or tablets may provide symptomatic relief. Severe cases are treated with a single dose or short course of systemic corticosteroids.

SKIN DISEASES CAUSED BY FUNGI

Dermatophytes and malasseziosis

Aetiology and pathogenesis

Superficial fungal infections by dermatophytes are cosmopolitan and affect any anatomical site, including scalp and nails; however, one of the commonest presentations occurs in one or both feet. Dermatophyte infections involve keratin only and do not penetrate living tissue, so the resultant inflammation is due to delayed hypersensitivity or due to metabolic products that are produced by the fungi. These fungi are transmitted to humans by direct skin contact from their habitat in the soil, vegetation, animals or other individuals. Local conditions on the skin such as a moist and hot environment are predisposing factors and therefore these infections are highly prevalent in tropical climates. The main genera involved in human infections are *Trychophyton*, *Epidermophyton* and *Microsporum*, and there are more than 25 pathogenic species. Common infections of the foot and toenails are particularly caused by *T. rubrum*, *T. mentagrophytes* and *E. floccosum*, whereas *Microsporum* and *Trychophyton* spp. are responsible for scalp infections. *E. floccosum* is the causative organism of tinea on the trunk, groin, hands and feet. Dermatophytes are keratinophilic organisms and exert their pathogenesis through attachment to the skin, nail or hair surfaces by the action of acid proteinases, keratinase, elastase and lipolytical enzymes.

Clinical findings and diagnosis

Individuals of both sexes and all age groups are affected by dermatophytes; however, children under the age of 10 rarely present with tinea pedis. The main clinical pictures are those of localized tinea pedis (Figure 19.22), intertriginous, plantar hyperkeratotic, and onychomycosis. Common names for these conditions include ringworm and athlete's foot. Dermatophyte infections can manifest as localized single (Figure 19.23) or multiple coalescing circinate plaques with erythema and variable degrees of scaling on the body in cases of tinea corporis (Figure 19.24). Athlete's foot can involve the dorsum or perimalleolar regions. Toe-web involvement is commonly bilateral, presenting with erythema, burning sensation, pruritus and scaling, particularly of the fourth interdigital toe-web space. Severe acute forms present with painful

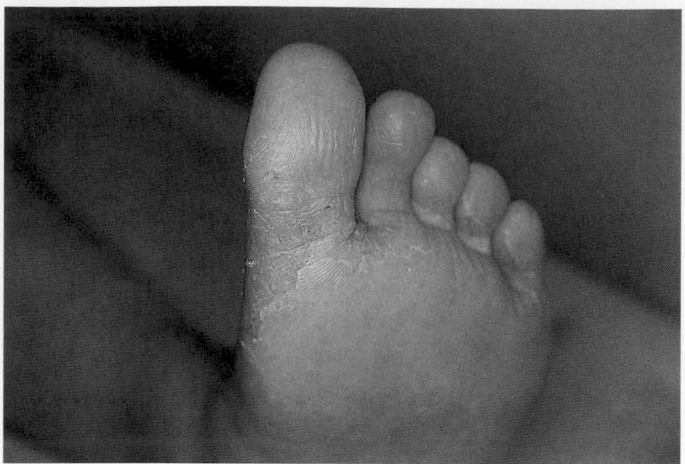

Figure 19.22 Scaling and diffuse erythema in tinea pedis.

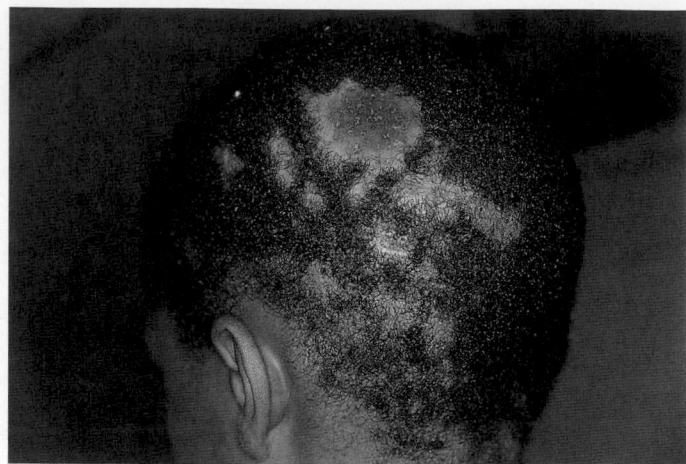

Figure 19.25 Non-scarring patchy alopecia and boggy inflammation in Celsus' kerion.

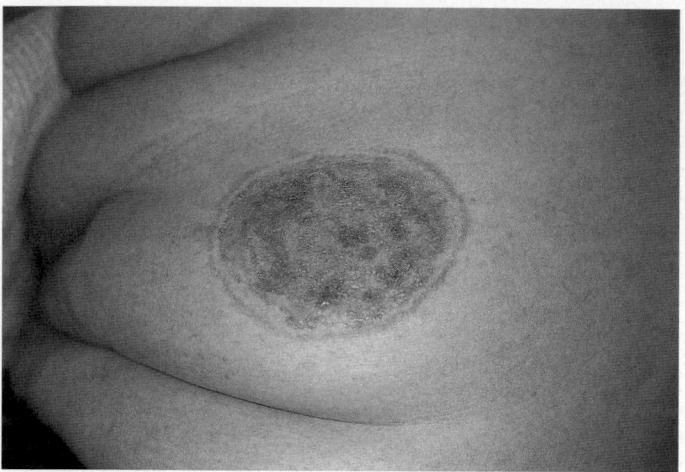

Figure 19.23 Pruritic erythematous and inflammatory localized plaque of tinea corporis.

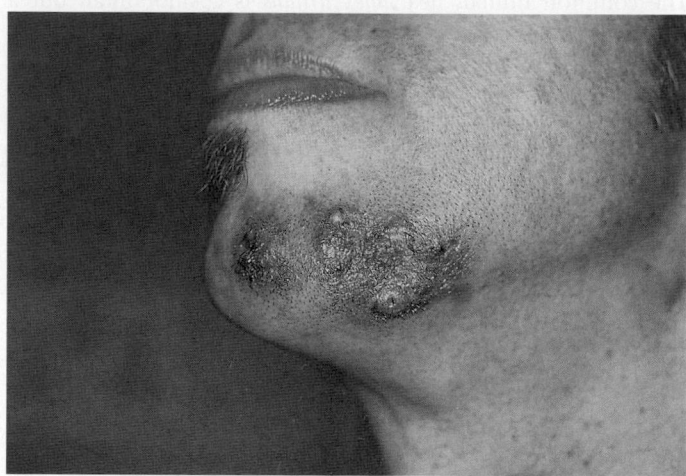

Figure 19.26 Erythematous plaque with nodules and pustules in tinea barbae caused by *Trichophyton mentagrophytes*.

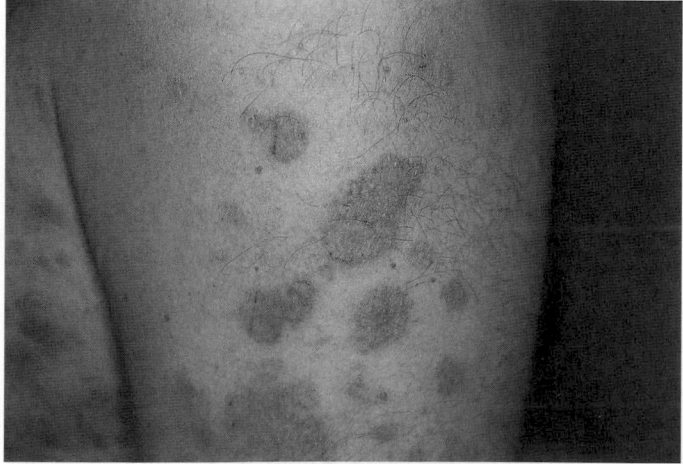

Figure 19.24 Coalescing small erythematous plaques with a microvesicular border in tinea corporis.

erythema and blistering in a similar pattern to that found in cases of acute eczema or pompholyx. Patients with a history of atopy are predisposed to superficial infections by dermatophytes, and in these cases erythematous inflammatory fungal lesions co-exist with patches of eczematous skin. Chronic plantar lesions develop asymptomatic large hyperkeratotic plaques, and a particular form of toenail infection by *T. rubrum* manifests clinically as a subungual white onychomycosis. Varying degrees of temporary disability may result from severe infections. Children manifest scalp infections under the kerion clinical form with patches of non-scarring alopecia and boggy inflammation of the skin (Figure 19.25). Less commonly, adults manifest granulomatous inflammation with varying degrees of scarring in pustular infections caused by other species of *Trichophyton* (Figure 19.26).

Discrete plaques of granuloma annulare have to be considered in the differential diagnosis of localized ringworm, whereas thickened plaques of plantar psoriasis may pose diagnostic difficulties with chronic hyperkeratotic infections by dermatophytes. Other

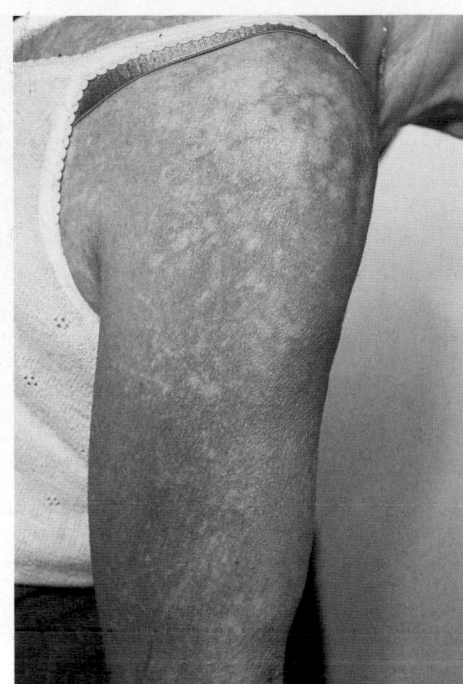

Figure 19.27 Hypo- and hyperpigmented small coalescing patches of pityriasis versicolor.

superficial skin and nail infections of the foot such as those caused by *Candida* and *Scytalidium* spp. may also represent a diagnostic difficulty. The returning traveller from the tropics is often referred to our specialized clinic with severe or recurrent superficial yeast infections by *Malassezia furfur* called pityriasis versicolor (Figure 19.27). This is characterized by small coalescing patches or plaques on upper truncal skin and shoulders showing hyper- or hypopigmentation and furfuraceous scaling.

The diagnosis of dermatophyte infection on the skin is made on clinical grounds. Additional diagnostic measures include direct microscopy of skin scrapings in 10–12% KOH solution,[46] and the identification by culture in Sabouraud's medium of the causative organism. A similar strategy is recommended for the laboratory diagnosis of pityriasis versicolor (malasseziosis) that requires special oily additives for a successful isolation in culture.

Management and treatment

The therapy of choice includes the use of topical and/or systemic azole or allylamine antifungal compounds. Localized infections require topical therapy for 3–4 weeks but cases with intertriginous athlete's foot may require up to 6–8 weeks. Topical steroids are often required to control the inflammatory picture, but are administered only when effective antifungal treatment is already in place. Oral therapy with antifungals is indicated in severe or disseminated skin infections, scalp ringworm and onychomycosis. Triazole and allylamine compounds have a similar efficacy in the treatment of tinea skin and nail infections; however, reports indi-

cate that triazoles induce less adverse side-effects and serious complications. Drug resistance rarely occurs with both groups of antifungals. *Malassezia furfur* infection responds to selenium sulfur topical preparations, ketoconazole shampoo, and other imidazolic or allylamine topical compounds applied for 6 weeks. Cases also respond to oral triazoles; however, recurrence is common. Other therapeutic measures should address the control of symptoms, secondary eczematization and superimposed bacterial infection. Measures of general hygiene and appropriate footwear can be useful to treat and prevent infections; however, the frequency of reinfections, particularly onychomycosis and athlete's foot, is a common problem in the tropics. Superficial lesions and broken skin on the lower limbs can be the port of entry for pyogenic or other bacteria and this is particularly dangerous in patients with diabetes and/or leprosy.

Sporotrichosis

Aetiology and pathogenesis

This infection is acquired by direct inoculation into the skin or subcutaneous tissue of mycelia or conidia from *Sporothrix schenckii*. Inhalation of infective organisms can also produce clinical disease and the accidental exposure takes place outdoors as a result of an accidental or professional contact involving splinters, thorns, straw, wood shavings or other sharp objects. This dimorphic fungus is ubiquitous in nature and lives in the soil, bark of trees, shrubs and plant detritus. This is a disease of temperate humid and tropical areas and represents a risk for travellers. *S. schenckii* has a low pathogenic potential and causes disease by virulence factors that include extracellular enzymes and polysaccharides as well as thermotolerance. The infective structures display a strong acid phosphatase activity and mannan compounds are capable of inhibiting phagocytosis by macrophages.

Clinical findings and diagnosis

Sporotrichosis may manifest as a systemic illness in pulmonary forms but in most cases the disease is limited to the skin, subcutaneous and lymphatic tissues. The upper and lower limbs are the usual sites of inoculation. Following the traumatic episode, the disease manifests with a localized skin nodule involving only the affected limb. This inoculation chancre develops a suppurative and granulomatous infection that remains fixed, or else disseminates proximally via the lymphatic system. Superimposed bacterial infection may occur and verrucous lesions show a tendency to ulceration. The gold standard of laboratory diagnosis is the identification of the fungus in culture, but direct microscopy and histopathological investigations also have some diagnostic value. Recently, enzyme-linked immunosorbent assay (ELISA) using mycelial-phase *S. schenckii* exoantigens has been demonstrated as being a very sensitive diagnostic tool for the serodiagnosis of sporotrichosis and can be used in combination with traditional methods of diagnosis, especially in cases where cross-reactions or false-positive results are seen with the serodiagnosis.[47] Outbreaks in parties of travellers require full epidemiological investigation.

Management

Potassium iodide in increasing daily oral doses from a saturated stock solution is the treatment of choice in the tropics; however, oral itraconazole or intravenous amphotericin B have also resulted in cure in a hospital context.[48] In view of the fact that the disease is acquired by direct inoculation into the skin, preventive measures are of the utmost importance. Protective footwear, clothing and avoidance of skin contact with splinters, rough bark, plant detritus and soil are the most efficient methods to prevent the disease. Activities such as tree-planting, gardening, hay-handling and soil removal carry a risk for infection either by direct skin inoculation or by inhalation of the infective forms.

Eumycetoma

Aetiology and pathogenesis

Madurella mycetomatis, *Pseudallescheria boydii* and *Leptosphaeria senegalensis* are the main aetiological agents of true fungal mycetoma, also known as eumycetoma. A generic term, 'Madura foot', is currently used to describe all forms of bacterial and fungal mycetoma (see 'Bacterial mycetoma' above). Madura foot is divided into eumycetoma caused by fungi and actinomycetoma caused by filamentous bacteria. Even though the term mycetoma suggests a fungal tumor, filamentous bacteria cause the majority of disease cases. The classic clinical triad is the presence of a subcutaneous mass, sinus tract formation, and granular discharge affecting particularly the foot (80% of cases) as well as other parts of the body.[49] Eumycetoma occurs in Sudan, Senegal and Saudi Arabia, particularly in arid or semi-arid regions. Cases also occur in India, Central and South America and in the south of the United States. Infective organisms penetrate the skin of the foot or other exposed regions by direct traumatic inoculation and in the host's tissue the agents multiply and infect adjacent structures. Changes in the fungus cell wall and melanin production are the main virulence factors involved in local pathogenesis.

Clinical findings and diagnosis

Eumycetoma affects predominantly young males between 20 and 50 years of age. It has been estimated that more than 70% of cases with eumycetoma manifest on one foot (Figure 19.28). Other anatomical regions for the accidental, professional or traumatic inoculation include the trunk, face and scalp. The perimalleolar region and the foot dorsum are the most commonly affected sites, but any region of the foot can suffer the direct inoculation of infective organisms. The characteristic clinical signs include a nodule or irregular swelling followed by sinus tract formation and discharge of purulent material containing the characteristic grains. Pigmentary changes of the skin and scarring result from the persistent and chronic inflammatory process over months or years. Periosteal involvement is the starting point of bone resorption, osteolysis and irreversible osteomyelitis.

The epidemiological context and characteristic clinical picture are diagnostic. This is confirmed by direct microscopy revealing pale or black grains that measure between 0.5 and 1 mm contain-

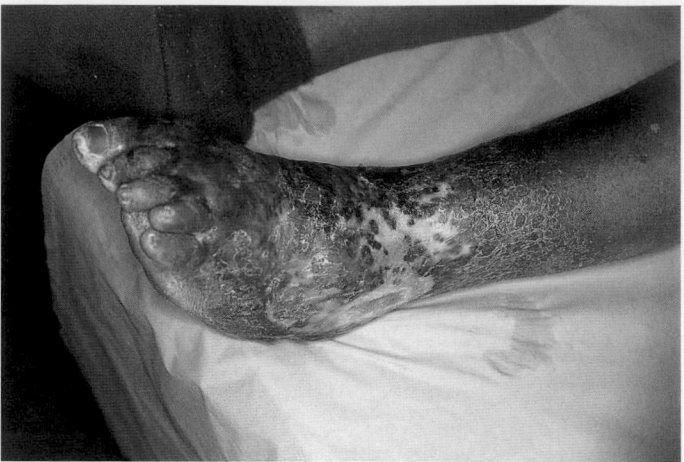

Figure 19.28 Deformity, atrophy, sinus tract formation, scarring and pigment disorder in fungal mycetoma.

ing fungal structures measuring 2–4 mm. This material grows in agar containing glucose and peptone, and the histological sections of deep skin specimens reveal the characteristic and in many cases pathognomonic grains of particular fungal species. Radiological investigation of the affected region discloses periosteal involvement, cortical resorption and osteolysis.

Management and treatment

In eumycetoma, a combination of medical and surgical approaches should be used. Surgical debridement together with medical therapy both before and after surgery is often the preferred therapeutic strategy.[50] Amputation carries the best chance of cure; however, this is disfiguring. Ketoconazole and itraconazole are the mainstays of therapy for eumycetoma.[51] A new azole, posaconazole, though not yet FDA-approved for this indication, has shown promising results in refractory cases.[52] Severe cases with bone involvement can only be cured by radical surgery. Education and use of protective footwear are the main strategies for prevention.

Chromoblastomycosis

Aetiology and pathogenesis

This is a chronic infection caused by pigmented fungi of *Fonsecaea*, *Cladosporium* and *Phialophora* spp. The disease is widely distributed in the tropics and affects predominantly agricultural workers, who acquire the infection through direct inoculation into the skin. Numerous cases have been reported mainly from Costa Rica, Cuba, Brazil, Mexico, Indonesia and Madagascar.

Clinical findings and diagnosis

The initial lesion starts as a papular or nodular inflammatory reaction that subsequently develops a warty appearance. In time, this lesion enlarges at a slow rate and becomes characteristically a large verrucous asymptomatic plaque. The commonest site affected in sporadic infections is the foot and the chronic verrucous plaque appears on the dorsum or the perimalleolar region. The plaque may become very thick in several years, and cause gross deformity of the affected foot. Varying degrees of disability and recurrent secondary infections and/or infestations are a common problem for the foot with chromoblastomycosis. Less characteristic clinical forms include psoriasiform, rupioid and sporotrichoid localized pictures.

The diagnosis is made on clinical–epidemiological grounds and confirmed by direct microscopy and mycological culture in glucose–peptone agar. The histopathology of skin specimens is characteristic, showing acanthosis with a granuloma formation and the presence of typical fungal structures known as fumagoid or muriform cells. ELISA has proved to be a valuable tool for the diagnosis and follow-up of patients with chromomycosis (due to *C. carrionii*).[53]

Management

Several months' treatment with itraconazole is the treatment of choice, often in combination with surgery as it is recognized that chromoblastomycosis is not easy to treat medically.[54] Localized and early cases respond successfully to complete surgical excision of the lesion, and thermosurgery has also been reported of benefit. A new antifungal compound, voriconazole, has shown efficacy in chromoblastomycosis.[55] All patients affected by chromoblastomycosis require follow-up by specialists in mycology, infectious diseases and/or dermatology.

Systemic mycosis manifesting on the skin

Infections by *Coccidioides immitis*, *Histoplasma capsulatum* and *Paracoccidioides brasiliensis* commonly manifest with disease of the lungs, but haematogenous dissemination results in the appearance of skin lesions.

Coccidioidomycosis is acquired through inhalation of infective spores in tropical but also subtropical desert regions of the world, particularly in the American continent. South and western states in the USA and north-western regions of Mexico represent well-recognized endemic regions, and the disease is acquired most commonly in urban areas. Travellers acquire the infection in urban areas where a high proportion of the resident population manifest a positive intradermal reaction on skin testing using coccidioidin. This systemic mycosis presents a risk particularly for the immunocompromised traveller. The skin becomes involved in a small proportion of cases and lesions manifest as erythematous, verrucous, scarring or scaling nodules on the face, trunk (Figure 19.29), upper or lower limbs. A history of exposure in endemic regions followed by an episode of erythema nodosum supports the diagnostic possibility. Other investigations such as serology, chest X-rays and culture for the isolation of the organism confirm the diagnosis. Culture of agents causing systemic mycoses should only be carried out in specialized laboratories as they represent a serious biological hazard. Systemic therapeutic options for coccidioidomycosis include amphotericin B and triazole compounds such as fluconazole and itraconazole, with surgical intervention sometimes being required as an adjunctive measure.[56]

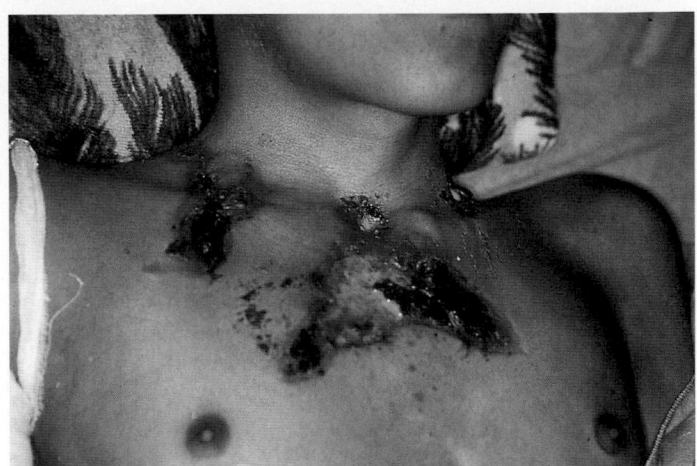

Figure 19.29 Ulcerated plaques and scarring of the trunk in coccidioidomycosis. (Courtesy of Dr Sergio González, Monterrey, Mexico.)

Histoplasmosis is highly prevalent in the American continent but species occur as saprophytes in other parts of the world. This fungus is found in birds' and bats' excreta (guano) and is highly prevalent in caves and abandoned mines. This infection is caused by the dimorphic fungus *Histoplasma capsulatum* var. *capsulatum* (American) or var. *duboisii* (African), acquired by inhalation. Most cases have been reported from the USA, Mexico, Colombia, Venezuela, Argentina and the Caribbean; however, the disease also occurs in the Far East, South-east Asia, India, Middle East, central and southern Africa, Europe, Australia and the South Pacific. Acute or chronic pulmonary forms may be asymptomatic or severe, with high mortality rates. The main differential diagnosis is pulmonary tuberculosis. A low proportion of chronic forms may result in haematogenous dissemination to the skin and mucosal regions, presenting as ulcerations or erythematous exudative nodules (Figure 19.30). Diagnosis is made by history of exposure, clinical picture, chest X-rays, direct microscopy and culture in Sabouraud's medium. Preferred systemic therapeutic agents include itraconazole and amphotericin B.[57] Immunocompromised individuals are at a higher risk for this infection.

Paracoccidioidomycosis occurs in Mexico, and Central and South America, predominantly affecting male individuals who live and acquire the infection in rural areas. Actual evidence of the mode of transmission is incomplete, but the respiratory route seems to be common in acquiring the infection. Following a chronic picture of lung involvement, weight loss and fatigue, the skin of the face, particularly periorificial, or else of other anatomical location on lower limbs, becomes affected. Painful nodular, haemorrhagic, ulcerated and verrucous lesions can be observed covered by a thick crust (Figure 19.31), and severe disability results in advanced forms of the disease. The diagnosis is based on the history of exposure in an endemic region and the clinical picture, supported by investigations to reveal the presence of the typical large budding yeast cells. These can be observed in direct microscopy from skin lesions, bronchoalveolar lavage and H&E preparations for histology, and are easily identified in culture. Effective systemic treatment has been reported with triazole compounds and amphotericin B.[49]

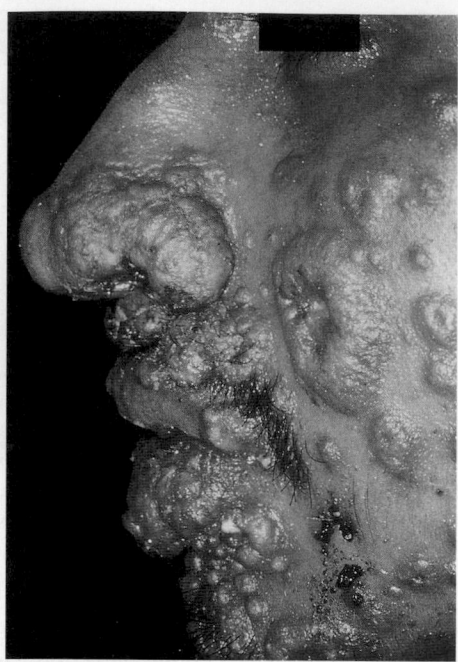

Figure 19.30 Nodular lesions and plaques with exudate on the face in a case with histoplasmosis. (Courtesy of Dr Alexandro Bonifaz, Mexico.)

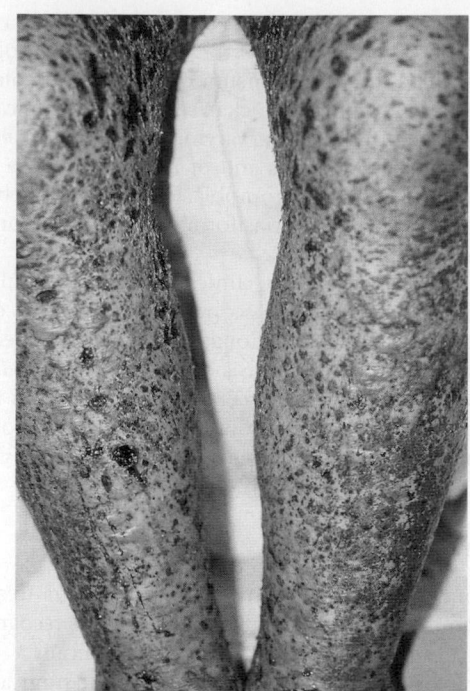

Figure 19.32 Disseminated blistering and crusting in a case of varicella infection.

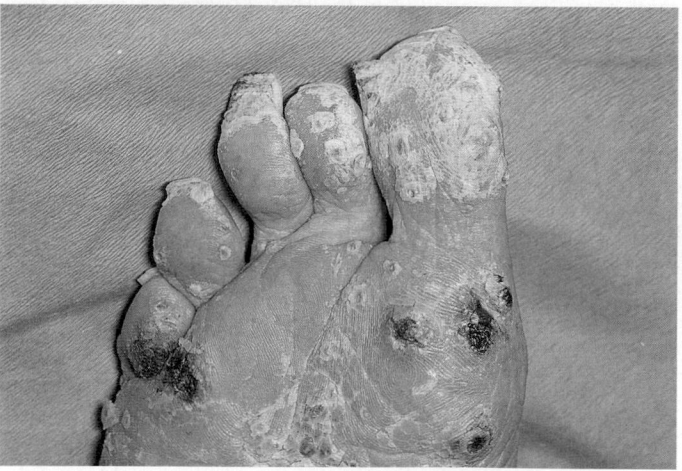

Figure 19.31 Hyperkeratotic, verrucous, ulcerated and crusted lesions on the feet in a patient with paracoccidioidomycosis.

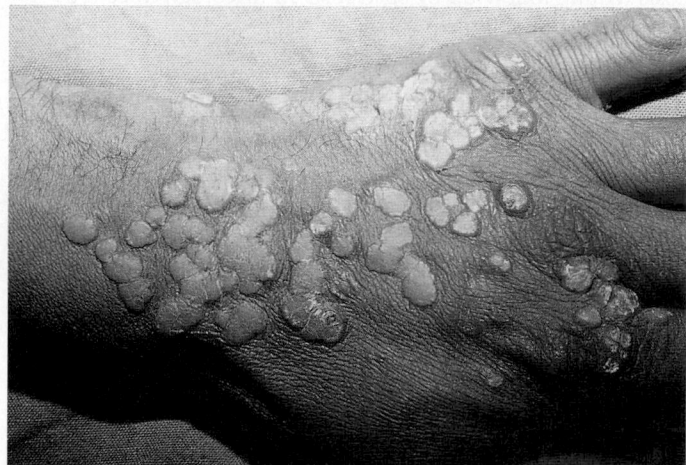

Figure 19.33 Chronic warty plaques on the dorsum of the hand caused by human papillomavirus in a patient with AIDS.

Patients with foot involvement from systemic fungal disease require immediate referral to an experienced hospital physician or specialist in mycology, infectious diseases or dermatology.

DISEASES CAUSED BY VIRUSES

Most common viral skin diseases are cosmopolitan, but the onset may coincide with a trip to the tropics and pose problems in the differential diagnosis of the returning traveller. Viral infections that are prevalent in the tropics include molluscum contagiosum in children, plantar warts in adults, Kaposi's sarcoma in patients with AIDS, and severe blistering forms by varicella (Figure 19.32). Severe cases require a full diagnostic protocol with specimens for culture, electron microscopy, serology and histopathology, followed by specialized treatment in tertiary referral centres.

For the last decade we have observed that 100% of our patients with HIV infection suffer from one or more skin conditions at some stage of their evolution. Severe forms of eczema, seborrheic dermatitis, recalcitrant viral warts (Figure 19.33) or worsening of psoriasis are commonly found in clinical practice. The frequency and number of skin problems increase with progressing AIDS-established illness. In the early to mid-1990s, prior to the introduction of new antiretroviral regimens, skin infections and vasculitis

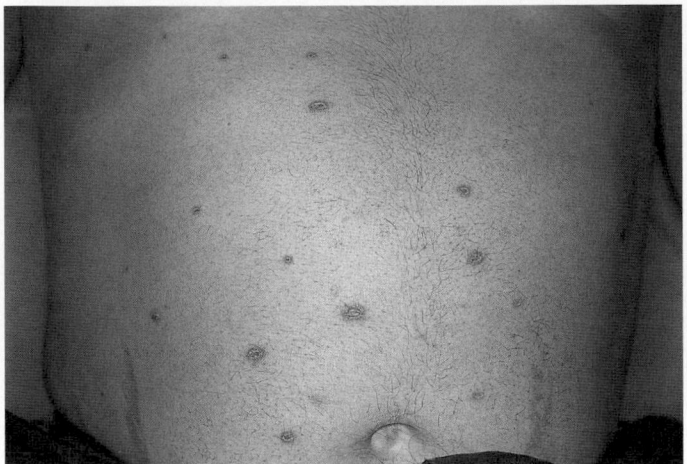

Figure 19.34 Erythematous lesions with central ulceration in cutaneous cryptococcosis.

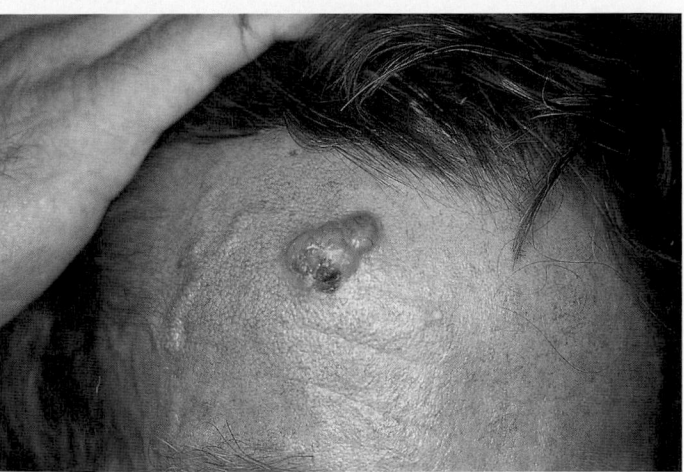

Figure 19.36 Large nodular basal cell carcinoma in a Caucasian patient with AIDS.

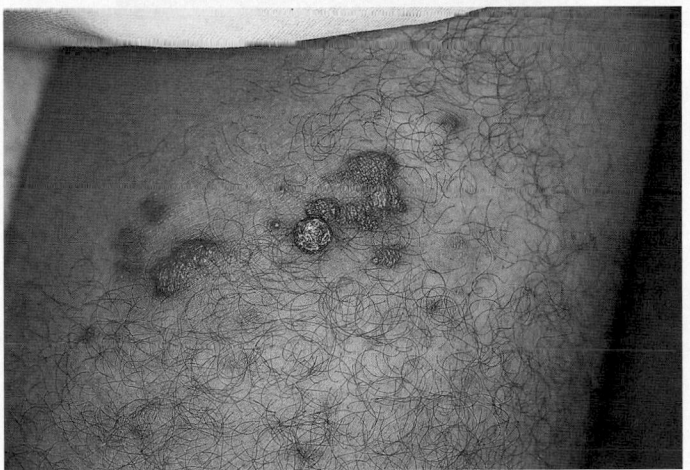

Figure 19.35 Violaceous plaques and nodules of Kaposi's sarcoma in a patient with AIDS.

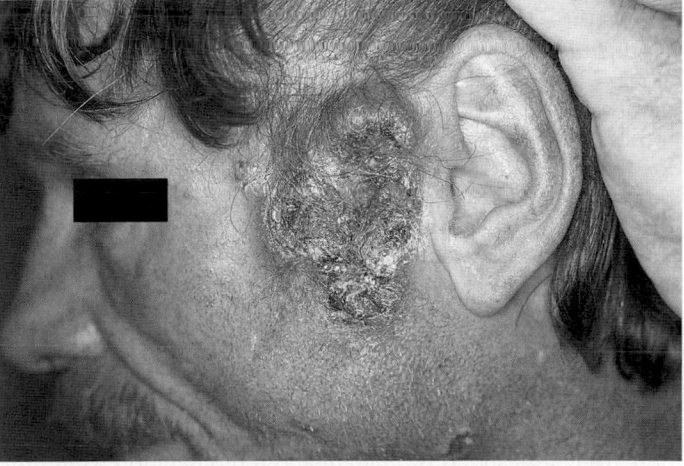

Figure 19.37 Ulcerated and exophytic large squamous cell carcinoma in a Caucasian patient with AIDS.

caused by cytomegalovirus were frequently observed. Severe dermatophyte infections, cutaneous cryptococcosis (Figure 19.34) and Kaposi's sarcoma (Figure 19.35) were more commonly diagnosed as well. However, in recent years where survival is approaching figures found in the general population without HIV infection, skin malignancy is expected to increase, particularly in Caucasian individuals of developed countries (Figures 19.36 and 19.37).

NON-INFECTIOUS SKIN PROBLEMS IN THE TROPICS

Cutaneous disorders in the tropics may vary according to the ethnic background of the patient. It is well recognized that the clinical expression of tropical diseases is dependent on genetic, socioeconomic and environmental factors, leading to a different presentation of common skin diseases and also a different approach to treatment.

Acne vulgaris

Acne vulgaris is the most common skin disease and affects 80% of all people at some time between the ages of 11 and 30 years. It begins from age 10–13 at a time when a child is undergoing puberty. It therefore can have far-reaching psychosocial consequences as well as result in permanent disfigurement.

Aetiology and clinical manifestations

Acne is a multifactorial disorder of the pilosebaceous unit and four pathophysiological interrelated factors are involved: excess sebum production, blockage of the pilosebaceous duct, *Propionibacteriun acnes* and inflammation.

The role of genetic predisposition in the development of acne is uncertain, but it is well known that the number and size of sebaceous glands and their subsequent activity is inherited. In addition, the concordance rate for the prevalence and severity of acne among identical twins is extremely high.

The adrenal glands mature in the prepubertal period and thereby produce increasing amounts of adrenal androgens. Gonadal development adds to this increased androgen production still further. The sebaceous gland contains the enzyme 5α-reductase, which converts testosterone to 5α-dihydroxytestosterone. There is good evidence to suggest that 5α-dihydroxytestosterone increases sebum production. Androgens may also have an important part in controlling ductal hyperproliferation, leading to blockage of the pilosebaceous duct. In addition, patients with acne seem to have decreased sebaceous linoleic acid; such a decrease is known to cause scaling of the skin in animal models and therefore it is thought that abnormal levels of linoleic acid in sebum may enhance accumulation of scale in the pilosebaceous duct and also lead to blockage. Clinically, this excess sebum production and blockage results in the formation of a microcomedone that evolves either into a comedone or an inflammatory lesion. The excess sebum and blockage of drainage is an ideal environment for the proliferation of *Propionibacterium acnes*, which results in the release of pro-inflammatory mediators resulting in the clinical expression of an inflammatory lesion. Therefore one can explain the clinical appearance of acne vulgaris with the comedones presenting as blackheads and whiteheads, and the inflammatory lesions presenting as inflamed papules, pustules and cystic nodules. A patient may have a mixture of all lesions or a predominance of either comedones or inflamed lesions. In the tropics the environment causes increased sebum production, and patients may find either an exacerbation or the first initial presentation of acne when they travel from a temperate zone to a tropical zone. There is a great deal of variation in the incidence of acne throughout the world, with South-east Asians having less sebaceous gland activity and tending to show a decreased incidence of acne as well as it being less severe. Black-skinned patients are more likely to form comedones, and white-skinned patients more likely to have inflammatory acne. It is thought that the pilosebaceous duct is more likely to respond by epidermal cell proliferation within the duct in black patients, whereas in white patients the pilosebaceous duct is more likely to disintegrate and rupture into the surrounding tissue and thereby produce an inflammatory reaction. Patients with black skin may respond to inflammatory acne by forming keloid scars which can result in gross disfigurement. The distribution of acne occurs where the density of sebaceous glands is greatest, namely the forehead, cheeks, chin (Figure 19.38), upper chest and upper back.

Management of acne vulgaris in the tropics

Early treatment of acne is essential for the prevention of lasting cosmetic disfigurement associated with scarring.

For an appropriate and effective treatment plan, the physician should consider: typology of the lesions, skin colour, and type of skin. Patients with oily skin tend to prefer gels and lotions, whereas those with drier skin type may prefer creams.

Mainly comedonal acne

This form of acne is very common in pre-teenage or early teenage years. Treatment at this stage may prevent further development

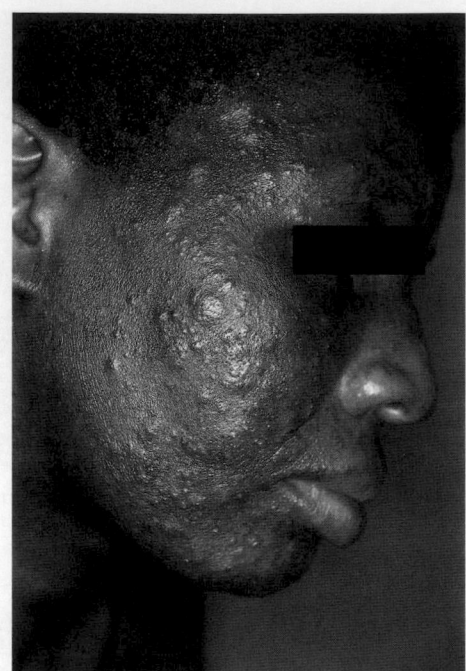

Figure 19.38 Papular, nodular and cystic facial late-onset acne.

of the acne: topical tretinoin or adapalene used once daily at night.[58] We prefer to use retinoids at night as they can photosensitize the skin and therefore are best washed off in the morning before going into the tropical sunshine. Topical retinoids are effective against comedogenesis and may also benefit patients with hyperpigmentation. If such retinoids are not available, salicylic acid up 2% in numerous formulations may be used as a comedolytic and mild antiinflammatory agent. Topical azelaic acid can also be effective. A specific form of comedomal acne that is very common in black patients is pomade acne, due to the application of waxes, greases and oils to the hair, resulting in pilosebaceous duct blockage and therefore comedogenesis. Ideally, the patient should cease from using such materials on the hair.

Mainly inflammatory acne

Mild inflammatory acne may be treated by either 5–10% benzyl peroxide on its own, or benzyl peroxide combined with erythromycin. This treatment is ideal as it is the most effective topical antimicrobial therapy. Topical clindamycin and erythromycin are also effective and can be used twice daily. More severe inflammatory acne will require systemic antibiotics such as erythromycin, tetracycline or its derivatives minocycline and doxycycline, or a combination of trimethoprim plus sulfamethoxazole. Systemic retinoids in the form of isotretinoin are the treatment of choice for severe cases. A 4–6-month course of 0.5–1.0 mg/kg per day causes complete remission in most cases.

Hormonal therapy can be very effective in female patients with acne, whether or not their serum androgens are abnormal. The most used is cyproterone acetate combined with an oestrogen.[59]

Eczema/dermatitis

It has to be appreciated that eczema is not a single disease, but rather a family of conditions. The hallmark of these conditions is epidermal oedema (spongiosis) and pruritus. This epidermal oedema may be caused by numerous factors, both endogenous and exogenous. Traditionally the eczemas have been classified into the exogenous and endogenous forms, although there is a great deal of interaction between the various factors. The main exogenous eczema is contact dermatitis, either primary irritant or allergic contact dermatitis. Primary irritant dermatitis occurs due to the application of a normally irritant substance to the skin and is most often occupationally related. Individuals vary in their susceptibility to such irritation and the vast majority of cases of contact dermatitis/eczema are of the primary irritant type. About a quarter of all contact dermatitis is due to allergy to a specific substance. In this case, epidermal spongiosis occurs due to the occurrence of a type IV hypersensitivity reaction (DTH) to the allergen. In such cases, patch testing has to be performed to identify the appropriate antigen. Endogenous causes of eczema include atopic dermatitis, seborrhoeic dermatitis, varicose eczema, xerotic eczema, discoid eczema and endogenous hand eczema.

Pruritus leads to chronic scratching and the epidermis becomes hyperkeratotic, thickened and more scaly. Acute eczema may have epidermal oedema which clinically manifests as vesicles; if these vesicles rupture onto the surface of the skin, the extracellular fluid accumulates and evaporation of water leaves protein behind, leading to crusting on the surface of the skin.

Atopic dermatitis

A typical atopic individual suffers from some combination of asthma, hayfever, atopic dermatitis and elevated serum IgE. The British prevalence of atopic dermatitis has been estimated to be from 10% to 15% of the population. Interestingly, migrant Asians or Africans tend to first express their atopic dermatitis when they arrive in Britain. Therefore it is thought that the incidence of atopic dermatitis is higher in Asians and Africans living in Britain than the incidence in their original countries of residence. In addition it seems to be a condition of more affluent groups and more common in urban environments than in rural environments.

Aetiology

Over 80% of patients with atopic dermatitis have a personal or family history of atopic disease. Twin and family studies have shown that the inheritance of atopic dermatitis is polygenic and that the clinical expression of atopy is dependent on the interaction of genetic and environmental factors. Currently there is evidence pointing to a genetic linkage between atopy and the IgE high-affinity receptor gene at chromosome 11q13. It is well recognized that there is an increase in both non-antigen-specific IgE levels and antigen-specific IgE levels in atopic dermatitis; therefore, it is postulated that genetic control is responsible for determining the overall risk for allergy and the total level of serum IgE, whereas environmental factors may be more important in determining antigen specificity. However, the immunohistological features of atopic dermatitis are more inconsistent with a type IV hypersensitivity reaction than a type I reaction. Indeed, epidermal

Langerhans cells in clinically involved skin of atopic dermatitis patients have been found to bind IgE. It is therefore hypothesized that cutaneous antigens may bind to allergen-specific IgE on the surface of these Langerhans cells and thereby present such antigens to T helper cells, leading to T lymphocyte activation and the eczematous reaction. The T cells that do proliferate have been found to have a Th2 predominance of clonal T cells, which produce cytokines such as IL-4, IL-5, IL-10 and IL-13. Such cytokines are meant to promote B cell proliferation and further IgE synthesis while at the same time suppressing the Th1 cell-mediated response. This diminished Th1-mediated response is expressed clinically by an increase in susceptibility of the atopic dermatitis patient to viral and bacterial infection. A particularly important bacterial colonization in exacerbations of atopic dermatitis is infection with *Staphylococcus aureus*. Staphylococcal superantigens have been implicated in stimulating a Th2 cell proliferation in the skin and also in inducing resistance to topical corticosteroid therapy. A small section of the atopic population may have reactions to *Malassezia furfur*, as specific IgE antibodies to such an organism have been found. Indeed, in some atopics, exacerbations may be controlled with oral ketoconazole or itraconazole. *Trichophyton rubrum* infection has been similarly implicated. Since fungal infections are extremely common in the tropics, fungal infection is an important factor in the exacerbation of atopic dermatitis and should not be overlooked. Much has been written about the role of food allergy in atopic dermatitis. Most cases of food allergy occur in children under 1 year of age, and almost certainly most children with dermatitis significantly affected by food allergy have lost such an association by the age of 4. Indeed, data from dietary restriction trials have shown little benefit from such manoeuvres in atopic dermatitis. This is important as the nutritional levels of patients in the tropics may already be low and dietary restriction may not only not help the atopic dermatitis but also further diminish the nutritional status of the patient.

Clinical manifestations

Presentation can be very varied or may be classic. When the lesions are characteristic and there is a personal or family history of atopy, a diagnosis is easily made. Most clinical manifestations of atopic dermatitis are a result of the secondary skin lesion caused by the patient continually scratching. The earliest manifestations of atopic dermatitis are dryness and transient redness of the skin. Acutely there is then the eruption of vesicles on an erythematous basis. These burst, leaving a honey-coloured crust on the surface. The accompanied scratching leads to thickening (lichenification) of the epidermis and results in accentuation of the normal skin lines as a result of this scratching. The distribution of atopic dermatitis is bilateral and symmetrical and varies with age at presentation. Infants have involvement of areas that are in contact with the floor by crawling and in areas where the infant can reach to scratch, such as the extensor extremities, the scalp, neck and face. Once the child is over 4 years old, facial involvement is uncommon and such children present with lesions in the antecubital and popliteal fossae, the neck, wrists and the ankles. Adult involvement tends to be flexural and less severe than in infants. In darker-skinned patients constant scratching may produce follicular papules instead of lichenification and it is important to note that in dark-skinned patients all the reaction may be follicular; such follicular papules are commonly found para-umbilically and on the extensor surface of the elbows. Darker-skinned patients may also undergo postinflammatory hyperpigmentation, which may take several years to resolve. The patient should be warned and educated about such pigmentation as it is often a cause of great concern.

Complications

These include eyelid dermatitis, atopic keratoconjunctivitis, anterior subcapsular cataracts, posterior cataracts (probably as a result of chronic corticosteroid usage) and retinal detachment. Abnormal cell-mediated immunity may lead to ocular herpes simplex virus infection and corneal damage. Generalized infection with herpes simplex virus can occur and can be rapidly fatal if not treated. Such an infection is called eczema herpeticum; the patient is unwell with a fever and has the appearance of numerous punched-out erosions on the skin.[60] Atopics are also susceptible to infection with molluscum contagiosum virus as well as the human papillomavirus. Acute exacerbations, as mentioned before, may be caused by infection with *S. aureus*, *M. furfur* and *T. rubrum*.

Management

Avoidance of precipitant factors for pruritus such as heat and perspiration is especially relevant in the tropical environment. Ninety per cent of patients are intolerant to wool and this should be avoided, with plain cotton being the cloth of choice. The most important foods which the patient may be intolerant to are eggs, cow's milk, soya beans, nuts and wheat, but this is more likely to be relevant in a child under the age of 4. There is some evidence to suggest that measures to decrease the amount of house dust mite may be of relevance, but the measures required to decrease them are extreme and the benefits quite marginal.

Topical therapy

Emollients should be used as a soap substitute and to moisturize the skin several times daily. Topical steroids are the mainstays of therapy for atopic dermatitis. They are classified into weak, moderate and potent strengths.[61] The patient is instructed to apply the required strength of topical steroid twice a day until the symptoms have subsided. Topical steroids are then slowly tapered to aim for treatment twice a week. In general, weaker steroids should be used on the face and flexures, with stronger steroids being used on the more lichenified areas. In adults, where flexures are more likely to be colonized by fungi, it may be wise to use a preparation that contains an antifungal component, such as Trimovate® or Daktacort®.

Unfortunately, steroids are associated with telangiectasias, striae, perioral dermatitis (when used on the face), cataracts and glaucoma (when used around the eyes). Tachyphylaxis and systemic absorption can also occur.

In recent years, macrolactams such as tacrolimus (FK 506) and pimecrolimus have been used systemically for the prevention of organ transplant rejection and have proven to be potent immunosuppressive and antiinflammatory drugs. Both agents have been tested topically for the treatment of atopic dermatitis.[62]

Tacrolimus and pimecrolimus are inhibitors of the phosphatase calcineurin enzyme, preventing the dephosphorylation activity crucial for the transcription of numerous cytokines involved in inflammation.

Exacerbating factors such as secondary infections require therapy with antifungals and/or antibiotics.

Systemic therapy

Antihistamines are commonly prescribed in atopic dermatitis; however, there is no role for non-sedating antihistamines in this condition.

Phototherapy with UVA combined with psoralen is called PUVA.[63] PUVA is very effective in atopic dermatitis but requires the use of specialized facilities often not available in the tropics. UVB therapies, both in a broad band and in a narrow band, have been used and are also effective, but these too require specialized equipment. However, one of the advantages of the tropics is that such radiation is freely available and, if cultural factors permit, the patient should be instructed to expose the body to sunlight, beginning with small periods of time such as 10–15 minutes and building up over weeks to 1 or 2 hours.

Azathioprine is reasonably safe and easy to monitor and is commonly used in the treatment of atopic dermatitis, although more extensive controlled clinical trials would aid understanding.[64] Doses of 50–150 mg per day are used and may, in very selected cases, be combined with systemic steroids in short courses.

Ciclosporin has been shown to be highly effective in both childhood and adult atopic dermatitis in clinically controlled trials. It is started at a dose of 2.5–5 mg/kg, and the dose adjusted according to clinical efficacy and safety.

Chinese herbal medicine has been found to be highly effective in atopic dermatitis but it is expensive and is found to be highly unpalatable by many patients. In addition, liver toxicity has been reported.

A promising approch is the use of prebiotics and optimal combinations of probiotics and prebiotics (synbiotics) in the treatment of atopic dermatitis.[65] **Probiotics** are dietary supplements containing potentially beneficial bacteria or yeast, with lactic acid bacteria (LAB). Some lactic acid bacteria, including *Lactobacillus plantarum*, *L. rhamnosus*, *L. casei* and *L. bulgaricus*, have demonstrated immunoregulatory effects that might help protect against some allergic disorders. There is some evidence that some of these probiotic strains can reduce the intestinal inflammation associated with some food allergies, including cow's milk allergy among neonates. Breast-fed infants of nursing mothers given *Lactobacillus* GG had significantly improved atopic dermatitis, compared with infants not exposed to this probiotic.

Contact dermatitis

This is divided into irritant and allergic contact dermatitis. All irritants when applied in sufficient concentration in frequent-enough applications should cause an irritant dermatitis. Therefore, those in professions which require immersion of hands in detergents, chemicals or dyes are more likely to get such a reaction. The commonest irritants are strong acids or alkalis and detergents. In such cases, considered advice about careers has to be given and all measures taken to avoid further irritation. Treatment requires avoidance of irritant or allergen as well as using emollients instead of soap, and topical steroids. A DTH reaction may occur in response to metal such as nickel (Figure 19.39), and fragrances. In Europe there is a standard battery of the commonest allergens in the form of a patch test. Patch tests are applied on a suitable anatomical location for a period of 48 hours and then removed. Any area of redness under each patch is graded as a positive result (Figure 19.40). Patches are then reviewed a further 48 hours later in order to identify a positive reaction. Latex products are commonly involved in contact dermatitis and a type I hypersensitivity reaction with urticaria and angio-oedema.

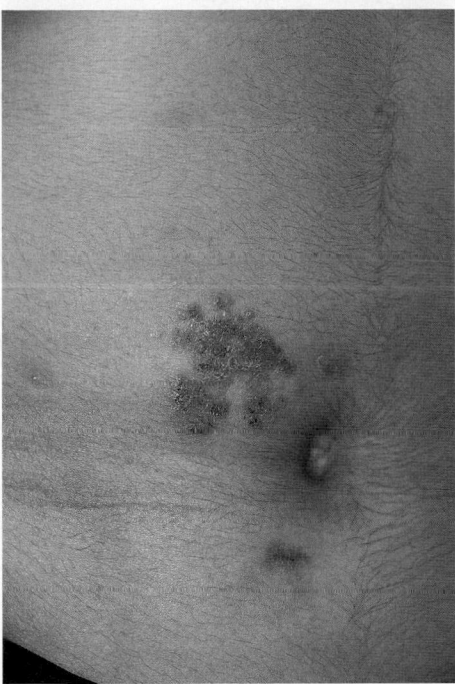

Figure 19.39 Acute allergic contact dermatitis to nickel from the metal button and buckle of blue jeans.

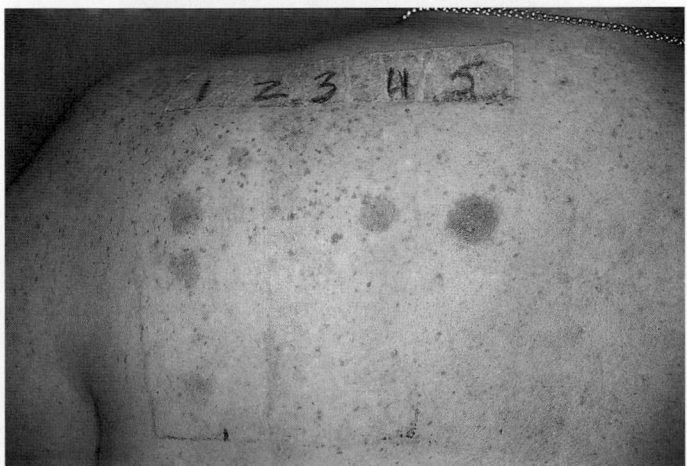

Figure 19.40 Erythema and induration of positive patch testing read at 96 hours.

Pompholyx

This is very common in the tropics, being associated with sweating of the hands and feet. The initial pathophysiological process of epidermal oedema causes superficial vesicles and since the keratin layer of the palmoplantar skin is especially thick they do not burst or form crusts. The condition is variably itchy and begins on the sides of the fingers and may be associated with atopy and other forms of endogenous eczema. Treatment is to avoid sweating of the hands, use of emollients instead of soap, and potent topical corticosteroids. Calcineurin inhibitors have been shown to be effective as well.[66] It should be noted that secondary fungal infection can be a complication.

Discoid eczema

This consists of a bilateral symmetrical itchy eruption. The lesions themselves are rather atypical of most eczemas in that they are well defined and up to 2 cm in diameter. When they first present as solitary lesions they may be mistaken for cutaneous fungal infection. They are commonly found on the arms and legs and vary in the degree of pruritus. There have been no aetiological factors described in this condition and treatment consists of emollients and topical steroids; it tends to respond to the same treatments as atopic dermatitis.

Keloid

The aetiology of keloid formation is unknown, although trauma may play a major part. Keloids are likely to occur after surgical procedures and are defined by their extension beyond the area first traumatized. Clinically, keloids are dense and hard with a shiny erythematous or hyperpigmented surface. The borders are usually smooth and they have claw-like extensions. The commonest sites are the earlobes, upper back, mid chest and shoulders. Symptomatically they can be painful and itchy.

Acne keloidalis nuchae is a chronic progressive keloidal scarring process on the nape of the neck that affects mainly black men. Patients present in their twenties and thirties and often after a short haircut. It is not associated with acne vulgaris. The initial pathophysiological process is follicular inflammation leading to a weak follicular wall and rupture of the hair follicle. This rupture elicits a foreign body inflammatory reaction in the dermis, where scarring leads to keloidal formation. The process may be exacerbated by superimposed infection. Clinically, a follicular pustular eruption is found on the nape of the neck. Unlike acne, comedones and blackheads are not seen. Such a process may cause a scarring alopecia.

Treatment of keloids may be medical and/or surgical. Keloid scars may be excised as long as there is not too much tension on the postoperative wound; however, the patient should be warned that such a procedure has a 50% recurrence rate. They may be shaved down to follicular level and then injected with potent intralesional steroids postoperatively with a single dose, followed up by four weekly injections until control of the scar is attained. Intralesional steroids may be used on their own in order to induce atrophy of smaller scars. Lesions of acne keloidalis nuchae may be excised, injected with intralesional steroid, or shaved with the postoperative injection of intralesional steroid. Active inflammation may also be controlled by tetracyclines combined with a topical dose of a potent topical steroid twice daily.

Psoriasis

Psoriasis is a chronic hyperproliferative condition of the skin of unknown aetiology. It can present in numerous morphological forms and it can affect a few areas up to total skin surface involvement.

Epidemiology and aetiology

Psoriasis is said to affect up to 1% of the whole world's population. Although it was thought to be less common in Africans and Afro-Caribbeans, it is now known that this is not the case, but that psoriasis is often less severe due to the therapeutic effects of a tropical environment. One-third of patients have a positive family history of psoriasis and it is in association with HLA-B13 and HLA-B17. It tends to develop in two different age groups: between 20 and 30 years, and between 50 and 60 years. It is postulated that activated T cells may play a major role in the pathogenesis of psoriasis and this is evidenced by the efficacy of ciclosporin therapy.

Clinical features

In making a diagnosis of psoriasis one has to consider the morphology of each lesion present as well as its distribution and extent of involvement. The condition tends to remit and exacerbate in a chronic manner throughout the patient's life. In some patients it may go into complete remission, whereas in others it may continue in a chronic form. The classic psoriasis lesion is well defined and raised. It has a red colour with a thick white silvery scale on its surface. Clinically, psoriasis may be divided into four general forms:

- Plaque psoriasis (psoriasis vulgaris). This is the commonest form, with involvement of the scalp, trunk (Figure 19.41), elbows and knees, the sacrum and the nails.
- Erythrodermic psoriasis. The skin is red and has a fine scale over the entire surface. There may be small areas of uninvolved skin but the vast majority will be affected. This form commonly arises in a patient with pre-existent plaque psoriasis but may occur as a first presentation. It may also occur as a result of medication with corticosteroids, lithium, β-blockers, nonsteroidal antiinflammatory drugs and antimalarials. The condition can be fatal and the patient should be hospitalized and kept warm, with particular attention paid to fluid and electrolyte imbalance as well as the risk of infection and septicaemia. Etanercept has been demonstrated to be an effective treatment, providing a safe and convenient alternative to current therapies.[67]
- Guttate psoriasis. This is characterized by the sudden onset of pink droplets or flat papules, which appear in crops principally on the trunk (Figure 19.42) and proximal extremities. It is strongly associated with recent or active β-haemolytic streptococcal infection.
- Pustular psoriasis. This may be a localized form on the palms and soles or it may be generalized. The palmoplantar form is

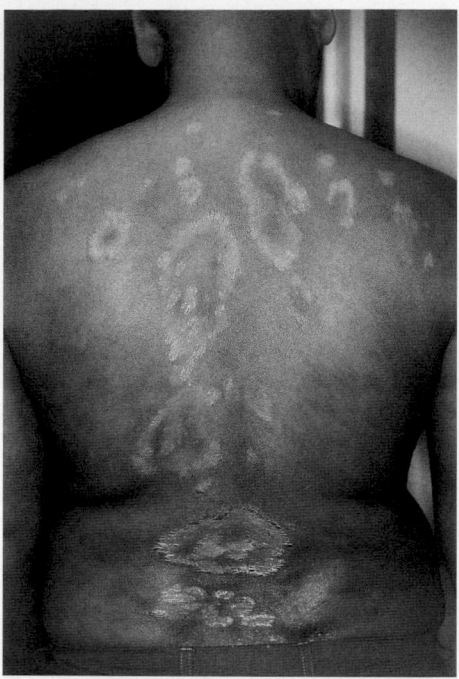

Figure 19.41 Circumscribed plaques of erythema, thickening and scale in plaque psoriasis.

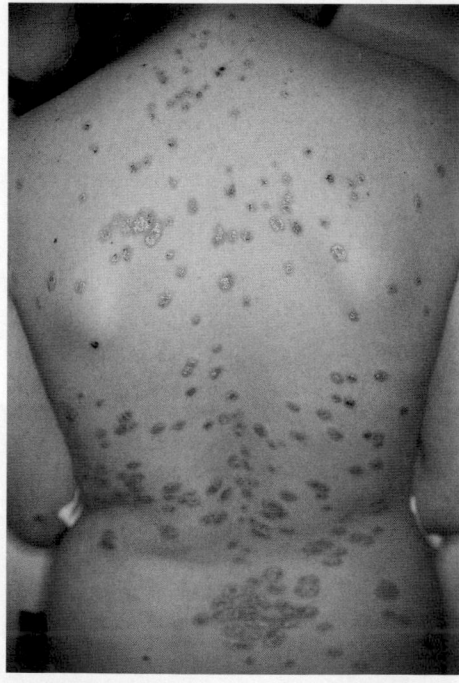

Figure 19.42 Guttate erythemato-scaling small plaques of guttate psoriasis.

relatively common, with the appearance of sterile yellow pustules on an erythematous background on the palms and soles (Figure 19.43). The generalized form can be fatal and it may be precipitated by treatment with corticosteroids or potent topical steroids if they are withdrawn rapidly. In the generalized

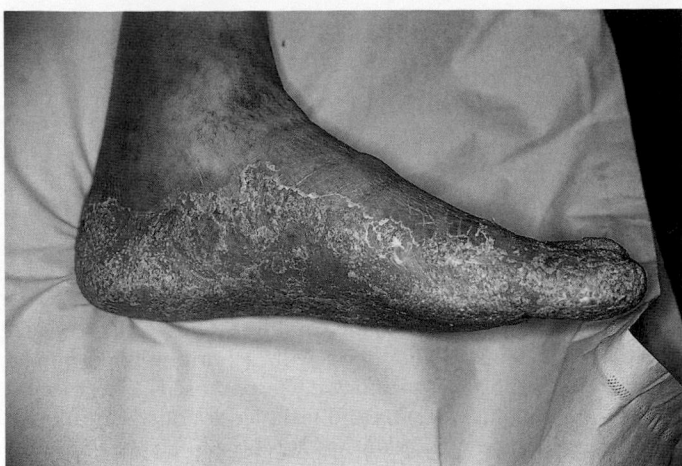

Figure 19.43 Erythema, scaling, hyperkeratosis and pustules in pustular plantar psoriasis.

form there are extensive sheets of sterile yellow pustules, which become painful and sore. The patient may have constitutional symptoms such as a fever and tachycardia.

Psoriatic arthropathy

There are five clinical patterns of joint involvement:

- An arthritis similar in distribution to osteoarthritis, with distal interphalangeal joint involvement and the clinical manifestations of Heberden's nodes.
- Rheumatoid arthritis distribution with involvement of the metacarpal and metatarsal joints.
- Mono- or oligo-arthropathy with one joint being involved, most commonly the knee or ankle.
- Arthritis mutilans. This is a particularly severe form of psoriatic arthritis where the phalanges are eroded leading to telescoping of the skin of the fingers and a destructive arthropathy.
- Sacroiliitis.

Treatment

It has already been mentioned that the tropical environment may be beneficial to psoriasis and all that patients may really need is an extended period of sun exposure. However, there are numerous treatments for psoriasis, reflecting the fact that none of them is a cure. Treatments are often used in combination and tailored to the anatomical distribution and extent of the disease and the availability of therapy. The patient should be instructed to stop using soap on the skin and to use an emollient instead. The patient is always instructed to moisturize the skin regularly with an emollient.

Tar has been used for several decades in a solution of 5%, 10% or 20% in some form of vehicle. A popular vehicle is Lassar's paste. This is applied once or twice daily but has the disadvantage of being extremely smelly and also tends to stain clothing. It can be especially effective in combination with ultraviolet therapy or simple sun exposure. It may be combined with a topical steroid for added potency.

Topical potent steroids should only be used for very small periods of time in psoriasis as rapid withdrawal can lead to a rebound effect with a more severe psoriasis. They are especially indicated for the face or the flexures, and scalp psoriasis.

Dithranol is derived from the bark of the aroroba tree. It has been used in psoriasis for several decades and is often made up in Lassar's paste in different concentrations varying from 0.1% to 1%, with higher concentrations being used for in-patients. The dithranol treatment may be applied for 24 hours and then washed off with arachis oil the next day. Other dithranol protocols require contact for 30 minutes and then the dithranol is washed off. This treatment has several disadvantages and causes erythema and burning, it stains clothing, and the patient's skin tends to have a characteristic staining which lasts for up to 2 weeks. It cannot be used in flexures or on pustular psoriasis.

Phototherapy with PUVA or UVB has been found to be effective in psoriasis. However, such treatment often is not available in the tropics and an alternative is graduated sun exposure if local traditions allow. If psoralens are available locally, a methoxypsoralen may be taken and the patient instructed to expose their skin to sunlight for 30–60 minutes three times weekly.

Calcipotriol is a vitamin D analogue and has to be used thickly twice a day on the psoriatic plaques. It may be combined with a weak topical steroid in order to increase its potency.

Systemic therapy for psoriasis involves the use of agents such as ciclosporin, methotrexate, hydroxyurea and micofenolate. Methotrexate has been highly effective in psoriasis for more than 25 years and is considered the gold standard of systemic therapy. Doses are given weekly, ranging from 2.5 mg to up to 25 mg per week. Baseline liver function tests and levels of procollagen peptide should be performed and monitored throughout therapy. A full blood count has to be performed regularly as methotrexate can cause bone marrow aplasia. Ciclosporin has been shown in a clinical controlled trial to be highly effective in psoriasis but it is very expensive and often not available in the tropics. Systemic retinoids have been used successfully in the form of acitretin at a daily dose of 30–40 mg daily; however, these are expensive drugs that require close monitoring for renal and liver toxicity. Teratogenesis is a main concern.

New developments in genetic engineering and biotechnology have allowed the creation of bioengineered molecules that target specific steps in the pathogenesis of psoriasis and psoriatic arthritis. A number of these agents are currently in clinical trials for psoriasis.

Alefacept (a leukocyte function-associated antigen-3 [LFA3]–IgG1 fusion molecule) and efalizumab (anti-CD11a) block T cell activation. Etanercept (a fully humanized fusion protein) and infliximab (a chimeric [human–mouse] monoclonal antibody) bind tumour necrosis factor-α (TNFα).[68]

Photosensitivity disorders

The photosensitivity diseases are a group of dermatoses characterized by the development of cutaneous eruption after exposure to UVB, UVA and/or visible light. In practice, the results of sun exposure are one of the commonest cutaneous disorders that patients will complain of after having visited a tropical environment. Photodermatoses can be classified into four main groups: idiopathic;

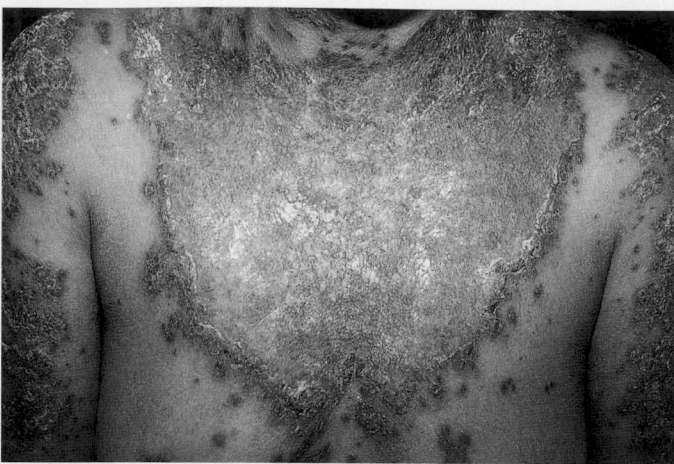

Figure 19.44 Severe erythema and inflammation on the neck 'V' following sun exposure in a case of photosensitive dermatosis.

those due to exogenous agents, such as phototoxicity and photo-allergy; those secondary to endogenous agents, such as the porphyrias; and dermatoses that are made worse by sunlight. The classic photoreactive eruption occurs on exposed sites such as the forehead, nose, cheeks, the V of the neck (Figure 19.44), the forearms and the dorsa of the hands.

Clinical evaluation in photosensitivity

Ask if the condition is photoexacerbated and ascertain the distribution of the eruption, the duration, the age of onset and whether the eruption occurs seasonally. It is also important to assess how much sun exposure is required to produce the eruption, how long after exposure the eruption occurs, and how long it lasts. Clues as to which wavelengths may be causing the photodermatosis may be sought as to whether the eruption occurs through window glass or in the presence of a UVB or broad-spectrum sunscreen. An occupational and social history should be taken to exclude any topical photosensitizers that have been applied. A family history is sought of autoimmune disorder, porphyrias or any genetic disorders. Physical examination has to obtain a description of the distribution of the rash. Morphology is a very good clue as to aetiology, with urticarial plaques being common in erythropoetic porphyria, and solar urticaria with papules, vesicles and plaques common in polymorphic light eruption. Vesicles, scarring and pigment disorder are commonly found in porphyria cutanea tarda.

Polymorphic light eruption

This is the most common idiopathic photodermatosis and it commonly occurs when patients go from a temperate environment to a tropical environment; it can also be caused by change in season within a temperate environment. Its onset is commonly from childhood to late adult life and is more common in women than in men. It is common in all races and skin types. It presents clinically with polymorphic lesions, including erythematous papules, vesicles, nodules, plaques, purpura and target-like lesions. Thankfully, only one type of lesion tends to predominate in any one patient. Unfortunately, it tends to recur indefinitely on sudden

exposure to sunlight. It is crucial that serology be performed to exclude systemic lupus erythematosus. Treatment includes photoprotection by covering up and sunscreens; as topical corticosteroids are only partially effective, systemic corticosteroids may be used for severe flares. UVB phototherapy may be used prophylactically and is to be preferred to PUVA therapy as it has fewer side-effects.[69] Antimalarials are disappointing and azathioprine has been used for severe cases.

Erythropoetic porphyria

This is an autosomal dominant condition with variable penetrance and presents in childhood with a burning and stinging sensation on exposure to sunlight. The photosensitive eruption consists of erythema, oedema and urticated lesions, with blisters only occurring rarely. The skin has a pebble-like appearance on the interphalangeal joint and there may be scar formation. There may be an associated anaemia and hepatic decompensation. The disorder is caused by a partial deficiency of the enzyme ferrochelatase, encoded by a single gene on chromosome 18. Investigations reveal elevated protoporphyrin in erythrocytes, with normal protoporphyrin in plasma, faeces and urine. The treatment is by photoprotection, β-carotenes, and liver transplantation in those who develop hepatic failure.

Porphyria cutanea tarda

This is the most common type of porphyria and is due to defective hepatic uroporphyrinogen decarboxylase activity. Most cases are sporadic, with a small amount being autosomal dominantly inherited. Precipitating factors may include alcohol, exogenous oestrogens, iron and chlorinated hydrocarbons. It may also be associated with hepatitis C and HIV infection. Clinically it presents with skin fragility, vesicles, milia on sun-exposed areas, periorbital hypertrichosis, mottled hyperpigmentation, hypopigmentation and sclerodermatous changes of the hands. Investigations reveal an elevated neuroporphyrin in the urine, and elevated isocoproporphyrin in the stool. Treatment is with phlebotomy, low-dose hydroxychloroquine, colestyramine and erythropoietin.[70]

Drugs that cause photosensitivity

There is a large group of drugs that may cause photosensitivity; the commonest are the tetracyclines, thiazide diuretics and sulfamide compounds.

SKIN MALIGNANCIES

Cutaneous cancer is rare in dark-skinned patients. Historical migrations of lighter-skinned peoples to the more tropical parts of the world have led to a large increase in the amount of skin cancer being diagnosed. Indeed, one of the major hazards of light-skinned people travelling even for short periods to the tropics is in fact skin carcinogenesis. The various skin cancers are easy to diagnose, often by morphology alone, with histology being the gold standard. Most commonly, cutaneous cancers are not fatal; however, those that arise from melanocytes are highly invasive and aggressive and are called malignant melanoma. Therefore it is practical to divide skin cancer into non-melanoma skin cancer and malignant melanoma skin cancer.

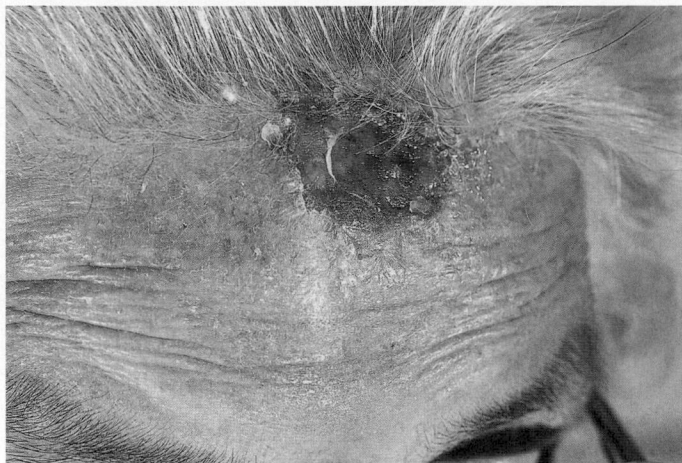

Figure 19.45 Erythema, superficial ulceration and scaling in actinic keratosis.

Non-melanoma skin cancer

The main and commonest groups are actinic keratoses, basal cell carcinomas and squamous cell carcinomas.

Actinic keratoses

These are poorly circumscribed erythematous macules and flat plaques variable in diameter from several millimetres to a few centimetres (Figure 19.45). A scale on the surface is adherent and rough. Lesions arising from the ears, dorsum of hands and forearms tend to be thicker and more hyperkeratotic than those on the face. Some actinic keratoses can be tender or hyperpigmented. Actinic keratoses arising on the lip present as confluent scaliness with focal erosion and fissures and loss of definition of the vermilion border. The natural history of actinic keratosis is controversial, but studies have shown that progression to squamous cell carcinoma is approximately 10%.[71]

Isolated lesions may easily be treated using cryotherapy, with two freeze/thaw cycles required for curative therapy. However, if the lesions are widespread, topical 5-fluorouracil (Efudix®) may be used once or even twice daily to the rough areas for 3 weeks. The patient should be warned that there is an intense inflammatory response as apoptosis of abnormal cells occurs and that this is a normal part of the treatment. The inflammation can be so intense as to extremely distress the patient. The patient should be reassured and, if the areas are painful, a moderate topical steroid may be used in the mornings, with the Efudix® being used at night. A more recent therapy has been the introduction of imiquimod 5% cream, which is a topical medication that up regulates a number of cytokines, which then invoke both a non-specific immune response and a specific immune response. It is applied two to three times a week for up to 4 months, although often 1 month is adequate.[72]

Squamous cell carcinoma (SCC)

This malignant tumour arises from epithelial keratinocytes whose cells usually show some degree of maturation toward keratin formation. The epidemiology of actinic keratoses mirrors that of SCC. The incidence of actinic keratoses and SCC is dependent on the combination of cumulative sun exposure and photosensitivity. Most actinic keratoses and SCCs occur in areas that receive the most solar radiation, with the vast majority occurring on the upper limbs, head and neck. Those with an outdoor job and those living closer to the equator are also more severely affected. The classic SCC is a hyperkeratotic, skin-coloured erythematous papule, nodule or plaque arising on sun-damaged skin. Invasive lesions may have a soft cutaneous extension.

Aetiology

Most actinic keratoses and SCCs will contain mutations of the *p53* tumour suppressor gene. p53 is a negative cancer regulator and normally acts to prevent cells from proliferating uncontrollably. It is hypothesized that ultraviolet radiation causes mutations in the *p53* gene, leading to clonal keratinocyte proliferation in an uncontrolled way. At the early stages of clonal expansion one would see the lesion clinically as an actinic keratosis. However, when the clonal proliferation advances, an SCC would develop.

Metastases and natural history

The actinic keratosis is the initial lesion in a disease continuum that progresses to in situ SCC (Bowen's disease) and invasive SCC. Eighty per cent of SCCs will have a concomitant actinic keratosis giving rise to or in close proximity to the SCC. Such high prevalence of concomitant actinic keratosis and cutaneous SCC suggests a strong correlation between these two lesions. Invasive SCC may grow slowly or rapidly and may metastasize, usually to the regional lymph nodes, with a metastatic rate of 5%, an overall mortality of 3% and a 70% mortality in the metastatic group. Local recurrence and regional metastasis are dependent on treatment modality, previous treatment, location, size, depth, histological differentiation, histological evidence of perineural involvement, precipitating factors other than ultraviolet light, and host immunosuppression. Lesions found on the ears and lip are known to be at higher risk of local recurrence and metastasis. SCCs presenting on the lip have an especially high local and metastatic rate, with 8% of patients presenting with clinically positive lymph node involvement with an overall 5-year mortality rate of 17%. Indeed, combined with poor histology the metastatic rate at presentation can be as high as 23%.

The surgical treatment of SCC requires a 4 mm margin; however, certain tumour characteristics are associated with a greater risk of subclinical tumour extension and include size of 2 cm or larger, aggressive histology – especially invasion of the subcutaneous tissue and perineural spread – and location in high-risk areas, in which case at least a 6 mm margin is recommended. However, carcinomas with a diameter of more than 20 mm involve a much higher risk of recurrence of 9.8%, because of local micrometastases, which require more generous local excision with a safety margin of about 10 mm.

Basal cell carcinoma (BCC)

This tumour is also called rodent ulcer or basal cell epithelioma and is a malignancy derived from the keratinocytes and stroma of the pilosebaceous follicle. BCCs are the most common human cancer, affecting an estimated 750 000 US inhabitants per year.

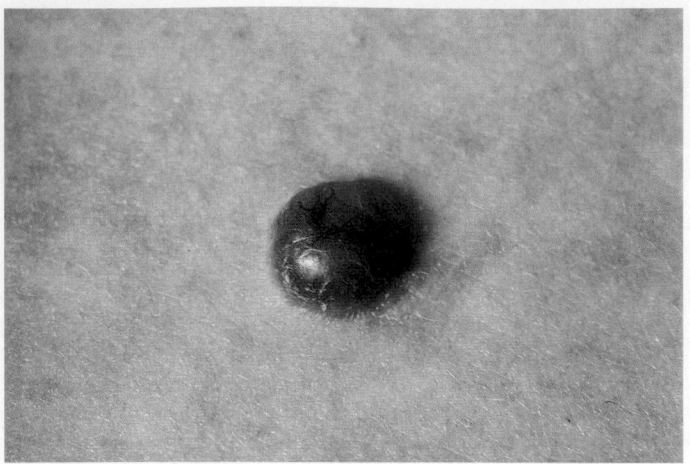

Figure 19.46 Nodular basal cell carcinoma on the chest.

Estimates predict that 28% of Caucasians born after 1994 will develop a BCC in their lifetime.

Aetiology

Epidemiological data implicate UV radiation exposure in BCC tumorigenesis. Sixty-six per cent of BCCs occur on the head and neck. The incidence is much greater in those with fair skin and they occur only very rarely in Africans. Most BCCs present on the face and upper trunk. The inner canthus and eyelids, which are more shielded from sunlight than other parts of the face, are frequently involved. Rare cases of vulval BCC also occur. This occurrence of BCCs in relatively sun-protected sites suggests that other co-factors may be important (Figure 19.46). Arsenic salts are a factor and arsenic-induced tumours are usually multiple and occur mainly on the trunk (see 'Arsenism', below). Molecular studies of the basal cell naevus syndrome and sporadic BCCs have led to the identification of an important tumour suppressor gene – the patched (*PTCH*) gene – which is thought to be crucial in the pathogenesis of BCCs. Inactivation of patched is believed to be a necessary step in the evolution of BCCs.

Metastasis, progress and clinical features

The course of BCCs is slow but steady, and progression results in local destruction of structures if left untreated. In immunosuppressed patients, tumours may be more aggressive. Metastases are extremely rare, with an estimated risk as low as 0.1%. There are six main clinical types of BCC.

- Rodent ulcer commences as a small papule that subsequently becomes nodular and undergoes central ulceration. The margins of the tumour are well defined, slightly raised with a rolled border and with a pearly, shiny appearance. Blood vessels traversing over the margin give it a telangiectatic appearance.
- Pigmented BCC is clinically similar to the rodent ulcer but the margins of the tumour are pigmented. Such pigmented BCCs may easily be mistaken clinically for malignant melanoma.
- Cystic BCC is a well-defined papule which attains a pearly-coloured lobulated appearance with a telangiectatic surface earlier on, with the central part of the tumour ulcerating later on in its evolution.

- Morphoeic (sclerosing) BCC may be difficult to eradicate, as clinically it is often impossible to determine the margins. Indeed, the tumour may have the clinical appearance of a scar; however, the pearly colour is maintained in certain areas of the tumour and telangiectasia is often present.
- Superficial BCC often occurs on the trunk or limbs. It is a well-defined, slightly raised red plaque with an adherent scaly surface. Most lesions are solitary and may be pigmented. Over many years, the lesion may thicken and appear more like the rodent ulcer; however, early on, the margin of the tumour does have a lightly rolled, pearly-looking border with the characteristic telangiectasia present. Such tumours, when multiple, may suggest arsenic ingestion as an aetiological factor.
- Linear BCC is an uncommon variant, first described in 1985. Clinically it is a linear, pearly and telengiectatic lesion and is located most often on the head and neck. On average this variant is thought to belong to a more aggressive subtype with subclinical dissemination.

Diagnosis and management of BCC

The diagnosis of BCC is based upon the clinical findings; however, if clinical doubt exists, a preoperative biopsy is advised. There are four generally accepted methods for obtaining tissue for diagnosis: shave biopsy, punch biopsy, cytology or definitive surgery. Almost all BCCs begin as small, easily managed lesions that can be treated in several different ways, resulting in minimal morbidity and a highly favourable outcome. Treatment by curettage and cautery, surgical excision, radiotherapy, cryotherapy and Moh's chemosurgery all have cure rates of well over 90%. Tumours in certain sites have a greater risk of recurrence, namely the nasae alae, nasolabial fold, tragus and retro-auricular area.

Follow-up

The main aims of follow-up are detection of tumour recurrence, and early detection and treatment of new lesions. Indeed, 36% of patients who have a previous BCC will develop a further BCC. Those especially at risk of BCCs are those with very fair skin and excess sun exposure. These patients with multiple BCCs are found in as many as 20% of such high-risk patients.

Most BCCs that will recur will do so within 3 years. It is a matter of the resources available, whether in an out-patient dermatology department or in general practice, as to how frequent or for how long the follow-up surveillance should be. Obviously, patients with multiple BCCs and at high risk of developing further BCCs should be followed up at least 6-monthly for the patient's remaining lifetime. However, it may not be economically justifiable to follow up every BCC, especially if it is a single isolated BCC in the older age group. One major advantage of regular follow-up is continued patient education regarding sun avoidance.

Malignant melanoma skin cancer

The incidence of malignant melanoma is increasing in developed countries and also in those fair-skinned persons who live in the tropics. Epidemiological studies suggest that sunlight is a major cause of melanoma. Worldwide the incidence of melanoma correlates inversely with latitude, with high rates closest to the equator and lower rates closer to the poles. Although pale-skinned patients are most at risk, rare forms such as the acral lentiginous malignant melanoma are equally distributed throughout all skin types. Five per cent of patients with a melanoma have a family history of malignant melanoma. Other risk factors are the existence of numerous dysplastic naevi, higher than average number of benign naevi, the existence of a congenital naevus, previous cutaneous melanoma, immunosuppression, excessive sun exposure and excessive sun sensitivity. Experimentally, melanocytes demonstrate resistance to UVB-induced apoptosis and therefore are at a higher risk of incorporating UV-induced mutations. Mutations have been found in susceptibility genes such as the *CDKN2A* gene or in genes implicated in control of the cell cycle or maintenance of cell integrity. However, the molecular basis of malignant melanoma still remains to be elucidated.

Metastasis and natural history of malignant melanoma

There is an inverse relationship between tumour thickness and survival. Therefore, the more superficial the lesion at presentation, the more likely is a cure. The thickness of the tumour is defined by the Breslow scale, which is measured in millimetres from the granular cell layer of the epidermis to the deepest tumour cells. Those tumours that have a Breslow thickness of 1.5 mm or less have a 93% 5-year survival rate, whereas those with a Breslow thickness of more than 3.5 mm have a 5-year survival rate of 37%. Metastasis is first to regional lymph nodes and then to lung, liver, brain, bone and peritoneum.

Clinical presentation

Most malignant melanomas appear de novo as pigmented lesions. A fifth of malignant melanomas are thought to arise from pre-existent naevi. Pigmented lesions that are asymmetric, have an irregular border, a variegated or dark colour, and a diameter of more than 0.6 cm and rapid elevation are all signs of malignant melanoma. Although most melanomas are typically asymptomatic, presentation may include itching and bleeding of existent naevi. There are four major types of malignant melanoma described clinically. These are superficial spreading malignant melanoma, lentigo maligna melanoma, acral lentiginous malignant melanoma and nodular melanoma. Lentigo maligna occurs in patients who are over 50 years old and is found mainly on sun-damaged skin of the head and neck. Clinically it appears as an irregularly bordered tan or brown macule which enlarges slowly over many years (Figure 19.47). It is commonly mistaken for another similar-looking lesion that occurs on the head and neck called a seborrhoeic keratosis and may even be mistaken for a solar lentigo. The prognosis of lentigo maligna is extremely good; however, if palpable areas develop within it, this means that this relatively non-aggressive tumour may have developed into a nodular malignant melanoma, which has a far worse prognosis. The superficial spreading malignant melanoma occurs after the age of 40; the lesions often have diameters more than 1 cm and are palpable. There is a great variability in the colour of these lesions, from shades of pink, red, brown and black (Figure 19.48). Since the prognosis of malignant melanoma is dependent on tumour thickness, this tumour has a very good prognosis. However, the appearance of nodular areas signifies the development of a

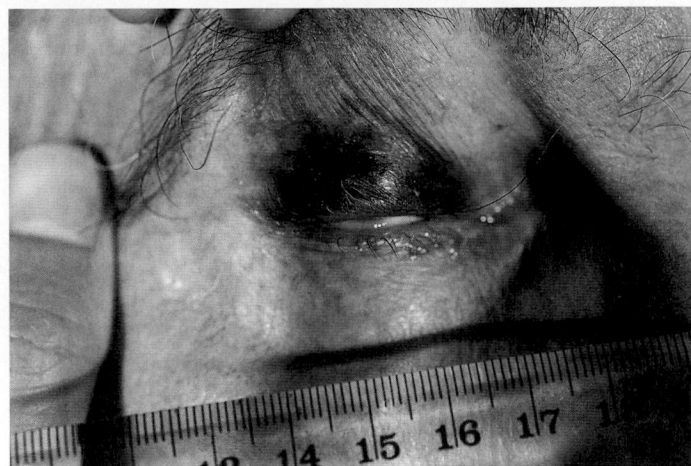

Figure 19.47 Chronic lentigo maligna melanoma on the upper eyelid of an elderly patient.

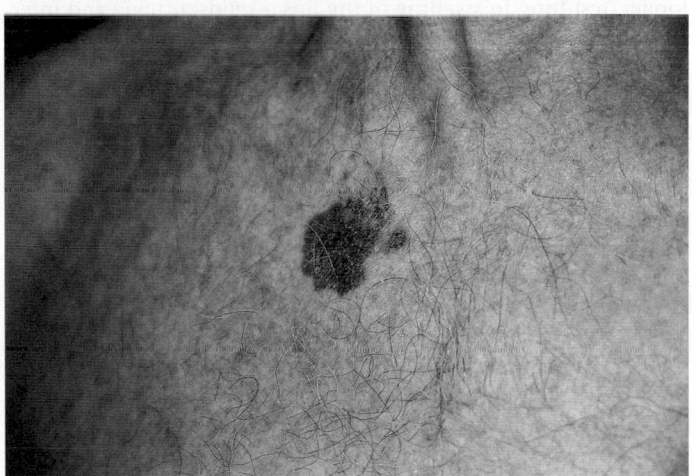

Figure 19.48 Superficially spreading malignant melanoma of the chest.

more aggressive tumour. Nodular malignant melanoma appears as a papule or a nodule and in men commonly occurs on the trunk and in women on the legs. It grows rapidly and is seen to elevate over a few months. Unfortunately this form of malignant melanoma has the worst prognosis. Acral lentiginous malignant melanoma is found on the palms, sole and nail-beds. Although this is a rare tumour, it is of equal incidence in all races and therefore may be seen in the tropics. This form of malignant melanoma has the poorest prognosis and it is vital that it is recognized early.

Management

The definitive treatment for malignant melanoma is excision. This means that diagnosis has to be made early in order to ensure a cure. The margins for excision should be of at least 1 cm and should include subcutaneous fat for thin melanomas of less than 1.5 mm. However, for the lentigo maligna a 2–5 mm margin of clinically normal skin should be sufficient. In cases of thick melanoma of 1.5 mm or more, it is suggested that a 2 cm margin of normal skin be used to ensure complete excision. Once the melanoma has metastasized there are no known therapies at present which affect long-term prognosis.

URTICARIA

This is a family of conditions characterized by the appearance of itchy wheals. Internationally, prevalence is thought to be as high as 20%. Clinically it can be divided into acute and chronic urticaria. The lesions themselves are transient and in the Caucasian patient they may be pink or red skin swellings surrounded by erythema. Such erythema and skin redness may not be apparent in the darker-skinned patient. The lesions vary considerably in shape and size and can occur anywhere on the body (Figure 19.49). By definition, an urticarial attack will last less than 24 hours. Another associated condition called angio-oedema may co-exist with urticaria and in this case the oedema is actually deeper in the dermis and subcutaneous tissues. The lesions last longer, resulting in swelling of the lips, eyelids, tongue and internal organs.

Acute urticaria

This is defined as urticaria occurring for less than 6 weeks. The commonest cause of acute urticaria is the ingestion or parenteral administration of drugs. The commonest involved drugs are antibiotics, sedatives, tranquillizers, analgesics, laxatives and diuretics. The pathogenesis of this process is thought to be IgE mediated, in which case they would need to be preformed IgE to the exposed allergen. However, drugs may cause acute urticaria in a non-immunological way, with opioid-type drugs being thought to release mast cell histamine by a direct mechanism. Other drugs such as aspirin and non-steroidal antiinflammatory drugs may also cause an acute angio-oedema. A minority of patients may have a food allergy and the commonest substances are nuts, fish, shellfish, eggs, milk, chocolate, tomatoes and certain food additives such as tartrazine and benzoic acid derivatives. When a patient's urticaria appears during spring and summer, the role of inhaled allergens such as pollens and spores should be considered as a cause of acute urticaria. Certain infectious agents such as viral infections and streptococcal pharyngitis in children may also cause a transient urticaria over weeks. The commonest acute contact urticarial reaction is to latex. This is especially a problem in healthcare workers, in which case non-latex gloves should be used.

Any possible precipitants or exacerbation factors such as drug therapy should be removed. The patient should be started on a non-sedating antihistamine and this is usually sufficient to treat an acute urticaria. If the patient is non-responsive to treatment or the whealing attacks seem to last longer than 6 weeks, then the patient should be treated as if they have a chronic urticaria.

Chronic urticaria

This is said to occur when whealing attacks last more than 6 weeks. By far the largest group are of the chronic idiopathic form with no immediate cause found. However, a careful history and examination should be carried out and appropriate tests performed in order to elicit a possible cause. The chronic urticarias may be divided into the physical urticarias, chronic idiopathic urticaria, angio-oedema and urticarial vasculitis.

Physical urticaria

This may be caused by physical pressure (Figure 19.50), vibration during exercise, periods in a hot environment, periods of cold and cooling of the skin, in response to sunlight, or aquagenic urticaria, where the wheals occur in response to contact with water. In most cases the type of physical urticaria can be elucidated by the detailed history, with pressure urticaria occurring under tight clothing and cholinergic urticaria occurring at times of emotion and sweating. Patients with cold urticaria may complain of lesions as soon as they exit a hot bath. Solar urticaria is very rare and occurs in response to natural or artificial sunlight. Cold urticaria may be tested for by placing an ice cube on the skin for 10 minutes and then observing a wheal appearing 5–10 minutes later.

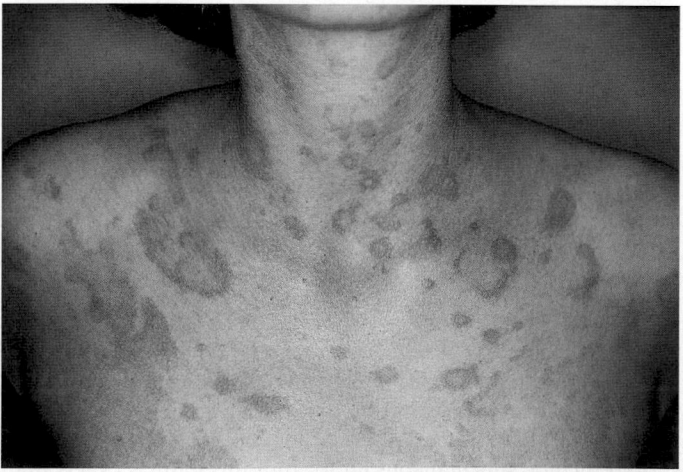

Figure 19.49 Pruritic urticarial wheals on the trunk.

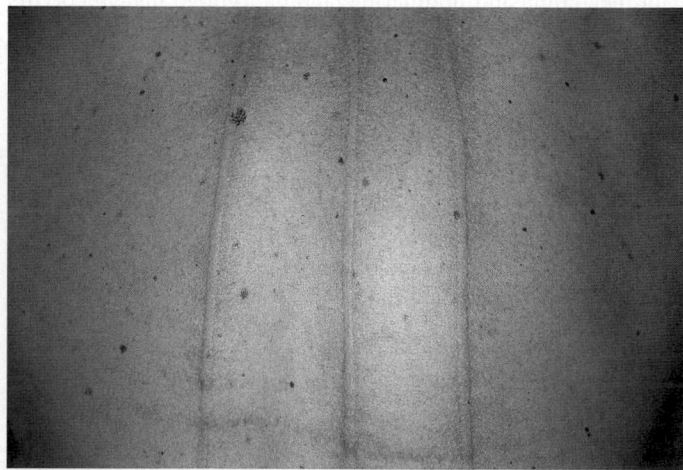

Figure 19.50 Pressure urticaria or dermographism.

Chronic idiopathic urticaria

This is a diagnosis made once all the previous aetiological factors have been excluded. However, in the tropics, common causes of long-standing urticaria may be hookworm, tapeworms and roundworms, and thus the stools should be examined in such patients. In addition the patient should be examined for evidence of trichinoses, dracunculosis, lymphatic filariasis and strongyloidiasis. A small minority of patients labelled as having chronic idiopathic urticaria may in fact have circulating histamine-releasing autoantibodies. In such patients, autologous serum injected intradermally produces an intense whealing reaction. Recent associations have been found with *Helicobacter pylori* infection and its eradication can lead to dramatic improvement in such urticaria.[73]

Angio-oedema

This is a deeper form of urticaria and may be associated with urticarial wheals. It results in swollen lips, eyelids, tongue, hands and feet, with involvement of the upper airways causing respiratory arrest and fatal respiratory failure. Less than 1% of cases of angio-oedema may be hereditary, in an autosomal dominant fashion, in which case a plasma complement C4 should be measured; if this is low, more detailed investigations of C1 esterase activity should be instituted.

Urticarial vasculitis

The lesions in this case may be painful and last for several days. Such an urticarial vasculitis should be investigated histologically and the biopsy should include both lesional and non-lesional skin. Biopsy will show a vasculitis or a leukocytoclastic vasculitis. A leukocytoclastic vasculitis is more likely to be associated with systemic diseases such as the autoimmune connective tissue diseases and the oral and parenteral administration of drugs.

Management of chronic idiopathic urticaria

Any identifiable causes should be removed and the patient should be educated to avoid drugs that may cause histamine release, such as aspirin, non-steroidal antiinflammatory drugs and the opioid drugs. The patient should be started on a non-sedating antihistamine; if there is a poor response, a further sedating antihistamine should be added at night. If the patient still has not responded, an H_2 antagonist such as cimetidine may be added. Resistant forms of urticaria may need short courses of systemic steroids and patients with hereditary angio-oedema or severe angio-oedema may need adrenaline (epinephrine) pens for emergency situations. Refractory cases may require immunosuppression with ciclosporin, intravenous immunoglobulin and even, in extreme cases, plasmapheresis.

OTHER NON-INFECTIVE DERMATOSES MAINLY LIMITED TO THE TROPICS

Arsenism

Although arsenic was commonly used in medications in the past, this had stopped by the first half of the twentieth century. Today, arsenic is widely used in its inorganic form in insecticides, fungicides, herbicides, and in the manufacture of glass and fireworks. Inorganic arsenic compounds exist in the form of arsenites and arsenates. Arsenites are thought to be the most toxic; such arsenites are normally detoxified in the liver and excreted in the urine. However, this detoxification process may be subject to genetic polymorphisms, resulting in the inability of a proportion of the population to detoxify arsenite, and thereby cause carcinogenicity and toxicity in humans. The commonest form of arsenism is now due to water contamination and cases have been reported in Chile, Taiwan, Mexico, Argentina, Thailand and the Ganges delta in India. Cutaneous changes begin with hyperpigmentation in the groin and areolae. These hyperpigmented areas may develop hypopigmented areas within them, giving rise to a characteristic raindrop appearance. As many as 30% of patients may have pigmentation in the oral cavity. Hyperkeratotic papules on the palms and soles occur in up to 70% of patients; patients may have an associated cutaneous malignancy such as Bowen's disease, BCC, SCC or keratoacanthomas. These tumours mainly occur on sun-exposed sites and suspicion of arsenism should be aroused as such tumours are rare in dark-skinned patients. The clinical management of these patients needs careful long-term monitoring for the development of cutaneous neoplasm and also associated internal malignancy. The hyperkeratotic areas on the palms and soles may be treated by a 10% salicylate ointment twice daily. In more affluent areas, systemic retinoids may be given to prevent the onset of cutaneous malignancy.

Brazilian pemphigus foliaceus (fogo selvagem – wild fire)

This is an autoimmune bullous dermatosis. It is characterized by antibodies to the epidermal desmosomes, specifically desmoglein 1 (Dsg1). It is clinically identical to the non-endemic form of pemphigus foliaceus, which is found throughout the world. Pemphigus foliaceus itself is a variant of pemphigus vulgaris, which is one of the commonest forms of blistering disease causing intraepidermal vesicles. Fogo selvagem, unlike the non-endemic form of pemphigus foliaceus, is endemic to certain regions of Brazil and some areas of Colombia, Bolivia, Paraguay and Argentina. It is associated with recent areas of colonization and cases tend to decrease with increasing urbanization. The sex and race incidence is the same within an endemic area. The vast majority of patients live near rivers and within flying range of black flies (*Simulium pruinosum*). Clinically, the lesions of fogo selvagem are superficial vesicles which can be mistaken for impetigo. The blisters rupture easily, leaving superficial erosions. The lesions begin on the face, scalp, upper chest and abdomen, and then spread to the limbs. Unlike in pemphigus vulgaris, oral or mucosal lesions are extremely uncommon in pemphigus foliaceus and fogo selvagem. The dermatosis evolves gradually over a period of several weeks or months. Fogo selvagem may present as a localized form of disease in which the seborrhoeic areas of the face and trunk are involved and this may lead to diagnostic confusion with discoid lupus erythematosus, but patients with fogo selvagem have no positive lupus serology and can be distinguished by skin biopsy. The localized form may stay localized or eventually become generalized. Patients with generalized fogo selvagem may present in one of three ways: an acute aggressive form; those with exfoliative erythroderma; and a more slowly aggressive form. Patients with the acute aggressive form have a predominance of blisters and it may be associated with fever, arthralgias and malaise. It is thought that patients who have this form of disease are susceptible to life-threatening herpes simplex virus infections. In those patients who develop exfoliative erythroderma the main clinical lesions are superficial erosions and crusting. The third form includes those patients in whom localized fogo selvagem has become generalized and clinically consists of keratotic plaques and nodular lesions in the seborrhoeic and acral areas. There is a rarer, hyperpigmented, form of fogo selvagem which often occurs when the patient is recovering from fogo selvagem after treatment.

It is especially important that this condition is diagnosed early in childhood as delay in diagnosis can lead to dwarfism and azoo-spermia as an adult. It is thought that fogo selvagem may also have psychiatric effects and may be associated with depression. This form may be differentiated from non-endemic pemphigus foliaceus by distinct epidemiological features. It may be distinguished from pemphigus vulgaris due to its lack of oral lesions. The gold test for diagnosis is indirect and direct immunofluorescence for Dsg1. However, if such investigations are not available, a Tzank smear may show acantholytic cells suggestive of fogo selvagem. Skin biopsy may also suggest the diagnosis.

Management

Left untreated, 40% of patients die within 2 years. High-dose systemic steroid is the treatment of choice and is slowly tapered in dosage according to response. Steroid-sparing agents such as azathioprine are useful and cyclophosphamide has been used with good results. Useful adjunctive therapies include antimalarials and dapsone. An important consideration before starting systemic corticosteroids is to rule out the possibility of concurrent tuberculosis. Fatal cases of disseminated strongyloidiasis have also been reported after steroid therapy for this condition.

Amyloid and amyloidosis

Amyloidosis is the abnormal extracellular deposition of a group of unrelated proteins that may show green birefringence on Congo red staining when viewed under polarized light. Light microscopy shows amyloid to be an amorphous homogeneous eosinophilic material. Electron microscopy shows it to be made of linear non-branching paired fibrils of protein arranged in a loose meshwork. Cutaneous lesions are common in patients with primary amyloid and myeloma-associated systemic amyloidosis. They may occur in up to 40% of patients. Clinically, these consist of waxy purpuric lesions on the skin and mucosae and should result in an investigation for a plasma cell dyscrasia. Associated features include carpal tunnel syndrome, macroglossia and hepatomegaly.

Cutaneous involvement in secondary systemic amyloidosis is uncommon, but, when it does occur, presents with petechiae, purpura and ecchymoses occurring spontaneously after minor trauma and is the result of amyloid infiltration of blood vessel walls. Purpuric lesions are likely to be found in flexural regions such as the eyelids, nasolabial folds, neck, axillae, umbilicus and anogenital area, as well as orally. A third form of amyloidosis is the group of localized cutaneous amyloidosis. This may present

Figure 19.51 Pruritic plaque of lichen amyloid on the shin.

as a nodular localized cutaneous amyloidosis, lichen amyloidosis or a macular amyloidosis.

Nodular localized cutaneous amyloidosis

This is uncommon and presents with single or multiple lesions on the limbs, face, trunk or genitalia. Clinically, the lesions may be identical to those of plasma cell dyscrasia and systemic amyloidosis. The lesions may vary in size from a few millimetres to several centimetres. Some patients develop a paraproteinaemia and overt systemic amyloidosis.

Lichen amyloidosis

This presents with an itchy eruption of multiple discrete hyperkeratotic papules distributed on the shins that coalesce to form plaques (Figure 19.51). Rarely, lesions may be found on the calves, ankles, dorsa of the feet and the thighs. There has been a great deal of debate as to the aetiology of lichen amyloidosis, with some researchers finding Epstein-Barr virus using in situ hybridization within the keratinocytes. It is also thought that it may occur as a result of an abnormal reaction to scratching, as most people with lichen amyloidosis have concomitant lichenified eczema around the plaques. Indeed, treatment with steroids, which decreases the itch, tends to improve the condition, although only minimally.

Macular amyloidosis

This is an itchy eruption of dusky brown-greyish macules, symmetrically distributed on the upper back and limbs. After constant scratching, the macules assume a rippled appearance. Macular amyloidosis and lichen amyloidosis may co-exist, leading to the hypothesis that they are the result of a single pathological process. Lichen amyloidosis is commoner among Chinese, whereas macular amyloidosis is commoner among Central and South Americans, Middle Easterners and South Asians. Familial cases have been described.

Treatment

Deposits of nodular primary localized cutaneous amyloidosis can be treated surgically, but they may recur locally. Lichen amyloidosis and macular amyloidosis are treated with a topical steroid, mainly under occlusion, but results are disappointing. There has been some success using dermabrasion as well as topical dimethylsulfonamide and systemic retinoids. However, none of these treatment methods totally eradicates lesions, which can recur.

Lichen planus and lichenoid eruptions

Lichen planus is a relatively common disease with a worldwide dermatology referral prevalence of 1–2%. The classic lesion presents on both skin and mucosae. Cutaneous lesions present with flat-topped, polygonal, pruritic shiny papules with a violaceous hue. In darker skin, purple, brown or black are more typical colours than violet (Figure 19.52). Postinflammatory hyperpigmentation is prominent and persistent in darker-skinned patients. It is thought that lichen planus itself is more common in darker-skinned patients. Variants of classical lichen planus include hypertrophic, atrophic and linear lichen planus. Classical lichen planus begins most frequently on the limbs, especially around the ankles and wrists, and a quarter of cases have involvement of the oral cavity, which may present in the form of white Wickham's striae or as erosive painful lesions (Figure 19.53). A quarter of patients have truncal involvement and a small number (5%) have face and neck involvement. The two types of lichen planus which are most relevant to the tropical physician are hypertrophic lichen planus and actinic lichen planus.

Hypertrophic lichen planus

This presents with red, brown or violaceous lichenified verrucous plaques which are extremely itchy. The lesions primarily occur on the lower legs and ankles. It is especially common in inhabitants of southern India and Sri Lanka.

Actinic lichen planus

This occurs in a photodistribution (see section on 'Photosensitivity disorders', above) and is induced by sun exposure. In countries such as India, actinic lichen planus forms as little as 5% of all cases of lichen planus, whereas in the Middle East it can be as high as 30–40% of cases. The main group of patients that are affected are children and young adults. There are three clinical presentations: annular, dyschromic and pigmented. The commonest form is the annular type, which presents as brownish plaques with an annular configuration, most commonly affecting the lateral aspects of the forehead, dorsum of the hands, forearms, lower lip, cheeks and the V-shaped area of the neck. With time, the annular lesion develops hypopigmentation centrally and some subtle atrophy. This form of lichen planus typically occurs in dark-skinned individuals, with women being affected more than men and occurring at a younger age of onset than classic lichen planus. It is not associated with positive autoimmune serology.

Treatment

Spontaneous remissions of cutaneous lichen planus occur in up to 70% of cases after 1 year. However, oral lesions tend not to resolve spontaneously, with the erosive form remission rate being as low as 3%. Other forms of oral involvement may last about 5 years and then resolve; however, such resolution only occurs in up to 40%.

Precipitant factors such as scratching or sun exposure should be avoided and patients advised to use a broad-spectrum, high factor sunscreen. Topical steroids, topical steroids with occlusion, and intralesional steroids are all used. Systemic steroids may be used when lichen planus is acute in onset and rapidly progressive. However, it is not recommended for long periods of treatment. Systemic retinoids have been used successfully in widespread lichen planus, as have ciclosporin, dapsone and antimalarials. Actinic lichen planus has been reported to respond particularly well to systemic antimalarials. Hypertrophic lichen planus can be treated with intralesional steroids and topical steroids under occlusion. The authors find that a potent steroid combined with 5% or 10% salicylate is particularly effective applied twice a day for a period of at least 4–6 weeks. Oral lichen planus, especially if it is erosive, will particularly require systemic treatments. Phototherapy can be used to treat most cutaneous forms of lichen planus apart from actinic lichen planus.

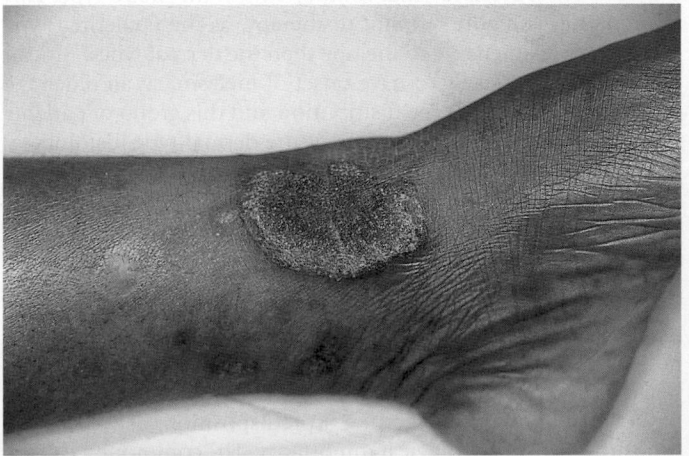

Figure 19.52 Isolated papules and large plaque of lichen planus with Wickham's striae.

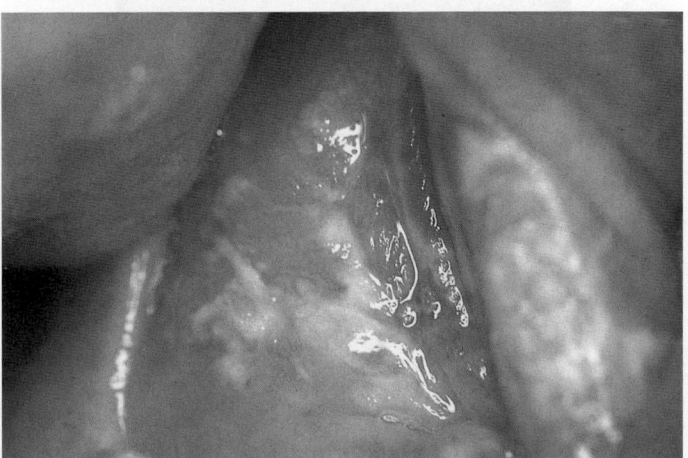

Figure 19.53 Erosive oral lichen planus.

Disorders of pigmentation

The majority of the world's population is brown skinned and therefore hyper- or hypopigmentation is of major concern to dermatologists worldwide and to tropical physicians. Inflammatory disease of the skin is extremely common and therefore postinflammatory hyperpigmentation is also common. The unfortunate and widespread use of depigmenting creams in Africa and parts of Asia in order to lighten the complexion has led to significant morbidity and in some cases permanent disfigurement. Treatment for hyperpigmentation disorders is difficult and prolonged and requires a great deal of patience and patient education.

Vitiligo

This is a condition characterized by the complete loss of pigment within skin. Initially it was thought that vitiligo was more common in dark-skinned patients, but it is much more likely that vitiligo is more clearly seen in such patients and therefore they are more likely to present. Males and females are equally affected and the condition most commonly occurs in the first to third decades, with congenital cases being described. It is thought that the aetiology of vitiligo is autoimmunity, because of its strong association with organ-specific autoimmune disease. Depigmentation starts suddenly, with the commonest sites being the hands, feet, genitalia, and periocular and perioral areas of the face. The pigmentation may form a generalized symmetrical pattern or a segmental pattern which follows a dermatome, and it ceases to progress after a year (Figure 19.54). The focal form may be an isolated lesion which progresses slowly. Vitiligo is usually symptomless but some patients may complain of pruritus. Diagnosis is clinical and confusion can sometimes be with pityriasis versicolor, postinflammatory hypopigmentation, scleroderma and lichen sclerosus et atrophicus.

Management

Unfortunately, due to the slow mobility of melanocytes, treatment of vitiligo can last more than a year. Melanocytes migrate from the margins and also from hair follicles. Therefore, when repigmentation occurs, it is around hair follicles and the periphery of the lesion. Unfortunately, most of the therapies for vitiligo are largely unsuccessful. However, potent topical steroids may cause repigmentation in between 15% and 55% of patients. A commonly used treatment is an oral psoralen with exposure to UVA radiation; this is, however, a prolonged treatment and risks the development of skin cancers in the depigmented areas. A newly developed treatment called narrow-band UVB has been found to be up to 60% successful in vitiligo.[74] Surgical treatments include minigrafting with melanocytes.

Melasma

There are three patterns of melasma that are recognized clinically: centrofacial, malar and mandibular. The lesions themselves are often symmetrical, uniformly hyperpigmented, sharply defined macules and patches on the face. They mainly occur on areas that are sun exposed, such as the upper lip, cheeks and forehead. Rarely, melasma can be more widespread, affecting the chest, upper back and the sun-exposed side of the arms. The centrofacial variant consists of lesions on the cheeks, forehead, upper lip, nose and chin, whereas in the malar variant the lesions are found on the cheeks and nose. When lesions are found on the ramus of the mandible, this is described as the mandibular distribution.

Melasma may be further subdivided into three different histological types. An increase predominantly in the basal and superbasal epidermis of melanin occurs in the epidermal type. In the dermal type there are melanin-laden macrophages in the superficial and deep dermis, with some of these melanin-laden macrophages being found in a perivascular distribution. The mixed type shows a histology that is a mixture of the previous two types. Clinically, the epidermal type of melasma is accentuated by Wood's light examination of the skin. Wood's light accentuation only occurs on the epidermal components in the mixed type. This examination is highly relevant to therapy, as the epidermal type is much more amenable to therapy than the dermal types. African women are more likely to have onset of melasma at an older age and to have the malar type distribution and this group of patients may also have a higher incidence of the dermal-type histology.

Epidemiology and aetiology

Ninety per cent of affected patients are women, although when men are affected the characteristics are identical in both sexes. The disease is most common in Hispanic, South Asian and South-east Asian people, and those who live in areas of high-intensity UV radiation. Black-skinned patients may be affected but melasma may not be easily noticed. Interestingly, up to 70% of patients can have a family history suggesting a predisposition, as well as UV exposure being of aetiological importance. The commonest causes, however, are oral contraceptives, hormone replacement therapy, pregnancy and, rarely, thyroid dysfunction. Some authorities have

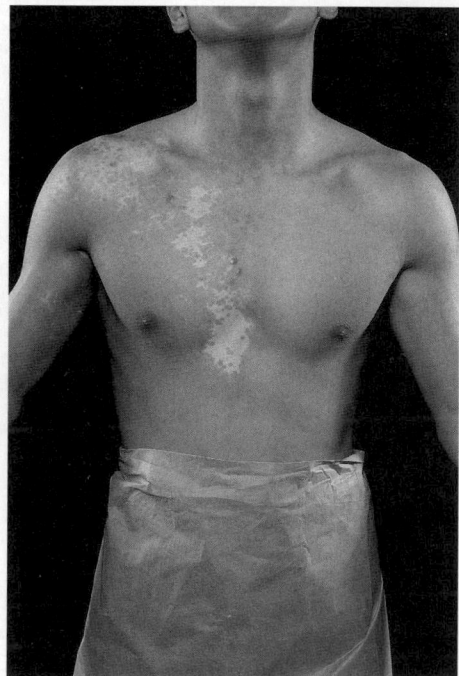

Figure 19.54 Segmental hypopigmentation of trunkal vitiligo.

found elevated levels of luteinizing hormone in a small group of patients and have suggested that subclinical ovarian dysfunction may be of significance.

Treatment

The most useful treatment is hydroquinone, which is a hydroxyphenolic chemical that inhibits the conversion of dopa to melanin by inhibiting the tyrosinase enzyme. Thankfully, this is widely available in the tropics and concentrations vary from 2% to 10%. It is suggested that the hydroquinone is used twice daily for 12 weeks. The authors cannot help but warn the reader that monobenzyl ether of hydroquinone, which is a permanent depigmentating agent, should never be used to treat melasma, as it causes irreversible loss of pigment. It is important to be aware of the side-effects of hydroquinone as it may cause local skin irritation and thereby lead to postinflammatory hyperpigmentation, making the skin appear worse. However, this is uncommon. The patient should be warned that if the hydroquinone happens to go onto surrounding normal skin, this may lighten as well, and may give the patient a sort of leopard-skin appearance. Exogenous ochronosis is thought to be a rare side-effect of hydroquinone therapy.

Hydroquinone may be combined with topical tretinoin and 1% dexamethasone in an ointment form and this is applied once a day at night for a minimum of 4–6 months. There may be an irritant dermatitis about which the patient should be warned. Azelaic acid may be used twice daily for 6 months and is tolerated very well, with very few side-effects.

The most important treatment for melasma is to remove any exacerbating causes such as medication and contraceptives; patients should be advised to wear a broad-spectrum sun block when going out and to cover up thoroughly, wearing a hat in the sun. More recent therapy for melasma has included glycolic acid peels, tretinoin peels and laser treatment.[75]

Postinflammatory hyperpigmentation

This is an acquired excess of pigment in skin that develops after an inflammatory dermatosis. The distribution of melanin synthesis is determined by the distribution of the preceding inflammation. Such inflammation may be caused by infections, allergic reactions, conditions such as eczema and psoriasis (Figure 19.55), reactions to medications, phototoxic eruptions and physical agents. The condition seems to be much worse in cases that disrupt the basement membrane layer, such as in discoid lupus erythematosus and lichen planus. As in melasma, the melanin may be epidermal, dermal or mixed, in which case a Wood's light examination is helpful. Treatment of postinflammatory hyperpigmentation may take 6–12 months and involves the use of hydroquinone, tretinoin cream, glycolic acid and azelaic acid.

Phrynoderma

This is a distinctive form of follicular hyperkeratosis, which was initially described in association with vitamin A deficiency. The condition presents as small papules and nodules with central intrafollicular plugs to large papules. Some of the larger papules may have massive hyperkeratosis which, when shed, leaves large crateriform lesions. Clinically, the lesions first appear on the extensor surfaces of the extremities, shoulders and buttocks, and some-

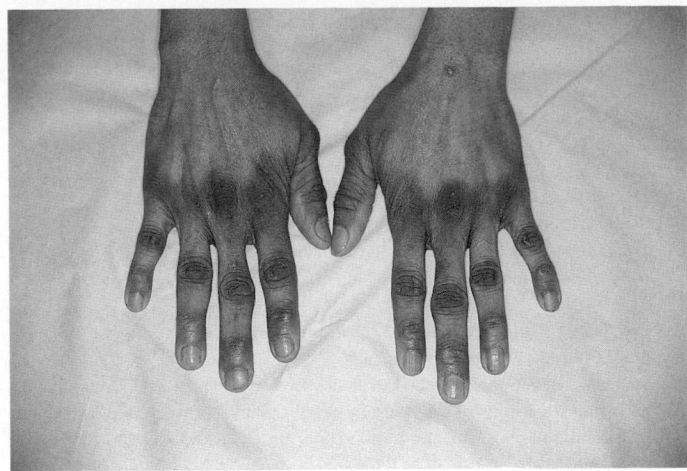

Figure 19.55 Postinflammatory hyperpigmentation of the hands in a patient with atopic eczema.

times may spread to most of the body. The lesions are flesh coloured but may be slightly hyperpigmented. Interestingly, the most recent and comprehensive study has shown that only 5% of patients have lower than normal serum vitamin A levels and these patients present with lesions localized around the knees and elbows only. Those patients with normal vitamin A levels had more widespread lesions. Unfortunately, there is no good evidence that adults with vitamin A deficiency respond to replacement therapy. However, children with phrynoderma seem to show signs of deficiency of both vitamin A and B; the B complex deficiency is more significant in Nigeria, whereas studies in India on affected children suggest an interaction of the vitamin B group and unsaturated fatty acids. Therefore it has been suggested that phrynoderma may be caused by a fat-soluble vitamin deficiency. A study from Thailand has shown that those children with vitamin deficiency respond well to vitamin A therapy. Those that do not have a vitamin A deficiency can be treated with a 5–10% salicylate ointment twice a day, a potent topical steroid on its own or in a combination with salicylate; 10–20% urea in a cream base has been used effectively. Most of the lesions tend to disappear before age 18 without treatment.

REFERENCES

1. Bisno AL, Stevens DL. Streptococcal infections of skin and soft tissues. *N Engl J Med* 1996; 334:240–245.
2. Elliott DC, Kufera JA, Myers RA. Necrotizing soft tissue infections: risk factors for mortality and strategies for management. *Ann Surg* 1996; 224:672–683.
3. Anaya DA, Dellinger EP. Necrotizing soft-tissue infection: diagnosis and management. *Clin Infect Dis* 2007; 44:705–710.
4. Goh BT. Syphilis in adults. *Sex Transm Infect* 2005; 81:448–452.
5. Mafart B. Goundou: a historical form of yaws. *Lancet* 2002; 360:1168–1170.
6. Farnsworth N, Rosen T. Endemic treponematosis: review and update. *Clin Dermatol* 2006; 24:181–190.
7. Laing RB, Flegg PJ, Watt B, et al. Antimicrobial treatment of fish tank granuloma. *J Hand Surg [Br]* 1997; 22:135–137.
8. Nackers F, Johnson RC, Glynn JR, et al. Environmental and health-related risk factors for *Mycobacterium ulcerans* disease (Buruli ulcer) in Benin. *Am J Trop Med Hyg* 2007; 77:834–836.

9. Wansbrough-Jones M, Phillips R. Buruli ulcer: emerging from obscurity. *Lancet* 2006; 367:1849–1858.

10. Ouattara D, Meningaud JP, Saliba F. Multifocal forms of Buruli ulcer: clinical aspects and management difficulties in 11 cases. *Bull Soc Pathol Exot* 2002; 95:287–291.

11. Casalini C, Matteelli A, Saleri N, et al. Nodular lesion of the skin as primary cutaneous tuberculosis. *J Travel Med* 2003; 10:306–308.

12. Thami GP, Kaur S, Kanwar AJ, et al. Lichen scrofulosorum: a rare manifestation of a common disease. *Pediatr Dermatol* 2002; 19:122–126.

13. Trindade MA, Fleury RN. Histological analysis of the Mitsuda reaction in contacts of multibacillary leprosy patients. *Int J Lepr Other Mycobact Dis* 1993; 61:109–110.

14. Coeytaux A, Truffert A, Mueller Y, et al. Leprosy, a neurologic disease. *Rev Med Suisse* 2007; 3:1178, 1180–1184.

15. Sousa AL, Stefani MM, Pereira GA, et al. *Mycobacterium leprae* DNA associated with type 1 reactions in single lesion paucibacillary leprosy treated with single dose rifampin, ofloxacin, and minocycline. *Am J Trop Med Hyg* 2007; 77: 829–833.

16. Mahaisavariya P, Chaiprasert A, Sivayathorn A, et al. Deep fungal and higher bacterial skin infections in Thailand: clinical manifestations and treatment regimens. *Int J Dermatol* 1999; 38:279–284.

17. Mendez-Tovar LJ, Serrano-Jaen L, Almeida-Arvizu VM. Combined cefotaxime and amikacin for immunomodulation in the treatment of actinomycetoma resistant to conventional treatment. *Gac Med Mex* 1999; 135:517–521.

18. Bonifaz A, Flores P, Saúl A, et al. Treatment of actinomycetoma due to *Nocardia* spp. with amoxicillin-clavulanate. *Br J Dermatol* 2007; 156: 308–311.

19. Serrano-Jaen L, Vega-Lopez F. Fulminating septicaemia caused by *Vibrio vulnificus*. *Br J Dermatol* 2000; 142:386–387.

20. Stanley JR, Amagai M. Pemphigus, bullous impetigo, and the staphylococcal scalded-skin syndrome. *N Engl J Med* 2006; 355:1800–1810.

21. Lee PL, Lemos B, O'Brien SH, et al. Cutaneous diphtheroid infection and review of other cutaneous Gram-positive *Bacillus* infections. *Cutis* 2007; 79:371–377.

22. Blackwell V, Vega-Lopez F. Cutaneous larva migrans: clinical features and management of 44 cases presenting in the returning traveller. *Br J Dermatol* 2001; 145:434–437.

23. O'Quinn JC, Dushin R. Cutaneous larva migrans: case report with current recommendations for treatment. *J Am Podiatr Med Assoc* 2005; 95:291–294.

24. Davies CR, Kaye P, Croft SL, et al. Leishmaniasis: new approaches to disease control. *BMJ* 2003; 326:377–382.

25. Ameen M. Cutaneous leishmaniasis: therapeutic strategies and future directions. *Expert Opin Pharmacother* 2007; 8:2689–2699.

26. Pasquau F, Ena J, Sanchez R, et al. Leishmaniasis as an opportunistic infection in HIV-infected patients: determinants of relapse and mortality in a collaborative study of 228 episodes in a Mediterreanean region. *Eur J Clin Microbiol Infect Dis* 2005; 24:411–418.

27. Sundar S, More DK, Singh MK, et al. Failure of pentavalent antimony in visceral leishmaniasis in India: report from the center of the Indian epidemic. *Clin Infect Dis* 2000; 31:1104–1107.

28. Thakur CP, Singh RK, Hassann SM, et al. Amphotericin B deoxycholate treatment of visceral leishmaniasis with newer modes of administration and precautions: a study of 938 cases. *Trans R Soc Trop Med Hyg* 1999; 93:319–323.

29. Thakur CP, Pandey AK, Sinha GP, et al. Comparison of three treatment regimens with liposomal amphotericin B (AmBisome) for visceral leishmaniasis in India: a randomized dose-finding study. *Trans R Soc Trop Med Hyg* 1996; 90:319–322.

30. Thakur CP, Narayan S, Ranjan A. Epidemiological, clinical & pharmacological study of antimony-resistant visceral leishmaniasis in Bihar, India. *Indian J Med Res* 2004; 120:166–172.

31. Debrah AY, Mand S, Marfo-Debrekyei Y, et al. Assessment of microfilarial loads in the skin of onchocerciasis patients after treatment with different regimens of doxycycline plus ivermectin. *Filaria J* 2006; 5:1.

32. Parola P, Caumes E. Gnathostomiasis. *Med Trop (Mars)* 2005; 65:9–12.

33. Ibanez-Bernal S, Velasco-Castrejon O. New records of human tungiasis in Mexico (Siphonaptera:Tungidae). *J Med Entomol* 1996; 33:988–989.

34. Beg MA, Saleem T, Zubari A, et al. Tungiasis: consequences of delayed presentation/diagnosis. *Int J Infect Dis* 2008; 12:218–219.

35. Heukelbach J, Franck S, Feldmeier H. Therapy of tungiasis: a double-blinded randomized controlled trial with oral ivermectin. *Mem Inst Oswaldo Cruz* 2004; 99:873–876.

36. Loong PT, Lui H, Buck HW. Cutaneous myiasis: a simple and effective technique for extraction of *Dermatobia hominis* larvae. *Int J Dermatol* 1992; 31:657–659.

37. Wild G. Cutaneous myiasis with *Dermatobia hominis* (human bot fly) larvae treated both conservatively and surgically. *J R Nav Med Serv* 2006; 92:78–81.

38. Dourmishev AL, Dourmishev LA, Schwartz RA. Ivermectin: pharmacology and application in dermatology. *Int J Dermatol* 2005; 44:981–988.

39. Hengge UR, Currie BJ, Jäger G, et al. Scabies: a ubiquitous neglected skin disease. *Lancet Infect Dis* 2006; 6:769–779.

40. Walton SF, Currie BJ. Problems in diagnosing scabies, a global disease in human and animal populations. *Clin Microbiol Rev* 2007; 20:268–279.

41. Dupuy A, Dehen L, Bourrat E, et al. Accuracy of standard dermoscopy for diagnosing scabies. *J Am Acad Dermatol* 2007; 56:53–62.

42. Strong M, Johnstone PW. Interventions for treating scabies. *Cochrane Database Syst Rev* 2007; (3):CD000320.

43. Heukelbach J, Feldmeier H. Scabies. *Lancet* 2006; 367:1767–1774.

44. Pitches DW. Removal of ticks: a review of the literature. *Euro Surveill* 2006; 11: E060817 4.

45. Duchemin JB, Fournier PE, Parola P. Fleas and diseases transmissible to man. *Med Trop (Mars)* 2006; 66:21–29.

46. Kannan P, Janaki C, Selvi GS. Prevalence of dermatophytes and other fungal agents isolated from clinical samples. *Indian J Med Microbiol* 2006; 24: 212–215.

47. Almeida-Paes R, Pimenta MA, Pizzini CV, et al. Use of mycelial-phase *Sporothrix schenckii* exoantigens in an enzyme-linked immunosorbent assay for diagnosis of sporotrichosis by antibody detection. *Clin Vaccine Immunol* 2007; 14:244–249.

48. Kauffman CA, Bustamante B, Chapman SW, et al. Clinical practice guidelines for the management of sporotrichosis: 2007 update by the Infectious Diseases Society of America. *Clin Infect Dis* 2007; 45:1255–1265.

49. Lupi O, Tyring SK, McGinnis MR. Tropical dermatology: fungal tropical diseases. *J Am Acad Dermatol* 2005; 53:931–951, quiz 952–954.

50. Fahal AH. Mycetoma: a thorn in the flesh. *Trans R Soc Trop Med Hyg* 2004; 98:3–11.

51. Rouphael NG, Talati NJ, Franco-Paredes C. A painful thorn in the foot: a case of eumycetoma. *Am J Med Sci* 2007; 334:142–144.

52. Negroni R, Tobón A, Bustamante B, et al. Posaconazole treatment of refractory eumycetoma and chromoblastomycosis. *Rev Inst Med Trop Sao Paulo* 2005; 47:339–346.

53. Oberto-Perdigon L, Romero H, Pérez-Blanco M, et al. An ELISA test for the study of the therapeutic evolution of chromoblastomycosis by *Cladophialophora carrionii* in the endemic area of Falcon State, Venezuela. *Rev Iberoam Micol* 2005; 22:39–43.

54. Lopez Martinez R, Mendez Tovar LJ. Chromoblastomycosis. *Clin Dermatol* 2007; 25:188–194.

55. Petrikkos G, Skiada A. Recent advances in antifungal chemotherapy. *Int J Antimicrob Agents* 2007; 30:108–117.

56. Blair JE. State-of-the-art treatment of coccidioidomycosis: skin and soft-tissue infections. *Ann N Y Acad Sci* 2007; 1111:411–421.

57. Wheat LJ, Freifeld AG, Kleiman MB, et al. Clinical practice guidelines for the management of patients with histoplasmosis: 2007 update by the Infectious Diseases Society of America. *Clin Infect Dis* 2007; 45:807–825.

58. Del Rosso JQ. Study results of benzoyl peroxide 5%/clindamycin 1% topical gel, adapalene 0.1% gel, and use in combination for acne vulgaris. *J Drugs Dermatol* 2007; 6:616–622.

59. Arowojolu AO, Gallo MF, Lopez LM, et al. Combined oral contraceptive pills for treatment of acne. *Cochrane Database Syst Rev* 2007; (1):CD004425.

60. Rerinck HC, Kamann S, Wollenberg A. Eczema herpeticum: pathogenesis and therapy. *Hautarzt* 2006; 57:586–591.

61. Brown S, Reynolds NJ. Atopic and non-atopic eczema. *BMJ* 2006; 332: 584–588.

62. Munzenberger PJ, Montejo JM. Safety of topical calcineurin inhibitors for the treatment of atopic dermatitis. *Pharmacotherapy* 2007; 27:1020–1028.

63. Comte C, Picot E, Peyron JL, et al. UVA-1 phototherapy: properties and indications. *Ann Dermatol Venereol* 2007; 134:407–415.

64. Schmitt J, Schäkel K, Schmitt N, et al. Systemic treatment of severe atopic eczema: a systematic review. *Acta Derm Venereol* 2007; 87:100–111.

65. Passeron T, Lacour JP, Fontas E, et al. Prebiotics and synbiotics: two promising approaches for the treatment of atopic dermatitis in children above 2 years. *Allergy* 2006; 61:431–437.

66. Wollina U, Abdel Naser MB. Pharmacotherapy of pompholyx. *Expert Opin Pharmacother* 2004; 5:1517–1522.

67. Esposito M, Mazzotta A, de Felice C, et al. Treatment of erythrodermic psoriasis with etanercept. *Br J Dermatol* 2006; 155:156–159.

68. Katugampola RP, Lewis VJ, Finlay AY. The Dermatology Life Quality Index: assessing the efficacy of biological therapies for psoriasis. *Br J Dermatol* 2007; 156:945–950.

69. Janssens AS, Pavel S, Out-Luiting JJ, et al. Normalized ultraviolet (UV) induction of Langerhans cell depletion and neutrophil infiltrates after artificial UVB hardening of patients with polymorphic light eruption. *Br J Dermatol* 2005; 152:1268–1274.

70. Kostler E, Wollina U. Therapy of porphyria cutanea tarda. *Expert Opin Pharmacother* 2005; 6:377–383.

71. Fuchs A, Marmur E. The kinetics of skin cancer: progression of actinic keratosis to squamous cell carcinoma. *Dermatol Surg* 2007; 33: 1099–1101.

72. Ooi T, Barnetson RS, Zhuang L, et al. Imiquimod-induced regression of actinic keratosis is associated with infiltration by T lymphocytes and dendritic cells: a randomized controlled trial. *Br J Dermatol* 2006; 154: 72–78.

73. Magen E, Mishal J, Schlesinger M, et al. Eradication of *Helicobacter pylori* infection equally improves chronic urticaria with positive and negative autologous serum skin test. *Helicobacter* 2007; 12:567–571.

74. Nicolaidou E, Antoniou C, Stratigos AJ, et al. Efficacy, predictors of response, and long-term follow-up in patients with vitiligo treated with narrowband UVB phototherapy. *J Am Acad Dermatol* 2007; 56:274–278.

75. Scheinfeld NS. Melasma. *Skinmed* 2007; 6:35–37.

Chapter 20 Christopher J. Hoffmann and
Richard E. Chaisson

HIV/AIDS and Opportunistic Illnesses

Introduction

Human immunodeficiency virus type 1 (HIV-1, or HIV) has emerged as a major cause of morbidity and mortality in many low and middle income countries around the world. Africa has the highest prevalence of HIV infection and the greatest number of individuals living with HIV. Although Africa accounts for 14% of the population in the world, 68% of all HIV-infected individuals live in sub-Saharan Africa.[1] In many hospitals in East and Southern Africa, over half of all in-patients are HIV infected, most suffering from complications of HIV.[2] Generalized epidemics are also occurring in parts of South-east Asia and the Caribbean, while the epidemic in Eastern Europe, Central Asia, China and India is currently concentrated in sub-populations, such as injection drug users or commercial sex workers. This chapter describes pathophysiology, epidemiology, complications and acute and chronic management of HIV disease.

Pathophysiology

The HIV virion is a 110 nm particle with a spherical lipid envelope and cone-shaped viral capsid.[3] Because the lipid envelope is sensitive to environmental degradation HIV is rapidly inactivated outside of the host. The approximately 10 000 base pair genome is organized into three major regions: *gag, pol* and *env*. The *gag* region contains the structural genes for HIV (i.e. matrix, capsid, nucleocapsid and two small peptides), the *pol* region contains the genes for the viral enzymes needed to carry out the life cycle (i.e. reverse transcriptase, integrase and protease) and the *env* region encodes the genes for the viral envelope proteins (i.e. gp160, which is cleaved by host proteases to gp120 and gp41).

HIV-1 has six regulatory genes: *tat* upregulates genome transcription; *rev* coordinates the expression of the regulatory and non-regulatory genes by facilitating the transport of spliced and unspliced RNA transcripts to the cell cytoplasm; *nef* helps with evasion of the host immune response by downregulating expression of CD4 and major histocompatibility complex (MHC) class I molecules on the cell surface; *vpu* reduces host cell CD4 expression; *vpr* is important for infection of quiescent cells by facilitating nuclear localization of the viral preintegration complex; and *vif* is important for virion assembly and inactivation of the host cell antiviral factor APOBEC3G.[4,5]

The first step in the life cycle is the attachment of the virus to the host target cell via binding of the HIV envelope surface protein (gp120) to the CD4 receptor on the host cell. For infection to proceed, cellular co-receptors (either of the chemokine receptors CCR5 or CXCR4) must bind gp120, causing a conformational change in gp120 and the exposure of the other HIV envelope protein, gp41 to the cell surface. The gp41 protein mediates fusion of the virus lipid envelope and host cell membrane. Sexually transmitted HIV typically involves strains with a gp120 structure that preferentially bind to CCR5 (i.e. R5-tropic strains). Over time (generally years), mutations in the gp120 allow binding to CXCR4 (X4-tropic strains). The shift to the X4-tropic phenotype is associated with more advanced HIV and more rapid progression of disease, although a causal relationship between X4-tropic and immune depletion has not been determined.

After the fusion of the viral and cellular membranes, the HIV reverse transcriptase enzyme, using host factors, converts the single-stranded HIV RNA into double-stranded DNA. The HIV reverse transcriptase is error-prone and produces mutations at a rate of approximately 1 in 10^4 base pairs, or about one mutation in every HIV RNA transcribed. In addition, during normal replication, the reverse transcriptase enzyme shifts from one strand of nucleic acid to another to complete the synthesis of daughter strands. This strand-shifting enables recombination between different viral strains infecting the same cell. Mutation and recombination generate a large pool of genetically related but distinct HIV strains called quasispecies. Most of these quasispecies have either fatal mutations or mutations that impair replication. However, strains with a mutation that provides a growth advantage in a particular environment (e.g. in the presence of specific antiretroviral drugs) will become the dominant strain.

After reverse transcription, the proviral DNA forms a complex with HIV integrase and localizes to the nucleus and becomes integrated as the HIV provirus into the host cell chromosome. Subsequently, cellular enzymes transcribe the provirus into spliced and non-spliced messenger RNA that encode the regulatory genes (*tat* and *rev*) and the structural genes. The late stages of viral replication involve assembly of the viral particles, with each viral core incorporating two copies of the viral RNA genome and the budding and release of the virions from the cell surface. The HIV protease enzyme plays an essential role by cleaving the *gag* polyprotein into smaller functional components required for the formation of a mature infectious virus.

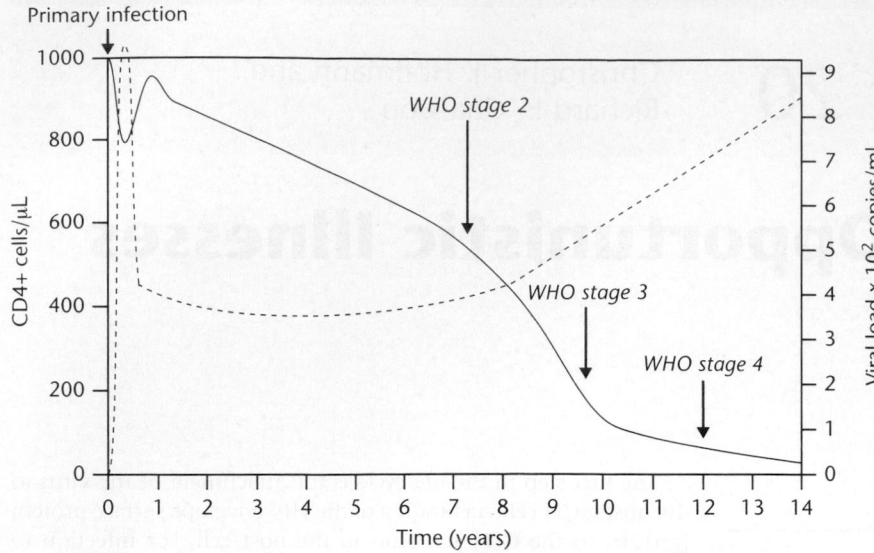

Figure 20.1 Natural history of untreated HIV-1 infection. WHO stage 2, minor symptoms and infections; stage 3, virulent and early opportunistic.

Within days to weeks of HIV infection, explosive expansion in HIV occurs in mucosal lymphoid tissue, especially within gut-associated lymphoid tissue (GALT). Up to 60% of memory CD4+ T cells in GALT are infected and die within weeks of infection.[6] Cell mediated response to this hyper-proliferation of HIV leads to symptoms of acute retroviral syndrome.[7] Within 6 months of primary HIV infection, the plasma level of HIV becomes fairly stable. This level, referred to as the 'set point', is determined by host and viral factors and varies from person-to-person, with the HIV-directed CTL response appearing to be among the most important factors.[8]

The second phase of CD4+ T cell depletion is marked initially by a steady state of both rapid T cell proliferation and rapid destruction, with the CD4 count maintained at relatively normal levels (800–1200 cells/mm³); this phase was formerly known as latent infection. Infected activated CD4 cells are quickly destroyed, with a half-life of 1–2 days. The paradox is that the total number of T cells infected with HIV is small compared with the total population experiencing rapid turnover.[9] Depletion of uninfected CD4 T cells appears to be driven by immune activation, possibly through interaction with the HIV gp120, leading to programmed cell death.[10] Eventually, CD4 cell destruction occurs faster than proliferation and the CD4 count declines rapidly (in the serum, 20–100 cells/mm³ per year).

During all periods of HIV replication, a small subset of infected CD4 cells escapes death and returns to a quiescent state. These cells remain latently infected and persist, with a half-life of up to 44 months,[11] forming a latent reservoir of HIV that can reactivate even after years of suppressive antiviral therapy. The persistence of this reservoir is the major obstacle to complete eradication of HIV from the body. Current estimates suggest that it would take >70 years to deplete all the latently infected quiescent memory T cells.[12] Because infected cells enter the latent reservoir whenever cycles of HIV replication are occurring, a genetic archive of all previous circulating HIV quasispecies is generated when HIV release and entry into uninfected cells is occurring. As a result, HIV

replication during non-suppressive antiretroviral therapy may lead to generation of drug-resistant viruses that are archived in a permanent reservoir that can re-emerge under conditions of selective pressure.[13,14]

The hallmark of HIV infection is the relentless decline in CD4 cells.[10,15] However, the rate of CD4 decline among HIV-infected individuals is highly variable, ranging from a rapid decline over 2 years to a slow decline over two decades. The rate of decline is dependent on multiple factors including HIV subtype,[16] HIV RNA plasma level ('viral load'), co-infections, nutritional status and other unidentified factors.[17–19] Studies of the natural history of HIV from Africa have suggested a similar rate of CD4 decline as in industrialized countries.[20–23] However, considerable inter-person variation exists in all regions. For example, a cohort study in Tanzania reported a range of progression from seroconversion to CD4 < 200 cells/mm³ between 4 and 13 years. The median CD4 decline from that study ranged from 18 to 52 cells/mm³/year.[24] Multiple factors including environmental, viral and host factors likely contribute to the heterogeneity of CD4 decline.[16,22] In low-income countries co-infection with malaria, Herpes simplex, tuberculosis and other endemic infections may also contribute to the rate of CD4 decline. While there is wide variation, the median time from infection to a CD4 of <200 cells/mm³ in the absence of treatment is approximately 8 years in both industrialized countries and low-income countries[25] (Figure 20.1).

As the CD4 count declines, infections normally cleared by cell-mediated immunity increase in frequency and severity. Notable pathogens include *Mycobacterium tuberculosis* (TB), non-tuberculosis mycobacteria, *Pneumocystis jiroveci*, *Cryptococcus neoformans*, cytomegalovirus (CMV) and other herpesviruses, endemic mycoses, such as *Histoplasma capsulatum* and *Penicillium marneffei* and bacteraemia from *Streptococcus pneumoniae* and *Salmonella spp*. When the CD4 is <200 cells/mm³ the risk of infection by these and other organisms rises significantly. Knowing the correlation between CD4 count and presentation of each opportunistic infection (OI) is especially useful in guiding diagnosis.[26]

EPIDEMIOLOGY

HIV subtypes and origin

AIDS was first described in 1981 among a group of five men who developed *Pneumocystis jiroveci* (then *carinii*) pneumonia and were found to have profound immunodeficiency.[27] Two years later, the causative agent of AIDS, human immunodeficiency virus (HIV), was first identified and serologic tests for antibodies as well as virus isolation methods were subsequently developed, permitting diagnosis of infection and identification of viral subtypes. Since that time, testing of stored serum specimens and analysis of geographical distribution of genetic HIV variants have helped traced the likely origins of the HIV epidemic. HIV-1 is believed to have jumped species from chimpanzees to bush-meat hunters in West Africa (likely Cameroon) through several independent events in the early twentieth century.[28,29] From there, it slowly spread along the trade routes to the cities of central Africa. The oldest identified serum specimen containing HIV-1 RNA was obtained in 1959 from an individual in Kinshasa, Democratic Republic of Congo. However, it was not until the spread to East Africa and the USA in the 1970s that an epidemic developed. In the years since the species jump, genetic changes have led to 10 distinct subgroups (A–J) and multiple circulating recombinant forms (CRF) between subgroups. Subgroup B predominates in North America, Europe and Australia and is the most extensively studied subgroup. However, more than half of all infections are from subgroup C, the predominant subgroup in Southern Africa and India (Figure 20.2). As research increases on non-subtype B HIV, it is likely that variations in pathogenesis and drug resistance mutation patterns will be identified. However, current evidence suggests similar natural history, development of opportunistic illnesses and response to antiretroviral therapy.

HIV-2, a retrovirus closely related to HIV-1, is believed to have jumped species from the sooty mangabey to humans early in the twentieth century.[30] Distribution of HIV-2 has mostly remained confined to West Africa. It causes slower progression to immunodeficiency. In addition, structural differences in the reverse transcriptase enzyme of HIV-2 compared with HIV-1, make it naturally resistant to the non-nucleoside reverse transcriptase inhibitor (NNRTI) class of antiretroviral agents (e.g. efavirenz and nevirapine).

Transmission

HIV is transmitted person-to-person from sexual contact, by transfusion of infected blood products, from women to their infants either in utero, intra-partum, or via breast milk, or by percutaneous injection with contaminated needles or other devices. Direct blood-to-blood contact, such as occurs with blood transfusion, venous puncture with a hollow-bore needle containing infected blood, or significant mucosal disruption during sexual activities, carries the highest risk. A number of biological factors are also associated with the risk of transmission, including size of the infectious inoculum, higher HIV viral load in the index case, genital ulcer disease in either the index case or recipient, mucosal abrasions or trauma and, possibly, immune activation in the

Table 20.1 Exposure and risk of HIV transmission[31–34]

Exposure route	Cases per 10 000 exposures
Blood transfusion	8200
Mother-to-child	2400
Needle sharing with intravenous drug use	80
Needlestick injury	30
Anal intercourse	
Receptive	30–80
Insertive	6
Vaginal intercourse	
Receptive	8–10
Insertive	5
Receptive oral sex	4

recipient. Overall, the risk of infection per exposure ranges from 60% from transfusion with infected blood to 0.04% from receptive oral sex (Table 20.1).

Global distribution

In 2007 UNAIDS estimated that 33.2 million people were alive with HIV, 2.1 million people died of AIDS-related causes that year and 2.5 million more individuals became infected.[1] Sub Saharan Africa has the highest prevalence of HIV; 68% of all HIV-infected adults, 90% of HIV-infected children and 76% of all AIDS deaths are in Africa. Southern Africa (Botswana, Lesothu, Mozambique, Namibia, South Africa, Swaziland, Zambia and Zimbabwe) has the highest prevalence of HIV, with the highest prevalence in Swaziland with 26% of the adult population (15–49 years) infected with HIV. South Africa is the country with the largest number of HIV-infected individuals with an estimated 5.5 million infected individuals. While several African countries reported declines in prevalence of HIV among women age 15–24 years seeking antenatal care, including Kenya, Cote d'Ivoire, Malawi and Zimbabwe, there was no evidence of a decline in South Africa, Mozambique, or Zambia.[1]

Most of the pandemic spread of HIV during the past decades has occurred through sexual exposure and injection drug use (IDU).[2] Sexual spread has been through heterosexual sex, men who have sex with men (MSM) and commercial sex work. In many regions, HIV first emerged among groups such as injection drug users, MSM, commercial sex workers (CSW), or migrant labourers.[35] In some regions, the epidemic has remained concentrated among these populations, whereas in other regions the epidemic has become generalized among the entire population. Because of the importance in understanding these differences in regional epidemics, the WHO has created definitions for concentrated and generalized epidemics. A 'concentrated epidemic' is defined as a region with >5% of at least one subgroup infected, but <1% of the general population infected. A 'generalized epidemic' is defined as HIV infection among >1% of the general population. A 'low level epidemic' is defined as HIV prevalence <5% in high risk sub-populations and <1% in the general population.[36] It is generally believed that an extensive transmission

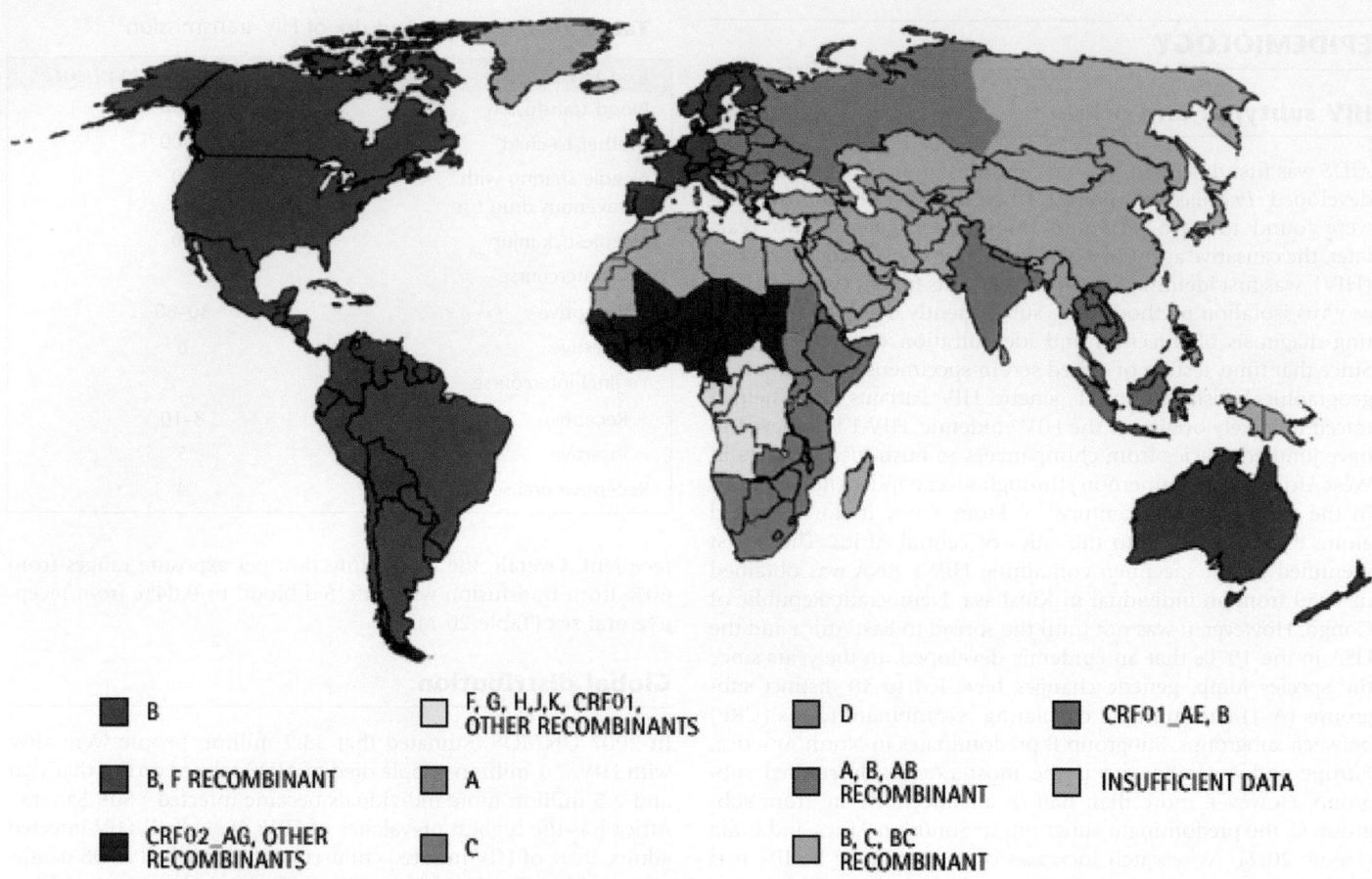

B

B, F RECOMBINANT

CRF02_AG, OTHER RECOMBINANTS

F, G, H,J,K, CRF01, OTHER RECOMBINANTS

A

C

D

A, B, AB RECOMBINANT

B, C, BC RECOMBINANT

CRF01_AE, B

INSUFFICIENT DATA

Figure 20.2 Global distribution of subgroups and circulating recombinant forms (CRF) of group M HIV-1. (From Francine E. McCutchan, Henry M. Jackson Foundation (Rockville, Maryland).)

network is needed to reach an HIV prevalence of 5% in either a sub-population or the general population. When the network within the general population is strong enough to support transmission throughout the population (and not just between sub-populations and their sexual partners in the general population) a generalized epidemic emerges. This may occur initially from spread from bridge groups among sub-populations, followed by spread within the general population. For example, in Southern Africa the early epidemic was likely concentrated among commercial sex workers, migrant labourers and long distance truck drivers.[2] However, because of the fluidity between these groups and the general population, HIV transmission began to be supported among the wider population, leading to the generalized epidemic. However, in central Asia, Eastern Europe and parts of South-east Asia, the majority of transmission continues to be among injection drug users and transmission among the general population has remained insufficient for a generalized epidemic. In parts of South-east Asia, however, most transmission has remained between commercial sex workers, their clients and other sexual partners, again, with insufficient transmission in the general population for a generalized epidemic to emerge.

It remains unclear why Southern Africa and East Africa have much higher HIV prevalence than other regions. However, several differences between Southern and East Africa and other regions of the world have been identified that may explain the difference. For example, men in Southern Africa have lower rates of circumcision and the population overall has higher prevalence of genital herpes infection, earlier sexual debut and greater gender inequality than West Africa.[37] Furthermore, while men and women in southern Africa have the same or fewer number of lifetime sexual partners as individuals in Asia or South America, they are more likely to have concurrent regular partners, unlike the serial monogamy reported from Thailand, for example.[38] Multiple concurrent sexual partners increases HIV transmission risk for two important and distinct reasons: (1) disease can spread rapidly through the extensive sexual network and (2) individuals are less likely to use condoms during sex with regular partners.[39,40] Geographical mobility with migration and urbanization are also likely important factors for the rapid spread in Southern Africa where migrant labour is common and transportation infrastructure is well developed. Specific heterosexual sexual practices have been implicated as contributing factors as well; these include the practice of so-called 'dry sex' and heterosexual anal intercourse.[41]

HIV PREVENTION

Very early in the AIDS epidemic it became clear that promotion of behavioural changes in individuals and groups at risk for the disease could be highly effective in prevention of transmission. Use of latex condoms during sex, reduction in the number of sexual partners, avoidance of high-risk sexual practices associated with mucosal trauma and stopping injection drug use or using sterile paraphernalia were all found to reduce the risk of transmitting and acquiring HIV. Community or national campaigns to promote behavioural change have had varying degrees of success. In Thailand, the '100% Condom' campaign, which included distribution of millions of condoms throughout the country and an emphasis on decreasing commercial sex transactions, was extraordinarily effective in reducing the incidence and prevalence of both HIV and other sexually transmitted infections. The success was partially a result of the nature of the epidemic being driven by transactional sex, a setting in which condom promotion has been most successful. Similar approaches in Brazil and other tropical countries have also helped contain emerging epidemics.

Interventions and campaigns to prevent HIV transmission have generally targeted uninfected individuals. However, in recent years, the importance of targeting interventions at HIV-infected people has become apparent. With >30 million people living with HIV infection, opportunities to interrupt transmission from these individuals to susceptible contacts are both abundant and critically important. HIV-infected individuals should be counselled on safer sexual practices including condom usage, avoiding needle/paraphernalia sharing, blood donation and other interventions. While modelling studies suggest that a large number of infections occur early in the course of HIV infection, before most individuals know they are infected,[42] a large number of infections are transmitted later, so that knowledge of serostatus accompanied by behavioural change can have a substantial impact on spread of the virus.[43]

Opportunities for prevention begin with local healthcare providers and rise to national and international levels. The best proven methods are prevention of mother-to-child transmission (PMTCT) and prevention of transmission via blood transfusion. Male circumcision has also been shown to reduce the risk of acquiring HIV in clinical trials, but scale-up is needed for a meaningful public health impact. As described above, condom promotion, behavioural change and reduction of multiple partners have had some success among certain sub-populations. Treatment of genital ulcer disease or chronic suppressive therapy of herpes simplex virus (HSV) have shown mixed results. Counselling and testing may also have a role in changing behaviour among individuals aware of being HIV infected. Among those who test negative, there is little evidence of impact on behaviour change.[44] For occupational and other high-risk exposures (such as rape) post-exposure prophylaxis (PEP) is a valuable means of prevention. Prevention methods such as vaccination, vaginal or rectal microbicides and pre-exposure prophylaxis are still in early experimental stages. Whether current basic research will lead to effective products in the future remains uncertain. HIV treatment is also an important method of reducing transmission to HIV discordant long-term partners. However, from a public health perspective, the small proportion of total HIV-infected individuals diagnosed and on antiretroviral therapy makes antiretroviral therapy unlikely to substantially reduce HIV incidence. Below, we highlight three of the methods requiring active participation by local healthcare providers.

Prevention of mother-to-child transmission (PMTCT)

The majority of HIV transmission from mother-to-child occurs during labour and delivery and postpartum, through breast-feeding. During these two periods, plasma HIV viral load is the strongest predictor of transmission. Other factors related to mother-to-child transmission are lower maternal CD4 count, acute HIV infection during pregnancy and presence of sexually transmitted diseases. Use of antiretroviral drugs can greatly reduce the risk of transmission during delivery, from 30% to <5%.[45,46] Diagnosis of HIV before or early in pregnancy can lead to the consideration of highly active antiretroviral therapy (HAART) for the mother. In general, initiation of HAART should follow guidelines for any HIV-infected adult (see below) with the exception that efavirenz should be avoided during the first trimester. It is also generally recommended that HAART should be delayed until the second trimester to reduce the risk of teratogenicity.[47]

Among women who are not HAART candidates, multiple single and multi-drug ART combinations have been evaluated. The simplest regimen is single dose nevirapine (nevirapine 200 mg once intrapartum followed by a single 2 mg/kg dose for the infant within 72 h of delivery). This regimen is convenient, can be instituted even if HIV is only diagnosed via rapid testing during labour and has a high rate of efficacy. The significant downside is that use of nevirapine as a single agent, even a single dose, can lead to the selection of and archiving of, resistant viruses due to the long serum half-life and low barrier to resistance of this agent. Although resistance develops rapidly, after removing the drug pressure, the majority of circulating HIV reverts to nevirapine sensitive forms and nevirapine would be expected to be equally effective for preventing transmission during subsequent pregnancies.[48,49] However, use of nevirapine is less likely to provide long-term success, especially if HAART is started within 6 months of single-dose nevirapine.[50] Several alternatives exist to single-dose nevirapine to reduce the risk of resistance. These include fully suppressive HAART continued indefinitely, monotherapy with zidovudine and various forms of short-term combination therapy including: (1) zidovudine 300 mg twice daily started at 14 to 36 weeks' gestation with zidovudine 2 mg/kg i.v. during labour, followed by continuous infusion of zidovudine 1 mg/kg per hour until delivery, followed by zidovudine 2 mg/kg every 6 h to the infant for 6 weeks; (2) single dose nevirapine to mother and infant followed by 7–14 days of zidovudine 300 mg and lamivudine 150 mg twice daily to the mother.

Following delivery, an uninfected infant has a 14% chance of infection via breast milk if the infected mother breast-feeds.[51,52] The risk of infection can be reduced by several strategies: (1) exclusive formula-feeding, (2) exclusive breast-feeding for the first 6 months followed by no further breast-feeding, (3) ART agents given to the infant to prevent infection (such as zidovudine and lamivudine) and (4) fully suppressive HAART to the mother.[53] Exclusive formula-feeding eliminates the chance of infection via breast milk but is logistically difficult in many low-income countries and increases the risk of diarrhoeal disease and malnutrition because of limited access to clean drinking water, use of diluted formula and the absence of maternal protective antibodies provided by breast-feeding. Exclusive breast-feeding appears to lower the risk of infection when compared with mixing breast-feeding with other foods.

Male circumcision

Three recently completed randomized clinical trials have proven the efficacy of circumcision to reduce HIV transmission during the first 12 months after circumcision. Across the three trials from South Africa, Kenya and Uganda, new cases of HIV were 60% less among the circumcised group vs the uncircumcised control group.[54-56] This effect appeared to become even larger over time from circumcision. Large scale male circumcision programmes in African countries with generalized epidemics and high prevalence of HIV could have a tremendous impact on reducing HIV incidence.

Post-exposure prophylaxis

Healthcare workers stuck by contaminated needles, and victims of rape, should be evaluated for post-exposure prophylaxis (PEP). Exposures considered to pose a risk of HIV transmission are percutaneous injury and contact of mucous membrane or non-intact skin with blood, tissue, semen, vaginal secretions, CSF, synovial fluid, pleural fluid, peritoneal fluid, pericardial fluid, or amniotic fluid from an individual with HIV. The risk of transmission is approximately 0.3% for percutaneous exposure and 0.09% for mucous membrane exposure, but varies depending on the volume of infectious fluid and the HIV RNA level of the source patient. The following are not considered infectious: faeces, nasal secretions, saliva, sputum, sweat, tears, urine and vomitus.[57]

Rapid implementation of PEP (from exposure via occupational exposure or rape) reduces the risk of transmission. Optimally, PEP should be initiated within 2 h of exposure and continued for 4 weeks. For lower-risk exposures, two-drug PEP is recommended: either zidovudine (300 mg twice daily) and lamivudine (150 mg twice daily) or tenofovir (300 mg daily) and emtricitabine (200 mg daily). Three-drug therapy is recommended for high-risk exposures, such as a needle stick from a hollow bore needle into a vein, using either of the above two nucleoside reverse transcriptase inhibitor (NRTI) regimens above with a protease inhibitor such as ritonavir-boosted lopinavir. The NNRTI efavirenz may also be used if pregnancy is unlikely, although the early neuropsychiatric side-effects can be problematic. *Nevirapine should be avoided because of the risk of hypersensitivity reactions and hepatic necrosis in patients with normal immune function.*[58] Frequent follow-up with laboratory testing and monitoring of side-effects is recommended, with HIV antibody testing repeated 6 months after exposure.

HIV CARE

HIV, laboratory medicine and clinical markers

HIV testing

HIV is diagnosed by detecting HIV specific antibodies with an enzyme linked immunoabsorbent assay (ELISA or EIA) or immunoblot, detection of HIV antigens (p24 or others), or detection of HIV RNA by polymerase chain reaction (PCR). Generally, the starting point to HIV testing is a laboratory based ELISA or a rapid immunoblotting detection kit. Rapid immunoblotting with point-of-care tests using either fingerstick blood or oral swabs has the advantage of being quick and is also highly sensitive and specific for chronic HIV infection. However, results vary with conditions and operator training. For example, review of results from a testing programme in Uganda found higher sensitivity when individuals with weakly positive tests who had been classified as 'HIV-positive' were classified as 'HIV-negative'.[59] To enhance the specificity of HIV testing, use of a confirmatory test following a positive immunoblot is recommended. When early or acute infection is suspected, ELISA and immunoblot tests may return false-negative results because humeral immune response to HIV infection takes usually takes 2–6 weeks and up to 3 months before it can be reliably detected. Thus when acute HIV is suspected, HIV RNA assays are far more sensitive. When HIV RNA testing is unavailable and the diagnosis remains in question, the ELISA should be repeated after 3 months.

Immunological testing

The absolute CD4+ T-cell count is the most important criterion for predicting short-term risk of opportunistic disease or death and is used widely in guidelines for initiation of HAART and prophylaxis for opportunistic infections.[60] Because CD4 testing is expensive and usually requires sophisticated laboratory facilities, efforts to identify surrogates of CD4 count have been intensively pursued. Despite a concerted effort, accurate clinical and laboratory surrogates have not been identified. One technique is to use total lymphocyte count <2000 cells/mm^3 as a cut-off for significant immunodeficiency. Unfortunately, this correlates poorly with absolute CD4 count. The sensitivity and specificity of other markers, such as weight loss, OIs and haemoglobin are also poor.[61-63] Large public health ART programmes need improved immunological testing to deliver on the promise of HIV care to all patients enrolled in their clinics. Fortunately, CD4 assay systems are becoming more widely available in many ART programmes and lower cost test systems are being developed.

Where CD4 count is unavailable, clinical staging by WHO stage should be used for decisions of prophylaxis and HAART initiation (see Table 20.7). However, this method has a major shortcoming because HAART is most successful when initiated before severe immune deficiency and ill health from opportunistic illnesses. Once individuals reach symptomatic AIDS, the risk of death, even after initiating ART, is high.[64]

HIV concentration (viral load)

The plasma HIV RNA level is an important marker of viral activity and the best measure of response to HAART. In patients not receiving antiretrovirals, the viral load predicts the rate at which the CD4 count will fall over time. While viral load is often measured in developed countries, the CD4 count is more often used for staging and following patients prior to initiating treatment in the developing world. Once antiretrovirals are initiated, however, viral load is a useful test for determining response to treatment. Viral load will rebound quickly when patients are non-adherent with therapy or when viral resistance has emerged and is a more sensitive indicator of treatment failure than CD4 count. Three methods are widely used for assaying HIV RNA levels: reverse transcriptase-polymerase chain reaction (RT-PCR; Amplicor HIV Monitor 1.5, Roche Diagnostics), nucleic acid sequence-based amplification (NASBA; NucliSens HIV QT assay, BioMerieux Inc.) and branched-chain DNA (bDNA; Versant HIV RNA 3.0 HIV assay in the USA, Quantiplex HIV RNA 3.0 assay in Europe, Bayer Corporation).[65,66] Each of these tests has variability within the same test of $\log_{10}$ 0.15 to 0.33 copies/mL; greater variability exists between tests. Because of variation between tests, the same test should be used consistently for monitoring a patient. All tests have been evaluated for all subtypes of genotype M and perform reasonably well, although there is less experience with the NASBA technique with multiple clades.[65,67,68] Research is ongoing to develop lower cost and more rapid testing for HIV viral load.

Resistance testing

HIV strains resistant to specific ART agents or classes of agents can emerge during non-suppressive therapy. Generally, mutations occur at characteristic locations in the HIV genome. Currently, resistance mutations are detected by sequencing regions of the HIV genome and identifying known mutations associated with resistance to specific ART agents. This test is costly, requires expert interpretation and is not available in most low-income countries. Lower cost alternatives such as real-time PCR and ELISA tests are under development. However, use of standard first and second-line therapies with predictable mutations at failure, reduces the importance of testing for specific HIV resistance mutations.

HIV Disease

Acute infection

Acute HIV presents as a mononucleosis-like syndrome with the most common presenting symptoms low-grade fever, malaise and headache. Symptoms usually last 1–4 weeks (median, 2 weeks) and may evolve to include maculopapular rash, lymphadenopathy, anorexia and weight loss.[69,70] Rarer findings include pharyngeal erythema, oral ulcerations and oropharyngeal candidiasis, meningoencephalitis, neuropathy, radiculopathy and Guillain–Barré syndrome. A similar acute illness develops in approximately 5% of patients after the discontinuance of suppressive HAART, as HIV RNA levels increase exponentially.[71,72] Symptoms occur 4–28 days after infection, corresponding to the peak in HIV viraemia.[73] In industrialized countries, symptoms occur among 20% to 90% of acutely infected individuals. However, a small study suggested a far lower rate of seroconversion illness (<20%) in Africa.[74] The lower rate may be a result of competing illnesses overshadowing the symptoms of acute HIV, less of a symptomatic response, or limitations in study design.

Chronic HIV

Chronic HIV is characterized by life-long infection involving a gradual decline in CD4 count leading to eventual overwhelming opportunistic infection. Appropriate use of HAART can halt the decline, lead to immune reconstitution and provide a near normal lifespan to an HIV-infected individual.[75–77] Unfortunately, many individuals with HIV are first diagnosed after the disease has progressed to advanced immunodeficiency and they present with opportunistic disease (AIDS). We begin by describing presentations of common opportunistic illnesses among individuals with HIV, organized by organ system involved.

Opportunistic Illnesses by organ system

The distribution of opportunistic illnesses is correlated with the CD4 count (Table 20.2). This relationship can be used to narrow a differential diagnosis when the CD4 count is known or to estimate the CD4 count when the opportunistic illness is known. In building the differential diagnosis, it is essential to remember that HIV-infected individuals often have multiple simultaneous processes. Thus, parsimony in developing an all-encompassing diagnosis is often not warranted. Furthermore, clinical deterioration despite appropriate therapy for known disease processes should lead to investigation for additional processes.

Systemic illness and fever

Fever with or without localization is a common presentation among individuals with HIV, especially among individuals with profound immunosuppression. The differential diagnoses of fever in an individual with HIV is long; however, a short and location-dependent list represents many of the causes (Table 20.3) encountered in low-income countries. This differential is especially relevant for fever lasting longer than a few days. In most low-income countries, TB is the most common cause of prolonged fever, followed by bacterial pneumonia, bacteraemia, malaria, cryptococcal disease, pneumocystis pneumonia and lymphoma (order of frequency varies by location).[78–81] This chapter briefly describes HIV-relevant aspects of diseases covered in greater depth in other chapters.

Tuberculosis (Mycobacterium tuberculosis complex and Mycobacterium kansasii)

TB is the leading cause of isolated fever or fever with respiratory symptoms among HIV-infected individuals in much of Africa, Asia and Latin America. HIV infection increases the risk of tuberculosis disease 100-fold,[82,83] leading to >50% of patients presenting with fever to be diagnosed with tuberculosis in some settings. The incidence of TB rises with declining CD4 count. In addition, extrapulmonary and miliary TB are more common at lower CD4 counts.[84] Thus tuberculosis should always be suspected in an HIV-infected individual with any of the following signs or symptoms: fevers, cough, weight loss, malaise, night sweats, chest pain, abdominal pain, or lymphadenopathy. Treatment must often be initiated empirically based on symptoms, examination, or radiographic findings because of diagnostic challenges in both extrapulmonary tuberculosis and pulmonary tuberculosis among HIV-infected individuals. However, even in areas with high TB prevalence and frequent use of empiric therapy for suspected TB, autopsy studies demonstrate that TB disease is often undiagnosed.[85]

Laboratory diagnosis of tuberculosis is a challenge. Sputum is <50% sensitive for diagnosis of pulmonary tuberculosis among HIV-infected individuals. Despite this limitation, 2 or 3 sputa should be obtained in any patient with a cough. In addition, HIV-infected patients with more advanced immunodeficiency

Table 20.2 Presenting CD4 range of opportunistic illnesses

CD4+ count (cells/mm³)	Infectious complications	Non-infectious complications
>500	Acute retroviral syndrome Candidal vaginitis	Persistent generalized lymphadenopathy Guillain–Barré syndrome Myopathy Aseptic meningitis
200–500	Pneumococcal and other bacterial pneumonias Pulmonary tuberculosis Herpes zoster Oropharyngeal candidiasis Kaposi sarcoma Oral hairy leukoplakia	Cervical neoplasia and cancer B-cell lymphoma Anaemia Mononeuropathy multiplex Idiopathic thrombocytopenic purpura Hodgkin lymphoma Lymphocytic interstitial pneumonia
<200	*Pneumocystis* pneumonia Disseminated histoplasmosis and coccidioidomycosis Miliary, pulmonary and extrapulmonary tuberculosis Progressive multifocal leucoencephalopathy	Wasting Peripheral neuropathy HIV-associated dementia Cardiomyopathy Vacuolar myelopathy Progressive polyradiculopathy Non-Hodgkin's lymphoma
<100	Disseminated herpes simplex Toxoplasmosis Cryptococcosis Cryptosporidiosis, chronic Microsporidiosis Candidal oesophagitis	
<50	Disseminated cytomegalovirus Disseminated *Mycobacterium avium* complex	

Table 20.3 Common causes of febrile illness among HIV-infected individuals

Tuberculosis
Bacteraemia (*Salmonella, Pneumococcal*)
Malaria
Cryptococcus neoformans
Pneumocystis jiroveci
Lymphoma
Mycobacterium avium complex (MAC)
Penicillium marneffei (Asia)
Visceral leishmania (most localized to Bangladesh, India, Brazil, Nepal, Sudan, Ethiopia)
CMV

(CD4 < 200 cells/mm³) very rarely develop cavitary lesions from pulmonary TB and are much more likely to have chest radiographs with atypical findings of lymphadenopathy, effusions, mid- and lower zone infiltrates, or miliary infiltrates.[86] Culture of sputum or other tissue in liquid media is far more sensitive than smear, but is expensive and results in diagnostic delays of up to several weeks. Nonetheless, the World Health Organization recommends that liquid cultures be obtained for HIV-infected patients with

suspect TB whose sputum smears are negative. Definitive diagnosis of extrapulmonary tuberculosis often requires invasive procedures to obtain fine needle aspirates or biopsies of lymph nodes or other organs. Pathology showing caseating granulomas and acid fast bacilli can confirm the diagnosis, as can culture.

Treatment of TB is effective among HIV-infected individuals and follows the same guidelines as for HIV-uninfected, with the exception that thiacetazone should not be used because of an increased risk of severe adverse events among HIV-infected individuals. TB treatment can complicate HIV treatment and ART regimens; however, this should not discourage the initiation, even empirically, of TB therapy (see below). A growing problem in many nations is multi-drug resistance TB (MDR) and extensively drug resistant TB (XDR), both of which may be more common in HIV-infected individuals.[87] MDR-TB is resistant to both isoniazid and rifampin. XDR-TB is resistant to isoniazid, rifampin and at least two classes of second-line drugs. Detection of drug-resistant TB requires culturing of the organism and performance of drug susceptibility tests, procedures often not performed in developing countries. Nevertheless, without such technology the diagnosis of MDR and XDR-TB is perilously unreliable.

In patients initiating treatment for TB who also receive antiretrovirals, approximately 5–20 % of individuals develop a paradoxical reaction or immune reconstitution disease (IRD).[88,89] IRD involves clinical or radiographic worsening of symptoms and signs and is often marked by fever, cough, lymphadenopathy and new infiltrates, pleural effusion, abscesses or central nervous system mass lesions.

Bacteraemia

Invasive bacterial infections are greatly increased among HIV-infected individuals, especially from *Streptococcus pneumoniae*, *Staphylococcus aureus* and *non-Typhi salmonella*. For example, HIV-infected individuals with pneumococcal pneumonia are also bacteraemic 95% of the time.[90–92] Symptoms of bacteraemia range from low-grade fevers for days or weeks to rigors, chills and sweats, to septic shock. Petechial rashes may be seen in staphylococcal, meningococcal, or pneumococcal sepsis and abdominal rose spots in typhoid fever, but generally rash is not a prominent feature of bacteraemia. Similarly myalgia is uncommon with bacterial sepsis. Both rash and myalgia are more commonly associated with viral and rickettsial diseases. Blood cultures are important for diagnoses of bacteraemia; however, many individuals arriving for evaluation may have already taken antibiotics, reducing the sensitivity of blood culture for diagnosis. Local guidelines for treating systemic infection and bacteraemia should be used to determine antibiotics and care plan. However, relapse of infection should be considered, especially for *Salmonella* bacteraemia, as relapse occurs in nearly 50% of *Salmonella* bacteraemia in some African settings.[93]

Malaria (focused on P. falciparum)

The symptoms of malaria in HIV-infected individuals are similar to those in the general population. However, HIV infection may increase risk for infection and severity of illness. Recent research has identified an increased risk of malaria at lower CD4 counts (2–4-fold increased risk with CD4 < 200 cells/mm^3 when compared with CD4 > 500 cells/mm^3)[94] and an increased risk of severe disease and death. In a study from South Africa, HIV-infection increased the risk of death from malaria 5-fold when compared with HIV-uninfected individuals, possibly because parasitaemia levels are higher with lower CD4 counts.[95] Common symptoms of malaria are similar to HIV-uninfected individuals: headache, malaise, myalgias, abdominal discomfort, anaemia, cough and, often, episodic rigors and fevers.[96]

Malaria should be suspected and managed as for the general population. However, as the immune system wanes, the competing risk from other infections including TB, invasive bacterial infection and cryptococcal disease rises much faster than malaria risk, making malaria a less common cause of febrile illness in individuals with advanced HIV. Among HIV-infected with fever in regions with high malaria incidence, malaria has been detected in <15%.[94] Because of the seemingly low rate of malaria among HIV-infected individuals, confirmation of a suspected malaria by blood smear or antigen testing with ELISA is important to avoid missed or delayed diagnosis of another cause of fever. Treatment of malaria among HIV-infected individuals is the same as for HIV-uninfected. Use of trimethoprim-sulfamethoxazole for PCP and bacterial pneumonia prophylaxis also effectively reduces the risk of malaria.

Mycobacterium avian *complex*

Mycobacterium avian complex (MAC) is a major cause of disease among profoundly immunosuppressed HIV-infected individuals in high-income countries. The incidence appears to be lower in Africa and Asia for unclear reasons. Environmental differences may play a role in different rates of exposure to high levels of the mycobacterium as may competing mortalities from other causes faced by individuals in low-income countries. Studies of hospitalized individuals with febrile illness in Africa have identified MAC among 5–10% of blood isolates, lower than *M. tuberculosis* isolation in those studies.[97,98] MAC infection rarely occurs with CD4 > 100 cells/mm^3 and usually with CD4 < 50 cells/mm^3. Symptoms are generally non-specific and usually include fever (78–84%), night sweats, weight loss, abdominal pain and diarrhoea.[99] Diarrhoea from MAC can be profound and chronic, leading to significant malabsorption and wasting. Diagnosis is made by mycobacterial culture from the blood, where available. In the many areas where mycobacterial culture is unavailable, there are few clinical or laboratory clues to suggest diagnosis. Anaemia, leucopenia and thrombocytopenia are common, but these may be normal. Alkaline phosphatase is often elevated, but this may also be normal and may be elevated in other disease states. In areas without mycobacterial culture facilities, some clinicians have used empiric therapy among individuals with CD4 count <50 cells/mm^3, fever and wasting (±diarrhoea) of unclear aetiology. However, response to therapy is generally slow (2–4 weeks for decrease in fever) and the treatment course is long; thus empiric treatment should be reserved for cases with high suspicion of MAC. Standard treatment is with either azithromycin (500–600 mg daily) or clarithromycin (500 mg twice daily) plus ethambutol (15 mg/kg daily) for at least 12 months. Success of therapy depends on immune reconstitution with antiretroviral therapy. Without antiretroviral therapy, survival, even with MAC treatment, is often <6 months.[99]

Cryptococcal disease

Infection with *Cryptococcus neoformans* usually causes isolated meningitis, without fever (50% of cases). However, it can also cause a disseminated febrile disease with fungaemia and umbilicated skin lesions or pneumonia. Serum cryptococcal antigen testing is diagnostic of systemic infection; CSF cryptococcal antigen testing is diagnostic of meningitis. Thus a lumbar puncture is indicated to evaluate for the presence of meningitis. Systemic infection without meningitis can be safely treated with fluconazole (200–400 mg p.o. daily) until immune reconstitution (CD4 > 200 cells/mL) has been achieved, while amphotericin B should be given for 10–14 days followed, by high dose fluconazole if meningitis is present (see Neurological disease below).

Penicillinosis

Penicillium marneffei is endemic in South-east Asia, southern China and north-eastern India. Cases occurring outside this region have been reported among returned travellers. In endemic areas, it is an important opportunistic infection and among the top five causes of subacute fever among individuals with CD4 < 100 cells/mm^3 (usually <50 cells/mm^3).[100,101] Symptoms are generally sudden onset of fever accompanied by anaemia, weight loss and characteristic skin lesions (a generalized papular rash with central umbilication, similar in appearance to molluscum contagiosum and cryptococcus). Individuals may also have a cough, generalized lymphadenopathy, hepatomegaly and diarrhoea.[102] Chest radiographs may reveal a diffuse reticulonodular or alveolar infiltrate. Diagnosis can be made based on characteristic skin lesions or by biopsy of skin lesions, liver, or bone marrow. Occasionally the intracellular organisms may be seen on blood smears. Standard therapy is amphotericin B (0.6 mg/kg daily) for 2 weeks followed by 10 weeks of itraconazole oral solution (200 mg twice daily). Secondary prophylaxis with itraconazole (200 mg daily) should be continued until immune reconstitution is achieved.

Lymphoma

Diffuse large B-cell lymphoma, primary effusion body lymphoma, Burkitt's lymphoma and primary CNS lymphoma are all increased among HIV-infected individuals. Among individuals with profound immunosuppression from HIV in industrialized countries, as many as 20% develop an AIDS-related malignancy. Reported rates of lymphoma in low-income countries are much lower, possibly a result of a combination of higher mortality from opportunistic infections and under-ascertainment.[103] Presentation is often a combination of B-symptoms (fevers (Pel-Ebstein), night sweats and weight loss). Peripheral lymphadenopathy may be present, but this finding is less common in HIV-associated lymphomas. However, visceral involvement is more common including pleural and peritoneal effusions. Detection often requires imaging and biopsies of affected organs. Treatment of lymphoma is based on locally available oncological care.

Visceral leishmaniasis

Visceral leishmaniasis is a disease caused by *Leishmania donovani*, Hodgkins lymphoma *L. braziliensis*, *L aethopica*, or *L. chagasi*, an organism transmitted by the bite of the *Phlebotomus* sand fly. Some 90% of cases occur in five countries: Bangladesh, Brazil, India, Nepal and Sudan.[104]. The classic presentation is fever (classically, a double quotidian fever), hepatosplenomegaly and pancytopenia. The fever may be persistent or remitting, usually lasting more than 2 weeks. The incubation period is up to 6 months; thus exposure may have occurred months prior while an individual was in an endemic area.[105] HIV-infected individuals have similar, although potentially more severe presentations than HIV-uninfected individuals that may also include weight loss, lymphadenopathy, diarrhoea, oesophagitis, splenomegaly and cutaneous lesions.[106–108] HIV increases the risk of developing visceral leishmaniasis 100–2000-fold, especially at CD4 < 200 cells/mm³. Diagnosis in HIV-infected individuals is best achieved by demonstrating amastigotes in blood or tissue biopsy, generally spleen or bone marrow. Antibody testing is helpful when positive; however, antibody response is muted among HIV-infected individuals and <50% sensitive. Treatment should follow the same guidelines for HIV-infected and HIV-uninfected individuals (Chapter 77). However, relapse is the rule unless immune recovery is achieved via HAART. Relapse usually occurs 1–8 months following therapy.

Cytomegalovirus (CMV)

CMV disease occurs among HIV-infected individuals with CD4 < 50 cells/mm³.[109] Most CMV disease is limited to the retina and causes rapidly progressive vision loss without fevers. Gastrointestinal and neurological involvement can also occur leading to colitis, polyradiculopathy, or encephalitis. Interstitial pneumonia from CMV among HIV-infected individuals is extremely rare. Fever may be associated with colitis or neurological disease. However, fever is rarely the dominant sign. Treatment with ganciclover or valganciclovir (900 mg twice daily for 4 weeks then daily).

Histoplasmosis

Histoplasma capsulatum is present on every continent except Antarctica. However, it has a varied distribution, favouring damp soil and bird guano and is rarely reported from Africa or Asia.[110] In individuals with low CD4 counts, disseminated histoplasmosis can present as weeks of malaise and fevers along with generalized lymphadenopathy, pancytopenia and pneumonia, with oral ulcers often present. Cutaneous findings of papules, ulcers, or plaques are present in one-third of patients. Diagnosis is made on histopathology of skin or organ biopsy or urine antigen test.[111] Amphotericin B (0.7 mg/kg daily) for 3–7 days is the treatment of choice for severe infection followed by itraconazole (200 mg twice daily followed by 200 mg daily until CD4 >150 for 6 months) or for 12 weeks (Chapter 71).

Immune reconstitution disease (IRD)

IRD is an exaggerated immune response to antigens from active or past infections. It occurs during immune reconstitution after HIV viral suppression with HAART. It usually occurs during the first 6 months of HAART as CD4 increases from a low nadir (usually <50 cells/mm³).[112] The presence of the underlying infection may be known at the time of HAART initiation or may be diagnosed after HAART initiation as symptoms emerge on therapy. High rates of endemic illness, OIs and the low CD4 count at HAART initiation have led to high rates of IRD in low-income countries.[113] Most troubling has been potentially fatal IRD associated with TB and cryptococcal meningitis. IRD with tuberculosis may present with fevers, lymphadenopathy or lymphadenitis, cold abscesses, worsening pulmonary status, or abdominal pain or bowel obstruction from abdominal lymphadenopathy. IRD associated with chronic hepatitis B infection may present as acute hepatitis, but is rarely fatal. There should be a high index of suspicion for IRD in patients recently started on ART who present with constitutional symptoms, lymphadenitis, soft tissue masses or abscesses, as IRD can be difficult to diagnose since there are no specific tests for it. Patients with severe presentation can be treated with a long, tapering course of systemic corticosteroids (e.g. prednisone 40 mg twice a day; however no standard regimens have been tested) along with continued HAART and specific therapy directed against the OI.

Neurological disease

Central nervous system disease can present either primarily with headaches, altered mental status, focal neurological deficits or seizures, or cognitive decline. Peripheral neurological disease can present with numbness, paraesthesias, or weakness.

Headache without focal neurological deficits

In HIV-infected persons with a CD4 count >200 cells/mm³, as in those without HIV infection, headache is often a result of conditions such as muscle tension, migraine, or sinusitis.[114] The differential diagnoses become broader if the CD4 count is

<200 cells/mm³ or if fever is present. Patients with CD4 < 200 cells/mm³ and especially <100 cells/mm³ presenting with a new or worsening headache (with or without fever) should be evaluated for cryptococcal meningitis with a lumbar puncture.[115] Cryptococcal meningitis is the most common cause of meningitis among HIV-infected individuals in many low-income regions and one of the most common CNS infections.[116–118] Among HIV-infected individuals cryptococcal meningitis generally has a subacute presentation with gradually worsening headaches from rising intracranial pressure because of debris from the cryptococcal polysaccharide capsule that interferes with normal cerebral spinal fluid (CSF) resorption in the arachnoid plexus. As the intracranial pressure rises headache worsens and cranial nerves may become involved, including the eighth nerve, leading to decreased hearing. Fever is often a minor symptom or absent. Meningismus is generally absent because there is usually little inflammation within the meninges. Patients with cryptococcal meningitis may also have disseminated disease with cutaneous lesions and choroiditis. Cutaneous lesions typically present as umbilicated lesions on the face and extremities with an appearance similar in appearance to *molluscum contagiosum*. However, shallow ulcerations may also be the primary cutaneous manifestation. Pulmonary involvement may cause a mild pneumonia. Cryptococcal meningitis is diagnosed by lumbar puncture. The opening pressure is usually high, the cell count normal (usually <20 white cells/hpf), glucose and protein normal and a cryptococcal antigen test positive. India ink can be used to stain CSF to identify organisms, but this has far lower sensitivity than antigen testing. Cryptococcus can also be cultured. Successful management of cryptococcal meningitis hinges on controlling intracranial pressure (ICP). This may require serial lumbar punctures or, in severe cases, placement of an intraventricular drain (elevated ICP is not a contraindication for lumbar puncture in this setting). Patients with cryptococcal meningitis should be treated with amphotericin B (0.7 mg/kg per day i.v.) and flucytosine (100 mg p.o.) for 14 days followed by fluconazole (400 mg p.o., q.d.) for 8 weeks and finally fluconazole (200 mg p.o. q.d.) prophylaxis indefinitely or until substantial immune recovery has occurred.

Other causes of headache include *Toxoplasma* encephalitis, primary CNS lymphoma, bacterial meningitis, viral encephalitis, coccidioidomycosis, histoplasmosis, tuberculosis meningitis, nocardiosis, neurocysticercosis and pyogenic brain abscess. TB is an important infectious cause of chronic headaches, usually accompanied by fevers, night sweats, weight loss, a CSF pleocytosis (>50 white blood cells, usually mononuclear) and elevated CSF protein. AFB staining and culture of the CSF are unreliable for diagnosis. Imaging generally demonstrates basilar meningeal enhancement; however, this may be absent and may be present with other processes.[119] Because of the difficulty with definitive diagnosis, empiric therapy is warranted when the diagnosis of TB meningitis is strongly suspected (Chapter 56). Bacterial meningitis, especially from *Streptococcus pneumoniae* and viral meningitis is also a common cause of fever and headache among HIV-infected individuals. These diagnoses may account for a third of meningitis in some HIV-infected populations.[120]

Focal neurological defects

The focal neurological lesions are suggested by asymmetrical weakness or paraesthesias or seizure with or without headaches,

fevers, or papilloedema. The most common causes in low-income countries are tuberculomas followed by CNS toxoplasmosis, neurocysticerosis, primary CNS lymphoma, progressive multifocal leucoencephalopathy and cryptococcomas.[119,121–123] Use of serology for toxoplasmosis can help to refine the differential diagnosis, as a negative serum toxoplasmosis IgG makes the diagnosis of toxoplasmosis unlikely.[124,125] Findings at additional sites, such as pulmonary infiltrates on chest radiography or lymphadenopathy suggestive of TB make tuberculomas the most likely diagnosis. Imaging, when available, can help to identify space occupying lesions and suggest diagnoses. TB, lymphoma, toxoplasmosis and cryptococcomas may all be ring enhancing, whereas, PML is not. A cystic mass is consistent with neurocysticerosis. Results from a lumbar puncture can also be helpful in guiding empiric therapy. If the CD4 count is <100 cells/mm³ and the CSF white count and protein are not highly elevated, empiric treatment for toxoplasmosis should be initiated (weight <60 kg: pyrimethamine 50 mg daily, leucovorin 10–20 mg daily and sulfadiazine 1 g four times a day; weight >60 kg: pyrimethamine 75 mg daily, folinic acid 10–20 mg daily and sulfadiazine 1.5 g four times a day (where leucovorin is unavailable this may be excluded from the regimen) for 6 weeks followed by lifelong prophylaxis with 50% of the dose for acute management). Response is usually rapid (within 1 week); failure to respond suggests an alternative diagnosis.[125] If the CSF has a pleocytosis and high protein, tuberculomas should be suspected and treatment of CNS TB initiated (Chapter 56). A positive cryptococcal antigen test should lead to treatment for cryptococcal disease. CSF positive for JC virus by PCR, lack of fever and focal neurologic deficits help make the diagnosis of PML. HAART may help if PML is suspected; however, there is no known effective therapy for PML.

Cognitive decline or impairment

Altered mental status is common in HIV infection. The approach to evaluation follows that used in the general population, with recognition of an increased risk of infectious and neoplastic causes. All of the CNS processes discussed previously can present as a change in mental status and several other diagnoses should be considered in the patient with advanced HIV disease. The most common cause is HIV-associated dementia (HAD), a condition that occurs in patients with advanced immunodeficiency. The incidence of HAD in low-income countries has not been well defined; however, in industrialized countries prior to the introduction of HAART, the annual incidence was nearly 10% and the lifetime prevalence was 15%.[126] HAD usually develops over months (rarely faster, although it may go unnoticed) and is characterized by cognitive, behavioural and motor dysfunction. In early stages, patients often present with fluctuating memory and concentration loss, loss of interest in activities, slowing of motor skills and intermittent ataxia. The first noted symptoms may be occasional loss of balance or stumbling. As HAD progresses, global dementia and paraplegia can develop. HAART may lead to partial reversal of HAD and some recovery of function.[127]

Extremity pain, numbness, or weakness

Peripheral neuropathy in HIV-infected patients may present as a distal sensory polyneuropathy, with symmetric numbness, tingling, burning, or pain in the feet or hands without motor weakness.[126] The two most common causes are toxic neuropathy from medications (usually stavudine, didanosine, or both) or HIV itself. Other causes or contributing factors can include alcoholism, thyroid disease, vitamin B_{12} deficiency, syphilis, CMV, diabetes mellitus, including diabetes caused by protease inhibitors. In drug-induced neuropathy, early interruption of the offending agent gradually leads to complete or near complete resolution of symptoms. However, several months may pass before any improvement is noted. CMV myelitis and polyradiculitis present as rapidly progressive weakness and numbness in the upper and lower extremities in patients with a CD4 < 50 cells/mm^3 (and usually only among individuals who also have CMV retinitis). Myopathy related to HIV or to medications (e.g. zidovudine) presents as muscle pain, usually in the thighs and shoulders and proximal weakness. It is usually associated with an increased serum creatine phosphokinase (CPK) level and can be definitively diagnosed by muscle biopsy.

Pulmonary disease

Pulmonary TB and community acquired bacterial pneumonia are the two most common diagnoses among HIV-infected individuals admitted to hospital in Africa with pulmonary symptoms.[110,128–131] *Pneumocystis jiroveci* is a cause of pulmonary infection when the CD4 count is <200 cells/mm^3, accounting for 5–10% of pulmonary infections in Africa and Asia.[128,132,133] Rarer pulmonary processes include infections from *Nocardia*, *Rhodococcus* equi, *M. kansasii*, *Cryptococcus* and viral pathogens and malignancy including Kaposi's sarcoma, lymphoma and primary lung cancer. When a patient with profound immunodeficiency develops a cavitary lesion, the differential diagnosis should be broadened to include pathogens such as *M. kansasii* and *Nocardia*. With the exception of lung cancer, TB and bacterial pneumonia, the processes listed usually occur at CD4 counts <100 cells/mm^3.

Signs and symptoms that suggest pulmonary infections are cough, fevers and dyspnoea. Pleuritic-type chest pain and haemoptysis and productive cough may also be present and are suggestive of either TB or pneumococcal pneumonia. Physical examination findings of areas of consolidation may be present with pulmonary TB, bacterial pneumonia, as well as other infectious pulmonary processes, but are rare with PCP. Rarer causes of dyspnoea include pleural effusions, pericardial effusions, congestive heart failure, acute severe anaemia and symptomatic lactic acidosis. Effusions most commonly occur as a result of extrapulmonary TB. Malignancy, including lymphoma and parapneumonic processes may also cause effusions.

Pulmonary TB (PTB)

The classic presentation of post-primary PTB is weeks to months of chronic cough (>2–3 weeks), weight loss, fatigue, fevers, night sweats and haemoptysis.[134] Fever is classically diurnal with an afebrile period early in the morning and a gradually rising temperature throughout the day, with a fever peak in the late afternoon or evening. Night-time defervescence is often accompanied by diaphoresis leading to drenching night sweats. Immunosuppression with advancing HIV disease may alter the presenting symptoms. For example, fever and non-specific symptoms, such as wasting and malaise, are more common among individuals

co-infected with HIV and pulmonary TB, while cough is less common.[135] HIV-infected individuals with pulmonary TB are more likely to also have extra-pulmonary sites of infection than individuals without HIV: 60% also have extra-pulmonary sites of infection compared with 28% of pulmonary TB patients without HIV.[84] The suspicion for pulmonary TB should be especially high among individuals with previously treated TB disease as both relapse and new infection are more frequent in this group.[136–138] However, diagnosis of recurrent TB can be complicated because pulmonary fibrosis and cavitary lesions from previous disease can obscure new infiltrates and complicate interpretation of chest radiographs.

Pulmonary TB is ideally diagnosed by AFB positive sputum smears with culture for confirmation. However, sputum smear is <50% sensitive for detecting pulmonary TB among HIV-infected individuals and mycobacterial culture, while far more sensitive, is slow and unavailable in much of the world. Clinical response to an empiric course of antibiotics for bacterial pneumonia has been used in some settings to exclude the diagnosis of TB. However, this approach is flawed for two reasons: (1) the natural history of PTB involves waxing and waning of symptoms and (2) both bacterial pneumonia and PTB may be present simultaneously. Thus, if this strategy is used, follow-up evaluations with AFB smear are essential.[139] However, failure to respond to a trial of antibiotics does indicate a high probability of pulmonary TB and can be used as a basis for an empiric diagnosis.

Bacterial pneumonia

Community-acquired pneumonia (e.g. from *Streptococcus pneumoniae*, *Haemophilus influenzae*, *S. aureus*, or *Pseudomonas aeruginosa*) occurs at a rate 25–200 fold higher than in the general population and is far more commonly accompanied by bacteraemia.[140,141] Classic signs and symptoms include abrupt onset, pleuritis chest pain, fevers, rigors and focal consolidation. Therapy should follow local guidelines for management of community acquired pneumonia. However, HIV-infected individuals may be sicker and progress in disease faster before responding to antibiotic therapy than non-HIV-infected individuals. Thus they warrant closer monitoring and follow-up.

Pneumocystis jiroveci *pneumonia*

Pneumocystis jiroveci pneumonia (PCP) can present as a subacute process of weeks to months of fevers, dry cough, worsening dyspnoea and weight loss in individuals with CD4 count <200 cells/mm^3. Fevers are usually a component of the presentation and may be the primary problem reported by a patient. Progressive dyspnoea, especially dyspnoea with exertion, is usually also present. On examination ronchi may be heard throughout the lungs. Chest radiography often reveals a bilateral diffuse interstitial infiltrate, but may be normal 20% of the time.[142] A history of adherence to trimethoprim-sulfamethoxazole or dapsone prophylaxis makes the diagnosis far less likely. PCP is very common in industrialized countries, but for unclear reasons it is less common in low-income countries. Diagnosis is based on the characteristics of fever for days or weeks, progressive dyspnoea on exertion and a dry (nonproductive) cough along with radiographic findings. Optimally, the organism is identified from sputum or bronchoalveolar lavage with immunofluorescent or Gomori–Methenamine silver staining. Standard treatment is trimethoprim-sulfamethoxazole 15–20 mg/kg (of trimethoprim) daily in three divided doses for 21 days. Oral therapy is two double strength tablets of trimethoprim-sulfamethoxazole three times a day. After initiation of treatment, an inflammatory reaction can develop to dead organisms, leading to a worsening of the respiratory status. The risk of severe decompensation can be reduced among individuals with baseline significant hypoxia (resting PaO2 <70) by use of corticosteroids (prednisone 40 mg twice daily ×5 days, 40 mg daily ×5 days, then 20 mg until therapy is completed).

Kaposi's sarcoma

Kaposi's sarcoma (KS) can present as a pulmonary syndrome with subacute progression of dyspnoea, dyspnoea on exertion, dry cough and wheezing. Fevers are usually absent.[143] Chest radiographic findings are often bilateral nodular infiltrates with or without pleural effusions; however, radiographic findings are highly variable and can also appear as focal consolidation. Most individuals with pulmonary KS have cutaneous or oropharyngeal lesions; however, 15% present without lesions identifiable on physical examination.[144] Diagnosis is by direct visualization of lesions via bronchoscopy. Biopsy is generally not necessary and risks significant bleeding. As KS is common in many regions in Africa, pulmonary KS is possibly under-diagnosed.

Gastrointestinal disease

Oral Lesions

Oropharyngeal candidiasis (thrush) is common in patients with CD4 < 300 cells/mm³. Patients with thrush may complain of oral discomfort, pharyngeal dysphagia or odynophagia, or fissured lips. Physical examination generally reveals white curd-like plaques, which can be easily scraped off, on the buccal mucosa, palate, tongue, or posterior pharynx. Treatment with clotrimazole troches (five lozenges a day for 7–14 days) or nystatin swish and swallow is usually effective.

Oral hairy leukoplakia (OHL) is found on the lateral margins of the tongue and appears as vertically oriented, white, linear plaques that cannot be scraped off with a tongue blade. OHL is associated with Epstein–Barr virus (EBV) infection and responds to effective HAART and immune restoration. Common aetiologies of ulcerative oral lesions include aphthous stomatitis and HSV, adenovirus and CMV infection. Oral lesions from syphilis, lymphoma and medications are less common.

Dysphagia and odynophagia

Dysphagia and odynophagia are very common symptoms in patients with advanced HIV disease and suggest oesophagitis. Candida is the most common cause when the CD4 is < 100 cells/mm³; therefore, empiric treatment with fluconazole (100–200 mg daily for 14–21 days) is appropriate. The likelihood of Candida oesophagitis is increased when oral thrush is also present, although thrush may be absent. The diagnosis of Candida oesophagitis is typically established by a response to fluconazole within days of starting treatment. If there is no response to empiric therapy within 3 to 4 days, the dose of fluconazole should be doubled.

Continued therapeutic failure suggests fluconazole resistant Candida spp. or alternative aetiologies (e.g. aphthous oesophagitis, CMV or HSV infection). Upper endoscopy with biopsy is helpful to evaluate for ulcerative diseases.[125]

Nausea and emesis

Nausea, vomiting and anorexia can be side-effects of medication (including antiretrovirals and antimicrobials) or may result from lactic acidosis, acute gastroenteritis, hypogonadism, pregnancy, depression (in the case of isolated anorexia), substance abuse, cholangitis, hepatitis, tuberculosis and lymphoma. Evaluation should include a detailed medication history and timing of onset of symptoms with respect to medication initiation. If the patient is taking stavudine, didanosine, or zidovudine, lactic acidosis should be considered and a serum lactic acid level should be obtained promptly. Additional signs and symptoms of lactic acidosis may include constitutional symptoms, nausea, dyspnoea, weight loss, myalgias and hepatitis.[145] The mortality associated with severe lactic acidosis (levels above 10 mmol/L) approaches 50%, so prompt withdrawal of combination antiretroviral therapy and institution of supportive care are critical. Normalization of serum lactic acid levels can take months. After recovery from lactic acidosis, patients should be treated with regimens that do not include stavudine or didanosine.

Diarrhoea

Diarrhoea is common in many low-income regions. HIV-infected individuals are at risk for diarrhoea from enteric viruses, Salmonella spp, Shigella spp, Campylobacter jejuni, Enterotoxigenic Escherichia coli, Giardia lamblia, Entamoeba histolytica, Strongyloides stercoralis, Ascaris lumbricoides and malaria. When the CD4 count is <200 cells/mm³ and especially when it is <100 cells/mm³, chronic diarrhoea from Cryptosporidium parvum, Strongyloides stercoralis, Isospora belli, Microsporidia spp, MAC and CMV becomes more common. Generally, when a cause of chronic diarrhoea is identified, Cryptosporidium is the most common followed by Strongyloides, Isospora, Salmonella and Mycobacterial infection.[146–150] One diagnostic approach is to assess carefully for systemic illness (malaria blood smears, TB sputum smears, blood cultures, mycobacterial blood cultures) and perform ova and parasite examination on stool. Patients who are acutely ill with blood or mucous in stool and negative ova and parasite examinations should be treated for bacterial gastroenteritis per local guidelines (for example ceftriaxone 1 g i.v. daily and metronidazole 500 mg orally three times a day). When no aetiology is identified for chronic diarrhoea, symptomatic management with loperamide or tincture of opium can improve comfort. Immune recovery with HAART may be required for resolution of diarrhoea.

Hepatitis

Hepatitis may be suspected based on findings of jaundice, abdominal pain, anorexia, or nausea. However, often the results of serum transaminase testing, with a markedly elevated ALT and AST and occasionally elevated bilirubin with only moderate elevation in alkaline phosphatase, alert to the presence of hepatic inflammation. Acute hepatitis can be the result of medications, infections, or metabolic causes. Some antiretroviral agents cause liver injury through direct toxicity; through inhibition of mitochondrial DNA polymerase gamma, leading to hepatic steatosis and lactic acidosis; and through idiosyncratic reactions, such as occur with nevirapine and abacavir.[151] Drug-induced hepatitis has been most strongly associated with nevirapine, especially when started in patients with higher CD4 counts (>250 for women and >400 for men).[152,153] Nevirapine-related hepatoxicity is often associated with a rash and occurs a median of 30 days after starting nevirapine.[154] Most protease inhibitors can cause hepatitis, especially in patients with chronic viral hepatitis. Both atazanavir and indinavir can cause an asymptomatic and benign indirect hyperbilirubinaemia without elevation in transaminase levels. In the case of atazanavir, jaundice, scleral icterus, or both can occur; however, it is benign and does not require discontinuation of therapy. Acute hepatitis from hepatitis A virus (HAV), hepatitis B virus (HBV), or hepatitis C virus (HCV) can occur among HIV-infected patients. Other conditions that can lead to transaminase elevations are leptospirosis, tuberculosis, lymphoma, autoimmune hepatitis and toxins (including alcohol and naturopathic medications). A patient presenting with a febrile illness, moderately to severely increased transaminase levels and an increased bilirubin level will most likely have tuberculosis or acute HAV or HBV infection, although other aetiologies, including acute drug reaction and obstructive cholelithiasis, are also possible. When HAART induced hepatotoxicity is suspected, generally therapy can be continued (except for abacavir and nevirapine), even with ALT and AST 5 to 10 times the upper limit of the normal reference range.[155] Exceptions are patients who are symptomatic or have elevated bilirubin along with high ALT and AST.

A cholestatic profile on serum chemistry raises the possibility of obstruction from stones or malignancy, lactic acidosis with hepatic steatosis, HIV cholangiopathy, infections such as tuberculosis or schistosomiasis, or medication-induced cholestasis (e.g. from TMP-SMX, amitriptyline, ampicillin, naproxen, or phenytoin). HIV cholangiopathy is the term that describes constriction of the biliary tract through strictures, papillary stenosis, or a sclerosing cholangitis-like pathology that usually occurs only among individuals with CD4 < 100 cells/mm³. Most patients have significant abdominal pain and a markedly elevated alkaline phosphatase.[156] Low-grade fevers and diarrhoea are often present. It is believed biliary tract infection from *Cryptosporidium*, *Microsporidia* spp., *Cyclospora cayetanensis*, or CMV leads to ductal changes. Abdominal ultrasonography is useful to make a diagnosis of a cholestasis process; however, endoscopic retrograde cholangiopancreatography (ERCP) is the optimal diagnostic tool as well as therapeutic tool if papillary stenosis is present.

Abdominal pain

Abdominal pain may be caused by pancreatitis, lactic acidosis, AIDS cholangiopathy, non-Hodgkin's lymphoma, abdominal tuberculosis, MAC lymphadenitis, CMV colitis and IRD.[157] Acute pancreatitis is usually associated with nausea and vomiting, may be seen at any CD4 count and is associated with didanosine and stavudine, especially when these two agents are taken together.[158] Alcohol, obstructive gallstones and hypertriglyceridaemia, which can be caused or exacerbated by some protease inhibitors, should also be considered as causes of pancreatitis. Abdominal imaging and serum chemistry studies are important for diagnosis.

Renal disease

Renal disease is common in patients with high HIV RNA and low CD4 counts who are not receiving HAART; 2–10% of such patients in industrialized countries are affected.[159] The prevalence in Africa and Asia has not been well described. The most common HIV-related renal disease is HIV-associated nephropathy (HIVAN). HIVAN is characterized by proteinuria, often nephrotic range (i.e. >3 g/dL), polyuria, minimal oedema and echogenic kidneys; biopsy shows collapsing focal and segmental glomerulosclerosis.[160] HIVAN is rare in patients with suppressed HIV RNA.[161] Complete suppression of HIV replication with HAART can reverse pathogenic changes and lead to recovery of renal function. In patients on HAART with suppressed HIV replication, hypertension and diabetes are important causes of kidney disease.

Dermatological disease

Dermatological complaints affected over 90% of HIV-infected patients in industrialized countries before the introduction of HAART. A common condition at lower CD4 counts is *prurigo nodularis*, characterized by highly pruritic, hyperpigmented and often excoriated papular lesions involving the extremities and torso. Over time, it may progress to *lichen simplex chronicum*. Emollients and high-potency topical corticosteroids can break the cycle of pruritus and excoriation, but symptom control is often difficult. HAART and immune restoration may lead to gradual resolution of symptoms. Eczematous conditions including seborrheic dermatitis, atopic dermatitis and xerotic eczema are also more common in HIV-infected patients.[162-165] Seborrheic dermatitis is characterized by erythematous, often pruritic, plaques with greasy scales and indistinct margins on the scalp, face and post-auricular area. Mid-potency steroids may be used for control of a flare; ketoconazole cream/shampoo or selenium shampoo may be effective for long-term management. Scabies should also be considered in the differential diagnosis of a pruritic skin rash and patients with more advanced immunosuppression are at risk for more severe, crusted (so-called Norwegian) scabies.

Papules may be caused by eosinophilic folliculitis, which presents as small, often pruritic, perifollicular papular and pustular lesions, usually on the upper body and proximal upper extremities and usually occurring with lower CD4 counts or during immune reconstitution.[166,167] Treatment with mid-potency corticosteroids may control symptoms. Larger, diffusely distributed papules and pustules may be caused by *S. aureus*, *Pseudomonas aeruginosa* and dermatophytes. Larger skin-coloured papules with central umbilication are caused by the pox virus, molluscum contagiosum, and are often distributed on the face and neck. Lesions can evolve into large disfiguring plaques. Disease is associated with advanced immunodeficiency. Treatment is immune restoration with HAART. Conditions that can have similar skin findings to *molluscum contagiosum* are disseminated cryptococcosis, blastomycosis and penicilliosis.

Varicella zoster (shingles), a reactivation of herpes zoster in the ganglion of a nerve, is a common cause of skin disease when the CD4 is <500 cells/mm³ and during immune reconstitution. Zoster presents as a painful vesicular rash in a dermatomal distribution; more rarely it may involve multiple dermatomes or become disseminated. Patients with advanced immunodeficiency may also present with extensive herpes simplex ulcerations appearing as painful, beefy red perineal and perianal ulcerations. Aciclovir or famciclovir are treatments of choice for both zoster and herpes simplex reactivation.

Violaceous plaques or nodules are caused by Kaposi's sarcoma (KS) (see below) and bacillary angiomatosis. Bacillary angiomatosis usually appears as a red or purple nodular or pedunculated lesion, is caused by *Bartonella* species and is associated with disseminated infection.[168] Bacillary angiomatosis can be confused with KS; however, the distinction between the two should be made, because it can be effectively treated (erythromycin 500 mg four times a day or doxycycline 100 mg twice a day for >3 months).

Drug reactions account for <5% of rashes in Africa.[165,169,170] The most well-known reactions are to sulphonamides, notably TMP-SMX and sulfadiazine. Other agents that commonly cause rash include abacavir (in the setting of a systemic hypersensitivity reaction), efavirenz, nevirapine and fosamprenavir. Drug reactions typically present as pruritic maculopapular, morbilliform, or urticarial eruptions, but they may also appear as erythema multiforme, erythema nodosum, or exfoliative dermatitis (toxic epidermal necrolysis and Stevens–Johnson syndrome). Manifestations of systemic involvement may include fever, elevated transaminase levels and interstitial nephritis. Management consists of symptomatic treatment, drug discontinuation and careful observation.

Malignancy

Major HIV-related malignancies are KS, non-Hodgkin's lymphoma, Burkitt's lymphoma and cervical cancer.[103] KS is a malignancy that can affect the skin, mucosal surfaces, lungs, gastrointestinal tract and internal organs, and remains the most common AIDS-defining malignancy, although most patients who develop Kaposi's sarcoma have not yet started HAART.[171] The incidence of cervical and anal squamous cell carcinoma is increased in HIV-infected persons and HIV-associated cervical cancer is more aggressive. For this reason, screening for cervical dysplasia with a Pap smear is important.

KS is among the leading opportunistic illnesses in many regions in Africa,[172] although rare in Asia and Latin America. It occurs via neoplastic transformation mediated by infection with human herpes virus 8 (HHV-8, also known as KSHV). It can develop in the dermis, deeper within soft tissue, within mucosal surfaces and within the lungs and viscera. It is commonly recognized as non-pruritic non-painful violaceous plaques or nodules on the pallet, groin, or lower extremities. As disease progresses, it can lead to obstruction of lymphatics and lymphoedema. KS of the lungs can lead to a respiratory syndrome and radiographic findings consistent with a bilateral pneumonia. KS of the gastrointestinal tract can lead to mild bleeding or obstruction. A diagnosis is either by visual inspection or biopsy and histopathology. Treatment response is poor with large lesions. Small lesions can resolve with immune reconstitution with HAART. Larger lesions may respond to a combination of HAART and chemotherapy (doxorubicin or daunorubicin are preferred, vinblastine, vincristine, or bleomycin may also reduce tumour burden). Radiation therapy may also help control tumour burden.

Long-term HIV care

Longitudinal HIV care begins at the time of HIV diagnosis. This should include a care package of psychological support, screening and prevention of opportunistic infections, nutritional support and planning for HAART. Each component of a care plan is important for both reducing morbidity and mortality and for improving quality of life (Figure 20.3). Such a package of services needs to be tailored to local needs but may include provision of safe drinking water, active screening for tuberculosis, TB prophylaxis among individuals without active TB (INH), micronutrient supplements, food packets, PMTCT, vaccinations, cotrimoxazole preventive therapy for PCP, malaria and bacterial infections, insecticide treated bed nets, psychological counselling, family HIV counselling and testing, management of opportunistic illnesses and HAART.[173,174]

Psychological support

Individuals infected with HIV may have higher rates of depression and increased social isolation and ostracism; furthermore, depression is likely under-appreciated in African HIV care programmes. However, it can impact on quality of life and medical adherence. Thus depression is optimally managed through a combination of psychiatric care, counselling and support groups. Inclusion of community leaders, religious figures and traditional diviners and healers in psycho-social support may reduce isolation and improve the sense of well-being. Antidepressants can be very valuable in controlling symptoms and improving quality of life.

Nutritional support

HIV infection is associated with increased resting energy expenditure, weight loss and malnutrition.[175] The combination of these underlying HIV factors and inadequate access to food makes nutrition an important aspect of HIV care in many low-income countries. Furthermore, after health improves with HAART, many patients experience an increase in appetite and may return to pre-HAART baseline weight if adequate nutrition is available. When food is scarce, an improved appetite can lead to hunger and compromise HAART adherence.[176] Thus, the issue of food security and access to food should be addressed within an HIV programme. Use of food supplements can improve the nutritional status, may improve immune status and can contribute to HAART adherence and continuation with HIV care.

The overall impact of micronutrients among adults within HIV treatment remains uncertain. Some studies have suggested benefit with supplementation of vitamins or minerals, whereas others have been equivocal.[177] While vitamin supplementation may have a role in HIV care, assuring the combination of adequate protein, energy and micronutrients (vitamin A, vitamin B_{12}, vitamin C, vitamin E, zinc) may be the best approach for HIV care for individuals living on the edge of food insecurity.

Screening for opportunistic infections

Initial and follow-up clinic evaluations of HIV-infected individuals are an opportunity to screen for opportunistic infections. A general review of symptoms can identify clues to suggest important diagnoses. New onset of headaches may suggest cryptococcal

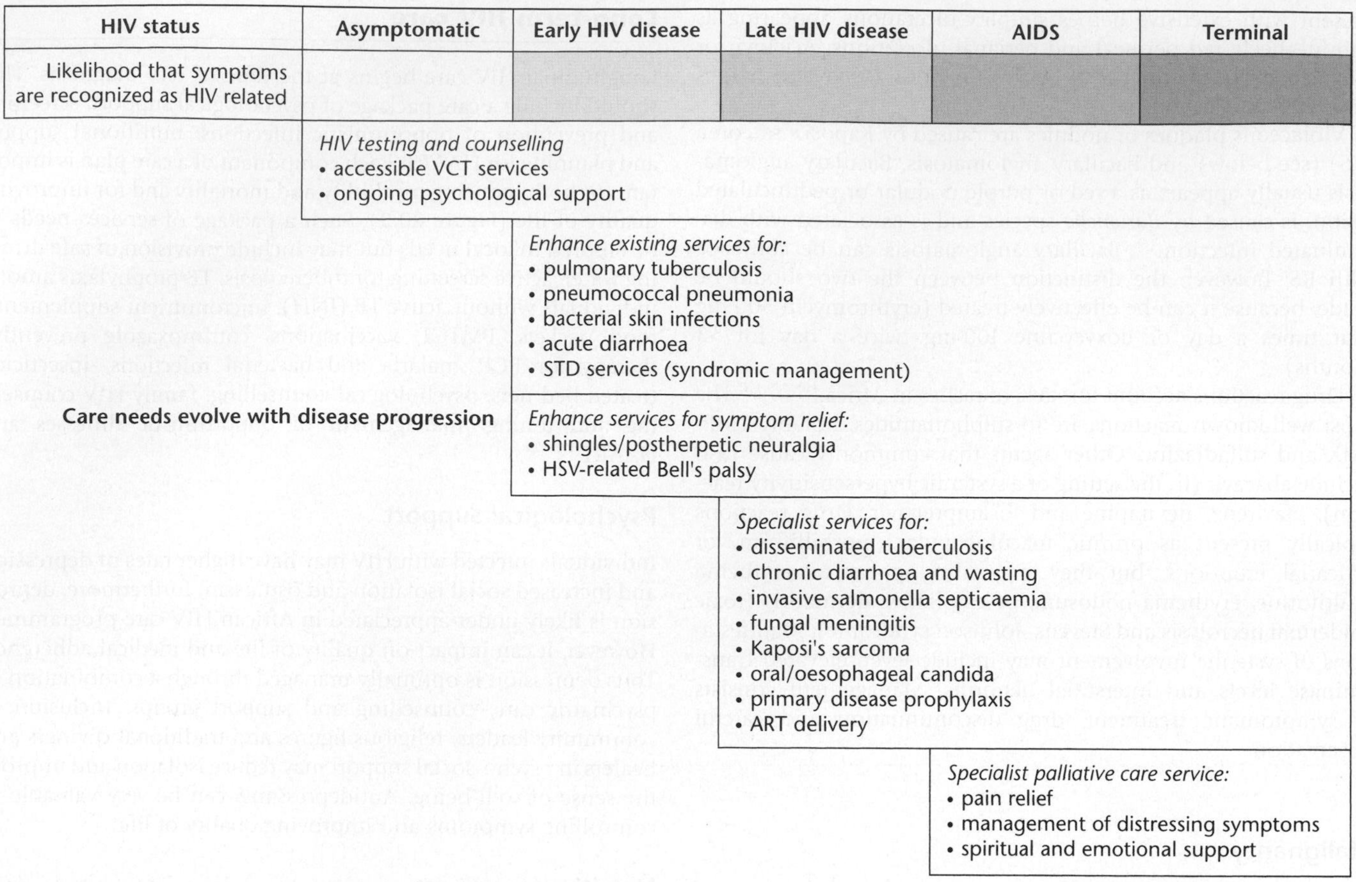

HIV status	Asymptomatic	Early HIV disease	Late HIV disease	AIDS	Terminal
Likelihood that symptoms are recognized as HIV related					

HIV testing and counselling
- accessible VCT services
- ongoing psychological support

Care needs evolve with disease progression

Enhance existing services for:
- pulmonary tuberculosis
- pneumococcal pneumonia
- bacterial skin infections
- acute diarrhoea
- STD services (syndromic management)

Enhance services for symptom relief:
- shingles/postherpetic neuralgia
- HSV-related Bell's palsy

Specialist services for:
- disseminated tuberculosis
- chronic diarrhoea and wasting
- invasive salmonella septicaemia
- fungal meningitis
- Kaposi's sarcoma
- oral/oesophageal candida
- primary disease prophylaxis
- ART delivery

Specialist palliative care service:
- pain relief
- management of distressing symptoms
- spiritual and emotional support

Figure 20.3 Evolving care needs with stage of HIV/AIDS disease. ART, antiretroviral therapy; HSV, herpes simplex virus; VCT, voluntary counselling and testing.

meningitis, odynophagia or dysphagia suggests candida oesophagitis, progressive dyspnoea on exertion suggest PCP, weight loss suggests a systemic illness or lactic acidosis for patients on stavudine and chronic productive cough and fevers suggests pulmonary TB.

Active case finding for TB is especially important during initial evaluation because of the complicated nature of co-treatment of HIV and TB and the high mortality from TB early after HAART initiation. Presence of one or more of the following symptoms should lead to further evaluation: cough for >2–3 weeks, sputum production, fevers, night sweats, or weight loss. If some of these symptoms are present, further investigation should include sputum smear and culture and chest radiography, where available. In individuals without evidence of active TB, use of isoniazid preventive therapy reduces developing TB disease.[178]

Prevention of opportunistic infections (Table 20.4)

Antiretroviral therapy

Although HAART is but one component of HIV care, it has proven to have the most significant impact on long-term survival and quality of life among individuals infected with HIV. HAART has fundamentally altered the previously grim prognosis of HIV and

has transformed it, in some settings, from a fatal disease to a chronic infection. As a result of effective HAART, the best predictor of long-term survival among HIV-infected individuals is successful long-term suppression of HIV replication.[179,180] Prior to the development of HAART, the estimated median survival from AIDS-defining condition to death was approximately 1.5 years.[181] HAART has extended this to ≥14 years.[75] Individuals able to maintain high levels of adherence to HAART have the potential for a life expectancy similar to that of uninfected individuals, especially when HAART is started at higher CD4 counts (around 350 cells/mm^3).[182] Success with HAART requires a structured care programme that can provide a continuous supply of medications, treatment monitoring and treatment support. When a structured programme is not in place, a patient should be referred to an established HAART programme. In places without established programmes a concerted effort should be made to put into place the infrastructure for HAART provision.

Principles of highly active antiretroviral therapy (HAART)

The goal of HAART is to inhibit replication of HIV to prevent further infection of uninfected cells. Success with this goal is reflected by a plasma HIV RNA below the level of detection by

Table 20.4 Prevention of opportunistic infection

Disease	When to initiate therapy	Therapy
Tuberculosis (TB)	After screening for active TB	Isoniazid 5 mg/kg daily for 6 months[178] BCG vaccination should not be given to HIV-infected children because of the risk of disseminated BCG disease
Tuberculosis (TB)	Always	Isolation of individuals with active pulmonary TB and good infection control practices in clinics (ventilation and minimizing crowding)
Pneumocystis jiroveci pneumonia (PCP) and bacterial pneumonia	Symptomatic HIV or CD4 < 500 cells/mm^3	TMP-SMX 400/80 2 tablets daily until immune restoration
Toxoplasmosis	Secondary prophylaxis after treating CNS toxoplasmosis	TMP-SMX 400/80 2 tablets daily until immune restoration
Malaria	Any CD4	Use of bed nets
Diarrhoeal disease	Any CD4	Clean water supplies, safe water storage, and use of home water chlorination
Cryptococcal meningitis	Secondary prophylaxis	Fluconazole 200 mg daily
Penicillinosis	Secondary prophylaxis	Itraconazole 200 mg daily

Because of the lower incidence of MAC in low-income countries, MAC prophylaxis is not recommended.

ultrasensitive assays (i.e. <50 copies/mL). However, successful HAART does not lead to the elimination of cells already infected at the time of HAART initiation. In these cells HIV persists and virions may be released, leading to low level viraemia (usually <10 copies/mL) and occasional 'blips' of viraemia with HIV RNA levels between 50 and 400 copies/mL.[183] Because some of the infected cells are long-lived memory T cells, some will survive for the life of the patient. These cells can be re-activated at any time leading to release of virions. If HAART is discontinued, HIV released from these cells will rapidly replicate leading to HIV levels often similar to pre-HAART levels. Thus HAART only provides benefit while it is being administered but cannot lead to cure of HIV. After initiation of HAART, if full HIV suppression is achieved, the absolute CD4 cell count typically rises and may return to normal levels.

Classes of antiretroviral agents

Each class of antiretroviral drug either targets a different step in the HIV life cycle or the same step via a different mechanism.[184] Currently, three classes of agents are generally available in low-income countries: nucleoside reverse transcriptase inhibitors (NRTIs), non-nucleoside reverse transcriptase inhibitors (NNRTIs) and protease inhibitors (PIs) (Table 20.5). Additional newer classes of antiretroviral drugs available in industrialized countries include entry inhibitors, integrase inhibitors and maturation inhibitors; however, these are rarely available in low and middle income settings and will not be discussed.

Nucleoside and nucleotide reverse transcriptase inhibitors (NRTIs)

NRTIs are nucleoside or nucleotide analogues that, after phosphorylation by host enzymes, are incorporated into the growing HIV nucleic acid chain. However, they prevent further chain elongation by HIV reverse transcriptase because they lack a 3' hydroxyl group. NRTI affinity for HIV reverse transcriptase is far higher than for human polymerases; nevertheless, inhibition of DNA synthesis by mitochondrial polymerase-γ is believed to contribute to adverse effects of some of the NRTIs, especially didanosine, stavudine and zidovudine. Most NRTIs are eliminated through the kidney and require dose adjustment in renal failure; the exception is abacavir, which undergoes hepatic metabolism.

Non-nucleoside reverse transcriptase inhibitors (NNRTIs)

NNRTIs act by directly binding HIV reverse transcriptase, causing a conformation change that inhibits its enzymatic activity. All current NNRTIs are metabolized via hepatic cytochromes P450 3A4 and 2B6 and have half-lives of 25–30 h and serum levels that remain detectable for weeks.[125] High-level resistance to first-generation NNRTIs develops rapidly because only a single point mutation is required to prevent NNRTI action.

Protease inhibitors

Protease inhibitors act by binding the active site of the protease enzyme, inhibiting the cleavage of viral peptides into structural proteins that required for mature virions. All protease inhibitors except nelfinavir are principally metabolized in the liver by cytochrome P450 3A4 (Cyp3A4). Nelfinavir is metabolized by both cytochromes 3A4 and 2C19. Inhibiting metabolism by Cyp3A4 has been harnessed as an important adjunct for maintaining higher trough serum concentrations of protease inhibitors. Ritonavir, originally developed as a protease inhibitor, is the most potent known pharmacological inhibitor of Cyp3A4. Because of its toxicity and poor tolerability at high doses, ritonavir is no longer used at full antiviral doses; however, low doses of ritonavir are now given along with most other protease inhibitors to

Table 20.5 Antiretroviral agents[125]

Name	Dose	Comments
NUCLEOSIDE REVERSE TRANSCRIPTASE INHIBITORS		
Abacavir (ABC)	300 mg twice a day or 600 mg daily	No food effect
Didanosine (ddI)	>60 kg: 400 mg daily <60 kg: 250 mg daily	Do not combine with tenofovir, stavudine, or atazanavir; Take 30 min before or 2 h after a meal
Emtricitabine (FTC)	200 mg daily	Do not combine with lamivudine; No food effect
Lamivudine (3TC)	150 twice a day or 300 mg daily	Do not combine with emtricitabine; No food effect
Stavudine (d4T)	30 mg twice a day	Do not combine with didanosine or zidovudine; No food effect
Tenofovir (TDF)	300 mg daily	Do not combine with didanosine; No food effect
Zidovudine (AZT)	300 mg twice a day	Do not combine with stavudine; No food effect
NON-NUCLEOSIDE REVERSE TRANSCRIPTASE INHIBITORS		
Efavirenz (EFV)	600 mg daily	Do not take with fatty meals
Nevirapine (NVP)	200 mg daily for 14 days then 200 twice a day (this is because induction of hepatic metabolism occurs)	No food effect; do not start in a women not on HAART with CD4 > 250 cells/mm³ or men with CD4 > 400 cells/mm³
PROTEASE INHIBITORS		
Atazanavir + ritonavir (ATV/r)	300 mg + 100 mg daily	Take with food, do not use with proton pump inhibitors; take 2 h apart from histamine 2 inhibitors (requires an acidic environment for absorption)
Fosamprenavir + ritonavir (FPV/r)	700 mg + 100 mg twice a day	No food effect
Indinavir + ritonavir (IDV/r)		No food effect
Lopinavir + ritonavir (co-formulated as Kaletra or Stochrin) (LPV/r)	Tablets (200 mg/50 mg) 2 tablets twice daily (3 tablets twice daily if taken with EFV or NVP) Capsules (133.3 mg/33.3 mg) 3 capsules twice a day (4 capsules twice a day when taken with EFV or NVP)	No food effect (for tablet formulation); capsules are taken with food
Nelfinavir (NFV)	1250 mg twice a day	Take with fatty food
Saquinavir + ritonavir (SQV/r)	1000 mg + 100 mg twice a day	Take within 2 h of meal

Note special adjustments are required for specific combinations of some protease inhibitors. Discussion of use of dual PIs is beyond the scope of this chapter.

increase trough concentrations and prolong half-lives of the PIs that are metabolized by Cyp3A4 (boosted PI).

Adverse effects from antiretroviral agents

Resistance

Partially suppressive therapy with HAART creates evolutionary pressure to favour replication competent mutants with partial or complete resistance to one or more HAART agents. A single amino acid substitution can cause high level resistance to nevirapine or efavirenz (K103N and others), to lamivudine and emtricitabine (M184V) or to tenofovir (K65R). Resistance from a single mutation coupled with the long half-life of nevirapine explains the risk of resistance emerging with a single dose of nevirapine (i.e. for PMTCT).[185] Fortunately other agents have higher barriers to resistance and require multiple mutations for high level resistance. For example, a collection of mutations known as thymidine analogue

mutations (M41L, D67N, K70R, L210W, T215Y) lead to significant resistance to zidovudine and stavudine and confer cross-resistance to other NRTIs.[186] Most protease inhibitors also require multiple mutations for resistance and have considerable cross-resistance within the class. Nelfinavir is an exception with a barrier to resistance. Protease inhibitors boosted with low-dose ritonavir have very high barriers to resistance especially if no protease inhibitor mutations are present when a boosted PI is initiated. However, even with a high barrier to resistance, incomplete adherence to pills will lead to incomplete HIV suppression, creating the optimal environment for resistance to emerge and treatment to fail. Unfortunately, once resistance mutations begin to emerge, the pathway leads to increasing resistance unless the failing regimen is changed to a new and fully suppressive regimen. As described above, once drug resistant quasispecies emerge, they remain permanently archived in resting CD4 cells and can rapidly re-emerge if the same agents are restarted.[14,183] The precise level of adherence required to maintain suppression of HIV varies by ART regimen; however, adherence of 90–95% is generally accepted as a minimum requirement for most regimens available in low-income regions.[187,188]

Failure of standard first-line regimens (AZT or d4T plus 3TC plus EFV or NVP) leads to predictable progression of resistance patterns when failure occurs as a result of resistance. With a standard first-line regimen of lamivudine, stavudine or zidovudine and nevirapine or efavirenz, the resistance pattern that emerges initially is a single mutation leading to lamivudine resistance (M184V) and one or more mutations leading to NNRTI resistance (to efavirenz or nevirapine, K103N and others). Resistance to stavudine or zidovudine develops more gradually and may not be present even after several months on a failing regimen. However, a long duration of treatment (>6 months) with a non-suppressive therapy will lead to gradual accumulation of thymidine analogue mutations and high-level resistance to zidovudine, stavudine and cross-resistance to all other NRTIs. During second-line therapy with a regimen of a boosted-PI, zidovudine and abacavir or tenofovir, resistance is most likely to develop initially against the NRTIs before failure of the boosted PI.

Transmitted resistance has the potential to undermine effectiveness of a regimen. In industrialized countries approximately 8% of individuals who are newly infected are infected with HIV with reduced susceptibility to at least one HAART agent.[189] Currently in low- and middle-income countries there is little transmitted resistance.[190] The future impact of transmitted resistance is unclear; however, poorly managed ART programmes with frequent interruptions to HAART delivery could lead to high levels of transmitted resistance, with NNRTI resistance likely to emerge first.

Adherence and follow-up

Few therapies are as dependent on daily adherence to pill taking as is HAART. Failure to maintain adherence allows for ongoing cycles of HIV replication leading to CD4 decline and, more ominously, the development of HIV escape mutants resistant to the HAART agents included in the regimen. When this happens, improving resistance will not lead to suppression. In regions with a limited selection of available HAART agents, often one or two regimens, loss of one regimen leaves an individual with but one HAART regimen to rely on. Loss of both regimens returns the individual to the position he or she was in prior to HAART, with the same grim prognosis. Thus, lifelong adherence is a must for HAART to help restore longevity.

Multiple factors affect adherence, including regimen simplicity, side-effects, social support, substance abuse, psychiatric illness, access to food, financial status, lack of understanding of HAART or HIV, lack of a sense of self-efficacy and other individual barriers.[191,192] Requiring payment for treatment is another major barrier.

Specific interventions for supporting adherence need to be tailored to local circumstances. A commonly used adherence strategy uses adherence counsellors to provide two or more education sessions (either group sessions or one-on-one) on HIV and HAART prior to HAART initiation. These sessions are then followed-up with further adherence sessions at regular scheduled intervals after HAART initiation. It is also vital for other care providers including

nurses, mid-level providers and physicians to reinforce the adherence message as a team, identify individual barriers to adherence and implement interventions to help overcome these barriers. General strategies for enhancing adherence include the use of pill boxes, pharmacy support programmes, cell phone reminder alarms, cell phone calls by treatment supporters, treatment of side-effects or switching therapy to minimize side-effects, improving convenience, patient education and empowerment, enlisting family and community supporters, treatment of substance abuse and management of depression.[193]

In an effort to improve adherence, some programmes have a structure of directly-observed therapy (DOT), taken as a model from tuberculosis control programmes and provide 'DOT-HAART' with community health workers, family members, neighbours, or others monitoring the taking of each dose and providing emotional support and reminders.[169,194]

The long-term success of HIV care requires lifelong ongoing contact between the HIV-infected individual and the healthcare system. Intermittent care or loss of contact with the healthcare system is associated with worse prognoses than routine follow-up. Unfortunately, loss to follow-up is very common in some HAART programmes in both industrialized and low-income countries. Published studies report loss to follow-up among 25–60% of individuals initiating HIV care.[195–198] Individual factors that increase loss to follow-up in industrialized countries include unstable housing, mental illness, drug abuse, recent clinic enrolment, not having an AIDS-defining illness at enrolment and personal beliefs regarding HIV.[170,199]

ART regimens

First- and second-line HAART regimens are selected based on toxicity profile, potency, laboratory monitoring requirements, cost, availability and ability to tolerate temperature extremes during transportation and storage, drug–drug interactions with other commonly used medications and safety during pregnancy. As a general rule HAART regimens contain two distinct NRTI agents combined with either a PI or an NNRTI. A third option is a three NRTI combination of lamivudine, zidovudine and abacavir. This has been advocated for use in some situations, such as pregnancy and during TB therapy; however, based on direct comparisons with NNRTI-based regimens, it is inferior. National guidelines should be adhered to when practical to facilitate transfer of care between clinics and predictable resistance patterns among first- and second-line HAART patients.

The first first-line regimen recommended by the WHO included stavudine, lamivudine and nevirapine. This regimen has been widely adopted and contributed to considerable increased survival. However, both stavudine and nevirapine can have significant side-effects (Table 20.6). Thus there has been a shift toward use of zidovudine in place of stavudine and efavirenz in place of nevirapine. Zidovudine can also have significant side-effects with suppression of bone marrow leading to anaemia and neutropenia.[202,203] However, studies from low-income countries have shown an overall increase in haemoglobin during treatment with zidovudine.[203]

After a patient is started on a first-line regimen, individual agents may need to be substituted in the setting of side-effects

Table 20.6 Adverse effects from antiretroviral agents[125]

Adverse effect	ART agents	Presentation and management
Abacavir hypersensitivity	ABC	Occurs 1 to 6 weeks after starting ABC. Fever and rash, often with respiratory symptoms that progressively worsen with continued ABC doses. Associated with HLA B*5701 (rare among Africans). ABC should be stopped and patient never rechallenged; on rechallenge may have fatal anaphylactic reaction
Anaemia	AZT, dapsone	May cause profound anaemia through bone marrow suppression, but investigate other causes. Can switch to d4T
Diarrhoea	ddI, PIs	Use symptomatic treatment after excluding infectious causes
Hepatotoxicity	All ART agents, TMP/SMX	Is higher in chronic HBV or with co-administration of TB therapy. It is also believed that some traditional remedies may cause hepatotoxicity; however, overall this has not emerged as a major problem. Hepatotoxicity likely also occurs commonly pre-HAART. If patient is asymptomatic and bilirubin is normal, may be able to continue therapy and monitor closely. Exceptions are NVP mediated hepatoxicity that occurs early after starting NVP (first 6 weeks) and is often accompanied by rash. NVP should be discontinued
Hyperbilirubinaemia	ATV, IDV	Benign isolated indirect hyperbilirubinaemia; if scleral icterus is bothersome to patient, can switch to another PI
Lactic acidosis	d4T, ddI (rarely with AZT and other NRTIs)	Caused by inhibition of mitochondrial DNA polymerase-γ. May present with abdominal pain, nausea, emesis, weight loss, dyspnoea. Up to 2/100 person years of therapy.[145] Point-of-care lactate testing can easily diagnose condition and reduce morbidity and mortality.[200] Always monitor symptoms when patients are on d4T. Discontinue all HAART and do not rechallenge with d4T or ddI
Lipodystrophy (lipoatrophy and lipohypertrophy)	d4T (other NRTIs) and PIs	Loss of subcutaneous fat, especially from extremities, increase in visceral fat in abdomen and breasts. Believed to be from mitochondrial toxicity. PIs associated with 'buffalo hump.' Switch to alternative agent (AZT, TDF, ABC) and increase physical activity[201]
Neuro-psychiatric	EFV	Sleep disturbances, vivid dreams, depression, fatigue, ataxia all may occur with EFV. These symptoms usually resolve within 12 weeks of HAART initiation
Neutropenia	AZT	Can cause profound neutropenia. Usually not associated with infections of neutropenia. Stop AZT and switch to another agent (d4T, TDF, ABC)
Pancreatitis	d4T, ddI	Nausea, emesis, left upper quadrant pain. Serum lipase or amylase or abdominal imaging helps to confirm diagnosis. Discontinue HAART and provide supportive care
Rash and drug eruptions	NVP, EFV, TMP/SMX	NVP and EFV cause benign self-limited maculopapular (NVP) or morbilliform (EFV) rash on trunk, face and extremities. Treatment need not be interrupted unless mucosal involvement occurs or hepatotoxicity is present (ALT should be assayed if rash occurs with NVP). EFV rarely needs to be discontinued due to rash
Nephrolithiasis	IDV, ATV	Colicky flank pain and haematuria, often when dehydrated. Encourage increased fluid consumption or switch PIs
Renal toxicity	TDF	Acute renal failure from renal tubular dysfunction. Usually occurs in setting of another renal insult
Peripheral neuropathy	d4T, ddI	Dysthaesia, hypersensitivity and decreased calcaneal tendon reflex. Same symptoms also occur with HIV-associated distal sensory polyneuropathy (DSP). May have similar pathophysiology as individuals with DSP are at higher risk for drug induced neuropathy. Start with amitriptyline or nortriptyline at night. If no improvement switch from d4T or ddI to alternative agent (AZT, TDF, ABC). Neuropathy very gradually improves after stopping agent

(Table 20.6). However, individual agents should not be substituted in the setting of virologic failure. If HIV is not suppressed and further adherence interventions have failed, it is time for a second-line regimen containing a new set of HAART agents.

The basic principle to selecting second-line regimens is to choose a potent regimen with limited cross-resistance with the first-line regimen. This can be achieved by using a protease inhibitor boosted with ritonavir. Such examples include the co-formulated lopinavir/ritonavir tablets and saquinavir, indinavir, or atazanavir boosted with ritonavir. There is some evidence that a fully active boosted PI may be sufficient to suppress and maintain suppression of the HIV replication, but efficacy is lower than for full HAART.[204,205] Thus second-line regimens should also include two NRTIs along with a boosted PI. Such a regimen may include lopinavir plus ritonavir, saquinavir plus ritonavir, or atazanavir plus ritonavir and two NRTIs such as didanosine or tenofovir plus abacavir or lamivudine, or zidovudine.

Third-line regimens available in low-income settings are often inadequate to achieve full suppression of HIV replication. However, merely reducing HIV RNA levels may slow CD4 decline. Thus options for individuals failing the second-line therapy include a number of combinations of non-suppressive HAART. It is generally believed that NNRTIs contribute little to a failing regimen.[206] However, NRTIs, especially lamivudine, do appear to slow CD4 decline.[207] Thus an individual who has failed both first- and second-line therapies remains a candidate for antiretroviral agents, only the goal must be shifted from full HIV suppression to slowing the CD4 decline. At a minimum, it is reasonable to include lamivudine in such a regimen. Adding a thymidine analogue such as zidovudine or adding tenofovir may add additional benefit due to the interactions between the lamivudine resistance mutation and TAMs or tenofovir resistance. Boosted PIs may also confer benefit although they have higher cost and can have significant toxicity.

Tuberculosis therapy and HAART regimen

Standard four-drug TB therapy includes rifampin, isoniazid, ethambutol and pyrazinamide. Rifampin is a powerful inducer of cytochrome P-450 oxidases, including 3A4, leading to greatly accelerated metabolism of PIs. As a result, standard dosing of all PIs, including nelfinavir, is inadequate to achieve therapeutic levels in the presence of rifampin.[208] When a PI is needed during therapy for TB, lopinavir plus ritonavir may be used with a double dose. However, drug levels are variable and this dose can be difficult to tolerate. Rifampin also induces metabolism of NNRTIs, reducing efavirenz levels by 25% and nevirapine levels by 50%.[209] Based on pharmacokinetics, use of higher doses of NNRTIs during concomitant TB treatment is a reasonable approach (efavirenz 800 mg daily). However, reports from Africa and Asia of use of standard doses of either agent as part of HAART during treatment of both TB and HIV have shown similar HIV RNA suppression between individuals receiving TB therapy and not receiving TB therapy.[210] When using this approach, it is important to consider local factors, such as body weight, when considering applicability to a specific setting. Based on this evidence, in individuals <70 kg it is appropriate to use standard doses of efavirenz (600 mg daily) or nevirapine (200 mg twice daily) among patients also receiving rifampin. Where available,

higher doses of efavirenz (800 mg daily) and avoidance of nevirapine when treating HIV and TB is prudent among heavier individuals.[210,211] An inferior alternative with lower rates of HIV RNA suppression is a combination of the three NRTIs, zidovudine, lamivudine and abacavir. This regimen should be considered when there are compelling reasons not to use efavirenz or nevirapine (possibly pregnancy).

Simultaneous use of TB medications and HAART increases risks for drug side-effects and reduced adherence.[208] Furthermore, if adverse reactions do occur, discerning the responsible agent is complicated for a patient on seven or more different medications. Thus general recommendations are to initiate TB therapy when TB is diagnosed and continue HAART if a patient is already on HAART. Patients not on HAART should be managed according to CD4 count or degree of illness. If the CD4 count is >350 cells/mm³, HAART should generally be deferred until after completing the 6-month TB therapy. Among individuals with CD4 200–350 cells/mm³ and who are not severely ill from HIV, HAART initiation should generally be deferred until after completing the induction phase of TB therapy (2 months). Partly because of toxicity and partly because of concerns about immune reconstitution inflammatory syndrome (IRD, see below), ART is often deferred, typically for two months, until the initial (intensive) phase of TB treatment is complete. However, delay in ART initiation may lead to further immunological decline and poor clinical outcomes, including increased mortality.[64,212] Severely ill individuals and those with CD4 counts <200 cells/mm³ are believed to have improved survival with earlier HAART initiation, although further study is needed. General recommendations are to delay HAART for 2 weeks to provide time to assess tolerance of the TB therapy. Monitoring, including clinical evaluation and liver enzyme tests, should be more frequent during TB and HAART co-administration. Bi-weekly monitoring of liver enzymes for the first 6–12 weeks of therapy is reasonable if resources are available.

Pregnancy and HAART regimen

Treatment of HIV during pregnancy may preserve the health of the mother and reduce risk of transmission to the infant. Current evidence suggests that HAART is safe and of low risk to the fetus.[213] However, non-human primate studies of efavirenz and tenofovir have suggested increased risk for neural tube defects and bone defects, respectively.[214] However, clinical experience with efavirenz has not identified a marked increase in birth defects among infants born to women receiving efavirenz during pregnancy.[215] In addition, after the first trimester, the neural tube has formed and use of efavirenz is likely to be as safe as any other HAART agent. If early pregnancy is detected in a women receiving efavirenz, it is prudent to switch to nevirapine. When HAART initiation is being considered, current guidelines recommend waiting until the second trimester for HAART initiation.

HIV RNA suppression with HAART close to the time of delivery greatly reduces the risk of mother-to-child transmission of HIV (2% risk vs 36% risk of transmission). Furthermore, HAART improves maternal health and survival. Thus HAART initiation is recommended during pregnancy in a women with a CD4 count <350 cells/mm³. Severely ill women with symptomatic HIV disease should have HAART initiated as soon as they are ready. For other women, waiting until after the first trimester is reasonable to reduce the teratogenic risk of HAART.

Hepatitis B co-infection and HAART regimen

Chronic hepatitis B (the persistence of hepatitis B surface antigen for more than 6 months) can lead to cirrhosis and hepatocellular carcinoma. Suppression of HBV replication among individuals with active chronic hepatitis B (evidence of liver disease, HBV DNA levels $>10^4$ copies/mL, or hepatitis e antigen positive) can reduce the progression of liver disease.[216] Three widely available HIV agents, lamivudine, emtricitabine and tenofovir, are active against HBV. Thus individuals with chronic HBV-HIV co-infection are likely to have better long-term outcomes if an HBV active ART agent is included in the regimen. Ideally, the first-line regimen of someone with chronic HBV includes lamivudine or emtricitabine and tenofovir. If the first-line HAART therapy fails for HIV suppression, an HBV suppressive agent should be continued in the subsequent therapy, even if it is unlikely to contribute substantially to suppression of HIV. For example, lamivudine or tenofovir can be continued along with other HAART agents selected for a second-line regimen. In addition to improving HBV outcomes, this reduces the risk of a hepatitis flare at the time of discontinuation of the suppressive agent.[217] Overall, tenofovir has the advantage of a much higher barrier to HBV resistance than lamivudine, HBV develops resistance to lamivudine at a rate of 25% per year.[218]

When to initiate HAART

HAART should be initiated in any individual with WHO stage III or IV HIV (Table 20.7) irrespective of CD4 count or total lymphocyte count (TLC). In asymptomatic individuals, HAART initiation should be considered once the CD4 count is <350 cells/mm³ or total lymphocyte count is <1200 cells/mm³. This is consistent with recommendations in industrialized countries as well as the guidelines of some non-governmental organizations in Africa;[47] however, the WHO current guidelines recommend starting HAART when the CD4 count is <200 cells/mm³.[60] Given poorer success with HAART when starting at low CD4 counts and the cost of managing opportunistic illnesses, both the health of a patient and the overall finances of a healthcare system may be better with HAART initiation before the CD4 count is <200 cells/mm³ (i.e. using <350 cells/mm³ as a cut-off for HAART initiation in asymptomatic individuals).[64,219–221] For reasons of medication cost, the WHO recommends HAART initiation at CD4 < 200 cells/mm³.

Before starting HAART, appropriate patient education is essential to increase the chance of adherence to therapy (see section on adherence). An approach of multiple (1–3) structured education and counselling sessions that provide education regarding HIV and HAART at a culturally and educationally appropriate level is important.

Clearly, any decision to start HAART must also involve the patient's desire and readiness for starting therapy. The WHO HIV/AIDS Programme HAART recommendations are an excellent resource for current and rapidly evolving recommendations regarding details of ART (http://www.who.int/hiv/pub/guidelines). National guidelines should be referred to for initiation and monitoring of ART.

Monitoring HAART

The goals of monitoring HAART are to: (1) reinforce adherence, (2) assess for side-effects, (3) assess for emergence of opportunistic illnesses, (4) assess success of HIV RNA suppression and (5) assess CD4 rise. Routine monitoring is vital for successful HAART therapy. Frequency of monitoring depends on local resources. The WHO recommends evaluation at least every 6 months. Table 20.8 shows a schedule for minimum assessments to identify HIV-related illness, treatment side-effects and treatment success or failure.

HIV suppression and determination of treatment success or failure

Treatment success and failure is best assessed by direct measure of circulating HIV. Direct testing usually means assaying viral load via PCR to measure serum HBV RNA levels. While this is the technique with which the most clinical experience has been amassed, assays of viral antigens (i.e. p24) are also reasonable measures of circulating HIV. Surrogate markers, such as CD4, weight change and new opportunistic illnesses lack sensitivity and specificity for failure of HIV suppression and, when they do indicate failure to suppress HIV, may lag behind the virologic failure by many months. For example, 5–10% of individuals without HIV suppression have initial increase in CD4 count.[222] Thus, the poor sensitivity and specificity of these techniques for monitoring leads to inappropriate switching to second-line regimens when there is no virologic failure, the development of potentially fatal opportunistic infections and the risk for the emergence of significant cross-resistant HIV mutations while on non-suppressive therapy that appears to be working but is not suppressing HIV.

Within days of starting HAART the HIV RNA level declines; within 2 weeks, a 2 $\log_{10}$ decline in HIV RNA occurs.[223] After this initial drop, there is a slower second phase of decline leading to an HIV RNA < 50 copies/mL by 24 weeks of HAART.

Failure to have an undetectable HIV RNA by 24 weeks or rise to detectable levels after achieving suppression is a result of inadequate adherence, malabsorption of HAART agents, drug resistance, or a combination of resistance and inadequate adherence. Laboratory error may also lead to erroneous results. However, there is currently no consensus on a definition for virologic failure for use in low-income regions. Creating a definition is complicated by 'blips' in HIV RNA that are likely clinically meaningless elevations in HIV RNA between 50 copies/mL and <400 copies/mL. An HIV RNA > 1000 copies/mL is a meaningful rise and should be considered a viral breakthrough. The WHO has recommended a cut-off of 10 000 copies/mL to define virologic failure.

We recommend that if a patient has an HIV RNA elevation >1000 copies/mL, treatment failure should be suspected and a management algorithm initiated. The first step is to reassess patient adherence and any illnesses occurring prior to HIV RNA testing that may have interfered with taking pills (e.g. acute gastroenteritis), to address barriers to adherence and to provide additional adherence counselling. We recommend follow-up testing 1–3 months after the first HIV RNA > 1000 copies/mL. A persistently elevated HIV RNA > 1000 copies/mL is suggestive of either HIV resistance or continued inadequate adherence. As a clinical

Table 20.7 WHO clinical staging of HIV

Clinical Stage 1	Asymptomatic Persistent generalized lymphadenopathy (lymphadenopathy >1 cm for >3 months without other explanation)
Clinical Stage 2	Unexplained weight loss (<10%) Recurrent upper respiratory tract infections Herpes zoster (shingles) Angular cheilitis Recurrent oral ulceration Papular pruritic eruptions Seborrheic dermatitis Fungal nail infections
Clinical Stage 3	Unexplained weight loss (>10%) Unexplained chronic diarrhoea (>1 month) Unexplained persistent fever Persistent oral candidiasis Oral hairy leukoplakia Pulmonary tuberculosis Severe bacterial infections (pneumonia, empyema, pyomyositis, bone or joint infections, meningitis, bacteraemia, pelvic inflammatory disease) Acute necrotizing ulcerating stomatitis, gingivitis, or periodontitis Unexplained anaemia (haemoglobin <8 g/dl), neutropenia (neutrophils $<0.5 \times 10^9$/L), or thrombocytopenia ($<50 \times 10^9$/L)
Clinical Stage 4	HIV wasting (>10% weight loss, plus either chronic diarrhoea or chronic fevers or night sweats without other explanation) *Pneumocystis jiroveci* pneumonia (PCP) Recurrent bacterial pneumonia (2+ episodes within 6 months) Chronic cutaneous herpes simplex Candida oesophagitis Extrapulmonary tuberculosis Kaposi's sarcoma Cytomegalovirus infection CNS toxoplasmosis HIV-associated dementia Extrapulmonary cryptococcosis Disseminated non-TB mycobacterial infection Progressive multifocal leukoencephalopathy Chronic cryptosporidiosis (>1 month) Chronic isosporiasis (>1 month) Disseminated coccidiomycosis or histoplasmosis Recurrent septicaemia Lymphoma Invasive cervical carcinoma Atypical disseminated leishmaniasis Symptomatic HIV-associated nephropathy or cardiomyopathy

Table 20.8 HAART monitoring schedule

	Entry into HIV care	Initiation of HAART	Week 2	Week 4	Week 6	Week 12	Every 6 months
History and physical	X	X	X	X	X	X	X
Haemoglobin	X	X		X		X	X
ALT	X	X				X	X
HIV RNA, CD4	X	X					X

note, an HIV RNA > 100 000 copies/mL suggests minimal, if any, pill taking and a lower risk for resistance. After reassessing adherence, it is appropriate to switch to a second-line HAART regimen. Because of the importance of achieving virologic success with this regimen, treatment supporters, an adherence programme, or 'DOT'-HAART should be considered when starting this second-line regimen. We recommend repeat HIV RNA assay at three months. Persistent elevation after regimen change is strongly suggestive of adherence problems; however, drug interactions and poor absorption can also contribute. Management can follow the same algorithm as for treatment failure with the first-line regimen.

CD4 response

Suppression of HIV replication usually leads to CD4 rise. This rise occurs in two phases. The first phase occurs during the first 3 months of HAART and represents a redistribution of memory CD4 cells from lymphoid tissue. Typical rise during this period is 2.5–5.5 cells/mm^3 per week.[224-227] The second phase is slower and is driven by the expansion of naïve CD4 cells. During this phase, the average increase is 0.73–3.1 cells/mm^3 per week.[224-227] This second phase continues for at least 4–6 years during suppressive HAART.[226,228]

Multiple factors contribute to CD4 response including treatment of other illnesses, such as TB, baseline CD4 count, nutritional status and development of intercurrent opportunistic illnesses. Furthermore, a subset of individuals has a discordant HIV RNA-CD4 response. Virologic suppression without CD4 rise occurs among 10–20% of patients started on HAART. Studies from industrialized countries have identified associations with older age, lower nadir CD4 count and lower baseline HIV RNA level.[222,229] However, individuals with HIV RNA suppression, even without CD4 rise, have improved survival and fewer opportunistic illnesses than those without HIV RNA suppression. Thus, the management strategy is to continue the HAART regimen, maximize nutrition and seek other infections, especially subacute or chronic illnesses such as TB. Some individuals have delayed recovery and continued HAART may lead to CD4 increase within 1 year among half of patients within initial discordant responses.

Stopping HAART

HAART should be stopped in the setting of severe HAART-related side-effects, patient desire to stop HAART, need to have nothing per mouth following major abdominal surgery and regimen failure. Stopping HAART in the setting of a suppressed HIV RNA level has specific considerations. NRTIs and PIs have a relatively short plasma half-life (0.5–17 h) and intracellular half-life (4–40 h except for tenofovir which has a half-life of 150 h). The half-life of NNRTIs is much longer (40–160 h). As a result, therapeutic levels of NNRTIs may persist in the serum long after elimination of co-administered agents. This leads to a risk of emergence of resistance to the NNRTI agent during the days to weeks it has significant plasma levels. Staggered stopping of treatment has the potential to reduce the development of resistance.[230] For example, the NNRTI component is stopped and the NRTI backbone continued for two additional weeks. Another option is to stop the NNRTI

and add a PI to the NRTI backbone to continue for 2–4 weeks after halting the NNRTI.

There is no role at present for structured treatment interruptions. Multiple studies have demonstrated worse outcomes among individuals in treatment interruption arms.[231,232]

Conclusions

The future success of HIV care in low-income countries depends on identifying a higher proportion of HIV-infected individuals and identifying them earlier in the disease course. This will allow earlier initiation of comprehensive HIV care. Currently in Africa, only an estimated 10% of HIV-infected individuals are aware of their HIV status.[233] An even smaller proportion are engaged in HIV care. However, expansion of care will not be able to keep pace with need unless significant successes are rapidly seen with prevention. A renewed commitment to prevention with use of circumcision, innovative social interventions, condom promotion and increased PMTCT is essential.

REFERENCES

1. UNAIDS. *AIDS Epidemic Update 2007*. Geneva: World Health Organization; 2007.
2. Simon V, Ho DD, Abdool KQ. HIV/AIDS epidemiology, pathogenesis, prevention and treatment. *Lancet* 2006; 368:489–504.
3. Greene WC. AIDS and the immune system. *Sci Am* 1993; 269:98–105.
4. Mangeat B, Turelli P, Caron G, et al. Broad antiretroviral defence by human APOBEC3G through lethal editing of nascent reverse transcripts. *Nature* 2003; 424:99–103.
5. Emerman M, Malim MH. HIV-1 regulatory/accessory genes: keys to unraveling viral and host cell biology. *Science* 1998; 280:1880–1884.
6. Derdeyn CA, Silvestri G. Viral and host factors in the pathogenesis of HIV infection. *Curr Opin Immunol* 2005; 17:366–373.
7. Koup RA, Safrit JT, Cao Y, et al. Temporal association of cellular immune responses with the initial control of viremia in primary human immunodeficiency virus type 1 syndrome. *J Virol* 1994; 68:4650–4655.
8. Walker BD, Goulder PJ. AIDS. Escape from the immune system. *Nature* 2000; 407:313–314.
9. Mattapallil JJ, Roederer M. Acute HIV infection: it takes more than guts. *Curr Opin HIV AIDS* 2006; 1:10–15.
10. Espert L, Denizot M, Grimaldi M, et al. Autophagy is involved in T cell death after binding of HIV-1 envelope proteins to CXCR4. *J Clin Invest* 2006; 116:2161–2172.
11. Siliciano JD, Kajdas J, Finzi D, et al. Long-term follow-up studies confirm the stability of the latent reservoir for HIV-1 in resting CD4+ T cells. *Nat Med* 2003; 9:727–728.
12. Chun TW, Fauci AS. Latent reservoirs of HIV: obstacles to the eradication of virus. *Proc Natl Acad Sci USA* 1999; 96:10958–10961.
13. Chun TW, Stuyver L, Mizell SB, et al. Presence of an inducible HIV-1 latent reservoir during highly active antiretroviral therapy. *Proc Natl Acad Sci USA* 1997; 94:13193–13197.
14. Finzi D, Hermankova M, Pierson T, et al. Identification of a reservoir for HIV-1 in patients on highly active antiretroviral therapy. *Science* 1997; 278:1295–1300.
15. Alimonti JB, Ball TB, Fowke KR. Mechanisms of CD4+ T lymphocyte cell death in human immunodeficiency virus infection and AIDS. *J Gen Virol* 2003; 84:1649–1661.
16. Laeyendecker O, Li X, Arroyo M, et al. The effect of HIV subtype on rapid disease progression in Rakai, Uganda. Abstract 44LB, 13th Conference on

Retroviruses and Opportunistic Infections, 5–8 February, 2006, Denver. Online. Available: www.retroconference.org/2006 27 April 2007.

17. Rodriguez B, Sethi AK, Cheruvu VK, et al. Predictive value of plasma HIV RNA level on rate of CD4 T-cell decline in untreated HIV infection. *JAMA* 2006; 296:1498–1506.

18. Sterling TR, Vlahov D, Astemborski J, et al. Initial plasma HIV-1 RNA levels and progression to AIDS in women and men. *N Engl J Med* 2001; 344:720–725.

19. Mellors JW, Rinaldo CR Jr, Gupta P, et al. Prognosis in HIV-1 infection predicted by the quantity of virus in plasma. *Science* 1996; 272:1167–1170.

20. Holmes CB, Wood R, Badri M, et al. CD4 decline and incidence of opportunistic infections in Cape Town, South Africa: implications for prophylaxis and treatment. *J Acquir Immune Defic Syndr* 2006; 42:464–469.

21. Morgan D, Mahe C, Mayanja B, et al. HIV-1 infection in rural Africa: is there a difference in median time to AIDS and survival compared with that in industrialized countries? *AIDS* 2002; 16:597–603.

22. Duvignac J, Anglaret X, Kpozehouen A, et al. CD4+ T-lymphocytes natural decrease in HAART-naive HIV-infected adults in Abidjan. *HIV Clin Trials* 2008; 9:26–35.

23. Minga A, Danel C, Abo Y, et al. Progression to WHO criteria for antiretroviral therapy in a 7-year cohort of adult HIV-1 seroconverters in Abidjan, Cote d'Ivoire. *Bull World Health Organ* 2007; 85:116–123.

24. Urassa W, Bakari M, Sandstrom E, et al. Rate of decline of absolute number and percentage of CD4 T lymphocytes among HIV-1-infected adults in Dar es Salaam, Tanzania. *AIDS* 2004; 18:433–438.

25. Fauci AS, Pantaleo G, Stanley S, et al. Immunopathogenic mechanisms of HIV infection. *Ann Intern Med* 1996; 124:654–663.

26. Hanson DL, Chu SY, Farizo KM, et al. Distribution of CD4+ T lymphocytes at diagnosis of acquired immunodeficiency syndrome-defining and other human immunodeficiency virus-related illnesses. The Adult and Adolescent Spectrum of HIV Disease Project Group. *Arch Intern Med* 1995; 155:1537–1542.

27. Twenty-five years of HIV/AIDS–United States, 1981–2006. *MMWR Morb Mortal Wkly Rep* 2006; 55:585–589.

28. Keele BF, Van HF, Li Y, et al. Chimpanzee reservoirs of pandemic and nonpandemic HIV-1. *Science* 2006; 313:523–526.

29. Sharp PM, Bailes E, Chaudhuri RR, et al. The origins of acquired immune deficiency syndrome viruses: where and when? *Philos Trans R Soc Lond B Biol Sci* 2001; 356:867–876.

30. Santiago ML, Range F, Keele BF, et al. Simian immunodeficiency virus infection in free-ranging sooty mangabeys (Cercocebus atys atys) from the Tai Forest, Cote d'Ivoire: implications for the origin of epidemic human immunodeficiency virus type 2. *J Virol* 2005; 79:12515–12527.

31. Baggaley RF, Boily MC, White RG, et al. Risk of HIV-1 transmission for parenteral exposure and blood transfusion: a systematic review and meta-analysis. *AIDS* 2006; 20:805–812.

32. Garcia PM, Kalish LA, Pitt J, et al. Maternal levels of plasma human immunodeficiency virus type 1 RNA and the risk of perinatal transmission. Women and Infants Transmission Study Group. *N Engl J Med* 1999; 341:394–402.

33. Vittinghoff E, Douglas J, Judson F, et al. Per-contact risk of human immunodeficiency virus transmission between male sexual partners. *Am J Epidemiol* 1999; 150:306–311.

34. Leynaert B, Downs AM, de Vincenzi I. Heterosexual transmission of human immunodeficiency virus: variability of infectivity throughout the course of infection. European Study Group on Heterosexual Transmission of HIV. *Am J Epidemiol* 1998; 148:88–96.

35. Buve A, Bishikwabo-Nsarhaza K, Mutangadura G. The spread and effect of HIV-1 infection in sub-Saharan Africa. *Lancet* 2002; 359:2011–2017.

36. UNAIDS. *Report on the Global AIDS Epidemic 2006.* Geneva: World Health Organization, 2006.

37. Auvert B, Buve A, Ferry B, et al. Ecological and individual level analysis of risk factors for HIV infection in four urban populations in sub-Saharan Africa with different levels of HIV infection. *AIDS* 2001; 15(suppl 4):S15–S30.

38. Halperin DT, Epstein H. Why is HIV prevalence so severe in southern Africa. *S Afr J HIV Med* 2007; 19–25.

39. Helleringer S, Kohler HP. Sexual network structure and the spread of HIV in Africa: evidence from Likoma Island, Malawi. *AIDS* 2007; 21:2323–2332.

40. Halperin DT, Epstein H. Concurrent sexual partnerships help to explain Africa's high HIV prevalence: implications for prevention. *Lancet* 2004; 364:4–6.

41. Myer L, Denny L, De Souza M, et al. Intravaginal practices, HIV and other sexually transmitted diseases among South African women. *Sex Transm Dis* 2004; 31:174–179.

42. Yerly S, Vora S, Rizzardi P, et al. Acute HIV infection: impact on the spread of HIV and transmission of drug resistance. *AIDS* 2001; 15:2287–2292.

43. Marks G, Crepaz N, Janssen RS. Estimating sexual transmission of HIV from persons aware and unaware that they are infected with the virus in the USA. *AIDS* 2006; 20:1447–1450.

44. Sherr L, Lopman B, Kakowa M, et al. Voluntary counselling and testing: uptake, impact on sexual behaviour and HIV incidence in a rural Zimbabwean cohort. *AIDS* 2007; 21:851–860.

45. Connor EM, Sperling RS, Gelber R, et al. Reduction of maternal-infant transmission of human immunodeficiency virus type 1 with zidovudine treatment. Pediatric AIDS Clinical Trials Group Protocol 076 Study Group. *N Engl J Med* 1994; 331:1173–1180.

46. Eshleman SH, Becker-Pergola G, Deseyve M, et al. Impact of human immunodeficiency virus type 1 (HIV-1) subtype on women receiving single-dose nevirapine prophylaxis to prevent HIV-1 vertical transmission (HIV network for prevention trials 012 study). *J Infect Dis* 2001; 184:914–917.

47. Panel of Antiretroviral Guidelines for Adults and Adolescents. Guidelines for the Use of Antiretroviral Agents in HIV-1-Infected Adults and Adolescents. Online. Available: http://www aidsinfo nih gov/ContentFiles/AdultandAdolescentGL.pdf 2008.

48. Gray GE, McIntyre JA. HIV and pregnancy. *BMJ* 2007; 334:950–953.

49. Dao H, Mofenson LM, Ekpini R, et al. International recommendations on antiretroviral drugs for treatment of HIV-infected women and prevention of mother-to-child HIV transmission in resource-limited settings: 2006 update. *Am J Obstet Gynecol* 2007; 197:S42–S55.

50. Lockman S, Shapiro RL, Smeaton LM, et al. Response to antiretroviral therapy after a single, peripartum dose of nevirapine. *N Engl J Med* 2007; 356:135–147.

51. Coovadia HM, Rollins NC, Bland RM, et al. Mother-to-child transmission of HIV-1 infection during exclusive breast-feeding in the first 6 months of life: an intervention cohort study. *Lancet* 2007; 369:1107–1116.

52. Dunn DT, Newell ML, Ades AE, et al. Risk of human immunodeficiency virus type 1 transmission through breast-feeding. *Lancet* 1992; 340:585–588.

53. Tonwe-Gold B, Ekouevi DK, Viho I, et al. Antiretroviral treatment and prevention of peripartum and postnatal HIV transmission in West Africa: evaluation of a two-tiered approach. *PLoS Med* 2007; 4:e257.

54. Auvert B, Taljaard D, Lagarde E, et al. Randomized, controlled intervention trial of male circumcision for reduction of HIV infection risk: the ANRS 1265 Trial. *PLoS Med* 2005; 2:e298.

55. Bailey RC, Moses S, Parker CB, et al. Male circumcision for HIV prevention in young men in Kisumu, Kenya: a randomised controlled trial. *Lancet* 2007; 369:643–656.

56. Gray RH, Kigozi G, Serwadda D, et al. Male circumcision for HIV prevention in men in Rakai, Uganda: a randomised trial. *Lancet* 2007; 369:657–666.

57. Panlilio AL, Cardo DM, Grohskopf LA, et al. Updated U.S. Public Health Service guidelines for the management of occupational exposures to HIV and recommendations for postexposure prophylaxis. *MMWR Recomm Rep* 2005; 54:1–17.

58. Patel SM, Johnson S, Belknap SM, et al. Serious adverse cutaneous and hepatic toxicities associated with nevirapine use by non-HIV-infected individuals. *J Acquir Immune Defic Syndr* 2004; 35:120–125.

59. Gray RH, Makumbi F, Serwadda D, et al. Limitations of rapid HIV-1 tests during screening for trials in Uganda: diagnostic test accuracy study. *BMJ* 2007; 335:188.

60. World Health Organization. *Antiretroviral therapy for HIV infection in adults and adolescents in resource-limited settings: towards universal access*, revised edn. Geneva: WHO; 2006.

61. Spacek LA, Gray RH, Wawer MJ, et al. Clinical illness as a marker for initiation of HIV antiretroviral therapy in a rural setting, Rakai, Uganda. *Int J STD AIDS* 2006; 17:116–120.

62. Dieye TN, Vereecken C, Diallo AA, et al. Absolute CD4 T-cell counting in resource-poor settings: direct volumetric measurements versus bead-based clinical flow cytometry instruments. *J Acquir Immune Defic Syndr* 2005; 39:32–37.

63. Mbanya D, Assah F, Ndembi N, et al. Monitoring antiretroviral therapy in HIV/AIDS patients in resource-limited settings: CD4 counts or total lymphocyte counts? *Int J Infect Dis* 2007; 11:157–160.

64. Badri M, Lawn SD, Wood R. Short-term risk of AIDS or death in people infected with HIV-1 before antiretroviral therapy in South Africa: a longitudinal study. *Lancet* 2006; 368:1254–1259.

65. Peter JB, Sevall JS. Molecular-based methods for quantifying HIV viral load. *AIDS Patient Care STDS* 2004; 18:75–79.

66. Schmitt Y. Performance characteristics of quantification assays for human immunodeficiency virus type 1 RNA. *J Clin Virol* 2001; 20:31–33.

67. Elbeik T, Alvord WG, Trichavaroj R, et al. Comparative analysis of HIV-1 viral load assays on subtype quantification. *J Acquir Immune Defic Syndr* 2002; 29:330–339.

68. McClernon DR, Vavro C, St.Clair M. Evaluation of a real-time nucleic acid sequence-based amplification assay using molecular beacons for detection of human immunodeficiency virus type 1. *J Clin Microbiol* 2006; 44:2280–2282.

69. Apoola A, Ahmad S, Radcliffe K. Primary HIV infection. *Int J STD AIDS* 2002; 13:71–78.

70. Schacker T, Collier AC, Hughes J, et al. Clinical and epidemiologic features of primary HIV infection. *Ann Intern Med* 1996; 125:257–264.

71. Mata RC, Viciana P, de A A, et al. Discontinuation of antiretroviral therapy in patients with chronic HIV infection: clinical, virologic and immunologic consequences. *AIDS Patient Care STDS* 2005; 19:550–562.

72. Kassutto S, Rosenberg ES. Primary HIV type 1 infection. *Clin Infect Dis* 2004; 38:1447–1453.

73. Daar ES, Moudgil T, Meyer RD, et al. Transient high levels of viremia in patients with primary human immunodeficiency virus type 1 infection. *N Engl J Med* 1991; 324:961–964.

74. Morgan D, Mahe C, Whitworth J. Absence of a recognizable seroconversion illness in Africans infected with HIV-1. *AIDS* 2001; 15:1575–1576.

75. Walensky RP, Paltiel AD, Losina E, et al. The survival benefits of AIDS treatment in the United States. *J Infect Dis* 2006; 194:11–19.

76. Lewden C, Chene G, Morlat P, et al. HIV-infected adults with a CD4 cell count greater than 500 cells/mm^3 on long-term combination antiretroviral therapy reach same mortality rates as the general population. *J Acquir Immune Defic Syndr* 2007; 46:72–77.

77. Lohse N, Hansen AB, Pedersen G, et al. Survival of persons with and without HIV infection in Denmark, 1995–2005. *Ann Intern Med* 2007; 146:87–95.

78. Lucas SB, Hounnou A, Peacock C, et al. The mortality and pathology of HIV infection in a west African city. *AIDS* 1993; 7:1569–1579.

79. Sok P, Harwell JI, McGarvey ST, et al. Demographic and clinical characteristics of HIV-infected inpatients and outpatients at a Cambodian hospital. *AIDS Patient Care STDS* 2006; 20:369–378.

80. Jowi JO, Mativo PM, Musoke SS. Clinical and laboratory characteristics of hospitalised patients with neurological manifestations of HIV/AIDS at the Nairobi hospital. *East Afr Med J* 2007; 84:67–76.

81. Etard JF, Ndiaye I, Thierry-Mieg M, et al. Mortality and causes of death in adults receiving highly active antiretroviral therapy in Senegal: a 7-year cohort study. *AIDS* 2006; 20:1181–1189.

82. Guelar A, Gatell JM, Verdejo J, et al. A prospective study of the risk of tuberculosis among HIV-infected patients. *AIDS* 1993; 7:1345–1349.

83. Selwyn PA, Hartel D, Lewis VA, et al. A prospective study of the risk of tuberculosis among intravenous drug users with human immunodeficiency virus infection. *N Engl J Med* 1989; 320:545–550.

84. Chaisson RE, Schecter GF, Theuer CP, et al. Tuberculosis in patients with the acquired immunodeficiency syndrome. Clinical features, response to therapy and survival. *Am Rev Respir Dis* 1987; 136:570–574.

85. Martinson NA, Karstaedt A, Venter WD, et al. Causes of death in hospitalized adults with a premortem diagnosis of tuberculosis: an autopsy study. *AIDS* 2007; 21:2043–2050.

86. Geng E, Kreiswirth B, Burzynski J, et al. Clinical and radiographic correlates of primary and reactivation tuberculosis: a molecular epidemiology study. *JAMA* 2005; 293:2740–2745.

87. Gandhi NR, Moll A, Sturm AW, et al. Extensively drug-resistant tuberculosis as a cause of death in patients co-infected with tuberculosis and HIV in a rural area of South Africa. *Lancet* 2006; 368:1575–1580.

88. Breen RA, Smith CJ, Bettinson H, et al. Paradoxical reactions during tuberculosis treatment in patients with and without HIV co-infection. *Thorax* 2004; 59:704–707.

89. Cheng VC, Ho P L, Lee RA, et al. Clinical spectrum of paradoxical deterioration during antituberculosis therapy in non-HIV-infected patients. *Eur J Clin Microbiol Infect Dis* 2002; 21:803–809.

90. Jover F, Cuadrado JM, Andreu L, et al. A comparative study of bacteremic and non-bacteremic pneumococcal pneumonia. *Eur J Intern Med* 2008; 19:15–21.

91. Feldman C, Glatthaar M, Morar R, et al. Bacteremic pneumococcal pneumonia in HIV-seropositive and HIV-seronegative adults. *Chest* 1999; 116:107–114.

92. Klugman KP, Madhi SA, Feldman C. HIV and pneumococcal disease. *Curr Opin Infect Dis* 2007; 20:11–15.

93. Kankwatira AM, Mwafulirwa GA, Gordon MA. Non-typhoidal salmonella bacteraemia–an under-recognized feature of AIDS in African adults. *Trop Doct* 2004; 34:198–200.

94. Byakika-Kibwika P, Ddumba E, Kamya M. Effect of HIV-1 infection on malaria treatment outcome in Ugandan patients. *Afr Health Sci* 2007; 7:86–92.

95. Hewitt K, Steketee R, Mwapasa V, et al. Interactions between HIV and malaria in non-pregnant adults: evidence and implications. *AIDS* 2006; 20:1993–2004.

96. Brentlinger PE, Behrens CB, Kublin JG. Challenges in the prevention, diagnosis and treatment of malaria in human immunodeficiency virus infected adults in sub-Saharan Africa. *Arch Intern Med* 2007; 167:1827–1836.

97. Gilks CF, Brindle RJ, Mwachari C, et al. Disseminated Mycobacterium avium infection among HIV-infected patients in Kenya. *J Acquir Immune Defic Syndr Hum Retrovirol* 1995; 8:195–198.

98. Pettipher CA, Karstaedt AS, Hopley M. Prevalence and clinical manifestations of disseminated Mycobacterium avium complex infection in South Africans with acquired immunodeficiency syndrome. *Clin Infect Dis* 2001; 33:2068–2071.

99. Roos F, Flepp M, Figueras G, et al. Clinical manifestations and predictors of survival in AIDS patients with disseminated Mycobacterium avium infection. *Eur J Clin Microbiol Infect Dis* 2001; 20:428–430.

100. Sirisanthana T. Penicillium marneffei infection in patients with AIDS. *Emerg Infect Dis* 2001; 7:561.

101. Supparatpinyo K, Khamwan C, Baosoung V, et al. Disseminated Penicillium marneffei infection in southeast Asia. *Lancet* 1994; 344:110–113.

102. Karp CL, Auwaerter PG. Coinfection with HIV and tropical infectious diseases. II. Helminthic, fungal, bacterial and viral pathogens. *Clin Infect Dis* 2007; 45:1214–1220.

103. Mbulaiteye SM, Katabira ET, Wabinga H, et al. Spectrum of cancers among HIV-infected persons in Africa: the Uganda AIDS-Cancer Registry Match Study. *Int J Cancer* 2006; 118:985–990.

104. Piscopo TV, Mallia AC. Leishmaniasis. *Postgrad Med J* 2006; 82:649–657.

105. Sinha PK, Pandey K, Bhattacharya SK. Diagnosis and management of leishmania/HIV co-infection. *Indian J Med Res* 2005; 121:407–414.

106. Pintado V, Martin-Rabadan P, Rivera ML, et al. Visceral leishmaniasis in human immunodeficiency virus (HIV)-infected and non-HIV-infected patients. A comparative study. *Medicine (Baltimore)* 2001; 80:54–73.

107. Pintado V, Lopez-Velez R. HIV-associated visceral leishmaniasis. *Clin Microbiol Infect* 2001; 7:291–300.

108. Russo R, Laguna F, Lopez-Velez R, et al. Visceral leishmaniasis in those infected with HIV: clinical aspects and other opportunistic infections. *Ann Trop Med Parasitol* 2003; 97(suppl 1):99–105.

109. Williams IG. Management of CMV disease in HIV infection. *Int J STD AIDS* 1999; 10:211–216.

110. Murray JF. Pulmonary complications of HIV-1 infection among adults living in Sub-Saharan Africa. *Int J Tuberc Lung Dis* 2005; 9:826–835.

111. McKinsey DS. Histoplasmosis in AIDS: advances in management. *AIDS Patient Care STDS* 1998; 12:775–781.

112. Hirsch HH, Kaufmann G, Sendi P, et al. Immune reconstitution in HIV infected patients. *Clin Infect Dis* 2004; 38:1159–1166.

113. Lawn SD, Myer L, Bekker LG, et al. Tuberculosis-associated immune reconstitution disease: incidence, risk factors and impact in an antiretroviral treatment service in South Africa. *AIDS* 2007; 21:335–341.

114. Holloway RG, Kieburtz KD. Headache and the human immunodeficiency virus type 1 infection. *Headache* 1995; 35:245–255.

115. Chayakulkeeree M, Perfect JR. Cryptococcosis. *Infect Dis Clin North Am* 2006; 20:507–vi.

116. Mwaba P, Mwansa J, Chintu C, et al. Clinical presentation, natural history and cumulative death rates of 230 adults with primary cryptococcal meningitis in Zambian AIDS patients treated under local conditions. *Postgrad Med J* 2001; 77:769–773.

117. French AL, Operskalski E, Peters M, et al. Isolated hepatitis B core antibody is associated with HIV and ongoing but not resolved hepatitis C virus infection in a cohort of US women. *J Infect Dis* 2007; 195:1437–1442.

118. Hakim JG, Gangaidzo IT, Heyderman RS, et al. Impact of HIV infection on meningitis in Harare, Zimbabwe: a prospective study of 406 predominantly adult patients. *AIDS* 2000; 14:1401–1407.

119. Modi M, Mochan A, Modi G. Management of HIV-associated focal brain lesions in developing countries. *QJM* 2004; 97:413–421.

120. Bergemann A, Karstaedt AS. The spectrum of meningitis in a population with high prevalence of HIV disease. *QJM* 1996; 89:499–504.

121. Bhigjee AI, Naidoo K, Patel VB, et al. Intracranial mass lesions in HIV-positive patients–the KwaZulu/Natal experience. Neuroscience AIDS Research Group. *S Afr Med J* 1999; 89:1284–1288.

122. Chadha DS, Handa A, Sharma SK, et al. Seizures in patients with human immunodeficiency virus infection. *J Assoc Physicians India* 2000; 48:573–576.

123. Amogne W, Teshager G, Zenebe G. Central nervous system toxoplasmosis in adult Ethiopians. *Ethiop Med J* 2006; 44:113–120.

124. Price P, Mathiot N, Krueger R, et al. Immune dysfunction and immune restoration disease in HIV patients given highly active antiretroviral therapy. *J Clin Virol* 2001; 22:279–287.

125. Bartlett JG, Gallant JE. *Medical Management of HIV Infection.* Baltimore: Johns Hopkins Medicine Health Publishing Business Group, 2007.

126. McArthur JC, Brew BJ, Nath A. Neurological complications of HIV infection. *Lancet Neurol* 2005; 4:543–555.

127. McArthur JC, Haughey N, Gartner S, et al. Human immunodeficiency virus-associated dementia: an evolving disease. *J Neurovirol* 2003; 9:205–221.

128. Sharma SK, Kadhiravan T, Banga A, et al. Spectrum of clinical disease in a series of 135 hospitalised HIV-infected patients from north India. *BMC Infect Dis* 2004; 4:52.

129. Anekthananon T, Ratanasuwan W, Techasathit W, et al. HIV infection/acquired immunodeficiency syndrome at Siriraj Hospital, 2002: time for secondary prevention. *J Med Assoc Thai* 2004; 87:173–179.

130. Klotz SA, Nguyen HC, Van PT, et al. Clinical features of HIV/AIDS patients presenting to an inner city clinic in Ho Chi Minh City, Vietnam. *Int J STD AIDS* 2007; 18:482–485.

131. Louie JK, Chi NH, Thao le TT, et al. Opportunistic infections in hospitalized HIV-infected adults in Ho Chi Minh City, Vietnam: a cross-sectional study. *Int J STD AIDS* 2004; 15:758–761.

132. van Oosterhout JJ, Laufer MK, Perez MA, et al. Pneumocystis pneumonia in HIV-positive adults, Malawi. *Emerg Infect Dis* 2007; 13:325–328.

133. Wong ML, Back P, Candy G, et al. Pneumocystis jirovecii pneumonia in African miners at autopsy. *Int J Tuberc Lung Dis* 2006; 10:756–760.

134. Garay SM. Pulmonary Tuberculosis. In: Rom WN, Garay SM, eds. *Tuberculosis*, 2nd ed. Philadelphia: Lippincott Williams & Wilkins; 2004:345–394.

135. Batungwanayo J, Taelman H, Dhote R, et al. Pulmonary tuberculosis in Kigali, Rwanda. Impact of human immunodeficiency virus infection on clinical and radiographic presentation. *Am Rev Respir Dis* 1992; 146:53–56.

136. Salaniponi FM, Nyirenda TE, Kemp JR, et al. Characteristics, management and outcome of patients with recurrent tuberculosis under routine programme conditions in Malawi. *Int J Tuberc Lung Dis* 2003; 7:948–952.

137. Verver S, Warren RM, Beyers N, et al. Rate of reinfection tuberculosis after successful treatment is higher than rate of new tuberculosis. *Am J Respir Crit Care Med* 2005; 171:1430–1435.

138. Sonnenberg P, Murray J, Glynn JR, et al. HIV-1 and recurrence, relapse and reinfection of tuberculosis after cure: a cohort study in South African mineworkers. *Lancet* 2001; 358:1687–1693.

139. Kudjawu Y, Massari V, Sow O, et al. Benefit of amoxicillin in differentiating between TB suspects whose initial AFB sputum smears are negative. *Int J Tuberc Lung Dis* 2006; 10:441–446.

140. Boyton RJ. Infectious lung complications in patients with HIV/AIDS. *Curr Opin Pulm Med* 2005; 11:203–207.

141. Janoff EN, Breiman RF, Daley CL, et al. Pneumococcal disease during HIV infection. Epidemiologic, clinical and immunologic perspectives. *Ann Intern Med* 1992; 117:314–324.

142. Kovacs JA, Gill VJ, Meshnick S, et al. New insights into transmission, diagnosis and drug treatment of Pneumocystis carinii pneumonia. *JAMA* 2001; 286:2450–2460.

143. Meditz AL, Borok M, MaWhinney S, et al. Gender differences in AIDS-associated Kaposi sarcoma in Harare, Zimbabwe. *J Acquir Immune Defic Syndr* 2007; 44:306–308.

144. Restrepo CS, Martinez S, Lemos JA, et al. Imaging manifestations of Kaposi sarcoma. *Radiographics* 2006; 26:1169–1185.

145. Bolhaar MG, Karstaedt AS. A high incidence of lactic acidosis and symptomatic hyperlactatemia in women receiving highly active antiretroviral therapy in Soweto, South Africa. *Clin Infect Dis* 2007; 45:254–260.

146. Mwachari CW, Meier AS, Muyodi J, et al. Chronic diarrhoea in HIV-1-infected adults in Nairobi, Kenya: evaluation of risk factors and the WHO treatment algorithm. *AIDS* 2003; 17:2124–2126.

147. Colebunders R, Lusakumuni K, Nelson AM, et al. Persistent diarrhoea in Zairian AIDS patients: an endoscopic and histological study. *Gut* 1988; 29:1687–1691.

148. Chhin S, Harwell JI, Bell JD, et al. Aetiology of chronic diarrhoea in antiretroviral-naive patients with HIV infection admitted to Norodom Sihanouk Hospital, Phnom Penh, Cambodia. *Clin Infect Dis* 2006; 43:925–932.

149. Andualem B, Kassu A, Moges F, et al. Diarrhoea-associated parasites in HIV-1 seropositive and sero-negative patients in a teaching hospital, Northwest Ethiopia. *Ethiop Med J* 2007; 45:165–170.

150. Tadesse A, Kassu A. Intestinal parasite isolates in AIDS patients with chronic diarrhoea in Gondar Teaching Hospital, North west Ethiopia. *Ethiop Med J* 2005; 43:93–96.

151. Kaplowitz N. Drug-induced liver injury. *Clin Infect Dis* 2004; 38 (suppl 2):S44–S48.

152. Sulkowski MS, Thomas DL, Chaisson RE, et al. Hepatotoxicity associated with antiretroviral therapy in adults infected with human immunodeficiency virus and the role of hepatitis C or B virus infection. *JAMA* 2000; 283:74–80.

153. Baylor MS, Johann-Liang R. Hepatotoxicity associated with nevirapine use. *J Acquir Immune Defic Syndr* 2004; 35:538–539.

154. Sanne I, Mommeja-Marin H, Hinkle J, et al. Severe hepatotoxicity associated with nevirapine use in HIV-infected subjects. *J Infect Dis* 2005; 191(6):825–829.

155. den Brinker M, Wit FW, Wertheim-van Dillen PM, et al. Hepatitis B and C virus co-infection and the risk for hepatotoxicity of highly active antiretroviral therapy in HIV-1 infection. *AIDS* 2000; 14:2895–2902.

156. Mahajani RV, Uzer MF. Cholangiopathy in HIV-infected patients. *Clin Liver Dis* 1999; 3:669–684, x.

157. Clarke DL, Thomson SR, Bissetty T, et al. A single surgical unit's experience with abdominal tuberculosis in the HIV/AIDS era. *World J Surg* 2007; 31:1087–1096.

158. Dassopoulos T, Ehrenpreis ED. Acute pancreatitis in human immunodeficiency virus-infected patients: a review. *Am J Med* 1999; 107:78–84.

159. Atta MG, Choi MJ, Longenecker JC, et al. Nephrotic range proteinuria and CD4 count as noninvasive indicators of HIV-associated nephropathy. *Am J Med* 2005; 118:1288.

160. Roling J, Schmid H, Fischereder M, et al. HIV-associated renal diseases and highly active antiretroviral therapy-induced nephropathy. *Clin Infect Dis* 2006; 42:1488–1495.

161. Estrella M, Fine DM, Gallant JE, et al. HIV type 1 RNA level as a clinical indicator of renal pathology in HIV-infected patients. *Clin Infect Dis* 2006; 43:377–380.

162. Coopman SA, Johnson RA, Platt R, et al. Cutaneous disease and drug reactions in HIV infection. *N Engl J Med* 1993; 328:1670–1674.

163. Maurer TA. Dermatologic manifestations of HIV infection. *Top HIV Med* 2005; 13:149–154.

164. Jensen BL, Weismann K, Sindrup JH, et al. Incidence and prognostic significance of skin disease in patients with HIV/AIDS: a 5-year observational study. *Acta Derm Venereol* 2000; 80:140–143.

165. Mbuagbaw J, Eyong I, Alemnji G, et al. Patterns of skin manifestations and their relationships with CD4 counts among HIV/AIDS patients in Cameroon. *Int J Derm* 2006; 45:280–284.

166. Myskowski PL, Ahkami R. Dermatologic complications of HIV infection. *Med Clin North Am* 1996; 80:1415–1435.

167. Eisman S. Pruritic papular eruption in HIV. *Dermatol Clin* 2006; 24:449–457, vi.

168. Tappero JW, Perkins BA, Wenger JD, et al. Cutaneous manifestations of opportunistic infections in patients infected with human immunodeficiency virus. *Clin Microbiol Rev* 1995; 8:440–450.

169. Farmer P, Leandre F, Mukherjee J, et al. Community-based treatment of advanced HIV disease: introducing DOT-HAART (directly observed therapy with highly active antiretroviral therapy). *Bull World Health Organ* 2001; 79:1145–1151.

170. Lanoy E, Mary-Krause M, Tattevin P, et al. Predictors identified for losses to follow-up among HIV-seropositive patients. *J Clin Epidemiol* 2006; 59:829–835.

171. Bower M, Palmieri C, Dhillon T. AIDS-related malignancies: changing epidemiology and the impact of highly active antiretroviral therapy. *Curr Opin Infect Dis* 2006; 19:14–19.

172. Jessop S. HIV-associated Kaposi's sarcoma. *Dermatol Clin* 2006; 24:509–520, vii.

173. Mermin J, Bunnell R, Lule J, et al. Developing an evidence-based, preventive care package for persons with HIV in Africa. *Trop Med Int Health* 2005; 10:961–970.

174. Mermin J, Ekwaru JP, Liechty CA, et al. Effect of co-trimoxazole prophylaxis, antiretroviral therapy and insecticide-treated bednets on the frequency of malaria in HIV-1-infected adults in Uganda: a prospective cohort study. *Lancet* 2006; 367:1256–1261.

175. Young T. Effects of micronutrient supplementation on morbidity and mortality among HIV-infected individuals – a summary of the evidence. *S Afr Med J* 2006; 96:1062–1064.

176. Hardon AP, Akurut D, Comoro C, et al. Hunger, waiting time and transport costs: time to confront challenges to ART adherence in Africa. *AIDS Care* 2007; 19:658–665.

177. Fawzi W. Micronutrients and human immunodeficiency virus type 1 disease progression among adults and children. *Clin Infect Dis* 2003; 37(suppl 2): S112–S116.

178. Golub JE, Saraceni V, Cavalcante SC, et al. The impact of antiretroviral therapy and isoniazid preventive therapy on tuberculosis incidence in HIV-infected patients in Rio de Janeiro, Brazil. *AIDS* 2007; 21:1441–1448.

179. Grabar S, Le M V, Goujard C, et al. Clinical outcome of patients with HIV-1 infection according to immunologic and virologic response after 6 months of highly active antiretroviral therapy. *Ann Intern Med* 2000; 133:401–410.

180. Piketty C, Weiss L, Thomas F, et al. Long-term clinical outcome of human immunodeficiency virus-infected patients with discordant immunologic and virologic responses to a protease inhibitor-containing regimen. *J Infect Dis* 2001; 183:1328–1335.

181. Gail MH, Tan WY, Pee D, et al. Survival after AIDS diagnosis in a cohort of hemophilia patients. Multicentre Hemophilia Cohort Study. *J Acquir Immune Defic Syndr Hum Retrovirol* 1997; 15:363–369.

182. Wang C, Vlahov D, Galai N, et al. Mortality in HIV-seropositive versus seronegative persons in the era of highly active antiretroviral therapy: implications for when to initiate therapy. *J Infect Dis* 2004; 190:1046–1054.

183. Haggerty CM, Pitt E, Siciliano RF. The latent reservoir for HIV-1 in resting CD4+ T cells and other viral reservoirs during chronic infection. *Curr Opin HIV AIDS* 2006; 1:62–68.

184. Samuel R, Bettiker R, Suh B. Antiretroviral therapy 2006: pharmacology, applications and special situations. *Arch Pharm Res* 2006; 29:431–458.

185. Jackson JB, Becker-Pergola G, Guay LA, et al. Identification of the K103N resistance mutation in Ugandan women receiving nevirapine to prevent HIV-1 vertical transmission. *AIDS* 2000; 14:F111–F115.

186. Kuritzkes DR. Preventing and managing antiretroviral drug resistance. *AIDS Patient Care STDS* 2004; 18:259–273.

187. Bangsberg DR, Acosta EP, Gupta R, et al. Adherence-resistance relationships for protease and non-nucleoside reverse transcriptase inhibitors explained by virological fitness. *AIDS* 2006; 20:223–231.

188. Bangsberg DR. Less than 95% adherence to nonnucleoside reverse-transcriptase inhibitor therapy can lead to viral suppression. *Clin Infect Dis* 2006; 43:939–941.

189. Ross L, Lim ML, Liao Q, et al. Prevalence of antiretroviral drug resistance and resistance-associated mutations in antiretroviral therapy-naive HIV-infected individuals from 40 United States cities. *HIV Clin Trials* 2007; 8:1–8.

190. Derache A, Traore O, Koita V, et al. Genetic diversity and drug resistance mutations in HIV type 1 from untreated patients in Bamako, Mali. *Antivir Ther* 2007; 12:123–129.

191. Mills EJ, Nachega JB, Buchan I, et al. Adherence to antiretroviral therapy in sub-Saharan Africa and North America: a meta-analysis. *JAMA* 2006; 296:679–690.

192. Roge BT, Barfod TS, Kirk O, et al. Resistance profiles and adherence at primary virological failure in three different highly active antiretroviral therapy regimens: analysis of failure rates in a randomized study. *HIV Med* 2004; 5:344–351.

193. Castro A. Adherence to antiretroviral therapy: merging the clinical and social course of AIDS. *PLoS Med* 2005; 2:e338.

194. Behforouz HL, Farmer PE, Mukherjee JS. From directly observed therapy to accompagnateurs: enhancing AIDS treatment outcomes in Haiti and in Boston. *Clin Infect Dis* 2004; 38(suppl 5):S429–S436.

195. Karcher H, Omondi A, Odera J, et al. Risk factors for treatment denial and loss to follow-up in an antiretroviral treatment cohort in Kenya. *Trop Med Int Health* 2007; 12:687–694.

196. Arici C, Ripamonti D, Maggiolo F, et al. Factors associated with the failure of HIV-positive persons to return for scheduled medical visits. *HIV Clin Trials* 2002; 3:52–57.

197. Nacher M, El G M, Vaz T, et al. Risk factors for follow-up interruption of HIV patients in French Guiana. *Am J Trop Med Hyg* 2006; 74:915–917.

198. Rosen S, Fox MP, Gill CJ. Patient retention in antiretroviral therapy programmes in sub-Saharan Africa: a systematic review. *PLoS Med* 2007; 4: e298.

199. Dalal RP, Macphail C, Mqhayi M, et al. Characteristics and outcomes of adult patients lost to follow-up at an antiretroviral treatment clinic in Johannesburg, South Africa. *J Acquir Immune Defic Syndr* 2008; 47:101–107.

200. Schutz C, Stead D, Meintjies G, et al. Trends in the presentation and mortality of severe hyperlactatemia at a public sector referral hospital in Cape Town, 2007. Abstract 740. 3rd South African AIDS Conference, June 2007 Durban, South Africa.

201. Morse CG, Kovacs JA. Metabolic and skeletal complications of HIV infection: the price of success. *JAMA* 2006; 296:844–854.

202. Curkendall SM, Richardson JT, Emons MF, et al. Incidence of anaemia among HIV-infected patients treated with highly active antiretroviral therapy. *HIV Med* 2007; 8:483–490.

203. Hoffmann CJ, Fielding KL, Charalambous S, et al. Antiretroviral therapy using zidovudine, lamivudine and efavirenz in South Africa: tolerability and clinical events. *AIDS* 2008; 22:67–74.

204. Pulido F, Arribas JR, Delgado R, et al. Lopinavir-ritonavir monotherapy versus lopinavir-ritonavir and two nucleosides for maintenance therapy of HIV. *AIDS* 2008; 22:F1–F9.

205. Delfraissy JF, Flandre P, Delaugerre C, et al. Lopinavir/ritonavir monotherapy or plus zidovudine and lamivudine in antiretroviral-naive HIV-infected patients. *AIDS* 2008; 22:385–393.

206. Deeks SG, Hoh R, Neilands TB, et al. Interruption of treatment with individual therapeutic drug classes in adults with multidrug-resistant HIV-1 infection. *J Infect Dis* 2005; 192:1537–1544.

207. Castagna A, Danise A, Menzo S, et al. Lamivudine monotherapy in HIV-1-infected patients harbouring a lamivudine-resistant virus: a randomized pilot study (E-184V study). *AIDS* 2006; 20:795–803.

208. McIlleron H, Meintjes G, Burman WJ, et al. Complications of antiretroviral therapy in patients with tuberculosis: drug interactions, toxicity and immune reconstitution inflammatory syndrome. *J Infect Dis* 2007; 196(suppl 1):S63–S75.

209. Autar RS, Wit FW, Sankote J, et al. Nevirapine plasma concentrations and concomitant use of rifampin in patients coinfected with HIV-1 and tuberculosis. *Antivir Ther* 2005, 10:937–943.

210. Manosuthi W, Sungkanuparph S, Thakkinstian A, et al. Plasma nevirapine levels and 24-week efficacy in HIV-infected patients receiving nevirapine-based highly active antiretroviral therapy with or without rifampicin. *Clin Infect Dis* 2006; 43:253–255.

211. Van Cutsem V, Cohen K, Bedelu M, et al. TB/HIV co-infected patients on rifampicin containing treatment have equivalent ART treatment outcomes and concurrent use of nevirapine is not associated with increased hepatotoxicity. Paper presented at the 3rd IAS Conference on HIV Pathogenesis and Treatment, 24–27 July, 2005, Rio de Janiero.

212. Lawn SD, Myer L, Bekker LG, et al. Burden of tuberculosis in an antiretroviral treatment programme in sub-Saharan Africa: impact on treatment outcomes and implications for tuberculosis control. *AIDS* 2006; 20:1605–1612.

213. Townsend CL, Tookey PA, Cortina-Borja M, et al. Antiretroviral therapy and congenital abnormalities in infants born to HIV-1-infected women in the United Kingdom and Ireland, 1990 to 2003. *J Acquir Immune Defic Syndr* 2006; 42:91–94.

214. Watts DH. Teratogenicity risk of antiretroviral therapy in pregnancy. *Curr HIV/AIDS Rep* 2007; 4:135–140.

215. Bussmann H, Wester CW, Wester CN, et al. Pregnancy rates and birth outcomes among women on efavirenz-containing highly active antiretroviral therapy in Botswana. *J Acquir Immune Defic Syndr* 2007; 45:269–273.

216. Liaw Y-F, Sung JJY, Chow WC, et al. Lamivudine for patients with chronic hepatitis B and advanced liver disease. *N Engl J Med* 2004; 351:1521–1531.

217. Hoffmann CJ, Thio CL. Clinical implications of HIV and hepatitis B co-infection in Asia and Africa. *Lancet Infect Dis* 2007; 7:402–409.

218. Benhamou Y, Bochet M, Thibault V, et al. Long-term incidence of hepatitis B virus resistance to lamivudine in human immunodeficiency virus-infected patients. *Hepatology* 1999; 30:1302–1306.

219. Uffic-Burban S, Losina E, Wang B, et al. Estimates of opportunistic infection incidence or death within specific CD4 strata in HIV-infected patients in Abidjan, Cote d'Ivoire: impact of alternative methods of CD4 count modelling. *Eur J Epidemiol* 2007; 22:737–744.

220. Badri M, Cleary S, Maartens G, et al. When to initiate highly active antiretroviral therapy in sub-Saharan Africa? A South African cost-effectiveness study. *Antivir Ther* 2006; 11:63–72.

221. Badri M, Bekker LG, Orrell C, et al. Initiating highly active antiretroviral therapy in sub-Saharan Africa: an assessment of the revised World Health Organization scaling-up guidelines. *AIDS* 2004; 18:1159–1168.

222. Goicoechea M, Smith DM, Liu L, et al. Determinants of CD4+ T cell recovery during suppressive antiretroviral therapy: association of immune activation, T cell maturation markers and cellular HIV-1 DNA. *J Infect Dis* 2006; 194:29–37.

223. Wei X, Ghosh SK, Taylor ME, et al. Viral dynamics in human immunodeficiency virus type 1 infection. *Nature* 1995; 373:117–122.

224. Kaufmann GR, Bloch M, Finlayson R, et al. The extent of HIV-1-related immunodeficiency and age predict the long-term CD4 T lymphocyte response to potent antiretroviral therapy. *AIDS* 2002; 16:359–367.

225. Bosch RJ, Wang R, Vaida F, et al. Changes in the slope of the CD4 cell count increase after initiation of potent antiretroviral treatment. *J Acquir Immune Defic Syndr* 2006; 43:433–435.

226. Hunt PW, Deeks SG, Rodriguez B, et al. Continued CD4 cell count increases in HIV-infected adults experiencing 4 years of viral suppression on antiretroviral therapy. *AIDS* 2003; 17:1907–1915.

227. Viard JP, Burgard M, Hubert JB, et al. Impact of 5 years of maximally successful highly active antiretroviral therapy on CD4 cell count and HIV-1 DNA level. *AIDS* 2004; 18:45–49.

228. Moore RD, Keruly JC. CD4+ cell count 6 years after commencement of highly active antiretroviral therapy in persons with sustained virologic suppression. *Clin Infect Dis* 2007; 44:441–446.

229. Dronda F, Moreno S, Moreno A, et al. Long-term outcomes among antiretroviral-naive human immunodeficiency virus-infected patients with small increases in CD4+ cell counts after successful virologic suppression. *Clin Infect Dis* 2002; 35:1005–1009.

230. Taylor S, Boffito M, Khoo S, et al. Stopping antiretroviral therapy. *AIDS* 2007; 21:1673–1682.

231. El-Sadr W, Neaton J. The SMART Study Investigators. Episodic CD4-guided use of antiretroviral therapy is inferior to continuous therapy: results of the SMART study, 2006.

232. DART Trial Team. Fixed duration interruptions are inferior to continuous treatment in African adults starting therapy with CD4 cell counts <200 cells/microL. *AIDS* 2008; 22:237–247.

233. WHO. HIV testing and counselling. Online. Available: http://www.who.int/hiv/topics/vct/en/index.html 2007. Accessed July 2008.

Chapter 21

John Richens and David C. W. Mabey

Sexually Transmitted Infections (Excluding HIV)

Sexually transmitted infections (STIs) are among the most common reasons for seeking medical care in developing countries, accounting for 10% or more of medical consultations in some parts of Africa.[1] Nevertheless, and in spite of their serious consequences (particularly for women and children), and extensive evidence that they facilitate the transmission of human immunodeficiency virus (HIV) through sexual contact,[2] they have often been accorded low priority by medical professionals and health planners. The consequent lack of good facilities for their management has led many patients with these conditions to seek treatment outside the formal health sector, with inadequate treatment regimens leading to increasing antimicrobial resistance among sexually transmitted pathogens. Because so few statistics are available for patients treated outside the formal health sector, the extent of the problem continues to be underestimated.

EPIDEMIOLOGY OF SEXUALLY TRANSMITTED DISEASES

Certain broad generalizations can be made about the epidemiology of sexually transmitted diseases (STIs). Clearly, they are diseases of the sexually active, although mother-to-child transmission also occurs. None of the sexually transmitted agents described in this chapter has an epidemiologically significant non-human reservoir. They are more common among young adults, among single people of both sexes, and among those who travel. Although no sexually active individual is immune, certain groups can be identified whose behaviour places them at higher risk than others. Such groups include sex workers and their clients, bar workers, adolescents, the military, truck drivers and sailors.

The behaviour of STIs within populations, as with other infectious diseases, can be predicted if information is available about the proportion of individuals who are susceptible to infection, the average efficiency of transmission per contact, the rates of contact between infected and uninfected persons and the average duration of infection. This is commonly expressed as the basic reproductive number (R_0), i.e. the average number of new cases arising from one infected person, with the equation $R_0 = \beta \times c \times d$ where β = the transmission efficiency, c = the rate of partner change and d = the duration of infection. The viral STIs which are persistent maintain themselves with ease, whereas some bacterial STIs such as chancroid, which are usually short-lived and require high rates of partner change to maintain themselves, can be brought under control relatively easily. Each of these factors is amenable to public health intervention, e.g. improving access to treatment, promoting delay in sexual debut and the use of barrier methods of contraception.

Accurate STI prevalence figures are not routinely available for any developing country, but much useful information has been gathered during limited surveys of antenatal women.[3] In a recent large research study in rural Uganda, a community-based survey of adults aged 15–59 years found the prevalence of syphilis to be 10%, of gonorrhoea 1.6% and of chlamydial infection 3%. A total of 24% of women had *Trichomonas vaginalis* infection, and 51% had bacterial vaginosis.[4] Table 21.1 shows a number of factors which may explain the higher incidence and prevalence of STIs in developing compared with industrialized countries. Lack of access to effective treatment probably explains much of the difference in the case of the curable STIs.

The relative importance of certain STIs is much greater in developing countries. For example, chancroid remains a common cause of genital ulceration in many African countries but has almost disappeared from Europe. Sporadic outbreaks among impoverished communities in North America in the 1980s suggest that this has more to do with socioeconomic factors than with climate. Donovanosis (granuloma inguinale) is highly prevalent in certain parts of Papua New Guinea, India and South Africa but appears to be rare outside these areas. The lack of reliable and cheap diagnostic tests for the three classical 'tropical STIs' – chancroid, donovanosis and lymphogranuloma venereum (LGV) – has hindered attempts to study their epidemiology.

Because of the lack of adequate diagnostic and treatment facilities for STIs in many developing countries, complications are commonly seen, particularly among women and children. Pelvic inflammatory disease (PID), due in the majority of cases to gonorrhoea or chlamydial infection, is the most common cause of admission to gynaecology wards in Africa.[5] Ectopic pregnancy as a sequela of PID is up to three times as common in Africa as in Europe, and tubal infertility, another common sequela, is widespread, with up to 20% of women affected in some regions of Africa.[6] The incidence of carcinoma of the cervix is extremely high in many developing countries. Some 2–3% of infants born in some African cities develop gonococcal ophthalmia neonatorum.

Table 21.1 Factors contributing to the high incidence of STIs in developing countries

1.	Demographic factors (high proportion of population are young adults)
2.	Rural–urban migration with breakdown of traditional customs
3.	Prostitution
4.	Lack of adequate medical services
5.	High prevalence of antibiotic-resistant strains of *Neisseria gonorrhoeae*, *Haemophilus ducreyi*
6.	Polygamy

Congenital syphilis has been an important cause of hospital admission among infants aged less than 3 months in Lusaka, Zambia,[7] and a recent study in Tanzania showed that syphilis was responsible for 50% of all stillbirths.[8]

Table 21.2 lists organisms transmissible by sexual contact and the diseases they cause. In this chapter, only those responsible for major morbidity in developing countries will be considered further.

CONTROL OF STIs

Strategies for the control of STIs include primary and secondary prevention, and, in the case of bacterial and protozoal infections, improving access to curative treatment. Primary prevention is health education given to young people before they are exposed to the risk of STIs, emphasizing the importance of delaying the onset of sexual activity, limiting the number of their sexual partners, and using condoms to reduce risk. Secondary prevention refers to health education given to individuals with STIs, aimed at reducing the risk to their sexual partners, and the likelihood of their becoming reinfected.

Improved case management, in which accessible, affordable and effective treatment is made available to patients with symptomatic STIs, is a cornerstone of STI control. Effective treatment should be given at the first visit, to reduce onward transmission and the likelihood of complications. The treatment of sexual partners of STI patients is also of critical importance for STI control. Since many STIs are asymptomatic, especially in women, screening programmes can play an important role in STI control; for example, screening of pregnant women is an important strategy for the prevention of congenital syphilis. Effective control of STIs cannot be achieved by health ministries in isolation. Coordinated multisectoral interventions which attempt to address broader societal issues that allow STIs to thrive (e.g. migrant labour and prostitution) also need to be tackled vigorously.[9]

STIS AND HIV INFECTION

There is no doubt that other STIs, by causing inflammation and ulceration of the genital tract, facilitate the transmission of HIV infection through sexual contact.[2] Ulcerative STIs, in particular, increase both the infectivity of HIV-positive individuals, and the susceptibility of HIV negatives, by a factor of 10–100 per sexual

exposure.[10] Gonococcal and chlamydial infection have been shown to increase the shedding of HIV at the cervix, and gonorrhoea to increase the shedding of HIV in seminal fluid.[11] An intervention trial in Tanzania showed that the incidence of HIV infection was reduced by 40% following the introduction of improved case management of STIs, using the syndromic approach, in rural health centres.[12] These studies have given renewed impetus to STI control programmes.

HISTORY-TAKING AND EXAMINATION IN THE STI CLINIC

It is not possible to provide a good clinical service for STIs unless one gains the confidence of the patient(s). This requires privacy and the avoidance of a moralistic attitude.

It is usually possible to take a history and examine a patient with an STI in 10 minutes. When taking a history, the following information should be collected[13]:
1. The nature and duration of the symptoms.
2. The nature of any treatment already taken for this condition.
3. A sexual history, which should indicate when and with whom the patient has had sexual intercourse. This information is essential in order to attempt contact tracing and/or partner notification. Information about the type of sexual activity and condom use will assist in examination, collection of specimens and preventive counselling.
4. Past medical history and history of previous STIs and HIV testing.
5. History of drug allergy.
6. In female patients a menstrual and obstetric history should be taken.

STI patients should always be counselled concerning risk reduction, including the promotion of condom use; the importance of compliance with the full course of treatment if directly observed single-dose treatment is not given; and the importance of referring sexual contacts for treatment.

The examination should be carried out in private in a good light. After examination of the mouth and palms, patients should be exposed from the umbilicus to the knees. The skin of the abdomen, groins and perineum should be examined in particular for evidence of scabies and pediculosis, and the inguinal glands palpated. In males the penis should be inspected, after retraction of the foreskin in uncircumcised patients. If a urethral discharge is not apparent, evidence of urethritis can be sought by milking the urethra forward and examining the meatus for discharge. The scrotum should be palpated for evidence of epididymitis. Female patients should be examined in the lithotomy position. The lower abdomen should be palpated for evidence of PID (masses and/or tenderness) and, after inspection of the vulva, a vaginal speculum should be passed. The cervix should be examined and the speculum then slowly withdrawn while the walls of the vagina are examined. Bimanual examination is used to identify pelvic masses and/or tenderness. The presence of pain on moving the cervix (cervical excitation tenderness) suggests the presence of PID. In both sexes the perianal skin should also be inspected, and proctoscopy may be performed to check for rectal infections.

The laboratory investigations requested will depend on the facilities available. In general they should be selected on the prin-

Table 21.2 Sexually transmitted infections in humans

	Agent	Disease
STIs PRODUCING GENITAL LESIONS		
Viruses	Herpes simplex virus	Genital herpes, disseminated and neonatal herpes infection
	Human papilloma virus	Genital warts, juvenile laryngeal papillomatosis, squamous carcinoma in anogenital area
	Molluscum contagiosum virus	Molluscum contagiosum
Bacteria	*Neisseria gonorrhoeae*	Gonococcal infections of urethra, epididymis, pharynx, rectum, conjunctiva, upper genital tract of women, disseminated gonorrhoeal infection
	Chlamydia trachomatis, serotypes D–K	As for gonorrhoea, except for disseminated infection; also infantile pneumonia and reactive arthritis
	Chlamydia trachomatis, L1,2,3 serotypes	Lymphogranuloma venereum
	Ureaplasma urealyticum	Non-gonococcal urethritis
	Mycoplasma genitalium	Urethritis, cervicitis and pelvic infection
	Haemophilus ducreyi	Chancroid
	Treponema pallidum	Syphilis
	Gardnerella vaginalis and anaerobes	Bacterial vaginosis
	Klebsiella (formerly *Calymmatobacterium*) *granulomatis*	Donovanosis (granuloma inguinale)
Fungi	*Candida albicans*	Genital candidiasis
Protozoa	*Trichomonas vaginalis*	Trichomoniasis
Arthropods	*Phthirus pubis*	Pediculosis
	Sarcoptes scabiei	Scabies
INFECTIONS WHICH CAN BE SEXUALLY TRANSMITTED BUT WHICH DO NOT GENERALLY PRODUCE GENITAL LESIONS		
Viruses	Hepatitis viruses	Hepatitis A–D
	Cytomegalovirus (CMV)	CMV infections of newborn and immunosuppressed
	HIV	Acquired immune deficiency syndrome
	HTLV-1	Tropical spastic paraparesis, T cell leukaemia/lymphoma
Bacteria	*Shigella* spp.	Shigellosis
	Campylobacter spp.	Campylobacter enteritis
	Salmonella spp.	Salmonellosis
	Group B streptococcus	Neonatal sepsis
Protozoa	*Giardia lamblia*	Giardiasis
	Cryptosporidium spp.	Cryptosporidosis
	Entamoeba histolytica	Amoebiasis*
Helminths	*Enterobius vermicularis*	Enterobiasis
	Strongyloides stercoralis	Strongyloidiasis
	Trichuris trichiura	Trichuriasis

*Occasionally produces anogenital ulceration in tropical countries.
Source: World Health Organization.

ciple that a patient with one STI is also at increased risk of other STIs; that is, they should not be limited to tests designed to identify the cause of the present symptoms. All patients with an STI should be screened for syphilis. Whether they should also be screened for HIV depends on the availability of counselling and of treatment for those found to be positive.

In settings where laboratory diagnosis is not feasible, the World Health Organization (WHO) recommends syndromic manage-ment, in which patients with a syndrome such as urethral discharge or genital ulcer are treated for all the likely causes of that syndrome.[14] Even when laboratory diagnosis is available, syndromic management has the advantage that treatment is given at the first visit, rather than relying on the patients to return for their results. Effective syndromic treatment depends on knowledge of local disease patterns and antimicrobial susceptibilities; a laboratory is required to monitor these, preferably in each country or

Table 21.3 Advantages and disadvantages of syndromic management of STIs

ADVANTAGES
Simple
Rapid
No laboratory required
Treatment given at first visit, preventing complications and further transmission
Simplifies reporting and supervision

DISADVANTAGES
Leads to over-treatment, especially in women
May lead to problems with partner notification, especially in women who are told they have an STI when they do not
Only symptomatic STIs treated

province.[15] WHO syndromic treatment flow charts for eight common STI syndromes are shown in Figure 21.1. The advantages and disadvantages of syndromic management are shown in Table 21.3. The flow chart for vaginal discharge is the least satisfactory, as many women with this complaint are not suffering from an STI. This not only leads to over-treatment, but can also jeopardize relationships if such women are asked to refer their partners for STI treatment.

DISEASES CAUSING A GENITAL DISCHARGE

Urethral discharge in males

Urethritis in males is either gonococcal, non-gonococcal or of mixed aetiology; the presence of gonococci is easily demonstrated by Gram stain. When the Gram stain is negative, the presence of >5 polymorphs per high-power field is accepted as evidence of non-gonococcal urethritis. In most developing countries, the majority of cases presenting to hospital are gonococcal. Up to 50% of cases of non-gonococcal urethritis are due to *Chlamydia trachomatis*; a proportion of the remaining cases are associated with *Mycoplasma genitalium*,[16-19] and a small percentage may harbour *Trichomonas vaginalis* or adenovirus.[20] According to the WHO syndromic management guidelines, men with urethral discharge should be treated for both gonorrhoea and chlamydial infection (this will also cover most cases of Ureaplasma and Mycoplasma infection). Cases in which it is possible to exclude gonorrhoea by microscopy of a Gram stain can be treated for chlamydial infection alone.

Gonorrhoea

Gonorrhoea is the most prevalent bacterial STI in the tropics. The causative organism, *Neisseria gonorrhoeae*, a Gram-negative oval diplococcus found only in man, is especially adept at colonizing the epithelial surfaces of the male and female urogenital tract, conjunctiva, pharynx, rectum and synovium.

Pathogenesis

Virulence is conferred by the presence of pili which mediate adherence, sufficient to withstand hydrodynamic forces within the urethra, and which also inhibit uptake by phagocytes. Invasion and multiplication have been demonstrated in mucus-secreting non-ciliated cells of the Fallopian tubes. No specific toxins produced by *N. gonorrhoeae* have been identified but the lipo-oligosaccharide and peptidoglycan components have been implicated in inhibition of ciliary function and the genesis of synovitis, respectively. *N. gonorrhoeae* is highly adept at avoiding the host immune response. The pilus antigens, the protein designated Por (formerly protein I, PI) and the lipo-oligosaccharide are all capable of antigenic variation sufficient to permit repeated reinfection of the same host within a short period. Antibodies to Rmp (formerly PIII) do not fix complement and can block bactericidal, complement-fixing antibodies to the lipo-oligosaccharide. The bacteria produce an IgA$_1$ protease which may impair the host mucosal immune response. The mucosal immune response to infection is characterized by the production of IgA, IgM and IgE, which can inhibit adherence and facilitate opsonization. These responses have been demonstrated in both infected and non-infected exposed contacts of infected individuals. Strains responsible for disseminated gonococcal infection have been shown to be less susceptible to killing by human serum, are less chemotactic to neutrophils and elicit greater amounts of blocking antibody.

Clinical features

The risk of contracting gonorrhoea after a single exposure is about 20% for males and probably higher for females. Typically men develop symptoms after a 2–5-day incubation period, with 90% of symptomatic infections manifesting within 14 days. Asymptomatic infections are frequent in women – up to 80% of infections are detected in contacts of symptomatic partners. Recent community-based studies from Tanzania have indicated much higher levels of asymptomatic gonorrhoea in males than previously recorded (about 85%).[21]

Symptomatic uncomplicated infections in males typically manifest as a thick, yellow urethral discharge. In females vaginal discharge or dysuria are the major symptoms. Accompanying symptoms include a variable degree of meatal itching, burning, dysuria, frequency and oedema. Infections of the pharynx and rectum (mostly asymptomatic) can result from orogenital and genitoanal sexual contact in males, but in females the rectum is easily infected by contamination from an infected vaginal discharge. Gonococcal infection may present as vulvovaginitis in children infected by sexual abuse or by infected fomites.

Complications in men

In males, spread of the infection to the epididymis, usually unilaterally, is the most common complication (20% of patients not receiving antibiotics). Acute epididymitis has initially to be distinguished from acute torsion. Because it is often difficult to establish an aetiological diagnosis, sexually active males should be given treatment that is effective for gonorrhoea and chlamydia. Some cases will be due to mumps virus infection, and in older men Gram-negative bacilli from the urinary tract may be responsible.

The older literature on gonorrhoea describes a number of complications seldom encountered in industrialized countries but which may still be seen in the tropics.[22] These include abscess and

Text continued on p. 417

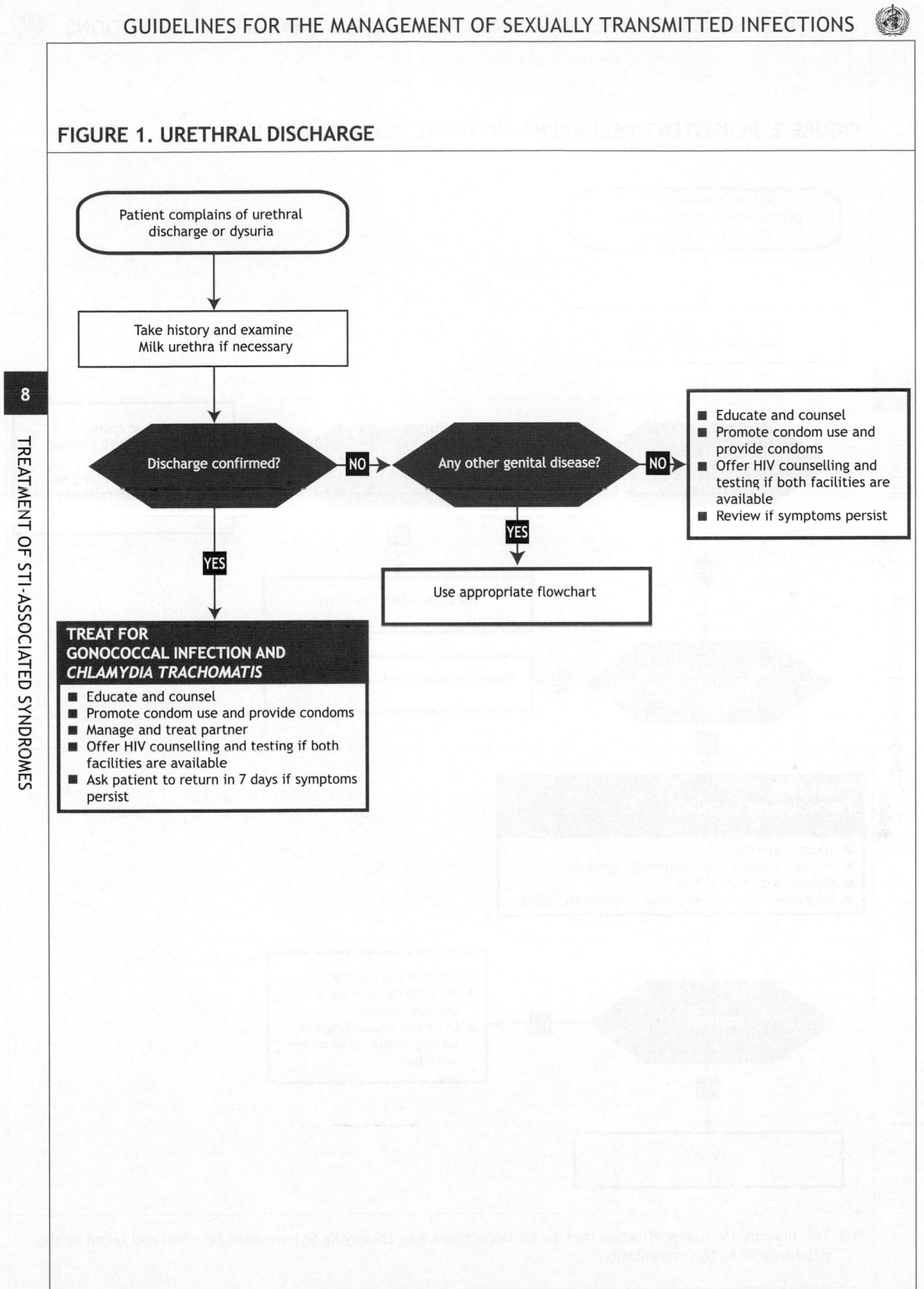

FIGURE 1. URETHRAL DISCHARGE

Patient complains of urethral
discharge or dysuria

Take history and examine
Milk urethra if necessary

8

TREATMENT OF STI-ASSOCIATED SYNDROMES

Discharge confirmed? —NO→ Any other genital disease? —NO→

- Educate and counsel
- Promote condom use and provide condoms
- Offer HIV counselling and testing if both facilities are available
- Review if symptoms persist

YES

YES

Use appropriate flowchart

**TREAT FOR
GONOCOCCAL INFECTION AND
*CHLAMYDIA TRACHOMATIS***

- Educate and counsel
- Promote condom use and provide condoms
- Manage and treat partner
- Offer HIV counselling and testing if both facilities are available
- Ask patient to return in 7 days if symptoms persist

Figure 21.1   WHO flow charts (1-1–1-9) for the management of common STI-associated syndromes (World Health Organization 2003).

GUIDELINES FOR THE MANAGEMENT OF SEXUALLY TRANSMITTED INFECTIONS

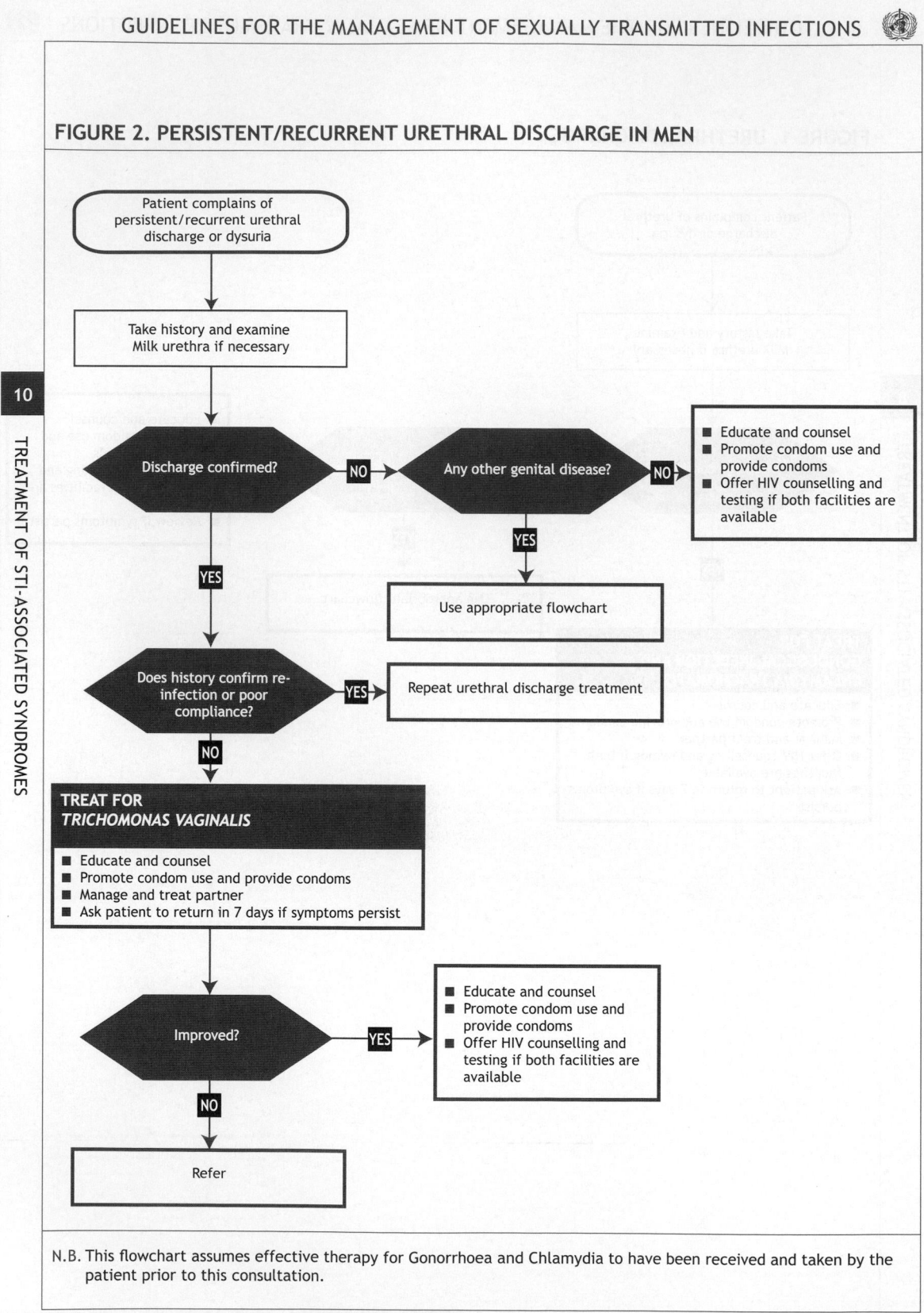

FIGURE 2. PERSISTENT/RECURRENT URETHRAL DISCHARGE IN MEN

10

TREATMENT OF STI-ASSOCIATED SYNDROMES

Patient complains of persistent/recurrent urethral discharge or dysuria

Take history and examine Milk urethra if necessary

Discharge confirmed? → NO → Any other genital disease? → NO →
- Educate and counsel
- Promote condom use and provide condoms
- Offer HIV counselling and testing if both facilities are available

YES (Any other genital disease?) → Use appropriate flowchart

YES (Discharge confirmed?)

Does history confirm re-infection or poor compliance? → YES → Repeat urethral discharge treatment

NO

TREAT FOR
TRICHOMONAS VAGINALIS

- Educate and counsel
- Promote condom use and provide condoms
- Manage and treat partner
- Ask patient to return in 7 days if symptoms persist

Improved? → YES →
- Educate and counsel
- Promote condom use and provide condoms
- Offer HIV counselling and testing if both facilities are available

NO

Refer

N.B. This flowchart assumes effective therapy for Gonorrhoea and Chlamydia to have been received and taken by the patient prior to this consultation.

Figure 21.1 Continued

GUIDELINES FOR THE MANAGEMENT OF SEXUALLY TRANSMITTED INFECTIONS

FIGURE 3. GENITAL ULCERS

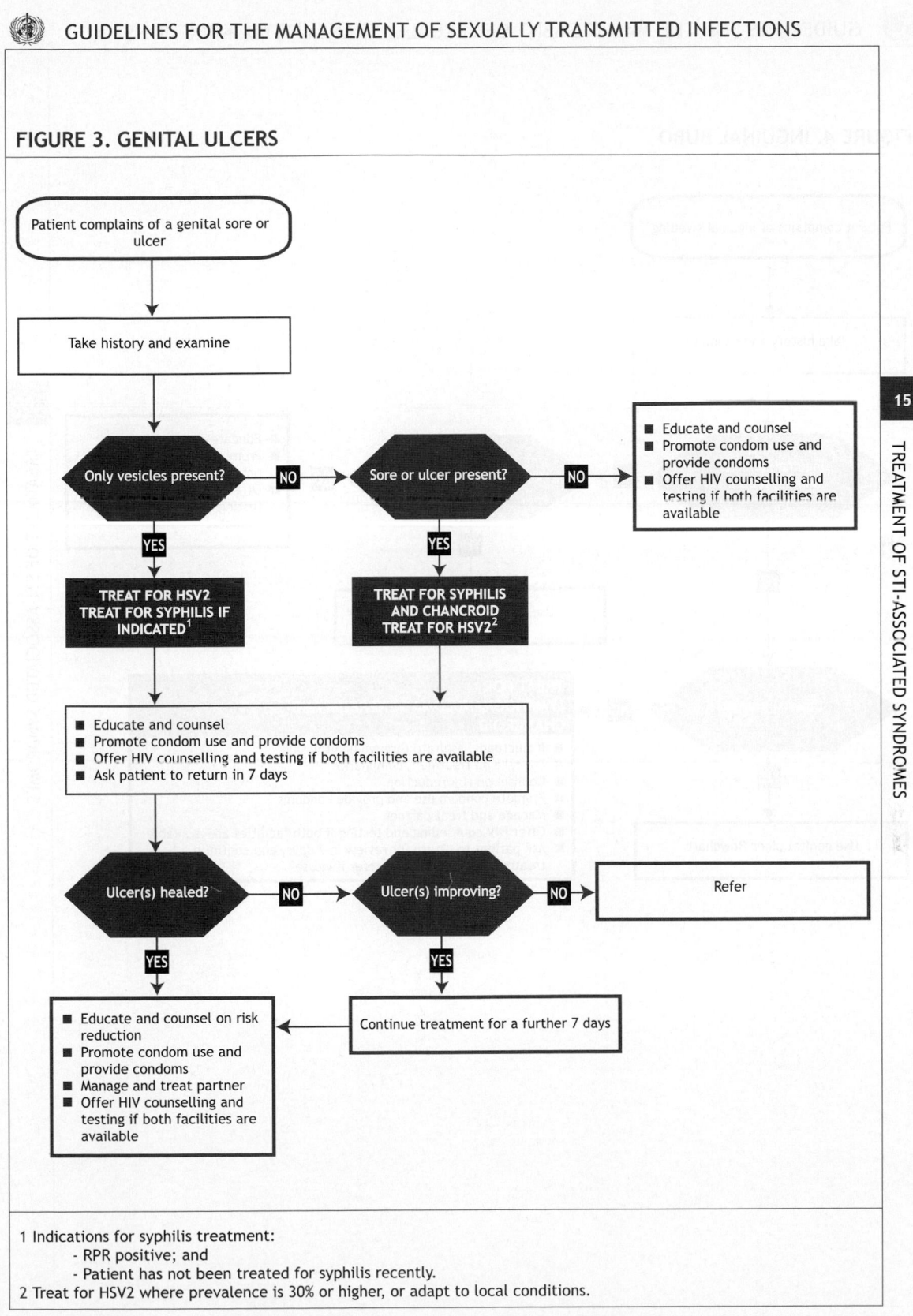

1 Indications for syphilis treatment:
 - RPR positive; and
 - Patient has not been treated for syphilis recently.
2 Treat for HSV2 where prevalence is 30% or higher, or adapt to local conditions.

Figure 21.1 Continued

15

TREATMENT OF STI-ASSOCIATED SYNDROMES

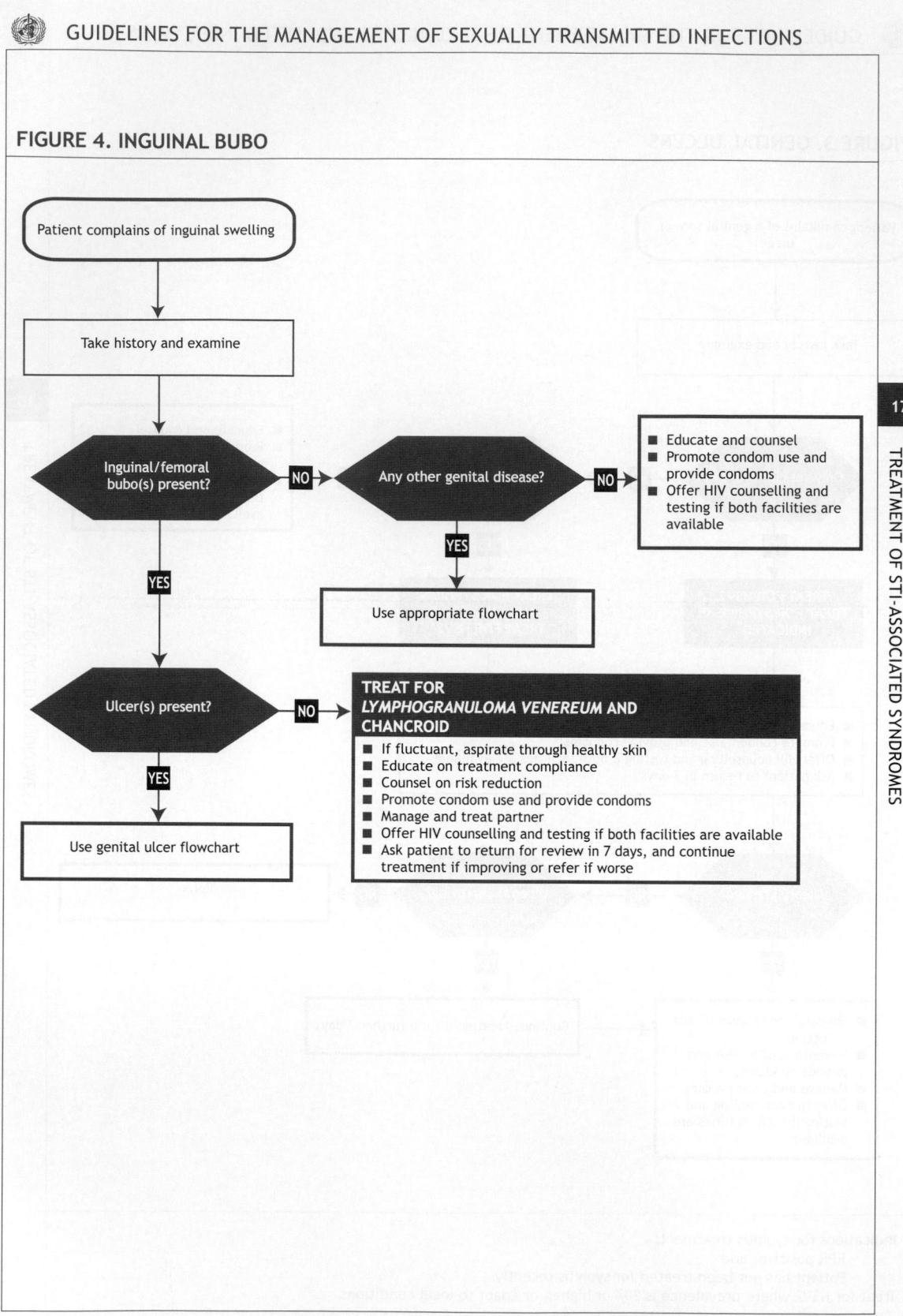

GUIDELINES FOR THE MANAGEMENT OF SEXUALLY TRANSMITTED INFECTIONS

FIGURE 4. INGUINAL BUBO

Patient complains of inguinal swelling

Take history and examine

Inguinal/femoral bubo(s) present?

NO → Any other genital disease? NO →
■ Educate and counsel
■ Promote condom use and provide condoms
■ Offer HIV counselling and testing if both facilities are available

YES ↓ (Any other genital disease?)

Use appropriate flowchart

YES (Inguinal/femoral bubo(s) present?) ↓

Ulcer(s) present? NO →

TREAT FOR
LYMPHOGRANULOMA VENEREUM AND CHANCROID
■ If fluctuant, aspirate through healthy skin
■ Educate on treatment compliance
■ Counsel on risk reduction
■ Promote condom use and provide condoms
■ Manage and treat partner
■ Offer HIV counselling and testing if both facilities are available
■ Ask patient to return for review in 7 days, and continue treatment if improving or refer if worse

YES ↓

Use genital ulcer flowchart

17

TREATMENT OF STI-ASSOCIATED SYNDROMES

Figure 21.1 Continued

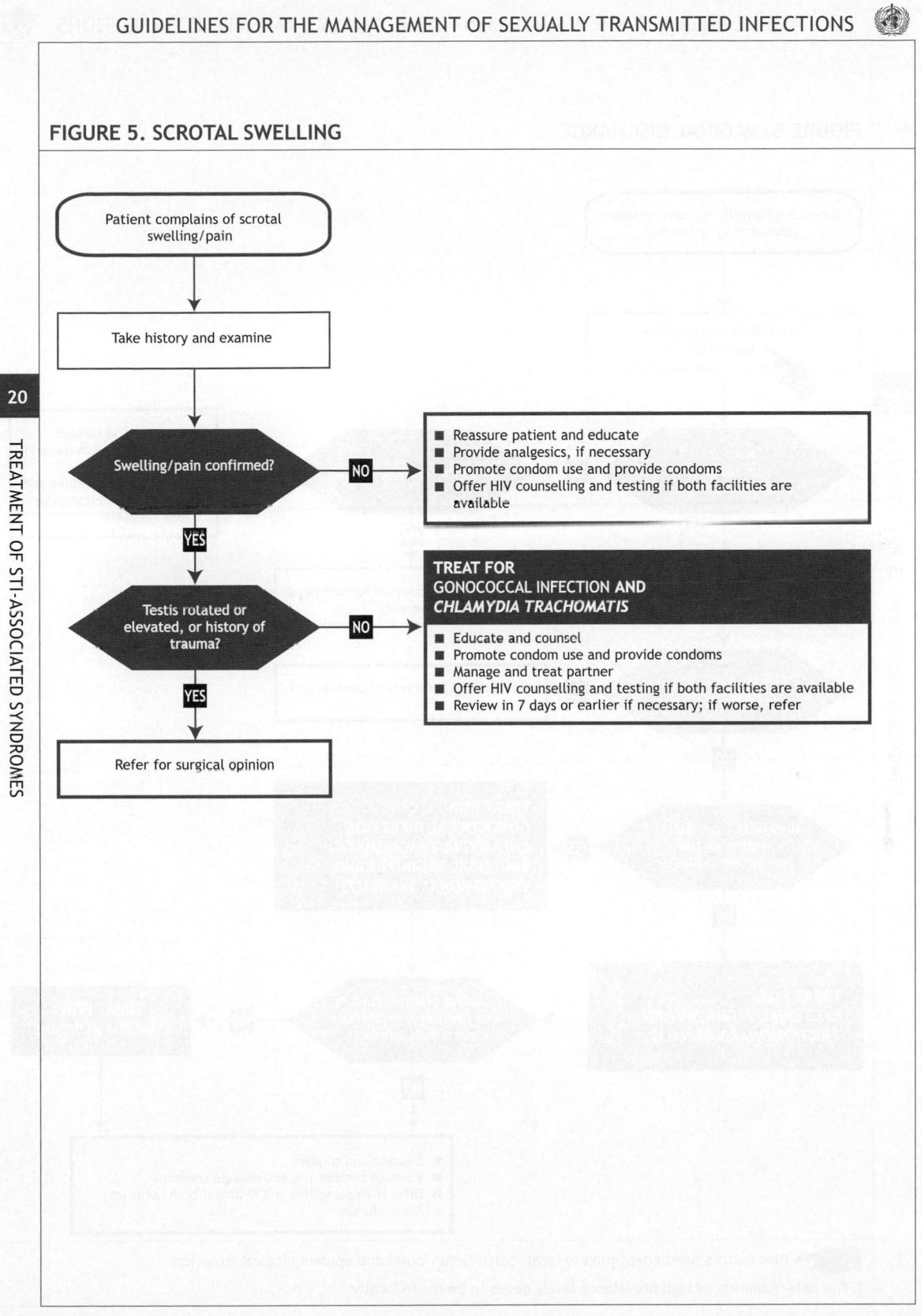

FIGURE 5. SCROTAL SWELLING

Patient complains of scrotal swelling/pain

Take history and examine

20

TREATMENT OF STI-ASSOCIATED SYNDROMES

Swelling/pain confirmed? — **NO** →

- Reassure patient and educate
- Provide analgesics, if necessary
- Promote condom use and provide condoms
- Offer HIV counselling and testing if both facilities are available

YES

Testis rotated or elevated, or history of trauma? — **NO** →

TREAT FOR GONOCOCCAL INFECTION AND *CHLAMYDIA TRACHOMATIS*

- Educate and counsel
- Promote condom use and provide condoms
- Manage and treat partner
- Offer HIV counselling and testing if both facilities are available
- Review in 7 days or earlier if necessary; if worse, refer

YES

Refer for surgical opinion

Figure 21.1 Continued

411

GUIDELINES FOR THE MANAGEMENT OF SEXUALLY TRANSMITTED INFECTIONS

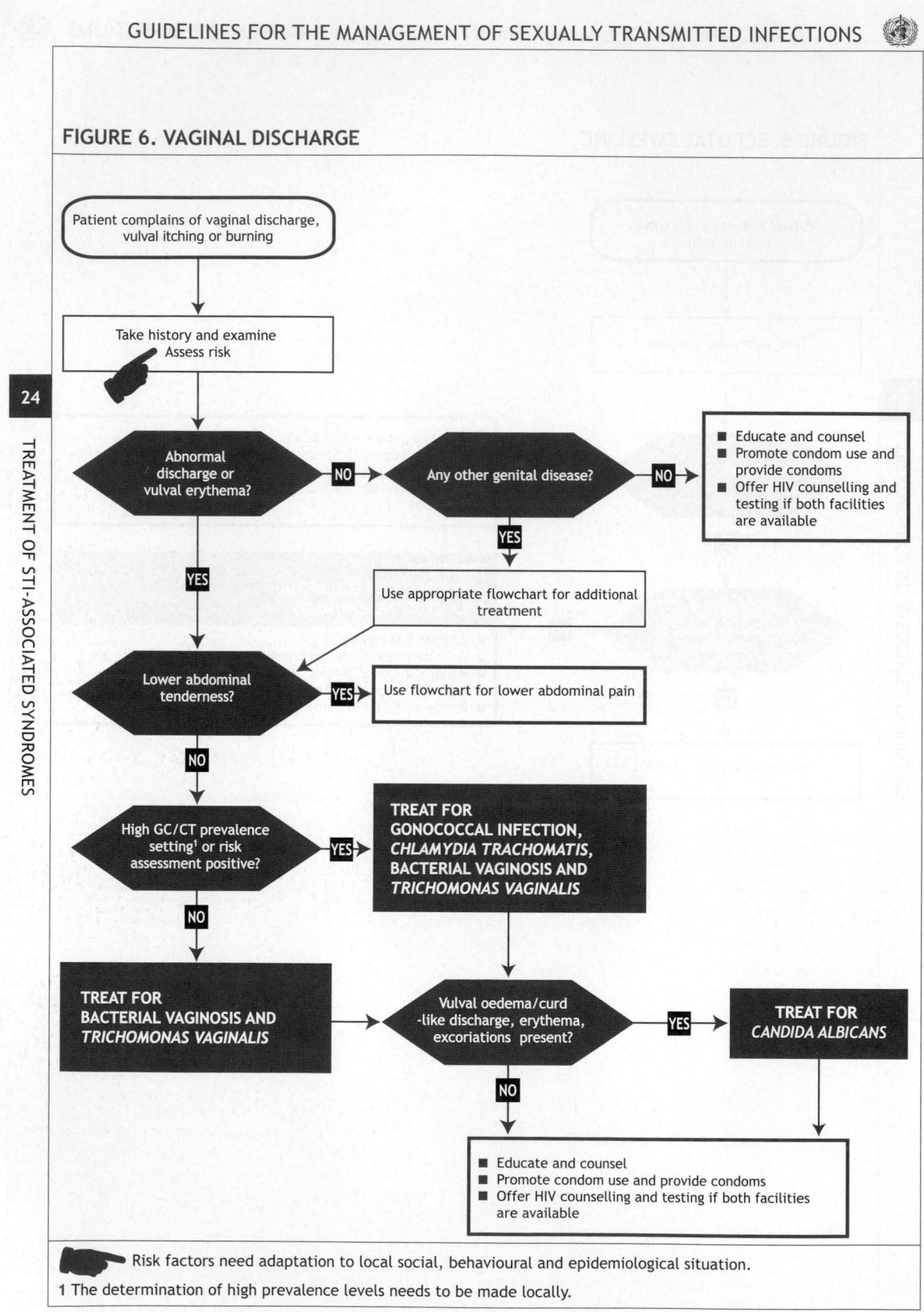

FIGURE 6. VAGINAL DISCHARGE

24

TREATMENT OF STI-ASSOCIATED SYNDROMES

Patient complains of vaginal discharge, vulval itching or burning

Take history and examine
Assess risk

Abnormal discharge or vulval erythema? — NO → Any other genital disease? — NO →
- Educate and counsel
- Promote condom use and provide condoms
- Offer HIV counselling and testing if both facilities are available

Any other genital disease? — YES → Use appropriate flowchart for additional treatment

Abnormal discharge or vulval erythema? — YES →

Lower abdominal tenderness? — YES → Use flowchart for lower abdominal pain

Lower abdominal tenderness? — NO →

High GC/CT prevalence setting[1] or risk assessment positive? — YES → **TREAT FOR GONOCOCCAL INFECTION, *CHLAMYDIA TRACHOMATIS*, BACTERIAL VAGINOSIS AND *TRICHOMONAS VAGINALIS***

High GC/CT prevalence setting[1] or risk assessment positive? — NO →

TREAT FOR BACTERIAL VAGINOSIS AND *TRICHOMONAS VAGINALIS* → Vulval oedema/curd-like discharge, erythema, excoriations present? — YES → **TREAT FOR *CANDIDA ALBICANS***

Vulval oedema/curd-like discharge, erythema, excoriations present? — NO →
- Educate and counsel
- Promote condom use and provide condoms
- Offer HIV counselling and testing if both facilities are available

Risk factors need adaptation to local social, behavioural and epidemiological situation.

1 The determination of high prevalence levels needs to be made locally.

Figure 21.1 Continued

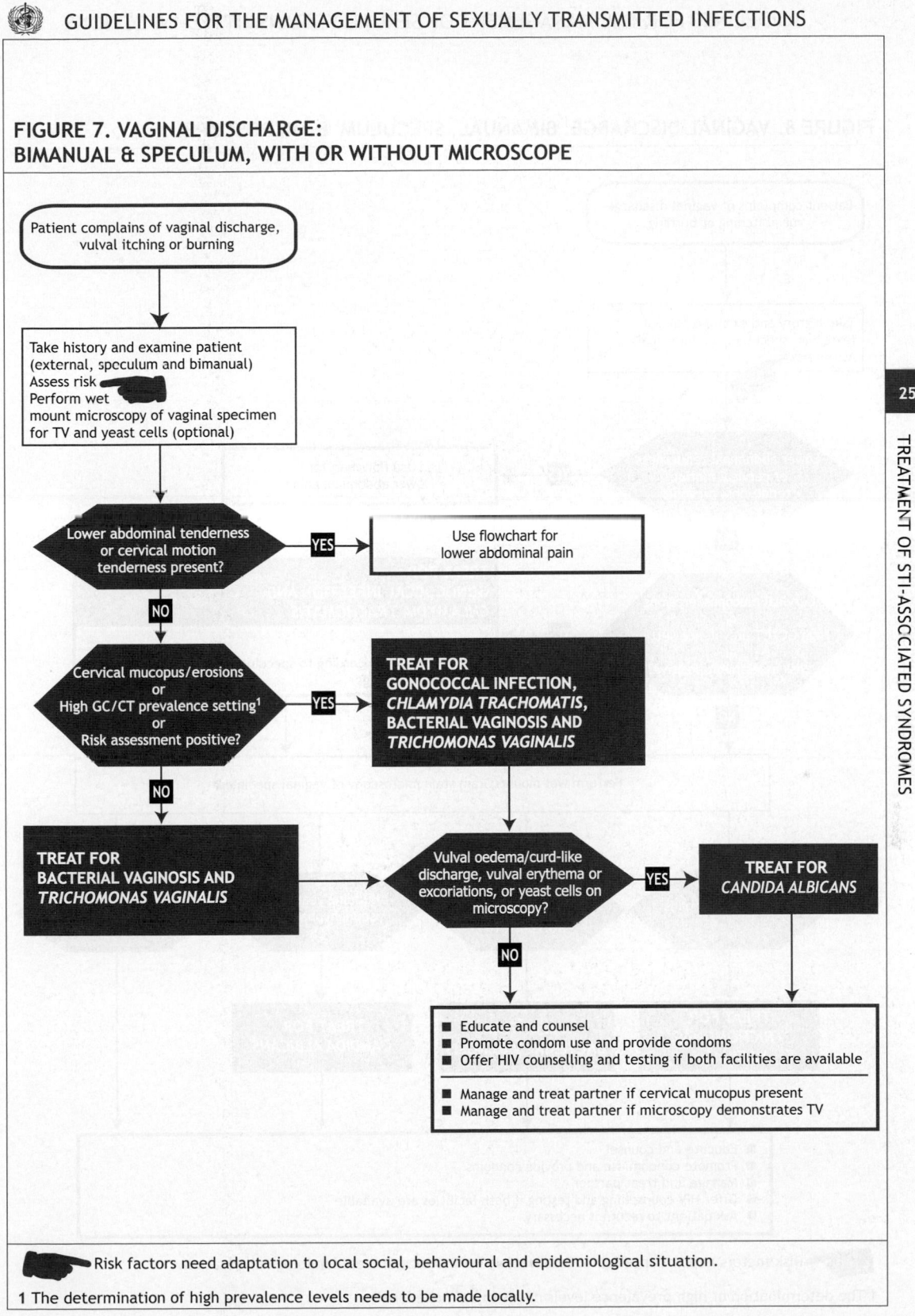

FIGURE 7. VAGINAL DISCHARGE:
BIMANUAL & SPECULUM, WITH OR WITHOUT MICROSCOPE

Patient complains of vaginal discharge, vulval itching or burning

Take history and examine patient (external, speculum and bimanual)
Assess risk
Perform wet mount microscopy of vaginal specimen for TV and yeast cells (optional)

Lower abdominal tenderness or cervical motion tenderness present? — **YES** → Use flowchart for lower abdominal pain

NO

Cervical mucopus/erosions
or
High GC/CT prevalence setting[1]
or
Risk assessment positive? — **YES** → TREAT FOR GONOCOCCAL INFECTION, *CHLAMYDIA TRACHOMATIS*, BACTERIAL VAGINOSIS AND *TRICHOMONAS VAGINALIS*

NO

TREAT FOR BACTERIAL VAGINOSIS AND *TRICHOMONAS VAGINALIS* → Vulval oedema/curd-like discharge, vulval erythema or excoriations, or yeast cells on microscopy? — **YES** → TREAT FOR *CANDIDA ALBICANS*

NO

- Educate and counsel
- Promote condom use and provide condoms
- Offer HIV counselling and testing if both facilities are available

- Manage and treat partner if cervical mucopus present
- Manage and treat partner if microscopy demonstrates TV

Risk factors need adaptation to local social, behavioural and epidemiological situation.

1 The determination of high prevalence levels needs to be made locally.

25

TREATMENT OF STI-ASSOCIATED SYNDROMES

Figure 21.1 Continued

GUIDELINES FOR THE MANAGEMENT OF SEXUALLY TRANSMITTED INFECTIONS

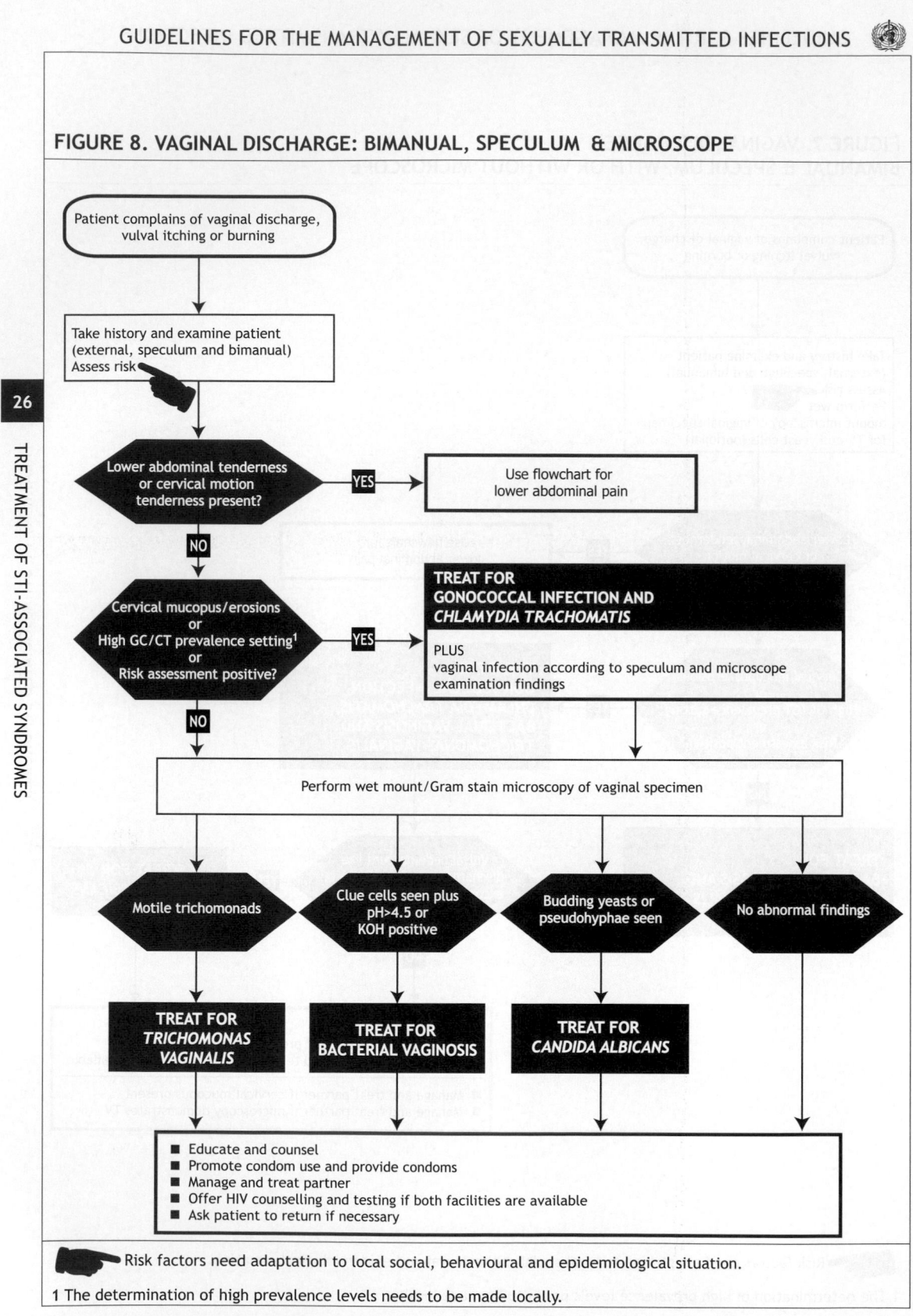

FIGURE 8. VAGINAL DISCHARGE: BIMANUAL, SPECULUM & MICROSCOPE

26

TREATMENT OF STI-ASSOCIATED SYNDROMES

Patient complains of vaginal discharge, vulval itching or burning

Take history and examine patient (external, speculum and bimanual) Assess risk

Lower abdominal tenderness or cervical motion tenderness present? — **YES** → Use flowchart for lower abdominal pain

NO

Cervical mucopus/erosions or High GC/CT prevalence setting[1] or Risk assessment positive? — **YES** → **TREAT FOR GONOCOCCAL INFECTION AND CHLAMYDIA TRACHOMATIS**

PLUS vaginal infection according to speculum and microscope examination findings

NO

Perform wet mount/Gram stain microscopy of vaginal specimen

Motile trichomonads → **TREAT FOR TRICHOMONAS VAGINALIS**

Clue cells seen plus pH>4.5 or KOH positive → **TREAT FOR BACTERIAL VAGINOSIS**

Budding yeasts or pseudohyphae seen → **TREAT FOR CANDIDA ALBICANS**

No abnormal findings

- Educate and counsel
- Promote condom use and provide condoms
- Manage and treat partner
- Offer HIV counselling and testing if both facilities are available
- Ask patient to return if necessary

Risk factors need adaptation to local social, behavioural and epidemiological situation.

1 The determination of high prevalence levels needs to be made locally.

Figure 21.1 Continued

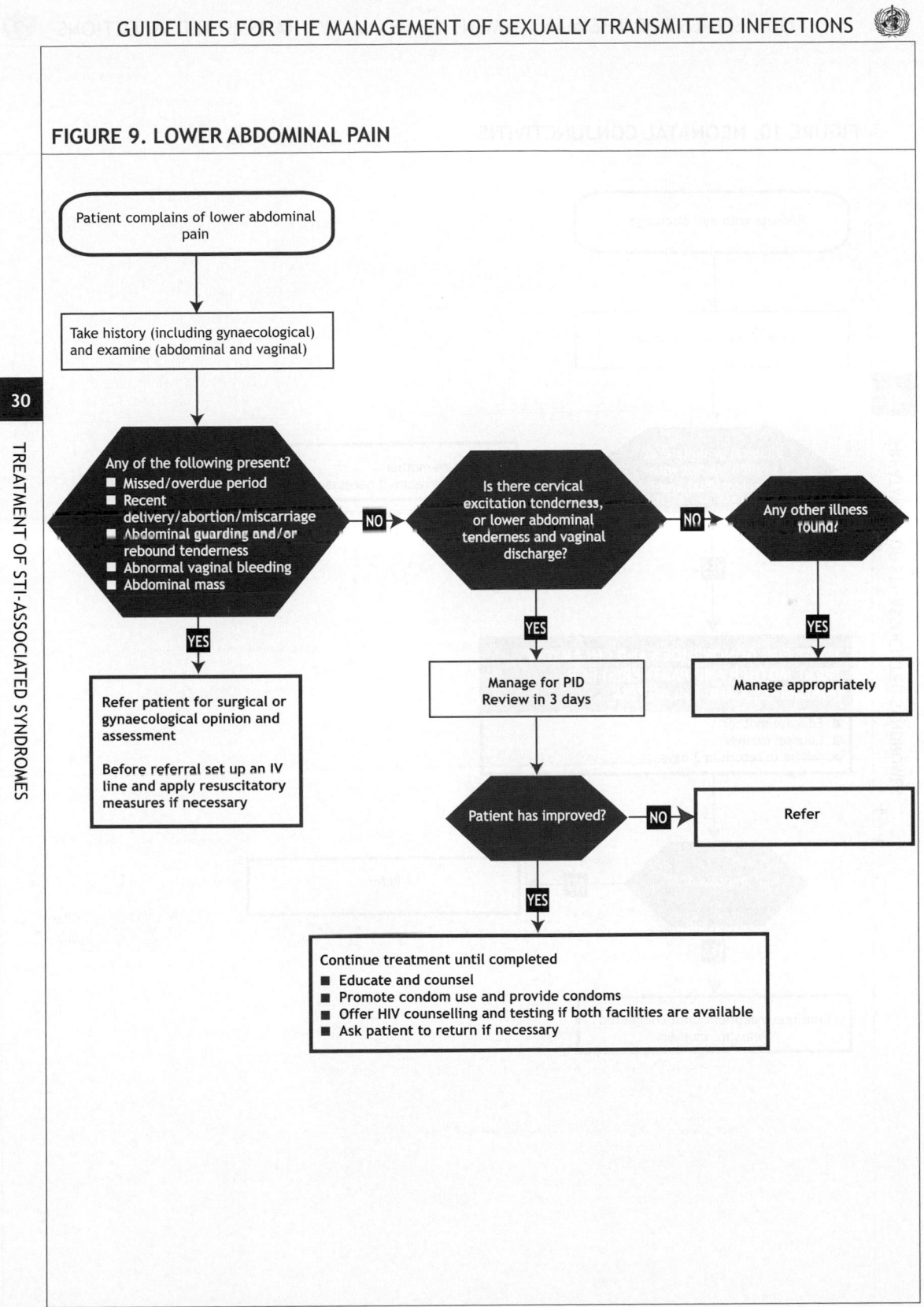

30

TREATMENT OF STI-ASSOCIATED SYNDROMES

FIGURE 9. LOWER ABDOMINAL PAIN

Figure 21.1 Continued

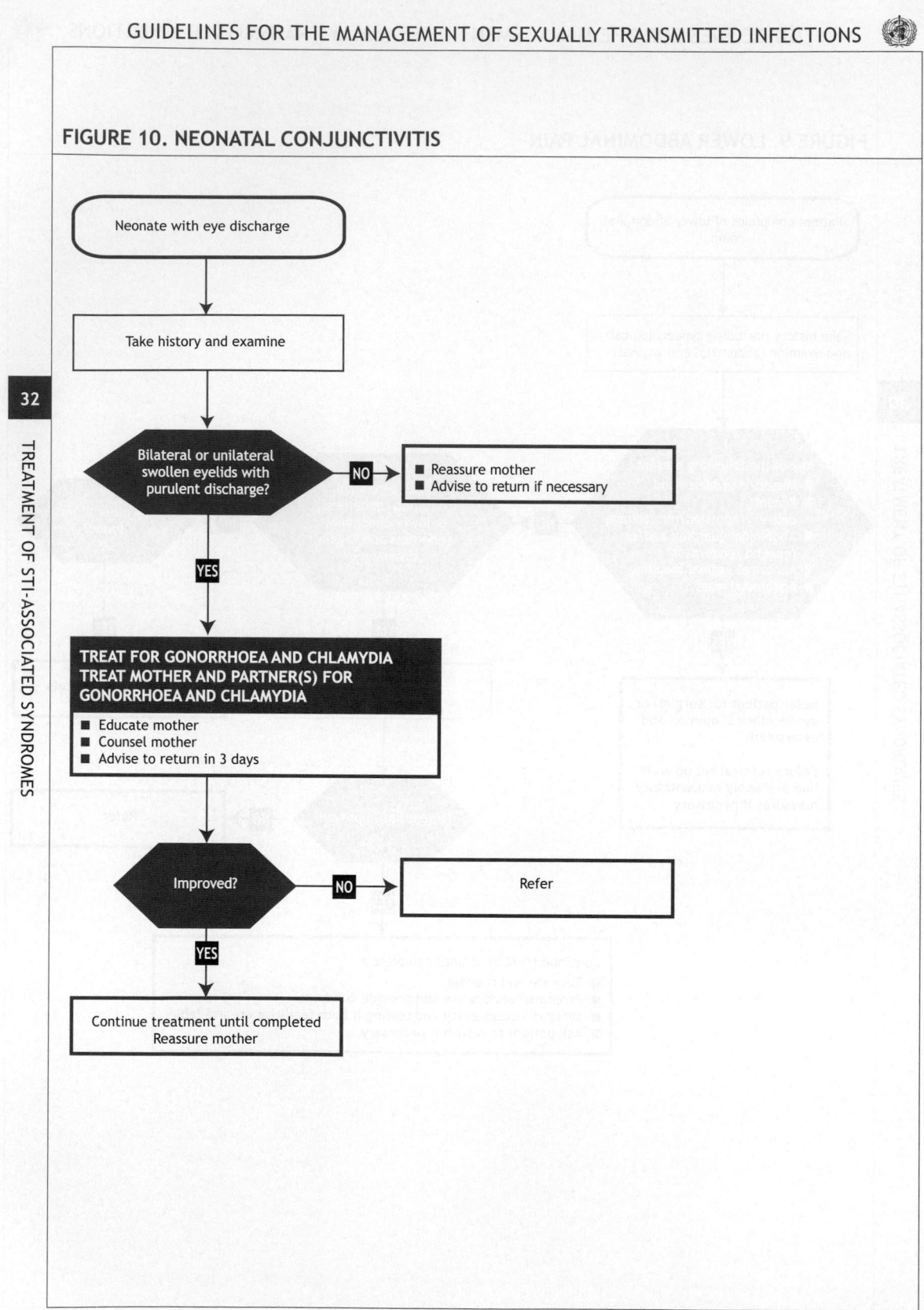

FIGURE 10. NEONATAL CONJUNCTIVITIS

Figure 21.1 Continued

fistula formation resulting from spread of infection to various glands associated with the genitourinary tract (prostate, glands of Tyson, Littré, Cowper). Ultimately, these may lead to urethral stricture, a difficult complication to manage, which appears to show marked geographical variation in the tropics.[23,24]

Complications in women

In women, common local complications are infections of the paraurethral (Skene's) glands and Bartholin's glands (Figure 21.2). Much more serious complications may ensue when infection spreads into the uterus and Fallopian tubes. Abortion, delivery and insertion of intrauterine devices are risk factors for ascending infection. Unusual uterine bleeding in sexually active women should prompt consideration of a possible gonococcal endometritis. Further spread may lead to acute complications such as acute salpingitis and abscess formation or long-term problems of chronic PID, and increased risk of ectopic pregnancy (increased 10-fold after one episode of salpingitis). Acute salpingitis has to be differentiated clinically from ectopic pregnancy (pregnancy test, ultrasonography) and acute appendicitis (laparoscopy).

Sterility may complicate both overt and silent infection in either sex. In a study from central Africa Fallopian tube occlusion was present in 83% of infertile women.[25] Acute salpingitis has been estimated to produce sterility in 17% of patients, the risk rising with multiple episodes of infection, in older patients and with more severe inflammation. Gonorrhoea in pregnancy has been associated with low birth weight,[26] premature rupture of membranes, chorioamnionitis and postpartum upper genital tract infection.[27] There is also a higher risk of disseminated gonococcal infection.

Disseminated infection

Disseminated gonococcal infection may arise in about 2% of patients with gonorrhoea. The local infection from which it originates is often asymptomatic. It manifests most often as an asymmetric oligoarthritis with a predilection for knees, ankles, and large and small joints of the upper limb. Tenosynovitis occurs frequently. The skin lesions (classically the tender necrotic pustule, but many other forms also occur) often noted in white skins are rare in dark-skinned patients. Gonococcal arthritis accounts for as much as 20% of acute arthritis in young adults in the tropics.[28] It has to be differentiated from other septic arthritides, and in particular from reactive arthritis, which is also often sexually acquired. Rarer manifestations of disseminated gonococcal infection include endocarditis and meningitis. Disseminated infections can no longer be expected to respond to penicillin as in the past. Treatment effective against penicillinase-producing strains is required. A total of 7 days therapy is recommended.

Ocular gonococcal infections

Ocular gonococcal infection in adults, which is presumed to follow autoinoculation with a contaminated finger in most cases, is a common and potentially blinding complication in developing countries.[29] It presents as an acute purulent conjunctivitis which may progress rapidly to corneal perforation in the absence of adequate systemic and topical antimicrobial treatment.

Ophthalmia neonatorum

Ophthalmia neonatorum is defined as an acute conjunctivitis occurring in the first month of life. The high prevalence of infection with N. gonorrhoeae and C. trachomatis among pregnant women in many tropical countries is reflected in a correspondingly high incidence of ophthalmia neonatorum, which occurs in 30–50% of children born to infected mothers if prophylaxis is not administered.

Ophthalmia neonatorum usually presents as an acute bilateral purulent conjunctivitis (Figure 21.3). Gonococcal infections frequently present in the first week and can lead to blindness. The diagnosis can often be made by microscopy (Gram stain for gon-

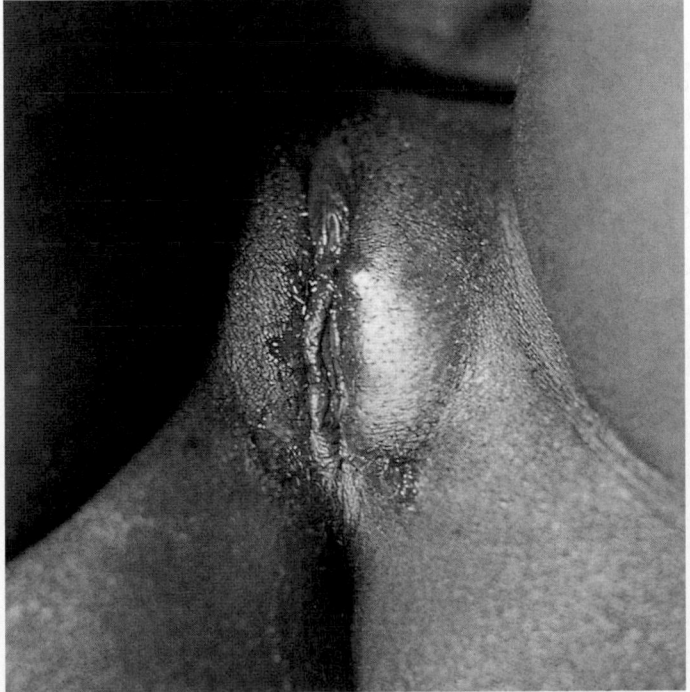

Figure 21.2 Acute bartholinitis due to gonorrhoea (Courtesy of D. Mabey).

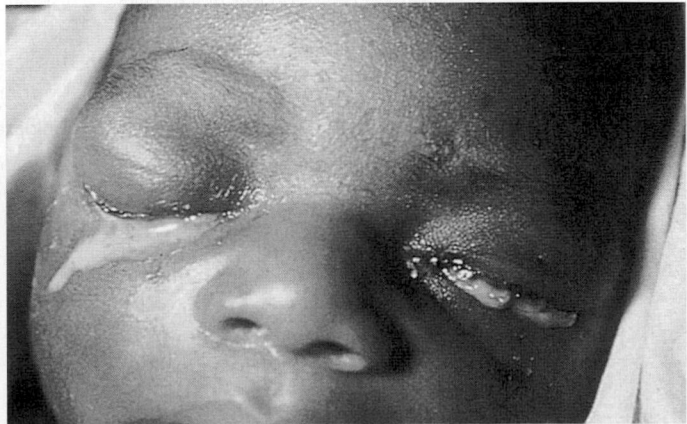

Figure 21.3 Gonococcal ophthalmia in a 7-day-old neonate (Courtesy of D. Mabey).

Table 21.4 Recommended treatment for STIs*

Disease	First-line antibiotics	Alternative antibiotics	Notes
Gonorrhoea	Cefixime 400 mg × 1 Ceftriaxone 125 mg or 250 mg injection × 1 Spectinomycin 2 g injection × 1	Ciprofloxacin 500 mg × 1 Ofloxacin 400 mg × 1	Resistance to penicillin, tetracyclines and quinolones is now widespread. Presumptive treatment for chlamydia co-infection is recommended. Disseminated infections require daily treatment for 1 week.
Gonococcal ophthalmia	Ceftriaxone 50 mg/kg injection × 1	Spectinomycin 25 mg/kg × 1 or kanamycin 25 mg/kg × 1	Special precautions need to be taken to avoid nosocomial spread of infection.
Chlamydia	Doxycycline 100 mg twice daily for 1 week Azithromycin 1 g × 1	Erythromycin 500 mg twice daily for 10–14 days Ofloxacin 200 mg or 400 mg daily for 7 days	Amoxicillin has been validated for use in pregnant women. Azithromycin is recommended for pregnant women by WHO but is not yet licensed for this use in the UK.
Chlamydial ophthalmia	Erythromycin syrup 50 mg/kg per day divided in 4 doses for 14 days		
Early syphilis	Benzathine penicillin 2.4 mU injection × 1 Azithromycin 2 g × 1	Doxycycline 100 mg twice daily for 14 days Tetracycline Erythromycin Ceftriaxone Procaine penicillin Erythromycin	Strains of *T. pallidum* with resistance to azithromycin have been reported in some parts of the world. Extended courses of penicillin are needed for late or complicated syphilis. Doses of benzathine are usually given half into each buttock.
Early congenital syphilis	Aqueous Benzylpenicillin 50 000 IU/kg 12-hourly i.v. for 7 days then 50 000 IU/kg 8-hourly i.v. for a further 3 days		
Chancroid	Ciprofloxacin 500 mg twice daily for 3 days Ceftriaxone 250 mg injection × 1 Azithromycin 1 g × 1	Erythromycin 500 mg 3–4 times daily for 7 days	Fluctuant inguinal buboes may require needle aspiration or incision and drainage.
Lymphogranuloma venereum	Doxycycline 100 mg twice daily for 21 days Azithromycin 1 g weekly for 3 doses	Erythromycin 500 mg 4 times daily for 21 days Tetracycline or minocycline	
Donovanosis	Azithromycin 1 g, then 500 mg daily or 1 g weekly Doxycycline 100 mg twice daily	Erythromycin 500 mg twice daily Ciprofloxacin 750 mg twice daily Tetracycline Co-trimoxazole	Treatment should be continued until lesions have re-epithelialized.
Trichomoniasis	Metronidazole 2 g × 1	Tinidazole 2 g × 1	
Bacterial vaginosis	Metronidazole 2 g × 1 or 4–500 mg twice daily for 5–7 days	Clindamycin 2% cream 5 g daily for 7 days	Treatment of sexual partners is not indicated.
Candidiasis	Clotrimazole 500 mg × 1 Fluconazole 150 mg × 1 Miconazole or clotrimazole 200 mg daily for 3 days	Nystatin	Treatment of sexual partners is not indicated.

Table 21.4 Continued

Disease	First-line antibiotics	Alternative antibiotics	Notes
Genital herpes (first episode)	Aciclovir 200 mg five times daily for 5–10 days	Famciclovir 250 mg three times daily for 7 days Valaciclovir 1 g twice daily for 7 days	Topical therapy is less effective than the oral route. Aciclovir treatment is less useful during recurrent episodes. If used, it needs to be started <24 h after the onset of lesions.
Genital herpes (suppression)	Aciclovir 400 mg twice daily	Valaciclovir 0.5–1 g daily Famciclovir 250 mg twice times daily	
Genital warts (self-treatment)	Podophyllotoxin Imiquimod 5% cream		
Genital warts (provider treatment)	10--25% podophyllin Cryotherapy with liquid nitrogen	80–90% trichloroacetic acid Surgical excision or electrosurgery	
Non-gonococcal urethritis	Doxycycline 100 mg twice a day for 7 days Azithromycin 1 g × 1	Erythromycin 500 mg twice daily for 14 days Ofloxacin 400 mg daily for 7 days	Treatment with metronidazole 2 g or azithromycin 1 g can be used in patients not responding to their first treatment.
Pelvic inflammatory disease	Treatment for gonorrhoea + doxycycline 100 mg twice daily + metronidazole 400 mg twice daily for 2 weeks	Clindamycin 900 mg i.v. 8-hourly + gentamicin 1.5 mg/kg i.v. 8-hourly	Treatment for gonorrhoea may be omitted in low prevalence settings where a culture has been taken. Intravenous treatment is indicated for more severe cases and is continued for 3 days after improvement and then followed with oral doxycycline for 14 days.
Epididymitis	Treatment for gonorrhoea + treatment for chlamydia	Ciprofloxacin 500 mg twice daily for 10 days Ofloxacin 200 mg twice daily for 7–14 days	Above the age of 40 epididymitis is less likely to be caused by STIs and treatment for other pathogens such as *E. coli* with ciprofloxacin or ofloxacin may be indicated. Severe cases may require intravenous antibiotics.
Genital scabies	Permethrin 5% Malathion 0.5%	Benzyl benzoate 25% Ivermectin 200 µg/kg repeated after 2 weeks	Ivermectin has proved useful in treatment of patients with crusted scabies.
Pediculosis	Malathion 0.5% Permethrin 1% Phenothrin 0.2%		If the eyelashes are involved a 10 min application of permethrin 1% lotion with the eyes closed can be used.

These recommendations are drawn from STI Treatment Guidelines published by the World Health Organization, Centers for Disease Control and the British Association for Sexual Health and HIV.

orrhoea, Giemsa stain for chlamydial inclusions). Cultures should be made when possible. Systemic and topical treatment (Table 21.4) should be administered to the neonate, and the mother and her sexual partner(s) should also be treated.

The use of ocular prophylaxis in countries where the prevalence of gonorrhoea in antenatal women exceeds 1% is highly cost-effective. A trial in Kenya showed that the instillation of 1% silver nitrate or 1% tetracycline ointment into the eyes of infants at delivery was equally effective in preventing gonococcal ophthalmia neonatorum,[30] but since it was conducted the prevalence of tetracycline-resistant strains of *N. gonorrhoeae* has increased greatly in developing countries; in some studies, 90% or more of strains were found to be resistant.[31] A later trial suggested that 2.5% povidone-iodine was as effective as 1% silver nitrate in preventing chlamydial and gonococcal ophthalmia.[32]

Laboratory diagnosis

The definitive diagnosis of gonorrhoea rests on the isolation of *N. gonorrhoeae*. In many health facilities in the tropics, this is not feasible. The demonstration of Gram-negative diplococci in urethral smears (Figure 21.4) has a sensitivity and specificity of >95% for the diagnosis of gonorrhoea in males, but both sensitivity and specificity are considerably lower in females, where culture is the method of choice. In disseminated infection specimens from joints, blood or skin lesions give a rather poor yield and the organism may be isolated more readily from the genital tract.

When cultures are to be made, the sites for swabbing should be determined by the history and examination findings. In males, it is best to obtain a urethral specimen by insertion and rotation

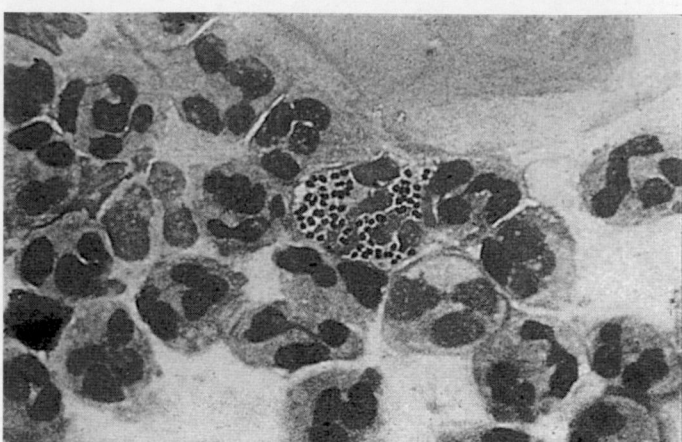

Figure 21.4 Appearance of *Neisseria gonorrhoeae* in a Gram-stained smear of urethral discharge.

of a swab in the urethra for 5 s. For women, the ectocervix should be wiped clean and a swab should be inserted into the cervical os and rotated for 10 s. Rectal swabs are best obtained through a proctoscope. *N. gonorrhoeae* is a delicate organism, highly susceptible to drying, and prompt inoculation of media and careful adherence to recommended laboratory technique is important to maximize isolation rates. Of newer reported methods for the diagnosis of gonorrhoea (e.g. antigen detection by immuno-fluorescence or enzyme immunoassay, serology, detection of gonococcal DNA), none has so far been shown to be superior to traditional methods.[33]

Treatment

Gonorrhoea is treated ideally with a single dose of supervised oral treatment (Table 21.4). The dose administered should give a serum level of at least three times the minimum inhibitory concentration for ≥8 h. Throughout the tropics an increasing proportion of isolates of *N. gonorrhoeae* show both plasmid- and chromosomally-mediated resistance to penicillin and other cheap antibiotics such as tetracycline and co-trimoxazole.[31] Penicillinase-producing *N. gonorrhoeae* (PPNG) accounts for more than 50% of isolates in many tropical countries. WHO recommendations for the treatment of uncomplicated gonorrhoea are shown in Table 21.4.[14] The value of the traditional test of cure has been questioned and is now rarely needed when evidence-based treatment and gonococcal strain surveillance are in place.

Treatment of contacts should extend to all individuals exposed within 2 weeks of the onset of symptoms in the index case and within 4 weeks of diagnosis of asymptomatic infected individuals. The issue of whether to give blind treatment for chlamydial infection to all patients with gonorrhoea is controversial but certainly worth serious consideration. This practice has been officially recommended in some developed countries.[34]

Prevention

The major obstacle to the control of gonorrhoea is the large reservoir of asymptomatic or clinically non-specific infections in women and the difficulty of establishing the diagnosis in women.

The greatly increased cost of effective treatment for PPNG is an added burden for tropical countries. Given these constraints it is more appropriate to direct resources to condom promotion and other safe sex messages than to costly strategies to increase case-finding and treatment. The development of vaccines for gonorrhoea has been hindered by the antigenic variation manifest by the organism.

Chlamydial infections

The demonstration in 1909 of chlamydial inclusions in cervical scrapings from the mother of an infant with inclusion conjunctivitis and in urethral scrapings from her male partner laid the basis for our understanding of genital chlamydial infections, but it was not until it became possible to isolate *C. trachomatis* in tissue culture in 1965 that the extent of the morbidity due to this organism became clear.

Epidemiology

C. trachomatis is the most prevalent sexually transmitted bacterial pathogen in industrialized countries,[35] and appears to be at least equally prevalent in developing countries (Table 21.1). Studies in industrialized countries have shown that genital chlamydial infection is more prevalent in younger age groups, even after taking account of differences in sexual activity, implying that some degree of protective immunity may develop after natural infection.

Aetiology

C. trachomatis is a Gram-negative bacterium which is an obligate parasite of eukaryotic cells. The genus *Chlamydia* has a unique life cycle. The metabolically inert infectious elementary body has a rigid cell wall and is adapted for extracellular survival. It appears to infect preferentially columnar epithelial cells, by which it is actively taken up. After entering the host cell it differentiates over a number of hours to the metabolically active reticulate body, which divides by binary fission until an intracellular inclusion is formed, which may contain several thousand organisms. The life cycle is completed when reticulate bodies condense to form elementary bodies, which are released from the inclusion after lysis of the host cell.

A number of serotypes of *C. trachomatis* have been identified by the microimmunofluorescence test of Wang and Grayston.[36] Serotypes A–C cause ocular infection in trachoma endemic areas, whereas serotypes D–K cause genital tract infections worldwide. Serotypes L1, L2 and L3 are more invasive both in vitro and in vivo, and cause lymphogranuloma venereum (LGV).

Pathology

The pathological hallmarks of infection with *C. trachomatis* are: (1) the subepithelial lymphoid follicle; and (2) fibrosis and scarring. The latter may progress for months and years even in the absence of chlamydial organisms demonstrable by conventional means. The host immune system is believed to play an important part in the pathogenesis of chlamydial infections, and a chlamydial heat shock protein of 57 kDa, which has been shown to elicit a delayed hypersensitivity reaction in previously infected animals may also be a determinant of immunopathology in humans.[37]

Clinical features

The clinical spectrum of disease due to chlamydial infection is similar to that seen in gonococcal infection. Although, in general, chlamydial infections are less likely than gonococcal to cause severe symptoms, they are more likely to cause serious sequelae, particularly in women.[38]

In males, chlamydial infection causes urethritis and, in a proportion of cases, epididymo-orchitis. It is possible that urethral stricture is a late sequela of chlamydial urethritis.

In females, chlamydial cervicitis is often asymptomatic. Sometimes patients will complain of vaginal discharge, and the finding of a mucopurulent discharge at the cervical os is suggestive of chlamydial or gonococcal cervicitis. Ascending infection of the female genital tract may lead to endometritis, salpingitis or PID and this is facilitated by trauma to the cervix, for example during childbirth, insertion of an intrauterine device or termination of pregnancy. Because the symptoms of chlamydial PID are often mild, patients may present only when the sequelae of irreversible damage to the Fallopian tubes (infertility, ectopic pregnancy) become apparent. Infection may track to the right upper quadrant, giving rise to a perihepatitis with characteristic adhesions between the liver capsule and peritoneum (Curtis–FitzHugh syndrome).

In both sexes, a sexually acquired reactive arthritis has been described as a sequel of chlamydial infection. This may involve both large and small joints and be accompanied by enthesitis and skin lesions (circinate balanitis and keratodermia blennorrhagica).

Some 30% of infants born to infected mothers become infected. In the majority of cases the only consequence of this is a self-limiting conjunctivitis presenting within the first 2 weeks of life, but occasionally chlamydial ophthalmia is more severe and if it persists it may give rise to conjunctival scarring. A small proportion of infected infants develop chlamydial pneumonitis, presenting usually between the ages of 6 weeks and 3 months with a paroxysmal cough and tachypnoea in the absence of fever. Rales may be heard on clinical examination, and a chest radiograph often reveals extensive bilateral pulmonary infiltrates with hyperinflation. There is characteristically a raised serum total IgG and IgM, and a mild eosinophilia.[39]

Diagnosis

Nucleic acid amplification tests (NAATS), such as the polymerase chain reaction (PCR) are now the gold standard for the diagnosis of genital chlamydial infection. Several are on the market, but they are expensive, and require expensive equipment as well as careful laboratory practice. NAATS are more sensitive than antigen detection tests or isolation, the sensitivity of which is only approximately 70%.[40] This means that the type of specimen taken is less critical. Whereas for culture and antigen detection it was essential to collect intra-urethral or endocervical samples, NAATS give good results in first-catch urine samples or self-administered vaginal swabs.

Serology has no place in the diagnosis of uncomplicated chlamydial infections, with the exception of the more invasive LGV, but may be helpful in the diagnosis of suspected PID and is the method of choice for the diagnosis of neonatal chlamydial pneumonia. It is only possible to distinguish between antibodies to the various species of Chlamydia by the micro-immunofluorescence test, which is subjective and labour intensive. Other serological tests may give positive results due to infection with the highly prevalent respiratory tract pathogen, Chlamydia pneumoniae.

Management

C. trachomatis remains sensitive to tetracyclines and macrolides, and single-dose treatment with azithromycin is effective in uncomplicated chlamydial infection (Table 21.4).[41]

Vaginal discharge

The three most prevalent causes of vaginal discharge are Candida albicans, Trichomonas vaginalis and bacterial vaginosis. Neisseria gonorrhoeae and Chlamydia trachomatis, which infect the endocervix rather than the vagina, are less commonly associated with symptomatic discharge. Unfortunately, it is not possible to distinguish reliably between these infections on clinical grounds, although the presence of mucopurulent discharge at the cervical os has been proposed as a marker of gonococcal or chlamydial infection. A wet preparation made from a swab collected from the posterior fornix, examined with a phase-contrast microscope, can usually distinguish between candidiasis, trichomoniasis and bacterial vaginosis. Sexual transmission is not considered important in vulvovaginal candidiasis and bacterial vaginosis, and treatment of sexual partners of affected women has not been shown help women who develop repeated episodes of these infections.

Vulvovaginal candidiasis

Candida albicans can be isolated from the vagina of up to 50% of sexually active women, the majority of whom are asymptomatic. Although sexual transmission may occur, the gastrointestinal tract has also been implicated as a source of infection. Symptomatic disease is associated with an increase in the number of yeasts present in the vagina; factors which predispose to this are pregnancy, antimicrobial therapy, oral contraceptive use, immunosuppression (e.g. HIV-related) and glycosuria. It has also been suggested that tight, poorly ventilated nylon underclothing, by increasing perineal moisture, may predispose to symptomatic disease.

The cardinal clinical features of vulvovaginal candidiasis are pruritus vulvae and vaginal discharge. The discharge is typically whitish, with curd-like plaques adhering to the vaginal wall, and does not smell. There may be erythema and/or oedema of the vulva and vaginal walls.

The diagnosis can be made on a wet preparation made from the vaginal discharge, the sensitivity of which can be increased by adding 10% potassium hydroxide. Typical mycelia and yeast cells are seen. For the treatment of vulvovaginal candidiasis, see Table 21.4.

Trichomoniasis

Trichomonas vaginalis (see Chapter 81) has been found in the vagina of up to 30% of antenatal clinic attenders in certain African centres.[3] Studies in the USA have shown that its prevalence is higher among women with many partners, and that it can be isolated from a high proportion of male contacts of infected women, suggesting that transmission is primarily through sexual contact. In males, most infections are believed to be asymptomatic and self-limiting, although occasionally it may give rise to urethritis. Recent studies using more sensitive diagnostic techniques have shown substantially higher rates of infection in males in developing countries.[42]

Up to 75% of women attending STI clinics with *T. vaginalis* infection complain of vaginal discharge. Pruritus vulvae, dyspareunia and dysuria are also common symptoms. On examination, a profuse yellow-green frothy discharge is typically noted. The vulva and vaginal walls may be excoriated and erythematous in severe cases, and punctate haemorrhages may be seen on the cervix.[43]

The diagnosis can be made on a wet preparation collected from the posterior fornix. Under phase contrast, increased numbers of polymorphonuclear leucocytes are usually seen, and motile flagellated parasites, slightly larger than polymorphonuclear leucocytes, are present. Compared with culture, direct microscopy is less than 80% sensitive, so that culture should also be performed when available. For the treatment of trichomoniasis, see Table 21.4.

Bacterial vaginosis

Bacterial vaginosis is a syndrome in which a malodorous vaginal discharge is associated with characteristic changes in the vaginal bacterial flora. There is an increase in numbers of anaerobes, *Gardnerella vaginalis* and *Mycoplasma hominis*, such that lactobacilli are no longer predominant. Bacterial vaginosis appears to be more prevalent among women with many sexual partners, but since it has been found in sexually inexperienced women it is not clear that it is a sexually transmitted condition.

The discharge of bacterial vaginosis is typically homogeneous and white-grey, and associated with increased vaginal pH (>4.5). The characteristic fishy smell is more easily detectable after the addition of a drop of 10% potassium hydroxide to a drop of discharge on a slide. Bacterial vaginosis has been shown to be associated with adverse pregnancy outcome (premature labour, chorioamnionitis and postpartum endometritis).[44]

The diagnosis of bacterial vaginosis can be made on Gram stain of a vaginal swab, according to Nugent's criteria, in which a score is given depending on the relative proportion of lactobacilli and Gram-negative rods and coccobacilli.[45] A simplified version of Nugent's criteria put forward by Hay and Ison is gaining in popularity and is easier to use than the criteria of Nugent. Essentially, this classifies the flora as either normal (predominantly lactobacilli), mixed flora, or BV (clue cells observed).[46] For the treatment of bacterial vaginosis, see Table 21.4.

DISEASES CAUSING GENITAL ULCERATION

Chancroid

Chancroid, or soft sore, was first distinguished from the hard chancre of syphilis by Ricord in 1838. In 1889, Ducrey, in Naples, showed that the inoculation of material from chancroidal ulcers into the skin of the forearm caused ulceration which could be serially passaged, and identified the causative organism which now bears his name. The development of defined solid media for the isolation of *Haemophilus ducreyi* in the 1970s enabled detailed epidemiological studies of chancroid to be carried out for the first time.[47,48]

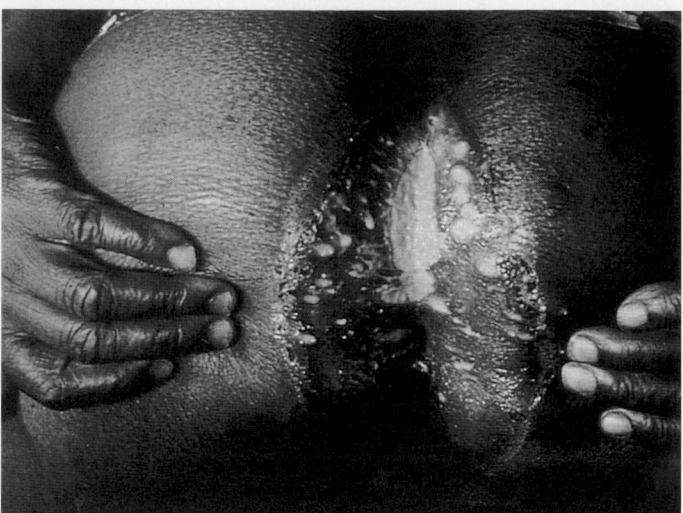

Figure 21.5 Extensive perianal ulceration resulting from a *Haemophilus ducreyi* infection in a sex worker (Courtesy of D. Mabey.).

Epidemiology

Chancroid is an important cause of genital ulceration in Africa. Before the HIV epidemic it accounted for more than 60% of genital ulcers seen in hospital, but in the 1990s hospital-based studies in several countries found that the proportion of ulcers due to *Herpes simplex* had increased, and that the proportion due to chancroid had decreased correspondingly.[49] Although generally rare in industrialized countries, there have been several well-documented outbreaks in North America since the 1970s. Characteristic features of these outbreaks have been a high male-to-female case ratio, the involvement of prostitutes and the low socioeconomic status of the populations affected. A study in Nairobi investigated the role of asymptomatic females in the transmission of the disease and concluded that they were of little importance.[50] Studies among Australian solders during the Vietnam war suggest that chancroid is more common among uncircumcised than circumcised males.[51]

The prevalence of chancroid is high among commercial sex workers in the cities of Africa (Figure 21.5), as is the prevalence of HIV infection. Prospective studies among both males and females at high risk of HIV infection in Nairobi have suggested that chancroid significantly increases the risk of transmission of HIV via heterosexual contact, either by increasing infectivity, susceptibility or both.[52,53] The unusually high rates of partner change required to sustain the transmission of chancroid make it a tempting target for local disease control campaigns and suggest that, compared to other STIs, it presents a relatively easy target for global elimination.[54]

Aetiology

Chancroid is caused by *Haemophilus ducreyi*, a small facultatively anaerobic Gram-negative bacillus which requires haemin (X factor), reduces nitrate to nitrite and forms typical streptobacillary chains on Gram stain. It is a fastidious organism which will only grow on enriched media and grows best at 30–33°C in an atmosphere of 5% carbon dioxide.

Pathogenesis

Histopathologically, chancroidal ulcers contain three distinct zones: a superficial zone consisting of necrotic tissue, fibrin and numerous bacteria; an intermediate zone showing oedema and new vessel formation; and a deep zone containing a dense infiltrate of neutrophils and plasma cells with fibroblastic proliferation.

Studies involving the inoculation of human volunteers have improved our understanding of the pathogenesis of chancroid.[55] The application of *H. ducreyi* to the human forearm does not produce a lesion unless the skin is traumatized. There is some evidence that virulent strains are relatively resistant to phagocytosis by human polymorphonuclear leucocytes and to complement-mediated killing by normal human and rabbit serum. An isogenic mutant lacking a receptor for haemoglobin showed reduced virulence in humans.[56] Two toxins have been characterized: one is a cell-associated haemolysin, similar to those produced by *Proteus mirabilis*, toxic to human foreskin fibroblasts but not to HeLa cells in tissue culture. The other is a soluble toxin, homologous to the cytolethal distending toxin produced by a number of enteric organisms, which is toxic to a variety of cell lines.[57] The suppurating lymphadenopathy of chancroid is notable for the large number of neutrophils and small number of bacilli present.

Clinical features

After an incubation period of 3–7 days, a papule appears at the site of inoculation which soon ulcerates. The typical ulcer of chancroid (Figure 21.6) is painful and soft, has a purulent base with an undermined edge, and bleeds on contact. Multiple ulcers are commonly present, and there is painful inguinal lymphadenopathy (Figure 21.7) in some 50% of cases, often unilateral. Atypical presentations are, however, common, and even in experienced hands chancroid cannot reliably be distinguished from primary syphilis on clinical grounds.[58] Herpes simplex, LGV and donovanosis must also be considered in the differential diagnosis of chancroid.

Chancroid may cause extensive local destruction (Figure 21.8), particularly in HIV-infected individuals who may fail to respond to antimicrobial treatment, but the infection does not disseminate.

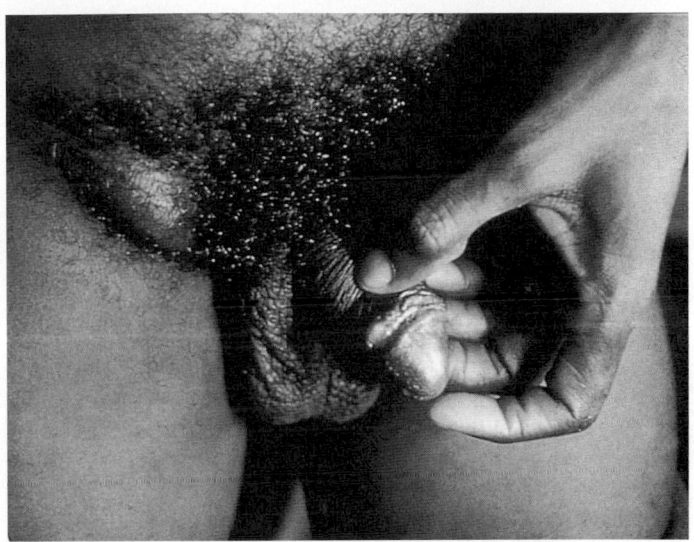

Figure 21.7 Chancroid: ulcer of corona accompanied by a painful bubo. (Courtesy of D. Mabey.)

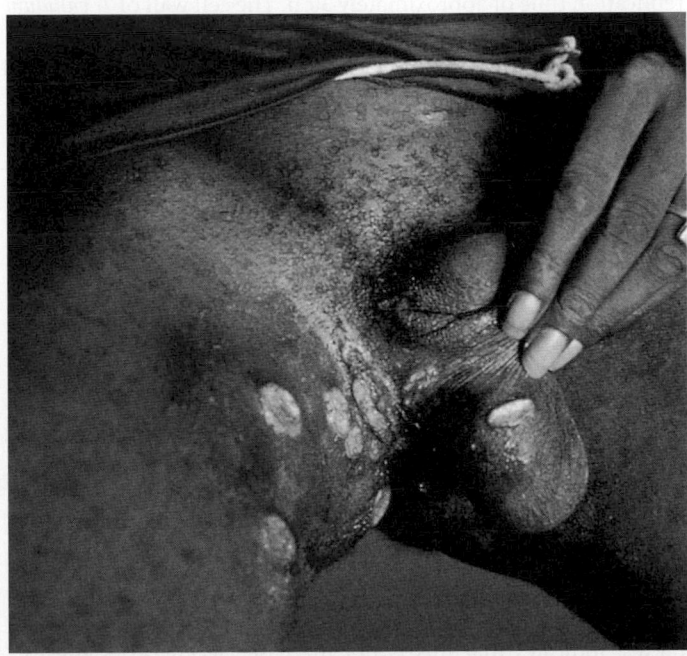

Figure 21.6 Chancroid: multiple soft painful ulcers. (Courtesy of D. Mabey.)

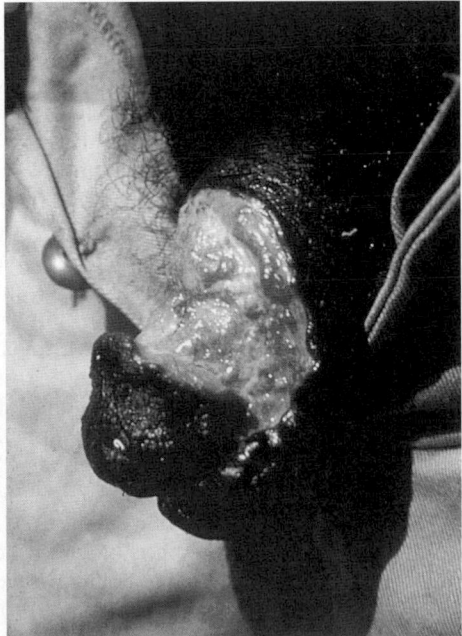

Figure 21.8 Phagedenic chancroid: destructive ulcer of penile shaft. (Courtesy of D. Mabey.)

Diagnosis

Gram stain of smears obtained from ulcers has been advocated in the past for the diagnosis of chancroid, but this lacks both sensitivity and specificity. Preferred methods for the laboratory diagnosis of chancroid are now either isolation of *H. ducreyi* from the ulcer or the use of NAATs. Swabs for culture should be taken from the ulcer base or its undermined edge and plated directly on appropriate blood-containing media enriched with fetal calf serum and Vitox and made selective with vancomycin. For optimal rates of isolation, media made up from both GC agar and Mueller–Hinton agar base should be inoculated. Plates should be incubated for at least 72 h in an atmosphere of 5% carbon dioxide at 33°C. *H. ducreyi* is identified by its typical colonial morphology (colonies are difficult to break up and can be moved intact across the surface of the agar), Gram stain and inability to ferment sugars.

Management

Chancroidal ulcers should be kept clean and dry, with regular washing in soapy water. The mainstay of antimicrobial treatment has, for a number of years, been co-trimoxazole or erythromycin in standard dosage given by mouth for 7 days (Table 21.4). However, an increasing proportion of strains worldwide are now resistant to sulfonamides, and many trimethoprim-resistant strains have been isolated in Thailand and Kenya. Ciprofloxacin 500 mg daily for 3 days by mouth and ceftriaxone 500 mg as a single intramuscular dose and azithromycin as a single 1 g oral dose appear to be effective alternatives, although in HIV-infected patients longer courses of treatment may be required.

Syphilis

History

Syphilis, a young shepherd boy, was the eponymous hero of a Latin poem written in 1530 by the Italian, G. Fracastorio. He succumbed to an apparently new disease which had swept across Europe a few years earlier in the wake of the French army's retreat from Naples. The timing of this epidemic led to the suggestion that syphilis had been brought back from the New World by Columbus and his men in 1493. An alternative hypothesis put forward by E. H. Hudson, a physician working in the 1930s in Mesopotamia (now Iraq), was that syphilis originated as an endemic infection of childhood (yaws) in the hot humid tropics, and that venereal transmission only became important when living standards improved sufficiently to prevent transmission in childhood giving rise to long-lasting immunity. This so-called unitarian hypothesis is supported by recent evidence of very close DNA homology between *Treponema pallidum* and *T. pertenue* (recently re-classified as *T. pallidum* subsp. *pertenue*).[59] Recent studies in animal models do however demonstrate different tissue tropisms between pallidum and pertenue strains of *T. pallidum*.[60] Although syphilis in all its clinical aspects had been described in detail by nineteenth-century physicians, notably Hutchinson in Britain and Fournier in France, it was not until 1905 that the causative organism, *T. pallidum*, was first identified by Schaudin and Hoffman; in 1906, Wasserman described the first serological test for the diagnosis of syphilis. Investigation of the *T. pallidum*

genome is yielding important insights into the extraordinary survival capability of *T. pallidum* following human infection.[61]

Epidemiology

The incidence of syphilis has declined steadily for most of the twentieth century in Western Europe and North America, with the exception of a brief rise during and immediately after each world war.

There are no reliable incidence figures for developing countries. Seroprevalence surveys have shown high rates of positivity among antenatal clinic attenders and in the general population in many African countries.[3] The relative rarity of late syphilis in parts of Africa where early syphilis is common has led to speculation that the disease has become more common in recent years, perhaps reflecting loss of herd immunity following the mass treatment campaigns against endemic treponemal disease in the 1950s and 1960s.

Transmission by sexual contact requires exposure to moist mucosal or cutaneous lesions; experiments in the rabbit suggest that an inoculum of some 50 organisms is sufficient to initiate infection. The rate of transmission from an infected partner is approximately 30%.

Aetiology

Syphilis is caused by *T. pallidum*, one of a small group of treponemes (of the order *Spirochaetales*) pathogenic to man. It cannot be distinguished morphologically from the agents responsible for yaws and pinta (*T. pallidum* subsp. *pertenue* and *T. carateum*, respectively). It is a spiral organism 6–15 mm in length and 0.15 mm in width, visible by light microscopy only under conditions of dark-field illumination, and cannot be grown on artificial media. In tissue culture and in animal models it divides slowly, with a replication time of approximately 30 h. The cell wall of *T. pallidum* is remarkable for a very low density of outer membrane proteins, which probably contributes to the organism's ability to persist in its host for lengthy periods. It is highly susceptible to drying.

Pathogenesis

T. pallidum has not been shown to produce either exotoxins or endotoxins. Following experimental infection in the rabbit, *T. pallidum* begins to replicate once it has passed through the epithelium. An initial polymorphonuclear leucocyte response at the lesion is soon replaced by an infiltrate of T and B lymphocytes. The primary chancre also contains mucoid material, mainly hyaluronic acid and chondroitin sulfate, which may modulate the host immune response. Both circulating *T. pallidum* – specific T cells and specific antibody can be found in the majority of cases of primary syphilis. At the same time as these are first noted, the number of organisms in the lesion decreases and the ulcer begins to heal, suggesting that the immune system is controlling the infection.

The appearance of secondary lesions some weeks later, due to the dissemination of organisms and circulating immune complexes, indicates that this is not the case. Recent work suggests that secondary syphilis coincides with the emergence of an antigenically distinct new strain which is no longer susceptible to antibodies directed at the infecting strain.[61] Much of the pathology of secondary syphilis may be immune complex mediated. High levels of antitreponemal antibody are present in the circulation, but cell-mediated immune responses are depressed.

Eventually cell-mediated immune responses to *T. pallidum* are restored as the lesions are brought under control, leading to the latent stage. Follow-up studies in the pre-penicillin era showed that relapse of infectious secondary lesions occurred in up to 25% of cases. The organism can survive in the body for many years thereafter, causing tertiary lesions characterized by the presence of a small number of organisms and a lymphocytic host response giving rise to an endarteritis.

Clinical features

After an incubation period of 10–70 days (median 21 days), a primary chancre (Figure 21.9) develops at the site of inoculation. The chancre is typically painless, indurated, with a clean base and a raised edge, and does not bleed on contact. There is usually only a single lesion; in the male it is most commonly on the glans, the foreskin, the coronal sulcus or the shaft of the penis, and in the female on the cervix or vulva. The primary chancre is often accompanied by inguinal lymphadenopathy; the glands are characteristically hard (the 'bullet bubo' of Hutchinson) and painless.

The primary chancre generally resolves spontaneously over several weeks. Between 3 and 6 weeks after its first appearance the features of secondary syphilis appear. The rash of secondary syphilis may take many forms: papular, macular or pustular; annular lesions are not uncommon. It often desquamates, but in moist areas of the body (e.g. perineum, axilla) soft raised condylomata lata may be seen (Figures 21.10, 21.11). It generally affects the palms (Figure 21.12) and soles, and does not itch. The mucous membranes may be involved, with mucous patches or oral ulceration sometimes in the form of the characteristic 'snail track' ulcer. In addition to its cutaneous manifestations secondary syphilis may cause systemic illness (fever, malaise),

generalized lymphadenopathy, nephritis, hepatitis, meningitis or uveitis.

The lesions of secondary syphilis generally resolve after several weeks, although relapses commonly occurred in the pre-antibiotic era. In the absence of adequate treatment the patient then enters the latent stage of the disease, and is liable to develop tertiary syphilis at some time in the future.

The lesions of tertiary syphilis fall into three categories: the gumma, cardiovascular disease and central nervous system disease. The classic Oslo study of untreated syphilis, in which some 1,400 patients were followed for up to 50 years, found that the most common manifestation was the gumma, a painless 'punched out' ulcer with little or no inflammatory reaction, which developed in 15%: 70% were cutaneous, 10% involved bone and rarely the viscera were involved. Most cases occurred in the first 15 years following infection. Cardiovascular lesions (aortitis, aortic valve disease or coronary ostial occlusion) were seen in 15% of males and 8% of females, with onset typically 30–40 years after infection. Neurological manifestations were seen in 9% of males and 5% of females, with meningovascular disease typically occurring after 15–20 years and tabes dorsalis or general paresis after 20–30 years.[62] The Tuskegee study of untreated black Americans showed similar results. It is therefore surprising that tertiary syphilis, and in particular neurosyphilis, appears rather uncommon in Africa in spite of the high incidence of early syphilis.

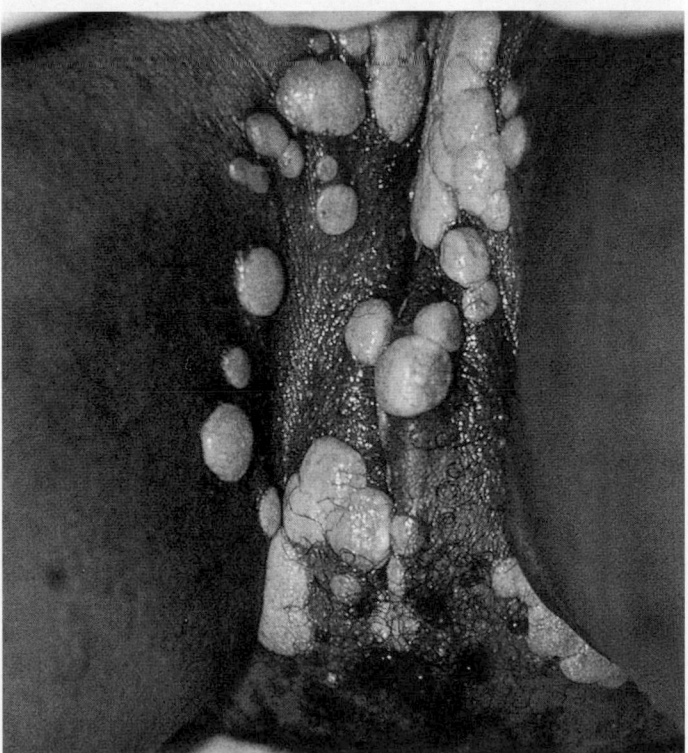

Figure 21.10   Secondary syphilis: condylomata lata. (Courtesy of J. Richens.)

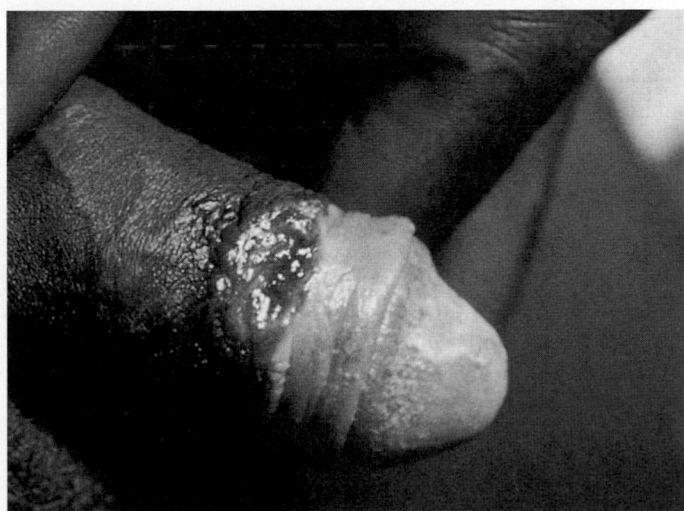

Figure 21.9   Syphilis: primary chancre. (Courtesy of D. Mabey.)

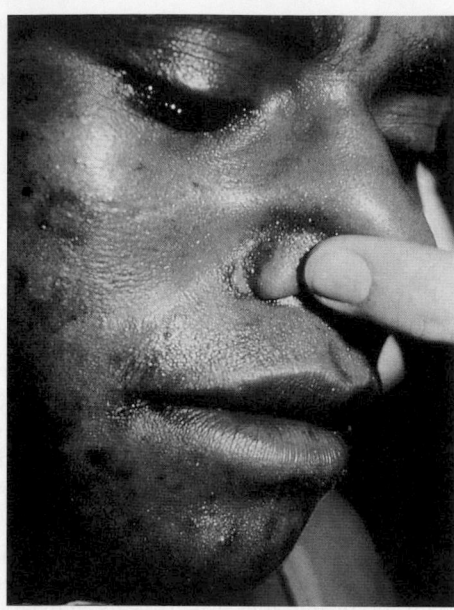

Figure 21.11 Secondary syphilis: condyloma abutting on ala nasi (Courtesy of J. Richens).

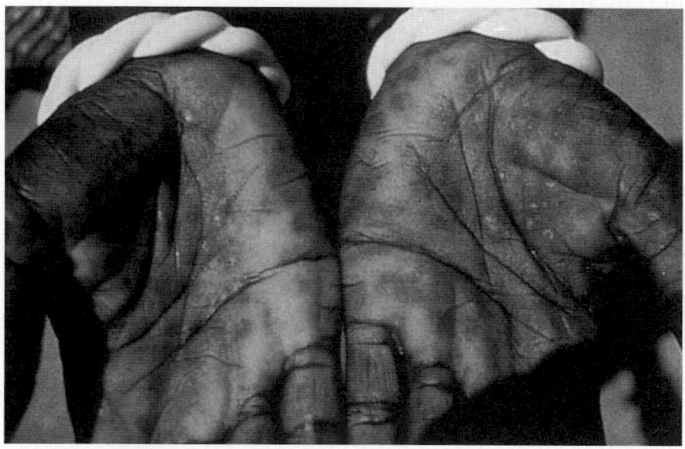

Figure 21.12 Secondary syphilis: typical palmar rash (Courtesy of J. Richens).

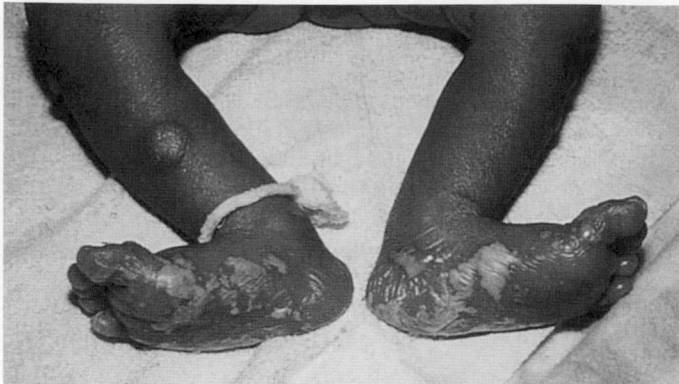

Figure 21.13 Congenital syphilis in a neonate: bullous lesions of feet. (Courtesy of D. McGregor.)

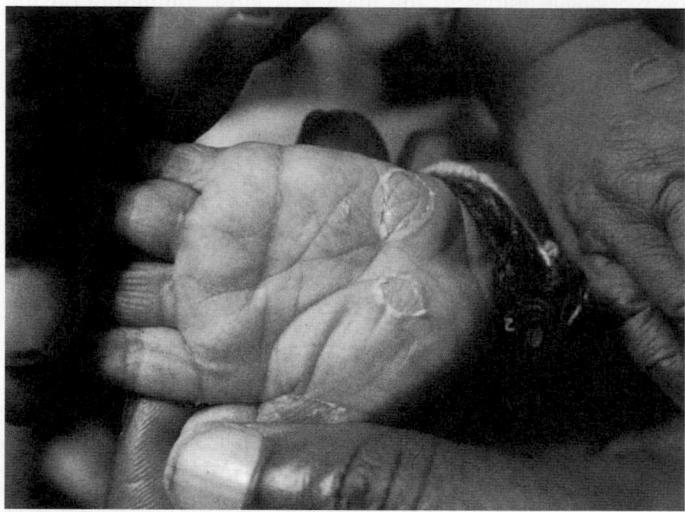

Figure 21.14 Congenital syphilis in a 3-month-old infant: desquamating lesion of palm (Courtesy of D. Mabey).

Congenital syphilis

Early congenital syphilis

Pregnant women with untreated early or latent syphilis are liable to give birth to congenitally infected infants. The risk is highest among those with primary or secondary syphilis during pregnancy, and diminishes as the duration of latent syphilis increases. Studies conducted in the pre-antibiotic era found that untreated early syphilis in the mother led to stillbirth in 25% of cases, neonatal death in some 15% of cases and a syphilitic infant in about 40% of cases. Corresponding figures for untreated late syphilis were 12%, 9% and 2%.[63] A recent study in Tanzania found that 25% of pregnant women with active syphilis (RPR titre >1:4)

delivered a stillbirth, 33% a low birth weight and 20% a premature infant.[8]

Signs of congenital syphilis in the neonate include a bullous rash (Figure 21.13), anaemia, jaundice and hepatosplenomegaly. The infant is often small for dates and may have feeding difficulties. The prognosis is poor in infants with signs of congenital syphilis at birth. More commonly, the syphilitic infant appears normal at birth, and presents in the first 3 months of life with: failure to thrive; a rash which resembles that of secondary syphilis, with desquamation usually involving the palms (Figure 21.14) and soles; persistent nasal discharge (sometimes blood-stained); and anaemia or hepatosplenomegaly (Figure 21.15). Periostitis of the long bones, with or without metaphyseal abnormalities, is radiologically evident in more than 90% of cases, and may present clinically as pseudoparalysis of one or more limbs. The prognosis is very much better in those presenting in the postnatal period.[7]

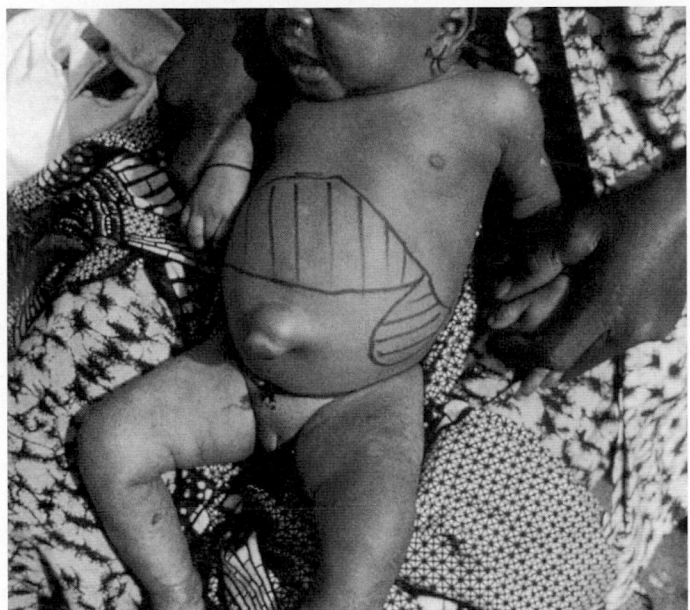

Figure 21.15 Congenital syphilis in a 3-month-old infant: hepatosplenomegaly. (Courtesy of D. Mabey.)

Late congenital syphilis

Late congenital syphilis in the child or adolescent corresponds to tertiary syphilis in the adult, although the cardiovascular system is seldom involved. Manifestations include bony and dental abnormalities (skull bossing, Hutchinson's teeth) and inflammatory lesions of the cornea (interstitial keratitis) and joints (Clutton's joints). Eighth nerve deafness is commonly seen, and symptomatic neurosyphilis may occur, corresponding to tabes dorsalis or general paresis in the adult. In view of the high incidence of early congenital syphilis in many African cities, late manifestations of the disease are surprisingly rare in Africa.

Diagnosis

Clinically, it may not be possible to distinguish a syphilitic primary chancre from other causes of genital ulceration. In most parts of Africa, herpes and chancroid are the most important differential diagnoses, but in areas where donovanosis is prevalent, this should also be considered. The primary chancre should also be distinguished from LGV, herpes and non-venereal causes of genital ulceration. Secondary syphilis may resemble a variety of other skin conditions, but rashes which do not itch and affect the palms and soles should be considered syphilitic until proved otherwise. Early congenital syphilis in the neonatal period may be confused with perinatally acquired herpes simplex on account of the bullous rash, or with other intrauterine infections causing hepatosplenomegaly, anaemia and jaundice (e.g. cytomegalovirus, toxoplasmosis, rubella).

Dark-field microscopy

T. pallidum may be demonstrated by dark-field microscopy in fluid from ulcerated or moist lesions of early syphilis, or in bulla fluid from lesions of early congenital syphilis. It can be distinguished from other spirochaetes that may be present under the foreskin, by its characteristic shape and motility. Dark-field microscopy is likely to be negative in patients who have applied antiseptics to the lesion or taken antibiotics.

Serological diagnosis

Two categories of test are available for the serological diagnosis of syphilis: non-specific or reagin tests (e.g. Venereal Disease Research Laboratory (VDRL), rapid plasma reagin (RPR)) and treponemal tests (*T. pallidum* haemagglutination (TPHA) or particle agglutination assays (TPPA), fluorescent treponemal antibody test (absorbed) (FTA)). The reagin tests are useful for monitoring the response to treatment because they exhibit a falling titre after successful therapy, but they may give false positive reactions in subjects with other chronic infections. The treponemal tests generally remain positive for life, and cannot therefore distinguish between a current and a past infection. They are more specific than the reagin tests but cannot distinguish between sexually acquired and endemic treponemal infections. The RPR and TPHA tests are simple to perform and do not require sophisticated laboratory equipment. In the neonate it is necessary to demonstrate IgM antibodies by the FTA test in order to distinguish between true infection and passively acquired maternal antibody; however, in an infant with signs of congenital syphilis, a positive maternal reagin test is sufficient grounds for treatment. A new generation of specific IgM EIA tests shows promise as a new tool for recognizing recently acquired active infection.[64,65]

Management

T. pallidum remains fully sensitive to penicillin. Because it is a slowly dividing organism it is necessary to ensure adequate circulating penicillin levels for at least 10 days. Recommended treatment regimens are shown in Table 21.4. It has been suggested that single-dose benzathine penicillin does not ensure adequate levels in the cerebrospinal fluid, and recent anecdotal evidence suggests that it may be ineffective in some HIV-infected patients and pregnant women. If it is possible to ensure compliance, 10 daily doses of aqueous procaine penicillin 1.2 million units may be preferable, although a recent randomized trial showed no differences in outcomes between patients treated with single-dose and extended high-dose penicillin, regardless of HIV status.[66] Epidemiological treatment is recommended for sexual contacts. A single 2 g dose of azithromycin has recently been validated as a useful oral alternative to benzathine penicillin in early syphilis but the emergence of macrolide resistance in syphilis may limit the usefulness of this option in the future.[67,68]

Early congenital syphilis should be treated with procaine penicillin 50 000 units/kg i.m. daily for 10 days. If compliance is considered unlikely, benzathine penicillin 50 000 units/kg i.m. as a single dose may be given, although this does not give therapeutic levels in the cerebrospinal fluid. The mother and her sexual partner(s) should be investigated and treated appropriately. If possible, infants should be followed up after 6 months to ensure that the RPR or VDRL test has reverted to negative.

Prevention

Congenital syphilis can be prevented by serological screening of pregnant women at antenatal clinics. Experience in Tanzania has shown that in a developing country setting, this is only successful if serological tests are performed in the clinic and treatment given immediately.[69]

Lymphogranuloma venereum

Lymphogranuloma venereum (LGV) is also known as lymphogranuloma inguinale, lymphopathia venereum, tropical or climatic bubo and Durand–Nicolas–Favre disease.

Epidemiology

The epidemiology of LGV is not well defined, owing to the lack of a sensitive and specific diagnostic test. The classical form of LGV is largely confined to the tropics, where in most places it accounts for only a small proportion of patients with STIs. The disease is seen more often in men than women. Since 2004, there has been a dramatic rise in LGV presenting with proctitis among homosexual HIV-positive males in Europe.[70]

Aetiology

LGV is caused by the invasive L1, L2 and L3 strains of *Chlamydia trachomatis*.

Pathology

The characteristic pathological features are a thrombolymphangitis and perilymphangitis with proliferation of the endothelial cells of the lymphatics. In the lymph nodes prominent migration of neutrophils leads to characteristic stellate abscess formation.

Clinical features

The disease is important, chiefly as a cause of bubo. When a sexually active adult presents with an inguinal bubo not associated with genital ulcer, LGV is an important diagnosis to consider. The initial event in infection, occurring 3–30 days after exposure, is typically a small, painless, usually herpetiform ulcer of the genitalia which may pass unrecognized and resolves spontaneously. It is thought likely that some patients develop asymptomatic infections of the urethra and cervix. The second phase of the illness is the development of increasingly painful lymphangitis and lymphadenitis, accompanied by fever and malaise. The infected nodes (bilateral in a third of cases) coalesce into a matted mass which may project outwards below or above the inguinal ligament to give the classical 'groove sign'. The nodes are liable to rupture, forming multiple sinuses. Untreated, the disease may cause extensive lymphatic damage, resulting in elephantiasis of the genitalia (Figure 21.16). The combination of elephantiasis with skin breakdown sometimes seen in late cases is referred to as esthiomène. An additional characteristic feature in long-standing cases is the development of fenestrations in the labia.

In women and homosexual men, the disease may present as an acute proctocolitis which, in a proportion of cases, leads to abscess formation, fibrosis, fistula and rectal stricture.[71] In the Caribbean,

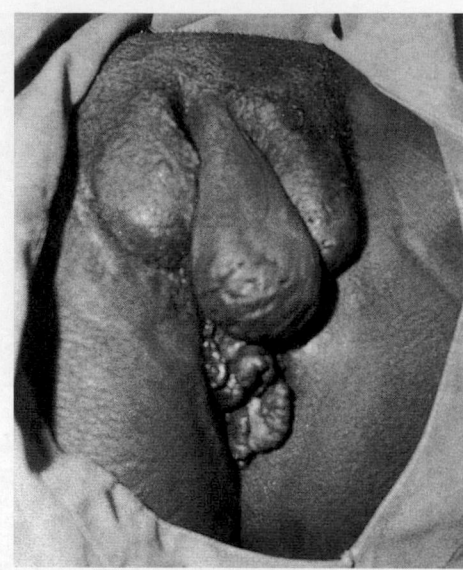

Figure 21.16 Lymphogranuloma venereum: elephantiasis in long-standing case. (Reproduced with permission from: Arya OP, Osoba AO, Bennett FJ. *Tropical Venereology*. Edinburgh: Churchill Livingstone; 1980.)

a high incidence of vulval carcinoma has been recorded among premenopausal women with scars of either LGV or donovanosis.[72] A substantial proportion of cases of rectal stricture may also develop carcinoma.

Diagnosis

The diagnosis of LGV can only be confirmed in specialist centres with facilities for the identification of *C. trachomatis* L1–3 strains using PCR methods, or the ability to perform the microimmunofluorescence serological test.[73,74] Serological tests show cross-reaction with other serovars of *C. trachomatis*, and with other species of Chlamydia, e.g. the prevalent respiratory tract pathogen *C. pneumoniae*. The protocols being used in the European outbreak involve initially detection of *C. trachomatis* using standard PCR methods, followed by a second PCR targeting LGV-specific DNA or alternatively amplification of the *omp*1 gene followed by restriction enzyme digestion to identify LGV serovars.[74] The presence of stellate abscesses in biopsy material is suggestive of LGV. Direct fluorescent antibody (DFA) staining may be used to demonstrate chlamydial elementary bodies in tissue or discharge from buboes. Additional laboratory findings include leucocytosis, an elevated erythrocyte sedimentation rate and increases in IgG and cryoglobulins.

Treatment

The drugs recommended for treatment of acute cases are of the tetracycline or macrolide groups, as for other chlamydial infections, but for a longer duration (21 days) (Table 21.4). Benefit in late cases, e.g. with rectal stricture, is slight. Plastic surgical operations may be of benefit in cases with extensive elephantiasis or deformity. Suspicious areas in healed scars should be biopsied for malignant change. Aspiration of buboes through adjacent healthy skin is usually advised.

Donovanosis

Synonyms are granuloma inguinale, granuloma venereum. It is important not to confuse this disease with lympho-granuloma venereum (see above) or to confuse Donovan bodies (see below) with Leishman–Donovan bodies (leishmaniasis). The disease was first recognized in India, where Donovan observed the bodies that bear his name in an oral lesion of the disease. Sir Patrick Manson did much to promote awareness of the disease by devoting a chapter to 'ulcerating granuloma of the pudenda' in the first edition of this textbook.

Epidemiology

Endemic areas are localized to a few specific areas of the tropics. The most important of these are currently India, Papua New Guinea (PNG), Brazil and eastern parts of South Africa. The disease is strongly associated with prostitution and low socioeconomic status. Major epidemics of donovanosis have been reported from PNG but are unlikely to be seen again. Outside PNG, the highest recently reported incidence of donovanosis has been in Durban, South Africa, where 16% of genital ulcers in men were due to donovanosis.[75] There is strong evidence that the disease is sexually transmitted in most patients. The risk of transmission to partners appears to be lower than for other STIs. Perinatal transmission is rare.

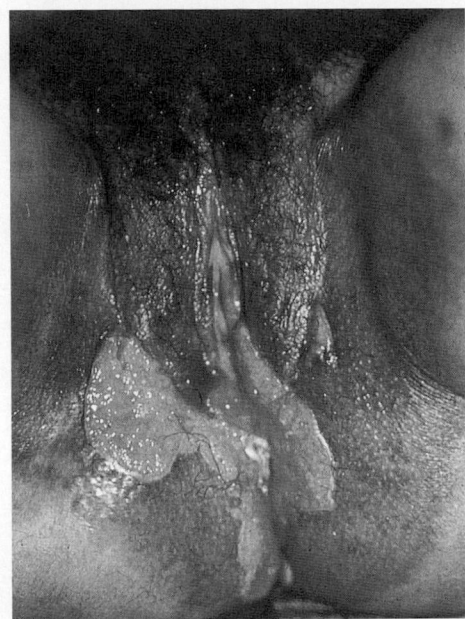

Figure 21.17 Donovanosis: slowly extending painless ulceration. (Courtesy of J. Richens.)

Aetiology

The disease is caused by a poorly characterized, encapsulated, Gram-negative coccobacillus, previously called *Calymmatobacterium granulomatis*, recently re-classified as a Klebsiella on the basis of ribosomal RNA sequences.[76] It is an intracellular parasite that can be grown in tissue culture.[77,78]

Pathology

The disease primarily attacks the skin. The bacteria are carried to inguinal nodes, where they occasionally cause a suppurating periadenitis ('pseudobubo') but more often they escape to produce ulcers in the overlying skin. The key histological features are (1) epithelial hyperplasia, (2) a dense dermal infiltrate of plasma cells, and (3) scattered large macrophages containing clusters of Donovan bodies. Donovan bodies stain poorly with haematoxylin and eosin but with Giemsa they typically display a capsule and bipolar densities which give a characteristic closed safety-pin appearance.

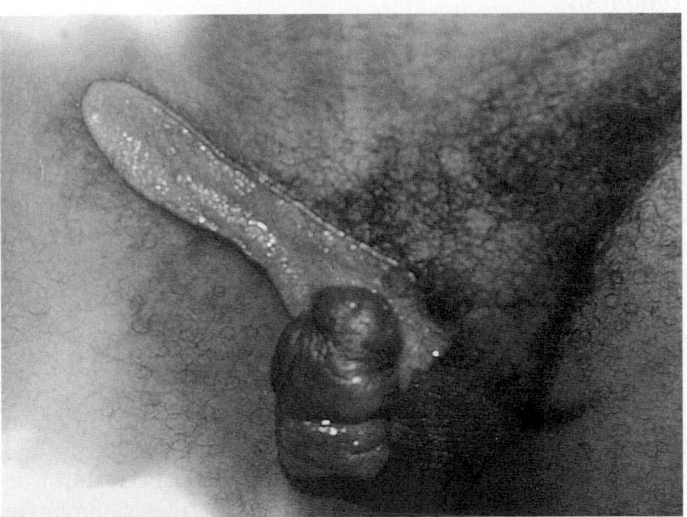

Figure 21.18 Donovanosis: lesion extending along inguinal fold. (Courtesy of J. Richens.)

Clinical features

The first manifestation, appearing after a 3–40-day incubation period, is usually a small papule, which ruptures to form a granulomatous lesion that is characteristically pain free, 'beefy-red' in colour, bleeds readily on contact and is often elevated above the level of the surrounding skin. The lesion has to be differentiated from other forms of genital ulcer. Most likely to cause confusion are chancroid,[79] condylomata lata, ulcerated warts and squamous carcinoma. Untreated, the ulcers slowly extend (Figure 21.17), particularly along skin-folds towards the groins (Figure 21.18) and anus. Special features are extragenital lesions (mostly neck and mouth), cervical lesions (resemble carcinoma or tuberculous cervicitis), involvement of uterus, tubes and ovaries (hard masses, abscesses, 'frozen pelvis', hydronephrosis) and rare cases of haematogenous dissemination to lung, liver, spleen and bone. Complications include rapid extension of lesions secondarily infected with fusospirochaetal organisms, scarring (in some populations very prominent), elephantiasis and the development of squamous carcinoma.

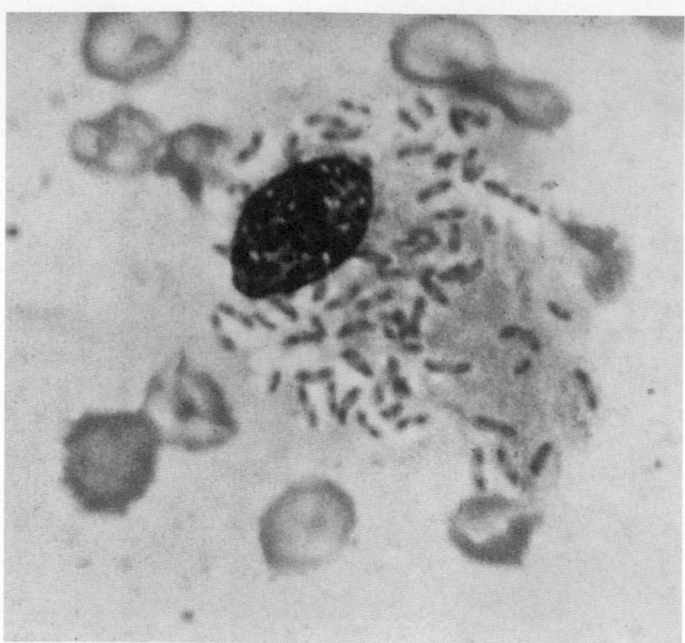

Figure 21.19 Donovan bodies: Giemsa-stained smear from genital ulcer demonstrating intracellular organisms with bipolar densities.

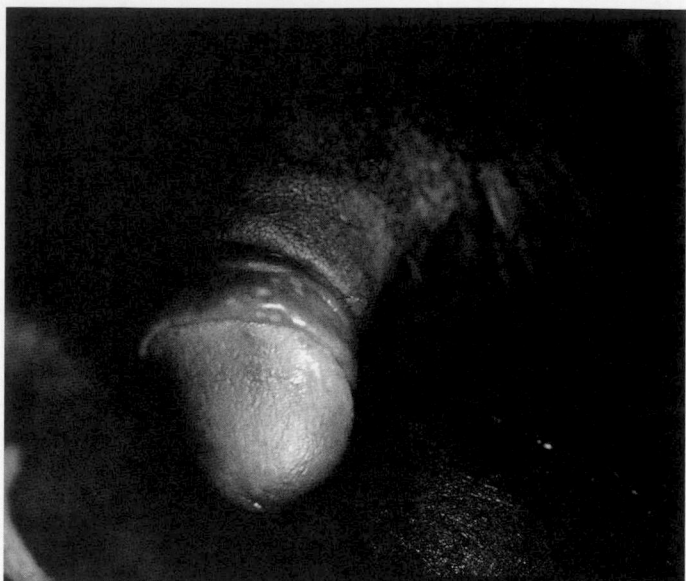

Figure 21.20 Recurrent genital herpes: cluster of small painful ulcers of corona.

Diagnosis

The diagnosis requires the demonstration of intracellular Donovan bodies (Figure 21.19) in either biopsy material (best stained with silver stains or Giemsa) or smears taken from active areas which can be stained by Giemsa or Leishman stains. For collection of specimens, a recommended technique is to thoroughly clean the lesions of surface debris, detach one to three 3–5 mm pieces of tissue by punch or snip biopsy, and then prepare a smear from one piece, followed by air-drying and fixation in 95% ethanol and fixing the remaining tissue in 10% formalin for histology.[80]

Management

The bacteria respond to many broad-spectrum antibiotics active against Gram-negative bacilli.[78] The most widely used in recent years have been azithromycin, doxycycline, co-trimoxazole and erythromycin. Fluorinated quinolones have also been shown to be of value, but experience in Australia suggests that azithromycin is the most useful treatment.[81] Treatment should be continued until lesions have resolved and, if possible, a little longer to reduce the risk of relapse. Plastic surgical procedures are required in some patients. Epidemiological treatment of contacts exposed within 40 days of the onset of symptoms in the index case may be recommended (Table 21.4).

Genital herpes

Genital herpes is an ulcerative STI caused principally by herpes simplex virus type 2 (HSV-2) and to a lesser extent by herpes simplex virus type 1 (HSV-1), the usual cause of oral herpes. Genital herpes accounts for a lower proportion of patients with genital ulcer in the tropics than it does in developed countries, although this pattern is changing rapidly in areas with high HIV incidence. Recent studies in Africa have demonstrated that HSV seroconversion is an especially important risk factor for HIV acquisition.[82] Prior infection with HSV-1 infection, which is almost universal by the age of puberty in many developing countries, reduces the severity and frequency of clinical recurrences in HSV-2 infection.[83]

Clinical features

The clinical picture is highly characteristic in many cases, with its localized clusters of vesicles, which break down to form ulcers (Figure 21.20), crust over and then resolve. Sites of involvement include the external genitalia, neighbouring skin, the urethra and cervix (both endocervix and ectocervix), pharynx and rectum. Tender lymphadenopathy may occur. During the primary attack, the virus ascends the peripheral nerves to local ganglia, where a latency is established, which is liable to be interrupted by periodic recurrences for the remainder of the patient's life. The primary attack is notably more severe than subsequent episodes, with lesions covering a wider and more symmetric area. HSV-2 causes substantially more severe primary disease than HSV-1 and is followed by more frequent relapse. The complications of genital herpes include a sacral radiculomyelopathy which may manifest with constipation and retention of urine as well as shooting pains down the legs. Other complications include aseptic meningitis, extragenital lesions and disseminated herpes. In pregnant women, recurrences and dissemination are more frequent and premature delivery may complicate primary attacks. Severe and intractable ulceration due to HSV-2 occurs in patients immunosuppressed by HIV.

Diagnosis

Clinical diagnosis alone is often sufficient. Genital herpes has to be distinguished from other STIs that cause painful genital ulcer and from non-infectious conditions such as Behçet's syndrome and Crohn's disease. The definitive diagnosis rests on viral isolation. Kits for antigen detection are available commercially, and DNA amplification tests have been successfully used to identify HSV-2 in symptomatic and asymptomatic shedders. Serological diagnosis is only of value in a primary attack.

Management

Specific treatment can rarely be offered in the tropics; nonetheless patients require explanation, reassurance and advice, just as elsewhere (Table 21.4). Patients need to be instructed to keep the lesions clean and dry. They should be told that the disease is likely to recur and that they will transmit the infection to others if they have sexual intercourse while they have lesions. Aciclovir has been shown to be of value in ameliorating symptoms of the primary attack, treatment of infected neonates and adults with immunosuppression or disseminated disease. Continuous prophylactic therapy has been found useful in ameliorating and preventing recurrences in patients particularly troubled by recurrent disease. Recent studies have demonstrated that periods of asymptomatic shedding commonly occur and that this shedding can be suppressed by aciclovir.[84] A recent study in Burkina Faso showed that suppressive treatment for herpes in HIV infected women reduced plasma HIV viral load and vaginal shedding.[85]

Herpes in pregnancy

Transmission from mother to child occurs in 50% of cases with a primary attack at term, is much lower in patients with recurrences (about 1%) and occasionally occurs as a result of asymptomatic viral shedding by the mother at term. Neonatal herpes carries a 60% mortality, which has changed little with the introduction of aciclovir. The presence of first-episode herpetic lesions of the cervix at term is an indication for caesarean section, although this operation does not fully protect against infection developing in the neonate. Aciclovir can be used in late pregnancy to reduce viral shedding among women recently diagnosed with herpes and as an alternative to caesarean for women who fear having a recurrence at term.

Genital warts

Epidemiology

In developed countries, genital infection with the human papillomavirus (HPV) is the most common viral STI and is four times as frequent as genital herpes. Using the most sensitive diagnostic methods infection can be demonstrated in as many as 40% of sexually active women.[86] In the tropics, HPV infections are common and cervical carcinoma is one of the commonest cancers of women.

Aetiology

Genital warts are caused by HPVs. The types most prevalent in genital lesions are designated HPV-6, -11 and -16. Of these, HPV-16 has been particularly associated with the development of cancer of the cervix, while HPV-6 and -11 have a lower potential for causing neoplasia and are more closely associated with exophytic (as opposed to flat) lesions and, rarely, with the development of respiratory papillomas in children born to infected mothers.

Pathology

The virus infects the basal layer of differentiating squamous epithelium and produces a pathognomonic large, clear, perinuclear zone known as koilocytotic atypia. Full assembly of viral particles is confined to the more superficial layers of the epithelium. HPV is very strongly implicated in the causation of cancer of the cervix.[87]

Clinical

The lesions produced by HPV vary from the well-known soft, fleshy, vascular condylomata acuminata with their frond-like appearance (Figure 21.21) to papular warts which resemble those seen on other parts of the body, pigmented and non-pigmented papules and leucoplakia. Warts may sometimes grow in the urethra. Recent research has shown that many patients have subclinical HPV infections that can only be visualized by colposcopy after application of 5% acetic acid or detected in tissue specimens by techniques such as PCR. In pregnancy, in immunosuppressed patients and in the presence of genital discharges there is a tendency for warts to grow rapidly. The lesions showing the greatest similarity to genital warts are lesions of molluscum contagiosum, condylomata lata of secondary syphilis, and anal skin tags.

Diagnosis and management

Biopsy confirmation of the diagnosis of condylomata acuminata warts is optional but cervical cytology, where available, is recommended for female patients and female contacts in order to detect progression of lesions to cervical intraepithelial neoplasia. Treat-

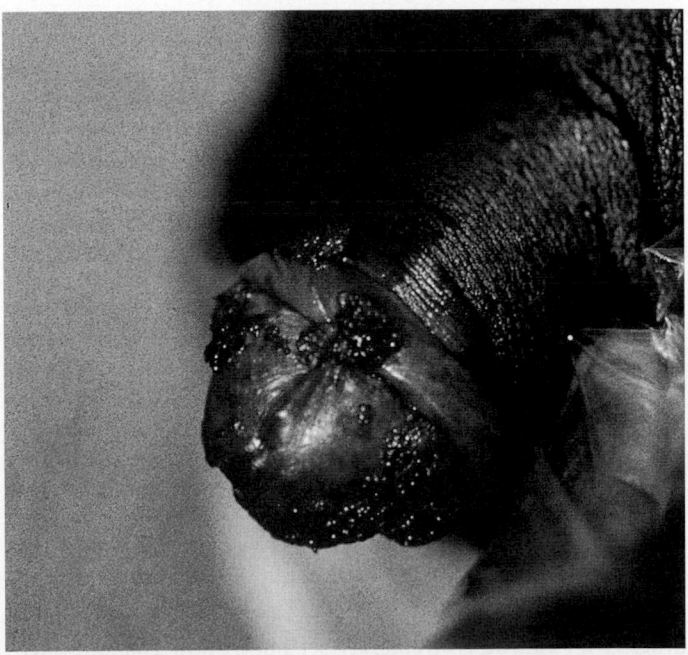

Figure 21.21 Genital warts: condylomata acuminata caused by human papillomavirus.

ment is generally reserved for macroscopic lesions because sub-clinical infections show high spontaneous regression rates and also show a strong tendency to relapse with currently available forms of treatment. Specific treatment for warts includes treatment with trichloroacetic acid and the traditional application of 20% podo-phyllin (maximum 0.5 mL) once or twice weekly.[88] Cure rates with podophyllin, at <50%, are not very satisfactory. Care is needed to avoid burning normal skin, which can be protected with glycerine. Podophyllin should be washed off after 4 h and is contraindicated in pregnant women. Larger warts can be removed with cryotherapy or diathermy. More modern treatments include the application of 5-fluorouracil cream, self-treatment with podophyllotoxin or imiquimod, and carbon dioxide laser treatment. Relapse rates of the order of 30% are seen with all forms of treatment.

The advent of highly effective vaccines against HPV[89] has raised the prospect of bringing cervical carcinoma under control across the world.[90]

THE MANAGEMENT OF STI CONTROL PROGRAMMES

The important components of an STI control programme are: (1) gathering of information, e.g. STI morbidity surveillance, special surveys on the aetiology of genital ulcer in a particular area, data on antibiotic sensitivities of local strains of *Neisseria gonorrhoeae* and *Haemophilus ducreyi*; (2) provision of management guidelines; (3) training programmes; (4) provision of healthcare to patients with STIs wherever they may present; (5) coordinated programmes of education about STIs for patients and the general public; and (6) management and supervision of the programme. Each of these will be discussed in more detail.

Information gathering

Morbidity surveillance in the tropics is often incomplete and unreliable. Given the rudimentary facilities available in many centres, it is often best to record numbers of patients by syndrome (ulcer, discharge, etc.) rather than by specific diagnosis. Good reporting from a few representative sentinel sites may be more useful than unreliable reports collated from the whole country. When possible, special surveys should be undertaken periodically, such as studies of the prevalence of gonorrhoea, chlamydial infection and syphilis in antenatal mothers. Statistics on ophthalmia neonatorum, congenital syphilis, PID, ectopic pregnancy and infertility may be useful for impressing upon health planners the full extent of STI morbidity.

Standard management guidelines for STIs

When a reasonable amount of information is available about the picture of STIs in a country and the antibiotic sensitivity patterns of local isolates, it is possible to draw up rational guidelines for local use, based on those recommended by the WHO.[14] These guidelines can be tailored to different levels of the health system according to the availability of supporting laboratory tests and drugs. They can be conveniently set out as flow charts or algorithms in pocket manuals which are supplied to all health workers who need to manage STIs. In view of the constantly changing

pattern of antibiotic sensitivities of *N. gonorrhoea* and *H. ducreyi*, it is important that guidelines are reviewed and revised at 3–4-yearly intervals.

Training

The high incidence of STIs in tropical populations makes it important for all health workers to acquire the basic skills to manage patients appropriately according to standard guidelines, to prevent ophthalmia neonatorum and congenital syphilis, and to promote the following health education messages which are important in STI prevention:
- reduction of the number of sexual partners
- avoidance of sex with high-risk partners
- use of condoms for protection against STIs
- knowledge of the symptoms, sequelae and transmissibility of STIs
- avoidance of sexual contact when symptoms are present
- knowledge of what AIDS is and how HIV is transmitted
- obtaining proper treatment promptly for STI symptoms
- ensuring that the patients' contacts are treated whether they have symptoms or not.

Provision of services for patients with STIs

The aim should be to maximize coverage and access of STI services for men and women and to have a way of referring problem cases. Costs to patients should be kept as low as possible and confidentiality safeguarded. Specialist STI clinics are valuable where the volume of patients is high, but in general, the provision of specialist clinics for the treatment of STIs, which has been successful in controlling these diseases in certain industrialized countries, is neither appropriate nor feasible in most developing countries, where patients with STIs should be managed at the primary healthcare level. Family planning and antenatal clinics provide opportunities for STI control activities which tend to be underutilized at present.

Education programmes

The appropriate content for education messages has been described above. These messages must be expressed in a sensitive manner after widespread consultation and careful pre-testing before they are disseminated by health workers, through posters and by the media. It is particularly important to target schoolchildren, sex workers and patients attending for treatment of STIs. Interest has recently focused on the use of peer educators to encourage people to listen to health messages. Condom promotion is of particular importance and the social marketing of condoms has shown promise in some countries.

Supervision and management of STI control

It is important for programmes of STI and AIDS control to be fully integrated because of their many shared objectives. The delegation of much routine STI treatment and control to the primary healthcare level is unlikely to succeed, unless the morale and commitment of healthcare workers responsible for treating patients with STIs are maintained by regular supportive visits by programme managers.

FURTHER READING

Holmes KK, Mårdh PA, Sparling PF, et al., eds. *Sexually Transmitted Diseases*. 4th edn. New York: McGraw-Hill; 2007.

Schulz KF, Cates W Jr, O'Mara PR. Pregnancy loss, infant death, and suffering: legacy of syphilis and gonorrhoea in Africa. *Genitourin Med* 1987; 63:320–325.

MMWR. 2006 Guidelines for Treatment of Sexually Transmitted Diseases Treatment. *Morbidity and Mortality Weekly Report* 2006; 55(RR11):1–94.

REFERENCES

1. Dallabetta G, Laga M, Lamptey P. *Control and Prevention of Sexually Transmitted Diseases: A Handbook for Design and Management of Programs*. Arlington: AIDSCAP/Family Health International; 2006.

2. Rottingen JA, Cameron DW, Garnett GP. A systematic review of the epidemiologic interactions between classic sexually transmitted diseases and HIV – How much really is known? *Sex Transm Dis* 2001; 28(10):579–597.

3. Mullick S, Watson-Jones D, Beksinska M, et al. Sexually transmitted infections in pregnancy: prevalence, impact on pregnancy outcomes, and approach to treatment in developing countries. *Sex Transm Infect* 2005; 81(4):294–302.

4. Wawer MJ, Sewankambo NK, Serwadda D, et al. Control of sexually transmitted diseases for AIDS prevention in Uganda: a randomised community trial. *Lancet* 1999; 353(9152):525–535.

5. Muir DG, Belsey MA. Pelvic inflammatory disease and its consequences in the developing world. *Am J Obstet Gynecol* 1980; 138(7):913–928.

6. Larsen U. Primary and secondary infertility in sub-Saharan Africa. *Int J Epidemiol* 2000; 29(2):285–291.

7. Hira SK, Bhat GJ, Patel JB, et al. Early congenital syphilis – clinico-radiologic features in 202 patients. *Sex Transm Dis* 1985; 12(4):177–183.

8. Watson-Jones D, Changalucha J, Gumodoka B, et al. Syphilis in pregnancy in Tanzania. I. Impact of maternal syphilis on outcome of pregnancy. *J Infect Dis* 2002; 186(7):940–947.

9. Blankenship KM, Friedman SR, Dworkin S, et al. Structural interventions: Concepts, challenges and opportunities for research. *J Ur Health-Bull NY Acad Med* 2006; 83(1):59–72.

10. Hayes RJ, Schulz KF, Plummer FA. The cofactor effect of genital ulcers on the per-exposure risk of HIV transmission in sub-Saharan Africa. *J Trop Med Hyg* 1995; 98(1):1–8.

11. Cohen MS, Hoffman IF, Royce RA, et al. Reduction of concentration of HIV-1, in semen after treatment of urethritis: Implications for prevention of sexual transmission of HIV-1. *Lancet* 1997; 349(9069):1868–1873.

12. Grosskurth H, Mosha F, Todd J, et al. Impact of improved treatment of sexually-transmitted diseases on HIV-infection in rural Tanzania – randomized controlled trial. *Lancet* 1995; 346(8974):530–536.

13. French P. Consultations requiring sexual history taking. British Association for Sexual Health and HIV 2006 National Guidelines 2007. Online. Available: *http://www.bashh.org/guidelines/2007/sexual_history_taking_0107.pdf* 6 Feb 2007.

14. Guidelines for the Management of Sexually Transmitted Infections. World Health Organization 2003. Online. Available: *http://www.emro.who.int/aiecf/web79.pdf*

15. Mayaud P, Mabey DCW. Managing sexually transmitted diseases in the tropics: is a laboratory really needed? *Trop Doc* 2000; 30(1):42–46.

16. Pepin J, Sobela F, Deslandes S, et al. Etiology of urethral discharge in West Africa: the role of Mycoplasma genitalium and Trichomonas vaginalis. *Bull WHO* 2001; 79(2):118–126.

17. Wikstrom A, Jensen JS. Mycoplasma genitalium: a common cause of persistent urethritis among men treated with doxycycline. *Sex Transm Infect* 2006; 82(4):276–279.

18. Morency P, Dubois MJ, Gresenguet G, et al. Aetiology of urethral discharge in Bangui, Central African Republic. *Sex Transm Infect* 2001; 77(2):125–129.

19. Ross JDC, Jensen JS. Mycoplasma genitalium as a sexually transmitted infection: implications for screening, testing, and treatment. *Sex Transm Infect* 2006; 82(4):269–271.

20. Bradshaw CS, Tabrizi SN, Read TRH, et al. Etiologies of nongonococcal urethritis: Bacteria, viruses, and the association with orogenital exposure. *J Infect Dis* 2006; 193(3):336–345.

21. Grosskurth H, Mayaud P, Mosha F, et al. Asymptomatic gonorrhoea and chlamydial infection in rural Tanzanian men. *Br Med J* 1996; 312(7026):277–280.

22. Pelouze PS. *Gonorrhoea in the Male and Female*. Philadelphia: WB Saunders; 1941.

23. Bewes PC. Urethroplasty for Stricture. *Trop Doc* 1986; 16(3):121–128.

24. Osegbe DN, Amaku EO. Gonococcal Strictures in Young-Patients. *Urology* 1981; 18(1):37–41.

25. Collet M, Reniers J, Frost E, et al. Infertility in Central-Africa – Infection is the cause. *Int J Gynecol Obstet* 1988; 26(3):423–428.

26. Elliott B, Brunham RC, Laga M, et al. Maternal gonococcal infection as a preventable risk factor for low-birth-weight. *J Infect Dis* 1990; 161(3):531–536.

27. Plummer FA, Laga M, Brunham RC, et al. Postpartum upper genital-tract infections in Nairobi, Kenya – epidemiology, etiology and risk-factors. *J Infect Dis* 1987; 156(1):92–98.

28. Stein CM, Hanly MG. Acute tropical polyarthritis in Zimbabwe – a prospective search for a gonococcal etiology. *Annals Rheum Dis* 1987; 46(12):912–914.

29. Kestelyn P, Bogaerts J, Meheus A. Gonorrheal keratoconjunctivitis in African Adults. *Sex Transm Dis* 1987; 14(4):191–194.

30. Laga M, Plummer FA, Piot P, et al. Prophylaxis of gonococcal and chlamydial ophthalmia neonatorum – a comparison of silver-nitrate and tetracycline. *N Engl J Med* 1988; 318(11):653–657.

31. Ison CA, Dillon JR, Tapsall JW. The epidemiology of global antibiotic resistance among Neisseria gonorrhoeae and Haemophilus ducreyi. *Lancet* 1998; 351:8–11.

32. Isenberg SJ, Apt L, Wood M. A controlled trial of povidone-iodine as prophylaxis against ophthalmia neonatorum. *N Engl J Med* 1995; 332(9):562–566.

33. Bignell C, Ison CA, Jungmann E. Testing guidelines for gonorrhoea. *Sex Transm Infect* 2006; 82(suppl 4):iv6–iv9.

34. Lyss SB, Kamb ML, Peterman TA, et al. Chlamydia trachomatis among patients infected with and treated for Neisseria gonorrhoeae in sexually transmitted disease clinics in the United States. *Annals Intern Med* 2003; 139(3):178–185.

35. Garnett GP, Bowden FJ. Epidemiology and control of curable sexually transmitted diseases – Opportunities and problems. *Sex Transm Dis* 2000; 27(10):588–599.

36. Wang SP, Grayston JT. Human Serology in Chlamydia-Trachomatis Infection with Microimmunofluorescence. *J Infect Dis* 1974; 130(4):388–397.

37. Peeling RW, Kimani J, Plummer F, et al. Antibody to Chlamydial hsp60 predicts an increased risk for chlamydial pelvic inflammatory disease. *J Infect Dis* 1997; 175(5):1153–1158.

38. Westrom L, Mardh PA. Chlamydial salpingitis. *Br Med Bull* 1983; 39(2):145–150.

39. Beem MO, Saxon EM. Respiratory-tract colonization and a distinctive pneumonia syndrome in infants infected with chlamydia-trachomatis. *N Engl J Med* 1977; 296(6):306–310.

40. Watson EJ, Templeton A, Russell I, et al. The accuracy and efficacy of screening tests for Chlamydia trachomatis: a systematic review. *J Med Microbiol* 2002; 51(12):1021–1031.

41. Lau CY, Qureshi AK. Azithromycin versus doxycycline for genital chlamydial infections – A meta-analysis of randomized clinical trials. *Sex Transm Dis* 2002; 29(9):497–502.

42. Watson-Jones D, Mugeye K, Mayaud P, et al. High prevalence of trichomoniasis in rural men in Mwanza, Tanzania: results from a population based study. *Sex Transm Infect* 2000; 76(5):355–362.

43. Wolnerhanssen P, Krieger JN, Stevens CE, et al. Clinical manifestations of vaginal trichomoniasis. *JAMA* 1989; 261(4):571–576.

44. Hillier SL, Nugent RP, Eschenbach DA, et al. Association between bacterial vaginosis and preterm delivery of a low-birth-weight infant. *N Engl J Med* 1995; 333(26):1737–1742.

45. Nugent RP, Krohn MA, Hillier SL. Reliability of diagnosing bacterial vaginosis is improved by a standardized method of Gram stain interpretation. *J Clin Microbiol* 1991; 29(2):297–301.

46. Ison CA, Hay PE. Validation of a simplified grading of Gram stained vaginal smears for use in genitourinary medicine clinics. *Sex Transm Infect* 2002; 78(6):413–415.

47. Hammond GW, Slutchuk M, Scatliff J, et al. Epidemiologic, clinical, laboratory, and therapeutic features of an urban outbreak of chancroid in North-America. *Rev Infect Dis* 1980; 2(6):867–879.

48. Morse SA. Chancroid and Hemophilus-Ducreyi. *Clin Microbiol Rev* 1989; 2(2):137–157.

49. O'Farrell N. Increasing prevalence of genital herpes in developing countries: implications for heterosexual HIV transmission and STI control programmes. *Sex Transm Infect* 1999; 75(6):377–384.

50. Plummer FA, Nsanze H, Karasira P, et al. Epidemiology of Chancroid and Hemophilus Ducreyi in Nairobi, Kenya. *Lancet* 1983; 2(8362): 1293–1295.

51. Hart G. Sexual behavior in a war environment. *J Sex Res* 1975; 11(3): 218–226.

52. Cameron DW, Dcosta LJ, Maitha GM, et al. Female to male transmission of human immunodeficiency virus Type-1 – risk-factors for seroconversion in men. *Lancet* 1989; 2(8660):403–407.

53. Plummer FA, Simonsen JN, Cameron DW, et al. Cofactors in male-female sexual transmission of human-immunodeficiency-virus type-1. *J Infect Dis* 1991; 163(2):233–239.

54. Steen R. Eradicating chancroid. *Bull WHO* 2001; 79(9):818–826.

55. Al Tawfiq JA, Thornton AC, Katz BP, et al. Standardization of the experimental model of Haemophilus ducreyi infection in human subjects. *J Infect Dis* 1998; 178(6):1684–1687.

56. Al Tawfiq JA, Fortney KR, Katz BP, et al. An isogenic hemoglobin receptor-deficient mutant of Haemophilus ducreyi is attenuated in the human model of experimental infection. *J Infect Dis* 2000; 181(3):1049–1054.

57. Stevens MK, Latimer JL, Lumbley SR, et al. Characterization of a Haemophilus ducreyi mutant deficient in expression of cytolethal distending toxin. *Infect Immun* 1999; 67(8):3900–3908.

58. Fast MV, Dcosta LJ, Nsanze H, et al. The clinical-diagnosis of genital ulcer disease in men in the tropics. *Sex Transm Dis* 1984; 11(2):72–76.

59. Hudson EH. *Non-venereal syphilis*. Baltimore: Williams and Wilkins; 1958.

60. Wicher K, Wicher V, Abbruscato F, et al. Treponema pallidum subsp pertenue displays pathogenic properties different from those of T-pallidum subsp pallidum. *Infect Immun* 2000; 68(6):3219–3225.

61. Lafond RE, Molini BJ, Van Voorhis WC, et al. Antigenic variation of TprK V regions abrogates specific antibody binding in syphilis. *Infect Immun* 2006; 74(11):6244–6251.

62. Gjestland T. The Oslo study of untreated syphilis. *Acta Derm Venereol Suppl* 1955; 35:1.

63. Ingraham NR. The value of penicillin alone in the prevention and treatment of congenital syphilis. *Acta Derm Venereol* 1951; 31(suppl 24): 60.

64. Young H. Guidelines for serological testing for syphilis. *Sex Transm Infect* 2000; 76(5):403–405.

65. Castro R, Prieto ES, Santo I, et al. Evaluation of an enzyme immunoassay technique for detection of antibodies against Treponema pallidum. *J Clin Microbiol* 2003; 41(1):250–253.

66. Rolfs RT, Joesoef R, Hendershot EF, et al. A randomized trial of enhanced therapy for early syphilis in patients with and without human immunodeficiency virus infection. *N Engl J Med* 1997; 337(5):307–314.

67. Riedner G, Rusizoka M, Todd J, et al. Single-dose azithromycin versus penicillin G benzathine for the treatment of early syphilis. *N Engl J Med* 2005; 353(12):1236–1244.

68. Holmes KK. Azithromycin versus penicillin for early syphilis – Reply. *N Engl J Med* 2006; 354(2):205.

69. Watson-Jones D, Oliff M, Terris-Prestholt F, et al. Antenatal syphilis screening in sub-Saharan Africa: lessons learned from Tanzania. *Trop Med Int Health* 2005; 10(9):934–943.

70. Van der Bij AK, Spaargaren J, Morre SA, et al. Diagnostic and clinical implications of anorectal lymphogranuloma venereum in men who have sex with men: A retrospective case-control study. *Clin Infect Dis* 2006; 42(2): 186–194.

71. Nieuwenhuis RF, Ossewaarde JM, Gotz HM, et al. Resurgence of lymphogranuloma venereum in western Europe: An outbreak of Chlamydia trachomatis serovar L-2 proctitis in The Netherlands among men who have sex with men. *Clin Infect Dis* 2004; 39(7):996–1003.

72. Sengupta BS. Vulval cancer following or co-existing with chronic granulomatous diseases of vulva – an analysis of its natural-history, clinical manifestation and treatment. *Trop Doc* 1981; 11(3):110–114.

73. Trama JP, Zimmerman JA, Mordechai E, et al. Detection of the Chlamydia trachomatis L serovars that cause lymphogranuloma venereum by real-time PC R. *J Molec Diagnostics* 2006; 8(5):643.

74. Herring A, Richens J. Testing guidelines for Lymphogranuloma venereum. *Sex Transm Infect* 2006; 82(suppl 4):iv23–iv25.

75. Ofarrell N, Hoosen AA, Coetzee KD, et al. Genital Ulcer Disease in Men in Durban, South-Africa. *Genitourinary Med* 1991; 67(4): 327–330.

76. Carter JS, Bowden FJ, Bastian I, et al. Phylogenetic evidence for reclassification of Calymmatobacterium granulomatis as Klebsiella granulomatis comb. nov. *Int J Systemat Bacteriol* 1999; 49:1695–1700.

77. Kharsany AB M, Hoosen AA, Kiepiela P, et al. Growth and cultural characteristics of Calymmatobacterium granulomatis – The aetiological agent of granuloma inguinale (Donovanosis). *J Med Microbiol* 1997; 46(7):579–585.

78. Richens J. The diagnosis and treatment of Donovanosis (Granuloma Inguinale). *Genitourinary Med* 1991; 67(6):441–452.

79. Verdich J. Hemophilus-Ducreyi infection resembling Granuloma Inguinale. *Acta Dermato-Venereologica* 1984; 64(5):452–455.

80. Bowden F. Donovanosis. In: Morse S, Holmes KK, eds. *Atlas of Sexually Transmitted Infections*. London: Mosby-Elsevier; 2003.

81. Bowden FJ, Mein J, Plunkett C, et al. Pilot study of azithromycin in the treatment of genital donovanosis. *Genitourinary Med* 1996; 72(1): 17–19.

82. Rodriguez MD M, Obasi A, Mosha F, et al. Herpes simplex virus type 2 infection increases HIV incidence: a prospective study in rural Tanzania. *AIDS* 2002; 16(3):451–462.

83. Reeves WC, Corey L, Adams HG, et al. Risk of recurrence after 1st episodes of genital herpes – relation to Hsv type and antibody-response. *N Engl J Med* 1981; 305(6):315–319.

84. Wald A, Zeh J, Barnum G, et al. Suppression of subclinical shedding of herpes simplex virus type 2 with acyclovir. *Annals Internal Med* 1996; 124(1):8–15.

85. Nagot N, Ouedraogo A, Foulongne V, et al. Reduction of HIV-1 RNA levels with therapy to suppress herpes simplex virus. *N Engl J Med* 2007; 356(8): 16–25.

86. Rando RF. Human papillomavirus – implications for clinical medicine. *Annals Internal Med* 1988; 108(4):628–630.

87. Sherman ME, Lorincz AT, Scott DR, et al. Baseline cytology, human papillomavirus testing, and risk for cervical neoplasia: A 10-year cohort analysis. *J Nat Canc Inst* 2003; 95(1):46–52.

88. Maw R. Critical appraisal of commonly used treatment for genital warts. *Int J Std Aids* 2004; 15(6):357–364.

89. Koutsky LA, Ault KA, Wheeler CM, et al. A controlled trial of a human papillomavirus type 16 vaccine. *N Engl J Med* 2002; 347(21): 1645–1651.

90. Kane MA, Sherris J, Coursaget P, et al. HPV vaccine use in the developing world. *Vaccine* 2006; 24:132–139.

Chapter 22   Adewale O. Adebajo

Musculoskeletal Diseases

There is a continuing recognition of the importance of musculoskeletal disorders in the tropics. Not only are these conditions associated with considerable morbidity and even mortality in the tropics, much of it is preventable. In addition, the study of these disorders in the tropics, can provide useful aetiopathogenetic clues.[1]

Musculoskeletal diseases are those disorders which affect muscles, tendons, ligaments, joints, the connective tissues and even bone. Unsurprisingly, many of these disorders in the tropics are of infectious origin. In addition, possibly due to factors such as increasing life expectancy and increasing adoption of western lifestyle and diet, even non-infectious musculoskeletal disorders such as gout, osteoarthritis, systemic lupus erythematosus and rheumatoid arthritis are being recognized as important socioeconomic problems in the tropics.[1,2]

DISEASES OF SKELETAL MUSCLE, TENDONS AND LIGAMENTS

Primary diseases of skeletal muscle are uncommon in the tropics. Muscle disorders are more commonly seen in association with another pathology, such as prolonged corticosteroids given therapeutically, endocrine disorders such as thyrotoxicosis, and in association with neoplasms such as hepatoma. The low prevalence of polymyalgia rheumatica in the tropics is of interest and remains unexplained.[3]

Polymyositis

Although this inflammatory disorder is uncommon in the tropics, it does occur.[3,4] Classical acute phase proteins, electromyographic and muscle biopsy changes are found. However, elevated serum creatinine kinase levels may occur in healthy black males[5] and must be interpreted with caution.

Infective pyomyositis

Pyomyositis is an acute inflammation of skeletal muscle mainly confined to the subtropics and tropics.[6,7] It occurs at any age but most frequently in children and young male adults. The initiating lesion may be a penetrating injury or crush injury, or it may be secondary to staphylococcal arthritis. Staphylococcus pyogenes is the usual infecting organism. It is possible that pyomyositis arises when the staphylococcus reaches a muscle recently damaged by a viral myositis, but malnutrition and various parasitic infections have also been implicated.

Muscular pain is usually the first symptom, followed within the next week by fever, localized induration and oedema. Any muscle group may be affected but most commonly the proximal limb muscles (gluteal and quadriceps) are involved. The erector spinae and shoulder girdle muscles can also be affected. The clinical features are those of a localized abscess with mild to moderate systemic features. If untreated, the condition will progress over subsequent weeks until there is extensive muscle destruction. Pus can often be aspirated from 10 days onwards. Occasionally, the systemic picture predominates and multiple muscle abscesses occur as a late finding. The more acute presentation and occurrence at peripheral sites make clinical differentiation from acute haematogenous osteomyelitis more difficult. There is often a minor degree of polymorphonuclear leucocytosis, and a moderate eosinophilia of about 10% is common.

Treatment involves the administration of an adequate dose of an appropriate antibiotic effective against penicillinase-producing organisms, given parenterally at least initially. Treatment for several weeks is often required and surgical drainage of fluctuant abscesses should be carried out. Despite the destruction of a large muscle bulk, functional and cosmetic recovery is usually remarkably good.

Parasitic pyomyositis

Several parasites can give rise to a myositis.[7] Trypanosomiasis causes an acute myositis, often with encephalomyelitis and myocarditis. The same is true of filariasis.

Soft tissue disorders

Diseases involving the musculoskeletal soft tissues (tendons and ligaments) present clinically in a manner identical to that found in the West. In contrast, however, patients with these problems in the tropics do not usually seek medical attention, as observed with shoulder lesions.[8] Similarly, back pain is very prevalent in the

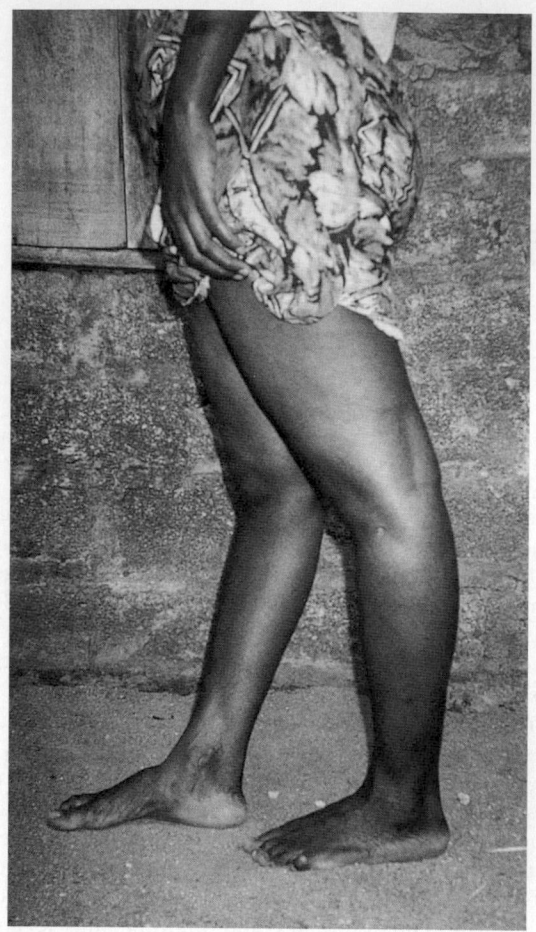

Figure 22.1 Hyperextensibility (hypermobility) of the knee in an African woman.

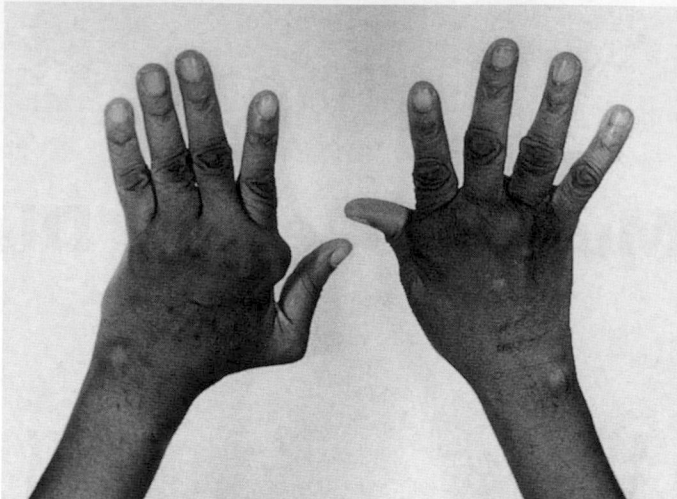

Figure 22.2 Hand deformity in an African woman with rheumatoid arthritis.

tropics, often in association with manual work. The fact that health insurance schemes and compensation claims for injuries are uncommon in many tropical countries may be one reason why only a small proportion of back pain sufferers seek medical attention. These various reasons might also explain why chronic widespread soft tissue pain (fibromyalgia) is less common in the tropics than the West, even when the same ethnic group is compared.[9]

Hypermobility

Hypermobility is due to laxity of the ligaments surrounding a joint as a result of genetic and/or environmental causes (Figure 22.1). Studies on hypermobility indicate that African populations have a higher prevalence of hypermobility than Caucasians, although this prevalence may be lower than amongst populations from the Indian subcontinent.[10,11]

DISEASES OF JOINTS

Diseases of joints form the bulk of the musculoskeletal disorders and particularly those seen in hospital clinics. Arthralgia refers to significant joint pain occurring in the total or virtual absence of any physical signs. Arthritis, on the other hand, refers to an inflammatory process of the joint lining, with the classical features of redness, warmth, swelling and limitation of function in addition to joint pain. Arthralgia occurs commonly in association with infectious diseases such as those due to arboviruses. Arthritis can be involved in a number of infective, immunological and metabolic conditions. Treatment usually involves the use of analgesics, non-steroidal antiinflammatory drugs, physiotherapy and, where appropriate, second-line or disease-modifying drugs. Public health measures such as improved sanitation can help in reducing the incidence of infective arthritis.[12]

Rheumatoid arthritis

Rheumatoid arthritis remains the most studied rheumatic disorder in the tropics. The disorder is a chronic inflammatory deforming and destructive polyarthritis usually affecting joints, often in a peripheral and symmetrical manner (Figure 22.2). In addition, it is a systemic disease affecting various organs and body systems. Rheumatoid factor autoantibodies are frequently found on serological testing although anti-cyclic citrullinated peptide antibodies are now considered more sensitive and specific.[13] Erosive changes are the hallmark of rheumatoid arthritis radiologically. The disorder is a relatively recent condition on the African continent.[14] The cause of this disease is unknown but there is a strong genetic association with the DR4 haplotype. Environmental factors may also be important.[14–17] There is some evidence to suggest that the disease is more prevalent in urban than rural areas.[16,17] In Southeast Asia and India, the disease appears to be slightly less prevalent than in the West and to follow a milder course, with systemic manifestations and subcutaneous nodules occurring rarely.[18] Interestingly, although the prevalence is seen to be less, morbidity and mortality are higher in South-east Asia, possibly due to socioeconomic conditions. In Jamaica there is a high prevalence of the disease but it is mainly mild and rheumatoid factor seronegative.[19] In East Africa and among urban but not rural black South Africans rheumatoid arthritis has a similar pattern to that in Caucasian

Table 22.1 Use of drugs for rheumatoid arthritis in the tropics

Drug	Potential problems
Chloroquine and hydroxychloroquine	Encourages malaria drug resistance
Sulfasalazine	High prevalence of glucose-6-phosphatase dehydrogenase deficiency in parts of the tropics
Methotrexate	Infection due to immunosuppression
Gold	Complicating infections due to regular injections
Ciclosporin	Infection due to immunosuppression and high cost
Leflunomide	High cost
Anti-TNF biological agents (e.g. Etanercept)	High cost and high infection risk
Prednisolone	Steroid side-effects

Table 22.2 Hip and knee joint involvement in Nigerian and British patients with osteoarthritis

Patients	Hip (%)	Knee (%)
Nigerian (Adebajo 1991)[35]	1.4	47.0
British (Cushnaghan and Dieppe 1991)[38]	19.0	41.2

From Cushnaghan & Dieppe, Study of 500 patients with limb joint osteoarthritis, 1. Analysis by age, sex and distribution of systematic joint sites. Ann Rheum Dis 1991; 50:8–13.

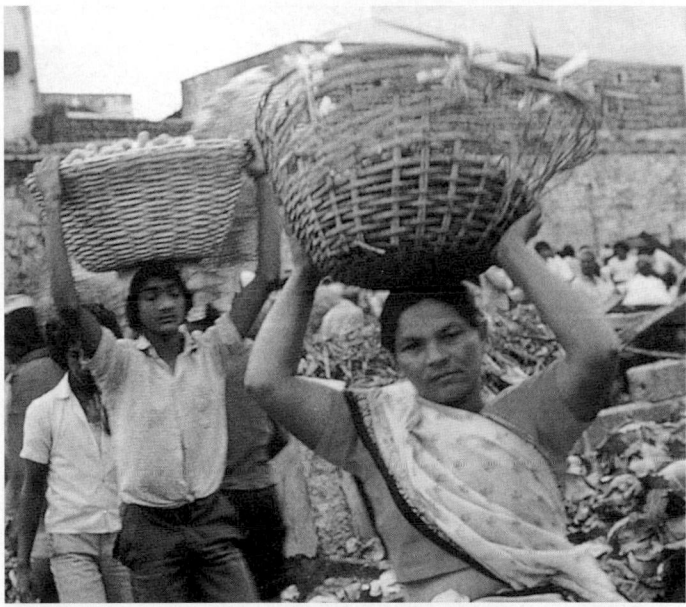

Figure 22.3 Carrying loads on the head is common in the tropics but is not associated with cervical spondylosis in the general population.

populations.[16,17,20,21] In West Africa, however, the disease is less common and milder.[22,23] A similar pattern has been found in some studies conducted in China.[24,25] The treatment of rheumatoid arthritis involves the use of second-line antirheumatoid drugs (Table 22.1). Adequate monitoring of any of these second-line antirheumatoid drugs can be difficult in many parts of the tropics and low-dose oral steroids are often the most pragmatic form of treatment. The importance of a multidisciplinary approach to treatment, involving physiotherapists, occupational therapists, nurses and others cannot be overemphasized.[26]

Spondyloarthropathies

Spondyloarthropathies such as ankylosing spondylitis are uncommon in Africans[27] and in the Middle East,[28] in keeping with the low prevalence of HLA-B27 in these areas. Ankylosing spondylitis is less common in the Chinese than in white populations[29] but its prevalence may be higher in rural parts of China.[24] Ankylosing spondylitis is characterized by limited spinal movement and sacroiliac joint tenderness. Peripheral joint involvement can also occur, particularly of lower limb joints. Radiologically, squaring of the vertebral bodies and ossification of the disc margins and longitudinal spinal ligaments resulting in a 'bamboo' spine as well as features of sacroiliitis are classically seen. Physiotherapy and nonsteroidal antiinflammatory drugs are the mainstay of treatment.

Reactive arthritis in general is common throughout the tropics and can be due to a number of organisms. It is commonly associated with Chlamydia trachomatis or enteric bacteria, such as *Shigella*, *Yersinia* and *Salmonella*. By definition, the organism is not found in the joint in reactive arthritis, unlike septic arthritis. Recent molecular techniques, such as polymerase chain reaction (PCR) are enabling particles from organisms to be identified even in reactive arthritis, thereby blurring the distinction between this and septic arthritis. Reiter's syndrome, comprising the triad of urethritis, conjunctivitis and arthritis, occurs predominantly after venereal disease in Africa and in Papua New Guinea.[30-32] Other seronegative arthropathies such as enteric associated arthritis (associated with Crohn's disease and ulcerative colitis), psoriatic arthritis and Behçet's disease are uncommon in the tropics.

Osteoarthritis

Osteoarthritis is a progressive joint disease characterized by destruction of articular cartilage and the generation of osteophytes. Osteoarthritis may be mono-, oligo- or polyarticular in joint distribution. Polyarticular disease is uncommon in many parts of the tropics.[33-35] Heberden's nodes (osteophytes involving the distal interphalangeal joints) are uncommon in Africans and Jamaicans.[36,37] Osteoarthritis of the hip joint is uncommon, in contrast with osteoarthritis of the knee (Table 22.2),[34,38] among Chinese,[39,40] Africans,[35,41] Indians[42] and in the Middle East.[28] Various sociocultural activities including squatting and kneeling, either in prayer or as a form of greeting, have been suggested as influencing this distribution of osteoarthritis. Developmental knee abnormalities from rickets, trauma or parasitic infections and a low prevalence of congenital hip abnormalities in many parts of the tropics may also determine the joint distribution. Interestingly, the habit of carrying loads on the head by some populations does not seem to predispose to cervical spondylosis (Figure 22.3). Increasing life expectancy in many parts of the tropics appears to be associated with an increase in the prevalence of osteoarthritis, with a concomitant increased demand for joint replacement surgery. Although joint replacement surgery has been shown to significantly improve the quality of life for appropriate patients, there are still major difficulties of availability of joint prostheses, cost and postoperative care in the tropics.[43]

An interesting degenerative arthropathy known as Mseleni's disease has been observed in southern Africa and was first described in 1970.[44,45] It is believed to be an unusual form of bone dysplasia and resembles dysplasia epiphysealis multiplex. A nutritional deficiency or toxin has been postulated to be the cause of this condition, although no environmental factor has as yet been identified. The disorder commonly affects females before the age of 40 years and most frequently involves the hip joint, although other joints – particularly the knees and ankles – can be affected. Laboratory investigations are usually normal. Radiological changes resemble osteoarthritis and, in addition, protrusio acetabuli with deformity and medial subluxation of the femoral head may be seen in the hip joints (Figures 22.4, 22.5). The clinical course is that of a slowly progressive disability and the treatment is as for osteoarthritis.

Arthritis of bacterial origin (septic arthritis)

Various organisms can give rise to septic arthritis. An acute pyogenic joint infection is one of the most common causes of joint disease in the tropics. It is commonly due to *Staphylococcus aureus*, although the source of the primary infection may not be evident. The hip joints are most commonly affected in infants and the knee joint in older children and adults.[46] Both healthy and previously damaged joints may be affected.

Salmonella joint infections are also common, particularly in those with sickle cell disease. Meningococcal arthritis can occur either as a localized suppurative arthritis or as generalized polyarthritis. Occasionally, the synovial fluid of affected joints may be sterile, indicating that immune complexes could play a large part in the pathogenesis of the disease.[47] Treatment of septic arthritis is a medical emergency involving initially broad-spectrum antibiotics until the specific antibiotic to which the organism is sensitive is known. Where significant pus is present, surgical drainage is recommended. Early intervention helps to prevent joint destruction.

Gonococcal arthritis can occur following spread of *Neisseria gonorrhoea* from the urogenital tract. It may mimic Reiter's syndrome (Figure 22.6) but, unlike the latter, the organism may be isolated from the synovial fluid on light microscopy and the condition responds to penicillin.

Tuberculosis remains an important cause of arthritis. It may affect any joint, particularly the hip or the knee, but is usually

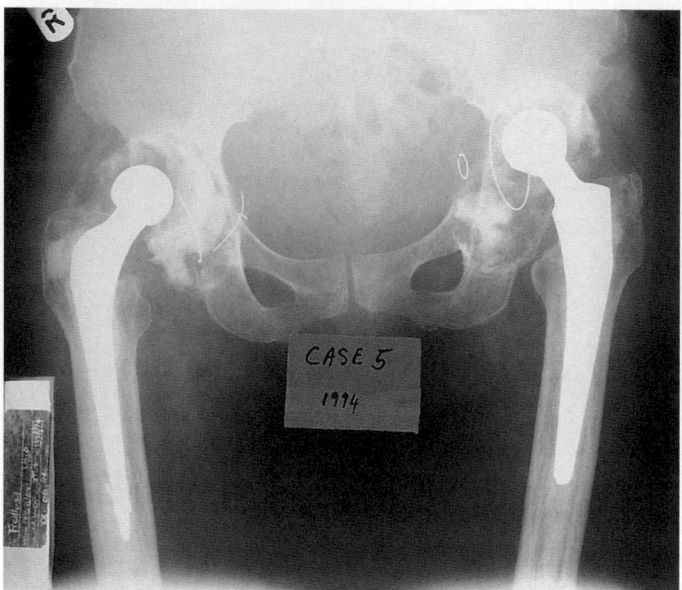

Figure 22.4 Hip joints of a man with Mseleni's disease after joint replacement surgery.

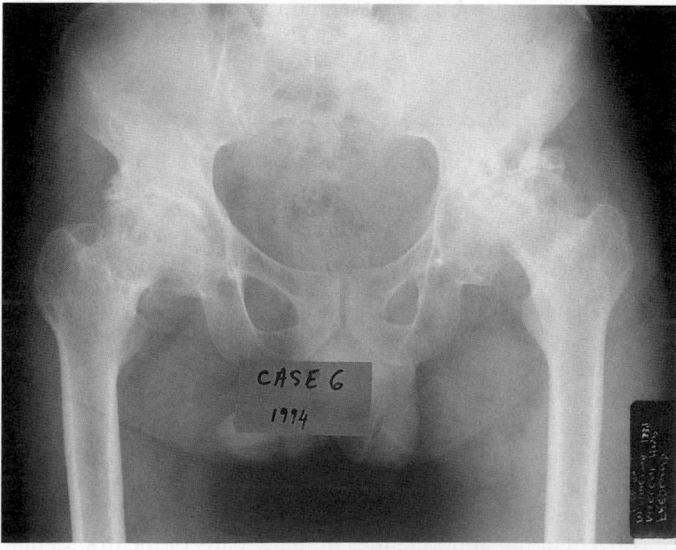

Figure 22.5 Hip joints of a man with Mseleni's disease before joint replacement surgery.

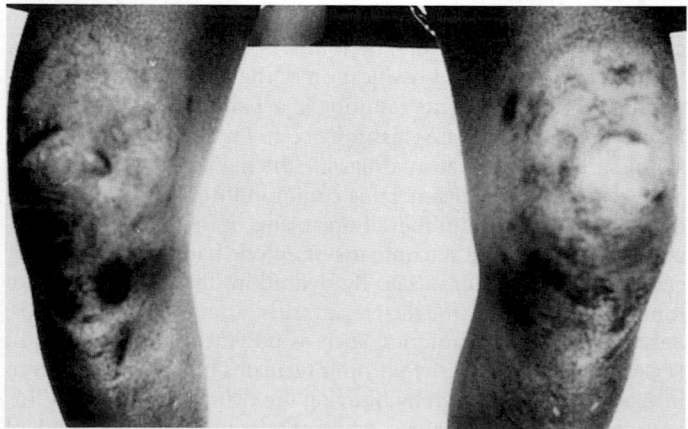

Figure 22.6 Left knee swelling in a young man with Reiter's syndrome.

monoarticular. There may also be other evidence of tuberculosis but diagnosis is often difficult and may require synovial biopsy. Once the diagnosis of tuberculosis has been made or there is a high index of suspicion, aggressive and appropriate antituberculosis therapy should be instituted. Surgical drainage and even excisional arthroplasty may be required.

Brucellosis occurs either as a local suppurative arthritis or a generalized non-suppurative polyarthritis in many parts of the tropics. Pastoral and nomadic populations are at particular risk.[48,49] As with spinal brucellosis and as with all forms of septic arthritis, treatment comprises appropriate antibiotics and adequate drainage.

Arthritis of viral origin

Arthralgia or arthritis can occur with most viral infections. In addition to such viruses as the hepatitis B virus, the arboviruses are particularly important as a cause of arthritis in the tropics (Table 22.3). The arboviral infections include o'nyong-nyong, Sindbis, chikungunya, dengue, Mayaro and yellow fever, among others.[50–54]

Table 22.3 Infectious agents particularly associated with rheumatic disorders in the tropics

VIRUSES
O'nyong-nyong
Dengue
Chikungunya
Hepatitis B
Yellow fever
Human immunodeficiency virus (HIV)
Sindbis
Ross river
SPIROCHAETES
Yaws
Syphilis
BACTERIA
Staphylococcus spp.
Salmonella spp.
Neisseria gonorrhoeae
Brucella spp.
PARASITES
Malaria
Schistosomiasis
Dracontiasis
Filariasis
Amoebiasis
FUNGI
Histoplasmosis
Madura foot

In general, these infections cause fever, a maculopapular or erythematous rash as well as arthralgia or arthritis. Diagnosis is usually made by identifying raised viral titres. Although in a few cases chronic arthralgia or arthritis may persist, the prognosis is usually good and analgesics are the mainstay of treatment. The need for awareness of these conditions, and in particular chikungunya, has recently been emphasized.[50]

Arthritis of parasitic and fungal origin

Various parasitic infections may be associated with arthritis, or more commonly arthralgia. Malaria is one of the most common causes of polyarthralgia in the tropics. Arthralgia and backache may occur as an extraintestinal symptom of amoebic dysentery and may even be a predominant symptom. Dracontiasis, schistosomiasis and filariasis have all been associated with joint problems. Usually there is arthralgia; however, arthritis may occur and the adult worm or larval form may be recovered from the joint fluid. Thus, in general, joint problems in association with these parasites may be due to several possibilities. The arthritis may be due to the invasion of the joint space by the parasite and in some cases discharge of larvae into the joint space, causing an inflammatory synovial fluid with microfilariae and eosinophilia. The arthritis may also be reactive, secondary to the localization of the parasite in surrounding tissues. Septic arthritis can occur due to secondary bacterial infection, as can happen with *Staphylococcus* complicating Guinea worm infestation. Onchocerciasis can be associated with disabling back pain.

Fungal infection due to *Histoplasma duboisii* as well as Madura foot may be associated with a periarthritis and even erosive changes.

With all of these parasitic infections, treatment generally comprises symptomatic treatment with non-steroidal antiinflammatory drugs and the use of the appropriate antiparasitic agent.

Acute tropical polyarthritis

Acute or idiopathic tropical polyarthritis is a condition which has generated considerable interest, as it is still uncertain as to whether it is a homogeneous entity. The declining frequency with which this diagnosis is being made would suggest that the entity is a diagnostic waste-paper basket for acute arthritis associated with unknown or undiagnosed tropical infections.[55–57] The condition appears to affect young adults of both sexes and usually involves large joints. Constitutional features including fever may be present and the erythrocyte sedimentation rate is raised. The white cell count, joint radiographs and synovial fluid analysis are normal. Spontaneous resolution of the condition commonly occurs and treatment is symptomatic.

Crystal arthropathies

Hyperuricaemia and gout are common in some Polynesian islands.[58] There is evidence that in some tropical countries gout is associated with urbanization, although both rich and poor may be affected.[59–61] Gout commonly affects the metatarsophalangeal joint of the large toe. Other joints that may be involved include the ankles, knees and small hand joints. Occasionally, polyarticular gout occurs which can mimic rheumatoid arthritis. Affected joints are acutely inflamed and very tender. Acute attacks may be precipitated by trauma or heavy drinking and thus may recur. Urate deposition into tissues leads to subcutaneous tophi, which is the hallmark of chronic gout. Other complications such as renal stones may also occur. In addition to these clinical features, the diagnosis is made by a raised serum uric acid level and evidence of uric acid crystals in synovial fluid. Radiographs may show areas of bone destruction around affected joints. Unfortunately, diagnostic delays frequently occur in the tropics. Colchicine or nonsteroidal antiinflammatory drugs are useful for acute attacks, while xanthine oxidase inhibitors such as allopurinol, which reduce uric acid synthesis, are used to lower the serum uric acid level and thereby prevent further acute gouty attacks.[59]

Chondrocalcinosis or pseudo-gout differs from gout in that calcium pyrophosphate crystals rather than uric acid crystals are deposited in the synovium and tissues. Pseudo-gout has been reported from the tropics.[62]

CONNECTIVE TISSUE DISORDERS

Connective tissue disorders such as systemic lupus erythematosus (a syndrome characterized by vasculitis, photosensitive skin rash, fever, nephritis and neuropsychiatric disturbances, in association with antinuclear antibodies) are not common in Africa.[63,64] Systemic lupus erythematosus is, however, common in China,[29] Malaysia,[65] India,[66] Puerto Rico[67] and the West Indies.[68] In Malaysia those of Chinese ethnic origin seem to be more vulnerable to systemic lupus erythematosus than Malays or those of Indian origin.[65,69] It has been suggested that tropical infections such as malaria may protect Africans against connective tissue diseases,[70] perhaps mediated through tumour necrosis factor.[64,71] This hypothesis has recently been developed further through the theory that implicates nitric oxide, of which there are abnormally high levels in malaria-parasitized, asymptomatic individuals (malaria tolerant). Increased nitrous oxide is then protective by minimizing proliferation of autoreactive T cells. This is in contrast to Africans living in the West, who do not have parasite-induced nitrous oxide protection.[72] A simple alternative explanation is that systemic lupus erythematosus and other connective tissue diseases are still being underdiagnosed in the tropics, at least in part due to the immunodiagnostic tests required. Diseases like tuberculosis may also mimic some of these connective tissue disorders.[63] Another problem is that autoantibodies that are usually found in patients with systemic lupus erythematosus may also occur in association with various tropical infections.[73] Malaria and tuberculosis, in particular, have been associated with a range of autoantibodies (Table 22.4), but not double stranded autoantibodies or extractable nuclear antigens.

Other connective tissue disorders such as scleroderma, systemic sclerosis, mixed connective tissue disease and vasculitides such as polyarteritis nodosa have all been reported from the tropics.[20,74–76]

Childhood arthropathies

Rheumatic fever remains an important cause of arthralgia in children, in the tropics.[77] Juvenile arthritis is also becoming increas-

Table 22.4 Autoantibodies associated with malaria and tuberculosis

Autoantibody	Malaria prevalence (%)	Tuberculosis prevalence (%)
Rheumatoid factor	22	20
Antinuclear	30	40
Single-stranded DNA	10	30
Antiphospholipid	35	43
ANCA	<5	<5

From Adebajo et al, Autoantibodies in malaria, tuberculosis and hepatitis B in a West African population. Clin Exp Immunol 1993; 92:73–76

ingly recognized in the tropics[78] as are haemophilia related arthritis,[79] HIV associated arthritis[78] and systemic lupus erythematosus[80] in children.

DISEASES OF BONE

Infections are the most common form of bone disease in the tropics but bone tumours, particularly Burkitt's lymphoma, are also found. Sickle cell disease can be complicated by bone lesions in those parts of the tropics where the disease occurs (mainly West Africa and the Caribbean). Rickets is still common in many parts of the tropics, but other metabolic bone diseases are less frequently seen. Congenital lesions of bone are rare.

Infective disease of bone

As with infective diseases of joints, many different organisms may be responsible. Acute osteomyelitis is commonly seen with or without any obvious focus of infection, such as skin sepsis. In patients with sickle cell disease, *Salmonella* organisms are common pathogens.[46] A chronic infection may develop with the formation of a sequestrum of dead bone, which can act as a nidus for the systemic spread of organisms. Acute infections are treated with antibiotics and drainage, while chronic infections often require prolonged antibiotics and excision of dead bone.

Tuberculosis can affect virtually any bone of the body. Tuberculosis of the vertebrae (Pott's disease) is a common problem in the tropics. The infection occurs most commonly in the thoracic spine, leading to vertebral collapse with a kyphosis. The spinal cord may be affected as a result of direct pressure of inflammatory tissue, or more commonly by occlusion of nutrient arteries. A paravertebral abscess may track around the abdominal or thoracic wall or in front of the psoas muscle to point in the groin as a psoas abscess. Spinal tuberculosis can be treated on an outpatient basis with antituberculous chemotherapy and, for the few cases where indicated, anterior decompression and fusion.[81]

Osteoarticular brucellosis is a major health problem in South America, the Middle East and the Mediterranean, reflecting the continued existence of the natural reservoir in animals in these regions for the coccobacillus *Brucella*. Humans are secondarily infected through the consumption of contaminated milk. *Brucella*

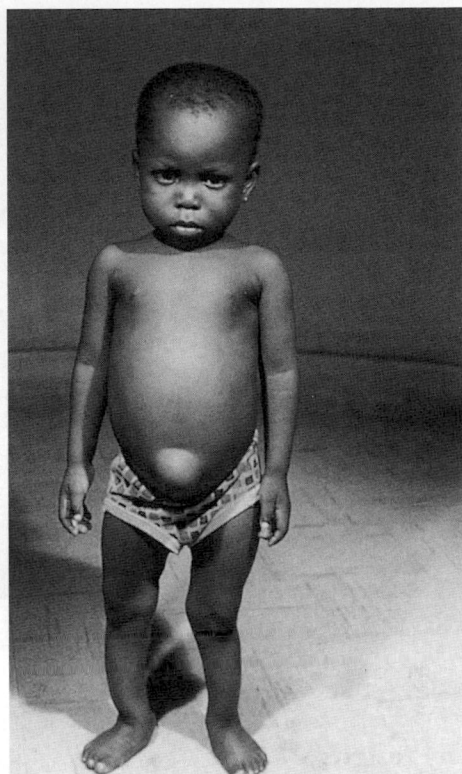

Figure 22.8   Child with rickets showing limb deformities.

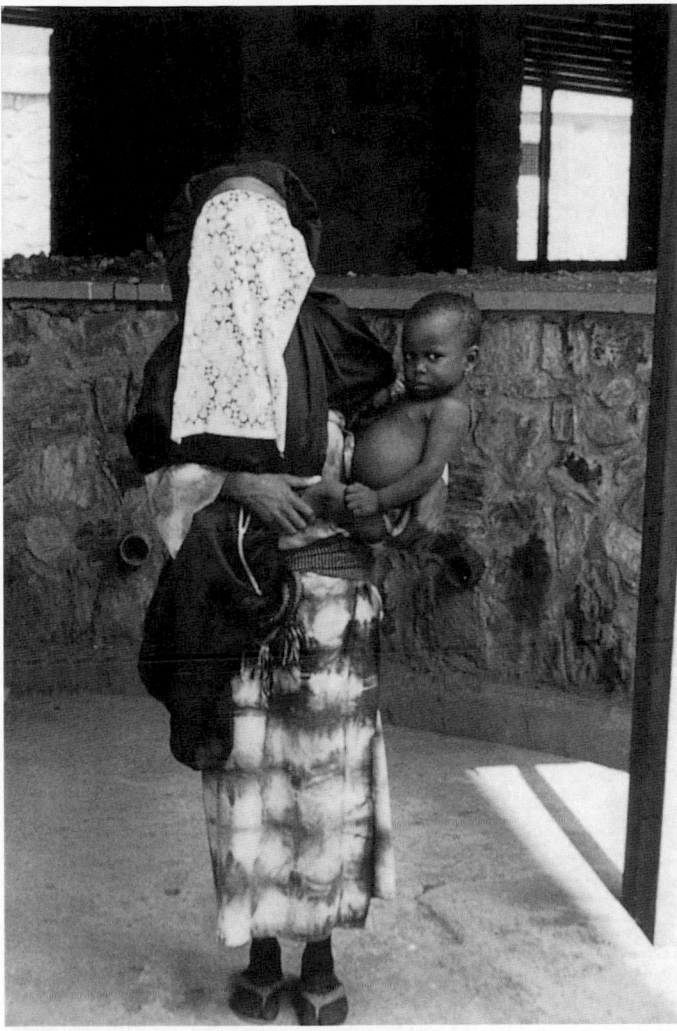

Figure 22.7   A mother in purdah; her child has rickets.

infection occurs most frequently in the lumbar spine but spinal cord damage is uncommon. Large peripheral joint articular pain, often with sterile effusions, is also frequently found. Radiographs show osteolytic lesions with new bone formation. Diagnosis is difficult but brucellosis should be considered in a patient with severe backache and radiological signs of bone destruction.[82] Treatment is with appropriate antibiotics, for example tetracycline or doxycycline for 6 weeks.

Arthritis is a common feature of leprosy, with joint symptoms present in up to 75% of patients. Direct joint infection causes joint destruction, possibly worsened by co-existing peripheral neuropathy. Joint inflammation representing a reactive arthritis may occur with *Mycobacterium leprae* not being present in the joints. The polyarthritis can mimic erosive rheumatoid and can become chronic, with predilection for hands and wrists.[83]

Bone tumours

Primary tumours of bone are uncommon, although osteogenic sarcomas may mimic acute osteomyelitis. Secondary deposits often arise from lymphomas or hepatocellular carcinomas.

Metabolic bone disease

Rickets remains a common problem in the tropics and is sometimes related to a poor diet as well as the wearing of purdah by mothers, which may lead to calcium deficiency in their babies (Figures 22.7–22.9).

Blount's disease occurs in parts of the tropics, mainly among blacks,[84] and is an osteochondrosis affecting the medial tibial physis, causing tibia vara. Treatment is by tibial osteotomy.

Osteoporosis and associated fractures are uncommon in many parts of the tropics,[85,86] possibly due to protection by both genetic and sociocultural factors – in particular exercise. A change in the incidence of osteoporosis in the tropics is likely, with increasing life expectancy.

Other metabolic bone diseases such as marble bone disease and Paget's disease appear to be uncommon in most parts of the tropics.

Haemoglobinopathies

Apart from osteomyelitis, bone lesions associated with haemoglobinopathies include bone crises as a result of infarction of bone(s), as well as bossing of the skull, biconcave vertebrae and dactylitis. Osteonecrosis or avascular necrosis of the bone epiphysis usually presents as a monoarthritis mainly affecting the hip, knee or shoulders and is especially seen in patients with haemoglobin SC or SS disease. Surgical intervention is occasionally required in addition to medical management.[43]

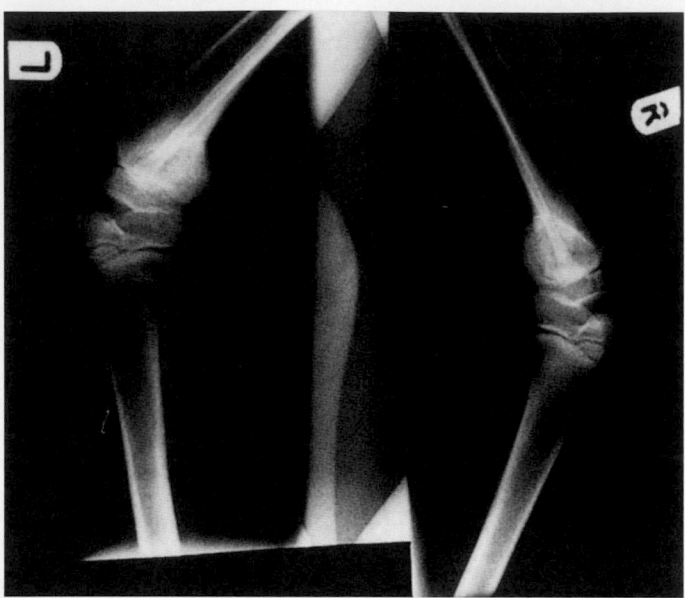

Figure 22.9 Radiograph of a child with rickets.

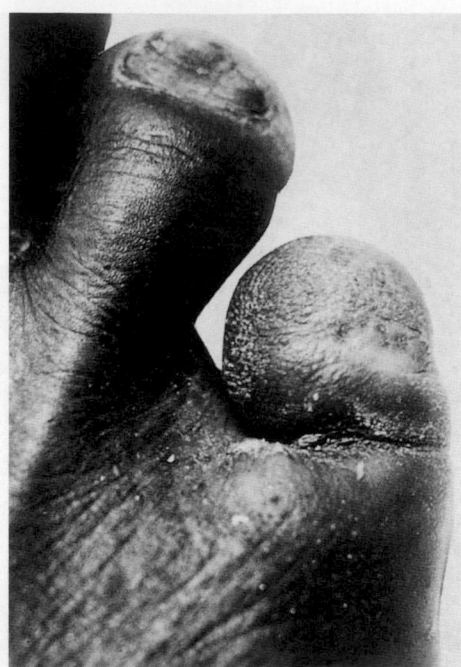

Figure 22.10 Ainhum at its height. (Courtesy of W. M. Meyers.)

Other bony lesions

Hypertrophic osteoarthropathy can occur in association with infections such as suppurative lung disease, or malignancy such as lung carcinoma.

Ainhum is a condition in which a stricture slowly develops between the fifth toe and the foot, leading to spontaneous amputation. It has its highest incidence in Africa, especially among women of the Transkei in South Africa,[87] but also occurs in people of African descent in the New World, Polynesians and Indians.[88] The aetiology is obscure and is considered as being due to abnormal fibrogenesis, angiodysplasia or a common toxic cause (possibly of plant origin) for both ainhum and phocomelia.[87,88] It is most common in people who walk barefoot. Clinically, there is a slow development of a constriction encircling the little toe at the level of the metatarsophalangeal joint(s). Pain may occur and the distal portion of the toe may swell. After some years the toe may remain attached to the foot by a fragile cutaneous pedicle only, and at this stage spontaneous or deliberate amputation usually occurs (Figures 22.10, 22.11). There is no proven treatment for the condition but when troublesome the affected toe should be amputated.

Transkei foot is a disorder consisting of marked lateral deviation of the fifth toe; it has been described in the Xhosa population of the Transkei and is possibly of genetic origin.[89]

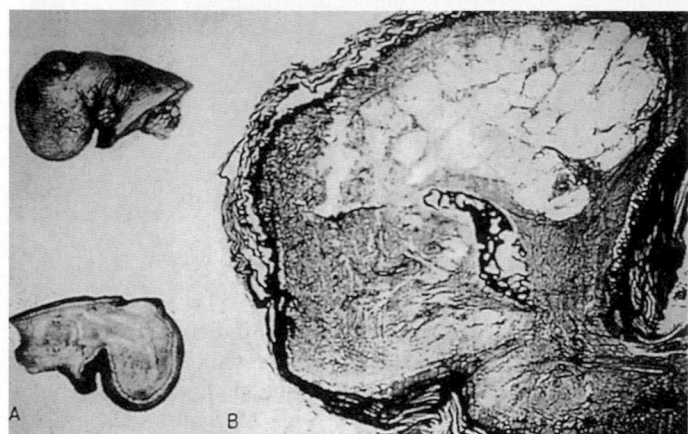

Figure 22.11 An amputated toe from a patient suffering from ainhum, showing constriction at the base. (Courtesy of B. H. Kean.)

REFERENCES

1. Muirden KD. Community oriented program for the control of rheumatic diseases: studies of rheumatic diseases in the developing world. *Curr Opinion Rheumatol* 2005; 17:153–156.
2. Rkain H, Allali F, Jroundi I, et al. Socioeconomic impact of rheumatoid arthritis in Morocco. *Revue du Rhumatisme* 2006; 73:278–283.
3. Stein M, Davis P. Rheumatic disorders in Zimbabwe: a prospective analysis of patients attending a rheumatic diseases clinic. *Ann Rheum Dis* 1990; 40:400–402.
4. Gelfand M, Taube F. Polymyositis in the African. *J Trop Med Hyg* 1966; 69:232–235.
5. Worrall JG, Phongsathorn V, Hooper RJL, et al. Racial variation in serum creatinine kinase unrelated to lean body mass. *Br J Rheumatol* 1990; 29: 371–373.
6. Levin MJ, Gardner P, Waldevogel FA. Tropical pyomyositis. *N Engl J Med* 1971; 284:196–198.
7. Chiedozi LC. Polymyositis: review of 205 cases in 112 patients. *Am J Surg* 1979; 137:255.

8. Adebajo AO, Hazleman BL. Soft tissue shoulder lesions in the African. *Br J Rheumatol* 1992; 31:275–276.

9. Njobvu P, Hunt I, Pope D, et al. Pain among ethnic minority groups of Pakistani Muslim origin in the UK: a review. *Rheumatology* 1999; 38: 1184–1187.

10. Beighton P, Solomon L, Seskilne CL. Articular mobility in an African population. *Ann Rheum Dis* 1973; 32:413–418.

11. Birrell F, Adebajo AO, Hazleman BL, et al. *Br J Rheumatol* 1994; 33:56–59.

12. Ashbolt NJ. Microbial contamination of drinking water and disease outcomes in developing regions. *Toxicology* 2004; 198:229–238.

13. Avouac J, Gossec L, Dougados M. Diagnostic and predictive value of anti-citrullinated protein antibodies in rheumatoid arthritis: a systematic literature review. *Ann Rheum Dis* 2006; 845:851.

14. Adebajo AO. Rheumatoid arthritis: a twentieth century disease in Africa. *Arthritis Rheum* 1991; 34:248.

15. Adebajo AO. Is rheumatoid arthritis an infectious disease? *BMJ* 1991; 303:786.

16. Solomon L, Robin G, Valkenburg HA. Rheumatoid arthritis in an urban South African negro population. *Ann Rheum Dis* 1975; 34:128–135.

17. Beighton P, Solomon L, Valkenburg HA. Rheumatoid arthritis in a rural South African negro population. *Ann Rheum Dis* 1975; 34:136–141.

18. Chopra A, Raghunath D, Singh A, et al. The pattern of rheumatoid arthritis in the Indian population: a prospective study. *Br J Rheumatol* 1988; 27:454–456.

19. Lawrence JS, Brenner JM, Bull JA, et al. Rheumatoid arthritis in a subtropical population. *Ann Rheum Dis* 1966; 25:59–66.

20. Lutalo SK. Chronic inflammatory rheumatic diseases in black Zimbabweans. *Ann Rheum Dis* 1985; 44:121–125.

21. Kalla AA, Tikly M. Rheumatoid arthritis in the developing world. *Best Pract Res Clin Rheum* 2003; 17:863–875.

22. Greenwood BM. Polyarthritis in Western Nigeria. I. Rheumatoid arthritis. *Ann Rheum Dis* 1969; 28:488–496.

23. Adebajo AO, Reid DM. The pattern of rheumatoid arthritis in West Africa and comparison with a cohort of British patients. *Q J Med* 1991; 292: 633–640.

24. Beasley P, Bennett PH, Lin CC. Low prevalence of rheumatoid arthritis in Chinese. *J Rheumatol* 1983; 10(suppl):11–15.

25. Moran H, Chen Shun-le, Muirden KD, et al. A comparison of rheumatoid arthritis in Australia and China. *Ann Rheum Dis* 1986; 45:572–578.

26. Solomon A, Christian BF, Dessein PH, et al. The need for tighter rheumatoid arthritis control in a South African public health care center. *Semin Arth Rheum* 2005; 35:122–131.

27. Chalmers IM. Ankylosing spondylitis in African blacks. *Arthritis Rheum* 1980; 23:1366–1370.

28. Rajapakse CN. The spectrum of rheumatic diseases in Saudi Arabia. *Br J Rheumatol* 1987; 26:22–23.

29. Chang NC. Rheumatic diseases in China. *J Rheumatol* 1983; 10(suppl): 41–45.

30. Maddocks I. Reiter's syndrome in Port Moresby Papua. *Br J Vener Dis* 1967; 43:280–283.

31. Hall L. Polyarthritis in Kenya. *East Afr Med J* 1966; 43:161–170.

32. Csonka GW. The course of Reiter's syndrome. *BMJ* 1958; i:1088–1090.

33. Bremner JM, Lawrence JS, Miall WE. Degenerative joint disease in a Jamaican rural population. *Ann Rheum Dis* 1968; 27:326–332.

34. Brighton SW, de la Harper AL, van Staden DA. The prevalence of osteoarthrosis in a rural African community. *Br J Rheumatol* 1985; 24: 321–325.

35. Adebajo AO. The pattern of osteoarthritis in a West African teaching hospital. *Ann Rheum Dis* 1991; 50:20–22.

36. Lawrence JS, Molyneux M. Degenerative joint disease among populations in Wensleydale, England and Jamaica. *Int J Biometeorol* 1968; 12:163–175.

37. Solomon L, Beighton P, Lawrence JS. Osteoarthrosis in a rural South African population. *Ann Rheum Dis* 1976; 35:274–278.

38. Cushnaghan J, Dieppe P. Study of 500 patients with limb joint osteoarthritis. I. Analysis by age, sex and distribution of symptomatic joint sites. *Ann Rheum Dis* 1991; 50:8–13.

39. Hoagkund FT, Yau A, Wong WL. Osteoarthritis of the hip and other joints in Southern Chinese in Hong Kong: incidence and related factors. *J Bone Joint Surg (Am)* 1973; 55:545–547.

40. Gunn DR. Don't sit-squat! *Clin Orthop* 1974; 103:104–105.

41. Solomon L. Pathogenesis of osteoarthritis. *Lancet* 1972; i:1072.

42. Mukhopadhaya B, Barooak B. Osteoarthritis of the hip in Indians: an anatomical and clinical study. *Indian J Orthop* 1967; 1:55–63.

43. Alonge TO, Shokunbi WA. The choice of arthroplasty for secondary osteoarthritis of the hip joint following avascular necrosis of the femoral head in sicklers. *J Nat Med Assoc* 2004; 96:678–681.

44. Wittman W, Fellingham SA. Mseleni. Unusual hip disease in remote parts of Zululand. *Lancet* 1970; 1:842–843.

45. Yach D, Botha JL. Mseleni joint disease in 1981: decreased prevalence rates, wider geographical location than before, and socioeconomic impact of an endemic osteoarthrosis in an underdeveloped community in South Africa. *Int J Epidemiol* 1985; 14:276–284.

46. Onyemelukwe G, Sturrock RD. Septic arthritis in Northern Nigeria. *Rheumatol Rehabil* 1979; 18:13–17.

47. Greenwood BM, Mohammed I, Whittle HC. Immune complexes and the pathogenesis of meningococcal arthritis. *Clin Exp Immunol* 1985; 59: 513–519.

48. Manson-Bahr PEC. Clinical aspects of brucellosis in East Africa. *J Trop Med Hyg* 1955; 59:103–106.

49. Ali-Rawi ZS, Al-Khateeb N, Khalifa SJ. Brucella arthritis among Iraqi patients. *Br J Rheumatol* 1987; 26:24–27.

50. Volpe A, Caramaschi P, Angheben A, et al. Chikungunya outbreak – remember the arthropathy. *Rheumatology* 2006; 45:1449–1450.

51. Nimmannitya S, Halstead SB, Cohen SN, et al. Dengue and chikungunya virus infection in man in Thailand. *Am J Trop Med* 1969; 17:107–111.

52. Adebajo AO. Dengue arthritis. *Br J Rheumatol* 1996; 35:909–910.

53. Haddow AJ, Ellice JM. Studies on bush-babies (Galago spp) with special reference to the epidemiology of yellow fever. *Trans R Soc Trop Med Hyg* 1964; 58:521–538.

54. Causey OR, Madbouly HM, Kemp GE, et al. Arbovirus surveillance in Nigeria, 1964–1967. *Bull Soc Pathol Exot* 1969; 62:249–259.

55. Editorial. Acute tropical polyarthropathy: homogeneous entity or diagnostic scrap heap? *Lancet* 1988; i:627–628.

56. Adebajo AO. Tropical polyarthritis. *Lancet* 1988; i:1103–1104.

57. Stein CM. Tropical polyarthritis. *Lancet* 1988; i:1103.

58. Prior IAM, Rose BS, Harvey HPB, et al. Hyperuricaemia, gout and diabetic abnormality in Polynesian people. *Lancet* 1966; i:333–338.

59. Darmawan J, Rasker JJ, Nuralim H. The effect of control and self-medication of chronic gout in a developing country. Outcome after 10 years. *J Rheumatol* 2003; 30:2437–2443.

60. Fleischmann V, Adadevoh BK. Hyperuricaemia and gout in Nigerians. *Trop Geogr Med* 1973; 25:255–261.

61. Mody GM, Naidoo PD. Gout in South African Blacks. *Ann Rheum Dis* 1984; 43:394–397.

62. Bejia I, Rtibi I, Touzi M, et al. Familial calcium pyrophosphate dihydrate deposition disease. A Tunisian kindred. *Joint, Bone, Spine* 2004; 71: 401–408.

63. Taylor HG, Stein CM. Systemic lupus erythematosus in Zimbabwe. *Ann Rheum Dis* 1986; 45:645–648.

64. Adebajo AO. Does tumour necrosis factor protect against lupus in West Africans? *Arthritis Rheum* 1992; 35:839–840.

65. Frank AO. Apparent predisposition to systemic lupus erythematosus in Chinese patients in West Malaysia. *Ann Rheum Dis* 1980; 39:266–269.

66. Malaviya A, Misra R, Banerjee S, et al. Systemic lupus erythematosus in Indian Asians: a prospective analysis of clinical and immunological features. *Rheumatol Int* 1986; 6:97–101.

67. Mendez-Bryan R, Gonsalez-Alcover R, Roger L. Rheumatoid arthritis: prevalence in a tropical area. *Arthritis Rheum* 1964; 7:171–176.

68. Harris EN, Williams E, Shah DJ, et al. Mortality of Jamaican patients with systemic lupus erythematosus. *Br J Rheumatol* 1989; 28:113–117.

69. Veerapen K, Wong F, Bosco J, et al. Systemic lupus erythematosus (SLE): a profile of 419 patients from Malaysia. *Br J Rheumatol* 1988; 27:40.

70. Greenwood BM, Herrick EM, Voller A. Can parasitic infection suppress autoimmune disease? *Proc Soc Med* 1970; 63:19–20.

71. Adebajo AO. Low frequency of autoimmune disease in tropical Africa. *Lancet* 1997; 349:361–362.

72. Clark IA, Al-Yaman FM, Cowden WB, et al. Does malaria tolerance, through nitric oxide explain the low incidence of autoimmune disease in Tropical Africa? *Lancet* 1996; 348:1492–1494.

73. Adebajo AO, Charles P, Maini RN, et al. Autoantibodies in malaria, tuberculosis and hepatitis B in a West African population. *Clin Exp Immunol* 1993; 92:73–76.

74. Buchanan WM, Gelfand M. Polyarteritis nodosa in the African. *Cent Afr J Med* 1970; 16:274–275.

75. Greenwood BM. Autoimmune disease and parasitic infections in Nigerians. *Lancet* 1968; ii:380–381.

76. Davis P, Stein M, Ley H, et al. Serological profiles in connective tissue diseases in Zimbabwean patients. *Ann Rheum Dis* 1989; 48:73–76.

77. Khriesat I, Najada A, Al-Hakim F, et al. Acute rheumatic fever in Jordanian children. *East Mediterr Health J* 2003; 9:981–987.

78. Chinniah K, Mody GM, Bhimma R, et al. Arthritis in association with human immunodeficiency virus infection in Black African children: causal or coincidental? *Rheumatology* 2005; 7:915–920.

79. Rodriguez-Merchan EC, Heim M. Haemophilia orthopedic management with emphasis on developing countries. *Sem Thrombosis Hemostasis* 2005; 31: 518–526.

80. Balkaran BL, Roberts LA, Ramcharan J. Systemic lupus erythematosus in Trinidadian children. *Ann Trop Paed* 2004; 24:241–244.

81. Abou-Raya S, Abou-Raya A. Spinal tuberculosis: overlooked? *J Intern Med* 2006; 260:160–163.

82. Rajapakse CN A, Al-Aska AK, Al Orainey I, et al. Spinal brucellosis. *Br J Rheumatol* 1987; 26:28–31.

83. Gibson T, Ahsan Q, Hussein K. Arthritis of leprosy. *Br J Rheumatol* 1994; 33:963–966.

84. Golding JS R, McNeil-Smith JD G. Observations on the etiology of tibia vara. *J Bone Joint Surg (Br)* 1963; 45:320–325.

85. Adebajo AO, Cooper C, Grimley Evans J. Fractures of the hip and distal forearm in West Africa and the United Kingdom. *Age Ageing* 1991; 20: 435–438.

86. Solomon L. Osteoporosis and fracture of the femoral neck in the South African Bantu. *J Bone Joint Surg (Br)* 1968; 50:2–13.

87. Daynes WE S. Ainhum: its possible causation by ingestion of plants. *S Afr Med J* 1973; 47:320–321.

88. Browne SG. Ainhum: a clinical and etiological study of 83 cases. *Ann Trop Med Parasitol* 1961; 55:314–320.

89. Schwartz PA, Shlugman D, Daynes G, et al. Transkei foot. *S Afr Med J* 1974; 48:961–962.

Chapter 23

Bernard J. Brabin, Stephen Owens
and James E. G. Bunn

Paediatrics in the Tropics

More than 10 million children younger than 5 years die every year and most deaths are due to preventable diseases: diarrhoea, pneumonia, measles, and vaccine preventable diseases.[1] Every day, it is estimated 28 000 children die before they reach their fifth birthday. Out of 60 developing countries, which account for 94% of child deaths, 20 have made no progress in reducing deaths among children aged under 5 years. The highest mortality rates are in Africa and South Asia (Table 23.1). Currently available interventions could prevent two-thirds of these deaths and eliminating healthcare coverage inequities is essential to reduce this high mortality. To address this situation, five strategies should be prioritized as recommended by Save the Children Fund.[2]

1. Ensure the well-being of mothers.
2. Invest in basic low cost solutions (breast-feeding, immunization and rehydration therapy, impregnated bednets, antibiotics for neonatal sepsis and pneumonia).
3. Expand availability of healthcare to the poorest (training health workers and providing basic newborn care).
4. Increase use of basic life-saving services.
5. Improve donor support for proven solutions.

The highest risk of death is in the young infant and 4 million babies die in the first few months of life. Neonatal deaths account for 65% of infant deaths in South Asia and approximately half of infant deaths in Africa, reflecting an urgent need for improvement in maternal health as well as health services and delivery systems. Maternal ill health, including malaria in pregnancy, other parasitic diseases, bacterial and viral infections including HIV, severe anaemia secondary to poor nutrition, sickle cell disease, rheumatic heart disease, severe malnutrition, hypertension in pregnancy and diabetes mellitus, contribute to stillbirths, low birth weight, premature birth, congenital infections and poor neonatal and infant outcomes. Adolescent health in girls is a neglected area of concern. It is clear that a very high proportion of girls enter motherhood at a young age, undernourished, undersized, underprivileged and uneducated. To make things worse, health services are often insensitive or unattractive to the adolescent.

AIDS is associated with relatively few deaths globally (3%), but in some countries in sub-Saharan Africa it causes 45–55% of childhood deaths. It was estimated in 2006 that 0.44–0.66 million children were newly infected with HIV, leading to 0.29–0.50 million child deaths. Nearly 90% of children who are born with HIV or infected through breast-feeding are from sub-Saharan Africa, largely as a consequence of high fertility rates, high HIV infection rates in women of the reproductive age group, and limited resources for HIV interventions to prevent mother-to-child transmission. A focus on child mortality should not diminish the need to address health issues related to disability and developmental delay in children who survive. Poor health and social determinants prevent at least 200 million children in low resource settings from achieving their developmental potential.

PERINATAL AND NEONATAL HEALTH

Most mortality and morbidity events in the perinatal and neonatal period are preventable.[3] The causes can be classified as maternal, obstetric, fetal and neonatal. Direct causes of stillbirths include hypoxia during labour, perinatal asphyxia and congenital infections such as syphilis, bacterial sepsis, malaria and HIV. Common fetal neonatal infections include pneumonia, tetanus, sepsis and diarrhoea. Low birth weight (<2500 g) is probably the most important indirect cause of early infant mortality. Other factors relate to poor maternal healthcare during pregnancy, inappropriate management of maternal complications or delivery, and lack of appropriate care for the newborn especially the resuscitation of mildly asphyxiated babies.

Improved perinatal and neonatal health will result from interventions starting with adolescent girls in order to improve the health of future mothers. These should aim to improve nutrition, discourage early marriage, improve female literacy and education and vaccinate girls against tetanus. Improved care of the pregnant woman is essential, including: reduction in anaemia, control of malaria in pregnancy and treatment of syphilis, treating pregnancy complications, e.g. pre-eclampsia, counselling on safe delivery and breast-feeding. The mother–baby package offers a minimum list of essential interventions (Table 23.2). The emphasis for these is on the birth attendant who can ensure carefully monitored deliveries and life-saving interventions.[4] Low-cost technologies for the newborn are especially important in developing countries. One of the cheapest appropriate technologies for low birth weight babies is close skin-to-skin contact with the mother. This is the basis of the kangaroo method, which can help in reducing perinatal mortality. Delayed cord clamping should also be promoted due to its influence in reducing infant anaemia.[5]

Table 23.1 Regional summary of infant and under 5 mortality rates

Region	UNDER 5 MORTALITY RATE (PER 1000 LIVE BIRTHS)			INFANT MORTALITY RATE (PER 1000 LIVE BIRTHS)			TOTAL POPULATION (×1000)	ANNUAL BIRTHS (×1000)
	1960	1998	2004	1960	1998	2004	2004	2004
Sub-Saharan Africa	261	173	171	156	107	102	697 561	28 263
Middle East/North Africa	241	66	56	153	51	44	371 384	9620
South Asia	239	114	92	146	76	67	1 459 305	37 052
East Asia and Pacific	201	50	36	133	38	29	1 937 058	29 932
Latin America/Caribbean	154	39	31	102	32	26	549 273	11 674
CEE/CIS and Baltic States	101	35	38	76	29	37	404 154	5570
Industrialized countries	37	6	6	31	6	5	956 315	10 939
Developing countries	216	95	87	138	64	59	5 166 574	119 663
Least developed countries	282	167	155	172	107	98	741 579	27 823
World	193	86	79	124	59	54	6 374 050	132 950

Source: State of the World's Children 2006, UNICEF, New York.

Table 23.2 Essential interventions for newborn care

At birth	After birth
Safe and clean delivery (hand washing)	Exclusive breast-feeding
Clean delayed cord cutting and tying	Maintain warmth
Dry, wrap and keep warm	Clean cord care
Early exclusive breast-feeding	Hand washing
Extra care if needed for resuscitation	Promote immunization and use of vitamin K
Prophylactic eye care	Recognize danger signs
	Treat infection early

Source: Staneki and Way 1997.

Congenital infections

Infection may be acquired through breast-feeding, poor delivery hygiene, blood transfusion or by the respiratory route from infected personnel in close contact with the infant. Pneumonia contributes to between 750 000 and 1.2 million neonatal deaths, many of which relate to gram-negative infections. For several infections there is a scarcity of information. Congenital syphilis, neonatal tetanus and congenital parasitic infections should be considered. Mother-to-child HIV transmission is discussed elsewhere.

Congenital syphilis

Congenital syphilis is a resurgent problem in tropical countries. Suspicion may arise in high-risk pregnancies, e.g. drug abusers.

Other clues include an unexplained large placenta, unexpected previous abortions and/or stillbirths, and ill-defined rashes or ulcerating lesions at unusual sites such as in the mouth, anus or breast. Most infants present at between 1 and 3 months, with pallor due to haemolysis, hepatosplenomegaly and skin lesions. Such lesions include peeling and involvement of the palms and soles, condylomata lata and perinatal rashes which may resemble a persistent nappy rash. Other features are persistent nasal discharge ('snuffles'), failure to thrive, pseudoparesis of one or more limbs secondary to syphilitic epiphysitis, delayed closure of fontanelles and frontal bossing. Symptomatic newborns are often jaundiced. The diagnosis of overt disease should not present a real diagnostic difficulty if syphilis is borne in mind. Positive serology in the presence of any of the classical clinical manifestations of congenital syphilis is diagnostic. Radiographic examination of the knees and legs will often reveal distinctive syphilitic pathology in children with indefinite clinical signs or who may be suspected on other grounds of having syphilis. This is particularly helpful when reliable serology is not available. When diagnostic laboratory facilities are lacking, as is often the case in the tropics, proof of diagnosis relies on response to treatment. Definitive serological diagnosis is usually based on a positive Venereal Disease Research Laboratory (VDRL) test with persistently high or rising titres or a persistent positive fluorescent antibody absorption test (FTA-ABS).

Penicillin is the drug of choice and is recommended in a dose of 50 000 units/kg of aqueous procaine penicillin, by intramuscular injection, daily for 7–10 days. A large dose of long-acting benzathine penicillin (at least 100 000 units/kg) given once, or preferably twice, a week apart, is recommended when daily treatment is not feasible or patient compliance is suspect. All children with syphilis should be followed to ensure recovery. Persistence of positive serology 6 months after treatment is an indication for a further course of treatment.

Neonatal tetanus

The majority of babies dying of tetanus are born in several high-risk countries (Bangladesh, Ethiopia, India, Nigeria, Pakistan, Somalia, Democratic Republic of Congo). As many as 200 000 newborns die annually from this condition and increased efforts are required for improved control through expanded maternal and adolescent tetanus immunizations and improved hygienic birth practices.

Congenital parasitic infections

Congenital parasitic infections are unusual, except for congenital malaria. Malaria may be symptomatic or asymptomatic, and in a proportion of cases only cord parasitaemia occurs. The risk of congenital symptomatic malaria is low (<1%) in babies born to women living under holoendemic conditions. If symptomatic at birth these babies present with anaemia, jaundice and splenomegaly and the diagnosis is frequently missed. Those with asymptomatic parasitaemia at birth may either suppress this spontaneously, or present with clinical symptoms in the late neonatal period.

Congenital infection with African trypanosomiasis has also been described. These infants may remain asymptomatic until the second year of life when they present with neurological sequelae and illness.[6] Congenital infection with South American trypanosomiasis ranges from 2% to 10% in some areas.

CHILDHOOD INFECTIONS

The current section highlights particular aspects of common infections relevant to their presentation and management in children.

Malaria

Nearly 600 000 children die of malaria each year, most of them in sub-Saharan Africa (see also Chapter 23 and 73). The clinical picture of malaria in children varies with the endemicity of the disease. Where malaria transmission is low or markedly seasonal, severe disease may occur at any age. Under conditions of persistent year-round transmission (stable or holoendemic malaria), severe disease occurs almost exclusively in very young children who, if they survive, develop a high degree of acquired immunity by 5–6 years of age which is sufficient to protect them thereafter from life-threatening malaria. In early infancy, transplacentally acquired maternal malaria antibody provides passive immunity which suppresses, but does not prevent, malarial infection in the infant. Exclusive breast-feeding may protect in a similar way, i.e. not by preventing infection but by reducing parasite density.

In some areas, *P. falciparum* prevalence approaches 100% by 12 months of age. There is a common misapprehension that in such areas clinical manifestations of malaria tend to occur after 6 months of age. This is not true. Life-threatening malaria can occur in infants under 6 months. Cases may present as early as 6 weeks, the incidence increasing gradually thereafter to reach a peak sometime after 6 months. Fever (usually without rigors), cough, vomiting, pallor and convulsions are the well-known presenting symptoms in childhood. Acute haemolytic episodes causing jaundice are unusual. The serious complications seen when severe infections present late include coma, cardiac failure from severe anaemia, haemoglobinuria and its associated renal problems, circulatory collapse, metabolic acidosis and respiratory distress, hypoglycaemia and rarely spontaneous bleeding.[7]

Cerebral malaria

The definition of cerebral malaria in children is the same as in adults: unrousable coma in *P. falciparum* malaria in the absence of an alternative or additional cause for altered consciousness. Peak prevalence occurs at 2–3 years and well-nourished children are more frequently and severely affected than malnourished. The condition is exceptionally rare in kwashiorkor. Clinical history is usually short, i.e. 1–2 days; convulsions preceded by alteration of consciousness and followed by coma is the most common mode of presentation. Headache and fever are common preceding complaints. The age incidence of 'febrile convulsions', which is 6 months to 5 years, overlaps precisely with the age incidence of cerebral malaria in holoendemic malarious areas, and this causes diagnostic difficulties in practice. Rapid recovery of full consciousness within half an hour of a convulsion virtually excludes cerebral malaria in childhood. Children with impaired consciousness or respiratory distress are at the highest risk of death.

A common clinical finding is hepatosplenomegaly, but not infrequently neither organ is enlarged. Opisthotonos may occur and suggests the diagnosis of meningitis or tetanus. Hypoglycaemia occurs quite commonly in young children and may aggravate and prolong coma if unrecognized and uncorrected. In West Africa, a popular traditional remedy for convulsions can cause hypoglycaemia and this is frequently given to children with cerebral malaria. The immediate administration of intravenous glucose is recommended for any child so treated who shows alteration of consciousness.

Case fatality is high (between 10% and 40%), with most deaths occurring within 24 h. Time from starting of treatment to resolution of coma in children is short (1–2 days). If the child recovers, neurological sequelae may occur. Cerebral malaria is the most severe neurological complication of malaria and following appropriate antimalarial therapy up to 11% may have gross neurological deficits on discharge, many of which persist.

The main parasitic causes of childhood fits, other than malaria, are neurocystercosis and toxoplasmosis. Cysticercosis prevalence is probably grossly underestimated in children with epilepsy living in areas with a high pork consumption. Among 88 epileptic patients (>15 years of age) in northern Togo (West Africa), 27 suffered from cysticercosis. Convulsions, intracranial calcification and hydrocephalus in the newborn point to the diagnosis of toxoplasmosis, although congenital cytomegalovirus infection may also be considered. In later childhood, epilepsy, mental retardation, microcephalus and cranial nerve palsies are other sequelae. Other parasitic causes of seizures include echinococcosis, cerebral paragonimiasis, African trypanosomiasis and *Schistosoma japonicum* infection.

Malaria and anaemia

Anaemia is a very frequent and often serious complication of *P. falciparum* malaria in early childhood, and young children are more likely to present with severe anaemia than cerebral malaria. There appears to be an inverse correlation between the degree of anaemia and cerebral involvement, i.e. the greater the degree of anaemia, the less the likelihood of cerebral malaria. The main cause of the anaemia appears to be dyserythropoiesis with a maturation arrest at the normoblast stage in bone marrow. Malarial anaemia responds very well to effective antimalarial treatment, but there is a lag period of 4–5 days before reticulocytosis occurs as a prelude to a rapid steady rise in haemoglobin concentration.

Quartan malaria

In terms of acute sickness, *P. malariae* quartan malaria is the most benign species of human malaria but it has the ability to compromise immune function(s). Quartan malarial nephrotic syndrome is the clinical expression of an immune complex nephritis caused by *P. malariae*, which is possibly the most common cause of chronic parenchymatous renal disease in childhood in the tropics. Patients present with classic signs of nephrotic syndrome such as oedema, massive albuminuria, hypoproteinaemia and hypercholesterolaemia, but with few exceptions do not show a satisfactory response to any form of treatment and eventually die from hypertension and renal failure. The use of corticosteroids in these cases is fraught and is only very rarely beneficial. Prednisolone in the management of this condition is only justified if the patient is under good clinical control that enables early detection of adverse effects and withdrawal of treatment if it is harmful.

Management of severe malaria

The management is similar to that in adults.[7] If a child has a convulsion, this is usually controlled with basic respiratory support, paraldehyde, 0.1–0.2 mL/kg body weight intramuscularly (given in a glass syringe), or a slow intravenous injection of diazepam, 0.15 mg/kg to a maximum of 10 mg. Diazepam, 0.5–1.0 mg/kg, can be given intrarectally if injection is not possible. The choice of antimalarial is the same as for adult malaria but weighing of children is mandatory and the dose of antimalarial should be calculated on a body weight basis. Rectal administration of artemisinin preparations appears to have acceptable therapeutic efficacy. A single rectal dose of artesunate is associated with rapid reduction of parasite density in children with moderately severe malaria. This option is useful for initial treatment if the child is unable to take oral medication, or if parenteral treatment is unavailable.[8] Hypoglycaemia should be treated with an intravenous bolus injection of 50% glucose (up to 1.0 mL/kg body weight), followed by a slow intravenous infusion of 10% glucose to prevent recurrence of hypoglycaemia. Blood transfusion is life-saving in severe malarial anaemia.[9] Respiratory distress is often a manifestation of metabolic acidosis. In children presenting with oliguria and dehydration, careful rehydration with isotonic saline is mandatory, with frequent re-examination of the jugular venous pressure and blood pressure. There is a high concurrence of septicaemia with severe malaria and a diagnosis of meningitis is often difficult to separate from one of cerebral malaria. The empirical use of a broad spectrum antibiotic should be considered in the treatment of severe malaria.

Measles

Measles is a leading cause of deaths in children in developing countries, with an estimated minimum of 350 000 children dying from measles in 2005. It is a disease of the under fives, with many cases in the first year of life and a peak incidence in 2–3 year-old children. The early phases of the disease are the same as classically described. The rash occurs after a prodromal period of 4 days and lasts 5–6 days. A haemorrhagic rash occasionally occurs and carries a poor prognosis. In malnourished children, skin desquamation following the exanthema is usually extensive, severe and prolonged for several weeks (Figure 23.1). Misdiagnosed patients with measles are often admitted to general wards where the disease then spreads to non-immune children with other serious diseases.

Multiple complications often occur. Bronchopneumonia is the most frequent and most important cause of death from measles. Stomatitis and other oral lesions, including cancrum oris (noma), and chronic diarrhoea with fluid and electrolyte disturbances are important complications. Acute measles encephalitis occurs not infrequently and subacute sclerosing panencephalitis occasionally. Activation of primary tuberculosis and miliary or bronchogenic spread are constant risks following measles. Otitis media and skin sepsis are very common, but rarely fatal complications. Chronic otitis may lead to hearing impairment. A necrotizing laryngotracheitis may lead to stridor. Severe measles is more frequent in poorly nourished children and those with HIV infection. All children in developing countries diagnosed with measles should receive 2 doses of vitamin A supplements given 24 h apart. Small frequent feeds are often required, with good attention to oral hygiene to ensure nutrition is maintained. Use antibiotics for clear indications. The current Expanded Programme on Immunization recommendations for increasing coverage remain crucial to improve measles control, and this should be complemented by mass supplemental immunization.[10]

Tuberculosis

In industrialized countries, tuberculosis in children has declined progressively over the decades, although it is still found in immi-

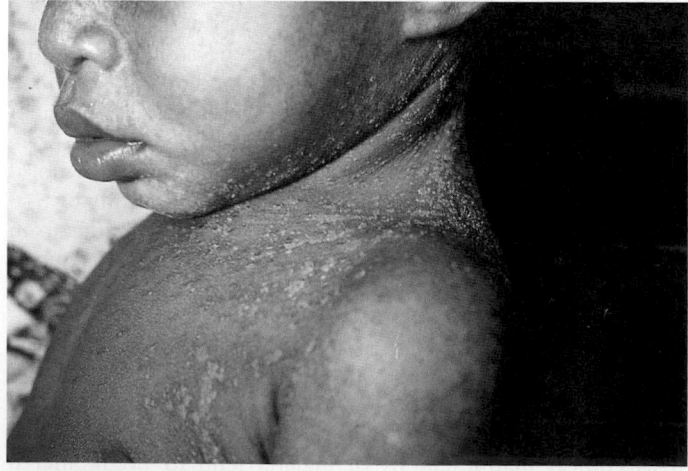

Figure 23.1 Measles desquamation in a Papua New Guinea child.

grants, minority groups and more recently in association with HIV infection (see Chapter 56). This decline is mainly associated with improved living conditions, contact tracing and individual case management. In developing countries, tuberculosis is a common problem among adults and children. Infants, adolescents and pregnant women have heightened susceptibility to tuberculosis. Susceptibility is also increased in malnutrition. Tuberculosis is a major problem in HIV-infected adults and children. A sentinel autopsy study from Central Africa of children dying of respiratory diseases has shown that bacterial pneumonia, tuberculosis, PCP and CMV are the top four causes of death in the HIV-positive group.[11] Recent evidence from South Africa, which found isoniazid prophylaxis improved mortality, would suggest TB is a larger problem in HIV than has previously been recognized.[12] However, in the few autopsy studies that have been reported[13] tuberculosis has not been found to be a common cause of death in this age group.

Tuberculosis in children mainly results from primary infection presenting usually as focal pulmonary disease (primary focus), followed by involvement of lymph nodes (primary complex), although tuberculosis can infect virtually all parts of the body. In developing countries where mothers bring their children late to the hospital, children may present with progressive and post-primary disease. Commonly observed manifestations of primary disease include pleural effusion, segmental collapse with consolidation, bronchopneumonia and pericarditis in younger children, and meningitis and bone or joint tuberculosis in older children. Disseminated tuberculosis (miliary tuberculosis) is usually seen in children with immunosuppression secondary to malnutrition or viral illness such as measles or chickenpox, and more recently in HIV infection.

The diagnosis of primary tuberculosis is based on a positive tuberculin test and enlarged nodes on chest radiograph with or without pulmonary infiltrates. In older children and adults, a wheal less than 5 mm in diameter that appears after tuberculin challenge is regarded as insignificant, 6–9 mm is likely to be associated with non-tuberculous mycobacteria, and greater than 10 mm is indicative of infection with *Mycobacterium tuberculosis*. Widespread BCG vaccination in infancy creates problems in interpreting tuberculin test results in infancy. After BCG the tuberculin response is usually less than 10–15 mm. A stronger response is suggestive of sensitivity to *M. tuberculosis*. A negative tuberculin test in children, however, does not exclude tuberculosis. In developing countries the tuberculin response may be negative in malnutrition, miliary tuberculosis, HIV, or following recent measles, chickenpox or kala azar. In infants and young children with clinical evidence of tuberculosis, in those with malnutrition or those in close contact with a case, an intermediate reaction of 6–9 mm may be significant. When the tuberculin response is negative in children with tuberculosis who are malnourished, it may become positive after 6–8 weeks when the nutritional status improves. The accelerated BCG response, in which local induration occurs within 48 h followed by ulceration and scab formation, was previously used for diagnosis, but this is now contraindicated, as it may cause disseminated BCG infection in immunosuppressed patients, particularly in children with AIDS. Newer T cell based γ-interferon assays appear more sensitive than the tuberculin test, can identify patients with previous TB infection, and can better differentiate TB from previous BCG or atypical mycobacteria infection. However, they do not distinguish active TB disease from previous primary infection. As with tuberculin tests there are still significant false negative rates. In a recent South African study the sensitivity in TB disease was reported to be 83% compared with 63% for the tuberculin test.[14]

Specimens for microscopy and culture are usually obtained from gastric lavage, induced sputum or a laryngeal swab. The yield of *M. tuberculosis* from different sources of specimens has been variable. Gastric aspiration performed in the morning in a fasting child on three consecutive mornings is positive by culture in about 40–50% of children with pulmonary tuberculosis.[15] Sputum induction has yielded a positive smear or culture in 28% of patients. Studies comparing gastric lavage with laryngeal swabs have yielded variable results. In a series involving Ugandan children, laryngeal swab cultures were positive in 63% of cases compared with 28% for gastric aspirates. Changes secondary to tuberculosis on chest radiograph include hilar adenopathy, or collapse consolidation, or pleural effusion or miliary opacities. In children co-infected with HIV, radiograph changes may not be typical. For example, HIV-infected children with lymphocytic interstitial pneumonitis (LIP) or chronic lung disease (CLD) have many features similar to tuberculosis, and in this group diagnosis is particularly difficult. The presence of finger clubbing in a child with chronic cough is more suggestive of LIP or CLD than TB.

The treatment of tuberculosis in children depends on the type and extent of the disease. The commonly used drugs are isoniazid (INH), rifampicin (R), pyrazinamide (PZA) and ethambutol (E) with streptomycin often added for TB meningitis or recurrence of disease. Isoniazid kills about 90% of the bacillary population during the first few days of chemotherapy. Rifampicin is essential for short treatment (6–9 month schedules), and a third or fourth drug usually is added for the first 2 months.

There is an additional consideration for children under 5 who are household contacts of a patient with TB or who have evidence of asymptomatic primary infection (a positive tuberculin test), with no clinical features of TB disease, and (where available) a normal chest radiograph. These can be treated with INH 'chemoprophylaxis' for 6 months or INH and rifampicin for 3 months, as there is a high probability of progression to active disease.

However, for those with symptomatic disease, or chest radiograph changes suggestive of tuberculosis, a full treatment course should be given. A typical regimen would consist of INH + R + PZA for 2 months followed by INH + R for 4 months. In severe disease, four drugs may be necessary.

In tuberculous meningitis, treatment should be for longer. Typically INH + RF + PZA for 2 months followed by INH + RF for 7 months. A fourth drug (ethambutol, ethionamide or streptomycin) can be added if the disease is severe or the child is wasted.

The above regimens are examples, but where available, national treatment protocols should be followed for TB treatment.

Corticosteroids are of benefit in tuberculous meningitis, and in TB pericarditis. Prednisolone (4 mg/kg per day) or dexamethasone can be given for up to 4 weeks and then the dose can be tapered off over 4–8 weeks.

Human immunodeficiency virus

Human immunodeficiency virus infection is a major emerging problem in many paediatric care facilities in tropical countries (see chapter 20). In sub-Saharan Africa, for example, half of HIV infection is in women, and paediatric AIDS constitutes 15–20% of AIDS cases compared with less than 4% in Europe. Children born from HIV-infected mothers may acquire HIV during pregnancy, labour or lactation. The HIV transmission rate from mother to infant without antenatal antiretroviral therapy has been estimated to be between 15 and 25% in industrialized countries and 20–45% in developing countries. The majority of infants acquire infection during labour.

Risk factors for transmission include high maternal viral load, low maternal CD4 cell count, maternal symptomatic HIV, newly acquired HIV infection, prematurity, vaginal delivery, prolonged rupture of membranes, chorioamnionitis and breast-feeding. Other factors with weaker evidence include viral characteristics, micronutrient deficiency and genetic factors. Risk factors for postnatal transmission during breast-feeding include mixed breast-feeding in the first 6 months of life,[15] newly acquired infection, sub-clinical or clinical mastitis, nipple disease including breast ulcers or abscess.

ARV treatment to mother and child in pregnancy or around the time of delivery significantly reduces the risk of transmission, and there are various regimens available. The choice is dependent on the complexity of regimen a country is able to deliver at a public health level. Promotion of exclusive breast-feeding is feasible and should be encouraged to 6 months of age.[16] Whether, or for how long a mother breast-feeds her infant depends on her ability to provide a breast-milk replacement safely. UNICEF and WHO have established the AFASS principles for this, which state that a mother should breast-feed unless an acceptable, feasible, affordable, sustainable and safe option to breast-milk is available.[17] These principles continue after 6 months, as breast-milk provides up to 50% of the calorie needs of the infant up to 1 year of age. Approximately 3–4% of HIV exposed infants will become infected in the first 6 months of exclusive breast-feeding,[16] and a further 3–4% if breast-fed from 6–12 months of life.[18]

The natural course of HIV in children is bimodal. Some of the children develop HIV in the first year of life, probably due to acquisition of infection during pregnancy. These children are known as rapid progressors. Other children survive several years before developing AIDS. Approximately one-third will die by their first birthday, half by 24 months and about 80% by 5 years.[19] The diagnosis of paediatric HIV infection should begin with identification of maternal HIV infection during or before pregnancy as most (>95%) paediatric HIV infections result from mother-to-child transmission (MTCT). This allows not only provision of preventive antiretroviral therapy in pregnancy and/or at delivery, but also early identification of at-risk babies for laboratory confirmation of HIV infection. Early diagnosis in the child will facilitate close clinical monitoring and cotrimoxazole preventive therapy for infections and provision of antiretroviral therapy (ART) from early infancy. Daily cotrimoxazole should be started from 6 weeks of age and continued to 18 months or until a child is known to be uninfected. In HIV-infected children, it should be continued indefinitely, as it is an effective means to reduce respiratory and other infections, and has been shown to halve the mortality in these children.[20]

In most tropical settings, HIV counselling and antibody testing (HCT) is not universal. In addition, paediatric infection cannot be confirmed using antibody tests alone under 18 months of age. A positive antibody test in this age group only confirms exposure to maternal infection, as maternal antibodies (IgG) persist for up to 15–18 months of age. The DNA polymerase chain reaction (PCR) test, recommended for early diagnosis of paediatric HIV, is not universally available in the tropics. It is expensive and requires both sophisticated equipment and experienced technologists.

The clinical presentation of paediatric HIV disease in children in the tropics often lacks specificity and usually mimics commonly observed clinical entities observed in children without HIV infection. Without specific clinical algorithms to aid front-line workers and with limited laboratory and other diagnostic facilities, arriving at a paediatric AIDS diagnosis is extremely difficult for most healthcare providers, especially in primary and secondary facilities, with most paediatric AIDS deaths occurring unconfirmed. WHO revised the paediatric classification for clinical staging in 2006[21] (Table 23.3), and has also re-defined the CD4 cut-offs for initiating ARVs where these are available. This uses CD4$^+$ cell count or percentage (preferred in children under 5 years) as a marker of immune status according to the child's age (Table 23.4). CD4$^+$ cell estimation has previously required complicated and expensive equipment; however, lower cost simplified technologies have recently become available and, with this, increasing availability in low resourced countries.

HIV clinical entities observed in children in the tropics differ from those in industrialized countries, with severe malnutrition a common presenting feature. Kaposi's sarcoma and rectovaginal fistula are well recognized specific entities strongly associated with HIV, and persistent diarrhoea, chronic lung disease, non-typhoidal salmonellosis, chronic ear discharge and TB infection are also common.

The Integrated Management of Childhood Illness (IMCI) has been adapted in many Southern African countries to include an HIV algorithm, and to identify children for referral for HCT.

Similarly there are algorithms for the presumptive diagnosis of HIV in children under 18 months of life (Table 23.5) who have positive HIV serology, and where PCR and/or CD4 confirmation are not available. It is important that any child who is seropositive under 18 months of age, and in whom a confirmatory PCR diagnosis has not been performed, is re-tested after 18 months of age to confirm their HIV status.

Pneumocystis jiroveci pneumonia (PCP) is the most frequent and severe cause of pneumonia affecting HIV-infected infants in industrialized countries. It was earlier reported that PCP was less common in Africa than in industrialized countries. However, both autopsy and clinical studies have shown that the prevalence of PCP is common in sub-Saharan Africa.[22] Clinically, a diagnosis of PCP should be considered in an infant less than 6 months of age with severe pneumonia characterized by marked hypoxia who does not respond to standard antibiotics. Laboratory confirmation is difficult. Immunofluorescent techniques on nasopharyngeal aspirates may be useful, but probably underestimate the diagnosis.[21]

Children with HIV commonly present with chronic respiratory symptoms, the cause of which may be difficult to determine. These children may have HIV-related LIP or chronic lung disease (CLD), but the diagnosis may be confused with pulmonary tuberculosis or Kaposi's sarcoma (KS) because of radiological features of the interstitial infiltrates with hilar prominence. The presence of finger clubbing points towards CLD and LIP. TB is suggested by a

Table 23.3 WHO clinical staging for infants and children with established HIV infection[21]

CLINICAL STAGE 1
Asymptomatic
Persistent generalized lymphadenopathy

CLINICAL STAGE 2[a]
Unexplained persistent hepatosplenomegaly
Papular pruritic eruptions
Fungal nail infections
Angular cheilitis
Lineal gingival erythema
Extensive wart virus infection
Extensive molluscum contagiosum
Recurrent oral ulceration
Unexplained persistent parotid enlargement
Herpes zoster
Recurrent or chronic upper respiratory tract infections (otitis media, otorrhoea, sinusitis, tonsillitis)

CLINICAL STAGE 3[a]
Unexplained moderate malnutrition or wasting not adequately responding to standard therapy
Unexplained persistent diarrhoea (14 days or more)
Unexplained persistent fever (above 37.5°C, intermittent or constant, for longer than 1 month)
Persistent oral candidiasis (after first 6–8 weeks of life)
Oral hairy leukoplakia
Acute necrotizing ulcerative gingivitis or periodontitis
Lymph node tuberculosis
Pulmonary tuberculosis

(continued)
Severe recurrent bacterial pneumonia
Symptomatic lymphoid interstitial pneumonitis
Chronic HIV-associated lung disease including bronchiectasis
Unexplained anaemia (<8.0 g/dL), neutropaenia (<0.5×10^9/L) and or chronic thrombocytopenia (<50×10^9/L)

CLINICAL STAGE 4[a,b]
Unexplained severe wasting, stunting or severe malnutrition not responding to standard therapy
Pneumocystis jiroveci pneumonia (PCP)
Recurrent severe bacterial infections (e.g. empyema, pyomyositis, bone or joint infection, meningitis, but excluding pneumonia)
Chronic herpes simplex infection; (orolabial or cutaneous of more than one month's duration, or visceral at any site)
Extrapulmonary tuberculosis
Kaposi sarcoma
Oesophageal candidiasis (or Candida of trachea, bronchi or lungs)
Cytomegalovirus (CMV) infection; retinitis or CMV infection affecting another organ, with onset at age over 1 month
Central nervous system toxoplasmosis (after the neonatal period)
Extrapulmonary cryptococcosis (including meningitis)
HIV encephalopathy
Disseminated endemic mycosis (extrapulmonary histoplasmosis, coccidiomycosis)
Chronic cryptosporidiosis (with diarrhoea)
Chronic isosporiasis
Disseminated non-tuberculous mycobacteria infection
Cerebral or B cell non-Hodgkin lymphoma
Progressive multifocal leukoencephalopathy
HIV-associated cardiomyopathy or nephropathy

[a] Unexplained, refers to where the condition is not explained by other causes.
[b] Some additional specific conditions can be included in regional classifications (e.g. disseminated Penicilliosis in Asia, HIV-associated rectovaginal fistula in Africa, and reactivation of American trypanosomiasis).

Table 23.4 WHO CD4 criteria for severe immunodeficiency in HIV infection. Age-specific CD4+ T lymphocyte counts and percentage of total lymphocytes to initiate ART[21]

	AGE OF THE CHILD			
	<11 months	12–35 months	35–59 months	6–12 years
CD$^+$/mm^3	<1500	<750	<350	<200
(%)	<25	<20	<15	<15

Table 23.5 WHO presumptive diagnosis criteria for paediatric AIDS in children <18 months where virological testing is not available[21]

- The infant is confirmed as being HIV antibody-positive
  and
- A stage 4 AIDS-indicator condition is diagnosed
  or
- The infant is symptomatic with two or more of the following:
  – oral thrush
  – severe pneumonia
  – severe sepsis
  and the above would be supported by a CD4 <20%

positive contact history, and a cough which does not improve on antibiotics. A tuberculin test may be positive. In lung KS, examination of the skin, lymph nodes, and palate will usually identify other KS lesions.

Immune reconstitution syndromes are increasingly being recognized after treatment for HIV, TB, and severe malnutrition, which may all be present in a child commencing ARVs. This commonly presents as a worsening of symptoms in the first months after starting ARVs, and the underlying cause should be sought and treated.

Treatment with ARVs has become simplified in recent years. It will generally consist of a 3-drug regime, usually as a combination tablet. Although adult tablets have been used for children, these have previously underdosed the nevirapine component, which has been a core component in most low resource settings. Newer specially formulated paediatric combination tablets are becoming available, the first of these being Pedimune baby and Pedimune junior (lamivudine, stavudine, and nevirapine). Suspensions may require refrigeration, and are therefore less easy to use in low resource countries. Adherence to treatment is critical, as it is in adults, otherwise resistance will develop to the first line regime. This field is rapidly changing, and reference should be made to current national and WHO guidelines to inform treatment choices.

Rheumatic fever

Rheumatic fever (see also Chapter 22) occurs exclusively in human beings and there are no known animal reservoirs. The greatest susceptibility is after 5 years of age and in adolescents.[23] Group A streptococcal infection always precedes rheumatic fever, and the most convincing evidence that this is the cause of the disease is that primary and secondary attacks can be prevented by the use of penicillin. The incidence is difficult to determine, as many cases may be sub-clinical. Disease results from auto-immunity as peptide sequences on the surface of the streptococcus are identical with that of collagen tissues in cardiac valves, joints and nervous tissue. Rheumatogenic streptococcal strains are associated with specific M-protein serotypes which can differ substantially in virulence. Clustering in families may reflect close contact and likelihood of spread, and this is one reason why the risk of rheumatic fever is higher in overcrowded conditions. Primary attacks of rheumatic fever are often not preceded by clinical pharyngitis and in about 20% there is no rise in the ASO titre. The site of infection in these children is unclear. The susceptibility of individuals relates to genetic factors due to the recognition that gene products of the human major histocompatibility complex are associated with rheumatic fever. Nearly all cases of rheumatic fever possess B lymphocyte allo-antigens before disease onset, and these are normally present in peripheral blood in only 1 in 5 of a population. In developing countries, improved socioeconomic conditions and less overcrowding partly explain the dramatic decline in the incidence since the 1950s where incidence is low (0.2–05/100 000). In contrast, the incidence rate in developing countries is high, with rates reaching 10–20 per 1000 population.

Clinical signs of rheumatic fever are similar wherever in the world the disease is encountered. Mitral valve involvement is commonest with a predominance of mitral regurgitation, especially in younger children. Isolated mitral stenosis in children is well described and occurs at a younger age in children in developing countries. If recurrences are prevented, a large proportion of children with pure mitral incompetence will have no heart disease after a decade. With a first attack about 50% of children will have carditis causing cardiac murmurs detectable by auscultation. The risk of carditis with recurrent attacks is much higher (>75%). In developing countries with inadequate prophylaxis, pure mitral regurgitation may progress to severe disease requiring cardiac surgery. These findings explain the high morbidity and mortality rates in less developed countries.

The most effective control is prophylaxis of recurrent streptococci pharyngitis with penicillin V (125–250 mg orally twice daily), or benzathine penicillin G (0.6–1.2 million units intramuscularly every 3 or 4 weeks according to body weight) is highly effective and should be continued until 25 years of age. This is best delivered as part of a coordinated programme. Patients with definite valvular disease will require life-time therapy.

Dengue haemorrhagic fever

The global incidence of dengue has increased exponentially over the past decade and is now endemic in many developing countries. In children, the infection is usually mild and non-specific. The presentation depends on age, with overt clinical dengue fever (DF) mainly apparent in children over 5 years old. There is an incubation period of 5–8 days following an infective mosquito bite. Clinical manifestations of DF include high continuous fever, headache, periorbital pain, myalgia, arthralgia, a maculopapular rash, leucopenia and, occasionally, haemorrhage.

The more severe dengue haemorrhagic fever (DHF) with plasma leakage and shock or haemorrhage occurs in individuals who have had previous infection with a different dengue serotype (of which there are four). This severe form therefore occurs mainly in areas where transmission of more than one serotype occurs, and commonly in children between 5 and 9 years of age. Clinical manifestations are the same as those of dengue fever, but in addition there may be evidence of plasma leakage (ascites and pleural effusion), a rising haematocrit hepatomegaly (with abnormal LFTs and clotting) and a low platelet count (<100 000/mm^3). Diagnosis is clinical and the tourniquet test can be helpful. The tourniquet test consists of applying an arm blood pressure cuff to the mean arterial pressure for 5 min, a positive test is more than 10 petechiae per square inch. Confirmation of dengue is usually by serology or positive viral culture.

The clinical course can be divided into a febrile phase (days 1–5), a haemorrhagic shock or toxic phase of 1–2 days duration (days 4–6), followed by a convalescent phase. The severity of the disease can be graded according to the presence of shock or bleeding.

Grade I: A febrile illness with non-specific constitutional symptoms and a positive tourniquet test.

Grade II: In addition to the above, there is haemorrhage in skin, gastrointestinal tract and other sites.

Grade III: Circulatory failure with rapid weak pulse, small pulse pressure, cold clammy extremities and hypotension.

Grade IV: Profound shock and moribund clinical state with undetectable pulse and blood pressure.

The management of DF and DHF is supportive, with antipyretics and analgesics. It is not advised to use non-steroidal antiinflammatory drugs. Fluid management is critical to success in DHF, and should be titrated against the haematocrit and clinical condition, to maintain effective circulation during the 48 h period of plasma leakage. The clinician walks a tightrope in managing DHF, as giving too much fluid may overload the circulation and can precipitate respiratory distress. Mortality rates of <1% have been achieved in experienced centres, and recovery is almost always complete.

The increasing geographical distribution of dengue haemorrhagic fever has meant that DHF is being encountered by clinicians with no previous experience in its management, with poorer outcomes initially for a disease which can carry a mortality rate of up to 50%. Vector control is the only preventative measure, in the absence of effective dengue virus vaccines, and recent outbreaks have been curtailed by these measures with variable success. Counselling mothers to recognize shock will improve earlier diagnosis and detection.

Pertussis

Pertussis (whooping cough) occurs worldwide and causes 300 000 deaths in children annually, mostly in developing countries.[24] The causative agent, *Bordetella pertussis*, is spread by aerosol droplet and the related *B. parapertussis* and *B. bronchiseptica* cause a similar illness.

The typical illness occurs classically in three stages, commencing with a 1–2 week coryzal stage clinically indistinguishable from other URTIs. This is followed by a 2–4 week paroxysmal stage when paroxysms of coughing (up to 10 staccato-like coughs) are followed by the characteristic high-pitched inspiratory whoop. Coughing may be followed by vomiting in younger children, cyanosis, apnoea and convulsions. With poor feeding and vomiting, rapid weight loss may be a problem, and rectal prolapse, subconjunctival haemorrhages and ulceration of the frenulum can occur. A convalescent stage usually of 1–2 weeks follows, but coughing can last for months and may be precipitated by intercurrent URTIs. The Chinese termed pertussis the '100 day cough'. In infants, classical disease is less common, and pertussis may present with apnoea, bradycardia, seizures or atypical cough with poor feeding.

Where available, a pernasal swab plated onto a Bordet–Gengou medium will confirm the diagnosis, but may not be positive in the paroxysmal stage of illness, when the clinical presentation is more helpful. The diagnosis is supported by finding blood lymphocytosis which occurs in the second to fifth weeks.

Management is mainly supportive, although erythromycin 50 mg/kg per day for 10–14 days if given during the catarrhal stage may shorten the clinical course. This is of most use in contacts that develop a coryzal illness. Prevention of paroxysms is best achieved by avoidance of the triggers and there is little benefit from cough suppressants or sedatives. Oxygen may be helpful and in infants may reduce apnoeic events. Maintenance of nutrition and hydration is important. Pneumonia is the commonest complication and may be from secondary bacterial infection or aspiration. Atelectasis due to obstruction of airways by tenacious secretions can occur and is often only apparent on radiography. Subsequent bronchiectasis may result. Encephalopathy is well rec-

ognized, and may be due to hypoxic brain injury, intracranial haemorrhage or toxin.

Treating cases with erythromycin and vaccinating unimmunized siblings may reduce transmission. Acellular and whole cell vaccines are both effective in preventing disease, with the more expensive acellular vaccine having fewer adverse reactions.

Diphtheria

Diphtheria (see Chapter 67) may occur as a mild or life-threatening illness usually presenting in young children, and before vaccination was available had epidemic cycles with 2–4 year intervals. Epidemics still occur in parts of Africa, South-east Asia and the newly independent states of the former Soviet Union.

A child with early tonsillar diphtheria may not appear ill initially, but within a few days may become very toxic with extensive membrane formation. All children with diphtheria require management in hospital. Nasal diphtheria, commonest in infants, may initially resemble a common cold with nasal discharge slowly becoming serosanguineous and then mucopurulent. Tonsillar and pharyngeal diphtheria tend to be more severe forms of disease, and within 1–2 days a patch or patches of grey–yellow membrane may cover the tonsils and pharyngeal walls, which may then extend to the uvula, soft palate or larynx and trachea. The breath may have a foul smell. Acute airways obstruction may resemble viral 'croup' in infants (pseudo croup). Cervical lymphadenitis is variable and when associated with soft tissue oedema, gives the appearance of a 'bull neck'. Bleeding diathesis (usually nasal) is associated with a poorer prognosis.

Complete heart block and myocarditis are not uncommon, and develop after the first week of illness. Neuropathy occurs between two and ten weeks into the illness, often when the child is getting better, and is reversible. Soft palatal paralysis occurs most commonly. Paralysis of the diaphragm and a bilateral and usual motor peripheral neuropathy may also occur. Cutaneous diphtheria is not uncommon in warmer climates, and can lead to immunity in children, and is one of the causes of tropical ulcer.

Mortality from diphtheria increases with delayed administration of antitoxin, so treatment (following a test dose) should be started on clinical suspicion of disease. Penicillin or erythromycin will render most patients non-infectious within 24 h, although resistance has been reported.

Prevention of diphtheria is by immunization, and although immunized persons can be infected by toxin-producing strains of diphtheria, systemic manifestations of diphtheria do not occur. Immunity may wane with time, particularly in communities where diphtheria is no longer present.

COMMON CHILDHOOD DISEASE ENTITIES IN THE TROPICS

Acute respiratory infections

This section deals with the causes and management of acute respiratory infections (ARI) in low resource countries, and not the management of upper respiratory tract infections (URTIs).

Of the 10.5 million children aged less than 5 years who die every year, almost one-third of the deaths are due to pneumonia.

Up to 50% of outpatient attendances are due to ARI of which two-thirds are URTIs. Some 30% of hospital admissions are for ARI, usually pneumonia. Outpatient management has been simplified through the development of a syndromic assessment strategy and standardized management protocols, which are now incorporated within the WHO Integrated Management of Childhood Illness (IMCI) programme.

Community-based studies from around the globe have shown a similar incidence of ARI with an average of six to eight episodes of ARI per year in urban areas. There is a much higher mortality rate from pneumonia in developing countries, with most deaths occurring in infants. Pneumonia not associated with measles accounted for 70% of the deaths due to ARI, followed by post-measles pneumonia (15%), pertussis (10%) and bronchiolitis and croup (5%) in 1983. This pattern has changed with improved immunization coverage for measles and pertussis, and as HIV-related pneumonia has become more common in certain regions.

Viruses are the primary cause of the majority of ARI, both of the upper and lower respiratory tract. Measles-related pneumonia carries a poor prognosis, and may be due to secondary staphylococcal infection. Respiratory syncytial virus (RSV) infection is seasonal worldwide; however, in most infants and children RSV bronchiolitis is a self-limiting illness. Human metapneumovirus has recently been identified as a common respiratory pathogen, second to RSV, to which it appears to have a similar disease spectrum, including URTI, bronchiolitis and viral pneumonia.[25] In some communities, *Chlamydia trachomatis* is a common pathogen in infancy. The vast majority of bacterial pneumonia (diagnosed through lung aspiration research studies) is caused by *Streptococcus pneumoniae* or *Haemophilus influenzae*. In children around 5 years of age mycoplasma infections also occur. In HIV-infected infants *Pneumocystis jiroveci* interstitial pneumonitis (PCP) (previously *carinii*) infection is common,[21] although most ARI remains due to organisms which normally cause community-acquired pneumonia. Children with severe malnutrition may also be infected with Gram-negative organisms such as non-typhoid *Salmonella* spp (NTS), *Klebsiella* spp and *Escherichia coli*. In infants under 2 months of age, Gram-negative organisms are also common. Factors that increase the incidence and severity of pneumonia include: young age, low birth weight, malnutrition, lack of breast-feeding, indoor smoke, and underlying disease.

The diagnosis of ARI and pneumonia is predominantly clinical, and with the promotion of IMCI, initiation of treatment on syndromic criteria is appropriate. Children usually present with cough and/or difficulty in breathing. Fever is common but not specific. It is important to identify the child with pneumonia who requires antibiotics and possibly hospital admission. A raised respiratory rate is consistently the most reliable clinical sign for pneumonia. More severe pneumonia is indicated by respiratory distress, with subcostal chest indrawing and possibly cyanosis or other 'danger signs'. These clinical signs of pneumonia have a lower predictive value in infants under 2 months, who may present with poor feeding, grunting, apnoea or hypothermia. Auscultation of the chest is often not helpful, especially in the young.

Chest radiographs are unreliable in differentiating viral from bacterial pneumonia, so do not generally help to determine specific treatment. They are best reserved for management failures and chronic cough. Blood cultures have a consistently low yield, and although nasopharyngeal culture may reflect the likely pathogen causing pneumonia in the community, it does not necessarily indicate the pathogen causing disease in an individual child. Lung aspiration remains a research tool.

Early treatment of pneumonia with appropriate antibiotics significantly reduces the morbidity and mortality rate attributed to ARI in developing countries. The choice of antibiotic for cases of pneumonia will depend on many factors, including drug availability, the likely aetiology, and the child's age and nutritional status. For children from 2 months up to 5 years of age, co-trimoxazole or amoxicillin are appropriate for the out-patient treatment of pneumonia, and for severe pneumonia parenteral benzylpenicillin (or ampicillin) should be used, and if very severe in combination with daily gentamicin. If there is no improvement within 48 h chloramphenicol should replace the penicillin. Depending on the likely aetiology, a macrolide, or addition of cloxacillin may be required. In children with malnutrition, or in those with HIV infection, Gram-negative organisms are relatively common, and antibiotic choice should reflect this, and where possible be informed by local sensitivity patterns. Oxygen concentrators (and pulse oximetry) are becoming more widely available, and oxygen should be given to children with severe indrawing of intercostal muscles, respiratory rates above 70/min, or who are hypoxic.

Infants who are infected with HIV are at risk of *Pneumocystis jiroveci* (carinii) interstitial pneumonitis (PCP), which typically presents in the first 6 months of life with severe respiratory distress, and severe persistent hypoxia; treatment should be with high-dose co-trimoxazole. The prognosis of PCP infection in HIV remains poor, particularly without intensive respiratory support. This infection can be prevented with daily prophylactic co-trimoxazole from 6 weeks of age in HIV exposed infants.

Diarrhoeal diseases

Children under 5 years old suffer around a billion episodes of diarrhoea each year. Diarrhoeal disease accounts for 17% of the mortality in this age group, causing the deaths of an estimated 2 million through dehydration. Only acute respiratory infections kill more children outwith the perinatal period. Those living in the poorest countries, where inadequate sanitation, lack of clean drinking water and malnutrition are endemic risk factors, carry the heaviest burden. A child living in the developing world can expect six or seven episodes of diarrhoea per year compared to one or two episodes for a child in the developed world.

The WHO defines diarrhoea as the passage of loose or watery stools at least three times in a 24 h period but also emphasizes the importance of parental perceptions of abnormal stool frequency or constituency in making the diagnosis. Acute diarrhoea typically has an abrupt onset, lasts less than 14 days and is infective in aetiology, with the presence of blood usually taken to signify dysentery. Chronic or persistent diarrhoea lasts at least 14 days, is more common in infancy and is frequently secondary to gastrointestinal infection complicating malnutrition, or poorly managed acute gastroenteritis. Less common causes of diarrhoea include the ingestion of drugs or toxins, hypersensitivity reactions and a range of congenital endocrine and metabolic abnormalities. It is also important to note that foci of infection outside the bowel may cause diarrhoea, for example pneumonia and otitis media.

Enteric infection is the most common and important cause of diarrhoea in tropical countries. Around 20 microorganisms (viruses, parasites and bacteria) cause diarrhoeal disease and the epidemiological significance of each varies according to age group, geographical location, nutritional status and the chronicity of illness. Rotavirus alone accounts for 60% of diarrhoeal episodes in developing countries and kills an estimated 600 000 children each year. Group A rotavirus infections are responsible for the majority of cases, which peak between 6 and 24 months of age and may produce epidemics in hot, dry seasons. Following an incubation period of 18–36 h, the virus invades the villi of mature enterocytes via apical receptors and calcium-dependent endocytosis. Lytic destruction of these cells may follow, leading to a loss of functional intestinal absorption and profuse, watery stools over the next 2–7 days. Immunity develops with repeated exposure and most disease is mild; however, severe dehydration and death are more likely in younger infants and the malnourished. Live, oral rotavirus vaccines have recently been licensed, and proven highly efficacious in trials. Intussusception was a reported complication of previous vaccines but appears to be less of a problem with newer formulations. Their introduction into vaccination schedules in the developing world would have a measurable impact on morbidity and mortality.

Pathogenic E. coli typify the bacteria causing diarrhoeal illness. They are classified into six groups according to their disease-forming properties but infection may remain asymptomatic. Enterotoxigenic E. coli (ETEC) is most commonly associated with disease and may also cause fever, abdominal pain and vomiting. The enterotoxin causes watery, secretory diarrhoea through the transduction of second messenger intracellular signal pathways. Spontaneous recovery usually occurs within 7 days but infection can persist if nutrition is compromised. Other relevant bacteria include Campylobacter spp, Salmonella spp and Yersinia spp. These organisms invade and disrupt the colonic mucosa, inducing an inflammatory response and resulting in ulceration and haemorrhage. Shigella spp are the most important causes of dysentery, however, accounting for 15% of all diarrhoeal deaths in the under-fives. Shigella dysenteriae type 1 is the leading cause of haemolytic–uraemic syndrome in tropical countries. Vibrio cholerae remains a major cause of epidemic diarrhoea, particularly in disaster areas but may also be endemic.

Giardia lamblia is frequently isolated from stool samples. Although this enteric parasite is an important cause of diarrhoea in malnourished children, its importance in other groups remains unclear, as carriage is frequently asymptomatic. Cryptosporidium parvum is commonly associated with HIV infection, severe wasting and chronic diarrhoea. Amoebic dysentery is caused by the protozoan parasite Entamoeba histolytica and tends to be more severe in the very young and those who are immuno-suppressed.

A precise aetiological diagnosis of diarrhoeal disease is often difficult. Stool culture is seldom available to clinical laboratories in tropical countries and quality control of such facilities is problematic. Fresh stool microscopy, which is more widely available, is required for the diagnosis of intestinal parasites, for which antimicrobial treatment is beneficial. Fortunately, the standard clinical management of acute diarrhoeal episodes is not otherwise dependent on microbiological investigations and most diarrhoeal disease resolves without the use of antibiotics. Dysentery is the exception to this general rule and cases should undergo stool culture and sensitivity testing if possible. Antibiotic resistant Shigella spp and Campylobacter spp are now a common problem.

Children with diarrhoea and no signs of dehydration may be managed at home, with an increase in normal fluid intake, continued feeding and careful monitoring. However, prompt recognition of the child who is deteriorating should lead to early contact with healthcare services and a rapid, accurate assessment of hydration status. Children with signs of severe dehydration or shock should be treated immediately with intravenous Ringers lactate solution, where available, or another crystalloid. Recent studies have shown that once significant hypovolaemia has been corrected, oral rehydration therapy (ORT) is as effective as ongoing intravenous fluid infusion. ORT, given by mouth or nasogastric tube, should be instituted as soon as a child can drink, with the aim of rehydrating within 4 h of presentation and maintaining that status until recovery. This requires periodic re-evaluation of the response to fluids and of stool output. Children with severe malnutrition, persistent vomiting, cholera and abdominal distension require additional consideration.

Reduced-osmolarity ORT appears to be broadly superior to standard ORT in the management of diarrhoeal dehydration. Variability in outcome measures between studies and insufficient data relating specifically to cholera merit a cautious interpretation of this conclusion. WHO currently recommends the universal use of ORT with an intermediate sodium content of 75 mmol/L.[26]

Malnutrition is a poor prognostic indicator in diarrhoeal disease and is also one of its main sequelae. This vicious cycle accounts for up to half of all diarrhoeal deaths in children. More frequent breast-feeding and early re-feeding with solids for older children is advised, once shock and dehydration have been corrected. There is substantial evidence that this is generally safe, well-tolerated and therapeutic. Caution is recommended only for non-exclusively breast-fed infants younger than 6 months and in those with very severe forms of diarrhoea. Although data are limited, the marked enteropathic changes in gut histology observed in this latter group suggest that re-feeding may be less successful.

Additional supplementation with zinc, and to a lesser extent with vitamin A, has been shown to reduce significantly the risk, duration and severity of chronic diarrhoea in children. The WHO recommends that all children admitted to hospital with diarrhoea be given zinc supplements soon after arrival and that these be continued for 2 weeks. Anti-diarrhoeal drugs, such as loperamide, kaolin or opiates have no role in the management of acute diarrhoea in children, may cause dangerous side-effects and should be avoided.

Bacterial meningitis

Bacterial or pyogenic meningitis is a widespread and common cause of paediatric mortality on the tropics.[27] For example, the African 'meningitis belt' defines an area from Senegal to Sudan, characterized by high endemicity and cyclical epidemics of meningococcal meningitis affecting up to 2% of the population. The majority of cases of bacterial meningitis are caused by Streptococcus pneumoniae (many serotypes), Neisseria meningitidis (serogroups A, B, C, Y, W135) and Haemophilus influenzae type b. The latter is uncommon in children over 5 years old, and has been largely eliminated from countries that have adopted universal immunization programmes. Meningococcal disease is more frequent in this age group and may occur in conjunction with severe septicaemia. Viral infections, dust, and smoke inhalation damage the upper respiratory tract, predisposing to invasive disease. A polyvalent meningococcal vaccine is available but lacks consistent immunogenicity in infants and young children. Haemoglobinopathies predispose to pneumococcal disease, together with traumatic head injury, otitis media and HIV infection. The introduction of the conjugated polyvalent pneumococcal vaccine should produce a significant decline in pneumococcal disease in countries implementing universal immunization in infancy.

In neonates, *Escherichia coli*, *Listeria monocytogenes*, pneumococci and the group B streptococci predominate while Staphylococci, *Salmonella* and *Klebsiella* are also potential causes. Preterm and low birthweight babies are at particularly high risk. Among HIV-infected children, non-typhoidal *Salmonella* and tuberculous meningitis are becoming more common.

Classical clinical features of meningitis in children include fever, vomiting, headache, photophobia and meningism (nuchal rigidity and severe pain on knee extension with hip flexion – Kernig's sign). Infants are more likely to present with a non-specific history of fever, vomiting, feed refusal, irritability and convulsions. Examination may reveal high-pitched crying or bulging fontanelle. Meningitis should always be considered in febrile infants with convulsions and in children with a diagnosis of cerebral malaria. The presence of a purpuric rash suggests meningococcal septicaemia and lesions should be sought carefully, especially on the buttocks and soles of the feet.

In the absence of focal neurological signs or cardiovascular instability, lumbar puncture with biochemical, microscopic and microbiological analysis of the cerebrospinal fluid should be performed to confirm the diagnosis. However, empirical antibiotics should be given early, before the results of the lumbar puncture are known. Third-generation cephalosporins are the treatment of choice for bacterial meningitis but are not commonly available in low resource settings. Monotherapy with parenteral chloramphenicol is also effective; the addition of ampicillin or benzylpenicillin, although often recommended, confers no additional benefit. Pathogen-specific therapy may be tailored later, when the results of laboratory analyses are known. The use of dexamethasone as an adjunct to prevent neurological sequelae or improve outcome in bacterial meningitis remains controversial. A large study in Malawi showed that steroid use conferred no additional benefit and other studies have shown harm.[28] Routine use of steroids in the treatment of childhood bacterial meningitis in developing countries is not recommended. Other aspects of supportive treatment include adequate oxygenation, careful fluid management, prevention of metabolic derangement and seizure control.

Mortality for meningitis varies with age and aetiology. Fatality rates as low as 2% have been reported in infants and children with meningococcal meningitis and as high as 20% in neonates with group B streptococcal infection. Mortality is also much greater for meningococcal septicaemia than for meningitis alone. Complications of bacterial meningitis are common and severe, including the syndrome of inappropriate antidiuretic hormone secretion (SIADH), subtotal emphysema, hemiplegia and hydrocephalus. In parts of West Africa, meningitis accounts for over one-third of cases of deafness.

INTEGRATED MANAGEMENT OF CHILDHOOD ILLNESSES

In 2005, 10.5 million children under 5 years of age died in developing countries, with 70% of these deaths being due to ARI (mostly pneumonia), diarrhoea, measles, malaria or malnutrition, or a combination of these. Most of these deaths would be averted if preventative measures and appropriate management were available at community level. At this level diagnostic support services such as radiology or laboratory services are minimal or not available, but despite this the majority of children can be allocated appropriate therapy using a syndromic approach to clinical assessment. For example, pneumonia requiring antibiotics or hospital admission can be identified with a high degree of sensitivity and reasonable specificity using a combination of a raised respiratory rate (age related), chest indrawing and the presence of 'danger signs'. Using this approach, children with fast breathing and fever may be allocated to receive both an anti-malarial and antibiotic, as for many sick children a single diagnosis may not be appropriate.

In 1997, the WHO initiated the 'Integrated Management of Childhood Illness' (IMCI), a strategy which combines the syndromic management of illness in the community with assessment and promotion of nutrition, immunization and other important factors influencing child health (Table 23.6). Through IMCI it is expected that death, and the frequency and severity of illness and disability will be reduced, and child growth and development will be improved.[29] Although IMCI focuses on the community care of children under 5 years, WHO has produced complementary materials,[30] which give guidelines for hospital care of children at first referral level in developing countries,

Table 23.6 Interventions included in the IMCI strategy[21]

Care pathway	Promotion of growth/prevention of disease	Response to sickness/curative care
Home	Community/home-based intervention to improve nutrition Insecticide-impregnated bednets	Early case management Appropriate care seeking Compliance with treatment
Health services	Vaccinations Complementary feeding and breast-feeding counselling Micronutrient supplementation	Case management of: diarrhoea, measles, malaria, malnutrition, ARI and other diseases Complementary feeding and breast-feeding counselling Iron treatment Anthelmintic treatment

and are consistent with the IMCI strategy and management plans for sick children.

With HIV an increasing problem in many sub-Saharan countries, WHO has developed and evaluated an adaptation to include HIV in the IMCI algorithms. This identifies specific symptoms and signs suggestive of HIV, and when three or more of these are present, prompts the health worker to refer the child and mother for HIV testing, and referral into HIV services.

IMMUNIZATION PROGRAMMES

The Expanded Programme on Immunization (EPI) was launched in 1974 by the WHO at a time when less than 5% of the world's children were immunized during their first year in life against the initial six target diseases: diphtheria, tetanus, whooping cough, polio, measles, and tuberculosis. Immunization with *H. influenzae* conjugate (Hib) vaccine and hepatitis B vaccine have been added to the infant schedule in many developing countries during the last decade (Table 23.7). These immunizations save more than 3 million lives a year. Despite this achievement, 30 million infants still have no access to basic immunization each year and the goal of reaching 80% coverage of the world's children has not yet been achieved.

At present, five contacts are needed during the first year of life (at birth, 6 weeks, 10 weeks, 14 weeks, and at 9 months) and in most low resource countries coverage rates decline progressively through this period. The schedule outlined in Table 23.7 is applicable for both HIV non-infected and asymptomatic infected children in developing countries. There are increasing efforts to expand services to include hepatitis B and Hib vaccines and to link these health contacts with delivery of vitamin A supplements and, if appropriate, intermittent preventive antimalarial treatment in infants against malaria (IPTi).

BCG

For further information on BCG, see Chapter 56.

Polio

Polio eradication is within reach, as there remain only four polio endemic countries in the world (Nigeria, India, Pakistan and Afghanistan). Under 1900 cases were reported in 2005. This success has been achieved through a global eradication strategy. This is four-pronged: high routine immunization coverage with oral polio vaccine (OPV); supplementary immunization in the form of National Immunization Days (NIDs); effective surveillance for acute flaccid paralysis and wild poliovirus; and door-to-door immunization ('mopping up' campaigns). The Americas were certified polio-free in 1994, the Western Pacific in 2000, and Europe in 2002.

While OPV vaccine is one of the safest vaccines available, one case of vaccine-associated polio occurs for every 2.5 million doses administered. In view of this some countries with no wild-type polio transmission are using inactivated poliovirus (IPV) in their EPI programmes. Unlike OPV, IPV vaccine induces low levels of immunity to enteric poliovirus, and although providing protection against systemic disease, cannot prevent the spread of wild

Table 23.7 The South African EPI schedule and method of vaccine administration

Age	Vaccine	Route of administration
Birth	BCG	Intradermal injection
	TOPV	Oral drops
6 weeks	TOPV	Oral drops
	DTP + Hib	Intramuscular injection to the left thigh
	Hepatitis B	Intramuscular injection to the right thigh
10 weeks	TOPV	Oral drops
	DTP + Hib	Intramuscular injection to the left thigh
	Hepatitis B	Intramuscular injection to the right thigh
14 weeks	TOPV	Oral drops
	DTP + Hib	Intramuscular injection to the left thigh
	Hepatitis B	Intramuscular injection to the right thigh
9 months	Measles	Intramuscular injection to the right thigh
18 months	TOPV	Oral drops
	DTP	Intramuscular injection to the left arm
	Measles	Intramuscular injection to the right arm
5–7 years (school entry)	TOPV	Oral drops
	Td	Intramuscular injection to the left arm
12–15 years (school leaving)	Td	Intramuscular injection to the left arm

BCG, Bacilli Calmete–Guerin (antituberculosis vaccine); TOPV, trivalent oral polio vaccine; DTP, diphtheria, tetanus, pertussis vaccine; Td, tetanus and diphtheria vaccine; Hib, *Haemophilus influenza* type b vaccine.

poliovirus. Use of OPV vaccines is central to the eradication of polio worldwide.

Measles

Globally, measles accounts for over half a million deaths in children under 5 years of age, often through the complications of pneumonia, diarrhoea and malnutrition. The majority of deaths occur in countries where immunization coverage for children is less than 50%. Measles vaccines have lower efficacy before 9 months of age, the EPI recommended age for vaccination, as the vaccine may be neutralized by maternal antibodies transplacentally acquired by the infant. For children at high risk of measles exposure, e.g. children in refugee camps or in hospital, the WHO recommends an initial dose of measles vaccine at six months as beneficial with a second dose at between 9 and 18 months.

Diphtheria

With good coverage, diphtheria has become rare in the industrialized world and also in many developing countries. Outbreaks in the newly independent states of the former Soviet Union relate to low vaccine coverage. With reduced boosting of immunity through natural exposure to diphtheria organisms, vaccine-induced immunity wanes over time, even in countries with consistently high levels of immunization coverage in infants. This allows groups of non-immune individuals to build up, creating the ideal conditions for epidemics, which may then occur if high coverage of infant immunization with diphtheria declines.

WHO recommends that at least 90% of children under the age of one are immunized with three doses of diphtheria vaccine, given as the combined DTP vaccine. In many developed countries a series of booster doses are also included in immunization schedules.

Pertussis

Loss of confidence in whole-cell pertussis vaccine due to a concern regarding vaccine-related encephalopathy in the 1970s reduced the uptake of this vaccine in a number of Western countries, resulting in a resurgence of infection, morbidity, and deaths. The disease is most dangerous in infants. WHO estimates indicated 17.6 million cases in 2003 and 279 000 deaths. Although establishing a link between this adverse event and the vaccine proved difficult to confirm, the public perception of the vaccine was damaged. As a result, a number of countries have incorporated the more expensive acellular vaccine in their immunization schedule, as this vaccine has similar efficacy but fewer side-effects, such as local reactions and fever. In countries where the incidence of pertussis has been considerably reduced by successful vaccination a booster dose administered 1–6 years after the primary series is warranted.

Hepatitis B

Hepatitis B infection is generally sub-clinical in infants and young children, and is predominantly acquired from mother to child, or by child-to-child transmission. The burden of disease develops in long-term carriers of Hepatitis B virus, and occurs in adult life as cirrhosis of the liver and liver cancer, which cause about a million deaths annually. This vaccine, now incorporated into the EPI schedule of over 150 countries, is unlikely to affect childhood morbidity, but it is expected to reduce one of the principal causes of cancer death in many parts of Africa, Asia, and the Pacific Basin. Where perinatal transmission of virus is common, e.g. in Southeast Asia, immunization is recommended at birth, 6 and 14 weeks, whereas in sub-Saharan Africa it is recommended at 6, 10 and 14 weeks. In the Gambia, the prevalence of chronic infection among children declined from 10% to 0.6% after implementation of universal hepatitis B vaccination.

Yellow fever

A single dose of the safe and highly effective yellow fever vaccine protects against disease for at least 10 years, and probably for life.

It is therefore recommended to be included in the EPI schedules of those countries at risk of yellow fever transmission, and is given at 9 months alongside measles immunization. As a strategy, it is almost certainly cheaper to prevent disease through immunization than to respond to outbreaks when they occur.

Other vaccines relevant to EPI immunization programmes

A number of vaccines are available but not widely used in developing countries. These include a vaccine against Japanese encephalitis, which in Thailand has been added to the EPI schedule. WHO recommends developing countries introduce the 7-valent pneumococcal conjugate vaccine (PCV7). The safety and efficacy of PCV7 has been well established, including in trials in developing countries which have shown a 16% reduction in all-cause mortality and a 65% reduction in invasive pneumococcal disease.[30,31] Similarly, rotavirus vaccines are also expected to have a significant impact on diarrhoeal deaths and malnutrition, but an initial vaccine introduced into the USA was subsequently shown to cause the rare adverse event of intussusception. The new rotavirus vaccines currently being tested are less likely to cause this complication.

There are many constraints to the delivery of effective immunization to communities in low-resource countries. These include effective maintenance of the 'cold chain', missed opportunities for immunization because of inappropriate contraindications and fear of side-effects, negative attitudes of healthcare workers, concerns about wastage of vaccine, and infrastructural difficulties in delivering vaccine at community level. HIV is not a contraindication to vaccination with the current EPI vaccines, apart from BCG, which is only contraindicated in symptomatic children with AIDS, but should still be given to neonates born to HIV-positive mothers. Achieving effective disease surveillance, sustainability and pricing are the main challenges for national and international organizations.

NUTRITIONAL DEFICIENCIES

Iron-deficiency anaemia

The World Health Organization estimates that over 40% of the world's children are iron deficient and regional prevalence figures for poor, high-risk populations frequently climb above 70%. Haematological indices, such as haemoglobin and serum ferritin concentrations are usually used as proxy measures of iron status but are in reality functional markers of iron bioavailability. The true prevalence of iron deficiency may be lower than that quoted. Nevertheless, iron deficiency represents an important public health problem in children because of its negative impacts on growth psychomotor development, cognition and the immune system. All of these effects may be modulated through iron deficiency anaemia. Recent work has demonstrated the importance of good maternal iron status from conception until delivery. The maternal-placental nutrient supply line must satisfy fetal demands for iron and provide the prenatal iron stores required by infants during early postnatal life.

Term infants with a normal birth weight are unlikely to become iron deficient during the first 6 months. However, breast-milk has low iron content, which despite being highly absorbed and utilized is inadequate for infants older than 6–9 months of age, when prenatal stores are exhausted. Prolonged exclusive breast-feeding beyond the first year and the provision of inadequate weaning foods thereafter contribute to the iron deficiency burden, which peaks in children under 2 years of age in poor countries. Dietary deficiency of iron is commonly exacerbated by poor absorption in the gut, secondary to the ingestion of dietary inhibitors (phytates, tannins, other divalent minerals) and/or gastroenteropathy. Chronic blood loss from intestinal helminthiasis and from the heavy menses of adolescent girls, are also particular risk factors.

The results from 26 randomized controlled trials of iron supplementation of children living in developing countries were recently reviewed.[32] Improved haematological indices and reductions in developmental deficits were observed in supplemented children with evidence of iron deficiency or anaemia at baseline. No consistent effects on growth were observed but in iron-replete children weight-gain was found to be adversely affected by supplementation. Most trials were too small to provide a reliable measure of morbidity and no overall effect was observed. A trial in eastern Africa described significant increases in mortality and serious adverse events secondary to malaria in children supplemented with iron compared with placebo.[33] Iron supplementation may best be targeted to those children with identified iron-deficiency anaemia rather than applied universally, especially in malaria-endemic regions.

Folate-deficiency anaemia

Folate deficiency occurs much more frequently in children in tropical countries than elsewhere. It is a well-recognized complication of kwashiorkor, sickle cell anaemia and other inherited haemolytic anaemias, goat's milk feeding in infancy, and malabsorption from many causes. Low birth weight babies are susceptible to folate deficiency, which should be suspected when these infants become anaemic and fail to thrive. Folate deficiency can cause persistent diarrhoea in infancy. Routine administration of folic acid, 400 μg daily, is recommended for the following conditions in childhood: sickle cell anaemia, thalassaemia and other inherited haemolytic anaemias; kwashiorkor; low birth weight babies; and children receiving long-term medication with drugs that have significant antifolate activity. Folate deficiency usually responds rapidly to treatment but megaloblastic anaemia in kwashiorkor may prove an exception.

Vitamin A deficiency

Between 125 and 250 million pre-school children are deficient in vitamin A, predominantly in South-east Asia and sub-Saharan Africa.[33] The definition of deficiency was previously expanded to include the full spectrum of vitamin A deficiency disorders (VADD). The categorization encompasses the various grades of xerophthalmia (Table 23.8 and Figure 23.2), down to subclinical deficiency (serum vitamin A concentration <0.7 mmol/L). Vitamin A deficiency is the leading cause of preventable blindness in children and at least half of the 500 000 children who become blind

Table 23.8 Clinical classification of xerophthalmia

Ocular sign	Classification
Night blindness	XN
Conjunctival xerosis	X1A
Bitot spot	X1B
Corneal xerosis	X2
Corneal ulcer/keratomalacia	X3
Corneal scar	XS
Xerophthalmia fundus	XF

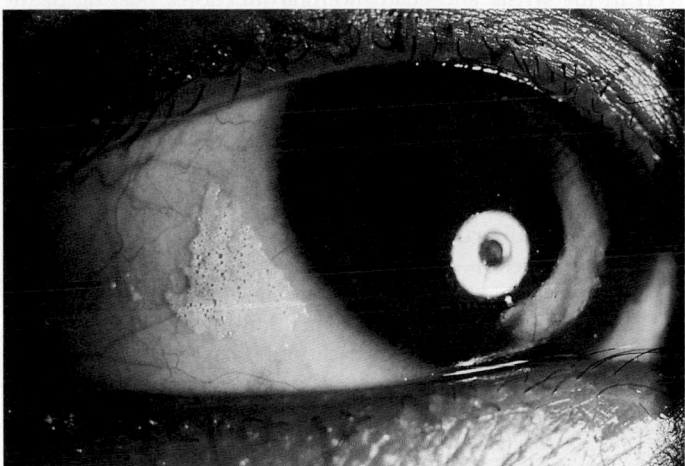

Figure 23.2 Pigmented conjunctival Bitot spot.

annually will die within a year of losing their sight.[34] Cheap, simple and highly effective supplementation programmes are now being implemented globally, which target children at risk between the ages of 6 months and 6 years. The administration of 200 000 IU of vitamin A every 4–6 months can reduce all-cause mortality by approximately 25% in high-risk children. Supplementation during acute measles reduces mortality by up to 50% and survivors recover more rapidly from diarrhoea and pneumonia. These programmes may be consolidated by a strong policy commitment to prolonged breast-feeding, which offers partial protection from clinical vitamin A deficiency to infants. Promotional campaigns on the dietary use of green leafy vegetables and food fortification campaigns, for example of sugar in Guatemala, have also proven successful. In infants under 6 months vitamin A supplementation schedules have been recommended, but there is controversy on dosage schedules.[35]

In older children, vitamin A is the treatment of choice for xerophthalmia. Retinyl palmitate or acetate, 200 000 IU in an oily solution is given orally on diagnosis, at 24 h and after 4 weeks (sooner if there is deterioration). Parenteral preparations are available in the event of vomiting or severe diarrhoea. Infants and children weighing less than 8 kg should be given half doses.

Vitamin D and calcium deficiency

Nutritional rickets (see also Chapter 30) occurs primarily in countries where for religious and/or social reasons, women and children are not exposed to the sun. It is quite common in Pakistan, Egypt, Somalia, Ethiopia the Middle East and West Africa, is considered rare in East Africa, but is well described in Nigeria.[36]

It commonly presents between 6 and 18 months of age and is increasingly recognized in very low birth weight babies. Rickets is a disease of growth and is infrequent therefore in severe malnutrition. Diagnosis is straightforward. The child may appear well nourished but restless and pale and a history of diarrhoea or respiratory infection may be given. Motor development is delayed, with poor linear growth. Infantile tetany may occur. Characteristic bony lesions in infancy include craniotabes, delayed closure of the fontanelles, delayed dentition, and epiphyseal enlargement best seen in the wrists and costochondral junctions. Bossing of the head, bow legs, knock knees and other limb deformities are common features in older children. Clinical diagnosis is confirmed by wrist radiographs and serum chemistry, which always shows raised alkaline phosphatase and depressed phosphate levels. Therapeutic vitamin D dose varies from 1500–5000 IU/day for 2–3 months, and the prophylactic dose is 400–600 IU/day. Where compliance with the long-term daily medication is poor and follow-up difficult, a single massive dose of vitamin D may be given by injection. This practice is quite common in the Middle East where the danger now exists that 'shopping around' for treatment may result in children receiving multiple doses of 100 000–200 000 IU of vitamin D. Breast milk may contain sufficient vitamin D to protect infants, but supplementation is required in high-risk infants, for those whose mothers keep them out of the sun and for those whose diet is a poor source of calcium.

Zinc deficiency

Zinc deficiency has a range of manifestations depending upon the severity of the restriction of the nutrient. Mild zinc deficiency would not be detected on clinical examination. Growth retardation and delayed development in children is one manifestation and it is recognized as having an important role in severe malnutrition when it may contribute to frank failure to thrive. Zinc deficiency has dermatological manifestations ranging from mild generalized drying to a specific hyperkeratosis in the areas of pressure and stress points. Diarrhoea may be present. There is laboratory evidence of immunosuppression. Diets rich in fibre and phytate may contribute to a reduced zinc status in many rural tropical populations. The consumption of zinc from breast milk is below recommended intakes, but there is a high efficiency of absorption. Rich sources of zinc include whole grains, poultry, lamb, liver, leafy and root vegetables. Daily regimens of zinc have been reported to prevent acute lower respiratory tract infection and diarrhoea, and to reduce child mortality.[37] In view of reductions in diarrhoea and pneumonia morbidity, zinc supplementation should be used as adjunct therapy for children with HIV-1 infection.[38]

Selenium deficiency

Evidence that selenium deficiency was responsible for human disease was reported when its association with a cardiomyopathy in Chinese children and women of child-bearing age was described. Oral supplementation with selenium is of value in preventing the disease. It has been shown that myxoedematous cretinism, which

occurs in regions of endemic goitre in tropical Africa, is related to a combined deficiency of selenium and iodine.

Iodine deficiency

It is estimated that iodine deficiency affects 35% of the world's population in 54 countries. Iodine is a component of the thyroid hormones, which are critical to the development of the central nervous system during the prenatal period and the first 3 years of postnatal life. Iodine deficiency can cause congenital hypothyroidism and is the commonest cause of mental retardation in children. It has been identified as one of the key modifiable risk factors for compromised childhood development in developing countries. Meta-analysis of trials conducted in China demonstrated that children living in severely deficient areas, who were supplemented with iodine prenatally and postnatally, scored higher on intelligence quotient testing than those who were not. Iodine fortification of salt is the usual means of supplementation and is most effective if given to pregnant women in the first half of pregnancy. Oral iodized oil is also an effective route as a single small dose is capable of correcting iodine deficiency for about a year.[39]

Interaction of nutrition and infection (see also Chapter 30).

Poor diets result in nutritional deficiencies associated with frequent infections and malnutrition. Malnutrition has a direct negative effect on the immune system leading to increased morbidity and mortality. Infection is a major force in the development of kwashiorkor. During weaning infections are more common, especially diarrhoea and respiratory infection and each infection results in growth faltering through energy depletion. Catch-up growth is usually incomplete and can lead through cumulative effects to severe malnutrition. The early introduction of complementary feeds worsens this problem.[40] The nutritional deficits from sequential infections accumulate, and a vicious cycle of infection-malnutrition results. These deficits are compounded by specific micronutrient and vitamin deficiencies. Nutrient supplementation of malnourished children may also alter infection risk. For example, iron supplementation may slightly increase the risk of death.[32] The alternatives of multi-micronutrient versus single nutrient supplementation for undernourished children should be considered in the development of preventative nutritional programmes during childhood. These targeted interventions should be developed in the context of community nutritional programmes.

REFERENCES

1. Black RE, Morris SS, Bryce J. Where and why are 10 million children dying every year? *Lancet* 2003; 361:2226–2234.
2. State of the World's Mothers 2007. *Saving the lives of children under 5*. London: Save the Children Fund; 2007.
3. Costello A, Manandhar D, eds. *Improving Newborn Infant Health in Developing Countries*. London: Imperial College Press; 2000.
4. WHO. *Postpartum Care of the Mother and Newborn: A Practical Guide*. Geneva: World Health Organization; 1998.
5. van Rheenen PF, Brabin BJ. A practical approach to timing and cord clamping in resource poor settings. *BMJ* 2006; 333:954–958.

6. Brabin L, Brabin BJ. Parasitic infections in women and their consequences. *Advan Parasitol* 1992; 31:1–81.

7. WHO. *Management of Severe Malaria: A Practical Handbook.* 2nd edn. Geneva: World Health Organization; 2000.

8. Barnes KI, Mwenechanya J, Tembo M, et al. Efficacy of rectal artesunate compared with parenteral quinine in initial treatment of moderately severe malaria in African children and adults: a randomised study. *Lancet* 2004; 363:1598–1605.

9. Njuguna PW, Newton CR. Management of severe falciparum malaria. *J Postgrad Med* 2004; 50:45–50.

10. Duke T, Mgone CS. Measles: not just another exanthema. *Lancet* 2003; 361:763–773.

11. Chintu C, Mudenda V, Lucas S, et al. Lung diseases at necropsy in African children dying of respiratory illnesses – a descriptive necropsy study. *Lancet* 2002; 360:985–990.

12. Zar HJ, Cotton MF, Strauss S, et al. Effect of isoniazid prophylaxis on mortality and incidence of tuberculosis in children with HIV: randomised controlled trial. *BMJ* 2007; 334:136–139.

13. Lucas SB, Peacock CS, Hounnou A, et al. Disease in children infected with HIV in Abidjan, Cote d'Ivoire. *BMJ* 1996; 312:335–338.

14. Liebershuetz S, Bamber S, Ewer K, et al. Diagnosis of tuberculosis in South African children with a T-cell-based assay: a prospective cohort study. *Lancet* 2004; 364:2196–2203.

15. Graham SM, Coulter JB S, Gilks CF. Pulmonary disease in HIV infected African children. *Int J TB Lung Dis* 2001; 5:12–23.

16. Coovadia HM, Rollins NC, Bland RM, et al. Mother-to-child transmission of HIV-1 infection during exclusive breastfeeding: the first six months of life. *Lancet* 2007; 369:1107–1116.

17. WHO. *HIV and infant feeding technical consultation consensus statement.* October 2006. Online. Available: http://www.who.int/child-adolescent-health/publications/NUTRITION/consensus_statement.htm

18. Coutsoudis A, Dabis F, Fawzi W, et al., for the Breastfeeding and HIV International Transmission Study Group. Late postnatal transmission of HIV-1 in breast-fed children: an individual patient data meta-analysis. *J Infect Dis* 2004; 189:2154–2166.

19. Marun LH, Tindyebwa D, Gibb B. Care of children with HIV infections and AIDS in Africa. *AIDS* 1997; 11(suppl B):S125–S135.

20. Chintu C, Bhat GJ, Walker AS, et al. Co-trimoxazole as prophylaxis against opportunistic infections in HIV-infected Zambian children (CHAP): a double-blind randomised placebo-controlled trial. *Lancet* 2004; 364:1865–1871.

21. WHO. *Antiretroviral Therapy for infants and children: Towards universal access. Recommendations for a public health approach.* Geneva: World Health Organization; 2006.

22. Graham SM, Mtitimila EL, Kamanga HS, et al. The clinical presentation and outcome of *Pneumocystis carinii* pneumonia in Malawian children. *Lancet* 2000; 355:369–373.

23. Carapetis J, McDonald M, Wilson N. Acute rheumatic fever. *Lancet* 2005; 366:155–168.

24. Crowcroft NS, Pebody RG. Recent developments in pertussis. *Lancet* 2006; 367:1926–1936.

25. Peiris JSM, Tang WH, Chan KH, et al. Children with respiratory disease associated with metapneumovirus in Hong Kong. *Emerg Infect Dis* 2003; 9:628–633.

26. King CK, Glass R, Bresee JS, et al. Managing acute gastroenteritis among children, oral rehydration, maintenance and nutritional therapy. *MMWR Recommendations and Reports* 2003; 52(RR16):1–16.

27. Peltola H. Burden of meningitis and other severe bacterial infections of children in Africa: Implications for prevention. *Clin Infect Dis* 2001; 31: 64–75.

28. Molyneux E, Wash A, Forsyth M, et al. Dexamethasone treatment in childhood bacterial meningitis in Malawi: a randomised controlled trial. *Lancet* 2002; 360:211–218.

29. WHO Division of Child Health and Development. Integrated management of childhood illness: conclusions. *Bull World Health Organ* 1997; 75(suppl 1):119–128.

30. WHO. *Management of the Child with a Serious Infection or Severe Malnutrition. Guidelines for Care at the First Referral Level in Developing Countries.* Geneva: World Health Organization, Department of Child Health and Adolescent Health; 2000:1–161.

31. Levine OS, O'Brien KL, Knoll M, et al. Pneumococcal vaccination in developing countries. *Lancet* 2006; 367:1880–1882.

32. Ianotti LL, Tielsch JM, Black MM, et al. Iron supplementation in early childhood: health benefit and risks. *Am J Clin Nutr* 2006; 84:1261–1276.

33. Sazwal S, Black RE, Ramsan M, et al. Effects of routine prophylactic supplementation with iron and folic acid on admission to hospital and mortality in preschool children in a high malaria transmission setting: community based, randomised, placebo-controlled trial. *Lancet* 2006; 367:133–143.

34. McLaren DS A, Frigg M. *Sight and life manual on vitamin A deficiency disorders.* Basel: Task Force Sight and Life; 2001.

35. Brabin BJ. Infant vitamin A supplementation: consensus or controversy. *Lancet* 2007; 369(9579):2054–2056.

36. Thacker TD, Fischer PR, Strand MA, et al. Nutritional rickets around the world: causes and future directions. *Ann Trop Paediatrics* 2006; 26:1–16.

37. Aggarwal R, Sentz J, Miller MA. Role of zinc and administration in prevention of childhood diarrhoea and respiratory illness: a meta-analysis. *Pediatrics* 2007; 119:1120–1130.

38. Bbat R, Coovadia H, Stephen C, et al. Safety and efficacy of zinc supplementation for children with HIV-1 infection in South Africa: a randomised double-blind controlled trial. *Lancet* 2005; 366:1862–1867.

39. Tonglet R, Bourdoux P, Minga T, et al. Efficacy of low oral doses of iodised oil in the control of iodine deficiency in Zaire. *N Engl J Med* 1992; 326: 236–241.

40. Kalanda BF, Verhoeff FH, Brabin BJ. Breast and complementary feeding practices in relation to morbidity and growth of Malawian infants. *Eur J Clin Nutr* 2006; 60:401–407.

Chapter 24   John. E. Jellis

Surgery in the Tropics

INTRODUCTION

There are some excellent surgical centres in the tropics but, situated in the cities and catering for the affluent, they are irrelevant to the two-thirds of the world's population that lacks proper surgical care.[1] In Third World countries, most surgeons work in the cities and are divorced from the large rural population by distance, cost of travel and the lack of workable referral systems.[2] Country-wide, more surgical operations are performed by general-duties doctors, clinical officers or nurses than by surgeons.[3] Fortunately, relatively few of the commonly performed surgical operations need 'specialist' expertise.[4] In some countries, surgeons visit up-country hospitals by road or air, or 'surgical camps' are organized, during which many operations are performed in a short time. These visiting surgeons can also teach the doctors more cost-effective methods of treatment for the common surgical problems of their country.[4–6]

Most tropical medical schools lack adequate funding and are chronically short of surgical teachers, nurses and paramedical staff because of economic migration to the health services of rich western nations. In Zambia for instance, 80% of medical graduates are working abroad and operating theatres lie idle for lack of nurses. Those who stay remain urbanized by the better economic, social and educational facilities of the towns.

Surgery is expensive and has a low priority in a poor nation's health budget. Donor aid programmes concentrate on preventive medicine, infectious diseases and, more recently, on the provision of antiretroviral drugs. Consequently, only a small percentage of necessary operations are performed.[7–9] Too often, the woman in obstructed labour, the man with a strangulated hernia, the patient with multiple injuries from a road traffic accident or the child with severe burns cannot find effective treatment. Surgery must become part of primary healthcare.

Tropical surgery is the realm of the truly general surgeon. Often working under austere conditions, he must operate on a host of surgical conditions which, in the West, fall within the realm of 'specialities'.[10] He is the 'district gynaecologist', dealing with ruptured ectopic pregnancy, obstructed labour and uterine ruptures. He will have to cope with trauma to all the systems of the body, including the eye, head, chest and abdomen, as well as fractures and dislocations of the limbs, pelvis and spine. Inevitably, he will be faced with locally common conditions outside the scope of his experience. Frustrated by failed attempts to refer such patients, he must seek appropriate training to tackle them himself.

A common attribute of surgeons in the tropics is their enthusiasm for the work. This contrasts markedly with colleagues in the West who take early retirement from repetitive work within a narrow field of expertise. Almost daily, the tropical surgeon faces the challenge of varied problems for which solutions must be found. He may never become rich but is respected and enjoys great job satisfaction.

In the cities, the affluent populations increasingly suffer from a 'western' pattern of surgical pathologies, often complicated by obesity, hypertension and diabetes. Patients from the urban poor and rural areas may have their fitness for major surgery compromised by concomitant 'tropical diseases' such as malnutrition, anaemia, malaria and bilharzia. In addition, there are many 'tropical' surgical pathologies, each needing special treatment. Fortunately, there is now a comprehensive 'Textbook of Tropical Surgery' (Kamel R, Lumley J, eds; see 'Recommended Reference Books'). This chapter attempts to direct the reader to successful management of the surgical problems commonly encountered in tropical countries.

THE INFLUENCE OF HIV DISEASE ON SURGERY IN THE TROPICS

Human immunodeficiency virus (HIV) and acquired immunodeficiency syndrome (AIDS) are widespread and add to the surgical workload. The free provision of antiviral drug combinations prolongs life for some patients, but, especially in rural areas, regular drug distribution and effective disease monitoring are often lacking. Tuberculosis and sepsis have become even more common and management of many conditions has had to change.

It is estimated that there are over 14 million people with HIV infection in Africa, 4 million in Asia and 2 million in South America.[11] In Zambia, HIV disease was first recognized in 1983.[12] By 1992, over 30% of adult patients admitted for trauma were HIV-positive[13] and some 40% of all surgical admissions were HIV-positive patients.[14]

A surgeon working in the tropics must be able to recognize HIV disease and the HIV-related pathologies. He must know how other pathologies have been influenced by the disease and be able to assess the risks of surgical operations in such patients. Lastly, universal precautions against the risk of surgical staff contracting infection in the operating theatre must be adopted.

Recognition of HIV-positive patients

HIV-positive patients are not a homogeneous group. A positive serological test for HIV only indicates the presence of antibodies. It tells the surgeon nothing about the patient's level of immune competence or fitness for surgery. These are assessed by examination, possibly supplemented by lymphocyte counts.

Every surgical patient should be examined undressed and in a good light, paying special attention to the mouth, lymph nodes (axillary, epitrochlear and posterior cervical), and for any skin signs.[15] The clinical classification proposed by the World Health Organization (WHO), modified as in Table 24.1, should be used.[16] Stage 0 has been added to classify the serologically HIV-positive patient with no clinical symptoms or signs. A total lymphocyte count or CD4 lymphocyte count will indicate the degree of immune compromise (Table 24.2).[17,18] Necessary surgery should not be withheld from HIV-positive patients, but the risks must be

Table 24.1 Staging of HIV-positive patients*

CLINICAL STAGE 0
Serologically HIV-positive but no signs or symptoms related to HIV infection
CLINICAL STAGE 1
Asymptomatic
Persistent generalized lymphadenopathy
CLINICAL STAGE 2
Weight loss, <10% of body weight
Minor mucocutaneous manifestations
Herpes zoster within the last 5 years
Recurrent upper respiratory tract infections
CLINICAL STAGE 3
Weight loss, >10% body weight
Unexplained chronic diarrhoea, >1 month
Unexplained prolonged fever, >1 month
Oral candidiasis or hairy leukoplakia
Pulmonary tuberculosis, within the past year
Severe bacterial infections
CLINICAL STAGE 4
AIDS: the HIV wasting syndrome
Severe opportunistic infections
Extrapulmonary tuberculosis
Lymphoma or Kaposi's sarcoma
HIV encephalopathy

* Based on 'An interim proposal for a WHO staging system for HIV infection and disease'[16] with modifications.

thoroughly assessed so that an appropriate operation can be planned and discussed with the patient.

Surgery on HIV-positive patients

HIV-positive patients suffer increased rates of postoperative wound, chest and urinary tract infections and the frequency of these complications increases with progression of their disease. In general terms, if a patient has no physical signs of HIV disease, their response to clean major surgery will approximate to that of HIV-negative patients. Where contamination exists (open fractures, bowel surgery, etc.), however, infection rates are likely to double and every precaution should be employed to minimize this risk. If major prosthetic surgery is a treatment option (hip and knee replacements, arterial grafts, etc.), preoperative counselling and testing is mandatory. Both the surgeon and patient must thoroughly appreciate the risks of such implants attracting untreatable haematogenous sepsis in the later stages of HIV disease and weigh them against the expected benefits of surgery. Only then can informed consent for operation be given.

Patients with physical signs of HIV disease need evaluation of their immune competence (CD4 or total lymphocyte counts) and their general fitness for operation, because the risks of delayed healing and sepsis are considerable. Their fitness, or otherwise, must be weighed against the risks and possible benefits of surgery. Obvious major 'damage control' operations (pus drainage, control of haemorrhage, relief of obstruction, etc.) should be undertaken, but 'cold surgery' (herniorrhaphy, correction of deformities, etc.) should not be contemplated. The internal fixation of fractures is very high-risk surgery in these patients. If such treatment is the only possible option, the implants should be removed as soon as the fracture has healed, to prevent intractable late bone infections.

Precautions against contracting HIV disease by inoculation while operating on HIV-positive patients

Surgeons commonly damage their gloves and skin from sharp instruments, needles, wires and bone fragments. All members of the theatre staff should take precautions to minimize the, admittedly small, risk of becoming infected with HIV.[19] Such precautions must be universally applied because it is impossible to know the HIV status of every patient. The most infectious patient is one in the viraemic phase of a recent infection, who would test HIV-

Table 24.2 Lymphocyte and CD4 cell counts in HIV disease*

Subdivision	Lymphocytes	CD4
(A)	>2000	>500
(B)	1000–2000	200–500
(C)	<1000	<200

* Based on 'An interim proposal for a WHO staging system for HIV infection and disease'[16] with modifications. Each clinical stage can be subdivided on the absolute or CD4 lymphocyte counts to give further evidence of immune status.

negative, and most HIV-positive patients undergoing surgery for trauma will have no clinical signs of HIV disease.[13]

Most precautions are simply common sense. Where blood spillage is expected (ruptured spleen, caesarean section, etc.) boots and an apron beneath an impervious gown with gauntlets, double gloves and an eye shield would be ideal. Ideal, that is, apart from the discomfort in tropical heat and humidity.

If sharp bone fragments are likely to be handled or wires used, an armoured glove is useful or a sterilized cotton (dermatological) glove should be worn over the rubber glove. Dexterity is somewhat reduced, but sharp fragments catch in the cotton, rather than penetrating through glove and skin. Eye protection is important, especially if an osteotome is in use, remembering that most fragments will fly towards the assistant.

Large incisions allow the surgeon to operate by sight more than by feel and assistants' fingers should be kept well clear of the operative field. Any sharp instrument should be handed to the surgeon in a dish and replaced in the dish after use. If a Mayo table is used, strict rules must be formulated to prevent the surgeon's hands meeting those of the scrub nurse while placing sharp instruments on the table.

Any injury should be reported and HIV tests conducted on both the patient and surgeon to confirm their pre-exposure status. Post-exposure prophylaxis with appropriate antiviral drugs should be commenced after significant injuries, pending these test results. A deep cut or needle stick with a blood-containing hypodermic needle is certainly significant, whereas a skin abrasion from a suture needle or instrument probably carries a lesser risk of transmission.

Blood transfusion in the tropics

It has become obvious that, although blood transfusion may be life-saving, it is also a dangerous procedure. Autologous blood floods the immune system with antigens reducing the patient's resistance to infections and tumour spread. Infections, such as HIV, hepatitis and malaria, are easily transmitted.[20] Even when every precaution is taken, viraemic HIV-negative donors may have been bled or bottles mislabelled.[21] Safe donated blood is in short supply and should be reserved for emergency situations.

Patients do well with haemoglobin levels well below the previously recommended minimum of 10 g/dL. A preoperative haemoglobin of 9 g/dL is acceptable for operations under tourniquet or when minimal blood loss is expected. After major surgery, haemoglobin levels down to 5 g/dL have been recorded without noticeably affecting respiration or wound healing.

When major surgery is planned and time permits, a patient may create a stock of his own blood by donating at weekly intervals, but this has disadvantages. If the patient is HIV-positive, the blood bank will refuse to store his blood. Once donated and tested, it is difficult to prevent the blood being used if a life-threatening emergency occurs and no other blood is available.

Acute euvolaemic haemodilution[22,23] overcomes many of these problems. Immediately before surgery, several units of blood may be taken from the patient, to be infused during any intraoperative haemorrhage or given back at the end of the operation. As each unit of blood is drawn, it is replaced by a double volume of intravenous saline. Each unit of blood taken will reduce the patient's haemoglobin by approximately 1 g/dL and the preoperative haemoglobin should not be allowed to fall below 9 g/dL. Haemodilution reduces blood viscosity and beneficially increases tissue perfusion.

In Lusaka, acute euvolaemic haemodilution has been used in major orthopaedic surgery for the last 10 years with satisfactory results. Rarely has additional banked blood been needed. As long as the blood is kept in contact with the patient, this practice has proved acceptable to Jehovah's Witnesses.

PATHOLOGIES ASSOCIATED WITH HIV DISEASE

Tuberculosis

Tuberculosis is the commonest and most virulent of the opportunistic infections associated with HIV disease. HIV specifically inhibits and destroys the tissue macrophages and thymic lymphocytes that are the body's main defence against *Mycobacterium tuberculosis*.[74] In many tropical countries there is a dual epidemic of HIV disease and tuberculosis.[24] Over 60% of adult patients with pulmonary[25] and bone and joint tuberculosis[26] are HIV-positive, as are 84% of those with tuberculous lymphadenitis.[27]

Extrapulmonary forms of tuberculosis, especially of the breast,[28] lymph nodes,[29] abdomen,[30] spine and major joints[26,31] are now common. HIV-associated tuberculosis does respond to standard antituberculous drug therapy, but the patient's prognosis depends more upon the stage of HIV disease than upon the extent of the tuberculous infection. Concomitant antiretroviral chemotherapy may be needed to improve the patient's immune response.

Lymphadenopathy

Although symmetrical chronic enlargement of the posterior cervical, axillary and epitrochlear lymph nodes is a sign of early HIV disease, asymmetrical enlargement of nodes merits investigation.[27] Possible pathologies include the reactive hyperplasia of HIV disease itself, tuberculosis, Kaposi's sarcoma, lymphoma and other metastatic tumour deposits. Bem[27,29] showed that the diagnosis can often be made on the naked-eye appearance of a cut node rather than waiting for a histology report. Aspiration cytology and imprint cytology are also useful diagnostic tools. With a little practice, the surgeon will have an immediate indication of the likely diagnosis.[32]

Empyema thoracis

Many HIV-positive patients, especially children and young adults, develop empyema and most have underlying tuberculosis.[33] Desai[34] showed that, if pus can easily be aspirated through a 21 F into a 10 mL syringe by one pull of the plunger, the empyema needs drainage through an intercostal tube and underwater-seal drain to prevent lung collapse. If, however, the pus is too thick to aspirate easily, 7.5 cm sections of two adjacent ribs over the most dependent part of the empyema should be resected for open drainage. Drainage is encouraged by the patient sleeping on the affected side, blowing up balloons or old surgical gloves, and irrigating the sinus with water. These patients can be discharged to home care within a week.

Adult haematogenous osteomyelitis

HIV-positive adults often present with chronic haematogenous osteomyelitis of insidious onset.[35] The disease mainly affects the metaphyses of the tibia (Figure 24.1) and femur and may symmetrically affect both legs. The infections are often staphylococcal, but salmonella and a variety of other 'bowel' flora have been found. Mixed infections occur, even before there is an open wound.

Despite treatment by drainage, sequestrectomy and wide debridement, the infection often progresses in an inexorable manner, causing much pain and suffering (Figure 24.2). Above-knee amputations, however, have healed well and have been followed by a worthwhile period of weight gain and better health for up to 5 years.[35]

Haematogenous infections commonly occur around joint prostheses, Kuntscher nails and other implants, years after their insertion, in patients reaching advanced stages of HIV disease.[35] Such infections may be controlled after removal of small implants, but have proved impossible to eradicate after removal of Kuntscher nails and hip prostheses.

Tropical pyomyositis

Pyomyositis is strongly associated with HIV disease in young adults.[36] In Uganda, 71% of sufferers of both sexes were HIV-positive[37] and, if abscesses were multiple, the association was 81%. The abscesses are mainly in the large muscles of the trunk and proximal compartments of the limbs. *Staphylococcus aureus* is still the usual organism grown, but a variety of other organisms have been found in HIV-positive patients. Whether there is a primary lesion in the muscle that becomes secondarily infected is still debated.[38]

These debilitated patients need good supportive care and systemic antibiotic therapy if the large volumes of pus are to be safely drained. After incision, careful palpation of the abscess cavity will differentiate pyomyositis from haematogenous osteomyelitis, in which bare bone devoid of periosteum will be felt in the base of the cavity.

Other musculoskeletal pathology and rheumatoid disease

Many HIV-positive patients present with non-specific backache and tenderness of the thoracic or lumbar spine. Acute rheumatoid arthritis, reactive arthritis (especially of the knees and ankles), erosive arthritis and enthesitis (especially of the tendo Achilles

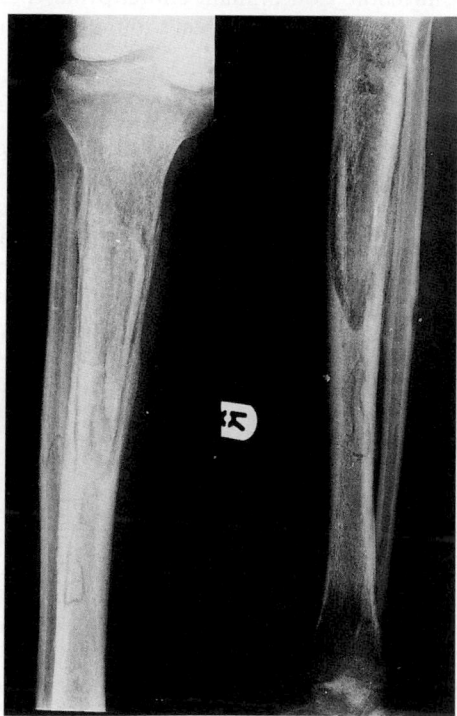

Figure 24.1 Radiograph of the tibia in a patient with HIV-related haematogenous osteomyelitis. There is bone destruction with very little new bone formation.

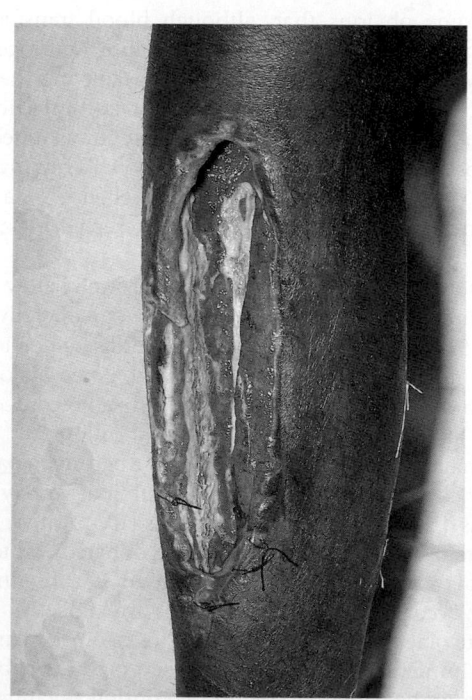

Figure 24.2 Non-healing wound after sequestrectomy for HIV-related haematogenous osteomyelitis of the tibia.

and plantar fascia) are now commonly seen in HIV-positive patients.[39]

Neurological manifestations of HIV infection

At least 40% of patients with HIV infection develop neurological manifestations at some stage, and over 80% have neuropathological findings at autopsy.[11] The protean effects of HIV range from acute neuropathy, myelopathy or encephalitis within 3 months of infection, to the AIDS-dementia complex occurring in late HIV disease. Cryptococcal meningitis, tuberculoma and other cerebral space-occupying lesions and progressive multifocal leukoencephalopathy may occur later.[11,40]

Necrotizing fasciitis

Necrotizing fasciitis (Fournier's gangrene) is a progressive, rapidly spreading synergistic infection with aerobic and anaerobic gas-forming organisms around the deep fascia. It has long been associated with diabetes mellitus, cancer, alcoholism and immunocompromised patients.[41] Now it is common in HIV-positive patients.

The disease carries a high mortality rate. Successful management demands early diagnosis, rapid resuscitation, aggressive surgical excision with frequent revision, coupled with high doses of broad-spectrum antibiotics and blood transfusion.[42]

Perianal infection

There is a strong association between HIV disease, fistula in ano and perianal abscess.[43,44] Experienced surgeons consider that fistula in ano and haemorrhoids should be treated conservatively in HIV-positive patients because anal wounds heal poorly, and both anal dilatation and sphincterotomy impair continence for fluid diarrhoea.[14]

Kaposi's sarcoma

Atypical aggressive Kaposi's sarcoma is now common in HIV-positive children and young adults of both sexes.[12] It affects the skin, lymph nodes and gastrointestinal tract as well as other organs and responds poorly to cytotoxic drugs.[45] Surgery is rarely indicated except to amputate a painful useless hand, foot or limb. If there is gastrointestinal involvement, the purple Kaposi tissue may be seen on the hard palate (Figure 24.3). Plaques in the small bowel may give rise to intussusception.[46]

TRAUMA

A surgeon working in the tropics needs to be capable of managing a very wide range of injuries with minimal equipment. Commonly, 60% of surgical in-patients have suffered trauma. They have major fractures, chest, abdominal, head and spinal injuries, wounds and burns.[1] In urban areas and near major roads, most

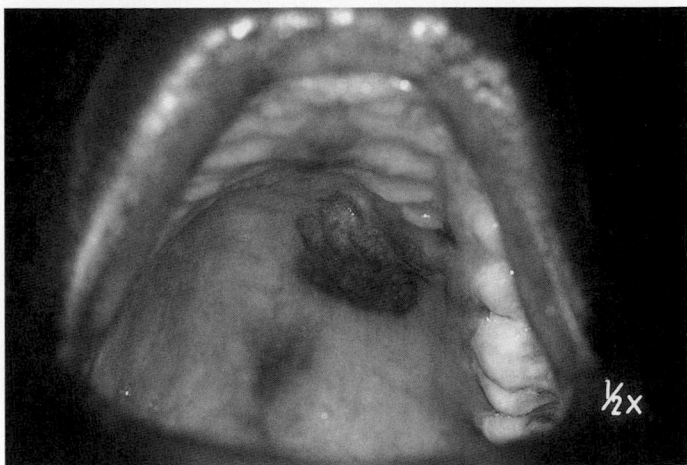

Figure 24.3 Purple plaque of Kaposi's sarcoma on the hard palate, indicating gastrointestinal involvement.

injuries result from road traffic accidents and interpersonal violence. In remote fishing communities, the major problems may be horrendous injuries from crocodiles.[47–49] Wars continue to maim many, and mutilating injuries from landmines continue years after the conflicts have ceased.

Late presentation to hospital is common because of distance and the lack of ambulance services. Patients may be dehydrated, hypothermic, shocked or anaemic and have established wound infections, peritonitis or pneumonia as they reach hospital. The management of neglected trauma is very different from the treatment appropriate soon after injury.[50]

Damage control

In severely injured patients, the restoration of normal physiology is much more important than early anatomical reconstruction. First, thorough but rapid resuscitation (ABC etc.) will save the life of the patient and help prevent further organ and tissue necrosis. Surgery should be limited to damage control: reconstruction can be undertaken later.[51] Bleeding must be controlled, dead tissue excised, pus drained, contaminated cavities and wounds lavaged, and fractures temporarily stabilized with casts, skeletal traction or external fixator.

If laparotomy is indicated for continued bleeding or peritonitis, only damage control should be performed. Severe bleeding from the liver is controlled by the four dry pack technique.[52] Severely damaged bowel is exteriorized or a proximal colostomy established and the distal bowel closed with a purse string. To save time, prevent the abdominal compartment syndrome[53,54] and allow an easy second look at 24 or 48 hours, the abdominal contents should be retained by sewing a plastic sheet to the edges of the incision (the Bagota bag).[55] Having got the patient off the operating table in the shortest possible time, physiology can be restored with warmth, blood and fluids as necessary.

Take the patient back to theatre for a second look at 24 or 48 hours if progress is unsatisfactory. Further tissue may have died or a perforation been missed, but, again, only control the damage. Success is a live patient: anatomical repair can be undertaken a week or so later.

Dislocations

Dislocations are a priority because they are easily reduced by manipulation soon after injury but can be very difficult several days later. Elbow dislocations may be reduced at up to 2 weeks, but it needs prolonged steady stretching to do so. Closed reduction of late-presenting hip dislocations is always worth trying[50] because open reduction can be a very difficult procedure.

Fractures

Because of the high cost and poor availability of implants, lack of orthopaedic surgeons and the prevalence of HIV disease, non-operative methods of management are appropriate in most situations.[1] Non-operative treatment has been neglected in the First World, but the innovative use of traction, casting, cast-bracing and external fixation has advanced in the tropics. Perkin's traction (Figure 24.4) and 90/90 traction for femoral fractures[5] are good examples of this. The skills of manipulative reduction and holding that reduction as swelling diminishes must be learned. Non-operative management is often more time-consuming than internal fixation but excellent results can be obtained.

Open fractures of the tibia are common and difficult to deal with because of the subcutaneous position of the bone. The injuries vary from a puncture wound produced by a fragment of bone from inside (grade 1) to the mangled limb (grade 4) which may need amputation. The principles of management are to treat the wound and to stabilize the fracture.

In moderate cases of soft tissue injury, the wound should be washed, debrided (with wide opening of the deep fascia to decompress damaged muscle compartments), lavaged with more than 10 L of tap water and dressed.[56] Temporary (7–21 days) stabilization can be provided with gentle (4 kg) calcaneal pin traction and elevation of the limb. This gives a window of opportunity in which the wound care can continue, swelling diminish and wounds closed (usually by split skin grafting) before the limb can be immobilized in a well-fitting cast to allow the patient to start partial weight bearing at 2 to 3 weeks.

With greater degrees of soft tissue damage, traction is inadequate and an external fixator (actual or improvised) should be applied immediately after the primary wound care. The stability provided promotes healing, reduces infection markedly, and allows easy access to the wounds for cleaning, dressings and early skin grafting. Knee and ankle exercises should be encouraged and the foot supported with a sling tied to the external fixator to prevent equinus deformity. The aim should be to start mobilizing the patient, partial weight bearing as soon as the wounds allow, hopefully at about 3 weeks.

Wound management

Only cleanly incised wounds seen within a few hours of injury should be sutured. Wounds that have an element of crush injury,

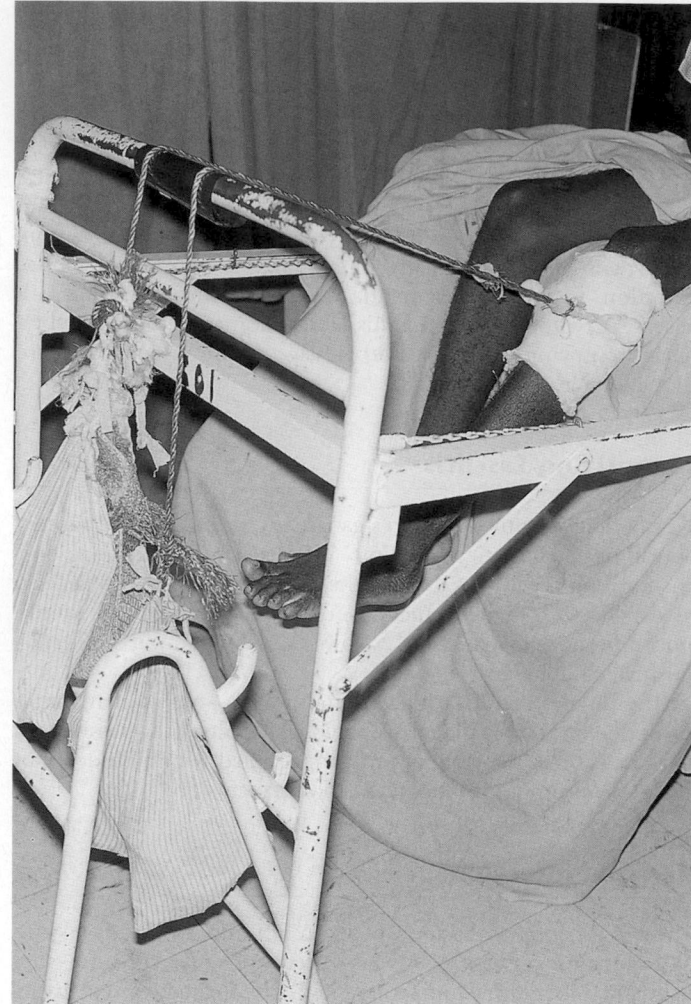

Figure 24.4 Patient exercising in Perkin's traction which encourages early union and prevents muscle wasting, knee stiffness and malrotation.

are contaminated or infected, or have presented late, should be cleaned, debrided, lavaged with copious amounts (>10 L) of tap water[56] and left open for suture or skin grafting several days later. Frequent washing of wounds is beneficial with the proviso that no substances toxic to cells are used. Never put in a wound what you would not put in your own eye! Great savings on antibiotic usage can be made if such regimens are followed.[57]

Dirty wounds with slough and obvious infection are common and can often be smelled on entering the side wards in which such patients are commonly sequestrated. There is no need for this scenario. Such wounds can be rendered odourless by excision of dead tissue and daily honey dressings. By next morning there will be no smell, and healthy granulation tissue ready for the application of split skin grafts will soon appear.

Hand injuries and infections

Whether a hand has been damaged by burning, crushing or infection, always remember that it must be kept in a functional position by dressings and splintage. Support must be improvised to keep the wrist extended (45°), the metacarpophalangeal joints flexed (as near 90° as possible) and the thumb opposed. Even if the tissue damage and subsequent scarring is severe, that hand will have useful function, in contrast to the useless spade or claw hand so often produced by thoughtless 'treatment' of the specific injury or infection alone.

Head injury and spinal injury

Many tropical countries do not have neurosurgical centres or they may be too distant for referral of injured patients. A good understanding of the principles of care for the unconscious or paraplegic patient will save many lives.[58,59] Burr holes or tracheostomy may be indicated early in head injury cases,[60,61] and should be done if the patient cannot reach specialist care within a very short time. Early operations on the spine are very rarely needed.[62-64] Cervical traction and reduction for neck fractures, positional reduction of others, 2-hourly turning of the patient and intermittent catheterization are the best treatment for patients with spinal injury.[1,64] Indwelling catheters are a potent source of urinary tract infection and urethral stricture, and should not be used in spinal injuries. If intermittent catheterization is needed for long periods, the patient's relative may be taught to introduce the catheter. Later, clean self-catheterization should be taught to the patient. In this way, much morbidity and possibly mortality may be avoided.

Burns

Severe burns are common in the tropics, especially in young children. Open fires are used for cooking and, especially on cold winter nights, become the focus of family life. Epileptic patients frequently fall into fires during their seizures. In many cultures they are thought to be spirit-possessed and will not be pulled clear until the fit has stopped.

Huts built of highly flammable material are often lit by primitive paraffin lamps which cause horrendous burns when they are knocked over or explode.[65] Burn injuries increase in the cold season and a heated burns ward may prevent deaths from hypothermia. A severe burn is any burn of over 10% body surface area in a child and over 15% in an adult. Prompt resuscitation with intravenous fluids as calculated by weight and age from the charts available in several books[66,67] should be monitored by urine output from an indwelling catheter.

A severely burnt patient not only loses his ability to regulate body temperature but also loses resistance to infection and may become severely anaemic from direct thermal damage and disseminated intravascular coagulopathy. These patients need very careful monitoring.[67] They have an increased metabolic rate and need extra food. Antibiotics and blood transfusion should be held in reserve for when signs of infection or anaemia appear. The burn wound should be treated with topical antibacterial agents such as silver sulphadiazine or a mixture of honey and ghee, both of which are inexpensive if made in the hospital.[68]

Priority should be given to the treatment of the hands, neck, perineum and the flexor surfaces of joints, where subsequent contracture will prove crippling. When not actively exercising, these areas should be splinted to prevent contracture. Deep circumferential limb and hand burns will need escharotomy to prevent distal ischaemic necrosis.[68] Very severe limb burns may require early amputation, and patients with deep burns covering more than 50% of body surface area do not survive.

Using such treatment methods (Figure 24.5),[68] superficial and partial thickness burns should be healed within 21 days. Unhealed areas should then be treated by split skin grafting without further delay. In babies with severe burns, maternal split skin may be used as graft material and meshing of grafts extends the area of cover considerably. Split skin grafts themselves will contract in the first 12 weeks after application, and splinting or plaster casts should be applied to prevent this as soon as the grafts are stable. Depigmented scar tissue, especially on areas of the body exposed to tropical sunlight, carries a very high risk of malignant change with epithelioma (squamous cell carcinoma; Marjolin's ulcer) developing within 10 years (Figure 24.6).

The release of burns contracture and excision and grafting of depigmented scars occupies a large place in reconstructive and plastic surgical work in the tropics.[69] This can be rewarding, but prevention is better than cure. All epileptic patients should be supplied with prophylactic anticonvulsants, which can be distributed by Psychiatric Clinical Officers and other health workers from government clinics.[70] This simple measure will largely prevent repeated expensive hospital admissions for these dreadful injuries.

FACTORS AFFECTING THE SAFETY OF SURGERY

The outcome of any surgical operation may be adversely affected by the condition of the patient. In the First World, old age, obesity, hypertension, ischaemic heart disease, diabetes and chronic bronchitis are common. In the tropics these are overshadowed by starvation, malnutrition, anaemia, malaria, sickle cell disease and HIV disease. A good history, thorough examination, haemoglobin determination and a blood slide for malaria are mandatory before surgery.

Starvation and malnutrition

Lack of food due to famine from natural catastrophes or displacement of populations by war occurs in many tropical countries (see Chapter 30). If surgery is needed, nutritional support will also be required.

Calorie/protein malnutrition or kwashiorkor can be recognized by the thin, sparse, silky brown hair, facial and peripheral oedema, pallor and swollen abdomen (Figure 24.7). Such children are often grossly anaemic, heavily parasitized and unfit for surgery. Preoperative transfusion, taking great care not to overload the circulation, will be necessary if emergency surgery is needed.

Anaemia

A haemoglobin of 9 g/dL is the lower limit acceptable for planned surgical operations. Of the many causes of anaemia, malnutrition, malaria and sickle cell disease are the most important (see Chapter

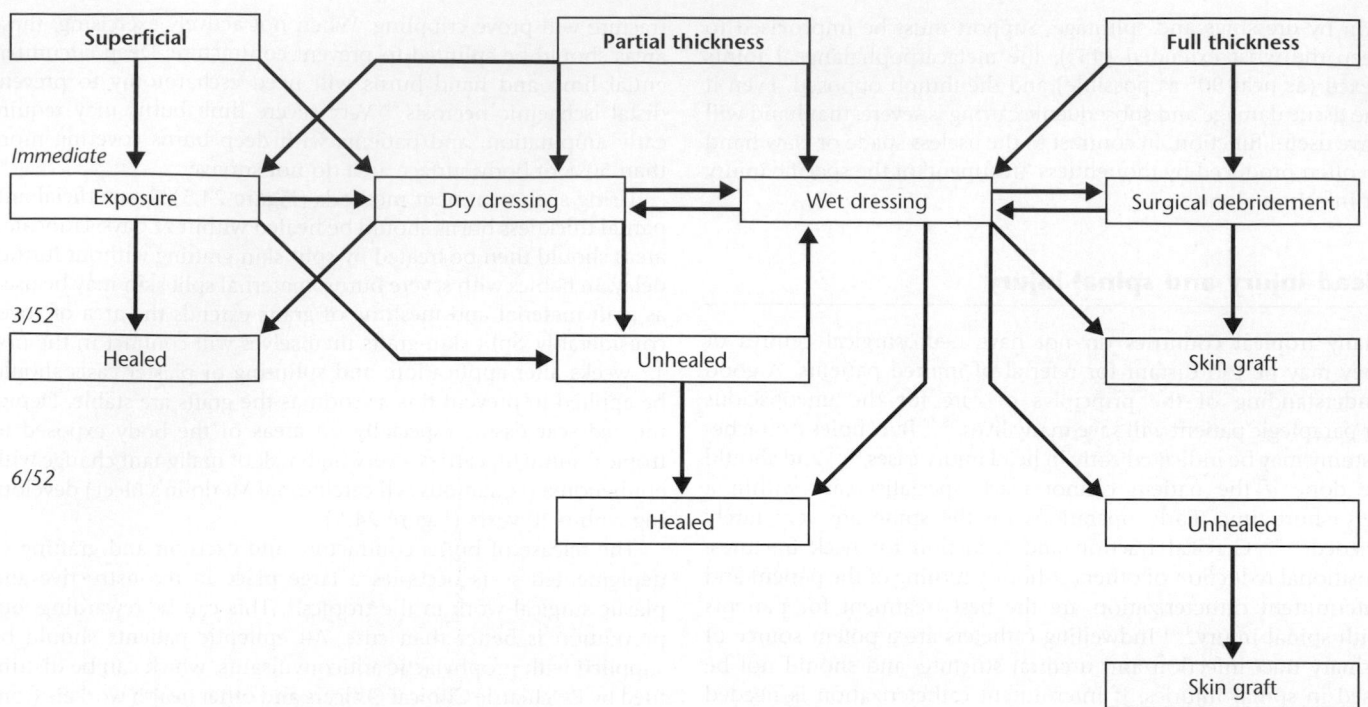

Figure 24.5 Scheme of burns management. (Redrawn with permission from James J. Treatment of the burn wound. *East Cent Afr J Surg* 1999; 5:61.)

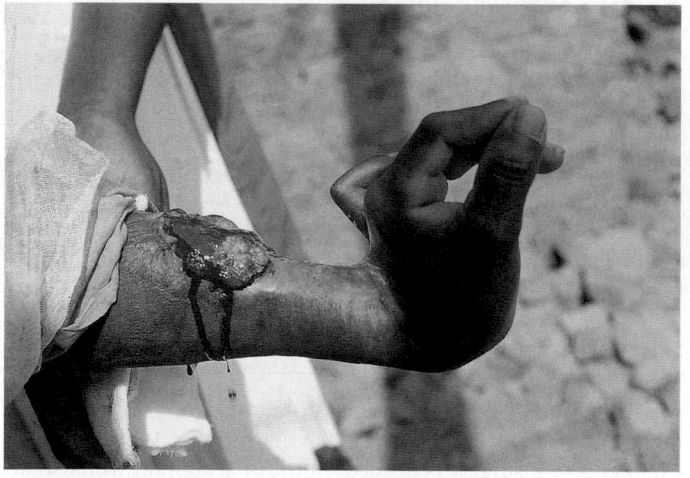

Figure 24.6 Squamous cell carcinoma in a burn contracture of the wrist.

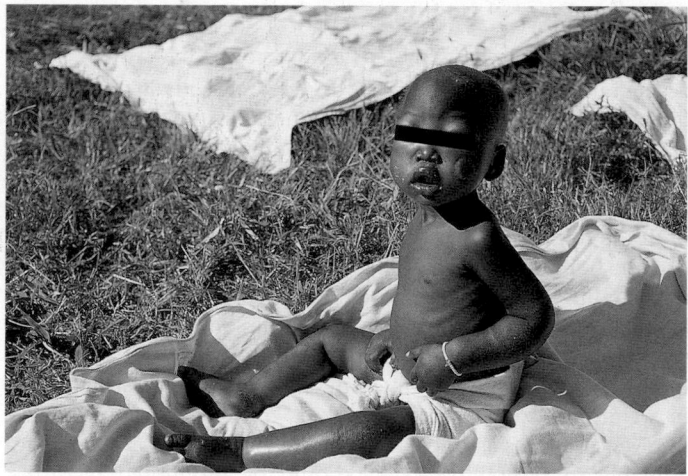

Figure 24.7 Kwashiorkor. The brown fine silky hair, distended abdomen and peripheral oedema are typical.

13). In adults, huge splenic enlargement (Figure 24.8) may cause chronic anaemia and thrombocytopenia. Splenectomy may be called for[71] but can be a hazardous undertaking.[72]

Sickle cell anaemia

In many sub-Saharan countries, up to 25% of the population carry the gene for sickle cell anaemia (HbS). Some offspring of these individuals will be afflicted with sickle cell disease (HbSS) and comprise about 1% of the population. They have a chronic haemolytic anaemia with periodic sickling crises characterized by severe anaemia, jaundice and painful infarcts in bone and other organs. Affected individuals are susceptible to infections such as otitis media, osteomyelitis and chest infections. In West Africa and Mediterranean countries, haemoglobin C disease and thalassaemia have similar, if less dramatic, effects. Those with the hetero-

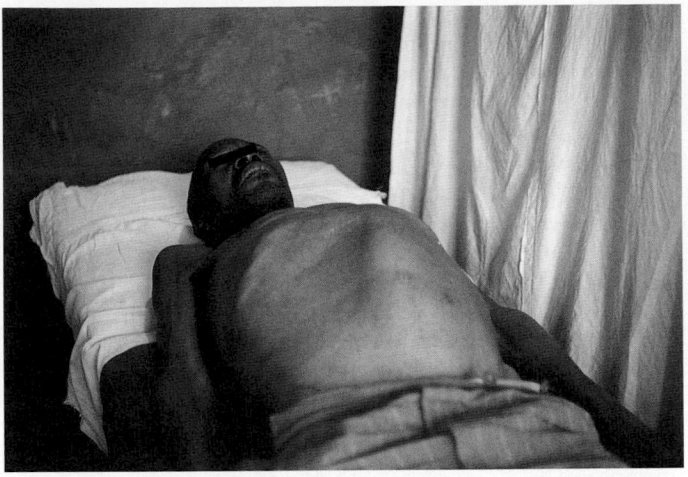

Figure 24.8 Patient with huge splenic enlargement. Splenectomy can be a formidable undertaking because of dense vascular adhesions.

zygous condition (HbS) do not suffer from such problems. See also Chapter 13.

In patients with sickle cell disease, the haemoglobin levels are usually between 5 g/dL and 8 g/dL, but during a sickling crisis drop much lower. If major surgery is needed, preoperative transfusion to bring the haemoglobin to at least 8 g/dL should be given and blood should be available to maintain this level throughout surgery and the postoperative period.

One potent cause of sickling is hypoxia. High pO_2 levels should be maintained throughout the operation and postoperative period. A pulse oximeter is a convenient way of monitoring this, but good oxygenation during surgery and oxygen by mask for 24 hours after surgery should be given in every case. Local nerve block analgesia should be considered because drugs that cause somnolence or depress respiration should not be used. Sudden collapse and death some hours after operation are a consequence of not observing these precautions.

The use of a tourniquet is controversial in patients with sickle cell disease. If bleeding is likely to be excessive or would prolong an operation by obscuring the anatomy, it is probably better to use a tourniquet. The limb should be properly exsanguinated with an Esmarch bandage before the arterial tourniquet is inflated, and high oxygen levels maintained when circulation to the limb is restored. The limb should be held elevated for at least 5 minutes after release of a tourniquet, to prevent pooling of blood or reactive haemorrhage. Adverse effects or a marked drop in the monitored pO_2 during such manoeuvres have not been encountered.

Malaria

Malaria is a common endemic or epidemic problem in many areas of the tropics and, with the emergence of resistant strains, control is difficult (see Chapter 73). Many patients, especially children, may remain fit to work and play but carry malarial parasites in their blood. The stress of surgery commonly provokes a severe attack of malaria with marked haemolysis and possibly cerebral involvement. Fever within 48 hours of surgery is most likely due either to atelectasis and chest infection or to malaria.

For planned surgery, especially in children, a haemoglobin check and a blood slide for malarial parasites should be done before surgery. Any patient with a haemoglobin of below 9 g/dL needs investigation. Those in whom malarial parasites are found should have a course of antimalarial treatment, and surgery should be delayed for several days. In an emergency situation, antimalarial drugs may be started soon after surgery.

COMMON 'TROPICAL' CONDITIONS

Haematogenous osteomyelitis

Haematogenous osteomyelitis is both a common and severe affliction of children in the tropics.[73] Many doctors find this a difficult pathology to understand and treat, so it is dealt with in some detail here.

Neonatal septic arthritis and osteomyelitis

Acute septic arthritis with adjacent osteomyelitis may develop within a few days of birth but the diagnosis, especially in the case of the hip joint, is often delayed. The neonatal response to severe infection is lethargy, failure to feed, subnormal temperatures and jaundice. Other causes of these symptoms, such as malaria and pneumonia, are often sought and treated until the mother reports that the child does not move one limb (pseudoparalysis) or gross swelling develops around a major joint. Aspiration of pus from the area will confirm septic arthritis and radiological changes of the adjacent bones are usually present by that time.

Treatment of this condition, with appropriate antibiotics, open drainage of the joint and splintage, is urgent if joint destruction is to be avoided. *S. aureus* and *Haemophilus influenzae* are both common organisms in this disease, so a combination of cloxacillin and ampicillin or other broad-spectrum antibiotics should be given by intravenous infusion pending the results of cultures. Hips should be splinted in abduction to prevent dislocation, an affected knee kept straight and the arm rested in a sling for shoulder and elbow pathology.

Because of late diagnosis, hip dislocation, destruction of the femoral head and severe damage to other joints are commonly seen. Other causes of neonatal joint swelling, such as birth trauma and congenital syphilis (producing *bilateral* periostitis), should be excluded by radiographs and diagnostic aspiration.

Haematogenous osteomyelitis in childhood

This common and serious condition produces prolonged morbidity, occasional deaths and life-long crippling. Bacteria are carried to the metaphyses of long bones, especially those of the tibia, femur and humerus, in the bloodstream. As blood flow slows in the medullary sinusoids, bacteria settle and produce acute inflammation. Intraosseous pressure rises, occluding the endosteal circulation and producing septic necrosis. The infection spreads to the diaphysis along the medullary cavity but the physeal plate usually prevents spread to the epiphysis. Pus eventually breaches the cortex, lifting the periosteum and depriving the bone of its remaining periosteal blood supply. The dead cortex becomes a sequestrum.

If the physeal plate is situated within the adjacent joint, as in the hip and elbow, infection will probably spread to the joint, producing septic arthritis. Eventually, pus will burst from beneath the periosteum into the soft tissues of the limb and through the skin to leave discharging sinuses. Recovery is by new periosteal bone forming an involucrum that eventually unites the unaffected regions of the bone, but, while sequestra remain, discharging sinuses will persist.

In the acute phase, which lasts for only 48 to 72 hours, the child has a high fever and much pain. The affected area of bone is tender and very painful on light percussion but the leg is not swollen. This is the only stage where effective treatment may cure the infection and stop progression to chronic osteomyelitis. The acute stage, however, often passes before admission to hospital.

The diagnosis is entirely clinical, there being no easily recognizable radiological signs, though oedema of the periosteum may be confirmed by ultrasonography.

Treatment in the acute phase is pain relief, high doses of intravenous antistaphylococcal antibiotics (e.g. cloxacillin 200 mg/kg/day), and decompression of the affected bone by drilling without periosteal stripping, followed by elevation and splintage of the limb. A radiograph at 14 to 21 days after onset will show the extent of disease. It may suggest resolution or show significant bone destruction.

Postacute haematogenous osteomyelitis

When pus lifts the periosteum, the intraosseous pressure is reduced. Although the leg now swells, the patient has less pain and the fever falls. This sign may erroneously suggest successful treatment of acute osteomyelitis rather than progression of the disease. Most children present at this postacute stage.

The same treatment is needed, but pus will be drained from the soft tissues rather than from the bone. The dead cortex (sequestrum) ensures that the disease will progress to chronic osteomyelitis. Radiographs will confirm death and destruction of bone and the need for protection of the limb from stress until the involucrum is strong enough to bear weight.

Chronic osteomyelitis

This is characterized by the history and presence of a swollen limb with a palpably enlarged bone and discharging sinuses. Radiographs will show sequestra and involucrum or a Brodie's abscess. Sequestrectomy should await the formation of enough involucrum to maintain integrity of the limb. A Brodie's abscess should be cleared by wide excision of the overlying cortex (saucerization). Antibiotics should be given at the time of surgery and for a week after sequestrectomy. Recurrent episodes of fever indicate the need for further drainage of pus and sequestrectomy rather than for antibiotic therapy.

Haematogenous osteomyelitis in sickle cell disease

This infection probably develops in areas of bone infarction. Often polyostotic and affecting the upper limbs as commonly as the lower, the infection is frequently diffuse throughout a given bone. Salmonellae are as common as staphylococcal infections and the antibiotic therapy must be adjusted accordingly. In general, surgery should be less radical and precautions (mentioned under sickle cell disease above) must be taken.

Sigmoid volvulus

Sigmoid volvulus is common in Africa, especially among men of Bantu race, and a high-bulk diet has been suggested as an aetiological factor.[74] Gakwaya, from Uganda, has described 16 patients (15 males, 1 female) with a syndrome of symptomatic redundant sigmoid colon that he considers the precursor of sigmoid volvulus.[75]

By the time of complete colonic volvulus, the colon has become hypertrophied and thick walled with lateral stretching of the taenia coli. Strangulation is comparatively late and, if no signs of peritonitis are present, the volvulus can often be decompressed by passing a soft rubber flatus tube through the twist at sigmoidoscopy with the patient in the knee–elbow position.[76] Once deflated, the flatus tube should be left in situ for several days. Unfortunately, there is a very high incidence of recurrence and sigmoid resection is needed to prevent this.[76] Surgeons expert in large bowel surgery often perform primary sigmoidectomy because many patients do not return for interval surgery.[77]

If peritonitis exists, flatus tube decompression should not be attempted. After rapid correction of dehydration and electrolyte imbalance and having given high doses of broad-spectrum antibiotics and metronidazole, the gangrenous sigmoid colon should be resected. These patients have deranged physiology and surgery should be limited to damage control. After a proximal colostomy and purse-string closure of the distal stump, the abdomen should be left open beneath a Bagota bag.[55]

Small bowel volvulus

In Africa and India, primary small bowel volvulus is an uncommon cause of acute intestinal obstruction[78] and, in children, is associated with ascariasis[79] and recent treatment with vermicide.[80] In parts of Nepal, however, it is common in men, and associated with large bulky high-fibre meals.[81] Adequate resuscitation of the patient before surgery will reduce the operative mortality.

Ileosigmoid knotting

This compound volvulus is not uncommon in the tropics and carries a high mortality rate.[82] The onset is acute, signs of peritonitis are already obvious at presentation, and gangrenous small bowel is usually present. Usually, both small and large bowel resections are necessary and surgery should not be delayed by efforts at referral. The principles of damage control should be followed using a Bagota bag.[51]

Helminthic intestinal obstruction

Infestation with the round worm, *Ascaris lumbricoides*, is a very common affliction of children in the tropics. A large mass of worms may block the ileum, causing intestinal obstruction. In 80% of such cases, conservative management with nasogastric

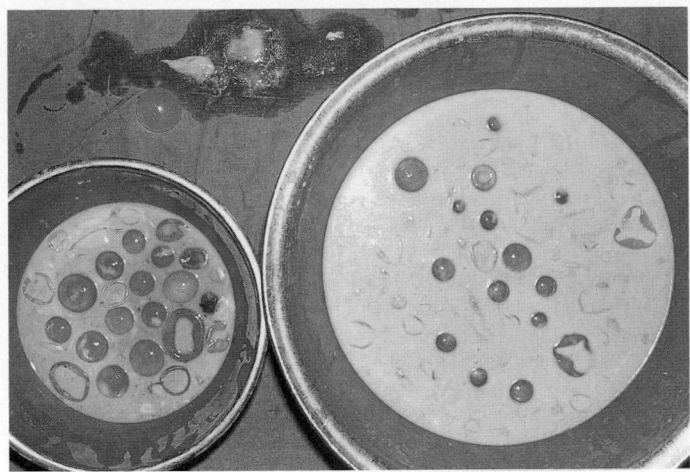

Figure 24.9 Pus and daughter cysts drained from an abdominal hydatid abscess.

suction and intravenous infusion is successful.[83] After the child is passing flatus or faeces, a vermifuge (either piperazine or a benzimidazole compound) should be given. Close observation is mandatory and laparotomy should be undertaken if signs of peritonitis or volvulus develop.[79] Worms in viable segments of the ileum may be 'milked' into the large intestine, but resection of any gangrenous segments of small bowel with the contained worms and primary anastomosis is the treatment of choice.[84] These small children are often debilitated and postoperative complications are common. Ileal perforation, appendicitis and biliary ascariasis may also be encountered.[85]

Hydatid disease

Liver abscess[86,87] and hydatid disease of the lung are common, and disease of the kidney,[88] brain,[89] bone[90] and other organs is not uncommon in many parts of the tropics where sheep and goats are the predominant livestock. The use of drugs such as albendazole and praziquantel and precautions against spillage of cyst contents (Figure 24.9) are the basis of successful treatment. See also Chapter 86.

OVERCOMING ISOLATION

Many tropical hospitals have only one doctor and may be 1000 km from the teaching hospital. How can the effects of such isolation be minimized?

First, assemble a reference library. The recommended surgical books are listed at the end of this chapter. To neglect such sources of wisdom and experience is to court disaster.[1] Many have cheap editions. Local service clubs (Rotary, Lions or Round Table, etc.) may help with book purchase and provide subscriptions to some of the relevant journals quoted in the references.

Some countries, such as Uganda, have continuing medical education (CME) programmes for up-country doctors, which publish literature on clinical problems common to the area. In East Africa, the flying doctor service (AMREF) sends surgical teams to remote rural areas, and similar outreach programmes exist in Zambia and

elsewhere. An invitation to visit is the first step in developing a very useful network of contacts.

Information technology is getting cheaper. A computer with CD-ROM and modem will give wide access if a telephone exists. Satellite phones are still expensive but invaluable in really remote regions. Many specialists are willing to advise on clinical problems, and acquisition of a simple digital camera makes the transmission of photographs and radiographs possible. Given a project proposal, charitable organizations should think the price reasonable for breaking down a doctor's isolation.

REFERENCES

1. Bewes PC. Third World trauma. *Trauma* 1999; 1:341–350.
2. Loefler IJP. Africa – surgery in an unstable environment. *ANZ J Surg* 2004; 74:1120–1122.
3. Bergstrom S. Who will do the caesareans when there is no doctor? Finding creative solutions to the human resource crisis. *BJOG* 2005; 112:1168–1169.
4. Watters DAK, Bayley AC. Training doctors and surgeons to meet the needs of Africa. *BMJ (Clin Res Ed)* 1987; 295:761–763.
5. King M, Bewes P. Fractures of the shaft of the femur. In: King M, Bewes P, eds. *Primary Surgery: Volume II. Trauma.* Oxford: Oxford Medical; 1987:313–321.
6. Jellis JE. Active conservative management of elbow injuries. *Proc Assoc Surg East Afr* 1991; 14:44–50.
7. Nordberg E. Incidence and estimated need of caesarean section, inguinal hernia repair and operation for strangulated hernia in rural Africa. *BMJ (Clin Res Ed)* 1984; 289:92–93.
8. Fenton PM. The epidemiology of District Surgery in Malawi: a two-year study of surgical rates and indices in rural Africa. *East Cent Afr J Surg* 1997; 3:33–41.
9. Nordberg E, Holmberg S, Kiugu S. Output of major surgery in developing countries. *Trop Geograph Med* 1995; 47:206–211.
10. Loefler IJP. Surgery in austere environments. In: Kamel R, Lumley J, eds. *Textbook of Tropical Surgery.* London: Westminster Publishing; 2004:154–155.
11. Rosenfield JV, Watters DAK. Neurological manifestations of HIV infection. In: Rosenfield JV, Watters DAK, eds. *Neurosurgery in the Tropics.* London: Macmillan; 2000:256–259.
12. Bayley AC. Aggressive Kaposi's sarcoma in Zambia, 1983. *Lancet* 1984; i:1318.
13. Kehoe NS, Jellis J E. The incidence of human immunodeficiency virus infection in injured patients in Lusaka. *Injury* 1994; 25:375–378.
14. Bayley AC, Jellis JE, Watters DK. Surgery for HIV-infected patients. In: Leaper DJ, Branicki FJ, eds. *International Surgical Practice.* Oxford: Oxford Medical; 1992:65–93.
15. Ansary MA, Hira SK, Bayley AC, et al. Cutaneous manifestations. In: *A Colour Atlas of AIDS in the Tropics.* London: Wolfe; 1989:28–54.
16. WHO. Interim proposal for a WHO staging system for HIV infection and disease. *Wkly Epidemiol Rec* 1990; 65:221–228.
17. Royer HD, Reinherz EL. T lymphocytes: ontogeny, function, and relevance to clinical disorders. *N Engl J Med* 1987; 317:1136–1142.
18. Creemers PC, O'Shaughnessy M, Boyko WJ. Analysis of absolute T helper cell numbers and cellular immune defects in HIV antibody positive and negative homosexual men. *AIDS Res Hum Retroviruses* 1988; 4:268–278.
19. Association of Surgeons of East Africa. Guidelines for the management of HIV infection in East and Southern Africa. *East Cent Afr J Surg* 1995; 1:53–58.
20. Wake DJ, Cutting WAM. Blood transfusions in developing countries: problems, priorities and practicalities. *Trop Doct* 1998; 28:4–8.
21. World Health Organization, Global Programme on AIDS, Global Blood Safety Initiative. *Guidelines for the Appropriate Use of Blood.* WHO/GPA/Inf/89:18 Geneva: WHO; 1989.
22. Nielsen CH. Perioperative euvolaemic haemodilution. *East Cent Afr J Surg* 1997; 3:81–82.
23. Liaw Y, Boon P, Deshpande S. Haemodilution study in major orthopaedic surgery. *Aust NZ J Surg* 1994; 64:535–537.

24. Chretien J. Tuberculosis and HIV: the cursed duet. *Bull Int Union Tuberc Lung Dis* 1990; 65:25–32.

25. Elliot AM, Luo N, Tembo G, et al. Impact of HIV on tuberculosis in Zambia: a cross sectional study. *BMJ* 1990; 301:412–415.

26. Jellis JE. Orthopaedic surgery and HIV disease in Africa. *Int Orthop* 1996; 20:253–256.

27. Bem C, Patil PS, Elliot AM, et al. The pathology of lymphadenopathy in Lusaka. *Proc Assoc Surg East Afr* 1990; 13:62–65.

28. Holcombe C, Weedon R, Llwin M. The differential diagnosis of breast lumps in the Tropics. *Trop Doct* 1999; 29:42–45.

29. Bem C. The value of naked eye examination of biopsied lymph nodes in the diagnosis of tuberculous lymphadenitis. *Trop Doct* 1996; 26:10–13.

30. Abdul-Ghaffar NUAMA, Ramadan IT, Marafie AA. Abdominal tuberculosis in Ahmadi, Kuwait: a clinico-pathological review. *Trop Doct* 1998; 28:137–139.

31. Govinder S, Annamalai K, Kumar KPS, et al. Spinal tuberculosis in HIV positive and negative patients: immunological response and clinical outcome. *Int Orthop* 2000; 24:163–166.

32. Dent AW, Seyfang M, Wallace S. Cytology and fine needle aspiration biopsy: appropriate technology, quick, safe and cheap. *Trop Doct* 1996; 37–39.

33. Desai G. Empyema thoracis in AIDS patients in the tropics. In: Zumla A, Johnson MA, Miller RF, eds. *AIDS and Respiratory Medicine*. London: Chapman & Hall; 1997:151–261.

34. Desai G, Mugala DD. Management of empyema thoracis at Lusaka, Zambia. *Br J Surg* 1992; 79:537–538.

35. Jellis JE. Orthopaedic infection associated with HIV disease. *Surgery* 1994; 12:175–177.

36. Sikasote CC, Erzingatsian K. Pyomyositis and HIV infection at the University Teaching Hospital. *East Cent Afr J Surg* 1998; 4:67.

37. Alidria-Ezati I. The association between pyomyositis and HIV infection in New Mulago Hospital. *Proc Assoc Surg East Afr* 1991; 14:91–94.

38. Ansaloni L. Tropical pyomyositis. *World J Surg* 1995; 20:613–617.

39. Njobvu P, McGill P, Kerr H, et al. Spondyloarthropathy and human immunodeficiency virus infection in Zambia. *J Rheumatol* 1998; 25:1553–1559.

40. Adeloye A. Neurological and neurosurgical manifestations of human immunodeficiency virus (HIV) infections in Africa. *East Cent Afr J Surg* 2000; 5:49–54.

41. McGeehan DF. Necrotising fasciitis: a biological disaster. *Today's Emergency* 1999; 5:27–28.

42. Loefler IJP. Fournier's gangrene. *Surgery* 2002; 20:2.

43. Muthuuri JM. AIDS in general surgical practice. *East Cent Afr J Surg* 1997; 3:31–36.

44. Bayley AC. Surgical pathology of HIV disease: lessons from Africa. *Br J Surg* 1990; 77:863–866.

45. Bayley AC. Kaposi's sarcoma. *Baillière's Clin Trop Medic Comm Dis* 1989; 3(2):311–327.

46. Korshid KA, Erzingatsian K, Watters DAK, et al. Intussusception due to Kaposi's sarcoma. *J R Coll Surg Edinb* 1987; 32:339–341.

47. Museru LM, Leshabari MT, Grob U, et al. The pattern of injuries seen in patients in the orthopaedic/trauma wards of Muhimbili Medical Centre. *East Cent Afr J Surg* 1998; 4:15–22.

48. Vanwersch K. Crocodile bite injury in Southern Malawi. *Trop Doct* 1998; 28:221–222.

49. Mekisic AP, Wardill JR. Crocodile attacks in the Northern Territory of Australia. *Med J Aust* 1992; 157:751–754.

50. Jellis JE. The management of neglected trauma. *East Cent Afr J Surg* 1999; 4:49–55.

51. Loefler IJP. Damage control and second look in emergency abdominal surgery. *East Afr Med J* 2001: 78:i–ii.

52. Krige JEJ, Terblanche J. Liver trauma. In: Kamel R, Lumley J, eds. *Textbook of Tropical Surgery*. London: Westminster Publishing; 2004:559–562.

53. Schein M, Wittman DH, Aprahamian CC, et al. The abdominal compartment syndrome: the physiological and clinical consequences of elevated intra-abdominal pressure. *J Am Coll Surg* 1995; 180:745–753.

54. Chang MC, Miller PR, D'Agostino R, et al. Effects of abdominal decompression on cardiopulmonary function and visceral perfusion in patients with intra-abdominal hypertension. *J Trauma* 1998; 44:440–445.

55. Fernandez L, Norwood S, Roettger R, et al. Temporary intravenous bag silo closure in severe abdominal trauma. *J Trauma* 1996; 40:258–260.

56. Fernandez R, Griffiths R, Ussia C. Water for wound cleansing. Cochrane Database Syst Rev 2002; (4):CD003861.

57. Loefler IJP. Antibiotics and the surgeon. *East Cent Afr J Surg* 1999; 4:45–48.

58. Watters DAK. Coma & head injuries. In: Watters DAK, Wilson IH, Leaver RJ, et al., eds. *Care of the Critically Ill Patient in the Tropics and Sub-tropics*. Basingstoke: Macmillan; 1991:159–173, 175–184.

59. Watters DAK, Sinclaire JR. Outcome of head injuries in Central Africa. *J R Coll Surg Edinb* 1988; 33:35–38.

60. Levy LF. The management of head injuries. *East Cent Afr J Surg* 1996; 2:49–62.

61. Rosenfield JV, Watters DAK. Head injury. In: Rosenfield JV, Watters DAK, eds. *Neurosurgery in the Tropics*. London: Macmillan; 2000:52–89.

62. Newcombe R, Merry G. The management of acute neurotrauma in rural and remote locations. A set of guidelines for the management of head and spinal injuries. *J Clin Neurosci* 1999; 6:85–93.

63. Jaffrey DC. The orthopaedic management of spinal injuries. *East Cent Afr J Surg* 1996; 2:63–66.

64. King M, Bewes P. The spine. In: King M, Bewes P, eds. *Primary Surgery: Volume II. Trauma*. Oxford: Oxford Medical; 1987:144–160.

65. Kumiponjera D. Burns caused by paraffin lamp explosion. *East Cent Afr J Surg* 2000; 5:82–83.

66. King M, Bewes P. Burns. In: King M, Bewes P, eds. *Primary Surgery: Volume II. Trauma*. Oxford: Oxford Medical; 1987:65–91.

67. Heywood AJ. Burns. In: Watters DAK, Wilson IH, Leaver RJ, et al., eds. *Care of the Critically Ill Patient in the Tropics and Sub-tropics*. Basingstoke: Macmillan; 1991:213–231.

68. James J. Treatment of the burn wound. *East Cent Afr J Surg* 1999; 5:61.

69. Nath S, Erzingatsian K, Simonde S. Management of postburn contracture of the neck. *Burns* 1994; 20:438–441.

70. Nzarubara GR. Risk factors for burns in Uganda and strategies for prevention. *East Cent Afr J Surg* 1999; 5:11–16.

71. Jameson JS, Thomas WM, Dawson S, et al. Splenectomy for haematological disease. *J R Coll Surg Edinb* 1996; 41:307–311.

72. Erzingatsian KL. The enlarged spleen and early post-splenectomy complications. *East Cent Afr J Surg* 1996; 2:29–33.

73. Jellis JE. Haematogenous osteomyelitis. *Surgery* 1992; 10:145–148.

74. Loefler IJP. Bantu volvulus. *Surgery* 1990; 84:1196–1198.

75. Gakwaya AM. The diagnosis and treatment of symptomatic redundant sigmoid colon. *Proc Assoc Surg East Afr* 1991; 14:88–90.

76. King M, Bewes PC, Cairns J, et al. Sigmoid volvulus. In: King M, Bewes PC, Cairns J, et al., eds. *Primary Surgery: Volume I. Non-Trauma*. Oxford: Oxford Medical; 1993:161–167.

77. Erzingatsian K. One-stage sigmoid colectomy in patients with volvulus. *East Cent Afr J Surg* 1996; 2:25–28.

78. Duke JH Jr. Primary small bowel volvulus. *Arch Surg* 1997; 112:685–688.

79. Holcombe C. Surgical emergencies in tropical gastroenterology. *Gut* 1995; 36:9–11.

80. Wiermsa R, Hadley GP. Small bowel volvulus and intestinal ascariasis. *Br J Surg* 1988; 75:86–87.

81. Parkes G. Primary small bowel volvulus in rural Nepal. *Trop Doct* 1997; 27:156–158.

82. Kamel R. Knotting of the bowel. In Kamel R, Lumley J, eds. *Textbook of Tropical Surgery*. London: Westminster Publishing; 2004:483–484.

83. Mokoena T, Luvuno FM. Conservative management of intestinal obstruction due to *Ascaris* worms in adult patients: a preliminary report. *J R Coll Surg Edinb* 1988; 33:318–321.

84. Hyde GA Jr, Kyambi JM. Gangrenous intestinal obstruction in children due to *Ascaris lumbricoides*: surgical management. *East Cent Afr J Surg* 1996; 2:17–19.

85. Pandit SK, Zarger HU. Surgical ascariasis in children in Kashmir. *Trop Doct* 1997; 27:13–14.

86. Fenton-Lee D, Morris DL. The management of hydatid disease of the liver: part I. *Trop Doct* 1996; 26:173–176.

87. Fenton-Lee D, Morris DL. The management of hydatid disease of the liver: part 2. *Trop Doct* 1997; 27:87–88.

88. Mehdiratta NK, Gupta SC, Misra V, et al. Renal hydatid disease. *Trop Doct* 1996; 26:33–34.

89. Rosenfeld JV, Clezy JKA, Watters DAK. Hydatid disease (cystic type). In: Rosenfeld JV, Watters DAK, eds. *Neurosurgery in the Tropics*. London: Macmillan; 2000:263–264.

90. Metcalfe JE, Grimer RJ. Tackling osseous hydatidosis using orthopaedic oncology techniques. *Ann R Coll Surg Engl* 2000; 82:287–289.

RECOMMENDED REFERENCE BOOKS

Ansary MA, Hira SK, Bayley AC, et al. *A Colour Atlas of AIDS in the Tropics*. London: Wolfe; 1989. ISBN 0-7234-1567-6.

Bewes P. *Surgery: A Manual for Rural Health Workers*. 2nd edn. Nairobi: AMREF; 2003. ISBN 9966-874-61-5.

British Medical Association Staff. *Appropriate Technology* (collected articles published in the *British Medical Journal*). London: BMJ Books; 1985. ISBN 0-7279-0157-5.

Dobson M. *Anaesthesia at the District Hospital*. Geneva: WHO; 1988. ISBN 0-92-4-154228-4.

Dobson M, Fisher R, eds. *Surgical Care at the District Hospital*. Geneva: WHO; 2003. ISBN 92-4-154575-5.

Kamel R, Lumley J, eds. *Textbook of Tropical Surgery*. London: Westminster Publishing; 2004. ISBN 0-9546855-0-4 (hardback), 0-9546855-1-2 (softback).

King M, ed. *Primary Anaesthesia*. Oxford: Oxford Medical; 1993. ISBN 0-19-261539-4.

King M, Bewes P, eds *Primary Surgery: Volume II. Trauma*. Oxford: Oxford Medical; 1987. ISBN 0-19-261599-8.

King M, Bewes P, Cairns J, et al., eds. *Primary Surgery: Volume I. Non-trauma*. Oxford: Oxford Medical; 1990. ISBN 0-19-261694-3.

Rosenfield JV, Watters DAK, eds. *Neurosurgery in the Tropics*. London: Macmillan; 2000. ISBN 0-333-68412-5.

Watters DAK, Wilson IH, Leaver RJ, et al., eds. *Care of the Critically Ill Patient in the Tropics and Sub-tropics*. Basingstoke: Macmillan; 1991. ISBN 0-33-353799-8.

Chapter 25   Yusuf Ahmed

Obstetrics in the Tropics

Pregnancy and childbirth are not diseases. However, an estimated 15% of pregnant women may develop potentially life-threatening complications directly related to complications of pregnancy, childbirth, and in the immediate postpartum period. This highlights the need to assure the availability, quality and utilization of emergency obstetric care and skilled attendants, particularly at the time of delivery. The outcome for both mother and fetus differs markedly across the world. Based on estimates for the year 2000, there were 529 000 maternal deaths in the world.[1] The vast majority of these deaths were almost equally divided between Africa (251 000) and Asia (253 000), with about 4% (22 000) occurring in Latin America and the Caribbean, and less than 1% (2500) in the more developed regions of the world. The levels of morbidity associated with pregnancy are difficult to calculate. For every woman who dies, 20 or more experience serious complications. These range from chronic infections and resulting infertility to severely disabling injuries such as obstetric fistula as a result of prolonged or obstructed labour. Some 50 000 to 100 000 new cases of *obstetric fistula* develop each year.[2]

Of the approximately 8 million babies that die each year before 1 year of age (infant mortality), about 50% occur at the time of delivery, or during the first week or month of life.[3] Ninety-eight per cent of the deaths take place in the developing world, and, like maternal mortality, rates are highest in sub-Saharan Africa and Asia. Of the almost 4 million babies who die in the first 4 weeks of life (neonatal mortality), 3 million occur in the early neonatal period – i.e. first week. Moreover, it is estimated that, additionally, more than 3.3 million babies are stillborn every year; one in three of these stillbirth deaths occurs during delivery. Early neonatal deaths in the first week have obstetric origins, similar to those leading to stillbirths, and could largely be prevented.

Responding to the world's main development challenges and to the calls of civil society, the Millennium Development Goals (MDGs) were adopted in the year 2000 to promote poverty reduction, education, maternal health, gender equality, and aim at combating child mortality, AIDS and other diseases.[4] The MDGs represent a global partnership that has grown from the commitments and targets established at the world summits of the 1990s. Two of the eight MDGs, to be achieved by 2015, include reducing child mortality (goal 4) and improving maternal health (goal 5). Since the majority of maternal and neonatal deaths are directly related to complications of pregnancy, childbirth, and the immediate postpartum period, an important strategy to achieve the MDGs is to assure the availability, quality and utilization of emergency obstetric care and skilled attendants at the time of delivery.

Details of the various conditions contributing to the complications of pregnancy, childbirth and newborn health are covered extensively in specialized textbooks of obstetrics. In addition there are a number of textbooks and manuals, including those published by the World Health Organization (WHO), relevant for adaptation and use by various categories of care givers in developing countries.[5–11]

STRATEGIES TO IMPROVE MATERNAL AND NEWBORN HEALTH

In this chapter, the conditions leading to the main causes of maternal mortality are summarized, particularly within the context of the tropics and much of the developing countries. Figures 25.1 and 25.2 illustrate the major causes of maternal and neonatal mortality worldwide, and highlight interventions that could prevent them.

The causes of maternal death are multifactorial and have been conceptualized according to a number of 'delays', which also allow potential interventions to be identified (Table 25.1).[12–14]

Interventions recommended by WHO for improving maternal and newborn health and survival are outlined in Tables 25.2 to 25.6. These include key interventions to be delivered through health services, family and the community to improve maternal and newborn health and survival.[11]

Table 25.2 lists interventions delivered to the mother during pregnancy, childbirth and in the postpartum period, and to the newborn soon after birth. Table 25.3 lists the places where care should be provided through health services, the type of providers required, and the recommended interventions and commodities at each level. Table 25.4 lists practices, activities and support needed during pregnancy and childbirth by the family, community and workplace. Table 25.5 lists key interventions provided to women before conception and between pregnancies. Table 25.6 addresses unwanted pregnancies.

HAEMORRHAGE

Obstetrical haemorrhage is a major cause of maternal morbidity and mortality and of perinatal death, requiring prompt medical

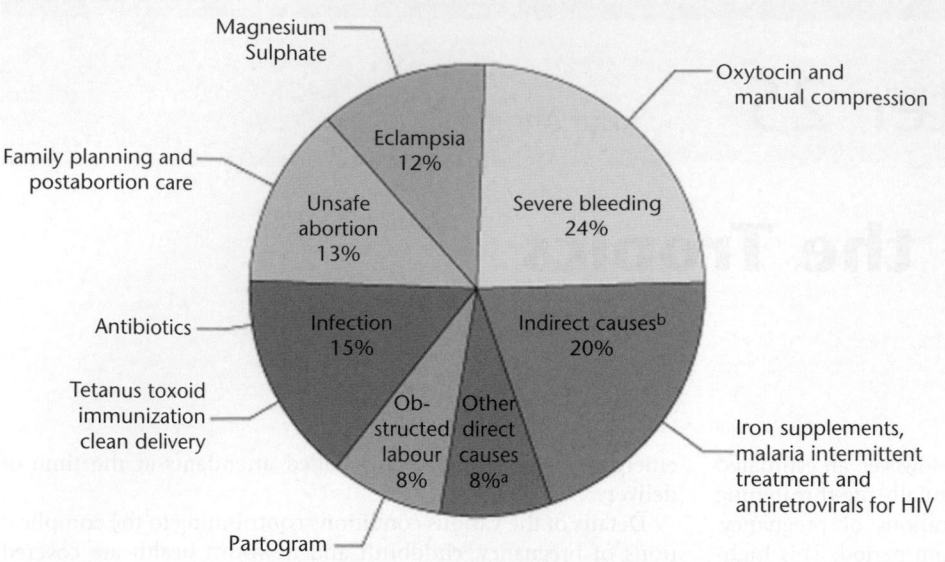

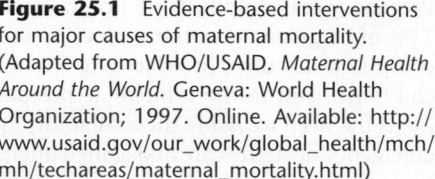

aOther direct causes include ectopic pregnancy, embolism, anaesthesia-related
bIndirect causes include anaemia, malaria, heart disease

Figure 25.1 Evidence-based interventions for major causes of maternal mortality. (Adapted from WHO/USAID. *Maternal Health Around the World.* Geneva: World Health Organization; 1997. Online. Available: http://www.usaid.gov/our_work/global_health/mch/mh/techareas/maternal_mortality.html)

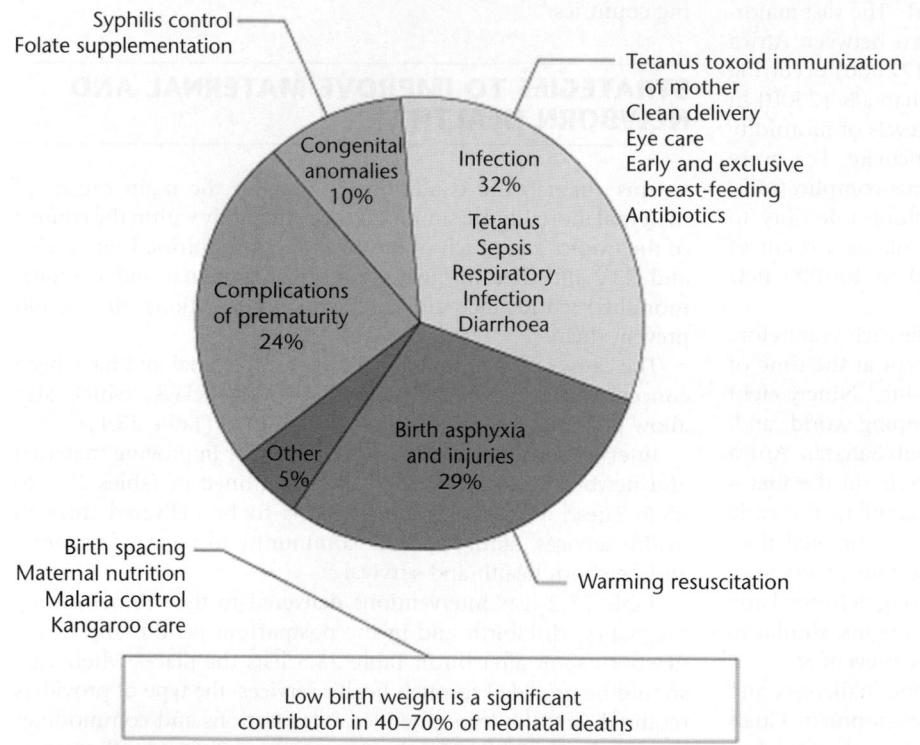

Figure 25.2 Major causes of neonatal death: evidence-based interventions. (Adapted from USAID at http://www.usaid.gov/our_work/global_health/mch/mh/techareas/neonatal_death.html)

intervention. Anaemia is an important contributory problem and many anaemic women will be at substantial risk, as even a relatively small volume of blood loss before, during or after delivery can pose a major risk. Blood loss can occur during pregnancy, labour, or postpartum.

Bleeding in the second half of pregnancy is termed antepartum haemorrhage (APH) and two common and potentially serious causes are abruptio placentae (premature separation of the placenta, which may be associated with pre-eclampsia) and placenta

praevia (abnormally low placental implantation that partially or completely covers the internal cervical os). A large retroplacental haemorrhage associated with separation of the placenta in abruptio placentae can lead to immediate fetal death and place the mother at risk due to hypotension, shock and possible disseminated intravascular coagulation (DIC). The signs of a tense, tender uterus, with the fetal parts difficult or impossible to palpate, and the fetal heart absent, may indicate abruptio placenta. Management includes prompt fluid replacement with plasma expanders

Table 25.1 Causes of maternal death – the 'four delays'

DELAY IN RECOGNIZING THE NEED FOR MEDICAL CARE
These are related to problem recognition and the lack of information about complications or pregnancy and childbirth and danger signs. Interventions include health education for the women and health providers. Traditional birth attendants can be encouraged to seek prompt referrals to a health facility.
DELAYS IN DECIDING TO SEEK CARE
Related to socio-cultural/economic factors and can be addressed through: couple communication and educating key decision makers, encourage the use of a birth plan, encourage and motivate greater use of skilled providers (midwives, physicians) either at home or in health centres.
DELAYS IN REACHING THE HEALTH FACILITY
Related to the availability and access of services. Interventions include improving the transportation system by working with local communities; develop maternity waiting homes near the health facilities; improve the community's knowledge regarding the nearest health facility and how to access their services.
DELAYS IN RECEIVING TREATMENT FROM THE HEALTH FACILITY
Related to the quality of care. Interventions include training of doctors and midwives in life-saving skills; ensure that equipment is functional; proper infection control practices are utilized; an inventory control system is in place to maintain a sufficient stock of drugs and medical supplies on a regular basis; promote 'mother friendly' environments.

Adapted from Maine 1987; Thaddeus and Maine, 1994; Ross, 1998.

or substitutes if blood is not available. An artificial rupture of the membrane generally expedites delivery and reduces the risk of DIC in the mother. Intervention by caesarean section may be necessary, but is considered with extreme caution because of the complications of DIC. In patients with placenta praevia, the maternal and fetal condition may remain satisfactory until haemorrhage is considerable. A diagnosis of placenta praevia is considered in the presence of a high presenting fetal part, commonly with unstable or transverse lie, and would require prompt intervention by caesarean section.

Postpartum haemorrhage (PPH) often begins immediately after birth. It is primarily due to failure of the uterus to contract (uterine atony). This may be associated with retention of the placenta for more than 30 minutes after delivery. Vaginal and cervical lacerations cause less severe bleeding but require repair as soon as possible to lessen blood loss. The risks of PPH are higher in mothers who have had an APH during the pregnancy, those of high parity, multiple pregnancy and a previous history of PPH. In the management of PPH, 'rubbing up' or massaging the uterus per abdomen may be effective in contracting an atonic uterus. Prompt resuscitation with intravenous fluids, plasma substitutes and blood, if available, decreases the risk to the mother. Active management of the third stage of labour reduces the risk of PPH. This entails administration of an oxytocic to the mother after the birth of the anterior shoulder of the baby and delivery of the placenta by controlled cord traction, once it is evident that the uterus has contracted and signs of separation of the placenta are evident.

ANAEMIA

Anaemia is defined as a haemoglobin concentration of less than 11 g/dL. However, in many communities it is common for women to have a haemoglobin level of <7 g/dL during pregnancy. As a consequence, anaemia can both be a cause of maternal death and contribute to the problems of haemorrhage and infection.

Anaemia is the end result of many factors in a woman's life. Poor nutrition in childhood may result in her starting her first pregnancy with low iron stores; repeated pregnancies too close together will deplete her iron, vitamin B12 and folate levels even further; and dietary traditions in pregnancy together with common infections such as hookworm and malaria compound the problem. Heavy periods prior to conceiving or intermittent blood loss during pregnancy may also be factors leading to anaemia.

Healthcare workers can be trained to recognize the clinical signs of anaemia by examination of the mucous membranes of the eyelids and lips. Investigation can be limited to measuring the haemoglobin and also to exclude any obvious underlying cause. Screening women for anaemia in the antenatal period with a haemoglobin level, preferably in the second trimester, can identify those who can derive most benefit from treatment. Haemoglobin levels can be checked again at follow-up visits, typically at 30 and 36 weeks. Along with nutritional advice, a daily dose of 30–60 mg of elemental iron for women with a normal iron store and 120–240 mg for those women with low iron stores, accompanied by 0.4 mg of folate, is usually sufficient. A rise in the level of haemoglobin should be seen within a month of commencing treatment. If there is no response, it may be due to an underlying disorder such as sickle cell disease or haemoglobinopathy, failure to comply with treatment, or failure to absorb the oral therapy. The problem of iron absorption can be overcome by the use of parenteral iron such as iron dextran given as a series of intramuscular injections or by total dose intravenous infusion. It is essential that the staff be trained to recognize and treat anaphylactic reactions, which may rarely occur with such administration. Between 0.5 and 1.0 ml of adrenaline (epinephrine) 1:1000 should be given subcutaneously if an anaphylactic reaction occurs. It must be emphasized that parenteral iron does not increase the haemoglobin level any more quickly than

Table 25.2 Care in pregnancy, childbirth and postpartum period for mother and newborn infant[11]

	Routine care (offered to all women and babies)	Additional care (for women and babies with moderately severe diseases and complications)	Specialized – obstetrical and neonatal care (for women and babies with severe diseases and complications)
Pregnancy care – 4 visits	• Confirmation of pregnancy	• Treatment of mild to moderate pregnancy complications:	• Treatment of severe pregnancy complications:
Essential	• Monitoring of progress of pregnancy and assessment of maternal and fetal well-being	– mild to moderate anaemia	– anaemia

	• Detection of problems complicating pregnancy (e.g. anaemia, hypertensive disorders, bleeding, malpresentations, multiple pregnancy)	– urinary tract infection
		  – vaginal infection
			– severe pre-eclampsia
			  – eclampsia
			  – bleeding

	• Respond to other reported complaints	• Post abortion care and family planning	– infection – other medical complications
	• Tetanus immunization, anaemia prevention and control (iron and folic acid supplementation)	• Pre-referral treatment of severe complications	• Treatment of abortion complications

	• Information and counselling on self care at home, nutrition, safer sex, breast-feeding, family planning, healthy lifestyle	– pre-eclampsia
		  – eclampsia
		  – bleeding	

	• Birth and emergency planning, advice on danger signs and emergency preparedness	– infection – complicated abortion	
	• Recording and reporting	• Support for women with special needs e.g. adolescents, women living with violence	
	• Syphilis testing	• Treatment of syphilis (woman and her partner)	
Situational	• HIV testing and counselling	• Prevention of mother-to-child transmission of HIV (PMTCT) by antiretroviral treatment (ART), infant feeding counselling, mode of delivery advice	• Treatment of severe HIV infection • Treatment of complicated malaria
	• Antimalarial Intermittent preventive treatment (IPT) and promotion of insecticide treated nets (ITN)	• Treatment of mild to moderate opportunistic infections	
	• Deworming	• Treatment of uncomplicated malaria	
	• Assessment of female genital mutilation (FGM)		

Adapted from WHO 2007[11]

		Treatment of uncomplicated malaria	Treatment of complicated malaria
Situational	• Promotion of ITN use	• Treatment of uncomplicated malaria	• Treatment of complicated malaria

Childbirth Care (labour, delivery, and immediate postpartum)
 	
 Essential
	• Care during labour and delivery
	   – Diagnosis of labour
	   – Monitoring progress of labour, maternal and fetal well-being with partograph
	   – Providing supportive care and pain relief
	   – Detection of problems and complications (e.g. malpresentations, prolonged and/or obstructed labour, hypertension, bleeding, and infection)
	   – Delivery and immediate care of the newborn baby, initiation of breastfeeding
	   – Newborn resuscitation
	   – Active management of third stage of labour
	 • Immediate postpartum care of mother
	   – Monitoring and assessment of maternal well-being, prevention and detection of complications (e.g. hypertension, infections, bleeding, anaemia)
	   – Treatment of moderate post-haemorrhagic anaemia
	   – Information and counselling on home self care, nutrition, safe sex, breast care and family planning
	   – Advice on danger signs, emergency preparedness and follow-up
	 • Recording and reporting
		• Treatment of abnormalities and complications (e.g. prolonged labour, vacuum extraction; breech presentation, episiotomy, repair of genital tears, manual removal of placenta)
		 • Pre-referral management of serious complications (e.g. obstructed labour, fetal distress, preterm labour, severe peri- and postpartum haemorrhage)
		 • Emergency management of complications if birth imminent
		 • Support for the family if maternal death
			• Treatment of severe complications in childbirth and in the immediate postpartum period, including caesarean section, blood transfusion and hysterectomy):
			   – obstructed labour
			   – malpresentations
			   – eclampsia
			   – severe infection
			   – bleeding
			 • Induction and augmentation of labour

Situational	• Vitamin A administration	• Prevention of mother-to-child transmission of HIV by mode of delivery, guidance and support for chosen infant feeding option	• Management of complications related to FGM

Postpartum maternal care (up to 6 weeks)
 	
 Essential
	• Assessment of maternal well-being
	 • Prevention and detection of complications (e.g. infections, bleeding, anaemia)
	 • Anaemia prevention and control (iron and folic acid supplementation)
	 • Information and counselling on nutrition, safe sex, family planning and provision of some contraceptive methods
	 • Advice on danger signs, emergency preparedness and follow-up
	 • Provision of contraceptive methods
		• Treatment of some problems (e.g. mild to moderate anaemia, mild puerperal depression)
		 • Pre-referral treatment of some problems (e.g. severe postpartum bleeding, puerperal sepsis)
			• Treatment of all complications
			   – severe anaemia
			   – severe postpartum bleeding
			   – severe postpartum infections
			   – severe postpartum depression
			 • Female sterilization

Continued

Table 25.2 Care in pregnancy, childbirth and postpartum period for mother and newborn infant—continued[11]

	Routine care (offered to all women and babies)	Additional care (for women and babies with moderately severe diseases and complications)	Specialized – obstetrical and neonatal care (for women and babies with severe diseases and complications)
Situational	• Promotion of ITN use	• Treatment of uncomplicated malaria	• Treatment of complicated malaria

Newborn care (birth and immediate postnatal)
 	
Essential
	• Promotion, protection and support for breast-feeding
	• Monitoring and assessment of well-being, detection of complications (breathing, infections, prematurity, low birthweight, injury, malformation)
	• infection prevention and control, rooming-in
	• Eye care
	• Information and counselling on home care, breast-feeding, hygiene
	• Advice on danger signs, emergency preparedness and follow-up
	• Immunization according to the national guidelines (BCG, HepB, OPV-0)
		• Care if moderately preterm, low birth weight or twin: support for breast-feeding, warmth, frequent assessment of well-being and detection of complications e.g. feeding difficulty, jaundice, other perinatal problems
		• Kangaroo Mother Care follow-up
		• Treatment of mild to moderate
		  – local infections (cord, skin, eye, thrush)
		  – birth injuries
		• Pre-referral management of infants with severe problems:
		  – very preterm babies and/or birth weight very low
		  – severe complications
		  – malformations
		• Supporting mother if perinatal death
			• Management of severe newborn problems – general care for the sick newborn and management of specific problems:
			  – preterm birth
			  – breathing difficulty
			  – sepsis
			  – severe birth trauma and asphyxia
			  – severe jaundice
			  – Kangaroo Mother Care (KMC)
			• Management of correctable malformations

Situational	• Promotion of sleeping under ITN	• Presumptive treatment of congenital syphilis
		• Prevention of mother-to-child transmission of HIV by ART
		• Support for infant feeding of maternal choice
			• Treatment of:
			  – congenital syphilis
			  – neonatal tetanus

Postnatal newborn care (visit from/at home)
Essential
	• Assessment of infant's well-being and breast-feeding
	• Detection of complications and responding to maternal concerns
	• Information and counselling on home care
	• Additional follow-up visits for high risk babies (e.g. preterm, after severe problems, on replacement feeding)
		• Management of:
		  – minor to moderate problems and
		  – feeding difficulties
		• Pre-referral management of severe problems:
		  – convulsions
		  – inability to feed
		• Supporting the family if perinatal death
			• Management of severe newborn problems:
			  – sepsis
			  – other infections
			  – jaundice
			  – failure to thrive

Table 25.3 Place of care, providers, interventions and commodities[11]

Healthcare	Level of healthcare	Venue / place	Provider	Interventions and commodities
Pregnancy (antenatal) care				
Routine	**Primary**	• Health centre in the community • Out-patient clinic of a hospital • Outreach home visit	• Health worker with midwifery skills*	• On site tests (Hb, syphilis) • Maternal health record • Vaccine • Basic oral medicines
Situational	**Primary**	• Health centre in the community • Out-patient clinic of a hospital • Outreach home visit	• Health worker with midwifery skills*	• On site tests (HIV) • Insecticide treated nets (ITN)
Additional	**Primary**	• Health centre in the community • Out-patient clinic of a hospital	• Health worker with midwifery and selected obstetric and neonatal skills*	• IV fluids • Parenteral drugs (antibiotics, MgSO4, antimalarial) • Manual Vacuum Aspiration (MVA) • Antiretroviral therapy (ART)
Specialized	**Secondary**	• Hospital	• Team of doctors, midwives and nurses	All of the above plus: • Blood transfusion • Surgery • Laboratory tests • Obstetric care
Childbirth (mother and baby)				
Routine	**Primary**	• Health centre in the community • Maternity ward of a hospital • Outreach home care	• Health worker with midwifery skills*	• Delivery set • Oxytocin • Partograph
Situational	**Primary**	• Health centre in the community • Maternity ward of a hospital • Outreach home care	• Health worker with midwifery skills*	• ART
Additional	**Primary**	• Health centre in the community • Maternity ward of a hospital	• Health worker with midwifery and selected obstetric and neonatal skills*	• Vacuum extraction • Manual removal of placenta • Repair of genital tears • IV fluids • MgSO4, parenteral uterotonics, and antibiotics • Newborn resuscitation
Specialized Mother	**Secondary**	• Hospital	• Team of doctors, midwives and nurses with neonatal care skills	All of the above plus: • Surgery • Blood transfusion
Specialized Newborn	**Secondary**	• Hospital	• Team of doctors and nurses with obstetric and nursing skills	• Oxygen • IV fluids • Parenteral antibiotics • Blood transfusion • Laboratory – biochemical and microbiology (small blood samples)

Adapted from WHO 2007[11]

Continued

Table 25.3 Place of care, providers, interventions and commodities—continued[11]

Healthcare	Level of healthcare	Venue / place	Provider	Interventions and commodities
Postpartum (mother), postnatal (newborn infant)				
Routine	**Primary**	• Health centre in the community • Out-patient clinic of a hospital • Outreach home visit	• Health worker with midwifery skills*	• On site tests (Hb, syphilis) • Vaccines • Basic oral medicines
Situational	**Primary**	• Health centre in the community • Out-patient clinic of a hospital	• Health worker with midwifery skills*	• On site tests (HIV) • ART
Additional	**Primary**	• Health centre in the community • Out-patient clinic of a hospital	• Health worker with midwifery and selected obstetric and neonatal skills*	• IV fluids • Parenteral drugs (antibiotics, MgSO4, antimalarial) • Manual removal of placenta
Specialized Mother	**Secondary**	• Hospital	• Team of doctors, midwives and nurses	All of the above plus: • Blood transfusion • Surgery • Laboratory tests • Obstetric care
Specialized Newborn	**Secondary**	• Hospital	• Team of doctors, midwives and nurses with neonatal skills	• Oxygen • IV fluids • Parenteral antibiotics • Blood transfusion • Laboratory – biochemical and microbiology (small samples)

*Health worker providing maternity care only or a health worker providing other services in addition to maternity care.
Adapted from WHO 2007[11]

oral therapy and should be reserved for those who cannot tolerate or absorb oral therapy.

For those patients who present in late pregnancy or in labour with a very low haemoglobin level, blood transfusion may be necessary, although in areas with endemic HIV infection this is an option that will be employed only as a last resort. Care must be taken to prevent cardiac failure when transfusing women with very low haemoglobin levels, as the anaemia may lead to inefficient cardiac action and fluid overload. The use of packed cells and use of intravenous diuretics reduces the risk of cardiac failure due to fluid overload. In rare circumstances, exchange transfusion may be employed.

Death due to cardiac failure may occur with haemoglobin levels below 4 g/dL. Women whose haemoglobin level is between 4 and 7 g/dL are also at greater risk of dying from infection due to poor resistance or from the effects of haemorrhage. Blood losses of 500 mL that may be easily tolerated by a woman with a normal haemoglobin level may be fatal in the presence of anaemia. Other effects of anaemia in pregnancy include stillbirth, intrauterine growth retardation and premature labour.

Prevention of anaemia in pregnancy can also be stressed by health workers in the promotion of a good diet, the composition of which will vary depending on the region but which should include green vegetables, staples, cereals and meat. Malaria prophylaxis is an important consideration in many parts of the world.

Counselling on family planning would ensure adequate spacing to allow a woman to replenish her iron stores after pregnancy and breast-feeding.

Hypertensive disorders of pregnancy

Hypertensive disorders of pregnancy (see Chapter 37) are common and complicate about 7–10% of all pregnancies. Almost 70% are due to pregnancy-induced hypertension (termed pre-eclampsia with the development of proteinuria and referred to as eclampsia when complicated by convulsions). Most of the other 30% are due to chronic hypertension, which is present before pregnancy or diagnosed early in pregnancy. Pregnancy-induced hypertension (PIH) occurs worldwide and is predominantly a disease of young primigravidae in the second and third trimesters of pregnancy, although it can occur in any age group and also in subsequent pregnancies. PIH in older patients probably reflects undiagnosed chronic hypertension. Severe cases of PIH, particularly in pregnant women without access to antenatal care, can progress to eclampsia characterized by convulsions and coma and are associated with a high maternal mortality rate.

The aetiology of PIH is still unknown and this contributes to the problems in classification of the disease, its diagnosis and management. However, much more is known about the pathophysiology of PIH. Although the main feature of PIH is the

Table 25.4 Home care, family, community and workplace support for the woman during pregnancy and childbirth and for the newborn infant[11]

	Home/family	Community and workplace
Pregnancy	• Safe and nutritive diet • Safe sexual practices • Support for quitting smoking • Protection from passive tobacco smoking • Support for avoiding hard work • Planning for birth, and emergencies – mother and baby • Knowledge and support for the birth and emergency plan • Recognition of labour and danger signs • Support for compliance with preventive treatments • Support / accompaniment for pregnancy care visits • Adolescent girls encouraged to continue going to school • Participation in improving quality of services • Participation in transport and financing scheme	• Maternity protection • Time off for antenatal care visits • Safe and clean workplace • Tobacco free working environment • Pregnant adolescents kept at school
Situational	• Support for taking ART and for coping with its side effects	• Support for HIV positive women
Childbirth	• Accompanying and supporting the woman in childbirth • Support and care for the rest of the family • Organize transport and financial support	• Support for the family during childbirth and immediate postpartum
Postpartum and beyond	• Support for exclusive breast-feeding/replacement feeding • Personal hygiene • Safe disposal / washing of pads • Suppprt for rest and lower work load • Safe and nutritive diet • Safe sexual practices • Motivation for prescribed treatments • Recognition of danger signs, including blues / depression • Optimal pregnancy spacing • Reporting birth and death (vital registration) • Participation in improving quality of services • Participation in transport and financing scheme	• Maternity leave • Breast-feeding breaks • Time off for postpartum and baby care visits • If mother referred to hospital, support that she is accompanied with the baby
Newborn and young infant	• Exclusive breast-feeding • Hygiene (cord care, washing, clothes) • Avoiding contacts with sick family members • Clean, warm and quiet place, tobacco and fire smoke free • Extra care for small babies (preterm, low birth weight) including KMC • Support for routine and follow-up visits • Motivation for home treatment of minor problems • Recognition of danger signs • Safe disposal of baby stool • Care seeking at health facility or hospital	• Promotion, protection and support for breast-feeding. • Keeping mother with the baby in hospital for breast-feeding • Supporting the family during maternal absence • Support for referral care for sick newborn
Situational	• Sleeping under ITN	

Adapted from WHO 2007[11]

Table 25.5 Care for the woman before and between pregnancies[11]

	Care by health services	Home/family	Community and workplace
Adolescence	• Immunization according to national policy (tetanus and rubella) • Family planning • HIV prevention including VCT	• Delayed childbearing • Healthy lifestyle • Balanced diet, including iodized salt • Optimal pregnancy timing	• Education • Information on prevention of HIV and STI infections
All women of reproductive age	• Family planning • Assessment and management of STIs • HIV prevention including testing and counselling		

Adapted from WHO 2007[11]

Table 25.6 Pregnant women not wanting child[11]

	Care by health services	Home/family	Community and workplace
Pregnant woman not wanting child	• Safe abortion (where legal) • Post-abortion care and family planning	• Care for unwanted pregnancy	

Adapted from WHO 2007[11]

development of hypertension (blood pressure greater than 140/90 mm Hg), the disease affects multiple systems and is progressive in nature. PIH is associated with a mild degree of disseminated intravascular coagulation, which may worsen with increasing severity of disease. Renal perfusion decreases and this can lead to renal failure. A syndrome of haemolysis, elevated liver enzymes and low platelet count (HELLP) has been noted in severe pre-eclampsia. Cerebral haemorrhage often complicates eclampsia and uncontrolled hypertension. Decreased uteroplacental flow due to the vasoconstrictive effects of pre-eclampsia leads to fetal growth restriction and fetal death. The perinatal mortality rate is increased in pre-eclampsia because of preterm delivery, uteroplacental insufficiency, abruptio placentae and unexplained fetal death. Preterm delivery is often necessitated by the fact that the definitive treatment of pre-eclampsia mandates termination of the pregnancy, regardless of the gestational age of the fetus.

Complications of the hypertensive disorders of pregnancy, including PIH, may be due to the disease itself, secondary to the convulsions in eclampsia, or to the side-effects of drugs or other treatment given. The main complications of treatment are related to respiratory depression and fluid overload. Regression of PIH only occurs after delivery of the fetus and placenta. The goals of management of a patient with PIH are to prevent deterioration to eclampsia, to prevent complications such as cardiovascular accidents, pulmonary oedema, renal failure, abruptio placentae and fetal death, and the timely delivery with minimal trauma to the mother. Mild and moderate forms of the disease can only be detected by monitoring the blood pressure during antenatal care, as the disease is symptomless at this stage other than the appearance of non-dependent oedema. Treatment is expectant at this stage, with admission to hospital if necessary. Labour can usually be induced without risk of prematurity to the fetus after 37 weeks' gestation. The objective of management prior to this time is to control blood pressure and monitor the maternal and fetal condition to ensure that deterioration does not occur. In the mild or moderate forms, treatment with antihypertensives under supervision may allow the pregnancy to be prolonged for a few weeks to allow for fetal maturation. Hypertension is just one sign of the

multisystem disorder, and control of the blood pressure does not imply cure of the disease. Control of blood pressure can be achieved with any of the standard antihypertensive agents such as methyldopa, hydralazine, nifedipine or labetalol (see Chapter 37). Beta-blockers such as propranolol are best avoided, as they tend to cause fetal bradycardia and hypoglycaemia in neonates.

The progress of PIH is extremely unpredictable. Some patients have only mild disease (with elevated blood pressure but no proteinuria) throughout the latter part of their pregnancy. Others progress rapidly within 24 hours from apparently mild disease to fulminating pre-eclampsia and eclampsia. Prior to the onset of convulsions in eclampsia, the woman may complain of frontal headaches, visual disturbances (e.g. 'flashing lights'), epigastric pain and vomiting. On examination, her reflexes tend to be exaggerated and urinary output decreased.

In areas with inadequate antenatal care provision or utilization, most women will present with severe pre-eclampsia or with eclampsia. Management in these circumstances is based on stabilizing the maternal condition and delivery of the fetus irrespective of gestation. Vaginal delivery may be possible following induction of labour by the use of prostaglandin analogues or rupturing the membranes and the judicious use of oxytocin. Careful monitoring of fluid intake and output is essential during this time as these patients are frequently oliguric and may develop pulmonary oedema. If the patient does not progress in labour, delivery by caesarean section may be necessary.

Magnesium suphate (intravenously or intramuscular) is the drug of choice for treating convulsions in eclampsia and preventing their recurrence, although diazepam and phenytoin are also used. Diazepam may cause maternal and neonatal respiratory depression. Magnesium sulphate may also cause respiratory and cardiac arrest if plasma magnesium levels become too high. Suppression of the reflexes occurs prior to respiratory or cardiac arrest, and decreased urine output would exacerbate toxicity. Care must be taken, therefore, when using magnesium sulphate, to check for adequate renal output and the presence of reflexes before giving a further dose. Its use in patients with severe pre-eclampsia to prevent eclampsia is still being evaluated. Phenytoin is less reliable in its action, is more expensive, and requires close monitoring of the patient. Patients can be at risk of eclamptic fits for up to 48 hours after delivery. During this time they should therefore receive intensive nursing in a semi-prone position in a quiet room. Antihypertensive and prophylactic anticonvulsant therapy with magnesium sulphate should be continued.

Obstructed labour

Prolonged labour increases the likelihood of fetal hypoxia and may result in stillbirth or neonatal death. When associated with prolonged labour, complications such as cephalopelvic disproportion, malpresentation (e.g. brow or shoulder presentation) and abnormal lie (e.g. transverse lie) will result in obstructed labour. In some cases vaginal delivery may still occur but at a cost not only of fetal death but also of serious maternal morbidity, such as vesicovaginal fistula due to pressure necrosis. In more extreme cases uterine rupture and subsequent maternal death will be the outcome.

The use of the partograph in the management of labour enables the health attendant to recognize when labour is not progressing normally, allowing for appropriate action to be taken. Where deliveries are conducted by traditional birth attendants they should be taught to recognize the signs which precede obstructed labour and encouraged to refer to an appropriate centre where medical staff and facilities are available. Midwives and nurses at primary health centres are encouraged to use the partograph to monitor the progress of labour to enable them to identify when there is failure of progress of labour and to refer to a hospital for further management. This may require the judicious use of oxytocin to improve uterine contractions, provided cephalopelvic disproportion and malpresentation have been excluded. Further lack of progress requires intervention by caesarean section that can then be performed early to ensure fetal survival and prevent maternal mortality and morbidity.

Puerperal sepsis

Puerperal sepsis contributes to some 15% of maternal deaths. Following delivery, the presence of a large denuded area of the uterus predisposes to the development of endometritis and subsequent puerperal sepsis. Sepsis may also occur secondary to laceration of the genital tract and in the presence of retained products of conception. The presence of untreated sexually transmitted diseases during pregnancy, poor hygiene on the part of the birth attendant, and poor sterilization of instruments inserted into the genital tract during delivery or abortion are a particular risk. The presence of a genital tract infection is suspected by the presence of foul-smelling lochia or discharge. Less specific symptoms include abdominal pain, vomiting, headache and loss of appetite. Examination reveals pyrexia and a tender bulky uterus. In more advanced stages of the disease, tender masses in the adnexa or in the posterior fornix may be found, suggesting the presence of tubo-ovarian or pouch of Douglas abscesses. Septicaemia may also occur.

Treatment in the early stages is by the use of broad-spectrum antibiotics followed by evacuation of the uterus after approximately 24 hours if retained products of conception are suspected.

In more advanced cases, following the administration of intravenous antibiotics, laparotomy to drain the tubo-ovarian abscesses is necessary, and in extreme cases hysterectomy and pelvic clearance may be required. Abscesses in the pouch of Douglas may be drained by colpotomy (via the vagina), but a significant proportion of such patients will subsequently require laparotomy.

Post-abortion care

Spontaneous abortion (miscarriage) can occur in as many as 15% of pregnancies, usually in the first trimester. If untreated, incomplete abortion frequently leads to continued vaginal bleeding and consequent anaemia. The retained products can also give rise to uterine sepsis. In many countries, management includes the common procedure of a sharp curettage of the uterine cavity, more frequently known as dilatation and curettage (D&C), which requires a physician, operating theatre and general anaesthesia. However, the manual vacuum aspiration (MVA) using a plastic cannula and syringe to create a vacuum is the preferred procedure because of its lower risk of complications. It can be performed under local anaesthesia and numerous countries have successfully trained nurse-midwives to conduct the procedure.

Induced abortion is illegal in many countries, but even where it is legal this does not ensure access to quality services. Consequently, a high proportion of women presenting with incomplete abortion may have associated sepsis due to self-abortion or the procedure having been performed by unskilled or untrained personnel. Some 13% of maternal mortalities occur due to complications of abortion (induced or spontaneous). Post-abortion care services provide for emergency care of complications which includes resuscitation, use of antibiotics, and evacuation of the uterus using MVA if possible. Strategies also include counselling related to recognition of symptoms and signs for the woman to look out for in the next few days. Further counselling and, if necessary, provision of other reproductive health services, particularly family planning, are also considered important.

Malaria in pregnancy

Malaria in general, and particularly infection with *Plasmodium falciparum*, is a major cause of morbidity and mortality in pregnancy, especially in the young primigravida in affected areas (see Chapter 73). Pregnant women living in endemic areas tend to lose their immunity to malaria, particularly during the second trimester, and are at increased risk of infection that tends to be more severe in pregnancy. The most serious effect of malaria in pregnancy is the development of haemolytic anaemia that, if severe enough, can lead to hypoxia of both the mother and fetus. The hepatorenal syndrome and cerebral malaria is often the cause of death. Other sequelae of malaria include miscarriage, intrauterine fetal growth restriction, fetal death and premature labour. In areas where malaria is holoendemic, it is an important cause of anaemia. The presentation of malaria in pregnancy, however, may be atypical and its presence should be suspected in any pregnant woman in endemic areas with fever or jaundice.

Medical treatment is dependent on the geographical area and the local pattern of drug resistance. *P. falciparum* and *P. vivax* account for the majority of cases. It is essential to follow local, national and regional treatment guidelines. Chloroquine is the treatment of choice in chloroquine-sensitive areas. However, chloroquine resistance is widespread and oral sulfadoxine/pyrimethamine or quinine salt can be used instead. Where multidrug-resistant *P. falciparum* limits treatment options, artesunate is used instead. In areas of mixed *falciparum–vivax* malaria, the proportions of malaria species and their drug sensitivity patterns vary, making reference to the local treatment guidelines especially pertinent. Chloroquine alone is the treatment of choice during pregnancy in areas with chloroquine-sensitive *vivax* malaria and chloroquine-sensitive *falciparum* malaria. Where there is chloroquine-resistant *falciparum* malaria, it is managed as a mixed infection with the addition of sulfadoxine/pyrimethamine.

Routine chemoprophylaxis is advocated for pregnant women, according to local guidelines. Regimens include weekly chloroquine (and daily proguanil) from 20 weeks' gestation onwards. In areas of high transmission in sub-Saharan Africa, the current strategy for malaria prevention is intermittent preventative treatment with sulfadoxine/pyrimethamine, once during the second trimester and once during the third trimester. In areas of high HIV prevalence, intermittent preventative treatment with sulfadoxine/pyrimethamine every month beginning in the second trimester appears to be optimal[15] (see also section on HIV in Pregnancy). In addition, insecticide-treated nets (ITN), or, more specifically, long-lasting insecticidal nets (LLIN), can achieve full coverage of populations at risk of malaria and further help reduce the risk of malaria.[16,17]

Tetanus

Maternal tetanus infection may occur as a result of abortion performed with improperly sterilized instruments or from delivery in unclean surroundings (see Chapter 64). Although maternal tetanus can occur as an ascending infection, neonatal tetanus is far more common. The neonate may get infected via the umbilicus, highlighting the need for umbilical cordcare and discouraging harmful practices. Treatment is described in Chapter 64, but mortality rates remain high. Training of birth attendants, particularly in the use of a clean delivery technique and use of sterilized equipment, can reduce the risk of infection. Antenatal programmes in developing countries now provide for tetanus immunization and aim to provide cover for the mother and also the neonate. To be effective, a pregnant woman needs to receive two doses of tetanus toxoid 4 weeks apart and at least 4 weeks prior to giving birth. The first dose should ideally be given at the first clinic visit.

HIV AND PREGNANCY

UNAIDS estimates that by 2007 over 33 million people were living with HIV with 22.5 million of them in sub-Saharan Africa.[18] Women constituted 15.4 million (46.4%) of the 30.8 million adults who were infected. In women of reproductive age, HIV in pregnancy has implications on the health of the mother and on mother-to-child transmission of HIV. Pregnancy appears to have little effect on the progress of infection in asymptomatic HIV-infected women or in those in the early stages of infection. In untreated women, however, adverse outcomes in early and late

pregnancy may be directly due to HIV or medical and social conditions that affect pregnancy. Compared with HIV-1, the prevalence of HIV-2, which is still found in parts of West Africa and some locations in Portugal and India, has been stable, is less common, has a slower clinical course, and mother-to-child transmission occurs less frequently.[19–21] This section only considers HIV-1.

HIV testing in pregnancy

The advantages to a woman knowing her HIV status prior to or during pregnancy includes the opportunity to facilitate early counselling and treatment; allows the implementation of strategies to prevent transmission to the child; enables the woman to take precautions to help prevent transmission to sexual partners; and enables sexual partners to be counselled and tested. Further, if the test is negative, women can be guided in appropriate HIV prevention measures and risk-reduction behaviour, where appropriate. The possible disadvantages of HIV testing in pregnancy include reported increased risk of violence, stigmatization by community and health workers, and higher levels of anxiety and psychological sequelae. In order to increase HIV testing to enable women to know their status, country programmes are adopting 'opt-out' policies, whereby an HIV test is performed unless the woman requests it not to be done. A variation is the 'provider-initiated' HIV testing and counselling in health facilities. Both strategies aim for wider knowledge of HIV status by women and to enable increased access to HIV treatment and prevention.[19,22]

Mother-to-child transmission of HIV

UNAIDS estimates that 420 000 children were newly infected with HIV in 2007 and nearly 90% of all HIV-infected children live in sub-Saharan Africa.[18] The primary mode of acquisition of HIV in children worldwide is through mother-to-child transmission (MTCT), which can occur during pregnancy, labour and delivery, or breast-feeding. In the absence of breast-feeding, about 30% of infant HIV infections occur in utero and 70% during labour and delivery.[23] In the presence of breast-feeding, one-third to one-half of perinatal HIV infections may be due to breast-feeding.[24,25] Risk factors for transmission include high maternal viral load, advanced maternal immune deficiency and prolonged rupture of membranes (>4 hours). Risk factors for breast-milk transmission include high viral load and subclinical mastitis.[26,27]

Without interventions to reduce MTCT, the estimated risk of transmission ranges from 15% to 25% in non-breast-feeding populations and 25% to 40% in breast-feeding populations.[28,29] In developed countries, the risk of MTCT has been reduced to under 2% by three main interventions: (i) use of antiretroviral therapy or as prophylaxis given to women during pregnancy and labour and to the infant in the first weeks of life; (ii) obstetrical interventions including elective caesarean delivery (prior to the onset of labour and rupture of membranes); and (iii) complete avoidance of breast-feeding.[30,31] In many resource-constrained settings, whereas programmes for antiretroviral prophylaxis (and therapy) are scaling up, elective caesarean delivery is not always feasible.[32] Further, alternatives to breast-feeding may also not be feasible for financial, logistical and cultural reasons. Research is ongoing to

Table 25.7 Maternal and neonatal antiretroviral regimens for treatment and PMTCT in resource-constrained settings – a tiered approach

	Maternal HAART indicated*	Maternal HAART not indicated*	No maternal antepartum antiretrovirals	No maternal antepartum or intrapartum antiretrovirals
Mother				
Antepartum period	HAART*	AZT twice a day at ≥28 wk	–	–
Intrapartum period	HAART	SD-NVP[†]+AZT/3TC	SD-NVP	–
Postpartum period	HAART	AZT/3TC twice a day ×7 d	AZT/3TC twice a day ×7 d	–
Infant	AZT × 7 d[‡]	SD-NVP + AZT twice a day ×1 wk[‡]	SD-NVP + AZT twice a day ×4 wk[§]	SD-NVP + AZT twice a day ×4 wk[§]

*Recommended for all HIV-infected pregnant women with WHO clinical stage 4, WHO clinical stage 3 and CD4 < 350 cells/mm³, WHO clinical stage 1 or 2 and CD4 < 200 cells/mm³. Recommended regimen: AZT + 3TC + NVP.
[†]If the woman receives at least 4 weeks of AZT during pregnancy, the omission of the maternal intrapartum NVP dose may be considered; in this case, the infant NVP dose must be given immediately at birth and received for 4 weeks, instead of 1 week of infant AZT; and the mother will not require 3TC during labour and AZT/3TC 'tail' postpartum.
[‡]If the mother receives <4 weeks of AZT during pregnancy, 4 weeks instead of 1 week of infant AZT is recommended.
[§]Data on the added efficacy of 4 compared to 1 week of infant AZT in this situation are limited.
3TC, lamivudine; AZT, zidovudine; HAART, highly active antiretroviral therapy; PMTCT, prevention of mother-to-child-transmission; SD-NVP; single-dose nevirapine.
Adapted from Dao et al.[29]

evaluate several new approaches to preventing HIV transmission during breast-feeding.[25] These include modification of infant feeding practices with exclusive breast-feeding for the infant's first few months of life followed by rapid weaning, treatments of expressed milk to inactivate the virus, and antiretroviral prophylaxis taken by the infant or mother during breast-feeding.[25]

Management of the HIV-infected pregnant woman

Antiretrovirals are not contraindicated in pregnancy. To take into consideration prevention of mother-to-child-transmission (PMTCT), antiretroviral regimens, particularly those developed by WHO (and summarized in Table 25.7), incorporate combinations for use by mothers whether maternal therapy was indicated or not.[19] Accordingly, these may vary in the antenatal, intrapartum and postnatal period. Regimens for the infant in the first week and to 4 weeks would similarly vary according to the maternal regimen. Furthermore, the regimens take into consideration situations where access to treatment is unavailable and PMTCT programmes are not fully established. The WHO recommendations for initiating antiretroviral treatment in pregnant women are based on clinical stage and availability of immunological markers (such as CD4 count).[19] Apart from serving the health needs of the pregnant woman herself and substantially reducing the risk of MTCT, such antiretroviral regimens minimize the consequences of resistance to nevirapine from the use of single-dose-nevirapine (SD-NVP)-containing antiretroviral prophylactic regimens that are commonly used for PMTCT in resource-constrained settings.

Most HIV-infected women will be asymptomatic and have no major obstetrical problems during their pregnancies and, apart from considerations of antimalarial and other prophylaxis, can receive similar antenatal care to that given to those uninfected. Where possible, invasive diagnostic procedures, such as chorion villus biopsy sampling, amniocentesis and cordocentesis, are best avoided due to a possible added risk of HIV transmission to the fetus. Similarly, external cephalic version of a breech fetus may be associated with potential maternal–fetal circulation leaks and the risk of HIV transmission.

Malaria in pregnancy has been shown to increase the risk of MTCT of HIV.[33] Intermittent preventative treatment with an effective, preferably a single dose, antimalarial drug should be made available to all primigravidae and secundigravidae in highly endemic areas. This is started in the second trimester and given at monthly intervals for HIV-infected pregnant women. In addition, there is benefit in the use of insecticide-treated nets (ITN), or, more specifically, long-lasting insecticidal nets (LLIN), to achieve full coverage of populations at risk of malaria.[16,17]

Prophylaxis for opportunistic infections is given in pregnancy as indicated by the clinical stage and according to local policy. This includes prophylaxis and treatment for tuberculosis. Of the antituberculosis drugs, streptomycin and pyrazinamide are not recommended during pregnancy. In resource-constrained settings, there is evidence to suggest that *Pneumocystis carinii* pneumonia (PCP) prophylaxis with co-trimoxazole (sulfamethoxazole/trimethoprim), in women with low CD4 counts, can also have indirect benefits for neonatal and infant health, in addition to the direct maternal benefit.[34] If a woman living with HIV is receiving co-trimoxazole prophylaxis and resides in a malarial zone, it is not necessary for her to have additional sulfadoxine/pyrimethamine-based intermittent presumptive therapy for malaria. Breast-feeding women should continue to receive co-trimoxazole prophylaxis.[35]

Management of labour and delivery remains the same as that for HIV-uninfected women. Prolonged rupture of membranes is avoided, as the risk of MTCT is increased where membranes are ruptured for more than 4 hours. The general rule is to avoid any procedure which breaks the baby's skin and/or increases the risk of contact with the mother's blood, such as scalp electrodes and fetal blood sampling. Episiotomy should not be a routine procedure, but should rather be reserved for those cases with an obstetrical indication. Caesarean section has been found to be associated with a decrease in transmission of HIV to the infant, although there are considerations of maternal complications. Nevertheless, prophylactic antibiotics are recommended for both elective and emergency caesarean sections.[36]

Postpartum care is similar to that for uninfected women. If untreated, HIV-infected women are more prone to postpartum infections, including urinary tract infections, chest infections, and episiotomy and caesarean section wound infections.

Counselling on breast-feeding includes discussing the risks and benefits of infant feeding choices. Mothers who chose to breast-feed are advised of the possible increased risk of transmission in the presence of cracked nipples, mastitis and breast abscess. Prevention of such problems can be achieved through adequate breast-feeding techniques. Reduced duration of breast-feeding and early cessation may be encouraged to reduce the risk of transmission if this can be safely achieved.[37] In resource-poor settings, alternatives to breast-feeding may not be feasible for financial, logistical and cultural reasons. Mothers should be given information on the advantages and disadvantages of breast-feeding and replacement feeding with regard to HIV infection and encouraged to make a fully informed decision about infant feeding. A consensus statement from a WHO HIV infant feeding technical consultation recommends that the most appropriate infant feeding option for an HIV-infected mother should continue to depend on her individual circumstances.[38] It states that exclusive breast-feeding is recommended for HIV-infected women for the first 6 months of life unless replacement feeding is acceptable, feasible, affordable, sustainable and safe for them and their infants before that time. Breast-feeding mothers of infants and young children who are known to be HIV-infected should be strongly encouraged to continue breast-feeding.

Contraceptive advice becomes important when a mother chooses not to breast-feed. She loses the contraceptive effects of breast-feeding, and information on alternative methods should be provided. In general, all methods are suitable for HIV-infected women in the postnatal period. In asymptomatic HIV-infected women or women clinically well on antiretroviral therapy, the advantages of initiating (or continuing) the intrauterine device (levonorgestrel- or copper-releasing) generally outweigh the theoretical or proven risks of increased sepsis. However, theoretical or proven risks usually outweigh the advantages of initiating the method in women with AIDS.[39,40]

REFERENCES

1. WHO, UNICEF, UNFPA. *Maternal Mortality in 2000: Estimates Developed by WHO, UNICEF and UNFPA.* Geneva: World Health Organization; 2004.

2. Lewis G, de Bernis L, eds. *Obstetric Fistula: Guiding Principles for Clinical Management and Programme Development.* Geneva: World Health Organization; 2006.

3. WHO. *Neonatal and Perinatal Mortality: Country, Regional and Global Estimates.* Geneva: World Health Organization; 2006.

4. United Nations. *UN Millennium Development Goals.* Online. Available: http://www.un.org/millenniumgoals/ 26 August 2008.

5. Lawson JL, Harrison KA, Bergström S, eds. *Maternity Care in Developing Countries.* London: RCOG Press; 2001.

6. Okonofua F, Odunsi K, eds. *Contemporary Obstetrics and Gynaecology for Developing Countries.* Benin City, Nigeria: Women's Health and Action Research Centre; 2003.

7. Schreuder GD. An approach to women's health in the tropics. In: Goldsmid JM, Leggat PA, eds. *Primer of Tropical Medicine.* Brisbane, Australia: The Australasian College of Tropical Medicine Publications; 2005; 17.1–17.12. Also available at: http://www.tropmed.org/primer/index.htm 26 August 2008.

8. WHO. *Pregnancy, Childbirth, Postpartum and Newborn Care: A Guide for Essential Practice.* Geneva: World Health Organization; 2006. Updated 2nd edn, 2007. Also available at : http://www.who.int/reproductive-health/publications/pcpnc/pcpnc.pdf 26 August 2008.

9. WHO. *Managing Complications in Pregnancy and Childbirth: A Guide for Midwives and Doctors.* Geneva: World Health Organization; 2003. Also available at: http://www.who.int/reproductive-health/impac/mcpc.pdf 26 August 2008.

10. WHO. *Managing Newborn Problems: A Guide for Doctors, Nurses and Midwives.* Geneva: World Health Organization; 2003. Also available at: http://www.who.int/reproductive-health/publications/mnp/mnp.pdf 26 August 2008.

11. WHO. *WHO Recommended Interventions for Improving Maternal and Newborn Health.* Geneva: World Health Organization; 2007. Also available at: http://whqlibdoc.who.int/hq/2007/WHO_MPS_07.05_eng.pdf 26 August 2008.

12. Maine D. *Studying Maternal Mortality in Developing Countries. A Guidebook: Rates and Causes.* FHE 87.7. Geneva: WHO; 1987.

13. Thaddeus S, Maine D. Too far to walk: maternal mortality in context. *Soc Sci Med* 1994; 38:1091–1110.

14. Ross SR. *Promoting Quality Maternal and Newborn Care: A Reference Manual for Program Managers.* Atlanta: CARE; 1998.

15. Parise ME, Ayisi JG, Nahlen BL, et al. Efficacy of sulfadoxine/pyrimethamine for prevention of placental malaria in an area of Kenya with a high prevalence of malaria and human immunodeficiency virus infection. *Am J Trop Med Hyg* 1998; 59:813–822.

16. Gamble C, Ekwaru JP, ter Kuile FO. Insecticide-treated nets for preventing malaria in pregnancy. *Cochrane Database Syst Rev* 2006; (2):CD003755.

17. Global Malaria Programme. *Insecticide-treated Mosquito Nets: A WHO Position Statement.* Geneva: World Health Organization; 2007. Also available at: http://www.who.int/malaria/docs/itn/ITNspospaperfinal.pdf 26 August 2008.

18. UNAIDS. *AIDS epidemic update: December 2007.*UNAIDS/07.27E / JC1322E (English original, December 2007). Online. Available: http://data.unaids.org/pub/EPISlides/2007/2007_epiupdate_en.pdf 26 August 2008.

19. WHO. *Antiretroviral Drugs for Treating Pregnant Women and Preventing HIV Infection in Infants: Towards Universal Access.* Geneva: World Health Organization; 2006. Also available at: http://www.who.int/hiv/pub/guidelines/pmtctguidelines3.pdf 26 August 2008.

20. Adjorlolo-Johnson G, De Cock K M, Ekpini E, et al. Prospective comparison of mother to child transmission of HIV-1 and HIV-2 in Abidjan, Ivory Coast. *JAMA* 1994; 272:462–466.

21. Cazein F, Hamers F, Alix J & Brunet JB. Prevalence of HIV-2 infection in Europe. *Euro Surveill* 1996; 1(3):21–23.

22. WHO. *Guidance on Provider-Initiated HIV Testing and Counselling in Health Facilities.* Geneva: World Health Organization; 2007. Online. Available: http://www.who.int/hiv/pub/guidelines/9789241595568_en.pdf 26 August 2008.

23. Mock PA, Shaffer N, Bhadrakom C, et al. Maternal viral load and timing of mother-to-child HIV transmission, Bangkok, Thailand. *AIDS* 1999; 13:407–414.

24. Wiktor SZ, Ekpini E, Nduati RW. Prevention of mother-to-child transmission of HIV-1 in Africa. *AIDS* 1997; 11(suppl B):S79–S87.

25. Kourtis AP, Jamieson DJ, de Vincenzi I, et al. Prevention of human immunodeficiency virus-1 transmission to the infant through breastfeeding: new developments. *Am J Obstet Gynecol* 2007; 197(suppl):S113–S122.

26. Semba RD, Kumwenda N, Hoover DR, et al. Human immunodeficiency virus load in breast milk, mastitis, and mother-to-child transmission of human immunodeficiency virus type 1. *J Infect Dis* 1999; 180:93–98.

27. UNICEF, UNAIDS, WHO, UNFPA. *HIV transmission through breastfeeding. A review of available evidence.* WHO 2004. Online. Available: http://www.who.int/reproductivehealth/docs/hiv_infantfeeding/breastfeeding.pdf 26 August 2008.

28. De Cock KM, Fowler MG, Mercier E, et al. Prevention of mother-to-child HIV transmission in resource-poor countries: translating research into policy and practice. *JAMA* 2000; 283:1175–1182.

29. Dao H, Mofenson LM, Ekpini R, et al. International recommendations on antiretroviral drugs for treatment of HIV-infected women and prevention of mother-to-child HIV transmission in resource-limited settings: 2006 update. *Am J Obstet Gynecol* 2007; 197(suppl):S42–S55.

30. European Collaborative Study. Mother-to-child transmission of HIV infection in the era of highly active antiretroviral therapy. *Clin Infect Dis* 2005; 40:458–465.

31. Dorenbaum A, Cunningham CK, Gelber RD, et al. Two-dose intrapartum/newborn nevirapine and standard antiretroviral therapy to reduce perinatal HIV transmission: a randomized trial. *JAMA* 2002; 288:189–198.

32. Stanton CK, Holtz SA. Levels and trends in cesarean birth in the developing world. *Stud Fam Plann* 2006; 37:41–48.

33. Bloland PB, Wirima JJ, Steketee RW, et al. Maternal HIV infection and infant mortality in Malawi: evidence for increased mortality due to placental malaria infection. *AIDS* 1995; 9:721–726.

34. Walter J, Mwiya M, Scott N, et al. Reduction in preterm delivery and neonatal mortality after the introduction of antenatal cotrimoxazole prophylaxis among HIV-infected women with low CD4 cell counts. *J Infect Dis* 2006; 194:1510–1518.

35. WHO. *Guidelines on co-trimoxazole prophylaxis for HIV-related infections among children, adolescents and adults in resource-limited settings. Recommendations for a public health approach.* World Health Organization 2006. Online. Available: http://www.who.int/hiv/pub/guidelines/ctxguidelines.pdf 26 August 2008.

36. The European Mode of Delivery Collaboration. Elective Cesarean section versus vaginal delivery in prevention of vertical HIV-1 transmission: a randomised clinical trial. *Lancet* 1999; 353:1035–1039.

37. UNAIDS,WHO,UNICEF. *HIV and Infant Feeding: A Guide for Health Care Managers and Supervisors.* Geneva, 1998. (UNAIDS/98.4, WHO/FRH/NUT/CHD/98.2, UNICEF/PD/NUT(J)98.2). Online. Available: http://data.unaids.org/publications/IRC-pub03/meetrev_en.pdf 26 August 2008.

38. WHO. *WHO HIV and infant feeding technical consultation held on behalf of the Inter-agency Task Team (IATT) on prevention of HIV infections in pregnant women, mothers and their infants. Geneva, October 25–27, 2006. Consensus statement.* Online. Available: http://www.who.int/reproductive-health/stis/mtct/infantfeedingconsensusstatement.pdf 26 August 2008.

39. WHO. *Medical Eligibility Criteria for Contraceptive Use.* 3rd edn. Geneva: World Health Organization; 2004. Online. Available: http://www.who.int/reproductive-health/publications/mec/mec.pdf 26 August 2008.

40. World Health Organization, Department of Reproductive Health and Research (WHO/RHR) and Johns Hopkins Bloomberg School of Public Health/Center for Communication Programs (CCP), INFO Project. *Family Planning: A Global Handbook for Providers* (Successor to the Essentials of Contraceptive Technology). Baltimore and Geneva: CCP and WHO; 2007. Online. Available: http://www.infoforhealth.org/globalhandbook/handbook.pdf 26 August 2008.

Eli Tumba Tshibwabwa,
Michael G. Kawooya and
Zeridah Muyinda

Chapter 26

Trends in Radiology and Imaging Services in the Tropics

Radiology is increasingly central to the investigation and treatment of patients in the developed world. The benefits that drive this shift in practice should be available to patients, and to planners of healthcare, in the tropics. Indeed, ironically, the benefits of minimally invasive therapy, as offered by interventional radiology, may be greater in the tropics where alternative treatments (long-term drug therapy, complex open surgery and so on) may not be available, or be prohibitively expensive.

While we should strive to place modern and dependable imaging ever more at the centre of provision of healthcare in the tropics, many practical considerations have to be tackled before this paradigm can be realized. In particular, we cannot simply translate from the model of radiology services in the developed world to the tropics. There are profound differences in the disease profiles between the two regions – trauma, various infections, and peripartum maternal or neonatal complications account for much of the pathology in the tropics rather than ischaemic heart disease or cancer.[1,2] Furthermore, the affluent areas in Europe and North America have comparatively large funds available for the provision of radiology equipment. Contrast this with the often impoverished regions in the tropics, which lack resources, equipment and personnel. The differential is exacerbated by a hostile topography and climate. Many areas are remote and sparsely populated, such that in many tropical countries resources are often concentrated in a few urbanized areas.[2,3]

SOME PRINCIPLES IN ESTABLISHING A RADIOLOGICAL SERVICE

The key to developing a sound radiological service is to match provision to demand (Box 26.1). Most of the cities and rural areas in Africa are blighted by a common group of pathologies.[1-3] HIV/AIDS and tuberculosis 'spearhead' the disease problem and there are other prevalent infections including those due to amoebiasis or helminths. Trauma accounts for a second major drain on limited healthcare resources. Thus, tropical imaging should be geared up for managing trauma, investigating and treating infection (e.g. percutaneous image-guided abscess drainage) and for obstetric care.

Plain radiography and ultrasound should form the core of any realistic imaging service. Computed tomography (CT), magnetic resonance imaging (MRI) and Positron Emission Tomography (PET) should be reserved for major centres alone.

A representative picture of radiological manpower and facilities has been built up for five sub-Saharan African countries (Box 26.2). This confirms that there is a desperate shortage of radiologists, radiographers and equipment, with most of the services located in the capital cities and few at rural hospitals. Information pertaining to radiology utilization in other tropical settings has been outlined in several articles.[2-4] Only 40% of countries in the sub-Saharan region have any CT scanners or high-resolution and/or Colour Doppler ultrasound machines and fluoroscopy. This is in contrast to the situation in the northern African region and in the Republic of South Africa, where academic radiology departments as well as other privately-owned departments are in addition better equipped and serviced with MRI and PET scanners. At present, major South African cities have hospitals which provide such high-tech imaging and management to patients from the neighbouring countries, and even from as far as central and eastern Africa, where the few existing CT scanners cannot cope with the patient load. At the University Teaching Hospital (UTH) of Lusaka (Zambia), the CT scanner has only recently been installed but the facility is already being outstripped by increasing demand for neurological investigations. One question that remains is whether the facilities and radiology services in major conurbations will be adequate or not for the size of the population, which fluctuates significantly as large numbers of people daily migrate from rural areas to cities in search of work and sustenance.

The measurement of the number of examinations per 1000 population in a year will serve as an indicator of radiological utilization in different countries and regions. We estimate the annual frequency of both simple and special procedures for the year 2005 as approximately 5, 10, 12 and 15 per 1000 population for the Democratic Republic of Congo, Zambia, Ethiopia and Uganda, respectively. These countries have been classified as countries with healthcare level III.[4] These figures suggest that fewer examinations have been performed than expected for a country with level III healthcare. By comparison, the annual frequencies of radiological examinations in South Africa (a healthcare level I country) range between 67 and 460 per 1000 population, respectively for 1000 blacks and 1000 whites.[4] The various radiological examinations performed for the white population in university teaching and main private establishments in South Africa appear

---

Box 26.1 Principles in establishing a radiological service

- Match provision to demand
- Core of imaging service: plain radiography and ultrasound
- Equipment should be reliable, durable and user-friendly, and most should be portable.

Box 26.2 Radiological manpower and facilities for sub-Saharan African countries

- Desperate shortage of radiologists, radiographers and equipment
- Most services are located in the capital cities with few at rural hospitals
- Only 40% of these countries have CT scanners or high-resolution ultrasound machines.

Box 26.3 A shift in the practice of tropical medicine

- Increasing availability of ultrasound machines has increased demand for ultrasound services, i.e. supply fuelled demand
- Wide range of ultrasound applications and their safety make it better suited to the budgets of a tropical setting.

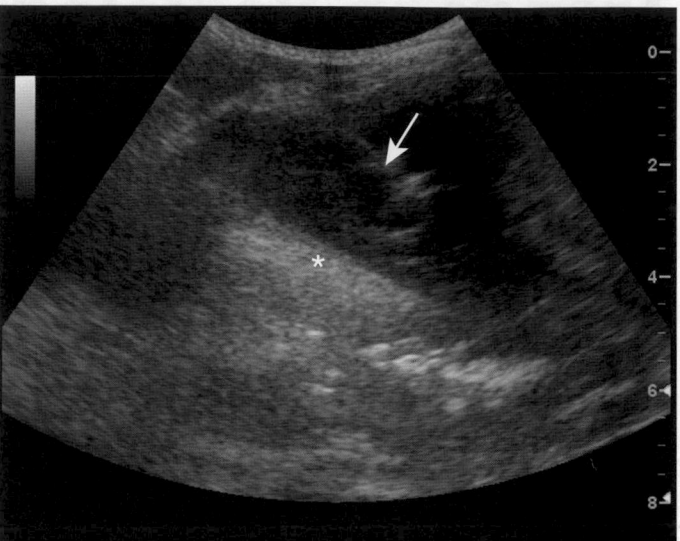

Figure 26.1 Ultrasound-guided left subphrenic abscess drainage; the collection is seen to have multiple loculations. Under sedation, local anaesthetic and ultrasound guidance, an 18-gauge needle was passed into the abscess. Some fluid was aspirated for culture and microscopy. An 8.5 French multipurpose drain was then inserted over the guidewire (arrow). The drain was left in and the procedure was uneventful (asterisk points to diaphragm overlying abcess).

to be comparable in numbers and variety to those in similar centres in the UK and USA.[4]

A SHIFT IN THE PRACTICE OF TROPICAL MEDICINE

The increasing availability of ultrasound machines, especially in tertiary hospitals such as UTH, or at competing private hospitals (and to a lesser extent at district hospitals), has led to an increase in the demand for ultrasound services (Box 26.3). Supply, in other words, has fuelled demand. Of course, this is in part because ultrasound is so suited to the investigation of many abdominal, traumatic, gynaecological and obstetrical conditions encountered in the tropics.[2,5,6] Moreover, there is an increasing awareness that ultrasound examinations can clinch an early diagnosis of disease, specifically when combined with ultrasound-guided intervention, such as aspiration and/or drainage of a collection or parenchymal biopsy (Figures 26.1–26.5). The wide range of ultrasound applications and the safety of this modality make it better suited to the budget of the tropical setting than any competing and more expensive high technology, such as digital radiography, CT or MRI equipment. Naturally, the benefits are obtained only when the machines are properly serviced and appropriate probes are available. Rather ironically, increasing demand in 'high-tech' developed-world intensive care units has prompted the manufacture of the hardware so that it is ideal for the rigours of the tropics: several high-quality yet small and affordable units are available which should function admirably in the intensive environments experienced in a tropical hospital.

In our experience of several departments in Africa, radiologists are fully responsible for daily diagnostic and interventional ultrasound, while residents carry out procedures under the supervision of a senior resident or staff radiologist. However, physicians, surgeons and radiographers who have been trained in ultrasound techniques (either from a local academic institution or abroad) and who have gained a satisfactory level in the practice of imaging and ultrasound-guided interventions are also a part of the radiological manpower outside university teaching hospitals. On the whole, the ultrasound service works, although there is a degree of concern from the established departments about users operating at private health centres that have not received adequate training. There is scope for misinterpretation which leads to inaccurate diagnosis. Another broad concern is that grey scale imaging is limited because limited resources prevent timely replacement of obsolete equipment. The inconsistency in operator and equipment and the consequent potential diagnostic errors become all the more worrying as the clinicians' reliance on ultrasound blossoms.

In this African setting, half of the patients referred for diagnostic ultrasound imaging present with large lesions. Patients may delay in seeking medical advice because of poverty, or because of traditional beliefs.[1] However, the remaining half of the patients do present to the radiology department at an earlier stage of the disease, and benefit from rapid treatment made possible by the speed and accuracy of ultrasound diagnosis and intervention.

RADIOLOGY IN THE WIDER CONTEXT OF HEALTHCARE

No amount of thought into the provision of the imaging equipment can on its own lead to a worthwhile imaging service. Imaging is only useful if it is coordinated with the clinical and pathological services within the hospital or within the region. There are two

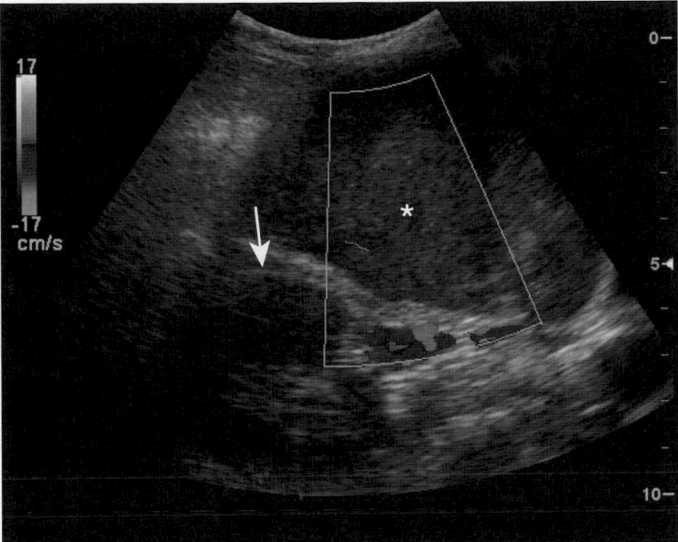

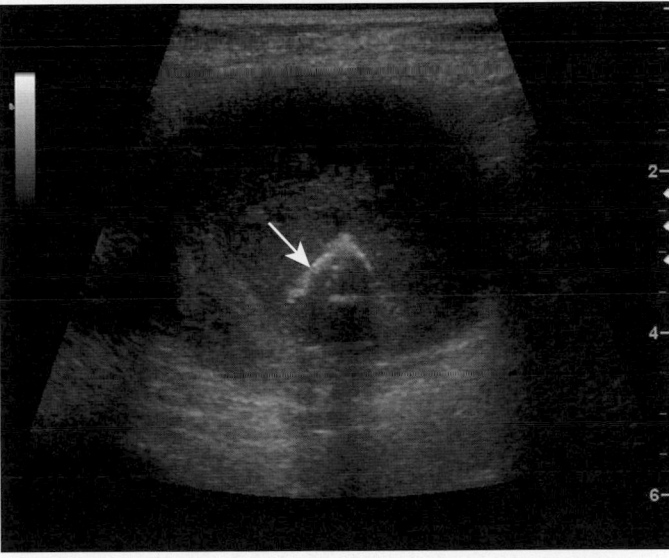

Figure 26.2 Ultrasound-guided focal liver biopsy. (A) Preliminary ultrasound confirms the presence of a focal hypoechoic lesion (asterisk) in liver segment (arrow points to right kidney). (B) Under ultrasound guidance, two 18-gauge core biopsies were obtained from the focal lesion. The procedure was well-tolerated under mild conscious sedation with no immediate complications (arrow points to the needle).

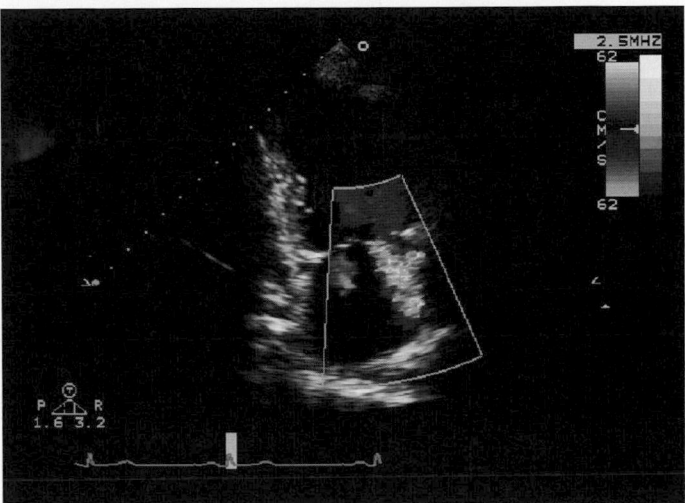

Figure 26.3 Mitral regurgitation. Apical two chamber view with Colour Doppler ultrasound showing the coloured mosaic pattern of regurgitation into the left atrium during systole.

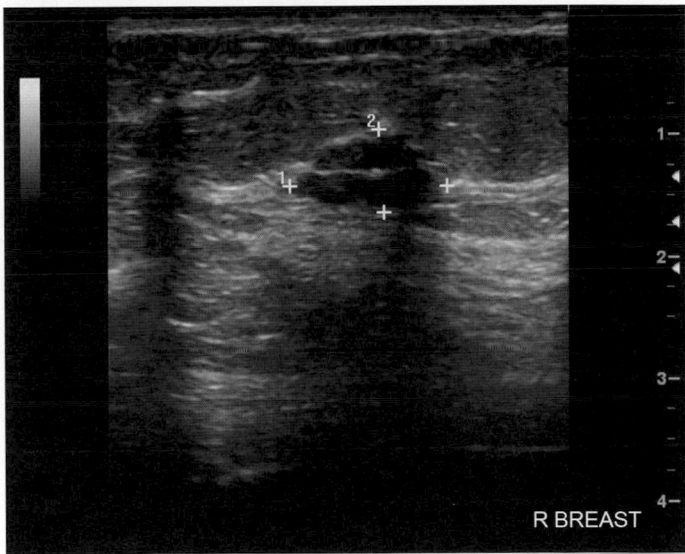

Figure 26.4 Right breast ultrasound. A well-defined lobulated nodule in the lower outer quadrant of the right breast is noted. The imaging features are in keeping with fibroadenomas and correlate with the biopsy finding.

Box 26.4 Radiology in the wider context of healthcare

- A radiographic study is only as good as the report it generates
- A radiograph or ultrasound scan of the highest quality still needs intelligent and clinically relevant interpretation.

Box 26.5 Transmission of digital ultrasound data globally

- The World Wide Web offers potential for image transfer and storage
- Teleradiology
- Simple imaging software packages for internet browsing of radiographs
- DICOM and PACS.

---

self-evident but nevertheless laudable statements which underpin this need for coordination: first, a radiographical study is only as good as the report it generates; and second, a report on its own is meaningless – it has worth only when it helps the physician managing the patient. In other words, a radiograph or ultrasound scan of the highest quality still needs intelligent and clinically relevant interpretation (Box 26.4).

We have to move away from the concept that this interpretation is to be provided at the site where the images have been obtained (Box 26.5). Dedicated landlines can be linked to inexpensive

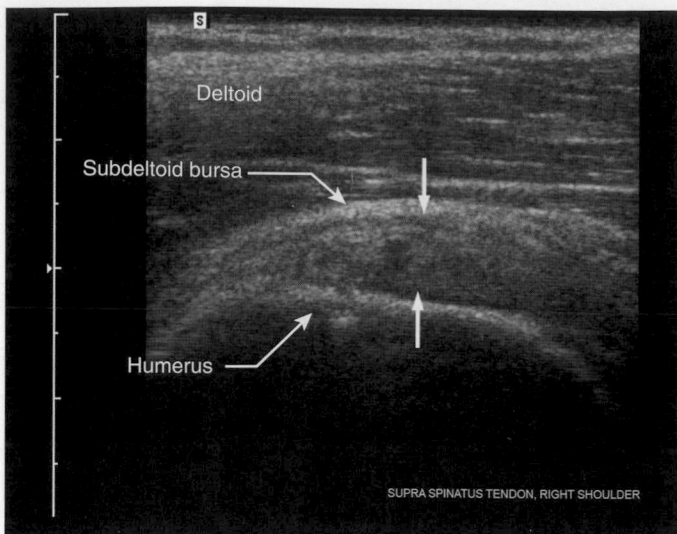

Figure 26.5 Right shoulder ultrasound showing mild to moderate tendinosis of the supraspinatus tendon (between arrows).

modems to permit transmission of digital ultrasound data across vast distances; on a more global scale, the World Wide Web offers potential for image transfer and storage. Teleradiology is coming of age. Several simple PC-based imaging software packages are available which allow internet browsing of radiographs. The film or study, in other words, can be moved from the 'spoke' to a 'hub'. Once the film has been read by a trained radiologist at the hub the report can be sent back by a landline connection to the remote spoke. Such teleradiology has also been used in India, Islamabad (Pakistan) and Tokelau (Pacific atoll), Colombia, Tomsk (Russia), Uganda, South Africa, and Nigeria.[7] Despite the current widespread use of Digital Imaging and Communications in Medicine (DICOM) and Picture Archiving and Communication System (PACS) in developed countries, these two types of digital technology are still under-utilized in sub-Saharan Africa.

INTERVENTIONAL RADIOLOGY

Radiology has moved resolutely from merely a diagnostic service to one in which it is pivotal in the treatment of numerous conditions (Box 26.6). This has been possible because of developments in catheter, guidewire and needle design, because of phenomenal advances in the technology (which has allowed real-time imaging to become commonplace) and because of several visionaries who have been very active in the past quarter of the century. Radiologists are at the forefront of minimally invasive therapy, with percutaneous techniques being employed in genitourinary, biliary, gastrointestinal and chest/vascular diseases. The more 'basic' techniques should certainly be available in the medium and larger centres within the tropics. Percutaneous drainage of abscesses and obstructed kidneys (renal stone disease is prevalent in hot countries) may be life-saving, and avoid the need for long-term antibiotic therapy. Many drains can be sited under ultrasound guidance as a 'single stick' procedure using only local anaesthetic and simple sedation (Figure 26.1). Techniques in fine needle aspi-

Box 26.6 Interventional radiology: from diagnostic service to treatment

- Catheter, guide wire and needle design developments
- Advances in technology
- Minimally invasive therapy, e.g. percutaneous techniques.

ration and biopsy may be equally important in the management of patients in the tropics (Figure 26.2A,B).

The limiting factor, of course, in the provision of such a service would be trained personnel.[2,3] Here, as in many other aspects concerning the delivery of healthcare in the tropics, resourcefulness is crucial.[1,3,4]

A TROPICAL SUCCESS STORY

In Kampala, the capital of Uganda, stands the Mulago University Teaching Hospital. In 1999, the Department of Radiology underwent major improvements with recruitment of appropriate staff at all levels and the establishment of high-resolution ultrasound, CT and gamma camera units.

A retrospective analysis for the 2 years preceding (2 January 2003 to 28 December 2004) and the 2 years following (2 January 2005 to 28 December 2006) revealed a total of 134 326 imaging examinations for the first period and 182 622 for the second period for Mulago hospital. Mulago is Uganda's, largest hospital and the National Referral and Teaching Hospital, with 2000 beds.

These figures show a 57% rise in workload for Mulago Hospital when compared with the workload of 116 150 examinations 1999 for the period January 1997 to December.

Statistics for the same period for Mengo Hospital, a 400-bed missionary private and not-for-profit hospital, also located in Kampala city, showed a total of 17 288 imaging examinations for the first period (2 January 2003 to 28 December 2004) and 18 259 for the second period (2 January 2005 to 28 December 2006).

The figures show a 59% rise in workload for Mengo Hospital when compared with the workload of 7500 examinations for the period 1997 January to 2000 December.

Ultrasound accounted for 23% of the imaging examinations for Mulago Hospital for the first period and 30% for the second period. For Mengo Hospital, ultrasound accounted for 51% of all the imaging studies for the first period and 58% for the second period. Both hospitals therefore registered an increasing reliance on ultrasound compared to other imaging examinations in this 4-year study period.

Ultrasound guided interventional studies rose from 200 examinations for the first period to 230 for the second period for Mulago hospital. For Mengo, they rose from 55 to 80 examinations for the same study period.

Fluoroscopy studies showed no change in the two hospitals and intravenous urography continues to decline to 1–2 per week.

CT, which is available in Mulago but not in Mengo, showed a climb from 1907 examinations in the first period to 10 962 in the second period. The frequent breakdown of CT machines may influence this trend.

Box 26.7 Mulago University Teaching Hospital, Kampala, Uganda: a model for delivery of imaging services in the tropics

- Commitment to continuing professional development
- Modernization of imaging equipment
- Quality control policy
- Increased reliance on ultrasound
- Use of teleradiology.

It can therefore be concluded that there is an increasing reliance on ultrasound examinations in the tropics, especially in hospitals where there are no CT services.

The ultrasound usage in Mengo hospital may be higher than Mulago because Mengo is a centre for ultrasound training. The ultrasound-training centre in Mengo Hospital (ECUREI) is affiliated to Thomas Jefferson University (JUREI) and Fontys University of Applied Science in the Netherlands. It attracts students from Uganda and several other African countries.

In the same time period, and in comparison to the findings in the UTH Department of Radiology, the frequency of imaging examinations performed at a local major private hospital with similar imaging facilities remained almost static, probably due to both small workload and prohibitive costs of radiology services in a two-tier system.

While conceding that there is always a need for improvement, the Mulago Hospital Department of Radiology is a model for delivery of imaging services in the tropics (Box 26.7). The department succeeds because:

- It is committed to continuing professional development. This encompasses visiting professor exchanges, conferences, journals, libraries, a well thought out radiology residency programme, and innovative curricula for the school of medicine and medical radiation sciences programme.
- Imaging equipment at the old Mulago Hospital has been modernized through a grant from the African Development Bank. Further resources underwritten by the Uganda Ministry of Health have helped procure equipment for basic and high-tech radiological services (even though no MRI units are available). A radiologist, however skilled and versatile, can function only within the limits of the available equipment.
- There is a quality control policy for radiological equipment and images.
- The increasing reliance on ultrasound imaging and ultrasound-guided interventions has been anticipated and hence accommodated.
- Resourcefulness has overcome the constraints imposed by scarcity of equipment and personnel. In particular, there is a widespread use of teleradiology for the delivery of training and diagnostic ultrasound services. A teleradiology link to district hospitals facilitates radiodiagnosis within the primary care level. After all, it deals with the same problems of abdominal/ chest infections, trauma and obstetrics as those encountered at Mulago Hospital.

Mengo hospital is also a model for maximizing benefits of ultrasound and interventional radiology for smaller hospitals which are equipped with X-ray, fluoroscopy and ultrasound.

The imaging needs of the communities in Kampala city are identical to those elsewhere in Africa or the tropics. Therefore, the principles underpinning the performance of radiology services at this Ugandan hospital should be extrapolated to and adopted by other tertiary hospitals in the tropics. The paradigm of delivering a modern and dependable imaging service, at the centre of tropical healthcare, may then be realized in many regions of the world. How the restrictions imposed by the World Bank and International Monetary Fund on the fragile economies of the developing countries – the majority of them being located in the tropics – will impede the development of a robust modern service in diagnostic and interventional radiology remains to be seen.

CONCLUSION

We must aim for a first-class imaging service which is global, not least because modern radiology is increasingly central to the diagnosis and treatment of numerous conditions. The many obstacles to establishing this service in the tropics can be overcome with clear thinking, resourcefulness, determination and sage investment: the university teaching hospital in Kampala sets an example. As a first step, all tropical imaging services should concentrate on infectious diseases, trauma and obstetric care. To this end, plain radiography and ultrasound must be developed: this demands investment in suitable equipment and investment in training and supporting personnel, wherever they are based.

REFERENCES

1. Tshibwabwa ET, Somers S, Jan E, et al. Tropical pulmonary radiology. In: Sharma O, ed. *Tropical Lung Diseases*. Series: Lung Biology in Health and Disease. New York: Taylor & Francis; 2006:37–62.
2. Dunser MW, Baelani I, Ganbold L. A review and analysis of intensive care medicine in the least developed countries. *Crit Care Med* 2006; 34: 1234–1242.
3. Rabinowitz DA, Pretorius E. Postgraduate radiology training in Sub-Saharan Africa: a review of current educational resources. *Acad Radiol* 2005; 12:224–231.
4. United Nations, Sources and Effects of Ionizing Radiation. 2000 Report to the General Assembly, Scientific Committee on the Effects of Atomic Radiation. New York: UN, Annex D (Medical radiation exposures); 2006:14 July.
5. Tshibwabwa ET, Mwaba P, Bogle-Taylor J, et al. Four year study of abdominal ultrasound in 900 Central African adults with AIDS referred for diagnostic imaging. *Abdom Imaging* 2000; 25:290–296.
6. Shaw JM, Bornman PC, Krige JEJ. Hydatid disease of the liver. *South African J Surg* 2006; 44:70–72.
7. Page D. *Teleradiology: Spreading the Health Demand for Medical Services in Remote Areas and Staffing Shortages Push Radiology to The Ends of the Earth*. 2003. Online. Available: http://home.earthlink.net/~douglaspage/id47.html 29 Jan 2007.

Chapter 27

Raman Bedi and Crispian Scully

Tropical Oral Health

INTRODUCTION

The importance of oral health as part of general health is now well established and this is true not only in industrialized countries but also tropical and subtropical climates. Oral health was notable by its absence in previous editions of *Manson's Tropical Diseases*, with the twentieth edition limiting the section on the mouth per se to little more than half a page.[1] Therefore, the decision to develop a whole chapter to the subject testifies to the growing importance and awareness of the impact oral health and the delivery of dental services can have on those who live in tropical and subtropical areas. The impact of the chapter in the twenty-first edition cannot be underestimated and international oral health as a specific discipline is beginning to take shape. In September 2005, during the UK's presidency of the European Union, Chief Dental Officers from around the world met in London to agree that child oral health should be given a priority. They, along with the WHO and World Dental Federation called for a global child dental health taskforce. This taskforce took shape in 2006 with a major donation from the UK government. Therefore, the focus for the early part of the twenty-first century for international oral health will be child oral health, and the commitment to eradicate (or at least confine to less than 10%) dental decay from the child cohort born in 2026.[2]

The term to be used in this chapter in this new edition to cover such geographical areas will be 'developing countries', and, as is custom, to have this description also cover transition countries. It is also recognized that tropical dentistry is not just dentistry (oral health) in the tropics, but that with migration and global travel, oral diseases traditionally restricted in some developing countries have manifested themselves within all areas of the global community.

DENTAL CARIES

Together with the common cold, dental caries is perhaps the most prevalent disease of modern man, but unlike the cold, its effects, invariably, leave behind defects that are permanent.[2] The general consensus of international epidemiological studies is that non-milk extrinsic sugars are the most important dietary factor in the aetiology of dental caries. The role of nutrition during tooth development is considered to be minimal in industrialized countries.[3,4] However, in tropical and subtropical areas where malnutrition is evident, delayed tooth eruption is observed, especially in the primary dentition,[5] but there is inconclusive evidence that malnutrition during tooth development can influence subsequent levels of dental caries.[6]

In the last few decades, there has been enormous progress in development. Since the 1960s, life expectancy in developing countries has risen from 46 to 64 years; infant mortality rates have halved; there has been an increase of more than 80% in the proportion of children enrolled in primary school; and there has been a doubling of access to safe drinking water and basic sanitation.[7] Such development is all too often coupled with increasing access to sugars, commonly in the form of confectionery or carbonated drinks. The World Health Organization's global data bank on oral health, established in 1969 and continuing to monitor dental caries levels across different countries, demonstrates two clear trends: first the ongoing decline in dental caries for the industrialized world and, second, the increasing prevalence of caries in the developing world.[6]

The treatment of dental caries has not essentially changed over the past few decades, although tooth cavity design and filling materials have changed the practical approach to dental restorative treatment. The Atraumatic Restorative Technique (ART) has produced promising results in developing countries, especially those with a shortage of suitably qualified manpower.[8,9]

There has been a number of studies that have demonstrated significant caries reductions as a result of fluoride toothpaste.[10] The major barrier to the provision of fluoride toothpaste to the developing world has been cost; however, the new WHO programmes to introduce locally produced affordable fluoridated toothpaste to many developing countries are producing encouraging results.[11]

The evidence base for addressing dental caries in children has been documented and the predictive models and policy options for managing this clarified.[2] It is clear that each health economy needs to document its fluoride policy and preferably adopt either water fluoridation or improving the child oral health.[2]

499

PERIODONTAL DISEASE

There is no evidence that periodontal disease in developed and developing countries is in principle different.[12] There are indeed more similarities in periodontal conditions globally, than differences.[12] Evidence shows that periodontal diseases are only more prevalent in developing countries in terms of poorer oral hygiene and greater calculus retention but not for periodontal destruction in adults.[12–14]

The WHO has recently published guidelines on prevention.[15] In addition, limited resources in many developing countries often inhibit the purchase of toothbrushes, and traditional cleaning materials such as the miswak chewing stick are still widely used.[16] The miswak are prepared from local tree roots or twigs, are commonly used in several African and Asian countries and have been shown to be effective tooth-cleaning agents.[16]

ORAL CANCER

Most oral cancer is squamous cell carcinoma (SCC), and it is customary to include cancers of the lip (ICD 140), tongue (ICD 141), gum (ICD 143), floor of the mouth (ICD 144) and unspecified parts of the mouth (ICD 145).[17] There is clear inter-country variation in both the incidence and mortality from oral cancer and also ethnic differences. These are attributed mainly to specific risk factors such as alcohol and tobacco (smoking and smokeless) and sunlight exposure, in the case of lip cancer, but dietary factors as well as the existence of genetic predisposition may play a part.[18] Variations in accessing care services are also evident.[18]

The incidence of oral cancer varies widely between countries and geographical areas of the world and is generally most common in developing countries. These variations have traditionally been explained by the exposure of these groups to specific risk factors, e.g. tobacco and alcohol use. Mouth cancer worldwide is the twelfth most common cancer but it is the eighth most common in males.[19] The gender ratio is 2:0 (M:F). Mouth cancer in men is most common in Western and Southern Europe, South Asia, Melanesia, southern Africa and Australia/NZ.[19] In females, it is most common in South-Central Asia, Melanesia and Australia/NZ. Lip cancer is particularly common in white Caucasians in the tropics and subtropics.[19]

The aetiology of oral cancer has been attributed to specific risk factors: tobacco[20] and/or alcohol in southern Africa, and 'betel quid' in South-Central Asia and Melanesia.[21] Annually there are 197 000 deaths worldwide from cancer of the mouth and pharynx, with the highest mortality from mouth cancer in Melanesia and South-Central Asia.[19,22]

Oral cancer appears most prevalent in areas with a high Asian population. Chinese have a lower risk of oral cancer than Indians do in Malaysia and a later age of onset.

There is a plethora of studies linking specific behaviours, such as tobacco and alcohol use, to oral cancer.[21] Smokeless (chewing) tobacco use is an important factor for South Asian populations. The areca (betel) nut habit is important in the development of oral submucous fibrosis and of mouth cancer.[23] Some chew the nut only and others prefer 'paan', which includes tobacco, and sometimes lime and catechu. Studies from India have confirmed the association between 'paan' tobacco chewing and oral cancer, particularly cancer of the buccal and labial mucosa.

There is growing evidence associating increased alcohol consumption with risk of oral cancer. The role of alcohol drinking is observed in a negative social class gradient and for many countries follows a similar pattern to tobacco use.

There is a considerable body of evidence indicating a protective effect on oral cancer and pre-cancer of diets rich in fresh fruits and vegetables and of vitamin A in particular.

The molecular changes found in oral carcinomas from Western countries (UK, USA, Australia), particularly p53 mutations, are infrequent in the East (India, South-East Asia), where the involvement of ras oncogenes, including mutation, loss of heterozygosity (H-ras) and amplification (K- and N-ras) is common, suggesting genetic differences. It is also evident that there can be genetic differences in the metabolism of pro-carcinogens and carcinogens by xenometabolizing enzymes or ability to repair the DNA damage in different ethnic groups.

Carcinomas present anywhere in the oral cavity, commonly on the posterolateral margin of the tongue and floor of mouth – the 'coffin' or 'graveyard' area – and in the buccal mucosa in betel users. It is crucial, therefore, not only to examine visually and manually the whole oral cavity, but also to take particular care to inspect and palpate the posterolateral margins of the tongue and the floor of mouth (Figure 27.1). There is usually solitary chronic:

- ulceration
- red lesion
- white lesion
- indurated lump
- fissure
- cervical lymph node enlargement.

Anterior cervical lymph node enlargement may be detectable by palpation. Some 30% of patients present with palpably enlarged nodes containing metastases and, of those who do not, a further 25% will go on to develop nodal metastases within 2 years.

Lip carcinoma presents with thickening, crusting or ulceration, usually of the lower lip. Potentially malignant lesions or conditions may include some:

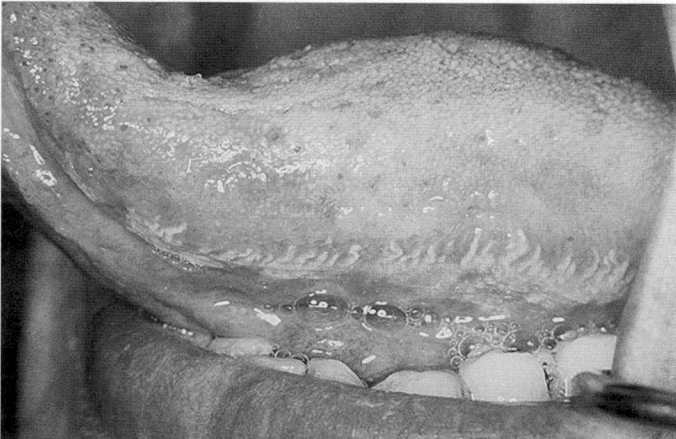

Figure 27.1 Hairy leukoplakia associated with HIV.

- erythroplasias
- dysplastic leukoplakias (about 50% of oral carcinomas have associated leukoplakia)
- lichen planus
- oral submucous fibrosis
- chronic immunosuppression.

Diagnosis

Too many patients with oral SCC present or are detected late, with advanced disease and lymph node metastases. The earlier the tumour is detected and treated:

- the less complicated is treatment
- the better are the cosmetic and functional results
- the greater is the improvement in survival.

There should be a high index of suspicion, especially of a solitary lesion present for over 3 weeks, particularly if it is indurated, there is cervical lymphadenopathy and the patient is in a high-risk group.

It is essential to confirm the diagnosis, and determine whether cervical lymph nodes are involved or there are other primary tumours, or metastases (Figure 27.2). Therefore almost invariably indicated are:

- lesional biopsy; an incisional biopsy is usually indicated but an oral brush biopsy is now available mainly for cases where there are widespread potentially malignant lesions, and for revealing malignancy in lesions of more benign appearance
- jaw and chest radiography
- endoscopy
- full blood count and liver function tests.

Management

Oral cancer is now treated largely by surgery and/or irradiation, though there have been few unequivocal controlled trials of treatment modalities. Combined clinics, with surgeons, oncologists and support staff, usually have an agreed treatment policy and offer the best outcomes. However, mortality rates for oral cancer have substantially increased in many countries. Although the effi-cacy of screening for oral cancer to increase survival and reduce mortality remains unproven,[24] it is believed that Cuba's ongoing oral cancer screening programme has resulted in a higher proportion of cancers being localized at diagnosis and a comparatively high survival rate.[25] A reduced incidence of oral pre-cancerous lesions has been reported in a primary prevention trial.[26] In addition, the abstinence of tobacco for a 6-week period resulted in the reversal of potentially pre-cancerous oral lesions.[27] The WHO has recently published guidelines on prevention.[28]

The prognosis is very site-dependent for:

- intra-oral carcinoma: 5-year survival may be as low as 30% for posterior lesions presenting late, as they often do
- lip carcinoma: there is often more than a 70% 5-year survival.

ERYTHROPLASIA (ERYTHROPLAKIA)

Erythroplasia is a rare, isolated, red, velvety lesion which affects patients mainly in the sixth and seventh decades. Erythroplasia usually involves the floor of the mouth, the ventrum of the tongue or the soft palate. This is one of the most important oral lesions because 75–90% of lesions prove to be carcinoma or carcinoma in situ, or are severely dysplastic. The incidence of malignant change is 17 times higher in erythroplasia than in leukoplakia. Erythroplasia should be excised and sent for histological examination.

Prevention is by avoidance of lifestyle habits of tobacco and alcohol use.[29]

LEUKOPLAKIA

All oral white lesions were formerly called leukoplakia and believed often to be potentially malignant. The term leukoplakia is now restricted to white lesions of unknown cause.

Most white lesions are innocuous keratoses caused by cheek biting, friction or tobacco, but also:

- infections (e.g. candidosis, syphilis, and hairy leukoplakia)
- dermatoses (usually lichen planus)
- neoplastic disorders (e.g. leukoplakias and carcinomas)
- other conditions, which must be excluded, usually by biopsy.

Keratoses are most commonly uniformly white plaques (homogeneous leukoplakia), prevalent in the buccal (cheek) mucosae, and are usually of low malignant potential. More serious are nodular and, especially, speckled leukoplakias, which consist of white patches or nodules in a red, often eroded, area of mucosa. The presence of severe epithelial dysplasia indicates a considerable risk of malignant development.

The overall prevalence of malignant change is 3–33% over 10 years, but a percentage (about 15%) regress clinically.

Diagnosis

It can be difficult to be certain of the precise diagnosis of a white patch, as even carcinoma can present as a white lesion. Incisional biopsy is indicated, sampling indurated, red, erosive or ulcerated areas rather than the more obvious whiter hyperkeratinized areas;

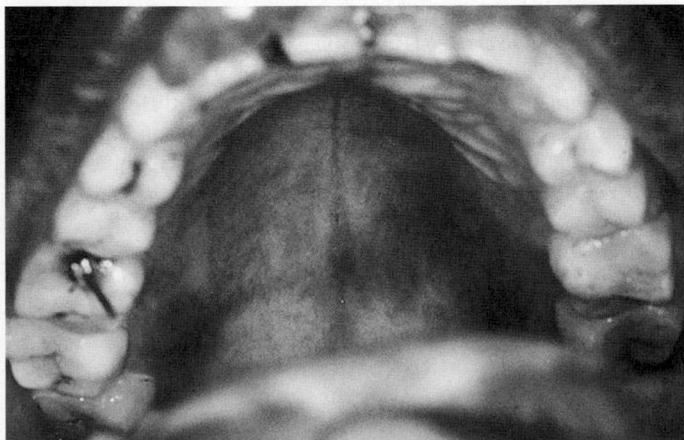

Figure 27.2 Kaposi's sarcoma associated with HIV.

staining with toluidine blue may help highlight the most appropriate area.

Management can be difficult, especially in extensive lesions of leukoplakia, and those with areas of erythroplasia. Obvious predisposing factors need to be reduced or eliminated. Prevention is by avoidance of lifestyle habits of tobacco and alcohol use.[29]

Some studies have shown regression of leukoplakia in over 50% of patients who stopped smoking for 1 year. Dysplastic lesions should certainly be excised and the patient should then be followed up regularly at intervals of 3–6 months. Unfortunately, more than one-third recur.

ORAL SUBMUCOUS FIBROSIS

Oral submucous fibrosis (OSMF), though not regarded as a connective tissue disease, has pathological changes closely similar to those of scleroderma. Unlike the latter, which has severe effects on the skin but minimal effects on the oral mucosa, OSMF causes severe and often disabling fibrosis of the oral tissues alone.

OSMF affects virtually only those from the Indian subcontinent.[30] There is some evidence it is premalignant.[31] The condition appears to be related to the chewing of areca nut and the 5A genotype of matrix metalloproteinase 3 (MMP3) promoter is associated with the risk of OSMF.[32] Iron deficiency anaemia may be present but this is not uncommon in Asians in the absence of submucous fibrosis. No consistent specific immunological abnormalities appear to be associated, although there is a greater prevalence of connective tissue diseases and serum immunoglobulin IgG, IgA and IgM levels are raised.[33]

Clinically, OSMF causes symmetrical fibrosis of such sites as the cheeks, soft palate or inner aspects of the lips. The fibrosis is often so severe that the affected area is almost white and so hard that it literally cannot be indented with the finger. Frequently, the buccal fibrosis causes such severe restriction of opening that dental treatment becomes increasingly difficult and finally impossible. Ultimately, tube-feeding may become necessary.

Management

Intralesional corticosteroids and regular stretching of the oral soft tissues with an interdental screw or Therabite may delay fixation in the closed position. Failing this, operative treatment may become necessary although some have found improvement with intralesional interferon-α.

INFECTIONS

Bacterial

Acute necrotizing ulcerative gingivitis

Acute necrotizing ulcerative gingivitis (ANUG) is characterized by painful ulceration of the gum between the teeth (interdental papillae) (Figure 27.3), a pronounced tendency to gingival bleeding and halitosis. Anaerobic fusiform bacteria and spirochaetes are implicated, predisposing factors including:

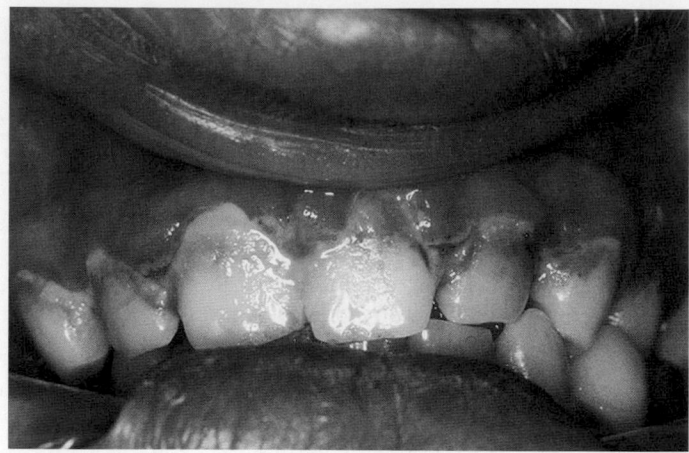

Figure 27.3 Acute necrotizing ulcerative gingivitis.

- poor oral hygiene
- smoking
- malnutrition
- immune defects including HIV and other viral infections and leukaemias.

ANUG is a problem in certain populations, particularly in those who are encountering significant poverty and malnourishment. It also impacts upon patients who are immunocompromised. ANUG not infrequently follows a respiratory tract infection, presumably being predisposed by the transient immune defect consequent upon some such infections, particularly viral. ANUG is increasingly seen in viral infections such as HIV disease; in some other persons with ANUG only more subtle immune defects, such as reduced salivary immunoglobulin A and neutrophil dysfunction, have been described. Worldwide, the major cause of immunodeficiency is still malnutrition and ANUG is indeed seen in malnutrition. However, there are patients who suffer from ANUG in the absence of any clear immune defect, malnutrition or other systemic factor and, in these, poor oral hygiene and tobacco-smoking may be factors. It is seen primarily in early childhood and young adults.[34]

ANUG is typically seen where plaque control is poor. A mixed flora dominated by fusobacteria and spirochaetes, such as *Treponema* species, *Bacteroides* (*Porphyromonas*) *melaninogenicus* species intermedius, *Fusobacterium* species, *Selenomonas* species and *Borrelia vincentii* is invariably present and the condition improves dramatically when treated with penicillin or metronidazole, suggesting a significant role for these bacteria. Viruses may play a role,[35] possibly also by inducing immune suppression.

Management includes:
- oral debridement and hygiene instruction
- peroxide or perborate mouthwashes
- metronidazole 200 mg t.d.s. for 3 days.

Gangrenous stomatitis (cancrum oris, noma)

Noma is derived from the Greek 'nomein', which means to 'devour'. Essentially it is a gangrenous stomatitis, which starts in the mouth as a benign oral lesion and rapidly destroys both the

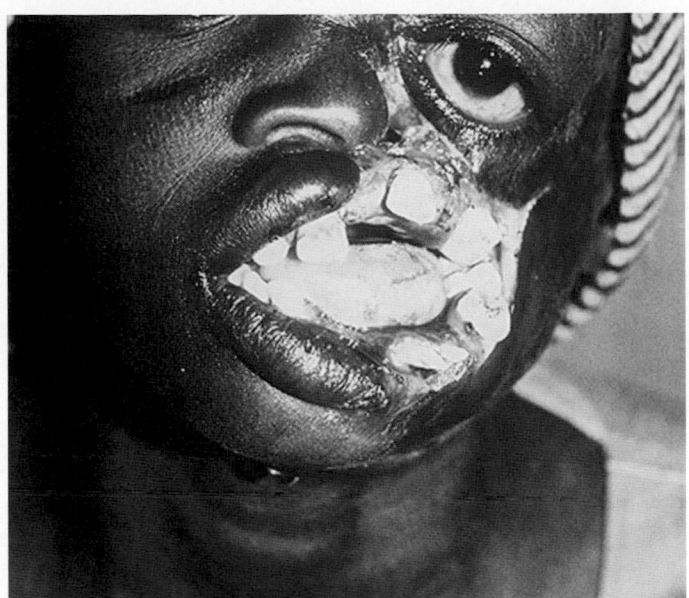

Figure 27.4 Noma.

soft and hard tissues of the mouth and face (Figure 27.4).[36] Most noma sufferers are under 6 years of age and it has been estimated that the case-fatality rate is probably between 70% and 90%. It is estimated that 100 000 African children under the age of 6 years contract noma every year.[36]

Noma is often an extension of an ANUG into the adjacent tissues, predominantly because of impaired host defences (Figure 27.5).[37] Other factors which predispose to the development of gangrenous stomatitis include protein-energy malnutrition and deficiencies of vitamins A, B, C, iron or magnesium. Therefore, poor living environment, exposure to debilitating childhood diseases, poor oral hygiene and malnutrition all appear to put children at risk for noma.[38]

The condition is seen especially in sub-Saharan Africa.[39] Nigeria probably has the highest incidence, although the Gambia, Algeria, Uganda, Senegal, Madagascar, South Africa, Sudan and Egypt are also areas of high prevalence, as are Afghanistan, India, the Philippines, China, Vietnam, Papua New Guinea and South America.[40] In the developed world, gangrenous stomatitis is rare, and typically seen in immunocompromised persons such as those with HIV infection, leukaemia and diabetes.[41-45]

Clinical features

The presenting feature may be a painful red or purplish-red spot (an indurated papule), usually on the gingiva in the premolar-molar region, which enlarges and ulcerates rapidly, spreading to the labiogingival or mucobuccal fold, and exposing the underlying bone. There is pain and often fetor. A blue–black area of discolouration appears on the skin and leads to a perforating wound. Sequestration of the exposed bone and loss of teeth are rapid and then the wound heals slowly by secondary intention, often leaving a defect. In former times, noma was often a lethal condition.

Management

Gangrenous stomatitis does not respond readily to treatment unless the underlying disease is controlled, especially nutritional rehabilitation. The wound should be cleaned regularly with chlorhexidine and/or saline and/or hydrogen peroxide. A soft cotton gauze or tulle gras dressing may be used but changed frequently. Any loose slough, loose teeth and bony fragments should be removed. Parenteral fluids should be given to correct any dehydration and electrolyte imbalance. Penicillin is the antimicrobial of choice. Folic acid, iron, ascorbic acid and vitamin B complex may be required.

Syphilis (venereal treponematosis)

In 1995, it was estimated that there were approximately 12 million new cases of syphilis among adults worldwide, with the greatest number of cases occurring in South and South-East Asia, followed by sub-Saharan Africa.[46]

Oral lesions

The lip is the most common extragenital site of primary infection with *Treponema pallidum*. It causes a chancre (primary, hard or Hunterian chancre) which begins as a small, firm, pink macule, changes to a papule and then ulcerates to form a painless round ulcer with a raised margin and indurated base. About 60% of oral cases affect the lip or may present at the angles of the mouth.[47] Other oral sites affected may include the tongue and to a lesser extent the gingivae and fauces. Lymph nodes in the submaxillary, submental and cervical regions are usually enlarged. Chancres heal spontaneously within 3–8 weeks. Secondary syphilis follows the primary stage after 6–8 weeks but a healing chancre may still be present. As in the primary stage, the mucosal lesions are highly infectious. The typical signs and symptoms are fever, headache, malaise, a rash (characteristically symmetrically distributed coppery maculopapules or lesions on the palms) and generalized painless lymph node enlargement. It is this stage that classically causes oral lesions.[48] Painless oral ulcers (mucous patches and snail-track ulcers) are the typical lesions and are slightly raised, greyish white, glistening patches seen on the fauces, soft palate, tongue, buccal mucosa and, rarely, gingivae.[49] Cervical nodes are enlarged and 'rubbery' in consistency. Latent syphilis follows secondary syphilis and persists until late syphilis (tertiary syphilis) develops. The characteristic lesion of tertiary syphilis is a localized midline granuloma ('gumma') varying in size from millimetres to several centimetres, which breaks down to form a deep punched-out painless ulcer (Figure 27.5). The most common oral site for a gumma is the hard palate[49] although the soft palate, lips or tongue are commonly involved. The gumma starts as a small, pale, raised area which ulcerates and rapidly progresses to a large zone of necrosis with denudation of bone and, in the case of a palatal gumma, may eventually perforate into the nasal cavity.[50]

Diagnosis

The presence of clinical manifestations, together with a history of contact may suggest the diagnosis but serodiagnostic

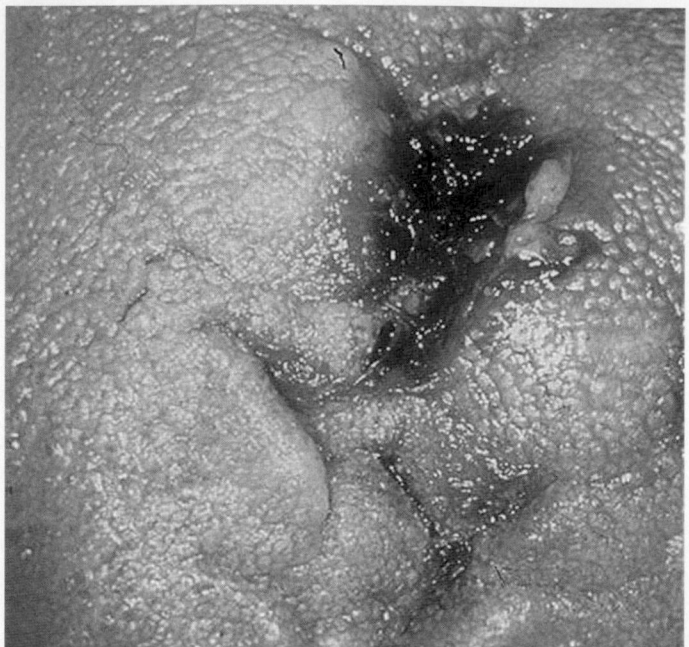

Figure 27.5 Oral lesion associated with syphilis.

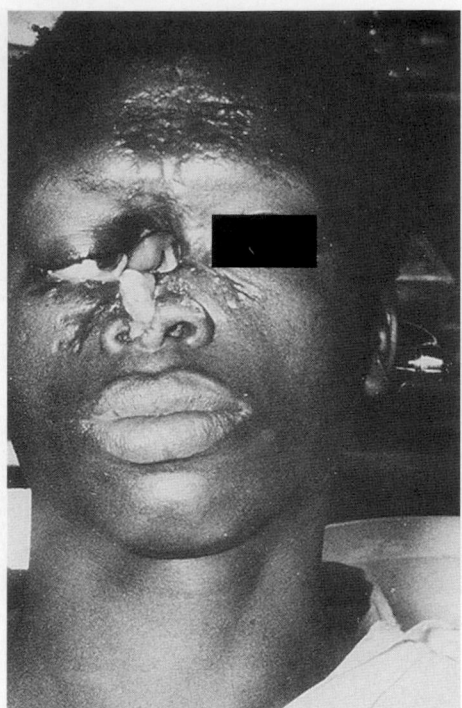

Figure 27.6 Yaws.

tests, and sometimes dark-field microscopy are required for confirmation.

Oral management

There is no specific oral management except general palliative care if there is soreness of oral soft lesions, but the general management is straightforward: procaine penicillin intramuscularly for 10 days (erythromycin for 14 days) should be given.

Non-venereal treponematoses (endemic treponematoses): endemic syphilis (bejel)

The early stage of bejel may present with mucous patches in the oronasopharyngeal region, and angular stomatitis. Late- or tertiary-stage disease is mainly gummatous and can involve the oral mucous membranes or bones and can lead to gross facial deformity (rhinopharyngitis mutilans).[51]

Diagnosis

Dark-field microscopy and serology are needed to confirm the diagnosis but differentiation from the other treponematoses is difficult.

Management

Penicillin is the drug of choice; tetracycline and erythromycin are alternatives.

Pinta

The primary slowly developing subcutaneous granulomatous lesion may involve the face. Secondary lesions (pintids) are papules, which develop into plaques with scaly and centrally pigmented areas. Facial skin is extensively affected but there are no oral lesions described.

Yaws (framboesia, pian, bouba)

The primary papule may appear around the body orifices including the mouth (Figure 27.6).[52] Gummatous nodular ulcerative lesions may develop.[52] The other type of lesion seen involving facial structures is basically a destructive lesion starting either on the soft palate, uvula or hard palate, eventually destroying parts of the nose (gangosa) and causing a 'saddle-nose' defect. Bone involvement may result in thickening of the face on either side of the bridge of the nose, giving rise to the characteristic facial appearance of 'goundou'.[53]

Diagnosis

Clinical features supported by dark-field microscopy, biopsy and serology are useful.

Management

This is using penicillin, erythromycin or tetracycline.

Gonorrhoea

Oral, pharyngeal and tonsil involvement is being reported with increasing frequency, particularly among homosexuals and heterosexuals practising oral sex. Infection of these sites is acquired primarily by fellatio and infrequently by cunnilingus. The tonsils become red and swollen with a greyish exudate and there is cervical lymphadenitis. Lesions in other parts of the mouth are described as showing fiery erythema and are sometimes oedematous, perhaps with painful superficial ulceration of the tongue, gingiva, buccal mucosa, hard or soft palate. The inflamed mucosa may also be covered with a yellowish or greyish exudate, which when detached may leave a bleeding surface.

Diagnosis

A throat swab should be taken for Gram staining to show polymorphs containing Gram-negative diplococci. Confirmation is by culture and sugar fermentation to aid differentiation of species. Rapid identification of gonococci by fluorescent antibody techniques is possible.

Management

Penicillin is the drug of choice, given as 2 g ampicillin plus 1 g probenecid as a single oral dose. Patients hypersensitive to penicillin can be treated with co-trimoxazole. Many strains are resistant to penicillin in parts of Africa and the Far East. Tetracycline, or cefazolin-probenecid and streptomycin or spectinomycin may be used.

Granuloma inguinale (Donovanosis)

A papule or nodule, usually in the inguinal or anogenital region, progresses to a destructive granulomatous ulcer. Most oral lesions are secondary to primary genital infection, can involve the periodontium, and are often misdiagnosed as actinomycosis.

Diagnosis

Direct examination of a piece of granulation tissue compressed between two slides and stained by Giemsa for the presence of Donovan bodies (clusters of bacilli lying within leucocytes) is the best method.

Management

Tetracycline, ampicillin or trimethoprim-sulfamethoxazole are first-line therapy.

Lymphogranuloma venereum

The tongue is the oral site most frequently affected in primary lymphogranuloma venereum (LGV) infections, usually with a painless vesicle. Lesions affecting the lips, cheeks, tongue, floor of mouth, uvula and pharynx but not gingivae have been described. As the disease progresses, the tongue enlarges with areas of scarring and deep grooves on the dorsum, which are intensely red with loss of superficial epithelium. Cervical lymphadenopathy is common, sometimes with no clinical oral lesions of LGV.

Diagnosis

Laboratory confirmation of the diagnosis includes isolation of *Chlamydia trachomatis* and serological tests. *C. trachomatis* is isolated on cell cultures of the yolk sac of chicken embryos. A skin test (Frei test) is available but not specific.

Management

LGV is treated by sulfonamides, tetracycline, erythromycin or rifampicin.

Actinomycosis

A breach in the continuity of mucosa caused either by trauma or surgery is the prerequisite for the majority of actinomycotic infections. Cervicofacial actinomycosis occurs predominantly in adult males following trauma either accidentally or, rarely, from dental treatment such as exodontia or endodontics.[54] Rarely, a periodontal pocket with suitable anaerobic conditions predisposes to the disease.[55] The perimandibular area appears to be the commonest site. A relatively painless reddish-purple indurated mass appears at the angle of the jaw or in the vicinity of the parotid gland. It may drain through sinuses, the material containing the so-called sulfur granules. Actinomycosis may rarely involve the oral cavity, tongue, mandible, maxilla, paranasal sinuses, eye, ear, face, neck or salivary glands.

Diagnosis

Sulfur granules may be seen by direct vision or after staining with Gram stain. Actinomycosis should be confirmed by the isolation of *A. israelii* in anaerobic culture.

Management

Penicillin is the first-choice antimicrobial. Alternatives include cephalosporin, clindamycin and lincomycin.

Nocardiosis

Nocardiosis is caused by bacteria of the family Nocardiaceae, usually *Nocardia asteroides*, *N. brasiliensis* or *N. caviae* and is seen mainly in Latin America. Dissemination may lead to oral involvement; nocardiosis of the cheek[56] and gingivae[57] has been reported.

Diagnosis

Smears should be examined for Gram-positive rods of coccal forms but culture is more useful in the diagnosis.

Management

Surgical drainage and a sulfonamide such as co-trimoxazole should be used.

Tuberculosis

It is estimated that over 1.5 million tuberculosis cases per year occur in sub-Saharan Africa.[58] HIV and tuberculosis speed each other's progress, with the latter contributing about 15% of AIDS deaths worldwide.[58]

Oral lesions are seen mainly in pulmonary tuberculosis although systemic symptoms suggestive of lung disease are by no means always present.[59] Apart from pain, typically the main symptom of tuberculosis is chronic ulcers or granular masses. These are usually on the dorsum/base of the tongue,[50-62] gingivae (Figure 27.7)[59] or occasionally in the buccal mucosa, floor of the mouth, lips and the hard and soft palates.[63-65]

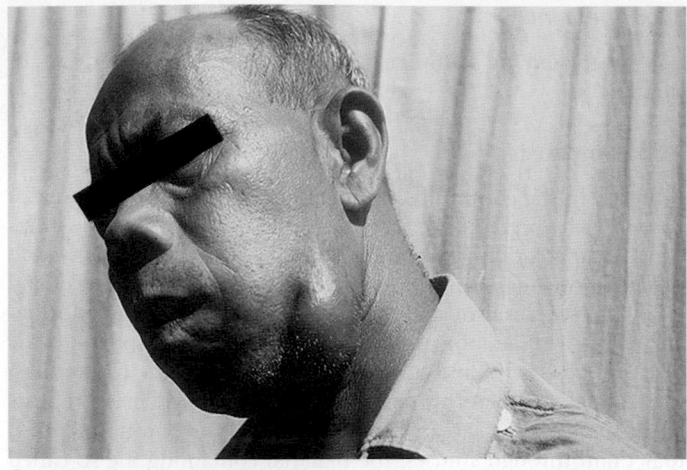

A

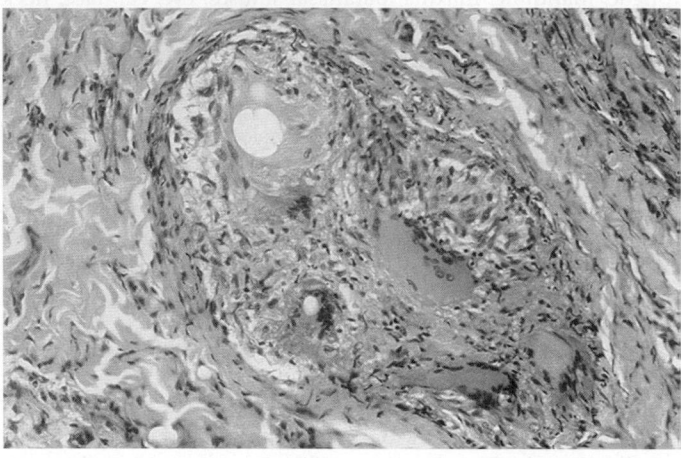

B

Figure 27.7 (A,B) Head and neck swelling associated with tuberculosis.

Primary oral lesions develop when bacilli are directly inoculated into the oral tissues of a person who has not acquired immunity. Primary tuberculosis of the mouth is more common in children and adolescents than adults. It usually presents as a single painless indolent ulcer, commonly on the gingiva with enlarged cervical lymph nodes,[66] or the gingivae, tooth extraction sockets and the buccal folds.[67]

Occasional cases of primary jaw tuberculosis have been reported,[68] usually resulting from extension of a gingival lesion, from an infected post-extraction socket, from an extension from a tuberculous granuloma at the apex of the tooth or haematogenous spread. Tuberculous osteomyelitis may involve the maxilla particularly, or the mandible. The same general pattern as seen in other affected bones is common, with a slow rarefying osteitis resulting in sequestration of bone.[69] Pain is not a prominent early feature but is seen later. Secondary infection may lead to difficulty in making a diagnosis. Tuberculous involvement of the mandible causes symptoms of pain, swelling, difficulty in eating, trismus, paraesthesia of the lower lip and enlargement of the regional lymph nodes.[68–74] The infection may spread throughout the jaw,

producing multiple sinuses, which drain intra- or extra-orally.[75–76] The posterior mandible and ascending ramus are typically affected, and radiographical appearances include irregular linear calcifications along the lower border and irregular radiolucencies within the jawbone.[68] In the maxilla the infra-orbital region, particularly in the young, is the usual site affected. Typically, a cold abscess develops and may eventually drain through fistulae[77] but occasionally a firm intra-bony lesion may be present.[78]

TB in AIDS may affect the salivary glands

Diagnosis

The diagnosis of pulmonary tuberculosis, suggested by a chronic cough, haemoptysis, loss of weight, night sweats and fever, is confirmed by physical examination, chest radiography, sputum smears and culture, and tuberculin testing (Mantoux or Heaf test).[79] A lesional biopsy should be examined histologically, and acid-fast stains and culture of the organism give the absolute proof of the disease.

Management

Conventional chemotherapy of tuberculosis consists of administering two or more active drugs for 18 months to 2 years. Isoniazid in combination with ethambutol, thiacetazone or para-aminosalicylic acid and, depending on the severity of the disease, streptomycin intramuscularly for a period of the first 2–3 months, may be necessary. Other available drugs include rifampin, pyrazinamide and ethionamide.

Non-tuberculous mycobacterial infections

Non-tuberculous (atypical) mycobacteria (NTM) include *Mycobacterium avium* and *M. intracellulare* (*M. avium-intracellulare* complex: MAC), *M. scrofulaceum* and *M. haemophilum*. Infections with NTM are being increasingly reported, especially in immunocompromised individuals.[80] Cervical lymphadenopathy is occasionally caused by NTM but oral lesions are rare.

Management

Atypical mycobacteria may be resistant to conventional antituberculous chemotherapy, although in children with cervical lymphadenitis caused by NTM conventional drug therapy alone[81] or cycloserine for very resistant cases may be effective, and only occasionally is surgical excision necessary.[82]

Leprosy

Accurate estimates of the number of cases of leprosy are difficult to obtain, but approximately 2.2 billion people live in areas where leprosy is an important problem, i.e. where the prevalence is such that the risk of contracting the disease is considered significant.[83]

Oral lesions are most commonly seen in lepromatous leprosy,[84–90] as nodules (lepromas) in the palate, tongue or elsewhere. These may eventually ulcerate and scar.[88,91–93] Lepromatous leprosy also affects nerves (eventually with hypoaesthesia), skin, lymph nodes and other tissues including bones, eyes, testes, kidneys and bone marrow. Tuberculoid leprosy causes thickening of cutaneous nerves, flat and hypopigmented or raised and erythematous skin lesions and enlarged lymph nodes.[50]

Diagnosis

The diagnosis is usually based on the presence of anaesthetic skin lesions and thickened peripheral nerves, confirmed by smears from an open lesion or biopsy. The lepromin test, a non-specific delayed type hypersensitivity skin test, is positive in many persons from endemic areas, whether leprotic or not.

Management

Dapsone is the standard treatment but clofazimine, rifampicin and prothionamide may be required if *M. leprae* is resistant.[94]

Fungal

Superficial mycoses

Candidosis

Candidosis (candidiasis) is the most common oral superficial mycosis. Caused mainly by *Candida albicans*, the condition typically reflects an underlying change in oral flora, depressed salivation, or immune defect. Increasingly, infections with variants of *C. albicans*, with other and sometimes new *Candida* species and of organisms resistant to antifungal agents, are now especially seen in immunocompromised persons.[95]

Pseudomembranous candidosis or thrush may be seen in neonates and among terminally ill patients, particularly in association with immunocompromising conditions (Figure 27.8).[96] Thrush is characterized by white patches on the surface of the oral mucosa, tongue, gingivae and elsewhere. The lesions form confluent plaques that resemble milk curds and can be wiped off the mucosa with a gauze. Oral candidosis in the form of thrush is classically an acute infection, but it may recur for many months or even years in patients using corticosteroids topically or by aerosol, in HIV-infected individuals and in other immunocompromised patients. The term chronic pseudomembranous candidosis has been used for chronic recurrence. Erythematous or atrophic candidosis is an uncommon and poorly understood condition. It may arise as a consequence of persistent acute pseudomembranous candidosis, when the pseudomembranes are shed, or in HIV infection may precede pseudomembranous candidosis. Erythematous areas are seen mainly on the dorsum of the tongue, palate, gingivae or buccal mucosa. Lesions on the dorsum of the tongue present as depapillated areas. Midline or median rhomboid glossitis, or glossal central papillary atrophy, is characterized by an area of papillary atrophy that is rhomboid in shape, symmetrically placed centrally at the midline of the tongue, anterior to the circumvallate papillae. Red areas are often seen in the palate in HIV disease. Hyperplastic candidosis (*Candida leukoplakia*) is typified by chronic, discrete raised lesions that are typically found at the commissures, rarely on the gingivae. Angular stomatitis (perlèche, angular cheilitis) is a clinical diagnosis of lesions that affect, and are restricted to, the angles of the mouth, characterized by soreness, erythema and fissuring, and is commonly associated with denture-induced stomatitis. Both yeasts and bacteria are involved, as interacting, predisposing factors. It is occasionally an isolated

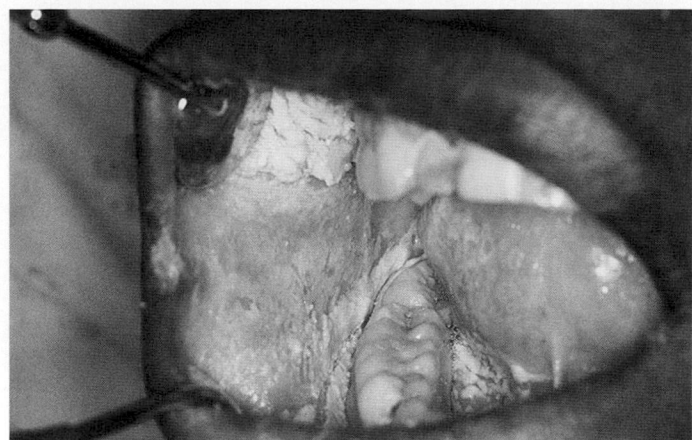

Figure 27.8 Thrush associated with HIV.

initial sign of anaemia or vitamin deficiency, and resolves when the underlying disease has been treated.[97] Angular stomatitis may also be seen in HIV disease and Crohn's disease.

Chronic multifocal oral candidosis is a term given when there are several lesions in the absence of predisposing drugs (except tobacco smoking) or medical conditions, typically angular stomatitis that is unilateral or bilateral, retrocommissural leukoplakia, which is the most constant component of the tetrad, median rhomboid glossitis, and palatal lesions where the lesions are of more than 1 month's duration.

Diagnosis

Clinical diagnosis can be supported by culture from saliva or an oral rinse.

Oral management

Antifungal therapy is initially with topical agents, especially the polyenes (nystatin, amphotericin), except in immunocompromised persons in whom the azoles, especially fluconazole, may be required systemically.

Systemic (deep) mycoses

The systemic mycoses are potentially serious, sometimes lethal fungal infections seen mainly in the developing world, or in those who have visited endemic areas. Cases have been recorded as long as 34 years after visits to endemic areas.[98] Infections are increasingly seen in immunocompromised persons,[99,100] especially in HIV infection.[101]

In otherwise healthy persons, infection with these fungi is typically subclinical although some have pulmonary infection. The increase in mycoses in immunocompromised persons is accompanied by significant morbidity and mortality and 'new' opportunists are appearing.[102]

Orofacial lesions are mainly chronic ulcers or maxillary sinus infection, which are typically associated with respiratory lesions. Most of the mycoses may mimic carcinoma or tuberculosis, and are diagnosed on the basis of a history of travel to endemic areas, or an immunocompromising state, confirmed by taking a smear, biopsy or culture of the affected tissues. Serodiagnosis, physical examination and chest radiograph may be indicated. Most systemic mycoses can be treated with systemic amphotericin or azoles.

Aspergillosis

Oral lesions are seen mainly in immunocompromised patients as invasive aspergillosis.[101] Yellow or black necrotic ulcers appear typically from antral invasion in the palate or occasionally are seen in the posterior tongue.[103–105]

Diagnosis

Diagnosis is confirmed by smear and lesional microscopy, staining with periodic acid-Schiff (PAS) or Gomori methenamine silver. Immunostains may help. Culture of tissue or fluids on Sabouraud's or Mycosel agar may be positive but this is not invariable as the organisms are ubiquitous, so that isolation of *Aspergillus* is not proof of disease.

Oral management

Invasive aspergillosis should be treated with surgery and systemic antifungals.[106] Topical ketoconazole or clotrimazole may clear superficial infections, but if there is no resolution in 72 h systemic amphotericin is needed.

Blastomycosis

Blastomycosis may disseminate to produce chronic proliferative mulberry-like ulcerated oral lesions,[107,108] and may mimic carcinoma or tuberculosis. The gingival or alveolar process are typical sites, but lesions are also seen particularly on the palate and lip.[107]

Diagnosis

Definitive diagnosis is based on smear or culture. Direct immunostaining is the most useful confirmation. DNA probes can give an answer in 2 h.

Oral management

Itraconazole is highly effective treatment, as is amphotericin.

Coccidioidomycosis

Oral lesions are rare verrucous lesions sometimes with infection of the jaw, typically secondary to lung involvement.[99,100]

Diagnosis is supported by histology (DNA probes are now available), serology, and the Spherulin or coccidioidin skin tests.

Oral management

Systemic amphotericin, sometimes supplemented with ketoconazole, itraconazole or fluconazole, is used.

Cryptococcosis

Oral *Cryptococcus* infection has presented mainly with non-healing extraction wounds, or chronic ulceration on the palate, gingivae or tongue[101] in disseminated disease. Wide dissemination is especially liable to occur in immunocompromised persons.[109] Most patients with disseminated cryptococcosis have cryptococcal meningoencephalitis at the time of diagnosis and, untreated, this is fatal in over 70% of cases.

Diagnosis

Diagnosis is confirmed by microscopy, staining with periodic acid-Schiff, mucicarmine or methenamine silver. Culture may help the diagnosis.

Oral management

Systemic amphotericin is effective therapy. Ketoconazole or itraconazole may also be used.

Histoplasmosis

Oral lesions are usually ulcerative or nodular, on the tongue, palate, buccal mucosa or gingiva, and occasionally the mandible or the maxilla,[101] may mimic carcinoma or tuberculosis, and are seen mainly in disseminated and potentially lethal histoplasmosis in immunocompromised persons (Figure 27.9).[110–112]

Diagnosis

Diagnosis of histoplasmosis is confirmed by microscopy. DNA probes are now available. Culture on Sabouraud's agar is also confirmatory. Complement fixation tests may be of value and several other serotests are available. The histoplasmin skin test is of little importance diagnostically.

Oral management

Amphotericin is given first for treatment, followed by ketoconazole.

Mucormycosis (zygomycosis: phycomycosis)

Mucoraceae can commonly be cultured from the throat and mouth of many healthy individuals but infection is virtually unheard of in otherwise healthy individuals. Immunocompromising conditions typically underlie zygomycosis.[101,113] It usually commences in the nasal cavity or paranasal sinuses with pain and nasal discharge, and fever, and may then invade the lip or palate to produce black necrotic oral ulcers.[114]

Diagnosis

Diagnosis is confirmed by smear or histology.

Oral management

Zygomycosis used to be almost uniformly fatal and still has a mortality approaching 20%. Control of underlying disease is essential if possible, together with systemic amphotericin and surgical debridement.

Paracoccidioidomycosis

Paracoccidioidomycosis caused by the dimorphic fungus *Paracoccidioides brasiliensis* is one of the most important systemic mycoses in Latin America (Figure 27.10).[115]

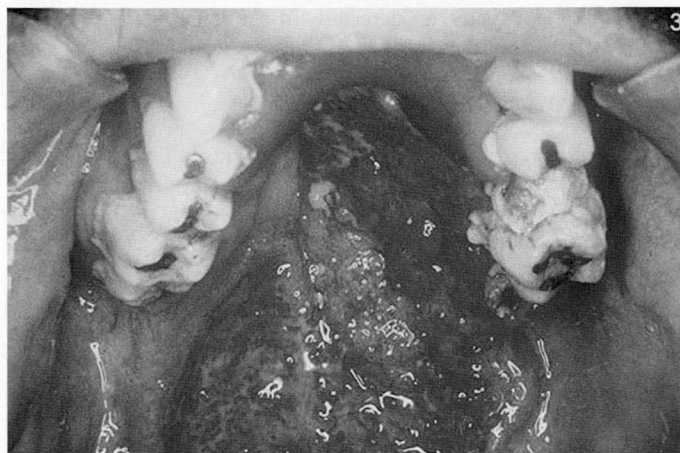

Figure 27.9 Histoplasmosis associated with HIV.

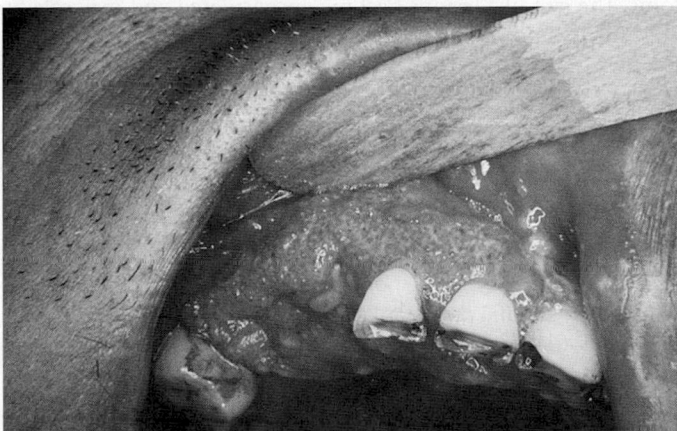

Figure 27.10 Paracoccidioidomycosis affecting the maxilla.

The disease causes cutaneous and/or respiratory tract mucosal lesions as well as lymph node enlargement. Involvement of the oral cavity and/or the nasopharynx/ larynx, either alone or in association with the lungs, is one of the commonest clinical presentations.[115] Oral lesions are often granular, exophytic and ulcerated and often affect the gingivae,[107,108,116] and may mimic carcinoma or tuberculosis.

Diagnosis

Pus or scrapings from the lesion, examined in potassium hydroxide, may show the rounded refractile cells of *P. brasiliensis* which may show characteristic multiple budding. Biopsy may be required for definitive diagnosis. Smear or culture can also be diagnostically useful but *P. brasiliensis* grows only extremely slowly. Serology may be helpful.[117]

Oral management

Systemic amphotericin alone can be curative but with sulfamethoxypyridazine is more effective. Sulfadiazine plus trimethoprim may be useful. Ketoconazole and itraconazole are superior since they can be given orally, but are expensive.

Rhinosporidiosis

Rhinosporidiosis, caused by *Rhinosporidium seeberi*, affects the nasal and other mucosae. Oral lesions are usually proliferative lumps on the palate.

Diagnosis

Diagnosis is by biopsy.

Management

Management is surgery.

Sporotrichosis

The primary lesion is a sporotrichotic chancre, which may ulcerate if in the mouth. Lesions may also then arise in lymphatics. Pulmonary and disseminated sporotrichosis is rare and of uncertain origin: antral and oral involvement has been described.

Diagnosis

Diagnosis is confirmed by histology and culture.

Oral management

Potassium iodide is effective treatment for superficial sporotrichosis, itraconazole or amphotericin for other forms.

Parasitic infections

Malaria is the most important parasitic disease of man, and like many parasitic infestations has few oral complications. However, the lack of reporting of oral lesions in parasitic infestations may simply be a reflection of their under-diagnosis.

Toxoplasmosis

Toxoplasma gondii is an intracellular parasite that may cause a glandular fever type of illness with fever and lymphadenopathy, which often causes cervical lymphadenopathy, sometimes with fever, rash, hepatosplenomegaly, myalgia and other minor features. These general non-specific signs and symptoms and the fact that commonly there is submandibular lymphadenopathy make the differential diagnosis of dental infections and toxoplasmosis a challenge. A number of cases have been reported in which children present to the dentist with apparent dental infection when the true problem is related to a parasitic infection.[118,119]

Diagnosis

The diagnosis of toxoplasmosis requires confirmation serologically by the Sabin-Feldman dye test, indirect fluorescent antibody test or indirect haemagglutination test. The organism may be demonstrable in tissue sections or smears.

Oral management

Treatment is not required for asymptomatic healthy persons who are not pregnant. For immunocompromised patients, treatment is a combination of pyrimethamine and sulfadiazine, together with folic acid, since pyrimethamine is a folate antagonist. Treatment may need to be carried on for at least 1 month after clinical resolution. Weekly full blood counts are essential.

Leishmaniasis (Donovanosis)

Transmitted by the bite of the infected female *phlebotomine* sandfly, the leishmaniases are a globally widespread group of parasitic diseases. Leishmaniasis is increasingly common in HIV disease. Leishmaniasis presents itself in humans in four different forms; visceral, mucocutaneous, cutaneous and diffuse cutaneous.

Oral lesions can be misdiagnosed as carcinoma or other malignant lesions, tuberculosis, or other chronic infections such as cellulitis, candidiasis or actinomycosis.[120–122]

Oral lesions are most frequent in mucocutaneous leishmaniasis; up to two-thirds of patients have oral lesions.[123] The mouth may be involved by direct extension from cutaneous leishmaniasis (oriental sore or chiclero ulcer).[124,125] However, oral lesions may occur years after skin lesions have healed and, occasionally, in people who have had no skin lesions.[126] In oral leishmaniasis, the hard palate is typically involved (espundia) but lesions can spread to the soft palate, uvula and pharynx or, less commonly, to involve the gingivae and upper lip. The lesions are typically raised and nodular but may be painless.[127] They may ulcerate and a mid-facial granulomatous destructive lesion may result.[50] Cutaneous leishmaniasis may cause lip[128] or facial swelling.[129]

Oral lesions seen in Sudan are typically caused by *L. donovani*[130,131] and present as fungating lesions. Oral symptoms in most patients centre upon pain or a sensation of a foreign body in the mouth, gingival bleeding or loosening of teeth.[130]

Leishmania/HIV co-infection is emerging as a serious and new disease.[132] Although people are bitten by sandflies that are infected with *Leishmania* protozoa, most do not develop the disease. However, among those who are immunosuppressed (e.g. HIV), cases can quickly evolve to a full clinical presentation of severe leishmaniasis. It is estimated that AIDS increases this risk by 100–1000 times in epidemic areas.[132]

In a similar way to HIV, leishmaniasis can be transmitted directly from person to person through the sharing of needles. This is important in developing countries where dental treatment is carried out by both trained and non-trained personnel, and where infection control procedures in the dental surgery can be variable.[133]

Diagnosis

There is no specific oral sign to help in the diagnosis of leishmaniases, and the approach to the clinical diagnosis is covered in the chapter dedicated to this disease.

Oral management

Essentially, the clinical and parasitological cures are implemented and oral ulcerations are managed via a palliative approach by altering the diet (i.e. changing its consistency by making it more bland and consuming it at tepid temperatures). However,

Leishmania-DNA can be detected in oral tissues years after apparently successful treatment of the infection.[134]

Trichinosis

Trichinella spiralis occurs in two forms: the adult *T. spiralis*, which is a white worm barely visible to the naked eye: and the cystic form, which is formed by the larva encapsulated by the host tissue. Since its transmission is by mouth from eating undercooked meat, it is not surprising that trichinosis is the most frequent roundworm infestation to affect the oral tissues. As in other parts of the body, encystations are commonly in the striated muscle, and in the oral cavity this is predominantly in the tongue and masseter muscle. The usual cycle of events is that they invade the tongue and masseter muscle, where calcification will take place after about 6 months and lead to the death of the larvae. The small intra-oral cyst-like lesions can commonly be confused as mucoceles; however, the latter are not associated with systemic symptoms. The cyst-like lesions become encapsulated and may calcify, at which time radiographically they appear as radiopaque nodules.[135]

Diagnosis

Diagnosis is clinical, supported by investigations and a history of ingestion of poorly cooked meat, and by serology.

Oral management

There is no specific oral management and treatment is similar to that of a trichinosis infection elsewhere in the body, namely treatment directed against the larvae and the immune reaction which they invoke. Prolonged oral high-dosage mebendazole or thiabendazole has been proved to be effective.

Echinococcosis (echinococciasis)

The larval stages of two small tapeworms, *Echinococcus granulosus* and *E. multilocularis*, cause the main forms of hydatid disease in man. In the oral tissues hydatid cysts are usually firm, round swellings of several months' duration, mainly in the tongue.[136]

Diagnosis

A history of possible exposure to infection may be elicited. A hydatid cyst may show a smooth round outline on radiography. Eosinophilia is merely suggestive of a parasitic disease and not specific. A definitive diagnosis is often made only by identifying the hydatid cyst at operation.

Oral management

As with the general management of this infection, high doses of mebendazole, albendazole or flubendazole interfere with growth of larvae but are not curative. The only curative treatment is surgery.

Cysticercosis

Cysticercosis is the infection by the small bladder-like larvae of the pork tapeworm, Taenia solium. Human cysticercosis is essentially a faecal-oral infection, acquired by ingesting eggs excreted in the faeces of a human tapeworm carrier. Although cysticerci are not uncommon in the striated muscles in the tongue and neck and subcutaneous tissues, morbidity of cysticercosis is almost entirely due to the central nervous system disease. A number of cases of children presenting with oral lesions of cysticercosis have been reported.[137,138] Oral lesions are typically well circumscribed, nodular, soft, elastic and fluctuant submucosal swellings situated in the dorsum of the tongue and buccal mucosa[139,140] Although such oral lesions may be present for a number of years, oral signs may be the first clinical sign of the infection.[138]

Diagnosis

Relies upon surgical removal of the parasite, the appearance of the translucent membrane with its central milky spot being characteristic.

Oral management

There is no reliable medical treatment but the general management approach is either albendazole or praziquantel (plus prednisolone can be curative).

Sparganosis

Larvae of the tapeworms of *Spirometra* species seen mainly in South-east Asia, especially Thailand, may rarely cause oral lesions.[141]

Larva migrans

Oral lesions have been recorded in relation to various worms, including *Ancylostoma* and *Gongylonema* species.

Oral management

Local application of 10% thiabendazole, ethyl chloride, chloroform, electrocoagulation and cryotherapy have all been tried. If the lesions are multiple, particularly in the mouth, thiabendazole is indicated but can produce adverse effects such as anorexia, nausea and rashes. Albendazole or mebendazole are alternatives.

Filariasis

The filariases result from infection with vector-borne tissue-dwelling nematodes called filariae. In public health terms, the two most important filariae are onchocerciasis and lymphatic filariasis, but dirofilariasis is also a problem.

Lymphatic filariasis, in humans, is estimated to infect 20% of the world's population and is the result of three species of filarial worms: *Wuchereria bancrofti*, *Brugia malayi* and *B. timori*.[142] It is fortunate that these species have rarely been found in the mouth.

Onchocerciasis (river blindness) is the result of infection with *Onchocerca volvulus*. The main clinical features of the infection are dermatitis, eye lesions and nodule formation. In Africa, 80% of nodules occur on the body prominences of the pelvic girdle. However, in Central America nodules are commonly found in the head and neck region. It is thought that this reflects the biting

habits of the vector flies.[143] Oral nodules are unusual, but when they occur they present as a rubbery nodule.

Dirofilariasis is widespread in southern and eastern Europe, Asia, and Florida USA. The nematodes are transmitted from dogs infected by mosquitoes. Rare human cases have been reported in the mouth.[144–148]

Diagnosis

The diagnosis is made by identifying the worm in biopsies.

Oral management

Nodulectomy has only limited use because many worms are present outside the nodules. However, it has been suggested that head nodules should be removed because their presence increases the risk of blindness.[143] The rationale for this procedure is that this will reduce the number of microfilariae which are produced. Nodulectomy campaigns have been attempted, although their impact has yet to be evaluated, but in Guatemala systematic campaigns were associated with decreased blindness.[143]

Gnathostomiasis

Gnathostomiasis may produce swellings in the skin or mouth, or occasionally bleeding. Skin tests and serodiagnosis help the diagnosis. Metronidazole may be of some benefit or the worm can be excised.

Myiasis

Myiasis is caused when fly maggots invade living tissue or when they are harboured in the intestine or bladder. In oral lesions they are seen mainly in the anterior maxillary or mandibular gingivae.[149–156] An opening burrow is usually patent, with induration of the marginal tissues and is raised, forming a dome-shaped 'warble', or an extraction wound may be effected. Often several larvae are present and there is severe inflammatory reaction in the surrounding tissues.

Diagnosis

Larvae can be seen with the naked eye.

Oral management

A few drops of turpentine oil or chloroform in light vegetable oil should be instilled in the lesion and the larvae removed with blunt tweezers. It may be prudent to give an antibiotic, as there is often a superimposed secondary infection. Ivermectin may be effective in some cases.[157]

Ciguatera poisoning

Ciguatera, the most common form of fish poisoning, occurring in most tropical and subtropical seas, may result in oral or peri-oral paraesthesiae or dysaesthesiae.[158–159]

Malaria

Oral features are rare in malaria and mainly iatrogenic ulcers on neuropathies.[160,–161]

REFERENCES

1. Cook GC. Tropical gastroenterological problems. In: Cook G, ed. *Manson's Tropical Diseases.* 20th edn. London: WB Saunders; 1998:29–30.
2. Beighton D, Edgar WN. Dental caries: aetiology and pathogenesis. In: Arens U, ed. *Oral Health: Diet and Other Factors.* Amsterdam: Elsevier; 1999.
3. Burt BA, Ismail AL. Diet, nutrition and food cariogenicity. *J Dent Res* 1986; 65:S1475–S1484.
4. Winter GB. Maternal nutritional requirements in relation to the subsequent development of teeth in children. *J Hum Nutr* 1976; 30:93–99.
5. Alvarez JO, Navia JM. Nutritional status, tooth eruption and dental caries: a review. *Am J Clin Nutr* 1989; 49:417–426.
6. Rugg-Gunn AJ. *Nutrition and Dental Health.* Oxford: Oxford University Press; 1993.
7. Department for International Development. *Eliminating World Poverty: Making Globalisation Work for the Poor. White Paper on International Development.* London: Stationery Office; 2000.
8. Frencken JE, Pilot T, Songpaisan Y, et al. Atraumatic restorative treatment (ART): rationale, technique and development. *J Public Health Dent* 1996; 56:135–140.
9. Holmgren CJ, Lo E CM, Hu D Y, et al. ART restorations and sealants placed in Chinese schoolchildren: results 3 years. *Community Dent Oral Epidemiol* 2000; 28:314–320.
10. Hansel-Petersson G, Bratthal D. The caries decline: a review of reviews. In dental caries: intervened-interrupted-interpreted. *Suppl Eur J Oral Sci* 1996; 104:436–443.
11. Adyatmaka A, Sutopo U, Carlsson P, et al. *School-Based Primary Preventive Programme of Children.* Geneva: World Health Organization; 1998.
12. Pilot T. The periodontal disease problem: a comparison between industrialised and developing countries. *Int Dent J* 1998 48(3 suppl 1): 221–232.
13. Ali RW, Johannessen AC, Dahlen G, et al. Comparison of the subgingival microbiota of periodontally healthy and diseased adults in northern Cameroon. *J Clin Periodontol* 1997 24(11):830–835.
14. Miyazaki H. A global overview of periodontal epidemiology. In: Pack ARC, Newman HN, eds. *Periodontal Needs of Developing Nations.* International Academy of Periodontology Symposium, 4 June 1995. Northwood: Science Reviews; 1996:1–7.
15. Petersen PE, Ogawa H. Strengthening the prevention of periodontal disease: The WHO Approach. *J Periodontol* 2005; 76(12):2187–2193.
16. Darout IA, Albandar JM, Skaug N. Periodontal status of adult Sudanese habitual users of miswak chewing sticks or toothbrushes. *Acta Odontol Scand* 2000; 58(1):25–30.
17. WHO. Manual of the International Statistical Classification of Diseases, Injuries and Causes of Death (based on the recommendations of the ninth revision conference). Geneva: World Health Organization; 1977.
18. Scully C, Bedi R. Ethnicity and oral cancer. *Lancet Oncol* 2000:1:37–42.
19. Parkin DM, Pisani P, Ferlay J. Estimates of the worldwide incidence of 25 major cancers in 1990. *Int J Cancer* 1999; 80:827–841.
20. International Agency for Research on Cancer. *IARC Monographs on the Evaluation of Carcinogenic Risks to Humans. Tobacco Smoking.* Vol. 38. Lyon: International Agency for Research on Cancer; 1986.
21. International Agency for Research on Cancer. IARC Monographs on the Evaluation of Carcinogenic Risks of Chemicals to Humans. *Tobacco Habits Other than Smoking: Betel Quid and Areca Nut Chewing and some Related Nitrosamines.* Vol. 37. Lyon: International Agency for Research on Cancer; 1986.
22. Sankarnarayanan R, Black RJ, Swaminathan R, et al. An overview of cancer survival in developing countries. In: Sankaranarayanan R, Black RJ, Parkin DM, eds. *Cancer Survival in Developing Countries.* IARC Scientific Publication No. 145. Lyon: Oxford University Press; 1998:135–157.
23. Van Wyk CW, Stander I, Padayachee A, et al. The areca nut chewing habit and oral squamous cell carcinoma in South African Indians: a retrospective study. *S Afr Med J* 1993; 83:425–429.
24. Mathew B, Sankaranarayanan R, Sunilkumar K, et al. Reproducibility and validity of oral visual inspection by trained health workers in the detection of oral cancer and precancer. *Br J Cancer* 1997; 76:390–394.
25. Fernandez Garrote L, Sankaranarayanan R, Lence Anta JJ, et al. An evaluation of the oral cancer control program in Cuba. *Epidemiology* 1995; 6:428–431.
26. Gupta PC, Mehta FS, Pindborg JJ, et al. Primary prevention trial of oral cancer in India: a 10 year follow-up study. *J Oral Pathol Med* 1992; 21: 433–439.
27. Martin GC, Brown JP, Eifler CW, et al. Oral leukoplakia status six weeks after cessation of smokeless tobacco use. *J Am Dent Assoc* 1999; 130:945–954.
28. Petersen PE. Strengthening the prevention of oral cancer: the WHO perspective. *Community Dent Oral Epidemiol* 2005; 33(6):397–399.
29. Jaber MA, Porter SR, Gilthorpe MS, et al. Risk factors for oral epithelial dysplasia – the role of smoking and alcohol. *Oral Oncol* 1999; 35: 151–156.
30. Bedi R. Betel-quid and tobacco chewing among the United Kingdom's Bangladeshi community. *Br J Cancer* 1996; 74(suppl XXIX):S73–S77.
31. Murti PR, Bhonsle RB, Pinborg JJ, et al. Malignant transformation rate in oral submucous fibrosis over a 17-year period. *Commun Dent Oral Epidemiol* 1985; 13:340–341.
32. Tu H F, Liu CJ, Chang CS, et al. The functional (−1171 5A → 6A) polymorphisms of matrix metalloproteinase 3 gene as a risk factor for oral submucous fibrosis among male areca users. *J Oral Pathol Med* 2006; 35(2):99–103.
33. Tilakaratne WM, Klinikowski MF, Saku T, et al. Oral submucous fibrosis: Review on aetiology and pathogenesis. *Oral Oncol* 2005; 42(6):561–568.
34. Horning GM, Cohen ME. Necrotizing ulcerative gingivitis, periodontitis, and stomatitis: clinical staging and predisposing factors. *J Periodontol* 1995; 66:990–998.
35. Contreras A, Falkler WA, Enwonwu CO, et al. Human Herpesviridae in acute necrotizing ulcerative gingivitis in children in Nigeria. *Oral Microbiol Immunol* 1997; 12:259–265.
36. WHO. *Noma, the Face of Poverty* (updated August). Geneva: World Health Organization; 2000.
37. Costini B, Larroque G, Dubosco JC, et al. Noma ou cancrum oris: aspects etiopathogeniques et nosologiques. *Med Trop* 1995; 55:263–273.
38. Idigbe EO, Enwonwu CO, Falker WA, et al. Living conditions of children at risk for noma: Nigerian experience. *Oral Dis* 1999; 5(2):156–162.
39. Ndiaye FC, Bourgeois D, Leclercq MH, et al. Noma: public health problem in Senegal and epidemiological surveillance. *Oral Dis* 1999; 5(2):163–166.
40. Enwonwu CO. Noma – the ulcer of extreme poverty. *N Engl J Med* 2006; 354(3):221–224.
41. Akula SK, Chreticos CM, Weldon-Linne CM. Gangrenous stomatitis in AIDS. *Lancet* 1989; i:955.
42. Giovannini M, Zuccotti GV, Fiocchi A. Gangrenous stomatitis in a child with AIDS. *Lancet* 1989; ii:1400.
43. Rotbart HA, Levin MJ, Jones JF, et al. Noma in children with severe combined immunodeficiency. *Pediatrics* 1986; 109:596–600.
44. Stassen LF, Batchelor AG, Rennie JS, et al. Cancrum oris in an adult Caucasian female. *Br J Oral Maxillofac Surg* 1989; 27:417–422.
45. Winkler JR, Murray PA, Hammerle C. Gangrenous stomatitis in AIDS. *Lancet* 1989; 2:108.
46. WHO. *Young People and Sexually Transmitted Diseases.* Fact Sheet No. 186, revised December. Geneva: World Health Organization; 1997.
47. Fiumara NJ, Berg M. Primary syphilis in the oral cavity. *Br J Vener Dis* 1974; 50:463–464.
48. Mani NJ. Secondary syphilis initially diagnosed from oral lesions. *Oral Surg Oral Med Oral Pathol* 1984; 58:47–50.
49. Manton SL, Egglestone SI, Alexander I, et al. Oral presentation of secondary syphilis. *Br Dent J* 1986; 160:237–238.
50. Ramos-e-Silva M. Facial and oral aspects of some venereal and tropical diseases. *Acta Dermatovenerol Croat* 2004; 12(3):173–180.
51. Erdelyi RL, Molla AA. Burned-out endemic syphilis (Bejel) facial deformities and defects in Saudi Arabia. *Plast Reconstr Surg* 1984; 74:589–602.

52. Furtado T. Some problems of late yaws. *Int J Dermatol* 1973; 12: 123–130.

53. Botreau-Roussel P. Goundou. In: Simons RDG, ed. *Handbook of Tropical Dermatology and Medical Mycology.* Amsterdam: Elsevier; 1952:6–76.

54. Stenhouse D, MacDonald DG, MacFarlane TW. Cervicofacial and intraoral actinomycosis: a 5 year retrospective study. *Br J Oral Surg* 1975; 13: 172–182.

55. Benoliel R, Asquith J. Actinomycosis of the jaws. *Int J Oral Surg* 1985; 14:195–199.

56. Roberts GD, Brewer WS, Hermans PE. Diagnosis of nocardiosis by blood culture. *Mayo Clin Proc* 1974; 49:293.

57. Rattner LJ. Case of suspected oral nocardiosis. *Oral Surg Oral Med Oral Pathol* 1958; 11:441.

58. WHO. *Tuberculosis.* Fact Sheet No. 104, revised April. Geneva: World Health Organization; 2000.

59. Eng HL, Lu S Y, Yang CH, et al. Oral tuberculosis. *Oral Surg* 1994; 81: 415–420.

60. Fujibayashi T, Takahasi Y, Yoneda T, et al. Tuberculosis of the tongue: a case report with immunologic study. *Oral Surg Oral Med Oral Pathol* 1979; 47:427–435.

61. Komet H, Scheffer RE, McHoney PL. Bilateral tuberculous granulomas of the tongue. *Arch Otolaryngol* 1965; 82:649–661.

62. Yusuf H. Oral tuberculosis. *Br Dent J* 1975; 138:470–472.

63. Michaud M, Blancette G, Tomich C. Chronic ulceration of the hard palate. first clinical sign of undiagnosed pulmonary tuberculosis. *Oral Surg Oral Med Oral Pathol* 1984; 57:63–67.

64. Rao TV, Satyanarayana CV, Sundareshwar B, et al. Unusual form of tuberculosis of lips. *J Oral Surg* 1977; 35:595–596.

65. Turbiner S, Giunta J, Maloney PL. Orofacial tuberculosis of the lip. *J Oral Surg* 1975; 33:443–447.

66. Agarwal MK, Gupta OP, Samant HC, et al. Tuberculosis of the tongue. *Ann Acad Med Singapore* 1979; 8:217–219.

67. Boyes J, Jones JDT, Miller FJW. The recognition of primary tuberculous infection of the mouth. *Arch Dis Child* 1956; 31:81–86.

68. Taylor RG, Booth DF. Tuberculous osteomyelitis of the mandible. *Oral Surg Oral Med Oral Pathol* 1964; 18:7–13.

69. Thilander H, Wennstrom A. Tuberculosis of the mouth and the surrounding tissues. *Oral Surg Oral Med Oral Pathol* 1956; 9:858–870.

70. Foster CF, Young WB. Tuberculosis infection of a fractured mandible: report of a case. *J Oral Surg* 1970; 38:686.

71. Ratliff DP. Tuberculosis of the mandible. *Br Dent J* 1973; 35:595–596.

72. Sachs SA, Eisenbund L. Tuberculous osteomyelitis of the mandible. *Oral Surg Oral Med Oral Pathol* 1977; 44:425–429.

73. Shengold MA, Shengold H. Oral tuberculosis. *Oral Surg Oral Med Oral Pathol* 1951; 4:239–250.

74. Weidman GM, MacGregor AJ. Tuberculous osteomyelitis of the mandible: report of a case. *Oral Surg Oral Med Oral Pathol* 1969; 28:632–635.

75. Bradnum P. Tuberculous sinus of the face associated with an abscessed lower third molar. *Dent Pract Dent Rec* 1961; 12:127–128.

76. Sowray JH. Tuberculous facial sinuses. *Br Dent J* 1967; 123:291–294.

77. Pratap VK, Samuel KC, Saxena H. Tuberculosis: manifestation at uncommon sites. *J Ind Med Assoc* 1972; 59:281–287.

78. Rosenquist JB, Beskow R. Tuberculosis of the maxilla: report case. *J Oral Surg* 1977; 35:309–310.

79. Rangel AL, Coletta RD, Almeida OP, et al. Parotid mycobacteriosis is frequently caused by Mycobacterium tuberculosis in advanced AIDS. *J Oral Pathol Med* 2005; 34(7):407–412.

80. Waldman RH. Tuberculosis and the atypical mycobacteria. *Otolaryngol Clin North Am* 1982; 15:581–586.

81. Ord RJ, Matz GJ. Tuberculous cervical lymphadenitis. *Arch Otolaryngol* 1974; 99:327–329.

82. Salyer KE, Votteler TP, Dorman GW. Surgical management of cervical adenitis due to atypical mycobacteria in children. *JAMA* 1968; 204:103–106.

83. Noorden SK, Pannikar VK. Leprosy. In: Cook GC, ed. *Manson's Tropical Diseases.* 20th edn. London: WB Saunders; 1996:1016–1044.

84. Barton RPE. Lesions of the mouth, pharynx and larynx in lepromatous leprosy. *Leprosy India* 1974; 46:130–134.

85. Moller-Christensen V, Bakke SN, Melsum RS, et al. Changes in the anterior nasal spine and the alveolar process of the maxillary bone in leprosy. *Int J Leprosy* 1952; 20:335–340.

86. Prahbu SR, Daftary DK. Atrophic lesions of the tongue in leprosy patients. *Odontostomatol Trop* 1982; V:75–85.

87. Reichart P. Facial and oral manifestations in leprosy. *Oral Surg Oral Med Oral Pathol* 1976; 41:385–399.

88. Reichart P. Pathologic changes in the soft palate in lepromatous leprosy. *Oral Surg Oral Med Oral Pathol* 1974; 38:898–904.

89. Scheepers A, Lemmer J, Lownie JF. Oral manifestations of Leprosy. *Leprosy Rev* 1993; 64(1):37–43.

90. Southam JC, Venkatraman BK. Oral manifestations of leprosy. *Br J Oral Surg* 1973; 10:272–274.

91. Girdhar BK, Desikan KV. A clinical study of the mouth in untreated lepromatous patients. *Leprosy Rev* 1979; 50:25–35.

92. Lighterman I, Watanabe Y, Hidaka T. Leprosy of the oral cavity and adnexa. *Oral Surg Oral Med Oral Pathol* 1962; 15:1178–1194.

93. Prabhu SR, Daftary DK. Clinical evaluation of orofacial lesions in leprosy. *Odontostomatol Trop* 1981; IV:83–95.

94. E-Silva R, Rebello PF. Leprosy: recognition and treatment. *Am J Clin Dermatol* 2001; 2(4):203–211.

95. Scully C, Monteil R, Sposto MR. Infectious and tropical diseases affecting the human mouth. In: Scully C, ed. *Oral Pathology and Medicine in Periodontics: Periodontology 2000.* Copenhagen: Munksgaard; 1998:47–70.

96. Scully C. Infectious diseases. In: Millard HD, Mason DK, eds. *1993 World Workshop on Oral Medicine.* Ann Arbor: University of Michigan; 1995.

97. Scully C, Cawson RA. *Medical Problems in Dentistry.* Bristol: Wright; 1987.

98. Chauvet E, Carreiro M, Berry A, et al. Oral histoplasmosis 34 years after return of Africa. *Rev Med Interne* 2003; 24(3):195–197.

99. De Almeida OP, Scully C. Oral lesions in the systemic mycoses. *Curr Opin Dent* 1991; 1:423–428.

100. Scully C, De Almeida OP. Orofacial manifestations of the systemic mycoses. *J Oral Pathol Med* 1992; 21:289–294.

101. Scully C, De Almeida OP, Sposto MR. Deep mycoses in HIV infection. *Oral Dis* 1997; 3(suppl 1):200–207.

102. Pfaller M, Wenzel R. Impact of the changing epidemiology of fungal infections in the 1990s. *Eur J Clin Microbiol Infect Dis* 1992; 11:287–291.

103. Napoli JA, Donegan JO. Aspergillosis and necrosis of the maxilla. *J Oral Maxillofac Surg* 1991; 49:532–534.

104. Rubin MM, Jui V, Sadoff RS. Oral aspergillosis in a patient with acquired immunodeficiency syndrome. *J Oral Maxillofac Surg* 1990; 48:997–999.

105. Shannon MT, Sclaroff A, Colm SJ. Invasive aspergillosis of the maxilla in an immunocompromised patient. *Oral Surg Oral Med Oral Pathol* 1990; 70:425–427.

106. Denning DW, Stevens DA. Antifungal and surgical treatment of invasive aspergillosis: review of 2,121 published cases. *Rev Infect Dis* 1990; 12: 1147–1201.

107. Sposto MR, Almeida OPD, Scully C, et al. Oral paracoccidioidomycosis: a study of 36 South American patients. *Oral Surg Oral Med Oral Pathol* 1993; 75:461–465.

108. Sposto MR, Mendes-Gianini MJ, Moraes RA, et al. Paracoccidioidomycosis manifesting oral lesions: a clinical cytological and serological investigation. *J Oral Pathol Med* 1994; 23:85–87.

109. Schmidt-Westhausen A, Grunewald T, Reichart PA, et al. Oral cryptococcosis in a patient with AIDS: a case report. *Oral Dis* 1995; 1(2):77–79.

110. Casariego Z, Kelly GR, Perez H, et al. Disseminated histoplasmosis with orofacial involvement in HIV-1-infected patients with AIDS: manifestations and treatment. *Oral Dis* 1997; 3(3):184–187.

111. Nittayananta W, Chungpanich S. Oral lesions in a group of Thai people with AIDS. *Oral Dis* 1997; 3(suppl 1):S41–S45.

112. Warnakulasuriya KA, Harrison JD, Johnson NW, et al. Localised oral histoplasmosis lesions associated with HIV infection. *J Oral Pathol Med* 1997; 26(6):294–296.

113. Jones AC, Bentsen TY, Freedman PD. Mucormycosis of the oral cavity. *Oral Surg Oral Med Oral Pathol* 1993; 75(4):455–460.

114. Thammayya A. Zygomycosis due to Conidiobolus coronatus in west Bengal. *Indian J Chest Dis Allied Sci* 2000 Oct–Dec; 42(4): 305–309.

115. De Castro CC, Bernard G, Ygaki Y, et al. MRI of head and neck paracoccidioidomycosis. *Br J Radiol* 1999; 72(859):717–722.

116. De Almeida OP, Jacks J, Scully C, et al. Orofacial manifestations of paracoccidioidomycosis (South American blastomycosis). *Oral Surg Oral Med Oral Pathol* 1991; 72:430–435.

117. Mendes-Giannini MJS. Serodiagnosis. In: Franco M, da Silva Lacaz C, Restrepo-Moreno A, et al., eds. *Paracoccidioidomycosis*. Boca Raton: CRC Press; 1994:345–357.

118. Azaz B, Milhem I, Hasson O, et al. Acquired toxoplasmosis of a submandibular lymph node in 13-year-old boy: case report. *Paediatr Dent* 1994; 16(5):378–380.

119. Macey-Dare LV, Kocjan G, Goodman JR. Acquired toxoplasmosis of a submandibular lymph node in a nine-year-old boy diagnosed by fine-needle aspiration cytology. *Int J Paediatr Dent* 1996; 6(4):265–269.

120. Clayton R, Grabczynska S. Mucocutaneous leishmaniasis presenting as facial cellulitis. *J Laryngol Otol* 2005; 119(7):567–569.

121. Azizi T, Sadeghipour A, Roohi A, et al. A 33-year-old male farmer with progressive gingival swelling and bleeding. *Ann Saudi Med* 2005 May–Jun; 25(3):262, 270–271.

122. Van Damme PA, Keuter M, Van Assen S, et al. A rare case of oral leishmaniasis. *Lancet Infect Dis* 2004; 4(1):53.

123. Sithequee MAM, Qazi AA, Ahmed GA. Study into leishmaniasis. *Br J Oral Maxillofac Surg* 1990; 28:43–46.

124. Gombos F, Laino G, Femiano F. Leishmaniosi muco-cutanea e del cavo orale. *Arch Stomatol* 1984; 25:349–357.

125. Meyruey M, Benkiran D, Landon A. Leishmaniose stomato-pharyngo-laryngee observee au Maroc. *Bull Soc Pathol Exot* 1974; 67:625–632.

126. Costa JW Jr, Milner DA Jr, Maguire JH. Mucocutaneous leishmaniasis in a US citizen. *Oral Surg Oral Med Oral Pathol Oral Radiol Endod* 2003; 96(5):573–577.

127. Aliaga L, Cobo F, Mediavilla JD, et al. Localized mucosal leishmaniasis due to Leishmania (Leishmania) infantum: clinical and microbiologic findings in 31 patients. *Medicine* (Baltimore) 2003; 82(3):147–158.

128. Sangueza OP, Sangueza JM, Stiller M, et al. Mucocutaneous leishmaniasis: a clinicopathological classification. *J Am Acad Dermatol* 1993; 28: 927–932.

129. Castling B, Layton SA, Pratt RJ. Cutaneous leishmaniasis: an unusual cause of facial swelling. *Oral Surg* 1994; 78:91–92.

130. El-Hassan AM, Meredith SE, Yagi HI, et al. Sudanese mucosal leishmaniasis: epidemiology, clinical features, diagnosis, immune responses and treatment. *Trans R Soc Trop Med Hyg* 1995; 89:647–652.

131. Goto H, Sotto MN, Corbett CEP, et al. A case of multiple lesion mucocutaneous leishmaniasis caused by Leishmania (Viannia braziliensis) infection. *J Trop Med Hyg* 1990; 93:48–51.

132. WHO. *The Leishmaniasis and Leishmania/HIV Co-infections*. Fact Sheet No. 116, revised May. Geneva: World Health Organization; 2000.

133. Littleton PA Jr, Kohn W. Dental public health and infection control in industrialised and developing countries. *Int Dent J* 1991; 41(6):341–347.

134. Premoli-de-Percoco G, Gonzalez N, Anez N, et al. PCR detection of specific Leishmania-DNA in patients with periodontal disease. *Pathologica* 2002; 94(1):28–31.

135. Hansen LS and Allard RH. Encysted parasitic larvae in the mouth. *J Am Dent Assoc* 1984; 108(4):632–636.

136. Bouckaert MM, Raubenheimer EJ, Jacobs FJ. Maxillofacial hydatid cysts. Oral *Surg Oral Med Oral Pathol Oral Radiol Endod* 2000; 89(3): 338–342.

137. Romero de Leon E, Aguirre A. Oral cysticercosis. *Oral Surg Oral Med Oral Pathol Oral Radiol Endod* 1995; 79(5):572–577.

138. Saran RK, Rattan V, Rajwanshi A, et al. Cysticercosis of the oral cavity: report of five cases and a review of literature. *Int J Paediatr Dent* 1998; 8(4):273–278.

139. Munjal S, Gujral M, Narang S. Lingual cysticercosis – a case report. *Indian J Pathol Microbiol* 2001; 44(4):459.

140. Roth B, Gocht A, Metternich FU. Cysticercosis as a rare cause of a tumor of the tongue. *Laryngorhinootologie* 2003; 82(8):564–567.

141. Iamaroon A, Sukontason K, Sukontason K. Sparganosis: a rare case of the oral cavity. *J Oral Pathol Med* 2002; 31(9):558–560.

142. Nigam S, Singh T, Mishra A, et al. Oral cysticercosis: reports of six cases. *Head and Neck* 2001; 23(6):497–499.

143. McMahon JE, Simonsen PE. Filariases. In: Cook GC, ed. *Manson's Tropical Diseases*. 20th edn. London: WB Saunders; 1996:1321–1368.

144. Tilakaratne WM, Pitakotuwage TN. Intra-oral Dirofilaria repens infection: report of seven cases. *J Oral Pathol Med* 2003; 32(8):502–505.

145. To EW, Tsang WM 7, Chan KF. Human dirofilariasis of the buccal mucosa: a case report. *Int J Oral Maxillofac Surg* 2003; 32(1):104–106.

146. Collins BM, Jones AC, Jimenez F. Dirofilaria tenuis infection of the oral mucosa and cheek. *J Oral Maxillofac Surg* 1993; 51(9):1037–1040.

147. Seddon SV, Peckitt NS, Davidson RN, et al. Helminth infection of the parotid gland. *J Oral Maxillofac Surg* 1992; 50(2):183–185.

148. Markopoulos AK, Trigonidis G, Papanayotou P. Submucous dirofilariasis involving the cheek. Report of a case. *Ann Dent* 1990; 49(1):34–5, 50.

149. Al-Ismaily MI, Scully C. Oral myiasis: report of two cases. *Int J Paediatr Dent* 1985; 5:177–179.

150. Bozzo L, Almeida ODP, Scully C. Oral myiasis caused by Sarcophagidae in an extraction wound. *Oral Surg Oral Med Oral Pathol* 1992; 74: 733–735.

151. Erfan F. Gingival myiasis caused by Diptera (Sarcophaga). *Oral Surg Oral Med Oral Pathol* 1980; 49:148–150.

152. Konstantinidis AB, Zamanis D. Gingival myiasis. *J Oral Med* 1987; 42: 243–245.

153. Gomez RS, Perdigao PF, Pimenta FJGS. Oral myiasis by screwworm Cochliomyia hominivorax . *Br J Oral Maxillofac Surg* 2003; 41: 115–116.

154. Ng K HL, Yip KT, Choi CH. A case of oral myiasis due to Chrysoma bezziana. *Hong Kong Med J* 2003; 9:454–456.

155. Aguiar AMM, Enwonwu CO, Pires FR. Noma (cancrum oris) associated with oral myiasis in an adult. *Oral Dis* 2003; 9:158–159.

156. Yazar S, Dik B, Yalcin S, et al. Nosocomial oral myiasis by Sarcophaga sp. in Turkey. *Yonsei Med J* 2005; 46(3):431–434.

157. Duque SFL, Valderrama HR, Gonzalez RJ. Treatment of oral myiasis with ivermectin; report of three cases caused by Cochliomyia hominivorax. *Rev Fac Odontol Univ Ant* 1998; 10:41–47.

158. Sanner BM, Rawert B, Henning B, et al. Ciguatera fish poisoning following travel to the tropics. *Z Gastroenterol* 1997; 35(5):327–330.

159. Heir GM. Ciguatera neurotoxin poisoning mimicking burning mouth syndrome. *Quintessence Int* 2005; 36(7–8):547–550.

160. Owotade FJ, Greenspan JS. Malaria and oral health. *Oral Dis* 2008; 14(4): 302–307.

161. Watt-Smith S, Mehta K, Scully C. Mefloquine-induced trigeminal sensory neuropathy. Oral Surg Oral Med Oral Pathol Oral Radiol Endod 2001; 92(2): 163–165.

Chapter 28 Ronald H. Behrens and Robert Steffen

Travel Health

Travel, especially to developing countries, is associated with an increased risk of morbidity and mortality. Travel health – the pre-travel segment of travel medicine – has become increasingly important for the 100 million residents of industrialized nations who travel annually to developing countries. Between 80% and 95% of these travellers are short-term tourists or persons visiting friends and relatives (VFR). Some travellers who work abroad may either make repeated short visits (airline crews or business persons) or reside for prolonged periods (missionaries, volunteer workers). Health risks differ between these groups and, depending on the environment and their behaviour, may vary within a single group.

The aim of pre-travel health advice is to reduce these risks by increasing the awareness of travellers and by promoting the use of preventive measures. The choice of these measures is guided by balancing the risk of illness or death against the risks, costs and benefits of prevention. Only frequent health risks will be considered for which epidemiological data are available. The reader should consult specific chapters for post-travel diagnostic and therapeutic measures and also for less common travel-associated infections such as leishmaniasis and schistosomiasis.

Interventions need to be tailor-made to the itinerary, individual's lifestyle, living conditions (environmental factors), allergies and other pre-existing medical conditions (host factors) (Table 28.1). An important prerequisite for accurately assessing risk and giving appropriate advice is up-to-date epidemiological data on travel mortality and morbidity (Figure 28.1).

The travel medicine practitioner must balance the recommendation of any intervention with the realistic risk of exposure to an infection or event, the consequences resulting from advice or prophylaxis, and the likely adherence of the patient. The highest priority must be given to health hazards that are common, treatable or avoidable, and those that are potentially fatal. These include illnesses such as malaria and hepatitis A, and hazards such as engaging in unprotected sex, road traffic accidents, or driving while intoxicated by drugs or alcohol. Health hazards that are rare, such as cholera or Japanese encephalitis, or those that have no effective prophylaxis, e.g. parasitic skin infections, have a lower priority. All travellers need to appreciate that any intervention is not 100% effective.

Travel medicine is a multi-disciplinary subject and includes many other areas apart from tropical medicine. Knowledge of infectious disease, pharmacology, public health, psychiatry, entomology, high-altitude physiology and behavioural sciences are all valuable to ensure effective advice. Pre-travel preparation is based on the promotion of appropriate behaviour to reduce risks; immunization, chemoprophylaxis, medication and the provision of advice for self-treatment of symptoms.

CONSULTATION AND RISK ASSESSMENT

In pre-travel consultations the prime consideration is to recognize that the potential traveller is not a patient. The collection of demographic information, including date of birth, is necessary at the start of a consultation. Medical details need to be obtained to assess, for example, the likely immune status of the person. The potential traveller should then describe in detail his or her travel plans.

Risk assessment

Risk assessment is important to rationalize pre-travel preparation, but the advice needs to reflect the health risk and not the interventions available. Risk assessment should be based on a broader view than administering drugs and vaccines.

Geographical risk

The geographical distribution of a number of infectious diseases means that travel through endemic regions or countries increases the exposure risk to these agents. The risk may vary by season and local environmental factors such as recent rainfall.

Personal risk

Age and pre-existing illness, including medication, will affect risks associated with travelling.

Age has an important influence on risk. Children are at higher risk of accidents and drowning, while teenagers have a higher risk of acquiring sexually transmitted infections. Older travellers are more likely to have pre-existing morbidity.

Risk associated with reason for travel

Long-term travellers and those visiting friends and relatives are more likely to encounter illness than are other groups of travellers.

Table 28.1 Essential questions to assess predisposing risks and host risk factors

- What is your destination(s) state: countries, city/resort/off-the-tourist-trail, itinerary?
- What is the purpose of your visit: tourism/business or other professional visit (specify)/visit (to relatives/expatriates), other reasons (military, airline crew, adoption, etc.)?
- What standard of hygiene do you expect throughout your visit: high (e.g. five-star hotels)/low (e.g. low-budget travel)?
- Are you planning any special activities: e.g. high-altitude trekking, diving, hunting, camping, etc.?
- What is your planned date of departure?
- How long do you intend to stay abroad?

Potential travellers should also answer at least the following set of questions on their health status and medical history:

- Do you currently use any medication? If yes, which ones?
- Are you currently unwell?
- Do you feel feverish? If yes, do you know what your temperature is?
- Do you suffer from any chronic illnesses? If yes, which ones?
- Are you allergic to eggs or medication? If yes, describe.
- Are you pregnant or breast-feeding? Provide details.
- Have you ever had seizures? Provide details.
- Have you ever had psychiatric or psychological problems? Provide details.
- Have you ever had jaundice or hepatitis? Provide details.
- Have you had a thymectomy?
- Are you or anybody in your household infected by HIV? Do you have any other immunodeficiency illness? Provide details.

Table 28.2 Strategies to reduce the risk of road traffic accidents

HOST/TRAVELLER FACTORS

Advise travellers to:

- Avoid alcohol before driving, avoid alcohol and food before swimming
- Use available safety equipment (seat belts, helmets, etc.)

VEHICLE FACTORS

Advise travellers to:

- Select safe cars – check availability of seat belts, good tyres
- Rent larger vehicles where possible, as passengers use rear seats
- Avoid using motorcycles and riding on the back of open trucks
- Avoid small, non-scheduled aircraft

ENVIRONMENTAL FACTORS

Advise travellers to:

- Avoid travel at night
- Employ a local driver who knows traffic and pedestrian patterns
- Carefully select swimming areas
- Know the local emergency medical system

In one study, tourists were found to be three times more likely than local drivers to be involved in a road traffic accident, and alcohol is often a contributing factor.[3] Drowning is also an important cause of death and accounts for 16% of all deaths from injuries in US travellers. Half of the fatalities were associated with recently consumed alcohol.[4] Drowning in coastal resorts is often linked to swimming in unsupervised beaches where currents and undertows result in travellers being swept out to sea. Assaults or terrorism are infrequent causes of death. Trauma (traffic accidents or criminal attacks) is the main reason for aeromedical evacuation from Africa, Asia and Latin America.[1] Table 28.2 lists the strategies that have been proposed to prevent accidents.

Among deaths due to infectious disease, HIV still, despite modern therapeutic options, has a place, although it does not appear in the usual statistics as it is a late consequence of infection abroad.[5]

Behaviour-related risks

Behaviour is associated with significant morbidity, particularly trauma and road traffic accidents.

Mortality occurring during travel is one of the most useful markers of serious and significant risk.

FATALITIES DURING TRAVEL

Accidents and cardiovascular events are the leading cause of death during intercontinental travel.[1] Cardiovascular deaths occur in older populations, but no data are available on whether the incidence is higher in travellers than in the general population and if therefore travel is a risk factor for a cardiovascular event. Fatalities due to injuries are two- to three-fold higher in travellers aged between 15 and 44 years than in similar age groups living in industrialized countries. Fatal accidents are predominantly due to motor vehicle accidents, with fatality rates in Africa reported to be as high as 20–118 deaths per 10 000 motor vehicles, and in Asia, 9–67 deaths per 10 000 motor vehicles. This compares to a fatality rate of 1.4 deaths per 10 000 motor vehicles in the UK (Figure 28.2).[2]

MORBIDITY DURING TRAVEL

More serious non-infectious morbidity is probably reflected by the mortality incidence, and is poorly described in the literature. Better described is the infectious disease prevalence associated with travel.

Studies of travellers describe that up to 62% of short-term travellers to malaria-endemic regions experience some new symptoms or illness during travel, of which only 21% may be attributable to their chemoprophylaxis and the remainder to morbidity associated with travel. Of these self-reported health problems, 7% were considered severe, although 2% were probably related to the chemoprophylactic drugs being used.[6,7] The most common infectious health impairment of travellers results from traveller's diarrhoea, upper respiratory tract infections, and skin sepsis which often follows an insect bite (Figure 28.3).

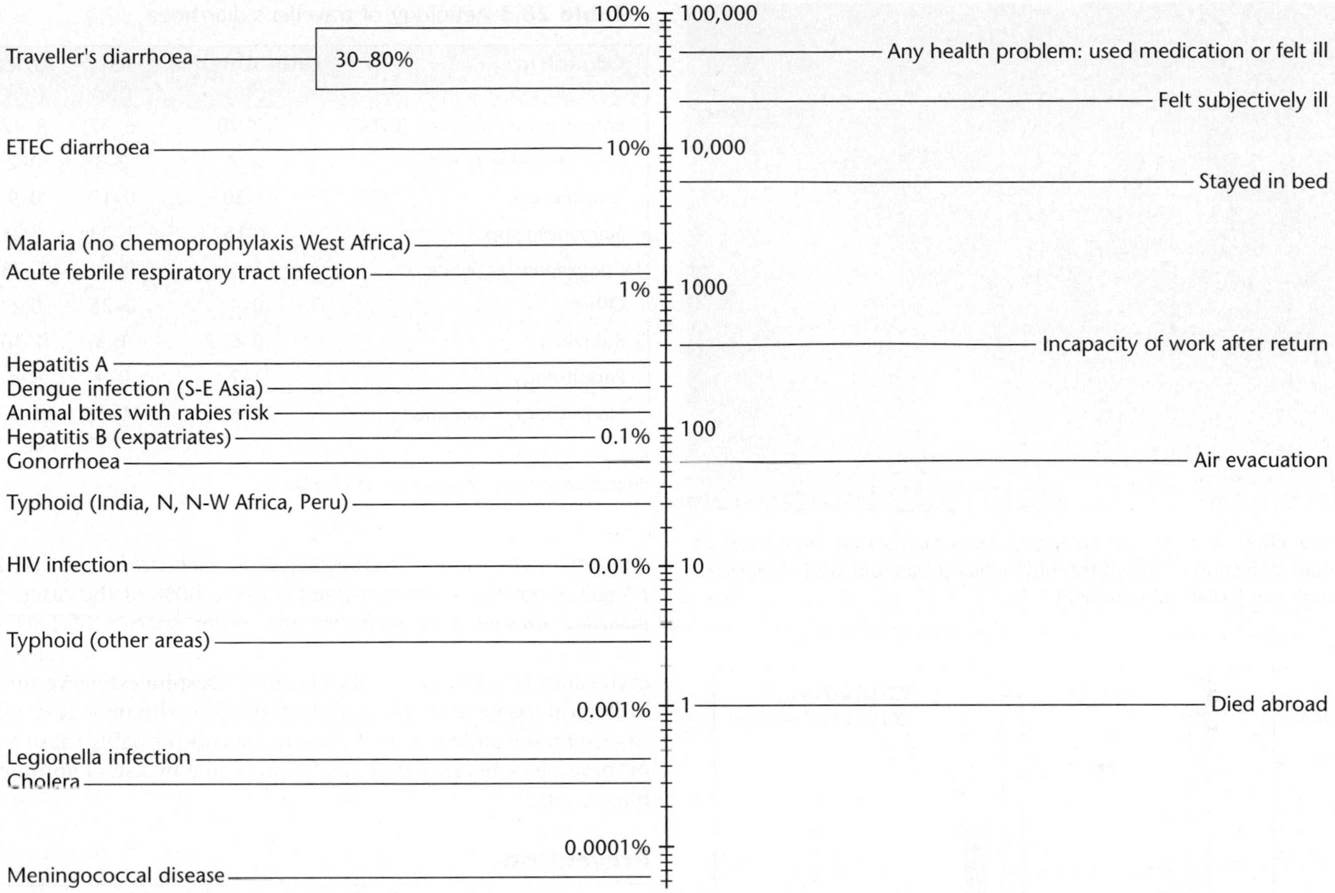

100%
100,000
Traveller's diarrhoea
30–80%
Any health problem: used medication or felt ill
Felt subjectively ill
ETEC diarrhoea
10%
10,000
Stayed in bed
Malaria (no chemoprophylaxis West Africa)
Acute febrile respiratory tract infection
1%
1000
Incapacity of work after return
Hepatitis A
Dengue infection (S-E Asia)
Animal bites with rabies risk
Hepatitis B (expatriates)
0.1%
100
Gonorrhoea
Air evacuation
Typhoid (India, N, N-W Africa, Peru)
HIV infection
0.01%
10
Typhoid (other areas)
0.001%
1
Died abroad
Legionella infection
Cholera
0.0001%
Meningococcal disease

Figure 28.1 Monthly incidence rates of health problems. Estimated incidence per month of travel, of health problems calculated from a number of studies using a logarithmic scale.

Zambia
Tanzania
South Africa
Kenya
India
UK
0
20
40
60
80
100
120
Fatalities/10 000 vehicles/year

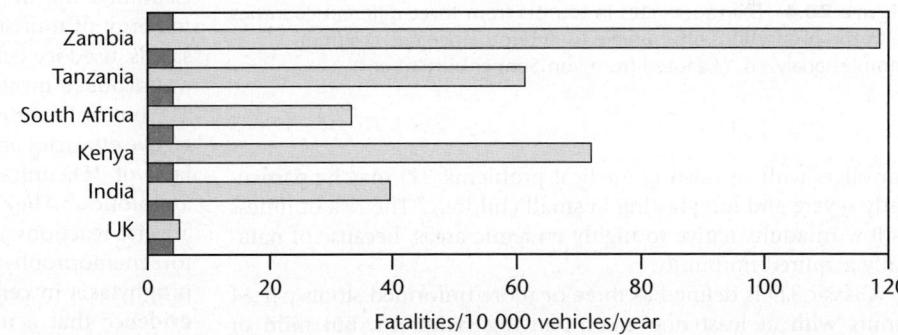

Figure 28.2 Road traffic fatalities per 10^4 vehicles/year in developing countries. Fatalities per 10 000 vehicles from published data, with UK rates as a reference population.

TRAVELLER'S DIARRHOEA

Epidemiology

There are three levels of risk for traveller's diarrhoea (TD): (i) travellers from industrialized countries spending 2 weeks in Canada, the United States, most parts of Europe, or Australia and New Zealand have a low diarrhoeal incidence of up to 8%; (ii) an intermediate incidence (8–20%) is identified among travellers to most destinations in the Caribbean, remote parts of eastern and southern Europe, Israel, Japan and South Africa; and (iii) rates of TD during visits to developing countries vary between 20% and 66% during the first 2 weeks of a stay (Figure 28.4).[8]

TD remains the most frequent infectious illness among travellers from industrialized countries visiting destinations in the developing world. Groups at particularly high risk of symptoms include infants, persons with an impaired gastric acid barrier, and

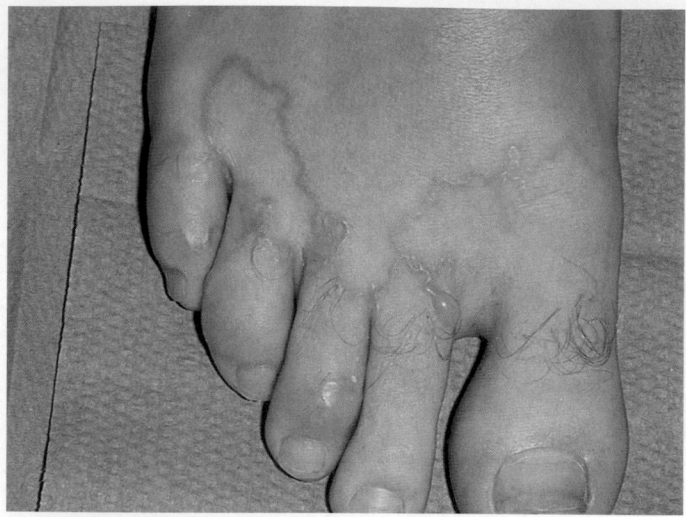

Figure 28.3 The track of cutaneous larva migrans on the dorsum of the foot. Infection occurred through walking barefoot while travelling through the Indian subcontinent.

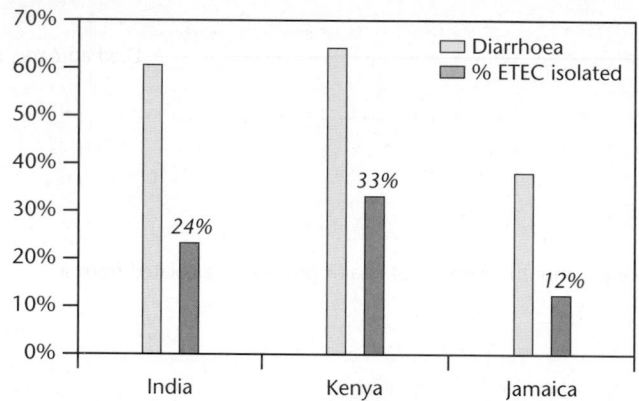

Figure 28.4 Diarrhoea rates in tourists from three different countries with the proportions attributable to enterotoxigenic *E. coli* from samples analyzed. (Adapted from von Sonnenburg et al.[8])

Table 28.3 Aetiology of traveller's diarrhoea

Organism	Latin America (%)	Asia (%)	Africa (%)
Enterotoxigenic *E. coli* (ETEC)	17–70	6–37	8–42
Enteroinvasive *E. coli*	2–7	2–3	0–2
Shigella spp.	2–30	0–17	0–9
Salmonella spp.	1–16	1–33	4–25
Campylobacter jejuni	1–5	9–39	1–28
Other	0–4	0–25	0–6
Rotavirus	0–6	1–8	0–36
Parasitology	1–2	0–9	0–4
No pathogen identified	24–62	10–56	15–53

From Ericsson.[14]
Proportion varies by destination and season.

enterotoxigenic and enteroaggregative *Escherichia coli* (ETEC, EAggEC), which are responsible for up to 60% of the cases. *Salmonella*, *Shigella*, *Campylobacter* and other species of bacterial pathogens, as well as *Giardia lamblia* and *Entamoeba histolytica*, each cause fewer than 5% of the cases.[12] Despite extensive microbiological assessment, the aetiology of approximately 20% of all cases remains undetermined. Bacterial agents probably cause most of these cases, because they can be prevented by use of antimicrobial agents.[13,14]

Prevention

There are various options to prevent TD. Parents with infants who intend to travel for pleasure to developing countries are advised to postpone their travel. Dietary restrictions using the rule of 'boil it, cook it, peel it, or forget it' may reduce the incidence of TD. These precautions are rarely complied with. Several studies which examined the impact of advice on behaviour revealed that the majority of tourists, despite advice to the contrary, still ate fresh salads, used ice cubes in their drinks, and chose to eat raw oysters or uncooked meats.[15] Many drugs have been proposed to prevent TD, but only antimicrobial agents have been shown to have protective efficacies above 80%.[16] The drugs of choice for the prophylaxis of TD, unless they are contraindicated, are the quinolone antibiotics.[12] They are not indicated for all travellers as the risk of adverse reactions and the cost restrict their widespread prescribing for chemoprophylaxis of TD. They should be considered for prophylaxis in certain circumstances (Table 28.4). There is now evidence that a non-absorbable rifamycin derivative, rifaximin, may reduce diarrhoea rates in travellers. However data on its use are limited and it is not currently licensed for chemoprophylaxis.[17]

Effective polyvalent immunization against TD is not yet available, and current vaccines against typhoid or cholera do not prevent TD at an acceptable level.[18]

Self-therapy

Because of the limitations of preventative strategies against TD, travellers should be offered a means of self-treatment while travelling. One option is to wait for symptoms to resolve spontane-

travellers with co-existing medical problems. TD may be particularly severe and long-lasting in small children.[9] The risk of illness is low in adults native to highly endemic areas, because of naturally acquired immunity.

Classic TD is defined as three or more unformed stools per 24 hours with at least one accompanying symptom, but mild or moderate TD may also result in incapacitation.[10] The symptoms of TD in tourists frequently start on the third day of the stay abroad, with second episodes beginning about a week after arrival in 20% of the cases. Untreated, the mean duration of TD is 4 days (median 2 days), and in 1% of cases the symptoms may persist for more than a month. Twenty-two per cent of patients show signs of mucosal invasive disease with fever and/or blood in the stools. There is now some evidence of an increased risk of developing longer-term irritable bowel syndrome following TD.[11]

TD is usually caused by faecal contamination of food and drink. Bacterial agents predominate (Table 28.3), especially

ously, while replacing fluid and electrolyte losses. Oral rehydration solution should always be used for infants, children and the older patient in whom dehydration may not be recognized and can lead to serious complications. Adult travellers often request and benefit from early use of curative or suppressive therapy. Loperamide, an antisecretory drug, is one of the fastest-acting agents to bring symptomatic relief in non-invasive TD.[19] Given alone, it is contra-indicated in invasive disease where there is fever and/or blood present in the stools, as it may aggravate symptoms in patients with dysentery.[20]

For general treatment, quinolone administered as a single dose (or a 3-day course) has been shown to significantly reduce the duration of diarrhoeal symptoms.[21]

Azithromycin is the drug of choice for diarrhoea acquired in South-east Asia. A combination of loperamide and quinolone has not been found to add any benefit to quinolone used alone. Thus, both loperamide and a quinolone antibiotic can be recommended for inclusion in the travel kit. Bismuth subsalicylate[20,22] and non-

Table 28.4 Indications for the chemoprophylaxis of traveller's diarrhoea

- Persons with increased susceptibility
  - History of severe traveller's diarrhoea on each trip
  - Impaired gastric acid barrier, including patients taking H2 antagonists and PPI drugs, and post-gastric surgery
  - Immune deficiency, e.g. HIV, etc.
- Persons with increased risk of complications
  - By dehydration: patients after TIA, stroke, diabetes
  - By electrolyte imbalance: patients on digitalis, etc.
- VIPs who have to accept whatever food is offered

absorbable antibiotics such as rifaximin[21,23] have also been found to reduce the duration of diarrhoeal symptoms. Rifaximin is licensed in North America and Italy for the treatment of non-dysenteric diarrhoea secondary to non-invasive *E. Coli* TD.

MALARIA IN TRAVELLERS

Malaria is transmitted in many tropical countries and is one of the most important causes of life-threatening morbidity in returning travellers. Approximately 9000–10 000 cases are reported annually in Europe, and there is an estimated 1.1% case fatality rate for those with *Plasmodium falciparum* malaria.[24]

Epidemiology

Using surveillance data and the numbers of travellers to the respective destinations, we can roughly estimate the risk of malaria in travellers visiting different countries (Figure 28.5). Malaria imported into Europe and the USA is predominantly *P. falciparum* (58–63%), and over a 10-year period an estimated 77 683 cases were reported in Europe.[24] Malaria rates in travellers to Kenya, a popular tropical destination, vary country by country. Malaria rates varied from 50 to 135 cases per 10 000 travellers. Mortality rates from malaria were also variable, with case fatality rates highest in Germany (3.6%) and lowest in the UK (0.65%). *P. falciparum* malaria rates in UK residents returning from visiting popular destinations in sub-Saharan Africa vary from 10 to 216 cases per 10 000 visits (Figure 28.5). The rates of imported malaria from the Indian subcontinent (India, Pakistan, Bangladesh and Sri Lanka) have fallen significantly and are now as low as 1 case per 1900 years exposed, warranting no chemoprophylaxis for most travellers.[25] Similar analysis of imported malaria from Central and South America suggests rates of malaria among travellers are of the same order of risk.

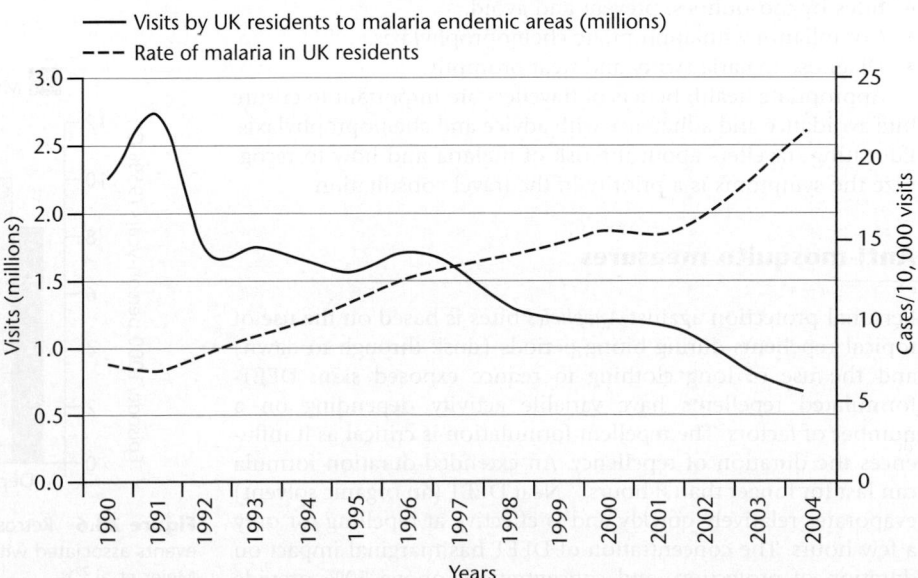

Figure 28.5 *P. falciparum* malaria rates in UK residents. Mean rates of 1989–1999. Rate of *P. falciparum* malaria per visit by UK residents, presented as a mean of the annual incidence. (Data by courtesy of the Malaria Reference Laboratory.)

Risk of infection

The risk of exposure to malaria depends on many factors relating to both vector and host behaviour. The selection of an appropriate antimalarial chemoprophylaxis is based on the risk of infection during the specific journey, the probability of side-effects, and the health beliefs and adherence of the traveller. Generally, without prophylaxis, the risk of malaria is highest in sub-Saharan Africa, intermediate in South Asia, and lowest in the Americas and South-east Asia, but it can be highly variable within countries. Any intervention that reduces the exposure to night-biting *Anopheles* mosquitoes, such as repellents and bed nets, will significantly reduce the risk of malaria. Other considerations include:

- Type of travel – backpacking versus air-conditioned, well-screened urban hotels.
- Traveller's exposure to bites, adherence with prophylaxis.
- Duration of stay – the cumulative risk of contracting malaria is proportional to the length of stay in the transmission area.
- Region visited.
- Altitude of destination – malaria is not transmitted above 2000 m.
- Season of travel – the rainy season is associated with higher transmission.

It is often useful to advise travellers about risk using the entomological inoculation rate (EIR). This is the annual number of infective *P. falciparum* mosquito bites received per person. The EIR in east Thailand is around 0.91, which is roughly equivalent to one infective mosquito bite a year, whereas in rural Tanzania a reported EIR of 667 is equivalent to two infective bites each night. In Kenya, the EIR ranges from 17 to 299.3 (one infective bite every 3 weeks to one bite a night).[26] The transmission rates in coastal resorts and cities appear to be significantly lower as compared with inland rural areas.

Prevention

Prevention of malaria is based on the acronym ABCD:
- *A*wareness: recognizing the risk.
- *B*ites by mosquitoes: prevent and avoid.
- *C*ompliance with appropriate chemoprophylaxis.
- *D*iagnose malaria swifty and treat promptly.

Appropriate health beliefs of travellers are important to ensure bite avoidance and adherence with advice and chemoprophylaxis. Educating travellers about the risk of malaria and how to recognize the symptoms is a priority in the travel consultation.

Anti-mosquito measures

Personal protection against *Anopheles* bites is based on the use of topical repellents during biting periods (dusk through to dawn) and the use of long clothing to reduce exposed skin. DEET-formulated repellents have variable activity depending on a number of factors. The repellent formulation is critical as it influences the duration of repellency. An extended-duration formula can last for longer than 8 hours.[27] Neat DEET (an organic solvent) evaporates relatively quickly and is effective at repelling for only a few hours. The concentration of DEET has marginal impact on duration of protection, and concentrations above 50% provide little added benefit. Highest concentrations should be avoided in infants and children.

Environmental measures include the use of insecticide sprays, vaporizers and nets. Sealed air-conditioned rooms provide a closed environment into which insects cannot enter and therefore anti-mosquito measures other than spraying to clear the room are unnecessary. Heated vaporizer mats clear a room of insects in around 30 minutes and remain effective for over 6 hours. Burning pyrethroid-impregnated coils is less effective and cosmetically less acceptable. In non-air-conditioned and poorly screened rooms, a pyrethroid-impregnated mosquito net is a very effective system for preventing bites. Limited compliance (35–70%) of travellers to one or more of these measures[28] puts many at risk of an infected bite. Optimal protection is provided when they are all used in combination. Oral vitamin B6, garlic and electric buzzers are of no proven value in bite prevention.

Chemoprophylaxis

Several drugs or drug combinations are available for travellers to areas with chloroquine-resistant malaria: mefloquine (Lariam®), doxycycline (Vibramycin®) and atovaquone–proguanil (Malarone®). Chloroquine and proguanil in combination have a limited protective efficacy of <70%[6] and are no longer considered adequate for areas of high transmission or resistance rates. The adverse event profiles of chemoprophylactic regimens have a significant bearing on travellers' acceptance and adherence with drugs. The reported adverse event rates of the differing regimens have varied depending on the study designs used. Blind control studies designed to identify adverse events in travellers have led to a more precise understanding of the tolerability and adverse event profiles of these drug regimens (Figure 28.6). The incidences of the more severe reactions are detailed in Table 28.5.

Mefloquine

Mefloquine, which has been available for over 20 years, remains a highly effective drug with a protective efficacy of >90% in sub-Saharan Africa. It has a weekly schedule and can be used in young

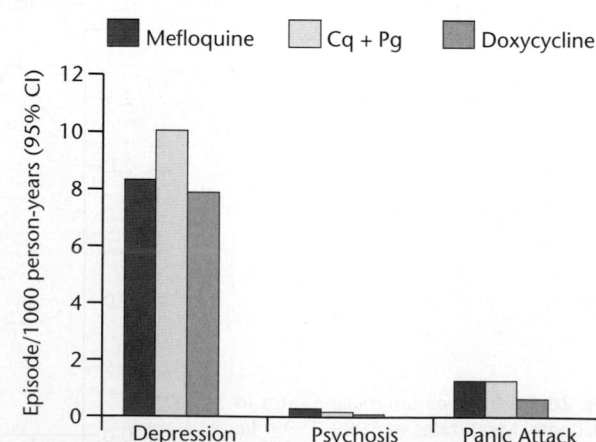

Figure 28.6 Retrospective analysis of neuropsychiatric adverse events associated with three prophylactic regimens. (Adapted from Meier et al.[29])

Table 28.5 Adverse events attributed to chemoprophylaxis, resulting in stopping medication[6,7]

Reported events	Atovaquone + proguanil	Chloroquine + proguanil	Mefloquine
Any treatment-limiting event (%)	1	2	5.5
Gastrointestinal (%)	0	2	1.5
Neuropsychiatric (%)	0.6	0	4

and elderly people, and during most of pregnancy. Nineteen per cent of travellers using mefloquine reported a drug-associated neuropsychiatric problem, predominantly vivid or strange dreams, although a small number reported depression and anxiety. Minor gastrointestinal symptoms also may occur. Neuropsychiatric problems are significantly more common among mefloquine users than among those taking any other prophylactic medication. Serious neuropsychiatric events (convulsions, psychosis, severe depression) attributable to chemoprophylaxis regimens were found to be similar in users of mefloquine as compared with users of proguanil and/or chloroquine, or doxycycline. Rates of psychosis in present and past mefloquine users were calculated at 1 case per 1000 years exposed, while panic attacks occurred in 3 per 1000 years exposed.[29]

Doxycycline

Doxycycline is an effective alternative for persons visiting areas of chloroquine or mefloquine resistance.[30] This drug is contraindicated for pregnant or breast-feeding women, and children under 12 years of age. Side-effects of doxycycline include monilial vaginitis, gastrointestinal symptoms in 37% of users (nausea or vomiting), and very rarely, phototoxicity after sun exposure.[31,32]

Atovaquone and proguanil

This is manufactured in a fixed-dose combination (Malarone®) and has been shown to be effective in the treatment and prophylaxis of malaria.[6,7,33] The combination of atovaquone and proguanil appears to have few side-effects. Occasional reports of mutations leading to therapeutic failure have been described. Cost may be a factor that will limit the wider use of this combination particularly for long-term use. Experience with long-term use of atovaquone and proguanil suggests no new or unexpected toxicity occurs when the drugs are used continuously for 6 months or longer.

Primaquine

Primary prophylaxis with primaquine at a dose of 30 mg daily starting 1 day before exposure and continuing for 1 week after departure from an endemic area provides a protective efficacy against *P. falciparum* of 95% and against *P. vivax* of 90%. Common side-effects following the use of primaquine are abdominal cramps and nausea, which occur in up to 10% of users. More serious is the potential for the drug to lead to acute intravascular haemolysis in people having a deficiency of G6PD. This needs to be excluded (through screening G6PD enzyme levels) before primaquine is prescribed. Primaquine is not licensed for use and is not widely available.

Table 28.6 Major drug regimens and estimated efficacy

Drug regimen and schedule	Estimated prophylactic effectiveness (%)
Atovaquone & proguanil daily	>95
Doxycycline daily	>95
Mefloquine weekly	>95
Primaquine primary prophylaxis	≥85
Primaquine post-exposure prophylaxis	≥90
Chloroquine & proguanil	~40

Terminal prophylaxis and radical therapy (PART) with primaquine is also effective. The recommended regimen is 30 mg daily for 14 days after exposure, and where the individual has been in a hyperendemic transmission region this should be supplemented with a blood schizonticide such as chloroquine or mefloquine. The same cautions apply to this dosing schedule as when used as primary prophylaxis.[34]

Chloroquine and proguanil

The combination of chloroquine and proguanil has been widely used for more than two decades. It has been shown to be safe in all age groups, during pregnancy and in long-term (>5 years) use. However, its protective efficacy has fallen in many parts of the world (Table 28.6), and breakthrough of *P. falciparum* malaria in compliant users is now a common problem. It is now no longer recommended for use in most of sub-Saharan Africa but has a role in regions with low levels of chloroquine resistance such as Central and South America.

Stand-by medication

Travellers to areas with a very low transmission rate of malaria may be advised to carry along a stand-by medication instead of using chemoprophylaxis.[35] Prescribing should always be supported by advice that drugs should be supervised by a health professional and with a laboratory diagnosis of malaria wherever possible. With careful instructions they should be able to self-treat if symptoms associated with malaria develop. The self-treatment can also be used if no medical care can be obtained within 12–24 hours after the onset of illness. Persons using mefloquine or doxycycline for prophylaxis need not carry stand-by medication. There are various concerns about advocating stand-by medication. Malaria symptoms are difficult to explain to untrained persons, and travellers do not always seek professional medical advice or

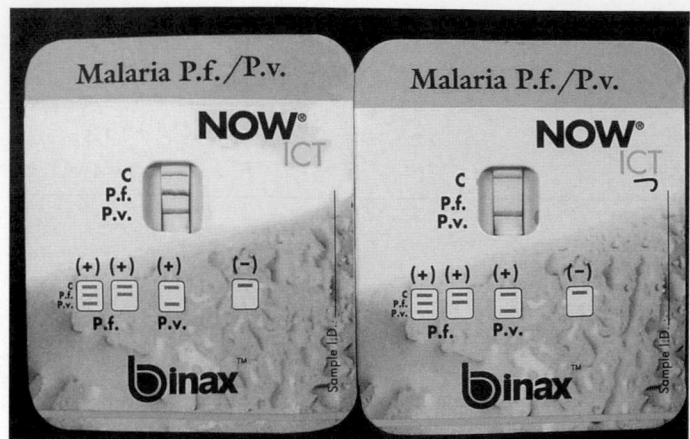

Figure 28.7 Positive HRP2 antigen tests for malaria. Two positive test cards. The left-hand card revealing evidence of a *P. falciparum* and the right-hand card non-*falciparum* (*P. vivax*) malaria. The appearance of a positive test with the control band confirms the test has functioned. The system contains antigen to detect *falciparum* and non-*falciparum* species. The test may be positive for some weeks after all viable parasites have been cleared, as antigen may continue to circulate.

utilize their stand-by treatment when they develop classical symptoms of malaria.[36] Current drugs recommended for use as stand-by medication include chloroquine (only in Central America), Fansidar® (exceptionally), Malarone® and the combination of lumefantrine and artemether (Riamet®). The indications for prescribing stand-by treatment include travel in regions of low transmission where chemoprophylaxis is not taken, or a long period of travel in a highly endemic area where chemoprophylaxis is not fully effective and where appropriate medical facilities are unavailable.

Self-administered diagnostic kits for malaria

Kits for self-diagnosis of *P. falciparum* malaria by travellers are on offer for use in remote areas where there is no access to diagnostic facilities (Figure 28.7). Histidine-rich protein (HRP2) or parasite lactose dehydrogenase (LDH) antigen-capture test-cards work reliably in the laboratory, and have been evaluated by infected travellers. One study found 32% of patients were unable to accurately perform the test,[37] while another study with simplified instructions found over 95% of sick patients successfully diagnosed their *falciparum* malaria.[38] The availability of these kits remains limited, but they could be of significant potential benefit to travellers prescribed stand-by malaria treatment whenever laboratory diagnosis of malaria is not possible.

SEXUALLY TRANSMITTED DISEASES

Casual sexual contacts abroad play an important role in the transmission of sexually transmitted disease (STD) infections.[39] Travel to tropical countries is an important factor in the spread of STDs. In spite of intensive anti-AIDS campaigns, some 5% of European or Canadian tourists have casual sexual contacts abroad. Among young British travellers, 10% reported casual sex while travelling, and 25% did not use condoms. Men's use of condoms was no different to that which they practised at home. Patterns of condom use by women varied according to their partners' backgrounds.[40] The prevalence of STDs is higher in tropical countries than in Western industrialized countries. More than 25% of cases of gonorrhoea treated in Switzerland from 1989 to 1991 were imported from abroad. The penicillin-producing *Neisseria gonorrhoea* (PPNG) strains isolated in Switzerland from 1989 to 1991 were mainly imported from abroad (60%).[41] The typical 'imported STIs' in Switzerland are chancroid, lymphogranuloma venereum and donovanosis. The clinical manifestations, laboratory and special examinations, and treatment of these diseases are described elsewhere. The most frequent STI from the so-called 'imported tropical STIs' is chancroid, which is also a major risk factor associated with the transmission of HIV infection. Data on sexual behaviour of short-term tourists and of long-term overseas workers are of concern.

Long-term male expatriates and workers frequently have casual sex with a local woman or prostitutes.[42] Similar risk behaviour was described in Dutch expatriates working in sub-Saharan Africa, where nearly one in three males had casual sexual contacts with the native population, and regular condom use was reported by less than one-quarter of them.[43] The World Health Organization (WHO) estimates that 75% of all HIV infections worldwide are sexually transmitted and that the efficiency of transmission per sexual contact ranges from 0.1% to 1%. The efficiency can be greatly increased by the presence of other STDs and genital lesions. In populations with a high prevalence rate of HIV and other STDs, as is often the case in female prostitutes in developing countries, the transmission probability of HIV is greatly enhanced. Studies indicate that the prevalence of HIV ranged from 0.4% in Dutch expatriates to 1.1% in Belgians and 8.6% in Danish volunteers. These rates are 100 to 500 times higher when compared to the native population in these countries.[42] Because of the risk of acquiring incurable viral STDs such as HIV, the emphasis should be on safe sex (i.e. always use a condom) for all those who travel and engage in casual sex. Other preventive measures include avoidance of inadequately screened blood. In some regions of West Africa, the risk of HIV infection per unit of blood transfused may be as high as 1%.[44] The use of sterile needles and syringes should be encouraged and these should be included in the travel kit. Hepatitis B in travellers is nearly always acquired through sexual exposure and not contaminated medical products or procedures.

VACCINE-PREVENTABLE DISEASES

Epidemiology

No recent morbidity and mortality data exist on the most frequent vaccine-preventable diseases (Figure 28.1). The incidence of hepatitis A and typhoid fever has significantly decreased from rates identified in the 1970s and 1980s. Recent estimates are that the incidence of hepatitis A in travellers has fallen 50-fold, with an incidence of the order of 10 to 30 per 100000 person-months exposed in all travellers[45] – hepatitis A is the most frequently administered travel vaccine. Typhoid rates are lower by a factor of

10–100 and cholera by a factor of 1000 in comparison to hepatitis A. The risk factors for exposure to these pathogens include duration of stay and hygiene associated with food and beverages (i.e. living with the local population versus in high-class hotels). Previous immunity to hepatitis A can be predicted by the traveller's age, history of previous stays or residence in highly endemic countries, history of jaundice, and immunization status. There is a mortality risk associated with each of these diseases, but it is rarely above 1%. A major risk factor for typhoid fever is a visit to the Indian subcontinent, especially by ethnic travellers when visiting friends and relatives (VFRs). Cholera infection may occur more frequently than reported[46] as it is predominantly symptomless or presents with few symptoms, similar to those of traveller's diarrhoea. It therefore poses no greater threat to travellers and responds to treatment with quinolone antibiotics. The last recorded case of polio in travellers occurred in the current decade, when hajj pilgrims from Africa infected others who in turn reintroduced the infection in Indonesia.

Hepatitis B is mostly diagnosed in expatriates in highly endemic countries, especially those in Asia. Tourists are rarely infected, despite deliberate or inadverent risk behaviour.[47]

The risk of rabies exposure can be significant, as shown in a study of contacts with dogs in Thailand. Nine per cent of respondents were licked and 2% bitten during an average 17-day visit to Thailand. The rate of exposure to animal bites is estimated to be 0.2–0.4% per month; in the majority of these incidents there was some concern about rabies infection.[48]

Yellow fever is extremely rare in travellers; however, several cases in unvaccinated travellers have been reported in the last 10 years, despite the fact travellers to endemic areas should have been immunized. Enhanced adverse event monitoring of yellow fever vaccine administration has brought to light a significant risk of vaccine-associated adverse events (and fatalities) in individuals over 60 years of age if unimmunized individuals or those who have thymus pathology. The prescribing of yellow fever vaccine requires a careful risk–benefit calculation to ensure that unnecessary toxicity is avoided.[49]

There are various other vaccine-preventable diseases about which few epidemiological data in travellers exist, as only anecdotal cases have been reported. The incidence rate of vaccine-preventable disease overall is probably less than 1 per million travellers per month. Outbreaks of meningococcal disease have occurred in situations in which travellers lived in crowded conditions, such as after trekking or after the Hajj to Mecca,[50] but due to compulsory immunization this has no longer been the case in the past few years. Although an increased endemicity of Japanese encephalitis has been observed lately in the indigenous population in an area including all Asian countries east and northeast of India, no more than one case of Japanese encephalitis per year among civilian visitors has been recorded in the literature. Only two cases of plague have been reported in international travellers since 1966.[51] The risk of acquiring a *Mycobacterium tuberculosis* infection during travel was reported as around 2.8 per 1000 person-months of travel. Working in healthcare significantly increased the risk of tuberculosis infection,[52] but even transmission during air, train or bus travel has been reported.[53]

Influenza is the most frequent vaccine-preventable infection associated with travel. Nearly 3% of Swiss travellers showed evidence of seroconversion following a journey[54] which occurred during travel outside the domestic influenza season. The presence and risk of H5N1 influenza for travellers at present is strictly theoretical.

Prevention

Immunizations required for international travel

According to the International Health Regulations, only yellow fever immunization may be required for international travel. Yellow fever vaccination is required for entry into many countries of tropical Africa or northern South America where the infection is endemic. In addition, some countries in Asia and in the Pacific require passengers that have transited through an infected or endemic area within the past 10 days to show proof of vaccination. Some experts also recommend yellow fever vaccination for endemic areas in which no cases of the infection have been detected for decades, such as in East Africa, since the vector is present and epidemics may theoretically occur. Yellow fever vaccination must be performed in centres that are approved by the national authorities, and it must be documented on an International Vaccination Certificate.

There is no valid indication for cholera vaccination, and even remote border posts have gradually realized that this can no longer be required. Saudi Arabia requires pilgrims to be immunized against meningococcal disease. Up-to-date information on mandatory immunizations can also be obtained from travel information manuals (e.g. TIM, TIMATIC) published by several airlines. However, the information regarding recommended immunizations published in these sources may be unreliable.

Routine immunizations

For reasons unrelated to travel, persons living in industrialized countries should be immune against poliomyelitis, tetanus and diphtheria, as well as against measles, mumps, varicella and rubella. As this applies even more for visits to the developing world, a medical consultation prior to departure makes it possible to administer the necessary booster doses, or sometimes to initiate vaccination against these infections.

Recommended immunizations

Hepatitis A immunization may be recommended to any non-immune traveller visiting developing countries (including northern Africa and Turkey for VFRs), but seems to be unnecessary for visits to the Caribbean (except Haiti and the Dominican Republic) or to southern Europe or the western seaboard of the USA. The seroprevalence of anti-HAV antibodies in Europeans is very low in those born after World War II, which makes pre-vaccination testing in this age group unnecessary (except when there is a history of jaundice).

Hepatitis B vaccination is indicated for residents and long-term or frequent travellers staying longer than 1 month in highly endemic countries.[35] It may also be considered for short-term visitors, particularly for young persons likely to travel frequently and those who intend to engage in high-risk activities, e.g. sex, tattooing and ear piercing (although this still leaves them unprotected against HIV infection!).

Vaccination against typhoid fever is indicated for persons who eat and drink in poor hygienic conditions or who have a prolonged stay in developing countries. It is also recommended for all visits to the Indian subcontinent, and long-term travel to Africa and South America.

Rabies vaccination should be considered for all long-term residents, particularly for children and those who will live in close contact with the local population in rabies endemic countries.

Other special-risk vaccinations are those against meningococcal disease using quadrivalent vaccine for stays in the Sahel zone during the winter months, particularly where there is close contacts with the local population and children. Japanese encephalitis vaccine may be recommended for persons who will stay for at least 4 weeks in rural areas in endemic countries. There is no common policy on recommending immunization against tuberculosis to long-term residents abroad; this is determined by local or national policies on the use of BCG.[55,56] In many countries this vaccine is no longer recommended to persons over 1 year of age. Unless any primary vaccination is needed which requires several doses, most vaccines may be given simultaneously during one single consultation.

CONCLUSION

Every physician or nurse who counsels future travellers must tailor specific recommendations to travellers based on a balance of the health risks to be expected during travel with the benefits and tolerance of protective measures. One should not protect or advise travellers against rare risks while failing to advise them against more likely or severe health threats. Four strategies are available to reduce health risks of foreign travel: (i) appropriate behaviour can prevent STIs, reduce the risks of malaria and diarrhoea, and reduce the danger of injuries; (ii) prophylactic drug use can prevent malaria; (iii) drug therapy for traveller's diarrhoea can reduce duration and morbidity of the illness; (iv) immunization can prevent disease without requiring compliance from the traveller.

REFERENCES

1. Hargarten SW, Baker TD, Guptill K. Overseas fatalities of United States citizen travelers: an analysis of deaths related to international travel 2. *Ann Emerg Med* 1991; 20:622–626.
2. Nordberg E. Injuries as a public health problem in sub-Saharan Africa: epidemiology and prospects for control. *East Afr Med J* 2000; 77(12 Suppl): S1–S43.
3. Petridou E, Askitopoulou H, Vourvahakis D, et al. Epidemiology of road traffic accidents during pleasure travelling: the evidence from the Island of Crete. *Accid Anal Prev* 1997; 29:687–693.
4. Centers for Disease Control and Prevention (CDC). Alcohol use and aquatic activities – United States, 1991. *MMWR Morb Mortal Wkly Rep* 1993; 42:681–683.
5. Hawkes S, Hart GJ, Johnson AM, et al. Risk behaviour and HIV prevalence in international travellers. *AIDS* 1994; 8:247–252.
6. Hogh B, Clarke PD, Camus D, et al. Atovaquone-proguanil versus chloroquine-proguanil for malaria prophylaxis in non-immune travellers: a randomised, double-blind study. *Lancet* 2000; 356:1888–1894.
7. Overbosch D, Schilthuis H, Bienzle U, et al. Atovaquone-proguanil versus mefloquine for malaria prophylaxis in nonimmune travelers: results from a randomized, double-blind study. *Clin Infect Dis* 2001; 33:1015–1021.
8. von Sonnenburg F, Tornieporth NG, Waiyaki P, et al. Risk and aetiology of diarrhoea at various tourist destinations. *Lancet* 2000; 356:133–134.
9. Pitzinger B, Steffen R, Tschopp A. Incidence and clinical features of travelers' diarrhea in infants and children. *Pediatr Infect Dis J* 1991; 10:719–723.
10. Steffen R, Collard F, Tornieporth N, et al. Epidemiology, aetiology and impact of travellers' diarrhea in Jamaica. *JAMA* 1999; 281:811–817.
11. Stermer E, Lubezky A, Potasman I, et al. Is traveler's diarrhea a significant risk factor for the development of irritable bowel syndrome? A prospective study. *Clin Infect Dis* 2006; 43:898–901.
12. Gomi H, Jiang ZD, Adachi JA, et al. In vitro antimicrobial susceptibility testing of bacterial enteropathogens causing traveler's diarrhea in four geographic regions. *Antimicrob Agents Chemother* 2001; 45:212–216.
13. Jiang ZD, Lowe B, Verenkar MP, et al. Prevalence of enteric pathogens among international travelers with diarrhea acquired in Kenya (Mombasa), India (Goa), or Jamaica (Montego Bay). *J Infect Dis* 2002; 185:497–502.
14. Ericsson CD. Travelers' diarrhea: epidemiology, prevention and self-treatment. *Infect Dis Clin North Am* 1998; 12:285–303.
15. Mattila L, Siitonen A, Kyronseppa H. Risk behaviour for travelers' diarrhea among Finnish travelers. *J Trav Med* 1995; 2:77–84.
16. DuPont HL, Ericsson CD. Prevention and treatment of travelers' diarrhea. *N Engl J Med* 1993; 328:1821–1827.
17. DuPont HL, Jiang ZD, Okhuysen PC, et al. A randomized, double-blind, placebo-controlled trial of rifaximin to prevent travelers' diarrhea. *Ann Intern Med* 2005; 142:805–812.
18. Peltola H, Siitonen A, Kyronseppa H, et al. Prevention of travellers' diarrhoea by oral B-subunit/whole-cell cholera vaccine. *Lancet* 1991; 338:1285–1289.
19. Wingate D, Phillips SF, Lewis SJ, et al. Guidelines for adults on self-medication for the treatment of acute diarrhoea. *Aliment Pharmacol Ther* 2001; 15:773–782.
20. Mattila L. Clinical features and duration of travelers' diarrhea in relation to its etiology. *Clin Infect Dis* 1994; 19:728–734.
21. De Bruyn G, Hahn S, Borwick A. Antibiotic treatment for travellers' diarrhoea (Cochrane review). *Cochrane Database Syst Rev* 2000; (3):CD002242.
22. Steffen R. Worldwide efficacy of bismuth subsalicylate in the treatment of travelers' diarrhea. *Rev Infect Dis* 1990; 12(suppl 1):S80–S86.
23. DuPont HL, Ericsson CD, Mathewson JJ, et al. Rifaximin: a nonabsorbed antimicrobial in the therapy of travelers' diarrhea. *Digestion* 1998; 59:708–714.
24. Muentener P, Schlagenhauf P, Steffen R. Imported malaria (1985–95): trends and perspectives. *Bull World Health Organ* 1999; 77:560–566.
25. Behrens RH, Bisoffi Z, Björkman A, et al. Malaria prophylaxis policy for travellers from Europe to the Indian Subcontinent. *Malar J* 2006; 5:1–7.
26. Hay SI, Rogers DJ, Toomer JF, et al. Annual *Plasmodium falciparum* entomological inoculation rates (EIR) across Africa: literature survey, internet access and review. *Trans R Soc Trop Med Hyg* 2000; 94:113–127.
27. Rutledge LC, Gupta RK, Mehr ZA, et al. Evaluation of controlled-release mosquito repellent formulations. *J Am Mosq Control Assoc* 1996; 12:39–44.
28. Schoepke A, Steffen R, Gratz N. Effectiveness of personal protection measures against mosquito bites for malaria prophylaxis in travellers. *J Trav Med* 1998; 5:188–192.
29. Meier CR, Wilcock K, Jick SS. The risk of severe depression, psychosis or panic attacks with prophylactic antimalarials. *Drug Saf* 2004; 27:203–213.
30. Ohrt C, Richie TL, Widjaja H, et al. Mefloquine compared with doxycycline for the prophylaxis of malaria in Indonesian soldiers. A randomised, double-blind, placebo-controlled trial. *Ann Intern Med* 1997; 126:963–972.
31. Frost P, Weinstein GD, Gomez EC. Phototoxic potential of minocycline and doxycycline. *Arch Dermatol* 1972; 105:681–683.
32. Schuhwerk M, Behrens RH. Doxycycline as first line malarial prophylaxis: how safe is it? *J Trav Med* 1998; 5:102.

33. Shanks GD, Kremsner PG, Sukwa TY, et al. Atovaquone and proguanil hydrochloride for the chemoprophylaxis of malaria. *J Trav Med* 1999; 6(suppl 1):S21–S27.

34. Hill DR, Baird JK, Parise ME, et al. Primaquine: report from CDC expert meeting on malaria chemoprophylaxis I. *Am J Trop Med Hyg* 2006; 75:402–415.

35. WHO. *International Travel and Health.* Geneva: World Health Organization; 2001.

36. Schlagenhauf P, Steffen R, Tschopp A, et al. Behavioural aspects of travellers in their use of malaria presumptive treatment. *Bull World Health Organ* 1995; 73:215–221.

37. Jelinek T, Amsler L, Grobusch MP, et al. Self-use of rapid tests for malaria diagnosis by tourists. *Lancet* 1999; 354:1609.

38. Whitty CJM, Armstrong M, Behrens RH. Self-testing for falciparum malaria with antigen-capture cards by travellers with symptoms of malaria. *Am J Trop Med Hyg* 2000; 63:295–297.

39. Mulhall BP. Sex and travel: studies of sexual behaviour, disease and health promotion in international travellers – a global review. *Int J STD AIDS* 1996; 7:455–465.

40. Bloor M, Thomas M, Hood K, et al. Differences in sexual risk behaviour between young men and women travelling abroad from the UK. *Lancet* 1998; 352:1664–1668.

41. Eichmann A. Sexually transmissible diseases following travel in tropical countries. *Schweiz Med Wochenschr* 1993; 123:1250–1255.

42. Bonneux L, Van der Stuyft P, Taelman H, et al. Risk factors for infection with human immunodeficiency virus among European expatriates in Africa. *BMJ* 1988; 297:581–584.

43. de Graaf R, van Zessen G, Houweling H, et al. Sexual risk of HIV infection among expatriates posted in AIDS endemic areas. *AIDS* 1997; 11:1173–1181.

44. Savarit D, De Cock KM, Schutz R, et al. Risk of HIV infection from transfusion with blood negative for HIV antibody in a west African city. *BMJ* 1992; 305:498–502.

45. Mutsch M, Spicher V, Gut C, et al. Hepatitis A virus infections in travelers, 1988–2004. *Clin Infect Dis* 2006; 42:490–497.

46. Mahon BE, Mintz ED, Greene KD, et al. Reported cholera in the United States, 1992–1994: a reflection of global changes in cholera epidemiology. *JAMA* 1996; 276:307–312.

47. Zuckerman JN, Steffen R. Risks of hepatitis B in travellers as compared to immunisation status. *J Trav Med* 2000; 7:170–174.

48. Bernard KW, Fishbein DB. Pre-exposure rabies prophylaxis for travellers: are the benefits worth the cost? *Vaccine* 1991; 9:833–836.

49. Khromava AY, Eidex RB, Weld LH, et al. Yellow fever vaccine: an updated assessment of advanced age as a risk factor for serious adverse events. *Vaccine* 2005; 23:3256–3263.

50. Taha MK, Achtman M, Alonso JM, et al. Serogroup W135 meningococcal disease in Hajj pilgrims. *Lancet* 2000; 356:2159.

51. Centers for Disease Control (CDC). Imported bubonic plague. *MMWR Morb Mort Wkly Rep* 1990; 39:895–901.

52. Cobelens FG, van Deutekom H, Draayer-Jansen IW, et al. Risk of infection with *Mycobacterium tuberculosis* in travellers to areas of high tuberculosis endemicity. *Lancet* 2000; 356:461–465.

53. Moore M, Valway SE, Ihle W, et al. A train passenger with pulmonary tuberculosis: evidence of limited transmission during travel. *Clin Infect Dis* 1999; 28:52–56.

54. Mutsch M, Tavernini M, Marx A, et al. Influenza virus infection in travelers to tropical and subtropical countries. *Clin Infect Dis* 2005; 10:1282–1287.

55. Lifson AR. *Mycobacterium tuberculosis* infection in travellers: tuberculosis comes home. *Lancet* 2000; 356:442–443.

56. Whitty CJM, Macallan DC, Lewis DJM. Use of BCG vaccination. *Lancet* 2000; 356:1609–1610.

Chapter 29   Kenneth J. Collins

Heat Stress and Associated Disorders

Human capacity to cope with the stress of hot environments is founded on an extremely efficient thermoregulatory system together with ancillary cardiovascular, osmotic, fluid balance and endocrine systems. Heat disorders appear when individuals are exposed suddenly to heat loads to which they are unaccustomed or with heat loads to which adaptation is not possible. This often occurs in heat waves or with increased physical exertion in hot conditions and when newcomers are first exposed to the tropics. Important factors increasing the risk of heat disorders include high environmental humidity, existing illness particularly cardiovascular or metabolic diseases, age, dehydration, medications affecting thermoregulation, and the lack of heat acclimatization. For many years, WHO Task Groups[1] have attempted to predict the potential health effects of global climatic change. As considered later in this chapter, disorders due to heat are increasingly likely to be one of the direct effects of global warming expected to influence human health both in the tropics and adjacent regions.

BODY TEMPERATURE REGULATION

Heat balance is maintained by the thermoregulatory system despite considerable heat loads imposed by heat stress from the environment and physical work.[2] Deep body temperature is, however, not held rigidly constant since temperature homeostasis allows body temperature fluctuations, normally about a ±0.3°C diurnal change at rest in a neutral environment, and ±2.0°C in more extreme ambient conditions and physical activity.

A rise in skin temperature and vasodilatation is an initial response to hot conditions brought about by vasomotor reflexes acting through the thermoregulatory centres in the brain and spinal cord and by the direct effects of heat on skin blood vessels. Much of the large increase in skin blood flow comes from opening of arteriovenous anastamoses deep to the skin capillaries. Dilatation of the large cutaneous vascular network causes a redistribution of blood from the body core to the skin and concomitantly a reduction in splanchnic blood flow. The compensatory fall in renal and hepatic blood flow produces oliguria in the heat and a reduced hepatic metabolic clearance. Skin temperature continues to rise in hot conditions and approaches 35°C over the whole body surface. At or near this point the deep body temperature is stabilized by the secretion of sweat. Sweating enhances body heat loss considerably, with 670 watts of power lost for every litre of sweat evaporated. Unevaporated sweat that drips from the body surface (which occurs particularly in humid environments) does not contribute to heat loss but simply adds to the loss of fluid. In extreme conditions with prolonged work, up to 10 L of hypotonic fluid may be lost during a day by profuse sweating, though this rate of sweating is usually not maintained. Serious dehydration is therefore a possible outcome within 24 h especially when water supplies are absent or scarce. With fluid loss by sweating there is also a loss of salt, which may pose another important problem – body salt depletion. Salt concentration in sweat may vary from about 1 g/L in heat-acclimatized personnel to 3 g/L in those who are not acclimatized. The rate of sweating, dietary intake of salt, and adrenal corticosteroid activity are all variables that determine sweat salt concentration and therefore the rate at which salt depletion occurs.

Cardiovascular strain develops with increasing demand for a higher cardiac output to transfer heat and water to vasodilated vascular beds. In resting conditions, extensive shunting of blood to the skin induces a fall in blood pressure and an increase in heart rate. With an adequate venous pressure, stroke volume is maintained and cardiac output increased. Dehydration as the result of excessive sweating, however, leads to a marked decrease in circulating blood volume, a reduction in stroke volume and an increased heart rate. Exercise in hot conditions presents a physiological dilemma to the body when blood must be shunted to working muscles as well as to the skin in order to maintain thermoregulation. In unacclimatized humans there is an initial period of cardiovascular instability which accompanies increasing body temperature and heart rate. Stability returns with acclimatization when plasma volume and stroke volume increase and heart rate decreases. Several standard works describe these and other general thermoregulatory responses to heat in greater detail.[3-5] Thermoregulation during exposure to heat and exercise differs between children and adults, mainly due to a lower sweating capacity and to metabolic, circulatory and hormonal disparities in children.[6]

Thermoregulation is integrated by a controlling system in structures in the brain and spinal cord which respond to the heat content of tissues. Receptors sensitive to thermal information from the skin, deep tissues and in the central nervous system itself provide feedback signals to this system. Principal centres reside in the hypothalamus where the temperature of blood perfusing the hypothalamus is a major drive to temperature control. Ideas on a putative hypothalamic 'set-point' have been developed in order to explain how body temperature is maintained at predetermined constant levels. The central thermoregulatory interface appears to consist essentially of two pathways from sensors with differing responses to thermal changes, and crossed inhibition between these two pathways. The effect may be to create a temperature null point or null zone.[7] Excessive increases in brain temperature are likely to affect the integrative function of central nervous structures and have profound deleterious consequences on the temperature control system. It has been postulated that some protection of the brain against hyperthermia may be provided by a countercurrent system in the blood supply of the face and head which permits selective cooling of the brain.[8]

Heat acclimatization and work performance

Writing more than 200 years ago on the heat hazard to newcomers to the tropics, Lind[9] pointed out that habituation to hot climates reduces the danger to health. The process of heat acclimatization was originally associated with an improved ability to perform work in the heat. In fact a useful degree of acclimatization to heat can be attained simply by hard physical training in a cool environment. The immediate physiological responses to acute heat stress give way to reduced signs of heat strain after a few days of work in hot conditions. Heart rate and deep body temperature do not rise so high and the sweating mechanism becomes more efficient. Total sweat rates of 0.5 to 1 L/h may increase to 2 L/h or more in a fully acclimatized man, though such high rates cannot be maintained for many hours. A major part of the improvement in sweat output is due to increased cellular secretory capacity of the sweat glands brought about by sweat gland 'training'. With the initial acclimatization process, the salt content of sweat is reduced in response to adrenal mineralocorticoids. Longer-term acclimatization to heat is associated with increments in blood volume, plasma volume, extracellular fluid volume and total body water content.

Heat tolerance can be achieved artificially by daily 1–2 h sessions of controlled hyperthermia or work-rest routines for 3–4 h in a climatic chamber (acclimation) or normal heavy daily physical work in a tropical environment (acclimatization). The adaptive process develops rapidly over the first 3 or 4 days and is virtually complete by 9 or 10 days (Figure 29.1). During this time, there is a progressive reduction in deep body temperature and heart rate with a concomitant increase in the amount of sweat produced. When exposure to heat and work ceases, the physiological adaptations are partly retained for up to 1 or 2 weeks but thereafter the benefits are rapidly lost.

Part of the longer-term process of heat adaptation involves behavioural adjustments, such as resting during the hottest part of the day. This is intuitive to tropical indigenes who normally will seek to avoid the stresses of hyperthermia, and in consequence may often not be fully heat acclimatized. Data drawn from physiological and anthropometric investigations tend to support the view that adult body form varies among populations so as to confer some advantage in the environment inhabited. The hot, dry climate that is the natural habitat of Nilotic people, for example, appears to confer morphological features of linearity and

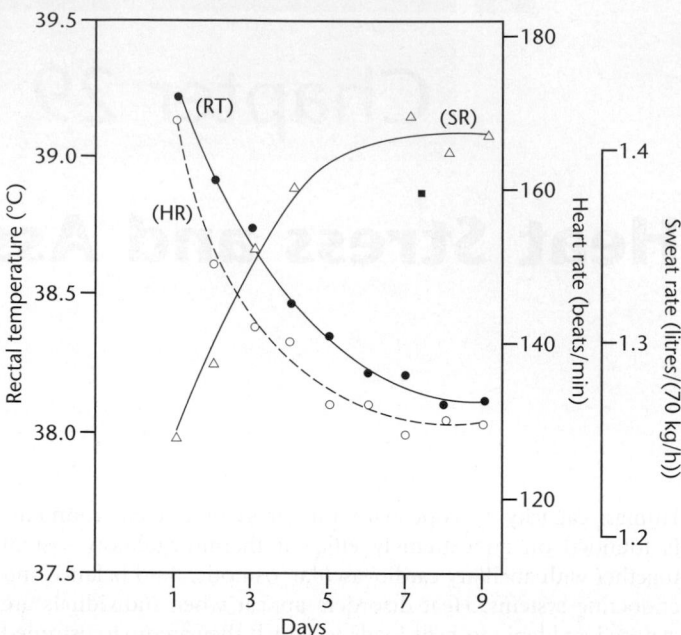

Figure 29.1 Typical mean rectal temperatures (•), heart rates (○) and sweat rates (△) in a group of men during the development of acclimatization to heat. (Adapted from Leithead and Lind 1964. All attempts at tracing copyright holder unsuccessful.)

high surface area to body weight. A process of selection in favour of smaller body size appears as an adaptive response to a hot, humid environment in equatorial forests where heat loss through sweating is less effective. Fitness and physical work capacity are regarded as fundamental determinants of human survival, and in many tropical populations agricultural work continues to underpin local economies. The relationship between working capacity, heat acclimatization and avoidance of heat disorders plays an important role in human ability to exploit the tropical habitat.[10]

HEAT STRESS

The heat stress of a given situation is measured by the combination of all those factors contributing to the heat gain of the body. It is therefore necessary to consider both climatic and non-climatic factors and, in some way, to evaluate their combined effects. Climatic factors include ambient temperature, humidity and air movement; non-climatic variables take account of physical activity and clothing. The resultant human thermal strain is usually assessed by two physiological measurements – core temperature and heart rate. Tolerance limits for work in adverse temperature conditions are commonly based on acceptable 'safe' levels of these two measurements, and in hot conditions the limits are usually 38.0°C core temperature and 180 beats per minute heart rate in normal healthy adults.

Heat stress indices provide a means of assessing hot environments and to predict their likely effect on people. Such indices provide the equivalence of various environmental factors,[11] usually with physical activity and clothing as independent variables. A number of different heat stress indices have been proposed which are divided broadly into those empirically derived and substantiated by the physiological effects on a test group of people, and those derived by theoretical consideration of the effects on the body's heat balance. No index or standard is universally applicable since all are affected to differing degrees by components of the thermal environment, clothing and metabolism. The wet bulb globe temperature (WBGT) index calculated from 0.7 wet bulb +0.2 globe (radiant) +0.1 dry bulb temperature is probably most widely used for outdoor activities where solar radiation is a component of the heat stress.[12] Safe physical activity schedules may be set according to the predicted environmental heat loads for the day, e.g. WBGT <18°C (low risk), WBGT >28°C (very high risk).[13] Better understanding of human thermoregulation and the processes of heat exchange have led to the development of mathematical models of human responses to hot environments, and the introduction of the digital computer has provided the opportunity for these relatively complex models to be conveniently used in practical applications.[14] In order to further improve the techniques for assessing the risks of heat disorders encountered during work in hot conditions European research teams have developed a 'heat strain model'.[15] This has now been accepted as the present international standard heat assessment method.[16]

HEAT DISORDERS

The pathological conditions associated with the effects of heat arise from four main aetiologies:
1. Circulatory instability
   a. Heat syncope
   b. Heat oedema
2. Heat-induced skin disorders
   a. Hidromeiosis
   b. Prickly heat (miliaria rubra)
   c. Anhidrotic heat exhaustion
3. Water and electrolyte imbalance
   a. Heat cramps
   b. Water-depletion heat exhaustion
   c. Salt-depletion heat exhaustion
4. Hyperthermic failure of thermoregulation
   a. Heat stroke.

Another category of heat disorder is sometimes described under the general heading of psychological effects of heat.[17] The predominant effects are characterized by deterioration in performance and loss of efficiency, presenting as 'acute heat neurasthenia' or 'tropical fatigue'. Heat neurotic syndromes are ill-defined and may not be attributable solely to the effects of heat.

Any factor that compromises the normal processes of thermoregulation may be implicated in the aetiology of heat disorders. Personnel most at risk have a history of heat intolerance, are overweight or physically unfit. Even in athletes, the combination of heat, humidity and exercise may sometimes result in heat illness.[18] There is sometimes failure on the part of the supervising authority, or the individuals themselves, to appreciate the potential dangers involved in exposure to severe heat stress.

Heat exposure may aggravate underlying pathology especially cardiovascular disease, and in this respect the elderly are particularly at risk. Occult infections have been observed to cause transient anhidrosis, and the influence of endogenous pyrogens can raise the 'set-point' around which body temperature is regulated.

Many heat stroke victims present with a previous history of infection or fever. Heat intolerance can also be extreme in cases of thyrotoxicosis, mucoviscidosis and congenital absence of sweat glands in ectodermal dysplasia.

Chemicals and medications may have direct effects on the control of body temperature, and some have indirect effects through induced toxicity reactions or drug interactions.[19] Special care is required in high temperature conditions with patients who have been prescribed diuretics, anticholinergics or central nervous stimulants or depressants.

It remains to say that there may be disorders other than those listed above which are causally related to heat stress. For example, it seems possible that environmental heat may be implicated in the pathogenesis of renal stones in hot countries where sub-clinical water-depletion is commonplace.

Minor heat disorders

Heat oedema

Mild swelling of the feet and ankles may be experienced by unacclimatized people arriving in the tropics, which with rest usually resolves within a few days. The aetiology is likely to be due to cutaneous vasodilatation and venous stasis in the legs. Mild oedema may also be a manifestation of an expansion of the extracellular space, influenced by aldosterone and antidiuretic hormone activity. Some newcomers to hot climates show their apprehension of the heat by overloading themselves with salt and water.

Heat syncope

It is common knowledge that fainting may follow prolonged standing, sudden postural changes or unaccustomed exercise, particularly in hot surroundings. Heat syncope occurs because of peripheral vascular pooling of blood and collapse of venomotor tone leading to hypotension and cerebral anoxia. The patient suddenly becomes pale with heart rate at first increasing and then slowing, and breathing is slow and sighing in nature. Consciousness is usually lost for a minute or so, but returns as cerebral circulation is restored when the patient is placed in the head-low position. Other causes of loss of consciousness must be excluded. Syncope may be the prelude to more serious heat disorders such as heat exhaustion or heat stroke.

Heat cramps

Heat-induced muscle cramps are probably due to a mild water intoxication or to salt depletion, occurring in people who are sweating profusely while at the same time drinking large amounts of unsalted fluids. Cramps may also be experienced by those who exercise regularly while adhering to a low-salt diet. The spasms usually last less than 1 min, occasionally for 2 or 3 min, but they may recur every few minutes for several hours. Heat cramps must be distinguished from tetany, which can sometimes occur in individuals with raised body temperature who may hyperventilate sufficiently to develop acute respiratory alkalosis.

Intravenous normal saline (0.5–1 L) can be given to treat severe cramps, or even a small quantity of 5% hypertonic saline. This should be followed by liberal quantities of salt in drinks until the urine contains at least 2–3 g chloride per litre. Heat cramps can usually be prevented in hot working conditions by the provision of salted drinks at the place of work.

Skin disorders with sweat suppression

Hidromeiosis

The term hidromeiosis is applied to a particular type of reduction in sweating associated with wetting the skin,[11] previously thought to represent 'sweat gland fatigue'. Sweat evaporation may diminish when there is wetting of the skin in hot, humid climates. In this case, suppression of sweating is caused by obstruction of sweat glands by swelling of the keratin layer of the skin and closure of sweat pores when water is absorbed at high skin temperatures. The process can be readily reversed by moving into a cool, dry environment. Hyperthermia develops more readily in hot humid conditions because of hidromeiosis and lack of effective evaporative cooling.

Prickly heat

This common skin complaint in hot climates causes considerable irritation and discomfort, also arising from prolonged wetting of the skin by sweat.[20] Maceration of the stratum corneum causes acute (*miliaria rubra*) or chronic (*miliaria profunda*) blockage of the sweat ducts. The pathogenesis therefore resembles that of hidromeiosis, but the sweat glands become more permanently blocked by plugs of mucopolysaccharide debris and there is distension of the sweat ducts. The rash of miliaria rubra (prickly heat) is an erythematous epidermal vesicular eruption that is pruritic, and it is accompanied by a prickling or tingling sensation when sweating is provoked. Subsequently miliaria profunda may develop, characterized by dermal vesicles without erythema or pruritus giving the affected skin area a gooseflesh appearance (Figure 29.2).[21] Secondary bacterial and fungal infections can occur.

Treatment consists of removing the patient to cool quarters if possible to avoid sweating, and removing tight-fitting clothing. Prickling can be relieved by a cool shower, thorough drying of the skin and application of calamine lotion or zinc oxide powder. Mildly astringent lotions such as those containing mercuric chloride may be useful, as are topical antimicrobial agents.

Anhidrotic heat exhaustion

Impairment of sweating by miliaria profunda or other skin disorders may lead to a state of heat exhaustion and heat intolerance affecting personnel exposed for several months to a hot climate. Humid heat is responsible for most cases but the disorder may occur in desert climates. Dyshidrosis is probably a more accurate term to describe the sweat suppression since complete absence of sweating does not usually occur. Exfoliative dermatitis and other atrophic skin disorders are sometimes involved. Patients are unable to perform even limited amounts of physical work without suffering undue fatigue and discomfort in the heat. Attempts to do so may precipitate other heat disorders, including heat stroke.

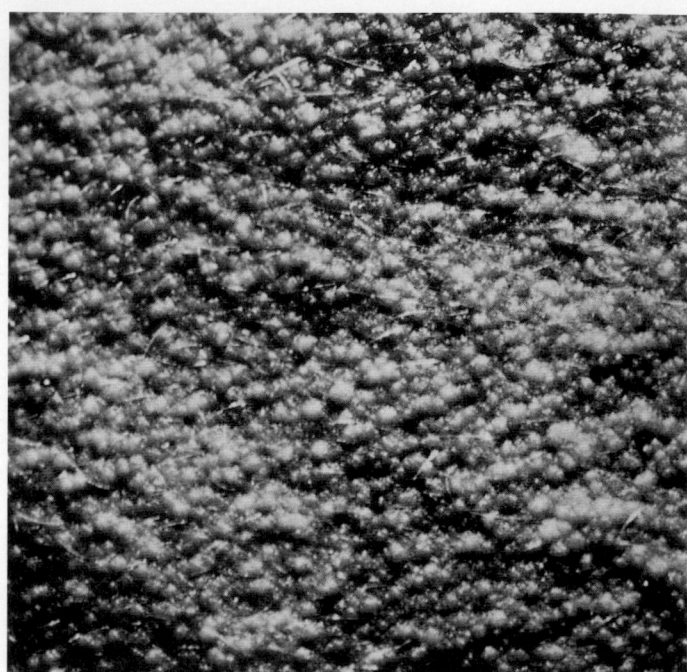

Figure 29.2 Miliaria profunda. Photographic enlargement of human skin. (From Horne and Mole 1951.[21])

Body fluid imbalance

Water-depletion heat exhaustion

People working in hot conditions frequently do not completely replace the volume of water lost by sweating (voluntary dehydration) and usually maintain a slight negative water balance averaging 1 or 2% of total body weight. This minor degree of dehydration, however, appears to be sufficient to impair maximum physical performance.[22] More serious degrees of dehydration develop when water supplies are scarce. Though water depletion is thought to cause mild reductions in thermal sweating, high sweat rates to defend body temperature appear to be possible during dehydration. The classic situations producing water-depletion heat exhaustion have been described among castaways at sea in the tropics, travellers stranded in the desert, labourers in hot mines and in service personnel. An accessory factor is often the additional loss of fluid due to vomiting and diarrhoea.

Dehydration due predominantly to water depletion is characterized by intense thirst, fatigue, weakness, anxiety and impaired judgement. Irritability and syncope appear as water loss approaches 6% of body weight. Urine is scanty and concentrated. Extracellular fluid volume is diminished, with increasing osmolality, and water moves from the cells into the extracellular compartment (Figure 29.3A,B). Haemoconcentration is slight at first and serum protein and sodium levels elevated. In severe water depletion the partial preservation of ECF at the expense of ICF is probably related to secondary aldosteronism.

It is important to decide whether heat exhaustion is due mainly to salt or water depletion, although there is usually a mixed depletion. The circumstances of onset are usually quite different. Sweat is hypotonic and a relatively far greater amount of water than salt

Table 29.1 Differential diagnosis of salt- and water-depletion heat exhaustion

	Predominant salt-depletion	Predominant water-depletion
Duration of symptoms	3–5 days	Often less than 3–5 days
Thirst	Not prominent	Prominent
Fatigue	Marked	Less marked
Giddiness	Prominent	Less prominent
Muscle cramps	In most cases	Absent
Vomiting	In most cases	Usually absent
Thermal sweating	Usually unchanged	Diminished
Haemoconcentration	Early and marked	Slight until late
Urine chloride	Negligible	Normal
Blood sodium	Below average	Above average
Mode of death	Oligaemic shock	Oligaemic shock; heat stroke

Leithead CS & Lind AR. Heat Stress and Heat Disorders. London: Cassell Plc; 1964. (All attempts at tracing copyright holder unsuccesful)

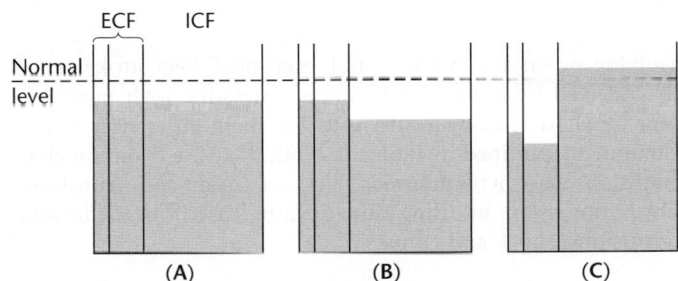

Figure 29.3 The effect of (A) mild water depletion, (B) severe water depletion, and (C) sodium depletion, on the partition of fluid between extracellular fluid (ECF) and intracellular fluid (ICF) compartments.

is lost so that progressive water depletion is always more rapid in development than salt depletion. Differential diagnosis may be established by the symptoms and signs shown in Table 29.1. In its most severe form, in individuals stranded in hot dehydrating desert conditions without water, the situation may become rapidly fatal within a day. Studies of dehydration in the desert suggest that death is ultimately due to oligaemic shock and to heat stroke due to loss of thermoregulatory control.[17]

Treatment consists of rest in cool surroundings with carefully controlled rehydration sufficient to ensure a net gain of 2–3 L over the first 24 h and 0.5–1 L/day subsequently. Excessively rapid correction of hypernatraemia may cause cerebral oedema, convulsive seizures and possibly death due to uncal herniation. Unconscious patients will require intravenous fluid replacement and if there is doubt whether the patient is predominantly water depleted or salt depleted, isotonic saline should be given; otherwise the fluid of choice is 5% glucose solution. Recovery is indicated by increased urine output but it is essential to avoid fluid overload if renal damage has occurred.

Salt-depletion heat exhaustion

In unacclimatized personnel, there is usually a higher salt content in sweat, and enough salt may be lost to cause a negative salt balance during the first few days of heat exposure. Daily losses in

5 L of sweat per day may amount to 15 g of salt and supplementation of dietary salt is required. Extra salt is usually unnecessary when heat acclimatization takes place since salt balance is restored after a few days by the salt-conserving action of aldosterone on the kidney and sweat glands.

Clinical findings in human salt deficiency include reduced plasma volume with haemoconcentration (Table 29.1). The concentration of sodium and chloride in urine is low. Extracellular fluid osmolality is reduced, causing hypovolaemia and a shift of fluid into the intracellular compartment (Figure 29.3C). Plasma sodium concentration may sometimes be deceptively normal but the sodium and chloride content of whole blood is reduced. Fatigue, giddiness, nausea and muscle cramps are common clinical features. Anorexia, diarrhoea and vomiting reduce the already inadequate intake of salt, establishing a vicious circle of events. Thirst is not a feature, unlike water depletion. In contrast to predominant water depletion, salt depletion does not generally predispose rapidly to heat stroke.

Treatment is usually easier than for water depletion and consists of bed rest in cool conditions with a high salt intake in the form of salted drinks. Salt should be added to cool fruit drinks (7 g/L) and salty food encouraged to achieve an intake of up to 20 g daily. Complete clinical recovery occurs usually only after 5–7 days bed rest and salt replacement, and is accompanied by the consistent appearance of significant amounts of chloride in urine. For comatose patients, isotonic saline may be given intravenously at the rate of 2–4 L during 12–24 h. When extreme hyponatraemia causes symptoms of water intoxication, rarely is hypertonic saline indicated. It is important to examine neck veins and lung bases during treatment for signs of circulatory overloading.

Heat stroke

Heat stroke, sometimes considered to be a tropical neurological disorder,[23] is caused by an excessive rise in deep body temperature due to thermoregulatory failure. It is characterized primarily by hyperthermia usually with core temperature above 40.6°C, central nervous system dysfunction resulting from tissue damage, metabolic derangement and coma. Heat stroke is the least common but most serious of heat disorders and it carries a high mortality

Table 29.2 Presentation of 'classical' and 'exertional' heat stroke

	'Classical'	'Exertional'
Age group	Infants, elderly	15–65 years old
Health status	Chronic illness	Usually healthy
History of febrile illness	Occasionally	Common
Activity	Sedentary	Usually highly active
Drug use	Diuretics, phenothiazines	Amphetamines, cocaine
Sweating	Usually absent	Usually present
Respiratory alkalosis	Dominant	Mild
Lactic acidosis	Absent or mild	Often marked
Rhabdomyolysis	Seldom severe	Severe
Creatinine phosphokinase/aldolase	Mildly elevated	Markedly elevated
Disseminated intravascular coagulation	Mild	Marked
Hypoglycaemia	Uncommon	Common

Knochel JP. Heat stroke and related heat disorders. Dis Mon 1989; 35:301-377.

rate if effective treatment is not given immediately. The high mortality in heat stroke may be secondary to multi-organ dysfunction.[24] For survivors, there is a risk of permanent neurological damage. In circumstances where heat disorders can be expected,[25] heat exhaustion syndromes usually occur up to ten times more frequently than heat stroke in the population at risk.

Epidemiology

Heat stroke occurs during heat waves even in temperate regions. Infants, the elderly and patients with heart disease are most at risk in the community during hot weather. Heat stroke also occurs in physically active people, e.g. service personnel, marathon runners during prolonged exercise or those engaged in hard work in hot conditions. Each year, a mass of people, currently about two million, gather at Mecca for the seven-day pilgrimage, the *Makkah Hajj*. There is high radiant heat and ambient temperature, aggravated by many people assembled in a restricted area. Lack of acclimatization, arduous physical rituals, and exposed spaces with limited or no shade pose a major heat threat to many pilgrims. Adequate fluid intake and seeking shade are essential.[26] During years when the *Hajj* takes place in seasons of mild weather conditions, there are very few heat-related hospital admissions.[27]

In many tropical countries precise statistics for morbidity and mortality are not available because of poor certification and the difficulty in defining the size and composition of the population at risk. In the South African gold mines, where the working population is homogeneous in its social background, heat stroke cases have been reported at rates of 0.3/1000 per year in environments of 32°C wet bulb temperature and 4.0/1000 per year at 34.4°C wet bulb.[28] Reported mortality ratios for heat stroke varied considerably at treatment centres during the 1980–82 Makkah Pilgrimages, ranging from 5% to 80%,[25] but it is not always clear whether treated cases have been included.

Aetiology

Two types of heat stroke have been described: 'classical' heat stroke associated with intolerably hot conditions or heat waves but not involving significant exertion, and 'exertional' heat stroke generally observed in younger individuals generating high metabolic loads by physical work in the heat. The main differences in presentation are outlined in Table 29.2, but there are common characteristics, e.g. hyperthermia, lack of heat acclimatization, dehydration, skin mottling and flushing, psychotic behaviour, convulsions, shock and coma.

Pathology

At about 42°C deep body temperature, hyperthermia causes denaturation of enzymes, liquefaction of membrane lipids, mitochondrial damage and destabilization of lipoproteins. The high temperature is primarily responsible for tissue damage, but cellular hypoxia, congestion, endotoxaemia and disseminated intravascular coagulation (DIC) are contributory.

Among the classically described anatomical changes found at autopsy are oedema of the brain and meninges, neuronal degeneration and petechial haemorrhages. The predominance of changes in cerebellar structures corresponds to the clinical picture of central nervous damage in patients who survive heat stroke. These patients often show cerebellar ataxia with marked dysarthria, polyneuropathy or dysmetria. Haemorrhages are also observed in serous cavities and in the heart, kidney, liver and gastrointestinal mucosa. Myocardial damage is common and, characteristically, subendocardial haemorrhages occur beneath the left interventricular septum. Skeletal muscle may show necrosis if rhabdomyolysis has accompanied heat stroke.[29] Liver damage is one of the most prominent features, with centrilobular fatty changes, congestion and degenerating hepatocytes resembling Councilman bodies. The kidneys are damaged and show hyperaemia and petechial haemorrhages. Deleterious effects in the blood include haemolysis, thrombocytopaenia, megakaryocyte damage, DIC and widespread fibrin deposition. DIC contributes to both the bleeding manifestations and shock syndrome.[25] As may be predicted, increased pro-inflammatory cytokine concentrations have been implicated in the pathogenesis of heat stroke.[30] Measurement of antibody against heat-shock proteins in patients with acute heat-induced illness may be one biomarker to evaluate susceptibility to excessive heat stress.[31]

Clinical features

In most cases of heat stroke the onset of delirium or coma is sudden but, in some cases, several days of ill-health precede the onset of coma and severe hyperthermia. With acute-onset heat stroke, prodromal symptoms lasting minutes or hours include headache, disorientation, stupor, emotional outbursts, dizziness, excessive thirst and locomotor changes.

Central nervous disturbances are typical presenting features. Often the patient is in coma with a rectal temperature of 40.6°C or more and there may be involuntary movements closely resembling epilepsy with tonic and clonic convulsions, and frequently urinary and faecal incontinence. Hyperpnoea with tetany[25] is sometimes observed. Sweating can be present at the stage of collapse, particularly in young active heat stroke casualties, so that anhidrosis with a hot, dry skin, thought to be a common feature of heat stroke cases, cannot therefore be regarded as pathognomic. On admission, the patient's pulse is thready and the face flushed or cyanotic. In some cases, blood pressure and pulse pressure may be increased, whereas in others there is profound hypotension and shock. The electrocardiogram often shows flattened or inverted t waves, transient conduction abnormalities and myocardial damage. Echocardiographic and Doppler studies reflect a hyperdynamic circulation with tachycardia and high cardiac output states in severe heat exposure.[32] Relative hypovolaemia and signs of peripheral vasoconstriction are more often present in heat stroke than in heat exhaustion. Gastrointestinal haemorrhage with haematemesis or melaena can sometimes occur as manifestations of coagulopathy.

Diagnosis

Heat stroke can be suspected in any patient who loses consciousness under conditions of heat stress. The diagnosis is highly probable if body temperature is above 40°C in the presence of clinical features described above. Measurement of rectal temperature is crucial but is often difficult in a struggling patient. High-reading, metal-cased thermometers or electronic probes should be made available where heat stroke is a known risk.

Cooling measures are urgently required, leaving little time for exploring alternative diagnoses. The possibility of high fevers from other causes, must, however, be kept under consideration. In the tropics, malaria is the most important differential diagnosis. High fevers from other causes such as meningitis, *salmonella* and arbovirus infections, encephalitis, bacterial pneumonia, septicaemia, tetanus and cerebral (pontine) haemorrhage are also to be considered. It is important to examine the skull for signs of injury which may have occurred during convulsions.

Laboratory findings include leucocytosis and thrombocytopaenia. Changes in plasma concentration of sodium, chloride and potassium are not consistent, though hypokalaemia has been frequently observed in heat stroke. Serum glutamic oxaloacetic transaminase, glutamic pyruvic transaminase, lactic dehydrogenase and creatine phosphokinase are usually elevated within 24 h of admission. The levels continue to rise for about 2 days and remain elevated for 12–14 days. Serum enzyme changes are of diagnostic

and prognostic significance. Severe renal involvement with rising urea nitrogen is evident in many fatal cases.

Treatment

In the field situation, the patient should be placed in the shade, clothing removed and the skin kept wet and fanned. An effective degree of conductive cooling can be attained simply by immersing the patient in a bath of cold water with the body and limbs massaged vigorously to promote skin circulation. In hospital, the patient may be placed on a slatted trolley, exposing the skin to good air movement from a fan and a fine spray of water. Alternatively, the patient can be cooled by tepid water sponging or by wrapping in a wet sheet and fanning.

The need to avoid vasoconstriction during cooling and yet enable the management of a violent, delirious, incontinent and vomiting patient has led to the development of a Body Cooling Unit (BCU) to treat heat stroke (Figure 29.4).[33] The method utilizes evaporative and convective cooling from sprays of atomized water at 20°C combined with a powerful flow of air at 45–50°C to maintain skin temperature above 31–32°C. Instrumentation has been developed to measure the combination of deep body and skin temperature of the individual patient and display the most effective temperature of air and water for cooling. The BCU has proved to be highly effective in the management of classical heat stroke patients among the *Hajj* pilgrims.[25]

Ice water immersion is a simple and available form of treatment which has been advocated since the first edition of this textbook was published in 1898.[34] The method, however, appears to deny a critical principle of heat dissipation by preventing cutaneous vasodilatation. However, it has been suggested that the hydrostatic pressure of water during immersion increases venous return to the heart in hypotensive heat stroke patients, and that

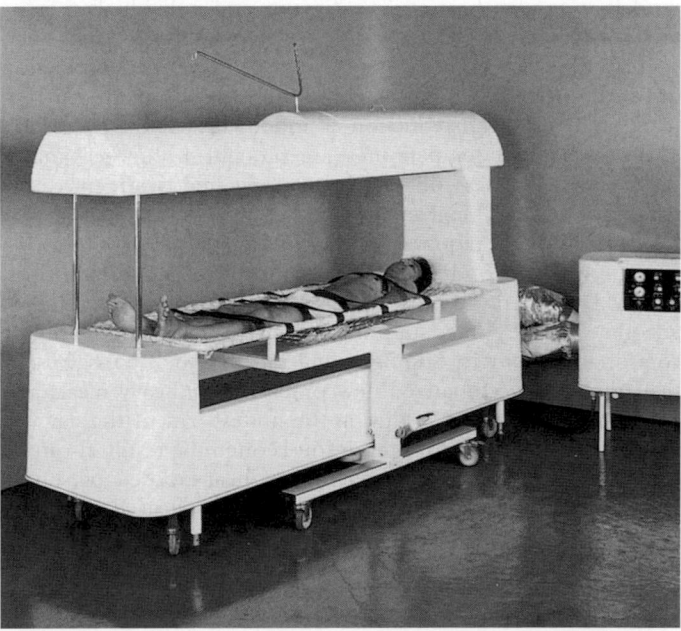

Figure 29.4 Body cooling unit for the treatment of hyperthermia and heat stroke (Photograph courtesy of Guardian Medical Products, see www.engments.co.uk).

pathological rather than physiological vasomotor responses occur, such that the core-shell insulative barrier may not increase at the onset of heat stroke.[35] It is also reported that no deaths had occurred during the treatment by ice water immersion in 252 heat stroke cases in Marine Corps recruits. A mean mortality of 12.1% using the BCU on the other hand was observed in *Hajj* pilgrims in 1982. However, there are obviously important differences between these two populations. The Marine Corps recruits were young, fit soldiers suffering from exertional heat stroke, all of whom were treated within 20 min of collapse. The *Hajj* pilgrims were often elderly or unfit, and were brought to treatment centres suffering from classical heat stroke at unknown periods after collapse.

With treatment, aspiration pneumonia must be avoided by keeping the airway clear and the patient nursed in a semi-lateral position. In addition to primary cooling procedures, intravenous chlorpromazine (20–50 mg) has been used to prevent shivering, though there is a danger that the drug may inhibit sweating. To treat dehydration, 5% glucose in normal saline can be given intravenously, which should be done with care in order to avoid circulatory overloading. Oxygen should be given while danger to the central nervous system persists. DIC has been successfully treated with heparin, though fresh plasma provides a safer alternative. Dextran should be avoided since it may impair platelet function.

PREVENTION OF HEAT DISORDERS

Recognition and prevention of the ill effects of heat stress, for health workers in the tropics, in industry, in the services and other situations where the heat risk exists, requires a working knowledge of the techniques for measuring heat stress, e.g. the use of the WBGT index for assessing heat stress and heat tolerance times or models to predict heat strain. Migrants and individuals moving into hot regions or those working in hot industries require supervision and advice on the effects of high temperatures. Prevention of the ill effects broadly involves the control of human activities in outdoor heat and reduction of indoor heat loads by control measures so that temperatures are brought within recognized safety limits. It is essential to have a prepared treatment centre where cooling can be given at once.

Special care is required when conditions are hostile, when escape from hot conditions is difficult or when water is in short supply. Due attention must therefore be paid to the provision of adequate potable water supplies, suitable clothing and thermally comfortable quarters. Supplemental salt may be necessary, particularly for unacclimatized newcomers. Large, heavy meals and excess alcohol, especially during the hottest part of the day, are to be avoided. Successful prevention is often the result of careful selection and continuous screening of heat-exposed personnel and, if possible, artificial acclimatization to heat beforehand. Regular exercise helps to provide a degree of heat adaptation.

CLIMATE CHANGE

An increase in the incidence of heat-associated disorders is likely to contribute to the potential health problems arising from climatic change. It is recognized that if global warming takes place, not all regions would be confronted by the same problems; extreme climatic events in different regions – heat waves, monsoons, droughts – may have a more profound impact than average climate change.[1] The direct effects of heat on individuals from increased heat stress in fact are likely to have less influence than indirect effects arising from complex changes in ecological infrastructure. Thus altered patterns of food production and the effects of inundation could lead to migration of large numbers of people into new zones. There are also likely to be changes in the distribution of vector-borne diseases in the tropics, subtropics and temperate climate zones. Since there are large areas of the world where water supplies and cooling systems are inadequate, in unusual heat wave conditions or prolonged periods of heat the availability of water may become the critical factor for survival.

Many scientists assert that global warming is now discernible, with forecasts of an increase in the average world temperature of between 1.0 and 3.5°C over the present century.[36,37] Others, including some climatologists who believe that current climate models do not accurately portray the atmosphere-ocean system, maintain that the reality of global warming is still uncertain.[38] This uncertainty appears to persist in spite of extensive testing of the predictive ability of Global Climate Models against historical climate measurements.[39]

Summer weather variability, rather than heat intensity, is regarded as the most important factor defining human vulnerability to heat.[40] People living in areas where summer climates are highly variable are poorly adapted to extreme heat, mainly because it occurs irregularly. There has, therefore, been a growing impetus to develop systems allowing urban health agencies to issue heat and health warnings taking into account climate, social structure and landscape. There are few paradigms useful for modelling the management of heat casualties occurring on a large scale. One, however, is the programme adopted at the *Hajj* pilgrimage where up to 7000 cases of heat-illness including heat stroke can be treated.[25]

The human species has a marked capacity for adapting to temperature changes and to survive under widely different climatic conditions. In most regions, the predicted increase in average surface temperature may be easily tolerated, though much greater sustained rises of temperature in the higher latitudes may have more serious consequences for populations, including heat-associated disorders.

REFERENCES

1. WHO. *Potential Health Effects of Climate Change: report of a WHO Task Group.* Geneva: World Health Organization; 1990.
2. Gagge A P, Gonzalez RR. Mechanisms of heat exchange: biophysics and physiology. In: Fregly MJ, Blatteis CM, eds. *Handbook of Physiology.* Section 4. Environmental Physiology. Vol. 1. New York: Oxford University Press; 1996:45–84.
3. Schönbaum E, Lomax P. Thermoregulation: Physiology and Biochemistry. Section 131. *International Encyclopedia of Pharmacology and Therapeutics.* New York: Pergamon; 1990.
4. Collins KJ. Regulation of body temperature. In: Tinker J, Zapol WM, eds. *Care of the Critically Ill Patient.* 2nd edn. Berlin: Springer Verlag; 1992:155–173.
5. Blatteis CM. Proceedings of the 19th International Symposium on Thermoregulation. *Annals NY Acad Sci* 1997; 813:1–878.

6. Falk B. Effects of thermal stress during rest and exercise in the paediatric population. *Sports Med* 1998; 25:221–240.

7. Bligh J. Mammalian homeothermy: an integrative thesis. *J Therm Biol* 1998, 23:143–258.

8. Cabanac M, Caputa M. Natural selective cooling of the human brain: evidence of its occurrence and magnitude. *J Physiol (Lond)* 1979; 286:255–264.

9. Lind J. *An Essay on Diseases Incidental to Europeans in Hot Climates*. London: Becket; 1768.

10. Collins KJ, Roberts DF. *Capacity for Work in the Tropics*. Cambridge: Cambridge University Press; 1988.

11. Kerslake DMcK. *The Stress of Hot Environments*. Cambridge: Cambridge University Press; 1972. Reprinted at Ann Arbor: University of Michigan Press; 2000.

12. ISO. *Hot environments: estimation of heat stress on working man, based on the WBGT Index (Wet bulb globe temperature)*. ISO 7243. Geneva: International Standards Organisation; 1989.

13. Shapiro Y, Saidman DS. Field and clinical observations of exertional heat stroke patients. *Med Sci Sports Exerc* 1990; 22:6–14.

14. Parsons KC. *Human Thermal Environments*. 2nd edn. London: Taylor and Francis; 2003.

15. Malchaire J, Kampmann B, Mehnert P, et al. Assessment of the risk of heat disorders encountered during work in hot conditions. *Int Arch Occup Environ Health* 2002; 75:153–162.

16. ISO. *Ergonomics of the thermal environment. Analytical determination and interpretation of heat stress using calculation of the predicted heat strain. BS EN ISO 7933*. Geneva: International Standards Organisation; 2004.

17. Leithead CS, Lind AR. *Heat Stress and Heat Disorders*. London: Cassell; 1964.

18. Coris EE, Ramirez AM, Van Durme DJ. Heat illness in athletes: the dangerous combination of heat, humidity and exercise. *Sports Med* 2004; 34:9–16.

19. Schönbaum E, Lomax P. Thermoregulation: pathology, pharmacology and therapy. Section 132. *International Encyclopedia of Pharmacology and Therapeutics*. New York: Pergamon; 1991.

20. Shaheen JA. Miliaria (prickly heat) – an update. *J Pak Assoc Dermatol* 2002; 12:197–201.

21. Horne GO, Mole RH. Mammillaria. *Trans Roy Soc Trop Med Hyg* 1951; 44:465–471.

22. Galloway SD. Dehydration, rehydration and exercise in the heat: rehydration strategies for athletic competition. *Canad J Appl Physiol* 1999; 24:188–200.

23. Sucholeiki R. Heatstroke. *Semin Neurol* 2005; 25:307–314.

24. Varghese GM, John G, Thomas K, et al. Predictors of multi-organ dysfunction in heatstroke. *Emerg Med J* 2005; 22:185–187.

25. Khogali M, Hales JRS. *Heat Stroke and Temperature Regulation*. New York: Academic Press; 1983.

26. Ahmed QA, Arabi YM, Memish ZA. Health risks at the Hajj. *Lancet* 2006; 367:1008–1015.

27. Al-Ghamdi SA, Akbar HO, Qari YA, et al. Pattern of admission to hospitals during Muslim pilgrimage (Hajj). *Saudi Med J* 2003; 24:1073–1076.

28. Wyndham CH. A survey of the causal factors in heat stroke and their presentation in the gold mining industry. *J S Afr Inst Min Metall* 1965; 66:125–155.

29. Gardner J W, Kark JA. Fatal rhabdomyolysis presenting as mild heat illness in military training. *Milit Med* 1994; 159:160–163.

30. Hammami MM, Bouchama A, Al-Sedairy S, et al. Concentrations of soluble tumor necrosis factor and interleukin-6 receptors in heat stroke and heat stress. *Critical Care Med* 1997; 25:1314–1319.

31. Wang ZZ, Wang CL, Wu TC, et al. Autoantibody response to heat shock protein 70 in patients with heatstroke. *Am J Med* 2001; 111:654–657.

32. Shahid MS, Hatle L, Mansour H, et al. Echocardiographic and Doppler study of patients with heat stroke and heat exhaustion. *Internat J Cardiac Imaging* 1999; 15:279–285.

33. Weiner JS, Khogali M. A physiological body cooling unit for treatment of heat stroke. *Lancet* 1980; i:507–508.

34. Manson P. *Tropical Diseases: A Manual of the Diseases of Warm Climates*. London: Cassell; 1898:211–213.

35. Costrini A. Emergency treatment of exertional heat stroke and comparison with whole body cooling techniques. *Med Sci Sports Exerc* 1990; 22:15–18.

36. Intergovernmental Panel on Climate Change (WGI). Houghton JT, Meira Filho LG, Callander BA, eds. *Climate Change 1995*. New York: Cambridge University Press; 1996.

37. McMichael AJ, Haines A. Global climate change: the potential effects on health. *BMJ* 1997; 315:805–809.

38. Michaels P. Conspiracy, concensus or correlation? What scientists think about the 'popular vision' of global warming. *World Climate Rev* 1993; 1:11.

39. Huntingford C, Hemming D, Gash JHC, et al. Impact of climate change on health: what is required of climate modellers? *Trans Roy Soc Trop Med Hyg* 2007; 101:97–103.

40. Kalkstein LS. Biometeorology – looking at links between weather, climate and health. *Biometeorology Bull* 2000; 5:9–18.

Chapter 30

Bernard J. Brabin and John B. S. Coulter

Nutrition-associated Disease

The interrelationship between nutrition, health and disease has long been recognized as fundamental to medical care. Diets in low resource areas are often unbalanced as well as being deficient in energy, and there is the added burden of bacterial and parasitic infections. These infections cause loss of appetite, maldigestion and malabsorption, which results in growth retardation, weight loss, micronutrient deficiencies and iron-deficiency anaemia. Seasonal and climatic variations have an enormous influence on disease transmission, agricultural potential and food security, which are all important factors affecting nutritional status. This concurrence can result in the 'hungry season', which describes the time between the exhaustion of the previous year's food stores and the new harvest which generates a state of nutritional stress in many developing countries. Traditional practices and cultural and religious food customs may lead to further dietary strictures.

MALNUTRITION IN CHILDREN

Malnutrition of variable degree is common in most developing countries. Over 50% of under-five-year-old (under-fives) child deaths are associated with malnutrition. The prevalence of severe acute malnutrition is around 2% in the least developed and 1% in other developing countries.[1] The interactions between infection and nutrition are key factors.[2,3]

Prevalence

The prevalence of malnutrition may be measured according to rates of stunting, underweight and wasting. Table 30.1 outlines the geographical distribution in developing countries. Approximately 38% of under-fives in developing countries are stunted.[4] Stunting is usually established by 3 years of age. Causes are multifactorial and reflect socioeconomic, educational and health status, and development and wealth of society. Prenatal factors and low birth weight are also important causes. Approximately 31% of under-fives are underweight.[4] Catch-up growth resulting in normal weight for height ratios is possible, but adults are often stunted. Wasting (low weight for age or weight for height ratios) affects approximately 9% of children and usually occurs between 6 months and 2 years. Rates increase in times of famine, war, forced migration and depression of the economy. Socioeconomic

causes of malnutrition vary geographically and are outlined in Table 30.2. Nutritional causes are difficult to assess. Wasting may be due more to deficient quantity and stunting to deficient quality of food.[2]

Severe acute malnutrition

Severe acute malnutrition is manifest by wasting and/or oedema. Major factors are nutritional deficiency and recurrent infections, both of which have underlying socioeconomic causes, particularly poverty and lack of hygiene and education (Table 30.2). Inadequate infant-feeding practices and complementary foods are compounded by infections associated with anorexia and increased metabolic demand. Many children with severe organic diseases, e.g. cardiac and renal disorders and mental and physical handicap, have variable degrees of malnutrition and are usually stunted and underweight. Neglect may also be an element in those who are disabled.

Measurement and classification

There are various methods of classifying malnutrition which depend on the type of information required and the prevalence of oedema; also the level of training of health workers undertaking measurements. Methods for assessment of underweight (WAZ), wasting (WHZ), stunting (HAZ), thinness (MUAC), and microcephali (head circumference) using Z-scores are available.[5] The National Centre for Health Statistics (NCHS)/WHO reference values are likely to be replaced by WHO standards.[6]

Weight for age

Weight for age as a percentage of the median standard is useful for assessment at child health clinics. Disadvantages include inaccuracy of age of the child for some uneducated mothers, and it also does not take into account lightness in weight due to stunting.

Mid upper arm circumference (MUAC)

This measurement is useful for screening children between 6 months and 5 years of age and only requires a measuring tape.

Table 30.1 Prevalence (%) of stunting, underweight and wasting for children under 5 years old in 1995 for UN regions

	Stunting	Underweight	Wasting
Africa	38.6	28.4	8.0
Asia	41.0	35.0	10.3
Latin America and Caribbean	17.9	9.5	3.0
Oceania	31.4	22.8	5.0

De Onis and Blossner 1997.[4]

Table 30.2 Socioeconomical causes of malnutrition

General	Food	Infection
Lack of education	Food insecurity	Poor hygiene and
Poverty	• general	sanitation
Frequent pregnancies	• seasonal	HIV infection
Low birth weight	Cultural practices	Failed measles
Intrafamilial	and taboos	immunization
• divorce, separation	Maldistribution	Tuberculosis
• working mothers	within the family	
• unemployment		
• sending a child away for care by a relative		
Inadequate medical and nutritional support		

Severe malnutrition is defined as <110 mm.[1] Standard deviations of MUAC in relation to age and standards for MUAC related to height (QUAC stick) are available.[1]

Weight for height

This is used in criteria for admission of children with acute malnutrition. It does not require age but is less 'user friendly' for health workers. It may be described as percentage of standard, standard deviations or standard deviation (or Z) scores.

Wellcome classification

This is used in areas such as sub-Saharan Africa, where oedematous malnutrition is still common (Table 30.3). The disadvantage is that it does not take stunting into account, e.g. low birth weight and stunted children may be classified as marasmus or marasmic kwashiorkor when weight for height is within normal limits. The weight of children after loss of oedema provides a record of the degree of wasting. The term oedematous malnutrition is now used more commonly to include both kwashiorkor and marasmic kwashiorkor.

WHO classification

This uses weight for height and presence of oedema. Those with oedema are described as oedematous malnutrition irrespective of weight (Table 30.4). In community-based nutrition programmes MUAC <110 mm is used as the sole criteria for therapeutic feeding in children 6–59 months. For infants <6 months visible severe wasting and oedema are used.[1]

Table 30.3 Wellcome classification

Weight (% of standard)[a]	OEDEMA	
	Present	Absent
60–80	Kwashiorkor	Underweight
<60	Marasmic kwashiorkor	Marasmus

[a]Median of National Child Health Statistics (NCHS)/WHO growth standards.

Table 30.4 WHO classification of severe malnutrition

Weight for height (SD or Z score)	Weight for height (median NCHS/WHO reference)	Oedema
<−3	<70%	Irrespective of weight or height

Adapted from WHO 1999.[7]

AETIOLOGY OF MALNUTRITION

Nutrient deficiency

Breast-feeding

In many traditional societies, prolonged breast-feeding for 1–2 years or longer is common. However, rarely is it exclusive;

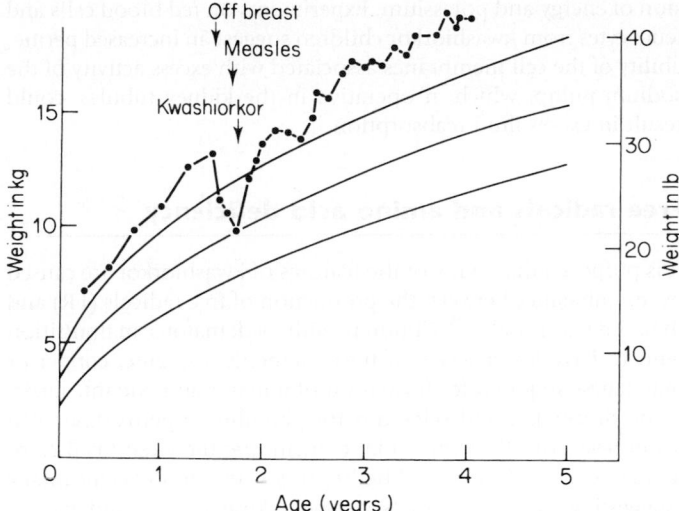

Figure 30.1 Effect of measles on weight gain. (From Morley 1968.[8])

additional foods/fluids may be introduced as early as the first month of life. In poor societies, absence of breast-feeding or cessation before 6 months of age is associated with early onset of malnutrition, especially wasting, and high mortality rates. Prolonged breast-feeding provides important sources of energy and animal protein, and anti-infective factors, but if not supplemented by complementary feeds the child's weight becomes static or falls. In the latter situation, severe malnutrition may follow quickly upon stopping of breast-feeding, commonly associated with recurrent infections, e.g. diarrhoea or measles (Figure 30.1).[8]

Infant diets

Diets often consist of single staples, e.g. millet, sorghum, maize or rice, which are usually bulky with high water content, low energy density and have high phytate levels (especially maize). High phytate concentrations reduce the bioavailability of nutrients such as zinc, iron and calcium. Contamination by pathogenic micro-organisms is common. Where the major component of diet is root crops, e.g. cassava, yams, potatoes or bananas, there is a low protein:energy ratio. Single-cereal diets may be deficient in a specific essential amino acids, e.g. tryptophan (maize) or lysine (cereals in general) and require to be balanced by a complementary plant protein source like legumes, e.g. beans, lentils, chickpeas and groundnuts, or even better, animal protein which has a high biological value, e.g. milk (human or animal), meat and eggs. Sick children require frequent meals during and for 2 weeks or more after the infection to assist catch-up growth.

Infection

Infection may cause severe weight loss through anorexia, catabolic loss and tissue depletion.[2,3] There are few prospective studies on the immunological effects of infection on growing children. Most studies are on hospitalized children with severe malnutrition. Of the latter, children with oedematous malnutrition tend to have more immune suppression than those with wasting only. Cell-mediated immunity is often severely depressed. Their B lympho-cytes and immunoglobulins are usually normal or raised due to recurrent infections (polyclonal stimulation), but the immune response to infections may be suboptimal. Complement is reduced. Activity of neutrophils in 'killing' ingested bacteria may also be depressed. An important factor in depression of the immune system associated with recurrent infections is failure of the system to recover because of nutrient deficiency, e.g. defective protein metabolism and micronutrient deficiency, especially zinc. Zinc is also important in promoting growth during rehabilitation[9] and in the prevention and management of persistent diarrhoea.[10]

Most children have gut and/or respiratory infections and bacteraemia is common, often due to Gram-negative bacteria, including *salmonellae*. Septicaemia and shock are important causes of death. Urinary tract infection is not infrequent. Tuberculosis and HIV may be underlying factors. Infections may be difficult to diagnose clinically as the temperature may be normal (or subnormal), the pulse not increased nor the neutrophil count raised and acute phase protein response is impaired. Hydration may be difficult to assess and clinical signs of pneumonia may be minimal despite radiological changes.[11]

HIV infection

HIV-infected children are more likely to be severely wasted than oedematous children and respond poorly to nutritional rehabilitation. Malnutrition occurs, despite apparently reasonable breast-milk intake. Chronic diarrhoea, often with lactose intolerance, persistent respiratory infections, tuberculosis and a variety of dermatological disorders, i.e. non-specific generalized dermatitis, are common. Their HIV-infected mothers may be symptomatic, depressed and have difficulty in coping.

EPIDEMIOLOGY

The onset of frank malnutrition frequently dates from the time that breast-feeding stopped and/or of a severe infection. If the infant is bottle-fed, onset is usually in the first 6 months of life, usually with wasting. Artificial or cow's milk is often over-diluted and infected. Otherwise, in breast-fed children malnutrition usually presents in the second and third years. However, malnutrition may occur in the first 6–12 months of age associated with tuberculosis and HIV infection despite apparent adequate breast-milk intake.

Geographical distribution

Kwashiorkor is associated with areas where staples have a low protein:energy ratio, e.g. root crops and bananas, or a maize diet (poor bioavailability of protein).[2] These foods may also be deficient in micronutrients. Kwashiorkor is not common in fish eating or cattle herding communities if diets are supplemented by animal protein. Comparison between village children in Keneba, The Gambia and the Baganda area of southern Uganda showed distinct differences in nutrition, growth and endocrine response.[12,13] In The Gambia, where the predominant type of malnutrition is marasmus, the main staple is a millet gruel which is low in energy. In the Baganda area of Uganda, kwashiorkor is the predominant type of malnutrition, the major staple is bananas (Matoke) and their diet has a lower protein:energy ratio than that in The Gambia. However, the energy intake was inadequate in both communities.

There are reports of kwashiorkor in middle-class American infants without significant infection, fed on low protein:energy ratio 'fad' diets.[14]

Season

In many parts of the world there is an increased rate of malnutrition in the wet (or hungry) season. There is deficiency of food as the previous year's crop has been consumed and families may have to survive on a meagre diet of fruits or vegetables while awaiting the harvest. Admissions for malnutrition often increase following an epidemic of measles. During the rains there is an increase in some infections, e.g. diarrhoea and malaria. The roads are often inaccessible and inhibit travel for medical care. Women are often busy working on the land and leave the younger children at home to be looked after and fed by siblings or relatives. They may only breast-feed at night or not at all.

AETIOLOGY OF KWASHIORKOR

The aetiology of hypoalbuminaemia and oedema in kwashiorkor has been debated since the 1930s when the simplistic theory of dietary protein deficiency was proposed by Cecily Williams who coined the name kwashiorkor.[15] Kwashiorkor is the name given by the Ga people in Ghana for 'the disease of the child displaced from the breast'. Recent associations include excess free radical generation,[16] deranged amino acid metabolism[17] and aflatoxin toxicity.[18,19] Essentially, in malnutrition there is adaptation to an inadequate diet by a reduction in metabolic activity, 'reductive adaption'. This adaptation is stressed and compromised by infection.

The cause of hypoalbuminaemia is multifactorial and includes: catabolism of albumin due to infection and stress, transient loss from capillary leak and in some cases from a damaged gut.[20,21] Malnourished children appear to maintain ability to synthetize albumin.[21] In nutritionally vulnerable children, a fall in serum albumin and lipoprotein levels commonly occurs in response to infections.[22] Tumour necrosis factor-α, interleukin (IL)-1 and IL-6 released from macrophages may depress albumin synthesis and divert amino acids to production of acute phase reactants. Capillary leak is associated with increased levels of leukotrienes.[20]

Oedema occurs essentially due to retention of sodium and water. Capillary leak may also be a factor during the initial stages associated with inflammation and release of cytokines.[23] However, the cause of sodium and water retention in hypoalbuminaemic states, e.g. oedematous malnutrition and the nephrotic syndrome, is still debated.[2,16,24,25]

In kwashiorkor, oedema may resolve during the initial stages of management on a low protein diet (0.6 g/kg) before serum albumin levels rise.[26] However, serum albumin may not reflect total vascular albumin mass or oncotic pressure.[25,27,28] Factors involved in clearance of established oedema may include restoration of homeostasis with stabilization of intracellular metabolism and cellular membranes of the kidney and other cells, and provi-

sion of energy and potassium. Experiments on red blood cells and leucocytes from kwashiorkor children suggest an increased permeability of the cell membranes associated with excess activity of the sodium pump, which, if operative in the kidney tubules, could result in excess fluid reabsorption.[24]

Free radicals and amino acid deficiency

It is proposed that many of the features of kwashiorkor are caused by an imbalance between the production of free radicals (FR) and their safe disposal.[16,29] Children with oedematous malnutrition tend to have lower levels of trace elements, e.g. zinc, copper or manganese required for formation of a major antioxidant, superoxide dismutase, and selenium for glutathione peroxidase; also lower levels of other antioxidants including the vitamins β carotene, E, C and riboflavin. Whether this is due to deficient intake (suggesting differential diets between kwashiorkor and marasmus), reduced binding capacity of serum proteins, maldistribution because of the metabolic disorder, or increased loss, is not certain. Free iron can catalyse FR reactions and high levels of stored or free iron are detected in severe malnutrition.[16,30] Reduced glutathione (γ-glutamylcysteineglycine or GSH) and glutathione peroxidase are important intracellular compounds in protection against FR damage, and low levels are considered to be a marker of FR activity. Lower erythrocyte levels of reduced GSH have been detected in kwashiorkor than marasmus and levels of thiobarbituric acid-reactive substances, a marker of lipid peroxidation, are raised in kwashiorkor.[16,31–34] These findings suggest there is more FR activity in children with kwashiorkor than marasmus. However, some studies have shown an overlap in reduced glutathione and glutathione peroxidase levels between kwashiorkor and marasmus.[32,33] In addition, there is a very slow restoration of reduced glutathione to normal levels despite a clinical response.[32] Conversely, low glutathione levels could be partly due to dietary deficiency of sulphur-containing amino acids, e.g. methionine, which are low in kwashiorkor.[17] Methionine is important for synthesis of cysteine. GSH is synthesized de novo from glycine, cysteine and glutamate. Methionine is also essential for functions of the Na$^+$/K$^+$/ATPase pump (sodium pump). Impaired sodium pump activity results in a large excess of intracellular sodium and a huge deficit in intracellular potassium. However, these intracellular electrolyte changes also occur in marasmus.

Decreased rates of synthesis of GSH have been demonstrated in children with oedematous malnutrition compared with non-oedematous patients.[34] Supplementation of oedematous children with N-acetylcysteine restored the synthesis rate of erythrocyte GSH and increased erythrocyte cysteine concentration.[35] This suggests that the low GSH levels in kwashiorkor may be, at least in part, due to limited availability of dietary essential amino acids and/or suppression of protein breakdown. However, a randomized placebo controlled trial of supplementation of 1–4 year olds in Malawi over a 5-month period with antioxidant powder containing riboflavin, vitamin E, selenium and N-acetylcysteine (three times the recommended dietary requirement of each micronutrient), failed to prevent development of oedematous malnutrition.[36] Although excess FR activity may have a role in the demise of sick children with severe malnutrition, these studies suggest that there other explanations for low GSH levels in kwashiorkor.

The difference in metabolism between children who develop oedematous and non-oedematous malnutrition (demonstrated in the recovered state) might support an interindividual genetic variation in susceptibility[37] but this would not explain the different geographical distribution of kwashiorkor and marasmus.

Aflatoxins

Aflatoxins are common contaminants of foods in tropical countries where the fungus *Aflatoxin flavus* thrives in the warm humid climate. Aflatoxins are commonly detected in urine of healthy adults and children in tropical countries, and they have also been detected in cord blood and breast milk.[18,19,38] Large doses administered to animals may be lethal and result in liver damage, profound metabolic disorders including hypoalbuminaemia and immunosuppression.

Studies in malnourished children in some (but not all) areas have demonstrated higher frequency and concentration of aflatoxins in blood of kwashiorkor than marasmus patients, and aflatoxical, a reversible derivative of aflatoxin B_1, has been detected in blood of kwashiorkor patients only.[18] Studies on autopsies[38] and biopsies[39] of livers from children have demonstrated that aflatoxin detection is virtually confined to oedematous children. The above findings suggest there is a clear difference in liver metabolism of aflatoxins between kwashiorkor and marasmus. This is most likely due to liver dysfunction in kwashiorkor. However, in sick kwashiorkor children aflatoxin toxicity may be an additional aetiological factor in the metabolic disturbance.

Growth difference between kwashiorkor and marasmus patients

Kwashiorkor patients tend to be taller, heavier (more fat) and have larger head circumference, and fewer delayed milestones than marasmic children.[40] This may be due to the chronicity of disease, poorer socioeconomic background and, in some cases, low birth weight in marasmus (and some marasmic kwashiorkor). However, the better growth of children predisposed to develop kwashiorkor may be a factor in aetiology by increasing the demand for energy, protein and micronutrients, thus making them more vulnerable when infection and acute deficits of nutrients occur.[13] Genetic factors may also be operative where the demand for nutrients may be higher in some children than others.[2]

Clinical features

In marasmus the main findings are growth failure with severe wasting of muscle and fat (Figure 30.2). There may be hair changes in longstanding cases. In kwashiorkor there is oedema, hair changes, skin changes (not always) and often an enlarged liver. Kwashiorkor tends to have an acute onset (Figure 30.3). Marasmic kwashiorkor has similar features to kwashiorkor, but there is more wasting and they are also more stunted and often have a higher mortality rate. The main biochemical difference between marasmus and kwashiorkor is hypoalbuminaemia (present in kwashiorkor). The following signs should be looked for:[11,40]

Sepsis and shock. Invasive bacteraemia and electrolyte imbalance are important causes of peripheral circulatory failure and death.

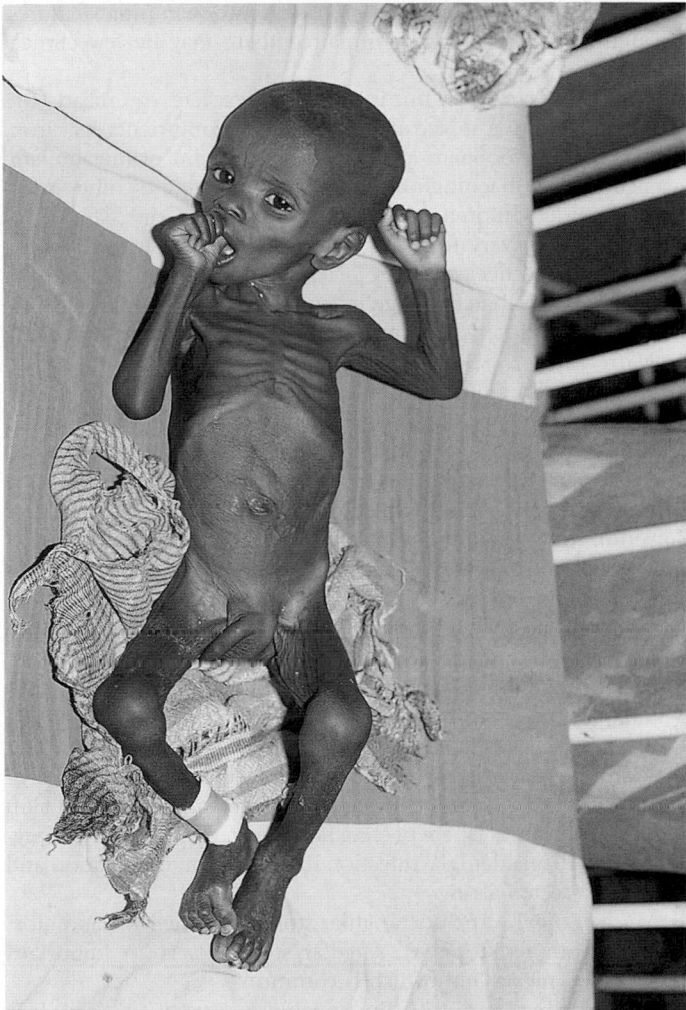

Figure 30.2 An 18-month-old Sudanese boy with marasmus. The mother has shaved his head because of hair changes.

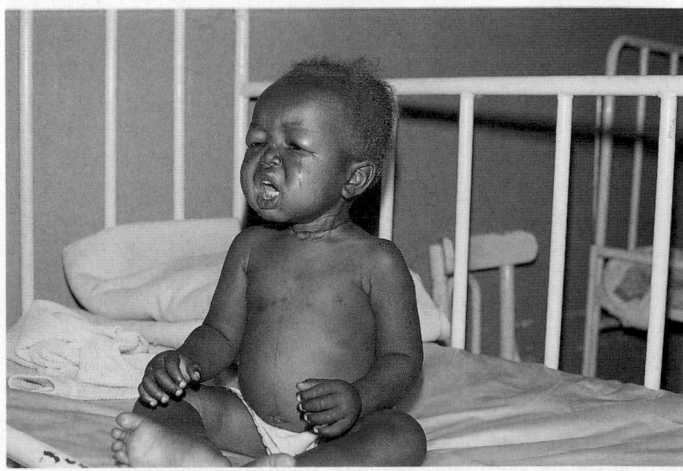

Figure 30.3 An 18-month-old Sudanese boy with acute kwashiorkor. Weight for age is above 80% of standard. There is retention of fat and no skin changes.

Lethargy and impaired consciousness are common features. Though cardiac function is impaired there may be few clinical signs.

Anaemia is common but is not usually severe, e.g. mean Hb8 g/dL. It is due to a mixed deficiency of micronutrients, e.g. iron, folic acid and riboflavin and general depression of metabolism. An acute fall in haemoglobin may follow malaria or other infections. In older children, hookworm may be a factor.

Oedema may vary from slight in the feet and legs with some swelling of the cheeks (moon facies) to marked and generalized. It can be exacerbated by giving excess oral rehydration fluid. Ascites is rare. Severe ileus may give an impression of ascites.

Hair changes, especially in colour, may antedate the florid appearance of malnutrition by some months. There may be dyspigmentation (change of colour to red or fair), sparseness (loss of hair), dry and thin hair fibres, loss of curls and easy-pluckability. The flag sign, alternating depigmented and normal hair, may be seen in children with long hair (not curly). Hair changes are common in longstanding malnutrition.

The *eyes* must always be examined. There may be conjunctivitis due to measles, herpes simplex, trachoma or bacterial infection. Xerophthalmia should be treated immediately.

Skin changes may vary from slight dryness and cracking or mild 'speckled' hyperpigmentation to marked hyperpigmentation with generalized peeling, e.g. flaky paint dermatosis (Figure 30.4). Ulcers may develop in flexures and around the perineum. Purpura may occur. Peeling is usually only seen in those with oedema or with a history of oedema. There may be generalized loss of skin pigment or in areas where peeling has occurred, localized hypopigmentation. Consider HIV infection if there is severe ulceration and multiple infected areas.

Mucosal changes include angular stomatitis, cheilosis and glossitis (smooth red tongue). Angular stomatitis is an important cause of anorexia. Oral thrush is common.

Liver size may vary from impalpable to grossly enlarged. It is more likely to be enlarged in those with oedema. In kwashiorkor, the liver is usually fatty (whether enlarged or not). Fatty change is considered to be due to reduced lipoprotein production and thus inability to transport lipids (triglycerides) from the liver. Fat clears spontaneously with rehabilitation and there is no residual liver damage. Serum bilirubin and transaminases are usually normal except in severe or lethal cases.

Lymphadenopathy is uncommon except in cases of local infection, e.g. tuberculosis or HIV infection. Other lymphoid tissues, e.g. tonsils, are also small.

Gut. There may be a chronic enteropathy, with variable degrees of villous atrophy due to infection, nutrient deficiency and possibly bacterial overgrowth. Protein loosing enteropathy may complicate measles and probably also other gut infections.

Brain. Mental changes vary from just irritability and lethargy to profound apathy (especially in kwashiorkor) or semi-consciousness. Reversible shrinkage of cerebral tissue has been demonstrated on brain imaging in kwashiorkor and less frequently in marasmus. Long-term effects are related to age of onset, longevity of malnutrition, poverty and lack of education and intellectual stimulation in the child's home environment.[41]

Management of acute severe malnutrition[1,7,42,43]

Community-based therapeutic care

An initial decision needs to be made regarding whether the child requires in-patient treatment or is suitable for community-based therapeutic care (CTC). CTC has recently been developed in a number of countries using ready-to-use therapeutic foods (RTUF).[1,42] Advantages of CTC include wide coverage, earlier presentation, reduced cost compared with in-patient care and a satisfactory outcome for most. Criteria for admission to in-patient care or an outpatient CTC program depends on severity of oedema and/or presence of complications (Table 30.5).

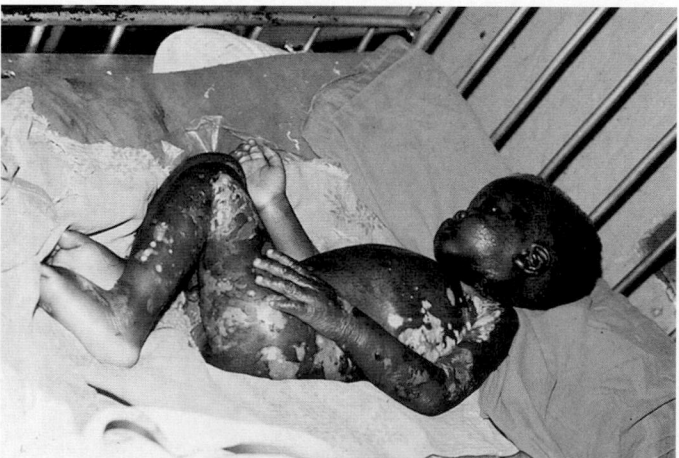

Figure 30.4 An 18-month-old apathetic Ugandan boy with kwashiorkor and persistent diarrhoea. There are widespread hyperpigmented, flaky-paint skin changes with underlying hypopigmented areas. His hair is dyspigmented, sparse, straight and easily 'pluckable'. The cheeks are puffy (moon facies).

Table 30.5 Criteria for in-patient or community-based therapeutic care in severe acute malnutrition

In-patient care for complicated cases	Out-patient care for uncomplicated cases
Generalized oedema *or*	MUAC <110 mm *or*
MUAC <110 mm + mild oedema *or*	MUAC ≥110 mm + mild oedema *and*
MUAC <110 mm or mild oedema *and one of the following*:	Alert Appetite present
Anorexia	Clinically well
Temperature >38.5°C	
Severe dehydration	
Pneumonia	
Severe anaemia	
Drowsy, lethargic or clinically unwell	

Adapted from Collins et al. 2006.[42]

Table 30.6 F-100 feed (in bold) and alternatives[a]

	Milk (g)	Sugar (g)	Vegetable oil (g)	Electrolyte/mineral mix (mL)	Water (mL)
Dried skimmed milk[b]	**80**	**50**	**60**	**20**	**to 1000**
Fresh cow's milk	880 (mL)	75	20	20	to 1000
Whole dried milk	110	50	30	20	to 1000

[a] If milk is unavailable a precooked corn-soya or wheat-soya blend (150 g) may be used with sugar (25 g), oil (40 g), electrolyte/mineral mix (20 mL) made up to 1000 mL water.
[b] Contains 2.9 g protein and 100 kcal/100 mL.

RTUFs are based on F-100 catch up feeds with the addition of peanut butter (Table 30.6). They have a greater energy and nutrient density than F-100. RTUFs are lipid-based pastes with a very low water activity and thus are resistant to bacterial contamination. They can be kept in silver foil packaging for several months unrefrigerated.

Children attend out-patients weekly or fortnightly and in addition to RTUFs (200 kcal/kg per day) receive a broad spectrum oral antibiotic, vitamin A, folic acid, anthelmintics and if required antimalarials. Patients are discharged after a minimum of 2 months when clinically well, free of oedema, with sustained weight gain and MUAC >110 mm. RTUFs are also appropriate for HIV-infected children either after discharge from in-patient care or primarily for care in the community. Weight gain is demonstrated in over 50% of HIV-infected patients.[42,44] RTUFs are also useful for supplemental feeds for children with moderate malnutrition and appear to be more effective than corn-soya flour diets.[45] Infants <6 months should not receive RUTFs or solid family foods.[1]

Although RTUFs are produced in low resource countries their cost and distribution are important factors in the sustainability of CTC programmes.

In-patient care

Two-thirds of deaths from acute severe malnutrition occur within the first week of admission. To reduce the mortality rate, special care has to be given during this period. The basic principle is, after initial resuscitation, to give high energy feeds with increased protein so that the child regains weight as rapidly as possible compatible with safety. Measles vaccination should be given to children >6 months of age who are not immunized or if the child is >9 months and has been immunized before 9 months. Delay immunization if the patient is in shock.

Resuscitation (first 1–7 days)

Avoid intravenous (i.v.) therapy if possible. Give modified WHO oral rehydration solution (ORS) (Table 30.7) over 4–10 h, 5 mL/kg every 30 min for 2 h, then 5–10 mL/kg hourly for 4–10 h. It has lower sodium than standard ORS and additional potassium and minerals. Great care must be taken to prevent overhydration. When hydrated (usually 4–6 h), commence Phase I with F-75 formula (Table 30.8), 130 mL/kg per day (100 mL/kg per day for oedematous children) as per the feeding regimen. If i.v. therapy is required, give Ringer lactate with 5% dextrose 15 mL/kg over 1 h, then 10 mL/kg per hour over the next 5 h or so. Whole

Table 30.7 Modified WHO oral rehydration solution (ORS): (low sodium)

Water	2 L
WHO–ORS	1 packet
Sugar	50 g
Electrolyte/mineral solution (Table 30.9)[a]	40 mL

[a] If electrolyte/mineral solution is not available give additional potassium, 40 mmol/L.

blood may be required for septic shock not responding to above. Also:

Diarrhoea usually settles over 3–5 days. Lactose intolerance may be treated with yoghurt and/or a cereal/oil/sugar mix (Table 30.8). In the rare situation where milk protein sensitivity is considered, alternative sources of protein include chicken, fish or soy protein. Give metronidazole if *Giardia lamblia* is detected or if treatment of anaerobic bacterial colonization of bowel is considered.

Hypothermia (rectal temp <35.5°C): Use a low reading thermometer. Clothe child, including the head, and keep in a warm room. Check for hypoglycaemia. Commence feeding as soon as possible.

Hypoglycaemia (blood glucose <3 mmol/L): Use glucose test strip. If able to drink, give 50 mL of 10% glucose solution or sugared water (1 teaspoon sugar to 3½ tablespoons of water) followed by the first feed of F-75. If blood glucose remains low repeat glucose or sugar solution. If unconscious/convulsing, give 5 mL/kg 10% dextrose i.v. or if unable to have i.v. access, give 50 mL of 10% glucose by nasogastric tube.

Infection: For mildly sick children showing no signs of infection, give co-trimoxazole for 5 days. For ill children give ampicillin (50 mg/kg parenterally 6-hourly for at least 2–3 days), then oral amoxicillin (15 mg/kg 8-hourly for 5 days) + once daily gentamicin (7.5 mg/kg) for 7 days. If still a poor response by 48 h, add chloramphenicol or cefotaxime. Consider tuberculosis or HIV infection in children who fail to respond to nutritional rehabilitation.

Blood transfusion: 10 mL/kg whole blood should be given over 3 h plus frusemide 1 mg/kg at commencement of transfusion, to anaemic children, i.e. Hb <4 g/dL or 4–6 g/dL in those who are very sick or have respiratory distress. If heart failure is suspected, give 10 mL/kg of packed cells.

Electrolytes and minerals: Potassium 6–8 mmol/kg per day should be given for 1–2 weeks or so. When high protein and

Table 30.8 F-75 feed (in bold) and alternatives[a]

	Milk (g)	Sugar[b] (g)	Vegetable oil (g)	Electrolyte mineral mix (mL)	Water (mL)
Dried skimmed milk[c]	**25**	**100**	**30**	**20**	**to 1000**
Fresh cow's milk	300 (mL)	100	20	20	to 1000
Whole dried milk	35	100	20	20	to 1000

[a] If milk is unavailable a precooked corn-soya or wheat-soya blend (50 g) may be used with sugar (85 g), oil (25 g), electrolyte/mineral mix (20 mL) made up to 1000 mL water.
[b] A low osmolar feed can be prepared by replacing 30 g sugar with 35 g cereal/flour solution which is cooked for 4 min. It is useful for osmotic diarrhoea.
[c] Contains 0.9 g protein and 75 kcal/100 mL.

Table 30.9 Electrolyte/mineral solution[a]

	Grams	Molar content of 20 mL (mmol)
Potassium chloride	224	24
Tripotassium citrate	81	2
Magnesium chloride	76	3
Zinc acetate	8.2	300
Copper sulphate	1.4	45

[a] Water: to 2500 mL.
Available from Nutriset, France.

Table 30.10 Vitamin A supplements

Age	Dose (IU)
Infants <6 months	50 000
Infants 6–11 months	100 000
Children >12 months	200 000

1 capsule = 50 000 IU Vitamin A. For measles or xerophthalmia repeat dose next day. For xerophthalmia give a third dose 5 weeks later.

energy formula is given only 1–2 mmol potassium supplements are then required. Where possible, magnesium 2–3 mmol/kg per day and other metals as per Table 30.9 should also be given. If this solution is unavailable, give zinc 2 mg/kg per day and one intramuscular (i.m.) injection of 50% magnesium sulphate 0.3 mL/kg (maximum 2 mL).

Vitamin A: If vitamin A has not been given in the last month, give as capsules as per the doses listed in Table 30.10. If unable to take orally, give 100 000 units (55 mg) i.m. (water miscible). Additional doses are required for measles and xerophthalmia.

Anti-malarials: Administer in endemic areas as clinically indicated.

Intestinal parasites: Mebendazole (500 mg, single dose or 100 mg b.i.d. for 3 days) may be indicated in children older than 12 months in areas where parasites such as hookworm and *Ascaris lumbricoides* are prevalent.

Rehabilitation

This is the phase of gradual increase in energy and protein intake until values such as 150–220 kcal/kg per day (normal require-ment 100–110 kcal) and protein 4–6 g/kg per day (normal 1.5–2 g/kg per day) are reached. To supply this amount of energy and protein without increasing the volume of fluid to excessive amounts, energy-rich foods, such as vegetable oil and sugar are added to the energy/protein source, which is preferably milk based (Tables 30.6 and 30.8).

Feeding regimen (Phase I and II)

In Phase I, F-75 formula is given 2-hourly, including during the night. Unless the child is able to take all the milk by cup, it should be given wholly or partly by nasogastric tube. Frequency of feeds is increased to 3–4-hourly over the next week or so. Mothers should be taught to give milk by spoon/syringe (Figure 30.5). A gradual change-over from Phase I to Phase II with F-100 should take approximately 3–4 days commencing after about 1 week. The volume of feed is gradually increased from 100 mL in Phase I, up to a maximum of around 200 mL/kg body weight in Phase II.

As soon as the child wants food, he is offered a normal diet in addition to his full requirement of F-100. Mothers should continue breast-feeding preferably after the formula feed. For infants under 6 months, if breast-milk is insufficient it can be supplemented by commercial infant formula or F-100 diluted with 1.5 L of water.

The mother should receive advice on infant feeding and health education and should be encouraged to participate as much as possible in the feeding of her child.

Additional treatment

Folic acid 5 mg on day 1 and 1 mg daily for 2–3 months. Iron-ferrous sulphate or gluconate 3 mg/kg per day for 3 months. Start iron 2 weeks after admission when the child has regained an appetite and starts to gain weight. Multivitamin solution should also be administered. Extra vitamin K should be given if purpura or bleeding tendency is present.

Discharge

When the child has regained an appetite and ideally is over 90% weight for height it is safe to discharge. However, this usually takes 4–6 weeks or more.[46] In practice, when the appetite returns, there is weight gain, infection is controlled, oedema is resolving and guardians are able to cope the child can be discharged to com-munity-based care (see above). Emotional (as well as medical)

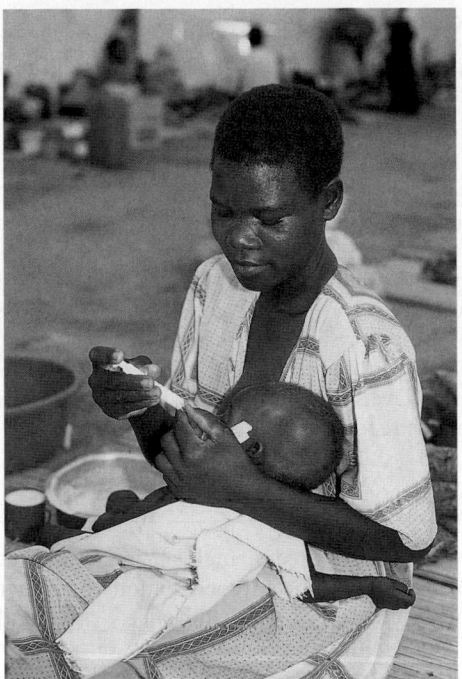

Figure 30.5 A mother tube-feeding her malnourished child by syringe in a rehabilitation unit in northern Uganda.

support for the child is essential during rehabilitation, especially in children of socially disrupted families. Encourage the family to stimulate and play with their child.

Prognosis

Case fatality rates may range from 5% to 50%, with a median of 20–30%.[47] The highest mortality rates occur in oedematous malnutrition, especially marasmic kwashiorkor and also in HIV-infected children. The aim should be around 5–10% mortality. High mortality rates reflect both the severity of malnutrition on admission and the management and prevalence of HIV infection.

Mortality rates after discharge may be 10% or more. This depends on a number of factors, including the condition of the child on discharge, the level of education of the mother, her ability to afford the necessary additional foods and nutrients for catch-up growth, and facilities for, and compliance with follow-up.

MALNUTRITION IN ADULTS

The aetiology of malnutrition in adults is similar to children, although clinical manifestations may differ, e.g. effusions into serous cavities and ascites may be seen in adults.[2] The stresses that cause malnutrition may also differ, e.g. the necessity to continue manual work despite dietary inadequacy and/or infections; prison and concentration camps; famine, where adults may have to continue to use energy in obtaining food and caring for the young; psychiatric disorders and in postsurgical or secondary malnutrition. In areas where kwashiorkor in children is common and

adults are subject to extreme dietary, physical and mental stress as in war, typical cases of kwashiorkor including skin changes, are seen in adolescents and adults.

A considerable amount of research has been undertaken on famine oedema in adults occurring during the First and Second World Wars in Europe and in Japanese prisoner camps and famines in Asia and Africa. The main controversy concerned the importance of hypoalbuminaemia.[2,16,48] When serum albumin levels are borderline, a dilute, salted vegetable diet may precipitate oedema, as may excess ORS in children with marasmus. Hypoalbuminaemia was less common in studies of oedematous subjects after the Second World War in Europe than in famine oedema in Asia and Africa. This may have been due to more prolonged dietary protein and micronutrient deficiency in the latter.[48] Other causes of oedema in adults include dropsy caused by consumption of contaminated cottonseed or mustard oil and beriberi.

IODINE DEFICIENCY DISORDERS

The term iodine deficiency disorders (IDD) replaces the terms 'endemic goitre' and 'cretinism' and emphasizes the wider spectrum of disorders which occurs as a result of iodine deficiency or the effect of goitrogens. The disorders include, apart from cretinism and varying degrees of brain damage, goitre and hypothyroidism in neonates, children and adults.

Epidemiology

Low iodine intake is related to lack of iodine in the environment. Areas of iodine deficiency are usually those far away from the sea, where iodine originally present in soil was leached by high rainfall and snow. The amount of iodine returned to the soil by rainwater is small and, as a result, many areas have insufficient iodine in the environment. It is estimated that globally 2.2 billion people live in areas with iodine deficiency and that this is the single most common cause of preventable mental retardation and brain damage in the world.[49] In the tropics it is found in Africa, Central and South America and in Asia and Papua New Guinea. Those exhibiting goitre are estimated at between 200 and 300 million. Goitre becomes endemic when the total goitre rate is 10% or more, or the visible goitre rate is 1% or more.

In western Africa, nearly all countries are affected by IDD, with an epicentre in Guinea.[50] It is a problem in the Atlas Mountains, Nile Valley, highland areas of Kenya, Tanzania, Rwanda, Burundi, Cameroon, and The Gambia. Central Africa contains some of the most severely affected populations in the world. Goitrogens in the diet, which interfere with thyroid metabolism, can be an important contributory cause, in particular thiocyanates which are found in the widely used tuber cassava (maniac). In Central and South America, IDD occurs widely. Ecuador, Peru and Bolivia are particularly affected. The most affected populations in Asia are China, India, Indonesia, Nepal, Myanmar and Bangladesh.

Aetiology

Inadequate intake of iodine leads to reduced production of thyroid hormone and stimulation of thyroid-stimulating hormone

(TSH) production. TSH increases thyroid hormone production resulting in the thyroid gland becoming hyperplastic and goitrous. The cause of endemic goitre is a failure of the thyroid gland to obtain adequate iodine to maintain its natural structure and function. Apart from iodine deficiency, other factors also influence iodine balance. Thiocyanate, a metabolic product of several factors, competitively inhibits active transport and is goitrogenic. Dietary goitrogens are found in cassava, lime beans, sweet potatoes, cabbage and broccoli and certain types of millets. Cassava has been implicated as an important contributing factor in Zaire. Goitrogenic factors seem to be superimposed on primary iodine deficiency.

Pathology

In the later chronic stages when iodine stores are exhausted, the thyroid gland becomes soft and enlarged (goitre) with a large number of colloid follicles. Nodular formation takes place and haemorrhage and calcification may occur. The gland does not become 'toxic' and malignancy does not occur.

The term 'endemic cretinism' refers to a combination of mental deficiency, deaf mutism and motor rigidity or, less commonly, to severe hypothyroidism. The two forms are often referred to as neurologic cretinism and hypothyroid cretinism, and can occur separately or together. They should be distinguished from 'sporadic cretinism' which results from congenital hypothyroidism and occurs worldwide. Endemic cretinism is associated with iodine deficiency that is sufficiently severe to cause goitre in 3% or more of the population, reaching 5–10% in areas with severe iodine deficiency. It appears that severe deficiency may be responsible for the impaired neurological development of the fetus from early in pregnancy.[51]

Clinical features

Goitre

Large goitres are easily recognized. Sizes are classified into three grades as shown below.[52] Tracheal pressure may interfere with the recurrent laryngeal nerve and produce hoarseness. Choking may occur with monstrous goitres. The patient is almost always euthyroid.

Classification of goitre:

0   No goitre
1A Goitre detectable only by palpation
1B Goitre palpable and visible when neck fully extended. Includes nodular glands if not goitrous
II Goitre visible with neck in normal position
III Very large goitre recognizable from a distance.

Endemic cretinism

This includes severe mental deficiency and there is a characteristic facies. Neurological cretinism includes defects of hearing, speech, squint and spastic dysplasia of varying degrees. Myxoedematous cretinism includes the predominant feature of profound hypothyroidism and short stature. Neuromotor deficits are less profound than in the neurological cretin and hearing is preserved.

Reproductive failure

There is higher risk of abortions, miscarriages, stillbirths, low birth weight and increased perinatal and infant mortality.

Diagnosis

Measurement of iodine in the urine is the most precise index of dietary iodine intake. Mild IDD occurs with iodine excretion ranging from 50–100 mg daily and in severe IDD the excretion is below 20 mg daily. In endemic goitre, serum T_4 levels are often low with a normal or slightly elevated serum T_3 and an increased TSH. In some countries newborns are screened for blood thyroxine and if low levels are identified immediate thyroxine replacement therapy is required.

Treatment

Cretinism with its associated mental deficiency cannot be reversed through treatment. For the myxoedematous type thyroxine and iodine supplementation reduce the effects of hypothyroidism. Goitres in older children and adults may disappear completely following iodine administration. Beneficial results will be observed in 4–6 weeks. Advanced goitres must be treated surgically if causing symptoms.

Prevention.

Fortification of salt for human and animal consumption is the method of choice for the prevention of IDD.[53] In Africa, virtually all edible salt is iodized in several countries. The level of iodine in salt must be enough to meet the minimum daily iodine requirement of 150 mg per person. Iodination of irrigation water has also been used in China.[54] Iodinized oil (lipiodol) is the major alternative and is the best option for severely afflicted areas. It is administrated by intramuscular injection or the oral route. The recommended dose is 480 mg iodine (1 mL) for subjects 1 year or older and 240 mg iodine in infants. This is effective for at least 1–2 years.[55] Priority should be given to improving the iodine status of adolescent girls and young women before they begin pregnancy.

SCURVY

The disease is due to lack of vitamin C, which is essential for collagen formation.

Epidemiology

Scurvy does not commonly affect any population as it did in the past, and therefore may be overlooked. Frank scurvy is uncommon and is most likely to occur in tropical areas where fresh fruit and vegetables are sparse. Babies are especially vulnerable when they are fed on dried cereals and boiled milk. Soldiers, prisoners and refugees in camps in dry desert areas are particularly vulnerable[56] and it can occur in epidemics in non-refugee populations.[57] The possibility of widespread subclinical deficiency in these areas cannot be ruled out. A form of scurvy has been extensively studied in South Africa among Bantu male labourers who developed haemachromatosis attributed to drinking large quantities of beer. It was thought that vitamin C in the body was irreversibly oxidized by large deposits of ferric iron in tissues.

Pathology

Vitamin C is required for the formation of fibrous collagen in connective tissue and bone. This leads to extravasation of blood, loosening of teeth and easily fractured bones with subperiosteal haemorrhage. Autopsy shows extensive haemorrhage in internal organs.

Clinical features

Infantile scurvy

The majority of cases present in the second half of the first year, especially in premature and artificially fed infants. The three main features are: irritability, leg tenderness and pseudoparalysis. The baby lies in a characteristic position with legs partially flexed at the knees and hips and internally rotated due to pain from subperiosteal haemorrhages. This may be mistaken for rheumatic fever, polio or osteomyelitis because of pain. These extravasations may be palpable at the proximal end of the tibia and distal end of the femur. Costochondral beading (scorbutic rosary) is also usually palpable. The arms are rarely involved. There may be bleeding around erupting teeth and gingival lesions. Bleeding into the skin is rarely a presenting sign. Hypochromic microcytic anaemia is commonly present. The anaemia may be megablastic due to accompanying folate deficiency resulting from lack of folate coenzymes associated with vitamin C. *Pyrexia* is frequent with associated infections, especially tuberculosis. The combination of gingival lesions, pseudoparalysis and irritability strongly suggests a diagnosis of scurvy.

Adult scurvy

There is an insidious onset with weight loss, progressive weakness and aching in bones, joints and muscles especially at night and characteristic stiffness in the leg muscles or other muscles in extensive use. Haematomas form in calf and thigh muscles. Perifollicular haemorrhages occur with subcutaneous petechiae on the limbs and trunk producing scorbutic purpura. Haemorrhage into the myocardium may be life threatening. Splinter haemorrhages may form a crescent on the fingernails. In extreme deficiency the gums become affected with swelling and sponginess of the alveolar margin, which is friable and bleeds readily. Secondary infection, gangrene and loose teeth supervene. Wounds fail to heal and scars break down.

Diagnosis

The main differential diagnosis is from rickets which may coexist as 'scurvy rickets'. Radiography reveals a characteristic ground glass appearance due to generalized osteoporosis and atrophy of the trabeculae. Epiphyseal ends are sharply outlined. Widening of the zone of provisional calcification causes a dense shadow at the end of the shaft (the white line of Frankel) and this is also seen at the periphery of ossification centres ('halo epiphysis' or pencilled effect). With treatment, even the grossest deformities resolve. The capillary permeability test of Hess using a sphygmomanometer to occlude venous return to the arm results in petechiae appearing. Laboratory tests on plasma or leucocyte levels of ascorbic acid are sensitive, although plasma levels are influenced by recent dietary intake.

Treatment

In infant scurvy ascorbic acid (50 mg four times daily) should be given for 1 week, followed by 50 mg twice daily for 1 month. In the adult, the usual dose is 100 mg administered three to five times daily until 4 g has been administered. If the patient is critically ill, 1 g can be given daily by intravenous infusion. Vitamin C may also be given as fresh daily orange juice. Severe weakness and bleeding rapidly resolve (48 h) and haematomas heal within 2 weeks. Radiological evidence may persist for years.

Prevention

Foods steamed and cooked rapidly retain much of their vitamin C which is destroyed by prolonged cooking. Artificially fed infants require supplements (e.g. fresh orange juice).

RICKETS AND OSTEOMALACIA

Nutritional rickets is still a major problem in many developing countries and is common in North Africa and the Middle East. The term 'rickets' and 'osteomalacia' refer to the histological and radiological abnormalities seen in a variety of vitamin D deficiency conditions.

Aetiology

Vitamin D deficiency results from inadequate dietary intake and/ or skin biosynthesis of vitamin D. Rickets describes the disordered growth and mineralization of the growth plate of the long bones. Osteomalacia describes abnormalities resulting from delayed and reduced mineralization of mature bone. Calcium deficiency has been implicated as a cause of rickets in African children with good exposure to sunlight. After weaning, the staple food of many young African children is maize porridge, which has low calcium and high fibre content. From 0 to 50 years, an adequate vitamin D intake is 200 IU(5 mg)/day.

Epidemiology

In the tropics, rickets may occur where sunlight is reduced by urban high-rise buildings, and in crowded areas of cities where there are few play areas. It is described in higher socioeconomic groups because these mothers tend to keep their babies indoors. Other factors are prolonged breast-feeding, weaning diets with inadequate vitamin D supplementation, high phytate diets, prematurity and low birth weight. Mothers with low sunshine exposure, vegetarians, dark-skinned mothers, cultural habits (e.g. purdah), and mothers with a low dietary intake of vitamin D whose breast-fed infants are at risk.[58]

Pathology

Defective calcification of developing long bones results in slowing of calcium and phosphorus precipitation in the newly formed matrix. A mass of uncalcified osteoid tissue causes enlargement of the growing ends of bone and a softening of all bones in both rickets and osteomalacia.

Clinical features

Rickets

The onset during the first 2 years of life is later than that in scurvy. The child becomes ill, pale, flabby and irritable, and prone to tetany and laryngeal stridor. There is general physical and mental retardation and deformity of ribs ('rachitic rosary'), spine, pelvis and limbs (widening of wrists and ankles) and short stature (Figure 30.6). Craniotabes occurs due to thinning of the outer table of the skull. The muscles are poorly developed and lack tone. In calcium deficient rickets neither muscle hypotonia nor bone pain are features and cases tend to be older (4–16 years of age). As the child grows, the skeletal changes heal, but marked deformities remain, such as pigeon chest, spinal curvature, knock-knees, and bow legs (Figure 30.7). Clinical rickets is less common in malnourished children, probably because they have less demand for calcium and phosphorus due to slow growth.

Osteomalacia

This occurs in women of child-bearing age, usually in their first pregnancy. The bones of the pelvic girdle, ribs and femora become soft, painful and deformed. The gait is characteristic. Tetany is common, anaemia is present and spontaneous fracture(s) occur. Fetal bones do not show signs of rickets.

Complications

Rickets may have severe consequences. It is strongly associated with pneumonia in young children in developing countries.[59] The relative risk of death for the children with rickets compared with those without is one in seven. Bony deformity of the pelvis in women leads to obstructed labour and increased perinatal morbidity and mortality rates.

Diagnosis

The distinction from infantile scurvy may be difficult, but rickets usually occurs in older infants and there are no subperiosteal haemorrhages; other possibilities are congenital syphilis, achondroplasia and osteogenesis imperfecta. Renal rickets does not respond to vitamin D. Radiographs show characteristic epiphyseal changes (cupping, fraying and decreased density; Figure 30.8). Early in vitamin D deficiency, the following values are typically seen: a normal fasting serum calcium; low-normal to low phosphorus; low 25 (OH) D; elevated levels of PTH, 1,25 (OH)₂D and alkaline phosphatase.

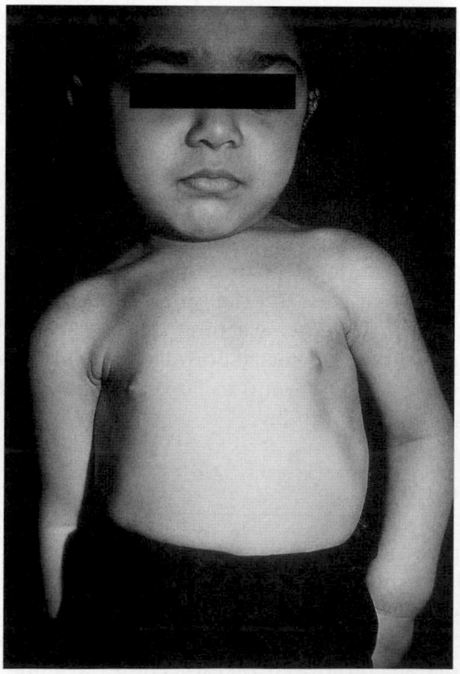

Figure 30.6 Rachitic rosary and chest deformity in a 2-year-old child.

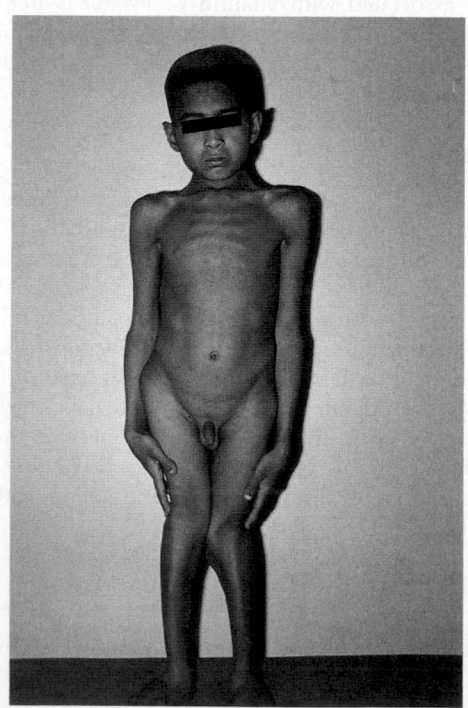

Figure 30.7 Stunting and limb deformity in a boy with Rickets from northern Pakistan.

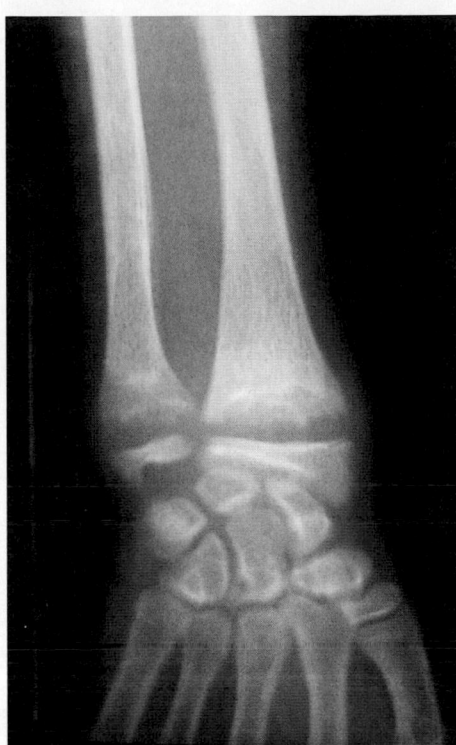

Figure 30.8 Radiological changes of rickets showing fraying, cupping and decreased density.

Treatment

Natural and artificial light are effective, but therapy is primarily based on providing an adequate calcium and vitamin D intake. The daily administration of 50–150 mg (2000–6000 IU) of vitamin D_3, or 0.5–2 mg of 1,25 $(OH)_2D$ will produce healing within 2–4 weeks. Calcium can be taken as milk, up to 500 mL daily. Administering 15 000 mg (600 000 IU) intravenously in a single dose may allow more rapid healing.

VITAMIN B₁ DEFICIENCY (BERIBERI)

Epidemiology

Until recently, beriberi was common in many tropical and subtropical areas and was endemic in countries of Asia and the Far East, where highly milled rice was the staple cereal. It was the scourge of plantations in Malaysia, China and Indonesia and caused enormous mortality and morbidity rates. Outbreaks have occurred in ships' crews, mining communities, institutions, such as mental homes, and among prisoners of war in the Far East. Endemic beriberi can show a seasonal pattern with increasing incidence in the pre-harvest farming months, possibly related to physical exertion at this time. Incidence has decreased with improved eating habits, but the reappearance of thiamin deficiency has been reported in Japan, The Gambia and South Africa. It remains endemic in Thailand, China, Myanmar, Laos and

Vietnam.[60] Cases of infantile beriberi have been frequently seen in refugee camps in Thailand. Antihistamine factors in the diet of breast-feeding mothers (e.g. freshwater fish) can increase the risk of infantile beriberi.

Aetiology

Thiamin is present in the tissues in the phosphorylated form and a continuous supply is required to satisfy the body's relatively high turnover rate as little is stored. It acts as a co-enzyme for carbohydrate metabolism in the Krebs citric acid cycle and exerts a role in the oxidative breakdown of pyruvic acid. Since the brain nervous tissue and heart muscle use large amounts of glucose, it is in these tissues that carbohydrate metabolism is especially deranged in thiamin deficiency. Thiamin is also involved in acetylcholine synthesis and in neurotransmission. Lactic acid accumulates with breakdown of the Krebs cycle, producing a metabolic acidosis.

The germ and bran portions of cereal grains contain the most thiamin. Highly milled rice is particularly low in thiamin (60 mg/100 g), although parboiling, prior to milling, retains much of the thiamin. The discovery that milling of rice was an aetiological factor was of great value in the prevention of beriberi. However, any factor leading to an increased thiamin demand may be aetiological. For example, young men are often affected possibly because they work hardest. Onset may be associated with fever,[61] infections including dysentery, and HIV infection; other factors such as pregnancy, lactation and rapid growth may exacerbate sub-clinical deficiency. Thiamin levels in the milk secreted by thiamin-depleted mothers will be inadequate to prevent beriberi in the suckling infant. Antithiamin factors (thiaminases) occurring in foods can alter thiamin structure and reduce biological activity. Thiaminases are found in raw freshwater fish and shellfish, in several microorganisms and in some vegetables, plants and tea.

True alcoholic beriberi is a form of oedematous cardiac disease with high output failure in severe alcoholics. It has been described as 'palm-wine tappers heart' in Gambia, as palm tappers work strenuously climbing trees and consume substantial quantities of fermenting sap. Drug-induced beriberi has been reported from the use of nitrofurazone (which interferes with pyruvate metabolism) in the treatment of trypanosomiasis.

Pathology

The pathological anatomy of beriberi involves changes in the nervous system, the heart and muscle fibres. Microscopically, the nerve trunks show changes ranging from slight medullary degeneration to complete neural destruction (Wallerian degeneration). In Wernicke's encephalopathy, foci of congestion and haemorrhage are scattered symmetrically in the grey matter of the brain stem, mamillary bodies and hypothalamic regions. There are also numerous perivascular haemorrhages and widespread degenerative brain changes.

In the heart, there is fatty degeneration of varying severity and loss of contractility due to water retention. The essential features of 'beriberi heart' are: a hyperkinetic circulation, peripheral vasodilation, right side enlargement and high output failure.[62] The cause of the hyperkinetic circulation deficiency is low peripheral arterial resistance from vasodilation due to loss of muscular arteriolar tone. Post-mortem appearances are those of severe right heart failure.

Clinical features

Beriberi assumes various clinical forms but can be grouped into five major types[63]:
1. Subacute cardiac (wet beriberi)
2. Acute fulminant
3. Neurological (dry beriberi)
4. Infantile
5. Wernicke's encephalopathy.

The two main forms, dry and wet beriberi, constitute the same disease and a mixture of the two forms is usual. The onset is insidious, but may be acute with death within hours without nervous system symptoms occurring.

Subacute cardiac beriberi

Symptoms include anorexia, fatigue, irritability, depression and abdominal discomfort. These may be associated with fever. Cardiovascular features are prominent with warm extremities, tachycardia, palpitations and breathlessness. Oedema may occur at the end of a working day and calf muscles have a sensation of fullness.

Acute fulminant beriberi

When heart failure appears, the hands may be cold. Blood pressure is low with a high pulse pressure producing a 'pistol shot' sound over larger arteries. There is cardiomegaly with right- and left-sided enlargement and a loud pansystolic murmur is audible over the pericardium (Figure 30.9). Atrial enlargement may cause paralysis of the recurrent laryngeal nerve. The liver is enlarged and tender. Pericardial effusion is unusual unless it is late-stage disease. Hydrothorax and ascites are frequent. The ECG shows inversion of T waves, a decreased P-R and increased Q-T interval, which rapidly revert to normal with treatment. Sudden cardiac failure is common. Death occurs from right heart failure and the patient usually dies fully conscious.

Neurological beriberi

The clinical features are those of a peripheral neuropathy of mixed motor and sensory type. There is peripheral neuritis with tingling, burning and paraesthesias of the feet. Glove and stocking anaesthesia may spread from the feet to the thighs or from the tips of the fingers. There is loss of vibration sense and tenderness and cramping of the leg muscles. The gait becomes ataxic due to loss of postural sensation. The cranial nerves are not involved, although ptosis of the eyelids may occur. Motor signs include: flaccid weakness and wasting with foot, toe and wrist drop, difficulty in standing from the squatting position and loss of tendon reflexes and deep sensation. Paralytic symptoms are more common in adults than children.

Infantile beriberi

This occurs in breast-fed infants of thiamin-deficient mothers, especially in those babies receiving a high carbohydrate diet.

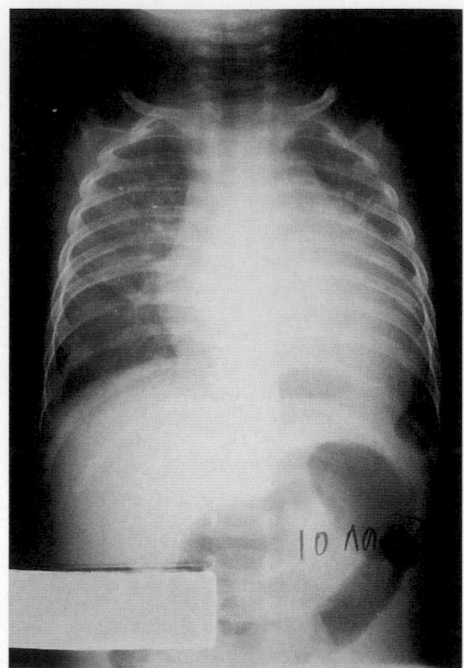

Figure 30.9 Chest radiograph showing cardiomegaly in an infant from Thailand.

Nearly all cases have infections before developing the symptoms of thiamin deficiency. These include pneumonia, diarrhoea, upper respiratory infections and cellulitis. The cases can be classified into three groups as: the cardiac form, the aphonic form and the pseudomeningitic form. It is not unusual to find features of two or three forms together. Characteristically, the cardiac form has its onset during the second or third month of life. The symptoms are dyspnoea, fever, cyanosis, vomiting and irritability with convulsions. The cardiorespiratory phase is most dramatic with rapid onset and physical examination reveals tachycardia, hepatomegaly and peripheral circulatory failure (Figure 30.9). Cardiac arrest may occur in a significant number of cases and infants may expire on the way to hospital. The overall mortality rate is between 5% and 20%. Blood chemistry shows metabolic acidosis. Survivors respond to parenteral thiamin within 24–48 h. The aphonic form occurs in slightly older infants (4–6 months). There is anorexia, weight loss and constipation. Left recurrent laryngeal nerve involvement from left atrial pressure gives rise to a characteristic cry (crying but no sound is heard). This may last a few days before restlessness, oedema and dyspnoea develop. The pseudomeningeal form occurs in older infants (6–12 months). There is vomiting and irritability. The infant develops nystagmus, a bulging fontanelle, twitching of muscles and convulsions followed by unconsciousness. The illness resembles meningitis or encephalitis but the CSF is normal.

Wernicke's encephalopathy

This is characterized by cerebellar degeneration, peripheral and optic neuropathy and is caused primarily by thiamin deficiency in alcoholics by causing reduced absorption of the vitamin from the gastrointestinal tract. Outbreaks of this disease, unrelated to alcohol, occurred in the Far East during the Second World War.

Diagnosis was established at autopsy by demonstration of mamillary body haemorrhages. Recent surveys suggest that the disease may have a prevalence of about 3% in all chronic alcoholics. Predisposing factors include diarrhoeal infections, sepsis and malaria. Clinical features of this syndrome include paralysis of one or more eye muscles, horizontal nystagmus, a wide gait, clouding of consciousness, insomnia, disorientation and semi-coma. Brain stem damage is associated with haemorrhage and necrosis and myelosis. Retinal haemorrhages occur. Wernicke's encephalopathy may be reversed with injection of thiamin, but the accompanying psychosis (Korsakoff's) is irreversible.

Laboratory diagnosis

The erythrocytes are among the first tissues affected in thiamin deficiency. The erythrocyte transketolase can be stimulated by TPP (thiamin pyrophosphate) and values >20% are found in deficient subjects. Urinary excretion of thiamin is low in subjects with thiamin deficiency but is not highly sensitive. The pyruvic acid concentration in blood is raised in acute beriberi and falls after thiamin administration.

Differential diagnosis

Wet beriberi must be must be distinguished from other causes of right heart failure with high output, e.g. severe anaemia and hookworm disease. Dry beriberi must be distinguished from other causes of flaccid paralysis and neuropathy: alcoholic, tabes dorsalis, chronic arsenic and lead poisoning, lathyrism, triorthocresyl phosphate paralysis in which there is a pure motor flaccid paralysis and nutritional neuropathies, e.g. vitamin B_{12} deficiency.

Treatment

In acute beriberi, patients may die without treatment. There is usually a dramatic improvement within hours of receiving parenteral thiamin (50 mg). In adult beriberi, oral treatment with 50 mg thiamin given three times daily should continue for some days followed by oral supplements of 10 mg/day for several weeks. In infants, 25 mg of thiamin should be given intravenously and a further 25 mg intramuscularly once or twice daily until symptoms have improved when oral supplements (10 mg) can be given daily.[54] Breast-feeding mothers should also be treated with 50 mg daily for several days.

Prevention

Health education and improved milling methods in which the germ is retained have reduced incidence in some Middle Eastern countries. Hand pounding of rice would improve thiamin content, but this traditional practice is unpopular and many rice eaters have strong preferences for particular types of milled rice. A maternal diet containing adequate thiamin prevents deficiency in breast-fed infants. Thiamin requirements increase with a high carbohydrate diet. General dietary improvement may increase intake, but this is not easy to achieve in poor developing countries. Mixed diets with other sources of thiamin are important, e.g. with pulses, groundnuts, whole wheat, vegetables and fruits.

PELLAGRA

Pellagra is a nutritional disease caused by the combined deficiency of the vitamin niacin and the essential amino acid tryptophan.

Epidemiology

While pellagra has vanished from most parts of the world where it was formerly present, it continues to be a problem in southern and central Africa. Recent reports of outbreaks in refugee camps and following civil strife[64] highlight that its presence often follows social disturbances with the establishment of large camps.

Aetiology

The spread of pellagra largely followed the introduction of maize as a dietary staple. The reason maize predisposes to pellagra is that the proteins of maize are poor in tryptophan required for nicotinic acid (niacin) synthesis. Pellagra has never been a problem in Central America, the original home of maize, because in preparation, rather than milling, maize is soaked in lime water which hydrolyses nicotinoylesters releasing nicotinic acid. It is likely that other factors play a role: marginal intakes of other vitamins (B_2 and B_6) required for endogenous synthesis of nicotinamide from tryptophan; prolonged exposure to mycotoxins which can deplete the body of nicotinamide; dietary excess of leucine causing an amino acid intolerance; and the impairment of tryptophan metabolism by oestrogens and progesterone which may be sufficient to precipitate pellagra more commonly in women than men. Pellagra may occur due to malabsorption, inborn errors of metabolism, following prolonged isoniazid treatment for tuberculosis (due to inhibition of kynureninase) and with faddist diets. It may follow intestinal surgery and be associated with gastrointestinal pathology, e.g. oesophageal stricture, carcinoma of the colon or stomach, Crohn's disease, chronic amoebiasis and tropical sprue). Alcoholic pellagra may complicate gastritis.

Pathology

The epidermis becomes hyperkeratotic and later becomes atrophic, and these changes are also present in the tongue, vagina and mucous membranes. The colonic mucous membrane is inflamed and pseudomembranes form; later, the mucosa atrophies. The viscera show fatty degeneration and a characteristic deep pigmentation. Haemorrhages may occur in the renal medulla. Nervous system changes occur late. Demyelination in the spinal cord may involve the posterior and lateral columns. Myelin degeneration in the peripheral nerves is common. Increased intracellular pigment is present in frontal lobes and basal ganglia.[65]

Clinical features

The main features comprise the triad: 'diarrhoea, dermatitis and dementia'. Since it is also fatal, a fourth 'D' is death. The classic symptoms are usually less well developed in infants and children.

Pre-pellagrin state

The early symptoms are vague: anorexia, lassitude, joint pains, dizziness and burning sensations which recur periodically for years. The complexion is 'muddy' with bluish leaden-coloured sclerae. The personality changes with irritability and character changes. There may be associated vitamin deficiencies and many people in endemic areas suffer from chronic ill-health. In children with parasites or chronic disorders manifestations may be severe.

Dermatitis

The cause of the photosensitive dermatitis in pellagra is unknown, but it may relate to low histidine levels in skin. This amino acid may absorb ultraviolet light and minimize skin damage from sunlight. Dermatological lesions appear on sites exposed to sun and/or pressure. An erythema initially occurs which may develop suddenly or insidiously; it is symmetric and can resemble sunburn. Mild cases may escape recognition. The lesions are usually sharply demarcated and are often on the neck (Casal's necklace), backs of the hands and feet (pellagrin glove or boot) (Figure 30.10), and sometimes on the scrotum, female genitalia or anus. The affected area is swollen, pruritic with burning sensations which become acute on exposure to the sun. Petechia, bullae and vesicles (wet type) may develop. The skin then becomes dry, rough, thickened, cracked with scaling a shiny surface and brown pigmentation (Figure 30.11). Erythema becomes blackish (or purplish) on black skin and is sepia in olive-skinned races. Hyperkeratosis may affect the malar or supraorbital regions and can involve the whole body. The cutaneous lesions are sometimes preceded by stomatitis, glossitis, vomiting, or diarrhoea. Swelling of the tongue may be followed by intense redness, ulceration, fissuring with atrophy of lingual papillae.

Diarrhoea

Diarrhoea is common in pellagrins, but is not a constant feature and in some cases there may be constipation. The cause is probably related to atrophy of intestinal mucosa. A characteristic symptom is pyrosis – a burning sensation in the oesophagus causing dysphagia. The stools are often pale, resembling those of tropical sprue.

Dementia

The psychiatric disturbances range from mild hallucinations with psychomotor retardation, insomnia, through confusion, to severe dementia, anxiety psychosis, intermittent stupor and possibly epileptiform convulsions and catatonia. Confusion and acute mania may herald death. The cause of the psychiatric disturbance is likely to be deficiency of tryptophan which is a precursor of the neurotransmitter serotonin. It has been estimated that 4–10% of patients with pellagra become permanently insane, and pellagrins were formerly numerous in lunatic asylums.[61]

The time of appearance of mental symptoms varies widely; they may be present from the start or occur during convalescence. In the later stages peripheral neuropathy, or ataxic or spastic paraplegia may develop. Tremors and rigidity (extra pyramidal) may occur. The cranial nerves may be involved (8th nerve deafness, retrobulbar neuritis, central scotomas). Some features of these late manifestations may be caused by vitamin B deficiencies. Corneal dystrophy and lens opacities may occur.

Acute encephalopathy is described to consist of cogwheel rigidity, clouding of consciousness, uncontrollable gasping and sucking. Stupor, delirium and acute psychotic symptoms may

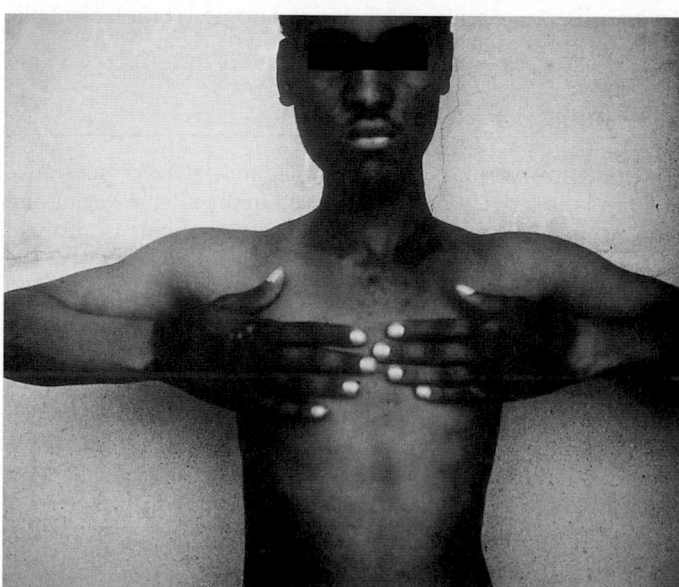

Figure 30.10 Pellagrin 'glove' skin changes. (Photo courtesy of the Liverpool School of Tropical Medicine.)

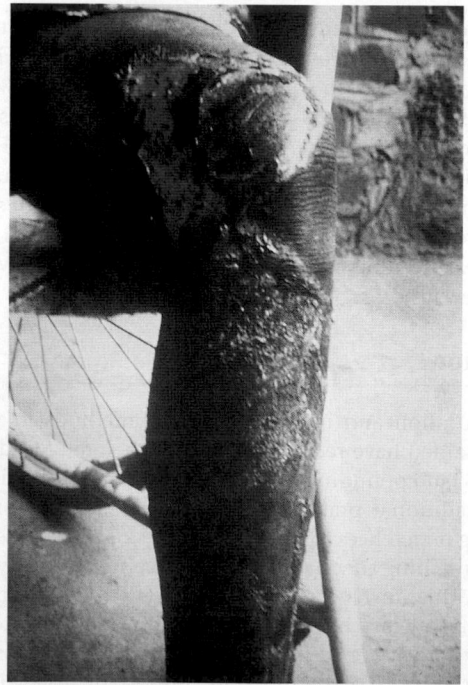

Figure 30.11 Limb dermatitis from pellagra.

be present and a mild pellagrin rash. These patients may respond dramatically to intravenous nicotinic acid.

Course

Symptoms may abate after 2–3 months although the skin remains dark and rough. It re-occurs the following year if the diet is similar. The eruption darkens and mental symptoms develop with melancholia, maniacal interludes and a suicidal tendency. The gait deteriorates and is of the paraplegic type. Body pains increase and may be acute with cramps, twitches and tremors. Symptoms may persist or deteriorate further unless treatment is given or the diet improved.

Diagnosis

This depends essentially on the history and physical examination. A rapid clinical response to niacin is an important confirming test. N-methylnicotinamide, a metabolite of niacin, is almost undetectable in urine in niacin deficiency (<0.5 mg/g creatinine).

Treatment

An adequate balanced diet is essentially supplemented with nicotinic acid at 50–150 mg daily for 2 weeks. In a severe case, or in cases of poor intestinal absorption, the dose can be doubled and 100 mg may be given intravenously. Administering large doses is usually followed within half an hour by sensations of local heat, flushing and burning of skin. Overdosage may cause numbness of the tongue and lower jaw. Intravenous nicotinic acid at high dose (1000 mg daily in divided doses) may produce rapid recovery in acute mania. Chronic psychotic and spinal symptoms respond poorly to nicotinic acid.

The diet should be supplemented with other vitamins especially riboflavin (1–3 mg daily). The diet of the cured pellagrin should be continuously supervised to prevent recurrence. Isoleucine (5 g daily) can counteract the metabolic effect of leucine on the metabolism of tryptophan and nicotinic acid. Leucine is present in large quantities in maize and sorghum. Sun exposure should be avoided during the active phase and skin lesions covered with soothing applications.

Prevention

Pellagra may be prevented through improved socioeconomic conditions among populations dependent on subsistence agriculture. In institutions, the diet should not be confined to maize meal but must include fresh fruit and vegetables, milk and eggs. Hard physical labour should be avoided.

ARIBOFLAVINOSIS

Epidemiology

Riboflavin deficiency without deficiencies of other vitamin B complex vitamins is rare. Deficiency is present in many developing countries and it was common in prisoner-of-war camps.

Aetiology

Riboflavin is not synthesized by higher animals and is therefore an absolute dietary requirement. The co-enzymes of flavin mono- and dinucleotide are synthesized from riboflavin, forming the prosthetic groups of several enzymes important in electron transport. Riboflavin is destroyed on exposure to light, and signs of deficiency occur if daily intake is less than 0.2–0.3 mg, although 2 mg is considered ideal for an adult. Riboflavin-poor staple diets, such as polished rice, are common in developing countries. Large amounts of riboflavin occur in liver, kidney, milk, cheese and eggs.

Clinical features

Cheilosis (sore red lips), vertical fissuring of lips (perlèche) and corners of the mouth (angular stomatitis), and a purplish raw, smooth tongue with loss of papillary structure are well-described features. Other features are scrotal dermatitis, keratitis, conjunctivitis, photophobia, corneal vasculation and seborrheic dermatitis. The skin has a roughened appearance due to hyperkeratosis (toad's skin or phrynoderma). Cheilosis epidemics occur in families and institutions on inadequate diets. A normocytic normochromic anaemia is common. Ariboflavinosis often complicates pellagra and PEM.

Diagnosis

Biochemical status estimates are based upon urinary excretion or measurements of erythrocyte glutathione reductase.

Treatment

Treatment consists of the oral administration of 3–10 mg of riboflavin daily. If no response occurs within a few days, intramuscular injections of 2 mg of riboflavin in saline may be used. Meat and fish are good sources of riboflavin and certain fruit and dark green vegetables.

VITAMIN A DEFICIENCY

SPECIAL GROUPS

Pregnant women

In addition to the usual requirements (see Chapter 25.), pregnancy incurs extra energy costs. It is, however, difficult to prescribe precise energy intakes for individual women, as their metabolic and behavioural responses (activity and food intake) cannot be predicted. Inadequate pregnancy weight gains have been associated with lower birth weights in undernourished women. It has long been recognized that pregnant and lactating women are especially vulnerable for mild xerophthalmia. Low vitamin A content of breast-milk will also contribute to the increased susceptibility of the infant. A high proportion of pregnant women in developing countries are at risk of inadequate intakes of zinc, iron, vitamin B_{12}, folic acid and other micronutrients. Improving the diets of pregnant women and adolescent girls before their first pregnancy is therefore important for primary prevention of nutritional disorders.[66] Practical methods include modifying the diets to improve bioavailability, and provision of appropriate micronutrient supplements during pregnancy which may yield substantial benefits. Maternal arm circumference can be used as an indicator of risk in non-pregnant and pregnant women because of its high correlation with maternal weight for height. A suitable cut-off for assessing risk in developing countries is less than 21–23.5 cm.

Vegetarians

In poor populations of tropical countries, the meat intake in the diet may be very low or absent. Despite this the macronutrient composition is unremarkable. Vegetarians are prone to iron deficiency due to low iron bioavailability. Combined deficiencies of vitamin B_{12} and folate can lead to megablastic anaemias. Consumption of unleavened breads such as chapattis, and brown rice may predispose to rickets and osteomalacia, particularly in Asian vegetarians. Leavening of bread with yeast destroys phytic acid which binds to calcium and this ameliorates this effect. Intake of high dietary fibre and phytates may modify zinc absorption. In general, vegetarians have lower rates of some cancers (mouth, prostate and possibly colon), but there is little evidence relating this to the absence of meat in the diet. The beneficial effects of a vegetarian diet may relate to cancer-preventive substances such as antioxidants and phytochemicals.

Refugees

Nutrition deficiencies in refugees and other uprooted people are well documented. Scurvy, xerophthalmia, anaemia, pellagra and beriberi are described in people dependent on refugee rations. Refugees are prone to anaemia because their food rations are often low in vitamin C which enhances iron absorption. Control of deficiency diseases among refugees has largely depended on the distribution of supplementary tablets and additional food, e.g. fruits, dried fish, meat. Nutrient fortification of bulk food to improve the quality of rations has been successfully exploited, e.g. micronutrients in cereals, vitamin A in oil and iron in sugar.[67]

REFERENCES

1. Prudhon C, Prinzo ZW, Briend A, et al. Proceedings of the WHO, UNICEF, and SCN informal consultation on community-based management of severe malnutrition in children. *Food Nutr Bull* 2006; 27(suppl 3):S99–S104.
2. Waterlow JC. *Protein-energy Malnutrition*. London: Edward Arnold; 1992.
3. Scrimshaw NS, San Giovanni JP. Synergism of nutrition, infection and immunity: an overview. *Eur J Clin Nutr* 1997; 66:464S–477S.
4. de Onis M, Blossner M. *WHO Global Database on Child Growth and Malnutrition*. WHO/NUT/97.4. Geneva: Programme of Nutrition, World Health Organization; 1997.
5. CDC. Epi info 2002. Atlanta: Centers for Disease Control and Prevention; 2002:computer program.
6. WHO. WHO child growth standards. *Acta Paediatr* 2006; 95(suppl): 1–101.
7. WHO. *Management of Severe Malnutrition: a Manual for Physicians and Other Senior Health Workers*. Geneva: World Health Organization; 1999.
8. Morley D. Prevention of protein-calorie deficiency syndromes. *Trans R Soc Trop Med Hyg* 1968; 62:200–208.
9. Golden M, Golden B. Effect of zinc supplementation on the dietary intake, rate of weight gain and energy cost of tissue deposition in children recovering from severe malnutrition. *Am J Clin Nutr* 1981; 34:900–908.
10. Cuevas LE, Koyanagi AI. Zinc and infection. *Ann Trop Paediatr* 2005; 25: 149–160.
11. Coulter JBS. Malnutrition related disease. *Curr Paediatr* 1999; 9:27–33.
12. Whitehead RG, Coward WA, Lunn PG, et al. A comparison of the pathogenesis of protein-energy malnutrition in Uganda and The Gambia. *Trans R Soc Trop Med Hyg* 1977; 71:189–195.
13. Lunn PG, Whitehead RG, Coward WA. Two pathways to kwashiorkor. *Trans R Soc Trop Med Hyg* 1979; 73:438–444.
14. Catto-Smith AG, Barr C, Fagan JE, et al. Non-dairy-creamer-induced kwashiorkor: 5 year follow-up. *J Pediatr Gastroenterol Nutr* 1991; 12:507–511.
15. Williams CD. Nutritional disease of childhood associated with a maize diet. *Arch Dis Child* 1933; 8:423–433.
16. Golden MHN. The development of concepts of malnutrition. *J Nutr* 2002; 132:2117S–2122S.
17. Roediger WE. New views on the pathogenesis of kwashiorkor: methionine and other amino acids. *J Pediatr Gastroenterol Nutr* 1995; 21:130–136.
18. Coulter JBS, Hendrickse RG, Lamplugh SM, et al. Aflatoxins and kwashiorkor: clinical studies in Sudanese children. *Trans R Soc Trop Med Hyg* 1986; 80: 945–951.
19. Hendrickse RG. Of sick turkeys, kwashiorkor, malaria, perinatal mortality, heroin addicts and food poisoning: research on the influence of aflatoxins on child health in the tropics. *Ann Trop Med Parsitol* 1997; 91: 787–793.
20. Mayatepek E, Becker K, Gana L, et al. Leukotrienes in the pathophysiology of kwashiorkor. *Lancet* 1993; 342:958–960.
21. Morlese JF, Forrester T, Badaloo A, et al. Albumin kinetics in edematous and non-edematous protein-energy malnourished children. *Am J Clin Nutr* 1996; 64:952–959.
22. Frood JD L, Whitehead RG, Coward WA. Relationship between patterns of infection and development of hypoalbuminaemia and hypo-b-lipoproteinaemia in rural Ugandan children. *Lancet* 1971; ii:1047–1049.
23. Sauerwein TRW, Mulder JA, Mulder L, et al. Inflammatory mediators in children with protein-energy malnutrition. *Am J Clin Nutr* 1997; 65: 1534–1539.
24. Patrick J. Oedema in protein energy malnutrition: the role of the sodium pump. *Proc Nutr Soc* 1979; 38:61–67.
25. Orth SR, Ritz E. Nephrotic syndrome. *N Engl J Med* 1998; 338: 1202–1211.
26. Golden MHN. Protein deficiency, energy deficiency, and the oedema of malnutrition. *Lancet* 1982; i:1261–1265.
27. Fiorotto M, Coward WA. Albumin and nutritional oedema. *Lancet* 1980; i:430.
28. Annotation. Nutritional oedema, albumin and vanadate. *Lancet* 1981; ii: 646–647.
29. Manary MJ, Leeuwenburgh C, Heinecke JW. Increased oxidative stress in kwashiorkor. *J Pediatr* 2000; 137:421–424.
30. Sive AA, Dempster WS, Malan H, et al. Plasma free iron: a possible cause of oedema in kwashiorkor. *Arch Dis Child* 1997; 76:54–56.
31. Jackson AA. Blood glutathione in severe malnutrition in childhood. *Trans R Soc Trop Med Hyg* 1986; 80:911–913.
32. Sive AA, Subotzky EF, Malan H, et al. Red blood cell antioxidant enzyme concentrations in kwashiorkor and marasmus. *Ann Trop Paediatr* 1993; 13: 33–38.
33. Becker K, Leichsenring M, Gana L, et al. Glutathione and associated antioxidant systems in protein energy malnutrition: results of a study in Nigeria. *Free Radical Biol Med* 1995; 18:257–263.
34. Reid M, Badaloo A, Forrester T, et al. In vivo rates of erythrocyte glutathione synthesis in children with severe protein-energy malnutrition. *Am J Physiol Endocrinol Metabol* 2000; 278:E405–E412.

35. Badaloo A, Reid M, Forrester T, et al. Cysteine supplementation improves the erythrocyte glutathione synthesis rate in children with severe edematous malnutrition. *Am J Clin Nutr* 2002; 76:646–652.

36. Ciliberto H, Ciliberto M, Briend A, et al. Antioxidant supplementation for prevention of kwashiorkor in Malawian children: randomised, double blind, placebo controlled trial. *BMJ* 2005; 330:1109–1111.

37. Marshall KG, Howell S, Reid M, et al. Glutathione S-transferase polymorphisms may be associated with risk of oedematous severe childhood malnutrition. *Br J Nutr* 2006; 96:243–248.

38. Lamplugh SM. Investigations into the presence of aflatoxins in human body fluids in tissues in relation to child health in the tropics. *Ann Trop Paediatr* 1998; 18:S41–S46.

39. Coulter JBS, Suliman GI, Lamplugh SM, et al. Aflatoxins in liver biopsies from Sudanese children. *Am J Trop Med Hyg* 1986; 35:360–365.

40. Coulter JBS, Suliman GI, Omer MIA, et al. Protein energy malnutrition in northern Sudan: clinical studies. *Eur J Clin Nutr* 1988; 42: 787–796.

41. Grantham-McGregor S, Powell C, Walker S, et al. The long-term follow-up of severely malnourished children who participated in an intervention program. *Child Develop* 1994; 65:428–439.

42. Collins S, Dent N, Binns P, et al. Management of severe acute malnutrition in children. *Lancet* 2006; 368:1992–2000.

43. Brewster DR. Critical appraisal of the management of severe malnutrition. *J Paediatr Child Health* 2006; 42:568–593.

44. Ndekha MJ, Manary MJ, Ashorn P, et al. Home-based therapy with ready-to-use therapeutic food is of benefit to malnourished, HIV-infected Malawian children. *Acta Paediatr* 2005; 94:222–225.

45. Patel MP, Sandige HL, Ndekha MJ, et al. Supplemental feeding with ready-to-use therapeutic food in Malawian children at risk of malnutrition. *J Health Pop Nutr* 2005; 23:351–357.

46. Heikens GT, Schofield WN, Dawson SM, et al. Long-stay versus short-stay hospital treatment of children suffering from severe protein-energy malnutrition. *Eur J Clin Nutr* 1994; 48:873–882.

47. Schofield C, Ashworth A. Why have mortality rates for severe malnutrition remained so high? *Bull World Health Organ* 1996; 74:223–229.

48. Waterlow JC. Protein-energy malnutrition: the nature and extent of the problem. *Clin Nutr* 1997; 16(suppl 1):3–9.

49. Walker SP, Wachs TD, Gardner JM, et al. Child development : risk factors for adverse outcomes in developing countries. *Lancet* 2007; 369: 145–157.

50. Konde M, Ingelbleek Y, Daffe M, et al. Goitrous endemic in Guinea. *Lancet* 1994; 344:1675–1678.

51. Xue-Yi C, Xin-Min J, Zhi-Hong D, et al. Timing of vulnerability of the brain to iodine deficiency in endemic cretinism. *New Engl J Med* 1994; 331: 1739–1744.

52. Dunn JT, Pretell EA, Daza CH, et al., eds. *Towards the Eradication of Endemic Goitre, Cretinism and Iodine Deficiency*. PAHO and WHO Scientific Publication No. 502. Geneva: World Health Organization; 1986.

53. WHO/UNICEF/ICCIDD. *Indicators for assessing iodine deficiency disorders and their control through salt iodisation*. WHO/NUT/94.6, Geneva: World Health Organization; 1994.

54. Delong GR, Leslie PW, Wang S-H, et al. Effect on infant mortality of iodination of irrigation water in a severely iodine-deficient area of China. *Lancet* 1997; 350:771–773.

55. Dunn JT, van der Haar F. *A practical guide to the correction of iodine deficiency: technical manual no 3*, ICCIDD-UNICEF-WHO. Wageningen: University of Wageningen; 1990.

56. Seaman J, Rivers JPW. Scurvy and anaemia in refugees. *Lancet* 1989; 336:1204.

57. Cheung E, Mutahar R, Essefa F, et al. An epidemic of scury in Afghanistan. *Food Nutr Bull* 2003; 24:247–255.

58. Thacher TD, Fisher PR, Strand MA, et al. Nutritional rickets around the world: causes and future directions. *Ann Trop Paediatr* 2006; 26:1–16.

59. Muhe L, Lulseged S, Mason KE, et al. Case-control study of the role of nutritional rickets in the risk of developing pneumonia in Ethiopian children. *Lancet* 1997; 349:1801–1804.

60. Mayxay M, Taylor AM, Khantharong M, et al. Thiamin deficiency and uncomplicated falciparum malaria in Laos. *Trop Med Int Health* 2007; 12: 363–369.

61. Cook GC. Nutrition-associated disease. In: Cook GC, ed. *Manson's Textbook of Tropical Diseases*. 20th edn. London: WB Saunders; 1996.

62. Cathcart AE, Thurnham DI. Beriberi. In: Sadler MJ, Strain JJ, Cabalhero B, eds. *Encyclopaedia of Human Nutrition*. San Diego: Academic Press; 1999.

63. Di Rocco M, Patrini C, Rimini A, et al. A 6-month old girl with cardiomyopathy who nearly died. *Lancet* 1997; 349:616.

64. Seal AJ, Creeke PI, Dibari F, et al. Low and deficient niacin status and pellagra are endemic in postwar Angola. *Am J Clin Nutr* 2007; 85:218–224.

65. Spillane JD, ed. *Tropical Neurology*. London: Oxford University Press; 1973.

66. Brabin L, Brabin BJ. The cost of successful adolescent growth and development in girls in relation to iron and vitamin A status. *Am J Clin Nutr* 1992; 55:955–958.

67. Weiso Prinzo Z, De Enoit B. Meeting the challenges of micronutrient deficiencies in emergency-affected populations. *Proc Nutr Soc* 2002; 61: 251–257.

Chapter 31   David A. Warrell

Venomous and Poisonous Animals

VENOMOUS BITES AND STINGS

Venoms are mixtures of proteins, polypeptides and other molecules that exert toxic, irritant or allergic properties when injected into prey or squirted at enemies. Possession of venom by an easily recognizable and sometimes highly coloured animal may confer protection both on its own species and on other harmless species which mimic its appearance or behaviour (Batesian or Müllerian mimicry). Venoms or poisons secreted on to the skin of some amphibians protect their moist respiratory integument against infection and are distasteful, poisonous and therefore deterrent to predators. Animals have evolved various methods of injecting venom. Mammals (e.g. monotremes, Insectivora and vampire bats), snakes, lizards, spiders, ticks, leeches and octopuses inject their venoms by biting with teeth, fangs, venom jaws, beaks or other hardened mouth parts; centipedes sting with modified limbs close to the jaws; male duck-billed platypuses are armed with venom-injecting spurs; fish, cnidarians (coelenterates), echinoderms, cone shells, insects and scorpions have different kinds of stinging apparatus. Some snakes, toads, scorpions and other arthropods can squirt their venom at enemies. Poisoning results from the ingestion of toxins from the skin of amphibians or the flesh and viscera of aquatic animals. Allergic reactions to injected venoms (e.g. of Hymenoptera – bee, wasp and ant venoms – and cnidarians) and ingested poisons (e.g. ciguatera fish poisons) are in some cases far more frequent and life-threatening than their direct toxic effects.

Venomous mammals

There is fossil evidence that some extinct mammals possessed venom-conducting teeth[1] and several living species have proved to be venomous.[2] The duck-billed platypus (*Ornithorhynchus anatinus*) is an aquatic egg-laying mammal (monotreme) of eastern Australia.[3] When males fight during the breeding season, they use venomous spurs on their hind limbs. Platypus venom contains four low-molecular-weight defensin-like peptides, a C-type natriuretic peptide B, an L-to-D-amino-acid-residue isomerase and hyaluronidase. Someone is stung by a platypus in Victoria almost every year.[3] There is agonizing local pain, relieved only by regional nerve block, persistent local swelling and inflammation with regional lymphadenopathy. No local necrosis or life-threatening envenoming has been reported. One patient experienced local weakness, stiffness and muscle wasting for more than 3 months after the sting. Experimentally, the venom is weakly haemolytic, coagulant and causes local haemorrhage, oedema and fatal hypotension in animals. Male echidnas (Tachyglossidae), monotremes of New Guinea and Australia, also have a spur and a vestigial venom apparatus that may not be functional.

Several species of Insectivora produce a venomous secretion from enlarged, granular submaxillary salivary glands that discharge at the base of the grooved lower incisors. The venom can immobilize invertebrate, amphibian or rodent prey and may be used, lethally, in internecine fights. Venomous species include the Haitian (*Solenodon paradoxus*) and Cuban (*S* [*Atopogale*] *cubanus*) solenodons, the European water shrew (*Neomys fodiens*), Mediterranean shrew (*N anomalous*) and short-tailed shrews of the eastern USA and Canada (*Blarina brevicauda, B. hylophaga, B. carolinensis*). The venom of *B brevicauda*, the most toxic, contains a kallikrein-like kininogen activator and vasodilator.[4] It can produce fatal cardiorespiratory and neurotoxic effects in rodents, lagomorphs and cats. In humans, bites by these species have occasionally caused local burning pain, swelling and inflammation.

The saliva of vampire bats (Desmodontinae) increases capillary permeability and inhibits platelet aggregation. Draculin, a glycoprotein, inhibits activated factors X and IX. An activator of plasminogen (vPA) is being developed as a thrombolytic drug. These activities serve to promote blood flow while the bat is feeding.

The slow loris (*Nycticebus coucang*) possesses brachial glands that secrete a toxin very similar in structure to Fel d 1 cat allergen, which the lorises suck up and can inject when they bite.[5] In humans, slow loris bites may be damaging, infective or toxic, causing pain, swelling and even anaphylaxis.

Venomous snakes[6]

Taxonomy, identification and distribution

Of the 2800 species of snakes, about 320 belong to the three families of venomous snakes, Atractaspididae, Elapidae (including sea snakes) and Viperidae. Only about 200 species have caused death or permanent disability by biting humans. Bites by more than 100 species of the largest family, Colubridae, once considered harmless, have caused mild envenoming in humans, but in the case of about 10 species, bites have resulted in human deaths.[6–8] The giant constrictors (family Boidae) are potentially dangerous to man. There are reliable reports of fatal attacks by South-east Asian (especially Indonesian) reticulated pythons (*Python reticulatus*), African rock pythons (*Python sebae*), South American anacondas (*Eunectes murinus*) and an Australian scrub python (*Morelia amethistina*). Some of the victims, even adults, were swallowed.

Snake taxonomy

Snakes are classified according to the numbers and arrangement of their scales (lepidosis), dentition, osteology, myology, sensory organs, the form of the hemipenes and, increasingly, by sequence analysis of DNA encoding important mitochondrial and other enzymes.[9,10]

Snake-like animals

Legless lizards, such as slow worms, glass lizards (family Anguidae), worm-like geckos (family Pygopodidae) and legless skinks, may be distinguished from snakes by their external ears, eyelids (in some cases), fleshy tongues, long friable tails and by the lack of enlarged ventral scales. Some have vestigial limbs. Amphisbaenid lizards have worm-like annular grooves along the length of their bodies and caecilians (legless amphibians) lack obvious eyes and scales. Eels (order Anguilliformes), especially snake eels (family Ophichthidae), and pipe-shaped fish must be distinguished from snakes by their gills and in most cases their fins.

Medically important snakes

Medically important snakes have one or more pairs of fangs in their upper jaw. These enlarged teeth have grooves or venom channels through which venom is injected through the skin of prey or human victims. Approximately 400 of the 1700 species of **Colubridae** have short, immobile opisthoglyphous (posteriorly placed) fangs or enlarged solid aglyphous (lacking groove or canal) teeth at the posterior end of the maxilla (Figure 31.1). The African and Middle Eastern burrowing asps or stiletto snakes (genus *Atractaspis*, family **Atractaspididae**), also known as burrowing or mole vipers or adders, false vipers, side-stabbing or stiletto snakes, have very long solenoglyphous (hinged erectile) front fangs on which they impale their victims by a side-swiping motion, the fang protruding from the corner of the partially closed mouth (Figure 31.2). The Natal black snake (*Macrelaps microlepidotus*) possesses two very large grooved opisthoglyphous fangs at the posterior ends of its maxillae. The **Elapidae** (cobras – *Naja*; kraits – *Bungarus*; mambas – *Dendroaspis*; shield-nosed snakes – *Aspidelaps*; Asian and American coral snakes – *Calliophis, Maticora, Sinomicrurus, Micrurus*; African garter snakes – *Elapsoidea*; terrestrial venomous Australasian snakes and sea snakes) have relatively short, fixed proteroglyphous (fixed erect) front fangs (Figure 31.3). The **Viperidae** (vipers, adders, rattlesnakes, moccasins, lance-headed vipers and pit vipers) have long, curved, hinged, solenoglyphous (hinged erectile) front fangs containing a closed venom channel (Figure 31.4). The subfamily **Crotalinae** (pit vipers) includes rattlesnakes (genera *Crotalus* and *Sistrurus*), moccasins (*Agkistrodon*) and lance-headed vipers (genera *Bothrops, Bothriechis, Porthidium, Lachesis*, etc.) of the Americas and the Asian pit vipers (genera *Gloydius/Agkistrodon, Deinagkistrodon*,

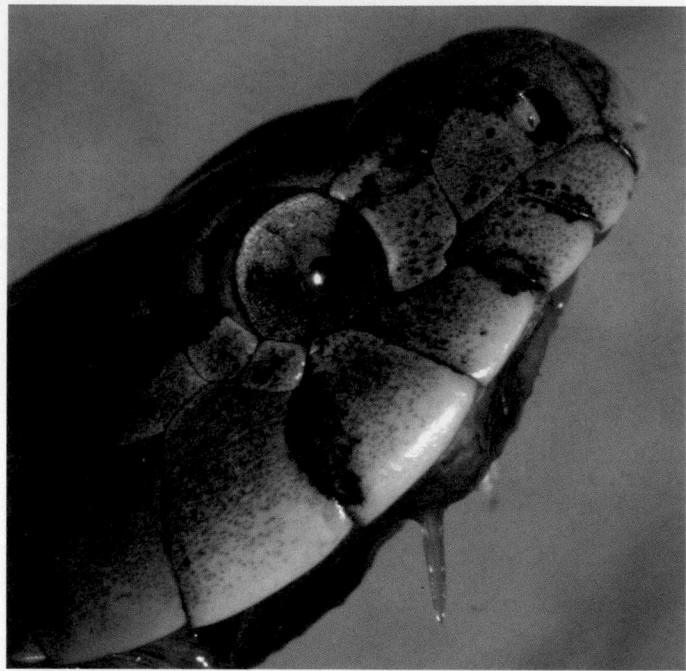

Figure 31.1 Rear fangs of the *Tomodon dorsatus*, a venomous South American colubrid snake. (Copyright D.A. Warrell.)

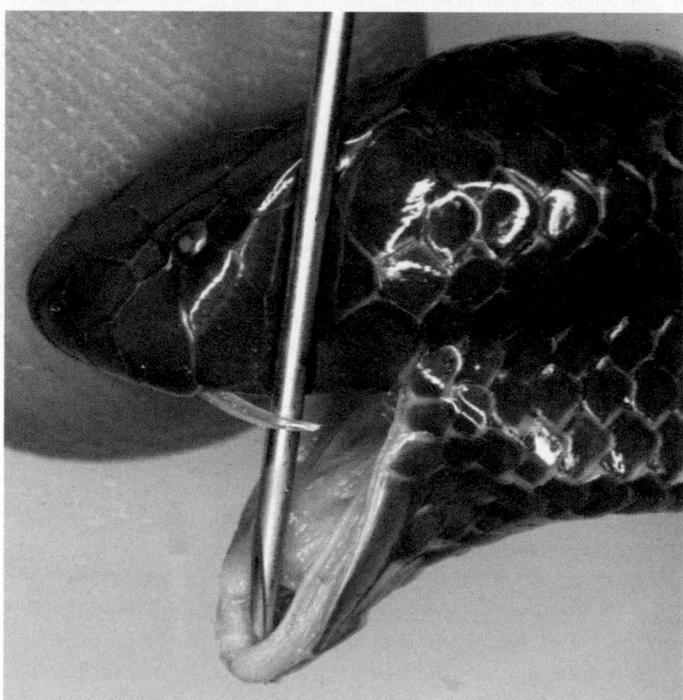

Figure 31.2 Very long front fang of a West African burrowing asp (*Atractaspis aterrima*: family Atractaspididae). (Copyright D. A. Warrell.)

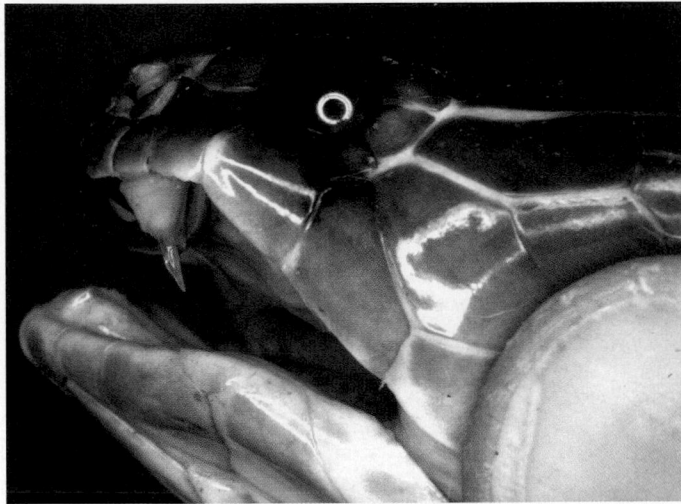

Figure 31.3 Short front fangs of the monocellate Thai cobra (*Naja kaouthia*: family Elapidae). (Copyright D. A. Warrell.)

Calloselasma, Hypnale, Trimeresurus – now divided into several different genera including *Paria, Cryptelytrops, Peltopelor, Viridovipera, Popeia, Himalayophis and Protobothrops*).[11]

The pit of crotaline snakes is an infrared/heat-sensitive organ, situated between the eye and nostril, which detects warm-blooded prey (Figure 31.5).[12] Snakes of the subfamily Viperinae, the Old World vipers and adders, lack this pit organ. The words viper (strictly a snake producing live young – ovoviviparous) and adder (laying eggs) are not used rigorously.

Snake identification

None of the care and skill lavished on the identification of parasites and their vectors has been devoted by medical staff to the identification of venomous snakes. There is no simple and reliable method of distinguishing venomous from non-venomous snakes. The snake's upper jaw can be examined for the presence of fangs, but these may be very small in elapids, and folded back inside a sheath in vipers. The shaft of a needle passed along the maxilla from the angle of the jaw to the snout may engage upon and reveal the fangs. The most dangerous species tend to be well known where they are important. The characteristic hood of cobras and some other elapids is erected only when the snake is rearing up in a defensive attitude (Figure 31.6). Vipers may be identifiable by their distinctive repeated and sometimes colourful dorsal pattern (Figure 31.7). Russell's vipers (*Daboia russelii* and *D. siamensis*) and puff adders (*Bitis arietans*) make a loud hissing sound by expelling air through their large nostrils; the saw-scaled or carpet vipers (genus *Echis*) and desert horned vipers (Cerastes) produce a characteristic rasping sound by rubbing their coils together (Figure 31.8); rattlesnakes produce an unmistakable sound like castanets; and king cobras (*Ophiophagus hannah*) 'growl'. Some harmless snakes are easily mistaken for the venomous species that they mimic: for example, *Telescopus* (cat snake) and *Dasypeltis* (egg-eating snake) mimic *Echis* (saw-scaled viper) species in Africa; *Boiga multomaculata* mimics *Daboia siamensis* in Thailand; various species of Dryocalamus, Dinodon and Lycodon

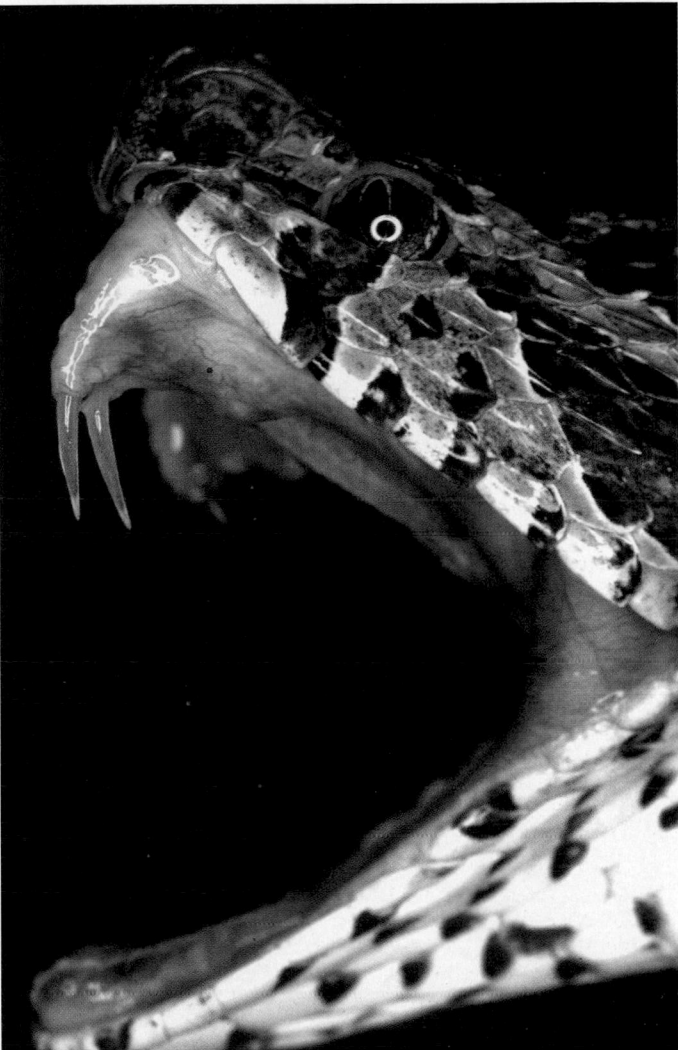

Figure 31.4 Long hinged front fangs, with reserve fang on its left side, enclosed in dental sheath, in a Thai Russell's viper (*Daboia siamensis*: family Viperidae; subfamily Viperinae). (Copyright D. A. Warrell.)

mimic the kraits *Bungarus candidus* and *B. caeruleus* in South Asia; *Xenodon severus* mimics *Bothrops atrox* and *B. brazili* in the Amazon region and the colourful venomous coral snakes (*Micruroides, Micrurus*) of the Western Hemisphere have many non-venomous mimics. The well-known adage 'red on yellow kills a fellow, red on black venom lack' is useful in separating corals from their mimics only in North America (Figure 31.9). Table 31.1 lists the species which, in each continent, are responsible for most snake bite deaths and severe morbidity. Some species notorious for the potency of their venom (e.g. sea snakes and the Australian inland taipan *Oxyuranus microlepidotus*), or their great size (e.g. king cobra, *Ophiophagus hannah* and Gabon vipers *Bitis gabonica* and *B. rhinoceros*), rarely bite humans. The African night adders (genus *Causus*) and burrowing asps (Atractaspis), Asian green pit vipers (genus *Trimeresurus* sensu lato), North American copperheads (*Agkistrodon contortrix*) and Latin American hog-nosed vipers (e.g.

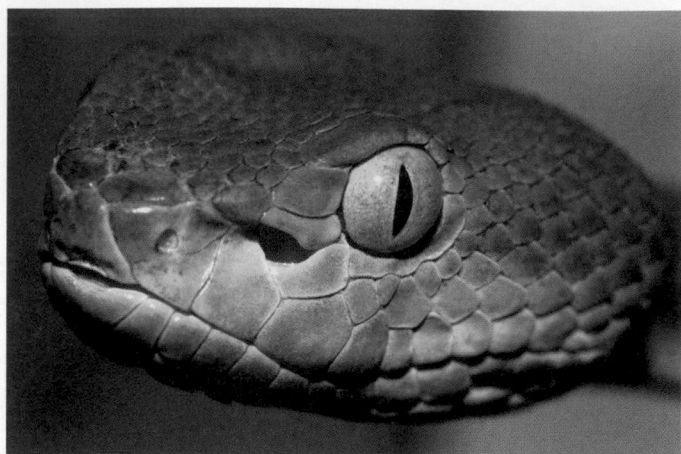

Figure 31.5 South-east Asian arboreal pit viper (*Trimeresurus* [*Cryptelytrops*] *macrops*: family Viperidae; subfamily Crotalinae) showing heat-sensitive pit organ between eye and nostril. (Copyright D. A. Warrell.)

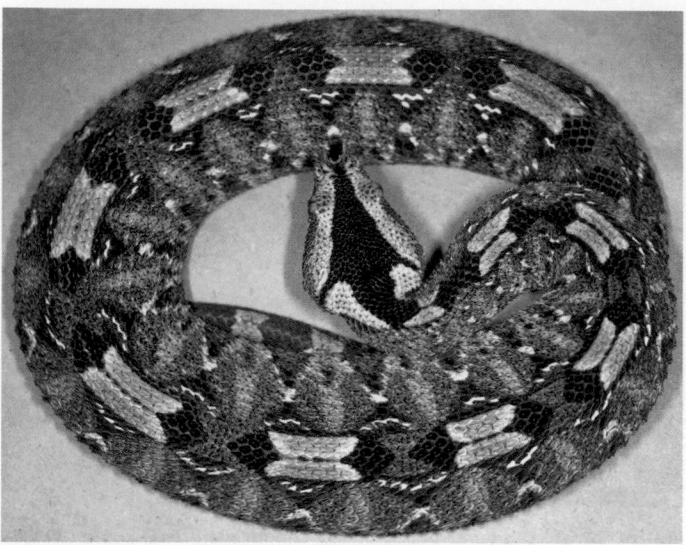

Figure 31.7 Rhinoceros or nose-horned viper of the African rain forest (*Bitis nasicornis*), showing distinctive repeated dorsal pattern. Specimen from Zimbabwe. (Copyright D. A. Warrell.)

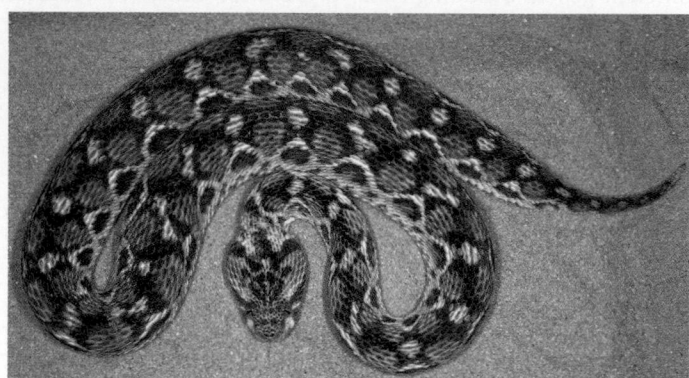

Figure 31.8 Saw-scaled or carpet viper (*Echis pyramidum*). Specimen 55 cm long from Saudi Arabia. (Copyright D. A. Warrell.)

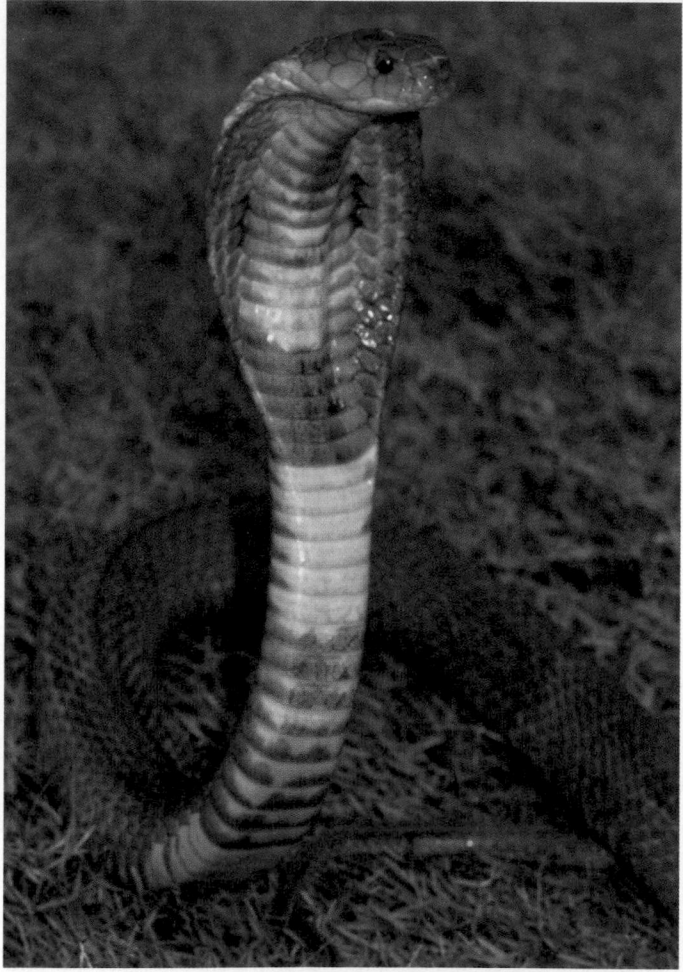

Figure 31.6 Thai spitting cobra, brown phase (*Naja siamensis*: family Elapidae), showing spread hood in threatening/defensive attitude. Specimen 1.3 m long from central Thailand. (Copyright D. A. Warrell.)

Porthidium nasutum) bite many people but rarely cause severe envenoming. Illustrated books, papers, keys and websites are available for the identification of venomous snakes in most parts of the world.

Distribution of venomous snakes

Venomous snakes are widely distributed especially in tropical countries, from sea level to altitudes of 4000 m (*Gloydius/Agkistrodon himalayanus*). The European adder (*Vipera berus*) enters the Arctic Circle. No other venomous species occur in cold regions such as the Arctic, Antarctic and north of about latitude 51°N in North America (Newfoundland, Nova Scotia). Also free from venomous snakes are most of the islands of the western Mediterranean, Atlantic and Caribbean (except in Martinique, Santa Lucia, Margarita, Trinidad and Aruba), New Caledonia, New Zealand, Hawaii and most other Pacific Islands, Crete, Ireland and Iceland.

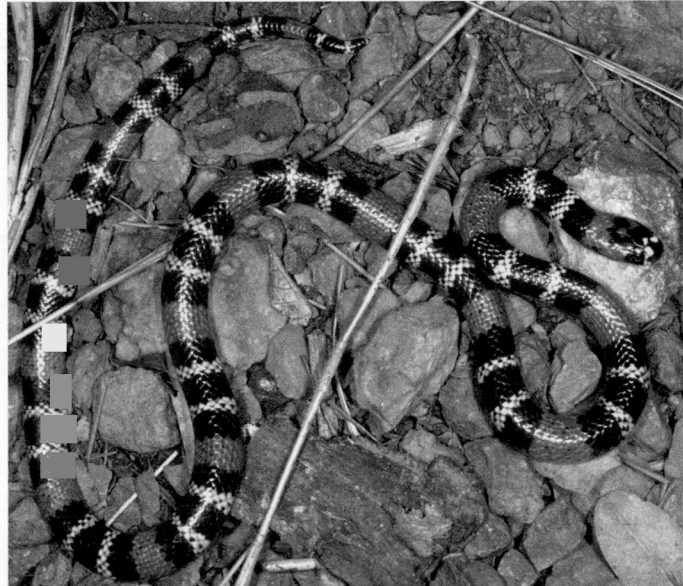

A

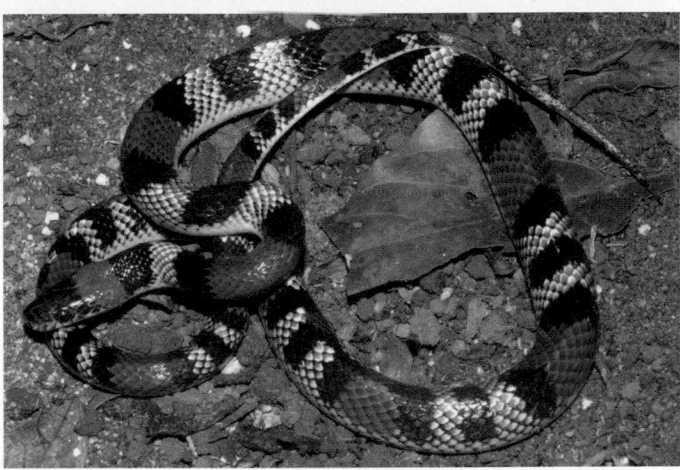

B

Figure 31.9 (**A**) South American coral snake (*Micrurus lemniscatus*: family Elapidae) and (**B**) one of its harmless mimics (*Oxyrophus trigeminus: family colubridae*). Specimens from Brazil. (Copyright D. A.Warrell.)

Madagascar and Chile have only mildly venomous colubrid snakes. Sea snakes exist in the Indian and Pacific Oceans between latitudes 30°N and 30°S, as far north as Siberia (*Pelamis platurus*) and as far south as Easter Island and the North Island of New Zealand and in estuaries, rivers and some freshwater lakes (e.g. *Hydrophis semperi* in Lake Taal, Philippines; *Enhydrina schistosa* in Ton Ley Sap, Cambodia).

Epidemiology of snake bite

The determinants of incidence and severity of snake bite are summarized in Table 31.2. In the tropical countries where snake bite is most common there are few reliable data. Most victims are treated by traditional methods and are lost to the official statistics. Hospital records, the sole source of most snake bite reporting, are likely to over-represent the more seriously envenomed patients,

and depend on the enthusiasm and workload of hospital staff. Population surveys give the most accurate picture of the incidence of snake bite in certain defined areas but cannot be extrapolated to provide national statistics.

In the past, death certification was imprecise because the International Classification of Diseases (ICD) did not distinguish snake bites from attacks by other animals. ICD10, published in 1990, classified snake bite as T63.0, while its revision in 2006 classified it as X20.

Asia

The highest recorded incidence was 162 deaths per 100 000 population per year, determined in the Eastern Terai of Nepal.[13] In this study, only 20% of the deaths occurred in hospitals. Increased risk of fatality was associated with being bitten inside the house while resting between 2400 and 0060 h, suggesting bites by the common krait (*Bungarus caeruleus*) (see below). Other risk factors were an initial visit to a traditional healer and delayed transport to the hospital. An estimated 15 000–20 000, but possibly as many as 50 000, people die each year from snake bite in India. In Barddhaman (Burdwan) District, West Bengal, a field survey in randomly selected villages suggested that among the total population of nearly 5 million people, nearly 8000 were bitten and 800 killed by snakes each year.[14] In the 1930s the annual snake bite mortality reported in Burma exceeded 2000 (15.4 per 100 000 population). Thirty years later it was still estimated to exceed 1000 (3.3 per 100 000) per year and Russell's viper (*Daboia siamensis*) bite was once the fifth most important single cause of all deaths in Burma. In Sri Lanka, about 900 snake bite deaths were recorded in 1984, an incidence of 6 per 100 000 per year. In 2002, the Ministry of Health recorded about 37 240 snake bite admissions to government hospitals, with 81 fatalities. However, comparison of hospital data with death certifications in Monaragala District during a 5-year period (1999–2003) revealed a 63% underestimate by hospital records of the true number of snake bite deaths,[15] partly explained by the fact that 36% of snake bite victims did not seek or achieve hospital treatment. In the Amami and Okinawa Islands of Japan, there were 5488 bites by the habu (*Trimeresurus flavoviridis*) resulting in 50 deaths during the 9 years from 1962 to 1970.[16] The highest incidence of bites on one of the islands was 4.6 per 1000 population per year.

Africa

In the Benue Valley of north-eastern Nigeria, the incidence of snake bites was found to be 497 per 100 000 population per year, with a mortality of 12.2%.[17] Most bites and deaths were attributed to saw-scaled vipers (*Echis ocellatus*). In Bandafassi, south-east Senegal, in a population of 10 509, snake bite mortality was 14 per 100 000 per year. Saw-scaled vipers (*E. ocellatus*), puff adders (*Bitis arietans*) and spitting cobras (*Naja katiensis*) were implicated.[18] A community survey of snake bites by the black-necked spitting cobra (*N. nigricollis*) in Malumfashi, northern Nigeria, found that in a population of 43 500 there were 15–20 bites per 100 000 per year. Only 8.5% of the victims had visited a hospital. The case fatality was 5% and 19% of survivors had persistent physical disability from the locally necrotic effects of the venom.[19] In Kenya, a preliminary survey based on Ministry of Health,

Table 31.1 Species of snake probably responsible for most human snake bite deaths and morbidity

Area	Scientific name	Common name
North America	*Crotalus adamanteus*	Eastern diamondback rattlesnake
	Crotalus atrox	Western diamondback rattlesnake
	Crotalus oreganus subspp.	Western rattlesnakes
Central America	*Crotalus simus* subspp.	Central American rattlesnakes
	Bothrops asper	Terciopelo
South America	*Bothrops atrox, B. asper*	Fer-de-lance, barba amarilla
	Bothrops jararaca	Jararaca
	Crotalus durissus subspp.	South American rattlesnakes, cascabel
Europe	*Vipera berus, V. aspis*	Vipers, adders
	Vipera ammodytes	Long-nosed or nose-horned viper
Africa	*Echis ocellatus, E. leucogaster, E. pyramidum*	Saw-scaled or carpet vipers
	Bitis arietans	Puff adders
	Naja nigricollis, N. Mossambica, etc.	African spitting cobras
	Naja haje	Egyptian cobra
Asia, Middle East	*Echis* spp.	Saw-scaled or carpet vipers
	Macrovipera lebetina	Levantine viper
	Daboia palaestinae	Palestine viper
	Naja oxiana	Oxus cobra
Indian subcontinent and South-east Asia	*Naja naja, N. kaouthia, N. siamensis*, etc.	Asian cobras
	Bungarus spp.	Kraits
	Daboia russelii, D. siamensis	Russell's vipers
	Calloselasma rhodostoma	Malayan pit viper
	Echis carinatus	Saw-scaled or carpet vipers
Far East	*Naja atra* etc.	Asian cobras
	Bungarus multicinctus	Chinese krait
	Trimeresurus (Protobothrops) flavoviridis	Japanese habu
	Trimeresurus (Protobothrops) mucrosquamatus	Cinese habu
	Gloydius blomhoffii subspp.	Mamushis
Australasia, New Guinea	*Acanthophis* spp.	Death adders
	Pseudonaja spp.	Brown snakes
	Notechis spp.	Tiger snakes
	Oxyuranus scutellatus subspp.	Taipans

Table 31.2 Determinants of snake bite incidence and severity of envenoming

Incidence of bites	Severity of envenoming
1. Frequency of contact between snakes and humans, depends on: (a) Population densities (b) Diurnal and seasonal variations in activity (c) Types of behaviour (e.g. human agricultural activities)	1. Dose of venom injected – depends on mechanical efficiency of bite and species and size of snake
	2. Composition and hence potency of venom – depends on species and, within a species, the geographical location, season and age of the snake
2. Snakes' 'irritability' – readiness to strike when alarmed or provoked – varies with species	3. Health, age, size and (?) specific immunity of human victim
	4. Nature and timings of first aid and medical treatment

hospital, clinic and dispensary records in Kakamega and western Kenya, Lake Baringo and Laikipia, Kilifi and Malindi and northern Kenya suggested an overall average frequency of snake bite of 14 (range 2–68) per 100 000 population per year with a minimum death rate of 0.45 per 100 000 per year. Puff adders, black mambas and spitting cobras were responsible for the fatalities.[20] However, a community-based study on the coast in Kilifi district discovered 15 adult snake bite fatalities per 100 000 population per year.[21]

Oceania

In Australia, there are 1000–2000 bites, with an average of three to four deaths, per year. In New Guinea, the incidence of bites was 215 and of deaths was 7.9 per 100 000 population per year in Central Province, while in Kairuku subprovince there were 526 bites per 100 000 per year.[22] The number of deaths may have increased recently because of inadequate antivenom supplies.

Europe

In Britain, there are more than 200 adder (*Vipera berus*) bites each year, but there have been only 14 deaths during the last hundred years, the last in 1975.[23] There were 44 deaths caused by this species in Sweden between 1911 and 1978; and, in Finland, 21 deaths in 25 years, with an annual incidence of almost 200 bites.

Americas

Snake bite is common in Latin America.[8] In Brazil, the case fatality of snake bites in the pre-antivenom era was thought to be about 25%, and the total number of bites 19 200 each year. By 1970, the estimated incidence was 51 026 bites and 1153 deaths per year, but, in 2005, 28 711 bites were reported with 114 deaths (0.4 %). In the USA there are 7000 bites by venomous snakes each year, with 12 to 15 deaths.

Some hunter–gatherer tribes are at high risk of snake bite. Two per cent of adult deaths among the Yanomamo of Venezuela, 5% among the Waorani of Ecuador and 24% among the Kaxinawa of Acré, Brazil, were attributed to snake bites.[24]

Snake bite as an occupational disease

In tropical countries, snake bite is an occupational disease of farmers, plantation workers, herders and hunters. Rice farmers in Burma, Sri Lanka and central Thailand tread on Russell's vipers or inadvertently pick them up in a handful of paddy during the harvest (Figure 31.10).[25] In the savannah of West Africa, farmers are bitten by *Echis* species as they dig the fields at the start of the rainy season.[17] Rubber-tappers in South-east Asia tread on Malayan pit vipers in the dark and are bitten as they make their early morning rounds of the rubber trees, and in the jungles of western Brazil the collectors of natural rubber ('seringueiros') are bitten by *Bothrops atrox*.[24]

Sea snake bites were an occupational hazard of fishermen in those parts of South-east Asia where hand nets were used. Records of 144 sea snake bites were collected in north-west Malaya in 1955–1956.[26] Mechanization of fishing methods in this region has resulted in a dramatic decrease in sea snake bites, but they still

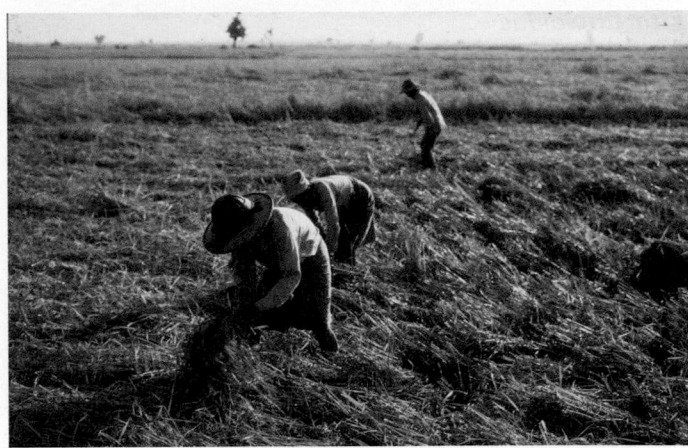

Figure 31.10 Burmese rice farmers harvesting the paddy, an occupation with a high risk of Russell's viper bite. (Copyright D. A. Warrell.)

occur along the coast of south Vietnam.[27] The beaked sea snake (*Enhydrina schistosa*) has caused most bites and deaths. Other common and medically important species are *Hydrophis cyanocinctus*, *H. spiralis* and *Lapemis curtus*.

In the more industrialized countries, venomous snakes are increasingly popular as exotic or 'macho' pets. Many are kept illegally.[23] Most bites are inflicted on the hands when the snakes are picked up, and, in the USA, 25% of bites resulted from snakes being attacked or handled. Unprovoked attacks are excessively rare, but snakes will bite if they are cornered or feel threatened. Some species, notably *Bungarus caeruleus* in India,[28] Nepal[13] and Sri Lanka, *B. candidus* in South-east Asia,[29] and *Naja nigricollis* in West Africa,[30] enter human dwellings at night in pursuit of their prey (rodents, lizards, toads) and may strike at someone who moves in their sleep. Epidemics of snake bite have resulted from a sudden increase in snake population density, for example after flooding in Colombia, Pakistan, India, Bangladesh, Nepal and Burma. In Togo in the 1950s there was an unprecedented increase in *Echis ocellatus* and bites that remain unexplained.[17] Invasion of the snake's habitat by large numbers of people may also be followed by an increased incidence of snake bite. This has happened during the building of new roads through jungles in South America and moving farmers to areas in the former dry zone of Sri Lanka made newly fertile by the Mahaweli irrigation scheme.

Venom apparatus[31]

Colubridae

The crudest venom apparatus is found in the back-fanged Colubridae. The posterior part of the superior labial gland (Duvernoy's gland) drains into a periodontal fold of buccal mucosa. The venom tracks down grooves in the anterior surfaces of the several enlarged posteriorly situated fangs (see Figure 31.1). This arrangement is effective for envenoming the natural prey, a chameleon in the case of the boomslang (*Dispholidus typus*), which is held in the snake's mouth until it is dead. Human envenoming is a rare accident, as the snake must seize and chew the finger of its victim, usually a herpetologist, in order to inject much venom.

Atractaspididae

The venom apparatus of Atractaspididae is unusual and the homology of the venom glands is uncertain.[31] The venom glands of *Atractaspis engaddensis* and *A. microlepidota* are very long, perhaps one-sixth of the snake's total length, as in some elapids (*Maticora*) and Viperidae (*Causus*). The fangs of *Atractaspis* are long. They are protruded out of the corner of the mouth to allow a side-swiping strike at their prey encountered underground in a burrow (see Figure 31.2).

Elapidae (including sea snakes) and Viperidae

The venom gland is situated behind the eye. Compressor muscles, principally the *adductor superficialis* in Elapidae, and the *compressor glandulae* in Viperidae, squeeze venom out of the gland through the venom duct to the base of the fang. Venom is transmitted to the tip of the fang through a partially or completely closed canal in the case of the Viperidae. In several elapid species, the African spitting cobras *Naja nigricollis*, *N. katiensis*, *N. pallida*, *N. ashei*, *N. nubiae*, *N. nigricinctus* and *N. mossambica*, the South African ringhals or rinkhals (*Hemachatus haemachatus*) and Asian spitting cobras (*N. sumatrana*, *N. siamensis*, *N. sputatrix*, etc.), the fang is modified to allow the snake to eject a spray of venom forwards for a metre or more, into the eyes of an aggressor. Instead of opening downwards at the tip of the fang, the venom channel is angled forward at its point of exit in the anterior surface of the fang, a few millimetres above its tip.[32,33]

The function of the venom apparatus has been studied in very few species. The Palestine viper (*Daboia palaestinae*) can inject doses of venom lethal to its natural prey at each of 10 or more consecutive strikes.[31] When a snake bites two or more humans in rapid succession, the second or third victims may, surprisingly, be more severely envenomed than the first. However, Russell's viper injects most of its available venom at the first strike.

Venomous snake bite without envenoming ('dry bites')

Between about 10% (in the case of *Echis ocellatus*) and 80% (Australian western brown snake *Pseudonaja textilis*) of people bitten by venomous snakes, with puncture marks proving that the fangs penetrated the skin, develop no signs of envenoming. Perhaps snakes can bite defensively without injecting venom, but there is little evidence that snakes can control the injected dose of venom: the strike is essentially a reflex 'all or nothing' action. The venom apparatus is evolved to deliver a lethal bite to the snake's natural prey. However, when the snake lashes out in reaction to being trodden upon or picked up, it is less likely, for purely anatomical and mechanical reasons, that an effective strike will be achieved on every occasion.

Venom composition[34,35]

Snakes have evolved the most complex of all venoms, each venom containing more than 100 different components. Snake venom should not be regarded as a single toxin. The variation of venom composition from species to species and within a single species throughout its geographical distribution, at different seasons of the year and as a result of ageing, contributes to the clinical diver-sity of snake bite. The evolutionary origin of snake venom toxins is of great interest.[36,37] More than 90% of the dry weight is protein, comprising a variety of enzymes, non-enzymatic polypeptide toxins and non-toxic proteins. Non-protein ingredients include carbohydrates and metals (often part of glycoprotein metallo-protein enzymes), lipids, free amino acids, nucleosides and biogenic amines such as serotonin (5-hydroxytryptamine) and acetylcholine.

Enzymes

Approximately 89–95% of viperid and 25–70% of elapid venoms consist of enzymes (molecular weight 13–15 kDa), including digestive hydrolases (proteinases, exo- and endopeptidases, phos-phodiesterases and phospholipases), hyaluronidase, and activa-tors or inactivators of the prey's physiological mechanisms. Most venoms contain L-amino acid oxidase, phosphomono- and di-esterases, 5′-nucleotidase, DNA-ase, NAD-nucleosidase, phospho-lipase A$_2$ and peptidases. Elapid venoms, in addition, contain acetylcholine esterase, phospholipase B and glycerophospha-tase, while viperid venoms have endopeptidase, arginine ester hydrolase kininogenase which releases bradykinin from brady-kininogen, thrombin-like serine proteases, and factor X- and pro-thrombin-activating enzymes. Phospholipases A$_2$ are the most widespread and extensively studied of all venom enzymes. Under experimental conditions, they damage mitochondria, red blood cells, leukocytes, platelets, peripheral nerve endings, skeletal muscle, vascular endothelium and other membranes, produce presynaptic neurotoxic activity, opiate-like sedative effects and the autopharmacological release of histamine. Hyaluronidase pro-motes the spread of venom through tissues. Proteolytic enzymes (endopeptidases or hydrolases) are responsible for local changes in vascular permeability leading to oedema, blistering and bruis-ing, and to necrosis. Metalloproteinases cause local and systemic haemorrhage and local myonecrosis, blistering and oedema through their actions on vascular endothelium, platelets,[38] muscle and other tissues. L-amino acid oxidase may have a digestive function.

Neurotoxins

Polypeptide toxins are low-molecular-weight, non-enzymatic proteins found almost exclusively in elapid venoms. Postsynaptic (curaremimetic) neurotoxins, or α-neurotoxins, are either 'short' (60–62 amino acids) or 'long' (66–74 amino acids), such as α-bungarotoxin and cobrotoxin. They bind to the α$_1$-component of nicotinic acetylcholine receptors at the motor end-plates of skeletal muscles, eventually causing generalized flaccid paralysis and death from bulbar and respiratory muscle weakness. They have a distinctive 'three-finger' structure, complementary in shape to their receptor, and have also been found in some colubrid venoms.[39] Presynaptic phospholipases A$_2$, or β-neurotoxins, such as β-bungarotoxin, crotoxin and taipoxin, contain about 120–140 amino acid residues and a phospholipase A subunit. These damage nerve endings at neuromuscular junctions, targeting voltage-gated potassium channels and causing sequential suppression, enhance-ment and finally complete failure of acetylcholine release. The resulting paralysis is clinically indistinguishable from that caused by postsynaptic toxins except that the latter may be ameliorated by anticholinesterases such as edrophonium or neostigmine. Some of the neurotoxic phospholipases A$_2$ and other phospholipases have myotoxic activity. Mamba (*Dendroaspis*) venoms contain a number of unusual neurotoxins.[34,35] Dendrotoxins (59-amino-acid proteins), which bind to voltage-gated potassium channels at nerve endings, causing acetylcholine release, and calciscludine, which blocks calcium channels, are both 'pear' fold structures. Two 'three-finger' neurotoxins are unique to mamba venoms. Fasciculins (61-amino-acid residues) inhibit some acetylcholinesterases, causing persistent muscle fasciculations, while calciseptine binds to calcium channels. Krait venoms have proved to be an important source of neurotoxins for experimental neuropharmacologists. They include presynaptic phospholipases A$_2$, β-bungarotoxins; and postsynaptic α-bungarotoxins and κ-bungarotoxins, which bind to some specific nicotinic acetylcholine receptors in the brain and various ganglia.

Biogenic amines

Biogenic amines such as histamine and serotonin, found particularly in viper venoms, may contribute to the local pain and permeability changes at the site of a snake bite.

Clinical features of envenoming[6]

Symptoms and signs in victims of snake bite are caused by fear, the direct action of the various venom components on tissues, indirect effects such as complement activation and autopharmacological release of endogenous vasoactive substances, effects of treatment and complications such as secondary infections.

Local swelling

In the bitten limb, increased vascular permeability and extravasation of plasma or blood causes swelling and bruising. Venom endopeptidases, metalloproteinase haemorrhagins, membrane-damaging polypeptide toxins, phospholipases, and endogenous autacoids such as histamine, serotonin and kinins are responsible. Venoms of some Viperidae, such as *Daboia* species, *V. berus* and *Crotalus* species, can produce a generalized increase in vascular permeability resulting in pulmonary oedema, serous effusions, conjunctival and facial oedema, and haemoconcentration.

Local tissue necrosis results from the direct action of venom myotoxins and cytotoxins, and ischaemia caused by thrombosis, compression of blood vessels by first-aid methods such as tight tourniquets, or by swollen muscle within a tight fascial compartment. Myotoxins are proteins that can damage the muscle cell plasma membrane directly. Most are phospholipases A$_2$, either enzymatically active (aspartate-49) or enzymatically inactive (lysine-49). Cobra 'cardiotoxins' are cytotoxic low-molecular-weight polypeptides.

Hypotension and shock

Acute profound hypotension with or without other features of anaphylaxis is part of the autopharmacological syndrome which may occur within minutes of bites by *Vipera berus*, *Daboia* species, *Bothrops* species, *Lachesis* species, *Actractaspis engaddensis* and *A. microlepidota*. Presumably this is caused by release of autacoids (eicosanoids, angiotensin, neurotensin, nitric oxide,

kinins, histamine, serotonin, endothelins, etc.). Oligopeptides in Viperidae venoms (e.g. *Bothrops* species) inhibit angiotensin-converting enzymes (ACEs) and enhance the activity of bradykinin-potentiating peptides. They were the model for synthetic ACE inhibitors used to treat hypertension.[40] Snake handlers may become sensitized to snake venoms and can develop life-threatening anaphylactic reactions within minutes of being bitten. Extravasation of plasma or blood into the bitten limb and elsewhere or massive gastrointestinal or uterine haemorrhage may cause hypovolaemia after viper bites. Vasodilatation, especially of splanchnic vessels, and a direct effect on the myocardium may contribute to hypotension after viper and rattlesnake bites.

Bleeding and clotting disturbances[41]

Incoagulable blood resulting from consumptive coagulopathy or venom anticoagulants, thrombocytopenia with platelet dysfunction, and vessel wall damage by haemorrhagins combine to cause life-threatening haemorrhage after snake bite. This group of venom activities is often referred to, inappropriately, as 'vasculotoxic', 'haematotoxic' or even 'haemolytic'. Anti-haemostatic effects are a feature of envenoming by vipers, pit vipers, Australasian elapids and colubrids.

Procoagulant enzymes activate intravascular coagulation which, combined with activation of endogenous fibrinolysis by plasmin, results in consumptive coagulopathy and incoagulable blood. Procoagulants in venoms of Colubridae, *Echis* species and Australian tiger snakes (*Notechis*) activate prothrombin, *Daboia* venoms contain factor V and X activators, and many pit viper (crotaline) venoms have a direct thrombin-like action on fibrinogen.

Activators of fibrinolysis: venoms of rattlesnakes such as *Crotalus atrox* and *C. adamanteus* cause defibrinogenation by activating the endogenous fibrinolytic system.

Venom anticoagulant action is attributable to phospholipases.

Platelet activators/inhibitors: thrombocytopenia is a common accompaniment of systemic envenoming but platelet function has rarely been investigated in human patients. Platelet activators include alboaggregin B (*Trimeresurus* [*Cryptelytrops*] *albolabris*], which activates platelets and promotes aggregation through receptors GPVI and GPIb. Aggretin (*Calloselasma rhodostoma*) activates platelets via receptors GPIb-IX-V and GPIa-IIa. Rhodocytin (or aggretin, *C. rhodostoma*) is a platelet agonist independent of GPIb, GPIa-IIa or GPVI, which activates via CLEC-2. Trimucytin (T. [*Protobothrops*] *mucrosquamatus*) activates platelets via GPIa-IIa, independent of the GPIa-IIa I domain (collagen-binding site). Convulxin (*Crotalus durissus terrificus*), ophioluxin (*Ophiophagus hannah*) and alborhagin (T. [*Cryptelytrops*] *albolabris*) activate platelets via GPVI. Proatherocytin (*Proatheris superciliaris*) is a platelet receptor PAR-1 agonist.

Platelet inhibitors include mocarhagin (*Naja mossambica*) and jararhagin (*Bothrops jararaca*), metalloproteinases which cleave GPIbα and GPIa-IIa, respectively, inhibiting platelet responses depending on these receptors. Rhodocetin (*Calloselasma rhodostoma*) inhibits platelets via interaction with GPIa-IIa. RGD-containing venom peptides are powerful inhibitors of GPIIb-IIIa, the fibrinogen receptor (trigramin, echistatin, contortrostatin, flavoviridin, etc). In patients bitten by Malayan pit vipers and green pit vipers (*T.* [*Cryptelitrops*] *albolabris*) there was initially inhibition of platelet agglutination followed by activation and the appearance of circulating clumps of platelets.[42] In the absence of trauma, defibrination induced by venom coagulants such as ancrod (Arvin, Arwin) from *C. rhodostoma* venom is a relatively benign state. Spontaneous systemic bleeding is attributable to distinct venom components, haemorrhagins, which damage vascular endothelium. These are zinc metallo-endopeptidases (reprolysins), some of which include disintegrin-like, cysteine-rich and lectin domains.

Intravascular haemolysis

Most snake venoms are haemolytic in vitro, but this effect is rarely of clinical significance. However, envenoming by some *Bothrops* species, *Daboia russelii* (in India and Sri Lanka), some Australasian elapids and members of the colubrid genera *Dispholidus*, *Thelotornis* and *Rhabdophis* may cause massive intravascular haemolysis contributing to renal failure. In victims of Sahara horned-viper (*Cerastes cerastes*),[43] Australian brown snake (*Pseudonaja*) and *Bothrops* envenoming, fragmented erythrocytes (schistocytes/helmet cells) are observed in the blood film, indicating microangiopathic haemolysis. This is associated with renal failure, a clinical picture so similar to haemolytic uraemic syndrome or thrombotic thrombocytopenic purpura that some patients have even been treated by plasmapheresis.

Complement activation and inhibition[44]

Elapid and some colubrid venoms activate complement via the alternative pathway ('cobra venom factor' is cobra C3b), whereas some viperid venoms activate the classical pathway. Complement activation may also affect platelets, the blood coagulation system and other humoral mediators.[41] Venom toxins from the Mojave rattlesnake (*Crotalus scutulatus*) and southern Pacific rattlesnake (*C. oreganus helleri*) inactivate both classical and alternative pathways.

Renal failure[45]

Renal failure is a potential complication of severe envenoming, even by species which usually cause relatively mild envenoming, such as *Trimeresurus* (*Cryptelytrops*) *albolabris*, the hump-nosed viper (*Hypnale hypnale*) and *Vipera berus*. However, it is a common event and causes many deaths following bites by Russell's vipers,[25] tropical rattlesnakes (*Crotalus durissus* subspecies) and sea snakes.[27] Mechanisms of acute tubular necrosis include prolonged hypotension and hypovolaemia, disseminated intravascular coagulation, a direct toxic effect of the venom on the renal tubule, haemoglobinuria, myoglobinuria and hyperkalaemia. Russell's viper venom produces hypotension, disseminated intravascular coagulation, direct nephrotoxicity[46] and, in Sri Lanka and India, intravascular haemolysis.[47] In Burmese patients envenomed by Russell's vipers (*D. siamensis*), high urinary concentrations of β_2-microglobulin, retinal binding protein and N-acetyl glucosaminidase suggested failure of proximal tubular reabsorption and tubular damage. High plasma concentrations of active renin suggested that renal ischaemia with activation of the renin–angiotensin system was involved in the development of renal failure. A massive transient capillary and glomerular leak of albumin was an early sign of oliguric renal failure. The mechanism of renal failure in victims of *Crotalus durissus* is most likely to be generalized rhabdomyolysis, combined with hypotension in some cases.[48] A variety of renal histopathological changes have been described after snake bite, including proliferative glomerulonephritis, toxic mesangiolysis with platelet agglutination, fibrin deposition, ischaemic changes, acute tubular necrosis, distal tubular damage ('lower nephron nephrosis') suggesting direct venom nephrotoxicity, and bilateral renal cortical necrosis with subsequent calcification.[45]

Neurotoxicity

The neurotoxic polypeptides and phospholipases of snake venoms cause paralysis by blocking transmission at peripheral neuromuscular junctions. Paralytic symptoms are characteristic of envenoming by most elapids, such as kraits, coral snakes, mambas and cobras, but not of the African spitting cobras (*Naja nigricollis*, *N. pallida*, *N. mossambica*, etc.) which, unusually among elapids, cause local tissue destruction without detectable neurotoxicity.[30] Venoms of terrestrial Australasian snakes, sea snakes and a few species of Viperidae, notably *Crotalus durissus terrificus*, mamushi (*Gloydius* [*Agkistrodon*] *blomhoffii* subspecies) in Japan, China, Korea and Russia, *Daboia russelii* in Sri Lanka and South Indian, the southern African berg adder (*Bitis atropos*), some other small *Bitis* species of southern Africa (*B. peringueyi*, *B. xeropaga*), and European *Vipera ammodytes* and *V. aspis* from southern France and the European Montpellier snake (*Malpalon monspessulanus*) are neurotoxic in humans. Patients with paralysis of the bulbar muscles may die of upper airway obstruction or aspiration, but the most common mode of death after neurotoxic envenoming is respiratory paralysis. Anticholinesterase drugs, by prolonging the activity of acetylcholine at neuromuscular junctions, may improve paralytic symptoms in patients bitten by snakes whose neurotoxins are predominantly postsynaptic in their action (e.g. Asian cobras,[49] Australasian death adders genus *Acanthophis*, Latin American coral snakes genus *Micrurus*). Some patients bitten by elapids or vipers become pathologically drowsy in the absence of respiratory or circulatory failure. This may be caused by endogenous opiates released by a venom component. Intracerebral injection of β-RTX (receptor-active protein) or 'vipoxin' from *Daboia russelii* venom produced sedation in rats.[50]

Rhabdomyolysis

Generalized rhabdomyolysis with release into the bloodstream of myoglobin, muscle enzymes, uric acid, potassium and other muscle constituents, is an effect in man of phospholipase A_2 presynaptic neurotoxins of most species of sea snakes,[27] many of the terrestrial Australasian elapids such as tiger snake (*Notechis scutatus* and *N. ater*), king brown or mulga snake (*Pseudechis australis*), taipan (*Oxyuranus scutellatus*), rough-scaled snake (*Tropidechis carinatus*) and small-eyed snake (*Cryptophis nigrescens*), at least one species of krait (*Bungarus niger*) and several species of Viperidae; tropical rattlesnake (*Crotalus durissus terrificus*),[48] canebrake rattlesnake (*Crotalus horridus atricaudatus*), Mojave rattlesnake (*Crotalus scutulatus*) and Sri Lankan Russell's viper (*Daboia russelii*).[47] Patients may die of bulbar and respiratory muscle weakness, from acute hyperkalaemia or later renal failure.

Venom ophthalmia[51]

Venoms of the spitting cobras and rinkhals are intensely irritant and even destructive on contact with mucous membranes such as the conjunctivae and nasal cavity. Corneal erosions, anterior uveitis and secondary infections may result.

Envenoming by different families of venomous snakes

Colubridae (back-fanged snakes)[7,8]

Severe or fatal envenoming has been reported in patients bitten by several species of back-fanged colubrid snake: in central and southern Africa – boomslang (*Dispholidus typus*), vine, twig, tree or bird snake (*Thelotornis* species); in Japan – yamakagashi (*Rhabdophis tigrinus*); in South-east Asia – red-necked keelback (*R. subminiatus*); in South America – Amazonian green racer (*Philodryas olfersii*), Argentine black-headed snake (*Phalotris lemniscatus*), *Tachymenis peruvianus* and the Amazonian false viper (*Xenodon severus*); and in Europe – Montpellier snake (*Malpolon monspessulanus*). Karl P Schmidt was killed by *Dispholidus typus* and Robert Mertens by *Thelotornis kirtlandi*. Both were distinguished herpetologists. Severe envenoming by colubrids is possible if the snake is able to engage its rear fangs and chew for 15 seconds or longer. All the species except *M. monspessulanus* give rise to similar symptoms, which may be delayed for many hours or even days after the bite. There is nausea, vomiting, colicky abdominal pain and headache. Bleeding develops from old and recent wounds such as venepunctures, and there is spontaneous gingival bleeding, epistaxis, haematemesis, melaena, subarachnoid or intracerebral haemorrhage, haematuria and extensive ecchymoses. Intravascular haemolysis and microangiopathic haemolysis have been described. Most of the fatal cases died of renal failure from acute tubular necrosis, many days after the bite. Local effects of the venom are usually trivial, but several patients showed some local swelling and one bitten by *Dispholidus typus* had massive swelling with blood-filled bullae. Investigations reveal incoagulable blood, defibrination, elevated fibrin(ogen) degradation products (FDPs), severe thrombocytopenia, anaemia, and complement activation by the alternative pathway.[52] These clinical features are explained by disseminated intravascular coagulation triggered by a venom prothrombin activator.

Other potentially dangerous colubrids include Blanding's tree snake (*Toxicodryas/Boiga blandingi*), Road Guarder (*Conophis lineatus*) of Middle America, and neotropical racers (*Alsophis* species and *Philodryas viridissimus*).

Atractaspididae (burrowing asps or stiletto snakes and natal black snake)

Seventeen species of the genus *Atractaspis* and one species of *Macrelaps* have been described in Africa and the Middle East. All are venomous, but fatal envenoming has been described by only three species: *A. microlepidota*, *A. irregularis* and *A. engaddensis*. Local effects include pain, swelling, blistering, necrosis, tender enlargement of local lymph nodes, local numbness or paraesthesiae. The most common systemic symptom is fever. Most of the fatal cases died within 45 minutes of the bite, after vomiting, producing profuse saliva and lapsing into coma.[53] Severe envenoming by *A. engaddensis* may produce violent autonomic symptoms (nausea, vomiting, abdominal pain, diarrhoea, sweating and profuse salivation) within minutes of the bite. One patient developed severe dyspnoea with acute respiratory failure; one had weakness, impaired consciousness and transient hypertension; and in three there were electrocardiographic changes (ST–T changes and prolonged PR interval).[54] Mild abnormalities of blood coagulation and liver function have also been described. *Atractaspis* venom has very high lethal toxicity. The venom of *A. engaddensis* contains four 21-amino-acid peptides, sarafotoxins, which show 60% sequence homology with endogenous endothelins. They cause coronary vasoconstriction and atrioventricular block.[55] The venom also contains haemorrhagic and necrotic factors but no true neurotoxins. Bites by *Macrelaps microlepidotus* are said to have resulted in collapse and loss of consciousness.

Elapidae (cobras, kraits, mambas, coral snakes, sea kraits and true sea snakes)

Local envenoming

In the case of kraits, mambas, coral snakes, most of the Australasian elapids (see below), some of the cobras (e.g. Philippine cobra, *Naja philippinensis*; Cape cobra, *N. nivea*) and sea snakes, local effects are usually mild. However, patients bitten by African spitting cobras (*N. nigricollis*, *N. pallida*, *N. katiensis*, *N. nubiae*, *N. mossambica* and *N. nigricincta*) and Asian cobras (*N. naja*, *N. kaouthia*, *N. siamensis*, *N. sumatrana*, *N. sputatrix*, *N. atra*, etc.) commonly develop tender local swelling, which may be extensive, and regional lymphadenopathy. A characteristic lesion may appear within 24–48 hours. Blistering often surrounds a demarcated pale or blackened anaesthetic area of skin (Figure 31.11(A)). The lesion smells putrid and eventually breaks down with sometimes extensive loss of skin and subcutaneous tissue (Figure 31.11(B)). Skip lesions, separated by areas of apparently normal skin, may extend proximally up the limb. Prolonged morbidity may result and some patients may lose a digit or the affected limb if there is secondary infection. Severe envenoming by the king cobra (*Ophiophagus hannah*) results in swelling of the whole limb and formation of bullae at the site of the bite, but local necrosis is minimal or absent.[56]

Neurotoxic effects

Descending flaccid paralysis is seen in patients envenomed by Asian cobras (it is the main feature in victims of *N. philippinensis*), king cobra and most other elapids, but has not been documented in victims of African spitting cobras. The earliest symptom of systemic envenoming is repeated vomiting, but the use of emetic herbal medicines may confuse the interpretation of this symptom. Other early pre-paralytic symptoms include contraction of the frontalis (before there is demonstrable ptosis), blurred vision, paraesthesiae especially around the mouth, hyperacusis, loss of sense of smell and taste, headache, dizziness, vertigo, and signs of autonomic nervous stimulation such as hypersalivation, congested conjunctivae and 'goose-flesh'. Paralysis is first detectable as ptosis and external ophthalmoplegia, as ocular muscles are most sensitive to neuromuscular blockade (Figure 31.12). These

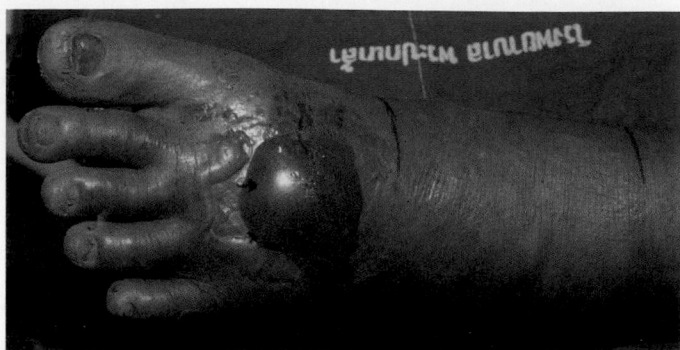

A

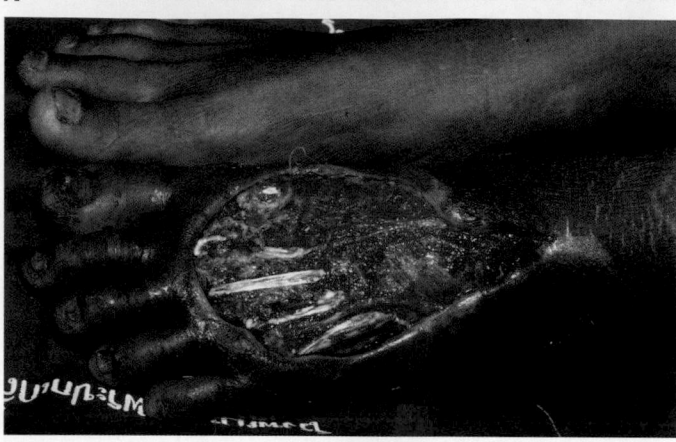

B

Figure 31.11 Characteristic local necrotic lesion produced by bites of African spitting cobras and Asian cobras. In this case, the patient was bitten by a monocellate Thai cobra (*Naja kaouthia*). (**A**) Four days after the bite, there is a darkened anaesthetic area at the site of the bite, surrounded by blisters. (**B**) Demarcated necrosis 1 week later. There was a characteristic smell of putrefaction. (Copyright D. A. Warrell.)

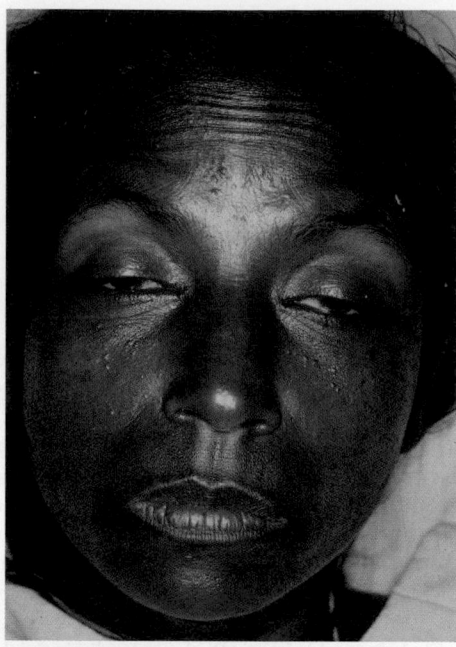

Figure 31.12 Severe ptosis, external ophthalmoplegia and inability to open the mouth, protrude the tongue or swallow in a Sri Lankan patient bitten by a common krait (*Bungarus caeruleus*). (Copyright D. A. Warrell.)

signs may appear as early as 15 minutes after the bite (cobras or mambas), but may be delayed for 10 hours or more following krait bites. Later, the facial muscles, palate, jaws, tongue, vocal cords, neck muscles and muscles of deglutition may become paralysed (Figure 31.13). The pupils are dilated. Many patients are unable to open their mouths, but this can be overcome by force. In a minority, the jaw is said to hang open. Respiratory arrest may be precipitated by obstruction of the upper airway by the paralysed tongue or inhaled vomitus. Intercostal muscles are affected before the limbs, diaphragm and superficial muscles, and, even in patients with generalized flaccid paralysis, slight movements of the digits may be possible, allowing the patients to signal. Loss of consciousness and generalized convulsions are usually explained by hypoxaemia in patients who have respiratory paralysis. However, drowsiness, before the development of significant paralysis, has often been described but remains unexplained. Drooping eyelids from tiredness may be misconstrued as ptosis, unless the extent of lid retraction with upward gaze is formally assessed. Patients with systemic envenoming suffer from headache, malaise and generalized myalgia. Intractable hypotension can occur in patients envenomed by Asian cobras, despite adequate respiratory support.

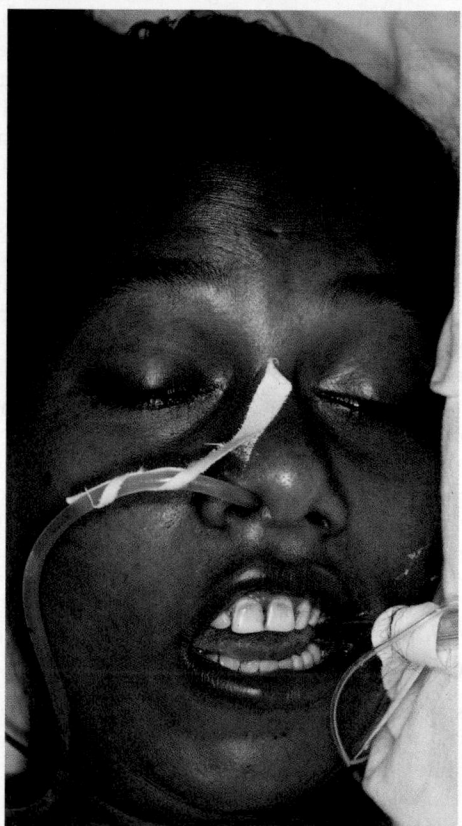

Figure 31.13 Ptosis and inability to open the mouth or protrude the tongue in a Sri Lankan patient bitten by a common krait (*Bungarus caeruleus*). (Copyright D. A. Warrell.)

Neurotoxic effects are completely reversible, either acutely in response to antivenom or (for example, in Asian cobra, South American coral snake and Australasian death adder bites) to anticholinesterases,[49] or they may slowly wear off spontaneously. In the absence of specific antivenom, patients supported by mechanical ventilators recover sufficient diaphragmatic movement to breathe adequately in 1–4 days. Ocular muscles recover in 2–4 days and there is usually full recovery of motor function in 3–7 days.

Bites by Australasian elapids[3,57,58]

Venoms of these snakes result in three main groups of symptoms: neurotoxicity similar to that seen with other elapid bites (Figure 31.14),[57–59] generalized rhabdomyolysis, and haemostatic disturbances. Local signs are usually mild, but extensive local swelling and bruising with necrosis has been reported, especially after bites by the king brown or mulga snake (*Pseudechis australis*). Painful and tender local lymph nodes are a common feature in patients developing systemic envenoming. Early symptoms include vomiting, headache and syncopal attacks similar to those experienced after some viper bites. Electrocardiographic changes were common in patients envenomed by taipans (*Oxyuranus scutellatus canni*) in Papua New Guinea, but only a few had raised cardiac troponin-T levels suggesting myocardial damage. In dogs, common brown snake (*Pseudonaja textilis*) venom caused myocardial depression attributed to disseminated intravascular coagulation and tiger snake (*Notechis scutatus*) venom caused formation of thrombi

within the heart leading to pulmonary and coronary artery thromboembolism.[3]

Persistent bleeding from wounds and spontaneous systemic bleeding from gums and gastrointestinal tract is found in association with incoagulable blood following bites by many Australasian species. Venoms of 15 out of 19 species exhibited procoagulant activity in vitro.[3] Some venoms (e.g. *Pseudonaja*, *Pseudechis* and *Micropechis ikaheka*, the New Guinean small-eyed snake) are anticoagulant. Haemostatic abnormalities are particularly frequent and serious in patients bitten by tiger snakes (*Notechis* species), taipans (*Oxyuranus* species) and brown snakes (*Pseudonaja* species), uncommonly with bites by black snakes (*Pseudechis* species) and rare with bites by death adders (*Acanthophis* species).

In the past, there has been some confusion between haemoglobinuria and myoglobinuria in patients passing dark urine. It is now clear, however, that haemoglobinaemia and haemoglobinuria can occur as a result of intravascular haemolysis (e.g. with envenoming by *Pseudechis australis*) but that myoglobinuria caused by generalized rhabdomyolysis is also a feature of envenoming by some species (e.g. *Notechis*, *Oxyuranus*, *Pseudechis australis*, etc). Renal failure may result from haemoglobinuria or myoglobinuria.

Snake venom ophthalmia[19,51]

Venom ophthalmia results when venom of spitting elapids enters the eye. There is intense local pain, blepharospasm, palpebral oedema and leukorrhoea (Figure 31.15). Slit-lamp or fluorescein examination reveals corneal erosions in more than half the patients spat at by *Naja nigricollis*.[51] Secondary infection of the corneal lesions may result in permanent opacities causing blindness or panophthalmitis with destruction of the eye. Rarely, venom is absorbed into the anterior chamber, causing hypopyon and anterior uveitis. Seventh (facial) cranial nerve paralysis is a rare complication.

Venom of other snakes, including Viperidae, may be forcibly ejected when striking, for example against the bars of a cage. There are reported cases of venom entering the eye under these circumstances and resulting in intense local pain and inflammation.

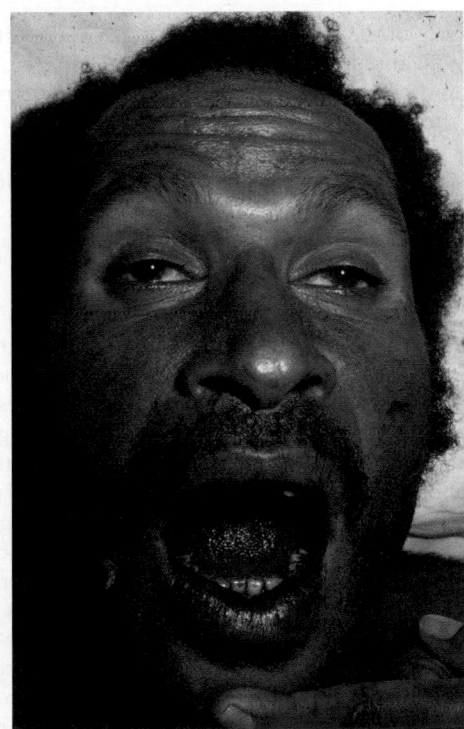

Figure 31.14 Ptosis, external ophthalmoplegia and bleeding gums in a Papua New Guinean man bitten by a taipan (*Oxyuranus scutellatus canni*). (Copyright D. A. Warrell.)

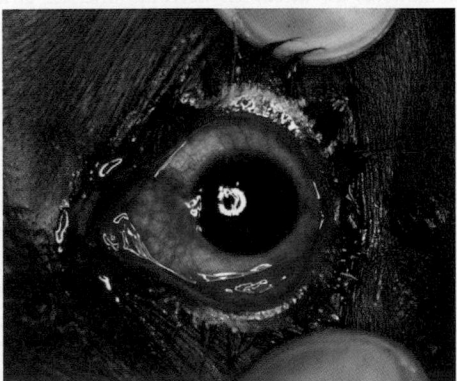

Figure 31.15 Intense conjunctivitis with leukorrhoea (and corneal erosions) in a patient 'spat' at 3 hours previously by an African black-necked or spitting cobra (*Naja nigricollis*). (Copyright D. A. Warrell.)

Bites by sea snakes[3,27,60]

The bite is usually painless and may not be noticed by the wader or swimmer. Teeth may be left in the wound. There is minimal or no local swelling, and involvement of local lymph nodes is unusual. Generalized rhabdomyolysis is the dominant effect of envenoming by these snakes. Early symptoms include headache, a thick feeling of the tongue, thirst, sweating and vomiting. Generalized aching, stiffness and tenderness of the muscles becomes noticeable between 30 minutes and $3^1/_2$ hours after the bite. Trismus is common. Passive stretching of the muscles is painful. Later, there is progressive flaccid paralysis starting with ptosis, as in elapid envenoming. The patient remains conscious until the respiratory muscles are sufficiently affected to cause respiratory failure. Myoglobinaemia and myoglobinuria develop 3–8 hours after the bite. These are suspected when the serum/plasma appears brownish and the urine dark reddish brown ('Coca-Cola-coloured'). 'Stix' tests will appear positive for haemoglobin/blood in urine containing myoglobin. Myoglobin and potassium released from damaged skeletal muscles may cause renal failure, while hyperkalaemia developing within 6–12 hours of the bite may precipitate cardiac arrest.

Viperidae (old world vipers and adders, new world pit vipers, rattlesnakes, moccasins and lance-headed vipers, asian pit vipers)

Local envenoming

Venoms of vipers and pit vipers usually produce more local effects than do other snake venoms. Swelling may appear within 15 minutes, but rarely is delayed for several hours. It spreads rapidly, sometimes to involve the whole limb and adjacent trunk. There is associated pain, tenderness and enlargement of regional lymph nodes. Bruising, especially along the path of superficial lymphatics and over regional lymph nodes, is common (Figure 31.16). There may be persistent bleeding from the fang marks. Swollen limbs can accommodate many litres of extravasated blood, leading to hypovolaemic shock. Blistering may appear at the bite site as early as 12 hours after the bite. Blisters contain clear or bloodstained fluid (Figure 31.17). Necrosis of skin, subcutaneous tissue and muscle (Figure 31.18) develops in up to 10% of hospitalized cases, especially following bites by North American rattlesnakes (e.g. *Crotalus adamanteus*, *C. atrox*, *C. horridus* and *C. viridis*), South American lance-headed vipers (genus *Bothrops*), bushmasters (genus *Lachesis*), Asian pit vipers (e.g. *Calloselasma rhodostoma*, *Deinagkistrodon acutus* and *Trimeresurus flavoviridis*), African vipers (genus *Bitis*), saw-scaled vipers (genus *Echis*) and Palestine viper (*Daboia palaestinae*). Bites on the digits and in areas draining into the tight fascial compartments, such as the anterior tibial compartment, are particularly likely to result in necrosis. High intracompartmental pressure may cause ischaemia which contributes, together with direct effects of the venom, to muscle necrosis.[61] Severe pain associated with tense swelling, segmental anaesthesia and pain on stretching the intracompartmental muscles (e.g. dorsiflexion of the foot in the case of the anterior tibial compartment) should raise the possibility of raised intracompartmental pressure. Sudden severe pain, absence of arterial pulses and a demarcated cold segment of limb suggest thrombosis of a major artery. Deep venous thrombosis has been described surprisingly rarely.

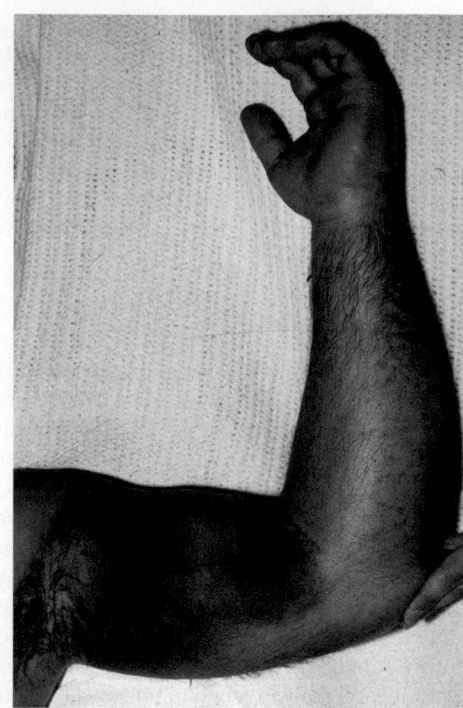

Figure 31.16 Bruising 48 hours after a bite on the hand by a Californian Pacific rattlesnake (*Crotalus oreganus helleri*). (Copyright D. A. Warrell.)

The absence of detectable local swelling 2 hours after a viper bite usually means that no venom has been injected. However, there are important exceptions to this rule: fatal systemic envenoming by the tropical rattlesnake (*Crotalus durissus terrificus*), Mojave rattlesnake (*Crotalus scutulatus*) and Burmese Russell's viper (*Daboia siamensis*) may occur in the absence of local signs. Victims of *C. d. terrificus* may develop local erythema, but rarely more than mild swelling.

Haemostatic abnormalities

These are characteristic of envenoming by Viperidae, but are usually absent in patients bitten by the smaller European vipers (*V. berus*, *V. aspis*, *V. ammodytes*, etc.) and some species of rattlesnakes. Persistent bleeding (>10 minutes) from the fang puncture wounds and from new injuries such as venepuncture sites and old partially healed wounds is the first clinical evidence of consumption coagulopathy. Spontaneous systemic haemorrhage is most often detected in the gingival sulci (Figure 31.19). Bloodstaining of saliva and sputum usually reflects bleeding gums or epistaxis. True haemoptysis is rare. Haematuria may be detected a few hours after the bite. Other types of spontaneous bleeding are ecchymoses, intracranial and subconjunctival haemorrhages, bleeding into the floor of the mouth, tympanic membrane, and gastrointestinal and genitourinary tracts, petechiae and larger discoid and follicular haemorrhages (Figure 31.20). Bleeding into the anterior pituitary (resembling Sheehan's syndrome) may complicate envenoming by Russell's vipers in Burma and India and, rarely, by

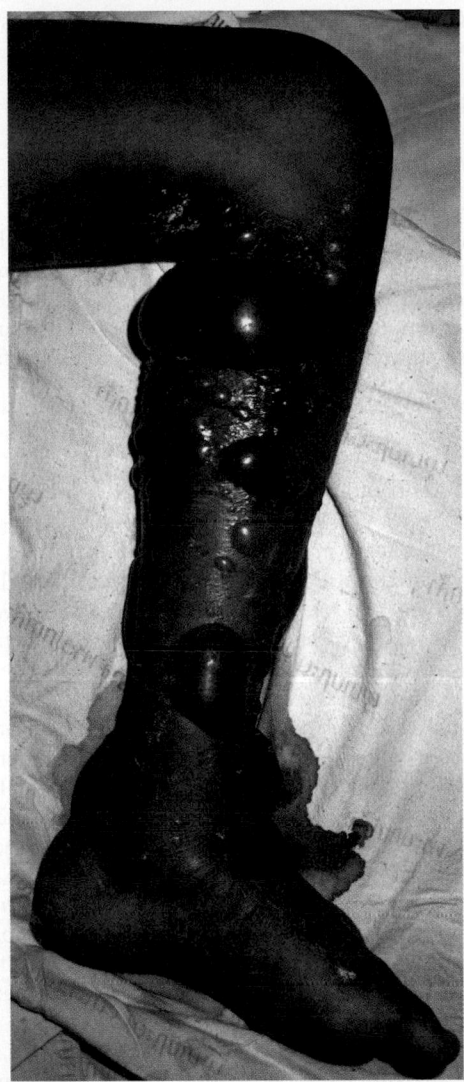

Figure 31.17 Massive swelling and bulla formation in a Thai patient 36 hours after being bitten by a Malayan pit viper (*Calloselasma rhodostoma*). (Copyright D. A. Warrell.)

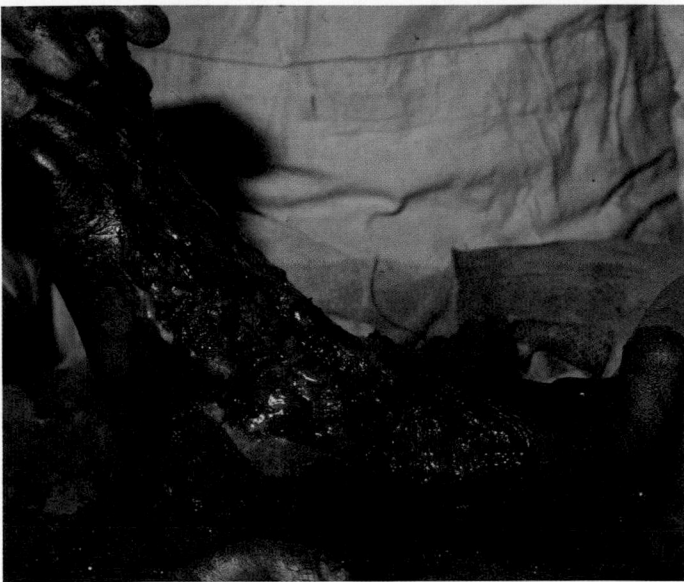

Figure 31.18 Necrosis of the skin and subcutaneous tissues in a Nigerian child 5 days after being bitten by a saw-scaled viper (*Echis ocelatus*). (Copyright D. A. Warrell.)

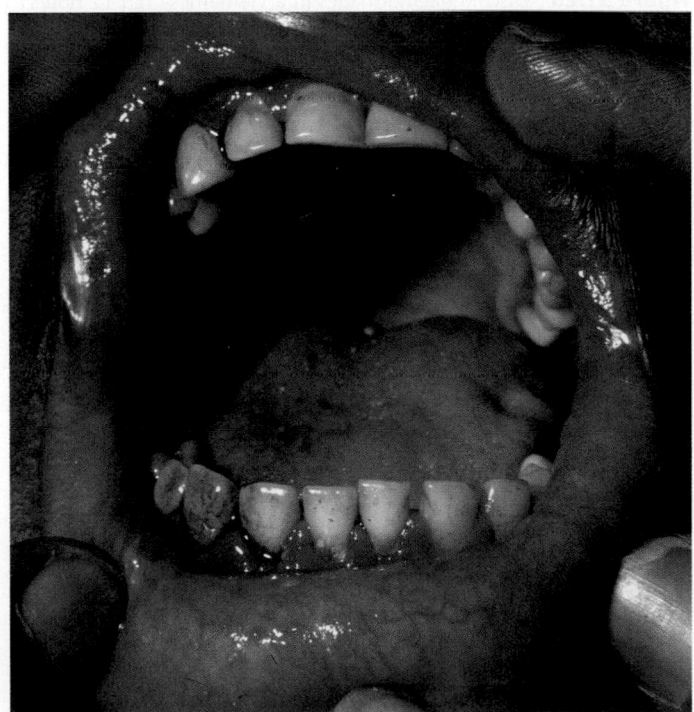

Figure 31.19 Bleeding from gingival sulci in a Nigerian patient bitten by a saw-scaled or carpet viper (*Echis ocellatus*). (Copyright D. A. Warrell.)

Bothrops species. Menorrhagia and antepartum and postpartum haemorrhage have been described after envenoming by vipers. Severe headache and meningism suggest subarachnoid haemorrhage; evidence of a developing central nervous system lesion (e.g. hemiplegia), irritability, loss of consciousness and convulsions suggest intracranial haemorrhage (Figure 31.21) or cerebral thrombosis. Abdominal distension, tenderness and peritonism with signs of haemorrhagic shock but no external blood loss (haematemesis or melaena) suggest retroperitoneal or intraperitoneal haemorrhage. Incoagulable blood resulting from defibrination or disseminated intravascular coagulation is a common and important finding in patients systemically envenomed by members of the following genera: *Atheris, Daboia, Vipera, Echis, Lachesis, Agkistrodon, Gloydius, Bothrops, Calloselasma, Crotalus, Deinagkistro-*

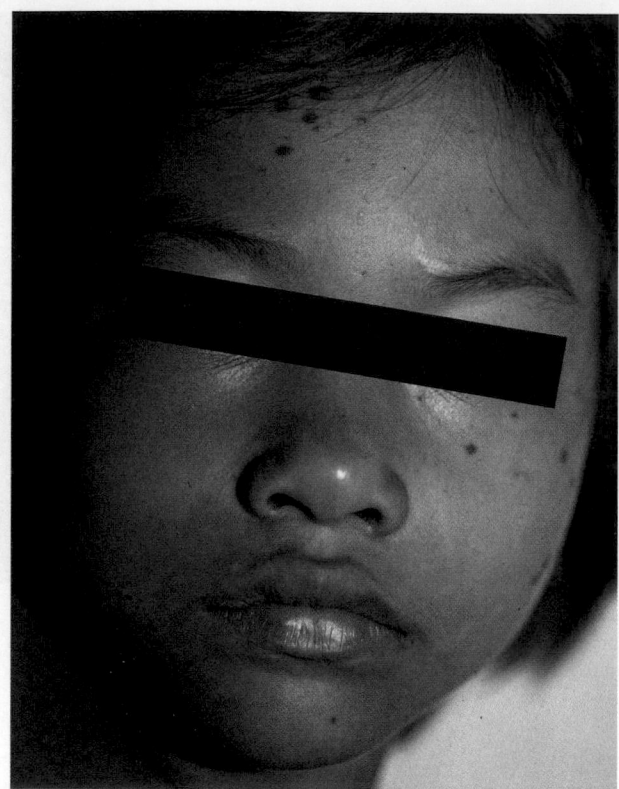

Figure 31.20 Discoid haemorrhages in a Vietnamese girl 12 hours after being bitten by a Malayan pit viper (*Calloselasma rhodostoma*). (Copyright D. A. Warrell.)

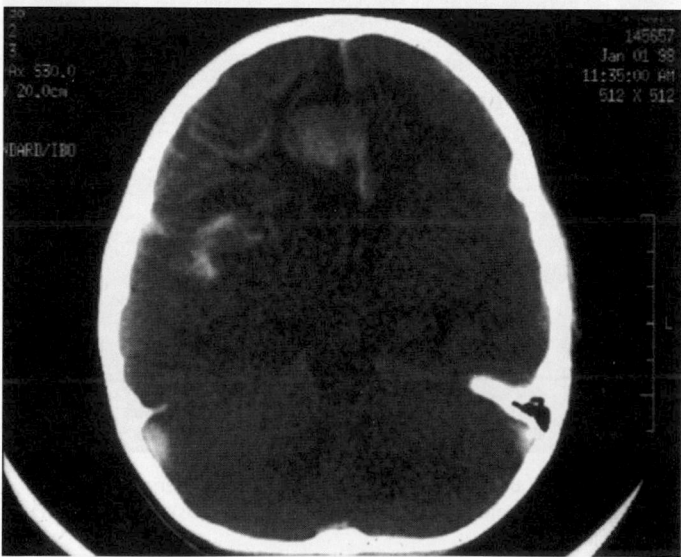

Figure 31.21 Cerebral CT scan of a 7-year-old Ecuadorian girl who had developed sudden headache followed by loss of consciousness 25 hours after being bitten by a *Bothrops atrox*. (Copyright D. A. Warrell.)

don and *Trimeresurus* sensu lato. In situ thrombosis of major arteries (cerebral, pulmonary, coronary, etc.) is an important feature of envenoming by the 'fer de lance' (*B. lanceolatus*) of Martinique and *B. caribbaeus* in adjacent St Lucia.[8]

Intravascular haemolysis

This presents as haemoglobinaemia (pink plasma) and black or greyish urine (haemoglobinuria or methaemoglobinuria). It has been described in patients bitten by Sri Lankan Russell's viper (*Daboia russelii*),[47] desert horned viper (*Cerastes cerastes*) and South American *Bothrops* species. Features of microangiopathic haemolysis with progressive severe anaemia and renal failure may result.

Circulatory shock (hypotensive) syndromes

A fall in blood pressure is a common and serious event in patients bitten by vipers, especially in the case of some of the North American rattlesnakes (e.g. *Crotalus adamanteus*, *C. atrox* and *C. scutulatus*), South American Crotalinae (e.g. *Lachesis muta*) and Old World Viperinae (e.g. *Daboia russelii*, *Daboia palaestinae*, *Vipera berus*, *Bitis arietans*, *B. gabonica* and *B. rhinoceros*). Sinus tachycardia suggests hypovolaemia resulting from external haemorrhage, blood loss into the tissues, or local or generalized increase in capillary permeability. Patients envenomed by Burmese Russell's viper (*Daboia siamensis*) may develop conjunctival oedema (Figure 31.22), serous effusions, pulmonary oedema (Figure 31.23), haemoconcentration and a fall in serum albumin concentration, evidence of increased vascular permeability.[25] The pulse rate may be slow or irregular if the venom is affecting the heart directly or reflexly (e.g. *Vipera berus*, *Bitis arietans*, *Calloselasma rhodostoma*). Vasovagal syncope may be precipitated by fear and pain. Early, repeated and usually transient syncopal attacks with features of anaphylaxis develop in patients bitten by some Viperidae (e.g. *Daboia palaestinae*, *V. berus*, *V. aspis* and *D. russelii*). Vomiting, sweating, colic, diarrhoea (with incontinence), shock, bronchospasm, urticaria and angio-oedema of the face, lips, gums, tongue and throat may appear as early as 5 minutes or as late as many hours after the bite. Hypotension is an important feature of anaphylactic reactions to antivenom (see below).

Renal failure

This can complicate severe envenoming by any species of snake, but it is common, and the most frequent cause of death in

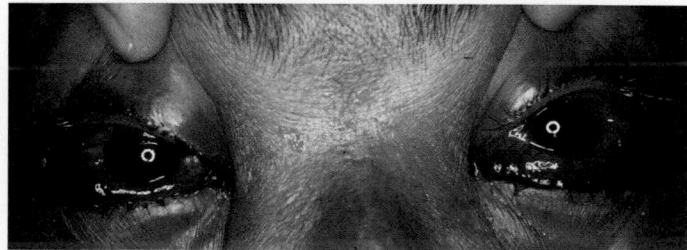

Figure 31.22 Intense bilateral conjunctival oedema (chemosis) in a Burmese man bitten 24 hours previously by a Russell's viper (*Daboia siamensis*). (Copyright D. A. Warrell.)

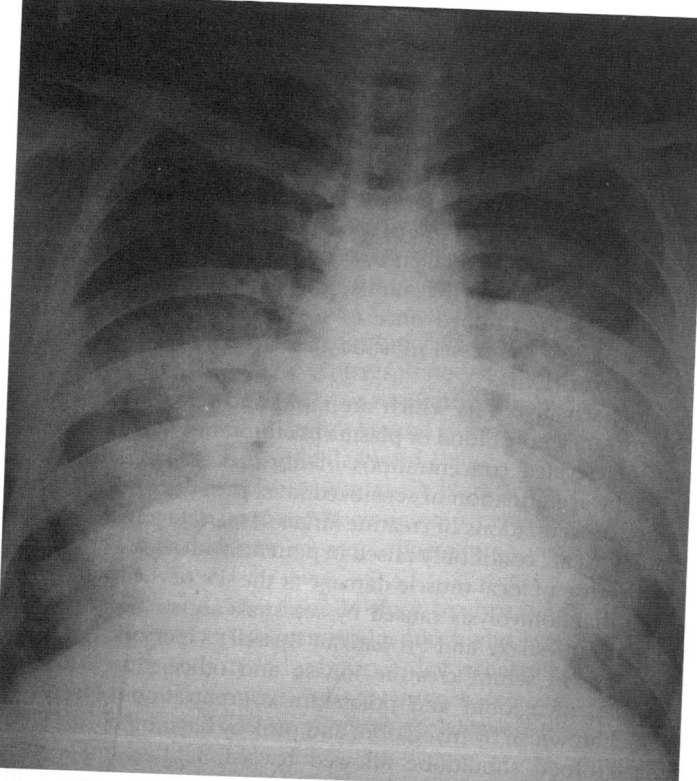

Figure 31.23 Chest radiograph of a Burmese man who developed pulmonary oedema after being bitten by a Russell's viper (*Daboia siamensis*). (Copyright D. A. Warrell.)

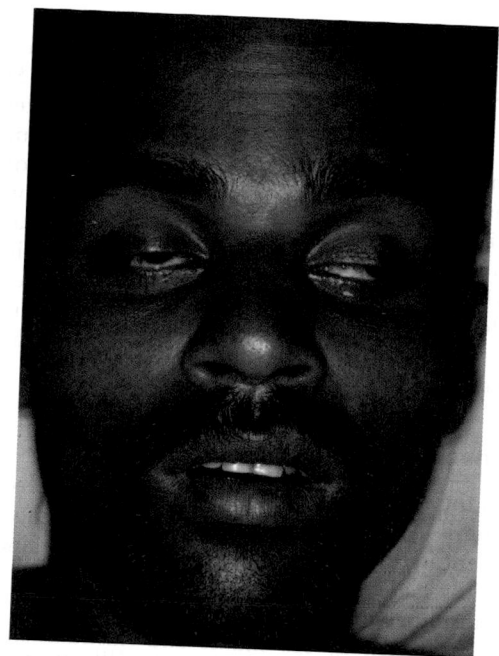

Figure 31.24 Sri Lankan man with neurotoxic envenoming by Russell's viper (*Daboia russelii*). There is ptosis, ophthalmoplegia and inability to open the mouth and protrude the tongue. (Copyright D. A. Warrell.)

victims of Russell's viper, tropical rattlesnake (*Crotalus durissus* subspecies) and some species of *Bothrops*. Patients bitten by Russell's vipers may become oliguric within a few hours of the bite. Loin pain and tenderness may be experienced within the first 24 hours and, in 3 or 4 days, the patient may become irritable, comatose or convulsing, with hypertension and evidence of metabolic acidosis.

Neurotoxicity

This is attributable to venom phospholipases A₂, and is a feature of envenoming by a few species of Viperidae (e.g. *Crotalus durissus terrificus*, *Agkistrodon blomhoffii*, *Vipera aspis*, *Bitis atropos* and other small South African *Bitis* species, and Sri Lankan Russell's viper). The clinical features are the same as with elapid envenoming (Figure 31.24). Progression to respiratory or generalized paralysis has been described. Associated generalized myalgia suggests the possibility of rhabdomyolysis. Pupillary dilatation, causing visual disturbance from loss of accommodation, is a feature of severe envenoming by tropical rattlesnakes and small *Bitis* species (e.g. *B. peringueyi*) and may be a permanent neurological sequela. In North America, distinctive patterns of neurotoxicity have been observed after rattlesnake bites. Severe envenoming by Mojave rattlesnakes (*Crotalus scutulatus scutulatus*) causes weakness and diffuse fasciculations often involving muscles innervated by cranial

nerves. Respiratory insufficiency may develop. Myokymia is reported after bites by timber rattlesnakes (*Crotalus horridus horridus*) and Western diamondback rattlesnakes (*C. atrox*). Venoms of some populations of Southern Pacific rattlesnakes (*C. oreganus helleri*) in south-west California and Baja California can cause dramatic neurotoxic clinical effects including a metallic taste in the mouth, generalized weakness, ptosis, diplopia, dysphagia, dysphonia, respiratory distress progressing to respiratory paralysis and persisting muscle fasciculations of the face, tongue, and upper extremities, as well as local swelling, shock, coagulopathy and rhabdomyolysis.[62,63]

Clinical course and prognosis

Local swelling is usually evident within 2–4 hours of bites by vipers and cytotoxic cobras, and may evolve very rapidly after rattlesnake bites. Swelling is maximal and most extensive on the second or third day after the bite. Resolution of swelling and restoration of normal function in the bitten limb may be delayed for months, especially in older people (e.g. after bites by the European adder *Vipera berus*). The earliest systemic symptoms such as vomiting and syncope may develop within minutes of the bite, but even in the case of rapidly absorbed elapid venoms, patients rarely die within 1 hour of the bite. Defibrination may be complete within 1–2 hours of the bite (e.g. saw-scaled or carpet viper *Echis ocellatus*).[64] Neurotoxic signs may progress to generalized flaccid paralysis and respiratory arrest within a few hours. If the venom is not neutralized by antivenom, these effects may be prolonged. Defibrination can persist for weeks (*Echis* species and *Calloselasma*

573

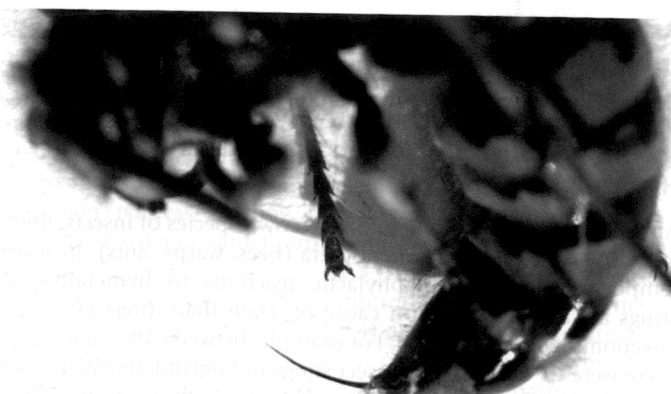

Figure 31.37 Stinger of the common European wasp (*Paravespula germanica*). (Copyright D. A. Warrell.)

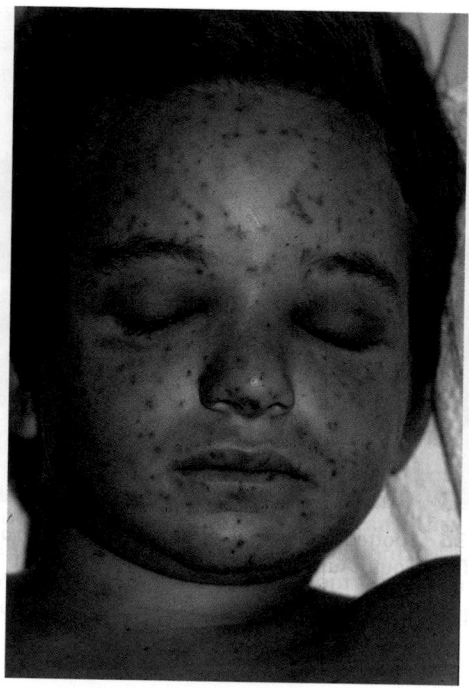

Figure 31.38 Multiple bee stings by Africanized honey-bees (*Apis mellifera scutellata*) causing severe envenoming in a 14-year-old Brazilian boy. (Copyright D. A. Warrell.)

diameter or last more than a few hours. Local effects are dangerous only if the airway is obstructed, for example following stings on the tongue.

In non-allergic subjects, fatal systemic toxicity can result from as few as 30 stings in children, while adults have survived more than 2000 stings by *Apis mellifera*. In some patients the clinical effects of massive envenoming resemble histamine overdose: vaso-dilatation, hypotension, vomiting, diarrhoea, throbbing headache and coma. However, mass attacks by Africanized bees in Latin America can cause intravascular haemolysis, generalized rhabdo-myolysis (causing grossly elevated serum creatine phosphokinase, aminopeptidases and myoglobin), hypercatecholinaemia (hyper-tension, pulmonary oedema, myocardial damage), bleeding, hepatic dysfunction and acute renal failure (Figure 31.38).[115] Hepatic dysfunction and rhabdomyolysis followed by myoglobin-uria and renal failure can occur after multiple hornet stings (*Vespa affinis*). Intravascular haemolysis with haemoglobinuria (*Vespa orientalis*), thrombocytopenic purpura, myasthenia gravis (*Polistes* species) and various renal lesions, including nephrotic syndrome, have also been described.

Allergic effects

Between 3% and 4% of the population may be hypersensitive to Hymenoptera venoms. Clinical suspicion of venom hypersensitiv-ity arises when systemic symptoms follow a sting. In England, sensitization to bee venom appears to require more stings (average, 81 on 23 occasions) than sensitization to wasp venom (average, four stings).[118] Most patients allergic to bee venom are bee-keepers or their relatives. Systemic symptoms include tingling scalp, flush-ing, dizziness, visual disturbances, syncope, wheezing, abdominal colic, diarrhoea and tachycardia developing within a few minutes of the sting. Over the next 15–20 minutes, urticaria, angio-oedema, oedema of the glottis, profound hypotension and coma may develop. Patients may die within minutes of the sting. Raised serum concentrations of mast-cell tryptase, which may persist for up to 6 hours, confirm the diagnosis of anaphylaxis. In a few cases, serum sickness develops a week or more after the

sting. Atopy does not predispose to sting allergy but asthmatics who are allergic to venom are likely to suffer severe reactions. Reactions are enhanced by β-blockers. The diagnosis of venom hypersensitivity can be confirmed by intradermal skin testing with dialysed venoms, or by detecting specific IgE antibodies in serum by the radioallergosorbent test (RAST). Whole body extracts of bees and wasps, traditionally used for skin testing, do not discriminate between hypersensitive patients and controls. A postmortem diagnosis of insect sting anaphylaxis is supported by detecting specific IgE in the victim's serum. Pathological findings in cases of fatal systemic anaphylaxis include acute pulmonary hyperinflation, laryngeal oedema, pulmonary oedema and intra-alveolar haemorrhage.

Treatment

The embedded bee sting should be removed as quickly as possible by any means. Domestic meat tenderizer (papain), diluted roughly 1 in 5 with tap water, is said to produce immediate relief of pain. Aspirin is an effective analgesic favoured from long experience by bee-keepers. Local antiseptics are acceptable but topical antihista-mines should not be used as they promote sensitization.

Toxic effects

In cases of severe systemic envenoming, large doses of parenteral antihistamines and corticosteroids should be given and, if needed, bronchodilators and adrenaline (epinephrine). Bee antivenoms have been developed but none is commercially available. As in crush syndrome, renal damage by myoglobinuria or haemoglobinuria should be prevented by correcting hypovolaemia and giving mannitol and bicarbonate. Acute tubular necrosis will require treatment with haemofiltration or renal dialysis.

Allergic effects

The most effective treatment for sting anaphylaxis is 0.1% adrenaline (epinephrine) in an adult dose of 0.5–1 mL, children 0.01 mL/kg, given by intramuscular injection. Patients known to be hypersensitive should wear an identifying tag (such as provided by Medic-Alert in Britain) as they may be discovered unconscious after a sting. They should be trained to give themselves adrenaline (epinephrine) intramuscularly and should always carry a pre-loaded syringe of adrenaline for this purpose (e.g. 'EpiPen' delivering 0.3 mg adult, or 0.15 mg child, doses of 0.1% adrenaline). Injection of a histamine H_1-blocker (e.g. chlorphenamine maleate, 10 mg intravenously or intramuscularly) will alleviate the mild urticarial symptoms, and an antihistamine should be given for the next 24–48 hours to combat the effects of histamine released during the reaction. The role of histamine H_2-blockers (e.g. cimetidine) is uncertain. Corticosteroid may prevent recurrence of anaphylaxis, said to occur after about 6 hours in up to 10% of cases. Severe reactions may require cardiorespiratory resuscitation. Salbutamol is an effective bronchodilator and large doses of hydrocortisone may help the resolution of massive oedema. Respiratory tract obstruction is the main cause of death. Stings in the mouth may cause serious airway obstruction even in people who are not hypersensitive to venom.

Prevention of Hymenoptera sting anaphylaxis

In 1978, a controlled trial proved that hyposensitization using pure venom was effective in protecting allergic patients against anaphylactic reactions to sting challenge.[119] However, immunotherapy is necessary only in patients with histories of systemic anaphylaxis and demonstrable venom-specific IgE. Most people are stung when they inadvertently crush the bee or wasp or interfere with their nests (i.e. bee-keepers). Wasps congregate where sweet things or meat are manufactured or consumed and in orchards and vineyards. Vespidae are attracted by brightly coloured floral patterns and perfumes. Some of the largest hornets (*V. veluntina* and *V. mandarinia*) are so aggressive that their territory cannot be cultivated until the nests have been destroyed.

Scorpion stings (order scorpiones)[113]

The 2000 species of scorpions (order Scorpiones) are distributed south of latitude 49°N, except in New Zealand and Antarctica. Those capable of inflicting fatal stings in humans are all members of the families Buthidae (thick-tailed scorpions) and Hemiscorpiidae (also known as Ischnuridae or Liochelidae) (rock, creeping or tree scorpions).[113] Examples of the most deadly species are:
- Family Buthidae – *Androctonus australis* (North Africa and Middle East), *A. crassicauda* (Turkey, Middle East and North Africa), *Buthus occitanus* (countries bordering the Mediterranean and Middle East), *Leiurus quinquestriatus* (North Africa and Middle East), *Parabuthus* species (South Africa), *Tityus trinitatis* (Trinidad and Venezuela), *T. serrulatus* (Figure 31.39) and *T. bahiensis* (Brazil, Argentina), *Centruroides (sculpturatus) exilicauda* (Cali-

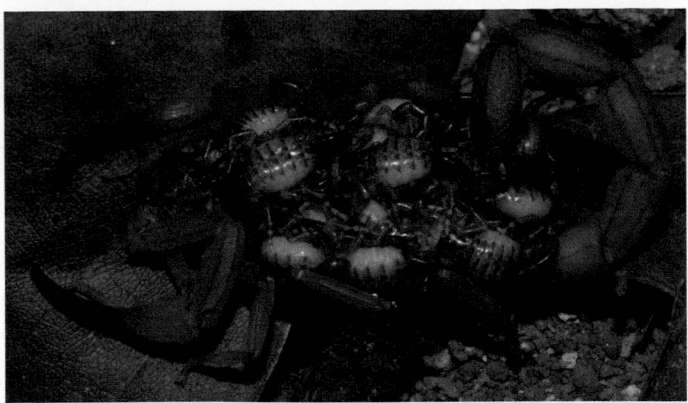

Figure 31.39 Brazilian scorpion (*Tityus serrulatus*; family Buthidae): female carrying its young. (Scale in centimeters.) (Copyright D. A. Warrell.)

fornia, New Mexico, Arizona and Baha California), *C. limpidus* and *C. suffusus* (Mexico) and *Mesobuthus tamulus* (India)
- Family Hemiscorpiidae – *Hemiscorpius lepturus* (Iran, Iraq, Pakistan-Balochistan, Yemen).

Epidemiology

Painful scorpion stings are a common event throughout the tropics. However, fatal envenoming is frequent only in parts of Latin America, North Africa, the Middle East and India. In southern Libya there were 900 stings with seven deaths per 100 000 population in 1979.[85] In Algeria there were 150 deaths in 1998 and 74 in 2005. In Tunisia there are about 40 000 stings with about 1000 hospital admissions and 100 deaths each year. In Khuzestan province, Iran, where 25 000 stings are treated each year, scorpion sting is the fourth major cause of death. *Hemiscorpius lepturus* is responsible for 12% of stings and more than 95% of fatalities. In India there are many cases of stings by the red scorpion (*Mesobuthus tamulus*), with fatalities in adults and children. There has been no death from scorpion sting in the USA since 1968. In Mexico, formerly there were between 1000 and 2000 deaths each year, with an incidence of 84 deaths per 100 000 per year in Colima state and a mere three deaths per 100 000 per year in the infamous Durango state. Case mortality was about 50% in children up to 4 years old.[120] Currently, about 250 000 stings are reported each year throughout the country but with only 70 fatalities. In Brazil, formerly the case fatality ranged from around 1% in adults to 15–25% in children less than 6 years old, but in 2005, among 36 558 reported stings there were only 50 deaths (0.14%).

Clinical features

Rapidly developing, excruciating local pain is the most common symptom. It is not true that stings by different species of scorpions result in the same systemic symptoms. Local signs such as swelling, redness, heat and regional lymph node involvement are never extensive. Local blistering and necrosis is most unusual except following stings by *Hemiscorpius lepturus* (Hemiscorpiidae). Sys-

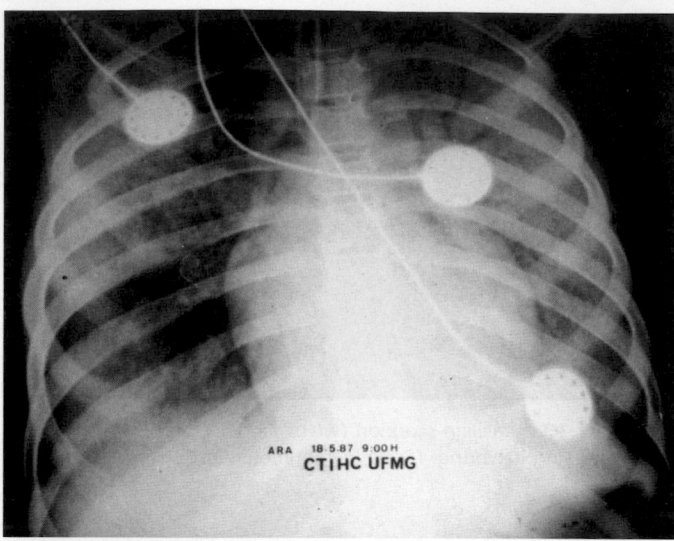

Figure 31.40 Chest radiograph of a Brazilian child envenomed by *Tityus serrulatus*, showing pulmonary oedema. (Courtesy of Dr Nilton Rezende, Belo Horizonte, Brazil.)

temic symptoms may develop within minutes, but may be delayed for as much as 24 hours. Features of autonomic nervous system excitation are initially cholinergic and later adrenergic. There is hypersalivation, profuse sweating, lacrimation, hyperthermia, vomiting, diarrhoea, abdominal distension, loss of sphincter control, and priapism. Massive release of catecholamines, as in phaeochromocytoma, produces piloerection ('gooseflesh'), tachycardia, hyperglycaemia, hypertension and toxic myocarditis with arrhythmias (most commonly sinus tachycardia), electrocardiographic S–T segment changes, cardiac failure and pulmonary oedema) (Figure 31.40). These cardiovascular effects are particularly prominent following stings by *Leiurus quinquestriatus*, *Tityus* species[121] and *Mesobuthus tamulus*.[122]

Neurotoxic effects such as fasciculation, muscle spasms that can be misinterpreted as tonic-clonic convulsive movements, and respiratory distress are a particular feature of stings by *Centruroides (sculpturatus) exilicauda*. *Parabuthus transvaalicus* envenoming is more likely to cause ptosis and dysphagia. Hemiplegia and other neurological lesions have been attributed to fibrin deposition resulting from disseminated intravascular coagulation, for example after stings by *Nebo hierichonticus*. Hypercatecholaminaemia could explain hyperglycaemia and glycosuria but, in the case of stings by the black scorpion of Trinidad (*Tityus trinitatis*), there is acute pancreatitis. Fifteen to 120 minutes after the initial searing pain of the sting, patients stung by this species begin to salivate, feel nauseated and vomit persistently, producing coffee-grounds or frank haematemesis. Hyperglycaemia, glycosuria and sometimes albuminuria can be detected a few hours after the sting. There is abdominal pain with distension and rigidity. Electrocardiographic abnormalities (T wave inversion, QRS segment abnormalities and QTc prolongation) are common and may last for 3–6 days. Other features include pyrexia, sweating, bradycardia, cardiac arrhythmias, hypotension and neuromuscular irritability. Acute oedema-

tous or haemorrhagic pancreatitis with development of pancreatic pseudocysts has been demonstrated at autopsy or laparotomy.

Treatment

The most effective treatment for pain is local infiltration with 1% lidocaine or xylocaine, ideally using digital block technique. Local injection of emetine is said to relieve the pain but may cause necrosis and can be dangerous if absorbed. Parenteral opiate analgesics such as pethidine and morphine may be required but are said to be dangerous in victims of *Centruroides (sculpturatus) exilicauda*.

The use of antivenom is recommended and is widely advocated in Middle and South America, North Africa and parts of the Middle East, although it has its opponents in India and Israel. Antivenoms are manufactured in many countries.[84]

Many accessory treatments have been suggested. For patients with cardiovascular symptoms (hypertension, bradycardia and early pulmonary oedema) vasodilators such as the α_1-blocker prazosin are recommended. In patients stung by *Mesobuthus tamulus*, priapism, dilated pupils, sweating and bradycardia indicate a high risk of progression to pulmonary oedema. Early energetic treatment with an an α_1-blocker may prevent this.[123] However, the use of atropine (except in cases of life-threatening sinus bradycardia), cardiac glycosides and β-blockers is controversial.[121]

Prophylactic immunization with scorpion venom toxoid has been considered in Mexico.

Spider bites (order Aranea)[124]

The spiders (order Aranea) are an enormous group containing more than 34 000 known species in 105 families. A single family, containing less than 1% of these species, is non-venomous. Only about 20 species are known to cause dangerous envenoming in humans, but many others have been suspected, usually wrongly, of inflicting harmful bites.[125] Spiders bite with a pair of fangs, the chelicerae (Figure 31.41), to which the venom glands are connected.[113] A central venom duct opens near the tip of the fang. In Brazil, in 2005, 19 634 spider bites were reported, with nine deaths (0.05%).

Clinical features

Two main clinical syndromes, 'necrotic loxoscelism' and 'neurotoxic araneism', are caused by spider bite.

Necrotic loxoscelism

Skin lesions, varying in severity from mild localized erythema and blistering to quite extensive tissue necrosis, have been falsely attributed to a variety of familiar peridomestic species, such as the Australian white-tailed spider (*Lampona cylindrata*), North American hobo spider (*Tegenaria agrestis*), European and South American wolf spiders (*Lycosa*, including the Italian 'tarantula' *L. terentula*) and cosmopolitan sac spiders (*Cheiracanthium*).[125] Only members of the genus *Loxosceles* (American recluse spiders) have proved capable of causing 'necrotic arachnidism/araneism'.[125] Many *Loxosceles* species are extending their geographical ranges. *Loxosceles laeta* (Figure 31.42) is widely distributed in Central and South America, especially in Chile and Peru, and *L. gaucho* is

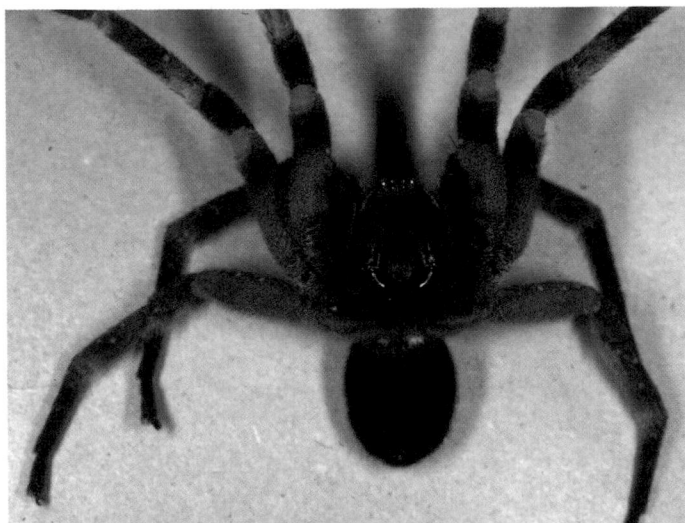

Figure 31.41 Brazilian 'banana', 'wandering' or 'armed' spider (*Phoneutria nigriventer*): threatening posture of a female. Note venom jaws. (Copyright D. A. Warrell.)

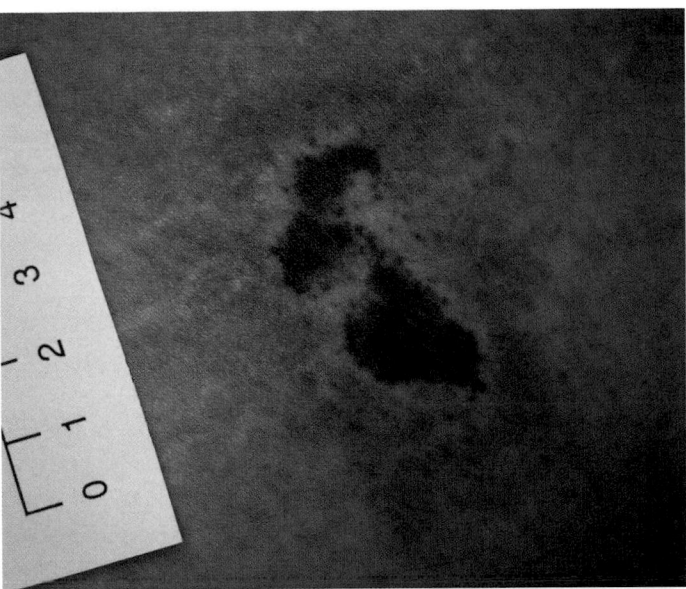

Figure 31.43 Early lesion at the site of the bite of a Brazilian spider (*Loxosceles gaucho*), showing the 'red-white-and-blue' sign. (Copyright D. A. Warrell.)

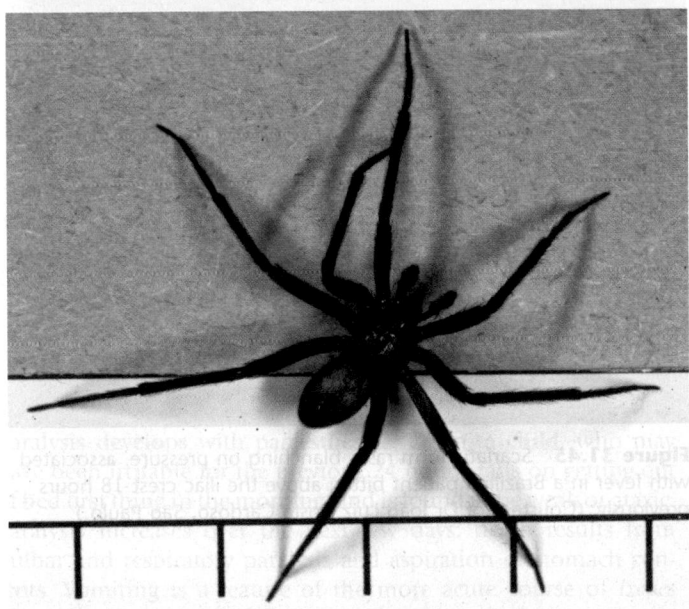

Figure 31.42 South American recluse spider (*Loxosceles laeta*): female, scale in cm. (Copyright D. A. Warrell.)

important in Brazil. *L. reclusa*, the brown recluse or violin spider, caused many bites but only six deaths in the USA in the twentieth century. *L. rufescens* occurs in the Mediterranean region, North Africa, Israel and elsewhere.

Eighty per cent of patients are bitten indoors, usually in their bedrooms while asleep or dressing, and in the USA a number of men were bitten on their genitals while they sat on outdoor lavatories in which the spiders had spun their webs. The bite may be painless initially but a burning pain develops at the site over the

next 12–36 hours with local oedema. An ischaemic lesion ('red-white-and-blue' sign), coloured red (vasodilatation), white (vaso-constriction) and blue (pre-necrotic cyanosis) appears (Figure 31.43) and, over the course of a few days, becomes a black eschar (Figure 31.44) which sloughs in a few weeks, sometimes leaving a necrotic ulcer. Rarely, the necrotic area may cover an entire limb. In 12% of cases there are systemic effects including fever, methae-moglobinaemia, haemoglobinuria and jaundice resulting from haemolytic anaemia, scarlatiniform rash (Figure 31.45), respiratory distress, collapse and renal failure. The average case fatality is about 5%.

Neurotoxic araneism

Members of the genus *Latrodectus* (widow, hour-glass, button or red-back spiders) are the most widespread and numerous of all venomous animals dangerous to man. *L. mactans* (black widow spider) occurs in the Americas. Sixty-three deaths were attributed to this species in the USA from 1950 to 1959. *L. tredecimguttatus*, widely but incorrectly known as 'tarantula', lives in fields in the Mediterranean countries, where it has been responsible for epidemics of bites. A total of 946 cases were reported in Italy between 1946 and 1951. *L. hasselti*, the Australian and New Zealand 'red-back spider' or 'katipo', causes up to 340 reported bites each year in Australia, where 20 deaths are known to have occurred. This adaptable species has settled in Japan, the Middle East and elsewhere. *L. mactans* and a related species, *L. geometricus*, also cause some bites in South and eastern Africa. *L. hasselti* bites produce local heat, swelling and redness, which is rarely extensive. Intense local pain develops in about 5 minutes; after 30 minutes, there is pain in local lymph nodes, and after about an hour, headache, nausea, vomiting and sweating occur. Tachycardia and hypertension may follow and there are muscle tremors and spasms which may be severe enough to demand artificial ventilation.

eye, intense conjunctivitis results and there may be corneal ulceration and even blindness. Skin lesions are initially stained brown or purple, blister after a few days, and then peel. First aid is generous irrigation with water. Eye injuries should be treated as for snake venom ophthalmia.

POISONING BY INGESTION OF MARINE ANIMALS[132–134]

A variety of illnesses, usually categorized as 'food poisoning', are caused by eating seafood. The best known are attributable to bacterial or viral infections. These include *Vibrio parahaemolyticus* (after eating crustaceans, especially shrimps), *V. cholerae* (crabs and molluscs), non-O1 *V. cholerae* (oysters), *V. vulnificus* (oysters), *Aeromonas hydrophila* (frozen oysters), *Plesiomonas shigelloides* (oysters, mussels, mackerel, cuttlefish), *Salmonella typhi* (molluscs), *Campylobacter jejuni* (clams), *Shigella* species (molluscs), hepatitis A virus (molluscs, especially clams and oysters), Norwalk virus (clams and oysters), and astro- and caliciviruses (cockles and other molluscs). Botulism has been reported in people eating smoked fish and canned salmon. Since 1953, approximately 100 000 Japanese are thought to have been affected by methyl mercury poisoning (Minamata disease) after eating fish and molluscs contaminated with methyl mercury derived from industrial waste dumped in Minamata Bay and at the mouth of the Agano River in Japan.[102] The victims developed severe central nervous system damage, with a mortality of 33% in the initial outbreak. Pregnant women exposed to methyl mercury gave birth to infants who were mentally retarded and had cerebral palsy and convulsions.

A number of clinical syndromes have been recognized which are related to the presence in the ingested flesh or viscera of marine animals of toxins either derived ultimately from marine microalgae or bacteria (e.g. ciguatera, tetrodotoxic or paralytic shellfish poisoning) or resulting from bacterial decomposition of fish during storage (scombrotoxic fish poisoning).

Gastrointestinal and neurotoxic syndromes

Nausea, vomiting, abdominal colic, tenesmus and watery diarrhoea may precede the development of neurotoxic symptoms. Paraesthesiae of the lips, buccal cavity and extremities are early symptoms. Other neurotoxic manifestations include a peculiar distortion of temperature perception so that cold objects feel hot (like dry ice) and vice versa, dizziness, myalgia, weakness starting with muscles of phonation and deglutition and progressing to respiratory paralysis and flaccid quadriplegia in some cases, ataxia, involuntary movements, convulsions, visual disturbances, hallucinations and psychoses, cranial nerve lesions and pupillary abnormalities. Cardiovascular abnormalities include hypotension and bradycardia and some patients develop florid cutaneous rashes.

Distinguishable within this general pattern of symptoms are a number of conditions related to the ingestion of a particular taxonomic group of animals. Some of the more important syndromes are described below.

Ciguatera fish poisoning

The word 'ciguatera' seems to derive from the Cuban word 'cigua' for a poisonous marine snail (*Livona pica*, the west Indian top

shell) which was coined by early Spanish settlers.[102] The term ciguatera is now applied to an illness resulting from the ingestion of any one of more than 400 species of warm-water, shore or reef fish between latitudes 35°N and 34°S, especially in the South Pacific and Caribbean (including Florida). These fish are now widely available in fish markets in temperate northern countries to meet the demands of immigrant populations. Overall, there must be more than 50 000 cases in the world each year, with an incidence of up to 2% of the population each year and a case fatality of about 0.1%. The fish most often associated with ciguatera are ray-finned fish (order Perciformes) of the families Serranidae (sea basses and groupers), Lutjanidae (snappers), Scaridae (parrot fish), Scombridae (mackerels, tunas, skipjacks and binitos), Sphyraenidae (barracudas) and Carangidae (jacks, pompanos, jack mackerels, scads), and eels (order Anguilliformes), notably Muraenidae (moray eels).

It is now known that the toxins responsible for ciguatera fish poisoning, the polyether ciguatoxins, maitotoxins and scaritoxins, originate from benthic dinoflagellates such as *Gambierdiscus toxicus*, which are ingested by herbivorous fish. These in turn are the prey of the carnivorous fish, which, when eaten by humans, may give rise to severe gastrointestinal, neurotoxic and cardiovascular symptoms. Ciguatoxins are concentrated in the intestine, gonads and viscera. The acquisition of toxin by fish cannot be predicted; there is no seasonal variation in its prevalence but the risk of poisoning is greater with some species, e.g. moray eels, and definitely increases as the fish gets larger. Three toxins, ciguatoxin, maitotoxin and scaritoxin (from the parrot fish *Scarus sordidus*) have been identified. Ciguatoxins excite Na^+ channels, while maitotoxin activates voltage-independent Ca^{2+} channels.

Clinical features

Exceptionally, symptoms first appear as early as minutes or as long as 30 hours after eating the poisoned fish; however, the usual interval is 1–6 hours. The earliest symptom is numbness or tingling of the lips, tongue, throat and extremities, a metallic taste, and a dry mouth or hypersalivation. Reversed perception of heat and cold is a distinctive symptom. In many cases, especially with milder poisoning, the earliest symptoms are gastrointestinal: sudden abdominal colic, nausea, vomiting and watery diarrhoea. Myalgia, ataxia, vertigo, visual disturbances and pruritic skin eruptions develop later. In severely neurotoxic cases, flaccid paralysis and respiratory arrest may develop. Gastrointestinal symptoms resolve within a few hours but paraesthesiae and myalgias may persist for a week, months or even years. Ciguatera poisoning from eating moray eels (*Gymnothorax* species) is particularly rapid and severe because of the high concentration of toxin in these animals.

Chelonitoxication results from the ingestion of marine turtles (Chelonia). Its clinical features resemble ciguatera poisoning. Most outbreaks have been in the Indo-Pacific area. The species usually implicated are green hawksbill and leathery turtles. The case fatality among reported cases is 28%.

Tetrodotoxic (puffer fish) poisoning

More than 50 species of tropical scaleless fish of the order Tetraodontiformes have proved poisonous. They include porcupine fish (*Chilomycterus*), molas or sunfish (*Mola*), and puffer fish or toadfish (Tetraodontidae – genera *Arothron*, *Fugu*, *Lagocephalus*, etc.). The flesh of the puffer fish (Japanese fugu) is particularly relished in Japan, where, despite the stringent regulations and skilful fugu cooks, tetrodotoxin poisoning continues to occur, causing around four deaths each year. Cases have been reported in Thailand and many other Indo-Pacific countries. Tetrodotoxin, an aminoperhydroquinazoline, is one of the most potent non-protein toxins known. It is concentrated in the fish's ovaries, viscera and skin. There is a definite seasonal variation in the toxin concentration, which reaches a peak during the spawning season (May to June in Japan). Tetrodotoxin impairs nervous conduction by blocking the sodium ion flux without affecting movement of potassium, producing neurotoxic and cardiotoxic effects. The origin of this toxin is unknown. It may be synthesized by *Pseudomonas* bacteria and acquired through the food chain. An identical toxin has been found in the skin of newts (genus *Taricha*), frogs (genus *Atelopus*) and salamanders, the saliva of octopuses (genus *Hapalochlaena*), in the digestive glands of several species of gastropod mollusc and in xanthid and horseshoe crabs, star fish, flat worms (*Planorbis*) and nemertine worms in Japan. Paralytic freshwater puffer fish poisoning attributable to saxitoxin has been reported in Thailand.

Clinical features

Paraesthesiae, dizziness and ataxia become noticeable within 10–45 minutes of eating the fish. Generalized numbness, hypersalivation, sweating and hypotension may develop. Some patients remain aware of their surroundings despite appearing comatose. Gastrointestinal symptoms may be completely absent. Death from respiratory paralysis usually occurs within the first 6 hours and is unusual more than 12 hours after eating the fish. Erythema, petechiae, blistering and desquamation may appear.

Paralytic shellfish poisoning

Bivalve molluscs such as mussels, clams (*Saxidomus*), oysters, cockles and scallops may acquire neurotoxins such as saxitoxins from the dinoflagellates *Alexandrium* species (formerly *Gymnodinium catenatum* and *Pyrodinium bahamense*) which occur between latitudes 30°N and 30°S. The dinoflagellates may be sufficiently abundant during the warmer months of May to October to produce a 'red tide'. The dangerous season is announced by the discovery of unusual numbers of dead fish and sea birds. Symptoms develop within 30 minutes of ingestion. They include perioral paraesthesia, gastrointestinal symptoms, ataxia, visual disturbances and pareses, progressing to respiratory paralysis within 12 hours in 8% of cases. Milder gastrointestinal and neurotoxic symptoms without paralysis have been associated with ingestion of molluscs contaminated by neurotoxic brevetoxins from *Gymnodinium breve*, which act on sodium channels. These microalgae also produce a 'red tide'.

Histamine syndrome (scombrotoxic poisoning)

The red flesh of scombroid fish such as tuna, mackerel, bonito and skipjack, and of canned non-scombroid fish such as sardines and pilchards, may be decomposed by the action of bacteria such as *Proteus morgani*, decarboxylating muscle histidine into histamine, saurine, cadaverine and perhaps other unidentified toxins. Toxic fish may produce a warning tingling or smarting sensation in the mouth when eaten. Between minutes and up to 24 hours after ingestion, flushing, burning, urticaria and pruritus of the skin, headache, abdominal colic, nausea, vomiting, diarrhoea, hypotensive shock and bronchial asthma may develop. Exogenous histamine may be detected in patients' plasma and urine and in the fish.[135] Identical symptoms have been described in Sri Lankan patients who ate fish while taking the antituberculosis drug isoniazid, which inhibits the enzyme normally responsible for inactivating histamine.

Poisoning by ingestion of carp's gallbladder[136]

In parts of the Far East, the raw bile and gallbladder of various species of freshwater carp (e.g. the grass carp *Ctenopharyngodon idellus*; Thai 'plaa yeesok' *Probarbus jullienii*) are believed to have medicinal properties. Patients in China, Taiwan, Hong Kong, Japan, Thailand and elsewhere have developed acute abdominal pain, vomiting and watery diarrhoea 2–18 hours after drinking the raw bile or eating the raw gallbladder of these fish. One patient developed flushing and dizziness. Hepatic and renal damage may develop, progressing to hepatic failure and oliguric or non-oliguric acute renal failure (acute tubular necrosis). The hepatonephrotoxin has not been identified, but is heat-stable and may be derived from the carp's diet.

Treatment of marine poisoning

The differential diagnosis includes bacterial and viral food poisoning and allergic reactions. No specific treatments or antidotes are available. If ingestion was recent, gastrointestinal contents should be gently eliminated by emetics and purges. Activated charcoal absorbs saxitoxin and other shellfish toxins. Atropine is said to improve gastrointestinal symptoms and sinus bradycardia in patients with gastrointestinal and neurotoxic poisoning. Oximes, such as pralidoxime and 2-pyridine aldoxime, have been claimed to benefit the anticholinesterase features of ciguatera poisoning, but the evidence is not convincing. Calcium gluconate may relieve mild neuromuscular symptoms. In scombroid poisoning, adrenaline (epinephrine), histamine H_1-blockers and H_2-blockers (e.g. cimetidine) corticosteroids and bronchodilators should be used, depending on severity. In cases of paralytic poisoning, endotracheal intubation and mechanical ventilation and cardiac resuscitation have proved life-saving. In Malaysia, a patient with tetrodotoxin poisoning developed fixed dilated pupils and brain stem areflexia, so appearing brain dead, but made a complete recovery after being mechanically ventilated.[137] The use of mannitol intravenously in acute ciguatera poisoning is not supported by convincing evidence. Gabapentin has been suggested as a treatment for chronic persisting paraesthesiae after ciguatera poisoning.

Prevention of marine poisoning

Ciguatera, tetrodotoxin and histamine are heat-stable, so cooking does not prevent poisoning. In tropical areas, the flesh of fish should be separated, as soon as possible, from the head, skin, intestines, gonads and other viscera, which may have high concentrations of toxin. All scaleless fish should be regarded as potentially tetrodotoxic, while very large fish carry an increased

90. Audebert F, Sorkine M, Bon C. Envenoming by viper bites in France: clinical gradation and biological quantification by ELISA. *Toxicon* 1992; 30:599–609.

91. Hutton RA, Looareesuwan S, Ho M, et al. Arboreal pit vipers (genus *Trimeresurus*) of Southeast Asia: bites by T. albolabris and T. macrops in Thailand and a review of the literature. *Trans R Soc Trop Med H* 1990; 84:866–874.

92. Lalloo DG, Trevett AJ, Owens D, et al. Coagulopathy following bites by the Papuan taipan (*Oxyuranus scutellatus canni*). *Blood Coagul Fibrinolysis* 1995; 6:65–72.

93. Warrell DA. Clinical snake bite problems in the Nigerian savanna region. Technische Hochschule Darmstadt. *Schriftenreihe Wissensch u-Technik* 1979; 14:31–60.

94. Theakston RDG, Phillips RE, Looareesuwan S, et al. Bacteriological studies of the venom and mouth cavities of wild Malayan pit vipers (*Calloselasma rhodostoma*) in southern Thailand. *Trans R Soc Trop Med Hyg* 1990; 84:875–879.

95. Jorge MT, Malaque C, Ribeiro LA, et al. Failure of chloramphenicol prophylaxis to reduce the frequency of abscess formation as a complication of envenoming by Bothrops snakes in Brazil: a double-blind randomized controlled trial. *Trans R Soc Trop Med Hyg* 2004; 98:529–534.

96. Garfin SR, Castilonia RR, Mubarak SJ, et al. Rattlesnake bites and surgical decompression: results using a laboratory model. *Toxicon* 1984; 22:177–182.

97. Sawai Y. Vaccination against snake bite poisoning. In: Lee CY, ed. *Snake Venoms. Handbook of Experimental Pharmacology*. Vol. 52. Berlin: Springer; 1979:881–897.

98. Russell FE, Bogert CM. Gila monster, venom and bite: a review. *Toxicon* 1981; 19:341–359.

99. [Anonymous]. Exenatide: AC 2993, AC002993, AC2993A, exendin 4, LY2148568. *Drugs R D* 2004; 5:35–40.

100. Raufman J-P. Review. Bioactive peptides from lizard venoms. *Regul Pept* 1996; 61:1–18.

101. Fry BG, Vidal N, Norman JA, et al. Early evolution of the venom system in lizards and snakes. *Nature* 2006; 439:584–588.

102. Halstead BW. *Poisonous and Venomous Marine Animals of the World*. 2nd edn. New Jersey: Darwin Press; 1988.

103. Williamson JA, Fenner PJ, Burnett JW, et al., eds. *Venomous and Poisonous Marine Animals: A Medical and Biological Handbook*. Sydney: University of New South Wales Press; 1996.

104. Smith WL, Wheeler WC. Venom evolution widespread in fishes: a phylogenetic road map for the bioprospecting of piscine venoms. *J Hered* 2006; 97:206–217.

105. Khoo HE. Bioactive proteins from stonefish venom. *Clin Exp Pharmacol Physiol* 2002; 29:802–806.

106. Castex MN. Freshwater venomous rays. In: Russell FE, Saunders PR, eds. *Animal Toxins*. Oxford: Pergamon Press; 1967:167–176.

107. Maretic Z. Some epidemiological, clinical and therapeutic aspects of envenomation by weeverfish sting. In: De Vries A, Kochva E, eds. *Toxins of Animals and Plant Origin*. Vol. 3. New York: Gordon & Breach; 1973:1055–1065.

108. Lee JY, Teoh LC, Leo SP. Stonefish envenomations of the hand – a local marine hazard: a series of 8 cases and review of the literature. *Ann Acad Med Singapore.* 2004; 33:515–520.

109. Barnes JH. Observations on jellyfish stingings in North Queensland. *Med J Aust* 1960; 2:993–999.

110. Seymour J, Carrette T, Cullen P, et al. The use of pressure immobilization bandages in the first aid management of cubozoan envenomings. *Toxicon* 2002; 40:1503–1505.

111. Alender CB, Russell FE. Pharmacology. In: Boolootian RA, ed. *Physiology of Echinodermata*. New York: Interscience; 1966:529–543.

112. Olivera BM. Conus peptides: biodiversity-based discovery and exogenomics. *J Biol Chem* 2006; 281:31173–31177.

113. Bettini S, ed. *Arthropod Venoms. Handbook of Experimental Pharmacology*. Vol. 48. Berlin: Springer; 1978.

114. Winston ML. *Killer Bees: The Africanized Honey Bee in the Americas*. Cambridge, MA: Harvard University Press; 1992.

115. França FOS, Benvenuti LA, Fan HW, et al. Severe and fatal mass attacks by 'killer' bees (Africanised honey bees – *Apis mellifera scutellata*) in Brazil: clinicopathological studies with measurement of serum venom concentrations. *Q J Med* 1994; 87:269–282.

116. Warrell DA. Taking the sting out of ant stings: venom immunotherapy to prevent anaphylaxis. *Lancet* 2003; 361:979–980.

117. Piek T. *Venoms of the Hymenoptera. Biochemical, Pharmacological and Behavioural Aspects*. London: Academic Press; 1986.

118. Ewan PW. Allergy to insect stings: a review. *J R Soc Med* 1984; 78: 234–239.

119. Hunt KJ, Valentine MD, Sobotka AK, et al. A controlled trial of immunotherapy in insect hypersensitivity. *N Engl J Med* 1978; 299: 157–161.

120. Mazzotti L, Bravo-Becherelle MA. Scorpionism in the Mexican Republic. In: Keegan HL, Macfarlane WV, eds. *Venomous and Poisonous Animals and Noxious Plants of the Pacific Region*. Oxford: Pergamon Press; 1963: 111–131.

121. Freire-Maia L, Campos JA, Amaral CFS. Treatment of scorpion envenoming in Brazil. In: Bon C, Goyffon M, eds. *Envenomings and their Treatments*. Lyon: Fondation Marcel Mérieux; 1996:301–310.

122. Bawaskar HS. Diagnostic cardiac premonitory signs and symptoms of red scorpion sting. *Lancet* 1982; i:552–554.

123. Bawaskar AS, Bawaskar PH. Severe envenoming by the Indian red scorpion (*Mesobuthus tamulus*): the use of prazosin therapy. *Q J Med* 1996; 89: 701–704.

124. Maretic Z, Lebez D. *Araneism*. Pula: Novit; 1979.

125. Isbister GK, White J, Currie BJ, et al. Spider bites: addressing mythology and poor evidence. *Am J Trop Med Hyg* 2005; 72:361–364.

126. Pauli I, Puka J, Gubert IC, et al. The efficacy of antivenom in loxoscelism treatment. *Toxicon* 2006; 48:123–137.

127. Murnaghan MF, O'Rourke FJ. Tick paralysis. In: Bettini S, ed. *Arthropod Venoms. Handbook of Experimental Pharmacology*. Vol. 48. Berlin: Springer; 1978:419–464.

128. Gothe R, Kunze K, Hoogstraal H. The mechanism of pathogenicity in the tick paralyses. *J Med Entomol* 1979; 16:357–369.

129. Pearn J. The clinical features of tick bite. *Med J Aust* 1977; 2:313.

130. Stone BF. Toxicoses induced by ticks and reptiles in domestic animals. In: Harris JB, ed. *Natural Toxins: Animal, Plant and Microbial*. Oxford: Clarendon Press; 1986:56–71.

131. Radford AJ. Millipede burns in man. *Trop Geogr Med* 1975; 27:279–287.

132. Salzman M, Madsen JM, Greenberg MI. Toxins: bacterial and marine toxins. *Clin Lab Med* 2006; 26:397–419, ix.

133. Sobel J, Painter J. Illnesses caused by marine toxins. *Clin Infect Dis* 2005; 41:1290–1296.

134. Daranas AH, Norte M, Fernández JJ. Review. Toxic marine micro-algae. *Toxicon* 2001; 39:1101–1132.

135. Morrow JD, Margolies GR, Rowland J, et al. Evidence that histamine is the causative toxin of scombroid-fish poisoning. *N Engl J Med* 1991; 324:716–720.

136. Lin YF, Lin SH. Simultaneous acute renal and hepatic failure after ingesting raw carp gall bladder. *Nephrol Dial Transplant* 1999; 14:2011–2012.

137. Loke YK, Tan MH. A unique case of tetrodotoxin poisoning. *Med J Malaysia* 1997; 52:172–174.

USEFUL WEB SITES

Envenoming

General, especially in Australasia: *http://www.toxinology.com/*

Snake bite in South and South-east Asia: *http://www.searo.who.int/en/Section10/ Section17/Section53/Section1024.htm*

Antivenoms

General

AFPMB: *http://afpmb.org/pubs/living_hazards/antiv.html*
Munich AntiVenomINdex (MAVIN): *http://toxinfo.org/antivenoms/*
http://globalcrisis.info/latestantivenom.htm
WHO: *http://www.who.int/bloodproducts/animal_sera/en/*

European antivenoms

Zagreb Immunology Institute in Croatia: *http://www.imz.hr/*

Australian antivenoms

http://www.csl.com.au/search.asp?qu=antivenom
http://www.toxinology.com/generic_static_files/cslavh_antivenom.html

South African antivenoms

http://www.savp.co.za/Products.htm

Venomous snake taxonomy updates

http://sbsweb.bangor.ac.uk/%7Ebss166/update.htm

Scorpions

http://www.ub.ntnu.no/scorpion-files/index.php

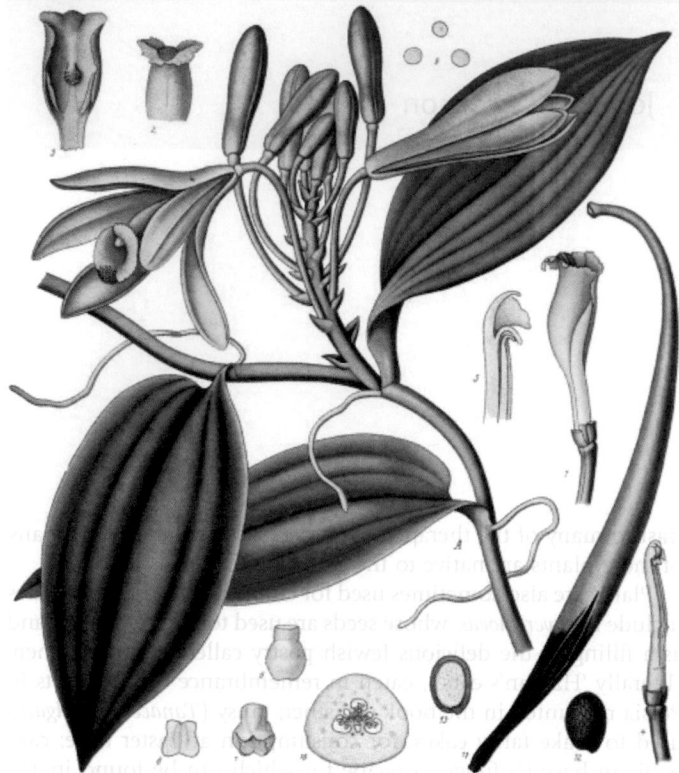

Figure 32.1 *Chondodendron tomentosum* (curare).

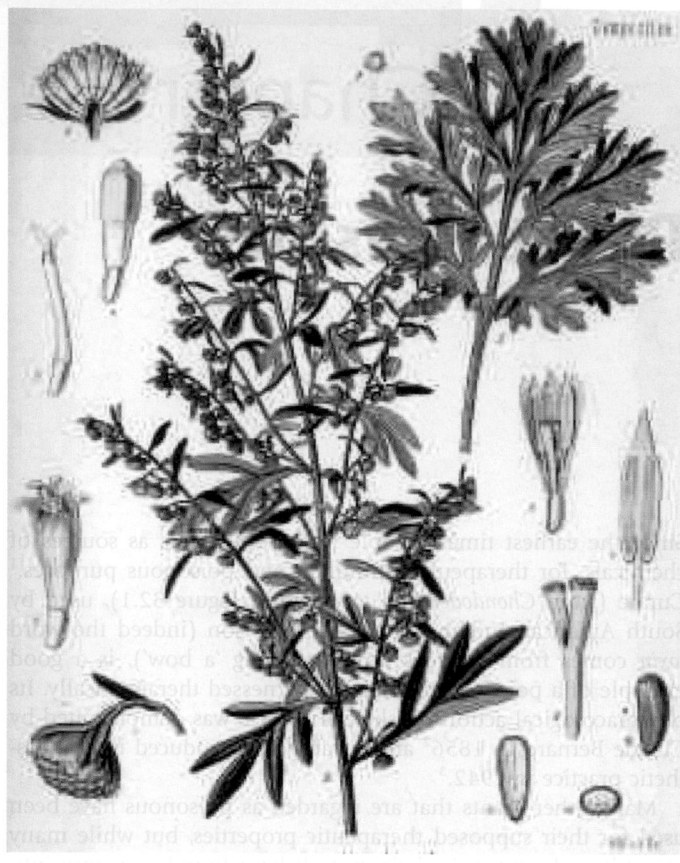

Figure 32.2 *Artemisia absinthium* (wormwood).

combination with allopathic drugs and the often unpredictable effects of such combinations add to the hazards.[15]

The frequency of exposure to poisonous pants is difficult to assess; many reports are anecdotal. In one series of 912 534 plant exposures in the USA, *Philodendron* spp. were the most commonly implicated, followed by *Dieffenbachia, Euphorbia, Capsicum* and *Ilex*.[16]

Plant poisoning can occur as a result of accidental, unknowing, or deliberate poisoning from contaminated foodstuffs or from toxic seeds and fruits; from the misuse of traditional or herbal medicines; or from the deliberate use of plants for their psychotropic properties. Contact dermatitis can occur from contact with irritant plants.[17] A report from the Uppsala Monitoring Centre of the WHO has summarized all suspected adverse reactions to herbal medicaments reported from 55 countries worldwide over 20 years.[18] A total of 8985 case reports were on record. Most originated from Germany (20%), followed by France (17%), the USA (17%) and the UK (12%). Allergic reactions were the most frequent serious adverse events and there were 21 deaths.

Not all parts or constituents of a poisonous plant are poisonous. The stalks of rhubarb can be eaten but the leaves contain toxic oxalates; all parts of the yew are poisonous except the fleshy red aril. The purgative castor oil is expressed from the beans of *Ricinus communis*, but the beans also contain the highly toxic alkaloid ricin. Ackee fruit is poisonous only when unripe. Furthermore, the amount of toxic ingredient in a single part of a plant varies from season to season.

Nor are all poisonous plants poisonous to all species. Goats, for example, can eat foxgloves and nightshade with impunity, since they eliminate their toxic ingredients rapidly; bees can harvest pollen from poisonous plants, such as rhododendrons, which contain grayanotoxins, and the honey so produced may be poisonous to man.[19] One should not be misled by seeing an animal feed on a plant into thinking that it is safe for human consumption.

There is no simple way of classifying poisonous plants, other than by their scientific names, and even those change from time to time. However, because many disparate plants contain compounds with similar effects, here I shall use headings that describe their pharmacological or clinical effects; when that is not possible I shall use the name of the plant or its chief constituent as a heading.

ALCOHOL

The history of alcohol is as ancient as human history and plants play a central part in its production. Rum (65–72% alcohol) is

Table 32.1 Some commonly used therapeutic agents that originally derived from plants (see also Table 32.2)

Drug	Example of medical use	Plant of origin
Artemether	Malaria	Qinghao (*Artemisia annua*)
Atropine	Anticholinergic	Deadly nightshade (*Atropa belladonna*)
Cannabinoids	Palliative care	Cannabis (*Cannabis sativa*)
Capsaicin	Painful neuropathies	Peppers (*Capsicum* spp.)
Cephaeline	Emetogenic	Ipecacuanha (*Cephaëlis ipecacuanha*)
Cocaine	Local anaesthetic	Coca (*Erythroxylon coca*)
Colchicine	Gout	Autumn crocus (*Colchicum autumnale*)
Curare	Anaesthesia	Pareira (*Chondrodendron tomentosum*)
Digoxin/digitoxin	Atrial fibrillation and heart failure	Foxgloves (*Digitalis lanata/purpurea*)
Ephedrine	Sympathomimetic	Sea-grapes (*Ephedra sinica*)
Gamolenic acid	Mastodynia	Evening primrose (*Oenothera biennis*)
Hyoscine	Anticholinergic	Thorn apple (*Datura stramonium*)
Ispaghula	Laxative	Ispaghula (*Plantago ovata*)
Opioid alkaloids	Analgesia	Poppies (*Papaver somniferum*)
Physostigmine	Myasthenia gravis	Calabar bean (*Physostigma venenosum*)
Pilocarpine	Glaucoma	Jaborandi (*Pilocarpus jaborandi*)
Quinine	Malaria	Cinchona (*Cinchona pubescens*)
Salicylates	Analgesics	Meadowsweet (*Spiraea ulmaria*)
		Willow (*Salix alba*)
		Wintergreen (*Gaultheria procumbens*)
Sennosides	Purgative	Senna (*Cassia acutifolia*)
Taxanes	Cytotoxic	Yew trees (*Taxus* spp.)
Theophylline	Asthma	Tea plant (*Camellia sinensis*)
Vinca alkaloids	Cytotoxic	Madagascar periwinkle (*Catharanthus rosea*)

distilled from fermented molasses in the West Indies and South America; arrack or sake (50–60%) is manufactured in India, China, Java, and Japan from fermented rice. Toddy, made from the sweet sap of various palms, such as coconut, is drunk in India, Sri Lanka, and West Africa. A potent drink, pulque, is made in South America from the juice of agaves.

Alcohol causes three main medical and psychiatric problems:

- acute alcohol intoxication
- chronic alcoholism
- alcohol withdrawal reactions (delirium tremens).

In the brain alcohol acts as a dose-dependent depressant, producing the well-known features of intoxication. At plasma concentrations of around 40 mg/dL (400 mg/L or 8.7 mmol/L) learned skills are impaired, including the ability to maintain self-restraint. Other early effects include loss of attentiveness, loss of concentration, and impaired memory, and there may be lethargy. At progressively higher concentrations there are further changes in mood, behaviour, and a variety of sensory and motor functions. The effects on mood depend on the individual's personality, mental state, and social environment. Commonly there is euphoria, but any kind of mood change can occur. Libido is often enhanced, but sexual performance impaired. Alcohol generally increases confidence, often resulting in aggressive or silly behaviour; loss of self-restraint leads to increased loquacity with immoderate speech content, such as swearing or the use of lewd language. Unsteadiness of gait, slurred speech, and difficulty in carrying out even simple tasks, with impaired coordination, become obvious at plasma concentrations of about 80 mg/dL (the concentration above which driving is illegal in the UK and many other countries). Driving skills are therefore impaired, and are affected even at concentrations below 80 mg/dL. Recovery from dazzle is delayed, which may impair night-time driving. Visual acuity, peripheral vision, colour vision, and visual tracking are impaired. Hearing and taste may also be impaired. The pain threshold is increased. At high concentrations there may be vertigo and nystagmus. Alcohol causes acute drowsiness and deep sleep; in high concentrations it causes coma and respiratory depression. In some individuals sleep may later be impaired. On waking there is the characteristic 'hangover', which usually consists of irritability, headache, thirst, abdominal cramps, and bowel disturbance. The cause of hangover is not known.

Delirium tremens is an acute withdrawal reaction that can be fatal. The symptoms come on within a few hours after the last drink and mount over the next 2–3 days. At first there is anxiety,

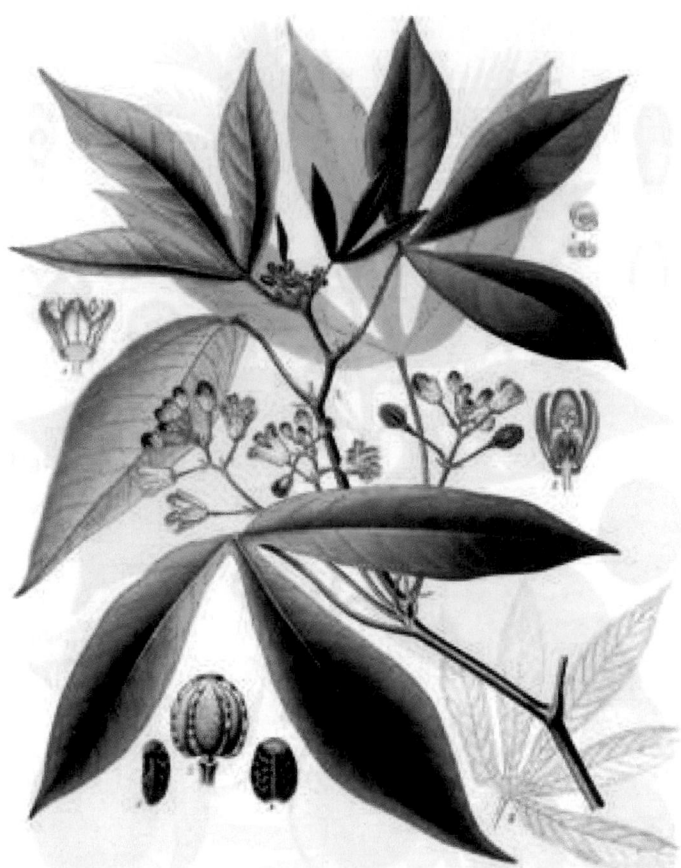

Figure 32.9 *Manihot esculenta* (cassava).

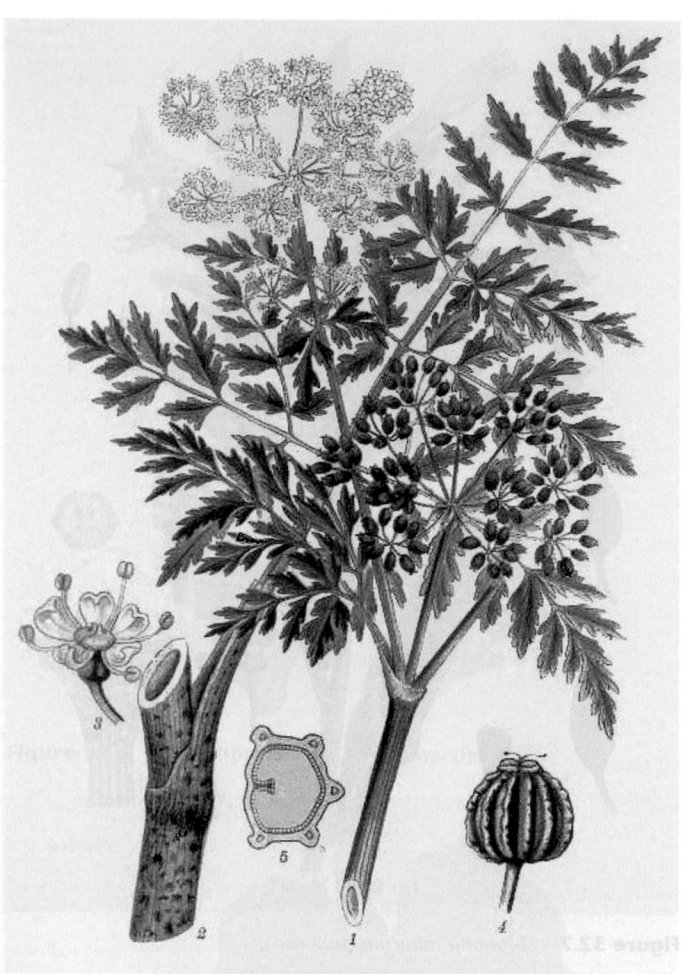

Figure 32.10 *Conium maculatum* (hemlock).

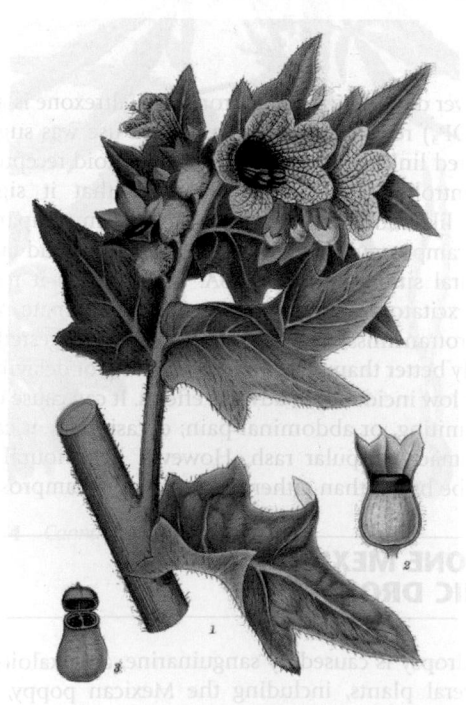

Figure 32.11 *Hyoscyamus niger* (henbane).

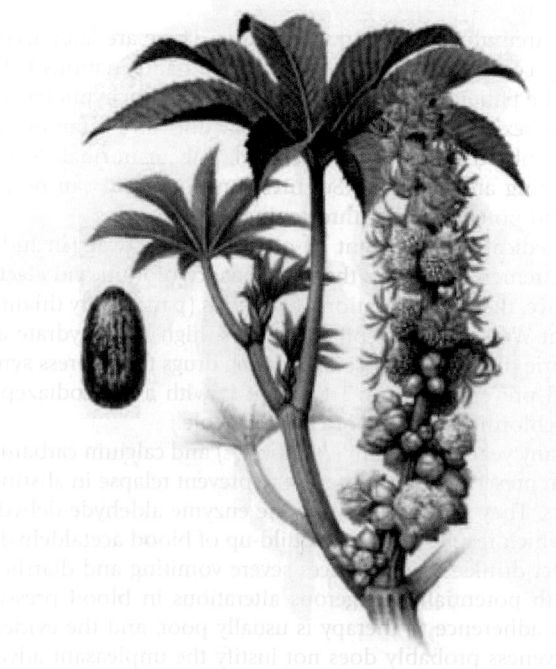

Figure 32.12 *Ricinus communis* (castor bean).

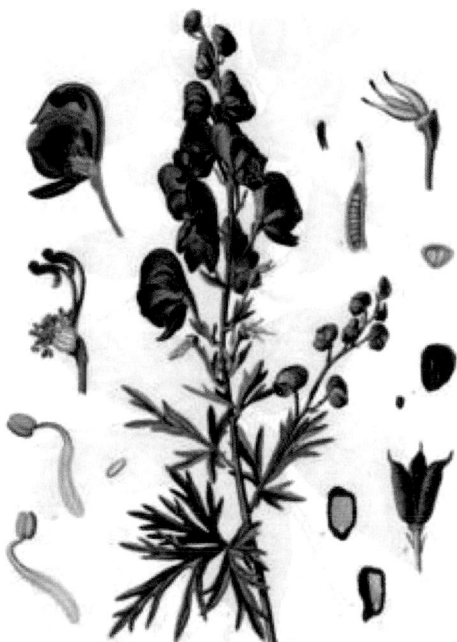

Figure 32.13 *Aconitum napellus* (Monkshood).

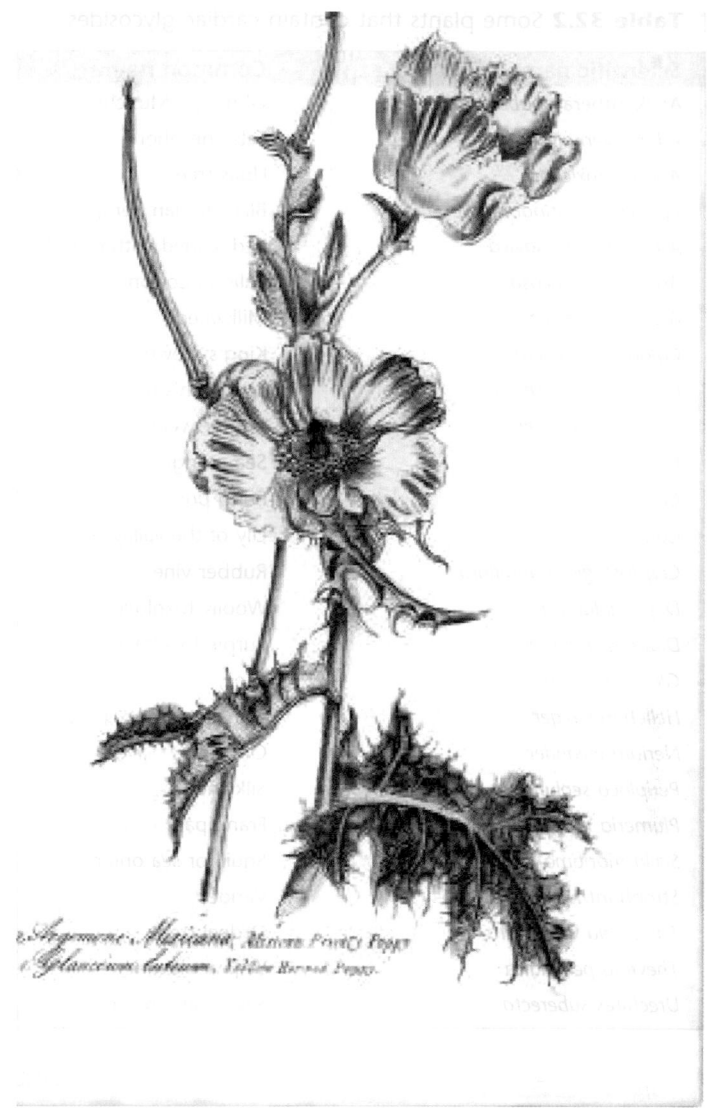

Figure 32.14 *Argemone mexicana* (Mexican poppy).

accidentally or by deliberate adulteration. Village boys in India can collect up to 8 kg of *Argemone* seeds a day in summer, and may sell them to unscrupulous dealers. As a contaminant of a widely used cooking oil derived from mustard seed, *Argemone* has led to outbreaks of so-called epidemic dropsy in many tropical countries. Sanguinarine is absorbed from the gut and through the skin if oil containing it is used for massage.[21] It causes capillary dilatation and increased permeability.

Epidemic dropsy is seen mostly in India,[22] but has also been reported in Mauritius, Fiji, South Africa, and Nepal.[23] It presents with gastrointestinal symptoms a week or so before the onset of pitting oedema of the legs, fever, and darkening of the skin, often with local erythema and tenderness. Perianal itching is common, and severe myocarditis and congestive cardiac failure can occur. Other features include hepatomegaly, pneumonia, ascites, glaucoma, alopecia, and sarcoid-like skin changes. Visual field disturbances can occur independent of any rise in intraocular pressure.[24] Haemolytic anaemia occurs when oxidative stress causes methaemoglobin formation by altering pyridine nucleotides and glutathione redox potential; treatment with antioxidants has been suggested to be effective.[25]

CARDIOTOXIC GLYCOSIDES IN PLANTS

The number of plants worldwide that contain cardiac glycosides (cardenolides or bufadienolides) is legion – the incomplete list given by Gibbs (1974)[26] runs to nearly 400 compounds and spans genera such as the Apocyanaceae, Asclepiadaceae, Cruciferae, Liliaceae, Moraceae, Ranunculaceae and Scrophulariaceae. Some examples are given in Table 32.2.

Some cardenolides (such as digoxin and digitoxin, obtained from foxgloves) are used therapeutically, and even then toxicity readily occurs, because these drugs have a low therapeutic index.[27] Poisoning with plants containing cardenolides is not uncommon. One example is the current epidemic of self-poisoning with the seeds of oleander trees in South India and Sri Lanka. In one series of 300 cases of self-poisoning with *Thevetia peruviana* (yellow oleander) (mostly women aged 11–20, of whom 97% took crushed seeds), the main symptoms were vomiting, palpitation, epigastric pain, a burning sensation in the abdomen, shortness of breath, and diarrhoea; sinus bradycardia, sinus arrest, sinoatrial block, and heart block were common.[28]

Other plants that have caused cardenolide poisoning include the pong pong (*Cerbera odollum*)[29] and the glory lily (*Gloriosa superba*).[30] In one series of 4556 cases of self-poisoning in Sri Lanka, 2.5% were caused by plants and mushrooms; *Gloriosa*

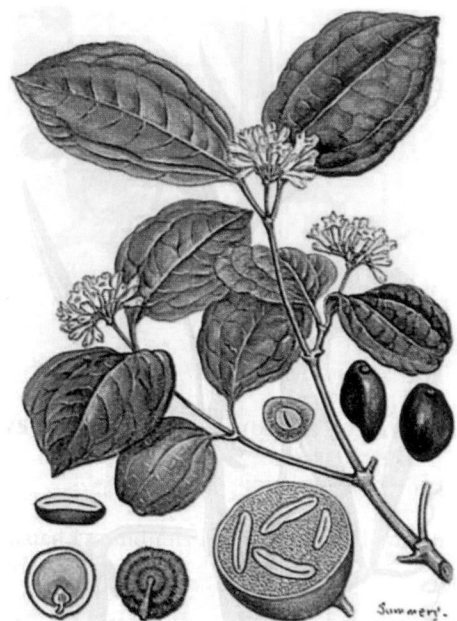

Figure 32.30 *Strychnos nux-vomica* (poison nut).

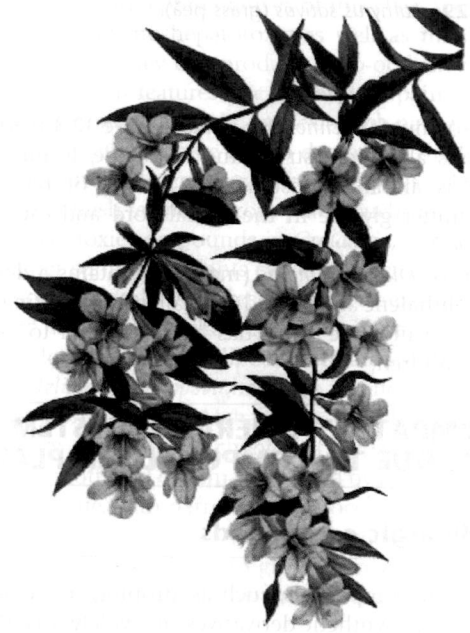

Figure 32.31 *Gelsemium sempervirens* (jessamine).

The thorn apple or Jimson weed, *Datura stramonium*, grows in most parts of the world and is a frequent cause of poisoning in cereal crops. The seeds contain alkaloids of the tropane series, notably hyoscyamine. One outbreak of poisoning in Tanzania involved the consumption of porridge made from millet distrib-

uted by a local branch of the National Milling Corporation.[83] Jimson weed has also been used as a drug of abuse.[84]

Other plants that can cause anticholinergic poisoning include angel's trumpet (*Brugmansia* spp., now called *Datura*),[85] found in Central and South America and prepared as a tea for its hallucinogenic effects, and jessamine (*Gelsemium sempervirens*, Figure 32.31),[86] which is native to North and Central America.

The seeds of various species of *Datura* have been used in cases of criminal poisoning in tropical countries. *D. fastuosa* was a favourite poison of practitioners of thagi in India; *D. sanguinea* is used in Colombia and Peru, *D. ferox* and *D. arborea* in Brazil, and the leaves of *Hyoscyamus fahezlez* by the Tuareg in the Sahara. The seeds of *D. stramonium* with *D. metel* have been used in East Africa for criminal purposes, as an inebriant to facilitate robbery, or to elicit confessions of witchcraft.[36]

Cholinergic compounds

Drugs can cause cholinergic effects either by stimulating acetylcholine receptors or by inhibiting acetylcholinesterase.

Drugs that stimulate acetylcholine receptors, of which nicotine and muscarine are the prototypes, are used therapeutically (e.g. pilocarpine in glaucoma) and are found in a wide variety of plants. The effects of poisoning are constricted pupils (miosis); hypersalivation and sweating; nausea, vomiting, and diarrhoea; bradycardia; and headache, vertigo, confusion, delirium, hallucinations, coma, and convulsions. Bronchorrhoea, bronchospasm and pulmonary oedema produce respiratory failure, the usual cause of death. Most cases of cholinergic poisoning with flowering plants have been reported with laburnum in temperate zones; other cases have been reported with hemlock (*Conium maculatum*).[87]

Many fungi contain cholinergic compounds, and muscarinic poisoning can occur with, for example, jack o'lantern (*Omphalotus olearius*), *Clitocybe* spp. and *Inocybe* spp. In severe cases of poisoning with *Amanita* spp. there may be cholinergic symptoms, but the main effects are due to the GABAergic compound muscimol.[88]

Anticholinesterases potentiate the actions of acetylcholine by inhibiting its breakdown. Solanine is one such compound, found in plants of the *Solanum* spp., including the unripe berries of the bittersweet nightshade (*S. dulcamara*) and greened tubers of potatoes (*S. tuberosum*). However, *S. dulcamara* poisoning can also present with anticholinergic effects.[89] Accidental or suicidal poisoning can occur with anticholinesterase organophosphorus insecticides;[90] treatment is with atropine[91] and cholinesterase reactivators, such as pralidoxime and obidoxime.[92]

PSYCHOTROPIC DRUGS IN PLANTS

Betel

Chewing betel, the leaves of *Piper betle* [sic], together with lime and areca (betel) nuts (*Areca catechu*) is a common practice in India, Sri Lanka and other Eastern countries. It may act by inhibiting GABA uptake. The mouth, lips and cheeks are stained bright red and the face is flushed; there is euphoria, heightened alertness, sweating, salivation, a hot sensation in the body, and an increased capacity to work; there are increases in heart rate, blood pressure, sweating, and body temperature.[93]

Cannabis

Cannabis sativa, the hemp plant, yields marijuana and hashish. A cannabis smoker inhales at least 60 mind-altering chemicals, but the main psychoactive ingredient is delta-9-tetrahydrocannabinol (delta-9-THC), an antiemetic, antispasticity agent, appetite stimulant, analgesic, anxiolytic, hypnotic and antipyretic, which also lowers intraocular pressure. However, its beneficial effects in terminal disease are disappointing.

Marijuana ('grass', 'weed', 'bush', 'herb') is the dried mixture of crushed leaves and stalks of the plant. The flowering tops of the plant secrete a resin that can be compressed to form hashish ('hash', 'blow', 'puff', 'draw', 'ganja', 'dope', 'pot'), or dissolved into an oil or tincture. Marijuana is usually rolled in home-made cigarettes ('spliffs', 'joints', or, if enormous, 'blunts'), with or without tobacco. Hashish is heated and crumbled on to tobacco in spliffs, or smoked in a wide variety of pipes. In many parts of the world cannabis is an ingredient of a range of culinary preparations.

Cannabis has physical and mental effects that begin within minutes. The physical effects include an increase in heart rate, peripheral vasodilatation, conjunctival suffusion, bronchodilatation, dryness of the mouth, and, in large doses, tremor, ataxia, nystagmus, nausea, and vomiting. The mental effects vary from person to person, depending on such variables as personality, mood, surroundings, expectations, and previous cannabis experience. Generally there is a feeling of well-being, accompanied by feelings of enhanced sensory perception. There may be drowsiness or hyperactivity. Ideas flow rapidly and may be disconnected. Time seems to pass slowly. Motor performance may be altered, as it may be by any sedative drug, and driving skills may be impaired.

There may be mild tolerance and a mild withdrawal syndrome, rather like a mild benzodiazepine withdrawal syndrome. Physical dependence does not seem to be a big problem, but psychological dependence does occur.

Heavy use of marijuana is associated with social apathy, but this often precedes drug use and may not be an adverse effect. Adverse psychological effects include anxiety, acute panic reactions, and paranoid ideas. Large doses can cause an acute toxic psychosis with confusion and hallucinations. There is controversy as to whether marijuana can produce a prolonged psychosis, but it can certainly aggravate pre-existing mental disease. Cannabis smoke contains more insoluble particulates and carcinogens than tobacco smoke, so lung and airways damage can be anticipated in heavy regular consumers. Birth defects occasionally follow use in pregnancy.

Coca

Erythroxylon coca (Figure 32.32) is widely grown in South America and India. The leaves are dried in the sun and are chewed with

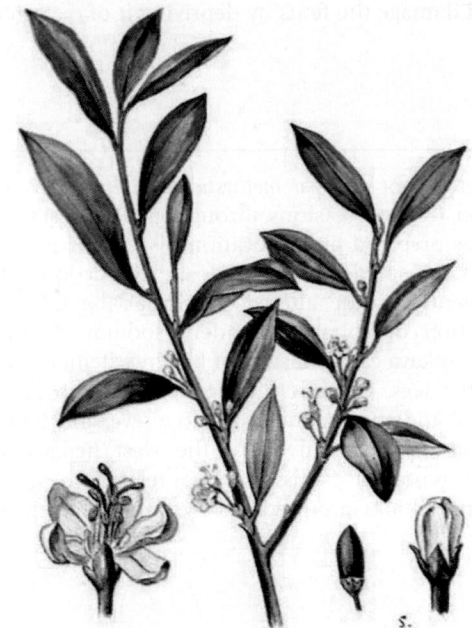

Figure 32.32 *Erythroxylon coca* (coca).

lime or, in India, with betel. Cocaine powder can be sniffed, prepared as a solution for intravenous injection, or separated from its hydrochloride and smoked as the free base or as 'crack' (so-called because of the popping and clicking of exploding impurities when it is burnt). Crack vaporizes at a much lower temperature than cocaine hydrochloride, so that the active ingredient escapes pyrolysis and reaches the lungs intact. Because the transfer from lung to brain is so fast, the impact of smoked cocaine gives a 'rush' comparable with that experienced after intravenous injection. However, the euphoriant effect also wears off quickly, producing a most unpleasant downswing of mood in many users, which they may attempt to fend off with repeatedly larger and larger doses.

The clinical effects of cocaine ('coke', 'snow', 'charlie', or 'crack') include euphoria, increased drive, increased confidence, increased sociability, loquacity, and increased physical and mental capacities. After chewing there is loss of sensation in the tongue and lips.

The tendency to repeat administration to fend off rebound effects, and the rapid tolerance that occurs to the euphoriant effects of cocaine, combine to cause a typical pattern of escalating doses terminating in 'crash', characterized by exhausted sleep followed by depressed mood, which fuels the initiation of the next binge. Termination of a binge comes about through physical or mental exhaustion, or through lack of money or further drug supplies. Repeated sniffing can cause perforation of the nasal septum. The use of prolonged and high dosages can lead to a cocaine-induced psychosis, not dissimilar from acute paranoid schizophrenia. There are no major physiological withdrawal phenomena from cocaine, but troublesome dysphoria and craving can persist for months or even years. When it is taken during pregnancy, cocaine can cause constriction of the uterine and placental blood vessels and damage the fetus by depriving it of oxygen and other nutrients.

Kava

The powdered root of *Piper methysticum*, prepared as a beverage, is drunk on festive occasions throughout Polynesia.[94] Formerly, the root was prepared by mastication by selected girls, a practice that caused the spread of tuberculosis. The actions of some of its constituents include altered activity at the GABA$_A$ receptor and inhibition of voltage-dependent sodium channels. Overindulgence in kava causes a state of hyperexcitement, with loss of power in the legs. Chronic intoxication leads to debility, with ataxia, visual and auditory defects, and a reversible ichthyosiform eruption (kava dermopathy). In the west hepatotoxicity has often been reported;[95] this may be related to the fact that western formulations are prepared by lipid rather than aqueous extraction.[96]

Khat

Khat (cafta, miraa, muiragi) is derived from a small tree, *Catha edulis*, indigenous to North Africa.[97] The leaves and twigs are chewed, infused, or smoked and produce euphoria and loquaciousness, with a misleading sensation of sharpened mental processes. Khat produces these effects because it contains cathinone and cathine, phenylalkylamines that are related to ephedrine and have amphetamine-like properties;[98] psychosis has been reported with heavy use. Other adverse effects include increased blood pressure and depression; long-term abuse can make you manic and aggressive; physical dependence does not occur but psychological dependence does. Chronic consumption may be genotoxic. The khat alkaloids are absorbed first from the oral cavity and then from the gut, justifying slow chewing.[99]

Nicotine

The leaves and flowers of *Nicotiana* spp. have been universally smoked, snuffed, or chewed for their stimulant effects. Preparations of the leaves applied to the chest to relieve respiratory complaints have sometimes given rise to toxic effects by percutaneous absorption of nicotine. However, nicotine is much more widespread in plants, and occurs in such diverse species as *Acacia* spp., *Aesculus hippocastanum*, *Asclepias* spp., *Duboisia* spp. *Echeviria* spp., *Erythroxylon coca*, *Juglans regia*, *Mucuna pruriens*, *Prunus* spp., *Sempervivum arachnoideum*, and *Urtica dioica*. During the nineteenth and early part of the twentieth century, Australian aborigines used pituri, a nicotine-containing preparation from the cured leaves of *Duboisia hopwoodii*.[100]

An unusual nostrum made by the Yoruba people of Nigeria is 'cow's urine mixture', which consists of green tobacco leaves, rock salt, citron (*Citrus medica*), the leaves of the bush basil, *Ocimum viride*, and cow's urine.[101] The remedy is swallowed or rubbed into the skin for the prevention and treatment of epileptic or eclamptic fits; the toxic effects are those of nicotine – central nervous excitation, with vomiting, diarrhoea, dehydration, and hypogly-

caemia, followed by depression and coma, sometimes with permanent neurological damage or death. Convulsions must be controlled and glucose given intravenously. The poison is removed by gastric lavage or cleansing of the skin; blood glucose, electrolytes, and fluid balance should be monitored.

Opium alkaloids and their derivatives

Opioid dependence is a worldwide public health menace associated with a great deal of criminal activity. Heroin ('smack', 'junk', 'gear', 'brown') is the opiate chosen by 75%, and heroin-related referrals are increasing by at least 15% per year. On initial use, there may be nausea, vomiting, and anxiety, but these symptoms disappear with subsequent use, and euphoria becomes predominant. As tolerance develops and the cost of the habit increases, the addict may switch to the intravenous route to maximize value for money. In an attempt to retain the euphoria (the 'rush') that results from rapidly increased concentrations of the drug in the brain, larger and larger doses will be used. Tolerance to constipation and pupillary constriction does not occur to any great extent. Eventually the addict becomes most concerned with combating withdrawal symptoms and needs a regular supply of the drug to avoid them.

Withdrawal symptoms begin at about 8 h after the last dose and reach a peak at about 36–72 h. Symptoms occur in the following order:

1. Psychological symptoms: anxiety, depression, restlessness, irritability, drug craving
2. Lacrimation, rhinorrhoea, mydriasis, yawning, sweating, tachycardia, and hypertension
3. Restless sleep, after which the above symptoms are accompanied by sneezing, anorexia, nausea, vomiting, abdominal cramps, diarrhoea, bone pain, muscle pain, tremor, weakness, chills and goose-flesh ('cold turkey'), twitching and jerking of the legs ('kicking the habit'), and insomnia. Hypotension, cardiovascular collapse, and convulsions occur rarely.

These symptoms gradually fade over about 5–10 days, during which time general malaise and abdominal cramps persist. This withdrawal syndrome is not as bad as has been widely depicted in literature and is not fatal.[102]

With methadone the onset of withdrawal symptoms is delayed for 24–48 h and peaks at 3–4 days; because of this slower effect, methadone is often used to help an addict withdraw, by substituting it for morphine or heroin.

TREATMENT OF POISONING[103]

This is not the place for a thorough description of the treatment of poisoning, but a few simple principles are summarized in Table 32.4.

DRUG INTERACTIONS WITH COMPOUNDS IN PLANTS

Drug interactions can occur between plant medicaments and allopathic medicines.[104,105,106] Some of these are summarized in Table 32.5. Many of these interactions are poorly attested, being anec-

Table 32.4 A summary of the management of acute self-poisoning

Target	Therapeutic action
1. Respiratory function	Check gag reflex
	Remove dentures
	Clear out oropharyngeal obstructions, debris, secretions
	Lay on the left side with head down
	Insert oral airway or, if cough reflex lost, an endotracheal tube
	Give oxygen if hypoxic
	Assist respiration if required
2. Circulatory function	Check heart rate and blood pressure
	If systolic blood pressure below 80 mmHg (young patients) or 90 mmHg (old patients):
	Raise end of bed If ineffective, give volume expanders
	If fluid overload and oliguria: Give dopamine and/or dobutamine
3. Renal function	Monitor urine output
4. Consciousness	Assess level of consciousness (Glasgow coma scale)
5. Temperature	Take temperature rectally; if below 36°C reheat slowly
	Warm all inspired air and intravenous fluids
6. Convulsions	Treat with diazepam, clomethiazole, phenytoin, or anaesthesia with assisted ventilation
7. Cardiac arrhythmias	Treat as required
8. Gastric lavage	Generally of no value after 1 h following poisoning
	Add non-specific or specific antidotes to lavage fluid or leave in stomach after lavage
9. Activated charcoal	A single dose after gastric lavage
	Repeated doses for some poisons
10. Fluid and electrolyte balance	Dehydration: oral fluids usually enough
	Unconscious patients: use intravenous fluids and insert a central venous line
	Treat hypokalaemia
11. Emergency measures	Specific to the poison
12. Chest radiography	In drowsy or comatose patients who vomit
	After endotracheal intubation
13. Collection of specimens	Gastric aspirate (drugs)
	Urine (drugs, renal function)
	Blood (drugs, arterial gases, electrolytes)

dotal. However, interactions with grapefruit and St John's wort are well described and are dealt with below.

Pharmacodynamic interactions

If a herbal medicine shares a pharmacological action with an allopathic remedy, it may potentiate its therapeutic or adverse effects; the following are examples:

- digitalis (Figure 32.33) and heart remedies containing cardioactive glycosides (*Strophanthus, Convallaria, Cytisus, Scilla*)
- antihypertensive drugs and hypotensive herbs (*Rauwolfia, Crataegus, Viscum*)
- oral hypoglycaemic drugs and karela, the fruit of *Momordica charantia*; karela, which has a hypoglycaemic action,[107] is used in curries and is a traditional Indian remedy for diabetes

- antiasthma drugs and betel nut, which is thought to have a bronchoconstricting effect
- ACE inhibitors and *Capsicum* spp.; ACE inhibitors increase the amount of bradykinin in the lung and enhance the cough response to capsaicin, which acts by depleting substance P from nerve endings; this is an example of an interaction enhancing an adverse rather than a therapeutic effect of a drug.

Anticoagulants

Table 32.5 is organized according to the plant product, but too many plants interact with oral anticoagulants (principally warfarin) to be included separately. The many plants and herbal products that have been reported to increase or reduce the actions of warfarin[108] include angelica root, anise, arnica flower, asafetida,

Table 32.5 Some reported drug interactions with plants and herbal products

Precipitant plant(s)	Object drug(s)	Outcome
Areca nut (*Areca catechu*)	Neuroleptic drugs	Exacerbation of extrapyramidal effects
Berberine (*Berberis aristata*)	Tetracycline	Prolonged diarrhoea in cholera
Bran, ispaghula husk (*Plantago ovale*)	Digoxin, iron, lithium, lovastatin, tricyclic antidepressants	Reduced absorption
Ginkgo biloba	Thiazide diuretics	Hypertension
Ginseng (*Panax ginseng*)	Antidepressants	Risk of mania
	Cocaine	Tolerance inhibited
	Digoxin	Increased plasma digoxin concentration
	Methamphetamine	Tolerance inhibited
	Opioids	Reduced pharmacological effects of opioids
	Phenelzine	Headache, tremulousness, hyperactivity
	Warfarin	Reduced anticoagulation
Grapefruit juice	Amiodarone	Risk of amiodarone toxicity (e.g. cardiac arrhythmias)
	Antihistamines (astemizole, terfenadine)	Prolongation of QT interval; risk of ventricular tachycardia
	Ciclosporin	Risk of ciclosporin toxicity (immunosuppression)
	Benzodiazepines (alprazolam, diazepam, midazolam, triazolam)	Increased drowsiness; altered psychometric tests
	Calcium channel blockers (felodipine, nifedipine, nisoldipine)	Reduced blood pressure, increased heart rate, headaches, flushing, light-headedness
	Lovastatin	Risk of lovastatin toxicity (including rhabdomyolysis and renal insufficiency)
	Quinidine	Prolongation of QT_c interval; risk of ventricular tachycardia
	Saquinavir	Risk of saquinavir toxicity
	Sertraline	Risk of sertraline toxicity (serotonin syndrome)
Guar gum (*Cyanopsis tetragonolobus*)	Digoxin, glibenclamide, metformin, phenoxylmethylpenicillin	Reduced absorption
Liquorice (*Glycyrrhiza glabra*)	Corticosteroids	Increased risk of hypokalaemia
	Spironolactone	Reduced potassium-sparing effect
Saint John's wort (*Hypericum perforatum*)	Amitriptyline, ciclosporin, digoxin, HIV protease inhibitors, irinotecan, oral contraceptives, phenprocoumon, theophylline, warfarin	Induction of metabolism by CYP3A4, causing reduced effects (e.g. increased risk of transplant rejection with ciclosporin, reduced anticoagulation with warfarin); induction of P glycoprotein, increasing intestinal and renal secretion
	Digoxin, indinavir	Induction of P glycoprotein, increasing clearance and reducing effects
	Serotonin re-uptake inhibitors	Serotonin syndrome
Shankhapushpi (an Ayurvedic mixture of herbs)	Phenytoin	Decreased concentrations of phenytoin, leading to seizures
Siberian ginseng (*Eleutherococcus senticosus*)	Digoxin	Increased plasma digoxin concentration
Tamarind (*Tamarindus indica*)	Aspirin	Increased systemic availability
Xaio chai hu tang (sho-salko-to)	Prednisolone	Reduced effect of prednisolone
Yohimbine (*Pausinystalia yohimbe*)	Tricyclic antidepressants	Increased risk of hypertension

Table 32.6 Some adulterants and contaminants that have been found in herbal products

Type of adulterant/contaminant	Examples
Allopathic drugs	Albendazole, analgesic and antiinflammatory agents (for example aminophenazone, cocaine, diclofenac, diethylpropion, indometacin, paracetamol, phenylbutazone), benzodiazepines, chlorphenamine, ephedrine, glucocorticoids, ketoconazole, sildenafil, sulfonylureas, tadalafil, thiazide diuretics, thyroid hormones
Botanicals	*Aristolochia* spp., *Atropa belladonna*, *Digitalis* spp. (see Table 32.2), *Colchicum*, *Rauwolfia serpentina*, pyrrolizidine-containing plants (see Table 32.3)
Fumigation agents	Ethylene oxide, methyl bromide, phosphine
Heavy metals	Arsenic, cadmium, lead, mercury
Microorganisms	*Escherichia coli*, *Pseudomonas aeruginosa*, *Salmonella* spp., *Shigella* spp., *Staphylococcus aureus*
Microbial toxins	Aflatoxins, bacterial endotoxins
Pesticides	Carbamate insecticides and herbicides, chlorinated pesticides (for example aldrin, dieldrin, heptachlor, DDT, DDE, HCB, HCH isomers), dithiocarbamate fungicides, organic phosphates, triazine herbicides
Radionuclides	^{134}Cs, ^{137}Cs, ^{131}I, ^{103}Ru, ^{90}Sr

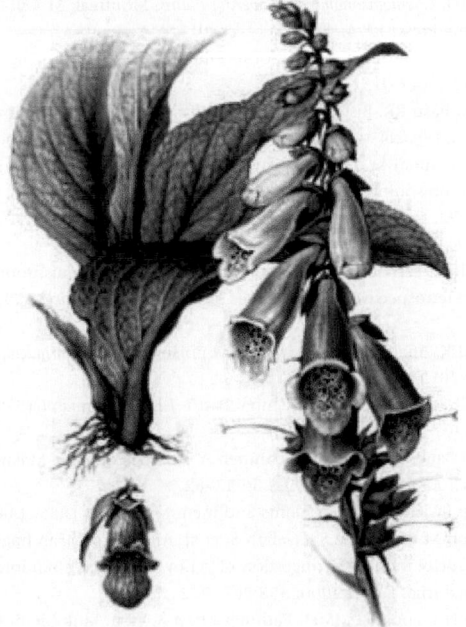

Figure 32.33 Digitalis purpurea (purple foxglove).

bogbean, borage seed oil, bromelain, capsicum, celery, chamomile, Chinese wolfberry (*Lycium barbarum*), clove, danshen (*Salvia miltiorrhiza*), devil's claw (*Harpagophytum procumbens*), dong quai (*Angelica sinensis*), fenugreek, feverfew, garlic, ginger, ginkgo, ginseng, green tea, horse chestnut, liquorice root, lovage root, meadowsweet, melilot, onion, papaya, parsley, passion-flower, poplar, quassia, red clover, rue, sweet clover (in which coumarin anticoagulants were originally discovered), sweet woodruff, tonka beans, turmeric, vitamin E, and willow bark. The mechanisms vary: for example, garlic reduces platelet aggregation; some plants (e.g. dong quai) contain anticoagulant coumarins; and some (e.g.

tonka beans) contain vitamin K, a natural antagonist of the actions of coumarin anticoagulants.

Citrus fruits

Various isoforms of the enzyme cytochrome P450 are responsible for the oxidative metabolism of many drugs.[109] One of these isoforms, CYP3A4, is responsible for the metabolism of several drugs in the gut wall while they are being absorbed after oral administration. Inhibition of the enzyme by something in grapefruits (*Citrus paradisi*)and Seville oranges (*Citrus bigaradia*) causes more of the drug to escape presystemic metabolism and enter the circulation unchanged, potentially leading to drug toxicity. The compounds in grapefruit juice and Seville oranges responsible for these interactions are not known. In some countries, a drug label has been introduced, alerting patients to potential drug interactions with grapefruit.[110] In the UK in 1997, the antihistamine terfenadine was withdrawn from over-the-counter sales because of cardiac arrhythmias,[111] and 1 year later another antihistamine, astemizole, was withdrawn for similar reasons.[112] Drugs whose effects can be increased by grapefruit juice, causing toxicity[113] are listed in Table 32.5.

Grapefruit juice probably also inhibits the P glycoprotein that is responsible for the intestinal secretion of many drugs,[114] and therefore other drug interactions are to be expected.

Ginseng

Reported drug interactions with ginseng (*Panax ginseng*) are listed in Table 32.5. The root has been used in China, Korea and Japan for centuries, in the belief that it counters fatigue and stress and confers health, virility and longevity; it is supposed to enhance immunity and to combat the effects of oxidative free radicals that cause chronic diseases and ageing.[115] The pharmacological basis for its reputation is slender, but ginseng is now in fashion world wide. It is often adulterated with *Eleutherococcus senticosus* (Siberian ginseng, Table 32.5), *Mandragora*, *Rauwolfia*, and other roots

623

of similar appearance. Ginseng contains a complex mixture of steroids and saponins; it can cause insomnia, tremor, headache, diarrhoea, hypertension, and oestrogen-like effects.[116] It may also increase the risk of gastric cancer.[117]

St John's wort[118]

As an antidepressant, St John's wort may enhance the effects of other antidepressants; since it is an inhibitor of 5-HT re-uptake, combination with serotonin reuptake inhibitors can cause the serotonin syndrome. Hyperforin, an ingredient of St John's wort (*Hypericum perforatum*) is an enzyme inducer and increases the metabolism of certain drugs, principally through CYP3A4, reducing their effects; St John's wort also induces intestinal P glycoprotein, leading to increased clearance of some drugs by intestinal and renal secretion.[119] Examples of these pharmacokinetic interactions are listed in Table 32.5.

ADULTERATION OF HERBAL PRODUCTS

There have been many reports that Chinese herbal remedies have been adulterated or contaminated with conventional drugs, heavy metals, and even other herbal substances not announced on the label.[120] Some examples are listed in Table 32.6.

REFERENCES

1. Lewin L. *Phantastica*. Berlin: Georg Stilke; 1924.
2. Bernard C. Analyse physiologique des propriétés des systèmes musculaires et nerveux au moyen du curare. *Comptes Rendus Acad Sci (Paris)* 1856; 43:825–829.
3. Griffith HR, Johnson GE. The use of curare in general anesthesia. *Anesthesiology* 1942; 3:418–420.
4. Cox PA. The ethnobotanical approach to drug discovery: strengths and limitations. *CIBA Found Symp* 1994; 185:25–36.
5. Anonymous. *Complementary Medicines*. London: Mintel International Group; 1997:13.
6. Institute of Medical Statistics Self-Medication International. *Herbals in Europe*. London: IMS Self-Medication International; 1998.
7. Brevoort P. The booming US botanical market. A new overview. *Herbalgram* 1998; 44:33–46.
8. Wohlmuth H, Oliver C, Nathan PJ. A review of the status of Western herbal medicine in Australia. *J Herb Pharmacother* 2002; 2:33–46.
9. Rudgley R. *The Alchemy of Culture. Intoxicants in Society*. London: British Museum Press; 1993.
10. Toklas AB. *The Alice B Toklas Cook Book*, revised edn. London: Brilliance Books; 1987.
11. Crompton R, Gall D. Georgi Markov-death in a pellet. *Med Leg J* 1980; 48:51–62.
12. Tai YT, But PP, Young K, et al. Cardiotoxicity after accidental herb-induced aconite poisoning. *Lancet* 1992; 340:1254–1256.
13. Watson G. *Theriac and Mithridatium. A Study in Therapeutics*. London: The Wellcome Historical Medical Library; 1966.
14. Garvey GJ, Hahn G, Lee RV, et al. Heavy metal hazards of Asian traditional remedies. *Int J Environ Health Res* 2001; 11:63–71.
15. Penn RG. Adverse reactions to herbal and other unorthodox medicines. In: D'Arcy PF, Griffin JP, eds. *Iatrogenic Diseases*, 3rd edn. Oxford: Oxford University Press; 1985:898–918.
16. Krenzelok EP, Jacobsen TD. Plant exposures . . . a national profile of the most common plant genera. *Vet Hum Toxicol* 1997; 39:248–249.
17. De Groot AC. Substances affecting the skin: contact allergy. In: Aronson JK, ed. *Meyler's Side Effects of Drugs. The International Encyclopedia of Adverse Drug Reactions and Interactions*, 15th edn. Amsterdam: Elsevier; 2006:3186–3201.
18. Farah MH, Edwards R, Lindquist M, et al. International monitoring of adverse health effects associated with herbal medicines. *Pharmacoepidemiol Drug Saf* 2000; 9:105–112.
19. Von Malottki K, Wiechmann HW. Akute lebensbedrohliche Bradykardie: Nahrungsmittelintoxikation durch turkischen Waldhonig. *Dtsch Med Wochenschr* 1996; 121:936–938.
20. Doggrell SA. Which treatment for alcohol dependence: naltrexone, acamprosate and/or behavioural intervention? *Expert Opin Pharmacother* 2006; 7:2169–2173.
21. Sood NN, Sachdev MS, Mohan M, et al. Epidemic dropsy following transcutaneous absorption of Argemone mexicana oil. *Trans R Soc Trop Med Hyg* 1985; 79:510–512.
22. Singh NP, Anuradha S, Dhanwal DK, et al. Epidemic dropsy – a clinical study of the Delhi outbreak. *J Assoc Phys India* 2000; 48:877–880.
23. Das M, Khanna SK. Clinicoepidemiological, toxicological, and safety evaluation studies on argemone oil. *Crit-Rev Toxicol* 1997; 27:273–297.
24. Singh K, Singh MJ, Das JC. Visual field defects in epidemic dropsy. *Clin Toxicol (Phil)* 2006; 44:159–163.
25. Babu CK, Khanna SK, Das M. Adulteration of mustard cooking oil with Argemone oil: do Indian food regulatory policies and antioxidant therapy both need revisitation? *Antioxid Redox Signal* 2007; 9:515–525.
26. Gibbs RD. *Chemotaxonomy of Flowering Plants*. Montreal: McGill-Queen's University Press; 1974.
27. Aronson JK, Hardman M. ABC of monitoring drug therapy. Digoxin. *BMJ* 1992; 305:1149–1152.
28. Bose TK, Basu RK, Biswas B, et al. Cardiovascular effects of yellow oleander ingestion. *J Indian Med Assoc* 1999; 97:407–410.
29. Narendranathan M, Das KV, Vijayaraghavan G. Prognostic factors in Cerbera odollum poisoning. *Indian Heart J* 1975; 27:283–286.
30. Aleem HM. Gloriosa superba poisoning. *J Assoc Phys India* 1992; 40:541–542.
31. Fernando R, Fernando DN. Poisoning with plants and mushrooms in Sri Lanka: a retrospective hospital based study. *Vet Hum Toxicol* 1990; 32:579–581.
32. Cassels BK. Analysis of a Maasai arrow poison. *J Ethnopharmacol* 1985; 14:273–281.
33. Bisset NG. Arrow poisons in China. Part I. *J Ethnopharmacol* 1979; 1:325–384.
34. Kopp B, Bauer WP, Bernkop Schnurch A. Analysis of some Malaysian dart poisons. *J Ethnopharmacol* 1992; 36:57–62.
35. Aronson JK. Glycosides of plants and men. *Med J Aust* 1986; 144:505–506.
36. Eddleston M, Rajapakse S, Jayalath S, et al. Anti-digoxin Fab fragments in cardiotoxicity induced by ingestion of yellow oleander: a randomised controlled trial. *Lancet* 2000; 355:967–972.
37. de Silva HA, Fonseka MMD, Pathmeswaran A, et al. Multiple-dose activated charcoal for treatment of yellow oleander poisoning: a single-blind, randomized, placebo-controlled trial. *Lancet* 2003; 361:1935–1938.
38. Vetter J. Plant cyanogenic glycosides. *Toxicon* 2000; 38:11–36.
39. Njoh J. Tropical ataxic neuropathy in Liberians. *Trop Geogr Med* 1990; 42:92–94.
40. Anonymous. Unproven methods of cancer management. Laetrile. *CA Cancer J Clin* 1991; 41:187–192.
41. Fisher AA. Poison ivy/oak dermatitis. Part I: Prevention – soap and water, topical barriers, hyposensitization. *Cutis* 1996; 57:384–386.
42. Fisher AA. Poison ivy/oak/sumac. Part II: Specific features. *Cutis* 1996; 58:22–24.
43. Park SD, Lee SW, Chun JH, et al. Clinical features of 31 patients with systemic contact dermatitis due to the ingestion of Rhus (lacquer). *Br J Dermatol* 2000; 142:937–942.
44. Tanaka T, Moriwaki SI, Horio T. Occupational dermatitis with simultaneous immediate and delayed allergy to chrysanthemum. *Contact Dermatitis* 1987; 16:152–154.

45. Guillet G, Helenon R, Guillet MH. La dermite du mancenillier. *Ann Dermatol Venereol* 1985; 112:51–56.

46. Sims JK, Brock JA, Fujioka R, et al. Vibrio in stinging seaweed: potential infection. *Hawaii Med J* 1993; 52:274–275.

47. Hinnen U, Willa-Craps C, Elsner P. Allergic contact dermatitis from iroko and pine wood dust. *Contact Dermatitis* 1995; 33:428.

48. Desjars P, Meignier M, Pinaud M, et al. Place du nitroprussiate de sodium dans les accidents ischémiques de l'ergotisme aïgu. *Nouv Presse Med* 1981; 10:2959–2961.

49. Kinamore PA, Jaeger R-W, De Castro FJ. Abrus and Ricinus ingestion: management of three cases. *Clin Toxicol* 1980; 17:401–405.

50. Olsnes S. The history of ricin, abrin and related toxins. *Toxicon* 2004; 44(4):361–370.

51. Kreitman RJ, Pastan I. Immunotoxins in the treatment of hematologic malignancies. *Curr Drug Targets* 2006; 7:1301–1311.

52. Hamilton RJ, Shih RD, Hoffman RS. Mobitz type I heart block after pokeweed ingestion. *Vet Hum Toxicol* 1995; 37:66–67.

53. Gardner DG. Injury to the oral mucous membranes caused by the common houseplant, Dieffenbachia. A review. *Oral Surg Oral Med Oral Pathol* 1994; 78:631–633.

54. Pusztai AJ. *Plant Lectins*. Cambridge: Cambridge University Press; 1991.

55. Addae JI, Melville GN. A re-examination of the mechanism of ackee-induced vomiting sickness. *West Indian Med J* 1988; 37:6–8.

56. Anonymous. Toxic hypoglycemic syndrome – Jamaica, 1989–1991. *MMWR Morb Mortal Wkly Rep* 1992; 41:53–55.

57. Morelli A, Grasso M, Meloni T, et al. Favism. Impairment of proteolytic systems in red blood cells. *Blood* 1987; 69:1753–1758.

58. Kitayaporn D, Charoenlarp P, Pataroarechachai J, et al. G6PD deficiency and fava bean consumption do not produce haemolysis in Thailand. *Southeast Asian J Trop Med Public Health* 1991; 22:176–181.

59. Saw JT, Bahari MB, Ang HH, et al. Potential drug-herb interaction with antiplatelet/anticoagulant drugs. *Complement Ther Clin Pract* 2006; 12:236–241.

60. Stickel F, Seitz HK, Hahn EG, et al. Hepatotoxizität von Arzneimitteln pflanzlichen Ursprungs. *Z Gastroenterol* 2001; 39:225–232, 234–237.

61. Kew MC. Hepatocellular cancer. A century of progress. *Clin Liver Dis* 2000; 4:257–268.

62. Aronson JK. Pyrrolizidine alkaloids. In: Aronson JK, ed. *Meyler's Side Effects of Drugs. The International Encyclopedia of Adverse Drug Reactions and Interactions*, 15th edn. Amsterdam: Elsevier; 2006:2989–2991.

63. Williams NA, Lee MG, Hanchard B, et al. Hepatic cirrhosis in Jamaica. *West Indian Med J* 1997; 46:60–62.

64. McDermott WV, Ridker PM. The Budd-Chiari syndrome and hepatic veno-occlusive disease. Recognition and treatment. *Arch Surg* 1990; 125:525–527.

65. Tandon BN, Tandon RK, Tandon HD, et al. An epidemic of veno-occlusive disease of liver in Central India. *Lancet* 1976; i:271–272.

66. Mohabat O, Srivastava RN, Younos MS, et al. An outbreak of hepatic veno-occlusive disease in Northwestern Afghanistan. *Lancet* 1976; ii:269–271.

67. Stickel F, Seitz HK, Hahn EG, et al. Hepatotoxizität von Arzneimitteln pflanzlichen Ursprungs. *Z Gastroenterol* 2001; 39:225–232, 234–237.

68. Vachvanichsanong P, Lebel L. Djenkol beans as a cause of hematuria in children. *Nephron* 1997; 76:39–42.

69. Areekul S, Muangman V, Bohkerd C, et al. Djenkol bean as a cause of urolithiasis. *Southeast Asian J Trop Med Public Health* 1978; 9:427–432.

70. Violon C. Belgian (Chinese herb) nephropathy: why? *J Pharm Belg* 1997; 52:7–27.

71. Nortier JL, Martinez MC, Schmeiser HH, et al. Urothelial carcinoma associated with the use of a Chinese herb (Aristolochia fangchi). *New Engl J Med* 2000; 342:1686–1692.

72. Massey LK, Roman-Smith H, Sutton RA. Effect of dietary oxalate and calcium on urinary oxalate and risk of formation of calcium oxalate kidney stones. *J Am Diet Assoc* 1993; 93:901–906.

73. Sanz P, Reig R. Clinical and pathological findings in fatal plant oxalosis. A review. *Am J Forensic Med Pathol* 1992; 13:342–345.

74. Sacks O. *Guam. The Island of the Colour-blind*. London: Picador; 1996:107–201.

75. Spencer PS, Hugon J, Ludolph A, et al. Discovery and partial characterization of primate motor-system toxins. *CIBA Found Symp* 1987; 126:221–238.

76. Spencer PS, Ludolph AC, Kisby GE. Neurologic diseases associated with use of plant components with toxic potential. *Environ Res* 1993; 62:106–113.

77. Yan ZY, Spencer PS, Li ZX, et al. Lathyrus sativus (grass pea) and its neurotoxin ODAP. *Phytochemistry* 2006; 67:107–121.

78. Smith BA. Strychnine poisoning. *J Emerg Med* 1990; 8:321–325.

79. Pattanapanyasat K, Panyathanya R, Pairojkul C. A preliminary study on toxicity of diospyrol and oxidized diospyrol from Diospyros mollis Griff. (Maklua) in rabbits eyes. *J Med Assoc Thai* 1985; 68:60–65.

80. Amlo H, Haugeng KL, Wickstrom E, et al. Forgiftning med piggeple. Fem tilfeller behandlet med fysostigmin. *Tidsskr Nor Laegeforen* 1997; 117:2610–2612.

81. Groszek B, Gawlikowski T, Szkolnicka B. Samozatrucie Datura stramonium. *Przegl Lek* 2000; 57:577–579.

82. Jones AL, Proudfoot AT. The features and management of poisoning with drugs used to treat Parkinson's disease. *Q J Med* 1997; 90:613–616.

83. Rwiza HT. Jimson weed poisoning; an epidemic at Usangi Rural Government Hospital. *Trop Geogr Med* 1991; 43:85–89.

84. Dewitt MS, Swain R, Gibson LB. The dangers of Jimson weed and its abuse by teenagers in the Kanawha Valley of West Virginia. *W Va Med J* 1997; 93:182–185.

85. Greene GS, Patterson SG, Warner E. Ingestion of angel's trumpet: an increasingly common source of toxicity. *South Med J* 1996; 89:365–369.

86. Blaw ME, Adkisson MA, Levin D, et al. Poisoning with Carolina jessamine (Gelsemium sempervirens [L.] Ait.). *J Pediatr* 1979; 94:998–1001.

87. Frank BS, Michelson WB, Panter KE, et al. Ingestion of poison hemlock (Conium maculatum). *West J Med* 1995; 163:573–574.

88. Hanrahan JP, Gordon MA. Mushroom poisoning. Case reports and a review of therapy. *J Am Med Assoc* 1984; 251:1057–1061.

89. Ceha LJ, Presperin C, Young E, et al. Anticholinergic toxicity from nightshade berry poisoning responsive to physostigmine. *J Emerg Med* 1997; 15:65–69.

90. Martin-Rubi JC, Yelamos-Rodriguez F, Laynez-Bretones F, et al. Intoxicaciones por insecticidas organofosforados. Estudio de 506 casos. *Rev Clin Esp* 1996; 196:145–149.

91. Fang Y, Pei ZI, Li Z. Study on observation indexes of rational dosage of atropine in treatment of acute organophosphorus insecticides poisoning. *Zhonghua Hu Li Za Zhi* 1997; 32:311–315.

92. Thiermann H, Mast U, Klimmek R, et al. Cholinesterase status, pharmacokinetics and laboratory findings during obidoxime therapy in organophosphate poisoned patients. *Hum Exp Toxicol* 1997; 16:473–480.

93. Chu NS. Effects of betel chewing on the central and autonomic nervous systems. *J Biomed Sci* 2001; 8:229–236.

94. Singh YN. Kava: an overview. *J Ethnopharmacol* 1992; 37:13–45.

95. Ernst E. Second thoughts about kava. *Am J Med* 2002; 113:347–348.

96. Singh YN, Devkota AK. Aqueous kava extracts do not affect liver function tests in rats. *Planta Med* 2003; 69:496–499.

97. Kalix P. Catha edulis, a plant that has amphetamine effects. *Pharm World Sci* 1996; 18:69–73.

98. Al-Motarreb A, Baker K, Broadley KJ. Khat: pharmacological and medical aspects and its social use in Yemen. *Phytother Res* 2002; 16:403–413.

99. Toennes SW, Harder S, Schramm M, et al. Pharmacokinetics of cathinone, cathine and norephedrine after the chewing of khat leaves. *Br J Clin Pharmacol* 2003; 56:125–130.

100. Watson PL, Luanratana O, Griffin WJ. The ethnopharmacology of pituri. *J Ethnopharmacol* 1983; 8:303–311.

101. Elegbe RA, Oyebola DDO. Cow's urine poisoning in Nigeria: cardiorespiratory effects of cow's urine in dogs. *Trans R Soc Trop Med Hyg* 1977; 71:127–132.

102. Dalrymple T. *Romancing Opiates: Pharmacological Lies and the Addiction Bureaucracy*. New York: Encounter Books; 2006.

103. Grahame-Smith DG, Aronson JK. *The Oxford Textbook of Clinical Pharmacology and Drug Therapy*, 3rd edn. Oxford: Oxford University Press; 2002:Ch. 35.

104. Griffin JP, D'Arcy PF. Drug interactions with remedies. In: *A Manual of Drug Interactions*, 5th edn. Amsterdam: Elsevier; 1997:537–548.

105. Fugh-Berman A. Herb-drug interactions. *Lancet* 2000; 355:134–138.

106. Gold JL, Laxer DA, et al. Herbal-drug therapy interactions: a focus on dementia. *Curr Opin Clin Nutr Metab Care* 2001; 4:29–34.

107. Welihinda J, Karunanayake EH, Sheriff MH, et al. Effect of Momordica charantia on the glucose tolerance in maturity onset diabetes. *J Ethnopharmacol* 1986; 17:277–282.

108. Heck AM, DeWitt BA, Lukes AL. Potential interactions between alternative therapies and warfarin. *Am J Health-Syst Pharm* 2000; 57:1221–1227.

109. Weber WW. *Pharmacogenetics*. New York: Oxford University Press; 1997.

110. Anonymous. Grapefruit warning label: now official in some countries. *Drugs Ther Perspect* 1998; 12:12–13.

111. Committee on Safety of Medicines, Medicines Control Agency. Terfenadine: now only available on prescription. *Curr Probl Pharmacovig* 1997; 23:9.

112. Committee on Safety of Medicines, Medicines Control Agency. Astemizole (Hismanal): only available on prescription. *Curr Probl Pharmacovig* 1999; 25:2.

113. Aronson JK. Forbidden fruit. *Nature Med* 2001; 7:7–8.

114. Ohnishi A, Matsuo H, Yamada S, et al. Effect of furanocoumarin derivatives in grapefruit juice on the uptake of vinblastine by Caco-2 cells and on the activity of cytochrome P450 3A4. *Br J Pharmacol* 2000; 130:1369–1377.

115. Kitts D, Hu C. Efficacy and safety of ginseng. *Public Health Nutr* 2000; 3:473–485.

116. Xie J-T, Mehendale SR, Maleckar SA, Yuan C-S. Is ginseng free from adverse effects? *Oriental Pharm Exp Med* 2002; 2:80–86.

117. Ahn YO. Diet and stomach cancer in Korea. *Int J Cancer* 1997(suppl 10):7–9.

118. Di Carlo G, Borrelli F, Izzo AA, Ernst E. St John's wort: Prozac from the plant kingdom. *Trends Pharmacol Sci* 2001; 22:292–297.

119. Henderson L, Yue QY, Bergquist C, et al. St John's wort (Hypericum perforatum): drug interactions and clinical outcomes. *Br J Clin Pharmacol* 2002; 54:349–356.

120. Ernst E. Herbal medicines. In: Aronson JK, ed. *Meyler's Side Effects of Drugs. The International Encyclopedia of Adverse Drug Reactions and Interactions*, 15th edn. Amsterdam: Elsevier; 2006:1609–1625.

FURTHER READING

Aronson JK, ed. Meyler's side effects of drugs. *The International Encyclopedia of Adverse Drug Reactions and Interactions*, 15th edn. Amsterdam: Elsevier; 2006.

Burkill HM. *The Useful Plants of West Tropical Africa*. 5 volumes. London: Crown Agents for Oversea Governments and Administrations; 1985, 1994, 1995, 1997, 2000.

Chopra RN. *Poisonous Plants of India*. Calcutta: Government of India Press; 1940.

Chopra RN. *Indigenous Drugs of India*, 2nd edn. Calcutta: Dhat; 1958.

Duke, James A. *Amazonian Ethnobotanical Dictionary*. Boca Raton: CRC Press; 1994.

Ellenhorn MJ, Schonwald S, Ordog G, et al. *Ellenhorn's Medical Toxicology*, 2nd edn. Baltimore: Williams & Wilkins; 1997.

Everist SL. *Poisonous Plants of Australia*, 2nd edn. Sydney: Angus & Robertson; 1981.

Felter HW, Lloyd JU. *King's American Dispensatory*. Online. Available: http://www.ibiblio.org/herbmed/eclectic/kings/main.html

Lampe KF, McCann MA. *AMA Handbook of Poisonous and Injurious Plants*. Chicago: American Medical Association; 1985.

Schmidt RJ. *Botanical Dermatology Database*. Online. Available: http://archive.uwcm.ac.uk/uwcm/dm/BoDD/index.html

Sodt J. *Ethnobotany Resources in the Western Libraries*. Western Washington University. Online. Available: http://www.library.wwu.edu/ref/subjguides/ethnobot.html

Watt JM, Breyer-Brandwijk MG. *The Medicinal and Poisonous Plants of Southern and Eastern Africa*, 2nd edn. Edinburgh: E & S Livingstone; 1962.

Chapter 33 Gordon C. Cook

Podoconiosis (Non-infectious Geochemical Elephantiasis)

Confusion has existed for many decades between elephantiasis caused by the lymphatic filariases (*Wuchereria bancrofti* and *Brugia malayi*) (Chapter 84) and endemic elephantiasis – which is not helminth-related. This latter disease is caused by microparticles of silica and aluminosilicates which enter the lymphatics of the lower limbs through the soles of the feet. It is a disease mainly associated with rural communities (often known locally as 'big foot disease') and affects individuals not accustomed to footwear. The term podoconiosis (Greek: *podos*, of the foot; *konion*, dust) has now gained widespread acceptance to describe the disease.[1,2]

HISTORY

Podoconiosis was probably described by the Latin philosopher Pliny, Augustine of Hippo (now Tunisia) and Isidore of Seville in Spain.[1] It was recognized as a 'specific' disease by the Persian physician Muhammed Ibn Zakariya (El Razi) in the tenth century AD; his original description in Arabic is (or was) housed at the Baghdad Medical School. He considered that 'if the disease is attended to at its onset and treated appropriately it can be cured or stopped and will not increase'; this differentiated it from filarial elephantiasis. Among early illustrations which probably depict podoconiosis is one in the thirteenth-century *Mappa Mundi* (map of the world) preserved at Hereford Cathedral,[3] a carved oak pew-end in the church at Dennington, Suffolk, and in the sixteenth-century *Cosmographia Universalis* of Munster.[1] Realization by Manson in the late nineteenth century that most cases of elephantiasis are associated with *W. bancrofti* (or *B. malayi*) infection[4,5] led to confusion regarding the aetiology of the disease, especially in parts of Africa where this helminthiasis seemed to be absent. In Guatemala there was apparently confusion with lepromatous leprosy.[1]

EPIDEMIOLOGY

In Africa, where most cases of the disease have been described, podoconiosis is most common in highland areas in east and central parts of the continent.[1,2,6] Here, the red clays are related to volcanism in prehistory.[7,8] In West Africa, highland areas are very limited, involving only Cameroon,[9,10] part of Nigeria and the Island of Malabo, Gabon, and Equatorial Guinea;[11] although *Onchocerca volvulus* is present in some highland areas, *W. bancrofti* is invariably absent. The disease has also been recorded in several volcanic oceanic islands: the Cape Verde Islands, Canary Islands, and Malabo Island (formerly Fernando Po),[11] and more recently in Sao Tome and Principe.[12] There is also a report for the Mount Elgon area of Uganda.[13] It has also been recorded in Central America, from Mexico to Colombia and Ecuador. Other descriptions are from Guatemala, Costa Rica, Puerto Rico, Surinam, French Guiana and Brazil. Reports also exist from north-west India[14] and Sri Lanka.

Most affected individuals are from families of barefooted agriculturalists; the disease is less common in pastoral areas.[1] The altitudes, climates, soil composition and particle size in areas endemic for podoconiosis have been studied extensively.[15,16] The soil is invariably volcanic and of red clay, which becomes extremely slippery after rain.[1,2,14,17] Electron diffraction analysis shows this to consist of aluminosilicate kaolinite, with ultrafine particles of amorphous silica and iron oxides. Thermoluminescence and exoemission studies indicate that the dynamic surface properties of endemic soils are important criteria in cytoxicity.

In summary, the physical characteristics of an endemic area are as follows:[1,2]

- a temperate or near-temperate climate situated within the tropics at an altitude >1500 m
- reddish-brown soil, of which approximately half (by weight) consists of microparticles <10 mm in diameter and one-third <2 mm
- microparticles with a predominance of silica in the 2–10 mm portion (silts), and of the aluminosilicate kaolinite in the <2 mm portion (clay)
- approximately half of the clay portion is <0.4 mm and often 0.1 mm; this presupposes that the local population is agrarian and walks barefooted.

PATHOGENESIS

Podoconiosis consists of a slowly progressive obstructive lymphopathy caused by particles of optimal size (in suitable soil) having penetrated the soles of the feet. This has been confirmed by analysis of biopsy specimens from the dermis, lymphatic vessels, lymph glands (by elemental analysis of incinerated residues) and by electron microscopic microanalysis of particles in thin tissue sections.[18]

The initial pathogenetic event is, therefore, entry of toxic mineral microparticles into the dermis of the foot; the pathological consequences are dependent on particle size.[16,19] This takes place to a greater extent in the soft thin skin of young people, and by the age of 10–15 years a sufficient load of toxic material is present in the foot to produce clinical evidence of tissue damage.[1,2] The lymphatic vessels leading from the dermis become fibrosed and, in some cases, completely obstructed. Regional lymph node involvement (in the groin) occurs subsequently. These events are followed by fibrotic changes. There seems to be a genetic predisposition to the disease.[20]

PATHOLOGY

Pathological features result from lymphatic obstruction and fibrosis. The anatomy and physiology of the lower limb lymphatics have been studied extensively. Associated lesions are 'pillowy' oedema, fibrous nodulation, hyperkeratosis, interdigital bacterial and fungal infection, tuberculous adenitis, and other changes which are a result of 'traditional' management.[1,2]

CLINICAL FEATURES

Podoconiosis commonly begins between the ages of 10 and 19 years in both sexes, but has been recorded as young as 5 and as late as 60 years of age.[1,2] A burning sensation of the sole following a long walk often heralds the disease; it may become worse in bed at night, after excessive alcohol intake, after prolonged exertion, during menstruation, and while standing in front of a fire. A local swelling of the foot, usually on the dorsum near the first toe cleft, slowly diminishes in size but recurs after further exertion. The lower part of the affected leg is progressively involved over a few months to several years, but the thigh is rarely affected. Both legs are, in fact, invariably affected, but the disease develops asymmetrically, so that the swelling of one leg usually increases whilst the other remains constant. Femoral lymphadenitis is common and a cluster of nodes may reach 5 cm in length and weigh 5–6 g. Recurrent acute febrile episodes are a usual, but inconstant, feature, and these lead progressively to lymphatic obstruction. The acute episodes are easily mistaken for a localized bacterial infection and in consequence an antibiotic is prescribed. After a varying period of time, lymphoedema (elephantiasis) becomes firmly established.

In an endemic area, early disease should be suspected in any young person complaining of discomfort in the lower legs and feet, especially in bed at night and after excessive exertion. Price[1] has summarized early signs indicating oedema of the dorsum of the foot and the plantar region:

- increased skin markings and indentation on pressure
- a large second toe
- a splayed forefoot
- lymph dampness of the forefoot skin
- hyperkeratosis ('mossy foot')

- 'block toes' (early oedema of the forefoot causes the toes to appear rigid, as if they were wooden and were nailed to the forefoot)
- plantar oedema
- persistent itching of a lower part of one or other leg.

In a fully developed case of podoconiosis, appearances vary from lymphoedema to thickened, rough and leathery skin of the foot, i.e. traditional elephantiasis.[1,2] In most cases, both features are present. In the oedematous form ('water bag' leg) the skin pits on pressure and can be pinched up with the fingers; it is smooth, with little hyperkeratotic change. There may be slight oozing of lymph, and skin hairs are usually lost. Secondary infection may supervene, and streptococcal lymphangitis may be a complication. In the fibrotic ('leathery' leg) form, the fibrotic dermis may be 3 cm or more in thickness and become fixed to the deep tissues; it does not pit and cannot be pinched up between the fingers. Hyperkeratosis is common and hyperpigmentation is present. Nodulation is common at the base of the toes or in front of the ankle. Inguinal nodes are usually prominent and tender, and abdominal nodes (sometimes tender) may be palpable on abdominal examination. In a minority of cases, the affected area may extend above the knee(s). Several conditions associated with prolonged lymphatic blockage (e.g. tuberculous adenitis) are described elsewhere in this book.

MANAGEMENT

Rhazes, writing in the ninth century AD, considered that 'This malady, if it takes hold, is incurable', but he continued, 'If it is treated at the beginning it can be stopped with no further advances'.[1] Those observations remain valid today because the pathogenic effect of silica and aluminosilicate penetration into the tissues of the foot causes slowly progressive but irreversible pathological change. Individuals living in endemic areas have for many centuries recognized an association with the soil, and have also been aware that migration away from an area of high prevalence to one free of the disease arrests its progress, and vice versa. Sections of the community afflicted by this disorder usually originate in the lower strata of society, in which financial resources for footwear, etc., are very limited.

Principles of management are as follows:[1] (1) the treatment of symptoms caused by early or established disease; (2) reduction of any additional load of silica particles in the dermis; and (3) either elevation of a limb and/or elastic stockings may help to assist in reducing the oedema. Obviously, use of footwear prevents further absorption of the responsible mineral particles. The use of matting to cover bare ground within residential huts should be encouraged. This controls the progress of early disease and prevents the mineral load reaching pathogenetic proportions in other (usually younger) members of the family. If possible, a young individual with early signs of the disease should be encouraged to take up residence in a non-endemic location, and may return to the site of high prevalence when footwear is available and is widely used. A change of occupation which reduces contact between the bare foot and soil is beneficial; home industries such as weaving and dressmaking may be encouraged. Oedema and fibrogenesis are interrelated; prolonged oedema produces fibrosis; similarly, prolonged fibrosis predisposes to oedema. Oedema can be reduced by elevation of the limb or by compression with bandages or a stocking. A variety of drugs have been used with the object of reversing established fibrosis; in Africa, various traditional plant derivatives have also been used, but to no avail.

Surgical procedures are unlikely to provide satisfactory results, even when the uptake of mineral microparticles has been arrested. No method is available by which particles can be removed from the dermis, lymphatic tissues of the lower leg and regional lymph nodes. Surgery is indicated in the following situations:[1]

- excision of 'nodules' on the foot
- removal of a femoral node which is subject to repeated attacks of adenitis
- removal of superfluous skin, after the use of compression methods, in the lymphoedematous type of swelling.

PREVENTION

Podoconiosis is a preventable disease. With greater recognition of its prevalence geographically in the future, exposure to pathogenic particles should be avoided. However, prevention is also heavily dependent on the raising of socioeconomic standards, and the provision of footwear.

ECONOMIC ASPECTS

In an assessment of productivity cost(s) attributable to podoconiosis, a group of workers in Ethiopia have concluded that it exerts 'enormous economic impact' in affected areas;[21] total productivity loss amounted to 45% of the working days each year.

REFERENCES

1. Price EW. Podoconiosis: Non-filarial Elephantiasis. Oxford: Oxford University Press; 1990.
2. Davey G, Tehola F, Newport MJ. Podoconiosis: non-infectious geochemical elephantiasis. Trans R Soc Trop Med Hyg 2007; 101:1175–1180.
3. Chancey M. Mappa Mundi. Hereford: Hereford Cathedral Publications; 1987.
4. Price EW. The elephantiasis story. Trop Dis Bull 1984; 81:R1–R12.
5. Cook GC. From the Greenwich Hulks to Old St Pancras: A History of Tropical Disease in London. London: Athlone Press; 1992:332.
6. Price EW. Endemic elephantiasis of the lower legs in Rwanda and Burundi. Trop Geogr Med 1976; 28:283–290.
7. Oomen AP. Studies on elephantiasis of the legs in Ethiopia. Trop Geogr Med 1969; 21:236–253.
8. Price EW. Endemic elephantiasis of the lower legs in Ethiopia: an epidemiological survey. Ethiop Med J 1974; 12:77–90.
9. Price EW, Henderson WJ. Endemic elephantiasis of the lower legs in the United Cameroon Republic. Trop Geogr Med 1981; 33:23–29.
10. Price EW, McHardy WJ, Pooley FD. Endemic elephantiasis of the lower legs as a health hazard of barefooted agriculturalists in Cameroon, West Africa. Ann Occup Hyg 1981; 24:1–8.
11. Corachan M, Tura JW, Campo E, et al. Podoconiosis in Equatorial Guinea: report of two cases from different geological environments. Trop Geogr Med 1988; 40:359–364.
12. Ruiz L, Campo E, Corachan M. Elephantiasis in Sao Tome and Principe. Acta Tropica 1994; 57:29–34.
13. Onapa AW, Simonsen PE, Pedersen EM. Non-filarial elephantiasis in the Mt. Elgon area (Kapehorwa District) of Uganda. Acta Tropica 2001; 78: 171–176.
14. Kalra NL. Non-filarial elephantiasis in Bikaner, Rajasthan. J Commun Dis 1976; 8:337–340.
15. Hirsch A. Handbook of Geographical and Historical Pathology. London: New Sydenham Society; 1886; 3.712.
16. Price EW, Plant DA. The significance of particle size of soils as a risk factor in the etiology of podoconiosis. Trans R Soc Trop Med Hyg 1990; 84:885–886.
17. Price EW. The association of endemic filariasis of the lower legs in East Africa with soil derived from volcanic rocks. Trans R Soc Trop Med Hyg 1976; 70: 288–295.
18. Heather CJ, Price EW. Non-filarial elephantiasis in Ethiopia: analytical study of inorganic material in lymph nodes. Trans R Soc Trop Med Hyg 1972; 66:450–458.
19. Spooner NT, Davies JE. Possible role of soil particles in the aetiology of non-filarial (endemic) elephantiasis: a macrophage cytotoxicity assay. Trans R Soc Trop Med Hyg 1986; 80:222–225.
20. Davey G, Gebrehanna E, Adeyemo A, et al. Podoconiosis: a tropical model for gene-environmental interactions? Trans R Soc Trop Med Hyg 2007; 101: 91–96.
21. Tekola F, Mariam DH, Davey G. Economic costs of endemic non-filarial elephantiasis in Wolaita Zone, Ethiopia. Trop Med Int Health 2006; 11: 1136–1144.

Chapter 34   Gordon C. Cook

Familial Mediterranean Fever (Recurrent Hereditary Polyserositis)

Familial Mediterranean fever is a clinical syndrome with a clear genetic basis which gives rise to recurrent febrile episodes associated with systemic manifestations, notably abdominal pain, pleurisy and arthropathy. It affects members of certain groups with an ethnic origin, usually but not always, from the Mediterranean littoral or the Middle East.[1,2] The major importance of this disease is that it forms an important differential diagnosis from other febrile illnesses. In addition, it gives rise to substantial morbidity (but not mortality) in those affected. In 1997, a new era opened up with cloning of the mutated gene (MEFV) responsible for this entity.[2]

HISTORY

The first description of a familial condition comprising 'recurring attacks of a peculiar nature' was made by Janeway and Mosenthal[3] in 1908: a 16-year-old Jewish schoolgirl 'without special neurotic inheritance' had suffered febrile bouts associated with abdominal pain, consisting of prodromal, crescendo and recovery phases, since the age of 2 weeks. Subsequent reports originated in the USA, and were dominated by accounts of individuals of Jewish origin.[4–6] Large series of cases were recorded involving Jewish residents of Israel,[7] Turks,[8] Armenians (most of them in the USA)[9,10] and 'fair-skinned' Arabs.[11] Many names have been applied to the syndrome, including:[1] benign paroxysmal peritonitis, periodic disease, periodic fever, periodic peritonitis, maladie dite périodique, épanalepsie méditerranéenne, familial paroxysmal polyserositis, recurrent polyserositis, paroxysmal peritonitis, familial Mediterranean fever (FMF), familial paroxysmal polyserositis, familial recurrent polyserositis, and recurrent hereditary polyserositis. Renal amyloidosis was first demonstrated in this condition by Mamou and Cattan[12] in 1952 (see below). In 1972, colchicine was first used successfully in FMF by Goldfinger,[13] and the first clear evidence that its administration prevents renal amyloid deposition was provided by Zemer and her co-workers[14] in Jerusalem in 1986.

EPIDEMIOLOGY

One estimate is that 2 million people suffer, or have suffered, from FMF, although the precise magnitude of the problem worldwide is impossible to ascertain. The major ethnic groups affected are Jews (both Sephardic, i.e. those descended from ancestors expelled from Spain in the fifteenth century, and Ashkenazi), Arabs, Armenians and Turks. In Sephardic and Iraqi Jews, an estimated gene frequency of 1:45 with a prevalence of 1:2000 homozygous individuals has been calculated.[1] Corresponding figures for Armenians in Lebanon are put at 1:32 and 1:1000. Gene frequencies varying between 1:52 and 0.032, in non-Ashkenazi Jews and Armenians, respectively, have been suggested.[10] Sporadic cases (with no clear family history of the disorder) have been recorded from many countries, including the UK, Ireland, France, Germany, Sweden, the former USSR, Japan and India.[1,15] Occasional reports of a comparable syndrome have also been made in Maoris. In many, but not all, of the reported series, a significant male predominance has been recorded,[7,11] the mean ratio being of the order of 1.7:1. Most studies have indicated Mendelian recessive transmission,[1,10] although a dominant mode of inheritance has been claimed by some. Prevalence rates around 18% have been recorded when both parents are healthy, and 36% when only one is affected. In the presence of full penetrance, the likely figures would be 25% and 50%, respectively. In one study, the number of offspring affected was significantly lower than that anticipated.[16] Incomplete penetrance might be more common in females; late appearance of the syndrome in a minority of individuals has been suggested as an explanation for this inequality.

AETIOLOGY AND PATHOGENESIS

Table 34.1 summarizes some of the numerous suggested aetiological and pathogenic bases for FMF.[2,5] Many investigators have concentrated on the likelihood of an immunological defect: suppressor T cell activity and chemotaxis are decreased in untreated disease, and these abnormalities are corrected after colchicine administration. A C5a-inhibitor deficiency in joint and peritoneal fluids may play a role in the acute inflammatory attacks.[17,18] However, none of these hypotheses has been confirmed.[2] Other suggested metabolic abnormalities include: a defect in one of the lipocortin proteins or a defect in the formation and elimination of circulating monohydroxy and dihydroxy fatty acids, and an inherited enzymatic error in catecholamine metabolism. There is no known relationship with another genetic marker; neither an

Table 34.1 Some of the formerly suggested aetiological and pathogenic bases for FMF, together with a selection of known precipitating factors[1]

Infective agent of unknown identity
'Immune defect'
'Allergen'
Dietary 'allergy'
Angioneurotic oedema
'Autoimmune'
C5a-inhibitor deficiency (joint/peritoneal fluid)
Inborn error of metabolism
Lipocortin-protein defect
Abnormal catecholamine metabolism
Endocrine
SOME ACKNOWLEDGED FACTORS, IN AN ACUTE ATTACK:
Stress/anxiety
Cold
Physical exercise
Menstruation

Table 34.2 Clinical features of uncomplicated FMF[1]

Abdominal pain (24–48 hours) + pyrexia (38–40°C) + tachycardia
Acute peritonitis (constipation common; diarrhoea unusual)
Pleurisy (+ effusion) (± 50%)
Arthropathy (large joints; symmetrical; usually non-destructive) (± 50%)
Dermatological lesions (usually resembling erysipelas) (10–70%)
Immune complex nephropathy

Table 34.3 Some less common clinical features of FMF[1]

Severe headaches
Pharyngitis
Pericarditis[23]
Myocarditis
Myalgia[24]
Panniculitis
Ophthalmic problems: colloid bodies, episcleritis
Acute orchitis-infertility
Mollaret's meningitis
Childhood growth retardation

ABO nor HLA link has been recorded. The fact remains, however, in the light of recent research, that the disorder must possess a definite genetic basis.[2,19–22] There is a notable absence of descriptions of this syndrome in historical texts (including the Bible and the Koran)[1] involving affected groups; this, therefore, leaves the possibility that a relatively recently introduced environmental factor (possibly dietary) might trigger the onset of the overt clinical syndrome.

PATHOLOGY

FMF is characterized by serosal inflammation and hyperaemic manifestations involving small blood vessels, venules and arterioles;[2,7] ultrastructural changes in the latter consist of basement membrane thickening, concentric layers being separated by ground substance. Serous membranes (precisely why they are the major targets of inflammation in FMF remains unexplained) exhibit both hyperaemia and an acute inflammatory exudate containing neutrophils, lymphocytes, monocytes, plasma cells and eosinophils. When present, adhesions are thin. Synovia are also affected. When present (see below), dermatological changes consist of mild acanthosis and hyperkeratosis with infiltration by neutrophils, lymphocytes and histiocytes around smaller blood vessels.

CLINICAL FEATURES

Approximately 50% of cases have an onset during the first decade of life; most present by the end of the second, and only about 1% at >40 years of age.[11] Table 34.2 summarizes the major clinical features of FMF. Vomiting in association with the abdominal pain is common, but diarrhoea is unusual. A high percentage of affected individuals have undergone a previous abdominal operation (usually an appendicectomy). Prevalence of symptoms and signs varies in different series; arthropathy seems to be more severe in Sephardic Jews. Dermatological lesions consist most commonly of erysipelas-like lesions involving the legs, ankles and dorsum of the feet. Schönlein–Henoch purpura, urticaria, bullous lesions and vasculitis have also been recorded. Symptoms are frequently alleviated during pregnancy.[6,9] A classical presentation of an uncomplicated case is described below:

A 46-year-old Arab man, who was born in Jerusalem, was referred to a London hospital on account of irregular bouts (usually at intervals of about 2 months) of abdominal pain since the age of 18 years. A clinical diagnosis of Crohn's disease was made and sulfasalazine prescribed. Fifteen years earlier he had been subjected to appendicectomy on account of his recurrent abdominal pain. His mother's sister's son (i.e. his cousin) had experienced similar attacks. Extensive investigation between attacks proved negative: erythrocyte sedimentation rate (ESR) 18 mm/h. Following initiation of colchicine chemotherapy (see below) he become totally asymptomatic, and has remained so after a follow-up period of several years.

Table 34.3 summarizes some less common clinical features of FMF, and Table 34.4 gives some differential diagnoses based on clinical criteria.[1,2]

Precise criteria for a clinical diagnosis of FMF are impossible to establish, but the following have been suggested: (1) more than four attacks (24–72 hours' duration) of peritonitis and/or pleurisy in the presence of fever, and, in many cases, arthropathy also; (2) absence of symptoms between attacks; and (3) lack of a known underlying aetiological and/or pathological factor. It is necessary to distinguish FMF from various rare clinical entities associated with recurrent febrile episodes.[2]

Table 34.4 Some clinical differential diagnoses of FMF[1]

Pyrexia of undetermined origin
Other inherited periodic 'febrile' diseases (rare)
Abdominal infection
Appendicitis
Cholecystitis
Perforated peptic ulcer
Diverticulitis
Relapsing pancreatitis
Acute intermittent porphyria
Pulmonary embolism/atelectasis
Septic arthropathy
Juvenile rheumatoid arthritis
Tuberculous arthritis
Systemic lupus erythematosus
Other causes of amyloidosis

An association has been recorded with vasculitis,[25] demyelination,[26] and intestinal obstruction.[27]

The most important complication of FMF is amyloid AA formation. The compound is deposited in many tissues, most importantly the kidneys (renal glomeruli),[17,28] but also involves the spleen, lung, heart, liver and intestine. This complication seems to be significantly more common in Sephardic Jews and Turks, although there might be selective errors in reporting.[29-32] Ashkenazi Jews, Armenians and Arabs are largely 'immune' from this complication. It seems possible that genetic mechanisms (as yet undefined) also protect some ethnic groups from amyloid formation.[29]

A protective effect against brucellosis (see Chapter 59) (very common in Middle East countries and populations) has been hypothesized.[33]

INVESTIGATIONS

Acute-phase reactants and ESR are elevated during an acute episode. However, this does not distinguish the syndrome from other conditions with an underlying inflammatory basis. Also, the polymorph leukocyte count is elevated. Transient haematuria may be present, and abnormalities can occur in both the electrocardiogram and electroencephalogram. Although initially considered to be of value, a metaraminol provocation test[34] and estimation of dopamine-β-hydroxylase concentration[35] have not stood the test of time. In summary, none of the formerly used laboratory tests for FMF has proved satisfactory.[2] In affected individuals, rectal/gum biopsy demonstrates amyloid deposition. The presence of amyloid can be confirmed in a renal biopsy specimen; however, renal biopsy is not without risk, as haemorrhage is a real possibility in the presence of amyloid deposition.

Since the cloning of *MEFV*, however, diagnosis of FMF has been revolutionized.[2,36-39] PCR primers can now be used to demonstrate the mutations responsible for the disease, three of which are present in 85% of FMF carrier chromosomes.

MANAGEMENT

Numerous therapeutic agents have been used historically in the management of FMF. These have included: para-aminobenzoic acid, chloroquine, corticosteroids, adrenaline (epinephrine), ephedrine, atropine, reserpine, nicotinic acid, and tuberculin desensitization. In addition, numerous analgesics, narcotics, antiemetics and non-steroidal antiinflammatory compounds have been used, with limited degrees of success. In some studies, a low-fat diet has been claimed effective, and one low in tyrosine has also been advocated. Successful management was heralded by the introduction of colchicine in 1972 (see above). Although the mode of its action is unknown, 0.5–1.5 mg daily is usually adequate to prevent attacks.[13,40,41] Unfortunately, this agent has been associated with male infertility. Following widespread use of colchicine in the prevention of acute episodes, clear evidence later emerged that this form of management also prevents the onset of the amyloid nephropathy.[14] Therefore, in high-risk groups (for amyloid deposition) it is of paramount importance that regular colchicine administration be continued indefinitely.

PROGNOSIS

This is entirely dependent on the presence or absence of amyloid AA deposition. Those in a low-risk group for this complication (Ashkenazi Jews and Armenians) and others successfully treated with colchicine should have a normal life expectancy.[1,2]

REFERENCES

1. Cook GC. Recurrent hereditary polyserositis or familial Mediterranean fever: an overview. *Ann Saudi Med* 1991; 11:576–584.
2. Ben-Chetrit E, Levy M. Familial Mediterranean fever. *Lancet* 1998; 351: 659–664.
3. Janeway TC, Mosenthal HO. An unusual paroxysmal syndrome probably allied to recurrent vomiting, with a study of the nitrogen metabolism. *Trans Assoc Am Phys* 1908; 23:504–518.
4. Alt HL, Barker MH. Fever of unknown origin. *J Am Med Assoc* 1930; 94: 1459–1461.
5. Reimann HA. Periodic disease: periodic fever, periodic abdominalgia, cyclic neutropenia, intermittent arthralgia, angioneurotic edema, anaphylactoid purpura and periodic paralysis. *J Am Med Assoc* 1949; 141:175–178.
6. Siegal S. Familial paroxysmal polyserositis: analysis of fifty cases. *Am J Med* 1964; 36:893–918.
7. Sohar E, Gafni J, Pras M, et al. Familial Mediterranean fever: a survey of 470 cases and review of the literature. *Am J Med* 1967; 43:227–253.
8. Ozedmir AI, Sokmen C. Familial Mediterranean fever among the Turkish people. *Am J Gastroenterol* 1969; 51:311–316.
9. Schwabe AD, Peters RS. Familial Mediterranean fever in Armenians: analysis of 100 cases. *Medicine (Baltimore)* 1974; 53:453–462.
10. Rogers DB, Shohat M, Petersen GM, et al. Familial Mediterranean fever in Armenians: autosomal recessive inheritance with high gene frequency. *Am J Med Genet* 1989; 34:168–172.
11. Barakat MH, Karnik AM, Majeed HWA, et al. Familial Mediterranean fever (recurrent hereditary polyserositis) in Arabs: a study of 175 patients and review of the literature. *Q J Med* 1986; 60:837–847.
12. Mamou H, Cattan R. La maladie périodique (sur 14 cas personnels dont 8 compliqués de néphropathies). *Sem Hop Paris* 1952; 28: 1062–1070.

13. Goldfinger SE. Colchicine for familial Mediterranean fever. *N Engl J Med* 1972; 287:1302.

14. Zemer D, Pras M, Sohar E, et al. Colchicine in the prevention and treatment of the amyloidosis of familial Mediterranean fever. *N Engl J Med* 1986; 314:1001–1005.

15. Yamane T, Uchiyama K, Hata D, et al. A Japanese case of familial Mediterranean fever with onset in the fifties. *Intern Med* 2006; 45:515–517.

16. Armenian HK. Genetic and environmental factors in the aetiology of familial paroxysmal polyserositis: an analysis of 150 cases from Lebanon. *Trop Geogr Med* 1982; 34:183–187.

17. Matzner Y, Brzezinski A. C5a-inhibitor deficiency in peritoneal fluids from patients with familial Mediterranean fever. *N Engl J Med* 1984; 311: 287–290.

18. Schwabe AD, Lehman TJA. C5a-inhibitor deficiency: a role in familial Mediterranean fever? *N Engl J Med* 1984; 311:325–326.

19. Booth DR, Gillmore JD, Booth SE, et al. Pyrin/marenostrin mutations in familial Mediterranean fever. *Q J Med* 1998; 91:603–606.

20. Ehrlich GE. Genetics of familial Mediterranean fever and its implications. *Ann Intern Med* 1998; 129:581–582.

21. Levin M. Genetics of familial Mediterranean fever. *Ann Intern Med* 1999; 130:780.

22. Booth DR, Gillmore JD, Lachmann HJ, et al. The genetic basis of autosomal dominant familial Mediterranean fever. *Q J Med* 2000; 93:217–221.

23. Odabas AR, Cetinkaya R, Selcuk Y, et al. Severe and prolonged febrile myalgia in familial Mediterranean fever. *Scand J Rheumatol* 2000; 29:394–395.

24. Kees S, Langevitz P, Zemer D, et al. Attacks of pericarditis as a manifestation of familial Mediterranean fever (FMF). *Q J Med* 1997; 90:643–647.

25. Balbir-Gurman A, Nahir AM, Braun-Moscovici Y. Vasculitis in siblings with familial Mediterranean fever: a report of three cases and review of the literature. *Clin Rheumatol* 2007; 26:1183–1185.

26. Akman-Demir G, Gul A, Gurol E, et al. Inflammatory/demyelinating central nervous system involvement in familial Mediterranean fever (FMF): coincidence or association? *J Neurol* 2006; 253:928–934.

27. Berkun Y, Ben-Chetrit E, Klar A, el al. Peritoneal adhesions and intestinal obstructions in patients with familial Mediterranean fever – are they more frequent? *Semin Arthritis Rheum* 2007; 36:316–321.

28. Mamou H. Maladie périodique amylogene. *Sem Hop Paris* 1955; 31:388–391.

29. Pras M, Bronshpigel N, Zemer D, et al. Variable incidence of amyloidosis in familial Mediterranean fever among different ethnic groups. *Johns Hopkins Med J* 1982; 150:22–26.

30. Yalinkaya F, Tekin M, Cakar N, et al. Familial Mediterranean fever and systemic amyloidosis in untreated Turkish patients. *Q J Med* 2000; 93:681–684.

31. Akar N, Hasipek M, Ozturk A, et al. Serum amyloid A1-13 T/C alleles in Turkish familial Mediterranean fever patients with and without amyloidosis. *J Nephrol* 2006; 19:318–321.

32. Touitou I, Sarkisian T, Medlej-Hashim M, et al. Country as the primary risk factor for renal amyloidosis in familial Mediterranean fever. *Arthritis Rheum* 2007; 56:1706–1712.

33. Ross JJ. Goats, germs, and fever: are the pyrin mutations responsible for familial Mediterranean fever protective against Brucellosis? *Med Hypotheses* 2007; 68:499–501.

34. Barakat MH, El-Khawad AO, Gumaa KA, et al. Metaraminol provocative test: a specific diagnostic test for familial Mediterranean fever. *Lancet* 1984; i: 656–657.

35. Barakat MH, Gumaa KA, Malhas LN, et al. Plasma dopamine-beta-hydroxylase: rapid diagnostic test for recurrent hereditary polyserositis. *Lancet* 1988; ii:1280–1283.

36. Eisenberg S, Aksentijevich I, Deng Z, et al. Diagnosis of familial Mediterranean fever by a molecular genetics method. *Ann Intern Med* 1998; 129:539–542.

37. Drenth JP, Van Der Meer JW. Periodic fevers enter the era of molecular diagnosis. *BMJ* 2000; 320:1091–1092.

38. Grateau G, Pecheux C, Cazeneuve C, et al. Clinical versus genetic diagnosis of familial Mediterranean fever. *Q J Med* 2000; 93:223–229.

39. Nir-Paz R, Ben-Chetrit E. Molecular diagnosis of familial Mediterranean fever. *N Engl J Med* 2000; 342:60.

40. Dinarello CA, Wolff SM, Goldfinger SE, et al. Colchicine therapy for familial Mediterranean fever: a double-blind trial. *N Engl J Med* 1974; 291:934–937.

41. Zemer D, Revach M, Pras M, et al. A controlled trial of colchicine in preventing attacks of familial Mediterranean fever. *N Engl J Med* 1974; 291:932–934.

Chapter 35

Alan E. Mills and John R. Sullivan

Malignant Disease

Of an estimated total world population of 6.2 billion, some 2.5 billion people, or more than 40%, are said to reside in the tropics. This broad geographical band, encompassing the entire circumference of the earth between 23°, 30 min on either side of the equator, is a vast terrain, with diverse climatic and topographical features. There is wide variation of demographic aspects, with numerous ethnic groups expressing a profusion of social and cultural practices. It is then clear, that 'Malignant disease' in the tropics cannot be condensed into a single chapter. Even an entire book, completely devoted to the topic, would barely scratch the surface of a study of cancers tending to afflict almost half of the entire world population.

This short overview will merely attempt to summarize some aspects of selected, commonly recognized tumours having a proclivity to occur in the tropics. Most of the chapter will be confined to common tropical cancers that have the potential for prevention, treatment or possible cure.

Many tropical countries are part of what was formerly termed the 'Third World', now more correctly referred to as 'developing nations,' as opposed to 'developed,' or 'First World' (mainly western or industrialized) nations. This dichotomy can result in marked disparity in the distribution of common cancers occurring in the two settings. The appellation 'developing' nation usually carries the implication of poverty, often resulting from overpopulation, with exploitation of human resources, attended by overcrowding, inadequate housing, and poor standards of education, resulting in unemployment, poor hygiene and malnutrition. Medical facilities are frequently meagre. Cancer sufferers often present with very advanced disease, usually at an incurable stage.[1] This contrasts with western societies, where malignancy is often diagnosed in the early and frequently curable stage. The strategy of 'screening' programmes for detection of common cancers is widely employed in affluent, developed countries, resulting in early identification of cancer sufferers and probable enhanced survival. Sadly, such facilities are rarely available in tropical regions.

There are wide global cancer incidence variations due to the fact that political boundaries rarely, if ever, comprise a population that is genetically, culturally and socioeconomically homogeneous. There is thus considerable variation of cancers observed in different regions of the world. Cancer of the cervix, for instance, the most common cancer in the developing countries, is the tenth most common in the developed countries. On the other hand, colorectal cancer, second only to lung cancer in the developed countries, is only eighth in the developing countries (Table 35.1). These data were extrapolated from Parkin et al.[2]

Many types of cancer in the tropics, and subtropics have a strong association with chronic infections. For instance, schistosomiasis with squamous cell carcinoma of the bladder, intestinal parasites with Mediterranean lymphoma and hepatitis B virus with liver cancer, to mention only a few.[1]

Tobacco use

Unfortunately, with increasing adoption of a Western lifestyle, especially smoking, the lung cancer incidence is expected to rise in developing countries. Such an increase has already been observed in Shanghai, China's largest city, in India and in Zimbabwe. The male lung cancer incidence recorded in Bulawayo, Zimbabwe, in 1963–1977 was 70.6/100 000 population.[3] The age standardized rate (ASR) for lung cancer in the capital, Harare, in 1990–1992, was 23.7/100 000 population. Such statistics call for an urgent need to counteract the ruthless and sophisticated smoking campaign launched by the tobacco companies. It is not enough to merely persuade individuals to give up smoking, or for governments to legislate against tobacco. There are powerful economic interests served by the production, promotion and sale of tobacco products, which seek to maximize consumption at all costs. Tobacco is the major source of foreign exchange revenue in some countries. The most prominent cancer risk factor is cigarette smoking, associated primarily with lung cancer but contributing considerably to cancers of the oropharynx, oesophagus and urinary bladder. It has been suggested that tobacco smoking is exacting a heavier toll in lives and dollars than cocaine, heroin, AIDS, traffic accidents, murder and terrorist attacks combined.[4] It is to be hoped that tobacco control policies, such as the WHO Framework Convention on Tobacco Control (FCTC), which came into being in 2005, will be widely supported by world governments.[5]

Other causes of cancer

Genetic factors are known to play an important role in the causation of certain cancers, notably increased incidence of skin cancers in individuals with defective capacity to repair DNA damage

Table 35.2 FIGO staging of carcinoma of the uterine cervix: 1988 update

Stage	Characteristics
0	Carcinoma in situ, intraepithelial carcinoma (cases of stage 0 should be included in statistics for invasive carcinoma)
I	Carcinoma strictly confined to the cervix
I-A1	Minimal, microscopically evident carcinoma of the cervix
I-A2	Lesion detected microscopically that can be measured. The lesion must invade less than 5 mm below the base of the surface or glandular epithelium and extend to no more than 7 mm in the horizontal plane
I-B	Lesions larger than stage I-A2. Preformed space involvement should not alter the staging but should be recorded
II	Carcinoma extends beyond the cervix but does not reach the pelvic wall. The carcinoma involves the vagina, but not the lower third
II-A	No obvious parametrical involvement
II-B	Obvious parametrical involvement
III	Carcinoma extends to the pelvic wall. On rectal examination there is no cancer-free space between the tumour and the pelvic wall. The tumour involves the lower third of the vagina. All cases with hydronephrosis or non-functional kidney should be included unless known to be due to other causes
III-A	No extension to the pelvic wall
III-B	Extension to the pelvic wall
IV	Carcinoma extending beyond the true pelvis or clinically involving the mucosa of the bladder or rectum
IV-A	Spread to adjacent organs
IV-B	Spread to distant organs

allograft recipients[34] and in patients with Hodgkin lymphoma[35] suggests a potential role of immunosuppression. However, the role of HIV immunosuppression in the development of cervical intraepithelial neoplasia (CIN) and the role of HIV in invasive cancer of the cervix remains unclear. Although invasive squamous cell carcinoma of the cervix was added to the Centers for Disease Control (CDC) AIDS definition in 1993,[36] the situation in Africa is far from clear. In most developing countries, and especially in sub-Saharan Africa, both HIV and cancer of the cervix are very common and by coincidence alone up to 35% of patients can have both. However, in such situations cervical carcinoma tends to run a rapid downhill course.

Exposure to sexually transmitted agents has been in the limelight for over three decades. Initial interest in the 1970s focused on herpes simplex virus type 2 (HSV-2). It was suggested that HSV-2 might be the initiating agent.[37] More recently human papilloma viruses (HPV) (especially HPV types 16 and 18) have emerged as the putative transmissible factor for cancer of the cervix. Walboomers and colleagues maintain that HPV is a necessary cause of invasive cervical carcinoma.[38] The viral transforming genes, E6 and E 7, of HPV 16 are thought to cause degradation of tumour suppressor proteins, such as p53 gene products (vide infra).[39] Degradation of another tumour suppressor gene, the retinoblastoma gene, pRb, has also been shown to be important in progression of cervical cancer.[40] The locus for p53 is on chromosome 17 (17 p13), and pRb is located on chromosome 13 (13 q14).

It is thought that p53 is inactivated by E6, and pRb is inactivated by E 7 viral oncoproteins, respectively.[40] HPV is a double-stranded DNA virus and is found in 95% of cervical condylomata acuminata.

The complete replication of chromosome ends, or telomeres, requires telomorase. In cancers, there is high telomorase activity. The human telomorase reverse transcriptase subunit (hTERT), which is the catalytic unit of telomorase, is upregulated, removing a barrier for unlimited cellular proliferation. This process is believed to be induced by the protein product of the proto-oncogene, c-myc, which promotes S phase activity in the mitotic cell cycle. The gene locus for c-myc is on chromosome 8 (8 q24). Increased c-myc expression is associated with cervical cancer.[41]

Certain histological variants seem to be associated with specific HPV types. HPV-16 appears commonly in squamous cell carcinoma, and its precursor lesion CIN. On the other hand, HPV-18 is seen frequently in adenocarcinoma and its precursor, C GIN (formerly AIS).

High risk HPV E7 oncoprotein has been suggested as a marker to detect cervical cancer.[42]

Staging

The staging system in wide use is the one recommended by the International Federation of Gynecology and Obstetrics (FIGO) (Table 35.2).

Pre-treatment evaluation and assignment of stage, in addition to history and physical examination, must include pelvic examination under anaesthesia, chest X-ray, intravenous pyelography, barium enema, cystoscopy and/or sigmoidoscopy. The stage is determined clinically and does not change on the basis of surgical findings. A recent study using computed tomography (CT) and magnetic resonance imaging (MRI) to determine the utility of these imaging techniques in detecting local or regional metastasis concluded that the 60% accuracy was too low to warrant routine use of these tests for staging.[43] The majority of patients present with advanced disease stage, with 80–90% being stages III and IV. The full pre-staging protocol proposed tends to be time consuming and expensive. A cost-effective protocol which omits some investigations without harming patients tends to be employed in developing countries.

Prognostic factors

The most reliable prognostic factors are stage at diagnosis, nodal status and size and grade of differentiation of primary tumour.

Prevention

Cancer of the cervix is both a preventable, and curable disease. Preventable because the pre-invasive in situ stage can be screen-detected, and is curable in the early stage. Screen detection has been based for over 50 years on Papanicolaou exfoliative cytology (Pap test), developed by Papanicolaou and Traut in 1943. It has been suggested that the time may be approaching when Pap testing can be replaced by molecular screening for HPV DNA.[44] However, for the time being, the Pap test remains the cornerstone of screening. The process of carcinogenesis from induction to development of invasive cancer is approximately 10 years. Precancerous changes can be detected several years before the development of invasive cancer by the Pap test, either by traditional smear, or liquid based ' thin prep' techniques. Cytological triage of women positive for HPV DNA, will determine those requiring colposopy.[45,48] Cytological screening as a sole method, may result in unnecessary colposcopy referrals.[46] Nevertheless, there is a need for screening in developing countries. However, it is recognized that Papanicolaou cytology has a low sensitivity. P16 is a surrogate marker for HPV infection, and can be used immunohistochemically, to detect HPV infected cells.[47] It has been suggested that screening can be improved by testing for DNA of oncogenic types of HPV on the same sample used for cytology.[47,48] Vaccination protection against HPV for young females, prior to sexual activity, has been referred to previously. Kahn and Burk have commented that papilloma vaccines have been shown to be highly effective.[49] Gardasil (or Silgard) is a quadrivalent vaccine active against HPV-16, HPV-18, HPV-6 and HPV-11. HPV types 16 and 18 are responsible for 70% of cervical cancers. HPV-31 and HPV-45 are more unusual causes of cervical cancer. HPV types 6 and 11 are mainly associated with genital warts. Cervarix is a bivalent vaccine, protecting against HPV types 16 and 18.[50] The vaccines are based on in vitro assembly of virus like particles (VLP), and synthesis of the major capsid protein, L1. The sub-unit vaccines, composed of VLP, are produced by recombinant technology, and as they contain no DNA, nor live products, are considered non-infectious.[51] It has been suggested that vaccination of 9–15-year-old girls could be extended to boys in the same age range, with some possible further advantage.[51] Anti-HPV vaccination may prevent about 70%, but not all cases of cervical cancer. It is therefore logical that vaccinated women should remain in a cervical cytology screening programme.

It has been suggested by some that cervical screening is not 'cost-effective'. Most of these observations reflect Western culture where cancer of the cervix is not common and it would therefore cost exorbitant sums of money to identify one case. The situation in the tropics is clearly different, and although cost-benefit analyses have not been systematically undertaken, the sheer numbers of victims would suggest that screening should be advocated.

Male circumcision has been previously alluded to.[29] Circumcision reduces penile HPV infection, and therefore probably reduces the risk of cervical cancer.

Management

Cervical screening, if successfully carried out, will reduce the incidence of clinically invasive squamous cell carcinoma and thus lower morbidity and mortality.

Carcinoma in situ (CIN 111 or stage 0), specifically in the third world situation, is best treated by abdominal hysterectomy, with or without vaginal cuff. If the patient wishes to retain fertility and she can be relied upon to return for regular review, then a cone biopsy may be adequate. The outcome for stage 0 is excellent, with <2% of patients developing recurrent cancer in situ or invasive carcinoma.[52] The treatment of stage I-A with minimal invasion is similar to that for stage 0. For stages I-B and II-A the treatment is either surgery (radical hysterectomy and pelvic lymphadenectomy) or radiotherapy, which consists of external beam irradiation and brachytherapy (temporary insertion of intrauterine and vaginal colpostats loaded with isotope, usually caesium-137). Surgery is the preferred approach for younger women who wish to retain ovarian function and avoid vaginal irradiation, which may result in stenosis. Radiotherapy is to be recommended for patients who are elderly and/or have surgical contraindications. The survival for the two approaches (radiation and surgery) is about equivalent, with survival at 5 years ranging from 80% to 90% under ideal conditions. Stages II-B and III patients are to be considered for radical hysterectomy and pelvic lymphadenectomy or external beam irradiation (4500–5500 cGy) followed by intracavitary brachytherapy. Patients with locally invasive stage IV-A or recurrence after radiotherapy may be considered for pelvic exenteration. Down-staging for patients with locally advanced disease is being advocated.

Role of chemotherapy

The main cause of death among women with cancer of the cervix is uncontrolled disease within the pelvis. The use of chemotherapy has several theoretical advantages. Given in a neoadjuvant fashion, it may result in down-staging and may facilitate surgical resection or enhance the effect of radiation. Chemotherapy may also act as a radiation sensitizer if used concurrently with radiotherapy. The possible mechanisms include: (1) the inhibition of repair of radiation-induced damage, (2) the promotion of synchronization of cells into radiosensitive phase of the cell cycle, and (3) the reduction of the hypoxic cell fraction that is known to be radio-resistant.

A number of randomized phase III trials have recently been published which support the use of chemotherapy for various stages of locally advanced cervical carcinoma. In one study a group of patients with bulky (>4 cm in diameter) node-negative, stage I-B were randomized to either receive radiation alone, or radiation together with 40 mg/m^2 of cisplatin given weekly for the 6 weeks

639

of radiation. This phase was followed 3–6 weeks later by adjuvant hysterectomy. The relative risk of progression was 0.51 (95% CI, 0.34–0.75) $p < 0.001$ and the overall survival was 0.54 (95% CI, 0.34–0.86) $p = 0.008$, both favouring combined treatment. As expected, there were more transient grades 3 and 4 haematological toxicity (21% vs 2%), and more gastrointestinal effects (14% vs 5%) in the combined treatment arm.[53] Another study was reported by Rose et al.,[54] which included previously untreated invasive squamous, adenosquamous or adenocarcinoma stages II-B, III or IV-A without pelvic node involvement. Patients with adequate marrow reserve (WBC $>3 \times 10^9$/L, platelets $> 100 \times 10^9$/L) and good renal function (creatinine < 177 μmol/L) were randomized in addition to radiotherapy to receive one of three treatment arms.

Various regimens of cisplatinum, with or without infusional 5 fluorouracil and hydroxyurea have yielded similar favourable outcomes.

The results of these and other studies led the United States National Cancer Institute to issue rare clinical announcements to the effect that 'strong consideration should be given to the inclusion of concurrent cisplatin-based chemotherapy with radiation therapy in women who require radiation therapy for treatment of cervical cancer'.[55]

The situation in Africa and most developing countries is such that the recommendations highlighted above may be inappropriate. Most patients present with disease at very advanced stage when even pelvic exenteration may not be possible. In many situations neither radiotherapy nor chemotherapy is available. Survival is difficult to ascertain as default rate is high. Most patients request for discharge to try alternative forms of therapy. Such pathetic situations underscore the need to develop comprehensive palliative care services, including pain control.

HEPATOCELLULAR CARCINOMA

Primary liver cancer includes hepatocellular carcinoma (HCC), which is very common, cholangiocarcinoma, which is quite uncommon, apart from parts of Asia, especially North East Thailand, and angiosarcoma of the liver, which is very rare. This discussion will concentrate on HCC. HCC is among the 10 most common cancers worldwide.[2] It is estimated that there are at least 260 000 new cases every year; the majority of these are to be found in sub-Saharan Africa, South-east Asia and the western Pacific. In Shanghai, the incidence rate is 34.4/100 000 males and 11.6/100 000 females. In the Philippines, the figures quoted are 17.5/100 000 males and 7.1/100 000 females.[20] In sub-Saharan Africa, primary liver cancer has, until the emergence of AIDS-associated Kaposi's sarcoma, been the most common cancer affecting men. The highest recorded incidence rate is in Mozambique, among the Mozambican Shangaans, and HCC accounts for $>^2/_3$ of all male and $^1/_3$ of female tumours, with an incidence rate of over 100/100 000 population.[56] A more recent survey in Mozambique recorded incidence rates ranging from 9.3 to 60.7/100 000 males and from 3.7 to 13.0/100 000 females.[57] The striking feature was the high rates in the very young, with estimated crude rates for those aged 20–29 years being 82.2/100 000 and for those aged 30–39 being 85.8/100 000.

Rates intermediate between those of the Far East and those of Europe and North America are reported in countries of the Middle East, the Caribbean and parts of South America.

Aetiology

HCC is multifactorial in aetiology and causal factors differ in different parts of the world. Hepatitis B virus (HBV) is believed to play a causal role in about 80% of patients with HCC worldwide. The incidence of HCC among HBV patients has been identified, using an automated data algorithm.[58] In low-risk populations about one-half of HCC cases in men and one-third in women can be attributed to a viral aetiology. Hepatitis C is spread similarly to HBV. The non-viral aetiological factors associated with HCC are iron overload, aflatoxin, cigarette smoking, oral contraceptives and alcohol ingestion.

Hepatitis B and C virus infection

About 80% of HCCs result from infection with HBV, a virus which causes other liver ailments as well, and is second only to tobacco as a known single cause of cancer. The evidence for its causal role in HCC is derived from epidemiological case-control and cohort studies, clinical data and laboratory investigations.[59] Follow-up of patients with chronic liver disease associated with HBV markers indicates that hepatitis B surface antigen (HBsAg)-positive individuals with chronic hepatitis and/or cirrhosis have a greater risk of developing HCC. The most convincing epidemiological evidence for the role of HBV as a causative agent for HCC comes from the prospective case-control surveillance of 22 000 middle-aged Chinese males in Taiwan observed for 75 000 man-years of follow-up. In the 15% who were HBsAg carriers there was a 223-fold excess risk of HCC over the non-carriers.[60] Integration of HBV DNA into human hepatocytes was first detected in a continuous cell line expressing HBsAg derived from a male HBV carrier with HCC. HBV DNA is now known to be incorporated into the host genome of HCC patients whether they have evidence of viral infection or not.[61]

Hepatitis C virus (HCV), is spread similarly to HBV. HCV is an enveloped single strand flavivirus. HCV infection leads progressively to cirrhosis, with many patients subsequently developing HCC. Cirrhosis is found in 86–100% of untreated anti-HCV-positive HCC patients. It is estimated that over 50% of cases of HCC diagnosed annually in Japan are probably HCV related. The role of HCV in the tropics is poorly defined. In Egypt, the prevalence may approach 20% of the population. However, the incidence of infection is probably significant in most tropical areas, and co-infection with HBV and/or HIV may worsen the prognosis, with acceleration of liver disease.[62,63]

Aflatoxin

Aflatoxin was first isolated in 1961 following an outbreak of fatal jaundice in turkeys. The 'turkey-X' disease was traced to poultry feed containing peanuts imported from Brazil contaminated with *Aspergillus flavus*. Subsequently aflatoxin B (so called because of its blue fluorescence) was found to be potently hepatotoxic and carcinogenic in a variety of animal species. Aflatoxins are a group of compounds produced by the mould *A. flavus*, which grows readily in warm, humid conditions. Although groundnuts are the substrate of choice for the mould, it can grow on other cereals, notably maize, millet, peas and sorghum.

People in some areas of the tropical world are frequently exposed to food contaminated with aflatoxin. In Mozambique 8% of prepared meal samples contain measurable aflatoxin. The average contamination level is 38.1 mg/kg wet food. The aflatoxin levels in food samples observed in Mozambique are the highest in the world.[57] In the Transkei the frequency of food sample contamination is much higher (25%) but the level of contamination is much lower than that in Mozambique.

The carcinogenic risk of aflatoxin has been evaluated and reported.[64] Laboratory research has demonstrated the hepatocarcinogenic properties of aflatoxin.[65,66] There is a clear correlation between HCC and the rate of aflatoxin ingestion.[57,67,68] Further confirmation of an aetiological role for aflatoxin in HCC has come from a case-control study in the Philippines where the mean contamination level of different dietary items was established and individual levels of consumption determined retrospectively.[69] Studies in Kenya[70] and Thailand have more or less found similar results. In Egypt, a country with a very low level of aflatoxin contamination because the climate is hot and dry, the incidence of HCC is relatively low. In Botswana, which is very dry, and Greenland, which is very cold, the incidence of HCC is low and presumably A. flavus growth in such unfavourable climates is inhibited.

The mechanism of carcinogenesis is not well understood, but several plausible explanations have been suggested. Aflatoxin B is metabolized by a microsomal mixed function oxidase system to produce aflatoxin B-2,3-epoxide, which is believed to be the carcinogen.[71] It has also been suggested that aflatoxin may suppress cell-mediated immunity and facilitate persistent HBV infection and eventually HCC.[72] There is a suggestion that aflatoxin only accumulates in the liver after the liver's ability to degrade aflatoxin has been impaired by persistent HBV infection.[73]

Cigarette smoking

Where studies have been done, in high-risk populations, as in South African blacks, the evidence supports the conclusion that cigarette smoking plays no aetiological role in HCC in South Africa.[74] In low-risk areas of the world, however, cigarette smoking is a significant risk factor with a relative risk ratio of >2.[75]

Alcohol

It is estimated that heavy alcohol consumption is another risk factor, especially in the low incidence areas. HCC is almost fivefold as common in men who imbibe more than 80 g of ethanol per day than in non-drinkers.[75] However, in tropical countries, most HCCs are associated with macronodular post-hepatitic rather than micronodular alcoholic cirrhosis.[76] There is very little evidence to implicate alcohol as playing a role in high-incidence areas of HCC.

Sex

Prevalence of HCC in men is higher than in women. The ratio of male to female cases of HCC is between 2:1 and 4:1. This may be a reflection of disturbance of the interleukin 6 (IL6) – myeloid differentiation factor 88 (MyD88) signalling mechanism. In the liver, IL6 is secreted by Kupffer cells, in response to hepatocyte injury and utilizes MyD88 as a messenger protein to transmit a signal to liver cell nuclei promoting cellular proliferation. Upregulation of IL6, in nitrosamine induced carcinogenesis in mice, is neutralized by oestrogen, which has a protective effect. This may perhaps provide an explanation for the sex bias?[77]

Iron overload

African iron overload, or nutritional haemosiderosis, are preferable terms to haemochromatosis which has become virtually synonymous with genetic or familial haemochromatosis. Genetic haemochromatosis, a common disorder of northern European kindreds, is related to mutation of the iron loading gene, HFE, located on chromosome 6. Single amino acid substitutions lead to the mutant genes, C282Y, or H63D, and more rarely, S65C. It is usually an autosomal recessive condition, but sometimes may be a complex heterozygous state. By contrast, African iron overload has been thought to be non-genetic, blamed on consumption of large amounts of iron in maize beer, which has a low pH, and is traditionally brewed in iron skillet pots. This theory seems to be reinforced by the observation that HCC seems to be declining, as more Africans are taking to commercially brewed beer, and western style alcoholic drinks. However, Gordeuk et al., have demonstrated that there is a genetic component associated with African iron overload.[78] This putative gene is not linked to the HLA locus. Other causes of iron overloading also exist in the tropics. These include transfusional siderosis, for transfusion dependent anaemia, such as sickle cell disease, other haemoglobinopathies, and thalassaemia, for instance.

Membranous obstruction of the inferior vena cava is an unusual condition, mainly confined to Southern Africa and Japan. It is said to result from incomplete resolution of thrombus leading to hepatic outflow obstruction, cirrhosis and subsequent carcinoma.[1]

Clinical features

The clinical and epidemiological features of HCC have recently been reviewed by Mazzanti et al.[57] HCC presents with right upper quadrant pain or discomfort, abdominal mass and distension. Physical examination reveals hepatomegaly in 90% of cases, wasting and ascites in 50%. Abdominal venous collaterals, if looked for, occur in 30% and icterus in 25%. A few patients may present with pathological fractures due to bone metastases. In Uganda, bone is the second most common site of metastases in HCC. Some patients have marked itching due to obstructive jaundice and about 10% may present with haematemesis and melaena following rupture of oesophageal varices in cases of advanced cirrhosis. Elevated alkaline phosphatase is detected in 75% of cases and AFP is above the normal level in 60%.

HCC affects young individuals, with remarkably high rates in the 10–29-year age group in Mozambique. In Uganda the peak incidence is observed during the third and fourth decades. The male to female ratio is 2–4:1. The clinical diagnosis of HCC in the tropics is relatively simple. This is because other tumours likely to metastasize to the liver are relatively rare. Thus in the tropics any young adult male presenting with abdominal pain and mass and found to have hepatomegaly has HCC until otherwise proven.

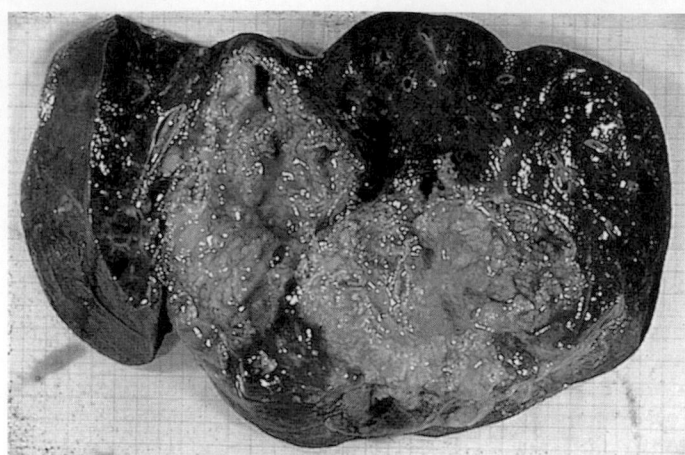

Figure 35.1 Hepatocellular carcinoma. Mass in liver.

If alkaline phosphatase is elevated this raises the suspicion even further. A positive AFP almost certainly confirms the diagnosis. However, if an intervention is contemplated a needle biopsy is recommended. The most common differential diagnosis in the tropics is an amoebic liver abscess.

Prognosis

HCC in the tropics runs a fulminant downhill course. The mean interval from onset to death in South African patients was 11 weeks.[79] In a study which included Algerian and French patients, the mean survival time of untreated patients was 73 days, suggesting the natural history of French patients may be similar to African and Asian patients with HCC.[80] Most patients present with a very advanced single massive tumour when first seen (Figure 35.1).

The fibrolamellar variant of HCC,[81] which occurs primarily in the young (peak in second to third decade), affects both male and female patients with non-cirrhotic livers and is rarely associated with positive AFP but has a better prognosis (average survival 44 months), is extremely rare in the tropics. No case of fibrolamellar HCC has been seen in South African blacks.[82]

Signs of poor prognosis include wasting, abdominal venous collaterals, ascites, elevated bilirubin and encephalopathy.[80,83–85]

Management

The treatment of HCC remains unsatisfactory. Surgical resection provides the only prospect for cure. However, <2% present at a stage when this approach is feasible. Even apparently early cases have advanced cirrhosis and recurrence in the remaining lobe after apparently curative resection is the rule rather than the exception.

The goal of treating most patients with HCC is palliation. Hepatic artery ligation is an effective way of relieving symptoms, especially pain, and in individuals who have had spontaneous intraperitoneal rupture, a common complication.[86] The rationale is based on the observation that liver tumours (primary and secondary) derive their blood supply from the hepatic artery, while normal liver is supplied from both the hepatic artery and the portal vein. Before hepatic artery ligation can be recommended the patency of the portal vein must be established.

Radiation therapy is rarely recommended because liver tissue is extremely sensitive even to low-dose radiation. However,[90] Y-labelled microspheres are undergoing clinical trials. Radiofrequency ablation (RFA), and direct injection of the lesion with alcohol have been used.

Chemotherapy appears to be an effective form of palliation. The best single agent seems to be the anthracycline doxorubicin.[85,87]

Several drug combinations have been tried, with disappointing results.[87,88] The combination of doxorubicin and cisplatin has been reported to result in a dramatic response, although it was complicated by the reactivation of hepatitis B infection.[89]

It should be stressed that in tropical areas the goal of treatment of HCC is to relieve symptoms and therefore the patient's quality of life is paramount. A recently completed quality of life-focused randomized clinical trial in Zimbabwe concluded that chemotherapy with doxorubicin, either at conventional monthly or weekly low doses, did not improve the quality of life or survival of patients so treated. While not practical in all tropical areas, liver transplantation for HCC in Asia has shown promising results.[90]

Prevention

Since 80% of HCC is attributed to HBV infection and an effective vaccine against the virus is now available, the prospect for cancer prevention is certainly in sight.[91] A vaccination trial sponsored by the World Health Organization was started in 1986 in The Gambia, West Africa, to determine its efficacy in preventing chronic liver disease and HCC in particular.[13] As HBV transmission in Africa occurs by horizontal spread, with a second wave of infection occurring at the time of school entry (5–6 years), it is possible to include HBV vaccine in the expanded programme of immunization. A pilot study started in the villages of Keneba and Manduar in Gambia in 1984 revealed that the overall vaccine efficacy in 1993 against HBV infection was about 95%. Despite rapidly falling antibody concentration in vaccinated children and the presence of viral variants, the efficacy of HBV vaccination against HBV and HbsAg carrier was maintained.[92] In unvaccinated children in the Far East, early infection with HBV leading to a carrier state results from vertical perinatal transmission from replicative carrier mothers. To prevent this, the first dose of the vaccine must be given soon after birth. This approach has greatly reduced the carriage rate in Asian children.

Screening using modern imaging techniques, CT and ultrasonography, as well as serial AFP testing, have been tried, but are not cost effective, in the tropical setting. The highest incidence of cholangiocarcinoma in the world is in north east Thailand. This has been related to infestation with the liver fluke, *Opisthorchis viverrini*, which is endemic in the region.[93]

SQUAMOUS CELL CANCER OF THE OESOPHAGUS

Squamous cell carcinoma of the oesophagus is relatively rare in most of Europe, apart from the French provinces of Brittany and Normandy, which have incidence rates in excess of 80/100 000 population. Outside Europe, high rates are recorded in Linxian province in northern China, in the province of Mazandarin in Iran on the Caspian sea, in east, central and southern Africa, India and Central America. In Linxian province of the Peoples' Republic of China the incidence rate is 130/100 000 population and oesophageal cancer is second only to stomach cancer as the leading cause of cancer deaths in China, according to the 1974–1976 statistics.

In most tropical areas, cancer of the oesophagus has an uneven geographical distribution. Both rural and urban dwellers appear to be equally affected. In South Africa, cancer of the oesophagus was a curiosity in the 1920s but it has now become one of the most common cancers affecting black males. The highest rates are recorded in the Transkei: up to 63/100 000 males and 65/100 000 females. More recently, high rates have been recorded in Zimbabwe, Zambia, Malawi, parts of Tanzania and in the region around Kisumu in Kenya. By contrast, oesophageal carcinoma appears to be rare in south-west Uganda, Democratic Republic of Congo and in West Africa. In all high incidence areas there is a strong male dominance but in recent years the tumour has been increasing in frequency in women in South Africa.

Oesophageal squamous cell carcinoma tends to occur in the mid oesophagus, and must be clearly distinguished from oesophageal adenocarcinoma, which occurs in the lower oesophagus, and is a completely separate entity.[94] Adenocarcinoma probably arises on a basis of dysplasia evolving from goblet cell, intestinal or so-called Barrett's metaplasia, which in turn is probably an acquired condition, initiated by gastro-oesophageal reflux disease (GERD). Barrett's oesophagus is thought to be a disease mainly affecting white Caucasian males of higher socioeconomic status.[95] That said, however, it is claimed the prevalence of Barrett's oesophagus in Eastern countries is rising to match the prevalence in the West.[96]

Aetiology

Alcohol and tobacco acting together have been established as the major cause of oesophageal squamous cancer in the industrialized world. Epidemiological studies in France show that those who smoke or drink heavily run a 44 times greater risk of oesophageal cancer than light drinkers and smokers. It has been postulated that alcohol might act as a solvent facilitating the passage of carcinogens into the inner layers of the oesophagus. The role of alcohol in the causation of cancer of the oesophagus in developing countries is not clearly documented. In Iran, for instance, it is not the custom of Turkoman people to drink and very few of the oesophageal cancer victims smoke. In China, of 527 patients 83% reported that they did not drink alcohol, and those who drank did so only on rare occasions. Gastric atrophy has emerged as a risk factor for oesophageal SCC.[97] The demographics of oesophageal squamous cell carcinoma and adenocarcinoma also have an East–West variation (as apposed to tropical–non-tropical differences), because in Japan more than 90 % of oesophageal cancers are of squamous cell type.[98] Abnormalities of chromosome 17 have been linked to oesophageal squamous carcinoma.[99] The tylosis oesophageal gene, mapped to chromosome 17q25, is a marker for oesophageal SCC. Tylosis is an uncommon autosomal recessive genodermatosis, in which hyperkeratosis of palms and soles occurs. It is associ-

ated with a high risk of oesophageal carcinoma. At variance with the usual pattern of risk factors in the West is the apparent lack of appreciable effects of alcohol usage on the disease in Zulus. Observations in South Africa appear to lend support to nutritional predisposing factors to cancer of the oesophagus. Dietary staples appear to be low in vitamins and minerals. This conforms with data from the Cancer Registry of Bulawayo, Zimbabwe, which established that low socioeconomic status / malnutrition is a significant risk factor.[100] The Cancer Registry of Bulawayo has also shown that bladder cancer frequency is also increased in low socioeconomic groups,[101] paralleling the situation with oesophageal carcinoma. In China and Iran, the so-called oesophageal cancer belt of south-central Asia, oesophageal cancer may also be related to nutritional factors. It has been demonstrated that victims of oesophageal cancer are malnourished and get neither vitamin A nor riboflavin requirements. One study showed over 40% consumed <10% in winter and <20% in spring and autumn of vitamin A requirements. A deficiency of vitamin A has been shown to lead to carcinogenesis, while an adequate intake of vitamin C has been shown to have an anticarcinogenic effect. In China, death from oesophageal cancer has been closely linked with ingestion of pickled vegetables.

Unfortunately, the addition of riboflavin, retinol and zinc had no effect on the high prevalence of precancerous oesophageal lesions.[102] There are several possible explanations for this negative result. First, the treatment may not have been given for a period long enough or the dosages were not large enough to effect change. Second, the precancerous oesophageal lesions, like gastritis, may be irreversible. Third, the hypothesis linking riboflavine/retinol deficiency with precancerous oesophageal lesions may not be correct.

Oesophageal carcinoma has been linked to exposure to silica dust in underground workers.[103]

Clinical features

In high-incidence areas, cancer of the oesophagus may be seen in the fourth and fifth decades of life. Men are two to three times more commonly affected, except in northern Iran, where women predominate, and in South Africa, where the frequency in women is on the increase. The disease often becomes symptomatic, with progressive dysphagia and severe weight loss and wasting.

Staging

Pre-treatment evaluation for accurate staging should include history, physical examination, barium swallow, upper gastrointestinal endoscopy and biopsy and a CT scan of the thorax and upper abdomen, and endoscopic ultrasound, if available. Direct laryngoscopy and bronchoscopy is advisable. Positron emission tomography (PET) scan has been shown to be a useful adjunct to conventional, non-invasive staging procedures. PET significantly improves the detection of stage IV disease and improves the diagnostic specificity for lymph nodes.[104] However, PET is not available as yet in many developing country cancer centres. Staging recommended by the American Joint Committee on Cancer (AJCC), as shown in Table 35.3 applies the tumour, node and metastasis (TNM) system. The following clinical, radiographic and

like jaws, orbits, ovaries, kidneys, adrenals, thyroid, testes and breasts and had concluded that they were all separate entities, it was Burkitt who felt that although the involved sites varied from patient to patient, a pattern emerged that suggested a unitary process. He then undertook a journey around Africa (the famous 'tumour safari') and was able to map out the geographical distribution of this tumour within Africa, the so-called 'lymphoma belt'. He further observed that the distribution was very similar to the malaria map and suggested that the tumour might be caused by an arthropod (mosquito)-borne virus. Subsequently, at a conference on lymphoreticular tumours held in Paris in 1963, it was unanimously agreed to give the tumour the eponym Burkitt's lymphoma in recognition of his pioneering work. Classification of non-Hodgkin's lymphoma has retained the eponym.[166]

Epidemiology

Endemic type A, or African BL is restricted to the geographical latitudes 10–15° north and south of the equator and to altitudes below 1500 m, occurring in Africa, and Papua New Guinea. It is rare in places where the diurnal temperature drops to below 16°C frequently and in places where the rainfall is <50 cm per annum. Outside tropical Africa BL is found in those areas of the tropical

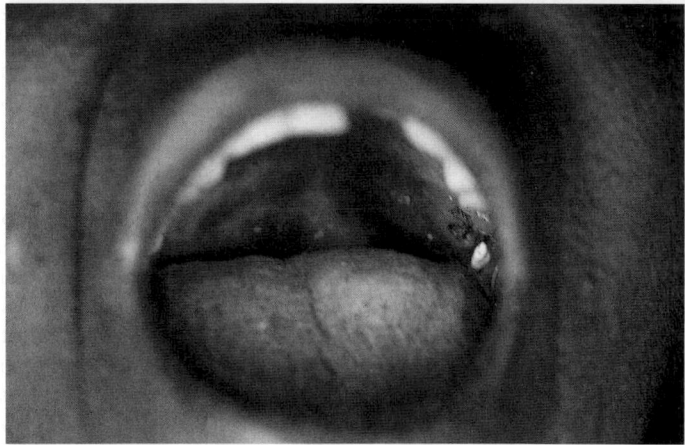

Figure 35.8 Epidemic AIDS-associated Kaposi's sarcoma. Note lesions on the hard palate.

belt with the above climatic conditions, namely Papua New Guinea. In these endemic regions BL accounts for more than 50% of childhood tumours.

The highest incidence of BL is in the West Nile district of Uganda, where the number recorded approaches 13/100 000 population. It is in the same area where time-space clustering has been recorded.[165] In most of the Westernized world, Type B, sporadic, non-endemic or American BL is a common childhood lymphoma, tending to present with bulky abdominal disease, centred on the ileo-caecal junction. A third variant of BL is immunodeficiency-associated BL, particularly occurring in association with AIDS, and tending to be node based. Variants include atypical or Burkitt-like lymphoma. This is the classification advocated by the WHO.[166] The clinical features of these non-endemic cases differ from those of the endemic forms (Table 35.4).

Aetiology

A cell line of endemic BL was established in which a hitherto unknown herpes virus was identified with electron microcopy by Epstein, Achong and Barr. This EBV virus bears two of their names.[167] EBV is known to transform human B lymphocytes in vitro; patients with BL have a significantly higher EBV serological response (viral capsid antigen, VCA; early antigen, EA; EB-determined nuclear antigen, EBNA) than controls and Burkitt's tumours carry footprints of the virus (EBV genome), detected either as EBV DNA or EBNA.[168] EBV infection, malaria, immunodeficiency and spontaneous mutation can all contribute to the origin of BL.[169]

It was originally thought that only B lymphocytes possessed the EBV receptor (CD21). However, there is now evidence that other cells, including oropharyngeal epithelium, and some T cell subsets, possess the appropriate epitopes.[170]

Two strains of EBV have been described. Type A, with a world wide distribution, and type B occurring mainly in tropical Africa and Papua New Guinea.

EBV is the major causative agent of infectious mononucleosis (human herpes virus type 6 or HHV-6 also can cause an identical syndrome). The epidemiology of EBV is complex. Based on VCA IgG titres, it appears that in Third World countries there is almost universal infection of young children, who exhibit a very high prevalence of IgG antibodies by 4 years of age. Infection of young children seems to be asymptomatic. Infectious mononucleosis is very rare in indigenous inhabitants of Africa. By contrast, in

Table 35.4 Comparison between endemic and sporadic Burkitt's lymphoma

Endemic	Sporadic
Related to climate	Unrelated to climate
Common in children	Common in children
>95% EBV associated	Less commonly EBV associated
Chromosomal translocation: invariable	Chromosomal translocation: invariable
Clinical features: Presents commonly with jaw tumour, nodal and marrow disease	Clinical features: Presents commonly with adominal mass. Nodal and marrow disease
Rare	Common

Western countries, the prevalence of infection is rare in young children, but infectious mononucleosis is common in adolescents and young adults.

EBV is strongly associated with the nasal form of angiocentric NK/T cell lymphoma, occurring in South-east Asia, especially Southern China and parts of South America, other forms of lymphoma, such as HIV-related and post-transplant large cell lymphoma, Hodgkin lymphoma, nasopharyngeal carcinoma and HIV-associated leiomyosarcoma.

The role of malaria in endemic BL may be to facilitate the development of lymphoma through either polyclonal B cell proliferation and/or T cell immunosuppression. Malaria prophylaxis was started in the North Mara province of Tanzania and this appeared to coincide with a downward trend. However, the curious geographical distribution of endemic BL in sub-Saharan Africa and in Papua New Guinea is best explained on the basis of malaria endemicity. In addition, studies in Uganda have suggested that other non-Burkitt, non-Hodgkin's lymphomas may also be related to malaria endemicity.[169,171]

Chromosomal abnormalities

Central to the evolution of BL, is amplification of the cellular oncogene, or so called proto-oncogene, c-myc, which is normally located on the long arm of chromosome 8 (8 q24). Manolov and Manolova first reported a characteristic chromosome abnormality in BL in 1972. Part of the long arm of chromosome 8 was translocated to the long arm of chromosome 14, i.e. t (8:14).[172] Some 90% of BL tumours have this translocation, which always involves the same bands of the two chromosomes, namely band q24 of chromosome 8 and band q32 of chromosome 14. The remaining 10% of BL tumours exhibited two variant translocations: a reciprocal translocation involving q24 of 8 with either band p11 of chromosome 2 or band q11 of chromosome 22, i.e. t (2:8), or t (8:22). These translocations were observed in all BL tumours irrespective of EBV genome status and whether they were endemic or non-endemic.

Tumour suppressor gene p53

The p53 gene is a recessive oncogene, also termed a tumour suppressor gene, or so-called anti-oncogene. It is located on the short arm of chromosome 17 (17p13), and is inactivated by deletion and/or point mutation in most solid tumours.[173] The p53 gene encodes for a 53 kilo dalton (kD) nuclear phosphoprotein involved in negative regulation of cell proliferation by promoting apoptotic cell death. The abnormal, inactive, overexpressed, mutant form in cancers has a long half-life, and unlike the native form, with a short half-life, may be detected immunohistochemically. The role of p53 in tumours has been reviewed.[174] In endemic and sporadic BL as well as L$_3$ ALL (Burkitt's acute lymphoblastic leukaemia) p53 mutation has been identified in the great majority of cases.[175]

Although p53 mutation is associated with features of poor prognosis, e.g. large tumour burden, low response to intensive chemotherapy and short survival in other haematological malignancies, notably acute myeloid leukaemia and myelodysplastic syndrome, this does not seem to be the case with either BL or L$_3$ALL.[176]

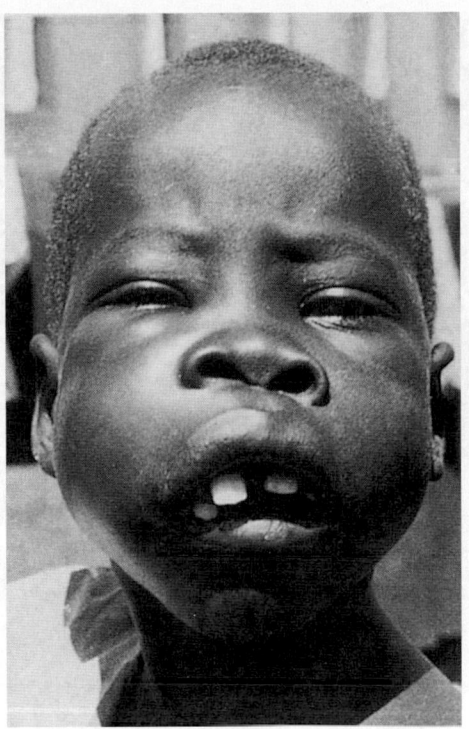

Figure 35.9 Burkitt's lymphoma. Jaw tumour.

Clinical features

Endemic BL presents usually with jaw swelling (75%), abdominal swelling (60%) and central nervous system involvement (30%). Patients with jaw swellings generally present with maxillary involvement more commonly than mandibular tumour. Maxillary tumours often spread upwards to involve the orbit (Figure 35.9). Bilateral maxillary tumour is common. Bilateral mandibular disease is rare unless all four quadrants are involved. Patients present complaining of loose teeth, and a lateral oblique radiograph of the jaw reveals loss of lamina dura. Abdominal swelling is a presenting feature in about 60% of patients, usually more so in females than in males. Almost any organ within the abdomen can and does get involved in the tumorous process and often malignant ascites is an accompanying feature. Central nervous system involvement is seen in about 30% of patients at presentation. This may be either as cranial nerve palsy (III, VI, VII commonly) or paraplegia or just malignant CSF pleocytosis alone. The peak age at presentation is 4–9 years. The tumour is unseen below 1 year, <1% under 2 years and peaks from 4 to 9 years, and then falls off such that <5% of patients are over 15 years of age.

The diagnosis of BL is often evident because of the clinical presentation in a child from an endemic area. However, histological confirmation must always be sought as other tumours, notably embryonal rhabdomyosarcoma, neuroblastoma, lymphoblastic lymphoma and Wilms' tumour, may all mimic BL. Histologically the classical 'starry sky' picture (Figure 35.10) is suggestive of BL and is due to the presence of large numbers of phagocytic macrophages among tumour cells.

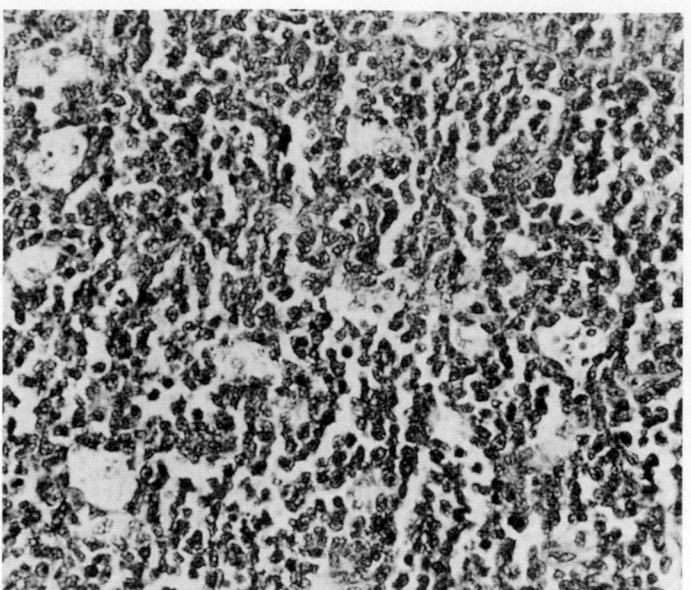

Figure 35.10 Burkitt's lymphoma. 'Starry sky' picture.

Staging

The staging system recommended by WHO for BL is based on the Murphy system.[166]

Cell kinetics

BL is a very rapidly growing tumour. It is the fastest-growing tumour in man and has been referred to as the human equivalent of the L1210 mouse model. It has a growth fraction of 100%, mean cell cycle time of 26 h and observed volume doubling time of 2.8 days. The cellular proliferation index, as assessed immuno-histologically by Ki 67 (Mib 1) immunostaining, approaches 100%.[166] This is histologically helpful in distinguishing BL from other high-grade non-Hodgkin lymphomas.[166]

Management

Because of the peculiar cell kinetics, BL is extremely responsive to drug therapy and is one of the early tumours noted to be curable by drugs alone. However, the management of this tumour requires a multidisciplinary approach. The role of surgery includes biopsy for diagnosis, spinal cord decompression and insertion of an Ommaya reservoir, but, most importantly, debulking. BL is one of the tumours where debulk surgery has been clearly shown to be beneficial.[177] An attempt should be made by the surgeon to remove as much tumour (>90%) as possible. In case of bilateral ovarian involvement, this means bilateral oophorectomy. Patients who have had >90% of their tumour taken out surgically have a survival advantage equal to those with early stage I or A disease. If the surgeon cannot remove sufficient tumour, removal of less tumour does not influence prognosis. BL is a radiosensitive tumour but because of its peculiar rapid growth conventional radiother-apy is ineffective as the tumour regrows between each day's

therapy. This problem is circumvented by superfractionation of each day's dose of irradiation into three treatments given 4 h apart. Such an approach is not practical in a busy radiotherapy department. However, prophylactic craniospinal irradiation failed to show any value in preventing or delaying central nervous system relapse.[178]

The treatment of choice for BL is chemotherapy. The single most effective agent is cyclophosphamide. Although single-agent cyclophosphamide is as effective as a three-drug combination consisting of cyclophosphamide, vincristine and methotrexate (COM), the combination is superior in preventing systemic relapse.[179] All in all about 80% of patients achieve complete tumour regression, 10% partial response. About 50% will relapse: those who relapse early, within 3 months, do poorly, while those who relapse late, after 3 months, respond well even to initial induction agents.[180] Patients remaining relapse-free after 1 year can be considered cured and the overall relapse-free survival at 10 years is 35–50%.[181]

Prevention

Epstein et al.[182] developed an EBV vaccine using the high molecu-lar weight glycoprotein component of EBV membrane antigen. This vaccine conferred 100% protection against a lymphomagenic dose of EBV in the cotton-top tamarind (a South American mar-moset). Further developments will hopefully yield safe vaccines capable of preventing infectious mononucleosis, and then BL and nasopharyngeal carcinoma[183] (vide infra). These may have a potential therapeutic role.[193]

NASOPHARYNGEAL CARCINOMA

Incidence and geographical distribution

Nasopharyngeal carcinoma (NPC) is an uncommon tumour in the white populations of Europe and North America, with an ASR of 1/100 000 population, but has long been recognized as an important problem in parts of the Far East, particularly southern China. In regions which have a high incidence the tumours are poorly differentiated, non-keratinizing squamous cell carcinomas and often show a heavy infiltration with lymphocytes and other inflammatory cells. This feature gave rise to the old term 'lympho-epithelioma'. These tumours appear to be aetiologically distinct from the well-differentiated squamous cell carcinomas that may occur anywhere in old people. The highest incidence rates are found in the southern provinces of China, particularly around Guandong, and in Hong Kong and Singapore, where rates of between 12 and 26/100 000 are recorded. There is also a high incidence in the Chinese population of Malaysia, Thailand, Indo-nesia and Hawaii. NPC is some 20 times more common in the Chinese population of Malaysia than in Indians living there. The incidence of NPC in South-east Asia is directly related to the degree of inbreeding within the immigrant populations from southern China.

Regions of intermediate frequency (from 1.5 to 9/100 000 a year) are found in several parts of Africa; these include the high-land areas of Kenya, and parts of the Sudan, Tunisia, Morocco and Algeria. In some of these countries the age distribution of the

Table 35.5 World Health Organization classification of nasopharyngeal carcinoma and EBV antibodies

Classification	EBV ANTIBODIES	
	IgG EA (%)	IgA VCA (%)
Type I Keratinizing squamous cell	35	16
Type II Non-keratinizing squamous cell	94	84
Type III Undifferentiated carcinoma	83	89

tumour shows two peaks, with the first occurring between 10 and 20 years.

Aetiology

The high incidence of NPC in peoples of southern Chinese descent who live in different environments, often contrasting with a low incidence in neighbouring ethnic groups, is suggestive of a genetic factor. HLA-typing has shown that Cantonese Chinese with A2, B17, BW46 haplotypes have an increased risk of developing NPC.

Epstein–Barr virus

Clinical disorders associated with EBV, as previously stated, include infectious mononucleosis, endemic BL and NPC, among other conditions. In infectious mononucleosis both IgG and IgM antibodies directed at the VCA are detected. Nuclear antigen antibodies are absent as these develop 2–6 months after initial infection. The relationship between NPC and EBV was postulated on the basis of the finding of antibodies to EBV in the serum and the identification of viral genomes by in situ hybridization of epithelial tumour cells.[184] In NPC IgG specific to EBV EA is often present as well as the IgA directed against VCA. These antibodies precede the appearance of the tumour and serve as a prognostic indicator of remission and relapse. Recently, plasma EBV DNA monitoring has been suggested as a tumour marker.[185] There is a correlation with the histological classification (Table 35.5), with the keratinizing squamous cell type (type I) having a much lower incidence of positive antibodies than the non-keratinizing or undifferentiated types.

EBV receptors have been demonstrated on, and virus binding to, the surface of oropharyngeal epithelial cells. Regardless of whether a patient with NPC lives in an area of endemic or sporadic incidence, the tumours contain EBV DNA.[186] Preinvasive lesions of NPC, including dysplasia and carcinoma in situ, are infected with EBV. The EBV is clonal, indicating that the lesions represent a focal cellular growth, which arose from a single cell infected with EBV. EBV infection appears to be an early and possibly an initiating event in the pathogenesis of NPC. The detection of EBV-transforming gene in all the neoplastic cells suggests that its expression is essential for the preinvasive epithelial proliferation associated with NPC.[187]

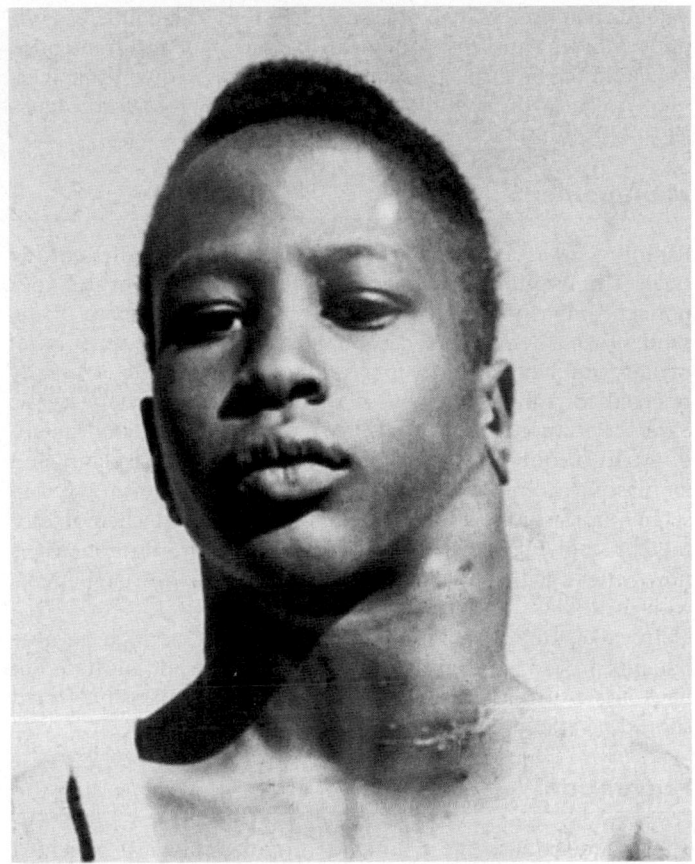

Figure 35.11 Nasopharyngeal carcinoma with massive cervical lymphadenopathy. (Courtesy of M. A. O. Malik.)

Dietary factors

It has been observed that ethnic differences in similar geographical regions (e.g. southern China) are associated with marked variations in the frequency of NPC and that these differences may be related to dietary habits. Evidence of the causative role of salted fish, especially if it is consumed early in life, has been postulated. Relatively high levels of nitrosamines have been identified in Cantonese salted fish and extracts have been shown to activate EBV in Raji cells (a BL cell line) in vitro.[188]

Clinical features

The diagnosis of NPC is often difficult because the nasopharynx is hard to visualize and the primary lesion tends to infiltrate submucosally and can easily be missed in a superficial biopsy.

Many cases of NPC are diagnosed late or remain undiagnosed until they present with clinical nodes without an obvious primary site.[189,190] The majority of patients seen with NPC in East Africa present with enlarged, often massive, cervical lymph nodes which may be mistaken for tuberculosis or malignant lymphoma (Figure 35.11). In some instances lymphadenopathy is a late phenomenon and such patients have, in addition, multiple cranial nerve palsies and pain due to tumour extension through the base of the skull. A small percentage (about 5%) present only with cranial nerve palsies. Because of the location of the primary tumour patients may present with blockage of the Eustachian tube, causing otitis media. Thus any adult with persistent or recurrent otitis media should be suspected of having NPC. Less frequently patients may present with nasal blockage or epistaxis. Serological diagnosis of NPC is proving promising.[191,192]

Management

Radiotherapy is the primary treatment of NPC regardless of the stage. The recommended dose is 6500–7000 cGy delivered to a port encompassing the nasopharynx as well as the base of the skull. Often a boost to the nasopharynx is considered, using intracavitary implants. Surgery plays a limited role and is usually reserved for salvage therapy of residual cervical nodal disease. Several cytotoxic agents show activity in NPC. These include methotrexate, bleomycin, 5-fluorouracil, doxorubicin, cisplatin and vinblastine. Combination chemotherapy has often been given in sequential fashion with radiotherapy. Concurrent chemoradiotherapy applying radiosensitizers, cisplatin and 5-fluorouracil is now better established, in the management of non-Asian patients with the disease.

In most tropical areas, mortality from NPC is high because patients present at a very advanced disease stage and most do not have access to radiotherapy facilities. Whenever possible, focus should be placed on prevention.

Prevention

Mirror and endoscopic examination, and serological screening should be considered for high-risk populations.

Prevention should also focus on dietary education. The prospect for vaccination is in sight. It has been suggested that a combined vaccine to both EBV associated Hodgkin's disease and nasopharyngeal carcinoma may be the path to follow, as prevention of Hodgkin's lymphoma will have more commercial appeal.[192] Duraiswamy and colleagues have developed an experimental polyepitope vaccine for EBV-associated Hodgkin's lymphoma, and nasopharyngeal carcinoma.[193]

ORAL AND OROPHARYNGEAL CARCINOMA

Incidence and geographical distribution

Mouth cancer is the most common cancer in South-east Asia, home to one-fifth of the world's population. Squamous cell carcinoma of the mucosa of the oral cavity and oropharynx is a tumour whose incidence is closely related to particular cultural habits. There is a high incidence in most of the populations of the Indian subcontinent and in peoples of Indian extraction living in other countries of the Far East, such as Singapore, Sri Lanka, Thailand and Vietnam. These types of cancer account for nearly 50% of cancer patients registered at the Tata Memorial Hospital in Bombay, and incidence rates of over 20/100 000 have been recorded in some districts of India. In Malaysia, these tumours account for 30% of all malignancies, and in Sri Lanka and India, approximately 35–40% of all cancers occur in the oral cavity, compared with only 2–3% in the UK and USA.

Aetiology

A high incidence of oropharyngeal tumour is related to the cultural practice of chewing betel quid and, less frequently, to smoking locally made cheroots called bidi. Betel quid consists of the young leaf of betel vine (Piper betel) mixed with slices of areca nut and varying quantities of slaked lime. Tobacco and spices are often added to this mixture. The resultant quid is held for long periods of time in the buccal sulcus. The development of squamous cell carcinoma is usually preceded by the development of precancerous leucoplastic changes in the oral epithelium. A high alcohol intake, vitamin A deficiency, dental caries and sepsis may be contributory factors in some patients. There is conflicting evidence as to the relative roles of tobacco and other constituents of the quid in the development of cancer.

Prevention and management

Oral pre-cancer and cancer meet the essential requirements of a screening programme. Up to 15 years may elapse before lesions in the mouth turn cancerous. Various studies in India have indicated a high prevalence of oral premalignant lesions. These are leukoplakia and oral submucous fibrosis. If these lesions, which are the first signs of danger, are detected in sufficient time for treatment, the disease is curable through surgery and radiotherapy. Unfortunately, most patients seek medical attention only when they are in pain, which is a late symptom, and therefore too late for any therapy but pain relief.

In a study using primary healthcare workers in Sri Lanka, it was demonstrated that the pre-cancerous lesions can be detected by this category of workers.[196] This approach has been found to be reliable and pragmatic, and since these primary healthcare workers outnumber dentists by a ratio of 10:1, they may give a lead on how to approach other cancers in remote populous tropical environments. Any improvement in general nutrition, particularly an adequate intake of vitamins, trace elements and animal protein, is likely to reduce the incidence in high-risk populations. Reduction of alcohol intake, and particularly tobacco consumption, should also be encouraged. Novel agents to target various growth factor receptor kinases, tyrosine kinase and serine/threonine kinase, which are major components of cell signalling pathways offer promise. Imatinib (Glivec), is the prime example of a drug of this class. Newer agents to treat oral cancer include ZD 1839 (Iressa), and erlotinib (Tarceva). Soulieres and colleagues report prolonged disease stabilization in a large group of patients with advanced head and neck cancer, treated with erlotinib.[194] Evaluation and staging of oral cancer has been suggested by Broumand and colleagues.[195] Preventative strategies are outlined by Kuriakose and Sharan.[196]

CARCINOMA OF THE URINARY BLADDER

Incidence and geographical distribution

Bladder cancer is the sixth most common form of cancer in the developed world (see Table 35.1), with an age-standardized rate of approximately 25/100 000. The majority of tumours are transitional cell carcinoma (TCC) in histological type and over 75% occur in elderly men. Within most of the tropics the rates are low for TCC, but in parts of east, central and southern Africa, Egypt and the Sudan and some regions of the Middle East rates are high for bladder cancer, of predominantly squamous cell carcinoma (SCC) type. In Bulawayo, Zimbabwe, for example, they are 17.9 and 9.5/100 000 in men and women, respectively[101].

Aetiology

The geographical distribution of high-incidence bladder cancer in the tropics parallels that of *Schistosoma haematobium* infection, an association that was first noted by Fergusson in Egypt in 1911. The aetiology, and natural history of squamous cell carcinoma of the urinary bladder has been reviewed by El Sebaie et al.[197] A clinicopathologic analysis of a large series of bladder squamous cell carcinoma has been reported by Lagwinski et al.[198] Estimated incidence rates in different districts and regions of east and central Africa show a close relationship between the prevalence and intensity of *S. haematobium* infection and high rates of bladder cancer.[3]

The mechanisms of carcinogenesis are uncertain. Heavy, chronic infection with *S. haematobium* leads to inflammation, fibrosis and calcification of the bladder with impairment of function and inadequate emptying. This predisposes to recurrent, mixed bacterial infections. In such patients, carcinogenic nitrosamines, which are formed from excreted nitrates, and nitrites have been detected.[199] It is thought that these substances acting on hyperplastic and metaplastic epithelium give rise to the characteristic squamous cell carcinomas. Lozano has demonstrated amplification of DNA *Schistosoma*-specific gene copy number by gene profiling, associated with bladder SCC in contrast to TCC.[200]

Human papilloma virus (HPV) infection has been suggested as being a co-player in vesical SCC, but a study from Egypt refutes this.[201]

Clinical features

Schistosomal bladder cancer occurs mostly in young individuals. It is commonly a well-differentiated squamous cell carcinoma and has less tendency to spread via the bloodstream and lymphatics. The mean age at presentation is about 45 years and in Egypt about 75% of the victims are under 50 years of age. It is rarely observed in the under-20 age group. This is in contradiction to non-schistosomal bladder cancer, where the mean age is about 65 years and <10% are under 50 years of age. The male to female ratio for schistosomal bladder cancer is 4–5 : 1. The male preponderance may be related to increased male exposure to schistosomal infection. Unfortunately the cardinal early sign of bladder cancer (painless terminal haematuria) is often ignored in schistosomal endemic areas as most of the populace will have had haematuria since childhood. For this and other reasons, the great majority of the cases present very late with symptoms of cystitis and obstructive uropathy. A plain radiograph of the abdomen may reveal a calcified outline of the urinary bladder. Cystoscopy and biopsy establishes the diagnosis. In centres such as the Cairo Cancer Institute, where investigators are experienced, urine cytology provides a fairly accurate diagnosis. Biopsy is still necessary to confirm the diagnosis, although 'aggressive biopsy' to determine the depth of tumour muscle invasion may cause perforation because of the advanced nature of most cases. Pre-staging work-up should include history and physical examination, urinalysis for cytology, and urine examination, to identify schistosomal eggs and malignant cells, and a plain radiograph of the abdomen. Urography should be followed by bimanual examination under anaesthesia. Cystoscopy and biopsy are essential. The currently recommended staging system is the TNM staging advocated by the International Union Against Cancer (UICC), for bladder cancer, including squamous cell carcinoma. This is a modification of the Jewiit Strong Marshall scheme.

Management

Radical surgery is the only curative treatment modality. However, radical cystectomy is associated with postoperative morbidity and mortality as high as 15–30% in some series. Adjuvant radiotherapy has been used postoperatively to prevent or delay recurrence. Radiotherapy as the sole treatment modality has been disappointing. This may be due to the massive tumour bulk associated with fibrosis and bacterial infection. Effective single cytotoxic agents include cisplatin, bleomycin, gemcitabine and methotrexate. The efficacy of combination chemotherapy or concurrent chemoradiotherapy has yet to be demonstrated. Unfortunately, most studies are patients with transitional cell carcinoma and the results cannot be extrapolated to include squamous cell carcinomas.

Prevention

The prevention of bladder cancer in those regions where schistosomiasis is endemic is dependent on effective schistosomal control. There is a minimum of 20 years lag period between infection and the development of bladder cancer. Schistosomal bladder cancer should therefore be amenable to screening. Screening has been advocated for high-risk populations in Egypt. Before such a practice is embarked upon on a wide scale, its cost-effectiveness needs to be carefully evaluated.

REFERENCES

1. Mills A. Cancer in the tropics and tropical cancers: an overview. *Ann Australasian College Trop Med* 2007; 2007:4–11.
2. Parkin DM, Bray F, Ferlay J, et al. Global cancer statistics, 2002. *CA Cancer J Clin* 2005; 55:74–108.
3. Parkin DM, Vizcaino AP, Skinner ME, et al. Cancer patterns and risk factors in the African population of southwestern Zimbabwe, 1963–1977. *Canc Epidemiol Biomarkers Prev* 1994; 3:537–547.
4. Bailey BJ. Tobaccoism is the disease–cancer is the sequela (editorial). *JAMA* 1986; 255:1923.
5. Anon. Editorial. Implementation of tobacco control policies proves hard. *Lancet* 2007; 369:2133.
6. Gul U, Kilic A, Gonul M, et al. Xeroderma pigmentosum: a Turkish case series. *Int J Dermatol* 2007; 46:1125–1128.
7. Friedberg EC, Wood RD. New insights into the combined Cockayne/xeroderma pigmentosum complex: human XPG protein can function in transcription factor stability. *Mol Cell* 2007; 27:162–164.

8. Miki Y, Swensen J, Shattuck-Eidens D, et al. A strong candidate for the breast and ovarian cancer susceptibility gene BRCA1. *Science* 1994; 266:66–71.

9. Ford D, Easton DF, Bishop DT, et al. Risk of cancer in BRCA1-mutation carriers. *Lancet* 1994; 343:692–695.

10. Wooster R, Bignell G, Lancaster J, et al. Identification of the breast cancer susceptibility gene BRCA2. *Nature* 1995; 378:789–792.

11. Goldstein NS. The gray area between hereditable and cancer somatic (tumor phenotype) molecular genetic testing of colorectal adenocarcinoma. *Am J Clin Pathol* 2006; 125:813–814.

12. Grave GF, Mills AE. Clinico-pathological study of thyroid diseased patients admitted to Mpilo Hospital. *Cent Afr J Med* 1980; 26:251–253.

13. Chang MH, Chen TH, Hsu HM, et al. Prevention of hepatocellular carcinoma by universal vaccination against hepatitis B virus: the effect and problems. *Clin Cancer Res* 2005; 11:7953–7957.

14. Silverberg MJ, Abrams DI. AIDS defining and non-AIDS defining malignancies: cancer occurrence in the antiretroviral therapy era. *Cur Opin Oncol* 2007; 19:446–451.

15. Tulvatana W, Bhattarakosal, Sansopha L, et al. Risk factors for conjunctival squamous cell neoplasia: a matched case control study. *Br J Ophthalmol* 2003; 87:396–398.

16. Newton R. A review of the aetiology of squamous cell carcinoma of the conjunctiva. *Br J Cancer* 1996; 74:1511–1513.

17. Deyrup AT, Lee VK, Hill CE, et al. Epstein Barr virus associated smooth muscle tumors are distinctive mesenchymal tumors reflecting multiple infection events: a clinicopathologic and molecular analysis of 29 tumors from 19 patients. *Am J Surg Pathol* 2006; 30:75–82.

18. Newell ME, Hoy JF, Cooper SG, et al. Human immunodeficiency virus-related primary central nervous system lymphoma: factors influencing survival in 111 patients. *Cancer* 2004; 100:2627–2636.

19. Kumari P, Schechter GP, Saini N, et al. Successful treatment of human immunodeficiency virus related Castleman's disease with interferon alpha. *Clin Infect Dis* 2000; 31:602–604.

20. Ferrazzo KL, Mesquita RA, Aburad AT, et al. EBV detection in HIV-related oral plasmablastic lymphoma. *Oral Dis* 2007; 13:564–569.

21. Aozasa K. Pyothorax associated lymphoma. *J Clin Hematop* 2006; 46:5–10.

22. Brimo F, Michel RP, Khetani K, et al. Primary effusion lymphoma: a series of 4 cases and review of the literature with emphasis on cytomorphologic and immunocytochemical differential diagnosis. *Cancer* 2007; 111:224–233.

23. Yang BH, Bray FI, Parkin DM, et al. Cervical cancer as a priority for prevention in different world regions: an evaluation using years of life lost. *Int J Cancer* 2004; 109:418–424.

24. Kamau RK, Osoti AO, Njuguna EM. Effect of diagnosis and treatment of inoperable cervical cancer on quality of life among women receiving radiotherapy at Kenyatta National Hospital. *East Afr Med J* 2007; 84:24–30.

25. Feyi-Wabosa P, Kamanu C, Aluka C. Awareness and risk factors for cervical cancer among women in Aba, south eastern Nigeria. *Trop J Obstet Gynaecol* 2005; 22:25–26.

26. Moscicki AB. HPV infections in adolescents. *Dis Markers* 2007; 23:229–234.

27. Brinton LA, Hamman RF, Huggins GR, et al. Sexual and reproductive risk factors for invasive cervical cell cancer. *J Natl Cancer Inst* 1987; 79:23–30.

28. Adami HO, Trichopoulos D. Cervical cancer and the elusive male factor. *Comment in N Engl J Med* 2002; 346:1160–1161.

29. Castellsague X, Bosch FX, Munoz N, et al. Male circumcision, penile human papilloma infection, and cervical cancer in female partners. *N Engl J Med* 2002; 346:1105–1112.

30. Appleby P, Beral V, Berrington de Gonzalez A, et al. Carcinoma of the cervix and tobacco smoking: collaborative reanalysis of individual data on 13,541 women with carcinoma of the cervix and 23,017 without carcinoma of the cervix from 23 epidemiological studies. *Int J Cancer* 2006; 118: 1481–1494.

31. Odida M, Schmauz R, Lwanga S. Grade of malignancy of cervical cancer in regions of Uganda, with varying malarial endemicity. *Int J Cancer* 2002; 99:737–741.

32. Piper JM. Oral contraceptives and cervical cancer. *Gynecol Oncol* 1985; 22:1–14.

33. Yach D, Townsend GS. Smoking and health in South Africa. *S Afr Med J* 1988; 73:391–399.

34. Halpert R, Fruchter RG, Sedlis A, et al. Human papillomavirus and lower genital neoplasia in renal transplant patients. *Obstet Gynecol* 1986; 68:251–258.

35. Katz RL, Veanattukalathil S, Weiss KM. Human papilloma infection and neoplasia of the cervix and anogenital region in women with Hodgkin's disease. *Acta Cytol* 1983; 27:220–224.

36. Anonymous. Centers for Disease Control 1993 revised classification system for HIV-infections and expanded surveillance case definition for AIDS among adolescents and adults. *Morbid Mortal Wkly Rep* 1992; 41:1–19.

37. Zur Hausen H. Condylomata acuminata and human genital cancer. *Cancer Res* 1976; 36:794.

38. Walboomers JM, Jacobs MV, Manos MM, et al. Human papillomavirus is a necessary cause of invasive cervical cancer worldwide. *Comment in J Pathol* 1999; 189:12–13.

39. Satish N, Abraham P, Peedicayil A, et al. Human Papilloma 16 E6/E7 transcript and E2 gene status in patients with cervical neoplasia. *Mol Diagn* 2004; 8:57–64.

40. Salcedo M, Taja L, Utrera D, et al. Changes in retinoblastoma gene expression during cervical cancer progression. *Int J Exp Pathol* 2002; 83:275–286.

41. Jeong Seo E, Jung Kim H, Jae Lee C, et al. The role of HPV oncoproteins and cellular factors in maintenance of hTERT expression in cervical carcinoma cells. *Gynecol Oncol* 2004; 94:40–47.

42. Ressler S, Scheiden R, Dreier K, et al. High risk human papillomavirus E7 oncoprotein detection in cervical squamous cell carcinoma. *Clin Cancer Res* 2007; 13:7067–7072.

43. Brodman M, Friedman F, Dottino P, et al. A comparative study of computerized tomography, magnetic resonance imaging and clinical staging for detection of early cervix cancer. *Gynecol Oncol* 1990; 36:409–412.

44. Runowicz CD. Molecular screening for cervical cancer. Time to give up Pap tests? *N Engl J Med* 2007; 357:1650–1653.

45. Irvin W, Evans SR, Andersen W, et al. The utility of HPV DNA triage in the management of cytological atypical glandular cells. *Am J Obstet Gynecol* 2005; 193:559–565.

46. Palma PD, Giorgi-Rossi P, Collina G, et al. The risk of false positive histology according to the reason for colposcopy referral in cervical screening: A blind revision of all histologic lesions found in the NTCC trial. *Am J Clin Pathol* 2008; 129:75–80.

47. Ekalaksananan T, Pientong C, Sriamporn S, et al. Usefulness of combined testing for p16 protein and human papillomavirus (HPV) in cervical carcinoma screening. *Gynecol Oncol* 2006; 103:62–66.

48. Franco EL. Commentary: Health inequity could increase in poor countries if universal HPV vaccination is not adopted. *BMJ* 2007; 335:378–379.

49. Kahn JA, Burk RD. Comment. Papillomavirus vaccines in perspective. *Lancet* 2007; 369:2135–2137.

50. Raffle AE. Challenges of implementing human papilloma (HPV) vaccination policy. *BMJ* 2007; 335:375–377.

51. Stanley M. Prophylactic HPV vaccines. *J Clin Pathol* 2007; 60:961–965.

52. Van Nagell JR Jr, Hanson MB, Donaldson ES, et al. Treatment of cervical intraepithelial neoplasma III by hysterectomy without intervening conization in patients with adequate colposcopy. *Cancer* 1985; 56:2737–2739.

53. Keys HM, Bundy BN, Stehman FB, et al. Cisplatin, radiation and adjuvant hysterectomy compared with radiation and adjuvant hysterectomy for bulky stage IB cervical carcinoma. *N Engl J Med* 1999; 340:1154–1161.

54. Rose PG, Bundy BN, Watkins EB, et al. Concurrent cisplatin-based radiotherapy and chemotherapy for locally advanced cervical cancer. *N Engl J Med* 1999; 340:1144–1153.

55. National Cancer Institute. Concurrent chemoradiation for cervical cancer. Clinical announcement, Washington DC, 22 February 1999.

56. Prates MD, Torres FO. A cancer survey in Lourenco Marques, Portuguese East Africa. *J Natl Cancer Inst* 1965; 35:729–757.

57. Mazzanti R, Gramantieri L, Bolondi L. Hepatocellular carcinoma: epidemiology and clinical aspects. *Mol Aspects Med* 2008; 29(1/2):130–143.

58. Ulcickas-Yood M, Quesenberry CP, Guo D, et al. Incidence of hepatocellular carcinoma among individuals with hepatitis B virus infection identified using an automated data algorithm. *J Viral Hepat* 2008; 15:28–36.

59. Jemal A, Siegel R, Ward E, et al. Cancer statistics, 2006. *CA Cancer J Clin* 2006; 56:106–130.

60. Beasley RP, Hwang LY, Lin CC, et al. Hepatocellular carcinoma and hepatitis B virus. *Lancet* 1981; ii:1129–1133.

61. Shafritz DA, Shouval D, Sherman NI, et al. Integration of hepatitis B virus DNA into the genome of liver cells in chronic liver disease and hepatocellular carcinoma. *N Engl J Med* 1981; 305:1067–1073.

62. Tibbs CJ. Hepatitis C. *Trans R Soc Trop Med Hyg* 1997; 91:107–120.

63. Tabor E, Kobayashi K. Hepatitis C virus, a causative infectious agent of non-A, non-B hepatitis: prevalence and structure. Summary of a conference of hepatitis C virus as a cause of hepatocellular carcinoma. *J Natl Cancer Inst* 1992; 84:86–90.

64. International Agency for Research on Cancer. Evaluation of carcinogenic risk of chemicals to man. *IARC Monogr* 1976; 10.

65. Newberne PM, Butler WH. Acute and chronic effects of aflatoxin on the liver of domestic and laboratory animals: a review. *Cancer Res* 1969; 29:230–235.

66. Carnaghan RBA. Hepatic tumours and chronic liver changes in rats following administration of aflatoxin. *Br J Cancer* 1967; 21:811–814.

67. Peers F, Bosch X, Kaldor J, et al. Aflatoxin exposure, hepatitis B virus infection and liver cancer in Swaziland. *Int J Cancer* 1987; 39:545–553.

68. Peers FG, Gilman GA, Linsell CA. Dietary aflatoxin and human liver cancer: a study in Swaziland. *Int J Cancer* 1976; 17:167–176.

69. Bulatao J, Almero EM, Castro Jardeleza Ma TR, et al. A case-control dietary study of primary liver cancer from aflatoxin exposure. *Int J Epidemiol* 1982; 11:112–119.

70. Linsell C. Aflatoxin and liver cancer. *Trans R Soc Trop Med Hyg* 1977; 7:471–473.

71. Campbell T, Hayes J. Role of aflatoxin metabolism in its toxic lesion. *Toxicol Appl Pharmacol* 1976; 35:195–222.

72. Lutwik L. Relations between aflatoxin, hepatitis B virus and hepatocellular carcinoma. *Lancet* 1979; i:755–757.

73. Coady A. The aflatoxin-hepatoma hepatitis B surface antigen story. *BMJ* 1975; 3:592–593.

74. Kew MC, Dibisceglie AM, Paterson A. Smoking as a risk-factor in hepatocellular carcinoma: a case-control study in Southern African blacks. *Cancer* 1985; 56:2315–2317.

75. Yu M C, Tong MJ. Non viral risk factors for hepatocellular carcinoma in low-risk population, the non-Asians of Los Angeles County, California. *J Natl Cancer Inst* 1991; 83:1820–1826.

76. Maynard EP, Sedikali F, Anthony PP, et al. Hepatitis-associated antigen and cirrhosis in Uganda. *Lancet* 1970; ii:1326–1328.

77. Wands J. Hepatocellular carcinoma and sex. *N Engl J Med* 2007; 357:1974–1976.

78. Gordeuk VR. African iron overload. *Semin Hematol* 2002; 39:263–269.

79. Kew MC, Kassianides C, Hodkinson J, et al. Hepatocellular carcinoma in urban born blacks: frequency and relation to hepatitis B virus infection. *BMJ* 1986; 293:1339–1341.

80. Attali P, Prod'homme S, Pelletier G, et al. Prognostic factors in patients with hepatocellular carcinoma. *Cancer* 1987; 59:2108–2111.

81. Sowl SH, Titelbaum DS, Gansler TS, et al. The fibrolamellar variant of hepatocellular carcinoma: its association with focal nodular hyperplasia. *Cancer* 1987; 60:3049–3055.

82. Van Tonder S, Kew MC, Hodkinson J, et al. Serum vitamin B_{12} binders in Southern African blacks with hepatocellular carcinoma. *Cancer* 1985; 56:789–792.

83. Vogel CL, Linsell CA. International symposium on hepatocellular carcinoma, Kampala, Uganda. *J Natl Cancer Inst* 1972; 48:567–571.

84. Primack A, Vogel CL, Kyalwazi SK, et al. A staging system for hepatocellular carcinoma: prognostic factors in Ugandan patients. *Cancer* 1975; 35:1357–1364.

85. Olweny CLM, Toya T, Katongole-Mbidde E, et al. Treatment of hepatocellular carcinoma with Adriamycin: preliminary communication. *Cancer* 1975; 36:1250–1257.

86. Chen M, Hwang T, Jeng L, et al. Surgical treatment for spontaneous rupture of hepatocellular carcinoma. *Surg Gynecol Obstet* 1988; 167:99–102.

87. Olweny CLM, Katongole-Mbidde E, Bahendeka S, et al. Further experience in treating patients with hepatocellular carcinoma in Uganda. *Cancer* 1980; 46:2717–2722.

88. Bezwoda WR, Weaving A, Kew M, et al. Combination chemotherapy of hepatocellular cancer. *Oncology* 1987; 44:207–209.

89. Olweny CLM, Johnson R. Rapid response to cisplatin and doxorubicin in hepatitis B virus reactivation. *J Gastroenterol Hepatol* 1987; 2:533–537.

90. de Villa V, Lo C M. Liver transplantation for hepatocellular carcinoma in Asia. *Oncologist* 2007; 12:1321–1331.

91. Prevention of hepatocellular carcinoma by immunization. *Bull World Health Organ* 1983; 61:731–744.

92. Whittle HC, Maine N, Pilkington J, et al. Long-term efficacy of continuing hepatitis B vaccination in infancy in two Gambian villages. *Lancet* 1995; 345:1089–1092.

93. Hughes NR, Pairojkul C, Royce SG, et al. Liver fluke associated and sporadic cholangiocarcinoma: an immunohistochemical study of bile duct, peribiliary gland and tumour cell phenotypes. *J Clin Pathol* 2006; 59:1073–1078.

94. Rohatgi PR, Swisher SG, Correa AM, et al. Comparison of clinical stage, therapy response and patient outcome between squamous cell carcinoma and adenocarcinoma of the esophagus. *Int J Gastrointest Cancer* 2005; 36:69–76.

95. Ford AC, Forman D, Dominic Reynolds P, et al. *Am J Epidemiol* 2005; 162:454–460.

96. Tu CH, Lee CT, Perng DS, et al. Esophageal adenocarcinoma arising from Barrett's epithelium in Taiwan. *J Formos Med Assoc* 2007; 106:664–668.

97. Iijima K, Koike T, Abe Y, et al. Extensive gastric atrophy: an increased risk factor for superficial esophageal squamous cell carcinoma in Japan. *Am J Gastroenterol* 2007; 102:1603–1609.

98. Takubo K, Aida J, Sawabe M, et al. Early squamous cell carcinoma of the oesophagus: the Japanese viewpoint. *Histopathology* 2007; 51:733–742.

99. Moodley R, Reddi A, Chetty R, et al. Abnormalities of chromosome 17 in oesophageal cancer. *J Clin Pathol* 2007; 60:990–994.

100. Vizcaino AP, Parkin DM, Skinner ME. Risk factors associated with oesophageal cancer in Bulawayo, Zimbabwe. *Br J Cancer* 1995; 72:769–773.

101. Vizcaino AP, Maxwell Parkin D, Boffetta P, et al. Bladder cancer: epidemiology and risk factors in Bulawayo, Zimbabwe. *Canc Causes Control* 1994; 5:517–512.

102. Munoz N, Wanrendorf J, Bang IJ, et al. No effect of riboflavin, retinol and zinc on prevalence of precancerous lesions of oesophagus. *Lancet* 1985; ii:111–114.

103. Yu I T, Tse LA, Wong TW, et al. Further evidence for a link between silica dust and esophageal cancer. *Int J Cancer* 2005; 114:479–483.

104. Flemen P, Lerut A, Van Cutsem E, et al. Utility of position emission tomography for the staging of patients with potentially operable oesophageal carcinoma. *J Clin Oncol* 2000; 18:3202–3210.

105. Ropp MB, Hawley D, Reising J, et al. Improved survival in squamous oesophageal cancer, preoperative chemotherapy and irradiation. *Arch Surg* 1986; 121:1330–1335.

106. Ellis FH, Maggs PR. Surgery for carcinoma of the lower oesophagus and cardia. *World J Surg* 1981; 5:527–533.

107. Orringer MB. Technical aids in performing transhiatal esophagectomy without thoracotomy. *Ann Thorac Surg* 1984; 38:128–132.

108. Hennessy TPJ. Choice of treatment in carcinoma of the oesophagus. *Br J Surg* 1988; 75:193–194.

109. Alexiou C, Khan OA, Black E, et al. Survival after esophageal resection for carcinoma: the importance of the histological cell type. *Ann Thorac Surg* 2006; 82:1073–1077.

110. Patel AN, Preskitt JT, Kuhn M, et al. Surgical management of esophageal carcinoma. *Proc (Bayl Univ Med Cent)* 2003; 16:280–284.

111. Rohatgi PR, Swisher SG, Correa AM, et al. Comparison of clinical stage, therapy response, and patient outcome between squamous cell carcinoma and adenocarcinoma of the esophagus. *Int J Gastrointest Cancer* 2005; 36: 69–76.

112. Earlam R, Cunha-Melo JR. Oesophageal squamous cell carcinoma: II. A critical review of radiotherapy. *Br J Surg* 1980; 67:457–461.

113. Launois B, Delarne D, Campion JP, et al. Preoperative radiotherapy for carcinoma of the oesophagus. *Surg Gynecol Obstet* 1981; 153: 690–692.

114. Kelsen D. Multimodality therapy of oesophageal carcinoma: still an experimental approach. *J Clin Oncol* 1987; 5:530–531.

115. Steiger Z, Franklin R, Wilson RF, et al. Complete eradication of squamous cell carcinoma of the oesophagus with combined chemoradiotherapy and radiotherapy. *Am J Surg* 1981; 47:95–98.

116. Leichman L, Steiger Z, Seydel HG, et al. Combined preoperative chemotherapy and radiation therapy for cancer of the oesophagus. *Semin Oncol* 1984; 11:178–185.

117. Poplon E, Fleming T, Leichman L, et al. Combined therapies for squamous cell carcinoma of the esophagus: a Southwest Oncology Group Study (SOGS-8037). *J Clin Oncol* 1987; 5:622–628.

118. Forastieve AA, Orringer MB, Perez-Tamayo C, et al. Concurrent chemotherapy and radiotherapy followed by transhiatal esophagectomy for local regional cancer of the oesophagus. *J Clin Oncol* 1990; 8:119–127.

119. Dewit L. Combined treatment of radiation and cisdiamine dichlonoplatinum (II): a review of experimental and clinical data. *Int J Radiat Oncol Biol Phys* 1987; 13:402–426.

120. Pfeffer MR, Teicher BA, Holder SA, et al. The interaction of cisplatin plus etoposide with radiation ± hyperthermia. *Int J Radiat Oncol Biol Phys* 1990; 19:1439–1447.

121. Walsh TN, Noonan N, Hollywood D, et al. A comparison of multimodal therapy and surgery for oesophageal adenocarcinoma. *N Engl J Med* 1996; 335:462–467.

122. Bossett GF, Gignoux M, Tribulet JP, et al. Chemoradiotherapy followed by surgery compared with surgery alone in squamous cell carcinoma of the oesophagus. *N Engl J Med* 1997; 337:161–167.

123. Cassarino DS, Derienzo DP, Barr RJ, et al. *J Cutan Pathol* 2006; 33(1/2): 191–206, 262–279.

124. Phan A, Touzet S, Dalle S, et al. Acral lentiginous melanoma: a clinicoprognostic study of 126 cases. *Brit J Dermatol* 2006; 155:561–569.

125. Vereecken P, Laporte M, Heenen M. Significance of cell kinetic parameters in the prognosis of malignant melanoma: a review. *J Cutan Pathol* 2007; 34:139–145.

126. Libberacht K, Husada G, Peeters T, et al. Initial staging of malignant melanoma by positron emission tomography and sentinel node biopsy. *Acta Chir Belg* 2005; 105:621–625.

127. Retsas S, Henry K, Mohammed MO, et al. Prognostic factors of cutaneous melanoma, and a new staging system proposed by the American Joint Committee on Cancer (AJCC). Validation in a cohort of 1284 patients. *Eur J Cancer* 2002; 38:511–516.

128. Page AJ, Carlson GW, Delman KA, et al. Prediction of nonsentinel lymph node involvement in patients with a positive sentinel node in malignant melanoma. *Am Surg* 2007; 73:674–678.

129. Balch CM, Soong S J, Bartolucci AA, et al. Efficacy of an elective regional node dissection of 1–4 mm thick melanomas for patients 60 years of age and younger. *Ann Surg* 1996; 224:255–266.

130. Gad D, Hoiland Carlsen PF, Bartram P, et al. Staging patients with cutaneous malignant melanoma by same-day lymphoscintigraphy and sentinel lymph node biopsy: a single institutional experience, with emphasis on recurrence. *J Surg Oncol* 2006; 94:94–100.

131. Kirkwood JM, Strawderman MH, Ernstoff MS, et al. Interferon alfa-2b adjuvant therapy of high-risk resected cutaneous melanoma. The Eastern Cooperative Oncology Group Trial EST 1684. *J Clin Oncol* 1996; 14:7–17.

132. Lee SM, Betticher DC, Thatcher N. Melanoma: chemotherapy. *Br Med Bull* 1995; 51:609–630.

133. Falkson CI, Falkson G, Falkson HE. Improved results with the addition of interferon alfa-2b to dacarbazine in the treatment of patients with metastatic malignant melanoma. *J Clin Oncol* 1991; 9:1403–1408.

134. Middleton MR, Grob JJ, Aaronson N, et al. Randomized phase III study of temozolomide versus dacarbazine in the treatment of patients with advanced metastatic malignant melanoma. *J Clin Oncol* 2000; 18:158–166.

135. Mills AE, Grave GF, Skinner MEG. *Kaposi Sarcoma in Childhood.* Sixth congress of the European Society of Pathology, London, September 1977, paper 338.

136. Harwood AR, Osoba P, Hostader SW, et al. Kaposi's sarcoma in recipients of renal transplants. *Am J Med* 1979; 67:759–765.

137. Du MQ, Bacon CM, Isaacson PG. Kaposi sarcoma-associated herpes virus/ human herpes virus 8 and lymphoproliferative disorders. *J Clin Pathol* 2007; 60:1350–1357.

138. Simonart T. Role of environmental factors in the pathogenesis of classic and African endemic Kaposi sarcoma. *Cancer Lett* 2006; 28:1–7.

139. Brown EE, Whitby D, Vitale F, et al. Virologic, hematologic and immunological risk factors for classic Kaposi sarcoma. *Cancer* 2006; 107:2282–2290.

140. Guttman-Yassky E, Dubnov E, Kra-Oz Z, et al. Classic Kaposi sarcoma. Which KSHV-seropositive individuals are at risk? *Cancer* 2006; 106:413–419.

141. Hbid O, Belloul L, Fajali N, et al. Kaposi sarcoma in Morocco: a pathological study with immunostaining for human herpesvirus-8 LNA-1. *Pathology* 2005; 37:288–295.

142. Ramos de Silva S, Elgui de Oliveira D, Borges L, Bacchi CE. Kaposi sarcoma associated herpes virus infection and Kaposi sarcoma in Brazil. *Braz J Med Biol Res* 2006; 39:573–580.

143. Deloose ST, Smit LA, Pals FT, et al. High incidence of Kaposi sarcoma associated herpesvirus infection in HIV related solid immunoblastic/ plasmablastic diffuse large cell lymphoma. *Leukemia* 2005; 19:851–855.

144. Viejo-Borbolla A, Schulz TF. Kaposi's sarcoma associated herpes virus (KSHV/ HHV8): key aspects of epidemiology and pathogenesis. *AIDS Rev* 2003; 5:222–229.

145. Shulz TF. The pleiotropic effects of Kaposi's sarcoma herpes virus. *J Pathol* 2006; 208:187–198.

146. Pauk J, Huang ML, Brodie SJ, et al. Mucosal shedding of human herpes virus 8 in men. *N Engl J Med* 2000; 343:1369–1377.

147. Reeve PA. HIV infection in patients admitted to a general hospital in Malawi. *BMJ* 1989; 298:1567–1568.

148. Lucas SB, De Cock KM, Hounnou A, et al. Contribution of tuberculosis to slim disease in Africa. *BMJ* 1994; 308:1531–1533.

149. Olweny CLM, Kaddu-Mukasa A, Atine I, et al. Childhood Kaposi's sarcoma: clinical features and therapy. *Br J Cancer* 1976; 33:555–560.

150. Grore JH. Kaposi's disease: report of an unusual case. *Radiology* 1955; 65:236–239.

151. Coetzee T, LeRoux CGJ. Kaposi's sarcoma presentation with intestinal obstruction. *S Afr Med J* 1967; 41:442–445.

152. Mitchell N, Feder A. Kaposi's sarcoma with secondary involvement of the jejunum, perforation and peritonitis. *Ann Intern Med* 1949; 31:324–329.

153. Novis BH, King N, Banks N. Kaposi's sarcoma presenting with diarrhoea and protein-losing enteropathy. *Gastroenterology* 1974; 67:996.

154. Khorshid KA, Erzingatsian K, Watters DAK, et al. Intussusception due to Kaposi's sarcoma. *J R Coll Surg Edinb* 1987; 32:339–341.

155. Cook J. The clinical features of Kaposi's sarcoma in the East African Bantu. *Acta Un Int Cancer* 1962; 18:388–398.

156. Slavin G, Cameron H McD, Forbes C, et al. Kaposi's sarcoma in East African children: a report of 51 cases. *Pathology* 1970; 100:189–199.

157. Krigel RL, Laubenstein LJ, Muggia FM. Kaposi's sarcoma: a new staging classification. *Cancer Treat Rep* 1983; 67:531–534.

158. Mitsuyasu RT, Groopman JE. Biology and therapy of Kaposi's sarcoma. *Semin Oncol* 1984; 11:53–59.

159. Taylor J, Afrasiabi R, Fahey JL, et al. A prognostically significant classification of immune changes in AIDS with Kaposi's sarcoma. *Blood* 1986; 67:666–671.

160. Kyalwazi SK. Chemotherapy of Kaposi's sarcoma: experience with Trenimon. *East Afr Med J* 1968; 45:17–26.

161. Olweny CLM, Sikyewunda W, Otim D. Further experience with Razoxane (ICRF 159-NSC 129943) in treating Kaposi's sarcoma. *Oncology* 1980; 37:174–176.

162. Olweny CLM, Toya T, Katongole-Mbidde E, et al. Treatment of Kaposi's sarcoma combination of actinomycin-D, vincristine and imidazole carboxamide (NSC 45388): results of a randomized clinical trial. *Int J Cancer* 1974; 14:649–656.

163. Olweny C, Borok M, Gudza I, et al. Treatment of AIDS associated Kaposi sarcoma in Zimbabwe: results of a randomised quality of life focused clinical trial. *Int J Cancer* 2005; 113:632–639.

164. Burkitt DP. A sarcoma involving the jaws in African children. *Br J Surg* 1958; 197:218–223.

165. Pike MC, Williams EH, Wright D. Burkitt's tumour in the West Nile district of Uganda. *BMJ* 1967; ii:395–399.

166. Diebold J, Jaffe ES, Raphael M, et al. World Health Organization: Classification of Tumours. Pathology and Genetics of tumours of Haematopoietic and Lymphoid Tissues. 2001; *Burkitt Lymphoma*, 181–184.

167. Epstein MA, Achong BG, Barr YM. Virus particles in cultured lymphoblasts from Burkitt's lymphoma. *Lancet* 1964; i:702–703.

168. Nonoyama M, Ragano JS. Homology between Epstein–Barr virus DNA and viral-DNA from Burkitt's lymphoma and nasopharyngeal carcinoma determined by DNA-DNA reassociation kinetics. *Nature* 1973; 242:44–47.

169. Brady G, MacArthur GJ, Farrell PJ. Epstein–Barr virus and Burkitt lymphoma. *J Clin Pathol* 2007; 60:1397–1402.

170. Birkenbach M, Tong X, Bradbury LE, et al. Characterization of an Epstein–Barr virus receptor on human epithelial cells. *J Exp Med* 1992; 178:1405–1414.

171. Schmauz R, Mugerwa JW, Wright DH. The distribution on non-Burkitt, non-Hodgkin's lymphomas in Uganda in relation to malaria endemicity. *Int J Cancer* 1990; 45:650–653.

172. Zech L, Haglund U, Nilsson K, et al. Characteristic chromosomal abnormalities in biopsies and lymphoid cell lines from patients with Burkitt and non-Burkitt lymphomas. *Int J Cancer* 1976; 17:47–56.

173. He X, He L, Hannon GJ. The guardian's little helper: micro RNAs in the p53 tumor suppressor network. *Cancer Res* 2007; 67:11099–11101.

174. Beuter M, Gasser M, Lebedeva T, et al. Influence of p53 on anti-tumour immunity. *Int J Oncol* 2006; 28:519–525.

175. Nagai J, Kigasawa H, Koga N, et al. Clinical significance of detecting p 53 protein in Burkitt lymphoma and B cell acute lymphoblastic leukemia using immunocytochemistry. *Leuk Lymphoma* 1998; 28:591–597.

176. Preudhomme C, Dervite I, Wattel E, et al. Clinical significance of p53 mutations in newly diagnosed Burkitt's lymphoma and acute lymphoblastic leukemia: A report of 48 cases. *J Clin Oncol* 1995; 13:812–820.

177. Magrath IT, Lwanga S, Carswell W, et al. Surgical reduction of tumour bulk in the management of abdominal Burkitt's lymphoma. *BMJ* 1974; ii:308–312.

178. Olweny CLM, Atine I, Kaddu-Mukasa A, et al. Cerebrospinal irradiation of Burkitt's lymphoma: failure in preventing central nervous system relapse. *Acta Radiol Ther Phys Biol* 1977; 16:225–231.

179. Olweny CLM, Katongole-Mbidde E, Kaddu-Mukasa A, et al. Treatment of Burkitt's lymphoma: randomized clinical trial of single versus combination chemotherapy. *Int J Cancer* 1976; 17:436–440.

180. Ziegler JL, Bluming AZ, Fass L, et al. Relapse patterns in Burkitt's lymphoma. *Cancer Res* 1972; 32:1267–1272.

181. Olweny CLM, Katongole-Mbidde E, Otim D, et al. Long-term experience with Burkitt's lymphoma in Uganda. *Int J Cancer* 1980; 26:261–266.

182. Epstein MA. Vaccination against Epstein–Barr virus: current progress and future strategies. *Lancet* 1986; i:1425–1427.

183. Taylor GS, Haigh TA, Gudgeon NH, et al. Dual stimulation of Epstein-Barr Virus (EBV) specific CD4+- and CD8 +-T cell responses by a chimeric antigen construct: potential therapeutic vaccine for EBV positive nasopharyngeal carcinoma. *J Virol* 2004; 78:768–778.

184. Wolf H, zur Hausen H, Becker V. Epstein–Barr virus genomes in epithelial nasopharyngeal cancer cells. *Nature (New Biol)* 1973; 244:245–247.

185. Ozyar E, Gultekin M, Alp A, et al. Use of plasma Epstein–Barr virus DNA monitoring as a tumor marker in follow up of patients with nasopharyngeal carcinoma preliminary results and reports of two cases. *Int J Biol Markers* 2007; 22:194–199.

186. Desgranges C, Wolf H, De-Thé G, et al. Nasopharyngeal carcinoma: presence of Epstein–Barr genomes in separated epithelial cells of tumours in patients from Singapore, Tunisia and Kenya. *Int J Cancer* 1975; 16:7–15.

187. Rathmanathan R, Prasad U, Sadler R, et al. Clonal proliferations of cells infected with Epstein-Barr virus in pre-invasive lesions related to nasopharyngeal carcinoma. *N Engl J Med* 1995; 333:693–698.

188. Shao YM, Poirier S, Ohshima H, et al. Epstein–Barr virus activation in Raji cells by extracts of preserved food from high risk areas for nasopharyngeal carcinoma. *Carcinogenesis* 1988; 9:1455–1457.

189. Agulnik M, Epstein JB. Nasopharyngeal carcinoma: Current management, future directions and dental implications. *Oral Oncol* 2008 (in press, Epub ahead of print).

190. Tang JW, Rohwader E, Chu IM, et al. Evaluation of Epstein–Barr virus antigen based immunoassays for serological diagnosis of nasopharyngeal carcinoma. *J Clin Virol* 2007; 40:284–288.

191. Paramita DK, Fachiroh J, Artama WT, et al. Native early antigen of Epstein–Barr virus, a promising antigen for diagnosis of nasopharyngeal carcinoma. *J Med Virol* 2007; 79:1710–1721.

192. Moss DJ, Khanna R, Bharadwaj M. Will a vaccine to nasopharyngeal carcinoma retain its orphan status?. *Dev Biol (Basel)* 2002; 110: 67–71.

193. Duraiswamy J, Sherritt M, Thomson S, et al. Therapeutic LMP 1 polyepitope vaccine for EBV associated Hodgkin disease and nasopharyngeal carcinoma. *Blood* 2003; 101:3150–3156.

194. Soulieres D, Senzer NN, Vokes EE, et al. Multicenter phase II study of erlotinib, an oral epidermal growth factor receptor tyrosine kinase inhibitor, in patients with recurrent or metastatic squamous cell cancer of the head and neck. *J Clin Oncol* 2004; 22:77–85.

195. Broumand V, Lozano TE, Gomez JA. Evaluation and staging of oral cancer. *Oral Maxillofac Surg Clin North Am* 2006; 18:435–444.

196. Kuriakose MA, Sharan R. Oral cancer prevention. *Oral Maxillofac Surg Clin North Am* 2006; 18:493–511.

197. El-Sebaie M, Zaghloul MS, Howard G, et al. Squamous cell carcinoma of the bilharzial and non-bilharzial urinary bladder: a review of etiological features, natural history, and management. *Int J Clin Oncol* 2005; 10:20–25.

198. Lagwinski N, Thomas A, Stephenson AJ, et al. Squamous cell carcinoma of the bladder: A clinicopathologic analysis of 45 cases. *Am J Surg Pathol* 2007; 31:1777–1787.

199. Hicks RM, Walters CL, el Sebai I, et al. Demonstration of nitrosamines in human urine: preliminary observations on a possible etiology for bladder cancer associated with chronic urinary infection. *Proc R Soc Med* 1977; 70:413–417.

200. Lozano JJ. Genomic imbalances in Schistosoma associated and non Schistosoma associated bladder carcinoma by comparative genomic hybridization analysis. *Cancer Genet Cytogenet* 2007; 177:16–19.

201. Helal Tel A, Fadel MT, El-Sayed NK. Human papilloma virus and p53 expression in bladder cancer in Egypt: relationship to schistomiasis and clinicopathologic factors. *Pathol Oncol Res* 2006; 12:173–178.

be rare in FCPD, have been reported from a number of centres. Macrovascular disease, however, appears to be an uncommon complication of FCPD.[54]

Despite clear clinical and pathologic descriptions of TCP and FCPD, the aetiology of the condition, including the relationship to malnutrition, remains unknown. Some of the difficulty in defining pathogenetic mechanisms relates to the lack of population-based epidemiology of the disease. Although early observations described the disease occurring predominantly in poor, malnourished communities, more recent studies have reported the occurrence of TCP and FCPD in persons of normal body weight (even in obese individuals) and in India the majority of affected persons are not underweight.[52] Furthermore, in many tropical countries where malnutrition is widespread, TCP and FCPD do not occur. Whether this relates to poor recognition of the disease or low incidence is, however, speculative without the support of population-based studies. This paucity of population-based data similarly hampers the understanding of MMDM, about which there is very little epidemiological, clinical or pathological information. Indeed the existence of an aetiological relationship between malnutrition and diabetes has been questioned and it may well be that malnutrition is a consequence of unrecognized and poorly treated diabetes, rather than an associated pathogenetic factor.[55]

A number of environmental and genetic factors have been studied in regard to the pathogenesis of TCP and FCPD. Although previously considered an aetiological factor, cassava toxicity is no longer regarded as a cause of TCP and FCPD. The evidence against cassava is largely epidemiological, with some substantiation by experimental studies. Pancreatic damage by free radicals, due to poor availability of antioxidant micronutrients, has also been proposed as a factor in the development of TCP by some authors.[52,55]

TCP appears to have a genetic basis and mutations in the serine protease inhibitor, Kazal type 1 (SPINK1) gene have been identified in affected subjects.[55] SPINK1 mutations are associated with a reduced capacity to inhibit activation of trypsinogen. More recently, polymorphisms in the cathepsin B (CTSB) gene have been found in association with TCP and the possible mechanism involved in the induction of pancreatitis is premature activation of trypsinogen.[56] MMDM, on the other hand, has been associated with polymorphisms in the MHC class 1 chain-related gene a (MIC-A) and with HLA *DR3-DQ2*, suggesting that the conditions are indeed separate and unrelated entities.[57-59] The genetic dichotomy suggests that FCPD develops as a consequence of chronic pancreatitis and the disease susceptibility is encoded in the genes responsible for premature activation of trypsinogen, whereas MMDM has features of an immune-mediated pathogenesis. More work is required to clarify whether MMDM is a form of autoimmune type 1 diabetes, with a distinctive phenotype that is influenced by nutritional deprivation.

Complications

From WHO estimates, the global excess mortality attributable to diabetes for the year 2000 is 2.9 million, equivalent to 5.2% of world all-cause mortality and similar in magnitude to those of HIV/AIDS in the same year, making diabetes the 5th leading cause of death in the world. Of the excess deaths, 1.9 million (65.5%) are from developing regions of the world where 1 in 10 excess deaths in economically productive individuals (35–65 years) can be attributed to diabetes; yet diabetes is perceived as a disease of affluent countries.[60]

The natural history and clinical course of diabetes in Africa are poorly understood and this is due in many instances to poor follow-up.[61] From the limited evidence, mortality rates are unacceptably high and the major contributors still include preventable acute metabolic complications and infective causes. Mortality rates of 5.0–11.8% have been reported from clinic studies and of 7.6–41% from outcome studies; the major causes of death were diabetic ketoacidosis (DKA) and infection. However, reports from Ethiopia and South Africa indicate that there is a changing pattern, with renal disease accounting for 30–50% of deaths in type 1 diabetes. From earlier necropsy studies, most deaths were due to DKA (34–54%) and infection was the second leading cause. However, the limitations of these studies were that they included mixed cohorts of subjects with type 1 and type 2 diabetes and varying diabetes duration.[61] Premature mortality related to type 1 diabetes has been highlighted in rural Mozambique where life expectancy after the diagnosis is drastically reduced to only 0.6 years, whereas in urban Zambia, life expectancy is an estimated 27 years.[63]

Previous impressions that chronic complications of diabetes are rare in Africa are likely related to the decreased survival from the disease and inadequate screening.[32,62,64] Clinic-based studies on mixed cohorts of type 1 and type 2 diabetes and varying diabetes duration have shown that, where examined, the prevalence of macrovascular disease is uncommon (peripheral vascular disease, 1.7–10%; angina 0.4–10.0%), hypertension is common (19–50%) and diabetic foot disease was reported in 0.6–36.6%. Regarding microvascular complications, the prevalence of retinopathy ranges from 2.9–57.1%, of nephropathy from 1.0–30.5%, and of neuropathy from 5.9–69.6%.[32,61,63]

The only population-based study, on the prevalence of microvascular complications in Egyptians with type 2 diabetes, showed rates among subjects with known diabetes and subjects with newly (survey) diagnosed diabetes of 41.5% and 15.7%, respectively, for retinopathy 6.7% and 6.8% for nephropathy, 21.9% and 13.6% for neuropathy, and 0.8% for both groups for foot ulcers. Each of the microvascular complications was significantly associated with increased blood glucose.[61]

Most of the data on long-duration disease in defined patient groups are from studies in type 1 diabetes; these data have shown rates of microvascular complications ranging from 40–50% for retinopathy, 20–40% for neuropathy, and 20–30% for nephropathy.[61] In South African Indians and Africans (Blacks) with long duration (>10 years) type 2 diabetes, retinopathy was found in 64.5%, nephropathy in 25%, treatment-requiring hypertension in 68%, abnormal serum creatinine in 25% and abnormal glomerular filtration rate in 42%. There was no significant ethnic difference for the prevalence of complications except for hypertension, which was more prevalent in Africans (84.8%) than in Indians (47.4%).[64]

Therefore, the available data indicate that with improving survival rates and the emergence of larger African populations with long-duration diabetes, the prevalence of chronic complications will approach that seen in the developed world. What needs to be established though is the apparent low frequency of macrovascular disease and the high prevalence of hypertension.

REFERENCES

1. National Diabetes Data Group. Classification and diagnosis of diabetes mellitus and other categories of glucose intolerance. *Diabetes* 1979; 28: 1039–1057.

2. WHO. WHO Expert Committee on Diabetes Mellitus, second report. *Technical Report Series*. No. 626. Geneva: World Health Organization; 1980.

3. WHO. Diabetes mellitus. Report of study group. *Technical Report Series*. No. 727. Geneva: World Health Organization; 1985.

4. King H, Rewers M, WHO Ad hoc diabetes Reporting Group. Global estimates for prevalence of diabetes mellitus and impaired glucose tolerance in adults. *Diabetes Care* 1993; 16:157–177.

5. Amos AF, McCarty DJ, Zimmet P. The rising global burden of diabetes and its complications. Estimates and projections to the year 2010. *Diabetic Med* 1997; 14(suppl 5):S1–S85.

6. King H, Aubert RE, Herman WH. Global burden of diabetes. Prevalence, numerical estimates and projections. *Diabetes Care* 1998; 21:1414–1431.

7. Wild S, Roglic G, Green A, et al. Global prevalence of diabetes. Estimates for the year 2000 and projections for 2030. *Diabetes Care* 2004; 27:1047–1053.

8. The Expert Committee on the diagnosis and classification of diabetes mellitus. Report of the Expert Committee on the diagnosis and classification of diabetes mellitus. *Diabetes Care* 1997; 20:1183–1197.

9. Alberti KG MM, Zimmet PZ, for the WHO Consultation. Definition, diagnosis and classification of diabetes mellitus and its complications. Part 1: diagnosis and classification of diabetes mellitus. Provisional report of a WHO consultation. *Diabetic Med* 1998; 15:539–553.

10. World Health Organization. *Definition and Diagnosis of Diabetes Mellitus and Intermediate Hyperglycaemia*. Report of a WHO/IDF Consultation. Geneva: WHO; 2006.

11. Hoet JJ, Tripathy BB. Report of the International Workshop on types of diabetes peculiar to the tropics. *Diabetes Care* 1996; 19:1014.

12. Rao RH, Yajnik CS. Commentary: time to rethink malnutrition and diabetes in the tropics. *Diabetes Care* 1996; 19:1014–1017.

13. Mauvais-Jarvis F, Sobngwi E, Porcher R, et al. Ketosis-prone type 2 diabetes in patients of sub-Saharan African origin: clinical pathophysiology and natural history of beta-cell dysfunction and insulin resistance. *Diabetes* 2004; 53: 645–653.

14. International Diabetes Federation. *Diabetes Atlas*. 3rd edn. Brussels: International Diabetes Federation; 2006.

15. Black RE, Morris SS, Bryce J. Where and why are 10 million children dying every year? *Lancet* 2003; 361:2226–2234.

16. The DIAMOND Project Group. Incidence and trends of childhood Type 1 diabetes worldwide 1990–1999. *Diabet Med* 2006; 23:857–866.

17. Achenbach P, Bonifacio E, Koczwara K and Ziegler A-G. Natural history of type 1 diabetes. *Diabetes* 2005; 54(suppl 2):S25–S31.

18. Redondo MJ, Eisenbarth GS. Genetic control of autoimmunity in type 1 diabetes and related disorders. *Diabetologia* 2002; 45:605–622.

19. Gorodezky C, Alaez C, Murguía A, et al. HLA and autoimmune diseases: type 1 diabetes (T1D) as an example. *Autoimmunity Rev* 2006; 5:187–194.

20. Onengut-Gumuscu S, Concannon P. The genetics of type 1 diabetes: lessons learned and future challenges. *J Autoimmunity* 2005; 25:34–39.

21. Knip M, Veijola R, Virtanen SM, et al. Environmental triggers and determinants of type 1 diabetes. *Diabetes* 2005; 54(suppl 2):S125–S136.

22. Pirie FJ, Hammond MG, Motala AA, et al. HLA class II antigens in South African Blacks with type 1 diabetes. *Tissue Antigens* 2001; 57:348–352.

23. Garcia-Pacheco JM, Herbut B, Cutbush S, et al. Distribution of HLA-DQA1, -DQB1 and DRB1 alleles in black IDDM patients and controls from Zimbabwe. *Tissue Antigens* 1992;40:145–149.

24. Mbanya JC, Sobngwi E, Mbanya DN. HLA-DRB1, -DQA1, -DQB1 and DPB1 susceptibility alleles in Cameroonian type 1 diabetes patients and controls. *Eur J Immunogenet* 2001; 28:459–462.

25. Cruz TD, Valdes AM, Santiago A, et al. DPB1 alleles are associated with type 1 diabetes susceptibility in multiple ethnic groups. *Diabetes* 2004; 53: 2158–2163.

26. Panz VR, Kalk WJ, Zouvannis M, et al. Distribution of autoantibodies to glutamic acid decarboxylase across the spectrum of diabetes mellitus seen in South Africa. *Diabet Med* 2000; 17:524–527.

27. Hawa MI, Picardi A, Costanza F, et al. Frequency of diabetes and thyroid autoantibodies in patients with autoimmune endocrine disease from Cameroon. *Clin Immunol* 2006; 118:229–232.

28. Goswami R, Kochupillai N, Gupta N, et al. Islet cell autoimmunity in youth onset diabetes mellitus in Northern India. *Diabetes Res Clin Pract* 2001; 53: 47–54.

29. Pardini VC, Mourao DM, Nascimento PD, et al. Frequency of islet cell autoantibodies (IA-2 and GAD) in young Brazilian type 1 diabetes patients. *Braz J Med Biol Res* 1999; 32:1195–1198.

30. Stumvoll M, Goldstein BJ, van Haefen TW. Type 2 diabetes: principles of pathogenesis and therapy. *Lancet* 2005; 365:1333–1334.

31. Bays H, Mandarino L, De Fronzo R. Role of adipocyte, free fatty acids, and ectopic fat in pathogenesis of type 2 diabetes: peroxisomal proliferator-activated receptor agonists provide a rational therapeutic approach. *J Clin Endocrinol Metabol* 2004; 89:463–478.

32. McLarty DG, Pollitt C, Swai ABM. Diabetes in Africa. *Diabetic Med* 1990; 7:670–684.

33. Motala AA, Omar MA, Pirie FJ. Diabetes in Africa. Epidemiology of type 1 and type 2 diabetes in Africa. *J Cardiovasc Risk* 2003; 10: 77–83.

34. The Expert Committee on the diagnosis and classification of diabetes mellitus. Follow up report on the diagnosis of diabetes mellitus. *Diabetes Care* 2003; 26:3160–3167.

35. Aspray TJ, Mugusi F, Rashid S, et al. Essential non-communicable disease health intervention project. Rural and urban differences in diabetes prevalence in Tanzania: the role of obesity, physical inactivity and urban living. *Trans R Soc Trop Med Hyg* 2000; 94:637–644.

36. Amoah AG, Owusu SK, Adjei S. Diabetes in Ghana: a community based prevalence study in Greater Accra. *Diabetes Res Clin Pract* 2002; 56: 197–205.

37. Ramaiya KL, Swai AB, McLarty DG, et al. Impaired glucose tolerance and diabetes mellitus in Hindu Indian immigrants in Dar-es-Salaam. *Diabetic Med* 1991; 8:738–744.

38. Swai AB, McLarty DG, Sherrif F, et al. Diabetes and impaired glucose tolerance in an Asian community in Tanzania. *Diabetes Res Clin Pract* 1990; 8(3): 227–234.

39. Omar MA K, Seedat MA, Dyer RB, et al. South African Indians show a high prevalence of NIDDM and bimodality in plasma glucose distribution patterns. *Diabetes Care* 1994; 17:70–73.

40. Levitt NS, Steyn K, Lambert EV, et al. Modifiable risk factors for Type 2 diabetes mellitus in a peri-urban community in South Africa. *Diabet Med* 1999; 16:946–950.

41. Levitt NS, Unwin NC, Bradshaw D, et al. Application of the new ADA criteria for the diagnosis of diabetes to population studies in sub-Saharan Africa. *Diabet Med* 2000; 17:381–385.

42. Levitt NS, Bradshaw D. The impact of HIV/AIDS on Type 2 diabetes prevalence and diabetes healthcare needs in South Africa: projections for 2010. *Diabet Med* 2006; 23:103–104.

43. Ramachandran A. Epidemiology of diabetes in India-three decades of research. *J Assoc Physicians India* 2005; 53:34–38.

44. Ramachandran A, Snehalatha C, Kapur A, et al. Diabetes Epidemiology Study Group in India (DESI). High prevalence of diabetes and impaired glucose tolerance in India: National Urban Diabetes Survey. *Diabetologia* 2001; 44:1094–1101.

45. Sadikot SM, Nigam A, Das S, et al. Diabetes India. The burden of diabetes and impaired fasting glucose in India using the ADA 1997 criteria: prevalence of diabetes in India study (PODIS). *Diabetes Res Clin Pract* 2004; 66:293–300.

46. Ramachandran A, Snehalatha C, Baskar AD, et al. Temporal changes in prevalence of diabetes and impaired glucose tolerance associated with lifestyle transition occurring in the rural population in India. *Diabetologia* 2004; 47:860–865.

47. Ramachandran A, Snehalatha C, Vijay V. Low risk threshold for acquired diabetogenic factors in Asian Indians. *Diabetes Res Clin Pract* 2004; 65: 189–195.

48. Banerji MA, Faridi N, Atluri R, et al. Body composition, visceral fat, leptin, and insulin resistance in Asian Indian men. *J Clin Endocrinol Metab* 1999; 84:137–144.

49. McKeigue PM, Shah B, Marmot MG. Relation of central obesity and insulin resistance with high diabetes prevalence and cardiovascular risk in South Asians. *Lancet* 1991; 337:382–386.

50. Umpierrez GE, Smiley D, Kitabchi AE. Narrative review: ketosis-prone type 2 diabetes mellitus. *Ann Intern Med* 2006; 144:350–357.

51. Sobngwi E, Vexiau P, Levy V, et al. Metabolic and immunogenetic prediction of long-term insulin remission in African patients with atypical diabetes. *Diabet Med* 2002; 19:832–835.

52. Barman KK, Premalatha G, Mohan V. Tropical chronic pancreatitis. *Postgrad Med J* 2003; 79:606–615.

53. Mohan V, Barman KK, Rajan VS, et al. Natural history of endocrine failure in tropical chronic pancreatitis: a longitudinal follow-up study. *J Gastroenterol Hepatol* 2005; 20:1927–1934.

54. Shelgikar KM, Yajnik CS, Mohan V. Complications in fibrocalculous pancreatic diabetes – the Pune and Madras experience. *Int J Diab Dev Countries* 1995; 15:70–75.

55. Balakrishnan V, Nair P, Lakshmi R, et al. Tropical pancreatitis – a distinct entity or merely a type of chronic pancreatitis? *Indian J Gastroenterol* 2006; 25:74–81.

56. Mahurkar S, Idris MM, Reddy DN, et al. Association of cathepsin B gene polymorphisms with tropical calcific pancreatitis. *Gut* 2006; 55: 1270–1275.

57. Chandak GR, Idris MM, Reddy DN, et al. Mutations in the pancreatic secretory trypsin inhibitor gene (PST1/SPINK1) rather than the cationic trypsinogen gene (PRSS1) are significantly associated with tropical calcific pancreatitis. *J Med Genet* 2002; 39:347–351.

58. Sanjeevi CB, Kanungo A, Berzina L, et al. MHC class I chain-related gene a alleles distinguish malnutrition-modulated diabetes, insulin-dependent diabetes and non-insulin-dependent diabetes mellitus patients from eastern India. *Ann NY Acad Sci* 2002; 958:341–344.

59. Kanungo A, Samal KC, Sanjeevi CB. Molecular mechanisms involved in the etiopathogenesis of malnutrition-modulated diabetes mellitus. *Ann NY Acad Sci* 2002; 958:138–143.

60. Roglic G, Unwin N, Bennett PH, et al. The burden of mortality attributable to diabetes. *Diabetes Care* 2005; 28:2130–2135.

61. Motala AA. Diabetes trends in Africa. *Diabetes Metab Res Rev* 2002; 18(suppl 3):S14–S20.

62. Beran D, Yudkin JS, De Courten M. Access to care for patients with insulin-requiring diabetes in developing countries. *Diabetes Care* 2005; 28:2136–2140.

63. Mbanya JC, Sobngwi E. Diabetes microvascular and macrovascular disease in Africa. *J Cardiovasc Risk* 2003; 10:97–102.

64. Motala AA, Pirie FJ, Gouws E, et al. Microvascular complications in South African patients with long-duration diabetes mellitus. *S Afr Med J* 2001; 91:987–992.

Chapter 37 Mohammed R. Essop and
Datshana P. Naidoo

Hypertension in the Tropics

INTRODUCTION

Almost one-half of the world's population resides in the tropics. Despite geographical uniformity, the region is characterized by much ethnic, cultural and socioeconomic diversity. Apart from Cuba, whose infant and adult mortality rates approximate those of the industrialized nations, overall mortality rates for the rest of the tropics are much higher. In the poorest regions of the tropics, much of the burden of disease is related to risk factors such as malnutrition, sanitation and hygiene. However, a large segment of the tropics characterized as lower-mortality, developing regions, where almost one-third of the global population live, shows a risk factor transition from mainly communicable diseases to those seen in established economies, including hypertension, hypercholesterolaemia, obesity and tobacco consumption. The increase in global burden of disease due to these risk factors, notably heart failure, coronary artery disease, stroke and renal failure, has largely occurred as a result of huge epidemiological changes in developing countries, with migration from rural areas to the cities, changes in diet, cigarette smoking, sedentary habits and psychosocial stresses.

The impact of hypertension on the global burden of disease was highlighted by the Comparative Risk Assessment Collaborating Group.[1] Worldwide, hypertension was the leading cause of death (12.78% of global mortality) and the third leading cause of disability-adjusted life years (64 million DALY), preceded only by childhood and maternal underweight (138 million DALY) and unsafe sex (92 million DALY). Furthermore, the global burden of hypertension is predicted to increase from 972 million (26.4% of the adult population) in 2000 to 1.56 billion in 2025 (29.2%).[2] Significantly, some two-thirds of the world's hypertensive population belongs to the developing countries.[2] Both at a global and regional level, hypertension presents a major public health challenge and will require an enormous effort directed at population- and individual-based interventions in order to stem the pandemic rise of cardiovascular disease.

DEFINITION AND CLASSIFICATION

The ability to measure blood pressure occurred just over 100 years ago with the introduction of the conventional sphygmomanometer by Scipione Riva-Rocci in 1896 and later modified by Nicolai

Korotkoff in 1905. For much of the first half of the twentieth century, elevated blood pressure was regarded to be compensatory and any attempt at lowering blood pressure frowned upon. Subsequent attempts to define the limits of normal blood pressure were severely hampered by lack of standardization in the technique of measurement, changes in blood pressure with age and geographical location, lack of consensus on the relative importance of systolic versus diastolic pressure, and, most importantly, the inherent biological variation of arterial pressure. Thus, physical and mental stress, and diurnal variation may result in fluctuations in blood pressure of 10–20% or more.

The current definition of hypertension as a blood pressure exceeding 140/90 mmHg is completely arbitrary, since there is a consistent, strong and graded relationship across the entire spectrum of systolic blood pressure, from levels as low as 110 mmHg, with several cardiovascular disease outcomes, including cardiovascular death, myocardial infarction, heart failure, stroke and renal dysfunction.[3] Furthermore, since hypertension is but one component of a number of risk factors which often cluster in a single individual, the decision to initiate treatment based on a threshold blood pressure alone may be inappropriate. This is reflected by most current guidelines on the treatment of blood pressure,[4–6] which emphasize therapy according to total calculated cardiovascular risk rather than an isolated threshold blood pressure.

The classification of hypertension is shown in Table 37.1.[4] The categories of normal and high normal blood pressure have been combined as prehypertension in the JNC 7 classification.[7] The reasons for this include the rapid progression from prehypertension to hypertension in many patients, the higher prevalence of other cardiovascular risk factors in prehypertensive as compared with normotensive individuals, and the increased incidence of cardiovascular disease in prehypertensive patients.[8] Isolated systolic hypertension is defined as a systolic pressure exceeding 140 mmHg with a diastolic pressure lower than 90 mmHg.

EPIDEMIOLOGY

Hypertension is as much a disease of populations as of individuals. In addressing the problem of hypertension, therefore, we need to consider why in some populations the entire distribution of blood pressure is shifted to the right, and the separate but related question of why some individuals within a population have blood

Table 37.1 Definitions and classification of blood pressure levels (mmHg)

Category	Systolic	Diastolic
Optimal	<120	<80
Normal	120–129	80–84
High normal	130–139	85–89
Grade 1 hypertension (mild)	140–159	90–99
Grade 2 hypertension (moderate)	160–179	100–109
Grade 3 hypertension (severe)	≥180	≥110
Isolated systolic hypertension	≥140	<90

When a patient's systolic and diastolic blood pressures fall into different categories, the higher category should apply. Isolated systolic hypertension can also be graded (grades 1, 2, 3) according to systolic blood pressure values in the ranges indicated, provided diastolic values are <90.
From the European Society of Hypertension–European Society of Cardiology.[4]

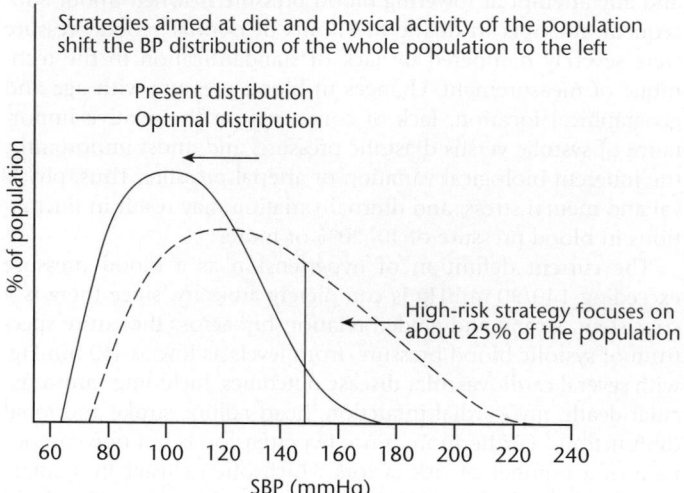

Figure 37.1 Current and optimal distribution of systolic blood pressure in populations. (Redrawn with permission from World Health Organization, International Society of Hypertension Writing Group.[6])

pressure levels at the upper tail of the normal distribution (Figure 37.1). It is accepted that the development of hypertension reflects a complex and dynamic interaction between environment and genetic factors. Differences in genetic susceptibility probably account for much of the blood pressure variation within populations exposed to a broadly similar environment, whereas differences in environmental factors largely determine variation in blood pressure levels between populations.

Apart from several rural and very isolated communities, a striking feature that is observed to a varying extent across all populations, whether defined by race, geographical location or gender, is the increase in blood pressure with age. Further, migration from rural to urban environs, and from developing to established market economies is associated with significant rises in blood pressure. Putative mechanisms include dietary changes with excess calories and obesity, increased salt and diminished potassium intake, physical inactivity and excess alcohol consumption.

Data on global estimates of blood pressure by age, sex and WHO subregions were published by Lawes et al.[9] Of note, mean systolic blood pressures were highest for Eastern Europe, followed closely by countries of West Africa, with lowest levels in the Southeast Asian and Western Pacific regions. In terms of the prevalence of hypertension, defined as blood pressure above 140/90 mmHg, a similar distribution has been observed.[2]

Although hypertension is more frequent in economically developed countries (37.3%) than in developing ones (22.9%), the absolute number of individuals affected – and therefore the population attributable risk – is much higher in the developing nations due to their larger populations.[2]

RISK FACTORS FOR HYPERTENSION

Age

Advancing age is the most predictable risk factor for increasing blood pressure. In the age group 30–44 years, mean systolic pressure is higher in males versus females. However, after 60 years, females tend to have higher systolic pressures than males, reflecting a steeper age–systolic pressure gradient in females.[9] However, blood pressure during childhood does not appear to correlate with blood pressure later in life.

Social gradient

An emerging phenomenon in tropical countries is that people of middle and upper socioeconomic class tend to have higher rates of hypertension than poorer groups. This excess is partly due to greater body mass, but other factors, including physical inactivity and nutritional influences, including alcohol consumption, and a high-salt diet with a low intake of potassium-rich foods, may also be involved.[10] Studies in developed societies show the opposite phenomenon, with an inverse relationship between social class and blood pressure. As urbanization and development in the tropics stabilize, this trend for hypertension and its complications to be more common in people of higher social class may reverse, as it did in the West about 50 years ago.

Obesity and insulin resistance

A series of abnormalities associated with insulin resistance, including hyperinsulinaemia, impaired glucose tolerance, obesity, increased plasma triglyceride levels, decreased high-density lipoprotein (HDL) concentrations and high blood pressure, have been reported in studies in Britain and the USA (see also Chapter 38). This constellation is now widely recognized as the metabolic syndrome. Most of these factors are independently related to the development of ischaemic heart disease. Based on these considerations, it has been suggested that insulin resistance and hyperinsulinaemia may be involved in the aetiology of hypertension.[11] Further support for this comes from two recently published studies that attempt to identify predictors of hypertension.[12,13] In the Strong Heart Study,[12] a population-based longitudinal cohort study of risk factors for hypertension in adults, not surprisingly, initial blood pressure was a strong predictor of incident hypertension. In patients with optimal blood pressure at baseline

(<120/80 mmHg), abdominal obesity, abnormal lipid profile and diabetes were significant predictors for the development of hypertension. The Physicians' Health Study[13] also found a powerful association between disturbed lipid metabolism and the risk for developing hypertension. Together, these observations underscore the potential role of dysregulated glucose and lipid metabolism for the development of hypertension.

However, the evidence for a relationship between insulin resistance and hypertension in non-European populations is inconsistent. For instance, hypertension rates are not increased in Pima Indians, Mexican Americans and several other ethnic groups with high rates of obesity and type II diabetes mellitus. Furthermore, there is only a weak association between blood pressure and insulin levels.[14]

Since there is still a low incidence of ischaemic heart disease in hypertensive patients in Africa, it could be argued that insulin resistance and its effects on lipid metabolism are less important. Animal fat intake in Africa is lower than in the West and this may explain the relative rarity of coronary heart disease, while hypertension-related strokes and renal failure are common. As in all populations, there is an excess of hypertension associated with diabetes mellitus. Community studies carried out in Cameroon and Madagascar put the association at between 20% and 30%. The association of raised blood pressure with non-insulin-dependent diabetes mellitus is associated with increased mortality rates from cardiovascular disease. Both risk factors are closely related to lifestyle, so their rising prevalence should be preventable.

Alcohol

Excess alcohol intake is a well-established risk factor for hypertension. It is of interest that the second-ever study reporting a relationship between alcohol and blood pressure was conducted in Bombay.[15] While earlier reports suggest that the risk of hypertension appeared at the level of about five drinks per day, recent data suggest that there is a relationship even at lower alcohol levels.[10] Epidemiological and clinical studies show that the alcohol–blood pressure relationship is rapidly reversible with moderation or cessation of drinking.

Sodium and potassium

Numerous studies have shown an important role for excess sodium and reduced potassium intake in the pathogenesis of hypertension.[16] Essential hypertension and the age-related increase in blood pressure almost never occur in populations with a daily consumption of sodium chloride of less than 50 mmol per day, and are observed mainly where daily salt intake exceeds 100 mmol. In the International Study of Salt and Blood Pressure (INTERSALT) of over 10 000 subjects across 52 countries, median 24-hour urinary excretion – an index of daily sodium intake – was 170 mmol per day.[10] A difference in mean sodium intake of 50 mmol/day was associated with a difference of 5 mmHg systolic and 3 mmHg diastolic blood pressure rise over 30 years. Furthermore, lower dietary potassium intakes are associated with an increased risk of hypertension. Both salt restriction and potassium supplementation can reduce blood pressure. INTERSALT demonstrated that hypertension is most common in populations with the lowest potassium consumption and the highest 24-hour urinary sodium excretion.[10] Thus, the ratio of potassium to sodium intake may be more important than the absolute intake of each.[16] In rural communities that ingest a diet rich in fruit and vegetables, the potassium:sodium ratio usually exceeds 3, whereas this ratio is less than 0.4 in industrialized countries.[16] Daily consumption of sodium and potassium impacts not only on blood pressure but also on other endpoints such as left ventricular hypertrophy and stroke.

Some of the electrolyte differences may be related to socioeconomic factors. Potassium-rich foods, which reduce blood pressure and hence strokes, are expensive and there is evidence, mainly from the USA, that their consumption in poor urban black communities is lower than in the rural populations and also lower than in white people.

Inter-individual variation in susceptibility to the pressor effect of salt loading, termed salt sensitivity, has been well documented. Salt sensitivity is affected by age, race and associated disease states, and hence is more common in the elderly, blacks and type II diabetics. Clinical studies in the USA have shown that black people are more sensitive to a given dietary salt load, exhibiting a greater rise in blood pressure and a delayed natriuresis when compared with whites.[17] Thus, black people may be more salt-sensitive even though they may consume similar amounts of salt. However, there is also evidence that a low-salt diet is more effective at reducing blood pressure in black compared with white hypertensives.

Physical activity

Although there are important health benefits associated with physical activity, there is surprisingly little good scientific evidence to show a significant reduction in blood pressure with exercise. A meta-analysis of eight randomized control trials showed a non-significant reduction in systolic/diastolic pressure of 0.8/3.7 mmHg in hypertensive and 0.2/0.1 mmHg in normotensive subjects.[18]

Psychosocial stress

While the association between psychosocial stress and blood pressure is controversial, the best evidence that anxiety may play a significant role is the observation of office hypertension with normal home or ambulatory blood pressure – the so-called white-coat effect, seen in almost one-third of patients. Diurnal variation with higher daytime pressures in day shift workers and nighttime pressures in night shift workers would also support the association between psychosocial factors and blood pressure. Finally, migrant studies may suggest a role for stress and the development of hypertension.[19] Unfortunately, there is very little evidence to show a beneficial effect on blood pressure of stress management techniques.

Birth weight and hypertension

The Barker hypothesis that birth weight and adult blood pressure are reciprocally related has had a considerable impact on how we now view exposure to factors in utero or in early postnatal life.[20,21] The association is consistent and has been found in many settings; it implies a causal relationship, although the mechanisms remain unclear. Disproportional impaired growth of the fetus and placenta appears to be a critical factor. Babies who were 'small for dates' are most at risk. A recent meta-analysis estimated the impact as 1 mmHg increase in systolic pressure per 500 g decrease in birth weight.[21] It remains unclear whether maternal nutritional status, specific placental nutrient supply, or poor placentation or placental function due to raised blood pressure underlies the association. Recently, both inadequate and excess 'catch-up' growth in childhood have been found to amplify the risk.[22]

The association is particularly relevant to analysis of ethnic differences in high blood pressure, because black populations, notably African Americans, continue to have average birth weights consistently some 200–300 g lighter than European Americans. The same applies to almost all other developing societies where hypertension as a chronic disease epidemic has emerged. There is evidence that population average birth weights are socioeconomically determined, with higher-status African-origin women having heavier babies, making a genetic basis unlikely.[23] There are few studies of the birth weight–later blood pressure question in African Americans, but a clear link has been reported in Jamaica[24] and India, where maternal undernutrition and low birth weight are common.

GENETICS OF ESSENTIAL HYPERTENSION

Essential hypertension is considered to be polygenic but the number of alleles and polygenes contributing to the hypertension phenotype is not yet known. Data from family and twin studies suggest that about 30–60% of blood pressure variability may be due to genetic mutations.[25] The expression of these genetic abnormalities depends on interaction with environmental factors such as salt intake, alcohol, obesity and stress. Although it is not known how many genes influence blood pressure, alleles at many different loci are suggested to contribute to the ultimate disease trait, and specific combinations of causative alleles may be different between individuals. In agreement with this observation, linkage or association analysis has consistently shown that blood pressure is not due to a single genetic variant.

SECONDARY HYPERTENSION

In a small minority of hypertensive patients, less than 5 %, a treatable underlying disease may be found which is the cause of raised blood pressure, and these are discussed in more detail elsewhere.[26] Intrinsic renal diseases such as glomerulonephritis and pyelonephritis are more common in Africa, but polycystic kidney disease, renal artery stenosis, endocrine diseases (Cushing's syndrome, primary aldosteronism, phaeochromocytoma and acromegaly) and coarctation of the aorta do not seem to occur with greater frequency. There is also an excess incidence of systemic lupus erythematosus in African-origin populations, which is an important cause of high blood pressure, especially in young women. Estimations of the prevalence of secondary hypertension are influenced by the availability of modern diagnostic facilities, and this presents problems for most tropical countries. Extensive investigation reveals that between 10% and 20% of patients with hypertension presenting to hospital in some African countries have evidence

of renal impairment, but this kidney damage may be a consequence rather than a cause of the hypertension.

Hypertension during pregnancy is an important problem in the tropics and is associated with increased maternal and fetal mortality. Perinatal and maternal mortality rates are high in developing countries and about one-third of these deaths may be due to hypertension. The diagnosis of pre-eclampsia is made on the presence of proteinuria and elevation of the blood pressure. If the diastolic blood pressure remains consistently below 100 mmHg, drug treatment should not be given. Many mothers develop gestational or pregnancy-induced hypertension in which blood pressure rises in pregnancy and falls after pregnancy is over. Where this elevation of blood pressure is mild, and not associated with proteinuria, drug treatment should not be given.

HYPERTENSION AND THE BURDEN OF DISEASE

Hypertension is an important public health challenge because it is frequent, is a major contributor – together with other risk factors including cholesterol, diabetes and obesity – to the epidemic of cardiovascular, cerebrovascular and kidney disease, and is modifiable. Currently, cardiovascular diseases, including myocardial infarction, heart failure and stroke, are responsible for 30% of global mortality, with an increasingly severe impact in emerging market economies where the middle-aged and economically productive are mostly affected.

Cardiovascular disease

The association between blood pressure, total cholesterol and body mass index and cardiovascular disease is continuous, linear, additive and evident across a broad range of values down to a systolic blood pressure of 115 mmHg, total cholesterol 3.8 mmol/L and body mass index 21 kg/m^2 (Figure 37.2). Also evident from the graph are, first, that over the range of values depicted, none of the risk factors show evidence of a plateau or J curve at the lower limits, and, second, much of the risk of blood pressure, cholesterol and weight occurs at levels much lower than what would be defined as normal.

Globally, non-optimal blood pressure is the major contributor to the cardiovascular disease burden, accounting for 45% of the attributable risk, followed by cholesterol (28%) and obesity (15%) (Figure 37.3). The burden of cardiovascular disease, even in the tropics, varies by geographical region, with deaths and DALYs due to stroke predominating in the Western Pacific and Africa subregions and cardiovascular disease the main burden elsewhere.[27,28] This may in part reflect the higher prevalence of hypertension in the stroke-prone areas[9] and elevated cholesterol in South-east Asian countries with high incidence of myocardial infarction. Despite these differences, in general, it would appear that the same risk factors for myocardial infarction are operational worldwide and that the approach to prevention can be based on similar principles in all regions.[29]

Cerebrovascular disease

Globally, some 15 million people succumb to strokes each year, of whom about a third die and another third are left permanently

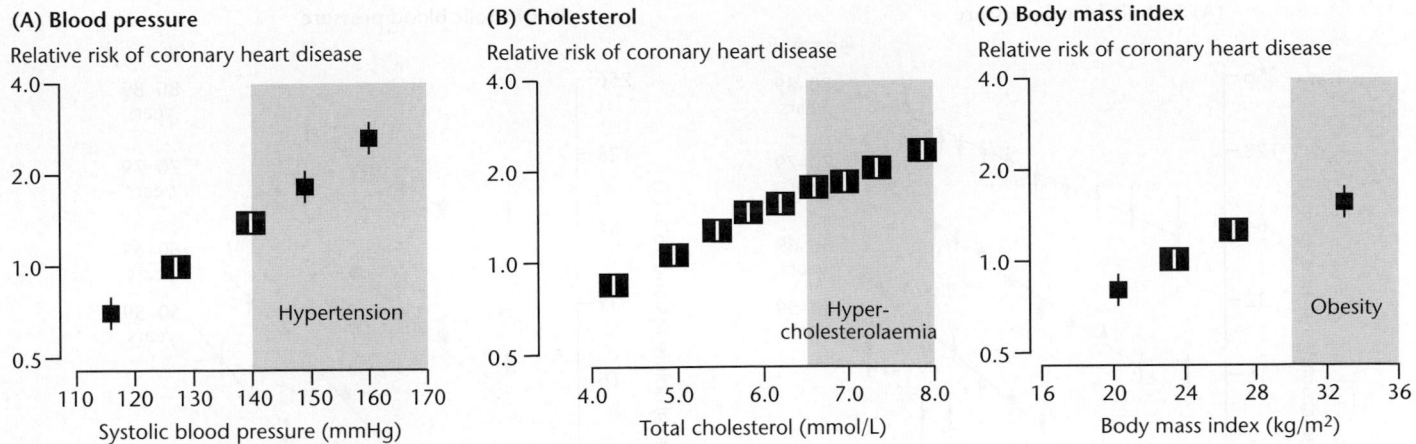

Figure 37.2 Continuous association of blood pressure, cholesterol and body mass index with coronary heart disease risk. (Redrawn with permission from Rodgers A, Lawes CMM, Gaziano TA, et al. The growing burden of risk from high blood pressure, cholesterol, and bodyweight. In: Murray CJL, Lopez AD, Mathers CD, et al., eds. *Disease Control Priorities in Developing Countries*. 2nd edn. New York: Oxford University Press; 2006.)

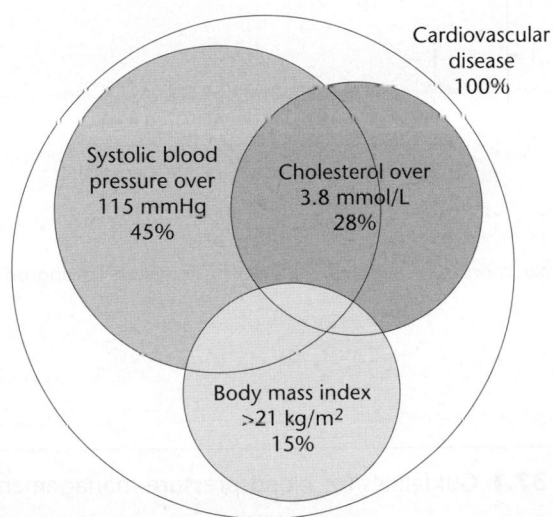

Figure 37.3 Contribution of blood pressure, cholesterol and body mass index to the global burden of cardiovascular disease. (Redrawn with permission from Rodgers A, Lawes CMM, Gaziano TA, et al. The growing burden of risk from high blood pressure, cholesterol, and bodyweight. In: Murray CJL, Lopez AD, Mathers CD, et al., eds. *Disease Control Priorities in Developing Countries*. 2nd edn. New York: Oxford University Press; 2006.)

disabled. Two-thirds of strokes occur in developing nations. Notably, cerebrovascular mortality exceeds coronary heart disease in China and sub-Saharan Africa.[28] Several non-modifiable (blacks, males, older age) and modifiable (smoking, excess alcohol, dyslipidaemia, carotid artery disease, atrial fibrillation) factors predispose to stroke. However, hypertension is by far the most powerful predictor of stroke, accounting for 60% of the population attributable risk. In a review of 61 cohort studies, the Prospective Studies Collaboration[3] showed a strong log-linear correlation without a threshold between stroke mortality and blood pressure, starting at levels of 115 mmHg systolic and 75 mmHg diastolic and con-

sistent across the age range of 50–89 years (Figure 37.4). Between the ages of 40 and 69 years, each difference in blood pressure of 20 mmHg systolic or 10 mmHg diastolic was associated with a more than two-fold difference in stroke mortality.

The proportion of cerebral haemorrhage to infarction is low (less then 10%) in western populations, but remains much higher in Africa and the Far East, although more precise data are not available.

Other complications of hypertension

Concentric left ventricular hypertrophy is an important cardiovascular phenotype that frequently accompanies hypertension and has been shown to be associated with an increased risk for several adverse clinical outcomes, including heart failure, myocardial infarction, stroke, arrhythmias and sudden death. It appears to be more frequent in long-standing severe hypertension and in blacks, and although most frequently diagnosed by ECG, is more accurately detected and quantified by means of echocardiography. Not surprisingly, it is the most frequent antecedent of heart failure, with population attributable risks of 40% for males and 60% for females in recent estimates from the Framingham study.[30] Acute pulmonary oedema, associated with severe hypertension and normal ejection fraction, is not infrequently encountered in sub-Saharan Africa and most likely is due to diastolic dysfunction.

Less common but potentially life-threatening complications of hypertension include aortic aneurysm and dissection. Equally catastrophic, and also not uncommon in Africa, is the syndrome of malignant hypertension with acute renal failure, heart failure, encephalopathy and papilloedema on fundoscopy. Prompt and aggressive control of blood pressure may reverse all of the abnormalities, including renal dysfunction, but 5-year mortality remains high at around 50%.

Hypertensive nephrosclerosis, with or without diabetes, is the most common cause of end-stage kidney disease and the need for dialysis. The distinction between hypertensive-induced renal dysfunction and hypertension secondary to some other primary renal

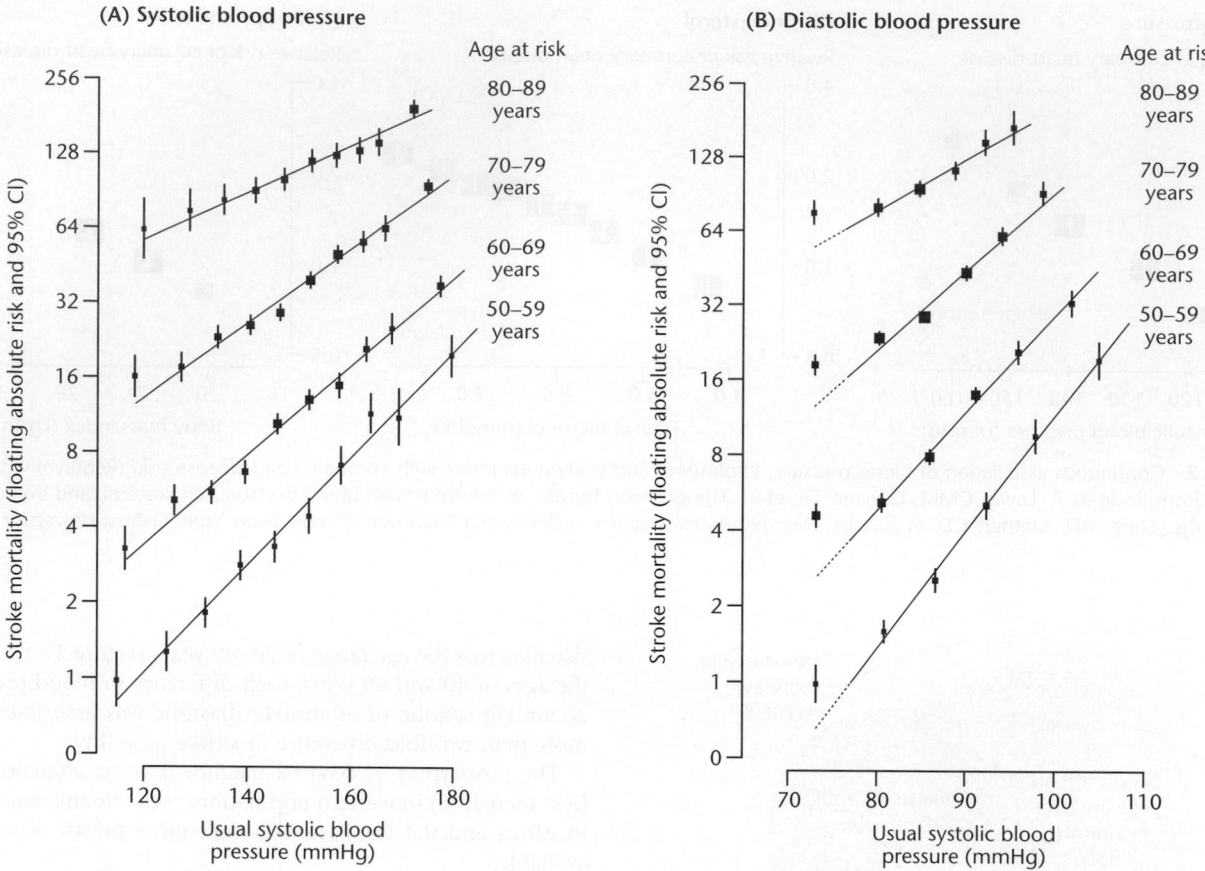

Figure 37.4 Age-specific relation of systolic and diastolic blood pressure with stroke mortality. (Redrawn with permission from Lewington et al.[3])

disease may be difficult, although certain factors such as black race, long history of antecedent hypertension, target organ involvement of the heart and eyes, and absence of any primary renal disease would support the former.

DIAGNOSIS OF HYPERTENSION

The frequency of hypertension, and the far-reaching implications for both the patient and society which has to shoulder the economic burden of treating this disease, make it imperative that the diagnosis is made simply, accurately and efficiently. Since symptoms are unusual and non-specific, the diagnosis rests entirely on accurate measurement of blood pressure. It is therefore crucial that appropriate guidelines be adhered to when measuring blood pressure (Box 37.1). Several national bodies have published detailed guidelines on the equipment and technique for measuring blood pressure, and for further information the reader is referred to these.[4–7]

The standard mercury manometer, when used properly, is still the gold standard for measuring blood pressure. Automated manometers are increasingly being used but may be problematic if not accurately calibrated. The manometer should be well main-

Box 37.1 Guidelines for blood pressure management

When measuring blood pressure, care should be taken to:

Allow the patients to sit for several minutes in a quiet room before beginning blood pressure measurements.

Take at least two measurements spaced by 1–2 minutes, and additional measurements if the first two are quite different.

Use a standard bladder (12–13 cm long and 35 cm wide) but have a larger and a smaller bladder available for fat and thin arms respectively. Use the smaller bladder in children.

Have the cuff at the heart level, whatever the position of the patient.

Use Phase 1 and V (disappearance) Korotkoff sounds to identify systolic and diastolic blood pressure, respectively.

Measure blood pressure in both arms at first visit to detect possible differences due to peripheral vascular disease. In this instance, take the higher value as the reference one, when the auscultatory method is employed.

Measure blood pressure 1 and 5 minutes after assumption of the standing position and in other conditions in which orthostatic hypotension may be frequent or suspected.

Measure heart rate by pulse palpitation (30 seconds) after the second measurement in the sitting position.

tained, with the mercury column vertical, and at rest the mercury should be at 0 mmHg. If the manometer is sloping away from the vertical, due to damaged hinges, this leads to overestimation of the pressure. The rubber bladder inside the arm cuff should encircle at least 80% of the upper arm. The use of too small a cuff leads to overestimation of blood pressure.

Blood pressures should normally be measured after at least 5 minutes of quiet sitting with the patient's feet on the floor and the arm supported at heart level. The arm should be slightly externally rotated and supported to avoid the isometric exercise required to hold the arm raised. The manometer cuff should be inflated to 15 mmHg above the level needed to occlude the brachial pulse and the stethoscope should be placed where the pulse was felt, on the medial side of the antecubital fossa. The column of mercury should be deflated slowly (2 mm/s). The systolic blood pressure is taken at the first appearance of Korotkoff sounds (phase I) and diastolic pressure at the final disappearance of sounds (phase V). Measurement of diastolic blood pressure at the phase of muffling of sounds (phase IV) is now obsolete.

The blood pressure recorded should be the average of two readings taken 1 minute apart; however, if the difference exceeds 5 mmHg, additional readings should be taken. In patients with mild hypertension, decisions on starting therapy should only be made after three repeat measurements taken on separate occasions within 2 months. Seated and standing blood pressure is important in the elderly and diabetics to exclude postural hypotension; and in patients seen for the first time, measurements should be taken in both arms to exclude coarctation.

In addition to measuring blood pressure in the clinic, home measurement using an automated device and 24-hour ambulatory blood measurement monitoring (ABPM) are increasingly being used. These devices cannot be routinely recommended in a resource-poor setting but do provide greater insight into the dynamics of blood pressure not apparent with clinic measurement alone. The 24-hour blood pressure load, absence of the normal nocturnal decline in blood pressure (non-dipping) and early morning surge of blood pressure are easily computed from ABPM and may refine the ability to predict cardiovascular risk and need for pharmacological therapy. In patients with treated hypertension, a higher ambulatory systolic or diastolic blood pressure is able to predict cardiovascular events even after adjustment for classic risk factors including office measurement.[31] Unfortunately, current guidelines on antihypertensive therapy are based entirely on clinic measurement, which remains the mainstay of clinical decision making. An additional problem with ABPM is the absence of a large body of data to define the limits of normality for daytime and nighttime blood pressure. Blood pressure measured by ABPM is typically lower than clinic pressure. Currently, ambulatory hypertension is defined as a pressure exceeding 130/80 mmHg over 24 hours, 135/85 mmHg for the daytime and 120/70 mmHg for nightime. A recent publication, in which diagnostic thresholds for ABPM were based on 10-year cardiovascular risk, suggests even lower limits for optimal ambulatory blood pressure.[32]

Occasionally, despite accurate measurements, office blood pressure may consistently over-estimate home or ambulatory blood pressure. This phenomenon, termed white-coat hypertension, is seen more commonly in the elderly, women, diabetics and during pregnancy. The diagnosis may be important since it is generally accepted that patients with white-coat hypertension are at relatively low risk and are unlikely to benefit from antihypertensive treatment.[33]

PATIENT EVALUATION

Further evaluation of the patient should aim to identify:
- secondary causes for the hypertension
- additional risk factors for cardiovascular disease
- target organ damage
- associated clinical conditions.

Based on this evaluation, which comprises a minimum of a clinical examination, blood and urine tests, and electrocardiogram, the patient is risk-stratified, with further management being dictated by the level of blood pressure and estimated cardiovascular risk.

Clinical examination

A thorough clinical examination includes assessment of height, weight, body mass index and waist circumference. The general appearance may suggest endocrine hypertension, such as thyrotoxicosis or Cushing's. Nicotine-stained fingers indicate a significant smoking history. Fundoscopy is essential and hypertensive retinopathy graded according to the classification of Keith–Wagener–Barker. Yellow nodules around the eye or tendon xanthomas are suggestive of dyslipidaemia. Radio-femoral delay may be the only clue to coarctation, and absent radial pulse with subclavian bruits, especially in Asian or black patients, may indicate Takayasu's arteritis. Evidence of left ventricular hypertrophy and heart failure should be sought. Abdominal examination should include auscultation for renal arterial bruits pointing to renovascular hypertension and palpation for polycystic kidney disease. Absent lower limb pulses and bruits point to the presence of peripheral vascular disease.

Laboratory investigations

Investigations depend on the severity of the hypertension and availability of facilities and are listed in Table 37.2. All patients receiving antihypertensive drug therapy should ideally have routine urine testing, and full biochemical profiling together with an ECG.

Haematuria and proteinuria may be due to hypertension or to underlying renal disease. For a given level of pressure, if there is proteinuria, mortality is approximately doubled. Haematuria may also be due to a neoplasm of the urinary tract. The measurement of microalbuminuria (urine albumin below 300 mg/L) is of value in diabetic hypertensives but its significance in other hypertensives is uncertain.

Current guidelines for the diagnosis of diabetes include symptoms of diabetes plus a fasting glucose greater than 7 mmol/L or a 2-hour postprandial glucose more than 11.1 mmol/L during an oral glucose tolerance test.

All patients should undergo at least one blood test to estimate plasma sodium and potassium levels. Serum potassium levels are low in both primary and secondary hyperaldosteronism, and if hypokalaemia is encountered this needs detailed investigation. The most common cause of hypokalaemia is diuretic therapy,

Table 37.2 Laboratory investigations in a patient with hypertension

ROUTINE TESTS
• Plasma glucose (preferably fasting)
• Serum total cholesterol
• Serum high-density lipoprotein(HDL)-cholesterol
• Fasting serum triglycerides
• Serum uric acid
• Serum creatinine
• Serum potassium
• Haemoglobin and haematocrit
• Urinalysis (dipstick test complemented by urinary sediment examination)
• Electrocardiogram
RECOMMENDED TESTS
• Echocardiogram
• Carotid (and femoral) ultrasound
• C-reactive protein
• Microalbinuria (essential test in diabetics)
• Quantitative proteinuria (if dipstick test positive)
• Funduscopy (in severe hypertension)
EXTENDED EVALUATION (DOMAIN OF THE SPECIALIST)
• Complicated hypertension: test of cerebral, cardiac and renal function
• Search for secondary hypertension: measurement of renin, aldosterone, corticosteroids, catecholamines; arteriography; renal and adrenal ultrasound; computer-assisted tomography (CAT); brain magnetic resonance imaging

From the European Society of Hypertension–European Society of Cardiology.[4]

which must be discontinued at least 4 weeks prior to testing. Serum urea or creatinine levels should be measured to obtain an estimate of renal function. The estimation of creatinine clearance is not valuable unless there is severe renal failure. Serum total, LDL and HDL cholesterol levels should be measured, preferably in the fasting state.

Haematological profiling with estimations of plasma viscosity or erythrocyte sedimentation rate (ESR) may provide evidence of connective tissue diseases which may cause high blood pressure. In such cases, proteinuria may also be present.

If renal impairment is present or there is unexplained hypokalaemia, more detailed investigation with renal ultrasound scanning is necessary. If one or both kidneys are found to be small but with a smooth outline, then the possibility of correctable renal artery stenosis should be borne in mind and renal angiography is worth considering. If the kidneys are small with an irregular outline, pyelonephritis is more likely and investigations should be conducted to exclude obstructive uropathy with vesicoureteric reflux. If hypokalaemia is present, patients should undergo estimation of plasma renin and aldosterone levels. In primary hyperaldosteronism, plasma renin is low, while concurrent plasma aldosterone levels are high. If these features are found, patients should proceed to computed tomography to detect an adrenal adenoma. In Conn's syndrome, removal of the aldosterone-secreting adenoma may lead to cure of hypertension.

Patients with symptoms of a paroxysmal nature with sweating, blanching, tachycardia, weight loss, constipation and panic attacks should be investigated to exclude phaeochromocytoma. This requires a 24-hour urine test for catecholamines, metanephrines or 4-hydroxy-3-methoxymandelic acid.

Electrocardiographic evidence of left ventricular hypertrophy, with the sum of the R wave in leads V5 or V6 and the S wave in V1 amounting to more than 35 mm, is specific but lacks sensitivity.

MANAGEMENT

Population-based strategies

Since elevated blood pressure is as much an affliction of populations as of the individual, it follows that a comprehensive strategy to combat this disease requires targeting not only the affected individual but also the whole population (Figure 37.1). Not only will a small reduction in blood pressure in the entire population be expected to have a far greater impact on the global burden of hypertension than would a large reduction in a small number of affected individuals, but also the benefits reaped will be at a far lower financial cost. The concept of a population-based strategy for the control of hypertension is founded on sound scientific and economic principles, but implementation requires a concerted effort on the part of governments, industry, the media, physician societies, schools and, ultimately, the practitioner. Implementation of a population-based strategy is even more urgently needed in developing regions – where two-thirds of the global at-risk population resides, financial resources are severely limited, and where many of the inhabitants are largely ignorant of the benefits of lifestyle modification.

Targets of a population-based strategy and the expected benefit in term of systolic blood pressure reduction are illustrated in Table 37.3. It should be emphasized that atherosclerotic vascular disease begins early in life and therefore many of these preventative strategies need to be initiated from childhood.

Patient-targeted strategies

In patients with hypertension, blood pressure-lowering therapy on average reduces the risk of stroke and myocardial infarction by only 35–40% and 20–25%, respectively. Much of this lack of success may be explained by the 'rule of halves' which states that only 50% of those with hypertension are detected, only half of those detected are treated, and of those treated, only half have their blood pressure adequately controlled (i.e. 12.5% of the total). However, an equally plausible explanation for the failure of antihypertensive therapy is the realization over the past decade that hypertension frequently clusters with other risk factors such as insulin resistance, diabetes and dyslipidaemia and that for each of these risk factors there is a linear relationship with cardiovascular risk.[34] By implication, a significant reduction in the burden of cardiovascular and cerebrovascular disease would require targeting all known risk factors and not only blood pressure. Also, in the presence of other risk factors, even milder forms of hypertension require aggressive management. Support for the concept of total cardiovascular risk comes from several studies. In the

Table 37.3 Lifestyle modifications and expected reduction in blood pressure*

MODIFICATION	RECOMMENDATION	APPROXIMATE SYSTOLIC BP REDUCTION, RANGE
Weight reduction	Maintain normal body weight (BMI, 18.5–24.9)	5–20 mmHg/10 kg weight loss
Adopt DASH eating plan	Consume a diet rich in fruits, vegetables and low-fat dairy products with a reduced content of saturated and total fat	8–14 mmHg
Dietary sodium reduction	Reduce dietary sodium intake to no more than 100 mEq/L (2.4 g sodium or 6 g sodium chloride)	2–8 mmHg
Physical activity	Engage in regular aerobic physical activity such as brisk walking (at least 30 minutes per day, most days of the week)	4–9 mmHg
Moderation of alcohol consumption	Limit consumption to no more than 2 drinks per day (1 oz or 30 mL ethanol [e.g. 24 oz beer, 10 oz wine or 3 oz 80-proof whiskey]) in most men and no more than 1 drink per day in women and lighter-weight persons	2–4 mmHg

BMI, body mass index calculated as weight in kilograms divided by the square of height in metres; BP, blood pressure; DASH, Dietary Approaches to Stop Hypertension.
*For overall cardiovascular risk reduction, stop smoking. The effects of implementing these modifications are dose and time dependent and could be higher for some individuals.
From the JNC 7 report.[7]

HOPE study,[35] intensive antihypertensive therapy with ramipril in patients with minimally elevated blood pressure but frequent additional cardiovascular risk factors produced a significant benefit in most endpoints. Similarly, in PROGRESS,[36] therapy with perindopril in patients with stroke resulted in significant reductions in rates of recurrent stroke and major vascular events, irrespective of blood pressure. In the ABCD trial,[37] intensive blood pressure lowering in normotensive diabetics produced significant reductions in stroke, proteinuria and retinopathy compared with a less aggressive strategy. Finally, in ASCOT,[38] lipid-lowering therapy in addition to antihypertensive treatment resulted in significant reduction in all endpoints.

Further refinements to the determination of cardiovascular risk are made by a search for evidence of target organ damage and associated clinical conditions (Table 37.4). Most national guidelines have embraced, to a greater or lesser extent, the principle of global risk assessment[4-7] and an example is shown in Table 37.5, from the ESH–ESC guidelines.[4] Based mainly on the Framingham data, patients are stratified by the 10-year risk of cardiovascular disease as low risk (<10%), medium risk (10–20%), high risk (20–30%) and very high risk (>30%). While there is consensus amongst the various guidelines regarding cardiovascular risk assessment, unfortunately, these guidelines have emerged solely from studies of western populations and their generalizability to most of the Asian subcontinent, Latin America and Africa is questionable.

THERAPEUTIC APPROACH

Lifestyle modification

Vigorous modification of lifestyle as outlined in Table 37.3 should be encouraged in all patients, irrespective of the severity of hypertension. Although there is no direct link between smoking and hypertension, patients should be advised to stop smoking in order to reduce the overall cardiovascular risk. While the INTERHEART study[29] confirmed that, in broad principle, the risk factors for cardiovascular disease and recommendations regarding lifestyle modification are universal, the emphasis might vary depending on racial, cultural, regional or other peculiarities. Thus, smoking is a significant problem in China but not India, excess dietary salt is frequent in Africa, obesity is endemic in African women, and lack of exercise is a significant problem in South-east Asia.

Drug therapy

Since the commitment to pharmacological treatment for hypertension is lifelong, great care has to be exercised before starting therapy. Most guidelines recommend antihypertensive therapy based on calculated cardiovascular risk.[4-6] Although similar in broad terms, a modification of the WHO cardiovascular disease risk management package for low- and medium-resource settings is appropriate for the tropics (Figure 37.5).[39] Patients judged to be at low or moderate risk should be started on drug therapy only if after an appropriate period of monitoring, blood pressure remains above 140/90 mmHg despite lifestyle modification. High-risk patients should be commenced on therapy immediately. A list of available drugs, dosages and frequency of administration are shown in Table 37.6, and guidelines for initial drug selection in Table 37.7.

General principles of drug therapy

Despite claims to the contrary, there is abundant clinical trial evidence that, in general, most classes of antihypertensive agents reduce a variety of cardiovascular outcomes to a similar extent and that the choice of a particular agent may not be as important as the effective lowering of blood pressure.[40] Furthermore, many patients will require two or more agents for effective blood pressure control, rendering the debate on class superiority less relevant. What is important is to choose an effective drug, with minimal side-effects, at the cheapest possible cost. The literature on hypertension is replete with mega-trials purporting to demon-

Table 37.4 Factors influencing prognosis in the patient with hypertension

Risk factor for cardiovascular disease used for stratification	Target organ damage (TOD)	Diabetes mellitus	Associated clinical conditions (ACC)
• Levels of systolic and diastolic BP • Men >55 years • Women >65 years • Smoking • Dyslipidaemia (total cholesterol >6.5 mmol/L, >250 mg/dL*, or LDL-cholesterol >4.0 mmol/L, >155 mg/dL*, or HDL-cholesterol M < 1.0, W < 1.2 mmol/L, M < 40, W < 48 mg/dL) • Family history of premature cardiovascular disease (at age <55 years M, <65 years W) • Abdominal obesity (abdominal circumference M ≥ 102 cm, W ≥ 88 cm) • C-reactive protein ≥1 mg/dL	• Left ventricular hypertrophy (electrocardiogram: Sokolow–Lyons >38 mm; Cornell >2440 mm/ms; echocardiogram: LVMI M ≥ 125, W ≥ 1 10 g/m²) • Ultrasound evidence of arterial wall thickening (carotid IMT ≥ 0.9 mm) or atherosclerotic plaque • Slight increase in serum creatine (M 115–133, W 107–124 µmol/L; M 1.3–1.5, W 1.2–1.4 mg/dL) • Microalbuminuria (30–300 mg/24 h; albumin–creatinine ratio M ≥ 22, W ≥ 31 mg/g; M ≥ 2.5, W ≥ 3.5 mg/mmol)	• Fasting plasma glucose 7.0 mmol/L (126 mg/dL) • Postprandial plasma glucose >11.0 mmol/L (198 mg/dL)	• Cerebrovascular disease: ischaemic stroke; cerebral haemorrhage; transient ischaemic attack • Heart disease: myocardial infarction; angina; coronary revascularization; congestive heart failure • Renal disease: diabetic nephropathy; renal impairment (serum creatinine M > 133, W > 124 µmol/L; M > 1.5, W > 1.4 mg/dL); proteinuria (>300 mg/24 h) • Peripheral vascular disease • Advanced retinopathy: haemorrhages or exudates, papilloedema

M, men; W, women; LDL, low-density lipoprotein; HDL, high-density lipoprotein; LVMI, left ventricular mass index; IMT, intima-media thickness.
*Lower levels of total and LDL-cholesterol are known to delineate increased risk, but they were not used in the stratification.
From the European Society of Hypertension–European Society of Cardiology.[4]

Table 37.5 Risk stratification of the hypertensive patient

Other risk factors and disease history	BLOOD PRESSURE (MMHG)				
	Normal SBP 120–129 or DBP 80–84	High normal SBP 130–139 or DBP 85–89	Grade 1 SBP 140–159 or DBP 90–99	Grade 2 SBP 160–179 or DBP 100–109	Grade 3 SBP ≥ 180 or DBP ≥ 110
No other risk factors	Average risk	Average risk	Low added risk	Moderate added risk	High added risk
1–2 risk factors	Low added risk	Low added risk	Moderate added risk	Moderate added risk	Very high added risk
3 or more risk factors or TOD or diabetes	Moderate added risk	High added risk	High added risk	High added risk	Very high added risk
ACC	High added risk	Very high added risk	Very high added risk	Very high added risk	Very high added risk

ACC, associated clinical conditions; DBP, diastolic blood pressure; SBP, systolic blood pressure; TOD, target organ damage.
From the European Society of Hypertension–European Society of Cardiology.[4]

strate superiority of one class of drugs over another. While these data may be informative, their broader applicability may be challenged given the limitations of trial design such as patient selection, variable endpoints, inadequate statistical power, inequalities in achieved blood pressure and short duration of follow-up. Bearing these limitations in mind, the choice of initial antihypertensive therapy may be influenced by associated features such as age, race, cardiovascular risk profile, target organ damage, and co-morbid diseases such as stroke, coronary disease, heart failure, diabetes, proteinuria and renal insufficiency.

Elderly patients

Elderly patients are characterized by a higher prevalence of hypertension (almost two-thirds), predominant systolic hypertension that is a more important risk factor than diastolic hypertension and more difficult to control, greater frequency of co-morbid disease, predisposition to postural hypotension, and are more likely to be on medication for other medical conditions. The benefits of antihypertensive therapy have been clearly demonstrated, and although diuretics and calcium channel blockers are the drugs of choice, all other classes of drugs may be effective,

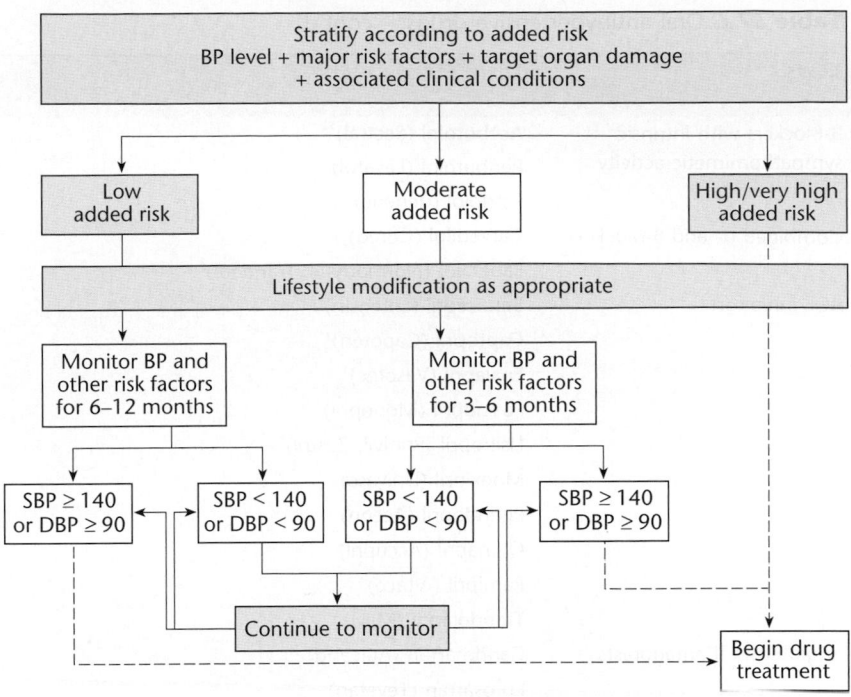

Figure 37.5 Management of the hypertensive patient according to added risk. (Redrawn with permission from the Joint National Hypertension Guideline Working Group 2006.[39])

Adapted WHO cardiovascular disease-risk management package for low-medium settings

Table 37.6 Oral antihypertensive drugs*

Class	Drug (Trade name)	Usual dose, range, mg/day	Daily frequency
Thiazide diuretics	Chlorothiazide (Diuril)	125–500	1
	Chlorthalidone (generic)	12.5–25	1
	Hydrochlorothiazide (Microzide, HydroDIURIL)[†]	12.5–50	1
	Polythiazide (Renese)	2–4	1
	Indapamide (Lozol)[†]	1.25–2.5	1
	Metolazone (Mykrox)	0.5–1.0	1
	Metolazone (Zaroxolyn)	2.5–5	1
Loop diuretics	Bumetanide (Bumex)[†]	0.5–2	2
	Furosemide (Lasix)[†]	20–80	2
	Torsemide (Demadex)[†]	2.5–10	1
Potassium-sparing diuretics	Amiloride (Midamor)[†]	5–10	1–2
	Triamterene (Dyrenium)	50–100	1–2
Aldosterone-receptor blockers	Eplerenone (Inspra)	50–100	1–2
	Spironolactone (Aldactone)[†]	25–50	1–2
β-Blockers	Atenolol (Tenormin)[†]	25–50	1
	Betaxolol (Kerlone)[†]	5–20	1
	Bisoprolol (Zebeta)[†]	2.5–10	1
	Metoprolol (Lopressor)[†]	50–100	1–2
	Metoprolol extended release (Toprol XL)	50–100	1
	Nadolol (Corgard)[†]	40–120	1
	Propranolol (Inderal)[†]	40–160	2
	Propranolol long-acting (Inderal LA)[†]	60–180	1
	Timolol (Blocadren)[†]	20–40	2

Continued

Table 37.6 Oral antihypertensive drugs*—cont'd

Class	Drug (Trade name)	Usual dose, range, mg/day	Daily frequency
β-Blockers with intrinsic sympathomimetic activity	Acebutolol (Sectral)[†]	200–800	2
	Penbutolol (Levatol)	10–40	1
	Pindolol (generic)	10–40	2
Combined α- and β-blockers	Carvedilol (Coreg)	12.5–50	2
	Labetalol (Normodyne, Trandate)[†]	200–800	2
ACE inhibitors	Benazepril (Lotensin)[†]	10–40	1–2
	Captopril (Capoten)[†]	25–100	2
	Enalapril (Vasotec)[†]	2.5–40	1–2
	Fosinopril (Monopril)	10–40	1
	Lisinopril (Prinivil, Zestril)[†]	10–40	1
	Moexipril (Univasc)	7.5–30	1
	Perindopril (Aceon)	4–8	1–2
	Quinapril (Accupril)	10–40	1
	Ramipril (Altace)	2.5–20	1
	Trandolapril (Mavik)	1–4	1
Angiotensin II antagonists	Candesartan (Atacand)	8–32	1
	Eprosartan (Tevetan)	400–800	1–2
	Irbesartan (Avapro)	150–300	1
	Losartan (Cozaar)	25–100	1–2
	Olmesartan (Benicar)	20–40	1
	Telmisartan (Micardis)	20–80	1
	Valsartan (Diovan)	80–320	1
Calcium channel blockers – non-dihydropyridines	Diltiazem extended release (Cardizem CD, Dilacor XR, Tiazac)[†]	180–420	1
	Diltiazem extended release (Cardizem LA)	120–540	1
	Verapamil immediate release (Calan, Isoptin)[†]	80–320	2
	Verapamil long-acting (Calan SR, Isoptin SR)[†]	120–360	1–2
	Verapamil-coer (Covera HS, Verelan PM)	120–360	1
Calcium channel blockers – dihydropyridines	Amlodipine (Norvasc)	2.5–10	1
	Felodipine (Plendil)	2.5–20	1
	Isradipine (Dynacirc CR)	2.5–10	2
	Nicardipine sustained release (Cardene SR)	60–120	2
	Nifedipine long-acting (Adalat CC, Procardia XL)	30–60	1
	Nisoldipine (Sular)	10–40	1
α₁-Blockers	Doxazosin (Cardura)	1–16	1
	Prazosin (Minipress)[†]	2–20	2–3
	Terazosin (Hytrin)	1–20	1–2
Central α₂-agonists and other centrally acting drugs	Clonidine (Catapres)[†]	0.1–0.8	2
	Clonidine patch (Catapres TTS)	0.1–0.3	1 weekly
	Methyldopa (Aldomet)[†]	250–1000	2
	Reserpine (generic)	0.05–0.25	1[‡]
	Guanfacine (generic)	0.5–2	1
Direct vasodilators	Hydralazine (Apresoline)[†]	25–100	2
	Minoxidil (Loniten)[†]	2.5–80	1–2

ACE, angiotensin-converting enzyme.
*Dosages may vary from those listed in the *Physicians' Desk Reference*, which may be consulted for additional information.
[†]Are now or will soon become available in generic preparations.
[‡]A 0.1 mg dose may be given every other day to achieve this dosage.
From the JNC 7 report.[7]

Table 37.7 Guidelines for selecting initial drug treatment of hypertension

Class of drug	Compelling indication	Possible indication	Absolute contraindication	Relative contraindication	Side-effects
Thiazide diuretics	Heart failure Elderly patients Systolic hypertension Blacks	Diabetes	Gout	Pregnancy Dyslipidaemia	Hypokalaemia Hyperglycaemia Hyperuricaemia Dyslipidaemia
β-Blockers	Angina Post infarction Heart failure Tachyarrhythmias	Diabetes	Heart block Asthma/COPD	Dyslipidaemia Metabolic syndrome Athletes Peripheral vascular disease Stroke prevention	Dyslipidaemia Impaired glucose tolerance Fatigue Impotence
ACE inhibitors	Heart failure Left ventricular dysfunction Post myocardial infarction Diabetes Chronic kidney disease Proteinuria Recurrent stroke prevention High coronary disease risk		Pregnancy Hyperkalaemia Bilateral renal artery stenosis		Cough Angio-oedema Hyperkalaemia Fetal malformations in pregnant women
Calcium channel blockers	Angina Elderly patients Systolic hypertension	Diabetes High coronary risk Peripheral vascular disease	Heart block (only with verapamil and diltiazem)	Heart failure Antiretroviral therapy	Headache Oedema Constipation Heart block (verapamil)
Aldosterone antagonists	Heart failure Post myocardial infarction		Renal failure Hyperkalaemia		Hyperkalaemia Gynaecomastia
Angiotensin receptor blockers	Heart failure Post myocardial infarction Diabetic nephropathy Proteinuria ACE cough		Pregnancy Bilateral renal artery stenosis Hyperkalaemia		Hyperkalaemia

with the exception of the β-blockers. While many of these patients may be on an α-blocker for prostate hypertrophy, the results of the large ALLHAT study,[41] in which the doxazosin arm was terminated early because of a higher incidence of combined cardiovascular disease events, are of some concern.

Race and ethnicity

Although cardiovascular risk factors in general are similar among most populations, it is well established that, at least in part, quantitative and qualitative differences segregate along racial and ethnic lines. The phenotypic expression of hypertension in black populations (including Afro-Americans, Afro-Caribbeans and Africans) is both more frequent and more aggressive, beginning at an earlier age and accompanied by greater target organ damage. Fundamental differences in pathogenetic mechanisms may also be present, since low-renin, salt-sensitive hypertension is much more frequent in blacks. Apart from hypertension, the prevalence of other cardiovascular risk factors is low. The cardiovascular disease burden is correspondingly characterized by a preponderance of stroke, non-ischaemic heart failure and chronic kidney

disease, although the incidence of coronary disease is on the rise. From a therapeutic standpoint, compared with whites and Asians, blacks respond poorly to β-blockers and angiotensin-converting enzyme (ACE) inhibitors as monotherapy, although this difference tends to disappear when combined with thiazide diuretics. The ALLHAT study[41] recruited more than 15 000 blacks of American and Afro-Caribbean ancestry with hypertension. Black patients randomized to receive the ACE inhibitor (lisinopril) had higher average follow-up blood pressure, a 40% higher risk of stroke and a 30% higher risk of heart failure as compared with those randomized to receive a diuretic. Despite this, black patients with heart failure, kidney disease or diabetes should not be denied the benefits of ACE inhibitor therapy. Diuretics and calcium channel blockers appear to be the most effective agents for the control of blood pressure in general and stroke in particular.[42]

South Asians have a particular predisposition to coronary artery disease. This appears to be explained by higher risk factor levels at younger ages.[43] The response to antihypertensive drugs in South Asians is broadly similar to that in whites. However, the high incidence of diabetes mellitus, glucose intolerance and hyperlipidaemia means that the thiazides, shown to be beneficial in hypertensive diabetics, should only be used in low dose (e.g. bendrofluazide up to 2.5 mg/day or hydrochlorothiazide up to 25 mg/day).

Although overall cardiovascular mortality rates in Chinese populations are similar to those in western populations, much of this can be attributed to stroke rather than coronary mortality.[44] Since almost 60% of the risk of stroke can be attributed to hypertension, aggressive strategies to manage blood pressure with any of the available drug classes are appropriate, although diuretics and calcium channel blockers may be more, and β-blockers less, effective. For secondary prevention of recurrent cerebrovascular events, most guidelines would recommend a combination of a diuretic (preferably indapamide) and an ACE inhibitor, based on the results of the PROGRESS study.[36]

Concomitant disease

Hypertension is frequently associated with additional abnormalities, both as a direct consequence of elevated blood pressure and the phenomenon of clustering of risk factors. These include diabetes, coronary heart disease, heart failure, cerebrovascular disease, proteinuria and chronic kidney disease. Therapeutic decisions in these patients should be formulated both to lower blood pressure and to prevent or ameliorate the associated abnormality.

The incidence of diabetes is increasing rapidly, more than half of all diabetics are hypertensive, and serious cardiovascular events are twice as common in patients who suffer from both as compared with either alone. The important issues in diabetics with hypertension include the potential adverse effects of certain antihypertensives on glucose tolerance and insulin sensitivity, the appropriate level of blood pressure at which antihypertensive therapy should be initiated, by how much blood pressure should be lowered, and the best choice of antihypertensive agent. Much of the controversy has centered on the association between thiazides and the development of diabetes. Although there is a clear relationship between exposure to thiazides and dysglycaemia, a vast body of literature has shown that they are as effective as any other agent for preventing cardiovascular events, and, more importantly, incident diabetes associated with their use carries no adverse prognosis (at least in the medium term). The risk of incident diabetes is also inversely related to potassium levels, suggesting that dietary supplementation may be useful. What has been clearly established, however, is that ACE inhibitors (or angiotensin receptor blockers) are effective in preventing incident diabetes, and, in patients with already-known diabetes, reduce proteinuria and retard the development of chronic kidney disease. A subanalysis of the ALLHAT study,[45] which is the largest study of the treatment of hypertension in diabetics, showed no superiority for the ACE inhibitor for the outcome of coronary events in diabetics, no inferiority for the use of the calcium channel blocker, and, most importantly, demonstrated the safety and efficacy of thiazides in this population group. The target blood pressure recommended by most guidelines is less than 130/80 mmHg, although studies are underway to determine if even lower targets would confer greater benefit.

With respect to coronary heart disease and stroke, it would appear that ACE inhibitors are preferable to calcium channel blockers for the former, but that the reverse is true for the latter.[46] For patients with heart failure, diuretics, β-blockers (metoprolol,

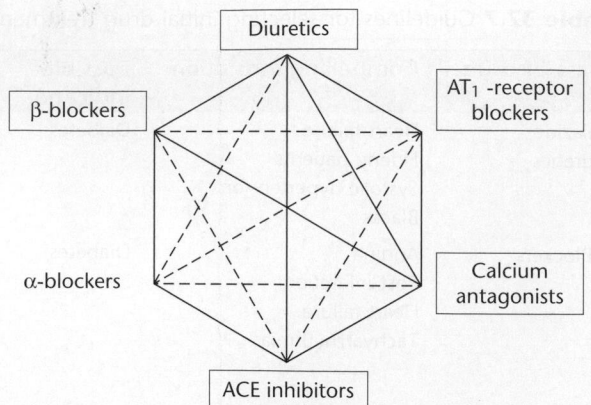

Figure 37.6 Preferred drug combinations for the treatment of hypertension. (Redrawn with permission from European Society of Hypertension–European Society of Cardiology Guidelines Committee.[4])

carvedilol and bisoprolol) and ACI inhibitors have a compelling indication based a large amount of documented evidence. However, calcium channel blockers may be detrimental and should only be used for significant associated hypertension refractory to other classes of drugs. Most guidelines recommend that patients who have hypertension and renal insufficiency, whether or not they are diabetic, should receive an ACE inhibitor. There is no cutoff value for serum creatinine at which ACE inhibitor therapy is inappropriate. Furthermore, a transient rise in creatinine may occur but this is not a reason to withhold therapy. As in the case of diabetics, the target blood pressure should be less than 130/80 mmHg.

Combination drug therapy

Most hypertensive patients will require more than one agent to achieve target levels of blood pressure. Rational drug combinations are depicted in Figure 37.6. The rationale for these preferred combinations includes synergism and mutual attenuation of side-effects. A classic example is the combination of a diuretic and ACE inhibitor, where the reflex activation of the renin–angiotensin system induced by the thiazide is countered by the ACE inhibitor. Furthermore, insulin resistance, hyperglycaemia, hypokalaemia and hyperuricaemia caused by thiazides are all attenuated by the ACE inhibitor.

Fixed drug combinations are an extension to the concept of combination therapy. In recognition of the effectiveness of combination therapy, the European Guidelines Committee[4] has recommended beginning therapy with fixed dose combinations in most patients, while the Joint National Committee[7] recommends this approach only in stage 2 or higher hypertension. The advantages of fixed dose combinations include fewer pills with better compliance, better tolerability due to lower individual doses, convenience, lower cost and more speedy attainment of target blood pressure.

Resistant hypertension

Resistant hypertension is defined as a blood pressure of at least 140/90 mmHg (or 130/80 mmHg in patients with diabetes and chronic kidney disease) despite treatment with full doses of at least three antihypertensive agents, one of which is a diuretic. The incidence is probably as high as 40% and is more frequent in the elderly. Potential causes include non-compliance, concomitant use of drugs that antagonize antihypertensive agents (ephedrine, steroids, cocaine, amphetamines, appetite suppressants, non-steroidal antiinflammatory agents, antidepressants, ciclosporin, tacrolimus and erythropoietin), significant alcohol abuse, excess salt intake, obesity and, finally, secondary causes of hypertension. Since many of these patients are volume overloaded, an increase in diuretic therapy or substitution of the thiazides with loop diuretics may ameliorate the blood pressure. If blood pressure remains refractory, additional therapy with aldosterone antagonists (spironolactone or eplerenone), combined α- and β-blockers (labetalol or carvedilol), centrally acting agents (clonidine or α_2-blockers), reserpine and direct vasodilators (hydralazine or minoxidil) may be necessary in some patients.

Hypertensive crises

Hypertensive crises may occur in three settings:
- marked elevation in blood pressure with severe headache and dyspnoea (hypertensive urgency)
- evidence of acute end-organ involvement such as grade 3 or 4 retinopathy, acute heart failure or coronary syndromes, encephalopathy or rapidly progressive renal dysfunction (hypertensive emergency)
- pregnant women with severe hypertension, proteinuria, neurological manifestations, renal failure, pulmonary oedema, thrombocytopenia or disseminated intravascular coagulation (eclampsia).

While blood pressure in hypertensive urgencies may be reduced slowly, in the case of hypertensive emergencies it should be lowered rapidly over a period of several hours. Therapy with nifedipine orally or intravenous treatment with nitroglycerin, nitroprusside, furosemide, hydralazine or labetalol may be effective.

CONCLUSION

Hypertension has become a disease of epidemic proportions. Control of hypertension, even in high-income countries, is unacceptably low. The tropical regions, apart from being poorly resourced, are in the grip of a double pandemic, one from infectious diseases and the other from cardiovascular disease. For this region, the most cost-effective strategy to manage the looming cardiovascular crisis is for all stakeholders, ranging from government to practitioners, to encourage a healthy lifestyle. While much may be achieved by education and advertisement, formal legislation to curb the sale of tobacco and limit the salt content of foods may be required.

Since hypertension is for the most part silent, screening programmes undertaken by primary healthcare givers may uncover larger numbers of people at risk. Furthermore, there is a dearth of data on risk factors for hypertension and cardiovascular disease and on best medical therapy in the developing regions of the world. Unfortunately, most of the studies in this field, and all of the guidelines, emanate from predominantly western populations and may not be appropriate to the tropics.

For the individual identified with hypertension, a concerted effort should be made to identify associated risk factors, clinical conditions and target organ damage. If pharmacological therapy is required, this should be with the most cost-effective drug, which, in most cases, would be the thiazide diuretics, since they are widely available, cheap and effective, with some metabolic side-effects the clinical relevance of which has not yet been established.

REFERENCES

1. Ezzati M, Lopez AD, Rodgers A, et al., and the Comparative Risk Assessment Collaborating Group. Selected major risk factors and global and regional burden of disease. *Lancet* 2002; 360:1347–1360.
2. Kearney PM, Whelton M, Reynolds K, et al. Global burden of hypertension: analysis of worldwide data. *Lancet* 2005; 365:217–223.
3. Lewington S, Clarke R, Qizilbash N, et al. Age specific relevance of usual blood pressure to vascular mortality: a meta-analysis of individual data for one million adults in 61 prospective studies. *Lancet* 2002; 360: 1903–1913.
4. European Society of Hypertension–European Society of Cardiology Guidelines Committee. 2003 European Society of Hypertension–European Society of Cardiology guidelines for the management of arterial hypertension. *J Hypertens* 2003; 21:1011–1053.
5. Williams B, Poulter NR, Brown MJ, et al. Guidelines for management of hypertension: report of the fourth working party of the British Hypertension Society, 2004-BHS IV. *J Hum Hypertens* 2004; 18:139–185.
6. World Health Organization, International Society of Hypertension Writing Group. 2003 World Health Organization (WHO)/International Society of Hypertension (ISH) statement on management of hypertension. *J Hypertens* 2003; 21:1983–1992.
7. Chobanian AV, Bakris GL, Black HR, et al., and the National High Blood Pressure Education Program Coordinating Committee. The Seventh Report of the Joint National Committee on Prevention, Detection, Evaluation, and Treatment of High Blood Pressure: the JNC 7 report. *JAMA* 2003; 289: 2560–2572.
8. Chobanian AV. Prehypertension revisited. *Hypertension* 2006; 48:812–814.
9. Lawes CMM, Vander Hoorn S, Law MR, et al. Blood pressure and the global burden of disease 2000. Part 1: Estimates of blood pressure levels. *J Hypertens* 2006; 24:413–422.
10. Intersalt Cooperative Research Group. Intersalt: an international study of electrolyte excretion and blood pressure: results for 24 hour urinary sodium and potassium excretion. *BMJ* 1988; 297:319–328.
11. Reaven GM. Role of insulin resistance in human disease. *Diabetes* 1988; 37:1595–1607.
12. de Simone G, Devereux R, Chinali M, et al., for the Strong Heart Study Investigators. Risk factors for arterial hypertension in adults with initial optimal blood pressure. *Hypertension* 2006; 47:162–167.
13. Halperin RO, Sesso HD, Ma J, et al. Dyslipidemia and risk of incident hypertension in men. *Hypertension* 2006; 47:45–50.
14. Collins VR, Dowse GK, Finch CF, et al. An inconsistent relationship between insulin and blood pressure in three Pacific Island populations. *J Clin Epidemiol* 1990; 43:1369–1378.
15. Shah WW, Kunjannam PV. The incidence of hypertension in liquor permit holders and teetotallers. *J Assoc Physicians India* 1959; 7:243–267.
16. Adrogue AJ, Madias NE. Sodium and potassium in the pathogenesis of hypertension. *N Engl J Med* 2007; 356:1966–1978.
17. Luft FC, Rankin LI, Bloch R, et al. Cardiovascular and humoral responses to extremes of sodium intake in normal white and black men. *Circulation* 1979; 60:697–706.
18. Ebrahim S, Smith GD. Lowering blood pressure: a systematic review of sustained effects of non-pharmacologic interventions. *J Public Health Med* 1998; 20:441–448.

19. James SA. Psychosocial precursors of hypertension: a review of the epidemiologic evidence. *Circulation* 1987; 76:160–166.

20. Barker DJP. *Mothers, Babies and Health in Later Life.* 2nd edn. Edinburgh: Churchill Livingstone; 1998.

21. Huxley R, Shiell AW, Law C. The role of size at birth and postnatal catch-up growth in determining systolic blood pressure: a systematic review of the literature. *J Hypertens* 2000; 18:815–831.

22. Eriksson JG, Forsen T, Tuomilehto J, et al. Catch-up growth in childhood and death from coronary heart disease: longitudinal study. *BMJ* 1999; 318:427–431.

23. David RJ, Collins JW. Differing birthweight among infants of US-born blacks, African-born blacks, and US-born whites. *N Engl J Med* 1997; 337:1209–1213.

24. Forrester TE, Wilks R, Bennett FI , et al. Fetal growth and cardiovascular risk factors in Jamaican schoolchildren. *BMJ* 1996; 312:156–160.

25. Binder A. A review of the genetics of essential hypertension. *Curr Opin Cardiol* 2007; 22:176–184.

26. Kaplan NM. *Clinical Hypertension.* 6th edn. Baltimore: Williams & Wilkins.

27. Lawes CMM, Vander Hoorn S, Law MR, et al. Blood pressure and the global burden of disease 2000. Part II: Estimates of attributable burden. *J Hypertens* 2006; 24:423–430.

28. Yusuf S, Reddy S, Ounpuu S, et al. Global burden of cardiovascular diseases. Part I: General considerations, the epidemiologic transition, risk factors, and impact of urbanization. *Circulation* 2001; 104:2746–2753.

29. Yusuf S, Hawken S, Ounpuu S, et al., on behalf of the INTERHEART Study Investigators. Effect of potentially modifiable risk factors associated with myocardial infarction in 52 countries (the INTERHEART study): case-control study. *Lancet* 2004; 364:937–952.

30. Lloyd Jones DM, Larson MG, Leip EP, et al. Lifetime risk for developing congestive heart failure: the Framingham Heart Study. *Circulation* 2002; 106:3068–3072.

31. Clement DL, De Buyzere ML, De Bacquer DA, et al., for the Office versus Ambulatory Pressure Study Investigators. Prognostic value of ambulatory blood pressure recordings in patients with treated hypertension. *N Engl J Med* 2003; 348:2407–2415.

32. Kikuya M, Hansen TW, Thijs L, et al., on behalf of the International Database on Ambulatory blood pressure monitoring in relation to Cardiovascular Outcomes (IDACO) Investigators. Diagnostic thresholds for ambulatory blood pressure monitoring based on 10-year cardiovascular risk. *Circulation* 2007; 115:2145–2152.

33. Pickering TG, Shimbo D, Haas D. Ambulatory blood pressure monitoring. *N Engl J Med* 2006; 354:2368–2374.

34. Mancia G. Total cardiovascular risk: a new treatment concept. *J Hypertens* 2006; 24(suppl 2):S17–S24.

35. Yusuf S, Sleight P, Pogue J, et al. Effects of an angiotensin converting enzyme inhibitor, ramipril, on cardiovascular events in high risk patients. *N Engl J Med* 2000; 342:145–153.

36. PROGRESS Collaborative Group. Randomised trial of a perindopril-based blood pressure lowering regimen among 6105 individuals with previous stroke or transient ischaemic attack. *Lancet* 2001; 358:1033–1041.

37. Schrier RW, Estacio RO, Esler A, et al. Effects of aggressive blood pressure control in normotensive type 2 diabetic patients on albuminuria, retinopathy and strokes. *Kidney Int* 2002; 61:1086–1097.

38. Sever PS, Dahlof B, Poulter NR, et al. Prevention of coronary and stroke events with atorvastatin in hypertensive patients who have average cholesterol concentrations, in the Anglo-Scandinavian Cardiac Outcomes Trial-Lipid Lowering Arm (ASCOT-LLA): a multicentre randomized control trial. *Lancet* 2003; 361:1149–1158.

39. Joint National Hypertension Guideline Working Group 2006: Seedat YK, Croasdale MA, Milne FJ, et al. South African hypertension guideline 2006. *S Afr Med J* 2006; 96:337–362.

40. Psaty BM, Lumley T, Furberg CD, et al. Health outcomes associated with various antihypertensive therapies used as first line agents: a network meta-analysis. *JAMA* 2003; 289:2534–2544.

41. The ALLHAT Officers and Coordinators for the ALLHAT Research Group. Major outcomes in high-risk hypertensive patients randomized to angiotensin-converting enzyme inhibitor or calcium channel blocker vs diuretic. The Antihypertensive and Lipid-Lowering Treatment to Prevent Heart Attack Trial (ALLHAT). *JAMA* 2002; 288:2981–2997.

42. Wright JT, Dun JK, Cutler JA, et al., for the ALLHAT Collaborative Research Group. Outcomes in hypertensive black and nonblack patients treated with chlorthalidone, amlodipine, and lisinopril. *JAMA* 2005; 293:1595–1608.

43. Joshi P, Islam S, Pais P, et al. Risk factors for early myocardial infarction in South Asians compared with individuals in other countries. *JAMA* 2007; 297:286–294.

44. Yusuf S, Reddy S, Ounpuu S, et al. Global burden of cardiovascular diseases. Part II: Variations in cardiovascular disease by specific ethnic groups and geographic regions and prevention strategies. *Circulation* 2001; 104:2855–2864.

45. Whelton PK, Barzilay J, Cushman WC et al., for the ALLHAT Collaborative Research Group. Clinical outcomes in antihypertensive treatment of type 2 diabetes, impaired fasting glucose concentration, and normoglycemia. *Arch Intern Med* 2005; 165:1401–1409.

46. Zhang H, Thijs L, Staessen JA. Blood pressure lowering for primary and secondary prevention of stroke. *Hypertension* 2006; 48:187–195.

Chapter 38

Nigel Unwin and Julia A. Critchley

Ischaemic Heart Disease

INTRODUCTION

Ischaemic heart disease (IHD) is the single largest cause of death worldwide and, with the exception of sub-Saharan Africa, is estimated to be responsible for around 1 in 8 of all deaths globally.[1,2] As populations age and lifestyles change, this burden will grow. This chapter aims to provide a description of the global distribution, risk factors, pathogenesis and clinical manifestations of this disease.

DEFINITION

Ischaemia refers to the situation where the oxygen supply to a tissue or organ is inadequate for its needs. IHD is the disturbance of cardiac function due to inadequate oxygen supply. Most commonly this is due to narrowing or complete occlusion of the coronary arteries caused by coronary atherosclerosis and associated thrombosis, and this chapter is concerned largely with ischaemia of atherosclerotic origin. There are, of course, many other causes of ischaemia related to either increased oxygen demand from the heart or decreased oxygen-carrying capacity of the blood. For example, ischaemia may also arise in severe ventricular hypertrophy due to hypertension or aortic stenosis, or in extremely severe anaemia. Quite commonly, two or more causes of ischaemia will co-exist, such as coronary atherosclerosis with increased oxygen demand due to the ventricular hypertrophy of hypertension.

GLOBAL DISTRIBUTION OF ISCHAEMIC HEART DISEASE AND RECENT TRENDS

Diseases of the cardiovascular system are found in populations at all stages of economic development. They are a significant contributor to morbidity and mortality in populations as diverse as those of rural Africa and North America. However, the types of cardiovascular disease that predominate differ with the level of economic development.[3] This changing pattern of cardiovascular diseases with economic development is part of a broader picture known as the 'epidemiological transition'.[4] This provides a useful framework for considering the interrelationships between demo-

graphy, disease patterns and social and economic conditions. The nature of the epidemiological transition and the relationships between these various factors are summarized in Figure 38.1. The figure illustrates the change from high fertility and high mortality, largely from infectious diseases that particularly afflict infants and children, to low fertility and low mortality, largely from chronic non-infectious diseases that particularly afflict adults and the elderly. The pace and details of change can and do vary greatly between populations and between subgroups, such as the rich and poor, within populations. The falling mortality and fertility is associated with huge changes in population age structure, from a very young age structure to that found in Western industrialized countries today. Four stages can be identified within this process according to the predominant disease patterns and life expectancy. Table 38.1 lists the predominant causes of death from cardiovascular disease at each of these stages. Table 38.1 illustrates the fact that IHD becomes a predominant contributor to mortality only in the later stages of the transition.

Global distribution of ischaemic heart disease

IHD is estimated to be the single largest cause of death worldwide.[1,2] Around 13% of all deaths globally are due to IHD. Some 75% of IHD deaths occur in low and middle income countries, partly reflecting the fact that 8 of 10 of all deaths worldwide occur in developing countries.[5]

There is marked regional variation in the importance of IHD as a cause of death (Figure 38.2). Thus, figures for the year 2000[6] in 'developed regions' (established market economies and former socialist economies) showed that around 23–28% of all deaths are due to IHD. In 'developing regions' (all other regions), the proportion varies from the lowest of 3% (sub-Saharan Africa) to the highest of just under 17% (Middle Eastern Crescent and India). Broadly, these differences represent different stages of the epidemiological transition described above. When the proportion of deaths due to IHD is examined by age group, in some developing regions, notably India and the Middle Eastern Crescent, IHD is found to contribute a similar, or in some age groups a greater, proportion of deaths than in developed regions. Estimates of age-specific death rates from IHD (Figure 38.3A, B) also suggest that these are higher in India and the Middle Eastern Crescent than in established market economies. In summary, most IHD deaths occur in developing countries and in some developing countries

IHD is now a more important contributor to mortality in adults than in developed regions.

Trends in 'developed' regions

The beginning of the twentieth century witnessed the start of an epidemic of IHD in most industrialized countries, particularly

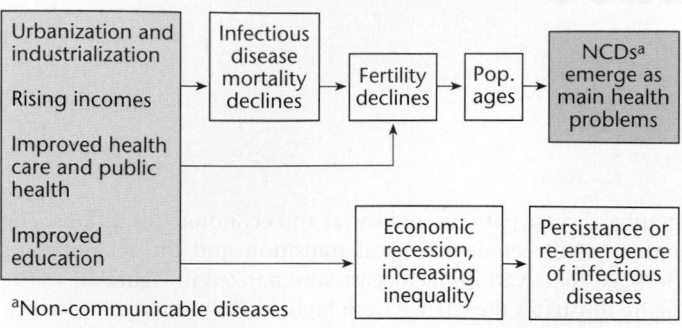

ªNon-communicable diseases

Figure 38.1 Representation of the epidemiological transition. The dashed line represents a 'protracted and polarized' transition, where persistent or new infectious disease (such as HIV) are found alongside rising levels of NCDs. This is the case in many of the world's poorest countries.

those of northern Europe, North America, Australia and New Zealand. This epidemic was most pronounced in men, in whom, even allowing for the contribution of artefacts such as changes in diagnostic practice, there was a very substantial rise in age-specific mortality rates from IHD over the first half of the twentieth century.[7] In women, for reasons not fully understood, increases in age-specific death rates were much less marked.[8] The evidence suggests that early in the epidemic, rates of IHD were highest in the socioeconomically better off but moved across socioeconomic groups to produce the current picture, where the least well off have the highest rates.[9]

In Western industrialized countries, age-specific mortality rates from IHD began to fall from around 1970. Declines of between 20% and 50% occurred between 1965 and 1990. The precise reasons for these declines remain the subject of debate, but are likely to represent a combination of falls in levels of risk factors and improvements in clinical care. Most estimates suggest that half or a little more of the decline can be attributed to trends in the major risk factors (smoking, dyslipidaemia and high blood pressure), and most of the rest to improvements in both the effectiveness and uptake of clinical care (particularly drug treatments for secondary prevention).[10–12]

In the former socialist economies of Russia and Eastern Europe, recent trends have been somewhat different, with rising age-specific death rates from these and other conditions in adults

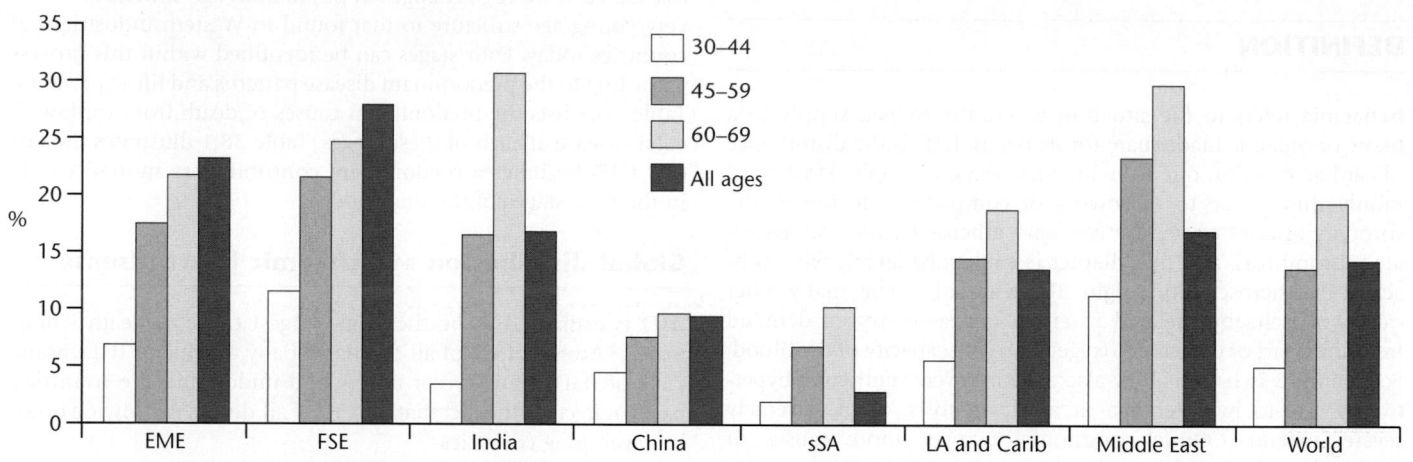

EME - established market economies; FSE - former socialist economies; sSA - sub Saharan Africa;
LA and Carib - Latin America and the Caribbean

Figure 38.2 Estimated percentage of deaths due to IHD in 2000 for men and women in different regions of the world. EME, established market economies; FSE, former socialist economies; sSA, sub-Saharan Africa; LA & Caribbean, Latin America and the Caribbean.[6]

Table 38.1 Deaths from cardiovascular disease (CVD) by stage of epidemiological transition[3]

Stage of transition	Deaths from CVD (%)	Main CVDs	Examples
Pestilence and famine	5–10	Rheumatic fever, infectious and nutritional cardiomyopathies	Sub-Saharan Africa, Rural India
Receding pandemics	10–35	As above + hypertensive heart disease and haemorrhagic stroke	China
Degenerative and human-made diseases	35–55	All stroke, IHD at relatively young ages	Urban India
Delayed degenerative diseases	<50	Ischaemic stroke and IHD at older ages	Western Europe, USA

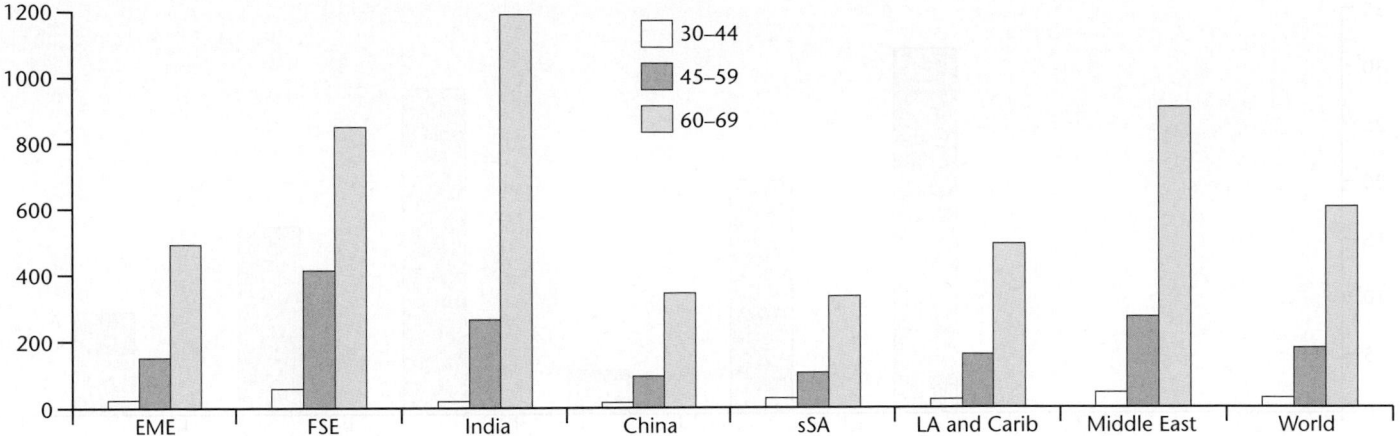

EME - established market economies; FSE - former socialist economies; sSA - sub Saharan Africa;

A LA and Carib - Latin America and the Caribbean

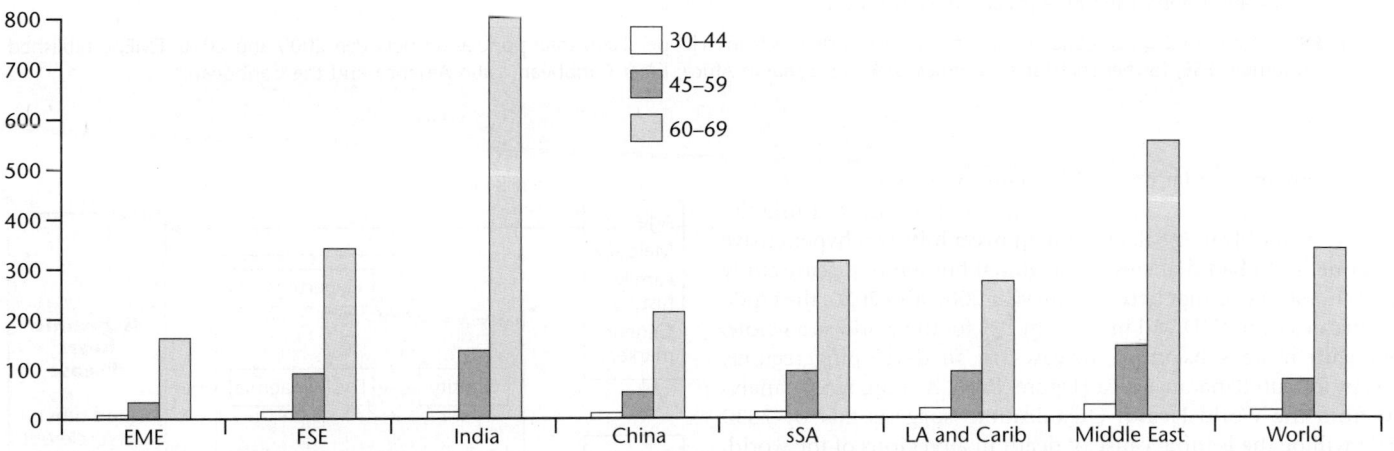

EME - established market economies; FSE - former socialist economies; sSA - sub Saharan Africa;

B LA and Carib - Latin America and the Caribbean

Figure 38.3   (A) Estimated annual age-specific death rates in men (per 100 000) from IHD in different world regions in 2000. (B) Estimated annual age-specific death rates in women (per 100 000) from IHD in different world regions in 2000. EME, established market economies; FSE, former socialist economies; sSA, sub-Saharan Africa; LA & Caribbean, Latin America and the Caribbean.[6]

during the 1980s.[13] This rise seemed to coincide with the end of the socialist system in these countries and may be related to increases in excessive alcohol consumption, falls in the consumption of fresh fruit and vegetables, and widening inequalities in income.[14] In some Eastern European countries, CHD mortality rates have now started to decline after peaking in the early 1990s (1990–94), (by about 3% per year in Poland, 2% per year in Hungary, and 5% per year in the Baltic states).[15] But in other countries, particularly in Russia, they remain very high, especially among males from lower socioeconomic groups. Some, but not all, of this high mortality rate may be related to alcohol consumption.[16]

Trends in 'developing' regions

The lack of good quality data means that trends in developing regions are often based on the earlier experience of developed regions. It is a safe prediction that crude IHD rates (e.g. per 1000 total population per year) will increase substantially over the coming years as the population age structure of developing regions grows older.[17] It also seems a safe prediction that in many – probably most – developing nations age-specific IHD rates will increase as the proportion of the population living in urban rather than rural areas increases. There are data from several developing regions, including India[17] and sub-Saharan Africa,[18] that demonstrate marked differences in IHD risk factor levels between rural and urban populations. Thus traditional rural lifestyles in developing countries tend to be associated with low levels of IHD risk factors (see below), with high complex carbohydrate diets, high levels of physical activity, and low levels of dyslipidaemia, obesity, hypertension and diabetes. In contrast, urban living is associated with high rates of obesity, physical inactivity, saturated fat intake, smoking, alcohol intake, dyslipidaemia, hypertension and diabetes. A recent study from Beijing showed a 50% increase in age-specific CHD mortality in men, and a 27% increase in women between 1984 and 1999; most of this increase was explained by considerable rises in total cholesterol levels and diabetes (reflecting substantial changes in traditional Beijing diets).[19]

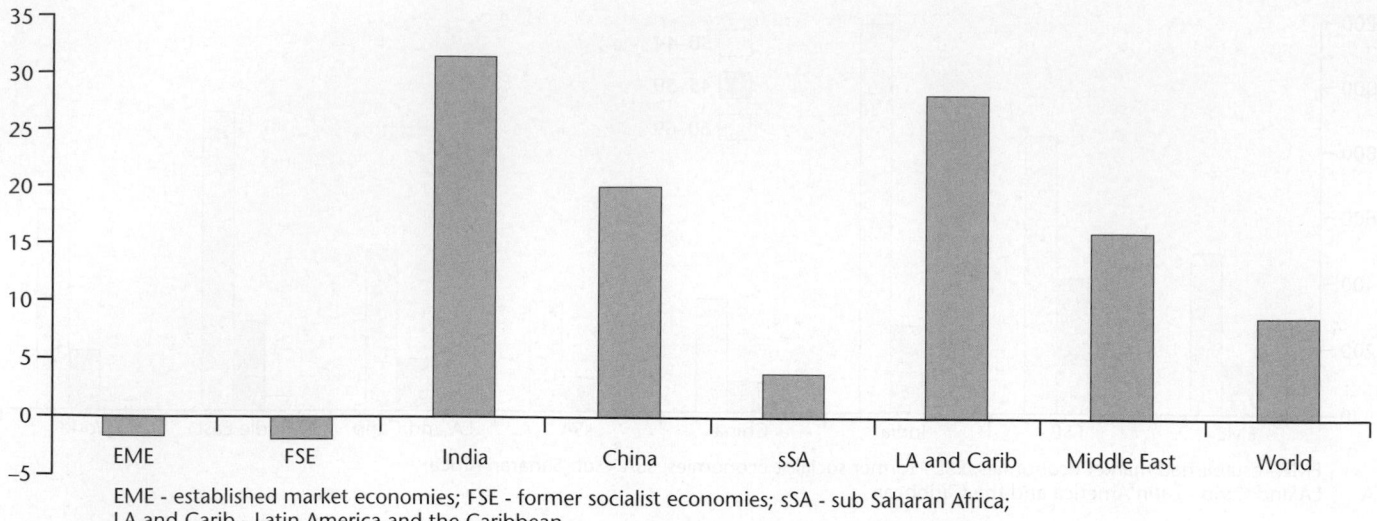

EME - established market economies; FSE - former socialist economies; sSA - sub Saharan Africa; LA and Carib - Latin America and the Caribbean

Figure 38.4 Estimated percentage change in number of deaths from IHD per 1000 total population between 2000 and 2020. EME, established market economies; FSE, former socialist economies; sSA, sub-Saharan Africa; LA & Caribbean, Latin America and the Caribbean.[6]

Contrary to popular perception, high levels of these risk factors are not limited to the urban wealthy. For example, in a middle-income area of Dar es Salaam, one in five adults was hypertensive and one in 20 had diabetes.[20] The global burden of disease study of 1996 estimated that between the year 2000 and 2020, the crude death rates from IHD will increase by 9% for the world as a whole, but with more substantial increases in all developing regions, except for sub-Saharan Africa (Figure 38.4). A more recent analysis from the World Health Organization[1] suggests that by 2030 IHD will be the leading cause of death in all regions of the world, including low income countries, and account for between 13% (low income countries) and 16% of all deaths (high income countries).

RISK FACTORS FOR ISCHAEMIC HEART DISEASE

A risk factor for ischaemic heart disease is simply an attribute or exposure that is associated with an increased probability of either having or developing the disease. More than 250 possible cardiovascular risk factors have been identified. However, a much smaller number has been shown consistently to be important (Figure 38.5).[21–24] Most risk factor studies have been carried out in developed countries, but the recent INTERHEART study (a case-control study of first myocardial infarction) took place globally in 52 countries throughout Asia, Europe, the Middle East, Africa, Australia, and North and South America.[25] The results were similar across the world, and suggested that about 90% of first heart attacks (myocardial infarction) can be attributed to nine risk factors, including cigarette smoking, an abnormal ratio of blood lipids, high blood pressure, diabetes, abdominal obesity, stress, a lack of daily consumption of fruits and vegetables, as well as a lack of daily exercise.

Risk factors are often grouped simply into those that cannot be changed (unmodifiable) and those that can be changed (modifi-

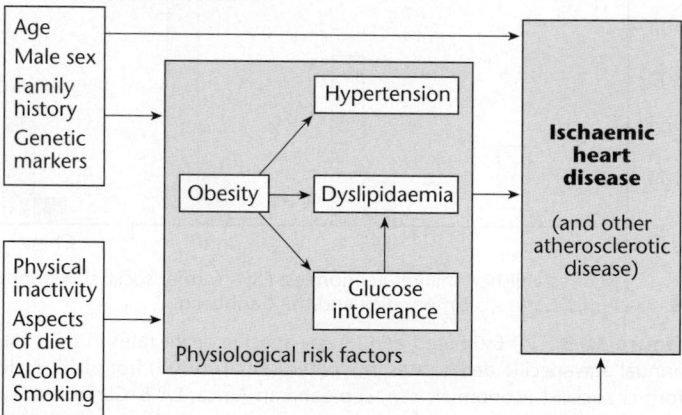

Figure 38.5 Established risk factors for ischaemic heart disease and their interrelationships.[3] See text for details.

able), and are thus of potential importance for the prevention of IHD. The major risk factors under these headings are described below.

Unmodifiable risk factors

Unmodifiable risk factors include increasing age, male sex, strong family history of IHD and genetic markers.

Age and sex

Death rates from IHD tend to increase exponentially with age in populations with both low and high rates of IHD. Rates are higher in men than in women in all populations. Below the age of 50 years, rates tend to be 4–5-fold higher in men compared with women. With increasing age above 50 years, rates in women approach but never reach those of men. This pattern of male to female rates is thought by most researchers to reflect premenopausal protective effects of oestrogen, mediated at least partly through higher levels of high density lipoprotein (HDL) cholesterol (see below), and the loss of these effects following the menopause.

Family history and genetic markers

A strong family history of IHD, often measured as a history of IHD in a first-degree relative below the age of 60 years, is associated with an increased risk over and above the effect of shared risk factors between family members. In the Framingham study, for example, such a family history was associated with a 30% increased risk independent of other risk factors.[23] At the time of writing, a limited number of genetic markers has been associated with an increased risk of IHD and it seems likely that the number will increase rapidly with the increasing use of genome wide association studies.[26] Two recent publications based on genome wide approaches have suggested that a region of chromosome 9 (p21) is associated with the risk of IHD and myocardial infarction.[26,27] However, in a disease as complex as IHD it is likely that a large number of genetic markers, for example reflecting aspects of such areas as lipid metabolism, blood pressure control and endothelial function, will be identified.

Modifiable risk factors

High total or low density lipoprotein (LDL) cholesterol (particularly when associated with low HDL cholesterol), high blood pressure and smoking have been shown to be the most important modifiable risk factors in most populations. Diabetes and lesser forms of glucose intolerance are also discussed here.

Dyslipidaemia

Total serum cholesterol concentration is strongly related to differences in IHD rates between and within populations. There is a strong and continuous relationship, for example, between the average serum cholesterol level in a population and that population's rate of IHD.[28] Within a population there is a strong and continuous relationship between an individual's cholesterol level and their risk of developing IHD. Total cholesterol is made up of several components, the most important of which are LDL and HDL cholesterol. The main atherogenic component of total cholesterol is LDL cholesterol, which is made particularly atherogenic through oxidation (see the section on pathogenesis). HDL cholesterol is independently related to a reduced risk of IHD. This is thought to be through its role in removing cholesterol from the tissues, including the arterial wall, and returning it to the liver. The single most predictive measures of dyslipidaemia that were found in the Framingham study are the ratios of LDL cholesterol:HDL cholesterol or of total cholesterol:HDL cholesterol. For example, a total HDL cholesterol ratio of 9.6 is associated with double the rate of IHD compared with a ratio of 5.0, which is associated with double the rate compared with a ratio of 3.4.[23] There is now substantial randomized controlled trial evidence of the benefits of lowering total or LDL cholesterol levels by means of pharmacological agents. The strongest evidence is for

the use of hydroxymethylglutaryl coenzyme A (HMG CoA) reductase inhibitors, the statins. These are highly effective at lowering total and LDL cholesterol levels, and several randomized controlled trials have found that they reduce coronary events by around one-third.[29] However, it is possible that not all of this effect is due to lowering LDL cholesterol levels, as intermediates of cholesterol synthesis are involved in the regulation of several functions, including the inflammatory response, which may also be important.[30]

Blood pressure

Raised blood pressure is a strong and independent risk factor for IHD. Prospective data on over 350 000 men in the USA, screened as part of the Multiple Risk Factor Intervention Trial (MRFIT),[31] demonstrated a continuous positive relationship between diastolic blood pressure from a level of 75 mmHg. With systolic blood pressure there was evidence of a plateau below 120 mmHg and a continuous positive relationship with IHD incidence above this. These and similar data suggest that a 5–6 mmHg reduction in diastolic blood pressure should lead to a 20–25% reduction in IHD events. A meta-analysis of 14 randomized controlled trials of blood pressure lowering, involving 37 000 individuals with diastolic hypertension, demonstrated a significant reduction in IHD events of around 14% in those receiving treatment.[32] The difference between this and the predicted value may reflect some unwanted effects of antihypertensive agents on lipid and glucose metabolism.

Left ventricular hypertrophy, often a consequence of prolonged hypertension, is also a risk factor for IHD events. Left ventricular hypertrophy is also associated with diabetes and obesity, and participants in the Framingham study with either electrocardiographic or echocardiographic evidence of this condition were at two to three times the risk of IHD.[23]

Smoking

There is overwhelming evidence for a causal role of cigarette smoking in IHD. Both the duration of smoking and the amount of tobacco smoked daily are directly related to the risk of IHD events. The relative risk associated with smoking varies by age, being highest in younger adults. For example, in a study of over 30 000 male British physicians, the risk of IHD death in those smoking ≥25 cigarettes a day was 15 times higher than in non-smokers. However, the risk was twice as high in those aged 55–64 years. Across all age groups, smokers of >25 cigarettes a day were 40% more likely to die from IHD than non-smokers.[33] Because smoking is common, it contributes substantially to IHD event rates. For example, smoking is estimated to be responsible for between one-sixth and one-fifth of all IHD deaths in North America and Britain, respectively.[34]

Although randomized controlled trial evidence is not available on the benefits of smoking cessation (apart from the practical difficulties, such a study would now be ethically unacceptable), there are many 'natural experiments' where people who stop smoking have been followed over time. For example, people who stop smoking after a myocardial infarction have around a 40% reduction in death rate compared with those who continue smoking.[35]

Diabetes and glucose intolerance

In the vast majority of populations studied, the incidence of IHD is higher in people with diabetes than in those without. In men it is roughly twice as high, and in women three times as high at all ages. The relative advantage in IHD rates that women have over men is lost in people with diabetes.[36] Some, but not all,[37] of the excess IHD incidence in people with diabetes is accounted for by higher levels of other risk factors, particularly dyslipidaemia and high blood pressure. Lesser forms of glucose intolerance, such as impaired glucose tolerance, are also associated with higher rates of IHD. Pooled prospective data from Europe with over 20 000 participants demonstrate that impaired glucose tolerance predicts IHD mortality independently of other major cardiovascular risk factors.[38]

Obesity, aspects of lifestyle and cardiovascular risk

Obesity and certain aspects of lifestyle, such as physical inactivity, alcohol consumption and aspects of diet, are risk factors for cardiovascular disease. Much of the effect of these is through their influence on the risk factors described above. For example, obesity is related to dyslipidaemia, particularly low HDL cholesterol and raised triglyceride levels, glucose intolerance, raised blood pressure and insulin resistance (a group of disorders referred to as the 'metabolic syndrome').[39] Physical inactivity is related to a similar group of disorders.[40] At a population level, the saturated fat content of the diet is the most important determinant of mean population total and LDL cholesterol levels. In individuals the relationship between saturated fat content and cholesterol concentration is less clear. This is probably because at the individual level dietary intake interacts with several different genetic factors to determine cholesterol level. There is evidence that other aspects of diet, such as fresh fruit and vegetable content, are also likely to be important in determining the risk of IHD. Likely mechanisms include the role of antioxidants in protecting against the oxidation of LDL cholesterol (see Pathogenesis below) and the beneficial effects of potassium, and the detrimental effects of sodium, on blood pressure. The protective effects of moderate alcohol consumption, around 2 units/day, on IHD in populations at high risk of the condition are well documented. At least part of this benefit is through the effect of alcohol on raising HDL cholesterol levels. An important caveat to the protective effects of alcohol is that these are associated with regular drinking, and that heavy binge drinking may have quite the opposite impact on cardiovascular outcomes.[41]

The interactive nature of risk factors

As would be expected, the greater the number of risk factors an individual possesses the higher is the probability of an IHD event, such as sudden death, myocardial infarction or the development of angina. The risk associated with a combination of risk factors is often greater than simply adding the risk associated with the individual risk factors together: it tends to be multiplicative. This is illustrated in Figure 38.6, which is based on a risk prediction formula from the Framingham study.[23] The figure shows how the risk of developing IHD in a 50-year-old man currently without

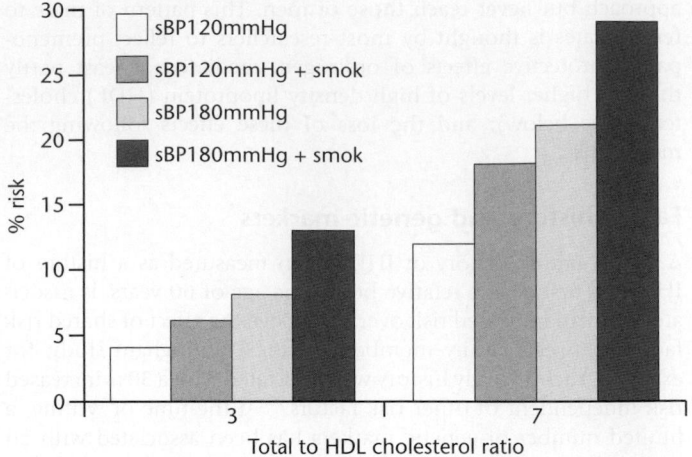

Figure 38.6 Risk of IHD over 10 years in a 50-year-old man with different levels of total to HDL cholesterol ratio, systolic blood pressure, and smoking status. See text for details.

IHD varies over seven-fold with different levels of the three main modifiable risk factors. Several scoring systems have been derived to provide an estimate of the risk of IHD within individuals based on their risk factor levels. Factors that are usually taken into account include age, sex, presence or absence of diabetes, blood pressure level, smoking status, and total:HDL cholesterol ratio. Such scoring systems are being promoted as aids to decision-making, for example to help determine who should receive lipid- or blood pressure-lowering medication, with the decision based on 'overall' or absolute risk of cardiovascular disease (expressed, for example as a percentage over the subsequent 10 years), rather than simply on high levels of one or more risk factors, and only on IHD, as in the past. A limitation of these systems is that they tend to be based on data from high-risk populations of European origin (in the past, the majority were based on data from one study, the Framingham study). There is evidence that the level of risk associated with both individual factors and combinations of factors varies between populations, depending both on their overall level of risk and the influence of less well understood IHD risk factors.[42-45] New scoring systems have recently been derived, including HEARTSCORE (based on a large European database of almost 3 million person-years of observation followed for almost 10 years with >7000 fatal cardiovascular events as an endpoint),[46] the Reynolds Risk score (designed specifically for women),[47] and ASSIGN (based on data from Scotland, including explicitly the effects of socio-economic deprivation on risk).[45] The Asia Pacific Studies Collaboration has also recently recalibrated a 'limited-information' version of the Framingham equations (which requires data only on age, systolic blood pressure, cholesterol and smoking status), for use in a low risk Asian population, and compared its performance with risk equations based on local (Chinese) cohorts. Both sets of equations discriminated cardiovascular risk well in Chinese cohorts.[48] Hence, there are now scoring systems more appropriate for both higher and lower incidence Western populations, and Asian populations, although the latter have not yet been widely used.

The 'only 50%' explanatory power of the major IHD risk factors

It is commonly stated that the major IHD risk factors described above can explain only about half the variation in IHD incidence.[7] In other words, within a population only about half the cases of IHD can be predicted by the above risk factors. Or, when comparing populations with different IHD rates, such as different socio-economic groups, only about half the difference in rates appears to be due to differences in smoking, lipid levels, blood pressure and diabetes. The 'only 50%' explanatory power has recently been challenged from several sources. A very large cohort study from the US found that non-smoking individuals with low blood pressure and low total cholesterol level had one-fifth or less the incidence of IHD compared with the rest.[44] Further, it is important to realize that both imprecision in measurement of a risk factor, and variation in measurement over time in the same individual can underestimate the importance of a risk factor (regression dilution bias). Analysis of data from the British Regional Heart Study has suggested that just three major risk factors (cigarette smoking, blood pressure, serum cholesterol) can account for 80% of variation in the risk of CHD events, after adjusting for this bias.[49] Nonetheless, the apparent inability of the major risk factors to explain much more than 50% of variation in IHD incidence has led to a huge research effort to identify other risk factors that may improve our ability to predict IHD. There is a very long list of putative risk factors under investigation.[24] The list includes new putative atherogenic factors, such as homocysteine. Clinical homocysteinuria is associated with very premature IHD, but epidemiological evidence suggests that levels of homocysteine within the general population are also related to increased risk of IHD, and that this risk is reduced by intake of vitamin B_{12} and folate, vitamins that promote the metabolism of homocysteine. Thrombogenic risk markers under investigation include fibrinogen, factor VII and plasminogen activator inhibitor. Markers and promoters of inflammation are also of interest and include C-reactive protein and interleukin 6, with the possibility that certain infections, such as Chlamydia pneumoniae, may increase the risk of atherosclerosis. Finally, a quite different category of risk markers that are being investigated are psychosocial stressors, such as psychological traits, working environment and social support. There is good observational evidence that some of these are associated with IHD risk,[50] although the biological mechanisms for such effects remain to be elucidated. The relative importance of each of most of these 'newer' risk factors is currently unclear.

Ethnic group differences in IHD risk factors

The associations between IHD and the major modifiable risk factors described above have been demonstrated in a wide variety of populations, whether defined by ethnic group or by geography. This has been confirmed by a recent collaboration, the Asia–Pacific Cohort study, which has carried out individual patient data meta-analysis from cohort studies (over 40) in the Asia-Pacific region to provide robust evidence about determinants of stroke, coronary heart disease and other common causes of death. Results have generally been very consistent between Asian and Pacific cohorts, and with studies elsewhere in the world. For example, they recently confirmed that smoking is a risk factor for IHD and stroke, independent of other confounders (such as BMI, blood pressure, and cholesterol levels) in Asia. The was no difference between Asian and Caucasian populations (in Australia and New Zealand), and the risk reduction on quitting was similar.[51]

In this respect, the evidence suggests that ethnic groups are much more alike than different in terms of the causes of IHD. Analyses of the predictive power of risk factors have found some differences between groups, for example between southern and northern European populations,[43] or between Japanese and white populations in the USA. Thus, for example, an analysis suggested that the risk prediction formula used to produce Figure 38.6 applies equally well to African and white Americans. However, some modification is needed to account for underlying differences in the prevalence of risk factors and the overall IHD rates before the formula can be applied to Japanese and native American groups.[42] The reasons for differences between ethnic groups are likely to be complex. Possible explanations include differences in exposures to lifestyle and environmental factors mediated by geography, socioeconomic status and culture. Differences in genetic background leading to differences in gene–environment interactions may also be important.

Migrant populations whose ancestral origins are from the Indian subcontinent suffer from particularly high rates of IHD compared with indigenous populations.[52] As with other groups, the major modifiable risk factors are important, but they do not appear to account for the higher rates of IHD,[53] and other factors have been suggested, including a higher prevalence of insulin resistance and metabolic syndrome.[54]

PATHOGENESIS OF ATHEROSCLEROSIS AND ISCHAEMIC HEART DISEASE

Atherosclerosis is a patchy, nodular type of arteriosclerosis (thickening and hardening of the arterial wall) that occurs mainly in large and medium-sized elastic and muscular arteries. It is characterized by lipid accumulation, hyperplasia and scarring in the arterial intima. These are reflected in the derivation of the term atherosclerosis, which comes from the Greek words 'athero' (meaning gruel or paste) and 'sclerosis' (hardness).

Atherosclerosis underlies the vast majority of ischaemic vascular disease, including IHD. Its major complications are myocardial, cerebral and peripheral (particularly lower limb) ischaemia and infarction. A broad spectrum of clinical disease is associated with atherosclerotic lesions in the coronary arteries. For example, atherosclerotic lesions may be silent and not give rise to any symptoms or signs. They may gradually lead to narrowing of a coronary artery giving rise to stable angina, or their surface may be disrupted leading to thrombus formation and the acute coronary syndromes of unstable angina and myocardial infarction. The evolution and behaviour of atherosclerotic lesions and their relationship to clinical disease are considered below.

Morphology and classification of atherosclerotic lesions

At the beginning of the twentieth century, two types of intimal lesion were recognized and associated with atherosclerosis. These

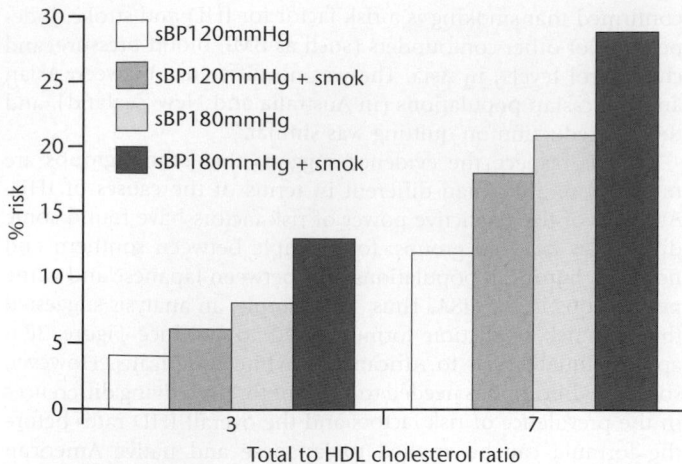

Figure 38.7 Types of atherosclerotic lesion.[56]

were the fatty streak (a thin lipid deposit in the intima in children) and the fibrous plaque (a thick lipid and fibrous lesion in adults). At this time it was not universally accepted that these two lesions were the early and advanced expressions of a single disease. By the 1950s, however, a classification that consisted of the sequence fatty streak, fibrous plaque and complicated lesion was widely used. The term 'complicated lesion' was used for a fibrous plaque that contained a haemorrhage or had ulcerated or fissured with associated thrombosis. The World Health Organization's classification, published in 1958, added the term 'atheroma' to these three terms.[55] This was added to distinguish advanced lesions with a predominantly lipid component (atheroma) from those with a predominantly collagenous component (fibrous plaque). More recently, the American Heart Association (AHA) reviewed the classification of lesions and using the latest available histological evidence proposed a classification based on six main types of lesion.[56,57] The classification essentially incorporates both the type and sequence of lesions described in previous classifications (Figure 38.7). Types I and II are early lesions and include the fatty streak. Types IV–VI are advanced lesions and include atheroma through to complicated lesions. Type III represents the transitory phase between early and advanced lesions.

Pathogenesis of atherosclerotic lesions

Exactly how atherosclerosis begins and evolves, and what factors drive and determine the direction of this whole process, is not fully known. However, any description of its pathogenesis must be able to account for the fact that lesions are not uniformly distributed throughout the arterial tree. Whether in human populations with a high or low incidence of atherosclerotic disease, or in animal models of atherosclerosis, the distribution of lesions is highly characteristic. They occur predominantly at bifurcation points and bends of the arteries. The 'response to injury hypothesis' suggests that endothelial and other cells within the arterial wall actively respond to a range of potential insults in a way that initiates and may promote the atherosclerotic process. One source of 'injury' is haemodynamic forces, and at arterial bifurcation points and bends there are low shear forces and turbulent blood

flow. In such regions there is increased residence time for circulating blood constituents, some of which may also be causes of injury.[58] In these regions, endothelial cells alter their normal homeostatic properties leading to increased adhesiveness for monocytes, T lymphocytes and platelets, and increased permeability to lipids. Their responses include the formation of vasoactive molecules, adhesion molecules, cytokines and growth factors. Such responses will be increased and sustained by the presence of other causes of injury and insult to the endothelium. These may include raised and modified LDL cholesterol levels, free radicals caused by cigarette smoking, hypertension and diabetes mellitus, raised plasma homocysteine concentrations and infectious microorganisms such as herpes viruses or *Chlamydia pneumoniae*.

Type 1 and type 2 atherosclerotic lesions (Figure 38.7) occur in all human populations studied, including those with a low incidence of IHD. These lesions, therefore, appear to represent a controlled, limited and universal inflammatory response to certain haemodynamic forces. The development of more advanced lesions seems to be dependent upon greater and continuing stimulation of this response.[59] Particularly central to this is the accumulation, within the arterial intima, of LDL cholesterol that has been mildly oxidized (oxLDL) when crossing the endothelial cell, and may be further modified within the intima. Accumulation of oxLDL acts as an attractant for monocytes and promotes their conversion to macrophages. Macrophages ingesting large amounts of oxLDL become foam cells. In addition, continuing inflammation sees migration, probably from the arterial media, and proliferation of smooth muscle cells. Smooth muscle cells are found in two main phenotypes: those of the contractile type, which are rich in myofilaments, and those of the synthetic type (derived from the contractile type in response to stimuli associated with injury), which are rich in rough endoplasmic reticulum. The synthetic phenotype of smooth muscle cells responds to various growth factors and secretes extracellular matrix components including collagen.

The lipid core of type IV lesions contains cholesterol and its esters,[57] some in crystalline form, and includes debris from macrophage and foam cell death. The lipid core is surrounded by macrophages. These are highly activated inflammatory cells, producing cell mediators such as tumour necrosis factor α, interleukins and metalloproteinases (connective tissue matrix degrading enzymes).[59] The connective tissue capsule surrounding the lipid core consists of collagen and matrix synthesized by smooth muscle cells, and as the size of the capsule increases and a fibrous cap clearly develops the lesion can be classified as a type V lesion.

Ulceration or fissuring of the fibrous cap is the precursor of complicated (type VI) lesions in which thrombus formation occurs (Figure 38.7). Highly activated macrophages are involved in both ulceration and fissuring. Ulceration is due to endothelial denudation exposing subendothelial connective tissue on which thrombus forms. Fissuring exposes the highly thrombogenic lipid core of the plaque. Thrombus forms initially within the plaque and may then extend into the arterial lumen.[60]

Relationship between coronary atherosclerosis and presentation of IHD

Clinically overt IHD is largely associated with type IV-type VI lesions.[57] Reduction in the diameter of the coronary artery by an atherosclerotic lesion can lead to ischaemia when the demands for blood supply through that artery are increased (e.g. by physical activity or emotion). Chronic stable angina and stable silent ischaemia (ischaemia without classical symptoms and detected through electrocardiography) are the clinical outcomes of this situation. Interestingly even large stable atherosclerotic lesions may not lead to symptoms. This is because much of the initial growth of the lesion occurs outwards, producing a bulging and remodelling of the arterial wall and leaving the cross-sectional area of the lumen untouched. Narrowing of the lumen starts to occur only when the lesion occupies >40% of the circumference.[61] Even then, the narrowing needs to be 50% or more before blood flow starts to decrease. One of the implications of these facts is that a coronary artery that appears normal on coronary arteriography may nonetheless be substantially diseased and, although not currently producing symptoms, may threaten an acute coronary syndrome (myocardial infarction or unstable angina).

Myocardial infarction and unstable angina arise from complicated (type VI) lesions. Thrombus formation, in response to plaque rupture or erosion of its surface, may occlude the lumen of the artery and thus lead to infarction of the heart muscle supplied by that artery. Unstable angina is associated with thrombus formation that neither fully occludes the artery nor fully resolves.[60] The thrombus thus severely restricts blood flow, producing symptoms without causing infarction.

CLINICAL SYNDROMES OF ISCHAEMIC HEART DISEASE

Classification and presentation of IHD

IHD can present in several ways. Figure 38.8 provides a classification based on how people with IHD may first come to the attention of clinicians. It is important to note that the categories are not mutually exclusive. For example, someone may present with the symptoms of myocardial infarction and cardiac insufficiency, and be subject to dysrhythmias. Similarly, once IHD has become manifest, an individual may through the course of the disease experience several of the categories shown in Figure 38.8. For example, they may be diagnosed with angina, suffer from episodes of silent ischaemia, be prone to dysrhythmias because of ischaemic damage to the conducting system of the heart, and develop cardiac insufficiency (heart failure) through accumulated ischaemic damage to the cardiac muscle.

Figure 38.9 shows the presentation of new cases of IHD in the Framingham study. In this cohort the first indication of IHD in around 15% of men and women was death as a result of the condition, with two-thirds of these deaths occurring within 1 h of the onset of symptoms (the definition of 'sudden death'). Women more commonly presented with angina than men, with a small proportion presenting with unstable rather stable angina. One-third of myocardial infarctions in men, and almost half in women, were unrecognized at the time (many presumably because they were painless) and picked up later by electrocardiographic changes.

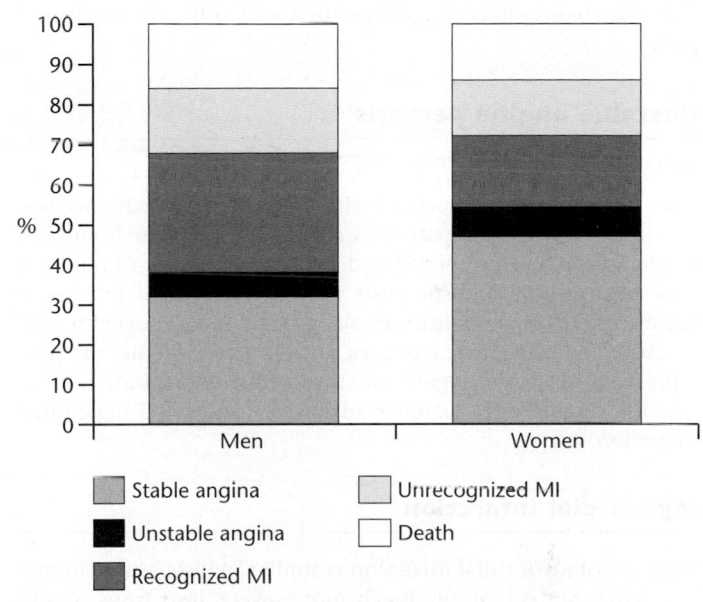

Figure 38.9 Presentation of new cases of IHD in men and women in the Framingham study.

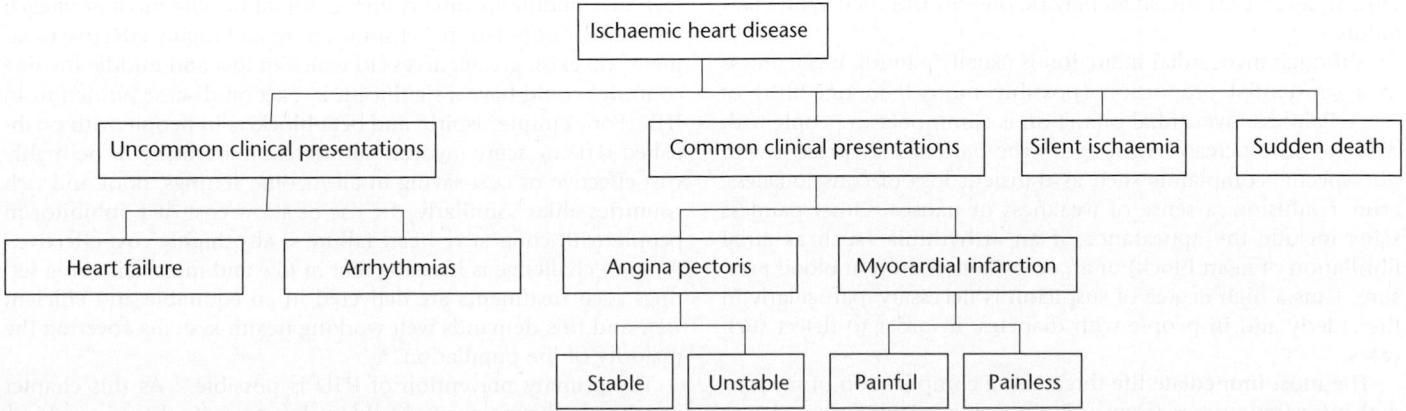

Figure 38.8 A classification of ischaemic heart disease based on its clinical presentation.

Stable or classical angina pectoris

The pain of stable angina pectoris is brought on by an increase in cardiac workload. Examples of activities that can result in angina include physical exertion, such as walking up hill, carrying a heavy load, emotion, eating a heavy meal or cold weather. The site of pain of angina pectoris is typically mid-sternal with radiation to the left arm. It may also radiate to the angle of the jaw and through to the back. It is usually described as a 'gripping' or 'tight' pain. Patients may describe it as like having a tight band around their chest. However, in some cases the pain is little more than a dull ache, and this may be felt only in the arm or jaw and not necessarily in the chest.

The pain of angina is typically relieved rapidly by rest. Thus, usually within 2 min or so of stopping exertion, the pain has gone. Another factor that should lead to rapid relief of the pain is the use of nitroglycerine tablets or spray (applied under the tongue). Indeed nitroglycerine is sometimes used to assist with diagnosis and to help distinguish angina pectoris from other causes of chest pain.

Unstable angina pectoris

Unstable angina is often also called 'angina at rest'. This is anginal chest pain that is not associated with exertion and which can come on suddenly while the patient is at rest. It may range from brief single episodes to prolonged and repeated episodes. Clinically it may be difficult to distinguish from a myocardial infarction, requiring further investigations such as electrocardiography and measurement of cardiac enzymes to determine whether the pain represents 'unstable angina' or 'myocardial infarction'. Indeed, unstable angina often signifies advanced disease and impending infarction.

Myocardial infarction

The pain of myocardial infarction is similar in distribution to that of angina, but is typically much more severe, lasts from 30 min to several hours, and is not relieved by rest or nitroglycerine. Patients often describe it as a crushing pain, as though a heavy weight or person was sitting on their chest. Nausea, vomiting and sweating may be present, especially at the start of the pain. With large infarcts, breathlessness may be present from left ventricular failure.

Although myocardial infarction is usually painful, it is painless in a substantial proportion (possibly more than one-fifth) of cases. Painless myocardial infarction is commoner in people with diabetes and increases with age.[62] The patient may present with non-specific complaints such as transient loss of consciousness, acute confusion, a sense of weakness or nausea. Other painless signs include the appearance of an arrhythmia (such as atrial fibrillation of heart block) or an unexplained drop in blood pressure. Thus a high degree of suspicion is necessary, particularly in the elderly and in people with diabetes, in order to detect such cases.

The most immediate life-threatening complication of myocardial infarction comes from arrhythmias, particularly ventricular fibrillation. Around 25–30% of people suffering a myocardial infarction die before they reach hospital, largely from ventricular fibrillation. This knowledge has led to great efforts in many countries both to reduce the time between the onset of symptoms and admission to hospital, and to make resuscitation equipment and people trained to use it more widely available in public places. Heart failure and clinical shock may ensue in the hours and days after large infarcts, with low blood pressure, low cardiac output and poor oxygenation of the blood. Other potential complications in the first few days include myocardial rupture, rupture of the interventricular septum, mitral regurgitation following damage to the papillary muscle, and systemic and pulmonary embolism. Typically a quarter of patients admitted to hospital with myocardial infarction die before discharge, although modern intensive therapy can reduce the mortality rate substantially.

Sudden cardiac death

By definition, 'sudden cardiac death' occurs within 1 h of the onset of symptoms. Sudden cardiac death is often associated with myocardial infarction leading to ventricular fibrillation, as described above. However, fatal arrhythmias may also occur in the absence of recent myocardial infarction, with a poorly functioning ventricle damaged by previous ischaemia being susceptible to arrhythmias including ventricular fibrillation.

Silent ischaemia

The widespread use of electrocardiography (ECG), including exercise ECG and continuous ambulatory monitoring, has identified people who have ECG evidence of ischaemia (S-T depression) on exertion but no symptoms. Such individuals are at an increased risk of coronary events, such as sudden death, myocardial infarction and clinical angina. Silent ischaemia is commoner in people with diabetes.

CONCLUSIONS AND CHALLENGES

This chapter aimed to provide a description of IHD, from its epidemiology to its pathogenesis. It has not aimed to cover treatment or prevention, although within these lie immense challenges, particularly in low- and middle-income countries. Much of the treatment given for IHD in richer countries is beyond the resources of low- and middle-income countries for all but the most privileged few of their population. Yet some cheap and highly effective treatments do exist, greater access to which in low and middle income countries could have a significant impact on disease burden from IHD. For example, aspirin and beta-blockers in people with established IHD or acute myocardial infarction are likely to be highly cost-effective or cost-saving in all income settings, poor and rich countries alike.[2] Similarly, the use of a low cost ACE inhibitor in people with congestive heart failure is also highly cost-effective.[2] A major challenge is insuring that in low and middle income settings such treatments are delivered in an equitable and efficient way, and this demands well working health systems covering the majority of the population.[63]

The primary prevention of IHD is possible.[64] As this chapter has shown, the major modifiable risk factors of tobacco smoking, high blood pressure, dyslipidaemia and glucose intolerance are consistent across different populations, and WHO has estimated that 80% of IHD is preventable based on current knowledge.[63] High blood pressure, dyslipidaemia and glucose intolerance arise from the common soil of an atherogenic diet (high in saturated fat and salt, low in fresh fruit and vegetables), physical inactivity and obesity. Methods appropriate to the cultural, social and economic contexts within each population will need to be developed and evaluated. Lessons should be learnt from the experience of population-based preventive measures in developed regions.[65,66] Approaches likely to be cost-effective in most contexts include broad-based policy and fiscal measures, particularly supporting tobacco control, the supply and marketing of certain food products and the design of environments and living arrangements conducive to physical activity.[63,67,68]

REFERENCES

1. Mathers CD, Loncar D. Projections of global mortality and burden of disease from 2002 to 2030. *PLoS Medicine/Public Library of Science* 2006; 3:e442.

2. Gaziano TA, Srinath Reddy K, Paccaud F, et al. Cardiovascular disease. In: Jamison DT, Breman JG, Measham AR, et al., eds. *Disease Control Priorities in Developing Countries*, 2nd edn. Washington/New York: World Bank/Oxford University Press; 2006:645–662.

3. Howson C, Reddy S, Ryan T, et al. *Control of Cardiovascular Diseases in Developing Countries. Research, Development and Institutional Strengthening.* Washington DC: National Academy Press; 1998.

4. Omran AR. The epidemiologic transition. A theory of the epidemiology of population change. *Milbank Memorial Fund Quarterly* 1971; 49:509–538.

5. World Health Organization. The World Health Report 2003. Geneva: WHO; 2003.

6. Murray C, Lopez A, Lopez A. *The Global Burden of Disease: a Comprehensive Assessment of Mortality and Disability from Diseases, Injuries, and Risk Factors in 1990 and Projected to 2020*, 1st edn. Geneva: World Health Organization; 1996.

7. Nieto FJ. Cardiovascular disease and risk factor epidemiology: a look back at the epidemic of the 20th century. *Am J Public Health* 1999; 89:292–294.

8. Lawlor D, Ebrahim S, Davey Smith G. Sex matters: secular and geographical trends in sex differences in coronary heart disease mortality. *BMJ* 2001; 323:541–545.

9. Marmot M. Coronary heart disease: the rise and fall of a modern epidemic. In: Marmot M, Elliott P, eds. *Coronary heart disease epidemiology: from aetiology to public health*. Oxford: Oxford University Press, 1992:3 19.

10. Capewell S, Morrison CE, McMurray JJ. Contribution of modern cardiovascular treatment and risk factor changes to the decline in coronary heart disease mortality in Scotland between 1975 and 1994. *Heart* 1999; 81:380–386.

11. Hunink MGM, Goldman L, Tosteson ANA, et al. The recent decline in mortality from coronary heart disease, 1980–1990. The effect of secular trends in risk factors and treatment. *JAMA* 1997; 277:535–542.

12. Vartiainen E, Puska P, Pekkanen J, et al. Changes in risk factors explain changes in mortality from ischaemic heart disease in Finland. *BMJ* 1994; 309V/94/E:23–27.

13. Chenet L, McKee M, Fulop N, et al. Changing life expectancy in central Europe: is there a single reason? *J Public Health Med* 1996; 18:329–336.

14. Ginter E. Cardiovascular risk factors in the former communist countries. Analysis of 40 European MONICA populations. *Eur J Epidemiol* 1995; 11:199–205.

15. Kesteloot H, Sans S, Kromhout D. Dynamics of cardiovascular and all-cause mortality in Western and Eastern Europe between 1970 and 2000. *Eur Heart J* 2006; 27:107–113.

16. Plavinski SL, Plavinskaya SI, Klimov AN. Social factors and increase in mortality in Russia in the 1990s: prospective cohort study. *BMJ* 2003; 326:1240–1242.

17. Reddy KS, Yusuf S. Emerging epidemic of cardiovascular disease in developing countries. *Circulation* 1998; 97:596–601.

18. Unwin N, Setel P, Rashid S, et al. Non-communicable diseases in sub-Saharan Africa: where do they feature in the health research agenda? *Bull World Health Organ* 2001; 79:947–953.

19. Critchley J, Liu J, Zhao D, et al. Explaining the increase in coronary heart disease mortality in Beijing between 1984 and 1999. *Circulation* 2004; 110:1236–1244.

20. Aspray TJ, Mugusi F, Rashid S, et al. Rural and urban differences in diabetes prevalence in Tanzania: the role of obesity, physical inactivity and urban living. *Trans R Soc Trop Med Hyg* 2000; 94:637–644.

21. Braunwald E. Shattuck lecture – cardiovascular medicine at the turn of the millennium: triumphs, concerns, and opportunities. *N Engl J Med* 1997; 337:1360–1369.

22. Gensini GF, Comeglio M, Colella A. Classical risk factors and emerging elements in the risk profile for coronary artery disease. *Eur Heart J* 1998; 19: A53–A61.

23. Kannel WB, Wilson PW. An update on coronary risk factors. *Med Clin North Am* 1995; 79:951–971.

24. Wood D, Force JEST. Established and emerging cardiovascular risk factors. *Am Heart J* 2001; 141(2 suppl):S49–S57.

25. Yusuf S, Hawken S, Ounpuu S, et al. Effect of potentially modifiable risk factors associated with myocardial infarction in 52 countries (the INTERHEART study). case control study. *Lancet* 2004; 364:937–952.

26. Psaty BM, Arnett D, Burke G. A new era of cardiovascular disease epidemiology. *JAMA* 2007; 298:2060–2062.

27. Topol EJ, Murray SS, Frazer KA. The genomics gold rush. *JAMA* 2007; 298:218–221.

28. Simons LA. Interrelations of lipids and lipoproteins with coronary artery disease mortality in 19 countries. *Am J Cardiol* 1986; 57:5G–10G.

29. LaRosa JC, He J, Vupputuri S. Effect of statins on risk of coronary disease. A meta-analysis of randomized controlled trials. *JAMA* 1999; 282:2340–2346.

30. Bellosta S, Ferri N, Bernini F, et al. Non-lipid-related effects of statins. *Ann Med* 2000; 32:164–176.

31. Neaton JD, Wentworth D. Serum cholesterol, blood pressure, cigarette smoking, and death from coronary heart disease. Overall findings and differences by age for 316,099 white men. Multiple Risk Factor Intervention Trial Research Group. *Arch Intern Med* 1992; 152:56–64.

32. Collins R, Peto R, MacMahon S, et al. Blood pressure, stroke, and coronary heart disease. Part 2, Short-term reductions in blood pressure: overview of randomised drug trials in their epidemiological context. *Lancet* 1990; 335:827–838.

33. Doll R, Peto R. Mortality in relation to smoking: 20 years' observations on male British doctors. *BMJ* 1976; 2:1525–1536.

34. Walters R, Whent H. *Health Update: Smoking*. London: Health Education Authority; 1996.

35. Critchley JA, Capewell S. Mortality risk reduction associated with smoking cessation in patients with coronary heart disease: a systematic review. *JAMA* 2003; 290:86–97.

36. Barrett-Connor EL, Cohn BA, Wingard DL, et al. Why is diabetes mellitus a stronger risk factor for fatal ischemic heart disease in women than in men? *JAMA* 1991; 265:627–630.

37. Haffner SM, Lehto S, Ronnemaa T, et al. Mortality from coronary heart disease in subjects with Type 2 diabetes and in nondiabetic subjects with and without prior myocardial infarction. *N Engl J Med* 1998; 339:229–234.

38. DECODE Study Group. Glucose tolerance and mortality: comparison of WHO and American Diabetes Association diagnostic criteria. The DECODE study group. European Diabetes Epidemiology Group. Diabetes epidemiology: collaborative analysis of diagnostic criteria in Europe. *Lancet* 1999; 354: 617–621.

39. Unwin N. The metabolic syndrome. *J R Soc Med* 2006; 99:457–462.

40. Whaley MH, Kampert JB, Kohl HW III, et al. Physical fitness and clustering of risk factors associated with the metabolic syndrome. *Med Sci Sports Exerc* 1999; 31:287–293.

41. Britton A, McKee M. The relation between alcohol and cardiovascular disease in Eastern Europe: explaining the paradox. *J Epidemiol Community Health* 2000; 54:328–332.

42. D'Agostino RB, Grundy S, Sullivan LM, et al.; CHD Risk Prediction Group. Validation of the Framingham coronary heart disease prediction scores: results of a multiple ethnic groups investigation. *JAMA* 2001; 286:180–187.

43. Menotti A, Lanti M, Puddu PE, et al. Coronary heart disease incidence in northern and southern European populations: a reanalysis of the seven countries study for a European coronary risk chart. *Heart* 2000; 84:238–244.

44. Stamler J, Stamler R, Neaton J, et al. Low risk-factor profile and long-term cardiovascular and noncardiovascular mortality and life expectancy: findings for 5 large cohorts of young adult and middle-aged men and women. *JAMA* 1999; 282:2012–2018.

45. Brindle PM, McConnachie A, Upton MN, et al. The accuracy of the Framingham risk-score in different socioeconomic groups: a prospective study. *Br Jf Gen Pract* 2005; 55:838–845.

46. De Backer G, Ambrosioni E, Borch-Johnsen K, et al. European guidelines on cardiovascular disease prevention in clinical practice. Third Joint Task Force of European and Other Societies on Cardiovascular Disease Prevention in Clinical Practice. *Eur Heart J* 2003; 24:1601–1610.

47. Ridker PM, Buring JE, Rifai N, et al. Development and validation of improved algorithms for the assessment of global cardiovascular risk in women: the Reynolds Risk Score. *JAMA* 2007; 297:611–619. [erratum *JAMA* 2007; 297:1433].

48. Asia Pacific Cohort Studies Collaboration, Barzi F, Patel A, Gu D, et al. Cardiovascular risk prediction tools for populations in Asia. *J Epidemiol Community Health* 2007; 61:115–121.

49. Emberson JR, Whincup PH, Morris RW, et al. Re-assessing the contribution of serum total cholesterol, blood pressure and cigarette smoking to the aetiology of coronary heart disease: impact of regression dilution bias. *Eur Heart J* 2003; 24:1719–1726.

50. Hemingway H, Marmot M. Psychosocial factors in the aetiology and prognosis of coronary heart disease: systematic review of prospective cohort studies. *BMJ* 1999; 318:1460–1467.

51. Woodward M, Lam TH, Barzi F, et al. Smoking, quitting, and the risk of cardiovascular disease among women and men in the Asia-Pacific region. *Int J Epidemiol* 2005; 34:1036–1045.

52. McKeigue PM, Miller GJ, Marmot MG. Coronary heart disease in south Asians overseas: a review. *J Clin Epidemiol* 1989; 42:597–609.

53. Lee J, Heng D, Chia KS, et al. Risk factors and incident coronary heart disease in Chinese, Malay and Asian Indian males: the Singapore Cardiovascular Cohort Study. *Int J Epidemiol* 2001; 30:983–988.

54. McKeigue PM, Shah B, Marmot MG. Relation of central obesity and insulin resistance with high diabetes prevalence and cardiovascular risk in South Asians. *Lancet* 1991; 337:382–386.

55. World Health Organization. Classification of Atherosclerotic Lesions: report of a Study Group. *WHO Technical Report Series*. Geneva: WHO; 1958.

56. Stary HC, Chandler AB, Glagov S, et al. A definition of initial, fatty streak, and intermediate lesions of atherosclerosis. A report from the Committee on Vascular Lesions of the Council on Arteriosclerosis, American Heart Association. *Circulation* 1994; 89:2462–2478.

57. Stary HC, Chandler AB, Dinsmore RE, et al. A definition of advanced types of atherosclerotic lesions and a histological classification of atherosclerosis. A report from the Committee on Vascular Lesions of the Council on Arteriosclerosis, American Heart Association. *Circulation* 1995; 92:1355–1374.

58. Gimbrone MAJ. Vascular endothelium, hemodynamic forces, and atherogenesis. *Am J Pathol* 1999; 155:1–5.

59. Ross R. Atherosclerosis – an inflammatory disease. *New Engl J Med* 1999; 340:115–126.

60. Davies MJ. The pathophysiology of acute coronary syndromes. *Heart* 2000; 83:361–366.

61. Glagov S, Weisenberg E, Zarins CK, et al. Compensatory enlargement of human atherosclerotic coronary arteries. *N Engl Jour Med* 1987; 316:1371–1375.

62. Vokonas PS, Kannel WB. Diabetes mellitus and coronary heart disease in the elderly. *Clin Geriatr Med* 1996; 12:69–78.

63. World Health Organization. Preventing chronic diseases: a vital investment: WHO global report. Geneva: WHO; 2005.

64. Lenfant C. Can we prevent cardiovascular diseases in low and middle income countries. *Bull World Health Organ* 2001; 79:980–987.

65. Ebrahim S, Davey Smith G. Exporting failure? Coronary heart disease and stroke in developing countries. *Int J Epidemiol* 2001; 30:201–205.

66. Nissinen A, Berrios X, Puska P. Community-based noncommunicable disease interventions: lessons from developed countries for developing ones. *Bull World Health Organ* 2001; 10:963–970.

67. Yach DM, Hawkes CP, Gould CLM, et al. The Global Burden of Chronic Diseases: Overcoming Impediments to Prevention and Control. *JAMA* 2004; 291:2616–2622.

68. Wipfli H, Stillman F, Tamplin S, et al. Achieving the Framework Convention on Tobacco Control's potential by investing in national capacity. *Tobacco Control* 2004; 13:433–437.

Chapter 39

Jane N. Zuckerman and Arie J. Zuckerman

Viral Hepatitis

Viral hepatitis is a major public health problem throughout the world affecting several hundreds of millions of people. Viral hepatitis is a cause of considerable morbidity and mortality in the human population, from both acute infection and chronic sequelae which include, with hepatitis B and hepatitis C infection, chronic active hepatitis, cirrhosis and primary liver cancer.

The hepatitis viruses include a range of unrelated and often unusual human pathogens:

- *Hepatitis A virus (HAV)*: a small unenveloped symmetrical RNA virus, which shares many of the characteristics of the picornavirus family. This virus has been classified in the hepatovirus genus, and is the cause of infectious or epidemic hepatitis transmitted by the faecal–oral route.
- *Hepatitis B virus (HBV)*: a member of the hepadnavirus group of double-stranded DNA viruses which replicate by reverse transcription. Hepatitis B virus is endemic in the human population and hyperendemic in many parts of the world.
- *Hepatitis C virus (HCV)*: an enveloped single-stranded RNA virus which appears to be distantly related (possibly in its evolution) to flaviviruses, although hepatitis C is not transmitted by arthropod vectors. Infection with this virus is common in many countries, and it is associated with chronic liver disease and also with primary liver cancer.
- *Hepatitis D virus (HDV)*: an unusual single-stranded circular RNA virus with a number of similarities to certain plant viral satellites and viroids. This virus requires hepadnavirus helper functions for propagation in hepatocytes, and is an important cause of acute and severe chronic liver damage in some regions of the world.
- *Hepatitis E virus (HEV)*: an enterically transmitted non-enveloped, single-stranded RNA virus which shares many biophysical and biochemical features with caliciviruses. Hepatitis E virus is an important cause of large epidemics of acute hepatitis in the subcontinent of India, central and South-east Asia, the Middle East, parts of Africa and elsewhere; this virus is responsible for high mortality during the third trimester of pregnancy.

HEPATITIS A

Outbreaks of jaundice have been described for many centuries and the term 'infectious hepatitis' was coined in 1912 to describe the epidemic form of the disease. HAV is spread by the faecal–oral route and is endemic throughout the world and hyperendemic in areas with poor standards of sanitation and hygiene. Common-source outbreaks are initiated most frequently by faecal contamination of food and water, and sporadic cases result from person-to-person contact. The seroprevalence of antibodies to HAV has declined since World War II in many industrialized countries. The exact incidence is difficult to estimate because of the high proportion of subclinical infections and infections without jaundice, differences in surveillance and differing patterns of disease. The extent of under-reporting is very high. Hepatitis A is recognized as an important travel-related infection in travellers from low prevalence areas to endemic countries.

The incubation period of hepatitis A is about 28 days. The virus replicates in the liver. Very large amounts of virus are shed in the faeces during the incubation period, before the onset of clinical symptoms and a brief period of viraemia occurs (Figure 39.1). The severity of illness ranges from asymptomatic to anicteric or icteric hepatitis and rarely fulminant hepatitis. The virus is non-cytopathic when grown in cell culture. Its pathogenicity in vivo, which involves necrosis of parenchymal cells and histiocytic periportal inflammation, may be mediated via the cellular immune response. By the time of onset of symptoms, excretion of virus in the faeces has declined and may have ceased and anti-HAV IgM, which is diagnostic of acute infection and appears late during the incubation period, increases in titre. Anti-HAV IgG may be detected 1–2 weeks later and persists for years. The virus does not persist and chronic excretion of HAV does not occur. There is no evidence of progression to chronic liver disease.[1]

Diagnostic tests are based mostly on enzyme-linked immunosorbent assays (ELISA).

Classification

Examination by electron microscopy of concentrates of filtered faecal extracts from patients during the incubation period reveals 27 nm unenveloped spherical particles typical of the Picornaviridae. The entire nucleotide sequence of the viral genome has been determined.

Comparison with other picornavirus sequences revealed limited homology to the enteroviruses or, indeed, the rhinoviruses; however, the structure and genome organization are typical of the

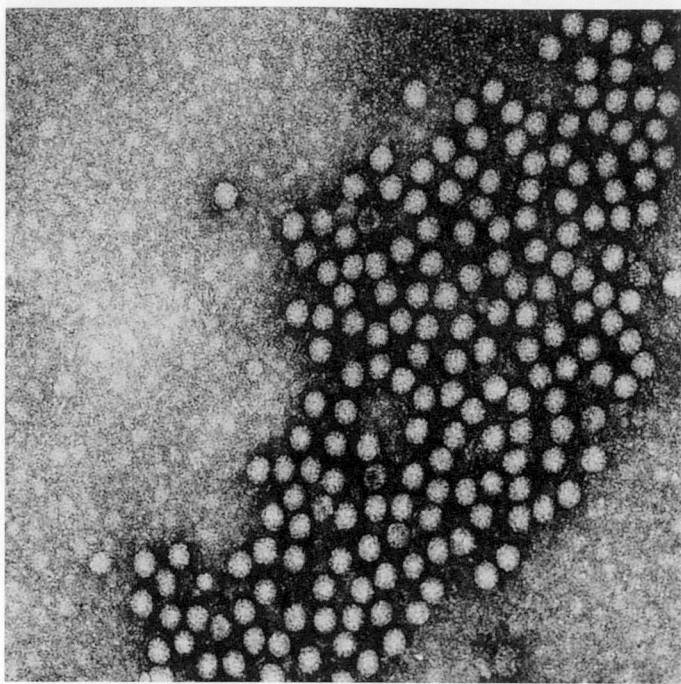

Figure 39.1 Electron micrograph showing the large number of hepatitis A virus particles in faeces during the incubation period of the infection. (Reduced from ×120 000. From a series by Anthea Thornton and A. J. Zuckerman.)

Picornaviridae. HAV is now considered as a separate genus (*Hepatovirus*) within the Picornaviridae as are the cardioviruses (of mice) and apthoviruses (foot and mouth disease viruses). There is one human serotype of HAV. Seven genotypes have been identified from wild-type strains, but all have a highly conserved single immunodominant epitope which generates neutralizing antibodies.

Organization of the HAV genome

The HAV genome comprises about 7500 nucleotides (nt) of positive sense RNA, which is polyadenylated at the 3′ end and has a polypeptide (VPg) attached to the 5′ end. A single, large open reading frame (ORF) occupies most of the genome and encodes a large polyprotein.

The viral polyprotein is processed to yield the structural (located at the amino terminal end) and non-structural viral polypeptides. Many of the features of replication of the picornaviruses have been deduced from studies of prototype enteroviruses and rhinoviruses, in particular poliovirus type 1. The virus replicates in the cytoplasm of hepatocytes.

HAV is stable at low pH and is resistant to degradation by environmental conditions.

Prevention and control of hepatitis A

Passive immunization

Control of hepatitis A infection is difficult. Since faecal shedding of the virus is at its highest during the late incubation period and the prodromal phase of the illness, strict isolation of cases is not a useful control measure. Spread of hepatitis A is reduced by simple hygienic measures and the sanitary disposal of excreta.

Normal human immunoglobulin, containing at least 100 IU/mL of anti-hepatitis A antibody, given intramuscularly before exposure to the virus or early during the incubation period, will prevent or attenuate a clinical illness. The dosage should be at least 2 IU anti-hepatitis A antibody/kg body weight, but in special cases, such as pregnancy or in patients with liver disease, that dosage may be doubled. Immunoglobulin does not always prevent infection and excretion of HAV, and inapparent or subclinical hepatitis may develop. The efficacy of passive immunization is based on the presence of hepatitis A antibody in the immunoglobulin, but the minimum titre of antibody required for protection has not yet been established. Immunoglobulin is used most commonly for close personal contacts of patients with hepatitis A and for those exposed to contaminated food. Immunoglobulin has also been used effectively for controlling outbreaks in institutions such as homes for the mentally handicapped and in nursery schools. Prophylaxis with immunoglobulin is recommended for persons without hepatitis A antibody visiting highly endemic areas. After a period of 6 months the administration of immunoglobulin for travellers should be repeated, unless it has been demonstrated that the recipient has developed his or her own hepatitis A antibodies. Active immunization (see below) is strongly recommended.

Active immunization: Hepatitis A vaccines

In areas of high prevalence most children have antibodies to HAV by the age of 3 years and such infections are generally asymptomatic. Infections acquired later in life are of increasing clinical severity. Less than 10% of cases of acute hepatitis A in children up to the age of 6 years are icteric but this increases to 40–50% in the 6–14 age group and to 70–80% in adults. Of 115 551 cases of hepatitis A in the USA between 1983 and 1987, only 9% of the cases, but more than 70% of the fatalities, were in those aged over 49. It is important, therefore, to protect those at risk because of personal contact with infected individuals or because of travel to highly endemic areas. Other groups at risk of hepatitis A infection include staff and residents of institutions for the mentally handicapped, day care centres for children, sexually active male homosexuals, intravenous narcotic drug abusers, sewage workers, healthcare workers, military personnel and members of certain low socioeconomic groups in defined community settings. Active immunization for travellers is strongly recommended. It is also recommended that food handlers should be immunized. In some developing countries the incidence of clinical hepatitis A is increasing as improvements in socioeconomic conditions result in infection later in life and strategies for immunization are yet to be agreed. Immunization against hepatitis A is also recommended for patients with chronic liver disease, and patients with chronic blood clotting disorders.

Hepatitis A vaccines

The foundations for a hepatitis A vaccine were laid in 1975 by the demonstration that formalin-inactivated virus extracted from the liver of experimentally infected marmosets induced protective antibodies in susceptible marmosets on challenge with live virus. Subsequently HAV was cultivated, after serial passage in marmosets, in a cloned line of fetal rhesus monkey kidney cells (FRhK6), thereby opening the way to the production of hepatitis A vaccines. Later it was demonstrated that prior adaptation in marmosets was not a prerequisite to growth of the virus in cell cultures and various strains of virus have been isolated directly from clinical material using several cell lines, including human diploid fibroblasts, and various techniques have been employed to increase the yield of virus in cell culture. The vaccines are inactivated, highly immunogenic and provide long-term protection against infection. Combined preparations of killed hepatitis A vaccines with hepatitis B vaccine and other vaccines are available or are under clinical trial. Combination vaccines are available: hepatitis A and B, hepatitis A and typhoid, and other polyvalent vaccines are under development.

HEPATITIS E

Retrospective testing of serum samples from patients involved in various epidemics of hepatitis associated with contamination of water supplies with human faeces led to the conclusion that an agent other than hepatitis A or hepatitis B was involved. Epidemics of enterically transmitted non-A, non-B hepatitis in the Indian subcontinent were first reported in 1980, but outbreaks involving tens of thousands of cases have also been documented in the former USSR, South-east Asia, northern Africa and Mexico. Infection has been reported in returning travellers. The average incubation period is longer than that for hepatitis A, with a mean of 6 weeks. The highest attack rates are found in young adults, and high mortality rates (up to 20%) have been reported in women in the third trimester of pregnancy.

Virus-like particles measuring 28–34 nm in diameter have been detected in faecal extracts of infected individuals by immune electron microscopy using convalescent serum. However, such studies have often proved inconclusive because a large proportion of the excreted virus may be degraded during passage through the gut. Cross-reaction studies between sera and virus in faeces associated with a variety of epidemics and other viral isolates in several different countries indicate that there are at least four major genotypes and phylogenetic and sequence analyses define at least nine different groups.

Studies on HEV have progressed following transmission to susceptible non-human primates. Man is the natural host of HEV.[2] A number of non-human primates such as chimpanzees, cynomolgus monkeys, rhesus monkeys, pigtail monkeys, owl monkeys, tamarins and African green monkeys are susceptible to natural (and experimental) infection with human strains of HEV. Swine strains have been identified and are able to infect humans. In endemic areas, antibodies to HEV acquired naturally have been found in 42–67% of domestic farm animals: cows, sheep and goats. In addition, there is evidence of widespread HEV or HEV-like infection in rodents in the USA, raising the possibility of reservoirs of HEV infection in industralized countries.

The problem of degradation of HEV in the gut was circumvented when the bile of infected monkeys was found to be a rich source of virus. This material permitted the molecular cloning of DNA complementary to the HEV (RNA) genome and the entire 7.5 kb sequence was determined. The organization of the genome is distinct from the Picornaviridae and the non-structural and structural polypeptides are encoded respectively at the 5' and 3' ends. HEV resembles the caliciviruses in the size and organization of its genome as well as in the size and morphology of the virion.

Laboratory tests

Sequencing of the HEV genome has resulted in the development of a number of specific diagnostic tests. For example, HEV RNA was detected, using the polymerase chain reaction (PCR), in faecal samples. An enzyme-linked immunosorbent assay (ELISA), which detects both IgG and IgM anti-HEV, has been developed using a recombinant HEV-glutathione-S-transferase fusion protein and used to detect antibodies in sporadic cases of infection in children and adults and during a number of epidemics. Epidemics are usually associated with warm weather and poor sanitation leading to faecal contamination of drinking water. Sporadic cases occur where HEV is endemic and also in Western countries in individuals without a history of travel to endemic countries.

Epidemiology

HEV is spread by the faecal-oral route. Consumption of drinking water contaminated with faecal material has led to epidemics, and the ingestion of raw or uncooked shellfish has caused sporadic infections and epidemics in endemic areas. The highest prevalence of infection occurs in regions with low standards of sanitation and non-chlorinated drinking water. The incubation period is 2–9 weeks, with an average of 6 weeks. Zoonotic spread of HEV appears likely, particularly from swine and possibly rodents. For example, although hepatitis E is not endemic in the USA and other developed countries, anti-HEV has been found in a significant proportion (up to 28% in some areas) of healthy persons in these countries. Subclinical infection might be the explanation. Infection in town dwellers might be caused by rodents. The prevalence of anti-HEV in blood donors (a highly selected sector of the population) in Central Europe and North America is 1.4–2.5%, in South Africa 1.4%, Thailand 2.8%, Saudi Arabia 9.5% and 24% in Egypt.

The prevalence of anti-HEV in endemic regions is 3–26%, which is much lower than expected, although HEV infections account for more than 50% of acute sporadic hepatitis in some highly endemic areas.

Virus is excreted from the liver via the bile duct into the intestine and faeces. Viraemia and shedding of HEV in the faeces reach a peak during the incubation period, and excretion in the faeces continues for up to 14 days after the onset of jaundice. The quantity of virus in the faeces is small, which is consistent with the low rate of secondary spread by person-to-person contact. There is no evidence for sexual transmission or for transmission by transfusion.

Clinical features

The clinical spectrum of infection with hepatitis E is similar to infection caused by other hepatitis viruses, and includes subclinical and anicteric infections, acute hepatitis with jaundice and fulminant hepatitis. Cholestatic features are common. Hepatitis E does not progress to chronic liver disease and there is no evidence of persistent infection. As with other forms of viral hepatitis, hepatitis E is more likely to be asymptomatic, subclinical and anicteric in young children.

Infection with hepatitis E is associated with a relatively high mortality of 1–4% of patients admitted to hospital from the general population. Fulminant hepatitis in pregnancy may lead to a mortality rate of 20% during the third trimester. Premature delivery and infant mortality of up to 33% have been observed.

Control and prevention

Outbreaks are more common in countries with a hot climate, and have been reported from many countries. Most outbreaks have occurred following heavy rain and flooding and contamination of drinking water, contamination of well water, and untreated sewage gaining access into city water treatment plants. Food-borne outbreaks have been associated with raw or uncooked shellfish. Therefore, the provision of safe (and chlorinated) drinking water and safe disposal of sanitary waste are essential, including safeguarding the water supply from animal waste from farm animals.

Smaller outbreaks and sporadic cases have been reported from many countries from South-East Asia, Central Asia, the Middle East, Northern and Western Africa, Mexico and also Italy and Spain. Sporadic cases have been reported from many other countries including Taiwan, Japan, the USA, South America and many countries in Europe among returning travellers and also among those who have not undertaken travel outside their own country.

In highly endemic areas, boiling is a good way of treating drinking water, and should be available both for drinking and for brushing teeth. Bottled water or water in sealed cans of well-known brand names should be used for drinking.

Raw or uncooked shellfish must be avoided, and the other usual elementary food hygiene precautions are recommended. These include not eating uncooked fruit or vegetables that are not peeled or prepared by the consumer.

Pregnant women travelling to countries where outbreaks have been reported and countries where HEV is endemic should be counselled and the importance of the precautions outlined above must be stressed.

Immunoprophylaxis

Passive protection with immunoglobulin prepared from pooled plasma obtained from blood donors from endemic countries does not afford protection. Several recombinant and subunit HEV vaccines are undergoing clinical trials.

HEPATITIS B

HBV was recognized originally as the cause of 'serum hepatitis', the most common form of parenterally transmitted viral hepatitis, and an important cause of acute and chronic infection of the liver in many countries. More than one-third of the world's population has been infected with HBV, and WHO estimates that it results in 1–2 million deaths every year. The incubation period of hepatitis B is variable, with a range of between 1 and 6 months. The clinical features of acute infection resemble those of the other viral hepatitides. Frequently, acute hepatitis B is anicteric and asymptomatic, although a severe illness with jaundice can occur and acute liver failure may develop. The virus persists in about 10% of infected immunocompetent adults and in as many as 90% of infants infected perinatally, depending on the ethnic group of the mother. About 350 million people worldwide are persistent carriers of hepatitis B. Liver damage is mediated by the cellular immune response of the host to the infected hepatocytes. Approximately 25% of all patients with chronic hepatitis will progress to cirrhosis and about 20% of those with cirrhosis will develop hepatocellular carcinoma. Hepatocellular carcinoma is one of the most common cancers worldwide.[3]

During the first phase of chronicity, virus replication continues in the liver and replicative intermediates of the viral genome may be detected in DNA extracted from liver biopsies. Markers of virus replication in serum include HBV DNA, the pre-S1 proteins (see below) and a soluble antigen, hepatitis B e antigen (HBeAg), which is secreted by productively infected hepatocytes. In those infected at a very young age this phase may persist for life but, more usually, virus levels decline over time. Eventually in most individuals there is immune clearance of infected hepatocytes associated with seroconversion from HBeAg to anti-HBe. During the period of replication the viral genome may integrate into the chromosomal DNA of some hepatocytes and these cells may persist and expand clonally. Rarely, seroconversion to anti-HBs follows clearance of virus replication but, more frequently, the surface antigen (HBsAg) persists during a second phase of chronicity as a result of the expression of integrated viral DNA.

Structure of the virus

The hepatitis B virion is a 42 nm particle comprising an electrondense nucleocapsid or core, 27 nm in diameter, surrounded by an outer envelope of the surface protein (HBsAg) embedded in membranous lipoprotein derived from the host cell (Figure 39.2). The surface antigen is produced in excess by the infected hepatocytes and is secreted in the form of 22 nm particles (initially referred to as Australia antigen) and tubular structures with the same diameter.

The 22 nm particles are composed of the major surface protein in both non-glycosylated (p24) and glycosylated (gp27) form in approximately equimolar amounts, together with a minority component of the so-called middle proteins (gp33 and gp36) which contain the pre-S2 domain, a glycosylated 55 amino acid N-terminal extension. The surface of the virion has a similar composition but also contains the large surface proteins (p39 and gp42) which include both the pre-S1 and pre-S2 regions. These large surface proteins are not found in the 22 nm spherical particles (but may be present in the tubular forms in highly viraemic individuals) and their detection in serum correlates with viraemia. The domain which binds to the specific HBV receptor on the hepatocyte resides within the pre-S1 region.

The nucleocapsid of the virion consists of the viral genome surrounded by the core antigen (HBcAg). The carboxy terminus of the core protein is arginine rich and this highly basic domain

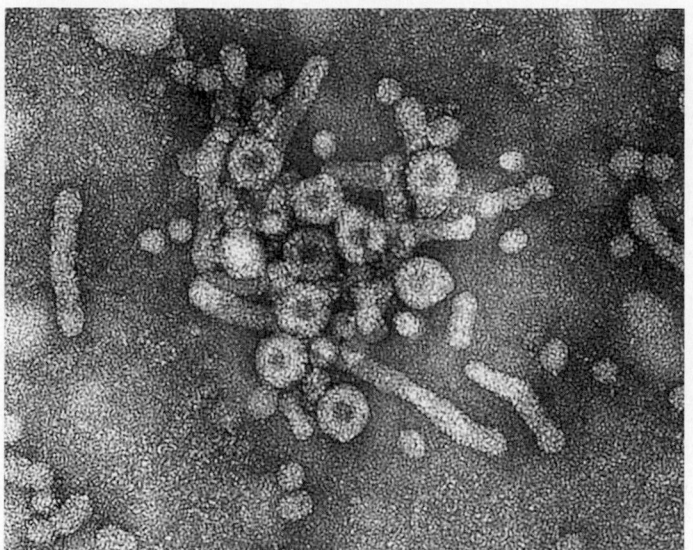

Figure 39.2 Hepatitis B virus. (Reduced from ×250 000. From a series by A. J. Zuckerman et al.)

is believed to interact with the genome. The genome, which is approximately 3.2 kb in length, has an unusual structure and is composed of two linear strands of DNA held in a circular configuration by base pairing at the 5′ end. One of the strands is incomplete and the 3′ end is associated with a DNA polymerase molecule which is able to complete that strand when supplied with deoxynucleoside triphosphates. In the past, this endogenous DNA polymerase reaction was used as a serological assay for the hepatitis B virion but this has now been superseded by DNA-DNA hybridization and PCR. The 5′ ends of both strands of the genome are modified. The 5′ end of the complete strand is covalently linked to a protein and the 5′ end of the incomplete strand is an oligoribonucleotide. In both cases these moieties seem to be primers for the synthesis of the respective strands during the genome replication. A motif of 12 base pairs is repeated directly in the genome near to the 5′ ends of the two strands (DR1 and DR2, respectively) and these sequences play an important role in replication.

Organization of the HBV genome

To date, the genomes of more than a dozen isolates of HBV have been cloned and the complete nucleotide sequences determined. Analysis of the coding potential of the genome reveals four ORFs, which are conserved between all of these isolates (Figure 39.3),

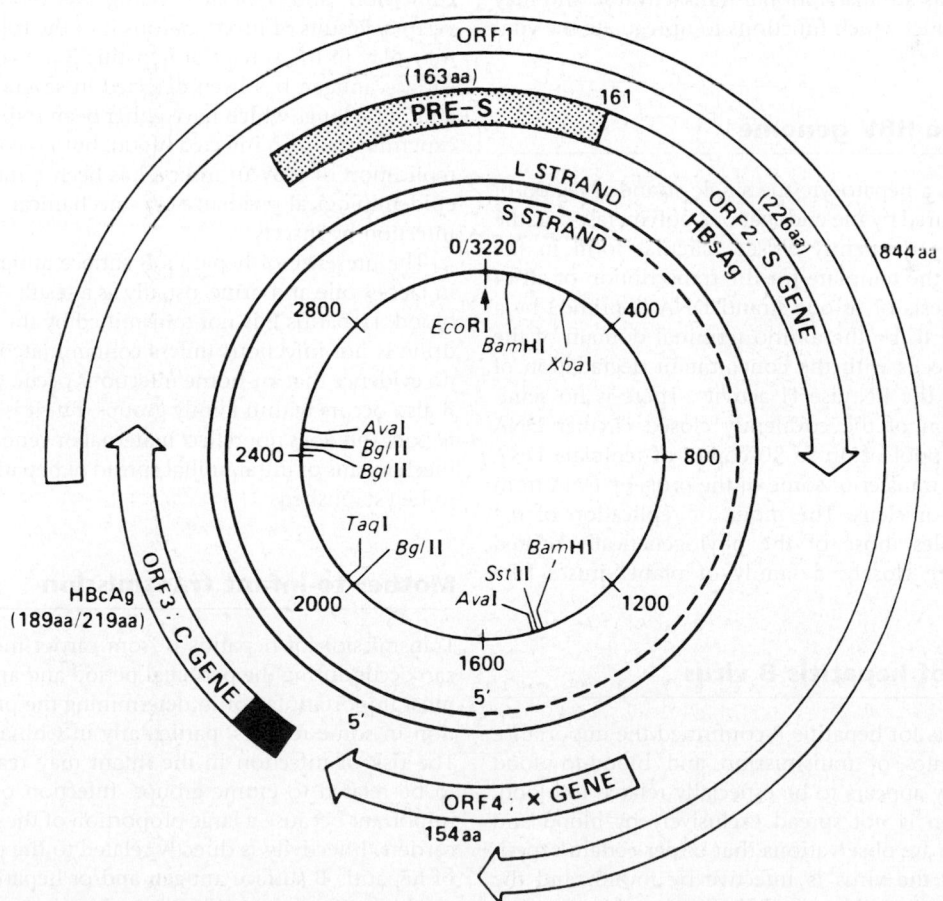

Figure 39.3 Organization of the genome of hepatitis B virus.

but there is some variation of sequence of up to 12% of nucleotides. These have the same polarity as the incomplete strand of genomic DNA, which therefore has been designated the plus strand.

The first ORF encodes the various forms of the surface protein and contains three in-frame methionine codons which are used for initiation of translation. Both the middle (gp33 and gp36) and major (p24 and gp27) proteins are translated from a family of 2.1 kb mRNAs transcribed from a promoter located in the pre-S1 region and polyadenylated in response to a signal sequence located just downstream from the start of the core ORF.

A second promoter is located upstream of the pre-S1 initiation codon. This directs the synthesis of a 2.4 kb mRNA which is co-terminal with the other surface messages and is translated to yield the large (pre-S1) surface proteins. This promoter seems to be weak (or may be downregulated) so that the message is of low abundance and relatively little of the large surface proteins is synthesized. Unlike the middle and major surface proteins, the large surface region is not secreted from the cell. In fact its synthesis inhibits the secretion of the smaller proteins and may be a signal for virus assembly.

The core ORF also has two in-phase initiation codons. The 'precore' region is highly conserved, has the properties of a signal sequence and is responsible for the secretion of HBeAg.

The third ORF, which is the largest and overlaps the other three, encodes the viral polymerase. The fourth ORF was designated 'x', but is now identified as a transcriptional transactivator, and may be an 'early' gene product which functions to upregulate the viral promoters.

Replication of the HBV genome

Following infection of a hepatocyte the single-stranded region of the virion DNA is repaired by the endogenous polymerase and the genome appears on a covalently closed, circular form in the nucleus. This DNA is the template for the transcription of all of the viral RNAs. Synthesis of minus strand DNA is primed by a protein, now believed to be the amino terminal domain of the polymerase, and proceeds with the concomitant degradation of the RNA template by the RNAase H activity. There is no semi-conservative replication of the covalently closed circular DNA in the nucleus and a pool of up to 30 copies of template DNA initially is built up by transfer of some of the progeny DNA from the cytoplasm to the nucleus. The mode of replication of the viral genome resembles those of the phylogenetically related retroviruses and, more closely, a family of plant viruses (the caulimoviruses).

Mode of spread of hepatitis B virus

Specific laboratory tests for hepatitis B confirmed the importance of the parenteral routes of transmission and blood-to-blood contact, and infectivity appears to be especially related to blood. However, the infection is not spread exclusively by blood and blood products. There are observations that under certain experimental circumstances the virus is infective by mouth and the infection may be endemic in closed and semi-closed institutions and in institutions for the mentally handicapped. It is more prevalent in adults in urban communities and among those living in poor socioeconomic conditions. Considerable differences in prevalence of the infection and of the carrier state exist in different geographical regions and between different ethnic and socioeconomic groups.

There is much evidence for the transmission of hepatitis B by intimate contact and by the sexual route. The sexually promiscuous, particularly active male homosexuals who change partners frequently, are at very high risk of infection with HBV. Hepatitis B surface antigen has been found in blood and in various body fluids such as saliva, menstrual and vaginal discharges, seminal fluid, colostrum and breast-milk and serous exudates, and these have been implicated as vehicles of transmission of infection. Contact-associated hepatitis is thus of major importance. Transmission of infection may result from accidental inoculation of minute amounts of blood or body fluids contaminated with blood, such as may occur during medical, surgical and dental procedures, immunization with inadequately sterilized syringes and needles, intravenous and percutaneous drug abuse; tattooing, ear-piercing and nose-piercing, and acupuncture with non-sterile equipment; laboratory accidents and accidental inoculation with razors, shared toothbrushes, bath brushes, towels and similar objects which have been contaminated with blood. Additional factors may be important for the transmission of hepatitis B infection in the tropics and in warm-climate countries. These include traditional tattooing and scarification, blood-letting, ritual circumcision and repeated biting by blood-sucking arthropod vectors. Results of investigations into the role which biting insects may play in the spread of hepatitis B are conflicting. Hepatitis B surface antigen has been detected in several species of mosquito and in bedbugs which have either been trapped in the wild or fed experimentally on infected blood, but no convincing evidence for replication of HBV in insects has been obtained, and there is no epidemiological evidence of mechanical transmission of the infection by insects.

The presence of hepatitis B surface antigen has been reported in faeces, bile and urine, usually as a result of contamination with blood. Hepatitis B is not transmitted by the faecal–oral route and urine is not infectious unless contaminated with blood. There is no evidence that air-borne infections occur. Clustering of hepatitis B also occurs within family groups, but it is not related to genetic factors and does not reflect maternal or venereal transmission. The mechanisms of intrafamilial spread of hepatitis B infection remain to be established.

Mother-to-infant transmission

Transmission of hepatitis B from carrier mothers to their babies can occur during the perinatal period and appears to be the single most important factor in determining the prevalence of the infection in some regions, particularly in China and South-east Asia. The risk of infection in the infant may reach 90% and appears to be related to ethnic groups. Infection of infants is especially important because a large proportion of these infants will become carriers. Infectivity is directly related to the presence of high titres of hepatitis B surface antigen and/or hepatitis B e antigen in the mother's circulation. When e antigen is present, as many as 95% of newborn children are infected, usually in the perinatal period.

The prevalence of e antigen among surface antigen maternal carriers, and thus the infectivity of mothers for their infants, varies markedly in different geographical areas and in different ethnic groups.

In some parts of Asia, particularly in South-east Asia, 30–50% of surface antigen carrier women of child-bearing age also carry e antigen in their blood, and perinatal infections may account for about half the carriers in the population. Perinatal transmission is of intermediate frequency in mothers of west Asian or Afro-Caribbean origin. In contrast, the carrier state and perinatal transmission are uncommon in Caucasian mothers. The pattern of mother-to-infant transmission and establishment of the carrier state is different in Africa, where e antigen is less frequent in carrier mothers and infection of infants occurs most commonly during the first 5 years of life as a result of horizontal transmission. Another mode of transmission of hepatitis B is infection of children of non-carrier mothers by contact with children who had been infected by their carrier mothers.

There is a substantial risk of perinatal infection if the mother has acute hepatitis B, particularly during the third trimester of pregnancy or within 2 months after delivery. Intrauterine infections are uncommon, since the virus does not cross the intact placenta and the few infections which occur in utero are probably the result of a leakage of maternal blood into the fetal circulation associated with a tear in the placenta.

Finally, the precise mechanism of perinatal infection is uncertain but it probably occurs during or shortly after birth as a result of a leak of maternal blood into the baby's circulation or its ingestion or inadvertent inoculation. Most of the children infected during the perinatal period become persistent carriers.

The carrier state

The carrier state is defined on the basis of longitudinal studies as persistence of the hepatitis B surface antigen in the circulation for more than 6 months. The carrier state may be life-long and may be associated with liver damage varying from minor changes in the nuclei of hepatocytes to persistent hepatitis, chronic active hepatitis, cirrhosis and hepatocellular carcinoma. In carriers of hepatitis B virus with or without histological evidence of liver disease, integration of the viral DNA may be at many sites or at a unique site in the host genome. Most of these carriers have circulating surface antigen with or without other viral markers such as e antigen or e antibody, DNA polymerase and HBV DNA, and it has been suggested that the continued expression of the surface antigen in patients may result from integrated viral DNA. Some carriers, however, may have hepatitis B viral DNA in their liver without expression of the surface antigen (latent viral infection). It is estimated that there are over 350 million carriers worldwide.

Several risk factors have been identified in relation to the development of the carrier state. It is commoner in males, more likely to follow infections acquired in childhood, as described above, than those acquired in adult life and more likely to occur in patients with natural or acquired immune deficiencies. A carrier state becomes established in approximately 5–10% of infected adults.

The prevalence of carriers among apparently healthy adults, particularly among blood donors, who have been studied most intensively, varies geographically. The world can be divided broadly into three zones according to the prevalence of infection with HBV:

- Hyperendemic regions where the infection is almost universal including many countries in South-east Asia (including China), the Western Pacific and sub-Saharan Africa. Carrier rates in these populations vary from more than 5% to 20%. In most of these countries infection in early life is very common.
- Intermediate endemic regions in which the overall prevalence of infection as judged by serological markers of HBV such as HBsAg, anti-HBs and anti-HBc ranges from 20% to 50% and carriers of HBsAg from 1% to 5% of the general population. These include countries of north Africa, the Middle East, parts of southern and eastern Europe and South America.
- Low-prevalence areas include northern Europe, most western European countries, the USA, Canada, Australia and New Zealand. In these countries less than 10% of the population have serological evidence of infection with HBV and the carrier rate is 0.1% or less. However, even in these countries the prevalence of infection and carriers may vary considerably within different groups of the population including the distribution of ethnic groups.

Age distribution and the prevalence of infection

Two different patterns of age distribution of infection are recognized. In populations with a high prevalence of hepatitis B virus, infection is usually acquired early in the life, and the highest infection and carrier rates are seen among children and young adults, with lower prevalence among older age groups. The e antigen has been found more commonly in young than in adult carriers, while the prevalence of e antibody is higher in older age groups. These findings suggest that young carriers could be the most infective.

In countries in which infection with hepatitis B virus is relatively uncommon, the highest prevalence of hepatitis B surface antigen is found in the 20–40 age group. The highest rates of infection are found among groups who have an increased risk of contact with blood or blood products, as outlined above, including healthcare personnel, certain categories of patients, intravenous drug abusers and male homosexuals who change partners frequently.

It should be noted that the prevalence of HBV infection and the age distribution of infection and the carrier rate are changing, and in some countries changing dramatically, with the implementation of a strategy of universal immunization against hepatitis B.

Prevention and control of hepatitis B

Hepatitis B virus has been classified into six genotypes designated A–F based on phylogenetic analysis of complete viral genomes. Genotypes A and D are disseminated widely throughout the Old World, while genotypes B and C are confined to the East Asian populations, and genotype E to sub-Saharan Africa. Genotype F is more divergent from the other genotypes and is found in aboriginal American populations. All six genotypes share a common immunodominant region on the surface antigen, termed the a determinant, which spans amino acids 124–147. The a determinant is hydrophilic and is believed to be in a form of two major and one minor loops with cysteine disulphide bonds. Neutralizing antibodies induced by immunization are targeted principally to the conformational epitopes of the a determinant, and evidence is reviewed below that amino acid substitutions within this region of the surface antigen can allow replication of HBV in vaccinated persons since antibodies induced by current vaccine do not recognize critical changes in the surface antigen domain.

The major response to immunization with the current hepatitis B vaccines is to the common *a* epitope of the virus with consequent protection against all subtypes of the virus.

Passive immunization

Hepatitis B immunoglobulin (HBIG) is prepared from pooled plasma with high titre of hepatitis B surface antibody (anti-HBs) and may confer temporary passive immunity under certain defined conditions. The major indication for the administration of HBIG is a single acute exposure to HBV, such as occurs when blood containing surface antigen is inoculated, ingested or splashed on to mucous membranes and conjunctivae. The optimal dose has not been established but doses in the range of 250–500 IU have been used effectively. It should be administered as early as possible after exposure and preferably within 48 h, usually 3 mL (containing 200 IU of anti-HBs/mL) in adults. It should not be administered 7 days following exposure. It is generally recommended that two doses of HBIG should be given 30 days apart.

Results with the use of HBIG for prophylaxis in babies at risk of infection with HBV are encouraging if the immunoglobulin is given as soon as possible after birth or within 12 h of birth, and the chance of the baby developing the persistent carrier state is reduced by about 70%. More recent studies using combined passive and active immunization indicate an efficacy approaching 90%. The dose of HBIG recommended in the newborn is 1–2 mL (200 IU of anti-HBs/mL).

Active immunization

Immunization against hepatitis B is required for groups which are at an increased risk of acquiring this infection. These groups include individuals requiring repeated transfusions of blood or blood products, prolonged in-patient treatment, patients who require frequent tissue penetration or need repeated access to the circulation, patients with natural or acquired immune deficiency and patients with malignant diseases. Viral hepatitis is an occupational hazard among healthcare personnel and the staff of institutions for the mentally handicapped and in some semi-closed institutions. High rates of infection with hepatitis B occur in narcotic drug addicts and drug abusers, male homosexuals who change partners frequently and prostitutes. Individuals working in high endemic areas are also at increased risk of infection. Women in areas of the world where the carrier state in that group is high are another segment of the population requiring immunization in view of the increased risk of transmission of the infections to their offspring. Young infants, children and susceptible persons living in certain tropical and subtropical areas where present socioeconomic conditions are poor and the prevalence of hepatitis B is high should also be immunized.

The failure to grow HBV in tissue culture has directed attention to the use of other preparations for active immunization. Since immunization with HBsAg leads to the production of protective surface antibody, purified 22 mm spherical surface antigen particles have been developed as vaccines. These vaccines have been prepared from the plasma of symptomless carriers. Trials on protective efficacy in high-risk groups have demonstrated the value of the vaccines and their safety. There is no risk of transmission of the acquired immune deficiency syndrome (AIDS) or any other infection by vaccines derived from plasma which meet the World Health Organization requirements of 1981, 1983 and 1987. Local reactions reported after immunization have been minor, occurring in less than 20% of immunized individuals, and consist of slight swelling and reddening at the site of inoculation. Temperature elevations of up to 38°C were observed in only a few individuals.

Site of injection for vaccination

Hepatitis B vaccination should be given intramuscularly in the upper arm or the anterolateral aspect of the thigh and not in the buttock. There are over 100 reports of unexpectedly low antibody seroconversion rates after hepatitis B vaccination using injection into the buttock. In one centre in the USA a low antibody response was noted in 54% of healthy adult healthcare personnel. Many studies have since shown that the antibody response rate was significantly higher in centres using deltoid injection than centres using the buttock. On the basis of antibody tests after vaccination, the Advisory Committee on Immunization Practices of the Centers for Disease Control, USA, recommended that the arm be used as the site for hepatitis B vaccination in adults, as have the Departments of Health in the UK.

A comprehensive study in the USA by Shaw et al.[4] showed that participants who received the vaccine in the deltoid had antibody titres that were up to 17 times higher than those of subjects who received the injections into the buttock. Furthermore, those who were injected in the buttock were two to four times more likely to fail to reach a minimum antibody level of 10 mIU/mL after vaccination. (Recent reports have also implicated buttock injection as a possible factor in a failure of rabies postexposure prophylaxis using a human diploid cell rabies vaccine.)

The injection of vaccine into deep fat in the buttocks is likely with needles shorter than 5 cm, and there is a lack of phagocytic or antigen presenting cells in layers of fat. Another factor may involve the rapidity with which antigen becomes available to the circulation from deposition in fat, leading to delay in processing by macrophages and eventually presentation to T and B cells. An additional factor may be denaturation by enzymes of antigen which has remained in fat for hours or days. The importance of these factors is supported by a finding at the Royal Free Hospital, London, and elsewhere, that thicker skin fold was associated with a lowered antibody response.

These observations have important public health implications, well illustrated by the estimate that about 20% of subjects immunized against hepatitis B via the buttock in the USA by March 1985 (about 60 000 people) failed to attain a minimum level of antibody of 10 mIU/mL and were therefore not protected.

Hepatitis B surface antibody titres should be measured in all individuals who have been immunized against hepatitis B by injection into the buttocks, and when this is not possible a complete course of three injections of vaccine should be administered into the deltoid muscle or the anterolateral aspect of the thigh – the only acceptable sites for hepatitis B immunization.

Intradermal immunization

The high cost of hepatitis B vaccines is a serious economic obstacle to extensive immunization against hepatitis B, which is needed in many countries in Africa and Asia. The possibility of reducing the amount of antigen required for immunization by reducing the dose of vaccine or by using the intradermal route has been explored. Presentation of antigen to the immune system intradermally results in a macrophage-dependent T lymphocyte response via specific epidermal cells, and the intradermal route has been used for immunization against tuberculosis, diphtheria, typhoid, cholera, influenza, rabies and other infections. A second reason for attempting to use hepatitis B vaccine intradermally is to accelerate the immune response in persons who suddenly experience a high risk of infection – for example, after accidental exposure to hepatitis B or infants born to carrier mothers.

A review of reports on the intradermal administration of hepatitis B vaccines raises several important and unresolved issues:

1. The immunogenicity of the plasma-derived vaccine given intradermally in doses of 0.1 mL (2.0 mg of antigen protein) has been clearly demonstrated. However, although the antibody titres after two intradermal or intramuscular doses given 1 month apart were similar, the booster injection at 6 months resulted in anti-HBs levels which were 10 times higher after intramuscular than intradermal inoculation.
2. Multi-site intradermal inoculation of a single reduced dose of rabies vaccine resulted in rapid seroconversion and antibody levels similar to those obtained with the extended intramuscular immunization route. However, after multi-site intradermal inoculation of a single reduced dose of hepatitis B vaccine, seroconversion was slower than that with intramuscular injection, and the antibody titres after the booster injection were also lower after intradermal than after intramuscular injections.
3. Intradermal inoculation requires skill, and subcutaneous injection into fat will result in a poor immune response.
4. Although adverse reactions after intradermal injection were not marked, local reactions at the site of administration of the vaccine (which contains aluminium hydroxide as adjuvant) frequently included the development of an erythematous macule 5–10 mm in diameter after 24–48 h; the lesion would subside after days or weeks, leaving a small pigmented macule, occasionally overlying a small palpable nodule.
5. The use of jet injectors for inoculation of hepatitis B vaccine has been considered. Current advice is that until further studies clarify the risk of transmission of infection (such as hepatitis B and the human immunodeficiency virus) by different types of jet injectors their use should be restricted to special situations where large numbers of persons need to be immunized within a short time. The use of jet injectors in the UK has been generally discouraged (although this does not apply to the use of jet injectors by individuals for self-administration of insulin or low-dose heparin).

Trials of intradermal hepatitis B vaccines in Gambian children illustrate many of the problems reviewed above. In the first trial 1 mg of a plasma-derived vaccine was given to neonates intradermally in the same syringe with BCG followed by two further doses of 1 mg of intradermal HBV vaccine. The trial was considered a failure because 19 of 32 neonates (59.4%) had a low response of less than 10 mIU/mL of anti-HBs compared with two of the 33 neonates who received the vaccine intramuscularly ($p < 0.01$). In the second trial in young children, two different regimens were used: two doses of 2 mg of the vaccine were given intradermally after a 20 mg intramuscular dose or three doses of 2 mg were given intradermally. In both cases the geometric mean antibody responses were significantly lower than in the control group who were given 20 mg intramuscularly followed by two 10 mg doses intramuscularly. Vaccine failures, defined as the presence of surface antigen or core antibody or the absence of surface antibody, were also significantly higher in the intradermal groups. In the third trial, 4 mg of vaccine were given intradermally with a multiple-orifice puncture gun to 20 young children and all had a good surface antibody response. It was pointed out, however, that this was a large dose, 40% of the recommended intramuscular dose, and might have been just as successful if it had been given intramuscularly. It was concluded that in an endemic area people soon become infected with hepatitis B virus and that at present the conventional intramuscular regimens using relatively large doses of vaccine are to be preferred, despite their considerable costs.[5] The overriding consideration is efficacy of protection. In most of the studies reported to date, those who received hepatitis B vaccine intradermally were young healthy subjects, in whom the antibody response is known to be good, and the vaccine was given by experienced staff under ideal conditions. There are no data on the longer-term duration of anti-HBs, on the subclass(es) of the antibody induced, or on antibody specificity and affinity. Furthermore, protective efficacy studies of intradermal immunization against hepatitis B have not been reported so far.

International and national requirements for vaccine manufacture and licence require assurance on safety, immunogenicity and protective efficacy of the recommended dosage and schedule of administration. It seems imprudent to ignore these requirements and recommendations. Careful evaluation and review of the intradermal route (and indeed of low-dose schedules) are essential, especially in countries where circumstances are not ideal either for storage or for accurate intradermal administration of a vaccine.

Immunization strategies and the kinetics of antibody production

Immunization strategies

Immunization against hepatitis B is recognized as a high priority in all countries, and strategies for immunization have been implemented. Universal vaccination of infants and adolescents is recommended, and more than 168 countries now offer hepatitis B vaccine to all children. A few countries with a low prevalence of hepatitis B (such as the UK) recommend at present immunization of only groups at an increased risk of acquiring this infection (see above).

There are three main approaches to developing new hepatitis B immunization strategies:

1. The introduction of universal antenatal screening to identify hepatitis B carrier mothers and vaccination of their babies. It

is important that any other strategies do not interfere with the delivery of vaccine to this group. Immunization of this group will have the greatest impact in reducing the number of new hepatitis B carriers. For children outside this group it is difficult to estimate the lifetime risk of acquiring a hepatitis infection.

2. Vaccinate all infants.

3. Vaccinate all adolescents. This approach delivers vaccination at a time close to the time when 'risk behaviour' would expose adolescents to infection. Vaccination could be delivered as part of a wider package on health education in general, to include sex education, the risk of AIDS, the dangers of drug abuse and smoking, and the benefits of a healthy diet and lifestyle.

The problems with this approach are as follows:

- Persuading parents to accept vaccination of the children against a sexually transmitted disease, a problem they may not wish to address at that time
- Ensuring that a full course of three doses is given
- Evaluating and monitoring vaccine coverage. The systems for monitoring uptake of vaccine in this age group may not operate efficiently.

The advantages of vaccinating infants are as follows:

- It is now known that effective hepatitis B vaccination can be delivered to babies
- Parents will accept vaccination against hepatitis B along with other childhood vaccinations, without reference to sexual behaviour.

The disadvantages are:

- It is not known whether immunity will last until exposure in later life (but see below). This may become less of a problem as more people are vaccinated and the chance of exposure to infection thereby reduced
- The introduction of another childhood vaccination may reduce the uptake of existing childhood vaccinations. The problem would be avoided if hepatitis B could be delivered in a combined vaccine containing DPT (diphtheria, polio, tetanus), and such preparations have been developed.

Vaccination of infants is preferable to vaccination of adolescents, as there are sufficient mechanisms to ensure, monitor and evaluate cover. A booster dose could be given in early adolescence, combined with a health education package. A rolling programme could be introduced, giving priority to urban areas.

It should also be stressed that in 31% of acute hepatitis B in the USA the mode of infection is not known (Centers for Disease Control, Atlanta, Georgia, 1992–1993) and this is therefore a powerful argument for universal immunization against hepatitis B.

Finally, travellers constitute an important group which is often overlooked. Susceptible adults and younger persons who have not been immunized are at risk of hepatitis B when travelling, particularly to areas where socioeconomic conditions are poor and the prevalence of hepatitis B is high, and should be immunized. A combined vaccine with hepatitis A is recommended.

The kinetics of anti-HBs response

The titre of vaccine-induced anti-HBs declines, often rapidly, during the months and years following immunization. The highest anti-HBs titres are generally observed 1 month after booster vaccination followed by rapid decline during the next 12 months and thereafter more slowly. Mathematical models have been designed and an equation was derived consisting of several exponential terms with different half-life periods. It is considered by some researchers that the decline of anti-HBs concentration in the serum of an immunized subject can be predicted accurately by such antibody kinetics and recommendations made on booster vaccination (reviewed by Zuckerman[6] and the European Consensus Group[7]). If the minimum protective level of anti-HBs is accepted at 10 IU/L, which is being debated, consideration should be given to the diversity of the individual immune response and the decrease in levels of anti-HBs as well as to possible errors in quantitative anti-HBs determinations. It would then be reasonable to define a level of >10 IU/L and <100 IU/L as an indication for booster immunization, particularly in certain risk groups (but see below). It has been demonstrated that a booster inoculation results in a rapid increase in anti-HBs titres within 4 days. However, even this time delay might permit infection of hepatocytes.

Several options should therefore be considered for maintaining protective immunity against hepatitis B infection:

1. Relying upon immunological memory to protect against clinical infection and its complications – a view which is supported by in vitro studies showing immunological memory for HBsAg in B cells derived from vaccinated subjects who have lost their anti-HBs but not in B cells from non-responders and by clinical data.

2. Providing booster vaccination to all vaccinated subjects at regular intervals without determination of anti-HBs. This option is not supported by a number of investigators because non-responders must be detected. In addition, while an anti-HBs titre of about 10 IU/L may in theory be protective, this level is not protective from a laboratory point of view since many serum samples may give non-specific reactions at this antibody level.

3. Testing anti-HBs levels after the first booster and administering the next booster before the minimum protective level is reached. A protective level of 100 IU/L seems to be appropriate.

The European Consensus Group,[7] however, concluded that long-term protection against clinically significant breakthrough hepatitis B infection and persistent carriage of the virus depends on immunological memory, which lasts for at least 15 years in the immunocompetent, allowing for a rapid and protective anamnestic antibody response, and therefore there is no need to administer booster doses of hepatitis B vaccine after the primary course of immunization had been completed. Groups at risk of hepatitis B infection need to be considered separately and several countries have a policy of administering booster doses. Boosters are required for immunocompromised patients, particularly when the antibody titre falls below 10 IU/L, and boosters may be used to provide reassurance of protective immunity, for example in healthcare workers undertaking invasive procedures. The group also concluded that long-term follow-up studies should continue to monitor groups of immunized individuals to determine if breakthrough infections occur or whether a carrier state develops.

Production of hepatitis B vaccines by recombinant DNA techniques

Recombinant DNA techniques have been used for expressing HBsAg and HBcAg in prokaryotic cells (*Escherichia coli* and *Bacillus subtilis*) and in eukaryotic cells, such as mutant mouse LM cells, HeLa cells, COS cells, CHO cells and yeast cells (*Saccharomyces cerevisiae*).

Recombinant yeast hepatitis B vaccines have undergone extensive evaluation in clinical trials. The results have indicated that this vaccine is safe, antigenic and free from side effects (apart from minor local reactions in a proportion of recipients). The immunogenicity is similar, in general terms, to that of the plasma-derived vaccine. Recombinant yeast hepatitis B vaccines are now being used in many countries. A vaccine based on HBsAg expressed in mammalian (CHO) cells is in use in the Peoples' Republic of China.

Mutations of hepatitis B surface antigen

The emergence of variants of hepatitis B virus, possibly due to selection pressure associated with extensive immunization in an endemic area, was suggested by the findings of hepatitis B infection in individuals immunized successfully.[8] These studies were extended subsequently by the finding of non-complexed HBsAg and anti-HBs and other markers of hepatitis B infection in 32 of 44 vaccinated subjects, and sequence analysis from one of these cases (AS) revealed a mutation in the nucleotide encoding the a determinant, the consequence of which was a substitution from glycine to arginine at amino acid position 145 (G145R).[9]

Various mutations and variants of HBsAg have since been reported from many countries including Italy, the UK, Holland, Germany, the USA, Brazil, Singapore, Taiwan, China, Japan, Thailand, India, west and South Africa and elsewhere. However, the most frequent and stable mutation was reported in the G145R variant. A large study in Singapore of 345 infants born to carrier mothers with HBsAg and HBeAg who received hepatitis B immunoglobulin at birth and plasma-derived hepatitis B vaccine within 24 h of birth and then 1 month and 2 months later revealed 41 breakthrough infections with HBV despite the presence of anti-HBs. There was no evidence of infection among 670 immunized children born to carrier mothers with HBsAg and anti-HBe, nor in any of 107 immunized infants born to mothers without HBsAg.[10] The most frequent variant was a virus with the G145R mutation in the a determinant. Another study in the USA of serum samples collected between 1981 and 1993 showed that 94 (8.6%) of 1092 infants born to carrier mothers became HBsAg positive despite postexposure prophylaxis with hepatitis B immunoglobulin and hepatitis B vaccine. Following amplification of HBV DNA, 22 children were found with mutations of the surface antigen, most being in amino acids 142–145; five had a mixture of wild-type HBV and variants, and 17 had only the 145 variant.[11]

The recent report from Taiwan[12] of the increase in immunized children in the prevalence of mutants of a determinant of HBV over a period of 10 years, from 8 of 103 (7.8%) in 1984 to 10 of 51 (19.6%) in 1989, and 9 of 32 (28.1%) in 1994, is of particular concern. The prevalence of HBsAg mutants among those fully immunized was higher than among those not vaccinated (12/33 vs 15/153, $p=0.0003$). In all 27 children with detectable mutants, the mean age of those vaccinated was lower than of those not vaccinated, and mutation occurred in a region with greatest hydrophilicity of the surface antigen (amino acids 140–149) and more frequently among those vaccinated than among those not vaccinated. More mutations to the neutralizing epitopes were found in the 1994 survey in Taiwan.

Another important aspect of the identification of surface antigen variants is the evidence that HBsAg mutants may not be detected by all of the blood donor screening tests and by existing diagnostic reagents. The detection of HBsAg mutants is influenced by the assay format and monoclonal antibody binding sites. Such variants may therefore enter the blood supply or spread by other means. This is emphasized by the finding in Singapore, between 1990 and 1992, of 0.8% of carriers of HBV variants in a random population survey of 2001 people. These findings add to the concern expressed in a study of mathematical models of HBV vaccination, which predict, on the assumption of no cross-immunity against the variant by current vaccines, that the variant will not become dominant over the wild-type virus for at least 50 years – but the G145R mutant may emerge as the common HBV in 100 or more years time.[13]

It is important therefore to institute epidemiological monitoring of HBV surface mutants employing test reagents which have been validated for detection of the predominant mutations; and consideration should be given to incorporating into current hepatitis B vaccines antigenic components which will confer protection against infection by the predominant mutant(s).

HBV precore mutants

When DNA–DNA hybridization replaced the less sensitive assay of the endogenous DNA polymerase activity as a method for detecting hepatitis B virions in serum, it became clear that some patients with anti-HBe were seropositive for virus. These and other early reports suggested that this finding was more common in Greece and other Mediterranean regions than elsewhere, raising the possibility of the involvement of a variant form(s) of HBV.

Vaudin et al.[14] reported the nucleotide sequence of the genome of a strain of HBV cloned from the serum of a naturally infected chimpanzee. A surprising feature was a point mutation in the penultimate codon of the precore region which changed the tryptophan codon (TGG) to an amber termination codon (TAG). The nucleotide sequence of the HBV precore region from a number of anti-HBe-positive Greek patients was investigated by direct sequencing PCR-amplified HBV DNA from serum.[15] An identical mutation of the penultimate codon of the precore region to a termination codon was found in seven of eight anti-HBe-positive patients who were positive for HBV DNA in serum by hybridization. In most cases there was an additional mutation in the preceding codon. Similar variants were found in an Italian study by amplification of HBV DNA from serum from a further seven anti-HBe-positive patients, one of whom seemed to be co-infected with wild-type virus. These variants are not confined to the Mediterranean region; the same nonsense mutation (without a second mutation in the adjacent codon) has been observed in patients from Japan and elsewhere, as well as rarer examples of defective precore regions caused by frameshifts or loss of the initiation codon for the precore region.

Patients without HBeAg with high levels of HBV replication from various geographical areas may be infected frequently by viruses with variant precore regions. Presumably, these can replicate without secretion of HBeAg. The majority of patients who are infected with these variants are anti-HBe positive, implying past infection with non-defective HBV. It is not clear whether these patients were infected originally with a mixture of wild-type and mutant viruses or whether the variants arose throughout the course of natural infection. The process of seroconversion from HBeAg to anti-HBe seems to select the variant viruses and this may be related to the expression of HBeAg on the surface of hepatocytes infected by the wild-type virus.

In many cases, precore variants have been described in patients with severe chronic liver disease and who may have failed to respond to therapy with interferon. This observation raises the question of whether they are more pathogenic than the wild-type virus. For example, a nosocomial outbreak of fatal fulminant hepatitis B in Israel was associated with transmission of mutant HBV from a common source to five individuals; and in a study of British patients with fulminant hepatitis B, precore mutants were found in eight of nine HBeAg-negative patients but in none of six who were HBeAg positive on presentation.

HBV and hepatocellular carcinoma

Regions of the world where persistent carriage of HBV is common have been found to coincide with a high prevalence of primary liver cancer. Furthermore, in these areas patients with the tumour are almost invariably seropositive for HBsAg. In a prospective study in Taiwan, 184 cases of hepatocellular carcinoma occurred in 3454 carriers of HBsAg at the start of the study, but only 10 such tumours occurred in 19 253 control males who were HBsAg negative.[16]

Southern hybridization of tumour DNA yields evidence of chromosomal integration of viral sequences in at least 80% of hepatocellular carcinomas from HBsAg carriers. There is no similarity in the pattern of integration between different tumours, and variation is seen both in the integration site(s) and in the number of copies or partial copies of the viral genome. Sequence analysis of the integrants reveals that the direct repeats in the viral genome often lie close to the virus-cell junctions, suggesting that sequences around the ends of the viral genome may be involved in recombination with host DNA. Integration seems to involve microdeletion of host sequences, and rearrangements and deletions of part of the viral genome may also occur. When an intact surface gene is present, the tumour cells may produce and secrete HBsAg in the form of 22 nm particles. Production of HBcAg by tumours is rare, however, and the core ORF is often incomplete and modifications such as methylation may also modulate its expression.

Cytotoxic T cell targeted against core gene products on the hepatocyte surface seems to be the major mechanism of clearance of infected cells from the liver, and cells with integrated viral DNA which are capable of expressing these proteins may also be lysed. Thus there may be immune selection of cells with integrated viral DNA which are incapable of expressing HBcAg.

The mechanism(s) of oncogenesis by HBV remains obscure. HBV may act non-specifically by stimulating active regeneration and cirrhosis, which may be associated with long-term chronicity. However, HBV-associated tumours occur occasionally in the absence of cirrhosis and it is difficult to explain the frequent finding of integrated viral DNA in tumours. In rare instances the viral genome has been found to be integrated into cellular genes such as cyclin A and a retinoic acid receptor. Translocations and other chromosomal rearrangements also have been observed. Although insertional mutagenesis of HBV remains an attractive explanation for oncogenicity, supportive evidence is lacking. In contrast to these findings in human hepatocellular carcinoma, liver cancer in woodchucks associated with persistent infection with the woodchuck hepatitis virus frequently involves integration of the viral genome in or near to cellular myc genes.

An alternative possibility is that tumour formation is associated with a viral gene product. The product of the x gene is known to be a transactivator of transcription and so may cause inappropriate upregulation of cellular genes. Truncated forms of HBsAg, which may be produced from incomplete surface ORFs integrated in tumour cells, can also have transactivating activity, perhaps through interaction with receptors in the cell membrane. Like many other cancers, the development of hepatocellular carcinoma is likely to be a multifactorial process. The clonal expansion of cells with integrated viral DNA seems to be an early stage in this process and such clones may accumulate in the liver throughout the period of active viral replication. In areas where the prevalence of primary liver cancer is high, virus infection usually occurs at an early age and virus replication may be prolonged, although the peak incidence of tumour is many years after the initial infection.

HEPATITIS D

Delta hepatitis was first recognized following the detection of a novel protein, delta antigen (HDAg), by immunofluorescent staining in the nuclei of hepatocytes from patients with chronic active hepatitis B. Hepatitis delta virus (HDV) requires a helper function of HBV for its replication. HDV is coated with HBsAg, which is needed for release from the host hepatocyte and for entry in the next round of infection.

Two forms of delta hepatitis infection are known. In the first, a susceptible individual is co-infected with HBV and HDV, often leading to a more severe form of acute hepatitis caused by HBV. Vaccination against HBV also prevents co-infection. In the second, an individual chronically infected with HBV becomes superinfected with HDV. This may accelerate the course of the chronic liver disease and cause overt disease in asymptomatic HBsAg carriers. HDV itself appears to be cytopathic and HDAg may be directly cytotoxic.

Delta hepatitis is common in some areas of the world with a high prevalence of hepatitis B infection, particularly the Mediterranean region, parts of eastern Europe, the Middle East, Africa and South America. It has been estimated that 5% of HBsAg carriers worldwide (approximately 15 million people) are infected with HDV. In areas of low prevalence for hepatitis B, those at risk of hepatitis B infection – particularly intravenous drug abusers – are also at risk of HDV infection.[17]

Structure and replication of HDV

The HDV particle is approximately 36 nm in diameter and is composed of an RNA genome associated with HDAg, surrounded by an envelope of HBsAg. The virus reaches higher concentrations in the circulation than HBV – up to 10^{12} particles per millilitre have been recorded. The HDV genome is a closed circular RNA molecule of 1679 nucleotides with extensive sequence complementarity that permits pairing of approximately 70% of the bases to form an unbranched rod structure. The genome thus resembles those of the satellite viroids and virusoids of plants, and similarly seems to be replicated by the host RNA polymerase II with autocatalytic cleavage and circularization of the progeny genomes via trans-esterification reactions (ribozyme activity). Consensus sequences of viroids which are believed to be involved in these processes are also conserved in the delta virus.

Unlike the plant viroids, however, HDV codes for a protein, HDAg. This antigen, which contains a nuclear localization signal, was originally detected in the nuclei of infected hepatocytes and may be detected in serum only after removing the outer envelope of the virus with detergent.

Prevention and control of HDV are similar to those for hepatitis B. Immunization against hepatitis B protects against HDV. The problem is protection against HDV superinfection of established carriers of hepatitis B. Specific HDV immunization based on HDV antigens is under development.

Laboratory diagnosis and epidemiology

Laboratory diagnosis of actue HDV infection is based on specific serological tests for anti-HDV IgM or HDV RNA or HDAg in serum. Acute infection is usually self-limited and markers of HDV infection often disappear within a few weeks.

Superinfection with HDV in chronic hepatitis B may lead to suppression of HBV markers during the acute phase. Chronic infection with HDV (and HBV) is the usual outcome in non-fulminant disease. Outbreaks of severe hepatitis with high mortality have been reported in native Indians of the Amazon Basin and in areas of Central Africa.

Antibody to delta hepatitis has been found in most countries, commonly among intravenous drug abusers, patients with haemophilia and those requiring frequent treatment with blood and blood products. A high prevalence of infection has been found in Italy and the countries bordering the Mediterrranean, Eastern Europe and particularly Romania; the former Soviet Union; South America and particularly the Amazon Basin, Venezuela, Columbia (hepatitis de Sierra Nevada de Santa Marta), Brazil (Labrea black fever) and Peru; and parts of Africa, particularly West Africa.

The ratio of clinical to subclinical cases of HDV and superinfection is not known; however, the general severity of both forms of infection suggests that most cases are significant clinically. A low persistence of infection occurs in 1–3% of acute infections and about 80% or higher in superinfection of chronic HBV carriers. The mortality rate is high, particularly in the case of superinfection, ranging from 2% to 20%.

Prevention and control

Prevention and control measures of HDV are similar to those for hepatitis B. Immunization against hepatitis B protects against HDV. The difficulty is protection against superinfection of the many millions of established carriers of hepatitis B. Studies are in progress to develop specific immunization in hepatitis B carriers against HDV based on HDAg.

Treatment with interferon at high doses for six months (or longer) results in biochemical and virological improvement. However, many patients relapse when treatment is stopped.

HEPATITIS C

Before the identification of hepatitis C virus (HCV), transmission studies in chimpanzees established that the main agent of parenterally acquired non-A, non-B hepatitis was likely to be an enveloped virus some 30–60 nm in diameter. These experimental studies provided a pool of plasma that contained a relatively high titre of the agent. In order to clone the genome, the virus was pelleted from the plasma. Because it was not known whether the genome was DNA or RNA, a denaturation step was included prior to the synthesis of cDNA so that either DNA or RNA could serve as a template. The resultant cDNA was then inserted into the bacteriophage expression vector l gt11 and the libraries screened using serum from a patient with chronic non-A, non-B hepatitis. This approach led to the detection of a clone (designated 5-1-1) which was found to bind to antibodies present in the sera of several patients with non-A, non-B hepatitis. This clone was used as a probe to detect a larger, overlapping clone in the same library. It was possible to demonstrate that these sequences hybridized to a positive-sense RNA molecule of around 10 000 nt which was present in the livers of infected chimpanzees but not in uninfected controls. By employing a 'walking' technique it was possible to use newly detected overlapping clones as hybridization probes in turn to detect further virus-specific clones in the library. Thus clones covering the entire viral genome were assembled and the complete nucleotide sequence determined. The organization of the genome closely resembles those of the pestiviruses and flaviviruses.

Detection of HCV infection

Since the 5-1-1 antigen was detected originally by antibodies in the serum of an infected patient it was an obvious antigen for the basis of an ELISA to detect anti-HCV antibodies. A larger clone, C100, was assembled from a number of overlapping clones and expressed in yeast as a fusion protein using human superoxide dismutase sequences to facilitate expression. This fusion protein formed the basis of first-generation tests for HCV infection. The 5-1-1 antigen comprises amino acid sequences from the non-structural, NS4, region of the genome and C100 contains both NS3 and NS4 sequences. It is now known that antibodies to C100 are detected relatively late following an acute infection. Furthermore, the first generation ELISAs were associated with a high rate of false positivity when applied to low-incidence populations and there were further problems with some retrospective studies on stored sera. Data based on this test alone should, therefore, be interpreted with caution.

Second and subsequent generation tests include antigens from the nucleocapsid and further non-structural regions of the genome. The former (C22) is particularly useful, and antibodies to the HCV core protein seem to appear relatively early in infection. These second-generation tests confirmed that HCV is the major cause of parenterally transmitted non-A, non-B hepatitis. Routine testing of blood donations is now in place in many countries and prevalence rates vary from 0.2–0.5% in northern Europe to 1.2–1.5% in southern Europe and Japan. Most of those with antibody have a history of parenteral risk, such as a history of transfusion or administration of blood products or of intravenous drug abuse. There is little evidence for sexual or perinatal transmission of HCV and the natural routes of transmission have yet to be identified.

The availability of the nucleotide sequence of HCV made the use of PCR possible as a direct test for the genome of the virus itself. The first step is the synthesis of a cDNA copy of the target region of the RNA genome using reverse transcriptase (primed by the antigenomic PCR primer or, better, by random hexamers) and the product of this reaction is then a suitable target for amplification. The concentration of virus in serum samples is often very low, so that the mass of product(s) from the PCR reaction is insufficient for visualization on a stained gel. Thus either a second round of amplification (with nested primers) or detection of the primary product by southern hybridization is required. There is considerable variation in nucleotide sequences among different isolates of HCV, and the 5′ non-coding region, which seems to be highly conserved, is the preferred target for the PCR.

Organization of the HCV genome

The genome of HCV (Figure 39.4) resembles those of the pestiviruses and flaviviruses in that it comprises around 10 000 nt of positive-sense RNA, lacks a 3′ poly A tract and has a similar gene organization. It has been proposed that HCV should be the prototype of a third genus in the family Flaviviridae. All of these genomes contain a single large ORF which is translated to yield a polyprotein from which the viral proteins are derived by post-translational cleavage and other modifications.[18]

There is a short, untranslated region at the 5′ end of the genomic RNA and a further untranslated region at the 3′ end, the large ORF accounting for over 95% of the sequence. The structural proteins are located forwards at the 5′ end and the non-structural proteins towards the 3′ end. The first product of the polyprotein is the non-glycosylated capsid protein, C, which complexes with the genomic RNA to form the nucleocapsid. As with the flaviviruses, a hydrophobic domain may anchor the growing polypeptide in the endoplasmic reticulum and facilitate cleavage by a cellular signalase, releasing the nucleocapsid precursor (anchored C). The amino acid sequence of the nucleocapsid protein seems to be highly conserved among different isolates of HCV.

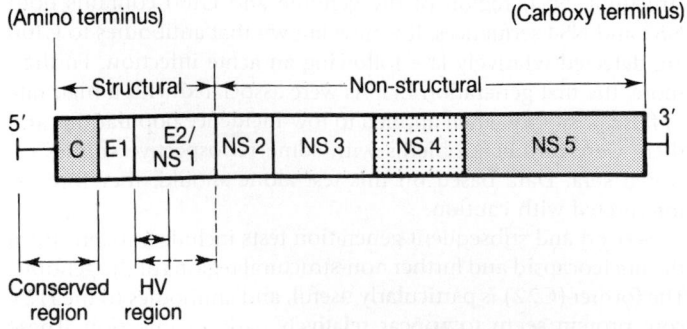

Figure 39.4 Hepatitis C viral genome. HV, hypervariable.

The next domain in the polyprotein also has a signal sequence at its carboxy terminus and may be processed in a similar fashion. The product is a glycoprotein which is probably found in the viral envelope and is referred to as E1/S or gp35. The third domain may be cleaved by a protease within the viral polyprotein to yield what is probably a second surface glycoprotein, E2/NS1 or gp70. These proteins are of considerable interest because of their potential use in tests for the direct detection of viral proteins and for HCV vaccines. Nucleotide sequencing studies reveal that both domains contain hypervariable regions. It is possible that this divergence has been driven by antibody pressure and that these regions specify important immunogenic epitopes.

The non-structural region of the HCV genome is divided into regions NS2-NS5. In the flaviviruses, NS3 has two functional domains: a protease which is involved in cleavage of the non-structural region of the polyprotein and a helicase which is presumably involved in RNA replication. Motifs within this region of the HCV genome have homology to the appropriate consensus sequences, suggesting similar functions. NS5 seems to be the replicase and contains the gly-asp-asp motif common to viral RNA-dependent RNA polymerases. The HCV protease is a major target for antiviral therapy.

Epidemiology and clinical features

Infection with HCV occurs throughout the world. Many of the seroprevalence data are based on blood donors, who represent a selected population. The prevalence of antibodies to HCV in blood donors varies from 0.02% to 1.25% in different countries. Higher rates have been found in southern Italy, Spain, central Europe, Japan and parts of the Middle East, with as many as 19% in Egyptian blood donors. Until screening of blood donors was introduced, hepatitis C accounted for the vast majority of non-A, non-B post-transfusion hepatitis. However, it is clear that, while blood transfusion and the transfusion of blood products are efficient routes of transmission of HCV, these account for a small proportion of cases of acute clinical hepatitis in a number of countries (with the exception of patients with haemophilia). Current data indicate that in 30% or more of patients in industrialized countries the source of infection cannot be identified; although transmission by contact with blood and contaminated materials is likely to be important, 35% of patients have a history of intravenous drug misuse; household contact and sexual exposure do not appear to be major factors in the epidemiology of this common infection (6–8%); and occupational exposure in the healthcare setting accounts for about 2% of cases. Transmission of HCV from mother to infant occurs in about 10% of viraemic mothers and the risk appears to be related to the level of viraemia. It should be noted, however, that information on the natural history of hepatitis C is limited because the onset of the infection is often unrecognized and the early course of the disease is indolent and protracted in most patients.

Most acute infections are asymptomatic: less than 30% of patients with acute infections have non-specific symptoms and some develop mild jaundice. Fulminant hepatitis has been described. Extrahepatic manifestations include mixed cryoglobulinaemia, membranous proliferative glomerulonephritis and porphyria cutanea tarda.

Between 50% and 80% of patients do not clear the virus by 6 months and develop chronic hepatitis. The majority have fluctuating abnormal alanine transaminase levels, but some 30% have normal levels. Histological examination of liver biopsies from asymptomatic HCV carriers (blood donors) reveals that none has normal histology and that up to 70% have chronic active hepatitis and/or cirrhosis. The rate of progression of chronic hepatitis is highly variable. The presence of antibodies to specific antigen components is variable and may or may not reflect viraemia, and in the case of interferon treatment there is a correlation between response and loss of specific antibodies to the E2 component.

Detection and monitoring of viraemia are important for management and treatment and sensitive techniques are available for the measurement of HCV RNA. The identification of specific types and subtypes is important, with observations suggesting an association between response to interferon and particular genotypes.

The response of the immune system to infection with HCV is complex and persistence of infection is common.[19]

Chronic hepatitis C infection leads to cirrhosis within two decades of the onset of infection in at least 20% of patients. Chronic infection is also associated with an increased risk of hepatocellular carcinoma, which occurs on a background of inflammation and regeneration related to chronic hepatitis over three or more decades. The risk of developing hepatocellular carcinoma (HCC) is estimated at 1–5% after 20 years, but this varies considerably in different areas of the world. It develops more commonly in men than in women.[20]

A vaccine against HCV is not available.

There is evidence that alcohol and hepatitis C may aggravate synergistically hepatic damage. Alcohol restriction is essential and abstinence from alcohol is strongly recommended.

Antiviral therapy for HCV infection is described below.

MANAGEMENT OF ACUTE VIRAL HEPATITIS

There is no specific treatment. General measures include bed-rest and a generally nutritious diet. Patients should be encouraged to exercise regularly if they feel well. Consumption of alcohol should be avoided during the acute phase and continue to be modest after convalescence.

Corticosteroids and non-steroidal antiinflammatory drugs are not indicated and should not be used.

TREATMENT OF CHRONIC HEPATITIS B INFECTION

Specific treatment is now available following the demonstration that interferon-α inhibits replication of HBV, and that prolonged treatment can lead to remission of the disease.

Antiviral therapy is aimed at patients with active disease and viral replication, preferably at a stage before signs and symptoms of cirrhosis or significant injury have occurred. Eradication of the disease is possible in only a minority of patients. Permanent loss of HBV DNA and HBeAg results in an improvement in necroinflammatory change(s), and reduced infectivity. It is possible that the accompanying histological improvement reduces the risk of cirrhosis and hepatocellular carcinoma.

Unfortunately, treatment of chronic hepatitis with interferon is effective in less than half of those treated. It is relatively expensive, requires administration by injection and is not free of side-effects. Nonetheless, recombinant interferon α has been licensed for treatment of chronic hepatitis B in the UK and several European countries.

The interferons act by interaction with specific membrane receptors, thereby inducing a number of enzymes and proteins, the best characterized of which are the 2′,5′-oligoadenylate synthetases (2′,5′- A synthetases) and protein kinases. The expression of the class I major histocompatibility antigen (MHC) genes is activated by all interferons, and those of class II by interferon-γ, to increase the expression of MHC at the cell surface, and thereby amplify viral antigen recognition and display. Interferons also modify the cellular and humoral immune response.

Three preparations of interferon-α are currently available, two of which are recombinant preparations and one of which is prepared from a lymphoblastoid cell line. Approximately 40%–50% of patients respond. Highest response rates are usually seen in carriers with higher baseline serum aminotransferase levels, lower levels of HBV DNA and without AIDS. Although these factors provide some predictive information, none of these criteria is absolute, and individual carriers, for example ethnic Chinese, with active disease or those patients with anti-HIV antibodies but normal CD4 lymphocyte counts may respond, making the prediction of treatment outcome somewhat difficult. The appropriate dose of interferon is not yet established, but 5–10 mU three times weekly for 3–4 months is currently prescribed.

The subclinical exacerbation of the hepatitis frequently seen in responders suggests that interferon acts by augmenting the immune response to HBV, perhaps triggered by the inhibition of viral replication as well as the effects of interferon on cytotoxic T cells. Although residual HBV DNA can be detected by PCR, the disease appears to be ameliorated. Approximately 20% of patients who respond to treatment with clearance of HBeAg will also clear HBsAg within a year of treatment, and up to 65% may later clear HBsAg after 6 years of follow-up.

Pulsed corticosteroid treatment and interferon may also be of benefit in patients without elevated serum aminotransferases. This treatment regimen should be used with caution in those patients with decompensated hepatitis B because of the risk of inducing severe hepatic necrosis.

The major early side-effects of interferon include an influenza-like illness. Later side-effects include malaise, muscle aches, headaches, poor appetite, weight loss, increased need for sleep, irritability, anxiety and depression, hair loss, thrombocytopenia and leucopenia. Unusual or severe side-effects include seizures, acute psychosis, bacterial infections, autoimmune reactions, thyroid disease, proteinuria, cardiomyopathy, skin rashes and interferon antibodies.

Pegylated interferon (PEG interferon) is used now.

Other antiviral drugs

A number of other agents have been used for the treatment of hepatitis B. These include interferon-γ, aciclovir (acycloguanosine), 6-deoxyaciclovir, ganciclovir, foscarnet (trisodium phosphonoformate), azido-3′-deoxythymidine triphosphate,

2',3'-dideoxycytidine and 2',3'-dideoxyinosine, adenine arabinoside 5'-monophosphate (ara-AMP), phyllanthrus amarus, interleukin 2, isoprinosine, thymosin, tumour necrosis factor, transfer factor, adenine arabinoside 5'-monophosphate conjugated with lactosaminated albumin, interferon-γ plus α, interferon-γ plus β, and aciclovir plus interferon. Few of these agents are useful clinically.

Lamivudine, a second-generation nucleoside analogue, inhibits both HBV DNA-dependent and RNA-dependent DNA polymerase activity. This may cause suppression of HBV DNA replication at four sites, and also has the indirect effect of restoring T cell hyporesponsiveness. The decline in viral titre is rapid and dose related, and maximum inhibition is observed with treatment with 100 mg by mouth once daily. While production of virus is inhibited rapidly, production of viral protein which is dependent on the presence of the RNA pregenome is unaffected by lamivudine. Reduction of viral protein concentrations depends on the destruction of infected liver cells, and with immune control of HBV replication viral protein production also declines.

Approximately 20% of patients clear HBeAg and HBV DNA within 1 year of starting treatment with lamivudine. Long-term therapy may be required, and extended therapy is feasible as, in contrast to interferon-α, lamivudine can be taken orally and is associated with a lower incidence of adverse events. Extended therapy with lamivudine has also been found to produce significant improvements in liver histology and increasing levels of seroconversion. In one cohort about 40% of patients seroconverted after 3 years. Seroconversion rates are likely to be enhanced if patients with alanine aminotransferase (ALT) elevations are selected (i.e. ALT levels >2× the upper limit of normal).

As with all antiviral agents, prolonged treatment with lamivudine is associated with a risk of HBV variants (mutants). The key variant with lamivudine therapy involves the highly conserved tyr-met-asp-asp (YMDD) motif, which forms part of the active site of the polymerase. Although experimental studies have shown that such YMDD variants confer resistance of lamivudine in vitro, they also have reduced replication competence both in vitro and in the clinical setting. As such their emergence is not a signal to stop treatment with lamivudine. In patients with HBeAg, 14% of patients developed the variant. While this was associated in one study with elevation of HBV DNA and ALT, these had not reached baseline levels by week 52, and the variant was not associated with any reduction in the histological response. The YMDD variants also emerged in anti-HBe patients, and while 40% of such patients have lost HBV DNA by 52 weeks, about 25% have the variant. In either case, the emergence of the variants is not a signal to stop treatment with lamivudine. Indeed, HBeAg seroconversion can still occur in patients with the YMDD variant.[21]

Nevertheless, in considering treatment options in the future for those who develop YMDD variants, other antiviral agents that do not share cross-resistance with lamivudine may be added. In vitro data suggest that lamivudine-resistant and famciclovir-resistant variants remain sensitive for example to adefovir, but combination therapy is yet to be evaluated clinically.

The introduction of lamivudine has made transplantation feasible in patients with decompensated liver disease with HBV DNA. It may also be of benefit in suppression of replication in non-decompensated patients prior to transplantation, and in post-transplant patients. The combination of lamivudine and hepatitis

B immunoglobulin is an effective prophylaxis against recurrent hepatitis B after transplantation, leading to improved graft and patient survival. Lamivudine is effective for the treatment of recurrent HBV infection after transplantation.

Other antiviral agents have also been developed including ganciclovir, famciclovir and adefovir dipivoxil. Combination therapy is also being used.[22]

The development of specific antiviral therapies offers a new opportunity to treat chronic carriers of hepatitis B virus, and while there is a need to define more precisely the indications for treatment, the costs of treatment and the logistics of screening for asymptomatic hepatitis B infection and assessment of active replicative HBV infection are substantial and constitute a major challenge particularly in countries where HBV is hyperendemic.

Several newer nucleoside analogues suppress hepatitis B in vitro, and these drugs are at present undergoing clinical trial in humans.

TREATMENT OF CHRONIC HEPATITIS C INFECTIONS

Treatment with pegylated interferon-alpha is indicated for patients with well-documented chronic hepatitis C in whom other causes of chronic hepatitis have been excluded, and who have at least a two-fold elevation of serum alanine aminotransferase. Interferon α ameliorates disease activity in approximately 50% of patients with hepatitis C after short courses (6 months) of treatment. Liver biopsy histology provides useful information regarding the extent of liver damage. Treatment should be started at a dose of 3×10^6 units, three times weekly, and administered subcutaneously for 6 months. Treatment can be discontinued after 3 months if no response has occurred. However, approximately 50% of responders relapse when treatment is stopped. Almost all of these relapses tend to re-respond to retreatment.

Ribavirin, a nucleoside analogue which is taken orally, has also been shown to inhibit HCV. This drug may be a better choice for patients with cirrhosis, who respond poorly to interferon, or it can be used in combination with pegylated interferon.

REFERENCES

1. Koff RS. Hepatitis A. *Lancet* 1998; 351:1643–1649.
2. Emmerson SU, Purcell RH. Hepatitis E Virus. *Rev Med Virol* 2003; 13: 145–154.
3. Zuckerman AJ, ed. *Hepatitis B in the Asian-Pacific Region*, vols 1–3. London: Royal College of Physicians; 1997, 1998, 1999.
4. Shaw FE Jr, Guess IJA, Roets JM, et al. Effect of anatomic site, age and smoking on the immune response to hepatitis B vaccination. *Vaccine* 1989; 7:425–430.
5. Whittle HC, Lamb WH, Ryder RW. Trials of intradermal hepatitis B vaccines in Gambian children. *Ann Trop Paediatr* 1987; 7:6–9.
6. Zuckerman JN. Protective efficacy, immunotherapeutic potential and safety of hepatitis B vaccines. *J Med Virol* 2006; 78:169–177.
7. European Consensus Group on Hepatitis B Immunity. Are booster immunisations needed for lifelong hepatitis B immunity? *Lancet* 2000; 355:561–565.
8. Zanetti AR, Tanzi E, Manzillo G, et al. Hepatitis B variant in Europe. *Lancet* 1988; 2:1132–1133.

9. Carman WF, Zanetti AR, Karayiannis P, et al. Vaccine-induced escape mutant of hepatitis B virus. *Lancet* 1990; 336:325–329.

10. Oon C-J, Lim G-K, Zhao Y, et al. Molecular epidemiology of hepatitis B virus vaccine variants in Singapore. *Vaccine* 1995; 13:699–702.

11. Nainan OV, Khristova ML, Bytm K, et al. Genetic variation of hepatitis B surface antigen coding region among infants with chronic hepatitis B infection. *J Med Virol* 2000; 68:319–327.

12. Hsu HY, Chang MH, Liaw SH, et al. Changes of hepatitis B surface antigen variants in carrier children before and after universal vaccination in Taiwan. *Hepatology* 1999; 30:1312–1317.

13. Wilson JN, Nokes DJ, Carman WF. The predicted pattern of emergence of vaccine-resistant hepatitis B: a cause for concern? *Vaccine* 1999; 17:973–978.

14. Vaudin M, Wolstenholme AJ, Tsiquaye KN, et al. The complete nucleotide sequence of the genome of a hepatitis B virus isolated from a naturally infected chimpanzee. *J Gen Virol* 1988; 69:1383–1389.

15. Carman WF, Jacyna MR, Hadziyannis S, et al. Mutation preventing formation of hepatitis B e antigen in patients with chronic hepatitis B infection. *Lancet* 1989; 2:588–591.

16. Tabor E, ed. *Viruses and Liver Cancer. Perspectives in Medical Virology.* Vol. 6. London: Elsevier; 2002:1–176.

17. Previsani N, Lavancy D, Rizzetto M. Hepatitis delta. In: Mushawar LK, ed. *Viral Hepatitis. Molecular Biology, Diagnosis, Epidemiology and Control. Perspectives in Medical Virology.* Vol. 10. London: Elsevier; 2004: 173–198.

18. Penin F, Dubuisson J, Rey FA, et al. Structural biology of hepatitis C virus. *Hepatology* 2004; 39:5–19.

19. Gremion C, Cerny A. Hepatitis C virus and the immune system. *Rev Med Virol* 2005; 15:235–268.

20. Report of a WHO Consultation. Global surveillance and control of hepatitis C. *J Viral Hepatitis* 1999; 6:35–47.

21. Schiff ER. Lamivudine for hepatitis B in clinical practice. *J Med Virol* 2000; 61:386–391.

22. Marcellin P, Asselah T, Boyer N. Treatment of chronic hepatitis B. In: Thomas HC, Lemon S, Zuckerman AJ, eds. *Viral Hepatitis.* Oxford: Blackwell; 2005:323–336.

Chapter 40

David W. Smith, Roy A. Hall,
Cheryl A. Johansen, Annette K. Broom
and John S. Mackenzie

Arbovirus Infections

Arboviruses (arthropod-borne viruses) are a diverse group of viruses that survive in nature by transmission from infected to susceptible hosts by certain species of mosquitoes, ticks, sand flies or biting midges.[1,2] These viruses multiply within the tissues of the arthropod to produce a high level of virus viraemia (extrinsic incubation period) and are then passed on to humans or other vertebrates by the bites of the insect. Most diseases caused by arboviruses are zoonoses, that is they are primarily infections of vertebrates other than humans; however, a number of these viruses can cause incidental infections in humans. Two major exceptions to this are o'nyong-nyong (ONNV) and dengue (DENV) viruses, whose only known vertebrate host is the human. However, for dengue virus, monkeys have been implicated as an alternative vertebrate host to man in rural settings and it is presumed that there is an unidentified vertebrate host for ONNV. Some viruses are classed as arboviruses even though they have not been associated with an arthropod vector.

The names by which these viruses are known are of mixed origin. Some are dialect names for the illnesses they cause (*chikungunya, o'nyong-nyong*), some are place names (West Nile, Bwamba) and some derive from clinical characteristics (Western equine encephalitis, yellow fever).[1,2]

In this chapter, we will concentrate on the medically important arboviruses. For more detailed information about the viruses and the diseases they cause, a number of major reviews of specific viruses are cited at the beginning of each section.

AETIOLOGY

There are over 500 arboviruses recognized worldwide[2] but only some are implicated in human disease. Some infect humans only occasionally or cause only mild illness, whereas others are of great medical importance and can cause large epidemics with considerable mortality (Table 40.1).

In this chapter, viruses are classified according to the eighth report of the International Committee on Taxonomy of Viruses.[3] Most arboviruses causing human disease belong to three major families: Togaviridae (genus *Alphavirus*), Flaviviridae (genus *Flavivirus*) and Bunyaviridae (*Bunyavirus, Orthobunyavirus, Nairovirus* and *Phlebovirus* genera). The alphaviruses and flaviviruses are enveloped, single-stranded, positive-sense RNA viruses. They are spherical particles, measuring from 40 to 70 nm.[4,5] The bunyaviruses are enveloped, negative-strand RNA viruses. They are generally spherical and measure 80–120 nm in diameter.

The flaviviruses are the most important group medically and three infections caused by viruses in this group, yellow fever virus (YFV), DENV and Japanese encephalitis virus (JEV), are sufficiently prevalent to be of global concern.[6] Other arboviruses, including tick-borne encephalitis virus (TBEV), Venezuelan equine encephalitis virus (VEEV), St. Louis encephalitis virus (SLEV) and West Nile virus (WNV), are usually restricted to specific regions. However, the spread of arboviruses across several regions may cause international health problems.[1] This has occurred most recently with WNV moving from Africa into North and South America, Rift Valley fever virus (RVFV) moving from Africa to the Middle East, JEV moving into the Australasian region and chikungunya virus (CHIKV) moving into islands in the south-west Indian Ocean. The major reasons for virus movement will be discussed later in the chapter.

EPIDEMIOLOGY

For effective arbovirus transmission to occur, three components are necessary: the vector (mosquito, tick, sandfly, biting midge), the vertebrate host(s) and suitable environmental conditions. Transmission cycles range from simple (involving one vector and one host) to the highly complex involving multiple vectors and hosts. The epidemiology of human arboviral diseases usually involves one of two transmission cycles. In the jungle or sylvatic cycle, an infected arthropod bites either a human or domestic animal that has strayed into the ecological niche of the virus/vector. This mode of infection results in small clusters of cases initiated at the same site. The second is the urban cycle where a person or domestic animal, infected via the sylvatic mode or moving from another area with urban activity, acts as an amplifier host in the transfer of the virus to other persons or domestic animals in the community. These cases occur as epidemics or epizootics in nature.[2] The vector species involved in the urban cycle may be the same or different to that in the sylvatic cycle. YFV is a good example of an arbovirus that undergoes both modes of transmission.[7]

Figure 40.1 shows examples of the types of transmission cycles that can occur in nature.

Table 40.1 Arboviruses

Virus[a]	Geographical distribution	Transmission	Fever	Clinical form	Rash
TOGAVIRIDAE					
Alphavirus genus					
Babanki	Africa	Mosquito			
Barmah Forest virus (BFV)[b]	Australia	Mosquito	+	A	+
Chikungunya virus (CHIKV)[b]	Africa, India, South-east Asia	Mosquito	+	H/A	+
Getah virus (GETV)	Asia, Australasia	Mosquito	+		
Mayaro virus (Uruma) (MAYV)[b]	South America	Mosquito	+		+
O'nyong-nyong virus (ONNV)[b]	Africa	Mosquito	+	A	+
Ross River virus (RRV)[b]	Australia, South Pacific	Mosquito	+	A	+
Sindbis virus (SINV)[b]	Africa, Asia, Europe, Australia	Mosquito	+	A	+ (Africa only)
Semliki Forest virus (SFV)	Africa, Russia	Mosquito	+		
Ockelbo virus (OCKV)[b]	Europe	Mosquito	+	A	+
Eastern equine encephalitis virus (EEEV)[b]	North and South America	Mosquito	+	E	
Western equine encephalitis virus (WEEV)[b]	North and South America	Mosquito	+	E	
Venezuelan equine encephalitis virus (VEEV)[b]	North and South America	Mosquito	+	E	
FLAVIVIRIDAE					
Flavivirus genus					
Mosquito-borne					
Banzi virus (BANV)	Southern Africa	Mosquito	+		
Bouboui virus (BOUV)	Central Africa	Mosquito			
Bussuquara virus (BSQV)	Central and South America	Mosquito	+	A	
Dengue virus-type 1–4[b]	Africa, Asia, America, the Caribbean and Pacific Islands, China, Taiwan, Indonesia, Australia	Mosquito	+	H	+
Edge Hill virus (EHV)	Australia	Mosquito	+	A	
Ilhéus virus (ILHV)	South and North America	Mosquito	+	E	
Japanese encephalitis virus (JEV)[b]	Asia, Australasia	Mosquito	+	E	
Karshi virus (KSIV)	Kazakhstan, Uzbekistan	Tick	+		
Kedougou virus (KEDV)	Senegal, Central Africa	Mosquito			
Kokobera virus (KOKV)	Australia, New Guinea	Mosquito	+	A	+
Koutango virus (KOUV)	Senegal	Mosquito	+	A	+
Kunjin virus (KUNV)[b]	Australia, Indonesia, Malaysia	Mosquito	+	A/E	+
Murray Valley encephalitis virus (MVEV)[b]	Australia, New Guinea	Mosquito	+	E	
Rocio virus (ROCV)[b]	Brazil	Mosquito	+	E	
Sepik virus (SEPV)	New Guinea	Mosquito	+		
Spondweni virus (SPOV)	South Africa	Mosquito	+	A	
St Louis encephalitis virus (SLEV)[b]	Americas	Mosquito	+	E	
Usutu virus (USUV)	Sub-Saharan Africa	Mosquito	+		+
Wesselsbron virus (WESSV)	Africa, Asia	Mosquito	+	E	+

Table 40.1 *Continued*

Virus[a]	Geographical distribution	Transmission	Fever	Clinical form	Rash
West Nile virus (WNV)[b]	Africa, the Middle East, India, Europe, North and South America	Mosquito	+	E	+
Yellow fever virus (YFV)[b]	Africa, South and Central America	Mosquito	+	H	
Zika virus (ZIKV)	Africa	Mosquito	+		+
Tick-borne					
Kyasanur Forest disease virus (KFDV)[b]	India	Ixodid tick	+	H/E	+
Langat virus (LANV)	Malaysia, Asia, Japan	Ixodid tick	+	E	
Louping ill virus (LIV)[b]	Britain, southern Europe	Ixodid tick	+	E	
Omsk haemorrhagic fever virus (OHFV)[b]	Siberia	Ixodid tick	+	H	+
Powassan virus (POWV)[b]	Canada, USA, Russia	Ixodid tick	+	E	
Tick-borne encephalitis virus (TBEV)[b]					
Far-Eastern subtype TBEV(RSSE)	Russia, Siberia, Asia	Ixodid tick	+	E	
European subtype TBEV	Europe	Ixodid tick	+	E	
Siberian subtype TBEV	Russia and Siberia	Ixodid tick	+	E	
Tyuleniy virus (TYUV)	Northern Europe, Russia, North America	Tick	+	A	
Other vectors					
Rio Bravo virus (RBV)	USA, Trinidad	Bat saliva?	+	E, meningitis	
BUNYAVIRIDAE					
Bunyavirus **genus**					
Bunyamwera virus (BUNV)	Africa, North and South America	Mosquito	+	E	
Caraparu virus (CARV)	South America, Panama	Mosquito	+		
Itaqui virus (ITQV)	South America	Mosquito	+		
Marituba virus (MTBV)	Trinidad, South/Central America	Mosquito	+		
Oriboca virus (ORIV)	South America	Mosquito	+		
California group					
California encephalitis virus (CEV)[b]	USA, Canada	Mosquito	+	E	
Inkoo virus (INKV)	Finland	Mosquito	+	Meningism	
La Crosse virus (LACV)[b]	USA, Canada	Mosquito	+	E	
Tahyna virus (Lumbo) (TAHV)[b]	Europe, Africa	Mosquito	+		
Trivattatus virus (TVTV)	USA	Mosquito	+		
Orthobunyavirus *genus*					
Bwamba virus (BWAV)	Africa	Mosquito	+		
Guaroa virus (GROV)	South and Central America	Mosquito	+		
Oropouche virus (OROV)[b]	South America	Mosquito/culicoides	+	E/A	
Guama virus (GMAV)	South America	Mosquito	+		
Catu virus (CATUV)	South America	Mosquito	+		
Nairovirus *genus*					
Crimean–Congo group					
Crimean–Congo haemorrhagic fever virus (CCHFV)[b]	Europe, Africa, Middle East, central Asia, Pakistan	Ixodid tick	+	H	+
Dugbe virus (DUGV)	Africa	Ixodid tick	+		
Nairobi sheep disease virus (NSDV)	Africa, India	Ixodid tick	+	A	

Table 40.1 *Continued*

Virus[a]	Geographical distribution	Transmission	Fever	Clinical form	Rash
Phlebovirus *genus*					
Sandfly fever virus (Naples, SFNV; Sicily, SFSV)[b]	Africa, Asia, central Europe	Sandflies	+		
Toscana virus (TOSV)	Italy, Portugal, Cyprus	Sandflies		E, meningitis	
Rift Valley fever virus (RVFV)[b]	Africa, Middle East	Mosquito	+	H/E	
Chandiru virus (CDUV)	Brazil	?	+		
Chagres virus (CHGV)	Panama	Phlebotomines/ mosquito?	+		
Other unassigned Bunyaviridae					
Bhanja virus (BHAV)	India, southern Europe	Tick	+		
Tataguine virus (TATV)	Nigeria	Mosquito	+		
REOVIRIDAE					
Coltivirus					
Colorado tick fever virus (CTFV)[b]	North America	Tick	+	H/E (in children)	+
Kemerovo complex	Former USSR and central Europe	Tick	+	E	
Orungo virus (ORUV)	Africa	Mosquito	+		

H, haemorrhagic; E, encephalitis; A, arthralgia.
[a] Classification of viruses according to virus taxonomy: 8th Report of the International Committee on Taxonomy of Viruses (2005).[3] For a complete list of mosquito vectors and the arboviruses they transmit, see Appendix IV.
[b] Of clinical importance.

The interactions of the vectors, hosts and environmental conditions that are necessary for virus transmission to occur will now be briefly discussed.

Vertebrate hosts

The major hosts for arboviruses are mammals and birds.[1] The potential for virus dispersal is dependent on the type of vertebrate host involved. Migratory birds can facilitate virus movement over large distances whereas most animal hosts are more sedentary and virus activity tends to be restricted to a particular region. These were reviewed elsewhere[8] and are summarized below.

Reservoir hosts

These include hosts that have previously been referred to elsewhere as either maintenance or amplifier hosts. These hosts are responsible for virus transmission and are essential for the continued existence of the virus. The immune status of the host species will affect the rates of transmission of arboviruses. Reservoir hosts become infected by the virus and produce high-titre viraemias to allow virus transmission to occur; however, they are generally not susceptible to disease. Arboviruses may have more than one host species involved in transmission cycles. An example of this is the flavivirus JEV, for which birds (particularly herons) are considered to be the major maintenance hosts in natural cycles. However, in Asia pigs are often kept in close proximity to

human dwellings and it has been shown that these animals amplify the virus to high titres and therefore can readily infect mosquitoes, which can then transmit the virus to humans. This is thought to have occurred in the Torres Strait (Australia) in 1995, when JEV was detected in the region for the first time.

Incidental hosts

These become infected but transmission does not occur with sufficient regularity for stable maintenance. Humans are usually an incidental host, often, but not always, being a dead end in the chain. Incidental hosts may or may not show symptoms.

Disseminating hosts

These host species may move virus from an area of active transmission to another location. Movement by viraemic waterbirds has been suggested as a mechanism of movement for a number of arboviruses including Murray Valley encephalitis virus (MVEV), JEV, WNV and Eastern equine encephalitis virus (EEEV). Arboviruses can also be introduced into new areas by the movement of humans, particularly as air travel now allows people to travel long distances during the few days that they are viraemic. This has been implicated in the spread of DENV between continents. Infected arthropod vectors may also disseminate disease if they are carried on air, marine, rail or road transport. This has been proposed as the most likely mechanism for introduction of WNV into the USA in 1999.

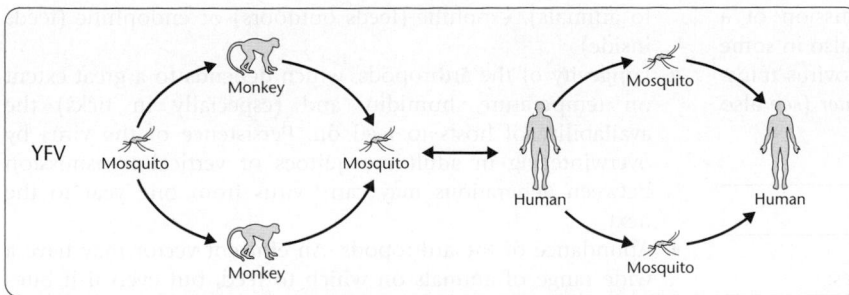

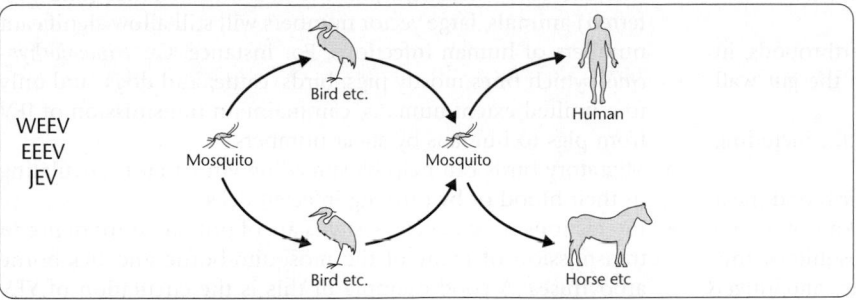

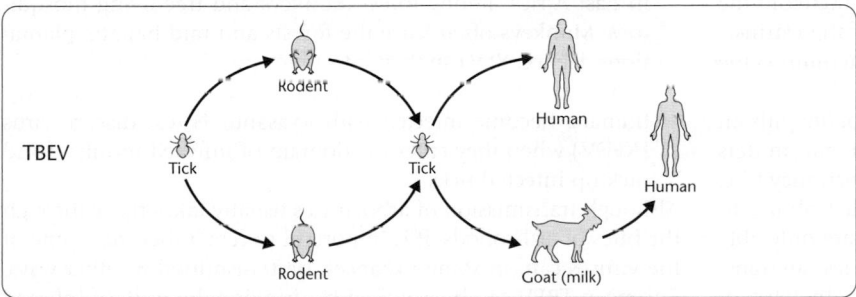

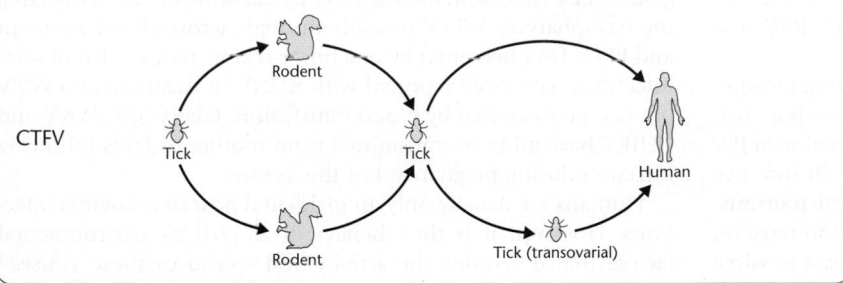

Figure 40.1 Transmission of some arboviruses. CTFV, Colorado tick fever virus; EEEV, Eastern equine encephalitis virus; JEV, Japanese encephalitis virus; TBEV, tick-borne encephalitis virus; WEEV, Western equine encephalitis virus; YFV, yellow fever virus.

Dead-end hosts

These species can become infected by the virus but do not develop a high enough viraemia to enable transmission to other vectors. Humans are thought to be a dead-end host for many arboviruses. Occasionally, one or a few abortive cycles of transmission may occur between these hosts and the vectors, but they cannot be sustained.

A wide variety of host species have been implicated in arbovirus diseases. These include birds, mammals (including primates), rodents, marsupials and bats. The host species associated with the major human and animal pathogens described in this chapter are included in the sections on the specific viruses.

Vectors/invertebrate hosts

Arthropod-borne viruses are distinguished from other animal viruses because of their ability to infect both vertebrate and invertebrate hosts. The virus replicates within the cells of the arthropod vector before being transferred to a susceptible host.[9] Occasionally, arthropods may also transmit viruses by a mechanical means whereby the vector simply transfers the virus from an infected to a susceptible host.

Invertebrate hosts include mosquitoes, sandflies, ticks and *Culicoides* (biting midges). Most arboviruses have been recovered from mosquitoes; a list of the vectors is given in Table 40.1 and

Appendix IV. Ixodid ticks are involved in transmission of a closely interrelated subgroup of the flaviviruses and also in some of the other groups. Genera of ticks involved in arbovirus transmission include *Haemaphysalis*, *Ixodes* and *Dermacentor* (see also Appendix IV).

TRANSMISSION

Transmission by arthropods involves several processes:
- Ingestion by the arthropods of virus in the blood (usually) or other body fluids of the vertebrate hosts
- Penetration of the viruses into the tissue of the arthropods, in the gut wall, or elsewhere after passing through the gut wall ('gut barrier')
- Multiplication of the viruses in the arthropod cells, including those of the salivary glands.[10]

The time interval between the ingestion of a viraemic blood meal and the ability of a vector to transmit the virus is known as the extrinsic incubation period of the disease. In mosquitoes this period is short: 10 days at 30°C (ambient temperature) and longer at lower temperatures. The quantity of blood, and therefore the amount of virus ingested, also affects the length of the extrinsic incubation period. This is extremely important in determining the transmission efficiency of a vector and may also vitally affect the course of an epidemic. Mosquitoes remain infective for life without any apparent ill-effects, and their effectiveness as transmitters depends upon longevity and the frequency with which they bite. Different species of female mosquitoes vary in their ability to transmit different arboviruses so that some species are only able to transmit a single virus, while other mosquito species can transmit many arboviruses (e.g. *Culex tarsalis* vectors both Western equine encephalitis virus, WEEV and SLEV, *Cx. annulirostris* vectors MVEV, JEV, Kunjin virus (KUNV), Ross River virus, RRV and Barmah Forest virus, BFV).

Viruses have been reported to persist in overwintering mosquitoes and this could be an important factor in virus survival. This has been shown to occur in *Cx. tritaeniorhynchus* infected with JEV and in *Cx. tarsalis* infected with WEEV (which remain infective by bite for up to 8 months). Transovarial or vertical transmission from one generation to the next via the desiccation-resistant eggs of some *Aedes* species has also been suggested as a possible mechanism of persistence for some arboviruses. However, Turell[11] suggests that other methods, including reintroduction of virus by migratory birds or survival in other vectors, may be more important in the long-term persistence of these viruses. Transmission of virus between the developmental stages (trans-stadial) is normal in ticks and transovarial passage has been observed in some species, and both are of great epidemiological importance. Some arboviruses may also persist for long periods in hibernating mammalian hosts.

Some important factors in transmission by arthopods include:
- Susceptibility of the arthropods to infection and ability to transmit
- Breeding habits of the arthropods and preferred habitats, whether near humans or other hosts of the virus
- Biting habits of the arthropods – in mosquitoes whether they are anthropophilic (attracted to humans) or zoophilic (attracted to animals), exophilic (feeds outdoors) or endophilic (feeds inside)
- Longevity of the arthropods, which depends to a great extent on temperature, humidity and (especially in ticks) the availability of hosts to feed on. Persistence of the virus by overwintering in adult mosquitoes or vertical transmission between generations may carry virus from one year to the next
- Abundance of the arthropods. An efficient vector may have a wide range of animals on which to feed, but even if it bites humans only infrequently in the presence of other (and preferred) animals, large vector numbers will still allow significant numbers of human infections. For instance, *Cx. tritaeniorhynchus*, which bites mostly pigs, birds, cattle, and dogs, and only to a limited extent humans, can maintain transmission of JEV from pigs to humans by sheer numbers
- Migratory birds can help by spreading virus that is circulating in their blood or by carrying infected ticks
- Interactions in ecological systems are of primary importance in transmission of many of the mosquito-borne and tick-borne arboviruses. A good example of this is the circulation of YFV in East Africa among forest monkeys and tree-living mosquitoes. Monkeys often leave the forests and raid banana plantations. Hence, YFV can then infect mosquitoes in these locations and from there can be transmitted to humans. Similarly, humans become infected with Kyasanur Forest disease virus (KFDV) when they enter the domain of infected monkeys and pick up infected ticks.

Although transmission of arboviruses usually takes place through the bites of arthropods, it is important to remember that some of the viruses can, in some instances, be transmitted in other ways. European TBEV can be acquired by drinking the milk of infected goats, VEEV (in cotton rats) apparently via urine or faeces infecting the nasopharynx, WEEV possibly through aerosol from a patient and EEEV (in pheasants) by one bird pecking another. Laboratory infections have been reported with KUNV in Australia and WNV has been transmitted by blood transfusion. DENV, JEV, WNV and CHIKV have all been transmitted from mother to fetus following infection during pregnancy, but this is rare.

Humans are usually only an incidental host in arbovirus infections. However, it is their behaviour as well as environmental factors that determine the activity and spread of these viruses.[1] Many human activities encourage transmission of these animal viruses to people. The construction of dams and extensive areas of irrigation often promotes the breeding of enormous numbers of mosquitoes. For instance, the development of rice fields encourages *Cx. tritaeniorhynchus* in Sarawak, spreading JEV, and *Mansonia uniformis* and *Anopheles gambiae* in Kenya spreading CHIKV, ONNV, possibly WNV and Sindbis virus (SINV). The seasonal cutting of old vegetation in Sarawak produces heavily polluted pools that support massive populations of culicines. The keeping of cattle driven into marginal forest areas in India promotes the growth and transport of ticks, and the intrusion of people into forest areas lays them open to infection with YFV and the tick-borne diseases. In many countries, the practice of using large containers for water storage has helped to increase the *Aedes aegypti* populations and hence has increased the transmission of DENV, CHIKV and other viruses vectored by this species.[12]

For a fuller discussion of the effect of human-related behaviour on arbovirus transmission, other reviews should be consulted.[13]

Environmental conditions

Environmental conditions, particularly rainfall, temperature and humidity, have an important role in arbovirus transmission cycles. Arbovirus activity is generally seasonal. For example, the alphaviruses transmitted by mosquitoes in temperate regions cause disease in summer during periods of increased vector activity.[14] In tropical areas, human infections caused by arboviruses usually occur during the wet season, with increased virus activity again coinciding with periods of high vector numbers.

Rainfall

Mosquito larvae and pupae are aquatic and hence require water for breeding.[15] The abundance of arthropod vectors is directly affected by the amount of rainfall and flooding in a particular region. Rainfall is also required to maintain permanent water bodies, or in some cases create temporary water bodies that provide a sanctuary and breeding grounds for waterbirds that act both as mechanisms for introducing the virus into that area and for amplifying the virus. A good example of the latter occurred in northern Australia during the 2000 wet season. This resulted in the unprecedented southerly spread of MVEV activity from areas of the tropical north of Western Australia to subtropical and temperate regions. High tides can also lead to increased mosquito breeding and hence increased activity of viruses that are vectored by salt-marsh mosquitoes.

Temperature

High external temperatures may have an adverse effect on vector survival. In addition, some mosquito species are temperature limited in their breeding. For example, *Cx. annulirostris*, the major vector of MVEV, RRV, and JEV in Australia, will not breed when the daily temperatures fall below 17.5 °C.[16] Temperature can also affect the length of the extrinsic incubation period and most studies have shown that the extrinsic incubation period for mosquitoes is shorter at 30 °C than at lower temperatures.[10] Hence the mosquito will become 'infectious' in a shorter time at higher temperatures.

Humidity

Increased humidity facilitates increased survival of mosquitoes.

Climate change

It is predicted that future climate changes such as those associated with global warming may affect arbovirus transmission cycles throughout the world. It has been suggested that global warming will affect the amount and extent of rainfall, frequency of high tides and actual tide heights, temperature, humidity, movement of vertebrate hosts and movement of human populations. The extent of these environmental changes is unknown but, because of the complex interactions between these viruses, their hosts and

vectors and the environment, it seems likely that even minor changes will affect arbovirus activity in different regions. This may result in an increased number of cases or a greater geographical spread of these viruses.[15,17]

IMMUNE RESPONSE TO ARBOVIRUS INFECTION[18,19]

After inoculation of an arbovirus into the skin of a vertebrate by the arthropod vector, the virus probably multiplies first in local tissues and regional lymph nodes where the earliest immune responses occur. As with most viral infections, non-specific innate responses occur during the first few days. These include the antiviral effects of macrophages, natural killer cells and virus-induced interferon. However, within 4–7 days after infection, the pathogen-specific humoral (antibody) and cell-mediated (T cell) immune responses come in to play. IgM antibodies are usually produced within the first few days after onset of illness, while IgG antibodies appear within 7–14 days. One of the characteristics of arbovirus infections is the long-term persistence of IgM, commonly for many months, therefore unlike many other infections, detection of IgM is not, of itself, a completely reliable indicator of recent infection. In general, antibody responses to arbovirus infections appear early and are long lasting, however, some viruses do not produce high antibody titres in humans while others produce short-lived or late responses.

A person who recovers from an arbovirus infection generally possesses life-long immunity against reinfection with the homologous virus. Neutralizing antibodies can be found as early as a few days after the beginning of the disease and persist for many years. This persistence of immunity does not depend upon re-exposure to the virus. While neutralizing antibodies are a good indication of protective immunity, antibodies that do not neutralize virus in vitro may also provide protection in vivo via other immune mechanisms such as complement-mediated cytolysis (CMC) or antibody-dependent cell-mediated cytotoxicity (ADCC). Non-neutralizing antibodies have also been implicated as a cause of more severe disease due to antibody dependent enhancement (ADE). The best known example of this is dengue haemorrhagic fever/dengue shock syndrome following secondary dengue infection with a heterologous serotype. This process may also have a role in the pathogenesis of arthritis following *alphavirus* infections.[20]

Flaviviruses are known to evoke very broad, cross-reactive antibody responses, particularly the IgG responses. Arboviruses are often grouped together according to antigenic similarity. For example, JEV, MVEV and WNV are all members of a single antigenic complex within the Flavivirus genus, while the four serotypes of DENV represent another. Infection with any flavivirus will usually result in antibody responses that react with antigens from a broad range of other flaviviruses, more so within the same antigenic complex. Indeed, recovery from an infection by one member of the group may provide a degree of resistance to a subsequent infection by another member of the same group; for instance, immunity to MVEV may provide subsequent protection against JEV, and vice versa. This may reduce the severity of clinical disease but is not yet proven. As mentioned above, cross-reacting non-neutralizing antibody may also increase disease severity due to ADE in dengue. The importance of antibodies in protecting against disease is illustrated by the ability of passively transferred immunoglobulin to protect against a range of flavivirus diseases in a mouse model. However, while immunoglobulin may protect against homologous virus, it can potentially enhance infection by related flaviviruses, as has been shown with MVEV and JEV infection.[21]

The role of the T cell-mediated immune response is not as clear as that of the antibody response. Broadly cross-reactive CD8+ cytotoxic T cells are induced by infection with flaviviruses and alphaviruses and are likely to have an important role in the clearance of the virus. Paradoxically however, the inflammatory responses and cytolysis caused by these cells contributes to the pathology of some, if not all, arbovirus infections.

It is also clear that host factors influence the susceptibility and severity of infections due to arboviruses. Severe manifestations of infection due to flaviviruses and the *alphavirus* CHIKV are more common in young children, the elderly and those with pre-existing illnesses. In contrast, the arthritic manifestations of alphavirus infections are less common in children. Genetic factors are also probably important. For example, genetically determined susceptibility to flaviviruses has been shown in mice, and persisting arthritis following RRV infection has been associated with HLA-DR7 positivity in humans.[20]

CLINICAL FEATURES IN GENERAL

Arbovirus infections are distributed throughout most of the world, and in areas with endemic or regular epidemic activity infection rates may be quite high within the human populations. However, the vast majority of infected individuals will have had either an asymptomatic or non-specific mild illness, and only a handful of those infected will develop one of the recognizable clinical syndromes. For the flaviviruses the case:infection ratio is usually very low (e.g. around 1:300 for encephalitis due to JEV) but varies depending on the virus. It may be higher during epidemic (rather than endemic) disease activity, and will be modified by host susceptibility factors. In particular, the major burden of disease is felt at the extremes of life – the very young and the elderly. For the alphavirus infections, particularly those causing arthritis, the ratio of symptomatic to asymptomatic infection is much higher, varying from 1:40 to 3:1.

If clinical manifestations arise after infection they do so after an intrinsic incubation period lasting from a few days to a week or more. During that time, the virus replicates at the site of in-oculation, then further amplifies within the reticuloendothelial system before it becomes viraemic and spreads to its target organs.

The most important clues to a possible arbovirus infection lie in a detailed travel and exposure history, coupled with a current knowledge of the viruses circulating in the potential area of exposure. That can be difficult if the patient is a returned traveller, especially if they have travelled through a number of countries during the potential period of infection. Information can be obtained from travel health websites such as those of the World Health Organization (http://www.who.int/topics/travel/en/) or the Centers for Disease Control in the USA (http://www.cdc.gov/travel/), or from commercial software programs. However, it may also be necessary to seek the advice of local experts to get the full picture in difficult cases.

The major clinical syndromes may be grouped as follows:
1. Systemic febrile disease
2. Arboviral haemorrhagic fever
3. Encephalitis
4. Polyarthralgic illness.

Systemic febrile disease

Arbovirus infection often produces a systemic febrile illness as part of the clinical illness. Fever is very common with flavivirus infections, whereas some symptomatic alphavirus infections produce fever in 50% or less. This illness may be completely non-specific or even suggest another viral illness, including gastrointestinal and respiratory infections, particularly in the early stages. There are some clinical features that are more characteristic of arbovirus infections. Headache is common and may be severe (even with the arboviruses that rarely, if ever, cause encephalitis) and accompanied by meningism. Muscle and joint aches are also common, especially with alphavirus infections where many also develop joint swelling and stiffness. Rash may be present and is usually generalized and maculopapular, although occasionally it is vesicular. Petechial rashes are less common and may be an early indicator of the haemorrhagic fevers. In the vast majority of cases the febrile illness is followed by recovery. In the remainder the illness progresses to one of the more serious forms of disease, sometimes following a few days of remission. Occasionally the infections have a fulminant course, particularly in young children, where the initial febrile illness is short and advances rapidly to severe illness.

The notable exception to the generally benign nature of the febrile illnesses is YF. This virus produces sufficient liver damage to cause clinical jaundice and a resulting severe febrile illness, even without progressing to haemorrhagic disease.

Haemorrhagic fever[22]

Most commonly caused by:
- Flaviviruses: DENV, YFV, KFDV, OHFV
- Alphaviruses: CHIKV
- Bunyaviruses: RVFV

These are the most serious manifestations of arbovirus infection. Haemorrhagic disease most often manifests as bleeding from the gums or gastrointestinal haemorrhage (haematemesis and melaena) and as cutaneous petechiae and purpura. The pathogenesis is complex and poorly understood for most. YF produces sufficient liver dysfunction to cause a reduction of the coagulation factors produced in that organ. However, in severe YF, there is also a consumptive coagulopathy (disseminated intravascular coagulopathy; DIC) due to complement and cytokine activation, resulting in a reduction of most coagulation factors and a rise in the levels of fibrin degradation products. There may also be platelet dysfunction.

DHF is associated with a marked thrombocytopenia and platelet dysfunction, and DIC may develop in severe disease. Complement activation is likely to be important in the induction of the coagulopathy, as is cytokine release from mononuclear cells. However, the major problem in DHF relates to endothelial cell damage and increased vascular permeability resulting in loss of fluid from the intravascular into the extravascular spaces. It appears that these processes are triggered by the host immune response, particularly uptake of virus into macrophages, followed by the release of cytokines and other inflammatory mediators from these cells and activated T cells, which in turn leads to complement activation and capillary leakage. There has been a lot of interest in the potential role of non-neutralizing antibodies in enhancing uptake of virus into macrophages (i.e. ADE) leading to this excessive immune response. With dengue, this may occur when past infection with one serotype results in cross-reactive non-neutralizing antibody if the person gets a subsequent infection with another serotype. This phenomenon has been widely observed in experimental systems with other flaviviruses and with some alphaviruses.

There is little information about KFDV, Omsk haemorrhagic fever virus (OHFV), RVFV and CHIKV, but DIC seems to be an important component of the severe haemorrhagic disease. It is likely that all the arbovirus haemorrhagic diseases will have a similar pathogenesis, but this is complex and not yet fully determined.

Treatment is directed mainly at control of the haemorrhage, maintenance of intravascular fluid volumes to prevent hypotension, and management of complications such as pneumonia and renal failure. Replacement of fluid loss in DHF is important and various solutions, such as 5% dextrose in saline, plasma, plasma substitutes or colloidal solutions may be used. If the haemoglobin level is falling, blood transfusion is needed.

Fresh frozen plasma may be used to provide coagulation factors, although they need to be used with caution owing to the potential for worsening DIC. In the early stages of YF when there is a selective decline in the hepatic coagulation factors, these can be replaced selectively. Vitamin K has also been suggested, but it is doubtful that the liver will be able to respond to this.

If significant bleeding is occurring as a result of thrombocytopenia, platelet transfusions may be necessary, but they should be used with caution when DIC is established.

There is some experimental evidence that ribavirin may be useful for RVFV, but clinical data are lacking.

Encephalitis[23]

Most commonly caused by:
- Alphaviruses: EEV, WEEV, VEEV
- Flaviviruses: JEV, MVEV, WNV, KUNV, SLEV, TBEV, LIV, KFDV
- Bunyaviruses: RVFV.

Many of the arboviruses are capable of infecting the central nervous system. It is assumed that they enter across the blood–brain barrier after the viraemic phase of infection. However, this has not yet been established and there is some evidence that entry via the olfactory bulb may be important. In either event, the resulting encephalitis has a fairly characteristic pattern of involvement. The major effects are seen within the central cerebral structures including the midbrain, basal ganglia and brainstem. The cerebellum and upper spinal cord are also often affected, particularly the anterior horn cells of the latter. As a result of the involvement of essential structures, encephalitis may result in coma, respiratory

failure and flaccid paralysis. Milder manifestations include cranial nerve palsies, tremor, cogwheel rigidity, cerebellar ataxia and upper limb weakness. The differential diagnosis in the early stages includes herpes simplex encephalitis, early bacterial cerebritis and tuberculous meningitis. Once signs of involvement of central cerebral structures appear, then it is more characteristic of arboviral encephalitis. Occasionally herpes simplex, post-infectious encephalitis, acute cerebral vasculitis and others may produce a similar picture.

The frequency and nature of sequelae varies with the virus, the severity of the initial illness and the age of the patient. Many survivors are left with mild residua and a few unfortunate ones with major intellectual and physical disabilities. Late neuropsychiatric manifestations are also prominent with the arboviral encephalitides, while other patients develop Parkinsonian-type features.

During the acute illness the CSF usually shows a mild to moderate lymphocyte pleocytosis (although a neutrophil predominance may be seen in early illness), accompanied by some increase in the levels of protein but a normal glucose concentration. Samples of serum and CSF should be collected for IgM testing as early as possible. If available, virus isolation and/or RNA detection by reverse transcriptase-polymerase chain reaction (RT-PCR) should also be performed on these samples. Computed tomography (CT) may show changes in the affected central structures, but magnetic resonance imaging (MRI) is more sensitive. Late scans in those with chronic disease show destructive changes in the thalamus and other central structures.

Limited data are available on treatment of arboviral encephalitis and no specific antiviral agents are currently available. Steroids have been shown to be ineffective in JE, but interferon-α may be beneficial. In view of the similarity of the different forms of arbovirus encephalitis, it seems likely that the same will apply to other flavivirus infections. Specific immunoglobulin has been used experimentally in mice with flavivirus infection, and successful treatment of a patient with WNV encephalitis has also been reported.[24]

However, treatment of these conditions is largely supportive in order to ensure that the patient does not succumb to respiratory failure or haemodynamic instability, or die from complications such as pneumonia that may arise with any serious illness.

Polyarthralgic Illness

Most commonly caused by:
- Alphaviruses: CHIKV, RRV, BFV, SINV, ONNV, MAYV
- Flaviviruses: KUNV, KOKV
- Bunyaviruses: OROV, Sandfly fever

A number of the *alphavirus* infections have polyarthralgia as a common and prominent component of the presenting illness. This is commonly accompanied by myalgia and fatigue, and may be accompanied by fever and/or rash. Typically, the small joints of the hands and feet, the wrists, elbows, shoulders and knees are involved. Symptoms may consist just of joint pain, but often there is evidence of true arthritis manifesting as joint swelling and morning stiffness. The tenderness and swelling are largely due to synovitis rather than effusions. Multiple joints are involved, usually in a symmetrical pattern. Back pain is common with some viruses, and neck or jaw pain may occur. Arthralgia is usually accompanied by myalgia and fatigue. Tendonitis and fasciitis may also be clinically evident, and paraesthesiae due to nerve entrapment also occur in the limbs. Most patients recover within a month, but prolonged arthralgia and myalgia is a feature of *alphavirus* infections, persisting for months or years in up to 50% of patients. There is mounting evidence that *alphavirus* arthritis is due to infection of synovial monocytes/macrophages and synovial cells resulting in release of inflammatory mediators and induction of a cytotoxic T cell response. The latter is probably important in viral clearance, but also contributes to the inflammatory response. Studies on RRV suggest that the chronic arthritis is due to persistence of the virus in a non-replicating form resulting in an ongoing inflammatory response. The persistence may be due to impaired antiviral cytokines as a result of antibody dependent enhancement of viral uptake into macrophages.

Flaviviruses less commonly produce polyarthralgia, with the exception of DENV, which causes joint pains but not a true arthritis. KOKV and KUNV are uncommon causes of an *alphavirus*-like polyarthritis.

The acute polyarthritis has a wide differential diagnosis. In some areas more than one arbovirus will be potentially responsible for the illness. In addition there are a number of other causes of polyarthritis with or without rash, including rubella, acute hepatitis B, parvovirus B19 (erythema infectiosum), human immunodeficiency virus (HIV) seroconversion illness, Henoch–Schoenlein purpura, drug-related serum sickness, and the acute onset of other non-infectious arthritides. Subacute or chronic disease following RRV or BFV infection may be confused with rubella or parvovirus B19 arthritis, as well as other chronic arthritides including rheumatoid arthritis, systemic lupus erythematosus and adult Still's disease.

Treatment is symptomatic with rest, gentle exercise, analgesics, and non-steroidal antiinflammatory drugs. There are no specific antiviral agents. Steroids have been used to treat some patients with RRV arthritis,[20] but they should be used with caution until further data emerge. Small uncontrolled trials have found a benefit for arthritis following CHIKV infection, consistent with its use for treatment of rheumatoid arthritis.

DIAGNOSIS

Virus detection

Viraemia lasts for a few days after the onset of illness and virus can be isolated from blood at that time. However, as it is technically demanding, limited in availability and often fails to yield a positive result, virus culture is rarely undertaken as a part of routine diagnosis. This should be reserved for unusual cases or rare pathogens. In cases of meningitis or encephalitis, culture from the CSF may also be undertaken, but with the same constraints as above. Where culture is attempted, blood and/or CSF should be collected as early as possible in the course of illness. Postmortem tissue may yield virus in the later stages of illness. Many will grow in a variety of cell lines, but maximum sensitivity for the mosquito-borne alphaviruses and flaviviruses is achieved by initially inoculating the sample on to a mosquito cell line (e.g., C6/36,

AP-61 or TRA-284) and incubating for 3–4 days at 28 °C. In order to obtain a cytopathic effect, this must be blind passaged to Vero, BHK, PS, chick embryo or various other cell lines and incubated at 37 °C for a few days. Virus can also be isolated by inoculation of specimen into suckling mouse brain or intrathoracic inoculation in appropriate mosquito species. Virus growth in mice manifests as paralysis and death after a few days, and is confirmed by identification of the virus in the brain. For the Bunyaviridae, suckling mouse brain inoculation or culture in mosquito cells (C6/36 or AP-61) is suitable. Coltiviruses grow in suckling mouse brain or in Vero or BHK-21 cell lines.

When an arbovirus is isolated in cell culture, it is most easily identified by monoclonal antibody binding in immunofluorescent antibody (IFA) or enzyme immunoassay (EIA) formats. Neutralization (N) with antisera or complement fixation (CF) assays are used less commonly. Specific reverse transcription PCR (RT-PCR) assays may also be used for identification, and sequencing of the product can provide detailed genetic mapping.

Virus may also be detected directly in clinical samples by amplification of viral RNA by RT-PCR or other nucleic acid amplification tests. Methods have been described for most of the flaviviruses and some of the alphaviruses. They are more sensitive and quicker to perform than virus culture and are now more accessible and, with real-time PCR protocols, results can be available within a few hours. Like culture, they can be performed on blood, CSF or tissues, and should be done as early as possible in the course of illness.

Postmortem tissues can be used for virus detection if available. The preferred site for sampling is dictated by the major sites of involvement. PCR can be performed on fixed tissues, even if paraffin embedded, but the sensitivity of detection for these samples is lower than fresh material. Amplified nucleic acid can be used for virus identification and characterization directly from patient samples using sequencing, DNA microarrays, or species-specific probes.

A variety of antigen detection methods have also been described, either by IFA or antigen capture EIA. They have been used for blood, CSF and tissues, but are less sensitive than the other virus detection methods and many have been replaced by PCR-based tests.

Serological diagnosis

This is the main routine diagnostic method for arboviral infections. Antibody may be detected by EIA, IFA, HI, N or CF assays. Most diagnosis is based on EIA and HI tests, with some use of IFA. The EIA and IFA tests can be formatted to detect either IgG or IgM, or both in the case of competitive EIA formats. HI will detect both IgG and IgM, and differentiation between them requires separation of the antibody classes by sucrose density centrifugation or in chromatography columns. They are now rarely used for IgM detection as they are less sensitive than EIA and IFA, and are more difficult to perform. N assays are regarded as the most specific of the tests, but are confined to specialized laboratories that are able to culture the viruses. More recently, epitope-defined blocking EIAs have come into use for identification of viral-specific antibody. These assays measure the inhibition of monoclonal antibody to virus-specific epitopes by serum antibody in a competitive format. If inhibition occurs then there is a significant amount of specific antibody in the patient's serum.

Recent infection is best diagnosed by an increase in antibody levels between acute and convalescent samples tested in parallel, but it may take 2–4 weeks before a diagnostic rise is detected. Detection of IgM is helpful in making an earlier diagnosis. IgM usually appears within a few days after onset of illness. A negative IgM using a sensitive test such as EIA or IFA in a sample collected a week or more into the illness makes recent infection very unlikely. For samples collected earlier in the illness or where there is a strong clinical suspicion despite the negative IgM finding, a second sample at least 2 weeks after onset is recommended. As IgM often persists for weeks or months, it does not reliably distinguish between acute infection and recent past infection. Therefore diagnosis of acute infection based on detection of IgM alone requires a clinically consistent illness and a suitable exposure history.

Cross-reactivity between antibodies within the major subgroups of arboviruses is a problem and may result in a misleading diagnosis. *Alphavirus* antibodies show limited cross-reactivity and standard tests are usually sufficient to identify the infecting virus, although it does depend on the particular alphaviruses circulating within that region. However, antibodies to the different flaviviruses generally cross-react widely, so that detection of IgM and/or IgG to one of these viruses in the routine tests is not definitive evidence of infection due to that virus rather than another flavivirus. The clinical and epidemiological circumstances may indicate that only one flavivirus is possible, for example detection of DENV antibody in a person with clinical dengue during a known epidemic. Otherwise specific serological tests, such as N or epitope-blocking EIA, are needed to identify the antibody.

Diagnosis may be further complicated by the phenomenon of 'original antigenic sin'. This occurs in people who have had a previous flavivirus infection, and who have a new infection with a different flavivirus. Owing to the antigenic similarities, they may mount a vigorous anamnestic antibody response to the original virus before they develop specific antibody to the new virus. As a result, serological tests may initially suggest recent infection with their previous virus. Late convalescent sera may clarify the situation, but sometimes it is not possible to determine the infecting virus. Occasionally a similar phenomenon is seen with closely related alphaviruses such as CHIKV and ONNV.

A detailed travel and exposure history is important for the accurate interpretation of arbovirus serology.

MANAGEMENT

There are no specific antiviral agents currently in use for the treatment of arboviral infections, nor are these likely in the near future. Treatment is supportive and symptomatic. Limited data on steroids, interferon, hydroxychloroquine and ribavirin are discussed under the relevant viruses.

IMMUNIZATION[18,19,25]

Highly effective vaccines have been developed against several arboviruses of public health significance. However, only vaccines against YFV, JEV, KFV and TBEV are licensed for use in the wider community.

The YFV 17D vaccine is one of the safest and most successful viral vaccines ever produced. This live vaccine was derived from a highly virulent strain of YFV (Asibi) that has been attenuated by in vitro serial passage in mouse embryonic tissue and chick embryo cells. After prolonged propagation in this medium, it was found that neurotropism and viscerotropism were both greatly reduced, but the virus retained its antigenic properties. The 17D vaccine is still widely used and highly effective, giving protection for at least 10 years, and probably longer. Less than 10% of vaccinees experience headache and malaise, while allergic reactions, liver function abnormalities and neurological complications are extremely uncommon. Nevertheless, recent reports have indicated that neurological complications may be more common than previously believed and, since 1996, a number of cases of disseminated infection due to vaccine strains have been reported. Estimates of the risk of neurological disease, mainly benign, are 1–16 per million, and of visceral disease, 2.5 per million doses. The vaccine is contraindicated for infants under 6 months of age for whom the frequency of neurological incidents is significantly increased. Depending on the relative risk of natural infection, immunization should also be avoided in pregnant women. Immunization against YFV is required by law before travellers are allowed into certain countries either for their protection or to prevent the importation of the disease to areas where *Ae. aegypti* is present.

Formalin-inactivated vaccines against JEV are licensed for use in several countries, one derived from infected mouse brain and the other cell culture of the attenuated S14-14-2 strain. Immunization is recommended for individuals living in endemic areas, or for travellers visiting regions that are experiencing current outbreaks. This vaccine is also used to immunize military personnel and laboratory workers who may be exposed to the virus. At least three doses of the vaccine at 7–14-day intervals are required to achieve more than 90% seroconversion, with booster doses recommended after 12 months. Minor side-effects such as local tenderness and mild systemic symptoms occur in 10–30% of vaccines, although more serious neurological complications are rare. Allergic responses, particularly in Western travellers, are not uncommon, with up to 1% of vaccinees experiencing reactions within 7 days of inoculation. A number of other vaccines, including live-attenuated, recombinant, virus-like particles and naked DNA vaccines are at various stages of development.

Inactivated vaccines against TBEV are used widely in several European countries. The highly purified Austrian vaccine induces seroconversion rates of more than 97% in the field with negligible side-effects. Immunization may be warranted for people living in endemic areas or those involved in high-risk activities, such as laboratory workers, military personnel, foresters, farmers or campers. Passive immunization with TBEV immunoglobulin is also used before or after exposure to tick bite in some European countries. As for JEV, a number of other types of vaccines are in development.

An inactivated RVFV vaccine has been shown to be safe and immunogenic in military personnel.[26] It is given as three subcutaneous doses (at 0, 7 and 28 days) and induces a greater than 90% seroconversion rate in recipients. It has been used for protection of the military and laboratory staff, but is not widely available.

There is a clear need for a safe and effective vaccine against DENV and a number of candidate vaccines are in development. However, to avoid vaccine-induced ADE of infection with heterologous serotypes, the vaccine must be delivered as a multivalent preparation so that immunization against each of the four serotypes is concurrent. Obtaining good immune responses to all four serotypes has been problematic.

WNV vaccines have been developed for veterinary use, but are not yet available commercially for humans.

Although no *alphavirus* vaccines have been licensed for widespread human use, several preparations have been used to protect laboratory workers or livestock. Inactivated EEEV and WEEV and VEEV whole-virus vaccines are available for restricted human use and have a veterinary application in horses. Vaccines for CHIKV, RRV and VEEV have had limited testing in volunteers and laboratory workers. There is ongoing commercial interest in *alphavirus* vaccines using new technologies, particularly for the encephalitis viruses, and some may become more widely available over the next few years.

CONTROL

Vector control

Vector control has been successful in some circumstances, for instance during the construction of the Panama Canal when, by strict discipline, all collections of water capable of breeding *Ae. aegypti* (and vectors of malaria) were eliminated from the area. Similar methods have been applied to cities and towns in South America under the threat of YFV. When DDT was introduced, extensive use in Guyana and elsewhere soon eradicated *Ae. aegypti* and with it the threat of urban YFV. In Africa, however, *Ae. aegypti* became resistant to DDT, and in some areas it is exophilic in habit, so that spraying dwellings with insecticide is ineffective. Forest mosquitoes, of course, are not susceptible to ordinary methods of spraying. Tick control by residual insecticides has, however, achieved some success in the former USSR. However, the problems of vector control, especially in rural areas, are formidable.

MEDICALLY IMPORTANT ARBOVIRUSES

The remaining sections describe the distribution, aetiology, transmission cycles, clinical features, diagnosis, treatment, control and epidemiology of individual medically important arboviruses in more detail.

ALPHAVIRUSES (FAMILY TOGAVIRIDAE, GENUS *ALPHAVIRUS*)

Barmah Forest virus (BFV)[27]

Geographical distribution

BFV is confined to the Australian mainland. It was first isolated in south-eastern Australia in 1974. Human infections have been described in all mainland states, but most disease occurs in the tropical north and the temperate coastal region of the south-west and northern and central parts of the east coast.

Aetiology

BFV is an *alphavirus* that occupies its own antigenic group.

Transmission

Transmission is similar to that of RRV.

Clinical features

Natural history

The incubation period is probably 7–9 days though it is likely that, like RRV, some patients will have a longer or shorter incubation period. Clinical illness is similar to the more common RRV infection, although joint pain is slightly less common (about 85%) and joint swelling or stiffness occurs in only about 30% of cases. Skin rash occurs in 50–100% of patients in different series. It is usually maculopapular, but may be urticarial or vesicular. Chronic illness has been reported in about 10% of patients. BFV disease occurs mainly between the ages of 20 and 60 years of age. Infection of children in endemic or epidemic areas is common, but clinical illness is infrequent.

Diagnosis

The diagnostic methods used are similar to those described for RRV. IgM may persist for many months following acute infection.

Management

In the absence of any controlled data, the infection is usually managed symptomatically, as recommended for RRV disease.

Epidemiology

BFV is found only on the Australian mainland and has an epidemiology similar to that of RRV, although it is less common. It is carried by the same mosquito vectors as RRV, probably uses the same marsupial vertebrate hosts as RRV and activity requires the same environmental conditions as RRV, but does not necessarily occur at the same time. BFV causes small epidemics as it enters a new area, with low level seasonal epidemics following that.

Chikungunya virus (CHIKV)[14,18,28–32]

Geographical distribution

CHIKV was first isolated from patients in Tanzania during an epidemic in 1952–1953. Its name is a local word meaning 'that which contorts or bends up'. Infection and human disease are widespread in Africa, and CHIKV is also present in Saudi Arabia, India (Calcutta and southern India), Thailand, Cambodia, Myanmar, Vietnam, Malaysia, Laos, Borneo, Indonesia and the Philippines (Figure 40.2). Large outbreaks have occurred in urban settings in many parts of Africa and Asia, and these may

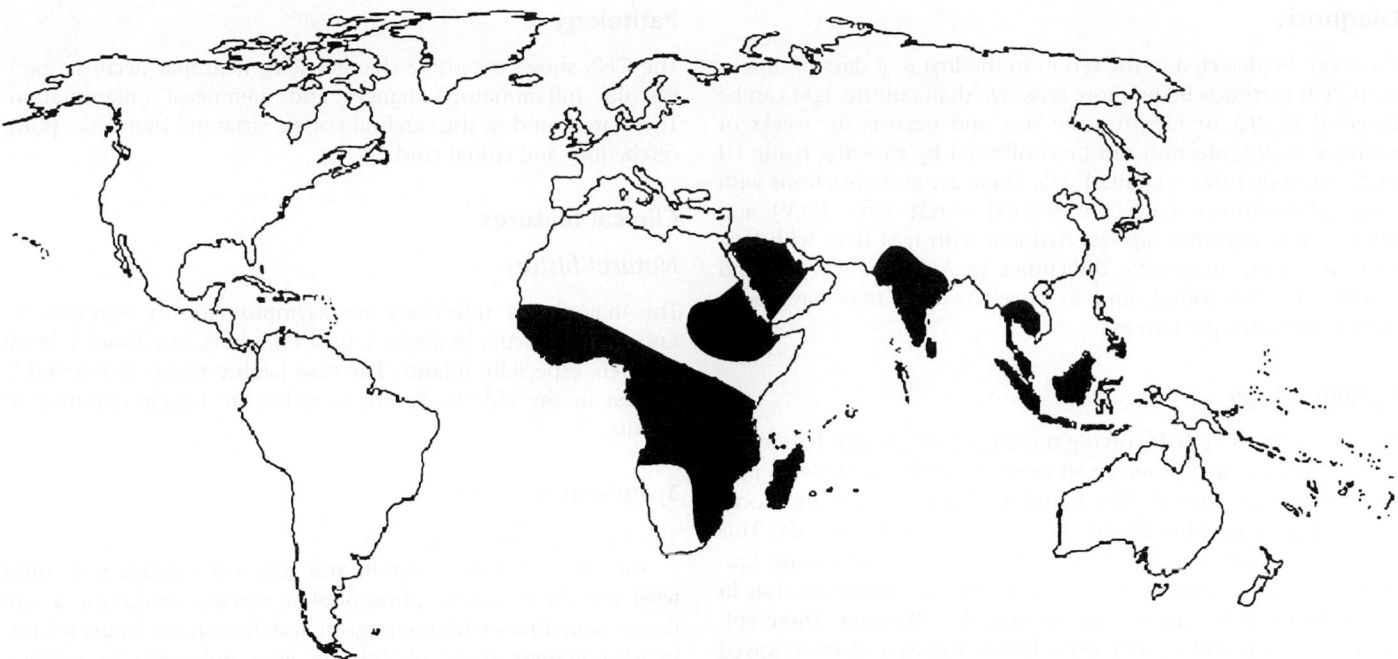

Figure 40.2 Geographical distribution of chikungunya virus.

extend over several years. At the beginning of 2005, CHIKV emerged in islands of the south-west Indian Ocean including the Comoros, Mayotte, Seychelles, La Réunion Island, Mauritius and Madagascar, spreading to India and causing imported cases of CHIKV disease in countries in Europe, North and South America, the Caribbean and Australia.[28] It has been estimated that more than 1.25 million cases have occurred in India alone, including several fatalities.[29]

There are two major lineages of the virus, one of which is found worldwide and is further subdivided into Asian and East African sublineages, and the other restricted to West Africa. However, CHIKV continues to evolve and large epidemics are usually due to a unique strain of the virus, as has been seen in the recent Indian Ocean outbreak.

Aetiology

CHIKV is an *alphavirus* in the Semliki Forest complex, and is most closely related to ONNV.

Transmission

The main vector to humans is *Ae. aegypti*, although a number of other species can transmit infection. *Ae. albopictus* was the most likely vector on La Réunion Island in 2005–2006. In Africa, the virus appears to be maintained in forest and savannahs in a cycle involving non-human primates and a variety of *Aedes* species and *Mansonia africana*. In Asia, *Ae. aegypti* is responsible for urban epidemics (Table 40.1 and Appendix IV). During the recent outbreak in the Indian Ocean, there was also evidence for non-vector early maternal–fetal transmission, possibly causing deaths in utero.[30]

Pathology

The pathology is not known, but is probably the same as for DENV.

Clinical features

Natural history

The incubation period is 3–12 days, with an average of 2–7 days. Classical illness begins with the rapid onset of severe arthralgia. Back pain may be prominent. There is associated myalgia, high fever, generalized lymphadenopathy and conjunctivitis. This usually improves after 2–3 days and is followed by the onset of a generalized maculopapular rash in about half. Fever may recur after a break of 1–2 days. Petechiae, bleeding from the gums and a positive tourniquet test have been described in many patients, so that the disease may clinically be mistaken for dengue. More severe haemorrhagic manifestations occur and are more common in children, but overall are rare. Some patients develop a febrile illness without rash or arthralgia. Most patients recover fully over a few weeks, although 5–10% experience chronic joint symptoms including pain, stiffness and swelling that may persist for years. The erythrocyte sedimentation rate is often mildly raised in acute and chronic disease.

In the past, severe and/or fatal illness has been due to haemorrhagic disease in children. However, in the recent Indian Ocean outbreak a number of fatalities in the elderly or those with pre-existing illnesses have occurred, as well as several cases of encephalitis. Children who are infected are less likely to develop the characteristic clinical illness.

There are no specific treatments though small, uncontrolled trials of hydroxychloroquine have shown a possible effect on the arthritis.

Diagnosis

Virus can be detected in the serum in the first 3–4 days of illness, with PCR methods being more sensitive than culture. IgM can be detected by IFA or EIA in acute sera and persists for weeks or months. Acute infection can be confirmed by showing rising HI or N antibody titres on paired sera. There are cross-reactions with other alphaviruses, especially Semliki Forest virus (SFV) and ONNV, although they are less frequent with IgM than with IgG. This may pose diagnostic difficulties in Africa where SFV and ONNV are also found, and in travellers who may have been exposed to multiple viruses.

Epidemiology

There is a forest cycle involving monkeys (vervets and baboons), transmitted by *Ae. africanus* and other mosquitoes. Rodents may also be hosts as they show a transient viraemia on being inoculated with virus, whereas monkeys show a high viraemia. This sylvatic cycle results in low level endemic human infections. Epidemic disease is associated with the wet season and with rises in the number of *Ae. aegypti* and, in Asia, *Ae. albopictus*. These epidemics are large, infrequent, often last 2–3 years and are followed by a prolonged absence from that area. It has been hypothesized that introduction of CHIKV into immunologically naïve populations and/or unique molecular changes that may have led to adaptation of CHIKV to mosquito vectors is the reason for the massive outbreak of disease in residents and visitors to islands in the south-west Indian Ocean and India in 2005–2006.[28,31]

Equine Encephalitides

Western equine encephalitis virus (WEEV)[14,18,33]

Geographical distribution (Figure 40.3)

WEEV is found in North America in Texas, Colorado and Saskatchewan where it causes disease in horses and humans. It is also found in Argentina, Brazil, Mexico and Guyana, where equine epizootics occur, but human infections have not been described.[33]

Aetiology

WEEV is an alphavirus that is in the same group as SINV. It has several antigenic variants, particularly among the South American strains.

Transmission

Transmission is by mosquitoes. *Cx. tarsalis*, which feeds readily on birds, transmits the infection in the western USA, and *Culiseta melanura* in areas where *Cx. tarsalis* does not occur (eastern USA) (see Appendix IV). Transplacental transmission can also occur in humans.

Immunity

Immunity is antibody mediated and protects against second attacks. Serological surveys show inapparent infections, and children are most affected in epidemics.

Pathology

The CNS shows extensive changes with neuronal necrosis, perivascular inflammatory changes and meningeal inflammation. These are found in the cerebral cortex, striatum, thalamus, pons, cerebellum and spinal cord.

Clinical features

Natural history

The majority of infections are asymptomatic or non-specific. Encephalitis occurs in about 1 in 1000 adults, but about 1 in 50 children, especially infants. The case fatality rate is 3–7% and is highest in the elderly. Severe sequelae are largely confined to infants.

Symptoms and signs

The incubation period is 5–10 days.

The onset in older children and adults is gradual, with mild fever, malaise, headache, photophobia, nausea, vomiting and sore throat, sometimes with meningism and drowsiness. In the minority who progress to encephalitis, the fever and headache increase, with deterioration of conscious state, possibly with flaccid or spastic paralysis. Infants have a much more rapid course with fever, convulsions and coma. There is a peripheral leucocytosis in the early stages and the CSF shows a pleocytosis with increased protein levels in those with CNS involvement. Most adults recover fully, although this may take months. Some have residual paralysis, intellectual disability, epilepsy or neuropsychiatric disease. High rates of residual paralysis and severe intellectual impairment are seen in infants, especially those under 3 months.

Diagnosis

The virus may be isolated from serum early in illness, but this is unusual. It can be isolated from postmortem brain and has been detected in the CSF in some cases. PCR-based tests have also been used successfully, but the diagnostic sensitivity is not yet known. Recent infection can be diagnosed by the detection of rising titres in HI or N tests. IgM detection by EIA is usually positive in the serum at the time of presentation.

Epidemiology

WEEV circulates in more than 75 species of wild birds and some domestic ones. The basic transmission cycle is between *Cx. tarsalis* and birds in the summer. Overwintering of the virus may occur in hibernating mammals but is more likely in overwintering mosquitoes. Epizootics in horses acting as amplifying hosts precede human epidemics. In humans, the highest attack rates are in infants and young males in a rural environment.

Control

Anti-mosquito measures are difficult in rural areas, but where small towns are involved 'fogging' with insecticide may terminate an epidemic. A non-neurotropic strain of virus isolated from birds has been used successfully as a vaccine, but only experimentally.

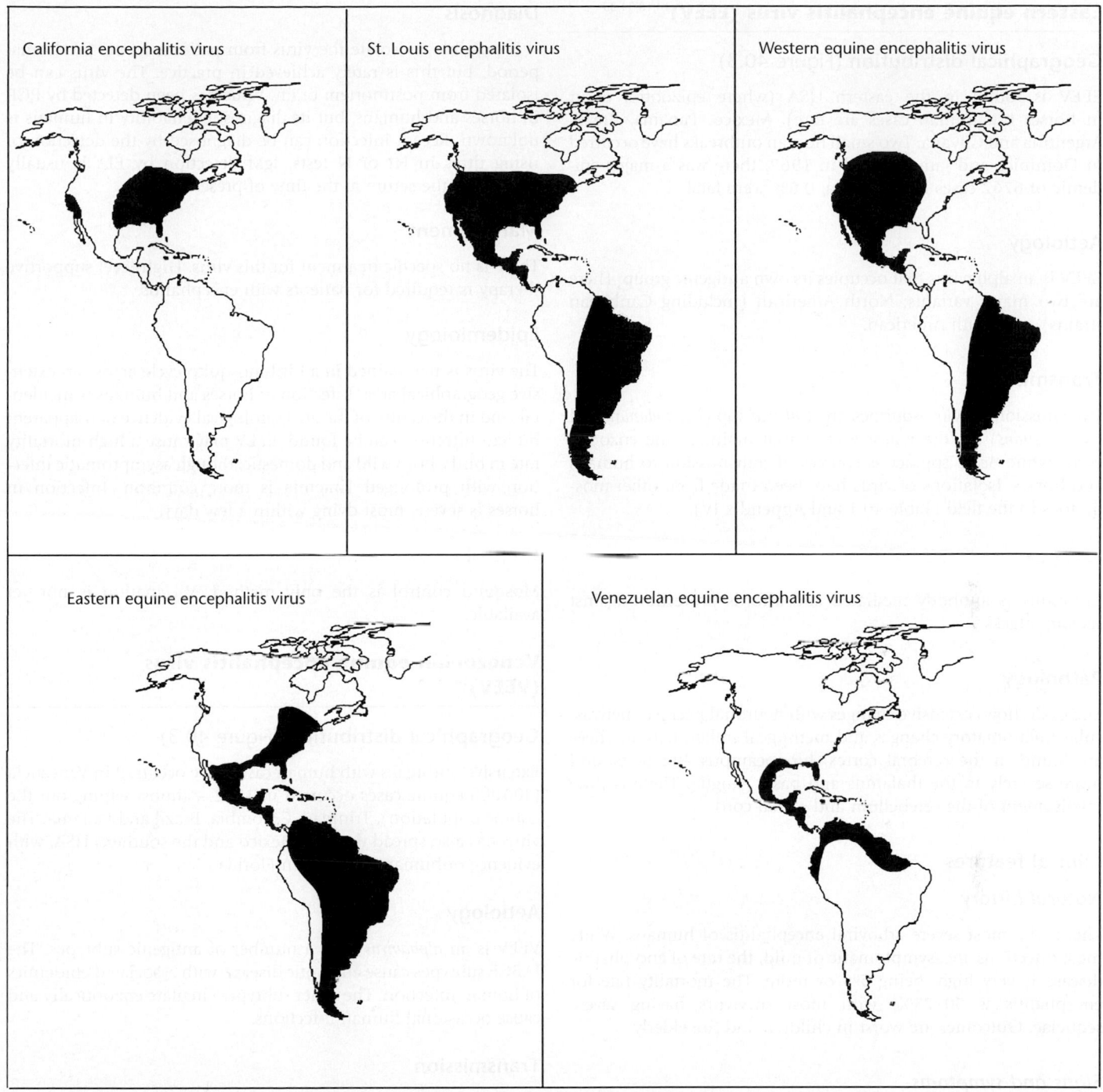

Figure 40.3 Geographical distribution of mosquito-borne encephalitis in the New World. California encephalitis virus, St Louis encephalitis virus, Western equine encephalitis virus, Eastern equine encephalitis virus, Venezuelan equine encephalitis virus.

Eastern equine encephalitis virus (EEEV)[14,18,34,35]

Geographical distribution (Figure 40.3)

EEEV is found in the eastern USA (where epizootics occur in horses but human cases are rare), Mexico, Panama, Brazil, Argentina and Guyana. Two small human outbreaks have occurred in Dominica and Jamaica, and in 1962, there was a major epidemic of 6762 cases in Venezuela; 0.6% were fatal.

Aetiology

EEEV is an alphavirus that occupies its own antigenic group. There are two major variants: North American (including Caribbean strains) and South American.

Transmission

Transmission is by mosquitoes; the *Culiseta* spp (*Cs. melanura* and *Cs. morsitans*) are the major vectors that maintain the enzootic cycle, while *Aedes* spp act as sources of transmission to humans and horses. Isolations of virus have been made from other mosquitoes in the field (Table 40.1 and Appendix IV).

Immunity

Immunity is antibody mediated and affords protection against second attacks.

Pathology

The CNS shows extensive changes with neuronal necrosis, perivascular inflammatory changes and meningeal inflammation. These are found in the cerebral cortex, hippocampus and pons, and more severely in the thalamus and basal ganglia. There is little involvement of the cerebellum and spinal cord.

Clinical features

Natural history

This is the most severe arboviral encephalitis of humans. While most infections are asymptomatic or mild, the rate of encephalitic disease is very high, being 5% or more. The mortality rate for encephalitis is 50–75%, with most survivors having severe sequelae. Outcomes are worst in children and the elderly.

Signs and symptoms

The incubation period is 7–10 days.

The illness begins as a febrile illness lasting up to 2 weeks. In most this resolves, but in about 2% of adults and 6% of children there is sudden onset of encephalitis. Headache, meningism and reduction of conscious state develop. This progresses to coma and convulsions, with most dying in the first few days. There is a peripheral leucocytosis in the early stages, and the CSF usually shows an early polymorph pleocytosis, with a mildly to moderately raised protein level. Those who recover usually have intellectual disability, neuropsychiatric illness and possibly paralysis.

Diagnosis

It is possible to isolate the virus from patients in the prodromal period, but this is rarely achieved in practice. The virus can be isolated from postmortem brain. Virus has been detected by PCR in horses and humans, but its diagnostic reliability in humans is unknown. Recent infection can be diagnosed by the detection of rising titres in HI or N tests. IgM detection by EIA is usually positive in the serum at the time of presentation.

Management

There is no specific treatment for this virus. High-level supportive therapy is required for patients with encephalitis.

Epidemiology

The virus is maintained in a bird-mosquito cycle across an extensive geographical area. Infection of horses and humans is incidental, and in the centre of the area serological evidence of inapparent human infection can be found. EEEV may cause a high mortality rate in birds, both wild and domestic, though asymptomatic infection with prolonged viraemia is more common. Infection in horses is severe, most dying within a few days.

Control

Mosquito control is the only method. Vaccination is not yet available.

Venezuelan equine encephalitis virus (VEEV)[14,18,36,37]

Geographical distribution (Figure 40.3)

Extensive outbreaks with human cases have occurred in Venezuela (100 000 equine cases occurred in 1962 – almost wiping out the equine population), Trinidad, Colombia, Brazil and Panama. The virus has also spread through Mexico and the southern USA, with evidence of human infection in Florida.

Aetiology

VEEV is an *alphavirus* with a number of antigenic subtypes. The IABCE subtypes cause epizootic disease, with associated epidemics of human infection. The other subtypes circulate enzootically and cause occasional human infections.

Transmission

The main vectors are *Culex* spp (particularly the subgenus *Melanoconion*), as well as *Mansonia*, *Psorophora* and *Aedes* species. Isolations have been made from about 40 other species (Table 40.1 and Appendix IV). *Simulium* spp. may transmit infections and there is a possibility of person-to-person spread by droplet infection; spread among horses can occur without an insect vector. Aerosol transmission to humans has occurred in laboratory settings.

Immunity

Immunity is antibody mediated and provides protection against second attacks. It therefore takes about 10 years to build up a susceptible population of humans and equines to sustain a new epidemic.

Clinical features

Natural history

Most infections are inapparent and the majority of the overt infections are mild and transient, although virulence may vary in epidemics.

Signs and symptoms

The incubation period is 2–5 days.

The onset is sudden, with fevers, rigors, headache and myalgia. A sore throat and upper respiratory symptoms are common, as are vomiting and conjunctivitis. Some also have diarrhoea. In some cases, and in about 4% of children under 15 years of age, symptoms progress with involvement of the CNS. Neck stiffness, convulsions, coma, and flaccid or spastic paralysis may develop. There is an initial leucopenia and sometimes thrombocytopenia, with pleocytosis and raised protein levels in the CSF. Long-term sequelae seem to be uncommon, but mental depression is common.

Aerosol spread can occur, so appropriate respiratory precautions should be used in hospitals to protect staff, visitors and other patients.

Diagnosis

Virus may be detected by culture or by RT-PCR from the blood in the acute phase, especially within 48 h of onset, and also from the throat. Recent infection can be diagnosed by the detection of rising titres in HI or N tests. IgM detection by EIA is usually positive in the serum within 1 week of onset.

Aerosol spread can occur and laboratory-acquired infections are well documented. The virus and samples likely to contain virus should be handled with extreme caution, and people working with the virus should be vaccinated.

Management

There is no specific treatment for this virus. High-level supportive therapy is required for encephalitis cases.

Vaccination

A live attenuated vaccine (TC-83) is available for primary immunization against the epidemic strains. It does not elicit good responses in people with previous *alphavirus* infections, nor is it very effective as a booster. An inactivated vaccine (C-84) seems to be better for these applications.

Epidemiology

VEEV circulates silently in small mammals and, with a high rainfall and an increase in the number of mosquitoes and their biting, horses become infected, acting as amplifying hosts. Equine cases precede human cases, most commonly children in whom the disease is more severe. A high proportion of equines develop immunity so that 10 years is necessary to build up another susceptible population.

Control

Mosquito control is difficult in rural conditions.

Mayaro virus (Mayv)[38]

MAYV is an *alphavirus* found initially in Trinidad and has since been recognized in Central America, northern South America and the Amazon basin. Two genotypes have been identified, one of which (Una virus) is restricted to northern Brazil. It is transmitted by *Haemagogus* mosquitoes, and wild vertebrates may serve as the animal hosts. Outbreaks are becoming more common as human populations move into forest areas. Clinically it resembles CHIKV and some develop persisting arthralgias (Table 40.1 and Appendix IV).

O'nyong-nyong virus (Onnv)[14,18,39,40]

Geographical distribution

ONNV is probably endemic in East Africa. A large epidemic beginning in 1959 involved over 2 million people in Uganda, Kenya, Tanzania, Zaire, Malawi, Mozambique, Senegal, Zambia and southern Sudan, and it has also been found in the Central African Republic and Cameroon. The next epidemic occurred in Kenya 35 years later. A variant, Igbo Ora virus is found in West Africa, including Nigeria, the Ivory Coast and the Central African Republic (Figure 40.4).

Aetiology

ONNV is an *alphavirus* closely related to CHIKV.

Transmission

Anopheles funestus is the major vector but *An. gambiae* is also involved (see Appendix IV). A non-human mammalian host has not yet been identified.

Clinical features

The clinical illness is very similar to CHIKV, with the exception that cervical lymphadenopathy is common, while fever is less prominent. Joint pains may persist for many months.

Epidemiology

There is no animal reservoir identified, though there is likely to be some form of animal–mosquito sylvatic cycle to maintain the virus. Large epidemics occur when the environmental conditions are supportive and there are enough susceptible subjects. Up to 70% of the population may be attacked, with all the age groups affected. Spread of the virus is believed to be by movement of viraemic humans.

Control

Avoidance of mosquito exposure by the use of protective clothing, mosquito nets and mosquito repellents is recommended during epidemic periods.

Ross river virus (RRV) disease[14,18,27,41]

Geographical distribution

RRV is named after the area in which it was first isolated from *Aedes vigilax* in 1974. Disease occurs throughout Australia, but most commonly in northern, north-eastern and south-western parts. Epidemics have occurred in Fiji, American Samoa, the Cook Islands and New Caledonia. Antibody studies have shown infection to be present in New Guinea, Solomon Islands, the Moluccas and Vietnam.

Transmission

Transmission is by a range of mosquito species including *Ae. vigilax, Ae. camptorhynchus, Cx. annulirostris, Ae. notoscriptus and Ae. sagax* in Australia[42] and *Ae. polynesiensis* in the Cook Islands.[43] *Ae. aegypti* and *Ae. albopictus* are efficient experimental vectors (Table 40.1 and Appendix IV).

Pathology

Arthritis is associated with a predominantly mononuclear inflammatory response in the synovium and the synovial fluid. Viral

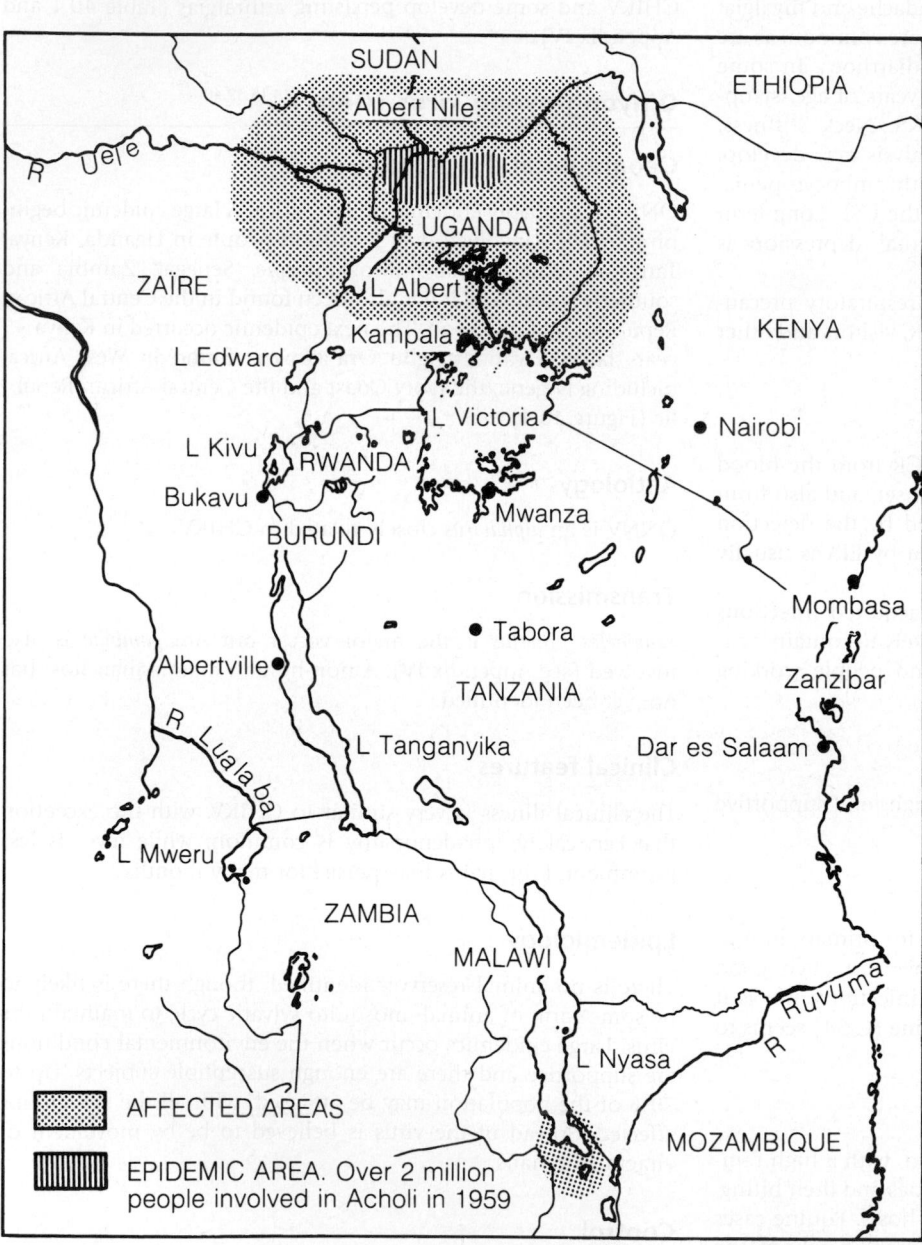

Figure 40.4 Geographical distribution of o'nyong-nyong fever. (Courtesy of the Department of Entomology, London School of Hygiene and Tropical Medicine.)

antigen and RNA have been found in joint tissue from patients and RRV is able to replicate in synovial macrophages in vitro. The pathogenesis of *alphavirus* arthritis is discussed earlier.

Clinical features

Natural history

The incubation period for RRV disease is usually 7–9 days but may vary from 3 to 21 days. Illness usually begins as joint pains (in a distribution typical of *alphavirus* arthritis) and myalgia, accompanied by lethargy in most patients and fever in about half. A generalized maculopapular rash occurs in 50%, usually after the onset of joint pains but sometimes preceding it. The rash is occasionally vesicular. Headache, photophobia, sore throat and lymphadenopathy may accompany the acute illness. Overall joint pains, swelling and stiffness develop in 80–90% of individuals. The swelling is largely due to synovitis without effusion. The lethargy may be profound and debilitating. The acute illness may resolve over weeks to months, but 10–25% will have joint pains, lethargy and myalgia persisting for over a year, and for several years in some. The chronic illness may follow a relapsing and remitting course.

Diagnosis

Viraemia lasts only a few days and infection is rarely diagnosed by virus isolation. RNA can be detected by PCR in acute serum, but is relatively insensitive. IgG and IgM can be detected by HI, EIA or IFA. There is some cross-reaction with antibody to other *alphaviruses* such as BFV, SINV and CHIKV, but IgM reactions are usually limited to the infecting virus. If necessary, specific antibody may be identified by N titres. IgM persists for many months after infection and is therefore only a presumptive indicator of recent infection. Demonstration of seroconversion or a significant rise in IgG levels is required to confirm recent infection.

Management

Treatment is symptomatic, with judicious use of non-steroidal antiinflammatory agents and simple analgesics for the relief of joint and muscle pains. Physiotherapy and graduated exercise programmes help some people. Corticosteroids provide relief of symptoms, but are not currently recommended until there are further data on long-term benefits and risks.

Epidemiology

Macropods (kangaroos and wallabies) are thought to be the natural vertebrate hosts, but in epidemics the virus can spread from humans to mosquitoes to humans. In Australia cases occur annually between summer and autumn. Explosive epidemics have occurred in Fiji, Samoa and the Cook Islands when the disease encountered a fresh non-immune population. Infection rates were 90%, with 40% of the population showing clinical attacks.

Sindbis virus (SINV)[14,18]

Geographical distribution

The virus was first isolated at Sindbis in Egypt, and has since been found to be widely distributed through sub-Saharan Africa, Europe, the Middle East, India, Asia, the Philippines, Australia and New Zealand. However, significant human epidemics occur only in Sweden (where it causes Ockelbo fever), Finland (Pogosta fever), adjacent parts of Russia (Karelian fever) and South Africa. There are two major antigenic lineages: the Oriental/Australian and the Paleoarctic/Ethiopian, with a third lineage being detected in south-western Australia.[44]

Aetiology

SINV is an *alphavirus* in the Western equine encephalitis serogroup. Ockelbo virus is a variant of SINV.

Transmission

A range of bird species, including migratory birds, are susceptible to SINV infection. Transmission to birds is via various *Culex* species, including *Cx. univittatus* and *Cx. pipiens*. Depending on the geographical region, humans may be infected by *Aedes*, *Culex*, *Culiseta* or *Mansonia* species.

Clinical features

Natural history

Descriptions of clinical illness are most detailed for Ockelbo and Pogosta diseases.[45] The incubation period is up to 1 week. Onset is usually joint pains typical of *alphavirus* infection, usually accompanied by a rash, malaise and fatigue. Fever is mild or absent. The rash is initially widespread and maculopapular. Chronic joint pains are common.

Diagnosis

SINV may be isolated form blood during acute illness and, more often, RNA can be detected by PCR. HI antibody can be detected but does cross-react with other alphaviruses. IgM can be detected by EIA and IFA, as well as HI.

Management

Treatment is symptomatic, as for other *alphavirus* arthritides.

Epidemiology

SINV is maintained primarily in a mosquito-bird cycle. Birds develop a prolonged viraemia, and infected migratory birds may be responsible for spread of the virus. The patterns of disease vary. Ockelbo outbreaks occur each summer/autumn, Pogosta occurs approximately every seven years, and irregular SINV epidemics occur in South Africa.

FLAVIVIRUSES (FAMILY FLAVIVIRIDAE, GENUS *FLAVIVIRUS*)

Dengue virus (DENV)

See Chapter 41 for information on Dengue virus.

Japanese encephalitis virus (JEV)[46–51]

Geographical distribution

The geographical range of JEV now extends from Japan, maritime Siberia and Korea in the north, through all except two provinces of China to the Philippines in the east, through South-east and southern Asia to Sri Lanka, India, Pakistan and Nepal in the west, and as far south as Indonesia, Papua New Guinea and far northern Queensland in Australia (Figure 40.5).

Aetiology

JEV is 50 nm in diameter and shares antigens with SLEV and MVEV.

Transmission

Culex tritaeniorhynchus, a rice-field breeding mosquito, is the main vector in north Asia and Japan. Other vectors include *Cx. annulirostris* in Guam and northern Australia, *Cx. gelidus* and *Cx. fusocephala* in India, Malaysia and Thailand, and *Cx. vishnui* in India (see Table 40.1 and Appendix IV). Vertical transmission of JEV in both *Culex* and *Aedes* mosquitoes has been demonstrated.

Pathology

After inoculation, the virus may replicate in the lymphatic tissues and possibly other organs before invading the CNS. In the brain there are areas of necrosis with small haemorrhages and perivascular cuffing in the grey matter of the cerebral cortex and in the thalamus, midbrain, cerebellum, brainstem and anterior horns of the spinal cord.

Immunity

An antibody-mediated immunity protects against second attacks and builds up resistance in the population.

Clinical features

Natural history

Many infections are asymptomatic or non-specific, with encephalitis estimated to occur in only 1 in 300 infections. Encephalitis has a mortality rate of 10–25%, but rises to 40–50% for comatose patients. Death is more common in children and in the elderly.

The incubation period is 6–16 days. The onset is sudden, although it may be preceded by gastrointestinal disturbance, especially in children. Fever, headache, altered mental state and, in children, convulsions are the main presenting features. Patients may show generalized weakness or paralysis, cranial nerve palsies and a coarse tremor. A characteristic attitude with head retracted, arms and knees bent, and shoulders pressed to the chest has been described (Figure 40.6). Some patients make a rapid and complete recovery, but generally severe depression of conscious state and/or evidence of respiratory paralysis are poor prognostic signs. If the acute stage is survived, recovery is slow and 25–50% will have neurological residua. These include paralysis, ataxia, Parkinsonism, mental deterioration, psychiatric disorders and speech difficulties.

The CSF usually shows a pleocytosis, initially due to neutrophils and later lymphocytes, while the protein concentration is normal or moderately raised. Electroencephalography (EEG) and CT findings are usually non-specific, though the latter may show thalamic and basal ganglia changes in severe cases. MRI has proven more useful in showing these changes.

JEV neurological disease may also present as benign aseptic meningitis, as polio-like acute flaccid paralysis, as an acute psychosis or without overt signs of encephalitis. A variety of psychiatric disturbances occur in many patients several months after recovering from the acute infection.

JEV infection in pregnancy is rare but can result in intrauterine infection and fetal death.

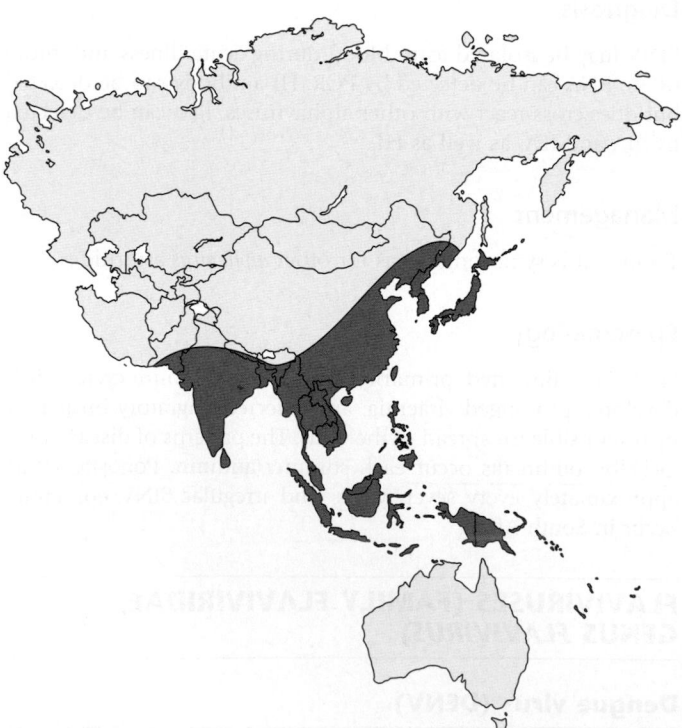

Figure 40.5   Geographical distribution of Japanese encephalitis virus.

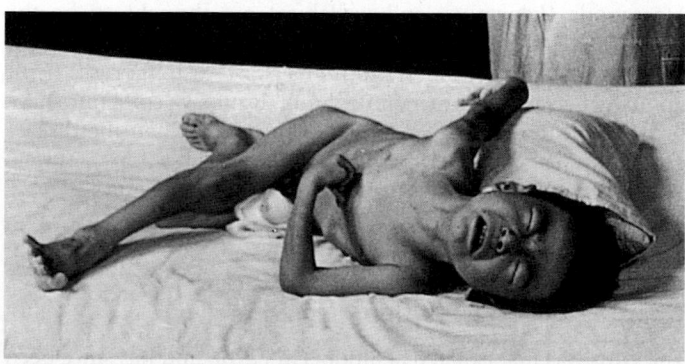

Figure 40.6   A 5-year-old boy with Japanese encephalitis virus.

Diagnosis

The virus has occasionally been cultured from human material, mainly CSF in severe cases. The viraemia is short lived so samples need to be collected early in infection. JEV will grow in mosquito cell lines, a wide range of mammalian cell lines and suckling mouse brain. A number of RT-PCR methods have been described and, if the test is available, it should be performed on early serum samples, CSF and brain tissue where collected. Antigen detection methods have also been used for virus detection in brain. Paired sera taken in the first few days after onset and 2–3 weeks later will show rising antibody levels by HI test, EIA or IFA. IgM is usually detected by EIA or IFA and is present in the serum in the early stages of illness in 80% of cases and virtually all by 10 days after onset. IgM may persist for weeks or months in the serum. It can be detected in CSF in most cases of encephalitis. IgM detection needs to be interpreted with caution in areas where other flavivirus infections occur as it may cross-react on tests. IgG antibodies will cross-react broadly with other flaviviruses. The specificity of antibody can be determined by N tests or by monoclonal antibody epitope blocking enzyme immunoassays.

Management

Treatment is supportive, and access to high-level support is important in the survival of severe cases. Neither dexamethasone nor interferon-α has been shown to influence the outcome.

Epidemiology

The main source of infection is rice fields where the vector *Cx. tritaeniorhynchus* breeds, becoming infected from pigs or birds. Three weeks after mosquito breeding begins in the spring, virus can be found in birds and pigs, but humans are not involved until there is a high density of mosquitoes. The virus is amplified by pigs and conveyed to humans. Birds (night herons and egrets) carry the infection from rural to urban areas. There is a seasonal summer incidence, with most activity occurring between June and September in temperate northern regions, with a longer period of transmission further south. In tropical areas transmission is often linked to local monsoonal weather patterns. Most cases are in children and elderly people, although visitors of any age are affected.

Control

An inactivated vaccine derived from the attenuated Nakayama strain grown in mouse brain is available, and is given in three injections at 0, 7 and 28 days. Boosters are required every 3 years. Local reactions to the vaccine are common. Serious hypersensitivity reactions occur in 1 in 200 people, and may be delayed for several days after administration. Several cases of acute encephalomyelitis have been reported following vaccination, but it is not yet certain that these are due to the vaccine. Two other vaccines are currently used extensively in China, including the live SA14/14/2 attenuated vaccine. Vector control using chemical larvicides and adulticides has been successful in many areas, although there are increasing problems with insecticide resistance.

Kyasanur Forest disease virus (KFDV)[52–54]

Local synonym: 'Monkey disease'

Geographical distribution

KFDV was first described in 1957 in the Kyasanur Forest of Mysore (now Karnataka) in south-western India, but has been gradually spreading from there (Figure 40.7). Alkhurma virus is a subtype of KFDV that has been found in Saudi Arabia.

Aetiology

KFDV is a flavivirus (Table 40.1) belonging to the Russian spring summer encephalitis virus group. It is antigenically related to OHFV and POWV, but there is no cross-immunity.

Transmission

KFDV is transmitted by the nymphal stages of ticks that have been infected in the larval stage from a rodent or monkey. The ticks are *Haemaphysalis spinigera*, *H. turturis* and *H. papuana* (kinneari). KFDV is also carried by *Ixodes petauristae* and *I. ceylonensis*, and has been recovered from *Dermacentor* nymphs (Table 40.1 and Appendix IV).

Pathology

There are degenerative changes in the large organs. The spleen shows reduction of malpighian corpuscles and erythrophagocytosis. There is focal haemorrhagic bronchopneumonia with focal necrosis of the liver and gastrointestinal tract. The kidneys show acute degeneration of the proximal and collecting tubules. Encephalitis has not been described in human cases.

Immunity

Immunity is antibody mediated. Little is known about immunity to second attacks, but monkeys that recover are immune. There is no cross-immunity to other flaviviruses.

Clinical features

Natural history

KFD is mainly a severe febrile illness with complete recovery following a prolonged convalescence. However, meningoencephalitis and/or haemorrhagic disease may develop in a small proportion of cases. The mortality rate is 3–5%, and no sequelae have been reported in survivors.

Signs and symptoms

The incubation period is 3–8 days after the infective tick bite. In about 20% of cases the disease is biphasic.

The onset is sudden with fever, headache, myalgia, cough, vomiting, diarrhoea, dehydration, hypotension and bradycardia. In the majority of cases there are no haemorrhages, but gastrointestinal bleeding and haemoptysis may occur. After 10 days the illness subsides. In 20% of cases, the fever returns 1–2 weeks after the first phase, lasting 1–7 days. There may then be symptoms of

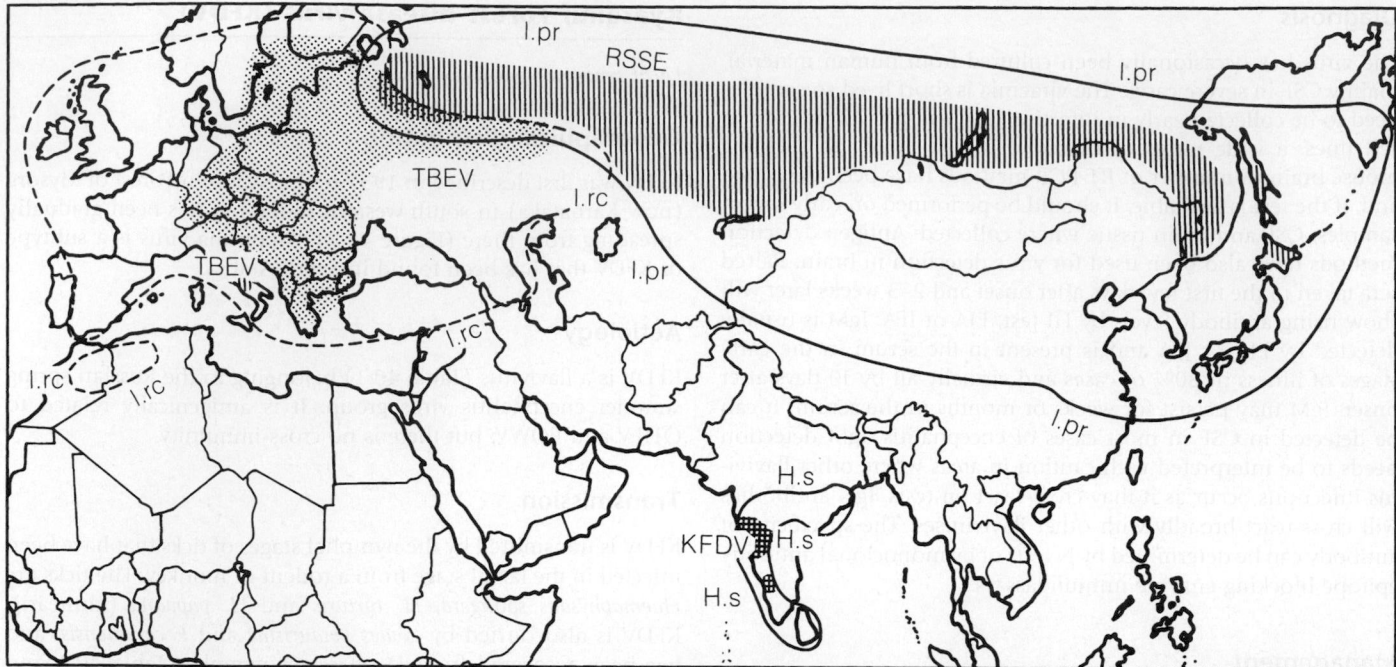

Figure 40.7 Geographical distribution of tick-borne encephalitis virus (TBEV) – RSSE, Russian spring-summer encephalitis (Eastern subtype TBEV); TBEV, European tick-borne encephalitis virus; KFDV, Kyasanur Forest disease virus – and the main vectors. I.pr, *Ixodes persulcatus*; I.rc, *Ixodes ricinus*; H.s, *Haemophysalis spinigera*. (Courtesy of the Department of Entomology, London School of Hygiene and Tropical Medicine.)

meningoencephalitis, with neck stiffness, mental disturbance, tremors and giddiness, lasting until the fever subsides. After recovery there is a prolonged convalescence, the patient remaining weak for some time. There is a marked leucopenia and a heavy albuminuria with casts in the urine. The CSF is normal in the first phase, but shows increased levels of protein but without cells in the second phase.

Diagnosis

Virus can be isolated from the blood up until the 12th day in suckling mice, hamster, monkey kidney or HeLa cells with cytopathic effect. Serological diagnosis can be made with rising antibody (IFA, HI and N) titres in acute and convalescent sera, as well as by EIA tests.

Management

Treatment is supportive. Care must be taken in the first 12 days to avoid exposure of medical and nursing staff to the patient's blood.

Epidemiology

KFDV circulates in forest rodents, especially the shrew (*Suncus murinus*) but also *Rattus wroughtoni*, *R. blandfordi* and a squirrel (*Funambulus tristriatus*), maintained mainly by larval ticks of *H. spinigera*, *H. turturis* and *H. papuana* (kinneari).

Langur monkeys (*Presbytes entellus*) and bonnet macaques (*Macaca radiata*) acquire larval ticks when foraging on the ground

and become infected. Many die, but some recover and are immune for life. When infected, the monkeys show a heavy viraemia. The larvae emerge from the ground as nymphs and come into contact with humans, to whom they transmit the infection as a dead-end infection.

Birds (grey jungle fowl and golden-backed woodpecker) are important in spreading the vector ticks, but are not thought to have a role in maintaining the infection in nature.

The risk of human infection has risen since humans moved into forest environments for rice cultivation, timber felling and cattle ranching. The cattle act as a good food source for the ticks, increasing the infection rates in monkeys and thus amplifying the virus and increasing the chance of human exposure.

Control

Control is essentially a breaking of the tick–human contact. Alteration of the environment and keeping cattle out of the forest are important. Personal protection involves regular (daily) de-ticking of the body and the use of repellents and protective clothing. A formalin-inactivated vaccine produced in chick embryo fibroblasts is now used in the endemic areas.

Kunjin virus (KUNV)[55,56]

KUNV is a flavivirus in the JE antigenic group and is a subtype of WNV. Human infection and disease have been demonstrated only in Australia, although the virus has been isolated from mosquitoes in South-east Asia. The distribution, reservoirs and transmission seem to be the same as for MVEV. Most infections are asymptomatic, although some produce a febrile illness with headache, with or without arthralgia, myalgia, fatigue and a maculopapular rash. Rare encephalitis cases occur that are clinically identical to MVEV but with a less severe disease and without fatalities.

Louping ill virus (LIV)[57,58]

LIV is a sheep virus transmitted by *Ixodes ricinus* and found in the UK and parts of southern Europe (Spain, Greece and Turkey). Tick-transmitted cases are rare, with the majority of naturally acquired human infections associated with occupational contact with infected animals. Laboratory acquired infections are common. It causes an illness very similar to the European subtype TBEV, and the vaccine for that virus will also protect against LIV.

Murray Valley encephalitis virus (MVEV)[55,59–62]

Geographical distribution

MVEV is found in Australia and New Guinea. Human disease has been identified mainly in the tropical northern areas of Australia, particularly the western and central areas of the north. Epidemic activity occasionally occurs outside these regions, and rarely it extends to the south eastern corner of the mainland.

Aetiology

MVEV is a flavivirus that lies in the JE antigenic group.

Transmission

Cx. annulirostris is the major mosquito vector. MVEV has also been isolated from a number of *Aedes* species and vertical transmission in these mosquitoes is proposed as a mechanism of persistence in many arid areas.

Pathology

The pathology of MVE is similar to that of JE, with perivascular cuffing in the grey matter, most marked in the thalamus and substantia nigra. These may extend into cerebral white matter, the cerebellum and spinal cord. In more advanced disease there is neuronal loss and areas of focal necrosis in the basal ganglia and thalamus. In severe residual disease these changes are more marked and thalamic necrosis may be seen.

Clinical features

The majority of infections are asymptomatic or non-specific. Only about 1 in 500 to 1 in 1000 develop encephalitis.

The incubation period is not well established, but is in the range of 1–3 weeks. Non-encephalitic illness consists of fever and headache, with or without arthralgia. It settles over 1–2 weeks, although full recovery may take some time. Encephalitic illness in children presents as fever of 1–2 days' duration, almost always with convulsions. Reduction of mental state and respiratory failure may follow. In adults, the encephalitic illness begins with headache, fever and altered mental state. Tremor may be apparent on examination and cranial nerve palsies may develop. The course may then vary from rapid recovery to a prolonged illness with respiratory paralysis or even death. Some patients recover rapidly, whereas others progress to more severe disease characterized by involvement of central brain structures, brain stem and possibly the spinal cord, often with respiratory paralysis. The mortality rate is around 25%, and about 50% of survivors have neurological residua varying from mild cranial nerve palsy to spastic quadraparesis. Death and severe residua are much more likely in the elderly and in infants.

In encephalitis cases the CT findings are usually unremarkable or show non-specific cerebral oedema, and the EEG shows non-specific changes. MRI in late disease has been reported to show thalamic destruction. Occasionally it mimics Herpes simplex encephalitis clinically, and may show temporal lobe changes on CT or MRI scan. The CSF shows a variable leucocyte pleocytosis, usually with lymphocyte predominance, and raised protein levels.

Diagnosis

The virus has rarely been cultured from human material, and the viraemia is likely to be short lived. It will grow in mosquito cell lines and suckling mouse brain. RT-PCR has been used to detect virus in the serum and CSF in the first few days of infection. Paired sera taken shortly after onset and 2–3 weeks later will show rising antibody levels by HI, EIA or IFA, although the HI test is the least sensitive and levels may rise late or not at all. IgM is nearly always present in the serum in the early stages of illness, and can also be detected in about 75% of CSF samples in encephalitis. IgM may persist for weeks or months in the serum. Antibody will cross-react with other flaviviruses, particularly KUNV and JEV, which may also cause encephalitis in the same geographical area. The specificity of antibody can be determined by N tests or epitope-blocking EIA, although misleading results may occur in patients who have had a previous flavivirus infection.

Management

Treatment is supportive, and access to respiratory support is important in the survival of severe cases. Based on the experience with JE, steroids are not recommended, although dexamethasone may be used to reduce intracranial pressure if needed. In contrast, preliminary data on the possible effectiveness of interferon-α for WNV infections suggest that this may be useful.

Epidemiology

The virus is maintained in a cycle involving water birds and mosquitoes. The vector *Cx. annulirostris* becomes infected with MVEV after feeding on birds, which can carry the infection widely by migration. There is also evidence for vertical transmission. A variety of wild and domesticated animals can be infected, but their role in the natural history is unclear (Table 40.1 and Appendix IV).

Immunization

There is no specific vaccine for MVEV. There are data from a mouse model that antibody induced by the inactivated JEV vaccine may enhance disease; this is a cause for concern in areas where both viruses may circulate.

Omsk haemorrhagic fever virus (OHFV)[52,58]

Geographical distribution

OHFV occurs in the Omsk and Novosibirsk regions of western Siberia.

Aetiology

OHFV is a flavivirus (Table 40.1), morphologically similar to but antigenically and genetically distinct from TBEV. The virus can be grown in HeLa cells or chick embryos.

Transmission

The virus is harboured by ticks – *Dermacentor reticulatus* and *D. marginatus* – with trans-stadial and transovarial transmission. The ticks transmit the infection to humans from rodents, mainly muskrats (Table 40.1 and Appendix IV). The mechanism of inter-rodent transmission in nature is not known, but mites may transmit the infection between muskrats and other rodents. Infection by direct contact with muskrat carcasses and pelts is common, and inter-human transmission occurs. There is some evidence of infection by the respiratory route.

Pathology

The pathology of fatal cases is that of haemorrhagic fevers with haemorrhage in tissues and necrotic areas in the liver. Immunity is antibody mediated; little is known about second attacks.

Clinical features

OHF is essentially a self-limiting acute infection in the majority of cases, although a small proportion develops haemorrhagic disease. The mortality rate is 1–3%.
The incubation period is 3–7 days.

Symptoms and signs

The illness is similar to KFD. Complete recovery is usual, although it may take several weeks. Some patients have a biphasic illness with pneumonia, neurological and/or renal disease.

Diagnosis

Virus can be isolated from the blood in the febrile period. Serological diagnosis is made by the CF, HI and N tests, and differentiation needs to be made with TBEV antibody.

Epidemiology and control

The reservoir of infection is the muskrat and ticks. Human infection depends upon muskrat–human contact, which may be via ticks or the handling of muskrat carcasses and pelts. When there is a great mortality of muskrats then contact is greater and outbreaks occur. TBEV vaccine may offer cross-protection against OHFV.

Powassan virus (POWV)[52,58]

Geographical distribution

POWV is found in Russia, the USA and Canada, and has been isolated from several tick species, including *Ixodes* species, *Dermacentor* species and *Haemophysalia longicornis*. The natural hosts are mainly wild rodents. Human infections are probably largely asymptomatic. However, some infected individuals develop a non-specific febrile illness that progresses to meningoencephalitis. The disease may resemble acute herpes simplex encephalitis, while other cases are similar to illness due to the Far-Eastern subtype of TBEV, with upper limb paralysis.

Rocio virus (ROCV)[63,64]

ROCV emerged as a cause of outbreaks of encephalitis in Brazil in 1975–1976 and since then sporadic cases have continued to be identified but there have not been further epidemics. It is probably carried by wild birds and transmitted by *Psorophora ferox* and *Aedes scapularis* mosquitoes (Table 40.1). It has an incubation period of 7–14 days, and illness begins with headache, fever, nausea and vomiting, sometimes with pharyngitis and conjunctivitis. Meningitis or encephalitis follows in many, with altered mental state and cerebellar tremor. Convulsions are uncommon. The mortality rate is about 10%. Death occurs in patients of all ages, and neurological sequelae are common. Gait distur-bances may appear in survivors. There is no specific therapy or vaccine.

St Louis encephalitis virus (SLEV)[64–67]

Geographical distribution

SLEV was the most important arbovirus in the USA prior to the introduction of WNV. It is widespread throughout North America but has also occurred in Trinidad, Central America, Brazil and Argentina (Figure 40.3).

Aetiology

SLEV is 30–40 nm in diameter and is antigenically related to JEV and WNV.

Transmission

The basic transmission cycle is between birds and several culicine mosquitoes with most activity in the summer months. This seasonal activity may be due to reintroduction of the virus by migratory waterbirds, or possibly over-wintering in hibernating bats, other mammals or mosquitoes. The main vectors for transmission to humans are *Cx. quinquefasciatus* in urban areas, and *Cx. tarsalis* and *Cx. nigripalpus* in rural areas. Transovarial transmission has been demonstrated in these three species (Table 40.1 and Appendix IV).

Pathology

The nervous system shows changes similar to the other flavivirus infections, with lymphocytic inflammation and neuronal degeneration in the basal ganglia, brainstem, cerebellum and spinal cord.

Clinical features

Natural history

The vast majority of infections are asymptomatic or non-specific. When clinically apparent, infection most often manifests as encephalitis, and less frequently as meningitis or as fever with severe headache. Children are less likely to develop symptomatic disease and it is usually mild. The overall mortality rate is 7%, but is age dependent with most deaths being in the elderly.

The incubation period is 6–16 days.

Onset is sudden, with fever and severe headache. Neck stiffness and photophobia may occur. Progression to CNS involvement is shown by drowsiness and confusion. Cerebellar ataxia, cranial nerve palsies and cogwheel rigidity may develop, and about 60% have intention tremor. Upper limb paralysis may occur. Convulsions are more common in children and, if severe and prolonged, are a poor prognostic sign. The CSF usually shows a mild to moderate lymphocyte pleocytosis and a raised protein concentration, though a neutrophil predominance may be seen in early infection. Changes in the basal ganglia may be seen on MRI scanning. Following recovery from the acute encephalitis, mild to serious sequelae may be found, particularly in the elderly. Parkinsonism, paralysis, tremor, confusion, gait disturbances and more general declines in cerebral function are seen. Neuropsychiatric disease is a relatively common late effect.

Diagnosis

Virus may be isolated from CSF in the early stages of the illness, but rarely from acute blood. It is best grown in newborn white mice, but also grows in hamster and chicken kidney cell cultures. Antigen may be detected by IFA in brain tissue or CSF mononuclear cells. Nucleic acid detection tests have also been used, but are usually negative by the time patients present. Serological diagnosis is achieved by showing rising antibody levels by HI, CF or N tests, and IgM detection by EIA helps to diagnose early infection. Detection of IgM in the CSF is a reliable indicator of encephalitis. IgM is relatively specific for the infecting virus, though possible cross-reactivity with WNV IgM should be considered. As with other flaviviruses, IgM persists in serum for several months after acute illness. To confirm the specificity of the antibody, N tests are required to differentiate it from antibody to other flaviviruses such as WNV.

Epidemiology

Cx. quinquefasciatus, being an urban mosquito, is responsible for urban outbreaks, while *Cx. tarsalis* and *Cx. nigripalpus* are responsible for rural outbreaks. In urban areas both children and adults are affected equally, but elderly people are most affected. In rural areas people with outdoors occupations are most at risk. Epidemics occur in the late summer and early autumn.

Treatment

Treatment is largely supportive, the level depending on the severity of disease. Interferon-α improves survival in a mouse model and, based on anecdotal experience with WNV encephalitis, it should be considered in severe cases.

Control

Surveillance and vector control are key to managing outbreaks of SLEV. 'Fogging' with insecticides may be necessary during epidemics.

Tick-borne encephalitis virus (TBEV)

This tick-borne flavivirus[52,58,68,69] has three subtypes: the Far-Eastern, the Siberian and the European, although there is considerable overlap. Other names include Russian epidemic encephalitis, Russian Far-East encephalitis, Russian spring-summer, central European encephalitis, Negishi virus and others.

Geographical distribution

The Far-Eastern subtype is seasonally epidemic in scattered foci in the far eastern part of the former USSR and extending across into China and Japan. The Siberian subtype occurs in the Urals, Siberia and far-eastern Russia, and the European subtype includes most virus isolates from Europe. The Siberian and Far-Eastern subtypes have also been detected in Europe (Figure 40.7).

Aetiology

TBEV is spherical, 50 nm in diameter, with a dense centre and surface membrane. It shares antigens with LIV, OHFV and KFDV, but not JEV.

Transmission

Ixodes ricinus is the major vector of European TBEV, while *Ix. persulcatus* is involved in transmission of the Siberian and Far-Eastern subtypes (see also Table 40.1 and Appendix IV). *Ix. ovatus*, *Ix. gibosus*, *Dermacentor* species and *Haemaphysalis* species have also been implicated. Viral infection is maintained by transovarial and trans-stadial transmission in ticks, as well as possible horizontal transmission by close proximity. In addition to tick bites, people may also become infected from drinking infected unpasteurized milk and less commonly by entry through injured skin or mucosa, such as crushing an infected tick on the skin. Rare aerosol transmission may occur.

Pathology

The virus enters via a tick bite, ingestion of infected milk or, rarely, through injured skin or mucosa or by inhalation. After multiplying at the site of injection it spreads through the reticuloendothelial system where it is further amplified. In some cases it then invades the CNS. It causes neuronal destruction in the cerebral cortex, basal ganglia, cerebellar cortex, brainstem and anterior horns of the spinal cord.

Clinical features

Natural history

The infection is often inapparent but when overt, is severe. The Far-Eastern subtype (mortality rate 20%) is more severe than the European (mortality rate 1–2%) and Siberian (mortality 1–3%) subtypes.

The incubation period is 3–14 days. Illness due to the Far-Eastern subtype usually presents with fever, headache, nausea, and myalgia. Up to 50% develop neurological signs such as meningitis, meningoencephalitis, ataxia, cranial and spinal nerve palsies, and paralysis. Rare haemorrhagic disease has occurred. The European subtype begins as an influenza-like illness that lasts a few days and may lead to a full recovery. In about one-third of cases a second phase begins several days later, with fever and a mild meningoencephalitis. Some have more severe disease resembling the Far-Eastern subtype. In rare cases a poliomyelitis-like syndrome with upper limb and respiratory paralysis occurs. The Siberian subtype produces a disease of intermediate severity. Residual neurological disease is common, such as neuropsychiatric disease, progressive weakness and Parkinsonism. The virus has been shown to persist in the brain for over 10 years in some patients.

Diagnosis

Virus can be isolated from the blood in the first week, but this is rarely done in practice. A number of RT-PCR assays have been developed and appear to be highly sensitive for detection of virus in the blood in early infection, prior to the appearance of antibody. Testing of CSF or of blood after the appearance of antibodies has a much lower yield.[70] IgM can be detected in acute serum and possibly the CSF. Serum IgM persists for many months. Paired acute and convalescent sera will show rising IgG levels by HI, CF, IFA, EIA or N tests. Specific antibody can be identified by N tests.

Treatment

Hyperimmune serum may be used in the first week, preferably within the first 3 days of onset of the initial illness, but its effectiveness is not clearly established. Otherwise, treatment is supportive.

Epidemiology

The virus circulates in small wild animals, chiefly rodents, and is transmitted by larval and nymphal ticks which, when they mature, feed on larger mammals, including humans. The incidence of the disease is seasonal – spring and early summer – occurring in small epidemics in the eastern part of the former USSR, where it is a disease of the forest and the taiga. In Europe it is a forest disease and occurs from late spring until early autumn, and outbreaks often follow a period when voles are numerous.

Control

Tick repellents and protective clothing may be of help. Pesticide treatment of large areas or restriction of access has been used.

Immunization

A formalin-inactivated vaccine grown in chick embryo cells is commercially available for the European subtype. The initial vaccine had a high rate of reactions, but that is not a problem with the current purified vaccines. It is 97–98% effective and has been used for mass vaccination in Austria and Germany. It is also recommended for people going to work in or visiting high-risk areas, and for laboratory personnel working with the virus. Hyperimmune globulin can also be used as prophylaxis before and after exposure.

Formalin-inactivated vaccines made from infected mouse brain and later from chick embryo cells have also been produced for the Far-Eastern subtype.

West Nile virus (WNV)[19,71]

Geographical distribution

Serological surveys, virus isolations and reports of disease outbreaks in humans and animals indicate that WNV is widely spread throughout Africa, the Middle East, southern Europe, Russia, southern India, parts of South-east Asia, North America and more recently South America (Figure 40.8). In addition, the Australian virus KUNV has now been recognized as a subtype of WNV.[72]

Virus morphology

WNV is a member of the JE antigenic complex within the *Flavivirus* genus. Similar to other flaviviruses, the virion is roughly spherical and approximately 40–50 nm in diameter. A lipid envelope encloses a nucleocapsid that contains the single-stranded, positive-sense RNA genome.

Transmission

Culex mosquitoes, particularly those that feed on birds, have a major role in the transmission of WNV. The virus has also been isolated from mosquitoes of other genera, including *Aedes* and *Mansonia*, which may also serve as natural vectors. WNV has also been isolated from several species of ticks, some of which have been shown to transmit the virus under laboratory conditions. These long-lived vectors may have an important role in the dispersal and overwintering of the virus.

WNV can also be transmitted via blood transfusion. Currently blood donations in the US are screened for the presence of WNV, and travel history to WNV endemic areas is used to screen donors in several countries. This approach has been effective in substantially reducing transfusion-transmission events. Other mechanisms of transmission include organ transplantation, percutaneous exposure, intrauterine infection and possibly via breast milk. Oral transmission occurs among animals by ingestion of infected animals or carcasses. There is some evidence to suggest faecal–oral transmission among confined animals.

Pathology

Following an infected mosquito bite, the virus replicates locally, probably in dendritic cells, then spreads via the reticuloendothelial system and the blood. In those who develop neurological disease, the virus infects neurones of the cerebral cortex, brainstem and spinal cord (especially the anterior horn), resulting in neuronal death. There are infiltrates of microglia and polymorphonuclear leucocytes, perivascular cuffing, neuronal degeneration, and neuronophagia. Immunohistochemical staining has demonstrated viral antigens in neurones, neuronal processes, and areas of necro-

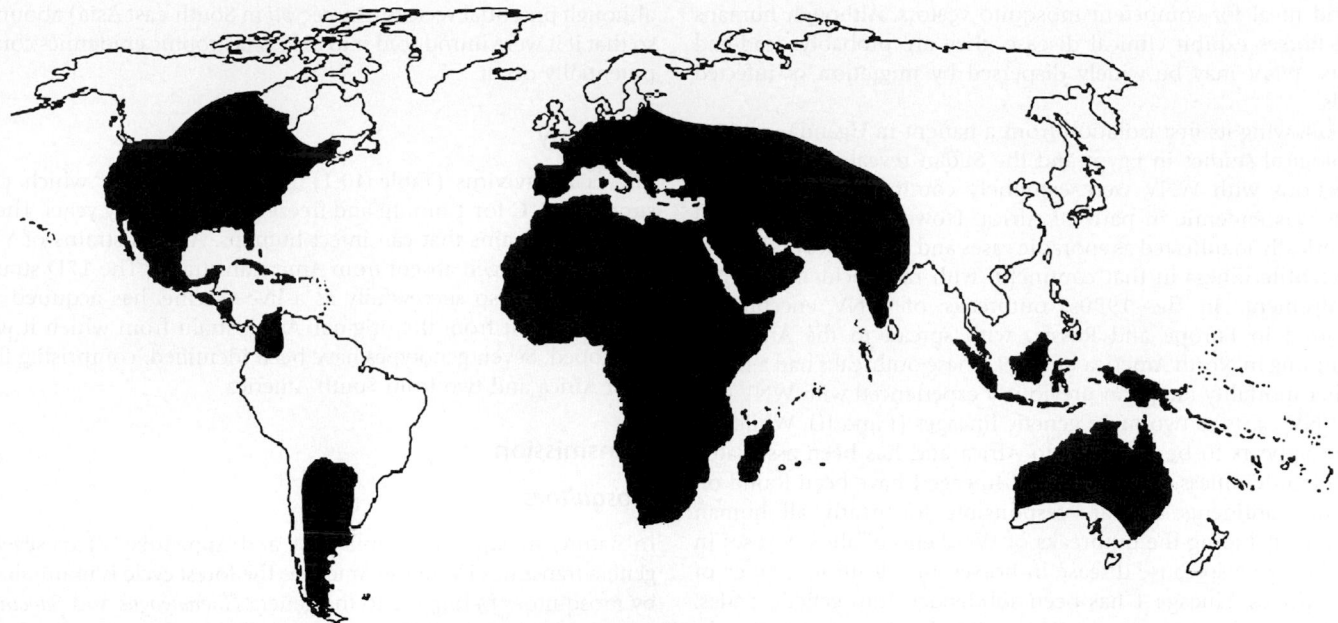

Figure 40.8 Geographical distribution of West Nile and Kunjin viruses.

sis. The histopathologic lesions and immunostaining are more prominent in the brainstem and spinal cord, which may explain the clinical manifestation of muscle weakness in some patients.[73] Virus has been detected in other organs in infected animals and in cancer patients, but this has not been demonstrated in immunocompetent humans.

Clinical features[73]

Natural history

In the great majority of cases WNV causes an inapparent infection; in others there is an acute dengue-like fever (for which it has often been mistaken) followed by recovery, but a few patients develop meningoencephalitis. Encephalitis has developed in about 1% of infected individuals in the USA, and is much more likely and more severe in adults than in children. The mortality rate from encephalitis is 10–40%.

The incubation period is 2–14 days. Historically, the disease has been typically mild, with fever, headache, myalgia, backache and anorexia. Generalized lymphadenopathy, maculopapular rash and nausea are also commonly reported. Other reported manifestations include hepatitis, myocarditis and rhabdomyolysis. Where progression to CNS involvement occurs, the patient develops severe headache, confusion and depression of conscious state, neck stiffness, cranial nerve palsies, tremors and generalized weakness. Presentations with a poliomyelitis-like syndrome and Guillain–Barré syndrome have both been reported. The CSF shows a mild pleocytosis, initially with neutrophil predominance and later lymphocytic, with a raised protein level. CT and MRI scans are usually not helpful in early disease and the EEG shows non-specific changes. Most survivors have significant neurological residua.

Diagnosis

Virus may be detected in clinical samples by isolation or RNA detection by PCR, especially in the first week after onset of illness.[74] A number of tests are now available for the detection of WNV-specific IgM in acute-phase serum of patients, and a positive result provides reliable evidence of recent infection. However, it is recommended to also test for IgM to other flaviviruses that may be present in the same area to exclude serological cross-reaction. Indeed, the initial diagnosis of index cases of WN in New York in 1999 was confounded by cross-reactions of WNV IgM with SLEV. Detection of IgM in CSF is a good indicator of encephalitis, but is absent in many cases. Recent infection results in seroconversion or a rise in IgG measured by HI, IFA or EIA. Specific WNV antibody can be identified using N titres or monoclonal antibody epitope-blocking enzyme immunoassays. It is not currently possible to serologically distinguish between antibody to the different lineages or sublineages of WNV, so KUNV infection is serologically identical to other WNV infections.

Treatment

Supportive therapy is the main component of patient management. Anecdotal experience with interferon-α in a small number of patients suggest that it may be useful, but further experience is needed.[75] Hyperimmune globulin has also been tried and may have some benefits.

Epidemiology

WNV is maintained in nature primarily in bird-mosquito cycles. Several species, including crows, bluejays and house sparrows, develop high titres of virus in the blood and provide an infectious blood meal for competent mosquito vectors. Although humans and horses exhibit clinical disease, they are probably dead-end hosts. WNV may be widely dispersed by migration of infected birds.

Following its first isolation from a patient in Uganda in 1937, serological studies in Egypt and the Sudan revealed that human infections with WNV were extremely common, indicating the virus was endemic in parts of Africa. However, the disease had historically manifested as sporadic cases and epidemics of dengue-like febrile illness in that continent, with rare incidents of CNS involvement. In the 1990s, outbreaks of WNV encephalitis occurred in Europe and Russia, with spread to the Americas, beginning in North America in 1999. These outbreaks had a much higher mortality rate than previously experienced with WNV.

WNV exists as two main genetic lineages (I and II). While the latter appears to be restricted to Africa and has been associated with febrile illness, virus strains of lineage I have been found on several continents and are responsible for nearly all human disease, including the outbreaks of WNV encephalitis. Viruses in this lineage also cause disease in horses and death in a range of bird species. Lineage 1 has been subdivided into genetic clades. Clade 1a strains appear to be responsible for the recent outbreaks of severe disease in humans, horses and birds, In contrast clade 1b stains, which are mainly confined to Australia where they are also called KUNV, rarely cause encephalitis and do not cause disease in animals or mortality in birds.

Immunization

Several candidate vaccines are in development or evaluation, including live vaccines, subunit vaccines, recombinant and chimeric vaccines. Immunogenicity, safety and protective efficacy have been shown in animals for some vaccines, but none are yet available for human use. There is also evidence that immunization with JE vaccine provides some cross-protection against WNV in mice. However, data suggesting possible enhancement of infection due to heterologous vaccine-induced antibody[21] mean that this approach requires careful evaluation.

Yellow fever virus (YFV)

Geographical distribution

YFV (see Chapter 40)[7,76,77] is found in the tropical forest areas of Africa and South America (Figure 40.9) and until early last century caused large epidemics in the Caribbean and the subtropical and temperate regions of North America as far north as Baltimore and Philadelphia. 'Jungle' YF still occurs in Brazil and there was an outbreak in Trinidad in 1978–1979, with 18 cases and eight deaths. Many other epidemics have occurred in South America, and a large epidemic in Ethiopia was responsible for many deaths in 1960–1962, and in Senegal in 1965–1966. YF has caused fatalities in tourists, especially in West Africa, who have not been vaccinated.

Genetic studies support the hypothesis that YFV probably originated in East and central Africa and was initially introduced into West Africa and then transported to South America, possibly by ships carrying infected mosquitoes in the post-Columbian period. YFV has never been established in Europe, Asia or Australasia

although potential vectors (*Ae. aegypti* in South-east Asia) abound, so that if it were introduced into Asia catastrophic epidemics could potentially occur.

Aetiology

YFV is a flavivirus (Table 40.1) 25–65 nm in size, which can survive at 4 °C for 1 month and freeze-dried for many years. There are several strains that can infect humans. African strains of YFV possess an antigen absent from American strains. The 17D strain, which is used so successfully as a live vaccine, has acquired an antigen absent from the original 'Asibi' strain from which it was developed. Seven genotypes have been identified, comprising five from Africa and two from South America.

Transmission

Mosquitoes

In nature, mosquitoes (Table 40.1 and Appendix IV) of several genera transmit YFV. In the Americas the forest cycle is maintained by mosquitoes belonging to the genera *Haemagogus* and *Sabethes*. *Ae. aegypti* is responsible for urban outbreaks. Virus has also been isolated from *Ae. fulvus* in Brazil. In Africa, *Ae. africanus* maintains the monkey-mosquito-monkey cycle in the forest, while *Ae. simpsoni*, which breeds close to humans in the axils of banana plants, becomes infected from monkeys raiding the plantations, and transmits YFV to people. Other *Aedes* involved in the forest cycle include *Ae. luteocephalus*, *Ae. opok*, *Ae. furcifer* and *Ae. taylori*. Vertical transmission of YFV from one generation to another in mosquitoes is thought to be important for virus survival during the dry season. In Africa the urban cycle is maintained by *Ae. aegypti*.

Mosquitoes can become infected from the first to third day of fever in the host. The intrinsic cycle in the mosquito is 4 days at 37 °C and 18 days at 18 °C. Mosquitoes remain infected for life. The possibility of transovarial transmission has already been mentioned.

Ticks

YFV has been isolated from *Amblyomma variegatum* in Brazil and trans-stadial transmission was demonstrated by infecting nymphs and passing on the infection to uninfected monkeys at the adult stage. The epidemiological significance of this is not clear.

Other methods

Other methods of transmission have not been identified in nature. However, the high level viraemia in infected humans and animals raises a potential for transmission though exposure to blood or infected tissues. Caution should be exercised in handling these materials.

Pathology

YFV replicates initially in the reticuloendothelial system before spreading to multiple organs, including liver, spleen, bone marrow, myocardium and skeletal muscle. Pathological changes are seen in all of these organs, characterized by cell damage. The kidneys show acute tubular necrosis, and there is damage of

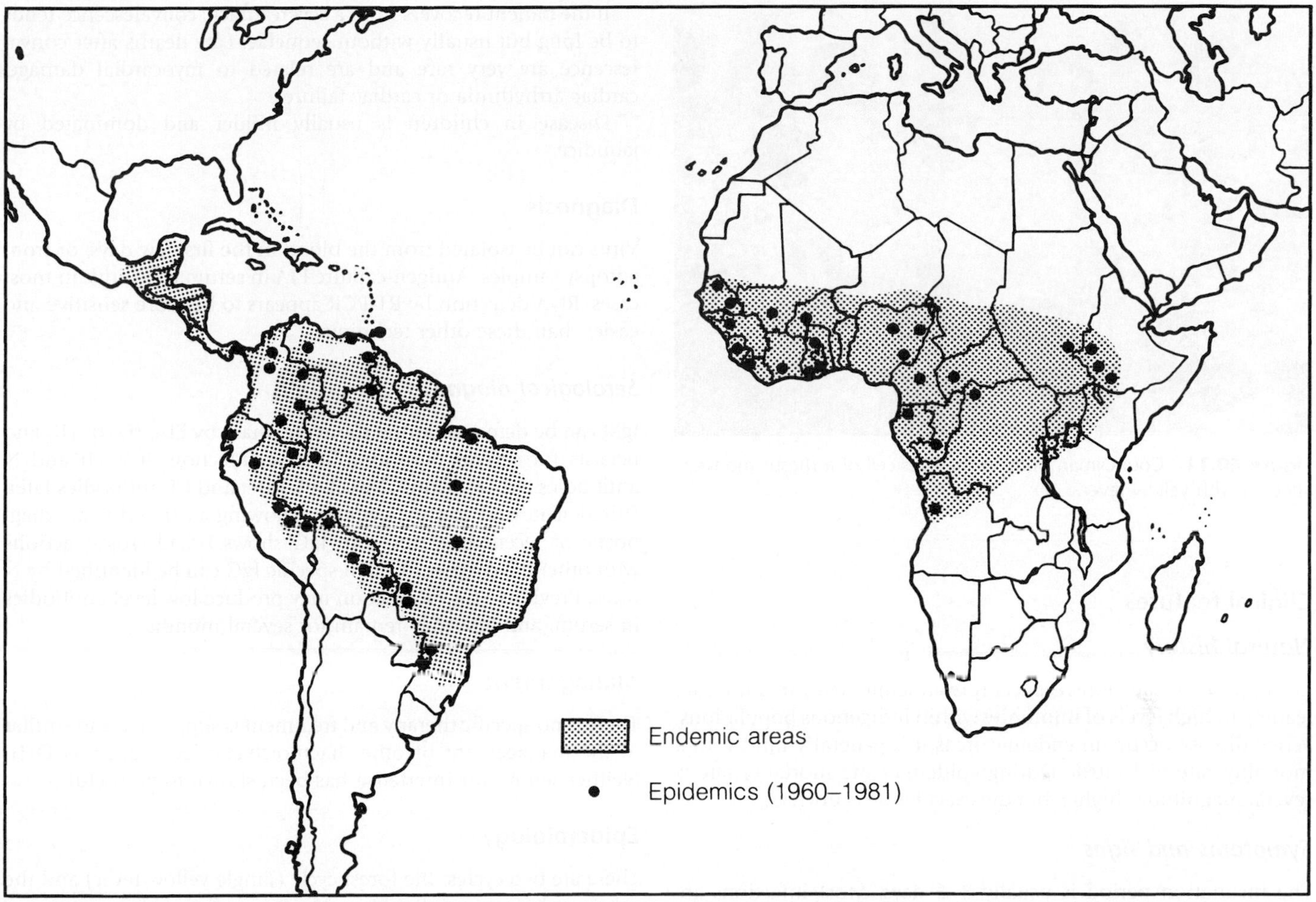

Figure 40.9 Geographical distribution of yellow fever virus.

myocardial cells. In the liver of acutely infected patients, YFV produces fatty degeneration of liver cells and central coagulative necrosis of the lobules with sparing of the borders (Figure 40.10). The nuclei of the liver cells are pyknotic and the coagulated contents of the cells stain deeply with eosin, the Councilman bodies resulting from this degeneration taking on a salmon-pink colour (Figure 40.11). These resolve completely in recovered cases. Cerebral changes may occur with oedema and petechial haemorrhages. Haemorrhages may also be seen in other organs such as the lungs, liver and spleen. The bleeding abnormalities are probably a result of a combination of reduced production of coagulation factors by the liver, combined with platelet dysfunction and DIC.

Death usually results from failure of the liver or kidneys or both, although cardiac damage may contribute.

Immunity

Immunity is antibody mediated, and lifelong immunity follows infection with YFV. In many endemic areas where contact with virus-carrying mosquitoes is constant (i.e. near the forest), infection in childhood is common, leading to reactivation in later life.

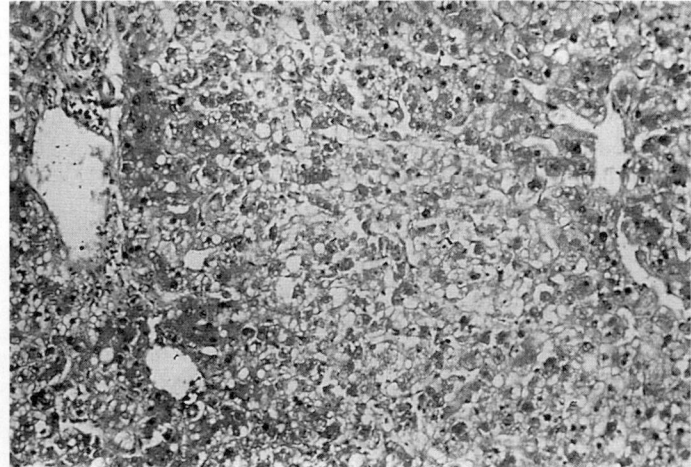

Figure 40.10 Postmortem appearance of the liver of a rhesus monkey with yellow fever, showing well marked mid-zonal necrosis and minimal inflammatory changes.

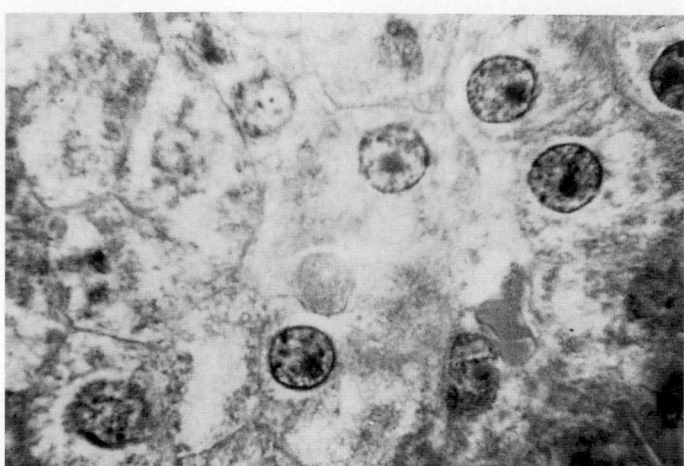

Figure 40.11 Councilman body in the liver cell of a rhesus monkey affected with yellow fever.

Clinical features

Natural history

Asymptomatic infections, especially in endemic areas, are common, leading to high levels of immunity within indigenous populations. When disease occurs in endemic areas it is generally mild with a mortality rate of 5–10%. During epidemics the mortality rate is several magnitudes higher, but the exact figure is unclear.

Symptoms and signs

The incubation period is usually 3–6 days. Most infections are asymptomatic or mild, with only a small proportion progressing to severe classical YF. The mild form is an acute febrile illness with sudden onset of fever and headache without other symptoms, lasting 48 h or less. In some other patients the headache is more severe, accompanied by myalgia, low back pain and slight protein-uria. The characteristic bradycardia in relation to temperature is present and the illness may last several days with recovery.

In severe illness the onset is abrupt with higher fever, severe headache, nausea, vomiting, abdominal pain and distressing pain in the back, loins and limbs. The patient is dehydrated with a dry tongue and foul breath. Early signs of jaundice may appear in the conjunctivae and skin, and minor bleeding from the gums and nose may be noted. This is called the 'period of infection' corresponding with the viraemia. It lasts about 3 days, and the patient may recover spontaneously after this. If they progress, there may be a 24-h period of apparent improvement, followed by rapid deterioration. Jaundice worsens and there is frank haemorrhaging from the gastrointestinal tract and other sites. Epigastric pain and vomiting develop and there is a deterioration of renal function and albuminuria. There can be hypotension and heart failure, with a characteristic prolongation of the PR and QT intervals on elec-trocardiography. The patient may recover rapidly after a period of 3–4 days, or recovery may take over 2 weeks. Death occurs in 20–50%, typically on the seventh to tenth day of illness. Bad prognostic signs are increasing proteinuria, haemorrhages, a rising pulse, hypotension, oliguria and azotaemia.

If the patient recovers from a severe attack, convalescence tends to be long but usually without sequelae. Late deaths after conva-lescence are very rare and are related to myocardial damage, cardiac arrhythmia or cardiac failure.

Disease in children is usually milder and dominated by jaundice.

Diagnosis

Virus can be isolated from the blood in the first few days, or from autopsy samples. Antigen-capture EIA in serum is positive in most cases. RNA detection by RT-PCR appears to be more sensitive and easier than these other techniques.

Serological diagnosis

IgM can be detected during the acute phase by EIA, IFA or HI, and persists for several months following infection. IFA, HI and N antibodies appear within 1 week of onset and CF antibodies later. Paired acute and convalescent sera showing a rising titre are diag-nostic of recent infection, but IgG shows broad cross-reactions with other flaviviruses, though specific IgG can be identified by N titres. Previous YFV vaccination may produce low level antibodies in serum, and IgM may remain for several months.

Management

There is no specific therapy and treatment is supportive and similar to the management of other haemorrhagic fevers such as DHF. Neither serum nor interferon has been shown to be useful.

Epidemiology

There are two cycles: the forest cycle (jungle yellow fever) and the urban cycle (urban yellow fever).

Forest cycle (jungle yellow fever)

In the Americas YFV is maintained in rainforests in a cycle involv-ing monkeys and marmosets and *Haemagogus* (tree-hole breeding) mosquitoes. Recurrent epizootics occur in howler (*Alouatta*) monkeys who die in large numbers, starting in Panama and spreading up the east coast of Central America to Guatemala, confirming the belief recorded by Balfour in 1914 that a 'silent forest' where all the howler monkeys had died denoted the pres-ence of YFV. A number of other monkey species also have a role: spider (*Ateles*) monkeys, squirrel (*Saimiris*) monkeys and owl (*Aotus*) monkeys develop fatal infections, while other species such as capuchin (*Cebus*) monkeys are asymptomatic but have viraemia sufficient to be infectious. Humans predominantly contract the disease when clearing forest areas; *Haemagogus* mosquitoes bite in and around houses in forest clearings. *Sabethes* (a drought-resistant mosquito) transmits infection during the dry season (see Appendix IV).

In the forests of West, Central and East Africa, a jungle cycle exists as an inapparent infection in monkeys, mainly *Cercopithecus* (vervet) monkeys. Other susceptible primates with asymptomatic infections include colobus (important in Ethiopia), mangabeys (*Cercocebus*) and baboons (*Papio*). In East Africa some species of bushbaby (*Galago*), which are susceptible to the virus, have been shown to have high levels of YFV antibodies and may be involved in transmission cycles. Several different *Aedes* spp. are important vectors of YFV in Africa (see the section on YFV transmission). Human infections generally follow the movement of humans into forested areas for agricultural purposes.

An endemic area population will show a rising percentage of positive antibody tests with age, whereas an epidemic situation will be shown by antibodies in the older age and none in the younger age groups.

Urban cycle (urban yellow fever)

When there is a high population of *Ae. aegypti*, intense transmission among humans occurs, with large epidemics where there are enough non-immunes in the population, which can be brought about by immigration, increased urbanization, poor maintenance of vaccination campaigns or a rising number of people born since the last epidemic. In the early years of the twentieth century huge epidemics of this nature frequently spread throughout the Caribbean and up the east coast of North America. Once *Ae. aegypti* was controlled, these epidemics ceased, and no urban cases of YF were described from the Americas for more than 40 years. However, urban cases continue to occur sporadically and the potential for future epidemics remains.

Regular YF epidemics continue in sub-Saharan Africa. In the Nuba mountains of southern Sudan in 1940 there was an epidemic (17000 cases; mortality rate 10%) and in south-western Ethiopia along the Omo River in 1960–1962 (15000–30000 deaths; mortality rate up to 85%). In 1965–1966 in Senegal there was an epidemic mainly affecting children under 10 years with a mortality rate of 15%. Since then activity has occurred in a number of countries in sub-Saharan Africa.

Control

Eradication and control of *Ae. aegypti* is the key to the prevention of urban YF in the Americas. This includes an attack on the breeding sites in water containers and tanks, and a monitoring system that gives an *Aedes* index of the numbers of *Aedes* mosquitoes. When this reaches a certain level an epidemic may result. In the presence of an epidemic, adult control by 'fogging' of towns and cities with insecticide will bring the epidemic to a halt. *Ae. aegypti* had been eradicated from the USA but has now returned to Louisiana, once a hotbed of YFV, in its previous numbers.

Vaccination

YF 17D is a safe, live, attenuated vaccine providing a long-lasting immunity. For purposes of certification, 10 years is considered the limit but immunity after 40 years has been documented and it may be lifelong. Vaccination to YFV is imperative for travellers to endemic areas and certificates are demanded for travellers from endemic areas to non-infected tropical areas. Immunity develops within 10 days of vaccination. Serious complications are rare. No consequences for the fetus have been recorded but pregnant women should avoid vaccination unless the risk from YFV is considered great. Vaccination is not recommended for children under 6 months of age, and especially children aged less than 4 months, because of an increased risk of encephalitis. It should also be avoided in immunosuppressed patients. The vaccine is prepared in chick embryos and people sensitive to egg protein may have reactions. Serious side-effects are rare with the 17D vaccine. Encephalitis, classical YF and severe multisystem illness have been reported. The risk of neurological disease is 1–16 per million doses, and of visceral disease is 2.5 per million doses.

BUNYAVIRUSES (FAMILY BUNYAVIRIDAE, GENUS *BUNYAVIRUS*)

California encephalitis virus (CEV)[78]

CEV was the first identified member of the California serogroup of bunyaviruses. It was identified as a cause of encephalitis in California in the 1940s, but rarely causes human infection (Figure 40.3). Human infections occur more commonly with the closely-related La Crosse virus and Jamestown Canyon virus. It infects rabbits and rodents, and is transmitted by *Aedes* species.

Oropouche virus (OROV)[78]

OROV is a member of the Simbu group of bunyaviruses (Table 40.1) and is a major cause of disease in the Amazon region of Brazil and Peru. It is transmitted by the midge *Culicoides paraensis* and some mosquito species. It is maintained in a jungle cycle involving sloths and monkeys. Disease onset is sudden, with fever, chills, headache, myalgia, arthralgia and photophobia being most common. The illness lasts 1–2 weeks and patients make a full recovery. Virus can be detected in blood in the first few days, but diagnosis is usually by serology.

Rift Valley fever virus (RVFV)[79–81]

Geographical distribution

RVFV was first recognized in Kenya in 1931 as causing a disease in sheep and humans. Until 1977 it was restricted to humans and domestic animals in sub-Saharan Africa, with epizootics in Kenya, South Africa, Zimbabwe, Sudan, Egypt, Uganda, Tanzania and Zambia. A similar virus (Zinga virus) was found to be present in West Africa (Mali, Nigeria and Zaire) and in Botswana and Mozambique, but without epizootics. In 1977 RVFV spread to Egypt where it caused massive epidemics and epizootics, and showed a capability to spread beyond sub-Saharan Africa (Figure 40.12). The Egyptian episode was centred largely in the Nile delta where approximately 600 human deaths are thought to have occurred. This was probably preceded by a massive epizootic along the Nile bank from Aswan in the south to Cairo in the north. RVF occurred again in Aswan in 1993 and several cases with ophthalmic complications have been seen in the Nile delta. The largest ever recorded outbreak of RFV occurred in Kenya and Somalia in 1997–1998 (when up to 89000 people were affected), and an outbreak was also recorded in the Arabian Peninsula in 2000.

Aetiology

RVFV is a member of the genus *Phlebovirus* in the Bunyaviridae family (Table 40.1). RVFV is an enveloped virus of up to

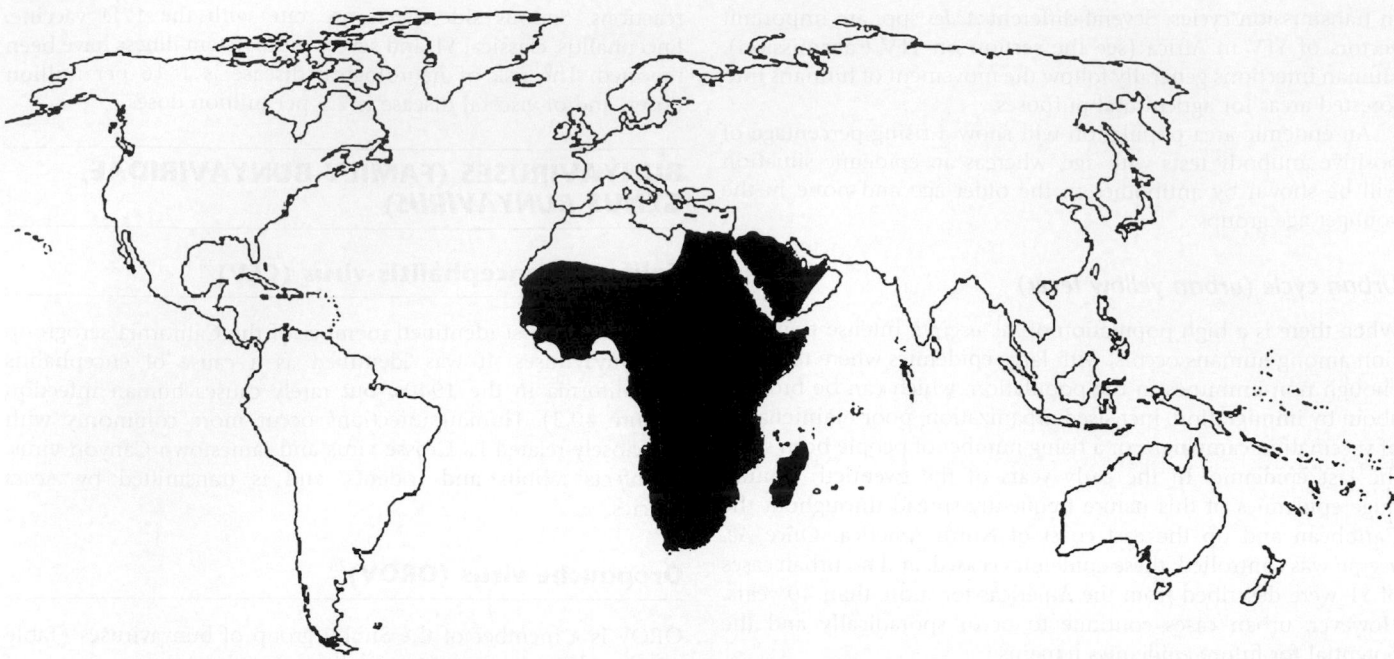

Figure 40.12 Geographical distribution of Rift Valley fever virus.

120 nm in size, and the RNA genome is divided into three segments.

Pathology

The pathogenesis of RVFV appears to be similar to that of YFV, with initial spread to lymphatic tissue and then to the liver, with necrotic change in the latter. In a small proportion this is followed by haemorrhage which is probably due to a combination of reduced production of coagulation factors and DIC. Cerebral invasion with encephalitis and retinitis may occur 1–4 weeks after recovery.

Transmission

The virus infects a large range of domestic animals. Transmission between the zoonotic hosts is by mosquitoes of the *Eretmapodites*, *Mansonia*, *Anopheles*, *Aedes* and *Culex* groups (Table 40.1 and Appendix IV), and possibly to humans by *Ae. caballus* and *Cx. theileri* in South Africa and *Cx. pipiens* in Egypt. Mechanical transmission may also occur by other biting insects including *Culicoides* and *Simulium* species. Direct transmission, especially during epidemics, is by the aerosol route from infected animal tissues. Person-to-person transmission does not occur but acute-phase blood and infected animal tissues are highly infectious, especially in abattoirs. Laboratory-acquired infections have been described and the virus should be handled with extreme caution.

Immunity

Active immunity

Immunity is antibody mediated and there is prolonged immunity to reinfection with homologous strains after recovery. Antibodies

formed are of the usual viral response (HI, CF and N). HI and CF antibodies are used in diagnosis, and N antibodies give specificity.

Passive immunity

A passive immunity can be transferred via the placenta to the child and lasts for several months; the possession of antibodies, especially N antibodies, can be used in treatment using convalescent sera.

Clinical features

Natural history

RVFV is a self-limiting disease in the great majority of infections, with a short, acute, febrile phase and complete recovery. However, in less than 5% of cases, encephalitis, retinal lesions, haemorrhage and hepatic disease develop.

Symptoms and signs

The incubation period is 2–6 days. The onset is abrupt with fever, headache, joint and muscle pains, conjunctivitis and photophobia. In the majority of cases this is followed by complete recovery. In a few cases there may be recrudescence of symptoms after the initial short illness and convalescence may be prolonged. Retinal disease develops in 5–10% of cases, between 1 and 3 weeks after the febrile illness, with macular exudates and, in some instances, retinal haemorrhages and vasculitis. About half of the patients are left with permanent impairment of vision. In a further 5%, encephalitis develops, but is rarely fatal. Haemorrhagic disease occurs in approximately 1% of cases and is very similar to YF. Mortality rates are in the region of 10%, but deaths are nearly always found in those with more severe forms of the disease.

Diagnosis

Virus can be detected in blood by culture or PCR in the first week of illness. Antigen detection methods are also available. Detection of IgM by EIA aids diagnosis of early infection.[82] Standard serological diagnosis is by HI test on paired sera, using a standard antigen from the World Health Organization. EIA has also been used for IgG and IgM detection, and the latter can assist early diagnosis. The N tests can be used to show RVF-specific antibody.

Management

High-level supportive care may be needed for the more serious cases. Ribavirin has activity against this virus in animal models and is recommended for treatment of haemorrhagic disease in humans.[83] Immune serum, if available, may also be tried for severe cases.

Epidemiology

RVFV is maintained in the forest in an enzootic fashion between vertebrates and the vector mosquito species. Spectacular epizootics in domestic animals are the result of large numbers of susceptible (European) breeds of cattle and sheep, high arthropod densities (resulting from heavy rainfall or irrigation), and spillover from the forest cycle. Originally restricted to domestic animals and humans in sub-Saharan Africa, since 1997 it has spread to Egypt, causing explosive epidemics in humans and domestic animals. The spread was possibly by camels from the Sudan carrying infection or arthropods, establishing new enzootic foci in the changing arthropod and vertebrate population after the construction of the Aswan High Dam. There is evidence in some areas that RVFV maintains endemnicity by transovarial transmission.

Control

Quarantine is not effective, but movements of animals should be controlled and sick animals should be allowed to die or recover, and not be slaughtered, to avoid spreading the infection in abattoirs. Control of abattoirs and vaccination of workers should be enforced. Vector control is also recommended.

Immunization

Vaccination of exposed laboratory workers and veterinary staff using a formalin-inactivated cell culture vaccine (expensive) should be performed.

Veterinary vaccines are the first line of defence against the spread of RVFV. Both live and inactivated vaccines have been used to control the spread in animals, with some success.

Sandfly fever

Geographical distribution

Sandfly fever (Sandfly fever Naples virus, SFNV; Sandfly fever Sicilian virus, SFSV)[84–86] is widespread throughout the Mediterranean and Middle East, Malta, Aegean Islands, Egypt and Iran, North Africa, Red Sea and Arabian Gulf; and in Asia in the Caucasus and Himalayas up to 4000 feet.

Aetiology

The viruses causing sandfly fever are phleboviruses. There are numerous antigenically distinct strains, only two of which, Sicilian and Naples, cause human disease. The others have been isolated from insects and animals.

Transmission

The sandfly responsible for transmission, *Phlebotomus papatasii*, becomes infective 6 days after feeding and remains infective for life. Transovarial transmission occurs so that newly emerged sandflies are capable of transmitting infection. It is possible that a parasitic mite of the sandflies acts as a reservoir.

Clinical features

Natural history

Sandfly fever is an acute self-limiting disease lasting 2–4 days, with complete recovery and immunity to further attacks, and no mortality.

The incubation period is 3–6 days.

Symptoms and signs

The onset is abrupt, with high fever, headache, myalgia, arthralgia and neck stiffness. After 3 (range 2–8) days the fever settles. Retro-orbital pain may be prominent and persist after resolution of fever. Mild neck stiffness develops in some patients. Occasionally there is a recrudescence (saddle back fever) lasting for 1–2 days. Rare cases of meningitis have been described.

Diagnosis

The viraemia lasts for only 24–36 h, so attempts at virus isolation from serum are unlikely to be successful. IgG and IgM enzyme immunoassays have been developed. Paired sera for HI and N antibody tests can show recent infection.

Management

There is no specific treatment.

Epidemiology

There are no animal reservoirs. In endemic areas transmission lasts from April to October. Epidemics occur among non-immune entrants to the community, especially military forces.

Tahyna virus (TAHV)

TAHV is a *bunyavirus* transmitted by *Aedes* species and causing occasional outbreaks of an influenza-like illness in central Europe (Table 40.1 and Appendix IV).

Toscana virus (TOSV)

TOSV[86-88] is a *Phlebovirus* currently recognized as a member of the SFNV serological complex. It is found in Italy, Portugal, France and Spain, and possibly occurs in other Mediterranean countries. It is transmitted by *Phlebotomus perniciosus* and *P. perfiliewi* and animal reservoir hosts are not known. TOSV causes a benign meningitis and occasional meningoencephalitis, with full recovery. Serological cross-reactivity occurs between TOSV and other serotypes of SFNV. Diagnosis is usually by serology, but virus can be detected in the CSF by culture and by RT-PCR.

COLTIVIRUSES (FAMILY REOVIRIDAE, GENUS *COLTIVIRUS*)

Colorado tick fever virus (CTFV)

CTF[89] is caused by a *coltivirus*, and is a member of the Reoviridae. It is found in the mountain regions of western USA and Canada, especially in the Rocky Mountain area in Colorado. Clinical illness consists of headache, fever, myalgia, arthralgia, retro-orbital pain, photophobia and neck stiffness, accompanied by a macular, maculopapular or petechial rash in about 10% of cases. It is biphasic in about half the patients, characterized by 2–3 days of illness, then 2 days of remission, followed by 2–3 days' more illness. Children may develop encephalitis. The most important hosts are the chipmunk and the golden-mantled ground squirrel, which infect immature ticks (*Dermacentor andersoni*). Other species of rodents may act as alternative secondary hosts of the virus.

MISCELLANEOUS ARBOVIRUSES

There are a large number of other arthropod viruses that only rarely cause human infection or whose role in human disease is uncertain.

Alphaviruses

Babanki virus (BBKV)

Babanki is related to SINV and has been found in West and Central Africa, and Madagascar. It has been isolated from humans, but its role as a cause of disease is uncertain.

Getah virus (GETV)

This mosquito-borne virus is closely related to RRV. It is distributed widely through Asia, South-east Asia and Australia. Human infection is rare and it is not clearly associated with any disease.

Semliki Forest virus (SFV)

This virus[90] is transmitted by various mosquito species in sub-Saharan Africa. Its role in human disease has not been established, but a laboratory-acquired case of fatal encephalitis has been reported.

Flaviviruses

Banzi virus (BANV)

BANV is a mosquito-borne rodent virus found in southern and eastern Africa and transmitted by *Culex* species. Febrile illness has been reported.

Bouboui virus (BOUV)

This mosquito-borne virus is found in central Africa and is closely related to BANV. Human infection is asymptomatic.

Bussuquara virus (BSQV)

This is a Central and South American rodent virus transmitted by *Culex* species; it causes fever, headache and arthralgia.

Edge Hill virus (EHV)

EHV has been isolated from *Ae. vigilax* and *Cx. annulirostris* mosquitoes and is widely distributed in Australia. Human infection occurs and a single possible case of polyarthralgic illness has been described.

Ilheus virus (ILHV)

This virus is found in numerous mosquito species. Disease and/or virus has been detected in people in Central and South America and in Trinidad. Rare cases of fever with headache, and a case of encephalitis, have been documented.

Karshi virus (KSIV)

KSV is a tick-borne virus that causes febrile illness. It has been found in Kazakhstan and Uzbekistan.

Kokobera virus (KOKV)

KOKV is found in Australia and New Guinea and is transmitted by *Ae. vigilax* and *Cx. annulirostris* mosquitoes. Human infections on the east coast of Australia have been documented in serosurveys. Kokobera virus can cause a polyarthralgic illness, sometimes with rash.

Kedougou virus (KEDV)

KEDV is a mosquito-borne virus that has been shown to infect children in Senegal and the Central African Republic. No illness has been identified.

Koutango virus (KOUV)

KOUV is a mosquito-borne virus found in Senegal. Natural human infection is not known to occur, but one laboratory-acquired infection caused fever, headache, arthralgia and rash.

Rio Bravo virus (RBV)

This is a flavivirus, but does not appear to be arthropod-borne. It is transmitted directly from bats to humans, with one case of febrile illness being reported.

Sepik virus (SEPV)

SEPV has been found in a variety of mosquito species in Papua New Guinea and has caused a case of fever with headache.

Spondweni virus (SPOV)

SPOV is transmitted by several mosquito species in South Africa. It may cause fever, headache and arthralgia. SPOV is closely related to ZIKV.

Tyuleniy virus (TYUV)

TYUV is a tick-borne virus, reported to have caused a single human infection with arthralgia and skin haemorrhages. Meaban virus and Saumarez Reef virus are closely related.

Usutu virus (USUV)

This virus is found in sub-Saharan Africa and Europe. It is primarily an avian virus transmitted by several mosquito species, causing fever and rash.

Wesselsbron virus (WESSV)

WESSV is found in sub-Saharan Africa and Thailand. It is transmitted by several mosquito species. Human illness is characterized by fever, hepatosplenomegaly, rash and sometimes encephalitis, with full recovery.

Zika virus (ZIKV)

This virus is transmitted by *Aedes* species in East, Central and West Africa, and maintained in a cycle similar to that of YFV. It causes fever, headache and rash. ZIKV is closely related to SPOV.

Bunyaviruses[91]

There is a large number of bunyaviruses that have been implicated in rare and mild human infection.

Nairoviruses

Congo-Crimean haemorrhagic fever virus (CCHFV)[58]

CCHFV is transmitted by *Hyalomma* species of ticks, especially *H. marginatum* and *H. anatolicum*, or by crushing those ticks. Nosocomial infection of medical workers after exposure to blood and secretions from patients occurs relatively frequently, and tertiary cases have occurred in family members of medical workers. Infection can also occur through butchering infected animals. This serious infection is discussed in Chapter 42 with the non-arthropod-borne viral haemorrhagic fevers.

Dugbe virus (DUGV)

This virus was found to cause a mild febrile illness in Nigeria and Central African Republic, with rare meningitis.

Nairobi sheep disease virus (NSDV)

NSDV infects sheep and goats and is transmitted by a number of tick species. Human infection has been reported from East Africa

and India, consisting of a fever and arthralgia. The illness is mild and recovery is full.

Orbiviruses

Kemerovo complex

This is a complex of a large number of viruses found in the former USSR and central Europe. They are tick-borne, and cause illnesses varying from fever to meningoencephalitis.

Orungo virus (ORUV)

Orungo virus is found in West and Central Africa and may be transmitted by a number of mosquito species. It is separated into four serotypes and causes fever and headache, with rare cases of encephalitis.

REFERENCES

1. WHO. Arthropod-borne and rodent-borne viral diseases. Report of a WHO Scientific Group. *World Health Organ Tech Rep Ser* 1985; 719: 1–114.
2. Bres P. Impact of arboviruses on human and animal health. In: Monath TP, ed. *The Arboviruses: Epidemiology and Ecology*. Vol. I. Florida. CRC Press, 1988:1–18.
3. Fauquet CM, Mayo MA, Maniloff J, et al. *Virus Taxonomy: 8th Report of the International Committee on Taxonomy of Viruses*. San Diego: Academic Press; 2005.
4. Harrison SC. Principles of virus structure. In: Knipe DM, Howley PM, eds. *Fields Virology*. Vol. 1. 5th edn. Philadelphia: Lippincott Williams & Wilkins; 2007:59–98.
5. Calisher CH, Karabatsos N. Arbovirus serogroups: definition and geographic distribution. In: Monath TP, ed. *The Arboviruses: Epidemiology and Ecology*. Vol. I. Florida: CRC Press; 1988:19–58.
6. Monath TP. Pathobiology of the flaviviruses. In: Schlesinger S, Schlesinger MJ, eds. *The Togaviridae and the Flaviviridae*. New York: Plenum Press; 1986: 375–440.
7. Barrett AD T, Higgs S. Yellow fever: a disease that has yet to be conquered. *Annu Rev Entomol* 2007; 52:209–229.
8. Scott TW. Vertebrate host ecology. In: Monath TP, ed. *The Arboviruses: Epidemiology and Ecology*. Vol. I. Florida: CRC Press; 1988: 257–280.
9. Porterfield JS. Comparative and historical aspects of the Togaviridae and Flaviviridae. In: Schlesinger S, Schlesinger MJ, eds. *The Togaviridae and the Flaviviridae*. New York: Plenum Press; 1986:1–19.
10. Hardy JL. Susceptibility and resistance of vector mosquitoes. In: Monath TP, ed. *The Arboviruses: Epidemiology and Ecology*. Vol. 1. Florida: CRC Press; 1988:87–126.
11. Turell MJ. Horizontal and vertical transmission of viruses by insect and tick vectors. In: Monath TP, ed. *The Arboviruses: Epidemiology and Ecology*. Vol. I. Florida: CRC Press; 1988:127–152.
12. Simpson DIH. Arbovirus diseases. *Br Med Bull* 1972; 28(1):10–15.
13. Dunn FL. Human factors in arbovirus ecology and control. In: Monath TP, ed. *The Arboviruses: Epidemiology and Ecology*. Vol. I. Florida: CRC Press; 1988: 281–290.
14. Calisher CH. Alphavirus infections (family Togaviridae). In: Porterfield JS, ed. *Kass Handbook of Infectious Diseases: Exotic Viral Infections*. London: Chapman & Hall; 1995:1–18.
15. Githeko AK, Lindsay SW, Confalonieri UE, et al. Climate change and vector-borne diseases: a regional analysis. *Bull World Health Organ* 2000; 78: 1136–1147.

16. Kay BH, Aaskov JG. Ross River virus (epidemic polyarthritis). In: Monath TP, ed. *The Arboviruses: Epidemiology and Ecology*. Vol. III. Florida: CRC Press; 1988:93–112.

17. McMichael AJ, Woodruff RE, et al. Climate change and human health: present and future risks. *Lancet* 2006; 367:859–869.

18. Griffin DE. Alphaviruses. In: Knipe DM, Howley PM, eds. *Fields Virology*. 5th edn. Vol. 1. Philadelphia: Lippincott Williams & Wilkins; 2007:1023–1067.

19. Gubler D, Kuno G, Markhoff L. Flaviviruses. In: Knipe DM, Howley PM, eds. *Fields Virology*. 5th edn. Vol. 1. Philadelphia: Lippincott Williams & Wilkins; 2007:1153–1262.

20. Suhrbier A, Linn ML. Clinical and pathological aspects of arthritis due to Ross River virus and other alphaviruses. *Curr Opin Rheumatol* 2004; 16:374–379.

21. Broom AK, Wallace MJ, Mackenzie JS, et al. Immunization with gamma globulin to Murray Valley encephalitis virus and with an inactivated Japanese encephalitis virus vaccine as a prophylaxis against Australian encephalitis: evaluation in a mouse model. *J Med Virol* 2000; 61:259–265.

22. WHO. *Dengue Haemorrhagic Fever: Diagnosis, Treatment, Prevention and Control*. 2nd edn. Geneva: World Health Organization; 1977.

23. Solomon T. Flavivirus encephalitis. *N Engl J Med* 2004; 351:370–378.

24. Agrawal AG, Petersen LR. Human immunoglobulin as a treatment for West Nile virus infection. *J Infect Dis* 2003; 188:1–4.

25. Pugachev KV, Guirakhoo F, Monath TP. New developments in flavivirus vaccines with special attention to yellow fever. *Curr Opin Infect Dis* 2005; 18:387–394.

26. Pittman PR, Liu CT, Cannon TL, et al. Immunogenicity of an inactivated Rift Valley fever vaccine in humans: a 12-year experience. *Vaccine* 1999; 18: 181–189.

27. Flexman AW, Smith DW, Mackenzie JS, et al. A comparison of the diseases caused by Ross River virus and Barmah Forest virus. *Med J Aust* 1998; 169:159–163.

28. Higgs S. The 2005–2006 Chikungunya Epidemic in the Indian Ocean. *Vector Borne Zoonotic Dis* 2006; 6:115–116.

29. WHO. Outbreak news. Chikungunya, India. *World Health Organization Weekly Epidemiological Record* 2006; 81:409–416.

30. Touret Y, Randrianaivo H, Michault A, et al. Early maternal-fetal transmission of the chikungunya virus. *La Presse Medicale* 2006; 35:1656–1658.

31. Schuffenecker I, Iteman I, Michault A, et al. Genome microevolution of Chikungunya viruses causing the Indian Ocean outbreak. *PLoS Medicine* 2006; 3:1–13.

32. Jupp PG, McIntosh BM. Chikungunya virus disease. In: Monath TP, ed. *The Arboviruses: Epidemiology and Ecology*. Vol. II. Florida: CRC Press; 1988: 137–158.

33. Reisen WK, Monath TP. Western equine encephalomyelitis. In: Monath TP, ed. *The Arboviruses: Epidemiology and Ecology*. Vol. I. Florida: CRC Press; 1988: 89–138.

34. Morris CD. Eastern equine encephalomyelitis. In: Monath TP, ed. *The Arboviruses: Epidemiology and Ecology*. Vol. III. Florida: CRC Press; 1988: 1–20.

35. Deresiewicz RL, Thaler SJ, Hsu L, et al. Clinical and neuroradiographic manifestations of eastern equine encephalitis. *N Engl J Med* 1997; 336: 1867–1874.

36. Walton TE, Grayson M. Venezuelan equine encephalomyelitis. In: Monath TP, ed. *The Arboviruses: Epidemiology and Ecology*. Vol. IV. Florida: CRC Press; 1988:203–231.

37. Linssen B, Kinney RM, Aguilar P, et al. Development of reverse transcription-PCR assays for specific detection of equine encephalitic viruses. *J Clin Microbiol* 2000; 38:1527–1535.

38. Tesh RB, Watts DM, Russell KL, et al. Mayaro virus disease: An emerging mosquito-borne zoonosis in tropical South America. *Clin Infect Dis* 1999; 28:67–73.

39. Johnson BK. O'nyong nyong virus disease. In: Monath TP, ed. *The Arboviruses: Epidemiology and Ecology*. Vol. III. Florida: CRC Press; 1988:217–223.

40. Shore H. O'nyong-nyong fever: an epidemic virus disease in East Africa. III. Some clinical and epidemiological observations in the northern province of Uganda. *Trans R Soc Trop Med Hyg* 1961; 55:361–373.

41. Mackenzie JS, Smith DW. Mosquito-borne viruses and epidemic polyarthritis. *Med J Aust* 1996; 164:90–92.

42. Russell RC. Vectors vs humans – who is on top down under? An update on vector-borne disease and research on vectors in Australia. *J Vector Ecol* 1998; 23(1):1–46.

43. Rosen L, Gubler DJ, Bennett PH. Epidemic polyarthritis (Ross River) virus infection in the Cook Islands. *Am J Trop Med Hyg* 1981; 30: 1294–1302.

44. Sammels LM, Lindsay MD, Poidinger M, et al. Geographic distribution and evolution of Sindbis virus in Australia. *J Gen Virol* 1999; 80: 739–748.

45. Laine M, Luukainen R, Toivanen A. Sindbis virus and other alphaviruses as a cause of human arthritic disease. *J Intern Med* 2004; 256: 457–471.

46. Burke DS, Leake CJ. Japanese encephalitis. In: Monath TP, ed. *The Arboviruses: Epidemiology and Ecology*. Vol. III. Florida: CRC Press; 1988: 63–92.

47. Solomon T, Vaughn DW. Pathogenesis and clinical features of Japanese encephalitis and West Nile virus infections. *Curr Top Microbiol Immunol* 2002; 267:171–194.

48. Halstead SB, Jacobson J. Japanese encephalitis. *Adv Virus Res* 2003; 61: 103–138.

49. Harinasatu C, Nimmanitya S, Titsa U, et al. A clinical trial of interferon-alpha on Japanese encephalitis in Thailand. *Southeast Asian J Trop Med Public Health* 1989; 20:656–657.

50. Kalita J, Misra UK. Comparison of CT scan and MRI findings in the diagnosis of Japanese encephalitis. *J Neurol Sci* 2000; 17:3–8.

51. Gajanana A, Samuel PP, Thenmozhi V, et al. An appraisal of some recent diagnostic assays for Japanese encephalitis. *Southeast Asian J Trop Med Public Health* 1996; 27:673–679.

52. Gaidamovich S. Tick-borne Flavivirus infection. In: Porterfield JS, ed. *Kass Handbook of Infectious Diseases: Exotic Viral Infections*. London: Chapman & Hall; 1995:203–222.

53. Pavri K. Clinical, clinicopathologic and hematologic features of Kyasanur Forest disease. *Rev Infect Dis* 1989; 11(suppl 4):S854–S859.

54. Pattnaik P. Kyasanur Forest Disease: an epidemiological view in India. *Rev Med Virol* 2006; 16:151–165.

55. Marshall ID. Murray Valley and Kunjin encephalitis. In: Monath TP, ed. *The Arboviruses: Epidemiology and Ecology*. Vol. III. Florida: CRC Press; 1988: 151–190.

56. Hall RA, Broom AK, Smith DW, et al. The Ecology and Epidemiology of Kunjin Virus. In: Mackenzie JS, Barrett AD T, Deubel V, eds. Japanese Encephalitis and West Nile Viruses. *Curr Top Microbiol Immunol* 2002; 267:253–269.

57. Davidson MM, Williams H, Macleod JA. Louping ill in man: a forgotten disease. *J Infect* 1991; 23:241–249.

58. Charrel RN, Attoui H, Butenko M, et al. Tick-borne virus diseases of human interest in Europe. *Clin Microbiol Infect* 2004; 10:1040–1055.

59. Mackenzie JS, Smith DW, Broom AK, et al. Australian encephalitis in Western Australia, 1978–1991. *Med J Aust* 1993; 158:591–595.

60. Burrow JN, Whelan PI, Kilburn CJ, et al. Australian encephalitis in the Northern Territory: clinical and epidemiological features, 1987–1996. *Aust NZ J Med* 1998; 28:590–596.

61. Cordova SP, Smith DW, Broom AK, et al. Murray Valley encephalitis in Western Australia in 2000, with evidence of southerly spread. *Comm Dis Intell (Aust)* 2000; 24:368–372.

62. Hall RA, Broom AK, Hartnett AC, et al. Immunodominant epitopes on the NS1 protein of MVE and KUN viruses serve as targets for a blocking ELISA to detect virus-specific antibody in sentinel animal serum. *J Virol Methods* 1995; 51:201–210.

63. Figueiredo LTM. The Brazilian flaviviruses. *Microbes Infect* 2000; 2: 1643–1649.

64. Luby JP. St. Louis encephalitis, Rocio encephalitis and West Nile fever. In: Porterfield JS, ed. *Kass Handbook of Infectious Diseases: Exotic Viral Infections*. London: Chapman & Hall; 1995:183–202.

65. Reisen WK. Epidemiology of St. Louis encephalitis virus. *Adv Virus Res* 2003; 61:139–183.

66. Brooks TJ, Phillpotts RJ. Interferon-alpha protects mice against lethal infection with St Louis encephalitis virus delivered by the aerosol and subcutaneous routes. *Antiviral Res* 1999; 41:57–64.

67. Southern PM, Smith JW, Luby JP, et al. Clinical and laboratory features of epidemic St Louis encephalitis. *Ann Intern Med* 1969; 71: 681–689.

68. Greskova M, Calisher CH. Tick-borne encephalitis. In: Monath TP, ed. *The Arboviruses: Epidemiology and Ecology*. Vol. IV. Florida: CRC Press; 1988: 177–202.

69. Dumpis U, Crook D, Oksi J. Tick-borne encephalitis. *Clin Infect Dis* 1999; 28:882–890.

70. Saksida A, Duh D, Lotric-Furlan S, et al. The importance of tick-borne encephalitis virus RNA detection for early differential diagnosis of tick-borne encephalitis. *J Clin Virol* 2005; 33:331–5.

71. Peterson LR, Roehrig JT. West Nile virus: a reemerging global pathogen. *Emerg Infect Dis* 2001; 7:611–614.

72. Hall RA. The emergence of West Nile virus: the Australian connection. *Viral Immunol* 2000; 13:447–461.

73. Sejvar JJ, Marfin AA. Manifestations of West Nile neuroinvasive disease. *Rev Med Virol* 2006; 16:209–224.

74. Tilley PA, Fox JD, Jayaraman GC, et al. Nucleic acid testing for West Nile virus RNA in plasma enhances rapid diagnosis of acute infection in symptomatic patients. *J Infect Dis* 2006; 193:1361–1364.

75. Sayao AL, Suchowersky O, Al-Khathaami A, et al. Calgary experience with West Nile virus neurological syndrome during the late summer of 2003. *Can J Neurol Sci* 2004; 31:194–203.

76. Digoutte J, Cornet M, Deubel V, et al. Yellow fever. In: Porterfield JS, ed. *Kass Handbook of Infectious Diseases: Exotic Viral Infections*. London: Chapman & Hall; 1995:67–98.

77. Marianneau P, Georges-Courbot M-C, Duebel V. Rarity of adverse events after 17D yellow fever vaccination. *Lancet* 2001; 358:84–85.

78. Schmaljohn CS, Nichol ST. Bunyaviridae. In: Knipe DM, Howley PM, eds. *Fields Virology*. Vol. II. 5th edn. Philadelphia: Lippincott Williams & Wilkins; 2007:1741–1789.

79. Meegan JM, Bailey CL. Rift Valley fever. In: Monath TP, ed. *The Arboviruses: Epidemiology and Ecology*. Vol. IV. Florida: CRC Press; 1988:51–76.

80. Jouan A, Le Guenno B, Digoutte, et al. A RVF epidemic in Mauritania. *Ann Inst Pasteur Virol* 1998; 139:307–308.

81. WHO. The use of veterinary vaccines for prevention and control of Rift Valley fever: memorandum from a WHO/FAO meeting. *Bull World Health Organ* 1983; 61:261–268.

82. Sall AA, Macondo EA, Sène OK, et al. Use of reverse transcriptase PCR in early diagnosis of Rift Valley fever. *Clin Diagn Lab Immunol* 2002; 9:713–715.

83. Bossi P, Tegnell A, Baka A, et al. Bichat guidelines for the clinical management of haemorrhagic fever viruses and bioterrorism-related haemorrhagic fever viruses. *Euro Surveill* 2004; 12:E11–12.

84. Verani P, Nicoletti L. Phlebovirus infections. In: Porterfield JS, ed. *Kass Handbook of Infectious Diseases: Exotic Viral Infections*. London: Chapman & Hall; 1995:295–318.

85. Tesh RB. Phlebotomus fevers. In: Monath TP, ed. *The Arboviruses: Epidemiology and Ecology*. Vol. IV. Florida: CRC Press; 1988:15–28.

86. Dionisi D, Esteri F, Vivarelli A, et al. Epidemiological, clinical and laboratory aspects of sandfly fever. *Curr Opin Infect Dis* 2003; 16:383–388.

87. Braito A, Corbisiero R, Corradini S, et al. Toscana virus infections of the central nervous system in children: a report of 14 cases. *J Pediatr* 1998; 132:144–148.

88. Charrel RN, Gallian P, Navarro-Mari JM, et al. Emergence of Toscana virus in Europe. *Emerg Infect Dis* 2005, 11:1567–1663.

89. Attoui H, Jaafar FM, de Micco P, et al. Coltiviruses and Seadorna viruses in North America, Europe and Asia. *Emerg Infect Dis* 2005; 11:1673–1679.

90. Willems WR, Kaluza G, Boschek CB, et al. Semliki forest virus: cause of a fatal case of human encephalitis. *Science* 1979; 201:1127–1129.

91. Calisher CH, Nathanson N. Bunyavirus infections. In: Porterfield JS, ed. *Exotic Viral Infections*. London: Chapman & Hall; 1995:247–260.

Chapter 41

Suchitra Nimmannitya

Dengue and Dengue Haemorrhagic Fever

Dengue infections caused by the four antigenically distinct dengue virus serotypes (DENV1, DENV2, DENV3, DENV4) of the family Flaviviridae are the most important arbovirus diseases in humans, in terms of geographical distribution, morbidity and mortality. The infection is transmitted from person to person by *Aedes* mosquitoes. Dengue infections may be asymptomatic or may lead to an undifferentiated fever (or viral syndrome), dengue fever or dengue haemorrhagic fever (DHF).[1] Each year there are an estimated 50–100 million dengue infections, 500 000 cases of DHF and 20 000 deaths, mainly children.

DENGUE FEVER

Geographical distribution

Dengue is a worldwide condition spread throughout the tropical and subtropical zones between 30°N and 40°S, where environmental conditions are optimal for dengue virus transmission by *Aedes* mosquitoes. There are 2.5 billion people living in these areas who are at risk of contracting dengue. It is endemic in South-east Asia, the Pacific, East and West Africa, the Caribbean and the Americas, where all dengue serotypes are prevailed.[2,3]

Aetiology

The dengue virus, a member of genus *Flavivirus* in the family Flaviviridae, is a single-stranded enveloped RNA virus, 30 nm in diameter, which can grow in a variety of mosquitoes and tissue cultures. There are four distinct but closely related serotypes (DENV1–4). They possess antigens that cross-react with other members in the same genus such as yellow fever, Japanese encephalitis and West Nile viruses. There is evidence from field and laboratory studies that there are distinct strain differences between dengue viruses. Recent development in molecular virology has led to increasing availability of viral gene sequence studies. It has been shown that there is abundant genetic variation within each serotype in the form of phylogenetically distinct clusters of sequences dubbed subtypes or genotypes.[4] At present, three subtypes can be identified in DENV-1, six in DENV-2 (one of which is only found in non-human primates), four in DENV-3 and four in DENV-4 (with another exclusive to non-human primates). A more notable observation is that subtypes often have differing geographical distributions, with some more widespread than the others. As for DENV-2, there are two subtypes apparently restricted to South-east Asia and another to America.[5] It has also been proposed that some subtypes differ in virulence, i.e. their capacity to cause severe disease as dengue haemorrhagic fever.[6]

Transmission

Dengue virus is transmitted from human to human by mosquito bites. Man is the main reservoir of the virus, though studies have shown that the monkey is the jungle reservoir in Malaysia and Africa.[2]

Ae. aegypti is the most efficient of the mosquito vectors because of its domestic habits. The female mosquito bites humans during the day. After feeding on a person whose blood contains the virus, the female *Ae. aegypti* can transmit dengue, either immediately by a change of host when its feeding is interrupted, or after an incubation period of 8–10 days during which time the virus multiplies in the salivary glands. Once infected, the mosquito host remains infective for life (30–45 days).

Other *Aedes* mosquitoes capable of transmitting dengue include *Ae. albopictus*, *Ae. polynesiensis* and several species of the *Ae. scutellaris* complex. Each of these species has its own particular geographical distribution and they are in general less efficient vectors than *Ae. aegypti*.

Transovarian transmission of dengue viruses has been documented but its epidemiological importance has not been established.[2]

Pathology

From experimental studies in rhesus monkeys, after inoculation the virus reaches the regional lymph nodes and disseminates to the reticuloendothelial system, in which it multiplies and from which it enters the blood.[7] Skin lesions in non-fatal, uncomplicated dengue fever seen in human volunteers were studied by biopsy. The chief abnormality occurred in and around small blood vessels and consisted of endothelial swelling, perivascular oedema and infiltration with mononuclear cells. Extensive extravasation of blood without appreciable inflammatory reaction was observed in the petechial lesions.[8]

Immunity

Immunity is antibody mediated. After an acute phase of infection by a particular dengue serotype there is an antibody response to all four dengue serotypes. There is a long-lasting immunity to the homologous serotype of the infecting strain. A cross-reactive heterotypic immunity has been reported by Sabin[8] to last for about 2 months in experimental human volunteers, while another community study reported a period of up to 1 year.[9] After infection by one serotype, the individual concerned will be immune to other serotypes for 2–12 months and become susceptible thereafter. A second attack of dengue has been reported.[10] The waning cross-reactive heterotypic antibody is implicated in the occurrence of DHF.[11]

Clinical features

The clinical features of dengue fever are age dependent: infants and children infected with dengue virus for the first time (i.e. primary dengue infection) usually develop a simple fever or undifferentiated febrile illness; dengue fever is most common in adults and older children and may be benign or may be a classical incapacitating disease (classical dengue fever) with severe muscle, joint and bone pain (break bone fever).[1]

Typically, after an incubation period of 5–8 days following an infective mosquito bite, the disease in adults begins with a sudden onset of fever with severe headache, and any of the following: chilliness, pain behind the eyes – particularly on eye movement or eye pressure-photophobia, backache, and pain in the muscles, bone and joints of the extremities.

The temperature is usually high (39–40°C); the fever may be sustained for 5–6 days and may occasionally have a biphasic course. As the disease progresses the patient becomes anorexic and may show marked weakness and prostration. Other common symptoms include sore throat, altered taste sensation, colicky pain and abdominal tenderness, constipation, dragging pain in the inguinal region and general depression. A relative bradycardia is common during the febrile phase. Symptoms vary in severity and usually persist for several days.

Several types of skin rash have been described. Initially, diffuse flushing, mottling or fleeting pinpoint eruptions may be observed on the face, neck and chest. These are transient in nature. A second type of skin rash is a conspicuous rash that may be maculopapular or scarlatiniform and appears on approximately the third or fourth day. This rash starts on the chest and trunk and spreads to the extremities and face and may be accompanied by itching and dermal hyperaesthesia.

There is generalized enlargement of the lymph nodes but the liver and spleen are not usually palpable. A positive tourniquet test and petechiae on extremities are not uncommon.

Towards the end of the febrile period or immediately after defervescence the generalized rash fades and localized clusters of petechiae may appear over the dorsum of the feet and on the legs, hands and arms. This confluent petechial rash is characterized by a scattered pale round area of normal skin (Figure 41.1).

Convalescence may be abrupt and uneventful but is often prolonged in adults, sometimes taking several weeks, and may be accompanied by pronounced asthenia and depression. Bradycar-

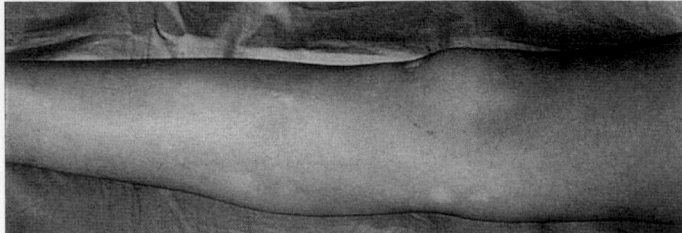

Figure 41.1 Dengue fever: convalescent rash – confluent petechial rash.

dia is common during this period. Loss of hair has been reported during convalescence.

Haemorrhagic complications such as epistaxis, gum bleeding, gastrointestinal haemorrhage, haematuria and hypermenorrhoea have been reported in many epidemics of dengue fever, and on rare occasions severe bleeding has caused deaths in some epidemics.[8,10]

Dengue fever with encephalitic signs but with normal cerebrospinal fluid has been reported in some epidemics.[10] Reye's syndrome associated with dengue infection is not uncommon.[12] Recently there has been an increase in reported cases of dengue encephalitis which was confirmed either by demonstration of virus, antigen or anti-dengue IgM antibody in cerebrospinal fluid.[13]

The most significant laboratory finding during the acute illness is leucopenia, which is usually noted 2–3 days after onset and lasts throughout the febrile phase. Mild to moderate thrombocytopenia is occasionally observed.[14]

Diagnosis

It is not possible to make a diagnosis of mild dengue or classical dengue fever from the clinical features as they resemble those of many other diseases, particularly chikungunya infection. Differential diagnosis includes malaria, leptospirosis and other viral, bacterial and rickettsial diseases. The presence of flushed face, a positive tourniquet test and leucopenia are helpful in differentiating dengue from other diseases. The diagnosis is best accomplished by serological tests for antibodies and virus isolation, or detection of dengue antigen by polymerase chain reaction (PCR).[1]

Virological diagnosis

See DHF below.

Management

This is entirely symptomatic and supportive.

Epidemiology

The first reported epidemics of dengue or dengue-like disease occurred in 1779 and 1780 in Egypt and Indonesia and in 1780 in the USA (Philadelphia).[10] It is clear that dengue and other arboviruses with similar ecology had a widespread distribution in the tropics as long as 200 years ago. Historically, Asia has been the area of highest endemicity, with all four dengue serotypes circulating in the large urban centres in most countries.[2,3]

During and after World War II, *Ae. aegypti* became more widespread in Asia and with an increased facility of communication and travel of susceptible foreigners into the endemic areas, together with the subsequent urbanization that occurred in most countries, the incidence of dengue infection increased dramatically. These changes coincided with the emergence of a newly described DHF in the 1950s. The advent of commercial jet air transport in the 1960s promoted the ideal mechanism for the carriage of dengue virus by persons who had visited endemic areas and were travelling during the incubation period. A trend of increased spread of dengue throughout the world has since developed. Increased epidemic activity was observed in the Pacific Islands and the Caribbean basin in the 1970s and epidemics of all four dengue serotypes were documented in both regions. Epidemiological changes in the American region have been the most dramatic; all four viruses are now endemic.[2,3]

In the 1980s increased dengue activity was observed in Africa, and all four dengue serotypes have now been documented in Africa.[2,3]

The incidence of dengue infection has increased markedly since the 1960s, first in Asia then in the Pacific and Americas and finally in Africa. It appears that most of the tropical world, with an estimated population of 2.5 billion, is at risk of infection with dengue.

Dengue transmission occurs throughout the year in endemic tropical areas; however, in most countries there is a distinct seasonal pattern, with increased transmission usually associated with the rainy season. While in some areas increases in dengue transmission coincide with periods of increased rainfall, the interactions between temperature and rainfall or variation in daily microclimates may be important determinants of dengue transmission.[2]

In dengue endemic areas with multiple serotypes children become infected early in childhood. Classical dengue fever is rare among indigenous people as most of the adults are immune. In these areas, both mild dengue illness and DHF occur mainly in children.

Control

See DHF below.

DENGUE HAEMORRHAGIC FEVER (DHF)

Geographical distribution

DHF (see also Chapters 40 and 41) is widespread in the South-east Asian and Western Pacific regions. Since its first epidermic in the Philippines in 1953–54 it is now occurring in most countries in tropical Asia. During the past two decades there has been a dramatic geographical expansion of epidemic DHF. DHF first appeared in Cuba in 1981 and since then it has been reported from 28 countries in Central and South America. To date, a DHF epidemic has not been reported in Africa or the Middle East, except a few imported cases reported from Saudi Arabia.[2,3]

Aetiology and pathogenesis

All four dengue serotypes are capable of causing dengue fever or DHF, depending on the immune status and probably age of the host, as DHF occurs almost exclusively in children under the age of 16 years and is associated with secondary dengue infection. A strong association between DHF and secondary dengue infection has led to Halstead's proposed concept of two sequential infections. Based on his in vitro and monkey studies, an antibody-dependent immune enhancement theory has been hypothesized by Halstead[11]: it is suggested that during the second infection with a heterotypic dengue virus which differs from the first one, pre-existing antibody from the first infection fails to neutralize and may instead enhance viral uptake and replication in the mononuclear phagocytes. Such infected cells may then become the target of an immune elimination mechanism which can trigger the production of mediators with activation of complement and the clotting cascade and eventually produce DHF.[11]

In Thailand, studies over the last 40 years have demonstrated transmission of all four dengue serotypes,[15] with dengue type 2 as the predominating serotype up to 1990.[16] The studies and experience in Thailand, as well as in Cuba, confirmed the suggestion that the interval between the two dengue infections and the sequences of infecting dengue serotypes, i.e. secondary infection with DENV2 following DENV1 infection may be important factors in determining the occurrence and severity of DHF.[11,17] The interval between the two infections was first suggested to be 1–5 years following Cuban experience with the first outbreak of DHF with DENV2 in 1981 which followed the outbreak of dengue fever with DENV-1 in 1977. The second outbreak of DHF in Santiago, Cuba in 1997 with DENV-2 after a period of apparent elimination of vectors and dengue virus for 16 years led to two important observations: (1) immune enhancement could occur after a long duration of 20 years and (2) primary DENV2 infection in children under 16 years did not cause DHF.[18] A study by Vaughn et al. revealed that increased dengue disease severity (dengue vs DHF) correlated with high viraemia titre, secondary dengue infection and DENV2 serotype.[19] The most recent study on the role of T cells in the pathogenesis of DHF has described a phenomenon of original antigenic sin.[20] The group has found a paradoxical T cell response in that many of the T cells had a relatively low affinity for the current infecting DENV serotype but showed higher affinity for serotypes which had been encountered before. This phenomenon resulted in delayed elimination of the secondary infecting serotype, allowing further proliferation and high viral load.[20]

Other theories involving a virulent strain of dengue virus[21] and genetic differences in the hosts[22,23] have been proposed. The association of the introduction of a specific (South-east Asian) genotype of DENV2 and the appearance of DHF in America suggested that a certain genotype has potential to cause severe dengue (DHF).[6] The finding that the same DENV2 genotype may cause dengue fever or DHF in Thailand suggested that both virus genotype and secondary infection are important contributing factors in the pathogenesis of DHF.[24]

Pathophysiology and pathology

The pathophysiological hallmarks of DHF are plasma leakage and abnormal haemostasis. Evidence supporting plasma leakage includes a rapid rise in haematocrit, pleural effusion and ascites, hypoproteinaemia and reduced plasma volume. A significant loss of plasma leads to hypovolaemic shock and death. The acute onset of shock and the rapid and often dramatic clinical recovery when the patient is treated properly, together with the absence of inflammatory vascular lesions, suggest a transient functional increase in vascular permeability that results in plasma leakage.

A disorder in haemostasis involves all major components:[14] (1) vascular change(s) including capillary fragility changes that lead to a positive tourniquet test and easy bruisability; (2) thrombopathy with impaired platelet function and moderate to severe thrombocytopenia; (3) coagulopathy, acute-type disseminated intravascular clotting (DIC) is documented in severe cases, often with prolonged shock and responsible for the severe bleeding. Evidence for DIC includes hypofibrinogen and the presence of fibrinogen degradation products (FDP) and D-dimer. The clotting factors II, V, VII, VIII, IX and XII are low. (4) Bone marrow changes include depression of all marrow elements, with maturation arrest of megakaryocytes during the early phase of the illness, which is readily reversed when the fever subsides and during the stage of shock.

Kidney studies in non-fatal cases show changes similar to glomerulonephritis but these are usually mild and transient.[1,25]

Postmortem studies show that serous effusions with high protein content, mostly found in pleural and peritoneal cavities, and widespread petechial haemorrhages in many organs are constant findings.[25] The sites of common haemorrhage include gastrointestinal tract, skin, heart, pleura and lungs, soft tissue, periadrenal tissue.[25]

Histological changes[1,25]

Significant changes are found in major organ systems:
- Vascular changes include vasodilatation, congestion, perivascular haemorrhage and oedema of arterial walls
- Proliferation of reticuloendothelial cells with accelerated phagocytic activity is observed frequently
- The lymphoid tissues show increasing activity of the B lymphocyte system with active proliferation of plasma cells and lymphoblastoid cells
- In the liver there is focal necrosis of the hepatic and Kupffer cells, with formation of Councilman-like bodies.

Dengue virus antigen is found predominantly in cells of the spleen, thymus and lymph nodes, in Kupffer cells and in the sinusoidal lining cells of liver and alveolar lining cells of the lung.

The pathogenetic mechanism of DHF is presumed to be immunological, involving both humoral and cell-mediated immune modulation. A constant finding in DHF is activation of the complement system with profound depression of C3 and C5 levels.[1] Immune complexes have been described in DHF cases associated with secondary infection, and they may contribute to complement activation. The C3a and C5a anaphylatoxins are released and their association with the time of leakage, shock and disease severity has been demonstrated.[26] They are the most likely vascular perme-ability-increasing mediators among the other as yet unidentified agents.

A most recent study in Thailand on the role of non-structural protein NS1 and complement in the pathogenesis of plasma leakage revealed that complement activation mediated by NS1 led to local and systemic generation of anaphylatoxin C5a and the terminal SC5b-9 complex. The plasma levels of NS1 and SC5b-9 complexes correlated with disease severity and they were present in the pleural fluid from patients with dengue shock syndrome (DSS). This is a novel finding that implicates the major role of NS1 as an important trigger for complete complement activation and the role of the terminal SC5b-9 complex in the pathogenesis of plasma leakage.[27] Notably, it was also shown in this study and by Libraty et al. that high circulating levels of NS1 that can be detected early in dengue illness are correlated with the development of DHF.[28]

Immunity

The immune status of the host appears to be the important component that determines the development of DHF as the disease occurs with high frequency in two immunologically defined groups: (1) children who have experienced a previous dengue infection; and (2) infants with waning levels of maternal dengue antibody. The acute phase of infection by a particular dengue serotype is believed to provoke long-lasting homotypic immunity. A cross-reactive heterotypic immunity has been reported to last about 2 months in one study of experimental infection,[8,10] while another community study presented epidemiological data suggesting that this cross-reactive heterotypic immunity might last up to 1 year.[9] It is hypothesized that this cross-heterotypic antibody, when weak and failing to neutralize the infecting dengue virus during the second infection, can enhance virus multiplication in the mononuclear phagocyte and trigger immune modulation and eventually produce DHF.[11] Passive IgG dengue antibody from the mothers of infants under the age of 1 year has been shown to be capable of enhancing virus replication when falling to below the neutralization level and to produce DHF during primary infection.[11,29]

A study of the cell-mediated immune response revealed that during a secondary dengue infection serotype cross-reactive dengue-specific T lymphocytes are activated and proliferate with production of lymphokines and monokines. It is suggested that this response, while contributing to recovery from infection, may also in some circumstances play a role in the immunopathogenesis of DHF.[30] Recently, it has been shown that cytokines, including tumour necrosis factor α (TNFα) interleukin 2 (IL-2), IL-6, IL-8 and interferons IFNγ, were released into the circulation during the early phase of DHF and their levels correlated well with disease severity.[31] The recently described T cell antigenic sin may lead to the complex series of events; slow clearance of the (second) infecting DENV leading to high virus load and massive T cell activation which will cause both direct T cell mediated cytotoxicity and the release of a variety of inflammatory cytokines. This in turn will lead to tissue damage and be involved in causing the leakage of plasma in DHF.[20]

A second attack of DHF is very rare: it has been shown to occur in about 0.5% of cases in a study over a 16-year period at the Children's Hospital in Bangkok.[32]

Clinical features

DHF is a severe form of dengue infection that is accompanied by haemorrhagic diathesis and a tendency to develop fatal shock (dengue shock syndrome: DSS) as a consequence of plasma leakage selectively into pleural and peritoneal cavities. The clinical course could be divided into febrile, critical and convalescence phases (Figure 41.2).

Typically, the disease begins with the febrile phase with an abrupt onset of high fever, accompanied by facial flush and headache. Some patients with an infected pharynx may complain of sore throat but rarely have rhinitis or cough. Anorexia, vomiting and abdominal pain are common. During the first few days of the febrile phase, which usually lasts for 2–7 days, the illness resembles dengue fever in many respects but a maculopapular rash and myalgia are less common. Occasionally the body temperature may be as high as 40–41 °C and febrile convulsions may occur.

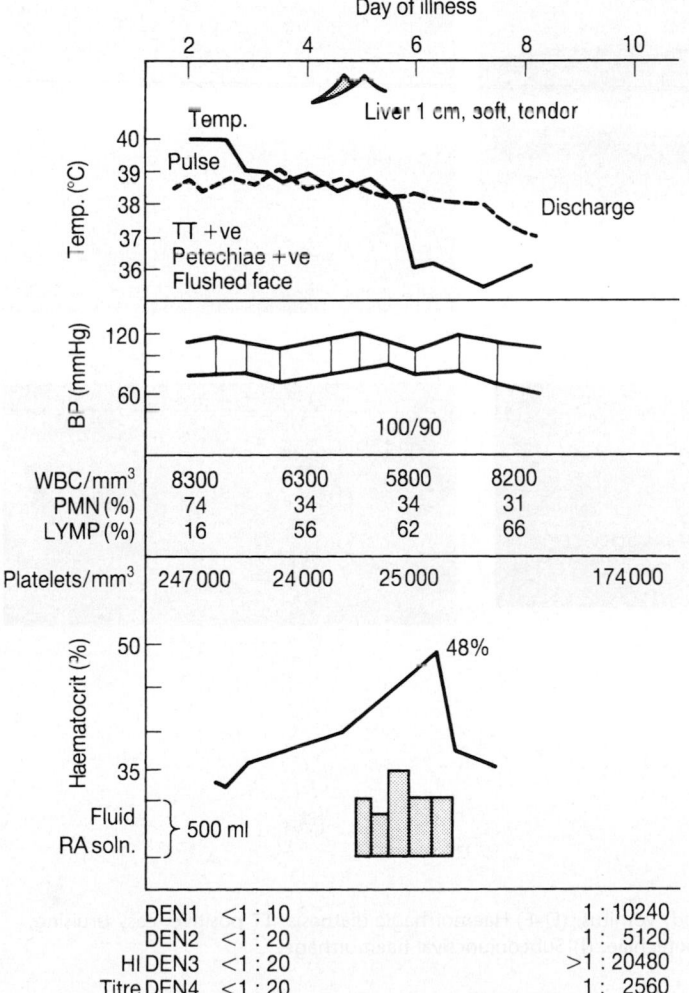

Figure 41.2 Dengue haemorrhagic fever: typical clinical course in a 9-year-old girl (with secondary dengue infection). TT, tourniquet test; PMN, polymorphonuclear leucocytes; LYMP, lymphocyte; RA, Ringer's acetate; HI, haemagglutination inhibition (antibody test by HI titres).

A haemorrhagic diathesis commonly presents in the febrile phase as scattered petechiae on extremities, axillae, trunk and face (Fig. 41.3). A positive tourniquet test and/or tendency to bruise at venepuncture sites are invariably present. Bleeding from the nose, gums and gastrointestinal tract are less common. Haematuria is extremely rare.

The liver is often enlarged, soft and tender but jaundice is not observed. Splenomegaly is rarely observed in small infants. Generalized lymphadenopathy is noted in about half of the cases.

The critical phase, which is the period of plasma leakage, is reached near or by the time the fever subsides. Accompanying, or shortly after, a rapid drop in the temperature there are varying degrees of circulatory disturbance. The patient is often sweating and restless and has cool extremities. In less severe cases (grade I, II) the changes in vital signs are minimal and transient; the patient recovers spontaneously or after a brief period of therapy. In more severe cases shock ensues. The skin is cold and clammy and the pulse pressure becomes narrow (≤20 mmHg) with a slight elevation of diastolic level, e.g. 100/80 mmHg. The course of shock is brief and stormy. If no treatment is given the patient deteriorates rapidly into the stage of profound shock with an imperceptible pulse and blood pressure and dies within 12–24 h. Prolonged shock is often complicated by metabolic acidosis and severe bleeding, which indicates a poor prognosis. However, if the patient is properly treated before irreversible shock has developed, rapid, often dramatic recovery is the rule. Infrequently, encephalitic signs associated with metabolic or electrolyte disturbances, intracranial haemorrhage or hepatic failure (a form of Reye's-like syndrome) occur and give rise to a more complicated course and grave prognosis.[12] The critical phase usually lasts 24–48 h.

The convalescence phase is usually short and uneventful. Sinus bradycardia is common. A characteristic confluent petechial rash with scattered round areas of pale skin, as described in dengue fever, which is frequently observed on the lower extremities is found in about 20–30%. The course of the illness is about 7–10 days in most uncomplicated cases.

A normal white blood count or leucopenia is common and neutrophils may predominate initially. Towards the end of the febrile phase there is a reduction in the number of total leucocytes and neutrophils shortly before or simultaneously with a relative increase in lymphocytes with the presence of atypical lymphocytes. The leucopenia usually reaches a nadir shortly before the temperature and platelets drop. This observation is valuable in predicting the end of the febrile period and the beginning of the critical phase. Thrombocytopenia and haemoconcentration are constant findings. The platelet count drops shortly before or simultaneously with the haematocrit rise (≥20%) and both changes occur before the subsidence of fever and before onset of shock. Clotting abnormalities are usually found, especially in severe cases with shock. Other changes include hypoproteinaemia, hypoalbuminaemia, hyponatraemia and mildly elevated alanine aminotransferase/aspartate aminotransferase levels.[33]

Disease severity is arbitrarily classified as 'non-shock' cases (grades I and II – grade II is more severe than grade I with the presence of spontaneous haemorrhage) and 'shock' cases (grades III and IV – the latter is a profound shock with imperceptible pulse and/or blood pressure).[1]

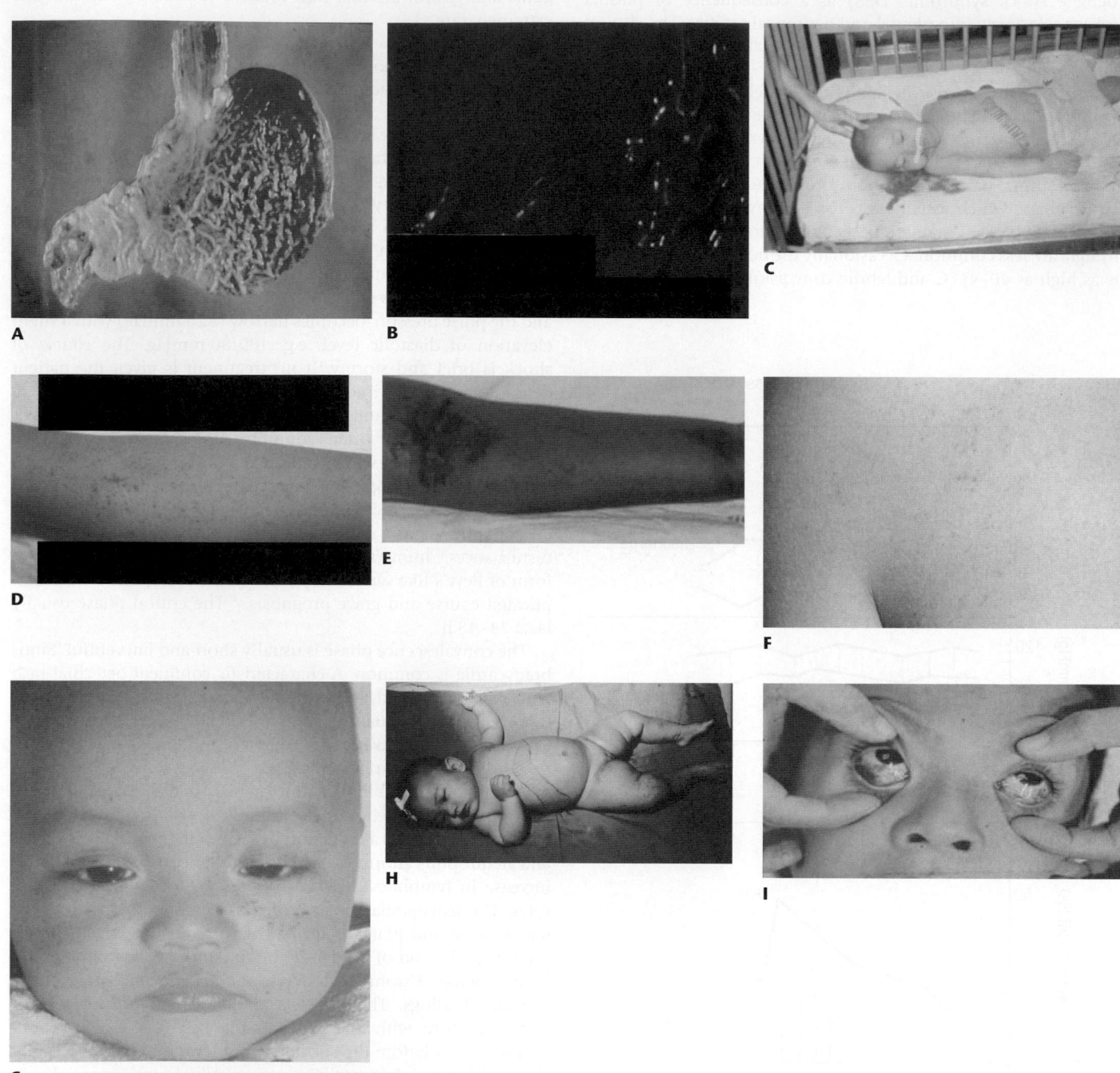

Figure 41.3 (A–B) Massive gastric bleeding. (C) Coffee ground (old blood) vomitus. (D–F) Haemorrhagic diathesis: TT positive, easy bruising, petechiae. (G,H) Haemorrhagic manifestations, most common on skin as petechiae. (I) Subconjunctival haemorrhage.

Diagnosis

The clinical features of DHF are rather stereotyped; thus it is possible to make a correct clinical diagnosis based on the major characteristic manifestations as described. The World Health Organization established criteria for clinical diagnosis:[1,33] high continuous fever for 2–7 days; a haemorrhagic diathesis; hepatomegaly and shock; together with two laboratory changes: thrombocytopenia ($\leq$100 000/mm^3) with concurrent haemoconcentration (haematocrit elevation of 20% or more). The time course relationship between the drop in platelet count and a rapid rise in haematocrit appears to be unique in DHF. These changes, which represent the major pathophysiological hallmarks of DHF, i.e. abnormal haemostasis and plasma leakage, clearly distinguish DHF from dengue fever and other diseases. Evidences of plasma leakage could be confirmed by chest X-ray at the right lateral decubitus position or by ultrasound to detect pleural effusion/ascites. A normal or low erythrocyte sedimentation rate (ESR) observed in DHF and DSS helps in differentiating DSS from septic shock.[34]

Virological diagnosis

Aetiological diagnosis can be confirmed by serological testing and virus detection by isolation or molecular technique from the blood during the early febrile phase. Antibodies to dengue virus antigens increase rapidly in patients with secondary dengue infection. A diagnostic (four-fold) increase in dengue antibody by the haemagglutination inhibition test can usually be demonstrated from paired sera obtained early in the febrile phase or on admission, and 3–5 days later. A third specimen 2–3 weeks after onset is, however, required to confirm diagnosis of primary dengue infection.[1]

Serological diagnosis by detection of anti-dengue IgM and IgG by enzyme-linked immunosorbent assay (ELISA) is now widely used to document primary and secondary infection. IgM antibody capture (MAC) – ELISA is a relatively new test. It is specific in distinguishing dengue from other flavivirus infections and has the advantage over the haemagglutination test in that a definite diagnosis can be made from an acute blood specimen alone, with a sensitivity of about 78%; when convalescent sera are tested the sensitivity is >97%.[35]

Recently an ELISA assay for dengue NS1 antigen detection has been developed and commercial test kits are now available.

Management

The management of DHF is entirely symptomatic and supportive and is principally aimed towards replacement of plasma loss during the period of active leakage of about 24–48 h. Prognosis depends on early clinical recognition and frequent monitoring for a drop in platelet count and rise in haematocrit. Early volume replacement when the haematocrit rises sharply ($\geq$20%) as plasma leaks out can prevent shock and/or modify severity.

The management of DHF during the febrile phase is similar to that of dengue fever. Usually DHF can not be distinguished from dengue fever until platelets drop, with a concurrent rise in haematocrit as plasma leakage starts by the end of the febrile phase. Therefore parents or care takers should be advised to observe for the warning signs of circulatory disturbance and bring the patients to the hospital for proper treatment. The warning signs include:

- refuse food or drinking water
- become drowsy or restless
- protracted vomiting
- acute abdominal pain
- oliguria/thirsty
- worsening of general condition when temperature drops
- any bleeding.

Antipyretics may be needed to control the high fever; aspirin and ibuprofen must not be used (to avoid gastric irritation and severe bleeding and as a precaution to prevent Reye's syndrome (aspirin) associated with dengue infection). Oral fluid and electrolyte therapy are recommended for patients who have anorexia and vomiting.

The critical period when plasma leakage occurs and shock may develop is at the transition from the febrile to the afebrile phase, which is varied according to the duration of febrile phase (2–7 days). Shock could develop as early as on the third day of illness in a patient whose febrile phase is two days. A drop in the platelet count to 100 000/mm^3 or less usually precedes a rise in the haematocrit. A rise in haematocrit of 20% or more (e.g. from baseline 35% to 42% or more) indicates significant plasma loss and intravenous fluid therapy is indicated. In mild to moderately severe cases (grades I and II) fluid therapy can be given for a period of 12–24 h at an out-patient clinic where there are facilities to monitor vital signs and haematocrit. Patients who continue to have high haematocrit or present with any warning signs should be admitted to the hospital.

As there is active and continuous leakage of plasma into the pleural and peritoneal cavities during the critical period, judicious volume replacement is mandatory.

Guiding principles for volume replacement in DHF:

- Intravenous fluid replacement is indicated when plasma leakage occurs, as indicated by rising haematocrit with concurrent thrombocytopenia
- The type of fluid used should be isotonic solution that has an electrolyte composition similar to plasma, e.g. 5% dextrose in normal saline solution (NSS) or Ringer's acetate solution. In case of massive leakage colloidal solution, e.g. Dextran 40 or other plasma expander may be needed
- The volume needed should be just sufficient to maintain effective circulation, which could be guided by vital signs, urine output and haematocrit level. The total volume needed during the period of leakage is approximately maintenance plus 5–6% deficit (similar to mild or moderate dehydration)
- The rate of fluid infusion must be adjusted according to the rate and extent of plasma leakage, which is more rapid during the 6–12 h around the time temperature drops
- The need for intravenous replacement usually lasts for no longer than 48 h, the time by which plasma leakage stops. Fluid replacement must be stopped when the haematocrit and vital signs become stable and return to normal and a diuresis ensues.

When shock has developed, satisfactory results have been obtained with the following regimen:

1. Immediately and rapidly correct hypovolaemia from plasma loss with isotonic salt solution at the rate of 10–20 mL/kg per hour until improvement in vital signs is apparent. In cases of profound shock with no blood pressure and/or pulse perceptible, a bolus of 10 mL/kg (1–2 bolus) should be given.

Colloidal solution may be needed if the haematocrit remains high after initial resuscitation. Oxygen should be given to all shock cases.

2. Continue to replace further plasma losses to maintain effective circulation for a period of 24–48 h. The rate of infusion should be reduced after initial resuscitation and adjusted according to rate of plasma leakage.

3. Correct metabolic and electrolyte disturbances e.g. metabolic acidosis, hypoglycaemia, hyponatraemia.

4. Blood transfusion is indicated in cases with significant clinical bleeding, most often with haematemesis and melena. Fresh whole blood is preferable and the blood should be given only in volume to achieve a normal red cell concentration. Blood components, e.g. concentrated platelets are rarely needed.

A case with persistent shock, despite adequate volume replacement and declining haematocrit level (e.g. from 50% to 40%), indicates significant (concealed) bleeding which requires prompt blood transfusion. It is a most difficult situation to recognize and estimate the degree of internal blood loss with the presence of haemoconcentration due to plasma loss. It is thus recommended to give fresh whole blood in small volumes (10 mL/kg) at a time. Then follow-up vital signs, haematocrit, for further bleeding.

Haematologic indicators such as coagulogram, prothrombin time, partial thromboplastin time, and thrombin time should be measured in all shock cases to document the onset and severity of DIC; results of these tests can provide valuable information for proper management and prognosis.

Fluid overload is the most common complication of fluid therapy in DHF/DSS. It is important to adjust the rate of intravenous infusion according to the rate of plasma leakage as guided by the haematocrit level, vital signs and urine output to avoid excessive fluid replacement. It must be emphasized that the total volume of fluid replacement should be just sufficient to maintain effective circulation during the period of leakage. Excessive fluid infusion will cause massive pleural effusion and ascites leading to respiratory compromise. Fluid replacement must be discontinued when leakage stops after 48 h. If further fluid replacement is given at this stage it can cause cardiac failure and/or acute pulmonary oedema when extravasated plasma is reabsorbed.[33]

With this regimen the fatality rate of DHF cases at the Children's Hospital in Bangkok has fallen to below 0.5%. There is no evidence that corticosteroids are of benefit in reducing the fatality rate or reducing the disease severity.[36] The efficacy of heparin in the treatment of cases with severe bleeding from disseminated intravascular coagulation has not been proved.[14,37]

Good nursing care with close observation 24 h a day is essential for management of patients with DHF/DSS.

Epidemiology

Since it was first recognized in the Philippines in 1954, DHF has occurred in Thailand, Malaysia, Singapore, Sri Lanka, Vietnam, India, Myanmar and Malaysia, several Pacific islands, China, Laos and Kampuchea. Between 1956 and 1995, there were 3 683 023 cases with 58 554 deaths reported from 12 Asian countries, the Pacific Islands, Cuba and Venezuela. The first outbreak of DHF to occur outside the South-east Asian and Western Pacific regions was in Cuba in 1981. Since then sporadic cases of DHF have been reported from the Caribbean and small outbreaks occurred in Venezuela in 1989 and Rio de Janeiro in 1991.[38] Between 1981 and 2005, DHF has emerged to become a major public health problem in 28 countries in tropical America. There were 34 739 reported cases of DHF with 514 deaths reported between 1981 and 1995. More adult cases were observed in these areas.[3,18] Recent outbreaks of DHF in adults who had DENV2 in 1997 following primary DENV1 infection in 1977 or 1981 in Cuba confirmed the role of secondary infection and sequence of DENV1–DENV2 infections as risk factors for the occurrence of DHF. It is noteworthy that DENV2 involved in the outbreak both in 1981 and 1997 in Cuba was of South-east Asian genotype.[6,18]

Outbreaks occur most frequently in areas where environmental conditions are optimal for dengue transmission and multiple types of dengue virus are simultaneously endemic or sequentially epidemic, and infections with heterologous types are frequent. In endemic areas where dengue infection is frequently asymptomatic and occurs in early childhood, classical dengue fever is rarely a recognizable disease among indigenous people. DHF occurs most frequently in children aged between 2 and 15 years. Older, and many of the younger, inhabitants are usually immune and escape DHF. However, cases in infants as young as 2 months and in young as well as aged adults have been increasingly reported. DHF is usually associated with secondary dengue infection but can appear during a primary infection, especially in infants under the age of 1 year, all of whom possess maternal IgG dengue antibody.[11] Notably, DHF in older children associated with primary infection caused by DENV-1 and DENV-3 is not uncommon. With increasing reports of dengue in adults, neonatal dengue cases including DHF as a result of vertical transmission have also been increasing.[39]

A seasonal incidence pattern usually coincides with the rainy season in many countries in tropical zones.

Prevention and control

The control of dengue depends on control of the vector, particularly *Ae. aegypti*, an anthropophilic domestic mosquito which lives intimately with its human host(s). These mosquitoes breed primarily in man-made containers such as those used for water storage, flower vases, old jars, tin cans and used tyres in and around human dwellings. Elimination of these breeding sites is an effective and definitive method of controlling the vector and preventing dengue transmission. The use of larvicides and insecticides during outbreaks has some limitations. Efforts are now focusing on health education and community participation in an attempt to control the vector(s) by eliminating or reducing the breeding sites.[1]

There is no dengue vaccine available for public health use at present. Research is in progress to develop an effective and safe tetravalent dengue vaccine. Many candidate dengue vaccines, e.g. live attenuated, inactivated whole virus, and recombinant vaccines are in the process of development. Some have been in phase 2 field trials.[40] In the absence of a dengue vaccine for public health use at present, prevention and containment of dengue outbreaks will require an effective long-term vector control with community participation and aggressive epidemiological surveillance.

REFERENCES

1. WHO. *Dengue Hemorrhagic Fever: Diagnosis, Treatment and Control.* Geneva: World Health Organization, 1997.
2. Gubler DJ. Dengue. In: Monath TP, ed. *The Arboviruses: Epidemiology and Ecology.* Boca Raton: CRC Press; 1988:223–260.
3. Gubler DJ. Dengue and dengue haemorrhagic fever: its history and resurgence as a global public health problem. In: Gubler DJ, Kuno G, eds. *Dengue and Dengue Haemorrhagic Fever.* Willingford: CAB International; 1997:1–22.
4. Rico-Hesse R. Molecular evolution and distribution of dengue virus type 1 and type 2 in nature. *Virology* 1990; 174:479–493.
5. Twiddy SS, Woelk CH, Holmes EC. Phylogenetic evidence for adaptive evolution of dengue viruses in nature. *J Gen Virol* 2002; 83:1679–1689.
6. Rico-Hesse R, Harrison LM, Salas RA, et al. Origin of dengue type 2 viruses associated with increased pathogenicity in the Americas. *Virology* 1997; 230:244–251.
7. Marchette NJ, Halstead SB, Falker WA Jr, et al. Studies on the pathogenesis of dengue infection in monkeys III: sequential distribution of virus in primary and heterologous infections. *J Infect Dis* 1973; 128:28–30.
8. Sabin AB. Dengue. In: Rivers TM, Horsfall FL, eds. *Viral and Rickettsial Infections of Man.* Philadelphia: Lippincott; 1959:361–373.
9. Winter PE, Nantapanich S, Nisalak A. Recurrence of epidemic dengue hemorrhagic fever in an insular setting. *Am J Trop Med Hyg* 1969; 18:573–579.
10. Schlesinger RW. *Dengue Viruses.* New York: Springer, 1977:90–91.
11. Halstead SB. The pathogenesis of dengue: the Alexander D Langmuir Lecture. *Am J Trop Med Hyg* 1981, 114.632–648.
12. Nimmannitya S, Thisyakon U, Hemserchart V. Dengue hemorrhagic fever with unusual manifestation. *Southeast Asian J Trop Med Public Health* 1987; 18:398–406.
13. George R, Lum LCS. Clinical spectrum of dengue infection. In: Gubler DJ, Juno G, eds. *Dengue and Dengue Haemorrhagic Fever.* Wallingford: CAB International; 1997:89–113.
14. Srickaikul T, Nimmannitya S. Haematology in dengue and dengue haemorrhagic fever. *Baillière's Clin Haematol* 2000:261–273.
15. Hoke CH, Nimmannitya S, Nisalak A, et al. Studies on dengue hemorrrhagic fever at Bangkok Children's Hospital 1962–1984. In: Pang T, Pathmanathan R, eds. *Proc Int Conf Dengue/DHF.* Kuala Lumpur: University of Malaysia Press; 1984.
16. Nisalak A, Endy TP, Nimmannitya S, et al. Serotype specific dengue virus circulation and dengue disease in Bangkok, Thailand from 1973 to 1999. *Am J Trop Med Hyg* 2003; 68(2):191–202.
17. Sangkawibha N, Rojanasuphots S, Ahandrik S, et al. Risk factors in dengue shock syndrome: a prospective epidemiological study in Rayong, Thailand. *Am J Epidemiol* 1984; 120:653–669.
18. Guzman MG, Kouri G, Vazquez S, et al. DHF epidemics in Cuba in 1981 and 1997: some interesting observations. *Dengue Bull* 1999; 23:39–43.
19. Vaughn DW, Green S, Kalayanarooj S, et al. Dengue viremia titer, antibody response pattern, and virus serotype correlate with disease severity. *J Infect Dis* 2000; 181:2–9.
20. Mongkolsapaya J, Dejnirattisai W, Xu XN, et al. Original antigenic sin and apoptosis in the pathogenesis of dengue hemorrhagic fever. *Nat Med* 2003; 9:921–927.
21. Rosen L. The Emperor's New Clothes revisited, or reflections on the pathogenesis of dengue hemorrhagic fever. *Am J Trop Med Hyg* 1977; 26:337–343.
22. Chiewsilp P, Scott RM, Bhamarapravati N, et al. Histocompatibility antigens and dengue hemorrhagic fever. *Am J Trop Med Hyg* 1981; 30:1100–1105.
23. Guzman MG, Kouri GP, Bravo J, et al. Dengue hemorrhagic fever in Cuba, 1981; a retrospective seroepidemiologic study. *Am J Trop Med Hyg* 1990; 42:179–184.
24. Rico-Hesse R, Harrison LM, Nisalak A, et al. Molecular evolution of dengue type 2 virus in Thailand. *Am J Trop Med Hyg* 1998; 58(1):96–101.
25. Bhamarapravati N, Tuchinda P, Boonyapaknavik V. Pathology of Thai haemorrhagic fever: a study of 100 autopsy cases. *Ann Trop Med Parasitol* 1967; 61:500–510.
26. Malasit P. Complement and dengue hemorrhagic fever/shock syndrome. *Southeast Asian J Trop Med Public Health* 1987; 18:316–320.
27. Avirutnan P, Punyadee N, Noisakran S, et al. Vascular leakage in severe Dengue virus infections: A potential role for the nonstructural viral protein NS1 and complement. *J Infect Dis* 2006; 193:1078–1088.
28. Libraty HD, Young PR, Pickering D, et al. High circulating levels of the dengue virus nonstructural protein NS1 early in dengue illness correlate with the development of dengue hemorrhagic fever. *J Infect Dis* 2002; 186.1165–1168.
29. Klick SC, Nimmannitya S, Nisalak A, et al. Evidence that maternal dengue antibodies are important in the development of dengue hemorrhagic fever in infants. *Am J Trop Med Hyg* 1988; 38:411–419.
30. Kurane I, Innis BL, Nimmannitya S, et al. Activation of T lymphocytes in dengue virus infections: high levels of soluble interleukin 2 receptor, soluble CD4, soluble CD8, interleukin 2, and interferon g in sera of children with dengue. *J Clin Invest* 1991; 88:1473–1480.
31. Green S, Vaughn DW, Kalayanarooj S, et al. Early immune activation in acute dengue illness is related to development of plasma leakage and disease severity. *J Infect Dis* 1999; 179:755–762.
32. Nimmannitya S, Kalayanarooj S, Nisalak A, et al. Second attack of dengue hemorrhagic fever. *Proc Int Conf Dengue/DHF,* 1–3 October 1990, Bangkok.
33. Nimmannitya S. Dengue haemorrhagic fever: Diagnosis and management. In: Gubler DI, Kuno G, eds. *Dengue and Dengue Haemorrhagic Fever.* Wallingford: CAB International; 1997:133–145.
34. Kalayanarooj S, Nimmannitya S. A study of erythrocyte sedimentation rate in dengue hemorrhagic fever. *Southeast Asian J Trop Med Public Health* 1989; 20:325–330.
35. Innis BL, Nisalak A, Nimmannitya S, et al. An enzyme linked immunosorbent assay to characterize dengue infections where dengue and Japanese encephalitis co-circulate. *Am J Trop Med Hyg* 1989; 40:418–427.
36. Sumarmo, Talogo W, Asrin A, et al. Failure of hydrocortisone to affect outcome in dengue shock syndrome. *Pediatrics* 1982; 69:45–49.
37. Nimmannitya S. Clinical spectrum and management of dengue hemorrhagic fever. *Southeast Asian J Trop Med Public Health* 1987; 18:392–397.
38. WHO. *Dengue Newsletter.* Vol. 17. Geneva: World Health Organization; 1992.
39. Chye JK, Lim CT, Ng KB. Vertical transmission of dengue. *Clin Infect Dis* 1997; 25:1374–1377.
40. Bhamarapravati N, Yoksan S. Live attenuated tetravalent dengue vaccine. In: Gubler DJ, Kuno G, eds. *Dengue and Dengue Haemorrhagic Fever.* Wallingford: CAB International; 1997:367–377.

Chapter 42
Tom Solomon and Gail Thomson

Viral Haemorrhagic Fevers

Few diseases create such fear among the general public and health-care community as the viral haemorrhagic fevers (VHFs). Although, in terms of the actual risks, this fear is often unfounded, there are many questions relating to the origin, pathogenesis, treatment and control of VHFs that remain to be answered. The term haemorrhagic fever dates back to the 1930s, when it was first used to describe an outbreak occurring in the region encompassing the Manchurian–Russian–Korean triangle in East Asia, which was probably caused by a hantavirus.[1]

EPIDEMIOLOGY

The haemorrhagic fever viruses are a diverse group of viruses from four viral families – the Arenaviridae, Filoviridae, Bunyaviridae and Flaviviridae – which are considered together because of the similarity of the clinical syndrome they produce (Table 42.1). There have important differences in their natural cycles, geographical distributions, and their potential for nosocomial transmission, which can be confusing. The epidemiology can be simplified by considering three questions (see Figure 42.1):
- How is the virus transmitted in its natural cycle – via arthropods, directly or unknown?
- How do human index cases get infected – via insects, directly or unknown?
- Is there nosocomial transmission from the human index case to secondary cases?

Most haemorrhagic fever viruses exist in enzootic (animal) cycles, causing little harm in their natural hosts. Humans become infected by these viruses coincidentally when they encroach upon this enzootic cycle. (Dengue is an important exception because humans *are* the natural host.) The viruses are transmitted naturally between host animals either via biting insects, or directly via excretions such as urine.[2] Those that are transmitted by insects – dengue, yellow fever, Crimean–Congo haemorrhagic fever (CCHF) and Rift Valley fever (RVF) – are labelled with the ecological term arboviruses (arthropod-borne viruses – Chapter 40). Viruses transmitted naturally via animal excreta include Lassa and Hantaan, the cause of haemorrhagic fever with renal syndrome (HFRS).

Some haemorrhagic fever viruses are particularly important because of their potential for direct transmission from one human to another, in blood and other secretions. This group includes Lassa fever, CCHF, and Ebola and Marburg – whose natural cycle remains unknown.

PATHOGENESIS

Although different pathophysiological processes occur in different VHFs, the following are common:
- vascular damage, which may be due to direct viral invasion of endothelial cells, complement and cytokine activation, and immune complex deposition
- disorders of coagulation, which may be due to thrombocytopenia (caused by bone marrow suppression and increased consumption), abnormal platelet function, impaired production of clotting factors by the liver, and disseminated intravascular coagulation (DIC)
- immunological impairment, which inhibits the immune response and allows uncontrolled viral replication
- end-organ damage, which is most often due to direct viral cytopathology (e.g. hepatic damage in yellow fever), or in some cases is due to the host inflammatory response (e.g. nephritis in HFRS).

CLINICAL FEATURES

The clinical manifestations that may result from these pathophysiological processes include:
- Increased vascular permeability which allows leakage of plasma from the vessels into the tissue and leads to two problems:
  - low blood pressure, which may manifest with cold clammy and sweaty skin, irritability, drowsiness, and, in children, a prolonged capillary refill time and a narrow pulse pressure (i.e. the difference between systolic and diastolic BP is less than 20 mmHg); if uncorrected, secondary complications of hypovolaemic shock occur, such as acidosis, renal failure, and other metabolic complications[3]
  - pulmonary oedema, pleural effusions, oedema of the face and neck (which can all contribute to respiratory failure); in some VHFs, pericardial and retroperitoneal effusions.
- Haemorrhagic manifestations are sometimes relatively minor, e.g. skin petechiae, bruising, oozing from venepuncture sites, gum or nose bleeding. More serious manifestations include gastrointestinal bleeding. However, for most VHFs, when shock occurs, it is a result of vascular leakage, not haemorrhage.
- Increased capillary fragility, determined by a positive tourniquet test (Figure 42.2).

Table 42.1 Overview of the major viral haemorrhagic fevers

Family	Genus	Virus	Disease	Geographical area	Natural cycle	Human disease
Arenaviridae	Arenavirus	Lassa	Lassa fever	Western Africa	*Mastomys* rodent	Direct transmission from rodent excreta and human-to-human spread. Mortality rate 2–15%. Treat with ribavirin
		Junin, Machupo, Guanarito	Argentine, Bolivian, Venezuelan haemorrhagic fevers	Localized areas in South America	*Calomys* and other rodents	Direct transmission from rodent excreta and human-to-human spread. Mortality rate 15–30%. Treat with ribavirin
Filoviridae	Filovirus	Ebola and Marburg	Ebola and Marburg haemorrhagic fevers	Sub-Saharan Africa	Unknown	Nosocomial spread common. Mortality rate 25–90%. No antiviral treatment
Bunyaviridae	Hantavirus	Hantaan, Dobrava, Seoul, Puumala	Haemorrhagic fever with renal syndrome	Far East, Europe	Various rural rodents	Direct transmission from rodent excreta. No human-to-human spread. Mortality rate 1–15%, depending on virus. Treat severe disease with ribavirin
	Nairovirus	Crimean–Congo haemorrhagic fever	Crimean–Congo haemorrhagic fever	Eastern Europe, Asia, Africa	*Hyalomma* ticks and livestock	Mosquito bites and direct transmission from blood of infected animals. Human-to-human spread. Mortality rate 15–30%. Treat with ribavirin
	Phlebovirus	Rift Valley fever	Rift Valley fever	Africa, Middle East	*Aedes* and other mosquitoes, and livestock	Tick bites and direct transmission from blood of infected animals. Human-to-human spread not documented, but possible. Most natural infections asymptomatic. Mortality rate 50% for VHF. Treat with ribavirin
Flaviviridae	Flavivirus	Dengue	Dengue fever, dengue haemorrhagic fever	Tropics and subtropics worldwide	*Aedes* mosquitoes and humans	Transmission from mosquito bites. No direct transmission. Mortality rate <1% with adequate fluid treatment. No antivirals
		Yellow fever	Yellow fever	Africa, South America	Various mosquitoes and monkeys	Transmission from mosquito bites. No direct transmission. Mortality rate 20–50%. No antivirals
		Omsk haemorrhagic fever	Omsk haemorrhagic fever	Western Siberia	Muskrats, other rodents, *Dermacentor* ticks	Direct contact with muskrats, and tick bites. Mortality rate 1–10%. No antivirals
		Kyasanur Forest disease	Kyasanur Forest disease	South-western India	*Haemaphysalis* ticks	Tick bites, no antivirals

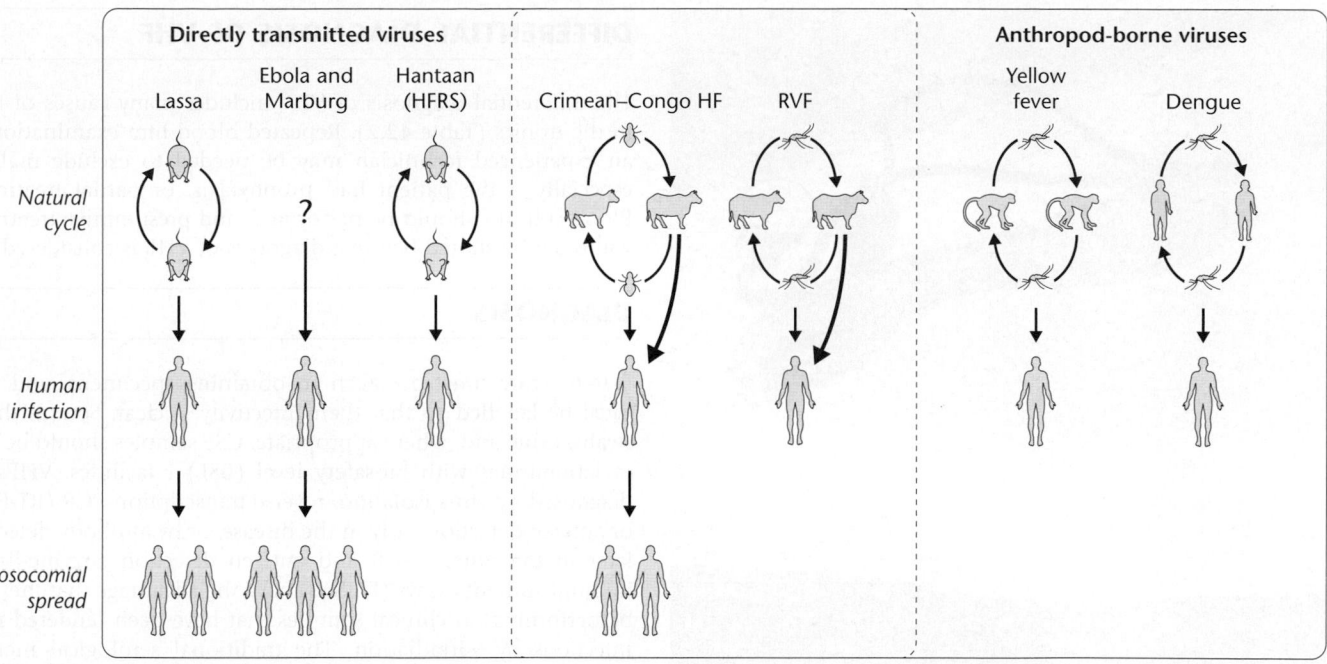

Figure 42.1 Ecological overview of viral haemorrhagic fevers, showing natural cycle, transmission to humans, and potential for nosocomial spread. Note the distinction between directly transmissible viruses, arboviruses, and those transmitted by both routes (CCHF and RVF). HF, haemorrhagic fever; HFRS, haemorrhagic fever with renal syndrome; RVF, rift valley fever.

- Hepatic failure, including mild hepatitis and jaundice or fulminant hepatic failure.
- Renal failure, which may be a consequence of hypovolaemia, or, in HFRS, direct renal damage.
- Encephalopathy, which may be secondary to the severe metabolic disturbances or, for some VHFs, caused by virus invading the central nervous system (CNS).[4]

MANAGEMENT OF VHF

Although the general principles are the same, the practicalities of managing a suspected case of VHF in a traveller returning from the tropics are different from those of managing a patient locally during a known epidemic. Specific issues for each disease are addressed later in the chapter. In general, management incorporates:

- identifying, diagnosing and treating a suspected VHF patient
- for the directly transmissible VHFs, limiting any further spread
- identifying others who may have been infected.

IDENTIFYING VHF CASES

Most patients with suspected VHF turn out to have malaria, typhoid, gastroenteritis or another non-transmissible disease. A travel history should include details of not only the countries visited, but also the regions of the country. Under natural circumstances, the directly transmissible VHFs are most often acquired in rural rather than urban areas. Because their importance may not be realized by the patient, specific questions should be asked about activities which could potentially have allowed exposure to haemorrhagic viruses, e.g. caving, exposure to monkeys, or to rat urine. In addition, it is important to ascertain whether they were in contact with any sick individuals, their tissues, or even those of sick animals. An interval of 3 weeks or more between the last possible exposure and onset of illness rules out the diagnosis of VHF. Many early symptoms are non-specific, but certain features should ring alarm bells (Figure 42.3). These include pharyngitis (especially if there are ulcers on the pharynx or it is severe enough to cause pain on eating), retrosternal chest pain, conjunctival injection, and prostration. Haemorrhagic manifestations may not be obvious initially. Look for gum bleeding, petechiae in the axillae and skin folds, and microscopic haematuria, and perform a tourniquet test (Figure 42.2). Vascular leakage may also not be apparent immediately. Ask relatives if they think the patient's face looks puffy around the eyes. A decubitus chest X-ray may reveal a small pleural effusion. Laboratory investigations that may suggest a VHF include a rising haematocrit (a consequence of increased vascular permeability, which is easily measured and a useful early marker of impending shock), leucopenia, thrombocytopenia, elevated transaminases, prolonged clotting times and proteinuria.

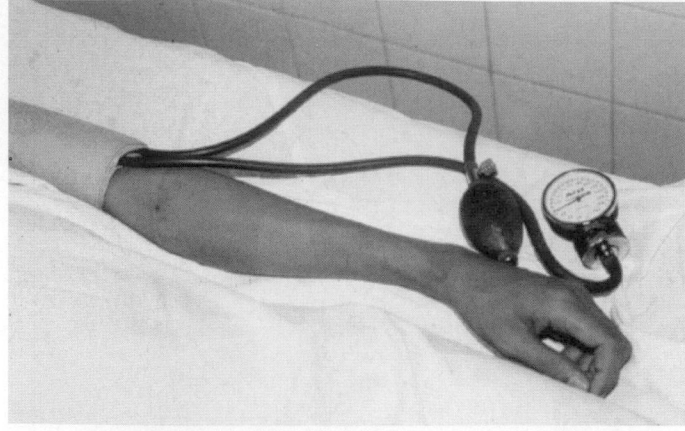

A

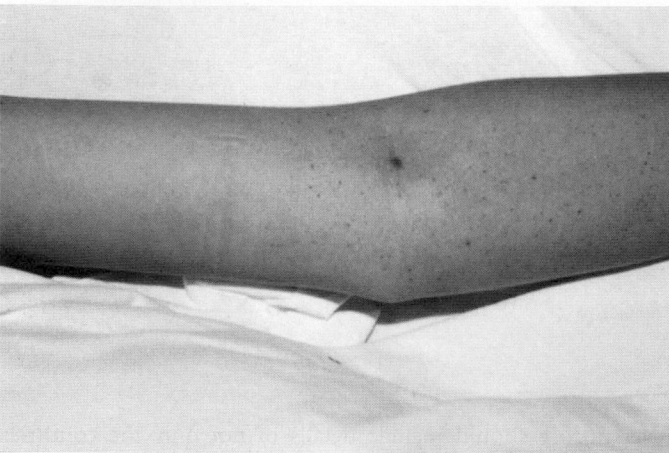

B

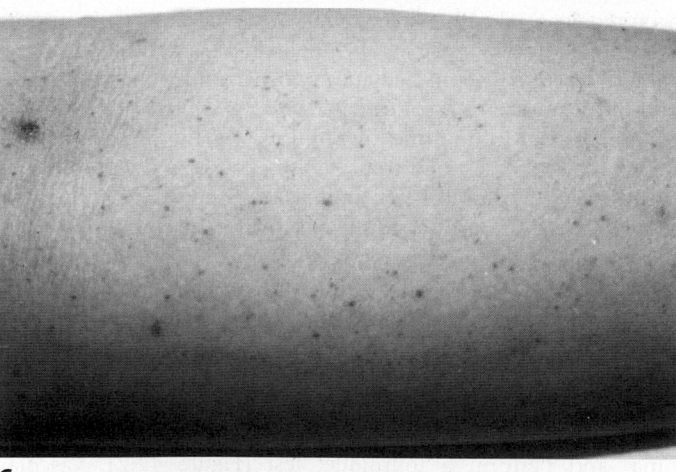

C

Figure 42.2 The tourniquet test of capillary fragility. A blood pressure cuff inflated to halfway between systolic and diastolic pressure for 5 minutes (**A**) causes more than 20 petechiae in a 2.5 cm square over the forearm (**B** & **C**). Note also bruising around a venepuncture site in the antecubital fossa. (Photo: Tom Solomon.)

DIFFERENTIAL DIAGNOSIS OF VHF

The differential diagnosis of VHF includes many causes of fever in the tropics (Table 42.2). Repeated blood film examination by an experienced technician may be needed to exclude malaria, especially if the patient had prophylaxis, or partial treatment. Blood cultures should be performed, and presumptive treatment will often be started before a diagnosis of VHF is considered.[5]

DIAGNOSIS

Extreme care must be taken in obtaining specimens, and they must be labelled so that their infectivity is clear. Serum, throat swabs, urine and, where appropriate, CSF samples should be sent to laboratories with biosafety level (BSL)-4 facilities. VHFs are diagnosed by virus isolation, reverse transcription PCR (RT-PCR) or antigen detection early in the disease, or by antibody detection later in the illness. PCR and antigen detection enzyme-linked immunosorbent assays (ELISAs) have the advantage that they can be performed on clinical samples that have been rendered non-infectious by γ-irradiation. The traditional serological method used for diagnosing many VHFs, the indirect fluorescent antibody test, has been replaced by IgM and IgG capture ELISAs.

TREATMENT

The antiviral drug ribavirin (a guanosine analogue) is effective in Lassa fever and CCHF, and, based on laboratory data and limited clinical data, it should also be used in severe RVF and HFRS. An intravenous (i.v.) loading dose of 30 mg/kg should be followed by 16 mg/kg i.v. every 6 hours for 4 days, then 8 mg/kg i.v. every 8 hours for 6 days.[3] All VHF patients should be given oxygen, pain relief and gentle sedation, if necessary, and supportive treatment for the complications of infection:

- Hypovolaemic shock: this occurs as a consequence of increased capillary permeability. Patients need to be rehydrated with intravenous colloid or crystalloid. However, injudicious use can lead to respiratory failure because of pulmonary oedema. For some VHFs, e.g. dengue haemorrhagic fever in children, treatment protocols have been published.[5] Intravenous crystalloid is recommended before colloid, though recent studies from Vietnam suggest earlier use of a colloid may be beneficial in patients who are severely shocked.[6–8] For Ebola and Marburg, treatment with oral rehydration solution is preferable to intravenous rehydration, where possible. It puts healthcare workers at less risk, and may be less likely to lead to oedema and hypokalaemia. However, many such patients are severely weakened, unable to sit up or hold a cup, and can only manage small sips. Yet, with extensive support from nursing staff or relatives, some patients will drink many litres of fluid in the first 24 hours, and subsequently survive. Daily provision of a 5 L plastic can of oral rehydration solution to each patient allows easy assessment of their fluid intake. Reducing the concentration to 80% and adding orange juice concentrate may improve patients' intake (Mardel S, personal communication). Ionotropes are useful in some VHFs, particularly late in the disease or if there is evidence of cardiac dysfunction.

	Directly transmissible VHF(a)					Non-directly transmissible VHF		
	Ebola/ Marburg	Lassa	South American VHFs	CCHF	RVF(b)	HFRS	DHF	Yellow fever

1. Obtain a travel history:

	Ebola/ Marburg	Lassa	South American VHFs	CCHF	RVF(b)	HFRS	DHF	Yellow fever
Africa	+	+		+	+		+	+
Middle East				+	+		+	
Asian subcontinent				+			+	
Europe				+		+		
Far East				+		+	+	
Americas			+				+	+

2. Ask about activities that may have caused exposure to virus:

	Directly transmissible VHF(a)					Non-directly transmissible VHF		
Exposure to human cases	Recent contact (< 3 weeks) with any sick individual with unexplained fever and bleeding					–	–	–
Exposure to animal reservoir	?Monkeys ?Bats	Rodent excreta (urban)	(rural)	Livestock		Rodent excreta	–	Monkeys
Activities undertaken	Jungle visits, caving	Cleaning basements, etc.	Farming, harvesting	Farming, abattoir work, rural activities		Rural, agricultural work	Urban mosquito exposure	Jungle mosquito exposure

3. Look for suggestive clinical features:

Early features	Pharyngitis	Rash	Facial oedema
	Conjunctival injection	Venepuncture oozing	Small pleural effusions
	Retrosternal chest pain	Petechial haemorrhages	Abdominal pain
	Prostration	Mucosal bleeding	Tender hepatomegaly

Late features	Shock	Haematemesis	Renal failure
	Pleural effusions	DIC	Encephalopathy
	Ascites	Hepatic failure	Acidosis
	Pericardial effusions		

4. Consider investigative findings common in VHFs:

Leucopenia	Proteinuria	Prolonged TT, APTT
Thrombocytopenia	Haematuria	Raised transaminase levels
Rising haematocrit	Renal impairment	

5. If malaria film and other tests negative and patient deteriorating despite presumptive treatment, suspect VHF:

For a directly transmissible VHF, begin isolation procedure; alert medical, nursing, laboratory, cleaning and laundry staff and public health officials	For non-transmissible VHF, ensure standard safe practices are being followed; inform public health authorities

6. Start intravenous ribavirin if likely to respond:

Ebola/ Marburg	Lassa	South American VHFs	CCHF	RVF(b)	HFRS	DHF	YF
–	+	+	+	+	+	–	–
Directly transmissible VHF					Non-directly transmissible VHF		

Notes:

a Directly transmissible between humans.

b Patients with VHF due to RVF should be treated as infectious, although direct transmission between humans has not yet been shown.

Figure 42.3 Algorithm for suspecting VHF in the febrile patient.

Table 42.2 Differential diagnoses of viral haemorrhagic fever

VIRAL HAEMORRHAGIC FEVERS (IN ORDER OF INCIDENCE)	FEVER WITH RASH DUE TO ARBOVIRUSES
Dengue haemorrhagic fever	Alphaviruses
Haemorrhagic fever with renal syndrome	Barmah Forest
Yellow fever	Chikungunya
Lassa fever	O'nyong nyong
Crimean–Congo haemorrhagic fever	Mayaro
Argentine, Bolivia, and Venezuelan haemorrhagic fevers	Ross River
Rift Valley fever	Sindbis
Kyasanur Forest disease and Omsk haemorrhagic fever	Bunyaviruses
Ebola and Marburg haemorrhagic fevers	Oropouche
	Coltiviruses
FEVER WITH RASH/HAEMORRHAGE DUE TO PARASITES/BACTERIA	Colorado tick fever
Parasites	**FEVER WITH RASH DUE TO NON-ARTHROPOD-BORNE VIRUSES**
Malaria	Enteroviruses
Bacteria	Coxsackieviruses
Meningococcus	Echoviruses
Typhoid	Enteroviruses 68–71
Septicaemic plague	Paramyxoviruses
Shigella	Measles
Any severe sepsis with DIC	Herpesviruses
Rickettsia	Herpes zoster virus
Tick and epidemic typhus	Human herpesvirus 6 and 7
Rocky mountain spotted fever	Orthomyxoviruses
Spirochaetes	Influenza A and B
Leptospirosis	Rubiviruses
Borrelia	Rubella
FULMINANT HEPATIC FAILURE	**MISCELLANEOUS**
Hepatitis viruses A–E	Drug reactions
Paracetamol and other drugs	Toxins
Reye's syndrome	Acute surgical emergencies (upper gastrointestinal bleeding)
Alcohol	

- Fluid overload is common, especially since in some VHFs the vascular permeability can return to normal rapidly. The rate of fluid infusion needs to be carefully tailored according to the vital signs, haematocrit, and urine output. Even cautious treatment may precipitate fluid overload. Central venous pressure monitoring using a line inserted via a compressible site, such as the internal jugular or femoral veins, or measurement of pulmonary capillary wedge pressure with a Swan-Ganz catheter, if possible, is helpful. Diuretics and ventilatory support are sometimes needed.
- Respiratory failure may occur secondary to swelling of the neck and larynx, pulmonary oedema or effusions.
- Bleeding diatheses: in many patients this presents as minor bleeding. Blood transfusions are therefore not required in most patients. Fresh frozen plasma is used in severely ill patients with deranged clotting. Although thrombocytopenia is common, it is not normally severe enough to require platelet transfusions. Intramuscular injections should be avoided, as should aspirin because of its antiplatelet effects, and potential to further damage the liver in a Reye's-like syndrome.
- Acid–base imbalance, renal failure, liver failure and encephalopathies are managed along standard lines.

RECOVERY

For survivors of VHFs, especially filovirus outbreaks, there are major issues to deal with in terms of their own psychological state, and being accepted back into the community. Witnessing other patients dying of Ebola was a major negative experience for some survivors in one outbreak.[9] World Health Organization (WHO) outbreak teams now include anthropologists, psychiatrists and psychologists. Something as simple as a letter stating it is now safe for a survivor to return to their village may be helpful.

PREVENTION OF NOSOCOMIAL SPREAD

Patients with suspected directly transmissible VHF should be isolated from other patients and strict barrier-nursing techniques practised. The risk of human-to-human transmission is highest during the later stages of the disease. Hospital staff coming into contact with patients should wear personal protective equipment (PPE) such as gowns, gloves, goggles and masks, which must not be reused unless disinfected. A 'buddy system' has proved a useful way of ensuring PPE is worn properly. Needlestick injuries carry the greatest risk of transmission to healthcare workers, and so extreme care should be taken. Thought also needs to be given to the 'administrative issues' and physical environment. Where possible, staff should work in a safe, well-lit building with a reliable water supply, and 'traffic control' of patient and staff movements. Staff should have regular rest time to reduce the risk of mistakes. There should be regular disinfection, and the patient should use a chemical toilet.

The risks of respiratory spread of VHFs between humans are low (possibly documented once only for Lassa fever[10]), but, in the West, patients are transferred to specialized isolation units with negative pressure or a tent facility.

Laboratory staff processing samples for routine investigations and for tests to rule out other causes (e.g. full blood count and blood film) must also be warned about the nature of the specimens. Particular attention should be paid to the disposal of clinical waste and sharps.

When patients die, preparation of the body by traditional healers can result in further spread of the virus.[11] Thus, an early priority in an outbreak is training personnel to become burial teams. Patients should be promptly buried or cremated by specialist teams trained to avoid the risk of further contamination.[12] However, allowing relatives to view the body in a safe manner before burial is important. In African settings where directly transmissible VHFs may occur, advance planning, which includes training staff in VHF procedures, and identifying a VHF coordinator, may save many lives in the event of an outbreak. Comprehensive manuals are available to facilitate such planning.[5]

Some have found the following algorithm useful to remind healthcare workers of the important points to prevent nosocomial spread (Mardel S, personal communication):

A – Alert – be alert to the possibility of a VHF
B – Barriers – use personal protective equipment and isolation facilities/practices
C – Clean and disinfect where appropriate
D – Disposal – safely dispose of all waste generated
E – Evaluate – keep all measures under constant evaluation.

Contact tracing

Contact tracing requires the identification of hospital personnel, family members and others who may have had contact with the patient (usually before the diagnosis was suspected). 'High-risk' contacts who were exposed to blood, secretions or body fluids, or had close physical contact with the patient should have their body temperature checked twice daily for 3 weeks after their last contact.

Any in whom the temperature rises above 38.5°C should be immediately hospitalized, isolated and ribavirin started if appropriate. Casual contacts who are only at low risk should be warned of their low risk of exposure and asked to report any fever.

The presence of VHFs in the community causes much fear and alarm. In the African setting, identifying community leaders and other resources to help educate about the risks of transmission can be very important. When VHF cases occur in the West, dealing with the media is one important and time-consuming aspect of the care.

ARENAVIRUSES

Arenaviruses cause chronic infections of rodents indigenous to Europe, Africa, America and possibly other continents. They are transmitted between rodents via their urine, and humans become infected when they come into contact with excreted viruses. For some there may then be secondary nosocomial transmission. Lymphocytic choriomeningitis virus (LCMV), the first arenavirus isolated, was discovered during a study of a St Louis encephalitis epidemic in 1933. It has received most attention as a model of viral immunology, being instrumental in developing concepts of immune tolerance, immune complex disease, and cytotoxic T cell function[13] LCMV is not typical of other arenaviruses in that in humans it causes occasional CNS, rather than haemorrhagic, disease. It is transmitted by the house mouse (*Mus* complex) and is widely distributed. Serosurveys have shown an antibody prevalence of 10% in parts of Europe and America.[14]

The first haemorrhagic arenaviruses isolated were Junin virus, which causes Argentine haemorrhagic fever, and then Machupo virus, which causes Bolivian haemorrhagic fever.[15] Lassa virus, the most important arenavirus to humans, was recognized in Africa in 1969.[16] In total, seven arenaviruses cause significant disease in humans and at least 11 others have been isolated (Table 42.3, Figures 42.4 & 42.5). The New World arenaviruses are each associated primarily with a single rodent host, and are focal in their geographical distribution. Phylogenetics studies have shown that they are closely related to each other, and group separately from the Old World arenaviruses.[17]

Virology

Arenaviruses (genus *Arenavirus*, family Arenaviridae) are small single-stranded RNA viruses, usually 100–130 nm in diameter (but ranging from 50 to 500 nm), with a lipid membranous envelope that contains projections on the surface. Within the virion are cellular ribosomes which resemble grains of sand on electron microscopy (*arena* = Latin for sand) and two circular nucleocapsid segments. The genome comprises two linear segments of single-stranded RNA: a long (L) segment, which encodes the viral RNA polymerase and a zinc-binding protein, and a small (S) segment, encoding the nucleoprotein (NP) and two glycoproteins (GP-1 and GP-2). Most of the genome is negative sense, but a small portion is positive sense, making it an *ambisense* virus.

Table 42.3 Arenaviruses pathogenic for humans*

Virus	Disease	Natural host	Geographical distribution
OLD WORLD ARENAVIRUSES			
Lassa	Lassa fever	*Mastomys* species	West Africa
Lymphocytic choriomeningitis	Aseptic meningitis	*Mus domesticus, Mus muluscus*	Europe, Americas, ?elsewhere
NEW WORLD ARENAVIRUSES			
Junin	Argentine haemorrhagic fever	*Calomys musculinus*	Argentine pampas
Machupo	Bolivian haemorrhagic fever	*Calomys callosus*	Beni region of Bolivia
Guanarito	Venezuelan haemorrhagic fever	*Zygodontomys brevicauda*	Plains of Venezuela
Sabia	Not yet named	Unknown	São Paulo, Brazil
Whitewater Arroyo	Not yet named	*Neotoma albigula*	Southern USA

*Arenaviruses isolated that are not significant pathogens for humans include the Old World viruses, Mopeia, Mobala and Ippy, and the New World viruses, Tacaribe, Amapari, Parana, Tamiami, Pichinde, Latino, and Flexel virus, which has caused two symptomatic laboratory infections.

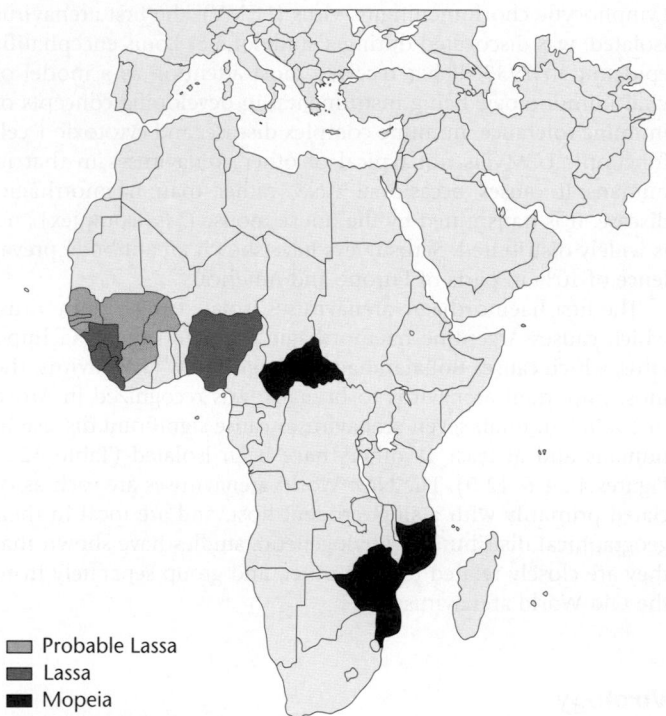

Figure 42.4 Geographical location of Lassa virus and the related Old World arenavirus, Mopeia.

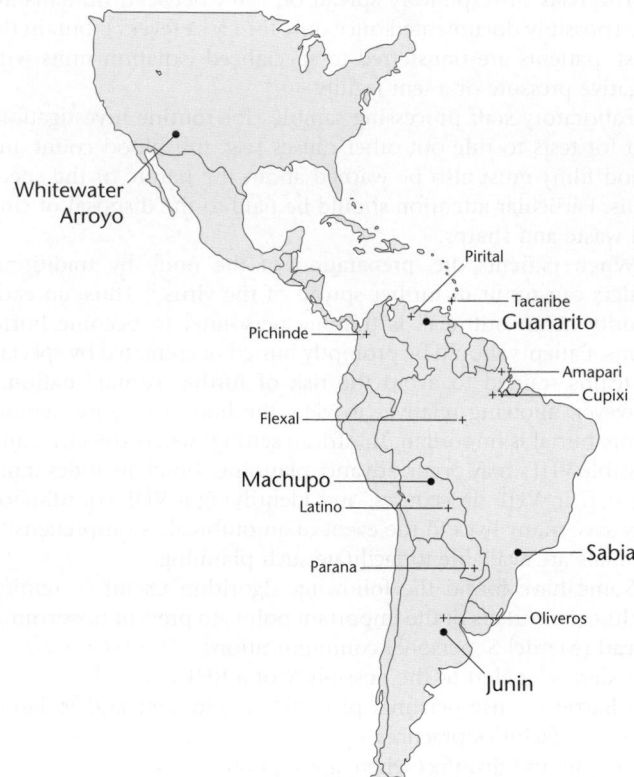

Figure 42.5 Geographical location of New World arenaviruses, including those that cause disease in humans (•), and those that are not significant human pathogens (+).[17]

Pathogenesis of Arenavirus infections

Following aerosol inhalation, arenaviruses are believed to initially replicate in the lung and hilar lymph nodes before disseminating.[17] The reticuloendothelial system, and particularly the macrophages, are major sites of replication throughout infection. Immunosuppression facilitates chronic infections in rodents, and probably contributes to the pathogenesis in humans. The exact mechanisms leading to haemorrhage and vascular leakage are incompletely understood, but pathological changes in the host tissues are relatively minor, and inflammatory cells are minimal

or absent.[18] Direct viral invasion of vascular endothelium has been demonstrated in vitro and, to a lesser extent, in vivo,[19] and may lead to damage of blood vessels.[20] Mild thrombocytopenia and disrupted coagulation may also contribute.[20,21]

Cytokines secreted from infected macrophages are thought to be responsible for many of the circulatory changes seen and are associated with a worse prognosis. Unlike other viral haemorrhagic fevers, activation of complement or coagulation pathways does not appear to be important in the pathogenesis. Immunological recovery from arenavirus infections is now thought to mostly be mediated by cellular immunity. Production of neutralizing antibodies is late and inefficient in Lassa fever, but may be more important with other arenaviruses.[18]

Pathology of Arenavirus infection

At autopsy of the liver there is a focal eosinophilic necrosis of hepatic cells with the presence of eosinophilic bodies resembling Councilman bodies (seen in yellow fever). The extent of necrosis is not thought to be sufficient to explain the observed hepatic insufficiency[22] but animal models show that histologically normal hepatocytes are also infected. The spleen shows lymphoid depletion with areas of eosinophilic necrosis; the lungs show pleural and peritoneal effusions and focal patches of pneumonitis, and the kidneys focal necrosis of renal tubules. There are interstitial haemorrhages in other organs. The CNS shows meningoencephalitis with oedema, congestion, neuronophagia and perivascular cuffing.

Lassa fever

In 1969, a nurse in a mission hospital in Lassa, north-eastern Nigeria, developed a febrile illness with haemorrhage, was transferred to a hospital in Jos, Nigeria, and subsequently died.[10] Two other nurses at the second hospital became ill, and a new arenavirus was isolated from one of them, who had been evacuated to New York, by arbovirologists at Yale University.[16,23] It has since been shown that Lassa virus is common in West Africa, and although Lassa fever can be fatal, and person-to-person transmission is a risk, neither the lethality nor the contagiousness is as pronounced as was initially suspected. However, during the 1970 outbreak, one of the physicians involved (Dr Jeanette Troup) died – thought to have become infected while performing an autopsy. Deaths of healthcare workers has sadly been a recurrent theme in the fight against this disease.[74]

Epidemiology

Lassa virus is enzootic in the ubiquitous West African multimammate mouse (*Mastomys natalensis*), in which it causes a chronic asymptomatic infection with constant excretion of virus in the urine, droppings and saliva. This peri-domestic rodent lives in or near human dwellings, breeds year round and is widely distributed across Africa (Figure 42.4). The virus is stable and infectious in aerosols, and is transmitted horizontally between rodents, as well as vertically to their offspring. Humans are thought to be infected by inhalation of the virus. In addition, excreta containing virus may be ingested with food, or enter through cuts. Secondary cases of Lassa fever may occur by nosocomial spread, mostly through needlestick injuries and other direct contact with infectious bodily fluids. Although air-borne transmission was postulated to be significant in one outbreak,[10] it is not generally thought to be a major risk.[25] Because of the high prevalence of Lassa virus, and its relatively long incubation period, it is the most common directly transmissible VHF of international travellers. Cases have occurred in the USA, the Netherlands, Japan, Israel Germany and the UK.[26]

Geographical distribution

Lassa fever is confined to West Africa, though related arenaviruses (not pathogenic for humans) occur in other parts of Africa (Figure 42.4). The virus has caused major outbreaks in Nigeria, Guinea, Liberia and Sierra Leone. In addition, antibody surveys and occasional confirmed cases implicate the Ivory Coast, Mali, Burkino Faso and Senegal. Serological surveys indicate that millions of West Africans have antibody. In most cases the infection causes a minor illness or inapparent infection.[27] However, recent estimates suggest that over 200 000 people are infected per year across West Africa, causing over 3000 deaths and leaving another 30 000 people with deafness.[28] Cases peak in the dry season, but outbreaks occur when human exposure to *Mastomys* increases. For example, major outbreaks were associated with the migration of nearly 100 000 people to the surface diamond mines in Sierra Leone.[27] More recently, armed conflicts in Sierra Leone and Liberia have created the circumstances for enhanced transmission to humans.

Clinical features

Patients typically present 7–14 days after exposure to the virus, though the incubation period may range from 5 days to 3 weeks. There is a gradual onset of non-specific fever with malaise and myalgia, followed by conjunctival injection, sore throat, cough, chest pain, and abdominal pain with vomiting and diarrhea.[29] The pharynx is often inflamed with characteristic white or yellow patches on the tonsils, and sometimes ulcers. The pain may be so severe that patients are unable even to swallow their saliva. In a case–control study performed over 2 years in Sierra Leone (1977–1979), a combination of fever, pharyngitis, retrosternal pain and proteinuria was found to be the best predictor of Lassa fever (predictive value together 0.81).[29] In patients with mild disease, these features resolve within 10 days. However, in a proportion, there is a rapid progression, with facial and laryngeal oedema (which causes stridor and respiratory distress), central cyanosis, a mild bleeding diathesis and shock. Once patients have overt bleeding, the chances of recovery are slim.[21] Pleural and pericardial effusions are common, and there may be bradycardia. There is often mild thrombocytopenia. Neurological complications include confusion, tremors, convulsions and coma, and carry a poor prognosis. Sensorineural deafness, which may be bilateral, occurs as a late complication in 30% of patients, and is thought to be immune-mediated.[30] About half of the patients show a near or complete recovery by 3–4 months after onset, but in others significant deafness persists and may become permanent. Infection with Lassa virus is also an important cause of admission among children.[31] Like other arenaviruses, Lassa crosses the placenta into the fetus, causing abortion and maternal death (particularly in the third trimester). The virus has also been isolated from milk, and may be a risk to breast-feeding infants. In one case–control study involving 1087 patients admitted with a febrile illness in Sierra Leone, 441 were confirmed as Lassa fever and the case fatality rate was 16.5%.[29]

Investigations reveal that the platelets are often reduced and have been shown in vitro to have dysfunction. The leukocyte count may be normal, low or even moderately elevated. The plasma aspartate amino transferase (AST) is usually elevated, and albuminuria is common.

Prognostic indicators

Approximately 15% of hospitalized patients die. A prospective clinical study found patients with vomiting, sore throat, tachpynoea, bleeding, diarrhoea or pyrexia (≥39°C) were more likely to die. The combination of fever, sore throat and vomiting carried five times the risk of death.[29] Other poor prognostic indicators include the peak viraemia, peak Lassa virus antigen level, and elevation in the plasma AST, above150 IU/mL.[32] Elevated viraemia and AST together carry a risk of death of nearly 80%.[28]

Differential diagnosis

The most important conditions in the differential include *falciparum* malaria, typhoid, other VHFs, meningococcaemia and septicaemia. (Table 42.2). In one study, concurrent infections occurred in 43% of patients.[20] In an endemic area of Sierre Leone, the combination of fever, exudative pharyngitis, retrosternal pain and proteinuria was able to distinguish Lassa fever from other febrile illness with a positive predictive value of 80%.[29]

Laboratory diagnosis

Lassa fever is confirmed by isolating virus from blood, throat swabs or urine in a BSL-4 laboratory, or by demonstrating antibody to the virus. Viraemia persists into the second week, and virus can also be isolated from urine and semen for 2–3 months (hence, precautions must be taken in convalescence). A new ELISA that detects Lassa virus antigen and RT-PCR allow more rapid diagnosis. The traditional technique for detecting antibodies, the indirect fluorescent antibody test, lacked specificity. It is being replaced by a new IgM ELISA, which has high sensitivity and specificity for acute infection, and an IgG ELISA that can be used to diagnose recent infection.[33]

Management

As with other VHFs, the issues in management are to treat the patient, identify others who may have been infected, and limit any further spread (see p. 765). Close monitoring for evidence of vascular leak, such as oedema, a rising haematocrit or proteinuria, is important, as these signs may indicate progression to severe disease.[20]

High-dose intravenous ribavirin administered during the first 6 days reduces the mortality significantly.[34] It has been used principally in patients with a poor prognosis (i.e. those with an AST >150 IU/mL). Oral ribavirin also has some effect, and has been used as prophylaxis for close contacts, or given at the first sign of fever. Immune convalescent serum with high antibody content has also been used, with apparent success. However, there are concerns about the transmission of infectious agents, including Lassa virus itself, during such treatment, as well as practical difficulties of collection and storage. The development of standardized monoclonal antibody directed against specific Lassa virus epitopes offers one possible future therapeutic approach. In the vast majority of cases, Lassa virus is not transmitted from a patient to secondary cases. Early in the disease and in mild cases, the risks of transmission are thought to be minimal. However, virus has been detected intermittently in the urine for up to 60 days after infection, and so the patients should be given appropriate advice to minimize the chance of infecting others. Nosocomial outbreaks and infection of multiple contacts is more likely for patients who are severely ill.

New treatments are in development. In human dendritic cells and macrophages, type I interferons or their inducers are involved in the control of Lassa virus replication.[35] In a hamster model of infection with the related arenavirus Pichinde, combined treatment with ribavirin and interferon alfacon-1 was effective.[36] The identification of α-dystroglycan as a receptor for Lassa virus,[37] as well as LCMV, may point the way towards new interventions, as may the discovery of a key structural protein, protein Z, as a crucial component in viral budding.[38]

Control

Although complete control of the rodent reservoir, *Mastomys*, is not possible, reducing their numbers (by trapping, poisoning and using cats) and their contact with humans may have some effect. An inactivated vaccine, despite producing high titres of antibody against all viral proteins, does not prevent virus replication and death in experimental animals – probably reflecting the importance of T cell immunity in controlling infection. Vaccination of macaque monkeys with vaccinia virus expressing Lassa virus structural nucleoproteins and glycoproteins protects against Lassa virus, and offers hope for the development of a human vaccine.[39]

Argentine haemorrhagic fever

Argentine haemorrhagic fever was first recognized in the 1950s, and the arenavirus responsible, Junin virus, was isolated in 1958.[17]

Epidemiology

The virus is enzootic in *Calomys* voles (particularly *Calomys musculinus*) which inhabit the maize fields of the pampas. Agricultural workers are exposed to the virus by contact with the rodent and its excretions, particularly at harvest times. At its peak, between 100 and 800 cases were diagnosed annually.

Clinical features

Patients present with a non-specific febrile illness. Within 3 to 4 days they may be prostrated and have signs of vascular damage, which include conjunctival injection, facial and neck flushing, mild hypotension, and petechiae in the axilla, soft palate and gingival margin.[15] Neurological signs are more common than in Lassa fever, and include irritability, lethargy, hyporeflexia, and tremor of the tongue and hands. In severe cases there is bleeding of the mucous membranes, haemorrhage, shock, anuria, coma and convulsions. Untreated, approximately 15–30% of hospitalized patients die.

Diagnosis

The diagnosis is confirmed in the first few days of illness by isolation of Junin virus from blood (in a BSL-4 laboratory), or antigen ELISA. Subsequently, IgM and then IgG antibodies are detected by ELISA.

Treatment

Immune treatment with convalescent plasma from patients who have recovered reduced the mortality of Argentine haemorrhagic fever from 15–30% to 1–2%. However, it is associated with a late neurological syndrome in 10% of patients. Preliminary studies with ribavirin have also been promising.[17] A range of other potential therapeutic agents have been identified by high-throughput screening, and are being assessed in animal models.[40] The recent identification of transferrin receptor 1 as a cellular receptor for Junin, and related New World Arenaviruses, may point the way towards new therapies.[41]

Prevention and control

Control of the rural rodent *Calomys* is not practical. A live attenuated Junin vaccine is effective[40] and has been used widely among adult males and, more recently, women and children. Its use in pregnant women should be avoided because of the risk to the fetus.[17]

Bolivian haemorrhagic fever

Bolivian haemorrhagic fever is caused by the arenavirus Machupo virus, which appears to be confined to the Beni, an isolated agricultural region in north east Bolivia. The clinical features are similar to those of Argentine haemorrhagic fever. The natural host is the rodent *Calomys callosus*, which lives in the grasslands and invades houses in villages and small towns. Urban cases have been reduced with rodent trapping, but rural cases continue. One of these was recently followed by six fatal secondary cases in family members.[17]

Venezuelan haemorrhagic fever

Guanarito virus was discovered in 1990 during investigations of VHF cases that followed the clearing of forests in the municipality of Guanarito on the plains of Venezuela (Figure 42.5). The cane mouse *Zygodonomys brevicauda* is thought to be the main natural host. However, the risk of infection is low even in those with high occupational exposure to appropriate hosts.[42] Clinically, Venezuelan haemorrhagic fever is similar to Argentine haemorrhagic fever, with thrombocytopenia, bleeding and, in some cases, neurological involvement.[43]

Sabia virus infection

This arenavirus was isolated from a patient with a fatal viral haemorrhagic fever, who was from Sabia, outside São Paulo, Brazil, in 1990. There was extensive liver necrosis, and yellow fever was initially suspected. Later, a laboratory worker and a virologist became infected. The latter was successfully treated with ribavirin.[44] The natural host of Sabia virus, presumed to be a rodent localized to this part of Brazil, has yet to be identified.

Whitewater Arroyo virus

This virus is a newly recognized North American arenavirus. It was first isolated from the white-throated woodrats (*Neotoma albigula*) collected from north-western New Mexico, but is widely distributed throughout the south-western United States.[45] To date, two human cases of VHF had evidence of acute Whitewater Arroyo virus infection.

FILOVIRUSES

In 1967, an outbreak of haemorrhagic fever occurred among employees of a viral laboratory in Marburg, and spread to medical personnel and their relatives. Similar events occurred in Frankfurt, and in Belgrade, former Yugoslavia, at around the same time. The outbreak was traced to African green (Vervet) monkeys (*Cercopithicus aethiops*) imported from Uganda. A long filamentous virus was isolated from both humans and monkeys, and named Marburg virus (see Figure 42.6).[46] Nine years later, two further epidemics of haemorrhagic fever occurred simultaneously in Africa (Table 42.4). One originated in villages near the Ebola river in the rainforests of the Democratic Republic of Congo (then known as Zaire), the other 600 km away in southern Sudan (see Figure 42.7). Secondary nosocomial spread was an important feature of both outbreaks. A virus, morphologically identical to but antigenically distinct from Marburg, was isolated from both sites and named Ebola.[47] Subsequently, the two distinct biotypes were designated Ebola Zaire and Ebola Sudan, the former appearing to have a higher mortality rate. Two further subtypes have been isolated since then, including one originating in the Philippines, which caused an outbreak in Reston outside Washington DC (see below) (Table 42.4). The natural host and ecology of the viruses have remained elusive despite extensive investigation. However, procedures for controlling outbreaks have been devised, and shown to be effective.[48]

The search for the filovirus reservoir

The natural reservoir of Ebola and Marburg viruses remains unknown. Primary infection in humans has always occurred in rural areas (sometimes bat-infested), or following contact with non-human primates. However, primates are unlikely to be the natural hosts, given that the virus causes disease in them, and they do not have latent infections. Studies in South Africa have shown that, following inoculation, bats have a prolonged asymptomatic viraemia, which one would expect for a natural host.[49] Similar experiments have failed to show filovirus replication in insects, reptiles or plants. It is presumed that the natural reservoir is a small mammal that has largely asymptomatic infection, and does not live in close association with humans.[50] Attempts to find evidence of natural infection have so far proved negative in more than 3000 vertebrates (including 500 bats) and 30 000 arthropods.[51] However, Ebola virus RNA has been detected in a small number of rodents and shrews from the Central African Republic, suggesting they have been exposed to the virus, even if they are not the natural reservoir.[52]

Virology

Filoviruses (*filo* = thread in Latin) appear as long, filamentous, U-, branch- or S-shaped rods, or more compact convoluted forms

Table 42.4 Outbreaks and cases of filovirus disease

Virus and subtype	Year	Location	No. of cases	Mortality rate (%)	Source and spread
MARBURG VIRUS					
Marburg	1967	Germany (Marburg and Hamburg), Yugoslavia (Belgrade)	32	23	First ever cases, from Vervet monkeys imported from Uganda
Marburg	1975	South Africa (Johannesburg)	3	33	Index case infected in Zimbabwe, travelled to South Africa; secondary cases in companion and nurse
Marburg	1980	Western Kenya (Nzoia) then Nairobi	2	50	Index case in Mount Elgin region; secondary case was in infected doctor who survived
Marburg	1987	Western Kenya (Kisumu)	1	100	Visited bat-infested cave in Mount Elgon region
Marburg	1999	DRC (Yambuku)	86	57	Community outbreak
EBOLA VIRUS					
Ebola Zaire	1976	DRC (Yambuku)	318	88	Unknown origin, nosocomial spread
Ebola Sudan	1976	Southern Sudan (Maridi)	284	53	Origin in a bat-infested cotton factory; nosocomial spread
Ebola Zaire	1977	Zaire (Tandala)	1	100	Sporadic case
Ebola Sudan	1979	Southern Sudan (Nzara and Yambio)	34	65	Site close to 1976 outbreak
Ebola Reston	1989	USA (Reston, Virginia)	4	0	Disease in monkeys imported from Philippines; humans asymptomatic
Ebola Reston	1990	USA (Reston, Virginia, and Texas)	0	0	Monkeys imported from Philippines only
Ebola Reston	1992	Italy (Sienna)	0	0	Monkeys imported from Philippines
Ebola Zaire	1994	Gabon (Minkouka)	44	63	Origin unknown; outbreak identified retrospectively in 1995
Ebola Côte d'Ivoire	1994	Ivory Coast (Tai Forest)	1	0	Conducted autopsy on dead chimpanzee, evacuated to Switzerland
Ebola Côte d'Ivoire	1994	Liberia	1	0	Serological diagnosis only
Ebola Zaire	1995	DRC (Kikwit)	315	77	Source unknown; secondary nosocomial and family cases
Ebola Zaire	1996	Gabon (Mayibout)	31	68	Contact with dead monkeys; secondary family cases
Ebola Zaire	1996	Gabon (Booué)	60	75	Index case a hunter; secondary nosocomial cases included doctor transferred to South Africa, and nurse infected there
Ebola Reston	1996	USA (Alice, Texas)	0	0	Monkeys imported from Philippines
Ebola Sudan	2000	Uganda (Gulu)	425	53	Community and nosocomial cases

DRC, Democratic Republic of Congo (formerly Zaire).

(Figure 42.6). They are composed of a lipid bilayer envelope with glycoprotein spikes, surrounding a helically wound nucleocapsid.[53] The virions are 80 nm in diameter, and may be as long as 14 000 nm. Within the nucleocapsid is a single strand of negative-sense RNA encoding seven structural proteins – NP, VP35, VP40, GP, VP30, VP24 and L. The viral envelope is composed of host-derived plasma membrane studded with a virally encoded type 1 glycoprotein (GP), which mediates viral entry into host cells. VP24 protein is also likely to be part of the envelope. The viral polymerase complex is composed of the large (L) protein and a phosphoprotein (VP35). Assembly of the replicated virus within the cell cytosol is thought to be led by VP40.[54]

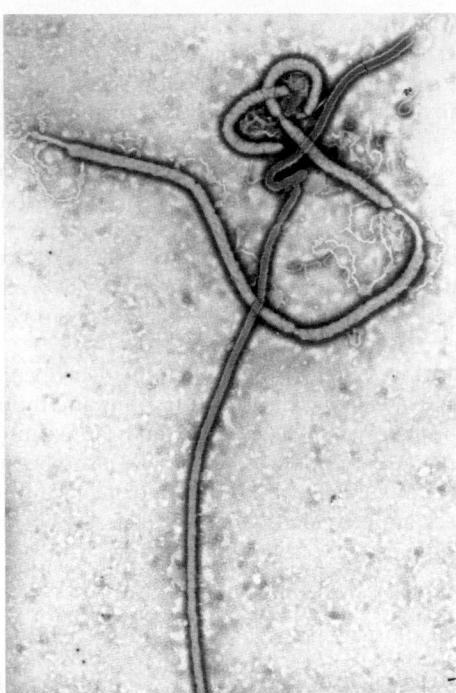

Figure 42.6 Electron micrograph of Ebola virus, showing the long filamentous forms. (Courtesy of Centers for Disease Control and Prevention.)

Pathogenesis and pathology of filovirus infections

The pathogenesis of filovirus disease appears to be a combination of direct viral cytopathology, cytokine-mediated vascular leakage, and an impairment of the host immune response (including an inflammatory response) that inhibits clearance of the virus.

Macrophages and monocytes are thought to be infected early, impairing the immune response, and disseminating the virus around the body. Viral particles are found in endothelial cells, macrophages and the parenchymal cells of almost all organs in the body.[55] The increased vascular permeability is thought to be a result of direct infection with virus, and the effects of elevated levels of cytokines. Tumour necrosis factor (TNF)-α, interleukin (IL)-2, IL-10, interferon (IFN)β and IFNγ are all elevated in filovirus infections.[56] Virus-like particles containing the Ebola virus transmembrane glycoprotein are potent activators of endothelial cells.[57] In vitro studies suggest the GP protein on the virus's outer coat may have a major role by inhibiting T cell proliferation and causing loss of endothelial cell adhesion.[58] In most fatal cases, no antibodies are detected. In prolonged cases and survivors, a delayed humoral response occurs, but a vigorous cell-mediated immune response is thought to be the major mechanism of viral clearance.[59]

More recent studies of cytokine and chemokine responses in fatal cases, survivors and asymptomatic infections (close contacts of cases who seroconverted) have helped elucidate the critical role of the inflammatory response. A transient early release of pro-inflammatory cytokines (IL-1β, IL-6, TNF-α, macrophage inflammatory protein [MIP]-1α and MIP-1β) is seen in survivors,[60] which is similar to that seen in asymptomatic infection,[61] but is not seen in fatal cases.[60] CD4 and CD8 T cells are important in virus clearance in a mouse model of Ebola infection.[62] When human CD4 and CD8 cells are infected in vitro, massive virus-mediated apoptotic cell death occurs,[63] and clinical studies have shown reduced T cells, including activated CD8 T cells, in fatal cases, compared with survivors.[64]

Pathologically there is extensive necrosis in the parenchymal cells of many organs, particularly the liver, spleen and kidneys, without much inflammatory infiltrate. Soluble glycoprotein from the virus has been shown to inhibit the inflammatory response.[57] In the liver, intracytoplasmic inclusion bodies (aggregates of viral nucleocapsid material) are seen in intact hepatocytes.

Transmission to humans

Secondary human cases of filovirus infection occur among those who come into contact with patients, their blood or other secretions. In the early outbreaks, the reuse of unsterilized needles and lack of barrier nursing led to rapid nosocomial spread. Family members who have contact with body fluids are also at risk. Occasionally, those who have just touched the skin have become infected (e.g. mourners at a burial services).[65] This may be explained by histological studies showing virus in the skin and in sweat glands. The exact route of entry is unknown for all secondary cases, but based on animal models is thought to be via cuts in the skin and contact with the conjunctivae. There is no firm evidence for aerosol spread in humans, though it has been shown in animals, and there is concern over large droplets and fomites.[66] Marburg virus has been isolated from semen, and sexual transmission has been documented. Serological surveys using ELISAs have revealed an antibody prevalence of around 10% among gold panners in Gabon and rural villagers in the Democratic Republic of Congo.

Ebola haemorrhagic fever

Epidemiology and geographical distribution

The first outbreaks of Ebola haemorrhagic fever occurred in 1976 simultaneously in northern Democratic Republic of Congo (then Zaire) and southern Sudan[47] (Figure 42.7). No clear index case was identified in the Congo outbreak, but in the Sudan outbreak the first patients came from a bat-infested cotton-weaving factory. In both outbreaks, subsequent spread to relatives, hospital staff and other patients occurred. In 1989, another Ebola subtype (Ebola Reston) was isolated from sick cynomoglus monkeys that had been imported to the USA from the Philippines, and were being kept at a holding facility in Reston, Virginia. There were no human cases, but serological evidence showed humans had had asymptomatic infection with Ebola Reston. On subsequent occasions, the same virus has been isolated from sick monkeys imported to the USA and Italy, which always originated from the same export facility in the Philippines. How the virus arrived at this facility is uncertain. In 1994, an ethnologist became sick after

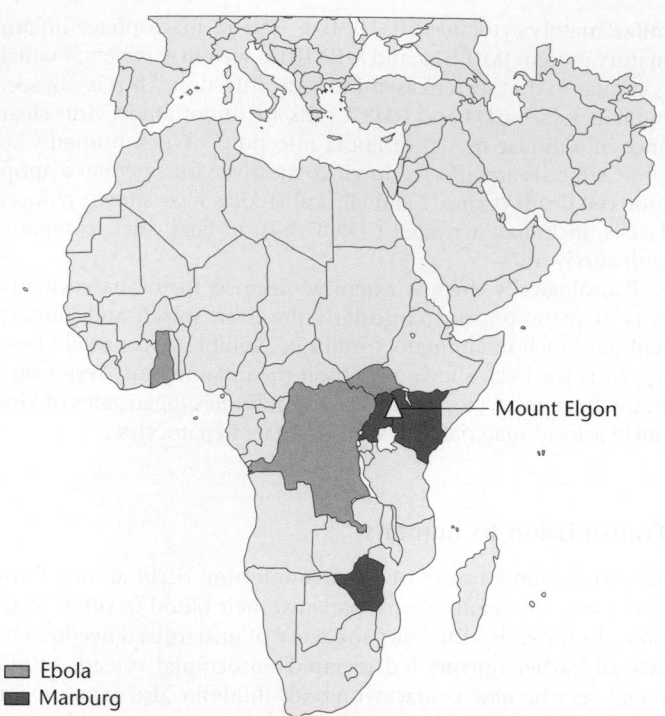

— Mount Elgon

▢ Ebola
■ Marburg

Figure 42.7 Location of outbreaks or isolated cases of Ebola and Marburg haemorrhagic fevers in Africa (Ebola subtype Reston has been isolated in monkeys from the Philippines).

performing a necropsy on a chimpanzee in the Ivory Coast. She was evacuated to Switzerland and the fourth Ebola species, Ebola Cote d'Ivoire, was isolated. Ebola Zaire caused a large outbreak around Kikwit, Democratic Republic of Congo, in 1995, with 325 cases (81% fatal), and in 2000–2001 there were 425 cases (53% fatal) of Ebola Sudan in Uganda. In December 2001, a new outbreak of Ebola haemorrhagic fever was confirmed in Gabon (65 cases, 50 fatal), with 37 cases in the neighbouring Republic of Congo (19 fatal). In 2002 there were a further 13 cases in the Republic of Congo, with further larger outbreaks in 2003 (one of 143 cases with 128 deaths, one 35 cases with 29 deaths). The last Ebola outbreak in the Republic of Congo was 2005, when there were 12 cases. After 20 years of no Ebola cases in Sudan, an outbreak occurred in 2004, when there were 17 cases of Ebola Sudan subtype. An outbreak occurred in the Democratic Republic of Congo and there is an outbreak ongoing in Uganda as this volume goes to press (December 2008).

Clinical features

After an incubation period of 4 to 10 days, patients present with an abrupt onset of fever, severe headache, myalgia, abdominal pain, diarrhoea and sore throat, with herpetic lesions on the mouth and pharynx.[67] Asthenia (lack of strength and energy) is also very common. There is severe conjunctival injection and gingival haemorrhages. A maculopapular rash may be evident

(especially on white skin). This is followed by bleeding with petechiae, echymosis, oozing from venepuncture sites, mucosal haemorrhage, haematemesis and bloody diarrhoea. In one outbreak, approximately 40% of patients had bleeding manifestations.[68] Neurological manifestations (hemiplegia, psychosis, coma, convulsions) are common. Later complications include shock, severe metabolic changes, and a diffuse coagulopathy. Death occurs most commonly around day 10. Tachypnoea was a better predictor of fatal outcome than was haemorrhage.[68] Mortality rates are higher for Ebola Zaire (60–90%) than Ebola Sudan (50–60%), and higher among patients who were infected by injection.[48,67]

Laboratory investigations reveal an initial leucopenia and lymphopenia, with a later increase in neutrophils and the appearance of large abnormal lymphocytes with dark cytoplasm (virocytes). There is a marked thrombocytopenia, and experiments in nonhuman primates have shown abnormal platelet function. Serum transaminases are elevated, whereas alakaline phosphatase and bilirubin are normal or only mildly elevated.

Differential diagnosis

The differential diagnosis for Ebola infection is broad. In patients with appropriate risk factors (travel to endemic areas, or potential contact with infected people or animals), the presence of fever, abdominal pain and bloody diarrhoea should arouse suspicion in the physician.

Laboratory diagnosis

Ebola infection is diagnosed early in the disease by virus isolation in Vero cells, RT-PCR or antigen-capture ELISAs. Higher viral loads are detected by RT-PCR in the blood of fatal cases than in that of survivors;[69] virus can also be detected in the saliva.[70] In those who survive long enough to make them, IgM and then IgG antibodies can be detected by ELISAs.[71]

Treatment

Patients are managed as for other VHFs (see p. 765), the emphasis being on providing compassionate care, whilst minimizing the risk to healthcare workers and other patients.

There is no established antiviral treatment. IFNα, although used in one patient, has little effect in vitro or in animal models. Convalescent serum has been used, as has whole blood transfused from convalescent patients, with some apparent improvement.[72] However, with no control patients, interpretation of these findings is difficult. Moreover, a neutralizing human monoclonal antibody, KZ52, which protects guinea pigs, was shown to have no effect on viral replication or outcome in rhesus macaque monkeys, even at very high doses.[73] Alternative approaches include modulating the host response to the infection, or using vaccines for postexposure treatment, similar to the approach used for rabies. rNAPc2 is a recombinant nematode anticoagulant protein that inhibits tissue factor-initiated blood coagulation, and provided some protection in the macaque model.[74] A recombinant vesicular stomatitis virus-based vaccine expressing Ebola virus glycoprotein protected small animals and macaques if given soon after exposure to the virus.[75] It might offer protection to those exposed in laboratory accidents, or in controlling secondary transmission during outbreaks.

Prevention and control

Since the source of Ebola virus and the means by which humans become infected are not known, primary prevention is not possible, although contact with sick or dead primates should be avoided. Control measures are therefore focused on limiting the spread from primary to secondary cases. This comprises containment of suspected cases, and contact tracing to identify further possible cases (see p. 769). In recent outbreaks there has been less nosocomial spread, probably because of better implementation of these practices. For example, in Zaire in 1995 nearly 30% of cases occurred in medical personnel, compared with less than 7% in Uganda in 2000.[48,67]

There is no vaccine for Ebola. However, the recombinant vesicular stomatitis virus-based vaccine, described above, is protective in a mouse model, when given orally as well as systemically.[76] Virus-like particle vaccines are also showing promise, providing protection in macaques,[77] and an adenovirus-based vaccine is protective in mice.[78]

Marburg haemorrhagic fever

Epidemiology

Marburg virus was the first filovirus identified, when, in 1967, it caused an outbreak of haemorrhagic fever in a polio vaccine laboratory in Marburg, Germany. It affected laboratory staff who handled blood tissue or cell cultures from African green monkeys. Secondary cases occurred in Marburg and Frankfurt and in Belgrade (former Yugoslavia).[46] There were 31 cases with seven deaths. The monkeys had been imported from the Kyoga region of Uganda, in a shipment that included sick monkeys. Excess deaths had also been seen among monkey colonies near Lake Kyoga to the east of Mount Elgon in Kenya (Figure 42.7). A few sporadic cases occurred in 1975 and 1987 (Table 42.4), and then in 1999 there was a large community outbreak in the Democratic Republic of Congo. This started among gold-mine workers in Durba and affected around 100 people, with 60% mortality.[79] In addition, up to four cases of suspected Marburg fever were reported from the Democratic Republic of Congo during March 2002. There was a large Marburg outbreak in Angola in 2005, with 374 cases, including 329 deaths. More recently, Marburg reappeared in Uganda, killing one.

Clinical features

The clinical features are similar to those of Ebola, but the mortality is around 25–30%. Uveitis complicated one case[80] and virus was isolated from the anterior chamber of the eye 80 days after onset. In one laboratory infection, the illness was mild and recovery complete after a long convalescence.

Diagnosis

Like Ebola virus, Marburg virus is diagnosed during the acute stage by virus isolation, PCR or antigen detection. Virus has been isolated from semen up to 3 months after the initial infection. In survivors, IgM and then IgG antibodies are subsequently elevated.

Control

Secondary control of Marburg infection is the same as that of Ebola: namely, barrier nursing to prevent, and tracing and monitoring of contacts.

BUNYAVIRIDAE

The family Buyaviridae is made up of five genera:
- the *Hantavirus* genus includes Hantaan virus, the cause of haemorrhagic fever with renal syndrome (HFRS)
- the *Nairovirus* genus includes Crimean–Congo haemorrhagic fever virus
- the *Phlebovirus* genus includes Rift Valley fever virus
- the *Bunyavirus* genus contains viruses that cause fever with rash (e.g. Oropouche) or CNS disease (e.g. La Crosse encephalitis) but not VHF, and so is not discussed further in this chapter
- the *Tospovirus* genus includes plant viruses but has no human pathogens.

Virological properties

All members of the family Bunyaviridae are spherical virions, 90–100 nm in diameter, with a lipid envelope that contains glycoprotein peplomers and encloses three circular nucleocapsids. The genome consists of three linear segments of single-stranded RNA, designated L (large), M (medium) and S (small), which code for a transcriptase (L protein), a nucleocapsid protein (N), and two glycoproteins (G1 and G2). Most have negative-sense genomes, but the S segment of Phleboviruses is ambisense.

Haemorrhagic fever with renal syndrome (HFRS)

During the Korean war of 1950–1952, more than 3000 United Nations troops developed a disease characterized by fever, haemorrhagic manifestations, acute renal failure and shock, with up to 10% mortality,[81] which was originally named Korean or epidemic haemorrhagic fever. In 1978, the virus which caused it was isolated from the field mouse (*Apodemus agrarius*),[82] and named Hantaan virus after the river where the original cases occurred. Similar diseases with different names had been recognized earlier in China, and the former Soviet Union. Later, three other hantaviruses were isolated and shown to be associated with similar clinical syndromes elsewhere: Dobrava virus causes a severe haemorrhagic fever syndrome in the Balkans, Seoul virus causes a milder syndrome in the Far East, and Puumula virus causes

Table 42.5 Summary of major hantaviruses causing disease in humans

Virus	Disease	Natural host	Geographical distribution
CAUSING HFRS			
Hantaan	HFRS (previously known as Korean or epidemic haemorrhagic fever)	*Apodemus agrarius*	Asia, Far East, Russia
Dobrava	Severe HFRS	*Apodemus flavicollis*	Balkans, Europe
Seoul	Mild HFRS	*Rattus norvegicus, R. rattus*	Worldwide
Puumala	HFRS with predominant renal disease: 'nephropathia epidemica'	*Clethrionomys glareolus*	Beni region of Bolivia
CAUSING HPS			
Sin Nombre	HPS	*Peromyscus maniculatus*	North America
Andes	HPS	*Oligoryzomys longicaudatus*	Argentina and Chile

HFRS, haemorrhagic fever with renal syndrome.
HPS, hantavirus pulmonary syndrome. At least 16 other hantaviruses, each associated with its own host in the Sigmodontinae rodent subfamily, have been isolated in the Americas; many of these viruses cause HPS.

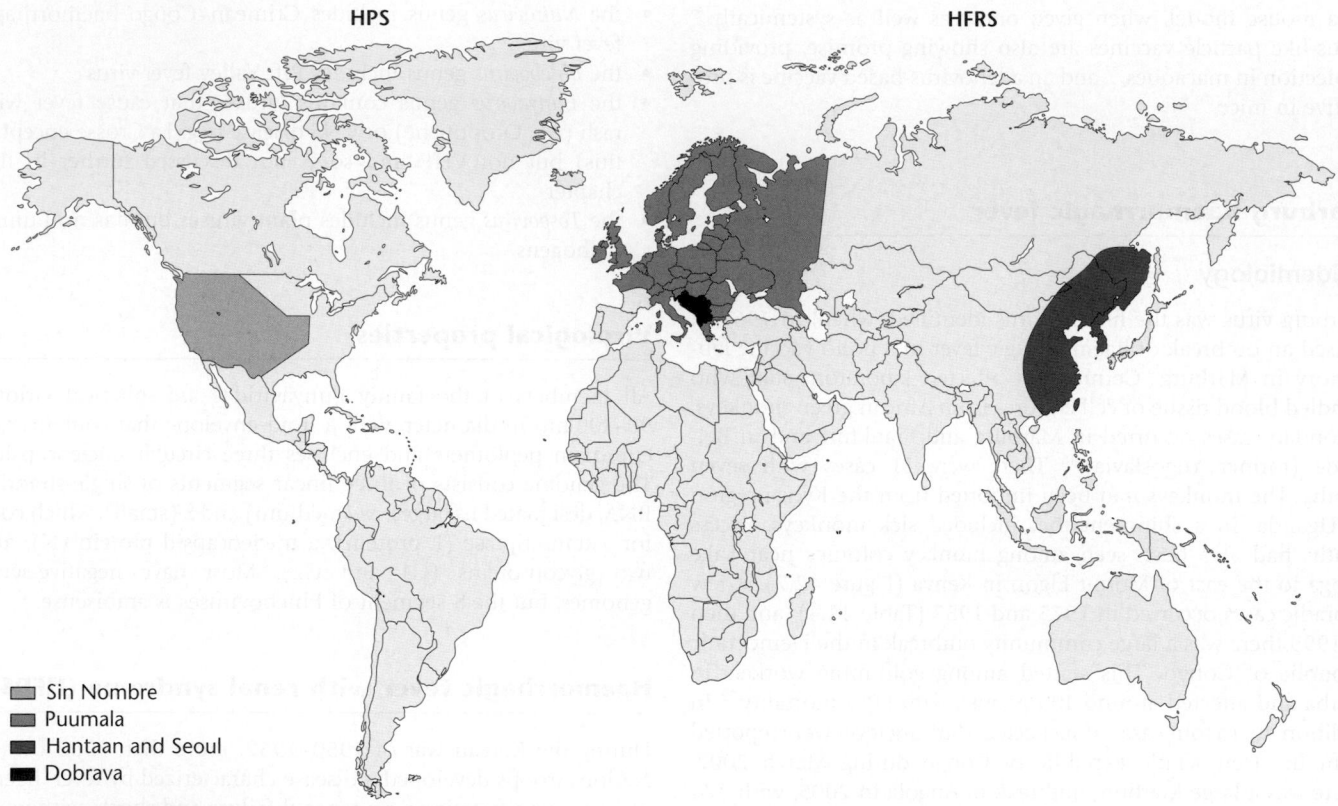

Figure 42.8 Location of major hantaviruses causing haemorrhagic fever with renal syndrome (HFRS) and hantavirus pulmonary syndrome (HPS).

'nephropathia epidemica' in Scandinavia (Table 42.5, Figure 42.8). Subsequently, these diseases have all been grouped together as haemorrhagic fever with renal syndrome (HFRS). In 1993, a new syndrome of fever, non-cardiogenic pulmonary oedema and shock was described in North America (hantavirus pulmonary syndrome – HPS). It is caused by Sin Nombre virus, transmitted by the common deer mouse (*Peromyscus maniculatus*). Related

hantaviruses transmitted by different rodents cause HPS through much of North and South America.

Epidemiology and geographical distribution

Following infection, rodents excrete hantaviruses in urine, faeces and saliva for several months. Transmission among rodents is thought to occur primarily by biting and scratching. Humans become infected following inhalation of infectious virus in rodent excretions.[83] There is no evidence of human-to-human transmission. Most cases of hantavirus disease are sporadic, but epidemics do occur (see below). Each hantavirus is associated with a unique rodent host, and its epidemiology and geographical distribution reflect that natural reservoir.

Hantaan virus causes epidemic HFRS in Korea, eastern China and far-eastern Russia. Because it is transmitted by a field mouse (*Apodemus agrarius*), agricultural workers are at greatest risk of infection. Most cases of HFRS occur in adult males, and peak in the autumn, possibly because virus-infected mice are abundant at this time, and exposure is increased during the harvest. Approximately 100 000 cases are reported annually from China, and up to 1000 in Korea.

Dobrava virus is transmitted by the rural *Apodemus flavicollis* and causes a similar severe HFRS in the Balkans and possibly other parts of Europe. Approximately 200 cases are seen annually. Epidemics have been seen in times of conflict, when rodent populations are high, and the number of troops and civilians living outside is increased. During 2005, more than 1000 cases were seen in Belgium, France, Germany, the Netherlands and Luxembourg.[84]

Seoul virus is transmitted by the domestic rat (*Rattus norvegicus* and *R. rattus*) and causes mild HFRS in urban areas. Although this rodent and the virus are found worldwide, for reasons that are unclear, Seoul virus-related HFRS is rare outside of China, Korea and laboratory institutions that house rats. Cases of HFRS due to Seoul virus peak in the spring and early summer, and are frequently related to cleaning barns or basements, or other activities that result in human exposure to rodent excreta.

Puumula virus causes *nephropathia epidemica* which is a milder disease, and is transmitted by the bank vole (*Calomys callosus*) across Scandinavia and northern Europe, including the UK.

Pathogenesis and pathology

Hantaviruses are thought to infect humans primarily via the respiratory mucosa, entry into cells being mediated by cell surface integrins. Viral DNA is detectable in patients' blood early in the disease. Viral antigens are subsequently found in endothelial cells throughout the body, particularly in the kidney in HFRS[85] and the lung in HPS. However, there are no viral cytopathic effects associated with these infected cells, and, unlike most VHFs, the damage is thought to be mediated by the host immune response. In HFRS, renal biopsies show acute tubulointerstitial nephritis, with a moderate inflammatory infiltrate, increased expression of cytokines (TNF-α, TGF-β, platelet-derived growth factor), upregulation of endothelial adhesion molecules (CD54, CD106, VCAM, CD31), and deposition of immune complexes. Similar changes are seen in the lung in HPS. As with other VHFs, the bleeding manifestations are thought to be due to a combination of increased vascular permeability (caused by a combination of viral infection, complement activation, the cytokine cascade, and immune complex deposition) and a reduced number of functionally impaired platelets. There is some evidence that certain HLA haplotypes (HLA-B8 DRB1*301) are associated with more severe disease.

Clinical features

Classically, patients with infected with Hantaan or Dobrava virus go through five phases. After an incubation period that is relatively long for VHFs (usually 2–3 weeks, but ranging from 2 days to 2 months), patients present with an acute flu-like illness. There is flushing of the face and neck, with conjunctival and pharyngeal injection, which are thought to reflect capillary dilatation. Lower back pain caused by retroperitoneal oedema is also common. The febrile phase is followed by a hypotensive phase, with mild shock lasting 1–2 days and haemorrhagic manifestations. These range from a mild petechial rash to major gastrointestinal bleeding, and are associated with marked thrombocytopenia and, in some patients, a low-grade DIC. An oliguric phase associated with hypertension and biochemical renal failure follows, contributing to about half the deaths if untreated.[81] At this stage there may also be pulmonary oedema and CNS signs. Patients who survive then have a diuretic phase that may last several months, followed by a convalescent phase. The mortality of patients with these classical features is 5–15%, though many patients with milder disease are probably not recognized. Laboratory findings include leukocytosis, thrombocytopenia, a rising haematocrit, deranged clotting and rising proteinuria.

Patients infected with Seoul virus tend to have milder HFRS, typically with just febrile and mild haemorrhagic manifestations. Hepatomegaly and hepatic impairment with mildly elevated serum transaminase levels is common. Puumula infection results in the mildest form of HFRS, with fever, mild hypotension, and petechiae rather than haemorrhage. Around the sixth day there is oliguria or renal failure, and this is often the cause of hospital admission (hence the pseudonym nephropathica epidemica). About 10% of patients require renal dialysis, and about 20% of patients have mild transient neurological features (e.g. confusion, dizziness).

Differential diagnosis

In endemic parts of Asia and northern Europe, any febrile patient with thrombocytopenia and renal impairment should be questioned about possible rodent exposure, and investigated for hantavirus infection. The differential includes leptospirosis, typhus, pyelonephritis, post-streptococcal glomerulonephritis, an acute abdomen and other haemorrhagic fevers.

Diagnosis

Since antibodies are almost always in evidence at presentation, hantavirus infections are diagnosed serologically. The indirect fluorescent antibody test has been replaced by IgM capture ELISAs which use infected cell preparations or recombinant nucleocapsid proteins as antigen. Attempts to isolate the virus are usually negative (presumably because of the strong host immune response), but RT-PCR has been used.

Treatment

In a double-blind placebo-controlled trial, ribavirin was shown to reduce the mortality and morbidity of HFRS in China.[86] Supportive treatment is similar to that for other VHFs (see p. 768),

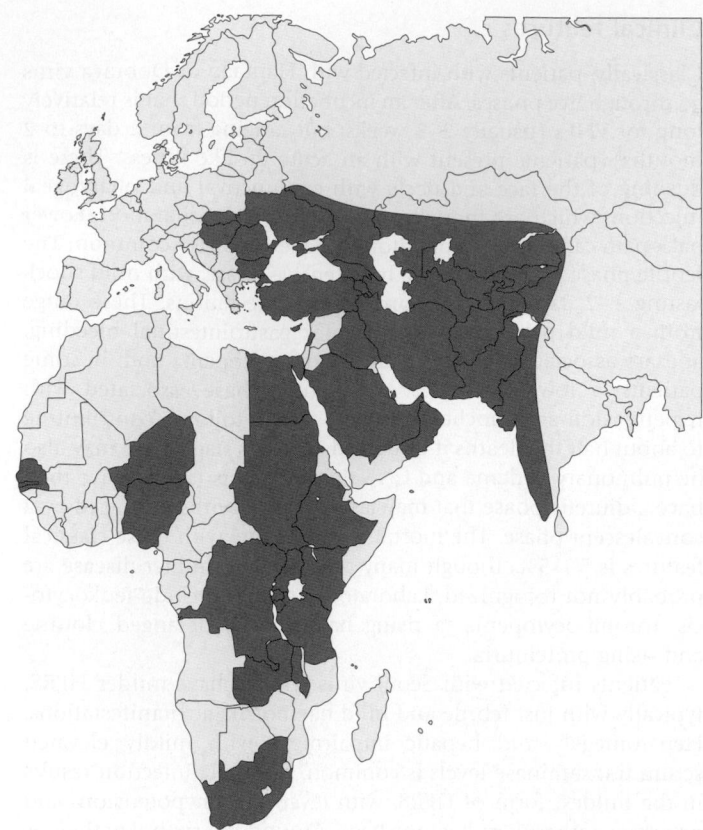

Figure 42.9 Distribution of Crimean–Congo haemorrhagic fever.

paying particular attention to fluid balance and the risk of renal failure. In the febrile phase, overhydration should be avoided; during the hypotensive phase, salt-poor plasma expanders and ionotropes should be used; during the oliguric phase, electrolyte balance and acid–base status should be carefully monitored. Severe hyperkalaemia, or fluid overload causing pulmonary oedema, should be treated with haemodialysis or peritoneal dialysis. Data from animal models suggest that a post-exposure prophylaxis regimen consisting of passive immunoprophyaxis and active vaccination might be effective for HPS, as has been shown for other viral diseases such as rabies, hepatitis A and B, and varicella.[87]

Prevention and control

Measures to minimize human exposure to rodent excreta include trapping rodents, rodent-proofing homes, correctly storing food, airing closed cabins, and removing rodent droppings. Several formalin-inactivated vaccines for Hantaan and Seoul viruses are used in Asia, and recombinant DNA vaccines are in development.[88]

Crimean–Congo haemorrhagic fever (CCHF)

CCHF is an arboviral infection, transmitted by ticks, which causes a severe viral haemorrhagic fever with high mortality and the potential for secondary nosocomial spread. Crimean haemorrhagic fever was first described in people bitten by ticks while harvesting crops in the Crimean peninsula in 1944, though descriptions of a compatible disease have existed since antiquity.[89] After the virus was isolated in 1967, it was shown to be identical to Congo virus, which had been isolated from a febrile child in 1956 in the Belgian Congo (now the Democratic Republic of Congo),[90] and the combined name has been used since. CCHF virus is a member of the *Nairovirus* genus (family Bunyaviridae), which contains at least 32 principally tick-borne viruses, though a few isolates have been made from culicoides flies and mosquitoes. The genus is named after the prototype, Nairobi sheep disease virus, which was isolated from sheep in 1910. This virus, along with Dugbe virus, causes occasional mild febrile disease in humans.

Epidemiology and geographical distribution

CCHF virus is maintained in nature in ixodid ticks, which are field-dwelling three-host ticks. Virus is transmitted vertically to the tick's offspring (via transovarial and trans-stadial transmission), venereally from males to females for some species, and horizontally to vertebrate hosts, when the ticks take a blood meal. Ticks of the genus *Hyalomma* appear to be the most important vectors for transmitting CCHF virus to vertebrates. The wide geographical distribution of CCHF in Eastern Europe, Asia and Africa coincides with the distribution of *Hyolamma* ticks (Figure 42.9). Small mammals such as hares are the preferred host for immature ticks, while adults prefer large herbivorous species, including sheep, goats, cattle and ostriches. Infection is usually inapparent in these animals.

Humans become infected with CCHF virus after being bitten by, or crushing, infected ticks, or by contact with blood from infected livestock or patients.[91] Thus, taking an occupational history is important. Direct transmission is thought to occur through contact of viraemic blood or other fluids with broken skin. Most nosocomial spread occurs before barrier nursing has been instituted. Needlestick injuries have been particularly implicated. Most patients are farmers, veterinarians or slaughtermen, but CCHF also occurs in town dwellers visiting the country, and health staff. The disease tends to occur sporadically in endemic countries, but in recent years there have been outbreaks in Afghanistan, Pakistan, the Russian Federation, Kosovo, Turkey and South Africa.

Pathogenesis and pathology

Viraemia and antigenaemia levels are high, and decline as antibody appears, after the first week.[92] In fatal cases there is little evidence of an antibody response.[93] Pro-inflammatory cytokines, IL-6 and TNF-α, were significantly higher in fatal cases than in survivors.[94] Histologically, necrotic lesions are seen in the liver, which are disproportionate to the amount of viral antigen demonstrated by immunofluorescence.[93]

Clinical features

Unlike with many other arboviruses, most infections with CCHF virus appear to cause symptoms. The incubation period is 1–3

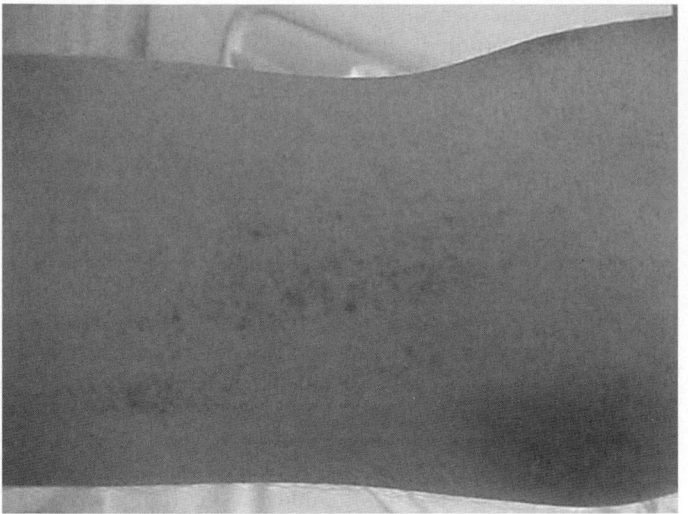

Figure 42.10 Petechial rash in a patient with Crimean–Congo haemorrhagic fever. (Courtesy of Professor Salih Ahmeti.)

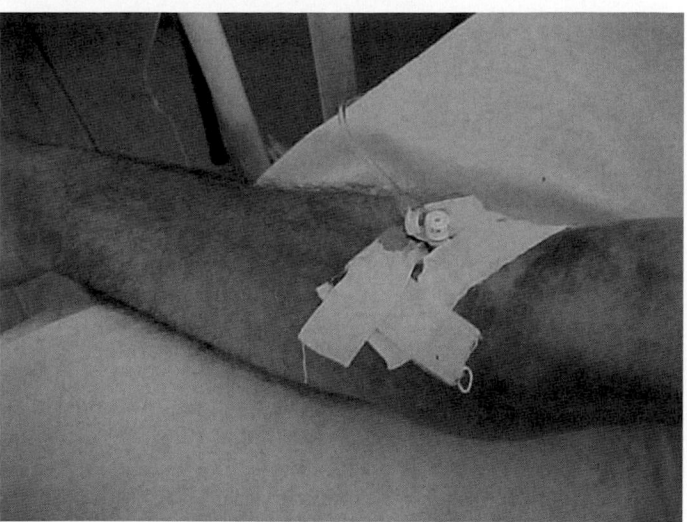

A

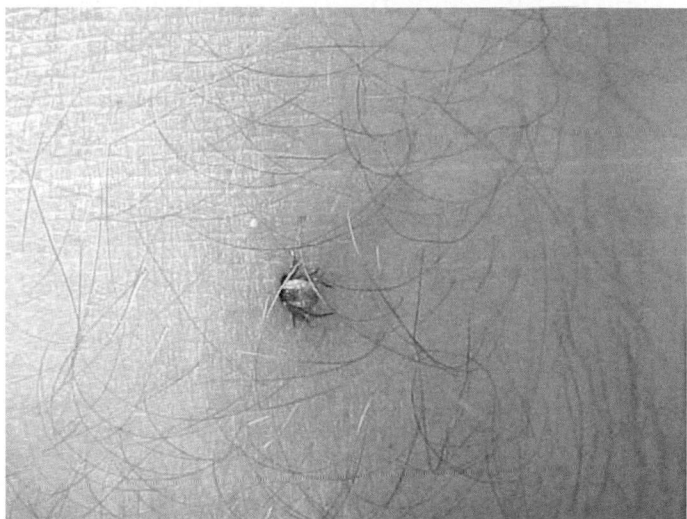

B

Figure 42.11 (**A**) Ecchymoses in a patient with Crimean–Congo haemorrhagic fever. (**B**) Hyalomma tick (the vector for Crimean–Congo haemorrhagic fever) engorging on the skin. (**A** & **B**, Courtesy of Professor Salih Ahmeti.)

days following a tick bite, or 5–6 days following exposure to infected blood. Patients present with a sudden onset of febrile illness with chills, headache, dizziness, neck pain and myalgia. Lymphadenopathy and tender hepatomegaly are common. This is followed by facial flushing and haemorrhage, which may range from petechiae to ecchymoses or major bleeds (Figures 42.10 & 42.11). Unlike in other VHFs, bleeding is more important than vascular leakage. Gastrointestinal bleeding may be profuse, and confused with surgical causes of bleeding.[95] The patients themselves may be confused or aggressive. Laboratory abnormalities include thrombocytopenia, leucopenia and elevated transaminases. Severely ill patients develop DIC, hepatic, renal and pulmonary failure, and coma. Approximately 30% of patients die. High viral load, leukocytosis $= 10 \times 10^9$/L, thrombocytopenia $= 20 \times 10^9$/L, aspartate aminotransferase (AST) $= 150$ U/L, activated partial thromboplastin time (APTT) $= 60$ seconds, and fibrinogen titre $= 110$ mg/dL have each been associated with a fatal outcome.[93,96]

Diagnosis

CCHF should be suspected in patients with an acute febrile illness and known exposure to tick bites or contact with livestock or their fresh products. The diagnosis is confirmed by virus isolation or antigen-detection ELISA, under BSL-4 conditions. Antibody may be detected by IgM ELISAs in patients who ultimately survive, but is rare in fatal cases.

Treatment

Ribavirin is effective against CCHF virus in vitro and in the mouse model. Oral ribavirin has been used successfully in Pakistan when surgeons were infected nosocomially while operating on a patient whose gastrointestinal bleeding turned out to be due to CCHF virus.[95] This remarkable paper includes the surgeons' personal accounts of their illness. Treatment with hyperimmune serum was also used in one outbreak, with apparent temporary improvements.[97]

Prevention and control

Exposure to tick bites is minimized by those in the agricultural and related industries by treating their clothing with pyrethroid preparations, and using insect repellents containing DEET on their skin. Workers in the livestock industry should wear appropriate clothing to reduce their exposure to potentially infected blood and tissue products. Patients with suspected CCHF should be barrier-nursed, and measures taken as for other directly transmissible

VHFs (see p. 769). Formalin-inactivated vaccines have been developed in Eastern Europe, but have not been widely used.[98]

Rift Valley fever (RVF)

RVF virus is an arbovirus transmitted by a range of mosquitoes (see p. 764), which is genetically related to the sandfly fever viruses (and hence a member of the *Phlebovirus* genus of the Bunyaviridae family). It is zoonotic in livestock, in which it causes abortions. Originally found in the Rift Valley of Kenya, the virus is distributed across sub-Saharan Africa, Egypt, Saudi Arabia and the Yemen.[99] Disease in animals follows the explosive increases in mosquito populations caused by heavy rains or new irrigation projects. Humans become infected by mosquitoes or contact with animal blood or other products. Although direct transmission between humans has never been documented, patients should be managed as for other directly transmissible VHFs. Most human infections cause a non-specific febrile illness, but about 2% cause retinitis, 1% cause CNS disease, and 1% result in VHF.[100] This is associated with hepatitis, and has a high mortality. Ribavirin treatment is probably effective, based on laboratory studies. Control measures include vaccination of livestock (with a live attenuated or inactivated vaccine), mosquito control, and personal protection of workers in the livestock industry.

FLAVIVIRUSES[101]

The VHFs caused by flaviviruses are all transmitted by mosquitoes or ticks, with no risk of nosocomial spread, and thus are discussed in detail in Chapter 40. The genus *Flavivirus* (family Flaviviridae) is named after the prototype, yellow fever virus (*flavus* = yellow in Latin). Its members include important causes of CNS disease, such as Japanese encephalitis virus,[102] as well as major causes of VHF.

Dengue haemorrhagic fever (DHF)

This is the most common VHF worldwide, and the one most likely to be seen in returning travellers. It is unusual among VHF viruses in that humans are the natural hosts. There are an estimated 100 million cases per year and 2.5 billion people at risk. Dengue has spread dramatically since the end of World War II, linked to a resurgence of the principal vector *Aedes aegypti*. Virtually every country between the Tropics of Capricorn and Cancer is now affected. Infection with one of the four serotypes of dengue virus can lead to a non-specific febrile illness, dengue fever (a fever–arthralgia rash syndrome) or DHF.[101]

DHF is characterized by a massive increase in vascular permeability, which leads to plasma leakage, an elevated haematocrit, oedema and effusions.[103] In addition there is thrombocytopenia and haemorrhagic manifestations (which may range from a few petechiae to frank bleeding). When the leakage is sufficient to cause shock, this is known as dengue shock syndrome. There is often also tender hepatomegaly, and sometimes neurological disease.[4] Diagnosis of DHF has been facilitated by new rapid diagnostic kits.[104] With early recognition and careful fluid management, the mortality of DHF has been reduced from around 30% to less than 0.02 %. Ringer's lactate is appropriate treatment for moderately severe dengue shock syndrome; in severe shock, a colloid solution should be used.[8] Control of *Aedes* mosquitoes is the main preventative measure. Tetravalent vaccines are currently undergoing clinical trials.

Yellow fever

Yellow fever virus is transmitted by mosquitoes between non-human primates in sylvatic cycles in South America and Africa. Humans become infected by entering this cycle, and may then carry the virus to populated areas. Here, *Aedes aegypti* spreads the disease, causing 'urban yellow fever'. In the savanna of Africa, smaller epidemics are known as 'intermediate yellow fever'. After a short incubation, there is an acute febrile illness, sometimes associated with a paradoxical slowing of the pulse (Faget's sign – indicating viral cardiac damage). After a brief period of remission, about 15% of patients develop VHF with mild jaundice (due to hepatitis) and impaired renal function. The mortality is 20–50%. The diagnosis is confirmed by ELISA, virus isolation or, in fatal cases, postmortem liver biopsy. There is no antiviral treatment. A live attenuated vaccine, available for very many years, was generally considered to be one of the safest vaccines known, though recently documented adverse events are prompting a rethink.[105,106]

Omsk haemorrhagic fever (OHF)

OHF virus is unusual among flaviviruses in that the vectors, *Dermacentor* ticks, are important reservoirs of the virus. It is found in the Omsk area of Siberia[107] and causes disease in many of the small mammals (including muskrats) to which it is transmitted. Muskrat hunters become infected by direct contact with infected carcasses, or tick bites. Most infections are asymptomatic, but there may be a papulovesicular eruption on the soft palate, and mucosal and gastrointestinal bleeding.

Kyasanur Forest disease

Kyasanur Forest disease is caused by a closely related tick-borne flavivirus found in forest rodents in south-western India. It is transmitted by *Haemaphysalis* ticks and causes annual outbreaks of febrile or haemorrhagic disease in monkeys and humans. A formalin-inactivated vaccine appears to be effective.[108] Other preventative measures include treatment of cows with acaricides to reduce the tick population, and the personal use of insect repellents.

REFERENCES

1. Mayer C. Epidemic hemorrhagic fever of the Far East or endemic hemorrhagic nephroso-nephritis. *Lab Invest* 1952; 1:291–311.
2. Solomon T. Emerging viral diseases. *Medicine (Baltimore)* 2001; 29:6–7.
3. Centers for Disease Control (CDC). Management of patients with suspected viral hemorrhagic fever. *MMWR Morb Mortal Wkly Rep* 1988; 37(suppl 3): 1–16.
4. Solomon T, Dung NM, Vaughn DW, et al. Neurological manifestations of dengue infection. *Lancet* 2000; 355:1053–1059.

5. Centers for Disease Control and Prevention and World Health Organization. *Infection Control for Viral Haemorrhagic Fevers in the African Health Care Setting.* Atlanta: Centers for Disease Control and Prevention; 1998.

6. Ngo NT, Cao XT, Kneen R, et al. Acute management of dengue shock syndrome: a randomized double-blind comparison of 4 intravenous fluid regimens in the first hour. *Clin Infect Dis* 2001; 32:204–213.

7. Dung NM, Day NP, Tam DT, et al. Fluid replacement in dengue shock syndrome: a randomized, double-blind comparison of four intravenous-fluid regimens. *Clin Infect Dis* 1999; 28:787–794.

8. Wills BA, Nguyen MD, Ha TL, et al. Comparison of three fluid solutions for resuscitation in dengue shock syndrome. *N Engl J Med* 2005; 353: 877–889.

9. De Roo A, Ado B, Rose B, et al. Survey among survivors of the 1995 Ebola epidemic in Kikwit, Democratic Republic of Congo: their feelings and experiences. *Trop Med Int Health* 1998; 3:883–885.

10. Carey DE, Kemp GE, White HA, et al. Lassa fever. Epidemiological aspects of the 1970 epidemic, Jos, Nigeria. *Trans R Soc Trop Med Hyg* 1972; 66:402–408.

11. Hewlett BS, Epelboin A, Hewlett BL, et al. Medical anthropology and Ebola in Congo: cultural models and humanistic care. *Bull Soc Pathol Exot* 2005; 98:230–236.

12. Lloyd ES, Zaki SR, Rollin PE, et al. Long-term disease surveillance in Bandundu region, Democratic Republic of the Congo: a model for early detection and prevention of Ebola hemorrhagic fever. *J Infect Dis* 1999; 179(suppl 1):S274–S280.

13. Buchmeier M, Welsh R, Dutko F, et al. The virology and immunobiology of lymphocytic choriomeningitis virus infection. *Adv Immunol* 1980; 30:275–331.

14. Ambrosio AM, Feulllade MR, Gamboa GS, et al. Prevalence of lymphocytic choriomeningitis virus infection in a human population of Argentina. *Am J Trop Med Hyg* 1994; 50:381–386.

15. Harrison LH, Halsey NA, McKee KT Jr, et al. Clinical case definitions for Argentine hemorrhagic fever. *Clin Infect Dis* 1999; 28:1091–1094.

16. Frame JD, Baldwin JM Jr, Gocke DJ, et al. Lassa fever, a new virus disease of man from West Africa. I. Clinical description and pathological findings. *Am J Trop Med Hyg* 1970; 19:670–676.

17. Buchmeier MJ, Bowen MD, Peters CJ. Arenaviridae: the viruses and their replication. In: Knipe DM, Howley PM, eds. *Fields Virology.* 4th edn. Philadelphia: Lippincott Williams & Wilkins; 2001:1635–1668.

18. Peters CJ, Jahrling PB, Liu CT, et al. Experimental studies of arenaviral hemorrhagic fevers. *Curr Top Microbiol Immunol* 1987; 134:5–68.

19. Jahrling P, Smith S, Hesse RA, et al. Pathogenesis of Lassa virus infection in guinea pigs. *Infect Immunol* 1982; 37:771–778.

20. Knobloch J, McCormick JB, Webb PA, et al. Clinical observations in 42 patients with Lassa fever. *Tropenmed Parasitol* 1980; 31:389–398.

21. White HA. Lassa fever. A study of 23 hospital cases. *Trans R Soc Trop Med Hyg* 1972; 66:390–401.

22. Walker DH, McCormick JB, Johnson KM, et al. Pathologic and virologic study of fatal Lassa fever in man. *Am J Pathol* 1982; 107:349–356.

23. Buckley SM, Casals J. Lassa fever, a new virus disease of man from West Africa. 3. Isolation and characterization of the virus. *Am J Trop Med Hyg* 1970; 19:680–691.

24. Bausch DG, Sesay SS, Oshin B. On the front lines of Lassa fever. *Emerg Infect Dis* 2004; 10:1889–1890.

25. Borio L, Inglesby T, Peters CJ, et al. Hemorrhagic fever viruses as biological weapons: medical and public health management. *JAMA* 2002; 287:2391–2405.

26. Anonymous. Lassa fever imported to England. *Commun Dis Rep CDR Wkly* 2000; 10:99.

27. Fraser DW, Campbell CC, Monath TP, et al. Lassa fever in the Eastern Province of Sierra Leone, 1970–1972. I. Epidemiologic studies. *Am J Trop Med Hyg* 1974; 23:1131–1139.

28. Fisher-Hoch SP, McCormick JB. Lassa fever vaccine. *Expert Rev Vaccines* 2004; 3:189–197.

29. McCormick JB, King IJ, Webb PA, et al. A case-control study of the clinical diagnosis and course of Lassa fever. *J Infect Dis* 1987; 155: 445–455.

30. Cummins D, McCormick JB, Bennett D, et al. Acute sensorineural deafness in Lassa fever. *JAMA* 1990; 264:2093–2096.

31. Sharp PC. Lassa fever in children. *J Infect* 1982; 4:73–77.

32. Johnson KM, McCormick JB, Webb PA, et al. Clinical virology of Lassa fever in hospitalized patients. *J Infect Dis* 1987; 155:456–464.

33. Bausch DG, Rollin PE, Demby AH, et al. Diagnosis and clinical virology of Lassa fever as evaluated by enzyme-linked immunosorbent assay, indirect fluorescent-antibody test, and virus isolation. *J Clin Microbiol* 2000; 38: 2670–2677.

34. McCormick JB, King IJ ,Webb PA. Lassa fever. Effective therapy with ribavirin. *N Engl J Med* 1986; 314:20–26.

35. Baize S, Pannetier D, Faure C, et al. Role of interferons in the control of Lassa virus replication in human dendritic cells and macrophages. *Microbes Infect* 2006; 8:1194–1202.

36. Gowen BB, Smee DF, Wong MH, et al. Combinatorial ribavirin and interferon alfacon-1 therapy of acute arenaviral disease in hamsters. *Antivir Chem Chemother* 2006; 17:175–183.

37. Cao W, Henry MD, Borrow P, et al. Identification of alpha-dystroglycan as a receptor for lymphocytic choriomeningitis virus and Lassa fever virus. *Science* 1998; 282.2079–2081.

38. Perez M, Craven RC, de la Torre JC. The small RING finger protein Z drives arenavirus budding: implications for antiviral strategies. *Proc Natl Acad Sci USA* 2003; 100:12978–12983.

39. Fisher-Hoch SP, McCormick JB. Towards a human Lassa fever vaccine. *Rev Med Virol* 2001; 11:331–341.

40. Maiztegui JI, McKee KT Jr, Barrera Oro JG, et al. Protective efficacy of a live attenuated vaccine against Argentine hemorrhagic fever. AHF Study Group. *J Infect Dis* 1998; 177:277–283.

41. Radoshitzky SR, Abraham J, Spiropoulou CF, et al. Transferrin receptor 1 is a cellular receptor for New World haemorrhagic fever arenaviruses. *Nature* 2007; 446:92–96.

42. Fulhorst CF, Milazzo ML, Armstrong LR, et al. Hantavirus and arenavirus antibodies in persons with occupational rodent exposure. *Emerg Infect Dis* 2007; 13:532–538.

43. de Manzione N, Salas RA, Paredes H, et al. Venezuelan hemorrhagic fever: clinical and epidemiological studies of 165 cases. *Clin Infect Dis* 1998; 26:308–313.

44. Barry M, Russi M, Armstrong L, et al. Treatment of a laboratory-acquired Sabiá virus infection. *N Engl J Med* 1995; 333:294–296.

45. Fulhorst CF, Bowen MD, Ksiazek TG, et al. Isolation and characterization of Whitewater Arroyo virus, a novel North American arenavirus. *Virology* 1996; 224:114–120.

46. Kissling RE, Robinson RQ, Murphy FA, et al. Agent of disease contracted from green monkeys. *Science* 1968; 160:888–890.

47. Johnson KM, Lange JV, Webb PA, et al. Isolation and partial characterisation of a new virus causing acute haemorrhagic fever in Zaire. *Lancet* 1977; i:569–571.

48. Anonymous. Outbreak of Ebola haemorrhagic fever, Uganda, August 2000–January 2001. *Wkly Epidemiol Rec* 2001; 76:41–46.

49. Swanepoel R, Leman PA, Burt FJ, et al. Experimental inoculation of plants and animals with Ebola virus. *Emerg Infect Dis* 1996; 2: 321–325.

50. Peterson AT, Carroll DS, Mills JN, et al. Potential mammalian filovirus reservoirs. *Emerg Infect Dis* 2004; 10:2073–2081.

51. Leirs H, Mills JN, Krebs JW, et al. Search for the Ebola virus reservoir in Kikwit, Democratic Republic of the Congo: reflections on a vertebrate collection. *J Infect Dis* 1999; 179(suppl 1):S155–S163.

52. Morvan JM, Deubel V, Gounon P, et al. Identification of Ebola virus sequences present as RNA or DNA in organs of terrestrial small mammals of the Central African Republic. *Microb Infect* 1999; 1:1193–1201.

53. McCormick JB, Fisher-Hoch SP. Filovirus infections. In: Porterfield JS, ed. *Exotic Viral Infections.* London: Chapman & Hall; 1995:319–328.

54. Paragas J, Geisbert TW. Development of treatment strategies to combat Ebola and Marburg viruses. *Expert Rev Anti Infect Ther* 2006; 4:67–76.

55. Sanchez A, Khan A, Zaki SR, et al. Filoviridae: Marburg and Ebola viruses. In: Knipe DM, Howley PM, eds. *Fields Virology*. Philadelphia: Lippincott Williams & Wilkins; 2001:1279–1304.

56. Villinger F, Rollin PE, Brar SS, et al. Markedly elevated levels of interferon (IFN)-gamma, IFN-alpha, interleukin (IL)-2, IL-10, and tumor necrosis factor-alpha associated with fatal Ebola virus infection. *J Infect Dis* 1999; 179(suppl 1):S188–S191.

57. Wahl-Jensen VM, Afanasieva TA, Seebach J, et al. Effects of Ebola virus glycoproteins on endothelial cell activation and barrier function. *J Virol* 2005; 79:10442–10450.

58. Yang ZY, Duckers HJ, Sullivan NJ, et al. Identification of the Ebola virus glycoprotein as the main viral determinant of vascular cell cytotoxicity and injury. *Nat Med* 2000; 6:886–889.

59. Nabel G J. Surviving Ebola virus infection. *Nat Med* 1999; 5:373–374.

60. Baize S, Leroy EM, Georges AJ, et al. Inflammatory responses in Ebola virus-infected patients. *Clin Exp Immunol* 2002; 128:163–168.

61. Leroy EM, Baize S, Volchkov VE, et al. Human asymptomatic Ebola infection and strong inflammatory response. *Lancet* 2000; 355:2210–2215.

62. Gupta M, Mahanty S, Greer P, et al. Persistent infection with Ebola virus under conditions of partial immunity. *J Virol* 2004; 78:958–967.

63. Gupta M, Spiropoulou C, Rollin PE. Ebola virus infection of human PBMCs causes massive death of macrophages, CD4 and CD8 T cell sub-populations in vitro. *Virology* 2007; 364:45–54.

64. Sanchez A, Lukwiya M, Bausch D, et al. Analysis of human peripheral blood samples from fatal and nonfatal cases of Ebola (Sudan) hemorrhagic fever: cellular responses, virus load, and nitric oxide levels. *J Virol* 2004; 78:10370–10377.

65. Roels TH, Bloom AS, Buffington J, et al. Ebola hemorrhagic fever, Kikwit, Democratic Republic of the Congo, 1995: risk factors for patients without a reported exposure. *J Infect Dis* 1999; 179(suppl 1):S92–S97.

66. Peters CJ, Jahrling PB, Khan AS. Patients infected with high-hazard viruses: scientific basis for infection control. *Arch Virol Suppl* 1996; 11:141–168.

67. Ndambi R, Akamituna P, Bonnet MJ, et al. Epidemiologic and clinical aspects of the Ebola virus epidemic in Mosango, Democratic Republic of the Congo, 1995. *J Infect Dis* 1999; 179(suppl 1):S8–S10.

68. Bwaka MA, Bonnet MJ, Calain P, et al. Ebola hemorrhagic fever in Kikwit, Democratic Republic of the Congo: clinical observations in 103 patients. *J Infect Dis* 1999; 179(suppl 1):S1–S7.

69. Towner JS, Rollin PE, Bausch DG, et al. Rapid diagnosis of Ebola hemorrhagic fever by reverse transcription-PCR in an outbreak setting and assessment of patient viral load as a predictor of outcome. *J Virol* 2004; 78:4330–4341.

70. Formenty P, Leroy EM, Epelboin A, et al. Detection of Ebola virus in oral fluid specimens during outbreaks of Ebola virus hemorrhagic fever in the Republic of Congo. *Clin Infect Dis* 2006; 42:1521–1526.

71. Saijo M, Niikura M, Morikawa S, et al. Enzyme-linked immunosorbent assays for detection of antibodies to Ebola and Marburg viruses using recombinant nucleoproteins. *J Clin Microbiol* 2001; 39:1–7.

72. Mupapa K, Massamba M, Kibadi K, et al. Treatment of Ebola hemorrhagic fever with blood transfusions from convalescent patients. International Scientific and Technical Committee. *J Infect Dis* 1999; 179(suppl 1): S18–S23.

73. Oswald WB, Geisbert TW, Davis KJ, et al. Neutralizing antibody fails to impact the course of Ebola virus infection in monkeys. *PLoS Pathog* 2007; 3: e9.

74. Geisbert TW, Hensley LE, Jahrling PB, et al. Treatment of Ebola virus infection with a recombinant inhibitor of factor VIIa/tissue factor: a study in rhesus monkeys. *Lancet* 2003; 362:1953–1958.

75. Feldmann H, Jones SM, Daddario-DiCaprio KM, et al. Effective post-exposure treatment of Ebola infection. *PLoS Pathog* 2007; 3:e2.

76. Jones SM, Stroher U, Fernando L, et al. Assessment of a vesicular stomatitis virus-based vaccine by use of the mouse model of Ebola virus hemorrhagic fever. *J Infect Dis* 2007; 196(suppl 2):S404–S412.

77. Warfield KL, Swenson DL, Olinger GG, et al. Ebola virus-like particle-based vaccine protects nonhuman primates against lethal Ebola virus challenge. *J Infect Dis* 2007; 196(suppl 2):S430–S437.

78. Patel A, Zhang Y, Croyle M, et al. Mucosal delivery of adenovirus-based vaccine protects against Ebola virus infection in mice. *J Infect Dis* 2007; 196(suppl 2):S413–S420.

79. Anonymous. Marburg fever, Democratic Republic of the Congo. *Wkly Epidemiol Rec* 1999; 74:145.

80. Gear JJS, Cassel GA, Gear AJ, et al. Outbreak of Marburg virus disease in Johannesburg. *BMJ* 1975; 4:489–493.

81. Earle DP. Symposium on epidemic hemorrhagic fever. *Am J Med* 1954; 16:617–709.

82. Lee HW, Lee PW, Johnson KM. Isolation of the etiologic agent of Korean hemorrhagic fever. *J Infect Dis* 1978; 137:298–308.

83. Tsai TF. Hemorrhagic fever with renal syndrome: mode of transmission to humans. *Lab Anim Sci* 1987; 37:428–430.

84. Heyman P, Cochez C, Ducoffre G, et al. Haemorrhagic fever with renal syndrome: an analysis of the outbreaks in Belgium, France, Germany, the Netherlands and Luxembourg in 2005. *Euro Surveill* 2007; 12:E15–E16.

85. Hung T, Zhou JY, Tang YM, et al. Identification of Hantaan virus-related structures in kidneys of cadavers with haemorrhagic fever with renal syndrome. *Arch Virol* 1992; 122:187–199.

86. Huggins JW, Hsiang CM, Cosgriff TM, et al. Prospective, double-blind, concurrent, placebo-controlled clinical trial of intravenous ribavirin therapy of haemorrhagic fever with renal syndrome. *J Infect Dis* 1991; 164:1119–1127.

87. Jonsson CB, Hooper J, Mertz G. Treatment of hantavirus pulmonary syndrome. *Antiviral Res* 2008; 78:162–169.

88. Hooper JW, Li D. Vaccines against hantaviruses. *Curr Top Microbiol Immunol* 2001; 256:171–191.

89. Hoogstraal H. The epidemiology of tick-borne Crimean-Congo hemorrhagic fever in Asia, Europe, and Africa. *J Med Entomology* 1979; 15:307–417.

90. Simpson DI, Knight EM, Courtois G, et al. Congo virus: a hitherto undescribed virus occurring in Africa. I. Human isolations – clinical notes. *East Afr Med J* 1967; 44:86–92.

91. Fisher-Hoch SP, McCormick JB, Swanepoel R, et al. Risk of human infections with Crimean-Congo hemorrhagic fever virus in a South African rural community. *Am J Trop Med Hyg* 1992; 47:337–345.

92. Shepherd AJ, Swanepoel R, Leman PA. Antibody response in Crimean-Congo hemorrhagic fever. *Rev Infect Dis* 1989; 11(suppl 4):S801–S806.

93. Swanepoel R, Gill DE, Shepherd AJ, et al. The clinical pathology of Crimean-Congo hemorrhagic fever. *Rev Infect Dis* 1989; 11(suppl 4): S794–S800.

94. Ergonul O, Tuncbilek S, Baykam N, et al. Evaluation of serum levels of interleukin (IL)-6, IL-10, and tumor necrosis factor-alpha in patients with Crimean-Congo hemorrhagic fever. *J Infect Dis* 2006; 193:941–944.

95. Fisher-Hoch SP, Khan JA, Rehman S, et al. Crimean Congo haemorrhagic fever treated with oral ribavirin. *Lancet* 1995; 346:472–475.

96. Cevik MA, Erbay A, Bodur H, et al. Viral load as a predictor of outcome in Crimean-Congo hemorrhagic fever. *Clin Infect Dis* 2007; 45:e96–100.

97. van Eeden PJ, van Eeden SF, Joubert JR, et al. A nosocomial outbreak of Crimean-Congo haemorrhagic fever at Tygerberg Hospital. Part II. Management of patients. *S Afr Med J* 1985; 68:718–721.

98. Ergonul O. Crimean-Congo haemorrhagic fever. *Lancet Infect Dis* 2006; 6:203–214.

99. Centers for Disease Control and Prevention. Outbreak of Rift Valley fever, Yemen, August–October 2000. *MMWR Morb Mort Wkly Rep* 2000; 49:1065–1066.

100. Laughlin LW, Meegan JM, Strausbaugh LJ, et al. Epidemic Rift Valley fever in Egypt: observations of the spectrum of human illness. *Trans R Soc Trop Med Hyg* 1979; 73:630–633.

101. Solomon T, Mallewa MJ. Dengue and other emerging flaviviruses. *J Infect* 2001; 42:104–115.

102. Solomon T. Japanese encephalitis. In Gilman S, Goldstein GW, Waxman SG, eds. *Neurobase*. San Diego: Medlink Publishing; 2000.

103. Bethell DB, Gamble J, Pham PL, et al. Noninvasive measurement of microvascular leakage in patients with dengue hemorrhagic fever. *Clin Infect Dis* 2001; 32:243–253.

104. Vaughn DW, Nisalak A, Solomon T, et al. Rapid serological diagnosis of dengue virus infection using a commercial capture ELISA that distinguishes primary and secondary infections. *Am J Trop Med Hyg* 1999; 60:693–698.

105. Monath TP. Dengue and yellow fever – challenges for the development and use of vaccines. *N Engl J Med* 2007; 357:2222–2225.

106. Vasconcelos PF, Luna EJ, Galler R, et al. Serious adverse events associated with yellow fever 17DD vaccine in Brazil: a report of two cases. *Lancet* 2001; 358:91–97.

107. Gaidamovich SY. Tick-borne flavivirus infections. In: Porterfield JS, ed. *Exotic Viral Infections*. London: Chapman & Hall; 1995:203–221.

108. Upadhyaya S, Dandwate CN, Banerjee K. Surveillance of formolized KFD vaccine administration in Sagar-Sorab Talukas district. *Ind J Med Res* 1979; 69:714–719.

Chapter 43

Hilary Williams and Dorothy H. Crawford

Epstein–Barr Virus and Associated Diseases

Epstein–Barr virus (EBV) was first isolated from cultures of Burkitt's lymphoma (BL) biopsy material and was rapidly shown to be a unique herpesvirus.[1] EBV is a ubiquitous human virus, infecting over 90% of the human population globally. This large DNA virus is normally transmitted via saliva; EBV is present in the oral secretions of most infected individuals and a naive host becomes infected through contact with infectious virus shed in saliva.[2] Most people undergo subclinical infection as infants; however, in the West delayed primary infection as a young adult may result in infectious mononucleosis (IM). After primary infection the virus persists for life; EBV infects memory B lymphocytes and these cells are the site of the long-term viral reservoir (latent infection).[3]

In the vast majority of healthy carriers EBV does not cause disease. This is because a delicate balance is maintained between the host immune system, which limits production of new virus, and the virus, which persists and is successfully transmitted in the face of host antiviral immunity. Disruption of this balance, due to primary or acquired abnormalities of the host's immune system, may lead to the development of EBV associated disease.

EBV plays a central role in the development of a number of lymphoid and epithelial cell-derived cancers. Viral-driven cell proliferation is thought to be key to the development of both BL and nasopharyngeal carcinoma (NPC), and, like other cancers driven by an infectious agent, these cancers are more common in the developing world than the West. Overall, infectious agents are responsible for 21% of all tumours in the developing world and 9% in the West. NPC comprises 0.7% of new tumours occurring on a worldwide basis each year.[4] The global HIV pandemic has caused significant changes in the profile of EBV-related conditions. Most crucially, EBV is associated with many non-Hodgkin's lymphomas and with oral hairy leukoplakia in HIV-positive individuals. Lymphocytic interstitial pneumonia may also be linked to EBV infection.

INFECTION IN HEALTHY INDIVIDUALS

Primary infection with EBV is commonly subclinical, occurs predominantly in early childhood, and gives rise to a lifelong carrier state.[5] In most populations, seropositivity increases with age, and over 90% of adults have persistent infection. However, the rate of seroconversion varies according to economic status, such that over 90% of children over the age of 2 years in developing countries have evidence of persistent infection,[6] whereas seroconversion may be delayed until adolescence in high socioeconomic groups of industrialized countries. It is thought that close family contact is the main route of spread in young infants, and that large family size and close proximity of living conditions are likely to aid spread. In the West, 5–10% of people remain EBV negative for life, whereas in Africa over 97% of the population carry the virus.[7] Most normal hosts carry only one of the two major virus subtypes of EBV, A or B (also called 1 and 2),[8] which have 70–80% sequence homology.[9] Type A is most common throughout the world; type B is rare, but is more prevalent in Africa and the Far East than the West.[10,11] In addition to EBV subtypes, minor sequence variants are classified as strains. It has recently been recognized that immunocompetent individuals may carry multiple strains of the virus, whereas previously multiple strain carriage was thought to be limited to the immunosuppressed.[12] Up until now there was no evidence that variation of either strain or type affected disease pathogenesis, but recent work on IM has revealed that type A more commonly gives rise to IM than type B, and this is not merely a reflection in the different geographical distribution of the 2 viral types.[13]

In healthy adults 1–50 B cells per million in peripheral blood are latently infected.[14] Significant numbers of these B cells can be identified in tonsils, where activation of virus-infected cells may lead to virus production (lytic infection) and continuous or intermittent low-level shedding of free virus in the oral cavity.[15] Infectious virus has also been recovered from male and female genital secretions (see later).

INFECTIOUS MONONUCLEOSIS

Infectious mononucleosis (IM) is an acute febrile illness, caused by primary infection with EBV, which presents with sore throat, fever, lymph node enlargement and severe fatigue.

Epidemiology

IM mainly affects affluent groups in the West, and is the commonest cause of prolonged illness in young army recruits in the USA.[16] In a recent study in the UK up to 25% of students entering university were seronegative for EBV,[17] and of those who seroconverted at university only 25% developed IM, which is lower than previously documented rates of approximately 45–65%.[18,19] The remaining primary infections are asymptomatic or non-specific, as in primary infection in young children. Until now it has not been clear what factors predispose to the development of clinical illness; however, a genetic link between HLA class I polymorphisms and risk of development of clinical IM has recently been recognized (KA McAulay, pers comm). Interestingly, these same polymorphisms have been associated with development of EBV-positive Hodgkin's disease.[20]

Transmission

IM is colloquially known as the 'kissing disease', and it is presumed that the initiation of sexual activity in adolescence places seronegative individuals at risk of contact with infectious virus in saliva. However, infectious virus is present in both male and female genital secretions of asymptomatic carriers[21,22] and recent evidence suggests that IM often results from spread during sexual intercourse.[23,24,25]

Pathogenesis and EBV

Primary infection occurs when virus particles infect B lymphocytes in the oropharynx (or possibly the genital tract) of EBV-negative individuals. It was originally thought that the initial site of infection was oropharyngeal squamous epithelial cells. However, it has not proved possible to identify EBV-infected epithelial cells in tonsils taken from patients with IM, although latent and lytic infection in B cells can be seen. Therefore, the consensus of opinion now is that the B cell is the site of both viral replication and persistence. The EBV major viral envelope glycoprotein (gp 350) binds to the CD21 receptor (also called complement receptor, CR2) on resting B cells, followed by fusion of the viral envelope with the cell membrane and release of the capsid into the cell. Once a cell is infected, the virus may replicate (lytic infection) with new virus production and cell death, or lie dormant in B cells (latent infection). During IM lytic infection predominates in the oropharynx, with large amounts of new virus produced and excreted into saliva. Individuals with IM may carry multiple strains of the virus.[26,27] In lytic infection nearly 100 viral proteins are transcribed which are important in modulating the host immune response, replicating viral DNA and forming the structural components of new virions.[28]

One of the ways the virus attenuates the host immune system is by producing virally encoded cytokines. The EBV BCRF1 protein has 70% homology with human interleukin 10.[29] This inhibits the production of interferon-γ (IFNγ), which is key to the host's response to early viral infection.

Neutralizing antibody to gp 350, the main viral envelope glycoprotein, is produced during primary infection, and there is increasing evidence that innate immune mechanisms, particularly natural killer cells, are important in controlling the early events in primary infection.[30]

The prolonged systemic symptoms of IM are thought to be caused by a dramatic cellular immune response to EBV-infected B cells, with large expansions of characteristic 'atypical' lymphocytes. These are predominantly, but not exclusively, CD8-positive cytotoxic effector cells. Large amounts of cytokines are released; IFNγ, tumour necrosis factor α (TNFα) and TNFβ have all been identified in IM tonsils.[31] Analysis of CD8 T cell antigen specificities from patients with acute IM has revealed that up to 50% of the total T cell numbers in peripheral blood are directed against single viral epitopes.[32] These virus-specific activated lymphocytes are thought to be essential in limiting virus spread to uninfected B cells.

After acute infection a state of viral persistence is established, with long-term cellular immunity provided by EBV-specific CD8 positive cytotoxic T lymphocytes. These cells can be detected in the circulation in all normal seropositive individuals.

Clinical features

It is estimated that IM occurs 30–50 days after exposure to the virus. The majority of patients experience fever, lymphadenopathy, sore throat and fatigue. Examination normally reveals marked tonsillar enlargement, sometimes with associated exudate and petechia, lymphadenopathy (which may be generalized or restricted to the cervical region) and splenomegaly. A degree of hepatomegaly and mildly abnormal liver function tests are also common, but jaundice is rare (<10%). Urticarial skin rashes can occur, most commonly associated with the use of ampicillin. Rare complications include acute liver necrosis, splenic rupture, pharyngeal or tracheal obstruction, and haematological disorders, including autoimmune thrombocytopenia and haemolytic anaemia.[33]

In the vast majority of cases IM is a benign and self-limiting disease with prolonged fatigue being the most disabling symptom, and full recovery after 6–8 weeks is the norm. Treatment is supportive, with advice to avoid both alcohol (particularly if hepatitis is present) and vigorous exercise, the latter because of the risk of splenic rupture. Steroids have long been advocated for serious complications of IM; however, a recent Cochrane review has identified a lack of evidence to support this, and in particular the lack of data on potential long-term side-effects.[34] Aciclovir inhibits viral replication but is ineffective in altering the clinical course of IM, since symptoms are not due to viraemia, but to the marked immune response to EBV, which is well established by the time of clinical presentation. IM cases may continue to harbour high EBV DNA loads in saliva, even up to 6 months after onset of symptoms, thus potentially remaining infectious.[35]

Relapses can occur in the first 6–12 months following infection, and IM may be a risk factor, in the short term, for the development of a prolonged fatigue syndrome and depression.[36] However, there is no evidence that the chronic fatigue syndrome is caused by an abnormal immunological response to EBV.[37]

It is likely that milder forms of the disease occur without detection, and a spectrum of clinical features exists ranging from mild sore throat to full-blown IM. Rare cases of IM have also been documented in children, middle-aged adults and the elderly.[38]

X-linked lymphoproliferative syndrome is a rare familial condition, in which primary infection with EBV leads to uncontrolled lymphoproliferation and usually death from subsequent hepatic or bone marrow failure. A few individuals survive primary infection, but later develop fatal EBV-driven lymphomas. The defect on the X chromosome underlying this disorder has been identified as mutations in SAP (signalling lymphocyte activation molecule (SLAM) associated protein).[39,40]

Chronic active EBV infection is another rare, but non-familial, disorder that again presents with inability to control primary EBV infection. Most identified cases have been in the Far East, and some of those affected develop severe EBV-linked organ failure or lymphoma. Treatment options are improving with the introduction of the use of etoposide and adoptive transfer of EBV-specific cytotoxic T lymphocytes.[41]

Laboratory diagnosis

The majority of individuals with IM have a profound lymphocytosis, with 'atypical' lymphocytes (activated T cells) in the peripheral blood. The presence of these cells is not diagnostic of IM because they are also found to a lesser extent in other infections, including HIV seroconversion illness, cytomegalovirus infection, viral hepatitis, toxoplasmosis, rubella, mumps and roseola.[42]

In the early stages of infection serum antibodies appear to a variety of viral antigens (Figure 43.1), but the gold standard for the diagnosis of IM is detection of IgM antibodies to viral capsid antigen (VCA). Most laboratories use an enzyme-linked immunosorbent assay (ELISA) as a screening method, but may supplement this with an indirect immunofluorescence assay as a more sensitive test.

Infection and activation of B cells by EBV results in polyclonal antibody production, leading to elevated titres of heterophile antibodies, which form the basis for the rapid monospot test used for diagnostic screening. This is positive in 85% of acute IM cases (Figure 43.1). On occasion, auto-antibodies, such as cold agglutinins, cryoglobulins, antinuclear antibodies or rheumatoid factor, arise. Two studies have found a positive relationship between increasing EBV DNA load and illness severity;[43,44] however, one much smaller study[45] found similar viral DNA loads in symptomatic and asymptomatic seroconvertors.

EBV-ASSOCIATED MALIGNANCIES

EBV infection is increasingly linked to a diverse group of lymphoid and epithelial cell-derived malignancies. Experimental infection of cotton-topped tamarins rapidly leads to lymphoid tumour development[46] and this, combined with EBV's ability to transform cultured B cells to continuously proliferating long-lived lymphoblastoid cell lines, has confirmed its oncogenic potential.[47] A limited set of viral gene products are expressed by these transformed B cells, and identification of their function, both in laboratory models and EBV-associated tumours, has been key to the understanding of viral driven oncogenesis. Our understanding of the role of EBV in the pathogenesis of these viral-associated tumours has increased substantially in the last 5 years. This has allowed us to exploit the relationship between the virus and the tumour to monitor treatment outcome more accurately and develop novel therapies. Unfortunately, the burden of these malignancies falls in the developing world, where access to even basic cytotoxic drugs and radiotherapy is very limited.[48]

However, we will only know how fundamental EBV infection is to tumour development if vaccination leads to a reduction in EBV-linked tumours.[49]

EBV-associated lymphoid malignancies

EBV DNA is present in approximately 95% of endemic Burkitt's lymphoma, and this was the first malignancy to be linked to EBV.[50] It is now recognized that EBV is linked to three groups of lymphoid tumours: non-Hodgkin's lymphoma (NHL), including Burkitt's lymphoma and AIDS-related NHL, Hodgkin's disease, and lymphoproliferative disease in the immunocompromised host. AIDS-related tumours will be discussed in the section on EBV and HIV.

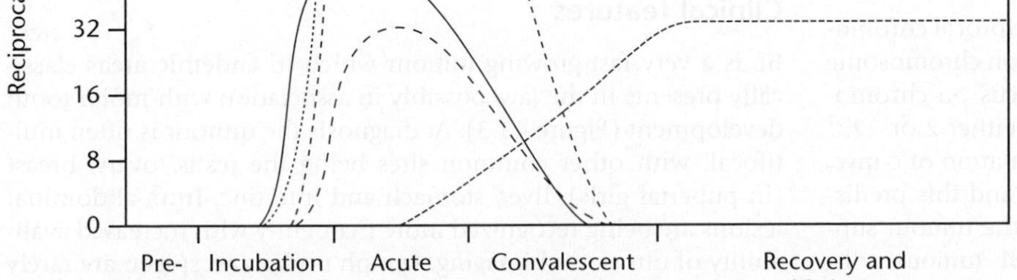
1024
512
256
128
64
32
16
8
0
Reciprocal antibody titre
Anti-VCA IgM
Anti-EA (D)
HA
Anti-VCA IgG
Anti-EBNA IgG
Pre-infection
Incubation period
Acute illness
Convalescent period
Recovery and life-long

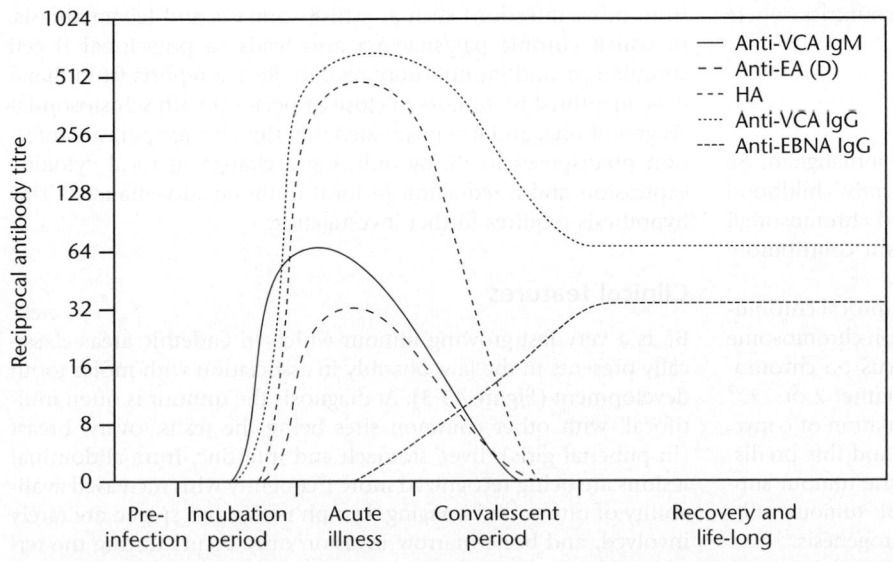

Figure 43.1 Profile of serum antibodies to EB virus-associated antigens before, during and after primary infection. EA(D), diffuse form of early antigen; VCA, viral capsid antigen; HA, heterophile antigen; EBNA, EB virus nuclear antigen.

Burkitt's lymphoma

Burkitt's lymphoma (BL) is a high-grade B-cell NHL, which commonly occurs in children.

Epidemiology (endemic, sporadic and intermediate)

The incidence of BL is categorized as high (endemic), low (sporadic) and intermediate.

Endemic BL is the most common childhood cancer in parts of equatorial Africa and Papua New Guinea (Figure 43.2A), with an annual incidence in Africa of 15–20 cases per 100 000 population.[51] Endemic BL occurs between the ages of 3 and 15 years, with a peak incidence at 5–7 years and a male predominance. The endemic areas, though geographically separate, have climatic features ideal for holoendemic malaria. These include an annual rainfall above 55 cm and a minimum temperature above 16.5°C.[52] In the Ivory Coast, West Africa, it has also been noted that the majority of children with BL live in rural communities, more often coming from forested areas (where tumour incidence is 5 : 100 000) than the savannah (where the incidence is less than 1 : 100 000).[53]

BL is not unique to endemic regions; the disease exists throughout the world at low incidence, and several areas of intermediate incidence have recently been recognized. In a series of children treated for NHL in north-east Brazil, 92 of 98 tumours were classified as being of Burkitt subtype, with 8 out of 11 cases studied being EBV-positive.[54] This area of tropical Brazil has a similar pattern of communicable disease and poverty to Africa.[55] Small studies of childhood lymphoma have also identified several other areas of intermediate incidence such as temperate South America, including Chile and Argentina, and Turkey. A review of cases in Turkey found that affected children were often from low socioeconomic groups.[56]

Childhood tumours with BL-like characteristics also occur in the West, but this sporadic form has an incidence which is 50–100 times lower than the endemic form, and an EBV association of 10–25%.[50] Further work is needed to clarify the epidemiology and patterns of disease in these different geographical areas. Of particular interest will be incidence in other countries where EBV-related tumours are common, e.g. China.

Pathogenesis and EBV

The transformation of a normal B lymphocyte to a malignant BL cell is a complex multi-step process, in which early childhood infection with EBV, chronic malaria infection and chromosomal translocation have all been identified as important contributory factors.

A constant feature of BL is the presence of a reciprocal chromosomal translocation between the c-myc oncogene on chromosome 8 and the immunoglobulin (Ig) heavy chain locus on chromosome 14 or, more rarely, the light chain loci on either 2 or 22.[57] This translocation event in B cells leads to deregulation of c-myc, a gene which normally drives cell proliferation, and this predisposes to lymphoma development. Mutations in the tumour suppressor gene p53 have also been identified in BL tumour cells, although these are thought to occur late in tumorogenesis.[58]

EBV DNA is present in up to 95% of tumours from endemic areas. The viral genome is clonal, indicating that virus infection was present in the initial tumour cell. Nearly all children in endemic areas are likely to have encountered EBV in early childhood. However, a prospective study of 42 000 children in Uganda found that those children who subsequently developed BL had a 10 times higher geometric mean IgG antibody titre to EB VCA than matched controls.[59] A similar pattern has been seen in more recent studies in Turkey.[60] In BL cells the only EBV protein expressed is EB viral nuclear antigen (EBNA)-1, which is required for viral replication and EBV genome maintenance. The classic EBV oncogenes, latent membrane protein (LMP)-1, EBNA-2 are not expressed, and the role of the virus in BL is therefore unclear. However, it is thought that this limited viral gene expression reduces recognition by the host immune system.[61]

At present it is not clear how early EBV infection, chronic parasitaemia and c-myc deregulation are linked in tumour pathogenesis. It is postulated that chronic parasite infection, be it malaria or other agents, leads to immunosuppression, altered cytokine profiles and polyclonal B cell stimulation. The increased turnover of B cells resulting from polyclonal activation increases the chance of a c-myc translocation occurring during Ig gene rearrangement, whereas the immunosuppression reduces EBV-specific cytotoxic T cell activity and allows a correspondingly higher number of circulating EBV-infected B cells to survive. This expanded pool of infected B cells also increases the chance of a translocation event occurring in a cell infected with EBV.

The role of malaria in BL is supported by the identification of high EBV DNA loads in serum of children, particularly those aged from 1–4, who live in holoendemic malaria regions[62] and that the treatment of malaria is associated with falling serum EBV DNA loads.[63] Additionally, the incidence of BL is known to fall in areas in which malaria has been eradicated.[64] It has also been postulated that sickle cell trait may reduce the risk of BL development as a consequence of its protection from malaria; however, epidemiological investigations have not reached statistical significance.[65] Though holoendemic malaria is thought to be an important co-factor in African BL, in other areas where a high rate of EBV-associated BL has been identified there is little Plasmodium falciparum malaria. In tropical Brazil young children commonly suffer from other infections such as schistosomiasis and leishmaniasis, in which chronic parasitaemia also leads to polyclonal B cell stimulation, and immunosuppression. Recent reports from Brazil have identified BL tumors in close association with schistosomiasis granuloma, and it is postulated that this chronic parasite infection predisposes to BL by inducing a change in local cytokine expression and a reduction in local immune surveillance.[55] This hypothesis requires further investigation.

Clinical features

BL is a very fast-growing tumour which in endemic areas classically presents in the jaw, possibly in association with molar tooth development (Figure 43.3). At diagnosis the tumour is often multifocal, with other common sites being the testis, ovary, breast (in pubertal girls), liver, stomach and intestine. Intra-abdominal lesions are being recognized more frequently with increased availability of ultrasound imaging. Lymph nodes and spleen are rarely involved, and bone marrow invasion only occurs during the ter-

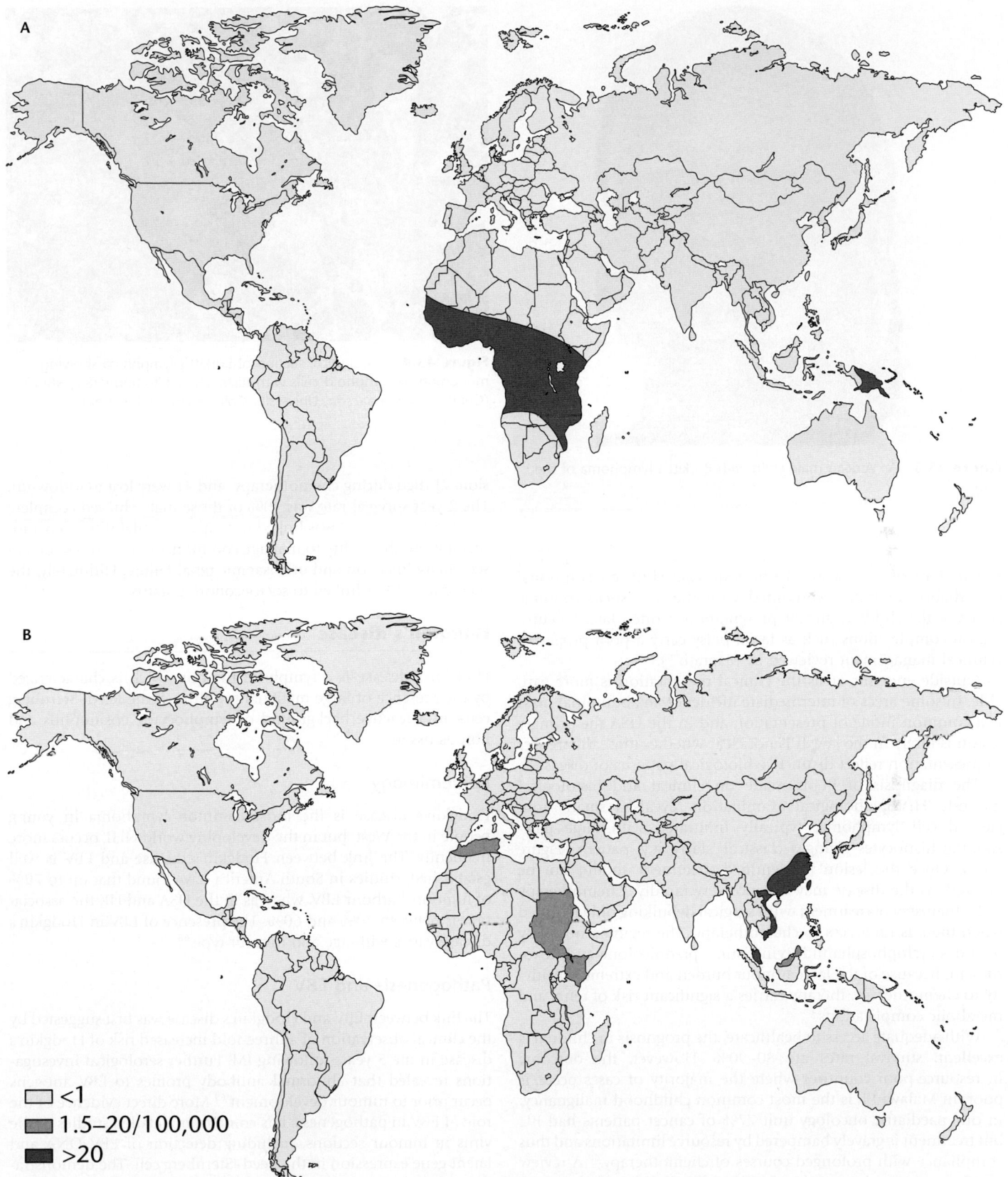

Figure 43.2 Worldwide distribution of incidence of EB virus-associated tumours: (A) Burkitt's lymphoma, and (B) nasopharyngeal carcinoma.

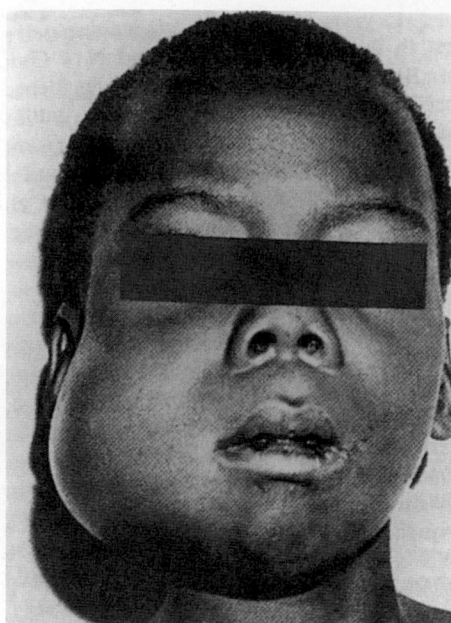

Figure 43.3 An African male child with Burkitt's lymphoma of the jaws.

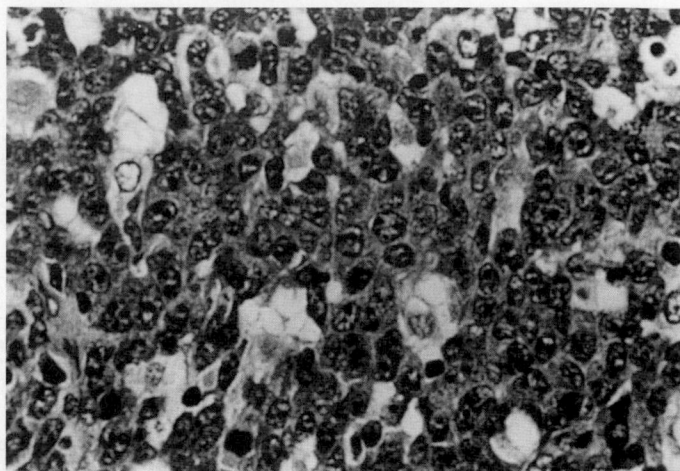

Figure 43.4 Histological section of Burkitt's lymphoma showing monomorphic lymphoid cells with histocytic infiltration (H&E, ×800). (Courtesy of P. Isaacson, University College Hospital, London.)

minal phase of the disease. The tumours cause little constitutional disturbance, and this, combined with the low socioeconomic status of the children, means presentation is often late.[53] Neurological complications such as facial palsy carry a poor prognosis (clinical management reviewed by Magrath[66]).

Outside endemic areas the clinical presentation is more variable. In some areas of intermediate incidence an abdominal mass is a common mode of presentation and in the USA the primary lesion is rarely in the jaw. It is not clear whether these differences in presentation reflect distinctive biological patterns of disease.[67]

The diagnosis of BL is made on clinical and histological grounds. Histopathological examination reveals a small, non-cleaved cell lymphoma, typically infiltrated with large pale-staining histiocytes giving a classical 'starry sky' pattern (Figure 43.4). Once the lesion is identified, treatment should not be delayed, as the disease may advance very rapidly. Chemotherapy is the mainstay of treatment, with surgical debulking only required when there is no access to chemotherapy. The regimen normally includes cyclophosphamide, vincristine, prednisolone and doxorubicin. Because of the large tumour burden and extreme sensitivity to chemotherapy, therapy carries a significant risk of renal and metabolic complications.[66]

With adequate access to healthcare, the prognosis in children is excellent; survival rates are 80–90%. However, the outcome in resource-poor countries where the majority of cases occur is poor. In Malawi BL is the most common childhood malignancy; in one paediatric oncology unit 77% of cancer patients had BL, but treatment is gravely hampered by resource limitations and thus compliance with prolonged courses of chemotherapy.[48] A review of 18 years' experience from the Côte d'Ivoire identified 433 BL patients, of whom only 219 completed systemic chemotherapy. Of these, 117 achieved complete remission, 40 achieved partial remis-

sion, 21 died during chemotherapy, and 41 were lost to follow-up. The 2-year survival rate was 70% of those that achieved complete remission.[53] Survival was linked not only to availability of chemotherapy, but the ability to manage common complications such as secondary infection and uricosaemic renal failure. Ultimately, the outcome of BL is linked to socioeconomic status.

Hodgkin's disease

Hodgkin's disease is a lymphoid tumour which is characterized by the presence of large malignant multinucleate Reed–Sternberg cells, in a reactive background of lymphocytes, eosinophils and fibrous tissue.

Epidemiology

Hodgkin's disease is the most common lymphoma in young people in the West, but in the developing world NHL occurs more frequently. The link between Hodgkin's disease and EBV is well established; studies in South America have found that up to 79% of tumours harbour EBV, whereas in the USA and UK the association is between 40% and 60%. The presence of EBV in Hodgkin's disease varies with age and tumour type.[68]

Pathogenesis and EBV

The link between EBV and Hodgkin's disease was first suggested by the clinical observation of a three-fold increased risk of Hodgkin's disease in the 5 years following IM. Further serological investigations revealed that abnormal antibody profiles to EBV antigens occur prior to tumour development.[69] More direct evidence of the role of EBV in pathogenesis has come from detailed studies of the virus in tumour sections, including detection of EBV DNA and latent gene expression in the Reed–Sternberg cell. The demonstration of viral clonality indicates that infection was present at the time of malignant transformation, suggesting that the virus contributes to the initial transformation event.[70] Extensive laboratory studies have identified expression of a number of key genes in EBV replication and oncogenesis. Of these EBNA-1, which is vital to replication, and LMP1, which is a viral oncogene, have both been identified in Hodgkin's disease.[71,72] As in other EBV-linked tumours, the restricted number of EBV genes expressed probably limits the ability of the immune system to identify aberrant malignant cells.

Another important clinical insight into the role of EBV in the disease is the increased incidence of Hodgkin's in those with HIV, even those on highly active antiretroviral therapy (HAART),[73] and the link with EBV is stronger in the immunosuppressed than the immunocompetent.[74]

Clinical features

Hodgkin's disease classically presents with lymph node enlargement and is treated with a combination of chemotherapy and radiotherapy. Prognosis is linked to stage, and age at presentation, but the overall 10-year survival is approximately 75–85% in the West. Early evidence from the UK, India and South Africa suggests that individuals with EBV-associated tumours have a better response to therapy, but it is not yet clear whether overall survival rates are also improved.[75,76,77] In the search for new treatment strategies, the presence of EBV in the tumour may be exploited to develop immunotherapy targeted at viral antigens.[78]

Post-transplant lymphoproliferative disease

Solid organ transplant recipients require long-term immunosuppression to prevent organ rejection. This places the recipient at risk of loss of immune control of persistent viruses as well as infection with new or unusual agents. EBV infection in this context, either as primary infection in children, or increased viral replication in adults, can predispose to the development of clonal B cell expansions and B cell lymphoma, collectively known as B cell lymphoproliferative disease (BLPD).[79] Between 1% and 10% of solid organ transplant recipients develop BLPD; the tumours are nearly always associated with EBV and usually follow an aggressive course. First-line treatment for BLPD is reduction of immunosuppression; however, recurrences often occur, and mortality remains high. Novel immunotherapies are currently being developed,[79] which may be extended for use in AIDS-related lymphoma and Hodgkin's disease.[78]

Epithelial cell tumours and EBV

Although there is no direct evidence of EBV infection of epithelial cells in the healthy host, EBV is able to infect epithelial cells in a number of pathological situations, both benign and malignant, oral hairy leukoplakia being an example of the former and nasopharyngeal carcinoma of the latter.[80,81]

Nasopharyngeal carcinoma

On a world wide basis, nasopharyngeal carcinoma (NPC) is one of the most common of the EBV-associated malignancies, and the one which is most consistently linked with EBV. NPC arises from squamous epithelial cells in the post-nasal space, and histopathologically it is subdivided into three categories: WHO I, II, III. WHO I is a keratinizing squamous carcinoma, WHO II is a non-

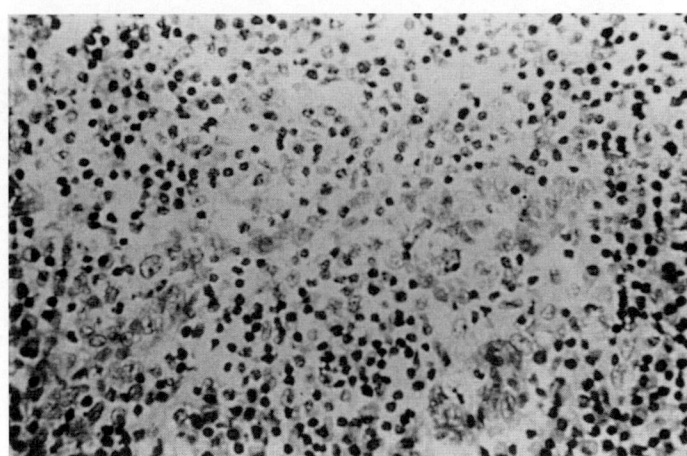

Figure 43.5 Histological section of undifferentiated nasopharyngeal carcinoma showing scattered malignant epithelial cells with heavy infiltrate of small lymphocytes (H&E, ×400).

keratinizing epidermoid type, and WHO III is undifferentiated or anaplastic (Figure 43.5). WHO III is invariably linked to EBV and is the most common type.[82]

Epidemiology

NPC has a distinct geographical pattern (Figure 43.2B): 44% of all NPC cases occur in China and 23% in South-east Asia. Endemic areas include southern China (Guangdong, Guanxi, Hunan and Fujian), where it is the most common tumour in men and the second commonest in women, and additionally Hong Kong, Thailand and Vietnam.[4] Outside Asia the incidence is lower, the only other high-risk population being the Inuit in Alaska and Greenland. The incidence is moderate in Morocco, Algeria, Sudan, Kenya and the Mediterranean basin, but NPC is rare in the rest of the world. In emigrés from endemic areas the incidence falls in one or two generations, but remains above that of low-risk populations.[83]

Pathogenesis and EBV

The presence of EBV DNA in malignant cells from nearly every case of undifferentiated NPC strongly suggests the virus has an essential role in oncogenesis. The events leading to malignant transformation are yet to be fully identified, but a number of important observations support a central role for the virus in the malignant process. Clonal EBV DNA has been identified in preinvasive NPC lesions, indicating that infection is a premalignant event.[84] The EBV oncogene LMP-1 is expressed in the malignant epithelial cells. Patients with NPC have abnormal EBV serology, typically with raised titres of IgA antibody against EBV early antigen (EA) and VCA which correlate with tumour burden.[82] Environmental and genetic co-factors are thought to be important in tumour development. The restricted geographical pattern of disease suggests that a genetic predisposition is important, and linkage to a HLA locus has been identified in Chinese populations at risk of NPC.[85] Childhood consumption of chemical carcinogens in preserved food has been suggested as a further risk factor in diverse geographical groups, including the Cantonese, Tunisians and Eskimos.[86]

Clinical features

NPC commonly occurs in the postnasal space and may present with non-specific symptoms such as nose bleeds or prolonged otitis media. However, the disease is often not symptomatic until spread to cervical lymph nodes or invasion of cranial nerves has occurred. The mainstay of treatment is radiotherapy, and 5-year survival rates following treatment are 80% for tumours limited to one site, but this is reduced to 20% for those with metastatic disease. Quantification of plasma EBV DNA may be a useful marker of disease burden in NPC, and had been shown to predict clinical outcome in patients with advanced disease.[87] Following the clinical success of EBV specific cytotoxic T cell therapy in PTLD[79] and Hodgkin's disease,[78] early trials have been reported for advanced NPC.[88,89]

Early detection is the best way to improve survival, and studies of EBV antigen-specific IgA in serum and saliva have proved useful for screening high-risk groups in southern China.[90] Rising antibody titres following treatment may herald a recurrence of disease; low or declining titres are indicative of a good prognosis.

Despite this clinical experience, a large population-based evaluation of screening strategies is warranted to establish the optimal panel of antibodies, as well as the sensitivity, specificity, cost effectiveness and timing of screening. The majority of survival data come from countries with adequate access to healthcare, with limited data from resource-poor countries. In one series of 150 patients in India the 5-year survival was only 13%.[91]

EBV and other cancers

Stomach cancer is the second most common cause of cancer death worldwide and EBV is associated with 4–18% of all stomach cancers, thus it represents the largest group of EBV-associated malignancies.[92] In tumours positive for the virus, EBV infection can be identified in every malignant cell and the DNA is clonal. These facts, as well as the identification of EBV in pre-malignant gastric lesions, suggest that EBV infection has a role in tumour pathogenesis.[93] EBV-positive gastric adenocarcinomas may be a distinct subset which have a lower frequency of lymph nodes metastasis;[94] however, larger studies are required. Other malignancies which have been linked to EBV include nasal T cell lymphoma, smooth muscle tumours in transplant recipients and salivary gland tumours.

EBV AND HIV

The immunodeficiency of HIV disturbs the tight control the host immune system has over quiescent persistent viral infections such as EBV, Kaposi's sarcoma-associated herpes virus, human papilloma virus and hepatitis C. Those with advancing HIV disease have decreased EBV-specific cytotoxic T cell activity, which allows increased viral replication and increased numbers of infected B cells, and results in high EBV loads in both blood and oropharyngeal secretions.[95,96] Reconstitution of EBV-specific T cells has been documented in patients on highly active antiretroviral therapy;

however, two small studies suggest that HAART does not substantially impact on EBV DNA load.[97,98] Diseases which occur in HIV have become some of the most common clinical problems associated with EBV.

Oral hairy leukoplakia

Oral hairy leukoplakia (OHL) is common in HIV-infected individuals throughout the world; in South Africa as many as 20% of those infected with HIV have evidence of OHL.[99] OHL presents as a white plaque with a characteristic ribbed appearance, typically on the lateral border of the tongue. It may occur as part of a seroconversion illness or as an early sign of progressive HIV disease.

Multiple strains of EBV infect the superficial layers of the squamous epithelium, resulting in epithelial cell hyperproliferation. In OHL the infected epithelial cells contain actively replicating virus, but there is no evidence that infection leads to malignant transformation.[80]

The lesions respond to a 2–3-week course of high-dose aciclovir, or to topical application of aciclovir cream or retinoic acid gel.

Lymphocytic interstitial pneumonitis

In lymphocytic interstitial pneumonitis (LIP) the lung alveolar septa are infiltrated by mononuclear cells leading to expansion of the lung interstitium. LIP is a common manifestation of HIV in children, particularly in Africa.[100] Like other opportunistic infections, the incidence of LIP has fallen in the West since the introduction of highly active antiretroviral therapy. LIP also occurs in those affected by autoimmune disease or treated with immunosuppressive therapies. Children usually present with hypoxia and the chest radiograph typically shows bilateral diffuse reticularnodular shadowing. Ideally, the diagnosis is confirmed by lung biopsy.

LIP in children has been linked to primary EBV infection, or may reflect increased viral replication due to reduced immune function. Examination of lung biopsy material has identified expansions of foci of B cells infected with EBV.[101] Further studies are warranted to clarify the role of EBV in the disease process.

EBV and AIDS-related cancers

Non-Hodgkin's lymphoma and EBV

AIDS-NHL are commonly aggressive high-grade B cell tumours, and are classified as an AIDS-defining illness. 'AIDS-related BL' and 'Burkitt-like lymphoma' (BLL) both have different epidemiological and biological characteristics from endemic childhood BL. BLL has morphological features intermediate between BL and large cell lymphoma, and commonly occurs in HIV, though not exclusively so.[102] Other AIDS-related NHL include AIDS-related primary central nervous system lymphoma (PCNSL) and AIDS-related diffuse large cell lymphoma (DLCL).

Epidemiology

NHL is the second commonest cancer in HIV-infected individuals, Kaposi's sarcoma being the most common,[103] and the aetiology of both cancers is linked to latent herpes virus infections. It is well established in the West that HIV-infected individuals have a much higher incidence of NHL, the risk of developing NHL being 60 times the risk of the general population.[104] In Africa, now that the median survival with HIV has increased to around 10 years,[105] the burden of AIDS-associated cancers has become apparent. In Uganda significant increases in incidence of NHL, including BL in children, have been identified.[106] In the West the incidence of NHL has fallen following the introduction of HAART. All types of AIDS-related NHL are linked to EBV, but the percentage of tumours in which EBV DNA can be identified varies with tumour type.[107] PCNSL is invariably linked with EBV, whereas 80% of DLCL are EBV positive and BL is only linked in around 50% of cases in the West.[70]

Pathogenesis and EBV

As in BL, the development of NHL in AIDS is a complex multi-step process, in which EBV infection may be one significant event. As already noted, HIV-infected individuals has impaired immune surveillance of EBV, and the combination of decreased cytotoxic T cells against EBV and increased viral load have been correlated with increased risk of AIDS DLCL. Persistent generalized lymphadenopathy (PGL) has long been recognized as being a common feature of HIV infection, and is caused by chronic B cell stimulation and expansion. The identification of EBV infection in PGL tissue may be a predisposing factor for the evolution of lymphoma.[108]

Clinical features

BL tends to occur quite early in the course of HIV, when the immune system is still relatively intact, and it typically occurs in young adults. It is not clear if the clinical course of BL in African children has changed in the context of marked immunosuppression.

In contrast to BL, primary cerebral NHL usually occurs with a CD4 count less than 50×10^6 and has a particularly poor prognosis. The majority of patients present with systemic features of weight loss, night sweats and fevers, combined with extranodal disease. Diagnosis may be confirmed by biopsy, but when this is not appropriate, identification of EBV in the cerebrospinal fluid of a patient with a cranial mass may help confirm the diagnosis of cerebral lymphoma.[109]

Primary effusion lymphoma is a rare variant of HIV-associated lymphoma in which there is no solid mass, but effusions in serosal cavities; both EBV and Kaposi's sarcoma-associated herpes virus can be often identified in the malignant cells.

The outcome for AIDS-related NHL remains poor, with the prognosis most critically linked to the degree of immunosuppression. Ideally, combination chemotherapy should be offered to those in the better prognostic groups. However, median survival even in the West is only 7–9 months, though outcomes have improved since the introduction of highly active antiviral therapy.[110]

Vaccine development

Both primary and persistent EBV infections are associated with significant pathology and this has led to interest in the development of an EBV vaccine. An ideal vaccine would prevent the main complication of late primary infection, IM, and prevent viral persistence, thereby potentially eradicating EBV-driven cancers.

Induction of neutralizing antibody to gp 350 should prevent virus binding to CD21, the key B cell receptor, and thus prevent infection. Gp 350 vaccines are under trial,[111] but it is not yet clear whether induction of an antibody response, possibly with induction of cytotoxic T cells to the same viral epitope, will provide sterile immunity.[112]

REFERENCES

1. Epstein MA, Achong BG, Barr YM. Virus particles in cultured lymphoblasts from Burkitt's lymphoma. *Lancet* 1964; 702–703.
2. Gerber P, Lucas S, Nonoyama M, et al. Oral excretion of Epstein–Barr virus by healthy subjects and patients with infectious mononucleosis. *Lancet* 1972; 11(2):988–999.
3. Lewin N, Aman P, Masucci MG, et al. Characterization of EBV–carrying B-cell populations in healthy seropositive individuals with regard to density, release of transforming virus and spontaneous outgrowth. *Int J Cancer* 1987; 39(4):472–476.
4. Pisani P, Parkin DM, Muñoz N, et al. Cancer and infection: estimates of the attributable fraction in 1990. *Cancer Epidemiol Biomarkers Prev* 1997; 6(6):387–400.
5. Henle W, Henle G, Lennette ET. The Epstein–Barr virus. *Sci Am* 1979; 241(1):48–59.
6. Haque T, Iliadou P, Hossain A, et al. Seroepidemiological study of Epstein–Barr virus infection in Bangladesh. *J Med Virol* 1996; 48(1):17–21.
7. Essers S, Schwinn A, ter Meulen J, et al. Seroepidemiological correlations of antibodies to human herpesviruses and human immunodeficiency virus type 1 in African patients. *Eur J Epidemiol* 1991; 7(6):658–664.
8. Dambaugh T, Beisel C, Hummel M, et al. Epstein–Barr virus (B95-8) DNA VII: molecular cloning and detailed mapping. *Proc Natl Acad Sci USA* 1980; 77(5):2999–3003.
9. Sample J, Young L, Martin B, et al. Epstein–Barr virus types 1 and 2 differ in their EBNA-3A, EBNA-3B, and EBNA-3C genes. *J Virol* 1990; 64(9): 4084–4092.
10. Zimber U, Adldinger HK, Lenoir GM, et al. Geographical prevalence of two types of Epstein–Barr virus. *Virology* 1986; 154(1):56–66.
11. Sculley TB, Apolloni A, Hurren L, et al. Coinfection with A- and B-type: Epstein–Barr virus in human immunodeficiency virus-positive subjects. *J Infect Dis* 1990; 162(3):643–648.
12. Srivastava G, Wong KY, Chiang AK, et al. Coinfection with multiple strains of Epstein–Barr virus in immunocompetent normal individuals; reassessment of the viral carrier state. *Blood* 2000; 95(7):2443–2445.
13. Crawford DH, Macsween KF, Higgins CD, et al. A cohort study among university students: identification of risk factors for Epstein–Barr virus seroconversion and infectious mononucleosis. *Clin Infect Dis* 2006; 43(3):276–282.
14. Miyashita EM, Yang B, Babcock GJ, et al. Identification of the site of Epstein–Barr virus persistence in vivo as a resting B cell. *J Virol* 1997; 71(7):4882–4891.
15. Ikeda T, Kobayashi R, Horiuchi M, et al. Detection of lymphocytes productively infected with Epstein–Barr virus in non-neoplastic tonsils. *J Gen Virol* 2000; 81(5):1211–1216.
16. Nikoskelainen J, Salmi HA, Laine MJ, et al. Epstein–Barr virus (EBV) infections in army recruits. *Acta Med Scand* 1974; 196(5):439–443.
17. Crawford DH, Swerdlow AJ, Higgins C, et al. Sexual history and Epstein-Barr virus infection. *J Infect Dis* 2002; 186(6):731–736.
18. Sawyer RN, Evans AS, Niederman JC, et al. Prospective studies of a group of Yale University freshmen. I. Occurrence of infectious mononucleosis. *J Infect Dis* 1971; 123(3):263–270.

19. Hallee TJ, Evans AS, Niederman JC, et al. Infectious mononucleosis at the United States Military Academy: a prospective study of a single class over four years. *Yale J Biol Med* 1974; 47(3):182–195.

20. Diepstra A, Niens M, Vellenga E, et al. Association with HLA class I in Epstein–Barr-virus-positive and with HLA class III in Epstein–Barr-virus-negative Hodgkin's lymphoma. *Lancet* 2005; 365(9478):2216–2224.

21. Israele V, Shirley P, Sixbey JW. Excretion of the Epstein–Barr virus from the genital tract of men. *J Infect Dis* 1991; 163(6):1341–1343.

22. Sixbey JW, Lemon SM, Pagano JS. A second site for Epstein–Barr virus shedding: the uterine cervix. *Lancet* 1986; ii(8516):1122–1124.

23. Thomas R, Macsween KF, McAulay K, et al. Evidence of shared Epstein–Barr viral isolates between sexual partners, and low level EBV in genital secretions. *J Med Virol* 2006; 78(9):1204–1209.

24. Higgins CD, Swerdlow AJ, Macsween KF, et al. A study of risk factors for acquisition of Epstein–Barr virus and its subtypes. *J Infect Dis* 2007; 195(4):474–482.

25. Pagano J. Is Epstein–Barr virus transmitted sexually? *Editorial Commentary.* JID 2007:195 (15 February): 469–447.

26. Sitki-Green DL, Edwards RH, Covington MM, et al. Biology of Epstein–Barr virus during infectious mononucleosis. *J Infect Dis* 2004; 189(3):483–492.

27. Tierney RJ, Edwards RH, Sitki-Green D, et al. Multiple Epstein–Barr virus strains in patients with infectious mononucleosis: comparison of ex vivo samples with in vitro isolates by use of heteroduplex tracking assays. *J Infect Dis* 2006; 193(2):287–297.

28. Cohen JI. Epstein–Barr virus infection. N Engl J Med 2000; 343(7):481–492.

29. Taga H, Taga K, Wang F, et al. Human and viral interleukin-10 in acute Epstein–Barr virus-induced infectious mononucleosis. *J Infect Dis* 1995; 171(5):1347–1350.

30. Parolini S, Bottino C, Falco M, et al. X-linked lymphoproliferative disease: 2B4 molecules displaying inhibitory rather than activating function are responsible for the inability of natural killer cells to kill Epstein–Barr virus-infected cells. *J Exp Med* 2000; 192(3):337–346.

31. Foss HD, Herbst H, Hummel M, et al. Patterns of cytokine gene expression in infectious mononucleosis. *Blood* 1994; 83(3):707–712.

32. Callan MF, Steven N, Krausa P, et al. Large clonal expansions of CD8+ T cells in acute infectious mononucleosis. *Nat Med* 1996; 2(8):906–911.

33. Epstein MA, Crawford DH. The Epstein–Barr virus. In: Weatherall DJ, Ledingham JGG, Warrell DA, eds. *Oxford Textbook of Medicine.* Oxford: Oxford University Press; 1996:352–356.

34. Candy B, Hotopf M. Steroids for symptom control in infectious mononucleosis. Cochrane Database Syst Rev 2006; 3 CD004402.

35. Fafi-Kremer S, Morand P, Brion JP, et al. Long-term shedding of infectious Epstein–Barr virus after infectious mononucleosis. *J Infect Dis* 2005; 191(6):985–989.

36. White PD, Thomas JM, Amess J, et al. Incidence, risk and prognosis of acute and chronic fatigue syndromes and psychiatric disorders after glandular fever. *Br J Psychiatry* 1998; 173:475–481.

37. Swanink CM, van der Meer JW, Vercoulen JH, et al. Epstein–Barr virus (EBV) and the chronic fatigue syndrome: normal virus load in blood and normal immunologic reactivity in the EBV regression assay. *Clin Infect Dis* 1995; 20(5):1390–1392.

38. Auwaerter PG. Infectious mononucleosis in middle age (clinical conference). *JAMA* 1999; 281(5):454–459.

39. Coffey AJ, Brooksbank RA, Brandau O, et al. Host response to EBV infection in X-linked lymphoproliferative disease results from mutations in an SH2-domain encoding gene. *Nat Genet* 1998; 20(2):129–135.

40. Sayos J, Wu C, Morra M, et al. The X-linked lymphoproliferative-disease gene product SAP regulates signals induced through the co-receptor SLAM. *Nature* 1998; 395(6701):462–469.

41. Maia DM, Peace-Brewer AL. Chronic, active Epstein–Barr virus infection. *Curr Opin Hematol* 2000; 7(1):59–63.

42. Klein G, Clifford P, Klein E, et al. Search for tumor-specific immune reactions in Burkitt lymphoma patients by the membrane immunofluorescence reaction. *Natl Acad Sci USA* 1966; 55:1628–1635.

43. Balfour HH Jr, Holman CJ, Hokanson KM, et al. A prospective clinical study of Epstein–Barr virus and host interactions during acute infectious mononucleosis. *J Infect Dis* 2005; 192(9):1505–1512.

44. Williams H, Macsween K, McAulay K, et al. Analysis of immune activation and clinical events in acute infectious mononucleosis. *J Infect Dis* 2004; 190(1):63–71.

45. Silins SL, Sherritt MA, Silleri JM, et al. Asymptomatic primary Epstein–Barr virus infection occurs in the absence of blood T-cell repertoire perturbations despite high levels of systemic viral load. *Blood* 2001; 98(13): 3739–3744.

46. Miller G, Shope T, Coope D, et al. Lymphoma in cotton-top marmosets after inoculation with Epstein–Barr virus: tumor incidence, histologic spectrum antibody responses, demonstration of viral DNA, and characterization of viruses. *J Exp Med* 1977; 145(4):948–967.

47. Pope JH, Horne MK, Scott W. Transformation of foetal human leukocytes in vitro by filtrates of a human leukaemic cell line containing herpes-like virus. *Int J Cancer* 1968; 3(6):857–866.

48. Philips JA. Is Burkitt's lymphoma sexy enough? *Lancet* 2006; 368: 2251–2252.

49. Rickinson AB. Epstein–Barr virus in action in vivo. *N Engl J Med* 1998; 338(20):1461–1463.

50. Ziegler JL, AnderssonM , Klein G, et al. Detection of Epstein–Barr virus DNA in American Burkitt's lymphoma. *Int J Cancer* 1976; 17(6): 701–706.

51. Williams EH, Smith PG, Day NE, et al. Space-time clustering of Burkitt's lymphoma in the West Nile district of Uganda: 1961–1975. *Br J Cancer* 1978; 37(1):109–122.

52. Burkitt DP, Wright DH. Geographical Distribution of Burkitt's Lymphoma. Edinburgh: Livingstone; 1970:186–197.

53. Plo KJ. Burkitt lymphoma in the Côte d'Ivoire from 1966 to 1995: a progress report. *Med Pediatr Oncol* 2000; 34(3):206–209.

54. Sandlund JT, Fonseca T, Leimig T, et al. Predominance and characteristics of Burkitt lymphoma among children with non-Hodgkin lymphoma in northeastern Brazil. *Leukemia* 1997; 11(5):743–746.

55. Araujo I, Foss HD, Bittencourt A, et al. Expression of Epstein–Barr virus-gene products in Burkitt's lymphoma in Northeast Brazil. *Blood* 1996; 87(12):5279–5286.

56. Ertem U, Duru F, Pamir A, et al. Burkitt's lymphoma in 63 Turkish children diagnosed over a 10 year period. *Pediatr Hematol Oncol* 1996; 13(2): 123–134.

57. Klein G. In defense of the 'old' Burkitt lymphoma scenario. Series title: *Advances in Viral Oncology.* New York: Raven Press; 1987; 207–211.

58. Gaidano G, Ballerini P, Gong JZ, et al. p53 mutations in human lymphoid malignancies: association with Burkitt lymphoma and chronic lymphocytic leukemia. *Proc Natl Acad Sci USA* 1991; 88(12):5413–5417.

59. de Thé G, Geser A, Day NE, et al. Epidemiological evidence for causal relationship between Epstein–Barr virus and Burkitt's lymphoma from Ugandan prospective study. *Nature* 1978; 274(5673):756–761.

60. Cavdar AO, Gözdaşoğlu S, Yavuz G, et al. Burkitt's lymphoma between African and American types in Turkish children: clinical, viral (EBV), and molecular studies. *Med Pediatr Oncol* 1993; 21(1):36–42.

61. Epstein MA, Crawford DH. Gammaherpesviruses: Epstein–Barr virus. In: Mahy BWJ, Collier L, eds. *Topley and Wilson's Microbiology and Microbial Infections.* Vol. 1. London: Arnold; 1998:351–366.

62. Moormann AM, Chelimo K, Sumba PO, et al. Exposure to holoendemic malaria results in suppression of Epstein–Barr virus-specific T cell immunosurveillance in Kenyan children. *J Infect Dis* 2007; 195(6): 799–808.

63. Clearance of circulating Epstein–Barr virus DNA in children with acute malaria after antimalaria treatment. *J Infect Dis* 2006; 193(7): 971–977.

64. Geser A, Brubaker G, Draper CC. Effect of a malaria suppression program on the incidence of African Burkitt's lymphoma. *Am J Epidemiol* 1989; 129(4):740–752.

65. Proceedings of the IARC Working Group on the Evaluation of Carcinogenic Risks to Humans. Epstein–Barr Virus and Kaposi's Sarcoma Herpesvirus/Human Herpesvirus 8. Lyon: France, 17–24 June 1997. *IARC Monogr Eval Carcinog Risks Hum* 1997; 70:1–492.

66. Magrath IT. Management of high-grade lymphomas. *Oncology* 1998; 12(10, Suppl 8):40–48.

67. Magrath I, Jain V, Bhatia K. Epstein–Barr virus and Burkitt's lymphoma. *Semin Cancer Biol* 1992; 3(5):285–295.

68. Chapman AL, Rickinson AB. Epstein–Barr virus in Hodgkin's disease. *Ann Oncol* 1998; 9(suppl 5):S5–S16.

69. Mueller N, Evans A, Harris NL, et al. Hodgkin's disease and Epstein–Barr virus: altered antibody pattern before diagnosis. *N Engl J Med* 1989; 320(11):689–695.

70. Weiss LM, Movahed LA, Warnke RA, et al. Detection of Epstein–Barr viral genomes in Reed-Sternberg cells of Hodgkin's disease. *N Engl J Med* 1989; 320(8):502–506.

71. Pallesen G, Hamilton-Dutoit SJ, Rowe M, et al. Expression of Epstein–Barr virus latent gene products in tumour cells of Hodgkin's disease. *Lancet* 1991; 337(8737):320–322.

72. Murray PG, Young LS, Rowe M, et al. Immunohistochemical demonstration of the Epstein–Barr virus-encoded latent membrane protein in paraffin sections of Hodgkin's disease. *J Pathol* 1992; 166(1):1–5.

73. Engels EA, Pfeiffer RM, Goedert JJ, et al. Trends in cancer risk among people with AIDS in the United States 1980–2002. AIDS. 2006; 20(12):1645–1654.

74. Carbone A, Gloghini A, Larocca LM, et al. Human immunodeficiency virus-associated Hodgkin's disease derives from post-germinal center B cells. *Blood* 1999; 93(7):2319–2326.

75. Murray PG, Billingham LJ, Hassan HT, et al. Effect of Epstein–Barr virus infection on response to chemotherapy and survival in Hodgkin's disease. *Blood* 1999; 94(2):442–447.

76. Naresh KN, Johnson J, Srinivas V, et al. Epstein–Barr virus association in classical Hodgkin's disease provides survival advantage to patients and correlates with higher expression of proliferation markers in Reed-Sternberg cells. *Ann Oncol* 2000; 11(1):91–96.

77. Engel M, Essop MF, Close P, et al. Improved prognosis of Epstein–Barr virus associated childhood Hodgkin's lymphoma: study of 47 South African cases. *J Clin Pathol* 2000; 53(3):182–186.

78. Rooney CM, Roskrow MA, Suzuki N, et al. Treatment of relapsed Hodgkin's disease using EBV-specific cytotoxic T cells. *Ann Oncol* 1998; 9(suppl. 5): S129–S132.

79. Haque T, Crawford DH. The role of adoptive immunotherapy in the prevention and treatment of lymphoproliferative disease following transplantation. *Br J Haematol* 1999; 106(2):309–316.

80. Greenspan JS, Greenspan D, Lennette ET, et al. Replication of Epstein–Barr virus within the epithelial cells of oral 'hairy' leukoplakia, an AIDS-associated lesion. *N Engl J Med* 1985; 313(25):1564–1571.

81. zur Hausen H, Schulte-Holthausen H, Klein G, et al. EBV DNA in biopsies of Burkitt tumours and anaplastic carcinomas of the nasopharynx. *Nature* 1970; 228(276):1056–1058.

82. Vokes EE, Liebowitz DN, Weichselbaum RR. Nasopharyngeal carcinoma. *Lancet* 1997; 350(9084):1087–1091.

83. Pagano PS. The Epstein–Barr virus and nasopharyngeal carcinoma. *Cancer* 1994; 74(9):2414–2424.

84. Raab-Traub N. Epstein–Barr virus and nasopharyngeal carcinoma. *Semin Cancer Biol* 1992; 3(5):297–307.

85. Simons MJ, Wee GB, Goh EH, et al. Immunogenetic aspects of nasopharyngeal carcinoma. IV. Increased risk in Chinese of nasopharyngeal carcinoma associated with a Chinese-related HLA profile (A2, Singapore 2). *J Natl Cancer Inst* 1976; 57(5):977–980.

86. West S, Hildesheim A, Dosemeci M. Non-viral risk factors for nasopharyngeal carcinoma in the Philippines: results from a case-control study. *Int J Cancer* 1993; 55(5):722–727.

87. Wei W, Sham W. Nasopharyngeal cancer. *Lancet* 2005; 365:2041–2054.

88. Straathof KC, Bollard CM, Popat U, et al. Treatment of nasopharyngeal carcinoma with Epstein–Barr virus- specific T lymphocytes. *Blood* 2005; 105(5):1898–1904.

89. Comoli P, Pedrazzoli P, Maccario R, et al. Cell therapy of stage IV nasopharyngeal carcinoma with autologous Epstein–Barr virus-targeted cytotoxic T lymphocytes. *J Clin Oncol* 2005; 23(35):8942–8949.

90. Chen HH, Prevost TC, Duffy SW. Evaluation of screening for nasopharyngeal carcinoma: trial design using Markov chain models. *Br J Cancer* 1999; 79 (11–12):1894–1900.

91. Koppikar SB, Advani SH, Gopal R, et al. Nasopharyngeal carcinoma in India: end-result analysis (1980–1984). *J Surg Oncol* 1988; 39(3):179–182.

92. Takada K. Epstein–Barr virus and gastric carcinoma. *Mol Pathol* 2000; 53(5):255–261, Review.

93. Yanai H, Takada K, Shimizu N, et al. Epstein–Barr virus infection in non–carcinomatous gastric epithelium. *J Pathol* 1997; 183(3):293–298.

94. van Beek J, zur Hausen A, Klein Kranenbarg E, et al. EBV-positive gastric adenocarcinomas: a distinct clinicopathologic entity with a low frequency of lymph node involvement. *J Clin Oncol* 2004; 22(4):664–670.

95. Birx DL, Redfield RR, Tosato G. Defective regulation of Epstein–Barr virus infection in patients with acquired immunodeficiency syndrome (AIDS) or AIDS-related disorders. *N Engl J Med* 1986; 314(14):874–879.

96. Kersten MJ, Klein MR, Howerda AM, et al. Epstein–Barr virus-specific cytotoxic T cell responses in HIV-1 infection: different kinetics in patients progressing to opportunistic infection or non-Hodgkin's lymphoma. *J Clin Invest* 1997; 99(7):1525–1533.

97. Piriou E, Jansen CA, van Dort K, et al. Reconstitution of EBV latent but not lytic antigen-specific CD4+ and CD8+ T cells after HIV treatment with highly active antiretroviral therapy. *J Immunol* 2005; 175(3):2010–2017.

98. Righetti E, Ballon G, Ometto L, et al. Dynamics of Epstein Barr virus in HIV-1 infected subjects on highly active antiretroviral therapy. *AIDS* 2002; 16(1):63–73.

99. Arendorf TM, Bredekamp B, Cloete C, et al. Oral manifestations of HIV infection in 600 South African patients. *J Oral Pathol Med* 1998; 27(4): 176–179.

100. Jeena PM, Coovadia HM, Thula SA, et al. Persistent and chronic lung disease in HIV-1 infected and uninfected African children. *AIDS* 1998; 12(10): 1185–1193.

101. Brodie SJ, de la Rosa C, Howe JG, et al. Pediatric AIDS-associated lymphocytic interstitial pneumonia and pulmonary arterio-occlusive disease: role of VCAM-1/VLA-4 adhesion pathway and human herpesviruses. *Am J Pathol* 1999; 154(5):1453–1464.

102. Davi F, Delecluse HJ, Guiet P et al. Burkitt-like lymphomas in AIDS patients: characterization within a series of 103 human immunodeficiency virus-associated non-Hodgkin's lymphomas. Burkitt's Lymphoma Study Group. *J Clin Oncol* 1998; 16(12):3788–3795.

103. International Collaboration on HIV and Cancer. Highly active antiretroviral therapy and incidence of cancer in human immunodeficiency virus-infected adults. *J Natl Cancer Inst* 2000; 92(22):1823–1830.

104. Beral V, Peterman T, Berkelman R, et al. AIDS-associated non-Hodgkin lymphoma. *Lancet* 1991; 337(8745):805–809.

105. Morgan D, Whitworth J. The natural history of HIV-1 infection in Africa. *Nat Med* 2001; 7(2):143–145.

106. Wabinga HR, Parkin DM, Wabire-Mangen F, et al. Trends in cancer incidence in Kyadondo County, Uganda, 1960–1997. *Br J Cancer* 2000; 82(9): 1585–1592.

107. Gaidano G, Capello D, Carbone A. The molecular basis of acquired immunodeficiency syndrome-related lymphomagenesis. *Semin Oncol* 2000; 27(4):431–441.

108. Shibata D, Weiss LM, Nathwani BN, et al. Epstein–Barr virus in benign lymph node biopsies from individuals infected with the human immunodeficiency virus is associated with concurrent or subsequent development of non-Hodgkin's lymphoma. *Blood* 1991; 77(7):1527–1533.

109. Bower M, Fife K. In: Gazzard B, ed. *Chelsea and Westminster Hospital AIDS Care Handbook*. London: Mediscript; 1999:102–110.

110. Vaccher E, Spina M, di Gennaro G, et al. Concomitant cyclophosphamide, doxorubicin, vincristine, and prednisone chemotherapy plus highly active antiretroviral therapy in patients with human immunodeficiency virus-related, non-Hodgkin lymphoma. *Cancer* 2001; 91(1):155–163.

111. Denis M, Haumont H, Bollen A. Vaccination against Epstein–Barr virus (EBV): Report of phase II studies using recombinant viral glycoprotein gp350 in healthy adults. Abstract 11th Biennial Conference of the International Association for research on Epstein–Barr Virus and Associated Diseases; September 2004, Regensburg, Germany.

112. Jackman WT, Mann KA, Hoffmann HJ, et al. Expression of Epstein–Barr virus gp350 as a single chain glycoprotein for an EBV subunit vaccine. *Vaccine* 1999; 17(7–8):660–668.

Chapter 44 Mary J. Warrell

Rabies

Rabies is a widespread infection of certain mammal species which is occasionally transmitted to man. Rabies is also known as hydrophobia, *la rage* in French, *la rabbia* in Italian, *la rabia* in Spanish, *la ravia* in Portuguese and *die Tollwut* in German.

HISTORY

Transmission of the infection from dogs' saliva was known to the Egyptians at the time of the Pharaohs, and suggested methods of treatment are found in Chinese manuscripts from the fifth century BC.[1] Animal rabies was described by Aristotle in the fourth century BC, and the Roman, Celsus, wrote of the human illness in the first century AD, when knowledge and fear of the disease were widespread. A sixteenth-century Italian physician, Fracastoro, described the clinical features of rabies.[2]

John Hunter initiated a scientific approach to rabies in 1793 and experiments on transmission of the infection were carried out in Germany by Zinke, and in France by Magendie early in the nineteenth century. Louis Pasteur's work in the 1880s demonstrated that rabies was an infection of the central nervous system. He repeatedly passaged virulent 'street' virus in rabbits, attenuating it to a 'fixed' laboratory strain, used to make the first rabies vaccine.[2]

Growth of the virus in tissue culture was achieved in the 1930s and the virus was first visualized by electron microscopy in the early 1960s.[3]

VIRUS

Rabies virus is a species of the genus *Lyssavirus* (Gk *lyssa*, rage/frenzy) of the large family of Rhabdoviridae (Gk *rhabdos*, rod). Seven genotypes are now recognized:[4] rabies genotype 1 and rabies-related viruses genotypes 2–7 (Table 44.1). All but one have caused fatal infection in man (see below). The lyssaviruses are divided into two phylogroups. Phylogroup II is relatively less pathogenic. Novel unclassified viruses have been identified in bats.[5] Other rhabdoviruses which very rarely cause disease in humans are: the vesicular stomatitis viruses, *Chandipura*, *Piry* and *Le Dantec* viruses.[6]

The bullet-shaped rabies virion (Figure 44.1) measures 180×75 nm, and contains a single strand of negative-sense RNA encoding five proteins. The genome combines with a nucleoprotein, a phosphoprotein and RNA polymerase to form a helical coil. This viral core, the ribonucleoprotein complex, is covered by a matrix protein and then by a glycoprotein bearing club-shaped spikes (Figure 44.1B) which project outward through a host cell-derived lipid bilayer.[7,8]

Inactivation

Rabies virus is rapidly inactivated by heat. At 56°C the half-life is less than 1 min, but at 37°C it is prolonged to several hours in moist conditions. At 4°C, there is little loss after 2 weeks.[9]

The lipid coat is disrupted by detergents or a simple 1% soap solution. Other virucidal agents include 45% ethanol, iodine solutions (1:10 000 available iodine) and 1% benzalkonium chloride, but phenol is not so effective.

GEOGRAPHICAL DISTRIBUTION

Rabies and rabies-related lyssaviruses are endemic worldwide with a few exceptions. Areas recently been reported to be rabies-free include: New Zealand; Papua New Guinea; Japan; Taiwan; Hong Kong Islands; Singapore; Peninsula Malaysia, Sabah, Sarawak, some islands of Indonesia (e.g. Bali), and in the Indian Ocean; many Pacific islands, e.g. Solomon Islands, Fiji, Samoa and Cook Islands; Ireland, Iceland, Finland, Sweden, Norway, Portugal, Italy, Greece, Mediterranean islands; some Caribbean islands (e.g. Barbados, Bahamas, Jamaica and Antigua); and Antarctica. The UK, along with other Western European countries and Australia, have rabies-related lyssaviruses in bats but not in terrestrial species. Although some countries have no canine or sylvatic rabies, infected wild animals cross land borders. Imported rabies is a universal risk.

The rabies virus occurs in separate cycles of transmission within dogs and wild mammal reservoir species. Infection sometimes spills over to other species, including domestic mammals and humans. Strains of virus from different species and locations can be identified by genetic sequence analysis or by antigenic typing using a panel of monoclonal antibodies. The enzootic in domestic dogs is of most importance to man, and is the cause of more than 95% of human rabies cases (Figure 44.2). The pattern of sylvatic (wildlife) rabies shows great geographical variation, and

Table 44.1 Classification of genus *lyssavirus* of the rhabdoviridae family

Lyssavirus genotype		Source	Known distribution
PHYLOGROUP I			
1. Rabies virus		Dog, fox, mongoose, raccoon, skunk etc., bats (in Americas only)	Widespread
4. Duvenhage		Insectivorous bat, e.g. *Nycteris thebaica*	South Africa, Zimbabwe (very rare)
5. European bat Lyssavirus	1a	bats, e.g. *Eptesicus serotinus*	Denmark, Germany, Netherlands, Russia, Poland, France, Hungary Czech Republic
	1b[a]	bats, e.g. *Eptesicus serotinus*	Netherlands, France, Spain
6. European bat Lyssavirus	2a	*Myotis dasycneme* bats	Netherlands, France (rare)
		Myotis daubentonii bats	UK
	2b	*Myotis daubentonii* bat	Switzerland (very rare)
7. Australian bat Lyssavirus		Flying foxes/fruit bats (*Pteropus* spp.); insectivorous bats	Australia
Unclassified[a,b]			
Irkut		*Murina leucogaster* bat	Siberia
Aravan		*Myotis blythi* bat	Kyrghyzstan
Khujand		*Myotis mystacinus* bat	Tajikistan
PHYLOGROUP II			
3. Mokola		Shrews (*Crocidura* spp.), cats[c], dogs[c]	Southern Africa, Nigeria, Cameroon, Ethiopia (rare)
2. Lagos bat virus[a]		Fruit bats, cats[c], dogs[c]	Africa (rare)
Unclassified[a,b]			
West Caucasian bat virus		*Miniopterus schreibersi* bat	Russia

[a] Viruses have *not* been detected in man.
[b] Single isolates only.
[c] Not reservoir species, but have been infected and are potential vectors.

knowledge of local current epizootics enables the prevention of human rabies fatalities (Figures 44.3–44.5). The distribution of dominant reservoir species is summarized in Table 44.2.[10–22]

INCIDENCE

In endemic tropical areas, especially where dogs are the dominant vector, the true incidence of human rabies is unknown because of under-reporting or lack of published figures. Estimates for Asia and Africa include an annual mortality of 55 000, with an incidence of $1.4/10^5$ population, but gross under-reporting is suspected and the figures may be 30-fold higher.[23] There is a high mortality, 20 000/year, in India and also in Bangladesh and Pakistan. Human deaths from dog rabies in China increased 30% between 2005 and 2006. Low mortalities persist in Latin America,[14] especially in Brazil, Colombia, El Salvador and Haiti, and in outbreaks of vampire bat rabies in Amazonian regions of Peru and Ecuador. In the USA, where sylvatic rabies is endemic, there have been 48 deaths over 16 years up to 2006. A total of 81% were indigenous, and 90% of these were due to infection from bats, although most do not report a bat bite. Recent European data show an average of 11 deaths annually, of which two are imported and the majority of indigenous cases are in Russia.

RABIES-RELATED VIRUS INFECTIONS

All lyssavirus genotypes[10,18] (Table 44.1) have caused human deaths, except for genotype 2: *Lagos bat virus. Mokola* virus, genotype 3, caused fatal encephalitis in a Nigerian child, while another recovered from pharyngitis and probably a febrile convulsion.[24,25] A laboratory worker recovered from an accidental infection.[26] *Duvenhage* virus is named after the first of three patients who had rabies-like encephalitis caused by the virus.[27,28]

European insectivorous bats harbour *European bat Lyssavirus* genotypes 5 (*EBLV 1*) and 6 (*EBLV 2*), and each is subdivided into subtypes a and b (Table 44.1).[21] Five human infections from bats have been reported in Europe. Two Russian girls died of rabies following bat bites.[29,30] In Finland in 1985, a Swiss zoologist bitten by a bat from an unknown source died in Finland of furious rabies-like encephalitis, due to *EBLV 2b*.[31] In 2002, a bat conservationist in Scotland, UK, died from infection with *EBLV 2a*,[32] and a Ukranian died from clinically diagnosed infection including hydrophobia after a bat bite.[33] A similar case occurred in China the same year.[34]

In Australia in 1996, flying foxes (fruit bats, genus *Pteropus*) were discovered to harbour the *Australian bat Lyssavirus* (genotype 7),[16,22] which has caused a rabies-like fatal illness in two women.

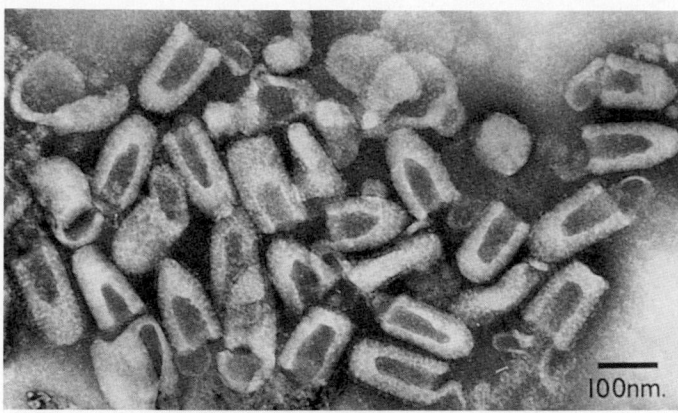

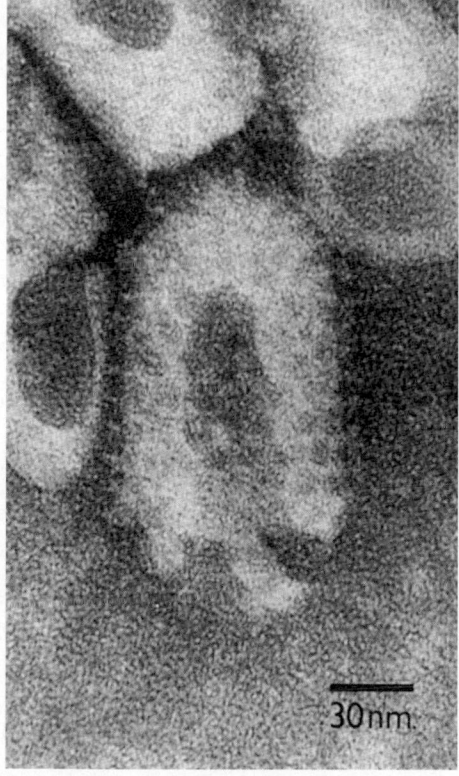

Figure 44.1 (A) and (B) Negatively stained electron micrographs of bullet-shaped rabies virions; (B) shows projections on the surface of the glycoprotein coat, covering all but the blunt end of the virion. (Courtesy of C. J. Smale and Joan Crick.)

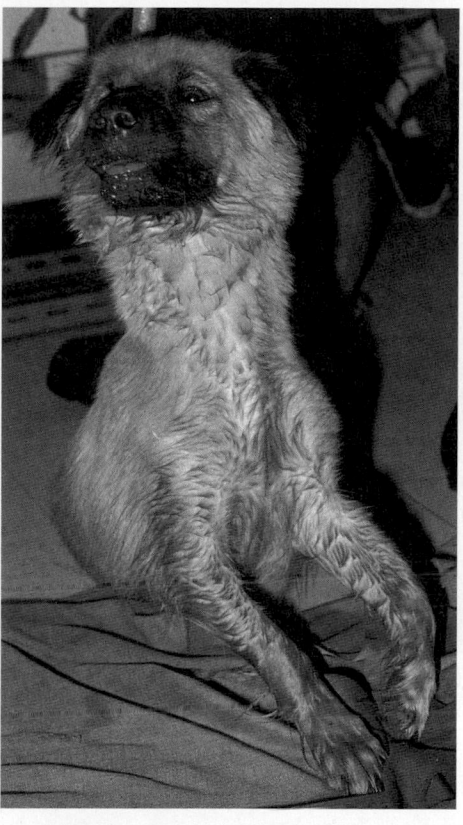

Figure 44.2 Domestic dog with paralytic rabies in Bangkok. Paralysis of neck and drooling of saliva. (©D. A. Warrell.)

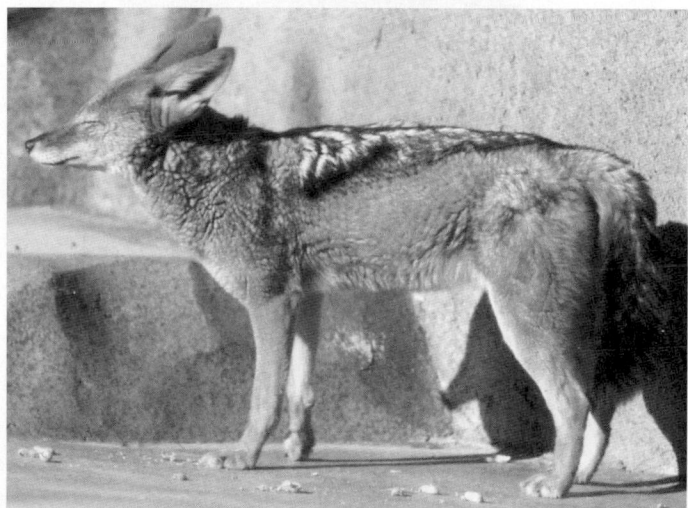

Figure 44.3 Black-backed jackal (*Canis mesomelas*), an important vector/reservoir of sylvatic rabies in Zambia, Zimbabwe and Namibia. (©D. A. Warrell.)

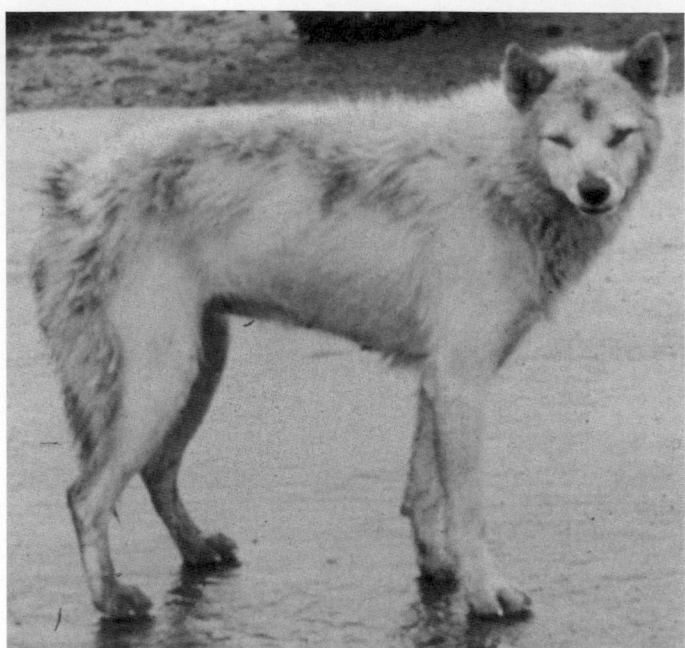

Figure 44.4 Rabid husky dog in Greenland. Probably infected with an arctic fox strain of virus. (©D. A. Warrell.)

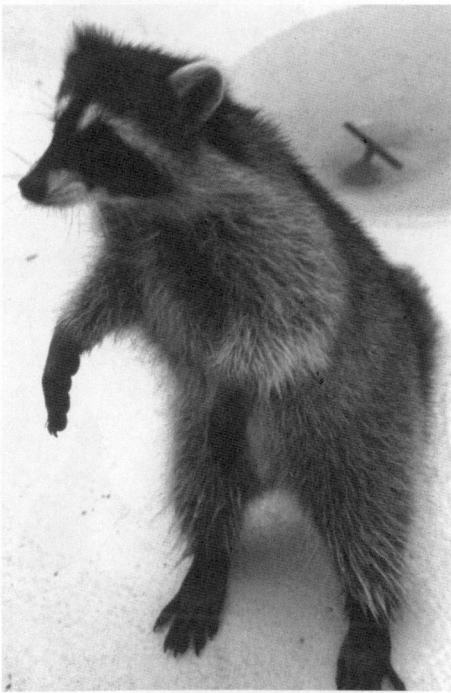

Figure 44.5 Raccoon (*Procyon lotor*), an important vector/reservoir of sylvatic rabies in North America. (©D. A. Warrell.)

Table 44.2 Distribution of important reservoir species of rabies genotype 1 and other lyssaviruses

Species	Distribution
AFRICA[10]	
Domestic dog[11]	Widespread dominant vector
Black-backed jackals (*Canis mesomelas*)[11]	Zambia, Zimbabwe, Namibia
Yellow mongoose (*Cynicitis penicillata*)[12]	South Africa
AMERICAS[13,14]	
Arctic fox (*Alopex lagopus*)	North-west Canada, Alaska
Striped skunk (*Mephitis mephitis*)	Central Canada and USA, California
Raccoon (*Procyon lotor*)	Mid-Atlantic states and south-east USA
Fox	Arizona, Texas and north-eastern USA, Canada
Coyote (*Canis latrans*)	Southern Texas
Insectivorous bats[15,16]	USA and South America
Domestic dog[14]	Widespread Mexico, Central and parts of South America
Vampire bat (*Desmodontidae*)[14,16]	Southern Texas, Mexico, Trinidad and Tobago, Central and South America south to Argentina and Chile
Mongoose (*Herpestes* species)[17]	Puerto Rico, Grenada, Cuba, Dominican Republic
ASIA[18]	
Domestic dog	Widespread dominant vector
Wolf	Iran, Iraq, Afghanistan
EUROPE AND MIDDLE EAST[18]	
Fox[19]	Widespread from France, east to Russian Federation
Arctic fox (*Alopex lagopus*)	Northern Russia
Raccoon dog (*Nycterentes procyonoides*)[20]	Baltic states, Russia, Poland, Ukraine
Wolf[20]	Russian Federation
Dog	Turkey, southern Russian states
Insectivorous bats[16,21,a]	Germany, Denmark, Netherlands, Russia, Poland, Spain, France, Czech Republic, Switzerland, Hungary, UK
AUSTRALIA[16,22]	
Fruit bats (flying foxes) (*Pteropus* spp.)[b]	Northern and Eastern coastal regions

All rabies virus genotype 1, except for [a]genotypes 5 and 6 in Europe (European bat Lyssavirus) and [b]genotype 7 in Australia (Australian bat lyssavirus).

Lyssavirus antibodies, some related to genotype 7, have been reported in bats in the Philippines, Cambodia, Thailand and Bangladesh. In Europe, *EBLV* seropositive bats with PCR-positive saliva indicate that bat infections are not always fatal. There is no evidence of chronic infection or virus excretion in bats.[35]

TRANSMISSION OF INFECTION

Animal contact

Humans are usually infected by virus-laden saliva, inoculated during the bite of a rabid dog. Inoculation of rabies virus into a wound or onto a mucous membrane may result in infection. This includes contamination of an unhealed lesion. Intact skin is a barrier against viral entry. The chance of developing rabies following exposure is revealed by data from the pre-vaccine era (see Efficacy of post-exposure prophylaxis, below).

Human-to-human

There are old anecdotal reports of infections from contact with human saliva, kissing, biting, sexual intercourse, breast-feeding and eating infected meat, but these routes remain unproven in man. Viraemia has not been detected.[36]

Transmission has occurred through *grafting of infected corneas*. Six virologically proven cases followed transplants from donors with unsuspected rabies. In Texas and in Germany, a mysterious encephalitis killed a total of seven *organ transplant* recipients. Liver, kidney, pancreas and even an iliac artery graft transmitted rabies virus from two donors aged 20 and 26 years old, who both died of undiagnosed neurological disease. Subsequent histories elicited a previous bat bite in the USA and contact with a dog in India.[37,38,39] Two cornea transplant recipients were given rabies post-exposure prophylaxis and remain healthy.[39]

Transplacental infection occurs in animals and a Turkish woman and her 2-day-old infant died of virologically confirmed rabies.[40] This is exceptional. Many mothers with rabies have been delivered of healthy babies.

Other routes

Two rabies infections resulted from inhaled aerosols of 'fixed' virus in laboratory accidents.[41,42] Two more people were possibly infected by inhalation of aerosolized virus in bat-infested caves, but direct bat contact was not excluded.[15]

PATHOGENESIS

The extraordinary journey of rabies virions along nerves up to the brain, and then outward to many organs, is gradually being unravelled.[8,43] It usually begins with the bite of a rabid animal inoculating virus-laden saliva through the skin, often into muscle. Experiments show viral replication occurring locally in striated muscle or mucous membrane, or directly invading a nerve cell. The virus can attach to several types of cell receptors. Neuronal infection may involve specific binding to the post-synaptic nicotinic acetylcholine receptor at neuromuscular junctions, and the neural cell adhesion molecule. Rabies enters the cell by glycoprotein-dependent endocytosis.[44]

Once inside a neurone the virus moves centripetally carried by retrograde axonal transport at a rate of 3 mm/h experimentally. There is evidence that attachment to dynein molecular motors may occur via the phosphoprotein on naked nucleocapsids or perhaps indirectly, via the p75 neurotrophin receptor (p75NTR), to the glycoprotein surface of a whole virion.[35] Its progress can be halted by sectioning nerves or by microtubule inhibitors, such as colchicine. Rabies ascends through ganglia, eventually reaching the brain by trans-synaptic spread, where intraneuronal replication occurs on a massive scale. Viral proteins accumulate in the cytoplasm, appearing as inclusions – the classical Negri bodies. Involvement of the limbic system causes aggressive behaviour and enables transmission from a vector species to another host. The often minimal histopathological changes do not account for the gross neuronal dysfunction, but there is evidence of viral influence on the expression of host genes accounting for suppression of immune responses and possibly altered neurotransmitter activity.

The rabies virus remains virtually confined to neurones as centrifugal dissemination progresses via autonomic and peripheral nerves. The virus has been isolated from human skeletal and cardiac muscle, skin, lung, kidney, adrenal, lacrimal and, of course, salivary glands.[36] Rabies antigen is found in neuronal tissue in most of these areas and around the gastrointestinal tract.[45]

In contrast to events in neurones, virus replication in acinar cells of the salivary glands produces large amounts of extracellular virus. Although there is no evidence of viraemia, rabies virus is shed in human lacrimal and respiratory tract secretions and possibly in urine[36] and in milk.

Rabies infection influences host neuronal gene expression, altering neuronal function and probably contributing to clinical effects. The virus evades immunological surveillance until a late stage of the disease. At the site of inoculation, some virus is briefly exposed, but once within the CNS virions and their antigens are hidden. During the final centrifugal phase of infection, when extracellular virus is produced, rabies antigens are expressed on cell membranes but if an immune response is induced, it is too late to combat the overwhelming infection (see Immunity, below).

PATHOLOGY

Cerebral congestion and a few petechial haemorrhages are usual findings in rabies encephalitis, but not gross cerebral oedema.[46,47] A lymphocytic perivenous infiltrate is common, and neutrophils are occasionally seen, perhaps only early in the disease. Eosinophilic cytoplasmic inclusions (Negri bodies) are found in 75% of cases, most frequently in large neurones of the hippocampus, Purkinje cells of the cerebellum and medulla.[48] Negri bodies contain eosinophilic rabies nucleoprotein matrix, occasional virions and small basophilic masses, probably fragments of host cell organelles, mechanically trapped during fusion of smaller inclusions.[3]

Neuronophagia, microglial reaction, foci of demyelination and perineural infiltration (Babès' nodules) also occur.[48] The brain stem and spinal cord are predominantly affected, but changes are often widespread. A meningeal reaction is common in children, and in paralytic disease the spinal cord is most severely affected. The extent of the histopathological change varies from complete disruption of neuronal structure and axonal degeneration of peripheral nerves following intensive care,[49] to an absence of any inflammation or degeneration.[46,47]

Extraneural pathology includes focal degeneration of salivary glands, liver, pancreas, adrenal medulla and lymph nodes,[50] and also interstitial myocarditis.[45,51]

IMMUNOLOGY

Response to infection

Following a rabid bite, no immune response is detectable in unvaccinated subjects before encephalitis has developed. Rabies antibody is first found in serum, then in cerebrospinal fluid (CSF) at least a week after the onset.[52] Neutralizing antibody may rise to a high level if life is prolonged. Specific rabies IgM antibody is occasionally found, but is unhelpful in diagnosis as it does not appear early and can also be present in postvaccinal encephalitis.[53]

There is little evidence of lymphocyte-mediated responses to encephalitis in man. Pleocytosis is observed in only 60% of patients, with a mean leucocyte count of 75/mm³,[52] Peripheral blood lymphocyte transformation has been shown in a few cases of furious rabies.[54] Very low levels of interferon have been found in the serum and CSF of about 30% of patients with rabies encephalitis.[55] Animal models show that clearance of virus from the CNS is dependent on CD4+ T lymphocytes by non-specific cytokine induction (e.g. γIFN) and as a B-cell helper to produce neutralizing antibody.[56] Survival following attenuated rabies infection is associated with increased neuronal apoptosis and cell surface expression of viral glycoprotein, features which are probably connected.[43,35]

Response to vaccine

The best available measure of immunity after vaccine treatment is the level of glycoprotein-induced neutralizing antibody, which usually appears 7–14 days after starting a primary vaccine course. The amount of antibody needed for protection against rabies in man cannot be determined, but the World Health Organization (WHO) recommends that a minimum neutralizing antibody level of 0.5 IU/mL should be attained to demonstrate unequivocal seroconversion.[57] The production of neutralizing antibody following rabies vaccine is influenced genetically. A relatively delayed, lower response occurred in up to 10% of vaccinees.[58] Increasing age (over 50 years) also impairs antibody production.[59]

The role of cell-mediated immunity in protection against disease is not clear. A small amount of interferon may be induced briefly following a first dose of rabies vaccine,[60] but it is very unlikely to afford significant protection in man.

CLINICAL FEATURES

Incubation period

The interval between inoculation and the onset of symptoms is between 20 and 90 days in at least 60% of cases,[61] but it has varied from 4 days[62] to 19 years.[63] It is reported to be over a year in 4–

6%.[61] In general, the nearer the bite is to the head, the shorter the incubation period.

Prodromal symptoms

Itching or paraesthesiae at the site of the healed bite wound are the only specific prodromal symptoms, occurring in about 40% of patients (Figure 44.6).[62] The wide range of non-specific features include fever, headache, myalgia, fatigue, sore throat, gastrointestinal symptoms, irritability, anxiety and insomnia. The disease progresses to either furious or paralytic rabies encephalomyelitis, usually within 1 week.[64]

Furious rabies

This familiar presentation is probably the more common in humans. Malfunction of the brain stem nuclei, limbic system, reticular activating system and higher centres results in the characteristic hydrophobic spasms. This is a reflex contraction of inspiratory muscles provoked by attempts to drink water, and later, through conditioning, even the sound or mention of water, and also sometimes by draughts of air (aerophobia), touching the palate, bright lights or loud noises.

Intense thirst forces patients to try to drink. They may have a tight feeling in the throat, the arm trembles, and jerky spasms of the sternomastoids, diaphragm and other inspiratory muscles lead to a generalized extension, sometimes with convulsions and opisthotonos (Figure 44.7).[64] There is an associated inexplicable feeling of terror which occurs during the first episode, and is not a learned response.[51] Respiratory or cardiac arrest following a hydrophobic spasm is fatal in one-third of cases.

Episodes of excitation, aggression, anxiety or hallucinations interspersed with periods of calm lucidity, during which no neurological abnormality may be detectable and patients realize their appalling predicament. Other features include cardiac arrhythmias, myocarditis, respiratory disturbances (e.g. cluster breathing), meningism, lesions of cranial nerves III, VII and IX, abnormal pupillary function, muscle fasciculation,[64] autonomic stimulation with lacrimation, salivation (Figure 44.8), labile blood pressure and temperature and rarely increased libido, priapism and spontaneous orgasms.[65,66] Low cerebral oxygen uptake suggests

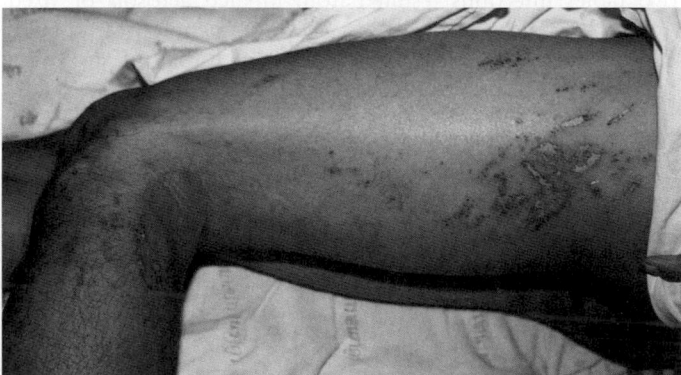

Figure 44.6 Intense itching of the bitten limb provoking scratching and excoriation, a common prodromal symptom of rabies encephalitis. (©D. A. Warrell.)

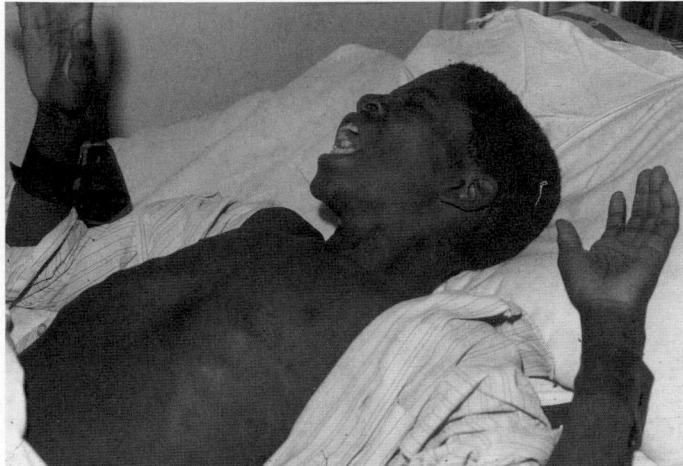

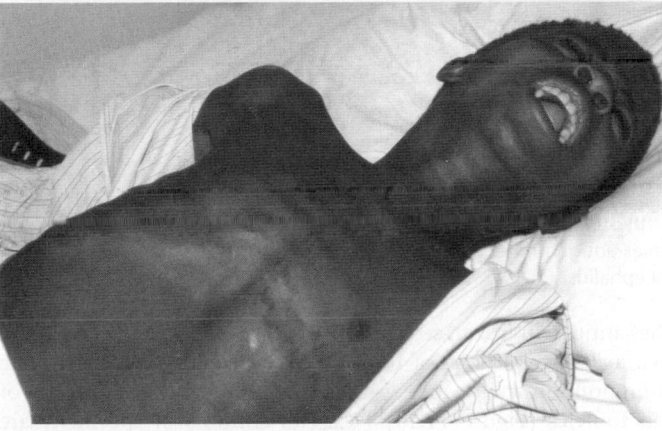

Figure 44.7 Progression of a hydrophobic spasm associated with terror in a Nigerian boy with furious rabies. (A) Note the powerful contraction of the diaphragm (depressing the xiphisternum) and sternocleidomastoid muscles. (B) The episode terminates in opisthotonos. (©D. A. Warrell.)

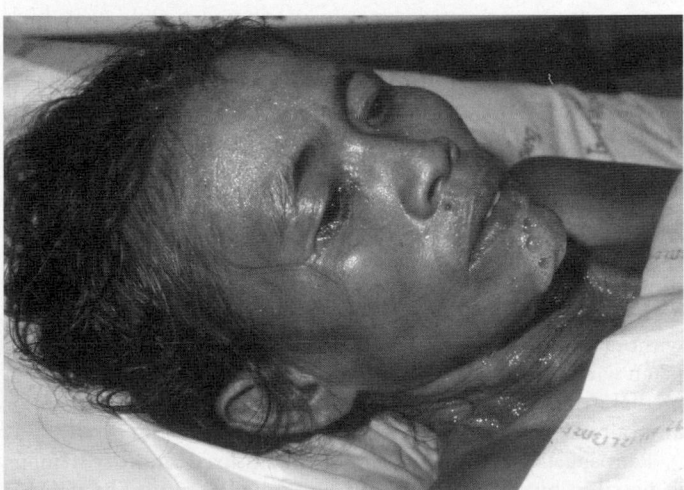

Figure 44.8 Hypersalivation and sweating in a Thai woman with furious rabies. (©D. A. Warrell.)

irreversible brain damage.[51] Coma eventually ensues, with flaccid paralysis, and the agonizing illness rarely lasts more than a week without intensive care.

Paralytic rabies

Less common than furious rabies, paralytic or 'dumb' rabies may be missed unless there is a high level of suspicion. Paralytic disease is characteristic of vampire bat-transmitted rabies[67] and it is more common following infections by attenuated viruses,[41,42,68] and perhaps after post-exposure vaccination.

Prodromal symptoms are followed by paraesthesiae or hypotonic weakness, commonly starting near the site of the bite and spreading cranially. Fasciculation or piloerection may be seen. The ascending paralysis results in constipation, urinary retention, respiratory failure and inability to swallow. Flaccid paralysis, especially of proximal muscles, is associated with loss of tendon and plantar reflexes, but sensation is often normal. Hydrophobic spasms may occur in the terminal phase and death ensues after 1–3 weeks.[64]

Management and complications

Patients with suspected rabies should be admitted to hospital and given adequate doses of sedatives and analgesics to relieve their agonizing symptoms. It remains a fatal infection, although rare recoveries have been reported (see below). Intensive care therapy can prolong life for 3–4 weeks, occasionally for months[42,69] and exceptionally for years (see below).[70,71]

During this time complications arise in every system. Cardiac arrhythmias are controlled by pacing, and respiratory failure requires ventilation. Full barrier nursing of the unconscious patient is needed, with specific treatment for likely complications such as convulsions, fluctuating blood pressure, pneumonia, pneumothorax, cerebral oedema, hyper- or hypopyrexia, inappropriate antidiuretic hormone secretion (diabetes insipidus) and haematemesis from stress ulceration.[64]

Treatment with hyperimmune serum and several antiviral agents, including intrathecal tribavirin (ribavirin) and interferon-α, have not been effective[6,55,72] and the success claimed for a regimen of sedation and multiple antiviral drugs in a girl infected by bat rabies in the USA[73] has not been confirmed in patients infected with canine or bat rabies viruses.[74]

Recovery from rabies

Two patients are claimed to have recovered completely from rabies encephalitis. They had been given post-exposure prophylaxis with nervous tissue vaccines and then intensive care.[75,76] Four further patients, given pre- or post-exposure tissue culture vaccines, survived months or years with profound neurological impairment: a microbiologist who inhaled fixed rabies virus,[42] two boys in Mexico[70,71] and a girl in India.[77] All the diagnoses were based on high rabies neutralizing antibody levels in the serum and CSF. No virus or antigen was identified. The first unvaccinated patient to survive rabies has returned to near normal life following intensive care and antiviral therapy.[73] This is reminiscent of a previous, vaccinated patient,[76] and both were infected by American insectivorous bat viruses which may have different pathogenesis, and hence reduced pathogenicity and virulence, from canine rabies strains.

Differential diagnosis

Rabies should be suspected if inexplicable neurological, psychiatric or laryngopharyngeal symptoms occur in those who have been to an endemic area. The animal contact may have been forgotten. The differential diagnoses include the following:[64]

• Tetanus, another wound infection, has a short incubation period, usually less than 15 days. The muscle rigidity is constant, without relaxation between spasms. The CSF is always normal
• Intoxications with drugs acting on the CNS, poisons and even delirium tremens could be confused with rabies
• Rabies phobia is a hysterical response, usually very soon after a bite, with aggressive behaviour and an excellent prognosis
• Guillain–Barré syndrome may present as paralytic rabies, and very rarely follows rabies tissue culture vaccine treatment
• Post-vaccinal encephalitis (see below), an allergic response to nervous tissue-containing rabies vaccine, can be clinically indistinguishable from paralytic rabies
• Other viral encephalomyelitides, including Japanese encephalitis, poliomyelitis and treatable herpes simiae B, from a monkey bite, should be considered.

DIAGNOSIS

Laboratory investigations are likely to be normal initially, except for a mild pleocytosis. A variety of non-specific EEG changes are reported. CT and MRI scans may be normal throughout,[32,73] but non-specific MRI changes have been seen especially in brainstem, or basal ganglia regions, and possibly in the spinal cord in paralytic disease.

Intravitam confirmation of human rabies encephalitis

The diagnosis of rabies can be made by virus isolation, rapid identification of antigen or, in unvaccinated people, antibody detection.[52]

Isolation of rabies virus

Culture of the virus is most successful during the first week of illness – from saliva, throat, tracheal or eye swabs, brain biopsy samples, CSF and possibly centrifuged urine.[52] Viraemia has not been detected. The method of inoculation of suckling mice yields results in 1–3 weeks, but tissue culture isolation in murine neuroblastoma cells takes about 2 days.[78,79]

Antigen detection[79]

Rabies diagnosis by polymerase chain reaction (PCR) tests on saliva, CSF[80] and skin biopsy are available in reference laboratories. A direct immunofluorescent antibody (IFA) test rapidly iden-

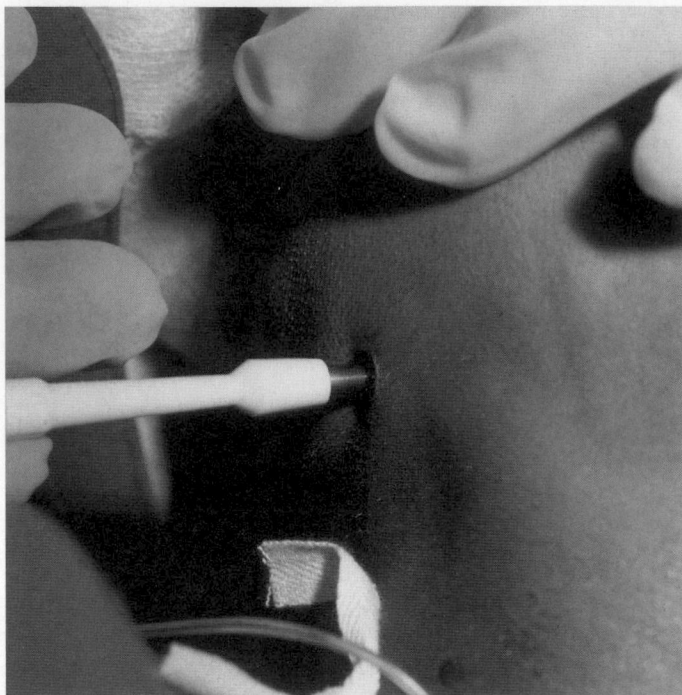

Figure 44.9 Punch biopsy of skin in the hairy nuchal region for rabies antigen detection in a patient with suspected rabies encephalitis. (©D. A. Warrell.)

tifies antigen in frozen sections of skin biopsies taken from a hairy area, usually the nape of the neck (Figure 44.9). Rabies-specific immunofluorescence appears in nerve twiglets around the base of hair follicles (Figure 44.10).[81] Careful controls of specificity are needed, but this method is 60–100% sensitive.[53,82] False positives have not been reported. The corneal smear test is too insensitive to be useful and false positives have occurred.[52,53,80]

Antibody detection

In unvaccinated patients, rabies seroconversion often occurs during the second week of illness and is diagnostic,[52] but many remain seronegative at death.[74] In vaccinated people, very high levels of antibody in the serum, and especially in the CSF, are needed to suggest the diagnosis.[70,71,73,76,77]

Postmortem diagnosis in humans

All the methods mentioned above may confirm the diagnosis postmortem, especially if the clinical illness was very short. Virus isolation from secretions is usually unsuccessful after 2 weeks of illness, but culture of brain tissue should be possible post mortem, even if the IFA staining is negative. Samples can be obtained without a full postmortem examination. Brain necropsies are taken with a Vim–Silverman or other long biopsy needle[83] via the medial canthus of the eye, through the superior orbital fissure or an occipital approach through the foramen magnum.

Retrospective diagnosis using formalin-fixed brain specimens is possible by trypsin digestion and labelled antibody staining with immunofluorescent, enzymatic or in situ-hybridization methods.

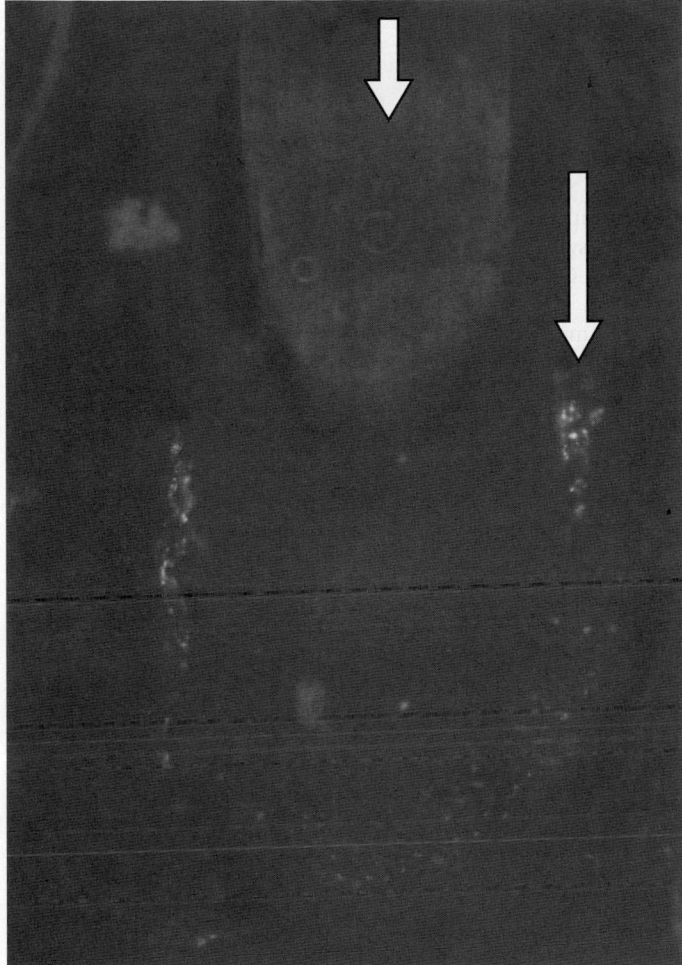

Figure 44.10 Diagnosis of rabies during life from a skin biopsy. Vertical section through a hair follicle. The small arrow shows the hair shaft. The bright fluorescence (large arrow) indicates rabies antigen in nerve cells around the follicle. (©M. J. Warrell.)

Diagnosis in the biting mammal

If laboratory facilities are available, suspect rabid animals should be killed immediately and their brains tested for rabies infection.[84] Observation in captivity is potentially dangerous and uncertain.[61] Ideally, samples of hippocampus, brain stem and cerebellum should be tested, but brain specimens can be obtained from dogs without craniotomy via the occipital foramen.[85] IFA staining of acetone-fixed impression smears takes 2–3 h[79] and is the usual method of diagnosis. It is about 98% sensitive compared with viral culture by the mouse inoculation test. The IFA test is unreliable in detecting rabies-related viruses. A commercial enzyme immunodiagnostic kit will test for antigen in brain tissue suspensions, but this is 2% less sensitive than the IFA test.[79]

No single test should be relied upon to make this important diagnosis. Virus isolation should be attempted on all IFA test-negative samples.

Strains of street rabies, or rabies-related viruses from different vector species or geographical areas, can be differentiated by genetic sequence analysis[13] or monoclonal antibody typing.[79]

CONTROL OF ANIMAL RABIES

The optimal method of protecting man from rabies infection or associated financial loss varies greatly in different endemic areas. The species of vector, its prevalence and interaction with man dictate whether elimination or vaccination of animals is appropriate and economically feasible.

Canine rabies

The control of endemic rabies in areas where dogs are the dominant vector[10,11,14,18] requires: epidemiological surveillance; laboratory diagnostic facilities; education to avoid unnecessary contact with animals, especially stray dogs, and vaccination of dogs, cats and humans.

The size of a population of stray dogs depends on available food and shelter. Attempts at control by killing dogs result in an increased reproduction rate and rapid restoration of numbers. There has been an impressive reduction in the number of local human cases following vector control campaigns, including dog population control, vaccination and removal of food and shelter by clearing street rubbish.[86] Mass vaccination campaigns, aimed at immunizing 80% of dogs, have eliminated canine rabies in Japan and Taiwan, and from densely populated urban areas of Argentina, Brazil and Peru.[87] Despite localized successes, there has been no evidence of a significant change in the overall incidence of animal rabies in most tropical endemic areas of Africa and Asia.

Efficient post-exposure vaccine treatment of dog-bite victims should be ensured, including a rapid animal diagnostic service and adequate supplies of vaccine and immune serum.

Sylvatic (wildlife) rabies

For some vector species active control is not attempted, owing to the low rate of transmission to other species and lack of effective methods. Insectivorous bats in North America and Europe are examples and simple measures are used to prevent contact with man. In contrast, where infection of domestic animals and humans is likely, as with fox rabies, campaigns for population control and vaccination have been mounted.

Trapping, gassing, poisoning and hunting are generally inefficient means of population reduction. Oral fox vaccine campaigns have been used to great effect. Live attenuated rabies virus vaccine or a live vaccinia recombinant vaccine expressing rabies glycoprotein disguised in baits has been distributed by hand or by aircraft over 18 European countries.[19] As a result, terrestrial rabies has been eliminated from seven Western countries. Oral vaccination is also used in the control of rabies in raccoons, coyotes and grey foxes in North America.[88] In Latin America, vampire bat rabies[14,16,88] is a major cause of death in cattle, with disastrous economic consequences. Specific control methods include bovine vaccination or treatment with anticoagulants, diphenadione or warfarin, to which bats, but not cattle, are highly sensitive.

RABIES PROPHYLAXIS IN HUMANS

Although prophylaxis is usually given post-exposure, as an emergency procedure after possible inoculation of the virus, there are advantages in immunizing people at risk of infection in advance, by pre-exposure vaccination.

Post-exposure prophylaxis

This treatment is needed after suspected contact with rabies virus through an open wound or mucous membrane (Figure 44.11). Intact skin is a barrier against infection. Post-exposure treatment is aimed at killing or neutralizing rabies virus in a wound before any virions enter a nerve ending. Once within the nervous system, the immune response is thought to be incapable of preventing disease. Post-exposure treatment has three components: wound treatment, active immunization and passive immunization with rabies immune globulin.

Assessing the risk of rabies infection

Knowledge of the local epidemiology of rabies vectors, the circumstances of the animal bite or contact, and the health and behaviour of the animal all contribute to assessment of the risk of exposure to rabies. An unprovoked attack by an unvaccinated sick animal indicates a high risk, but so does contact with a paralysed or unusually tame wild mammal. Vaccinated animals have also transmitted rabies. In endemic areas, strenuous efforts should be made to have the biting animal put down and its brain examined for rabies.[84] If the animal has escaped or there is any doubt, post-exposure prophylaxis should be given, irrespective of the length of time since the bite. The official WHO recommendations are summarized in Table 44.3.

Wound treatment

Immediate cleaning of the wound or site of contact with a rabid animal is imperative (Figure 44.12) by scrubbing with concentrated soap solution or detergent and copious running water. If possible, swab with a virucidal agent: iodine solutions or 40–70% alcohol.[89] Quaternary ammonium compounds are neutralized by soap and are not generally recommended.[90] Energetic wound cleaning may require local or even general anaesthesia. Suturing should be delayed or avoided to prevent inoculation of virus deeper into the tissues.[84]

Tetanus prophylaxis may be required, and other bacterial infections associated with mammal bites may be treated with antibiotics; for example, *Pasteurella multocida* is usually sensitive to ampicillin, tetracycline and co-trimoxazole.

Active immunization: vaccine treatment

All current human rabies vaccines contain inactivated whole virus which has been grown on a variety of substrates. The original tissue culture vaccine, human diploid cell vaccine (HDCV) was introduced 30 years ago. It is expensive to make, so other cell lines are now used. Two vaccines are widely exported: a German purified chick embryo cell vaccine (PCECV) and a French purified vero cell vaccine (PVRV) (Table 44.4). Tissue culture vaccines are also made, mainly for local use, in China, India, Japan and Russia.

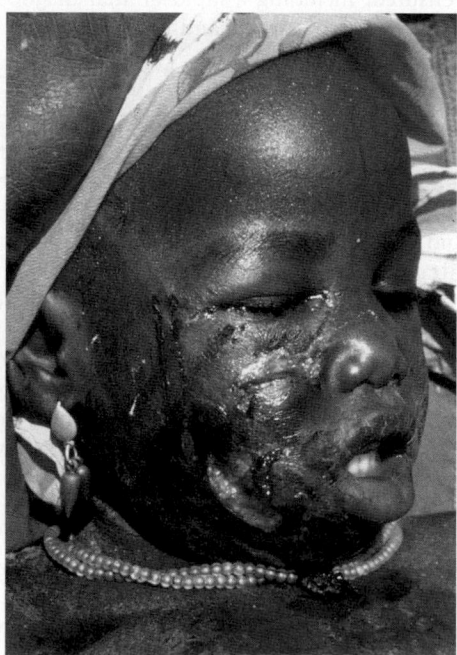

Figure 44.11 Facial bites inflicted by a rabid dog in Nigeria. (©D. A. Warrell.)

Table 44.3 Specific post-exposure prophylaxis for use in a rabies endemic area (following contact with a domestic or wild rabies vector species, whether or not the animal is available for observation or diagnostic tests)

Exposure	Treatment
MINOR: WHO CATEGORY II	
Including scratches or abrasions without bleeding	Start vaccine administration immediately
	Stop treatment if domestic cat or dog remains healthy for 10 days
	Stop treatment if animal's brain proves negative for rabies by appropriate laboratory tests
MAJOR: WHO CATEGORY III	
Including licks of mucosa or broken skin, minor bites or major bites (multiple or on face, head, fingers or neck)	Immediate rabies immune globulin and vaccine
	Stop treatment if domestic cat or dog remains healthy for 10 days
	Stop treatment if animal's brain proves negative for rabies by appropriate laboratory tests

Adapted from WHO publications.[84,91]

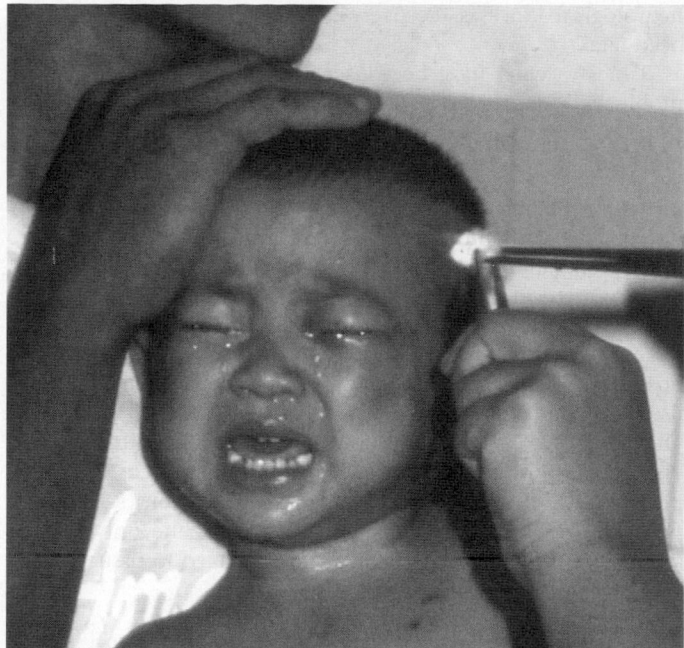

Figure 44.12 Thorough wound cleaning following an attack by a rabid dog (as in this Thai boy) is an essential part of post-exposure prophylaxis. (©D. A. Warrell.)

Table 44.4 Human rabies vaccines fulfilling WHO requirements

Vaccine	Abbreviation	Virus	Origin	i.m. vial
Human diploid cell vaccine	HDCV	PM1503	France	1.0 mL
Purified vero cell rabies vaccine	PVRV	PM1503	France	0.5 mL
Purified chick embryo cell	PCECV	LEP	Germany and India	1.0 mL

Post-exposure vaccine regimens

Tissue culture vaccines

Rabies vaccines (Table 44.4) fulfilling WHO requirements: PCECV, PVRV and HDCV should be used with the following post-exposure regimens (Table 44.5):[84,91,92]

1. The standard intramuscular (i.m.) 5-dose regimen is as follows:
   - Days 0, 3, 7, 14 and 28: 1 vial (PCECV and HDCV 1.0 mL, or PVRV 0.5 mL) i.m. into the deltoid (or anterolateral thigh in children, but never the buttock).[92]
2. An alternative method is a *2-1-1 i.m. regimen*:
   - Day 0: 2 i.m. doses (deltoids)
   - Days 7 and 21: 1 i.m. dose (deltoid)
   A total of 4 doses, but the antibody level is likely to fall more rapidly.[93]
   The prohibitive cost of i.m. treatment may be reduced using economical multisite intradermal (i.d.) methods. Two i.d. regimens are approved by the WHO: an eight-site regimen and a two-site regimen.
3. The *eight-site i.d. economical regimen*.[84,94] This method is used with PCECV and HDCV (whose i.m. dose is 1 mL). It has a wide margin of safety, and consists of:
   - Day 0: 0.1 mL injected i.d. at eight sites (right and left deltoid, suprascapular, thigh and lower lateral abdominal areas) using up the whole 1.0 mL ampoule
   - Day 7: 0.1 mL i.d. at four sites (deltoids and thighs)
   - Days 28 and 91: 0.1 mL i.d. at one site (deltoid).
   The distribution of sites is designed to stimulate many different groups of lymph nodes. Neutralizing antibody induction is rapid.[94] Less than two ampoules of vaccine are needed – a 60% reduction of the i.m. regimen. Four visits to the clinic are required, which reduces the cost of travel and time off work for patients. This regimen cannot be used economically with PVRV as the vial contains 0.5 mL.
4. *The two-site i.d. economical regimen* has been tested post-exposure, with immune globulin.[95] Using PVRV (0.5 mL/ampoule) each i.d. dose is 0.1 mL per i.d. site. With other,

Table 44.5 Rabies vaccine regimens

Regimen	Route	Days of injection (number of injection sites)						Total number of vials of vaccine
Pre-exposure	i.m. or i.d.[a]	0		7		21 ← **28**		3 or 0.3/0.6
Post-exposure[b]								
Standard i.m.	i.m.	0	3	7	14	28		5
Alternative i.m.	i.m.	0 (2)		7		21		4
Two-site ID	i.d.[c]	0 (2)	3 (2)	7 (2)		28 (1)	90 (1)	<2
Eight-site ID	i.d.[a]	0 (8[d])		7 (4)		28 (1)	90 (1)	<2 (not PVRV)
Four-site ID[e]	i.d.[c]	0 (4[d])		7 (2)		28 (1)	90 (1)	<2

[a] i.d. dose is 0.1 mL/site.
[b] Rabies immune globulin also given on day 0 with all regimens.
[c] Volume of i.d. dose is 0.1 ml/site with PVRV, 0.2 mL/site with PCECV and HDCV is preferred, but 0.1 mL/site is also used.
[d] Using whole vial of vaccine, Divided between eight or four sites.
[e] New regimen, not yet considered by WHO.

1.0 mL vaccines, PCECV and HDCV, the equivalent i.d. dose is 0.2 mL, although 0.1 mL/site is also used.

- Days 0, 3 and 7: 0.1/0.2 mL i.d. at two sites (deltoids)
- Days 28 and 91: 0.1/ 0.2 mL i.d. at one site (deltoid).

WHO now advises that double the dose can be given on day 28, and the day 91 dose omitted.[96] The two i.d. regimens use the same amount of vaccine. Sharing of ampoules of vaccine needs great care. Opened ampoules must be kept in the refrigerator and used within 8 h. A separate syringe and needle must be used for every patient to prevent cross-infection.

A comparison of these i.d. regimens[97] showed that the eight-site method induces neutralizing antibody more rapidly and to higher levels than the two-site regimen, and it has been recommended for use when no immune globulin is available.[84]

There is evidence that a *four-site i.d. regimen*[98,99] is also highly immunogenic:

- Day 0: 0.1/ 0.2 mL approx. i.d. injections at four sites (deltoids, thighs), using the entire contents of the vial
- Day 7: 0: 0.1/ 0.2 mL i.d. at two sites (deltoids)
- Days 28 and 90: 0: 0.1/ 0.2 mL i.d. at one site (deltoid).

This has several advantages: it requires only four or perhaps three visits (days 0, 7 and 28 with an optional day 90). Injecting a whole ampoule of vaccine divided between i.d. sites on day 0 is more practicable for widespread use and is safer, especially in inexperienced hands. Unlike the 8-site method, it can be used economically with all three vaccines (0.1/ 0.2 mL per site).

The manufacturer's instructions should be followed for all other vaccines.

Post-exposure treatment for those who have had previous vaccination

Wound care and booster doses of vaccine are still vital and urgent. Provided that a full pre- or post-exposure course of one of the recommended vaccines (Table 44.4) has been given, or if at least 0.5 IU/mL of rabies neutralizing antibody has been documented following any other treatment, a short course of two doses of vaccine given i.m. on days 0 and 3 is recommended.[84] Passive immunization is not required. Otherwise, a full course of vaccine and rabies immune globulin is needed.

Side-effects of tissue culture vaccines

Minor local reactions occur in 2–74% of vaccinees, and include pain, erythema, swelling, aching and paraesthesia. Multiple-site i.d. injections cause local itching in 7–64% in different studies. Mild systemic reactions, reported by 3–40% of vaccinees, consist of influenza-like symptoms, headache, fever, malaise, myalgia, nausea, dizziness or a rash.[84]

Booster doses of HDCV, usually about a year after previous treatment, have caused systemic allergic reactions in 6% of American vaccinees. After 3–13 days, urticaria, rash, angio-oedema and arthralgia appear, but always respond promptly to symptomatic treatment.[100] This is likely to be an immune response to non-viral vaccine constituents.[92] Other more highly purified vaccines may not have this complication.

Extremely rare neurological illness following HDCV is either Guillain–Barré-like (in four patients) or local limb weakness (in two patients).[101] PCECV has also been implicated in two neurological illnesses. Recovery is usually rapid, and none has been fatal.

Rabies vaccines have been used widely in pregnancy without problems.

Nervous tissue vaccines (NTVs)

Although they are being phased out, these inactivated homogenates of infected animal brains are still in use in some countries in Asia, Africa and South America. Sheep brain Semple vaccine, first produced in 1911, is used in Bangladesh and Pakistan. Seven to 14 daily injections are given subcutaneously over the anterior abdominal wall, a large area able to accommodate the 2–5 mL doses of vaccine. Fuenzalida's suckling mouse brain vaccine is used in Vietnam and in parts of South America and Africa. The potency of NTVs is variable, and treatment failures occur. They should not be used for pre-exposure prophylaxis. Although post-vaccinal encephalitis is a serious complication (see below), post-exposure treatment is urgent, so if it is the only vaccine available, treatment can be started and changed to tissue culture vaccine at any time.

Post-vaccinal encephalomyelitis following nervous tissue vaccines[6,101]

This is an inflammatory, demyelinating, autoimmune response due to sensitization by myelin and other neural antigens contained in the vaccine. Estimates of its incidence vary with different products, but the frequency is up to 1:220 recipients of Semple vaccine, with a mortality rate of 3%. Symptoms usually appear within 2 weeks of starting the course, but may not appear until 2 months later.[6] Suckling mouse brain vaccines have a lower complication rate (1:8000 to 1:27000) but peripheral nervous system signs, such as Guillain–Barré-like syndrome, frequently predominate and are fatal in 22% of cases.

A wide variety of neurological signs include polyneuritis, often involving limbs, transverse myelitis, ascending paralysis, and meningoencephalitis. Corticosteroid therapy (e.g. prednisolone 40–60 mg/day) is conventional, and cyclophosphamide in addition has been suggested. Recovery often occurs within 2 weeks and is usually complete, but residual neurological deficits can ensue.

Post-vaccinial encephalitis can be clinically identical to paralytic rabies, and the diagnosis must be made by exclusion. The skin biopsy technique of rabies antigen detection has proved a useful rapid method.[53] No further nervous tissue vaccine must be given, but the course completed with a tissue culture vaccine.

Passive immunization

Rabies immune globulin (RIG) provides passive protection during the first 7–10 days of a primary post-exposure course of vaccine, when no neutralizing antibody is detectable. This not only neutralizes virus in the wound, but also may enhance the presentation of vaccine antigens to T lymphocytes.[102]

The efficacy of RIG treatment combined with rabies vaccine has been proved by animal studies and natural experiments when wolves have bitten groups of people in Iran[103] and China.[104] The mortality from head wounds was reduced five-fold by the addition of immune serum to vaccine treatment.[105]

A dose of 40 IU/kg of *equine RIG* or 20 IU/kg of *human RIG* should ideally accompany every primary post-exposure vaccine course, but it is essential following severe bites: that is, on the head, neck or hands and multiple or deep bites. RIG is infiltrated around the wound if anatomically possible, and any remaining injected i.m. at a site remote from the vaccine, but not into the buttock. RIG given days or even hours before the vaccine is started impairs the immune response.[106] The dose must not be exceeded because RIG may reduce the immunogenicity of the vaccine.

RIG is prohibitively expensive. In Asia and Africa, Human RIG costs approximately US$110, and equine RIG US$25 per person. RIG is unobtainable in large areas including some whole countries.

A large study showed an incidence of reactions to equine and human RIG of 1.8% and 0.09%, respectively, and serum sickness occurred in 0.72% and 0.007% of recipients.[107] An intradermal skin test does not predict anaphylaxis[107] or most other reactions[84] and RIG should be given, despite a positive result.[84,96] The test should be abandoned. Adrenaline should always be at hand in case of anaphylaxis.

Efficacy of post-exposure prophylaxis

The untreated mortality from rabid animal bites depends on the part of the body affected and the severity of the bite. Data from the pre-vaccine era give an estimate of the chance of infection from suspect rabid dogs. The mortality from multiple bites on the head was 60–80%, from a single facial bite 30%, and from bites on the hand 15–67%.[108,109] In India, the overall mortality from proven rabid dog bites was 35–57%,[110,111] but no information on wound treatment was given in these studies.

If wound treatment, tissue culture vaccine and RIG are given on the day of the bite in the correct manner, prophylaxis is virtually 100% effective. Nevertheless, patients are known to have died of rabies after receiving these vaccines.[112] This mortality has been attributed to human or circumstantial failure to deliver optimum treatment, and not to reduced antigen content or other failure of the vaccine.

Possible reasons for failure of post-exposure prophylaxis are as follows:

1. Any delay in starting vaccine increases the chance of the rabies virus entering neurones before the immune response is generated. The mortality following head wounds from Iranian rabid wolves doubled if vaccine was delayed beyond 8 days.[105] Treatment is urgent, and it is never too late to begin. Vaccine and RIG should be used even if the bite occurred months before.
2. Failure to give rabies immune globulin or to infiltrate the wound, especially with severe exposure.
3. Injecting vaccine into the buttock instead of the deltoid.
4. Inability of the patient to mount an immune response due to chronic disease (e.g. HIV infection, cirrhosis) or immuno-suppressive drugs (e.g. steroids).[112]

Rabies genotype 1 virus strains show a high degree of homology with the strains used in vaccine production, but there is great antigenic diversity within the genus. Vaccine is effective against Australian bat Lyssavirus[22,113] but the protection afforded against other Phylogroup I lyssaviruses is less efficient than that

against genotype 1 viruses,[21] and there is little if any protection against Mokola virus.[113]

PRE-EXPOSURE PROPHYLAXIS[84,92]

No deaths from rabies have been reported in anyone who has had pre-exposure treatment and booster injections after exposure. Pre-exposure prophylaxis is advisable for anyone likely to be in contact with a rabid animal. This may include veterinarians, animal handlers, laboratory staff, zoologists, wildlife enthusiasts, health workers, travellers and residents in endemic areas where dogs are the dominant vector species.

A pre-exposure vaccine course is three doses of one of the recommended vaccines (Table 44.5), given i.m. on days 0, 3 and 28. The third dose may be advanced towards day 21 if short of time. An economical alternative is i.d. injections of 0.1 mL at the same intervals.[84,92] If the injection is too deep, withdraw the needle and repeat the procedure. A separate syringe must be used for each patient. Chloroquine taken as malaria prophylaxis can suppress the antibody response to i.d. primary pre-exposure treatment,[114] so the vaccine must be given i.m. with this drug. Vaccinees must keep a record of their immunization.

A booster dose 1–2 years after the primary course increases the persistence of antibody to 10 years in 96% of people in a study of i.m. treatment.[115] Although the titre of antibody falls more rapidly after i.d. than i.m. inoculation, the response to a booster dose is similar, whatever the original route. Confirmation of seroconversion is unnecessary unless immunosuppression is suspected.[92]

Booster doses may be given intradermally or intramuscularly at intervals depending on the risk of infection.[115] Boosters are not necessary if the rabies neutralizing antibody level is at least 0.5 IU/mL.

Laboratory staff handling rabies virus should have a serology test or booster injection every 6 months,[84,92] but others may require booster doses after 2–10 years according to their risk of exposure. Travellers who will have rapid access to vaccine if exposed need not have further immunization. However, if medical resources will be unreliable, booster vaccination may be advisable before departure, if 3–5 years have elapsed since the last dose.

REFERENCES

1. Théordoidès J. *Histoire de la Rage, Cave Canem*. Paris: Masson; 1986.
2. Wilkinson L. The development of the virus concept as reflected in corpora of studies on individual pathogens. 4. Rabies: two millennia of ideas and conjecture on the aetiology of a virus disease. *Med Hist* 1977; 21:15–31.
3. Matsumoto S. Rabies virus. *Adv Virus Res* 1970; 16:257–301.
4. Badrane H, Bahloul C, Perrin P, et al. Evidence of two Lyssavirus phylogroups with distinct pathogenicity and immunogenicity. *J Virol* 2001; 75(7):3268–3276.
5. Kuzmin IV, Hughes GJ, Botvinkin AD, et al. Phylogenetic relationships of Irkut and West Caucasian bat viruses within the Lyssavirus genus and suggested quantitative criteria based on the N gene sequence for Lyssavirus genotype definition. *Virus Res* 2005; 111(1):28–43.
6. Warrell MJ, Warrell DA. Rhabdovirus infections of man. In: Porterfield JS, Tyrrell DA J, eds. *Handbook of Infectious Diseases*. Vol. 3. Exotic viral infections. London: Chapman & Hall; 1995:343–383.

7. Wunner WH. Rabies virus. In: Jackson AC and Wunner WH, eds. *Rabies.* 2nd edn. London: Academic Press; 2007.

8. Finke S, Conzelmann KK. Replication strategies of rabies virus. *Virus Res* 2005; 111(2):120–131.

9. Michalski F, Parks NF, Soko F, et al. Thermal inactivation of rabies and other rhabdoviruses: stabilization by the chelating agent EDTA at physiological temperatures. *Infect Immun* 1976; 14:135–143.

10. Nel LH, Rupprecht CE. Emergence of lyssaviruses in the Old World: the case of Africa. *Curr Top Microbiol Immunol* 2007; 315:161–193.

11. Bingham J. Canine rabies ecology in southern Africa. *Emerg Infect Dis* 2005; 11(9):1337–1342.

12. Nel LH, Sabeta CT, von Teichman B, et al. Mongoose rabies in southern Africa: a re-evaluation based on molecular epidemiology. *Virus Res* 2005; 109(2):165–173.

13. Hanlon CA, Niezgoda M, Rupprecht CE. Rabies in terrestrial animals. In: Jackson AC, Wunner AH, eds. *Rabies.* 2nd edn. London: Elsevier; 2007; 201–258.

14. Belotto A, Leanes LF, Schneider MC, et al. Overview of rabies in the Americas. *Virus Res* 2005; 111(1):5–12.

15. Messenger SL, Smith JS, Rupprecht CE. Emerging epidemiology of bat-associated cryptic cases of rabies in humans in the United States. *Clin Infect Dis* 2002; 35(6):738–747.

16. Kuzmin IV, Rupprecht CE. Bat rabies. In: Jackson AC, Wunner AH, eds. *Rabies.* 2nd edn. London: Elsevier; 2007; 259–307.

17. Everard COR, Everard JD. Mongoose rabies. *Rev Inf Dis* 1988; 10:S610–S614.

18. Nel LH, Markotter W. Lyssaviruses. *Crit Rev Microbiol* 2007; 33:301–324.

19. Cliquet F, Aubert M. Elimination of terrestrial rabies in Western European countries. *Dev Biol (Basel)* 2004; 119:185–204.

20. Cherkasskiy BL. Roles of the wolf and the raccoon dog in the ecology and epidemiology of rabies in the USSR. *Rev Infect Dis* 1988; 10:S634–S636.

21. Fooks AR, Brookes SM, Johnson N, et al. European bat lyssaviruses: an emerging zoonosis. *Epidemiol Infect* 2003; 131:1029–1039.

22. Warrilow D. Australian bat lyssavirus: a recently discovered new rhabdovirus. *Curr Top Microbiol Immunol* 2005; 292:25–44.

23. Knobel DL, Cleaveland S, Coleman PG, et al. Re-evaluating the burden of rabies in Africa and Asia. *Bull World Health Organ* 2005; 83(5):360–368.

24. Familusi JB, Moore DL. Isolation of a rabies related virus from the CSF of a child with 'aseptic meningitis'. *Afr J Med Sci* 1972; 3:93–96.

25. Familusi JB, Osunkoya BO, Moore DL, et al. A fatal human infection with Mokola virus. *Am J Trop Med Hyg* 1972; 21:959–963.

26. Crick J. Rabies. In: Gibbs EPJ, ed. *Virus Diseases of Food Animals,* vol. II. London: Academic Press; 1981:469–516.

27. Meredith CD, Rossouw AP, van Praag Koch H. An unusual case of human rabies thought to be of chiropteran origin. *S Afr Med J* 1971; 45:767–769.

28. Paweska JT, Blumberg LH, Liebenberg C, et al. Fatal human infection with rabies-related Duvenhage virus, South Africa. *Emerg Infect Dis* 2006; 12:1965–1967.

29. Selimov MA, Tatarov AG, Botvinkin AD, et al. Rabies related Yulivirus: identification with a panel of monoclonal antibodies. *Acta Virol (Praha)* 1989; 33:542–546.

30. King A, Crick J. Rabies-related viruses. In: Campbell JB, Charlton KM, eds. *Rabies.* Boston: Kluwer; 1988:177–199.

31. Lumio J, Hillbom M, Roine R, et al. Human rabies of bat origin in Europe. *Lancet* 1986; i:378.

32. Nathwani D, McIntyre PG, White K, et al. Fatal human rabies caused by European bat Lyssavirus type 2a infection in Scotland. *Clin Infect Dis* 2003; 37(4):598–601.

33. Botvinkin AD, Selnikova OP, Antonova AB, et al. Human rabies case caused from a bat bite in Ukraine. *Rab Bull Eur* 2005; 29(3):5–7. Online. Available: http://www.who-rabies-bulletin.org/Journal/Archive/Bulletin_2005_3.PDF 26 Feb 2007.

34. Tang X, Luo M, Zhang S, et al. Pivotal role of dogs in rabies transmission, China. *Emerg Infect Dis* 2005; 11(12):1970–1972.

35. Warrell MJ, Warrell DA. Rabies and other Lyssavirus diseases. *Lancet* 2004; 363(9413):959–969.

36. Helmick CG, Tauxe RV, Vernon AA. Is there a risk to contacts of patients with rabies? *Rev Infect Dis* 1987; 9:511–518.

37. Srinivasan A, Burton EC, Kuehnert MJ, et al. Transmission of rabies virus from an organ donor to four transplant recipients. *N Engl J Med* 2005; 352(11):1103–1111.

38. Burton EC, Burns DK, Opatowsky MJ, et al. Rabies encephalomyelitis: clinical, neuroradiological, and pathological findings in 4 transplant recipients. *Arch Neurol* 2005; 62(6):873–882.

39. Rabies Bulletin Europe. Rabies infections in organ donor and transplant recipients in Germany (2005) 2005; 29(3):8–9. Online. Available: http://www.who-rabies-bulletin.org/Journal/Archive/Bulletin_2005_3.PDF 26 Feb 2007.

40. Sipahioglu U, Alpaut S. Transplacental rabies in humans. *Mikrobiyol Bül* 1985; 19:95–99.

41. Winkler WG, Fashinell TR, Leffingwell L, et al. Airborne rabies transmission in a laboratory worker. *JAMA* 1973; 226:1219–1221.

42. Centers for Disease Control. Rabies in a laboratory worker: New York. *MMWR* 1977; 26:183–184.

43. Dietzschold B, Schnell M, Koprowski H. Pathogenesis of rabies. *Curr Top Microbiol Immunol* 2005; 292:45–56.

44. Lafon M. Rabies virus receptors. *J Neurovirol* 2005; 11(1):82–7.

45. Jackson AC, Ye H, Phelan CC, et al. Extraneural organ involvement in human rabies. *Lab Invest* 1999; 79:945–951.

46. Tangchai P, Yenbutr D, Vejjajiva A. Central nervous system lesions in human rabies: a study of twenty-four cases. *J Med Assoc Thai* 1970; 53:471–486.

47. Dupont JR, Earle KM. Human rabies encephalitis: a study of forty-nine fatal cases with a review of the literature. *Neurology* 1966; 15:1023–1034.

48. Perl DP. The pathology of rabies in the central nervous system. In: Baer GM, ed. *The Natural History of Rabies.* Vol. I. New York: Academic Press; 1975:235–272.

49. Maton PN, Pollard JD, Newsom-Davies J. Human rabies encephalomyelitis. *BMJ* 1976; i:1038–1040.

50. Sandhyamani S, Roy S, Gode GR, et al. Pathology of rabies: a light and electronmicroscopical study with particular reference to the changes in cases with prolonged survival. *Acta Neuropathol (Berl)* 1981; 54:247–251.

51. Warrell DA, Davidson N Mc D, Pope HM, et al. Pathophysiologic studies in human rabies. *Am J Med* 1976; 60:180–190.

52. Anderson LJ, Nicholson KG, Tauxe RV, et al. Human rabies in the United States, 1960 to 1979: epidemiology, diagnosis and prevention. *Ann Intern Med* 1984; 100:728–735.

53. Warrell MJ, Looareesuwan S, Manatsathit S, et al. Rapid diagnosis of rabies and post-vaccinal encephalitides. *Clin Exp Immunol* 1988; 71:229–234.

54. Hemachudha T, Phanuphak P, Sriwanthana B, et al. Immunologic study of human encephalitic and paralytic rabies: preliminary report of 16 patients. *Am J Med* 1988; 84:673–677.

55. Merigan TC, Baer GM, Winkler WG, et al. Human leucocyte interferon administration to patients with symptomatic and suspected rabies. *Ann Neurol* 1984; 16:82–87.

56. Lafon M. Modulation of the immune response in the nervous system by rabies virus. *Curr Top Microbiol Immunol* 2005; 289:239–258.

57. World Health Organization, Working Group II. Vaccine potency requirements for reduced immunization schedules and pre-exposure treatment. *Dev Biol Stand* 1978; 40:268–270.

58. Kuwert EK, Barsenbach C, Werner J, et al. Early/high and late/low responders among HDCS vaccinees? In: Kuwert EK, Wiktor TJ, Koprowski H, eds. *Cell Culture Rabies Vaccines and their Protective Effect in Man.* Geneva: International Green Cross; 1981:160–167.

59. Anderson LJ, Winkler WG, Smith JS, et al. Post-exposure rabies prophylaxis with 5 doses of a tri-N-butyl phosphate inactivated human diploid cell vaccine. In: Kuwert EK, Wiktor TJ, Koprowski H, eds. *Cell Culture Rabies Vaccines and their Protective Effect in Man.* Geneva: International Green Cross; 1981:300–306.

60. Nicholson KG, Kuwert EK, Werner J, et al. Interferon response to human diploid cell strain rabies vaccines in man. *Arch Virol* 1979; 61:35–39.

61. Editorial. Human rabies: strain identification reveals lengthy incubation. *Lancet* 1991; 337:822–823.

62. Vibulbandhitkij S. Data of rabies patients from Bhamrasnaradura Hospital between 1971–1977. In: Tongcharoen P, ed. *Rabies*. Bangkok: Aksornsamai Press; 1980.

63. Gavrila I, Iurasog G, Luca E. La rage chez l'homme. Observations personnelles sur la séroprophylaxie, l'incubation prolongée et les essais thérapeutiques. *Ann Inst Past* 1967; 112:504–515.

64. Warrell DA. The clinical picture of rabies in man. *Trans R Soc Trop Med Hyg* 1976; 70:188–195.

65. Talaulicar PM. Persistent priapism in rabies. *Br J Urol* 1977; 49:462.

66. Udwadia ZF, Udwadia FE, Rao PP, et al. Penile hyperexcitability with recurrent ejaculations as the presenting manifestation of a case of rabies. *Postgrad Med J* 1988; 64:85–86.

67. Hurst EW, Pawan JL. An outbreak of rabies in Trinidad, without history of bites, and with the symptoms of acute ascending myelitis. *Lancet* 1931; ii:622–628.

68. Pará M. An outbreak of post-vaccinal rabies (rage de laboratoire) in Fortaleza, Brazil in 1960: resistant fixed virus as the etiological agent. *Bull World Health Organ* 1965; 33:172–182.

69. Emmons RW, Leonard LL, De Genaro F, et al. A case of human rabies with prolonged survival. *Intervirology* 1973; 1:60–72.

70. Alvarez L, Fajardo R, Lopez E, et al. Partial recovery from rabies in a nine-year-old boy. *Pediatr Inf Dis J* 1994; 13:1154–1155.

71. Alvarez L, Lomeli HM MB, Baer GM, et al. Human rabies: partial recovery in two Mexican children. *Abstr 7th Int Cong Inf Dis, Hong Kong* 1996; No. 59.002.

72. Warrell MJ, White NJ, Looareesuwan S, et al. Failure of interferon alfa and tribavirin in rabies encephalitis. *BMJ* 1989; 299:830–833.

73. Willoughby RE Jr, Tieves KS, Hoffman GM, et al. Survival after treatment of rabies with induction of coma. *N Engl J Med* 2005; 352(24):2508–2514.

74. Hemachudha T, Sunsaneewitayakul B, Desudchit T, et al. Failure of therapeutic coma and ketamine for therapy of human rabies. *J Neurovirol* 2006; 12(5):407–409.

75. Porras C, Barboza JJ, Fuenzalida E, et al. Recovery from rabies in man. *Ann Intern Med* 1976; 85:44–48.

76. Hattwick MA W, Weis TT, Stechschulte CJ, et al. Recovery from rabies: a case report. *Ann Intern Med* 1972; 76:931–942.

77. Madhusudana SN, Nagaraj D, Uday M, et al. Partial recovery from rabies in a six-year-old girl. *Int J Infect Dis* 2002; 6(1):85–86.

78. Rudd RJ, Trimarchi CV. Development and evaluation of an in vitro virus isolation procedure as a replacement for the mouse inoculation test in rabies diagnosis. *J Clin Microbiol* 1989; 27:2522–2528.

79. Bourhy H, Sureau P. *Laboratory Methods for Rabies Diagnosis*. Paris: Institut Pasteur; 1990.

80. Crepin P, Audry L, Rotivel Y, et al. Intravitam diagnosis of human rabies by PCR using saliva and cerebrospinal fluid. *J Clin Microbiol* 1998; 36:1117–1121.

81. Bryceson AD M, Greenwood BM, Warrell DA, et al. Demonstration during life of rabies antigen in humans. *J Infect Dis* 1975; 131:71–74.

82. Blenden DC, Creech W, Torres-Anjel MJ. Use of immunofluorescence examination to detect rabies virus antigen in the skin of humans with clinical encephalitis. *J Infect Dis* 1986; 154:698–701.

83. Marsden PD. Correspondence. *Am J Trop Med Hyg* 1970; 19:740.

84. World Health Organization. WHO recommendations on rabies post-exposure treatment and the correct technique of intradermal immunization against rabies. 1997: WHO/EMC/ZOO.96.6. Online. Available: http://whqlibdoc.who.int/hq/1996/WHO_EMC_ZOO_96.6.pdf

85. Hirose JA, Bourhy H, Sureau P. Retro-orbital route for brain specimen collection for rabies diagnosis. *Vet Rec* 1991; 129:291–292.

86. Reece JF, Chawla SK. Control of rabies in Jaipur, India, by the sterilisation and vaccination of neighbourhood dogs. *Vet Rec* 2006; 159(12):379–383.

87. Larghi OP. Perspectives for rabies control and eradication from domestic species in developing countries. *Dev Biol (Basel)* 2004; 119:205–212.

88. Rupprecht CE, Hanlon CA, Slate D. Oral vaccination of wildlife against rabies: opportunities and challenges in prevention and control. *Dev Biol (Basel)* 2004; 119:173–184.

89. Kaplan MM, Cohen D. Studies on the local treatment of wounds for the prevention of rabies. *Bull World Health Organ* 1962; 26:765–775.

90. Anderson LJ, Winkler WG. Aqueous quaternary ammonium compounds and rabies treatment. *J Infect Dis* 1979; 139:494–495.

91. World Health Organization WHO Expert Consultation on rabies. WHO Technical Report Series 931, First Report. 2006. Online Available: http://www.wpro.who.int/NR/rdonlyres/B1ED8443-0993-408C-BF09-D1D06A6E1B45/0/FINALTEXTWHOTechnicalReportSeries090605.pdf

92. Centers for Disease Control. Human rabies prevention – United States, 1999: Recommendations of the Advisory Committee on Immunization Practices (ACIP). *MMWR* 1999; 48:RR1–21.

93. Lang J, Simanjuntak GH, Soerjosembodo S, et al. Suppressant effect of human or equine rabies immunoglobulins on the immunogenicity of post-exposure rabies vaccination under the 2-1-1 regimen: a field trial in Indonesia. MAS054 Clinical Investigator Group. *Bull World Health Organ* 1998; 76(5):491–495.

94. Warrell MJ, Nicholson KG, Warrell DA, et al. Economical multiple site intradermal immunisation with human diploid-cell-strain vaccine is effective for post-exposure rabies prophylaxis. *Lancet* 1985; i:1059–1062.

95. Chutivongse S, Wilde H, Supich C, et al. Post-exposure prophylaxis for rabies with antiserum and intradermal vaccination. *Lancet* 1990; 335:896–898.

96. WHO. Rabies vaccines. WHO position paper. *Wkly Epidemiol Rec* 2007; 82:425–435. Online. Available: http://www.who.int/wer/2007/wer8249_50.pdf

97. Madhusudana SN, Anand NP, Shamsundar R. Evaluation of two intradermal vaccination regimens using purified chick embryo cell vaccine for post-exposure prophylaxis of rabies. *Natl Med J India* 2001; 14:145–147.

98. Ambrozaitis A, Laiskonis A, Balciuniene L, et al. Rabies post-exposure prophylaxis vaccination with purified chick embryo cell vaccine (PCECV) and purified Vero cell rabies vaccine (PVRV) in a four-site intradermal schedule (4-0-2-0-1-1): an immunogenic, cost-effective and practical regimen. *Vaccine* 2006; 24(19):4116–4121.

99. Warrell MJ, Riddell A, Yu L-M, et al. A simplified 4-site economical intradermal post-exposure rabies vaccine regimen: a randomised controlled comparison with standard methods. *PLoS Negl Trop Dis* 2008; 2(4): e224. doi: 10.1371/journal.pntd.0000224.

100. Dreesen DW, Bernard KW, Parker RA, et al. Immune complex-like disease in 23 persons following a booster dose of rabies human diploid cell vaccine. *Vaccine* 1986; 4:45–49.

101. Warrell M. Rabies encephalitis and its prophylaxis. *Pract Neurol* 2001; 1:114–129.

102. Celis E, Wiktor TJ, Dietzschold B, Koprowski H. Amplification of rabies-virus induced stimulation of human T-cell lines and clones by antigen-specific antibodies. *J Virol* 1985; 56:426–433.

103. Baltazard M, Bahmanyar M. Practical trial of antirabies serum in people bitten by rabid wolves. *Bull World Health Organ* 1955; 13:747–772.

104. Fang-tao L, Shu-beng C, Guan-Fu W, et al. Study of the protective effect of the primary hamster kidney cell rabies vaccine. *J Infect Dis* 1986; 154:1047–1048.

105. Fathi M, Sabeti A, Bahmanyar M. Séroprophylaxie antirabique chez les sujets mordus par loups enragés en Iran. *Acta Med Iran* 1970; 13:5–9.

106. Wiktor TJ, Lerner RA, Koprowski H. Inhibitory effect of passive antibody on active immunity induced against rabies by vaccination. *Bull World Health Organ* 1971; 45:747–753.

107. Suwansrinon K, Wilde H, Benjavongkulchai M, et al. Survival of neutralizing antibody in previously rabies vaccinated subjects: a prospective study showing long lasting immunity. *Vaccine* 2006; 24(18):3878–3880.

108. Babès V. *Traité de la Rage*. Paris: Baillière; 1912.

109. Suzor R. Hydrophobia. An account of M Pasteur's system containing a translation of all his communications on the subject, the techniques of his method, and the latest statistical results. London: Chatto & Windrush; 1887.

110. Cornwall JW. Statistics of antirabic inoculations in India. *BMJ* 1923; 298.

111. Veeraraghavan N. Annual report of the Director 1969 and scientific report 1970. Coonoor: Pasteur Institute of Southern India; 1971.

112. Editorial. Rabies vaccine failures. *Lancet* 1988; i:917–918.

113. Nel LH. Vaccines for lyssaviruses other than rabies. *Expert Rev Vaccines* 2005; 4(4):533–540.

114. Pappaioanou M, Fishbein DB, Dreesen DW, et al. Antibody response to pre-exposure human diploid-cell rabies vaccine given concurrently with chloroquine. *N Engl J Med* 1986; 314:280–284.

115. Strady A, Lang J, Lienard, et al. Antibody persistence following preexposure regimens of cell-culture rabies vaccines: 10-year follow-up and proposal for a new booster policy. *J Infect Dis* 1998; 177:1290–1295.

Chapter 45 C. Anthony Hart, Nigel A. Cunliffe and Osamu Nakagomi

Diarrhoea Caused by Viruses

The gastrointestinal tract is the commonest portal of entry for a variety of pathogens, including viruses, but not all these viruses are causally associated with diarrhoeal disease. Among the viruses that infect enterocytes, or at least use them as a portal of entry, there are two major groups. The first group comprises those viruses that cause systemic infections after entering into the body through the gastrointestinal tract, and diarrhoea, if ever present, is not a major feature of infection. This group includes many enteroviruses, including poliovirus and coxsackieviruses, hepatitis A and E viruses, and some adenoviruses. The second group comprises the viruses that infect the upper small intestine and cause non-inflammatory diarrhoea. It is generally perceived that the enteropathogenic viruses do not normally cause systemic infection. While these viruses are difficult to grow in cell culture, there are often enormous numbers of virions shed into stool, which can be identified by direct electron microscopy or immune electron microscopy. There are currently five genera of viruses recognized as established causes of gastroenteritis in humans, i.e. *Rotavirus*, *Norovirus*, *Sapovirus*, *Astrovirus*, and group F adenovirus.

ROTAVIRUS

Human rotavirus was first discovered in 1973 on thin-section electron microscopy of duodenal biopsies from a child with acute gastroenteritis, and named duovirus.[1] The virus was subsequently found in large numbers in faeces as demonstrated by direct negative-stain electron microscopy[2] and significant antibody titre rises were shown between acute and convalescent sera from diarrhoeal children by immune electron microscopy.[3] The virus was named rotavirus because of its characteristic wheel-shaped (*rota* is Latin for a wheel) morphology on electron microscopy (Figure 45.1).

Geographical distribution

Virtually all children are infected with rotavirus (group A rotavirus) by the age of 3–5 years, whether they live in developing or developed countries.[4,5] Thus, rotavirus is distributed evenly across the world. However, the consequences of infection are markedly different depending on where the child lives, and the majority of deaths due to rotavirus diarrhoea occur in the developing

countries of the Indian subcontinent and sub-Saharan Africa (Figure 45.2).[5,6]

Epidemiology

Rotavirus diarrhoea occurs at an earlier age in children in developing countries than in children in developed countries (Figure 45.3).[7] The median age of children hospitalized with rotavirus diarrhoea in many African and Asian counties is 6–9 months, and up to 80% are less than 1 year old.[8] In contrast, the median age in developed countries is 13–16 months and the highest proportion of cases occurs in the second year of life.[7] Nevertheless, in both developing and developed countries, rotavirus is the major cause of severe gastroenteritis requiring hospitalization and, where access to medical intervention is limited, of death. It has been estimated that, from 1986 to 1999, a median of 22% (range 17–28%) of acute diarrhoea cases in children less than 5 years of age were due to rotavirus,[5] but this proportion has nearly doubled recently (from 2000 to 2004) to become 39% (range 29–45%).[6] The estimated annual global mortality due to rotavirus diarrhoea among children less than 5 years of age has also been increased to 611000 (range 454000–705000), reflecting the increasing detection rate of rotavirus as the cause of severe diarrhoea.[6] Included among countries where the disease burden is estimated to be the highest are Afghanistan (1:90 children), Democratic Republic of Congo (1:130) and Nigeria (1:140), and the cumulative incidence of rotavirus diarrhoeal deaths in developing countries is estimated to be on average 1:250.[9] On the other hand, in developed countries, hospitalization due to rotavirus in children under 5 years of age is estimated as between 1:20 and 1:80.[7] In temperate countries, rotavirus infections peak in the winter and early spring, with fewer cases at other times. In tropical countries, rotavirus infections occur throughout the year, although more cases are observed in the cooler and drier months (Figure 45.4).

Virology

Rotavirus is a genus within the family Reoviridae, and within the genus there are seven groups (A to G), each of which represents a separate species, e.g. *Rotavirus A*, *Rotavirus B*, etc. Only group A, B and C rotaviruses are established as human pathogens. Group A rotavirus has much greater medical importance and, unless mentioned otherwise, rotavirus usually means group A rotavirus. Group B rotavirus infection is rare and affects both adults and children, causing both outbreaks and sporadic infections, primarily in China, India and Bangladesh.[10,11] Group C rotaviruses tend to affect older children than group A rotavirus, and up to a third of adult humans have serological evidence of infection with group C rotavirus.[12,13]

By conventional negative-stain electron microscopy, rotavirus has a characteristic double capsid structure measuring approximately 75 nm in diameter (Figure 45.1), but cryoelectron micro-

scopic studies have shown that a rotavirus virion consists of a triple-layered capsid with 60 spikes protruding from its surface, making its overall diameter nearly 100 nm. As shown in Figure 45.5, the outermost layer (outer capsid) consists of proteins, VP4 and VP7, each of which independently serves as a neutralization antigen. The serotype defined by the VP4 protein is called the P type, for protease-sensitive protein (because VP4 is proteolytically cleaved into VP8* and VP5*), and the serotype defined by the VP7 protein is called the G type, for glycoprotein. The inner capsid or the middle layer consists of the most abundant viral protein, VP6, which is the major protein against which antibodies are raised during infection with rotavirus. These antibodies are, however, non-neutralizing. The core or the innermost layer consists of VP2, a scaffolding protein, and inside this layer are VP1 (viral RNA-dependent RNA polymerase) and VP3 (guanyltransferase), which is present in association with the 11 segments of double-stranded genomic RNA. In addition to these five structural proteins, there are six non-structural proteins (NSPs), each of which is encoded by a single genome segment, except for NSP5 and NSP6, which carry out various functions during replication and morphogenesis. NSP4 works as a chaperone protein enabling the subviral particle to acquire the outer capsid proteins VP4 and VP7 during the later phases of viral morphogenesis. NSP4 also acts as viral enterotoxin, causing diarrhoea in newborn mice.[14–16]

Rotavirus genomic RNA can be extracted directly from clinical specimens and separated by polyacrylamide gel electrophoresis (PAGE). With this, two major RNA migration patterns are recognized in which genome segments 10 and 11 of long RNA pattern

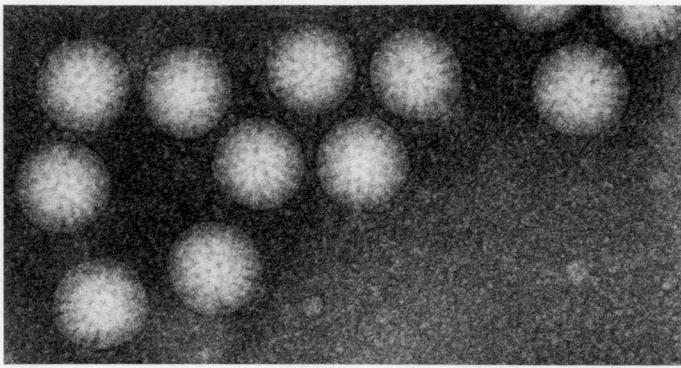

Figure 45.1 Negative-stain electron micrograph of rotavirus particles. (×200 000.)

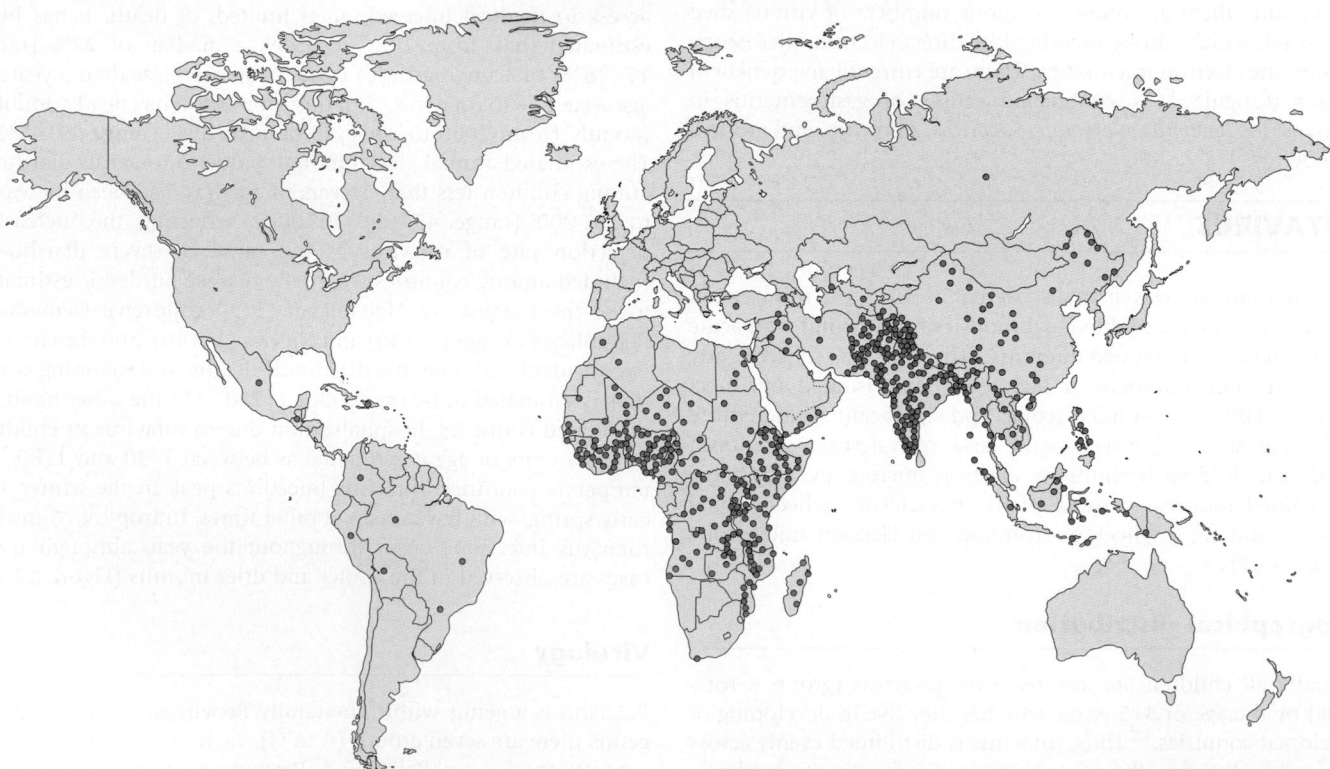

Figure 45.2 Map showing global distribution of rotavirus mortality in children less than 5 years of age. Each dot represents 1000 deaths. (Reprinted from Parashar et al.[6])

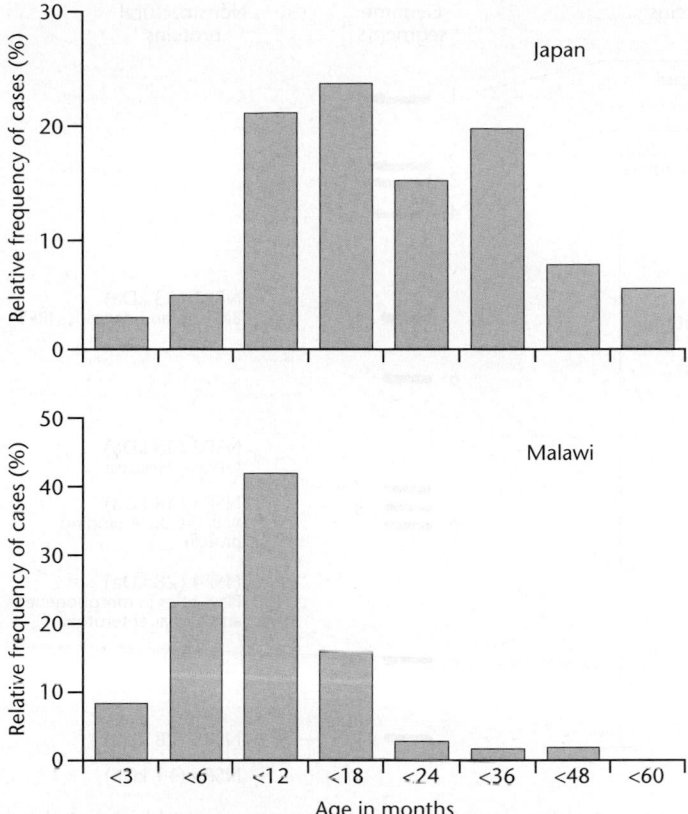

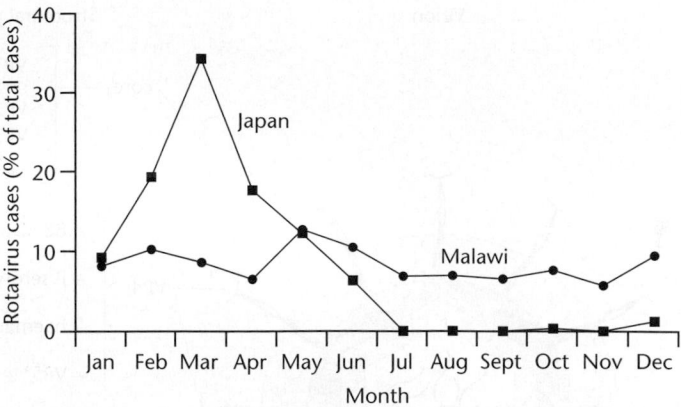

Figure 45.4 The contrasting seasonality of rotavirus diarrhoea occurring in Malawi (as an example of a country in the tropics) and in Japan (temperate climate). Rotavirus gastroenteritis peaks in winter to early spring in temperate countries, while the disease is year-round in the tropics. (Data taken from Nakagomi et al.[7] and Cunliffe et al. [unpublished].)

Figure 45.3 Two contrasting patterns of age distribution of rotavirus diarrhoea occurring in Malawi (as an example of a developing country) and in Japan (as an example of a developed country). There is a clear difference in the median ages of children hospitalized with rotavirus diarrhoea in the two countries. (Data taken from Nakagomi et al.[7] and Cunliffe et al. [unpublished].)

viruses migrate faster than do those of short RNA pattern viruses (Figure 45.6).[17] The precise migration pattern is characteristic for each rotavirus strain and is called an 'electropherotype', which has been extensively used in molecular epidemiological studies.[18]

The serotype is the most important antigenic determinant of rotavirus and is defined traditionally by serological assays. However, serological assays are now being replaced by molecular typing. While there is an exact correlation between G serotype and G genotype, thereby allowing the use of the same numbering system, different numbering systems are adopted to designate P serotype and P genotype. In the latter, a number for P genotype is designated within a squared bracket. Thus, the serotype of prototype human rotavirus strain Wa is described as G1P1A[8]. There are currently 16 G serotypes and 26 P serotypes described in the literature, but the G and P type combinations (Figure 45.7) detected in human rotaviruses are mostly limited to G1P[8], G2P[4], G3P[8], G4P[8] and G9P[8].[19,20] However, previously rare G[12] strains appear to have emerged across the world,[17,21] and G8 strains with either P[6] or P[4] account for a significant proportion of human rotavirus strains in Africa.[22] Such genetic diversity seems to be generated by frequent reassortment of the genome segments and interspecies transmission of rotaviruses between humans and animals.[23,24]

Further discrimination between group A rotaviruses is based on subgroup (I, II, I+II, neither I nor II) antigens that are carried on the VP6 protein, and subgrouping rotavirus isolates is sometimes used in epidemiological studies.

Pathogenesis

Large amounts of rotavirus (up to 10^{11} virus particles per gram) are excreted in faeces during the acute phase of infection, and the shedding continues after the symptoms cease, sometimes for more than 1 month, albeit detectable only by sensitive reverse-transcription (RT) PCR assays.[25] Children with severe diarrhoea excrete more virus than do children with less severe diarrhoea.[26] The minimum infective dose is as low as 10^2–10^3 virus particles in adult volunteers.[27] Person-to-person spread by the faecal–oral route is most likely, but there are possibilities for air-borne and water-borne transmission of rotavirus. The incubation period is usually 1–3 days. Rotavirus exclusively infects the mature differentiated villous enterocytes of the small intestine. Unlike parvovirus, rotavirus cannot infect the immature villous crypt cells, hence stem cells are spared, nor does rotavirus infect colonic enterocytes. Rotavirus attaches to its cellular receptors (sialoglycoprotein and integrins) via the VP4 protein, but whether the virus enters the cells by endocytosis or direct penetration has not been determined. Three mechanisms have been described for the pathogenesis of rotavirus diarrhoea. In the first 12–24 hours post infection, enterocytes are intact but levels of the brush border disaccharidases (sucrase, maltase, lactase) are greatly decreased.[28] This is apparently due to interference with transport of the enzymes to the brush border.[29] As a result, disaccharides in the diet cannot be hydrolysed to monosaccharides and thus cannot be absorbed, producing an osmotic diarrhoea. Second, NSP4 has an effect in opening calcium channels in the enterocyte. This causes an efflux of sodium and water, and a secretory diarrhoea.[14] Finally, the raised intra-enterocyte calcium concentration causes enterocytes to die by oncosis.[30] The rate of death of the mature villous tip

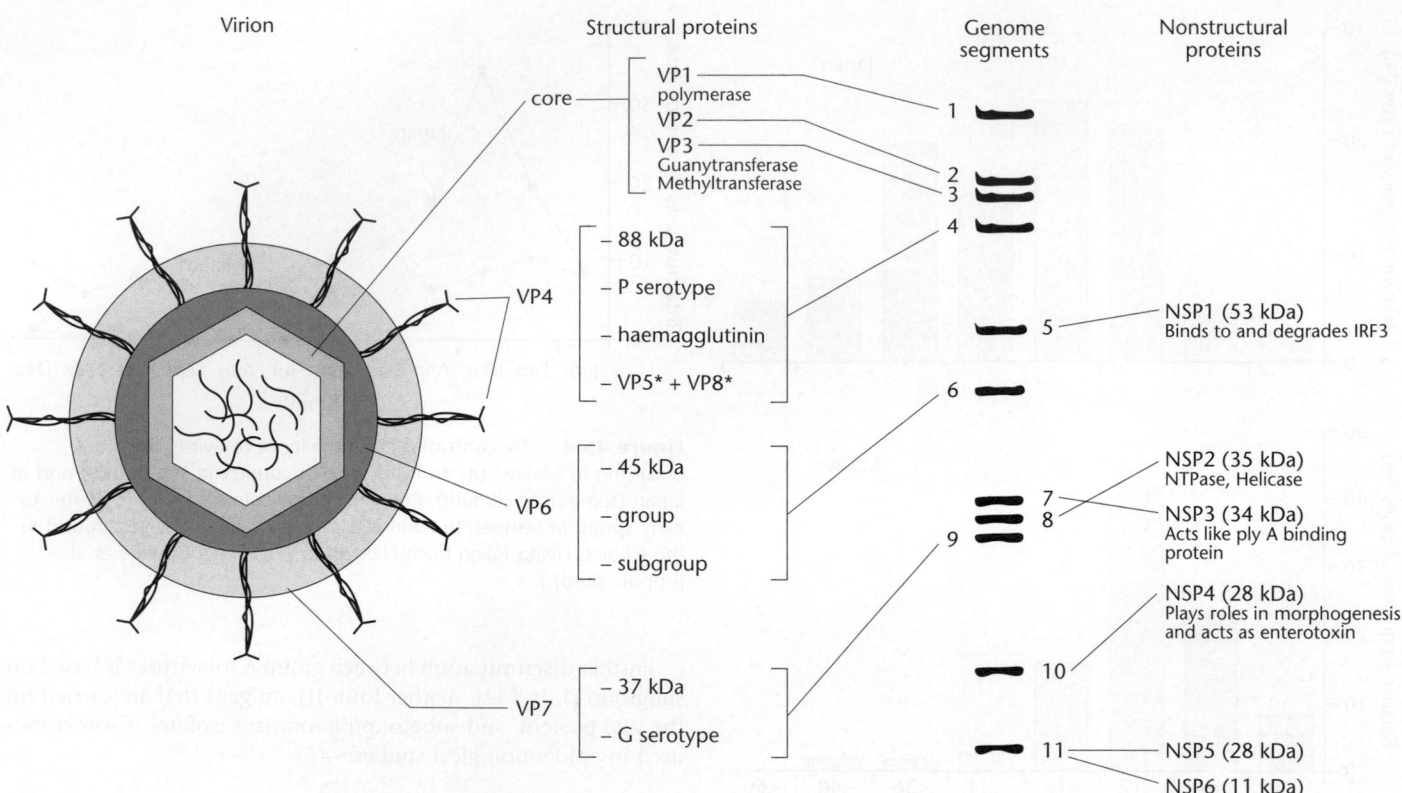

Figure 45.5 A schematic diagram showing the relationships between the structure of the rotavirus virion and the genomic double-stranded RNA segments. IRF3, interferon regulatory factor 3; NTPase, nucleotide triphosphatase.

enterocytes exceeds the rate of growth of immature enterocytes that are regenerated from the stem cells in the crypt, causing villous blunting and thus malabsorption. Infection resolves both as the virus runs out of susceptible mature enterocytes and an immune response is generated. Generally speaking, it is on only the first two or three occasions that disease occurs. However, it is now increasingly recognized that otherwise healthy adults can have rotavirus diarrhoea and elderly people appear to become more susceptible as their immunity wanes.[31,32] Recently, rotavirus antigen has been detected in the blood of immunocompetent infants as well as in experimentally infected animals.[33] The clinical significance of this finding is being investigated.

Immunity

In general, one or more episodes of rotavirus infection confers protection against subsequent severe rotavirus diarrhoea but not against asymptomatic reinfection or mild to moderate diarrhoea. In a cohort study in Mexico, children who had experienced one, two or three episodes of rotavirus diarrhoea had adjusted relative risks of experiencing a further attack of rotavirus diarrhoea of 0.23, 0.17 and 0.08, respectively, but of asymptomatic rotavirus infection of 0.62, 0.40 and 0.34, respectively.[34] Infection with one serotype provides serotype-specific (homotypic) protection, and repeated infections lead to partial cross-serotype (heterotypic) protection. Thus, serotype matters but it does not seem to be the sole determinant in providing protective immunity. Cellular

immunity appears to be important in resolution of rotavirus infection and appears to be cross-protective between the different G serotypes.[35]

Protection of neonates against rotavirus infection appears to be by both transplacentally acquired maternal antibody[36,37] and by antibodies and other factors in breast milk.[38] However, a study in Bangladesh showed that hospitalized children with rotavirus diarrhoea were more likely to be breast-fed than were children with diarrhoea due to other infectious agents.[39] Interestingly, rotavirus infection in neonates often results in asymptomatic infection, unless novel serotypes emerge, and rotavirus can circulate silently in neonatal units. Since such asymptomatic neonatal infections induce protection against subsequent severe rotavirus gastroenteritis,[40] the use of neonatal strains as vaccine candidates has been pursued. However, a recent study in India showed that neonatal infection with a G10P[11] strain that resembles a neonatal vaccine candidate did not confer protection against subsequent rotavirus infection or diarrhoea of any severity.[41]

Clinical features

The outcome of rotavirus infection varies from asymptomatic, through mild short-lived watery diarrhoea, to an overwhelming gastroenteritis with dehydration leading to death. Severe disease and death are more common in children who are already malnourished or have measles. The onset of symptoms is abrupt after a short incubation period of 1–2 days. Fever, vomiting and watery

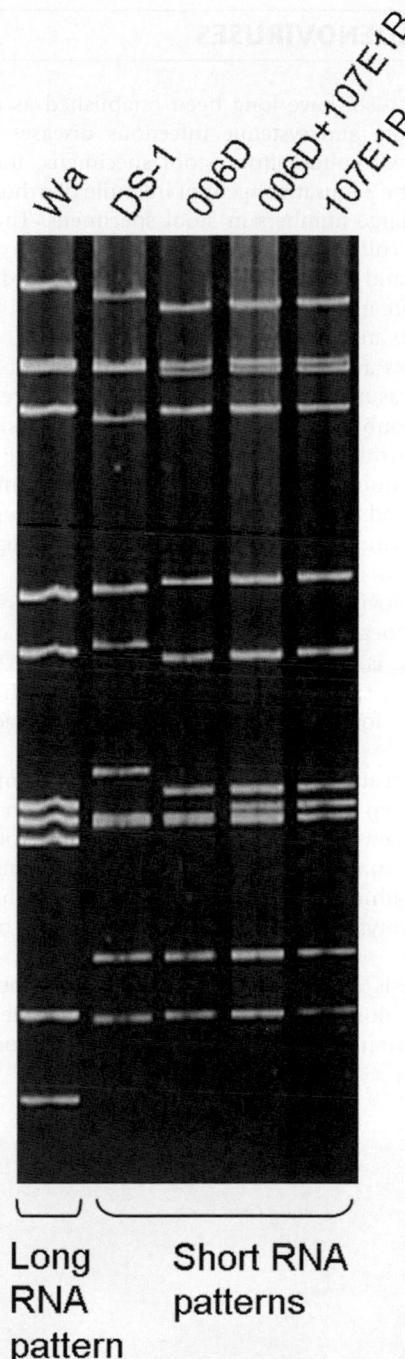

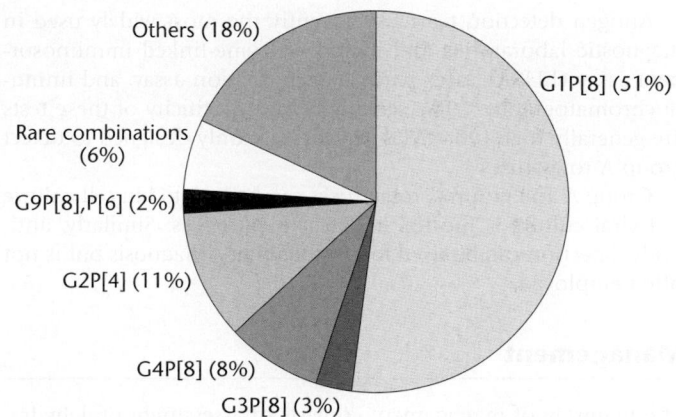

Figure 45.7 Relative frequencies of rotavirus genotypes detected globally among human rotaviruses over the period 1994–2003. (Adapted from Gentsch et al.[19])

Figure 45.6 Separation of rotavirus genomic RNA into 11 bands by polyacrylamide gel electrophoresis. Two RNA patterns, long and short, are represented by prototype strains Wa and DS-1, respectively. Strains 006 and 107E1B have similar but distinct RNA electropherotypes. The differences in migration of segments 7, 8, and 9 are clearly demonstrated by co-electrophoresis in which RNAs from both 006 and 107E1B were loaded on the same lane. (Adapted from Nakagomi, et al.[17])

diarrhoea are seen in the majority of infected children and last for 2–6 days. Rotavirus diarrhoea tends to be more severe than that due to other common enteropathogens[42] but co-infection with another pathogen does not increase disease severity.[43] Respiratory signs are often found during rotavirus gastroenteritis but its aetiological association with rotavirus infection is not clear. Extraintestinal manifestations during rotavirus gastroenteritis, including encephalopathies, have captured much attention since it was recently shown that rotavirus causes viraemia.[33,44] It is not possible to distinguish rotavirus gastroenteritis from other viral causes of non-inflammatory diarrhoea solely on clinical grounds. The stools are usually pale and watery or loose, and are seldom blood-stained. In hospitalized patients, the duration of diarrhoea is from 2 to 23 days, with a median of 6 days.[45] Patients continue to excrete virus for extended periods of time[25,46] and may thus be a reservoir for infecting others. The cause of death is dehydration, which can be hypo- or hypernatraemic and is often associated with metabolic acidosis.

Diagnosis

Rotavirus can be detected in stool specimens by a number of techniques, including electron microscopy, PAGE, antigen detection assays, RT-PCR and virus isolation. Electron microscopy is still a valuable diagnostic tool since it is a catch-all technique that will also detect other potential viral enteropathogens. PAGE is also a convenient diagnostic tool for the detection of rotavirus RNA extracted directly from stool specimens (Figure 45.6). The assay also allows detection of non-group A rotaviruses which fail to react in most antigen detection assays. This technique is relatively simple with good specificity (100%) and sensitivity (80–90%), and can be performed in tropical countries relatively cheaply.[47] It has an added advantage of providing epidemiological information because the electrophoretic migration pattern of the 11 segments of the double-stranded RNA genome is specific to each rotavirus strain.[18,48] Detection of viral genome by RT-PCR is a research tool which provides information on the G and P genotypes of the circulating strains[49–51] and the duration of viral shedding in stool.[25,46]

Antigen detection tests are currently the most widely used in diagnostic laboratories and include enzyme-linked immunosorbent assay (ELISA), latex particle agglutination assay, and immunochromatography.[52] The sensitivity and specificity of these tests are generally high (90–95%) but they are only designed to detect group A rotaviruses.

Group A and group C rotaviruses can be isolated in cell culture but viral culture is limited to research purposes. Similarly, antibody detection can be used for establishing a diagnosis but is not often employed.

Management

The mainstay of management consists of assessment of dehydration and replacement of lost fluid by oral rehydration with fluids of specified electrolyte and glucose composition. Intravenous rehydration therapy is indicated for patients with severe dehydration, shock or reduced levels of consciousness. Human or bovine colostrum and hyperimmune human serum immunoglobulin have been used to manage chronic rotavirus infection in immunocompromised children. Administration of probiotics such as *Lactobacillus casei* GG also appears beneficial. Recently, the antiprotozoal drug nitazoxanide was shown to decrease the median duration of rotavirus gastroenteritis by 44 hours in a randomized double-blind placebo-controlled trial in Egyptian children.[53] How this agent would be used in children in developing countries is unclear.

Prevention and control

Since virtually all children will have experienced rotavirus infection by the age of 3–5 years in both developing and developed countries, it is clear that the high standards of hygiene and sanitation practised in developed countries are not sufficient to prevent the spread of rotavirus infection within the community. Thus, prophylaxis of severe rotavirus gastroenteritis by vaccines remains as the only practical preventive measure.[4,54] The first licensed rotavirus vaccine, a rhesus monkey rotavirus-based tetravalent human reassortant vaccine (RotaShield®), was withdrawn after this live, oral vaccine was associated with the development of intestinal intussusception in approximately 1 : 10 000 vaccine recipients in the USA. Two new rotavirus vaccines, Rotarix® (GlaxoSmithKline Biologicals) and Rotateq® (Merck & Co.), have recently completed phase III clinical trials, each involving more than 60 000 infants. Both vaccines were found to be safe when given to infants under 3 months of age and were >85% efficacious in preventing severe gastroenteritis due to rotavirus.[55,56] Rotarix® is a monovalent human rotavirus vaccine of serotype G1P1A[8], whereas Rotateq® is a pentavalent bovine–human reassortant vaccine comprising types G1, G2, G3, G4 and P[8]. Updated disease burden estimates and economic justification will be needed wherever vaccine introduction is considered. Further confirmation of the safety profile of either vaccine will depend on post-licensure evaluation. Assessment of the ability of each vaccine to provide protection against an increasingly diverse population of rotavirus strains will require continuous global strain surveillance. Rotavirus does not produce more severe disease in HIV-infected infants,[57] so use of live-reassortant rotaviruses in populations with a high prevalence of HIV should not pose a risk.

ENTERIC ADENOVIRUSES

While adenoviruses have long been established as the cause of some respiratory and systemic infectious diseases and can be recovered in cell culture from stool specimens, they were not considered to be a causative agent of infantile diarrhoea until they were seen in large numbers in stool specimens. These adenoviruses were not cultivatable in cells used for the more conventional adenoviruses, and were thus called 'enteric' or 'fastidious' adenoviruses. They are now readily grown in 293 cells and are classified as serotypes 40 and 41 in group F adenoviruses.

Adenoviruses are unenveloped DNA viruses with an icosahedral capsid measuring 70–75 nm in diameter (Figure 45.8). Their genomes are double-stranded linear DNA of 33–45 kilobase pairs. Family Adenoviridae has now been divided into the genus *Mastadenovirus* (mammalian adenoviruses, to which human adenoviruses belong) and the genus *Aviadenovirus* (adenoviruses of birds). Human adenoviruses are further divided into six subgenera (A–F) and 51 serotypes.

Enteric adenoviruses account for approximately 5% of cases of infantile diarrhoea, occurring most often in children under 2 years of age.[58] There is no apparent seasonality to infection. Enteric adenoviruses are spread from person to person by the faecal–oral route. Neither food-borne nor water-borne spread has been described.

The clinical features of enteric adenovirus gastroenteritis do not differ greatly from those of rotavirus but the duration of diarrhoea tends to be longer in adenovirus infection than in rotavirus infection.[59,60] Other than gastroenteritis, adenovirus is implicated as a cause of idiopathic intussusception in infants.[61,62] These adenoviruses are of serotypes 1, 2, 3 and 5, and rarely of 40 or 41 (enteric adenoviruses).

The diagnosis of adenovirus infection is by visualization of characteristic virions in stool specimens under the electron microscope; demonstration of adenovirus antigens in stool by ELISA,

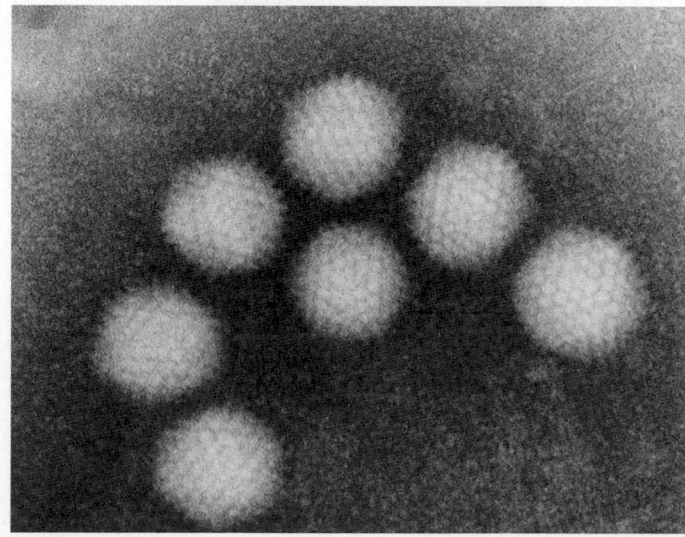

Figure 45.8 Negative-stain electron micrograph of enteric adenovirus. (×200 000.)

latex agglutination assay or immunochromatography; or detection of the genome by DNA hybridization (mostly in tissues) and PCR.

Treatment of adenovirus diarrhoea is by managing dehydration. There is neither a specific therapeutic intervention nor a vaccine.

ASTROVIRUS

Astrovirus was first described in 1975 and is now established as an important cause of gastroenteritis in children and adults. The family Astroviridae can infect a variety of animal species, including humans. Astrovirus is an unenveloped virus measuring 28–30 nm in diameter. Under the electron microscope it has a characteristic star shape 'stamped' on its surface, a five- or six-pointed star with an electron-dense centre (*astron* is Greek for a star) (Figure 45.9). It has a positive-sense single-stranded RNA genome approximately 7 kb in length which encodes an RNA polymerase (ORF1a), a serine protease (ORF1b) and three capsid proteins (ORF2).

There are at least eight serotypes (serotypes 1–8) of human astroviruses and serotype 1 is the most frequently detected.[63] However, other serotypes can be responsible for outbreaks of food-borne infections and there appears to be a greater diversity of serotypes in developing countries.[64] The importance of astrovirus gastroenteritis has only recently been recognized with the development of improved diagnostic tests such as ELISA. Astrovirus infections predominate in young children aged between 4–5 months and 4 years, and account for between 2% and 10% of cases of diarrhoea in children. The disease tends to be milder and more frequently encountered in community-based studies.[65] One such study in Mexico estimated the incidence rate of astrovirus gastroenteritis to be 0.1 episodes per child per year.[66] Sero-epidemiological studies have demonstrated that more than 90% of children in the USA will have experienced astrovirus infections by the age of 6–9 years.[67] Astrovirus has been detected in all countries where sufficiently sensitive detection methods have been used, including Malawi,[68] Mexico,[66] South Africa,[69] and Egypt.[70] In temperate countries it shows a similar seasonal distribution to rotavirus but peaks a month earlier.

Astrovirus is transmitted faeco-orally either directly or by ingestion of food. Astrovirus infects the upper small intestine but the mechanism of diarrhoea is not known. The features of the illness are similar to those of rotavirus but may be milder and its duration is 4–5 days on average. However, in Bangladesh, astrovirus was found to be associated with prolonged diarrhoea.[64]

Diagnosis used to be solely by electron microscopy, but this is now being replaced by more sensitive and easy-to-perform ELISA or latex agglutination assays, or by detection of the genome by RT-PCR. Treatment is by managing dehydration. There is no vaccine available and little is known of immunity to infection other than that children with immunodeficiency excrete the virus for long periods.[71]

CALICIVIRUSES

Norovirus and *Sapovirus* are two different genera of viruses that belong to the family Caliciviridae and are major causative agents of acute gastroenteritis in children and adults. The Norwalk agent, the prototype of *Norovirus*, was first identified by immune electron microscopy as 27 nm virus particles with a feathery-ragged outline (Figure 45.10) in stool specimens of volunteers who were challenged with the clinical specimens collected during a gastroenteritis outbreak in Norwalk, Ohio, USA.[72] In addition, stool examination by negative-stain electron microscopy has demonstrated the presence of 'typical' calicivirus-like particles (Figure 45.11), now classified as *Sapovirus* (the prototype was found in Sapporo, Japan), in the stool specimens of children. These exhibit the 'classical' distinct cup-shaped depressions (*calyx* is Greek for a cup) on the surface of the virion.[73,74] Molecular cloning of these viruses has confirmed that both noroviruses and sapoviruses are members of Caliciviridae but each constitutes a distinct genus within the family.[75]

Norovirus

Norovirus has an unenveloped virion with icosahedral symmetry, measuring 27–30 nm in diameter. Its genome is positive-sense, single-stranded RNA, approximately 7 kb in length, with a stretch of poly A sequence at its 3′ terminus. The genome contains three

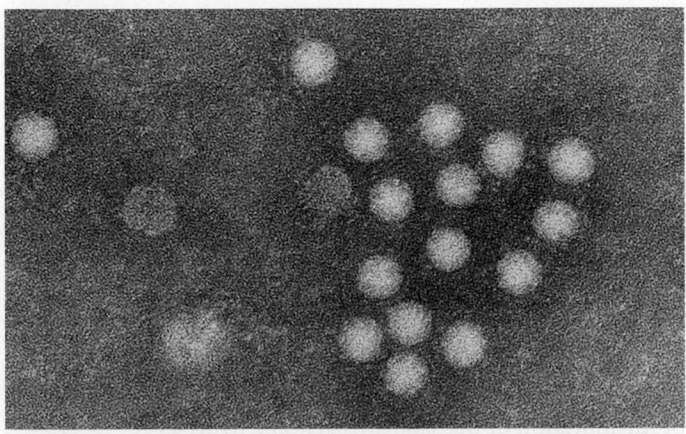

Figure 45.9 Negative-stain electron micrograph of enteric astrovirus. (×200 000.)

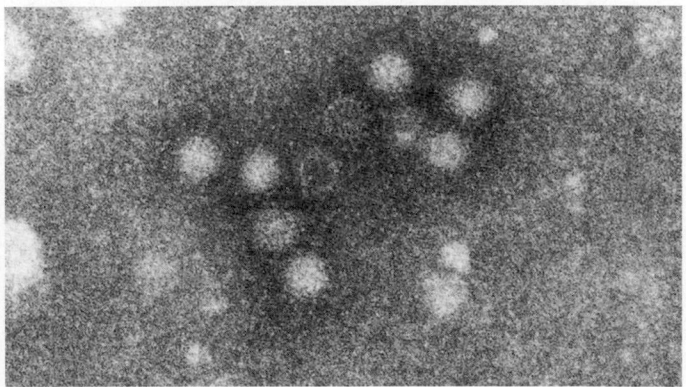

Figure 45.10 Negative-stain electron micrograph of norovirus with a feathery-ragged outline. (×200 000.)

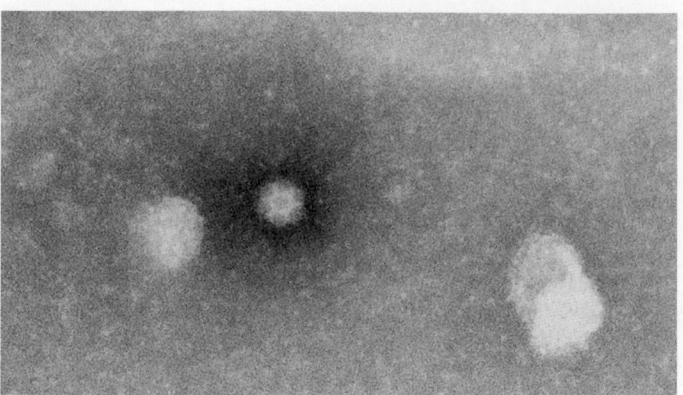

Figure 45.11 Negative-stain electron micrograph of a sapovirus with the classical 'Star of David' morphology. (×200 000.)

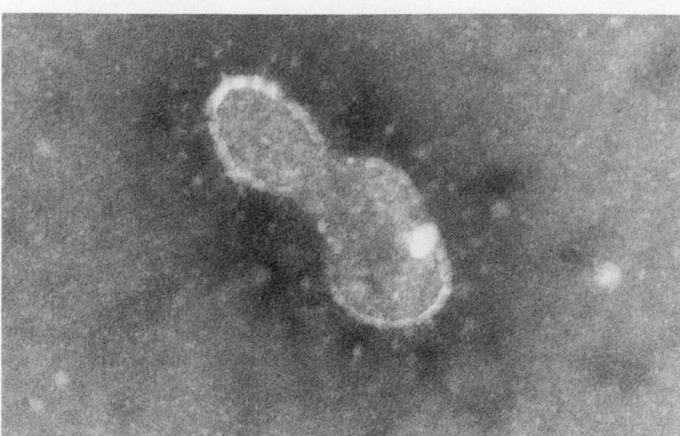

Figure 45.12 Negative-stain electron micrograph of an enteric coronavirus. (×200 000.)

ORFs, of which ORF2 encodes a single polypeptide of 59 kDa on which the antigenicity of a virus strain is expressed. Since neither animal model nor cell culture systems are available to test the infectivity of norovirus other than volunteer challenge studies, serotypes of norovirus have not been established. The genome of norovirus exhibits a great diversity and there are multiple genotypes that are distributed into four genogroups (GI–GIV).[76]

Norovirus is spread faeco-orally, and causes an illness with an abrupt onset of vomiting, diarrhoea and abdominal pain after a short incubation period of 1–2 days. While transmission via the respiratory route has not been established, it has been suggested from epidemiological observations that aerosolized saliva or vomitus can be the source of infection.[77] The illness is generally mild and fever rarely exceeds 38 °C. Recovery follows within 1–3 days, but the excretion of norovirus into stool lasts longer, sometimes up to 2 weeks. Approximately half of those infected with norovirus remain asymptomatically infected. In temperate countries, norovirus gastroenteritis tends to show a winter seasonality. Infection can occur as point-source food-borne outbreaks or sporadically.

Norovirus was initially thought solely to be the cause of epidemic gastroenteritis limited to older children and adults, but it is now known that norovirus is also a major cause of infantile diarrhoea. In a study in Finnish children, norovirus was responsible for 20% of cases of gastroenteritis. In comparison, sapovirus was detected in 9%, astrovirus in 10%, enteric adenovirus in 6%, and rotavirus in 31% of the cases.[78]

Electron microscopy is relatively insensitive except in the first days of the illness and the definitive diagnosis needs to be made based on either antigen detection or identification of the norovirus genome by RT-PCR.[79] Recently, commercial antigen detection kits have been developed, which are less sensitive than genomic detection by RT-PCR but the specificity is close to 100%.

Following infection, patients produce serum and faecal antibody to viral capsid proteins but their role in protective immunity is not fully defined. Recently, considerable progress has been made in understanding the relationships between norovirus and tissue antigens, including the ABO blood groups.[80] Norovirus appears to use secreted blood group (H) antigens expressed on the mucosal surface of the enterocytes as viral receptors; thus, non-secretors, in whom such antigens are not expressed on the intestinal mucosa, are resistant to norovirus infection.[81]

There is no specific therapy nor are vaccines available.

Sapovirus

Sapovirus has an unenveloped virion with icosahedral symmetry, measuring 30–35 nm in diameter. Negative-stain electron microscopy reveals characteristic particle morphology with cup-like depressions, often described as the 'Star of David' (Figure 45.11). Its genome is positive-sense, single-stranded RNA of approximately 7 kb in length with a stretch of poly A sequence at its 3′ terminus. Unlike norovirus, sapovirus encodes the capsid protein contiguous with the large non-structural polyprotein (ORF1). The junction that corresponds to ORF1 and ORF2 of norovirus consists of a one- or four-nucleotide overlap between the stop codon of ORF1 and the first AUG codon of ORF2. This creates a −1 frameshift. The 3′ end of ORF1 encodes a single polypeptide of 62 kDa.

Illness due to sapovirus tends to predominate in young children, and virtually all children appear to have experienced infection by sapovirus by the age of 5 years. In temperate countries, sapovirus gastroenteritis occurs more frequently in winter. Sapovirus accounts for approximately 5% of cases of infantile diarrhoea, the detection rates being similar to those of adenovirus and astrovirus. Sapovirus rarely causes outbreaks of food-borne gastroenteritis.

Sapovirus spreads faeco-orally and infects, and causes predominantly diarrhoea in infants and young children. Protective immunity appears to follow infection, since, unlike with norovirus, adults rarely get sapovirus gastroenteritis.

While a typical calicivirus-like morphology under the electron microscope strongly suggests the presence of sapovirus, the definitive diagnosis needs to be made based on either antigen detection or identification of the sapovirus genome by RT-PCR.[79]

Treatment is by management of dehydration. There is neither specific antiviral chemotherapy nor a vaccine available.

OTHER VIRUSES

A number of other viruses, including coronavirus[82] (Figure 45.12), torovirus,[83] picobirnavirus[84,85] and pestivirus,[86] have been detected in stool specimens of patients with acute gastroenteritis, but their significance as aetiological agents of diarrhoea remains to be established.

REFERENCES

1. Bishop RF, Davidson GP, Holmes IH, et al. Virus particles in epithelial cells of duodenal mucosa from children with acute non-bacterial gastroenteritis. *Lancet* 1973; ii:1281–1283.

2. Bishop RF, Davidson GP, Holmes IH, et al. Detection of a new virus by electron microscopy of faecal extracts from children with acute gastroenteritis. *Lancet* 1974; i:149–151.

3. Kapikian AZ, Kim HW, Wyatt RG, et al. Reovirus like agent in stools: association with infantile diarrhea and development of serologic tests. *Science* 1974; 185:1049–1053.

4. Cunliffe NA, Nakagomi O. A critical time for rotavirus vaccines: a review. *Exp Rev Vaccines* 2005; 4:521–532.

5. Parashar UD, Hummelman EG, Bresee JS, et al. Global illness and deaths caused by rotavirus disease in children. *Emerg Infect Dis* 2003; 9:565–572.

6. Parashar UD, Gibson CJ, Bresse JS, et al. Rotavirus and severe childhood diarrhea. *Emerg Infect Dis* 2006; 12:304–306.

7. Nakagomi T, Nakagomi O, Takahashi Y, et al. Incidence and burden of rotavirus gastroenteritis in Japan as estimated from a prospective sentinel hospital study. *J Infect Dis* 2005; 192(suppl 1):106–110.

8. Cunliffe NA, Kilgore PE, Bresee JS, et al. Epidemiology of rotavirus diarrhoea in Africa: a review to assess the need for rotavirus immunization. *Bull World Health Organ* 1998; 76:525–537.

9. Glass RI, Bresee JS, Turcios R, et al. Rotavirus vaccines: targeting the developing world. *J Infect Dis* 2005; 192(suppl 1):160–166.

10. Hung T, Chen GM, Wang CG, et al. Rotavirus-like agent in adult non-bacterial diarrhoea in China. *Lancet* 1983; 5; ii:1078–1079.

11. Sen A, Kobayashi N, Das S, et al. The evolution of human group B rotaviruses. *Lancet* 2001; 357:198–199.

12. Kuzuya M, Fujii R, Hamano M, et al. Seroepidemiology of human group C rotavirus in Japan based on a blocking enzyme-linked immunosorbent assay. *Clin Diagn Lab Immunol* 2001; 8:161–165.

13. Riepenhoff-Talty M, Morse K, Wang CH, et al. Epidemiology of group C rotavirus infection in Western New York women of childbearing age. *J Clin Microbiol* 1997; 35:486–488.

14. Ball JM, Tian P, Zeng CQ, et al. Age-dependent diarrhea induced by a rotaviral nonstructural glycoprotein. *Science* 1996; 5:272:101–104.

15. Horie Y, Nakagomi O, Koshimura Y, et al. Diarrhea induction by rotavirus NSP4 in the homologous mouse model system. *Virology* 1999; 262:398–407.

16. Sasaki S, Horie Y, Nakagomi T, et al. Group C rotavirus NSP4 induces diarrhea in neonatal mice. *Arch Virol* 2001; 146:801–806.

17. Nakagomi T, Gentsch JR, Das BK, et al. Molecular characterization of serotype G2 and G3 human rotavirus strains that have an apparently identical electropherotype of the short RNA pattern. *Arch Virol* 2002;147:2187–2195.

18. Holmes IH. Development of rotavirus molecular epidemiology: electropherotyping. *Arch Virol* 1996; 12(suppl):87–91.

19. Gentsch JR, Laird AR, Bielfelt B, et al. Serotype diversity and reassortment between human and animal rotavirus strains: implications for rotavirus vaccine programs. *J Infect Dis* 2005; 192(suppl 1):146–159.

20. Santos N, Hoshino Y. Global distribution of rotavirus serotypes/genotypes and its implication for the development and implementation of an effective rotavirus vaccine. *Rev Med Virol* 2005; 15:29–56.

21. Castello AA, Arguelles MH, Rota RP, et al. Molecular epidemiology of group A rotavirus diarrhea among children in Buenos Aires, Argentina, from 1999 to 2003 and emergence of the infrequent genotype G12. *J Clin Microbiol* 2006; 44:2046–2050.

22. Cunliffe NA, Gentsch JR, Kirkwood CD, et al. Molecular and serologic characterization of novel serotype G8 human rotavirus strains detected in Blantyre, Malawi. *Virology* 2000; 274:309–320.

23. Cunliffe NA, Bresee JS, Gentsch JR, et al. The expanding diversity of rotaviruses. *Lancet* 2002; 359:640–642.

24. Nakagomi O, Nakagomi T. Genomic relationships among rotaviruses recovered from various animal species as revealed by RNA-RNA hybridization assays. *Res Vet Sci* 2002; 73:207–214.

25. Richardson S, Grimwood K, Gorrell R, et al. Extended excretion of rotavirus after severe diarrhoea in young children. *Lancet* 1998; 351: 1844–1848.

26. Kang G, Iturriza-Gomara M, Wheeler JG, et al. Quantitation of group A rotavirus by real-time reverse-transcription-polymerase chain reaction: correlation with clinical severity in children in South India. *J Med Virol* 2004; 73:118–122.

27. Ward RL, Bernstein DI, Young EC, et al. Human rotavirus studies in volunteers: determination of infectious dose and serological response to infection. *J Infect Dis* 1986; 154:871–880.

28. Batt RM, Embaye H, van de Waal S, et al. Application of organ culture of small intestine to the investigation of enterocyte damage by equine rotavirus. *J Pediatr Gastroenterol Nutr* 1995; 20:326–332.

29. Jourdan N, Brunet JP, Sapin C, et al. Rotavirus infection reduces sucrase-isomaltase expression in human intestinal epithelial cells by perturbing protein targeting and organization of microvillar cytoskeleton. *J Virol* 1998; 72:7228–7236.

30. Perez JF, Chemello ME, Liprandi F, et al. Oncosis in MA104 cells is induced by rotavirus infection through an increase in intracellular Ca2+ concentration. *Virology* 1998; 252:17–27.

31. Nakajima H, Nakagomi T, Kamisawa T, et al. Winter seasonality and rotavirus diarrhoea in adults. *Lancet* 2001; 357:1950.

32. Anderson EJ, Weber SG. Rotavirus infection in adults. *Lancet Infect Dis* 2004; 4:91–99.

33. Blutt SE, Kirkwood CD, Parreno V, et al. Rotavirus antigenaemia and viraemia: a common event? *Lancet* 2003; 362:1445–1449.

34. Velazquez FR, Matson DO, Calva JJ, et al. Rotavirus infections in infants as protection against subsequent infections. *N Engl J Med* 1996; 335: 1022–1028.

35. Heath RR, Stagg S, Xu F, et al. Mapping of the target antigens of the rotavirus-specific cytotoxic T cell response. *J Gen Virol* 1997; 78:1065–1075.

36. Ramachandran M, Vij A, Kumar R, et al. Lack of maternal antibodies to P serotypes may predispose neonates to infections with unusual rotavirus strains. *Clin Diagn Lab Immunol* 1998; 5:527–530.

37. Widdowson MA, van Doornum GJ, van der Poel WH, et al. Emerging group-A rotavirus and a nosocomial outbreak of diarrhoea. *Lancet* 2000; 356:1161–1162.

38. Jayashree S, Bhan MK, Kumar R, et al. Protection against neonatal rotavirus infection by breast milk antibodies and trypsin inhibitors. *J Med Virol* 1988; 26:333–338.

39. Glass RI, Stoll BJ, Wyatt RG, et al. Observations questioning a protective role for breast-feeding in severe rotavirus diarrhea. *Acta Paediatr Scand* 1986; 75:713–718.

40. Bishop RF, Barnes GL, Cipriani E, et al. Clinical immunity after neonatal rotavirus infection. A prospective longitudinal study in young children. *N Engl J Med* 1983; 309:72–76.

41. Banerjee I, Gladstone BP, Le Fevre AM, et al. Neonatal infection with G10P[11] rotavirus did not confer protection against subsequent rotavirus infection in a community cohort in Vellore, South India. *J Infect Dis* 2007; 195:625–632.

42. Perez-Schael I, Garcia D, Gonzalez M, et al. Prospective study of diarrheal diseases in Venezuelan children to evaluate the efficacy of rhesus rotavirus vaccine. *J Med Virol* 1990; 30:219–229.

43. Unicomb LE, Faruque SM, Malek MA, et al. Demonstration of a lack of synergistic effect of rotavirus with other diarrheal pathogens on severity of diarrhea in children. *J Clin Microbiol* 1996; 34:1340–1342.

44. Nakagomi T, Nakagomi O. Rotavirus antigenemia in children with encephalopathy accompanied by rotavirus gastroenteritis. *Arch Virol* 2005; 150:1927–1931.

45. Hart CA, Cunliffe NA. Viral gastroenteritis. *Curr Opin Infect Dis* 1999; 12: 447–457.

46. Wilde J, Yolken R, Willoughby R, et al. Improved detection of rotavirus shedding by polymerase chain reaction. *Lancet* 1991; 337:323–326.

47. Herring AJ, Inglis NF, Ojeh CK, et al. Rapid diagnosis of rotavirus infection by direct detection of viral nucleic acid in silver-stained polyacrylamide gels. *J Clin Microbiol* 1982; 16:473–477.

48. Watanabe M, Nakagomi T, Koshimura Y, et al. Direct evidence for genome segment reassortment between concurrently-circulating human rotavirus strains. *Arch Virol* 2001; 146:557–570.

49. Gouvea V, Glass RI, Woods P, et al. Polymerase chain reaction amplification and typing of rotavirus nucleic acid from stool specimens. *J Clin Microbiol* 1990; 28:276–282.

50. Gentsch JR, Glass RI, Woods P, et al. Identification of group A rotavirus gene 4 types by polymerase chain reaction. *J Clin Microbiol* 1992; 30:1365–1373.

51. Gunasena S, Nakagomi O, Isegawa Y, et al. Relative frequency of VP4 gene alleles among human rotaviruses recovered over a 10-year period (1982–1991) from Japanese children with diarrhea. *J Clin Microbiol* 1993; 31:2195–2197.

52. Thomas EE, Puterman ML, Kawano E, et al. Evaluation of seven immunoassays for detection of rotavirus in pediatric stool samples. *J Clin Microbiol* 1988; 26:1189–1193.

53. Rossignol J-F, Abu-Zekry M, Hussein A, et al. Effect of nitazoxanide for treatment of severe rotavirus diarrhoea: randomised double-blind placebo-controlled trial. *Lancet* 2006; 368:124–129.

54. Glass RI, Parashar UD, Bresee JS, et al. Rotavirus vaccines: current prospects and future challenges. *Lancet* 2006; 368:323–332.

55. Ruiz-Palacios GM, Perez-Schael I, Velazquez FR, et al. Safety and efficacy of an attenuated vaccine against severe rotavirus gastroenteritis. *N Engl J Med* 2006; 354:11–22.

56. Vesikari T, Matson DO, Dennehy P, et al. Safety and efficacy of a pentavalent human-bovine (WC3) reassortant rotavirus vaccine. *N Engl J Med* 2006; 354:23–33.

57. Cunliffe NA, Gondwe JS, Kirkwood CD, et al. Effect of concomitant HIV on presentation and outcome of rotavirus gastroenteritis in Malawian children. *Lancet* 2001; 358:550–555.

58. Barnes GL, Uren E, Stevens KB, et al. Etiology of acute gastroenteritis in hospitalized children in Melbourne, Australia, from April 1980 to March 1993. *J Clin Microbiol* 1998; 36:133–138.

59. Yolken RH, Lawrence F, Leister F, et al. Gastroenteritis associated with enteric type adenovirus in hospitalized infants. *J Pediatr* 1982; 101:21–26.

60. Kotloff KL, Losonsky GA, Morris JG, et al. Enteric adenovirus infection and childhood diarrhea: an epidemiologic study in three clinical settings. *Pediatrics* 1989; 84:219–225.

61. Montgomery EA, Popek EJ. Intussusception, adenovirus and children: a brief reaffirmation. *Hum Pathol* 1994; 25:169–174.

62. Bines JE, Liem NT, Justice FA, et al. Intussusception Study Group. Risk factors for intussusception in infants in Vietnam and Australia: adenovirus implicated, but not rotavirus. *J Pediatr* 2006; 149:452–460.

63. Sakamoto T, Negishi H, Wang QH, et al. Molecular epidemiology of astroviruses in Japan from 1995 to 1998 by reverse transcription-polymerase chain reaction with serotype-specific primers (1 to 8). *J Med Virol* 2000; 61:326–331.

64. Unicomb LE, Banu NN, Azim T, et al. Astrovirus infection in association with acute, persistent and nosocomial diarrhea in Bangladesh. *Pediatr Infect Dis J* 1998; 17:611–614.

65. Maldonado Y, Cantwell M, Old M, et al. Population-based prevalence of symptomatic and asymptomatic astrovirus infection in rural Mayan infants. *J Infect Dis* 1998; 178:334–339.

66. Guerrero ML, Noel JS, Mitchell DK, et al. A prospective study of astrovirus diarrhea of infancy in Mexico City. *Pediatr Infect Dis J* 1998; 17:723–727.

67. Mitchell DK, Matson DO, Jiang X, et al. Molecular epidemiology of childhood astrovirus infection in child care centers. *J Infect Dis* 1999; 180:514–517.

68. Pavone R, Schinaia N, Hart CA, et al. Viral gastro-enteritis in children in Malawi. *Ann Trop Paediatr* 1990; 10:15–20.

69. Steele AD, Basetse HR, Blacklow NR, et al. Astrovirus infection in South Africa: a pilot study. *Ann Trop Paediatr* 1998; 18:315–319.

70. Naficy AB, Rao MR, Holmes JL, et al. Astrovirus diarrhea in Egyptian children. *J Infect Dis* 2000; 182:685–690.

71. Cox GJ, Matsui SM, Lo RS, et al. Etiology and outcome of diarrhea after marrow transplantation: a prospective study. *Gastroenterology* 1994; 107:1398–1407.

72. Kapikian AZ, Wyatt RG, Dolin R, et al. Visualization by immune electron microscopy of a 27-nm particle associated with acute infectious nonbacterial gastroenteritis. *J Virol* 1972; 10:1075–1081.

73. Madeley CR, Cosgrove BP. Caliciviruses in man. *Lancet* 1976; i:199–200.

74. Chiba S, Sakuma Y, Kogasaka R, et al. An outbreak of gastroenteritis associated with calicivirus in an infant home. *J Med Virol* 1979; 4:249–254.

75. Jiang X, Graham DY, Wang K, et al. Norwalk virus genome cloning and characterization. *Science* 1990; 250:1580–1583.

76. Radford AD, Gaskell RM, Hart CA. Human norovirus infection and the lessons from animal caliciviruses. *Curr Opin Infect Dis* 2004; 17: 471–478.

77. Becker KM, Moe CL, Southwick KL, et al. Transmission of Norwalk virus during football game. *N Engl J Med* 2000; 343:1223–1227.

78. Pang XL, Honma S, Nakata S, et al. Human caliciviruses in acute gastroenteritis of young children in the community. *J Infect Dis* 2000; 181(suppl 2):288–294.

79. Atmar RL, Estes MK. Diagnosis of noncultivatable gastroenteritis viruses, the human caliciviruses. *Clin Microbiol Rev* 2001; 14:15–37.

80. Moreno-Espinosa S, Farkas T, Jiang X. Human caliciviruses and pediatric gastroenteritis. *Semin Pediatr Infect Dis* 2004; 15:237–245.

81. Lindesmith L, Moe C, Marionneau S, et al. Human susceptibility and resistance to Norwalk virus infection. *Nat Med* 2003; 9:548–553.

82. Zhang XM, Herbst W, Kousoulas KG, et al. Biological and genetic characterization of a hemagglutinating coronavirus isolated from a diarrhoeic child. *J Med Virol* 1994; 44:152–161.

83. Jamieson FB, Wang EE, Bain C, et al. Human torovirus: a new nosocomial gastrointestinal pathogen. *J Infect Dis* 1998; 178:1263–1269.

84. Ludert JE, Liprandi F. Identification of viruses with bi- and trisegmented double-stranded RNA genome in faeces of children with gastroenteritis. *Res Virol* 1993; 144:219–224.

85. Wakuda M, Pongsuwanna Y, Taniguchi K. Complete nucleotide sequences of two RNA segments of human picobirnavirus. *J Virol Methods* 2005; 126:165–169.

86. Yolken R, Dubovi E, Leister F, et al. Infantile gastroenteritis associated with excretion of pestivirus antigens. *Lancet* 1989; i:517–520.

Chapter 46

J. S. Malik Peiris and Charles R. Madeley

Respiratory Viruses

No individual can survive without a functioning respiratory tract. It is frequently invaded by infective agents of all kinds, including viruses and bacteria. The consequences depend not only on the particular agent but also on the individual patient. Pre-existing impairment of the tract by congenital malformations or damage from previous episodes of infection or trauma, as well as the circumstances of the individual as a whole (malnutrition, poverty, overcrowding, sanitation, etc.), will profoundly affect the outcome. This chapter primarily concerns viruses but other microorganisms may be involved, alone or in combination. The respiratory tract may also be involved in part of a more extensive disease process which may itself be due to a virus. Infection of one part of the respiratory tract should therefore not be seen in isolation; the wider implications must be considered.

Acute respiratory infections are estimated to cause approximately 1.9 million childhood deaths annually, 70% of them in Africa and South-east Asia.[1] The contribution of acute respiratory infections to overall childhood mortality ranges from <5% in the developed countries to 25% in some developing countries. Bacterial infections in general have a higher case fatality than acute viral infections, but viruses are far more common causes of acute respiratory infection. Overall they contribute to at least one-third of the deaths caused by acute respiratory infection in the developing world.[2]

CLINICAL PICTURE

The respiratory tract can be divided into upper and lower parts, with the boundary at the lower end of the larynx. Viral infections confined to the upper part (upper respiratory tract infection, URTI) are rarely life-threatening, with the exception of croup. They can be uncomfortable but do not usually call the individual's future into question. These infections do not automatically spread to the lower respiratory tract, but where the lower respiratory tract is involved the process is extensive and rarely confined to one lobe or even one lung. This contrasts with pneumococcal pneumonia, which is typically confined to one lobe of one lung (see also Chapter 11).

Although widespread, the clinical consequences of viral infection are usually less severe than those seen in bacterial pneumonia; otherwise, such infections would be much more lethal. Severe Acute Respiratory Syndrome (SARS) and disease due to avian influenza subtype H5N1 are notable exceptions, where disease severity and mortality from a virus infection is particularly high. The most common manifestations of a lower respiratory tract infection (LRTI) are bronchiolitis (in infants) or an atypical pneumonia. Even when an LRTI occurs, the upper tract is also usually involved and the causative virus can usually be recovered from it.

There are no clear-cut differences between the clinical presentation(s) of any viruses in the respiratory tract. For example, although respiratory syncytial virus (RSV) is the most common cause of bronchiolitis worldwide, this clinical condition may also be caused by parainfluenza viruses, influenza viruses, adenoviruses or rhinoviruses. Consequently, it must not be assumed that two patients with similar clinical illnesses will have been infected by the same virus. This is particularly so in babies and young children. Conversely, the same virus may cause a range of clinical manifestations in different patients.[3]

THE VIRUSES

Table 46.1 lists those viruses generally associated with the respiratory tract. Nevertheless, other viruses may be present as part of a generalized process in which the respiratory component is only a (small) part.

Table 46.1 is divided into two sections: section A lists those viruses usually associated with respiratory tract disease. Confirming their presence will usually identify the cause of the illness, although dual and even triple infections can occur, particularly in the compromised host. The viruses are listed in approximately descending order of importance in terms of numbers of cases annually and their potential severity. By almost any criterion RSV would head the list but the others could be ranked in a different order, depending on the age, time of year and geographical location of the population. Section B lists another three viruses which may be found in the respiratory tract of clinically normal individuals, especially children. Nonetheless, enteroviruses are increasingly recognized as aetiological agents of respiratory disease. Herpes simplex virus, too, may cause no overt lesions in the respiratory tract, although its presence indicates a potential to cause damage if the opportunity occurs – particularly in compromised patients. Reoviruses are not proven pathogens in the respiratory tract, although they are frequently isolated from the throats of

Table 46.1 Viruses infecting the respiratory tract

Virus	No. of serotypes	Group antigen?	Common disease presentation[a]
A. USUALLY PATHOGENIC IN THE RESPIRATORY TRACT			
RSV	1 (2 subtypes: A and B)	Yes[b]	Bronchiolitis in <2 years and in elderly (also URTI, failure to thrive, febrile fits)
Influenza A	Genetically unstable → sequential variants[c]	Yes	URTI, influenza
Influenza B	Genetically unstable → sequential variants[c]	Yes	URTI, influenza, may include abdominal pain
Human metapneumovirus	1 (2 subtypes: A and B)	Yes	Bronchiolitis in <2 years, and in elderly (also URTI, failure to thrive, febrile fits)
Parainfluenza	1–4a,b	No	URTI, croup, bronchiolitis
Adenovirus	47[d]	Yes	URTI, acute respiratory disease
Rhinovirus	>100	No	URTI ('common cold')
Coronavirus[e]	229E, OC43, NL63, HKU1	No	URTI ('common cold'), LRTI, croup, pneumonia
SARS-coronavirus	1	Yes	Severe and often fatal pneumonia
Epstein–Barr virus	1	Yes[b]	Glandular fever
Cytomegalovirus	1	Yes[b]	Various (in the immunocompromised only)[f]
Measles	1	Yes[b]	Measles[g]
Hantaviruses	Several	No	Hantavirus pulmonary syndrome
Bocavirus	Only 1 known	?	–
B. MAY BE RECOVERED FROM THE RESPIRATORY TRACT BUT ROLE IN RESPIRATORY DISEASE UNCERTAIN			
Enteroviruses	68	No	–
Herpes simplex (hominis)	1	Yes[b]	–[h]
Reovirus	3	No	–[i]

[a] Although this column lists the more common presentations, there is considerable overlap in clinical signs and symptoms between respiratory viruses.
[b] There is only one serotype. This is used as a group antigen for diagnostic purposes.
[c] The RNA of influenza A and B viruses is constantly undergoing mutation which is reflected antigenically, causing 'drift' in both influenza A and B and 'shift' in influenza A.
[d] Most respiratory infections are due to types 1–7.
[e] Coronavirus 229E, OC43, NL63 and HKU1 viruses are now recognized.
[f] Usually no overt illness in the immunocompetent, except congenital damage and for some examples of glandular fever.
[g] Rash may be absent in the immunocompromised.
[h] Causes stomatitis and may be a cause of pneumonitis in compromised patients.
[i] No identified disease in man.

children. Important features of each virus, and infection with it, are discussed below.

Respiratory syncytial virus (RSV)

This virus is distributed worldwide and is found wherever it has been sought. It is frequently associated with bronchiolitis in babies – with a peak incidence at about 6 months – and is the most common virus detected, especially in children under 1 year of age who are hospitalized with respiratory infections. Large epidemics occur annually at the same season, but the seasonality of RSV epidemics may vary in different geographical regions (see Epidemiology, below). The starting date and extent of the epidemic may vary but the annual epidemic occurs reliably. For diagnostic purposes there is only one serotype, but two subtypes (A and B) have been described and they may co-circulate, with

one usually predominating in any given year. No obvious differences in disease severity or pathogenesis have been documented.[3]

RSV causes a substantial but variable LRTI disease burden in tropical countries.[4] In a population-based study of infants in Kenya it was found that RSV was common, approximately 36% of infections led to LTRI, 23% were severe and 3% of infected children were hospitalized.[5] More recently, it is becoming clear that RSV causes significant morbidity in the elderly as well as in infants.[6]

Influenza A and B viruses

Antigenically, these are the most variable of the respiratory viruses. Both exhibit antigenic 'drift', in which the surface antigens of the virus change gradually in the face of immunological pressure from the host species, with one or two variants predominating at a given time. In showing this progressive and 'directional' antigenic change, they are unique among respiratory viruses. In addition, influenza A, but *not* influenza B, shows occasional major antigenic changes in the surface antigenic structures (haemagglutinin and/ or neuraminidase), and called 'antigenic shift', which may lead to a pandemic. Such pandemic influenza viruses are derived from avian influenza viruses through genetic re-assortment with animal or human strains. This results in the incorporation of new viral surface antigens to which the human population is immunologically naïve. The timing, extent and direction of either 'drift' or 'shift' have so far been completely unpredictable. However, when viruses with antigenic shift appear in the human population, a worldwide pandemic of influenza A becomes possible; memorable examples occurred in 1918 ('Spanish flu'), in 1957 ('Asian flu') and in 1968 ('Hong Kong flu'). With no animal reservoirs to provide such new antigens, shift does not occur in influenza B.

Smaller-scale influenza epidemics associated with antigenic drift contribute to mortality in the elderly and in those with pre-existing conditions such as chronic cardiopulmonary or renal disease, diabetes, immunosuppression or severe anaemia. The risk of Reye's syndrome is increased following influenza in children on long-term aspirin therapy. While the morbidity and excess mortality associated with influenza in temperate regions is well documented,[6] the more diffuse seasonality (see Epidemiology, below) obscures the disease burden due to influenza in the tropics. Nevertheless, recent studies in Hong Kong and Singapore have revealed that influenza-associated mortality and morbidity in tropical settings is as significant as in temperate climates.[7] Interestingly, influenza-associated mortality is not restricted solely to respiratory complications. A small proportion of cardiovascular mortality also appears to be triggered by influenza.[7]

Avian influenza virus (H5N1) is currently endemic in poultry in a number of countries in Asia and Africa and has repeatedly been transmitted zoonotically to humans, often with fatal consequences.[8,9] The associated disease was unusual in that previously healthy young adults and children are among those most severely ill. The disease presents as a rapidly progressive viral pneumonia with severe leucopenia and lymphopenia, progressing to Acute Respiratory Distress Syndrome and multi-organ dysfunction that fail to respond to standard antibiotic therapy for the pathogens causing community acquired pneumonia. Some patients also manifest a watery diarrhoea and moderate liver dysfunction. Most, though not all, patients have a history of recent exposure to sick poultry. Transmission remains zoonotic although occasional instances of limited and, so far, unsustained human-to-human transmission following close family-type contact have been reported. Early diagnosis and treatment with oseltamivir is lifesaving (see Treatment, below).

Other avian influenza A viruses (e.g. subtypes H9N2, H7N7) have also caused human infection. H9N2 and H7N7 have caused mild flu-like illness or conjunctivitis (H7N7). But one fatal respiratory illness caused by H7N7 virus is documented.

The continued zoonotic transmission of these avian viruses does not imply that they are inevitably likely to lead to another pandemic. However, the unusual severity of H5N1 disease in humans gives cause for concern, because one cannot assume that the acquisition of human-to-human transmissibility (if it ever occurs) will always be associated with a significant loss of virulence. Irrespective of whether or not a putative pandemic threat becomes reality, it is clear that H5N1 viruses have already had a significant impact on the poultry industry, on human economic and social well-being and consequently on human health.

Human metapneumovirus

This virus, which resembles respiratory syncytial virus (RSV), was discovered in 2001 by van den Hoogen and colleagues in The Netherlands.[10] It is now recognized to be a separate virus in its own right, although the disease it causes, its world wide distribution and seasonality are similar to those of RSV.[11,12] It, too, may cause infections in the elderly as well as in babies under 1 year old, and its discovery has accounted for some of the diseases in these age-groups for which no cause had been found hitherto. Retrospective serology, though, has shown that this is not a new pathogen, even for man, but has been around for a long time.

Parainfluenza virus

There are four serotypes of parainfluenza, with type 4 possessing two subtypes: 4a and 4b. Types 1 and 2 typically cause croup, a high-pitched barking cough in children which is profoundly irritating to their parents. Type 3 can cause bronchiolitis or pneumonia and, less often, croup. In temperate countries, types 1 and 2 (together with RSV) are more prevalent in the winter months, whereas type 3 is unusual (among respiratory viruses) in occurring more often in spring and early summer. This dissociation between the peaks of activity of parainfluenza type 3 and RSV has also been observed in tropical regions.[13]

Adenovirus

There are 51 different serotypes but the majority of respiratory infections involve types 1–7. Types 1, 2, 5 and 6 are usually associated with endemic disease in temperate regions, and types 3, 4 and 7 with epidemics. The higher-numbered serotypes appear in the respiratory tract from time to time but the majority of them have been found only in the gut (see Chapter 46).

Adenoviruses are unusual in that prolonged carriage (up to 2 years in some cases) may occur in the tonsils of children, often with no continuing illness. The clinical significance of adenoviruses isolated from the throats of children must therefore be interpreted cautiously, especially if the strain has not been typed. However, they may cause a primary and severe pneumonia in debilitated children, in whom it may be rapidly fatal, and in some immunocompromised patients.

Rhinoviruses

These are frequent causes of the 'common cold', itself a frequent winter and summer illness in temperate countries but they have a year-round seasonality in the tropics.[14] They can be difficult to grow in culture and are very under-reported, mainly because diagnosis is often not attempted. With over 100 serotypes, serological diagnosis is impracticable. Molecular diagnosis based on conserved parts of the viral genome has revealed that rhinoviruses are detected in a substantial number of children hospitalized with acute respiratory disease in both temperate and tropical regions.[14] However, in a proportion of cases, a rhinovirus is detected together with other respiratory pathogens and the relative contribution of rhinovirus to the illness is unclear. A better understanding of the epidemiology of rhinoviruses in apparently asymptomatic children (and adults) is needed. Rhinoviruses are now also recognized to be a significant precipitating factor in exacerbations of asthma and chronic obstructive airways disease in both children and adults.[15] They have also occasionally been the sole pathogens present in the lungs of immunocompromised patients dying with respiratory signs and symptoms.

Coronaviruses

Human coronavirus (HCoV) strains 229E and OC43 have been long recognized as the second main cause of the common cold. More recently, three other coronaviruses have been detected in humans, SARS CoV (see below), HCoV-NL63 and HCoV-HKU1. The HCoV 229E, OC43, NL63 and HKU1 viruses are ubiquitous and are regularly detected in respiratory specimens of a small proportion (1–10%) of children hospitalized with acute respiratory disease and in many parts of the world.[16-18] Infection with these human coronaviruses presents as an upper respiratory tract infection, asthma exacerbation, acute bronchiolitis, pneumonia, febrile seizures and also as croup (especially NL63). HKU1 can be associated with URTI, LRTI (especially in those with underlying diseases of the respiratory tract) and with febrile seizures in children.[17] HCoV are not readily cultivable and require molecular methods (such as reverse transcription polymerase chain reaction, RT-PCR) for detection (see Diagnosis, below).

SARS-coronavirus

In 2003, a coronavirus causing a severe and often fatal pneumonia emerged in southern China. Within weeks of its spread to Hong Kong, the disease had also spread worldwide to affect over 30 countries across five continents; a dramatic illustration of how rapidly a newly emerging respiratory disease can spread.[19] It was unusual in that it caused severe disease, which was also readily transmitted to those caring for the patients. Unlike many other respiratory viral infections, viral load in the upper respiratory tract did not peak until the second week of illness and, consequently, transmission was rare within the first 5 days from onset of illness. This allowed public health measures of early case recognition and isolation to interrupt transmission within the community. SARS was a disseminated infection and not one confined to the respiratory tract.[19] Virus was detectable in the faeces and urine and these may also contribute to transmission under some circumstances.

The virus originated as a zoonosis. The precursor virus is present in bats (*Rhinolophus* spp).[20] Civet cats and other small mammals within live game-animal markets in southern China provided a reservoir and amplifier of the virus and probably provided the opportunity for adaptation to humans.[21] While the transmission of the human-adapted virus that caused the global outbreak in 2003 has been interrupted, it is possible that the disease may reappear, either through the escape of the human-adapted SARS CoV from a laboratory or by the re-adaptation of the animal virus to efficient human transmission.

Measles

Measles (see also Chapters 43 and 47) is often not recognized as a major cause of LRTI morbidity or mortality, and there are a number of factors that may account for this underassessment.[22] Children with measles may not always be admitted to a general paediatric ward, the aetiology may be attributed to a super infecting pathogen rather than to measles, and some patients with measles (especially when immunocompromised as a result of malnutrition, cytotoxic drug treatment or for other reasons) will fail to develop the typical rash. In patients who do not manifest typical clinical features, both clinical and laboratory diagnosis of measles is difficult, even in the developed world. Where the diagnosis has been actively sought in developing countries, measles is found to be a major cause of LRTI, accounting for 6–21% of morbidity and 8–50% of the mortality attributed to LRTI. The effects of the virus on the respiratory tract can be direct (giant cell pneumonitis) or indirect. The latter includes the depressive effects of the virus on the host immune system, stores of vitamin A and overall nutritional status. All of these can lead to an increased risk of super-infection with other viral or bacterial pathogens.

Other viruses causing disease in the respiratory tract

Human *Boca* viruses belong to the family Parvoviridae are associated with a proportion of lower respiratory tract disease and wheezing in children, especially those aged 6 months–2 years.[23,24] The viral DNA is also detectable in the serum but it is not clear whether this represents infectious virus. Enteroviruses have been known for many years as causes of a range of clinical manifestations. Their role in respiratory infections is now being increasingly investigated.[25]

Hantavirus pulmonary syndrome (HPS) is a rare but important cause of severe respiratory illness in the North and South American continents. Their role in respiratory disease was first recognized in May 1993, when an outbreak of a severe, and frequently fatal, respiratory disease occurred in the area in the USA where the four states Arizona, Colorado, New Mexico and Utah abut. The causative agent was found to be a hantavirus, later called *Sin Nombre* virus. The natural host was found to be the deer mouse, *Peromyscus maniculatus*, the local population of which had recently increased rapidly, bringing them and their excreta more into contact with humans, and allowing the virus to cross the species gap. Related viruses causing a similar disease syndrome have since been isolated in North (e.g. New York, Bayou, Black Creek Canal viruses) and South (e.g. Andes virus) Americas, but with different species of natural rodent hosts.[26] These viruses all belong to the same hantavirus genus as those causing haemorrhagic fever with renal syndrome (HFRS) in the Old World: Hantaan, Seoul and Puumala viruses. Both HFRS and HPS have a similar febrile prodrome with thrombocytopenia and leucocytosis. In HPS, the key differences are that the capillary leakage which follows is localized to the lungs and that, with *Sin Nombre* virus, renal dysfunction is minimal. There was no evidence of human-to-human transmission in this outbreak, but there is evidence that some of the South American hantaviruses causing HPS may be transmitted between humans in a nosocomial setting.

Viruses causing respiratory disease in the immunocompromised

A detailed analysis of the respiratory complications of the immunocompromised patient (oncology, leukaemia, transplantation) is outside the compass of this book but some mention is necessary of opportunistic infections in patients who have been immunodepressed by the human immunodeficiency virus (HIV) or who have the acquired immune deficiency syndrome (AIDS) (see also Chapter 20). They are likely to contract any of the viruses already mentioned and may have difficulty in eradicating them due to the lack of functioning cellular immunity. However, viral respiratory infections are not in themselves necessarily a life-threatening problem in patients with AIDS, with three exceptions: cytomegalovirus, measles and varicella-zoster virus.

Cytomegalovirus is an opportunist pathogen in immunocompromised patients in whom it can cause serious or even fatal respiratory complications. It is more important as an opportunist pathogen of transplant recipients (especially bone marrow transplants) than those immunocompromised through AIDS. Perinatal cytomegalovirus infection may occasionally present as pneumonitis in the newborn and (together with *Chlamydiae*) must be considered in the differential diagnosis. Apart from such occasional illnesses, most cytomegalovirus infections are clinically silent, although serological surveys have shown positivity rates approaching 100% in some overcrowded populations. It is also a cause of congenital malformations, especially sensorineural deafness, following maternal infection in pregnancy (see also Chapter 47).

In the immunocompromised, giant cell pneumonitis due to measles can be fatal, and may occur even in patients who have past immunity (naturally derived or vaccine induced). Chickenpox is usually trivial in school-age children but may be severe and include respiratory complications in adults and in the immunocompromised.

Other non-viral 'atypical' pathogenic agents

The diagnosis of several other agents has been undertaken in virus laboratories because these agents cause respiratory infections which overlap clinically with those due to viruses, and they are diagnosed serologically (see below). They include psittacosis, Q fever and mycoplasmosis, where isolation of the causative organism is either difficult or dangerous. They also include *Chlamydia pneumoniae* (TWAR), which is recognized as a cause of community-acquired pneumonia although diagnostic tests are not yet widely available.

The activities of these agents are under-recorded in most parts of the world. Since they are amenable to antibiotic therapy, it is important that they are diagnosed.

EPIDEMIOLOGY

The aetiology and epidemiology of acute respiratory infections have been intensively studied in the temperate areas of the world. Information from tropical regions is more scanty, but what evidence there is suggests that the viruses responsible for respiratory disease in the tropics are no different from those found in temperate zones.[5,13,27-30] However, the severity of illness and its sequelae, as well as their seasonality, may be markedly different from those in the developing world.[31]

The data on respiratory infections obtained by Jacob John and his colleagues[13] in Vellore, India, and shown in Tables 46.2 and 46.3, confirm a range of aetiological agents familiar to workers in temperate zones though with different seasonality. In temperate regions, respiratory infections have generally been shown to increase in the autumn and winter, although the exact mechanisms are still not fully understood. A similar periodicity is shown in tropical regions but this may be related to fluctuations in rainfall or humidity rather than temperature.[31] In contrast to temperate regions, influenza in the tropics may occur in the summer months or all year round, and RSV in subtropical Hong Kong is a *summer* disease.

Table 46.2 Frequency of virus detection, by age, in 809 subjects with acute respiratory infection

	NO. OF CHILDREN OF INDICATED AGE IN WHOM VIRUS DETECTED				
Virus	<1 year (*n*=359)	1 year (*n*=226)	2 years (*n*=92)	3 years (*n*=74)	≥4 years (*n*=58)
RSV	108	32	16	6	1
Influenza A	6	3	2	4	1
Influenza B	3	2	3	2	4
Parainfluenza 1	9	7	4	3	2
Parainfluenza 2	1	4	0	3	2
Parainfluenza 3	29	18	7	4	4
Adenovirus	9	13	1	6	2
Other viruses positive[a]	23	10	12	3	1
Total No. (%)	177 (49)	79 (35)	42 (46)	29 (39)	15 (26)

[a] Two different viruses were isolated in 11, 10, 3 and 1 children of <1, 2, 3 and ≥4 years of age, respectively.
Reproduced with permission from Jacob John et al. 1991.[13]

Table 46.3 Frequency of virus detection, by syndrome, in 331 children with lower respiratory tract infection (LRTI)

Type of LRTI	No. of children	No. (%) positive for virus	NO. IN WHOM VIRUS WAS DETECTED				
			RSV	Influenza	Parainfluenza	Adenovirus	Other[a]
Pneumonia	178	65 (37)	34	3	15	6	11
Bronchiolitis	116	83 (72)	67	1	13	4	3
Tracheobronchitis	14	7 (50)	2	1	2	2	0
Croup	8	4 (50)	0	0	5	0	1
Other[b]	15	4 (27)	3	0	1	0	0
Total	331	163 (49)	106	5	36	12	15

Two viruses were detected in four children with pneumonia, five with bronchiolitis, two with croup.
[a] Enterovirus (21 children), herpes simplex (13), measles virus (7), mumps virus (1), unidentified virus (7).
[b] Acute exacerbation of bronchial asthma (8), tropical pulmonary eosinophilia (2), tuberculosis (2), foreign body aspiration (2) and membranous tracheitis (1).
Reproduced with permission from Jacob John et al. 1991.[13]

The activities of influenza A and B remain impossible to predict and can fluctuate greatly from year to year. The appearance of a 'new' strain of either A or B can be associated with an epidemic the size of which is likely to be greater as the size of the antigenic change increases, although other, so far unidentified, virulence factors may be even more influential. Recently, with detection of H5N1 influenza A strains in migratory birds, and fatal infections in domestic poultry and a high mortality where the virus has been transmitted to humans,[8] there has been widespread anxiety that a human pandemic will follow. So far this has not happened and predicting whether, when and where this might happen is impossible. With no shift changes in influenza B, major epidemics are less common.

Even where high-quality, competent diagnostic services are available, not every clinical respiratory disease yields unequivocal evidence of infection by a virus or other microorganism. The proportion in which a positive diagnosis is made varies from a quarter to a half, depending on laboratory, area, population and time of year. The recent discoveries of a number of newly recognized respiratory viruses (e.g. human metapneumovirus, bocavirus, novel coronaviruses and novel hantaviruses) has highlighted the fact that there are probably still more viruses to be uncovered.

With the development and application of new methods to detect pathogens, novel respiratory viruses are likely to be increasingly recognized in the respiratory tract. It is essential, however, to differentiate asymptomatic viral carriage from infections of aetiological significance, a task that requires careful epidemiological studies including the relevant controls.

Hospitalized vs community patients

Berman[2] has summarized the data from developing countries and found that the percentage of hospitalized patients who were virus positive was about twice the figure found in those attending as outpatients. This difference is not surprising and probably reflects both the greater opportunity to make a specific diagnosis in the hospitalized patient and the greater severity of their disease. The majority of trivial episodes (head colds and increased nasal secretions) are not subjected to virus diagnosis and the causative viruses are unconfirmed.

Other factors

As with most other diseases, respiratory infections are made worse by other components of the patient's environment. Poverty, malnutrition, pollution and overcrowding (common in urban environments everywhere in the world) are well recognized to contribute to the frequency and severity of respiratory illness. The effects may be direct or indirect through the presence of other disease, poor sanitation and poor personal hygiene (Figure 46.1).

Nevertheless, although a poor, malnourished child in a densely populated and economically deprived urban area will have many respiratory illnesses, viruses are no respecters of persons and his or her better-off cousin in a wealthy environment may also have a considerable number of infections. Where the difference lies is that the latter will be able to cope better and will have fewer longer-term sequelae, which include chronic respiratory impairment, wheezing, asthma, bronchitis and bronchiectasis.

LABORATORY DIAGNOSIS

There are three main reasons for providing a laboratory diagnosis of viral respiratory infections: for individual patient diagnosis to aid clinical management (specific therapy, stopping antibiotic therapy, infection control); to monitor routine virus activity in the community (epidemiology, e.g. vaccine strain selection for influenza); or for research investigations.

Rapid diagnosis of viral respiratory infections (i.e. in less than 3 h) has been shown to reduce antibiotic use and to be cost-effective.[32] In addition, such confirmation of the cause is useful in hospital infection control (e.g. in cohorting similar cases) and, occasionally, in deciding whether to use antiviral drugs in selected high-risk patients (see Treatment, below). The new antineuraminidase drugs for treating influenza provide an additional incentive

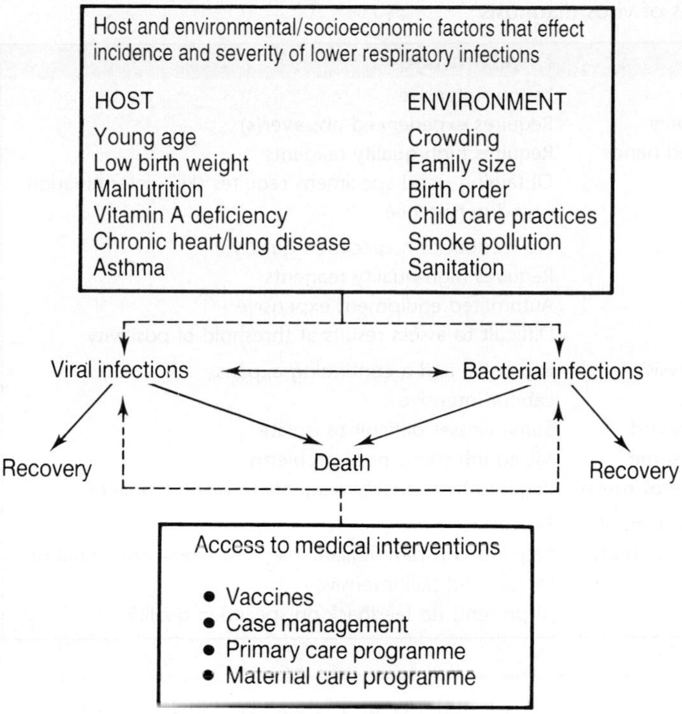

Host and environmental/socioeconomic factors that effect incidence and severity of lower respiratory infections

HOST
Young age
Low birth weight
Malnutrition
Vitamin A deficiency
Chronic heart/lung disease
Asthma

ENVIRONMENT
Crowding
Family size
Birth order
Child care practices
Smoke pollution
Sanitation

Viral infections ← → Bacterial infections

Recovery   Death   Recovery

Access to medical interventions

- Vaccines
- Case management
- Primary care programme
- Maternal care programme

Figure 46.1 Aetiology and epidemiology of lower respiratory tract infections in developing countries. (Reproduced with permission from Berman 1991.[2])

for making rapid diagnoses in, for example, an outbreak situation, although their cost may yet deter their widespread use.

It is self-evident that individual diagnosis must be quick if it is to influence clinical management. Rapidity of diagnosis is also important in epidemiological studies because the clinician will lose interest in sending specimens if there is no equally rapid feedback on the cause of the patient's illness. It is not surprising that epidemiological data are patchy, but they can reflect year-by-year variations if the population on which the studies are performed remains approximately constant.

Diagnosis of respiratory infection is achievable within 2–3 h using techniques such as antigen detection (see below).[33–35] However, these techniques are not universally available, even in hospitals in the developed world, mainly because they are labour- and expertise-intensive. In the developing world this is compounded by a shortage of staff experienced in the use of such techniques, but these objections are surmountable. Enzyme immunoassays in 'kit format' which are relatively simple to perform are available for the diagnosis of influenza A and B and for respiratory syncytial virus. They are, however, expensive. They have adequate positive and negative predictive value of infection during influenza epidemics but have poor predictive values during periods of low influenza activity.[36] They also have poor sensitivity for the diagnosis of avian influenza (H5N1) disease in humans.[9]

The increasing need to provide diagnosis for avian influenza H5N1 which is best done by sensitive molecular (e.g. RT-PCR) methods (because other options are less sensitive and virus culture necessitates biosafety level 3 facilities) is increasing the need for establishing this technology in reference laboratories investigating

respiratory infections, even in a developing country setting. This may in time permit more utilization of multiplex molecular tests for investigation of a wider range of respiratory pathogens (Multiplex PCR).[37] However, these methods remain resource and expertise intensive and need to be well controlled with regular quality control exercises. Microarray methods with the potential to detect a range of pathogens in a single test are in development on a research basis but it is unclear if they have adequate sensitivity for virus detection in clinical specimens (in contrast with virus isolates where high titres of nucleic acid are present). These methods however have potential for the detection of novel pathogens and also for greater recognition of co-infection by multiple pathogens.

Methods of viral diagnosis

Laboratory diagnosis of respiratory virus infections depends on the demonstration of either virus or viral components in the patient at the acute stage of the illness, or subsequently an immune (serological) response to the virus.

Demonstration of virus

There are several approaches to this. They include demonstration of: (1) viral antigens by immunofluorescence[33,34] or enzyme immunoassays,[35] (2) viral infectivity by growth in cell culture; or (3) viral nucleic acid by various techniques. Details of the techniques are not given here, but the advantages and disadvantages of each are indicated in Table 46.4. Before setting up a diagnostic laboratory, the aims of the operation should be clearly thought out. If the catchment population is very large, the number of specimens may also be large and the advantages of automation (e.g. in machine-based nucleic acid amplification or enzyme immunoassays) may be decisive. However, this level of abundance is rare and the number of available specimens may be too few. Automation may then be less advantageous and is often minimal except for serology (see below). Except for special studies, most of the specimens will come from hospitalized patients because of the practical difficulties of collecting and delivering specimens from the community. Virology specimens are perishable and must be delivered to the laboratory without delay.

Such methods of diagnosis depend on good-quality specimens being taken from the patient. It is easier to take a bad specimen than a good one, and close cooperation with the laboratory will help to raise the positivity rate.

Demonstration of an immune response

This, at present, means demonstrating an antibody response in the serum to the stimulus provided by the virus. Seeking responses in cellular immunity or antibody in other body fluids remain research techniques only.

For a valid diagnosis, a convalescent specimen of serum (taken after enough time for a response has elapsed) is needed but may be difficult to collect 2 weeks after the onset from patients who may by then be totally recovered and unwilling to oblige the investigator's interest. This is particularly true with children. Nevertheless, unless an antibody response can be demonstrated

Table 46.4 Advantages and disadvantages of various techniques of virus diagnosis

Technique	Advantages	Disadvantages
Immunofluorescence	Rapid, i.e. same day	Labour-intensive
	Allows assessment of specimen quality	Requires experienced observer(s)
	Sensitive and specific in experienced hands	Requires high-quality reagents
		Obtaining good specimens requires skill, determination and persistence
Enzyme immunoassay	Relatively rapid	No feedback on specimen quality
	Suitable for large numbers	Requires high-quality reagents
	Can be semiautomated	Automated equipment expensive
	Detects incomplete virus particles	Difficult to assess results at threshold of positivity
Culture	Provides more virus for further analysis	Expensive and a continuing expense
	Confirms presence of infective virus	Labour-intensive
	Generally regarded as the gold standard	Some viruses difficult to isolate
	Only currently feasible method for some viruses (e.g. rhinoviruses and enteroviruses)	Mixed infections pose problems
		Requires high-quality reagents to identify isolates
Detection of nucleic acid by amplification (e.g. PCR, RT-PCR, NASBA, etc.)	Can be made both very sensitive and specific	Expensive
	Can detect virus in the presence of antibody	Requires constant vigilance against cross-contamination
		Labour and skill intensive
		At present, no feedback on specimen quality

(seroconversion or a rising titre) some uncertainty over the validity of the result will remain. The alternative is to demonstrate an IgM-class response but this suffers from the twin disadvantages that such tests are not available for all viruses and the sample (to be reliably positive) may have to be taken after the acute illness is over, with the problem(s) already mentioned.

Serology remains the routine choice for some respiratory agents which, although not viral in nature, are traditionally diagnosed by virus laboratories. These include: psittacosis, Q fever and *Mycoplasma pneumoniae* infection. All cause an illness with an insidious onset and are difficult and/or dangerous to isolate. Since all, therefore, are susceptible to antibiotics, a diagnosis is important and can be life-saving. The role of *Chlamydia pneumoniae* is poorly documented at present in the absence of an easily used test.

Diagnosis of respiratory viral infections in the immunocompromised host

The diagnosis of chickenpox is usually clinically obvious, but measles may present problems because the skin rash is often absent in the immunocompromised patient. Immunofluorescent examination of nasopharyngeal secretions for measles-infected cells provides a rapid diagnosis, but this is unlikely to be widely available. Cytomegalovirus can be cultured from the sputum (voluntary or induced) or detected in bronchoalveolar lavage/lung biopsy specimens, if available. Adenoviruses in the immunocompromised may be detected by culture or molecular methods in the respiratory tract, blood, urine and faeces. Detection in multiple sites is evidence of disseminated disease and is an indicator of poor prognosis and for urgent antiviral therapy.

NOSOCOMIAL INFECTION

RSV and influenza viruses are particularly infectious, and are notorious causes of cross-infection in hospitals. This may pose par-

ticular hazards to patients at higher risk, such as those with underlying heart or lung disease (e.g. congenital heart damage or bronchopulmonary dysplasia). Transmission of RSV (as with most other respiratory viruses) is by direct contact or via infected surfaces or fomites. Influenza A, on the other hand, is efficiently spread by large droplets and occasionally via small droplets.

Precautions that may help reduce the risk of cross-infection include the isolation and/or cohort nursing of infected patients and scrupulous care in hand-washing between patients. It is essential to remember that viruses can also infect medical and other hospital staff (RSV may be asymptomatic or cause a 'common cold' in adults) and be transmitted by and through them. SARS was indeed a frightening reminder that hospitals may serve as a venue for amplification and dissemination of virus infections.

TREATMENT

Amantadine, and its alternative rimantadine, were options for the prevention (in outbreaks within closed communities of high risk individuals) and less convincingly for the treatment of influenza A.[38] However, since 2003, increasing resistance of both H3N2 and H1N1 subtypes of influenza A virus has now led to its withdrawal as an option for the treatment of seasonal influenza. Neuraminidase inhibitors such as zanamivir and oseltamivir, which inhibit the viral enzyme neuraminidase from both influenza A and B (concerned with release of the virus from infected cells) are effective for the treatment and prophylaxis of influenza but have to be given within 48 h of onset for apparent clinical benefit. They are expensive and are best used on those most at risk of serious illness – those at the extremes of life. They are also effective against other influenza A virus subtypes including avian influenza A H5N1. While either zanamivir (given by inhaler) or oseltamivir (given orally) can be used for prophylaxis of H5N1 influenza disease, given the potential for dissemination of this virus beyond the respiratory tract, the systemically active oseltamivir is the preferred option for treatment. However, experience with human cases of H5N1 avian influenza has shown that resistance develops rapidly and may be a major problem in widespread prophylactic or therapeutic use. These drugs are not active on other respiratory viruses, even those with viral neuraminidases.

Generally, the management of viral respiratory infections is essentially symptomatic and is dealt with elsewhere (Chapter 11). Antibiotics are not routinely indicated for viral respiratory infections unless secondary bacterial superinfection occurs. The 'atypical' bacterial infections mentioned above (Q fever, mycoplasmosis and chlamydiosis) are amenable to antibiotic therapy. (T)ribavirin given as an aerosol inhalation is claimed to reduce the severity of RSV infection in infants, but this remains controversial. It is a very expensive drug, but may be life-saving in those with congenital heart and/or lung damage for whom RSV infection may be the final insult which pushes them into heart or lung failure. (T)ribavirin may have some effect in influenza but the evidence is minimal. It has also been used in hantavirus pulmonary syndrome but, again, the evidence of efficacy is minimal.

Aciclovir (given i.v.) is effective in the treatment of varicella or herpes simplex infections of the respiratory tract in the immunocompromised patient. It should also be used in an immunocompetent patient (usually an adult) with varicella pneumonia. Ganciclovir and foscarnet are useful in cytomegalovirus infection in the immunosuppressed, but a detailed discussion of this problem is beyond the scope of this chapter.

PREVENTION

With the cells of the target organ immediately accessible to viruses, it is proving difficult to produce effective vaccines to respiratory tract viruses.[39] Other than in measles, which has a systemic phase, vaccines have had only limited success. In the tropics, even the measles vaccine has limitations because much of the impact of this virus on morbidity and mortality is during infancy, and existing measles vaccines are not effective at inducing immunity in the presence of passive maternal antibody. Newer measles vaccines, including one using canarypox virus as a vector, have been explored but not yet adopted. A second dose of conventional vaccine has also been suggested but cost makes this impractical in many countries.

Influenza vaccine is used for persons at high risk (e.g. patients with underlying heart, respiratory or immunocompromising diseases, patients on dialysis, the elderly) and contains antigens from two current influenza A subtypes (H3N2 and H1N1) and from influenza B. The constituents are modified as the prevalent strains vary. The conventional influenza vaccine is formalin-killed egg-grown virus and has provided useful protection, particularly in the elderly and those with pre-existing lung damage in whom even minimal protection may be enough to prevent death. An alternative approach of a live attenuated vaccine containing cold-adapted influenza strains has shown some efficacy and such vaccines are now available.

The possible emergence of an H5N1 avian strain adapted to man has stimulated research into new ways to produce vaccines (e.g. using reverse genetics or a disabled adenovirus as a vector

for influenza antigens) and for new antiviral drugs. Phase 2/3 clinical trials with such H5N1 candidate vaccines are in progress and have shown that the conventional approaches used in seasonal vaccines are poorly immunogenic with the avian H5 haemagglutinin. Therefore, novel adjuvants and whole virus vaccines are now being tried. In mathematical simulations of a new pandemic, vaccines have been shown to be the intervention with the greatest public health impact but until the virus does adapt, we do not know whether any of these novel approaches will be effective in controlling a pandemic. An experimental enteric coated vaccine to adenovirus 14 was developed for use in the US Army to combat epidemics in recruit camps but has found no application elsewhere. Prevention of RSV, severe measles and varicella in susceptible (immunocompromised or severely malnourished) contacts may also be achieved by passive immunization. There is evidence that humanized mouse antibodies or hyperimmune gamma-globulin may give some protection from, or reduce the severity or duration of, RSV infections in the more vulnerable (e.g. premature) babies, but these preparations are very expensive and their use should be confined to those in whom infection will be life-threatening on standard management.[40] Normal human gamma globulin is effective in preventing/attenuating measles if administered within 3 days of contact. For the prophylaxis of varicella, high-titre varicella-zoster human immune globulin (ZIG) must be used. Maximum protection (from severe disease, but not from infection) follows administration within 48 h of contact, but some benefit may accrue if given within 10 days of exposure.

SUMMARY

Respiratory infections are very common throughout the world and are worse where social conditions are inadequate. Much childhood respiratory tract disease is either totally due to viruses or is virus-initiated, and the same viruses appear to be involved in all regions, tropical or temperate. Epidemiological data are incomplete everywhere (but more so for the poorer parts of the world) and come mostly from hospitalized patients.

Nevertheless, RSV is a universal childhood pathogen, found everywhere it has been sought. The numbers of virologically confirmed diagnoses each year (most them in patients in hospital) in the Newcastle and Tyneside area in the UK (population about 1 million) and from Hong Kong island (population about 0.7 million) are remarkably similar: 500–600 and 500–700 cases, respectively. There are likely to be many more in the crowded cities of India, China, the Philippines, Brazil and elsewhere. The effects of RSV (and other viruses) are exacerbated by overcrowding, malnutrition, air pollution, poor sanitation, minimal medical care, etc.

A pandemic of influenza A (similar to the one that swept the world in 1918/9) will be a major health problem. Whether and when it may happen is unpredictable but current preparative measures may help to reduce its impact. Respiratory disease, like diarrhoea, results in significant morbidity and mortality in the developing world, has significant economic consequences and will require an enormous commitment of resources to abate. Viruses and bacteria are both involved and there are few effective vaccines at present.

REFERENCES

1. Williams BG, Gouws E, Boschi-Pinto C, et al. Estimates of world-wide distribution of child deaths from acute respiratory infections. *Lancet Infect Dis* 2002; 2:25–32.
2. Berman S. Epidemiology of acute respiratory infections in children of developing countries. *Rev Infect Dis* 1991; 13(suppl 6):S454–S462.
3. Treanor JJ. Respiratory infections. In: Richman DD, Whitley RJ, Hayden FG, eds. *Clinical VirologyI*. 2nd edn. Washington DC: ASM Press; 2002:7–26.
4. Robertson SE, Roca A, Alonso P, et al. Respiratory syncytial virus infection: denominator-based studies in Indonesia, Mozambique, Nigeria and South Africa. *Bull World Health Organ* 2004; 82:914–922.
5. Nokes DJ, Okiro EA, Ngama M, et al. Respiratory syncytial virus epidemiology in a birth cohort from Kilifi district, Kenya: infection during the first year of life. *J Infect Dis* 2004; 190:1828–1832.
6. Falsey AR, Walsh EE. Viral pneumonia in older adults. *Clin Infect Dis* 2006; 42:518–524.
7. Wong CM, Chan KP, Hedley AJ, et al. Influenza-associated mortality in Hong Kong. *Clin Infect Dis* 2004; 39:1611–1617.
8. Peiris JS, De Jong M, Guan Y. Avian influenza A H5N1: A threat to human health. *Clin Microbiol Rev* 2007; 20(2):143–267.
9. Abdel-Ghafar AN, Chotpitayasunondh T, Gao Z, et al. Update on avian influenza A (H5N1) virus infection in humans. *N Engl J Med* 2008; 358: 261–273.
10. van den Hoogen BG, van Doornum GJ, Fockens JC, et al. Prevalence and clinical symptoms of human metapneumovirus infection in hospitalized patients. *J Infect Dis* 2003; 188:1571–1577.
11. Fouchier RA, Rimmelzwaan GF, Kuiken T, et al. Newer respiratory virus infections: human metapneumovirus, avian influenza virus, and human coronaviruses. *Curr Opin Infect Dis* 2005;18:141–146.
12. Banerjee S, Bharaj P, Sullender W, et al. Human metapneumovirus infections among children with acute respiratory infections seen in a large referral hospital in India. *J Clin Virol* 2007; 38:70–72.
13. Jacob John T, Cherian T, Steinhoff MC, et al. Etiology of acute respiratory infections in children in tropical Southern India. *Rev Infect Dis* 1991; 13(suppl 6):S463–S469.
14. Miller EK, Lu X, Erdman DD, et al. New Vaccine Surveillance Network. Rhinovirus-associated hospitalizations in young children. *J Infect Dis* 2007; 195:773–781.
15. Gern JE, Busse WW. Association of rhinovirus infections with asthma. *Clin Microbiol Rev* 1999; 12:9–18.
16. van der Hoek L, Sure K, Ihorst G, et al. Human coronavirus NL63 infection is associated with croup. *Adv Exp Med Biol* 2006; 581:485–491.
17. Lau SK, Woo PC, Yip CC, et al. Coronavirus HKU1 and other coronavirus infections in Hong Kong. *J Clin Microbiol* 2006; 44:2063–2071.
18. Chiu SS, Chan KH, Chu KW, et al. Human coronavirus NL63 infection and other coronavirus infections in children hospitalized with acute respiratory disease in Hong Kong, China. *Clin Infect Dis* 2005; 40:1721–1729.
19. Peiris JS, Yuen KY, Osterhaus AD, et al. The severe acute respiratory syndrome. *N Engl J Med* 2003; 349:2431–2441.
20. Lau SK, Woo PC, Li K S, et al. Severe acute respiratory syndrome coronavirus-like virus in Chinese horseshoe bats. *Proc Natl Acad Sci US A* 2005; 102:14040–14045.
21. Guan Y, Zheng BJ, He YQ, et al. Isolation and characterization of viruses related to the SARS coronavirus from animals in southern China. *Science* 2003; 302:276–278.
22. Markowitz LE, Nieburg P. The burden of acute respiratory infection due to measles in developing countries and the potential impact of measles vaccine. *Rev Infect Dis* 1991; 13(suppl 6):S555–S561.
23. Allander T, Jartti T, Gupta S, et al. Human bocavirus and acute wheezing in children. *Clin Infect Dis* 2007; 44:904–910.
24. Anderson LJ. Human bocavirus: a new viral pathogen. *Clin Infect Dis* 2007; 44:911–912.
25. Ruohola A, Meurman O, Nikkari S, et al. Microbiology of acute otitis media in children with tympanostomy tubes: prevalences of bacteria and viruses. *Clin Infect Dis* 2006; 43:1417–1422.
26. Schmaljohn C, Hjelle B. Hantaviruses: a global disease problem. *Emerg Infect Dis* 1997; 3:95–103.
27. Bale JR, ed. Symposium on etiology and epidemiology of acute respiratory tract infection in children in developing countries. *Rev Infect Dis* 1990; 12(suppl 8):S861–S1083.
28. Assaad F, Cockburn WC. A seven year study of WHO virus laboratory reports on respiratory viruses. *Bull World Health Organ* 1974; 51:437–445.
29. Forgie IM, Campbell H, Lloyd-Evans N, et al. Etiology of acute lower respiratory tract infections in children in a rural community in The Gambia. *Paediatr Infect Dis J* 1992; 11:466–473.
30. McIntosh K, Halonen P, Ruuskanen O. Report of a workshop on respiratory viral infections: epidemiology, diagnosis, treatment and preventions. *Clin Infect Dis* 1993; 16:151–164.
31. Shek LP, Lee BW. Epidemiology and seasonality of respiratory tract virus infections in the tropics. *Paediatr Respir Rev* 2003; 4:105–111.
32. Woo PC Y, Chiu SS, Seto WH, et al. Cost-effectiveness of rapid virus diagnosis of viral respiratory tract infections in pediatric patients. *J Clin Microbiol* 1997; 35:1579–1582.
33. Gardner PS, McQuillin J. *Rapid Virus Diagnosis: Application of Immunofluorescence*, 2nd edn. London: Butterworth, 1980.
34. Madeley CR. Respiratory viruses. In: Caul EO, ed. *Immunofluorescence Antigen Detection Techniques in Diagnostic Microbiology*. London: Public Health Laboratory Service; 1992:33–48.
35. Arstila PP, Halonen P. Direct antigen detection. In: Lennette EH, Halonen P, Murphy FA, eds. *Laboratory Diagnosis of Infectious Diseases: Principles and Practice*. Vol. II. New York: Springer; 1988:60–75.
36. Grijalva CG, Poehling KA, Edwards KM, et al. Accuracy and interpretation of rapid influenza tests in children. *Pediatrics* 2007;119:e6–e11.
37. Freymuth F, Vabret A, Cuvillon-Nimal D, et al. Comparison of multiplex PCR assays and conventional techniques for the diagnostic of respiratory virus infections in children admitted to hospital with an acute respiratory illness. *J Med Virol* 2006; 78:1498–1504.
38. Hayden FG. Antivirals for influenza: historical perspectives and lessons learned. *Antiviral Res* 2006 71:372–378.
39. Gillim-Ross L, Subbarao K. Emerging respiratory viruses: challenges and vaccine strategies. *Clin Microbiol Rev* 2006;19:614–636.
40. Anonymous. Prevention of respiratory syncytial virus infections: indications for use of palivizumab and update on the use of RSV-IGIV. American Academy of Pediatrics Committee on Infectious Diseases and Committee of Fetus and Newborn. *Pediatrics* 1994; 102:1211–1262.

Chapter 47

Gordon C. Cook and Alimuddin I. Zumla

Cutaneous Viral Diseases

The skin is a common site of lesions resulting from systemic diseases as well as localized skin infections.[1] Tables 47.1 and 47.2 summarize medically important RNA and DNA viral infections of the skin in adults and children together with the diseases they cause. With the advent of the human immunodeficiency virus (HIV) pandemic, the incidence, severity and clinical presentations of cutaneous viral infections have changed over the past two decades. Cutaneous manifestations of these viral diseases often lead to a diagnosis of HIV or the underlying immunosuppressive disease.

RNA VIRUSES CAUSING CUTANEOUS DISEASE

A large number of RNA viruses cause skin manifestations in humans (Table 47.1). This section considers only measles and rubella. Diseases due to other RNA viruses are dealt with elsewhere in this book.

Measles

Geographical distribution

Measles has a worldwide distribution. Its introduction to many countries that had previously been free, such as Fiji, Tasmania, Greenland, and many tropical areas where isolated people had had no previous contact with the disease, frequently had disastrous results. Measles remains a leading vaccine-preventable cause of child mortality worldwide, particularly in sub-Saharan Africa where almost half of the estimated 454 000 measles deaths in 2004 occurred.[2] It is one of the most prevalent infectious diseases of the tropics, and certainly one of the most serious of the acute childhood communicable illnesses.[3] However, great progress in measles control has been made in resource-poor countries through improved measles-control efforts.

Aetiology

The causative agent, which is closely related to rinderpest and canine distemper, is a single-stranded RNA virus with a pleomorphic appearance on electron microscopy (120–250 nm in size); it consists of two components, an outer envelope with short projections and an inner nucleocapsid of RNA and a glycoprotein. There is only one strain and no known antigenic variation; alterations in virulence worldwide are due to underlying host and environmental factors. The virus grows slowly in human and monkey cell cultures. Viraemia occurs 4–5 days before the appearance of the rash, and abates within 24–48 h. The virus can also be isolated from the throat in the coryzal stage.

Transmission

Measles is one of the most contagious of infections; approximately 90% of susceptible individuals will contract the disease after contact with a case. Transmission is direct, from secretions from the respiratory tract – by droplet spread. Cases are infectious only in the early stages, when virus can be isolated from the throat. Transplacental spread does not seem to occur and, although it is possible that fetal damage may follow measles contracted during pregnancy, this is not proven.

Pathology

Infection begins in the nose and throat from which, following limited multiplication, the virus spreads (via leucocytes) to the cells of the reticuloendothelial system; here it attacks the lymphocytes of the immune system. Further multiplication precedes the viraemic phase; epithelial cells are affected and the clinical signs and symptoms of measles develop after an incubation period of 10–14 days. Virus multiplication occurs in the reticuloendothelial system, in which it produces the appearance of large multinucleate giant cells. Target organs affected are the skin, conjunctivae, mouth, larynx, bronchial tree, and gastrointestinal tract. The essential lesion is 'catarrhal' inflammation of the respiratory and gastrointestinal tracts, the initial inflammation of epithelial cells being rapidly followed by fatty degeneration and exfoliation of dead cells. Complete resolution with recovery is the rule, although widespread denudation of epithelium in the gastrointestinal tract may result in significant enteropathy (see Chapter 10).

Immunity

Immunity to measles is both antibody and cell mediated; following an acute attack, this is lifelong. Antibodies appear simultaneously with the rash and IgM concentration peaks at 10 days, disappearing after 1 month; a resulting increased IgG

Table 47.1 Aetiology and cutaneous manifestation of diseases caused by to RNA viruses

Family	Virus	Cutaneous disease
Paramyxovirus	Respiratory syncytial virus (RSV)	Skin rash
	Measles virus	Measles (rubeola)
	Mumps virus	Mumps
	Retroviruses HIV-1, HIV-2	AIDS; dermatitis
Picornavirus	Enterovirus	Herpangina; hand, foot and mouth disease
	Coxsackie	Exanthem
	ECHO virus	
Togavirus	Rubivirus	Rubella (German measles)
	Group A arboviruses	Haemorrhagic fevers
Flavivirus	Group B arboviruses	Haemorrhagic fevers
Arenaviruses	Machupo virus	Haemorrhagic fevers
	Junin virus	
	Lassa virus	

Table 47.2 Aetiology and cutaneous manifestation of diseases caused by DNA viruses

Family	Virus	Cutaneous disease
Pox viruses	*Variola*	Smallpox
		Monkey pox
		Orf
		Cowpox
		Tanapox
	Molluscum	*Molluscum contagiosum*
Herpesviruses	Herpes simplex virus (HSV) type 1	Orofacial herpes
	Herpes simplex virus (HSV) type 2	Genital herpes
	Varicella-zoster virus (VZV)	Chickenpox; shingles
	Cytomegalovirus (CMV)	Ulcers, exanthem
	Epstein–Barr virus (EBV)	Infectious mononucleosis
	Human herpesvirus (HHV)	
	HHV-6	*Exanthema subitum*
	HHV-7	*Roseola infantum* or 'sixth disease'
	HHV-8 (KSAHV)	Kaposi's sarcoma
Adenoviruses	Adenovirus	Adenovirus dermatitis in the immunosuppressed
Papovavirus	Human papilloma virus (HPV)	Warts
Parvoviruses	Parvovirus B19	Erythema infectiosum (fifth disease)
Hepadnaviruses	Hepatitis B virus	Macular skin rash

concentration decreases slowly over 6 months. Passive immunity (transferred from mother to infant transplacentally) lasts for the first few months of life and evidence of inapparent infection during months of declining maternal antibody can be found in one-quarter of older children. Cell-mediated immunity plays an important role in virus elimination. Resultant on its action on the cells of the reticuloendothelial system, measles depresses cell-mediated immunity, which can also be reduced simultaneously by malnutrition, which accounts for the severity of the disease in many tropical countries. Depressed cell-mediated immunity also reactivates tuberculosis and allows secondary infections, which are common in patients with measles, to develop.

Clinical features

Natural history

Measles consists of an acute self-limiting infection; recovery occurs in the majority of cases. In tropical populations it may be complicated by severe bronchopneumonia, diarrhoea, malabsorption, malnutrition, severe conjunctivitis and blindness, gangrene of limbs and death. The case mortality rate in the tropics is estimated to be about 5% (sometimes reaching 10% in rural areas).[3,4] In some village epidemics, 40% of children die as a result of infection; a combination of pertussis and measles is particularly dangerous.

Symptoms and signs

The incubation period is 10–14 days. Onset is gradual; prodromal fever and coryzal symptoms appear within 24 h. Severe conjunctivitis and cough follow; this prodromal phase lasts for 3–4 days. Within 3 days of onset (and 24 h before the rash), Koplik's spots can be visualized as blobs of bright red with a small bluish-white

centre on the buccal mucous membrane. The exanthem (Figure 47.1) appears 24 h later, first on the forehead and neck, spreading to invade the trunk over 3–4 days. The lesions are at first reddish and maculopapular, later becoming brown, and in dark skin appearing totally different to lesions in pale skins, with a diffuse deep red or purple rash followed by severe desquamation 2–4 days later. This may lead to patchy depigmentation and, occasionally, boils. Haemorrhagic measles with a purpuric rash and accompanied by bleeding from mucous membranes is rare; it carries a very high mortality rate.

Other systems

The mouth becomes sore, interfering with sucking and eating; this can lead to malnutrition and cancrum oris. Laryngitis is common; this is followed by bronchopneumonia, which carries a high mortality rate. Diarrhoea, sometimes accompanied by tenesmus and faecal blood and mucus in the stool, leads to dehydration; parenteral replacement may be necessary to prevent death.

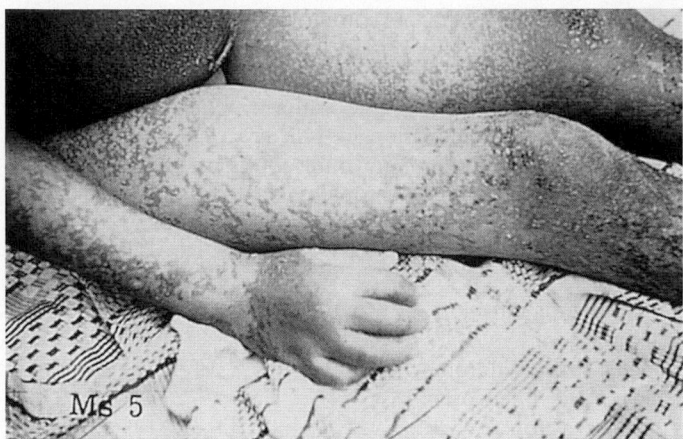

Figure 47.1 Measles rash near the knee in an African child. In a pigmented skin the rash has a deep bluish colour. (Courtesy of David Morley.)

Central nervous system

The most common manifestation is a short, generalized convulsion early in the course of infection, from which recovery is complete.

Encephalitis

Measles encephalitis is associated with generalized convulsions. The risk increasing with age; the course is variable. Onset is usually 4–7 days after appearance of the rash (48 h to 2 weeks after onset) and is characterized by fever, irritability, meningism and coma. The cerebrospinal fluid shows moderate pleocytosis and an increase in protein concentration. The mortality rate can be as high as 10–15%; one-quarter of affected children are left with a permanent neurological deficit. This phenomenon probably has an immunological basis, as shown by the histological changes, perivascular cuffing, demyelination and gliosis.

Complications

Subacute sclerosing panencephalitis

This complication is caused by a persistent viral infection within the brain. It usually manifests 5–10 years after infection, and pursues a slow degenerative course, starting with personality change(s) and deterioration of intellect (with signs of mental deterioration), and progressing to a state of decerebrate rigidity. Very high levels of antibody to measles virus are present in cerebrospinal fluid.

Depression of cell-mediated immunity can give rise to giant cell pneumonia, also seen in patients with defective cell-mediated immunity. Severe ulcerative herpes of the mouth and eye results from cell-mediated immune depression. Severe conjunctivitis, often associated with vitamin A deficiency,[5–7] causes corneal perforation and blindness. Respiratory complications are common and sometimes fatal. Bronchitis, bronchiolitis, 'croup' and giant cell bronchopneumonia occur. Measles is one of the most common causes of blindness in the tropics (see Chapter 18). Gangrene of the extremities may develop. Malnutrition associated with measles can precipitate kwashiorkor and marasmus. Otitis media can lead to mastoiditis and a hearing deficit. Measles exerts a major impact on infant and child development.

Diagnosis

The association of fever, cough, conjunctivitis, coryza, Koplik's spots in the mouth, and a morbilliform rash is usually diagnostic, but other conditions with dermatological manifestations have often been mistaken for measles; tick-borne and louse-borne typhus, meningococcaemia, scarlet fever and infectious mononucleosis are also associated with a morbilliform rash. There is a leucocytosis in the early stage(s), followed by an increase in lymphocytes – some of the Turk type.

During the prodromal phase large multinucleate (giant) cells can be visualized in stained smears of sputum or urine, or of Koplik's spots on the buccal mucosa. Serological tests on acute (IgM measles antibody) and convalescent sera reveal haemagglutination-inhibiting (HI) and neutralizing (N) antibodies, with a four-fold rise in titre following the initial infection. Immunofluorescent staining of cells may demonstrate measles antigen in smears from the nasopharynx or Koplik's spots.

Management

No chemotherapeutic agent influences the course of the viraemia. Food and fluid intake should be maintained, and rehydration undertaken.[8] Antibiotics are essential when otitis media, bacterial pneumonia and skin infections are present. Temperature control may lead to a reduction in febrile convulsions.

Epidemiology

Homo sapiens is the sole reservoir of infection. The incidence of measles worldwide is diminishing in developed countries, where the mean age of onset is now over 5 years. As infant immunization becomes more widely practised, the mean age of infection is rising; consequently, unprotected individuals and visitors to developing countries that do not have an immunization programme are at increased risk.

In developing countries, children generally develop the disease at 18–30 months; epidemics occur during the dry season when festivals and concourses of people usually take place. In isolated (e.g. nomadic) populations measles may occur at any age if the last exposure was many years previously. In large cities measles is endemic throughout the year; in smaller towns childhood epidemics occur every 2–3 years and infection spreads to the villages.

Control

Both passive immunization with human immunoglobulin and active immunization with a live attenuated vaccine are highly successful.[9–14]

Passive immunization

Passive immunization (human gamma globulin 0.25 mg/kg) is effective if given within 5 days of exposure. In one study, passive immunization of children on admission to hospital gave complete protection, which was immediate.

Active immunization

A live attenuated strain of the virus is used; this gives a 98% sero-conversion rate under ideal conditions. Fever of moderate severity and a mild rash occur rarely. Encephalitis is a rare complication. Immunization programmes now incorporate this vaccine into a triple vaccine containing live attenuated mumps, measles and rubella (MMR). MMR is given to children in the second year of life with a booster at school entry. Immunity appears long lasting but the effect of immunizing HIV-positive children is not yet known. A high uptake of the vaccine may lead to increased herd immunity to a level where few susceptible hosts remain for the three viruses to survive in the community.

Contraindications to measles immunization include; pregnancy, immunodeficiency states and hypersensitivity to eggs.

Maternal antibody is transferred transplacentally and this inhibits vaccine efficacy up to the age of 6 months. Normally, vaccination is aimed at children of 9 months of age,[13] but vaccination at 6 months, despite a lower seroconversion rate, is used in areas of high risk, sometimes in conjunction with a booster dose 1 year later. In order to eradicate the disease, immunization uptake rates of 90–95% are required.[14]

A 49% reduction in mortality rate in African children hospitalized with pneumonia and gastroenteritis has been recorded when measles vaccine was given as a routine admission procedure. Human immunoglobulin should be combined with measles vaccine in malnourished children.

Live vaccines are rapidly inactivated at room temperature, and the difficulty of maintaining this 'cold chain' is a major handicap to its use in most tropical countries. Monitoring of seroconversion rates should be a feature of all anti-measles campaigns.

An aerosol-administered vaccine has been successfully developed; it can be administered by anyone (with minimum qualifications) by hand pump, and should prove a great advance compared with previous methods of mass immunization. A heat-stable vaccine is under development. A major problem is that measles vaccination campaigns have to be repeated regularly; it is essential that measles vaccine is incorporated into the regular healthcare system for rural areas, together with other immunizations.

Rubella (German measles)

Rubella is a mild systemic viral infection, with skin rashes as the cutaneous manifestation. The clinical importance of rubella lies in the potentially disastrous consequences of infection in early pregnancy leading to severe congenital malformations.

Epidemiology

Rubella is less infectious than measles, and transmission occurs via the air-borne route, by person to person contact. The incubation period from exposure to development of fever is 14–21 days. A person with rubella remains infectious from 7 days before the onset of rash to 4–5 days afterwards.

Clinical features

After an incubation of 2–3 weeks, the patient may develop a mild pharyngitis, gritty feeling in the eyes due to mild conjunctivitis, and fever. A macular skin rash appears on the second or third day;

petechiae or papules are not common. The rash spreads over the face and behind the ears. A skin rash may not be present in all cases and thus the diagnosis may be difficult. The macules diffuse into one another, forming a generalized 'blush' by 2 days, and fading without desquamation in 4–5 days. Painful joints of the hands and feet are common in young adults, and suboccipital and posterior cervical lymphadenopathy are common. Differential diagnosis of a rubelliform skin eruption includes:

- Parvovirus infection
- Measles
- Enterovirus infection
- Scarlet fever
- Toxic shock syndrome
- Acute HIV infection
- Drug reaction.

Complications

Complications of rubella include: (a) idiopathic thrombocytopenic purpura, (b) encephalitis and (c) arthralgia. This thrombocytopenia is transient, lasting from 1 to 3 weeks. If the case is severe, intravenous immunoglobulin and steroids may be required. Encephalitis occurs in 1 in 5000 cases and is variable in severity.

Diagnosis

The following laboratory investigations are valuable in the diagnosis of rubella:

1. Serology. Two serological tests have been used widely:
   a. detection of rubella-specific IgM by enzyme-linked immunosorbent assay (ELISA) or particle agglutination.
   b. four-fold rise in haemagglutinin inhibition antibodies in paired sera.
2. Viral culture.
3. Detection of rubella-specific RNA fragments using polymerase chain reaction (PCR).

Other tests used for detection of immunity (before infection or post-vaccination immunity) in pregnant women include: (a) a single radial haemolysis test and (b) a passive haemagglutination test.

Prevention

Rubella vaccine is a live attenuated preparation of the virus. Live rubella vaccine is contraindicated in people with immunosuppression and in pregnancy. Rubella is a notifiable disease. Children should be excluded from school for at least 7 days after onset of the rash. Contact with pregnant women should be avoided and, where contact occurs during the first trimester of pregnancy, serological testing of the mother should be carried out to determine previous immunity to rubella.

Congenital rubella

Rubella is potentially teratogenic if contracted by a pregnant woman in the first 16 weeks of pregnancy. The main defects caused by rubella in the fetus are a triad of: (a) cataract, (b) nerve deafness and (c) heart abnormalities (e.g. patent ductus arteriosus, ventricular septal defect (VSD), pulmonary artery stenosis, or Fallot's tetralogy). Affected infants also have a generalized infection which, together with the congenital defects, is termed the rubella syndrome. The physical signs may include: (a) hepatosplenomegaly; thrombocytopenic purpura, low birth weight, intellectual impairment, jaundice, anaemia, and lesions in the metaphysis of the long bones.

Diagnosis of maternal rubella

Recent infection is diagnosed by detection of rubella-specific IgM antibodies using ELISA or immunofluorescence. PCR may detect rubella-specific RNA fragments.

Management

Antenatal women less than 16 weeks pregnant with rubella are best advised to terminate the pregnancy. Those who find this unacceptable may be given passive immunization with immunoglobulin, which may have some attenuating or prophylactic effect.

DNA VIRUSES CAUSING CUTANEOUS DISEASE

Table 47.2 lists DNA viruses that cause cutaneous disease in humans.

Diseases due to pox viruses

Orthopox viruses

Poxviruses are DNA viruses that are especially adapted to epidermal cells.[15] The orthopox viruses are DNA double-stranded viruses, brick or ovoid shaped, and 200–250 nm in size; they are all antigenically related and include cowpox, ectromelia (mice), monkey pox, Turkmenia rodent pox and vaccinia. The only members of the group that have infected humans are *variola* (smallpox), *vaccinia*, monkey pox and cowpox. Tanapox, although not an orthopox virus, is closely related.

Smallpox

Smallpox was formerly a devastating, severe, febrile illness characterized by an extensive, profuse, vesicular rash and a high mortality rate.[16] Survivors were left with severe disfiguring facial scars. The human smallpox virus was one of the most fatal of all viral infections and it is probably the only infectious disease that has been eradicated globally. The success of this eradication programme was based on several factors:
1. Human beings were the sole hosts.
2. An effective vaccine inducing solid immunity was available.
3. Governments were committed to vaccination programmes. This was backed up the World Health Organization's 'search and containment' campaigns where cases were isolated and contacts traced and vaccinated.
The world has been free from naturally occuring smallpox since 1977 and the eradication campaign is heralded as one of the most successful carried out by the WHO. In 2008, smallpox has again become a concern to both physicians and the general

public since it has been suggested that it could be used for bioweapons programmes in current global conflicts. For more details about smallpox, see the review on smallpox by Moore and colleagues.[15]

Monkey pox

Geographical distribution

This disease is confined to tropical Africa (Figure 47.2). Although monkey pox has been recorded since 1958 in captive monkeys, the first human case was recognized in Zaire in 1970;[16,17] since then, more than 200 cases have been reported, mainly in Zaire, but also in Liberia, Nigeria, Ivory Coast, Cameroon and Sierra Leone. Monkey pox has been reported only rarely outside these areas of tropical rainforest.

Aetiology

The causative agent is a 'brick-shaped' orthopox virus (200–250 nm in size) which forms cytoplasmic inclusions and is morphologically indistinguishable from variola. It can be readily distinguished in culture because the pocks on chick chorioallantoic membrane are slightly larger and more haemorrhagic than those caused by variola. Unlike variola, monkey pox virus is pathogenic in rabbits, and has a higher temperature ceiling for growth. It grows readily in the green monkey and rodent cell cultures. Four strains of poxviruses have been isolated from monkey kidney cells and from rodents; these differ from monkey pox, but are closely related to variola, from which they can be distinguished by DNA analysis. These are known as 'whitepox' viruses; their relation to human infection is unknown.

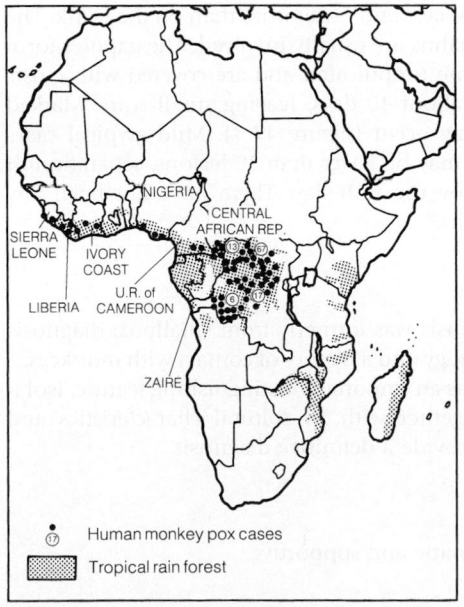

Figure 47.2 Geographical distribution of human monkey pox showing cases reported from 1970 to 1984. (Courtesy of the World Health Organization.)

Transmission

The usual mode of transmission from monkey to humans is unclear, but infection is sometimes direct, resulting from handling dead monkeys for eating, or by droplet spread via the respiratory tract.[16] Transmission by a chimpanzee bite has also been recorded. The disease is not readily transmitted from person to person, but secondary cases have been recorded. Little tertiary spread occurs, and epidemics are not a feature.

Pathology

Few individuals are known to have died from monkey pox; no autopsies have been performed, and therefore histopathological information is not available. It seems likely that pathological changes resemble those previously attributable to smallpox.

Immunity

There is well defined immunity to reinfection, and complete cross-immunity with variola and vaccinia. Monkey pox has never been recorded in an individual vaccinated for smallpox.[16]

Natural history

Monkey pox infection in humans is a dead-end infection, manifesting itself as a typical smallpox-like illness. It possesses a 2–3-day prodromal period, and the smallpox-like rash evolves over 2–4 days. The illness is usually mild, and is followed by complete recovery. When rarely death has occurred, it has usually been in children.

Clinical features

The incubation period is 5–17 days. The onset is abrupt with fever and a prodromal illness lasting 2–3 days.[16] On the third day, a rash appears; this consists of a single crop of discrete papules, more abundant on the face and extremities than on the trunk. The soles of the feet and palms are usually involved. The papules form pustules which become umbilicated and are covered with crusts which separate after about 10 days, leaving small scars. Marked lymphadenopathy may occur (Figure 47.3). Mild atypical cases occur in which there may be fewer than 10 lesions, separation of the crusts occurring by the fifth day. There have not been any recorded complications.

Diagnosis

The differential diagnosis was formerly from smallpox; diagnosis is based on epidemiology and a history of contact with monkeys.[16] Lymphadenopathy was an important distinguishing feature. Isolation of the virus, together with its cultural characteristics and antigenic structure, provide a definitive diagnosis.

Management

Treatment is symptomatic and supportive.

Epidemiology

It is not known whether the primary maintenance hosts are chimpanzees, other primates or small mammals. Most patients give a

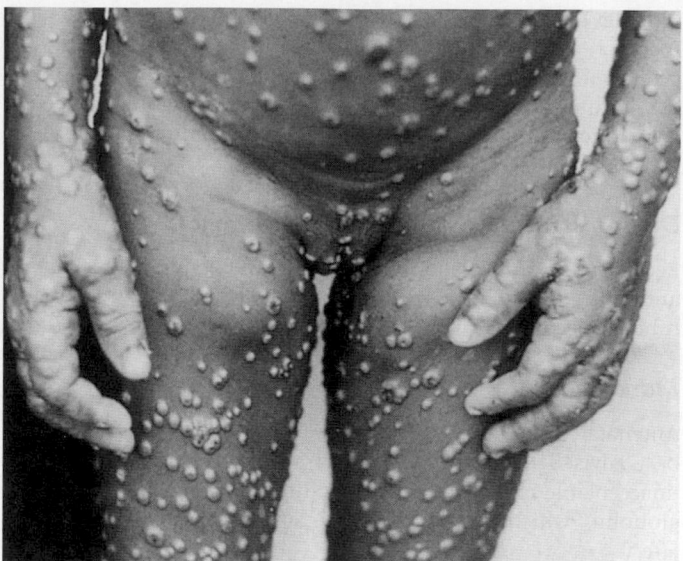

Figure 47.3   Monkey pox, showing characteristic inguinal and femoral lymphadenopathy. (Reproduced with permission from Breman JG, Kalisa-Ruti, Steniowski MV, et al. Human monkeypox, 1970–79. *Bull World Health Organ* 1980; 58(6):849–868.)

clear account of contact with monkeys which they have caught and/or eaten.[16–18] Most cases occur during the dry season. Children are affected more than adults. The attack rate is 10% in susceptible individuals in close contact with a primary case, in contrast to smallpox infection in which it was 20%. Secondary spread occurs in families, but tertiary transmission is rare and epidemics are not a feature. Now that smallpox vaccination level in communities has fallen dramatically, human monkey pox may become more common.

Tanapox

Tanapox[19] was first described in 1957 and 1962 in epidemics in the lower Tana River of Kenya. Serological surveys have shown continuing transmission along the lower Tana River. Human infections have since been recorded in the forest area of Zaire. A closely-related virus has been isolated from outbreaks in primate colonies in the USA, and in contacts of human cases.

Aetiology

Tanapox virus is not an orthopox virus; with the Yabapox virus it forms a distinct subgroup of poxviruses. It cannot be cultured on chick chorioallantoic membrane, but grows well on green monkey kidney cell and Vero cell cultures.

Transmission

Epidemiological studies suggest that the virus is transmitted from monkeys to humans by mosquitoes; outbreaks in humans have occurred in low-lying country near the Tana River after floods had isolated wild animals, humans and their domestic animals on islands in the flood water, on which *Mansonia uniformis* and *M.*

africanus had proliferated in immense numbers. There is no evidence of direct person-to-person spread.

Pathology

Pathology is limited to the epidermis where the pock forms. There are few or no destructive changes. Hypertrophied epidermal cells containing acidophilic inclusion bodies predominate; cellular infiltration is mild, and the dermis remains intact.

Immunity

Virtually nothing is known about second attacks. Antibodies that develop in infected individuals and monkeys persist for some years. There is no cross-immunity with *vaccinia*; recently-vaccinated individuals can develop the disease.

Clinical features

The infection is usually mild; fever heralds the appearance of one or two pock-like lesions. Complete recovery follows.

Symptoms and signs

The incubation period is unknown. Onset is abrupt with fever lasting 3–4 days, accompanied in some cases by severe headache and prostration. Prevalence is open to doubt because histories have usually been recorded retrospectively, long after the event. During the febrile episode, one or two (but never more) pock-like lesions appear on the skin, resembling those formerly caused by smallpox. Lesions become umbilicated; they never proceed to pustule formation, but form firm cheesy centres instead (Figure 47.4). The pocks occur mainly on exposed surfaces: upper arms, face, neck and trunk, but never on the hands, legs or feet. Recovery takes place rapidly; no scars are left and there are no residual complications.

Diagnosis

Tanapox had formerly to be distinguished from modified smallpox in a vaccinated person; the character of the pock (which at first resembles smallpox) differs in its larger size, firm, solid nature and absence of postulation. Electron microscopical appearances are similar to those previously associated with smallpox. Virus can be isolated by culture in green monkey kidney or Vero cells, and is clearly distinguished by antigenic structure from orthopox viruses. Serum antibodies develop slowly, but complement fixation and neutralizing tests on both human and monkey sera show antibody at low titre; this persists for some years and can be used for a retrospective diagnosis.

Management

Treatment is not required and patients make a complete recovery.

Epidemiology

The epidemiology is poorly understood. The primary maintenance hosts are unknown; many monkeys, especially vervet

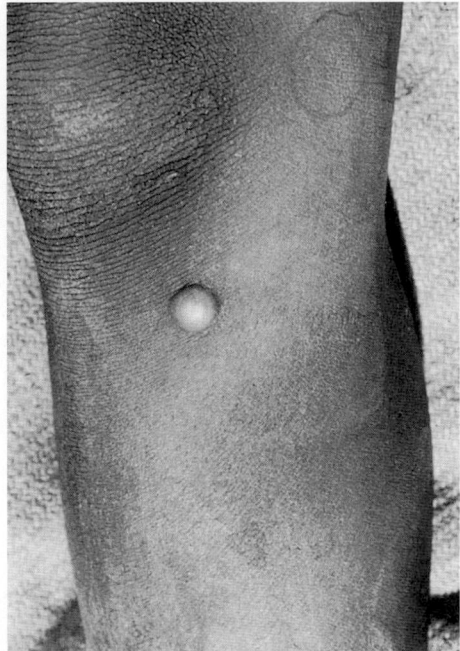

Figure 47.4 Tanapox. Solid pock containing firm cheesy material.

(*Cercopithecus aethiops*) are susceptible, and are common in endemic area(s). Small outbreaks have occurred after flooding, but transmission was shown to be continuing along the lower Tana River in serological surveys carried out in 1971 and 1976; infection has persisted since 1962. Antibodies were detected in 9.2% of the population, and in children between the ages of 2 and 12 years. There is no evidence of direct person-to-person transmission.

Molluscum contagiosum (MC)

MC causes a wart-like skin condition and is produced by a poxvirus infection of the prickle cell layer of the skin.[20] Infection is transmitted by contact. The infected cells proliferate, vacuolate, enlarge and protrude above the skin surface as pearly, umbilicated lesions. The central cavity of the lesion contains white, pulpy material with infectious vacuolated cells. Accumulation of the molluscum bodies in the cytoplasm causes compression of the nucleus to the periphery of the cell, leading to rupture and thus infecting adjacent cells.

The lesions occur in groups, on the face, arms or near genitalia, and their appearance is diagnostic. The number of lesions in HIV-positive individuals can exceed 100 (Figure 47.5), leading to coalescence of lesions forming large plaques with many smaller lesions ('agminate form'). In some cases, MC infection can induce localized dermatitis known as molluscum dermatitis.

In immunocompetent individuals, the lesions are self-limiting and regress spontaneously with time (6–12 weeks). Lesions in HIV-positive individuals do not usually resolve spontaneously, persisting for months or even years, although marked improvements in MC are now being observed in patients receiving highly active antiretroviral therapy (HAART).

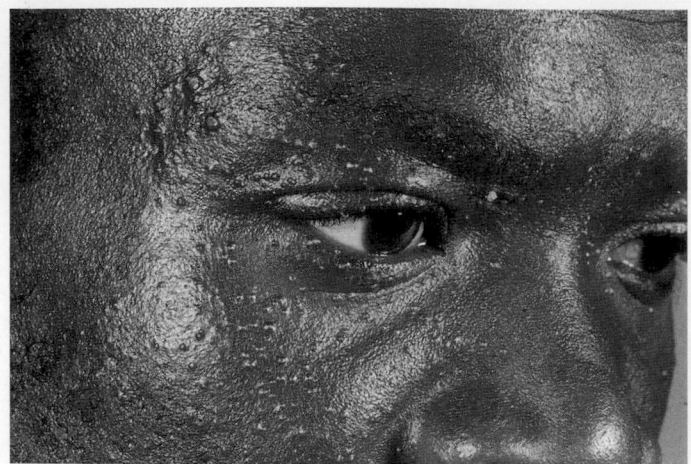

Figure 47.5 *Molluscum contagiosum*; multiple facial lesions.

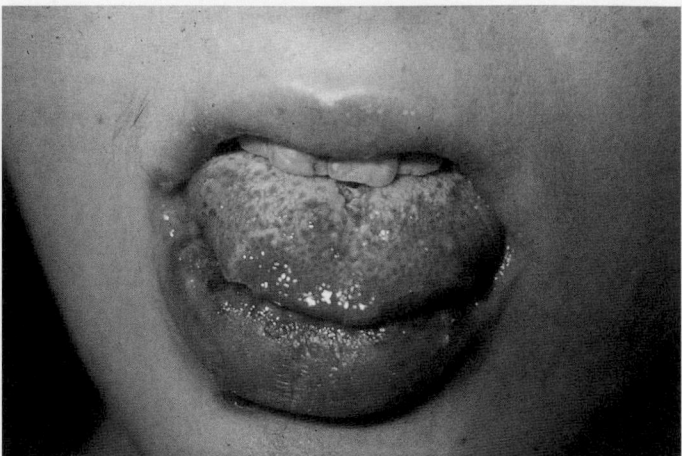

Figure 47.6 Herpes simplex lesions around the mouth (gingivostomatitis).

Diagnosis

The diagnosis of MC is usually on clinical grounds; however, HIV-positive patients may have other lesions of similar appearance, such as those caused by cryptococcosis, cutaneous pneumocystosis and other infectious disorders. Solitary MC lesions may resemble other entities (e.g. pyogenic granuloma, keratoacanthoma and basal cell carcinoma). A biopsy will exclude more serious conditions.

Management

Treatment of persisting lesions is by physical means, including cryotherapy, electrosurgery, topical keratolytic preparations, cantharidin and curettage. These methods may be effective; however, they can be very painful and may lead to scarring and discolouration of the skin. An orange stick dipped in 80% phenol solution is sometimes used to pierce the umbilicated centre. This must not be used on the face or near the genitalia. Other treatment modalities that have been used with moderate success include wax stripping and application of salicylic acid pastes.

Human herpesviruses

The human herpesvirus family[21] includes eight viruses that cause disease in *Homo sapiens* (Table 47.3). All herpesviruses are enveloped double-stranded DNA viruses that have the property of remaining latent in viable form within host cells after primary infection. The herpesviruses can reactivate from time to time from the latent state to produce recurrent clinical lesions, many of which have cutaneous manifestations.

Herpes simplex viruses (HSV)

Herpes simplex viruses[22] are unusual among viruses in causing a wide variety of clinical syndromes. Two types of herpes simplex virus cause human disease:
1. Herpes simplex virus type 1 (HSV-1).
2. Herpes simplex virus type 2 (HSV-2).
The basic pathological lesions are cutaneous or mucocutaneous vesicles, and transmission of HSV involves direct contact with

Table 47.3 Human herpesviruses

HHV-1	Herpes simplex virus (HSV) type 1
HHV-2	Herpes simplex virus (HSV) type 2
HHV-3	Varicella-zoster virus (VZV)
HHV-4	Epstein–Barr virus (EBV)
HHV-5	Cytomegalovirus (CMV)
HHV-6	Human herpesvirus 6
HHV-7	Human herpesvirus 7
HHV-8	Human herpesvirus 8 (KSAHV)

either active lesions on skin or mucous membranes, or areas of asymptomatic viral shedding from saliva, semen or cervical secretions. Diseases due to herpes simplex viruses can be grouped into two categories:
1. Primary disease.
2. Reactivation disease.

Primary HSV infections

Primary clinical disease occurs when the virus is first encountered. Transmission is by contact (kissing or touching). Most primary infections are asymptomatic. When primary infection causes disease, a range of clinical manifestations can occur. HSV-1 usually causes lesions affecting the orofacial region, whereas HSV-2 usually causes lesions affecting the anogenital region; HSV-1 can, in a small proportion of cases, cause anogenital lesions while HSV type 2 can cause orofacial lesions.

Clinical syndromes due to HSV type 1 (orofacial)

1. Gingivostomatitis (vesicles or ulcers in and around gums and mouth) (Figure 47.6).
2. Ocular herpes: keratoconjunctivitis (vesicles or ulcers on eyelids, conjunctiva, cornea) (Figure 47.7).
3. Meningoencephalitis.

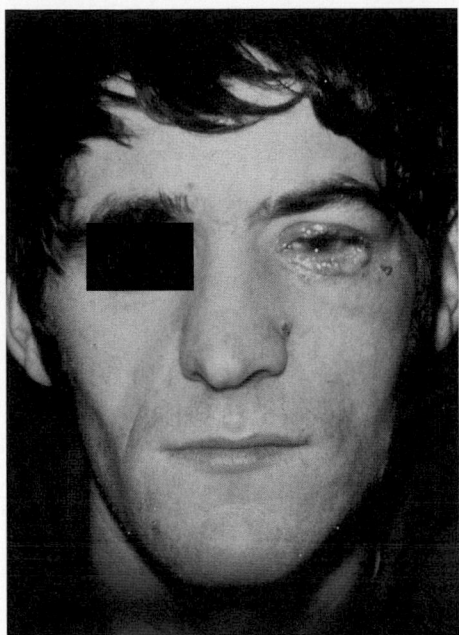

Figure 47.7 Herpes simplex virus ocular lesions (keratoconjunctivitis).

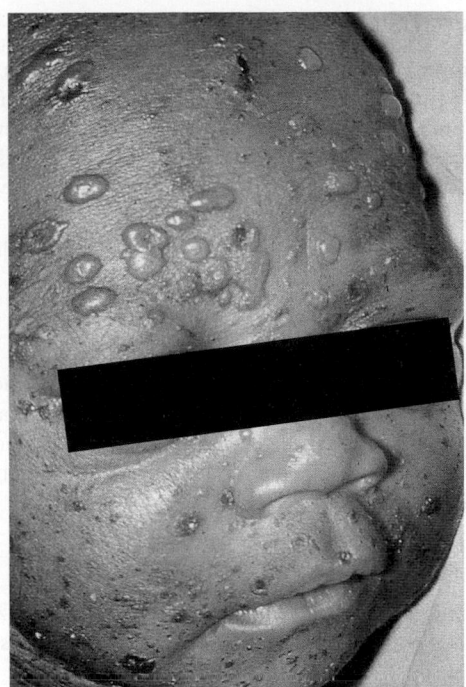

Figure 47.8 Generalized herpes simplex vesicular skin lesions.

Clinical syndromes due to HSV type 2 (anogenital)

1. Balanoposthitis (vesicles or ulcers on prepuce and glans penis).
2. Vulvovaginitis (vesicles or ulcers on vulva and vaginal mucosa).
3. Anoproctitis (vesicles or ulcers around the anal skin and in the anus).

Other clinical cutaneous syndromes due to herpes simplex

1. Herpetic 'whitlow' is the term given to herpes simplex vesicles on fingertips. This is an occupational hazard of doctors, nurses and anaesthetists who deal with unconscious patients; herpes infection is acquired through fingertip contamination. The lesion looks similar to a staphylococcal 'whitlow', but the exudate is serous rather than purulent.
2. Kaposi's varicelliform eruption. This is a superinfection by herpes simplex of eczematous skin, seen mainly in young children. It may progress to a serious disease with a significant mortality rate.
3. Neonatal infection. Primary genital infection in the mother (HSV-2) can give rise to severe generalized infection in the neonate (Figure 47.8). Affected children may have jaundice, hepatosplenomegaly, thrombocytopenia and large vesicular lesions on the skin. There is a high case fatality rate.

Latency

Following a primary mucocutaneous infection, HSV enters nerve endings underlying the skin lesion and travels up the peripheral nerve to nerve cell bodies in the dorsal root ganglion (DRG). HSV then enters a latency stage in the DRG for days to years.

Reactivation can occur as a result of immunosuppression, physical or emotional stress, fever (e.g. orofacial herpes is common in patients with lobar pneumonia and malaria), skin damage, menstruation, fatigue or ultra-violet light. During reactivation, HSV is transmitted back to the primary mucocutaneous site via efferent nerves. Reactivation may recur sporadically throughout life.

Primary HSV infections in HIV-infected individuals

Up to half of HIV-positive patients have clinical manifestations of a herpesvirus infection in the course of the disease, and these tend to be more severe and persistent than recurrences in normal host individuals.[20,23] In HIV-positive individuals, primary infections may be so severe that they are life threatening, or may manifest as chronic ulcerative mucocutaneous lesions, verrucous plaques or hyperplastic nodules. Painful and often deep, these chronic ulcers usually present around the perianal area, penis and lips.[24] HSV can affect other areas in HIV-positive patients, such as the cornea, tracheobronchial tree, oesophagus, lung, pericardium, liver and brain.

As one of the leading causes of genital ulcers, HSV may enhance acquisition of HIV infection via reduced epithelial barriers and by localizing CD4+ cells, the primary target of HIV, to the ulcers. It is hypothesized that antigenic stimulation of mucosal sites by reactivation of HSV can potentially increase HIV-1 replication on mucosal surfaces.

The differential diagnosis of HSV includes all causes of ulceration. Ulcerated lesions can mimic: (a) aphthous ulcers, (b) cytomegalovirus (CMV) ulcers, (c) drug reactions, (d) opportunistic atypical mycobacterial infections, (e) fungal infections and (f) traumatic ulcers. Verrucous-appearing lesions can mimic such entities as warts and epithelial neoplasms.

843

Diagnosis of HSV infections

Confirmation can be made from: (1) smears of lesions, (2) vesicular fluid (which can be obtained by placing a small needle into the vesicle and aspirating) and (3) tissue biopsy and several laboratory investigations. These include: (a) culture of virus, (b) electron microscopic visualization, (c) serology (complement fixation test; immunofluorescence for antigen and antibody detection; ELISA for anti-HSV IgM antibodies) and (d) DNA amplification tests (e.g. PCR).[25]

Treatment of HSV infections

Antiviral drugs are rarely required in primary infections in an immunocompetent individual. Topical aciclovir preparations may provide relief from a tingling sensation and shorten the duration of lesions. Treatment of HSV infections in immunocompromised individuals is described below.

Varicella-zoster virus infections

Varicella (chickenpox) and zoster (shingles or herpes zoster) are different diseases caused by an identical virus. Varicella is a primary illness, whereas zoster is a reactivation disease.

Varicella (chickenpox)

Chickenpox is a systemic viral infection with a characteristic cutaneous vesicular rash. The primary infection usually occurs in young children and is always symptomatic; in the majority of cases recovery is complete. The disease may be severe and fatal in infants aged less than 2 weeks, in adults and in the immunosuppressed.

Incubation period and transmission

The incubation period for chickenpox is 12–24 days, averaging 15–18 days. Chickenpox is transmitted by person-to-person contact, or by air-borne spread of respiratory secretions or vesicular fluid. The infectious period is usually 1–2 days before and up to 6 days after appearance of the rash. This may be prolonged in the presence of immunodeficiency.

Clinical features

Children rarely have prodromal symptoms, whereas adults may experience fever, headache and myalgia. The appearance of a skin rash on the trunk is often the first sign of disease. The macule rapidly progresses to a papule and forms a clear vesicle; vesicles are oval, with their long axis along creases of skin. These evolve to opaque pustules and may become umbilicated as they dry and crust. New waves of lesions occur as the older ones evolve (cropping). Successive crops of lesions are smaller and eventually fail to develop. Lesions appear most densely on the trunk and face; the hands and feet are relatively spared. Lesions may affect the conjunctivae, buccal mucosa, intestinal mucosa, and lungs.

In immunosuppressed individuals (post-transplantation, corticosteroid therapy, HIV/AIDS), primary chickenpox infection may cause a serious clinical disease with extensive cutaneous and systemic manifestations (Figure 47.9).[26] Treatment is with intravenous antiviral agents.

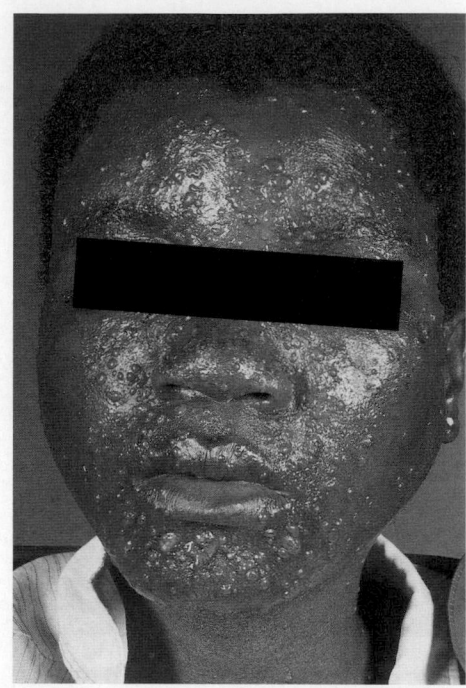

Figure 47.9 Severe chickenpox lesions in an immunosuppressed patient.

Complications

Systemic involvement

Widespread systemic involvement may sometimes occur. Chickenpox pneumonia, disseminated intravascular coagulation, and abnormal renal and hepatic function may result in a life-threatening illness. Patients with chickenpox pneumonia may have secondary bacterial infections. Those who survive chickenpox pneumonia may have calcified lesions on chest radiography. Post-chickenpox encephalitis can occur, and is mild and self-limiting leading to a complete recovery in most cases. Patients may present with a cerebellar disturbance (ataxia, nystagmus). Thrombocytopenia may occur, manifesting clinically as purpura and haematuria, and the rash may be haemorrhagic (Figure 47.10).

Secondary bacterial infections

As the skin vesicles burst leaving an itchy surface, secondary infection with *Staphylococcus aureus* or *Streptococcus pyogenes* may occur. These may sometimes progress to toxic shock syndrome, scarlet fever or erysipelas.

Diagnosis of chickenpox

Diagnosis of chickenpox is usually obvious on clinical examination. Confirmation can be made by subjecting smears of vesicular lesions, vesicular fluid (which can be obtained by placing a small needle into a vesicle and aspirating) and tissue biopsy to several laboratory investigations: (a) culture of virus, (b) electron microscopic visualization, (c) serology (complement fixation test; immunofluorescence for antigen and antibody detection; ELISA) and (d) DNA amplification (e.g. PCR).

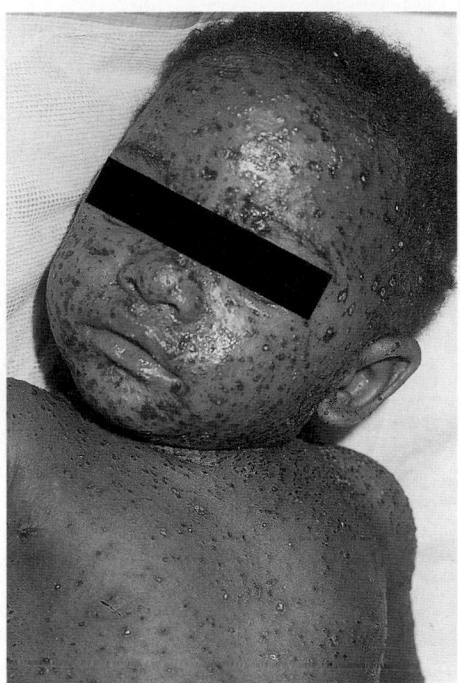

Figure 47.10 Haemorrhagic chickenpox in a child.

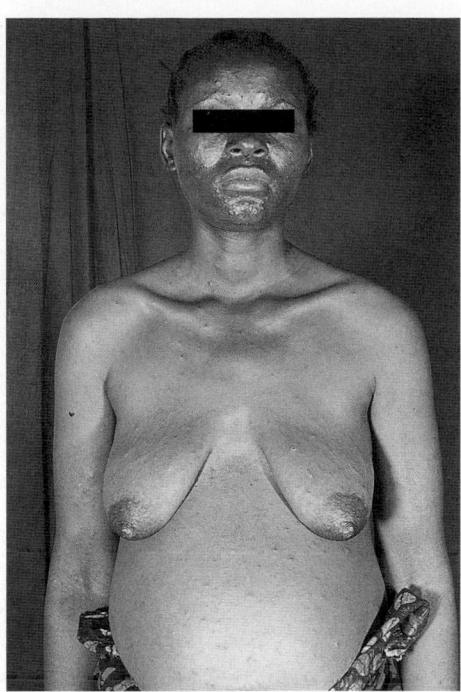

Figure 47.11 Chickenpox in a pregnant woman.

Management

Most patients recover without specific treatment. Pruritus may be reduced by antihistamines. Oral aciclovir (10 mg/kg five times a day for 5 days) reduces the duration of fever and active rash (from 6.5 to 5.7 days). Aspirin (acetylsalicylic acid) should not be used for reduction of fever, or analgesia because of an association with Reye's syndrome.

Treatment of chickenpox pneumonia requires an early infusion with aciclovir (10 mg/kg 8-hourly i.v.), being given slowly over 1 h to avoid nephrotoxicity, which is related to peak levels. Urea, creatinine and electrolytes must be monitored during therapy. Secondary bacterial infections are common and thus broad-spectrum antibiotics with anti-staphylococcal activity must be used. Arterial oxygen saturation should be monitored where possible; patients with falling oxygen saturations may require assisted ventilation. Newer antiviral agents, effective against all herpesviruses, are described below. Thrombocytopenia can be managed by a short course of corticosteroids and/or immunoglobulin. Platelet transfusion should be given, depending on the platelet count.

Prevention and control

Live varicella vaccines have been developed and highly effective.[27]

Passive immunization using varicella-zoster immunoglobulin (VZIG) is indicated for use in: (a) leukaemic and other immunosuppressed patients who do not have a previous history of chickenpox, and have been in contact with patients with chickenpox or zoster; (b) neonates whose mothers develop chickenpox (Figure 47.11) 7 days before or after delivery; and (c) non-immune pregnant contacts.

Children with chickenpox should be excluded from school for 1 week after the appearance of the rash. Patients are no longer infectious when the lesions are dry and scabbed. Because of the risk to other susceptible patients, all patients with zoster and chickenpox should be isolated.

Shingles or zoster

Varicella-zoster virus produces lifelong latency and may reactivate later in life, causing the clinical entity 'shingles'. The varicella-zoster virus (VZV) remains dormant in the dorsal root ganglia until reactivation, at which time it travels down the nerve to manifest the typical cutaneous lesions of zoster (shingles), which presents as a vesicular eruption along the distribution of one or two dermatomes served by a dorsal root ganglion (Figure 47.12). The mechanism of reactivation is unclear, although it is related clinically to stress, ageing, underlying malignancy and immunosuppression.

Clinical features

Patients with herpes zoster typically experience a prodromal phase which may manifest as pain, numbness, tingling and/or itching in a specific dermatomal distribution on any part of the body. This is commonly followed by an eruption of vesicles in the dermatomal distribution, on an erythematous base. Often the prodromal pain can be so severe as to lead to a misdiagnosis of myocardial infarction or an abdominal emergency. The usual dermatomal distribution is unilateral in appearance; however, many cases of multidermatomal zoster (Figure 47.13) are seen in patients infected with HIV infection. Zoster generally appears within 2–7 years of HIV seroconversion, most commonly during the asymptomatic phase. In these cases, it is more severe, more

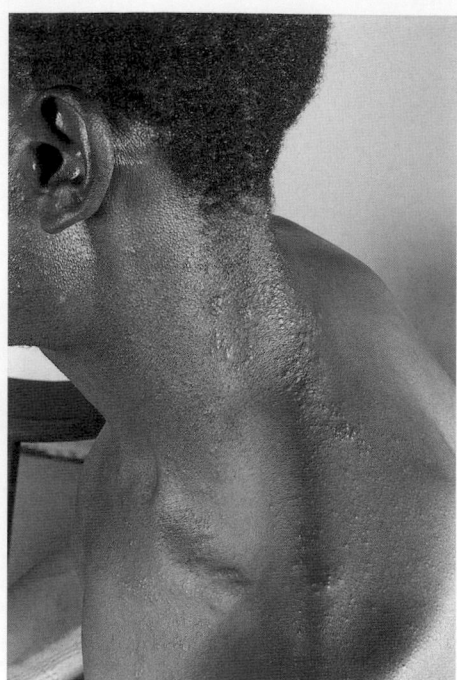

Figure 47.12 Herpes zoster (shingles) affecting a single dermatome.

intense and more difficult to treat, leaving serious scarring. Shingles is now frequently seen in HIV-positive children (Figure 47.14).

Complications

Ophthalmic zoster must be treated aggressively and watched carefully because there is a high likelihood of eye involvement resulting in conjunctivitis and blindness. The risk of post-herpetic neuralgia tends to increase with age but not with immunosuppression, and pain may continue for months or even years (post-herpetic neuralgia).

Complications of zoster in immunocompromised individuals include dissemination over large areas of the skin with possible secondary infection, potentially fatal pulmonary involvement, and encephalitis. Zoster also tends to have a higher rate of recurrence (5–23%) in HIV-infected individuals, compared with less than 5% in normal individuals. In addition to the severe pain experienced by patients with postherpetic neuralgia, crusted, punched-out ulcerations that leave painful atrophic scars (Figure 47.13) may also occur. Verrucous plaques can also occur in zoster; these are chronic and often resistant to therapy with aciclovir.

Diagnosis of zoster

The diagnosis is usually a clinical one. Confirmation can be made using the laboratory investigations described below.

Epstein–Barr virus

The clinical disease 'infectious mononucleosis' or 'glandular fever' is caused by the Epstein–Barr virus (EBV). EBV is shed in pharyngeal secretions, and transmission occurs via close contact (e.g.

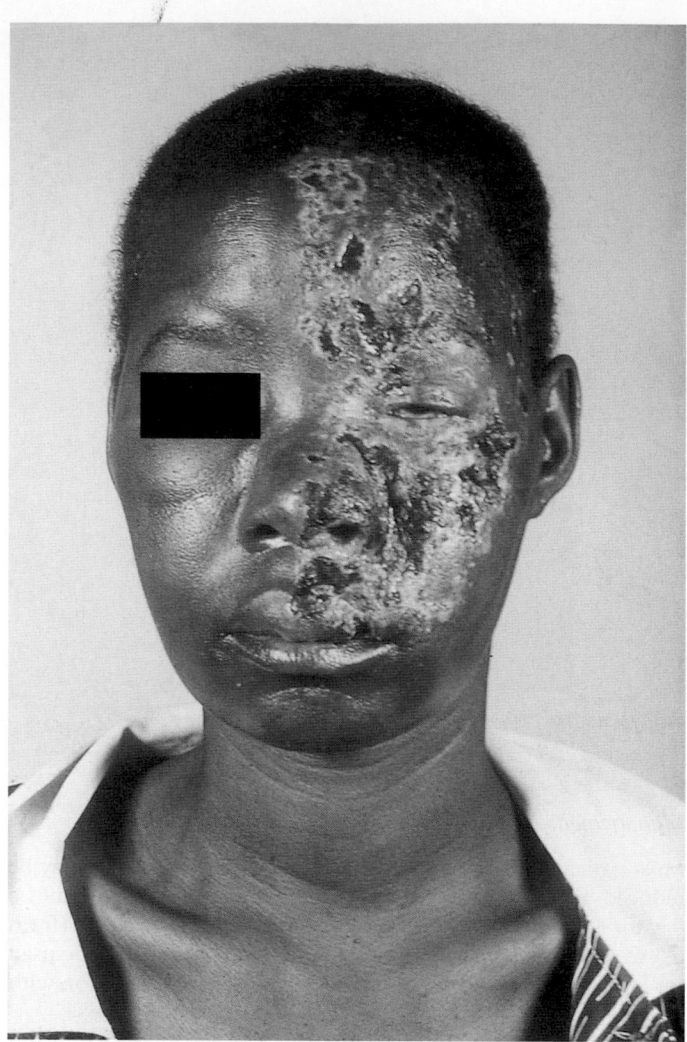

Figure 47.13 Multidermatomal herpes zoster in a patient with AIDS.

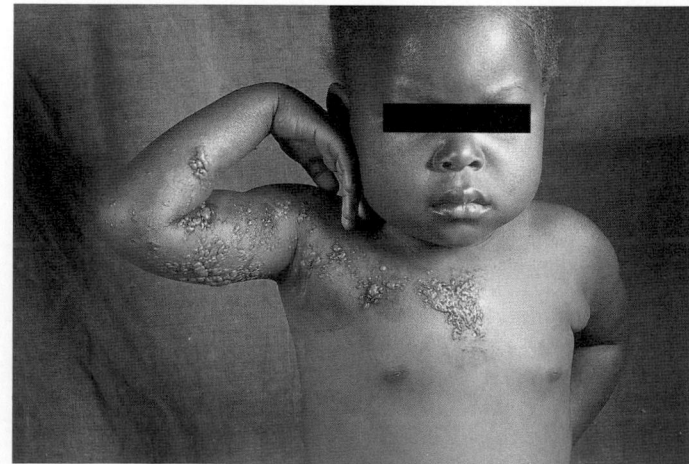

Figure 47.14 Herpes zoster in an HIV-positive child.

kissing). Primary EBV infection begins in oropharyngeal epithelium, where EBV virions are replicated and released from the epithelial cells to saliva. The virions carrying gp350/220 infect B cells via CD21 molecules, or receptors for the C3d in oropharyngeal areas, and form an episome in the nucleus (atypical mononuclear cells). Although major target cells of EBV are human B cells, epithelial cells, salivary gland duct cells, T cells, natural killer (NK) cells, macrophages/monocytes, smooth muscle cells and endothelial cells are found to be infected. The EBV-infected B cells express various EBV-associated antigens that are the target molecules recognized by the host immune response. When the immune surveillance system fails, reactivation of EBV-infected B cells occurs with subsequent polyclonal proliferation and dissemination of EBV to other tissues. Over 50% of healthy adults have been previously infected with EBV or human herpesvirus 4, which usually remains in a latent phase.

Clinical features

In primary infection, the virus selectively infects B lymphocytes as well as certain types of squamous epithelia; this manifests as infectious mononucleosis. The virus replicates primarily in the oropharyngeal epithelium, followed by entry into the B-cell system, where it remains latent until reactivation or dissemination to other sites. In HIV-infected individuals with severe immunodeficiency, viral replication leads to the clinical manifestations of: hairy leukoplakia, Burkitt's lymphoma or EBV-associated large cell lymphoma (see Chapter 35).

Cutaneous manifestations of EBV infection

In immunocompetent patients the cutaneous manifestations of infectious mononucleosis may include a petechial skin rash (due to thrombocytopenia) or a macular skin one due to use of ampicillin. The mucocutaneous manifestations of EBV in HIV-infected patients[28] include oral hairy leukoplakia (OHL),[29] correlating with moderate to advanced immunodeficiency. As with zoster, OHL has been linked with an advance from HIV infection to AIDS, and manifests as whitish plaques on the inferolateral margins of the tongue (Figure 47.15). The surface of the plaques may be smooth, corrugated or folded with thick hair-like projections. Lesions of OHL can mimic other mucous membrane lesions such as tobacco-associated leukoplakia and candidiasis. Lesions caused by OHL cannot be dislodged by a tongue depressor. They are asymptomatic and cause few problems; however, they occasionally become verrucous and may lead to dysphagia.

Differential diagnosis

OHL must be distinguished from candidiasis by the absence of hyphae in a microscopic examination of scrapings. Lesions caused by OHL can also mimic tobacco-associated leukoplakia, squamous cell carcinoma, condyloma acuminatum, lichen planus, white sponge naevus, leukokeratosis oris, mucous patches of syphilis and aphthous ulcers.

EBV and human cancer

EBV has been linked epidemiologically with two human cancers: (a) Burkitt's lymphoma and (b) nasopharyngeal carcinoma (see Chapter 35).

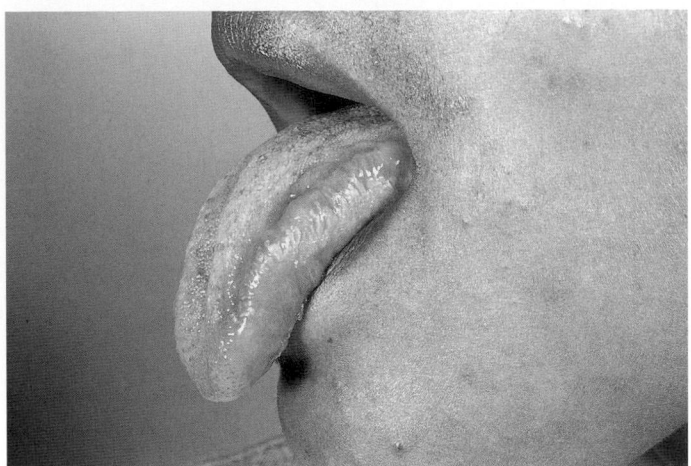

Figure 47.15 Hairy leukoplakia of the tongue.

Diagnosis

Diagnosis is made by detection of viral capsid antigen (VCA) and anti-IgM anti-EBV capsid antibody. A monospot (Paul Bunnell) test to detect heterophile antibodies may be useful in diagnosing glandular fever. Molecular methods using PCR may detect EBV DNA in peripheral blood mononuclear cells.

Management

Treatment is palliative: no specific treatment is available.

Cytomegalovirus

Human cytomegalovirus (CMV or human herpesvirus HHV-5) is a ubiquitous member of the herpes family of viruses.[30] More than 80% of healthy adults are seropositive for CMV, indicating previous exposure. After primary infection, usually asymptomatic, CMV, like other herpes viruses, undergoes latency, persisting in the infected individual. It is not clear which types of cell can harbour the virus and support an on going infection, nor is it clear whether leucocytes behave as specific carriers of the virus during a systemic infection, or represent a reservoir of replicating virus or a possible site of latency. The mechanism underlying reactivation is unknown. Although dermatologists are generally familiar with cutaneous manifestations of infection with herpes simplex virus and varicella-zoster virus, CMV infection has seldom been discussed.

CMV rarely causes symptomatic disease in the immunocompetent individual. It became a significant clinical problem, however, after the introduction of transplantation and associated immunosuppressive therapy.[31] Nowadays, about 90% of patients with AIDS develop acute active CMV infection at some point during their illness; it is one of the most common opportunistic viral infection in patients with AIDS.[32,33] About 95% of HIV-positive patients with a CD4 count of less than 100 cells/mm^3 have clinical manifestations of CMV.

Clinical features

A typical CMV viraemia is associated with basophilic intranuclear inclusions, or 'owl's eyes' (Figure 47.16), in urine, tears, breast

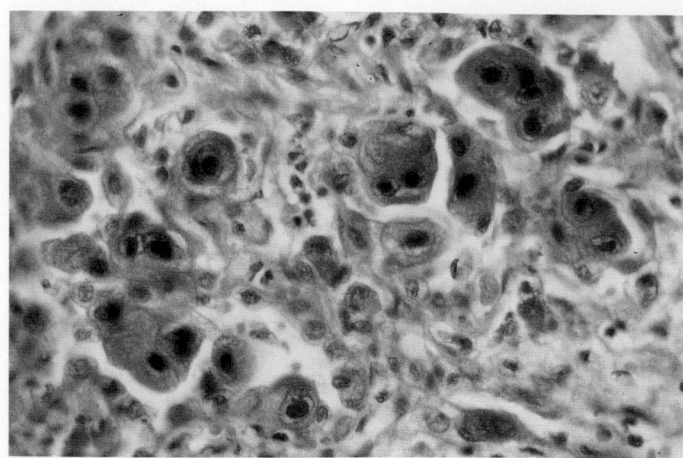

Figure 47.16 Intranuclear inclusions in a CMV infection.

milk, faeces, semen, cervical secretions, blood, bronchoalveolar lavage specimens and saliva. This viraemia is usually followed by infection of the vascular endothelium of every organ, skin rash, vasculitis and ulceration of mucosal surfaces.

Cutaneous lesions of CMV can have a varied presentation, including:

1. Localized and diffuse ulceration
2. Keratotic verrucous lesions
3. Palpable purpuric papules
4. Vesicular, bullous and generalized morbilliform eruptions
5. Hyperpigmented indurated plaques
6. Generalized bullous toxic epidermal necrolysis-like eruption associated with CMV hepatitis.

Other clinical manifestations of a CMV infection include retinitis and gastroenteritis in about 50% of all patients with AIDS. Up to 10% of patients have a serious CMV pneumonia, CMV retinitis (increasing to 30% at autopsy), oesophagitis, colitis or proctocolitis causing perianal ulceration,[26] which is believed to be a contiguous spread to the skin from the gastrointestinal tract. Lesions caused by CMV can also appear ulcerated, and must be distinguished from other ulcerated lesions as described for HSV.

Diagnosis

Cutaneous manifestations of CMV infection are not sufficiently distinctive to allow the diagnosis to be made on clinical grounds alone. The diagnosis of cutaneous CMV involvement has usually been established by microscopic examination. Cytomegalic inclusions, CMV antigens or CMV DNA detected in skin biopsy specimens have been considered a significant criterion to diagnose cutaneous CMV infection. However, whether CMV detected in skin biopsy specimens is responsible for the pathogenesis of the cutaneous manifestations is still controversial, because characteristic cytomegalic cells in biopsy specimens taken from uninvolved skin have been detected in a patient with AIDS.

There are no laboratory assays that are diagnostic in recent infection. Standard methods applied to all herpes viruses are used in the diagnosis of CMV.

Microscopy

Historically, the detection of characteristic intranuclear inclusions known as 'owl's eyes' has been considered to be an indicator of active CMV disease. However, the detection of inclusions by microscopic examination may be an inadequate method for establishing the diagnosis, because these intranuclear inclusions can also be caused by other viruses.

Viral culture

Routine cell culture of samples obtained from body fluids to confirm characteristic cytopathic effects takes a long time, because of the slow growth of this virus.

Serological diagnosis

Serological diagnosis, by use of complement fixation test, and detection of IgM and IgG antibodies may be helpful – they are widely used to determine previous infection. Demonstration of a four-fold rise in IgM antibody titres in the serum of ill patients could be interpreted as an indication of a primary infection with CMV. Useful findings for acute CMV infection in normal adults are: culture of blood and tissue biopsies for CMV and CMV-specific IgG seroconversion. Nevertheless, it is difficult to distinguish between primary infection and reactivation.

Immunohistology

Immunohistochemical study of samples with antibodies against specific viral antigens of CMV may reveal cell-inclusions. Although the DNA hybridization assay was expected to be useful for the diagnosis of CMV infection, because of the insensitivity of hybridization, this assay has failed to achieve widespread use.

Molecular methods

Recent developments in the fields of CMV diagnosis are exciting. Molecular amplification methods such as the PCR have been utilized to study CMV infection with samples such as urine, leucocytes, plasma, serum and paraffin-embedded sections. This method has been used with almost uniform success in most clinical settings. Nevertheless, positive results in PCR studies should be viewed with caution, because such a sensitive procedure may demonstrate the presence of viruses totally unrelated to the aetiology of diseases. Precautions have also to be adopted to avoid contamination that may yield false-positive results.

The most rapid available approach to the diagnosis of CMV infection is the direct detection of CMV antigen in nuclei of peripheral blood leucocytes, an assay known as the pp65 direct antigenaemia test. Monoclonal antibodies directed against the CMV lower matrix protein pp65 (UL83) are used for the direct detection of CMV in circulating polymorphonuclear leucocytes by use of immunoperoxidase techniques. The predictive value of this test rests on the capacity to quantify the number of pp65-positive cells, thus providing an estimate of viral burden. This assay is one of the most rapid and reliable tests for the diagnosis of CMV disease in both patients with AIDS and organ transplant recipients.

Management

The usual treatment for clinical disease caused by CMV is intravenous ganciclovir (dihydroxypropylguanine, DHPG). Cidofovir, foscarnet and fomivirsen are also approved for the treatment of CMV retinitis in patients with AIDS.

Human herpesviruses 6 and 7

HHV-6 and HHV-7 have been recently discovered and are prevalent in humans with a tropism for CD4+ lymphocytes.[34] Primary infection with HHV-6 has been associated with exanthema subitum (roseola or sixth disease) in children, and febrile illnesses with seizures. Other clinical associations made with this virus include: (a) multiple sclerosis, (b) infectious mononucleosis-like illness and (c) drug-induced hypersensitivity syndrome. More recently, HHV-6 has been recognized as an opportunistic pathogen in patients with HIV infection and in transplant recipients, causing fever, skin rash and malaise.

The clinical characteristics of HHV-7 are not well defined, although some cases of exanthema subitum have been linked with this virus.

Human herpesvirus 8

This herpesvirus was first discovered in 1994 and was named Kaposi's sarcoma-associated herpesvirus (KSAHV) because it was found in almost 100% of Kaposi's sarcomas (KS) from patients with AIDS.[35] This virus is now commonly referred to as human herpesvirus 8 (HHV-8) and has subsequently been found in peripheral blood mononuclear cells of patients with KS, in body cavity-based lymphomas in HIV-positive patients without KS, in classical KS and in other forms of KS. HHV-8 DNA has also been detected in patients with pemphigus vulgaris, pemphigus foliaceus, carcinoma and lymphoma.

Diagnosis of herpesvirus infections

Usually, diagnosis of herpesvirus infections is made on clinical grounds. However, because of the varied appearance of lesions in HIV-positive individuals, laboratory investigations may aid diagnosis. The main laboratory analyses of patient samples for the diagnosis of herpesviruses include:

- Electron microscopy
- Viral culture ('gold standard')
- Immunofluorescence (antigen detection)
- Histopathological examination of biopsied lesions (Tzanck smear with the presence of multinucleated giant cells can help diagnose HSV or VZV but cannot distinguish between HSV-1, HSV-2 and VZV)
- In situ hybridization of biopsied lesions
- Immunoperoxidase stains of biopsied lesions for EBV, CMV, HSV
- PCR for detecting viral DNA
- ELISA to detect virus-specific IgM (acute) and IgG (chronic) antibodies.

Management of herpesvirus infections

Several antiviral drugs and immunomodulatory agents are now available for treating herpesvirus infections.[36-39]

Aciclovir (ACV)

ACV is the most widely used medication for herpesvirus infections. It is a safe, systemic antiviral agent.

Oral ACV stimulates herpesvirus-infected cells to produce thymidine kinase (TK), an enzyme that sequentially phosphorylates ACV to an active triphosphate form which inhibits viral DNA polymerase, resulting in chain termination. First-episode genital herpes requires a 200-mg dose of ACV given orally five times a day for 10 days. Recurrent herpes necessitates 200 mg of ACV five times per day for a period of 5 days or longer, depending on the clinical response. ACV has an intracellular half life of 1 h, so frequent dosing is necessary. Greater convenience can be achieved by dosing ACV at a dose of 400 mg three times daily instead of five times daily.

Acute herpes zoster requires a dosage of ACV 800 mg given orally five times per day for 7–10 days. This dose regimen reduces the duration of postherpetic neuralgia symptoms from 62 to 20 days for immunocompetent patients treated with placebo versus ACV, respectively.

Topical ACV is also available; however, it is not commonly used because of its low efficacy, although it does appear to reduce the pain and tingling sensation if used early.

Dosing of ACV in HIV-infected patients is similar to the schedule described above but variations occur. Because of the low bioavailability of ACV in the oral form, patients with HIV and severe HSV disease may require the intravenous (i.v.) form, especially when both dissemination and visceral organ involvement are present.

Ophthalmic preparations including idoxuridine, trifluridine and vidarabine are in use for herpes keratitis and keratoconjunctivitis.

Two other agents, valaciclovir and famciclovir, have been approved for treatment of herpes in order to provide both easier convenience and higher bioavailability.

Valaciclovir (VACV)

VACV is the valyl ester of ACV with a five times greater bioavailability (54%) than oral ACV, reaching plasma levels of ACV similar to the level attained with intravenous ACV. First-episode genital herpes is usually treated with 500 mg of VACV given twice daily for 10 days. Recurrent episodes of genital herpes are treated with 500 mg of VACV twice daily for 5 days. VACV can be used at a dose of 500 mg once daily for suppression of recurrent genital herpes in immunocompetent individuals with fewer than 10 episodes per year. It has been approved for the treatment of acute herpes zoster at a dose of 1000 mg three times daily for 7 days. This therapy is as safe as oral ACV.

VACV has been safe and well-tolerated for both short- and long-term use in immunocompromised patients, including HIV-positive patients. The dose schedule for HIV-positive patients is similar to that described above; however, patients may require 500 mg of VACV twice daily, or 1000 mg once daily for suppression of chronic recurrent genital herpes.

Famciclovir (FCV)

FCV is the oral prodrug form of the nucleoside penciclovir. As with ACV, FCV must be phosphorylated to a triphosphate form in order to be active. As with VACV, FCV has greater bioavailability (77%) than ACV. It is approved for the episodic treatment of recurrent genital herpes at a dose of 125 mg twice daily for 5 days. Single dose treatment regimens show promise in clinical trials.

FCV can be used for first-episode genital herpes at a dose of 250 mg three times daily for 10 days. Recently, approval was granted by the US Food and Drug Administration (FDA) for FCV at a dose of 250 mg twice daily for recurrent genital herpes suppression. Also, FCV can be used for acute herpes zoster infection at a dose of 500 mg three times daily for 7 days. At this dose, it has been shown to decrease the healing time of cutaneous manifestations of herpes zoster, and to significantly reduce the duration of postherpetic neuralgia (PHN).

FCV can also be used in immunocompromised individuals including those infected with HIV. In HIV-infected patients, FCV is effective for the suppression of symptomatic as well as asymptomatic HSV reactivation; duration of symptoms is decreased by 65% and there is an 81% reduction in viral shedding. Suppressive dosing of FCV (500 mg twice daily) is as effective as ACV (400 mg five times a day) for recurrent genital herpes in HIV-infected individuals at a more convenient dosing regimen.

Evidence for resistance to ACV in HIV-infected individuals has recently emerged. Most ACV-resistant HSV isolates can be treated and are susceptible to certain other antivirals not requiring thymidine kinase activation.

Foscarnet

Foscarnet is an FDA-approved pyrophosphate analogue that directly inhibits HSV DNA polymerase without activation; it is administered for treatment of ACV-resistant HSV at a dose of 40 mg/kg i.v. every 8 h. Its use is limited owing to significant renal toxicity.

Cidofovir (CDV)

CDV is a nucleotide analogue of deoxycytidine monophosphate that requires phosphorylation to an active metabolite by host cellular enzymes, rather than the virus-specific enzymes used by the other antivirals. This agent has broad-spectrum anti-DNA virus activity. The gel formulation has been evaluated for treatment of ACV-resistant mucocutaneous HSV infection in patients with AIDS; significant benefits in lesion healing, pain reduction and virological effects have been demonstrated.

Post herpetic neuralgia treatment

PHN can be treated symptomatically with topical analgesic agents such as capsaicin, which may be helpful in some cases. Other schemes for treating PHN that have been shown to be effective include: (a) amitriptyline, (b) carbamazepine, (c) nerve blocks, (d) Triavil, (e) lidocaine (lignocaine) and (f) fentanyl patches.

Oral hairy leukoplakia treatment

Usually OHL requires no treatment; however, several therapeutic agents have been tried, including: ACV, topical podophyllin resin, topical isotretinoin, as well as local destructive measures.

Papovaviruses

Human papillomavirus

Human papillomavirus (HPV) causes cutaneous warts at any site on the body.[40] HPV is transmitted by contact and is an asymptomatic infection in the majority of immunocompetent persons who acquire the infection. In a small proportion of individuals, HPV causes warts, which vary in size and number; these are in most cases self-limiting.

Various causes of immunodeficiency are associated with an increased incidence of HPV infection.[40,41] Penile and perianal warts are twice as common in HIV-seropositive men than in individuals with a normal immune system. Depressed cell-mediated immunity in HIV-seropositive persons is associated with an increased prevalence of HPV infection. The incidence of genital warts in HIV-seropositive women has been reported to be increased by as much as 10-fold. Severe HPV infections involving multiple portions of the anogenital area are common in HIV-seropositive persons. These cutaneous lesions are increased in number and severity, and are difficult to treat. Many recur after treatment.

Invasive cervical cancer, which is closely associated with oncogenic HPV, is considered an AIDS-defining illness in HIV-seropositive women.[41] Cervical cancer is the second most common cancer killer of women worldwide. The high prevalence of HIV in Third-World women and the increasing incidence in those in industrialized countries are adding to the cervical cancer epidemic.[41]

Anogenital warts in people with a normal immune response usually do not contain oncogenic HPV and are thus not considered to be premalignant. In HIV-seropositive persons, however, anogenital warts often harbour multiple HPV types including some considered to be oncogenic.

Management

Depending on their size, extent and location, warts can be treated by topical agents (podophyllin; imiquimod), surgery (excision or cautery) or cryotherapy using a cryoprobe.

Surgical therapy of HPV-related lesions in HIV-seropositive patients carries the risk of transmission of HIV to the surgeon. Laser surgery and electrosurgery carry a risk of transmission of both HIV and HPV from the aerosolized wart tissue. High recurrence rates of warts in HIV-positive patients receiving surgical therapy are recorded.

Experimental cytokine therapy for warts

Interferon (IFN) α was the first FDA-approved antiviral agent for genital warts, and has also been reported as useful adjunctive treatment for HIV.[42,43] Owing to systemic side-effects (i.e. influenza-like syndrome) of IFN, the need for multiple intralesional injections, high cost and relatively slow rate of lesion resolution, exogenous IFN therapy has been used in combination with other methods.

Imiquimod[44] can be used as a topical (5% cream) self-applied therapy for condyloma acuminatum. Imiquimod acts by inducing endogenous production of IFNα and a spectrum of other cytokines. Thus, imiquimod is an immunomodulatory agent that also acts via antiviral mechanisms. It has proved safe and efficacious in the treatment of condyloma acuminatum in otherwise healthy persons when used overnight on alternating nights, three times a weekly for up to 16 weeks.

Cidofovir is a broad-spectrum antiviral agent with activity against all human herpes viruses and HPV.

Parvovirus infections

Human parvovirus B19

The cutaneous manifestations of human parvovirus B19 infection include a petechial eruption in a 'glove and stocking' distribution, reticular truncal erythema and the 'slapped cheek sign'.[45] The dermatopathology of B19 infection suggests that tissue injury is mediated by delayed-type hypersensitivity, antibody-dependent cellular immunity directed at microbial antigenic targets in the epidermis and endothelium, and by circulating immune complexes in the setting of leucocytoclastic vasculitis. These findings appear to portray a picture of connective tissue disease. Topical cidofovir has been used successfully given intralesionally against HPV-associated skin lesions.[46]

REFERENCES

1. Dyer JA. Childhood viral exanthems. *Pediatr Ann* 2007; 36:21–29.
2. Moss WJ, Griffin DE. Global measles elimination. *Nature Rev Microbiol* 2006; 12:900–908.
3. Fetuga MB, Jokanma OF, Ogunfowora OB, et al. A ten year study of measles admissions in a Nigerian Teaching Hospital. *Niger J Clin Pract* 2007; 10(1): 41–46.
4. Uyirwoth GP. Measles in Mashonaland Central Province: Zimbabwe. *East Afr Med J* 1993; 70:455–459.
5. Hussey GD, Klein M. Routine high-dose vitamin A therapy for children hospitalized with measles. *J Trop Pediatr* 1993; 9:342–345.
6. Latham MC. Vitamin A and childhood mortality. *Lancet* 1993; 342:549.
7. Huiming Y, Chaomin W, Meng N. Vitamin A for treating measles in children. *Cochrane Databas Syst Rev* 2005; 4:CD001479.
8. Foster SO, Spiegel RA, Mokdad A. Immunization, oral rehydration therapy and malaria chemotherapy among children under 5 in Bomi and Grand Cape Mount counties, Liberia, 1984 and 1988. *Int J Epidemiol* 1993; 22(suppl 1): S50–S55.
9. Garenne M, Leroy O, Beau JP, et al. Efficacy of measles vaccine after controlling for exposure. *Am J Epidemiol* 1993; 138:182–195.
10. Longini IM Jr, Halloran ME, Haber M, et al. Measuring vaccine efficacy from epidemics of acute infectious agents. *Stat Med* 1993; 12:249–263.
11. Tulchinsky TH, Ginsberg GM, Abed Y, et al. Measles control in developing and developed countries: the case for a two-dose policy. *Bull World Health Organ* 1993; 71:93–103.
12. Orenstein WA, Markowits LE, Atkinson WL, et al. Worldwide measles prevention. *Isr J Med Sci* 1994; 30:469–481.
13. Aaby P, Andersen M, Sodemann M, et al. Reduced childhood mortality after standard measles vaccination at 4–8 months compared with 9–11 months of age. *BMJ* 1993; 307:1308–1311.
14. Burstrom B, Aaby P, Mutie DM. Child mortality impact of a measles outbreak in a partially vaccinated rural African community. *Scand J Infect Dis* 1993; 25:763–769.
15. Moore ZS, Seward JF, Lane JM. Smallpox. *Lancet* 2006; 367:425–435.
16. Diven DG. An overview of poxviruses. *J Am Acad Dermatol* 2001; 44:1–16.
17. Parker S, Nuara A, Buller RM, et al. Human monkeypox: an emerging zoonotic disease. *Future Microbiol* 2007; 2:17–34.
18. Cook GC. Human monkeypox: a viral disease with an uncertain future in Africa. *Trop Dis Bull* 1988; 85:R1–R16.
19. Knight JC, Novembre FJ, Brown DR. Studies on Tanapox viruses. *Virology* 1989; 172:116–124.
20. Yen-Moore A, Straten MV, Carrasco D, et al. Cutaneous viral infections in HIV-infected individuals. *Clin Dermatol* 2000; 18(4):423–432.
21. Roizman B. Herpesviridae. A brief introduction. In: Fields BN, Knipe DM, Howley RM, et al., eds. *Fields Virology*. 5th edn. Philadelphia: Lippincott-Williams & Wilkins; 2007.
22. Corey L. Herpes simplex virus. In: Mandell GL, Bennett JE, Dolin R, eds. *Principles and Practice of Infectious Diseases*. 5th edn. Philadelphia: Churchill Livingstone; 2000:1564–1580.
23. Safran S, Ashley R, Houlihan C, et al. Clinical and serological features of herpes simplex virus infection in patients with AIDS. *AIDS* 1991; 5: 1107–1110.
24. Siegal FP, Lopez C, Hammer GF, et al. Severe acquired immunodeficiency in male homosexuals manifested by chronic perianal ulcerative herpes simplex lesions. *N Engl J Med* 1981; 305:1439-1444.
25. Jain S, Wyatt D, McCaughey C, et al. Nested multiplex PCR for the diagnosis of cutaneous herpes simplex and herpes zoster infections and a comparison with electronmicroscopy. *J Med Virol* 2001; 63(1):52–56.
26. Jura E, Chadwick EG, Josephs HS, et al. Varicella zoster virus infections in children infected with human immunodeficiency virus. *Pediatr Infect Dis J* 1989; 8:856–890.
27. Arvin AM. Varicella vaccine-the first six years. *N Engl J Med* 2001; 344: 1007–1009.
28. Iwatsuki K, Xu Z, Ohtsuka M, et al. Cutaneous lymphoproliferative disorders associated with Epstein-Barr virus infection: a clinical overview. *J Dermatol Sci* 2000; 22:181–195.
29. Reichart PS, Langford A, Gelderblom HR, et al. Oral hairy leukoplakia: observations in 95 cases and review of the literature. *J Oral Pathol Med* 1989; 18:410–415.
30. Drago F, Aragone MG, Rebora A. Cytomegalovirus infection in normal and immunocompromised humans: a review. *Dermatology* 2000; 200: 189–195.
31. Choi YL, Kim JA, Jang KT, et al. Characteristics of cutaneous cytomegalovirus infection in non-AIDS immunocompromised patients. *Br J Dermatol* 2006; 155:977–982.
32. Nico MM, Cymbalista NC, Hurtado YC, et al. Perianal cytomegalovirus ulcer in an HIV infected patient: case report and review of literature. *J Dermatol* 2000; 27:99–105.
33. Kano Y, Shiohara T. Current understanding of cytomegalovirus infection in immunocompetent individuals. *J Dermatol Sci* 2000; 22: 196–204.
34. Kosuge H. HHV-6, 7 and their related diseases. *J Dermatol Sci* 2000; 22: 205–212.
35. Chang Y, Cesarman E, Pessin MS, et al. Identification of herpesvirus-like DNA sequences in AIDS-associated Kaposi's sarcoma. *Science* 1994; 266: 1865–1869.
36. Herne K, Cirelli R, Lee P, et al. Advances in antiviral therapy. *Curr Opin Dermatol* 1996; 3:195–201.
37. Tyring S, Barbarash RA, Nahlik J, et al. Famciclovir for the treatment of acute herpes zoster: Effects on acute disease and postherpetic neuralgia. *Ann Intern Med* 1995; 123:89–96.
38. Lalezari JP, Stagg RJ, Jaffe HS, et al. A preclinical and clinical overview of the nucleotide-based antiviral agent cidofovir (HPMPC). In: Mills J, Corey L, eds. *Antiviral Chemotherapy*. New York: Plenum; 1996.
39. Conant A. Immunomodulatory therapy in the management of viral infections in patients with HIV infection. *J Am Acad Dermatol* 2000; 43:S27–S30.
40. Tyring SK. Human papillomavirus infections: epidemiology, pathogenesis and host immune response. *J Am Acad Dermatol* 2000; 43:S18–S26.

41. Palefsky J. Human papillomavirus-associated malignancies in HIV-positive men and women. *Curr Opin Oncol* 1995; 7:437–441.

42. Semprini AE, Stillo A, Marcozi S, et al. Treatment with interferon for genital HPV in HIV-positive and HIV-negative women. *Eur J Obstet Gynecol Reprod Biol* 1994; 53:135–137.

43. Rockley PF, Tyring SK. Interferons alpha, beta, and gamma therapy of anogenital human papillomavirus infections. *Pharmacol Ther* 1995; 65:265–287.

44. Edwards L, Ferenczy A, Eron L, et al. Self-administered topical 5% imiquimod cream for external anogenital warts. *Arch Dermatol* 1998; 134:25–30.

45. Magro CM, Dawood MR, Crowson AN. The cutaneous manifestations of human parvovirus B19 infection. *Hum Pathol* 2000; 31(4):488–497.

46. Bonatti H, Aigner F, DeClerq E, et al. Local administration of cidofovir for human papilloma virus associated skin lesions in transplant recipients. *Transpl Int* 2007; 20:238–246.

Chapter 48   Sandra Amor

Virus Infections of the Central Nervous System

Although virus infections of the central nervous system (CNS) are relatively rare, they are responsible for some of the most devastating and diverse effects of disease in humans and animals. Nevertheless, almost all the families of viruses have members associated with CNS disorders in humans. In this chapter we also briefly discuss prion diseases although these diseases are not strictly 'viral'.

CNS viral infections were first reported in Babylonian times, and trepanning in early times was possibly the earliest treatment for such diseases. Fortunately, the explosion in advances in the field of virus isolation techniques, immunology and molecular biology in addition to detailed knowledge of viral replication have enabled the rational control of CNS viral infections by prophylactics such as immunization and vector control, or following pharmacological intervention.

The broad spectrum of clinical manifestations of CNS infections (outlined in Table 48.1) poses the clinician not only a problem of prompt diagnosis but also that of treatment and aggressive management to allow recovery with little chance of sequelae. In many cases CNS diseases due to viral infections were thought to be more common in tropical regions but are now posing serious problems in Europe in recent years. With the increase in travel and changing climates due to global warming humans are becoming increasingly exposed to infections that were otherwise specific of tropical regions. This is particularly true for West Nile virus (WNV) disease, Toscana virus (TOSV) disease, avian influenza virus (H5N1) as well tick-borne encephalitis virus and arboviruses that have been frequently reported in several European countries.

Viral spread to the CNS

Consideration of how viruses enter the CNS is paramount to developing therapies through determining the methods by which such potential infections may be avoided or controlled. Space does not allow detail on entry of viruses and the reader is referred to Berger and Nash 2003[1] and *Fields Virology* by Knipe et al. 2007.[2]

For a virus to enter the CNS, it must first enter the host. The skin is the most extensive barrier to the entry of viruses but once it is broached by injury or piercing, for example by arthropod bites, viruses may rapidly invade. Similarly, entry may be via the mucosal surfaces of the respiratory, gastrointestinal and genitourinary tracts, which form the most formidable barrier due to mucous film and secretory immunoglobulin but may, nevertheless, be permeable to acid-resistant viruses, such as the enteroviruses. The major portals of entry of viruses causing human CNS infections are summarized in Table 48.2.

Following entry into the host and assuming the infection is not adequately controlled by the innate and adaptive immunity, the virus may gain access to the CNS either through the neural route via axonal transport, through the olfactory route, or via the blood across the blood–brain barrier (BBB).

Neural route

Retrograde transmission along the axon is a well-recognized route for rabies virus and has since been described for several other neurotropic viruses such as, varicella zoster and herpes simplex viruses (HSV), Herpes B virus and polio. For rabies, the neurological disease often precedes widespread dissemination in the host and the site of entry determines the incubation period. Moreover, experimental rabies and polio are prevented when the infected nerve is severed. Both retrograde and anterograde transneuronal and non-neuronal (ependymal cells and cerebrospinal fluid) pathways are utilized by vesicular stomatitis virus (VSV) within the CNS.

Olfactory route

Olfactory transmission of viruses to the CNS is well-known.[3] Experimental intranasal infection with HSV and togaviruses such as Semliki Forest virus (SFV) shows that virus is spread to the CNS via the olfactory route. In contrast to rabies virus and HSV-1, VSV does not use the trigeminal nerve for entry into the brain, as the trigeminal ganglion remains virus free following intranasal infection. Rather VSV has a tropism for olfactory receptor cells, using them for entry into the CNS.

Haematogenous route

The majority of viruses that induce CNS infection are acquired from the blood and must cross the BBB – an anatomical structure composed of endothelial cells joined by tight junctions, pericytes that form a discontinuous layer around the endothelial cells and astrocytic foot processes that surround the pericytes. The first

Table 48.1 Clinical manifestations of viral infections of the CNS

Disease	Duration	Clinical signs	Examples
Acute meningitis	Days	Rapid onset of high fever, stiff neck, altered mental state, photophobia, raised intracranial pressure	Viral meningitis
Chronic meningitis	Months	Gradual onset of signs associated with the above	Enteroviruses
Acute encephalitis	Days	Association with systemic illness, nausea, vomiting, seizures. Specific signs associated with tropism of virus, e.g. temporal lobe lesions following HSV infection	Measles, herpes simplex
Chronic encephalitis	Months to years	Gradual onset of signs as above, progressing to severe disability and death. General debility and dementia may develop	SSPE, HIV encephalitis
Post-infectious	Days to weeks	Onset of signs following recovery from viral infection. Such signs include the development of chronic fatigue syndrome or Guillain–Barré syndrome	Post-infectious encephalomyelitis
Slow viruses	Months to years	Progressive signs of neuronal destruction. Observed following immunosuppressive therapy	PML
Prion diseases	Months to years	Progressive signs of neurological dysfunction. Not associated with conventional virus	Creutzfeldt–Jakob disease, Kuru

HSV, herpes simplex virus; SSPE, subacute sclerosing panencephalitis; HIV, human immunodeficiency virus; PML, progressive multifocal leukoencephalopathy.

Table 48.2 Routes of entry of neurotropic viruses

Route of entry	Example
Inoculation	
Arthropod bite	Arboviruses
Animal bite	Rabies
Blood transfusion	Cytomegalovirus
Transplantation	Creutzfeldt–Jakob disease
Respiratory	Influenza
Enteric	Polio
Venereal	HIV
Transplacental	Cytomegalovirus

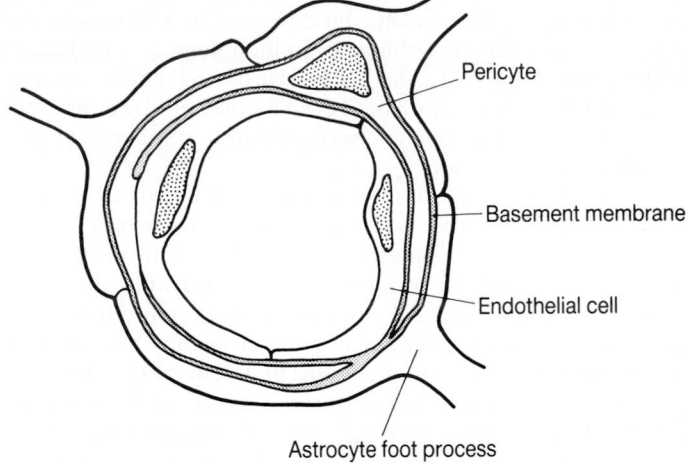

Figure 48.1 The blood–brain barrier.

description of the BBB was made in the late nineteenth century by Paul Ehrlich, who noticed that certain dyes stained all organs except the brain in an intact animal. A diagrammatic representation of the BBB is shown in Figure 48.1.

In general, the physical and chemical nature of the molecule determines its ability to cross the BBB; for example, lipid-soluble molecules are readily transferred across the BBB whereas charged non-lipid-soluble molecules are less effective. The BBB also forms a barrier for the entry of viruses; nevertheless, most viruses invade the CNS. Transfer of viruses across the BBB may take place either after infection of leukocytes, as is observed for measles and mumps virus, or following adherence of virus to erythrocytes, as is seen with togaviruses and paramyxoviruses. The infected cells migrate across the BBB and although such traffic is limited in the normal situation, it is severely augmented during injury or infection.[4] Alternatively, viruses may be taken up by receptors, induce the formation of pinocytotic vesicles on the endothelial cells and be actively transported, as in Semliki Forest virus infection (Figure 48.2).

Spread within the nervous system

Whether viruses reach the CNS via the haematogenous, olfactory or neural route, the progression of clinical signs is dependent on the subsequent spread of virus within the tissue. Additionally, the tropism of viruses for different cells determines the characteristic clinical signs and manifestation of disease associated with specific viruses (Table 48.1). For example, the spread of HSV within the temporal lobes leads to temporal lobe seizures, whereas infection of oligodendrocytes by JC papovavirus induces lesions of demyelination.

Attachment of viruses to cells prior to entry is obviously important in the development of disease, and binding domains or receptors for numerous viruses have been identified, such as the

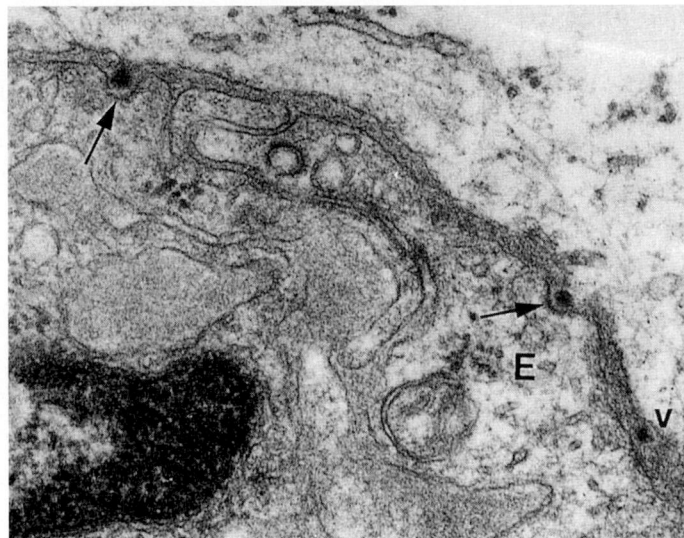

Figure 48.2 Brain capillary endothelial cell (E) showing the formation of coated vesicle containing mature virus (arrows). Mature virus (V) is also present in the basement membrane. Semliki Forest virus ×60 000. (Kindly provided by L. Pathak, St Thomas's Hospital.)

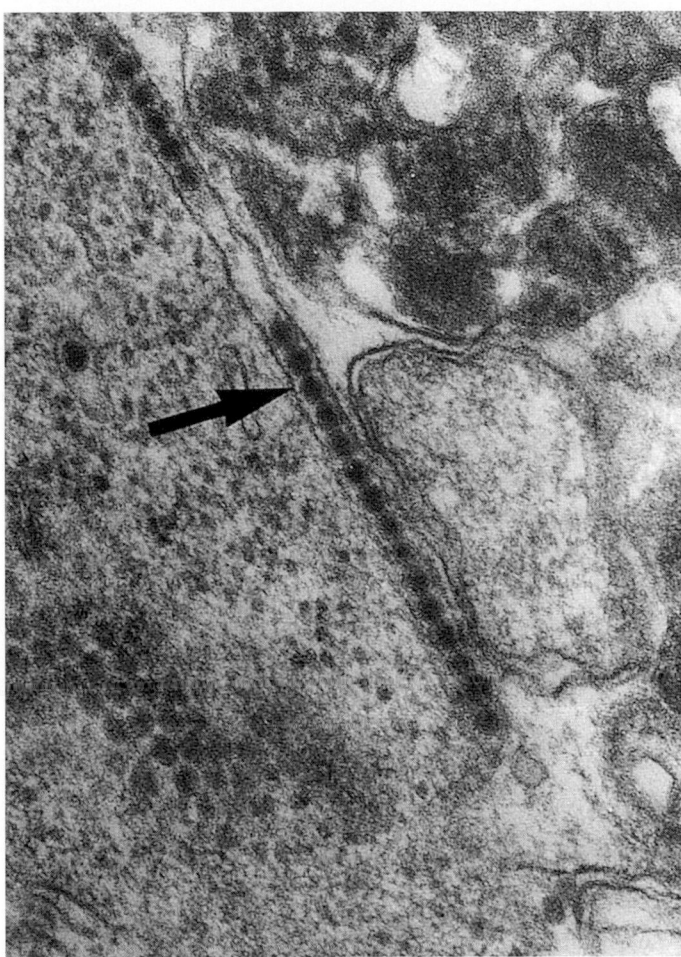

Figure 48.3 Langat virus (family Flaviviridae) (arrow) within the extracellular space of CNS tissue.

β-adrenergic receptor for reoviruses. The utilization of neurotransmitter receptors by viruses and interference in the functioning of specific neurones may explain why viruses have been implicated in chronic fatigue syndrome.[5] Other receptors include the CD4 receptor for the human immunodeficiency virus (HIV), acetylcholine receptor for rabies virus, and fibroblast growth factor receptor for HSV-1.

Once the virus has gained entry into the cell, replication and dissemination are necessary for progression of disease. Although cell-to-cell spread is the most obvious, there is little evidence for any virus that this occurs. Viruses have been observed in the extracellular spaces (Figure 48.3) and reduction of togavirus titres by specific antibody[6] suggests that extracellular movement must occur. Alternatively, transport via glial cells and axons has been suggested.[7]

As with entry of viruses into the CNS, the infiltrating leukocytes may be important in the spread of virus within the tissue. This is observed in human herpesviruses and especially with cytomegalovirus (CMV). Additionally, the role of the immune response in the progression of the disease must be considered, since autoimmune responses initiated by viruses are an important phenomenon.

ADENOVIRIDAE

While adenoviruses have been found in patients with encephalitis, these have often been cases of meningoencephalitis in immunocompromised hosts and rarely in immunocompetent patients.[8] Such associations have been carried out using nested polymerase chain reaction (PCR) and genotypes using partial gene sequence analysis to detect presence of virus in the brain or CSF, while virus in the brain was also identified by immunohistochemical staining.

ARBOVIRUSES

The vast majority of CNS infections are due to viruses transmitted by arthropod vectors, such as mosquitoes, ticks, fleas and midges, that are termed arboviruses (*ar*thropod-*bo*rne viruses). The arbovirus group, which includes over 550 viruses, spans both DNA and RNA viruses belonging to several families: i.e. Bunyaviridae, Togaviridae, Flaviviridae, Reoviridae, Rhabdoviridae and Orthomyxoviridae (Table 48.3). These arboviruses and viruses of other families implicated in CNS disorders are discussed under the virus family heading(s).

ARENAVIRIDAE

The name is derived from the Latin arena, meaning 'sand', to describe the granules observed inside the virions. The two major groups within this family are the lymphocytic choriomeningitis (LCM) group, comprised of LCM and Lassa, in which aseptic meningitis, encephalomyelitis and meningoencephalomyelitis have been described, and the Tacaribe complex, which are distinguished on the basis of antigenic reactivity. These viruses are single-stranded RNA viruses of various sizes.

855

Table 48.3 Arthropod-borne viruses responsible for CNS diseases

Arbovirus	Genus	Family
California encephalitis	Bunyavirus	Bunyaviridae
La Crosse	Bunyavirus	Bunyaviridae
Crimean haemorrhagic fever	Nairovirus	Bunyaviridae
Tensaw	Bunyamwera group	
Bunyaviridae		
Rift Valley fever	Phlebovirus	Bunyaviridae
Toscana	Phlebovirus	Bunyaviridae
Inkoo		Bunyaviridae
Oropouche		Bunyaviridae
Colorado tick fever	Orbivirus	Reoviridae
Chikungunya	Alphavirus	Togaviridae
Eastern equine encephalitis (EEE)	Alphavirus	Togaviridae
O'nyong-nyong	Alphavirus	Togaviridae
Semliki Forest	Alphavirus	Togaviridae
Venezuelan equine encephalitis (VEE)	Alphavirus	Togaviridae
Western equine encephalitis	Alphavirus	Togaviridae
Rubella	Rubivirus	Togaviridae
Dengue		Flaviviridae
Ilheus		Flaviviridae
Japanese B		Flaviviridae
Kunjin		Flaviviridae
Kumlinge		Flaviviridae
Langat		
Flaviviridae		
Louping III		Flaviviridae
Kyasanur Forest Disease		Flaviviridae
Murray Valley encephalitis		Flaviviridae
Negishi		Flaviviridae
Powassan		Flaviviridae
TBE – western subtype; Russian spring–summer encephalitis		Flaviviridae
TBE – eastern subtype		Flaviviridae
Rocio		Flaviviridae
St Louis encephalitis		Flaviviridae
West Nile		Flaviviridae
Wesselsbron		Flaviviridae
Yellow fever		Flaviviridae
Thogoto	Ungrouped	

Lymphocytic choriomeningitis (LCM) group

LCM virus (LCMV) was the first virus isolated from aseptic meningitis in humans. The other members of this complex, namely Ippy, Mopeia and Mobala, are not associated with human disease.

Epidemiology and mode of transmission

LCMV is transmitted to humans by rodents such as the common house mouse, via exposure of open wounds or by contamination of food by infected animal excrement. Human-to-human contact is not common although it has recently been described following organ transplant[9] and is also recognized as an emerging cause of congenital defects in children and abortions.[10] Due to the nature of transmission, animal handlers or those living in impoverished conditions are at higher risk. Although LCMV infections are rare, the seroprevalence varies worldwide, one of the highest being 36% in Croatia and the lowest in France of 0.33% (in 2007). LCMV infection in humans ranges from asymptomatic infection, mild systemic illness to CNS involvement. The severity of the illness may depend on dose, route of infection and host immunogenetic background. In mice fetal infection, in the absence of a sufficient immunological response induces a persistent infection. The damage within the CNS is primarily due to the immunopathological effect.

Clinical features

The incubation period in humans is approximately 10 days and disease begins with fever, malaise, weakness, headache and myalgia, which is most severe in the lumbar region. Anorexia, nausea and dizziness are also common and the patients may have any combination of sore throat, vomiting and arthralgia with chest pain and pneumonitis. In some cases, haematological disturbances such as leucopenia are observed. The second phase occurs after a few days, with headache, stiff neck and typical signs of encephalitis in approximately 15% of infections, of which some are severe encephalitis and the mortality rate is <1.0%.

The white blood cell count is often 3000/mm^3 or less, with a mild thrombocytopenia. CSF from patients with meningeal signs contains several hundred white cells, predominantly lymphocytes (>80%), with increased protein and occasionally low sugar levels. Virus is often found in the spinal fluid during acute disease.[11] Convalescence is prolonged, with persistent fatigue and dizziness although most people recover completely.

Prevention

All persons in contact with rodents should practise safe handling procedures, avoiding eating and drinking around pets and washing and cleaning up thoroughly. Children should be educated to avoid hand to mouth contact around pets.

Lassa fever

Epidemiology

Lassa fever[12] was first described in West Africa in the 1950s, although the virus was not isolated until 1969. The only known reservoir of Lassa fever virus in Central and West Africa is *Mastomys natalensis*, one of the most commonly occurring rodents in Africa. The virus is rapidly spread from person to person by direct contact with blood tissues or needle-stick, giving rise to a mortality rate of 30–66%. Consequently, knowledge of the pathological features is limited. Rates of seroconversion to Lassa virus range from 5% to 20% in populations of Sierra Leone villages with the highest rates in crowded, highly mobile, populations. In recent years Lassa fever has reached Europe and the USA due to air travel from Africa. Clinically, infection gives rise to haemorrhage, nephropathy, myocarditis and encephalitis.

Pathogenesis and pathology

The most common and consistently observed lesions in fatal human Lassa fever are focal necroses of the liver, adrenal glands and spleen.[13,14] Although high virus titres occur in other organs, such as the brain, ovary, pancreas, uterus and placenta, no lesions have been reported in humans, while infected monkeys have been reported to have CNS lesions.

Clinical diagnosis

Lassa fever begins 7–18 days after primary infection, leading to onset of fever, headache and malaise. Patients with Lassa fever show features of anxiety and there is a raised respiratory rate. In 15–20% of patients, bleeding occurs from gums and nose. Oedema of the face and neck are commonly seen in severe cases. Important clinical events in fatal disease are intractable hypovolaemic shock and/or severe CNS involvement, bleeding and oedema of the face. There is also endothelial and platelet dysfunction and mild thrombocytopenia.

Prevention

The ideal method of prevention is to prevent contact between rodents and humans. This can be achieved by improving the housing and food storage, which might reduce the domestic rodent population. There are two vaccines for arenaviral diseases. A live attenuated vaccine has been used extensively. A second vaccine has been made by cloning and expressing Lassa virus glycoprotein gene into vaccine virus. This vaccine has proven highly successful in preventing severe disease and death in challenged monkeys and may be relevant for treating humans.[15] Ribavirin can prevent death in Lassa fever when given at any point in the illness, but is more effective when given early and administered intravenously.[16]

Bornaviridae

In the seventeenth century, Borna disease was known as the 'disease of the head' affecting horses and was later ascribed to Borna disease virus (BDV), an unsegmented, single- and negative-stranded, enveloped RNA virus. In humans the virus has been associated with psychiatric diseases. This has been based on studies in rats infected with BDV that show behavioural changes and emotional and learning deficits and by the presence of viral nucleic acid in the blood or brain.

Table 48.4 Genera and serogroups within the family Bunyaviridae

Genus	Serogroups
Orthobunyavirus	*Anopheles A.*, *Anopheles B.*, Bunyamwera, Bwamba
(Bunyavirus)	California, Capim, Gamboa, Guama, Koongol, Olifantsvlei, Patois, Simbu, Teteu, Turlock
Nairovirus	Crimean–Congo, Dera Gharzi Khan, Hughes, Nairobi SD, Qalyub, Sakhalin Uukuniemi
Phlebovirus	Phlebotomus
Hantavirus	*Hantaan* and *Sin Nombre*
Tospovirus	Does not infect mammals

Bunyaviridae

The Bunyaviridae family is taxonomically divided into five genera: Hantavirus, Nairovirus, Orthobunyavirus, Phlebovirus and Tospovirus, and viruses that are not assigned. The family is comprised of over 250 viruses (Table 48.4) between 90 and 100 nm in size that have a lipid envelope derived from the host cell membranes during maturation. (For more information on the structure and replication of Bunyaviruses, see references.[2,17])

This section will concentrate on those viruses within the genera that are important with respect to causing significant human disease involving the CNS.

Orthobunyaviruses

The most important serogroup with respect to induction of human diseases is the California (CAL) group, which includes California encephalitis (CE) and La Crosse (LAC) viruses. This group of viruses has 14 serotypes, the prototype virus being La Crosse virus, first isolated from a child in La Crosse, Wisconsin, in 1960.[18]

Epidemiology and mode of transmission

Members of the CE virus serogroup were first recognized in California in 1943 and have since been isolated in Canada, the USA, Trinidad, Europe, Africa and Finland, although each has a very narrow host range and geographical distribution. More recently in western Europe, two viruses of the California group – Tahyna virus and Inkoo virus – have been associated with CNS involvement, such as encephalitis.

Animals such as chipmunks and squirrels are commonly involved. La Crosse virus, the prototype virus, is transmitted by the mosquito *Aedes triseriatus*, which is the most important vector in California, although other *Aedes* species may be involved. Children and young adults aged 1–19 years are at greatest risk of exposure to this vector, which is a woodland mosquito, during activities such as camping and hiking.[19]

La Crosse infection is the second most prevalent mosquito-borne viral infection in the USA and accounts for approximately 75 definite cases a year, although seroprevalence may reach 20% in older persons. La Crosse virus is transmitted mainly by *Ae.*

triseriatus, a treehole-breeding woodland mosquito that frequently feeds on small mammals, particularly chipmunks and squirrels.[20] An alternative mosquito habitat is provided by discarded tyres that hold rainwater on which egg rafts may be laid. This virus produces acute encephalitis in children. The acute illness lasts 10 days or less in most cases. The first symptoms are non-specific and last for 1–3 days, followed by involvement of the CNS. The symptoms include stiff neck, lethargy and seizures. Earlier examination shows high counts of both polymorphonuclear neutrophil leukocytes and mononuclear cells in about 65% of patients. The most important sequela of La Crosse encephalitis is epilepsy, which occurs in about 10% of the children, and learning disabilities and other objective cognitive deficits have been reported in a small proportion of patients. A few patients (2%) have persistent paresis.

Pathology

The lesions induced by bunyaviruses are typical of acute viral encephalitis. Examination of the CNS reveals perivascular cuffing of mononuclear cells and, in severe cases, necrotic areas. Histopathologically the lesions, which consist of scattered glial nodules, perivascular cuffs, mild leptomeningitis and occasional areas of focal necrosis, are found more often in the cerebral cortex and to a lesser extent in the brain stem and medulla.

Clinical features

Following an incubation period of 3–7 days, features associated with acute encephalitis are observed. Brief 'flu-like' symptoms and primary viraemia, which follow the arthropod bite, are observed. The secondary phase is marked by fever and a secondary viraemia coinciding with CNS involvement. Clinical expression includes headache, fever and meningoencephalitis, with upper motor neuronal signs and occasionally chorea. Neurological sequelae may occur, in which persistent seizures are observed, although lasting cognitive deficits are rare. Onset of seizures may be rapid with no other signs of disease. Acute arthritis is observed, with Tahyna virus, whereas respiratory system involvement is more commonly seen in Jamestown Canyon virus infections.

Diagnosis

Clinical diagnosis of La Crosse virus may be made as a result of localization of neurological lesions. Specific diagnosis is based on complement fixation (CF) or haemagglutination inhibition (HI) assays, although neutralization tests (NTs) are also used. Artsob[21] has described an enzyme-linked immunosorbent assay (ELISA) for serotyping. Isolations in suckling mice and Vero cells have been used for virus typing.

Prevention and control

To date, apart from mosquito repellents, no specific prevention is available. Anticonvulsants are used to control seizures. Recently, reports in mice have suggested that plasmid DNAs, encoding either of the virus surface glycoproteins G1 and G2, efficiently blocked the spread of virus from the primary replication site to the brain, suggesting that such approaches may be beneficial in patients.

Phleboviruses

Rift Valley fever

Rift Valley fever (RVF) virus is a prototype Bunyavirus and the most notable virus in the genus Phlebovirus. It was first reported after an epidemic of fever and myalgia in which a few people developed encephalitis in Egypt in 1979.[22] Additional outbreaks have been observed throughout Africa, including Nigeria, Egypt, Sudan and Kenya. More than 20 species of mosquitoes have been implicated as possible vectors. *Culex pipiens*, *Cx. theileri*, *Ae. caballus* and other mosquitoes of the *Culex* and *Aedes* group may be involved. The major sources of reservoirs are animals such as cows, sheep, and goats, although camels and antelopes can be infected. Transmission of the virus from animal to animal during epidemics may result from biting flies.

Clinical features

RVF in the human illness is biphasic. The primary phase is associated with fever, back and joint pains, and headaches that last about 1 week. After 1–2 days' remission, the second phase consists of similar symptoms for 1–2 days, with nausea and sometimes a haemorrhagic diathesis with evidence of liver and renal damage. The mortality rate is <1.0%. Occasionally disturbed vision, with evidence of a retinitis and cotton-wool exudates in the region of the macula, is observed. Altered levels of consciousness are observed with, in some cases, persistent fever. Meningeal irritation occurs, with focal motor signs and hallucinations.[23]

Diagnosis

Identification of increasing levels of IgM-specific antibodies in the CSF is used for the specific diagnosis.

Treatment and prevention

No specific treatment exists for Rift Valley fever, although a formalin-inactivated vaccine may be of use for laboratory workers and troops who may be exposed to this virus. More recently an inactivated RVF vaccine TSI-GSD-200 has been found beneficial. Ribavirin may be effective if administered in time and passive neutralizing antibody is effective in protecting from disease.

Hantaviruses

Epidemiology and mode of transmission

Hantaviruses are human pathogens that are prevalent worldwide and consist of more than 16 different viruses including Puumala, Hantaan, Dobrava-Belgrade, Seoul, Sin Nombre. The predominant serotype is Puumala (PUUV), which causes encephalitis and is endemic in western Russia, Finland, Sweden, France, Belgium, Germany and former Yugoslavia but has also been reported in Denmark, Norway, the Netherlands and Austria. Puumala virus is spread by rodents and is transmitted to humans by inhalation or ingestion of food contaminated with rodent excreta. The seroprevalence in Finland is 5% and 1.8% in Austria. The incidence of NE in a cyclic fashion, with peaks occurring every 3rd to 4th year, coinciding with peaks in vole populations.

Pathology

Infection with PUUV may also lead to neurological symptoms including meningoencephalitis, polyradiculitis, seizures, cerebral haemorrhage, urinary bladder paralysis, and hypopituitarism.

Clinical features

The most common symptoms of PUUV infection are red throat, fever, nausea, vomiting, headache, stomach ache and back pain usually associated with kidney infection. Most patients recover in 7–10 days without sequelae and the mortality is less than 0.2%.

Diagnosis

Diagnosis is by an immunocytochemistry test called immunochromatographic rapid test (POC PUUMALA) by Erilab Ltd, Kuopio, Finland, that uses a highly purified baculovirus-expressed PUUV nucleocapsid protein antigen to detect IgM to PUUMV in the blood.

Treatment and prevention

Aside from avoiding contact with infected animals there is little in terms of control and treatment. A vaccine against PUUV, as well as specific treatment for the encephalitis, is still lacking.

CALICIVIRIDAE

The Caliciviridae family is comprised of Norwalk virus and hepatitis E virus. Norwalk-like viruses are the major cause of gastroenterovirus although to date only one case of encephalopathy has been possibly linked with Norwalk virus infection when the viral genome was detected in CSF by reverse transcription PCR.

CORONAVIRIDAE

Members of the Coronaviridae family are pleomorphic RNA viruses, 80–130 nm in diameter, which replicate within the cytoplasm. The family includes several animal viruses, including murine hepatitis virus known to induce demyelination in the CNS of infected mice. The neurotropic strain of mouse hepatitis virus, JHM, was first isolated from a spontaneously paralysed mouse. The virus induces lesions of acute demyelination in the brain and spinal cord.[24] The relevance of this to human disease is the finding of coronaviruses in the CNS of some patients with multiple sclerosis. More recently, the outbreak of severe acute respiratory syndrome (SARS) due to the human coronavirus (SARS-CoV) has also been associated with virus in the CNS.[25]

FILOVIRIDAE

The family Filoviridae contains a single genus *Filovirus* with subgroups *Marburg* and *Ebola*, both associated with severe haemorrhagic fevers (see Chapter 42). The mortality is high and varies between 30% and 90%, in which clinical signs develop early, with death occurring between days 6 and 16. Due to the high pathogenicity few tissues have been studied. In *Ebola*-infected monkeys, coagulation is seen in the brain and in human patients, haemorrhages in the brain induce strokes.

FLAVIVIRIDAE

Formerly classified as Group B arboviruses, the Flaviviridae were re-classified as an independent family. The family Flaviviridae are composed of the genera Flavivirus, Hepacivirus and Pestivirus. The genus Flavivirus comprises the largest group of viruses known to induce CNS diseases and is subdivided according to the mode of transmission, i.e. mosquitoes or ticks (Table 48.5).[26] Further serological subgroups may be distinguished on the basis of reactivity in HI and neutralization assays. Flaviviruses are small icosahedral enveloped viruses that replicate and mature cytoplasmically, deriving the lipid envelope from the internal membrane of the host cell. While yellow fever virus, the prototype Flavivirus (*L. flavus* = yellow), is a serious haemorrhagic disease inducing heart and kidney failure – its name derived from the jaundice induced following infection – very few reports describe encephalitis. Rather, encephalitis following vaccination with the attenuated yellow fever Asibi 17D virus is described in the elderly and immunocompromised patients.[27]

Vector control by water drainage is not feasible in most cases due to the terrain, i.e. jungle areas, but has been used successfully in urban areas when combined with insecticides. Inactivated vaccines, live attenuated vaccines and subunit vaccines using recombinant DNA technology have been utilized and developed for several Flaviviruses. Ongoing research has identified possible targets for inhibition, including binding and uptake of the virus to cells together with the viral proteases and some factors governing replication, and these may be useful in the future development of antiviral therapeutic strategies.

As seen in Table 48.5, many Flaviviruses induce CNS diseases, some of which are discussed in other chapters.

Dengue virus

Dengue and Dengue haemorrhagic fevers (see Chapter 41) also involve the CNS and several reports suggest that the incidence of Dengue fever is rising. For example, in Vietnam the death rate for Dengue fever increased by 83% in 2006. The encephalitis is confirmed by CSF microscopy, immunoglobulin in the CSF, as well as MRI, CT and EEG changes, although in some patients no alteration was observed in the CSF.[28]

Japanese encephalitis

A disease resembling Japanese encephalitis (JE) was recorded as early as 1871. In 1935, an infectious agent was recovered from the brain of a person in Tokyo and was virologically and serologically established as the prototype (Nakayama) strain. JE virus is the prototype of the JE antigenic complex. The complete nucleotide sequence of the JE viral genome has been determined. Antibody adsorption HI, CF, kinetic neutralization, agar gel diffusion and monoclonal antibody analysis have demonstrated antigenic variations. At least two immunotypes have been identified: Nakayama and JaGAr-01 (isolated from *Culex* mosquitoes). The virus replicates in a number of primary and continuous cell cultures of

Table 48.5 Classification of neurotropic Flaviviruses where known

Genus: Flavivirus	Neurotropic	B. TICK-BORNE VIRUSES	
A. MOSQUITO-BORNE VIRUSES		**Mammalian tick-borne virus group**	
Aroa virus group		Gadgets Gully virus (GGYV)	
Aroa virus (AROAV)		Kadam virus (KADV)	
Dengue virus group		Kyasanur Forest disease virus (KFDV)	Humans, mice
Dengue virus (DENV)	Humans	Alkhurma haemorrhagic fever virus (AHFV)	Humans
Kedougou virus (KEDV)		Langat virus (LGTV)	Mice, humans
Japanese encephalitis virus group		Omsk haemorrhagic fever virus (OHFV)	
Cacipacore virus (CPCV)		Powassan virus (POWV)	Humans
Koutango virus (KOUV)		Tick-borne encephalitis virus (TBEV)	Humans
Japanese encephalitis virus (JEV)	Humans	Eastern type – Russian Spring-Summer (RSSE)	Humans, macaques
Murray Valley encephalitis virus (MVEV)	Humans	Western type	
Alfuy virus (ALFV)		Royal Farm virus (RFV)	
St Louis encephalitis virus (SLEV)		Louping ill virus (LIV)	Sheep, goats
Usutu virus (USUV)	Owls	**Seabird tick-borne virus group**	
West Nile virus (WNV)	Humans	Meaban virus (MEAV)	
Yaounde virus (YAOV)		Saumarez Reef virus (SREV)	
Rocio (ROC)	Humans	Tyuleniy virus (TYUV)	
Kokobera virus group		**C. VIRUSES WITH NO KNOWN ARTHROPOD VECTOR**	
Kokobera virus (KOKV)		**Entebbe virus group**	
Ntaya virus group		Entebbe bat virus (ENTV)	
Bagaza virus (BAGV)		Yokose virus (YOKV)	
Ilheus virus (ILHV)	Humans	**Modoc virus group**	
Israel turkey meningoencephalomyelitis virus (ITV)	Turkeys	Apoi virus (APOIV)	
		Cowbone Ridge virus (CRV)	
Ntaya virus (NTAV)		Jutiapa virus (JUTV)	
Tembusu virus (TMUV)		Modoc virus (MODV)	Experimental hamsters, mice
Spondweni virus group		Sal Vieja virus (SVV)	
Zika virus (ZIKV)		San Perlita virus (SPV)	
Yellow fever virus group		**Rio Bravo virus group**	
Banzi virus (BANV)	Sheep, experimental mice	Bukalasa bat virus (BBV)	
Bouboui virus (BOUV)		Carey Island virus (CIV)	
Edge Hill virus (EHV)		Dakar bat virus (DBV)	
Jugra virus (JUGV)		Montana myotis leukoencephalitis virus (MMLV) small rodents	
Saboya virus (SABV)			
Sepik virus (SEPV)		Phnom Penh bat virus (PPBV)	
Uganda S virus (UGSV)		Rio Bravo virus (RBV)	
Wesselsbron virus (WESSV)	Goats, cows		
Yellow fever virus (YFV)	Mice (vaccine in humans)		

hamster, pig, monkey, Vero and mosquito. JE virus produces lethal encephalitis in infant mice by any route, whereas weanling mice succumb to intracerebral virus inoculation. Hamsters and monkeys die after intracerebral inoculation but develop asymptomatic viraemia after intraperitoneal inoculation. JE virus does not cause death in rabbits and guinea pigs after inoculation by any route.

Epidemiology

JE continues to be the major type of encephalitis in eastern, southeastern and southern Asia including Japan, the Far East, Guam, the former USSR, Malaysia, India and western Pacific island areas. In endemic areas, children are affected most, with attack rates in the 3–15 years age group 5–10 times higher than those in older people because of the higher incidence of protective immunity in older age groups. Among factors that influence mortality are age, different virus strains and cross-protective immunity to other flaviviruses, especially dengue. The *Cx. tritaeniorhynchus* and *Cx. vishnui* mosquitoes are the most important vectors. Other species of *Culex, Aedes, Anopheles* and *Mansonia* have been implicated. Pigs and many birds, including herons and egrets, may be the chief source of virus. Other domestic animals can become infected and humans may play a part in epidemics. More recently, the emergence of flaviviruses including JE has been reported in Europe.[29]

Clinical illness

Clinical illness is characterized by headache, fever and other signs of meningitis. Convulsions occur in children. Upper motor neurone involvement with extrapyramidal disturbances is a feature of this disease. The mortality rate of those with meningoencephalitis is around 20% in children and up to 50% in those over 50 years of age. Motor and psychological disturbances are common sequelae.

Pathogenesis and pathology

Pathogenicity in mice varies with different strains of JE virus. During the acute stage, oedema and small haemorrhages are found in the brain. Destruction of cerebellar Purkinje cells may occur. Lesions include neuronal degeneration and necrosis, glial nodules and perivascular inflammation. These changes occur mainly in grey matter and predominantly affect diencephalic, mesencephalic and brain stem structures. In the extraneural tissue a variety of pathological features, including hyperplasia of germinal centres of lymph nodes, enlargement of malpighian bodies in the spleen, interstitial myocarditis and focal haemorrhages in the kidneys, are seen. Transplacental infection in swine results in abortion and stillbirth. Pregnant mice inoculated intraperitoneally also transmit JE virus to the fetus, with subsequent abortion.

Diagnosis

The IgM-capture ELISA is especially well suited for diagnosis by detection of locally synthesized antibody in the CSF. The HI, CF assays and NT are applicable. More recently, the potential application of JE non-structural protein (NS) 1-specific indirect ELISA to differentiate infection from vaccination has been described. More specifically imaging of the brain using MRI has proven useful to examine the impact of JE infection.

Prevention and control

Formalin-inactivated vaccines for use in humans are prepared from infected adult mouse brains or infected primary hamster kidney cell cultures in Japan and China, respectively.[30–32] Primary immunization requires two doses at a 7–14-day interval. Booster vaccinations are given during the first year after primary immunization and then at 3–4-year intervals. A bivalent vaccine has been developed incorporating Nakayama and JaGAr-01 (the two subtypes of JE virus). This vaccine has also proved to be effective although it may not provide complete protection. Vaccination of horses with formalin-inactivated vaccines has been successful. Use of pesticides in rice-growing areas has reduced populations of *Cx. tritaeniorhynchus*. Spraying of residual insecticides in livestock pens has reduced the case incidence in China.[32] Treatment consists of good general management and nursing care, especially in the semicomatose and comatose patient. Hyponatraemia secondary to inappropriate antidiuretic hormone secretion is managed with water restriction. Increased intracranial pressure should be considered in severely ill patients with deepening coma and loss of brain stem reflexes. Anticonvulsant therapy may be required.

Murray Valley encephalitis virus

Between 1917 and 1925 and from 1950 to 1951 severe encephalitis called Australian X disease outbreaks occurred in the Murray Valley region. In 1951 Murray Valley encephalitis (MVE) virus was first isolated from human brain and found to be a member of the JE antigenic complex. The host range of MVE virus is wide, being found in humans,[33] monkeys, horses, sheep and some birds, that all develop encephalitis after intracerebral inoculation. A closely related virus, Kunjin, has also been implicated in encephalitis in the same region as MVEV.

Epidemiology

MVE virus is endemic to tropical North Australia, particularly Western Australia and the Northern Territory, but can occur in other parts of Australia, and Papua New Guinea. *Cx. annulirostris* is the major mosquito vector. *Ae. normanensis* may be involved. Birds, including herons, cormorants and other water birds, are the major reservoir of this virus.

Clinical illness

Onset is sudden, with headaches, fever and symptoms of a meningoencephalitis. Paresis of both upper and lower motor neurones may occur and breathing and swallowing may become impaired. With modern intensive care the fatality rate has been reduced dramatically to 20%. However, as a result of the increased survival rate, the number of people with both upper and lower motor neurone and psychiatric sequelae has increased.[33]

Prevention and control

Detection of flavivirus seroconversions in sentinel chicken flocks has been used as an early warning of increased levels of MVE and Kunjin virus activity. No specific treatment for MVE exists although vector control is as with other members of this family, and massive insecticide programmes are deployed when vector breeding is increased.

St Louis encephalitis virus

St Louis encephalitis (SLE) virus was first identified as the cause of human encephalitis in 1933 in Missouri and since then many outbreaks have been reported. SLE virus is transmitted by the mosquitoes *Cx. tarsalis* and *Cx. pipiens*, giving rise to one of the most common and important epidemic arbovirus infections in the USA. Since the 1930s numerous outbreaks have been described in Texas, Ohio and Florida. Occasional cases have been reported in Canada and Mexico.

Epidemiology

SLE in central USA is commonly dependent on *Cx. pipiens* and *Cx. quinquefasciatus*, whereas in Florida *Cx. nigripalpus* is the principal vector. The virus is transmitted from mosquitoes that are infected by feeding on birds. In western USA *Cx. tarsalis* is the major vector. Epidemic outbreaks appear every 10 years and appear to be dependent on the breeding of *Cx. pipiens*. Disease occurs in late summer and early autumn, and the number of affected humans ranges from 0.1% to 8%.

Clinical illness

SLE induces febrile headache, aseptic meningitis and encephalitis. Although persons of all ages are affected, morbidity and mortality is seen more commonly in the elderly. Following a 3–4-day incubation a generalized illness is observed, with malaise, fever, myalgia, headache and vomiting.[34] After a similar period the symptoms may resolve or progress to clinical findings indicative of neurological involvement. Of patients with neurological signs, 50% die within 7 days of exhibiting signs and a further 30% succumb in the second week. Many patients who survive neurological involvement have persistent headaches and memory loss, and others have overt neurological sequelae such as speech or sensory disturbances.

Diagnosis

Patients exhibiting signs of encephalitis in SLE endemic areas, particularly in late summer and early autumn, should be investigated for SLE. Virus isolation from biological specimens such as blood and urine may be difficult, although virus has been isolated from brain tissue. Confirmation of SLE infection is made by HI or CF tests. IgM-capture ELISA is useful for diagnosis.

Prevention and control

There is no specific treatment or vaccine for SLE. Education of individuals within infected areas and vector control have been shown to be useful following detection of SLE virus activity.

West Nile virus

Epidemiology

West Nile Virus (WNV) is widely distributed in Africa, Europe, Asia,[33] Mexico, the Caribbean islands and Colombia and has emerged as the most common cause of epidemic meningoencephalitis in North America. A study in Germany showed that migrating birds have been in contact with WNV although no outbreaks have been reported in Europe. The outbreak in New York City in 1999 was the first time WNV was detected in the Western hemisphere and led to 20 000 confirmed cases. Given the subsequent rapid spread of the virus, which led to the hospitalization of 59 patients, of whom 37 (63%) had clinical signs of encephalitis and seven (12%) died, this infection should now be considered as a serious threat. From 1999–2005. more than 8000 cases of neuroinvasive WNV disease were reported in the US, resulting in over 780 deaths.

The vector for WNV is *Culex* species and other ornithophilic mosquitoes. Birds, including domestic poultry, are the reservoirs and horses and dogs have also been reported to develop WNV. In 2002, WNV transmission through blood transfusion and organ transplantation, and intrauterine transmission were first documented.

Clinical illness

Following WNV infection symptoms including fever, headaches, retrobulbar and muscular pain, sore throat, nausea and vomiting occur. Development of a maculopapular rash on the trunk, face and limbs may be seen. Occasionally arthralgia may occur and involvement of ophthalmic tracts has been reported. The disease is usually mild in the young, but in older age groups a second phase with mild meningoencephalitis may develop with no sequelae. Many patients with WNV neurological disease have abnormal MRI in the basal ganglia, thalamus, cerebellum, and brainstem. In some cases movement disorders have been described due to lesions in the substantia nigra. Examination of the CSF reveals increased cell counts with predominance of neutrophils. WNV disease has also been reported in immunosuppressed patients. Recovery from neurological sequelae of WNV infection including cognitive deficits and weakness may be prolonged and incomplete.[34,35]

Diagnosis

Since clinical manifestations are difficult to differentiate from other infections, diagnosis should be made from WNV-specific IgM detectable in the CSF and serum, which is nearly 100% positive after the 8th day of infection and can persist for up to 16 months. CT and MRI again cannot accurately diagnose WNV infection although the virus does have predilection for the brainstem.

Prevention and control

Although there is no proven therapy for WNV disease, several vaccines and antiviral therapy with antibodies, antisense oligonucleotides, and interferon preparations are currently undergoing human clinical trials. As with other mosquito-borne diseases, insect repellents are crucial to prevent infection and avoidance of areas where infected mosquitoes may be present is advisable. Arboviral surveillance and vector control programmes are essential.

Rocio encephalitis

Epidemiology

In March 1975, an outbreak of encephalitis was recorded in São Paulo, south-east Brazil, in 465 cases with 61 deaths recorded.[36]

The majority of those affected were workers who frequented the forest areas; this was suggestive of an arbovirus infection. In 1975, an unknown arbovirus was isolated from the cerebellum and spinal cord of a 39-year-old farmer and referred to as Rocio virus. Further analysis identified 47 arbovirus isolates in an area previously unknown for arbovirus infections. Rocio (ROC) virus is typical of flaviviruses, being spherically shaped with a diameter of 43 nm and cross-reacting with other members of the group (i.e. SLE, Ilheus, JE and MVE virus). Since 1980, no human disease caused by this virus has been diagnosed.

Pathogenesis

The pathology has been detailed by Rosenberg.[37] Interstitial mononuclear infiltration, microglial proliferation and perivascular cuffing are observed. In acute disease neuronophagia is evident with a distinctive topographical pattern in which the dentate nucleus is more susceptible and the brainstem less so.

Clinical diagnosis

In humans the incubation period is between 7 and 14 days. The clinical features include headache, fever, vomiting, anorexia and nausea, hyperaemia of the oropharynx and conjunctivae, and photophobia. Involvement of the CNS includes meningeal irritation, alteration in consciousness, motor abnormalities and abnormalities in cranial nerve function.

Diagnosis

Epidemiological background and clinical history are paramount. Diagnosis is by cytochemical analysis of the CSF and isolation of the virus in 2-day-old mice from infected tissue. Haemagglutination, CF and plaque reduction techniques in Vero cells, IgM antibody-capture ELISA and ultimately histological examination confirm infection.

Prevention and control

The use of larvicides in ditches and flooded areas, and sanitary measures to drain stagnant waters, have decreased the incidence of infection. Formalin-treated extract of infected mouse brain is used as a vaccine.

Tick-borne encephalitis

The tick-borne encephalitis (TBE) virus complex consists of 14 antigenically closely related viruses, eight of which cause human disease. Russian spring-summer encephalitis (RSSE) and central European encephalitis virus (CEE) are very closely related antigenically and are considered to be subtypes of the same virus. They are separated on the basis of kinetic HI and CF tests and at the molecular level. Peptide maps of both the E and the largest non-structural protein (NS-5) of the two subtypes show some differences.

TBE complex viruses grow in a variety of cell cultures, including pig, bovine and chick embryo, HeLa, human amnion, Hep2, Vero, and primary reptilian and amphibian cells.[38] Cytopathic effect and plaquing are variable. TBE viruses cause encephalitis in rats, guinea pigs, sheep, monkeys and swine after intracerebral inoculation.

Infant and weanling mice develop fatal encephalitis by all routes of inoculation. Experimental inoculation of wild vertebrate species, including rodents, foxes, birds, hares and bats, results in viraemia and antibody formation. Cows, goats and sheep infected by inoculation or tick bite develop viraemia and secrete virus in their milk. The Far Eastern virus type (RSSE) is more virulent for sheep and monkeys inoculated intracerebrally than the Western (CEE) subtype virus.

Epidemiology

TBE encompasses a wide area including Siberia across to Scandinavia, through Vienna into Belgium, to Scotland and Northern Ireland, across Canada, the USA and Japan. The disease occurs in areas that are favourable for ticks. The virus is maintained in nature in a cycle involving ticks and wild vertebrate hosts. Small rodents such as shrews, moles and hedgehogs are believed to be important reservoirs. Large mammals, such as goats, sheep and cattle, serve as host for adult Ixodes ticks. *I. ricinus* and *I. persulcatus* are responsible for transmission in Europe and the former Soviet Union, respectively.[39] Other tick species, of the genera Dermacentor and Haemaphysalis, have been implicated in transmission, especially in areas that do not support *Ixodes* ticks. Transmission to humans occurs mainly in adults over 20 years old, who come in contact with infected animals. The disease occurs in two peaks (May–June and September–October) coinciding with the activity of adult *Ixodes* ticks. Small outbreaks involving all age groups result from consumption of raw sheep or goat's milk or cheese.

Pathogenesis and pathology

In monkeys, the anterior horn cells of the spinal cord and cerebellar cortex appear to be more affected than other neuronal cells. Members of the TBE complex cause persistent infection in experimental animals. For instance, CEE virus has been isolated from monkey tissues by co-cultivation and explant techniques long after infection. Mice infected with Kyasanur Forest virus are shown to survive for months, with paralysis, low titres of virus in the brain and absence of detectable neutralizing antibodies.[40] Monkeys infected with TBE complex develop chronic encephalitis with degenerative spongiform lesions and astrocytic proliferation. Chronic progressive human encephalitis and seizure disorders have been associated with RSSE virus.

Histopathological findings consist of meningeal and perivascular inflammation, neuronal degeneration and necrosis, and glial nodule formation in areas such as the cerebellar cortex, brainstem, basal ganglia, cerebrum and spinal cord. The anterior horn cells of the cervical cord are especially vulnerable, which may result in the lower motor neurone paralysis seen in many cases.

Clinical features

The clinical characteristics of TBE infection in humans vary depending on the age of the patient.[41] Most of the tick-borne viruses have been associated with human disease, but there is a gradation of virulence. The Far Eastern (Siberian) strains (formerly called RSSE virus) cause severe encephalitis, often with bulbar and cervical cord involvement, a high fatality rate and frequent sequelae. The disease seen in central Europe is frequently biphasic, with influenza-like symptoms and signs of mild encephalitis.

Diagnosis

Definitive diagnosis depends on virus isolation or serology. The virus may be isolated from the blood during the first phase of illness and from brain tissue of patients dying early in the infection. Suckling mice, embryonated eggs and chick embryo cell cultures (with detection of virus by interference assay or immunofluorescence) have been used for virus isolation. Serological diagnosis including HI, CF, single radial haemolysis and NT have been used. Diagnosis by estimation of IgM antibodies is valuable for rapid diagnosis and is applicable to both serum and CSF.

Prevention and control

In the former USSR, formalin-inactivated mouse brain vaccines were used before World War II (1939–1945). Recently, vaccines have been produced in embryonated eggs or chick embryo cell cultures. However, the most effective vaccine is derived from chick embryo cell culture-grown virus which is highly purified and inactivated by formalin. The vaccine produces serological conversions in over 95% of recipients and has provided 99% protection in field trials. Preventive measures include pasteurization or boiling of raw milk, avoidance of tick bite by use of repellents and protective clothing. More recently, as with other viral therapeutic strategies, DNA vaccine encoding TB viral components has been shown to be effective in mice and offers the possibility of rational therapy in humans.[42]

Other tick-borne viruses

Kyasanur forest disease (KFD) caused by KFD virus (KFDV) was first recognized as a febrile illness in the Karnataka state of India in the 1950s it induces a haemorrhagic disease in human beings in which encephalopathy is observed in some patients. A variant of KFDV, Alkhurma haemorrhagic fever virus (AHFV), has been recently identified in Saudi Arabia. KFD is known to be encephalitogenic in mice and rodents.

Langat virus (LGT) is a naturally attenuated member of the tick-borne encephalitis virus (TBEV) complex. While LGT infects humans; there are no cases of disease recorded from tick bites. In the 1970s, Langat was briefly used as a live vaccine against more virulent tick-borne encephalitis viruses in Russia but caused encephalitis complications in about one of every 10 000 people. Injection of LGT virus in mice induces severe encephalitis.

Omsk haemorrhagic fever virus (OHFV) is principally restricted to western Siberia and is seen mostly in muskrat trappers. The disease is manifested by fever, chills, headache, pain and rash on the soft palate. CNS abnormalities develop after 1–2 weeks. The disease is fatal in up to 10% of people. To date, there are no antivirals available.

Powassan virus (POWV) was first identified in Powassan, Ontario, Canada, in 1958 and only 12 cases were reported between 1958 and 1999 and four cases were fatal. The disease, transmitted by tick bites, leads to inflammation of the brain.

Louping ill virus (LIV) infects sheep reared in Scotland, northern England, Wales and Ireland. The virus is excreted in faeces and saliva. The first report of human infection was in 1934 and to date 31 cases of human infection have been reported. Encephalitis in man is seen with LIV.[43]

HERPETOVIRIDAE

Herpesviruses are double-stranded DNA viruses approximately 100–110 nm in diameter and able to establish latency and reactivation. Of the nearly 100 herpesviruses that have been characterized at least partially, the following have been associated with CNS infections particularly in humans:[44]

- Herpes simplex virus 1 (HSV-1) (HHV-1)
- Herpes simplex virus 2 (HSV-2) (HHV-2)
- Varicella-zoster virus (VZV) (HHV-3)
- Epstein-Barr virus (EBV) (HHV-4)
- Human cytomegalovirus (HCMV) (HHV-5)
- Human herpesvirus 6 (HHV-6)
- Human herpesvirus 7 (HHV-7)
- Human herpesvirus 8 (HHV-8)

The simian herpesvirus, B virus (*Cercopithecine* herpesvirus-1 herpes simiae) in macaque monkeys results in severe pathogenesis and often death in untreated humans.[45]

Herpes simplex virus (HHV-1 and HHV-2)

Infections caused by HSV have been known since the time of ancient Greece, where the name herpes was used to mean 'creep' or 'crawl' and probably described the spreading nature of some of the skin lesions resulting from infections. Mouth ulcers and lip vesicles associated with fever were referred to as *herpes febralis* by the Roman scholar Herodotus. It was only later that herpetic lesions and genital infections were associated and by the late nineteenth century the vesicular nature of the lesions was characterized. Histological descriptions of herpes infections were identified in the early twentieth century including the encephalitogenicity of herpesviruses.[44]

Epidemiology

HSV are distributed worldwide by humans, who are deemed the sole reservoir for transmission during close personal contact. There is no seasonal variation in infections and, because of the nature of infection, it is estimated that more than one-third of the world's population is infected. Antibody prevalence studies have demonstrated that geographical location, socioeconomic status and age influence the frequency of infection. HSV-1 encephalitis is the more common and has a high mortality while HSV-2 is involved in 4–6% of cases.[45]

Pathogenesis

The pathogenesis of both HSV types is unclear, although it is apparent that both primary and recurrent HSV infection may result in CNS disease. Experiment has shown that HSV gains entry to the CNS via the olfactory and trigeminal nerves although whether primary or recurrent HSV is reactivated within the CNS are unknown in humans. In mice HSV-1 has been shown to be transmitted vertically, possibly explaining how neonatal infection occurs that causes severe disease and death in newborns.[46]

Pathology

Acute necrotizing encephalitis is the most common type of acute encephalitis and is observed in all age groups, with the exception of young children. The gross appearance of the brain in adults shows acute inflammation, congestion and softening. The necrosis is widespread and asymmetrical, associated predominantly with the temporal lobes. The necrotic tissue is sometimes haemorrhagic. In patients who survive for more than several weeks, the brain tissue starts to disintegrate. Severe microglial reactivity is observed and in cases of disseminated HSV infection mononuclear infiltrates and perivascular cuffing are observed. Viral inclusion bodies may be detected in the nuclei of neurones and to a lesser extent in oligodendrocytes and astrocytes.

Clinical features

The effects of HSV encephalitis on the CNS vary with the type of infection. Patients present with the sudden onset of an acute febrile encephalitic illness characterized by headaches, confusion and meningeal irritation. This is rapidly followed by deterioration in consciousness and may include focal epilepsy and focal motor neurological signs. Disseminated HSV infection is commonly observed in neonates and is related to HSV-2.

Diagnosis

Patients presenting with neurological involvement and suspected herpes simplex encephalitis may be evaluated by scanning procedures such as computed tomography or magnetic resonance imaging, together with CSF analysis. Imaging often shows evidence of oedema and a midline shift in cortical structures. However, virus isolation remains the definitive diagnosis for HSV and allows for typing of the virus. The most commonly used tests are CF, NT and ELISA although the use of polymerase chain reaction (PCR) gives definitive confirmation of infection in the CSF.

Prevention and control

Owing to the high risk of infection during birth in women with active genital HSV, infants born to such mothers should be isolated and cultures obtained at intervals to exclude infection; otherwise therapy should be administered.

HSV infections may be controlled by avoidance of infectious secretions, vaccination or antiviral therapy. Patients thus presenting with obvious HSV sores should avoid contact with persons at risk, particularly neonates. The antiviral agents, vidarabine and aciclovir,[47] have proved useful in the therapy of HSV encephalitis, although the outcome is dependent on factors of age, level of consciousness and disease duration. Such agents have also been suggested to be of use prophylactically for the newborn and for women at the onset of labour. Vaccination remains the preferred method for the prevention of virus infection, although recurrent episodes of infection occur in the presence of antibody and this introduces problems. However, protection from life-threatening infections has been achieved in experimental animal models.[48]

Varicella-zoster virus (VSV; HHV-3)

VZV causes two distinct diseases: chickenpox and 'shingles'. Chickenpox (varicella) is the primary disease, generally of children, and results in a highly contagious, generalized exanthem which occurs in epidemics. (The disease should not be confused with smallpox (variola) with which there is no relation.) The name 'chickenpox'

is thought to be derived from the French chick (chickpea), referring to the appearance of the vesicle or pox. Shingles (herpes zoster) is a less common disease that occurs in immunocompromised or older individuals and is characterized by dermatomal vesicular rashes. Herpes zoster is regarded as a secondary infection associated with the reactivation of VZV that has remained latent since an earlier attack of varicella. The name 'shingles' is derived from the Latin cingulum, meaning girdle, which is the appearance of the lesions on the dermatome.

The association between varicella and zoster was described in 1888 by von Bókay, who noted the appearance of chickenpox in a family after exposure to zoster. Furthermore, serological testing could not distinguish between the viruses and the ultimate confirmation came from studies by Weller and Stoddard,[49] who isolated virus from varicella lesions and zoster lesions, and determined that the recovered viruses were identical.

Epidemiology

Varicella is endemic in the population and epidemic in late winter and early spring. The disease affects 90% of children under the age of 10 years and intimate contact is necessary for infection. In contrast, zoster infections are a consequence of reactivation of VZV. Patients at greatest risk are those with Hodgkin's and non-Hodgkin's lymphoma and immunosuppressive conditions, such as AIDS. The incidence of CNS complications following varicella is unknown but has been reported as between 0.1 and 0.75%.[50] In contrast, the incidence of encephalitis following zoster is much higher, particularly in immunosuppressed patients.

Pathogenesis

Primary infection with VZV results from respiratory droplet transmission. The virus enters the mucosa of the upper respiratory tract, and to a lesser extent the conjunctiva, and disseminates via the blood. Cycles of replication occur, giving rise to a secondary viraemia from which the virus becomes widespread before the formation of cutaneous lesions. The complications of neurological involvement following varicella infection are classified into: (1) cerebellar ataxia, (2) generalized meningoencephalitis, (3) transverse myelitis, and (4) aseptic meningitis. The pathogenesis of these conditions is unknown, although immunological mechanisms of tissue damage, as a result of infection, have been suggested.[51] In general, the CNS involvement following zoster infections is associated with higher mortality rates than varicella. Complications following infection include encephalitis, ophthalmic zoster, myelitis, multifocal leukoencephalopathy, Guillain–Barré syndrome, and cranial and peripheral nerve palsies. VZV has been isolated from several patients with zoster encephalitis, and inclusions have been found in the glial cells and neurones. Antiviral antibodies have been demonstrated in the CSF of such patients.

Pathology

The neuropathological changes observed in varicella or zoster virus infections depend on the complication induced. In fatal varicella encephalitis, mononuclear infiltration and demyelination have been reported.[52] More detailed pathological findings have been reported for zoster complications because of the higher incidence of death. Zoster meningoencephalitis includes mononuclear infiltration of the meninges, necrosis and axonal degeneration. Degeneration may also involve the posterior columns where neurophagia is observed.

Clinical features

The incubation period for varicella in children is between 14 and 15 days, and is associated with malaise and mild fever. Anorexia and a sore throat are additional clinical features of adult varicella infection. The rash proceeds to the characteristic vesicles that crust. CNS involvement occurs more often in children who present with cerebellar ataxia a few days after the onset of the rash.[50]

The rash of zoster is preceded by pain in the dermatome affected. The lesions, which resemble varicella, appear unilaterally and generally do not cross the midline. Crusts appear up to 1 week after eruption and last for approximately 2 weeks. Neurological complications of zoster may precede the appearance of the rash or appear as late as 10 months afterwards. Complications are observed in immunosuppressed patients as a result of persistence of virus within the CNS.

Diagnosis

The onset of neurological signs concomitant with appearance of varicella or zoster rash would suggest such infection of the CNS. However, infection is not usually verified by virus isolation from the brain tissue, the exception being at necropsy. The new guidelines recommend that where CNS infection due to VZV is suspected, the CSF should be analysed by PCR for VZV DNA. As VZV antibodies may be present in the CSF in the presence or absence of detectable VZV DNA, CSF should also be analysed for VZV-specific antibody.[53]

Prevention and control

There is generally no specific treatment, apart from antipyretics (not aspirin) for varicella in the immunocompetent host. Neurological complications of varicella, particularly in the immunocompromised host, are important because of the high morbidity and mortality rates. Although α-interferon is effective, two nucleoside analogues, vidarabine and aciclovir, are also employed, although side-effects have been reported. The possibility that immune-mediated reactions contribute to the CNS manifestations has given rise to the use of corticosteroids as a treatment of CNS involvement. In contrast, as evidence suggests active viral replication within the CNS, it would appear that antiviral agents should be employed.

Epstein–Barr virus (HHV-4)

Epstein–Barr virus (EBV) (see also Chapter 43) gives rise to CNS complications such as meningoencephalomyelitis, encephalitis and neuropsychiatric syndromes, although the frequency of such manifestations is extremely low. The CSF of patients with CNS disorders following EBV infection shows an increased protein level. In patients dying from EBV infection, the CNS is more often affected and shows perivascular cuffing, oedema and demyelination. In the X-linked lymphoproliferative disease (Duncan syndrome), a rare inherited disorder, patients are unable to clear Epstein–Barr virus infection. In these patients EBV encephalitis is observed as well as CNS lymphoproliferative disease, and lymphoma. EBV seropositivity has also been linked with multiple sclerosis.

Other herpesvirus infections

Human cytomegalovirus (HCMV) (HHV-5). HCMV is the most frequent infectious cause of developmental brain disorders and causes brain damage in immunocompromised individuals; for example, HCMV infection of the CNS occurs in at least 50% of AIDS patients. Although the brain is one of the main targets of CMV infection, little is known about the neuropathogenesis of the brain disorders caused by CMV in humans because of the limitations in studying human subjects. For diagnosis, the PCR recommended for viral DNA is performed on CSF. Treatment should be directed toward the prevention of CMV disease using ganciclovir.

Human herpesvirus 6 (HHV-6). Like other herpesviruses, HHV-6 infects virtually all children within the first few years of life and establishes latency after primary infection. In immunocompromised hosts HHV-6 has been linked with CNS disease. In particular, longitudinal studies have established a correlation between systemic HHV-6 reactivation and CNS dysfunction such as limbic encephalitis and temporal lobe epilepsy.

Human herpesvirus 7 (HHV-7). Infections of the CNS have rarely recently been reported in children although, like HHV-6, there are several reports linking these infection with multiple sclerosis, chronic fatigue syndrome and epilepsy.

Human herpesvirus 8 (HHV-8). This has also been linked with demyelinating diseases using PCR to detect virus in the blood of patients.

Cercopithecine herpesvirus 1 (B virus)

The non-human primate Cercopithecine herpesvirus 1 (B virus) is highly pathogenic to humans. Originally transmitted by the bite of rhesus or macaque monkeys, the virus is now thought to be transmitted from person to person. In 1932, following the bite from a monkey, a physician developed a localized reaction, lymphangitis, lymphadenitis and transverse myelitis, and died. The virus was subsequently recovered from the CNS of the patient and found to be lethal to rabbits following injection.

Epidemiology

The B virus is indigenous to Old World monkeys. Although B virus has been reported in only 22 human cases and is generally transmitted via a bite, individuals in Florida have been affected (two fatally), suggesting person-to-person spread of the virus.[54] Virus is secreted in the saliva and stools of infected animals and these must therefore be considered as potential sources of infection for humans.

Pathogenesis

After the bite, a local reaction occurs, followed by lymph node involvement. The course of the disease is dependent on the route of inoculation (as determined from animal studies), although transverse myelitis is a prominent neurological finding before invasion of the CNS. As with other herpesviruses, the B virus becomes latent and may be reactivated under certain conditions.[55] Virus spread to the brain is suggested to occur via the neural routes, as with HSV.

Pathology

All regions of the brain may be infected by B virus and show haemorrhagic foci, necrosis and inflammation in the form of perivascular cuffing of mononuclear cells. Motor neurones are affected and show degeneration. Astrocytosis is observed, with gliosis.

Clinical features

Incubation of B virus varies from 2–3 to 24 days. The neurological involvement is observed 3–7 days after the appearance of the vesicular rash. Death may ensue within 10–14 days, although the progression of the disease depends on the age, site of bite and immunological status of the patient. Clinically, the patients present with a localized inflammatory reaction at the site of the bite, or with a respiratory illness: such responses have been described in two individuals.

Diagnosis

Although serological tests demonstrate the presence of B virus, a significant problem is the cross-reactivity with HSV antigens. Diagnosis is therefore dependent on the isolation of virus, particularly from the CSF of humans suspected of being infected, and the use of cell lines susceptible to B virus infection. These include rabbit kidney cells or cell lines such as BSC or LLC-RK1. Definitive diagnosis may be made using molecular methods and neutralization of isolates in serological assays.

Prevention and management

Procedures that limit the transmission of the virus should be adhered to. These include limited contact with macaque monkeys and the routine screening of such animals. The use of hyperimmune serum has not proved effective in controlling human infection, although some success has been achieved in experimental infections.[56] Antiviral therapy has concentrated on the nucleoside analogues: vidarabine, aciclovir and ganciclovir. The use of aciclovir in humans has been reported to slow the infection.[57]

ORTHOMYXOVIRIDAE

Orthomyxoviruses (Greek 'myxa' meaning mucus) are large enveloped RNA viruses and include the influenza A, B and C viruses which infect swine, horses, seals and a large variety of birds as well as humans. Influenza type A viruses are divided into subtypes based on two proteins on the surface of the virus, the haemagglutinin (H) and neuraminidase (N). There are 15 different haemagglutinin subtypes and nine different neuraminidase subtypes, all found among influenza A viruses in wild birds. Genetic reassortment produces subtypes that give rise to epidemics of highly contagious, acute respiratory illness afflicting humans.

Epidemiology

Influenza viruses are unique among the respiratory tract viruses in that they undergo significant antigenic variation. Antigenic drift involves minor antigenic changes in H and N proteins. Wild birds are the primary natural reservoir for all subtypes of influenza A viruses and are thought to be the source of influenza A viruses in all other animals. Most influenza viruses cause asymptomatic or mild infection in birds; however, the range of symptoms in birds varies greatly depending on the strain of virus. Infection with certain avian influenza A viruses (e.g. some strains of H5 and H7 viruses) can cause widespread disease and death among some species of wild and especially domestic birds such as chickens and turkeys. In May 1997, a young child in Hong Kong died of complications of influenza H5N1 – the first case in humans. The subtype H5 causes lethal avian influenza (bird flu) but did not cause an epidemic in humans since it was thought that the strain was poorly adapted to humans.

Pathogenesis and pathology

A wide spectrum of CNS involvement has been shown during influenza A virus infection in humans, ranging from irritability, drowsiness and confusion to more serious manifestations of psychosis and coma. There are two specific CNS syndromes: influenza encephalopathy and postinfluenza encephalitis. Encephalopathy occurs at the height of the influenza illness and may progress to death.[58] Histological changes are minimal. The CSF is usually normal and the brain shows severe congestion at autopsy. The post-encephalitis syndrome is extremely rare and occurs 2–3 weeks after recovery from influenza. The CSF findings suggest that inflammatory changes have occurred. Influenza A virus has only rarely been isolated from the brain or CSF. It has been suggested that the syndrome of encephalitis lethargica followed by post-encephalitic Parkinson's disease was associated with the influenza epidemics of 1918.[59]

Clinical features

Influenza A virus infections in avian species vary with the strain of the virus. Infections with most strains of influenza virus are asymptomatic. However, some strains cause chronic respiratory infections and a minority lead to a rapidly fatal infection accompanied by CNS involvement, with death occurring within 1 week. Febrile convulsion may occur in children with and without underlying CNS abnormalities. Pregnant women in the second or third trimester also have an increased risk of developing fatal influenza disease,[60] and increased incidences of congenital abnormalities and haematological malignancies have been reported following influenza virus infection in pregnancy.[61] Acute necrotizing encephalopathy manifesting with coma, convulsions and hyperpyrexia has been associated with Influenza B in children.[62]

Prevention and control

Antivirals

Several antiviral drugs are used for influenza virus infections e.g. amantadine hydrochloride is effective against all subtypes of influenza A virus but not B or C viruses.[63,64] The antiviral activity is exerted after adsorption, penetration and uncoating have taken place but before primary transcription.[65] Zanamivir is the first widely approved neuraminidase inhibitor for the treatment of influenza. It is delivered directly to the primary site of viral replication, the respiratory tract, and is well tolerated and effective in the treatment of both influenza A and B. Oseltamivir is the second antiviral drug, after amantadine, to be marketed in the European Union for the prevention of influenza in children aged from 1 to 12 years.[66]

Vaccines

Inactivated influenza A and B virus vaccines are designated either whole virus (WV) or split product (SP). The WV vaccines contain intact formalin-treated virus, whereas SP vaccines contain purified formalin-treated virus disrupted with chemicals that solubilize the lipid-containing viral envelope. In addition, experimental vaccines containing the isolated haemagglutinin (HA) and neuraminidase (NA) surface proteins are called subunit vaccines. Other types of vaccine are those that contain a monovalent influenza A H1N1 virus of a mixture of H1N1, H3N2 and B viruses.

PAPOVAVIRIDAE

The family Papovaviridae is divided into the two subfamilies: polyomaviruses and papillomaviruses, which, although they share several properties, are not related immunologically or genetically.

Polyoma viruses

The first human disease associated with a polyomavirus was a rare demyelinating disease of the CNS, progressive multifocal leukoencephalopathy (PML). The disease is observed in immunodeficient individuals and was suggested, in 1961, to be due to a common virus which in the immunocompromised host runs an atypical course of infection. In 1971 two viruses implicated in PML were isolated from the brain (JC virus) of a patient with PML and the urine (BK virus) of a renal transplant patient.[67] JC and BK viruses are contracted in early childhood, persist in the host and are reactivated in cases of immunocompromise, such as in AIDS.

Epidemiology

Polyomaviruses are widely distributed in many species of animals, although they are generally species specific. BK and JC viruses do not naturally infect species other than humans. Antibody titres to BK virus are acquired by 50% of children by 3 years of age and against JC virus by 50% at 6 years of age.[68] It is estimated that 60–80% of adults in Europe and the USA have antibodies to JC virus. PML is worldwide in distribution and occurs as a complication in lymphoproliferative disorders, and chronic disease such as sarcoidosis, in immunodeficiency diseases and in patients on long-term immunosuppressive therapy. Reactivation of both JC and BK viruses is also known to occur in pregnancy, diabetes, chronic disorders and old age. Approximately 20% of patients with PML have AIDS, whereas PML is reported to occur in as many as 3.8% of patients with AIDS presenting with neurological disorders.[69] More recently, PML has been identified in some patients with MS prescribed Tysabri.[69]

Pathogenesis

Primary JC infections of healthy individuals are not associated with illness, although BK virus has been linked with mild respiratory illness. The mode of transmission of BK and JC viruses is unknown, although the rapid acquisition of antibodies has been suggested to be consistent with respiratory disorders. Following primary infection the virus remains latent in the kidney and is reactivated under immunosuppression.

Pathology

The PML brain is characterized by foci of demyelination that are widespread and vary in size. In advanced cases the areas may be necrotic. The lesions occur in the absence of inflammatory cells and are more frequent in the white matter of the cerebrum. Nuclear changes in the oligodendrocytes at the edge of the demyelinated plaques are associated with the presence of JC virus. The lesions are also marked with bizarre giant astrocytes and oligodendrocytes with enlarged nuclei which, at light microscopical level, are deeply basophilic and may contain inclusion bodies. Neurones are unaffected.

Clinical features

Symptoms such as cognitive changes, ataxia, aphasia and sensory deficits characteristic of a multifocal brain disease observed without signs of raised intracranial pressure in an immunocompromised host suggest PML. Generally, people with PML deteriorate rapidly and death occurs within 6 months, although in rare cases patients experience fluctuating symptoms over 2–3 years.

Diagnosis

Computed tomography or magnetic resonance imaging of the brain will detect lesions of demyelination. Verification of PML may be carried out following examination of brain tissue in which JC virus may be identified by electron microscopy, immunohistological identification as well as in CNS sections, cultivation of the virus in fetal glial cells and characterization of viral DNA by in situ hybridization and PCR.[70]

Management and control

There is no certain treatment for PML, although the accepted regimen is to discontinue the immunosuppressive therapy in combination with the use of antiviral drugs. Attempts at treatment with nucleic acid-based analogues have been reported. See also under HIV infections, as PML is more prevalent in patients with AIDS.

Papillomaviruses

While not commonly associated with CNS diseases, recently pregnant women infected with the human papilloma virus may give birth to children with pathologies of the nervous system.

PARAMYXOVIRIDAE

The Paramyxoviridae family consists of negative-stranded enveloped RNA viruses classified as three genera: *Morbillivirus*, *Para-*

myxovirus, and *Pneumovirus*, and includes four important human pathogens: measles, mumps, parainfluenza (types 1–4) and respiratory syncytial viruses.

Morbillivirus

The Morbillivirus genus is important in that it contains the human neurotropic virus measles and the canine distemper virus.

Measles

Measles (see also Chapter 47) as a disease was first described by Sydenham in the early seventeenth century and the implication that this was a virus infection was established in the 1920s. The disease is generally a childhood illness and is not fatal, although it may be serious in the very young or elderly. Great epidemics of measles have been described, such as the 'black measles' of the eighteenth century. Waves of measles infection are occasionally observed, with the greatest incidence between November and March.

Epidemiology

In the less developed countries, measles is the most important cause of death between the ages of 1 and 5 years. Death occurs predominantly from respiratory and CNS complications. Measles does not have animal reservoirs and no vectors are involved. The principal mode of transmission is via droplets of infected respiratory tract secretions inhaled as a consequence of face-to-face exposure. However, air-borne transmission may be important in certain settings, including schools, hospitals and other institutions. Virus is present in respiratory secretions and in the conjunctivae during the latter part of the incubation period. Viraemia is also present during this time and virus is present in the urine for 4 or more days after the onset of rash.[71] Patients are considered infectious from the onset of symptoms through the fourth day of rash. Maternal antibodies provide protection during the first 6 months of life and, although cell-mediated immunity is required to clear measles virus infection, both humoral and cell-mediated immunity are able to prevent disease in normal individuals. The slow infection of measles in humans (i.e. subacute sclerosing panencephalitis, SSPE) is a rare disease in which virus persists in the CNS. The incidence of SSPE is more common in males than females, and is more prevalent in rural areas. The average age of onset is between 5 and 15 years, and infection with measles before the age of 15 years increases the risk of developing SSPE. In the USA the mean annual incidence rate of SSPE was estimated at 0.06 cases per million (aged under 20 years) in 1980.

Clinical features

Measles begins, after an incubation period of 8–12 days, with fever, malaise and anorexia followed by conjunctivitis and cough. The infection then spreads to the epithelial surfaces of the mouth, nasopharynx, respiratory tract and gastrointestinal tract. Two to three days before the onset of the rash, Koplik's spots appear on the buccal mucosa. Koplik's spots are small (1–3 mm), irregular, bright red spots, each of which has a minute bluish-white speck at its centre. The temperature reaches 39.4–40.6°C at the height of the eruption on the 5th day of the illness. The rash starts around day 3 or 4 of prodromal symptoms and spreads downward over the face, neck and trunk, continuing downwards until it reaches the feet by the third day. Cough and coryza follow as a result of an intense inflammatory reaction that involves the mucosa throughout the respiratory tract. The most common complications involve the middle ear, CNS, eyes and skin.[72]

The three forms of measles encephalitis are:

1. Acute post-infectious measles encephalitis; the most common neurological complication of measles. Children under the age of 2 years are rarely affected but it occurs in older children in the ratio of 1 in 1000. It appears a short time after the rash. Between 10% and 20% die and the majority of the survivors have some neurological sequelae. Histopathological examination shows perivascular inflammatory changes and demyelination.
2. Acute progressive infectious encephalitis which is generally observed in immunosuppressed patients. Exposure to measles leads to seizures, motor and sensory deficits, and lethargy. The clinical progress and pathology are a result of unrestricted cytolytic replication of the virus.[73]
3. Late complication of measles. The symptoms develop over months, reflecting loss of cerebral cortical function.[74] In the early stage subtle mental changes and diminishing intellectual capacity are seen. Later, myoclonic jerks occur and progress to choreoathetosis, ataxia and finally coma. Focal retinitis occurs in the majority of the cases, leading to blindness.

Pathogenesis and pathology

Measles virus replicates initially in the respiratory mucosa and spreads, perhaps carried intracellularly in pulmonary macrophages and other cells, to draining lymph nodes where further replication occurs. Virus then enters the bloodstream and from here dissemination of the virus throughout the reticuloendothelial system takes place. This results in a secondary viraemia that disseminates the infection to tissues throughout the body. The most striking feature of measles virus infection in vivo and in vitro is the formation of multinucleated giant cells which result from the fusion of infected cells with the adjacent cells.[75] In tissue culture these giant cells contain eosinophilic cytoplasmic inclusion bodies and their nuclei show condensation of chromatin at the nuclear membrane. The CNS of patients with SSPE shows inflammation of the meninges and perivascular cuffing in both grey and white matter. In the later stages of disease, demyelination and gliosis are observed. Although the mechanisms of myelin damage are unknown, it may be a result of either neural damage or the involvement of an autoimmune response, as T lymphocyte reactivity to the myelin constituent, myelin basic protein, has been observed.[76]

Diagnosis

Most measles infections are easily recognizable by the distinctive Koplik's spots, rash and catarrhal symptoms. Effective tests for laboratory diagnosis are available and include virus isolation in primary human or monkey cells and antibody determination by simple HI test and by ELISA.[77] Serological tests are effective in identifying cases of SSPE. Patients with this disease have increased serum antibody titres, which are 10–100 times higher than those seen in late convalescent-phase sera. There is also a pronounced local production of oligoclonal measles virus antibodies in the CNS.[78] Viral antigen can be identified by immunofluorescence.

Prevention and control

No effective treatment is available, although in vitro measles virus replication is sensitive to interferon and ribavirin treatment. No treatment is presently available but pooled immunoglobulin can be administered for postexposure prophylaxis up to 5 days after exposure. Live attenuated vaccines are widely used and it is aimed to eradicate measles worldwide.[79] The rate of seroconversion after vaccination exceeds 90%. Vaccine complications are very rare. Encephalitis occurs at the same rate as in non-vaccinated individuals and the frequency of occurrence of SSPE is reduced by a factor of at least 10 in vaccinated persons. Recently, early administration with intrathecal high-dose interferon-α and intravenous ribavirin has been shown to be effective in the treatment of SSPE.

Canine distemper virus

Canine distemper virus (CDV) deserves mention in this chapter because of its relationship with measles virus and implication in the human neurological disease, multiple sclerosis. This virus gives rise to a chronic relapsing disease of dogs in which demyelination lesions are observed.[80] Furthermore, several studies have suggested associations between the incidence of multiple sclerosis and canine distemper in the dog population.[81]

Paramyxoviruses

Mumps

Mumps has been recognized from the fifth century BC when Hippocrates described the disease as one of swellings behind the ears accompanied by swelling of the testes. However, the first description of neurological involvement was that by Hamilton[82] in the eighteenth century. Transfer of disease from filtered secretions of an affected patient into experimental animals suggested the disease had a viral aetiology.

Epidemiology

Mumps infection increases in the winter months. Immunity to mumps is usually acquired between the ages of 5 and 14 years, with maximal humoral antibody occurring between 4 and 7 years of age.[83] Mortality from mumps is related primarily to the complications of meningitis/encephalitis and orchitis. These occur as age- and sex-specific hazards, with a peak risk in post-pubertal males. The incidence of CSF pleocytosis is reported in 30% of patients with mumps parotitis, whereas encephalitis occurs in as many as 35% of cases.[84]

Clinical features

The most characteristic feature of mumps is the swelling of the salivary glands which occurs in up to 95% of all symptomatic cases. The parotid glands are often involved. A moderate febrile response is present at the time of the disease onset. A wide variety of other organs have been involved and include the testes, CNS,

epididymis, prostate, ovaries, liver, pancreas, spleen, thyroid, kidneys, eyes, thymus, heart and joints. The onset of mumps meningitis is marked by fever, with vomiting, neck stiffness, headache and lethargy. Seizures occur in 21–30% of patients with CNS symptoms. In cases of CNS involvement about one-third of all patients have evidence of intrathecal IgG synthesis and the presence of oligoclonal immunoglobulins during the first week of CNS symptoms. Examination of the CSF shows abnormalities in the vast majority of cases. The protein content in the CSF is markedly increased in 60–70% of all cases. This may be due to a damaged BBB, as indicated by high albumin indices that do not normalize for several weeks to months after the onset of the CNS symptoms. The CSF glucose content is depressed to 17–41% of the serum value in 6–29% of all cases.[85]

Pathogenesis and pathology

Natural infection is initiated by droplet spread with primary viral replication in nasal mucosa or upper respiratory mucosal epithelium and the time to first clinical symptoms is about 18 days. Virus is actively shed in saliva 6 days before symptoms, during which the virus multiplies in the upper respiratory mucosa and spreads to draining lymph nodes with subsequent transient plasma viraemia. Plasma viraemia is terminated by the developing humoral antibodies as early as 11 days after experimental infections of humans. Mumps virus has been shown to infect human lymphocytes in vitro and appears preferentially to infect activated cells of the T lymphocyte subset. This could imply that cell-associated viraemia may be another mode of virus dissemination. Viral replication in the parotid glands is accompanied by periductal interstitial oedema and a local inflammatory reaction involving lymphocytes and macrophages. Once within neurones, virus is able to distribute widely along neuronal pathways.

Viral invasion of the CNS occurs across the choroid plexus, although rarely is mumps meningoencephalitis fatal. CNS pathology is restricted to perivascular infiltration with mononuclear cells, scattered foci of neuronophagia and microglial proliferation.[86] Perivascular demyelination also occurs; this may be the result of an autoimmune attack on the brain tissue. Persistence of mumps virus has been suggested within the CNS of humans. Deafness is probably the result of direct damage to the cochlea and, to a lesser extent, cochlear neurones.[87] Most cases of mumps meningitis resolve without sequelae. However, ataxia and behavioural disturbances may be slow to resolve following mumps meningoencephalitis.[88,89]

Diagnosis

The clinical diagnosis of mumps is seldom problematic in the presence of parotitis. Laboratory diagnosis includes determination of virus-specific IgM and IgG levels. Mumps meningitis can be confirmed on the basis of a raised CSF serum antibody ratio.

Management and control

Hyperimmune γ-globulin to modify the course of mumps is used in selected cases. Two general types of vaccine have been used. Recently controversy over the links with autism and measles-mumps-rubella (MMR) vaccination has led to the idea of single vaccines. However, the most widely used are the live attenuated mumps virus preparations given as the triple MMR vaccine; killed mumps virus antigens have a more restricted use.[90]

PARVOVIRIDAE

To date parvoviruses have rarely been implicated in human CNS disease[91] although infections of experimental animals with parvoviruses are well-known to induce cerebellar ataxia and affect the development of the cerebellum during the perinatal period.

PICORNAVIRIDAE

The Picornaviridae family consists of small RNA viruses and comprises nine genera: *Enterovirus*, *Rhinovirus*, *Hepatovirus*, *Aphthovirus* and *Cardiovirus*, *Parechovirus*, *Erbovirus*, *Kobuvirus* and *Teschovirus*. Those in which neurological disease has been reported are given in Table 48.6.

Enteroviruses

The enteroviruses multiply throughout the alimentary tract and tend to be resistant to known antibiotics and chemotherapeutic agents. The host range of the enteroviruses is varied and may be readily induced to yield variants, which has led to the development of attenuated polio vaccine strains. The enteroviruses which are important CNS pathogens of humans are polioviruses and coxsackie. For more detailed studies on enteroviruses, the reader is referred to *Fields Virology*.[2]

Poliovirus

The disease poliomyelitis (see also Chapter 16) has existed since ancient times, although the fact that the causative agent was a virus was first demonstrated only in 1909 by Landsteiner and Popper.[92] Studies in monkeys and the adaptation to tissue culture resulted in the development of methods of purification and the production of reliable vaccines through which infection can now be controlled. Poliomyelitis may be caused by one of three strains of virus: polio types 1, 2 or 3. Three forms of clinical disease have been recognized: paralysis, aseptic meningitis and minor febrile illness.

Epidemiology

Poliovirus was, until very recently, endemic worldwide, infecting susceptible infants and producing paralytic poliomyelitis in those who were not protected by maternal antibody. In 1916, 80% of cases were in those under 5 years of age. The changes in sanitation and hygiene in the late nineteenth century, with industrialization in the north of Britain, decreased the incidence in infants but resulted in a higher incidence of paralytic poliomyelitis in later childhood due to delay in exposure to the virus. In the epidemics of 1950 the peak age was 5–9 years, although about one-third of cases and two-thirds of deaths were in those over 15 years. Since 1985, most of the cases of polio worldwide have been in developing countries, although the number of deaths due to other diseases may mask the true incidence of infantile paralysis. Nevertheless, there are still outbreaks and the polio eradication programme aims to achieve its goal by the end of 2008.[93]

Pathogenesis

Following ingestion, poliovirus replicates in the pharynx and intestines, from which it is excreted. Transmission is by the faecal-oral route and thus the necessity for hygiene is paramount. After initial replication in the lymphoid tissue of the pharynx and gut, which leads to viraemia, the virus infects the CNS via the blood. Neural spread has been demonstrated in children following tonsillectomy.

Pathology

The anterior horn cells of the spinal cord are susceptible to infection with poliovirus and are damaged or, in severe cases, completely destroyed.[94] The lesions observed in the CNS may extend to the hypothalamus and thalamus. Neuronophagia is commonly observed, with inflammation being secondary to neuronal attack. In less severe cases oedema, which results in temporary disturbance of neural functions, subsides and the cells recover completely.

Clinical features

Following infection, approximately 1% of patients present with clinical disease. Abortive poliomyelitis is the most common form of the disease in which fever, malaise, drowsiness, headache and sore throat are experienced to varying degrees. The signs abate within a few days. Stiffness and pain in the back of the neck may also be experienced, in which case non-paralytic poliomyelitis, or aseptic meningitis, is diagnosed. The disease may become biphasic, whereby a minor illness is followed by a remission, but which subsequently develops into a major severe illness.

Diagnosis

Antibodies are usually present by the time paralysis occurs and a viraemia may be detected and used to determine the subtype using

Table 48.6 Picornaviruses implicated in human neurological disease

Genus	Virus	Disease
Enteroviruses	Human polio	Paralysis, aseptic meningitis, febrile illness
	Human coxsackie (groups A and B)	Aseptic meningitis, paralysis, meningoencephalomyelitis
	Echovirus	Aseptic meningitis, paralysis, encephalitis, ataxia or Guillain–Barré syndrome
	Enteroviruses (types 70, 71)	Paralysis, meningoencephalitis
Cardiovirus		Encephalomyocarditis

serological techniques. More recently, molecular biological techniques have been used to demonstrate poliovirus in CSF.

Prevention

In 1952, Salk developed an inactivated poliovirus vaccine[95] which became generally available in 1955, and by 1959, oral polio vaccines were developed using live attenuated virus which today consists of a mixture of three strains. The oral vaccine protects by producing both systemic antibody and local secretory IgA which would block virulent virus, preventing spread from the gut. These vaccines have the advantages over killed preparations of ease of administration and long-lasting immunity, although they have the 'disadvantage' of being excreted and thus have the potential to spread to non-vaccinated persons.[96]

Coxsackie and echoviruses

Of the non-polioenterovirus infections, echovirus 9 is the most frequent cause of enterovirus disease and the most common virus to be isolated in epidemics. The chief viruses implicated in CNS disease are coxsackie B1-6, A7 and A9, although many echoviruses have been associated with meningitis, as has enterovirus type 70. Of all the enteroviruses, Coxsackie B is responsible for more than half the cases of aseptic meningitis in children less than 3 months. Severe CNS disease has been observed in enterovirus 71 infections in the 1975 epidemic in Bulgaria, where antibodies to enterovirus 71 were detected in 72% of patients with paralysis and virus was isolated from the CNS. Of the seven reported epidemics with enterovirus 71, all reported evidence of CNS involvement.[97]

Other picornaviruses

Hepatitis A infection has also been linked with CNS involvement in which a child presented with seizures.[98] Also human parechovirus infections have been linked with transient paralysis and encephalitis.

More recently, a newly identified picornavirus, Ljungan virus, isolated from rodents, induces encephalitis in rodents, while a porcine teschovirus has been associated with encephalitis in pigs.

POXVIRIDAE

The family name is taken from the major clinical symptom of these viruses, namely pox – an elevated skin lesion – and includes variola and vaccinia. Neurological complications of poxvirus infections are generally associated with vaccination, namely postvaccination encephalitis. The pathogenesis and pathology resemble other post-infectious encephalitides and include perivascular cuffing, mononuclear infiltration and demyelination.

REOVIRIDAE

The family REOviridae (Respiratory Enteric Orphan viruses) is comprised of 12 genera. The genus Coltivirus contains Colorado tick virus; Orbivirus, the Blue tongue virus that infects cattle and African horse sickness virus; the genus Rotaviruses contains viruses that cause diarrhoea. Seadornavoiruses are emerging pathogens

from South-east Asia and contain Banna virus isolated from humans with encephalitis.[99] Rotaviruses have been rarely associated with encephalopathy in children and encephalitis was observed in four people as a result of accidental exposure to a vaccine of the Orbivirus, African horse sickness virus.

Coltiviruses

The genus Coltivirus are tick-borne viruses such as Colorado tick fever virus, associated with patients with flulike syndromes, meningitis, encephalitis, and other severe complications. Another coltivirus, Eyach virus, isolated from ticks in France and Germany, has been associated with febrile illnesses and neurological syndromes.[99]

Colorado tick fever

Colorado tick fever (CTF) was first described in the mid-nineteenth century in the Rocky Mountain States and associated with infections from the tick Dermacentor andersoni.[100]

Epidemiology

This disease is confined to the geographical distribution of the adult Dermacentor andersoni tick in the Rocky Mountain States and in parts of north-western Canada; it is a common infection in hikers and foresters during May and June.

Pathogenesis

Infection with CTF virus gives rise to little or no disease in the natural host and induces a prolonged or persistent viraemia in vertebrate hosts such as ground squirrels and chipmunks that serve as amplificatory rodents. CTF virus is involved in bone marrow precursor cells and its presence in erythrocyte precursors renders the host susceptible to haemorrhagic disorders. The onset of disease occurs 3–6 days after the tick bite.

Pathology

CTF virus infections do not generally result in death and thus pathological features are not well described. However, following experimental infections of mice, the cerebellum shows widespread necrosis and cellular infiltration.

Clinical features

A febrile illness develops, with headache and myalgia. A maculopapular rash is seen in about 50% of patients. Colorado tick fever is a benign disease but in very rare cases a bleeding diathesis may develop and, particularly in children, there may be a typical meningoencephalitic illness. Resolution of the acute phase may take 5–10 days. Infection in the CNS may be observed as a mild meningeal reaction to severe encephalitis. The frequency of CNS involvement ranges from 1 to 10%.[100]

Diagnosis

Abnormalities include leucopenia and thrombocytopenia; virus may be isolated from the blood owing to its persistence in the erythrocytes. Some time after disease onset, CF and neutralizing antibodies may be detected in the blood[101] although PCR is more efficient and sensitive. CSF findings are typical of encephalitis.

Prevention and control

At present, there is no treatment for CTF, although health awareness when hiking in the affected areas may help to limit exposure to tick bites.

RETROVIRIDAE

Several features of retroviruses, such as their unique replication cycle, oncogenic ability and the wide variety of interactions with the host, including their ability to remain latent, have led to the intense scientific attention these viruses have received. Retroviruses are classified into the three subfamilies: Oncovirinae, Lentivirinae – lentiviruses (e.g. maedi-visna, which results in chronic inflammation of the CNS and human immunodeficiency viruses which result neurologically in AIDS dementia and demyelination) – and Spumavirinae.

Lentiviruses

In contrast to viruses that cause acute disease and where virus is finally eliminated, the lentiviruses include those that are able to escape such elimination and persist in the host. These include the maedi-visna of sheep, which give rise to chronic neurological disorders, and human immunodeficiency viruses in which neurological damage has been recognized.

Maedi-visna

Maedi-visna (*maedi* = laboured breathing, *visna* = wasting and paralysis – Icelandic translations) is the prototype lentivirus in which the slow onset of clinical disease results from prolonged incubation of the virus.

Epidemiology

The disease was first recognized in Iceland[101] but is observed in most countries with large sheep populations. Early transmission studies in Iceland showed that the disease could be transmitted from infected sheep to naive sheep by intracerebral inoculation. Many strains of visna have been obtained which vary in their ability to, for example, be propagated in tissue culture.

Pathogenesis

Virus is isolated from many tissues, particularly the lymphatics, spleen and peripheral blood leukocytes. Higher titres are isolated from the brain and lung. Conversion of the maedi illness to visna may occur as a result of infected peripheral blood leukocytes crossing the BBB and subsequently infecting the CNS.

Pathology

Following experimental infection, severe meningitis and encephalitis are observed, coinciding with perivascular lesions of inflammatory cells. The inflammatory cells observed in the CNS consist of monocytes/macrophages, plasma cells and T lymphocytes.

Depending on the duration of the disease, the brain may show large areas of focal demyelination. Additionally, inflammatory lesions and/or demyelination may occur in the presence of areas of necrosis and gliosis.[102]

Clinical features

Clinical disease is observed as lymphadenopathy, pneumonia and CNS involvement. The sheep appear dyspnoeic with loss of flesh. The appearance of clinical disease is dependent on the strain of animal and dose of inoculation.[103]

Prevention and control

Due to the expense of developing vaccines for animals, very few studies on controlling infection have been attempted. However, sheep hyperimmunized with disrupted virus are known to develop neutralizing antibodies which are able to confer some protection against homologous virus infection.

Human immunodeficiency virus

The human immunodeficiency viruses (see also Chapter 20) consist of HIV-1 and HIV-2 and are typical lentiviruses. This chapter will concentrate only on the CNS diseases in HIV infections which are important because they are commonly seen during all stages of the disease and contribute to the outcome of the disease despite therapy.[104] The variations in clinical manifestation are dependent on both the stage of HIV disease and opportunistic infections, whether viral, such as JC infection giving rise to PML, or bacterial (e.g. *Listeria* monocytogenes meningitis).

The gross clinical features observed in neurological complications of HIV infections are classified by the neuroanatomical localization, i.e. whether the brain or cord is involved and whether the lesions are focal or non-focal. With regard to the neurological complications, these may be categorized depending on the stage of the disease: (1) during acute HIV infection of the CNS; (2) asymptomatic infection; (3) aseptic meningitis and headache; and (4) AIDS dementia complex (ADC). CNS syndromes of children give rise to a fifth syndrome resulting in abnormal neurological development and arrested intellectual and motor function.

HIV infection of the CNS

HIV may enter the brain across the BBB or by infecting monocytes (macrophages and microglia) which are productively infected by virtue of having surface CD4 molecules. Such macrophages may then cross the BBB, thus allowing the HIV access to the CNS. During the asymptomatic phase CNS involvement is common and at least 40% of all persons with HIV have abnormal CSF, with increased cell counts and protein levels. Anti-HIV antibodies are detectable in the CSF and in some patients oligoclonal bands are observed. It has been suggested that aseptic meningitis and headache, AIDS dementia complex and progressive encephalopathy of children are due to the direct effects of HIV infection.

The common neurological symptoms of early or primary HIV-1 infection are headaches and photophobia, which may be either acute or chronic. Although the cause of such clinical symptoms is not known in all patients, headaches have been related to systemic disease such as Pneumocystis carinii infection. Such features may subside or progress to encephalitis, meningitis or ataxia. Aseptic meningitis affects 5–10% of HIV-infected patients; HIV may be diagnosed by positive virus culture or p24 antigen in the serum or CSF.

AIDS dementia complex

ADC is commonly observed in the later stages of HIV-1 infection in relation to major systemic infections, although in a small group of patients ADC occurs in the absence of opportunistic infections and may be related to HIV-1 infection of the brain. Infection and disease are not synonymous. ADC may be classified into five major stages ranging from stage 0, which encompasses normal mental and motor functions, to stage 4, in which the patient demonstrates rudimentary levels of intellectual and social comprehension and is paraparetic or paraplegic.

Epidemiology

The progression of HIV-1 infection to ADC is related, in general, to the level of immunosuppression in the patient. In early disease with opportunistic infections, approximately 10–30% of patients exhibit ADC stage 1, while 5–15% exhibit severe neurological disturbances (stage 2–3). In contrast, in the late stages of infection the majority of patients with AIDS show severe disability (stage 4).

Pathology

Pathological changes in the CNS of patients with ADC are most prominent in the subcortical regions, correlating with the observed subcortical clinical abnormalities. The most common changes include: (1) pallor of the white matter and demyelination; (2) gliosis, necrosis and mild neuronal loss; (3) multinucleated giant cells, which may be observed in the later stages of disease; and (4) spongiform changes, which are related to severity of dementia.[105]

Clinical features

Patients with ADC show distinct cognitive changes associated with subcortical, as opposed to cortical, changes. There is general mental slowing, including apathy, impaired concentration and features associated more with depression than CNS infection. Confusion, hallucinations, impaired memory and problem-solving deficiencies are common prior to obvious dementia. ADC may progress in steps or with sudden deterioration associated with systemic infection.

Diagnosis

In patients with ADC, computed tomography and magnetic resonance imaging show cerebral atrophy, although such a finding is non-specific. The CSF of ADC patients contains HIV-specific cytotoxic T cells, increased protein, oligoclonal bands and soluble intercellular adhesion molecule 1 (ICAM-1), which may serve as a marker for disease.[106]

Prevention and control

Zidovudine (formerly AZT) has been shown to improve neuropsychological performance and reduce the incidence of ADC, as has the antiinflammatory alkaloid cepharanthine.[107] Psychiatric disorders such as mania may be treated with lithium, as in non-infected patients.

CNS syndromes in children

Mother-to-child transmission accounts for 80% of HIV infections in children. Infected children present with encephalopathy, either progressive or static, that may be seen from the age of 2 months. The children with progressive encephalopathy become inactive and may develop paralysis and, if untreated, die within 1 year. The CSF may show an increased protein concentration and high levels of HIV-specific antibodies. Antibody levels in the serum (as a means of diagnosis) may be difficult to interpret owing to the presence of transplacental maternal antibodies. The brains of HIV-infected children are atrophic and contain perivascular inflammation, and the small vessels show calcification.

Opportunistic viral infections of the CNS

Although a variety of opportunistic CNS infections occur with HIV infection, only viral infections will be considered in this section. The major infections are observed with JC virus that gives rise to PML (see under Papovaviruses) and cytomegalovirus (CMV). PML occurs in 2–5% of patients with AIDS; its effects are observed as dementia and/or focal neurological signs. Herpesvirus infections, in the form of CMV, VZV and HSV-1 and -2, give rise to 'secondary viral encephalomeningitides'. CMV may result in encephalitis and retinal infiltration, which is observed in approximately 20% of patients with AIDS. As a result of immunosuppression VZV may be reactivated, giving rise to neurological syndromes such as hydrocephalus or ventriculitis. Like VZV, Human cytomegalovirus (HCMV) causes disease after both primary and recurrent infections. The former is more serious, particularly in pregnant women, who may transmit the virus to their offspring, with a high risk of intellectual impairment and deafness. Various experimental vaccines are in development, ranging from live, attenuated HCMV, subunit envelope glycoprotein, poxvirus vectors with CMV genes inserted, and plasmid DNA.

RHABDOVIRIDAE

The family Rhabdoviridae is divided into six genera, including *Lyssavirus*, which contains rabies virus, and *Vesiculovirus*, containing vesicular stomatitis virus (VSV). The name Rhabdoviridae is derived from the Greek 'rhabdos', meaning rod, reflecting the rod or bullet-shaped virus.

Vesiculovirus

While not commonly associated with neurological disorders, *Chandipura*, a vesiculovirus was associated with an outbreak of encephalitis in India in 2003 affecting 349 children with 55% mortality.[108]

Lyssaviruses

The name of this genus is derived from the Greek 'lyssa', meaning rage or frenzy, and includes rabies virus. The Duvenhage and Mokola viruses of this genus are also associated with human disease.

The rabies virus has a helical nucleocapsid with a lipid bilayer from which protrude 10-nm protein spikes. Of the five proteins identified, those designated G and N have been characterized most extensively. The G protein is the only viral protein that induces virus-neutralizing antibody and is also a target for T helper and T cytotoxic lymphocyte reactivity. The importance of such antigenic determination offers an approach for the development of vaccines.

Rabies infections have been recorded since before 2000 BC and mentioned in historical documents of Democritis, Aristaeus and Artemis. Six important events in the history of rabies since the 1880s include the application of the human rabies vaccine (1885) and the finding of the pathognomonic Negri bodies for diagnosis (1903). In the 1940s a mass application of potent rabies vaccine for dogs was introduced, which greatly diminished the spread of disease. More recently the introduction of oral vaccination of foxes has resulted in the virtual elimination of rabies from Switzerland. Rabies hyperimmune antiserum was used in addition to the human vaccine regimen (1954) and the adaptation of rabies virus to cell culture and the development of a fluorescent antibody test for diagnosing infected animal brains (1958) have resulted in a dramatic improvement in the control of the disease.

Epidemiology

Rabies virus is capable of infecting all warm-blooded animals, but there is a hierarchy for susceptibility. Most susceptible are foxes, coyotes, jackals and wolves. The opossum is the least susceptible species. Moderately susceptible animals include dogs, the most frequent vector for transmission to humans, as well as cats, raccoons and skunks. An increasing source of rabies is observed in bat populations[109] and accounts for approximately 10% of rabies-infected animals in the USA. The epidemiology of human rabies parallels that in the animal population. The annual number of deaths worldwide caused by rabies is estimated at approximately 55 000 by the World Health Organization. A higher incidence is observed in areas where public health programmes are not implemented, such as in India and Mexico where the incidence is 3.3 cases per 100 000. Rabies has recently been reported following organ transplantation in four patients.[110]

Pathogenesis

The major route of infection is invariably via the bite from a rabid animal, although transmission by aerosols and as a result of corneal grafts must be taken into account. Once introduced, rabies virus is quickly sequestered. It was thought that the virus stayed in the nervous tissue close to the wound site, although later studies indicated that the virus replicates in muscle tissue before progressing to the peripheral nervous tissue via the neuromuscular connections. That rabies virus travels to the central nervous tissue via the nerves has been demonstrated experimentally: when the sciatic nerve was severed prior to injection of rabies virus in the foot of an animal, disease was prevented. The incubation period of the disease varies and may be as short as 2 weeks but is more commonly 1–3 months, and in a few cases more than 1 year.[111] Although it is widely accepted that the incubation period is related to the distance between the site of the bite and proximity to the CNS, a study by Dupont and Earle[112] did not support this view.

Pathology

Human rabies pathology, apart from the pathognomonic Negri body, consists of perivascular cuffing, some neuronophagia and limited neuronal necrosis. The limited pathology does not match the marked symptoms of hydrophobia, aerophobia, excitation and coma. There is pathology in other organs, and Negri bodies have been found in the cornea and adrenal glands.

Clinical features

Development of infection depends on the severity of the exposure, the site of the bite and possibly other factors. Neurological findings may be classified as either 'furious' or 'paralytic' and are not exclusive. Furious rabies is far more common and is characterized by spasms in response to tactile, auditory, visual and olfactory stimuli (e.g. aerophobia and hydrophobia). Such symptoms alternate with periods of lucidity, agitation, confusion and autonomic dysfunction. The alternative form of paralytic rabies ranges from paralysis of one limb to quadriplegia. Disease progresses to coma with neurological complications associated with abnormal hormonal homeostasis, alterations in temperature and inability to control blood pressure.

Diagnosis

Clinical diagnosis of rabies may be difficult in patients presenting with a paralytic or Guillain–Barré-like syndrome, and the World Health Organization (WHO) Committee on Rabies[113] has emphasized that rabies must be included in the differential diagnosis of all persons presenting with neurological involvement.

The laboratory diagnosis of rabies may be performed by fluorescent antibody techniques, on smears or frozen sections, and by the use of ELISA. A rapid rabies enzyme immunodiagnosis assay allows the antigen to be visualized by the naked eye and is thus a test that can be carried out in the field (with a special test kit). Molecular tests, such as the polymerized chain reaction, are available. Virus isolation can be performed using a murine neuroblastoma cell line (NAC1300), which reduces the time taken for diagnosis by 2 days.

Prevention and control

Rabies is 100% preventable and mortality can be reduced by preventing exposure to the virus, aborting infection and thereby preventing illness, or curing clinical disease. The WHO committee has stressed the importance of the adoption and establishment of international and regional surveillance systems in combination with dog control. In over 80 countries rabies is prevalent in dogs, the most dangerous reservoir. Each year approximately 4 million people in these areas receive treatment after exposure to rabies and in 99% of all human cases the virus is transmitted by dogs. Furthermore, 90% of people who receive postexposure treatment live in areas of canine rabies.[114]

Vaccination

The control of rabies is through oral immunization of domestic and, more recently, wild animals. Recombinant vaccines that make use of poxvirus, baculovirus and adenoviruses are possible. The vaccines available for human immunization are: (1) brain tissue vaccine (possible side-effects of autoreactivity to brain tissue); (2) purified duck embryo vaccine inactivated with b-propiolactone; and (3) tissue culture vaccines. For animal vaccination, nervous tissue-derived virus has been shown to be effective in mass vaccination of the canine population in North Africa. In contrast, cell culture-derived virus (either inactivated or modified live virus) for canine rabies has been used in a combined vaccination programme with distemper, hepatitis, parvo and leptospirosis vaccines. Combined vaccines with foot and mouth vaccine are used for cattle, sheep and goats. For feline control, the rabies vaccine is combined with panleucopenia virus, feline calicivirus and feline parvovirus vaccines.

The vaccine virus is collected from infected human diploid cells (HDC), inactivated, and stored in a freeze-dried state. The vaccine (HDCV) contains no preservatives and must be used immediately once reconstituted.

Monoclonal antibodies

Post exposure treatment with murine monoclonal antibodies, and more recently murine–human chimeric antibodies and humanization of monoclonal antibodies, offers a more specific treatment regimen.

Interferon and interferon inducers

Administration of recombinant α-interferon with vaccines decreases rabies virus in subhuman primates. Exogenous interferon has already been shown to be effective in a patient given a corneal transplant from a patient with rabies.

TOGAVIRIDAE

The family Togaviridae comprises the genera alphaviruses and is based on various characteristics such as size, mode of replication and transmission by mosquitoes. The name togavirus is derived from the structure of the virus which consists of a ribonucleic acid within a lipid envelope (*Latin toga* = coat).

Alphaviruses

The knowledge of the structure and replication of alphaviruses has been based on the prototype virus Sindbis (SIN) as well as Semliki Forest viruses (SFV) which are discussed briefly in this section. Of the alphaviruses that are important encephalitogenic agents, eastern equine encephalitis (EEE), Venezuelan equine encephalitis (VEE) and western equine encephalitis (WEE) viruses are the most important. However, chikungunya virus (CHIK) infection is also known to induce neurological complications (Table 48.3). Other members such as Ross River Virus and O'nyong'nyong induce polyarthritis.

Chikungunya

The word chikungunya, meaning 'to contort or bend', was used by a tribe in Tanzania to describe the clinical manifestations (arthritis) of a virus epidemic of 1952–1953. Because this virus invariably results in crippling arthritis, CHIK infection was probably responsible for the epidemic in 1779 in Indonesia.

Epidemiology

CHIK is found in Africa, including Tanzania, Zimbabwe, Transvaal, Zambia and the Congo, and India, Sri Lanka and South-east Asia, including Vietnam and Thailand.[115] More recently, an outbreak in 2006 on Reunion Island led to over 200 deaths[116] and it has re-emerged in Malaysia in 2007.[117] The disease is transmissible by mosquitoes. *Ae. aegypti* and various *Culex* species are the vectors

in urban epidemics in Asia. In Africa, the vector involved in forest areas is *Ae. africanus* and in Sudan *Ae. leuteocephalus*.

Clinical illness

The disease is biphasic. In the first phase, symptoms include fever and severe joint, limb, and spine pains. This phase can last 6–10 days. The second phase occurs after a febrile period of 2–3 days and is associated with an irritating maculopapular rash over the body, particularly on the extensor surface of the limbs. Joint pains may persist occasionally, without fever, for up to 4 months. In some cases myocarditis and peripheral circulatory failure have been seen. In this second phase, encephalitis and manifestations of neurological involvement are occasionally observed.[118] The mortality rate is estimated at 0.4%, but in patients under 1 year old it may be as high as 2.8% and similarly in those aged over 50 years the death rate may increase.

Diagnosis

Definitive diagnosis is by specific serological analysis such as HI, CF and ELISA and RT PCR[119] although the combination of febrile illness and rheumatic manifestations in a patient returning from sub-Saharan Africa or parts of Asia is a characteristic feature of CHIK infection.

Management and control

Supportive care for patients with CHIK infections is important with respect to the arthralgia. In severe cases, chloroquine phosphate may be administered. Inactivated virus vaccines have been shown to be effective but vaccination is restricted to laboratory workers, although a live attenuated virus is undergoing trials in experimental animals. The live CHIK vaccine TSI-GSD-218 has been reported to be promising in humans.[120]

Eastern equine encephalitis

Epidemiology

Eastern equine encephalitis (EEE) was first isolated in 1933[121] and retrospective studies of epidemics are suggestive of EEE as early as 1931 EEE virus is endemic along the eastern coast of the USA, Canada, Trinidad, Guyana, Mexico, Panama, Brazil, Peru, Columbia and Argentina. In most areas the virus is transmitted between marsh birds and Culiseta melanura mosquitoes, which do not feed on large vertebrates. With alterations in the conditions of the marshes or swamps, the virus is transmitted to other host mosquitoes that feed on small rodents, reptiles and amphibians. *Culex* species are considered to be the vectors for transmission of EEE virus in South America.[122] Human and equine cases are seen only when the spread becomes endemic.

Pathogenesis and pathology

Viraemia occurs soon after infection and may be accompanied by a febrile prodrome. Virus gains access to the nervous system and results in severe encephalitis. HI and neutralizing antibody are present in samples taken during the first 3–5 days of encephalitis.[123] However, this effective humoral immune response does not eradicate the virus from the brain, and neural destruction continues through direct cytopathic effect, inflammatory damage and vasculitis. The primary pathological features of EEE are confined to the CNS.[124] Lesions are scattered throughout the cortex and are particularly severe in basal ganglia and the brainstem; the cerebellum and spinal cord are minimally involved. Virions are present in oligodendrocytes and there is extensive neuronal damage as well as thrombosis of arterioles and venules. Inflammatory cells are widespread in lesions, perivascular areas and meninges. The cells are predominantly polymorphonuclear in the first week, but later mononuclear cells may predominate.

Clinical illness

Human infections are rare. In children the ratio is estimated to be from 2 : 1 to 8 : 1; in adults it is from 4 : 1 to 50 : 1. In severe cases the onset is abrupt, with high fever followed by all the features of meningitis, including coma, convulsions and neurological damage. Age is not a major factor in mortality but severe sequelae are more pronounced in children under 10 years of age.

Diagnosis and investigation

The abrupt onset of a severe febrile CNS illness is suggestive of this disease, and death in horses associated with hot, wet summers and the proximity of salt marshes give further credence to EEE infection.

The virus may be isolated from serum during the initial infection but most cases are diagnosed by testing paired sera in conventional HI or NT. Very high CF titres occur in most people convalescing from EEE. IgM antibodies are readily detected in acute sera by ELISA.[109] Virus may be isolated at autopsy.

Prevention and control

A vaccine inactivated by formalin treatment is available for use in laboratory workers or others at high risk of exposure. The same vaccine is used to protect endangered whooping cranes, which are susceptible to lethal visceral infection.[125]

Venezuelan equine encephalitis

This virus was first isolated by Beck and Wyckoff[126] from equine encephalitis epizootics in Venezuela. Viral strains belonging to the VEE group are pathogenic for horses and have been involved in human infections; the most important are designated subtype 1, variants A, B and C.

Epidemiology

VEE is endemic in Central and South America and parts of North America, and has occurred particularly in Venezuela, Colombia, Equador, Panama, Brazil, Mexico, Florida, Texas and Trinidad. Mosquitoes of both the *Aedes* and *Culex* genera are involved. *Cx. melanoconion* and *Deinocereites* species are the main vectors in rodent-to-rodent transmission. Horses are a major reservoir of infection and transmission of the virus can occur from horse to horse as well as transplacentally. More than 150 different animal species, including domestic and wild dogs and pigs, have been found to be infected with this virus. Birds have low viraemias but could infect mosquitoes, which may spread the disease and cause new epidemics.

Pathogenesis

Conventional serological methods show that the viruses grouped into the VEE complex are all closely related. The viruses in this group were further divided into subtypes and variants by Young et al.[127] using the HI test, and it seems that these minor distinctions are responsible for the fundamental differences in pathogenicity and biochemical significance.

The earliest humoral immune response appears around day 5 in hamsters and is directed to virion surface component. An epitope on E2 is shown to produce the most dominant protective neutralizing antibodies. In the mouse model, cell transfer experiments suggest that T helper lymphocyte activity is important in protection.

Clinical illness

The clinical disease in humans resembles an influenza-like syndrome, with fever lasting for 1–4 days. Occasionally this is complicated by shock and coma, in which case there appears to be widespread destruction of lymphoid tissues. Meningoencephalitis can occur, particularly in children, but is much less common in adults. Approximately 4% of patients develop CNS infections with convulsions, coma and paralysis. The overall mortality is <1% but in children with meningitis this may rise to 20% and is more frequent in undernourished populations and in the absence of medical care.

VEE should be suspected in any person suffering from febrile myalgic illness 6 days after being exposed to an enzootic biotope.

Prevention and control

Patients who develop CNS disease require anti-convulsants. Vaccinia virus recombinants containing genes encoding the VEE virus structural gene regions (C-E3-E2-6 K-E1) protect mice against virulent VEEV, but provide only partial protection against air-borne challenge. VV recombinants encoding the structural genes E3-E2-6 K-E1, E3-E2-6 K or 6 K-E1 also demonstrate the importance of E2 in protection. The experimental vaccine TC-83 is a live attenuated vaccine and the C-84 a formalin inactivated vaccine based on TC-83. Alpha interferon and the interferon producer PolyICLC have proved useful for postexposure prophylaxis.

Western equine encephalitis

Epidemiology

WEE virus is found in the USA but human infections are limited to the western two-thirds of the country. It is also found in Canada, particularly Manitoba, Saskatchewan, Alberta and British Columbia, and in South America. The disease is transmitted by various species of mosquito vectors. These include *Cx. tarsalis*, *Culiseta melanura* and other mosquitoes of these two genera. *Aedes* and *Anopheles* species may be slightly involved. The natural cycle is between *Cx. tarsalis* mosquitoes and wild birds. *Culex* mosquitoes readily feed on large vertebrates, so equine and human cases occur annually. The number of cases is dependent on rainfall because mosquito breeding is largely in ground pools.

Pathogenesis and pathology

The pathogenesis of WEE virus in humans resembles that of EEE. However, WEE is less neuroinvasive and neurovirulent, in both humans and laboratory animals. Infected cynomolgus macaques show multiple foci of necrosis, and cellular infiltrate,[128] found predominantly in areas such as the striatum, globus pallidus, cerebral cortex, thalamus and pons. In some areas polymorphonuclear infiltrates occur. There is widespread perivascular cuffing and meningeal reaction. The pathogenesis in rodents is similar to that of other alphaviruses.

Clinical illness

WEE is characterized by sudden onset of fever, headache and general symptoms of meningoencephalitis which can be clinically severe but rarely fatal. Neurological and psychological sequelae are seen primarily in children under 2 years of age. The ratio of inapparent to apparent clinical infection is estimated at 50 : 1–8 : 1 in children and more than 1000 : 1 in adults.

Prevention and control

Social activities such as screening of windows and doors and avoiding external pursuits are necessary to avoid infection. An inactivated vaccine is available for workers at risk from infection. More recently a DNA vaccine plasmius pVHX-6 has shown some efficacy in rodent infections.[115]

Semliki Forest virus

Although SFV has been assumed not to infect humans, the death of a scientist from whom SFV was isolated may suggest otherwise. More recently mild febrile illness has been reported in humans in Africa and was suggested to be due to SFV. The fact that SFV is known to induce neurological disease in experimental animals, with perivascular infiltrates and demyelination (Figure 48.4), warrants mention of this virus in this chapter. SFV was originally isolated in Uganda in 1944. Experimentally the virus induces encephalitis in a variety of laboratory rodents. Infection of mice with the A7 or M9 strains of SFV gives rise to lesions of demyelination in the CNS.

RUBIVIRUSES

History

The sole member of the rubivirus genus, rubella virus, was initially described in the early 1800s.[129] Although it is primarily a childhood illness, the disease is endemic worldwide and serious complications such as encephalomyelitis and post-infectious encephalopathy have been reported in adults and children. The large number of studies by German scientists have given rubella virus the synonym 'German measles', although the organism is unrelated to measles virus.

Epidemiology

Unlike most other togaviruses, rubella has no known vertebrate host and the only natural reservoir is humans. Rubella virus infections are found worldwide and in the temperate regions the epi-

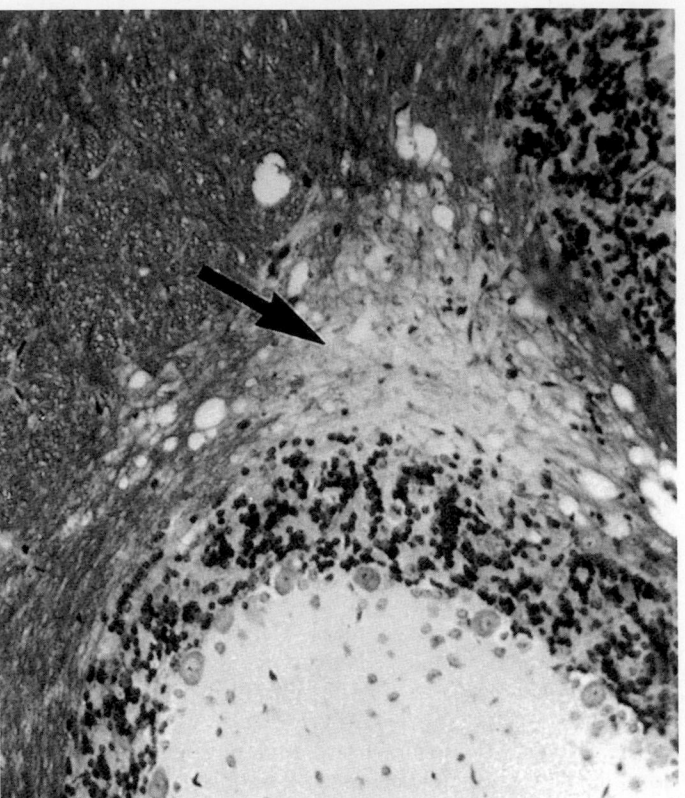

Figure 48.4 Demyelination (arrow) within the cerebellum of a mouse infected with Semliki Forest virus.

demics occur in late winter and early spring. Periods of increased incidence every 6–9 years occur, with major epidemics every 10–30 years. Such epidemics are related to the susceptibility of individuals and factors that increase the transmission. Infection is generally acquired in childhood and approximately 60% of the population have antibodies by the age of 14 years. With the introduction of the rubella vaccine in 1969,[129] the incidence of rubella has decreased, although the seroprevalence rates approach 90–95%. The incidence of infection is higher in the tropics. Postinfectious encephalopathy or encephalomyelitis is estimated to occur in 1 in 6000 cases of natural rubella.

Pathogenesis and pathology

The pathology resulting from rubella infection is dependent on the mode of infection, i.e., whether it is due to maternal–fetal transmission or is acquired postnatally. The effect on the fetus depends on the gestation period. In the first trimester there is a high risk of infection and developmental growth is arrested, although the mechanism of damage is unknown. Maternal infection after the first trimester does not appear to damage the fetus, although the risk of congenital disease is known to increase before birth. Delayed neurological disease has been reported following late-onset rubella infection and may be associated with either congenital rubella or a rare complication of natural rubella acquired in childhood.

The pathological features of CNS involvement, particularly in the adult, include perivascular lesions of mononuclear cells and demyelination. In childhood encephalopathy, neural degeneration is more apparent than in the adult, whereas perivascular infiltrates and demyelination are less common. The suggestion that autoreactivity may play a role in the pathology of late-onset rubella encephalitis, often referred to as progressive rubella panencephalitis, chronic progressive panencephalitis or non-congenital rubella, comes from studies in which lymphocytes proliferate in response to CNS proteins such as myelin basic protein.[130]

Clinical features

Rubella infection in early childhood or adult life is usually mild and asymptomatic. Symptoms of post-infectious rubella encephalopathy are observed shortly after the onset of the rash of typical rubella. The clinical features of encephalitis are similar to those of other forms of encephalitis, including headache, vomiting, stiff neck, fevers and convulsions, and altered levels of consciousness. The mortality rate is approximately 20%, with death occurring within a few days of the onset of symptoms. The late-onset rubella encephalitis is similar to other slow virus infections of the CNS. Following a prolonged asymptomatic period, neural degeneration is observed, usually in the second decade of life. Symptoms include behavioural changes, ataxia and seizures. Death usually results within 8 years of onset.

Diagnosis

The common symptoms of rubella, such as low-grade fever and maculopapular rash, should not be confused with other such infections. Confirmation of rubella may be made following isolation of the virus or by specific serological assays such as ELISA. The CSF cell count of patients with rubella encephalitis is high (50/mm^3); the majority of the cells are lymphocytes. The electroencephalogram is abnormal, oligoclonal bands are observed in the CSF[131] and rubella virus may be isolated.[132]

Management and prevention

Treatment of rubella encephalitis with corticosteroids has been reported.[133] Rubella vaccines, developed in the 1960s, have been used to vaccinate both school-aged children (USA) and women of child-bearing age (UK) in an attempt to decrease the incidence of congenital rubella infection. The attenuated viruses used are capable of infecting the fetus and thus vaccination of pregnant women is not recommended. More recently the policy of including the combined MMR vaccination procedure for all schoolchildren has been implemented in the UK. Future development of subviral vaccines may be necessary to counter the side-effects of vaccination using attenuated virus.

PRION DISEASES

Several so-called 'slow virus infections' of the CNS, although transmissible, are not conventional virus infections but rather classified as prion diseases or subacute spongiform encephalopathies (Table 48.7).

Prion diseases have a unique characteristic in being devoid of nucleic acid and yet able to transfer disease. Transmission of disease does not occur if the agents are treated with proteases.

Table 48.7 Prion disease of humans and animals

Host	Disease
Humans	Kuru
	Creutzfeldt–Jakob Disease, Classic (CJD)
	Variant Creutzfeldt–Jakob Disease (vCJD)
	Gerstmann–Sträussler–Scheinker Syndrome
	Fatal familial insomnia
Animals	Bovine spongiform encephalopathy (BSE)
	Chronic wasting disease of mule deer and elk
	Scrapie
	Transmissible mink encephalopathy
	Feline spongiform encephalopathy
	Ungulate spongiform encephalopathy

Additionally, attempts at molecular cloning are negative and nucleic acid antagonists have been shown to be ineffective. The term prion is derived from *pr*otein and *in*fection, meaning that the infectious agent is protein devoid of nucleic acid. This 'protein only' hypothesis is still under debate.

Of particular importance is the presence of a normal form of the protein found on all cells, particularly neurones. The two forms of prion proteins (PrP) (normal and infectious) are identical in terms of amino acid sequences but differ in their conformations. Furthermore, the normal protein is broken down by enzymes, whereas the abnormal prion protein (PrP^{sc}) is resistant to attack by enzymes and found in the CNS only during disease where the protein accumulates in the cell.

Kuru

Kuru was restricted to the population of villages in the highland of Papua New Guinea. The disease, which means shaking or shivering in the Fore language, is characterized by tremors that progress to lack of motor control and complete cerebellar ataxia. The clinical course of the disease generally results in death within 1 year of onset, although prolonged disease has been reported.[134] The disease was more common in children and females than in males, and was thought to be due to the practice of certain tribal rituals. The changes in ritual cannibalism and treatment of corpses have halted the contact of persons with infected brain tissue, resulting in a virtual cessation in the incidence of disease. In a recent review 11 patients were identified with Kuru between 1999 and 2004; the incubation times have been suggested to be as long as 56 years.[135]

The pathological picture is restricted to the CNS and is characterized by diffuse neuronal degeneration and astrocytic hypertrophy. The term 'spongiform encephalopathy' is derived from the large vacuolation of the large neurones of the striatum. In many cases amyloid-containing plaques are observed and electron microscopy reveals scrapie-associated fibrils common to other diseases in this group.

Creutzfeldt–Jakob disease and Gerstmann–Sträussler–Scheinker syndrome

Patients with Creutzfeldt–Jakob disease (CJD) present with rapidly progressive dementia and motor dysfunction; like Kuru, it is usually fatal within 1–2 years following onset. The incidence of CJD is low (prevalence of 1 per million) and is generally sporadic, although there is evidence for a familial trait in 10% of all cases. Mutations in the natural PrP segregate with disease. The disease is transmissible experimentally, as shown in laboratory animals,[136] or as a result of 'accidental transmission' to humans following surgery.[137] Although the average age of CJD onset is in middle to late life, the disease has been described in young (4–19 years) patients undergoing growth hormone therapy. In these transmissions the disease resembled Kuru rather than typical CJD, suggesting that Kuru may have originated in New Guinea as a result of contamination of tissue from a patient with CJD.

Gerstmann–Sträussler–Scheinker syndrome (GSS) is a variant of CJD in which patients present with progressive cerebellar ataxia, giving rise to a longer period from onset to death compared with CJD. Again, several mutations in the PrP have been described and the disease is transmissible to laboratory animals.

Prevention and control

The resistance of the CJD/GSS prion to common sterilization procedures, such as boiling or the use of ultraviolet light, has resulted in a change in operating procedures and the use of hypochlorate and sodium hydroxide for sterilization.[138] To date, no treatment for the human diseases has been effective. Future therapeutic regimens will possibly include drugs that interfere with the PrP^{sc}, preventing it from accumulating in the cell, or gene therapy to switch off production of the protein.

More recently, studies directed towards blocking infective prion protein migration have been seen to be dependent on B-cells. In addition, therapeutic strategies using antibodies directed against the conformational forms of PrP are currently under investigation.

Animal prion diseases

Scrapie was observed in the 1930s following the use of louping ill virus vaccine produced in scrapie-contaminated brain tissue, although the disease has been recognized in sheep breeders for more than two centuries. The disease is a chronic disease in which affected animals present with progressive ataxia tremor and wasting. The name 'scrapie' is derived from the necessity of animals to rub or scrape as a result of the disease. Susceptibility to scrapie is dependent on the strain of sheep and is linked to polymorphisms in ovine PrP.

The disease, like the human prion infections, is characterized histologically by the presence of vacuolated neurones and spongiform changes, and may be induced experimentally in laboratory mice and guinea pigs. The use of transgenic mice, in which mutations in the PrP are deliberately introduced with resulting neurological defect, supports the role of this protein in initiating disease. Furthermore, transgenic mice lacking the gene that codes for the natural PrP are resistant to infection with the scrapie PrP.[139] The use of experimental prion disease has allowed the investigation of potential therapies and, although no effective treatment is available, the use of amphotericin B has been shown to reduce the concentration of scrapie PrP during the preclinical phase and to prolong the incubation period of the disease.[140]

Transmissible mink encephalopathy, which is very similar to scrapie, is spread through mink colonies as a result of fighting and cannibalism, and is thought to have originated from contaminated food derived from cattle. Infected tissue can transfer disease. Likewise bovine spongiform encephalopathy, first described in England in 1986, was possibly a result of feeding scrapie-contaminated food.[141]

REFERENCES

1. Berger JR, Nath A. *Clinical Neurovirology.* New York: Marcel Dekker; 2003.
2. Knipe DM, Howley PM, Griffin DE, et al. *Fields Virology.* 5th edn. Philadelphia: Lippincott Williams & Wilkins; 2007.
3. Mori I, Nishiyama Y, Yokochi T, et al. Olfactory transmission of neurotropic viruses. *J Neurovirol* 2005; 11:129–137.
4. Maslin CL, Kedzierska K, Webster NL, et al. Transendothelial migration of monocytes: the underlying molecular mechanisms and consequences of HIV-1 infection. *Curr HIV Res* 2005; 3:303–317.
5. Webb HE, Parsons LM. Treatment of the postviral fatigue syndrome-rationale for the use of antidepressants. In: Jenkins R, Mowbray J, eds. *Post Viral Fatigue Syndrome.* New York: Wiley; 1991:297–303.
6. Levine B, Hardwick JM, Trapp BD, et al. Antibody-mediated clearance of alphavirus infection from neurons. *Science* 1991; 254:856–860.
7. Mazarakis ND, Azzouz M, Rohll JB, et al. Rabies virus glycoprotein pseudotyping of lentiviral vectors enables retrograde axonal transport and access to the nervous system after peripheral delivery. *Hum Mol Genet* 2001; 10:2109–2121.
8. Amor S, Scallan MF, Morris MM, et al. Role of immune responses in protection and pathogenesis during Semliki Forest virus encephalitis. *J Gen Virol* 1996; 77:281–291.
9. Sauter C, Sauter BV. LCMV transmission by organ transplantation. *N Engl J Med* 2006; 355:1737.
10. Jamieson DJ, Kourtis AP, Bell M, et al. Lymphocytic choriomeningitis virus: an emerging obstetric pathogen? *Am J Obstet Gynecol* 2006; 194:1532–1536.
11. Warkel RL, Rinaldi DF, Bancroft WH, et al. Fatal acute meningoencephalitis due to lymphocytic choriomeningitis virus. *Neurology* 1973; 23:198–203.
12. Gunther S, Lenz O. Lassa virus. *Crit Rev Clin Lab Sci* 2004; 41:339–390.
13. Monath TP, Casals J. Diagnosis of Lassa fever and the isolation and management of patients. *Bull World Health Organ* 1975; 52:707–715.
14. Walker DH, McCormick JB, Johnson KM, et al. Pathologic and virologic study of fatal Lassa fever in man. *Am J Pathol* 1982; 107:349–356.
15. Fisher-Hoch SP, McCormick JB. Towards a human Lassa fever vaccine. *Rev Med Virol* 2001; 11:331–341.
16. McCormick JB, King IJ, Webb PA, et al. Lassa fever. Effective therapy with ribavirin. *N Engl J Med* 1986; 314:20–26.
17. Soldan SS, Gonzalez-Scarano F. Emerging infectious diseases: the Bunyaviridae. *J Neurovirol* 2005; 11:412–423.
18. Thompson WH, Kalfayan B, Anslow RO. Isolation of Californian encephalitis group virus from a fatal human illness. *Am J Epidemiol* 1965; 81:245–253.
19. McJunkin JE, de los Reyes EC, Irazuzta JE, et al. Crosse encephalitis in children. A. *N Engl J Med* 2001; 344:801–807.
20. Grimstad PR, Craig GB, Ross QE, et al. Aedes triseriatus and La Crosse virus: geographical variation in vector susceptibility and ability to transmit. *Am J Trop Med Hyg* 1977; 26:990–996.
21. Artsob H. Distribution of California serogroups and virus infection in Canada. In: Calisher CH, Thompson WH, eds. *California Serogroup Viruses.* New York: Alan R Liss; 1983:277–292.
22. Meegan JM. The Rift Valley fever epizootic in Egypt 1977–1978. 1. Description of the epizootic and virological studies. *Trans R Soc Trop Med Hyg* 1979; 73:618–623.
23. Maar SA, Swanepoel R, Gelfand M. Rift Valley fever encephalitis. A description of a case. *Cent Afr J Med* 1979; 25:8–11.
24. Lampert PW, Sims JK, Kniazeff AJ. Mechanism of demyelination in JHM virus encephalomyelitis. Electron microscopic studies. *Acta Neuropathol (Berl)* 1973; 24:76–85.

25. Lau KK, Yu W C, Chu CM, et al. Possible central nervous system infection by SARS coronavirus. *Emerg Infect Dis* 2004; 10:342–344.

26. Gritsun TS, Lashkevich VA, Gould EA. Tick-borne encephalitis. *Antiviral Res* 2003; 57:129–146.

27. Centers for Disease Control and Prevention (CDC). Adverse events associated with 17D-derived yellow fever vaccination – United States, 2001–2002. *MMWR* 2002; 51:989–993.

28. Kalita J, Misra. UK EEG in dengue virus infection with neurological manifestations: a clinical and CT/MRI correlation. *Clin Neurophysiol* 2006; 117:2252–2256.

29. Gould EA, Higgs S, Buckley A, et al. Potential arbovirus emergence and implications for the United Kingdom. *Emerg Infect Dis* 2006; 12: 549–555.

30. Hsu TC, Hsu ST. Supplementary report. Effectiveness of Japanese encephalitis vaccine. Study in the second year following immunisation. In: Hammon W McD, Kitaoka M, Downs WG, eds. *Immunisation for Japanese Encephalitis.* Baltimore: Williams & Williams; 1971:266–267.

31. Srivastava AK, Putnak JR, Lee SH, et al. A purified inactivated Japanese encephalitis virus vaccine made in Vero cells. *Vaccine* 2001; 19:4557–4565.

32. Huang CH. Studies of Japanese encephalitis in China. *Adv Virus Res* 1982; 27:71–101.

33. Burrow JN, Whelan PI, Kilburn CJ, et al. Australian encephalitis in the Northern Territory: clinical and epidemiological features, 1987–1996. *Aust N Z J Med* 1998; 28:590–596.

34. Finley K, Riggs N. Convalescence and sequelae. In: Monath TP, ed. *St Louis Encephalitis.* Washington, DC: APHA; 1980:535–550.

35. Davis LE, DeBiasi R, Goade DE, et al. West Nile virus neuroinvasive disease. *Ann Neurol* 2006; 60:286–300.

36. de Souza Lopes O, de Abreu Sacchetta L, Coimbra TL, et al. Emergence of a new arbovirus disease in Brazil. II. Epidemiological studies on 1975 epidemic. *Am J Epidemiol* 1978; 108:394–401.

37. Rosenberg S. Neuropathology of Sao Paulo south coast epidemic encephalitis (Rocio encephalitis). *J Neurol Sci* 1980; 45:1–12.

38. Pudney M, Varma MGR. The growth of some tick-borne arboviruses in cell cultures derived from tadpoles of the common frog, Rana temporaria. *J Gen Virol* 1971; 10:131–138.

39. Shope RE. Medical significance of togaviruses: an overview of diseases caused by togaviruses in man and in domestic and wild vertebrate animals. In: Schlesinger RW, ed. *The Togaviruses: Biology, Structure, Replication.* New York: Academic Press; 1980:47–82.

40. Chiba N, Iwasaki T, Mizutani T, et al. Pathogenicity of tick-borne encephalitis virus isolated in Hokkaido, Japan in mouse model. *Vaccine* 1999; 17:779–787.

41. Logar M, Bogovic P, Cerar D, et al. Tick-borne encephalitis in Slovenia from 2000 to 2004: comparison of the course in adult and elderly patients. *Wien Klin Wochenschr* 2006; 118:702–707.

42. Zent O, Broker M. Tick-borne encephalitis vaccines: past and present. *Expert Rev Vaccines* 2005; 4:747–755.

43. Davidson MM, Williams H, Macleod JA. Louping ill in man: a forgotten disease. *J Infect* 1991; 23:241–249.

44. Kleinschmidt-DeMasters BK, Gilden DH. The expanding spectrum of herpesvirus infections of the nervous system. *Brain Pathol* 2001; 11: 440–451.

45. Skoldenberg B. Herpes simplex encephalitis. *Scand J Infect Dis Suppl* 1996; 100:8–13.

46. Burgos JS, Ramirez C, Guzman-Sanchez F, et al. Hematogenous vertical transmission of herpes simplex virus type 1 in mice. *J Virol* 2006; 80: 2823–2831.

47. Kennedy PG. Viral encephalitis. *J Neurol* 2005; 252:268–272.

48. Mohamedi SA, Heath AW, Jennings R. A comparison of oral and parenteral routes for therapeutic vaccination with HSV-2 ISCOMs in mice; cytokine profiles, antibody responses and protection. *Antiviral Res* 2001; 49:83–99.

49. Weller TH, Stoddard MB. Intranuclear inclusion bodies in cultures of human tissue inoculated with varicella vesicle fluid. *J Immunol* 1952; 68:311–319.

50. Johnson R, Milborne PE. Central nervous system manifestations of chickenpox. *Can Med Assoc J* 1970; 102:831–834.

51. Applebaum E, Rachelson MH, Dolgopol VB. Varicella encephalitis. *Am J Med* 1953; 15:223–230.

52. Heppleston JD, Paerch KM, Yates PO. Varicella encephalitis. *Arch Dis Child* 1959; 34:318–321.

53. Gilden D. Varicella zoster virus and central nervous system syndromes. *Herpes* 2004; 11(suppl 2):89A–94A.

54. Centers for Disease Control. Herpes B encephalitis – California. *MMWR* 1973; 22(40):333–334.

55. Vizoso AD. Latency of herpes simiae (B virus) in rabbits. *Br J Exp Pathol* 1975; 56:489–494.

56. Buthala DA. Hyperimmunised horse anti-B virus globulin: preparation and effectiveness. *J Infect Dis* 1962; 111:101–106.

57. Boulter EA, Thornton B, Bauer EJ, et al. Successful treatment of experimental B virus (herpesvirus simiae) infection with acyclovir. *BMJ* 1980; 280:681–683.

58. Delorme L, Middleton PJ. Influenza A virus associated with acute encephalopathy. *Am J Dis Child* 1979; 133:822–824.

59. Ravenholt RT, Foege WH. Before our time. 1918 influenza, encephalitis lethargica, parkinsonism. *Lancet* 1982; ii:860–864.

60. McKinney WP, Volkert P, Kaufman J. Fatal swine influenza pneumonia during late pregnancy. *Arch Intern Med* 1990; 150:213–215.

61. Randolph VL, Heath CW Jr. Influenza during pregnancy in relation to subsequent childhood leukemia and lymphoma. *Am J Epidemiol* 1974; 100:399–409.

62. Huang SM, Chen CC, Chiu PC, et al. Acute necrotizing encephalopathy of childhood associated with influenza type B virus infection in a 3-year-old girl. *J Child Neurol* 2004; 19:64–67.

63. Consensus Development Conference at National Institutes of Health. Amantadine: does it have a role in the prevention and treatment of influenza? *Ann Intern Med* 1980; 92:256–258.

64. Zlydnikov DM, Kubar OI, Kovaleva TP, et al. Study of rimantadine in the USSR: a review of the literature. *Rev Infect Dis* 1981; 3: 408–421.

65. Dolin R, Reichman RC, Madore HP, et al. A controlled trial of amantadine and rimantadine in the prophylaxis of influenza A infection. *N Engl J Med* 1982; 307:580–584.

66. Anon. Oseltamivir: new indication. Prevention of influenza in at-risk children: vaccination is best. *Prescrire Int* 2007; 16:9–11.

67. Gardner S. The new human papovaviruses: their nature and significance. In: Waterson AP, ed. *Recent Advances in Clinical Virology.* New York: Churchill Livingstone; 1977:93–115.

68. Doerries K. Human polyomavirus JC and BK persistent infection. *Adv Exp Med Biol* 2006; 577:102–116.

69. Berger JR, Houff S. Progressive multifocal leukoencephalopathy: lessons from AIDS and natalizumab. *Neurol Res* 2006; 28:299–305.

70. Flaegstad T, Sundsfjord A, Arthur AA, et al. Amplification and sequencing of the control regions of BK and JC virus from human urine by polymerase chain reaction. *Virology* 1991; 180:553–560.

71. Lee MS, Nokes DJ, Hsu HM, et al. Protective titres of measles neutralising antibody. *J Med Virol* 2000; 62:511–517.

72. Krugman S, Katz SL, Gershon AA, et al. Measles (rubeola). In: Mosby CV, ed. *Infectious Diseases of Children.* St Louis: Mosby; 1985:152–166.

73. Markowitz LE, Chandler FW, Roldan EO, et al. Fatal measles pneumonia without rash in a child with AIDS. *J Infect Dis* 1988; 158:480–483.

74. Font RL, Jenis EH, Tuck KD. Measles maculopathy associated with subacute sclerosing panencephalitis. *Arch Pathol* 1973; 96:168–174.

75. Pinkerton H, Smiley WL, Anderson WAD. Giant cell pneumonia with inclusions: lesion common to Hecht's disease, distemper and measles. *Am J Pathol* 1945; 21:1–23.

76. Fleischer B, Kreth HW. Clonal expansion and functional analysis of virus-specific T lymphocytes from cerebrospinal fluid in measles encephalitis. *Hum Immunol* 1983; 7:239.

77. Kleiman BM, Blackburn LK, Zimmerman ES, et al. Comparison of enzyme linked immunosorbent assay for acute measles with hemagglutination inhibition, complement fixation and fluorescent antibody methods. *J Clin Microbiol* 1981; 14:147–152.

78. Vandvik B, Norrby E. Oligoclonal IgG antibody response in the central nervous system to different measles virus antigens in subacute sclerosing panencephalitis. *Proc Natl Acad Sci USA* 1973; 70:1060–1063.

79. Moss WJ, Griffin DE. Global measles elimination. *Nat Rev Microbiol* 2006; 4:900–908.

80. Raine CS. On the development of CNS lesions in natural canine distemper encephalomyelitis. *J Neurol Sci* 1976; 30:13–28.

81. Cook SD, Dowling PC, Russell WC. Neutralising antibody to canine distemper and measles virus in multiple sclerosis. *J Neurol Sci* 1979; 41:61–70.

82. Hamilton R. An account of a distemper, by the common people in England, vulgarly called the mumps. *London Med J* 1790; 11:190–211.

83. Galazka AM, Robertson SE, Kraigher A. Mumps and mumps vaccine: a global review. *Bull World Health Organ* 1999; 77:3–14.

84. Koskiniemi M, Donner M, Pettay O. Clinical appearance and outcome in mumps encephalitis in children. *Acta Paediatr Scand* 1983; 72:603–609.

85. Wilfert CM. Mumps meningoencephalomyelitis with low cerebrospinal-fluid glucose, prolonged pleocytosis and elevation of protein. *N Engl J Med* 1969; 280:855–859.

86. Taylor FB, Toreson WE. Primary mumps meningoencephalitis. *Arch Intern Med* 1963; 112:114–119.

87. Lindsay JR, Davey PR, Ward PH. Inner ear pathology in deafness due to mumps. *Ann Otol Rhinol Laryngol* 1960; 69:918–935.

88. Spataro RF, Lin SR, Horner FA, et al. Aqueductal stenosis and hydrocephalus: rare sequelae of mumps virus infection. *Neuroradiology* 1976; 12:11–13.

89. Thompson JA. Mumps: a case of acquired aqueductal stenosis. *J Paediatr* 1979; 94:923–924.

90. Bonnet MC, Dutta A, Weinberger C, et al. Mumps vaccine virus strains and aseptic meningitis. *Vaccine* 2006; 24:7037–7045.

91. Bilge I, Sadikoglu B, Emre S, et al. Central nervous system vasculitis secondary to parvovirus B19 infection in a pediatric renal transplant patient. *Pediatr Nephrol* 2005; 20:529–533.

92. Landsteiner K, Popper E. Ubertragung der Poliomyelitis acuta auf Affen. *Z Immunitatsforsch Orig* 1909; 2:377–390.

93. Lahariya C, Pradhan SK. Prospects of eradicating poliomyelitis by 2007: compulsory vaccination may be a strategy. *Indian J Pediatr* 2007; 74:61–63.

94. Melnick JL. Current status of poliovirus infections. *Clin Microbiol Rev* 1996; 9:293–300.

95. Salk J, Salk D. Control of influenza and poliomyelitis with killed virus vaccines. *Science* 1977; 195:834–837.

96. Furesz J. Developments in the production and quality control of poliovirus vaccines – historical perspectives. *Biologicals* 2006; 34:87–90.

97. Melnick JL. Enterovirus type 71 infections: a varied clinical pattern sometimes mimicking paralytic poliomyelitis. *Rev Infect Dis* 1984; 6:387–390.

98. Cam S, Ertem D, Koroglu OA, et al. Hepatitis A virus infection presenting with seizures. *Pediatr Infect Dis J* 2005; 24:652–653.

99. Attoui H, Mohd Jaafar F, de Micco P, et al. Coltiviruses and seadornaviruses in North America, Europe, and Asia. *Emerg Infect Dis* 2005; 11:1673–1679.

100. Bowen GS, McLean RG, Shriner RB, et al. The ecology of Colorado tick fever in Rocky Mountain National Park in 1974. II. Infection in small mammals. *Am J Trop Med Hyg* 1981; 30:490–496.

101. Sigurdsson B. Observations on three slow infections of sheep, maedi, paratuberculosis, rida, a slow encephalitis of sheep with general remarks on infections which develop slowly and some of their special characteristics. *Br Vet J* 1954; 110:255–270.

102. Nathanson N, Georgsson G, Lutley R, et al. Pathogenesis of visna in Icelandic sheep: demyelinating lesions and antigenic drift. In: Mims CA, Cuzner ML, Kelly RE, eds. *Viruses and Demyelinating Diseases*. London: Academic Press; 1983:111–124.

103. Straub OC. Maedi-Visna virus infection in sheep. History and present knowledge. *Comp Immunol Microbiol Infect Dis* 2004; 27:1–5.

104. Riedel DJ, Pardo CA, McArthur J, et al. Therapy Insight: CNS manifestations of HIV-associated immune reconstitution inflammatory syndrome. *Nat Clin Pract Neurol* 2006; 2:557–565.

105. Everall IP, Hansen LA, Masliah E. The shifting patterns of HIV encephalitis neuropathology. *Neurotox Res* 2005; 8:51–61.

106. Heidenrich F, Arendt G, Jander S, et al. Serum and cerebrospinal fluid levels of soluble intercellular adhesion molecule 1 (sICAM) in patients with HIV associated neurological diseases. *J Neuroimmunol* 1994; 52:117–126.

107. Okamoto M, Ono M, Baba M. Suppression of cytokine production and neural cell death by the anti-inflammatory alkaloid cepharanthine: a potential agent against HIV-1 encephalopathy. *Biochem Pharmacol* 2001; 62:747–753.

108. Rao BL, Basu A, Wairagkar NS, et al. A large outbreak of acute encephalitis with high fatality rate in children in Andhra Pradesh, India, in 2003, associated with Chandipura virus. *Lancet* 2004; 364:869–874.

109. Calisher CH, El-Kafrawi AO, Al-Deen Mahmud MI, et al. Complex-specific immunoglobulin M antibody patterns in humans infected with alphaviruses. *J Clin Microbiol* 1986; 23:155–159.

110. Burton EC, Burns DK, Opatowsky MJ, et al. Rabies encephalomyelitis: clinical, neuroradiological, and pathological findings in 4 transplant recipients. *Arch Neurol* 2005; 62:873–882.

111. Dietzschold B, Schnell M, Koprowski H. Pathogenesis of rabies. *Curr Top Microbiol Immunol* 2005; 292:45–56.

112. Dupont JR, Earle KM. Human rabies encephalitis: a study of forty-nine cases with a review of the literature. *Neurology* 1966; 15:1023–1034.

113. WHO Expert Committee on Rabies. *WHO Tech Rep Ser* 1992; 824:1–84.

114. Rupprecht CE, Willoughby R, Slate D. Current and future trends in the prevention, treatment and control of rabies. *Expert Rev Anti Infect Ther* 2006; 4:1021–1038.

115. Nagata LP, Hu W G, Masri SA, et al. Efficacy of DNA vaccination against western equine encephalitis virus infection. *Vaccine* 2005; 23:2280–2283.

116. Pialoux G, Gauzere BA, Strobel M. Chikungunya virus infection: review through an epidemic. *Med Mal Infect* 2006; 36(5):253–263.

117. AbuBakar S, Sam IC, Wong PF, et al. Reemergence of endemic Chikungunya, Malaysia. *Emerg Infect Dis* 2007; 13:147–149.

118. Halstead SB, Nimmannitya S, Margiotta MR. Dengue and Chikungunya virus infection in man in Thailand 1962–1964. Observations on disease in out-patients. *Am J Trop Med Hyg* 1969; 18:972–978.

119. Parida MM, Santhosh SR, Dash PK, et al. Rapid and real-time detection of Chikungunya virus by reverse transcription loop-mediated isothermal amplification assay. *J Clin Microbiol* 2007; 45:351–357.

120. Edelman R, Tacket CO, Wasserman SS, et al. Phase II safety and immunogenicity study of live chikungunya virus vaccine TSI-GSD-218. *Am J Trop Med Hyg* 2000; 62:681–685.

121. Hayes RO. Eastern and western encephalitis. In: Steele JH, Beran GW, eds. *Handbook Series in Zoonoses, Section B: Viral Zoonoses*. Vol. 1. Boca Raton: CRC Press; 1981:29–57.

122. Downs WG, Aitkin THG, Spence L. Eastern equine encephalitis virus isolated from Culex nigripalpus in Trinidad. *Science* 1959; 130:1471.

123. Goldfield M, Taylor BF, Welsh JN. The 1959 outbreak of eastern encephalitis in New Jersey. 3. Serological studies of clinical cases. *Am J Epidemiol* 1968; 87:18–22.

124. Bastain FO, Wende RD, Singer DB, et al. Eastern equine encephalitis. Histopathological and ultrastructural changes with isolation of the virus in a human case. *Am J Clin Pathol* 1975; 64:10–13.

125. Strizki JM, Repik PM. Differential reactivity of immune sera from human vaccinees with field strains of eastern equine encephalitis virus. *Am J Trop Med Hyg* 1995; 53:564–570.

126. Beck CE, Wyckoff RWG. Venezuelan equine encephalomyelitis. *Science* 1938; 88:530.

127. Young NA, Johnson KM, Gauld LW. Viruses of the Venezuelan equine encephalomyelitis complex. *Am J Trop Med Hyg* 1969; 18:290–296.

128. Reed DS, Larsen T, Sullivan LJ, et al. Aerosol exposure to western equine encephalitis virus causes fever and encephalitis in cynomolgus macaques. *J Infect Dis* 2005; 192:1173–1182.

129. Polk BF, Modlin JF, White JA. A controlled comparison of joint reactions among women receiving one of two rubella vaccines. *Am J Epidemiol* 1982; 115:19–25.

130. Johnson RT, Griffin DE, Hirsch RL, et al. Measles encephalomyelitis – clinical and immunological studies. *N Engl J Med* 1984; 310:137–141.

131. Vandvik B, Weil ML, Grandien M, et al. Progressive rubella panencephalitis: synthesis of oligoclonal virus-specific IgC antibodies and homogenous free light chains in the central nervous system. *Acta Neurol Scand* 1978; 57: 53–64.

132. Squadrini F, Taparelli F, DeRienzo B, et al. Rubella virus isolation from cerebrospinal fluid in postnatal rubella encephalitis. *BMJ* 1977; ii:1329–1330.

133. Neveh Y, Friedman A. Rubella panencephalitis successfully treated with corticosteroids. *Clin Pediatr* 1975; 22:143–148.

134. Gajdusek DC. Kuru. *Trans R Soc Trop Med Hyg* 1963; 57:151–169.

135. Collinge J, Whitfield J, McKintosh E, et al. Kuru in the 21st century – an acquired human prion disease with very long incubation periods. *Lancet* 2006; 367:2068–2074.

136. Gajdusek DC, Gibbs CJ Jr. Transmission of two subacute spongiform encephalopathies of man (kuru and Creuzfeldt-Jakob disease) to New World monkeys. *Nature* 1971; 230:588–591.

137. Anonymous. Rapidly progressive dementia in a patient who received cadaveric dura mater graft. *MMWR* 1987; 36:49–50.

138. Brown P, Rohwer RG, Gajdusek DC. Sodium hydroxide decontamination of Creutzfeldt-Jakob disease virus. *N Engl J Med* 1984; 310:727.

139. Weissmann C, Bueler H, Fischer M, et al. Susceptibility to scrapie in mice is dependent on PrPC. *Philos Trans R Soc Lond [Biol]* 1994; 343: 431–433.

140. Amor S, Mehta S. Prions, viruses and antiviral drugs. *Lancet* 1993; 342:545.

141. Ferguson-Smith MA. BSE and variant CJD. Assumption that BSE originated from scrapie in sheep led to misjudgment. *BMJ* 2001; 322:1544–1545.

Chapter 49

George O. Cowan, Göran Friman and
Göran Günther

Rickettsial Infections

The typhus group and 'spotted' fevers are caused by bacteria of the family *Rickettsiaceae*,[1] which are obligate, intracellular, Gram-negative, non-flagellate small pleomorphic coccobacilli (0.3–0.6 × 0.8–2.0 μm). Rickettsiae are often carried to humans by insects from animal reservoirs or by the insects themselves, in which the bacteria may be maintained transovarially.

The species of the genus *Rickettsia* are divided into:

* The typhus group, containing *R. prowazekii*, the agent of classical epidemic typhus transmitted by the human body louse, and *R. typhi* (*mooseri*), the cause of endemic murine typhus carried by the rat and rat fleas.
* The 'spotted fever' group (SFGR), containing a large number of species (*R. rickettsii*, *R. conorii*, *R. africae*, etc.) transmitted from rodents and other animals by ticks (except *R. akari*, which is transmitted by mouse mites).
* Scrub typhus, caused by *Orientia tsutsugamushi* and transmitted by mite larvae (chiggers) of the genus *Trombicula*.

The genus previously named *Rochalimaea* has been reclassified in the family *Bartonellaceae*[2] and contains more than 20 named species, several of which have been implicated in human disease, including *Bartonella quintana*, the cause of trench fever, *B. henselae*, the agent of cat-scratch disease, and *B. vinsoni* and *B. elisabethae*, both being occasional causes of endocarditis. (South American bartonellosis caused by *B. bacilliformis* is described in Chapter 61.)

Coxiella burnetii, the only species of its genus, causes Q fever.

The tribe Ehrlichieae has been reclassified into four genera: *Ehrlichia* and *Anaplasma* associated with ticks; *Neorickettsia* with helminths; and *Wolbachia* with both arthropods and helminths.[3] For instance, *E. chaffeensis* and *A. phagocytophila* can cause disease in humans, whereas *Neorickettsia* and *Wolbachia* spp. have not been associated with human disease.

HISTORY

'Typhus' is derived from *tyfos*, the ancient Greek word for 'fever with stupor' or 'smoke', cognate with the Sanskrit word for 'smoke', dhupa.

The earliest reference to epidemic typhus is in the account by Thucydides of the Great Plague of Athens in 430 BC, although a recent medical historian has deemed measles or smallpox to be more likely causes.[4] The historical centres of the disease were in the Middle East, North Africa and the Levant. In the eleventh century AD, epidemics occurred in Sicily and Bohemia, but it was not until siege warfare on a large scale became common in the late fifteenth century that epidemics spread through armies to the civilian population.

The earliest medical accounts of typhus were written by Cardano[5] and Fracastoro[6] from Venice.

Epidemics flourished in Europe in the armies of the Thirty Years' War (1618–1648). In the eighteenth century, physicians recognized that armies, ships and prisons were fertile sources of 'spotted' fever.

Damaging outbreaks of typhus occurred on both sides in the American War of Independence in 1776 and in Napoleon's Grand Army in Russia in 1812. Notably, *R. prowazeki* DNA was recently found by PCR in the dental pulps of French soldiers buried in Vilnius at that time.[7]

Gerhard in 1832 in Philadelphia first described the pathological differences between typhus and typhoid fevers.

Cober[8] proposed in 1685 that the body louse was involved in the spread of typhus, which was proven by Nicolle[9–12] in 1910. Da Rocha Lima (1916)[13] described the organism and proposed the name *Rickettsia prowazekii* to honour Howard Taylor Ricketts and Stanislaus von Prowazek, who had both recently died from typhus acquired during their research efforts.

Louse-borne typhus caused large epidemics in the First World War in Serbia, Poland, eastern Germany and Mesopotamia, and in the Second World War in the Balkans, Naples, Russia and Germany, especially in the concentration camps at Belsen, Auschwitz and Buchenwald.

Flea-borne (murine) typhus had been described in Mexico in 1570 by Bravo,[14] and the complicating myocarditis was to kill Ricketts there in 1910. It was described clinically in grain silo workers in South Australia by Hone in 1923, but the final bacteriological separation from *R. prowazekii* did not occur until studies by Maxcy (1926)[15] and Mooser (1928),[16] the organism being named *R. mooseri* or *R. typhi*.

Earlier work by Ricketts was on Rocky Mountain spotted fever (RMSF), which had first been described in 1872 in the Bitter Root Valley of western Montana and on the Snake River in Idaho in the USA.[17] He identified the causative organism in 1906, and demonstrated that ticks were its vector,[18] the first bacterial disease proved to be transmitted by an insect. The organism was named *R. rickettsii*.

Old World tick-borne typhus was not described until 1910, by Conor and Bruch[19] in Tunisia. The species was named *R. conorii*.

Scrub typhus, or Japanese river fever, was known in Japanese folklore to be associated with the jungle mite or chigger, which was named 'dangerous bug' (tsutsu ga mushi). The illness was described by Hashimoto in 1810 and again in 1879 by Baelz and Kawakami.[20]

In 1925 the disease was reported in Malaya,[21] and in 1931 Ogata[22] isolated the organism and named it *Orientia tsutsugamushi*.

Trench fever was first described in 1915 in soldiers on the Western Front, and in 1916 in the Volhynia region of Poland.[23] Töpfer (1916)[24] isolated the organism from body lice. It was named *Rochalimaea quintana*, later changed to *Bartonella quintana*. In 1992, Regnery et al. found *Rochalimaea henselae*, currently *Bartonella henselae*, to be implicated in cat-scratch disease and characterized the organism,[25,26] which can also cause other serious conditions, particularly in immunocompromised persons, including AIDS patients. Cats seem to be the most important reservoir for *B. henselae*, which exists on all continents. Almost 20 additional *Bartonella* species have so far been described, less than half of which are currently suspected or proven causes of disease.

Rickettsialpox was described in New York State, by Sussman[27] in 1946 and the organism was named *R. akari*.

Q fever (query fever) was reported by Derrick[28] in abattoir workers in Brisbane, Australia, in 1937, and the organism subsequently named *Coxiella burnetii*.

The earliest crude vaccine against *R. typhi* was made by Weigl in 1924 and used widely until a purified version devised by Cox and Bell[29] in 1940 superseded it for use against epidemic and endemic typhus. Fulton and Joyner[30] in 1945 developed a vaccine for scrub typhus. In 1947, chloramphenicol was introduced for treatment and prophylaxis, initially for scrub typhus in Malaya, and soon the tetracyclines were found to be effective in all types of typhus, both these drug classes remaining in use today, generally with doxycycline as the first choice.

PATHOGENESIS

The rickettsial diseases consist of acute fevers accompanied by general constitutional symptoms and especially by headache and, in severe cases, neurological disturbances, and often by a skin rash, either macular or haemorrhagic. Other complications, such as myocarditis, pneumonia and renal insufficiency may also occur. In some types of rickettsiosis the site of inoculation may form a characteristic skin ulcer with a black crust (eschar).

The rickettsial pathogenesis is not explained in detail. There is a lack of evidence as to whether all results found in vitro also apply in vivo. The rickettsial transmission occurs by inoculation from feeding ticks, by deposition through scratches of infected faeces from lice or fleas, or by inhalation of dry faeces in aerosol. The portal of entry is thus through the skin, mucosal membranes (e. g. the conjunctiva) or respiratory tract. The spread is believed to occur via lymphatic vessels at the entry site to regional lymph nodes (still under debate) and then by the bloodstream throughout the body. The target cells are endothelial cells, macrophages

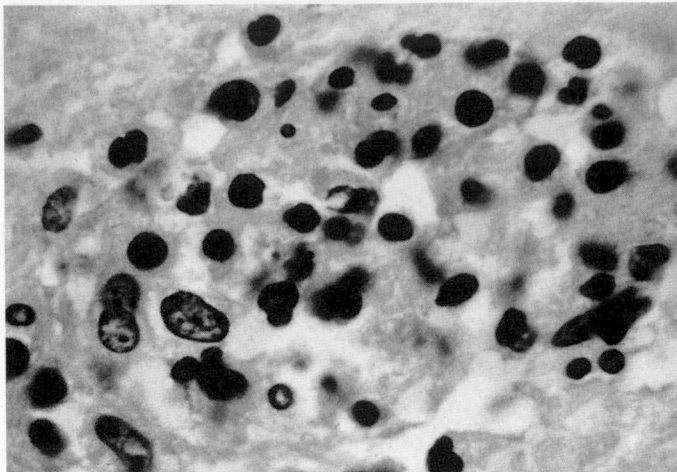

Figure 49.1 Typhus, or Wohlbach's nodule.

and, presumably, hepatocytes. Endothelial cells become denuded, and viable infected endothelial cells circulate during human rickettsioses. They may provide a protective vehicle for rickettsiae so that they can establish new foci of infection in the capillaries where they lodge. Disseminated infection of endothelial cells may take place in all organs, although brain and lungs are often critically affected vital organs. Reactive oxygen species (ROS) produced by the infected endothelial cells play an important role in the cell damage. The pathogenic mechanism that causes the damage and increased vascular permeability is as yet unexplained. Interestingly, disseminated intravascular coagulation does not occur and thrombotic disease is not a part of the pathogenesis leading to severe illness and organ failure.

The early part of the febrile illness represents a period of proliferation of rickettsiae in the blood and on the endothelial surface of small blood vessels. The endothelial cell integrity is damaged, leading to leakage of fluid into tissues and to platelet aggregation and proliferation of polymorphonuclear leukocytes and monocytes within the vessel wall and in the perivascular spaces. This results in a focal occlusive end-angiitis of small venules and arterioles leading to microinfarction, producing the characteristic histological appearances of the 'typhus nodule' described by Fränkel and Wohlbach[31] (Figure 49.1). In the latter part of the fever phase, if significant rickettsaemia persists, excessive immune complex deposition may occur within the skin, kidneys and other tissues. Immunity to rickettsiae is generally long-lasting. The immune response is both humoral and cell-mediated. Viable rickettsiae may remain latent in host tissues after the acute infection. The clearance of rickettsiae is mediated by cytotoxic T lymphocytes. In humans, IFNγ, TNF-α, IL-1b and Rantes activate rickettsicidal activity. Natural killer cells are also important in the early course of the disease. Antibodies to epitopes of OmpA and OmpB, but not lipopolysaccharides, also render help to the strong immune response and protection.

DIAGNOSIS

Serological diagnosis was pioneered in 1916 by Weil and Felix,[32] who described heterophilic antibody agglutination of the OX-2 and OX-19 strains of *Proteus mirabilis* by typhus sera; this was extended to scrub typhus in 1926 by Fletcher and Lesslar,[21] who named an agglutinated variant strain OX-K. The old Weil–Felix reaction demonstrating heterophilic antibodies to *Proteus* strains OX-19 and OX-2 based on cross-reactivity with the rickettsiae is insensitive and unspecific and may be considered outdated; however, it is still in use in laboratories with poor resources.

Rickettsia spp. grow in guinea-pigs injected with infected human blood but *Rickettsia*, *Anaplasma*, *Ehrlichia* and *Coxiella* spp. are extremely difficult to culture in vitro, whereas *Bartonella* spp. are slow-growing. Although newer serological methods exist and PCR methodologies are under development, the diagnosis of all these diseases remains a challenge to the physician.

First, there are problems with cross-reactions among *Rickettsia* spp., especially among the spotted fever rickettsiae, and also among the *Bartonella* and within the *Anaplasma*/*Ehrlichia* group of pathogens. Second, antibodies appear relatively late in the clinical course of the disease, at the earliest 7–14 days after onset, such as in epidemic louse-borne rickettsiosis and RMSF, but often 3 weeks or more after onset, such as in African tick bite fever. For the rickettsioses, the reference method is indirect microimmunofluorescence assay (IFA), with a high degree of sensitivity and specificity. Indirect IFAs exist for both specific IgM and IgG. Threshold titres for positivity vary between laboratories. Preferably, serum specimens should be obtained at least 2–3 weeks apart to examine for a four-fold or greater increase in antibody titre. This is the most appropriate approach to confirm tick-borne rickettsial disease. Where enzyme-linked immunosorbent assay (ELISA) tests are available, they should be used qualitatively only.[33] Although PCR methods are generally relatively insensitive in their standard performances, they may be used on biopsies from eschars. A new, so-called 'suicide' PCR with improved sensitivity has been launched as an alternative, hitherto used on blood samples.[34] For the anaplasmosis/ehrlichiosis, PCR on blood samples is appropriate, although a negative result does not exclude the diagnosis,[33] whereas the mainstay for the diagnosis of the bartonelloses is antibody testing by indirect IFA.

THERAPY

Overall, the treatment of rickettsial disease is not controversial. The challenge is to recognize and diagnose rickettsial infections early in order to start antibiotic therapy as soon as possible after the onset of the first symptoms, i.e. on the basis of history and symptomatology only. If treatment is delayed, severity and mortality increase significantly in many rickettsioses and the patient may die before serological data are available. Thus, RMSF mortality is significantly reduced by early antibiotic treatment. The drug of first choice is doxycycline, in an adult dose of 200 mg daily (4 mg/kg body weight per day in children), intravenously (i.v.) or orally (p.o.), preferably in two divided doses, for a minimum of 5 days, although 7–10 days are generally recommended. Alternatively, chloramphenicol in an adult dose of 500–750 mg 6-hourly (75 mg/kg per day divided 6-hourly in children) p.o. or i.v. for 7 days can be used in rickettsioses but is not considered to be effective in anaplasmosis/ehrlichiosis. Both drugs are rickettsiostatic. The i.v. route should be used if the patient is seriously ill or unable to take oral medication because of nausea and vomiting. Fluoro-

quinolones are generally less efficient, but can be considered if the first-line drugs should be avoided; levofloxacin has been used successfully in the dosage 500 mg i.v. or p.o. once daily for 2 weeks. The macrolide azithromycin has been proven effective in vitro.

Doxycycline is the recommended treatment even in children, although fluoroquinolones may be an alternative. The risk of teeth staining must be considered when treating children with tetracyclines, but that risk is less with short-term use and considered acceptable in potentially serious rickettsioses such as RMSF. For pregnant women, chloramphenicol is considered the best choice. However, late in pregnancy the risk of 'grey baby syndrome' in the neonatal period must be taken into consideration. Fluoroquinolones should be avoided due to the risk of fetal complications. In life-threatening disease, doxycycline is always the first-line therapy in rickettsioses, irrespective of pregnancy or age of the patient, as well as in anaplasmosis and ehrlichiosis, where chloramphenicol is generally considered ineffective.

Passive administration of antibodies, used preferentially in experimental situations against typhus-group rickettsioses and scrub typhus, is not sufficient to control the infection, although phagocytosis of the rickettsiae may be enhanced by antibody coating.[35]

PROPHYLAXIS

Early removal of the tick, using tweezers or specific tick removers, is an important measure to prevent tick-borne diseases. The technique is to grip the tick as close to its mouth parts as possible and pull directly out. It is important not to twist the tick while pulling it out, as this manoeuvre may break its mouth parts, leaving material in the skin that may cause a local skin infection. Some commercially available mosquito repellents have been shown to have preventive effects against ticks. Considered most effective is N, N-diethyl-meta-toluamide (DEET), which can also be used in combination with permethrin.[36] Prophylactic antibiotic treatment after tick bites in endemic areas is generally not indicated.

Since the 1920s, attempts have been made to produce a sufficiently active vaccine. Both live and killed vaccines have been developed. However, both types of vaccines suffered from major drawbacks concerning quality of the vaccines, and severe adverse reactions occurred. Also, subunit vaccines produced with modern molecular-based techniques have not been succesful. Today, no original vaccines against the typhus group or the spotted fever group rickettsiae are licensed for use.[35]

TYPHUS GROUP

Epidemic (louse-borne) typhus

Epidemiology

R. prowazekii is transmitted by the human body or clothing louse *Pediculus humanus* from person to person. There is no evidence that head lice act as vectors of this infection. Rickettsiae from the blood of a human case are ingested by the biting louse and multiply in the gut of the insect so that its faeces are heavily infected. Scratching of a subsequent bite inoculates the organisms, which can also enter the body through rubbing into the conjunctival membrane. Infected lice may die from the disease but can transmit the rickettsiae to other lice through ingestion of faeces. Transovarial vertical transmission does not occur in lice. Air-borne infection may occur in crowded conditions by the inhalation of dried louse faeces. Blood transfusion has rarely transmitted the disease. Laboratory infection is a major risk. Specimens suspected of containing rickettsiae must be treated as for a 'dangerous pathogen'. In the USA, *R. prowazekii* has also been isolated from flying squirrels (*Glaucomys volans*) and is transmitted between them by their lice and fleas and occasionally to humans, primarily in the winter when flying squirrels enter buildings.

The genome of *R. prowazekii* has recently been sequenced, providing new and fascinating evidence of an evolutionary relationship between rickettsiae and intracellular mitochondria in general.[37]

Foci of endemic human infection from which epidemic spread can occur in times of famine, war, migration and overcrowding exist mainly in the cooler mountainous regions of tropical countries, such as Rwanda, Burundi, Uganda, Ethiopia, Lesotho, Transkei, Ciskei, Transvaal, Namibia, Nigeria, Kurdistan, northern India and Pakistan, China, Papua New Guinea, the Andes Mountains, Guatemala, Mexico, and Serbia and Greece (Figure 49.2).

Typical circumstances prevailed in the Burundi epidemic of 1995, which began with cases in a prison and spread to the mal-

nourished inmates of refugee camps in the central highlands, causing over 50 000 cases, with a mortality rate of 2.6%.[38,39]

Chronic human carriage of *R. prowazekii* may result in later relapses of typhus fever, a phenomenon first described by Brill[40] in 1910 in Jewish migrants from the Balkans to New York, and subsequently confirmed by Zinsser[41] (Brill–Zinsser disease). Such patients are thought to form a source of potential infection when louse infestation becomes common in prisons and refugee camps or in other insanitary crowded conditions.

Clinical description

In the populations at risk of epidemic typhus fever, nutrition and general immunity to infection are inadequate, so that the illness is often severe, with a mortality rate of up to 20% overall, and greater than 50% in the weak and aged. The incubation period averages 12 days. There is an abrupt onset of fever, prostration and severe headache, with pain in the limbs, especially the shins, and nausea and vomiting. Fever rises rapidly to 39–40°C, and remains high until death or resolution by 'crisis' towards the end of the second week, if untreated. The conjunctivae are suffused, the face congested, and the patient looks vacant and depressed as if drugged or drunk (Figure 49.3). Delirium may ensue and a mid-brain ischaemic syndrome of akinetic mutism can occur. There is fetor

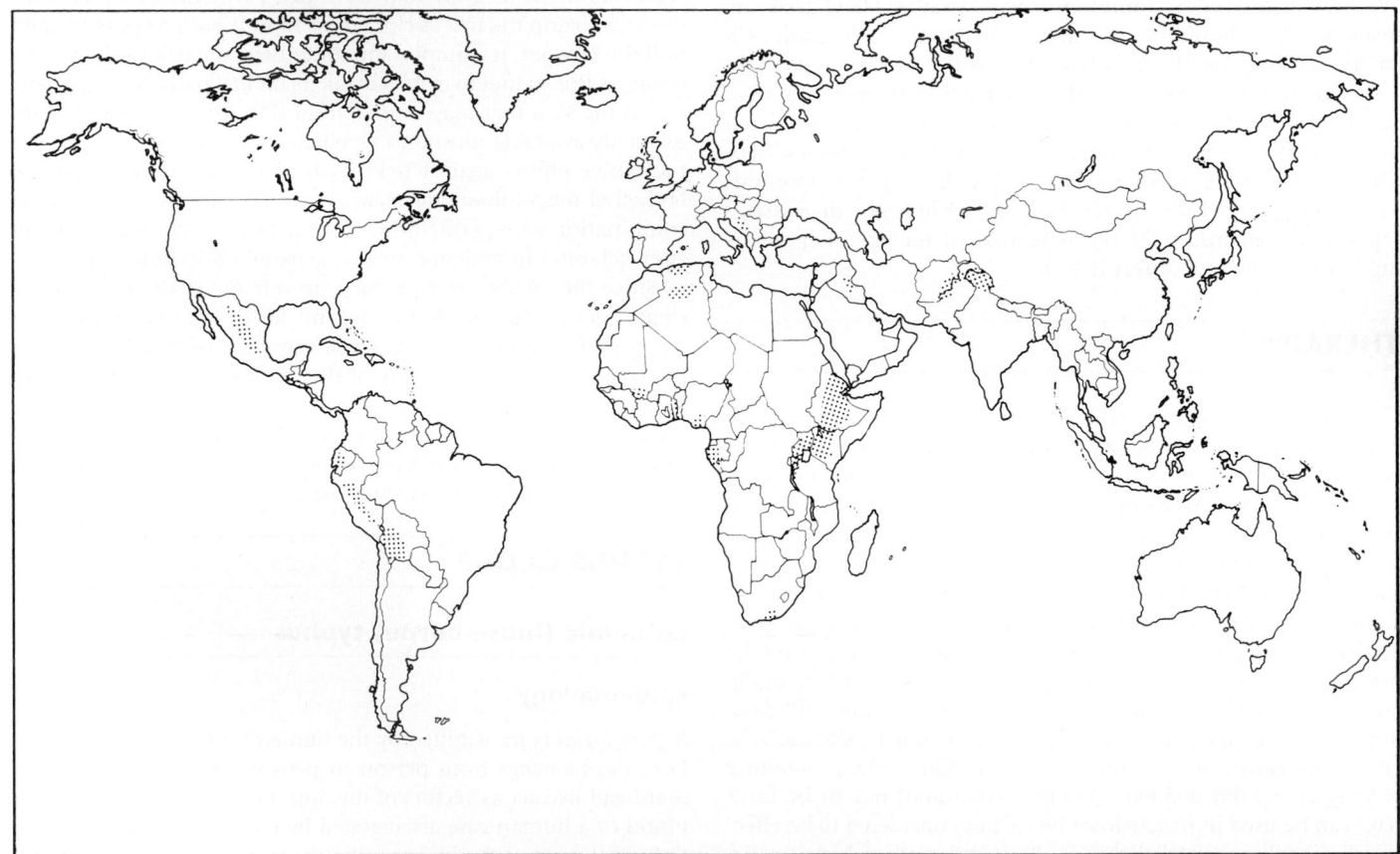

Figure 49.2 Endemic foci of louse-borne typhus (*R. prowazekii*). (Courtesy of the Department of Entomology, London School of Hygiene and Tropical Medicine.)

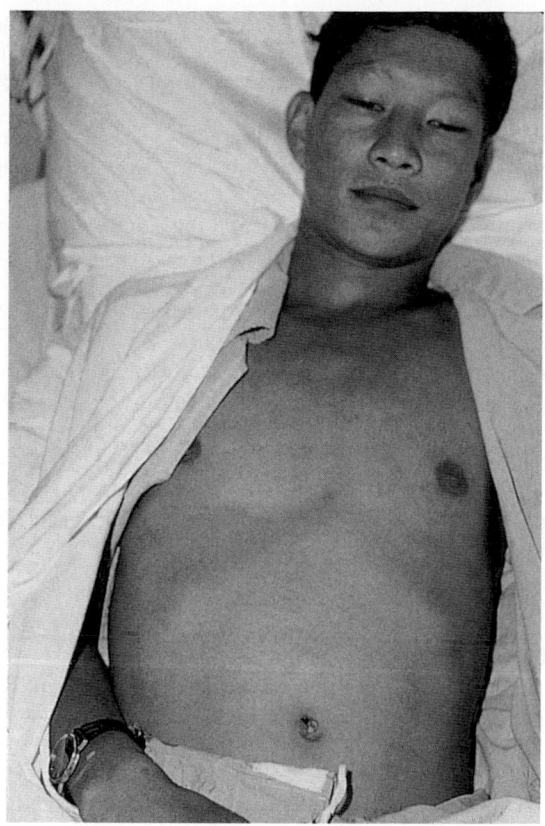

Figure 49.3 A patient with mild typhus encephalitis.

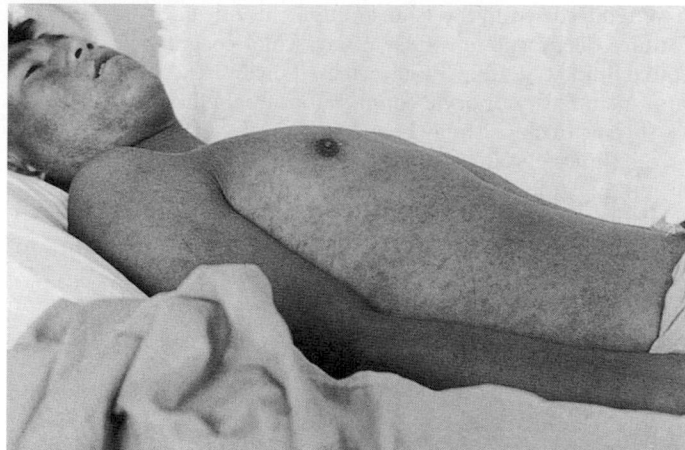

Figure 49.4 The rash of typhus fever. (Courtesy of G. W. Brown.)

oris, and epistaxis and a dry cough are common. Splenomegaly is usual. The typhus rash appears on the second to fourth day of fever, mainly on the trunk and proximal limbs (Figure 49.4). It consists of small irregular pink macules which rapidly darken to a mulberry or purple colour, and rarely become frankly petechial (Figure 49.5). Coalescence to a generalized patchy purple mottling under the skin may occur a few days later. There is no eschar at the site of inoculation. Patients are said to smell of mice, boot polish or rifle-barrel washings. Constipation is usual, and paralytic ileus may occur.

In up to 50% of severe cases, a meningoencephalitis ensues, with meningism, tinnitus and hyperacusis followed by deafness, dysphagia, dysphoria, agitated delirium and coma. Survivors may suffer transverse myelitis, hemiparesis, peripheral neuropathy with hyperaesthesia, and prolonged psychiatric disturbances.

Other possible complications include secondary infection leading to bronchopneumonia, suppurative parotitis or otitis media, and peripheral blood vessel occlusion resulting in leg vein thrombosis and peripheral gangrene, for instance of digits. An important further complication is myocarditis, which can occur during recovery with or without specific treatment. This presents with hypotension, tachycardia and low-output cardiac failure or sudden arrhythmic collapse.

Diagnosis

Routine blood investigations in typhus are unhelpful, with a normal total and relative white blood cell count. More severe cases

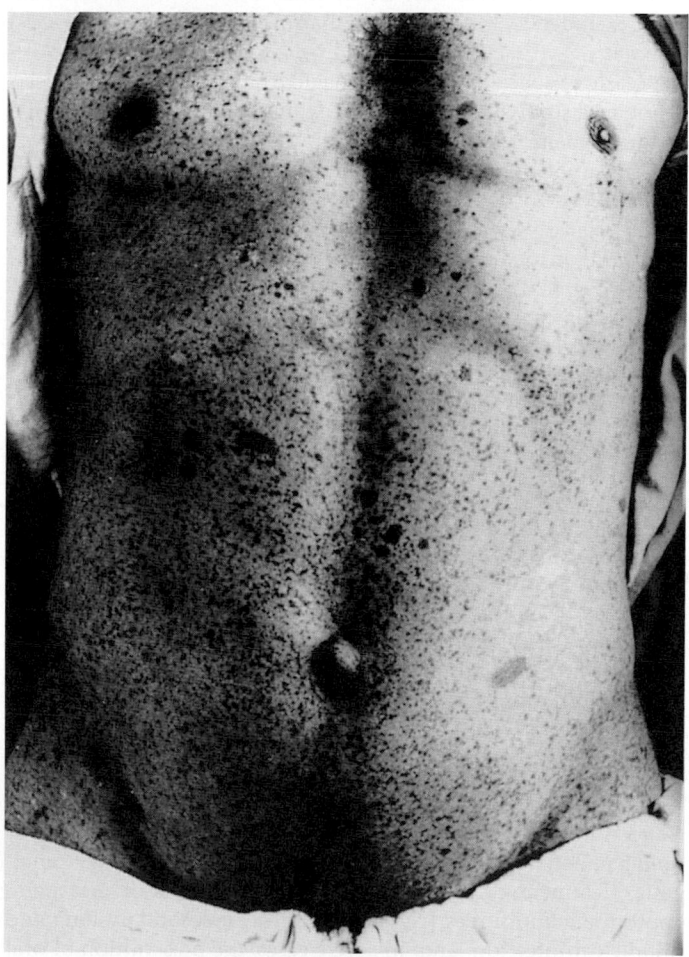

Figure 49.5 Typhus rash in the second week, showing the typical distribution. The dark-coloured areas are petechial; the lighter-coloured, discrete areas disappear on pressure.

889

have reduced serum levels of sodium, chloride and albumin, and features diagnostic of diffuse intravascular coagulation. Cerebrospinal fluid (CSF) may be at increased pressure, with modest rises in protein and monocyte count, but normal glucose content.

Specific diagnosis may be made:

- on clinical grounds, in an epidemic situation, confirmed by rapid response to specific treatment
- serologically, usually by indirect IFA
- serologically, by ELISA; the ELISA test can also be modified for field use by application to filter paper.

The diagnosis may also be made in the early acute stage in specialized laboratories:

- by PCR of blood or tissue
- by isolation of rickettsiae by inoculation of blood or tissue in shell vial cell culture
- by antigen detection by immunofluorescence on skin biopsy.

Differential diagnosis

The differential diagnosis of epidemic typhus includes:

- Typhoid fever. This may be clinically very similar and should be excluded by blood or bone marrow culture(s) for *Salmonella typhi*.
- Measles, especially if haemorrhagic. The rash of measles affects the face severely, unlike that of typhus.
- Viral haemorrhagic fevers (e.g. dengue, Rift Valley fever, Crimean–Congo haemorrhagic fever and yellow fever). These may need to be excluded by PCR, if the patient is febrile, or serologically.
- Meningococcal septicaemia. This can be excluded by culture of blood or CSF.
- Louse-borne relapsing fever. This may be very similar clinically, but with a haemorrhagic rash. This diagnosis is established by the demonstration of borreliae in the peripheral blood of febrile patients, e.g. by examining acridine orange-stained smears using fluorescence microscopy.[42]
- Leptospirosis. This may be clinically similar in the early stages of the illness. Distinguishing features include marked skeletal muscle tenderness and peripheral blood polymorphonuclear leukocytosis. PCR is of great value for rapid diagnosis.[43] Also, leptospires can be isolated from blood and CSF during early disease.
- *Plasmodium falciparum* malaria, especially if cerebral involvement has occurred. Blood films should be stained to exclude this, although rashes and skin haemorrhage are rare in malaria.

Management

General medical and nursing care is important, with attention to fluid balance, mouth toilet, avoidance of bed sores, adequate analgesia, treatment of agitation with judicious doses of diazepam, appropriate antibiotics (e.g. amoxicillin) for secondary lung and middle ear infection, and, in severe cases, the prescription of oral prednisolone 40 mg initially and 20 mg daily for several days, followed by reducing doses. Oliguria and anuria may require peritoneal or haemodialysis.

Specific chemotherapy should be with one of the following:

- Doxycycline: adult dose of 200 mg daily (4 mg/kg body weight per day for children), preferably in two divided doses, for 7–10

days. If there is a shortage of drugs, 200 mg or 100 mg in a single oral dose for adults and children, respectively, repeated once later if necessary, or a short course of 100–200 mg daily for 3 days will cure most cases.[44]

- Chloramphenicol: adult dose of 500–750 mg 6-hourly (in children, 75 mg/kg per day, divided 6-hourly), orally or intravenously, for 7 days.
- Tetracycline: adult dose of 300–500 mg 6-hourly (in children, 50 mg/kg per day, divided 6-hourly), orally or intravenously, for 7 days.

Rapid defervescence should be anticipated within 48 hours if the diagnosis is correct.

Measures directed against the louse vector are essential. On admission, patients should be stripped of clothing and washed thoroughly with soap and water. Clothing should be incinerated or autoclaved. Delousing powder (1% malathion) can be applied to hospital clothing and bed sheets. Treatment of medical and nursing attendants with delousing powder once weekly is also desirable.

Prevention and control

Epidemic typhus should be controlled by:

- Delousing of patients and all members of closed communities (e.g. refugee camps, prisons) where infection occurs—using 1% malathion powder.
- Consideration of single-dose (200 mg) doxycycline treatment of all contacts and residents of infected areas, and medical and nursing attendants.

No safe vaccine is currently commerciably available.

Murine (endemic or flea-borne) typhus

Epidemiology

Murine typhus is caused by *R. typhi* (*R. mooseri*), which is transmitted to humans by *Xenopsylla cheopis* fleas living on *Rattus rattus* (the black rat), *Rattus norvegicus* (the brown rat) and various species of mouse, and between rats by the louse *Polyplax spinulosa* and the mite *Liponyssus bacoti*. Flea faeces infected with rickettsiae contaminate the flea bite, which is then scratched, so inoculating the infection, or may be inhaled when dried or rubbed into the conjunctival membrane. Rodents with rickettsaemia of this type do not suffer serious illness and so act as a reservoir of infection. Humans are infected by close contact with rodents and their fleas in granaries, breweries, shops and food stores, and domestically in developing countries. Garbage workers are at special risk.

The geographical distribution of human cases of murine typhus is shown in Figure 49.6.

Clinical description

The incubation period is similar to that of louse-borne typhus, and the illness is also similar, but generally much less severe, with a mortality rate of only 1–2%. Headache and muscular pains are the predominant symptoms. There is no eschar at the site of inoculation, and the rash of fine red macules is less extensive than in epidemic typhus or may be absent. Serious neurological, renal and other complications are unusual.

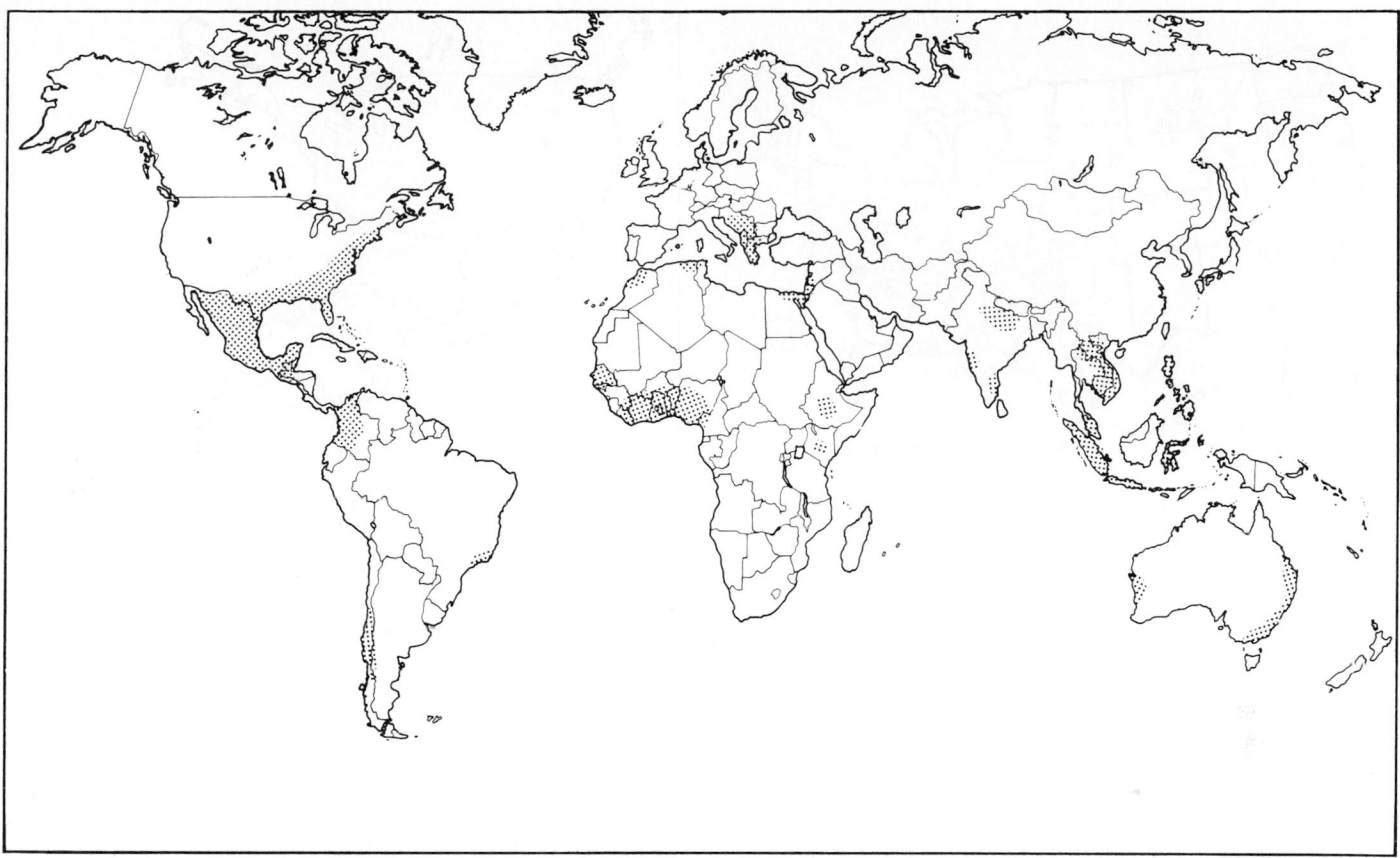

Figure 49.6 Geographical distribution of flea-borne (murine) typhus (*R. mooseri*). (Courtesy of the Department of Entomology, London School of Hygiene and Tropical Medicine.)

Diagnosis

The diagnosis is made by the same method(s) as in louse-borne typhus.

Serology by indirect IFA and specific *R. typhii* antigen turns positive in approximately 50% of cases within 1 week and in virtually all patients within 15 days of onset of illness.[45]

Serology is cross-reactive between *R. typhi* and *R. prowazekii* and can be distinguished by absorption only.

Differential diagnosis

The differential diagnosis of murine typhus includes:
- Typhoid fever—excluded by blood or bone marrow culture
- Louse-borne and scrub typhus—distinguished only by specific serological tests, and treated identically anyway
- Arbovirus infections with a macular rash (e.g. dengue and chikungunya)—distinguished serologically
- Relapsing fever, transmitted by lice or ticks—established by the demonstration of borreliae in the peripheral blood of febrile patients, e.g. by examining acridine orange-stained smears with the fluorescence microscope[42]
- Leptospirosis—distinguished by exquisite muscle tenderness and polymorphonuclear leukocytosis and established by isolation or PCR
- Malaria—excluded by stained blood films

- Other causes of fever with macular rash, e.g. Epstein-Barr virus, primary HIV infection—distinguished serologically.

Management

The general and specific treatment of murine typhus is the same as for louse-borne typhus. Steroid treatment is needed only exceptionally.

Prevention and control

The prevention of murine typhus has to depend on reducing human contact with rodents and their fleas by:
- urban and domestic rodent control using warfarin
- proofing of grain and other food stores against rodents
- the wearing of protective clothing by garbage workers.

RICKETTSIAL SPOTTED FEVERS

These infections are caused by a large number of rickettsial species, all of which, except *R. akari*, are transmitted to humans by the bite of animal ticks or by inoculation of tick faeces or body fluids if the attached tick is crushed. Many other species of tick-borne rickettsiae exist (in animal reservoirs) that have yet to be characterized or identified.

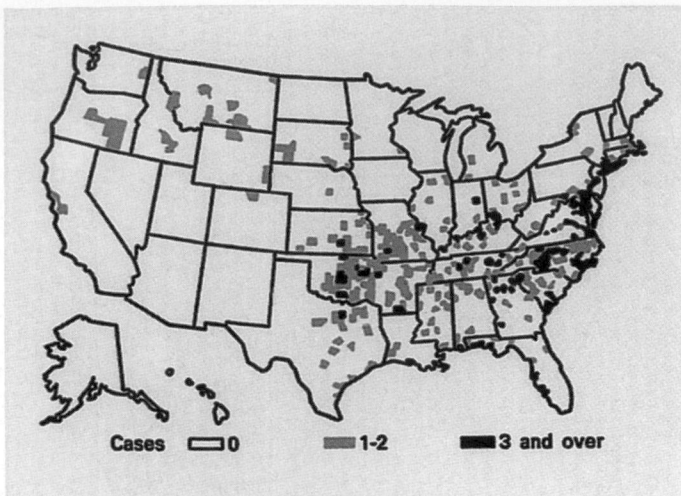

Figure 49.7 Typhus fever—tick-borne (Rocky Mountain spotted fever). Reported cases by country—USA, 1988.

Rocky Mountain spotted fever

Epidemiology

Rocky Mountain spotted fever (RMSF), due to *R. rickettsii*, is a potentially life-threatening infection. Following its original description in the mountain states of north-west USA in the late nineteenth century and the demonstration of the organism in its tick vector by Ricketts in 1906, RMSF has since been recognized as an important cause of illness throughout the USA, especially now in the south-eastern states and on the eastern seaboard. In all, several hundreds of cases are reported annually in the USA (Figure 49.7). It also occurs in Canada, Mexico, Colombia and Brazil, especially in the area of São Paulo.

The ixodid tick vectors are:

- *Dermacentor andersoni* (wood tick)—western USA
- *Dermacentor variabilis* (dog tick)—western USA
- *Amblyomma americanum* (lone-star tick)—south and south-eastern USA
- *Amblyomma cajennense*—Brazil and Colombia
- *Haemaphysalis leporispalustris*—this rabbit tick does not bite humans but transmits the infection between rabbits, which act as a reservoir for transmission to human-biting ticks (Figure 49.8).

Transovarial transmission of rickettsiae occurs in ixodid hard ticks, which are thus the main reservoir of infection.

Dermacentor andersoni ticks normally live on goats, sheep, badgers, lynx and black bears, and their larvae on squirrels. *Dermacentor variabilis* and *Amblyomma* ticks live on domestic dogs, rabbits, foxes, opossums, gophers and racoons, and their larvae on field mice.

Clinical description

Surprisingly, in RMSF there is rarely an eschar at the site of the tick bite. After an inoculation period of 6–10 days, there is an abrupt onset of fever with severe headaches and muscle pains, and

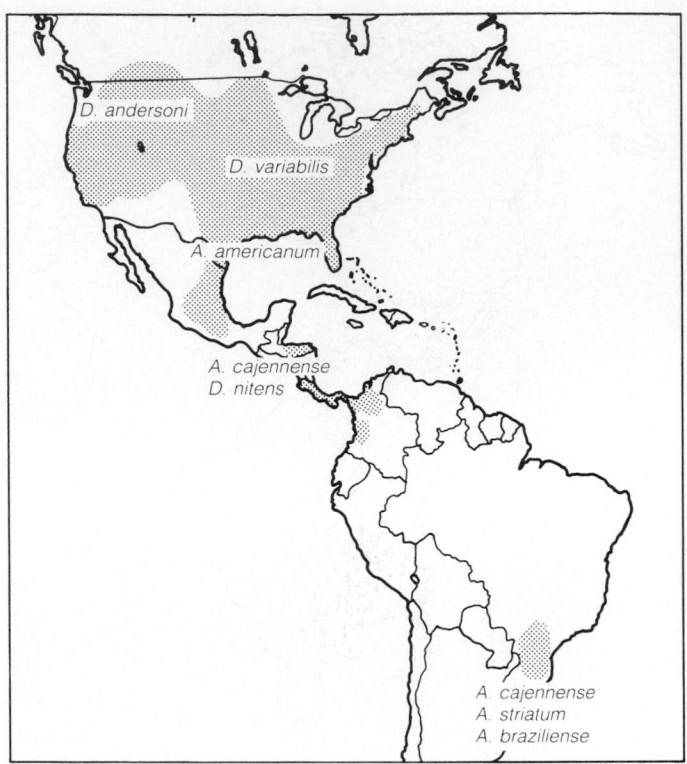

Figure 49.8 Geographical distribution of Rocky Mountain spotted fever (*R. rickettsii*). (Courtesy of the Department of Entomology, London School of Hygiene and Tropical Medicine.)

a dry cough. The unspecific symptoms at this early stage often cause a delay in diagnosis and treatment, resulting in an increased risk of serious complications and even death. After 2–3 days, the typhus rash of fine pink macules develop (Figure 49.9), which in this disease is most marked on the soles of the feet, wrists and forearms. In more severe infections, the rash quickly spreads and becomes petechial with large ecchymoses and the potential for gangrene of digits and pressure areas. The overall mortality rate is 7–10%, and in young children and elderly adults the rate is up to 25%. Meningoencephalitis is common in severe cases and, as the illness progresses, the stuporose or comatose patient will become hypotensive, oliguric or anuric, and uraemic. Other complications are similar to those seen in severe louse-borne typhus and include bronchopneumonia, otitis media, parotitis and intestinal ileus. In severe cases, disseminated intravascular coagulation is a common accompaniment.

Diagnosis

The total white blood cell count (WBC) is typically normal, but increased numbers of immature bands are generally observed. Thrombocytopenia, mild elevations of hepatic transaminases and hyponatraemia exist in a proportion of cases.[33] The diagnosis of RMSF is based on similar methods to those used in epidemic typhus. Indirect IFA for specific antibodies is the most sensitive and specific test. Enzyme immunoassay methods are also considered reliable, whereas PCR testing for bacteria in blood most often turns out negative.

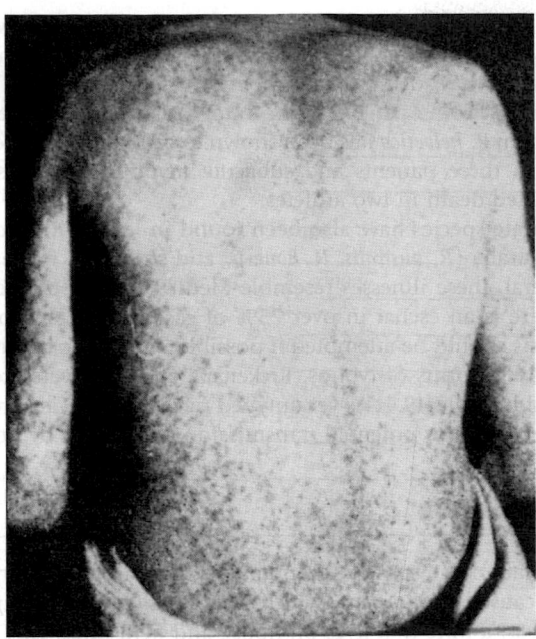

Figure 49.9 The rash of Rocky Mountain spotted fever.

Differential diagnosis

Before the appearance of rash, a variety of acute infectious diseases will have to be considered, including respiratory tract infections and various viral infections, and also:

- Typhoid and paratyphoid fever—diagnosed by blood culture.
- Malaria (if in endemic area)—diagnosed by blood smears
- Lyme disease—diagnosed by serology
- Tick-borne relapsing fever—diagnosed by the demonstration of borreliae in blood smears[42]
- Tularaemia—diagnosed mainly by serology or, if an ulcer is present, by PCR/culture
- Purulent meningitis—diagnosed by CSF and blood culture

Following the onset of rash, the latter three diseases will still have to be ruled out, and several others, including drug reactions, infectious mononucleosis, etc.

Management

Specific chemotherapy should be given with a tetracycline, preferably doxycycline 100 mg twice daily to adults for at least 7 days and continued for 2 days after the patient has become afebrile. The physician should not hesitate to initiate presumptive treatment, i.e. before the diagnosis has become evident or confirmed. Single-day treatment is not recommended. Although associated with a higher case fatality rate,[46] chloramphenicol is preferred to tetracyclines during pregnancy, because of concerns for the fetal teeth and bones. However, for children, a single course of doxycycline (4 mg/kg/day) or tetracycline (50–75 mg/kg/day) for a similar period of time as in adults is recommended because of the life-threatening nature of the disease and the associated low risk of teeth stains with such a limited course of treatment.

Prevention and control

It is not possible to eradicate the infection in ticks and animals, but the number of human cases can be reduced by avoiding tick bites. Thus:[33]

- Limit exposure to tick-infested habitats, including woody and grassy areas; walk on cleared trails; avoid brushing against tall grass and other vegetation.
- Wear protective clothing, including a hat, long-sleeved shirts, trousers, socks and closed-toe shoes, to prevent ticks from reaching the skin and attaching.
- Use products containing DEET for application on exposed skin and clothing to repel ticks. Products containing permethrin can be used to treat outer clothing but should not be applied to skin. Clothing should be allowed to completely dry before being worn.
- Check for tick attachment after episodes of exposure to animal contact and forest habitats; remove attached ticks gently with tweezers, as described earlier in this chapter under Prophylaxis (p. 3).
- Check domestic dogs and other pets for ticks; insecticide powders may be used.

There is no useful vaccine available for the prevention of RMSF.

Brazilian spotted fever

Brazilian spotted fever is caused by *R. rickettsii* with *Amblyomma cajennense* as the vector tick. An eschar at the site of the tick bite is usual; the illness is otherwise similar to RMSF.

Mediterranean spotted fever

Mediterranean spotted fever (fièvre boutonneuse), caused by *R. conorii*, occurs throughout the coastal countries of the Mediterranean but also in many other countries, including Ukraine, Russia, Georgia, India, Ethiopia, Kenya and South Africa. *R. conorii* is transmitted by the dog tick *Rhipicephalus sanguineus*, and the main reservoir of infection is in domestic dogs, rabbits and rodents. The illness is similar to RMSF, with the possibility of a haemorrhagic rash and renal and cerebral involvement, but in most cases it is less severe.

There is almost always an eschar (tache noire) at the site of the tick bite, with regional adenitis (Figure 49.10).

Among the differential diagnoses, African tick bite fever caused by *R. africae* should be considered in cases occurring in sub-Saharan Africa, where that disease is prevalent. In such cases, as in cases in other areas, typhoid, meningococcal septicaemia, measles and viral haemorrhagic fevers should also be considered. Diagnostic serological tests are similar to those for other forms of spotted fevers. Management is as for other forms of typhus. Prevention depends on methods similar to those for RMSF to reduce tick bites. There is no vaccine.

Israeli tick typhus

Israeli tick typhus, which is caused by a variant organism, *R. sharoni*, is transmitted by *Rhipicephalus* dog ticks, but eschar formation is unusual.

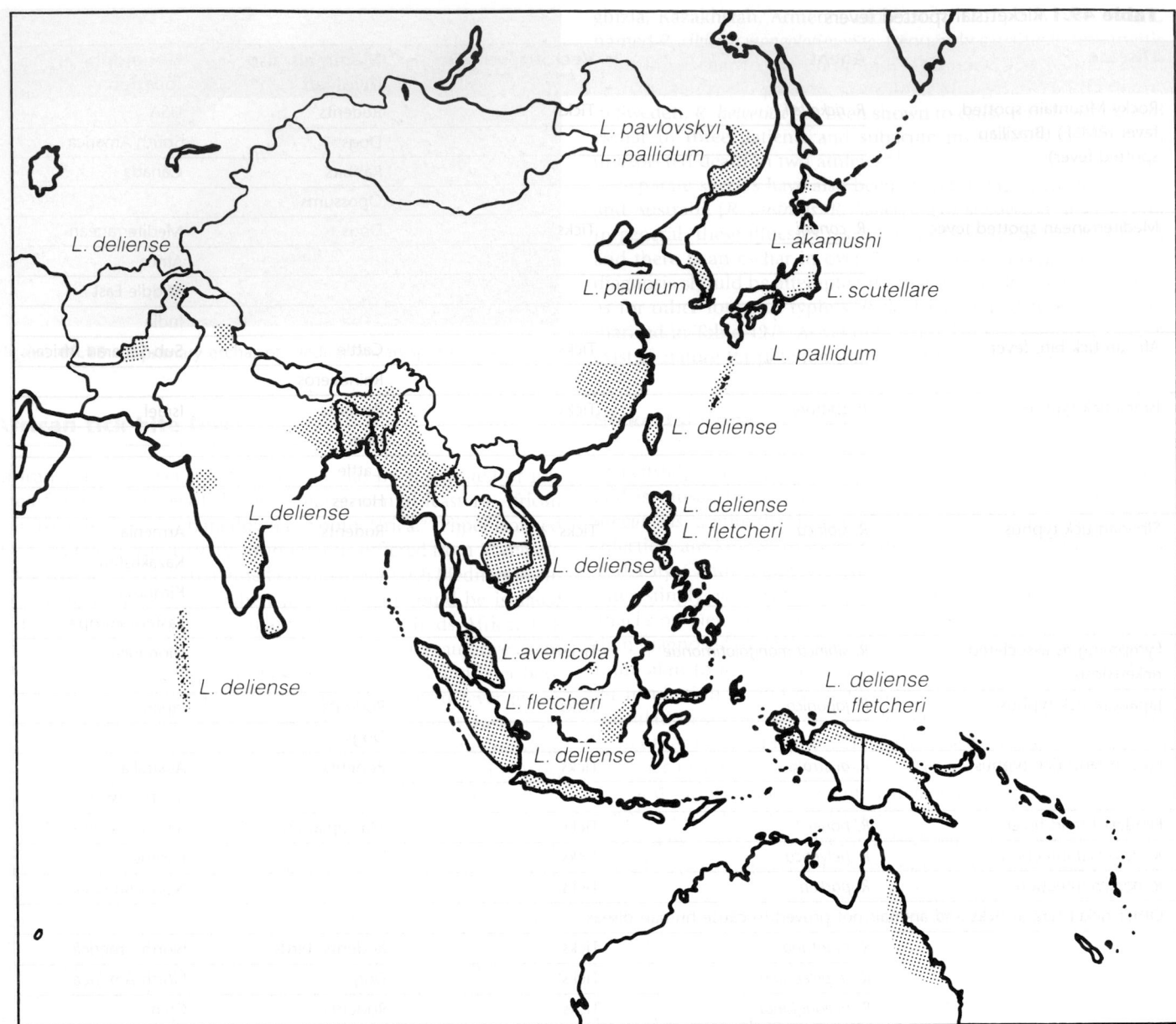

Figure 49.11 Geographical distribution of scrub (mite-borne) typhus (*as reflected in the distribution of the various species of Leptosporidium mites carrying Orientia tsutsugamushi*). (Courtesy of the Department of Entomology, London School of Hygiene and Tropical Medicine.)

and has the usual typhus accompaniments of suffused conjunctivae and face, severe headache, drowsiness, apathy, pain in the shins and other muscles, and, more characteristically, generalized lymphadenopathy and hepatosplenomegaly. Other symptoms may include nausea and vomiting, tinnitus and hyperacusis followed by deafness, constipation, epistaxis and a dry cough.

The rash is similar to that of louse-borne typhus and occurs mainly on the arms, thighs and trunk. In severe cases, meningoencephalitis ensues with neck stiffness, delirium, focal signs, papilloedema and coma. Myocarditis may complicate this phase, and oliguria with uraemia is common in severe cases. Adult respiratory distress syndrome (ARDS) and septic shock have also been reported.

Indigenous peoples of areas endemic for scrub typhus commonly have a less severe illness, often without any rash or eschar. This is one of the most common causes of 'pyrexia of unknown origin' in such areas, after malaria is excluded, but severe pneumonia has also been described.[55]

Immunity to scrub typhus following an attack is remarkably short-lived, lasting only a few months, and is specific to each strain of the organism, so that further attacks are common.

Diagnosis

As in other forms of typhus, routine blood examinations are unhelpful. IFA and specific immunoperoxidase have sufficient

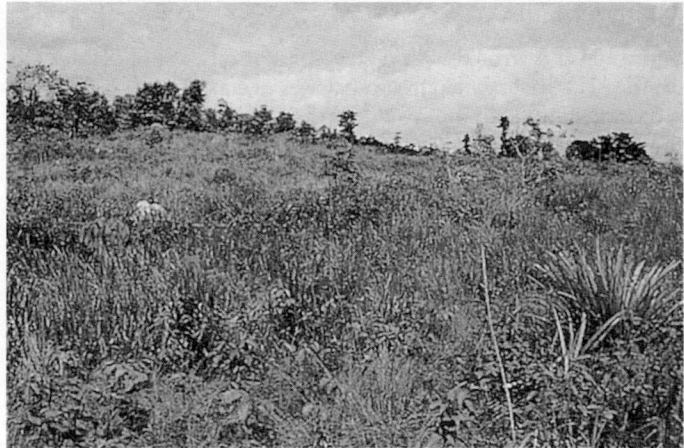

Figure 49.12 Typical scrub typhus country. (Courtesy of G. W. Brown.)

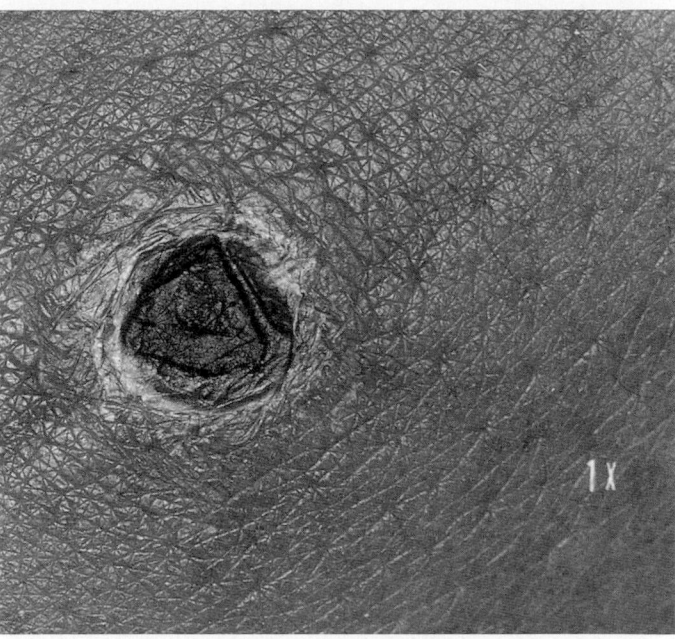

Figure 49.14 The eschar of scrub typhus, close-up view. (Courtesy of G. W. Brown.)

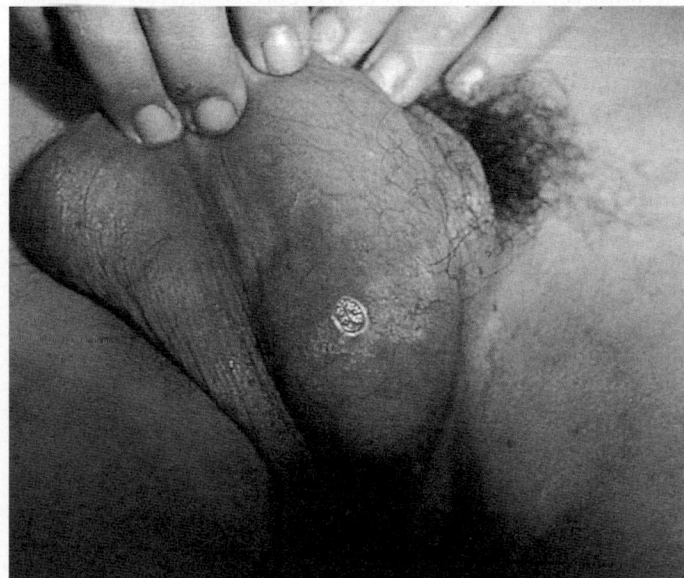

Figure 49.13 The eschar of scrub typhus. (Courtesy of G. W. Brown.)

sensitivity and specificity. PCR testing of blood, lymph node or eschar samples is useful but less often available. Commonly, the clinical diagnosis is based on the geographical history and physical signs, and confirmed by the rapid response to specific chemotherapy.

Differential diagnosis

Scrub typhus should be distinguished from:
- Malaria—by stained blood films
- Arbovirus infections (e.g. dengue)—by serological methods. The macular rash of dengue fever is much finer and often accompanied by marked thrombocytopenia

- Leptospirosis—by PCR if available[43] or blood or CSF culture
- Meningococcal disease—by blood and CSF cultures
- Typhoid—by blood and bone marrow cultures
- Infectious mononucleosis.

Management

A single oral dose of doxycycline, 200 mg for adults or 4 mg/kg body weight for children, or, in more severe cases, that dosage continued for 3–7 days, is the preferred treatment. In the small proportion of patients in whom, having received one single dose, the usual rapid defervescence is followed by a relapse of fever 5–7 days later, another single such dose is given. Alternatively, continuous chloramphenicol or tetracycline therapy can be given for 7 days, as in louse-borne typhus, unless the patient is oliguric or anuric; in the latter cases, doxycycline is safe.

O. tsutsugamushi seems as yet to be the only member of the *Rickettsia* tribe that has been shown to have developed antibiotic resistance, in northern Thailand, to chloramphenicol and tetracycline.[56] Alternative drugs include azithromycin, rifampicin and the quinolones. Importantly, rifampicin should never be used alone, because of the risk of resistance development, and ciprofloxacin, recently used in pregnant women in India, was ineffective and caused stillbirth or abortion.[57]

Prevention and control

Scrub typhus can be partly prevented or controlled by protective clothing and repellents when walking in terrain of endemic areas.

TRENCH FEVER

Epidemiology

Trench fever (His-Werner disease, Wolhynia fever) was first described as an epidemic disease in the First World War and many cases occurred also in the Second World War. Subsequently, this disease seems to have disappeared in its classical form. Instead, it reappeared in the 1990s, then causing bacteraemia and endocarditis among homeless men in France, USA. and Finland. The causative organism, *Bartonella quintana*, is closely related to the rickettsiae but is not an obligate intracellular parasite and can thus be cultured on blood agar although it is slow-growing. It is transmitted by the human body louse, *Pediculus humanus*. No non-human vertebrate reservoir has yet been identified.

Clinical description

Classical trench fever is described as a fever of sudden onset, often, but not always, accompanied by severe headache, leg and lumbar muscle pains, dizziness, nausea and vomiting. However, the illness can be fairly mild, which is believed to be the situation in a majority of cases. There is usually a sparse macular rash, but no eschar. The patient may have a single episode of fever lasting a few days, or suffer recurrent fever at intervals of about 5 days (quintan fever), or a more prolonged 'typhoidal' fever. Full recovery is usual and the mortality rate negligible, although some patients suffer prolonged debility with dyspnoea on exertion, but without objective evidence of myocarditis by the diagnostic methods used.

By contrast, the trench fever of homeless and alcoholic men, as diagnosed by blood culture in the 1990s, is characterized by a paucity of clinical signs, e.g. lack of significant fever and low antibody titres in most cases. In a minority of cases showing increasing levels of antibodies, endocarditis was diagnosed.[58] Blood culture positivity may persist for several years in some patients with trench fever. Furthermore, *B. quintana* infection may be a complication in HIV infection, where bacillary angiomatosis characterized by subcutaneous and lytic bone lesions, but without peliosis hepatis, may develop.[59]

Diagnosis

The mainstay for the clinical diagnosis of the bartonelloses, including trench fever, is antibody testing by indirect IFA. Also, *Bartonella* spp. can be isolated from blood by prolonged incubation on blood agar in a carbon dioxide-enriched environment or in endothelial cell lines.

Differential diagnosis

Trench fever should be distinguished from:
- Louse-borne typhus, although the treatment is identical
- Louse-borne relapsing fever—by the demonstration of borreliae in the peripheral blood of febrile patients, e.g. by examining acridine orange-stained smears with the fluorescence microscope[42]
- Typhoid—by blood and bone marrow cultures
- Brucellosis—by serological methods
- Q fever—by serological methods.

Management

Trench fever is treated with doxycycline or other tetracyclines—as for the rickettsial spotted fevers. In cases of endocarditis, an aminoglycoside should be administered for 2 weeks. During that time and for another 4 weeks, ceftriaxone with or without doxycycline should be given.

Prevention and control

No accumulations of classical trench fever have been reported after the World Wars. The recently re-emerged subacute urban trench fever would require hygienic intervention, including washing and delousing.

CAT-SCRATCH DISEASE

Epidemiology

B. henselae was genetically characterized in 1992[25,26] and could then be established as the cause of cat-scratch disease,[25,26] currently the most common zoonosis in the USA. *B. henselae* is globally endemic, primarily because infection of domestic cats, who remain asymptomatic, is worldwide and with a higher prevalence in warm, humid climates. Especially kittens are bacteraemic. It is suspected that the cat flea, which carries *B. henselae*, may have a role in the transmission.

Clinical description and management

The classical clinical manifestation is the development of a papule or pustule at the site of a cat scratch and a swollen regional lymph node. The condition is subacute and the swollen lymph node may persist for several months. The clinical diagnosis is confirmed by IFA. Antimicrobial chemotherapy is usually not required. However, as in *B. quintana* infection, the immunocompromised state is associated with an increased severity and complication rate. Thus, bacillary angiomatosis, including peliosis hepatis, and endocarditis are well-known manifestations in *B. henselae* infection.[60] These complications require antimicrobial chemotherapy as in trench fever.

Q FEVER

Epidemiology

Q fever was so named by Derrick in 1937 as 'query fever' before the causative organism was discovered, and not after Queensland where he discovered it. The strange name has persisted, despite the discovery and naming of the causative agent *Coxiella burnetii*. The disease has also been known as 'Balkan grippe', 'Red River fever' (Zaire) and 'Nine Mile fever' (from a creek in the Rocky Mountains). *C. burnetii* is a 0.3–0.7 μm-long pleomorphic Gram-negative coccobacillus. A spore stage exists, which explains why *C. burnetii* is particularly resistant to heat and drying. *C. burnetii* undergoes a phase variation. The virulent phase I exists in nature and in laboratory animals; and, due to chromosomal deletions,[61] the avirulent phase II develops following repeated passage of phase I bacteria in embryonated chicken eggs. In nature, *C. burnetii* exists in arthropods, rodents, birds and even fish, and arthropods,

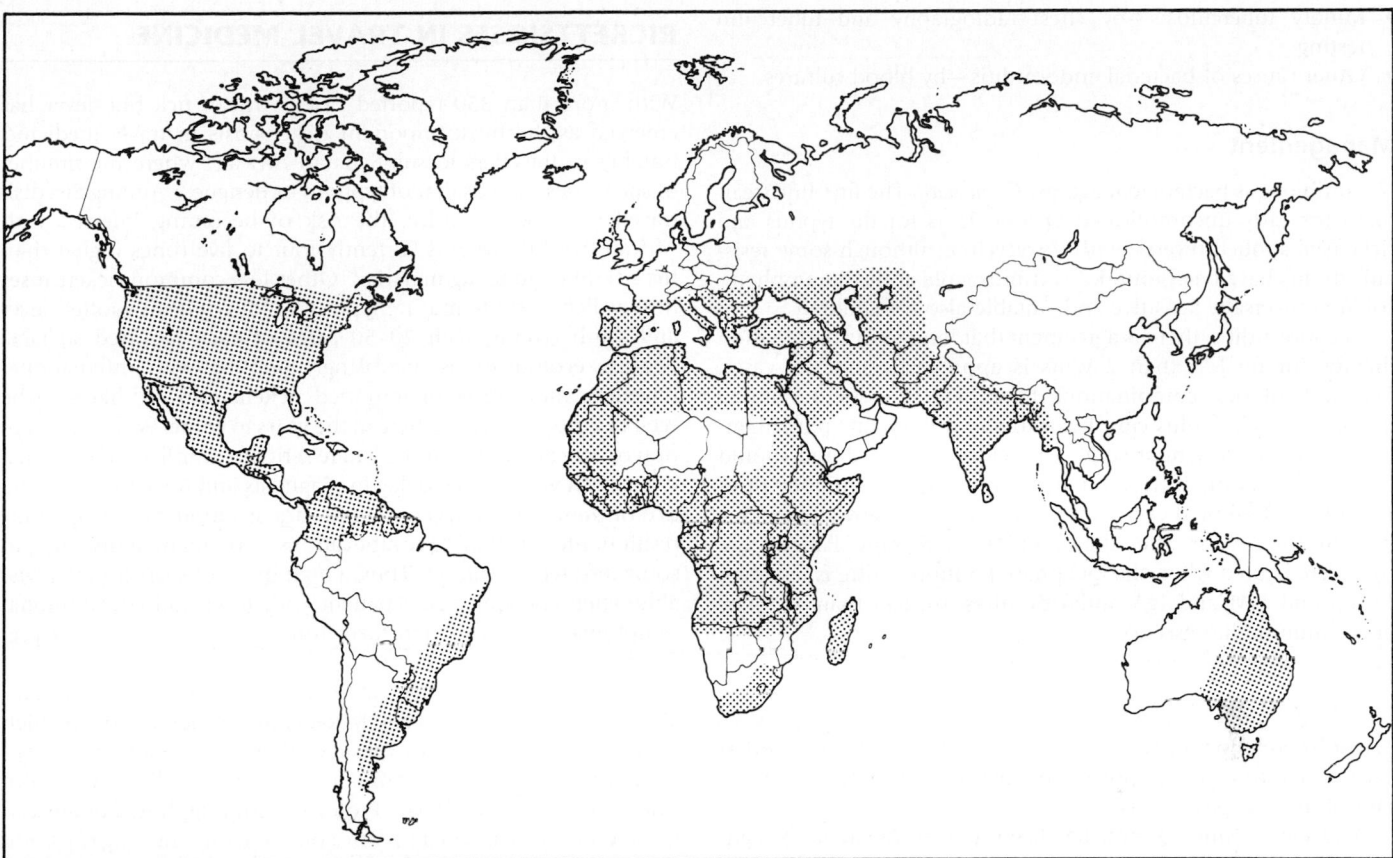

Figure 49.15 Geographical distribution of Q fever.

including ticks, transmit bacteria to domestic goats, sheep and cattle. Humans are not usually infected by arthropods but directly through milk, placental products and dried faeces in dust that is inhaled. Infective dust can be spread by winds over rather long distances and result in human cases. Q fever is primarily an occupational disease among farmers, abbatoir workers and veterinarians. Human-to-human transmission is extremely rare. It has a worldwide geographical distribution (Figure 49.15) and is an important cause of abortion in domestic goats and cattle.

C. burnetii produces an intracytoplasmic infection, especially in splenic histiocytes and the Kupffer cells of the liver, where it elicits a granulomatous response.

Clinical description

Q fever may pass as an inapparent infection with seroconversion through a mild brief fever to a distinct clinical presentation, including pneumonia, hepatitis, osteomyelitis or endocarditis.[62] The pneumonia is commonly 'atypical'. Even neurological manifestations may develop. The mortality rate was 2.4% in one large series.[63] The infection may pass into a chronic stage, in which endocarditis is the most consistent manifestation, occurring in up to 80% of such cases. A complicating endocarditis may not be apparent from the usual clinical features until many months have elapsed. Most commonly, valves affected were initially abnormal or prosthetic.

Diagnosis

The diagnosis of Q fever is frequently made by complement fixation (CF) test on paired sera. However, circulating immune complexes sometimes interfere with the CF test, making CF results difficult to interpret. This can be circumvented by applying an ELISA or microimmunofluorescence test using fixed C. burnetii antigen of phase I as well as phase II.[64]

Liver biopsy may show 'doughnut granuloma' considered typical to Q fever.[65]

Differential diagnosis

Q fever should be distinguished from:
- Typhoid—by blood and bone marrow culture
- Other causes of atypical pneumonia (e.g. viruses, *Mycoplasma pneumoniae*, *Chlamydia pneumoniae*, *Chlamydia psittaci*)—by appropriate serological methods
- Viral hepatitis—by serology
- Other viral infections, including Epstein-Barr, HIV and cytomegalovirus—by appropriate serology
- Brucellosis and Lyme disease—by serology
- Leptospirosis—distinguished by exquisite muscle tenderness and polymorphonuclear leukocytosis and established by isolation or PCR

- Miliary tuberculosis—by chest radiography and tuberculin testing
- Other causes of bacterial endocarditis—by blood cultures.

Management

No antibiotic is bactericidal against *C. burnetii*. The first-line treatment for early uncomplicated Q fever is as for the typhus and rickettsial spotted fevers—with doxycycline, although some resistant strains have been found. Co-trimoxazole and chloramphenicol are universally sensitive and suitable also for children.

In endocarditis, there is agreement that long-term combination therapy for no less than 2 years is appropriate in most cases. Several antibiotic combinations have been successful—among them, doxycycline plus ciprofloxacin and doxycycline plus rifampicin. Valve replacement surgery is seldom required and should be considered only if haemodynamically needed. Antibody titres should be monitored every 6 months during therapy and every 3 months for 2 years after the cessation of therapy. Patients are considered cured when the IgG phase I antibody titre is less than 1:800 and IgM and IgA antibody titres are less than 1:50 by microimmunofluorescence.[66]

Prevention and control

Aerosol dissemination of *C. burnetii* is very difficult to prevent because control of the disease in domestic animals is difficult. Milk should be pasteurized.

A vaccine against Q fever has been used in Australia for agricultural and abbatoir workers, veterinarians, etc., according to the National Q Fever Management Program.[67] Vaccine may currently be available at the US Army Medical Research Institute of Infectious Diseases (USAMRIID), Fort Detrick, Frederick, MD, USA.

EHRLICHIOSIS AND ANAPLASMOSIS

Human monocytic ehrlichiosis (HME), caused by *Ehrlichia chaffeensis*, is a tick-borne zoonosis. Thousands of cases have been diagnosed in the USA and cases have also been reported from Korea. The disease is a mild to severe febrile illness. Headache, malaise, myalgia, chills, rigors and anorexia are common symptoms. Also, leucopenia, thrombocytopenia and liver involvement are common, but less than half of the patients develop a rash.[68] Severe complications develop in a minority and include renal insufficiency, meningoencephalitis and coagulopathy. HME is diagnosed serologically by IFA on paired sera. Morulae within circulating leukocytes is a classical, although relatively rare, finding in HME.

Human granulocytotropic anaplasmosis (HGA) is well documented in the USA and Europe. HGA is generally milder than HME, and especially so in Europe. Morulae within blood leukocytes are more common in HGA than in HME. The diagnosis is serological.

HME and HGA respond to treatment with doxycycline 100 mg twice daily or tetracycline 25 mg/kg/day in four divided doses, but chloramphenicol is ineffective. The prevention of HME and HGA is limited to preventing tick bites and removing ticks as early as possible.

RICKETTSIOSES IN TRAVEL MEDICINE

With more than 350 reported cases, African tick bite fever has emerged as the most important rickettsiosis in travel medicine, notably in travellers to sub-Saharan Africa,[69] where the number of such cases exceeds that of typhoid or dengue.[70] Among Swedish travellers to South Africa, the risk of becoming infected with African tick bite fever is currently four to five times higher than the risk of contracting malaria.[71] Other less common rickettsioses in travellers include murine typhus, Mediterranean spotted fever and scrub typhus, with 20–50 cases of each reported so far.[69] Because ecotourism is increasingly popular with international travellers, more cases of imported rickettsioses are likely to be seen in Europe and elsewhere in the years to come. With the exception of African tick bite fever, where serious complications are rare, it has been warned that delay in diagnosis and the common practice of prescribing β-lactam antibiotics as empirical therapy may result in life-threatening complications or permanent disability in some infected travellers.[72] Thus, a high index of suspicion is advisable when encountering a patient with fever and constitutional symptoms after having returned from an endemic area. For prevention, weekly 200 mg doses of doxycycline can prevent scrub typhus[73] and possibly other rickettsioses, and may thus be a valuable option for backpackers, trekkers and other visitors at high risk. However, African tick bite fever has been reported in safari travellers despite the concomitant use of tetracycline hydrochloride as malaria prophylaxis.[69] Protective clothing should be advised for travellers to sub-Saharan Africa on safari and hunting trips, and topical repellents, such as DEET, should be used on exposed skin; notably, frequent application is required because of the short-lasting effect against the ticks that transmit African tick bite fever.[69]

REFERENCES

1. Raoult D, Fournier PE, Eremeeva M, et al. Naming of Rickettsiae and rickettsial diseases. *Ann N Y Acad Sci* 2005; 1063:1–12.
2. Brenner DJ, O'Connor SP, Winkler HH, et al. Proposals to unify the genera *Bartonella* and *Rochalimaea*, with descriptions of *Bartonella quintana* comb. nov., *Bartonella vinsonii* comb. nov., *Bartonella henselae* comb. nov., and *Bartonella elizabethae* comb. nov., and to remove the family *Bartonellaceae* from the order Rickettsiales. *Int J Syst Bacteriol* 1993; 43:777–786.
3. Dumler JS, Barbet AF, Bekker CP, et al. Reorganization of genera in the families *Rickettsiaceae* and *Anaplasmataceae* in the order *Rickettsiales*: unification of some species of *Ehrlichia* with *Anaplasma*, *Cowdria* with *Ehrlichia* and *Ehrlichia* with *Neorickettsia*, descriptions of six new species combinations and designation of *Ehrlichia equi* and 'HGE agent' as subjective synonyms of *Ehrlichia phagocytophila*. *Int J Syst Evol Microbiol* 2001; 51: 2145–2165.
4. Cunha BA. The cause of the plague of Athens: plague, typhoid, typhus, smallpox, or measles? *Infect Dis Clin North Am* 2004; 18:29–43.
5. Cardano G. *De malo recentiorum medicorum medendi usu libellus*. Venetiis, apud O. Scotum 1536.
6. Fracastoro G. *De sympathia et antipathia rerum liber unus. De contagione et contagiosis morbis et curatione*. 1546; Venetiis, apud heredes L. Iuntae.
7. Raoult D, Woodward T, Dumler S. The history of epidemic typhus. *Infect Dis Clin North Am* 2004; 18:127–140.
8. Cober T. *Observationum medicorum Castrensium Hungaricarum Helmstadii*. F. Linderwald 1685.

9. Nicolle CJH. Recherches experimentales sur le typhus exanthematique. *Ann Inst Pasteur* 1910; 24:243–275.

10. Nicolle CJH. Recherches experimentales sur le typhus exanthematique. *Ann Inst Pasteur* 1911; 25:97–144.

11. Nicolle CJH. Recherches experimentales sur le typhus exanthematique. *Ann Inst Pasteur* 1912; 26:250–280.

12. Nicolle CJH. Recherches experimentales sur le typhus exanthematique. *Ann Inst Pasteur* 1912; 26:332–350.

13. da Rocha-Lima H. Zür Aetiologie des Fleckfebers. *Berl Klin Wochenschr* 1916; 53:567–569.

14. Bravo F. *Opera Medicinalia*. Mexico: Ocharte; 1570:1–90.

15. Maxcy KF. Clinical observations on endemic typhus in southern United States. *Public Health Rep* 1926; 41:1213–1220, 2967–2995.

16. Mooser H. Experiments relating to the pathology and etiology of Mexican typhus (tabardillo). *J Infect Dis* 1928; 43:241–272.

17. Maxey EE. Some observations on the so-called spotted fever of Idaho. *Med Sentinel (Portland, OR)* 1899; 7:433–438.

18. Ricketts HT. The transmission of Rocky Mountain spotted fever by the bite of the wood tick (*Dermacentor occidentalis*). *JAMA* 1906; 47:358.

19. Conor ALJ, Bruch A. Un lèvre éruptive. *Bull Soc Pathol Exot* 1910; 3: 45–96.

20. Baelz E, Kawakami K. Das japanische Fluss-oder-Ueberschwemmungs-feber, eine acute Infections-Krankheit. *Virchows Arch Pathol Anat* 1879; 78:373–420, 528–530.

21. Fletcher W, Lesslar JE. *The Weil-Felix Reaction in Sporadic Tropical Typhus*. London: John Bale; 1926.

22. Ogata N. Aetiologie der Tsutsugamushi-Krankheit; *Rickettsia tsutsugamushi*. *Zentralbl Bakteriol (Abt Orig)* 1931; 122:249–253.

23. His W. Ueber eine neue periodische Feberkrankung (Febris Wolhynica). *Berl Klin Wochenschr* 1916; 53:322–323.

24. Töpfer HW. Zür Ursache und Uebertragung des Wolhynischen Febers. *Munch Med Wochenschr* 1916; 63:1495–1496.

25. Regnery RL, Olson JG, Perkins BA, et al. Serological response to 'Rochalimaea henselae' antigen in suspected cat-scratch disease. *Lancet* 1992; 339: 1443–1445.

26. Regnery RL, Anderson BE, Claridge JE, et al. Characterization of a novel *Rochalimaea* species, *R. henselae* sp. nov., isolated from blood of a febrile, human immunodeficiency virus-positive patient. *J Clin Microbiol* 1992; 30:265–274.

27. Sussman LN. Kew Gardens spotted fever. *N Y Med* 1946; 2:27–28.

28. Derrick EH. Q fever, a new fever entity; clinical features and laboratory investigations. *Med J Aust* 1937; 2:281–299.

29. Cox HR, Bell EJ. Epidemic and endemic typhus. Protective value for guinea-pigs of vaccines prepared from infected tissues of the developing chick embryo. *Public Health Rep* 1940; 55:110–115.

30. Fulton F, Joyner L. Cultivation of *Rickettsia tsutsugamushi* in lungs of rodents. Preparation of a scrub typhus vaccine. *Lancet* 1945; ii: 729–734.

31. Wohlbach SB. *The Aetiology and Pathology of Typhus*. Cambridge, MA; Harvard University Press; 1922.

32. Weil E, Felix A. Zür serologischen Diagnose des Fleckfebers. *Wein Klin Wochenschr* 1916; 29:33–35.

33. Chapman AS, Bakken JS, Folk SM, et al. Diagnosis and management of tickborne rickettsial diseases: Rocky Mountain spotted fever, Ehrlichioses, and Anaplasmosis – United States: a practical guide for physicians and other health-care and public health professionals. *MMWR Recomm Rep* 2006; 55: 1–29.

34. Brouqui P, Bacellar F, Baranton G, et al. Guidelines for the diagnosis of tick-borne bacterial diseases in Europe. *Clin Microbiol Infect* 2004; 10: 1108–1132.

35. Richards AL. Rickettsial vaccines: the old and the new. *Expert Rev Vaccines* 2004; 3:541–555.

36. Wilson ME. Prevention of tickborne bacterial diseases. *Med Clin North Am* 2002; 86:219–238.

37. Anderson SGE, Zomorodipour A, Anderson JO, et al. The genome sequence of *Rickettsia prowazekii* and the origin of mitochondria. *Nature* 1998; 396: 133–140.

38. Raoult D, Ndihokubwayo JB, Tissot-Dupont H, et al. Outbreak of epidemic typhus associated with trench fever in Burundi. *Lancet* 1998; 348:86–89.

39. Ndihokubwayo JB, Raoult D. Epidemic typhus in Africa—a review. *Med Trop* 1999; 59:181–192.

40. Brill NE. An acute infectious disease of unknown origin. A clinical study based on 221 cases. *Am J Med Sci* 1910; 139:484–502.

41. Zinsser H. Varieties of typhus vaccine and the epidemiology of the American form of European typhus fever (Brill's disease). *Am J Hyg* 1934; 20:513–532.

42. Sciotto CG, Lauer BA, White WL, et al. Detection of *Borrelia* in acridine orange-stained blood smears by fluorescence microscopy. *Arch Pathol Lab Med* 1983; 107:384–386.

43. Brown PD, Gravekamp C, Carrington DG, et al. Evaluation of the polymerase chain reaction for early diagnosis of leptospirosis. *J Med Microbiol* 1995; 43:110–114.

44. Maurin M, Raoult D. *Rickettsia prowazekii*. In: Mann J, Crabbe MJC, eds. *Bacteria and Antibacterial Agents*. Baltimore: Williams & Wilkins; 2001: 558–561.

45. Dumler JS, Taylor JP, Walker DH. Clinical and laboratory features of murine typhus in south Texas, 1980 through 1987. *JAMA* 1991; 266:1365–1370.

46. Holman RC, Paddock CE, Curns AT, et al. Analysis of risk factors for fatal Rocky Mountain spotted fever: evidence for superiority of tetracyclines for therapy. *J Infect Dis* 2001; 184:1437–1444.

47. Jensenius M, Fournier PE, Kelly P, et al. African tick bite fever. *Lancet Infect Dis* 2003; 3:557–564.

48. Fournier PE, Gouriet F, Brouqui P, et al. Lymphangitis-associated rickettsiosis, a new rickettsiosis caused by *Rickettsia sibirica mongolotimonae*: seven new cases and review of the literature. *Clin Infect Dis* 2005; 40:1435–1444.

49. Nilsson K, Lukinius A, Pahlson C, et al. Evidence of *Rickettsia* spp. infection in Sweden: a clinical, ultrastructural and serological study. *APMIS* 2005; 113:126–134.

50. Uchida T, Yu X, Uchiyama T, et al. Identification of a unique spotted fever group rickettsia from humans in Japan. *J Infect Dis* 1989; 159:1122–1125.

51. Stenos J, Roux V, Walker D, et al. *Rickettsia honei* sp. nov—the agent of Flinders Island spotted fever. *Int J Syst Microbiol* 1998; 48:1399–1404.

52. Paddock CD, Zaki SR, Koss T, et al. Rickettsialpox in New York City: a persistent urban zoonosis. *Ann N Y Acad Sci* 2003; 990:36–44.

53. Tamura A, Ohashi N, Urakami H, et al. Classification of *Rickettsia tsutsugamushi* in a new genus *Orientia* gen. nov. as *Orientia tsutsugamushi* comb. nov. *Int J Syst Microbiol* 1995; 45:589–591.

54. Tay ST, Ho TM, Rohani MY, et al. Antibodies to *Orientia tsutsugamushi*, *Rickettsia typhi* and spotted fever group rickettsiae among febrile patients in rural areas of Malaysia. *Trans R Soc Trop Med Hyg* 2000; 94:280–284.

55. Tsay RW, Chang FY. Serious complications in scrub typhus. *J Microbiol Immunol Infect* 1998; 31:240–244.

56. Watt G, Chouriyagune C, Ruangweerayrnd R, et al. Scrub typhus infections poorly responsive to antibiotics in northern Thailand. *Lancet* 1996; 348: 86–89.

57. Mathai E, Rolain JM, Verghese L, et al. Case reports: scrub typhus during pregnancy in India. *Trans R Soc Trop Med Hyg* 2003; 97:570–572.

58. Brouqui P, Lascola B, Roux V, et al. Chronic *Bartonella quintana* bacteremia in homeless patients. *N Engl J Med* 1999; 340:184–189.

59. Koehler JE, Sanchez MA, Garrido CS, et al. Molecular epidemiology of bartonella infections in patients with bacillary angiomatosis-peliosis. *N Engl J Med* 1997; 337:1876–1878.

60. Relman DA, Loutit JS, Schmidt TM, et al. The agent of bacillary angiomatosis. *N Engl J Med* 1990; 323:1573–1580.

61. Hoover TA, Culp WE, Vodkin MH, et al. Chromosomal DNA deletions explain phenotypic characteristics of two antigenic variants, phase II and RSA 514 (crazy), of the *Coxiella burnetii* nine mile strain. *Infect Immun* 2002; 70: 6726–6733.

EPIDEMIOLOGICAL ASPECTS

The prevalence of different enteropathogens varies with the age of the individual, how the diarrhoea is acquired (e.g. food poisoning or traveller's diarrhoea), between acute and chronic diarrhoea, and with the state of the host's immunity (Table 50.2).

Age

In general, paediatric diarrhoea is most often due to viral enteropathogens (see Chapter 45). Up to 60% of cases in most hospital-based surveys are due to viruses, with rotavirus accounting for a large proportion of cases, followed by adenovirus 40/41 and then astrovirus, but it is now clear that noroviruses are important causes of outbreaks of disease. Bacterial enteropathogens such as enteropathogenic *Escherichia coli* (EPEC), enteroinvasive *E. coli* (EIEC), enterotoxigenic *E. coli* (ETEC), enteroaggregative *E. coli* (EAggEC), salmonellae, *Campylobacter jejuni* and shigellae and the protozoan *Cryptosporidium parvum* and *C. hominis* are responsible for the majority of the remaining cases where a pathogen is found.

In adults, bacteria assume greater importance, although viral gastroenteritis does occur, due, for example, to unusual serogroups of rotavirus, norovirus or astrovirus.[18,19] For instance, it is estimated that *C. jejuni* is responsible for 17–20% of episodes of adult diarrhoea.

Environmental factors

In temperate countries, viruses, except for noroviruses, produce peaks of disease in the cold dry weather of winter,[20] whereas in tropical Africa the seasonality is blurred but with an upsurge in cases in the dry season.[21] In contrast, bacterial and protozoal diarrhoeas tend to occur in the wetter seasons in the tropics and summer in temperate countries. In temperate countries, cryptosporidiosis peaks in spring with a lesser peak in autumn, but, for example, in Gaza, most cases occur in the hottest and driest parts of the year, perhaps when water availability and quality is compromised.[22] On a more global scale, during the 1997–1998 El Nino, when mean ambient temperatures were 5°C higher than normal, in Peru the number of daily hospital admissions with gastroenteritis doubled.[23]

Table 50.1 Paediatric diarrhoea in developed and developing countries

Feature	Developed countries	Developing countries
Episodes per annum	<1	3–10
Seasonality	Winter	None
Severe dehydration	Rare	Frequent
Nutritional sequelae	Rare	Usual
Measles associated	Non-existent	15–63%
Epidemic	Rare	Frequent
Polymicrobial	Unusual	>20%
Case fatality rate	<0.01%	0.6%

After Kumate & Isibasi.[9]

Table 50.2 The relative importance of enteropathogens in childhood diarrhoeal disease

	Mexico	Multicentre	China	Philippines	Malawi	Canada	Chile	Australia
Reference	(10)	(11)	(12)	(13)	(14)	(15)	(16)	(17)
No. of subjects	271	3640	186	236	168	206	90	4637
Survey duration	4.5 months	24 months	22 months	25 months	2 months	24 months	12 months	13 years
Setting	Community	Out-patient	In-patient	In-patient	Out-patient	In-patient	Out-patient	In-patient
	% Positive	% Positive	% Positive	% Positive	% Positive	% Positive	% Positive	% Positive
Rotavirus	3.7	16	56	65	42	3.9	1.1	39.6
Astrovirus	61	NT	8.5	0.4	1.2		5.6	NT
Adenovirus 40/41	12.9	4	2.5	0.4	4.2	} 3.9	1.1	6%
Caliciviruses*	NT	3	7.6	0.4	1.2		NT	NT
Toroviruses	NT	NT	NT	0	0	3.5	NT	NT
Total viruses	77.6	23	74.6	66.2	48.6	42.8	7.8	45.6
Total bacteria	20.3	51	NT	23.4	NT	NT	32.2	9.2
Total protozoa	NT	3.3	NT	2.1	4.2	NT	3.3	NT
Mixed infection	7.4[†]	0	0	7[†]	0	NT	30[†]	0
No pathogen detected	NA	22.7	25.4	1.2	NA	NA	42	43.5

NT, not tested; NA not applicable.
* Includes noroviruses and sapoviruses.
[†] Predominantly viruses.

Table 50.3 Clinical features of inflammatory and non-inflammatory diarrhoea

	Non-inflammatory	Inflammatory
Symptoms	Nausea, vomiting, abdominal pain, but fever not a major feature	Abdominal pain, tenesmus, fever
Stool	Voluminous, watery	Frequent, small volume; blood-stained, pus cells present, mucus
Site	Proximal small intestine	Distal ileum, colon
Mechanism	Osmotic or secretory	Invasion of enterocytes leading to mucosal cell death and inflammatory response

Table 50.4 Pathogens in inflammatory and non-inflammatory diarrhoea

	Inflammatory	Non-inflammatory
Viruses (see Chapter 45)	Nil	Rotavirus Adenovirus 40/41 Astrovirus Norovirus Sapovirus Coronavirus Torovirus Bredavirus Picobirnavirus
Bacteria (see Chapter 51)	Enteroinvasive *E. coli* (EIEC) Enterohaemorrhagic *E. coli* (EHEC), e.g. 0157 Enteroaggregative *E. coli* (EaggEC) *Aeromonas hydrophila* *Campylobacter* spp. *Salmonella* spp. *Shigella* spp. *Yersinia enterocolitica* *Clostridium difficile* *Laribacter hongkongensis*	Enterotoxigenic *E. coli* (ETEC) Enteropathogenic *E. coli* (EPEC) *Vibrio cholerae* *Vibrio parahaemolyticus* *Campylobacter* spp. *Salmonella* spp. *Plesiomonas shigelloides* *Bacillus cereus* *Clostridium perfringens* *Clostridium difficile*
Protozoa (see Chapter 79)	*Entamoeba histolytica* *Balantidium coli*	*Cryptosporidium hominis* *Giardia intestinalis (lamblia)* *Cyclospora cayetanensis* *Blastocystis hominis* *Isospora belli* *Enterocytozoon bieneusi* (Microsporidia)

Food poisoning

Diarrhoeal disease following ingestion of food or water contaminated by bacteria, toxins or protozoa is still an important problem in both developed and developing countries. Although high-intensity animal rearing is important in the maintenance of human enteropathogens in developed countries, in developing countries human-derived enteric pathogens such as *Salmonella* spp. and *C. jejuni* and enterohaemorrhagic *E. coli* (EHEC) may still be implicated in outbreaks of food poisoning. Recently, water-borne outbreaks of *C. parvum* have been assuming greater importance.

Traveller's diarrhoea (turista, Aztec two-step, Montezuma's revenge, Delhi belly, etc.)

It is estimated that approximately 16 million people will travel annually from their domicile in industrialized countries to less-

developed countries. Approximately one-third of these will develop diarrhoeal disease and in the majority of cases this will be due to an infective agent.[24] A large number of different entero-pathogens have been implicated, but in most surveys ETEC are the predominant pathogens (Table 50.5), followed by *C. jejuni* and *Salmonella* spp. The aetiological agents vary considerably according to the countries visited; for example, *C. parvum* and *C. hominis* have recently been shown to be important in visitors to the Caribbean[25] and Africa.[26] Viral enteropathogens can cause traveller's diarrhoea but have, for example, been more frequently associated with shipboard epidemics, in which astrovirus and norovirus have been implicated.

Immunocompromised host

In tropical countries, the immune compromises due to malnutrition and HIV are of major importance; both affect the frequency

Table 50.5 Enteropathogens in traveller's diarrhoea

Pathogen	Prevalence (%)
Enterotoxigenic *E. coli*	30–80
Campylobacter jejuni	c. 20
Shigella spp.	5–15
Salmonella spp.	3–15
Giardia lamblia	0–3
Cryptosporidium spp.	?
Entamoeba histolytica	0–3
Rotavirus	10
Astrovirus	1
Norovirus	1
Unknown	10–15

Table 50.6 Clinical assessment of rehydration

Severity	Body weight loss (%)	Clinical state	Signs
Mild	<5	Not unwell	Thirsty, mucous membranes dry
Moderate	5–10	Apathetic	Sunken eyes, sunken fontanelle, tachypnoea, oliguria, loss of skin turgor
Severe	10–15	Shocked	Hypotensive, peripheral circulatory failure
Critical	>15	Moribund	Severely shocked, comatose

and severity of diarrhoeal disease. With the appearance of AIDS, diarrhoeal disease due to previously unrecognized pathogens, such as *C. parvum, Isospora belli, Enterocytozoon bieneusi* and *Mycobacterium avium-intracellulare*, has assumed increasing importance, albeit more often causing chronic diarrhoea.[27] Interestingly, rotavirus—the major cause of infantile gastroenteritis—appears to be no more severe in HIV-infected than in HIV-uninfected children.[28]

MANAGEMENT OF ACUTE DIARRHOEA

The mainstay of management of diarrhoeal disease is the assessment of dehydration (Figure 50.1) and the appropriate replacement of fluid and electrolytes.[29] Although diarrhoeal disease can produce dehydration at any age, its impact is greatest in those under 5 years old. This is because, as a result of their relatively greater surface area and thus greater fluid loss through skin, infants require 2.5 times more water per kilogram body weight than older individuals. Fluid and electrolyte loss is also greatly exacerbated by vomiting. Both the initial degree of dehydration and the response to rehydration therapy should be monitored clinically (Table 50.6).

Originally, rehydration was exclusively intravenous. This resulted in a tremendous drop in fatality rates – for example, in cholera, from 40% to less than 1% when properly administered. A major advance was made when an effective oral rehydration regimen was devised.

Oral rehydration therapy

Early oral rehydration solutions (ORS) contained only electrolytes and water and it was not until it was realized that glucose or sucrose was required to enhance sodium absorption that effective oral rehydration therapy became available. Glucose and sodium transport into enterocytes are coupled. Sucrose, a dimer of glucose and fructose, must be cleaved by brush-border sucrase for it to be absorbed. Nevertheless, glucose and sucrose seem to be equally effective in ORS,[30] although there may be minor advantages with glucose.[31]

There is also some debate over the use of bicarbonate or citrate to correct acidosis. Both are equally effective, but citrate is more

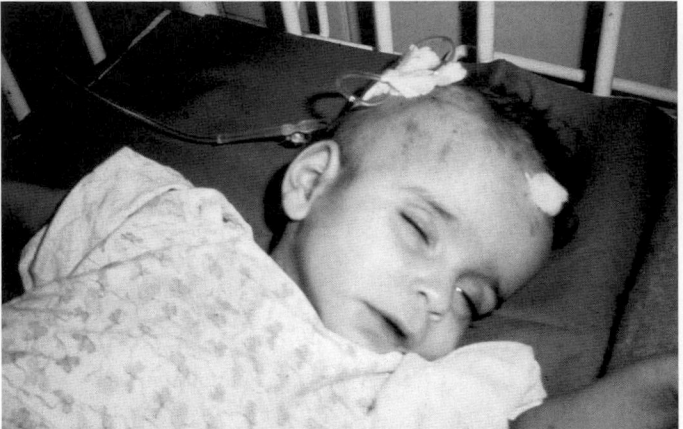

Figure 50.1 A child with severe dehydration being rehydrated intravenously.

stable and has replaced bicarbonate in World Health Organization (WHO) solutions. A further modification has been the incorporation of glycine, which is taken into the enterocyte by a specific amino acid transport system. Glycine, when present in ORS at a concentration of 111 mmol/L, was found to decrease both duration of diarrhoea and stool volume.[32] The composition of various ORS is shown in Table 50.7. ORS can be obtained in packets from UNICEF or can be made up locally. They should contain sodium chloride (3.5 g), potassium chloride (1.5 g) and glucose monohydrate (22 g), made up to 1 L with potable water (sucrose, 40 g, may replace glucose, and trisodium citrate dehydrate, 2.9 g, sodium bicarbonate). To be fully effective ORS should be available at the village level so therapy can be initiated as rapidly as possible. This will require the solution(s) to be available either prepacked or in bulk, with appropriate measuring spoons, a method of providing the correct volume of potable water, and instructions on use as well as to discard unused solution within 24 hours. Studies have shown that when properly instructed 98% of mothers can prepare ORS with a sodium range of 30–110 mmol/L.[33] Recently, rice powder-based ORS have been investigated, since these are more readily available. Rice powder at 30–50 g/L is an effective substitute for glucose. It tastes better than simple electrolyte–glucose ORS and is thus more acceptable to children. A recent meta-analysis of 13 randomized trials of rice-based versus glucose-based oral rehydration therapy demonstrated the superiority of the rice-based solution in cholera diarrhoea, although the benefit was considerably smaller for children with acute non-cholera diarrhoea.[34] During the initial phase of oral rehydration therapy, while the patient is dehydrated, adults can consume 750 mL/h and children up to 300 mL/h. Maintenance therapy of 20 mL solution per kilogram body weight should be started as soon as signs of dehydration have gone. ORS are suitable for rehydration of all except severely dehydrated infants and those with shock (Table 50.8). Decreased-osmolarity ORS (178–268 mmol/L) has been shown to be as safe and effective as conventional ORS (311 mmol/L).[35]

Intravenous rehydration

Approximately 98% of children will respond to oral rehydration therapy. The remainder are generally infants with severe dehydration or those with profuse vomiting or a high purging rate. These will require rehydration by the intravenous route. Suitable solutions include: Ringer's lactate (Hartman's), consisting of NaCl 6.2 g, KCl 0.4 g, Na lactate 2.3 g and 2 mL 50% glucose per litre of solution; Dacca solution (NaCl 5 g, NaHCO$_3$ 4 g, KCl 1 g and 2 mL 50% glucose per litre of solution); or acetate solution (NaCl 5 g, KCl 1 g, Na acetate 6.5 g and 2 mL 50% glucose per litre of solution). Oral rehydration therapy should be started as soon as

possible following institution of intravenous rehydration; however, if signs of severe dehydration persist, it may be necessary to continue using Ringer's lactate at 100 mL/kg body weight per 4 hours.

Adjunctive therapy

Other potential therapeutic interventions include antimicrobial agents, antimotility drugs and antisecretory drugs. They have varying degrees of efficacy and some are absolutely contraindicated for certain conditions.

Antimicrobial drugs

In general, infants with acute watery diarrhoea are best managed without recourse to antibiotics. However, if there is evidence of systemic spread, cholera or dysentery, then antimicrobials will shorten the course of diarrhoea and ameliorate its effects. With the advent of the fluoroquinolones such as ciprofloxacin and ofloxacin, the debate on the use of antimicrobials has been reopened. First, there is no doubt that the widespread indiscriminate use of antimicrobials, often in subtherapeutic regimens, encourages resistance in both pathogens and normal enteric flora.[36] On the other hand, even with ETEC, early treatment with co-trimoxazole[37] or ciprofloxacin can decrease the severity of diarrhoea. This is preferred to the widespread prophylactic use of these antimicrobials, which will certainly produce resistant bacteria.

In cholera, tetracycline or ciprofloxacin decreases the duration of diarrhoea and shedding of bacteria. In countries where *Shigella* spp. dysentery is endemic or when epidemics occur, antimicrobials are of benefit, but development of resistance during the course of epidemics occurs with monotonous regularity.[36] Metronidazole (or tinidazole) is valuable in the treatment of giardiasis or amoebic dysentery.

Antimotility drugs

These should be avoided.

Antisecretory drugs

These will of course only be effective if there is a secretory component to the diarrhoea. The value of loperamide as an adjunct in treating diarrhoea in well-nourished children has been demonstrated[38] but these authors warned against its use in malnourished children.

Compounds such as kaolin or charcoal which, it is postulated, act by absorbing toxins, have had little effect in controlled trials.

Table 50.7 Composition of oral rehydration solutions

Component	CONCENTRATION (MMOL/L WATER)		
	Citrate ORS	Bicarbonate ORS	Glycine ORS*
Sodium	90	90	90
Potassium	20	20	20
Chloride	80	80	80
Citrate	10	—	—
Bicarbonate	—	30	30
Glucose	111	111	111
Glycine	—	—	111

* May contain either bicarbonate or citrate.

Table 50.8 Guidelines for rehydration

Degree	Age group	Type of fluid	Volume (mL/kg body weight)	Timing
Mild	All	ORS	50	Every 4 hours
Moderate	All	ORS	100	Every 4 hours
Severe	Infants	i.v. (Hartman's)	70	Every 4 hours
Severe and shock	All	i.v. (Hartman's)	70–100	Every 4 hours

Nutritional supplements

Micronutrient deficiencies have been associated with increased incidence, severity and duration of diarrhoeal and other diseases. Micronutrient supplementation trials have yielded varying results. For example, a trial of vitamin A supplementation in Haiti demonstrated an increased 2-week prevalence of diarrhoea post supplementation,[39] whereas a trial of zinc supplementation in India has demonstrated clinically important decreases in the severity and duration of diarrhoea.[40]

There is increasing interest in the value of administering commensal bacteria (probiotics) to ameliorate diarrhoeal disease.[41] In trials in Pakistan and Thailand, administration of one such probiotic, *Lactobacillus casei* GG, decreased the duration of diarrhoea and reduced stool frequency in children with acute watery diarrhoea.[42,43]

CONTROL OF DIARRHOEAL DISEASE

In industrialized countries, it has been the separation of human and animal excreta from potable water and foodstuffs that has contributed to the great decline in the incidence of diarrhoeal disease. In addition, improvements in facilities for personal hygiene within the home have decreased the intrafamilial spread of enteropathogens. To implement these measures in developing countries will need a massive input from industrialized countries. Other simpler and more locally applicable measures to prevent diarrhoeal disease include development of technologies and practices that interrupt disease transmission by muscid flies.[44,45] Recently it has been shown that exposure of drinking water (in plastic bottles) to tropical sunlight decreased diarrhoeal disease in Maasai children in Kenya.[46]

There is little doubt that measles and malnutrition increase the morbidity and mortality of diarrhoeal disease, and control of measles by immunization should be possible. Finally, it is unlikely that spread of some enteric pathogens, such as rotavirus, can be prevented completely by public health and good hygiene. A safe and effective vaccine would be of major benefit.

Morbidity

Malnutrition greatly affects immunity[47,48] and the incidence and severity of diarrhoeal disease. Similarly, diarrhoeal disease will greatly exacerbate malnutrition, thus creating an inexorable downward spiral. Acute diarrhoeal disease can become chronic, and chronic diarrhoea, for example that due to *C. parvum* or *C. hominis*, can become greatly prolonged.[49] Disaccharide (principally lactose) intolerance following certain types of diarrhoea has been a source of great controversy. Certain pathogens such as rotavirus or EPEC produce a great decrease in small-intestinal disaccharidase levels. Some consider that infants should not be given their normal diet because of the problem of disaccharide intolerance. Most evidence now suggests that infants should return to their normal diet within 24 hours of onset of diarrhoea unless there are specific contraindications.[50]

CONCLUSIONS

Diarrhoeal disease is still a major cause of mortality even though it has been shown that introduction of oral rehydration therapy can decrease mortality to less than 0.5% in defined study areas.

Editors regret to announce the untimely death of Professor Tony Hart whose contributions to Manson's were invaluable.

REFERENCES

1. Murray CJL, Lopez AD. Mortality by cause for eight regions of the world: global burden of disease study. *Lancet* 1997; 349:1269–1276.
2. Bern C, Martines J, de Zoysa I, et al. The magnitude of the global problem of diarrhoeal disease: a ten year update. *Bull World Health Organ* 1992; 70: 705–714.
3. Hart CA, Cunliffe NA. Diagnosis and causes of viral gastroenteritis. *Curr Opin Infect Dis* 1996; 9:333–339.
4. WHO/CDD/VID/84.4 *Diarrhoeal Disease Control Programme. Report of the Third Meeting of the Scientific Working Group on Viral Diarrhoeas. Microbiology, Epidemiology, Immunology and Vaccine Development.* Geneva: WHO; 1984:8–14.
5. Mata L, Simhon A, Urrutia J, et al. Epidemiology of rotavirus in cohort of 45 Guatemalan Mayan Indian children from birth to age 3 year. *J Infect Dis* 1984; 148:452–461.
6. Black RC, Lopez de Romana G, Brown KH, et al. Incidence and etiology of infantile diarrhea and major routes of transmission in Huascar, Peru. *Am J Epidemiol* 1989; 129:785–799.
7. Gurwith M, Wenman W, Hinde D, et al. A prospective study of rotavirus infection in infants and young children. *J Infect Dis* 1981; 144:218–224.
8. de Wit MAS, Koopmans MPG, Kortbeek LA, et al. Gastroenteritis in sentinel practices, The Netherlands. *Emerg Infect Dis* 2001; 7:82–91.
9. Kumate J, Isibasi A. Pediatric diarrheal diseases: a global perspective. *Pediatr Infect Dis J* 1986; 5(suppl):S21–S28.
10. Maldonaldo Y, Cantwell M, Old M, et al. Population-based prevalence of symptomatic and asymptomatic astrovirus infection in rural Mayan infants. *J Infect Dis* 1998; 178:834–839.
11. Hulian S, Zhen LG, Mathan MM, et al. Etiology of acute diarrhoea among children in developing countries: a multicentre study in five countries. *Bull World Health Organ* 1992; 69:549–555.
12. Qiao HP, Nilsson M, Abreu ER, et al. Viral diarrhea in children in Beijing, China. *J Med Virol* 1999; 5:390–396.
13. Pajé-Vilar E, Co BG, Caradang EH, et al. Non-bacterial diarrhoea in children in the Philippines. *Ann Trop Med Parasitol* 1994; 88:53–58.
14. Pavone R, Schinaia N, Hart CA, et al. Viral gastroenteritis in children in Malawi. *Ann Trop Paediatr* 1990; 10:15–20.
15. Jamieson FB, Wang EL, Bain C, et al. Human torovirus: a new nosocomial gastrointestinal pathogen. *J Infect Dis* 1998; 178:1263–1269.
16. Gaggero A, O'Ryan M, Noel JS, et al. Prevalence of astrovirus infection among Chilean children with acute gastroenteritis. *J Clin Microbiol* 1998; 36: 3691–3693.
17. Barnes GL, Uren E, Stevens KB, et al. Etiology of acute gastroenteritis in hospitalized children in Melbourne, Australia from April 1980 to March 1993. *J Clin Microbiol* 1998; 36:133–138.
18. Krishnan T, Sen A, Choudhury JS, et al. Emergence of adult diarrhea rotavirus in Calcutta, India. *Lancet* 1999; 353:380–381.
19. Glass RI, Noel J, Mitchell D, et al. The changing epidemiology of astrovirus-associated gastroenteritis: a review. *Arch Virol* 1996; 12(suppl):287–300.
20. Hart CA, Cunliffe NA. Viral gastroenteritis. *Curr Opin Infect Dis* 1999; 12: 447–457.
21. Cunliffe NA, Kilgore PE, Bresee JS, et al. Epidemiology of rotavirus diarrhea in Africa: a review to assess the need for rotavirus immunization. *Bull World Health Organ* 1998; 76:525–537.

22. Sallon S, El Showaa R, El Masri M, et al. Cryptosporidiosis in children in Gaza. *Ann Trop Paed* 1990; 11:277–281.

23. Checkley W, Epstein LD, Gilman RH, et al. Effects of El Nino and ambient temperature on hospital admissions for diarrhoeal diseases in Peruvian children. *Lancet* 2000; 355:442–450.

24. Steffan R, van der Linde F, Gyre K, et al. Epidemiology of diarrhea in travellers. *JAMA* 1983; 249:1176–1180.

25. Ma P, Kaufman DC, Helmick CG, et al. Cryptosporidium in tourists returning from the Caribbean. *N Engl J Med* 1985; 312:647–648.

26. Soave R, Ma P. Cryptosporidium: traveller's diarrhea in two families. *Arch Intern Med* 1985; 145:70–72.

27. Smith PD. Gastrointestinal infections in AIDS. *Ann Intern Med* 1992; 116: 63–77.

28. Cunliffe NA, Gondwe JS, Kirkwood CD, et al. Effect of concomitant HIV infection on presentation and outcome of rotavirus gastroenteritis in Malawian children. *Lancet* 2001; 18:550–555.

29. Cash RA. Oral rehydration therapy. In: Farthing MJG, Keusch GT, eds. *Enteric Infection*. London: Chapman & Hall; 1989:441–451.

30. Sack DA, Chowdhury AMAK, Eusof A, et al. Oral rehydration in rotavirus diarrhoea: a double blind comparison of sucrose with glucose electrolyte solution. *Lancet* 1978; ii:280–283.

31. Nalin DR, Levine MM, Mata L, et al. Comparison of sucrose with glucose in oral therapy of infant diarrhoea. *Lancet* 1978; ii:277–279.

32. Mahalanabis D, Patra FC. In search of a super oral rehydration solution: can optimum use of organic solute-mediated sodium absorption lead to the development of an absorption promoting drug? *J Diarrhoeal Dis Res* 1983; 1:76–81.

33. Bhatia S, Cash RA, Cornaz I. Evaluation of the oral therapy expansion program (OTEP) of the Bangladesh rural advancement committee (BRAC). *Swiss Development Cooperation and Humanitarian Aid* 1983; January 24–February 12.

34. Gore SM, Fontaine O, Pierce NF. Impact of rice based oral rehydration solution on stool output and duration of diarrhoea: meta-analysis of 13 clinical trials. *BMJ* 1992; 304:287–291.

35. Murphy C, Hahn S, Volmink J. Reduced osmolarity oral rehydration solution for treating cholera. *Cochrane Database Syst Rev* 2004; (4):CD003754.

36. Kariuki S, Hart CA. Global aspects of antimicrobial resistant enteric bacteria. *Curr Opin Infect Dis* 2001; 14:576–586.

37. DuPont HR, Randall RR, Galindo E, et al. Treatment of traveller's diarrhea with trimethoprim/sulfamethoxazole and with trimethoprim alone. *N Engl J Med* 1982; 307:841–844.

38. Diarrhoeal Diseases Study Group (UK). Loperamide in acute diarrhoea in childhood: results of a double blind placebo controlled multicentre clinical trial. *BMJ* 1984; 298:1263–1267.

39. Stansfield SK, Muller P-L, Lerebours G, et al. Vitamin A supplementation and increased prevalence of childhood diarrhoea and acute respiratory infections. *Lancet* 1993; 342:578–582.

40. Sazawal S, Black RE, Bhan MK, et al. Zinc supplementation in young children with acute diarrhea in India. *N Engl J Med* 1995; 333:839–844.

41. MacFarlane GT, Cummings JH. Probiotics and prebiotics: can regulating the activities of intestinal bacteria benefit health? *BMJ* 1999; 318: 999–1003.

42. Raza S, Graham SM, Allen SJ, et al. *Lactobacillus* GG promotes recovery from acute non-bloody diarrhea in Pakistan. *Pediatr Infect Dis J* 1995; 14:107–111.

43. Pant AR, Graham SM, Allen SJ, et al. *Lactobacillus* GG and acute diarrhoea in young children in the tropics. *J Trop Pediatr* 1996; 42:162–165.

44. Chavasse DC, Shier RP, Murphy OA, et al. Impact of fly control on childhood diarrhoea in Pakistan: community randomised trial. *Lancet* 1999; 353:22–25.

45. Emerson PM, Lindsay SW, Walraven GEL, et al. Effect of the fly control on trachoma and diarrhoea. *Lancet* 1999; 353:1401–1403.

46. Conroy RM, Elmore-Meegan M, Joyce T, et al. Solar disinfection of drinking water and diarrhoea in Maasai children: a controlled field trial. *Lancet* 1996; 348:1695–1696.

47. Chandra RK. Nutrition, immunity and infection: present knowledge and future directions. *Lancet* 1983; i:688–691.

48. Dowd P, Heatly R. The influence of undernutrition on immunity. *Clin Sci* 1984; 66:241–248.

49. Sallon S, Deckelbaum RJ, Schmid II, et al. *Cryptosporidium*, malnutrition and chronic diarrhea in children. *Am J Dis Child* 1988; 142:312–315.

50. Committee on Nutrition. Use of oral fluid therapy and posttreatment feeding following enteritis in children in a developed country. *Pediatrics* 1985; 75:358–361.

Chapter 51

C. Anthony Hart and Paul Shears

Bacterial Enteropathogens

The adult human comprises some 10^{14} cells but only 10% of these are mammalian. The remaining 9×10^{13} consists of the bacteria, fungi, protozoa and even multicellular parasites that make up normal flora. The gastrointestinal tract is the major reservoir for these flora. Although bacteria can be found in the stomach and small intestine, they are present in low numbers ($10^2–10^4$ colony forming units [cfu]/mL) and are usually transient(s). In contrast, the lower ileum and colon contain large numbers of bacteria ($\approx 10^{12}$ cfu/mL), weighing 1–2 kg. To detect small numbers of pathogens in this mass of normal flora can therefore be problematic and has led to the formulation of selective media, which work with varying degrees of success.

HELICOBACTER PYLORI

Since the beginning of the 1900s, histopathologists have described spiral bacteria in the stomach. It was not until 1983 that a bacterium was grown, rather serendipitously.[1] This microorganism was originally named *Campylobacter pyloridis*, renamed *C. pylori* for grammatical reasons, and was finally designated *Helicobacter pylori*.[2,3] It is now accepted that *H. pylori* causes acute and chronic non-autoimmune gastritis and is probably the commonest bacterial infection of mankind. It is responsible for up to 80% of gastric and 95% of duodenal ulcers (odds ratios 3–12). In 1994, *H. pylori* was classified as a grade 1 carcinogen, by the International Agency for Research on Cancer, the only bacterium to be so classified. It causes gastric carcinoma (odds ratios 2–12) and is estimated to be involved in up to 60% of gastric carcinomas but only after long-term infection (30–40 years). It is also associated with intestinal mucosa-associated lymphoid tumours (MALTomas) (odds ratio >10).

Epidemiology

Infection with *H. pylori* is present in all areas of the world surveyed.[2,3] In developed countries, approximately 10% of healthy individuals under 30 years of age have serological evidence of infection and this rises to 60% in those over 60. In developing countries, infection is highly prevalent and develops at a younger age. For example, in the Gambia, 15% of infants under 20 months and 46% of those under 5 years had antibodies to *H. pylori*;[4] in Peru, 48% of children aged 2 months to 12 years have evidence of infection.[5] In most developing countries, virtually 100% of individuals are seropositive by early childhood.[6] It is accepted that infection is usually acquired in the first 5 years of life but that improving hygienic and socioeconomic conditions in developed and some developing countries has led to a decreased rate of acquisition and an apparent birth cohort effect. Humans appear to be the major reservoir for *H. pylori* and it has been grown or its genome detected in saliva, dental plaque, vomitus, gastric juice and faeces.[7] How it is transmitted is unclear. Person-to-person spread via endoscopes, pH electrodes or nasogastric feeding tubes[3,7] has been documented, but this is unlikely to be a major mode of transmission. Close contact promotes spread; for example, families of infected children have a higher incidence of infection, as have gastroenterologists who are endoscopists.[8,9] Family clusters of infection are related to socioeconomic status,[10] and infection is most readily transmitted between siblings, especially if their age gap is small.[11] The faecal–oral route is the most likely mode of spread and *H. pylori* DNA and antigen have been detected in faeces, but others have suggested that interoral spread is most important and some have suggested that the oral cavity is a permanent reservoir of *H. pylori*.[12] The domestic fly (*Musca domestica*) can become colonized by *H. pylori*, and *H. pylori* DNA has been detected in houseflies from three continents.[13] This raises the possibility of fly contamination of food leading to food-borne infection. *H. pylori* does not grow in foods but does survive, providing it is kept cool, moist and is not too acid. Water-borne spread has also been suggested as a major factor in developing countries.[5] Finally, some animal species, including the macaque, sheep and pig, have been shown to harbour *H. pylori*, suggesting the possibility of zoonotic spread.[7] *H. pylori* has even been detected in sheep's milk. A number of other *Helicobacter* species have been detected in a variety of animals, but only *H. heilmanii* is found in the human stomach.

Microbiology

H. pylori is a sinusoidal Gram-negative bacterium approximately 3.5 μm long by 0.5–1 μm in diameter (Figure 51.1). It has a smooth surface and four to six sheathed flagella with terminal bulbs (unlike *Campylobacter* spp.). The bacterium produces a

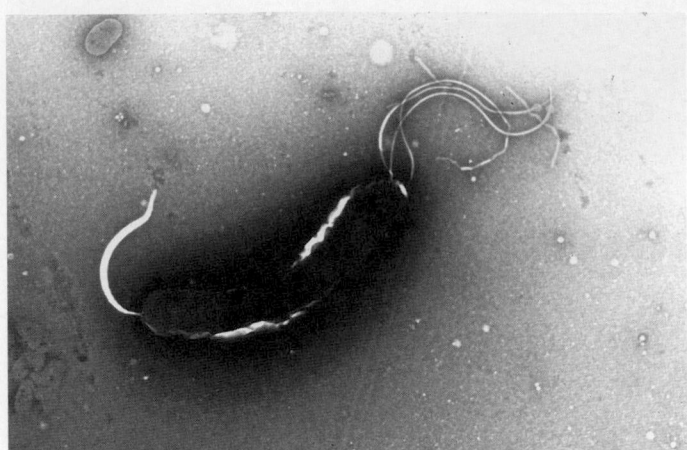

Figure 51.1 Negative-stain electron micrograph of *Helicobacter pylori* showing sheathed flagella with a terminal bulb.

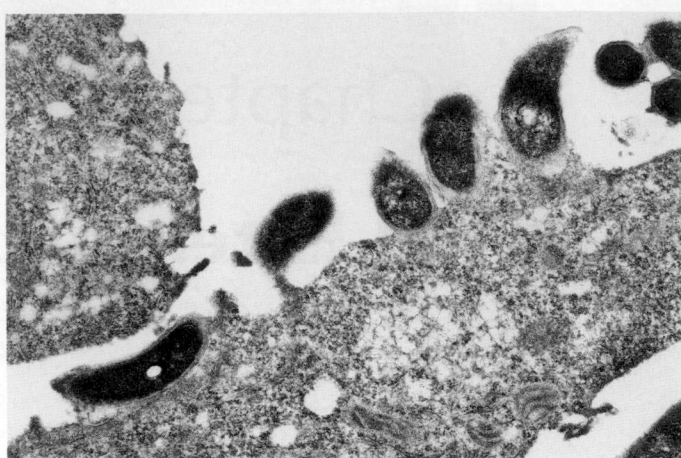

Figure 51.2 Thin-section electron micrograph of *H. pylori* intimately attached to a gastric enterocyte.

powerful urease and seems well adapted to living beneath the mucous layer attached to the surface of gastric enterocytes. *H. pylori* is fastidious and slow-growing. It requires enriched selective media for isolation from clinical specimens. Growth is optimal at 37°C under humidified microaerophilic conditions in 10% carbon dioxide and takes 4–6 days.

Pathogenesis

Koch's postulates have been largely accepted for an association of *H. pylori* and antral non-autoimmune (type B) gastritis both in adults and in children.[2,3,14,15] There is also a strong association between *H. pylori* and peptic ulceration.[2] In feeding experiments, doses of between 10^5 and 10^9 cfu have established infection, but the minimum dose has not been determined. *H. pylori* appears to be able to survive an acidic gastric pH to penetrate the mucus covering the gastric epithelial cells. It has been postulated that the bacterium's spiral morphology and flagella are important in this aspect of pathogenesis.[9] The bacteria can exist free in the mucous layer or firmly attached to the epithelial cells (Figure 51.2). *H. pylori* then elaborates a powerful urease which helps to neutralize the acidic pH, a cytotoxin which causes vacuolation (Vac A), a protease which hydrolyses mucus, and other factors which stimulate gastric acid secretion. Recently it has been found that certain strains of *H. pylori* are more likely to produce inflammation. These tend to possess a 40 kb pathogenicity island (a region of chromosomal DNA acquired by horizontal transmission) called the *cag* pathogenicity island (PAI).[2] This region encodes a secretion system (type IV) that transports a protein, cag, across both bacterial membranes and injects it into host cells. Cag is also encoded in the PAI and once inside the gastric enterocyte induces the secretion of pro-inflammatory cytokines including interleukin-8.[16] The pathogenesis of MALToma production appears to involve chronic antigenic stimulation, and elimination of *H. pylori* is associated with cure of the lymphomas. Infected individuals mount a systemic and local humoral immune response to the bacterium. *H. pylori*-specific secretory IgA can be detected both in saliva and gastric juice. What role this plays in immunity is unclear since antibody is detectable in patients who are colonized or infected.

Pathology

H. pylori is strongly associated with chronic antral gastritis and with its active phase. Although macroscopic inflammation is usually not present, examination of biopsies reveals *H. pylori* in close apposition to the gastric mucosa which shows an infiltrate with mono- and polymorphonuclear leukocytes. *H. pylori* and evidence of inflammation may also be found in areas of gastric metaplasia in the oesophagus (Barrett's oesophagus) or duodenum.

Clinical features

Chronic epigastric pain is very common in the populations of many developing and developed countries. In sub-Saharan Africa, non-ulcerous dyspepsia and duodenal ulcer are the most common causes of epigastric pain.[17,18] Infection with *H. pylori* was found in 141 (88%) of adult Malawians undergoing gastroscopy for chronic epigastric pain.[18] Other features associated with *H. pylori* gastritis include nausea, vomiting and flatulence. Similar features may also be seen in children with *H. pylori* infection.[15] The clinical features of gastritis relapse and remit, thus it is possible to detect *H. pylori* infection in individuals who have histological evidence of gastritis but no signs or symptoms.

Duodenal ulceration is associated with chronic antral gastritis. *H. pylori* can be detected in both antrum and duodenal ulcer tissue, but it will not colonize the duodenum except in areas of duodenal metaplasia.[19]

Diagnosis

Specific diagnosis may be reached by invasive or non-invasive techniques (Table 51.1).

Invasive techniques

Gastroscopic biopsies from the antrum, duodenal ulcer(s) or other areas of potential colonization are examined by culture and histology and for urease activity. Two biopsy specimens from the antrum are sufficient to detect *H. pylori*.[18] Histological samples may be stained by Giemsa, silver impregnation or acridine orange

Table 51.1 Invasive and non-invasive tests for the diagnosis of *H. pylori* infection

Test	Sensitivity (%)	Specificity (%)	Cost	Comment
NON-INVASIVE				
Antibody detection – ELISA	84–95	80–95	+	Can be used for proof of cure
Antibody detection – rapid	60–75	88–92	+	Can be used for proof of cure
Stool antigen detection	90–100	92–95	++	Becomes rapidly negative after therapy
^{13}C breath test	90–96	99	+++	Needs specialized equipment
^{14}C breath test	90–96	99	+++	Needs specialized equipment
INVASIVE				
Histology	80–90	93–100	+++	Takes time
Culture	75–90	100	+	Takes 3–4 days
Urease	85–95	99	+	Rapid test
Gram or other stain	75–90	80–90	+	Rapid but not ideal
PCR	95–100	95–99	+++	Very sensitive, takes 4–5 hours

for detection of *H. pylori*. This is more sensitive than culture in most surveys.

For culture, biopsy specimens are either rolled on the surface of an appropriate culture medium (e.g. brain–heart infusion-enriched Columbia blood agar incorporating Skirrow's antibiotics) or homogenized and similarly applied. In tropical countries it is advisable to incorporate an antifungal such as amphotericin B into the medium. A '1 minute' urease test, in which the biopsy is immersed in a urea (10% deionized water) solution containing a pH indicator (phenol red), has proved highly sensitive and specific.[18]

Non-invasive techniques

Detection of antibody to *H. pylori* in serum or saliva is possible using an enzyme-linked immunosorbent assay (ELISA). Such tests have proved highly sensitive[14,15] but the specificity is variable since it is possible to detect antibody in those who are no longer infected.[18]

Breath tests which, for example, involve administering [^{13}C] urea and measuring the release of the isotope in the patient's breath have proved useful in developed and developing countries.[5] They depend upon the presence of *H. pylori* urease, which hydrolyses the urea with release of $^{13}CO_2$.

Recently, an antigen-capture ELISA has been developed for detection of *H. pylori* in stool. It has proved sensitive and specific[20] and is useful as a test of cure. It is rapid and easy to carry out. It costs less than £10 per test,[21] which is about half the cost of a breath test but still unaffordable in most developing countries.

Management and treatment

Often, non-ulcer dyspepsia is not treated other than by symptomatic management. *H. pylori* is susceptible in vitro to a wide range of antimicrobials, including ampicillin, quinolones, cephalosporins, nitroimidazoles and macrolides, but all fail as monotherapy in vivo. Combinations of tripotassium dicitratobismuthate and ampicillin or metronidazole achieve 40% and 80% eradication rates, respectively,[22] but require 2–4 weeks' administration. Unfor-

tunately, resistance of *H. pylori* to metronidazole is high in African countries.[18]

Although treatment with H_2-blockers heals most duodenal ulcers, the majority (70–80%) relapse within 12 months. A combination of bismuth salts with amoxicillin and metronidazole with or without H_2 blockers is associated with ulcer healing, eradication of *H. pylori* and a greatly decreased relapse rate.[22,23] Current optimal regimens are based on the macrolide clarithromycin combined with proton pump inhibitors or ranitidine bismuth citrate with or without amoxicillin.[24] However, these will need to be evaluated locally.

Complications

In Gambian children, an association between *H. pylori* and chronic diarrhoea and malnutrition has been described.[4] *H. pylori* gastritis was associated with protein-losing enteropathy in South African children.[25] Co-infection with *H. pylori* and *Vibrio cholerae* 01 was found frequently in Peruvian children and elderly adults, suggesting that hypochlorhydria induced by acute and chronic *H. pylori* infection might increase susceptibility to cholera.[26] Finally, epidemiological studies have suggested a link between current infection with *H. pylori* and atherothrombogenesis.[27]

Prevention and control

Infection with *H. pylori* is ubiquitous throughout the world but highly localized in individuals. Until more is known about the mode of spread, pathogenesis and immunity, prevention and control are impossible. The decrease in infection in children in developed countries suggests that improving socioeconomic and hygienic conditions should help. However, experimental vaccines are currently being tested.[2]

ESCHERICHIA COLI

Escherichia coli is the major aerobic component of the normal intestinal flora ($\approx 10^7$ cfu/mL) but is also a major cause of diarrhoeal

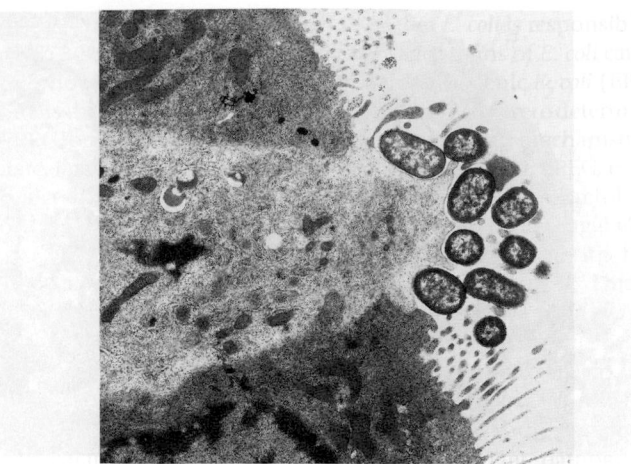

Figure 51.5 Thin-section electron micrograph of duodenal mucosa showing loss of brush border and intimately attached enteropathogenic *E. coli* (attaching/effacement).

charidase enzymes are integral proteins in the microvillous membrane, levels of these enzymes are markedly depressed.[44,45] The disaccharides sucrose, lactose and maltose in the diet must be hydrolysed to monosaccharides to be absorbed. Because of loss of the brush border, the disaccharides cannot be cleaved and are thus not absorbed. They pass to the colon and cause a non-inflammatory osmotic diarrhoea, although in some cases there also appears to be a secretory component.[38]

Clinical features

EPEC tend to produce more severe and prolonged diarrhoea which may remit and relapse. There is initially vomiting, with fever and profuse diarrhoea with mucus but no blood. Fatality rates in epidemics range from 30% to 50%, but with oral rehydration and antibiotic therapy mortality rates have decreased to less than 8%.[46]

Treatment and prevention

The initial treatment should be to rehydrate. Because the diarrhoea can be prolonged, enteral or parenteral nutrition and antibiotics may be indicated. Ampicillin is unlikely to be effective even if the EPEC are sensitive. Administration of oral non-absorbable antibiotics such as neomycin or polymyxin B is effective. Oral absorbable antibiotics such as fluoroquinolones or trimethoprim may also be of benefit. However, antibiotic resistance to most antibiotics has been observed in EPEC.

A vaccine is not available for prevention of infection.

Enterohaemorrhagic *E. coli* (EHEC)

EHEC were first described in Canada in 1983, when they were linked to cases of haemorrhagic colitis[47] and haemolytic–uraemic syndrome.[48] Infections were caused by a newly emerged (in the late 1970s) bacterium, *E. coli* O157. Subsequently, a number of other *E. coli* O serogroups and other coliforms (*Enterobacter cloacae* and *Citrobacter freundii*), have caused disease in humans.

Epidemiology

Infections with EHEC were initially described in industrialized countries. Here they tend to cause outbreaks of infection usually as the result of the consumption of incompletely cooked beef or pork.[49] EHEC can be part of the normal enteric flora of cattle, pigs, sheep, goats, cats and dogs, in which they cause no disease.

An initial survey of adults in Thailand with diarrhoea showed that 2% of 458 patients were infected by EHEC.[50] There have recently been large outbreaks of haemorrhagic colitis caused by EHEC in southern Africa, associated with animal contamination of open water supplies in drought affected areas in Swaziland and among Mozambiquan refugees in Malawi.[51,52] However, because the infective dose is low (<10^2 cfu), person-to-person spread also occurs.

Pathogenesis

EHEC produce attaching effacement, limited to the terminal ileum and colon, and have most of the genes in the LEE pathogenicity island of EPEC. In addition, they release one or both of the toxins originally named verocytotoxins (VT) 1 and 2. These toxins are now called Shiga-like toxins (SLT) 1 and 2; they inhibit protein synthesis and are cytotoxic.[53] They are subunit toxins that bind to globoside receptors (the P-blood group antigen) on cells. The receptors are more densely expressed on renal endothelial cells and in children. In the colon they kill enterocytes, leading to an inflammatory haemorrhagic colitis. If they enter the systemic circulation, they can damage renal endothelial cells and precipitate the haemolytic–uraemic syndrome.[49]

Clinical features

Haemorrhagic colitis presents with abdominal cramps and watery diarrhoea that is followed by a haemorrhagic discharge resembling a colonic bleed. There is rarely an accompanying fever. Haemolytic-uraemic syndrome is one of the commonest, if not the most common, cause of acute renal failure in childhood in industrialized countries. In an Indian study, EHEC were implicated in 19 of 28 cases of haemolytic–uraemic syndrome and *Shigella* spp. in only six.[54] Haemolytic–uraemic syndrome presents with acute renal failure, thrombocytopenia, coagulopathy and evidence of microangiopathic haemolytic anaemia. With peritoneal dialysis the outlook is good, with the fatality rate falling from 50% to less than 10%.

Diagnosis

The first strains of *E. coli* associated with haemorrhagic colitis and haemolytic–uraemic syndrome were of serogroup O157; and sorbitol non-fermenters. Thus, serogrouping and sorbitol MacConkey agar are used to diagnose infections. However, other serogroups (Table 51.1) are also implicated. The toxins SLT1 and SLT2 are transferable between bacteria on promiscuous bacteriophages. Thus, specific diagnosis depends upon detection of SLT or its genes (by DNA hybridization or PCR) or of EHEC plasmid encoded fimbrial adhesin genes.[50] Excretion of EHEC beyond the period of diarrhoea is short lived. For retrospective diagnosis it is possible to detect serum antibody to SLT.[55]

Treatment and prevention

The treatment of haemorrhagic colitis is essentially treatment of dehydration. Antibiotics have no role and in some cases (as with *Sh. dysenteriae* 1) may increase the risk of complications.[56] For haemolytic–uraemic syndrome, peritoneal dialysis is the most important intervention. No vaccine is currently available.

Enteroaggregative *E. coli* (EAggEC)

EAggEC are the most recently discovered pathogenic group.[57] They are named for their characteristic pattern of adherence to tissue culture cells: in large aggregates.

EAggEC can cause both acute and persistent diarrhoea. In a survey of EAggEC infection in India, the most notable clinical features were fever, vomiting, overt blood in the stool and a mean duration of diarrhoea of 17 days.[58] How diarrhoea is produced is not known, but intestinal inflammation appears to be linked to stimulation of interleukin-8 secretion.[59]

Diagnosis is by culture of *E. coli* that produce a distinctive aggregative pattern on cultured cells and that contain EAggEC pathogenicity genes detectable by PCR.[60]

CAMPYLOBACTER JEJUNI

The genus *Campylobacter* is a major cause of gastroenteritis in both developed and developing countries. Although *C. fetus* was recognized as an opportunist pathogen as early as 1947, the full role of *Campylobacter* species as major enteric pathogens was not realized until appropriate selective media were devised.[61,62]

A related genus, *Arcobacter* (principally *A. butzleri*), is increasingly recognized as an enteropathogen with similar pathogenic potential to *Campylobacter*.[63,64]

Epidemiology

The major enteric pathogens in the genus are *C. jejuni* (I and II), *C. coli* and *C. lari*, although *C. upsaliensis* is increasingly recognized. Of these, *C. jejuni* is the most common (≈ 90% of cases of campylobacteriosis) cause of gastroenteritis. All can be normally present in the gastrointestinal tract of domestic and wild animals and birds, which act as the major reservoir for infection. *C. lari*, in particular, can be part of the normal intestinal flora of birds. Campylobacters can survive for 2–5 weeks in cow's milk or water kept at 4°C but they do not multiply. Infection is spread faeco-orally, human-to-human or animal-to-human (there have even been cases of human-to-animal spread), either directly or indirectly in food and water.

- *Animal-to-human.* Close contact with animals, such as that in villages in developing countries where poultry, goats, cattle and dogs roam freely, increases the risk of infection.
- *Human-to human.* Transmission may occur from infected individuals or from convalescent carriers, especially young children. Epidemics of infection can occur in nurseries or paediatric wards.
- *Food.* Contamination can occur during preparation of food from the animal's intestinal content(s) or by incomplete cooking.

- *Milk.* Consumption of raw unpasteurized milk is strongly associated with illness,[65,66] as is contamination of bottled milk following attack by birds.[67]
- *Water.* Excreta from wild and domesticated animals can contaminate surface water, and water-borne transmission is important in developing countries.

The incubation period is 2–5 days[66] with an infective dose of 500 cfu. The median duration of excretion of *C. jejuni* following cessation of diarrhoea is 2–3 weeks.

Infection is most common in those under 1 year old, with a decrease in attack rate with increasing age. Data on Campylobacter infection in tropical areas is limited, partly because of the difficulty of isolating the organism with limited laboratory facilities. Its prevalence has been shown from studies in India,[68] Egypt,[69] and southern Africa.[70]

Bacteriology

Campylobacters are Gram-negative bacteria with a single polar flagellum (Figure 51.6). They are spiral or bent rods, 0.2–0.5 μm in diameter and 1.5–3.5 μm long. They are thermophilic and will grow at 42°C but prefer a microaerophilic atmosphere. *C. jejuni* can hydrolyse hippurate, which distinguishes it from *C. coli* and *C. lari*. *C. coli* is sensitive to nalidixic acid but *C. lari* is resistant. All can be cultivated on simple media.

Pathogenesis

Campylobacters can produce both inflammatory diarrhoea and non-inflammatory diarrhoeas. How campylobacters cause diarrhoea is unclear but does involve attachment to the intestinal mucosa, and is also dependent on motility by means of flagella.[71] Other factors include iron acquisition, invasion of enterocytes and possibly toxin production.

Immunity to infection is acquired following one or more infective episodes, but duration of immunity is unknown. Following infection, serum and secretory antibodies to *Campylobacter* flagella, enterotoxin, lipolysaccharide and other surface antigens that are involved in attachment are produced. In developing countries, antibodies are acquired in early life[72,73] – perhaps because of

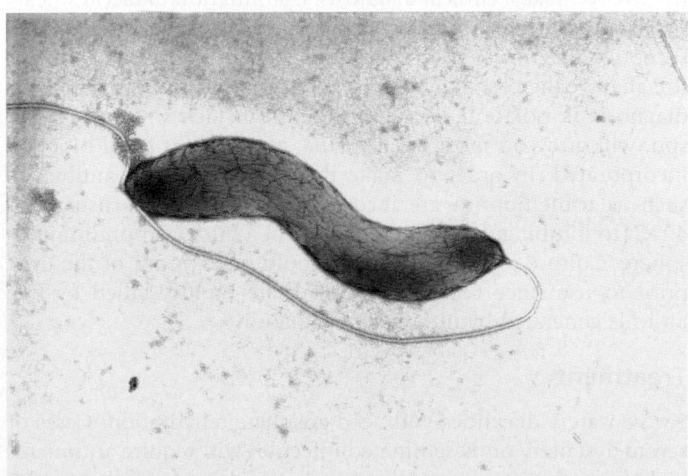

Figure 51.6 Negative-stain electron micrograph of *Campylobacter jejuni.*

continuous exposure from animals. This may account for the lower prevalence of infection in adults in developing countries compared with developed countries, and the higher prevalence of asymptomatic infection in the former. It is probable that the presence of secretory IgA against *Campylobacter* spp. is the main determinant of immunity.

In a small proportion of those infected, usually the immuno-incompetent, bacteria translocate from the intestinal lumen, causing bacteraemia.

Pathology

In the dysentery-like illness, inflammatory infiltrates into the lamina propria and crypt abscesses can be seen in the rectal, colonic and terminal ileal mucosa. This is a similar finding to that seen in shigellosis and salmonellosis, Crohn's disease or ulcerative colitis.

Clinical features

In developing countries, Campylobacter enteritis is generally less severe than that in developed countries. It is more likely to be of the non-inflammatory type, without fever or bloody diarrhoea.[73] However, severe bloody diarrhoea resembling bacillary dysentery can occur and will also occur in travellers acquiring infection in developing countries. In general, diarrhoea is self-limiting and resolves in 2–7 days.

Disseminated infection can occur and predisposing factors include: malnutrition, hepatic dysfunction, malignancy, diabetes mellitus, renal failure and immunosuppression. Extraintestinal and rare forms of infection include: asymptomatic bacteraemia, meningitis, deep abscesses and cholecystitis. Reactive arthritis may follow campylobacteriosis enteritis in genetically susceptible individuals (HLA-B27). Campylobacter enteritis is one of the commonest precipitating causes of Guillain–Barré syndrome, resulting from antigenic cross-reactivity between the bacterial surface and neuronal glycolipids.

Diagnosis

The features of Campylobacter infection are not sufficiently distinctive to make a clinical diagnosis. Examination of faecal smears by Gram stain or dark-field microscopy can provide a rapid presumptive diagnosis. Where laboratory facilities are not optimal, this may be the best diagnostic tool. However, the basis of specific diagnosis is isolation of the bacteria from faeces. *Campylobacter* spp. will grow on most basal media, especially if lysed blood is incorporated. In order to make the media selective, antibiotics such as trimethoprim are incorporated.[74] Culture is usually at 42°C (to inhibit gut commensals) and in a microaerophilic atmosphere. Culture plates and swabs should be kept out of the light prior to use since *Campylobacter* spp. are rapidly killed by free radicals generated by ultraviolet irradiation.

Treatment

Severe watery diarrhoea will need adequate rehydration. Cases of severe dysentery or disseminated infection will require antimicrobial chemotherapy. *C. jejuni* is usually sensitive to erythromycin, but increased resistance has been reported,[69] and quinolones such as ciprofloxacin may be required.

Prevention and control

There is no vaccine for prevention of infection; thus, non-specific methods for prevention such as improvements in sanitation, provision of clean potable water and good food hygiene are important.

YERSINIA ENTEROCOLITICA

The genus *Yersinia* comprises *Y. pestis*, the cause of plague, *Y. pseudotuberculosis* and *Y. enterocolitica*. Of these, *Y. enterocolitica* is the only important cause of diarrhoea.[75]

Epidemiology

Although Yersinia infection is said to have a worldwide distribution, it is found much more commonly in temperate zones than in the tropics. Even in temperate countries, infection is more prevalent in colder climates and is more common in winter.[75] In most surveys of acute diarrhoeal disease where *Y. enterocolitica* was sought, it was either absent, or present in less than 1% of cases.[76] However, cases of generalized infection have been recorded in South Africa[77] and other studies have shown infection in West Africa[78] and Ethiopia.[79]

The reservoir for *Y. enterocolitica* is a variety of animal species, including birds, frogs, fish, snails, oysters and most mammals. The organism is excreted in faeces from pigs and cattle and can persist in lakes, streams, soil and vegetables. Patient-to-patient spread is rare except by blood transfusion. The incubation period is 1–11 days and bacteria are excreted for 14–97 (mean, 42) days.

Bacteriology

Y. enterocolitica is a small Gram-negative rod with peritrichous flagella. It will grow on simple media and is lactose non-fermenting on MacConkey agar. It is psychrophilic, and isolation from clinical samples often involves a cold enrichment step. O serogrouping is used to subdivide strains.

Pathogenesis

Pathogenic strains of *Y. enterocolitica* carry a large plasmid which encodes surface proteins and lipopolysaccharides mediating cell attachment, resistance to phagocytosis and serum resistance. Chromosomal genes (*inv, ail*: attaching invasion locus) encode the ability to invade epithelial cells. Although *Y. enterocolitica* produces a toxin similar to LT, its role in pathogenesis is unclear. *Y. enterocolitica* invades ileal enterocytes and M cells in Peyer's patches, where it multiplies. This produces an inflammatory diarrhoea. Bacteria may pass to local lymph nodes, thence to produce systemic disease.

In addition to disease produced directly by *Y. enterocolitica*, there are a number of autoimmune phenomena which present in a proportion of patients after initial infection. These include: erythema nodosum, reactive arthropathy, Reiter's syndrome and glomerulonephritis. In addition, there is a linkage with thyroid disorders, in that patients with Hashimoto's thyroiditis have high titres of *Y. enterocolitica*-agglutinating antibodies. It is noteworthy that the surface of *Y. enterocolitica* has receptors for thyroid-stimulating hormone.

Clinical features

Most symptomatic infections are in children under 5 years of age.[75] Characteristically, clinical features consist of diarrhoea, low-grade fever and abdominal pain. The diarrhoeic stool will be frankly blood-stained in a quarter of cases. Nausea, vomiting, headache and pharyngitis are minor presentations. The abdominal pain may be present alone or with mild diarrhoea and is often termed the pseudoappendicular syndrome. Infection may spread elsewhere to produce bacteraemia, peritonitis, hepatic, renal and splenic abscesses, pyomyositis and osteomyelitis.[75,77,78] These are more likely to occur in patients who are immunocompromised or who have iron overload—as in haemochromatosis.[77] The extraintestinal manifestations are more likely to occur in adults, as are the autoimmune phenomena. Of those with reactive arthritis, 80% are of HLA-B27 histocompatibility type.

Diagnosis

Y. enterocolitica can be isolated from stool, appendix, mesenteric lymph nodes, blood and other focal sites of infection, using simple media. Strategies for isolation include MacConkey agar incubated at 25–30°C for 48 hours or selective media such as cefsulodin–irgasan–novobiocin (CIN) agar at 37°C. For isolation from food or water, cold enrichment in phosphate-buffered saline for up to 4 weeks at 4°C prior to plating on to CIN agar greatly increases the yield of both pathogenic and non-pathogenic *Yersinia* spp. Speciation is obtained by biochemical tests and it is noteworthy that all non-pathogenic *Y. enterocolitica* have pyrizinamidase activity. Pathogenic *Y. enterocolitica* all possess the virulence plasmid. For retrospective diagnosis, serology using ELISA, whole cell agglutination, or complement fixation tests can be performed. They can be difficult to interpret and cross-reactions, for example *Y. enterocolitica* 0:9 with *Brucella abortus*, *E. coli*, *Morganella morganii* and *Salmonella* spp., do occur. The specificity of the test can be improved by detecting a greater than four-fold increase in titre between acute and convalescent sera.

Treatment and control

In children with uncomplicated diarrhoea, antimicrobial treatment is of little benefit.[80] In complicated infection, cotrimoxazole, tetracycline or chloramphenicol should be effective. Although natural infection with *Y. enterocolitica* produces immunity, no vaccine is available.

CLOSTRIDIUM SPP.

Clostridia are anaerobic sporing Gram-positive rods (Figure 51.7). Two species, *Cl. perfringens* and *Cl. difficile*, are associated with diarrhoeal disease.

Clostridium perfringens

Two forms of diarrhoeal disease are associated with *Cl. perfringens* (formerly *welchii*). The first is a food-poisoning illness due to ingestion of *Cl. perfringens* type A or the α toxin (enterotoxin) it produces. Although this is a common cause of food poisoning in industrialized countries, it produces mild, short-lived disease and is extremely uncommon in the tropics.

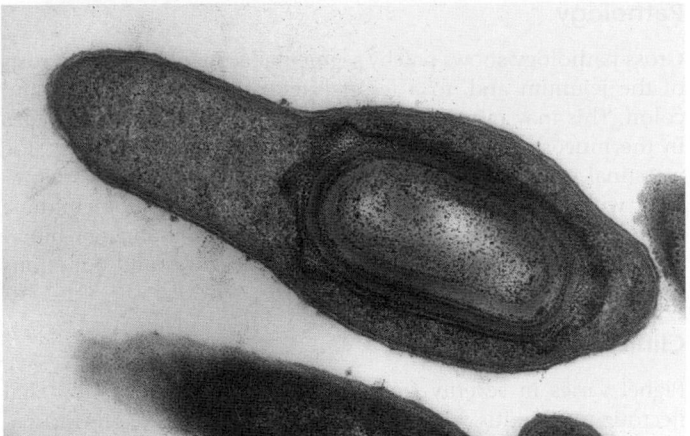

Figure 51.7 Thin-section electron micrograph of *Clostridium perfringens* showing its endospore.

Cl. perfringens type C, in contrast, is common in certain areas of the tropics and produces a severe necrotic enteritis.

Epidemiology

Cl. perfringens type C has been implicated in enteritis necroticans (Darmbrand) seen in malnourished individuals in Northern Europe after World War II[81] and 'pigbel' in the highlands of Papua New Guinea.[82] A similar disease has been described in Uganda,[83] Malaysia, Thailand, Indonesia, China,[84] and, more recently, in India.[85]

Infection can occur sporadically[83,84] but also in epidemics.[81,82] It occurs at any age but is more likely to present as acute toxic or acute surgical problems in children under 10 years old.[82,84] In Papua New Guinea, pigbel is associated with large 'pig feasts' that occur every 3–10 years. Infection is more common in males than females; whether this represents a true difference in susceptibility or male greed is unclear. *Cl. perfringens* type C can be found in the human normal intestinal flora, in pig excreta and in soil.

Microbiology

Cl. perfringens type C produces both α and β toxins, which, it is presumed, are responsible for disease manifestations.

Pathogenesis

Since *Cl. perfringens* type C can be found as part of the normal intestinal flora, it is considered that host-dependent factors are also involved. First, the bulk of the normal anaerobic flora is found in the large bowel and one hypothesis is that overgrowth of *Cl. perfringens* type C in the jejunum might be related to development of disease. A more attractive hypothesis links malnutrition and type of diet with disease. The β toxin is readily inactivated by intestinal proteases. Protein deficiency decreases intestinal protease levels; in addition, the sweet potato, which is a staple diet in highland Papua New Guinea, contains heat-stable trypsin inhibitors. Thus, consumption of meat contaminated by *Cl. perfringens* type C or its β toxin in an individual with low intestinal protease activity due to malnutrition or dietary protease inhibitors would allow the toxin to produce intestinal damage.[84,86]

Pathology

Gross pathology shows patchy segmental acute ulcerative necrosis of the jejunum and, to a lesser extent, the ileum, caecum and colon. This may rapidly progress to segmental gangrene with gas in the mucosa, mesentery or lymph nodes. Microscopically, the intestinal wall shows separation of the mucosa from the submucosa, with large denuded areas covered with a pseudomembrane of dead enterocytes and infiltrating neutrophils and red blood cells. Healing occurs with fibrosis, and strictures and adhesions may form later.

Clinical features

Pigbel varies in severity from mild diarrhoea to a rapidly fatal necrotizing enteritis, with high mortality (up to 85%). The incubation period is approximately 48 hours after the feast but can vary from 24 hours to up to a week.

Disease has been classified into four main presentations.[82,83] Type I (acute toxic) presents with fulminant toxaemia and shock. Type II (acute surgical) presents as mechanical and paralytic ileus, acute strangulation, perforation and peritonitis. Type III (subacute surgical) presents later, with complications of mild type II. Finally, type IV (mild or trivial) presents with mild diarrhoea but may rarely progress to type III. Type I disease occurs most commonly in young children and has the highest mortality (85%). Type II disease has a 42% mortality; type III, 44% mortality; and type IV is never fatal. In type II and type III disease, a palpable segment of thickened intestine may be found. The stool will contain blood and pus cells and there is a neutrophil leukocytosis in peripheral blood. The differential diagnosis includes: acute causes of inflammatory diarrhoea, peritonitis, acute abdominal obstruction, acute pancreatitis, acute amoebic colitis, and sickle cell crises.

Diagnosis

Cl. perfringens can be cultured from faeces, peritoneal fluid or other infected sites by plating on to neomycin blood agar and incubating anaerobically. *Cl. perfringens* type C is differentiated from other *Cl. perfringens* by serological techniques, including immunofluorescence and type C antibody-coated silica beads.[87] Interpretation of results can be difficult since *Cl. perfringens* type C is also found in normal individuals. Detection of antibodies to the toxin can be useful in reaching a diagnosis in survivors.[82]

Treatment

Acute resuscitation is by fluid and electrolytes intravenously, together with bowel decompression by restricting oral intake and nasogastric intubation. Antibiotics will be needed if there is extraintestinal spread of the organism (e.g. peritonitis), and metronidazole, ampicillin, chloramphenicol or penicillin should be of value. Administration of *Cl. perfringens* type C antiserum is also beneficial.[82] Surgical intervention will be necessary if there is persisting obstruction, increasing signs of toxaemia, or signs of peritonitis or of strangulation. There is some evidence that early surgical intervention can decrease mortality.[82]

Prevention

Active immunization with a toxoid prepared from *Cl. perfringens* type C toxins has decreased the incidence of pigbel in children.[88]

Clostridium difficile

Cl. difficile is the cause of antibiotic-associated colitis, and of pseudomembranous colitis. The organism and toxins can be detected in asymptomatic infants but their finding in older individuals is related to disease. The bacterium can be found worldwide but its role as a cause of diarrhoeal disease in developing countries is probably underestimated.[89,90] The new hypertoxin-producing O27 strain of *Cl. difficile* is thus far confined to developed countries.

AEROMONAS AND *PLESIOMONAS*

These two genera within the Vibrionaceae family are both aquatic microorganisms and can be readily isolated from fresh and salt water, fish, soil and food.

Aeromonas hydrophila

Epidemiology

A. hydrophila has been associated with gastroenteritis in many countries throughout the world.[91] In tropical countries, it can be isolated from healthy as well as diarrhoeic individuals. In Thailand, *Aeromonas* spp. were isolated from 9% of cases of gastroenteritis and were second in importance only to ETEC.[92]

Microbiology

The genus *Aeromonas* encompasses three motile species: *A. hydrophila*, *A. caviae* and *A. sobria*. A fourth, non-motile species, *A. salmonicida*, is a fish pathogen and will not grow above 30°C. They are oxidase-positive and will grow on most simple media. *Aeromonas* produces a wide range of extracellular factors including: proteases, elastases, esterases, DNase, haemolysins, cytotoxins and enterotoxins.

Pathogenesis

Aeromonas is associated with both inflammatory and non-inflammatory diarrhoea. It possesses both fimbrial and non-fimbrial adhesins for attachment to the intestinal mucosa. It produces an enterotoxin which has a similar mode of action to *E. coli* LT but uses a different receptor. The haemolysins of *Aeromonas* are also cytotoxic for cultured cells. Finally, *Aeromonas* can invade cells in vitro and in vivo, and this property might be related to production of inflammatory diarrhoea.

Clinical features

Gastroenteritis associated with *Aeromonas* spp. can vary from acute watery diarrhoea with fever to chronic dysentery with fever and abdominal cramps.

Diagnosis

Aeromonas can be isolated from faeces using selective media such as ampicillin blood agar. Prior enrichment in alkaline peptone water increases the sensitivity of isolation. Since *Aeromonas* spp. can be isolated from normal individuals, isolation does not prove causation. For the future, it may be necessary to detect pathogenicity factors (toxins, adhesins or invasiveness) to link isolation with the disease in a particular patient.

Treatment

Rehydration is usually the only intervention needed. If infection becomes disseminated or there is chronic dysentery, antimicrobials such as fluoroquinolones might be of benefit.

Plesiomonas shigelloides

This bacterium has been associated with food-borne (usually fish) gastroenteritis in Mali and India,[93,94] and there has even been a case of snake-to-human transmission.[95]

SHIGELLOSIS (BACILLARY DYSENTERY)

Dysentery has been a disease of poor and crowded communities throughout history, and continues to be a major cause of morbidity and mortality in the tropics. Dysentery bacilli were first demonstrated by Shiga in 1898, and subsequent studies showed that four species, *Shigella dysenteriae*, *Sh. flexneri*, *Sh. boydii* and *Sh. Sonnei*, were responsible for the disease described as bacillary dysentery. *Sh. dysenteriae* and *Sh. flexneri* are responsible for most infections in the tropics, with case fatality rates of up to 20%.[96] Shigellosis occurs both endemically and as epidemics. In many tropical countries, endemic infection is largely due to *Sh. flexneri* and is more commonly a disease of children. Studies in Thailand[97] and Bangladesh[98] have shown *Shigella* spp. to be isolated from up to 50% of children presenting with bloody diarrhoea. Case fatality rates among children with shigellosis may be as high as 30% in those with severe complications, particularly the haemolytic–uraemic syndrome.[99]

Bacteriology

Shigella species are members of the Enterobacteriaceae, and are aerobic, Gram-negative, non-motile bacilli. They are typically non-lactose fermenting, lysine-decarboxylase-negative and do not produce gas from glucose. The exceptions are *Sh. sonnei*, which ferments lactose slowly, and *Sh. flexneri* 6 and *Sh. boydii* 13, which produce gas from glucose. *Sh. dysenteriae*, *Sh. flexneri* and *Sh. boydii* are each divided into a number of serotypes (Table 51.3).

Serotype (O) antigens are located on the outer polysaccharide chains of the lipopolysaccharide component of the cell wall. *Shigella* spp. are non-motile and do not possess H antigens.

For epidemiological studies, serotypes may be subdivided by molecular methods such as plasmid and chromosomal DNA restriction endonuclease digests.[100]

In pure growth, *Shigella* spp. are readily cultured on non-selective media, but for isolation from clinical specimens, selective media such as MacConkey and xylose lysine deoxycholate (XLD) are necessary.

Pathogenesis

Shigella dysentery is characterized by invasion of the colonic mucosa, local spread of the infecting organism, and death of intestinal epithelial cells. In a proportion of cases, extraintestinal complications occur, including seizures, hyponatraemia and hypoglycaemia, septicaemia, Reiter's syndrome, encephalopathy, and the haemolytic–uraemic syndrome. A number of pathogenic factors and their genetic determinants have been described. Invasion is associated with specific outer membrane proteins that are encoded on a plasmid (extrachromosomal) DNA of size 220 kb. Strains not containing these plasmids have been shown to be non-virulent. The lipopolysaccharide component of the cell membrane, which includes the polysaccharide side-chains specific to different O antigenic types, is a further virulence factor.[101] The lipid A component has endotoxic activity and contributes to the systemic effects of infection. The O antigen polysaccharides provide the bacteria with resistance to host defence mechanisms, including opsonization, phagocytosis and intracellular killing. O polysaccharide genes are generally chromosomally encoded. However, in *Sh. sonnei* the genes are present on a 180 kb plasmid, and in *Sh. dysenteriae* 1, a 9 kb plasmid, in conjunction with chromosomal genes, is associated with O-antigen synthesis. Genes responsible for invasion (*ipa* genes), intracellular spread (*ics* genes) and virulence regulatory genes (*virR*) have been described, and increasing understanding of their role may contribute to vaccine development. In addition to these virulence factors, *Sh. dysenteriae* 1 produces a toxin, Shiga toxin (Stx). Stx inactivates ribosomal RNA, inhibiting protein synthesis, and leads to cell death. Stx is composed of A and B subunits, the genes being chromosomally located, and is the same as SLT1 and SLT2 produced by EHEC. The cytotoxic effects of Shiga toxin are involved both in the haemorrhagic intestinal manifestations and in the haemolytic–uraemic syndrome.

Pathology and immunology

The characteristic pathology is an acute, locally invasive, colitis, ranging from mild inflammation of the mucous membranes of the distal colon to severe necrosis of much of the large bowel. Sigmoidoscopy reveals a red, bleeding mucosa with patches of necrotic membrane, which may separate to leave ulcerated areas. The inflammatory process may extend through the submucosa to

Table 51.3 Classification of *Shigella* serotypes

Species	No. of serotypes	Glucose	Mannitol (fermentation)	Lactose
Sh. dysenteriae	10	+	−	−
Sh. flexneri	6	+	+	−
Sh. boydii	15	+	+	−
Sh. sonnei	1	+	+	Late

31. Guerrant RC, Kirchhoff LV, Nations MK, et al. Prospective study of diarrhoeal illness in north eastern Brazil. *J Infect Dis* 1983; 148:986–987.

32. Black RE, Merson MH, Rahman ASMM, et al. A two year study of bacterial viral and parasitic agents associated with diarrhoea in rural Bangladesh. *J Infect Dis* 1980; 142:660–665.

33. Merson MH, Sack RB, Islam S, et al. Disease due to enterotoxigenic *E. coli* in Bangladesh adults. Clinical aspects and a controlled trial of tetracycline. *J Infect Dis* 1980; 141:702–711.

34. DuPont HL, Reves RR, Galindo E, et al. Treatment of traveller's diarrhoea with trimethoprim/sulfamethoxazole and trimethoprim alone. *N Engl J Med* 1982; 307:841–844.

35. Peltola H, Siitonen A, Kyronseppa H, et al. Prevention of traveller's diarrhoea by oral B-subunit/whole cell cholera vaccine. Lancet 1991; 338:1285–1289.

36. Taylor DN, Echeverria P, Sethabutre O, et al. Clinical and microbiologic features of *Shigella* and enteroinvasive *Escherichia coli* infections detected by DNA hybridization. *J Clin Microbiol* 1988; 26:1362–1366.

37. Pal T, Pasca S, Emody L, et al. Antigenic relationship among virulent enteroinvasive *Escherichia coli*, *Shigella flexneri* and *Shigella sonnei* detected by ELISA. *Lancet* 1983; ii:102.

38. Levine MM, Berquist EJ, Nalin DR, et al. *Escherichia coli* strains that cause diarrhoea but do not produce heat-labile or heat-stable enterotoxins and are non-invasive. *Lancet* 1978; i:1119–1122.

39. Edelman R, Levine MM. Summary of a workshop on enteropathogenic *Escherichia coli*. *J Infect Dis* 1983; 147:1108–1118.

40. Echeverria P, Taylor DN, Bettelheim KA, et al. HeLa cell-adherent enteropathogenic *Escherichia coli* in children under 1 year of age in Thailand. *J Clin Microbiol* 1987; 25:1472–1475.

41. Senerwa D, Olsvik O, Mutanda LN, et al. Enteropathogenic *Escherichia coli* serotype O111:HNT isolated from preterm neonates in Nairobi Kenya. *J Clin Microbiol* 1989; 27:1307–1311.

42. Vallance BA, Finlay BB. Exploitation of host cells by enteropathogenic *Escherichia coli*. *Proc Natl Acad Sci USA* 2000; 97:8799–8806.

43. Embaye H, Batt RM, Saunders JR, et al. Interaction of enteropathogenic *Escherichia coli*: O111 with rabbit intestinal mucosa in vitro. *Gastroenterology* 1989; 96:1079–1086.

44. Embaye H, Hart CA, Getty B, et al. Effects of enteropathogenic *Escherichia coli* on microvillar membrane proteins during organ culture of rabbit intestinal mucosa. *Gut* 1992; 33:1184–1189.

45. Taylor CJ, Hart CA, Batt RM, et al. Ultrastructural and biochemical changes in human jejunal mucosa associated with enteropathogenic *Escherichia coli* (O111) infection. *J Pediatr Gastroenterol Nutr* 1986; 5: 70–73.

46. Rothbaum R, McAdams AJ, Giannella R, et al. A clinicopathologic study of enterocyte-adherent *Escherichia coli*: a cause of protracted diarrhoea in infants. *Gastroenterology* 1982; 83:441–454.

47. Riley LW, Remis RJ, Helgerson SD, et al. Hemorrhagic colitis associated with a rare *Escherichia coli* serotype. *N Engl J Med* 1983; 308:681–685.

48. Karmali MA, Steele BT, Petric M, et al. Sporadic cases of haemolytic-uraemic syndrome associated with faecal cytotoxin and cytotoxin-producing *Escherichia coli* in stools. *Lancet* 1983; i:619–620.

49. Karmali MA. Infection by verocytotoxin-producing *Escherichia coli*. *Clin Microbiol Rev* 1989; 2:15–38.

50. Bettelheim KA, Brown JE, Lolekha S, et al. Serotype of *Escherichia coli* that hybridized with DNA probes for genes encoding Shiga-like toxin I, Shiga-like toxin II and serogroup O157 enterohaemorrhagic *E. coli* fimbriae isolated from adults with diarrhoea in Thailand. *J Clin Microbiol* 1990; 28: 293–295.

51. Isaacson M, Canter PH, Effler P, et al. Haemorrhagic colitis epidemic in Africa. *Lancet* 1993; 341:961.

52. Cunin P, Tedjouka E, Germani Y, et al. An epidemic of bloody diarrhea: *Escherichia coli* emerging in Cameroon. *Emerg Infect Dis* 1999; 5:285–290.

53. Roe AJ, Gally DJ. Enteropathogenic and enterohaemorrhagic *Escherichia coli* and diarrhoea. *Curr Opin Infect Dis* 2000; 13:511–517.

54. Kishore K, Rattan A, Bagga A, et al. Serum antibodies to verotoxin-producing *Escherichia coli* (VTEC) strains in patients with haemolytic uraemic syndrome. *J Med Microbiol* 1993; 37:364–367.

55. Chart H, Smith HR, Scotland SM, et al. Serological identification of *Escherichia coli* O157:H7 infection in haemolytic uraemic syndrome. *Lancet* 1991; 337:138–140.

56. Kimmitt PT, Harwood CR, Barer MR. Toxin gene expression by shiga toxin-producing *Escherichia coli*: the role of antibiotics and the bacterial SOS response. *Emerg Infect Dis* 2000; 6:458–465.

57. Nataro JP, Steiner T, Guerrant RL. Enteroaggregative *Escherichia coli*. *Emerg Infect Dis* 1998; 4:251–261.

58. Bhan MK, Raj P, Levine MM, et al. Enteroaggregative *Escherichia coli* associated with persistent diarrhoea in a cohort of rural children in India. *J Infect Dis* 1989; 159:1062–1064.

59. Steiner TS, Lima AAM, Nataro JP, et al. Enteroaggregative *Escherichia coli* produce intestinal inflammation and growth impairment and cause interleukin-8 release from intestinal epithelial cells. *J Infect* 1998; 177: 88–96.

60. Dutta S, Pal S, Chakrabarti S, et al. Use of PCR to identify enteroaggregative *Escherichia coli* as an important cause of acute diarrhoea among children living in Calcutta, India. *J Med Microbiol* 1999; 48:1011–1016.

61. Butzler JP, Dekeyser P, Detrain M, et al. Related vibrio in stools. *J Pediatr* 1973; 82:493–496.

62. Skirrow MB. Campylobacter enteritis: a 'new' disease. *BMJ* 1977; 2:9–11.

63. Prouzet-Mauleon V, Labadi L, Bouges N, et al. *Arcobacter butzleri*: underestimated enteropathogen. *Emerg Infect Dis* 2006; 12:307–309.

64. Samie A, Obi CL, Barrett LJ, et al. Prevalence of *Campylobacter* species, *Helicobacter pylori* and *Arcobacter* spp in stool samples from the Venda region, Limpopo, South Africa: studies using molecular diagnostic methods. *J Infect* 2007; 54:558–566.

65. Potter ME, Blaser MJ, Sikes RK, et al. Human Campylobacter infection associated with certified raw milk. *Am J Epidemiol* 1983; 117:475–483.

66. Korlath JA, Osterholm MT, Judy LA, et al. A point source outbreak of campylobacteriosis associated with consumption of raw milk. *J Infect Dis* 1985; 152:592–596.

67. Southern JP, Smith RMM, Palmer SR. Bird attack on milk bottles: possible mode of transmission of *Campylobacter jejuni* to man. *Lancet* 1990; 336: 1425–1427.

68. Rajan DP, Mathan VI. Prevalence of *Campylobacter fetus* subsp. *jejuni* in healthy populations in southern India. *J Clin Microbiol* 1982; 15:749–751.

69. Putnam SD, Frenck RW, Riddle MS, et al. Antimicrobial susceptibility trends in Campylobacter jejuni and Campylobacter coli isolated from a rural Egyptian community with diarrhea. *Diagn Microbiol Infect Dis* 2003; 47: 601–608.

70. Samie A, Ramalivhana J, Igumbor EO, Obi I. Prevalence and antibiotic susceptibility profiles of Campylobacter spp. isolated from human diarrhoeal stools in Vhembe District, South Africa. *J health Poplu Nutr* 2007; 25: 406–413.

71. Altekruse SF, Stern NJ, Fields PJ, et al. *Campylobacter jejuni* – an emerging foodborne pathogen. *Emerg Infect Dis* 1999; 5:28–35.

72. Glass RI, Stoll BJ, Juq MI, et al. Epidemiologic and clinical features of endemic *Campylobacter jejuni* infection in Bangladesh. *J Infect Dis* 1983; 148:292–296.

73. Black RF, Levine MM, Brown KH, et al. Immunity to *Campylobacter jejuni* in man. In: Pearson DA, Skirrow MB, Lior H, et al., eds. *Campylobacter III*. London: Public Health Laboratory Service; 1985:129.

74. Butzler JP, Skirrow MB. Campylobacter enteritis. *Clin Gastroenterol* 1979; 8:737–765.

75. Cover TL, Aber RC. *Yersinia enterocolitica*. *N Engl J Med* 1989; 321:16–24.

76. Gomes TAT, Rassi V, MacDonald KC, et al. Enteropathogens associated with acute diarrhoeal disease in urban infants in Sao Paulo, Brazil. *J Infect Dis* 1991; 164:331–337.

77. Rabson AR, Hallett AF, Koornhof HJ. Generalized *Yersinia enterocolitica* infection. *J Infect Dis* 1975; 131:447–451.

78. Awunor-Renner C, Lawande RV. Yersinia and chronic glomerulopathy in the savannah region of Nigeria. *BMJ* 1982; 285:1464–1465.

79. Andualem B, Geyid A. The prevalence of Yersinia enterocolitica isolates in comparison to those of commonly encountered enteropathogens causing diarrhoea among Ethiopian patients in Addis Ababa. *Ethiop Med J* 2003; 41:257–266.

80. Pai CH, Gillis F, Tuomanen E, et al. Placebo-controlled doubled-blind evaluation of trimethoprim sulfamethoxazole treatment of *Yersinia enterocolitica* gastroenteritis. *J Pediatr* 1984; 104:308–311.

81. Jeckeln E. Uber 'Darmbrand': das pathologisch antatomische Bild des Darmbrandes. *Dtsch Med Wochenschr* 1947; 11:105.

82. Murrell TGC, Roth L, Egerton J, et al. Pigbel: enteritis necroticans. A study in diagnosis and management. *Lancet* 1966; i:217–222.

83. Foster WD. The bacteriology of necrotising jejunitis in Uganda. *East Afr Med J* 1966; 45:550.

84. Shann F, Lawrence G, Jun-Bi P. Enteritis necroticans in China. *Lancet* 1979; i:1083–1084.

85. Gupta SC, Mishra V, Mishra SP, et al. Necrotizing enteritis stimulating Pig-Bel disease in northern India. *Indian J Gastroenterol* 1994; 13:109–111.

86. Lawrence G, Walker PD. Pathogenesis of enteritis necroticans in Papua New Guinea. *Lancet* 1976; i:125–126.

87. Lawrence G, Brown R, Baters J, et al. An affinity technique for isolation of *Clostridium perfringens* type C from man and pigs in Papua New Guinea. *J Appl Bacteriol* 1984; 57:333–338.

88. Lawrence G, Shann F, Freestone DS, et al. Prevention of necrotising enteritis in Papua New Guinea by active immunisation. *Lancet* 1979; i:227–230.

89. Albert MJ, Faruque ASG, Faruque SM, et al. Case-control study of enteropathogens associated with childhood diarrhea in Dhaka, Bangladesh. *J Clin Microbiol* 1999; 37:3458–3464.

90. Simango C. Prevalence of Clostridium difficile in the environment in a rural community in Zimbabwe. *Trans R Soc Trop Med Hyg* 2006; 100:1146–1150.

91. Ljungh A, Wadstrom T. Aeromonas and Plesiomonas. In: Farthing MJG, Keusch G, eds. *Enteric Infections*. London: Chapman & Hall; 1989: 169–181.

92. Echeverria P, Seriwatana J, Taylor DN, et al. A comparative study of enterotoxigenic *Escherichia coli*, *Shigella*, *Aeromonas* and *Vibrios* as etiologies of diarrhoea in north eastern Thailand. *Am J Trop Med Hyg* 1985; 34:547–554.

93. Vandepitte J, VanDamme L, Fofana Y, et al. *Edwardsiella tarda* et *Plesiomonas shigelloides*: leur rôle comme agents de diarrhées et leur épidémiologie. *Bull Soc Pathol Exot* 1980; 73:139–149.

94. Sakazaki R, Tamura K, Prescott LM, et al. Bacteriological examination of diarrhoeal stools in Calcutta. *Indian J Med Res* 1971; 59:1025–1034.

95. Davis WA, Chretien JH, Gargarusi VF, et al. Snake to human transmission of *Aeromonas (Pl.) shigelloides* resulting in gastroenteritis. *South Med J* 1978; 71:474–476.

96. Bennish ML. Potential lethal complications of shigellosis. *Rev Infect Dis* 1991; 13(suppl 4):S319–S324.

97. Taylor DN, Bodhidatta L, Echeverria P. Epidemiological aspects of shigellosis and other causes of dysentery in Thailand. *Rev Infect Dis* 1991; 13(suppl 4): S231–S237.

98. Ahmed F, Clemens JD, Rao MR, et al. Epidemiology of shigellosis among children exposed to cases of Shigella dysentery: a multivariate analysis. *Am J Trop Med Hyg* 1997; 56:258–264.

99. Nathoo KJ, Porteous JE, Siziya S, et al. Predictors of mortality in children hospitalized with dysentery in Harare, Zimbabwe. *Cent Afr J Med* 1998; 44:272–276.

100. Kariuki S, Muthotho N, Kimari J, et al. Molecular typing of multi-drug resistant *Shigella dysenteriae* type 1 by plasmid analysis and pulsed field gel electrophoresis. *Trans R Soc Trop Med Hyg* 1996; 90:712–714.

101. Lindberg AA, Karnell A, Weibtraub A. The lipopolysaccharide of Shigella bacteria as a virulence factor. *Rev Infect Dis* 1991; 13(suppl 4): S279–S284.

102. Usman J, Aziz S, Karamat KA, et al. Shigella septicaemia in an infant. *J Pak Med Assoc* 1997; 47:150–151.

103. Boyce JM, Hughes JM, Alim AR, et al. Patterns of Shigella infections in families in rural Bangladesh. *Am J Trop Med Hyg* 1982; 31: 1015–1020.

104. Hassain MA, Albert JM, Hassan KZ. Epidemiology of shigellosis in Teknaf, a coastal region of Bangladesh: a 10 year survey. *Epidemiol Infect* 1990; 105: 41–49.

105. Mache A, Mengistu Y, Cowley C. Shigella serogroups identified from adult diarrhoeal patients in Addis Ababa: antibiotic resistance and plasmid profile analysis. *East Afr Med J* 1997; 74:179–182.

106. Milleliri JM, Soares JL, Signoret J, et al. Epidemic of bacillary dysentery in the Rwanda refugee camps of the Goma region (Zaire, North Kivu) in August 1994. *Ann Soc Belg Med Trop* 1995; 75:201–210.

107. Ries AA, Wells JG, Olivola D, et al. Epidemic *Shigella dysenteriae* type 1 in Burundi: panresistance and implications for prevention. *J Infect Dis* 1994; 169:1035–1041.

108. Karas JA, Pillay DG, Naicker T, et al. Laboratory surveillance of *Shigella dysenteriae* type 1 in KwaZulu-Natal. *S Afr Med J* 1999; 89:59–63.

109. Bhimma R, Rollins NC, Coovadia HM, et al. Post dysenteric haemolytic uraemic syndrome in children during an epidemic of Shigella dysentery in KwaZulu-Natal. *Paediatr Nephrol* 1997; 11:560–564.

110. WHO. *Recommended Surveillance Standards, 1999*. WHO/CDS/CDR/ISR 99.2. Geneva: World Health Organization; 1999.

111. NCCLS. *Performance Standards for Antimicrobial Disc Susceptibility Tests*. 6th edn. NCCLS Document M2-A6. Pennsylvania: NCCLS; 1997.

112. Vinh H, Wain J, Chinh MT, et al. Treatment of bacillary dysentery in Vietnamese children: two doses of ofloxacin versus 5-days nalidixic acid. *Trans R Soc Trop Med Hyg* 2000; 94:323–326.

113. Anonymous. Vaccine research and development. New strategies for accelerating Shigella vaccine development. *Wkly Epidemiol Rec* 1997; 72: 73–79.

114. Colombo MM, Mastrandrea S, Santoni A, et al. Distribution of ace zot and ctx-a toxin genes in clinical and environmental *Vibrio cholerae*. *J Infect Dis* 1994; 88:298–299.

115. Rahman MH, Biswas K, Hossain MA, et al. Distribution of genes for virulence and ecological fitness among a diverse Vibrio cholerae population in a cholera endemic area: Tracking the evolution of pathogenic strains. *DNA Cell Biol* 2008; 27: Epub doi:10.1089/dna.2008.0737

116. Islam MS, Miah MA, Hassan MK, et al. Detection of non-culturable Vibrio cholerae 01 associated with a cyanobacterium from an aquatic environment in Bangladesh. *Trans R Soc Trop Med Hyg* 1994; 88:298–299.

117. Siddique AK, Baqui AH, Eusof A, et al. Survival of classic cholera in Bangladesh. *Lancet* 1991; i:1125–1127.

118. Goma Epidemiology Group. Public health impact of Rwandan refugee crisis: what happened in Goma, Zaire in July 1994. *Lancet* 1995; i: 339–344.

119. Griffith DC, Kelly-Hope LA, Miller MA. Review of reported cholera outbreaks worldwide, 1995–2005. *Am J Trop Med Hyg* 2006; 75:973–977.

120. WHO. *Guidelines for Cholera Control, 1993*. WHO/CDD/SER/80.4. Geneva: World Health Organization; 1993.

121. Patra FC, Mahalanbis D, Jalan KV, et al. Is oral rice-water electrolyte solution superior to glucose electrolyte solution in infantile diarrhoea? *Arch Dis Child* 1982; 57:910–912.

122. Clemens JD, Sack DA, Harris JR, et al. Field trial of oral cholera vaccines in Bangladesh: results of a three year follow up. *Lancet* 1990; 335: 270–273.

123. Trach DD, Clemens JD, Ke NT, et al. Field trial of a locally produced, killed oral cholera vaccine in Viet Nam. *Lancet* 1997; 349:231–235.

124. WHO. *Oral cholera Vaccine use in Complex Emergencies: Report of a WHO Meeting, Cairo 2005*. WHO/CDS/NTD/IDM/2006.2. Geneva: World Health Organisation;2006.

125. Woo PCJ, Lau SKP, Teng JLL, et al. Current status and future direction for *Laribacter hongkongensis*, a novel bacterium associated with gastroenteritis and traveller's diarrhoea. *Curr Opin Infect Dis* 2005; 18:413–419.

Chapter 52   Claire Jenkins and Stephen H. Gillespie

Salmonella Infections

BACTERIOLOGY

The genus *Salmonella*, part of the family of Enterobacteriacieae (see Chapter 10), comprises three species, *Salmonella bongori*, *Salmonella subterranea* and *Salmonella enterica*, which is divided into six subtypes: enterica, salamae, arizonae, diarizonae, houtenae and indica.[1-4] The taxonomic group contains more than 2463 serovars, and these are given names as if they were different species, e.g. *Salmonella typhimurium*, when, strictly speaking, it should be described as *Salmonella enterica* subsp. *enterica* serovar Typhimurium, or abbreviated to *Salmonella* Typhimurium. The serovars are defined on the basis of the somatic O (lipopolysaccharide) and flagellar H antigens (Kaufmann–White scheme).[2] Further differentiation of strains within individual serotypes by bacteriophage typing and DNA fingerprinting helps epidemiological investigations. They include organisms that typically cause localized enteritis and organisms such as *S. enterica* subsp. *enterica* serovar Typhi that causes the systemic infectious disease.

On the basis of host preference and disease manifestations in man, the salmonellae can be conveniently placed into two clinical categories:
- *S.* Typhi, *S.* Paratyphi A, *S.* Paratyphi B (Schotmulleri) and *S.* Paratyphi C (Hischfeldii). These serotypes are primarily host-adapted to man and cause a bacteraemic illness also known as enteric fever in which diarrhoea rarely plays a major role.
- Other serotypes. These are host-adapted to animals, and infection in man is usually confined to the bowel and presents as acute diarrhoea, but sometimes causes life-threatening bacteraemia. The serotypes of enterica subspecies account for most human and warm-blooded animal infections, and are grouped on the basis of sharing of a common O antigen. Examples of commonly occurring groups of enterica subspecies serotypes are given in Table 52.1.

TYPHOID AND PARATYPHOID FEVERS OR ENTERIC FEVER

Typhoid fever was so named because its symptoms and signs resembled typhus. The confusion between the two was resolved only with the publication in 1850 of William Jenner's book *On the Identity or Non-Identity of Typhoid and Typhus Fevers*.[5]

Epidemiology

Typhoid and paratyphoid fevers are endemic in the Indian subcontinent, South-east and East Asia, the Middle East, Africa, and Central and South America. Although the overall ratio of disease caused by *S.* Typhi to that caused by *S.* Paratyphi is about 10 to 1, the proportion of *S.* Paratyphi infections is increasing in some parts of the world.[6] A low level of endemicity also exists for paratyphoid B infections in the southern and eastern parts of Europe. In the rest of Europe, North America and Australasia, enteric fevers occur almost exclusively as imported infections.[7] Paratyphoid C is rare, with occasional cases in Guyana and Eastern Europe.

Transmission

Typhoid is an exclusively human disease and the organisms that are responsible for infection are transmitted through food or water contaminated with faeces or urine of a patient or carrier. Paratyphoid infections are less often water-borne, because they need a higher infective dose, which is unlikely to be found in water as multiplication does not occur. Raw fruit and vegetables are important vehicles in some countries where human faeces are used as a fertilizer or where contaminated water is used to make fruit look attractive in the market. Shellfish harvested in coastal water polluted by raw sewage may cause outbreaks.[3]

Pathogenesis

Natural infection in enteric fever occurs by ingestion, followed by penetration through the intestinal mucosa. Disease production is dependent on several factors: number of organisms swallowed; state of gastric acidity; and possession of Vi antigen by the organisms. The infecting dose of *S.* Typhi needs to be large to produce illness in healthy individuals. In volunteers, a dose of 10^9 organisms induced disease in most (95%) but a dose of 10^3 rarely did so. Some 25% of the volunteers became ill after ingesting 10^5 organisms.[8] Possession of Vi capsular antigen is linked with increased infectivity: Vi antigen-positive strains caused illness more commonly than non-Vi variants in healthy volunteers.[8] Gastric acidity is an important defence against enteric infections, and gastric hypoacidity from any cause (e.g. antacids, H_2 antagonists) will allow a greater number of organisms to enter the small

Table 52.1 Some examples of commonly occurring *Salmonella* serotypes and the groups to which they belong

Group	Serotype
A	S. Paratyphi A
B	S. Paratyphi B
	S. Stanley
	S. Saintpaul
	S. Agona
	S. Typhimurium
C	S. Paratyphi C
	S. Cholerae-suis
	S. Virchow
	S. Thompson
D	S. Typhi
	S. Enteritidis
	S. Dublin
	S. Gallinarum

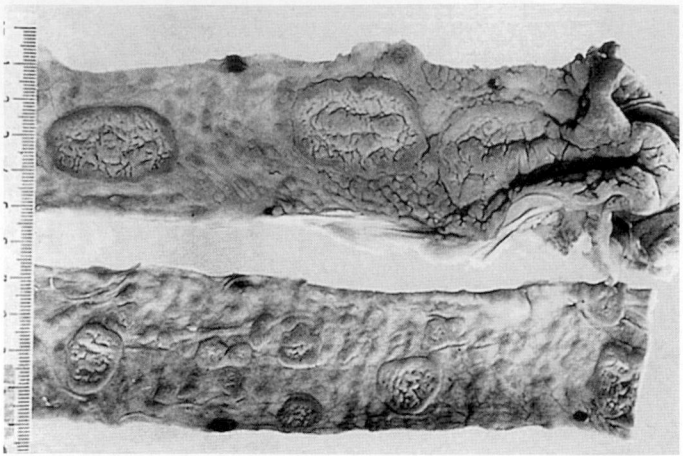

Figure 52.1 Typhoid ulceration of the small intestine. (Courtesy of the Wellcome Tropical Institute Museum (WTIM).)

intestine. Also, the infective dose is reduced if it comes in food where the organisms are protected from gastric acid. Once in the small intestine, the organisms penetrate rapidly through the intestinal mucosa. Organisms multiply in the lumen for a short period and stools can be culture-positive during the first 4 days of the incubation period.[3,8]

From the submucosa, invading bacteria are taken up by macrophages,[9] and the organisms travel to mesenteric lymph nodes. After a brief period of multiplication here, the organisms enter the bloodstream via the thoracic duct (transient primary bacteraemia) and are transported to the liver and spleen. After a period of further multiplication at these sites, huge numbers of organisms enter the bloodstream, marking the onset of clinical illness (secondary bacteraemia). During this secondary bacteraemia, which continues for the greater part of the illness, very few organs escape invasion but the involvement of the gallbladder and Peyer's patches in the lower small intestine have important clinical significance. The gallbladder is probably infected via the liver and the resultant cholecystitis is usually subclinical. The infected bile renders stool cultures positive. Pre-existing gallbladder disease predisposes to chronic biliary infection, leading to chronic faecal carriage.

Invasion of the Peyer's patches occurs either during the primary intestinal infection or during the secondary bacteraemia, and further seeding occurs through infected bile. The Peyer's patches become hyperplastic, with infiltration of chronic inflammatory cells. Later, necrosis of the superficial layer leads to formation of irregular, ovoid ulcers along the long axis of the gut, so that stricture formation does not occur after healing (Figure 52.1). When an ulcer erodes into a blood vessel, severe haemorrhage results and transmural perforation leads to peritonitis.

Molecular basis of pathogenesis

To be effective pathogens, salmonella must be able to invade epithelial cells, and for organisms to cause enteric fever, they have

to be adapted to survive inside cells of the reticuloendothelial system.

Epithelial invasion

The target of salmonella invasion is the M cell but the bacteria must cross the epithelial layer to achieve this.[9] Salmonellae invade the intestinal epithelial cells by a complex mechanism which includes triggering active rearrangements, formation of pseudopodia, and phagocytosis of the bacterium into the cells. Membrane ruffling then returns to normal after the bacterium has invaded. The ruffling–internalization process is controlled by a type III secretion system encoded by genes found in the *inv* locus (containing genes *inv A–H*).[10] These genes are located on a pathogenicity island, SPI-1 (*Salmonella* pathogenicity island 1), which encodes all of the genes necessary for the invasion of intestinal epithelial cells. SPI-1 activity is downregulated after a few hours of invasion and the type III secretion system encoded on SPI-2 is activated.[11]

Intracellular survival

Salmonella serotypes that cause enteric fever must be able to survive and replicate within the host macrophage system so that they may establish a systemic infection.[11] Once inside these locations they are shielded from the effect of human immunity, but to do this they must overcome the nutrient-poor environment within the macrophage and defeat its bactericidal mechanisms.[12] Salmonella genes necessary for survival inside macrophages are constituents of a two-component response regulator termed phoP/phoQ. Genes activated by this phoP/phoQ are known as *pag* genes, of which *pag A–C* have been characterized. The *pag* genes are expressed within the macrophage phagosome and are required for survival within it.[13] Conversely, the phoP repressed genes switch off in the phagosome and include components of the SPI-1. Mutants that are phoP null or with constitutive expression of phoP are avirulent, suggesting that proper timing of switching on and off of these mechanisms is critical in ensuring successful invasion and survival.

More recently, a second type III secretion mechanism necessary for survival inside macrophages has been described in a second pathogenicity island, SPI-2. This system activates within the phagosome and translocates bacterial effector proteins from the phagosome into the macrophage cytosol.[11]

Mechanism of immunity

Production of humoral antibody appears to play little role in recovery from acute infection, as the patient often continues to deteriorate despite the appearance of O, H and Vi antibodies. Cell-mediated immunity is probably the key factor in recovery. The ability of Vi antibody to prevent infection is demonstrated by the efficiency of Vi antigen vaccine. However, protection afforded by phenolized-killed vaccine, which does not contain Vi antigen, indicates a role for other antibodies. Local gut immunity is probably important in preventing reinfection. Specific secretory IgG and IgA antibodies have been demonstrated in gut.[14]

In the endemic countries, enteric fevers have the highest prevalence in the young, adults having acquired substantial immunity through previous exposure(s).

Clinical manifestations

The incubation period of typhoid fever varies with the size of the infecting dose[5] and averages from 10 to 20 (range 3–56) days. In paratyphoid fever it ranges from 1 to 10 days.

The duration of illness in untreated cases of average severity is usually 4 weeks. In the first week the features are non-specific, with headache, malaise and a rising remittent fever. Constipation and a mild non-productive cough are common. During the second week the patient looks toxic and apathetic with sustained high temperature. The abdomen is slightly distended and splenomegaly is common. In about 50% of cases, crops of 2–4 mm-diameter pink papules (rose spots), which fade on pressure, develop on the upper abdomen and lower chest, between the 7th and 12th days. They are difficult to detect in dark-skinned individuals. Rose spots may also occur in invasive salmonellosis and shigellosis. The spots are caused by bacterial embolization and rose-spot cultures may be positive, although this is rarely performed. Relative bradycardia, a pulse lower than anticipated in a febrile patient, is common during the first 2 weeks.

With the onset of the third week the patient becomes more ill and is febrile. A continuous high fever persists and a delirious confusional state sets in (typhoid state). Abdominal distension becomes pronounced, with scanty bowel sounds. Diarrhoea is common, with liquid, foul green–yellow stools. The patient is weak with a feeble pulse and rapid breathing; crackles may develop over the lung bases. Death may occur at this stage from overwhelming toxaemia, myocarditis, intestinal haemorrhage or perforation. Considerable weight loss is common. In patients who survive into the 4th week, the fever, mental state and abdominal distension slowly improve over a few days but intestinal complications may still occur. Convalescence is usually a slow process. However, with the use of antibiotics this disease evolution is rarely seen.

Variation in the clinical picture is common, and mild and inapparent infections are frequent. Diarrhoea may occur even during the first week[15] and children may present with a high fever and febrile convulsion(s). Chronic or recurrent fever with bacteraemia

may occur in association with concurrent schistosomiasis, as salmonellae are able to survive within the parasites, protected from the body's defences.[15]

The diagnosis of typhoid fever, particularly in the developing world, is usually made on clinical grounds. The symptoms sometimes mimic other common illnesses, such as malaria, sepsis with other bacterial pathogens, tuberculosis, brucellosis, tularaemia, leptospirosis and rickettsial disease. Viral infections such as dengue, acute hepatitis and infectious mononucleosis are also included in the differential diagnosis.[16]

Relapse

Between 10% and 20% of patients treated with antibiotics suffer a relapse after initial recovery, whereas in the pre-antibiotic era the incidence used to be somewhat lower (8–12%). A relapse typically occurs a week or so after stopping therapy, but occurrence after 70 days has been reported. The blood culture is positive again, even in the presence of high serum levels of H, O and Vi antibodies, and rose spots may reappear. A relapse is generally milder and shorter than the initial illness. The incidence of relapse after treatment with fluoroquinolones (1.5%) or broad-spectrum cephalosporins (5%) is lower than after treatment with chloramphenicol, trimethoprim-sulfamethoxazole and ampicillin.[17] Rarely, second or even third relapses may occur.

Complications

Extra-intestinal infectious complications can occur and recognition of these can prevent a delay in diagnosis.[18]

Intestinal

The two most serious complications of enteric fever are intestinal haemorrhage and perforation, which usually occur when the sloughs overlying the Peyer's patches separate during the late second or early third week of the illness. Clinical signs of haemorrhage are a sharp fall in body temperature and blood pressure, and sudden tachycardia. The blood passed per rectum is usually bright red but may be altered if intestinal stasis is present. Sometimes there may not be any passage of blood – when frank ileus is present.[19]

Management of haemorrhage is conservative, with sedation and transfusion unless there is evidence of perforation, when surgery is indicated.

Unlike other causes of intestinal perforation, typhoid perforation occurs in a patient who already had a vaguely tender distended abdomen with scanty bowel sounds. Therefore, recognition of perforation can be difficult.[20,21] Usually, pain and tenderness worsen, the pulse rises and the temperature falls suddenly. However, abdominal rigidity may not be a prominent sign and bowel sounds may not disappear altogether. The discovery of free fluid in the abdomen may be the only sign of perforation. Demonstration of gas under the diaphragm by X-ray is a valuable aid to diagnosis.

The treatment of choice for typhoid perforation is surgical intervention, although conservative management with nasogastric suction, antibiotic therapy directed against anaerobes and Enterobacteriaciae, and general supportive care will reduce the mortality to 30%.[22,23] Most surgeons prefer simple closure of perforation

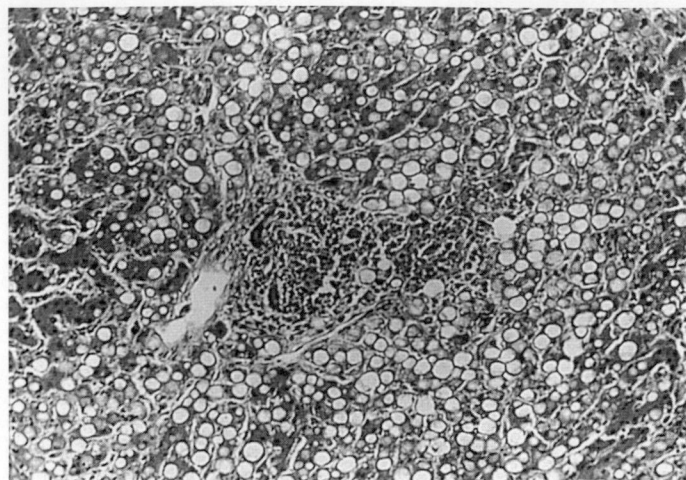

Figure 52.2 Typhoid nodule in portal tract of liver. (Courtesy of WTIM.)

with drainage of the peritoneum, and reserve small-bowel resection for patients with multiple perforations. Early diagnosis, energetic resuscitation and rapid, simple surgery are the key to lower mortality. The prognosis is clearly related to the time elapsed between perforation and surgery.

Liver, gallbladder and pancreas

Mild jaundice may occur in enteric fever and may be due to hepatitis, cholangitis, cholecystitis or haemolysis. Biochemical changes indicative of hepatitis are common during the acute stage.[24] Liver biopsy in such cases often shows cloudy swelling, balloon degeneration with vacuolation of hepatocytes, moderate fatty change and focal collection of mononuclear cells – 'typhoid nodules' (Figure 52.2). Intact typhoid bacilli can be seen at these sites. Pancreatitis has also been reported.[25]

Cardiorespiratory

Toxic myocarditis and endocarditis occur in 1–5% of cases and represent a significant cause of death in endemic countries.[23] Both occur in severely ill toxaemic patients and is characterized by tachycardia, weak pulse and heart sounds, hypotension and electrocardiographic abnormalities. Respiratory symptoms, such as cough and mild bronchitis, occur in 11–86% of cases[23] and bronchopneumonia or lobar consolidation may develop rarely.

Nervous system

A toxic confusional state, characterized by disorientation, delirium and restlessness, is characteristic of late-stage typhoid but occasionally these and other neuropsychiatric features may dominate the clinical picture from an early stage.[18] Facial twitching or convulsion(s) may be the presenting feature; sometimes, paranoid psychosis or catatonia may develop during convalescence.[26] Meningism is not uncommon but bacterial meningitis caused by *S.* Typhi is a rare, but recognized, complication. Encephalomyelitis may develop and the underlying pathology may be that of demyelinating leukoencephalopathy.[27] Rarely, transverse myelitis, polyneuropathy or cranial mononeuropathy may develop.

Haematological and renal

Subclinical disseminated intravascular coagulation occurs commonly in typhoid fever; this rarely manifests as haemolytic–uraemic syndrome.[28] Haemolysis may also be associated with glucose 6-phosphate dehydrogenase (G6PD) deficiency. Immune complex glomerulitis has been reported and IgM immunoglobulin, C3 and *S.* Typhi antigen can be demonstrated in the glomerular capillary wall.[29] Nephrotic syndrome may complicate chronic *S.* Typhi bacteraemia associated with urinary schistosomiasis.[29]

Musculoskeletal and other systems

Skeletal muscle characteristically shows Zenker's degeneration (a hyaline degeneration of muscle fibres), particularly affecting the abdominal wall and thigh muscles; clinically evident polymyositis may occur.[30]

Localization may occur in almost any organ/system, and involvement of bones, joints, meninges, endocardium, spleen and ovary have all been reported, but such cases are rare.[31]

Comparison of typhoid fever and paratyphoid fever

In general, the illness in paratyphoid B infection is milder and of shorter duration than in typhoid fever and complications are less frequent.[32] It can also present as acute gastroenteritis. Paratyphoid A and C fall between typhoid and paratyphoid B fevers in severity.

Laboratory findings

Mild leukocytosis may develop initially, but, with disease progression, leucopenia and neutropenia commonly develop. Even in uncomplicated cases, low-grade normocytic anaemia, mild thrombocytopenia, modestly elevated serum transaminases and mild proteinuria are common.

Diagnosis

The definitive diagnosis of enteric fever requires isolation of the organism from blood or bone marrow.[3] Isolation from stool or urine provides strong presumptive evidence only in the presence of a characteristic clinical picture.

Blood and bone marrow culture

The definitive diagnosis of typhoid is by the isolation of the organism from a sterile site. Isolation of the organism from the stool is useful information but may be a false positive due to long-term carriage. Thus, in patients with suspected typhoid, blood or bone marrow cultures should be performed. Modern automated systems rapidly detect the presence of the organism, but conventional non-automated methods also have a high diagnostic yield.

In untreated patients, blood cultures are usually positive in about 40–60% of cases, usually early in the course of disease.[33] A success rate of about 90% is obtained from bone marrow culture.[34] Prior antibiotic therapy makes positive blood culture less likely but the bone marrow culture often remains positive in the face of antibiotic therapy.[34] A high yield (60%) has also been reported from rose-spot cultures in such a situation.[34]

Faecal and urine cultures

With modern techniques, faecal cultures are often positive even during the first week, though the percentage positivity rises steadily thereafter. Urine cultures are positive less often.

Serology

The traditional Widal test measures antibodies against flagellar (H) and somatic (O) antigens of the causative organism. In acute infection, O antibody appears first, rising progressively, later falling and often disappearing within a few months. H antibody appears a little later but persists for longer. Rising or high O antibody titre generally indicates acute infection, whereas raised H antibody helps to identify the type of enteric fever. However, the Widal test has many limitations. Raised antibodies may have resulted from previous typhoid immunization or earlier infection(s) with salmonellae sharing common O antigens with S. Typhi or S. Paratyphi. In endemic countries, patients have higher H antibody titres. This is a particular problem in developing countries, where background antibodies mean that the Widal test lacks sensitivity. Some patients show a poor or negligible antibody response to active infection. Vi antibody is often raised during acute infection and persists afterwards during chronic carriage. However, its use as a screening test for the carrier state is limited because of the frequency of false positives and false negatives.[35]

Newer diagnostic methods

Newer tests that directly detect IgM antibodies to a wide range of specific S. Typhi antigens have been developed, such as Typhidot and Tubex, and these have compared favourably with the Widal test. [36] Some of these tests have been adapted to a simple dipstick technique using whole bacteria antigens to detect IgM antibody and are beneficial in situations where a laboratory is not available.[37] Urinary Vi antigen ELISAs and PCR-based assays are under development.[38,39]

Carrier state in enteric fever

Faecal carrier

After clinical recovery, faecal cultures remain positive in a high proportion of patients during the immediate convalescent period, but stools rapidly become negative, although up to 3% of patients will still be positive by the end of the third month. Between 1% and 3% will continue to excrete organisms in their stools for more than a year and will be designated as chronic carriers – they are likely to remain so for the rest of their lives. The incidence of chronic carriage is higher in women and in the elderly. A similar situation exists with paratyphoid infections.

Urinary carrier

In the absence of urinary tract pathology, persisting urinary carriage is rare after the third month, but it is common in countries where urinary schistosomiasis is endemic.

Treatment

Patients should be managed under strict enteric precautions, with attention to adequate hand washing and safe disposal of faeces and urine. They should receive adequate rest and nutrition and correction of fluid and electrolyte imbalance. Antibiotic therapy is essential and should begin empirically if the clinical suspicion of an enteric fever is strong. Patients should also be monitored for complications and clinical relapse.

Choice of antimicrobial agents in enteric fever

Ciprofloxacin and other 4-quinolone drugs

Ciprofloxacin has proved to be highly effective in the treatment of typhoid and paratyphoid fevers. Defervescence occurs in 3–5 days; convalescent carriage and relapses are rare (less than 2%).[33,40] Other 4-quinolone drugs such as ofloxacin, norfloxacin and pefloxacin are equally effective.[41] Ciprofloxacin is usually given orally 500 mg twice daily for 14 days, but there are reports that courses of 7 days may be adequate.[42] If vomiting or diarrhoea is present, the drug should be given intravenously, 200–400 mg twice daily. The 4-quinolone drugs are highly effective against multi-drug-resistant (MDR) strains and trials have shown this in comparison with chloramphenicol.[41]

The 4-quinolone drugs are not currently recommended for use in children and pregnant women because of their observed potential for causing cartilage damage in growing animals. However, extensive experience of these drugs in children has shown no evidence of bone or joint toxicity.[42] For children with severe infection with a strain that is likely to be multi-resistant, the balance of risk shifts towards treatment with quinolones.[43]

Third-generation cephalosporins

Cefotaxime, ceftriaxone and cefoperazone have excellent in vitro activity against S. Typhi and other salmonellae and have acceptable efficacy in the treatment of typhoid fever.[44] Only intravenous formulations are available. Cefotaxime is given 1 g three times daily (in children: 200 mg/kg daily in divided doses) for 14 days. Ceftriaxone has an advantage of only requiring a single dose daily. The cephalosporins are not active against many MDR strains and this limits their use in empirical treatment when resistant typhoid is likely.

Chloramphenicol

Since its introduction in 1948, chloramphenicol has proved to be remarkably effective in the treatment of enteric fever worldwide. It produces a rapid improvement in the patient's general condition, followed by defervescence in 3–5 days. The recommended adult dose is 500 mg every 4 hours till defervescence, then 6-hourly for a total course of 14 days. The drug is given orally unless the patient is nauseous or having diarrhoea, when the intravenous route should be used initially. The intramuscular route should be avoided as this gives unsatisfactory blood levels and may delay defervescence. The disadvantages of chloramphenicol are: rare marrow toxicity and aplastic anaemia; higher relapse rate following its use (5–15%);[33] and emergence of resistant strains of S. Typhi. S. Typhi strains with plasmid-mediated resistance to chloramphenicol began to appear in the 1960s and later became widespread in many of the endemic countries of the Americas and South-east Asia, highlighting the need for alternative therapeutic agents.

Ampicillin and amoxicillin

Although ampicillin is distinctly inferior to chloramphenicol, its close relative amoxicillin is at least as effective as chloramphenicol in respect of defervescence and relapse rate (4–8%),[33] and convalescence carriage occurs perhaps less commonly. It is usually given orally four times daily for 14 days.

Co-trimoxazole

This combination of trimethoprim and a sulphonamide amide is also as effective as chloramphenicol in terms of defervescence and relapse rate, and is given orally 960 mg twice daily but can be given parenterally if necessary.

Azithromycin

Azithromycin is a macrolide antibiotic which produces high tissue concentrations but low serum concentrations because of its unique pharmacokinetic properties. The antibiotic is concentrated within cells, making it ideal for the treatment of infection by an organism with an intracellular lifestyle. Animal models have shown that azithromycin is highly effective against *S*. Typhi and non-typhoidal *Salmonella*. It has now been shown to be effective in a series of open and randomized control trials. Oral administration is a benefit, and the results of clinical studies demonstrate that it is as effective as chloramphenicol, cefriaxone and ciprofloxacin. It was also effective in cases of MDR typhoid. This provides a useful alternative for the management of children with uncomplicated typhoid in developing countries.[45]

Emergence of multi-resistant typhoid fever

Since 1989 there has been a rapid emergence and spread of *S*. Typhi strains with simultaneous plasmid-mediated resistance to chloramphenicol, ampicillin and co-trimoxazole in the Indian subcontinent and parts of South-east Asia (see also Chapter 53). Quinolones and azithromycin are possible alternatives for treatment of infection with these organisms. Quinolone-resistant strains are now emerging as a clinical problem and it has been suggested that treatment regimens should restrict the use of further second- and third-line antibiotics for treating typhoid.[46] Recent studies led the authors of a Cochrane review of antimicrobial treatment of typhoid fever to conclude that satisfactory cure rates can be achieved in drug-sensitive cases with first-line antibiotics, such as chloramphenicol.[47] Increasing resistance in strains of *S*. Paratyphi A have been seen in travellers to the Indian subcontinent.[48]

Current therapeutic strategy

Because of the efficacy and low relapse and carrier rates associated with their use, the 4-quinolone drugs are now the drugs of choice in the treatment of adult typhoid, certainly in areas where multi-resistant typhoid fever has been reported.[40,49] However, because of its cheapness, chloramphenicol will continue to be used in other areas where the local strains are sensitive, although azithromycin may in the future be a useful alternative, especially in children.

In areas of high ciprofloxacin resistance, a third-generation cephalosporin, e.g. cefotaxime, will be the preferred drug if 4-quinolone drugs are to be avoided. Azithromycin is another potential alternative that combines oral availability with intracellular penetration and activity against the pathogen. A third-generation cephalosporin, or azithromycin, is the recommended regimen for children. However, their cost and the need for intravenous administration are significant disadvantages, particularly in the developing countries, and ciprofloxacin is being used increasingly in children with typhoid.[50]

Corticosteroid therapy

High-dose dexamethasone (initially 3 mg/kg body weight, followed by eight doses of 1 mg/kg 6-hourly) reduces mortality in severely ill patients with depressed levels of consciousness or shock.[51]

In the non-endemic countries, patients should be kept under bacteriological surveillance after clinical recovery until six consecutive negative faecal and urine cultures are obtained.

Management of chronic carriers

Prolonged courses of amoxicillin or co-trimoxazole may be effective, but the failure rate is high if there is chronic gallbladder disease. Ciprofloxacin (750 mg twice daily) and norfloxacin (400 mg twice daily) have been much more effective, with cure rates of 78% and 83%, respectively.

Cholecystectomy is not always successful, because of persisting hepatic infection. It is a major operation which should be performed only if strictly indicated for the patient's gallbladder disease, but not for the sole purpose of eradicating the carrier state.

Chronic urinary carriers should be investigated for urinary tract abnormalities, including schistosomiasis.

Prognosis

Early antibiotic therapy has transformed a previously life-threatening illness of several weeks duration with a mortality rate approaching 20% into a short-lasting febrile illness with negligible mortality. The high mortality rates which continue to be reported from some endemic countries are undoubtedly related to delayed diagnosis and/or inappropriate treatment.

Prevention

In the endemic countries, the most cost-effective strategy for reducing the incidence of enteric fever is the institution of public health measures to ensure safe drinking water and sanitary disposal of excreta. The effects of these measures are long lasting and will also reduce the incidence of other enteric infections which are a major cause of morbidity and mortality in those areas. In the absence of such a strategy, mass immunization with typhoid vaccines at regular intervals will also reduce the incidence of infections considerably.[52] The typhoid vaccines currently in use are described in Box 52.1. The need to administer multiple doses has led to attempts to develop single-dose oral vaccines. Phase I and

Box 52.1 Typhoid vaccines currently in use

1. Vi capsular polysaccharide antigen vaccine

This is a single parenteral dose vaccine from the Merieux Institute. Observed overall protection rates of 75% in Nepal,[53] 64% in South Africa[54] and 70% in China[55] compare favourably with the efficacy of the killed vaccine and it has the advantage of minimal side-effects. Revaccination is necessary every 3 years to maintain protection. It is not suitable for children under 18 months of age as polysaccharide antigens evoke a weak antibody response. The Vi vaccine can be given simultaneously with other vaccines relevant for international travellers.[56]

2. Vi-conjugate vaccine

Revaccination using the Vi vaccine does not elicit a booster effect because the immune response against polysaccharides does not involve T cells. To overcome this limitation, the Vi vaccine has been conjugated to a non-toxic recombinant *Pseudomanas aeruginosa* exotoxin A[57] and recently evaluated in Vietnam and shown to have 91.5% protective efficacy. This vaccine is suitable for children.[58]

3. Live attenuated vaccines

An oral vaccine containing live attenuated *S.* Typhi Ty21a strains in an enteric-coated capsule is now commercially available. It is well tolerated and an overall protective efficacy of 67–80% has been demonstrated for up to 7 years after three doses given on alternate days. There is also evidence of indirect protection (herd immunity), possibly due to the vaccine causing significant reduction in excretion of virulent Salmonella and fewer temporary carriers.[57] A four-dose schedule, which appears to give better protection,[59] is preferred in the USA. However, only 42% efficacy was recorded in Indonesia, suggesting that the vaccine may not be as effective in areas where exposure is intense.[6]

II clinical trials have been successful in a number of these novel typhoid fever vaccines.[60,61]

Although some studies have shown some cross-reactive cell-mediated immunity, Vi vaccines are generally regarded as ineffective against *S.* Paratyphi A, B and C, as these serotypes lack the Vi antigen.[54] However, this reduced efficacy against *S.* Paratyphi serotypes has an important implication in areas where there is increasing incidence of *S.* Paratyphi A.

Typhoid vaccination is recommended for travellers to highly endemic areas in Asia, Africa and the Americas. However, the protection is partial and travellers should be made aware of this and encouraged to pay close attention to personal, food and water hygiene.

OTHER SALMONELLA INFECTIONS (SALMONELLOSIS)

Although human salmonellosis occurs worldwide, it has become a major public health problem in developed countries. Individual cases and outbreaks in the community and in institutions are common. Of the large number of *Salmonella* serotypes, only a few account for the vast majority of human infections. Worldwide, examples of common human isolates are *S.* Enteritidis, *S.* Typhimurium, *S.* Virchow, *S.* Newport, *S.* Hadar, *S.* Heidelberg, *S.* Agona and *S.* Indiana; the order of prevalence is variable according to geography and time.[3,4]

Epidemiology

The organisms are widely distributed in the animal kingdom. Domestic animals, notably cattle, pigs and poultry, are frequent excretors and many wild animals are also infected. Household pets such as dogs, cats, birds and turtles are all potential, albeit rare, sources of human infection. Human cases and convalescent carriers are also important sources. Transmission is faecal–oral, usually through ingestion of contaminated foods such as improperly prepared poultry, meat and egg. The carcass of an animal harbouring salmonella in its gut becomes contaminated during evisceration, and infection spreads to other non-infected carcasses during large-scale storage. Thus, inadequately cooked meat or pre-cooked food contaminated from raw meat in the kitchen are important vehicles of transmission. Salmonella may survive deep freezing, and adequate thawing is essential before cooking. Fresh shell hen eggs infected through vertical transmission continue to be an important source of *S.* Enteritidis infection, although since 1999 most infections have been associated with eggs imported from abroad.[62]

The factors that are responsible for the dramatic rise of salmonella infections in developed countries in recent years are the adoption of large-scale intensive farming methods for rearing food animals and the use of bulk-imported infected animal feeds, both of which create conditions suitable for rapid spread of infection among the animals. The rising incidence of drug-resistant salmonellae has been linked to the extensive and poorly controlled use of antimicrobials in farm animals. The decrease in infections in the UK has been attributed to vaccination in poultry and to improvements in the microbiological quality of food, the 'farm to fork' approach.[63]

Transmission from a human source is infrequent; convalescent excretors with adequate standards of personal hygiene rarely transmit infection once their stools are formed. However, infected asymptomatic food-handlers have caused a number of restaurant-associated outbreaks. Institutional outbreaks are usually food related, but outbreaks in maternity, neonatal and geriatric units have followed admission of patients with an undiagnosed salmonella infection.

Unpasteurized milk is a recognized source in some countries. Unusual sources include pharmaceutical or diagnostic products of animal origin. In the developing countries, the epidemiological pattern is different, as large-scale rearing of food animals is not common and methods of cooking are different. Salmonellosis is an important cause of childhood infection, although rare in adults.[64]

Infection is more common and may be more severe in those who are predisposed to infection. This includes patients with reduced gastric acid or who have been prescribed antibiotic agents. Immunocompromise, most notably with HIV, predisposes to salmonellosis. Splenectomy and sickle cell disease also predispose to invasive salmonellosis.[4]

Pathogenesis

Site of invasion

Most of our understanding about the mechanisms of disease production by salmonella infection in man has come from work in animals and is described in detail above.

Mechanism of diarrhoea production

The exact mechanisms responsible for diarrhoea are unclear. Mucosal invasion and inflammation are clearly important, at least accounting for the bloody, mucoid type of stools which occur commonly, but do not explain the copious watery stools in the early stages. Observations in experimental animals of an enteropathy with water and electrolyte transport defects suggest the existence of secretory mechanisms.[65] Production of prostaglandin-like secretagogues and other mediators by the inflammatory tissues and toxin production by the organisms have been suggested. Salmonellae produce an enterotoxin and a cytotoxin. The enterotoxin activates adenylate cyclase and has some physicochemical characteristics in common with cholera toxin but limited antigenic homology.

Infecting dose

The size of the infecting dose is important to the outcome of a salmonella infection. The rarity of water-borne outbreaks of salmonellosis suggests the necessity of a large infecting dose that can usually be found only in food following multiplication. Limited experimental evidence in volunteers suggests an infecting dose of 10^5 in the production of clinical illness.[4] However, very small infecting doses, possibly as low as 17 organisms, have caused outbreaks. The size of the infecting dose is clearly influenced by the infectivity of the organism and host factors such as age, immune status, underlying debilitating disease or stress factors, and the physiological state of the stomach and upper small intestine at the precise time of intake of the organism. Gastric acidity is a significant barrier to enteric infection, and hypoacidity or increased transit time increase the susceptibility to infection.

Virulence of the organism

The serotypes vary greatly in their potential to produce invasive illness outside the gastrointestinal tract. Although any serotype can cause invasive disease, some are more invasive than others. S. Cholerae-suis regularly produces septicaemic or metastatic illnesses, and less commonly gastroenteritis. Other serotypes with increased invasiveness are S. Virchow and S. Dublin.[66] The multiresistant S. Typhimurium strains which have caused large outbreaks in Africa, India and the Middle East produce a high incidence of septicaemia and metastatic organ involvement. What governs this virulence potential is unclear, but in animal models serotypes bearing high-molecular-weight plasmids (virulence plasmids) have the ability to spread beyond the initial site of infection in the intestine. Virulence plasmids may be important in the pathogenesis of bacteraemia in humans.[67]

Clinical manifestations

There is wide variation in both the severity and the nature of manifestations of salmonellosis. Two often overlapping clinical syndromes are seen: acute enterocolitis (most common) and invasive salmonellosis with septicaemia or metastatic extraintestinal localization of infection. The incubation period is usually between 12 and 48 hours, but longer incubation periods of up to 72 days have been reported.

Acute enterocolitis

This is the preferred term to describe the acute diarrhoea of salmonellosis because both small and large intestines are involved in the disease process. The illness begins with nausea and vomiting, often associated with malaise, headache and fever. Very soon, cramp-like abdominal pains and diarrhoea supervene. Initially, the stools are of large volume and watery without visible blood or mucus; later, the volume may decrease as blood and mucus appear, indicating development of colitis. This may be associated with localization of pain over the left iliac fossa and some degree of rebound tenderness may develop. The severity of diarrhoea is quite variable, from a mild attack of several loose stools for a day to voluminous watery stools every half-hour or so over several days – leading to dehydration. The elderly, particularly those with debilitating illnesses, and individuals with gastric hypoacidity are prone to develop severe diarrhoea; this may have a cholera-like intensity in patients with a partial gastrectomy.

Occasionally, colitis may dominate the clinical picture, with the passage of frankly blood-stained stools containing pus. Toxic dilatation may complicate the picture. Sigmoidoscopy shows mucosal oedema, hyperaemia, petechial haemorrhages and, in severe cases, friable mucosa with ulcerations. Histological features include dilatation and congestion of capillaries in the mucosa and submucosa, with focal collections of polymorphonuclear leukocytes in the lamina propria (Figure 52.3A). In others there may also be a diffuse increase in chronic inflammatory cells in the lamina propria (Figure 52.3B). Crypt abscesses may be seen, but crypt architecture is usually normal with a normal goblet cell population; however, in severe cases, crypt distortion with mucus depletion may occur and distinction from inflammatory bowel disease is difficult (Figure 52.3C). Barium enema usually shows features of diffuse colitis, but segmental involvement may occur, mimicking Crohn's disease.

Alternatively, ileal involvement may be the predominant feature, with pain and tenderness localized over the right lower abdomen; this may be misdiagnosed as appendicitis.

Invasive salmonellosis

Bacteraemia is not uncommon in salmonella infection, even in previously healthy individuals, and its frequency depends on the serotype of the organism and host factors. Overall, bacteraemia rates of 8% have been observed, with higher rates for some serotypes, e.g. S. Cholerae-suis, S. Virchow and S. Dublin, and in the very young. Apart from age, other host factors are: immune suppression, malignancy, gastric hypoacidity, debilitating disease, bartonellosis and sickle cell disease.

In previously healthy individuals, bacteraemia is usually a transient event, but in a minority of patients, particularly those with the risk factors outlined, bacteraemia may be significant and characterized by either a septicaemic illness (swinging fever, rigors and general toxicity complicating the diarrhoeal illness) or a typhoid-like illness (sustained fever, splenomegaly and even rose spots but minimal diarrhoea) or evidence of metastatic localization in the meninges, bone and joints, lungs, endocardium and arteries, liver, spleen, ovary and kidneys.[31] Soft tissue localization can also occur. Metastatic infections may be unassociated with a diarrhoeal illness, as in S. Cholerae-suis infections. Meningitis occurs almost exclusively in neonates and children under 2 years of age, and reports of high incidence have come from a number of the devel-

Figure 52.3 (**A**), (**B**) and (**C**) are from rectal biopsies from patients with *Salmonella* spp. infection. (**A**) Milder lesions: focal inflammation of mucosa with polymorphonuclear leukocytes in the lamina propria and mucosal capillaries, but no increase in chronic inflammatory cells. (H&E, ×80.) (**B**) More severe lesions: severe acute inflammation with polymorphs in the lamina propria infiltrating the crypt epithelium and present on the mucosal surface. There is an increase in chronic inflammatory cells but the goblet cell population is well preserved. (H&E, ×135.) (**C**) Severe focal abscesses tending to be localized in the crypt: there is marked depletion of mucus but crypt architecture is not distorted. The surface epithelium is flattened. (H&E, ×150.) (**D**) Normal mucosa. (H&E, ×120.) (**A**), (**B**) and (**C**) are reproduced from Day et al. The rectal biopsy appearances in Salmonella colitis. *Histopathology* 1978; 2:117–131, with permission of the authors and the editor of *Histopathology*; (**D**) is reproduced by courtesy of B. C. Morson. (Reproduced with permission from Turnbull PCB. Food poisoning with special reference to salmonella: its epidemiology, pathogenesis and control. *Clin Gastroenterol* 1979; 8(3).)

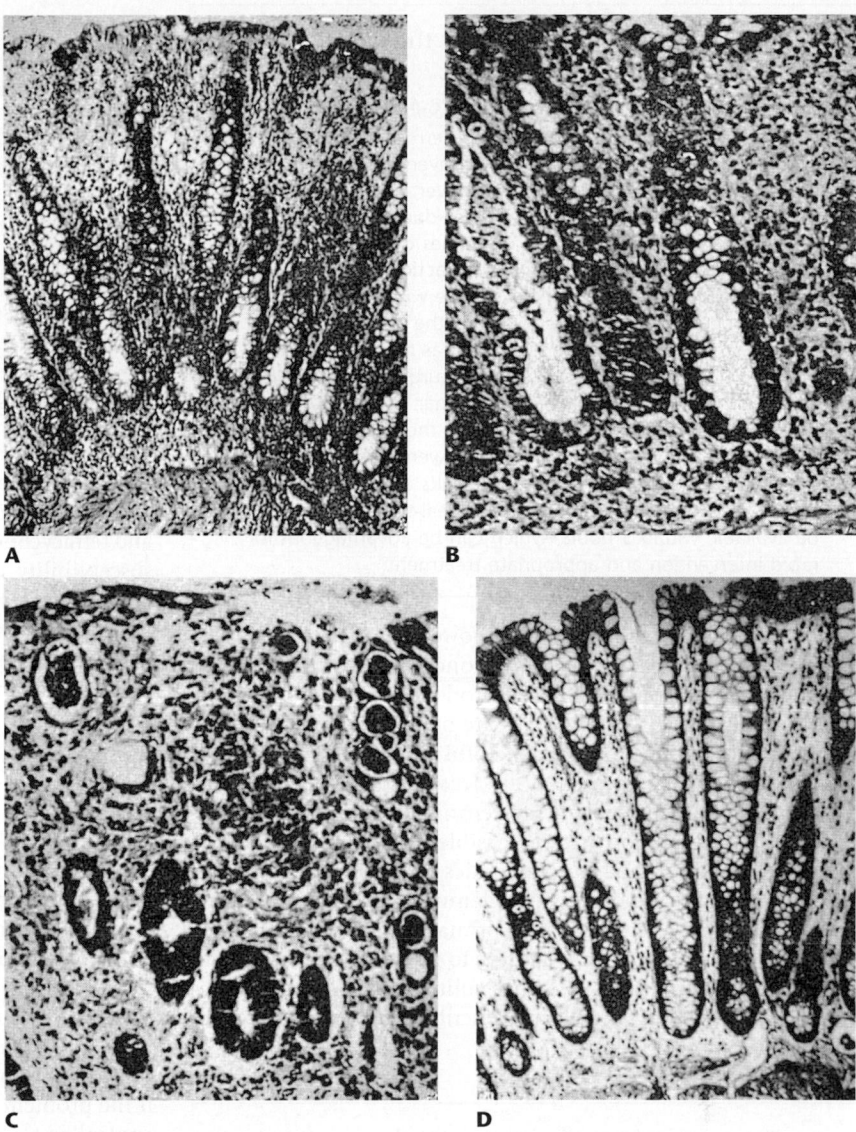

oping countries. Salmonella infection accounts for most cases of aortic and other vascular infections in the elderly. Atherosclerotic aneurysms of the abdominal aorta or iliac vessels, or prosthetic valves and grafts may all be infected. Normal arteries are affected very rarely. Children with sickle cell disease are particularly prone to developing osteomyelitis. Patients with chronic schistosomiasis are prone to suffer from recurrent bacteraemia from salmonella organisms living within the helminth.[68] HIV infection is an important predisposing factor for invasive salmonella infections, especially in sub-Saharan Africa where the HIV epidemic coincides with conditions of poor sanitation.[69,70] Infection is associated with prolonged excretion of the organisms and an enhanced risk of invasive disease. In adults with documented bacteraemia, *Salmonella* was identified in 35%.[69]

Reactive arthritis

Sterile synovitis may follow salmonella infection, particularly in HLA-B27-positive individuals. The symptoms usually develop 1–2 weeks after the acute infection. Any joint may be affected, although the knees and ankles are most frequently involved. Occasionally, there is migratory polyarthritis, resembling acute rheumatic fever, or bilateral proximal interphalangeal joint involvement, as in rheumatoid arthritis. Acute iridocyclitis may complicate the picture. Deposition of salmonella polysaccharide in the synovial cells may be an important factor in the pathogenesis of reactive arthropathy.

Carrier state

Adults recovering from salmonellosis usually continue to excrete the organism(s) for 4–8 weeks; infants and the elderly excrete for longer periods. Chronic carriage beyond 1 year occurs in far fewer than 1% of cases.

Diagnosis

Definitive diagnosis of salmonella enterocolitis requires positive faecal isolation. Blood cultures should be done in all severely ill

---

Box 52.2 Molecular techniques for the detection of *Salmonella*

Molecular techniques for the detection of *Salmonella* spp., such as PCR, have considerable advantages in terms of specificity, speed and standardization over the conventional methodologies described above. However, it is difficult to perform PCR directly on faecal samples due to the presence of inhibitory substances and large quantities of bacterial DNA other than the target DNA.[71] DNA extraction from faeces can be improved by pre-treating the sample with polyvinyl pyrrolidone (PVP). Commercial kits for the detection of *Salmonella* spp. by real-time PCR, such as the RealArt™ *Salmonella* PCR kit (Artus GmbH, Hamburg, Germany), are available but are not used routinely. Amar et al. (2004)[72] found that culture and PCR methods used for the detection of *Salmonella* from clinical faecal samples were of similar sensitivity. However, using culture, results are available within 2–3 days, whereas those obtained by real-time PCR assays can be available within 3 hours, which can be advantageous for rapid intervention and appropriate treatment.

---

patients. Coincidental inflammatory bowel disease should be suspected if bloody diarrhoea persists beyond 2 weeks despite the use of an appropriate antibiotic (e.g. ciprofloxacin). Sigmoidoscopic and barium contrast study findings are not discriminatory at this stage, but rectal biopsy is often helpful as crypt distortion and prominent goblet cell depletion are features of ulcerative colitis and are very rarely present in severe primary salmonella colitis. When such a distinction is not possible, the patient should be treated with prednisolone and antibiotics continued. In those who respond promptly, the diagnostic dilemma can be resolved only by a repeat biopsy after 6 weeks. In primary salmonella colitis the rectal biopsy histology usually returns to normal by this time, but this is quite uncommon in ulcerative colitis. Molecular techniques for the detection of *Salmonella* are described in Box 52.2.

Treatment

Most patients with salmonella enterocolitis have a short-lasting, self-limiting illness and require only increased fluid intake.

Antibiotics such as neomycin, colistin, ampicillin, chloramphenicol and co-trimoxazole do not influence the clinical illness and may prolong the duration of intestinal carriage, possibly due to the antibiotics suppressing the protective effects of the commensal intestinal flora. However, the 4-quinolone drugs (e.g. ciprofloxacin 500 mg twice daily for 5 days) have been shown to shorten the duration of the illness and should be used in patients who are at high risk of developing severe enterocolitis and/or invasive illness, i.e. the elderly, patients who are immunocompromised or have gastric hypoacidity, aortic aneurysm, vascular graft(s), valve prosthesis or debilitating diseases. Antibiotics are definitely indicated in patients with suspected or confirmed septicaemia and/or metastatic infection(s). Severe colitis is another indication for therapy.

Chloramphenicol, co-trimoxazole and amoxicillin are also effective against invasive disease if the infective organism is sensitive. However, the incidence of infection due to salmonella organisms resistant to one or more of these drugs has increased in many parts of the world, including the UK and the USA. There is much geographical variation in the prevalence of the resistant strains and local knowledge of such is essential if these drugs are to be used (see Chapter 53).

Third-generation cephalosporins (e.g. cefotaxime, ceftriaxone and cefoperazone) are highly effective, and resistance to these drugs is rare. They are particularly suitable for use in children if 4-quinolone drugs are to be avoided.

The complication of colonic dilatation usually resolves without surgery. Aortic salmonellosis generally requires surgical intervention.

Ciprofloxacin is also useful in eradicating persisting faecal carriage and should be given to food-handlers.

Antibiotic resistance

There is increasing incidence of multiple drug resistance in *Salmonella*, with reports of *S.* Typhimurium with resistance to ampicillin, chloramphenicol, trimethoprim–sulfamethoxazole, streptomycin and tetracycline.[73] More recently there have been reports of reduced susceptibility to ciprofloxacin.[74] Much of the resistance in nontyphoidal *Salmonella* is due to the use of antibiotics in animal husbandry. For example, enrofloxacin is a quinolone antibiotic used in veterinary medicine that may be related to the increased incidence of quinolone resistance. Although rare, resistance to extended-spectrum cephalosporins has now also been reported, narrowing the options when antibiotic therapy is indicated.[75]

Prevention

The main control measures are directed at maintaining high standards of hygiene in slaughterhouses and all areas of food preparation and distribution – both commercial and private. Raw meat and cooked food must be stored and handled separately. Thorough cooking of raw meat after adequate thawing is essential. Eggs should be boiled for 5 minutes and liquid egg for commercial use should be pasteurized. In the developing countries, adequate infection control procedures are essential in paediatric hospitals if the problem of endemic *Salmonella* spp. cross-infection is to be controlled.[76] Control of infection in the animal reservoir is a much more difficult problem. However, heat treatment of animal feeds, better standards of animal care and hygiene on the farm, and raising of infection-free flocks are some of the measures which will lower the contamination rates of flesh foods destined for human consumption.

Asymptomatic excretors who are handlers of unwrapped food meant for consumption without further cooking or reheating should be free of infection before returning to work. Others may do so or return to school once their diarrhoea has settled, provided their hygiene standards are adequate.

REFERENCES

1. Heyndrickx M, Pasmans F, Ducatelle R, et al. Recent changes in *Salmonella* nomenclature: the need for clarification. *Vet J* 2005; 170:275–277.
2. Brenner FW, Villar RG, Angulo FJ, et al. Salmonella nomenclature. *J Clin Microbiol* 2000; 38:2465–2467.
3. Jenkins C, Gillespie SH. Salmonella. In: Gillespie SH, Hawkey PM, eds. *Principles and Practice of Clinical Bacteriology*. 2nd edn. Chichester: Wiley; 2006:367–376.

4. Hohmann EL. Nontyphoidal salmonellosis. *Clin Infect Dis* 2001; 32:263–269.

5. Christie AB. *Infectious Diseases: Epidemiology and Clinical Practice*. 3rd edn. Edinburgh: Churchill Livingstone; 1980.

6. Ochiai RL, Wang X, von Seidlein L, et al. Salmonella paratyphi A rates, Asia. *Emerg Infect Dis* 2005; 11:1764–1766.

7. Cooke FJ, Day M, Wain J, et al. Cases of typhoid fever imported into England, Scotland and Wales (2000–2003). *Trans R Soc Trop Med Hyg* 2007; 101: 398–404.

8. Hornick RB, Greiseman SE, Woodward TE, et al. Typhoid fever: pathogenesis and immunological control. *N Engl J Med* 1970; 283:686–691.

9. Wain J, House D, Parkhill J, et al. Unlocking the genome of the human typhoid bacillus. *Lancet Infect Dis* 2002; 2:163–170.

10. Galan JE. Salmonella interactions with host cells: type III secretion at work. *Annu Rev Cell Dev Biol* 2001; 17:53–86.

11. Waterman SR, Holden DW. Functions and effectors of the Salmonella pathogenicity island 2 type III secretion system. *Cell Microbiol* 2003; 5: 501–511.

12. Eriksson S, Lucchini S, Thompson A, et al. Unravelling the biology of macrophage infection by gene expression profiling of intracellular *Salmonella enterica*. *Mol Microbiol* 2003; 47:103–118.

13. Pegues DA, Hantman MJ, Behlau I, et al. PhoP/PhoQ transcriptional repression of *Salmonella typhimurium* invasion genes: evidence for a role in protein secretion. *Mol Microbiol* 1995; 17:169–181.

14. Sarasombath S, Banchuin N, Sukusol T, et al. Systemic and intestinal immunities after natural typhoid infection. *J Clin Microbiol* 1987; 25: 1088–1093.

15. Bhan MK, Bahl R, Bhatnagar S. Typhoid and paratyphoid fever. *Lancet* 2005; 366:749–762.

16. Bhutta ZA. Current concepts in the diagnosis and treatment of typhoid fever. *BMJ* 2006; 333:78–82.

17. Wain J, Hien TT, Connerton P, et al. Molecular typing of multiple-antibiotic-resistant *Salmonella enterica* serovar Typhi from Vietnam: application to acute and relapse cases of typhoid fever. *J Clin Microbiol* 1999; 37:2466–2472.

18. Huang DB, DuPont HL. Problem pathogens: extra-intestinal complications of *Salmonella enterica* serotype Typhi infection. *Lancet Infect Dis* 2005; 5:341–348.

19. Lee JH, Kim JJ, Jung JH, et al. Colonoscopic manifestations of typhoid fever with lower gastrointestinal bleeding. *Dig Liver Dis* 2004; 36:141–146.

20. Van Basten JP, Stockenbrugger R. Typhoid perforation: a review of the literature since 1960. *Trop Geogr Med* 1994; 46:336–339.

21. Hosoglu S, Aldemir M, Akalin S, et al. Risk factors for enteric perforation in patients with typhoid fever. *Am J Epidemiol* 2004; 160:46–50.

22. Dutta TK, Beeresha, Ghotekar LH. Atypical manifestations of typhoid fever. *J Postgrad Med* 2001; 30:1225–1237.

23. Su CP, Chen YC, Chang SC. Changing characteristics of typhoid fever in Taiwan. *J Microbiol Immunol Infect* 2004; 37:109–114.

24. Khosla SN. Typhoid hepatitis. *Postgrad Med J* 1990; 66:923–925.

25. Hermans P, Gerard M, Laethem YV, et al. Pancreatic disturbances and typhoid fever. *Scand J Infect Dis* 1991; 23:201–205.

26. Breaky WR, Kala AK. Typhoid catatonia responsive to ECT. *BMJ* 1977; ii: 357–359.

27. Krishna KK, Mitra DK, Diwan AG, et al. Acute disseminated encephalomyelitis with typhoid fever. *J Assoc Physicians India* 1999; 47:1017–1019.

28. Albaqali A, Ghuloom A, Al Arrayed A, et al. Hemolytic uremic syndrome in association with typhoid fever. *Am J Kidney Dis* 2003; 41:709–713.

29. Boonpucknavig V, Soontornniyomkij V. Pathology of renal diseases in the tropics. *Semin Nephrol* 2003; 23:88–106.

30. Naidoo PN, Yan CC. Typhoid polymyositis. *S Afr Med J* 1975; 49:1975–1976.

31. Cohen JI, Bartlett JA, Corey GR. Extra-intestinal manifestations of Salmonella infections. *Medicine (Baltimore)* 1987; 66:349–388.

32. Gadeholt H, Madsen ST. Clinical course complications and mortality in typhoid fever as compared with paratyphoid B. A survey of 2647 cases. *Acta Med Scand* 1963; 174:753.

33. World Health Organization Department of Vaccines and Biologicals. *Background document: the diagnosis, prevention and treatment of typhoid fever.* Geneva: WHO; 2003:19–23. (www.who.int/entity/vaccine_research/documents/en/typhoid_diagnosis.pdf)

34. Gilman RH, Terminel M, Levine MM, et al. Relative efficacy of blood, urine, rectal swab, bone-marrow and rose-spot cultures for recovery of *Salmonella typhi* in typhoid fever. *Lancet* 1975; i:1211–1213.

35. Dutta S, Sur D, Manna B, et al. Evaluation of new-generation serologic tests for the diagnosis of typhoid fever: data from a community-based surveillance in Calcutta, India. *Diagn Microbiol Infect Dis* 2006; 56:359–365.

36. Olsen SJ, Pruckler J, Bibb W, et al. Evaluation of rapid diagnostic tests for typhoid fever. *J Clin Microbiol* 2004; 42:1885–1889.

37. House D, Wain J, Ho VA, et al. Serology of typhoid fever in an area of endemicity and its relevance to diagnosis. *J Clin Microbiol* 2001; 39:1002–1007.

38. Fadeel MA, Crump JA, Mahoney FJ, et al. Rapid diagnosis of typhoid fever by enzyme-linked immunosorbent assay detection of Salmonella serotype typhi antigens in urine. *Am J Trop Med Hyg* 2004; 70:323–328.

39. Prakash P, Mishra OP, Singh AK, et al. Evaluation of nested PCR in diagnosis of typhoid fever. *J Clin Microbiol* 2005; 43:431–432.

40. Parry CM. Typhoid fever. *Curr Infect Dis Rep* 2004; 6:27–33.

41. Arnold K, Hong CS, Nelwan R, et al. Randomized comparative study of fleroxacin and chloramphenicol in typhoid fever. *Am J Med* 1993; 94: 195S–200S.

42. Leibovitz E. The use of fluoroquinolones in children. *Curr Opin Pediatr* 2006; 18:64–70.

43. Dutta P, Rasaily R, Saha MR, et al. Ciprofloxacin for treatment of severe typhoid fever in children *Antimicrob Agents Chemother* 1993; 37:1197–1199.

44. Soe GB, Overturf GD. Treatment of typhoid fever and other systemic salmonellosis with cefotaxime, ceftriaxone, cefoperazone and other newer cephalosporins. *Rev Infect Dis* 1987; 9:719–736.

45. Frenck RW Jr, Mansour A, Nakhla I, et al. Short course azithromycin for the treatment of uncomplicated typhoid fever in children and adolescents. *Clin Infect Dis* 2004; 38:951–957.

46. Okeke IN, Klugman KP, Bhutta ZA, et al. Antimicrobial resistance in developing countries. Part II: strategies for containment. *Lancet Infect Dis* 2005; 5:568–580.

47. Thaver D, Zaidi AK, Critchley J, et al. Fluoroquinolones for treating typhoid and paratyphoid fever (enteric fever). *Cochrane Database Syst Rev* 2005; (2): CD004530.

48. Threlfall EJ, Day M, de Pinna E, et al. Drug-resistant enteric fever in the UK. *Lancet* 2006; 367:1576.

49. Ferreccio C, Morris JG Jr, Valdivieso C, et al. Efficacy of ciprofloxacin in the treatment of chronic typhoid carriers. *J Infect Dis* 1988; 157:1235–1239.

50. Basnyat B. Typhoid and paratyphoid fever. *Lancet* 2005; 366:1603.

51. Hoffman SL, Punjabi NH, Kumala S, et al. Reduction of mortality in chloramphenicol treated severe typhoid fever by high dose dexamethasone. *N Engl Med J* 1984; 310:82–87.

52. Bodhidatt L, Taylor DN, Thisyakorn U, et al. Control of typhoid fever in Bangkok, Thailand, by annual immunization of school children with parenteral typhoid vaccine. *Rev Infect Dis* 1987; 9:841–845.

53. Acharya IL, Lowe CU, Thapa R, et al. Prevention of typhoid fever in Nepal with the Vi capsular polysaccharide of *Salmonella typhi*: a preliminary report. *N Engl J Med* 1987; 317:1101–1104.

54. Levine MM, Ferreccio C, Black RE, et al., and the Chilean Typhoid Committee. Large scale field trial of Ty21a live oral typhoid vaccine in enteric-coated capsules: a field trial in an endemic area. *Lancet* 1987; i:1049–1052.

55. Yang HH, Wu CG, Xie GZ, et al. Efficacy trial of Vi polysaccharide vaccine against typhoid fever in south-western China. *Bull World Health Organ* 2001; 79:625–631.

56. Proell S, Maiwald H, Nothdurft HD, et al. Combined vaccination against hepatitis A, hepatitis B, and typhoid fever: safety, reactogenicity, and immunogenicity. *J Travel Med* 2002; 9:122–126.

57. Guzman CA, Borsutzky S, Griot-Wenk M, et al. Vaccines against typhoid fever. *Vaccine* 2006; 24:3804–3811.

58. Lin FY, Ho VA, Khiem HB, et al. The efficacy of a *Salmonella typhi* Vi conjugate vaccine in two-to-five-year-old children. *N Engl J Med* 2001; 344:1263–1269.

59. Ferreccio C, Levine MM, Rodriguea H, et al., and the Chilean Typhoid Committee. Comparative efficacy of two, three or four doses of Ty21a live oral typhoid vaccine in enteric-coated capsules: a field trial in an endemic area. *J Infect Dis* 1989; 159:766–769.

60. Tacket CO, Pasetti MF, Sztein MB, et al. Immune responses to an oral typhoid vaccine strain that is modified to constitutively express Vi capsular polysaccharide. *J Infect Dis* 2004; 190:565–570.

61. Kirkpatrick BD, McKenzie R, O'Neill JP, et al. Evaluation of *Salmonella enterica* serovar Typhi (Ty2 aroC-ssaV-) M01ZH09, with a defined mutation in the Salmonella pathogenicity island 2, as a live, oral typhoid vaccine in human volunteers. *Vaccine* 2006; 24:116–123.

62. PHLS. Public Health Investigation of *Salmonella* Enteritidis in raw shell eggs. *CDR Weekly* 2002; 12(50):3–5.

63. Ward LR, Maguire C, Hampton MD, et al. Collaborative investigation of an outbreak of *Salmonella enterica* serotype Newport in England and Wales in 2001 associated with ready-to-eat salad vegetables. *Commun Dis Pub Health* 2002; 5:301–304.

64. Jones TF, Ingram LA, Fullerton KE, et al. A case-control study of the epidemiology of sporadic Salmonella infection in infants. *Pediatrics* 2006; 118:2380–2387.

65. Coburn B, Grassl GA, Finlay BB. Salmonella, the host and disease: a brief review. *Immunol Cell Biol* 2007; 85:112–118.

66. Acheson DWK. Enterotoxins in acute infective diarrhoea. *J Infect* 1992; 24:225–245.

67. Fierer J, Krause M, Tauxe R, et al. *Salmonella typhimurium* bacteraemia: association with the virulence plasmid. *J Infect Dis* 1992; 166:639–642.

68. Young SW, Higashi G, Kamel R, et al. Interactions of salmonellae and schistosomes in host-parasite relations. *Trans R Soc Trop Med Hyg* 1973; 67:797–802.

69. Kankwatira AM, Mwafulirwa GA, Gordon MA. Non-typhoidal salmonella bacteraemia – an under-recognized feature of AIDS in African adults. *Trop Doct* 2004; 34:198–200.

70. Graham SM, Molyneux EM, Walsh AL, et al. Nontyphoidal Salmonella infections of children in tropical Africa. *Pediatr Infect Dis J* 2000; 19: 1189–1196.

71. Wilson IG. Inhibition and facilitation of nucleic acid amplification. *Appl Envir Microbiol* 1997; 63:3741–3751.

72. Amar CFL, East C, Maclure E, et al. Blinded application of microscopy, bacteriology culture, immunoassays and PCR to detect gastrointestinal pathogens from faecal samples of patients with community-acquired diarrhoea. *Eu J Clin Microbiol Infect Dis* 2004; 23:529–534.

73. Helms M, Ethelberg S, Molbak K. DT104 Study Group. Typhimurium DT104 infections, 1992–2001. *Emerg Infect Dis* 2005; 11:859–867.

74. Hopkins KL, Davies RH, Threlfall EJ. Mechanisms of quinolone resistance in *Escherichia coli* and Salmonella: recent developments. *Int J Antimicrob Agents* 2005; 5:358–373.

75. Miriagou V, Tassios PT, Legakis NJ, et al. Expanded-spectrum cephalosporin resistance in non-typhoid Salmonella. *Int J Antimicrob Agents* 2004; 23: 547–555.

76. Food Standards Agency. Salmonella outbreaks prompt agency to issue hygiene alert (Press Release). London: FSA; 15 October 2002. (http://www.food.gov.uk/news/newsarchive/salmonellaoutbreaknews)

Chapter 53   Eric John Threlfall

Resistant Gut Bacteria

Resistance to antimicrobial drugs, including both resistance to key antimicrobials and multiple resistance (to four or more unrelated antimicrobials), is now a major problem in bacterial enteric pathogens in both developing and developed countries throughout the world. The problem affects *Salmonella enterica*, including not only *S. enterica* serotypes Typhi and Paratyphi, but also a range of other serovars, notably Typhimurium in developing countries and Typhimurium, Virchow, Hadar and Newport in developed countries. Resistance to therapeutic antimicrobials is also an increasing problem in *Shigella*, especially *Sh. dysenteriae* 1 (Shiga's bacillus), but also in *Sh. flexneri* and *Sh. boydii* in developing countries and *Sh. sonnei* in developed countries. Resistance to therapeutic antimicrobials has also been reported in *Vibrio cholerae* O1, O139 and non-O1, non-O139 strains, and increasingly in *Escherichia coli*. Since the early 1990s, resistance to key antimicrobials has also been reported in *Campylobacter* spp. Resistance in this organism is increasing and has been linked to the use of antimicrobials in animal husbandry.

SALMONELLAE

The occurrence of resistance is of particular concern in *Salmonella* Typhi and S. Paratyphi infections where treatment with an appropriate antibiotic is essential, and should commence as soon as clinical diagnosis is made. The increasing occurrence of both resistance to key antimicrobials and multiple resistance in serotypes other than Typhi has also had a profound effect, particularly in developing countries, in the treatment of salmonella septicaemia in infants and young children, where, since 1980, multi-resistant strains have been implicated in numerous outbreaks in hospital paediatric units.

Salmonella Typhi and Paratyphi

Salmonella Typhi

Typhoid fever is a systemic illness caused by *S. enterica* serotype Typhi and is a significant cause of morbidity and mortality among children and adults in developing countries. The organism remains endemic in developing countries in Africa, South and Central America, and the Indian subcontinent, and the World Health Organization (WHO) estimates that 22 million illnesses and 200 000 deaths are attributable to S. Typhi each year.[1] In contrast, in developed countries such as the UK or USA, the incidence of S. Typhi is much lower, and the majority of cases are in travellers returning from endemic areas. For example, in the UK, between 150 and 300 cases occur each year, with at least 70% of cases in patients with a history of recent foreign travel.[2] Similarly in the USA, 293 infections were reported in the 12-month period from 1 June 1996 to 31 May 1997, of which 81% were recorded in patients with a history of recent travel to endemic areas.[3]

For patients with typhoid fever, the administration of an effective antibiotic is essential. Ideally, treatment should commence as soon as clinical diagnosis is made, without recourse to the results of antimicrobial sensitivity tests. From 1948 to the mid-1970s, chloramphenicol was the first-line drug of choice and in developed countries the use of chloramphenicol resulted in a reduction in the mortality rate from 10% to less than 2%. Following the occurrence of extensive outbreaks of typhoid fever in Mexico and India in the early and mid-1970s, in which the epidemic strains were resistant to chloramphenicol, there were fears that the efficacy of this antimicrobial had been seriously jeopardized. Alternative drugs which were then used for typhoid fever included ampicillin and trimethoprim. Since 1989, strains of S. Typhi with resistance to ampicillin and trimethoprim in addition to chloramphenicol, streptomycin, sulphonamides and tetracyclines (= MRSTY) have been isolated with increasing frequency in several countries, particularly in the Indian subcontinent (India, Pakistan, Bangladesh, Nepal) but also in several other countries in South-east Asia (Kuala Lumpar, the Philippines, Vietnam) as well as Egypt and several countries in the Arabian Gulf, particularly those with a significant proportion of immigrant workers from the Indian subcontinent.[4] In India the most common S. Typhi phage type implicated in outbreaks caused by MRSTY since 1990 has been Vi-phage type E1, with outbreaks of infection reported in major conurbations in the north, east, south and west of the country.[5,6] In contrast, the predominant multi-resistant Vi-phage type in Pakistan from 1989 to 1992 was M1, and over this period there was an extensive outbreak in Rawalpindi caused by strains of this phage type.[7] More recently, MRSTY Vi-phage type M1 has been replaced by MRSTY phage type E1 in Pakistan, with several outbreaks reported since the mid-1990s.[4] In addition, MRSTY of different phage types have been isolated in Egypt, Canada and

Table 53.1 Outbreaks of multi-resistant *Salmonella enterica* serovar Typhi, 1989–2002

Year	Country or area	Phage type	R-type	Plasmid type
1989	Pakistan	M1	ACSSuTTm	HI1
1990–1995	India	E1, 51, O	ACSSuTTm	HI1
1990–1995	Arabian Gulf	E1, 51, O	ACSSuTTm	HI1
1990–1993	Kuala Lumpur	E1	ACSSuTTm	HI1
1991	UK	M1	CSTTm	HI1
1991	South Africa	A	ACKSSuT	HI1
1991–1992	Egypt	E2, C1, D1-N	ACSSuTTm	HI1
1992–1994	Vietnam	?	ACSSuTTm	HI1
1993–1994	Philippines	?	CKSSuTTm	?
1994, 1998	Bangladesh	E1	ACSSuTTm	HI1
1994–1998	Pakistan	E1	ACSSuTTm	HI1
1993–1998	Vietnam	?	ACSSuTTm (Cp$_L$)	HI1
1997–1999	Kenya	?	ACSSuTTm	HI1
1997–1998	Nigeria	?	ACSSuTTm	?
1998–1999	Tajikistan	UVS	ACSSuTTmCp$_L$	HI1
2002	Nepal	?	ACSSuTTmCp$_L$	HI1

Resistance symbols: A, ampicillin; C, chloramphenicol; K, kanamycin; S, streptomycin; Su, sulphonamides; T, tetracyclines; Tm, trimethoprim; Cp$_L$, decreased susceptibility to ciprofloxacin (MIC: 0.25–1.0 mg/L) ?, not known.

South Africa (Table 53.1). Since 1997, MRSTY have also become increasingly common in Africa, with isolations reported from countries as far apart as Nigeria and Kenya.[8,9] Strains from these countries have been resistant to chloramphenicol, ampicillin and co-trimoxazole, with a significant proportion of isolates from Nigeria also showing resistance to nalidixic acid. Examples of outbreaks caused by MRSTY that have occurred since 1989 are shown in Table 53.1.

An increasing problem in the Indian subcontinent has been the rapid appearance of strains with resistance to nalidixic acid and with concomitant decreased susceptibility to ciprofloxacin (minimal inhibitory concentration [MIC]: 0.25–1.0 mg/L).[10,11] Such strains may also be resistant to chloramphenicol, ampicillin and trimethoprim.[12] A similar picture has emerged in several European countries,[13] where the majority of infections with *S.* Typhi are in travellers recently returned from endemic areas.

Ciprofloxacin became the drug of choice for infections with MRSTY in 1991.[14-16] Although the level of resistance to ciprofloxacin in strains with decreased susceptibility is below the recommended treatment level, numerous cases of treatment failure have been reported in widely separated areas.[17-20] Since 1993, strains of *S.* Typhi with decreased susceptibility to ciprofloxacin have also been isolated with increasing frequency in Vietnam.[19] In 1997 there were over 6000 recorded cases in an extensive epidemic in Tajikistan of nalidixic acid-resistant *S.* Typhi with decreased susceptibility to ciprofloxacin.[20] In both Vietnam and Tajikistan, treatment failures with fluoroquinolone antibiotics were common.[19,20] In 2002, a total of 5963 cases of typhoid fever were reported in an outbreak in Nepal; in this outbreak the causative strain exhibited decreased susceptibility to ciprofloxacin.[21] Despite the low level of resistance, treatment failures have been noted in all areas where such strains have caused infections.[18-22] A new development

has been the appearance of strains of *S.* Typhi with resistance to ciprofloxacin at therapeutic levels.[23,24] Although such strains have as yet not been implicated in outbreaks, the emergence of high-level resistance to the primary first-line drug is of major concern.

Because the vast majority of cases of typhoid fever in the UK are in travellers returning mainly from the Indian subcontinent,[25] the situation in the UK has mirrored that seen in India and Pakistan, with MRSTY strains and strains with decreased susceptibility to ciprofloxacin accounting for 49% of isolates in 2004.[26] In cases of treatment failure with ciprofloxacin, alternatives such as ceftriaxone or cefotaxime have been used with some success. In this respect it is reassuring that all strains of *S.* Typhi from cases of typhoid fever so far tested in the UK have been sensitive to these antimicrobials.[27] Azithromycin, a macrolide antibiotic, has also been evaluated in the treatment of infections caused by both MRSTY and *S.* Typhi with decreased susceptibility to ciprofloxacin, with encouraging results.[28] To date, no strains of azithromycin-resistant *S.* Typhi have been reported, but the expense of this antibiotic, and that of the third-generation cephalosporins listed above, may preclude their widespread usage in developing countries.

Irrespective of phage type or country of origin, in all strains of *S.* Typhi with resistance to chloramphenicol, ampicillin and trimethoprim, the complete spectrum of multiple resistance has been encoded by plasmids of approximately 150 kilobases (kb) belonging to the HI1 incompatibility group.[4,29] Evolutionary diversity within this incompatibility group has been recently observed among HI1 plasmids from multi-resistant strains of *S.* Typhi isolated in Vietnam in the late 1990s.[30] In contrast, decreased susceptibility to ciprofloxacin has resulted from mutations within *gyrA* in the bacterial chromosome. Four different mutations have been identified within GyrA in strains of *S.* Typhi of different phage types originating in India,[31] indicating that such strains are not clonal in respect of phage type or ciprofloxacin susceptibility.

Salmonella Paratyphi A

Infections caused by S. Paratyphi A, although in general not as severe as typhoid fever, may also require antimicrobial intervention before the results of susceptibility tests are available. Multiple drug resistance has been reported to be increasing in S. Paratyphi A in India since 1990, often coupled with decreased susceptibility to ciprofloxacin.[32,33] An increase in strains of S. Paratyphi A with decreased susceptibility to ciprofloxacin was reported in 10 European countries in 2000,[13] and in 2005 84% of 221 isolates of S. Paratyphi A from patients in the UK exhibited such resistance.[26] This resistance has been attributed to the widespread use of ciprofloxacin and ciprofloxacin derivatives in developing countries to treat many human infections irrespective of prescription. To maintain the efficacy of fluoroquinolones it is essential that such antimicrobials are reserved for the treatment of invasive diseases and are not used for prophylaxis or for the treatment of uncomplicated gastroenteritis.

Resistance to fluoroquinolone antibiotics in Salmonella Typhi and S. Paratyphi A

The British Society for Antimicrobial Chemotherapy and the Clinical and Laboratories Standards Institute zone size equivalents for ciprofloxacin resistance in Enterobacteriaceae in disc diffusion tests are 2.0 and 4.0 mg/L, respectively. At these levels decreased susceptibility to ciprofloxacin (MIC: 0.20–1.0 mg/L) is often undetected, sometimes leading to delay in the administration of an effective antibiotic. Because of treatment failures in cases where the levels of resistance are below 2.0 mg/L, it has been suggested that consideration be given to lowering the breakpoint recommendations.[34] Similarly, to ensure detection of decreased susceptibility, it has been recommended that nalidixic acid be used as a primary screen and that organisms exhibiting resistance to this antimicrobial be subjected to testing for ciprofloxacin resistance/susceptibility by MIC, with appropriate controls.[18,26]

Other salmonella serovars

On a global scale it has been estimated that there are about 1.3 billion cases of acute gastroenteritis due to non-typhoidal salmonellae per annum, resulting in 3 million deaths.[35] The proportion of salmonella infections caused by antimicrobial-resistant strains has steadily increased around the world over the last 20 years, and now represents 20–40% of all isolates from cases of human infection. In developed countries such as the UK, the majority of countries in Western Europe and the USA, salmonella infections, excluding those with S. Typhi and S. Paratyphi A, are primarily zoonoses. When resistance is present, in the majority of instances it has been acquired prior to transmission of the organism through the food chain to humans. Such resistance acquisition has often been linked to the use of antimicrobials in animal husbandry. Long term, the most important serotypes in the UK, Europe and

the USA are Enteritidis, Typhimurium and Virchow, and the main method of spread is through contaminated food. In the USA S. Newport has been an increasing problem since the late 1990s and S. Heidelberg has also been a commonly isolated serotype. In general, person-to-person transmission is not of major importance in the spread of these serotypes. In most cases the clinical presentation is that of mild to moderate enteritis, the disease is usually self-limiting and antimicrobial therapy is seldom required. In contrast, in developing countries, particularly in the Indian subcontinent, South-east Asia, South and Central America and Africa, serotypes such as Typhimurium, Wien, Johannesburg and Oranienburg have undergone changes in both their epidemiology and their clinical disease. An additional feature of these strains has been the possession of plasmid-mediated multiple drug resistance, often with resistance to seven or more antimicrobial agents.

Developing countries

Since 1970, multi-resistant salmonellae have caused extensive outbreaks in many developing countries. The common pattern has been for several hospitals, often situated many miles apart, to be involved. The majority of outbreaks have occurred in neonatal and paediatric wards, but community outbreaks in villages and small towns have also been reported. The clinical disease has been severe, with enteritis frequently accompanied by septicaemia, and in several outbreaks a mortality rate of up to 30% has been reported. Serotypes involved include, notably, Typhimurium in the Middle East and the Indian subcontinent, and Wien in Southern Europe, North Africa and India, although infections caused by multi-resistant strains belonging to several other serotypes have also been reported. Strains have been resistant to up to 10 antimicrobials. Examples of such outbreaks are shown in Table 53.2. For a review, see Rowe and Threlfall.[36] A disturbing development in recent years has been the emergence in developing countries of strains of multi-resistant non-typhoidal salmonellae with high-level resistance to nalidixic acid (MIC >100 mg/L) and with reduced susceptibility to ciprofloxacin (MIC 0.25–1.0 versus <0.01 mg/L for nalidixic acid-sensitive strains). This has been particularly noticeable in countries such as India, not only for S. Typhimurium[37] but also for S. Senftenberg[38] and other serotypes.

A particular feature of infections with multi-resistant non-typhoidal salmonellae in developing countries has been the lack of involvement of food animal reservoirs. Spread has been by person-to-person contact and antibiotic resistance has developed as a result of the use of antibiotics in human medicine, particularly in those countries where there is little control over the use of antibiotics. An example of the type of epidemic caused by multi-resistant salmonellae is that which has occurred throughout India since 1977.[39] The serotype involved was Typhimurium and strains have belonged to closely related phage types. Outbreaks occurred both in communities and in hospitals, particularly amongst neonates, although older children and adults have also been affected. The most common presentation has been severe enteritis, and cases of septicaemia have also been reported. Mortality was high in at least five outbreaks. The majority of strains have been characterized by plasmid-mediated resistance to at least seven antimicrobials, including ampicillin, chloramphenicol, gentamicin, kanamycin, streptomycin, sulphonamides, tetracyclines and trim-

Table 53.2 Examples of outbreaks of multi-resistant non-typhoidal *Salmonella enterica* in developing countries, 1969–2000

Year	Country or area	Serotype	Phage type	R-type	Plasmid type
1969–1972	North Africa, Southern Europe, India	Wien	–	ACSSuT	FI$_{me}$
1972–1980	Middle East	Typhimurium	208, UT	ACSSuT, ACGKSSuT	FI$_{me}$
1974–1978	South Africa	Johannesburg	–	ACKSSuT	FI$_{me}$
1974–1996	Turkey	Typhimurium	UT	ACGKSSuTTm	FI$_{me}$
1976–1980	Kenya	Typhimurium	NC	ACSSuT	FI$_{me}$
1979–1990	India	Typhimurium	66/122	ACSSuT, ACGKSSuTTmNx	FI$_{me}$
1990–1999	Albania, Italy	Typhimurium	?	ACKSSuTTm	FI$_{me}$
1990–2000	India	Senftenberg	–	ACGKSSuTTmNx	FI$_{me}$

Resistance symbols: See Table 53.1; G, gentamicin; Nx, nalidixic acid. UT, untypable; NC, non-conforming; ?, not known; –, not applicable.

ethoprim. Chromosomally-mediated resistance to furazolidone and nalidixic acid, accompanied by decreased susceptibility to ciprofloxacin, has also been common.

Plasmids

With the exception of resistance to furazolidone and nalidixic acid/ciprofloxacin, all resistances in such strains have been plasmid-mediated and have been encoded by high molecular mass, transmissible plasmids belonging to incompatibility group FI$_{me}$ (inc FI$_{me}$).[40] In addition to coding for multiple drug resistance, such plasmids also carry genes coding for the production of the hydroxamate siderophore aerobactin, which is a known virulence factor for some enteric and urinary tract pathogens. This plasmid type was first identified in a strain of *S.* Typhimurium definitive phage type (DT) 208 which caused numerous epidemics in Middle Eastern countries in the 1970s.[40] It was subsequently identified in unrelated phage types of *S.* Typhimurium which have caused similar outbreaks throughout the Middle East and in several countries in Africa, and in a multi-resistant strain of *S.* Wien responsible for a massive epidemic which started in Algeria in 1969 and spread rapidly through paediatric and nursery populations in many countries throughout North Africa, Western Europe, the Middle East and eventually the Indian subcontinent over the next 10 years.[41,42] Similar plasmids have also been identified in strains of *S.* Typhimurium isolated in Italy and originating in Albania.[43] A 30-year retrospective molecular study of this group of plasmids has demonstrated that the plasmids have evolved through sequential acquisition of integrons, which are themselves highly mobile genetic elements capable of horizontal transfer between different bacterial strains, carrying different arrays of antibiotic resistance and virulence genes.[44]

Alarming developments with non-typhoidal salmonella infections in developing countries have recently been reported. In Taiwan a highly virulent strain of *S.* Cholerae-suis displaying high-level resistance to ciprofloxacin and plasmid-mediated resistance to ceftriaxone caused a fatal infection in a patient in 2003.[45] Fortunately the strain did not spread and no further infections were reported. Since the late 1980s there have been a growing number of reports of isolates of *Salmonella* spp. with resistance to third-

generation cephalosporin antimicrobials. Such strains produce either extended-spectrum β-lactamases (ESBLs) or a plasmid-mediated AmpC β-lactamase. Such strains are now widespread in North Africa,[46] and may be endemic in other parts of Africa, India, the Western Pacific region[47] and parts of South America.[48] Strains with resistance to ESBLs have also been isolated increasingly in Europe. For example, CTX-M-9, -15, and -17 to -18 have recently been reported in six different serovars from humans in England and Wales,[49] and although often associated with foreign travel, isolates from patients without a history of such travel are being increasingly identified.[50] CTX-M-like enzymes have also been identified in *S.* Virchow in Spain,[51] and *S.* Anatum in Taiwan.[52] A further development is the emergence of strains of salmonella with plasmid-mediated resistance to fluoroquinolones, particularly with the quinolone resistance determinant qnrS1.[53,54] As with strains producing ESBLs, such strains are mostly associated with infections in patients who acquired their infections in developing countries, or as a result of consuming food products exported from such countries.[54]

Antimicrobial therapy

Antimicrobial therapy is often essential for the treatment of infections caused by these multi-resistant strains, particularly when such strains cause extra-intestinal infections. Ciprofloxacin and some of the newer fluoroquinolone antibiotics have been used extensively for this purpose in developing countries, although their efficacy is now being eroded following the emergence of strains with decreased susceptibility and high-level resistance. Alternative antimicrobials such as ceftriaxone have been used for individual patients, but the emergence of resistance to such antimicrobials means that their efficacy for the treatment of serious disease is rapidly being eroded.

Developed countries

In contrast to the situation in developing countries, in developed countries such as those in Western Europe and North America, salmonella septicaemia is rare in other than a few serotypes of limited epidemiological importance. Indeed, over the 10-year period from 1981 to 1990, the occurrence of bloodstream invasion for the two most common serovars, Enteritidis and Typhimurium, in England and Wales, was less than 2%.[55] A similar situation was observed in strains isolated in the 3-year period from 1995 to 1997.[56]

Since the late 1980s the most important multi-drug-resistant strains in developed countries have been S. Typhimurium DT 104 (MR DT 104), with a worldwide distribution,[57] and in the USA, S. Newport with AmpC-mediated ESBL resistance in addition to resistance to a range of other antimicrobials.[58] MR DT 104 first appeared in the UK in 1984, when it was isolated from gulls and exotic birds imported from the Far East. By 1989 the strain was increasingly becoming isolated from cattle and also from cases of human infection. In England and Wales, isolations of MR DT 104 from humans increased from about 200 in 1990, peaking at over 4000 in 1996. By the early 1990s MR DT 104 had also become common in poultry, particularly turkeys, pigs and sheep.[57] Although there have been no indications of increased virulence of the organism in cases of human infection in the UK,[56] in some countries there have been reports of an apparent predilection of the organism to cause serious disease.[59]

MR S. Typhimurium DT 104 is characterized by chromosomally encoded resistance to five antimicrobials – ampicillin, chloramphenicol/florphenicol, streptomycin, sulphonamides and tetracyclines (ACSSuT). Such resistances are contained within a 46 kb resistance island (Salmonella genomic island 1 [SGI1]). The resistance locus consists of the floR (chloramphenicol/florphenicol) and tetG (tetracyclines) resistance genes flanked by two Class 1 integons, the first containing the aadA2 gene conferring resistance to streptomycin, in addition to the sul1 gene conferring resistance to sulphonamides, and the second the β-lactamase gene bla$_{PSE-1}$ conferring resistance to ampicillin, in addition to sul1.[60] Although chromosomally located, in recent years SGI1 has been identified in several different salmonella serotypes, including Agona, Albany, Derby, Kentucky and Paratyphi B variant Java. Such strains have caused infections in humans and cattle,[61] and there has been speculation that the resistance island originated in the Far East, possibly in ornamental fish.[62]

It should be realized that multiple resistance in salmonellae in developed countries is not confined to S. Typhimurium DT 104 and related strains containing SGI1. In Spain, emergent multi-resistant strains of S. enterica serotype [4,5,12:i:-] have been associated with an increasing number of human infections since the mid-1990s.[63] Such strains have also caused infection in humans in the UK[64] and Denmark. Similarly in Greece, multi-resistant strains of S. Blockley have caused numerous infections in humans since 1996.[65] It should be emphasized that, although the most common presentation has been gastroenteritis in infections caused by both S. enterica serotype [4,5,12:i:-] and S. Blockley, in some cases patients have not responded to antimicrobial treatment, possibly as a consequence of the wide resistance spectrum of the organisms concerned. Of note in Europe at the present time is a substantive increase in isolations of S. Enteritidis with resistance to nalidixic acid with concomitant decreased susceptibility to ciprofloxacin. In 2000, 13% of isolates of S. Enteritidis from 14 636 cases of infection in 10 European countries exhibited such resistance.[66] In the UK, strains of S. Enteritidis exhibiting such resistance have been linked to imported eggs, and it has been suggested that the use of fluoroquinolones in poultry production has contributed to the emergence of such strains.[67]

SHIGELLAE

Developing countries

Following extensive outbreaks of multi-resistant strains of Shigella spp., particularly Sh. dysenteriae (Shiga's bacillus), in many countries in Central America, Africa and the Indian subcontinent from 1969 (for a review, see Rowe and Threlfall[36]), with many deaths, outbreaks of Sh. dysenteriae with a continually expanding spectrum of resistance are being increasingly reported from developing countries throughout the world. The first major international outbreak was that which occurred in Central America from 1969 to 1972. The causative strain was resistant to chloramphenicol, streptomycin, sulphonamides and tetracyclines (R-type CSSuT). Resistances were plasmid encoded by a plasmid of incompatibility group B. The second major international outbreak occurred in Central Africa (Zaire, Rwanda, Burundi) from 1979 to 1982, with over 13 000 cases reported in eastern Zaire between 1981 and 1982, and with over 1700 deaths. In this outbreak the strain was of R-type ACSSuT (A, ampicillin) and, although resistances were plasmid encoded, the plasmids were of different incompatibility groups to those identified in the Central American strain, and in strains which had caused outbreaks in India in the 1970s.[68] Following the discontinuation of the use of tetracyclines and the introduction of co-trimoxazole in Zaire early in 1981, plasmid-mediated resistance to the latter antimicrobial soon emerged.[69] Nalidixic acid was subsequently introduced in Zaire in November 1981 for the treatment of Shiga dysentery, and the use of this antimicrobial resulted in a drop in the case fatality rate from 4.6% to 2.0%. Subsequent to these outbreaks in the 1980s, serious epidemics of multi-resistant Sh. dysenteriae 1 were reported in the 1990s in Zimbabwe,[70] Zambia,[71] Kenya,[72] Dakar,[73] KwaZulu-Natal[74] and Sierra Leone.[75] The causative strains were resistant to a wide range of antimicrobials, including ampicillin, chloramphenicol, tetracyclines, trimethoprim and nalidixic acid.

Since 1984 there have been increasing reports of epidemics and outbreaks in the Indian subcontinent of bacillary dysentery caused by multi-resistant Sh. dysenteriae type 1.[76] Initially, strains were resistant to ampicillin, chloramphenicol, tetracyclines and co-trimoxazole. Because of the appearance in such strains of resistance to ampicillin and co-trimoxazole – at that time the drugs of choice for first-line treatment of bacillary dysentery in India – nalidixic acid became the first-line alternative treatment in the 1980s. Strains with resistance to nalidixic acid rapidly emerged in the Indian subcontinent,[77] thus undermining the efficacy of this antimicrobial for the treatment of bacillary dysentery in that area. Resistance to ciprofloxacin in Sh. dysenteriae 1 has recently been reported in both India[78] and Bangladesh.[79] This development has undermined the efficacy of fluoroquinolones for treatment, which had been found to be highly effective when coupled with standard rehydration therapy.[80]

Strains of multi-resistant Sh. dysenteriae 1 are now becoming commonplace in other developing countries, not only in Central America, India and Africa but also in the Middle East. For example, in the 5-year period comprising 1990–1993 and 1996, Sh. dysenteriae accounted for 5% of shigella strains isolated in Kuwait.[81] All isolates were multi-resistant. Once more, because of multi-resistance the therapeutic options for oral therapy were severely restricted.[81]

An increasing problem in many developing countries in recent years has been the appearance and spread of multi-resistant strains of *Sh. flexneri*. Outbreaks with such strains have been reported in many countries in South-east Asia and the Indian subcontinent,[82] and treatment problems have been recorded in infections in many countries. Strains have often been resistant to at least five antimicrobials, including ampicillin, chloramphenicol and trimethoprim, with an increasing number of strains from the Indian subcontinent showing resistance to nalidixic acid. In strains from Tanzania, resistance to ampicillin has been related to integron-mediated OXA-1 and TEM-1 β-lactamases.[83]

Britain

Between 1983 and 1987 the incidence of resistance to ampicillin in *Sh. dysenteriae*, *Sh. flexneri* and *Sh. boydii* infections in England and Wales increased from 42% to 65% and the incidence of resistance to trimethoprim from 6% to 64%. Furthermore, of 1524 strains tested in 1995–1996, 46% were resistant to both these antimicrobials.[84] Resistance to nalidixic acid was uncommon and only a very small number of strains were resistant to ciprofloxacin. On the basis of these observations it was concluded that, if it should be necessary to commence treatment before the results of laboratory-based sensitivity tests were available, the best options would be to use nalidixic acid for children and a fluoroquinolone antibiotic such as ciprofloxacin for adults. It is important to note that *Sh. dysenteriae*, *Sh. flexneri* and *Sh. boydii* are not indigenous in England and Wales, and the majority of infections have been identified in patients either with a history of recent foreign travel, particularly to the Indian subcontinent, or who have had contact with recent travellers. Thus, resistance in these serotypes does not reflect the use of antibiotics for the treatment of shigellosis in Britain.

In 2002, 10% of shigellae of subgroups A, B and C, and 13% of isolates of subgroup D (*Sh. sonnei*) from patients in England and Wales were resistant to nalidixic acid.[85] These findings suggested that the choice of antimicrobial for the first-line treatment of shigellosis was becoming increasingly limited, and it was recommended that, for children under 10 years of age, strains should be tested for resistance to this antimicrobial before commencing treatment. This recommendation is in line with information from other countries, where in some instances nalidixic acid has been abandoned as a therapeutic option for acute shigellosis.

Recommendations for therapy

Until 1984, ampicillin was widely regarded as the drug of choice for the treatment of severe bacillary dysentery, with trimethoprim the drug of choice for patients infected with ampicillin-resistant strains. More recently, because of the increased prevalence of strains resistant to ampicillin and trimethoprim, nalidixic acid has been used increasingly in developing countries as a primary alternative. If *Sh. dysenteriae* type 1 infection is suspected or nalidixic acid-resistant strains of *Shigella* have been identified, treatment with pivmecillinam has been recommended.[86] For children, treatment with pivmecillinam or ceftriaxone has been suggested, although reservations have been expressed both about the cost of these antibiotics and about the non-availability of an oral formulation of ceftriaxone.[86] It has also been recommended that in

developing countries the newer quinolone drugs should be held in reserve for the treatment of strains resistant to nalidixic acid and pivmecillinam. For developed countries where resistance to ampicillin and co-trimoxazole is less common, it has been recommended that, if antibiotic therapy is indicated, children should continue to be treated with ampicillin or trimethoprim–sulfamethoxazole, and that adults should be treated with one of the new quinolone drugs. Because of the rapidly increasing range of resistance in shigella strains, it has been strongly recommended that, whenever possible, antibiotic sensitivities should be determined before commencing treatment, as the choice of antibiotic for initial treatment is becoming increasingly limited. This is particularly the case in the UK (see above), where it has been recommended that the best options would be to use nalidixic acid for children and a fluoroquinolone antibiotic such as ciprofloxacin for adults until the results of laboratory-based sensitivity tests are available.[85]

VIBRIO CHOLERAE

Vibrio cholerae O1

The first protracted outbreak of *V. cholerae* O1 with multiple drug resistance was that which occurred in Tanzania in 1977.[87] The strains were of R-type ACKSSuT (K, kanamycin) and the appearance of resistance was attributed to the extensive use of tetracyclines for cholera prophylaxis in Tanzania. Major outbreaks of drug-resistant strains of *V. cholerae* O1 have subsequently been reported in Bangladesh in 1979–1980 and 1981, in Zaire in 1982–1983, in Tanzania in 1983 and in Kenya in the late 1990s.[88] A variety of R-types has been identified and, in addition to the resistances listed above, strains with resistance to gentamicin and trimethoprim have been identified in Bangladesh and Zaire. In 1993, strains of *V. cholerae* O1 with resistance to ampicillin, chloramphenicol, kanamycin, sulphonamides, tetracyclines and trimethoprim were identified in epidemic cholera in Ecuador, South America,[89] and it has been subsequently reported that up to 36% of strains from this epidemic were multi-resistant.[90] In 1995, multi-resistant strains of *V. cholerae* O1 were reported to have caused outbreaks in the Horn of Africa (Ethiopia and Somalia) in epidemics in the 1980s,[91] and multi-resistant strains have subsequently been reported in Uganda,[92] Albania and Italy,[93] India[94] and Guinea-Bissau.[95]

When studied, in all multi-resistant strains of *V. cholerae* O1 from outbreaks in Africa, the Indian subcontinent and South America the complete spectrum of resistance has been encoded by plasmids of the inc C group.[89] It would therefore appear that plasmids of the inc C group have an affinity for *V. cholerae* similar to that shown by inc HI1 plasmids for *S.* Typhi (see above). In these inc C plasmids, resistance to trimethoprim and aminoglycosides is contained within class I integrons.[92,94] Such integrons are similar to those identified in multi-resistant *S.* Typhimurium and *Sh. flexneri* (see above). Thus it is possible that resistance genes contained on these inc C *V. cholerae* plasmids may have originated in other Gram-negative bacteria.

Although the therapy of choice for cholera is oral rehydration, when antimicrobial therapy is indicated, doxycycline, a long-acting form of tetracycline, is recommended for adults and co-trimoxazole for children, with furazolidone, erythromycin and chloramphenicol considered to be effective alternatives.[96] The appearance in countries with low standards of hygiene of strains with resistance to three of the drugs of choice for the treatment of cholera is of some concern, and reappraisal of the use of antimicrobials in some outbreak situations may now be necessary. Indeed, because of the development of resistance to tetracyclines in epidemic strains, in some developing countries fluoroquinolone drugs have been used in combination with oral rehydration therapy. Regrettably, the emergence of intermediate resistance to norfloxacin in an outbreak in Malda, West Bengal, in 1997,[97] and the appearance of clinical resistance to norfloxacin and ciprofloxacin in V. cholerae O1 in an epidemic in and around Hubli, South India in 2002[98] suggests that the efficacy of such antimicrobials for V. cholerae has already been jeopardized.

Vibrio cholerae O139

Since early 1993 there have been reports of outbreaks of cholera caused by V. cholerae O139 in the Indian subcontinent.[99] A limited study of strains isolated in the UK from travellers known to have returned recently from the Indian subcontinent demonstrated that these strains were resistant to streptomycin, sulphonamides and trimethoprim.[100] As with infections caused by V. cholerae O1, the therapy of choice for infections caused by non-O1 V. cholerae is oral rehydration, and the occurrence of resistance to streptomycin, sulphonamides and trimethoprim should have little effect on treatment regimens. Regrettably, in the epidemic in Hubli, South India in 2002 (see above), 47% of isolates of V. cholerae O139 were resistant to ciprofloxacin,[98] indicating that the efficacy of this antimicrobial is jeopardized.

ESCHERICHIA COLI

The occurrence of antibiotic resistance in pathogenic E. coli responsible for gastrointestinal illness has been documented elsewhere[36,101] and will not be discussed at length in this chapter. Plasmids have been identified that code for antibiotic resistance and the production of both heat-stable (ST) and heat-labile (LT) toxin, and in a study of drug resistance among toxin-producing strains isolated in the Far East in 1978, 72% of strains were reported to be drug resistant and 44% multi-resistant.[102]

For Vero cytotoxin-producing E. coli O157 (VTEC O157) 23% of 1087 isolates from people in England and Wales were drug resistant but only 2% were multi-resistant; the most common resistance patterns were streptomycin, sulphonamides and tetracyclines, and sulphonamides and tetracyclines.[103,104] Until 1999, resistance to fluoroquinolone antibiotics had not been identified in VTEC O157 from humans in infections associated with foods or food animals in the UK. It should be realized that, in general, antimicrobials are not recommended for the treatment of VTEC O157 infections in humans. Indeed, the use of quinolone antibiotics may stimulate the production of toxin-encoding bacteriophages from strains of Shiga toxin-producing E. coli and thereby potentially exacerbate the disease syndrome in humans.[105]

A newly emerging problem in the UK is a substantive increase in E. coli with plasmids encoding CTX-M-15 β-lactamases in cases of urinary tract infection.[106] These strains have caused serious disease, with significant mortality. Although there is as yet no indication that such strains may be linked to organisms originating in the gut, the occurrence of strains of CTX-M-producing E. coli from cattle in the UK[107] suggests that such strains may be widely disseminated in the environment, and possibly in foods.

The use of antibiotics for the treatment of E. coli gut infections is also a contentious issue. There is little doubt that a number of antibiotics reduce the incidence and duration of diarrhoea in travellers,[108] and both ciprofloxacin[109] and norfloxacin[110] have been reported to be particularly effective. However, concern has been expressed that the widespread use of these antimicrobials for prophylaxis may in the long term reduce their efficacy.[111]

CAMPYLOBACTER SPP.

Campylobacter jejuni is recognized as the most common cause of bacterial gastroenteritis in many developed countries.[112,113] Because Campylobacter enteritis is usually a self-limiting disease, antibiotics are not usually administered except to septicaemic patients and those with other underlying complications. When antibiotics have been indicated, until the mid-1990s erythromycin has been the drug of choice.[114,115] Gentamicin, tetracyclines, chloramphenicol and furazolidone have also been used with some success, and gentamicin and chloramphenicol have been recommended for the treatment of patients with erythromycin-resistant strains.[116]

The use of fluoroquinolone drugs for the treatment of a variety of acute diarrhoeal diseases, including Campylobacter enteritis, has recently been advocated.[117] Therefore, of potential importance for therapy was a reported increase of up to 11% in the incidence of fluoroquinolone resistance in campylobacters isolated from humans in The Netherlands in 1990 following the extensive use of enrofloxacin in the poultry industry in that country.[118] Similarly, in England and Wales in 1997, 11% of 5400 isolates were resistant to ciprofloxacin at greater than 8 mg/L.[119] More recently, quinolone-resistant strains of C. jejuni isolated from patients in the USA were shown by molecular methods to be indistinguishable from similar strains isolated from poultry.[120] These findings have given rise to concern that the injudicious use of fluoroquinolone-containing products in the poultry industry in Europe, and more recently in the USA, has resulted in the emergence of strains of Campylobacter spp. with resistance to ciprofloxacin. It is important not to overlook the role of foreign travel, as in the USA study quoted above a substantial number of quinolone-resistant isolates were associated with patients with a recent history of foreign travel, particularly to Mexico.[120]

CONCLUSION

Multiple drug resistance and resistance to key antimicrobials are now common in pathogenic gut bacteria in both developing and developed countries throughout the world. The rapid emergence of resistance to the drugs of choice for diseases such as typhoid fever, bacillary dysentery and cholera is of particular concern. Although for the most part such resistance is plasmid mediated, a recent development is the emergence of strains with chromosomal resistance, not only to antibiotics such as chloramphenicol, ampicillin and trimethoprim, but also to nalidixic acid and some of the fluoroquinolone drugs such as ciprofloxacin, which are now the first-line choice for the treatment of invasive disease. Additionally, resistance to the newer cephalosporins is now becoming commonplace, with resistance to ESBLs in organisms such as *Salmonella* and *E. coli* being reported in both developed and developing countries, in strains from food production animals, foods and cases of human infection. To preserve the efficacy of such drugs for the treatment of life-threatening infections, it is essential that their usage be strictly regulated. Thus, whenever possible, drugs such as the fluoroquinolones and third-generation cephalosporins should be reserved for the treatment of severe infections that do not respond to more conventional antimicrobials. In developed countries, where resistance is often associated with the use of antimicrobials in food-producing animals, such usage should be strictly regulated and the unnecessary prophylactic use of antimicrobials avoided wherever possible.

REFERENCES

1. Crump JA, Luby SP, Mintz ED. The global burden of typhoid fever. *Bull World Health Organ* 2004; 82:346–353.
2. Anonymous. Typhoid and paratyphoid fevers. *OPCS Monitor* 1985; MB2 85/2:9–11C.
3. Ackers ML, Puhr ND, Tauxe RV, et al. Laboratory-based surveillance of *Salmonella* serotype Typhi infections in the United States: antimicrobial resistance on the increase. *JAMA* 2000; 283:2668–2673.
4. Rowe B, Ward LR, Threlfall EJ. Multiresistant *Salmonella typhi* – a world-wide epidemic. *Clin Infect Dis* 1997; 24(suppl 1):S106–S109.
5. Prakash K, Pillai PK. Multidrug-resistant *Salmonella typhi* in India. *APUA Newslett* 1992; 1:1–3.
6. Jesudasan MV, John TJ. Multiresistant *Salmonella typhi* in India. *Lancet* 1990; 36:256.
7. Karamat KA. Multiple drug resistant *Salmonella typhi* and ciprofloxacin. In: *Proceedings of the Second Western Pacific Conference on Infectious Diseases and Chemotherapy*. Thailand: Infectious Disease Association of Thailand, Western Pacific Society of Chemotherapy; 1990:480.
8. Akinyemi KO, Coker AO, Olukoya DK, et al. Prevalence of multi-drug resistant *Salmonella typhi* among clinically diagnosed typhoid fever patients in Lagos, Nigeria. *Z Naturforsch* 2000; 55:489–493.
9. Kariuki S, Gilks C, Revathi G, et al. Genotypic analysis of multidrug-resistant *Salmonella enterica* serovar Typhi, Kenya. *Emerg Infect Dis* 2000; 6:649–651.
10. Rahman MM, Haq JA, Morshed MA, et al. *Salmonella enterica* serovar Typhi with decreased susceptibility to ciprofloxacin – an emerging problem in Bangladesh. *Int J Antimicrob Agents* 2005; 25:345–346.
11. Mehta G, Randhawa VS, Mohapatra NP. Intermediate susceptibility to ciprofloxacin in *Salmonella typhi* strains in India. *Eur J Clin Microbiol Infect Dis* 2001; 20:760–761.
12. Rahman M, Siddique AK, Shorma S, et al. Emergence of multidrug-resistant *Salmonella enterica* serotype Typhi with decreased ciprofloxacin susceptibility in Bangladesh. *Epidemiol Infect* 2006; 134:433–438.
13. Threlfall EJ, Fisher IST, Berghold C, et al. Trends in antimicrobial drug resistance in *Salmonella enterica* serotypes Typhi and Paratyphi A isolated in Europe, 1999–2001. *Int J Antimicrob Agents* 2003; 22:487–491.
14. Rowe B, Ward LR, Threlfall EJ. Treatment of multiresistant typhoid fever. *Lancet* 1991; 337:1422.
15. Mandal BK. Modern treatment of typhoid fever. *J Infect* 1991; 22:1–4.
16. Rowe B, Ward LR, Threlfall EJ. Ciprofloxacin and typhoid fever. *Lancet* 1992; 339:740.
17. Umasankar S, Wall RA, Berger J. A case of ciprofloxacin-resistant typhoid fever. *CDR Rev* 1992; 2:R139–R140.
18. Threlfall EJ, Ward LR, Skinner JA, et al. Ciprofloxacin-resistant *Salmonella typhi* and treatment failure. *Lancet* 1999; 353:1590–1591.
19. Parry C, Wain J, Chinh NT, et al. Quinolone-resistant *Salmonella typhi* in Vietnam. *Lancet* 1998; 351:1289.
20. Murdoch DA, Banatvala NA, Bone A, et al. Epidemic ciprofloxacin-resistant *Salmonella typhi* in Tajikistan. *Lancet* 1998; 351:339.
21. Lewis MD, Serichantalergs O, Pitaeangsi C, et al. Typhoid fever: a massive single-point source, multidrug-resistant outbreak in Nepal. *Clin Infect Dis* 2005; 40:554–561.
22. Kadhiravan T, Wig N, Kapil A, et al. Clinical outcomes in typhoid fever: adverse impact of infection with nalidixic acid-resistant *Salmonella typhi*. *BMC Infect Dis* 2005; 5:37.
23. Renuka K, Sood S, Das BK, et al. High-level ciprofloxacin resistance in *Salmonella enterica* serotype Typhi in India. *J Med Microbiol* 2005; 54:999–1000.
24. Ahmed D, D'Costa LT, Alam K, et al. Multidrug-resistant *Salmonella enterica* serovar typhi isolates with high-level resistance to ciprofloxacin in Dhaka, Bangladesh. *Antimicrob Agents Chemother* 2006; 50:3516–3517.
25. Threlfall EJ, Rowe B, Ward LR. Occurrence and treatment of multi-resistant *Salmonella typhi* in the UK. *PHLS Microbiol Digest* 1992; 8:56–59.
26. Threlfall EJ, Day M, de Pinna E, et al. Drug-resistant enteric fever in the UK. *Lancet* 2006; 367:1576.
27. Threlfall EJ, Ward LR. Decreased susceptibility to ciprofloxacin in *Salmonella enterica* serotype Typhi, United Kingdom. *Emerg Infect Dis* 2001; 7:448–450.
28. Wallace MR, Yousif AA, Habib NF, et al. Azithromycin and typhoid fever. *Lancet* 1994; 343:1497–1498.
29. Kidgell C. Genetic variation in *Salmonella enterica* subspecies *enterica* serotype Typhi. PhD thesis. University of London, 2005.
30. Wain J, Diem Nga LT, Kidgell C, et al. Molecular analysis of incHI1 antimicrobial resistance plasmids from *Salmonella* serovar Typhi strains associated with typhoid fever. *Antimicrob Agents Chemother* 2003; 47:2732–2739.
31. Walker RA, Skinner JA, Ward LR, et al. LightCycler gyrA mutation assay (GAMA) identifies heterogeneity in GyrA in *Salmonella enterica* serotypes Typhi and Paratyphi A with decreased susceptibility to ciprofloxacin. *Int J Antimicrob Agents* 2003; 22:622–625.
32. Chandel DS, Chaudhry R, Dhawan B, et al. Drug resistant *Salmonella enterica* serotype Paratyphi A in India. *Emerg Infect Dis* 2000; 6:420–421.
33. Mandal S, Mandal MD, Pal NK. Antibiotic resistance of *Salmonella enterica* serovar Paratyphi A in India: emerging and reemerging problem. *J Postgrad Med* 2006; 52:163–166.
34. Aarestrup FM, Wiuff C, Mølbak K, et al. Is it time to change the break points for fluoroquinolones for *Salmonella* spp.? *Antimicrob Agents Chemother* 2003; 47:827–829.
35. Pang T, Bhutta ZA, Finlay BB, et al. Typhoid fever and other salmonellosis: a continuing challenge. *Trends Microbiol* 2005; 3:253–255.
36. Rowe B, Threlfall EJ. Drug resistance in Gram-negative aerobic bacilli. *Br Med Bull* 1984; 40:68–76.
37. Lewin CS, Nandivada LS, Amyes SGB. Multiresistant salmonella and fluoroquinolones. *J Antimicrob Chemother* 1991; 27:147–149.
38. Gupta V, Ray P, Sharma M. Ciprofloxacin-resistant *Salmonella senftenberg* in north India. *Indian J Gastroenterol* 1999; 18:42.
39. Rowe B, Frost JA, Threlfall EJ. Spread of a multiresistant clone of *Salmonella typhimurium* phage type 66/122 in South-East Asia and the Middle East. *Lancet* 1980; i:1070–1071.
40. Anderson ES, Threlfall EJ, Carr JM, et al. Clonal distribution of resistance plasmid-carrying *Salmonella typhimurium*, mainly in the Middle East. *J Hyg (Camb)* 1977; 79:429–448.
41. Le Minor S. Apparition en France d'une épidémie à *Salmonella wien*. *Med Mal Infect* 1972; 2:441–448.
42. McConnell MM, Smith HR, Leonardopoulos J, et al. The value of plasmid studies in the epidemiology of infections due to drug-resistant *Salmonella wien*. *J Infect Dis* 1979; 139:178–190.

43. Colonna B, Nicoletti M, Visca P, et al. Composite IS1 elements encoding hydroxamate-mediated iron uptake in FIme plasmids from epidemic *Salmonella* spp. *J Bacteriol* 1985; 162:307–316.

44. Carattoli A. Plasmid-mediated antimicrobial resistance in *Salmonella enterica*. *Curr Issues Mol Biol* 2003; 5:113–122.

45. Chiu C, Su LH, Chu C, et al. Isolation of *Salmonella enterica* serotype Choleraesuis resistant to ceftriaxone and ciprofloxacin. *Lancet* 2004; 363:1285–1286.

46. Ben Hassen A, Fournier G, Kechrid A, et al. Enzymatic resistance to cefotaxime in 56 strains of *Klebsiella* spp., *Escherichia coli* and *Salmonella* spp. at a Tunisian hospital (1984–1988). *Path Biol (Paris)* 1990; 38: 464–469.

47. Bradford PA. Extended-spectrum beta-lactamases in the 21st century: characterisation, epidemiology, and detection of this important resistance threat. *Clin Microbiol Rev* 2001; 14:933–951.

48. Rossi MS, Tokumoto M, Couto E, et al. Survey of the levels of antimicrobial resistance in Argentina: WHONET program – 1991 to 1994. *Int J Antimicrob Agents* 1995; 6:103–110.

49. Batchelor M, Hopkins KA, Threlfall EJ, et al. *bla* CTX-M genes in clinical isolates of *Salmonella* recovered from humans in England and Wales from 1992 to 2003. *Antimicrob Agents Chemother* 2005; 49:1319–1322.

50. Batchelor M, Threlfall EJ, Liebana E. Cephalosporin resistance among animal-associated Enterobacteria: a current perspective. *Expert Rev Anti-infective Ther* 2005; 3:403–417.

51. Simarro E, Navarro F, Ruiz J, et al. *Salmonella enterica* serovar virchow with CTX-M-like beta-lactamases in Spain. *J Clin Microbiol* 2000; 38: 4676–4678.

52. Su LH, Chiu CH, Chu C, et al. In vivo acquisition of ceftriaxone resistance *Salmonella enterica* serotype anatum. *Antimicrob Agents Chemother* 2003; 47:563–567.

53. Kehrenberg C, Friederichs S, de Jong A, et al. Identification of plasmid-borne quinolone resistance gene qnrS in *Salmonella enterica* serovar Infantis. *J Antimicrob Chemother* 2006; 58:18–22.

54. Hopkins KL, Wootton L, Day MR, et al. Plasmid-mediated quinolone resistance determinant qnrS1 found in *Salmonella enterica* strains isolated in the UK. *J Antimicrob Chemother* 2007; 59:1071–1075.

55. Threlfall EJ, Hall MLM, Rowe B. Salmonella bacteraemia in England and Wales, 1981–1990. *J Clin Pathol* 1992; 45:34–36.

56. Threlfall EJ, Ward LR, Rowe B. Multiresistant *Salmonella typhimurium* DT 104 and salmonella bacteraemia. *Lancet* 1998; 352:287–288.

57. Threlfall EJ. Multiresistant *Salmonella typhimurium* DT 104: a truly international multiresistant clone. *J Antimicrob Chemother* 2000; 46:7–10.

58. Zhao S, Qaiyumi S, Friedman S, et al. Characterization of *Salmonella enterica* serotype newport isolated from humans and food animals. *J Clin Microbiol* 2003; 41:5366–5371.

59. Helms M, Vastrup P, Gerner-Schmidt P, et al. Excess mortality associated with antimicrobial drug-resistant *Salmonella typhimurium*. *Emerg Infect Dis* 2002; 8:490–495.

60. Briggs CE, Fratamico PM. Molecular characterization of an antibiotic resistant gene cluster of *Salmonella typhimurium* DT104. *Antimicrob Agents Chemother* 1999; 43:846–849.

61. Evans SJ, Davies RH, Binns SH, et al. Multiple antimicrobial resistant *Salmonella enterica* serovar Paratyphi B variant Java in cattle: a case report. *Vet Rec* 2005; 166:343–346.

62. Musto J, Kirk M, Lightfoot D, et al. Multi-drug resistant *Salmonella* Java infections acquired from tropical fish aquariums. *Commun Dis Intell* 2006; 30:222–227.

63. Guerra B, Laconcha I, Soto SM, et al. Molecular characterisation of emergent multiresistant *Salmonella enterica* serotype [4,5,12:i:-] organisms causing human salmonellosis. *FEMS Microb Lett* 2000; 190:341–347.

64. Walker RA, Lindsay E, Woodward MJ, et al. Variation in clonality and antibiotic resistance genes among multiresistant *Salmonella enterica* serotype Typhimurium phage type U302 (MR U302) from humans, animals and foods. *Microb Drug Resist* 2001; 7:13–21.

65. Tassios PT, Chadjihristodoulou C, Lambiri M, et al. Molecular typing of multidrug-resistant Salmonella Blockley outbreak isolates from Greece. *Emerg Infect Dis* 2000; 6:60–64.

66. Threlfall EJ, Fisher IST, Bergold C, et al. Antimicrobial drug resistance in isolates of *Salmonella enterica* from cases of salmonellosis in humans in Europe in 2000: results of international multi-centre surveillance. *Euro Surv* 2003; 8:41–45.

67. Threlfall EJ, Day M, De Pinna E, et al. Assessment of factors contributing to changes in the incidence of antimicrobial drug resistance in *Salmonella enterica* serotypes Enteritidis and Typhimurium from humans in England and Wales in 2000, 2002 and 2004. *Int J Antimicrob Agents* 2006; 28:389–395.

68. Frost JA, Rowe B, Vandepitte J, et al. Plasmid characterisation in the investigation of an epidemic caused by multiply-resistant *Shigella dysenteriae* type 1 in Central Africa. *Lancet* 1981; ii:1074–1076.

69. Frost JA, Rowe B, Vandepitte J. Acquisition of trimethoprim resistance in epidemic strains of *Shigella dysenteriae* type 1 from Zaire. *Lancet* 1982; i:963.

70. Mason PR, Nathoo KJ, Wellington M, et al. Antimicrobial susceptibilities of *Shigella dysenteriae* type 1 in Zimbwabe – implications for the management of dysentery. *Cent Afr J Med* 1995; 41:132–137.

71. Tuttle J, Ries AA, Chimba RM, et al. Antimicrobial resistant epidemic *Shigella dysenteriae* type 1 in Zambia; modes of transmission. *J Infect Dis* 1995; 171:371–375.

72. Iverson ER, Colding H, Petersen L, et al. Epidemic *Shigella dysenteriae* in Mumias, western Kenya. *Trans R Soc Trop Med Hyg* 1998; 92:30–31.

73. Sow AI, Camara B, Sow O, et al. Place and resistance of epidemic strains of *Shigella dysenteriae*-1 isolated at the Fann Hospital from 1995 to 1999. *Dakar Med* 2002; 47:234–238.

74. Chopra M, Wilkinson D, Stirling S. Epidemic shigella dysentery in children in northern KwaZulu-Natal. *S Afr Med J* 1997; 87:48–51.

75. Guerin PJ, Brasher C, Baron E, et al. Case management of a multidrug-resistant *Shigella dysenteriae* serotype 1 outbreak in a cris context in Sierra Leone, 1999–2000. *Trans R Soc Trop Med Hyg* 2004; 98:635–643.

76. Pal SC. Epidemic bacillary dysentery in West Bengal, India. *Lancet* 1984; i:1462.

77. Sen D, Dutta P, Deb BC, et al. Nalidixic acid-resistant *Shigella dysenteriae* type 1 in Eastern India. *Lancet* 1988; ii:911.

78. Chunder N, Bhattacharya SK, Biswas D, et al. Isolation of fluoroquinolone resistant *Shigella dysenteriae* strain from Calcutta. *Indian J Med Res* 1997; 106:494–496.

79. Naheed A, Kalluri P, Talukder KA, et al. Fluoroquinolone-resistant *Shigella dysenteriae* type 1 in northeastern Bangladesh. *Lancet Infect Dis* 2004; 4: 607–608.

80. Bhattacharya SK, Battacharya MK, Dutta D, et al. Single dose ciprofloxacin for shigellosis in adults. *J Infect* 1992; 25:117–119.

81. Jamal WY, Rotimi VO, Chugh TD, et al. Prevalence and susceptibility of *Shigella* species to 11 antibiotics in a Kuwait teaching hospital. *J Chemother* 1998; 10:285–290.

82. Sohail M, Sultana K. Antibiotic susceptibilities and plasmid profiles of *Shigella flexneri* isolates from children with diarrhoea in Islamabad, Pakistan. *J Antimicrob Chemother* 1998; 42:838–839.

83. Navia MM, Capitano L, Ruiz J, et al. Typing and characterisation of mechanisms of resistance of *Shigella* spp. isolated from feces of children under 5 years of age from Ifakara, Tanzania. *J Clin Microbiol* 1999; 37:3113–3117.

84. Cheasty T, Skinner JA, Rowe B, et al. Increasing incidence of antibiotic resistance in shigellas from humans in England and Wales: recommendations for therapy. *Microb Drug Resist* 1998; 4:57–66.

85. Cheasty T, Day M, Threlfall EJ. Increasing incidence of resistance to nalidixic acid in shigellas from humans in England and Wales: implications for therapy. *J Clin Microbiol* 2004; 10:1033–1035.

86. Bennish ML, Salam MA. Rethinking options for the treatment of shigellosis. *J Antimicrob Chemother* 1992; 30:243–247.

87. Mhalu MS, Mmari PW, Ijumba J. Rapid emergence of El Tor *Vibrio cholerae* resistant to antimicrobial agents during first month of fourth cholera epidemic in Tanzania. *Lancet* 1979; i:345–347.

88. Scrascia M, Maimone F, Mohamud KA, et al. Clonal relationships among *Vibrio cholerae* O1 El Tor strains causing the largest cholera epidemic in Kenya in the late 1990s. *J Clin Microbiol* 2006; 44:3401–3404.

89. Threlfall EJ, Said B, Rowe B, et al. Emergence of multiple drug resistance in *Vibrio cholerae* El Tor from Ecuador. *Lancet* 1993; 342:1173.

90. Weber JT, Mintz ED, Canizares R, et al. Epidemic cholera in Ecuador: multidrug-resistance and transmission by water and seafood. *Epidemiol Infect* 1994; 112:1–11.

91. Coppo A, Colombo M, Pazzani C, et al. *Vibrio cholerae* in the horn of Africa: epidemiology, plasmids, tetracycline resistance gene amplification, and comparison between O1 and non-O1 strains. *Am J Trop Med Hyg* 1995; 53:351–359.

92. Kruse H, Sörum H, Tenover FC, et al. A transferable multiple drug resistance plasmid from *Vibrio cholerae* O1. *Microb Drug Resist* 1995; 1:203–210.

93. Falbo V, Carattoli A, Tosini F, et al. Antibiotic resistance conferred by a conjugative plasmid and class I integron in *Vibrio cholerae* O1 El Tor strains isolated in Albania and Italy. *Antimicrob Agents Chemother* 1999; 43:693–696.

94. Garg P, Chakraborty S, Basu I, et al. Expanding multiple antibiotic resistance among clinical strains of *Vibrio cholerae* isolated from 1992–1997 in Calcutta, India. *Epidemiol Infect* 2000; 124:393–399.

95. Dalsgaard A, Forslund A, Peterson A, et al. Class 1 integron-borne multiple-antibiotic resistance encoded by a 150-kilobase conjugative plasmid in epidemic *Vibrio cholerae* strains isolated in Guinea-Bissau. *J Clin Microbiol* 2000; 38:3774–3779.

96. WHO. *Guidelines for Cholera Control.* Geneva: World Health Organization; 1993.

97. Bhattacharya MK, Ghosh S, Mukhopadhyay AK, et al. Outbreak of cholera caused by *Vibrio cholerae* O1 intermediately resistant to norfloxacin in Malda, West Bengal. *J Indian Med Assoc* 2000; 98:389–390.

98. Krishna BV, Patil AB, Chandrasekhar MR. Fluoroquinolone-resistant *Vibrio cholerae* isolated during a cholera outbreak in India. *Trans R Soc Trop Med Hyg* 2006; 100:224–226.

99. Basu A, Garg P, Datta S, et al. *Vibrio cholerae* O139 in Calcutta, 1992–1998: incidence, antibiograms, and genotypes. *Emerg Infect Dis* 2000; 6:139–147.

100. Cheasty T, Rowe B, Said B, et al. *Vibrio cholerae* serogroup O139 in England and Wales. *Lancet* 1993; 307:1007.

101. Weber MA, Piddock LJV. Antibiotic resistance in *Escherichia coli*. In: White DG, Alkeshun MN, McDermott PF, eds. *Frontiers in Antimicrobial Resistance; a Tribute to Stuart B. Levy.* Washington DC: ASM Press; 2005:374–386.

102. Echeverria P, Verhaert L, Ulangco CV, et al. Antimicrobial resistance and enterotoxin production among isolates of *Escherichia coli* in the Far East. *Lancet* 1978; ii:589–592.

103. Willshaw GA, Cheasty T, Frost JA, et al. Antimicrobial resistance of O157 VTEC in England and Wales. *Notiziario dell' Istituto Superiore di Sanita* 1996; 9(suppl 3):3–4.

104. Threlfall EJ, Ward LR, Frost JA, et al. The emergence and spread of antibiotic resistance in food-borne bacteria. *Int J Food Microbiol* 2000; 62:1–5.

105. Zhang X, McDaniel AD, Wolf LE, et al. Quinolone antibiotics induce Shiga toxin-encoding bacteriophages, toxin production, and death in mice. *J Infect Dis* 2000; 181:664–670.

106. Karisik E, Ellington MJ, Pike R, et al. Molecular characterisation of plasmids encoding CTX-M-15 beta-lactamases from *Escherichia coli* strains in the United Kingdom. *J Antimicrob Chemother* 2006; 58: 665–668.

107. Liebana E, Batchelor M, Hopkins KL, et al. Longitudinal farm study of extended-spectrum beta-lactamase resistance. *J Clin Microbiol* 2006; 44: 1630–1634.

108. Gross RJ. *Escherichia coli* diarrhoea. In: Smith G, ed. *Topley and Wilson's Principles of Bacteriology, Virology and Immunity.* Vol. 3. 8th edn. London: Edward Arnold; 1990: 470–487.

109. Ericsson CD, Johnson PC, DuPont HL, et al. Ciprofloxacin or trimethoprim-sulfamethoxazole as initial therapy for travellers' diarrhoea. A placebo-controlled, randomized trial. *Ann Intern Med* 1987; 106:216–220.

110. Wistrom J, Jertborn M, Hedstrom SA, et al. Short-term self-treatment of travellers' diarrhoea with norfloxacin: a placebo-controlled study. *J Antimicrob Chemother* 1989; 23:905–913.

111. Wood MJ. The use of antibiotics in infections due to *Escherichia coli* O157: H7. *PHLS Microbiol Digest* 1991; 8:18–21.

112. Frost JA. Current epidemiological issues in human campylobacteriosis. *Symp Ser Soc Appl Microbiol* 2001; 30:85S–95S.

113. Tauxe RT. Epidemiology of *Campylobacter jejuni* infections in the United States and other industrialized nations. In: Nachamikin I, Blaser MJ, Tomkins LS, eds. *Campylobacter jejuni: Current Status and Future Trends.* Washington, DC: American Society for Microbiology; 1992:9–19.

114. McNulty CAM. The treatment of campylobacter infections in man. *J Antimicrob Chemother* 1987; 19:281–284.

115. Bibhat K, Mandal P, De Mol P, et al. Clinical aspects of Campylobacter infection in humans. In: Butzler J-P, ed. *Campylobacter Infection in Man and Animals.* Boca Raton: CRC Press; 1984:22–30.

116. Rowe B, Gross RJ. Salmonellosis, *Campylobacter* enteritis and *Shigella* dysentery. In: Goodwin CS, ed. *Microbes and Infections of the Gut.* Oxford: Blackwell; 1984:47–77.

117. Dupont HL, Corrado M, Sabbaj J. Use of norfloxacin in the treatment of acute diarrheal disease. *Am J Med* 1987; 82(suppl 6B):79–83.

118. Endtz HP, Ruijs GJ, van Klingeren B, et al. Quinolone resistance in campylobacter isolated from man and poultry following the introduction of fluoroquinolones in veterinary medicine. *J Antimicrob Chemother* 1991; 27:199–208.

119. Thwaites RT, Frost JA. Drug resistance in *Campylobacter jejuni*, *C. coli* and *C. lari* isolated from humans in north west England and Wales, 1997. *J Clin Pathol* 1999; 52:812–814.

120. Smith KE, Besser JM, Hedberg CW, et al. Quinolone-resistant *Campylobacter jejuni* infections in Minnesota, 1992–1998. *N Engl J Med* 1999; 20: 1525–1532.

Chapter 54   Neil French

Pneumococcal Diseases

INTRODUCTION

Streptococcus pneumoniae, the pneumococcus, is a ubiquitous human respiratory bacterial pathogen, well known for its association with pneumonia and meningitis. It causes disease in all age groups, particularly at the extremes of infancy and old age and is a major cause of morbidity and mortality in the tropics. The pneumococcus is the leading cause of acute lower respiratory infections, which are an important cause of death and the principal cause of global morbidity assessed in disability adjusted life years.[1] In addition, the epidemiology of pneumococcal infection in many regions of the tropics has been profoundly altered by the interaction of the pneumococcus with the human immunodeficiency virus, leading to a much increased disease burden. Antibiotic resistance amongst pneumococci continues to evolve and this threatens to undermine the basic principles of affordable management.

Set against these concerns has been a renewed interest in prevention of pneumococcal disease, driven by developments in conjugate vaccine technology. The first trial of a pneumococcal polysaccharide-based vaccine was undertaken in South African gold miners during the early twentieth century, and it was perhaps fitting that the first successful efficacy trial of conjugate pneumococcal vaccine in the tropics was reported from South Africa in 2003.[2] However, widespread vaccine-based control of pneumococcal disease does not appear to be an immediate prospect and the pneumococcus will continue to be a leading public health and clinical problem.

EPIDEMIOLOGY

No significant animal reservoir of infection exists and pneumococcal transmission is a consequence of human contact and an inescapable fact of human life. The overwhelming majority of human–bacteria encounters will result in asymptomatic nasopharyngeal carriage, which will persist for days or months. In only a few of these human–bacteria interactions will clinical disease develop – by local mucosal spread to the sinuses, middle ear or bronchial tree. Rarely, the bacteria will invade tissue to produce bacteraemia, meningitis and other metastatic infections.

Young children and elderly adults are typically at greatest risk of serious pneumococcal infection. However, in regions of high HIV prevalence invasive disease has become a feature of young adults. Males have higher rates of disease than females at all ages and this is a consistent phenomenon in geographically and historically diverse reports. Pneumococcal infections also show seasonality. In the temperate regions of the globe, infection rates increase during the winter months and decline in the summer. In the tropics, rates of disease rise and fall at different times of the year and while these fluctuations show a relationship to rainfall and humidity, these relationships are not consistent in different regions. As such, the observed climate relationships may be more to do with spread of respiratory viruses (co-factors for colonization and disease) as a consequence of human mobility than with climate parameters *per se*.

Pneumococci can be subtyped by determining the seroreactivity of their bacterial polysaccharide capsule against a set of standard antisera – so called serotypes. Ninety one serotypes have been identified and serotyping has been used as a tool for epidemiological surveillance. The predominant serotypes causing disease vary by age and by region,[3] with some notable for causing serious disease in children (serotype 1) and in adults (serotype 3), while other serotypes are associated with multiple antibiotic resistance (6B, 14, 19F and 23F). More sophisticated molecular epidemiology tools have been developed and provide greater discriminatory power than serotyping[4] and have been used to map the global spread of antibiotic resistant bacterial clones.

Epidemiology of carriage

Nasopharyngeal carriage is critical to the maintenance and spread of pneumococci. Evidence from several sites in the tropics would suggest that early colonization is more intense than that found in developed countries. Point prevalence studies in infants and children throughout the tropics have recorded high rates of carriage, typically 60–80% and very often with multiple serotypes.[5-8] These rates fall in older children and adults when 20% carriage rates are more typical. Nevertheless, these rates are still higher than those found in age-matched populations in the developed world. Defects in the mucosal immune response may contribute to these higher rates of carriage, but a more likely explanation is that there is continued high exposure to pneumococci at all stages of life. Carried serotypes tend to be those associated with lower virulence, but are often the serotypes implicated in mucosal disease in children.[9] Carriage may be increased in adults with underlying

HIV-disease – carriage point prevalence was 50% greater (29% vs 19%) in HIV-infected age-matched adults in two separate studies in Nairobi (Gilks C, unpublished data) and Entebbe.[10] There are no data from the tropics describing carriage rates in the elderly.

Childhood epidemiology

Serious manifestations of pneumococcal disease are highly prevalent in paediatric populations across the tropics. *S. pneumoniae* is a leading blood culture isolate from most reported bacteraemia studies in infants and children globally,[11-14] although notably infrequent in reports from South-east Asia.[15,16] Community-based incidence data from Africa consistently report high rates of disease. Studies from Soweto in South Africa,[17] The Gambia[11] and coastal Kenya[18] measured rates of invasive disease in under-fives of 130, 240 and 111 per 100 000 child-years, respectively, rates several-fold higher than those in the developed world (c.f. 20 per 100 000 child-years in the UK in under-fives).[19] Peak rates are found in those under one year old and in The Gambia exceeded 500 per 100 000 child-years. Moreover, the rates of pneumococcal pneumonia are almost certainly significantly higher and may contribute between 40% and 60% of all childhood pneumonia.[20-22] Meningitis is the most lethal of the clinical syndromes associated with pneumococcal infection. Outside of the meningococcal epidemics of the central African meningitis belt, the pneumococcus is the leading cause of meningitis in children. Between 5% and 25% of all invasive disease will be accounted for by meningitis.[5,23]

The explanation for these high rates of disease is undoubtedly multifactorial. Lowbirth weight, poor nutrition, micronutrient and vitamin deficiencies and increased pneumococcal exposure have all been suggested. In a formal case-control study in The Gambia overcrowding, parental education and occupation showed no clear association with risk but passive smoking, cooking indoors and preceding illness were significant risk factors.[24]

Acute otitis media is the most frequent manifestation of pneumococcal disease in children in the developed world but little is known about its epidemiology in the developing world. Hearing impairment and chronic suppurative ear problems are a frequent finding in children in the tropics[25,26] and the long-term consequences of this in terms of failure of language skills and education are poorly understood. The pneumococcal-attributable contribution to acute and subsequent chronic ear disease remains to be established. Prevention of acute pneumococcal otitis media is not currently a priority for pneumococcal vaccine strategies in the developing world. With more data on disease burden, priorities may change.

Adult epidemiology

Limited community based incidence rates of pneumococcal disease exist for adult populations in the tropics. Little of this is properly stratified by age and the additional disease burden in the elderly is not well characterized. The best available estimates would suggest rates between 20 and 300 cases of invasive (bacteraemia and/or meningitis) pneumococcal disease per 100 000 adult-years.[27,28] The lower level estimates are similar to the rates of invasive disease in elderly populations in the UK.[19] In otherwise healthy adults, bacteraemia complicates pneumonia in about one quarter of cases; thus the rates of pneumococcal pneumonia may be four times greater.

Outside the African meningitis belt, the pneumococcus is the leading cause of bacterial meningitis, a situation that has been worsened by the impact of HIV. Within those regions contained in the meningitis belt, pneumococcal disease remains important and at times mimics the severe outbreaks of meningococcal disease. Well characterized epidemic outbreaks of pneumococcal meningitis have occurred with high case-fatality.[29,30] These outbreaks appear to be a consequence of the arrival of specific pneumococcal strains to which there is only limited immunity.

The higher rates of pneumococcal infection in otherwise fit and well adults, particularly in sub-Saharan Africa, compared with adults in the developed world, are incompletely understood. Environmental and social factors are believed to play a leading part and it is perhaps important to note the similarities in rates of disease today in the tropics to those measured in the industrialized world in the 1920s and 1930s.[31] Host genetic factors are also believed to be important. Studies in the USA have found rates of pneumococcal infection to be higher amongst African-Americans than European-Americans, a finding incompletely accounted for by social and environmental confounding.[32] The dynamics of carriage and the intensity of exposure to serotypes not previously encountered may also contribute to disease rates. Pneumococcal disease is more likely to occur when an individual is exposed to a new pneumococcal serotype, and this will happen more frequently in an environment of intense transmission. This was an important factor in the epidemics of pneumococcal disease in South African gold miners, which drove the initial studies of pneumococcal vaccination, and outbreaks in crowded conditions continue to be described.[33]

The use of tobacco in the developing world, a predisposing factor for invasive pneumococcal disease in the industrialized world,[34] is on the increase. There is every reason to suspect that this adverse effect of smoking will also contribute to an increased burden of disease as smoking rates rise in the developing world. However, of greatest importance as a risk factor for developing pneumococcal disease is human immunodeficiency virus (HIV) infection.

HIV-associated pneumococcal disease

HIV increases the risk of pneumococcal pneumonia by between 6 and 20 times.[27,35] Bacteraemia complicates pneumonia in 80% of cases. Thus rates of invasive disease are from 10–100 times more frequent in age-matched HIV-infected than the HIV-uninfected. Even with optimal antiretroviral therapy HIV-infected adults remain at significantly elevated risk of disease.[36] It is estimated that HIV is the cause of over 80% of all invasive pneumococcal events in adults in sub-Saharan Africa and over half of all pneumonia cases are HIV-co-infected.[37] Community-based incidence data from East Africa have recorded rates of invasive disease in HIV-infected adults between 1700 and 4200 per 100 000 person-years.[28,38] Rates of disease show a strong association with HIV-related immunosuppression; higher rates at lower CD4+ T-cell counts. Furthermore, reinfection rates are extremely high at up to 25 000 per 100 000 person-years.[38] In Malawi, HIV accounted for 95% of hospital admissions with pneumococcal bacteraemia during 1997/98,[39] this in a region with an underlying adult HIV seroprevalence estimated at 15–20%. Within this case series the proportion of meningitis cases was also high. This is also a feature of the HIV/pneumococcal interaction in this region.[40] The impact of HIV on pneumococcal disease in children in the tropics is less well described, but the risk of bacteraemic disease is increased,[18] and this comes on the back of a much increased background rate of disease.

MICROBIOLOGY

Streptococcus pneumoniae is a Gram-positive bacterium, which grows in chains in liquid media, but is more characteristically seen as pairs in clinical specimens. The term lanceolate is used to describe this paired appearance, the organisms appearing egg shaped, with their flatter ends opposed. A source of H_2O_2 is required for growth and consequently pneumococci grow better in the presence of catalase. In the diagnostic laboratory this is usually achieved by growing the organism in the presence of blood on a blood agar or heated blood agar (chocolate agar) plate. They grow best at $37°C$ (growth range 25–40°) in the presence of 5%–10% CO_2, conditions which can be achieved in a candle-extinction jar. Horse blood is typically used in media preparation. When this is not readily available sheep or goat blood provides a suitable alternative. Human or cow blood is best avoided, not only for the infection risks associated with handling human blood products, but growth may be suboptimal. Liquid media appropriate for use in manual blood culture systems to recover pneumococci are nutrient broth, tryptone soya broth and brain heart infusion broth. Further information on media and reagent preparation relevant to laboratory practice in the developing world is available in Cheeseborough's *Medical Laboratory Manual for Tropical Countries*.[41]

On a blood agar plate, pneumococci form colonies that are usually opaque, 1–2 mm in diameter with central umbilication which are surrounded by a characteristic green zone (α-haemolysis) as a result of the action of an exotoxin, pneumolysin, producing a pigment from haemoglobin. Production of a polysaccharide capsule by the bacteria is responsible for the opaque appearance. Colonies may appear mucoid if the bacteria produce large quantities of capsule. Failure to produce a significant capsule leads to the growth of transparent colonies. These phenotypic characteristics may be important in pathogenesis (see later). Pneumococci readily undergo autolysis and death, and this explains the umbilicated characteristics of the colonies, with the centre of the colony collapsing. This characteristic may hinder diagnosis. Pneumococci grown in liquid media will produce turbidity that may then clear on further culture in as little as 16 h. Although less of a problem with modern continually monitored blood culturing systems, laboratories using manual systems need to time visual inspections and sub-culturing to avoid this pitfall. A zone of 'haemolysis' above the sedimented red cells in a manual system will provide additional evidence of bacterial growth.

Pneumococci must be differentiated from other α-haemolytic *Streptococci* by demonstrating sensitivity to optochin (ethyl hydrocupreine, a quinine derivative, once used for therapy but withdrawn because of toxicity) and solubility when cultured after exposure to bile salts. Antibiotic sensitivity testing should be performed when available. This is particularly crucial for managing meningitis when knowledge of penicillin sensitivity is key to appropriate therapy (see later). Penicillin sensitivity is best assessed with a 1 µg oxacillin disc. Not only is oxacillin more stable and storage-friendly than low strength penicillin discs, it is relatively precise in predicting reduced susceptibility to penicillin (zone diameter ≤ 19 mm). Accurate determination of the susceptibility characteristics of pneumococci will require measurement of the minimal inhibitory concentration (MIC) by a broth or agar dilution method or the use of a graduated antibiotic-impregnated plastic strip, E-test® (AB Biodisk, Sweden). Serotyping of pneumococci is unnecessary for routine clinical diagnostic work, but may be performed for epidemiological surveillance. The Quellung reaction remains the standard. A suspension of pneumococci is incubated with capsular-type-specific antiserum and methylene blue for 10 min. If there is recognition of the capsule by the antiserum present, the resultant capsular-antibody complex leads to a change in the refractive index of the capsule that stands out and contrasts (often referred to as swelling) against the methylene blue-stained intracellular contents. A phase-contrast microscope is needed to correctly view these changes and a positive control should be available for comparison as the reactions are often difficult to assess.

BACTERIAL ANATOMY AND PHYSIOLOGY

The membranous and external structures of the pneumococci are made up of a triple layered cell membrane, cell wall and a polysaccharide capsule (Figure 54.1). These structures confer the principal mechanisms underlying the pathogenicity and virulence of the bacteria. Exotoxin production is more limited than in other streptococcal species, and tissue damage as a consequence of pneumococcal infection is primarily the consequence of the inflammatory response triggered by cell wall and capsular components.

The cell wall is made up of a combination of peptidoglycan bound covalently to teichoic acid which protrudes deep into the capsule. This is the C-polysaccharide and is unique (with the exception of a few *Viridans streptococci*) to the pneumococcus. C-polysaccharide activates complement either by the alternative pathway or by the classical pathway in the presence of anti-C-polysaccharide antibody and also leads to the production of inflammatory cytokines.

The pneumococcal capsule is formed from the polymerization of oligosaccharides, which are bound to the bacterial cell wall. Permutations in the monosaccharides used in the production of the oligosaccharide macro-molecules lead to antigenic diversity. Genetic control of capsule production depends on the use of several genes combined into a single translational unit,[42] but importantly bacteria may possess or acquire additional capsule-related genes and thus can change their capsular characteristics.[43] This does not appear to be a common process,[44] but under vaccine-induced immune pressure may become so and have implications for long-term vaccine-induced control of disease (see later).

The polysaccharide capsule is critical to the organism's virulence and in the absence of type-specific opsonizing antibody the capsule blocks phagocytosis. The mechanism by which the capsule does this is not clear. It is probably in part related to its ability to cover and hide cell wall bound complement and immunoglobulin

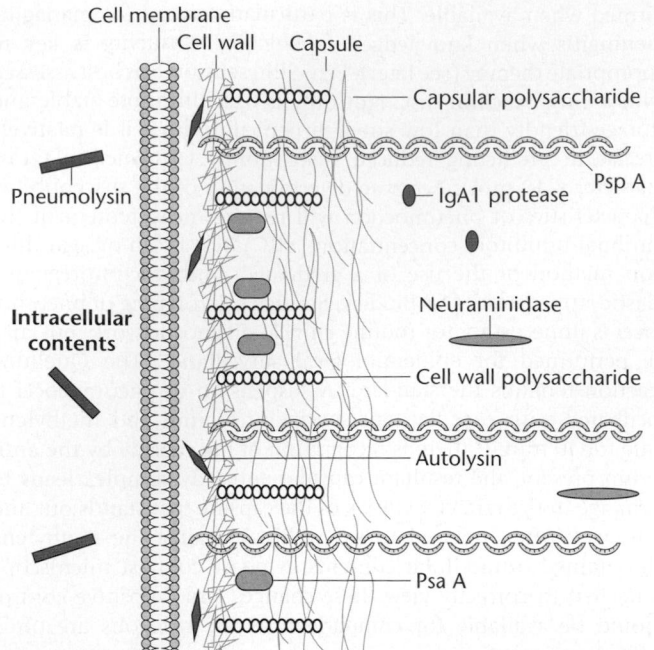

Cell membrane
Cell wall   Capsule

Pneumolysin

Intracellular
contents

Capsular polysaccharide

Psp A

IgA1 protease

Neuraminidase

Cell wall polysaccharide

Autolysin

Psa A

Figure 54.1 Schematic structure of pneumococcal cell membrane, wall and capsule. PspA protrudes through the capsule and may act to stabilize the capsular structure. PspA is highly variable with over 40 serotypes recognized and marked genetic heterogeneity but with a number of stable immunologically cross-reactive molecular epitopes. PsaA is genetically and antigenically conserved across most capsular serotypes. Its anatomical localization within the surface components is unclear. Cell wall polysaccharide consists of teichoic acid, peptidoglycan and phosphorylcholine. When bound to a lipid molecule it is able to extend in to the lipid rich cell membrane and is then known as the Forssmann or F-antigen.

which would otherwise act as opsonins and thereby prevent phagocytosis. Other cell surface components have been identified and are likely to play a role in pathogenesis. Pneumococcal surface protein A (Psp A) and pneumococcal surface adhesin A (Psa A, although not physiologically an adhesion molecule) are the two best described members of a family of choline binding proteins. Bacteria deficient in these proteins show reduced virulence.

Pneumolysin and autolysin are exotoxins, which contribute to virulence. The former is cytotoxic for phagocytic and respiratory epithelial cells and is pro-inflammatory by activating complement, the latter is involved in cell wall remodelling. Other bacterial components, e.g. neuraminidase and hyaluronidase may also contribute to virulence/pathogenicity but their role in human disease awaits clarification. Although somewhat esoteric, the specific interest in these proteins comes from their possible use as a vaccine or vaccine component.[45]

HOST SUSCEPTIBILITY

For pneumococcal disease to develop several critical events must take place. The bacteria must gain entry to the nasopharynx (or rarely to the female genital tract) and adhere to the epithelial cells. Subsequently they must spread to susceptible anatomical sites

i.e. sinuses, middle ear, bronchial tree (peritoneum), reproduce freely and finally may breach endothelial surfaces and invade the blood stream and other distant sites. In broad terms, the host defends itself against pneumococcal mucosal infection by preventing mucosal attachment and spread, using the mucociliary system that lines the respiratory tract and adaptive mucosal immune responses. Defence against invasive disease is critically dependent on the presence of opsonizing anti-capsular antibodies and a functioning phagocytic system. A list of conditions pre-disposing to pneumococcal infection is shown in Table 54.1.

Anatomical defences

The immature development of the Eustachian tube and the inability to clear secretions and bacteria from the middle ear are believed to underlie the susceptibility of young children to otitis. Similarly, other factors which interfere with mucociliary function will predispose to infection: cigarette smoking; smoke inhalation from poorly ventilated fires; and preceding viral infection leading to direct destruction of ciliated epithelium in the upper respiratory mucosa. In addition, viral infections may upregulate the mucosal expression of ligands for the choline binding proteins on the surface of the pneumococci, improving mucosal attachment. This may be particularly relevant for allowing access of more virulent pneumococcal serotypes, which may have a decreased capacity for carriage but a high propensity for invasion once attached. Pneumococci of the transparent phenotype (see earlier) produce little capsule but have a phosphatidylcholine-rich cell wall and are believed to bind upper respiratory epithelium more effectively than their capsulate counterparts. They are never found as invasive isolates as a capsule is essential for this. Furthermore, inflammatory changes, mucus hyper-secretion and the subsequent postnasal drip which often accompanies 'colds and flu' will predispose to aspiration of pneumococci through the larynx and into the bronchial tree.

Mucosal immune response

Innate and adaptive immune system responses contribute to prevention of carriage or spread of pneumococci across mucosal surfaces. Lactoferrin, lysozyme, lactoperoxidase and Mannose Binding Protein (MBP) are components of the innate immune system and act by binding and opsonizing pneumococci for clearance by mucosally associated phagocytes. C-reactive protein (CRP), another agent of the innate immune response, acts in a similar way, but during systemic infection. Polymorphisms in the genes encoding MBP are associated with invasive pneumococcal disease and have been described in African populations.[46] It has been postulated that the evolutionary persistence of CRP is a direct consequence of its ability to protect against pneumococcal disease.

Secretory IgA, the predominant human immunoglobulin at mucosal surfaces, has the ability to prevent binding of pneumococci (and possibly neutralize pneumolysin) and opsonize bacteria for phagocyte recognition. Of the two IgA isotypes, IgA2 is the most important as it is resistant to an IgA protease secreted by the pneumococcus that is able to disrupt IgA1. Animal studies have confirmed the defensive properties of IgA; however, the importance of IgA in the overall scheme of protection against

Table 54.1 Conditions that predispose to pneumococcal infection in the tropics by mechanism of susceptibility

	Defective antibody	Reduced mucosal clearance[a]	Anatomical defects	Complement deficiency	Increased exposure	Phagocyte dysfunction	Comments
IMPORTANT							**COMMON CONDITION OR STRONG ASSOCIATION WITH RISK**
HIV infection	X	X					Debility interferes with respiratory secretion clearance in late stages
Sickle cell disease	X			X		X	
Infancy and ageing	X	X			X		High carriage rates in siblings of infants lead to increased exposure
Alcoholism		X				X	
Chronic chest disease		X	X			X	Tuberculosis, asthma and bronchiectasis
Malnutrition	X	X					
Diabetes						X	
Smoking		X				X	Mucociliary interference and direct toxicity on alveolar macrophages
Poverty					X		Overcrowding and usually co-existent nutritional deficiencies
LESS IMPORTANT							**LESS COMMON CONDITION OR WEAK ASSOCIATION**
Kidney disease	X			X			
Liver cirrhosis			X			X	
Lymphoproliferative disease	X						
Visceral leishmaniasis (and other parasitic infections)	X			X		X	Complex immune defects and abnormalities of splenic function

[a] By virtue of immobility, bed-ridden or defective mucociliary action.

pneumococci in humans remains unclear. Selective deficiencies of IgA are not clearly associated with pneumococcal infection and are believed to be uncommon in non-Caucasian populations. Moreover pneumococci may use cleaved IgA to assist with attachment and translocation across mucosa.[47]

The principal (and most studied) phagocyte in the respiratory tract is the human alveolar macrophage. These cells are able to rapidly destroy pneumococci following phagocytosis. The pneumococcus, unlike *Mycobacterium tuberculosis* for instance, possesses little in its armamentarium to prevent phagolysosomal digestion. Central to the competent functioning of the macrophage is appropriate activation of the cell and opsonization of the pneumococcal target.[48] Cellular mucosal immune responses may also play a part in protection against carriage[49] but much remains to be understood about mucosal defences in general.

Systemic immune response: Critical to protection against invasive disease is the presence of capsule-specific opsonizing antibodies and an intact phagocytic cell system in the liver and particularly spleen.

The central role of serum in protection was identified in the late nineteenth century, when protection could be achieved in animal models by the infusion of immune serum. In the 1920s, further discoveries led to the realization that the antibody conferring protection was directed against the pneumococcal capsule. Subsequently, passive vaccination or serum therapy using serotype-specific antisera formed the basis of early therapeutic successes in treating pneumococcal disease. Recent studies have confirmed the association between low levels/decreased activity of capsule specific IgG and risk of disease.[50,51] Unfortunately, the absolute level of capsule-specific immunoglobulin in isolation is not a wholly reliable predictor of protection or susceptibility. This is in part due to the measurement of low affinity or cross-reactive antibodies and the 'quality' of the antibody to opsonize and stimulate phagocytosis is also important.

Diseases that lead to under-production of immunoglobulins are associated with an increased risk of pneumococcal disease. This is perhaps most dramatic in the primary and acquired hypogammaglobulinaemias, in which repeated episodes of otitis, sinusitis, pneumonia and invasive disease occur. The high rates of invasive pneumococcal disease in early childhood are in part related to underproduction of an IgG isotype, IgG2, the principal isotype contributing to anti-capsular antibodies in adults. An IgG2 response is produced when derivatives of the complement factor C3, which is an important opsonin of pneumococcal polysaccharide, bind a co-receptor on the B cell (complement receptor 2:CR2: CD21) in association with B-cell receptors binding polysaccharide. Importantly, children under 2 years of age do not adequately express complement receptor 2 on B-cells, and consequently little IgG produced is of the IgG2 isotype.

Deficient capsule-specific IgG production underpins the increased susceptibility of HIV-infected individuals to pneumococcal disease. Massive and progressive B-cell destruction is a feature of uncontrolled HIV infection. HIV has a selective preference for destruction of B cells which use the VH3 family of genes to produce their immunoglobulin heavy chain variable regions. In healthy adults it is B cells expressing antibodies of this VH3 idiotype that make up the majority of those active against pneumococci. Thus HIV destroys the humoral immune response that protects against pneumococcal infection. No other HIV-associated immune defect has been clearly shown to be linked to risk of disease, although carriage of pneumococci increases with decreasing CD4 count, suggesting a possible role of the cellular response in protection.

Malnutrition, old age, chronic liver disease including alcohol related disease and renal failure are associated with pneumococcal disease. Although impaired immunoglobulin production to a greater or lesser extent is a feature of these conditions, other factors play a part in increasing susceptibility, e.g. overcrowding, impaired cough reflex, immobility, phagocyte defects, presence of ascites and orthostasis.

In addition to immunoglobulin, complement will also opsonize pneumococci. In vitro studies confirm the value of complement in stimulating phagocytosis of pneumococci and, as mentioned above, complement is able to modulate B cell responses to polysaccharides. Gram-positive organisms are able to resist the effects of the terminal membrane attack complex (C5–C9); consequently it is the early complement factors that are implicated in defence. Perhaps surprisingly, there are few reports of specific complement deficiency states associated with pneumococcal infection, although the increased risk of disease in nephrotic syndrome is believed to be due to hypocomplementaemia as a consequence of deposition and consumption of the early complement factors in the kidneys.

Once opsonized, pneumococci must be removed from circulation and killed by phagocytes. Polymorphonuclear leucocytes and macrophages in the liver and spleen undertake this task. Surprisingly, primary defective functioning of phagocytes either by chemotaxis or impaired oxidative killing is not associated with increased rates and severity of pneumococcal disease, although neutropaenic individuals are at greater risk. Likewise, individuals who lack a spleen (following splenectomy) or are functionally asplenic (homozygous sickle cell disease) suffer high rates of pneumococcal disease, which is in large part due to the reduction in phagocytic function, although other factors including abnormal antibody production and loss of the key marginal zone of the spleen contribute to increased susceptibility. Other phagocytic defects occur as a result of variation in phagocyte-expressed Fc receptors, particularly FcγRIIa. These have been associated with increased susceptibility to respiratory infections in children. However, the importance of polymorphisms in these receptors and risk of pneumococcal disease in African or Asian populations remains to be established.

CLINICAL SYNDROMES

Pneumonia

Pneumonia is the most important presentation of pneumococcal disease by virtue of its frequency, accounting for 80–90% of all pneumococcal disease in adults, and its significant mortality. In the pre-antibiotic era case-fatality was 40–50%. In the antibiotic era, case-fatality in adults of 10% remains typical for bacteraemic disease.[52] Delayed presentation as a consequence of compromised health-seeking behaviour through poverty or lack of access to healthcare, markedly influences case-fatality rates. Mortality rates in children were similarly high but early access to antibiotic therapy dramatically improves outcome from pneumococcal pneumonia and mortality rates of 1–2% are achievable,[53] but not necessarily typical.[54] A clear understanding of the presentation, management and expected outcome of pneumonia is essential knowledge for basic healthcare provision in the tropics.

Clinical presentation

Presentation is typically acute with a 2 or 3 day history of cough, fever, dyspnoea and purulent sputum production. A more prolonged course may occur if the pneumonia has been partially treated or if there is underlying chronic chest disease, in particular tuberculosis. Other symptoms which may be prominent include: haemoptysis – the classic 'rusty sputum,' is characteristic when present (the pigmentary effect of exotoxins on haemoglobin), but infrequent; pleuritic chest pain; headache, often severe and associated with meningism without confirmed meningitis; and diarrhoea, which may occasionally be the primary presenting complaint and lead to confusion with acute gastroenteritis.

Patients appear unwell and will be tachycardic and tachypnoeic. Cyanosis, if present, indicates more severe disease but is difficult to assess in individuals with black skin. Chest signs of consolidation (dullness to percussion, bronchial breathing and aegophony) or more commonly coarse inspiratory crackles consistent with retained secretions are usually heard on auscultation. A pleural rub may also be present and does not necessarily predict complicated pleural disease. Diagnostic confusion may occur if the presentation is hyperacute with abrupt onset of rigors, when malaria, other bacterial septicaemic illness or fulminant viral illness may then head the list of differential diagnoses. Presentations with acute psychosis, confusion, hypothermia, jaundice and abdominal pain may lead to diagnostic confusion.

The presentation, recognition and assessment of pneumonia in children are detailed in Chapter 23.

Investigations

Pneumonia is confirmed by finding consolidation in a lobar, segmental or sub-segmental distribution on chest radiography. Chest radiography is not a requirement when the clinical presentation is clear but will often resolve diagnostic confusion (Figure 54.2). Confirmation of a pneumococcal aetiology can be made

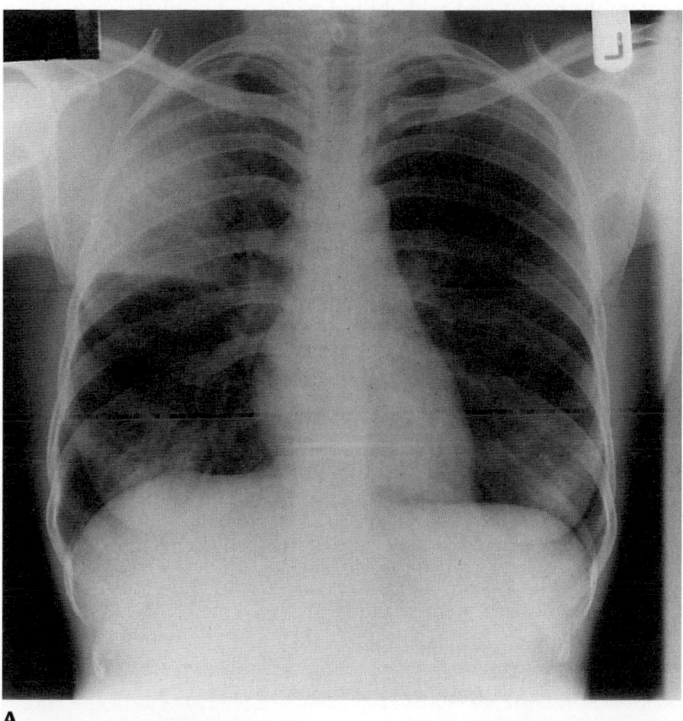
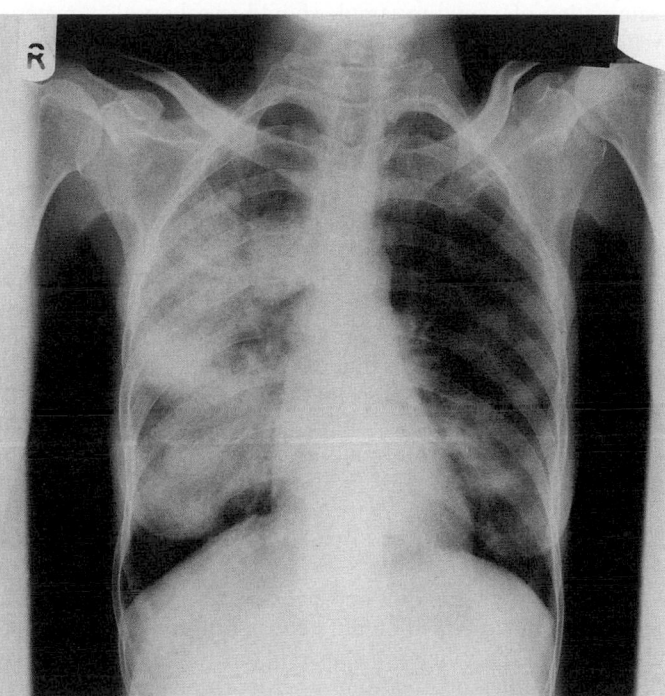
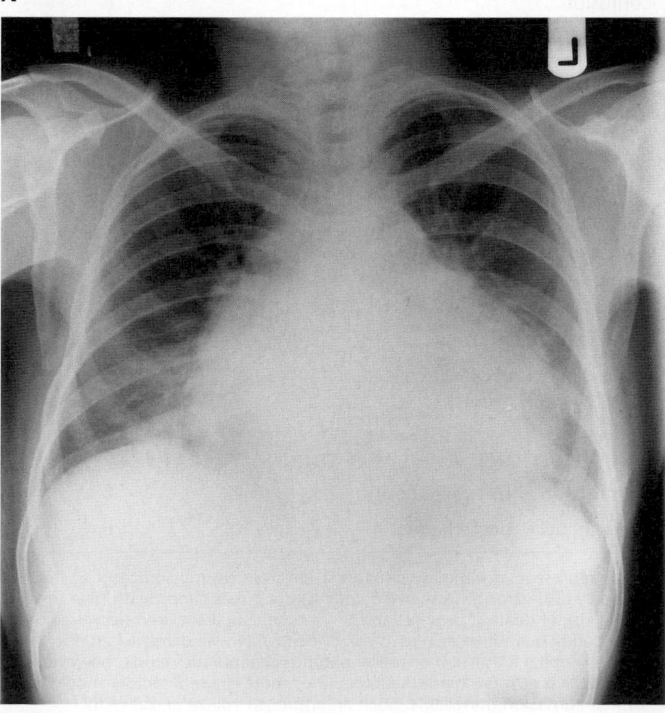
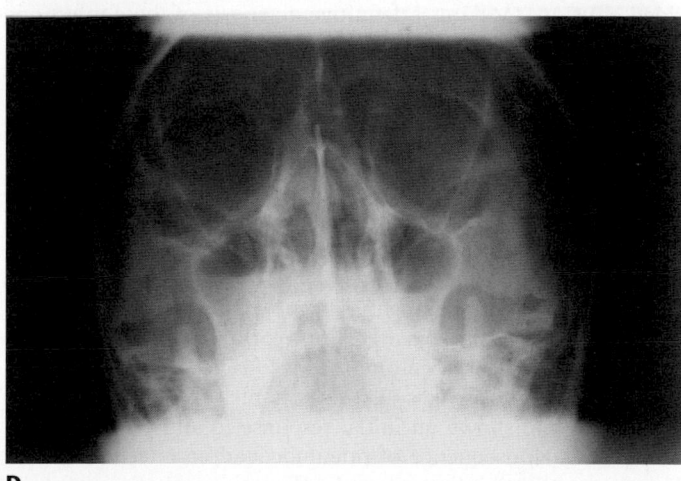

Figure 54.2 Radiographic appearances of pneumococcal disease: (A) Classical right upper lobe pneumococcal pneumonia in a 32-year-old HIV-infected Kenyan woman; (B) Bilateral pulmonary consolidation particularly in the right lung as a consequence of *S. pneumoniae*/*M. tuberculosis* co-infection in a 26-year-old HIV-infected Kenyan woman; (C) Pneumococcal pericarditis and pericardial effusion in a 34-year-old Ugandan male of uncertain HIV status; (D) bilateral maxillary sinus fluid levels in a 28-year-old HIV-infected Kenyan with pneumococcal bacteraemia and no pulmonary focus.

definitively by the recovery of pneumococci from blood culture or from a trans-thoracic needle lung aspirate. This latter technique has proved a safe and valid technique in both adults and children when aspiration is performed on consolidated pulmonary tissue using a small gauge needle. Sputum is often the most readily available clinical specimen. Interpretation of Gram-stain examination and culture results requires some caution. Pneumococci carried in the nasopharynx may contaminate expectorated sputum specimens and lead to a false-positive diagnosis. Macroscopic examination of a sputum sample should reveal purulent material (yellow/green mucus). Gram-positive diplococci in association with 10–20 pus cells and no epithelial cells per high powered field (×100 oil immersion objective) provides good supporting evidence of pneumococcal aetiology. Examination of the sputum for acid and alcohol-fast bacilli should be performed because of the frequent co-existence of tuberculosis with pneumococcal pneumonia. Commercial kits for the identification of pneumococcal capsular polysaccharide in blood or urine are available but have variable sensitivity and are usually an unjustifiable cost for basic diagnostic laboratories. Likewise, serological tests based on pneumolysin-immune complexes or rising antibody titres to Psa A do not have a place in routine clinical practice at present.

Subsidiary investigations including white cell counts, arterial blood gases, electrolyte measurements and liver function tests are not particularly helpful in establishing a diagnosis, but may be used as measures of severity.

Differential diagnosis

When respiratory symptoms and signs are lacking, pneumococcal pneumonia may need to be differentiated from a wide range of febrile conditions. When a diagnosis of pneumonia is established, the primary differential is from other infectious agents of pneumonia, and occasionally typhoid or amoebic liver abscess (right-sided effusion). Making a definitive diagnosis of these infections is in many ways more difficult than pneumococcal disease. Many are not readily identifiable (e.g. Chlamydia, Mycoplasma, Rickettsial, Viral) or investigations are difficult to interpret (i.e. Gram-negative organisms in sputum). Tuberculosis is the most critical differential diagnosis to consider. It may present as an acute pneumonic illness or as a co-infection with the pneumococcus. *M. tuberculosis* may be implicated in 5–15% of adult CAP in sub-Saharan Africa,[55] the association being particularly important in HIV-infected adults.[52] Ziehl–Neelsen staining of sputum samples will help in making the diagnosis; however, in up to half the cases of *M. tuberculosis* infection reported in a series of CAP from the Kenyan coast, culture for Mycobacteria was required to establish a diagnosis. It is also important to note that many of these cases had shown an initial response to anti-pneumococcal therapy as a consequence of pneumococcal co-infection.[52] Poor response to antibiotics, pleural effusions, cavitation of lung lesions, cervical or other giant lymphadenopathy or incomplete resolution of pneumonia at follow-up should raise the suspicion of *M. tuberculosis* infection.

Management and therapy

With overcrowded in-patient facilities, the threshold for admission to hospital will be towards more severe disease and an assessment of suitability for out-patient oral therapy or the need for in-patient parenteral therapy is required. Indicators of poor outcome are listed in Table 54.2.[56] Further indicators of the suitability of oral therapy involve an assessment of gastrointestinal symptoms and microbial factors. Vomiting or profuse diarrhoea are relative contraindications to oral therapy as antibiotic absorption may be impaired.

In addition to antimicrobial therapy, other supportive treatment should be initiated. Supplemental oxygen if available, and preferably monitored with blood gases or peripheral saturation measurements, should be provided when hypoxia is present. Clearance of respiratory secretions by changing posture, suctioning and provision of moist air may also be necessary. Maintenance of appropriate hydration (with i.v. fluids if necessary) and nebulized saline may be particularly helpful at preventing desiccation

Table 54.2 Associations of severe disease and poor outcome in pneumonia

	Severity grading
DEMOGRAPHIC FEATURES	
Age >55 years	A
Use of traditional healer	A
Increasing distance from health centre	B
Recent migration/refugee camps	B
CLINICAL FEATURES	
Confusion	B
Diastolic blood pressure <60 mmHg	A
Respiratory rate >30 breaths/min	A
Pulse rate >120 bpm	A
Cyanosis	B
Extra-pulmonary infection	B
Jaundice	B
Reduced body mass index/wasted	B
INVESTIGATIONS: AVAILABLE AT INITIAL ASSESSMENT	
Multilobar disease	B
White cell count <4000 cells/μL	A
White cell count >18000 cells/μL	B
INVESTIGATIONS: AVAILABLE DURING THERAPY	
Co-infection with tuberculosis	B
Pneumococcal bacteraemia	B

The table represents a summary of information from several sources.[56] Factors are graded as A – strongly associated with severe disease and death (five times or greater risk of death if present) and B – moderately associated (less than 5 times or poorly quantified increased risk of death). No validated scheme to determine hospital admission or use of parenteral antibiotics exists; however, the presence of two or more grade A factors, 3 or more grade B factors should lead to hospital admission if available. Such an approach will be sensitive for identifying severe disease but will lack specificity.

of respiratory and pharyngeal secretions and assist expectoration. Assisted ventilation, when available, will be necessary for some cases when respiratory muscle fatigue develops, heralded by a rising partial pressure of CO_2 and more latterly altered conscious level, blood pressure instability and decreasing respiratory effort.

Complications

Pneumococcal pneumonia may be further complicated by metastatic spread of infection and empyema. Osteomyelitis, arthritis, endocarditis, suppurative pericarditis and other localized infections are unusual. Empyema complicates 2–3% of pneumonic episodes and may be more common with particular strains of pneumococci. Inadequate or sub-therapeutic antibiotic therapy may predispose to this complication. Management of pleural effusions/empyema should be active from the outset to avoid the late sequelae of chronic empyema. Pleural fluid should be examined. Parapneumonic effusions may be left whilst infected effusions/empyema should be drained. Differentiating between the two may be problematic. Biochemical measures can assist in determining the likelihood of infection (low pH, low glucose and high lactate dehydrogenase), but macroscopic appearance and microscopy will provide broad indicators of infection, the presence of bacteria being a clear indicator of infection. If empyema is diagnosed, drainage of fluid/pus by use of a chest drain or at least with a needle and syringe should be performed, with the intention of removing as much fluid as possible.

Meningitis

Meningitis is the most lethal syndrome associated with pneumococcal infection and high rates of serious complications are present in survivors. Case fatality in children has been measured in excess of 60% and similar rates are recorded in adults.[57,58] These rates are substantially higher than those seen in the developed world. It is unlikely that the difference is wholly down to therapy. Even in study settings when access to therapy is good, high case fatality rates are recorded. Meningitis occurs after haematogenous seeding of the central nervous system and it is probable that meningitis reflects the consequence of late presentation of a bacteraemic illness.

Clinical presentation

Pneumococcal meningitis in adults follows the typical pattern of headache and fever in association with neck stiffness, progressive alteration in conscious level and features of disseminated sepsis, with symptoms evolving over 12–48 h. Preceding or superimposed pneumonia is also common. Difficulties in diagnosis arise when neck stiffness is absent, which may be associated with advanced disease, infancy, old age and immunosuppression, and the diagnosis may be missed or confused with cerebral malaria.

Investigations

Examination of cerebrospinal fluid (CSF) is important to confirm a diagnosis. CSF findings will show the characteristics of a bacterial infection, polymorphonuclear leucocyte pleocytosis, raised protein, low sugar and a Gram stain demonstrating Gram-positive lanceolate diplococci. White cell counts can however be low in the immunosuppressed or those with overwhelming infection. In such circumstances Gram stain evidence of bacteria is usually found. In the absence of a confirmatory Gram stain or following antibiotic therapy, it may be possible to detect pneumococcal antigen in CSF to provide a rapid diagnosis. Definitive proof of pneumococcal aetiology relies on culture and laboratory characterization. In the absence of evidence of pneumococcal aetiology, empiric therapy should always include an agent effective against pneumococci. In laboratories able to perform sensitivity testing, this should be performed on all isolates from CSF as reduced susceptibility to penicillin is critically important in determining therapy for meningitis (see later).

The risks of performing a lumbar puncture must be balanced against the value of the information obtained. However, only basic laboratory equipment is required to perform a CSF examination (microscope, counting chamber, slides, Gram stain) and this will often rapidly establish an aetiological diagnosis. The presence of a focal neurological deficit (present in 20% of cases of bacterial meningitis), altered conscious level (>60% of cases), papilloedema (<1% of cases), seizures (30% of cases) and suppurative ear disease should necessitate a reconsideration of the need for lumbar puncture, but are not absolute contraindications.

Differential diagnosis

This includes: other bacterial meningitis (Chapter 55), the meningococcus being the most important; falciparum malaria; rickettsial infections; relapsing fever; viral meningo-encephalitis; and cryptococcal meningitis. Tetanus, hypertensive crisis, poisoning and sub-arachnoid haemorrhage may also need to be considered. Differentiation relies on CSF examination. Blood cultures should also be performed on all cases of suspected meningitis when available. Bacterial growth will occur within 24 h and this is a particularly valuable investigation when lumbar puncture is contraindicated. Antibiotic therapy prior to performance of a blood culture will dramatically reduce sensitivity.

Management and therapy

Therapy for meningitis should be given as soon as a diagnosis is considered but after blood cultures have been taken. Parenteral therapy is obligatory. In addition to antimicrobial agents other supportive therapy will be needed. These are aimed at: treating the complications of bacteraemia with intravenous fluids and supplemental oxygen if available; preventing the complications of immobility by good nursing care; and minimizing the rise in intracranial pressure by nursing in a head up position. High dose corticosteroids are recommended for the treatment of pneumococcal meningitis based on clinical trial findings from Europe.[59,60] However, two large trials from Malawi in children and adults do not support this approach in settings where HIV is prevalent and where presentation may be delayed.[61,62]

Complications

Outcome following pneumococcal meningitis is poor. In survivors convalescence may be prolonged and residual neurological deficit and disability is common, notably deafness, stroke and blindness.

antibiotic penetration is decreased. Increased penicillin dosing cannot be used in the treatment of meningitis caused by resistant pneumococci. CSF concentrations of penicillin are usually 1–5% of serum levels and maintaining a concentration above the MIC for at least 40% of the dosing interval (a figure required for therapeutic success with β-lactams in animal studies) is unachievable. Where resources are available, a third generation cephalosporin should be used as the initial therapy of meningitis, and modified on the basis of sensitivity testing. In the absence of cephalosporins, chloramphenicol may be appropriate to use. However, the association of chloramphenicol with penicillin resistance may make this approach inappropriate. Local sensitivity knowledge will assist with these decisions, but in the absence of laboratory information the combination of penicillin and chloramphenicol represents the most pragmatic approach. Other agents with anti-pneumococcal activity which have been used to treat penicillin resistant pneumococcal meningitis include carbapenems (e.g. Meropenem), glycopeptides (e.g. Vancomycin), oxazolidinones (e.g. Linezolid) and Rifampicin. These agents are expensive and less readily available than cephalosporins and with the exception of Rifampicin, none are included in the WHO essential drugs list. Rifampicin is widely available as a combination tablet with other antituberculous drugs but more difficult to find as a single agent and resistance rapidly develops when used alone. The aminoglycosides gentamicin and streptomycin should not be used as single agents, as achievable tissue concentrations are below the MICs of even the most sensitive organisms. The use of these antibiotics in synergy with a β-lactam has been suggested for penicillin resistant pneumococcal infections, but this approach has no role in meningitis due to the minimal CSF penetration of aminoglycosides.

PREVENTION

Prevention of pneumococcal disease and pneumonia in children by the use of pneumococcal protein conjugate vaccine has now been demonstrated in several large and convincing randomized controlled trials, two of these in African settings.[2,73] Notwithstanding, there is little structured approach to the prevention of pneumococcal disease in the tropics, despite its clear importance as a public health and clinical problem. The current high cost of the available vaccines and the lack of appreciation by health planners of the importance of pneumococcal infection may be reasons why wide-scale vaccination has not yet started. Chemoprophylaxis continues to have a key role in specific conditions.

Polysaccharide vaccine

These vaccines have been available in some form for the past 90 years. The current formulations contain capsular polysaccharide from the 23 commonest disease-causing pneumococcal serotypes. Depending on geography and the prevalent disease-causing serotypes, they will provide potential coverage against 85–95% of pneumococcal disease events. Vaccination is given as a single intramuscular injection. The efficacy of these vaccines is debatable and whilst they have been used widely in North America and Europe, use of the vaccine elsewhere and particularly in the tropics has been very limited. The vaccine provides protection against invasive pneumococcal disease in immunocompetent adults par-

ticularly in settings of epidemic pneumococcal spread but has not been shown to be effective in immunocompromised groups. The vaccine has never been shown to convincingly reduce pneumonia or function in infants. Thus current recommendations for use of the vaccine in the tropics are somewhat limited but extend to individuals with sickle cell disease, or other causes of functional or anatomic asplenia. Moreover, the uncertainty over the vaccine's effectiveness and its unsuitability as a component of the childhood EPI programme have led to the 23-valent polysaccharide vaccine being unavailable in much of the tropics.

Protein conjugate pneumococcal vaccine

The development of protein conjugate vaccines was driven by the ineffectiveness of polysaccharide vaccines in young children and an understanding that by attaching the polysaccharide to a polypeptide 'carrier' the vaccine becomes T cell dependent. T cell dependent responses are present from birth, unlike responses to pure polysaccharide. With T cell involvement not only does the vaccine become immunogenic in infants, there is also the production of functionally competent, affinity-matured antibodies and the creation of long-lived memory B lymphocytes.

Two large randomized controlled trials of a nine-valent vaccine (three doses given with standard infant vaccines) have reported highly significant reductions in vaccine-serotype invasive pneumococcal disease, all cause pneumonia and in the study undertaken in The Gambia a 15% decrease in all-cause infant mortality.[2,73] Moreover, in the South African study the vaccine was shown to be safe and effective in HIV-infected children, although to a lesser extent than in the HIV-uninfected. These were impressive results and followed on from studies in the USA, which had also convincingly demonstrated protection against vaccine-serotype disease and pneumonia. A further key outcome from use of these vaccines in national vaccine programmes has been a dramatic indirect protective effect as a consequence of herd immunity. Unvaccinated adults and children in the USA have seen falls in rates of vaccine serotype pneumococcal disease,[74] the effect being so large that more pneumococcal disease has been prevented through this mechanism than directly to the vaccine recipients.

Introduction of conjugate pneumococcal vaccine would therefore appear to be an essential next step in the evolution of infant vaccines in the tropics. There has been much discussion about the need to introduce these conjugate vaccines more widely but problems remain. The commercially available vaccines were developed to meet US requirements and provide a high percentage of coverage for US serotypes, in excess of 80%. Coverage in paediatric populations in Africa is reduced, with between 40–60% coverage.[75] This degree of coverage would be welcome, particularly in the light of the mortality reductions reported in The Gambian study. However non-vaccine serotype disease will increase following the introduction of conjugate vaccines. This has been described in the USA but the effect to date has not significantly offset the net benefit of vaccine except in HIV-infected adults. In this group decreases in vaccine serotype disease through indirect benefits of vaccine have been completely offset by non-vaccine serotype replacement. This effect will be larger in regions of high HIV prevalence but whether this would limit the overall programmatic benefits of vaccine introduction or limit the long-term durability of vaccination is doubtful. A further concern has been uncertainties over efficacy of specific serotype conjugates within the vaccines, particularly serotypes 3 and 1. This suggests that there may be problems extending conjugate technology to cover all serotypes and this will be more of a problem in regions where these serotypes are in greater circulation. However, all of these problems are relative (and potentially solvable with modifications to vaccines and increased serotype coverage) and it is the economics of vaccination that is currently limiting widespread introduction. Conjugate vaccines are expensive and will remain so given the technical difficulties of production. Set against this is the lack of information on the economic and quality of life costs of pneumococcal disease with which to make appropriate public health policy. The situation is, however, evolving and it is to be hoped that by the next edition of Manson widespread pneumococcal vaccination will be routine.

The role of conjugate vaccines in adult populations and in HIV-related immunosuppression is uncertain, although studies to investigate their efficacy are underway. It may well be that widespread introduction of infant vaccination will have the same effect as direct vaccination of high-risk adults.

Other vaccine candidates

Concerns over the high production costs of conjugate vaccines and their serotype-specific limitations have led the search for other vaccine candidates.[45] Several pneumococcal peptides are under investigation of which pneumolysin, pneumococcal surface adhesin A (Psa A) and BVH-3 are at present the most likely alternatives. They are attractive because they provide a relatively homogeneous antigenic structure and are independent of capsular serotype, and may be significantly easier to produce with modern cloning technology. Several of these peptides have reached human studies, but it is unclear as to which if any products will reach phase 3 trials at this time.

Chemoprophylaxis

The use of penicillin prophylaxis (oral phenoxymethyl penicillin 125–250 mg twice daily or i.m. benzathine penicillin 1.2 MU 4-weekly) is recommended for the prevention of pneumococcal disease in sickle cell disease sufferers and in individuals without a spleen. Prophylaxis should continue at least up until the age of 5 years in SCD and for a minimum of 5 years post-splenectomy. More prolonged prophylaxis may be beneficial as the true morbidity and mortality of late pneumococcal sepsis in these conditions is uncertain. The increasing prevalence of penicillin resistant pneumococci may decrease the value of this approach in the future. Alternative agents for prophylaxis include erythromycin or azithromycin.

Co-trimoxazole is recommended by the WHO for HIV-infected (adults and children) individuals. This recommendation is distinct from its use as an agent to prevent *Pneumocystis carinii* pneumonia and strongly based on studies from Côte D'Ivoire that showed the benefits of this approach in reducing several morbid end points including pneumonia in adults.[76] Outside of West Africa, there have now been several studies confirming the benefits

of co-trimoxazole in reducing mortality, but only one study from Zambia in children, where this effect seems to be modulated by a reduction in pneumonia.[77] High rates of co-trimoxazole resistance in pneumococci found in east and southern Africa limit the impact of this approach on pneumococcal and respiratory disease in HIV-infected adult populations in these regions.

Antiretroviral therapy

Antiretroviral therapy reduces rates of primary and recurrent pneumococcal disease in HIV-infected adults in North America and Europe, although rates of disease remain substantially higher than in the HIV-uninfected.[36] As antiretroviral therapy becomes more widely available it is expected that a similar effect will be seen in developing countries but other prophylactic strategies will still be needed.

REFERENCES

1. WHO/OMS. *World Health Report* 2000. Geneva 2000.
2. Klugman KP, Madhi SA, Huebner RE, et al. A trial of a 9-valent pneumococcal conjugate vaccine in children with and those without HIV infection. *N Engl J Med* 2003; 349:1341–1348.
3. Hausdorff WP, Feikin DR, Klugman KP. Epidemiological differences among pneumococcal serotypes. *Lancet Infect Dis* 2005; 5:83–93.
4. Enright MC, Spratt BG. A multilocus sequence typing scheme for Streptococcus pneumoniae: identification of clones associated with serious invasive disease. *Microbiology* 1998; 144(Pt 11):3049–3060.
5. Greenwood B. The epidemiology of pneumococcal infection in children in the developing world. *Philos Trans R Soc Lond B Biol Sci* 1999; 354:777–785.
6. Coles CL, Rahmathullah L, Kanungo R, et al. Nasopharyngeal carriage of resistant pneumococci in young South Indian infants. *Epidemiol Infect* 2002; 129:491–497.
7. Jain A, Kumar P, Awasthi S. High nasopharyngeal carriage of drug resistant Streptococcus pneumoniae and Haemophilus influenzae in North Indian schoolchildren. *Trop Med Int Health* 2005; 10:234–239.
8. Hill PC, Akisanya A, Sankareh K, et al. Nasopharyngeal carriage of Streptococcus pneumoniae in Gambian villagers. *Clin Infect Dis* 2006; 43: 673–679.
9. Sleeman KL, Griffiths D, Shackley F, et al. Capsular serotype-specific attack rates and duration of carriage of Streptococcus pneumoniae in a population of children. *J Infect Dis* 2006; 194:682–688.
10. French N, Watera C, Moi K, et al. *Pneumococcal Carriage is Higher in Ugandan Adults Infected with HIV than in the Uninfected, Shows Seasonal Variation and is Directly Associated with Pneumococcal Disease Rates.* 4th ISPPD, Helsinki, Finland 9–14 May 2004.
11. Hill PC, Onyeama CO, Ikumapayi UN, et al. Bacteraemia in patients admitted to an urban hospital in West Africa. *BMC Infect Dis* 2007; 7:2.
12. Enwere G, Biney E, Cheung YB, et al. Epidemiologic and clinical characteristics of community-acquired invasive bacterial infections in children aged 2–29 months in The Gambia. *Pediatr Infect Dis J* 2006; 25: 700–705.
13. Brent AJ, Ahmed I, Ndiritu M, et al. Incidence of clinically significant bacteraemia in children who present to hospital in Kenya: community-based observational study. *Lancet* 2006; 367:482–488.
14. Nimri LF, Rawashdeh M, Meqdam MM. Bacteremia in children: etiologic agents, focal sites, and risk factors. *J Trop Pediatr* 2001; 47:356–360.
15. Shwe TN, Nyein MM, Yi W, et al. Blood culture isolates from children admitted to Medical Unit III, Yangon Children's Hospital, 1998. *Southeast Asian J Trop Med Public Health* 2002; 33:64–71.

16. Chierakul W, Rajanuwong A, Wuthiekanun V, et al. The changing pattern of bloodstream infections associated with the rise in HIV prevalence in northeastern Thailand. *Trans R Soc Trop Med Hyg* 2004; 98:678–686.

17. Karstaedt AS, Khoosal M, Crewe-Brown HH. Pneumococcal bacteremia during a decade in children in Soweto, South Africa. *Pediatr Infect Dis J* 2000; 19:454–457.

18. Berkley JA, Lowe BS, Mwangi I, et al. Bacteremia among children admitted to a rural hospital in Kenya. *N Engl J Med* 2005; 352:39–47.

19. Sleeman K, Knox K, George R, et al. Invasive pneumococcal disease in England and Wales: vaccination implications. *J Infect Dis* 2001; 183: 239–246.

20. Wall RA, Corrah PT, Mabey DC, et al. The etiology of lobar pneumonia in the Gambia. *Bull World Health Organ* 1986; 64:553–558.

21. Scott JA. The preventable burden of pneumococcal disease in the developing world. *Vaccine* 2007; 25:2398–2405.

22. Madhi SA, Klugman KP. World Health Organization definition of 'radiologically-confirmed pneumonia' may under-estimate the true public health value of conjugate pneumococcal vaccines. *Vaccine* 2007; 25: 2413–2419.

23. Campbell JD, Kotloff KL, Sow SO, et al. Invasive pneumococcal infections among hospitalized children in Bamako, Mali. *Pediatr Infect Dis J* 2004; 23:642–649.

24. O'Dempsey TJ, McArdle TF, Morris J, et al. A study of risk factors for pneumococcal disease among children in a rural area of west Africa. *Int J Epidemiol* 1996; 25:885–893.

25. Hatcher J, Smith A, Mackenzie I, et al. A prevalence study of ear problems in school children in Kiambu district, Kenya, May 1992. *Int J Pediatr Otorhinolaryngol* 1995; 33:197–205.

26. Westerberg BD, Skowronski DM, Stewart IF, et al. Prevalence of hearing loss in primary school children in Zimbabwe. *Int J Pediatr Otorhinolaryngol* 2005; 69:517–525.

27. Jones N, Huebner R, Khoosal M, et al. The impact of HIV on Streptococcus pneumoniae bacteraemia in a South African population. *AIDS* 1998; 12:2177–2184.

28. Gilks CF, Ojoo SA, Ojoo JC, et al. Invasive pneumococcal disease in a cohort of predominantly HIV-1 infected female sex-workers in Nairobi, Kenya. *Lancet* 1996; 347:718–723.

29. Leimkugel J, Adams FA, Gagneux S, et al. An outbreak of serotype 1 Streptococcus pneumoniae meningitis in northern Ghana with features that are characteristic of Neisseria meningitidis meningitis epidemics. *J Infect Dis* 2005; 192:192–199.

30. Yaro S, Lourd M, Traore Y, et al. Epidemiological and molecular characteristics of a highly lethal pneumococcal meningitis epidemic in Burkina Faso. *Clin Infect Dis* 2006; 43:693–700.

31. Heffron R. *Pneumonia with Special Reference to Pneumococcus Lobar Pneumonia.* Cambridge, MA: Harvard University Press; 1939.

32. Robinson KA, Baughman W, Rothrock G, et al. Epidemiology of invasive Streptococcus pneumoniae infections in the United States, 1995–1998: Opportunities for prevention in the conjugate vaccine era. *JAMA* 2001; 285:1729–1735.

33. Sanchez JL, Craig SC, Kolavic S, et al. An outbreak of pneumococcal pneumonia among military personnel at high risk: control by low-dose azithromycin postexposure chemoprophylaxis. *Mil Med* 2003; 168: 1–6.

34. Nuorti JP, Butler JC, Farley MM, et al. Cigarette smoking and invasive pneumococcal disease. Active Bacterial Core Surveillance Team. *N Engl J Med* 2000; 342:681–689.

35. Gilks CF. Royal Society of Tropical Medicine and Hygiene meeting at Manson House, London, 12 December 1996. HIV and pneumococcal infection in Africa. Clinical, epidemiological and preventative aspects. *Trans R Soc Trop Med Hyg* 1997; 91:627–631.

36. Heffernan RT, Barrett NL, Gallagher KM, et al. Declining incidence of invasive Streptococcus pneumoniae infections among persons with AIDS in an era of highly active antiretroviral therapy, 1995–2000. *J Infect Dis* 2005; 191:2038–2045.

37. French N. Community acquired pneumonia in Africa – the contribution of HIV. *Int J Tuberc Lung Dis* 2003; 7:s133–s134.

38. French N, Nakiyingi J, Carpenter LM, et al. 23-valent pneumococcal polysaccharide vaccine in HIV-1-infected Ugandan adults: double-blind, randomised and placebo controlled trial. *Lancet* 2000; 355:2106–2111.

39. Gordon MA, Walsh AL, Chaponda M, et al. Bacteraemia and mortality among adult medical admissions in Malawi – predominance of non-typhi Salmonellae and Streptococcus pneumoniae. *J Infect* 2001; 42:44–49.

40. Klugman KP, Madhi SA, Feldman C. HIV and pneumococcal disease. *Curr Opin Infect Dis* 2007; 20:11–15.

41. Cheesbrough M. *Medical Laboratory Manual for Tropical Countries.* Oxford: Butterworth-Heinemann and Tropical Health Technology; 1992.

42. Bentley SD, Aanensen DM, Mavroidi A, et al. Genetic analysis of the capsular biosynthetic locus from all 90 pneumococcal serotypes. *PLoS Genet* 2006; 2: e31.

43. Coffey TJ, Enright MC, Daniels M, et al. Recombinational exchanges at the capsular polysaccharide biosynthetic locus lead to frequent serotype changes among natural isolates of Streptococcus pneumoniae. *Mol Microbiol* 1998; 27:73–83.

44. Meats E, Brueggemann AB, Enright MC, et al. Stability of serotypes during nasopharyngeal carriage of Streptococcus pneumoniae. *J Clin Microbiol* 2003; 41:386–392.

45. Swiatlo E, Ware D. Novel vaccine strategies with protein antigens of Streptococcus pneumoniae. *FEMS Immunol Med Microbiol* 2003; 38:1–7.

46. Lipscombe RJ, Beatty DW, Ganczakowski M, et al. Mutations in the human mannose-binding protein gene: frequencies in several population groups. *Eur J Hum Genet* 1996; 4:13–19.

47. Weiser JN, Bae D, Fasching C, et al. Antibody-enhanced pneumococcal adherence requires IgA1 protease. *Proc Natl Acad Sci USA* 2003; 100: 4215–4220.

48. Gordon SB, Molyneux ME, Boeree MJ, et al. Opsonic phagocytosis of Streptococcus pneumoniae by alveolar macrophages is not impaired in human immunodeficiency virus-infected Malawian adults. *J Infect Dis* 2001; 184:1345–1349.

49. Malley R, Trzcinski K, Srivastava A, et al. CD4+ T cells mediate antibody-independent acquired immunity to pneumococcal colonization. *Proc Natl Acad Sci USA* 2005; 102:4848–4853.

50. Musher DM, Phan HM, Watson DA, et al. Antibody to capsular polysaccharide of Streptococcus pneumoniae at the time of hospital admission for Pneumococcal pneumonia. *J Infect Dis* 2000; 182:158–167.

51. French N, Moore M, Haikala R, et al. A case-control study to investigate serological correlates of clinical failure of 23-valent pneumococcal polysaccharide vaccine in HIV-1-infected Ugandan adults. *J Infect Dis* 2004; 190:707–712.

52. Scott JA, Hall AJ, Muyodi C, et al. Aetiology, outcome, and risk factors for mortality among adults with acute pneumonia in Kenya. *Lancet* 2000; 355:1225–1230.

53. Usen S, Adegbola R, Mulholland K, et al. Epidemiology of invasive pneumococcal disease in the Western Region, The Gambia. *Pediatr Infect Dis J* 1998; 17:23–28.

54. Roca A, Sigauque B, Quinto L, et al. Invasive pneumococcal disease in children <5 years of age in rural Mozambique. *Trop Med Int Health* 2006; 11:1422–1431.

55. Allen SC. Lobar pneumonia in Northern Zambia: clinical study of 502 adult patients. *Thorax* 1984; 39:612–616.

56. Feldman C. Prognostic scoring systems: which one is best? *Curr Opin Infect Dis* 2007; 20:165–169.

57. Gordon SB, Walsh AL, Chaponda M, et al. Bacterial meningitis in Malawian adults: pneumococcal disease is common, severe, and seasonal. *Clin Infect Dis* 2000; 31:53–57.

58. Molyneux E, Riordan FA, Walsh A. Acute bacterial meningitis in children presenting to the Royal Liverpool Children's Hospital, Liverpool, UK and the Queen Elizabeth Central Hospital in Blantyre, Malawi: a world of difference. *Ann Trop Paediatr* 2006; 26:29–37.

59. de Gans J, van de BD. Dexamethasone in adults with bacterial meningitis. *N Engl J Med* 2002; 347:1549–1556.

60. Schaad UB, Lips U, Gnehm HE, et al. Dexamethasone therapy for bacterial meningitis in children. Swiss Meningitis Study Group. *Lancet* 1993; 342: 457–461.

61. Molyneux EM, Walsh AL, Forsyth H, et al. Dexamethasone treatment in childhood bacterial meningitis in Malawi: a randomised controlled trial. *Lancet* 2002; 360:211–218.

62. Scarborough M, Gordon SB, Whitty CJM, et al. Steroids for bacterial meningitis in adults with HIV in sub-Saharan Africa. *N Engl J Med* 2007; 357:2441–2450.

63. Feldman C, Glatthaar M, Morar R, et al. Bacteremic pneumococcal pneumonia in HIV-seropositive and HIV-seronegative adults. *Chest* 1999; 116:107–114.

64. French N, Williams G, Williamson V, et al. The radiographic appearance of pneumococcal pneumonia in adults is unaltered by HIV-1-infection in hospitalized Kenyans. *AIDS* 2002; 16:2095–2096.

65. Gwanzura L, Pasi C, Nathoo KJ, et al. Rapid emergence of resistance to penicillin and trimethoprim-sulphamethoxazole in invasive Streptococcus pneumoniae in Zimbabwe. *Int J Antimicrob Agents* 2003; 21:557–561.

66. Fleming AF. The presentation, management and prevention of crisis in sickle cell disease in Africa. *Blood Rev* 1989; 3:18–28.

67. Kizito ME, Mworozi E, Ndugwa C, et al. Bacteraemia in homozygous sickle cell disease in Africa: is pneumococcal prophylaxis justified? *Arch Dis Child* 2007; 92:21–23.

68. Aken'ova YA, Bakare RA, Okunade MA. Septicaemia in sickle cell anaemia patients: the Ibadan experience. *Cent Afr J Med* 1998; 44:102–104.

69. Yu V L, Chiou CC, Feldman C, et al. An international prospective study of pneumococcal bacteremia: correlation with in vitro resistance, antibiotics administered, and clinical outcome. *Clin Infect Dis* 2003; 37:230–237.

70. Parry CM, Duong NM, Zhou J, et al. Emergence in Vietnam of Streptococcus pneumoniae resistant to multiple antimicrobial agents as a result of dissemination of the multiresistant Spain(23F)-1 clone. *Antimicrob Agents Chemother* 2002; 46:3512–3517.

71. Felmingham D. Comparative antimicrobial susceptibility of respiratory tract pathogens. *Chemotherapy* 2004; 50(suppl 1):3–10.

72. Bryan CS, Talwani R, Stinson MS. Penicillin dosing for pneumococcal pneumonia. *Chest* 1997; 112:1657–1664.

73. Cutts FT, Zaman SM, Enwere G, et al. Efficacy of nine-valent pneumococcal conjugate vaccine against pneumonia and invasive pneumococcal disease in The Gambia: randomised, double-blind, placebo-controlled trial. *Lancet* 2005; 365:1139–1146.

74. Whitney CG, Farley MM, Hadler J, et al. Decline in invasive pneumococcal disease after the introduction of protein-polysaccharide conjugate vaccine. *N Engl J Med* 2003; 348:1737–1746.

75. Gordon SB, Kanyanda S, Walsh AL, et al. Poor potential coverage for 7-valent pneumococcal conjugate vaccine, Malawi. *Emerg Infect Dis* 2003; 9:747–749.

76. Anglaret X, Chene G, Attia A, et al. Early chemoprophylaxis with trimethoprim-sulphamethoxazole for HIV-1-infected adults in Abidjan, Cote d'Ivoire: a randomised trial. Cotrimo-CI Study Group. *Lancet* 1999; 353:1463–1468.

77. Chintu C, Bhat GJ, Walker AS, et al. Co-trimoxazole as prophylaxis against opportunistic infections in HIV-infected Zambian children (CHAP): a double-blind randomised placebo-controlled trial. *Lancet* 2001; 364:1065–1071.

Chapter 55

C. Anthony Hart and Luis E. Cuevas

Bacterial Meningitis

Bacterial meningitis is a medical emergency and is common in many areas of the tropics. It has a significant mortality, especially in children (see also Chapter 16). The bacteria causing meningitis vary with geographical and climatic conditions, with immunosuppression, with age, availability and usage of vaccines and whether the illness is chronic or acute (Tables 55.1, 55.2). Outside the neonatal period the three major pathogens are: *Streptococcus pneumoniae, Haemophilus influenzae* and *Neisseria meningitidis*. Neonatal meningitis may also be caused by these organisms[1] but other bacteria such as *Escherichia coli*, *Str. agalactiae* (Group B streptococcus) and *Klebsiella pneumoniae* tend to predominate. The relative importance of *H. influenzae*, pneumococci and meningococci outside the neonatal period varies according to country; for example, in humid low lying regions *Str. pneumoniae* and *H. influenzae* predominate, whereas in dryer regions, for example the meningitis belt of sub-Saharan Africa, the meningococcus causes vast spreading epidemics.[2] *H. influenzae* meningitis is rare in individuals over 7 years of age. In addition to a high mortality rate, bacterial meningitis carries a high risk of neurological sequelae.

NEONATAL MENINGITIS

With improvements in, and the more widespread availability of neonatal intensive care, neonates of increasing prematurity have a chance of survival. The premature neonate is not only immature in terms of pulmonary, alimentary and renal function but is also an immune-compromised host. This means that the neonate, and especially the premature neonate, is at increased risk of infection. Early bacterial meningitis is usually part of a syndrome of sepsis neonatorum with few specific signs in the premature neonate.[3] Once infection is established, convulsions, bulging fontanelle and neck stiffness may be detected.

Geographical aspects

Although some geographical variations in the incidence and microbiology of neonatal meningitis are reported, the variability relates more to the presence of neonatal intensive care units and thus whether the infection is hospital or community acquired. For example, in Nigeria, *Salmonella* spp. and *Staphylococcus aureus* are the major pathogens[4,5] whereas in neonatal intensive care units in South Africa Group B Streptococci, *Klebsiella* spp. and *E. coli* are predominant (Table 55.3).[6-10]

Epidemiology

The incidence of neonatal meningitis varies according to the degree of prematurity and in some areas is apparently decreasing. In Durban, the incidence was 2.27/1000 live births in 1981 and had fallen to 0.22/1000 live births in 1987.[6] Over the period 1981–92 the overall incidence of neonatal meningitis was 0.72/1000 live births but for low birth weight neonates (<2500 g) was 1.69/1000 in another part of South Africa.[7] A survey in Oman has revealed an incidence of 1/1000 live births.[11] In Ethiopia an incidence of 0.97/1000 live births was found in term neonates but in pre-term neonates it was 3.66/1000.[9]

Bacteriology

The bacteria causing neonatal sepsis have altered considerably over the past 60 years.[12] This change, in part, reflects the changes in neonatal intensive care and in the availability of antibiotics of increasing potency and breadth of spectrum. In the first part of the twentieth century, group A β-haemolytic streptococci, followed by *Staph. aureus*, were the major pathogens. After the introduction of penicillins Gram-negative bacteria such as *E. coli* and *Klebsiella* spp. emerged as significant pathogens. Then in the 1970s the importance of the group B streptococcus (*Str. agalactiae*) was realized and antibiotic-resistant coliforms emerged. Latterly, low-virulence pathogens such as *Staph. epidermidis* have been shown to be capable of causing septicaemia and meningitis.[3] In tropical countries this evolution has only been apparent in centres with neonatal intensive care units. Elsewhere, primary pathogens such as *Salmonella* spp., *Str. agalactiae* and *Listeria monocytogenes* are more important. For example, in Malawi non-typhoidal *Salmonellae* (NTS) account for 33% of cases of neonatal meningitis.[13] It must not be forgotten that the classical bacterial pathogens, *Str. pneumoniae*, *H. influenzae* and *N. meningitidis* can also cause neonatal meningitis (Table 55.3). Finally, in endemic areas unusual pathogens such as *Burkholderia pseudomallei* can cause meningitis.[14]

ably refers only to meningococcal disease. The meningococcus was first isolated in 1887 at autopsy and in 1896 in life. Thereafter, the individual pathogens were gradually isolated and the disease more clearly defined.

Geographical aspects

Acute bacterial meningitis is found throughout the world but the relative contribution of the three main pathogens varies considerably. The reasons for this variation are still unclear. In the meningitis belt of sub-Saharan Africa (Figure 55.1) epidemics of meningococcal meningitis can occur with 2–14 year cycles. During epidemics the incidence rises to over 400 cases/100 000 population per year but even between epidemics the endemic rate is often over 50 cases/100 000 per year.[29] These cases are most often due to group A meningococci. Occasionally group C meningococci can cause epidemics but more recently groups W135, X and Y have emerged in various countries in the belt.[30,31] In recent years the classic meningitis belt has expanded to include Tunisia and Algeria to the north and Somalia, Kenya, Tanzania, Zambia, Uganda and Rwanda to the east and south.[2,32] Over the last 10 years, epidemics have also been reported from Angola, Namibia, Mozambique, the South of the Democratic Republic of Congo, (DRC: previously Zaire) and Botswana (Figure 55.2). A common feature for the occurrence of epidemics is the 300–1100 mm mean annual rainfall isohyets. Thus climatic changes may govern the distribution of the meningitis belt. In contrast, in certain parts of Africa such

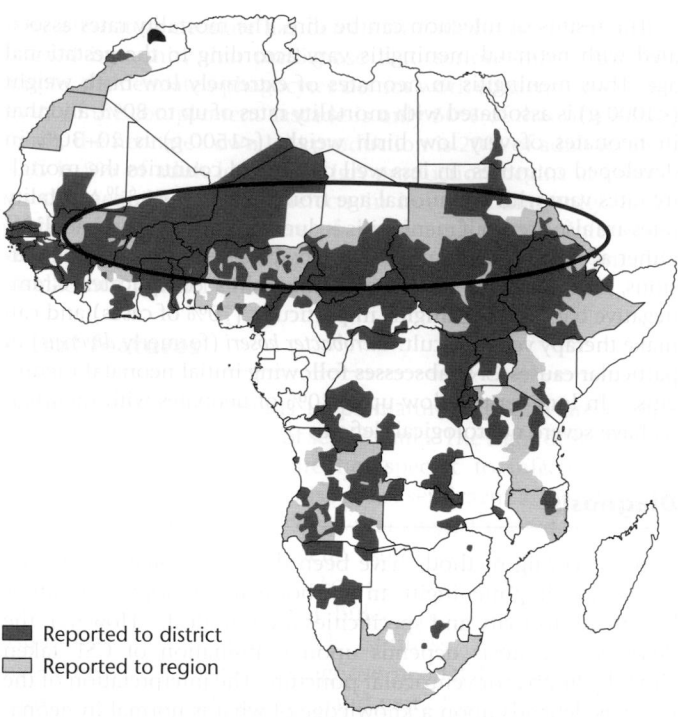

■ Reported to district
□ Reported to region

Figure 55.1 'The classical meningitis belt' of sub-Saharan Africa (circle) where epidemics occur in 2–14 year cycles and the districts affected by epidemics in the twentieth century.

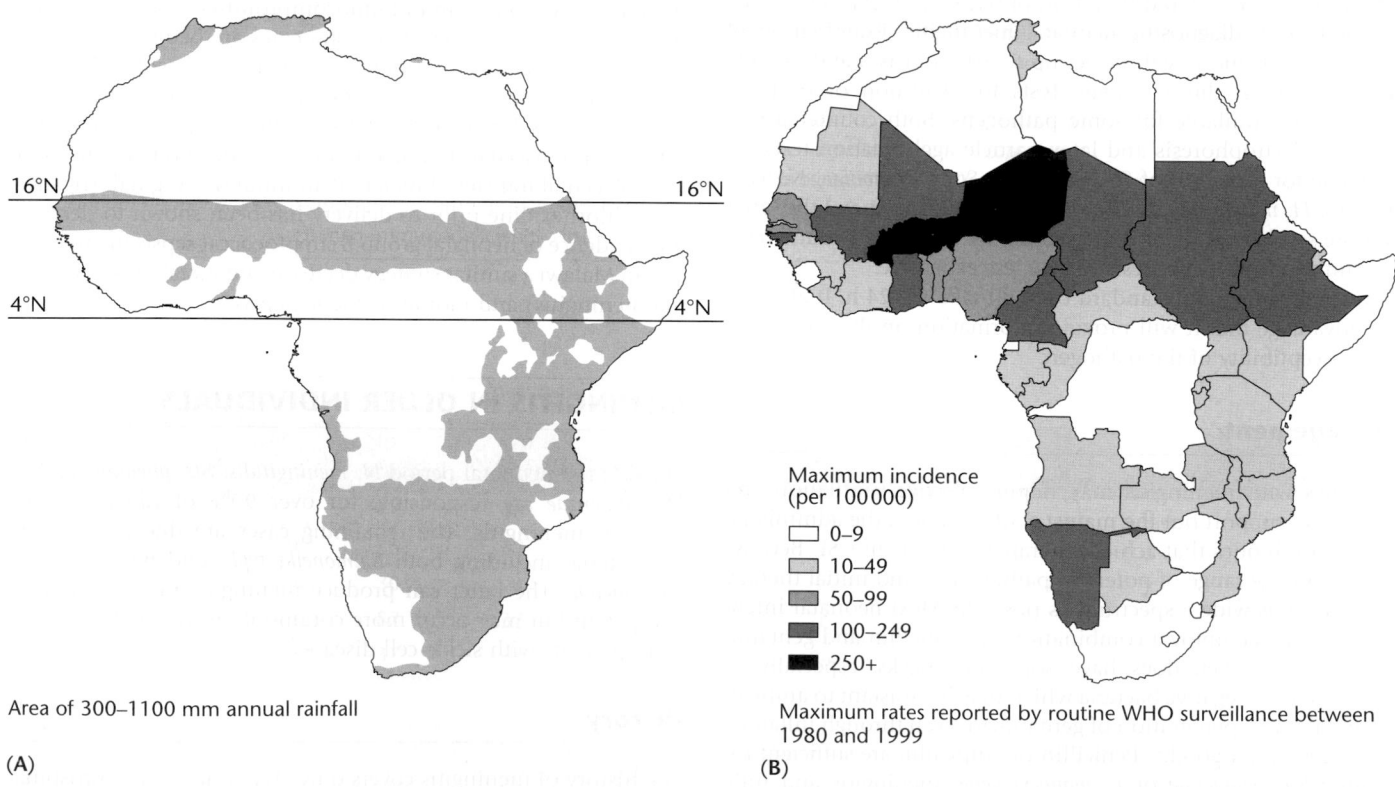

Area of 300–1100 mm annual rainfall

(A)

Maximum incidence
(per 100 000)

□ 0–9
▨ 10–49
▨ 50–99
▨ 100–249
■ 250+

Maximum rates reported by routine WHO surveillance between 1980 and 1999

(B)

Figure 55.2 Area of 300–1100 mm annual rainfall. Maximum rates of meningococcal meningitis reported to WHO 1980–1999.

Table 55.4 Relative importance of meningeal pathogens

	CASES OF MENINGITIS (%)[a]				
	N. meningitidis	*S. pneumoniae*	*H. influenzae*	Population	Years
AFRICA					
South Africa[33]	31	22	16	M	1980–1982
Malawi[34]	4	54	38	C	1983
Malawi[35]	47	42	11	M	1983–1989
Zambia[36]	23	38	6.3	M	1978–1981
Zaire[37]	1.6	33	46	C	1958–1977
Nigeria[38]	16	39	28	C	1976–1979
Ivory Coast[39]	6.4	39	17	M	1971–1975
Libya[40]	10	18	27	C	1981–1984
Senegal[41]	11	29	20	M	1970–1979
Algeria[42]	30	11	19	M	1969
ASIA					
India[43]	0	61	7	M	1972–1980
Malaysia[44]	5.6	24	54	C	1985–1987
Thailand[45]	5.6	47	39	C	1967–1968
AUSTRALASIA					
Papua New Guinea[46]	36	59	4	A	1974–1979
Vanuatu[47]	35	33	23	C	1983–1988
CARIBBEAN					
Jamaica[48]	4.1	38	30	M	1965–1980
Puerto Rico[49]	1.4	10	74	C	1976–1982
AMERICA					
Brazil[50]	40	21	28	A	1973–1982
Chile[51]	8.6	33	58	C	1972–1981
Panama[52]	14	14	0	A	1975–1982
EUROPE					
UK (Merseyside)[53]	57	14	30	C	1981–1990
Denmark	41	19	8	A	1966–1976

A, adults; C, children; M, children and adults.
[a] Percentage of bacteriologically proven cases.

Epidemiology

as in the Congo basin of DRC (Table 55.4)[33-53] and in temperate industrialized countries epidemics with group A meningococci are rarely reported. In low lying regions such as DRC pneumococci are the major meningeal pathogens in all age groups.[37] *H. influenzae* is responsible for cases of meningitis in children under 5 years old in all regions of the world where the conjugate vaccine is not routinely used.

For each of the three main pathogens spread is by droplet or exchange of saliva. Spread is facilitated by close contact. For example, household contacts of a case of meningococcal disease run a risk of developing infection which is 1245 times greater than that for the general population.[54] In most cases, colonization of the nasopharynx precedes invasive disease. The incubation period can be as short as 2–3 days but secondary cases of meningococcal disease have been reported as long as 4 months after contact. However, in studies of secondary cases in households with an index case of meningococcal disease, 70% of secondary cases occur within the first week of contact, 13% in the second week, 6% in the 3rd week and the remaining 11% from the 4th to 10th week.[54]

Although the incidence of pneumococcal and *H. influenzae* meningitis remains relatively constant, *N. meningitidis* is able to produce epidemics spreading through many parts of the world.[29,32]

For example, a clone of group A *N. meningitidis* (III-1) produced an epidemic of disease in China in the 1970s which spread to Nepal and India in 1982, causing an epidemic in 1983–1984. The same clone was responsible for epidemics in New Delhi (1985) and Pakistan (1985). It was then brought by *hadjis* to Mecca in 1987 (Figure 55.3). Clone III-1 was then disseminated throughout the world by *hadjis* returning home. In the African meningitis belt it initiated a wave of epidemics in 1988 but in other areas such as Europe and USA, despite up to 11% of returning pilgrims being carriers, it rarely caused secondary cases. However, recent epidemics in 2004 and 2005 have been due to serogroup W135 and with this, secondary cases did occur when pilgrims returned to Europe.[55]

Although, in Africa, epidemic meningococcal disease occurs in the dry season this is not the sole determinant. Person-to-person spread of the meningococcus occurs as readily throughout the year and it is thought the seasonality of disease is related to increased invasiveness. This may reflect an effect of the dust storms, extreme dryness and heat on the host's mucosal defences.[2,29,32]

Bacteriology

Neisseria meningitidis

Meningococci are small (0.8 × 0.6 µm), non-motile Gram-negative cocci arranged in pairs with contiguous sides flattened.

Optimal growth of meningococci is achieved on enriched media (blood or chocolatized agar) in CO_2 (10%) in air at 37°C.

Small convex greyish mucoid colonies are produced after 18–24 h incubation. All pathogenic meningococci are piliated (protein spikes for attachment to epithelial and endothelial cells) and capsulate. The capsules are acidic polysaccharides that allow the bacteria to evade phagocytic killing. There are at least nine different capsular serogroups (A,B,C,D,X,Y,Z,W-135 and 29E being mostly responsible for human disease). Groups A, B and C are associated with most cases of meningitis. Groups A and C are associated with epidemics and group B with sporadic and endemic disease and hyper-endemicity in some areas such as New Zealand. Groups B and C may be further subdivided on the basis of outer membrane proteins to provide further epidemiological information. Group A meningococci may be further subdivided by means of multilocus enzyme electrophoresis,[56] and more recently by multi-locus sequence typing.[57]

Haemophilus influenzae

This is a small pleomorphic (1.5 × 0.4 µm) non-motile Gram-negative coccobacillus. It requires chocolatized blood agar and an atmosphere of CO_2 (10%) in air for growth and produces small convex greyish mucoid colonies after 18–24 h. Only one of the capsulate strains of *H. influenzae* is able to produce invasive disease in the immunocompetent. This is *H. influenzae* (b) which possesses a polyribitol phosphate capsule. Although *H. influenzae* meningitis is rare in those over 5–7 years old, it can still occur in adults.[36,40,43]

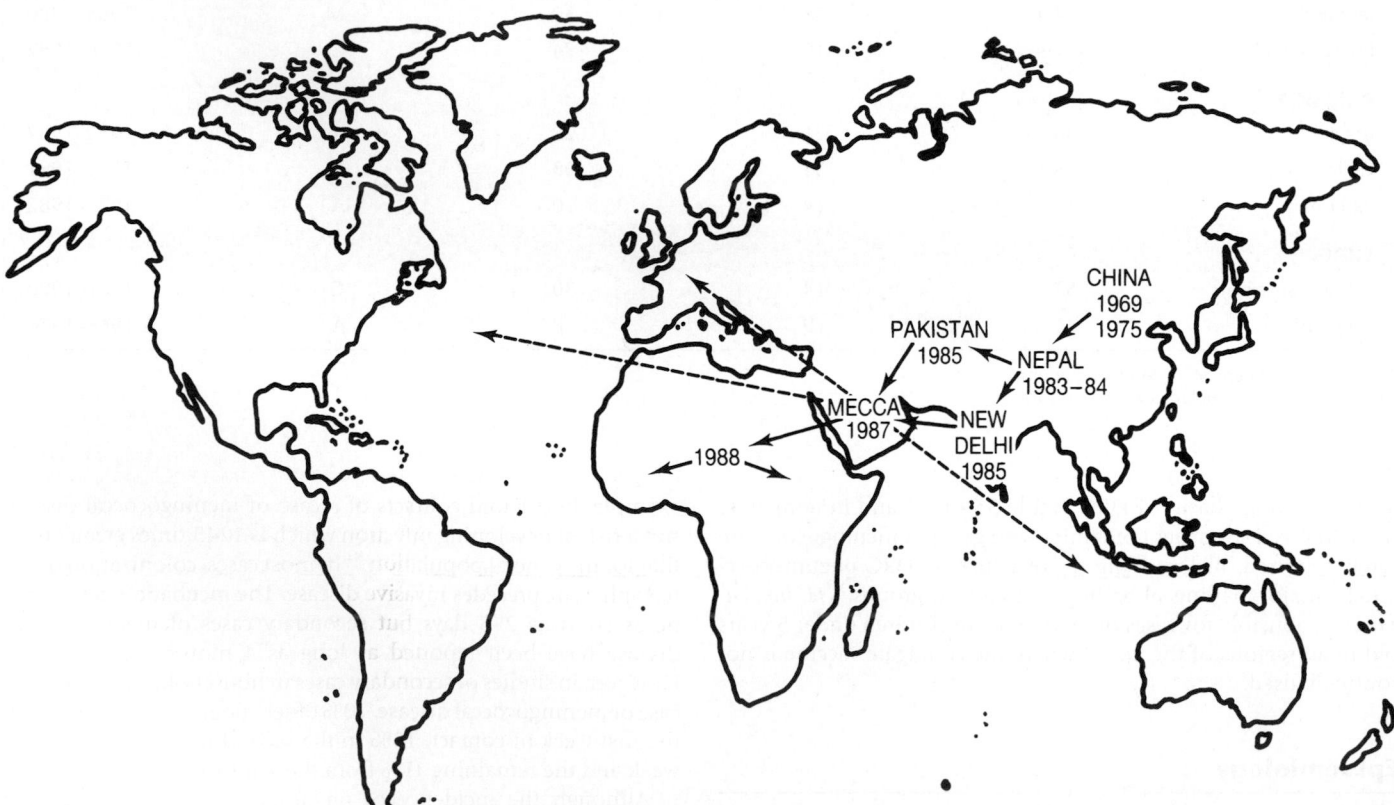

Figure 55.3 Intercontinental spread of clone III-1 of group A *N. meningitidis*.

Streptococcus pneumoniae

These are lanceolate Gram-positive cocci ($0.8 \times 1.0\ \mu m$), usually arranged in pairs. They grow best on blood agar in CO_2 (10%) in air, where they produce either small draughtsman-like colonies or large transparent mucoid (like drops of water) α-haemolytic colonies. The latter are the more virulent strains. Pneumococci are sensitive to optochin which differentiates them from other α-haemolytic streptococci. There are over 80 different capsular types but the 23 included in the current capsular vaccine are responsible for 90–95% of cases of invasive disease. Pneumococci also produce an exotoxin, pneumolysin.

Pathogenesis

Each of the three main pathogens is able to colonize the nasopharynx. There is evidence to suggest that the risk of disease is greatest in the period immediately after colonization. Bacteria in the nasopharynx then translocate to enter the circulation. How this occurs is not clear, but for the meningococcus there is an association between respiratory tract infection with viruses or mycoplasma and meningitis.[58] The bacteria localize in the pia and arachnoid maters and set up an inflammatory response in the meninges and cerebrospinal fluid. The presence of capsule allows bacteria to survive longer in the circulation and meninges. Various components of the bacterial cell surface, such as teichoic acid in pneumococci, lipopolysaccharide (endotoxin) in meningococci and H. influenzae and peptidoglycan in all of them, induce secretion of a variety of factors such as tumour necrosis factor (TNF), interleukins 1 and 6 (IL-1, IL-6), eicosanoids, and platelet activating factor (PAF). This results in potentiation of inflammation, further activation of neutrophils, further complement activation and increased permeability of the blood–brain barrier. This can then produce cerebral vessel thrombosis and vasculitis, cerebral oedema, intracranial hypertension and cerebral infarction. Finally, the activated neutrophils consume large amounts of glucose and oxygen and deprive neuronal tissues of these essential components, driving the brain into anaerobic respiration and production of lactate which is also neurotoxic.

Pathology

The pathological features of acute bacterial meningitis are similar for each of the pathogens and have been well reviewed.[59] The principal feature is of a purulent exudate in the subarachnoid space which often damages the pia mater and the underlying superficial cortex. There is cerebral vessel vasculitis and thrombosis with neuronal damage and superficial encephalitis. There may also be damage to cranial and spinal nerves as they traverse the subarachnoid space.

Clinical features

The signs and symptoms of bacterial meningitis are those of infection and of inflammation of the meninges. The onset is sudden with fever in most cases but is often preceded by symptoms of upper respiratory tract infection. Meningeal irritation will become manifest by nausea, vomiting, headache, irritability, confusion, back pain and neck stiffness. In addition it may be possible to elicit Kernig's (pain on attempting to extend the knee with the hips flexed) or Brudzinski's (neck flexion producing flexion of the hips and knees) signs. It is unusual for all of these features to be present at once, especially in young patients or in the early stages of disease. For example, in a review of over 1000 children with meningitis 1.5% showed no signs of meningeal irritation throughout their infection.[60]

Even early in infection there may be some evidence of mental dysfunction, ranging from drowsiness and lethargy to coma in fulminant infection. Convulsions may occur, especially in children. These are reported in up to 20% of children prior to admission and in 26–30% overall. There may be signs of raised intracranial pressure reflected by headache, and in infants by bulging fontanelle or even diastasis of sutures. Papilloedema is not common in children. Finally, inappropriate secretion of antidiuretic hormone is a common occurrence (in up to 80% of cases) in childhood meningitis. This leads to water retention and may lead to a further rise in intracranial pressure.

Pneumococcal meningitis in particular is more likely to be associated with focal signs on admission.

DIFFERENTIAL DIAGNOSIS

Meningitis can be missed in its early stages, especially in children when there may be only subtle signs of meningism. It should be considered in any child with febrile convulsions or in patients suddenly becoming confused. Similar clinical features may be seen in cerebral malaria, typhus, relapsing fever and cerebral tumours. Viral, fungal or tuberculous meningitis may also present in a similar fashion. Examination of CSF will help to differentiate bacterial meningitis from the rest.

COMPLICATIONS

The mortality rates associated with bacterial meningitis vary according to the age of the patient and the infecting microorganisms. For example, in one survey in Brazil the overall mortality in non-neonatal meningitis was 32% but rose to 48% in those aged 2–6 months and 40% in those aged from 6 months to 2 years.[50] The mortality rate from pneumococcal meningitis (57%) is highest, followed by H. influenzae meningitis (38%) with meningococcal meningitis (14%) having the lowest mortality. Overall mortality rates were much lower (19%) in a series reported from Malaysia.[44]

The acute and later sequelae of H. influenzae meningitis are shown in Table 55.5. Unfortunately, there are few long-term follow-up studies of bacterial meningitis in the tropics and most of the information is extrapolated from temperate zones. However, in one study in Malaysia, 47% of children attending follow-up at least once had neurological sequelae.[44] The incidence of sequelae in H. influenzae and pneumococcal meningitis is similar and higher than that encountered in meningococcal meningitis. A proportion of children with H. influenzae meningitis re-develop pyrexia at day 5–6 of therapy. This can represent the formation of subdural effusion of abscesses but most often no reason is found.

Table 55.5 Complications of *H. influenzae* meningitis

Complication	Cases (%)
EARLY	
Recurrent or persistent pyrexia	35–40
Subdural effusions	33
Inappropriate antidiuretic hormone secretion	50–80
Paralysis	16
LATE	
Persistent paralysis	2–3
Relapse of meningitis	4
Visual impairment	2–3
Hearing deficit	10–15
Hypertension	2–3
Hydrocephalus	<1
Epileptic fits	7

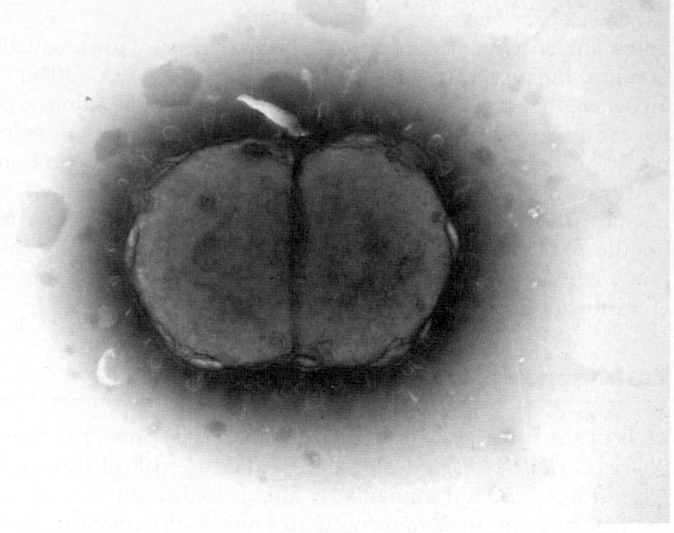

Figure 55.4 Transmission electron micrograph of *N. meningitidis* showing pili and loss of the outer membrane by 'blebbing'.

MENINGOCOCCAL DISEASE

Although the mortality from meningococcal meningitis is relatively low, its mortality in the meningitis belt is higher during endemic periods and the early stages of an epidemic, with the lowest mortality occurring at the end of an epidemic. In addition, if infection is complicated by septicaemia it can prove rapidly fatal. The meningococcus continuously blebs off part of its outer membrane (Figure 55.4). Approximately 25% of the lipid in the outer membrane is lipo-oligosaccharide (LOS). This is a powerful endotoxin, and release of endotoxin produces activation of clotting and complement factors, activation of neutrophils and macrophages, with release of IL-1 (endogenous pyrogen), and TNF vasculitis. This can result in profound shock and bleeding from capillaries. On the skin this produces petechiae, purpura and ecchymoses which together with adrenal haemorrhage constitute the Waterhouse–Friedrichsen syndrome. The onset of disease is sudden with fever and progression through shock, purpura and coma, and death can be rapid (as fast as 2 h). It is important to distinguish meningococcal meningitis from meningococcal meningitis with septicaemia or septicaemia alone,[61] since the management and progression of the two differ. Defects in the terminal components of the complement cascade (C6-9) and properdin predispose to the development of fulminant meningococcal septicaemia. The proportion of cases of meningococcal disease with a septicaemic component appears to be significantly lower in the meningitis belt. For example, only 4 of 112 (4%) cases of meningococcal disease had septicaemia in one study in Sudan[62] and we observed only 11 cases of septicaemia out of 329 cases of meningococcal disease (3.3%) in Malawi.[2] A similarly low incidence of meningococcal septicaemia (5%) was observed in Nigeria.[63] In contrast only 19% of cases of meningococcal disease on Merseyside had no septicaemic component and in tropical countries outside the African meningitis belt over two-thirds of cases have a septicaemic component at presentation.[61] Whether this difference represents a true difference in susceptibility to meningococcal septicaemia, or is a reflection of the difficulties of recognizing a petechial rash on a dark skin (Figure 55.5), or patients in Africa with septicaemia are dying prior to reaching hospital is unclear. However the former seems more likely.[2]

Complications of meningococcal septicaemia include gangrene of the skin and extremities and arthritis, which can be purulent or immunologically mediated. There is also evidence of some neurological deficit.[64]

Diagnosis

The definitive diagnosis of bacterial meningitis depends upon examination of CSF (Table 55.6). The CSF is usually turbid due to the presence of large numbers of neutrophils. However, in early infection low cell counts (200/mm³) may cause the CSF to appear clear. A high CSF neutrophil count and protein concentration and low CSF glucose reflect the extent of inflammation and indicate a poorer prognosis. A specific aetiological diagnosis can be obtained rapidly by examining a Gram-stained smear of centrifuged CSF deposits. This will provide a specific diagnosis in 80–85% of cases. A useful, if expensive, adjunct to diagnosis is detection of bacterial capsular antigens (acidic polysaccharides). Countercurrent immunoelectrophoresis is less sensitive than latex particle agglutination, which has a sensitivity and specificity of 85–100% and 96–100%, respectively, for detection of the appropriate microorganism.[65,66]

CSF culture will take 18–24 h but has the advantage of being relatively cheap and providing data on the antimicrobial susceptibility of the bacterium. Blood culture, if facilities are available, is a useful adjunct to diagnosis. Detection of antigen in urine or serum can also be of value for diagnosis of pneumococcal or *H. influenzae* meningitis but is less useful in meningococcal meningitis.[66] However, a recent study from Kenya estimates that the diagnosis of acute childhood bacterial meningitis is likely to be missed in about one-third of cases in the absence of adequate and reliable laboratory support.[67]

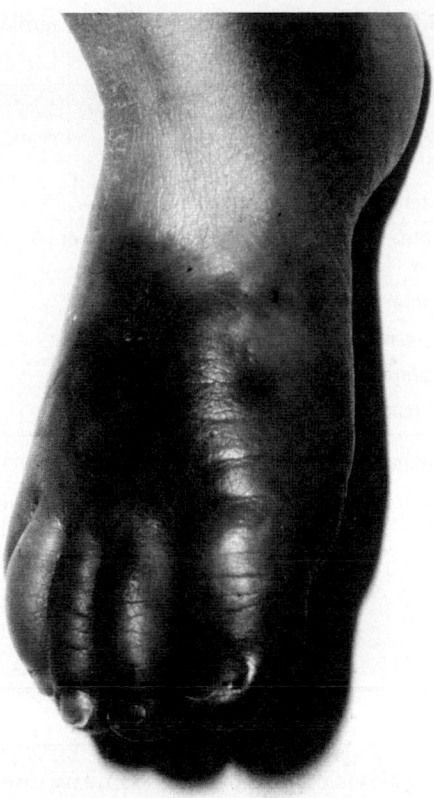

Figure 55.5 An African child with meningococcal septicaemia.

Management

Patients with meningitis should, where possible, be managed in hospital. Blood pressure and respiratory and pulse rates should be monitored regularly. The unconscious patient should be nursed so as to maintain an open airway. Fluid intake should be monitored to prevent dehydration (due to fever and poor fluid intake) or overhydration (due to inappropriate antidiuretic hormone secretion). If fits occur, appropriate anticonvulsants should be administered, bearing in mind that hepatic microsomal enzyme inducers such as phenobarbitone or phenytoin might increase the rate of conjugation of chloramphenicol and decreased blood levels. In studies in the USA and Europe high dose intravenous dexamethasone (0.15 mg/kg 6-hourly for children or 12 mg/12 h for adults) has been shown to decrease mortality in pneumococcal meningitis[68] and decrease neurological sequelae and inflam-mation in *H. influenzae* meningitis.[68] However, results of trials of dexamethasone in developing countries have not been uniformly positive.[68–72] For example, in one study in Pakistan there was a mortality rate of 25% in children receiving dexamethasone compared with 12% in those receiving placebo.[70]

The efficacy of antimicrobial chemotherapy depends upon the penetration of the antibiotic into CSF (Table 55.7) and the susceptibility of the infecting microorganism.

For blind initial therapy chloramphenicol has been shown to be as effective as a chloramphenicol–penicillin combination[73] and a long-acting oily suspension of chloramphenicol as effective as ampicillin.[74] The oily suspension has the benefits of providing treatment even for those who abscond from hospital and is particularly useful in epidemics of meningococcal meningitis.[75] Early antibiotic treatment even prior to hospital admission has been shown to improve outcome in bacterial meningitis.[76]

Table 55.6 Cerebrospinal fluid in meningitis

	Normal	Bacterial meningitis	Aseptic meningitis
Volume (mL)	40–120	–	–
Appearance	Clear	Turbid	Clear to opalescent
Pressure (mmH$_2$O)	<180–200	Raised	Normal
Protein (g/L)	0.15–0.4	0.5–6.0	0.5–1.0[b]
Mononuclear cells (×10^6/L)	0–5	Can be raised	15–500
Neutrophils (×10^6/L)	0	100–6000	<15
Glucose (mmol)[a]	2.2–3.3	0–2.2	2.2–3.3[b]

[a] Must be compared with blood glucose (should be 50–60% of blood glucose level).
[b] In tuberculous meningitis the CSF protein is often high and glucose low.

Table 55.7 Penetration of antibiotics into cerebrospinal fluid

Antibiotic	Serum level in CSF (%)	Therapeutic Level
PENICILLINS		
Penicillin	2–6	+
Ampicillin	10	+
CEPHALOSPORINS		
Cephalothin	1–5	±
Cefuroxime	5–10	+
Cefotaxime	10–25	+
Ceftazidime	20	+
Ceftriaxone	5–10	+
AMINOGLYCOSIDES		
Gentamicin	10–30	–
Netilmicin	20–25	–
OTHERS		
Sulphadiazine	50–80	+
Sulphamethoxazole	25–30	±
Trimethoprim	30–50	+[a]
Tetracycline	25	+
Chloramphenicol	90	+
Ciprofloxacin	5–20	+[b]

[a] Not effective against *N. meningitidis*.
[b] Not effective against *Str. pneumoniae*.

Meningococcal meningitis

Benzylpenicillin (300 000 units/kg per day) should be given i.v. or i.m. 6-hourly for up to 7 days. Chloramphenicol (75–100 mg/kg per day) is a useful alternative given 6-hourly orally or i.m. There are sporadic reports of penicillin insusceptible meningococci,[77] but most are still exquisitely sensitive. Of the cephalosporins, ceftriaxone, which is now off patent and thus less expensive, is probably the most appropriate. In sub-Saharan Africa, where epidemics can overwhelm health services, the World Health Organization recommends using a short-course of long-acting oily chloramphenicol. However, the production of this drug is uncertain given the low demand for stockpiles during inter-epidemic years. A single-dose treatment of ceftriaxone has been shown to be as effective as oily chloramphenicol and guidelines for its wider use are currently under development.

Pneumococcal meningitis

Benzylpenicillin (400 000 units/kg per day) is given 6-hourly i.v. or i.m., usually for 10 days. Chloramphenicol, but not oily chloramphenicol, can also be used in a regimen, as for meningococcal meningitis. The emergence of penicillin-resistant pneumococci is an increasing problem worldwide.[78–80] Meningitis due to such strains is unlikely to be treatable successfully by penicillin. In some cases these penicillin-resistant pneumococci, although susceptible to chloramphenicol in vitro, are not eradicated by chloramphenicol in vivo.[79]

H. influenzae meningitis

Chloramphenicol (75–100 mg/kg per day) should be given every 6 h parenterally and subsequently may be given orally. Treatment is usually continued for 10 days. Ampicillin (200 mg/kg per day)is an alternative although this may be associated with higher morbidity. Strains of H. influenzae (b) resistant to ampicillin (5–10%) or chloramphenicol (5%) and even to both antibiotics[81] are emerging.

Although penicillin and chloramphenicol have the advantage of cheapness and ready availability in tropical countries, a recent randomized open study in Finland demonstrated that cephalosporins such as cefotaxime or ceftriaxone had a clear advantage over chloramphenicol.[82] However, these cephalosporins can be expensive and none of the antibiotics was associated with a 100% cure rate.

Meningococcal septicaemia

The treatment of fulminant meningococcal septicaemia is difficult and requires intensive management. Clinical scoring systems such as the Glasgow Meningococcal Septicaemia Prognostic Score[83] are of value in assessing the severity of disease and identifying those at greatest risk of dying (Table 55.8). Its use has also been validated in a tropical setting.[84] If possible, patients should be artificially ventilated electively and given plasma and inotropes, such as dobutamine as well as penicillin. Dexamethasone does not alter the course of endotoxic shock.

Table 55.8 Glasgow Meningococcal Septicaemia Prognostic Score (GMSPS)

	Points[a]
Systolic blood pressure: <4 years, <75 mmHg; >4 years, <85 mmHg	3
Skin/rectal temperature difference >3°C	3
Modified coma scale score[b] <8 or deterioration of >3 points in 1 h	3
Deterioration in hour prior to scoring	2
Absence of *meningism*	2
Extending purpuric rash or widespread ecchymoses	1
Base deficit (capillary or arterial) >8.0	1

[a] A GMSPS of >8 predicts mortality with a sensitivity of 100% and specificity of 95%.
[b] Modified coma score. (1) *Eyes open*: spontaneously, 4; to speech, 3; to pain, 2; none, 1. (2) *Best verbal response*: orientated 6; words, 4; vocal sounds, 3; cries, 2; none, 1. (3) *Best motor response*: obeys commands, 6; localized pain, 4; moves to pain, 1; none, 1. Add scores in (1) (2) and (3) to obtain coma score.

Prevention

Chemoprophylaxis is used to prevent secondary cases of meningococcal and *H. influenzae* meningitis in household contacts of an index case. There is no evidence that it is beneficial in pneumococcal meningitis. Most trials of chemoprophylaxis use eradication of nasopharyngeal carriage of meningococci or *H. influenzae* as their endpoint and demonstrate benefit.[85]

N. meningitidis

Reports from the USA prior to the availability of vaccination and chemoprophylaxis show that secondary attack rates of 4–10% within households were common.[86] More recently it has been shown that 10% of patients presenting with meningococcal meningitis in Nigeria were secondary cases.[87] Two strategies are employed. In the first, phenoxymethyl-penicillin or amoxicillin is given as pre-emptive therapy for 7 days. The rationale for this is that most secondary cases occur in the first week after contact.[54] This will not affect nasopharyngeal carriage nor will it prevent secondary cases after therapy has ceased.

The second strategy aims to eradicate nasopharyngeal carriage. Antibiotics that are effective in eradicating susceptible nasopharyngeal meningococci include sulphadiazine, minocycline, rifampicin, ciprofloxacin or ceftriaxone.[85,88] Resistance to sulphonamides limits the value of these agents and minocycline has a high incidence of side-effects and cannot be used in children, pregnancy or lactation.

Rifampicin has been used in Africa[89] and does eradicate carriage. It is given as a 2-day regimen orally (600 mg twice daily for adults, 10 mg/kg per day for children of 1–12 years and 5 mg/kg per day for children under 1 year). Disadvantages include emergence of resistant meningococci during treatment[88] and the possibility of compromising the use of rifampicin as a first-line drug in tuberculosis. Ciprofloxacin (500–700 mg orally) or ceftriaxone

(125 mg i.m.) are given as single dose regimens and are as effective as rifampicin in eradicating carriage.[85] Unless sulphonamides are used, chemoprophylaxis can be expensive. To use vaccines would be much more cost-effective; however, vaccines are of no value in the immediate protection of household contacts since it will take 2 weeks or more to develop protective antibody levels.

H. influenzae

In the USA secondary attack rates in households by invasive *H. influenzae* in children under 5 years are 500–800 times greater than the endemic rate.[90] Chemoprophylaxis is by means of a 4-day regimen of rifampicin (20 mg/kg per day once daily). This is given to all household members where there is an index case and a child under 3 years, except for pregnant or lactating women and those with severe hepatic impairment.

Vaccine

The acidic capsular polysaccharides of each of the three bacteria are highly immunogenic and vaccines are available for all of them. The problem in using polysaccharide antigens is that they are T cell-independent antigens, which means that the antibody response is predominantly IgM and IgG_2 and immunological memory is poor.

The immunogenicity of such vaccines is particularly poor in infants and young children. For example, in children under 4 years old the group A meningococcal polysaccharide vaccine produced persistent protective antibody 1 year after immunization in 100%, in 52% after 2 years and 0% after 3 years, whereas in children of 4 years or older the corresponding figures were 85%, 75% and 67% respectively.[91] This, however, was with only one dose of vaccine and there is evidence that for Group A vaccine two or more doses are better.[92]

H. influenzae (b)

The capsular polysaccharide of *H. influenzae* (b) (Hib) is polyribitol phosphate. The problem of poor immunogenicity of the capsular antigen has been overcome by conjugating it to a protein (diphtheria or tetanus toxoid). This significantly improves the quantity and duration of antibody response, even in those under 2 years old.[93] The Hib vaccine can be given together with the triple (diphtheria, pertussis, tetanus) vaccine with no deleterious effects. Hib vaccine has been shown to have 74% efficacy in preventing invasive Hib infection and 76% efficacy in preventing Hib meningitis in children aged 18–59 months.[94] Routine immunization of infants in The Gambia with Hib conjugate vaccine reduced the annual incidence of Hib meningitis from over 200/100 000 children aged younger than 1 year (1990–93) to 0/100 000 in 2002, and from 60 to 0 in children <5 years old. It also eliminates oropharyngeal carriage and thus provides herd immunity.

N. meningitidis

A meningococcal vaccine incorporating groups A and C capsular polysaccharides (as well as Y and W 135) is available. Its use has proved effective in controlling epidemics of meningococcal disease in Asia, Africa and Latin America. Protective antibodies persist for up to 5 years in adults but only 1–2 years in children under 4 years old when given as a single dose regimen. The vaccine does not affect nasopharyngeal carriage[95] and thus does not provide herd immunity.

Recently, both conjugate Group A and conjugate Group C meningococcal vaccines have been introduced, which induce long-term immunological memory when given to infants.[96] The conjugate group C meningococcal vaccine was introduced into routine use in the UK and has been shown to have 92% and 97% protective efficacy in infants and adolescents respectively.[97] A conjugate A, C, W135 and Y vaccine is available in the USA, but as for other conjugate polysaccharide vaccines, they are much more expensive than the polysaccharide alone and not available for use in high incidence areas. Whether a conjugate Group A vaccine is needed has been questioned,[92] especially since in outbreaks in the meningitis belt adolescents and young adults represent the peak of the age spectrum. How the vaccine should be used in the meningitis belt has been an area of intense discussion for decades. Ideally a vaccine, probably conjugate, would be given to all infants to give life-long immunity.[98] A conjugate A vaccine is currently under development and is expected to be licensed by 2009. Although this vaccine is likely to change the characteristics of these epidemics, this is not possible at present and mass emergency immunization with the non-conjugate polysaccharide vaccine at the start of an epidemic is current WHO policy.[99] This policy requires good surveillance which is not always available and sets thresholds for interventions. In populations of over 30 000 an incidence of five cases per 100 000 population per week is an alert threshold when investigation and confirmation of cases is required and surveillance should be enhanced. If there have been no epidemics in the region, and vaccine coverage is less than 80% or it is early in the dry season, then mass immunization is introduced when the incidence reaches 10 cases/100 000 per week; otherwise the vaccination threshold is 15 cases per 100 000 per week. For populations under 30 000 the alert is two cases per week and vaccination threshold five cases per week or doubling of the number of cases in a 3-week period. In addition, alert thresholds become epidemic thresholds if there is an epidemic in a neighbouring area. Introduction of mass immunization is a major undertaking. It requires transport of vaccine, needles and syringes to the epidemic area, mobilization of large numbers of healthcare workers and gaining access to the population. If the thresholds are too high then the mass vaccination campaign may not begin until the epidemic is past its peak, if too low there may be false alarms. Others have concluded that an alert threshold of five cases/100 000 per week allows time to prepare for an epidemic and 10 cases/100 000 per week should signal mass vaccination.[100] Being able to predict when epidemics might occur based on satellite and meteorological data could be of great benefit in the meningitis belt until we are able to deliver conjugate vaccines as part of routine childhood immunization.[30]

The group B meningococcal capsule is a homopolymer of *N*-acetylneuraminic acid (as is the *E. coli* K1 capsule) and is a self-antigen being found on human neuronal glycoproteins and glycolipids. Thus there is no group B capsular vaccine. Vaccines incorporating group B meningococcal outer membrane proteins have worked well in Cuba[101] and New Zealand but less well in Chile or Norway.[102]

Str. pneumoniae

The pneumococcal polysaccharide vaccine incorporates 23 of the 84 pneumococcal capsular polysaccharides. These 23 serogroups are responsible for 90–95% of invasive pneumococcal disease. The vaccine is not widely used and suffers from the same problems as other polysaccharide vaccines. Its use is confined to those who are about to have splenectomy or in patients with sickle cell disease. Seven-valent and nine-valent polysaccharide conjugate vaccines have been developed which incorporate serogroups important in invasive disease and otitis media in developed countries, some of which are also important in the tropics.[103] Clinical trials so far have been directed towards prevention of otitis media and of bacteraemia and there are no data on prevention of pneumococcal meningitis in the tropics.

REFERENCES

1. Holt DE, Halket S, de Louvois J, et al. Neonatal meningitis in England and Wales: 10 years on. *Arch Dis Child Fetal Neonatal Ed* 2001; 84:F85–F89.
2. Hart CA, Cuevas LE. Meningococcal disease in Africa. *Ann Trop Med Parasitol* 1997; 91:777–785.
3. Hensey OJ, Hart CA, Cooke RWI. Serious infection in a neonatal intensive care unit. *J Hyg* 1985; 95:289–297.
4. Barcley B. High frequency of *Salmonella* species as a cause of neonatal meningitis in Ibadan, Nigeria. *Acta Paediatr Scand* 1971; 60:540–544.
5. Longe AC, Omene JA, Okolo AA. Neonatal meningitis in Nigerian infants. *Acta Paediatr Scand* 1984; 74:477–481.
6. Coovadia YM, Mayosi B, Adhikari M, et al. Hospital acquired neonatal meningitis: the impacts of cefotaxime usage on mortality and of amikacin usage on incidence. *Ann Trop Paediatr* 1989; 9:233–239.
7. Nel E. Neonatal meningitis: mortality, cerebrospinal fluid, and microbiological findings. *J Trop Pediatr* 2000; 46:237–239.
8. Chang Chien HY, Chiu NC, Li W C, et al. Characteristics of neonatal bacterial meningitis in a teaching hospital in Taiwan from 1984–1997. *J Microbiol Immunol Infect* 2000; 33:100–104.
9. Gebremariam A. Neonatal meningitis in Addis Ababa: a ten year review. *Ann Trop Paediatr* 1998; 18:279–283.
10. Molyneux E, Walsh A, Phiri A, et al. Acute bacterial meningitis in children admitted to the Queen Elizabeth Central Hospital, Blantyre, Malawi in 1996–1997. *Trop Med Int Health* 1998; 3:610–618.
11. Rajab A, de Louvois J. Survey of infection in babies at the Khoula Hospital, Oman. *Ann Trop Paediatr* 1990; 10:39–43.
12. Freedman RM, Ingram DL, Gross I, et al. A half century of neonatal sepsis at Yale: 1928 to 1978. *Am J Dis Child* 1981; 135:140–144.
13. Molyneux EM, Walsh AL, Malenga G, et al. *Salmonella* meningitis in children in Blantyre, Malawi, 1996–1999. *Ann Trop Paediatr* 2000; 20:41–44.
14. Halder D, Zainal N, Wah CM, et al. Neonatal meningitis and septicaemia caused by *Burkholderia pseudomallei. Ann Trop Paediatr* 1998; 18:161–164.
15. De Moraes Pinto MI, Verhoeff F, Milligan P, et al. Placental antibody transfer: influence of maternal HIV-infection and placental malaria. *Arch Dis Child Fetal Neonatal Ed* 1998; 79:F202–F205.
16. Overall JC. Neonatal bacterial meningitis: analysis of predisposing factors and outcome compared with matched control subjects. *J Pediatr* 1970; 76:499–508.
17. Berman PH, Bank BQ. Neonatal meningitis: a clinical and pathological study of 29 cases. *Pediatrics* 1996; 38:6–18.
18. McCracken GH, Shinefield HR. Changes in the pattern of neonatal septicaemia and meningitis. *Am J Dis Child* 1966; 112:33–41.
19. McCracken GH, Mize SG. A controlled study of intrathecal antibiotic therapy in Gram negative enteric meningitis of infancy. *J Pediatr* 1976; 89:66–74.
20. Doran TI. The role of Citrobacter in clinical disease of children: review. *Clin Infect Dis* 1999; 28:384–394.
21. Weber MW, Carlin JB, Gatchalain S, et al. Predictors of neonatal sepsis in developing countries. *Pediatr Infect Dis J* 2003; 22:711–716.
22. Sarff LD, Platt LH, McCracken GH. Cerebrospinal fluid evaluation in neonates. Comparison of high risk infants with and without meningitis. *J Pediatr* 1976; 88:473–479.
23. McCracken GH, Mize SG, Threlkeld N. Intraventricular gentamicin therapy in Gram negative bacillary meningitis of infancy. *Lancet* 1980; i:787–791.
24. Daoud AS, Batieha A, Al-Sheyyab M, et al. Lack of effectiveness of dexamethasone in neonatal bacterial meningitis. *Eur J Pediatr* 1999; 158:230–233.
25. Gray KJ, Bennett SL, French N, et al. Invasive group B streptococcal infection in infants, Malawi. *Emerg Infect Dis* 2007; 13:223–229.
26. Burman LG, Christensen P, Christensen K, et al. Prevention of excess neonatal morbidity associated with group B streptococci by vaginal chlorhexidine disinfection during labour. *Lancet* 1992; 340:65–69.
27. Taha TE, Biggar RJ, Broadhead RL, et al. Effect of cleansing the birth canal with antiseptic solution on maternal and new-born morbidity and mortality in Malawi: clinical trial. *BMJ* 1997; 315:216–220.
28. Webb DKH, Serjeant GR. Systemic Salmonella infections in sickle cell anaemia. *Ann Trop Pediatr* 1989; 3:169–172.
29. Moore PS. Meningococcal meningitis in sub-Saharan Africa: a model for the epidemic process. *Clin Infect Dis* 1992; 14:515–525.
30. Savory EC, Cuevas LE, Yassin MA, et al. Evaluation of the meningitis epidemics risk model in Africa. *Epidemiol Infect* 2006; 134:1047–1051.
31. Gagneux SP, Hodgson A, Smith T, et al. Prospective study of a serogroup X *Neisseria meningitidis* outbreak in Northern Ghana. *J Infect Dis*; 185: 618–626.
32. Molesworth AM, Thomson MC, Connor SJ, et al. Where is the meningitis belt? Defining an area at risk of epidemic meningitis in Africa. *Trans Roy Soc Trop Med Hyg* 2002; 96:242–249.
33. Liebowitz LD, Koornhof HJ, Barrett M, et al. Bacterial meningitis in Johannesburg—1980–1982. *S Afr Med J* 1984, 66:677–679.
34. Borgstein A. Pyogenic meningitis in children at Queen Elizabeth Central Hospital Blantyre. *Malawi Med Quart J* 1984; 17:26–27.
35. Cuevas LE, Hart CA. Acute bacterial meningitis in Malawi. *Malawi Med J* 1991; 7:2–6.
36. Dube SD, Shenderov BA. Incidence and pattern of bacterial meningitis in Lusaka. *Cent Afr J Med* 1983; 29:100–103.
37. Omanga U, Nethihinyurwa M, Shako D, et al. Aspects étiologiques et évolutifs des méningites purulentes de l'enfant à Kinshasa: analyse de 471 cases. *Méd d'Afrique Noire* 1980; 27:25–34.
38. Babalola AA, Coker AO. Pyogenic meningitis among Lagos children: causative organisms, age, sex and seasonal incidence. *Cent Afr J Med* 1982; 28:14–18.
39. Couprie F, Chippaux-Hyppolite C. Les méningites purulentes à Abidjan. *Méd Armées* 1977; 5:823–828.
40. Elzouki AY, Vesikari T. First international conference on infections in children in Arab countries. *Pediatr Infect Dis* 1985; 4:527–531.
41. Cadoz M, Denis F, Diop Mar I. Etude épidémiologique des cas de méningites purulentes hospitalisés à Dakar pendant la décennie 1970–79. *Bull World Health Organ* 1981; 59:575–584.
42. Behhassine M, Mered B. Les méningites purulentes en Algérie: étude bactériologique de 133 cas. *Arch Inst Pasteur Algér* 1969; 47:13–26.
43. Bhat BV, Verma IC, Puri RK, et al. Prognostic indicators in pyogenic meningitis. *Indian Pediatr* 1987; 24:977–983.
44. Choo KF, Ariffin WA, Ahmad T, et al. Pyogenic meningitis in hospitalized children in Kelantan Malaysia. *Ann Trop Paediatr* 1990; 10:89–98.
45. Sunakorn P, Lexomboon U, Sindhurat S. Acute bacterial meningitis at the children's hospital Bangkok. *J Med Assoc Thai* 1969; 52:1001–1011.

46. Naraqi S. Aetiology of acute bacterial meningitis in the highlands and islands of Papua New Guinea. *Papua New Guinea Med J* 1980; 23:108–110.

47. McKay T. Experience of changing antibiotic protocol in childhood bacterial meningitis in Vanuatu. *Trop Doct* 1989; 19:158–159.

48. Sharma A, Sharma D, Prabhakar P. Infectious meningitis at the university hospital of the West Indies. Review of clinical and laboratory findings (1965–1980). *West Indian Med* 1984; 33:14–30.

49. Munoz AI. Bacterial meningitis in pediatric patients: a five year experience. *Bol Assoc Med PR* 1982; 74:62–65.

50. Bryan JP, de Silva Hr, Ravares A, et al. Etiology and mortality of bacterial meningitis in North Eastern Brazil. *Rev Infect Dis* 1990; 12:128–135.

51. Juliet C, Rodriguez G, Marti A, et al. Meningitis bacteriana en el nino: experiencia con 441 casos. *Rev Med Chil* 1983; 111:690–698.

52. Cherigo-Quiros EZ, Rodriguez-French A. Meningitis bacteriana en Hospital Santo Tomas (1975–1982). *Rev Med Panama* 1984; 9:35–44.

53. Bohr V, Hansen B, Jessen O, et al. Eight hundred and seventy five cases of bacterial meningitis. I: Clinical data, prognosis and the role of specialized hospital departments. *J Infect* 1983; 7:21–30.

54. De Wals P, Hertoghe L, Boree-Grimee I, et al. Meningococcal disease in Belgium. Secondary attack rate among household, day-care nursery and pre-elementary school contacts. *J Infect* 1981; 3(suppl I):53–61.

55. Taha MK, Achtman M, Alonso JM, et al. Serogoup W135 in meningococcal disease in Hajj pilgrims. *Lancet* 2000; 356:2159.

56. Caugant DA, Froholm LO, Bovre K, et al. Intercontinental spread of a genetically distinctive complex of clones of *Neisseria meningitidis* causing epidemic disease. *Proc Natl Acad Sci USA* 1986, 83.4927–4931.

57. Maiden MCJ, Bygraves JA, Foil E, et al. Multilocus sequence typing: A portable approach to the identification of clones within populations of pathogenic microorganisms. *Proc Natl Acad Sci USA* 1998; 95: 3140–3145.

58. Moore PS, Hierholzer J, De Witt W, et al. Respiratory viruses and mycoplasma as cofactors for epidemic group A meningococcal meningitis. *JAMA* 1990; 264:1271–1275.

59. Adams RD, Kubik CS, Bonner FJ. The clinical and pathological aspects of influenzal meningitis. *Arch Pediatr* 1948; 65:354–376.

60. Geisler PJ, Nelson KE. Bacterial meningitis without clinical signs of meningeal irritation. *South Med J* 1982; 75:448–450.

61. Riordan FAI, Marzouk O, Thomson APJ, et al. Changing presentation of meningococcal disease. *Eur J Pediatr* 1995; 154:472–474.

62. Salih MAM, Ahmed HS, Karrar ZA, et al. Features of a large epidemic of group A meningococcal meningitis in Khartoum, Sudan in 1988. *Scand J Infect Dis* 1990; 22:161–170.

63. Whittle HC, Greenwood BM. Meningococcal meningitis in the northern savanna of Africa. *Trop Doct* 1976; 6:99–104.

64. Fellick JM, Sills JA, Marzouk O, et al. Neurodevelopmental outcome in meningococcal disease: a case-control study. *Arch Dis Child* 2001; 85:6–11.

65. Cuevas LE, Hart CA, Mughogho G. Latex particle agglutination tests as an adjunct to the diagnosis of bacterial meningitis: a study from Malawi. *Ann Trop Med Parasitol* 1989; 83:375–379.

66. Holland SJ, Marzouk O, Thomson APJ, et al. Sensitivity and specificity of serum antigen detection for diagnosis of meningococcal disease in children. *Serodiagn Immunother Infect Dis* 1990; 4:345–349.

67. Berkley JA, Mwangi I, Ngetsa CJ, et al. Diagnosis of acute bacterial meningitis in children at a district hospital in sub-Saharan Africa. *Lancet* 2001; 357:1753–1757.

68. McIntyre PB, Berkey CS, King SM, et al. Dexamethasone as adjunctive therapy in bacterial meningitis. A meta-analysis of randomized clinical trials since 1988. *JAMA* 1997; 278:925–931.

69. Girgis NI, Farid Z, Mikhail IA, et al. Dexamethasone treatment for bacterial meningitis in children and adults. *Pediatr Infect Dis J* 1989; 8:848–851.

70. Qazi SA, Khan MA, Mughal N, et al. Dexamethasone and bacterial meningitis in Pakistan. *Arch Dis Child* 1996; 75:482–488.

71. Macaluso A, Pivetta S, Maggi RS, et al. Dexamethasone adjunctive therapy for bacterial meningitis in children: a retrospective study in Brazil. *Ann Trop Paediatr* 1996; 16:193–198.

72. Shembesh NM, Elbargathy SM, Kashbur IM, et al. Dexamethasone as adjunctive treatment of bacterial meningitis. *Ind J Pediatr* 1997; 64: 517–522.

73. Shann F, Barker J, Poore P. Chloramphenicol alone versus chloramphenicol plus penicillin for bacterial meningitis in children. *Lancet* 1985; ii:681–701.

74. Pecoul B, Varine F, Keita M, et al. Long acting chloramphenicol versus intravenous ampicillin for treatment of bacterial meningitis. *Lancet* 1991; 388:862–866.

75. Lewis RF, Dorlencourt F, Pinel J. Long-acting oily chloramphenicol for meningococcal meningitis. *Lancet* 1998; 352:823.

76. Gedde-Dahl TW, Hoiby EA, Eskerud J. Unbiased evidence on early treatment of suspected meningococcal disease. *Rev Infect Dis* 1990; 12:973–992.

77. Esso DV, Fontanals D, Uriz S. *Neisseria meningitidis* strains with decreased susceptibility to penicillin. *Pediatr Infect Dis* 1987; 6:438–439.

78. Allen KD. Penicillin-resistant pneumococci. *J Hosp Infect* 1991; 17:3–13.

79. Friedland IR, Klugman KP. Failure of chloramphenicol therapy in penicillin-resistant pneumococcal meningitis. *Lancet* 1992; 339:405–408.

80. Yomo A, Subramanyam VR, Fudzulani R, et al. Carriage of penicillin-resistant pneumococci in Malawian children. *Ann Trop Paediatr* 1997; 17:239–243.

81. Coovadia YM, Coovadia HM, van den Ende J. Meningitis due to beta-lactamase producing, chloramphenicol resistant *Haemophilus influenzae* type b in South Africa. *J Infect* 1986; 12:247–249.

82. Peltola H, Anttila M, Renkonen OK. Randomized comparison of chloramphenicol, ampicillin, cefotaxime and ceftriaxone for childhood bacterial meningitis. *Lancet* 1989; i:1281–1287.

83. Thomson APJ, Sills JA, Hart CA. Validation of the Glasgow Meningococcal Septicaemia Prognostic Score. A ten year retrospective survey. *Crit Care Med* 1991; 19:26–30.

84. Silva PSL, Fonseca MCM, Iglesias SBO, et al. Comparison of two different severity scores (Paediatric Risk of Mortality [PRISM] and the Glasgow Meningococcal Prognostic Score [GMSPS]) in meningococcal disease. *Ann Trop Paediatr* 2001; 21:135–140.

85. Correia JB, Hart CA. Meningococcal disease. *Clinical Evidence Concise* 2006; 16:344–347.

86. French MR. Epidemiological study of 383 cases of meningococcal meningitis in the city of Milwaukee, 1927, 1928 and 1929. *Am J Public Health* 1931; 21:130–138.

87. Greenwood BM, Bradley AK, Cleland PG. An epidemic of meningococcal meningitis at Zaria, Northern Nigeria. *Trans R Soc Trop Med Hyg* 1979; 73:557–573.

88. Cuevas LE, Hart CA. Chemoprophylaxis of bacterial meningitis. *J Antimicrob Chemother* 1993; 31:79–91.

89. Blakebrough IS, Gilles HM. The effect of rifampicin on meningococcal carriage in family contacts in northern Nigeria. *J Infect* 1980; 2:137–143.

90. Glode MP, Daum RS, Goldmann DA, et al. *Haemophilus influenzae* type b meningitis: a contagious disease in children. *BMJ* 1980; i:899–901.

91. Reingold AC, Broome CV, Hightower AW, et al. Age specific differences in duration of clinical protection after vaccination with meningococcal polysaccharide A vaccine. *Lancet* 1985; ii:114–118.

92. Robbins JB, Schneerson R, Gotschlich EC. A rebuttal: epidemic and endemic meningococcal meningitis in sub-Saharan Africa can be prevented now by routine immunization with group A meningococcal capsular polysaccharide vaccine. *Pediatr Infect Dis J* 2000; 19:945–953.

93. Booy R, Moxon ER. Immunization of infants against *Haemophilus influenzae* type b in the UK. *Arch Dis Child* 1991; 66:1251–1254.

94. Wenger JD, Pierce R, Deaver KA, et al. Efficacy of *Haemophilus influenzae* type (b) polysaccharide-diphtheria toxoid conjugate vaccine in US children aged 18–59 months. *Lancet* 1991; 338:395–398.

95. Blakebrough IS, Greenwood BM, Whittle HC, et al. Failure of meningococcal vaccination to stop the transmission of meningococci in Nigerian schoolboys. *Ann Trop Med Parasitol* 1983; 77: 175–178.

96. MacLennan J, Obaro S, Deeks J, et al. Immunologic memory 5 years after meningococcal A/C conjugate vaccination in infancy. *J Infect Dis* 2001; 183:97–104.

Table 56.1 Historical clinical descriptions of tuberculosis

Description	Clinical type of tuberculosis
Consumption	Pulmonary
Pthisis	Pulmonary
Tabes pulmonalis	Pulmonary
Tissic	Pulmonary
Hectic fever	Pulmonary
Asthenia	Pulmonary
Galloping consumption	Pulmonary
Scrofula	Cervical lymphadenitis
Struma	Cervical lymphadenitis
King's evil	Cervical lymphadenitis
Hydrocephalus (acute or infantile)	Tuberculous meningitis
Pott's disease	Spinal/vertebral tuberculosis
Tuberculous chancre	Skin
Scrofuloderma	Skin
Lupus vulgaris	Skin

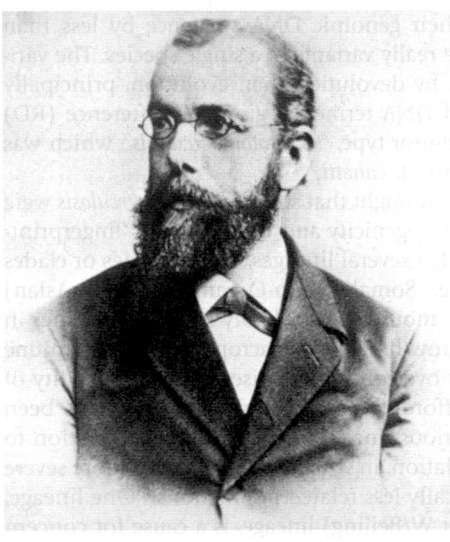

Figure 56.1
Professor Robert Koch, discoverer of *Mycobacterium tuberculosis*.

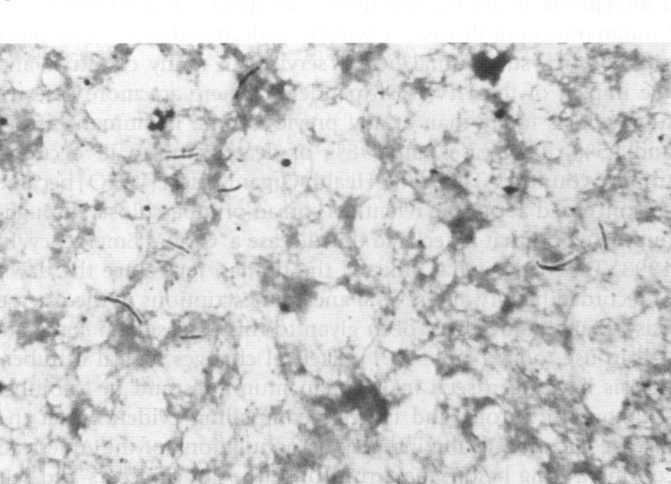

A

B

Figure 56.2 (A) Ziehl–Neelsen staining of a sputum sample and (B) a bronchoalveolar lavage washing showing acid-fast bacilli.

PATHOGENESIS

Infection of humans with *M. tuberculosis* occurs by inhalation, ingestion or traumatic inoculation. Intrauterine infection resulting in congenital tuberculosis is extremely rare.

In most cases infection is by inhalation of small droplets of cough spray containing a few bacilli. These particles, around 5 μm in diameter, lodge in the alveolae or small airways, mostly in the lower regions of the lung. The usual sources of such infectious particles are other human beings with open pulmonary tuberculosis but those working with cattle may be infected by *M. bovis* in the cough spray of diseased animals. A less frequent mode of infection is consumption of milk or food contaminated by *M. bovis*, in which case the bacilli often lodge in the tonsil or intestinal wall. Rarely, tubercle bacilli enter the skin through cuts and abrasions (Figure 56.3) and primary skin tuberculosis was an occupational hazard of butchers, anatomists and pathologists.

Traditionally, tuberculosis has been divided into two forms, primary and post-primary. In the past it was usually assumed that post-primary tuberculosis was always the result of endogenous reactivation of latent or dormant primary lesions but DNA fingerprinting has shown that many cases, particularly among immunosuppressed persons, are due to exogenous reinfection.[5]

The natural history of infection with *M. tuberculosis* and its sequelae are shown diagrammatically in Figure 56.4. Most people infected by tubercle bacilli do not develop symptoms and the primary infection may go unnoticed. In most cases, effective immune responses lead to containment of the disease process and

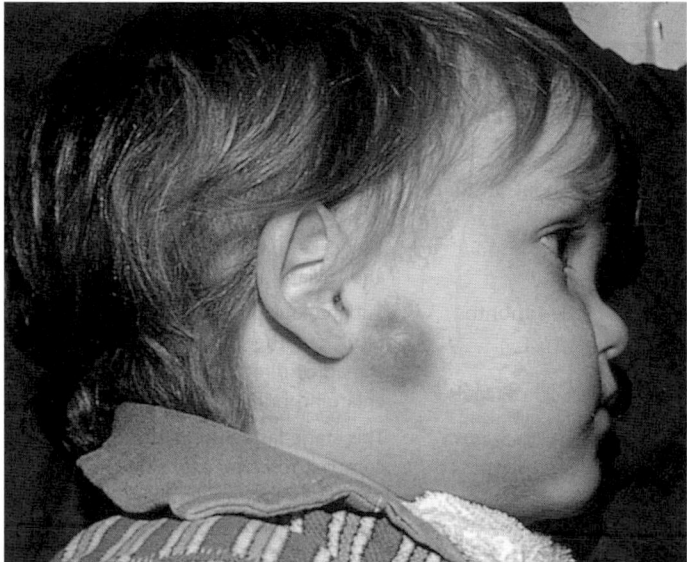

Figure 56.3 Primary tuberculous lesion of the skin.

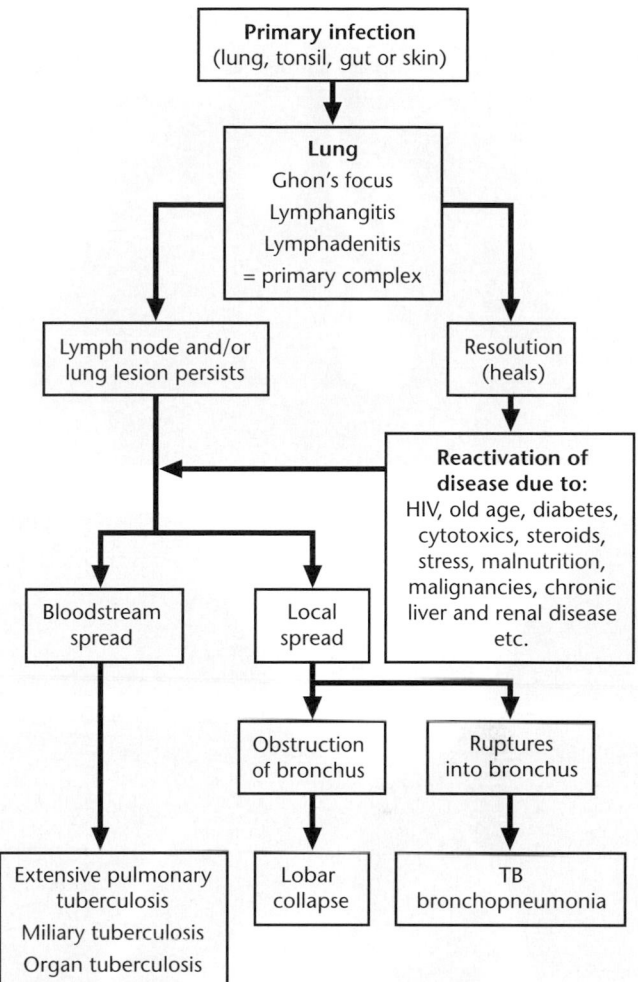

Figure 56.4 Natural history and sequelae of tuberculosis infection.

life-long immunity. As a general rule, 2–5% of persons infected develop clinically evident primary tuberculosis and a further 2–5% subsequently develop post-primary disease. Little is known of the early events following initial infection and our limited understanding is derived from experimental observations in animals. In the case of pulmonary infection, the bacilli are initially engulfed by alveolar macrophages in which they multiply, eventually killing the cell. Additional blood-borne phagocytic cells, both macrophages and polymorphonuclear leucocytes, aggregate around the focus of infection and form a foreign body granuloma termed the *primary focus* or, in the older literature, the *Ghon focus*. Some bacilli are transported to the regional lymph nodes (the mediastinal, paratracheal and, occasionally, the supraclavicular nodes when the primary focus is in the lung) where secondary lesions develop. The combination of the primary focus and the local lymphatic component – lymphangitis and lymphadenopathy – is termed the *primary complex* (Figure 56.5). Bacilli may subsequently enter the bloodstream and lodge in various organs of the body and cause the various non-pulmonary forms of primary tuberculosis.

In most cases in which the immune response enables the primary complex to contain the infection, the lesions become fibrotic and may subsequently become calcified but tubercle bacilli are able to persist within these dormant lesions, and also possibly in surrounding normal tissue, for years or decades. The nature of these 'persisters' has generated much speculation. Some researchers postulate that they are truly dormant until reactivated by a 'wake-up call' while others suggest that they replicate, albeit slowly, but are destroyed by immune mechanisms at roughly the same rate.

In a minority of those infected, overt primary tuberculosis manifests in a number of ways (Figure 56.6) and local or systemic spread may occur. Primary foci at the periphery of the lung may rupture into the pleural cavity, causing a self-limiting pleural effusion or a much more serious empyema. Diseased mediastinal lymph nodes may rupture into the pericardial cavity, causing tuberculous pericarditis, or into a bronchus, causing a spreading endobronchial infection. Enlarged mediastinal lymph nodes may, particularly in young children, press on the major bronchi, causing partial or total obstruction and pulmonary collapse, a condition termed epituberculosis (Figure 56.7). The primary lesion may progress to tuberculous pneumonia with tissue destruction, especially when immunity is compromised. Alternatively, it may gradually enlarge to form a circular 'coin lesion' which may progress to a characteristic post-primary lesion or heal with calcification. Concentric rings of calcification, resulting from alternating periods of progression and healing, may be seen. Primary lesions in the tonsils spread to cervical nodes (Figure 56.8), from which local and systemic spread may occur.

Haematogenous dissemination following infection leads to serious, often fatal, non-pulmonary disease, principally involving the central nervous system, bones and kidneys. Observations in the pre-antituberculosis therapy era, notably by Wallgren,[6] revealed a sequence of events, or 'timetable', of primary tuberculosis, as shown in Table 56.2. This is only a rough guide and many individual variations occur. Young children are very prone to overt disease following infection but those between the age of 5 years and the onset of puberty appear to be relatively protected – the 'safe school age'.

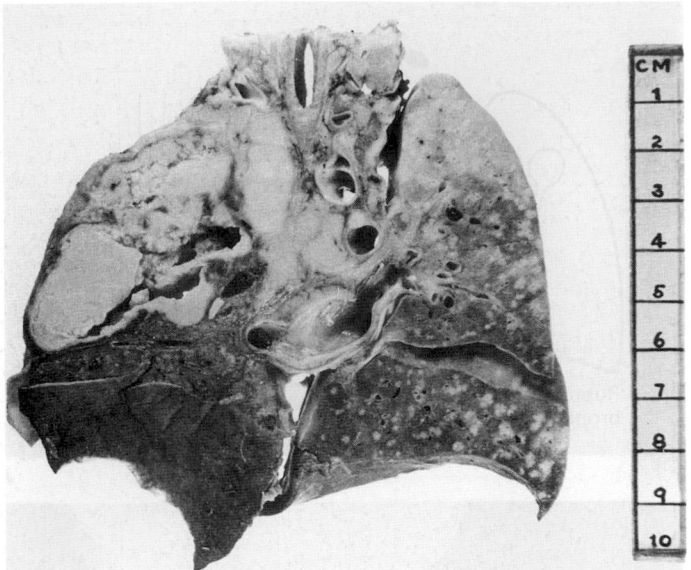

Figure 56.7 Progressive primary tuberculosis. Postmortem specimen of the lungs of a 6-month-old child showing extensive caseous necrosis, enlarged hilar lymph nodes and numerous tuberculous lesions throughout the lung fields.

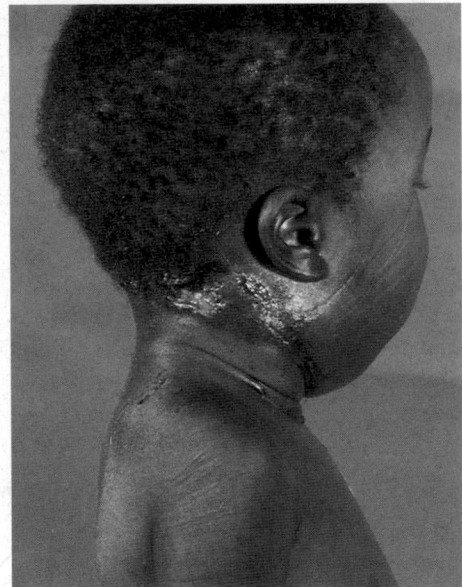

Figure 56.8 Caseating cervical lymph nodes in child with tuberculosis.

When bacilli gain access to the bronchi and are expectorated in the sputum, the patient becomes infectious and is said to have open tuberculosis. Bacilli escaping from the cavities may infect other parts of the same and the other lung by endobronchial spread. A typical radiological appearance of post-primary pulmonary tuberculosis is of one or more apical cavities and numerous smaller lesions in the other lung fields (Figure 56.9). Bacilli in the sputum may also lodge in the larynx, causing tuberculous laryngitis, or may be swallowed and cause indurating ulcers in the intestinal tract and, rarely, anal fistulae. In contrast to primary tuberculosis, the post-primary lesions are usually so walled off by fibrosis that lymphatic and haematogenous dissemination of disease is unusual. Both cavity formation and the localization of disease are due to immune processes and, as described below, are compromised in immunosuppressed patients.

PATHOLOGY OF TUBERCULOSIS

A wide spectrum of pathological manifestations is seen in tuberculosis. The initial host response to infection consists of an acute inflammatory reaction with an influx of polymorphonuclear neutrophil leucocytes. If this acute inflammatory response is unable to limit the infectious process, a progressive infiltration with macrophages occurs. The macrophages have a pale eosinophilic cytoplasm and elongated nuclei and as they resemble epithelial cells they are called epithelioid cells. Some macrophages fuse to form multinucleated 'Langhans giant cells'. A zone of lymphocytes and fibroblasts surrounds this compact cellular structure which is termed the 'tubercle' as it resembles a small potato tuber (Figure 56.10A). The tubercle is an example of a granuloma, a characteristic feature of chronic infections. Within 2 weeks, caseous necrosis is seen in the centres of the granulomas but this is also seen in other chronic infections, including deep-seated fungal infections (e.g. *Histoplasma capsulatum*) and thus a specific diagnosis, based on the determination of the aetiological agent, is important.

Granuloma formation is a central event in the immune response against *M. tuberculosis*, but while the granuloma restricts the spread of the infection, it is a space-occupying lesion that can damage surrounding normal tissues. Granulomas are dynamic structures characterized by the accumulation of activated macrophages and an infiltration of T lymphocytes. The extent and morphological features of the granuloma vary considerably from person to person so that a wide spectrum of granulomatous reactions is seen in tuberculosis. At one end of this spectrum, characterized by compromised immune responses, there is poor granuloma formation and extensive areas of tissue necrosis containing large numbers of mycobacteria. At the other end, in which immune responses are relatively intact, indolent non-caseating granulomas containing few organisms are seen. The latter are typically seen in chronic skin tuberculosis (lupus vulgaris) and histologically the lesions resemble those seen in tuberculoid leprosy and sarcoidosis. Most tuberculosis patients fall between these two extremes.

The tuberculous process may involve serous cavities, usually the pleural cavities but sometimes the pericardial cavity. Such involvement appears to be primarily due to a hypersensitivity reaction to antigens of the tubercle bacillus and is characterized by an inflammatory, fibrin-rich exudate containing lymphocytes and polymorphonuclear leucocytes. Epithelioid and Langhans giant cells are scanty.

In the majority of cases, effective immune responses limit the progression of the primary complex which heals by fibrosis and

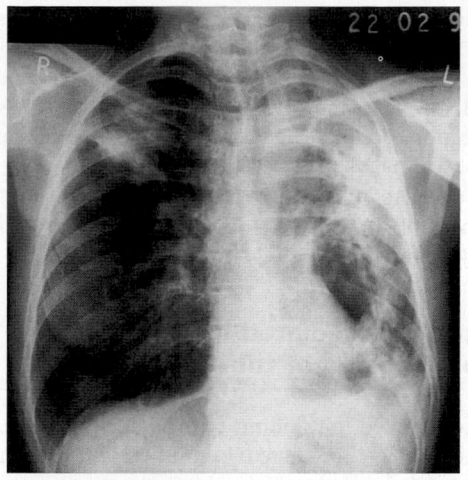

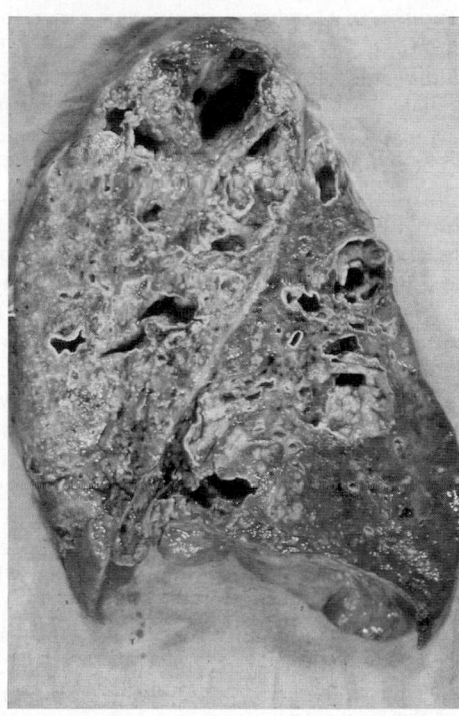

Figure 56.9 (A) Extensive pulmonary tuberculosis with cavitation. (B) Postmortem lung showing several cavities and extensive lung involvement due to tuberculosis.

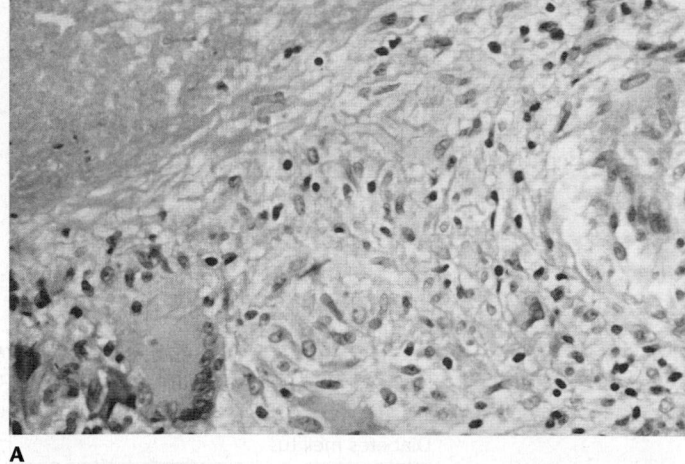

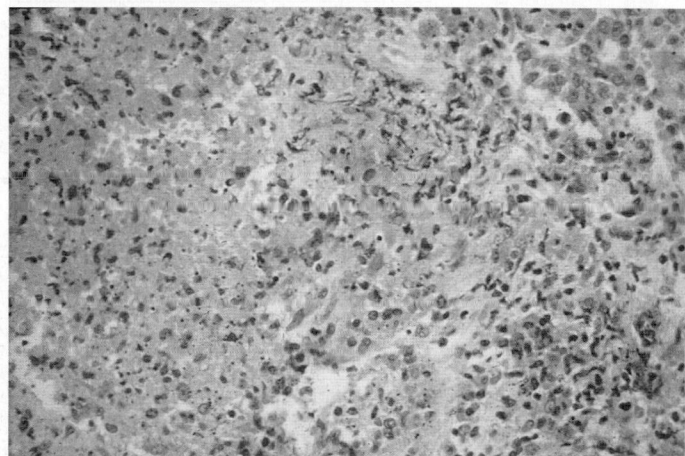

Figure 56.10 (A) Classical caseating granuloma due to *M. tuberculosis*. Note the central area of caseous necrosis surrounded by a rim of epithelioid cells, Langhans giant cells and lymphocytic infiltrate. (B) Lung histopathology illustrating an 'anergic response' to infection with *M. tuberculosis* in a lung of a patient with AIDS. There is widespread granular necrosis and a non-reactive 'anergic' cellular response with a few lymphocytes and epithelioid cells and no Langhans giant cells.

may eventually calcify. Alternatively, it may soften and enlarge with individual necrotic foci tending to coalesce, resulting in large areas of necrotic debris. The surrounding granulomatous reaction and associated scarring assist in localization of the infection.

Expression of clinical disease

The variety of clinical presentations of pulmonary tuberculosis seen in clinical practice reflects a complex series of interactions between mycobacteria, cells of the immune system and their secreted cytokines. Mild and self-limiting disease is associated with protective cellular immune responses whereas advanced disease is associated with immune suppression and inappropriate cell-mediated hypersensitivity reactions which cause tissue damage and immunopathology.

HOST IMMUNE RESPONSES TO *M. TUBERCULOSIS*

Many factors including host genetics, microbial virulence and disturbances in host immunity (Table 56.3) determine whether infection by *M. tuberculosis* is contained or progresses to overt disease, whether it follows an acute or chronic course and whether lesions

Table 56.3 Factors affecting susceptibility to tuberculosis

Age	Extremes of age: below the age of 5 years, and old age
Geographical origin	Asians, Africans, North American Indians
Immune suppression	HIV infection
	Protein-calorie malnutrition
	Steroid therapy
	Cytotoxic drugs
	Congenital immunodeficiencies
	Vitamin D deficiency
Medical conditions	Liver failure
	Cancer
	Diabetes mellitus
	Smoking-related lung damage
	Industrial dust disease of the lungs, e.g. silicosis, asbestosis
	Renal failure
	Measles
	Schistosomiasis
	Gastrectomy
Genetic factors	HLA-DR allele, NRAMP gene, vitamin D receptors
Stress	Excess corticosteroid production
Environmental factors	Exposure to populations of environmental mycobacteria
Mycobacterial factors	Strain variation in virulence

Adapted from Zumla A, Mwaba P, Rook G, et al. Tuberculosis. In: James DG, Zumla A, eds. *The Granulomatous Disorders*. Cambridge: Cambridge University Press; 1999:132–160.

are localized or widespread.[7] There is a constant battle between the various immune defence mechanisms of the host and strategies developed by the pathogen for evading these mechanisms. Although in recent years much light has been shed on what is clearly a very complex interplay of specific and non-specific immune phenomena in tuberculosis, the reasons why the immune system in most people is capable of preventing active disease but is not capable of clearing the infection are not fully understood. Many basic questions remain unanswered regarding the host-organism interactions:

1. What are the mechanisms of protective immunity to *M. tuberculosis*?
2. Why do only a small proportion of people who are infected go on to develop clinical disease?
3. In those who develop disease, why does tuberculosis manifest as a spectrum of clinical forms?
4. Why can mycobacteria survive for such long periods of time in host tissues?
5. Why do some patients with apparently normal immune systems develop disease?

Both non-specific and specific effector mechanisms appear to play a role in protective immunity to tuberculosis.

Non-specific immune effector mechanisms

When *M. tuberculosis* bacilli are inhaled they pass through the upper and lower respiratory tract and reach the alveoli, where initial infection occurs. The mycobacteria are phagocytosed by alveolar macrophages, phagocytosis being facilitated by surfactant apoprotein A. This initial interaction can result in destruction of the organism or persistence and replication of the organism within the macrophage.

Protective cell-mediated immunity and immunopathology in tuberculosis

It is now recognized that killing of mycobacteria in humans is a manifestation of cell-mediated immunity rather than antibody production and that helper T lymphocytes are of crucial importance in the induction of such protective immunity. Although antibody responses to *M. tuberculosis* antigens occur, their role in protective immunity, if any, is unclear. As well as mediating protective immunity, it has long been recognized that T lymphocytes may also mediate harmful tissue-destroying hypersensitivity reactions that favour progression of disease. The paradox of a single type of cell mediating such different immune phenomena was resolved by the discovery that T helper cells mature along at least two different pathways to produce populations of Th1 and Th2 lymphocytes. The Th1 and Th2 lymphocyte subsets produce or induce quite different cytokines termed, respectively, type 1 and type 2. The former include the interleukins IL-2, IL-12 and interferon-gamma (IFNγ) and the latter include IL-4, -5, -6, -10 and -13.

Studies on animal models and humans show that type 1 cytokines are responsible for the activation of macrophages and granuloma formation. IFNγ plays a major role in the activation of macrophages, the principal effector cells in the killing of mycobacteria. Macrophage activation also requires vitamin D, which explains the higher incidence of tuberculosis in those with low levels of this vitamin, a phenomenon seen particularly in vegetarians a few years after migrating from sunny countries to more gloomy and dismal environments, such as the UK.[8] Factors contributing to the aggregation of activated macrophages and other cells into the compact structure termed the granuloma are not clearly defined but animal models show that cytokines play a prominent role. In tuberculosis, the type 1 cytokines IL-2 and IFNγ and also tumour necrosis factor alpha and beta (TNFα and TNFβ) are essential for granuloma formation.

By contrast, type 2 cytokines are, directly or indirectly, associated with impaired granuloma formation. Also, a Th2 response appears to lead to the gross tissue necrosis that is so characteristic of tuberculosis, particularly the post-primary type. If mice are pre-immunized so that they have a mixed response that is mostly Th1 but includes a Th2 component they are more susceptible to the disease than are non-immunized controls. Although TNFα is essential for granuloma formation, in the presence of even small amounts of type 2 cytokines it has the opposing property of causing the tissue damage. An excess of TNFα appears to account for several symptoms of tuberculosis, including fever, lassitude and the characteristic wasting (consumption or cachexia) and an older name for TNFα is cachectin. Evidence that these symptoms may indeed depend on TNFα in human tuberculosis has come from the experimental use of thalidomide, which decreases the half-life of the mRNA for this cytokine. Patients treated with thalidomide show rapid symptomatic relief and weight gain.

Thus, depending on the pattern of cytokines generated by the immune responses in tuberculosis, TNFα has the opposing effects of aiding protective granuloma formation and mediating harmful immunopathological phenomena.

There is some evidence that other mechanisms contribute to protective immunity in tuberculosis, including CD8+ cytotoxic T lymphocytes, γ/δ T cells and natural killer (NK) cells. These may protect by causing programmed cell death, or apoptosis, of infected macrophages, a process accompanied by metabolic changes that destroy at least some of the contained bacilli.

Factors determining the nature of the immune response in tuberculosis

The findings that the immune responses, protective or harmful, are determined to a major extent by the Th1 and Th2 responses raise the question of which factors regulate the patterns of T lymphocyte maturation. Although details are far from clear, hormonal and environmental factors appear to have key roles.

Hormonal factors in tuberculosis

Before the age of 5 years, children are highly susceptible to tuberculosis but they tend to develop consolidation and pneumonia, without cavitation or caseous necrosis. Between the ages of 5 and 10 (i.e. during adrenarche) children appear to be resistant to the disease in spite of an increasing incidence of tuberculin test positivity indicative of continuing exposure to infection in this age group. This interval between the ages of 5 and 10 was known as the 'safe school age' in nineteenth-century Europe, and the phenomenon is currently observed in high-incidence areas such as Cape Town, South Africa. Susceptibility returns at puberty, but the type of disease now resembles that seen in adults, with typical cavitation and necrosis. These temporal changes suggest an underlying endocrinological cause. A reasonable hypothesis, for which there are supportive animal data, is that the three periods correspond to age-related changes in the ratio of cortisol to the anti-glucocorticoid hormone, dehydroepiandrosterone (DHEA).[9] In this context, there is evidence that a preponderance of cortisol, relative to DHEA, is able to induce a drift of T lymphocyte maturation towards the Th2 type. Excess cortisol production is a feature of stress and this may account for the many reports in the older literature of a link between stress and a higher risk of active tuberculosis.

Environmental factors

From the time of birth, humans are exposed to a huge range of microorganisms in the environment, including many species of saprophytic mycobacteria and members of related genera. Contact with these is able to modify the pattern of immune responsiveness to pathogenic mycobacteria and to BCG vaccine. Indeed, such environmental contact provides the most likely explanation for the considerable geographical variation in the protective efficacy of BCG vaccination (p. 1033). Recent observations suggest that

environmental mycobacteria and related species modify immune responses by activating Toll-like receptors (TLRs): a group of cell membrane proteins that bind to certain commonly occurring microbial components, termed adjuvants.[10] Activation of TLRs plays a key role in the maturation and correct functioning of the various cells that process epitopes and present them to the relevant T cell populations, thereby determining the subsequent maturation pathways of the T lymphocytes. This raises the possibility of using bacterial or synthetic adjuvants to modify the pattern of immune responsiveness in tuberculosis and possibly other diseases for therapeutic purposes.[11]

Role of macrophages

As mentioned above, cytokine-activated macrophages play a key role in the destruction of mycobacteria, although the precise mechanisms involved are not clear. Likely mechanisms involve the generation of toxic oxygen- and nitrogen-derived products including superoxide anions, hydrogen peroxide, and nitric oxide (NO) and peroxynitrites produced by the interaction of NO and oxygen/reduction products.

It is also likely that the entire granuloma has greater antimycobacterial properties than the isolated activated macrophage, as the centres of the granulomas are acidic, anoxic and contain high levels of free fatty acids, all of which inhibit mycobacterial growth. Once a cavity has formed and the anoxic and acidic contents have been replaced by air enriched with carbon dioxide, bacterial growth increases enormously.

Mycobacterial factors

Mycobacteria have evolved several strategies for avoiding the various host defence mechanisms and a large number of determinants of virulence have been described in M. tuberculosis.[12] Some of these are involved in early events after infection and others are of more importance at later stages. It is probable that the relative importance of determinants of virulence varies according to the lineage or family of the bacillus as they appear, at least in the mouse, to elicit different patterns of immune responsiveness. Of prime importance is the ability of mycobacteria to avoid being killed by phagocytes (Figure 56.11). Within the macrophage, survival of mycobacteria depends principally on their ability to inhibit phagosome maturation and to block phagosome-lysosome fusion.[13]

Advances in genomic analysis have revealed the molecular basis of differences between the attenuated BCG vaccine strains and virulent tubercle bacilli. Several regions of the genome are missing from BCG and one of these contains three genes associated with virulence, two of which code an immunodominant antigen ESAT-6 (Early Secretory Antigenic Target, 6 kDa), which is involved in tissue invasion.[14]

EPIDEMIOLOGY OF TUBERCULOSIS

As discussed above, not all those who are infected develop overt tuberculosis, and the interval between infection and disease may be years or decades. On the basis of skin-testing surveys, the WHO has estimated that one-third of the world's human population,

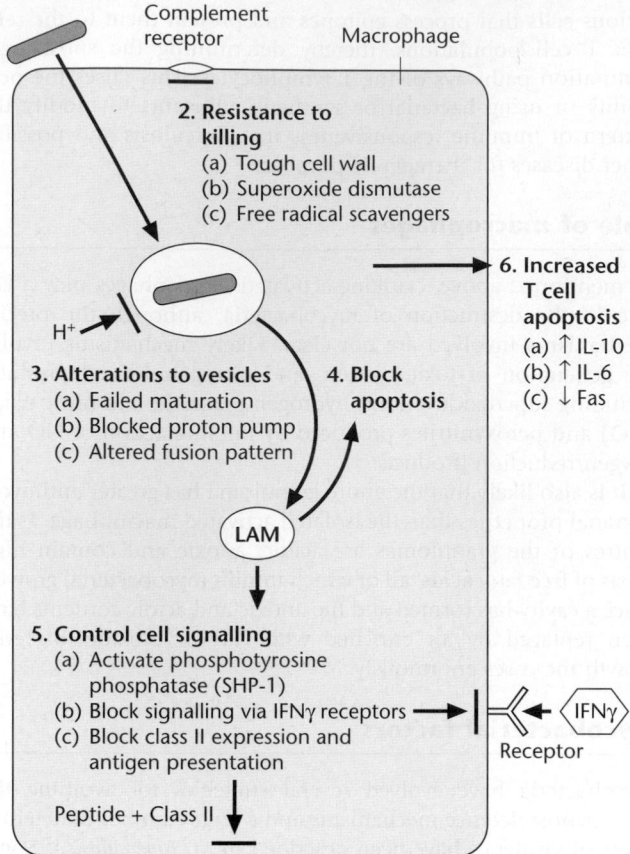

1. Blocking uptake mechanism
(a) Via Mannose receptor
(b) Block Ca^{2+} signalling by complement receptor

2. Resistance to killing
(a) Tough cell wall
(b) Superoxide dismutase
(c) Free radical scavengers

3. Alterations to vesicles
(a) Failed maturation
(b) Blocked proton pump
(c) Altered fusion pattern

4. Block apoptosis

5. Control cell signalling
(a) Activate phosphotyrosine phosphatase (SHP-1)
(b) Block signalling via IFNγ receptors
(c) Block class II expression and antigen presentation

6. Increased T cell apoptosis
(a) ↑ IL-10
(b) ↑ IL-6
(c) ↓ Fas

Figure 56.11 Mechanisms of survival of *M. tuberculosis* in macrophages. *M. tuberculosis* avoids the killing mechanisms in macrophages and blocks apoptosis of macrophages, presumably because apoptosis also can lead to death of the contained bacteria. Bad is a pro-apoptotic protein, inactivated when phosphorylated. LAM has multiple roles, including activation of SHP-1, a phosphotyrosine phosphatase intimately involved in cell signalling pathways. Downregulation of Fas, together with increased expression of Fas ligand, may lead the macrophage to signal apoptosis to Fas-positive T cells. Short thick lines indicate blocked pathways. IFN, interferon; IL, interleukin; LAM, lipoarabinomannan; TGF, transforming growth factor; TNFr2, tumour necrosis factor receptor 2.

around 2000 million people, are infected by tubercle bacilli. The percentage of the population infected varies from region to region: in Western Europe, around 11% are infected, mostly elderly persons, while in some tropical countries over half may be infected, including a much higher proportion of younger people.

Infection is spread predominantly by those with 'open', cavitating, post-primary pulmonary tuberculosis. Thus those positive on microscopy are much more likely to be infectious than those who are negative. Only a small minority of children are infectious. The number of persons infected by a source case is termed the *contagion parameter*. On average, an untreated source case infects between 10 and 15 people every year but the actual number varies greatly and is affected by many factors including crowding and ventilation.

Table 56.4 shows the estimated rates of tuberculosis incidence by WHO region in the year 2004 (Figure 56.12).[15] In that year, an estimated 8.9 million new cases (140 per 100 000 population) of tuberculosis arose from the infected pool, 95% of them in the developing nations Around 1.9 million cases occurred in the West Pacific Region, 2.6 million in Africa and almost 3 million, a third of all cases, in South-east Asia. Half of all cases of tuberculosis occur in six Asian countries: Bangladesh, China, India, Indonesia, Pakistan and the Philippines. Owing to the chronic nature of the disease and the limited resources for effective diagnosis and treatment in many countries, the prevalence of active disease is much higher than the incidence of new cases. In 2004, there were an estimated 14.6 million people with active tuberculosis, of whom 6.1 million had infectious forms of the disease and infected some 100 million people, over 1% of the world's population. In the same year, an estimated 1.7 million people, principally young adults, died of tuberculosis, with 98% of deaths occurring in the developing nations. This amounts to around 5000 deaths every day.

MOLECULAR EPIDEMIOLOGY OF TUBERCULOSIS

Until about a decade ago, the only bacterial markers available to study the epidemiology of tuberculosis were drug susceptibility profiles and bacteriophage types. In recent years, a number of methods have been introduced to 'fingerprint' tubercle bacilli.[16] The most widely used DNA fingerprinting technique is restriction fragment length polymorphism (RFLP) analysis which relies on the presence of several copies of insertion sequences ('jumping genes') in the genome of *M. tuberculosis*. The most commonly used insertion sequence is IS6110 which is almost specific for *M. tuberculosis* and is present in most but not all isolates, with up to 25 copies throughout the chromosome. The mycobacterial DNA is extracted and then cleaved with restriction endonucleases, and subsequent electrophoresis and hybridization with labelled IS6110 DNA probes gives a series of bands, the number and position of which distinguishes between different strains.

This technique forms the basis of what is now termed the molecular epidemiology of tuberculosis and has been used to determine routes of transmission in a community, to understand the dynamics and clustering of specific outbreaks of tuberculosis, to determine to what extent new cases are due to endogenous reactivation or exogenous reinfection, to study the characteristics of MDRTB outbreaks in conjunction with the determination of drug resistance patterns and to detect multiple infections in a single patient. On a global scale, it has been used to delineate families or clades of *M. tuberculosis* that appear to differ in virulence. As mentioned above, the Beijing lineage, which is spreading globally, appears to be of relatively high virulence.

Although RFLP analysis based on IS6110 is the standard typing method for *M. tuberculosis*, it is technically laborious and requires large quantities of high-quality genomic DNA. Several alternative typing methods are in use, including spacer oligonucleotide typing, or 'spologotyping' for short, which, being PCR based, may be con-

Table 56.4 The estimated incidence, prevalence and mortality of tuberculosis, 2004

| WHO region | INCIDENCE | | | | PREVALENCE | | MORTALITY | |
| | ALL FORMS | | SMEAR-POSITIVE | | | | | |
	Number – thousands (% of global total)	Per 100 000 population	Number – thousands	Per 100 000 population	Number – thousands	Per 100 000 population	Number – thousands	Per 100 000 population
Africa	2573 (29)	356	1098	152	3741	518	587	81
The Americas	363 (4)	41	161	18	466	53	52	5.9
Eastern Mediterranean	645 (7)	122	289	55	1090	206	142	27
Europe	445 (5)	50	199	23	575	65	69	7.8
South-east Asia	2967 (33)	182	1327	81	4965	304	535	33
Western Pacific	1925 (22)	111	865	50	3765	216	307	18
Total	8918 (100)	140	3939	62	14 602	229	1692	27

Data from WHO.[15]

ducted directly on clinical samples. This is based on a structurally unique part of the mycobacterial genome, of unknown function, termed the direct repeat (DR) locus and consisting of repetitive 36 base pair (bp) units of DNA separated by non-repetitive 34–41 bp spacer oligonucleotides which can be amplified by PCR employing just one pair of primers. There are thousands of possible combinations of these oligonucleotides in the *M. tuberculosis* complex, providing a highly discriminative typing system.[17]

IMPACT OF THE HIV/AIDS EPIDEMIC

Over the last quarter of a century, the epidemiological trends of tuberculosis have been adversely affected by the HIV/AIDS pandemic and infection by HIV is now the most important predisposing factor for the development of active tuberculosis.[18] While, as described above, a non-immunocompromised person who has overcome the primary infection has about a 5% chance of developing post-primary tuberculosis later in life, the chance rises to 50% in an HIV-positive person. The annual risk of a person co-infected with the tubercle bacillus and HIV developing tuberculosis is around 50 times higher than in an HIV-negative person. The chance of an HIV-positive person developing tuberculosis after a primary infection or reinfection is very high, especially in those with AIDS, in whom the risk approaches 100%. In addition, the progression from infection to overt disease is very rapid, the time-scale being 'telescoped' from several years to a few months. These factors have led to a number of explosive mini-epidemics of tuberculosis in centres caring for AIDS patients.

At the end of 2006, there were an estimated 39.5 million HIV-positive persons worldwide; 4.3 million had been newly infected in that year and 2.9 million died. In 2004, an estimated 741 000 of the 8.9 million new cases of tuberculosis, and 248 000 of the 1.7 million who died of tuberculosis were co-infected with HIV. Tuberculosis is the single most prevalent cause of death in those infected with HIV and kills at least 11% and, in some regions,

possibly as many as 50% of AIDS patients.[15,18] At present, the greatest impact of HIV-related tuberculosis is felt in sub-Saharan Africa, where 70% of the world's cases occur and where, in many regions, 75% of adults and children with tuberculosis are co-infected with HIV and where the number of cases of tuberculosis is rising by 4% each year. This dual infection is having a devastating effect on health services and on societal structure in this region. In Zambia, for example, one in four pregnant women is infected with HIV and tuberculosis is now among the top non-obstetric causes of maternal death in that country.[19]

Countries with a high burden of HIV disease often lack facilities for making significant impacts on the control of tuberculosis. In 2005, only four of the 25 countries with the highest HIV prevalence achieved targets for treatment outcomes under the WHO DOTS strategy (p. 1032) for tuberculosis control. In African countries with a high prevalence of HIV infection, only one in three tuberculosis patients receives a full course of antituberculosis therapy. Until there is a much greater implementation of the effective and cost-effective DOTS strategy together with key HIV prevention and treatment measures, it is unlikely that the countries with a high prevalence of HIV infection will be able to make a significant impact on the incidence of HIV-related tuberculosis.[20]

A huge potential public health problem is posed by the rapid spread of HIV infection in Asia where, owing to the huge population, most of the world's cases of tuberculosis occur. Unless the spread of HIV is checked by public health measures or by the advent of effective vaccination or therapeutic strategies, the problems currently facing Africa will be experienced on a much greater scale in those regions.

IMPACT OF DRUG AND MULTI-DRUG RESISTANCE

Effective control of tuberculosis is threatened by the emergence of strains of *M. tuberculosis* resistant to one or more of the standard

these 53 (44 HIV positive) had XDRTB. Despite anti TB therapy including concomitant antiretroviral agents, all except one died within a few weeks of diagnosis.

FACTORS AFFECTING DYNAMICS OF TUBERCULOSIS IN POPULATIONS

An epidemic wave of tuberculosis in England began in the sixteenth century and reached its peak around 1780, at the time of the Industrial Revolution. Similar peaks were seen in Western Europe in the early 1800s and in Eastern Europe around 80 years later. This wave pattern has led some workers to propose that the disease rapidly rises to epidemic proportions in genetically susceptible populations and declines as a more resistant population develops by natural selection. There is, in fact, very little evidence for such a selection. Although a number of genetic factors affecting resistance to tuberculosis have been described, these appear much less important than environmental ones in determining the prevalence of the disease in a community.[24] The decline in the incidence of tuberculosis in the industrially developed nations is more likely to have been due to socioeconomic factors than to evolutionary selection. In this context, however, the inverse relationship between the incidence of tuberculosis and the improvement of social conditions is by no means straightforward. While some workers claim that the decline in the incidence of tuberculosis is a natural and predictable consequence of better nutrition and living and working conditions, others argue that the decline is the cumulative result of many specific public health measures introduced only after intense political lobbying.[25] The distinction is a crucial one as proponents of the first view claim that tuberculosis will decline as socioeconomic conditions improve worldwide while those holding the second view stress the need for specific tuberculosis control measures and health advocacy.

RISK FACTORS FOR TUBERCULOSIS

The principal factors predisposing to tuberculosis are listed in Table 56.3. In recent years, HIV infection has, as described above, emerged as the most important and widespread risk factor for the development of active tuberculosis. Other infections such as measles, whooping cough and chronic malaria and causes of lung damage, such as exposure to silicon and other industrial dusts, are also risk factors. Smoking has clearly been shown to be a major risk factor. An extensive retrospective study in India has shown that men who smoke are between four and five times more likely to develop tuberculosis than non-smokers and that, in that country, smoking accounts for 200 000 deaths from tuberculosis each year, many victims being young men (most Indian women are too sensible to smoke).[26]

Other predisposing conditions are those that compromise immune responsiveness and include malnutrition, alcoholism and other substance abuse, diabetes, renal failure (particularly if haemodialysis is required), treatment with immunosuppressive drugs and steroids (see below), liver failure and cancers, especially haematological malignancies. Transmission of infection is facilitated by overcrowding, poor ventilation and low levels of ultraviolet light – conditions frequently linked to poverty.

Tuberculin reactivity

Tuberculin reactivity is a risk factor for the development of tuberculosis as it is usually indicative of past infection by the tubercle bacillus, but the relation between such reactivity and risk of disease is not straightforward. In general, small reactions imply no increased risk, or even a degree of protection, but large reactions imply increased risk, though considerable regional variations in the risk in relation to reaction size occur.

Immunosuppressive drugs and steroids

Patients receiving post-transplant or other immunosuppressive therapy are prone to develop tuberculosis which is often insidious in onset, and miliary or cryptic disseminated forms of the disease (p. 1006) are common. Prophylaxis against tuberculosis should be considered, particularly for tuberculin negative patients who receive an organ from a tuberculin positive donor. Disease due to environmental mycobacteria (Chapter 57) is also common in these patients and poses diagnostic difficulties. There is a widespread belief that treatment with steroids predisposes to tuberculosis although the evidence for this is weak. Nevertheless, isoniazid chemoprophylaxis for 1 year is recommended for patients on long-term steroid therapy with one or more of the following: a history of inadequately treated tuberculosis, an abnormal chest radiograph, a tuberculin reaction of 10 mm or more in diameter and recent exposure to a tuberculosis patient.[27]

Age and sex

As outlined above, children up to the age of 5 years are highly susceptible to tuberculosis, especially miliary tuberculosis and tuberculous meningitis, but those between the age of 5 years and the onset of puberty appear relatively resistant. In developing countries the great majority of cases occur between the ages of 15 and 59 years. Surveys in several countries show that more males than females are diagnosed with tuberculosis but it is not clear whether this is affected by gender-related differences, lifestyle factors such as smoking or ability to access healthcare. Studies on the effect of pregnancy on tuberculosis are confusing, with reports variously claiming no effects, protective effects or a worsening of the disease.[28] Yet other reports suggest protection during pregnancy but an exacerbation after delivery – a phenomenon also observed in leprosy. This subject is in urgent need of investigation as tuberculosis is a major cause of death of pregnant women in sub-Saharan Africa, being responsible for more loss of life than obstetric complications.[16] The added impact of HIV infection on pregnancy-related mortality due to tuberculosis is also poorly understood.

CONTACT TRACING AND EXAMINATION

Most tuberculosis is spread within households, although 'mini-epidemics' occur in schools, prisons, hospitals and other situations where people at risk are crowded together. Household contacts of smear-positive patients should be examined: screening of casual contacts only yields a further 1% of cases and is usually not justified. Although children with primary tuberculosis are rarely infectious, household screening will often reveal a sputum-positive source case. Procedures for contact tracing vary according to local facilities and the prevalence of tuberculosis in the community. Tuberculin testing is useful in young children and, when indicated, chest radiography.

DIAGNOSIS OF TUBERCULOSIS

The success of tuberculosis control programmes depends critically on the quality of diagnostic services. Detailed accounts of the establishment and management of tuberculosis laboratories, the collection of specimens and subsequent laboratory procedures are available.[29,30]

Diagnosis in a community may either be active – involving a deliberate search for cases – or passive, relying on patients with symptoms presenting for treatment. The latter approach requires much less investment in time and personnel but its success depends on public education and the availability of user-friendly facilities.

Diagnosis of tuberculosis is based on a high index of clinical suspicion (described in relevant sections below), appropriate clinical and radiological examinations and laboratory investigations. The following investigations help to confirm the diagnosis and monitor treatment:

1. *Bacteriological examinations* include detection of acid-fast bacilli by microscopy and culture of the causative organism from appropriate clinical specimens such as sputum, bronchial aspirates and brushings, gastric aspirates, pleural, peritoneal and pericardial fluids, cerebrospinal fluid (CSF), blood, bone marrow and tissue aspirates or biopsies.
2. *Imaging techniques* including radiology, ultrasound, computed axial tomography (CAT) scanning, magnetic resonance imaging (MRI) and radioisotope scans.
3. *Molecular techniques* utilizing nucleic acid amplification systems – the polymerase chain reaction (PCR) and related techniques.
4. *Haematological and biochemical investigations* such as haemoglobin levels, erythrocyte sedimentation rate (ESR) and liver function tests may be required in overall patient management but have limited diagnostic roles.
5. *Tuberculin skin tests* and other immunological tests including interferon-γ assays.

In resource-poor settings, clinical acumen and simple microscopy are the mainstay of diagnosis and in many cases a trial of therapy is commenced on clinical suspicion only. One of the most frustrating challenges in tuberculosis management has been the lack of a specific, sensitive, inexpensive, and rapid point-of-care test for the diagnosis of tuberculosis. For individual patients, the cost, complexity and potential toxicity of 6 months of standard treatment demands certainty in diagnosis. For communities, the risk of transmission from undetected cases requires widespread access to diagnostic services and early detection. Unfortunately, current diagnostic services in most endemic settings fail both the individual and the community. Patients are commonly diagnosed after weeks to months of waiting, at substantial cost to themselves, and at huge cost to society as TB goes unchecked. Many patients are missed altogether, and contribute to the astonishing number of annual deaths from tuberculosis worldwide. Some of this failure could be corrected by better implementation of existing standards of clinical and laboratory practice. The World Health Organization (WHO) and its member states have made great gains in the expansion of the DOTS (Directly Observed Treatment, Short course) strategy to control tuberculosis, with an important rise in rates of cure. Improving case detection rates has proven more difficult, in large part because of limitations of existing diagnostic technologies. As many as 3 million cases of tuberculosis each year present as sputum smear-negative pulmonary disease and extra-pulmonary disease, for which sputum smear microscopy is inadequate.

As an indicator of the difficulty of implementing quality microscopy services, fewer than 45% of predicted incident smear-positive cases of tuberculosis are currently detected and notified. Paediatric and multi-drug-resistant (MDRTB) and extensively drug resistant (XDRTB) cases pose additional diagnostic challenges not addressed by sputum-smear microscopy. Diagnostics need to be driven by the reality of health systems infrastructure; well-engineered, simplified tests are needed at the point-of-care, at district hospital laboratories, and at central laboratories. Different diagnostic strategies sputum concentration methods, fluorescence microscopy, improved mycobacterial culture system also need to be evaluated for their impact on case detection. Diagnostic algorithms, including the use of empiric antibiotic trials to exclude TB, need to be carefully reassessed and improved. Implementation research can also assess the potential of integrating health service at district and health centre levels as a means of overcoming infrastructural and manpower impediments to operationalizing case detection services. Key factors to study include transportation, user fees, hunger, work and gender discrimination, and other barriers to accessing care. Better clinical diagnostic algorithms and case definitions are required for diagnosing tuberculosis in HIV-infected individuals and children. Thus, precisely in the areas of the world where microscopy has the poorest performance, the need for new early detection tests is the greatest. Current diagnostics research priorities are:

- To replace or improve microscopy with a simpler, point-of-care technology to detect smear-positive tuberculosis
- To develop a faster alternative to culture to detect smear-negative tuberculosis
- To develop and evaluate tests for rapid antibiotic susceptibility testing
- To develop tests for detecting latent infection at risk for relapse.

Bacteriological identification

Microscopy

In most laboratories, clinical specimens are examined by light microscopy for acid-fast bacilli after staining by the Ziehl–Neelsen method. Fluorescence microscopy, although requiring more expensive equipment which must be carefully maintained, is more sensitive as larger areas of the material on the microscope slide can be scanned at low-power magnification. Differentiation of species is not possible on microscopy and reports should only state whether acid-fast bacilli are or are not seen.

In practice, the great majority of specimens are sputum and more than one specimen should be examined. Ideally these include a 'spot' specimen obtained when the patient attends the

penetrate the skin and held in place for 10 s so that the dried PPD dissolves in the tissue fluids. Results are more variable than with the other test methods but it has some advantages when very few people are tested.

Interferon-γ assays

To overcome the problem of specificity encountered with tuberculin testing, the production of interferon-gamma by peripheral blood lymphocytes when exposed to antigens of *M. tuberculosis* in vitro has been utilized for the development of commercially available diagnostic tests. Increased specificity is achieved by selecting antigens present in *M. tuberculosis* but not in BCG or environmental mycobacteria. Studies to date indicate that these assays are of potential value but more extensive evaluations in a range of populations and settings are required for the confirmation of their usefulness and benefits and their ability to distinguish active from latent disease.[38]

TUBERCULOSIS IN CHILDREN

There are many differences between the pathological, clinical, radiological and epidemiological features of tuberculosis in children (see also Chapter 23) and adults. Children are usually infected by the aerogenous route and develop primary pulmonary complexes as described below. The most usual source is an adult with tuberculosis in the family. Less frequently they are infected by drinking milk containing *M. bovis*, usually with implantation of the bacilli in the tonsil or intestinal wall. Primary inoculation lesions due to infection of cuts and abrasions and congenital tuberculosis resulting from intrauterine infection are rarely encountered. Guidelines for the management of tuberculosis in children, including those who are infected with HIV, are available from the WHO.[39]

Clinical presentations of tuberculosis in children

Many children with primary tuberculosis have no obvious symptoms or signs and may go unnoticed for a while. Thus a high index of suspicion is essential throughout the tropical countries and other regions where tuberculosis is common. Bacteriological investigations are usually regarded as being of limited use for the diagnosis of pulmonary tuberculosis in children since obtaining sputum samples is more difficult than in adults. Even when specimens are obtained, acid-fast bacilli are only demonstrable in a minority of cases, especially in regions where facilities for extensive modern bacteriological investigations are not available. Bacteriological investigations are essential for the diagnosis of non-pulmonary disease, especially tuberculous meningitis. In view of the diagnostic difficulties, clinical algorithms have been developed,[40] and a flow diagram that has been in use for some time for diagnosis is shown in Figure 56.14.

Primary pulmonary tuberculosis

Clinical features are usually non-specific and include a failure to gain weight or loss of weight, a lack of energy, a persistent cough and/or wheeze and an unexplained fever for more than 1 week. A study in Cape Town, South Africa, of children with a cough of more than 2 weeks duration showed that a persistent and non-remitting cough and persistent fatigue of recent origin were sensitive and specific indicators of pulmonary tuberculosis.[41] Persistent fever and chest pain were also specific indicators but were present in only a quarter of children with tuberculosis. The tuberculin test is usually positive and the primary focus and/or enlarged intrathoracic lymph nodes may be seen on X-ray. It is not uncommon for children with primary pulmonary tuberculosis to have normal chest X-rays, although a computed tomography (CT) revealed enlarged mediastinal nodes in 60% of such radiologically normal children.[42]

Gross enlargement of the intrathoracic lymph nodes or endobronchial spread of the disease causes obstruction of the bronchi and the children present with cough and wheezing. Partial blockage of a major bronchus may limit exhalation, resulting in hyperinflation of the lung and clinically detectable mediastinal shift. Involvement of paratracheal nodes may cause stridor, sometimes requiring emergency tracheostomy.

Endobronchial spread of the disease process results in a range of clinical and radiological changes including pulmonary collapse, consolidation and hyperinflation and, in severe cases, widespread bronchopneumonia, particularly in younger children. In most cases, the lesions resolve clinically and radiologically on effective treatment although a few are left with residual bronchiectasis.

Congenital tuberculosis

This is a very rare condition and the mother always has tuberculosis, although sometimes in a form that is not clinically or radiologically obvious, such as renal tuberculosis.[43] There are two main types resulting from, respectively, transplacental infection and aspiration or inhalation of infected amniotic fluid.

Transplacental infection causes primary hepatic lesions and the infant presents with hepatic enlargement, fever and failure to gain weight. Jaundice is common. Respiratory infection leads to extensive lung involvement resulting in respiratory distress and cyanosis and diffuse nodular opacities on chest X-ray. Intrathoracic lymphadenopathy, sometimes extensive enough to cause respiratory obstruction, and miliary disease are common. The tuberculin test is often negative but there are numerous tubercle bacilli in the lungs and/or liver which are usually demonstrable by examination of tracheal or gastric aspirates or fine-needle liver biopsies. Mortality is high, as many as one-half die, and therapy should be commenced on suspicion of the disease. Treatment with corticosteroids may be life-saving in seriously ill children.

Hypersensitivity reactions

Primary tuberculosis in childhood is sometimes associated with hypersensitivity reactions: phlyctenular conjunctivitis and erythema nodosum (Figure 56.15).

Phlyctenular conjunctivitis is characterized by conjunctival itching or pain, lacrimation and photophobia, usually in one eye. Small, grey, translucent nodules are seen near the limbus of the cornea and the blood vessels in the adjacent conjunctiva are dilated. A leash of small blood vessels extends to the edge of the conjunctival

PATIENT'S DETAILS

Name
Age   yrs
(d.o.b.   /   /   )
Sex   MF
Weight   kg
BCG scars   0/1/2/3

HOSPITAL OR PHC LOCATION

Date
Scored by:

Nurse/Health Ass/Doctor

SCORE CHART   (Circle box and write in score)

Children suspected of having tuberculosis

FEATURE	0	1	3	
LENGTH OF ILLNESS	LESS THAN 2 WEEKS	2–4 WEEKS	MORE THAN 4 WEEKS	
NUTRITION (WEIGHT)	ABOVE 80% FOR AGE	BETWEEN 60% AND 80%	LESS THAN 60%	
FAMILY TUBERCULOSIS PAST OR PRESENT	NONE	REPORTED BY FAMILY	PROVED SPUTUM POSITIVE	

SCORE FOR OTHER FEATURES IF PRESENT

Positive tuberculin test	3
Large painless lymph nodes; firm, soft, sinus in neck, axilla, groin	3
Unexplained fever, night sweats, no response to malaria treatment	2
Malnutrition, not improving after 4 weeks	3
Angle deformity of spine	4
Joint swelling, bone swelling or sinuses	3
Unexplained abdominal mass or ascites	3
CNS: change in temperament fits or coma (send to hospital if possible)	3

TOTAL SCORE

When score is 7 or more treat for tuberculosis – see notes.

A

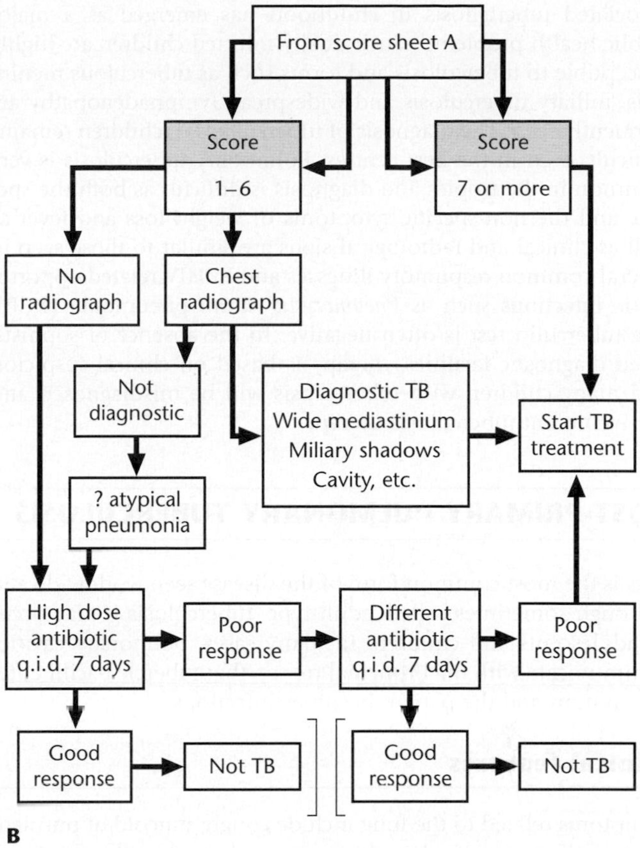

Flow chart B:

From score sheet A → Score 1–6 / Score 7 or more

Score 1–6 → No radiograph / Chest radiograph

Chest radiograph → Not diagnostic → ? atypical pneumonia

Chest radiograph → Diagnostic TB / Wide mediastinium / Miliary shadows / Cavity, etc. → Start TB treatment

Score 7 or more → Start TB treatment

No radiograph / ? atypical pneumonia → High dose antibiotic q.i.d. 7 days → Poor response → Different antibiotic q.i.d. 7 days → Poor response → Start TB treatment

High dose antibiotic q.i.d. 7 days → Good response → Not TB

Different antibiotic q.i.d. 7 days → Good response → Not TB

B

Figure 56.14   (A,B) Paediatric tuberculosis management flow chart.

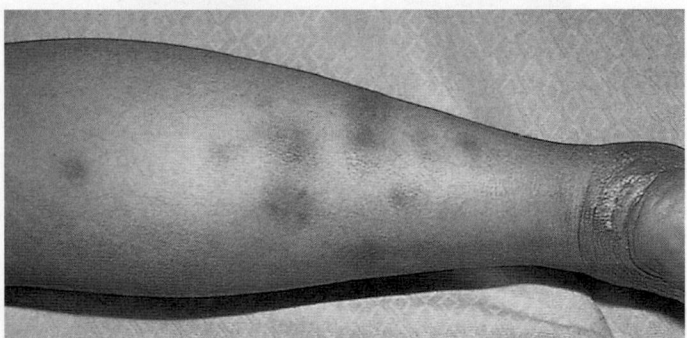

Figure 56.15   Erythema nodosum due to tuberculosis.

sac. Occasionally corneal ulceration occurs. More usually, the condition regresses over several days but recurrent attacks may occur. The condition occurs most frequently in children aged between 5 and 10 years and is much more frequent in girls than in boys. Some cases have followed BCG vaccination and streptococcal infection. It usually occurs soon after primary infection but a few cases have been reported in children with calcified primary complexes.

Erythema nodosum also usually occurs in association with primary tuberculosis and affects a similar age group as phlyctenular conjunctivitis. It is more common in girls and in those with fair skin. It is characterized by erythematous, indurated, painful plaques or nodules, usually on the lower limbs, and may be accompanied by fever and joint pain. The ESR is raised and, if the cause is tuberculosis, the tuberculin test is strongly positive. Resolution usually occurs within 2 weeks although the skin may remain discoloured for several weeks. Treatment, other than that of the underlying condition, is unnecessary, although corticosteroids may be given if joint pain is severe. The condition is not unique to tuberculosis as it also occurs in streptococcal infections, sarcoidosis, leprosy, systemic fungal infections, lymphoproliferative disorders and after treatment with certain drugs, notably sulphonamides.

Tuberculosis in HIV-infected children

HIV infection is increasingly encountered in children as the risk of an HIV-positive mother transmitting the virus to her child during pregnancy or at birth is between 24% and 40%, and even higher if the mother has AIDS. In sub-Saharan Africa HIV-associated tuberculosis in childhood has emerged as a major public health problem.[44] Such dually infected children are highly susceptible to tuberculosis and forms such as tuberculous meningitis, miliary tuberculosis and widespread lymphadenopathy are frequently seen. The diagnosis of tuberculosis in children remains difficult, even in the best centres. Pulmonary tuberculosis is very common in the tropics and diagnosis is difficult as both the specific and the non-specific symptoms of weight loss and fever as well as clinical and radiological signs are similar to those seen in several common respiratory illnesses and in HIV-related opportunistic infections such as *Pneumocystis carinii* pneumonia (PCP). The tuberculin test is often negative. In the absence of sophisticated diagnostic facilities, therapy is based on clinical suspicion and many children with tuberculosis will be misdiagnosed and receive no antituberculosis therapy.

POST-PRIMARY PULMONARY TUBERCULOSIS

This is the most common form of the disease seen worldwide and although sometimes called 'adult-type' tuberculosis it may occur in adolescents and children. In many cases, pulmonary cavities communicate with the bronchial tree so that tubercle bacilli enter the sputum and the patient becomes infectious.

Clinical features

Symptoms related to the lung include cough, mucoid or purulent sputum, haemoptysis, breathlessness and chest wall pain. More general and non-specific constitutional symptoms include fever and sweating (particularly at night), weight loss, general malaise and anorexia. None of these symptoms are specific for tuberculosis and some patients, even those with quite extensive disease, may have no apparent symptoms at all. Physical chest signs may be absent or limited to fine apical crackles. In more advanced cases there may be areas of dullness on percussion or localized wheezing. Clubbing of the finger is rare but is sometimes seen in severe cases of advanced disease with bronchiectasis. Clinical signs are often less obvious than would be expected from the radiological picture.

Diagnosis

Diagnosis is usually made by examination of sputum smears by microscopy and, where facilities are available, bacteriological culture and radiological examination (Figures 56.16–56.20). Advanced imaging techniques where available are useful in localizing pathology in cryptic sites (Figure 56.21–56.23).

Complications

The complications of post-primary pulmonary tuberculosis include pleural effusion and empyema, pneumothorax or pyopneumothorax due to formation of a bronchopleural fistula, tuberculous laryngitis and indurated intestinal ulcers due to implantation of tubercle bacilli in swallowed sputum. Occasionally an empyema or an intercostal node ruptures into the chest wall to form a cold abscess. Spread to other organs by the haematogenous or lymphatic route is uncommon when patients are relatively immuno-

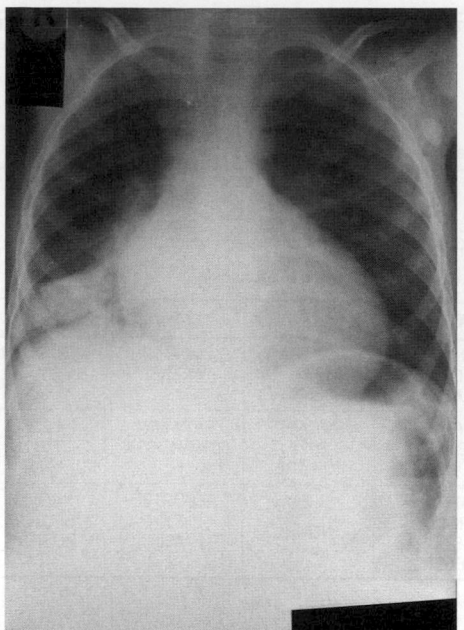

Figure 56.16 Chest X-ray showing right lower lobe consolidation due to tuberculosis.

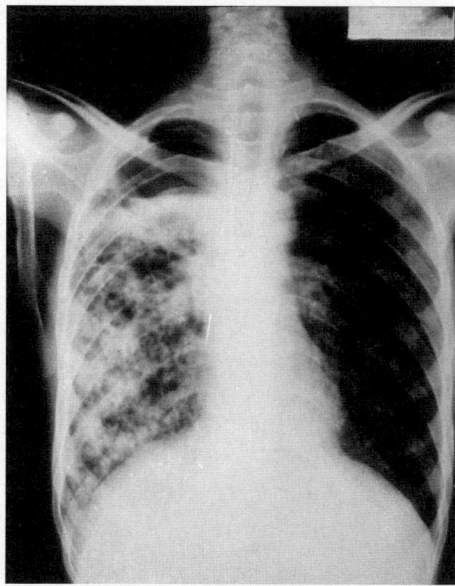

Figure 56.17 Chest X-ray with extensive patchy consolidation in the right lung fields. Sputum examination revealed acid-fast organisms confirmed on culture to be *M. tuberculosis*.

competent, but it is seen in many patients infected with HIV or with other conditions compromising their immunity. A late complication is chronic obstructive airways disease and cor pulmonale secondary to extensive pulmonary fibrosis. Other, much rarer, late complications include aspergillomas (Figure 56.24) developing in healed cavities and amyloidosis.

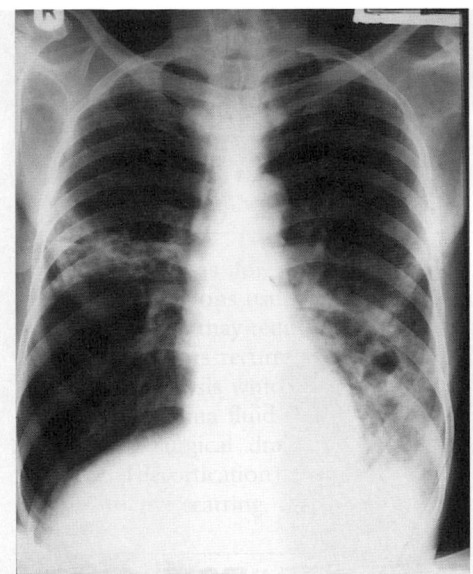

Figure 56.18 Chest X-ray of an HIV-positive patient with cavitating tuberculous consolidation in the right middle and left lower lung fields.

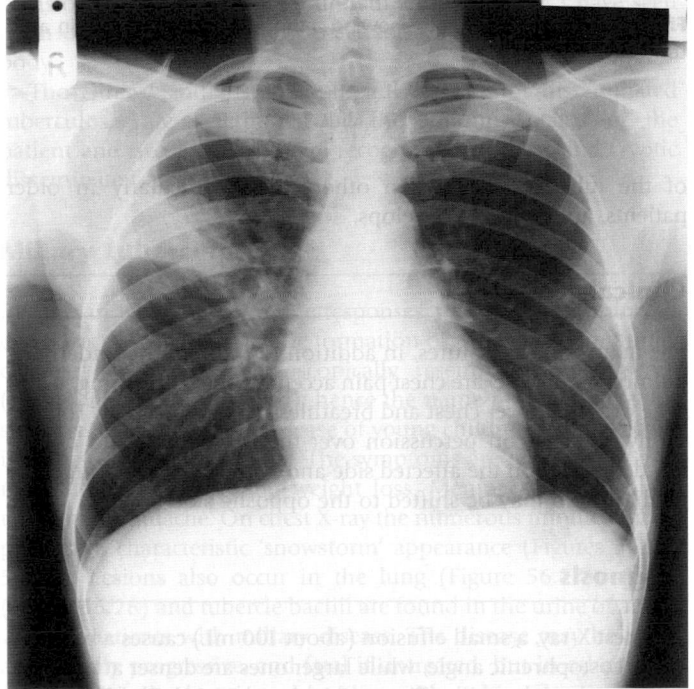

Figure 56.19 Post-primary tuberculosis. Right upper lobe tuberculous consolidation in a 15-year-old HIV-positive patient.

Differential diagnosis

The principal conditions with which pulmonary tuberculosis may be confused are community acquired unresolved pneumonias, carcinoma of the lung, Kaposi's sarcoma, helminth infections of the lung (hydatid, schistosomiasis, paragonimiasis), pulmonary

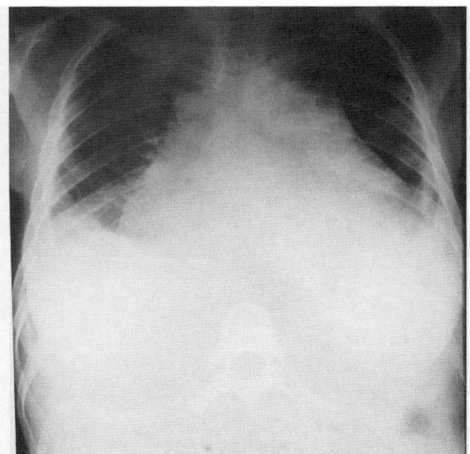

Figure 56.20 Post-primary tuberculosis. Pleural and pericardial effusions in a 44-year-old HIV-positive patient. *M. tuberculosis* was isolated from pleural fluid.

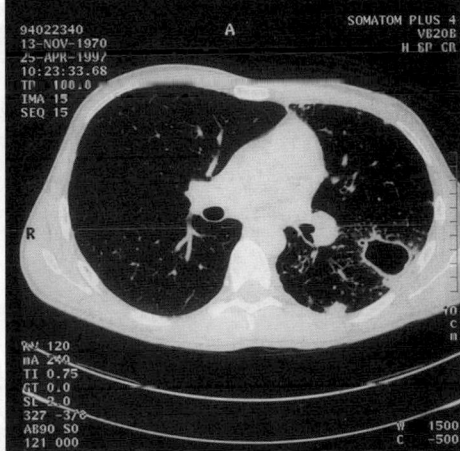

Figure 56.21 CT of the chest showing tuberculous cavity.

fibrotic lung disease secondary to sarcoidosis or industrial dust disease and pulmonary infarct. Lung cancers, pulmonary amoebiasis and abscesses of unresolved pneumonia, especially when caused by *Staphylococcus aureus* or *Klebsiella pneumoniae*, and cysts of *Paragonimus westermanii* may appear as cavitating lesions on chest X-ray. The absence of acid-fast bacilli on microscopy may suggest one of these other causes and, in the case of unresolved pneumonia, the causative organisms may be isolated by the appropriate bacteriological examinations. A therapeutic trial with a suitable antibiotic(s) may also differentiate tuberculosis from atypical pneumonia and pulmonary abscesses. The cachexia and malaise of advanced tuberculosis resemble that seen in AIDS, disseminated cancer and diabetes mellitus.

Management

The management of pulmonary tuberculosis involves prescription of an appropriate antituberculosis drug regimen, management of

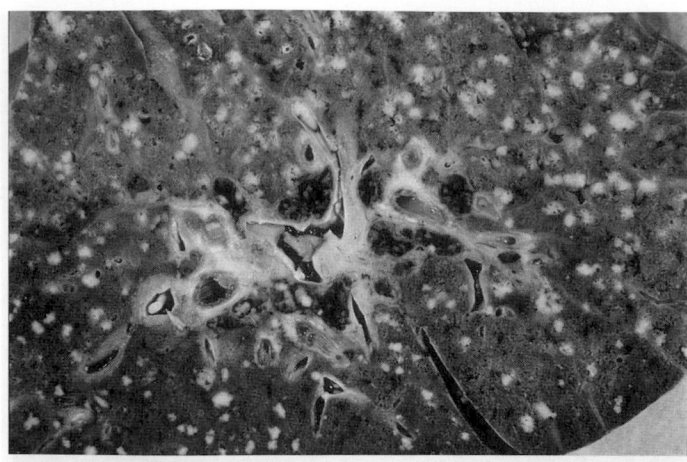

Figure 56.27 Postmortem lung specimen showing miliary tuberculosis.

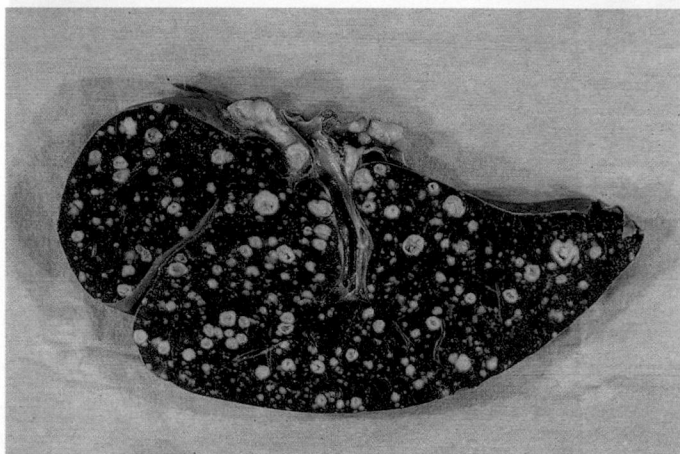

Figure 56.28 Miliary tuberculosis involving the spleen.

Figure 56.29 Grouped erythematous papules on the skin of the face in miliary tuberculosis.

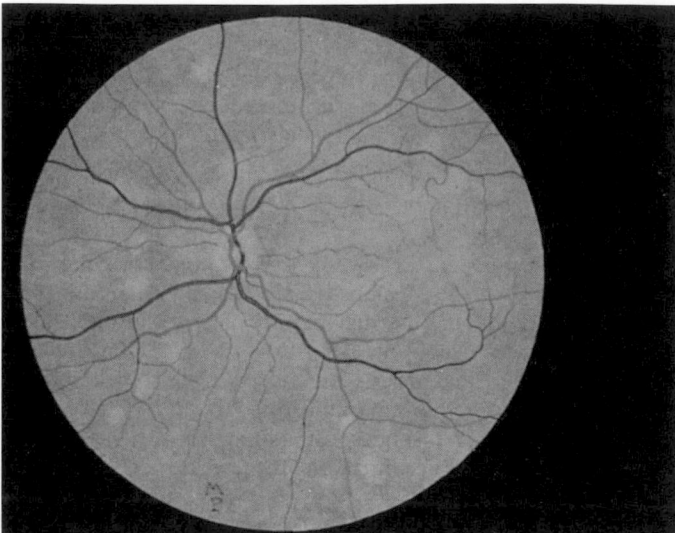

Figure 56.30 Choroidal tubercules.

in cases of suspected miliary tuberculosis and, indeed, in anyone with an unexplained fever. The differential diagnosis includes viral or mycoplasmal pneumonia, histoplasmosis and coccidioidomycosis.

Miliary tuberculosis responds well to antituberculosis therapy but corticosteroid therapy may be life-saving in seriously ill patients.

Cryptic disseminated tuberculosis

This form of tuberculosis is common in HIV-positive adults and children, particularly in the more profoundly immunosuppressed, as well as in others whose immune responses are suppressed, or weakened due to old age. In contrast to miliary tuberculosis, the widespread lesions show very little cellular infiltration but consist of minute necrotic foci teeming with acid-fast bacilli. The lesions are usually too small to be visible on chest X-ray which is often deceptively normal, hence the name cryptic disseminated tuberculosis for this form of the disease. The diagnosis is often missed as patients present with non-specific features such as fever, weight loss and anaemia and the tuberculin test is almost always negative. Many cases are therefore only detected at autopsy Patients are usually extremely ill on presentation and, without therapy, rapidly die. Biopsy of the lung, liver or bone marrow may provide the diagnosis after staining for acid-fast mycobacteria, culture for *M. tuberculosis* or identification of mycobacterial DNA by PCR.

BONE AND JOINT TUBERCULOSIS

This is the result of haematogenous dissemination of bacilli from a primary focus and, in the tropics, it is a common manifestation of tuberculosis in children. Most cases present 6 months to 3 years after the initial infection. Any bone or joint may be affected but the most frequent site is the spine, involved in half the cases, followed in frequency by the large joints of the lower limb (hip, knee and ankle) and then the large joints of the upper limb (shoulder, elbow and wrist). Multiple lesions, often cystic, may occur in disseminated tuberculosis and are easily mistaken for metastatic carcinoma.[45]

Spinal tuberculosis

Spinal tuberculosis, also termed Pott's disease, after Sir Percival Pott (1713–1788), a surgeon at St Bartholomew's Hospital, London, is a cause of severe deformity and handicap. Although any part of the spine may be affected, lesions most often occur at or near the 10th thoracic vertebra. The disease process usually begins in an intervertebral disc and subsequently involves the anterior parts of the adjacent vertebrae (Figure 56.31). Erosion of the bone by the disease process causes vertebral collapse with anterior wedging and, in severe cases, the characteristic angular spinal deformity or 'gibbus' (Figure 56.32). 'Cold' abscesses are common and may track along fascial planes and emerge at the skin surface well away from the site of disease. Thus psoas abscesses secondary to disease in the lumbar vertebrae may emerge in the thigh below the inguinal ligament. Tuberculosis of the cervical spine may present as a retropharyngeal abscess.

The usual presenting feature is chronic back pain, often with stiffness and limitation of movement. An unwillingness to pick something off the floor is a characteristic sign. Clinical features may, however, be minimal and non-specific and diagnosis is often delayed. Neurological signs due to pressure on, or vasculitis of, the spinal cord occur in about half the cases and paraplegia develops in severe cases. Clinical examination may reveal muscular spasm and rigidity, cold abscesses, sinuses and spinal deformity.

On radiological examination lesions may be confused with those of pyogenic osteomyelitis. Features suggesting tuberculosis include a relative sparing of the disc space, a fragmentary pattern of bone destruction and large paraspinous abscesses with dense rims and, in some cases, calcification within them.[46] Radiological signs may, however, be minimal and give an underestimate of the extent of the disease and, where available, CT, MRI or radionuclide bone scans (Figure 56.33) permit a more accurate assessment of the extent of the disease. Biopsies or fine-needle aspirates, conducted by those with adequate experience, may establish the diagnosis. Histological as well as bacteriological examination is essential as there may be too few acid-fast bacilli in the biopsy material for them to be detectable microscopically. The tuberculin test is usually positive although it may be negative in malnourished or immunosuppressed patients.

The differential diagnosis includes bacterial osteomyelitis and blood tests for staphylococcal and streptococcal infections and for typhoid, paratyphoid and brucellosis may help to rule these infections out. Spinal tuberculosis may resemble tumours and care should be taken not to confuse the combination of opacities on chest X-ray and osteolytic lesions of the spine with metastatic lung cancer.

Surgical intervention is required for patients with marked spinal deformity and severe neurological signs but most patients can be managed by standard therapy alone.[47] The most effective form of surgery for correction of deformity and relief or prevention of paraplegia is radical excision of diseased tissue and anterior spinal fusion – the so-called 'Hong Kong operation'. This, however, calls for surgical skills and resources that are not widely available.

Tuberculosis of other bones and joints

Tuberculosis of other bones and joints mimics a wide range of other conditions, especially the various forms of arthritis, and diagnosis is not easy. Disseminated lesions in many bones may mimic metastatic carcinoma. Tuberculosis of the skull usually

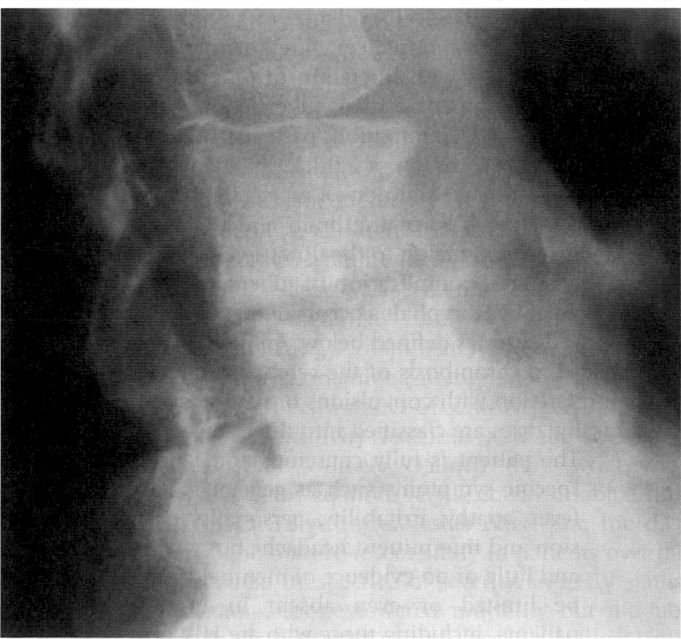

Figure 56.31 Spinal tuberculosis. Note involvement of two adjacent vertebrae and loss of joint space.

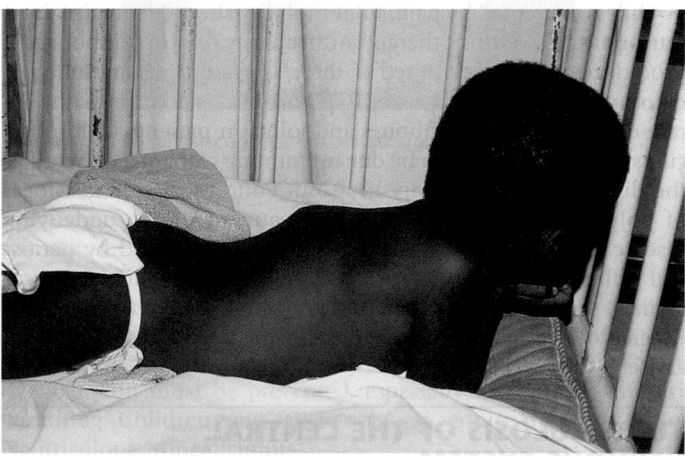

Figure 56.32 Pott's disease of the spine: spinal tuberculosis in a child showing a visible, palpable lump (gibbus) over the spine. The nappy was being used for urinary incontinence caused by spinal cord involvement.

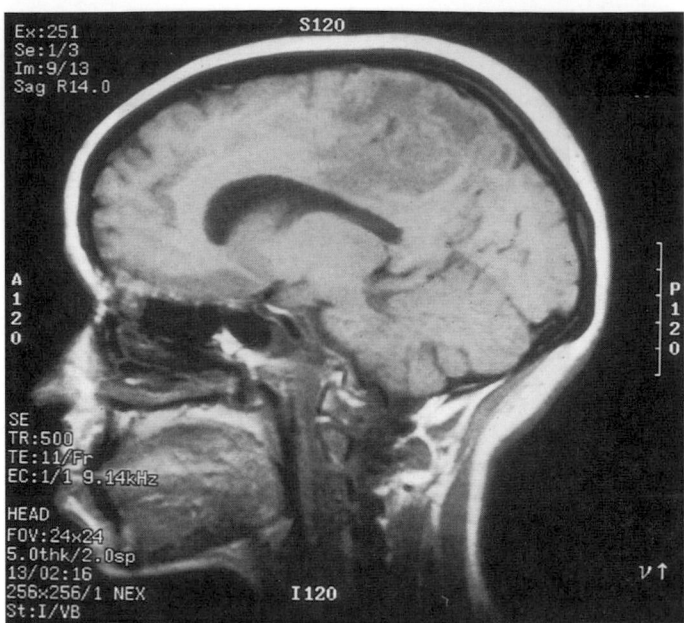

Figure 56.37 T1-weighted MRI, pre-contrast. Multiplanar reformation (coronal, left column, sagittal, right column) is 'as routine as' conventional axial images. Enhancement patterns mirror those of CT scan. The patient has cerebral tuberculosis.

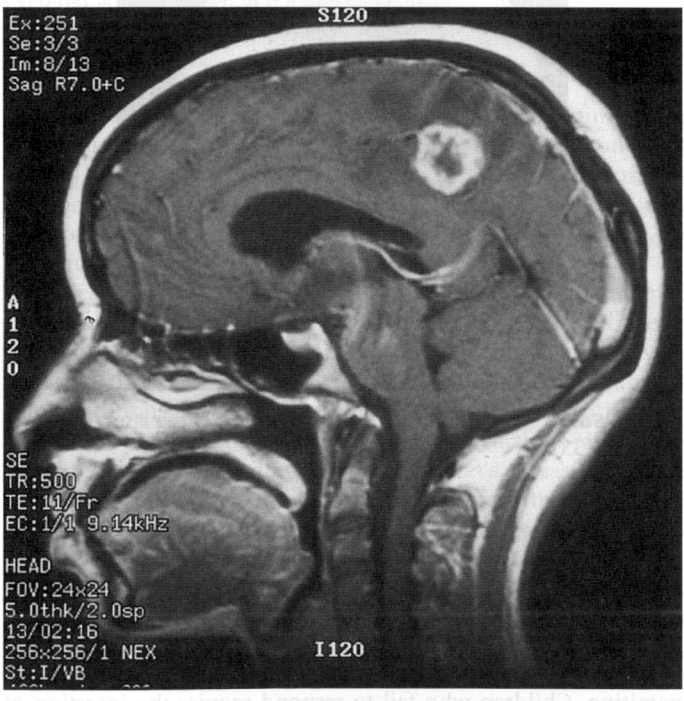

Figure 56.38 T1-weighted MRI, post-contrast. (see also Figure 57.37).

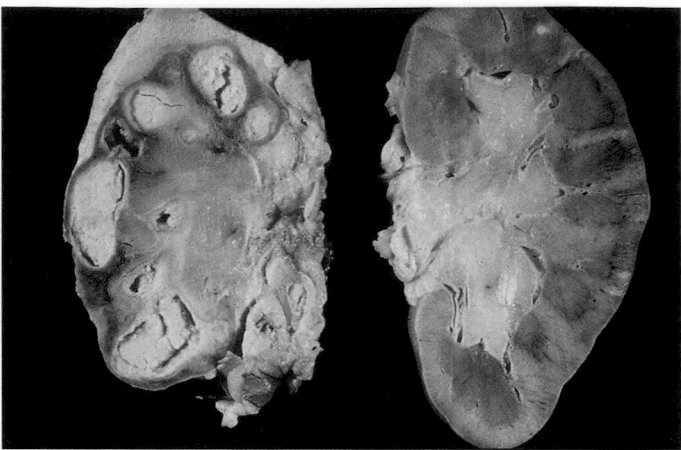

Figure 57.39 Postmortem kidney specimens showing caseating tuberculous lesions.

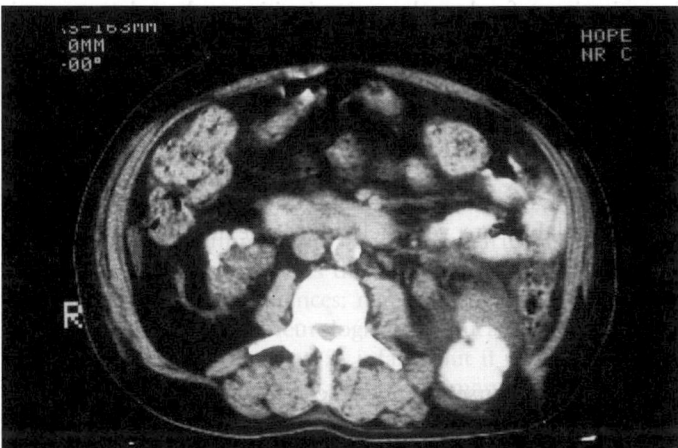

Figure 56.40 Non-enhanced CT scan through the lower abdomen. Large parenchymal deposits of calcification involving both kidneys as a result of earlier tuberculous infection.

URINARY AND GENITAL TRACTS

Tuberculosis of the kidney is a common form of extrapulmonary tuberculosis and autopsy studies indicate that it is commoner than expected in AIDS patients. Renal tuberculosis is usually a late manifestation of haematogenous spread from a primary focus of tuberculosis, presenting 6–15 years after the initial infection.[52] The disease, which may be unilateral or bilateral, usually commences in the renal cortex and progresses towards the medulla (Figures 56.39, 56.40). Lesions may eventually rupture into the renal pelvis with release of tubercle bacilli into the urine, causing secondary lesions in the ureters and bladder and, in males, in the epididymis, testis, seminal vesicles and prostate.[53] Although usually secondary to tuberculosis of the kidney, some cases of tuberculous epididymitis appear to be due to direct haematogenous spread from primary foci of disease. In advanced disease, an entire kidney may be replaced with caseous material – a condition termed 'cement kidney'.

Symptoms, including frequency, dysuria, nocturia, suprapubic pain and haematuria, resemble those of non-acid-fast bacterial cystitis.[54,55] In other cases, symptoms are of a vague 'orthopaedic' nature. Renal colic is uncommon, occurring in less than 10% of patients and constitutional symptoms are also uncommon. Secondary infection of the kidney, with renal pain and fever, may develop or if, as is often the case, diagnosis is delayed, ureteric obstruction, shrinkage and fibrosis of the bladder and even renal failure may develop. About 40% of patients have subclinical impairment of renal failure indicated by raised serum creatinine levels and about 10% have mild hypertension, which resolves on antituberculosis therapy. A male patient may present with a swollen epididymis or testis or with infertility.

An insidious form of renal tuberculosis termed tuberculous interstitial nephritis may lead to advanced renal failure without the usual tissue destruction and anatomical distortion.[56] Renal biopsies reveal an interstitial granulomatous infiltrate with limited caseation and scanty acid-fast bacilli. Diagnosis is not easy as it is unusual to find acid-fast bacilli in the urine. As tuberculosis is common in the tropics, it should be considered in all cases of renal failure when there are no other obvious causes.[57]

Tuberculosis of the female genital tract is, in contrast to the disease in males, almost always the direct result of haematogenous dissemination from the primary focus. Sexually transmitted tuberculosis is exceedingly rare. The disease usually commences in the epithelium of the Fallopian tubes (Figure 56.41) and spreads to the endometrium or to the peritoneal cavity, causing tuberculous peritonitis. Presenting features include infertility, pelvic pain and either excessive menstrual bleeding or amenorrhoea.

Diagnosis

Examination of the urine may reveal a few white cells, red cells and protein. Care is required in the interpretation of acid-fast bacilli seen in urine as various environmental mycobacteria occur as contaminants of the lower urethra and external genitalia. Diagnosis is confirmed by cultivation of tubercle bacilli in urine, for which purpose up to six specimens, preferably taken in the early morning, should be examined.

Radiology of the urinary tract (Figure 56.42) is useful for the detection of urinary obstruction and other forms of gross tissue damage. Being a late manifestation of primary tuberculosis, appearances suggestive of pulmonary tuberculosis are only seen in 5% of cases but patients may give a history of tuberculosis. Ultrasonography may reveal renal calyceal dilatation and more overt evidence of obstruction. Between 50% and 75% of males with genital tuberculosis have radiological abnormalities in the urinary tract, so the appropriate radiological investigations should be undertaken.

Diagnosis of tuberculosis of the female genital tract is made by histological and bacteriological examination of endometrial biopsies and culture of cervical secretions and menstrual blood.

Management

Treatment of all forms of genitourinary tuberculosis is by standard short-course antituberculosis therapy. Surgical intervention may

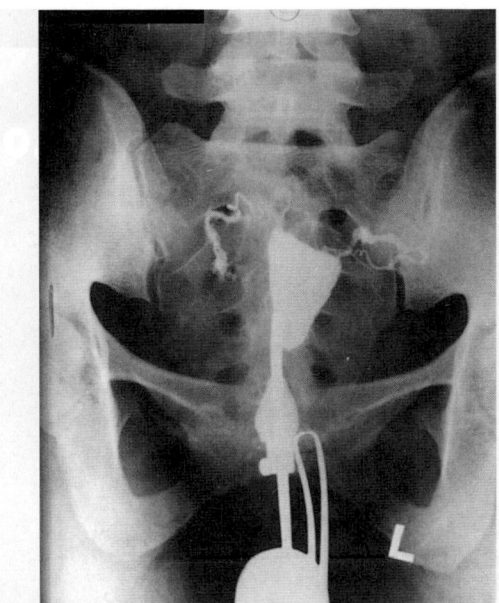

Figure 56.41 Hysterosalpingogram showing distortion of Fallopian tubes due to chronic tuberculous salpingitis.

be required for relief of ureteric or urethral obstruction, shrunken bladders or, rarely, for the removal of grossly damaged and nonfunctioning kidneys in the presence of symptoms. Ureteric obstruction may respond to treatment with steroids.

ABDOMINAL TUBERCULOSIS

This is divisible into intestinal and peritoneal disease. The former is either a primary infection, usually due to drinking milk containing *M. bovis* or a manifestation of post-primary disease as a result of swallowing sputum containing tubercle bacilli. The latter is the result of lymphatic or haematogenous dissemination from a primary focus, usually pulmonary, or to spread from an infected intra-abdominal organ such as the intestine or a Fallopian tube.

Primary intestinal tuberculosis usually involves the ileocaecal region and results in mucosal hypertrophy which, together with enlarged lymph nodes, presents as a tender mass in the right iliac fossa. Complications including malabsorption, intestinal obstruction, fistulae, peritonitis and, rarely, massive rectal bleeding which may be life-threatening. The stomach and small intestine are the usual sites of post-primary lesions and ulceration, rather than hypertrophy, is characteristic, with a risk of intestinal perforation leading to peritonitis.

The principal groups of patients developing tuberculous peritonitis are young women and elderly alcoholic men. It is a common cause of ascites: in a study in Lesotho it was found to account for 42% of all cases of ascites and there was a mortality rate of 26% among elderly alcoholic patients.[58] Diagnosis is difficult, especially in elderly alcoholics, as the symptoms and signs are non-specific. The 'doughy abdomen' cited in many textbooks as a classical sign is an uncommon manifestation of advanced disease. Tubercle bacilli in swallowed bacilli may enter anal fissures and lead to local granulomatous lesions and fistula formation.

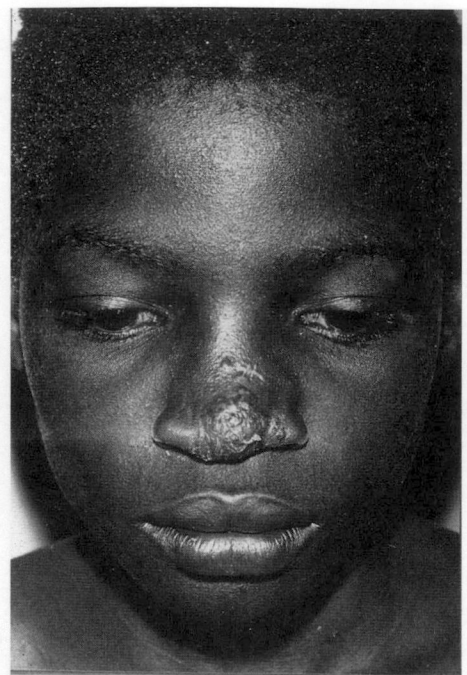

Figure 56.49 Lupus vulgaris of the face. Chronic ulcerating granulomatous lesion due to *M. tuberculosis*.

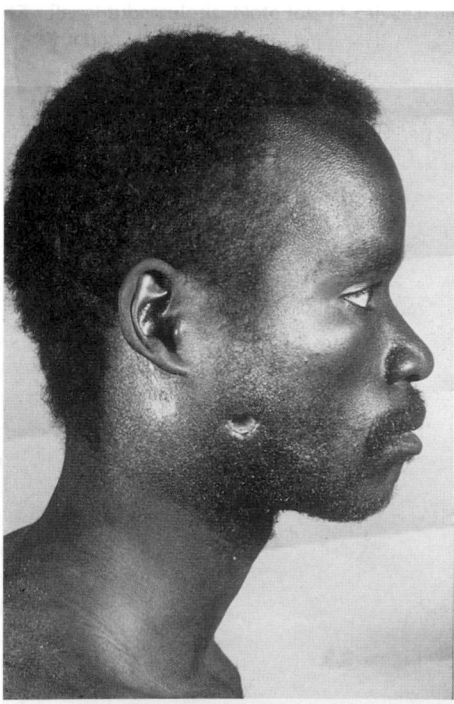

Figure 56.50 Chronic ulcerating lesion with parotid fistula due to parotid gland tuberculosis.

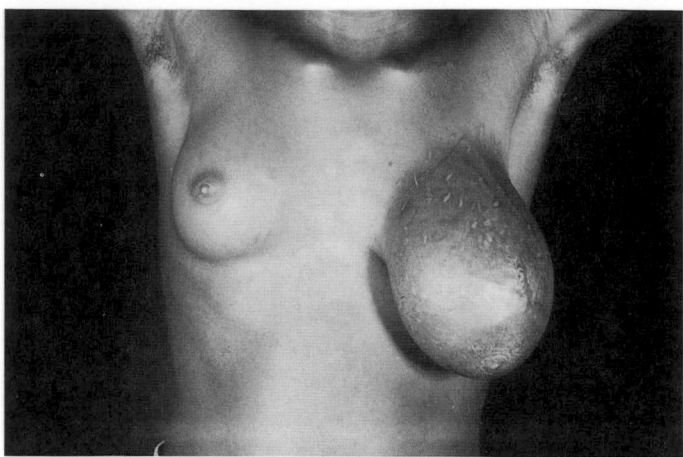

Figure 56.51 Tuberculous mastitis affecting the left breast.

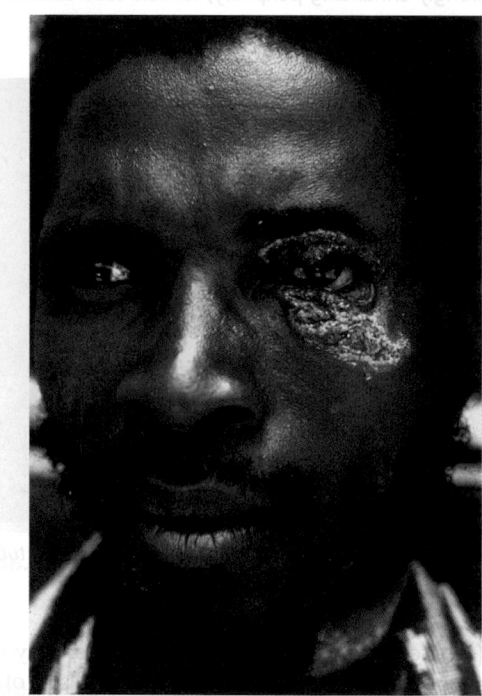

Figure 56.52 Chronic granulomatous skin lesions on the face due to *M. tuberculosis* (lupus vulgaris).

Extension of disease from underlying structures results in sinus formation. The usual cause is a spread from an underlying tuberculous lymph node: a condition termed 'scrofuloderma'.

Lupus vulgaris is a very slowly progressive and chronic form of skin tuberculosis that usually occurs on the nose, cheeks or neck and, if untreated, may cause severe disfigurement (Figures 56.47, 56.49 and 56.52). It is characterized by red-brown semi-translucent nodules which may subsequently coalesce and ulcerate. When compressed with a glass slide the nodules often have an opalescent 'apple jelly' appearance. It is due either to haematogenous dissemination of tubercle bacilli from internal organs or to secondary spread from scrofuloderma. There is some evidence to suggest that lupus vulgaris is more likely to be caused by *M. bovis* than *M. tuberculosis*. The skin may be involved in disseminated tuberculosis, and small skin papules may be seen in cases of miliary tuberculosis (Figure 56.29).

The tuberculides are uncommon and poorly understood skin lesions associated with tuberculosis.[63] Two main types have been described: lichen scrofulosorum and papulonecrotic tuberculide. The former is characterized by non-necrotic dermal granulomas with epithelioid and giant cells and the latter by tissue necrosis, sometimes extensive, due to an obliterative vasculitis. The aetiology of the tuberculides is unknown but it has been suggested that they are due to hypersensitivity reactions to blood-borne whole tubercle bacilli, bacillary debris or antigens. The rarely encountered erythema induratum (Bazin's disease) and tuberculosis-associated idiopathic gangrene of the extremities may be due to similar necrotic hypersensitivity reactions in larger blood vessels. Lupus vulgaris occasionally develops at the site of a tuberculide, indicating the presence of viable tubercle bacilli.

SUPERFICIAL LYMPH NODES

Tuberculous lymphadenitis is well documented in early literature in which it is referred to, for unknown reasons, as scrofula (Figures 56.8, 56.53–56.57). The usual site is the neck and two main types have been described: that due to primary inoculation of bacilli, usually milk-borne *M. bovis*, into the pharynx and that secondary to intrathoracic primary complexes. Lymphadenopathy also occurs as a component of disseminated tuberculosis in HIV-positive patients. Lymphadenopathy in children aged 5 years or below is occasionally caused by other mycobacterial species (see Chapter 57).

Lymphadenopathy associated with a primary pharyngeal lesion usually affects the tonsillar and pre-auricular nodes, while the supraclavicular nodes are involved when the disease is due to an upward extension of an intrathoracic primary complex. The latter is more common in females than males. In early disease, affected nodes are discrete, rubbery in texture and usually painless. Constitutional symptoms occur in less than half the patients. Subsequently, the affected glands may undergo necrosis and become fluctuant, and the disease may invade the surrounding tissues and ultimately the skin with the formation of sinuses. The disease

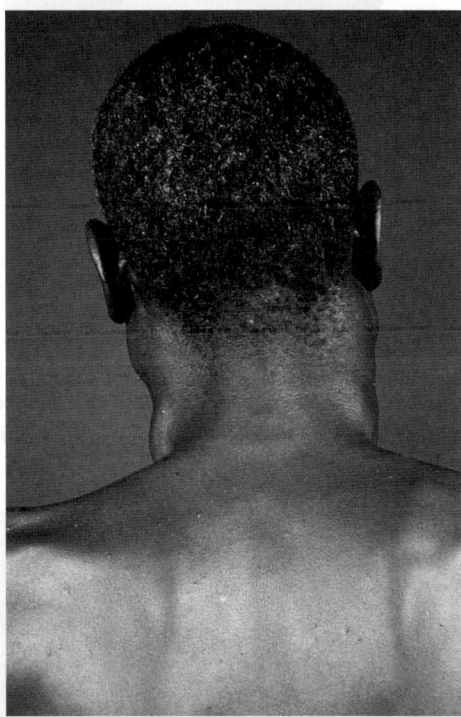

Figure 56.54 Cervical lymphadenopathy due to tuberculosis in an HIV-positive Zambian adult.

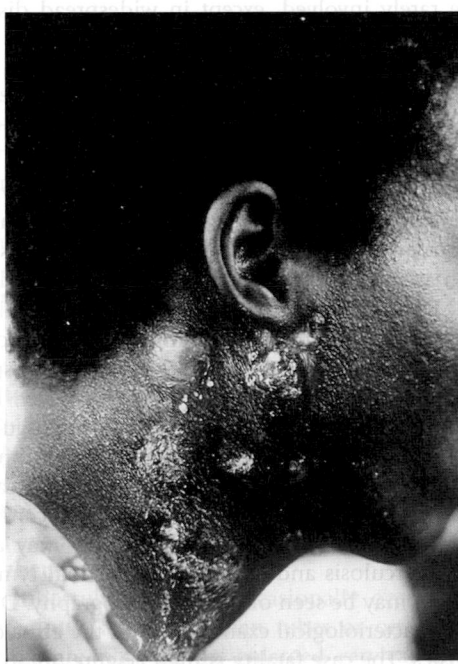

Figure 56.53 Enlarged tuberculous cervical lymph nodes exuding caseous material ('open tuberculosis').

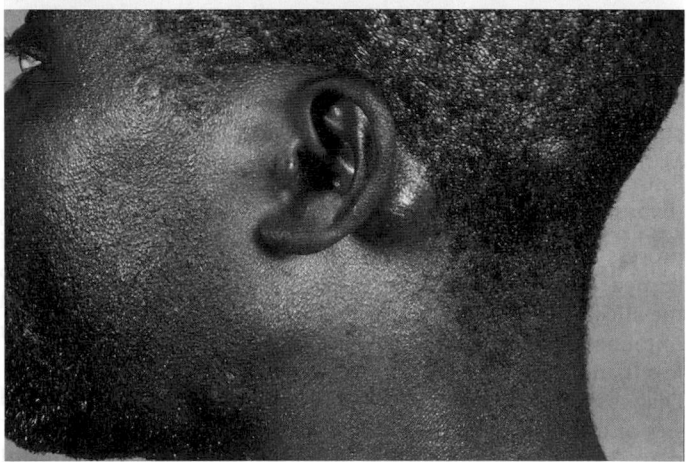

Figure 56.55 Enlarged posterior auricular lymph node in an HIV-positive adult. *M. tuberculosis* was isolated from a lymph node aspirate.

HIV infection, tuberculosis leads to a lowering of the CD4+ T cell count and to a marked increase in the viral load in HIV-infected patients.[70] Increased IL-2, IL-6 and TNFα (type 2 cytokines) generated by infection with *M. tuberculosis* may be responsible for these increases in HIV burden.

Pathology of tuberculosis in HIV infection

Autopsy studies in Africa show that between one-third and one-half of those dying of an AIDS-defining condition had active tuberculosis, many showing fibrous and calcified lesions of tuberculosis adjacent to recent active lesions containing viable tubercle bacilli. These new lesions may be due to endogenous reactivation of primary complex lesions but DNA fingerprinting indicates that many are due to exogenous reinfection. In HIV-infected patients a range of histological features related to the extent of immunosuppression are seen.[71] For practical purposes, there are three identifiable histological stages of cellular immune responses which correlate well with the stage of HIV disease – granulomatous response, hyporeactive response and anergic response. The susceptibility to, and clinical characteristics of, tuberculosis show only a partial correlation with the CD4+ lymphocyte counts as qualitative as well as quantitative defects of these cells compromise protective immune functions such as macrophage maturation and granuloma formation.

Patients showing a granulomatous response have relatively intact cellular immune responses, a relatively high CD4+ lymphocyte count and develop typical, well-formed granulomas containing abundant epithelioid cells and Langhans giant cells, clusters of CD4+ T cells and low numbers of acid-fast bacilli. Macrophages show abundant cytoplasm and markers of maturation.

With progressive immunosuppression and decline of CD4+ T cell counts, there is a hyporeactive response with loss of Langhans giant cells and, subsequently, of epithelioid cells. The proportion of macrophages with abundant cytoplasm is also decreased. Intracellular killing of mycobacteria is compromised and therefore the number of acid-fast bacilli increase (Figure 56.60). The

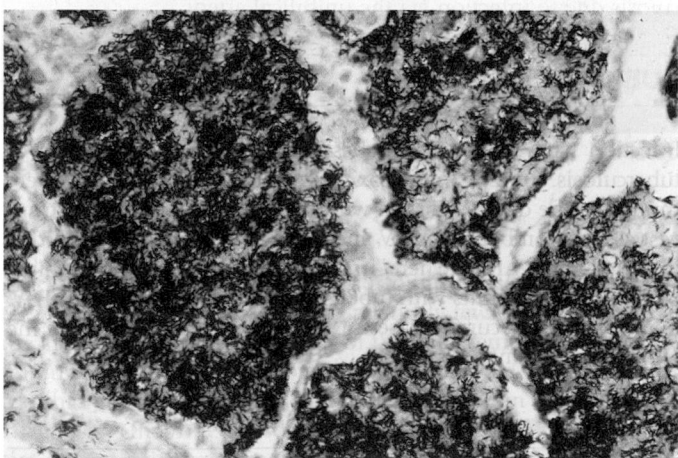

Figure 56.60 Lung histopathology of an AIDS patient who died of tuberculosis. Note the vast number of acid-fast tubercle bacilli in the alveolar necrotic exudate.

caseous centres enlarge centrifugally and lesions coalesce. A mixture of suppurative and caseous necrosis is seen.

Finally, in the late stages of AIDS, disseminated anergic tuberculosis develops and is often only detected at autopsy. While no relative decrease in the number of macrophages in the tuberculous lesion is seen, they show little or no maturation. Epithelioid cells are scanty, Langhans giant cells are absent, there are few CD4+ T cells in the lesions and granuloma formation is not seen (Figures 56.10A and B). Caseous necrosis is replaced by suppuration, coagulative necrosis and large amounts of apoptotic debris. Large numbers of mycobacteria are present within macrophages and in the necrotic areas.

Clinical manifestations of HIV-related tuberculosis

Pulmonary tuberculosis occurs in patients with a wide spectrum of immunodeficiency but, as mentioned above, the risk and clinical manifestations are not entirely dependent on the degree of depletion of CD4+ lymphocytes. Around 30% of cases of tuberculosis in HIV-positive patients are extrapulmonary. If tuberculosis occurs in the early stages of HIV infection when immunity is only slightly compromised, the clinical characteristics are similar to post-primary tuberculosis occurring in HIV-negative persons. Thus disease is often localized to the apices of the lungs; there is lung destruction and cavitation and abundant acid-fast bacilli are seen on sputum microscopy. HIV-positive patients with more advanced immunodeficiency present with atypical pulmonary disease characterized by extensive pulmonary infiltrates with limited or no cavitation, involvement of all parts of the lung especially the lower lobes, enlargement of the hilar and mediastinal lymph nodes and few or no acid-fast bacilli seen in sputum smears. Dissemination of the disease beyond the lung is common.

Diagnosis of pulmonary tuberculosis in HIV-positive adults

As the proportion of patients with smear-negative pulmonary tuberculosis is greater in those co-infected with HIV than in those who are not, the diagnosis of tuberculosis in an HIV-positive patient with a chronic cough, night sweats, weight loss but negative sputum smears for acid-fast bacilli is a challenge for the clinician. In studies in HIV-positive African patients with respiratory illness and negative sputum smears, bronchoscopy with bronchoalveolar lavage or induction of sputum demonstrated that about one-third had tuberculosis. Another third had other respiratory diseases including *Pneumocystis carinii* pneumonia (PCP), bacterial pneumonia due to a wide range of pathogens, Kaposi's sarcoma, nocardiosis and fungal infections. Even where facilities exist for more extensive investigations (e.g. bronchoscopy with bronchoalveolar lavage and biopsy, sputum culture and molecular methods) the bacteriological confirmation of tuberculosis may be difficult. In most developing country health centres, the diagnosis of pulmonary tuberculosis is based on simple techniques only: sputum smear microscopy and, possibly, chest radiography.

There is a large range and variety of radiological appearances.[72] In those with relatively intact immunity, the appearances are those

Table 56.7 Comparison of the clinical and radiological characteristics of post-primary tuberculosis in non-immunosuppressed and immunosuppressed persons

Characteristic	Non-immunosuppressed	Immunosuppressed
Pulmonary cavitation	Prominent	Diminished or absent
Localization by fibrosis	Marked	Limited
Intrathoracic lymphadenopathy	Uncommon	Common
Pleural effusions	Present	Very common
Miliary disease	Uncommon	Common
Atelectasis	Uncommon	Common
Lymphatic and haematogenous dissemination	Uncommon	Common
Adverse drug reactions	Uncommon	Common
Tuberculin test	Positive	Small reaction or negative
Relapse following therapy	Uncommon	Frequent
Mortality rate	Low	Increased

of typical pulmonary tuberculosis but in the more profoundly immunosuppressed atypical appearances are common, including vague, spreading opacities suggestive of pneumonia, predominantly lower lobe disease, pleural effusions, air-fluid levels, widespread pulmonary mottling and intrathoracic lymphadenopathy. On the other hand, there is significantly less cavitating disease and atelectasis. Radiological features may change rapidly in appearance. Classical miliary lesions are seen in a minority of HIV-positive patients with disseminated disease, as in most cases the formation of these granulomatous lesions is suppressed. The X-rays may therefore appear deceptively normal. The atypical clinical and radiological features seen in the more profoundly immunosuppressed patients are summarized in Table 56.7. Further details on the clinical aspects of HIV-related tuberculosis are available from the WHO.[73]

Extrapulmonary tuberculosis in HIV-positive adults

Frequent manifestations of extrapulmonary tuberculosis seen in HIV-infected persons in sub-Saharan Africa include pleural disease, lymphadenopathy (usually asymmetrical), pericardial disease and widely disseminated disease. Tuberculosis affecting the CNS, genitourinary tract and bone marrow is, in contrast to the industrialized countries, infrequently reported but this probably reflects patient selection and differences in the availability of diagnostic facilities. Patients usually present with non-specific constitutional symptoms (fever, night sweats and weight loss) and local symptoms and signs related to the site of disease. Lymphadenopathy is a frequent manifestation of tuberculosis in HIV-infected persons and can present in a variety of ways. While usually chronic and cryptic, it may also occasionally be acute and resemble an acute pyogenic infection. Diagnosis of lymph node tuberculosis can be made by simple techniques such as staining needle aspirates for acid-fast bacilli, naked eye inspection of biopsied lymph nodes for macroscopic caseation and microscopy of smears from the cut surface of a lymph node. The CSF may be normal or near-normal in HIV-infected patients with tuberculous meningitis and clinical features can easily be confused with those of cryptococcal meningitis (a common HIV-related infection), making the diagnosis very difficult. Empirical treatment may have to be given on clinical suspicion alone.

Management considerations in HIV-positive persons

There are several specific management issues which arise in the treatment of HIV-infected persons with tuberculosis. These patients overall tend to have:

- Increased morbidity rates
- Increased mortality rates
- Increased number of drug side-effects
- Serious interactions between antiretroviral drugs and antituberculosis drugs
- Immune reconstitution inflammatory syndrome (IRIS)
- Increased recurrence rates after completion of treatment.

Increased morbidity rates

Clinical response to antituberculosis treatment, clearing of chest X-ray abnormalities and sputum conversion rates occur at the same rates during treatment in both HIV-positive and HIV-negative patients with tuberculosis. On the other hand, HIV-positive patients on treatment for tuberculosis often have other opportunistic infections and tumours and thus commonly suffer from recurrent fever, chest infections, recurrent diarrhoea, oral candidiasis, bacteraemia, cryptococcosis and Kaposi's sarcoma. These other conditions require appropriate drug treatment, rendering the care more expensive than is the case with HIV-negative patients. Delays in the diagnosis and treatment of tuberculosis compromise the chances of individual cure in HIV-positive patients. Untreated tuberculosis in HIV-infected persons accelerates the decline in immunocompetence and the progression to severe immunodeficiency.

Increased mortality rates

HIV-positive patients not receiving antiretroviral therapy have a much higher mortality during and after antituberculosis treatment compared with HIV-negative patients. In sub-Saharan Africa,

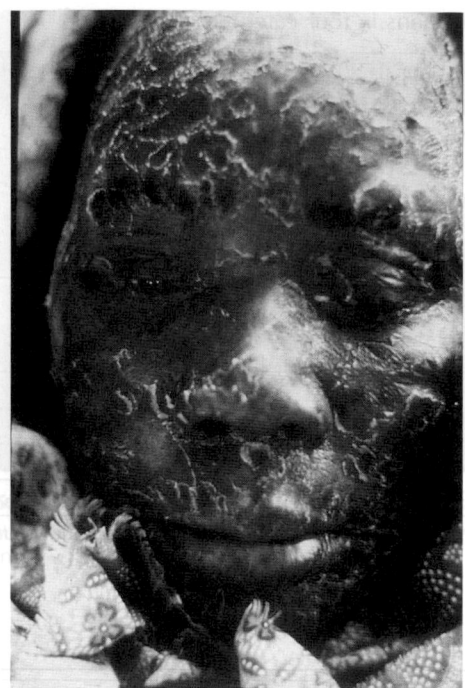

Figure 56.64 Extensive skin reaction due to isoniazid.

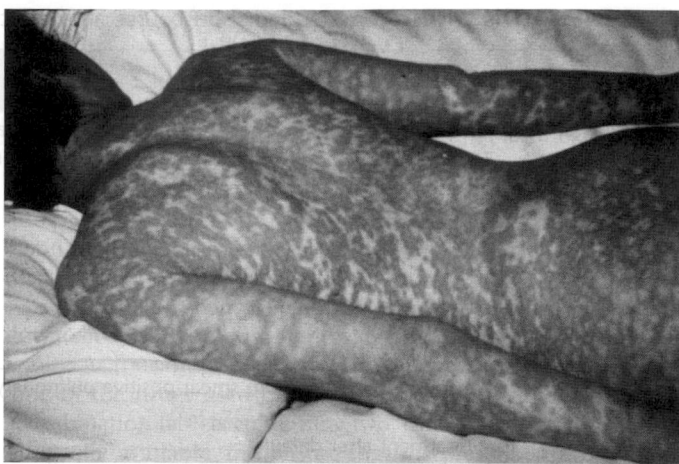

Figure 56.65 Erythema multiforme skin reaction due to rifampicin.

10 mg/day and this has become standard practice in many countries. Some national programmes recommend the routine prescription of pyridoxine to patients with liver disease, renal failure requiring dialysis, pregnant women, alcoholics, HIV-positive patients, the malnourished and the elderly.

Rifampicin (rifampin in the USA)

This, a member of the rifamycin group of antibiotics, is readily absorbed from the gastrointestinal tract and effective concentrations are obtained in all tissues, with moderate levels in the CSF. Cross-resistance to other classes of antituberculosis drugs does not occur. It is red coloured and patients should be warned that it imparts this colour to urine, tears and sweat.

Adverse reactions include mild and usually self-limiting skin rashes, erythema multiforme (Figure 56.65) and itchiness of the skin. Gastrointestinal upsets occur in some patients and are reduced by giving it with food. Impairment of liver function may be seen in patients with pre-existing liver disease and a history of alcoholism and, if possible, assay of serum bilirubin and other liver function tests should be done monthly on such patients. Another adverse effect is the so-called 'flu syndrome', characterized by fever, chills and headache, aching bones and, in some cases, a mild thrombocytopenic purpura. For unknown reasons, the flu syndrome is more frequent in those on intermittent treatment than in those given rifampicin daily.

Much rarer, but serious, adverse events usually associated with intermittent dosing include respiratory shock syndrome, thrombocytopenic purpura, haemorrhages, haemolytic anaemia and renal failure. Rifampicin must be stopped immediately if one of these serious adverse reactions develops and must never be given

again. Corticosteroid therapy may be required for the respiratory shock syndrome.

Ethambutol

This has bactericidal activity in the early, intensive, phase of treatment and is reported to enhance the activity of other antituberculosis agents by increasing mycobacterial cell wall permeability. Resistance is uncommon. It is concentrated in the alveolar macrophages. It does not diffuse through healthy meninges but CSF levels of 25–40% of the plasma concentration, with considerable variation between patients, are achieved in tuberculous meningitis.

The most important side-effect is optic neuritis, which may become irreversible and lead to blindness. This rarely occurs if no more than 25 mg/kg is given daily for no longer than 2 months. National codes of practice for detection and prevention of ocular toxicity should be followed. Patients should be instructed to stop therapy and to seek medical advice if they notice any change in visual acuity, peripheral vision or colour perception. Ethambutol should not be given to young children and others unable to comply with this advice. Other adverse effects include peripheral neuritis, joint pain due, in some cases, to hyperuricaemia, rashes and, rarely, thrombocytopenia and jaundice.

Pyrazinamide

Pyrazinamide is only active in acidic environments and is therefore principally effective against intracellular tubercle bacilli and those in acidic, anoxic inflammatory lesions. It freely enters the CSF, where levels achieved are similar to those in the plasma. Resistance is uncommon.

Despite early reports of hepatotoxicity, pyrazinamide is usually well tolerated and skin rashes occur rarely (Figure 56.66). Although moderate elevations of serum transaminases occur early in treatment, severe hepatotoxicity is uncommon except in patients with pre-existing liver disease. Its principal metabolite, pyrazinoic acid, inhibits renal excretion of uric acid, occasionally resulting in gout requiring treatment with allopurinol. An unrelated arthralgia, notably of the shoulders and responsive to analgesics, also occurs.

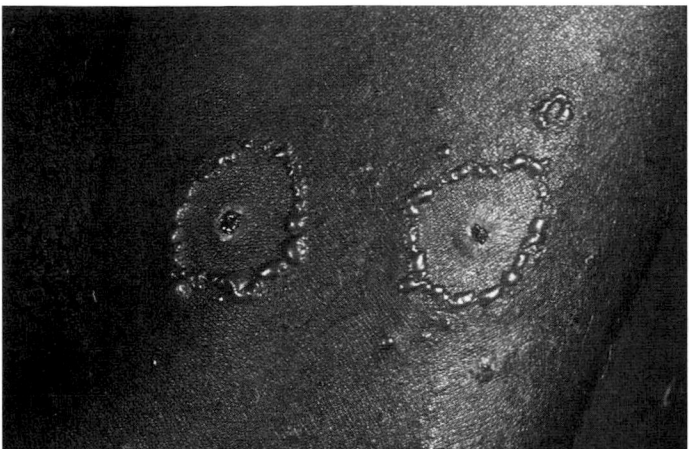

Figure 56.66 Reaction to antituberculosis drugs: 'Target lesions' due to pyrazinamide.

Other side-effects include anorexia, nausea and photosensitization of the skin.

Second-line drugs

These are indicated in cases of drug resistance and, very occasionally, when the use of a first-line drug is prevented by adverse drug reactions. In general, they are less effective, more toxic and more expensive than the first-line drugs. As mentioned above, there are six classes of second-line drugs, namely: aminoglycosides, thioamides, fluoroquinolones, polypeptides, p-aminosalicylic acid and cycloserine.[23] In addition, a few experimental agents are being evaluated.[82]

Thiacetazone is no longer included as, although once widely used, the WHO strongly recommends that it should be abandoned on account of its poor activity, widespread resistance to it and the high risk of severe and sometimes fatal skin reactions, including exfoliative dermatitis and Stevens–Johnson syndrome, particularly in those who are infected with HIV.

Aminoglycosides

Streptomycin was the first effective antituberculosis drug but is no longer a first-line drug as it has the disadvantage that it is not absorbed from the intestine and must therefore be given by intramuscular injection. This raises the associated danger of transmission of HIV and other viruses by contaminated needles. The principal side-effects involve the vestibular apparatus of the inner ear and manifest as unsteadiness and vertigo. This complication is more likely in older patients and the damage may be permanent if the drug is not stopped immediately when the symptoms commence. Deafness occasionally occurs and, if an aminoglycoside is given during pregnancy, it can lead to impaired hearing in the child. A further uncommon complication is anaphylaxis. Other aminoglycosides active against tubercle bacilli are kanamycin and amikacin which, in common with streptomycin, must be given by intramuscular injection and are ototoxic and nephrotoxic.

Thioamides – ethionamide and prothionamide

These are bacteriostatic drugs structurally related to isoniazid, although no cross-resistance occurs. Their use is restricted by a high incidence of gastric irritation, although this undesirable effect is reduced by commencing with a low dose and gradually increasing to the full dose and by taking the drugs at bedtime.

Fluoroquinolones

Clinical trials on several fluoroquinolones including ofloxacin, ciprofloxacin, ofloxacin, levofloxacin and moxifloxacin have been or are currently being evaluated in clinical trials.[83]

Although not currently recommended as first-line drugs for the treatment of drug-susceptible tuberculosis (although preliminary reports suggest that they could reduce the length of standard therapy) these agents are included in regimens for MDRTB. Further studies to compare the efficacy of the various fluoroquinolones and to establish their optimum use are required.

Polypeptides – capreomycin and viomycin

In common with the aminoglycosides, they must be given by intramuscular injection and are ototoxic and nephrotoxic. They show partial cross-resistance with the aminoglycosides. Viomycin is no longer obtainable in many countries.

p-Aminosalicylic acid

This was one of the early antituberculosis drugs but is now rarely used as it has only bacteristatic activity, commonly causes gastrointestinal upsets and is of limited availability.

Cycloserine

This is a bacteriostatic drug which has unpleasant side-effects including headache, dizziness and psychiatric complications. It is usually the last drug of choice.

Other (including experimental) agents

After three decades of neglect, there is now a Gates Foundation-funded Global Alliance for TB Drug Development, which has considerable interest and activity in the development of new antituberculosis drugs. Among the rifamycins, rifabutin is used as an alternative to rifampicin in HIV-positive patients receiving antiretroviral therapy (p. 1026). There is anecdotal evidence for efficacy of the antileprosy drug clofazimine and of amidopenicillins in combination with β-lactamase inhibitors, such as amoxicillin with sulbactam. Groups of novel agents being evaluated in pre-clinical and clinical studies include diarylquinolones, nitroimidazoles, quinazolines and ethambutol analogues.[82] More detailed accounts of the antituberculosis drugs are available in other texts.[84–86]

Immunotherapy

The use of adjunct immunotherapy to treat tuberculosis is a subject of growing interest. Administration of exogenous IFNγ or

In January 2006, the GPSTB published its ambitious, yet realistic, global plan for control of tuberculosis between 2006 and 2015.[104] The aim of the plan, in common with that of the Millennium Development Goals, is to halve the prevalence of, and deaths due to, tuberculosis from the 1990 baseline by the year 2015. This will require the successful treatment of 50 million patients, including 800 000 with MDRTB or XDRTB and three million co-infected with HIV who will also receive antiretroviral therapy under the UNAIDS plan for universal access. The estimated cost will be US$50 billion and will therefore require an enormous and sustained advocacy effort but it has the potential to save at least 14 million lives. Other key elements of the plan are to develop and deploy, by 2015, new and effective vaccines and also therapeutic regimens that will reduce the treatment time to 1–2 months, be suitable for the cure of MDRTB and XDRTB and be compatible with antiretroviral therapy. It is noted in the plan that a particular effort will be required in the African and Eastern European WHO regions due, respectively, to the high incidence of HIV infection and MDRTB and XDRTB.

The WHO DOTS strategy

In the expanded DOTS framework for effective tuberculosis control published in 2002,[103] the five elements of the DOTS strategy are defined as:

- Sustained political commitment to increase human and financial resources and to make tuberculosis control a nationwide activity integral to national health systems
- Access to quality-assured tuberculosis sputum microscopy for case detection among people presenting with, or found through surveys to have, symptoms of tuberculosis (most importantly, prolonged cough). Special attention is necessary for case detection among HIV-infected people and other high-risk groups, such as people in institutions
- Standardized short-course therapy for all cases of tuberculosis under proper case-management conditions, including direct observation of therapy. Proper case-management conditions imply technically sound and socially supportive treatment services
- Uninterrupted supply of quality-assured drugs with reliable procurement and distribution systems
- Recording and reporting system enabling outcome assessment of each and every patient and assessment of the overall programme performance.

Case finding

This may be active, involving a deliberate enquiry of symptoms, usually a history of a cough of more than 3 weeks' duration, sometimes by means of door-to-door surveys. Passive case finding relies on patients with symptoms presenting at a clinic. The efficiency of the latter approach critically depends on public health education, the proximity of the clinic from the patients' homes and the reputation of the clinic in the region. In some regions, poor people prefer attending private practitioners even though they can ill afford them, as the state-sponsored centres have a poor reputation for caring and competence.

Diagnosis

This is usually based on sputum microscopy. As case holding is of key importance, the number of times that a patient has to attend a clinic should be kept to a minimum. A commonly adopted policy is to examine a sputum sample produced by the patient on his or her first visit, an early morning specimen brought to the clinic the following day and a third specimen collected on that visit. As mentioned above (p. 998) there are differing opinions on the value of the third specimen.

The efficiency and accuracy of sputum microscopy critically depend on the skill and dedication of the microscopist. As microscopical examination of sputum smears is tedious work, it is important to give laboratory staff a variety of examinations to undertake and no member of staff should examine more than 20 sputum smears each day. Quality control, training and attention to job satisfaction are important factors to be attended to in the management of microscopy services. The organization and practice of microscopy and other aspects of the tuberculosis laboratory are discussed in detail elsewhere.[29,30]

Supply of drugs

It is essential that a regular supply of good-quality drugs is maintained and that these are available to the patients at no cost to them. Intermittent supplies of drugs are a major cause of treatment failure, the emergence of drug resistance and a loss of public confidence in the treatment services. Combination preparations, containing two or more antituberculosis drugs, must only be purchased from manufacturers approved by the WHO, as poorly formulated preparations may not allow adequate levels of the drugs to be absorbed, with a risk of treatment failure and the development of drug resistance.

Supervision of therapy

As a result of the effectiveness of modern short-course therapy, and the rapid loss of infectiousness, patients with no complicating factors can be treated as out-patients and pursue normal occupational and social activities. As hospitalization is thus the exception rather than the rule in many regions, the question of supervision of therapy must be addressed. This, of the five points of the WHO, DOTS strategy, is the one that calls for particular care and attention in its planning and application.[105,106] While non-compliance with therapy is one of the major reasons for the global failure to control tuberculosis, dogmatic assertions on the need for every dose to be taken in the presence of a qualified health worker may well add to the problems. In some countries, patients accept a restrictive discipline of attending regularly for their medicine but in others this may prove counterproductive. Good results have been obtained by the use of volunteer supervisors chosen from the local community as this encourages a relationship between equals – concordance rather than compliance with 'authority'. Various incentives may enhance adherence to therapy. In one successful programme, patients pay a nominal fee at the commencement of therapy which is reimbursed, with interest, on successful completion of therapy.[107] Supervision strategies must be 'user-friendly', and must respect the dignity and human rights of the patient. In this respect, it is important to organize services on the basis of local attitudes and related factors and not on dogma.[108–110]

Tuberculosis, especially HIV-related tuberculosis, carries a definite stigma which may hinder treatment-seeking and adherence, and should be addressed in health education activities.[111]

Monitoring of tuberculosis control services

This is essential to ascertain whether the above strategies are effective and cost-effective in a given circumstance. For this purpose, record-keeping is essential and patients reaching the end of therapy should be followed up to detect early bacteriological relapse due to inadequate supervision of therapy.

When adopted and applied, the DOTS strategy is able to make a significant impact on tuberculosis and in 2005 about 45% of all tuberculosis patients received treatment under this strategy. Between 2002 and 2003 the global incidence of new cases of tuberculosis rose by 1% but, as a result of improved case finding and treatment, the prevalence declined by 5% and deaths dropped by 2.5% overall and 3.5% among those not infected with HIV.[15]

DOTS-plus

A necessary addition to the DOTS strategy is the effort to detect and treat multi-drug resistant tuberculosis (MDRTB) which can be cured in the majority of cases, even in relatively poor nations, if the required facilities for diagnosis and supervised treatment are available. To achieve effective control, the so-called DOTS-Plus strategy is required,[112] and the GPSTB has established a 'green light committee' to assess and facilitate pilot projects and publishes guidelines for establishing such pilot projects.[93,113]

Projects being evaluated include those based on empirical treatment regimens and the more costly but more effective ones based on individualized treatment regimens according to drug susceptibility patterns determined in the laboratory. DOTS-Plus strategies are in a state of evolution, and up-to-date WHO publications should be consulted for developments and guidelines. It is important that DOTS-Plus programmes are only introduced in regions where optimal DOTS strategies are already in place. The establishment of a DOTS-Plus programme at the expense of a DOTS programme can have a detrimental effect on overall tuberculosis control.

Global strategies for control of tuberculosis and HIV

The WHO DOTS strategy is the best way of controlling tuberculosis in regions with a high prevalence of HIV infection. Effective antituberculosis therapy is a highly effective and cost-effective way of prolonging life and improving the quality of life in those with HIV-related tuberculosis. In view of the particular stigma associated with HIV infection and the ways that this differs from region to region, operations research is essential to ensure that tuberculosis is diagnosed promptly and that therapy is completed. It is, however, becoming apparent that DOTS alone is insufficient to control tuberculosis in areas with a high prevalence of HIV infection and that additional strategies are required. To this end the GPSTB established a TB/HIV Working Group in 2001 to coordinate activities aimed at reducing the burden of tuberculosis in those infected with HIV and the burden of HIV-related problems in those with tuberculosis. There is increased collaboration between WHO groups involved in tuberculosis and HIV and a key aim is to make antiretroviral agents more widely available.[114]

BACILLE CALMETTE–GUÉRIN VACCINATION

The only vaccine currently available for the prevention of tuberculosis is Bacille Calmette–Guérin (BCG), named after Albert Calmette and Camille Guérin, the French investigators who developed the vaccine from a strain of *M. bovis* early in the twentieth century. This live attenuated vaccine was intended for oral administration in neonates to mimic protection conferred by milk-borne *M. bovis* infection but without the risk of disease. Following a tragedy at the German city of Lübeck in 1930, when children were accidentally vaccinated with a virulent strain of *M. tuberculosis* with the death of over 70, the vaccine was prepared in central facilities and freeze-dried for intradermal use.

The mode of action of BCG vaccination is poorly understood. It prevents disseminated forms of primary tuberculosis, such as tuberculous meningitis, in children but it has only a small impact on post-primary, infectious, pulmonary tuberculosis. It is therefore of limited value in global control strategies. A major problem in its use is that, as shown in Table 56.14, its efficacy has been

Table 56.14 Protection afforded by BCG vaccination in nine major trials

Country	Year of commencement of trial	Age range at time of vaccination	Protection afforded (%)
North America	1935	0–20 years	80
Chicago, USA	1937	3 months	75
Great Britain	1950	14–15 years	78
Puerto Rico	1949	1–18 years	31
South India	1950	All ages	31
Georgia, USA	1950	5 years	14
Illinois, USA	1948	Young adults	0
South India[a]	1968	All ages	0
Malawi	1978	All ages	0

[a] No protection at 7.5-year follow-up but some protection at 15-year follow-up in those vaccinated in infancy.

3. Kremer K, Glynn JR, Lillebaek T, et al. Definition of the Beijing/W lineage of *Mycobacterium tuberculosis* on the basis of genetic markers. *J Clin Microbiol* 2004; 42:4040–4049.

4. Toungoussova OS, Caugant DA, Sandven P, et al. Impact of drug resistance on fitness of *Mycobacterium tuberculosis* strains of the W-Beijing genotype. *FEMS Immunol Med Microbiol* 2004; 42:281–290.

5. Glynn JR, Crampin AC, Yates MD, et al. The importance of recent infection with *Mycobacterium tuberculosis* in an area with high HIV prevalence: a long-term molecular epidemiological study in northern Malawi. *J Infect Dis* 2005; 192:480–487.

6. Wallgren A. The time table of tuberculosis. *Tubercle* 1948; 29:245–251.

7. Rook GAW, Zumla A. Advances in the immunopathogenesis of pulmonary tuberculosis. *Curr Opin Pulm Med* 2001; 7:116–123.

8. Wilkinson RJ, Llewelyn M, Toossi Z, et al. Influence of vitamin D deficiency and vitamin D receptor polymorphisms on tuberculosis among Gujarati Asians in west London: a case-control study. *Lancet* 2000; 355: 618–621.

9. Hernandez-Pando R, de la Luz Streber M, Orozco H, et al. Emergent immunoregulatory properties of combined glucocorticoid and anti-glucocorticoid steroids in a model of tuberculosis. *QJM* 1998; 91: 755–766.

10. Iwasaki A, Medzhitov R. Toll-like receptor control of the adaptive immune response. *Nature Immunol* 2004; 5:987–995.

11. Means TK, Jones BW, Schromm AB, et al. Differential effects of a Toll-like receptor antagonist on *Mycobacterium tuberculosis*-induced macrophage responses. *J Immunol* 2001; 166:4074–4082.

12. Smith I. *Mycobacterium tuberculosis* pathogenesis and molecular determinants of virulence. *Clin Microbiol Rev* 2003; 16:463–496.

13. Deretic V, Singh S, Master S, et al. *Mycobacterium tuberculosis* inhibition of phagolysosome biogenesis and autophagy as a host defence mechanism. *Cell Microbiol* 2006; 8:719–727.

14. Pym AS, Brodin P, Majlessi L, et al. Recombinant BCG exporting ESAT-6 confers enhanced protection against tuberculosis. *Nature Med* 2003; 9: 533–539.

15. WHO. *Global Tuberculosis Control: Surveillance, Planning, Financing*. WHO Report. Geneva: World Health Organization; 2006: WHO/HTM/TB/2006.34962.

16. Van Soolingen D. Molecular epidemiology of tuberculosis and other mycobacterial infections: main methodologies and achievements. *J Int Med* 2001; 249:1–26.

17. Groenen PM, Bunchoten D, van Soolingen D, et al. Nature of DNA polymorphism in the direct repeat cluster of *Mycobacterium tuberculosis* and its use as an epidemiological tool. *Mol Microbiol* 1993; 10:1057–1065.

18. UNAIDS/Stop TB Partnership. *Information pack on TB/HIV*. Geneva: World Health Organization; 2006.

19. Ahmed Y, Mwaba P, Chintu C, et al. A study of maternal mortality at University Teaching Hospital, Lusaka, Zambia: the emergence of tuberculosis as a major non-obstetric cause of maternal death. *Int J Tuberc Lung Dis* 1999; 3:675–681.

20. WHO. *Progress Report on the Global Plan to Stop Tuberculosis*. Geneva: World Health Organization; 2004: WHO/HTM/STB/2004.29.

21. WHO. *Anti-Tuberculosis Drug Resistance in the World*. Report No. 3. Geneva: World Health Organization; 2004: WHO/HTM/2004.343.

22. Mitchison DA. How drug resistance emerges as a result of poor compliance during short course chemotherapy of tuberculosis. *Int J Tuberc Lung Dis* 1998; 2:10–15.

23. Centers for Disease Control. Emergence of *Mycobacterium tuberculosis* with extensive resistance to second-line drugs – worldwide, 2000–2004. *MMWR* 2006; 55:301–305.

24. Davies RPO, Tocque K, Bellis MA, et al. Historical declines in tuberculosis in England and Wales: improving social conditions or natural selection? *Int J Tuberc Lung Dis* 1999; 3:1051–1054.

25. Grange JM, Gandy M, Farmer P, et al. Historical declines in tuberculosis – nature, nurture and the biosocial model. *Int J Tuberc Lung Dis* 2001; 3: 208–212.

26. Gajalakshmi V, Peto R, Kanaka TS, et al. Smoking and mortality from tuberculosis and other diseases in India: retrospective study of 43 000 adult male deaths and 35 000 controls. *Lancet* 2003; 362:507–515.

27. American Thoracic Society, Centers for Disease Control. Treatment of tuberculosis and tuberculosis infection in adults and children. *Am J Respir Crit Care Med* 1994; 149:1359–1374.

28. Grange JM, Ustianowski A, Zumla A. Tuberculosis and pregnancy. In: Diwan V, Thorson A, Winkvist A, eds. *Gender and Tuberculosis*. Göteborg: Nordic School of Public Health; 1998:77–88.

29. Collins CH, Grange JM, Yates MD. *Tuberculosis Bacteriology: Organization and Practice*. 2nd edn. London: Butterworth-Heinemann; 1997.

30. International Union Against Tuberculosis and Lung Disease. *Management of Tuberculosis: A Guide for Low Income Countries*. 5th edn. Paris: IUATLD; 2000.

31. Rieder HL, Chiang CY, Rusen ID. A method to determine the utility of the third diagnostic and the second follow-up sputum smear examinations to diagnose tuberculosis cases and failures. *Int J Tuberc Lung Dis* 2005; 9:384–391.

32. Leonard MK, Osterholt D, Kourbatova EV, et al. How many sputum specimens are necessary to diagnose pulmonary tuberculosis? *Am J Infect Control* 2005; 33:58–61.

33. Saglam L, Akgun M, Aktas E. Usefulness of induced sputum and fibreoptic bronchoscopy specimens in the diagnosis of pulmonary tuberculosis. *J Int Med Res* 2005; 33:260–265.

34. Olu Osoba A. Microbiology of tuberculosis. In: Madkour M, ed. *Tuberculosis*. Berlin: Springer; 2003:115–132.

35. Andreu J, Caceres J, Pallisa E, et al. Radiological manifestations of pulmonary tuberculosis. *Eur J Radiol* 2004; 51:139–149.

36. Shamputa IC, Rigouts L, Portaels F. Molecular genetic methods for diagnosis and antibiotic resistance detection of mycobacteria from clinical specimens. *APMIS* 2004; 112:728–752.

37. Fitzgerald JM, Menzies D. Interpretation of the tuberculin skin test. In: Davies PDO, ed. *Clinical Tuberculosis*. 3rd edn. London: Arnold; 2003:323–336.

38. Dheda K, Udwadia ZF, Huggett JF, et al. Utility of the antigen-specific interferon-gamma assay for the management of tuberculosis. *Curr Opin Pulm Med* 2005; 11:195–202.

39. WHO. Guidance for national tuberculosis programmes on the management of tuberculosis in children. Geneva: World Health Organization; 2006: WHO/HTM/TB/2006.371.

40. Fourie PB, Becker PJ, Festenstein F, et al. Procedures for developing a simple scoring method based on unsophisticated criteria for screening children for tuberculosis. *Int J Tuberc Lung Dis* 1998; 2:116–123.

41. Marais BJ, Gie RP, Obihara CC, et al. Well defined symptoms are of value in the diagnosis of childhood pulmonary tuberculosis. *Arch Dis Child* 2005; 90:1162–1165.

42. Delacourt C, Mani TM, Bonnerot V, et al. Computed tomography with normal chest radiograph in tuberculous infection. *Arch Dis Child* 1993; 69:430–432.

43. Smith KC. Congenital tuberculosis: a rare manifestation of a common infection. *Curr Opin Infect Dis* 2002;15:269–274.

44. Marais BJ, Donald PR, Gie RP, et al. Diversity of disease in childhood pulmonary tuberculosis. *Ann Trop Paediatr* 2005; 25:79–86.

45. Ormerod LP, Grundy M, Rathman MA. Multiple tuberculous bone lesions resembling metastatic disease. *Tubercle* 1989; 70:305–307.

46. Joseffer SS, Cooper PR. Modern imaging of spinal tuberculosis. *J Neurosurg Spine* 2005; 2:145–150.

47. Nene A, Bhojraj S. Results of nonsurgical treatment of thoracic spinal tuberculosis in adults. *Spine J* 2005; 5:79–84.

48. Thwaites G, Chan TT, Mai NT, et al. Tuberculous meningitis. *J Neurol Neurosurg Psychiatry* 2000; 68:289–299.

49. Johansen IS, Lundgren B, Tabak F, et al. Improved sensitivity of nucleic acid amplification for rapid diagnosis of tuberculous meningitis. *J Clin Microbiol* 2004; 42:3036–3040.

50. Prasad K, Volmink J, Menon GR. Steroids for treating tuberculous meningitis. *Cochrane Database Syst Rev* 2000; CD002244.

51. Thwaites GE, Nguyen DB, Nguyen HD, et al. Dexamethasone for the treatment of tuberculous meningitis in adolescents and adults. *N Engl J Med* 2004; 351:1741–1751.

52. Ustvedt HJ. The relationship between renal tuberculosis and primary infection. *Tubercle* 1947; 28:22–25.

53. Petersen L, Mommsen S, Pallisgaard G. Male genitourinary tuberculosis: report of 12 cases and review of the literature. *Scand J Urol Nephrol* 1993; 27:425–428.

54. Eastwood JB, Corbishley CM, Grange JM. Tuberculosis and the kidney. *J Am Soc Nephrol* 2001; 12:1307–1314.

55. Eastwood JB, Corbishley CM, Grange JM. Renal tuberculosis and other mycobacterial infections. In: Davidson AMA, Cameron JS, Grunfeld J-P, et al., eds. *Oxford Textbook of Nephrology*. 4th edn. Oxford: Oxford University Press; 2004;7.3.

56. Morgan SH, Eastwood JB, Baker LRI. Tuberculous interstitial nephritis: the tip of an iceberg. *Tubercle* 1991; 71:5–6.

57. Eastwood JB, Zaidi M, Maxwell JD, et al. Tuberculosis as primary renal diagnosis in end-stage uraemia. *J Nephrol* 1994; 7:290–293.

58. Menzies RI, Alsen H, Fitzgerald JM, et al. Tuberculous peritonitis in Lesotho. *Tubercle* 1986; 67:47–54.

59. Tshibwabwa–Tumba E, Mwaba P, Bogle-Taylor J, et al. Four year study of abdominal ultrasound in 900 Central African adults with AIDS referred for diagnostic imaging. *Abdominal Imaging* 2000; 25:290–296.

60. Akgun Y. Intestinal and peritoneal tuberculosis. Changing trends over 10 years and a review of 80 patients. Canadian Journal of Surgery 2005; 48: 131–136.

61. Falkner MJ, Reeve PA, Locket S. The diagnosis of tuberculous ascites in a rural African community. *Tubercle* 1985; 66:55–59.

62. Grange JM, Noble WC, Yates MD, et al. Inoculation mycobacterioses. *Clin Exp Dermatol* 1988; 13:211–220.

63. Morrison JGL, Fourie ED. The papulonecrotic tuberculide from Arthus reaction to lupus vulgaris. *Br J Dermatol* 1974; 91:273–277.

64. Lau SK, Wei WI, Hsu C, et al. Efficacy of fine needle aspiration in the diagnosis of tuberculous cervical lymphadenopathy. *J Laryngol Otol* 1990; 104:24–27.

65. Strang JI. Tuberculous pericarditis in Transkei. *Clin Cardiol* 1984; 7:667–670.

66. Dinning WJ, Marston S. Cutaneous and ocular tuberculosis: a review. *J R Soc Med* 1985; 78:576–581.

67. Rosen PH, Spalton DJ, Graham EM. Intraocular tuberculosis. *Eye* 1990; 4:486–492.

68. Alevritis EM, Sarubbi FA, Jordan RM, et al. Infectious causes of adrenal insufficiency. *South Med J* 2003; 96:888–890.

69. Glynn JR, Crampin AC, Yates MD, et al. The importance of recent infection with *Mycobacterium tuberculosis* in an area with high HIV prevalence: a long-term molecular epidemiological study in Northern Malawi. *J Infect Dis* 2005; 192:480–487.

70. Schon T, Wolday D, Elias D, et al. Kinetics of sedimentation rate, viral load and TNF-alpha in relation to HIV co-infection in tuberculosis. *Trans R Soc Trop Med Hyg* 2006; 100:483–488.

71. Lucas SB, Peacock CS, Hounnou A, et al. Disease in children infected with HIV in Abidjan, Cote-d'Ivoire. *BMJ* 1996; 312:335–338.

72. Tshibwabwa-Tumba E, Mwinga A, Pobee JOM, et al. Radiological features of pulmonary tuberculosis in 963 HIV-infected adults at three Central African hospitals. *Clin Radiol* 1997; 52:837–841.

73. WHO. *TB/HIV. A Clinical Manual*. 2nd edn. Geneva: World Health Organization; 2004.

74. Lawn SD, Bekker LG, Wood R. How effectively does HAART restore immune responses to *Mycobacterium tuberculosis*? Implications for tuberculosis control. *AIDS* 2005; 19:1113–1124.

75. Grimwade K, Sturm AW, Nunn AJ, et al. Effectiveness of cotrimoxazole prophylaxis on mortality in adults with tuberculosis in rural South Africa. *AIDS* 2005; 19:163–168.

76. WHO HIV/AIDS Programme. Antiretroviral therapy for HIV infection in adults and adolescents in resource-limited settings: towards universal access. Recommendations for a public health approach. 2006 Revision. Geneva: World Health Organization; 2006.

77. WHO Global Tuberculosis Programme and UNAIDS. *Policy Statement on Preventive Therapy against Tuberculosis in People Living with HIV*. Geneva: WHO, 1998.

78. Cosivi O, Grange JM, Daborn CJ, et al. Zoonotic tuberculosis due to *Mycobacterium bovis* in developing countries. *Emerg Infect Dis* 1998; 4:59–70.

79. Kazwala RR, Daborn CJ, Sharp JM, et al. Isolation of *Mycobacterium bovis* from human cases of cervical adenitis in Tanzania: a cause for concern? *Int J Tuberc Lung Dis* 2001; 5:87–91.

80. Mitchison DA. The role of individual drugs in the chemotherapy of tuberculosis. *Int J Tuberc Lung Disease* 2000; 4:796–806.

81. WHO. *Treatment of Tuberculosis: Guidelines for National Programmes*. 3rd edn. Geneva: WHO; 2003: WHO/CDS/TB2003.313.

82. Onyebujoh P, Zumla A, Ribiero I, et al. Treatment of tuberculosis: present status and future prospects. *Bull WHO* 2005; 83:857–865.

83. Ziganshina LE, Vizel AA, Squire SB. Fluoroquinolones for treating tuberculosis. *Cochrane Database Syst Rev* 2005; 3:CD004795.

84. Grange JM, Zumla A. Antituberculosis agents. In: Cohen J, Powderly WG, eds. *Infectious Diseases*. London: Elsevier Health Sciences. 2nd edn. Section 7. 2003; 1851–1867.

85. Grange JM. Antimycobacterial agents. In: Finch RG, Greenwood D, Norrby SR, et al., eds. *Antibiotic and Chemotherapy*. 8th edn. Edinburgh: Churchill Livingstone; 2003:426–440.

86. Peloquin CA. Clinical pharmacology of antituberculosis drugs. In: Davies PDO, ed. *Clinical Tuberculosis*. 3rd edn. London: Arnold; 2003:171–190.

87. Johnson JL, Kamya RM, Okwera AM, et al. Randomised controlled trial of *Mycobacterium vaccae* immunotherapy in non-immunodeficiency virus-infected Ugandan adults with newly diagnosed pulmonary tuberculosis. *J Infect Dis* 2000; 181:1304–1312.

88. Stanford JL, Stanford CA, Grange JM, et al. Does immunotherapy with heat-killed *Mycobacterium vaccae* offer hope for multi-drug-resistant pulmonary tuberculosis? *Respir Med* 2001; 95:444–447.

89. Yew WW. Clinically significant interactions with drugs used in the treatment of tuberculosis. *Drug Saf* 2002; 25:111–133.

90. Launay-Vacher V, Izzedine H, Deray G. Pharmacokinetic considerations in the treatment of tuberculosis in patients with renal failure. *Clin Pharmacokinet* 2005; 44:221–235.

91. Chan ED, Laurel V, Strand MJ, et al. Treatment and outcome analysis of 205 patients with multidrug-resistant tuberculosis. *Am J Respir Crit Care Med* 2004; 169:1103–1109.

92. Nathanson E, Lambregts-van-Weezenbeek C, Rich ML, et al. Multidrug-resistant tuberculosis management in resource-limited settings. *Emerg Infect Dis* 2006; 12:1389–1397.

93. WHO. *Guidelines for the Programmatic Management of Drug-Resistant Tuberculosis*. Geneva: World Health Organization; 2006: WHO/HTM/TB/2006.361.

94. Farmer P, Kim JY. Community based approaches to the control of multidrug resistant tuberculosis: introducing 'DOTS-plus'. *BMJ* 1998; 317:671–674.

95. Alzeer AH, FitzGerald JM. Corticosteroids and tuberculosis: risks and use as adjunct therapy. *Tubercle Lung Dis* 1993; 74:6–11.

96. Israel HL. Chemoprophylaxis for tuberculosis. *Respir Med* 1993; 87:81–83.

97. Blumberg HM, Leonard MK, Jasmer RM. Update on the treatment of tuberculosis and latent tuberculosis infection. *J Am Med Assoc* 2005; 293:2776–2784. (Erratum in *J Am Med Assoc* 2005; 294:182; dosage error in text).

98. Shiraishi Y, Nakajima Y, Katsuragi N, et al. Resectional surgery combined with chemotherapy remains the treatment of choice for multidrug-resistant tuberculosis. *J Thorac Cardiovasc Surg* 2004; 128:523–528.

99. The Winterthur Health Forum. *Massive Effort Advocacy Forum Report. Massive Effort Against Diseases of Poverty*. Geneva: World Health Organization; 2000. Online. Available: www.winterthurhealthforum.org

100. Grange JM, Zumla A. Tuberculosis and the poverty-disease cycle. *J R Soc Med* 1999; 92:105–107.

101. UN Millennium Project. *Investing in Development: A Practical Plan to Achieve the Development Goals*. New York: UNDP; 2005.

Table 57.1 The Runyon classification of the environmental mycobacteria

Group	Pigment types	Characteristics	Examples
I	Photochromogens	Producing pigment only on or after exposure to light	*M. kansasii, M. marinum*
II	Scotochromogens	Producing pigment in the dark	*M. scrofulaceum, M. gordonae*
III	Nonchromogens	Producing no pigment	*M. avium* complex, *M. malmoense, M. nonchromogenicum*
IV	Rapid growers[a]	Rapid growth and any of the above	*M. chelonae, M. fortuitum, M. vaccae*

[a]Most isolates from cases of human disease, on which the classification was based, are non-pigmented. Rapid growers isolated from the environment, e.g. *M. vaccae*, are mostly chromogenic.

Table 57.2 The usual environmental mycobacteria causing human disease according to category of disease

Disease	Causative agent
Lymphadenopathy	*M. avium* complex[a]
	M. scrofulaceum
Skin lesions	
Post-trauma abscesses	*M. chelonae*
	M. abscessus
	M. fortuitum
	M. peregrinum
	M. terrae group[b]
Swimming pool granuloma	*M. marinum*
Buruli ulcer	*M. ulcerans*[c]
Pulmonary disease	*M. avium* complex
	M. celatum
	M. gordonae
	M. kansasii
	M. malmoense
	M. simiae
	M. szulgai
	M. xenopi
Disseminated disease	
AIDS related	*M. avium* complex
	M. genevense
Non-AIDS related	*M. avium* complex
	M. abscessus
	M. chelonae
	M. haemophilum[d]

[a]Human pathogens in this group are *M. avium avium* and *M. avium intracellulare*.
[b]Includes *M. terrae, M. nonchromogenicum* and *M. triviale*.
[c]Includes strains named *M. shinshuense*.
[d]A rare cause of skin lesions in renal transplant patients and lymphadenopathy in children.

stood, clinically significant isolates of MAC from HIV-positive patients usually belong to the group defined by DNA analysis as *M. avium avium*, whereas a broader distribution of types is found in HIV-negative patients and in the environment.[8] Other members of the species are *M. avium lepraemurium*, the cause of a leprosy-like disease of rodents and cats, *M. avium sylvaticum*, a cause of disease in wood pigeons and *M. avium paratuberculosis*, the cause of hypertrophic enteritis or Johne's disease in cattle.

Some species of EM grow very poorly, or not at all, on standard culture media and some require nutritional supplements for growth. Thus some MAC, especially strains of *M. avium paratuberculosis* and *M. avium sylvaticum*, require the addition of mycobactin, a lipid iron-chelating agent found in the cell walls of most mycobacteria, and *M. haemophilum* requires the addition of haem or other sources of iron to the culture medium.

Only a few of the rapid-growing species cause human disease and the three most usually encountered are *M. abscessus*, *M. chelonae* and *M. fortuitum*. Uncommon causes are *M. flavescens* and *M. peregrinum*. Little is known about the determinants of virulence of the EM causing human disease. One species, *M. ulcerans*, produces a toxin, as described below.

EPIDEMIOLOGY AND PREDISPOSING FACTORS

Except, perhaps, in extreme environments, such as deserts and the polar regions, the human population is regularly exposed to EM, yet disease resulting from such contact is very uncommon. On the other hand, various immune responses induced by exposure to EM provide the most plausible explanation for the wide geographical variations in the efficacy of BCG vaccination as discussed in Chapter 56.

There has been a recent increase in the prevalence of disease due to EM in some regions as a result of HIV disease and other forms of immune suppression. An increase in prevalence has also been observed in non-HIV infected persons in some regions.[9] This observed increase could be the result of greater clinical awareness and improvements in microbiological technique but this may not be the complete explanation. One particular disease, Buruli ulcer (see below), has certainly increased in prevalence in parts of Africa and this has been attributed to environmental changes. On the other hand, HIV-related MAC disease was common in Europe before the introduction of antiretroviral therapy (ART) but, although the organisms are present in the African environment, such disease is rare in that continent where ART is, at present, not widely available.

An inverse relationship between the incidence of tuberculosis and disease due to EM has been observed, suggesting that the former may induce protective immunity against the latter. Likewise, BCG vaccination may also protect against disease due to EM. Thus a substantial increase in the incidence of lymphadenopathy due to EM in children has been shown to occur in countries where neonatal BCG vaccination has been terminated.[10]

Patients with pulmonary and disseminated disease due to EM often have underlying predisposing conditions such as cancer (including lymphoproliferative disorders such as Hodgkin's disease and hairy cell leukaemia), autoimmune disease, renal failure, post-transplant immunosuppressive therapy, high-dose corticosteroid therapy, overt congenital immunodeficiencies and HIV disease. Lung disease, including bronchiectasis, cystic fibrosis and industrial disease, is a predisposing factor. A minority of patients have no detectable local or general predisposing factors.

There is evidence that those exposed to aerosols containing mycobacteria through the use of showers, aerated hot tubs and spas are at risk of pulmonary disease.[1,2,11] Miners are exposed to the dual predisposing factors of dust and contaminated aerosols and, in a study of South African gold miners in 1995, mycobacteria were cultured from sputum from 505 miners: 425 cultures yielded M. tuberculosis, seven yielded a mixed growth of M. tuberculosis and EM and 73 yielded just EM. Of the latter, 51 of the 73 were judged to have disease due to EM on the basis of the American Thoracic Society criteria described below. Patients with EM disease were less likely to be HIV-positive (35%) than those with tuberculosis (49%) and the commonest cause of disease was M. kansasii (34 of 51).[12] A subsequent study confirmed that M. kansasii was the predominant cause of EM disease among South African gold miners and it was noted that this species has been associated with mining and pneumoconiosis in other countries, notably Czechoslovakia.[13]

As mentioned above, patients with HIV disease are, for reasons that are not understood, particularly susceptible to disease due to a restricted range of genotypes of the MAC. A small proportion of cases of pulmonary disease due to EM occur in patients who are apparently otherwise healthy, although there is evidence that many such patients have low levels of cytokines involved in protective immunity to mycobacterial disease.[14] Most children with cervical lymphadenopathy due to EM appear to be otherwise healthy but a small minority have various forms of congenital immune defects and are prone to develop disseminated mycobacterial disease.

In addition to the predisposing factors discussed above, the risk of disease due to EM depends on the number and types of EM in the environment. Some species of EM causing disease, such as the MAC, are found worldwide while others, including M. xenopi, M. malmoense and M. ulcerans, are more restricted in their geographical distribution. In addition, the relative preponderance of EM in a given environment varies over time and this is reflected in changes in the observed type of disease.[11] Thus in the USA, the predominant EM causing lymphadenitis in children has changed from M. scrofulaceum to MAC.

Infection is directly from the environment: human-to-human transmission leading to disease, if it occurs at all, is extremely rare

and the few reported clusters of cases could well have resulted from exposure to a common environmental source. Thus the incidence of disease due to EM in a given region is independent of that of tuberculosis, which is spread principally by human-to-human transmission.

Owing to a lack of suitable laboratory services, very little is known of the prevalence of disease due to EM in the tropics. In Lagos, Nigeria, culture of sputum from 668 patients with persistent symptoms of lower respiratory tract infection yielded 102 mycobacteria, of which 87 were M. tuberculosis, 4 were M. bovis and 11 were EM: 6 MAC, 4 M. kansasii and 1 M. fortuitum.[15] In Guinea-Bissau, mycobacteria were isolated from 206 patients with suspected tuberculosis: 189 (36 HIV positive) yielded M. tuberculosis and 17 (2 HIV positive) yielded MAC.[16] In the absence of facilities for culture, the disease would have been misdiagnosed in up to 10% of patients, but it is not known whether these findings are representative of other tropical countries.[17]

DIAGNOSIS

The only disease due to EM with clear-cut pathognomonic features is Buruli ulcer. The other dermatological, pulmonary and disseminated manifestations of EM disease are non specific and require differentiation from tuberculosis and other infectious and non-infectious conditions with which they may be confused. Diagnosis is usually based on isolation and identification of the causative organism although, as mentioned above, EM are ubiquitous in nature. Thus, their isolation from clinical specimens, especially sputum and urine, that are likely to be contaminated with various bacteria, does not itself indicate that they are causing disease.

It is not unusual to obtain single isolates of EM from sputum and, more especially, from urine.[18] Thus, as a general rule, several cultures of an EM from sputum – at least two, but preferably three or four, cultures yielding a heavy growth at least 1 week apart – with compatible clinical features and careful exclusion of other causes, including tuberculosis, are required for diagnosis of pulmonary disease.[19] Criteria for the diagnosis of pulmonary disease due to EM proposed by the American Thoracic Society are listed in Table 57.3.

As the external genitalia and lower urethra are frequently contaminated by EM, and as renal disease due to them is very rare, even stricter criteria for diagnosis are required, including histological demonstration of granulomas in, and isolation of the EM from, the lesion itself.

As mentioned above, all specimens must be collected directly into sterile containers to avoid a false diagnosis. Where available, fibreoptic bronchoscopy is a useful technique for obtaining aspirates or biopsies directly from suspicious pulmonary lesions,[20] but false diagnoses have resulted from the use of inadequately sterilized endoscopes.[21]

Once isolated, EM are usually identified in reference laboratories, as described above. The use of reagents prepared from a range of EM have been used in differential skin testing for the diagnosis of disease due to EM,[22] but the British Thoracic Society concludes that more research is needed before this diagnostic method can be recommended.[23]

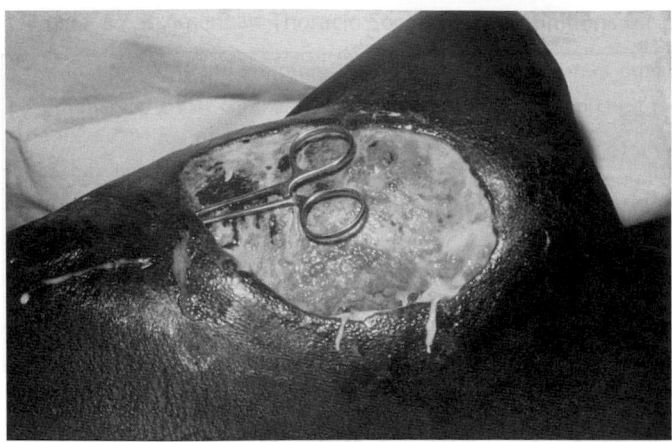

Figure 57.4 Buruli ulcer: large and deeply undermined ulcer overlying the left shoulder. The inserted 'Spencer Wells' forceps illustrates the extensive undermining of the ulcer.

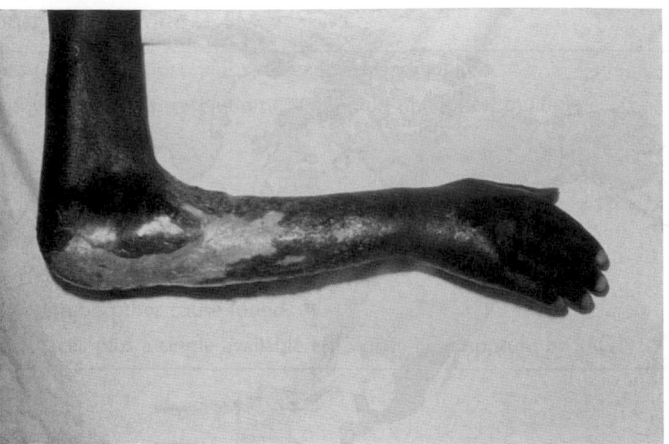

Figure 57.7 Buruli ulcer: healed lesion with extensive scarring leading to a fixed elbow joint. The skin is thin and easily traumatized. Note the oedematous hand due to a compromised lymphatic drainage.

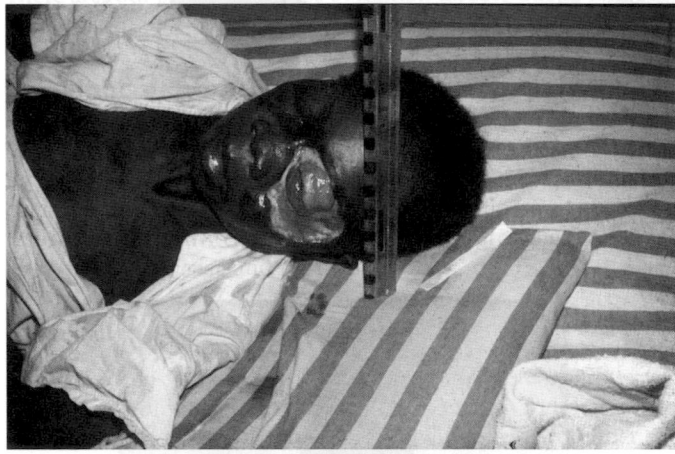

Figure 57.5 Buruli ulcer: lesion involving the left eye and orbit. The lesion eventually resolved, unfortunately with loss of vision in the eye.

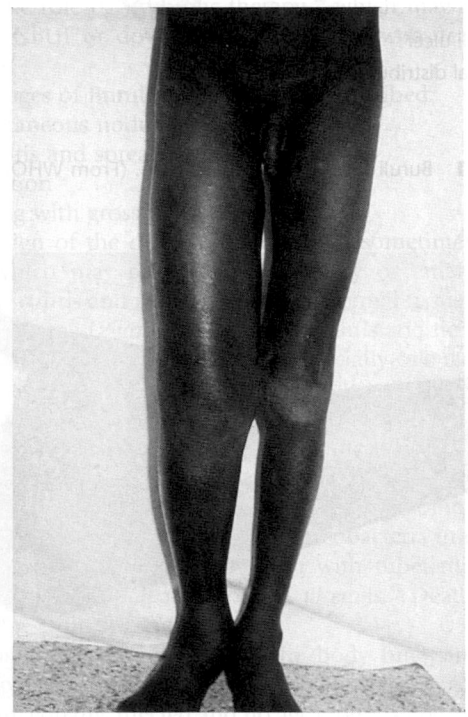

Figure 57.8 Buruli ulcer: Diffuse, non-ulcerating form of the disease in a Congolese child with lower limb swelling.

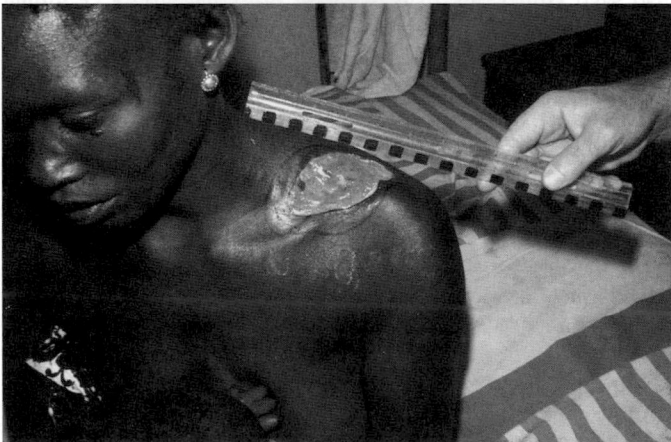

Figure 57.6 Buruli ulcer: a resolving ulcer on the left shoulder. Note the granulating base and absence of trophic changes in the surrounding skin.

tropical ulcers, cutaneous diphtheria, actinomycosis, cancrum oris, bacterial abscesses, skin tuberculosis and cutaneous leishmaniasis.

Diagnosis is made on clinical features, demonstration of acid-fast bacilli in smears from the bases of progressive ulcers, biopsy and demonstration of *M. ulcerans* by conventional culture or, where available, PCR.

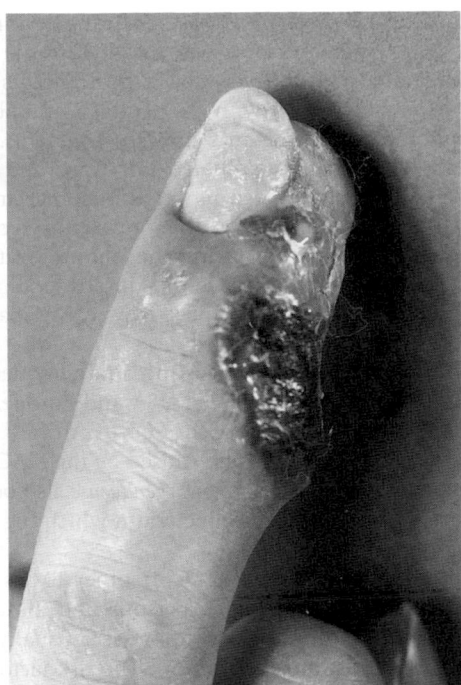

Figure 57.9 'Fish tank granuloma' due to *M. marinum* infection.

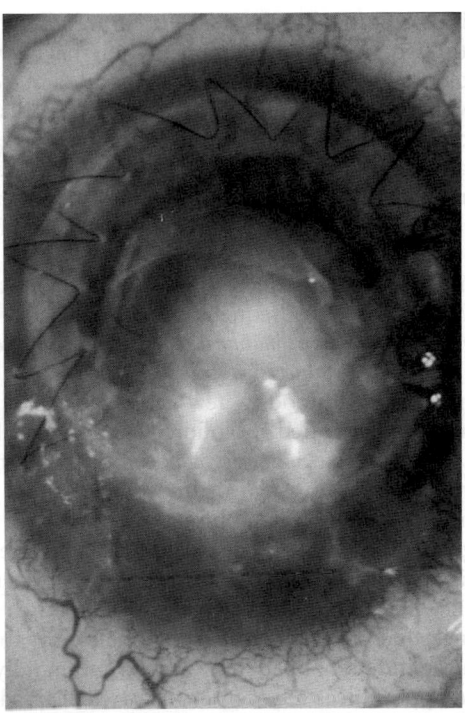

Figure 57.10 Keratitis due to *M. chelonae* following corneal transplant. Note the characteristic 'cracked windscreen' appearance.

Swimming pool granuloma

Also called fish tank granuloma, this disease is caused by *M. marinum*, a water-borne EM that enters cuts and abrasions acquired while swimming in pools or handling tropical fish tanks.[37,38] Cases have also occurred among fishermen. The condition is characterized by the development of warty skin lesions resembling those of skin tuberculosis at the site of inoculation (Figure 57.9). Secondary lesions often develop along the draining lymphatics, resembling those seen in the fungal disease sporotrichosis and thus termed sporotrichoid spread. Rare complications include carpal tunnel syndrome, osteomyelitis and disseminated disease. Uncomplicated lesions usually heal spontaneously after a few months but treatment, described below, accelerates resolution.

Other forms of post-inoculation EM disease

Three main types of lesion are encountered – superficial warty lesions similar to those of swimming pool granuloma, localized post-injection abscesses and deeper lesions following more serious penetrating injuries or surgical procedures.

Superficial warty lesions

These have occasionally been caused by *M. kansasii*, *M. szulgai*, *M. chelonae* and unidentified slow-growing scotochromogens and in some cases there is sporotrichoid spread.[39] Outbreaks of skin ulcers associated with non-cultivable mycobacteria have been reported on the USA/Canada border and in Brazil and are termed Feldman-Hershfield ulcers, after the workers who first described them.[40]

Post-injection abscesses

These are mostly caused by the rapid-growing species *M. abscessus*, *M. chelonae*, *M. fortuitum* and, rarely, *M. flavescens* and *M. peregrinum*. Abscesses may occur sporadically, especially when dirty needles are used, and are a cause of 'sterile' post-injection abscesses, so called because cultivation on standard media yields no bacterial growth. There have also been small outbreaks of abscesses after injection of contaminated material, such as vaccines, from multidose containers.[41,42] Abscesses develop 1–12 months after the injection and may reach an enormous size, up to 8 cm in diameter. Many abscesses remain localized and resolve after surgical drainage, curettage or excision but a spreading cellulitis requiring antimicrobial therapy may develop, especially in immunosuppressed persons and insulin-dependent diabetics. Corneal ulcers and abscesses due to *M. abscessus*, *M. chelonae* and *M. fortuitum* have followed abrasions or penetrating injuries of the cornea (Figure 57.10).[43]

Deeper lesions

Serious and life-threatening post-traumatic lesions due to *M. abscessus*, *M. chelonae* and *M. fortuitum* have followed cardiac surgery involving the insertion of bioprosthetic heart valves and, rarely, other forms of surgery involving the insertion of prosthetic devices,[44] and peritonitis due to the accidental introduction of EM has occurred in patients on intermittent peritoneal dialysis.[18]

Pulmonary disease

Most cases occur in middle-aged or elderly men who often have a history of smoking, bronchiectasis, healed tuberculosis or expo-

trials are awaited. There is also preliminary evidence that nitrogen oxide-generating creams limit the progression of disease.[58]

Swimming pool granuloma

Lesions due to *M. marinum* usually resolve spontaneously but recovery is accelerated by systemic treatment with minocycline, trimethoprim with sulfamethoxazole (co-trimoxazole) or a combination of ethambutol with either rifampicin or clarithromycin.[37] Small lesions may also be cured by surgical excision.

Disease due to slowly growing EM

The newer macrolides azithromycin or clarithromycin form the basis of the modern treatment for all forms of disease due to MAC, *M. kansasii*, *M. malmoense* or *M. xenopi*, irrespective of the site of disease and the immune status of the patients.[59] One of the macrolides is given with at least one companion drug, preferably ethambutol but alternatively rifabutin or a quinolone. Some reports state that the addition of rifabutin to the macrolide–ethambutol regimen improves the clinical response. Serious cases with high fever may require treatment with intravenous amikacin. The macrolide–ethambutol regimen is also the treatment of choice for pulmonary disease due to the species mentioned above in non-HIV-infected patients.[59] The duration of therapy depends on the clinical response. Disease due to the less common mycobacteria must be treated empirically; for example, *M. genavense* infections are treated with the drug combinations used for MAC. Surgery is used for localized pulmonary lesions that fail to respond to antimicrobial therapy.

Antiretroviral therapy (ART) is more important in the treatment of AIDS-related EM disease than antimycobacterial therapy and should be given when available.[60] Rifabutin causes fewer drug interactions with ART than rifampicin but treatment with a macrolide with ethambutol is preferable. Some patients receiving ART and antimycobacterial therapy develop the immune reconstitution inflammatory syndrome (IRIS).[61]

Disease due to rapidly growing EM

Localized post-injection and post-traumatic abscesses caused by the rapid growers *M. abscessus*, *M. chelonae* and *M. fortuitum* usually respond to excision, curettage or drainage, but multiple abscesses or spreading cellulitis, as are sometimes seen in insulin-dependent diabetics and immunocompromised persons, require antimicrobial therapy. Information on treatment is derived from anecdotal experience, which indicates that useful agents for localized disease include erythromycin with trimethoprim and/or doxycycline and, for spreading or disseminated disease, various combinations of amikacin, gentamicin, cephalosporins, clarithromycin, imipenem and fluoroquinolones. The outcome of therapy is very unpredictable and no guidelines on length of therapy can usefully be given.

Pulmonary disease due to the above rapidly growing EM, as occurs for example in children with cystic fibrosis, responds in a very unpredictable manner to therapy, which is based on the drugs described above for post-injection and post-traumatic lesions.

The rare cases of serious wound infection due to *M. abscessus*, *M. chelonae* or *M. fortuitum* in both HIV and non-HIV infected persons should be treated empirically as described above for disseminated disease due to these species.

Lymphadenopathy

Disease involving a single lymph node in an otherwise healthy child is usually curable by total excision if that can be achieved without damaging the facial nerve or other important structures. If total excision is not possible, antimicrobial therapy appropriate for the causative organism as described above is required. Opinions differ on the need for routine antimicrobial therapy for cases in which surgical excision appears complete. Nodes should not be merely incised and drained as this predisposes to chronic sinus formation.

NOCARDIAL DISEASE

Many species of nocardiae are found in the environment, notably in soil, and over 30 species have been shown to be associated with opportunist disease in humans, termed nocardiasis or nocardiosis. The principal causes of disease are *Nocardia asteroides* (including *N. cyriacigeorgica*) so named because of their star-shaped colonies. Other causes of disease are *N. farcinica*, *N. brasiliensis*, *N. abscessus*, *N. otitidiscaviarum*, *N. nova* and *N. transvalensis*. The other species are rarely encountered ones recently identified by molecular technology and isolated from profoundly immunosuppressed patients with a wide range of unusual presentations.[62]

Pathogenesis

As with mycobacterial disease, infection usually occurs by inhalation of the bacilli or, occasionally, by traumatic inoculation into the skin. Nocardiae are uncommon causes of opportunist pulmonary disease that usually, but not always, occurs in immunocompromised individuals, including those with HIV disease or those receiving chemotherapy for cancer or post-transplant immunosuppressive therapy.[63-68] Therapy with corticosteroids is a strong risk factor. As a result, the frequency and diversity of clinical manifestations of nocardial disease has increased in recent years. Pre-existing lung disease, especially alveolar proteinosis, also predisposes to nocardial disease. A few cases of aspiration pneumonia due to nocardiae following near-drowning have been reported, including cases of the recently described Tsunami lung – a chronic necrotizing pneumonia presenting about 1 month after immersion.[69] In a minority of cases, ranging from 10–25% in published reviews, no underlying predisposing disease or immunosuppressive condition was detected.[67]

The clinical and radiological features of nocardial pulmonary disease are non-specific and variable so that diagnosis is not easy and is often delayed or missed. Radiology usually reveals multiple confluent abscesses with little or no surrounding fibrous reaction. Local spread may cause pleural effusions, empyema and invasion of the bones of the thoracic cage. The course of the disease is very variable, from very chronic to rapid spread through the lungs. Secondary abscesses in the brain and, less frequently, in other organs due to haematogenous dissemination occur in about one-third of patients with pulmonary disease.[70] Widespread dissemination with skin abscesses and lesions in many organs is seen in those with AIDS and other causes of profound immunosuppression.[68]

Nocardiae cause primary post-traumatic, post-operative or post-inoculation cutaneous infections (primary cutaneous nocardiasis). This is usually caused by *N. brasiliensis* and, less often, by *N. asteroides*, *N. otitidiscaviarum*, *N. transvalensis* and, rarely, by some recently described species including *N. abscessus*, *N. africana* and *N. veterana*. Cutaneous infections may result in fungating tumour-like masses resembling mycetomas.

Laboratory diagnosis

Microscopical examination of sputum usually reveals numerous lymphocytes and macrophages, some of which contain pleomorphic Gram-positive and weakly acid-fast bacilli. Extracellular branching filaments may also be seen. The Gram–Weigert and Gomori methenamine silver methods are useful for demonstrating nocardiae in sections of tissue biopsies. Nocardiae grow on a range of laboratory media including Löwenstein–Jensen medium, with colonies visible between 2 days and 1 month after inoculation. Identification of nocardiae at the species level is not easy, especially as many newly described species, though genetically distinct, are very similar in their phenetic characteristics.[62] Thus identification is undertaken in specialist laboratories by molecular methods including PCR restriction enzyme analysis and 16S rRNA sequencing.

Treatment

The nocardiae, especially the more recently described ones, have variable drug susceptibilities but the more common ones, including *N. asteroides*, usually respond to treatment with sulphamethoxazole with trimethoprim (co-trimoxazole) for 3 or more months, although this prolonged course often causes adverse drug reactions and may be inadequate for severe and disseminated disease. An alternative regimen is high dose imipenem with amikacin, usually for 4–6 weeks. Limited experience indicates that various combinations of minocycline, third generation cephalosporins and linezolid (a member of the oxazolidinone class of synthetic antimicrobial agents for oral or intravenous use) are also effective. Strains of *M. farcinica* are often resistant to many antimicrobial agents including co-trimoxazole and cephalosporins, but one reported case of an extensive brain abscess responded well to moxifloxacin.[71] Drug susceptibility testing is subject to several variables and no standardized methods have been proposed. Mycetomata, even long-standing and extensive cases, respond well to antimicrobial therapy.

CONCLUSIONS

Relative to tuberculosis, disease due to EM is uncommon in tropical countries, although in some countries, notably some in West Africa, Buruli ulcer is becoming a major health problem. Although often associated with various forms of immunosuppression, some forms of EM disease such as post-inoculation lesions and lymphadenitis in children occur in otherwise healthy persons. Diagnosis is usually made by bacteriological techniques. There are relatively few firm guidelines to therapy, although several clinical trials are underway. If control measures succeed in reducing the prevalence in tuberculosis worldwide, disease due to EM, which is acquired by environmental exposure rather than human-to-human spread, will continue as a challenge to the physician. Nocardiosis, although uncommon, must be added to the list of infections that immunocompromised people are subject to and it poses yet another diagnostic and therapeutic challenge, especially in those with HIV disease.

REFERENCES

1. Collins CH, Grange JM, Yates MD. Mycobacteria in water. *J Appl Bacteriol* 1984; 57:193–211.
2. Primm TP, Lucero CA, Falkinham JO. Health impacts of environmental mycobacteria. *Clin Microbiol Rev* 2004; 17:98–106.
3. Zumla A, Grange JM. Infection and disease due to environmental mycobacteria. *Curr Opin Pulm Med* 2002; 8:166–172.
4. Runyon EH. Anonymous mycobacteria in pulmonary disease. *Med Clin North Am* 1959; 43:273–290.
5. Collins CH, Grange JM, Yates MD. *Tuberculosis Bacteriology: Organization and Practice.* 2nd edn. London: Butterworth-Heinemann, 1997.
6. Kirschner P, Springer B, Vogel U, et al. Genotypic identification of mycobacteria by nucleic acid sequence determination: report of a 2-year experience in a clinical laboratory. *J Clin Microbiol* 1993; 31: 2882–2889.
7. Arbeit RD, Slutsky A, Barber TW, et al. Genetic diversity of *Mycobacterium avium* strains causing monoclonal and polyclonal bacteremia in patients with the acquired immunodeficiency syndrome (AIDS). *J Infect Dis* 1993; 167:1384–1390.
8. Guthertz LS, Damsker B, Bottone EJ, et al. *Mycobacterium avium* and *Mycobacterium intracellulare* infections in patients with and without AIDS. *J Infect Dis* 1989; 160:1037–1041.
9. Marras TK, Daley CL. Epidemiology of human pulmonary infection with nontuberculous mycobacteria. *Clin Chest Med* 2002; 23:553–567.
10. Romanus V, Halalander HO, Wahlen P, et al. Atypical mycobacteria in extrapulmonary disease among children: incidence in Sweden from 1969 to 1990, related to changing BCG-vaccination coverage. *Tubercle Lung Dis* 1995; 76:300–310.
11. Falkinham JO. The changing pattern of nontuberculous mycobacterial disease. *Can J Infect Dis* 2003; 14:281–286.
12. Corbett EL, Blumberg L, Churchyard GJ, et al. Nontuberculous mycobacteria. Defining disease in a prospective cohort of South African miners. *Am J Respir Crit Care Med* 1999; 160:15–21.
13. Sonnenberg P, Muray J, Glynn JR, et al. Risk factors for pulmonary disease due to culture-positive *M. tuberculosis* or nontuberculous mycobacteria in South African gold miners. *Eur Respir J* 2000; 15:291–296.
14. Greinert U, Schlaak M, Rüsch-Gerdes S, et al. Low in vitro production of interferon-γ and tumour necrosis factor-α in HIV-seronegative patients with pulmonary disease caused by non-tuberculous mycobacteria. *J Clin Immunol* 2000; 20:445–452.
15. Idigbe EO, Anyiwo CE, Onwujekwe DI. Human pulmonary infections with bovine and atypical mycobacteria in Lagos, Nigeria. *J Trop Med Hyg* 1986; 89:143–148.
16. Koivula T, Hoffner S, Winqvist N, et al. *Mycobacterium avium* complex sputum isolates from patients with respiratory symptoms in Guinea-Bissau. *J Infect Dis* 1996; 173:263–265.
17. Zumla A, Grange JM. Non-tuberculous mycobacterial pulmonary infections. *Clinics in Chest Medicine* 2002; 23:369–376.
18. Eastwood JB, Corbishley CM, Grange JM. Renal tuberculosis and other mycobacterial infections. In: Davidson AMA, Cameron JS, Grunfeld J-P, et al.,

Chapter 58 Stephen G. Withington

Leprosy

INTRODUCTION

Leprosy is a chronic granulomatous disease caused by infection with *Mycobacterium leprae*. It is primarily characterized by an insidious process of direct infection of skin and nerves and associated immunological damage. Nerve involvement is responsible for repeated ulceration and paralysis affecting hands, feet and eyes. On a global scale leprosy is an important cause of physical disabilities, commonly affecting people in their most productive stage of life. The disability and related social stigma associated with leprosy and its complications result in significant barriers to full participation in society, and in considerable socioeconomic burden to those affected and society as a whole.

EPIDEMIOLOGY

Accurate information on leprosy is difficult to obtain, considering delays in diagnosis caused by the insidious onset of disease and fear of stigmatization, inaccuracies in treatment registry data, and incompleteness of reporting, particularly in regard to disability caused by leprosy. Almost 300 000 new cases of leprosy were reported in 2005, the vast majority occurring in South and Southeast Asia, South America and Africa, and nearly 220 000 were registered on treatment on 31 December, 2005 as shown in Table 58.1.[1] A total of 115 countries reported on leprosy in 2005, among which India, Brazil, Indonesia, Democratic Republic of the Congo, and Bangladesh reported the most new leprosy cases. Leprosy prevalence, measured in cases registered for treatment per 10 000 population, was highest in Mozambique, Nepal, Democratic Republic of the Congo, Brazil, Tanzania and Madagascar. Only these six countries remained above the WHO target for elimination of leprosy as a public health problem, defined as a registered prevalence of less than 1/10 000, at the end of 2005. For many years, two-thirds of all new cases of leprosy have been reported from India alone. In recent years there has been a significant fall-off in new cases in India and overall global trends reflect this, though elsewhere there is little or no evidence of a decline in new cases.

The global registered prevalence of leprosy has decreased markedly in the 20 years since 1985, when around 5.4 million were on treatment registers. Interpretation of prevalence and incidence trends is, however, complicated by significant reductions in duration of treatment, the widespread updating of treatment registers, and large scale public health campaigns. In addition, recent changes in health system management of leprosy, particularly the integration of leprosy into general health services in many countries, notably India, have necessitated a major simplification of guidelines, and a decreased focus on leprosy. Over 14 million people have been cured of leprosy since 1985; however, a significant proportion of these have ongoing disability as a result of leprosy-related nerve damage. Data on disability due to leprosy are scarce, but it is probable that 3 million or more people are currently living with leprosy-related physical impairments and disabilities. Many are suffering stigmatization as a result, including both felt and enacted stigma.

Distribution

Leprosy is known to occur at all ages, with incidence rates peaking in young adulthood. Disability due to leprosy is associated with increasing age at diagnosis. Males are more commonly diagnosed with leprosy than women in many, though not all countries, often in the ratio of 2 : 1. Since the diagnosis of leprosy is highly sensitive to operational issues involved in case finding, decreased access for women to health information and health services needs to be considered as a possible explanation for the sex ratio observed. There are also questions about differential risks of exposure for men and women related to social customs of mobility in relation to gender. The development of clinical leprosy is associated with poverty, though it can affect people of every socioeconomic status. Leprosy had virtually disappeared from some historically endemic pockets of leprosy, such as Western Europe, prior to the era of effective chemotherapy, presumably related to socioeconomic development.

Incidence among contacts

In general, people with known leprosy-affected contacts are in the minority among new cases and the vast majority of those in close contact with leprosy-affected people will not develop leprosy. Nevertheless, attack rates for contacts are higher than in the surrounding population, five to ten times higher in contacts of multibacillary index cases (who have multiple lesions corresponding to more bacilli as in Figure 58.1), and two to four times higher in

Table 58.1 Distribution of leprosy cases by WHO region (excluding Europe), 2005

WHO region	Registered cases	Prevalence per 10 000 on 31 December, 2005	New cases detected	Case detection per 100 000 in 2005
Africa	40 830	0.56	42 814	5.9
Americas	32 904	0.39	41 780	5.0
South-east Asia	133 422	0.81	201 635	12.2
East Mediterranean	4 024	0.09	3 133	0.7
West Pacific	8 646	0.05	7 137	0.4
Total	219 826		296 499	

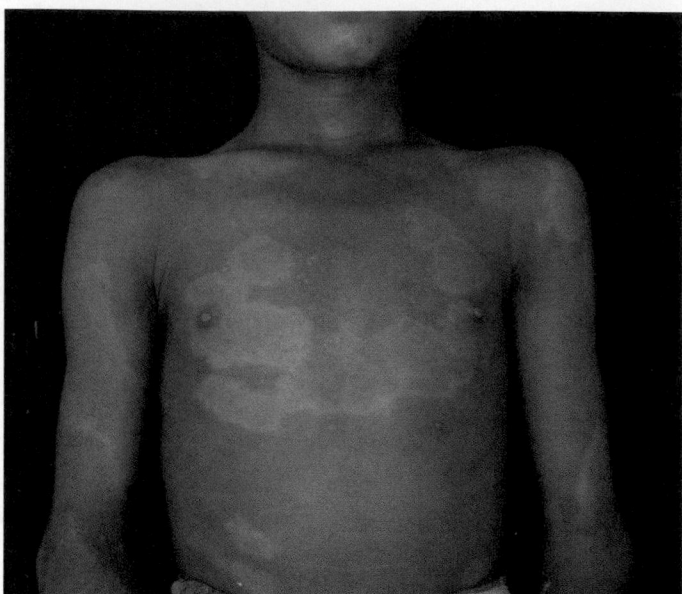

Figure 58.1 Multiple lesions of multibacillary leprosy.

paucibacillary cases. There appears to be a gradient in susceptibility depending on how physically or socially distant the contact is, along with a persisting genetic effect that is independent of physical distance.[2]

Transmission

The aetiological agent in leprosy is *Mycobacterium leprae*, which was first identified microscopically by Armauer Hansen in Norway in 1873. Humans are the only known significant reservoir of infection in leprosy. People with untreated lepromatous leprosy may harbour billions of organisms per gramme of tissue and are believed to be the key factor in transmission of leprosy. Non-lepromatous cases, though more frequent, have a much smaller bacillary load, not easily detectable by routine microscopy. The carriage of *M. leprae* by healthy subjects in nasal mucosa may also play a role in the transmission of leprosy. Rates of population nasal carriage of *M. leprae* based on PCR studies are much higher than registered prevalence rates of leprosy.[3] The natural occurrence of disease due to *M. leprae* in wild, nine-banded armadillos is of negligible relevance to human leprosy globally though leprosy has occasionally been reported in armadillo handlers.

Portal of exit

Nasal secretions are believed to be the main portal of exit in leprosy, while the role of desquamating skin is less certain. Large numbers of viable organisms can be detected in the nasal secretions of those with untreated lepromatous leprosy. By contrast, despite presence of large number of bacilli in deeper layers of the skin, it has generally proved difficult to detect acid-fast bacilli in desquamating epithelium of such patients, though Job has recently reported *M. leprae* in more superficial layers.[4]

Viability outside the host

The discharge of large numbers of *M. leprae* from nasal mucosa in secretions or droplet form raises the question of organism viability in the environment. *M. leprae* is known to survive for many days and possibly months under optimal conditions of high humidity and low sunlight.

Portal of entry

The portal of entry for *M. leprae* is uncertain but the only seriously considered sites are the upper respiratory tract and skin. Rees and McDougall succeeded in experimentally infecting immuno-deficient mice through aerosols containing *M. leprae*[5] and the nasal route is generally thought to be most important. Experimental models and clinical examples of transmission through the skin have, however, also been reported.[6]

Host susceptibility

It has long been accepted that host susceptibility plays a significant role in the development of clinical leprosy. The mechanisms by which lower socioeconomic status predisposes to an increased susceptibility to leprosy remain unclear. BCG vaccination has a protective effect, though studies in different countries have reported different rates of protection.[7-9] HIV infection has not been associated with an increased risk of developing leprosy, or of developing more serious forms of leprosy.[10] Leprosy reactions may, however, be increased in HIV-positive individuals with leprosy. Studies into genetic susceptibility have suggested a two stage process, whereby non-HLA genes may have a significant effect on the development of leprosy, while clinical subtype is partially controlled by HLA genes and partially by other genes.[11] Studies have identified a locus on chromosome region 6q25 in Vietnamese patients significantly linked to leprosy susceptibility.[12] A mutation in the intracellular portion of Toll-like receptor 2 (TLR-2) was found to be associated with lepromatous leprosy in 10 of 45 Korean patients, but was not found in 41 tuberculoid patients or 45 healthy controls.[13] Downstream signalling for immune response to M. leprae cell wall components was also abolished in in-vitro studies using the same TLR-2 mutation.[14]

Incubation period

The incubation period for leprosy is both difficult to define and extremely variable. Onset is usually insidious, subclinical infection common, detection often delayed, and immunological tools inadequate to determine onset of disease. The average incubation period is generally agreed to be from 3–5 years, though rarely infants have been reported with leprosy in the first few months of life, and war veterans exposed in endemic areas up to 30 years earlier may develop leprosy. The reported average delay to diagnosis from onset of clinical symptoms varies greatly but is often in excess of two years. The lengthy combined period of incubation and delay to diagnosis implies significant spread of leprosy prior to treatment, and makes decreasing transmission through early diagnosis and treatment a difficult prospect.

Modelling transmission

The transmission of leprosy under several future scenarios has been modelled, based on observed trends in new case diagnosis globally and in specific countries where data collection is good, relying on a number of assumptions and adjustment of relevant variables. The SIMLEP model[15] predicts a gradual decline in leprosy incidence on current trends, though with a significant risk of future increase in leprosy incidence if BCG vaccination coverage declines or if global diagnostic and treatment services for leprosy deteriorate leading to further treatment delay. To some extent increased delay in diagnosis is inevitable with decline in prevalence, and has been associated with extensive disability at diagnosis in low prevalence countries such as the UK.[16]

MICROBIOLOGY

Mycobacterium leprae is a strongly acid-fast bacillus, with parallel sides and rounded ends, closely resembling Mycobacterium tuberculosis. Under electron microscopy the bacillus shows a great variety of forms, the most common being a slightly curved filament, 3–10 μm in length. Organisms may be identified in stained biopsies, smears of nasal secretions, or more commonly from slit skin smears. Bacilli are often grouped together in slides of smears from lepromatous patients like bundles of cigars known as palisades, and are occasionally present in large intracellular or extracellular clumps known as globi. It is thought that only the few solid staining organisms are viable while the vast majority of organisms, which show patchy staining and fragmented morphology, are non-viable. The proportion of solidly staining organisms (known as the

Morphological Index or MI) is often around 4–5% in untreated lepromatous leprosy patients and falls dramatically within a few days of commencing standard leprosy chemotherapy.

Growth characteristics

Mycobacterium leprae is extremely fastidious in regard to growth requirements and is yet to be successfully cultured on artificial media. It is cultured in a small number of laboratories worldwide in laboratory mice using Shepard's hind footpad inoculation method. Antibiotic sensitivities are determined through the ability of the organism to grow in mice fed different concentrations of antibiotic. The organism generation time is extremely long, around 14 days on average, thus the determination of antibiotic sensitivity takes several months. In normal mice maximum growth occurs during a period of up to 6 months to around 10^6 organisms from an initial inoculum of around 10^4 bacilli. In immunodeficient, thymectomized, irradiated (TR) mice microbial growth continues beyond 6 months with yields of up to 10^9 organisms, giving a model analogous to lepromatous leprosy with broad dissemination of bacteria beyond the footpads.[17] This method can be used to culture small numbers of viable bacilli from patient specimens, which would not be possible using normal mice.

The nine-banded armadillo (Dasypus novemcinctus), in addition to being a natural host for M. leprae, has become the principal source of the organism for immunological and biochemical research. The animal's primitive immune system and low body temperature make for ideal incubation conditions for M. leprae. Disseminated disease follows intravenous inoculation, and bacterial yields from liver and spleen can reach 10^{12} organisms per gramme of tissue.

Genome

The genomic sequence of M. leprae has been mapped using a combination of automated DNA sequence analysis of selected cosmids and whole-genome 'shotgun' clones. Investigation into the genome of M. leprae in comparison with M. tuberculosis reveals an extreme case of reductive evolution. The genome of M. leprae is over 25% smaller than M. tuberculosis, amounting to a reduction of 1200 protein sequences, despite evidence for a common ancestor. Recent evidence suggests that many of the genes that were present in the genome of M. leprae have truly been lost.[18] Less than half of the genome contains functional genes and whole metabolic pathways together with their regulatory circuits have been eliminated.[19] This likely explains the organism's extreme generation time, and the inability to culture it in vitro. Research is now underway to develop diagnostic skin tests based on information from the completed genome, to better understand mechanisms of nerve damage and drug resistance and to identify novel targets and drugs for new therapeutic regimens.

PATHOGENESIS

Point of entry

Evidence for an entry point for Mycobacterium leprae primarily via the nasal cavity is enhanced by nasal endoscopic and biopsy

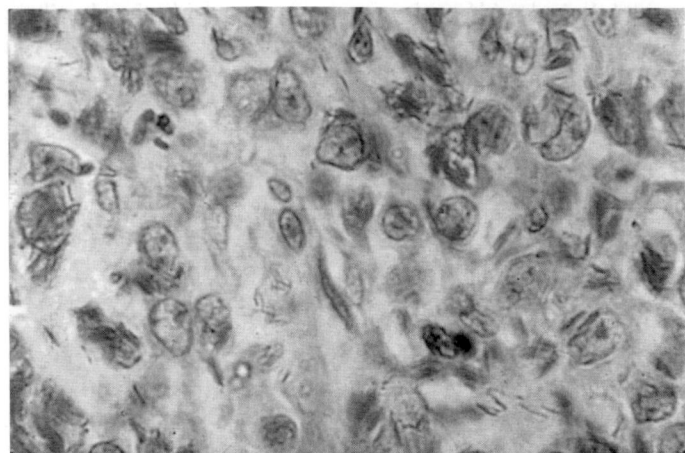

Figure 58.3 Skin lesions of lepromatous leprosy (high power) showing the lepra cellular tissue. (Courtesy of the late S. G. Browne.)

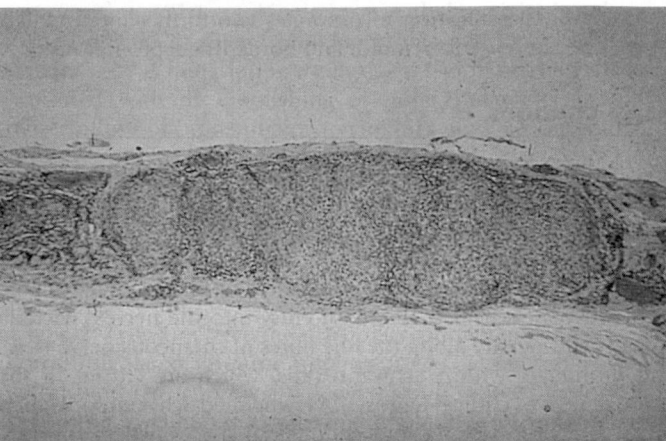

Figure 58.4 Nerve lesions (low power) of tuberculoid leprosy. (Courtesy of the late S. G. Browne.)

Histoid leprosy is a rare nodular form of lepromatous leprosy which usually occurs in relapsed patients who have secondary resistance to dapsone, but may also occur with primary dapsone resistance. The histopathological features consist of well-formed lesions surrounded by a pseudocapsule, with variously arranged spindle-shaped, polygonal and foamy histiocytes, and a large number of solid staining acid-fast bacilli.[28]

Borderline leprosy

Histologically, borderline leprosy shows features intermediate between those of lepromatous and tuberculoid leprosy. An inflammatory reaction is seen in the superficial layers of the dermis, consisting of small round cells, histiocytes and clumps of epithelioid cells but without giant cells. Depending on which immunological pole the patient response leans towards, nerves may show large numbers of bacilli or epithelioid cells with few bacilli, i.e. they may resemble nerves in tuberculoid or lepromatous disease (Figures 58.4, 58.5). Borderline leprosy is unstable, with potential for sharp immunological upgrading towards the tuberculoid pole of the spectrum (known as a reversal or type 1 reaction) or a more gradual drift to the lepromatous pole, sometimes referred to as downgrading.

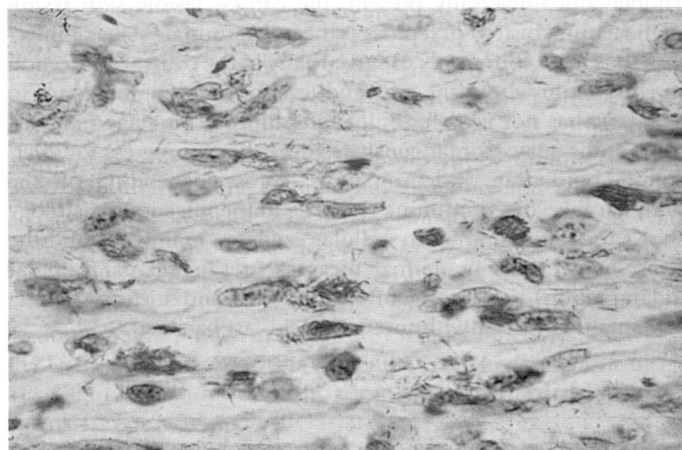

Figure 58.5 Nerve lesions (high power) of lepromatous leprosy. (Courtesy of the late S. G. Browne.)

CLINICAL MANIFESTATIONS

Infection with *Mycobacterium leprae* is far more common than the expression of clinical disease and the majority of early leprosy lesions resolve without treatment. The natural history of leprosy is highly variable. A small minority of cases with a weak cell-mediated immune response develop polar lepromatous leprosy, a chronic, progressive and disseminated infection with multiple demonstrable acid-fast bacilli in skin smears and nasal secretions. A larger proportion mount a stronger immune response and develop tuberculoid leprosy, a highly localized disease characterized by primarily immunological damage to skin and nerves. In the spectrum between these two immunological and clinical poles, and prone to swing one way or the other, fall the majority of cases with borderline leprosy. A further group of patients have early, indeterminate leprosy and are undifferentiated immunologically.

Symptoms and signs

The mode of onset of leprosy is usually insidious, an absence of toxicity being characteristic of leprosy, even where bacterial load is enormous. Nevertheless, local inflammatory reactions to *M. leprae* may appear unpredictably, sometimes accompanied by systemic manifestations of inflammation. The onset of clinical disease may be precipitated by another acute disease or physiological stress, such as puberty, childbirth or menopause.

The diagnosis of leprosy is usually based on clinical signs and symptoms alone, identifiable by appropriately trained health workers. Common presentations are changes in the appearance of the skin, tenderness, tingling or thickening of nerves, localized areas of anaesthesia with insensitivity to trauma, and numbness and tingling of extremities. Only rarely are laboratory investigations required to confirm the diagnosis of leprosy.

Tuberculoid leprosy is confined to skin and/or nerve, being localized to one or a few asymmetric areas. In lepromatous leprosy, negligible immune resistance results in the wide dissemination of *M. leprae* throughout skin, nerves and the reticuloendothelial system. Invasion of eyes, testes, bones and mucous membranes of the upper respiratory tract also occurs in some. Borderline leprosy occurs in those with levels of immune resistance intermediate between tuberculoid and lepromatous leprosy and generally affects both skin and nerve. Distribution is therefore less widespread and symmetrical than in lepromatous leprosy but more than in tuberculoid forms.

Skin

Typical leprosy skin lesions are either less pigmented than surrounding skin or they may have a reddish or coppery hue. Macules or papules are most common, single or multiple, and ranging in size from just under 1 cm in diameter to very large. Lesions can be found anywhere on the body, but are uncommon in hairy areas such as the scalp. The most common sites are the face, buttocks and extremities. Palms and soles are not spared, but lesions are very rare in the axillae and groin. Sensory loss within skin lesions is a typical feature of leprosy, tested usually by light touch and/or pin prick. Skin infiltration is also a common presentation, either as a feature of defined skin lesions or as a diffuse phenomenon, particularly affecting the face. *Indeterminate leprosy* is an early phase in the natural history of leprosy, usually presenting as a single hypopigmented macule (Figure 58.6) with uncharacteristic histology and absence of bacilli.

Skin lesions in *tuberculoid leprosy* appear as macules or plaques. Either erythematous or hypopigmented, tuberculoid macules often have a dry, rough surface with lack of sweating. They have well-defined borders, and loss of sensation is clearly demonstrable. Tuberculoid leprosy plaques are usually erythematous, sometimes with a coppery, brownish or even purple hue. Plaque surface is dry, rough, and sometimes scaly and irregular. Edges are well defined and raised, while the centre of lesions may become flat-tened and sometimes have evidence of healing, appearing like normal skin. Skin lesions of tuberculoid leprosy are more common on the face, extensor surfaces of limbs, back and buttocks (Figure 58.7). A few small 'satellite' lesions may be seen alongside a tuberculoid plaque. Thickened cutaneous nerves may also be palpated in the vicinity of the lesions and the edge of lesions should be palpated to detect such cutaneous nerves.

Skin lesions in *lepromatous leprosy* are generally multiple, small and symmetrically distributed. Sensory impairment within the lesions is often but not always detectable. A variety of morphologies of skin lesions are seen, including macules, plaques (infiltrations), papules and nodules. Sometimes all of these may be present at the same time in well advanced disease. The earliest skin lesions are macules, which are small, circular or elliptical, and are often ignored by the patient through lack of pain or itching. Hypopigmentation (not depigmentation) of these macules is usual, though erythematous lesions in light skins and coppery lesions in dark skins are also common. The surface of lesions is smooth and shiny, and edges are generally indistinct. Infiltrated plaques are raised above the skin, particularly centrally, and give a sensation of thickening on palpation. As a rule, infiltrated lesions are not anaesthetic. Papules and nodules are more advanced and often occur on the face. The ears should always be carefully examined by close inspection and palpation. The earlobes are more constantly affected than any other part of the body, and appear thickened quite early in the course of the disease, later becoming nodular (Figure 58.8). Significant infiltration of facial skin accentuates normal wrinkles into deep furrows giving rise to characteristic leonine ('lion-like') facies. Early infiltration may be difficult to detect. Nodules may occasionally undergo necrosis and ulceration. Large ulcers may also form distally on the lower limbs secondary to lymphatic occlusion by bacillary invasion in advanced lepromatous disease. Trophic changes to digits may

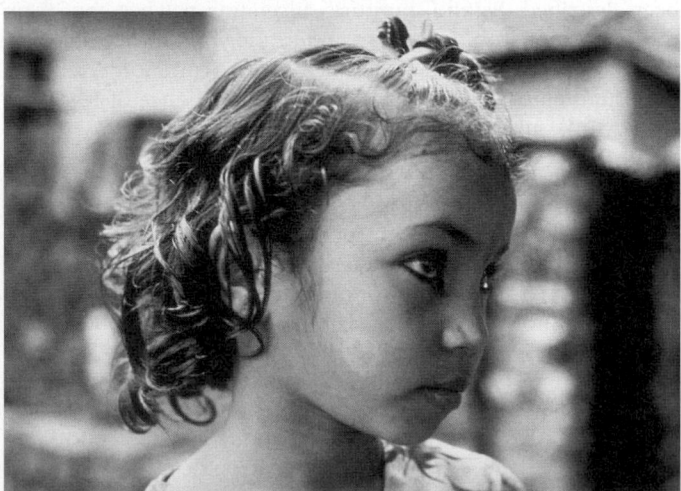

Figure 58.6 Early indeterminate lesion of paucibacillary leprosy.

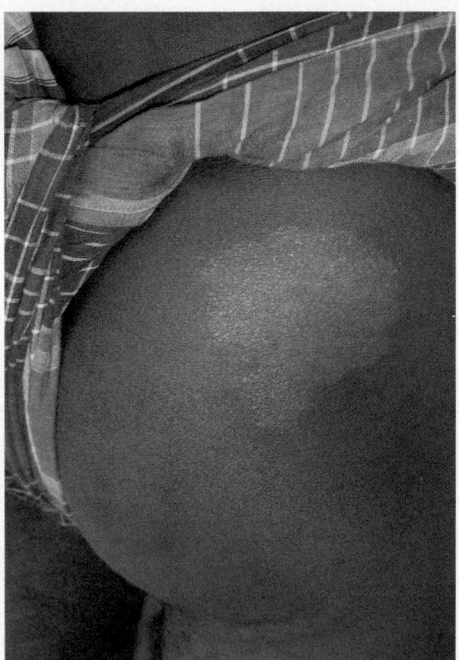

Figure 58.7 Tuberculoid leprosy macule on buttock.

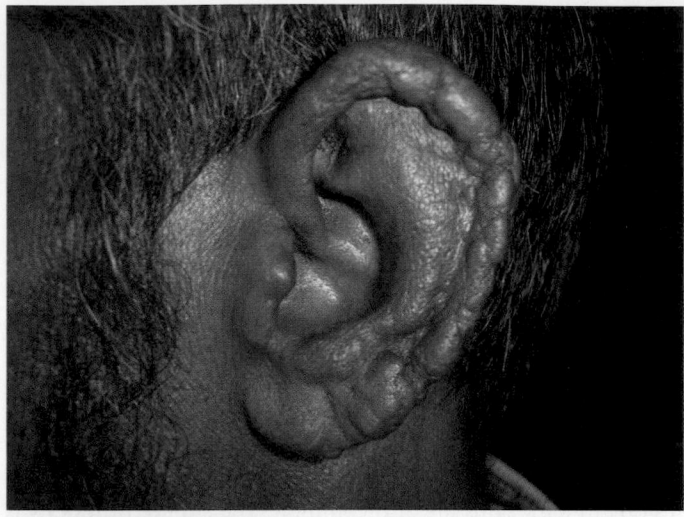

Figure 58.8 Nodular changes in ear lobe in lepromatous leprosy.

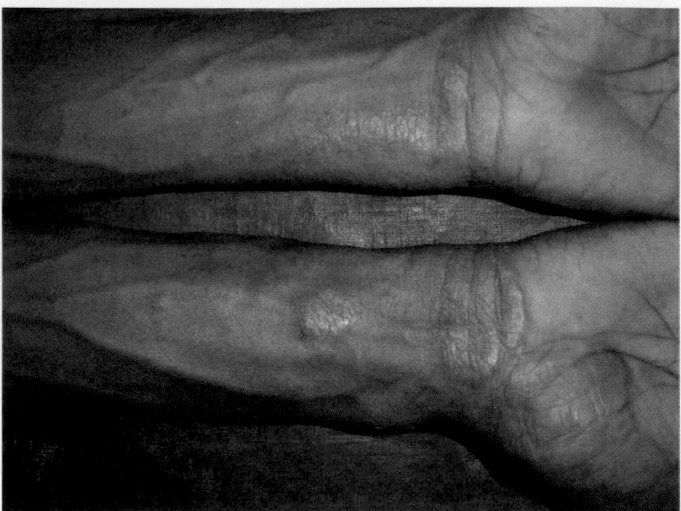

Figure 58.10 Borderline tuberculoid leprosy plaques.

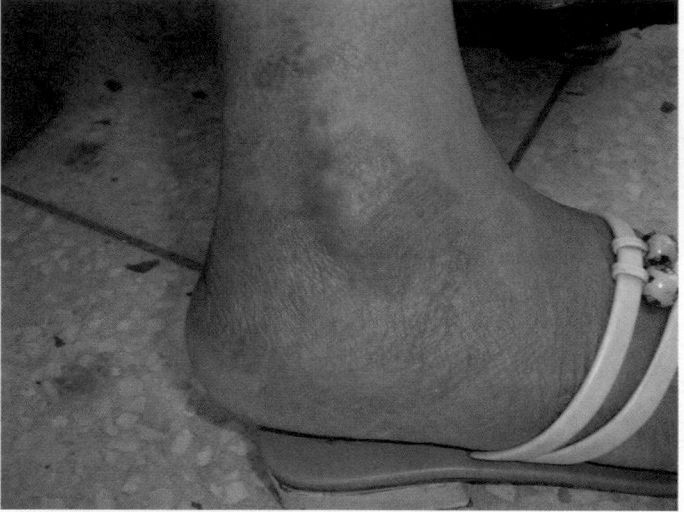

Figure 58.9 Erythematous borderline tuberculoid leprosy macule with satellite lesions.

result in nails of fingers and toes becoming dry, dull, narrow and ridged longitudinally. Hair follicles of eyebrows and eyelids are frequently damaged, if not obliterated, by skin invasion by *M. leprae* in lepromatous leprosy. The resulting thinning of the eyebrows commences in the lateral half and sometimes progresses to complete loss of eyebrows and eyelashes, known as superciliary and ciliary madarosis, respectively.

Skin lesions in *borderline leprosy* are either macular lesions (Figure 58.9) or infiltrated plaques (Figure 58.10), or combinations of these. Sensory impairment can be detected in some if not all macular lesions, while plaques are invariably anaesthetic. Lesions have their own distinctive features in which the hypoaesthetic characteristics of the two polar types (lepromatous and tuberculoid) are merged. Lesions are moderate in number and asymmetrical in distribution. The surface is often smooth and

shiny and slopes away peripherally from a raised centre to edges which are well defined in places and indefinite in others. Annular lesions are a characteristic form of borderline leprosy. An oval area of anaesthetic skin of normal appearance is surrounded by a band of infiltrated, raised tissue of varying width. The inner edge of this band is raised and clear-cut, giving the central area a punched-out appearance, while the outer border merges gradually with the surrounding skin. Sometimes an oval band of infiltrated tissue occurs within annular lesions giving the impression of a target. Plaques may be found on any non-hairy part of the body, but favour the limbs and buttocks.

A rare variant of lepromatous skin infiltration was described by Lucio and Alvarado in Mexico in 1852. The entire skin is diffusely infiltrated with no discrete lesions seen, and becomes stiff and smooth, similar to scleroderma. Loss of eyebrows and eyelashes occurs, and nasal destruction, alopecia and loss of body hair may develop. Widespread small telangiectases are also described. In such patients, a unique and very rare form of lepra reaction known as 'Lucio's phenomenon' (or type 3 reaction) has been described. Painful, purpuric, ulcerating patches appear on the skin, later becoming crusted and healing by scarring. This may be differentiated from the much more common erythema nodosum leprosum (ENL) reaction by the absence of fever and leucocytosis, and absence of tender subcutaneous lesions.

Ulceration

In established leprosy, where peripheral sensory nerve damage is well advanced, leprosy may present with trophic skin ulcers, due to a lack of self-protection from burns, sharp object trauma, and repetitive minor trauma. Ulcers are most common on the plantar aspect of the feet over pressure areas – toes, metatarsal heads, heel, and lateral foot border. Hands may also be involved with ulcers, commonly involving the fingers and palm, especially due to burns. Repetitive minor injury results in gradual absorption and shortening of digits of fingers and toes. Trophic ulcers also occur on anaesthetic patches if they occur at trauma-prone sites, e.g. on buttocks or elbows.

Leprosy skin reactions

Type 1 skin reactions typically begin as redness, swelling, warmth and, occasionally, tenderness arising suddenly within existing leprosy skin lesions (Figure 58.11). Occasionally, new skin lesions that were not previously apparent are 'unmasked' through the upgrading in cell-mediated immune responses characteristic of type 1 reactions. These reactions are most common in the first few months following institution of antibiotic therapy for leprosy, but can occur before and after treatment. Generalized swelling of hands, feet and ankles may also accompany the more localized changes within leprosy skin lesions. Associated damage to involved nerves is another common manifestation of type 1 reactions. Treatment of HIV infection with highly active antiretroviral therapy in people with leprosy has been associated with the development of type 1 reactions as part of an immune reconstitution inflammatory syndrome.[29,30]

Type 2 skin reactions are characterized by small (5–10 mm) subcutaneous nodular lesions, which may occur at any body site, but rarely on the face, and are known as erythema nodosum leprosum (ENL). When severe, these lesions may ulcerate and become pustular. ENL occurs in approximately 5% of multibacillary cases of leprosy and is characteristically associated with a systemic inflammatory response including fever, tachycardia and malaise.

Nerves

Leprosy affects peripheral mixed nerves and cutaneous nerves. The most common peripheral nerves affected, in order of frequency, are the posterior tibial, ulnar, median, lateral popliteal (common peroneal), facial, and radial nerves. The trigeminal nerve, especially the ophthalmic branch, may also be affected, causing loss of corneal sensation. Enlargement of involved nerves at particular sites, notably the ulnar nerve at the elbow and the lateral popliteal at the head of the fibula, is characteristic of leprosy and requires training and practice to detect reliably. Peripheral nerve trunks should be formally examined for enlargement and for loss of function at diagnosis and on a regular basis to detect any deterioration. Cutaneous nerve thickening usually affects small nerves

adjacent to leprosy skin lesions. Particular regional cutaneous nerves may also be enlarged, notably the greater auricular nerve (Figure 58.12), supraclavicular nerves, ulnar cutaneous nerve, radial cutaneous nerve, superficial peroneal nerve, and the sural nerve. Enlargement is sometimes graded as 1+ (mild) to 3+ (severe). It may be nodular rather than uniform thickening. Sensory loss is usually more prominent than motor function loss. Nerve thickening by itself, without associated sensory loss and/or muscle weakness, is suspicious but not a reliable sign of leprosy, hence other diagnostic features need to be sought to confirm a clinical diagnosis.

Subjective symptoms of paraesthesiae, hyperaesthesiae, and hyperalgesia may signal sensory nerve function impairment, though frequently the impairment of light touch, temperature or pain sensation develops 'silently'. Loss of position sense, vibration sense and tendon reflexes is rare. Motor nerve function impairment also often develops in the absence of other signs of nerve inflammation. Muscle wasting may ensue, if motor function loss and paralysis becomes established. Resulting deformities (Figure 58.13), such as claw hand (ulnar nerve), 'ape thumb' (median nerve), drop foot (common peroneal nerve) and facial palsy (facial nerve) are all too frequent complications. Autonomic nerve involvement may be signalled by mild oedema of the hands and feet, which later may become dry, puffy and cyanosed.

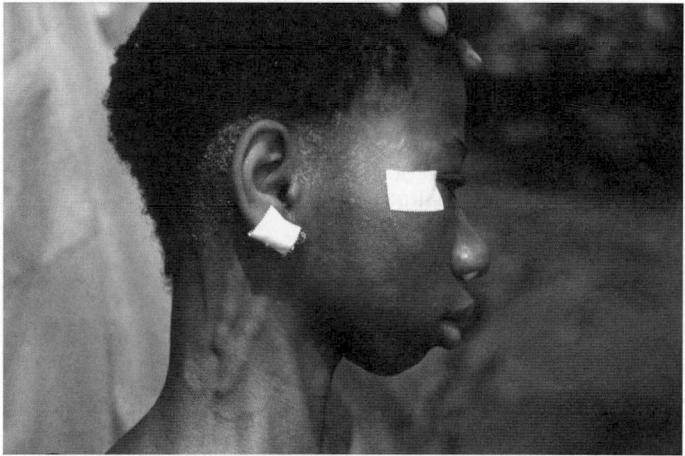

Figure 58.12 Leprosy patient with enlarged cutaneous nerves.

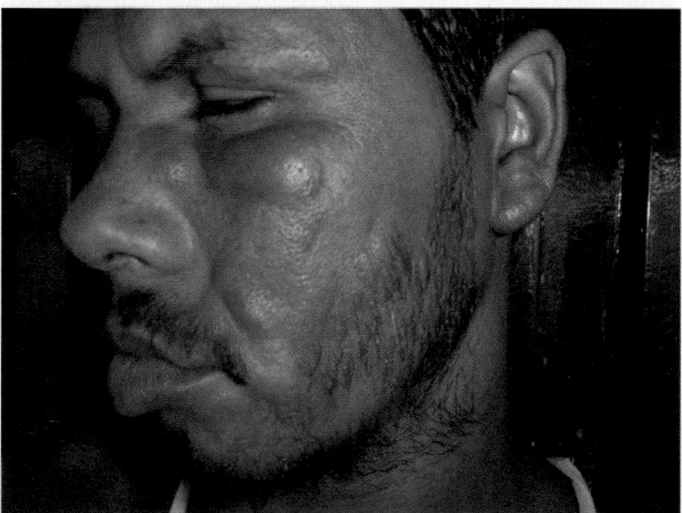

Figure 58.11 Borderline leprosy skin lesions in type 1 reaction.

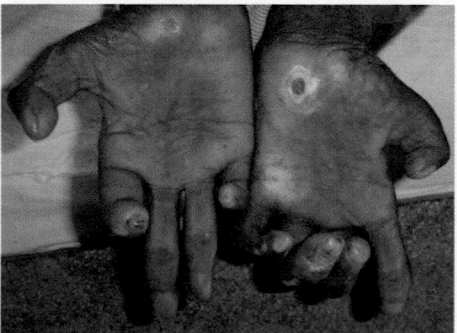

Figure 58.13 Typical leprosy hand deformities: ulnar claw, 'ape thumb' and pressure ulceration.

Nerve thickening and associated dysfunction occurs more slowly in *lepromatous leprosy* than in other forms of leprosy due to the weaker immune response, but may involve multiple nerves. As with skin involvement, nerve thickening tends to be bilateral and symmetrical. Glove and stocking loss of sensation is common in established lepromatous leprosy.

Affected nerves in *tuberculoid leprosy* are thickened, often irregularly, and associated sensory, motor or autonomic nerve function may be impaired. Sensory disturbances are most common. Motor changes are shown by muscle weakness or wasting and should always be examined for in the face, the intrinsic muscles of the hand and the dorsiflexors of the foot. It is rare for the dorsiflexors of the wrist to be affected, as the radial nerve is less commonly affected.

Nerve involvement can very often be demonstrated in *borderline leprosy*. Symptoms such as paraesthesiae and hyperalgesia often precede the clinical detection of skin lesions. Nerves are involved asymmetrically. As in tuberculoid leprosy, other body tissues are not affected directly by *M. leprae* but only indirectly, through reactions, nerve damage, and secondary infection.

Reactions involving nerves

Acute nerve swelling and/or tenderness may accompany neuritis due to lepra nerve reactions, though silent neuritis is also common. In the AMFES study in Ethiopia, 55% of 594 new cases of leprosy had nerve impairment at diagnosis, and a further 12% developed new impairment after starting treatment.[31] Most reactions occur in the first year after diagnosis but can be delayed and/or recurrent. Occasionally nerve abscesses are found. 'Cold' nerve abscesses are not uncommon in tuberculoid leprosy, occurring as part of lepra reactions. Culture of pus from such abscesses is almost always sterile. Neuropathic pain due to leprosy is increasingly recognized.

Testing nerve function

Detection of nerve damage is an important issue, especially considering the frequency of silent neuritis. Light touch, pin prick and temperature sensation can be differentially affected and, ideally, should all be tested. In practice, careful and repeated testing using one modality such as light touch is usually adequate. Testing sensation using graded nylon monofilaments has become more widely used in clinical practice, with good sensitivity and reproducibility, though more sophisticated tests of nerve function may reveal more widespread subtle abnormalities. Testing of sensation using a ball-pen is convenient and widely used in field practice, though the correlation with graded monofilament-defined thresholds for normal and for protective sensation in hands and feet is highly operator dependent, and prone to underdetection.[32] Clinical voluntary muscle testing underestimates leprosy-related deficits compared with nerve conduction studies, but regular testing using the MRC grading system will detect important changes in motor function. Sensory and motor nerve testing at diagnosis helps to stratify patients in terms of level of risk of further nerve function impairment. Regular testing, preferably on a monthly basis, is recommended for up to 12 months in paucibacillary patients and 24 months in multibacillary patients.

Eyes

Leprosy is a leading cause of blindness worldwide. The anterior portion of the eye is primarily involved in leprosy. Visual impairment and blindness are common in patients with advanced lepromatous leprosy. Cornea, iris and lens can all be directly involved by *M. leprae* infection. Lagophthalmos (Figure 58.14), i.e. the failure of eye closure due to facial nerve damage, leads to exposure keratitis and predisposes to corneal trauma. Reduced or absent corneal sensation due to involvement of the ophthalmic branch of the trigeminal nerve is an additional potent cause of corneal ulceration and scarring, and goes unrecognized by the patient due to lack of corneal irritation. The eyes may also be involved in tuberculoid or borderline leprosy as a secondary consequence of damage to the facial and trigeminal nerves.

Iridocyclitis occurs as part of the type 2 reaction in lepromatous leprosy and may be an acute or chronic process. Acute iridocyclitis is signalled by pain, photophobia, and a red eye. Conjunctival vascularity is increased in a peri-corneal distribution. Untreated acute iridocyclitis may become chronic, and the development of posterior synechiae leads to a small irregular pupil. A more insidious form of chronic iridocyclitis also occurs in lepromatous leprosy and regular tests for visual acuity are recommended as a screening test. Slit lamp examination shows 'flare' (cloudiness of aqueous fluid) and cells in the anterior chamber. Later, iris atrophy develops and a regular pinpoint pupil without posterior synechiae formation. Cataract formation is also increased in lepromatous leprosy. Chronic iridocyclitis is a common cause of cataract as is the use of long term systemic steroids for lepra reactions.

Mucous membranes

Mucous membranes are frequently involved in lepromatous leprosy, especially in the upper respiratory tract. Nasal discharge, possibly blood-stained, and nasal stuffiness may occur. Examination reveals hyperaemia and swelling of the mucosa. Nasal septal ulceration may progress to perforation, cartilage destruction, and nasal bridge collapse causing the characteristic 'saddle-nose' deformity. Nodules and subsequent ulceration may also occur elsewhere throughout the upper respiratory tract. Laryngeal involvement is a very rare and serious complication, characterized by hoarse cough, husky voice and stridor. Urgent tracheotomy has been performed for those with oedema of the glottis, as a result of reactions in those with laryngeal lesions.

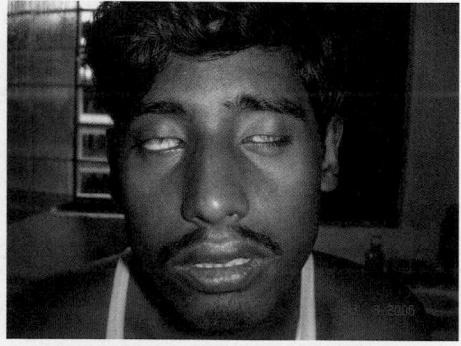

Figure 58.14 Lagophthalmos due to leprosy.

Bones

Extensive bony changes are common in lepromatous leprosy, particularly in the hands and feet, and are multifactorial in origin. Repeated trauma resulting from analgesia and secondary infection from trophic ulceration with resultant osteomyelitis are the major causes. Severe sensory loss may lead to the development of Charcot joints in fingers, toes, wrists and ankles. Infiltration of *M. leprae* bacilli, neurotrophic atrophy, disuse due to paralysis and contractures, and generalized osteoporosis also contribute to bony damage. Bone cysts and aseptic necrosis may be seen. Periostitis of the tibia, fibula and ulna has also been described. In the proximal phalanges the diaphyses may become gradually thinned until only a fine needle of bone remains, or the bone disappears altogether. Atrophy in metatarsal bones begins distally, leading to a thin, pointed, 'sucked candystick' appearance.

Rarely, generalized osteoporosis may follow defective production of testosterone as a result of testicular damage in lepromatous leprosy, but is more common as a complication of long-term steroid use in the management of reactions. Facial deformities result from a combination of aseptic necrosis of the anterior nasal spine and alveolar maxillary processes due to endarteritis in lepromatous leprosy, and secondary pyogenic osteomyelitis as a result of extensive mucosal ulceration of the nose. Nasal collapse, loss of incisor teeth and, rarely, perforation of the palate may result.

Symmetrical bony changes in hands and feet are less common in tuberculoid and borderline than lepromatous leprosy due to a lack of bacillary invasion of bone and small vessels. Disuse atrophy resulting from muscle wasting and paralysis, and neuropathic atrophy arising from sensory nerve involvement are, however, well recognized but are usually asymmetrical. Trophic ulceration of the feet and hands is common.

Reticuloendothelial system

Rubbery, painless enlargement of lymph nodes of the limbs may occur, and occasionally one or more nodes become swollen and inflamed as part of a lepra reaction, or more commonly in response to secondary infection of ulcers. Lymphoedema, especially of the lower legs, may occur. Spleen, liver and bone marrow may also be invaded by *M. leprae* in disseminated lepromatous leprosy.

Testes

Gynaecomastia and infertility may result from testicular invasion by *M. leprae* and resulting testicular atrophy in lepromatous leprosy.

Kidneys

Renal involvement in lepromatous leprosy occurs rarely, but is probably under-diagnosed. Glomerulonephritis, interstitial nephritis, pyelonephritis, and renal amyloidosis have been described. The latter appears to be related to the severity and frequency of type 2 lepra reactions, in which disseminated antigen-antibody immune complex deposition occurs.

DIAGNOSIS

Early diagnosis and treatment of leprosy is essential to minimizing disability, and potentially limiting disease spread. Delay in diagnosis has been associated with a significant increase in nerve damage at diagnosis. Leprosy is primarily a clinical diagnosis. Biopsy is rarely required to confirm the diagnosis where leprosy is commonly encountered. In an endemic area, any one of the classic triad of cardinal signs of leprosy (Table 58.3) is enough to establish a diagnosis.

Clinical classification for treatment

For treatment purposes a simple clinical classification is generally employed (Table 58.4). In an effort to simplify leprosy diagnosis and therefore decentralize leprosy services to primary health units as much as possible, WHO has emphasized clinical diagnosis on the basis of skin findings alone. This has allowed significant simplification of diagnosis and treatment allocation. Those with up to five skin lesions due to leprosy are classified as *paucibacillary* (PB) while those with more than 5 skin lesions are classified as *multibacillary* (MB). A recent study of 5439 patients in South India suggests that this cut-off of 5 lesions is the best option for sensitivity (88.6%) and specificity (86.7%) for detection of MB cases compared with the gold standard of slit skin smear.[33]

There is no doubt that leprosy control service coverage and access to treatment has improved as a result of such simplification of diagnosis. Nevertheless, there is debate about the potential for cases to be missed or diagnosis delayed under this simplified diagnostic regime. In one major study almost 50% of skin smear positive cases did not have a skin lesion with definite sensation loss.[34] Such skin smear positive cases represent the greatest public health risk. In patients for whom a skin smear has been performed which is positive for acid-fast bacilli, the disease is automatically considered MB. Such patients represent 25–50% of all clinical MB cases where skin smear testing is routinely done. Some programmes consider nerve involvement, demonstrated by peripheral and cutaneous nerve enlargement to be additional

Table 58.3 The three cardinal signs of leprosy

Hypopigmented or erythematous skin lesions showing definite reduction in sensation, or
Enlarged and clinically impaired nerves at sites characteristic of leprosy, or
Acid-fast bacilli in slit skin smears.

Table 58.4 A guide for treatment classification of leprosy

Paucibacillary (PB) leprosy	Multibacillary (MB) leprosy
Up to five skin lesions	Over five skin lesions
Up to one nerve trunk may be involved	Many nerve trunks may be involved
Slit skin smear (if performed) is negative	Slit skin smear (if performed) may be positive

REFERENCES

1. WHO. Global leprosy situation, 2005. *Weekly Epidemiol Rec* 2005; 80(34):289–296.
2. Moet FJ, Pahan D, Schuring RP, et al. Physical distance, genetic relationship, age, and leprosy classification are independent risk factors for leprosy in contacts of patients with leprosy. *J Infect Dis* 2006; 193(3): 346–353.
3. Hatta M, van Beers SM, Madjid B, et al. Distribution and persistence of Mycobacterium leprae nasal carriage among a population in which leprosy is endemic in Indonesia. *Trans R Soc Trop Med Hyg* 1995; 89:381–385.
4. Job CK, Jayakumar J, Aschhoff M. 'Large numbers' of Mycobacterium leprae are discharged from the intact skin of lepromatous patients; a preliminary report. *Int J Lepr* 1999; 67:164–167.
5. Rees RJW, McDougall AC. Airborne infection with Mycobacterium leprae in mice. *J Med Microbiol* 1977; 10:63–68.
6. Brandsma JW, Yoder L, MacDonald M. Leprosy acquired by inoculation from a knee injury. *Lepr Rev* 2005; 76(2):175–179.
7. Cunha SS, Rodrigues LC, Pedrosa V, et al. Neonatal BCG protection against leprosy: a study in Manaus, Brazilian Amazon. *Lepr Rev* 2004; 75:357–366.
8. Karonga Prevention Trial Group. Randomised controlled trial of single BCG, repeated BCG, or combined BCG and killed Mycobacterium leprae vaccine for prevention of leprosy and tuberculosis in Malawi. *Lancet* 1996; 348:17–24.
9. Fine PE, Smith PG. Vaccination against leprosy – the view from 1996. *Lepr Rev* 1996; 67:249–252.
10. Gebre S, Saunderson P, Messele T, et al. The effect of HIV status on the clinical picture of leprosy: a prospective study in Ethiopia. *Lepr Rev* 2000; 71(3): 338–343.
11. Buschman E, Skamene E. Leprosy susceptibility revealed. *Int J Lepr* 2003; 71(2):115–118.
12. Mira MT, Alcaïs A, Van Thuc N, et al. Chromosome 6q25 is linked to susceptibility to leprosy in a Vietnamese population. *Nat Genet* 2003; 33: 412–415.
13. Kang TJ, Chae GT. Detection of Toll-like receptor 2 (TLR2) mutation in the lepromatous leprosy patients. *FEMS Immunol Med Microbiol* 2001; 31:53–58.
14. Bochud P, Hawn TR, Aderem A. Cutting edge: a Toll-like receptor 2 polymorphism that is associated with lepromatous leprosy is unable to mediate mycobacterial signaling. *J Immunol* 2003; 170:3451–3454.
15. Meima A, Smith WCS, van Oortmarssen GJ, et al. The future incidence of leprosy: a scenario analysis. *Bull World Health Organ* 2004; 82(5): 373–380.
16. Lockwood DN, Reid AJ. The diagnosis of leprosy is delayed in the United Kingdom. *Quarterly J Med* 2001; 94(4):207–212.
17. Rees RJW, Waters MFR, Weddell AGM, et al. Experimental lepromatous leprosy. *Nature* 1967; 215:599–602.
18. Cole ST, Eiglmeier K, Parkhill J, et al. Massive gene decay in the leprosy bacillus. *Nature* 2001; 409:1007–1011.
19. Cole ST, Brosch R, Parkhill J, et al. Deciphering the biology of Mycobacterium tuberculosis from the complete genome sequence. *Nature* 1998; 393: 537–544.
20. Martins AC, Castro JC, Moreira JS. A ten-year historic study of paranasal cavity endoscopy in patients with Leprosy. *Revista Brasileira de Otorrinolaringologia* 2005; 71(5):609–615.
21. Suneetha S, Arunthathi S, Job A, et al. Histological studies in primary neuritic leprosy: changes in the nasal mucosa. *Lepr Rev* 1998; 69(4):358–366.
22. Ekambaram V, Sithambaram M. Self-healing in non-lepromatous leprosy in the area of the ELEP Leprosy Control Project Dharmapuri (Tamil Nadu). *Lepr India* 1977; 49(3):387–392.
23. Makino M, Maeda Y, Ishii N. Immunostimulatory activity of major membrane protein-II from Mycobacterium leprae. *Cellular Immunology* 2005; 233(1): 53–60.
24. Krutzik SR, Ochoa MT, Sieling PA, et al. Activation and regulation of Toll-like receptors 2 and 1 in human leprosy. *Nature Medicine* 2003; 9(5):525–532.
25. Ridley DS, Jopling WH. Classification of leprosy according to immunity. A five-group system. *Int J Lepr* 1966; 34:255–273.
26. Spierings E, de Boer T, Wieles B, et al. Mycobacterium leprae-specific, HLA class II-restricted killing of human Schwann cells by CD4+ Th1 cells: a novel immunopathogenic mechanism of nerve damage in leprosy. *J Immunol* 2001; 166:5883–5888.
27. Abulafia J, Vignale RA. Leprosy: pathogenesis updated. *Int J Dermatology* 1999; 38:321–334.
28. Sehgal VN, Srivastava G, Beohar PC. Histoid leprosy – a histopathological reapparel. *Acta Leprologica* 1987; 5(2):125–131.
29. Singal A, Mehta S, Pandhi D. Immune reconstitution inflammatory syndrome in an HIV seropositive leprosy patient. *Lepr Rev* 2006; 77:76–80.
30. Trindade MAB, Manani MIP, Masetti JH, et al. Leprosy and HIV co-infection in five patients *Lepr Rev* 2005; 76:162–166.
31. Saunderson P, Gebre S, Desta K, et al. The pattern of leprosy-related neuropathy in the AMFES patients in Ethiopia: definitions, incidence, risk factors and outcome. *Lepr Rev* 2000; 71(3):285–308.
32. Koelewijn LF, Meima A, Broekhuis SM, et al. Sensory testing in leprosy: comparison of ballpoint pen and monofilaments. *Lepr Rev* 2003; 74:42–52.
33. Norman G, Joseph G, Richard J. Validity of the WHO operational classification and value of other clinical signs in the classification of leprosy. *Int J Lepr* 2004; 72(3):278–283.
34. Saunderson P, Groenen G. Which physical signs help most in the diagnosis of leprosy? A proposal based on experience in the AMFES project, ALERT, Ethiopia. *Lepr Rev* 2000; 71(1):34–42.
35. Suneetha S, Arunthathi S, Kurian N, et al. Histological changes in the nerve, skin and nasal mucosa of patients with primary neuritic leprosy. *Acta Leprologica* 2000; 12(1):11–18.
36. Smith WCS, Smith CM, Cree IA, et al. An approach to understanding the transmission of Mycobacterium leprae using molecular and immunological methods: results from the MILEP2 study. *Int J Lepr* 2004; 72(3) 269–277.
37. Honore N, Cole S. Molecular basis of rifampin resistance in Mycobacterium leprae. *Antimicrob Agents Chemother* 1993; 37:414–418.
38. Manandhar R, LeMaster JW, Butlin CR, et al. Interferon-gamma responses to candidate leprosy skin-test reagents detect exposure to leprosy in an endemic population. *Int J Lepr* 2000; 68(1):40–48.
39. Ji B, Jamet P, Perani EG, et al. Bactericidal activity of single dose of clarithromycin plus minocycline, with or without ofloxacin, against Mycobacterium leprae in patients. *Antimicrob Agents Chemother* 1996; 40:2137–2141.
40. Single-lesion Multicentre Trial Group. Efficacy of single dose multidrug therapy for the treatment of single-lesion paucibacillary leprosy. *Indian J Lepr* 1997; 69(2):121–129.
41. WHO. Expert Committee on Leprosy. *World Health Organ Tech Rep Ser* 1998; 874:1–43.
42. Jamet P, Ji B; the Marchoux Chemotherapy Study Group. Relapse after long-term follow up of multibacillary patients treated by WHO multidrug regimen. Marchoux Chemotherapy Study Group. *Int J Lepr* 1995; 63:195–201.
43. Girdhar BK, Girdhar A, Kumar A. Relapses in multibacillary leprosy patients: effect of length of therapy. *Lepr Rev* 2000; 71:144–153.
44. Rao PS, Sugamaran DS, Richard J, et al. Multi-centre, double blind, randomized trial of three steroid regimens in the treatment of type-1 reactions in leprosy. *Lepr Rev* 2006; 77:25–33.
45. Van Brakel WH, Anderson AM, Withington SG, et al. The prognostic importance of detecting mild sensory impairment in leprosy: a randomized controlled trial (TRIPOD 2). *Lepr Rev* 2003; 74:300–310.
46. Richardus JH, Withington SG, Andersen A, et al. Treatment with corticosteroids of long-standing nerve function impairment in leprosy: a randomized controlled trial (TRIPOD 3). *Lepr Rev* 2003; 74:311–318.
47. Smith WC, Anderson AM, Withington SG, et al. Steroid prophylaxis for prevention of nerve function impairment in leprosy: randomised placebo controlled trial (TRIPOD 1). *BMJ* 2004; 328(7454):1459.
48. Gahalaut P, Pinto J, Pai GS, et al. A novel treatment for plantar ulcers in leprosy: local superficial flaps. *Lepr Rev* 2005; 76:220–231.

49. Nicholls PG, Bakirtzief Z, Van Brakel WH, et al. Risk factors for participation restriction in leprosy and development of a screening tool to identify individuals at risk. *Lepr Rev* 2005; 76:305–315.

50. Croft RP, Nicholls PG, Steyerberg EW, et al. A clinical prediction rule for nerve-function impairment in leprosy patients. *Lancet* 2000; 355(9215):1603–1606.

51. Bakker MI, Hatta M, Kwenang A. Prevention of leprosy using rifampicin as chemoprophylaxis. *Am J Trop Med Hyg* 2005; 72(4):443–448.

52. WHO. Global strategy for further reducing the leprosy burden and sustaining leprosy control activities (2006–2010): Operational guidelines. New Delhi: World Health Organization; 2006:SEA/GLP/2006.2.

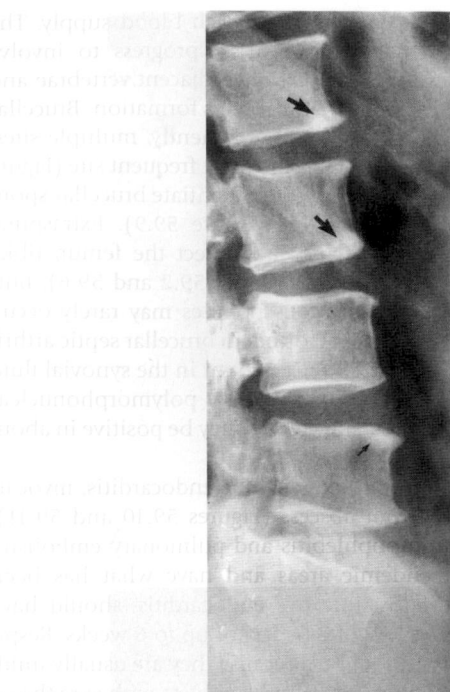

Figure 59.8 Early brucellar spondylitis. There is sclerosis at the anterior aspect of the superior end-plate of L4. Similar areas are seen in the inferior end-plates of L1 and L2. Note the normal disc spaces.

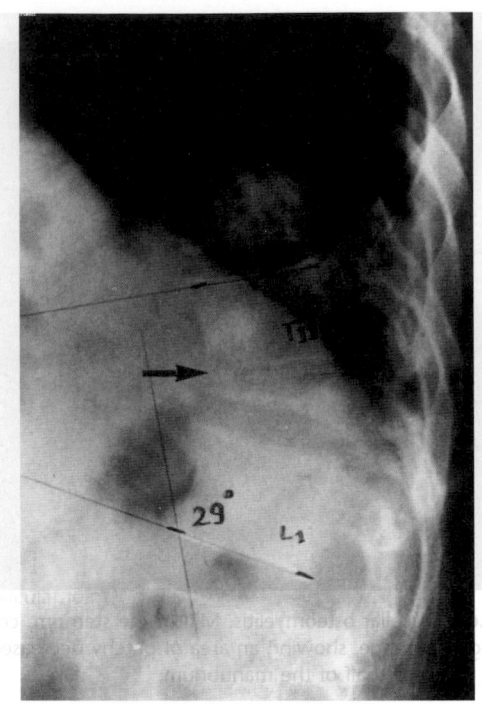

A

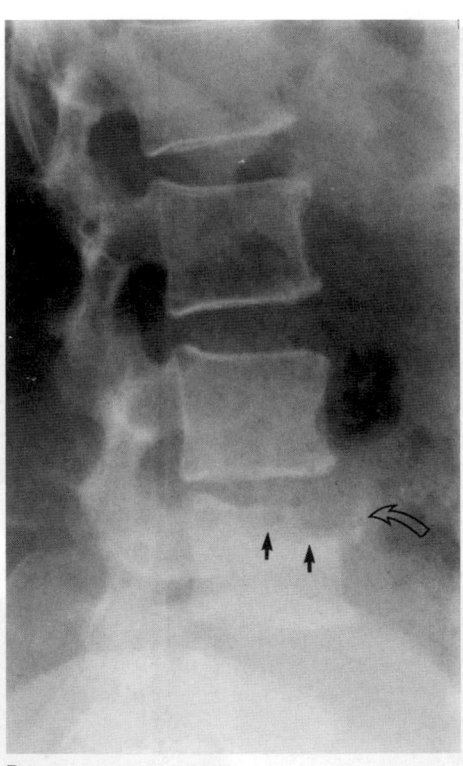

B

Figure 59.9 Comparative image features of plain radiography of tuberculous and brucellar spondylitis.

losis may be caused by direct blood-borne invasion by *Brucella* organisms, pressure from destructive spinal lesions, vasculitis, or an immune-related process. In meningoencephalitis the cerebrospinal fluid (CSF) pressure is usually elevated and the fluid may look clear, turbid or, rarely, haemorrhagic; the protein content and number of cells (predominantly lymphocytes) are raised, while glucose may be reduced or normal. *Brucella* organisms may be cultured from CSF. *Brucella* agglutinins in CSF are usually raised but occasionally may not be detected.

In endemic areas, the outcome of pregnancy in humans is similar to that noted in animals; this includes normal delivery of healthy infants, abortion, intrauterine fetal death, premature delivery, or retention of the placenta and other products of conception, as well as transmission to infants through breast milk.

Skin manifestations are uncommon. They include maculopapular eruptions and contact dermatitis, particularly among veterinarians and farmers assisting animal parturition. Other dermatological manifestations include erythema nodosum, purpura and petechiae, chronic ulcerations, multiple cutaneous and subcutaneous abscesses, vasculitis, superficial thrombophlebitis, discharging sinuses, and, rarely, pemphigus.

Direct splashing of live brucella vaccine into the eyes may cause conjunctivitis. Keratitis, corneal ulcers, uveitis, retinopathies, subconjunctival and retinal haemorrhages, retinal detachment, and endogenous endophthalmitis with positive vitreous cultures are well documented.

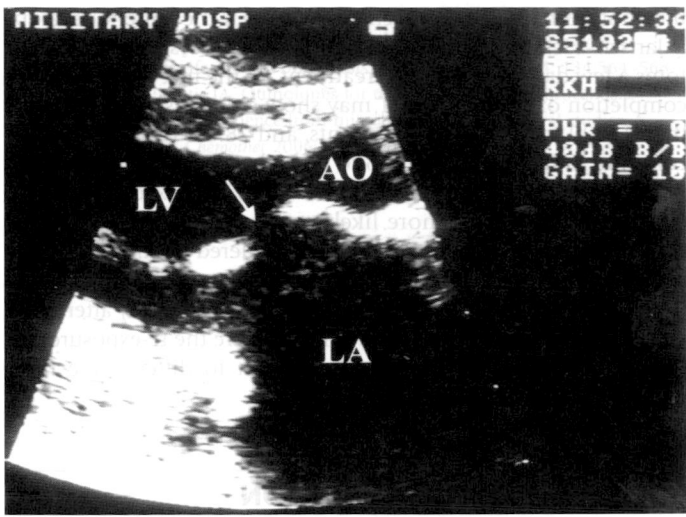

Figure 59.10 Brucellar endocarditis with perforation of the anterior mitral valve leaflet (arrow) depicted by 2-D transthoracic echocardiography.

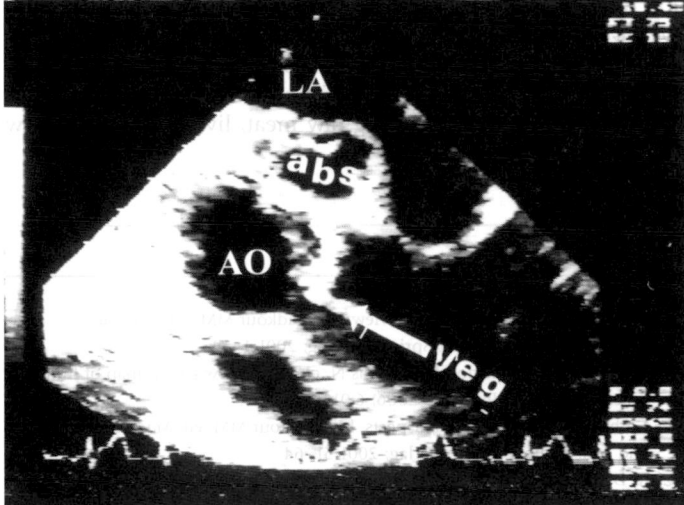

Figure 59.11 Brucellar aortic root abscess and aortic valve vegetation demonstrated in this horizontal transoesophageal endocardiography view.

DIAGNOSIS

Definite diagnosis of brucellosis requires the isolation of the organism from the blood, body fluids or tissues. Positive blood culture yield ranges between 40% and 70%. Identification of specific antibodies against bacterial lipopolysaccharide and other antigens can be detected by the standard agglutination test (SAT), rose bengal, 2-mercaptoethanol (2-ME), antihuman globulin (Coombs') and indirect enzyme-linked immunosorbent assay (ELISA). SAT is the most commonly used serological test in endemic areas. An agglutination titre of 1:160 or higher is considered significant in non-endemic areas and 1:320 or higher in endemic areas.

Due to the similarity of the O polysaccharide of *Brucella* to that of various other Gram-negative bacteria (e.g. *Francisella tolerensis*, *E. coli*, *Salmonella* Urbana, *Yersinia enterocolitica*, *Vibrio cholera*, *Xanthomanas maltophilia*) the appearance of cross-reactions of class M immunoglobulins may occur. The inability to diagnose *B. canis* by SAT due to lack of cross-reaction is another drawback. False-negative SAT may be caused by the presence of blocking antibodies (the prozone phenomenon) in the α_2-globulin (IgA) and in the α-globulin (IgG) fractions. Dipstick assays are new and promising, based on the binding of *Brucella* IgM antibodies, and found to be simple, accurate and rapid.

ELISA typically uses cytoplasmic proteins as antigens. It measures IgM, IgG and IgA with better interpretation and overcomes some of the shortcomings of SAT. PCR is fast and specific. Many varieties of PCR have been developed (e.g. nested PCR, real-time PCR and PCR-ELISA) and found to have superior specificity and sensitivity. Other laboratory findings include normal peripheral white cell count, and occasional leucopenia with relative lymphocytosis. The serum biochemical profiles are commonly normal.[9]

TREATMENT

Treatment of brucellosis is still far from ideal. Two classical regimens – a combination of doxycycline plus streptomycin (DS) or doxycycline plus rifampicin (DR) – recommended by WHO, have been used all over the world, as an out-patient management, for many years and remained effective. Doxycycline (preferred to other tetracyclines) is the most effective agent for the treatment of brucellosis. Doxycycline has increased activity in the acidic environment of the phagolysosomes in the macrophages. Regimens containing doxycycline are more efficient, with fewer therapeutic failures and relapses, than other regimens. The streptomycin-containing regimen is slightly more efficacious in preventing relapses, as rifampicin downregulates doxycycline levels in the serum. Doxycycline is given in an oral dose of 100 mg 12-hourly for 6 weeks. Streptomycin is administered intramuscularly, in a single daily dose of 15 mg/kg for 2–3 weeks. Rifampicin is used in a single oral daily dose of 600–900 mg for 6 weeks. Patients with localizations such as spondylitis, endocarditis, neurobrucellosis, and abscess formations in body organs may require hospitalization for possible surgery and triple antibiotics (doxycycline, aminoglycoside and rifampicin) should be used for a longer period of up to 6 months. Urgent valve replacement or drainage of abscesses may also be required with antibiotics. The overall therapeutic failure and relapse rates with DS and DR regimens range between 3% and 10%. The parenteral administration of aminoglycoside, nephrotoxicity and ototoxicity require adequate monitoring in the healthcare system. Monotherapy has been abandoned because of the unacceptably high rates of therapeutic failure and relapses.

Alternative regimens have been used over the past two decades. Gentamicin and netilmicin are alternative aminoglycosides, which

of patients and in these, immunosuppression may allow the development of gastrointestinal symptoms.[41] The classical triad of weight loss, diarrhoea and malabsorption may or may not be present. Patients are often non-specifically unwell with low-grade fever and lymphadenopathy. Laboratory investigations usually reveal malabsorption with a raised erythrocyte sedimentation rate.[8,10] Apart from the classical changes in the bowel, patients may have seronegative arthralgia and uveitis. Synovium may be positive for *T. whipplei* by molecular probe[42,43] or culture.[44] In the cardiovascular system, heart valves (including xenografts) and coronary arteries may be involved, and rarely a patient may have myocarditis with focal fibrosis.[45] Although now well-described in a number of case reports, culture-negative endocarditis is extremely rare compared with the more conventional causes.[46] Often patients with endocarditis are afebrile.[47] The vegetations show fibrosis, infiltration with mononuclear cells and minimal inflammation.[48]

Whipple disease is a rare cause of non-specific global encephalopathy[49] and dementia and may be diagnosed by brain biopsy or PCR on cerebrospinal fluid. Rarely, a patient may have a discrete tumour masquerading as glioma[50] or may have arteritis.[51] A comprehensive review in 2002 of 12 local cases of central nervous system disease in France revealed 122 case reports.[52]

Disseminated disease may present as a lymphoma-like illness with infected macrophages present associated with non-caseating granulomas in the bone marrow.[53,54]

Diagnosis

Classical disease is diagnosed by histopathological examination of intestinal biopsies, which reveal heavy deposits of periodic acid-Schiff (PAS) – positive material. Sampling error may lead to failure to identify abnormalities, although tissues are still positive by molecular methods.[55] Histopathologists should perform PAS and diastase staining for the bacteria when confronted by non-specific granulomatous inflammation. Bacteria similar to those seen in the intestine can be found in the coronary arteries of patients who have died with classical Whipple disease.[56] Clumps of bacteria, some intracellular, have been associated with the arterial media, and atheroma, sometimes, although not always, with evidence of local inflammation. Changes like sarcoidosis have been seen in affected lymph nodes positive for *T. whipplei* 16S RNA.[57] With the sequencing of the genome,[58] candidate protein antigen determinants have been identified, which may make serodiagnosis possible in the near future.[59] Similarly, immunostaining of tissues may be applicable in the future.[60,61] Molecular diagnosis of tissues in reference centres is likely to be the diagnosis of choice.[62] Contamination of reusable biopsy instruments such as flexible endoscopes is not properly removed by conventional methods of decontamination. Theoretically, the organism could therefore be passed from one patient to another or specimens for PCR could be contaminated.[63]

Management

The treatment of choice at present, based on empirical studies, is co-trimoxazole, which should be continued for at least 1 year.[64] Gerard and co-workers (2002)[52] suggest repeated examination of

the CSF in individuals with CNS disease on treatment and non-discontinuation of treatment until the PCR is negative. However, breakthrough infections have been described. Some give 2 weeks of intravenous cephalosporin (such as ceftriaxone or cefotaxime) before using co-trimoxazole. There is little evidence for the efficacy of this strategy. The organism was found to be sensitive in vitro to many antibiotics including doxycycline and hydroxychloroquine, a combination used in the treatment of coxiellosis.[65,66] It is resistant to trimethoprim, suggesting that the active component of co-trimoxazole is the sulphonamide.

REFERENCES

1. Weese WC, Smith JM. A study of 57 cases of actinomycosis over a 36 year period. *Arch Intern Med* 1975; 135:1562–1568.
2. Brock DW, Georg LK, Brown JM, et al. Actinomycosis caused by Arachnia propionica. Report of 11 cases. *Am J Clin Pathol* 1973; 59:66–77.
3. Vyas JM, Kasmar A, Chang HR, et al. Abdominal abscesses due to actinomycosis after laparoscopic cholecystectoy: case reports and review. *Clin Infect Dis* 2007; 44:e1–4.
4. Spence MR, Gupta PK, Frost JK, et al. Cytologic detection and chemical significance of Actinomyces israelii in women using intrauterine contraceptive devices. *Am J Obstet Gynecol* 1978; 131:295–298.
5. Pritt B, Mount SL, Cooper K, et al. Pseudoactinomycotic granules of the gynecologic tract: a potential diagnostic pitfall. *J Clin Pathol* 2006; 59: 17–20.
6. Slack JM, Gerencser MA. Two new serological groups of Actinomyces. *J Bacteriol* 1970; 103:265–266.
7. Slack JM, Landfried S, Gerencser MA. Identification of Actinomyces and related bacteria in dental calculus by the fluorescent antibody technique. *J Dent Res* 1971; 50:78–82.
8. Whipple GH. A hitherto undescribed disease characterised anatomically by deposits of fat and fatty acids in the intestinal and mesenteric lymphatic tissues. *Bull John's Hopkins Hosp* 1907; 18:382–391.
9. LaScola B, Fenollar F, Fournier PE, et al. Description of Tropheryma whipplei gen. nov., sp. nov., the Whipple's disease bacillus. *Int J Syst Evol Microbiol* 2001; 51:1471–1479.
10. Maizel H, Ruffin JM, Dobbins WO III. Whipple's disease. A review of 19 patients from one hospital and review of the literature since 1950. *Medicine (Baltimore)* 1970; 49:175–205.
11. Vitel-Durand D, Lecomte C, Cathebras P, et al. Whipple disease: clinical review of 52 cases. *Medicine (Baltimore)* 1997; 76:170–184.
12. Caples SM, Petrovic LM, Ryu JH. Successful treatment of Whipple disease diagnosed 36 years after symptom onset. *Mayo Clin Proc* 2001; 76: 1063–1066.
13. Razman NN, Loftus E Jr, Burgart LJ, et al. Diagnosis and monitoring of Whipple disease by polymerase chain reaction. *Ann Intern Med* 1997; 126:520–527.
14. Relman DA, Schmidt TM, MacDermott RP, et al. Identification of the uncultured bacillus of Whipple's disease. *N Engl J Med* 1992; 327:293–301.
15. Raoult D, Birg ML, La Scola B, et al. Cultivation of the bacillus of Whipple's disease. *N Engl J Med* 2000; 342:620–625.
16. Dobbins WO III. *Whipple's Disease.* Springfield, Illinois: Charles C Thomas, 1987.
17. Yardley JH, Hendrix TR. Combined electron and light microscopy in Whipple's disease. Demonstration of 'bacillary bodies' in the intestine. *Bull John's Hopkins Hosp* 1961; 109:80–98.
18. Chears WC, Ashworth CT. Electron microscopy study of the intestinal mucosa in Whipple's disease. Demonstration of encapsulated bacilliform bodies in the lesion. *Gastroenterology* 1961; 41:129–138.
19. Wilson KH, Blitchington R, Frothingham R, et al. Phylogeny of the Whipple's disease-associated bacterium. *Lancet* 1991; 338:474–475.

20. Schoedon G, Goldenberger D, Forrer R, et al. Deactivation of macrophages with interleukin-4 is the key to the isolation of Tropheryma whipplei. *J Infect Dis* 1997; 176:672–677.

21. Raoult D, La Scola B, Lecocq P, et al. Culture and immunological detection of Tropheryma whipplei from the duodenum of a patient with Whipple disease. *JAMA* 2001; 285:1039–1043.

22. Maiwald M, Von Herbay A, Lepp PW, et al. Organisation, structure, and variability of the rRNA operon of the Whipple's disease bacterium (Tropheryma whipplei). *J Bacteriol* 2000; 182:3292–3297.

23. Hinrikson HP, Dutly F, Nair S, et al. Detection of three different types of Tropheryma whipplei directly from clinical specimens by sequencing, single-strand conformation polymorphism (SSCP) analysis and type-specific PCR of their 16S-23S ribosomal intergenic spacer region. *Int J Syst Bacteriol* 1999; 49:1701–1706.

24. Hinrikson HP, Dutly F, Altwegg M. Evaluation of a specific nested PCR targeting domain III of the 23S rRNA gene of 'Tropheryma whipplei' and proposal of a classification system for its molecular variants. *J Clin Microbiol* 2000; 38:595–599.

25. Feule GE, Dorken B, Schopf E, et al. HLA-B27 and defects in the T-cell system in Whipple's disease. *Eur J Clin Invest* 1979; 9:385–389.

26. Ectors N, Geboes K, De Vos R, et al. Whipple's disease: a histological, immunocytochemical and electron microscopic study of the immune response in the small intestinal mucosa. *Histopathology* 1992; 21:1–12.

27. Marth T, Roux M, von Herbay A, et al. Persistent reduction of complement receptor 3 alpha-chain expressing mononuclear blood cells and transient inhibitory serum factors in Whipple's disease. *Clin Immunol Immunopathol* 1994; 72:217–226.

28. Dobbins WO III. Is there an immune deficit in Whipple's disease? *Dig Dis Sci* 1981; 26:247–252.

29. Bjerkness R, Odegaard S, Bjerkvig R, et al. Demonstration of a persisting monocyte and macrophage dysfunction. *Scan J Gastroenterol* 1988; 23:611–619.

30. Marth T, Kleen N, Stallmach A, et al. Dysregulated peripheral and mucosal Th1/Th2 response in Whipple's disease. *Gastroenterology* 2002; 123:1468–1477.

31. Schneider T, Stallmach A, von Herbay A, et al. Treatment of refractory Whipple's disease with interferon-gamma. *Ann Intern Med* 1998; 129:875–877.

32. Desnues B, Raoult D, Mege JL. IL-16 is critical for Tropheryma whipplei replication in Whipple's disease. *J Immunol* 2005; 175:4575–4582.

33. Ghigo E, Capo C, Aurouze M, et al. Survival of Tropheryma whipplei, the agent of Whipple's disease, requires phagosome acidification. *Infect Immun* 2002; 70:1501–1506.

34. Maiwald M, Schuhmacher F, Ditton HJ, et al. Environmental occurrence of the Whipple's disease bacterium (Tropheryma whipplei). *Appl Environ Microbiol* 1998; 64:760–762.

35. Raoult D, Lepidi H, Harle JR. Tropheryma whipplei circulating in blood monocytes. *N Engl J Med* 2001; 345:548.

36. Ehrbar HU, Bauerfeind P, Dutly F, et al. PCR-positive tests for Tropheryma whipplei in patients without Whipple's disease. *Lancet* 1999; 353:2214.

37. Street S, Donoghue HD, Neild GH. Tropheryma whipplei DNA in saliva of healthy people. *Lancet* 1999; 354:1178–1179.

38. Amsler L, Bauernfeind P, Nigg C, et al. Prevalence of Tropheryma whipplei DNA in patients with various gastrointestinal diseases and in healthy controls. *Infection* 2003; 31:81–85.

39. Maiwald M, von Herbay A, Persing DH, et al. Tropheryma whipplei DNA is rare in the intestinal mucosa of patients without other evidence of Whipple disease. *Ann Intern Med* 2001; 134:115–119.

40. Rolain JM, Fenollar F, Raoult D. False positive PCR detection of Tropheryma whipplei in the saliva of healthy people. *BMC Microbiol* 2007; 7:48.

41. Mahnel R, Kalt A, Ring S, et al. Immunosuppressive therapy in Whipple's disease patients is associated with the appearance of gastrointestinal manifestations. *Am J Gastroenterol* 2005; 100:1167–1173.

42. Puechal X, Saad R, Poveda JD. Tropheryma whipplei in synovial tissue and blood. *Ann Intern Med* 1999; 131:795–796.

43. Schilling D, Adamek HE, Kaufmann V, et al. Arthralgia as an extraintestinal symptom of Whipple's disease. Report of five cases. *J Clin Gastroenterol* 1997; 24:18–20.

44. Puechal X, Fenollar F, Raoult D. Cultivation of Tropheryma whipplei from the synovial fluid in Whipple's arthritis. *Arthritis Rheum* 2007; 56:1713–1718.

45. McGettigan P, Mooney EE, Sinnott M, et al. Sudden death in Whipple's disease. *Postgrad Med* 1997; 73:509–511.

46. Houpikian P, Raoult D. Blood culture-negative endocarditis in a reference centre: etiological diagnosis of 348 cases. *Medicine (Baltimore)* 2005; 84:162–173.

47. Richardson DC, Burrows LL, Korithoski B, et al. Tropheryma whippelii as a cause of culture-negative endocarditis: the evolving spectrum of Whipple's disease. *J Infect* 2003; 47:170–173.

48. Lepidi H, Fenollar F, Dumler JS, et al. Cardiac valves in patients with Whipple endocarditis: microbiological, molecular, quantitative histologic and immunohistochemical studies of 5 patients. *J Infect Dis* 2004; 190:935–945.

49. Anderson M. Neurology of Whipple's disease. *J Neurol Neurosurg Psychiatry* 2000; 68:2–5.

50. Lohr M, Stenzel W, Plum G, et al. Whipple Disease confined to the central nervous system presenting as a solitary frontal tumour. *J Neurosurg* 2004; 101:336–339.

51. Peters G, du Plessis DG, Humphrey PR. Cerebral Whipple's disease with a stroke-like presentation and cerebrovascular pathology. *J Neurol Neurosurg Psychiatry* 2002; 73:336–339.

52. Gerard A, Sarrot-Reynauld F, Liozon E, et al. Neurological presentation of Whipple disease: report of 12 cases and review of the literature. *Medicine (Baltimore)* 2002; 81:443–457.

53. Walter R, Bachmann SP, Schaffner A, et al. Bone marrow involvement in Whipple's Disease: rarely reported, but really rare? *Br J Haematol* 2001; 112:677–679.

54. Krober SM, Kaiserling E, Horny HP, et al. Primary diagnosis of Whipple's disease in bone marrow. *Hum Pathol* 2004; 35:522–525.

55. Lynch T, Odel J, Fredericks DN, et al. Polymerase chain reaction-based detection of *Tropheryma whipplei* in central nervous system Whipple's disease. *Ann Neurol* 1997; 42:120–124.

56. James TN. On the wide spectrum of abnormalities in the coronary arteries of Whipple's disease. *Coron Art Dis* 2001; 12:115–125.

57. Gras E, Matias-Guiu X, Garcia A, et al. PCR analysis in the pathological diagnosis of Whipple's disease: emphasis on the extraintestinal involvement or atypical morphological features. *J Pathol* 1999; 188:318–321.

58. Raoult D, Ogata H, Audic S, et al. Tropheryma whipplei Twist: a human pathogenic Actinobacteria with a reduced genome. *Genome Res* 2003; 13:1800–1809.

59. Kowalczewska M, Fenollar F, Lafitte D, et al. Identification of candidate antigen in Whipple's disease using a serological proteomic approach. *Proteomics* 2006; 6:3294–3305.

60. Fenollar F, Raoult D. Molecular techniques in Whipple's disease. *Expert Rev Mol Diagn* 2001; 1:299–309.

61. Baisden BL, Lepidi H, Raoult D, et al. Diagnosis of Whipple disease by immunohistochemical analysis: a sensitive and specific method for the detection of Tropheryma whipplei in paraffin-embedded tissue. *Am J Clin Pathol* 2002; 118:742–748.

62. Sloan LM, Rosenblatt JE, Cockerill FR 3rd. Detection of *Tropheryma whipplei* DNA in clinical specimens by LightCycler real-time PCR. *J Clin Microbiol* 2005; 43:3516–3518.

63. La Scola B, Rolain JM, Maurin M, et al. Can Whipple's disease be transmitted by gastroscopes? *Infect Control Hosp Epidemiol* 2003; 24:191–194.

64. Garas G, Cheng WS, Abrugiato R, et al. Clinical relapse in Whipple's disease despite maintenance therapy. *J Gastroenterol Hepatol* 2000; 15:1223–1226.

65. Boulos A, Rolain JM, Raoult D. Antibiotic susceptibility of *Tropheryma whipplei* in MRC5 cells. *Antimicrob Agents Chemother* 2004; 48:747–752.

66. Boulos A, Rolain JM, Mallet MN, et al. Molecular evaluation of antibiotic susceptibility of *Trophyrema whipplei* in axenic medium. *J Antimicrob Chemother* 2005; 55:178–181.

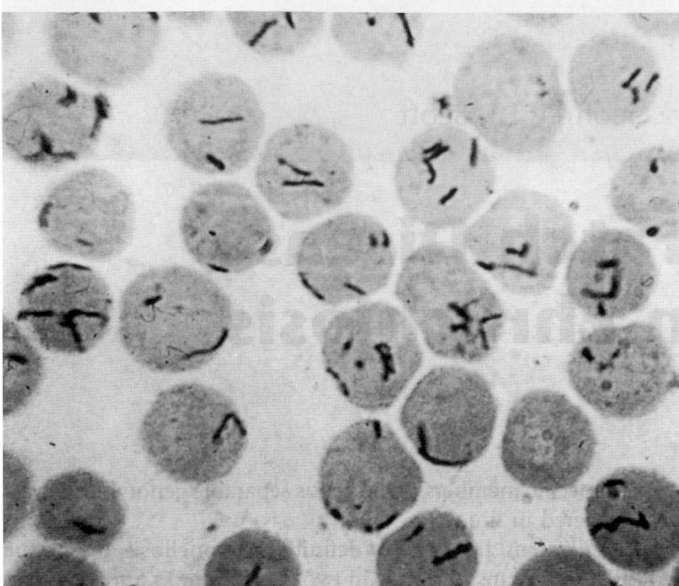

Figure 61.1 *Bartonella bacilliformis* in blood.

Introduction

Carrión, a medical student, infected himself with tissue from verruga peruana in 1885, a cutaneous eruption of haemangioma-like growths. He developed Oroya fever, an acute febrile haemolytic illness, and died, thus establishing the intimate link between these two disparate clinical conditions.[16]

Geographical distribution

Classical bartonellosis has a remarkable focal distribution, occurring between latitudes N05 and S16, between altitudes 800 and 3000 m on the western slopes of the Andes in Columbia, Peru and Ecuador.[17,18] Furthermore, the infection tends to cause outbreaks only in narrow valleys (quebradas) where the vector proliferates.

Experimental transmission: bartonellosis as a zoonosis?

Intravenous injection of *B. bacilliformis* into macaque monkeys causes irregular fever and anaemia, while the organisms can be demonstrated in the blood cells. The monkeys are often asymptomatic unless splenectomized, and then the blood from a patient with Oroya fever is fatal.[14] Intradermal inoculation into the supraorbital tissues gives rise to verrugous nodules. After inoculation of grey squirrels (*Citellus tridecemlineatus*) the organism could be recovered only for the first 24–48 h, and the animals were asymptomatic. Verruga can be conveyed by inoculation to puppies and rabbits, and *B. vinsonii* occurs as a natural infection in native American Indian dogs. It is possible that human infection is a zoonotic disease depending on a natural animal reservoir, although in the case of Oroya fever this has not been established with certainty.

Human reservoir

It is likely that the main reservoir consists of asymptomatic human cases. *Bartonella* was cultured from seven of 81 students and three of these seven were asymptomatic. In the verruga zone, 10–15% of people have been shown to be chronic carriers with positive blood cultures.[14,19] *B. bacilliformis* can be seen in the endothelial cells of cutaneous verruga nodules, suggesting that they could act as a source of continuing infection to sandflies.

Sandfly transmission

The only proven vectors in humans are New World sandflies, *Lutzomyia* spp.: *L. verrucarum* is the definitive vector.[20] Evidence incriminating *L. noguchii* (and *L. verrucarum*) was obtained when insects were collected in a verruga district of Peru and sent to New York, where they were ground up in saline and injected intradermally into monkeys.[21] An outbreak of Oroya fever in the Mantaro valley of Peru occurred in the absence of *L. verrucarum*, but *L. pescei* (rare below 2400 m) and *L. bicornutus* (rare above 2600 m) were identified as being prevalent in the area of the epidemic. The former species was thought to be more likely to be responsible for the outbreak because the cases occurred at higher altitudes. In the Narino department of south-western Colombia, the habits of *L. colombianus* are so like those of *L. verrucarum* that it may be a vector in this area. *L. noguchii* and *L. peruensis* are also suspected vectors.

The organisms adhere to the midgut of the sandfly in moderate numbers after feeding on infected patients and have been found occasionally on the proboscis of wild-caught sandflies, suggesting that transmission may be by mechanical inoculation during biting.

Pathology

Red blood cells

The organisms bind to multiple surface glycoproteins of erythrocyte membranes.[22,23] They invade erythrocytes, in which they multiply, causing destruction of the cells.[24] In severe cases, the red cell count may drop in 3 or 4 weeks to 500 000/mm³. There is an associated polymorphonuclear leukocytosis, but without eosinophilia. The anaemia is typically normocytic and hypochromic but may be macrocytic because of reticulocytosis or if there is associated dietary folate deficiency.[25] Destruction of the red cells is due to intravascular haemolysis; 50% of labelled erythrocytes have a half-life of 6 days (normal median survival 120 days). However, those red cells that survive this period have a normal survival rate. Normal erythrocytes injected into patients in the febrile anaemic phase behaved similarly, but red cells from a patient with verruga peruana survived normally, suggesting that the patient had acquired resistance to the haemolytic process after cessation of the febrile stage.

Reticuloendothelial system

The organisms invade the cells of the reticuloendothelial system causing hyperplasia in the lymph glands, with proliferation of Kupffer cells of the liver and histiocytes in the spleen, bone marrow, kidneys, adrenals, pancreas, thyroid and testes. They also parasitize the endothelial lining cells of the blood and lymph vessels, which may be so distended by closely packed masses of the bacteria that infected cells can be detected on low-power microscopic examination of lymph glands, spleen, liver and intestine.[22] Marked changes are present in the liver, spleen and bone marrow. In the liver, areas of degenerative and central necrosis are found around the hepatic veins. In the centre of the necrotic areas, a yellow pigment resembling haemosiderin is present in abundance. The spleen is invariably enlarged and contains necrotic areas with pigment. The lymph glands contain large macrophage endothelial cells studded with bacteria. The bone marrow shows proliferation, necrosis and marked phagocytosis of the large endothelial cells. The malpighian bodies are not affected.

Verruga stage

The verrugous eruption is a sequela to the lesions in the reticuloendothelial system.[26] There is proliferation of the endothelium of the lymphatic channels which become obstructed by plasma cells and fibroblasts, but the structure is much more vascular than that of yaws, which it otherwise resembles. The capillary blood vessels become dilated so that the granulomatous tumours are vascular, almost cavernous, and apt to bleed profusely. Nodules of angioblasts around the blood vessels are characteristic of the disease. *B. bacilliformis* is seen in considerable numbers in the endothelial cells of cutaneous verruga nodules, but distension of the cells is less than that seen in cases of Oroya fever. Scanty bacteria may be found in blood corpuscles.

Immunity

Recovery from the disease in any of its forms confers lasting immunity but this is not solely dependent on the presence of specific agglutinins in the blood.[27] Passage from Oroya fever to the verruga stage, which is a change in the host–parasite relationship resulting from the development of immunity, is accompanied by a diminution of symptoms. It was shown that graduated inoculation of verrugous material induces an artificial immunity.[22] In monkeys infected with verruga tissue, splenectomy reverses the process and produces Oroya fever.

Serum antibodies that agglutinate the organism in titres from 10 to 80 have been found in patients in both the Oroya fever and verruga stages.[27,28] Cross-reactions occur with *Proteus* sp. OX19, OXK and OX2 (another tenuous link with rickettsiae). A strong agglutinating serum can be prepared for laboratory identification of *B. bacilliformis*.

Prophylactic inoculation with a formalinized suspension of *B. bacilliformis* resulted in partial immunity so that subsequent attacks of Oroya fever were modified.[27]

Clinical features[17]

Natural history

The spectrum of disease ranges from common asymptomatic carriage, to the severe and often fatal Oroya fever and on to verruga peruana.

OROYA FEVER

The incubation period of Oroya fever is about 3 weeks.[17,29] Onset of the fever is insidious, and marked by malaise, soon followed by a rapidly developing anaemia and an irregular remittent pyrexia, associated with very severe pains in the head, joints and long bones. The bone pains are probably connected with disturbances in the haemopoietic system. The initial fever is like that of malaria, and the most severe illness resembles fulminant typhus and is known as the 'severe fever of Carrión'. The liver, spleen and lymph nodes are enlarged and tender.

A characteristic anaemia develops with a tendency to macrocytosis with nucleated red cells and a high reticulocytosis. In the febrile phase, most of the red cells contain numerous bacilliform organisms and there is a polymorphonuclear leukocytosis.

The death rate varies from 10% to 40%, death coming within 2–3 weeks of the onset of the disease. A terminal delirium is often noted. In cases that proceed to the verruga stage, the fever may have lasted for 3–4 months. Superinfection with *Salmonella typhimurium* may prove fatal.[30]

Verruga peruana stage (localized bartonellosis or eruptive stage)

The latent interval subsequent to the development of Oroya fever is 30–40 days. Although verruga is usually a sequel of Oroya fever, it may arise spontaneously as long as 2 months after exposure. The initial stages are characterized by rheumatic-like pains together with fever, the pains being like those of yaws only more severe. As in yaws, the constitutional symptoms subside on the appearance of the skin lesions. The eruption may be sparse or abundant, discrete or confluent. Some granulomas fail to erupt, others subside rapidly, and others may continue to increase and then, after remaining stationary for a time, gradually wither, shrink and drop off without leaving a scar.

Two types of eruption are seen. The miliary eruption (Figure 61.2), not exceeding the size of a small pea, is found most abundantly on the face and extensor aspects of the extremities, less commonly on the trunk. A pink macule first appears, later darkening and becoming nodular. The verruga artificially produced in monkeys by injection of *Bartonella* bodies is bright cherry-pink. The nodules, which are flat or somewhat pedunculated, are vascular and may develop on mucous surfaces in the mouth, oesophagus, stomach, intestine, bladder, uterus and vagina; hence dysphagia is a common symptom, with occasional haematemesis, melaena, haematuria and bleeding from the vagina.

The Oroya fever and verruga stages frequently co-exist and relapses of both the fever and the eruption may occur.

The nodular eruption (Figure 61.3) is rarer but more chronic than the miliary form. Individual lesions can grow to the size of a pigeon's egg and may become strangulated and a source of danger as a result of haemorrhage. This type does not invade the mucous membranes and is usually confined to the regions of the knees and elbows. It appears in crops and lasts 2–3 months. The mortality rate from verruga is practically nil.

occur without lymph node involvement[59,60] and may be very long lasting.[61]

Patients without lymphadenopathy tend to have persistent fever and systemic complications. This type of response is more common in the elderly. Rarely recognized presentations of disseminated bartonellosis include 'gastroenteritis'[62] or mesenteric adenitis with acute ileitis.[63] Spread to the liver and spleen via the portal system leads to hepatosplenic syndrome,[64] granulomatous hepatitis[65] and splenic abscess.[66,67] Infections may simulate pyogenic conditions such as osteomyelitis,[68–72] parotitis,[73] breast mass[74] or even bacillary angiomatosis on an area of burned skin.[75] Endocarditis is now well recognized.[76] There is a tantalising relationship between Henoch–Schönlein purpura and positive *B. henselae* serology.[77] Late immunological complications include IgA nephritis,[78] or necrotizing crescentic glomerulonephritis.[79]

Differential diagnosis

Local lymphadenitis is usually considered at first to be due to tuberculosis, and the nodular skin lesions in patients with AIDS are usually confused with Kaposi's sarcoma. A history of animal contact is valuable but not essential. The differential diagnosis of fever with disseminated lymphadenopathy is so wide that serology must simply be borne in mind. Granuloma formation may occasionally lead to hypercalcaemia, as in sarcoid. Biopsy of persistently enlarged nodes and masses involving other organs is therefore essential to differentiate these diseases, and the histological findings are likely to be a surprise. It is wise to keep some biopsy material fresh and unfixed, preferably frozen, so that appropriate cultures and DNA studies can be set up once histological examination is completed.

Beyond classical cat-scratch disease, the manifestations of infection with *B. henselae* are so diverse and the differential disease is so wide that patients are often thought to have serious disease, including malignancy[80] or tuberculosis, and the diagnosis is usually delayed.

Diagnosis

Diagnosis may be made serologically[81] and the histopathological changes are characteristic although not pathognomonic. Serological kits are available[82] but of variable sensitivity.[83] Culture in the conditions suggested above for bartonellosis may be positive but caution has to be taken if reliance is placed on binding to polyclonal antiserum, which may react with *Chlamydia* spp.[84] Differentiation of *B. henselae* from *B. quintana* may be made with specific monoclonal antibodies,[10,85,86] with polymerase chain reaction-restriction fragment length polymorphism (PCR-RFLP) and then using appropriate restriction endonucleases.[87] DNA amplification methods are likely to be the method of diagnosis of choice in the future.[88,89] A skin test preparation has been described but is not properly validated and not available commercially.

Pathology

B. henselae does not bind to human red cells like *B. bacilliformis*, but intraerythrocyte growth in cat red cells occurs. Both *B. henselae*

and *B. quintana* grow in human epithelial cells and stimulate the proliferation of endothelial cells.[90] The organism survives in endosomes and inhibits lysosome fusion.[91] Cat-scratch disease is characterized by a necrotizing and coalescent granulomatous reaction to the infection.[66] This differs from other granulomas in having some neutrophil infiltration and clumps of bacteria. Bacillary angiomatosis is a proliferation of new vessels lined with cuboidal epithelium and a neutrophil infiltrate (Figure 61.4) mediated by interleukin-8 and its receptor on endothelial cells.[92] Microcolonies of bacteria can be seen by Giemsa or silver stain, or on electron microscopy. Bacillary peliosis is characterized by blood-filled lacunae up to several millimetres in size, lined with discontinuous endothelial cells lying in a stroma loaded with clumps of bacteria (Figure 61.5), with inflammatory cells and capillaries. Although

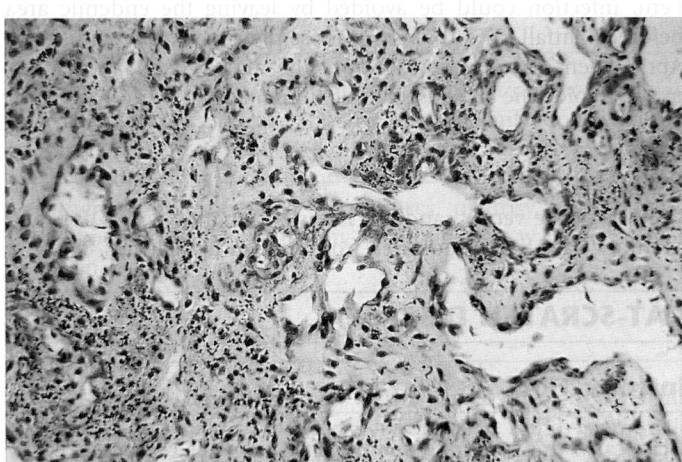

Figure 61.4 Histological appearance of cutaneous angiomatosis (H&E stain). (Courtesy of S. Lucas.)

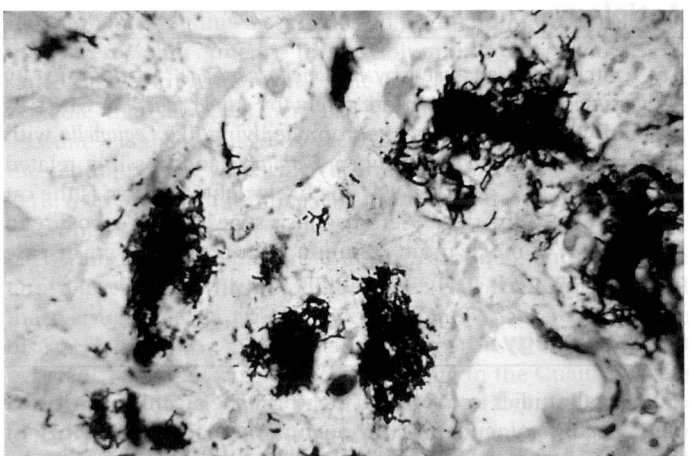

Figure 61.5 Peliosis hepatitis (silver stain). (Courtesy of S. Lucas.)

generally recognized in the liver, they may be seen in other organs of patients with AIDS. The organism will grow on special media, provided enough time is allowed, which probably accounts for low yields from routine methods.

Management

Bartonellae are sensitive to many antimicrobials in vitro, including penicillins and cephalosporins, co-trimoxazole, tetracyclines, rifampicin and fluoroquinolones. Spontaneous resolution is the norm but one placebo-controlled trial with azithromycin showed more rapid resolution of large lymph nodes.[93]

TRENCH FEVER

'. . . my servant and one other, are the only non-verminous bodies in the platoon; not to say licentious'
(Wilfred Owen, letters, 1917)

Introduction

Louse-borne bartonellosis is caused predominantly by *B. quintana*.[94] This disease was described in World War I. Chronic carriage is possible and some patients develop endocarditis.

History

The term trench fever was coined by Hunt and Rankin,[95] who described 30 cases. In 1916, His and Werner described the disease in German troops on the Eastern front, calling it Wolhnyian fever, and McNee et al.[96] wrote a detailed description from the Western Front. Gratzer, an experienced army physician, said it had been endemic in Eastern Front troops since 1914. It was the cause of 20–30% of troop wastage on both sides in the Great War.[97] Recent molecular studies found evidence of *B. quintana* in lice and dental pulp of soldiers of Napoleon's army who died and were buried in Lithuania.[98] The disease is found in patients infested with body lice, although not head lice, even though the latter have been shown to support the organism. The infectious nature of this disease was established by experimental transmission of the aetiological agent in volunteers.[99]

Clinical presentation

In experimental trench fever, the incubation period is usually 7–9 days but it may be much longer, depending on the inoculum – whether whole blood, the red cell fraction or extracts of infected lice or louse faeces. Although biting by lice may cause disease, this is less efficient than rubbing louse faeces into scarified skin. Classically, the patient develops sudden-onset general influenza-like illness with a high fever (>39°C), retro-orbital headache and lower limb pain. Severe and persistent anterior tibial pain is a classical, although unexplained, feature. Hyperaesthesia of thoracic and lumbar dermatomes and an analogy to tabes dorsalis, with a lack

of periosteal or muscle inflammation, suggest that the pain is neurological in origin. Patients often have a transient erythematous rash. Splenomegaly is not unusual. The fever lasts a matter of 2–8 days, resolves suddenly with all symptoms, but classically relapses after a few more days. The height of the fever in the relapse may be the same as that in the presenting phase but is often less marked and may become chronic. Some patients have a prolonged relapsing-remitting fever and convalescence may be prolonged. Patients returned to base hospitals from the front were unfit for duty for an average of 60–70 days, and some 10% of these became semi-permanent invalids. Blood remains infectious to volunteers and positive on culture for many weeks. However, the disease is rarely fatal.

Many carriers are asymptomatic. Alcoholics with bacteraemia are likely to have headaches, severe leg pain, pruritic lesions and reduced platelet counts.[100] *B. quintana* may cause retinal artery occlusion and peripapillary angiomata with severe loss of vision.[101]

Endocarditis

B. quintana is now recognized as an important cause of 'culture negative' endocarditis.[102–105] Duke criteria may not be fulfilled.[106] Serological studies and special attention to the blood cultures are essential when preliminary investigations prove negative. A history of urban homelessness and likely exposure to lice is very important.[102]

It is not certain whether different clinical manifestations of infection are more determined by host variation or genetic diversity of strains.[107]

Differential diagnosis

When the disease was first recognized, it was quite clear to experienced physicians that this was something different from rheumatic fever (which was surprisingly rare in the troops), enteric and typhus fevers, and influenza. Most cases were initially called suspected typhoid fever, a diagnosis not confirmed on blood culture. The characteristics of the remitting fever with severe limb pain were quite unlike typhoid. Patients with typhus were severely ill with a high mortality rate, and tended to have a purpuric rash.

Management

There is a dearth of information about antimicrobial treatment and its effects. The organism is sensitive to many antibiotics in vitro. It is likely that the most effective agents are tetracyclines or macrolides. Patients who have endocarditis should probably be treated by valve replacement.[105]

Diagnosis

The diagnosis may be made serologically, by culture and histologically with specific PCR on infected tissues such as heart valve. Blood culture is slow. The organism can be seen by acridine

35. Hertig M, Fairchild GB. Control of Phlebotomus in Peru with DDT. *Am J Trop Med* 1948; 28:207–230.

36. English CK, Wear DJ, Margileth AM, et al. Cat-scratch disease: isolation and culture of the bacterial agent. *JAMA* 1988; 259:1347–1352.

37. Gerber MA, Sedgwick AK, MacAlister TJ, et al. The aetiological agent of cat scratch disease. *Lancet* 1985; i:1236–1240.

38. Giladi M, Avidor B, Kletter Y, et al. Cat scratch disease: the rare role of Afipia felis. *J Clin Microbiol* 1998; 36:2499–2502.

39. La Scola B, Raoult D. Afipia felis in hospital water supply in association with free-living amoebae. *Lancet* 1999; 353:1330.

40. Sander A, Zagosek A, Bredt W, et al. Characterization of Bartonella clarridgeiae flagellin (FlaA) and detection of antiflagellin antibodies in patients with lymphadenopathy. *J Clin Microbiol* 2000; 38:2943–2948.

41. Tsukahara M, Tsuneoka H, Iino H, et al. Bartonella henselae infection from a dog. *Lancet* 1998; 21:1682–1683.

42. Del Prete R, Fumaola D, Fumarola L, et al. Prevalence of antibodies to Bartonella henselae in patients with suspected cat scratch disease (CSD) in Italy. *Eur J Epidemiol* 1999; 15:583–587.

43. Arvand M, Klose AJ, Schwartz-Porsche D, et al. Genetic variability and prevalence of *Bartonella henselae* in cats in Berlin, Germany, and analysis of its genetic relatedness to a strain from Berlin that is pathogenic for humans. *J Clin Microbiol* 2001; 39:743–746.

44. Chang CC, Chomel BB, Kasten RW, et al. Bartonella spp. isolated from wild and domestic ruminants in North America. *Emerg Infect Dis* 2000; 6:306–311.

45. Schouls LM, Van de Pol I, Rijpkema SG, et al. Detection and identification of Ehrlichia, Borrelia burgdorferi sensu lato, and Bartonella species in Dutch Ixodes ricinus ticks. *J Clin Microbiol* 1999; 37:2215–2222.

46. Chang C, Yamamoto K, Chimel BB, et al. Seroepidemiology of Bartonella vinsonii subsp. berkhoffii infection in California coyotes, 1994–1998. *Emerg Infect Dis* 1999; 5:711–715.

47. Roux V, Eykyn SJ, Wyllie S, et al. Bartonella vinsonii subsp. berkhoffii as an agent of febrile blood culture-negative endocarditis in a human. *J Clin Microbiol* 2000; 38:1698–1700.

48. Reynolds MG, Holman RC, Curns AT, et al. Epidemiology of cat-scratch disease hospitalizations among children in United States. *Pediatr Infect Dis J* 2005; 24:700–704.

49. DeBoit PE, Berger TG, Egbert BM, et al. Epithelioid haemangioma-like vascular proliferation in AIDS: manifestation of cat scratch disease bacillus infection? *Lancet* 1988; i:960–964.

50. Plettenberg A, Lorenzen T, Burtsche BT, et al. Bacillary angiomatosis in HIV-infected patients – an epidemiological and clinical study. *Dermatology* 2000; 201:326–331.

51. Massei F, Messina F, Talini I, et al. Widening of the clinical spectrum of Bartonella henselae infection as recognized through serodiagnostics. *Eur J Pediatr* 2000; 15:416–419.

52. Tsukahara M, Tsuneoka H, Iino H, et al. Bartonella henselae infection as a cause of fever of unknown origin. *J Clin Microbiol* 2000; 38:1990–1991.

53. Massei F, Messina F, Massmetti M, et al. Pseudoinfectious mononucleosis: a presentation of Bartonella henselae infection. *Arch Dis Child* 2000; 33:443–444.

54. Grando D, Sullivan LJ, Flexman JP, et al. Bartonella henselae associated with Parinaud's oculoglandular syndrome. *Clin Infect Dis* 1999; 28:1156–1158.

55. Lohmann CP, Gabler B, Kroher G, et al. Disciform keratitis caused by Bartonella henselae: an unusual ocular complication in cat scratch disease. *Eur J Ophthalmol* 2000; 10:257–258.

56. Thompson PK, Vaphiades MS, Saccente M. Cat-scratch disease presenting as neuroretinitis and peripheral facial palsy. *J Neuroophthalmol* 1999; 19:240–241.

57. Rosen BS, Barry CJ, Nicoll AM, et al. Conservative management of documented neuroretinitis in cat scratch disease associated with Bartonella henselae infection. *Aust NZ Ophthalmol* 1999; 27:153–156.

58. Ormerod LD, Dailey JP. Ocular manifestations of cat-scratch disease. *Curr Opin Ophthalmol* 1999; 10:209–216.

59. Salgado CD, Weisse ME. Transverse myelitis associated with probable cat-scratch disease in a previously healthy pediatric patient. *Clin Infect Dis* 2000; 31:609–611.

60. McNeill PM, Verrips A, Mullaart R, et al. Chronic inflammatory demyelinating polyneuropathy as a complication of cat scratch disease. *J Neurol Neurosurg Psychiat* 2000; 68:797.

61. Stockmeyer B, Schoerner C, Frangou P, et al. Chronic vasculitis and polyneuropathy due to infection with Bartonella henselae. *Infection* 2007; 35:107–109.

62. Liapi-Adamidou G, Tsolia M, Magiakou AM, et al. Cat scratch disease in two siblings presenting as acute gastroenteritis. *Scand J Infect Dis* 2000; 32:317–319.

63. Massei F, Massimetti M, Messina F, et al. Bartonella henselae and inflammatory bowel disease. *Lancet* 2000; 356:1245–1246.

64. Arisoy ES, Correa AG, Wagner ML, et al. Hepatosplenic cat-scratch disease in children: selected clinical features and treatment. *Clin Infect Dis* 1999; 28:778–784.

65. Lenoir AA, Storch GA, Deshryver-Kecskemeti K, et al. Granulomatous hepatitis associated with cat scratch disease. *Lancet* 1988; i:1132–1136.

66. Ventura A, Massei F, Not T, et al. Systemic Bartonella henselae infection with hepatosplenic involvement. *J Pediatr Gastroenterol Nutr* 1999; 29:52–56.

67. Mehanna D, Peck N, Arnot R, et al. Cat scratch disease presenting as splenic abscess. *Aust NZ J Surg* 2000; 70:622–624.

68. Krause R, Wenisch C, Pladerer P, et al. Osteomyelitis of the hip joint associated with systemic cat-scratch disease in an adult. *Eur J Clin Microbiol Infect Dis* 2000; 19:781–783.

69. Ruess M, Sander A, Brandis M, et al. Portal vein and bone involvement in disseminated cat-scratch disease: report of two cases. *Clin Infect Dis* 2000; 31:818–821.

70. Hussain S, Rathmore MH. Cat scratch disease with epidural extension while on antimicrobial treatment. *Pediatr Neurosurg* 2007; 43:164–166.

71. deKort JG, Robben SG, Schrander JJ, et al. Multifocal osteomyelitis in a child: a rare manifestation of cat scratch disease: a case report and systematic review of the literature. *J Pediatr Orthop B* 2006; 15:285–288.

72. Hajjaji N, Hocqueloux L, Kerdraon R, et al. Bone infection in cat-scratch disease: a review of the literature. *J Infect* 2007; 54:417–421.

73. Malatskey S, Fradis M, Ben-David J, et al. Cat-scratch disease of the parotid gland: an often mis-diagnosed entity. *Ann Otol Rhinol Laryngol* 2000; 109:679–682.

74. Fortune SM, Kaelin CM, Gulizia JM, et al. Cat scratch disease presenting as a breast mass. *Obstet Gynecol* 2000; 95:1027.

75. Karakas M, Baba M, Aksungur VL, et al. Bacillary angiomatosis on a region of burned skin in an immunocompetent patient. *Br J Dermatol* 2000; 143:609–611.

76. Gouriet F, Lepidi H, Habib G, et al. From cat scratch disease to endocarditis, the possible natural history of Bartonella henselae infection. *BMC Infect Dis* 2007; 7:30.

77. Robinson JL, Spady DW, Prasad E, et al. *Bartonella* seropositivity in children with Henoch-Schonlein purpura. *BMC Infect Dis* 2005; 5:21.

78. Hopp L, Eppes SC. Development of IgA nephritis following cat scratch disease in a 13 y-old boy. *Pediatr Nephrol* 2004; 19:682–684.

79. Bookman I, Scoley JW, Jassal SV, et al. Necrotising glomerulonephritis caused by Bartonella henselae endocarditis. *Am J Kidney Dis* 2004; 43:e25–e30.

80. Millot F, Tailboux L, Paccalin M, et al. Cat-scratch disease simulating a malignant process of the chest wall. *Eur J Pediatr* 1999; 158:403–405.

81. Cimolai N, Benoit L, Hill A, et al. Bartonella henselae infection in British Columbia: evidence for an endemic disease among humans. *Can J Microbiol* 2000; 46:908–912.

82. Harrison TG, Doshi N. Serological evidence of *Bartonella* spp. infection in the UK. *Epidemiol Infect* 1999; 123:233–240.

83. Vermeulen MJ, Herremans M, Verbakel H, et al. Serological testing for Bartonella henselae infections in The Netherlands: clinical evaluation of immunofluorescence assay and ELISA. *Clin Microbiol Infect* 2007; 13:627–634.

84. Maurin M, Raoult D. Isolation in endothelial cell cultures of Chlamydia trachomatis LGV (serovar L2) from a lymph node of a patient with suspected cat scratch disease. *J Clin Microbiol* 2000; 38:2062–2064.

85. Sander A, Penno S. Semiquantitative species detection of Bartonella henselae and *Bartonella quintana* by PCR-enzyme immunoassay. *J Clin Microbiol* 1999; 37:3097–3101.

86. Liang Z, Raoult D. Species-specific monoclonal antibodies for rapid identification of Bartonella quintana. *Clin Diagn Lab Immunol* 2000; 7: 21–24.

87. Matar GM, Koehler JE, Malcolm G, et al. Identification of Bartonella species directly in clinical specimens by PCR-restriction fragment length polymorphism analysis of a 16S rRNA gene fragment. *J Clin Microbiol* 1999; 37:4045–4047.

88. Del Prete R, Fumarola D, Ungari S, et al. Polymerase chain reaction detection of Bartonella henselae bacteraemia in an immunocompetent child with cat scratch disease. *Eur J Pediatr* 2000; 159:356–359.

89. Maas M, Schreiber M, Knobloch J. Detection of Bartonella bacilliformis in cultures, blood and formalin preserved skin biopsies by use of the polymerase chain reaction. *Trop Med Parasitol* 1992; 43:191–194.

90. Maeno N, Oda H, Yoshiie K, et al. Live *Bartonella henselae* enhances endothelial proliferation without direct contact. *Microb Pathog* 1999; 27: 419–427.

91. Kyme PA, Haas A, Schaller M, et al. Unusual trafficking pattern of Bartonella henselae-containing vacuoles in macrophages and endothelial cells. *Cell Microbiol* 2005; 7:1019–1034.

92. McCord AM, Resto-Ruiz SI, Anderson BE. Autocrine role for interleukin-8 in Bartonella henselae-induced angiogenesis. *Infect Immun* 2006; 74: 5185–5190.

93. Conrad DA. Treatment of cat scratch disease. *Curr Opin Pediatr Dis* 2001; 13:56–59.

94. Foucault C, Brouqui P, Raoult D. Bartonella quintana characteristics and clinical management. *Emerg Infect Dis* 2006; 12:217–223.

95. Hunt GH, Rankin AC. Intermittent fever of obscure origin, occurring among British soldiers in France: the so-called 'trench fever'. *Lancet* 1915; ii: 1133–1136.

96. McNee JW, Renshaw A, Brunt EH. Trench fever: a relapsing fever occurring with the British forces in France. *BMJ* 1916; i:225–234.

97. Swift HF. Trench fever. *Arch Intern Med* 1920; 26:76–98.

98. Raoult D, Dutour O, Houhamdi L, et al. Evidence for louse-transmitted diseases in soldiers of Napoleon's Grand Army in Vilnius. *J Infect Dis* 2006; 193:112–120.

99. Vinson JW, Varela G, Molina-Pasquel C. Trench fever 3: Induction of clinical disease in volunteers inoculated with Rickettsia quintana propagated on blood agar. *Am J Trop Med Hyg* 1969; 18:713–722.

100. Brouqui P, Lascola L, Roux V, et al. Chronic Bartonella quintana bacteremia in homeless patients. *N Engl J Med* 1999; 340:184–189.

101. Gray AV, Reed JB, Wendel RT, et al. Bartonella henselae infection associated with peripapillary angioma, branch retinal artery occlusion and severe vision loss. *Am J Ophthalmol* 1999; 127:223–224.

102. Drancourt M, Mainardi JL, Brouqui P, et al. Bartonella (Rochalimaea) quintana endocarditis in three homeless men. *N Engl J Med* 1995; 332: 419–423.

103. Barbe KP, Jaeggi E, Ninet B, et al. *Bartonella quintana* endocarditis in a child. *N Engl J Med* 2000; 342:1841–1842.

104. Ohl ME, Spach DH. Bartonella quintana and urban trench fever. *Clin Infect Dis* 2000; 31:131–135.

105. James EA, Hill J, Uppal R, et al. Bartonella infection: a significant cause of native valve endocarditis necessitating surgical management. *J Thorac Cardiovasc Surg* 2000; 119:171–172.

106. Simon-Vermont I, Altwegg M, Zimmerli W, et al. Duke criteria-negative endocarditis caused by *Bartonella quintana*. *Infection* 1999; 27:283–285.

107. Schulte B, Linke D, Klumpp S, et al. Bartonella quintana variably expressed outer membrane proteins mediate vascular endothelial growth factor secretion but not host cell adherence. *Infect Immun* 2006; 74:5003–5013.

108. Patel R, Newell JO, Procop GW, et al. Use of polymerase chain reaction for citrate synthase gene to diagnose *Bartonella quintana*. *Am J Clin Pathol* 1999; 119:36–40.

109. Rahimian J, Raoult D, Tang YW, et al. Bartonella quintana endocarditis with positive serology for *Coxiella burnetti*. *J Infect* 2006; 53:151–153.

110. Azad AF, Sacci JB Jr, Nelson WM, et al. Genetic characterization and transovarial transmission of a typhus-like rickettsia found in cat fleas. *Proc Natl Acad Sci USA* 1992; 89:43–46.

111. Woolley MW, Gordon DL, Wetherall BL. Analysis of the first Australian strains of *Bartonella quintana* reveals unique genotypes. *J Clin Microbiol* 2007; 45:2040–2043.

112. Roux V, Raoult D. Body lice as tools for diagnosis and surveillance of reemerging diseases. *J Clin Microbiol* 1999; 37:596–599.

113. Raoult D, Birtles RJ, Montoya M, et al. Survey of three bacterial louse-associated diseases among rural Andean communities in Peru: prevalence of epidemic typhus, trench fever and relapsing fever. *Clin Infect Dis* 1999; 29:434–436.

114. Seki N, Sasaki T, Sawabe K, et al. Epidemiological studies on Bartonella quintana infections among homeless people in Tokyo, Japan. *Jpn J Infect Dis* 2006; 59:31–35.

115. Fukuda T, Kitao T, Keida Y. Studies on the causative agent of 'hyuganetsu' disease. I. Isolation of the agent and its inoculation trial in human beings. *Med Biol* 1954; 32:200–209.

116. Maeda K, Markowicz N, Hawley RC, et al. Human infection with Ehrlichia canis, a leukocytic rickettsia. *N Engl J Med* 1987; 316:853–856.

117. Chen S-M, Dumler JS, Bakken JS, et al. Identification of a granulocytotropic Ehrlichia species as the etiologic agent of human disease. *J Clin Microbiol* 1994; 32:589–595.

118. Dawson JE, Anderson BE, Fishbein DB, et al. Isolation and characterization of an Ehrlichia sp. from a patient with human ehrlichiosis. *J Clin Microbiol* 1991; 29:2741–2745.

119. Buller RS, Arens M, Hamiel SP, et al. Ehrlichia ewingii, a newly recognised agent of human ehrlichiosis. *N Engl J Med* 1999; 341:195–197.

120. Hotopp JC, Lin M, Madupu R, et al. Comparative genomics of emerging human ehrlichiosis agents. *PLoS Genet* 2006; 2:e21.

121. Perez M, Bodor M, Zhang C, et al. Human infections with Ehrlichia canis accompanied by clinical signs in Venezuela. *Ann NY Acad Sci* 2006; 1078:110–117.

122. Fishbein DB, Dawson JE, Robinson LE. Human ehrlichiosis in the United States, 1985–1990. *Ann Intern Med* 1994; 120:736–743.

123. Lotrick-Furlan S, Petrovec M, Avsic-Zupanc T, et al. Human ehrlichiosis in central Europe. *Wien Klin Wochenschr* 1998; 110:894–897.

124. Bjoersdorff A, Berglund J, Kristiansen BE, et al. Varying clinical picture and course of human granulocytic ehrlichiosis. Twelve Scandinavian cases of the new tick-borne zoonosis are presented. *Lakartidningen* 1999; 96: 4200–4204.

125. Aguero-Rosenfeld M, Horowitz HW, Wormser GP, et al. Human granulocytic ehrlichiosis (HE): a series from a single medical center in New York State. *Ann Intern Med* 1996; 125:904–908.

126. Telford SR, Dawson JE, Katavolos P, et al. Perpetuation of the agent of human granulocytic erhlichiosis in a deer tick-rodent cycle. *Proc Natl Acad Sci USA* 1996; 93:6209–6214.

127. Fritz CL, Bronson LR, Smith CR, et al. Clinical, epidemiologic and environmental surveillance for ehrlichiosis and anaplasmosis in an endemic area of northern California. *J Vector Ecol* 2005; 30:4–10.

128. Thompson C, Spielman A, Krause PJ. Coinfecting deer-associated zoonoses: Lyma disease, Babesiosis and Ehrlichiosis. *Clin Infect Dis* 2001; 33:676–685.

129. Rikihasa Y. Clinical and biological aspects of infection caused by *Ehrlichia chaffeensis*. *Microbes Infect* 1999; 1:367–376.

130. Rikihisa Y. *Ehrlichia* subversion of host innate responses. *Curr Opin Microbiol* 2006; 9:95–101.

131. Klein MB, Hu S, Chao CC, et al. The agent of human granulocytic ehrlichiosis induces the production of myelosuppressing chemokines without induction of pro-inflammatory cytokines. *J Infect Dis* 2000; 182:200–205.

Water-borne infection

The infection is maintained among rodents, mainly in water. The water is contaminated by dead animals[10] and excreta, and large numbers of rodents may be infected and die in this way.

Ingestion

Carnivores are infected chiefly from the consumption of sick, infected rodents which are easy to catch. Domestic cats may become infected in this way and then transmit the organisms to humans by biting.[11-13]

Insect vectors

A wide variety of ticks can act as vectors. The nymph stages feed on small rodents and adults feed on larger mammals, including humans. The infection persists during the development of the tick, but infection is also transmitted transovarially. By this method infection can be maintained through the winter.

Dermacentor andersoni (wood tick), *D. variabilis*, *D. occidentalis*, *D. reticulates*, *Ixodes ricinus* and *Haemaphysalis leporispalustris* (rabbit tick) can all transmit the infection. *D. andersoni* is particularly important in the USA and *F. tularensis* is found in the intestinal lumen, in the cells of the gut wall, in the body fluids and in the faeces. The organism can also be transmitted by biting fleas, the deer-fly (*Chrysops discalis*) as well as the stable fly (*Stomoxys calcitrans*), the squirrel flea (*Ceratophyllus acutus*), the rabbit louse (*Haemodipus ventricosus*) and the mouse louse (*Polyplax serratus*). The bacteria may be found in bed bugs or mites, but it is not certain how important these are in transmission. *Aedes* and *Theobaldia* spp. mosquitoes have been shown to transmit *F. tularensis* under experimental conditions, and in Sweden *Aedes cinereus* does so in nature. Mosquitoes transmit the infection to and between birds.

PATHOLOGY

As the disease is rarely fatal in humans, the pathology is best seen in infected animals. The pathological appearances of infected guinea pigs and rabbits at autopsy resemble those of plague. In an experimentally infected guinea pig, there is haemorrhagic oedema at the site of inoculation, blood-stained peritoneal exudate and a diffusely enlarged spleen with characteristic small necrotic foci. Similar lesions may be detected in the liver. On microscopic section of these organs, a dense infiltration with polymorphonuclear cells can be found, but the organisms can be detected only with difficulty. In the spleen of the mouse, on the other hand, little or no leukocytic response occurs and *F. tularensis* can be demonstrated in large numbers. In the few recorded autopsies in humans, nodules have been found in the lung and spleen.

IMMUNITY

There is a great deal of interest in the immunopathology of tularensis, a typical intracellular infection where cell-mediated immunity plays an important part in response to infection.[14-17] The organism replicates in the cytosol of the macrophage, having inhibited the respiratory burst and escaped from the phagolysosome.[18] Persistence in macrophages is determined by genes which code for a protein secretory system.[19] Other virulence properties include capsule, pili and lipopolysaccharide (which is relatively inert and poorly recognized by conventional LPS binding systems[20]) and determinants (membrane, stress response and metabolic proteins coded by a host of genes).[21] The organism stimulates upregulation of IL23 and IL12, the former inducing IFN-gamma.[22] Infected macrophages secrete prostaglandin E2 which inbits T cell proliferation.[23] Non-immune mice given neutralizing antibodies to tumour necrosis factor alpha (TNFα) and interferon gamma (IFNγ) are rendered defenceless against sublethal doses of *F. tularensis*.[24] Similarly, Toll-like receptor 2-deficient mice are more susceptible to infection. Virulent strains with capsules consume complement, leading to resistance to the bactericidal activity of serum.[25] Infection induces long-lasting immunity in humans and there is no record of a second generalized attack. However, local reinfection may occur and persistent infection in those treated with bacteriostatic antibiotics is not infrequent. Agglutinating antibodies appear in the serum in the second week and reach a maximum level between the fourth and eighth weeks, after which there is a gradual fall, but they may persist for as long as 11 years. Serum antibodies can be used in diagnosis, but cross-reactions occur with *Brucella melitensis* and *B. abortus* (23% of tularaemia sera cross-react with *B. melitensis* and *B. abortus*, and 35% of *B. melitensis* and *B. abortus* with tularaemia). In 13% of cases of tularaemia, the serum agglutinates *Proteus* OX19 at a titre of 80 or over.

Type IV hypersensitivity can be demonstrated by an intradermal test employing a suspension of killed organisms, and peripheral lymphocytes proliferate in response to *F. tularensis* antigens[26] and heat-shock protein chaperone 60.[27]

CLINICAL FEATURES

Subclinical infections

Seroprevalence surveys during outbreaks and in areas of hyperendemicity reveal that the majority acquire *F. tularensis* asymptomatically or without a characteristic infection. In Sweden, up to 23% of a population studied had been infected, the infection being subclinical in one-third of those with positive reactions. The disease presents in a number of ways, depending on the route of infection. The incubation period is 1–10 days.

Cutaneous (ulceroglandular) form (approximately 60% of cases)[28]

Local cutaneous disease results from the bite of an infected tick or fly, or an animal,[11-13] or from direct contact of the broken skin with an infected source. An inflamed papule develops at the site of infection, which becomes pustular with a necrotic centre. This separates, leaving a punched-out ulcer (Figure 62.1), which is replaced by a scar on healing. Small sores on the hands are usually not diagnosed as tularaemia. However, there may be painful enlargement of the local lymph glands which may suppurate after 1–2 months and may remain enlarged for 2–3 months. A

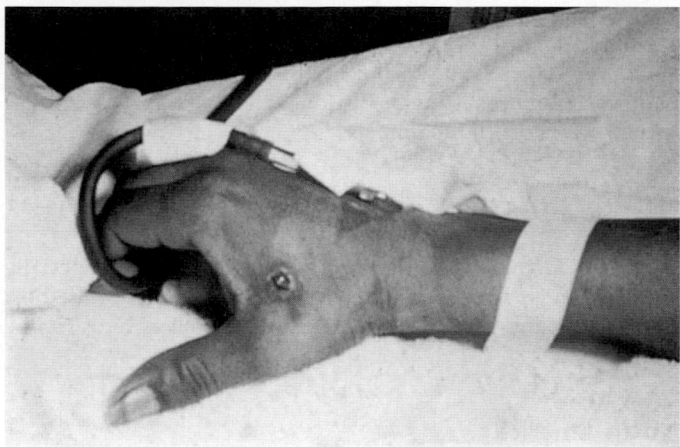

Figure 62.1 An ulcer on the hand of a patient with tularaemia. (Courtesy of the Tropical Resources Unit.)

glandular form of the disease may be seen (in about 15% of cases) without any sore. Sometimes the local lesion is associated with general signs of infection such as fever and prostration.

Ophthalmic (oculoglandular) form (1% of cases)

The site of entry of infection is the conjunctival sac, which is usually involved unilaterally. The patient may have rubbed the eyes while handling infected material or have been bitten on the eyelid by an infected insect. There is itching, lacrimation, photophobia and pain in the eye with swelling of the preauricular, parotid, submaxillary and cervical lymph glands. The eyelids become swollen and the conjunctiva red and covered with small discrete nodules and grey exudate. Punched-out ulcers develop and last for 2–3 weeks. Suppuration of the glands is common. Dacryocystitis and corneal ulcers occur, and permanent impairment of vision may follow.

Oral and abdominal form

This follows ingestion of infected meat or other food or water contaminated by rodent excreta. There is a necrotizing pharyngitis with abscesses on the roof of the mouth, fever, enlargement of local lymph glands and sometimes abdominal pain, vomiting and diarrhoea. Peritonitis may develop with persistent ascites, appendicitis or intestinal haemorrhage.

Pneumonic and typhoidal (septicaemic) forms

These forms may arise primarily from infection via the respiratory route or as a late result of dissemination from a local infection. The onset is sudden with severe headache, vomiting, chills and fever. Myalgia and arthralgia are common. The initial rise in temperature is above 40°C, with generalized weakness, aching, prostration, sweats and loss of weight. The fever may show an initial rise followed by remission and a secondary rise or a continuous course lasting usually for 10–15 days, and rarely 3–4 weeks. Petechial, roseolar, papular and pustular rashes are seen. A slightly

tender enlargement of the spleen is found in one-third of cases. There may be a moderate polymorphonuclear leukocytosis of $12–15 \times 10^9$/L but more often in this infection the white count is normal.

In one-half of the cases (some 10–20% of the total in the USA[29]), pulmonary symptoms develop, particularly dyspnoea and pleuritic pain. Milder forms resemble atypical pneumonia but may last for a month and there may be a solitary pulmonary nodule. There may be pleurisy, effusion, pneumonic consolidation or lobular bronchopneumonia with abscess and cavitation in severe cases and occasionally pericarditis. The effusion mimics that seen in tuberculosis.[30] There is an associated enlargement of the bronchial and mediastinal glands.

Dissemination may lead to meningitis, which mimics tuberculous meningitis, or osteomyelitis or even endocarditis on native[31] or prosthetic material.[32] The disease may present with lone neurological symptoms suggestive of encephalitis.[33] These presentations are all rare.[34]

Course

The infection is rarely fatal but in a series of severe untreated cases there was a mortality rate of 62% in pulmonary and 20% in typhoidal forms of the disease. The mean duration of fever in untreated cases is 26 days and adenopathy may last for 3–4 months. In one-third of cases, recovery is slow, the debilitating effect being very marked and lassitude persisting for months. *F. tularensis* may remain dormant intracellularly for years.

DIAGNOSIS

The diagnosis is suspected only by a keen clinical awareness of behavioural risk in the patient and local geographical pathology. The differential diagnosis of the local form must be made from anthrax, plague, tick typhus and rat bite fever.[34] The organism is isolated from an ulcer or lymph node aspirate on enriched agar or broth or by inoculation into guinea pigs, mice or rabbits, from whose tissues the organism may be isolated on special media as described. The organisms are rarely present in the blood[35] but may be isolated from sputum.[36] A serological diagnosis may be attempted using agglutination tests with cultures of *F. tularensis* from the spleens of infected mice in a formalinized citrate suspension, but cross-reactions with undulant and typhus fevers may occur. Half of patients with culture-proven tularaemia are seronegative. Recently, diagnostic polymerase chain reaction (PCR) has been tried with limited success (sensitivity 73%), from the ulcers of patients with serologically proven tularaemia.[37] From other specimens, PCR has roughly the same sensitivity as culture.[38]

The differential diagnosis of the pulmonary form of tularaemia[39] includes all the causes of atypical pneumonia, including legionellosis, psittacosis, Q fever, *Mycoplasma pneumoniae* and *Chlamydophila pneumoniae*.

TREATMENT

Streptomycin is extremely effective: 1 g intramuscularly daily for 7 days will terminate the infection. Gentamicin is a suitable and less toxic alternative. The patient should be kept in bed for a time after subsidence of the fever and convalescence should be prolonged. More recently, tetracycline (250 mg four times daily for 2 weeks) has been preferred, but there may be a relapse. Although erythromycin may be selected empirically to treat atypical pneumonia, and has been successful in tularaemia,[40] it is worth noting that some strains are constitutively resistant. Doxycycline and ciprofloxacin were both effective in an animal model of virulent tularaemia.[41] The fluoroquinolones are very active in vitro[42] and have been successful in treating the few cases where they have been tried.[13,43–47]

EPIDEMIOLOGY

Tularaemia in humans is essentially a rural infection and has a varying epidemiology according to the area in which it occurs and the method of transmission (Table 62.1). Several important methods of acquisition have been identified:

1. *Vector-borne*: by ticks, tabanid flies and mosquitoes.
2. *Trapping*: from the skins of infected rodents, muskrats and rabbits.
3. *Hunting*: from the consumption of rabbit meat.
4. *Water-borne*: from the water of streams infected by dead rats; well water infected by mice and field voles.
5. *Agricultural*: from working in haystacks contaminated by field voles and mice; processing of agricultural products; air-borne transmission by contaminated dust.
6. *Domestic*: use of grain and other products contaminated by mice; from bites by domestic cats.

Table 62.1 Areas of human tularaemia infection and associated species

Area	Species
USA	Wandering shrew, grey fox, dog, cat, various ground squirrels (Pirote, Wyoming, Beechey's and Columbian), chipmunk, beaver, wood rat, white-footed mouse, meadow mouse and varieties (Sawatch and Tule) of muskrat and brown rat (*Rattus norvegicus*), varying hare, jack rabbit, black-tailed jack rabbit, cotton-tail rabbit, sheep, calves, ruffed grouse, sharp-tailed grouse, bobwhite quail and horned owl.
Canada	Richardson's ground squirrel, Osgood's white-footed mouse, Drummond meadow mouse, varying hare, white-tailed jack rabbit, deer mice and Franklin's gull.
Sweden	Lemming and varying hare.
Central Europe	Rabbit and hare.
USSR (former)	Introduced muskrat, little ground squirrel, steppe lemming, water rat, continental vole, large water vole, house mouse, long-tailed field mouse and hamster.
Asia Minor	Continental vole, house and harvest mouse.
Japan	Local rabbit.

7. *Laboratory infections*: presumably by the aerosol route or by accidental ingestion.
8. *Wartime*: trench and foxhole outbreaks.

Outbreaks in humans invariably follow natural epizootics in different species of wild mammals.

Natural infections

F. tularensis occurs as a natural infection of wild rodents, especially rats, field mice, hares and rabbits. It has an extremely wide host range and many other species of animals as well as birds can be infected.[48]

North America

In North America, the most important reservoirs of infection are the jack rabbit, hare and their relatives. The infection is found in Wyoming and Montana in streams contaminated by dead beavers, which have been found in large numbers. Humans acquire the infection from skinning infected animals after hunting, and preparing carcasses for cooking, and also after tick and deer fly (*Chrysops discalis*) bites. Occasionally, contact with sheep is a source of infection. The disease is most prevalent during the months of June to August.[49] The disease is also present in wild animals in the East, as illustrated by seroprevalence studies in cats.[50] 59 cases presumed of air-borne origin and associated with grass mowing originated in Martha's Vineyard, MA, USA between 2000 and 2006.[51]

Europe

In Sweden, the lemming and varying hare are the main reservoirs and tularaemia is known as 'lemming fever'; it is caused by contact with infected water contaminated by the bodies and excreta of infected lemmings. Outbreaks have occurred in peasant women who go barefoot in summer and are bitten by numerous mosquitoes (*Aedes cinereus*). A very large outbreak involving 676 identified cases occurred in Sweden in the winter of 1966, in which the likely source was air-borne dust from hay contaminated by vole faeces.[52] In Austria, the Czech and Slovak Republics, and in Poland, the rabbit and hare are the main reservoirs. Between 1997 and 2005, a grumbling outbreak in Bulgaria affected 285 people. The new strain was different from one isolated in 1962.[53] In France, the infection has become much more common since the introduction of hares from central Europe for sporting purposes. In northern Europe, cases occur from July to October and in southern Europe from June to August.

F. tularensis subsp. *holarctica* caused an outbreak in free living marmosets in a research institute in Munich.[54]

The former USSR

In Russia, the water rat and introduced muskrat, which spread widely in the Ukraine after the disturbance caused by the great tank battles of World War II (1939–1945), are the main reservoirs. There was a great increase in the number of human infections after World War II (1945 onwards). In central Asia, *Microtus* and *Arvicola* are the predominant rat hosts.

PREVENTION

Prevention depends upon avoidance of the circumstances leading to infection in the various endemic areas. Rabbits should not be skinned without gloves, and sick rabbits should not be eaten. However, proper cooking destroys the organism, as does prolonged freezing. Experimental work with *F. tularensis* in the laboratory must be undertaken with great caution, and staff in routine laboratories are discouraged from handling the organism. Killed and live attenuated vaccine strains have been used in the former Soviet Republics for over 50 years.[55] Live attenuated vaccines are much more effective than killed ones; they induce cell-mediated immunity[26,56] and protective antibodies against lipopolysaccharide.[57] They do not reduce the risk of ulceroglandular disease but simply the danger from bacteraemia. A vaccine is not currently universally available.[55]

REFERENCES

1. Ohara Y, Sato T, Homma M. Arthropod-borne tularaemia in Japan: clinical analysis of 1374 cases observed between 1924 and 1996. *J Med Entomol* 1998; 35:471–473.

2. Ohara Y, Sato T, Homma M. Epidemiological analysis of tularaemia in Japan (yato-byo). *FEMS Immunol Med Microbiol* 1996; 13:185–189.

3. Bellido-Casado J, Perez-Casrillon JL, Bachiller-Luque P, et al. Report on five cases of tularaemic pneumonia in a tularaemic outbreak in Spain. *Eur J Clin Microbiol Infect Dis* 2000; 19:218–220.

4. Eigelsbach HT, McGann VG. Genus Francisella. In Krieg NR, Holt JG (eds) *Bergey's Manual of Systemic Bacteriology.* Vol. 1. Baltimore: Williams & Wilkins; 1984:394–399.

5. Uhari M, Syrjala H, Salminen A. Tularaemia in children caused by *Francisella tularensis* biovar *palaearctica. Pediatr Infect Dis J* 1990; 9:80–83.

6. Gurycova D. First isolation of *Francisella tularensis* subsp tularensis in Europe. *Eur J Epidemiol* 1998; 14:797–802.

7. Johansson A, Ibrahim A, Goransson I, et al. Evaluation of PCR-based methods for discrimination of *Francisella* species and subspecies and development of a specific PCR that distinguishes the two major subspecies of *Francisella tularensis. J Clin Microbiol* 2000; 38:4180–4185.

8. Chaudhuri RR, Ren CP, Desmond L, et al. Genome sequencing shows that the European isolates of *Francisella tularensis* subspecies tularensis are almost identical to US laboratory strain Schu S4. *PLoS ONE* 2007; 2:e352.

9. de la Puente-Redondo VA, del Blanco NG, Gutierrez-Martin CB, et al. Comparison of different PCR approaches for typing of *Francisella tularensis* strains. *J Clin Microbiol* 2000; 38:1016–1022.

10. Berdal BP, Mahl R, Haaheim H, et al. Field detection of *Francisella tularensis. Scand J Infect Dis* 2000; 32:287–291.

11. Liles WC, Burger RJ. Tularaemia from domestic cats. *West J Med* 1993; 158:619–632.

12. Cappelan J, Fong IW. Tularaemia from a cat bite: case report and a review of feline-associated tularaemia. *Clin Infect Dis* 1993; 16:472–475.

13. Arav-Boger R. Cat-bite tularaemia in a seventeen-year-old girl treated with ciprofloxacin. *Paediatr Inf Dis J* 2000; 19:583–584.

14. Tarnvik A. Nature of protective immunity to *Francisella tularensis. Rev Infect Dis* 1989; 11:440–451.

15. Surcel HM. Diversity of *Francisella tularensis* antigens recognised by human T lymphocytes. *Infect Immun* 1990; 58:2664–2668.

16. Karttunen R, Surcel HM, Andersson G, et al. *Francisella tularensis*-induced in vitro gamma interferon, tumor necrosis factor alpha, and interleukin 2 responses appear within two weeks of tularaemia vaccination in human beings. *J Clin Microbiol* 1991; 29:753–756.

17. Tarnvok A, Ericsson M, Golovliov I, et al. Orchestration of the protective immune response to intracellular bacteria; *Francisella tularensis. FEMS Immunol Med Microbiol* 1996; 13:221–225.

18. McCaffrey RL, Allen LA. *Francisella tularensis* live vaccine strain evades killing by human neutrophils via inhibition of the respiratory burst and phagosome escape. *J Leukoc Biol* 2006; 80:1224–1230.

19. Barker JR, Klose KE. Molecular and genetic basis of pathogenesis in *Francisella tularensis. Ann NY Acad Sci* 2007.

20. Barker JH, Weiss J, Apicella MA, et al. Basis for the failure of Francisella tularensis lipopolysaccharide to prime human polymorphonuclear leukocytes. *Infect Immun* 2006; 74:3277–3284.

21. Su J, Yang J, Zhao D, et al. Genome-wide identification of *Francisella tularensis* virulence determinants. *Infect Immun* 2007; 75:3089–3101.

22. Butchar JP, Rajaram MV, Ganesan LP, et al. *Francisella tularensis* induces IL-23 production in human monocytes. *J Immunol* 2007; 178:4445–4454.

23. Woolard MD, Wilson JE, Hensley LL, et al. *Francisella tularensis*-infected macrophages release prostaglandin E2 that blocks T cell proliferation and promotes in Th2-like responses. *J Immunol* 2007; 178:2065–2074.

24. Sjostedt A, North RJ, Conlan JW. The requirement of tumour necrosis factor-alpha and interferon-gamma for the expression of protective immunity to secondary murine tularaemia depends on the size of the challenge inoculum. *Microbiology* 1996; 142:1369–1374.

25. Sorokin VM, Pavlovich NV, Prozorova LA. *Francisella tularensis* resistance to bactericidal action of normal human serum. *FEMS Immunol Med Microbiol* 1996; 13:249–252.

26. Waag D, Galloway A, Sandstrom G, et al. Cell mediated and humoral responses induced by scarification vaccination of human volunteers with a new lot of the live vaccine strain of *Francisella tularensis. J Clin Microbiol* 1992; 30:2256–2264.

27. Ericsson M, Golovliov I, Sandsrom G, et al. Characterisation of the nucleotide sequence of the groE operon encoding heat shock proteins chaperone-60 and -10 of *Francisella tularensis* and determination of the T-cell response to the proteins in individuals vaccinated with F. tularensis. *Infect Immun* 1997; 65:1824–1829.

28. Rohrbach BW, Westerman E, Istre GR. Epidemiology and clinical characteristics of tularaemia in Oklahoma, 1979–1985. *South Med J* 1991; 84:1091–1096.

29. Gill V, Cunha BA. Tularaemia pneumonia. *Semin Respir Infect* 1997; 12: 61–67.

30. Pettersson T, Nyberg P, Nordstrom D, et al. Similar pleural fluid findings in pleuropulmonary tularaemia and tuberculous pleurisy. *Chest* 1996; 109: 572–575.

31. Tancik CA, Dillaha JA. *Francisella tularensis* endocarditis. *Clin Infect Dis* 2000; 30:399–400.

32. Cooper CL, Van Caeseele P, Canvin J, et al. Chronic prosthetic device infection with *Francisella tularensis. Clin Infect Dis* 1999; 29:1589–1591.

33. Le Doux MS. Tularaemia presenting with ataxia. *Clin Infect Dis* 2000; 30: 211–212.

34. Kostman JR, DiNubile MJ. Nodular lymphangitis: a distinctive but often unrecognised syndrome. *Ann Intern Med* 1993; 118:883–888.

35. Hoel T, Scheel O, Nordahl SH, et al. Water- and air-borne *Francisella tularensis* biovar palaearctica isolated from human blood. *Infection* 1991; 19:348–350.

36. Fredricks DN, Remington JS. Tularaemia presenting a community-acquired pneumonia. Implications in the era of managed care. *Arch Intern Med* 1996; 156:2137–2140.

37. Sjostedt A, Eriksson U, Berglund L, et al. Detection of *Francisella tularensis* in ulcers of patients with tularaemia by PCR. *J Clin Microbiol* 1997; 35: 1045–1048.

38. Johansson A, Berglund L, Eriksson U, et al. Comparative analysis of PCR versus culture for diagnosis of ulceroglandular tularaemia. *J Clin Microbiol* 2000; 38:22–26.

39. Scofield RH, Lopez EJ, McNabb SJ. Tularaemia pneumonia in Oklahoma 1982–1987. *J Okla State Med Assoc* 1992; 85:165–170.

40. Harrell RE Jr, Simmons HF. Pleuropulmonary tularaemia: successful treatment with erythromycin. *South Med J* 1990; 83:1362–1364.

41. Russell P, Eley SM, Fulop MJ, et al. The efficacy of ciprofloxacin and doxycycline against experimental tularaemia. *J Antimicrob Chemother* 1998; 41:461–465.

42. Ikaheimo I, Syrjala H, Karhukorpi J, et al. In vitro antibiotic susceptibility of *Francisella tularensis* isolated from humans and animals. *J Antimicrob Chemother* 2000; 46:287–290.

43. Syrjala H, Schildt R, Raisaninen S. In vitro susceptibility of *Francisella tularensis* to fluoroquinolones and treatment of tularaemia with norfloxacin and ciprofloxacin. *Eur J Clin Microbiol Infect Dis* 1991; 10:68–70.

44. Scheel O, Hoel T, Sandvik T, et al. Susceptibility pattern of Scandinavian *Francisella tularensis* isolates with regard to oral and parenteral antimicrobial agents. *Acta Pathol Microbiol Immunol Scand* 1993; 101:33–36.

45. Chocarro A, Gonzalez A, Garcia I. Treatment of tularaemia with ciprofloxacin. *Clin Infect Dis* 2000; 31:623.

46. Johansson A, Berglund L, Gothefors L, et al. Ciprofloxacin for treatment of tularaemia in children. *Pediatr Infect Dis J* 2000; 19:449–453.

47. Limaye AP, Hooper CJ. Treatment of tularaemia with fluoroquinolones: two cases and a review. *Clin Infect Dis* 1999; 29:922–924.

48. Burrough AL, Holdenreid R, Longanecker DS, et al. A field study of latent tularaemia in rodents with a list of all known naturally infected vertebrates. *J Infect Dis* 1945; 76:115–119.

49. Cumming HS. La tularémie aux Etats-Unis. *Bull Off Int Hyg Publique* 1937; 29:2532–2535.

50. Magnarelli L, Levy S, Koski R. Detection of antibodies to *Francisella tularensis* in cats. *Res Vet Sci* 2007; 82:22–26.

51. Matyas BT, Neider HS, Telford SR. Pneumonic tularaemia on Martha's Vineyard: clinical, epidemiologic and ecological characteristics. *Ann NY Acad Sci* 2007.

52. Dahlstrand S, Ringertz O, Zetterburg B. Airborne tularaemia in Sweden. *Scan J Infect Dis* 1971; 3:7–16.

53. Kantardjiev T, Ivanov I, Velinov T, et al. Tularemia outbreak, Bulgaria, 1997–2005. *Emerg Infect Dis* 2006; 12:678–680.

54. Splettstoesser WD, Matz-Rensing K, Seibold E, et al. Re-emergence of *Franciselle tularensis* in Germany: fatal tularaemia in a colony of semi-free-living marmosets (Callithrix jacchus). *Epidemiol Infect* 2007; 19:1–10.

55. Fortier AH, Slayter MV, Ziemba R, et al. Live vaccine strain of Francisella tularensis: infection and immunity in mice. *Infect Immun* 1991; 59: 2922–2928.

56. Waag DM, Sandstrom G, England MJ, et al. Immunogenicity of a new lot of *Francisella tularensis* live vaccine strain in human volunteers. *FEMS Immunol Med Microbiol* 1996; 13:205–209.

57. Conlan JW, Oyston P. Vaccines against *Francisella tularensis*. *Ann NY Acad Sci* 2007.

GENERAL READING

Review: Proceedings of the First International Conference on Tularaemia, Sweden, 1995. *FEMS Immunol Med Microbiol* 1996; 13:179–260.

Chapter 63

Geoffrey M. Scott

Anthrax

Anthrax (Greek: black) is a disease of domestic herbivores caused by the bacterium *Bacillus anthracis*, which lives in topsoil and is ingested by the animals when grazing. Infection in humans is rare considering the potential exposure to the organism, and it presents as a local cutaneous lesion, gastrointestinal infection or with overwhelming pneumonia and disseminated disease. The toxins are carried on plasmids. Other species rarely identified as the cause of typical anthrax-like cutaneous infections include *B. pumilus*,[1] and *B. cereus* has been implicated in cases of inhalational disease.[2]

GEOGRAPHICAL DISTRIBUTION

Anthrax occurs worldwide but is 'endemic' in herbivorous livestock in certain regions. Domestic carnivores (dogs and cats) may be infected by eating contaminated carcasses. Human disease is most likely to occur in endemic regions (e.g. Iran,[3] Central Africa, South America, Russia) by direct contact with infected carcasses. Industrial cases may occur anywhere and reflect exposure to imported animal carcass products, such as bone meal (which used to be used for making glues) or hides.

AETIOLOGY AND PATHOGENESIS

Bacillus comprises a diverse and complex genus of air-borne aerobic spore-bearing organisms.[4] *B. anthracis* is a large, non-motile, brick-shaped, aerobic, Gram-positive rod which has the capacity to make heat- and dry-resistant spores under adverse conditions. The spore is central and does not expand the bacterium. Spores survive for decades in topsoil and resist high temperatures (e.g. 140°C in dry heat for 3 h, and 100°C in moist heat for 10 min). The organism may be provisionally identified by Gram staining of pus aspirated from a lesion and will grow in air within 24 h to give large irregular colonies on simple media. The edge of the colony is sometimes likened to Medusa's head, and the colony has a ground-glass appearance and adheres to the loop. The organism is then distinguished from other *Bacillus* spp. on non-motility, microscopical appearance of spores; isolates tend not to be haemolytic and are tyrosine deaminase negative.

Virulence is conferred by a capsule, coded by pX02, (which develops soon after germination in vivo and inhibits phagocyto-

sis) and a complex exotoxin pX01, which are plasmid determined. Over expression of pX02 inhibits sporulation. The toxin has three components which are not toxic in their own right but combine at the surface of mammalian cells which bear receptors.[5] Activated 'Protective Antigen' (PA) heptamerizes, binds to receptors and then organizes binding of the other factors, a metalloproteinase 'lethal factor' (LF) and an adenylyl cyclase 'oedema factor' (OF). A heptameric pore is drilled into endosome membrane allowing the OF-LF complex into the cytosol.[6] OF is toxic to mice and causes adrenal haemorrhage; it also inhibits platelet aggregation.[7] Small amounts of OF sensitize mice to LF.[8,9] LF is a protein kinase which cleaves mitogen-induced protein kinases: LF-treated *ex vivo* mouse and human macrophages gradually die by apoptosis, in part by poisoning mitochondria.[10,11] OF and PA upregulate cyclic AMP intracellularly and increase *antx*R expression, enhancing internalization of the three factors.[12] The exotoxins are released by germinating spores at damaged epithelium and replicating organisms.[13] It is presumed that they act on cells locally where the organisms first invade, then in the local lymph nodes and then at distant sites as the patient becomes bacteraemic. After inhalation, alveolar macrophages cannot kill the bacterium when exposed to LT, implying a failure of innate immune response and possibly a failure of early recruitment of neutrophils to alveolar sites. Other important virulence factors include potent siderophores.[14,15]

The toxin-binding receptor is coded by *antr*X and autosomally recessive inherited mutations of *antr*X2 lead to a curious and very rare condition of systemic hyalinosis.[16,17]

EPIDEMIOLOGY AND TRANSMISSION

The sequence of events leading to the manifestation of anthrax in animals (and, usually subsequently, in humans) is complex and not completely understood. In areas of endemicity, the soil may be heavily contaminated by spores. These spores originated from vast numbers of organisms shed from animals who died from the disease. The bacteria have to compete with other soil bacteria, and rapid sporulation encouraged at high ambient temperature is critical to their survival. Vegetative forms die. Germination of spores occurs in conditions of high humidity, again encouraged by high temperature. In temperate conditions, although very humid, the temperature is rarely high enough to encourage either sporulation or germination, so it is rare for the topsoil to become

10. Alileche A, Squires RC, Muehlbauer SM, et al. Mitochondrial impairment is a critical event in anthrax lethal toxin-induced cytolysis of murine macrophages. *Cell Cycle* 2006; 5:100–106.

11. Muehlbauer SM, Evering TH, Bonuccelli G, et al. Anthrax lethal toxin kills macrophages in a strain specific manner by apoptosis or caspase-1-mediated necrosis. *Cell Cycle* 2007; 6:758–766.

12. Maldonado-Arocho FJ, Fulcher JA, Lee B, et al. Anthrax oedema toxin induces anthrax toxin receptor expression in monocyte derived cells. *Mol Microbiol* 2006; 61:324–337.

13. Bischof TS, Hahn BL, Sohnle PG. Characteristics of spore germination in a mouse model of cutaneous anthrax. *J Infect Dis* 2007; 195:888–894.

14. Cendrowski S, MacArthur W, Hanna P. *Bacillus anthracis* requires siderophore biosynthesis for growth in macrophages and mouse virulence. *Mol Microbiol* 2004; 51:407–417.

15. Abergel RJ, Wilson MK, Arceneasux JE, et al. Anthrax pathogen evades the mammalian immune system through stealth siderophore production. *Proc Natl Acad Sci USA* 2006; 103:18499–18503.

16. Shieh JT, Swidler P, Martignetti JA, et al. Systemic hyalinosis: a distinctive early childhood-onset disorder characterised by mutations in the anthrax toxin receptor 2 gene. *Pediatrics* 2006; 118:e1485–e1492.

17. Liu S, Leung HJ, Leppla SH. Characterisation of the interaction between anthrax toxin and its cellular receptors. *Cell Microbiol* 2007; 9:977–987.

18. McKendrick DRA. Anthrax and its transmission in humans. *Cent Afr J Med* 1980; 26:126–129.

19. Turner M. Anthrax in humans in Zimbabwe. *Cent Afr J Med* 1980; 26:160–161.

20. Heyworth B, Ropp ME, Meinel H, et al. Anthrax in the Gambia: an epidemiological study. *BMJ* 1975; iv:79–82.

21. Fendall NRE, Grounds JG. The incidence and epidemiology of disease in Kenya. I. Some diseases of social significance. *J Trop Med Hyg* 1965; 68:77–84.

22. Karakas HM, Bayindir Y, Firat AK, et al. Cerebral diffusional changes in the early phase of anthrax: is cutaneous anthrax only limited to the skin. *J Infect* 2006; 52:354–358.

23. Kyriacou DN, Yarnold PR, Stein AC, et al. Discriminating inhalational anthrax from community-acquired pneumonia using chest radiograph findings and a clinical algorithm. *Chest* 2007; 131:489–496.

24. Ichhpujani RL, Rajagopal V, Bhattachaya D, et al. An outbreak of human anthrax in Mysore (India). *J Commun Dis* 2004; 36:199–204.

25. Sirisanthana T, Navachareon N, Tharavichitkul P, et al. Outbreak of oral-oropharyngeal anthrax: an unusual manifestation of human infection with *Bacillus anthracis. Am J Trop Med Hyg* 1984; 33:144–150.

26. Babamahmoodi F, Aghabarari F, Arjmand A, et al. Three rare cases of anthrax from the same source. *J Infect* 2006; 53:175–179.

27. Reissman DB, Whitney EA, Taylor TH Jr, et al. One-year health assessment of adult survivors of *Bacillus anthracis* infection. *JAMA* 2004; 291:1994–1998.

28. Peterson JW, Comer JE, Noffsinger DM, et al. Human monoclonal anti-protective antigen antibody completely protects rabbits and is synergistic with ciprofloxacin in protecting mice and guinea pigs against inhalational anthrax. *Infect Immun* 2006; 74:1016–1024.

29. Holty JE, Bravata DM, Liu H, et al. Systematic review: a century of inhalational anthrax cases from 1900 to 2005. *Ann Intern Med* 2006; 144:270–280.

30. Sejvar JJ, Tenover FC, Stephens DS. Management of anthrax meningitis. *Lancet Infect Dis* 2005; 5:287–295.

31. Hirsh MI, Cohen V. Chloroquine prevents T lymphocyte suppression induced by anthrax lethal toxin. *J Infect Dis* 2006; 194:1003–1007.

32. Kunanusont C, Limpakarnjanarat K, Foy HM. Outbreak of anthrax in Thailand. *Ann Trop Med Parasitol* 1990; 84:507–512.

33. Sekhar PC, Singh RS, Sridhar MS, et al. Outbreak of human anthrax in Ramabhadrapuram village of Chittar district of Andhra Pradesh. *Indian J Med Res* 1990; 91:448–452.

34. Turnbull PC. Anthrax vaccines: past, present and future. *Vaccine* 1991; 9:533–539.

35. Zeng M, Xu Q, Pichichero ME. Protection against anthrax by needle-free mucosal immunisation with human anthrax vaccine. *Vaccine* 2007; 25:3588–3594.

36. Ivins BE, Welkos SL, Knudson GB, et al. Immunization against anthrax with aromatic compound-dependent (Aro-) mutants of *Bacillus anthracis* and with recombinant strains of *Bacillus subtilis* that produce anthrax protective antigen. *Infect Immun* 1990; 58:303–308.

37. Iacono-Connors LC, Welkos SL, Ivins BE, et al. Protection against anthrax with recombinant virus-expressed protective antigen in experimental animals. *Infect Immun* 1991; 59:1961–1965.

38. Stokes MG, Titball RW, Neeson BN, et al. Oral administration of a *Salmonella enterica*-based vaccine expressing *Bacillus anthracis* protective antigen confers protection against aerosolized *B. anthracis. Infect Immun* 2007; 75:1827–1834.

39. Klietmann WF, Ruoff KL. Bioterrorism: implications for the clinical microbiologist. *Clin Microbiol Rev* 2001; 14:364–381.

40. Meselson M, Guillemin J, Hugh-Jones M, et al. The Sverdlovsk anthrax outbreak of 1979. *Science* 1994; 266:1202–1208.

Chapter 64

Catherine L. Thwaites and Lam Minh Yen

Tetanus

Tetanus is a disease characterized by muscle rigidity and spasms. It derives its name from the Greek word 'tetanos' meaning 'to contract'. Despite the World Health Organization's efforts to eradicate the disease by 1995, tetanus remains one of the world's major preventable causes of death, with an estimated incidence of 700 000 to 1 million cases a year, causing an estimated 213 000 deaths.[1,2]

People have recognized the association between wounds and subsequent rigidity, spasms and death since ancient times. The Edwin Smith papyrus (1000 BC) outlines the case of a man with a scalp wound who developed trismus and muscle rigidity. Hippocrates (400 BC) describes a similar case of a man who, having sustained a penetrating wound to the back, experienced trismus and muscle spasms then died on the second day of the illness. However, it was not until 1880 that Nicolaier demonstrated that soil contamination of wounds resulted in tetanus. Nicolaier also discovered identical bacilli in the wounds, but it was Kitasato who isolated the first pure culture of *Clostridium tetani* 9 years later. In 1890, Faber discovered tetanus toxin, the same year as von Berhring and Kitasato produced the first antitoxin. Then, using formaldehyde, Ramon succeeded in detoxifying tetanus toxin, yet still preserving its antigenicity. In 1926, he performed the first successful vaccination of humans.[3]

The availability of a tetanus vaccine has enabled developed countries to virtually eliminate the disease. However, *C. tetani* will never be eradicated from the soil and so wherever vaccination programmes are ineffective or inadequate, tetanus will continue to occur.

EPIDEMIOLOGY

C. tetani is a ubiquitous organism, present in the soil and in human and animal faeces. The disease it causes is now primarily confined to developing countries as a consequence of inadequate immunization. In 2004, an estimated 27 million children did not complete their primary immunization course.[1] Neonatal tetanus usually arises from contamination of the umbilical stump. Infection is linked to delivery on unclean surfaces, traditional midwifery practices such as cutting the umbilical cord with bamboo and applying soil, cow dung, clarified butter or even engine oil to the umbilical stump.[4] Ritual surgery such as ear-piercing or circumcision may also cause infection. Neonatal tetanus is prevented

by maternal immunization, yet with an estimated 40 million unimmunized pregnant women in 2004 the WHO's desired eradication remains elusive.[1] Even after maternal immunization, the infant is still at risk in many countries, as malaria and HIV reduce placental transfer of protective antibody.[5,6]

In children and adults, lacerations to feet and hands are common injuries associated with tetanus.[7] Otitis media is an important portal for the disease in children. Tetanus arising from injections (either therapeutic medical or via drug abuse) carries an especially poor prognosis, as does tetanus arising from other internal sites of infection.[7]

In the developed world, tetanus is rare: in 2002 there were six cases in the UK.[8] Similarly US data from 1998–2000 shows an average of 43 cases/year.[9] Most cases occur in the elderly – a group at increased risk due to declining protective antibody levels. However, recent studies have shown that younger people are also vulnerable due to missed immunizations or additional risk factors.[10] In 2004, an outbreak of tetanus occurred in drug users in the UK – the exact reasons for this remains unclear, but it appears that many had an incomplete vaccination history or used a high-risk administration method known as 'skin popping'.[11] Heroin users are known to be particularly at risk from tetanus. Heroin is sometimes mixed with quinine which causes local necrosis, a favourable environment for *C. tetani* multiplication as well as its low pH facilitating toxin entry into nerves.

BACTERIOLOGY

C. tetani is a strictly anaerobic Gram-positive bacillus found in soil and animal faeces. When subjected to adverse conditions, rounded terminal spores are formed: this gives the classical 'drumstick' appearance to the bacillus, although this is not always seen. *C. tetani* is described as Gram-positive, but from cultures >24 h old, it is readily decolourized and thus can appear to be Gram-negative. It is motile by means of numerous flagella and when cultured on blood agar, this results in swarming, giving a film with a feathery margin on the surface of the agar. Increasing the concentration of agar in the medium will inhibit swarming. Discrete colonies are flat, translucent and show a narrow zone of haemolysis.

The biochemical activity of *C. tetani* is limited. In general it does not ferment sugars, although some strains will ferment glucose. Gelatin is slowly hydrolysed but other proteins used in

Table 64.1 Tetanus severity score (TSS), calculated from the total of individual section scores

	Score
Age (years)	
≤70	0
71–80	5
>80	10
Time from 1st symptom to admission (days)	
≤2	0
3–5	−5
>5	−6
Difficulty breathing on admission	
No	0
Yes	4
Co-existing medical conditions[a]	
Fit and well	0
Minor illness or injury	3
Moderately severe illness	5
Severe illness not immediately life-threatening	5
Immediately life-threatening illness	9
Entry site[b]	
Internal or injection	7
Other (including unknown)	0
Highest systolic blood pressure recorded during 1st day in hospital (mmHg)	
≤130	0
131–140	2
>140	4
Highest heart rate recorded during 1st day in hospital (b.p.m.)	
≤100	0
101–110	1
111–120	2
>120	4
Lowest heart rate recorded during 1st day in hospital (b.p.m.)	
≤110	0
>110	−2
Highest temperature recorded during 1st day in hospital (°C)	
≤38.5	0
38.6–39	4
39.1–40	6
>40	8

[a]Defined according to ASA physical status scale.
[b]'Internal' site includes postoperative/postpartum or open fractures; 'injection' includes intramuscular, subcutaneous or intravenous injections.
Source: Thwaites CL, Yen LM, Glover C, et al. Predicting the clinical outcome of tetanus: the tetanus severity score. *Trop Med Int Health* 2006; 11:279–287.

MANAGEMENT

Management of tetanus is essentially supportive. It involves three main strategies: to prevent further toxin release, to neutralize any unbound toxin and to minimize effects of already-bound toxin while maintaining the airway and adequate respiration.

Prompt debridement of the wound is essential to prevent further multiplication and toxin release of *C. tetani*. Metronidazole is the antibiotic of choice, although penicillin is still widely used. Patients treated with metronidazole have fewer spasms and require less sedation than those treated with penicillin.[28] Penicillin is similar in structure to GABA, and although it does not readily cross the blood-brain barrier, in high doses it can act as a central GABA competitive antagonist, thus exacerbating the effects of tetanus toxin.

Unbound toxin should be neutralized with antitoxin. Historically, equine anti-tetanus serum has been used, but it is associated with a high incidence of anaphylactic reactions. In many countries it has now been replaced by the human tetanus immune globulin (HTIG). Much debate has centred on the best route of administration of antitoxin. Results of animal experiments almost 100 years ago suggested that intrathecal administration of antitoxin may be superior. A recent study has once again suggested that intrathecal immunoglobulin may indeed reduce progression to more severe disease and reduce hospital stay and length of mechanical ventilation.[29] Furthermore, its results have been supported by a recent meta-analysis.[30]

Good nursing care is crucial to the outcome of patients with tetanus. All patients should be nursed in quiet, dark rooms to minimize provoked spasms. Frequent turning is necessary to prevent the development of pressure sores, although truncal rigidity of the patients makes this difficult. Patients who are unable to swallow will require a nasogastric tube. Close attention should be paid to fluid balance, as tetanus patients have greatly increased insensible fluid losses, especially in the presence of autonomic dysfunction.

Benzodiazepines are the mainstay of treatment in mild to moderate tetanus. As inhibitors of an endogenous inhibitor at the $GABA_A$ receptor, they oppose the effects of tetanus toxin on the GABAergic neurones. Diazepam is the most commonly used although its long half-life, and those of its metabolites, may cause prolonged effects. It can be given orally in mild cases, or intravenously in more severe disease.[31] Doses up to 100 mg/h have been reported, and up to 200 mg/day is common. Intravenous infusion of midazolam may be a preferred option by virtue of its shorter half-life, although prolonged use will still lead to accumulation. The anaesthetic agent, propofol, has been used to provide sedation and additional muscle relaxation. It is non-cumulative and has a short duration of action, making it an attractive adjunct.[32]

If spasms persist despite benzodiazepine therapy, then paralysis and mechanical ventilation should be instituted. Non-depolarizing muscle relaxants with minimal cardiovascular effects, such as vecuronium or cisatracurium, are the muscle relaxants of choice. Older agents, such as pancuronium, may exacerbate autonomic instability. Tracheostomy is the usual means of securing the airway, allowing ventilation and secretion clearance. Patients with laryngeal spasm may require urgent tracheostomy. For this reason, all tetanus patients should be nursed under close supervision with appropriately skilled personnel at hand to deal with any emergencies.

Tetanus literature contains many reports of the use of other agents used to treat spasticity: dantrolene has been used to reduce spontaneous muscular spasms, but it is potentially hepatotoxic if used for prolonged periods. The $GABA_B$ agonist baclofen has also successfully suppressed spasticity.[33]

In patients with autonomic instability, the usual manifestation is a tachycardia accompanied by hypertension. First-line therapy in this situation has been intravenous or intramuscular morphine. It inhibits sympathetically mediated vasoconstriction and induces peripheral arteriolar vasodilatation by inhibiting central sympathetic discharge. Other opioid agents with shorter half-lives have also been reported to be beneficial, although no randomized controlled trials have been performed.[34] Peripheral β-adrenoceptor blockade alone is usually insufficient to gain satisfactory cardiovascular control in severe cases of tetanus. The relatively long duration of action of most agents has been associated with subsequent refractory hypotension and cardiac arrest. The combined α- and β-blocker labetalol may confer some advantages, but its duration of action is still too long to be a useful alternative. The new short-acting β-blocker esmolol, however, has been used successfully.[35] Peak effects are observed within 6–10 min of injection, and have almost completely disappeared after 20 min. Chlorpromazine, clonidine and epidural bupivacaine have all been used with success in the past.[36] Recent interest has surrounded magnesium sulphate-α vasodilator and muscle relaxant that offers the potential to control both muscle spasms and autonomic instability. An initial series reported such benefits that the authors suggested it as an alternative to benzodiazepines as a first-line agent,[37] however a larger randomized controlled trial has not shown such convincing benefits, although it does indeed appear to have beneficial effects in controlling spasms and reducing autonomic instability.[38]

Hypotension may be treated by head-down positioning, noxious stimulation or inotropic agents. Bradyarrhythmias require atropine.

Finally, the amount of toxin circulating in natural disease is insufficient to provoke an immunizing antibody response. Therefore, all patients should receive a course of tetanus toxoid to prevent recurrences.

PREVENTION

The prevention of tetanus depends on primary immunization and the thorough management of wounds in those people who have not been immunized or whose immune status is thought to be inadequate. In addition, health education and improved socioeconomic conditions are important: for example, the use of aseptic techniques in the management of the umbilical cord and the provision of adequate protective footwear.

Tetanus toxoid is produced by formaldehyde treatment of the toxin (plain toxoid). Although it is a relatively good immunogen, the duration of antibody response is much improved by adsorption with aluminium hydroxide as an adjuvant. It may be given alone, or preferably in combination with diphtheria toxoid. Tetanus toxoid is considered very safe, even in immunocompromised individuals.

The WHO recommends a six-part primary immunization programme with five childhood doses (three under 1 year, and boosters aged 4–7 years and 12–17 years) with one further dose in adult life – for example at first pregnancy or military service.[1]

In the UK, the first dose is given at 2 months of age, followed by the second and third doses at 4-week intervals. Adsorbed toxoid is available in combination with diphtheria toxoid and pertussis vaccine (DTP) for use in these immunization schedules of young children. Two booster doses of tetanus and diphtheria toxoids (DT) are given at 3–5 years of age and at 13–18 years of age. In the USA, an initial four-dose schedule is recommended with intervals of 4–8 weeks between the first three doses and the fourth dose 6–12 months later. A booster is given at 4–6 years old and again 10 years later.[39] In the USA, the advice is to give additional booster doses of adsorbed tetanus toxoid every 10 years. However, in the UK, more recent advice is that five doses (primary course plus two boosters) are sufficient and additional booster doses are not recommended unless a tetanus-prone wound occurs.

Neonatal tetanus may be prevented by immunization of women during pregnancy. In women with incomplete or unknown vaccination history, two or preferably three doses of adsorbed toxoid should be given, with the last dose at least 2–4 weeks prior to delivery.[1] Immunity is passively transferred to the fetus and the antibodies will remain long enough to protect the baby during the neonatal period. In subsequent pregnancies, a single booster can be given at 6 months' gestation, but if pregnancies are frequent, boosters should only be given every 5 years. Special care should be taken to ensure those with HIV or living in malaria-endemic areas receive a full course of vaccination.

Prevention of tetanus also depends on the effective management of wounds. It is most important that wounds are thoroughly cleaned, all foreign material removed and non-viable tissue débrided. Particular attention should be given to tetanus-prone wounds. These include puncture wounds, burns, animal and human bites, wounds contaminated with soil or faeces, and any wound where treatment is delayed. These wounds should not be sutured: packing, frequent inspection and delayed primary closure is preferable. Antibiotic chemoprophylaxis is of secondary importance to good surgical management and immunoprophylaxis. When indicated, a long-acting penicillin can be given. If the wound is infected with β-lactamase-producing staphylococci an appropriate alternative antibiotic such as erythromycin or flucloxacillin should be used.

A history of previous immunization should be sought, as this will determine the exact type of immunoprophylaxis to be given. If the patient has received a full course or a booster of tetanus toxoid within 10 years, a further dose is not required. If the last dose was >10 years ago, a further dose should be given. Where there is doubt about previous immunization or a full course was never completed, a full course of adsorbed tetanus toxoid should be commenced.[40]

Passive immunization with HTIG (250 units) should also be given for tetanus-prone wounds occurring in people with inadequate immunization status (i.e. incomplete, unknown or a booster >10 years ago). Even where immunization is adequate (the last dose within 10 years) a dose of HTIG may be given if the risk of developing tetanus is high. If HTIG is not available, equine antiserum (1500 units) is an alternative. Very high-risk wounds

dependent coagulase is produced during infection of the flea, which causes clotting of blood in the proventriculus. As a consequence of this blockage of the flea's foregut, blood containing many organisms is regurgitated during subsequent attempts to feed. The coagulase is most active at temperatures below 30°C but is inactive at 35°C or above. Fleas are cold blooded and these observations may explain why transmission of plague ceases in the hot seasons in endemic areas. Fraction 1 antigen is a capsular glycoprotein, which enables the organism to evade phagocytosis; it is produced at 37°C but not below 27°C. Thus in the flea and when first inoculated into humans these organisms express F1 antigen poorly and are easily phagocytosed, but not killed, by neutrophils and monocytes. However, subsequent generations express F1 antigen fully, which together with pH6 antigen and the Yop virulon, enables them to avoid phagocytosis. *Y. pestis* also possess the ability to survive and replicate within the phagolysosome of macrophages.

V antigen, which is present within the cytoplasm or secreted from the cell, is an essential virulence factor and is highly immunogenic. The exact function of V antigen is not known, but it appears to suppress pro-inflammatory cytokines[6] and inhibit neutrophil chemotaxis.[7]

Table 65.1 Cases of human plague reported to the World Health Organization (1994–2003)

Location	Cases (*n*)	Mortality (%)
Africa – total	25 096	7.1
Madagascar	8416	
Democratic Republic of Congo	3619	
Tanzania	3527	
Mozambique	2387	
Americas – total	754	6.1
Peru	631	
Asia – total	2675	6.9
Vietnam	1331	
Worldwide – total	28 530	7

Other virulence factors include plasminogen activator, haemin storage system and classical lipopolysaccharide endotoxin. The largest plasmid also encodes for a murine toxin, which is essentially lethal for mice and rats only.[4]

PATHOLOGY

The essential feature of plague in man is the bubo – an enlarged, congested and centrally necrotic lymph node. *Y. pestis* can be demonstrated in abundance in these lesions. Congestion and haemorrhage may be seen in most organs of the body, and extensive haemorrhages may be present in the mucosa of the gastrointestinal tract. In pneumonic plague the findings are of a haemorrhagic pneumonia and blood-stained fluid in the pleural cavities (Figure 65.3).

CLINICAL MANIFESTATIONS

Historical accounts suggest that plague is one of the most virulent infections known to man, but subclinical cases are not uncommon and bubonic plague can be of mild or moderate severity. The incubation period is generally 2–5 days but may be up to 15 days. In a small proportion of cases, there is a prodromal stage of fever,

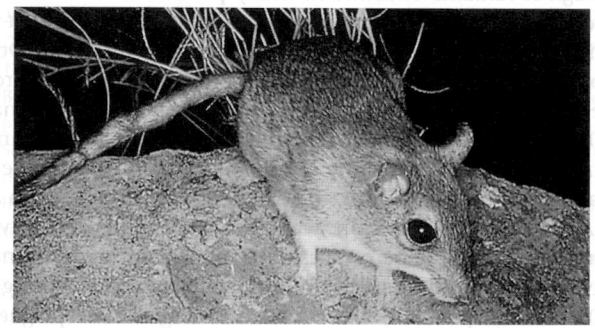

Figure 65.2 *Tatera robusta.* Several gerbils from this genus have been found infected with *Y. pestis* in East and South Africa, as well as in India where they are associated with focal outbreaks in humans.

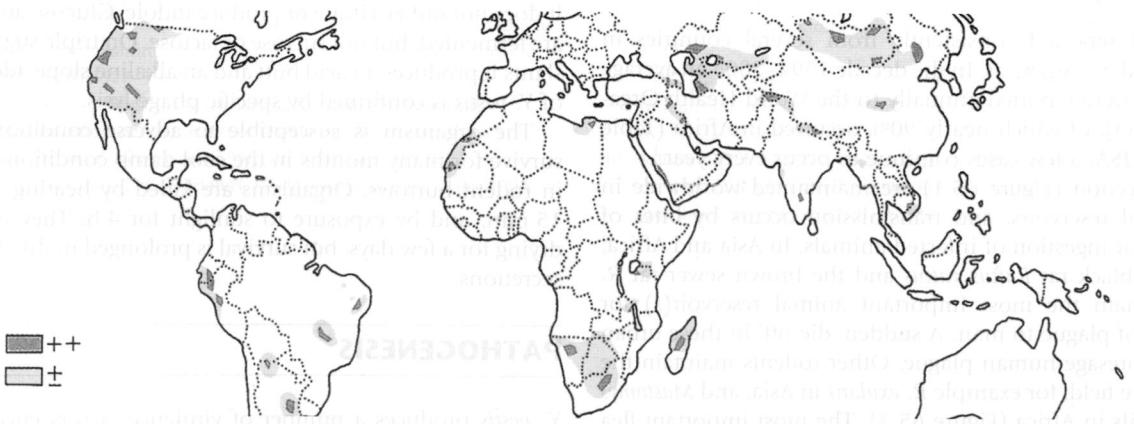

Figure 65.1 Known and probable foci of plague. ++, Frequent transmission; ±, infrequent or suspected transmission.

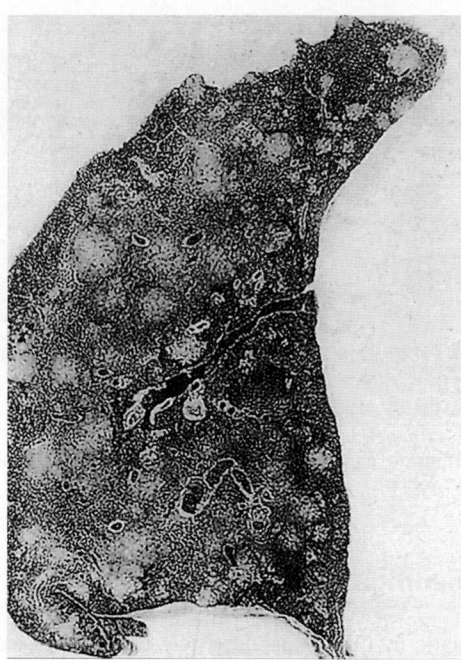

Figure 65.3 The lung from a fatal case of pneumonic plague. The lower lobe shows intense hyperaemia and haemorrhage with necrotic nodules. The upper lobe contains only necrotic nodules with compensatory emphysemal changes.

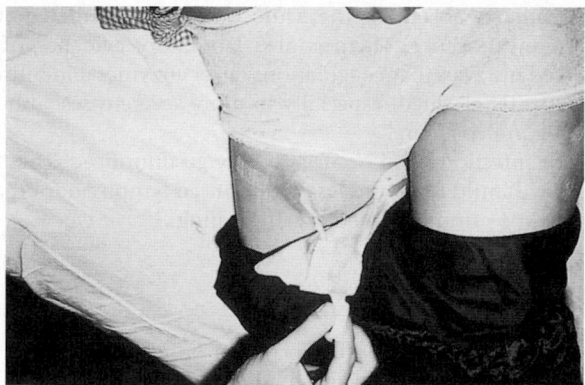

Figure 65.4 Bubonic plague. Fever and regional lymphadenopathy with suppuration, especially in the inguinal and axiliary regions, commence after an incubation period of less than 1 week.

weakness and anorexia. The initial manifestations are usually due to lymphadenitis in the nodes draining the site of a flea bite.

Bubonic plague

This is the most common form of plague and has a characteristic clinical picture. Typically, bubonic plague presents with a short prodrome of fever, malaise, anorexia and headache. Sometimes there is a dull ache at the site of future buboes, which will develop within 24 h. The primary buboes will be found in different locations depending on the site of inoculation. The most common site is the groin (70–80%), with the femoral nodes more often involved compared with the inguinal nodes (Figure 65.4).[8] Other primary sites are the axilla (14–20%), the cervical and submaxillary regions, and very rarely the clavicular, popliteal and epitrochlear nodes. Cervical and submaxillary node involvement is more often present in children. Buboes usually affect only one site but very occasionally two or more may be involved.

Development of the bubo is characterized by severe pain, swelling and marked tenderness of the affected lymph node. Individual nodes may attain the size of a hen's egg; sometimes clusters of nodes form a larger, more irregular swelling. There is surrounding oedema and the overlying skin is warm, reddened and adherent. The mass is immoveable and non-fluctuant, although, particularly if not treated with antibiotics, suppuration and abscess formation will occur during later stages. The buboes are generally so tender that the patient will hold the associated limb, or head, in such a position as to relieve the pressure.

The onset of fever in plague is often abrupt with the temperature rising rapidly to 39–40°C, or even higher. Prostration and

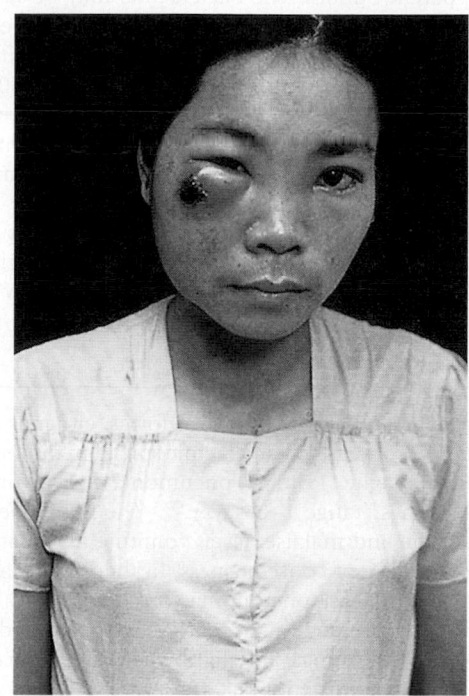

Figure 65.5 A young woman with eschar of an infected flea bite and local facial carbuncle.

lethargy are marked. Sometimes there is agitation or even delirium. Vomiting and diarrhoea occur occasionally. Hepatomegaly is common, but the spleen, although slightly enlarged, is not usually palpable.

In some patients, small skin lesions, such as vesicles and pustules may be seen in the region drained by the affected nodes. These may ulcerate or form an eschar (Figure 65.5), or rarely a carbuncle. *Y. pestis* can be isolated from these lesions. Although uncommon, perhaps the best-known skin manifestation is a patchy purpuric dermal necrosis, which gave rise to the popular name 'Black Death'.

Laboratory findings include an elevated leukocyte count (12000–22000/mm³) and toxic granulation of neutrophils.

Eosinophilia is absent in the acute phase but is often noticed during convalescence. There is also laboratory evidence of disseminated intravascular coagulation.[9] Liver enzymes and bilirubin are frequently elevated, especially in more severe cases, although clinical jaundice is rare.

Minor infections also occur and may go unnoticed. They may present with mild fever and less pronounced lymph node enlargement ('pestis minor'), which is self-limiting.

Septicaemic plague

Episodes of bacteraemia often occur in bubonic plague: in one study, quantitative culture of small volumes of blood detected bacteraemia in 40% of cases.[10] Densities greater than 10^2/mL were associated with higher mortality.

The term 'septicaemic plague' denotes a severe acute illness characterized by a high density of organisms in the blood, without clinically apparent buboes. The bacteraemia may be so high (up to 10^7/mL) that organisms are detectable in a peripheral blood smear. Septicaemic plague accounted for 11% of cases in the USA during the 1970s.[11] However, in New Mexico from 1980 to 1984, 25% of the 71 cases reported were septicaemic.[12] This was more likely to occur in people aged over 40 years. Symptoms include fever, rigors, malaise and headache. Gastrointestinal symptoms of nausea, vomiting, diarrhoea and abdominal pain are more frequent than in bubonic plague. The duration of illness is shorter than in bubonic plague and, if not treated appropriately, the patient rapidly becomes shocked and dies within a few days.

Pneumonic plague

Pneumonia in plague can occur in two forms, either as a primary pneumonia or secondary to bacteraemic spread in bubonic plague or septicaemic plague. Primary pneumonia has an incubation period of 2–4 days (range 1–6 days).[13,14] The illness begins with intense headache and malaise, fever, vomiting and marked prostration and clouding of consciousness. In the initial stages, there may be little to suggest pneumonia, but cough and dyspnoea develop with the production of watery, blood-stained sputum. Physical signs in the lungs are slight; there are reduced breath sounds and coarse crepitations at the bases. Respiratory failure ensues and the patient rapidly dies. Chest radiography shows evidence of multilobar consolidation or bronchopneumonia; there may be minimal pleural effusions. The discrepancy between gross radiographic abnormalities and minimal physical signs in the chest is characteristic. The mortality rate in both types of plague pneumonia is extremely high, and appropriate antibiotic treatment must be given within 24 h of onset if the mortality rate is to be reduced.

Pneumonic plague is generally very uncommon, but it is the one form that may result in human-to-human transmission via infected droplets. This usually requires close contact with cases who have a productive cough. Where the climate is cool and humid, allowing infectious particles to persist, epidemics of pneumonic plague have occurred, such as that in Manchuria in 1910–1911. It is also a potential risk in laboratory workers handling cultures of Y. pestis. Pneumonic plague is probably not as contagious as it is commonly believed.[14] An analysis of past outbreaks

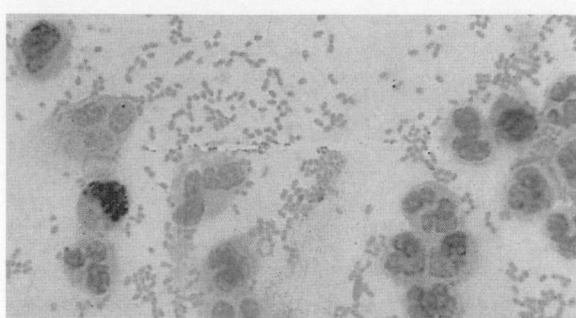

Figure 65.6 *Yersinia pestis* in cerebrospinal fluid taken from a patient with meningitis.

estimated that the average number of secondary cases per primary case (R_0) was only 1.3, even before control measures are implemented.[13]

Plague meningitis

Primary plague meningitis is extremely rare. Most cases of meningeal involvement have occurred as a complication of inadequately treated bubonic plague, typically after 9–15 days. There is an association between the presence of axillary buboes and the development of meningitis.[10] It is postulated that this may be due to spread by the lymphatic route, but bacteraemia is considered to be the means of spread from other sites.

Plague meningitis presents with symptoms and signs common to all types of pyogenic meningitis, including fever, headache, vomiting and neck stiffness. Examination of cerebrospinal fluid will show a predominately neutrophil leukocytosis, and Y. pestis may be demonstrated by Gram stain (Figure 65.6). Mortality is higher than in uncomplicated bubonic plague.

Pharyngeal or tonsillar plague

This is a rare variety of plague that results from ingestion[15] or possibly inhalation of the organism. Usually the tonsils become swollen and inflamed. There is anterior cervical lymphadenopathy and swelling of the parotid area, with surrounding oedema. Y. pestis can be isolated from the throat.

Asymptomatic plague

Asymptomatic infections are probably not uncommon in endemic areas as demonstrated by serological surveys.[16] Asymptomatic carriage of the organism in the throat has also been documented.[17]

DIAGNOSIS

The diagnosis of plague must be considered in anyone presenting with fever and localized lymphadenitis, without another obvious cause of infection, if they live in, or have returned from, an endemic area. Once plague is suspected, laboratory confirmation should be sought as quickly as possible, so that appropriate therapy is given. The definitive diagnosis of plague requires culture of Y. pestis from a clinical specimen, or a four-fold rise in antibody titre.[18]

In most cases, aspiration of a bubo will provide material for microscopic examination and culture. If no fluid or pus is obtained, a small amount of saline can be injected and reaspirated. Smears may be stained with Wayson, Giemsa or Gram stains. A presumptive diagnosis of plague is made by demonstration of bipolar staining coccobacilli, with rapid identification by immunofluorescence using F1-specific antibodies labelled with fluorescein. Blood cultures should always be taken, and in suspected pneumonic or meningeal plague specimens of sputum or cerebrospinal fluid should be processed in the same way as bubo aspirates. Specimens for culture should be inoculated on to blood agar and MacConkey agar, and may also be placed into an enrichment broth, with subculture after 24–48 h.

Serological diagnosis is possible but antibodies may not be detectable when the patient first presents; however it is useful in culture-negative cases. Haemagglutinating antibodies to F1 antigen appear after 1 week and may be detected by the passive haemagglutination test (PHA). A single titre of ≥16 is very suggestive of plague, whereas a fourfold rise in paired sera is diagnostic. Enzyme immunoassays (EIA) have been applied to the detection of serum antibody[19] and F1 antigenaemia.[20] Both appear to be useful diagnostic tests.

A significant recent advance in the diagnosis of plague has been the development of a hand-held, immunochromatographic test, which detects F1 antigen in a range of sample types, with good sensitivity and specificity.[21] It holds promise as a rapid bedside test, even in remote areas that do not have access to other means of diagnosis.

Several methods of DNA detection using polymerase chain reaction (PCR) have been developed recently. One clinical study to determine the diagnostic value of PCR on bubo aspirates found that, although very specific, it was not as sensitive as culture or F1 antigen detection.[22]

DIFFERENTIAL DIAGNOSIS

Although the picture of severe bubonic plague is distinctive, other infections can cause acute lymphadenitis. Staphylococcal and streptococcal infections will usually be associated with an obvious suppurative lesion or an area of lymphangitis in the region drained by the affected lymph nodes. In the USA tularaemia may cause confusion. Lymphogranuloma venereum and chancroid also cause inguinal lymphadenopathy; however, the buboes are less painful and often fluctuant, and there are usually mild constitutional features.

Primary septicaemic plague and meningeal plague are generally indistinguishable from other Gram-negative septicaemias and other types of pyogenic meningitis, respectively. Pneumonia in plague has to be differentiated from the 'adult respiratory distress syndrome' that may occur in bubonic and septicaemic forms. Pharyngeal or tonsillar plague should be distinguished from other common causes of acute tonsillitis and diphtheria.

TREATMENT

In clinically suspected cases, appropriate antibiotic therapy should be started as soon as specimens have been taken for microbio-logical confirmation. Even bubonic plague can evolve quickly into a life-threatening disease. Streptomycin, tetracycline and chloramphenicol are the antibiotics traditionally used in the treatment of plague, and they remain highly effective today. The response to treatment is dramatic provided the patient is not already moribund. Patients with pulmonary involvement are highly infectious and must be kept in strict isolation, with precautions against airborne spread, until at least three days of antibiotic treatment has been given and the patient is clinically improved.

Streptomycin was established as the treatment of choice over 40 years ago; the regimen is 30 mg/kg per day in two divided doses, given intramuscularly, for 10 days. This drug is potentially ototoxic and nephrotoxic. In elderly patients and those with renal impairment, the frequency of administration and total dosage should be reduced. Renal function should be monitored and blood taken for streptomycin levels, if available. Newer aminoglycosides have very good in vitro and in vivo activity,[23,24] and a recent clinical trial showed that gentamicin (2.5 mg/kg intramuscularly, twice daily, for 7 days) was very effective in treating plague in adults and children.[25]

Tetracycline (250–500 mg four times daily, for 10 days) is a satisfactory alternative, especially in milder cases when an oral drug is required. Doxycycline has better in vitro activity[23] and is also very effective clinically (adult dose 100 mg twice daily for 7 days).[25] The tetracyclines are useful when prophylaxis is considered necessary. They should not be given to pregnant women or children up to 8 years of age, and should also be avoided in renal failure.

Chloramphenicol is the drug of choice for plague meningitis because it achieves good concentrations in the cerebrospinal fluid. An initial loading dose of 25 mg/kg is given intravenously, followed by 100 mg/kg per day in four divided doses. When the clinical condition permits, it can be administered orally for a total course of 10 days.

Susceptibility studies show that the fluoroquinolone compounds and third-generation cephalosporins are the most active antimicrobial agents against Y. pestis in vitro.[23,24] In murine models of infection, the fluoroquinolones are also highly active against Y. pestis,[26,27] suggesting that they will be effective in treating human disease. However, the newer cephalosporins gave poor results,[26] so they cannot be recommended for treatment until more data are available.

Until recently, all strains of Y. pestis were remarkably sensitive to a wide range of antibiotics. In 1995, two distinct strains, with antibiotic resistance, were isolated from patients in different areas of Madagascar. One was resistant to streptomycin alone. However, the other strain was resistant to streptomycin, tetracycline, chloramphenicol and sulphonamides, but remained susceptible to trimethoprim, fluoroquinolones and cephalosporins. In both cases, the resistance was mediated by a plasmid, which could be transferred easily to other strains of Y. pestis.[28]

PROGNOSIS

The mortality rate from plague before the antibiotic era ranged from 50% to 95%. With the advent of effective antibiotic therapy the mortality rate fell dramatically. The overall fatality rate in cases reported more recently is approximately 7%.[1] In uncomplicated bubonic plague this may be as low as 5%, but in septicaemic plague documented in New Mexico the case fatality rate was 33%.[12] The prognosis is much worse in patients with pulmonary involvement and, in particular, primary pneumonia invariably remains fatal if treatment is delayed more than 24 h.

PREVENTION

Plague is subject to the International Health Regulations and confirmed cases should be reported to WHO. The control of plague depends upon public education, active surveillance and rodent and flea control measures. During an outbreak, active case finding and follow-up of contacts are essential.[18]

Surveillance should be undertaken to assess the potential for epizootic plague and the risk of transmission to man. This includes bacteriological monitoring of dead or sick rodents and the serological testing of 'sentinel animals', such as carnivores and dogs, which are more likely to have contact with plague-infected rodents.[18] EIA techniques have advantages over PHA for serological surveillance. Flea indices should be established; this involves determining the number and species of fleas per host animal, as well as the percentage of hosts infested. DNA detection, using PCR, has been applied to the identification of Y. pestis in fleas and is more sensitive than mouse inoculation.[29]

The presence of food sources and shelter in areas of human habitation encourages rodents and may be associated with outbreaks of plague. There should be proper disposal of food and refuse; unused out-buildings, wood piles and other forms of shelter for rats should be removed. People should be educated to avoid activities that will bring them into contact with rodents and their fleas. In areas of sylvatic plague, pet cats and dogs should be treated periodically with insecticides.

Specific rodent and flea control measures with the use of rodenticides and effective insecticides, although important, are most likely to be successful in the control of urban plague, rather than sylvatic plague (which may cover a large area). Attempts at rodent control must be preceded by flea control measures because of the potential risk of increasing human exposure to plague-infected fleas.[18] Rat control on ships and in docks, by fumigation, poisoning and trapping, is very important in preventing the dissemination of plague.

The inactivated vaccine, which consisted of formalin-killed Y. pestis is no longer available; there were doubts about this vaccine's efficacy in preventing pneumonic plague. New subunit vaccines based on F1 and V antigens are being developed and show much greater efficacy in mice.[30]

Chemoprophylaxis with oral tetracycline or doxycycline, for 7 days, is recommended for persons in close contact with plague pneumonia, and individuals contaminated in laboratory accidents. Ciprofloxacin should be a suitable alternative as it has proved to be protective against experimental pneumonic infection in mice.[27]

REFERENCES

1. [Anonymous]. Human plague in 2002 and 2003. *Weekly Epidemiol Rec* 2004; 79:301–306.

2. Gage KL, Dennis DT, Orloski KA, et al. Cases of cat-associated human plague in the western US, 1977–1998. *Clin Infect Dis* 2000; 30: 893–900.

3. Chanteau S, Ratsifasoamanana L, Rasoamanana B, et al. Plague, a reemerging disease in Madagascar. *Emerg Infect Dis* 1998; 4:101–104.

4. Brubaker RR. Factors promoting acute and chronic diseases caused by Yersiniae. *Clin Microbiol Rev* 1991; 4:309–324.

5. Zhou D, Han Y, Yang R. Molecular and physiological insights into plague transmission, virulence and etiology. *Microbes Infect* 2006; 8: 273–284.

6. Nakajima R, Brubaker RR. Association between virulence of Yersinia pestis and suppression of gamma interferon and tumor necrosis factor alpha. *Infect Immun* 1993; 61:23–31.

7. Welkos S, Friedlander A, McDowell D, et al. V antigen of Yersinia pestis inhibits neutrophil chemotaxis. *Microb Pathog* 1998; 24:185–196.

8. Butler T. A clinical study of bubonic plague: observations of the 1970 Vietnam epidemic with emphasis on coagulation studies, skin histology and electrocardiograms. *Am J Med* 1972; 53:268–276.

9. Butler T, Bell WR, Linh NN, et al. Yersinia pestis infection in Vietnam. I. Clinical and hematologic aspects. *J Infect Dis* 1974; 129:S78–S84.

10. Butler T, Levin J, Linh NN, et al. Yersinia pestis infection in Vietnam. II. Quantitative blood cultures and detection of endotoxin in the cerebrospinal fluid of patients with meningitis. *J Infect Dis* 1976; 133:493–499.

11. Kaufmann AF, Boyce JM, Martone WJ. Trends in human plague in the United States. *J Infect Dis* 1980; 141:522–524.

12. Hull HF, Montes JM, Mann JM. Septicemic plague in New Mexico. *J Infect Dis* 1987; 155:113–118.

13. Gani R, Leach S. Epidemiologic determinants for modeling pneumonic plague outbreaks. *Emerg Infect Dis* 2004; 10:608–614.

14. Kool JL. Risk of person-to-person transmission of pneumonic plague. *Clin Infect Dis* 2005; 40:1166–1172.

15. Bin Saeed AA, Al-Hamdan NA, Fontaine RE. Plague from eating raw camel liver. *Emerg Infect Dis* 2005; 11:1456–1457.

16. Legters LJ, Cottingham AJ Jr, Hunter DH. Clinical and epidemiologic notes on a defined outbreak of plague in Vietnam. *Am J Trop Med Hyg* 1970; 19:639–652.

17. Marshall JD, Quy DV, Gibson FL. Asymptomatic pharyngeal plague infection in Vietnam. *Am J Trop Med Hyg* 1967; 16:175–177.

18. Dennis DT, Gage KL, Gratz N, et al. *Plague Manual: Epidemiology, Distribution, Surveillance and Control*. Geneva: World Health Organization; 1999.

19. Rasoamanana B, Leroy F, Boisier P, et al. Field evaluation of an immunoglobulin G anti-F1 ELISA assay for serodiagnosis of plague in Madagascar. *Clin Diagn Lab Immunol* 1997; 4:587–591.

20. Spettstoesser WD, Rahalison L, Grunow R, et al. Evaluation of a standardized F1 capsular antigen capture ELISA test kit for the rapid diagnosis of plague. *FEMS Immunol Med Microbiol* 2004; 41:149–155.

21. Chanteau S, Rahalison L, Ralafiarisoa L, et al. Development and testing of a rapid diagnostic test for bubonic and pneumonic plague. *Lancet* 2003; 361:211–216.

22. Rahalison L, Vololonirina E, Ratsitorahina M, et al. Diagnosis of bubonic plague by PCR in Madagascar under field conditions. *J Clin Microbiol* 2000; 38:260–263.

23. Smith MD, Vinh DX, Hoa NT T, et al. In vitro antimicrobial susceptibilities of strains of Yersinia pestis. *Antimicrob Agents Chemother* 1995; 39: 2153–2154.

24. Hernandez E, Girardet M, Ramisse F, et al. Antibiotic susceptibilities of 94 isolates of Yersinia pestis to 24 antimicrobial agents. *J Antimicrob Chemother* 2003; 52:1029–1031.

25. Mwengee W, Butler T, Mgema S, et al. Treatment of plague with gentamicin or doxycycline in a randomized clinical trial in Tanzania. *Clin Infect Dis* 2006; 42:614–621.

26. Byrne WR, Welkos SL, Pitt ML, et al. Antibiotic treatment of experimental pneumonic plague in mice. *Antimicrob Agents Chemother* 1998; 42: 675–681.

27. Steward J, Lever MS, Russell P, et al. Efficacy of the latest fluoroquinolones against experimental Yersinia pestis infection. *Int J Antimicrob Agents* 2004; 24:609–612.

28. Galimand M, Carniel E, Courvalin P. Resistance of Yersinia pestis to antimicrobial agents. *Antimicrob Agents Chemother* 2006; 50:3233–3236.

29. Engelthaler DM, Gage KL, Montenieri JA, et al. PCR detection of Yersinia pestis in fleas: comparison with mouse inoculation. *J Clin Microbiol* 1999; 37:1980–1984.

30. Titball RW, Williamson ED, Dennis DT. Plague. In: Plotkin SA, Orenstein WA, eds. *Vaccines*. 4th edn. Philadelphia: WB Saunders; 2004:999–1010.

Chapter 66 — David A. B. Dance

Melioidosis

INTRODUCTION

Melioidosis is the name used to describe any infection of humans and a wide range of other animals caused by the saprophytic environmental bacterium Burkholderia (formerly Pseudomonas) pseudomallei. Originally identified by Whitmore and Krishnaswami in Rangoon, Burma, in 1911,[1] it is increasingly recognized as an important indigenous infection in many tropical and sub-tropical regions, but is probably greatly under-diagnosed.[2,3] This increasing recognition, including travel-associated cases, along with its potential as a biological weapon, has seen a surge of interest in the disease in recent years.[3–5]

EPIDEMIOLOGY AND MODE OF TRANSMISSION

Melioidosis is widely endemic in south- and east-Asia, especially Thailand, and northern Australia, although it is unevenly distributed within these areas.[2,3] In north-east Thailand, the average annual incidence has been estimated as 4.4/100 000, although this is probably an underestimate, and B. pseudomallei accounts for almost 20% of community-acquired septicaemia.[3,4] In northern Australia, where in some places melioidosis is the commonest cause of fatal community-acquired bacteraemic pneumonia, rates as high as 41.7/100 000 have been reported.[3] Recent cases in Brazil have highlighted the presence of the disease in the Americas,[6] but the position in Africa is unclear, although sporadic cases have been reported there.[2,3,7] During the 1970s, an unusual epizootic also occurred in France.[2–4]

In endemic areas, B. pseudomallei is readily isolated from mud and surface water, particularly rice paddy.[8] Melioidosis is most common in people who have close contact with soil and water (e.g. rice farmers in Thailand, aboriginals in Australia), although in most cases the precise mode of acquisition is unclear. It is usually assumed that most infections result from inoculation, although inoculation events can only be identified in 5–25% of cases.[3,9] Occasional cases follow immersion in, or aspiration of, fresh water, such as occurred during the Asian tsunami of 2004.[3,10] More recently, mounting evidence suggests that inhalation is an important mode of acquisition, especially during severe weather events.[11,12] Other recent outbreaks have been traced to contaminated potable water supplies and contaminated disinfectants or detergents.[3] Iatrogenic and laboratory-acquired infections have occurred occasionally,[2,3] but transmission through direct contact with infected humans or animals, including transplacental transmission and mother-to-infant spread via breast milk, has been described only rarely.[2,3]

Melioidosis is highly seasonal, with 75–85% of cases presenting during the rainy season,[3,4,9,11,12] presumably reflecting recent exposure to the organism in the environment. When a specific exposure can be identified, the incubation period is usually 1–21 days (mean 9 days).[3] However, B. pseudomallei has the unusual ability to remain latent for periods of up to 62 years,[13] which has given rise to the nickname 'Vietnamese time-bomb'. The proportion of seropositive persons who are latently infected is unknown.

MICROBIOLOGY

B. pseudomallei is an ovoid, oxidase-positive, motile Gram-negative bacillus which often exhibits marked bipolarity microscopically. It grows readily on most routine culture media, often forming rugose colonies, and giving off a sweet earthy smell. Other important characteristics include arginine dihydrolase and gelatinase activity, growth at 42°C, the ability to use a wide range of carbon and energy sources, and intrinsic resistance to aminoglycosides, polymyxins and the early beta-lactams, but susceptibility to co-amoxiclav. The species is antigenically homogeneous, but a number of molecular techniques, most usefully multilocus sequence typing, can distinguish between isolates.[3,5] The genome has been sequenced and comprises two chromosomes of 4.07 and 3.17 megabase pairs, associated with core and accessory functions, respectively, with a high proportion of genomic islands.[3,5,14] Burkholderia mallei, the causative agent of glanders, appears to be a clone of B. pseudomallei that has lost genetic material in association with adaptation to equine hosts. Another closely related but avirulent soil organism, Burkholderia thailandensis, has proved useful for the study of B. pseudomallei virulence determinants.[15]

PATHOGENESIS

Although severe melioidosis may occur in apparently normal individuals, up to 80% of cases have underlying diseases, most frequently diabetes mellitus or chronic renal failure.[3–5,15] Steroid therapy, alcohol abuse and liver disease, chronic lung disease (including cystic fibrosis), kava consumption, malignant disease, thalassaemia, chronic granulomatous disease and pregnancy may also predispose to melioidosis but, surprisingly, infection with HIV does not appear to.[3-5] Recrudescence of latent infection also usually occurs at times of intercurrent stress.[16]

The result of exposure to *B. pseudomallei* in the environment varies markedly from case to case, ranging from asymptomatic seroconversion (the commonest outcome) to fulminant sepsis and death. Which route is followed in any individual depends on a balance between the size and route of the inoculum and the virulence of the infecting strain on the one hand, and the host response on the other. This topic has recently been comprehensively reviewed.[3-5,15,16] A range of bacterial factors, including an antiphagocytic polysaccharide capsule, quorum sensing mechanisms, a type III secretion system associated with intracellular growth and spread, bacterial components such as lipopolysaccharide, flagella, pili, secreted products (e.g. protease, lipase, lecithinase, various toxins) and a siderophore ('malleobactin') have all been associated with virulence,[3-5,15] but the relative contributions of individual virulence factors to the disease process have not been well characterized. The ability of the organism to survive and grow intracellularly or become metabolically inactive within granulomas probably contributes to the recalcitrant and persistent nature of the infection.[16] On the host side, innate immune mechanisms, macrophage and neutrophil function, and both cellular and humoral responses probably all play a role in defence against the organism.[3,4,15,17] An exaggerated host response may also be damaging.[3,4,15]

PATHOLOGY

The microscopic appearance of lesions is not pathognomonic and forms a spectrum from abscess to granuloma depending on the duration of the illness and the response of the individual. Multinucleate giant cells, often containing 'globi' of bacteria, in a background of acute necrotizing inflammation, are a characteristic feature.[18]

CLINICAL MANIFESTATIONS

The variable course and manifestations have made it difficult to develop a satisfactory clinical classification of melioidosis. Since 60–70% of the population in endemic areas have antibodies to *B. pseudomallei* by the age of 4 years,[19] yet few acquire clinically-apparent melioidosis, and the majority of infections are presumably mild or asymptomatic. Seroconversion has been associated with a flu-like illness.[20] Some of the more common clinically apparent forms are described below.

Septicaemic melioidosis

Some 46–60% of cases of culture-positive melioidosis are bacteraemic, and the majority of these are clinically septicaemic.[3,4,21] Patients usually have a short history (median 6 days; range 1 day to 2 months) of fever and rigors.[21] Some 4% of cases in Australia are thought to represent recrudescent latent infections.[3] Approxi-

mately half have evidence of a primary focus of infection, usually pulmonary or cutaneous.[3,4,21] Diminished consciousness, jaundice and diarrhoea may also be prominent features. Initial investigations usually reveal anaemia, a neutrophil leukocytosis, coagulopathy and evidence of renal and hepatic impairment. Deterioration is often rapid, with the development of widespread metastatic abscesses, particularly in the lungs, liver (Figure 66.1), spleen and prostate, and metabolic acidosis with Kussmaul's breathing. Mycotic aneurysms are being recognized with increasing frequency.[22] Cutaneous or subcutaneous abscesses occur in approximately 10% of cases and an abnormal chest radiograph is found in 80% of patients, the most common pattern being widespread, nodular shadowing (Figure 66.2).

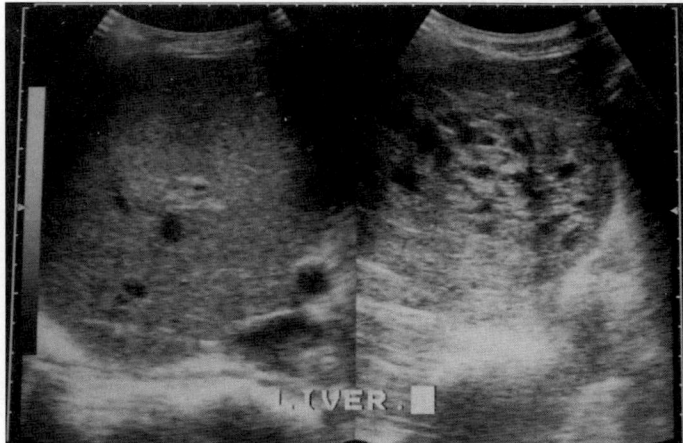

Figure 66.1 Ultrasound of liver showing multiple abscesses in a patient with septicaemic melioidosis (©Dr S. Peacock).

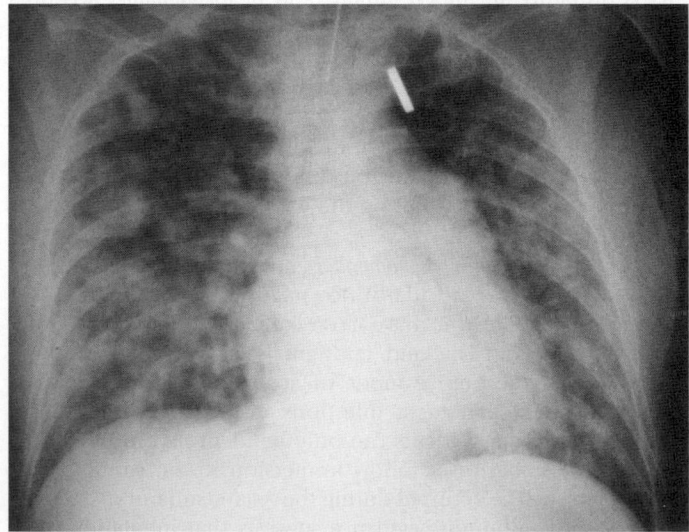

Figure 66.2 Septicaemic melioidosis. Widespread nodular shadowing representing blood-borne pneumonia (©Professor N. J. White).

Localized melioidosis

The lung is the most common site for localized melioidosis. The most frequent form is a cavitating pneumonia accompanied by profound weight loss, which is often confused with tuberculosis or lung abscess (Figure 66.3), although mild bronchitis or bronchopneumonia may be the only manifestations. Any lung zone may be affected, although there is a predilection for upper lobe involvement.[23] Localized complications include pneumothorax, empyema and purulent pericarditis, whilst progression to septicaemia is not uncommon.

Localized *B. pseudomallei* infection may occur in any organ. Well described presentations include: cutaneous and subcutaneous abscesses, suppurative parotitis, lymphadenitis, osteomyelitis and septic arthritis, liver and/or splenic abscesses (Figure 66.4), cystitis, pyelonephritis, prostatic abscesses, epididymo-orchitis, keratitis, meningoencephalitis, and brain abscesses.[3,4] For reasons

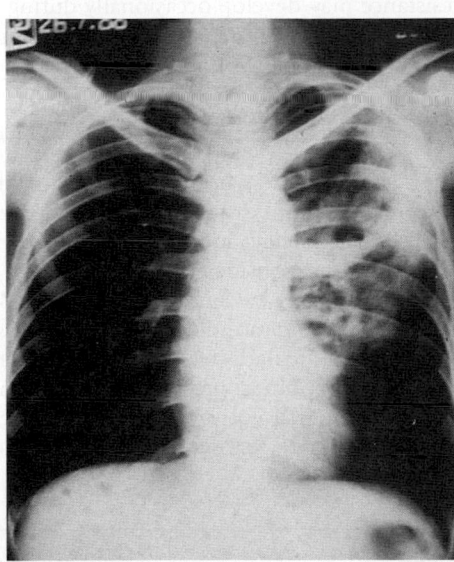

Figure 66.3 Cavitating pneumonia in melioidosis, with an air-fluid level.

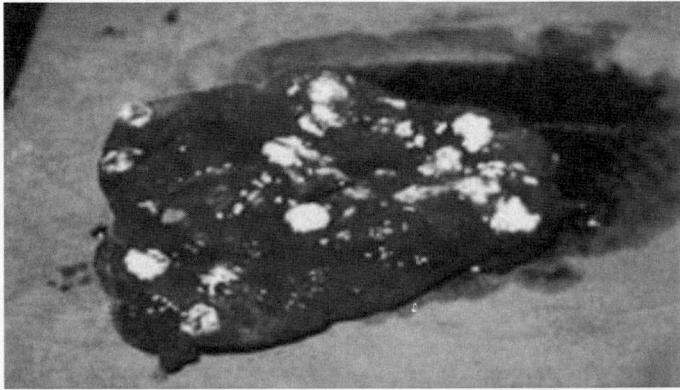

Figure 66.4 Spleen removed from a patient with chronic melioidosis showing multiple abscesses (©Professor N. J. White).

that have yet to be explained, parotitis in children is common in Thailand but not Australia, whereas prostatic abscesses and neurological melioidosis are reported more frequently from Australia than Thailand.[3,4]

DIAGNOSIS

Melioidosis should be considered in any patient who has ever visited an endemic area who presents with septicaemia and/or abscesses, especially if they have a strongly associated predisposing condition, such as diabetes. It is difficult to make a clinical diagnosis with confidence. A failure to defervesce on empirical treatment with penicillin and gentamicin, a combination often used to treat patients with septicaemia in the tropics, is useful supporting evidence, but usually the diagnosis depends on the isolation of *B. pseudomallei*, the detection of its antigens or nucleic acid, or the presence of specific antibodies. Microscopy of pus, sputum or urine may reveal bipolar or unevenly staining Gram-negative rods, but this appearance is not specific for *B. pseudomallei*. The most useful rapid diagnostic tool is immunofluorescence on pus or secretions, but this is not generally available.[24] Numerous PCR assays for *B. pseudomallei* have been developed and some have shown promise in small scale evaluatons,[3,5,25] but none is in widespread use.

The organism should be sought in blood, pus, urine, sputum or any other specimen indicated by the patient's clinical presentation. The laboratory should be notified when melioidosis is suspected, since selective techniques increase the isolation rate,[3–5] and the organism may be overlooked or discarded as a contaminant by the unwary. The antibiotic susceptibility pattern described above is a useful clue. The organism is classified as a 'category 3' pathogen because of the potential for infection among laboratory staff, although this has rarely occurred. Commercial *B. cepacia* medium compares favourably with other media designed to grow *B. pseudomallei*, and is more likely to be available outside endemic areas, but commercial identification kits may give misleading results,[5] so possible isolates should always be sent to a Reference Laboratory for confirmation by those who rarely encounter the organism.

There is no standard assay for serodiagnosis of melioidosis. An indirect haemagglutination (IHA) test, using a crude mixture of poorly characterized antigens, is the test most widely used in endemic areas, although many other assays have been described. Most tests have disappointing sensitivity and specificity, particularly in endemic areas where background seropositivity rates are high.[3–5] A commercial immunochromatographic test produced in Australia has given variable results in field evaluations.[3,5] Serology may be useful in patients from non-endemic areas, in whom a single IHA titre of >1:40 at presentation is suggestive of melioidosis. In patients from endemic areas, only a rising or very high titre in a patient with a compatible illness can be taken as presumptive evidence of melioidosis.

Differential diagnosis

With such variable manifestations that it has been nicknamed 'the remarkable imitator', the range of differential diagnoses of melioidosis is very wide, and varies considerably from patient to patient depending on the site of infection. Common differentials in acute severe cases include any bacterium causing community-acquired septicaemia, pneumonia or abscesses, particularly *Staphylococcus aureus*. Chronic pulmonary cases must be distinguished from tuberculosis and anaerobic lung abscesses, and hepatic cases from mixed bacterial or amoebic liver abscesses.

MANAGEMENT

General

Patients with septicaemic melioidosis require aggressive supportive treatment, with particular attention to correction of volume depletion and septic shock, respiratory and renal failure, and hyperglycaemia or ketoacidosis. Severe cases should ideally be managed in an intensive care unit. Abscesses should be drained surgically whenever possible in both disseminated and localized disease.

Antimicrobial therapy

Several prospective randomized comparisons of antimicrobial therapy for melioidosis have been undertaken over the past 20 years, resulting in a good evidence base for treatment, which has been summarized in recent reviews.[3–5,26] The standard approach to chemotherapy of severe disease is to use at least 2 weeks of parenteral treatment initially, followed by 12–20 weeks of oral 'eradication' therapy to reduce the risk of relapse. Mild cases may be treated with oral drugs alone. Preferred regimens are given in Table 66.1. Co-amoxiclav and cefoperazone-sulbactam have also been used for parenteral treatment, but experience is more limited.

Encouraging results using G-CSF for adjunctive treatment of melioidosis septic shock have been reported in an uncontrolled study from northern Australia,[3,5] but this did not achieve statistical significance in a prospective randomized trial.[27] In vitro resistance

Table 66.1 Preferred regimens for antimicrobial therapy for melioidosis

Agent	Dose
Acute parenteral phase (at least 2 weeks and longer if persistent fever, undrained abscesses etc.)	
Imipenem or meropenem	60 mg/kg per day i.v. in three divided doses
Ceftazidime	120 mg/kg per day i.v. in three divided doses
Oral eradication phase (12–20 weeks)	
Co-trimoxazole plus	10/50 mg/kg per day in two divided doses
Doxycycline	4 mg/kg per day in two divided doses
Amoxicillin-clavulanate	60/15 mg/kg per day in three divided doses

Adjust doses as necessary in renal impairment. Amoxicillin-clavulanate preferred for oral treatment in children ≤8 years or pregnant women.

to co-trimoxazole, which can only reliably be determined by 'E-test', is not uncommon, but it is not known whether this increases the risk of relapse or should alter the choice of treatment.[5,28]

PROGNOSIS

Even with optimal antibiotic treatment, the mortality of severe melioidosis is 19% in Australia and 40% in Thailand, death within the first 48 h of hospital admission being common.[3–5] Even in those that recover, the response to therapy is often slow (median time to resolution of fever 9 days).[4,21] Poor prognostic features include hypotension, absence of fever, leucopenia, azotaemia, abnormal liver function tests, a high level of bacteraemia, raised levels of a range of pro-inflammatory cytokines, and positive urine or sputum cultures.[3–5] Relapse occurs in 9.7% overall, and is commoner in those with disseminated infections who receive less than 12 weeks of treatment.[29] Surprisingly, reinfection also appears to occur in 3.4% of survivors followed-up for long periods of time.[29] Antibiotic resistance may develop occasionally during the course of treatment, although this is rare (<1%) with β-lactams.

PREVENTION

No *B. pseudomallei* vaccine has been developed for human use, although experimental vaccines are under development.[30] Antibiotic prophylaxis has been attempted following laboratory exposures and would be considered in the event of deliberate release, but there is limited evidence of its efficacy.[3] Prevention is thus limited to the avoidance of contact with *B. pseudomallei* in the environment, particularly by 'at-risk' individuals such as diabetics, the removal of point sources and adequate chlorination of water supplies. The risk of cross-infection appears to be very low, but cases may be barrier nursed where facilities are available.

REFERENCES

1. Whitmore A, Krishnaswami CS. An account of the discovery of a hitherto undescribed infective disease occurring among the population of Rangoon. *Indian Med Gazette* 1912; 47:262–267.
2. Dance DAB. Melioidosis: the tip of the iceberg? *Clin Microbiol Rev* 1991; 4: 52–60.
3. Cheng AC, Currie BJ. Melioidosis: epidemiology, pathophysiology, and management. *Clin Microbiol Rev* 2005; 18:383–416.
4. White NJ. Melioidosis. *Lancet* 2003; 361:1715–1722.
5. Peacock SJ. Melioidosis. *Curr Opinion Infect Dis* 2006; 19:421–428.
6. Inglis TJJ, Rolim DB, Sousa ADQ. Melioidosis in the Americas. *Am J Trop Med Hygiene* 2006; 75:947–954.
7. Borgherini G, Poubeau P, Paganin F, et al. Melioidosis: an imported case from Madagascar. *J Trav Med* 2006; 13:1195–1982.
8. Inglis TJJ, Sagripanti J-L. Environmental factors that affect the survival and persistence of *Burkholderia pseudomallei*. *Appl Environ Microbiol* 2006; 72: 6865–6875.
9. Suputtamongkol Y, Hall AJ, Dance DAB, et al. The epidemiology of melioidosis in Ubon Ratchatani, Northeast Thailand. *Int J Epidemiol* 1994; 23:1082–1090.
10. Chierakul W, Winothai W, Wattanawaitunechai C, et al. Melioidosis in 6 tsunami survivors in southern Thailand. *Clin Infect Dis* 2005; 41:982–990.

11. Currie BJ, Jacups SP. Intensity of rainfall and severity of melioidosis, Australia. *Emerg Infect Dis* 2003; 9:1538–1542.

12. Cheng AC, Jacups SP, Gal D, et al. Extreme weather events and environmental contamination are associated with case-clusters of melioidosis in the Northern Territory of Australia. *Int J Epidemiol* 2006; 35:323–329.

13. Ngauy V, Lemeshev Y, Sadkowski L, et al. Cutaneous melioidosis in a man who was taken as a prisoner of war by the Japanese during World War II. *J Clin Microbiol* 2005; 43:970–972.

14. Holden MG, Titball RW, Peacock SJ, et al. Genomic plasticity of the causative agent of melioidosis, *Burkholderia pseudomallei*. *Proc Natl Acad Sci* 2004; 101:14240–14245.

15. Wiersinga WJ, van der Poll T, White NJ, et al. Melioidosis: insights into the pathogenicity of *Burkholderia pseudomallei*. *Nature Rev Microbiol* 2006; 4: 272–282.

16. Gan Y-H. Interaction between *Burkholderia pseudomallei* and the host immune response: sleeping with the enemy? *J Infect Dis* 2005; 192: 1845–1850.

17. Easton A, Haque A, Chu K, et al. A critical role for neutrophils in resistance to experimental infection with *Burkholderia pseudomallei*. *J Infect Dis* 2007; 195:99–107.

18. Wong KT, Putucheary SD, Vadivelu J. The histopathology of human melioidosis. *Histopathology* 1995; 26:51–55.

19. Wuthiekanun V, Chierakul W, Langla S, et al. Development of antibodies to *Burkholderia pseudomallei* during childhood in melioidosis-endemic northeast Thailand. *Am J Trop Med Hygiene* 2006; 74:1074–1075.

20. Ashdown LR, Johnson RW, Koehler JM, et al. Enzyme-linked immunosorbent assay for the diagnosis of clinical and subclinical melioidosis. *J Infect Dis* 1989; 160:253–260.

21. Chaowagul W, White NJ, Dance DAB, et al. Melioidosis: a major cause of community-acquired septicemia in Northeastern Thailand. *J Infect Dis* 1989; 159:890–899.

22. Low JGH, Quek AML, Sin YK, et al. Mycotic aneurysm due to *Burkholderia pseudomallei* infection: case reports and literature review. *Clin Infect Dis* 2005; 40:193–198.

23. Dhiensri T, Puapairoj S, Susaengrat W. Pulmonary melioidosis: clinical and radiologic correlation in 183 cases in northeastern Thailand. *Radiology* 1988; 166:711–715.

24. Wuthiekanun V, Desakorn V, Wonsuwan G, et al. Rapid immunofluorescence microscopy for diagnosis of melioidosis. *Clin Diag Lab Immunol* 2005; 12:555–556.

25. Meumann EM, Novak RT, Gal D, et al. Clinical evaluation of a type III secretion system real-time PCR assay for diagnosing melioidosis. *J Clin Microbiol* 2006; 44:3028–3030.

26. Samuel M, Ti T Y. Interventions for treating melioidosis. *Cochrane Database of Systematic Reviews* 2002; 4:CD001263.

27. Cheng AC, Limmathurotsakul D, Chierakul W, et al. A randomised controlled trial of granulocyte colony-stimulating factor for the treatment of severe sepsis due to melioidosis in Thailand. *Clin Infect Dis* 2007; 45:308–314.

28. Chaowagul W, Chierakul W, Simpson AJ, et al. Open-label randomized trial of oral trimethoprim-sulfamethoxazole, doxycycline, and chloramphenicol compared with trimethoprim-sulfamethoxazole and doxycycline for maintenance therapy of melioidosis. *Antimicrob Agents Chemother* 2005; 49:4020–4025.

29. Limmathurotsakul D, Chaowagul W, Chierakul W, et al. Risk factors for recurrent melioidosis in northeast Thailand. *Clin Infect Dis* 2006; 43:979–986.

30. Warawa J, Woods DE. Melioidosis vaccines. *Expert Rev Vaccines* 2002; 1: 477–482.

Chapter 67

Nicholas J. White and Tran Tinh Hien

Diphtheria

DEFINITION

Diphtheria is an acute infectious disease of the tonsils, pharynx, larynx or nose, and occasionally of other mucous membranes or skin, caused by *Corynebacterium diphtheriae*. The word diphtheria originates from the term 'diphtherite', which has a Greek root meaning skin or hide, and refers to the leathery appearance of the characteristic pharyngeal membrane.[1] The disease is caused by the local effects of destructive infection (usually in the nasopharynx) and the distal effects of diphtheria toxin on the heart, peripheral nerves and kidneys. Death results from airways obstruction, myocarditis or polyneuritis. Diphtheria has declined dramatically in affluent countries over the past 80 years,[2,3] but it remains an important disease in many parts of the tropics and there has been a recent resurgence of the disease in the West. Between 1990 and 1999, over 158 000 cases and 4000 deaths were reported in the countries of the former Soviet Union. Approximately 100 years ago, 1% of all medical publications were on diphtheria. Now there is very little clinical research on diphtheria. Most new developments are in vaccine formulations.

BACTERIOLOGY

The diphtheria bacillus was first grown in pure culture by Loeffler in 1884. The causative organism, *C. diphtheriae* is a non-motile, non-capsulated, non-spore-forming aerobic bacillus. Although it is described as Gram-positive, it is easily decolourized during the staining procedure and may appear Gram-negative. On microscopy, *C. diphtheriae* exhibits considerable pleomorphism, ranging from the classical club shape to long slender bacilli. The arrangement of organisms on a smear often resembles Chinese letters. The presence of metachromatic granules when stained by Loeffler's methylene blue or Albert's stain is characteristic, although this should not be relied upon for identification.

C. diphtheriae grows well on blood agar, but tellurite blood agar (Hoyle's medium) is recommended as this inhibits other respiratory flora and allows the characteristic colonial morphology of the three biotypes (gravis, intermedius and mitis) to develop.[4] Although, as the name implies, toxigenic gravis strains are generally associated with more severe disease, in vitro mitis strains often produce more toxin than gravis or intermedius strains. Toxin production is very dependent on the composition of the growth medium. The iron content is particularly important. Young organisms produce more toxin than older organisms, and thus increased toxin production is associated with rapid growth. The association between biotype and severity is not constant. *C. diphtheriae* is further identified by biochemical reactions: acid is produced from glucose and maltose but only very rarely from sucrose; urea is not hydrolysed. The gravis biotype ferments starch.[5] Simple screening tests have been developed for identification of the pathogenic corynebacteria, which do not produce pyrazinamidase, but do produce cystinase (seen as a brown halo around colonies, when cystine is incorporated into modified Tinsdale's agar).[6]

PATHOGENESIS

The potentially lethal effects of diphtheria in humans are caused by an exotoxin. The toxigenicity of *C. diphtheriae* depends on the presence of a tox+ phage (α lysogenic β-phage) which induces the organism to produce toxin. Harmless non-toxigenic strains of *C. diphtheriae*, lacking the tox+ β-phage, can be converted to pathogenic toxigenic strains by infection with a lysogenic phage (in vitro). This process may also occur in vivo.[7]

Toxin production by corynebacteria is usually detected by Elek's test[5] or guinea pig inoculation, but recently enzyme immunoassays have been developed which are cheaper and easier.[8] Diphtheria toxin can also be produced by *C. ulcerans* and this has resulted in clinical diphtheria.[9]

Diphtheria exotoxin is a 62 000 Da polypeptide which includes two segments: the active toxin moiety (A) and the binding (B) segment, which binds to specific receptors on susceptible cells. The binding B portion attaches to the cell membrane, allowing the active A portion to enter the cells where it catalyses a reaction that inactivates the transfer RNA (tRNA) translocase 'elongation factor 2' (EF-2), in eukaryotic cells. This factor is essential for reactions that transfer triplet codes from messenger RNA to amino acid sequences via tRNA. Thus EF-2 inactivation stops synthesis of the polypeptide chains. The diphtheria toxin affects all human cells, but the most profound effects are on the myocardium (myocarditis), peripheral nerves (demyelination) and kidneys (acute tubular necrosis).

the muscles of accommodation together with paralysis of the pharynx, larynx and respiratory muscles. The IXth and Xth cranial nerves are most commonly affected, followed by the VIIth nerve, the nerves to the external ocular muscles (III, IV and VI).[19] Quadriparesis is common, and death from respiratory failure may result either from paralysis of the respiratory muscles or paralytic closure of the larynx. Limb weakness occurs in about half of those with neuropathy. Sensory deficit affects proprioception in particular. Autonomic dysfunction is common, and sudden hypotension may occur between the fourth and seventh weeks of disease. The evolution of the neurological deficit is often asynchronous such that cranial nerve deficits may be improving while peripheral nerve deficits worsen.[19] In comparing diphtheria with Guillain–Barré syndrome (GBS), diphtheric polyneuropathy is much more likely than GBS to have a bulbar onset, to lead to respiratory failure, to evolve more slowly, to take a biphasic course, and to cause death or long-term disability. In a recent series of adults with diphtheria from Latvia, 41% of those with limb weakness still could not work at their 1-year follow-up. Antitoxin seems ineffective in preventing neuropathy if administered after the second day of diphtheritic symptoms.[20]

Other complications

Less common complications of diphtheria include acute tubular necrosis, disseminated intravascular coagulation, endocarditis and secondary pneumonia. The overall mortality rate of diphtheria is approximately 5–10%, with relatively higher rates in infancy and old age.

DIAGNOSIS

In many parts of the world, especially in developing countries, diphtheria is still a common disease. It should be considered in any patient with the following symptoms: tonsillitis and/or pharyngitis with pseudomembrane, hoarseness and stridor, cervical adenopathy or cervical swelling (bull neck), unilateral bloody nasal discharge or paralysis of the palate. Direct smears of infected areas of the throat are often made, but these are unreliable. The diagnosis is confirmed by isolation and identification of *C. diphtheriae* from infected sites, but cultures are often negative, particularly if the patient has received antibiotics before admission to hospital. The differential diagnosis includes streptococcal or viral pharyngitis and tonsillitis, and Vincent's angina. Common and sometimes tragic errors are to diagnose tonsillar diphtheria as infectious mononucleosis, or a case of 'bull neck' (malignant diphtheria) as mumps. If possible, cardiac enzymes or troponins should be monitored along with the electrocardiogram to anticipate myocardial dysfunction and conduction disturbances.

MANAGEMENT

Emergency tracheostomy should be performed to anticipate or relieve respiratory obstruction in laryngeal diphtheria.[21,22] The procedure must not be delayed until the patient develops cyanosis. Agitation and the use of the accessory respiratory muscles are indications for immediate tracheostomy. As the mortality rate of diphtheria increases with delay in antitoxin administration, treatment with diphtheria antitoxin should be started on clinical suspicion, without waiting for definitive laboratory confirmation. The dose of antitoxin depends on the site of primary infection, the extent of pseudomembrane, and the delay between the onset and the antitoxin administration: 20 000–40 000 units for faucial diphtheria of less than 48 h duration, or cutaneous infection; 40 000–80 000 units for faucial diphtheria of more than 48 h duration, or laryngeal infection; 80 000–100 000 units for malignant diphtheria (bull neck, toxic state). Adrenaline (epinephrine) should be available to cope with rare anaphylactic reactions to the antitoxin.

Antibiotics will stop toxin production and prevent further spread of organisms in the host. *C. diphtheriae* is susceptible to a variety of antibiotics including penicillin, cephalosporins, erythromycin and tetracycline. In a randomized comparison in Vietnam, the use of penicillin was associated with shorter fever clearance (median 27 h) compared with 46 h for erythromycin recipients and, whereas there was no penicillin resistance, 27% of the *C. diphtheriae* isolated were resistant to erythromycin.[23] The recommended antibiotic treatment regimen is therefore penicillin G, 50 000 units/kg daily in four divided doses, with erythromycin, parenterally or orally, 5 mg/kg four times daily as an alternative for penicillin-allergic patients. Antibiotic susceptibility should be checked when cultures are positive. Erythromycin is considered to be more effective in eliminating the carrier state, although there are limited data to support this.

Bed rest is recommended during the acute phase, but there is no proof of its benefit. Close electrocardiographic monitoring is indicated, particularly after the first week, to detect early signs of cardiac involvement. Angiotensin-converting enzyme inhibitors (captopril) have been used in patients, but there have been no randomized trials. If there is high-grade or complete heart block, then temporary pacing should be performed, although again there have been no large trials to determine whether these measures influence outcome. One study has suggested that carnitine may be beneficial by decreasing the incidence of myocarditis,[24] but additional evidence of its efficacy is required. The administration of corticosteroids may benefit laryngeal diphtheria by reducing swelling,[25] but otherwise is of no benefit.[26]

Insertion of a temporary pacemaker is indicated in complete heart block with bradycardia, although the mortality remains high.[27,28]

PREVENTION

Diphtheria is readily preventable by vaccine administration. This is included in the triple vaccine: diphtheria, tetanus and pertussis vaccine (DTP) or the quintuple diphtheria, tetanus, pertussis, polio and HiB vaccine. The recommended primary course of immunization of children aged up to 7 years consists of three doses: the first at 6–8 weeks of age, the second at 3 months and the third at 4 months. A booster dose of diphtheria, tetanus, pertussis, and polio (dTaP/IPV or DTaP/IPV) vaccine is given between 40 months and 5 years of age. A final immunization with diphtheria, tetanus, polio (Td/IPV) vaccine is given between 13 and 18 years of age. If primary immunization is delayed until 7 years of age, or is interrupted, a series of three doses of tetanus and diphtheria toxoid adsorbed (DT ads), which contains less diphtheria toxoid than DTP, should be completed, giving the second dose 4–8 weeks after the first, and the third 6–12 months later. Research continues into combination vaccines and the intranasal delivery route. Patients with diphtheria should receive active immunization after recovery. Close contacts should be screened for *C. diphtheriae* with throat swab culture. If the immunization status is unclear, they should be treated with an appropriate antibiotic if culture positive, and receive primary immunization according to their age. Immunity following immunization can be assessed by means of the Schick test. A standardized sterile diluted filtrate from a culture of *C. diphtheriae* (the Schick test toxin) is injected intradermally (0.2 mL) into the flexor surface of the left forearm. An equal volume (0.2 mL) of heat-inactivated filtrate (Schick test control) is injected intradermally into the right forearm. The injection sites are inspected after 24–48 h and again at 5–7 days. A lack of inflammation indicates adequate antitoxic immunity. Sometimes non-specific reactions (pseudoreactions) occur, but these are usually equal in both arms (i.e. toxin and control elicit an equal inflammatory reaction). Schick-negative patients are either resistant to disease or, with gravis and intermedius strains, they may sometimes develop mild disease.

REFERENCES

1. English PC. Diphtheria and theories of infectious disease: centennial appreciation of the critical role of diphtheria in the history of medicine. *Pediatrics* 1985; 76:1–9.
2. Kwantes W. Diphtheria in Europe. *J Hyg (Camb)* 1984; 93:433–347.
3. Dixon JMS. Diphtheria in North America. *J Hyg (Camb)* 1984; 93:419–432.
4. Noble WC, Dixon JMS. Corynebacterium and other coryneform bacteria. In: Parker TM, Duerden BI, eds. *Topley and Wilson's Principles of Bacteriology, Virology and Immunity*. Vol. 2. 8th edn. London: Edward Arnold; 1990:103–118
5. Brooks R, Joynson DHM. Bacterial diagnosis of diphtheria. *J Clin Pathol* 1990; 43:576–580.
6. Coleman G, Weaver E, Efstratiou A. Screening tests for pathogenic corynebacteria. *J Clin Pathol* 1992; 45:46–48.
7. Pappenheimer AM, Murphy JH. Studies on the molecular epidemiology of diphtheria. *Lancet* 1983; ii:923–926.
8. Hallas G, Harrison TG, Samuel D, et al. Detection of diphtheria toxin in culture supernates of Corynebacterium diphtheriae and C. ulcerans by immunoassay with monoclonal antibody. *J Med Microbiol* 1990; 32:247–253.
9. Meers PD. A case of classical diphtheria due to Corynebacterium ulcerans. *J Infect* 1979; 1:139–142.
10. Krumina A, Logina I, Donaghy M, et al. Diphtheria with polyneuropathy in a closed community despite receiving recent booster vaccination. *J Neurol Neurosurg Psychiatry* 2005; 76:1555–1574.
11. Hong NT, Phu VT, Hien TT. *A study of 2597 cases of diphtheria treated at Cho Quan Hospital during 10 years (1976–85)*. Annual Scientific Report of Cho Quan Hospital, Vietnam 1985:65–78.
12. Naiditch MJ, Bower AG. Diphtheria. A study of 1433 cases observed at the Los Angeles County Hospital. *Am J Med* 1954; 17:229–245.
13. Boyer NH, Weinstein L. Diphtheritic myocarditis. *N Engl J Med* 1948; 239:913–919.
14. Loukoushkina EF, Bobko PV, Kolbasova EV, et al. The clinical picture and diagnosis of diphtheritic carditis in children. *Eur J Pediatr* 1998; 157: 528–533.
15. Kneen R, Dung NM, Solomon T, et al. Clinical features and predictors of diphtheritic cardiomyopathy in Vietnamese children. *Clin Infect Dis* 2004; 39:1591–1598.
16. Bethell DB, Dung MN, Loan HT, et al. Prognostic value of electrocardiographic monitoring in severe diphtheria. *Clin Infect Dis* 1995; 20:1259–1265.
17. Walshe FMR. On the pathogenesis of diphtheritic paralysis. *Quart J Med* 1917–18; 11.191–204
18. Walshe FMR. On the pathogenesis of diphtheritic paralysis. Part 2. *Quart J Med* 1917–18; 12:14–19.
19. Piradov MA, Pirogov VN, Popova LM, et al. Diphtheritic polyneuropathy: clinical analysis of severe forms. *Arch Neurol* 2001; 58:1438–1442.
20. Logina I, Donaghy M. Diphtheritic polyneuropathy: a clinical study and comparison with Guillain–Barré syndrome. *J Neurol Neurosurg Psychiatry* 1999; 67:433–438.
21. Kadirova R, Kartoglu HU, Strebel PM. Clinical characteristics and management of 676 hospitalized diphtheria cases, Kyrgyz Republic, 1995. *J Infect Dis* 2000; 181(suppl 1):S110–S115.
22. Rakhmanova AG, Lumio J, Groundstroem K, et al. Diphtheria outbreak in St. Petersburg: clinical characteristics of 1860 adult patients. *Scand J Infect Dis* 1996; 28:37–40.
23. Kneen R, Giao PN, Solomon T, et al. Penicillin versus erythromycin in the treatment of diphtheria. *Clin Infect Dis* 1998; 27:845–850.
24. Ramos ACMF, Elias PRD, Barrucand L, et al. The protective effect of carnitine in human diphtheric myocarditis. *Pediatr Res* 1987; 18:815–819.
25. Havaldar PV. Dexamethasone in laryngeal diphtheritic croup. *Ann Trop Paediatr* 1997; 17:21–23.
26. Thisyakorn U, Wongvanich J, Kumpeng V. Failure of corticosteroid therapy to prevent diphtheric myocarditis or neuritis. *Pediatr Infect Dis* 1984; 3: 126–128.
27. Stockins BA, Lanas FT, Saavedra JG, et al. Prognosis in patients with diphtheric myocarditis and bradyarrhythmias: assessment of results of ventricular pacing. *Br Heart J* 1994; 72:190–191.
28. Dung NM, Kneen R, Kiem N, et al. Treatment of severe diphtheritic myocarditis by temporary insertion of a cardiac pacemaker. *Clin Infect Dis* 2002; 35: 1425–1429.

Chapter 68   Moses S. Kapembwa

Endemic Treponematoses

The endemic or non-venereal treponematoses include yaws, endemic syphilis and pinta. Their causative organisms, *Treponema pallidum* subsp. *pertenue* for yaws, *T. pallidum* subsp. *endemicum* for endemic syphilis and *T. pallidum* subsp. *carateum* for pinta, have remained until recently morphologically and antigenically indistinguishable from *T. pallidum* subsp. *pallidum*, which causes venereal syphilis (see Chapter 21). Likewise, there are no differences in serology or response to penicillin. Nevertheless, there are significant clinical and epidemiological differences among these treponematoses.

The discrepant manifestations of these biologically 'similar' organisms has generated considerable interest leading to academic disputes and much speculation and argument among medical historians. Hudson[1] recognized only *T. pallidum* and believed in an all-embracing concept (unitarian theory): all the treponematoses were due to the same organism and the differences were determined by the socioenvironmental conditions, such as age, microclimate of skin, temperature and humidity. Others, including Hackett,[2] believe that these conditions are separate entities caused by different organisms. Whereas PCR amplification has provided ample evidence in support of species specificity,[3] no genetic differences have been shown to distinguish between the non-venereal treponemal sub-species. Subtle differences are possible and remain to be characterized. In one study, for example, *Treponema pallidum* subsp. *pertenue* and *T. pallidum* subsp. *pallidum* were reported to differ in at least one nucleotide.[4] The differences with regard to experimental infections by these treponemes in laboratory animals have also been described.[5] Humans are the only proven reservoirs for the non-venereal treponemes and, although similar organisms have been isolated from primates in Africa, their significance with regard to human disease is unclear.[6]

Endemic treponematoses were among the most predominant diseases in the pre-antibiotic era. Thus, in the mid-twentieth century, there were an estimated 50 million cases of yaws worldwide (half in Africa), over 1 million cases of endemic syphilis (mostly in North Africa and the eastern Mediterranean basin) and about 1 million cases of pinta confined to Central and South America. Discovery of long-acting penicillin preparations, which were cheap, safe and curative with a single intramuscular injection, made a cost-effective eradication programme possible. Consequently, in 1948, the World Health Organization, in conjunction with UNICEF and many national governments, established a global control programme, first against yaws and later extended to include endemic syphilis and pinta. Mobile teams were formed, and over 50 million individuals were treated of the 160 million examined in 46 countries. As a result, these diseases were brought under control and even eliminated from some areas. However, dismantling of the mobile teams and lack of active surveillance led to the persistence of endemic foci in some countries. From 1980, not surprisingly, reports began to appear of an alarming resurgence, notably of yaws and endemic syphilis, particularly in West Africa, Central Africa, and to a lesser extent, south-East Asia and the western Pacific.[7-11] In some parts of the Central African Republic, the pygmy population has been suggested to harbour the main focus of yaws.[12] Sporadic cases were also being reported from some countries in the Americas.[13,14] The geographical distribution of the endemic treponematoses in the early 1990s is shown in Figure 68.1. In some tropical areas, when yaws came under control, venereally acquired syphilis had apparently become more prevalent, possibly because of immunological and sociocultural factors. Thus, both yaws and venereally acquired syphilis were being encountered in these areas, giving rise to diagnostic problems.

In addition to the similarities mentioned above, the endemic treponematoses have some other common characteristics, including non-venereal transmission (mainly in childhood), a predominantly rural distribution associated with poverty, overcrowding, the absence of congenital transmission and the lack of involvement of cardiovascular and central nervous systems. The occasional reports purporting to show evidence of involvement of cardiovascular and central nervous systems have attracted little support, and positive serological tests in the newborn may be due to passive transplacental transfer of IgG. Their differentiation, therefore, at the present time, is dependent on clinical and epidemiological aspects. The incubation period of endemic treponematoses is similar to that of venereal syphilis.

YAWS

Yaws is also known by other names: Framboesia (German), Pian (French), Buba (Spanish), Parangi and Paru (Malay).

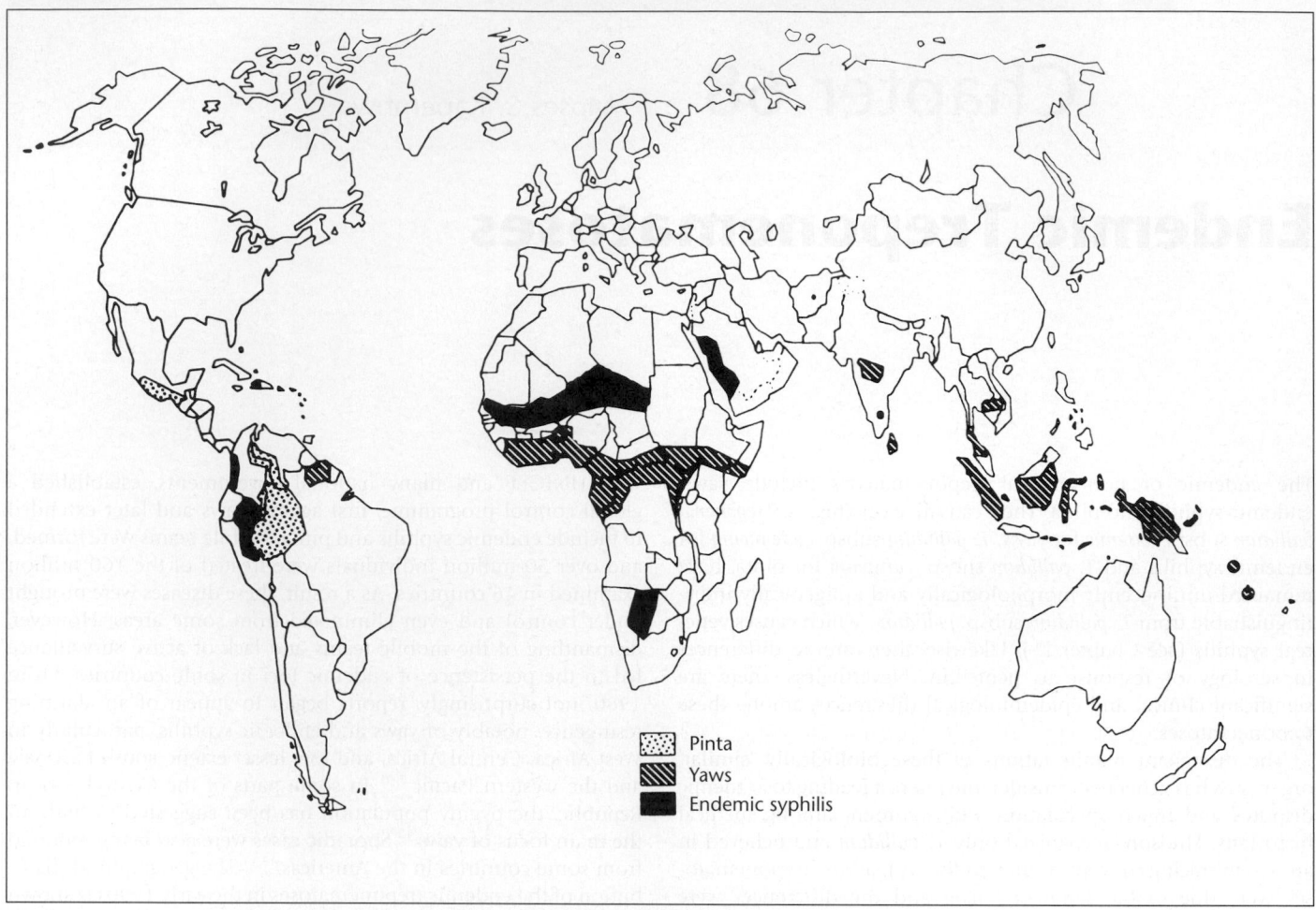

Figure 68.1 Geographical distribution of the endemic treponematoses in the early 1990s. (From *Clinics in Dermatology* 1999; 17:144; courtesy of Dr Herman Jan H. Engelkens.)

Pinta
Yaws
Endemic syphilis

Epidemiology and mode of transmission

Yaws is found in the warm, humid, tropical, predominantly rural areas of Africa, Central and South America, the Caribbean, and equatorial islands of South-east Asia, notably Indonesia and Papua New Guinea, with a limited distribution in some remote parts of India and Thailand. In endemic areas, the prevalence of infectious yaws increases during the rainy season, when skin lesions tend to be more numerous.

Yaws occurs commonly among children aged 2–15 years who live in poor, overcrowded and insanitary conditions. Direct personal skin-to-skin contact is the major route of transmission of yaws. The reproducibility of yaws in humans by inoculation with secretions from patients with framboesia was demonstrated by Paulet in 1848 and by Charlouis in 1881, well before the identification of *T. pertenue* by Castellani in 1905.[15-17] A lack of soap and water, clothes and footwear facilitates the spread of the disease. Infectivity occurs particularly under humid tropical conditions. Indirect transmission of treponemal infection by formites and insects settling on open moist lesions is theoretically possible

but no evidence exists.[18] Sexual transmission does not, as a rule, play a role in endemic treponematoses.

Clinical features

The course of yaws may be divided into early, latent (during which infectious relapses may occur) and late (tertiary) non-infectious stages.

Early stage

Early yaws comprises the primary and secondary stages. After an average incubation period of 21 (range 9–90) days, the initial or primary lesion ('mother yaw') appears at the site of entry of the organisms, usually on the exposed parts of the body, such as the legs, arms, face and neck. The lesion manifests as a round or oval papule, 2–5 cm in diameter, and may develop into a large papilloma (Figure 68.2). Early-stage skin lesions are often itchy, leading to excoriation and ulceration. Such lesions contain numerous treponemes and are, therefore, highly infectious.

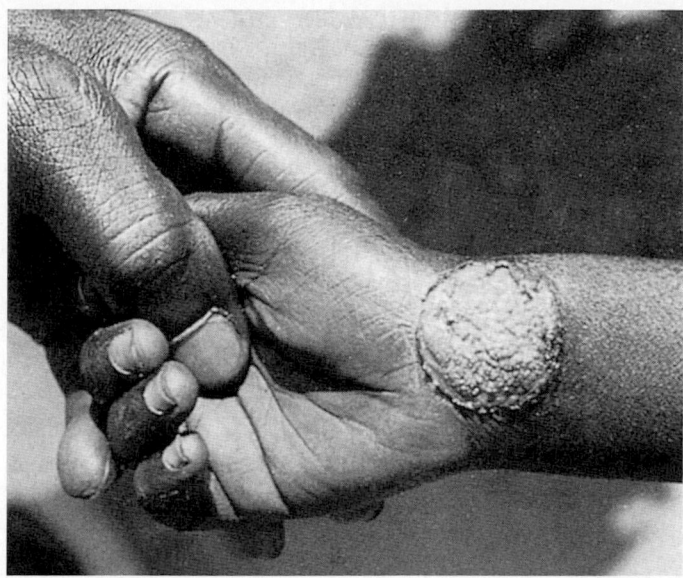

Figure 68.2 Yaws: initial lesion 'mother yaw'. (Courtesy of C. J. Hackett.)

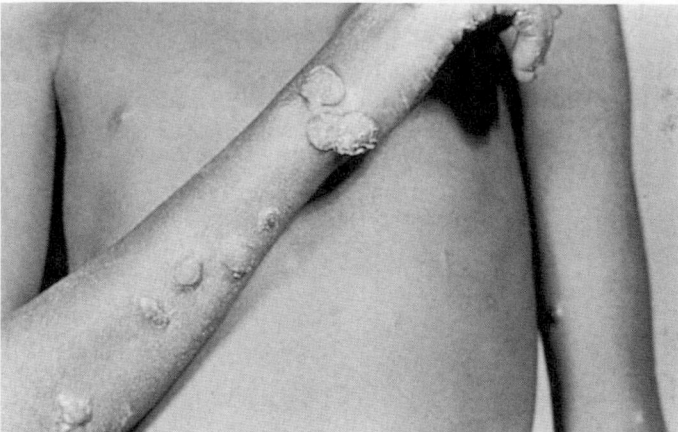

Figure 68.4 Cutaneous early yaws: papillomas on the arm. (Courtesy of C. J. Hackett.)

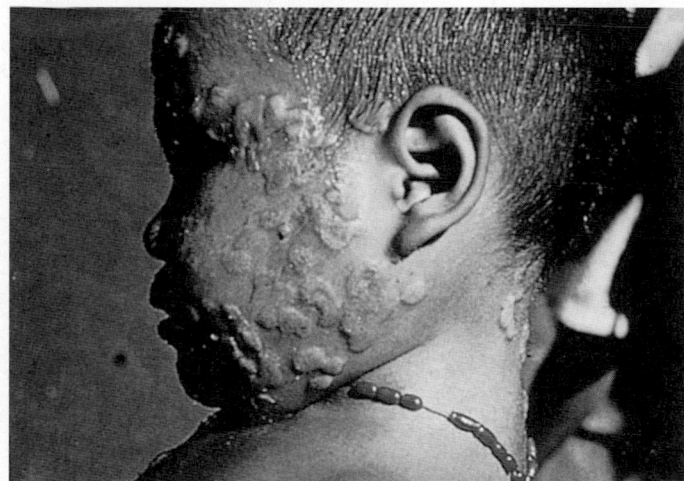

Figure 68.3 Cutaneous early yaws: papillomas. (Courtesy of C. J. Hackett.)

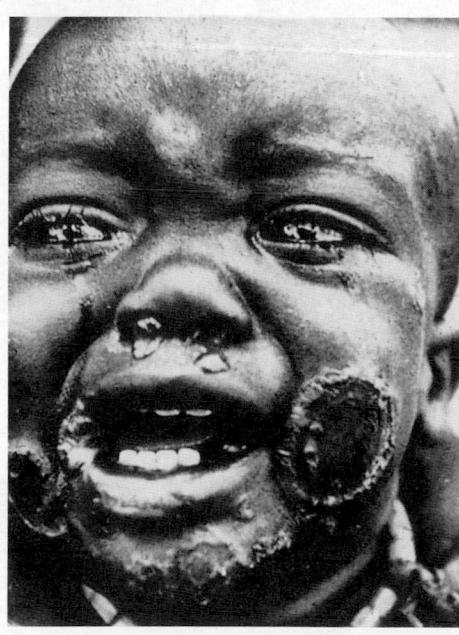

Figure 68.5 Cutaneous early yaws: discoid papillomas. (Courtesy of C. J. Hackett.)

The primary lesion may last for 3–6 months and heal with or without scar formation. Lymphatic spread may lead to lesions in the neighbouring areas, and haematogenous spread of the organisms may produce lesions elsewhere in the body.

Secondary lesions usually appear a few weeks to up to 2 years after the appearance of the primary lesion, and may be preceded or accompanied by fever, arthralgia, malaise and generalized lymphadenopathy. The skin manifestations resemble the initial lesion but are more disseminated. They may become crusted and removal of the yellow crust reveals raspberry granulomas (framboesides) (Figures 68.3, 68.4). Annular, discoid (Figure 68.5), crescentic or irregularly shaped papules and nodules can also be seen. The palms of the hand and soles of feet show hyperkeratotic plaques. Plantar papillomas, in particular, take longer to erupt than those elsewhere on the skin and may make walking painful, resulting in a sideways 'crab-like' gait (crab yaws) (Figure 68.6). Lesions occurring on the moist areas of the body or at the mucocutaneous junctions may resemble the condylomata lata of syphilis. The secondary lesions, which tend to occur in crops, may last for up to 6 months and heal without any scars, except when ulcerated and secondarily infected.

Bone involvement is manifested by osteitis and periostitis; the affected bones are painful (worse at night) and tender. Dactylitis

(i.e. osteoperiostitis of the proximal phalanges of the fingers; Figure 68.7) and swelling of the ulna, as well as involvement of the long bones of the legs, are common in children. Plain radiography is usually sufficient to identify early bone changes.[19] In very rare cases, there is hypertrophic osteitis of the nasal process of the maxillae, giving rise to the swellings on both sides of the bridge of the nose, called goundou (Figure 68.8). In untreated cases, the swellings may grow and obstruct the nostrils.

Attenuated yaws is a milder clinical presentation that is recognized in areas of low prevalence, comprising transient, dry, flat cutaneous lesions confined to intertriginous areas of the body.[20]

Latent stage

The disease may then progress to latency, resulting eventually in spontaneous cure or persistent latency. Serological tests may remain positive, usually at low titres. An estimated 10% of patients develop late lesions after 5 or more years of untreated infection.

Late stage

Late stage yaws is characterized by necrotic destructive lesions of the skin (Figure 68.9), gummatous lesions of the bones (Figure 68.10) and overlying tissues resulting in varying degrees of scarring and deformity. These lesions are similar to those of venereal syphilis (Chapter 21). The late manifestations include: hyper-

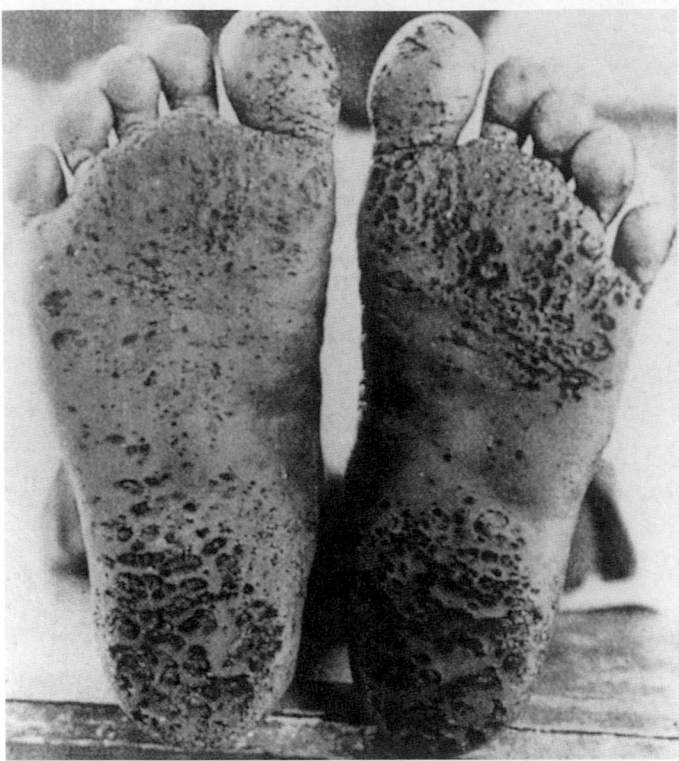

Figure 68.6 Indeterminate yaws: plantar hyperkeratosis (crab yaws).

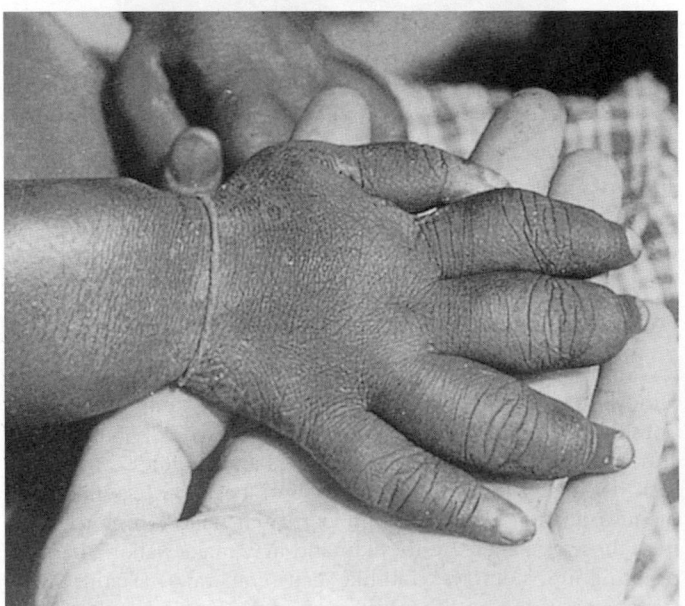

Figure 68.7 Early yaws: polydactylitis.

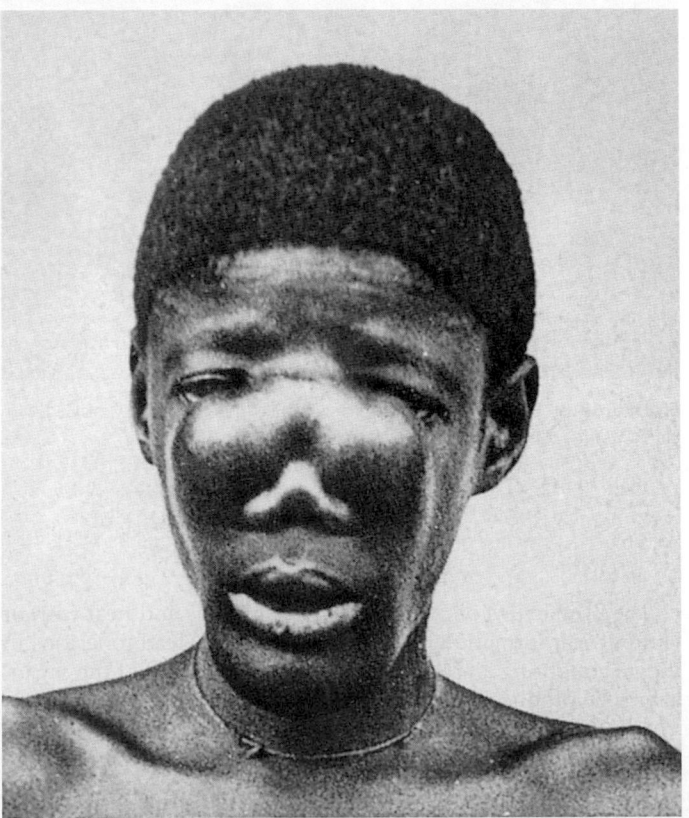

Figure 68.8 Early yaws: goundou. (Courtesy of C. J. Hackett.)

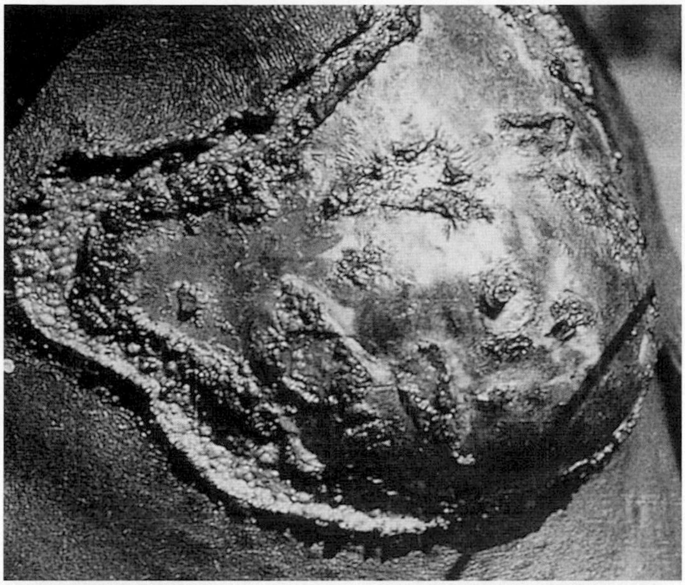

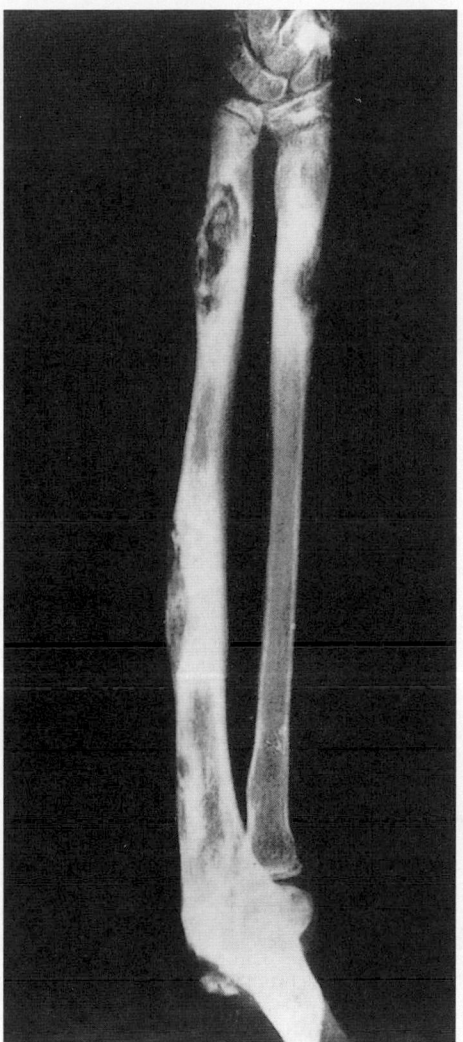

Figure 68.9 Late yaws: gumma of the right breast. (Courtesy of C. J. Hackett.)

Figure 68.10 Late yaws: gummatous osteitis of radius and ulna. (Courtesy of C. J. Hackett.)

keratosis of palms and soles with deep fissuring; juxta-articular subcutaneous fibrous nodules around the elbows and knees; bursitis (Figure 68.11); disfiguring lesions of the nasopharynx (rhinopharyngitis mutilans or gangosa) (Figure 68.12) as a result of ulceration of the palate or nasal septum progressing to perforation of the turbinates and pharynx; offensive discharge. In addition, hypertrophic osteoperiostitis gives rise to bowing of the tibia (sabre tibia, Figure 68.13). Hyperkeratosis of palms and soles (see Figure 68.6) and goundou (see Figure 68.8) tend to be more pronounced in late yaws. The former may be accompanied by fissures and may be very painful. Eventually, there may be scarring and disfiguration of the hands and feet.

Congenital transmission does not occur, and the cardiovascular and nervous systems are considered not to be affected. However, in one study, ocular and neurological abnormalities were noted in patients presumed to be suffering from late yaws.[21] Other indirect evidence of yaws causing idiopathic myeloneuropathy has led to suggestions that the potential sequelae of yaws are identical to those of venereal syphilis.[22]

Histopathology

In early yaws, papillomatous epidermal hyperplasia is the main feature and treponemes can be demonstrated in specimens stained by silver impregnation technique[23] or immunofluorescence.[24] It is generally believed that the basic pathology in yaws is the same as that in venereal syphilis. However, in yaws, endothelial proliferation seems to be much less marked; obliterative changes in the vessels are not encountered and acanthosis is more prominent.[23]

Studies have been carried out to localize treponemes and characterize inflammatory infiltrate in skin biopsies from patients with early venereal syphilis and early infectious yaws.[25] Treponemes in yaws cases (from West Sumatra) were found to be mostly, but not exclusively, confined to the epidermis as opposed to early venereal

syphilis lesions – in which the organisms were demonstrated largely in the dermal-epidermal junction as well as in the dermis. Using specific monoclonal antibodies, these same authors were also struck by the paucity of T and B lymphocytes in yaws specimens.

Diagnosis and differential diagnoses

Dark-field examination of exudates from primary and secondary skin lesions will reveal motile treponemes which must be differentiated from saprophytic spirochaetes. Serological tests behave as in the case of venereal syphilis (Chapter 21).

Clinical diagnosis of yaws in the presence of classical lesions is straightforward in endemic areas, but differentiation from endemic syphilis may occasionally be difficult. The common skin conditions to be differentiated include chronic scabies, verrucae, fungal infections, impetigo, lichen planus, sarcoidosis, psoriasis, eczema and tungiasis. Gummatous lesions should be differentiated from: tropical ulcer, fungating mycotic lesions, cutaneous leishmaniasis,

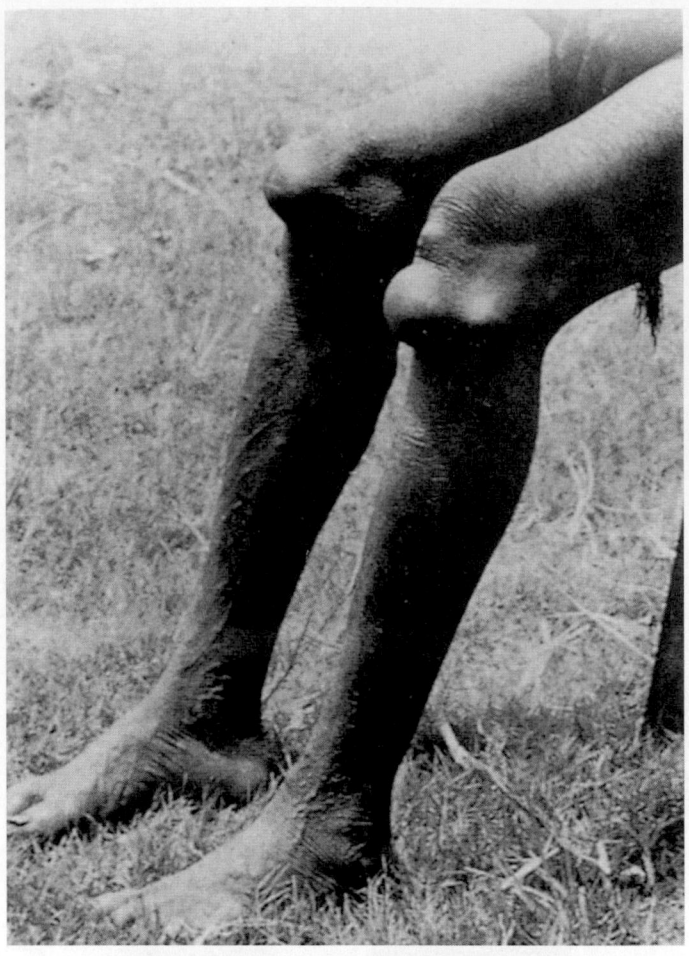

Figure 68.11 Late yaws: chronic bilateral prepatellar bursitis.

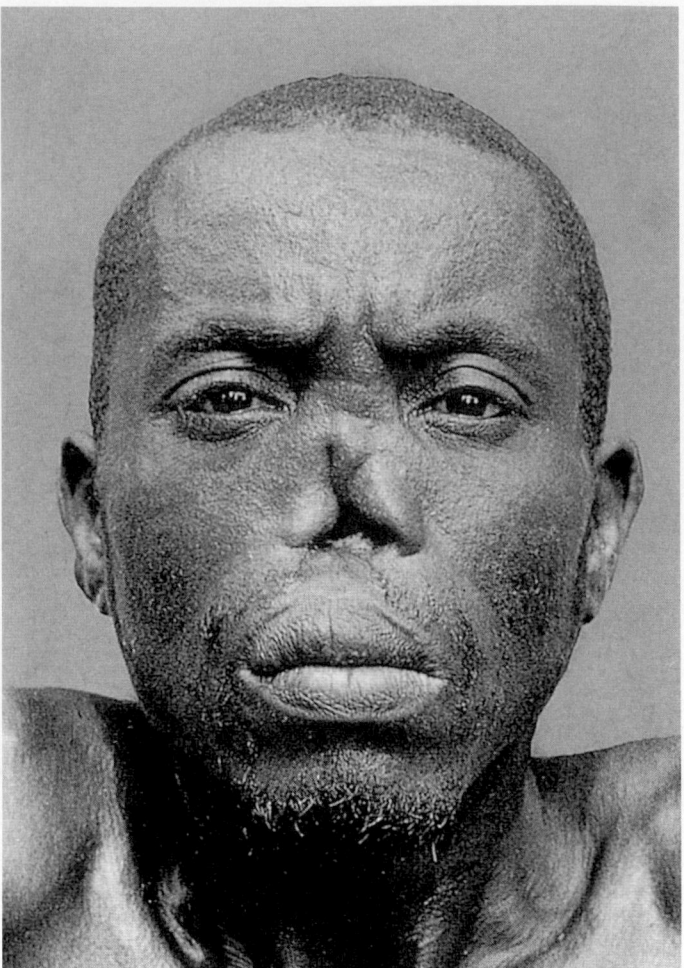

Figure 68.12 Late yaws: gangosa. (Courtesy of C. J. Hackett.)

leprosy, neoplasm(s) and possibly other conditions. Juxta-articular nodules of onchocerciasis and dactylitis of tuberculosis and sickle cell disease should be distinguished by appropriate tests. Radiography will demonstrate bone lesions but these may be identical to those of venereal and endemic syphilis.

If differentiation from venereal syphilis is difficult, especially in latent cases – as may happen when an immigrant presents at a clinic in a country with a temperate climate and the adequacy of any previous treatment is in doubt – the person should be treated as for syphilis. However, in view of the social implications, special care should be taken in communicating the diagnosis to the patient, who should be given a full explanation.

Management and control

See later in this chapter.

ENDEMIC SYPHILIS

Epidemiology and mode of transmission

Endemic syphilis, also known as Bejel, Firjal, Loath, Njovera, Dichuchwa, Siti, is a chronic childhood infection of skin, bone and cartilage. The disease is endemic in the arid Sahelian areas of West Africa, with foci also in Zimbabwe (Njovera) and Botswana (Dichuchwa), and to a lesser extent among the nomadic people in the Arabian Peninsula and the aborigines of central Australia. The disease primarily affects people in poor rural communities living in unhygienic and overcrowded conditions. The majority of early cases are found in children aged 2–15 years, who are the main reservoir of infection. The initial lesion is usually on the oral mucosa and transmission is by direct contact through kissing or by indirect contact through eating and drinking utensils. The infection spreads easily among family groups from infected children to other children and previously uninfected adults. The role of flies acting as vectors remains unproven. There is no proof that congenital transmission occurs in endemic syphilis.

Clinical features

A primary lesion is rarely present in endemic syphilis. The earliest lesions encountered are the mucous patches which are shallow painless ulcers on the lips (Figure 68.14) and in the oropharynx. The latter may give rise to sore throat and hoarseness of the voice due to laryngitis. Other early manifestations of the disease are

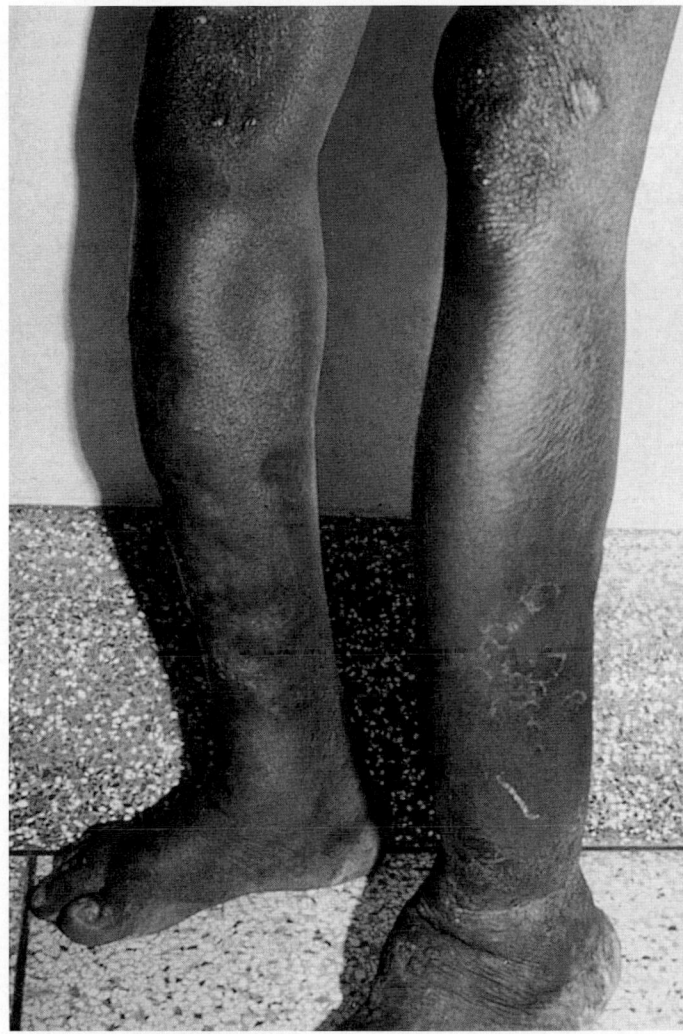

Figure 68.13 Late yaws: sabre tibia. (Reproduced with permission from Arya OP, Osoba AO, Bennett FJ, eds *Tropical Venereology*. 2nd edn. Edinburgh: Churchill Livingstone; 1988:138.)

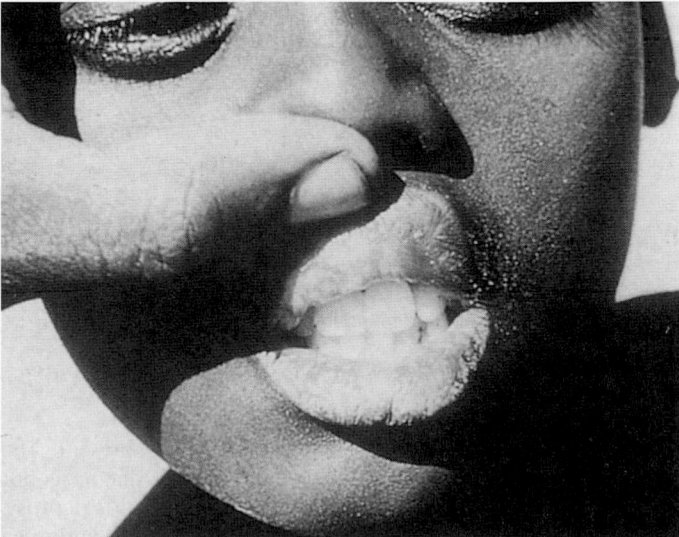

Figure 68.14 Early endemic syphilis: mucous papules on the buccal surface of the upper lip.

osteoperiostitis of the long bones causing nocturnal bone pains as in yaws, condylomata lata occurring in the moist areas of the body (e.g. anogenital area; Figure 68.15), axillae, angular stomatitis and split papules including, occasionally, a generalized maculopapular and other forms of rash, as in venereal syphilis. Generalized lymph gland enlargement may also be encountered.

In untreated patients, the early lesions tend to undergo healing with or without scarring, and the patient passes into the latent phase of the disease. Secondary relapses are uncommon. The period of latency is usually prolonged, after which some patients develop late lesions, such as osteoperiostitis and gummatous lesions. These result in ulceration and destruction of the skin and bones. As in yaws, destruction of the maxilla, palate and nasal bones results in gangosa. Severe plantar and palmar keratosis may be encountered, with ulceration and disability. Juxta-articular nodules also occur. There is, as yet, no convincing evidence of the involvement of cardiovascular and nervous systems in endemic syphilis. One report described ocular manifestations in 17 patients (age range 37–73 years) with clinical findings consistent with bejel.[26]

As with attenuated yaws, a seemingly less virulent form of bejel has been reported in Saudi Arabia and attributed to improved nutrition and hygiene.[27]

Diagnosis and differential diagnosis

These are essentially the same as those for yaws.

Management and control

See later in this chapter.

PINTA

Epidemiology and mode of transmission

Pinta, also referred to as Azul, Carate, Mal De Pinto is the mildest of the non-venereal treponematoses and occupies a unique position in having principally skin manifestations. The disease is confined to the underdeveloped rural areas of northern South America, namely, the western area of Brazil, Columbia, Bolivia[28,29] and Mexico in the states of Oaxaca, Guerrero, Michoacan and Chiapas.[30] However, there is a paucity of data with regard to the current prevalence of pinta.

The infection is acquired in childhood or early adolescence among people living in unhygienic conditions. Those aged 15–30 years with long-standing skin lesions comprise the main reservoir. Treponemes persist in these lesions for many years. The lesions tend to be dry but are itchy, and scratching may release serum with abundant treponemes. Transmission, as in the case of yaws, is believed to be by direct lesion-to-skin contact, facilitated by a breach in the recipient's skin. As in the case of other treponematoses, the role of flies in the transmission of pinta remains uncertain.

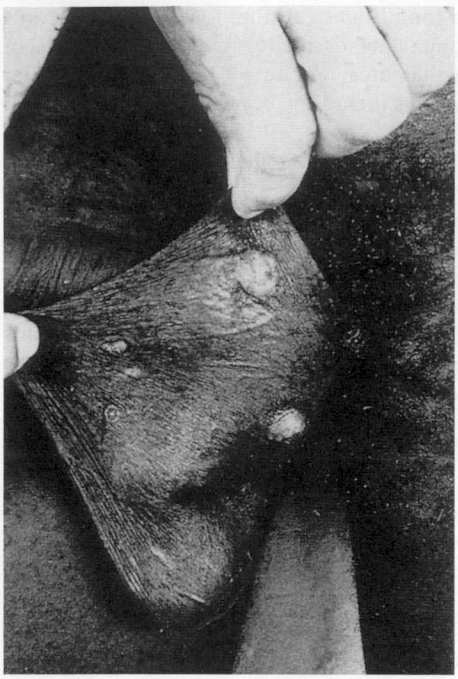

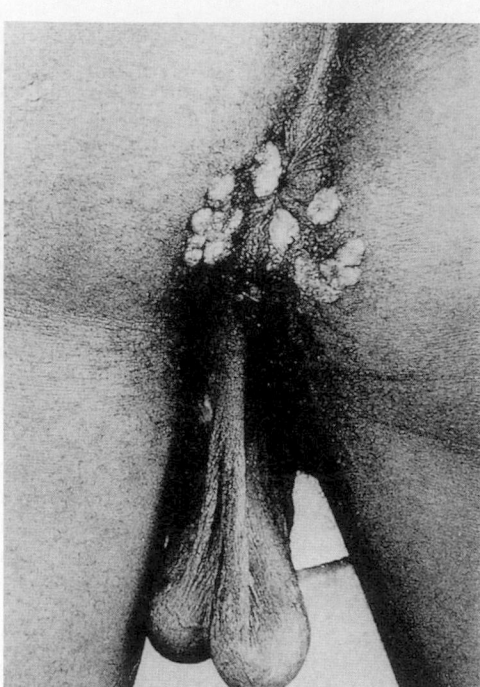

A   B

Figure 68.15 Early endemic syphilis: moist papules involving the (A) scrotum and (B) anus. (Courtesy of P. D. Marsden.)

Clinical features

The primary lesion appears at the site of entry of the organisms, usually located on the exposed parts of the body such as arms, legs or face. It starts as an erythemato-squamous papule which enlarges slowly and is accompanied by satellite lesions. The initial lesion may become pigmented, hyperkeratotic and scaly. The regional lymph nodes are enlarged and painless.

The secondary stage develops several months after the initial lesion, with the appearance of more extensive, often smaller, plaques either around the primary lesion or disseminated to other areas. These 'pintids' are painless but itchy. They undergo a variety of colour change(s) from red to copper colour, lead-grey and bluish-black. Such lesions, which may remain present for years or reappear in recurrences, are to be found anywhere on the body.

The late lesions are characterized by varying degrees of pigmentary changes, hypochromia and atrophy around dyschromic lesions (Figure 68.16). Hyperkeratosis of the palms and soles, including juxta-articular nodes, is occasionally encountered. However, some experts dispute this and consider that these patients may in fact be suffering from yaws. Leucoderma is the main complication and this may result in social stigmas. There is no reliable evidence of systemic involvement.

Diagnosis and differential diagnosis

Diagnostic tests are the same as those for other endemic treponematoses, i.e. dark-field examination of the material from the early lesions and serological tests. The histopathological picture is largely similar to that of yaws. In addition, the basal cells show loss of melanin and many melanophages may be present in the dermis.[31] A moderate dermal inflammatory infiltrate consisting

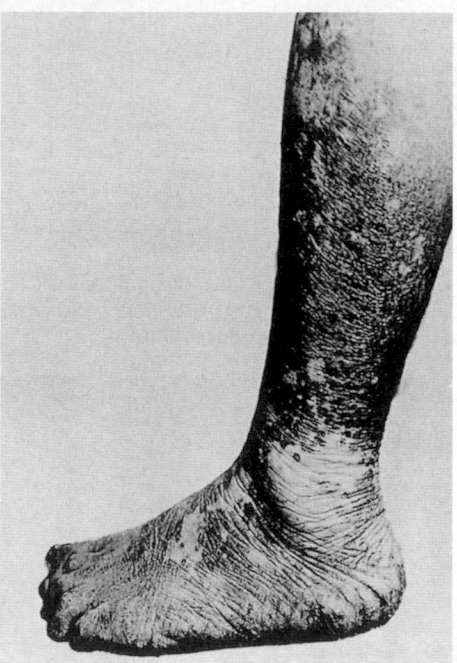

Figure 68.16 Late pinta: depigmentation of the lower leg. (Courtesy of L. A. Leon.)

mainly of plasma cells and lymphocytes may be present. The characteristic colour changes provide a clue to the diagnosis but other conditions, such as vitiligo, pityriasis versicolor, leprosy, discoid lupus erythematosus, chronic pellagra, psoriasis and tinea corporis should be excluded.

HUMAN IMMUNODEFICIENCY VIRUS INFECTION AND ENDEMIC TREPONEMATOSES

No information is at present available on the relationship between human immunodeficiency virus (HIV) infection and endemic treponematoses. However, immunological abnormalities associated with HIV infection have been reported to alter the course of syphilis, albeit in a minority of patients. These abnormalities may reactivate latent infection, decrease the latent period before onset of neurosyphilis, increase the severity of manifestations, alter serological responses and render conventional therapy inadequate.[32-34] It is highly likely that HIV infection will have similar influences on endemic treponematoses. The modified clinical manifestations and serological responses may cause difficulties in diagnosis.

Ulcerative lesions caused by syphilis are believed to facilitate HIV transmission. Likewise, yaws lesions may also enhance the risk of acquiring and transmitting HIV.

MANAGEMENT OF ENDEMIC TREPONEMATOSES

A long-acting penicillin preparation is the drug of choice. Benzathine penicillin G is given as a single intramuscular injection in the upper outer quadrant of the buttock. The dose is 600 000 units for children and contacts under 6 years of age, 1.2 million units for those aged 6–15 years, and 2.4 million units for adults.

Treatment in the early stage(s) will result in cure and complete resolution of manifestations but will not reverse the damage caused by late stage disease. The lesions become non-infectious within 24 h after administration of the antibiotic.

Erythromycin or tetracycline, 500 mg by mouth four times daily for 15 days is recommended for those allergic to penicillin. Children between the ages of 8 and 15 years should receive half that dose. Tetracycline should not be given to pregnant women or to children below 12 years of age.

Follow-up

After adequate treatment, in the great majority of patients, non-treponemal tests, namely the rapid plasma reagin (RPR) or Venereal Disease Research Laboratory (VDRL) test, titres either decline or become negative in due course. However, in a minority of patients, especially if treated in the late stages, these tests may remain positive at low titre (below 1 : 8). This is not an indication for further treatment. The specific tests such as *T. pallidum* haemagglutination (TPHA) or fluorescent treponemal antibody absorption (FTA-ABS), which remain reactive throughout life, play no part in assessment of the adequacy of treatment.

CONTROL OF ENDEMIC TREPONEMATOSES

Following the successful mass detection and treatment campaigns of the 1950s and 1960s, surveillance for the endemic treponematoses diminished and a resurgence of yaws has now been documented in Papua New Guinea and Guyana.[35,36] Millions of people are again at risk of contracting these infections due to the ever increasing frequency of worldwide travel, migration and poverty in the developing world. Development of a treponemal vaccine in the foreseeable future and the prospect of eradication of the non-venereal treponematoses seem unlikely. The main method of control will, therefore, lie in identification and treatment of infectious cases, including treatment of immediate contacts. Despite isolated reports of apparent treatment failure, there is no evidence of emergence of penicillin-resistant treponemes. However, this situation could change at any time; hence, the control of endemic treponematoses should be a priority. The principal intervention strategies for control include clinical surveillance (requiring dark-field microscopy and RPR or VDRL tests) to detect cases of infection, detection of latent disease using serological tests and effective mass treatment programmes.

The treatment policies recommended by the World Health Organization[37] are as follows:

1. If the prevalence of clinically active infection in the community is over 10%, give benzathine penicillin G to the entire population.
2. If the prevalence of clinically active cases is 5–10%, give benzathine penicillin G to the patients, their contacts and to all children below the age of 15 years.
3. If the prevalence of clinically active infection is under 5%, treat all active cases as well as household and other obvious contacts with benzathine penicillin G.

Economic considerations may necessitate integration of treponematosis control activities into other public health programmes including health education.

The standards of living and personal and environmental hygiene must be improved. Sustained surveillance, integrated into strengthened primary healthcare, must be maintained to detect and treat new or missed cases including their contacts, and treatment failures.

REFERENCES

1. Hudson EH. *Non-venereal Syphilis. A Sociological and Medical Study of Bejel.* Edinburgh: Livingstone; 1958.
2. Hackett CJ. On the origin of the human treponematoses. *Bull WHO* 1963; 29:7–41.
3. Norris SJ. Polypeptides of Treponema pallidum: progress toward understanding their structure, functional and immunologic roles. Treponema Pallidum – Polypeptide Research Group. *Microb Rev* 1993; 57:750–779.
4. Noordhoek GT, Hermans PWM, Paul AN, et al. Treponema pallidum subspecies pallidum (Nichols) and Treponema pallidum subspecies pertenue (CDC 2575) differ in at least one nucleotide: comparison of two homologous antigens. *Microb Pathog* 1989; 6:29–42.
5. Turner TB, Hollander DH. *Biology of the Treponematoses.* WHO Monograph Series, No. 35. Geneva: World Health Organization; 1957.
6. Fribourg-Blanc A, Mollaret HH. Natural treponematoses of the African primate. *Primates Med* 1969; 3:113–121.
7. Editorial. Yaws again. *BMJ* 1980; 281:1090.
8. Editorial. Endemic treponematoses in the 1980s. *Lancet* 1983; ii:551–552.
9. Agadzi VK, Aboagye-Atta Y, Nelson JW, et al. Resurgence of yaws in Ghana. *Lancet* 1983; ii:389–390.

10. Proceedings of inter-regional meeting on yaws and other endemic treponematoses, Cipanas, Indonesia, 22–24 July 1985. *Southeast Asian J Trop Med Public Health* 1986; 17(suppl 4):1–96.

11. Noordhoek GT, Engelkens HJ, Judanarso J, et al. Yaws in West Sumatra, Indonesia: clinical manifestations, serological findings and characterisation of new Treponema isolates by DNA probes. *Eur J Clin Microb Infect Dis* 1991; 10:12–19.

12. Herve V, Kassa Kelembho E, Normand P, et al. Resurgence of yaws in Central African Republic. Role of the pygmy population as a reservoir of the virus. *Bull Soc Pathol Exot* 1992; 85:342–346.

13. St John RK. Yaws in the Americas. *Rev Infect Dis* 1985; 7(suppl 2):266–272.

14. Guderian RH, Guzman JR, Calvopina M, et al. Studies on a focus of yaws in the Santiago Basin, Province of Esmeraldas, Ecuador. *Trop Geogr Med* 1991; 43:142–147.

15. Paulet P. Memoire sur le yaws, pian ou framboesia; de son traitement, et des moyens de faire disparaitre cette maladie des contrees ou elle sevit. *Arch Gen Med* 1848; 17:385–405.

16. Charlouis M. Ueber Polypapilloma tropicum (Framboesia). *Vierteljahrsschrift fur Dermatologie und Syphilis* 1881; 8:431–466.

17. Castellani A. On the presence of Spirochaeteae in two cases of ulcerated parangi (yaws). *J Trop Med* 1905; 8:253.

18. Goncalves AP, Basset A, Maleville J. Tropical treponematoses. In: Canizares O, Harman RRM, eds *Clinical Tropical Dermatology*. 2nd edn. Oxford: Blackwell Scientific; 1992:129–150.

19. Engelkens HJH, Ginai AZ, Judanarso J, et al. Radiological and dermatological findings in 2 patients suffering from early yaws in Indonesia. *Genitourin Med* 1990; 66:259–263.

20. Vorst FA. Clinical diagnoses and changing manifestations of treponemal infection. *Rev Infect Dis* 1985; 7:S327–S331.

21. Lawton Smith J, David NJ, Indgin S, et al. Neuro-ophthalmological study of late yaws and pinta: II. The Caracas project. *Br J Vener Dis* 1971; 47:226–251.

22. Román GC, Román LN. Occurrence of congenital cardiovascular, visceral, neurologic, and neuro-ophthalmologic complication in late yaws; a theme for future research. *Rev Infect Dis* 1986; 8:760–770.

23. Engelkens HJH, Vuzevski VD, Judanaso J, et al. Early yaws; a light microscopic study. *Genitourin Med* 1990; 66:264–266.

24. Lever WF, Schaumburg-Lever G. Treponemal diseases. In: Lever WF, Schaumburg-Lever G, eds. *Histopathology of the Skin*. 7th edn. Philadelphia: JB Lippincott; 1992:353–359.

25. Engelkens HJH, ten Kate FJW, Judanarso J, et al. The localisation of treponemes and characterization of the inflammatory infiltrate in skin biopsies from patients with primary or secondary syphilis, or early infectious yaws. *Genitourin Med* 1993; 69:102–107.

26. Tabbara KF, Al Kaff AS, Fadel T. Ocular manifestations of endemic syphilis (bejel). *Ophthalmology* 1989; 96:1087–1091.

27. Pace JL, Csonka GW. Endemic non-venereal syphilis (bejel) in Saudi Arabia. *Br J Vener Dis* 1984; 60:293–297.

28. Hopkins DR, Florez D. Pinta, yaws, and venereal syphilis in Columbia. *Int J Epidemiol* 1977; 6:349–355.

29. Pecher SA. Immunologia da pinta terciaria. *Med Cutan Ibero Lat Am* 1988; 16:111–114.

30. Meheus A, Antal GM. The endemic treponematoses: not yet eradicated. *World Health Stat Q* 1992; 45:228–237.

31. Marquez F. Pinta. In: Canizares O, ed. *Clinical Tropical Dermatology*. Oxford: Blackwell Scientific; 1975:86–92.

32. Johns DR, Tierney M, Felsenstein D. Alterations in the natural history of neurosyphilis by concurrent infection with the human immunodeficiency virus. *N Engl J Med* 1987; 316:1569–1572.

33. Hicks CB, Benson PM, Lupton GP, et al. Seronegative secondary syphilis in a patient infected with the human immunodeficiency virus (HIV) with Kaposi sarcoma: a diagnostic dilemma. *Ann Intern Med* 1987; 107:492–495.

34. Musher DM, Hamill RJ, Baughn RE. Effect of human immunodeficiency virus (HIV) infection on the course of syphilis and on the response to treatment (review). *Ann Intern Med* 1990; 113:872–881.

35. Manning LA, Ogle GD. Yaws in the periurban settlements of Port Moresby, Papua New Guinea. *P N G Med J* 2002; 45:206–212.

36. Scolnik D, Aronson L, Lovinsky R, et al. Efficacy of a targeted, oral penicillin-based yaws control programme among children living in rural South America. *Clin Infect Dis* 2003; 36:1232–1238

37. World Health Organization. Treponemal infections. *World Health Organ Tech Rep Ser* 1982; 674:16–20.

GENERAL READING

Perine PL, Hopkins DR, Niemel PLA, et al. *Handbook of Endemic Treponematoses: Yaws, Endemic Syphilis and Pinta*. Geneva: World Health Organization; 1984.

Antal GM, Lukehart SA, Meheus AZ. The endemic treponematoses. *Microbes Infect* 2004; 4:83–94.

Farnsworth N, Rosen T. Endemic treponematoses: review and update. *Clin Dermatol* 2006; 24:181–190.

Chapter 69

Gordon C. Cook

Other Spirochaetal Diseases (excluding *Treponema* spp. and *Leptospira* spp.)

There are several examples of tick-borne diseases of *Homo sapiens*;[1,2] the most topical at present is Lyme disease.

LYME DISEASE

This consists of a tick-borne zoonosis (in its natural cycle, rodents and hard ticks of the *Ixodes ricinus* complex are involved) caused by *Borrelia burgdorferi*;[3–5] clinical manifestations can be divided into acute and chronic forms involving the skin, joints, nervous system, and pericardium, endocardium and myocardium. Deer and other mammals form a reservoir of infection.

History

The disease was first described in the mid-1970s in the USA, following an outbreak in children at Lyme, Connecticut. However, it occurs throughout much of the Northern Hemisphere and is the most common 'tick-borne' diseases are seen in Europe, Russia and, to a lesser extent, Asia (especially South-east Asia). Suspected but unsubstantiated cases of Lyme borreliosis have been documented in sub-Saharan Africa, South America and Australia. Since 1980, several outbreaks have occurred in the eastern USA, and circumstantial evidence suggests that the infection is becoming more common in both northern America and Europe, although it is impossible to exclude increased awareness and greater recognition.

Aetiology

The spirochaetes were first identified in the mid-gut of the adult black-legged tick *Ixodes scapularis* (Figure 69.1). They were subsequently isolated from blood, skin and cerebrospinal fluid (CSF) of patients with early Lyme disease.

B. burgdorferi was taxonomically described in 1984; it is a flagellated, helical, spirochaetal bacterium. Surface membrane proteins are specific for individual strains; a prominent 41 kDa antigen is located on the flagellum. Arthropathy is more common with the predominant strain in North America, and cutaneous and neurological complications with the European and Asian strains.

Humans are incidental hosts of *B. burgdorferi* and are usually infected in late spring and early summer. The ticks responsible for this infection require a shady environment of high humidity, and ready access to appropriate vertebrate hosts. These vary enormously – from the white-footed mouse in coastal north-eastern USA, the chipmunk (in the eastern USA), to deer in much of Europe and Asia. Transmission of *B. burgdorferi* to *Homo sapiens* is via saliva of feeding ticks. There is no person-to-person transmission, although there is some evidence of transplacental infection. The organism can survive for long periods in stored blood, although transfusion-acquired infection has not been recorded.

Pathology

Lyme disease consists of an inflammatory process with non-specific histological changes; the causative agent is extremely sparse in infected tissue and is difficult to identify, even in silver-stained sections. The most striking histological changes are in joints, in both the acute and chronic stages. There is very little information on neuropathological changes histologically.

B. burgdorferi has been isolated from the myocardium of a patient with a long-standing cardiomyopathy; the organism has also been documented in the myocardium of a patient who suffered from both Lyme disease and babesiosis.

Clinical features

Lyme disease can affect all age groups of both sexes,[6] but the highest rates have been recorded in children aged less than 15 years and in adults aged 40 years or more.

The portal of entry is the dermis; following inoculation by the infected tick, spread of infection is via cutaneous, lymphatic or haematogenous routes. The incubation period is typically 7 to 14 days, but may be as short as 3 days or as long as 30 days. Early infection is either localized or disseminated: the former consists of a slowly expanding, annular, erythematous rash (Figure 69.2) (which is not always remembered by the patient), and, in the latter, the skin, nervous system, musculoskeletal system and/or heart are involved. Late disseminated infection occurs weeks or months after initial infection, assuming the patient has not

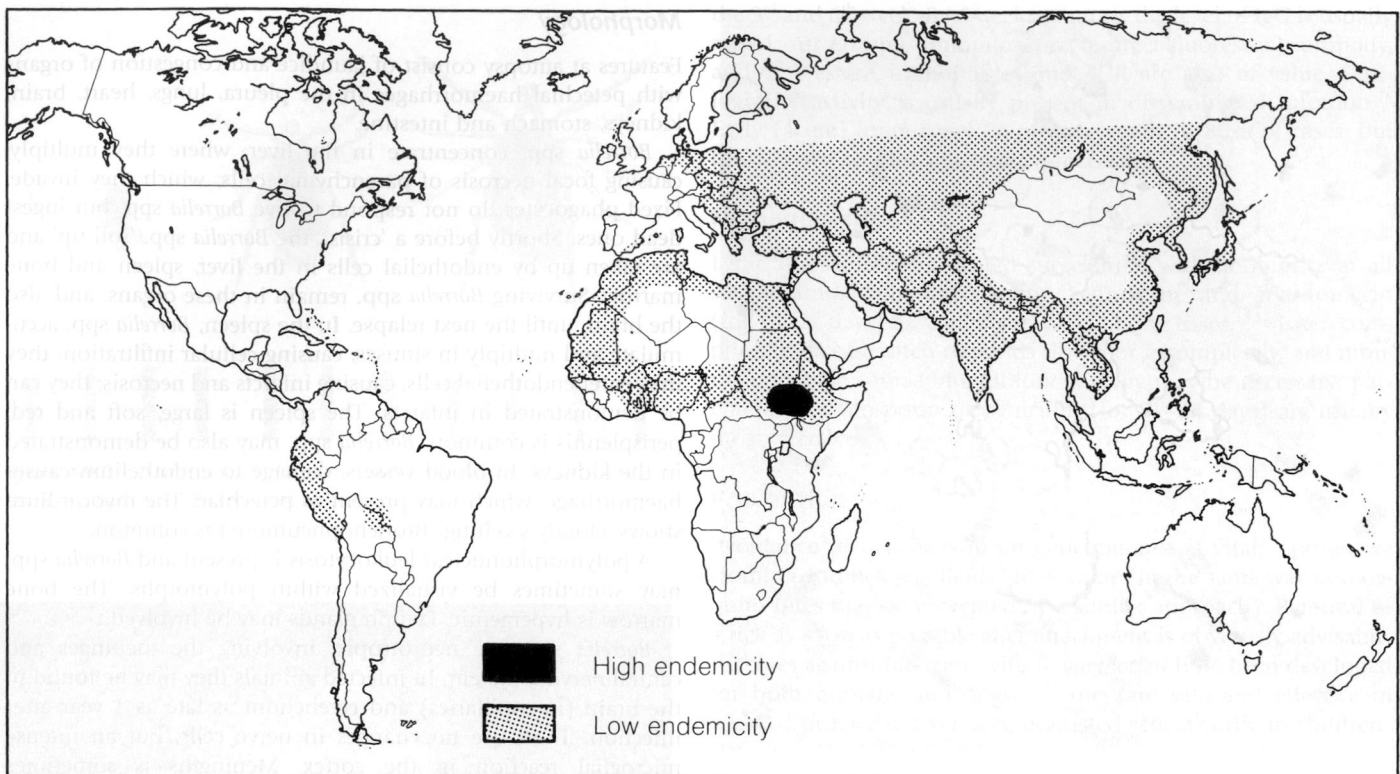

Figure 69.4 Geographical distribution of louse-borne relapsing fever (*Borrelia recurrentis*). (Courtesy of the Department of Entomology, London School of Hygiene and Tropical Medicine.)

Transmission

Louse transmission

Homo sapiens constitutes the only known mammalian host, and the disease is transmitted from person to person by the body (*Pediculus humanus* var. corporis) and head (*P. h.* var. capitis) louse. Lice can be infected only by feeding on blood during a pyrexial episode. Spirochaetes are taken into the stomach and disappear from there in 24 hours at 28°C; they cannot be detected again until 6 days later, when they appear in the body cavity (haemocoele), where they increase rapidly in numbers to involve all organs, except the ovaries, salivary glands and intestinal tract. The louse remains unaffected; spirochaetes can escape only by injury to the body or limbs. Lice are not infective until 6 days after a feed, and humans are infected by crushing lice on the skin – not by a bite. There is no transovarian transmission.

Congenital transmission

Transplacental transmission and abortion are not uncommon.

Transmission by blood transfusion

This has been recorded, albeit rarely.

Clinical features

Natural history

Louse-borne relapsing fever can manifest as a severe disease, consisting of a febrile illness characterized by a primary attack of fever, followed by up to four relapses. There is a great variation in the degree of severity, varying from an asymptomatic parasitaemia to a severe febrile illness with death resulting from hepatic or cardiac failure. In some epidemics, a mortality rate of 70% or more has been recorded.

Incubation period

This is 2–10 (usually 4–8) days.

Symptoms and signs

Onset is sudden, with chills and fever (temperature rises rapidly to 40.5°C or even higher) and the patient may become delirious.[25,26] The patient sits or lies on the bed or ground, silent, with a glazed expression and apathetic manner, and is mentally dull or confused. There is associated dizziness, severe headache,[25,26] and pain in the back, chest, abdomen, legs (especially the calves) and joints. Nausea, vomiting and dysphagia are common. Dyspnoea is often present; it is loud and hissing, and can be heard for some distance away from the patient; the diagnosis may be suspected from a distance. Cough is common; the sputum may contain *Borrelia* spp. The spleen becomes enlarged,[25] occasionally to such a degree that spontaneous rupture occurs. Hepatomegaly is present; jaundice is common. Bleeding often occurs into the skin (petechial rash),[25] over the flanks and shoulders, and into mucous membranes; epistaxis is common. During a first attack, an erythematous rash may appear over the upper part of the body, resembling that of typhoid fever (see Chapter 52). Conjunctival vessels are congested and may bleed (clumps of adherent *Borrelia* spp. become impacted in capillaries, where they enmesh red cells, causing capillary rupture followed by haemorrhage). There may be widespread intravascular coagulation. Heavy albuminuria is usually present.

Fever lasts for 5–7 days; temperature falls by crisis to 36°C or even lower (when there may be a state of collapse) and is accompanied by profuse sweating, diarrhoea, weakness and relief from associated symptoms. Rarely, the infection presents as a febrile illness in travellers; one such case occurred in a French patient returning from Mali.[29] Tick-borne relapsing fever has been misdiagnosed as malaria in Swedish travellers returning from Togo.[30]

Relapse occurs 5–9 days after the first attack in two-thirds of patients (Figure 69.5); it is less severe and there is no rash. A second relapse occurs in one-quarter of those infected, but more than four relapses are exceedingly unusual.

Liver function tests reflect extensive hepatocellular dysfunction.[25] Anaemia is present and a marked polymorphonuclear leukocytosis (15–30 × 10⁹/L) is apparent on a peripheral blood film. CSF pressure is often raised; a lymphocytic pleocytosis is common and *Borrelia* spp. may be present.

Complications

Complications include pneumonia (of lobar distribution),[24,25] which may be a major clinical feature, and nephritis, parotitis, diarrhoea, arthritis, neuropathy, acute ophthalmitis and iritis, meningoencephalitis, meningitis or meningism.

Cardiac involvement

Myocardial involvement[25] is common on the day of crisis; this is accompanied by a prolonged QTc, altered T waves, tachycardia greater than 100/min, systolic blood pressure of 90 mmHg or less, gallop rhythm, and reversed splitting of the second sound in the pulmonary area. A phase of critically low cardiac output (resulting from myocardial damage) may ensue; this usually resolves after treatment.

Prognosis

The case mortality rate varies; it is usually around 2–9% but occasionally reaches 12%. Death usually occurs during the first febrile attack, as a result of prothrombin deficiency, hepatic coma, myocarditis or disseminated intravascular coagulation. During the initial crisis, death may result from hyperpyrexia, with convulsions, heart failure, shock or cerebral oedema. Death is usually sudden and unexpected, and may occur shortly after initiation of treatment.

Differential diagnosis

In parts of East Africa, epidemics of febrile illness in which jaundice[25] is a feature often result from louse-borne relapsing fever. During the initial attack, other causes of febrile jaundice can present similarly: yellow fever (which does not usually present with jaundice as a major feature), viral hepatitis, leptospirosis, severe *Plasmodium falciparum* infection, typhoid fever, louse-borne typhus fever (with which it sometimes co-exists), trench fever and cerebrospinal meningitis (CSF has been known to reveal meningococci and *Borrelia* spp. in the same microscopical field). After the initial attack, and during relapses,[25,26] other differential diagnoses are relapsing typhoid fever, relapsing malaria (*Plasmodium vivax*), pyelonephritis, gallstones and kala-azar.

Diagnosis

Borrelia spp. are usually detected in thick blood films obtained during a febrile attack. They may be isolated at any time by

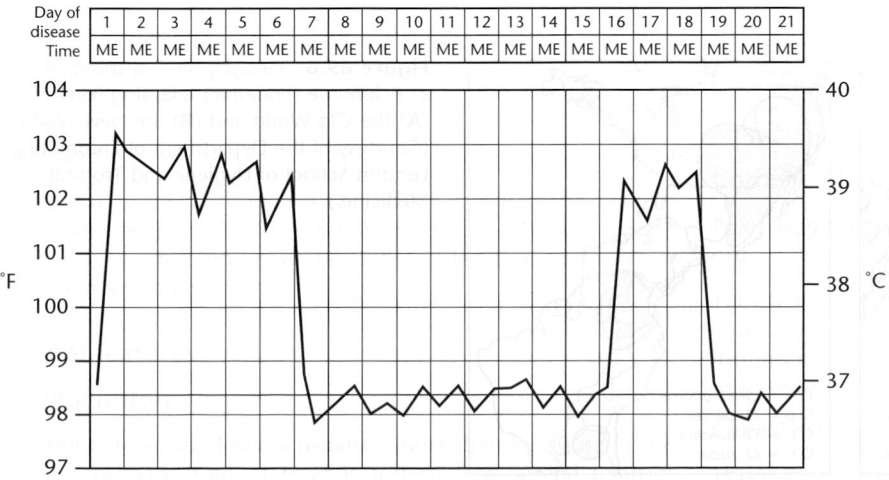

Figure 69.5 Temperature chart in a case of louse-borne relapsing fever. There is usually one relapse, and not more than four.

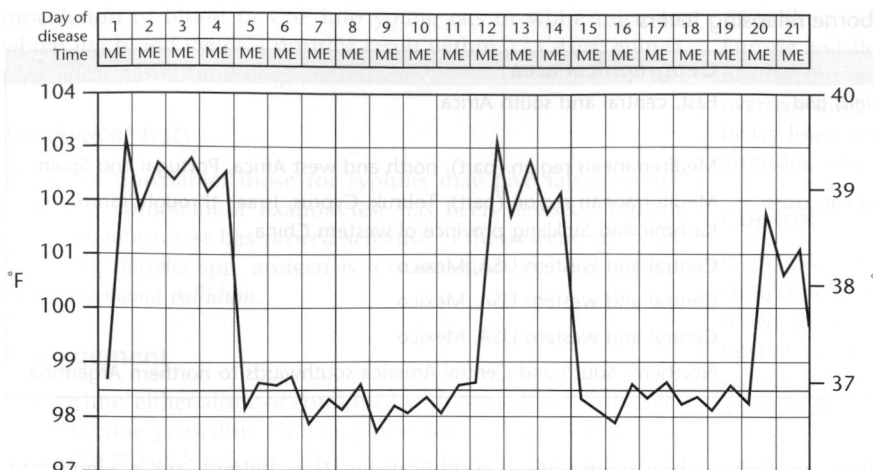

Figure 69.7 Temperature chart in tick-borne relapsing fever. There are usually three to six relapses; as many as 11 have been recorded.

the 3rd, 4th, 5th, 6th (with ophthalmoplegia) and 8th (with deafness) cranial nerves may also be affected.

Meningitic form

Lymphocytic meningitis, and occasionally subarachnoid haemorrhage, may occur. The CSF is under pressure; a pleocytosis is frequently present. This form is not uncommon in expatriates in the Dakar area.

Other cerebral syndromes

Hemiplegia, aphasia, encephalitis, optic atrophy, iritis and iridocyclitis are by no means uncommon. The spinal nerves may be involved, especially in *O. moubata* and *O. tholozani* infections. There may be sciatic neuralgia, with anaesthesia. Most cerebral complications resolve without a residual deficit.

Other complications

Bronchitis, hepatic failure and arthritis may occur.

Differential diagnosis

Other fevers should be distinguished, and distinction made between louse-borne relapsing fever and other relapsing fevers (rat bite fevers); major differences between tick-borne and louse-borne forms are summarized in Table 69.2.

Diagnosis

In the febrile phase, *Borrelia* spp. can be visualized in a peripheral blood film; they are fewer than in the louse-borne form, and inoculation into mice and rats may be required for demonstration. Diagnosis is often difficult in the afebrile period; a history of travel and residence in a known infected camp or village is of value, and, in a subsequent relapse, *Borrelia* spp. can be demonstrated at the onset and peak of the febrile episode. Serological tests may be useful, as in louse-borne relapsing fever.

Management

Treatment is the same as for louse-borne relapsing fever: tetracycline (single 500 mg dose) or procaine penicillin (300 mg). Dox-

Table 69.2 Major differences between tick-borne and louse-borne relapsing fevers

	Tick-borne	Louse-borne
Parasites in peripheral blood	Scanty	Numerous
Paroxysms	Relatively short – not more than 5–7 days. Often chronic, irregular fever	Relatively long – up to 10 days
Relapses	Two or more	Two or fewer, often none
Vomiting	Only with meningitis	At any stage
Other symptoms	Lethargy, loss of weight, debility	Diarrhoea, jaundice, coma, severe haemorrhage
Neurological complications	Common. Cranial nerve palsies	Infrequent
Ocular complications	Papilloedema with meningitis	Infrequent
Illness	Less severe	More severe
Mortality	Less than 10%	May be high – up to 50%

After Cogill NF. *J R Army Med Corps* 1949; 93:2.

ycycline has also been used.[28,31] The Jarisch–Herxheimer reaction is not a common complication, but can occur.[28]

Epidemiology

Tick-borne relapsing fever is an endemic disease found only in certain locations. In Central, East and South Africa, where humans are the sole reservoir, it is present in human habitations and wherever people live collectively (i.e. in certain types of house, staging camps for migrant workers and old camping sites). In East Africa, *O. moubata* consists of two types: one preferring to feed on chickens (which are not important in transmission) living in hot humid conditions, and the other preferring humans and found in cooler, wetter locations (highlands), where it is an important vector.

O. moubata porcinus, which is widely distributed in dwellings at all altitudes in East Africa, feeds on humans and favours a higher rainfall and a high relative humidity; it is a superior vector than O. moubata. O. savignyi prefers a hot, dry climate and infects marketplaces and cattle byres around wells; here it comes into contact with humans.

In North Africa, the eastern Mediterranean, central Asia, and North and South America, rodents constitute the major reservoir; infection is transmitted to humans incidentally. Ticks live in animal burrows and caves, and, in North America, in holiday homes – where chipmunks live in roofs.

Control

Control of infection (where dwellings are the source of infection) is achieved by the construction of concrete floors and improved walls so that ticks lack access. Ticks can be killed by most insecticides but are relatively unaffected by DDT; they are, however, susceptible to BHC (20 mg per 900cm^2) used to dust the floor. Old camping sites and mud houses should be avoided. Travellers must never sleep on the floor.[28]

RAT BITE FEVERS[32]

Two forms have been described:
- sodoku (sokosho),[33,34] named by Japanese workers and caused by *Spirillum minus* (*S. morsus-muris*)
- Haverhill fever (infectious erythema), named by American workers, and caused by *Actinobacillus muris* (formerly *Streptobacillus moniliformis*).

These are not strictly tropical diseases; their inclusion here is because they are 'relapsing' diseases and may be confused with other infections.

Sodoku

Geographical distribution

Most recorded cases have occurred in Japan; the condition also occurs in Australia, Africa, the Americas and Europe.

Aetiology

Spirillum minus is a short spiral organism (2–4 μm long), rather thick, and with regular rigid spirals and pointed ends continued into one or more flagella. It moves rapidly, resembling a vibrio, and is readily stained by methylene blue or Giemsa.

S. minus can be cultivated; subcultivation has been successful. It can be grown by intraperitoneal inoculation into guinea pigs, mice and rats.

Transmission

S. minus parasitizes rats, which are healthy carriers. Transmission is from rat to human, although infection can be caused by the bite of cats, ferrets and bandicoots. Rat urine contaminating food constitutes a further vehicle of transmission.

Pathology

The organism enters at the site of the bite; local inflammation and even necrosis may be present. It is transmitted to regional lymph glands. In fatal cases, neuronal degeneration has been recorded in brain, and degenerative changes in liver and kidneys.

Clinical features

Natural history

Sodoku consists of a relapsing fever that may subside spontaneously or continue for many months. It is usually a relatively mild disease, but the mortality rate is about 10%.

Incubation period

This varies from 5 to 30 days, the average being 5–10 days.

Symptoms and signs

There is usually a history of a bite,[33] which heals but may later break down to form an ulcer (Figure 69.8). Later, the scar and sometimes the surrounding tissues become inflamed, with formation of blebs and even necrosis. The local lymphatics are involved and regional glands become swollen and tender. Onset of fever is characterized by rigors and malaise; body temperature gradually rises over 3 days to a maximum of 39.4–40°C; after a further 3-day period this ends in a crisis, accompanied by profuse sweating.

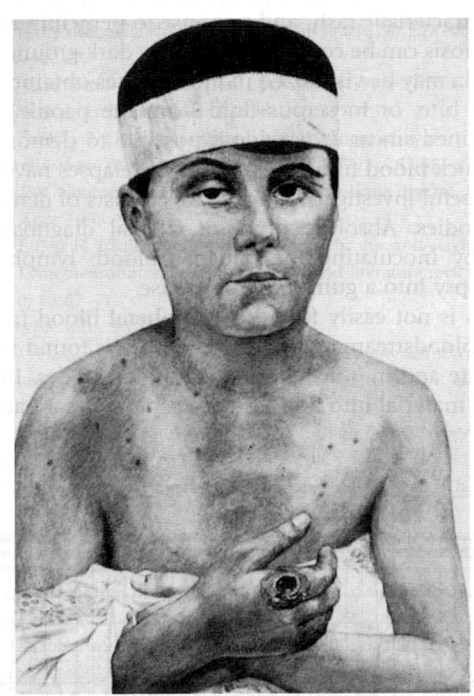

Figure 69.8 Rat bite fever produces an initial lesion at the site of the bite; this is followed by relapsing fever and rash. (Courtesy of Tropical Resources Unit.)

21. Morshed MG, Konishi H, Nishimura T, et al. Evaluation of agents for use in medium for selective isolation of Lyme disease and relapsing fever *Borrelia* species. *Eur J Clin Microbiol Infect Dis* 1993; 12:512–518.

22. Cutler SJ, Fekade D, Hussein K, et al. Successful in-vitro cultivation of *Borrelia recurrentis. Lancet* 1994; 343:242.

23. Cadavid D, Bundoc V & Barbour AG. Experimental infection of the mouse brain by a relapsing fever *Borrelia* species: a molecular analysis. *J Infect Dis* 1993; 168:143–151.

24. Almaviva M, Hailu B, Borgnolo G, et al. Louse-borne relapsing fever epidemic in Arssi Region, Ethiopia: a six months survey. *Trans R Soc Trop Med Hyg* 1993; 87:153.

25. Borgnolo G, Denku B, Chiabrera F, et al. Louse-borne relapsing fever in Ethiopian children: a clinical study. *Ann Trop Paediatr* 1993; 13: 165–171.

26. Borgnolo G, Hailu B, Ciancarelli A, et al. Louse-borne relapsing fever. A clinical and an epidemiological study of 389 patients in Asella Hospital, Ethiopia. *Trop Geogr Med* 1993; 45:66–69.

27. Sundnes KO, Haimanot AT. Epidemic of louse-borne relapsing fever in Ethiopia. *Lancet* 1993; 342:1213–1215.

28. Colebunders R, De-Serrano P, Van-Gompel A, et al. Imported relapsing fever in European tourists. *Scand J Infect Dis* 1993; 25:533–536.

29. Gallien S, Sarfati C, Haas L, et al. Borreliosis: a rare and alternative diagnosis in travellers' febrile illness. *Travel Med Infect Dis* 2007; 5:247–250.

30. Nordstrand A, Bunikis I, Larsson C, et al. Tickborne relapsing fever diagnosis obscured by malaria, Togo. *Emerg Infect Dis* 2007; 13:117–123.

31. Spach DH, Liles WC, Campbell GL, et al. Tick-borne diseases in the United States. *N Engl J Med* 1993; 329:936–947.

32. Dow GR, Rankin RJ, Saunders BW. Rat-bite fever. *N Z Med J* 1992; 105:133.

33. Hinrichsen SL, Ferraz S, Romeiro M, et al. Sodoku – a case report. *Rev Soc Bras Med Trop* 1992; 25:135–138.

34. Bhatt KM, Mirz NB. Rat bite fever: a case report from a Kenyan. *East Afr Med J* 1992; 69:542–543.

35. Fordham JN, McKay-Ferguson E, Davies A, et al. Rat bite fever without the bite. *Ann Rheum Dis* 1992; 51:411–412.

36. Konstantopoulos K, Skarpas P, Hitjazis F, et al. Rat bite fever in a Greek child. *Scand J Infect Dis* 1992; 24:531–533.

37. Rygg M, Bruun CF. Rat bite fever (*Streptobacillus moniliformis*) with septicemia in a child. *Scand J Infect Dis* 1992; 24:535–540.

38. Vasseur E, Joly P, Nouvellon M, et al. Cutaneous abscess: a rare complication of *Streptobacillus moniliformis* infection. *Br J Dermatol* 1993; 129:95–96.

39. Kornbluth CM, Destian S. Imaging of rickettsial, spirochetal, and parasitic infections. *Neuroimaging Clin North Am* 2000; 10:375–390.

Chapter 70

Geoffrey M. Scott and Timothy J. Coleman

Leptospirosis

Leptospirosis is a zoonosis that occurs in many parts of the world but most frequently in tropical and subtropical regions. Most cases are mild or asymptomatic but the most severe illness, often referred to as Weil's disease, characterized by a severe febrile illness with bleeding, jaundice and renal failure, may be associated with death through renal failure or pulmonary haemorrhage.[1-5] It is known by many different local names (e.g. mud, swamp, sugar cane, Fort Bragg and Japanese autumnal fevers). Overall, the major maintenance hosts are rodents and the organism is passed in their urine for long periods of time, even for the lifetime of the animal. Leptospires can survive for up to a few weeks in fresh water depending on the pH, but they remain viable for a much shorter period in brackish water. Humans are infected through direct or indirect contact with the urine of infected animals.

AETIOLOGY

The organism

The causative agents belong to the genus *Leptospira*, fine spiral bacteria of 0.1 μm in diameter and 6-20 μm in length.[6] Under dark ground microscopy, the organism appears straight with one or both ends hooked (Figure 70.1). Spinning motility around their long axis may disguise the spiral nature of the organisms.[7]

Classification

The family of Leptospiraceae has been subdivided into three genera – the *Leptospira*, *Leptonema* and *Turneria* (previously *Leptospira parva*). The genus *Leptospira* comprises two species: *L. interrogans* (pathogenic) and *L. biflexa* (saprophytic).

The species *L. interrogans* is divided into serogroups (e.g. *canicola*) and then into many serovars, and strains are identified by cross-agglutination – absorption with known strains using homologous antisera raised in rabbits. The test is labour intensive and therefore expensive. Major and unique antigens are currently being defined by raising monoclonal antibodies and these may be applied to the identification of certain specific serovars. New serovars may be found occasionally.[8]

Analysis of whole-cell DNA digests may also be used to show dissimilarities between strains.[9,10] This welcome move away from (potentially variable) antigen characterization may well reveal even more strains contained in what are termed 'geno' and 'subgeno' groups. However, at present, classification based on serological differences rather than DNA relatedness is often the most practical for clinical usage.

L. interrogans comprises the parasitic and pathogenic strains that can cause disease in humans and animals, whereas *L. biflexa* includes those that are considered non-pathogenic. The species *L. interrogans* can be divided into more than 200 recognized serovars. The severity of infection is probably as much to do with dose and host susceptibility as with the strain involved, because any serovar has the ability to cause mild to severe disease in different hosts. Some serovars tend to show a particular geographical distribution and differences in the major maintenance host. For example, in the UK, *L. hardjo* is particularly associated with cattle, explaining the observed increased risk of infection with this serovar in dairy farmers. Social and economic changes and alterations of working practices may occasionally result in a serovar that had previously been identified only in animals causing disease in humans.[11]

Free-living saprophytic strains (*L. biflexa*) do not cause disease in humans but their presence in the environment indicates that conditions exist under which strains pathogenic to humans can survive. *L. biflexa* strains are not pathogenic to hamsters and grow at 13°C and in the presence of 8-azaguanine, both of which are inhibitory to *L. interrogans*.

Requirements for culture

L. interrogans is an obligate aerobe that can be grown on various media that incorporate vitamins B_1 and B_{12}, long-chained fatty acids (= C_{15}) and ammonium salts. The optimal growth conditions are pH 7.2–7.6 with media enriched with fresh serum or albumin, with incubation at a temperature of 28–30°C. The organism survives in anticoagulated (but not citrated) blood for many days and, for a few days, in some commercial blood culture bottles.[12] As most blood cultures are incubated at 37°C, leptospires are unlikely to survive for subsequent culture in the case of a late suspected diagnosis made after more frequent causes of bacteraemia have been excluded. However, it is unusual for clinicians and laboratories routinely to undertake blood culture specifically to detect leptospires, unless they are in a centre of endemic or epidemic infection.

diately raise the question of leptospirosis. Renal failure is the usual cause of death but myocarditis, adrenal failure, haemorrhage and cerebral artery thrombosis may also be contributory. In those who survive without renal support, the creatinine concentration begins to fall at the end of the second week of the illness, indicating rapid resolution of the tubular necrosis. All renal function parameters will have returned to normal by 6 months except urinary concentrating ability.[48]

Abdominal pain may occur with sufficient increases in the level of amylase and lipase, despite renal failure, to suggest that pancreatitis is the cause, especially in younger patients.[49,50]

Central nervous system involvement

A patient may present, especially in the first phase of the illness, predominantly with meningitis; the CSF contains moderate numbers of lymphocytes and mildly raised protein levels without altered glucose concentration. Rarely, there is acute encephalomyelitis or a psychiatric syndrome characterized by mania. The presence of myalgia, conjunctival suffusion, slight jaundice and occasional petechiae can be clues to help move the diagnosis away from enterovirus infection. Cerebral arteritis is an unusual late complication – moyamoya syndrome is caused by obstruction of the internal carotid arteries near the circle of Willis.

Eye involvement

The eyes are suffused and there may be subconjunctival haemorrhages during acute leptospirosis. Pathogenic leptospires may invade the eye during the acute febrile phase and this may be followed by uveitis weeks or months after recovery. More commonly, a mild anterior iridocyclitis, blurring of the vitreous and haemorrhages in the retina can occur and result in disturbance to vision.[51]

DIFFERENTIAL DIAGNOSIS

Jaundice and renal failure with an acute febrile illness should immediately include leptospirosis in the differential diagnosis, and a full history of occupational, recreational and animal exposure must be taken. In practice, most cases of jaundice will at first be thought to be due to viral hepatitis: a raised bilirubin level with relatively unchanged enzymes and polymorphonuclear leukocytosis with negative viral serology should point away from viral in-fection. However, many other acute fevers are associated with jaundice (e.g. malaria, acute schistosomiasis, visceral leishmaniasis, melioidosis, plague, tularaemia and relapsing fever). The most important clinical clue is the link with renal failure. The haemolytic–uraemic syndrome may be caused by toxins produced by gut pathogens such as *Shigella* spp. and *Escherichia coli* (serotype O157), but dysentery is a prominent feature in such cases. In one series from Mumbai, leptospirosis presented as acute liver failure in 5/28 patients.[52] If petechiae are present, meningococcal disease must be excluded. Examination of the CSF is, therefore, very important when there is any hint of meningitis. Any patient with acute lymphocytic meningitis must have a full history for possible exposure to leptospirosis taken.

DIAGNOSIS

It is unlikely that the early non-specific illness of leptospirosis will be diagnosed unless there is a clear suggestion of the diagnosis in some occupational or recreational exposure, or if there is an outbreak. Clinical clues that may suggest the diagnosis of leptospirosis over other causes of acute fever are disproportionate myalgia, jaundice, conjunctival suffusion, pretibial rash and lymphocytic meningitis. If the diagnosis is suspected at this early stage, it is important to liaise with the microbiologist to arrange for appropriate specimens to be examined.[3] However, rapid results are not always possible: cultures may take 2–3 weeks to prove positive and antibodies are unlikely to be detected until at least 5–6 days after the onset of symptoms. Diagnosis using dark-field microscopy requires considerable experience; many artefacts (e.g. red blood cell membranes) may resemble leptospires when blood cultures are viewed directly. Culture into special media is more sensitive than direct microscopy. The chance of detecting leptospires in blood cultures declines rapidly when the specimen is taken after day 4 of the illness.[53]

The urine will be negative in the bacteraemic phase, so is not worth testing until the illness has been under way for some 10 days; but by then serological tests will be positive. Therefore, it is not often worthwhile directly examining urine if serum is available. If urine is submitted, it must be examined fresh since the leptospires will die if it is acidic. A simple way of alkalinizing the urine is to give potassium citrate mixture, for example as Cystopurin, one sachet (equivalent to 3 g) three times/day for 2 days, or sodium bicarbonate, 3 g every 2 h, until the urine pH > 7. Some confusion will occur if there are protein fibrils in the urine associated with renal tubular damage – they look surprisingly like immobile leptospires. The viability and motility of the bacteria are therefore particularly important.

When the patient is jaundiced, the bilirubin level is markedly raised but transaminase and alkaline phosphatase concentrations may not rise much beyond the upper limit of normal. The liver shows steatosis. The urine contains bilirubin and urobilinogen with some protein. The creatine phosphokinase[54] and amylase[50] levels are often raised. There is also a polymorphonuclear leukocytosis, which is useful in distinguishing leptospirosis from acute viral hepatitis. The haemoglobin level may fall, partly due to the infection and partly to haemorrhage. As the illness develops, the albumin level falls and the globulin and triglyceride concentrations rise. The bleeding time is prolonged: the clotting is normal and bleeding is due to capillary fragility.[36] There is no consumption of clotting factors. Later a rise in prothrombin time reflects hepatocyte failure. The erythrocyte sedimentation rate rises in the second week.

Serological detection of antibodies to leptospires is usually the investigation of choice after symptoms have been present for 5–6 days.[2,55] Early tests in non-specific febrile illness are not usually positive.[56] After this, a single high titre (such as a micro-agglutination titre >800) may be of help[57] but a rising titre is diagnostic. Reference laboratories may provide differentiation of the antibody into IgM and IgG, and perform more specific tests including one of a variety of enzyme-linked immunosorbent assay (ELISA) techniques or microscopic agglutination against live or formalized organisms (MAT), which aids differentiation of serogroups and serovars.[58,59] Various assays have been compared including microscopic agglutination (MAT) versus IgM-ELISA;[60] the latter may become positive somewhat earlier than the former. Rapid latex agglutination and dipstick assays are currently under evaluation.[61–64] Crude agglutination or complement fixation tests using a standardized polyvalent antigen are performed in some local laboratories. A commercially available 'LeptoDipstick' detects IgM in serum and urine but may be oversensitive compared to conventional diagnostic tests.[65] Therefore any positive results should be confirmed by alternative tests. New tests are being developed using recombinant antigens.[66] Theoretically molecular diagnostic tests should be helpful but they are experimental at the moment and unlikely to be available where leptospirosis is most common or where it is very rare.[67] DNA amplification from urine is difficult.[68] Several groups have identified suitable DNA segments for amplification (e.g. in gyrase subunit B or ompL1 or multi-locus sequence typing of housekeeping genes) which can detect and discriminate between some serovars and may eventually prove useful in diagnosis.

SYNDROMES ASSOCIATED WITH OTHER SEROVARS

There are no serovar-specific syndromes of leptospirosis. Any of the serovars of L. interrogans can cause any of the syndromes mentioned, and the illness can be of any seriousness. Serovar L. lai was first recognized in association with pulmonary haemorrhagic syndrome; this was then recognized as being an occasional feature of other serovars. Recognition of disease, dynamic epidemiology, virulence and predominant strains are all subject to variation, according to changes in climate and animal hosts. Nevertheless, there have been some striking associations with particular serovars.

Canicola fever

Serovar canicola is more likely to cause lymphocytic meningitis than the hepatorenal syndrome and is rarely fatal.[69] If acquired in pregnancy, the fetus may abort. The disease is usually acquired from domestic dogs, which can excrete the organism in the urine for years. Dogs may fall ill themselves on acquiring the infection and should be immunized against leptospirosis as puppies. A common symptom in the infected dog is polyuria, and the history of contact with dogs, other pets or farm animals must be sought from any patient with lymphocytic meningitis (or other symptom complex suggestive of leptospirosis). Pigs sometimes also acquire L. canicola but are usually asymptomatic.

Other serovars

Outbreaks of infection with other serovars are geographically focal and become well recognized locally. Most cause symptoms that are non-specific (headache, myalgia, fever, perhaps with mildly raised bilirubin levels but rarely with overt jaundice). However, infection with L. autumnalis is particularly associated with a Fort Bragg fever: Curious pretibial, raised 2–4-cm erythematous patches, which are much less tender than erythema nodosum and

occur at the height of the illness.[70] Pretibial fever may also occur with other serovars (e.g. L. pomona) and there has been some confusion with legionellosis. Serovar pomona, a parasite predominantly of pigs, causes swineherd's disease, first described in Australia and then in Switzerland, and behaves in humans like canicola fever. Serovar australis group antibodies that were not cross-reactive with canicola and icterohaemorrhagiae were shown in beagles with chronic hepatitis.[71]

Serovar grippotyphosa causes swamp or mud fever, and bataviae causes rice-field disease, described in outbreaks first in Indonesia and later in Italy.

MANAGEMENT

Penicillin and other related β-lactam antibiotics are active against experimental leptospirosis in animals.[72] Tetracyclines are also effective and there is some controversy as to whether penicillin is preferable to tetracyclines. Macrolides (azithromycin and clarithromycin) and the ketolide telithromycin are also active in animal challenge experiments.[73] However, penicillin (1.2G benzylpenicillin intravenously or intramuscularly every 4–6 h) is probably the drug of choice in patients suspected of having leptospirosis, yet it is a widely held view that this would be ineffective if delayed beyond the first few days of the illness.[74] This is, perhaps, explained by the fact that after this time the manifestations of the disease are immunologically mediated. However, whereas recent placebo-controlled studies suggest that there may still be a small advantage in giving penicillin late (that is, beyond the fourth day of the illness),[75] a systematic review revealed only three trials that were acceptable for analysis that failed to prove any benefit for antibiotic treatment at all.[76] A more recent randomized trial of penicillin vs placebo after day 4 in Brazil showed a non-significant trend to reduction in mortality (15/125 to 8/128) in line with previous tantalizing results.[77] Tetracycline (e.g. doxycycline 100 mg orally every 12 h)[78] or erythromycin (500 mg orally every 12 h) are alternatives in patients who are allergic to penicillin, but are not more likely to be effective. Ceftriaxone was not better than penicillin in a small open-label study.[79] There were no differences in outcome in patients with possible leptospirosis empirically treated with either penicillin, cefotaxime or doxycycline in an open-label study of 264 patients (confirmed) in northern Thailand, although the tetracycline was usefully active against rickettsial infection which affected 132 additional patients.[80] For possible concurrent malaria with leptospirosis, doxycycline, azithromycin and clindamycin show in vitro activity.[81]

For very ill patients, intensive care support may be necessary. Specific support therapy is required for anaemia due to bleeding and for renal failure. Haemodiafiltration is now favoured if resources permit, but when resources are limited, peritoneal dialysis should be instituted to tide the patient over until the tubular necrosis has begun to resolve. A tendency to bleeding is not a contraindication to haemodialysis.

For the acute pulmonary syndrome, pulsed methylprednisolone may be effective. A small non-randomized study showed a significant reduction in mortality when the steroid was started soon after the onset of the pulmonary syndrome.[82] Parenteral feeding is important because of the hypercatabolic state of the febrile patient in renal failure.[34]

There are negligible risks to healthcare workers of acquiring the disease from an infected patient.

CONTROL AND PREVENTION

With more than 200 pathogenic serovars and the fact that all animals may become infected, some chronically, the eradication of leptospirosis is clearly impossible. However, there are three main ways in which the risk of leptospirosis in humans can be reduced. First, domestic farm animals and pets can be immunized. This does not completely abolish the risk of an animal acquiring infection but significantly reduces the overall risk to humans.[83] Secondly, risks in occupational and recreational exposure can be identified and addressed. Although classically described in sewer workers, leptospirosis is now rare in this group in many countries because protective clothing and simple hygienic precautions have been introduced. In general, farmers tend not to take similar precautions because of a misconception in some parts of the world that the disease is not particularly associated with farming. However, specific measures can be taken; e.g. burning cane fields prior to harvest reduces the risk of the sharp young shoots cutting hands. Other simple measures, such as removing rubbish from work and domestic environments, will reduce the rodent population. Improved education of people at particular risk (e.g. farmers and those taking part in water sports) and healthcare staff increases awareness and may enable earlier diagnosis and treatment. Thirdly, chemoprophylaxis (e.g. with doxycycline) can be used in groups at particularly high risk.[84–87]

A Cochrane database review found only two properly controlled prophylactic trials of doxycycline (and in one of these the method of blinding was not described) involving 1022 subjects. The risk of leptospirosis in the treated groups was 0.6% (3 of 509) compared with 4.9% (25 of 513) in those who received no treatment. It was calculated that prophylaxis in 24 subjects (95% confidence intervals 17–43) was needed to prevent disease in one subject. Side-effects were recorded in 3% of those receiving doxycycline, compared with 0.2% of control subjects, and this has to be taken into account when deciding on a prophylaxis strategy at times of high risk and special circumstances.[88]

REFERENCES

1. Turner LH. Leptospirosis I. *Trans R Soc Trop Med Hyg* 1967; 61:842–855.
2. Turner LH. Leptospirosis II. *Trans R Soc Trop Med Hyg* 1968; 62:880–899.
3. Turner LH. Leptospirosis III. *Trans R Soc Trop Med Hyg* 1970; 64:623–646.
4. Edwards GA, Domm BM. Human leptospirosis. *Medicine* 1960; 39:117–156.
5. Heath CW Jr, Alexander AD, Galton MM. Leptospirosis in the United States. Analysis of 483 cases in man 1949–1961. *N Engl J Med* 1965; 273:857–864.
6. Johnson RC, Faine S. Leptospiraceae. In: Krieg NR, Holt JG, eds. *Bergey's Manual of Systemic Bacteriology*. Vol. 1. Baltimore: Williams, Wilkins; 1984: 62–67.
7. Cox PJ, Twigg GI. Leptospiral motility. *Nature* 1974; 250:260–261.
8. Rosetti CA, Liem M, Samartino LE, et al. Buenos Aires, a new *Leptospira* serovar of serogroup *Djasiman*, isolated from an aborted dog fetus in Argentina. *Vet Microbiol* 2005; 107:241–248.
9. Hookey JV, Waitkins SA, Jackman PJH. Numerical analysis of Leptospira DNA-restriction endonuclease patterns. *FEMS Microbiol Lett* 1985; 29:185–188.
10. Robinson AJ, Ramadass P, Lee A, et al. Differentiation of subtypes within *Leptospira interrogans* serovars *hardjo*, *balcanica* and *tarassovi* by bacterial restriction-endonuclease DNA analysis (BRENDA). *J Med Microbiol* 1982; 15:331–338.
11. Peterson AM, Boyce K, Blom J, et al. First isolation of *Leptospira fainei* serovar *Hurstbridge* from two human patients with Weil's syndrome. *J Med Microbiol* 2001; 50:96–100.
12. Palmer MF, Zochowski WJ. Survival of leptospires in commercial blood culture systems revisited. *J Clin Pathol* 2000; 53:713–714.
13. Johnson MA, Smith H, Joeph P, et al. Environmental exposure and leptospirosis, Peru. *Emerg Infect Dis* 2004; 10:1016–1022.
14. Romero EC, Bernardo CC, Yasuda PN. Human leptospirosis: a twenty-nine-year serological study in Sao Paulo, Brazil. *Rev Inst Med Trop Sao Paulo* 2003; 45:245–248.
15. Thai KT, Binh TQ, Giao PT, et al. Seroepidemiology of leptospirosis in southern Vietnamese children. *Trop Med Int Health* 2006; 11:738–745.
16. Lopes AA, Costa E, Costa YA, et al. Comparative study of the in-hospital case-fatality rate of leptospirosis between paediatric and adult patients of different age groups. *Rev Inst Med Trop Sao Paulo* 2004; 46:19–24.
17. Hutchinson JH, Pippard JS, White MH G, et al. Outbreak of Weil's disease in the British Army in Italy. *BMJ* 1946; i:81–86.
18. Vinetz JM, Glass GE, Flener CE, et al. Sporadic urban leptospirosis. *Ann Intern Med* 1996; 15:794–798.
19. Kupek E, de Sousa Santos Faversini MC, de Souza Phillippi JM. The relationship between rainfall and human leptospirosis in Florianopolis, Brazil, 1991–1996. *Braz J Infect Dis* 2000; 4:131–134.
20. Trevejo RT, Rigau-Perez JG, Ashford DA, et al. Epidemic leptospirosis associated with pulmonary haemorrhage-Nicaragua, 1995. *J Infect Dis* 1998; 178:1457–1463.
21. Sanders EJ, Rigau-Perez JG, Smits HL, et al. Increase of leptospirosis in dengue-negative patients after a hurricane in Puerto Rico in 1996. *Am J Trop Med Hyg* 1999; 61:399–404.
22. Russell KL, Motiel Gonzalez MA, Watts DM, et al. An outbreak of leptospirosis among Peruvian Military recruits. *Am J Trop Med Hyg* 2003; 69:53–57.
23. Hadad E, Pirogovsky A, Bartal C, et al. An outbreak of leptospirosis among Israeli troops near the Jordan River. *Am J Trop Med Hyg* 2006; 74:127–131.
24. Anonymous. Leptospirosis outbreak in Eco Challenge 2000 participants. *Commun Dis Rep CDR Wkly* 2000; 22:341.
25. Anonymous. Update: leptospirosis and unexplained acute febrile illness among athletes participating in triathlons – Illinois and Wisconsin, 1998. *MMWR Morb Mortal Wkly Rep* 1998; 47:673–676.
26. Anonymous. Outbreak of leptospirosis among white-water rafters – Costa Rica, 1996. *MMWR Morb Mortal Wkly Rep* 1997; 46:577–579.
27. Friman G, Wesslen L. Special features for the Olympics: effects of exercise on the immune system: infections and exercise in high-performance athletes. *Immunol Cell Biol* 2000; 78:510–522.
28. Holk K, Nielsen SV, Ronne T. Human leptospirosis in Denmark 1970–1996: an epidemiological and clinical study. *Scand J Infect Dis* 2000; 32:533–538.
29. Karande S, Gandhi D, Kulkarni M, et al. Concurrent outbreak of leptospirosis and dengue in Mumbai, India, 2002. *J Trop Pediatr* 2005; 51:174–181.
30. Sejvar J, Tangkanakul W, Ratanasang P, et al. An outbreak of leptospirosis, Thailand – the importance of the laboratory. *Southeast Asian J Trop Med Public Health* 2005; 36:289–295.
31. Arean VM. The pathologic anatomy and pathogenesis of fatal human leptospirosis (Weil's disease). *Am J Pathol* 1962; 40:393–423.
32. Ramos-Morales F, Díaz-Rivera RS, Cintrón-Rivera AA, et al. The pathogenesis of leptospiral jaundice. *Ann Intern Med* 1959; 51:861–878.
33. Sitprija V. Renal involvement in human leptospirosis. *BMJ* 1968; ii:656–658.
34. Kennedy ND, Pusey CD, Rainford DJ, et al. Leptospirosis and acute renal failure: clinical experiences and a review of the literature. *Postgrad Med J* 1979; 55:176–179.
35. Lai KN, Aarons I, Woodroffe AJ, et al. Renal lesions in leptospirosis. *Aust NZ J Med* 1982; 12:276–279.

36. Edwards CN, Nicholson GD, Hassell TA, et al. Thrombocytopenia in leptospirosis: the absence of evidence for disseminated intravascular coagulation. *Am J Trop Med Hyg* 1986; 35:352–354.

37. Younes Ibrahim M, Buffin-Meyer B, Cheval L, et al. Na,K-ATPase: a molecular target for *Leptospirosis interrogans* endotoxin. *Braz J Med Biol Res* 1997; 30: 213–233.

38. Abuldaker RC, Seguro AC, Malheiro PS, et al. Peculiar electrolyte and hormonal abnormalities in acute renal failure due to leptospirosis. *Am J Trop Med Hyg* 1996; 54:1–6.

39. Yang CW, Hung CC, Wu M S, et al. Toll-like receptor 2 mediates early inflammation by leptospiral outer membrane proteins in proximal tubule cells. *Kidney Int* 2006; 69:815–822.

40. Yang GG, Hsu YH. Nitric oxide production and immunoglobulin deposition in leptospiral haemorrhagic respiratory failure. *J Formos Med Assoc* 2005; 104:759–763.

41. Salkade HP, Divate S, Deshpande JR, et al. A study of autopsy findings in 62 cases of leptospirosis in a metropolitan city in India. *J Postgrad Med* 2005; 51:169–173.

42. Nicodemo AC, Duarte MI, Alves VA, et al. Lung lesions in human leptospirosis: microscopic, immunohistochemical and ultrastructural features related to thrombocytopenia. *Am J Trop Med Hyg* 1997; 56:181–187.

43. Nally JE, Chow E, Fishbein MC, et al. Changes in lipopolysaccharide O antigen distinguish acute versus chronic Leptospira interrogans infections. *Infect Immun* 2005; 73:3251–3260.

44. Sharma A, Joshi SA, Srivastave SK, et al. Leptospirosis in the causation of hepato-renal syndrome in and around Pune. *Indian J Pathol Microbiol* 2000; 43:337–341.

45. Rao P, Sethi S, Sud A, et al. Screening of patients with acute febrile illness for leptospirosis using clinical criteria and serology. *Natl Meb J India* 2005; 18:244–246.

46. Martinez-Garcia MA, de Diego Damia A, Menendez Villanueva R, et al. Pulmonary involvement in leptospirosis. *Eur J Clin Microbiol Infect Dis* 2000; 19:471–474.

47. Yersin C, Bovet P, Merien F, et al. Pulmonary haemorrhage as a predominant cause of death in leptospirosis in Seychelles. *Trans R Soc Trop Med Hyg* 2000; 94:71–76.

48. Daher Ede F, Zanetta DM, Abdulkader RC. Pattern of renal function recovery after leptospirosis acute renal failure. *Nephron Clin Pract* 2004; 98:c8–14.

49. O'Brien MM, Vincent JM, Person DA, et al. Leptospirosis and pancreatitis: a report of ten cases. *Pediatr Infect Dis J* 1998; 17:436–438.

50. Daher EF, Brunetta DM, de Silva GB, et al. Pancreatic involvement in fatal human leptospirosis: clinical and histopathological features. *Rev Inst Med Trop Sao Paolo* 2003; 45:307–313.

51. Rathinam SR. Ocular leptospirosis. *Curr Opin Ophthalmol* 2002; 13:381–386.

52. Deepak NA, Patel ND. Differential diagnosis of acute liver failure in India. *Ann Hepatol* 2006; 5:150–156.

53. Smith J. Weil's disease in the north-east of Scotland. *Br J Ind Med* 1949; 6:213–220.

54. Johnson WD, Silva IC, Rocha H. Serum creatine phosphokinase in leptospirosis. *JAMA* 1975; 233:981–982.

55. Cursons RT M, Pyke PA, Penniket J. The serological diagnosis of leptospirosis. *N Z J Med* 1982; 95:26–37.

56. Cohen AL, Dowell SF, Nisalak A, et al. Rapid diagnostic tests for dengue and leptospirosis: antibody detection is insensitive at presentation. *Trop Med Int Health* 2007; 12:47–51.

57. Katz AR, Effler PV. 'Probable' versus 'confirmed' leptospirosis: an epidemiologic and clinical comparison utilizing a surveillance case classification. *Ann Epidemiol* 2003; 13:196–203.

58. Pappas MG, Ballou WR, Gray MR, et al. Rapid serodiagnosis of leptospirosis using the IgM-specific dot-ELISA: comparison with the microscopic agglutination test. *Am J Trop Med Hyg* 1985; 34:346–354.

59. Watt G, Alquiza LM, Padre LP, et al. The rapid diagnosis of leptospirosis: a prospective comparison of the dot enzyme linked immunosorbent assay and the genus-specific microscopic agglutination at different stages of illness. *J Infect Dis* 1988; 157:840–842.

60. Cumberland P, Everard CO, Levett PN. Assessment of the efficacy of an IgM-ELISA and microscopic agglutination test (MAT) in the diagnosis of acute leptospirosis. *Am J Trop Med Hyg* 1999; 61:731–734.

61. Smits HL, van de Hoorn MA, Goris MG, et al. Simple latex agglutination assay for rapid serodiagnosis of human leptospirosis. *J Clin Microbiol* 2000; 38:1272–1275.

62. Ramadass P, Samuel B, Nachimuthu K. A rapid latex agglutination test for detection of leptospiral antibodies. *Vet Microbiol* 1999; 70: 137–140.

63. Yersin C, Bovet P, Smits HL, et al. Field evaluation of a one-step dipstick assay for the diagnosis of human leptospirosis in the Seychelles. *Trop Med Int Health* 1999; 4:38–45.

64. Smits HL, Hartskeerl RA, Terpstra WJ. International multi-centre evaluation of a dipstick assay for human leptospirosis. *Trop Med Int Health* 2000; 5: 124–128.

65. Manocha H, Goshal U, Singh SK, et al. Frequency of leptospirosis in patients of acute febrile illness in Uttar Pradesh. *J Assoc Physicians India* 2004; 52: 623–625.

66. Dey S, Madhan Mohan C, Ramadass P, Nachimuthu K. Recombinant antigen-based latex agglutination test for rapid serodiagnosis of leptospirosis. *Vet Res Commun* 2007; 31:9–15.

67. Levett PN, Morey RE, Galloway RL, et al. Detection of pathogenic leptospires by real-time PCR. *J Med Microbiol* 2005; 54:45–49.

68. Lucchesi PM, Arroyo GH, Etcheverria AI, et al. Recommendations for the detection of Leptospira in urine by PCR. *Rev Soc Bras Med Trop* 2004; 37: 131–134.

69. McIntyre WI, Seiler HE. The epidemiology of canicola fever. *J Hyg (Camb)* 1953; 51:330–339.

70. Fraser DW, Glosser JW, Francis DP, et al. Leptospirosis caused by serotype Fort Bragg. *Ann Intern Med* 1973; 79:786–794.

71. Adamus C, Buggin-Daubie M, Izembart A, et al. Chronic hepatitis associated with leptospiral infection in vaccinated beagles. *J Comp Pathol* 1997; 117: 311–328.

72. Alexander AD, Rule PL. Penicillins, cephalosporins and tetracyclines in treatment of hamsters with fatal leptospirosis. *Antimicrob Agents Chemother* 1986; 30:835–839.

73. Moon JE, Ellis MW, Griffith ME, et al. Efficacy of macrolides and telithromycin against leptospirosis in a hamster model. *Antimicrob Agents and Chemother* 2006; 50:1989–1992.

74. Christie AB, ed. Leptospiral infections. In: *Infectious Diseases*. Vol. 2. 4th edn. Edinburgh: Churchill Livingstone; 1982:1173.

75. Watt G, Padre LP, Tuazon ML, et al. Placebo controlled trial of intravenous penicillin for severe and late leptospirosis. *Lancet* 1988; i:433–435.

76. Guidugli F, Castro AA, Atallah AN. Antibiotics for treating leptospirosis. *Cochrane Database Syst Rev* 2000; 2:CD001306.

77. Costa E, Lopes AA, Sacramento E, et al. Penicillin at the late stage of leptospirosis: a randomised controlled trial. *Rev Inst Med Trop Sao Paulo* 2003; 45:141–145.

78. McClain JBL, Ballou WR, Harrison SM. Doxycycline therapy for leptospirosis. *Ann Intern Med* 1984; 100:696–698.

79. Panaphut T, Domrongkitchaiporn S, Vibhagool A, et al. Ceftriaxone compared with sodium penicillin G for the treatment of severe leptospirosis. *Clin Infect Dis* 2003; 36:1507–1513.

80. Suputtamongkol Y, Niwattayakul K, Suttinont C, et al. An open, randomised controlled trial of penicillin, doxycycline, and cefotaxime for patients with severe leptospirosis. *Clin Infect Dis* 2004; 39:1417–1424.

81. Murray CK, Ellis MW, Hospenthal DR. Susceptibility of *Leptospira* serovars to antimalarial agents. *Am J Trop Med Hyg* 2004; 71:685–686.

82. Shenov VV, Nagar VS, Chowdhury AA, et al. Pulmonary leptospirosis: an excellent response to bolus methylprednisolone. *Postgrad Med J* 2006; 82: 602–606.

83. Feigin RD, Lobes LA Jr, Anderson D, et al. Human leptospirosis from immunized dogs. *Ann Intern Med* 1973; 79:777–785.

84. Takafuji ET, Kirkpatrick JW, Miller RN, et al. An efficacy trial of doxycycline prophylaxis against leptospirosis. *N Engl J Med* 1984; 310:497–500.

85. Sehgal SC, Sugunan AP, Murhekar MV, et al. Randomized controlled trial of doxycycline prophylaxis against leptospirosis in an endemic area. *Int J Antimicrob Agents* 2000; 13:249–255.

86. Gonsalez CR, Casseb J, Monteiro FG, et al. Use of doxycycline for leptospirosis after high-risk exposure in Sao Paulo, Brazil. *Rev Inst Med Trop Sao Paulo* 1998; 40:59–61.

87. Sejvar J, Bancroft E, Winthrop K, et al. Leptospirosis in 'Eco-Challenge' athletes, Malaysian Borneo, 2000. *Emerg Infect Dis* 2003; 9:702–707.

88. Guidigli F, Castro AA, Atallah AN. Antibiotics for preventing leptospirosis (Cochrane review). *Cochrane Database Syst Rev* 2000; 4:CD001305.

GENERAL READING

McBride AJ, Athanazio DA, Reis MG, et al. Leptospirosis. *Curr Opin Infect Dis* 2005; 18:376–386.

Chapter 71

Roderick J. Hay

Fungal Infections

The fungi are recognized causes of disease in all parts of the world. The commonest of the infections caused by these eukaryotic organisms are superficial, and include diseases such as dermatophytosis or ringworm and candidosis. However, extensive, deforming and potentially fatal deep or systemic fungal infections can also occur.[1] Fungal cells are similar to animal cells but are characterized by the presence of a polysaccharide-based cell wall. There are two principal types of fungi: the yeasts, single cells which reproduce by a process of bud formation to give rise to single daughter cells; and the mycelial or mould fungi, which form chains of contiguous cells, hyphae. Some fungi, the dimorphic fungi, exist as either yeasts or mycelia at different stages of their life cycles. Examples of dimorphic organisms include most of the major respiratory pathogens such as *Histoplasma capsulatum* and *Coccidioides immitis*. The formation of specialized reproductive structures or spores (conidia) is also typical of fungi, although this usually only occurs under laboratory conditions. Fungi can cause human disease in a number of different ways, through the production of toxins, sensitizing antigens (allergens) or by the invasion of tissue. Invasive diseases caused by fungi are known collectively as the mycoses: the superficial, subcutaneous or systemic mycoses.

The distribution of mycoses is affected by a number of factors: the presence of the organisms in the environment, host immunity, frequency and route of exposure and the use of invasive or immunosuppressive medical technology. These influence the spread of fungal disease in the tropics as well as in temperate climates. The main superficial mycoses are common in the tropics. The subcutaneous infections, which occur through implantation of pathogenic organisms via injury, are largely confined to the tropics and subtropics. The main systemic mycoses due to respiratory pathogens, such as *Histoplasma capsulatum*, also occur in the tropics, while systemic opportunistic infections caused by organisms such as *Aspergillus* are probably more common in temperate areas where there is a greater reliance on therapeutic immunosuppression.

SUPERFICIAL MYCOSES

Superficial infections caused by fungi are common in all environments, particularly the tropics. While, on occasions, this is due to the existence of endemic foci of specific species, such as the causes

of tinea imbricata or tinea capitis, there is also a real increase in prevalence of certain infections. Factors such as climate, humidity of the skin surface and the PCO_2 concentration may all affect the expression of these diseases.

The main superficial infections are dermatophytosis or ringworm, superficial candidosis and pityriasis (tinea) versicolor (Table 71.1). However, other conditions, such as foot infections caused by *Scytalidium dimidiatum* as well as the hair shaft infections, white and black piedra, and tinea nigra are also seen. Otomycosis, a superficial infection of the external auditory meatus, is also common. Oculomycosis, in particular mycotic keratitis, occurs in temperate as well as tropical environments but poses a frequent and difficult management problem in the tropics (see Chapter 18).

Dermatophytosis

The dermatophyte or ringworm fungi are common causes of superficial infections.[2] They are mould fungi which became adapted to parasitize the skin by attacking the keratin through the production of proteases with keratin specificity. They can invade epidermis but remain confined to the stratum corneum as well as the hair shaft or nail plate. There are three pathogenic genera of dermatophyte in humans: *Trichophyton*, *Microsporum* and *Epidermophyton*. These organisms normally cause exogenous infections originating from outside the human host. There are three main sources: other humans, animals or soil, known respectively as anthropophilic, zoophilic or geophilic. Examples of possible animal hosts are cats and dogs (*M. canis*), cattle (*T. verrucosum*), monkeys (*T. simii*) and rodents (*T. mentagrophytes*).

Pathogenesis

The fungi invade after adhering to stratum corneum cells. Factors which encourage fungal invasion include increased environmental humidity and CO_2 content, both of which may occur in a tropical environment and in the presence of occlusion. Less is known about those factors which determine human susceptibility; generally it is thought that most individuals are susceptible to infection.[3] The presence of medium chain length fatty acids in sebaceous material may, however, prevent hair shaft invasion by dermatophytes in postpubertal children. There is evidence that

Tinea pedis

Dermatophytosis affecting the feet is very common in most temperate climates; although less common in developing countries, it none the less occurs. The most common sites of infection are the interdigital spaces or the soles. The main symptoms are itching and occasionally pain. There may be erosions affecting web spaces. If there are severe erosive changes, particularly if there is greenish discolouration of the area, Gram-negative bacteria, such as *Pseudomonas* species, may be implicated. Other possibilities include *Candida* and *Scytalidium* species or erythrasma, a bacterial infection caused by *Corynebacterium minutissimum*. *Scytalidium* infections which are indistinguishable from those due to *T. rubrum* are encountered frequently in West Africa.

The usual treatment for toe-web dermatophytosis is a topically applied antifungal. Good results can be obtained with a range of compounds including Whitfield's ointment, azoles such as clotrimazole or miconazole, or terbinafine. For infections of the sole requiring treatment, oral therapy with griseofulvin, terbinafine or itraconazole is preferable. Scytalidium infections respond poorly to current antifungals.

Onychomycosis

Nail plate invasion caused by dermatophytes is common in temperate countries, where it may affect up to 15% of the population. The prevalence of this infection in the tropics is unknown. It normally occurs together with sole or web-space infections and is most common in the toe-nails. The usual causes are anthropophilic fungi, such as *Trichophyton rubrum*. The affected nails become thickened and opaque; distal erosion of the nail plate occurs in long-standing cases[29] (Figure 71.4). Superficial invasion of the nail plate caused by dermatophytes, such as *T. interdigitale*, or moulds such as *Acremonium* or *Fusarium* species, is seen more frequently in the tropics.[30] This is called superficial white onychomycosis. Therapy is difficult, with few nail infections responding to topical antifungals, although in the early stages some will clear with tio-

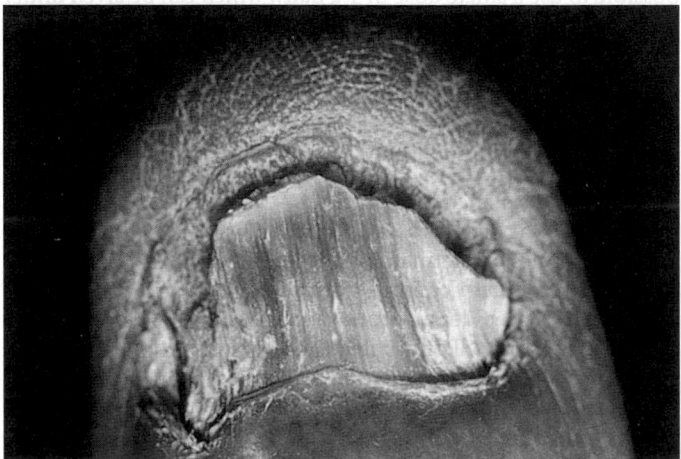

Figure 71.4 Onychomycosis due to a dermatophyte.

conazole or amorolfine nail solutions. The cheapest oral treatment, griseofulvin, is associated with a high relapse rate when toe-nails are involved. It may have to be used for 12–18 months. Other oral drugs, terbinafine (250 mg daily)[31] or itraconazole (400 mg daily for 1 week per month ×3),[32] produce higher recovery rates in shorter periods (3 months). They are also more expensive than griseofulvin.

Superficial candidosis

Superficial infections due to *Candida* species are common in a tropical environment and include oral and vaginal as well as skin infections.[33] The principal pathogen is *C. albicans*, although other species, such as *C. tropicalis*, *C. parapsilosis*, *C. krusei* and *C. glabrata* may also cause human infections. *C. albicans* forms filaments or hyphae during the process of tissue invasion. The disease is seen worldwide, although some clinical varieties such as interdigital candidosis are more common in warm climates.[14]

Pathogenesis and epidemiology

Candida albicans is a normal commensal of the mouth, gastrointestinal tract and vagina. Carriage rates vary but 15–60% of normal individuals have commensal carriage in the mouth. Somewhat lower percentages have colonization of the gastrointestinal tract or vagina.[34] Survival of the organisms in these sites depends on a variety of factors, including their ability to adhere to mucosal cells and compete with commensal bacteria. Factors which disturb this balance favour either elimination or growth and subsequent invasion by the organism. They can usually be explained logically. For instance, use of antibiotics eliminates other members of the commensal flora of the mouth and bowel and allows *Candida* to invade. Depression of either T lymphocyte or neutrophil-mediated immunity allows the organisms to grow and invade following inhibition of normal control mechanisms. The main exception is vaginal candidosis, where most women with this common infection have no detectable predisposition.

Clinical features

The main clinical forms of superficial disease are oropharyngeal, vaginal and cutaneous candidosis. In addition, chronic mucocutaneous candidosis is a condition which may appear as a rare chronic infection in predisposed patients. Systemic candidosis is a serious infection generally confined to compromised patients. It will be discussed elsewhere.

Oropharyngeal candidosis

Oral infection is seen in all countries, particularly in infants, the elderly and immunocompromised patients, including those with AIDS.[35] It occurs in breast-fed and bottle-fed infants and may be a complication of malnutrition, in which it can affect the reintroduction of feeding because of soreness of the mouth. As a complication of human immunodeficiency virus (HIV) infection, the appearance of oropharyngeal candidosis is a common and early manifestation of the development of AIDS.

There are a number of different clinical types of oropharyngeal candidosis.[36,37] These are largely distinguished by their chronicity and clinical appearances. Acute pseudomembranous candidosis presents with white plaques on the epithelium that are inflamed and easily detached. The scattered nature of these appearances is suggestive of the speckling on a thrush's breast, hence its common name 'thrush'. This may present as an acute infection in infants, the elderly or in patients who are immunocompromised, such as those with AIDS. In the last group and in patients with chronic mucocutaneous candidosis the condition is often persistent and refractory to therapy – chronic pseudomembranous candidosis.

In some individuals, plaques are not formed but the mucosal surface appears red and glazed – acute erythematous candidosis, also known as acute atrophic oral candidosis. This may occur in patients with AIDS.[37,38] In patients presenting with inflammatory changes and oral discomfort associated with dentures (denture sore mouth), persistent erythema associated with *Candida* is a common feature – chronic erythematous candidosis. In smokers, chronic candidosis may have additional features such as the appearance of irregular white plaques, which cannot be detached, on the tongue and other areas of the mouth–chronic plaque-like candidosis. Histologically, this contains epithelial atypia and, in some patients, oral carcinomas have developed. A few patients with chronic oral *Candida* infection may develop a pebbly appearance on the mucosa – chronic nodular candidosis.

Any of the above changes can be accompanied by splitting at the corners of the mouth (angular cheilitis), which in these cases may be due to *Candida* infection. This is an important and common sign of candidosis.

In most patients the main focus of infection is the buccal mucosa, but in severely infected individuals there is involvement of the tongue or pharynx, as well as the oesophagus. Oesophageal candidosis is mainly seen in patients with AIDS, leukaemia or chronic mucocutaneous candidosis. While it may present with retrosternal pain on swallowing, it is often silent. Secondary oral infection due to *Candida* may occur in patients with epithelial abnormalities, such as hyperkeratosis or ulceration due to lichen planus, pemphigus and other conditions such as oral submucous fibrosis, mainly seen in patients from the Indian subcontinent.

Vaginal candidosis

Vaginal *Candida* infection is normally caused by *C. albicans*, although other *Candida* species, such as *C. glabrata* or *C. tropicalis* have also been cultured.[33] While it can occur in pregnant women or diabetics, one of the features of this condition is that there is usually no underlying abnormality to be found. Severely immunocompromised women do not usually show a higher frequency of persistent vaginal infections than appropriate control groups, although persistent vaginal infection has been reported in some women with AIDS.

The main clinical forms of vaginal candidosis are similar to those seen in the oral mucosa, most commonly an acute (pseudomembranous or erythematous) form.[34] However, chronic relapsing or persistent vaginal candidosis and secondary vaginal candidosis can all occur.[39] The symptoms of the acute types vary from a creamy discharge to itching and dyspareunia. Recurrent infections are unfortunately common and occasionally they are persistent. The clinical appearances are varied but the main varia-

tions are the presence or absence of soft white plaques (thrush). Secondary candidosis may occur in those with underlying mucosal disease, such as pemphigoid, lichen planus or Behçet's syndrome.

Candida *intertrigo*

The skin is only indirectly involved in vaginal infection when there is spread of infection to the vulva and the perineum. In this case, a prominent red rash in the groin and on the upper surface of the thighs may appear, together with satellite pustules and papules. The same can occur in other sites such as beneath the breasts and around the umbilicus. In some cases, there is no underlying skin abnormality, although groin candidosis in males and females is more common in diabetic subjects. Eczema or psoriasis affecting the skin flexures may be accompanied by secondary candidosis.

Interdigital candidosis

Infection of the finger- or toe-web spaces by *Candida* is more common in hot climates. It may be the most common type of foot infection in army groups in the tropics. Lesions are white with soggy-looking skin, which is superficially eroded. *Candida* may be a secondary invader of interdigital dermatophytosis. Lesions between the fingers are mainly seen in women and a relationship between repeated washing and cooking has been suggested; it is also more common in the overweight.

Candida *infection and nappy dermatitis*

Nappy rash in infants is a form of irritant eczema, which is often secondarily infected with, among other organisms, *C. albicans*. The presence of yeasts may be suspected by the appearance of satellite pustules and this is confirmed by culturing the organisms from swabs of the area.

Candidosis of the nails

Paronychias are acute or chronic infections of the nail folds caused by *Candida* species, such as *C. albicans* or *C. parapsilosis*.[40] These are common in the tropics. They occur in patients who are likely to immerse their hands frequently in water or whose occupations involve cooking. In addition to swelling of the nail fold, pain and intermittent discharge of pus, the lateral border of the nail may be undermined with onycholysis (Figure 71.5). Other causes of paronychia are staphylococcal and Gram-negative bacterial infections. The latter often co-exist with *Candida* species. However, in many chronically affected patients, this disease is complicated by irritant dermatitis and eradication of the organisms alone will not effect recovery.

Chronic mucocutaneous candidosis

The rare syndrome of chronic mucocutaneous candidosis (CMC) usually presents in childhood or infancy with oral, nail and cutaneous candidosis which recurs despite treatment.[41] Other chronic skin infections, such as warts (papilloma viruses) and dermatophytosis may also appear. An adult form also exists.

The oral lesions are usually of the chronic pseudomembranous or plaque types. The skin may be covered with crusted plaques –

Tinea nigra is an infection of palmar or plantar skin caused by a black yeast, *Phaeoannelomyces werneckii*. It is mainly seen in the tropics but can present in Europe and the USA. The main differential diagnosis is an acral melanoma as it presents as a flat pigmented mark on the hands or feet. If the lesion is scraped with a glass slide or scalpel it can be shown to be scaly. Lesions are usually solitary. The presence of pigmented hyphae in skin scrapings is typical. Tinea nigra responds to a variety of treatments including Whitfield's ointment and azole creams.

Alternaria species cause a rare form of skin granuloma, often presenting with ulceration in normal or immunocompromised patients. The lesions are most often located over exposed sites, such as the dorsum of the hands. It has been seen in patients with AIDS.

A variety of different fungi, such as *Fusarium*, *Aspergillus* and *Pyrenochaeta*, also occasionally cause onychomycosis. *Acremonium* and *Fusarium* species, in particular, are sometimes associated with superficial nail-plate invasion (superficial white onychomycosis) in the tropics.

Otomycosis

Otomycosis or otitis externa caused by fungi is seen in most tropical areas. The most common cause is *Aspergillus niger*,[54] which forms a dense mat in the external auditory meatus, with loss of hearing and serous secretion. This can be removed carefully with a wax hook through an otoscope.

SUBCUTANEOUS MYCOSES

Subcutaneous fungal infections are mainly confined to the tropics and subtropics (Table 71.2). While they are seldom common, their diagnosis and management are difficult and it is important to establish the correct diagnosis. These infections are generally caused by direct introduction of organisms through the skin into the dermis or subcutaneous tissues and for this reason, they are often called 'mycoses of implantation' (Table 71.3). They generally remain confined to their site of introduction, only spreading locally; however, there are rare examples where the infection disseminates beyond this area to affect distal sites. In addition, the disease sporotrichosis has both a subcutaneous and a systemic form, in the latter instance the infection spreading from a primary pulmonary focus.

Mycetoma

Mycetoma (Madura foot) is a chronic subcutaneous infection caused by actinomycetes or fungi in which the organisms form into aggregates (called grains), attracting an inflammatory response in the deep dermis and subcutaneous tissue and leading to the development of draining sinuses communicating with the overlying skin and causing osteomyelitis.[55] Those mycetomas caused by actinomycetes are called actinomycetomas; those caused by fungi, eumycetomas (mycotic mycetomas) (Table 71.4).

Table 71.2 Causes of mycetoma

Organism	Colour of grain	Common distribution
Fungi		
Madurella mycetomatis	Black	Africa, Middle East, India
M. grisea	Black	Central and South America, Caribbean
Scedosporium apiospermum	White/yellow	Anywhere, USA and Europe
Fusarium or *Acremonium* spp.	White/yellow	Anywhere
Aspergillus nidulans	White/yellow	Sudan, elsewhere
Neotestudina rosati	White/yellow	Africa
Actinomycetes		
Actinomadura madurae	White/yellow	Africa, Middle East, elsewhere
A. pelletieri	Red	Africa, India, elsewhere
Streptomyces somaliensis	White/yellow	Africa, Middle East, elsewhere
Nocardia spp.	Small white/yellow	Americas, elsewhere

Table 71.3 Subcutaneous mycoses

Mycetoma
Chromoblastomycosis (chromomycosis)
Sporotrichosis
Lobomycosis
Subcutaneous zygomycosis
due to *Basidiobolus*
due to *Conidiobolus*

Table 71.4 Causes of chromoblastomycosis

Fonsecaea pedrosoi
Cladophialophora carrionii
F. verrucosa
Rhinocladiella aquaspersa

Epidemiology

Mycetoma is generally a disease seen in the tropics or subtropics, although cases are described from other zones.[55,56] It is more often seen in areas where there is a low annual rainfall. The main sites for this infection are Mexico, Central and northern South America, Africa, the Middle East and India. Cases are reported less frequently in the Far East. The main causes of mycetoma are shown in Table 71.3. Organisms prevalent in certain areas are shown; however, cases may rarely be seen outside these endemic zones. As a general principle, the main causes of mycetoma in Central America are *Nocardia* species,[57] whereas in most African countries and the Indian subcontinent *Madurella mycetomatis* is the most common cause. The causes of mycetoma are generally classified according to organism, namely fungi (eumycetoma) or actinomycetes (actinomycetoma), and by grain colour – black, red or pale, e.g. red grain actinomycetoma is an infection caused by *Actinomadura pelletieri*. The proportion of pale grain eumycetomas is higher in temperate areas and in addition many of the fungi isolated are sterile moulds which cannot be identified because of a lack of distinguishing characteristics.

Mycetoma is more common in males than females and generally affects adults. It is also mainly seen in agricultural workers, although this is not invariable. The majority of patients appear to have no predisposing illness. There is evidence that the organisms are spread from the environment via a penetrating injury such as a thorn prick. The fungal causes of mycetoma have been isolated from plants, plant debris and soil; *Nocardia* species have been isolated from soil. It appears that the organisms possess mechanisms that aid survival in the human host allowing them to evade defences. Some of the mechanisms of adaptation include the deposition of intra- or extracellular melanin, cell wall thickening and immunomodulation.[58]

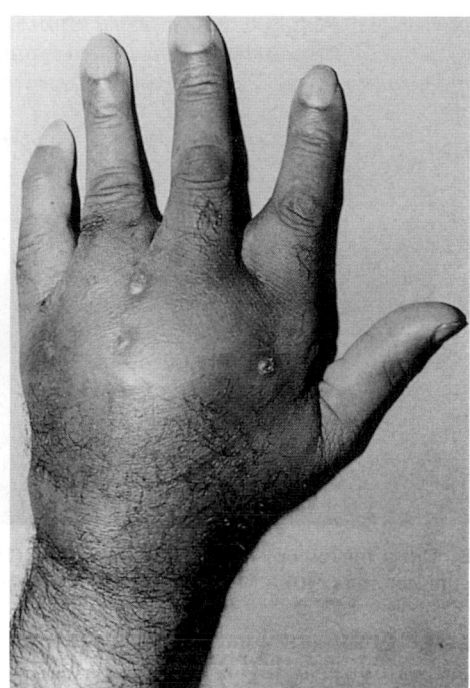

Figure 71.7 Mycetoma affecting the hand due to *Madurella grisea*.

Clinical features

The earliest sign of a mycetoma is the appearance of a small symptom-free dermal or subcutaneous swelling.[55,56] It is difficult to give an accurate estimate of incubation periods as few patients give a history of a penetrating injury. However, it may take several years before the first sign of disease, a painless subcutaneous nodule, is seen. With time, this slowly enlarges and sinuses appear on its upper surface (Figure 71.7). Pain may occur prior to rupture of sinuses on to the skin surface and in the early stages these dry up. Chronically discharging sinuses may be formed in well-established lesions. At this stage there is considerable woody swelling affecting the site, accompanied by deformity.

The main areas affected are those subject to trauma such as the feet, lower legs and hands. Nocardia species are prominent among causes of lesions on the chest and back; *Streptomyces somaliensis* is the most common cause of head and neck lesions. Dissemination is rare, although some infections may become very extensive and spread widely over a limb. The only threat to life is where they involve the skull.

Radiological changes include cortical thinning or hypertrophy, periosteal proliferation and lytic lesions.[59] Magnetic resonance imaging (MRI) is the most accurate method of delineating the extent of lesions.

Differential diagnosis

Mycetomas may be mistaken for osteomyelitis caused by bacteria or actinomycosis. Actinomycosis is an infection caused by *Actinomyces israelii*, *A. bovis* or other actinomycetes, such as *Arachnia propionica*. The infections are usually located close to the sites where these organisms can be carried, such as the oral cavity, chest, and within the abdominal cavity, around the caecum.

Laboratory diagnosis

The laboratory diagnosis of mycetoma depends on the demonstration of grains of the organisms.[60] These are generally obtained by opening a sinus where there is a small amount of pus beneath the skin surface, using a sterile needle. The grains can usually be seen with the naked eye in the pus and blood coming from the sinus tract. They can be processed as follows:

Direct microscopy. Grains are mounted in 5–10% potassium hydroxide (Figure 71.8). They are gently squashed. As a general rule, if the filaments can be seen with the ×40 objective the cause is a fungus. However, if these are not visible, the cause is likely to be an actinomycete.

Grains can be taken directly from sinuses for histology and embedded after formalin fixation. The pathology laboratory should be shown the grains, otherwise they may be discarded prior to fixation.[61] The appearance of many grains is typical in haematoxylin and eosin stained sections and the use of special fungal stains, such as periodic acid–Schiff or methenamine silver is not strictly necessary.

Grains can be cultured on a variety of media and the appearances of the fungi or actinomycetes is typical, although a specialist laboratory will be needed for their identification.

If grains cannot be obtained by this method, a deep and wide biopsy is necessary and the specimen submitted for histology and culture.

A main aim of laboratory diagnosis is to separate fungal and actinomycete causes because the treatment of each is different.

Management

The treatment of mycetoma depends on knowing whether the cause is an actinomycete or a fungus.[62] The actinomycetes respond

blastomycosis is most often seen in the tropics. The main sites of dissemination are the skin and bones. Skin lesions may be ulcers, abscesses, granulomas or crusted plaques which heal with scar formation. The bones involved are principally axial skeletal bones, such as vertebrae, and spinal cord compression may occur as a result of this infection. Dissemination also occurs in the immunocompromised patient.[91]

Laboratory diagnosis

The diagnosis of this infection is based on direct microscopy at suitable sites as well as sputum and culture. *B. dermatitidis* is a dimorphic fungus which grows as a mould at room temperature but as a yeast at 37°C. Histological changes of blastomycosis are typical as the yeasts produce a characteristic broad-based bud.

Management

Therapy of blastomycosis involves the use of either itraconazole (200–400 mg daily) or intravenous amphotericin B is an alternative (0.6–1.0 mg/kg daily).

Coccidioidomycosis

This infection is caused by *Coccidioides immitis* or its very close relative *C. posadasii* which are soil organisms, geographically confined to semi-desert areas of the New World.[92] The infection consists of a respiratory disease which may spread to other sites. Coccidioidomycosis may affect both healthy and immunocompromised patients.

Epidemiology

This infection is seen mainly in a geological zone known as the lower Sonoran life zone, where there is a low annual rainfall and a characteristic vegetation including cacti and creosote bushes. The disease is confined to the semi-desert areas of the New World in the USA, Central America (Honduras, Guatemala), Colombia, Venezuela, Argentina and Paraguay. The infecting form is an arthrospore, which is inhaled but is transformed in the host into a spore-like structure, the spherule. This is a large 50–80 mm diameter spore containing small endospores which are released by rupture of the spherule; they can develop into further spores.

Clinical features

Infection follows inhalation. Once again in the endemic area, a significant proportion of the populace appear to be subclinically sensitized, e.g. up to 70% in California.[93] The primary infection, when it is symptomatic, may present with fever, weight loss, cough and chest pains. Arthralgia, conjunctivitis and erythema nodosum or erythema multiforme may all develop. The radiological changes vary from minimal focal consolidation to pleural effusion to massive hilar adenopathy. This clinical type is usually self-resolving, although progression is much more likely in American Indians, Blacks or mestizos. Pregnant women are also at risk from dissemination. An extensive pneumonia may follow infection in patients with depressed T lymphocyte function, such as those who have received organ transplants. Chronic pulmonary nodules or cavitation may also occur.[92] The latter is char-

acteristically thin-walled on radiography. Dissemination is also seen. Dissemination of coccidioidomycosis often affects the joints or meninges, but skin and other organs may also be affected. Skin changes include ulcers and granulomas as well as warty papules and nodules. Meningitis is a chronic process which clinically mimics tuberculous infection. It is notoriously difficult to treat. In patients with AIDS prolonged pneumonia and disseminated infections can both occur.[94]

Laboratory diagnosis

The diagnosis depends on the identification of spherules in smears, biopsies or sputum as well as on the growth of the organism. *Coccidioides* is a white mould fungus which is easily spread by aerosol: the two species can only be distinguished by molecular genetic techniques. It is therefore a potential laboratory hazard and laboratory staff should be forewarned if this is being considered diagnostically. There are also a number of useful serological tests (complement fixation, immunodiffusion and immunoelectrophoresis).

Management

The treatment of coccidioidomycosis has been changing in recent years, with an increasing reliance on the use of itraconazole and fluconazole. Intravenous amphotericin B is an alternative. Posaconazole may also prove to be an effective therapy. The responses of widely disseminated infection and meningitis to these treatments are often poor.

Paracoccidioidomycosis

Paracoccidioidomycosis or South American blastomycosis is a systemic fungal infection, which is confined to Central and South America.[95] It causes a range of pulmonary and systemic symptoms but is a sporadically occurring infection caused by the dimorphic fungus *Paracoccidioides brasiliensis*. Yeast phase organisms can be found in tissue.

Epidemiology

The main areas where this disease is present are Colombia, Venezuela, Ecuador, Brazil and Argentina, but other South and Central American countries may be involved. Skin testing reveals that the distribution of sensitization in the community is patchy, and seldom more than 25% have positive skin tests. Both sexes may be sensitized but this infection is more common in men than women. The process of transformation from hyphal (environmental) phase to yeast phase *P. brasiliensis* is partly regulated by an intracytoplasmic oestrogen receptor. The natural source of the organism is probably soil.

Clinical features

The presence of a small group of healthy individuals in an endemic area with positive skin test reactions suggests that there is a subclinical form of this disease.[96] The main clinical types are named after those parts of the body predominantly affected, such as pulmonary, lymphonodular, mucocutaneous or mixed. In chronic pulmonary infection there is often widespread and extensive infiltration followed by severe fibrosis. There is also dissemination to other sites such as the oral or nasal mucosa or lymph nodes.[97] These are the mucosal (mucocutaneous) or lymphatic forms, respectively, but the most common variety is a mixed type where there are multiple foci of infection. Usually all are only slowly progressive. On mucosal surfaces this infection produces large erosions and ulcers, less commonly warty papules. All these forms of infection are virtually confined to males. While in most patients paracoccidioidomycosis is an indolent infection, an aggressive widespread form of disease occurs occasionally in younger patients. Paracoccidioidomycosis is rare in patients with AIDS.

Laboratory diagnosis

The infection is diagnosed by demonstrating presence of the characteristic yeast forms in sputum, smears or biopsies. These yeasts form multiple buds, often appearing around the periphery of a parent cell. The organism is a dimorphic fungus which can be isolated in culture. At room temperature it grows as a mycelial form and has to be converted on enriched agar into the yeast phase at 37°C. Immunodiffusion and complement fixation tests are also available.

Management

The main treatments are itraconazole (100–200 mg daily) or ketoconazole (200 mg daily), but intravenous amphotericin B is an alternative. The latter may be necessary in the widespread aggressive forms of infection.

Infection due to *Penicillium marneffei*

P. marneffei is a fungus which is a pathogen of bamboo rats of the genus Canomys, found in China and South-east Asia. It causes a disease which grossly resembles histoplasmosis in both otherwise healthy and immunocompromised patients.[98,99] It is common in AIDS patients. The endemic areas extend from parts of Malaysia through Thailand to Myanmar and Assam and north to South China, Taiwan and Hong Kong. Infections are commoner after the rains and it is assumed that the main portal of entry is the lung.

The main sites affected are the lungs, skin, liver, spleen and bone marrow. Most patients have disseminated disease, although occasionally the infection is localized. Skin lesions occur in about 60% of cases with AIDS and consist of umbilicated papules, small ulcers of nodules. They are very prominent on the face.

The organisms resemble *Histoplasma* species but do not form buds, individual cells being divided by septa. Cells may also be curved. The organism has a characteristic appearance in culture and often produces a diffusible red pigment.

The main therapeutic agents are itraconazole or amphotericin B. In AIDS patients the initial treatment is amphotericin B followed by long-term suppressive treatment with itraconazole. Again, itraconazole can be withdrawn with caution after 4–6 months, especially in patients on antiretrovirals

SYSTEMIC OPPORTUNISTIC PATHOGENS

The main opportunistic fungi are listed in Table 71.7. In industrialized countries they are a major problem in severely ill patients,

Table 71.7 Opportunistic systemic mycoses

Systemic *candidosis*
Aspergillosis
Mucormycosis
Cryptococcosis
Less common
Systemic infections due to *Trichosporon, Fusarium, Bipolaris*

particularly those with neutropenia and those receiving solid organ or bone marrow transplants. They are also seen in intensive care units. In addition to these, some infections, such as cryptococcosis, are present in patients with AIDS. In the tropics less attention has been paid to some of these opportunists, such as *candidosis* and *aspergillosis*, with some important exceptions;[100] by contrast, cryptococcosis is recognized to be a common and increasingly important problem everywhere. For more detailed information on these infections the reader is referred to other texts.[101]

Systemic candidosis

Systemic *Candida* infections occur in a variety of patients, particularly those who are neutropenic, such as leukaemia patients, those who have received major surgery and patients receiving long-term intravenous feeding. The importance of these infections in the tropics is largely unknown.[101]

Aspergillosis

Aspergillosis is a disease caused by species of the genus *Aspergillus*, principally *A. fumigatus*, *A. flavus* and *A. niger*. There are a number of different clinical syndromes caused by these fungi, which occur in temperate and tropical climates alike. *Aspergilli* are well-recognized causes of allergic pulmonary disease, either when inhaled as spores (extrinsic asthma) or when growing within airways where, in susceptible individuals, they may cause a form of intrinsic asthma known as allergic bronchopulmonary aspergillosis.[102] The latter causes reversible bronchoconstriction in the early stages but thereafter irreversible pulmonary damage may occur. This type of disease has been recorded in India, among other tropical areas. A form of aspergillosis seen regularly in tropical areas is the development of a fungus ball in patients with pulmonary cavitation, usually secondary to tuberculosis.[103] This fungus ball may elicit an inflammatory response and in a minority of patients (15%) will cause severe haemoptysis.[104] The other mode of pathogenesis by *Aspergillus* is through invasion of tissue. This is mainly a problem in the severely neutropenic patient. However, there is one invasive *Aspergillus* syndrome that is mainly seen in the tropics: invasive paranasal *Aspergillus* granuloma.

Invasive *Aspergillus* granuloma of the paranasal sinuses is a slowly progressive infection affecting the sinuses, orbit and brain.[101,105] It is seen mainly in Africa and the Middle East and in most patients is caused by *A. flavus*. The patient presents with headache, nasal obstruction and orbital swelling with, in some cases, proptosis. In later stages, invasion of the brain may ensue.

1185

20. Vanbreusegehem R. Trichophyton soudanense infection in and outside Africa. *Br J Dermatol* 1968; 80:140–148.

21. Verhagen AR. Distribution of dermatophytes causing tinea capitis in Africa. *Trop Geogr Med* 1973; 26:101–120.

22. Wright S, Robertson VJ. An institutional survey of tinea capitis in Harare, Zimbabwe and a trial of miconazole cream versus Whitfield's ointment in its treatment. *Clin Exp Dermatol* 1986; 11:371–377.

23. Pomeranz AJ, Sabnis SS, McGrath GJ, et al. Asymptomatic dermatophyte carriers in the households of children with tinea capitis. *Arch Pediat Adoles Med* 1999; 153:483–486.

24. Babel D, Baughman SA. Evaluation of the adult carrier state in juvenile tinea capitis caused by Trichophyton tonsurans. *J Am Acad Dermatol* 1989; 21:1209–1212.

25. Elewski B. Tinea capitis: a current perspective. *J Am Acad Dermatol* 1999; 42:1–20.

26. Davies RR. Griseofulvin. In: Speller DCE, ed. *Antifungal Chemotherapy.* Chichester: Wiley, 1980:149–182.

27. Gupta AK, Sauder DN, Shear NH. Antifungal agents: an overview. *J Am Acad Dermatol* 1994; 30(Part I):677–698, (Part II):911–933.

28. Clayton YM, Connor BL. Comparison of clotrimazole cream, Whitfield's ointment and nystatin ointment for the topical treatment of ringworm infections, pityriasis versicolor, erythrasma and candidiasis. *Br J Dermatol* 1973; 89:297–303.

29. Baran R, Hay RJ, Haneke E, et al. *Onychomycosis: A Current Approach to Current Diagnosis and Treatment.* London: Martin Dunitz; 2005.

30. Zaias N. Superficial white onychomycosis. *Sabouraudia* 1966; 5:99–103.

31. Caceres-Rios H, Rueda M, Ballona R, et al. Comparison of terbinafine and griseofulvin in the treatment of tinea capitis. *J Am Acad Dermatol* 2000; 42:80–84.

32. Terrell CL. Antifungal agents. Part II. The azoles. *Mayo Clin Proc* 1999; 74:78–100.

33. Fidel PL, Wozniak KL. Superficial candidiasis. In: Merz W, Hay RJ, eds. *Medical Mycology. Topley and Wilsons Microbiology and Microbial Infections.* Vol. 5. London: Edward Arnold; 2005:256–272.

34. Gough PM, Warnock DW, Turner A, et al. Candidosis of the genital tract in non-pregnant women. *Eur J Obstet Gynecol Reprod Biol* 1985; 19:237–246.

35. Torssander J, Morfeldt-Mauson L, Biberfeld G, et al. Oral *Candida* albicans in HIV infection. *Scand J Infect* 1987; 189:291–295.

36. Samaranayake LP, MacFarlane TW, eds. *Oral Candidosis.* London: Wright; 1990.

37. Pindborg JJ. Classification of oral lesions associated with HIV infection. *Oral Surg Oral Med Oral Pathol* 1989; 67:292–295.

38. Greenspan D, Komaroff E, Redford M, et al. Oral mucosal lesions and HIV viral load in the Women's Interagency HIV Study (WIHS). *J Acquir Immune Defic Syndr* 2000; 25:89–104.

39. Sobel JD. Pathogenesis and treatment of recurrent vulvovaginal candidiasis. *Clin Infect Dis* 1992; 14:S148–S153.

40. Hay RJ. Yeast infections. In: Elgart ML, ed. *Cutaneous Mycology. Dermatologic Clinics.* Philadelphia: WB Saunders; 1996:113–124.

41. Dwyer JM. Chronic mucocutaneous candidiasis. *Annu Rev Med* 1981; 32:491–497.

42. Cha R, Sobel JD. Fluconazole for the treatment of candidiasis: 15 years experience. *Expert Rev Antiinfect Ther* 2004; 2:357–366.

43. Jones HE, ed. *Ketoconazole Today: A Review of Clinical Experience.* Manchester: ADIS Press; 1987.

44. Pierard GE, Arrese JE, Pierard-Franchimont C. Itraconazole. *Expert Opin Pharmacother* 2000; 1:287–304.

45. Hay RJ, Moore MK. Clinical features of superficial fungal infections caused by Hendersonula toruloidea and Scytalidium hyalinum. *Br J Dermatol* 1984; 110:677–683.

46. Gugnani HC, Nzelibe FK, Osunkwo IC. Onychomycosis due to Hendersonula toruloidea in Nigeria. *J Med Vet Mycol* 1986; 24:239–241.

47. Moore MK. Morphological and physiological studies of isolates of Hendersonula toruloidea Nattrass cultured from human skin and nail samples. *J Med Vet Mycol* 1988; 26:25–39.

48. Ashbee HR. Recent developments in the immunology and biology of Malassezia species. *FEMS Immunol Med Microbiol* 2006; 47:14–23.

49. Roberts SO. Pityriasis versicolor: a clinical and mycological investigation. *Br J Dermatol* 1969; 81:315–326.

50. Crespo-Erchiga V, Florencio VD. Malassezia species in skin disease. *Curr Opin Infect Dis* 2002; 15:133–142.

51. Kaiter DC A, Tschen JA, Cernoch PL, et al. Genital white piedra: epidemiology, microbiology and therapy. *J Am Acad Dermatol* 1986; 14: 982–993.

52. Lassus A, Kanerva L, Stubbs S, et al. White piedra. *Arch Dermatol* 1982; 118:208–211.

53. Adam BA T, Soo-Hoo TS, Chong KC. Black piedra in West Malaysia. *Austr J Dermatol* 1977; 18:45–47.

54. Kaur R, Mittal N, Kakkar M, et al. Otomycosis : a clinicomycologic study. *Ear Nose Throat J* 2000; 79:606–609.

55. Fahal AH. Mycetoma: a thorn in the flesh. *Trans Roy Soc Trop Med Hyg* 2004; 98:3–11.

56. Mariat F, Destombes P, Segretain G. The mycetomas: clinical features, pathology, etiology and epidemiology. *Contrib Microbiol Immunol* 1977; 4: 1–39.

57. Mahe A, Develoux M, Lienhardt C, et al. Mycetomas in Mali: causative agents and geographic distribution. *Am J Trop Med Hyg* 1996; 54:77–79.

58. Wethered DB, Markey MA, Hay RJ, et al. Ultrastructural and immunogenic changes in the formation of mycetoma grains. *J Med Vet Mycol* 1986; 25: 39–46.

59. Abd El Bagi ME. New radiographic classification of bone involvement in pedal mycetoma. *Am J Roentgenol* 2003; 180:665–668.

60. Khatri ML, Al-Halali HM, Fouad Khalid M, et al. Mycetoma in Yemen: clinicoepidemiologic and histopathologic study. *Int J Dermatol* 2002; 49:586–593.

61. Destombes P. Histological diagnosis of mycetoma granules. In: *Proceedings of the First International Symposium on Mycetoma,* Venezuela; 1978:80–94.

62. Hay RJ, Mahgoub ES, Leon G, et al. Mycetoma. *J Med Vet Mycol* 1992; 30(suppl. 1):41–49.

63. Minotto R, Bernardi CD, Mallmann LF, et al. Chromoblastomycosis: a review of 100 cases in the state of Rio Grande do Sul, Brazil. *J Am Acad Dermatol* 2001; 44:585–592.

64. Banks IS, Palmieri JR, Lanoie L, et al. Chromomycosis in Zaire. *Int J Dermatol* 1985; 24:302–307.

65. Silva JP, de Souza W, Rozental S. Chromoblastomycosis: a retrospective study of 325 cases in Amazonic Region (Brazil). *Mycopathologia* 1999; 143:171–175.

66. Esterre P, Andriantsimahavandy A, Raharisolo C. Natural history of chromoblastomycosis in Madagascar and the Indian Ocean. *Bull Soc Pathol Exot* 1997; 90:312–317.

67. McGinnis MR. Chromoblastomycosis and phaeohyphomycosis: new concepts, diagnosis and mycology. *J Am Acad Dermatol* 1983; 8: 1–16.

68. Lyon GM, Zurita S, Casquero J, et al. Population-based surveillance and a case-control study of risk factors for endemic lymphocutaneous sporotrichosis in Peru. *Clin Infect Dis* 2003; 36:34–39.

69. Carvalho MT, de Castro AP, Baby C, et al. Disseminated cutaneous sporotrichosis in a patient with AIDS: report of a case. *Revista Da Sociedade Brasileira de Medicina Tropical* 2002; 35:655–659.

70. Quintal D. Sporotrichosis infection on mines of the Witwatersrand. *J Cutan Med Surg* 2000; 4:51–54.

71. Kauffman CA. Sporotrichosis. *Clin Infect Dis* 1999; 29:231–236.

72. Itoh M, Okamoto S, Kanya H. Survey of 260 cases of sporotrichosis. *Dermatologica* 1986; 172:203–213.

73. Silva-Vergara ML, Maneira FR, De Oliveira RM, et al. Multifocal sporotrichosis with meningeal involvement in a patient with AIDS. *Med Mycol* 2005; 43:187–190.

74. Baker RD, Seabury JH, Schneidau JD. Subcutaneous and cutaneous mucormycosis and subcutaneous phycomycosis. *Lab Invest* 1962; 11: 1091–1102.

75. Martinson FD. Clinical, epidemiological and therapeutic aspects of entomophthoromycosis. *Ann Soc Belg Med Trop* 1972; 52:329–342.

76. Segura JJ, Gionzale K, Berrocal J, et al. Rhinoentomophthoromycosis; report of the first two cases observed in Costa Rica (Central America) and review of the literature. *Am J Trop Med Hyg* 1981; 30:1078–1084.

77. Thammayya A. Zygomycosis due to Conidiobolus coronatus in west Bengal. *Ind J Chest Dis Allied Sci* 2000; 42:305–309.

78. Kamalam A, Thambiah AS. Muscle invasion by Basidiobolus haptosporus. *Sabouraudia* 1984; 22:273–277.

79. Baruzzi RG, Marcopito LF. Lobomycosis. *Baillière's Clin Trop Med Commun Dis* 1989; 4:97–112.

80. Taborda PR, Taborda VA, McGinnis MR. Lacazia loboi gen. nov., comb. nov., the etiologic agent of lobomycosis. *J Clin Microbiol* 1999; 37:2031–2033.

81. Wheat LJ, Kaufman CA. Histoplasmosis. *Infect Dis Clin North Am* 2003; 17:1–19.

82. Gugnani HC. Histoplasmosis in Africa: a review. *Ind J Chest Dis Allied Sci* 2000; 42:271–277.

83. Goodwin RA, Shapiro JL, Thurman GH, et al. Disseminated histoplasmosis. *Medicine* 1980; 59:1–33.

84. Wheat J, Sarosi G, McKinsey D, et al. Practice guidelines for the management of patients with histoplasmosis. Infectious Diseases Society of America. *Clin Infect Dis* 2000; 30:688–695.

85. Barton EN, Roberts L, Ince WE, et al. Cutaneous histoplasmosis in the acquired immunodeficiency syndrome: a report of three cases from Trinidad. *Trop Geogr Med* 1988; 40:153–157.

86. Lemos LB, Guo M, Baliga M. Blastomycosis: organ involvement and etiologic diagnosis. A review of 123 patients from Mississippi. *Ann Diagn Pathol* 2000; 4:391–406.

87. Klein BS, Vergeront JM, Weeks RJ, et al. Isolation of Blastomyces dermatitidis in soil associated with a large outbreak of blastomycosis in Wisconsin. *N Engl J Med* 1986; 314:529–534.

88. Emerson PA, Higgins E, Branfoot A. North American blastomycosis in Africans. *Br J Dis Chest* 1984; 78:286–291.

89. Kingston M, El-Mishad MM, Ashraf AM. Blastomycosis in Saudia Arabia. *Am J Trop Med Hyg* 1980; 29:464–466.

90. Randhawa HS, Khan ZV, Gaur SN. Blastomyces dermatitidis in India: first report of its isolation from clinical material. *Sabouraudia* 1983; 21:215–221.

91. Chapman SW, Bradsher RW Jr, Campbell GD Jr, et al. Practice guidelines for the management of patients with blastomycosis. Infectious Diseases Society of America. *Clin Infect Dis* 2000; 30:679–683.

92. Ampel NM. Coccidioidomycosis. *Semin Respir Infect* 2001; 16:229–296.

93. Gifford J, Catanzaro A. A comparison of coccidioidin and Spherulin skin testing in the diagnosis of coccidioidomycosis. *Am Rev Respir Dis* 1981; 124:440–444.

94. Bronniman DA, Adam RD, Galgiani JN, et al. Coccidioidomycosis in the acquired immunodeficiency syndrome. *Ann Intern Med* 1987; 106:373–379.

95. Franco M, Lacaz CS, Restrepo A, et al., eds. *Paracoccidioidomycosis*. Boca Raton, Florida: CRC Press, 1994.

96. Benard G, Duarte AJ. Paracoccidioidomycosis: a model for evaluation of the effects of human immunodeficiency virus infection on the natural history of endemic tropical diseases. *Clin Infect Dis* 2000; 31:1032–1039.

97. Tobon AM, Agudelo CA, Osorio ML, et al. Residual pulmonary abnormalities in adult patients with chronic paracoccidioidomycosis: prolonged follow-up after itraconazole therapy. *Clin Infect Dis* 2003; 37:898–904.

98. Sirisanthana T, Supparatpinyo K. Epidemiology and management of penicilliosis in human immunodeficiency virus-infected patients. *Int J Infect Dis* 1998 3:48–53.

99. Ranjana KH, Priyokumar K, Singh TJ, et al. Disseminated Penicillium marneffei infection among HIV-infected patients in Manipur state, India. *J Infect* 2002; 45:268–271.

100. Hay RJ. Opportunistic fungal infection in the tropics. *Baillière's Clin Trop Med Commun Dis* 1989; 4:249–267.

101. Warnock D, Richardson MD, eds. *Fungal Infections in the Compromised Patient*. Chichester: Wiley; 1989.

102. Attapattu MC. Allergic bronchopulmonary aspergillosis in a chronic asthmatic. *Ceylon Med J* 1983; 28:251–270.

103. Bovornkitti S, Pacharee P, Chatvanich K, et al. Aspergilloma in a bronchogenic cyst: a case report. *J Med Assoc Thai* 1984; 53: 211–215.

104. Martinson FD, Ali AF, Clarke BM. Aspergilloma of the ethmoid. *J Laryngol Otol* 1970; 84:857–861.

105. Veress B, Malik OA, El Tayeb AA, et al. Further observations on the primary paranasal aspergillus granuloma in the Sudan. *Am J Trop Med Hyg* 1973; 22:765–772.

106. Bahadur S, Ghosh P, Chopra P, et al. Rhinocerebral phycomycosis. *J Laryngol Otol* 1983; 97:267–270.

107. Perfect JR, Cox GM. Cryptococcosis. In: Merz W, Hay RJ, eds. *Medical Mycology. Topley and Wilsons Microbiology and Microbial Infections*. Vol. 5. London: Edward Arnold; 2005:637–658.

108. Dupont B. Cryptococcosis. *Baillière's Clin Trop Med Commun Dis* 1989; 4:113–124.

109. Naka W, Masuda M, Konohana A, et al. Primary cutaneous cryptococcosis and Cryptococcus neoformans serotype D. *Clin Exper Dermatol* 1995; 20:221–225.

110. Kovacs JA, Kovacs AA, Polis M, et al. Cryptococcosis in the acquired immunodeficiency syndrome. *Ann Intern Med* 1985; 103:533–538.

111. Odhiambo FA, Murage EM, Ngare W, et al. Detection rate of Cryptococcus neoformans in cerebrospinal fluid specimens at Kenyatta National Hospital, Nairobi. *East Afr Med J* 1997; 74:576–578.

112. Thomas PA, Geraldine P. Oculomycosis. In: Merz W, Hay RJ, eds. *Medical Mycology. Topley and Wilsons Microbiology and Microbial Infections*. Vol 5. London: Edward Arnold; 2005:273–344.

Chapter 72 Robert F. Miller

Pneumocystis jiroveci Infection

INTRODUCTION

Different species of the ascomycetous fungus *Pneumocystis* asymptomatically infect a wide range of mammalian hosts and may cause a pneumonia, known as PCP (from PneumoCystis Pneumonia). In humans, *Pneumocystis* pneumonia is caused by *Pneumocystis jiroveci* (previously called *Pneumocystis carinii*).[1]

Pneumocystis was first described by Chagas in 1909, but it was not until 1951 that it was identified as the cause of interstitial plasma cell pneumonitis. This had been described in Europe in the late 1930s and 1940s in premature and malnourished children, especially those in orphanages. In the 1960s *Pneumocystis* pneumonia occurred largely in children with congenital defects of the immune system and in both children and adults with acquired immune defects secondary to malignancy or its treatment.[2] With organ transplantation it became apparent that *Pneumocystis* pneumonia was associated with the immunosuppression used to prevent organ rejection. With prophylaxis (see below), case rates fell in those populations. In 1980, clusters of *Pneumocystis* pneumonia in previously healthy men precipitated a search for underlying immunosuppression and subsequently the acquired immune deficiency syndrome (AIDS) was defined.[2]

EPIDEMIOLOGY AND MODE OF TRANSMISSION

Most patients who develop *Pneumocystis* pneumonia have abnormalities of T lymphocyte function or numbers; rarely *Pneumocystis* pneumonia occurs in patients with isolated B cell defects and in persons without underlying immunosuppression (Table 72.1).[3-5] Irrespective of the nature or intensity of the underlying immunosuppression, glucocorticoid therapy is an independent risk factor for development of *Pneumocystis* pneumonia in non-HIV immunosuppressed individuals.[3-5]

Before the introduction of prophylaxis, attack rates for *Pneumocystis* pneumonia in children varied from 25% in those with rhabdomyosarcoma and 22–43% in those with acute lymphoblastic leukaemia to 27–42% in those with severe combined immunodeficiency.[3-5] After organ transplantation, attack rates in adults for *Pneumocystis* pneumonia vary from 4–10% following renal transplantation to 16–43% after heart or heart–lung transplantation, if prophylaxis is not given.[3,5]

The CD4+ T lymphocyte count is used in HIV-infected patients to determine the risk of *Pneumocystis* pneumonia in an individual and also when to start prophylaxis (see below). The CD4+ T lymphocyte count may also be useful in determining risk of *Pneumocystis* pneumonia in non-HIV-infected immunosuppressed patients.

Pneumocystis pneumonia remains a common AIDS-defining diagnosis in Europe, North America and Asia, but is largely confined to patients unaware of their HIV status at presentation and to those who are non-compliant with or intolerant of prophylaxis and antiretroviral therapy.[6]

Pneumocystis pneumonia had been regarded as uncommon in HIV-infected patients in Africa,[7-9] in contrast to the high incidence reported in developed countries in the early stages of the HIV epidemic. Data emerging from central Africa about the significance of *Pneumocystis* pneumonia in adult patients with HIV infection have been conflicting.[10,11] Differences in patient selection criteria, difficulties in diagnosing *Pneumocystis* pneumonia or true geographical variation in the prevalence of *Pneumocystis* might have accounted for such differences. More recently, several studies have shown that *Pneumocystis* is an important pathogen causing much morbidity and mortality in African adults and children infected with HIV.[12-16]

Based on its morphology and lack of response to antifungal drugs, *Pneumocystis* was previously regarded taxonomically as a protozoan. *Pneumocystis* is now known to be an ascomycetous fungus.[1] Pneumocystis cannot be reliably cultured in vitro. *Pneumocystis* from humans and other mammalian host species shows antigenic, karyotypic and genetic heterogenicity.[1,17,18] Cross-infection between host species has not been achieved, suggesting host specificity and that *Pneumocystis* infection in humans is not a zoonosis.[1,18] Lower levels of genetic diversity are seen among human-derived *Pneumocystis* than occur among *Pneumocystis* derived from different mammalian hosts.[1,17,19]

The majority of healthy children and adults have antibodies to *Pneumocystis*, suggesting that *Pneumocystis* pneumonia in an immunosuppressed individual arises by reactivation of a childhood-acquired, symptomless, latent infection.[1,2] However, this hypothesis is challenged by the failure to find *Pneumocystis* in bronchoalveolar lavage fluid or autopsy lung tissue from immune-competent individuals[18] and by the observation that *Pneumocystis*-specific DNA is detectable at low levels using the polymerase chain reaction (PCR) in less than 25% of HIV-positive patients with CD4+ T lymphocyte counts lower than 200 cells/μL who present

Table 72.1 At-risk groups for *Pneumocystis* pneumonia

Sporadic disease

    Patients receiving chemotherapy

        Acute lymphoblastic leukaemia

        Hodgkin lymphoma

        Rhabdomyosarcoma

    Organ transplant recipients

        Allogeneic bone marrow

        Heart, heart–lung

        Liver

        Renal

    Immunosuppression for inflammatory disorders

        Wegener granulomatosis

        Collagen vascular disease

    Congenital immunodeficiency

        Severe combined immunodeficiency syndrome

        Hypogammaglobulinaemia

Epidemic disease

    HIV infection

No apparent risk factors

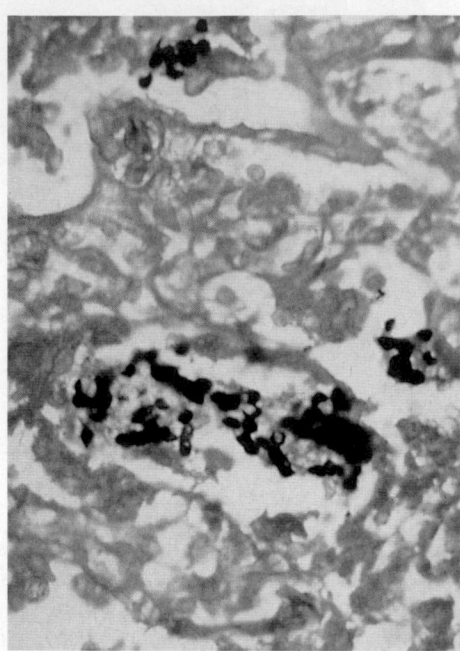

Figure 72.1 Transbronchial biopsy showing cysts of *Pneumocystis carinii* (Grocott's methenamine silver, ×200).

with respiratory episodes and diagnoses other than *Pneumocystis* pneumonia. *Pneumocystis* pneumonia in humans is now thought to arise by de novo infection from an exogenous source; this model is supported by the finding of different *Pneumocystis* genotypes in each episode in patients with recurrent pneumonia.[20,21] Recent molecular data also suggest that transmission of *Pneumocystis* from infected patients to susceptible immunocompromised individuals may occur, although there are insufficient data to support routine isolation of patients with suspected or proven *Pneumocystis* pneumonia.[22–25] Pneumocystis-specific DNA may be detected in respiratory samples from patients without clinically-apparent *Pneumocystis* pneumonia who have minor levels of immunosuppression induced by HIV infection, non-HIV infected patients receiving long-term glucocorticoid therapy and also in immune competent individuals with chronic pulmonary disease.[26] These observations suggest that asymptomatic carriage or 'colonization' by *Pneumocystis* may occur.

PATHOGENESIS

Pneumocystis is inhaled and deposited in the alveoli, where the trophic form attaches to type 1 pneumocytes. The organism is eliminated by immune-competent individuals; in the immunodeficient host, *Pneumocystis* pneumonia will develop. The major surface glycoprotein (MSG) of *Pneumocystis* binds macrophages, induces proliferation of T lymphocytes and secretion of tumour necrosis factor alpha (TNFα), interleukin (IL) 1 and IL-2.[27] Monocytes respond to MSG by releasing IL-8 and TNFα. *Pneumocystis* induces changes in pulmonary surfactant: the phospholipid level is reduced and total cholesterol, phosphatidylglycerol and phospholipase A$_2$ levels are increased.[28]

PATHOLOGY

Pulmonary infection with *Pneumocystis* is characterized by an eosinophilic foamy intra-alveolar exudate which is associated with a plasma cell interstitial infiltrate.[29] Two forms of *Pneumocystis* may be identified morphologically. By using Grocott's methenamine silver, toluidine blue O or cresyl violet stains, thick-walled cystic forms (6–7 μm in diameter), each containing four to eight sporozoites, are seen to lie freely within the alveolar exudate (Figure 72.1). The exudate itself consists largely of thin-walled, irregularly shaped, single nucleated trophic forms (2–5 μm in diameter) which are shown with Giemsa stain or electron microscopy. Both forms of *Pneumocystis* may also be demonstrated by use of indirect immunofluorescence with monoclonal antibodies raised against *Pneumocystis*. Unusually, interstitial fibrosis, granulomatous inflammation, diffuse alveolar damage, cavitary lesions and pneumatocele formation may occur.[30] Rarely, *Pneumocystis* infection may extend beyond the alveoli and extrapulmonary pneumocystosis involving liver, spleen or gut may occur.[31]

CLINICAL MANIFESTATIONS

Clinical presentation is non-specific. Patients typically present with progressive exertional dyspnoea, a non-productive cough and fever of several days' or weeks' duration, which is often associated with a sensation of inability to take in a deep breath.[32] In patients immunosuppressed by HIV infection, symptoms are usually of longer duration than in patients immunosuppressed as a result of other causes.[33] Auscultation of the chest is usually normal; rarely, fine inspiratory crackles may be heard. Table 72.2

Table 72.2 Presentation of *Pneumocystis* pneumonia

Typical features	Atypical features
Symptoms	
Progressive exertional dyspnoea over days or weeks	Sudden onset of dyspnoea over hours
Cough: non-productive, or productive of mucoid sputum	Cough productive of purulent sputum
Tachypnoea	
Inability to take in a deep breath, not due to pleuritic pain	Pleuritic chest pain
Fever ± sweats	Haemoptysis
Signs	
Normal breath sounds or fine end-inspiratory basal crackles	Signs of focal consolidation, pleural effusion or wheeze
Investigations	
Chest radiograph	
Normal	
or	⎫ Early presentation
perihilar haze	⎭
Bilateral interstitial shadowing	⎫
or	⎪
alveolar-interstitial changes	⎬ Later presentation
or	⎪
'white out' (marked alveolar consolidation)	⎭

Arterial blood gases		
PaO₂	PaCO₂	
Normal	Normal or hypocarbia	Early presentation
Hypoxaemia	Normal or hypercarbia	Later presentation

Reproduced from Malin AS, Miller RF. *Pneumocystis carinii* pneumonia: presentation and diagnosis. *Rev Med Microbiol* 1991; 3:80–87.

shows typical and atypical features for patients presenting with *Pneumocystis* pneumonia.

DIAGNOSIS

Non-invasive investigations

These investigations have moderate to high sensitivity but lack specificity.

Chest radiology

In early pneumonia, the chest radiograph may be normal; with later presentations, and with more severe disease, diffuse perihilar interstitial infiltrates are seen (Figure 72.2). These appearances

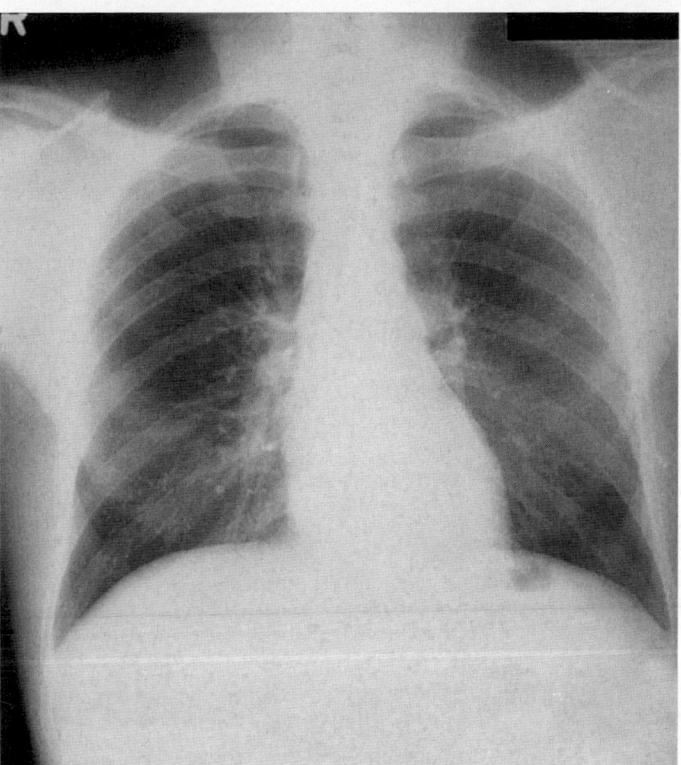

Figure 72.2 Chest radiograph showing perihilar shadowing in a patient with early *Pneumocystis* pneumonia.

may progress to diffuse bilateral air space (alveolar) consolidation resembling pulmonary oedema (Figure 72.3).[32] With delayed presentation or untreated severe disease, there may be confluent alveolar shadowing ('white out') throughout both lungs, with sparing of the costophrenic angles and apices. The chest radiographic appearances in *Pneumocystis* pneumonia may change rapidly from being normal at presentation to markedly abnormal over a period of only 2–3 days.[32] Atypical radiographic features are seen in up to 20% of patients with *Pneumocystis* pneumonia; these include cystic air space and pneumatocele formation, unilateral consolidation, lobar infiltrates, nodules, mediastinal lymphadenopathy, pleural effusions and upper zone infiltrates resembling tuberculosis (Figure 72.4).

Although the chest radiograph is a very sensitive way of detecting *Pneumocystis* pneumonia, these typical and atypical radiographic appearances may also occur in other fungal, mycobacterial and bacterial infections, and in non-infectious conditions, such as pulmonary Kaposi sarcoma (KS) and non-specific interstitial pneumonitis (NIP).

With treatment, improvements in the chest radiographic appearances are not usually apparent for 7–10 days. After treatment and clinical recovery, some radiographs remain abnormal for many months in the absence of symptoms; others show residual fibrosis or post-infectious bronchiectasis.

High-resolution computed tomography

This may be useful in the symptomatic patient with a normal or equivocal chest radiograph. Patches of 'ground glass' shadowing

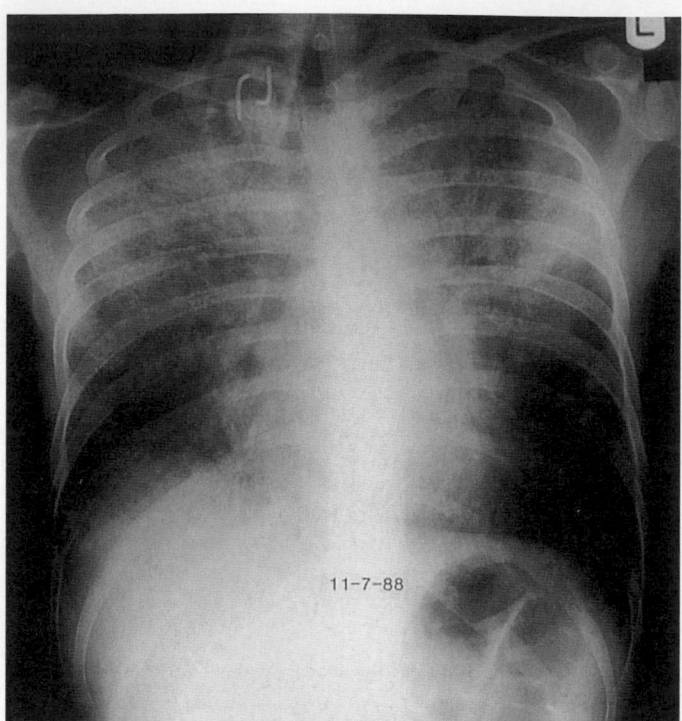

Figure 72.3 Chest radiograph showing extensive bilateral shadowing in a patient with severe *Pneumocystis* pneumonia.

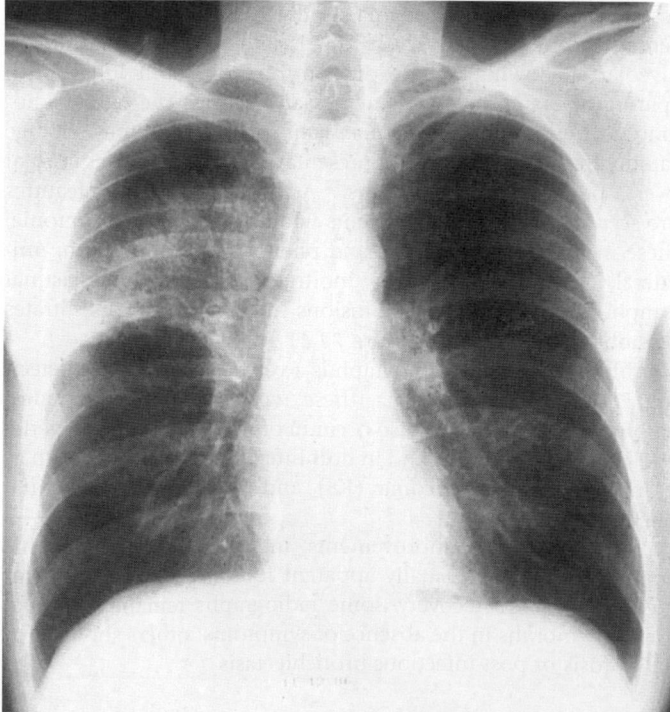

Figure 72.4 Chest radiograph showing atypical appearances of upper lobe consolidation, mimicking tuberculosis, in a patient with *Pneumocystis* pneumonia.

indicate active pulmonary disease caused by *Pneumocystis* or by cytomegalovirus or fungal pneumonia.

Arterial blood gases

In early *Pneumocystis* pneumonia, even though the arterial oxygen tension (PaO_2) may be normal or near normal, hypocarbia (indicating hyperventilation) may be present. With progression of the pneumonia, hypoxia may occur (Table 72.2).[32] The occurrence of hypercarbia in the hypoxaemic patient with *Pneumocystis* pneumonia is an ominous sign and implies severe respiratory compromise. By performing arterial blood gas analysis the alveolar-arterial oxygen gradient $A - aO_2$ may be calculated. The $A - aO_2$ gradient is widened in over 90% of patients with *Pneumocystis* pneumonia. Both hypoxaemia and a widened $A - aO_2$ gradient may also occur in bacterial and mycobacterial infections, NIP and KS.[32]

Exercise oximetry

In immunosuppressed patients with respiratory symptoms, normal or near-normal chest radiographs and normal resting PaO_2 values, exercise-induced arterial desaturation is a sensitive and specific method of detecting *Pneumocystis* pneumonia. A normal exercise test (with no desaturation) virtually excludes the diagnosis.

Invasive investigations

Sputum induction

Immunosuppressed patients with suspected *Pneumocystis* pneumonia rarely expectorate sputum spontaneously, but sputum may be obtained by inhalation of an aerosol of hypertonic (2.7%, 0.44 mol/L) saline generated by an ultrasonic nebulizer. The success rate for this technique varies considerably between centres.[34] Careful patient preparation (in particular rigorous cleansing of the mouth before the procedure) and deployment of an experienced nurse or physiotherapist to supervise the procedure increase the success rate.[34] *Pneumocystis* is usually found in clear 'saliva-like' samples. Purulent samples suggest a bacterial infection. The sensitivity varies between 55% and 90%; a negative result from sputum induction for *Pneumocystis* should prompt referral for bronchoscopy. Some patients find sputum induction is unpleasant and experience cough, nausea and retching, or dyspnoea. Unpredictable arterial blood desaturation may occur during inhalation of saline and persist for up to 20 min after the procedure.[35] The patient's arterial oxygen saturation should be measured with an oximeter during sputum induction. The procedure should be carried out away from other patients and healthcare workers, ideally in a 'negative pressure' room to avoid the risk of nosocomial transmission of tuberculosis.[36]

Fibreoptic bronchoscopy

Fibreoptic bronchoscopy with bronchoalveolar lavage (BAL) and transbronchial biopsy (TBB) have a high diagnostic yield when used in the investigation of immunocompetent and immunosuppressed patients with radiographically diffuse pneumonia. Early in the AIDS epidemic both BAL and TBB were used routinely in order to diagnose *Pneumocystis* pneumonia and to identify other pathogens. With the realization that BAL alone has a sensitivity of 90% or greater for detection of *Pneumocystis* and that TBB adds very little additional diagnostic information, yet is associated with pneumothorax (in up to 20% of cases), haemorrhage and sudden falls in PaO$_2$ which occasionally require ventilatory support, the technique has been used less frequently.[37] At bronchoscopy the majority of AIDS centres now routinely perform only BAL. Treatment should never be deferred pending results of bronchoscopy in a patient with suspected *Pneumocystis* pneumonia as significant clinical deterioration may occur. The yield for diagnosis of *Pneumocystis* from BAL fluid is not reduced for up to 10 days after starting antimicrobial therapy.

Open lung biopsy

The high yield from bronchoscopy and BAL for diagnosis of *Pneumocystis* pneumonia means that this technique is now rarely necessary. Open lung biopsy is still occasionally performed in immunosuppressed patients with diffuse pneumonia and negative results from two or more bronchoscopies, and in patients who deteriorate despite treatment for a bronchoscopically-confirmed pathogen.[38]

Molecular detection tests

Detection of *Pneumocystis*-specific DNA using the polymerase chain reaction (PCR) in BAL fluid and induced sputum is superior to histochemical staining,[39,40] but specificity is less than 100%. *Pneumocystis* DNA may also be detected in oropharyngeal samples obtained by gargling with 10–15 mL normal saline.[40,41] Molecular detection tests are not currently available commercially.

Empirical therapy

Some physicians have suggested that it is not necessary to perform invasive tests, including bronchoscopy, in HIV-infected patients presenting with symptoms, chest radiographic and arterial blood gas abnormalities typical of *Pneumocystis* pneumonia, and that such patients may be treated empirically,[42] with bronchoscopy reserved for those who fail to respond by day 5 or deteriorate on therapy and for those who have presentations atypical for *Pneumocystis* pneumonia.[43] Others have argued strongly that bronchoscopic confirmation of the diagnosis is mandatory in every case. Both strategies appear to be equally effective in clinical practice.[44]

TREATMENT

An assessment of the severity of the pneumonia, using the history, examination findings and results of arterial blood gas estimations and the chest radiograph (Table 72.3), will enable decisions to be made about choice of therapy; some drugs are unproven or ineffective in severe disease.[45,46] Severity stratification also identifies patients who will benefit from adjunctive glucocorticoids (see below). Patients with glucose 6-phosphate dehydrogenase deficiency should not receive co-trimoxazole, dapsone or primaquine as they increase the risk of haemolysis.[45,46]

THERAPY

Co-trimoxazole

High-dose co-trimoxazole (100 mg/kg daily of sulfamethoxazole and 20 mg/kg daily of trimethoprim) given in two to four divided doses orally or intravenously is first choice therapy for *Pneumocystis* pneumonia of all grades of severity. In HIV-infected patients treatment is given for 21 days because shorter courses are associated with treatment failure.[46] In patients with other causes of immunosuppression, shorter courses (e.g. 14–17 days) are often given.[46] In patients with moderate or severe disease, co-trimoxazole is given intravenously for the first 7–10 days, then orally; in patients with mild disease oral co-trimoxazole may be given throughout. Adverse reactions to co-trimoxazole, which are usually first evident at 6–14 days of treatment, are common and include neutropenia and anaemia in up to 40% of patients, rash in 25%, fever in over 20% and abnormal liver function in approximately 10%.[46]

Co-administration of folic or folinic acid does not reduce or prevent haematological toxicity and may be associated with increased therapeutic failure. Dose reduction of co-trimoxazole, to 75% of the dose given above, is associated with a reduced toxicity profile but may be associated with reduced efficacy.[46] It is not clear why there is such a high frequency of adverse reactions to co-trimoxazole in patients immunosuppressed by HIV infec-

Table 72.3 Grading of severity of *Pneumocystis* pneumonia

	Mild	Moderate	Severe
Clinical features	Increasing exertional dyspnoea ± cough and sweats	Dyspnoea on minimal exertion, occasional dyspnoea at rest, fever ± sweats	Dyspnoea at rest, tachypnoea at rest, persistent fever, cough
Arterial blood gas (room air)	PaO$_2$ normal, SaO$_2$ falling on exercise	PaO$_2$ = 8.1–11 kPa	PaO$_2$ < 8.0 kPa
Chest radiograph	Normal or minor perihilar infiltrates	Diffuse interstitial shadowing	Extensive interstitial shadowing ± diffuse alveolar shadowing ('white out'), sparing costophrenic angles and apices

SaO$_2$, arterial oxygen saturation, measured with a *transcutaneous oximeter.*
Reproduced with permission from the BMJ publishing group: From Miller RF, Mitchell DM. *Pneumocystis carinii* pneumonia. *Thorax* 1992; 47:305–314.

Table 72.4 Treatment of *Pneumocystis* pneumonia

	Mild	Moderate	Severe
First choice	Co-trimoxazole	Co-trimoxazole	Co-trimoxazole
Second choice	Clindamycin–primaquine	Clindamycin–primaquine	Clindamycin–primaquine
Third choice	Dapsone–trimethoprim or Atovaquone	Dapsone–trimethoprim or Atovaquone	i.v. Pentamidine
Fourth choice	i.v. Pentamidine	i.v. Pentamidine	–
Adjunctive glucocorticoids	Unproven benefit	Yes	Yes

tion compared with patients immunosuppressed by other causes, but it may be due to HIV-induced changes in acetylator status, accumulation of toxic metabolites such as hydroxylamines, or glutathione deficiency.[46]

Alternative therapy

Several other treatments are available if co-trimoxazole is not tolerated by the patient or if treatment fails (Table 72.4).[45,46]

Clindamycin with primaquine

This combination was originally only used to 'salvage' patients with mild and moderately severe *Pneumocystis* pneumonia who failed to respond to co-trimoxazole or pentamidine. It is now used as alternative therapy in patients with pneumonia of all grades of severity.[46] Clindamycin 450–600 mg four times daily with primaquine 15 mg daily (by mouth) are used. Higher doses of primaquine confer no therapeutic advantage and are associated with a greater risk of methaemoglobinaemia.[46] Treatment is for 21 days regardless of the type of underlying immunosuppression. Clindamycin is usually given intravenously for the first 7–10 days, then orally in moderate and severe disease; the treatment may be given orally throughout in patients with mild disease. Clindamycin-primaquine is as effective as co-trimoxazole or dapsone-trimethoprim (see below) when given as initial treatment for patients with *Pneumocystis* pneumonia of mild and moderate severity[47] and is superior to intravenous pentamidine when used in patients intolerant of, or who are failing treatment with, co-trimoxazole.[46,47] Almost two-thirds of patients develop a rash and approximately 25% develop diarrhoea. If diarrhoea occurs during clindamycin-primaquine therapy, the stool should be analysed for the presence of *Clostridium difficile* toxin.

Dapsone with trimethoprim

In patients with mild or moderately severe *Pneumocystis* pneumonia, the combination of dapsone (100 mg per day) and trimethoprim (20 mg/kg daily) is as effective as co-trimoxazole (doses as above) and is better tolerated.[46,48] Rash, nausea and vomiting, and asymptomatic methaemoglobinaemia (due to dapsone) are the major side-effects with this combination. Approximately 50% of patients develop mild hyperkalaemia (<6.1 mmol/L), which is due to trimethoprim. This combination has not been shown to be effective in severe disease.

Atovaquone

Atovaquone 750 mg twice daily, orally for 21 days, is less effective than either oral high-dose co-trimoxazole or intravenous pentamidine for treatment of mild and moderate severity *Pneumocystis* pneumonia, but is better tolerated than either drug.[46,49] It is ineffective in patients with severe pneumonia. Common adverse reactions include rash, nausea and vomiting, and constipation. Absorption of the drug from the gastrointestinal tract is variable; taking the suspension with food may increase its absorption.

Parenteral pentamidine

Intravenous pentamidine is now seldom used in mild and moderately severe disease because of its toxicity profile and because other less toxic treatments have equivalent efficacy. It continues to be used in patients with severe pneumonia.[46,50] It is given at a dose of 4 mg/kg daily, by intravenous infusion for 21 days. Intramuscular pentamidine is no longer used because of the risk of sterile abscess at the injection site. Compared with high-dose co-trimoxazole, intravenous pentamidine is of almost equivalent efficacy but has a greater toxicity profile. Up to 60% of patients receiving pentamidine develop nephrotoxicity, which is usually manifested as an isolated increase in the serum creatinine level; approximately half develop leucopenia. Hypotension and nausea/vomiting both occur in up to 25% of patients.[46] Hypoglycaemia occurs in approximately 20% of patients. Reduction of the dose of pentamidine (to 3 mg/kg daily) does not compromise efficacy and reduces toxicity.[50] There are no therapeutic advantages if high-dose co-trimoxazole and intravenous pentamidine are combined; indeed the combination has a much higher toxicity profile than when either drug is used alone.

Nebulized pentamidine

This form of therapy is no longer recommended for the treatment of *Pneumocystis* pneumonia.[46] Patients given nebulized pentamidine (600 mg/day) for 21 days respond to therapy very slowly; reductions in fever and dyspnoea and improvements in radiographic appearances and blood gases may take more than 14 days.[46,51] There is a greater rate of relapse of *Pneumocystis* pneumonia in patients treated with nebulized pentamidine when compared to those given parenteral therapy.[51] Development of extrapulmonary pneumocystosis may not be suppressed by this form of treatment as very little of the inhaled pentamidine is absorbed systemically.

Corticosteroids

Adjunctive therapy with glucocorticoids for patients with moderate and severe *Pneumocystis* pneumonia has been shown to reduce the likelihood of respiratory failure (by half) and death (by one-third) in HIV-infected patients.[52,53] In the non-HIV-infected immunosuppressed population, adjuvant steroids reduce the duration of time on mechanical ventilation and overall time in the intensive care unit.[4,54] Corticosteroids probably act by reducing the body's intrapulmonary inflammatory response to *Pneumocystis*. It is recommended that glucocorticoids are given to HIV-infected patients with proven or suspected *Pneumocystis* pneumonia who have a PaO$_2$ < 9.3 kPa or A − aO$_2$ = 4.7 kPa (both measured while the patient is breathing room air).[52,53] No specific recommendations exist for non-HIV-infected patients, but the above criteria are often used in clinical practice.

Corticosteroid treatment should begin at the start of specific anti-*Pneumocystis* therapy. Clearly, in some patients treatment will begin on a presumptive basis and it is necessary to confirm the diagnosis as soon as possible. Several regimens have been used, the most common being oral prednisolone 40 mg twice daily for 5 days, thereafter 40 mg once daily for days 6–10 and then 10 further days of 20 mg daily. Intravenous methylprednisolone may be given at 75% of these doses; alternatively, higher doses may be given for a shorter period of time, such as methylprednisolone 1 g once daily for 3 days and 0.5 g on days 4–6, followed by oral prednisolone 40 mg once daily reducing to zero over 20 days.[45,46,52,53] There is no evidence that adjunctive corticosteroids are of benefit in patients with mild *Pneumocystis* pneumonia.

General management

Patients with mild *Pneumocystis* pneumonia may be treated with oral co-trimoxazole as out-patients under close supervision of a physician. All patients with moderate and severe *Pneumocystis* pneumonia should be treated in hospital with intravenous co-trimoxazole, clindamycin with primaquine, or pentamidine and adjunctive corticosteroids. If the patient does not respond by 7–10 days, or deteriorates before this time, he or she should be switched to alternative therapy.[46]

All hypoxaemic patients with *Pneumocystis* pneumonia should receive supplemental oxygen therapy via a tight-fitting face mask in order to maintain the PaO$_2$ = 8.0 kPa. If an inspired oxygen concentration of 60% fails to maintain the PaO$_2$ = 8.0 kPa, non-invasive ventilatory support with continuous positive airways pressure (CPAP) ventilation, either by nasal or face mask, may be used. If CPAP ventilation fails to maintain oxygenation, or the PaCO$_2$ rises, or the patient becomes tired, mechanical ventilation should be considered. The prognosis of patients with severe *Pneumocystis* pneumonia with respiratory failure has improved in recent years, as a consequence of general improvements in ICU management of respiratory failure.[55] Most centres would mechanically ventilate patients with a first or second episode of *Pneumocystis* pneumonia and those who rapidly deteriorate following bronchoscopy. The timing of starting antiretroviral therapy in relation to treatment of *Pneumocystis* pneumonia is uncertain.[56,57]

PROGNOSIS

Several clinical and laboratory features are thought to predict a poor outcome in an HIV-infected patient with *Pneumocystis* pneumonia[32,55] but, unfortunately, studies are inconsistent, as not all provide prognostic information.[32,55] Prognostic factors include patient's age at admission, lack of knowledge of HIV status, presentation with a second or subsequent episode of *Pneumocystis* pneumonia, evidence of poor oxygenation (PaO$_2$ < 7.0 kPa or A − aO$_2$ = 4.0 kPa), marked chest radiographic abnormalities, peripheral blood leukocytosis (white blood cell count >10.8 × 10^9/L), a low serum albumin concentration (<35 g/L) and raised serum lactate dehydrogenase (LDH) enzyme levels (>300 IU/L). After admission and investigation, identification of a co-pathogen in induced sputum or BAL fluid, the presence of neutrophilia >5% in BAL fluid and raised serum LDH enzyme levels (that remain increased despite treatment), need for mechanical ventilation and/or development of a pneumothorax are also predictive of a poor outcome.[32,55]

CHEMOPROPHYLAXIS

With progressive immunosuppression and falls in CD4+ T lymphocyte counts, HIV-infected individuals are at increased risk of developing *Pneumocystis* pneumonia. Primary prophylaxis, to prevent a first episode of *Pneumocystis* pneumonia, is given when the CD4+ T lymphocyte count falls below 200 cells/μL or the CD4 total lymphocyte ratio is less than 1:5, to patients with HIV-related constitutional symptoms such as unexplained fever of 3 weeks or more in duration, or oral candida regardless of CD4 count, and to patients with other AIDS-defining diagnoses, such as KS.[46,58] Secondary prophylaxis is given in order to prevent a recurrence.[46,58] In individuals immunosuppressed by other causes, prophylaxis is given to those with high attack rates for *Pneumocystis* pneumonia, for example children with acute lymphoblastic leukaemia or severe combined immunodeficiency syndrome, adults with Hodgkin disease, rhabdomyosarcoma or Wegener granulomatosis and to individuals following organ transplantations such as allogenic bone marrow, renal, heart or heart–lung, or liver.[2,4,59]

Co-trimoxazole 960 mg once daily is the first-choice regimen for both primary and secondary prophylaxis. Lower doses, 960 mg three times weekly or 480 mg once daily, may be equally effective and have fewer side-effects.[58] Co-trimoxazole may also protect against bacterial infections and reactivation of cerebral toxoplasmosis. Rash, with or without fever, occurs in up to 20% of patients. Desensitization should be attempted in those unable to tolerate co-trimoxazole.[46] Alternatively, other less effective agents may be used for prophylaxis. These include nebulized pentamidine, 300 mg once per month, via a jet nebulizer (once per fortnight if the CD4+ T lymphocyte count is <50 cells/μL), dapsone, 100 mg daily with pyrimethamine 25 mg once weekly (pyrimethamine may protect against cerebral toxoplasmosis), atovaquone, 750 mg twice daily, or azithromycin 1250 mg once a week.[46,58]

1197

Chapter 73

Nicholas J. White

Malaria

Malaria is the most important parasitic disease of man. Approximately 5% of the world's population is infected, and it causes over 1 million deaths each year. The disease is a protozoan infection of red blood cells transmitted by the bite of a blood-feeding female anopheline mosquito. Malaria, or ague as it was commonly known, has been described since antiquity. Hippocrates is usually credited with the first clear description among occidental writers: In *Epidemics*, he distinguished different patterns of fever, and in his *Aphorisms* he describes the regular paroxysms of intermittent fever. In Europe, seasonal periodic fevers were particularly common in marshy areas, and were frequently referred to as 'paludial' (*L. palus* marshy ground; *Fr. paludisme*). In the early nineteenth century, miasmatic influences were believed to cause a variety of diseases. Malaria was thought by Italian writers to be caused by the offensive vapours emanating from the Tiberian marshes.[1] The word 'malaria' comes from the Italian, and means literally 'bad air'. Indeed the cause of the seasonal periodic fevers was a continuous source of debate until the late nineteenth century.[2] The work of Meckel, Virchow and Frerichs had established that the pigment (mistakenly thought to be melanin) observed in the blood of some patients with periodic fever resulted from the destruction of red blood corpuscles. This same pigment caused the characteristic grey discolouration of the internal organs in patients dying from this disease. In the 1870s, medicine slowly moved towards the germ theory of disease, following the pioneering work of Koch. In 1879, Edwin Klebs and Corrado Tommasi-Crudelli reported the identification of a bacterial cause of malaria. Recovery of the 'organism', *Bacillus malariae*, from patients with malaria was confirmed by several influential Italian physicians and pathologists – and similar reports began to appear in the USA. It was not surprising, therefore, that the report of a French Army surgeon working in Algeria, claiming that malaria was caused by a parasite, was treated initially with some scepticism.[3] On 20 October 1880 (or in a later publication he gives the date as 6 November), Charles Louis Alphonse Laveran was examining the fresh blood of a patient with ague, and observed moving bodies (he was probably watching gametocyte exflagellation) which he surmised correctly were parasites of the red blood cells. The transmissability of the infection in blood was proved 4 years later, by Gerhardt, but the route of natural infection was not discovered until the next decade. Following the suggestion of Patrick Manson, a young Scottish physician in the Indian Medical Service, Ronald Ross, began to investigate the possibility that malaria could be transmitted by mosquitoes. In 1897, after many months of failure, he reported the presence of pigmented bodies in the gut of a certain species of brown 'dapple winged' mosquito fed on patients with malaria.[4] He speculated that these might represent the parasite stage in the mosquito (he was in fact describing the oocysts) but, because of difficulties in obtaining these 'unusual' mosquitoes and his transfer to Calcutta, he was unable to characterize the complete life cycle, i.e. transmission from human to mosquito to human. After many years of study, Ross finally proved the existence of the complete life cycle involving a mosquito in the malaria of canaries.[5] He identified the anopheles mosquito as the vector of human malaria, although by the time Ross finally had the opportunity to demonstrate *Plasmodium falciparum* sporogony in anopheline mosquitoes in Sierra Leone, Bignami and his colleagues[6] in Rome, following the pioneering work of Grassi, had succeeded in infecting a healthy volunteer with *P. falciparum* from mosquito bites. Both Laveran and Ross received Nobel Prizes for their respective discoveries.

Understanding of the biology of malaria was further advanced by a third Nobel-prize winning discovery. In 1883, the Viennese psychiatrist Julius Wagner–Jarregg became interested in the relationship between fever and mental illness. Between 1888 and 1917, he experimented on a number of methods of inducing fever to treat patients with General Paralysis of the Insane (GPI is a form of neurosyphilis). On 14 June 1917, he inoculated blood from a soldier with tertian fever into two patients with GPI.[7] So began the era of malariatherapy of neurosyphilis. This became standard treatment practice throughout the world until the introduction of penicillin 30 years later. Overall, at a time when GPI accounted for 10% of all mental hospital in-patients in Europe, malaria therapy gave approximately 30% of patients a full, and 20%, a partial remission of this debilitating and ultimately lethal infection.

Until the nineteenth century, malaria was found in northern Europe, North America and Russia – and transmission in parts of Southern Europe was intense. Since then it has been eradicated from these areas, and the number of cases in the Middle East, China, and parts of Asia and South America has fallen, but elsewhere in the tropics there has been a resurgence of the disease[1] and between 1970 and 2000 the number of cases worldwide and the number of deaths steadily increased. Approximately 270 million people suffer from malaria, and there are over one million deaths each year. Most of these deaths are in African children

the number of times each day that the mosquito bites man, and the tenth power of the probability of the mosquito surviving for 1 day. The model described by MacDonald has certain theoretical limitations (it has been refined in recent years to accommodate these[21]), but it does illustrate certain fundamental points of practical relevance to control or eradication programmes. Vector longevity in determining transmission is clearly great and focuses control measures on the adult mosquito. At very high levels of transmission, there is considerable reserve in the system and large reductions in transmission reduce malaria by a negligible amount (e.g. a reduction in transmission of 90% from 300 infectious bites/year to 30 bites/year will make very little difference to the prevalence of malaria) – but as r_0 approaches the critical value of 1 (below which the disease dies out), small reductions in r_0 have very large effects on the amount of malaria. Thus malaria is very vulnerable in low transmission settings. Control programmes can be very effective in these circumstances, and can eradicate malaria – as indeed they did in Europe where r_0 was certainly low in many areas, and the vector rested inside houses and could be attacked with residual insecticides. The value of r_0 has been much debated, although there is good reason to believe it is generally low (e.g. <10). This gives hope to those developing vaccines and other interventions aimed at reducing transmission of malaria. Vectors differ considerably in their natural abundance (particularly with season of the year), feeding and resting behaviours, breeding sites, flight ranges, choice of blood source (many anopheline vectors also bite animals), and vulnerability to environmental conditions and insecticides.

There is also considerable variation in the ability of anopheline mosquitoes to transmit malaria (the vectorial capacity). There are nearly 400 species of anopheline mosquitoes and many are species complexes. Confusingly, the taxonomy continually changes as differences within species complexes are characterized. Approximately 80 anopheline species can transmit malaria, 66 are considered natural vectors, and about 45 are considered important vectors.[16] Each vector has its own behaviour patterns and even within species these can vary between geographical areas. For example, in South-east Asia mosquitoes of the *Anopheles dirus* complex are highly effective vectors, and are an important cause of 'forest and forest fringe' malaria. They breed in the tree collections of water, and are consequently vulnerable to deforestation, or too little or too much rainfall, but they are very difficult to attack with insecticides. *A. sundaicus* (recently subspeciated into *A.sundaicus* [Indonesia] and *A.epiroticus* [mainland SE Asia]) is found near the coast as it breeds in brackish water but human biting times vary considerably within the species complex. *A. stephensi*, the principal vector in the Indian subcontinent, breeds in wells or stagnant water and can be controlled by treating breeding sites with insecticides or polystyrene balls. The most effective malaria vectors (such as the *A. gambiae* complex) are hardy, long-lived, naturally occur in high densities, and bite humans frequently. Malaria is often seasonal, coinciding with the rainy season which provides water for mosquito breeding and increased humidity favouring mosquito survival. Other factors, which are not well understood, also influence mosquito populations and lead to fluctuations in the prevalence of malaria.

The human host

The behaviour of man also plays an important role in the epidemiology of malaria. There must be a human reservoir of viable gametocytes to transmit the infection. In areas where there is a long dry season, and malaria is highly seasonal, the reservoir for malaria transmission is in people who asymptomatically harbour parasites for long periods until the next rainy (transmission) season. In areas of high transmission, infants and young children are more susceptible to malaria than the more immune older children and adults. Parasite densities are higher and gametocytaemia is detected more frequently in children. In endemic areas the relative contributions to overall transmission of the younger age group, who have higher parasite densities, become ill more often, and are therefore more likely to receive drugs, versus the older asymptomatic individuals who have more immunity, lower parasite densities, and are less likely to receive antimalarial treatment, are unclear. The endemicity of malaria is best defined by the entomological inoculation rate (EIR), or number of infectious mosquito bites received per person per year, but is defined traditionally in terms of the spleen or parasite rates in children aged between 2 and 9 years (Box 73.1).[22]

In areas which are holoendemic or hyperendemic for *P. falciparum*, such as much of tropical Africa or coastal New Guinea, people are infected repeatedly throughout their lives. There is considerable morbidity and mortality during childhood. In The Gambia, where people were infected once each year on average,[20] malaria was estimated to cause 25% of deaths between 1 and 4 years of age. The effects of insecticide-treated nets on death rates in children (average reduction in all-cause mortality in children under 5 years old of approximately 20%) across sub-Saharan Africa are further testament to the impact of malaria on child survival. But eventually, if the child survives, a state of 'premunition' is achieved where infections cause little or no problem to the host. Thus a form of immunity develops which is sufficient to control, but not prevent the infection. The slow rate at which premunition is acquired may be a function of age. Non-immune adults entering an area of intense transmission acquire premunition more rapidly than children.[23] *Falciparum* malaria infections are more severe in pregnancy, particularly in primigravidae,[24–26] and appear to be augmented by iron supplementation.[27–29]

Malaria mortality and morbidity

It is difficult to be precise about how many people die each year from malaria, as the disease is most prevalent where health

---

Box 73.1 Traditional classification of malaria epidemiology

- Hypoendemic: spleen rate or parasite rate 0–10%.
- Mesoendemic: spleen or parasite rate 10–50%.
- Hyperendemic: spleen or parasite rate 50–75% and adult spleen rate is also high.
- Holoendemic: spleen or parasite rate over 75%, and adult spleen rate low. Parasite rates in the first year of life are high.

services are lacking. But in recent years, a considerable effort has gone into deriving estimates of the global burden of disease.[30–32] The Disease Control Priorities Project estimated 42 280 000 disability adjusted life years (DALYs) and 1 124 000 deaths from malaria in 2000. It is widely quoted that 90% of the deaths from malaria in the world are in African children, but recent studies suggest that the burden of malaria in Asia may have been underestimated.[18] The setting up of standardized demographic surveillance systems in many malaria endemic areas will result in more accurate data, and more accurate measurement of the impact of interventions.

Clinical epidemiology

Babies develop severe malaria relatively infrequently (although, if they do, the mortality is high). The factors responsible for this include passive transfer of maternal immunity,[33] and the high haemoglobin F content of the infants' erythrocytes which retards parasite development.[34] In holoendemic areas the baby is inoculated repeatedly with sporozoites during the first year of life, but the blood stage infection is seldom severe.[19] People may receive up to three infectious bites per day. In this epidemiological context, the main clinical impact of *falciparum* malaria is to cause severe anaemia in the 1–3-year age group (Figure 73.2). With less intense or more variable or unstable transmission the age range affected by severe malaria extends to older children, and cerebral malaria becomes a more prominent manifestation of severe disease.[35–37] Although mortality falls with decreasing transmission intensity, it remains substantial until the EIR falls well below one. In hyperendemic and holoendemic areas indigenous adults never develop severe malaria, unless they leave the transmission area and return years later (and even then malaria is seldom life-threatening). Immunity is constantly boosted and effective premunition prevents parasite burdens reaching dangerous levels. Most infections in adults are asymptomatic.

Where transmission of malaria is low, erratic, markedly seasonal, or focal, symptomatic infections are more common. A state of premunition is often not attained. Symptomatic disease occurs at any age, and cerebral malaria is a prominent manifestation of severe disease at all ages. This is termed 'unstable' malaria. In many areas, the transmission of malaria varies considerably over short distances, and severe disease is common when non-immune individuals enter these areas (e.g. woodcutters in South America and South-east Asia where malaria is of the 'forest fringe' type or highland refugees in Burundi descending into malarious lowlands).

Malaria is usually a 'rainy season disease' coinciding with increased mosquito abundance. In some areas, parasite rates (i.e. the proportion of people with positive blood smears) are relatively constant throughout the year, but the majority of cases still do occur during the wet season.[38] In Europe, before eradication, *falciparum* malaria was common in spring and in late summer and autumn, and was termed 'aestivo-autumnal malaria'.[39] The intensity of transmission or 'endemicity' can change. For example in Africa, the sub-Sahelian drought has reduced rainfall and mosquito transmission in countries such as Senegal and The Gambia. In the 1960s transmission was intense, and severe disease was rare in children over 3 years of age.[40,41] Today, transmission has fallen to levels found in areas of unstable endemicity, such as some areas of South-east Asia[42] and cases of cerebral malaria occur occasionally in indigenous adults. Deforestation, population migration, and changes in agricultural practice have profound effects on malaria transmission. Urban malaria is becoming an increasing problem in many countries.

In low transmission settings malaria can behave as an epidemic disease carrying a high mortality. Epidemics are caused by migrations (i.e. introduction of susceptible hosts), the introduction of new vectors, or changes in the habits of the mosquito vector or the human host. Epidemics have occurred in North India, Sri Lanka, South-east Asia, Ethiopia, Madagascar, Brazil (when the formidable African vector A. *gambiae* was inadvertently imported from Africa in the 1930s) and more recently in Burundi and KwaZulu Natal where drug resistance was also a contributory factor.

Increasing international air travel and worsening antimalarial drug resistance have led to an increase in imported cases of malaria in tourists, travellers and immigrants. With the recent exception of some of the former Soviet republics in East Europe and West Asia, this has not led to the reintroduction of malaria to areas from where it had earlier been eradicated (although the vector, and thus the potential, remains). The incidence of malaria has risen markedly in several African countries, India, and Bangladesh over recent decades. Imported malaria is often misdiagnosed, leading to delays in treatment and severe presentations of *falciparum* malaria are not uncommon. Malaria may also be transmitted by blood transfusion, transplantation, or through needle-sharing among intravenous drug addicts.

MALARIA PARASITE LIFE CYCLE

Pre-erythrocytic development

Infection with human malaria begins when the feeding female anopheline mosquito inoculates plasmodial sporozoites at the time of feeding.[43] The small motile sporozoites are injected during the phase of probing as the mosquito searches for a vascular space

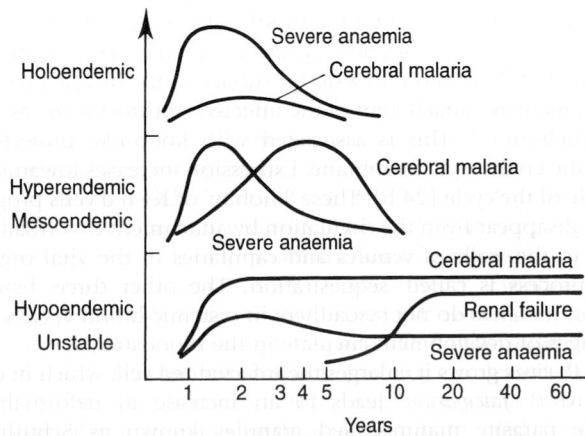

Figure 73.2 The relationship between age and the clinical presentations of severe malaria at different levels of malaria transmission.

transmit the infection. The process of gametocytogony takes about 7–10 days in *P. falciparum*. Thus there is an interval of approximately 1 week between the peaks of asexual and sexual stage parasitaemia in acute falciparum malaria. In contrast *P. vivax* begins gametocytogenesis immediately, and the process of gametocytogony in the blood stage infection takes only 4 days. Symptomatic *P. vivax* infections are therefore more likely to present with patent gametocytaemia and to transmit before treatment than acute *P. falciparum* infections. The male-to-female gametocyte sex ratio for *P. falciparum* is approximately 1 : 4.[62] One male (containing 8 microgametes) and one female (macrogamete) are required per mosquito blood meal (approximately 2 μL) for infection to occur. Thus gametocyte densities of 1 per μL are theoretically sufficient to infect mosquitoes, a density beneath the limit of detection for most routine microscopy. Following ingestion in the blood meal of a biting female anopheline mosquito, the male and female gametocytes become activated in the mosquito's gut. The male gametocytes undergo rapid nuclear division and each of the eight nuclei formed associates with a flagellum (20–25 μm long). The motile male microgametes separate and seek the female macrogametes. Fusion and meiosis then takes place to form a zygote. For a brief period, the malaria parasite genome is diploid. Within 24 h the enlarging zygote becomes motile and this form (the ookinete) penetrates the wall of the mosquito mid-gut (stomach) where it encysts (as an oocyst). This spherical bag of parasites expands by asexual division to reach a diameter of approximately 500 μm, i.e. it becomes visible to the naked eye. During the early stage of oocyst development there is a characteristic pigment pattern and colour that allows speciation (it was this that caught the eye of its discoverer, Ronald Ross, in 1894), but these patterns become obscured by the time the oocyst has matured to contain thousands of fusiform motile sporozoites. The oocyst finally bursts to liberate myriads of sporozoites into the coelomic cavity of the mosquito. The sporozoites then migrate to the salivary glands to await inoculation into the next human host during feeding. The development of the parasite in the mosquito is termed sporogony, and takes between 8 and 35 days depending on the ambient temperature and species of parasite and mosquito. The longevity of the mosquito is a critical factor in determining its vectorial capacity (see above).

Molecular genetics

Inheritance in *Plasmodium* is similar to that in other eukaryotes. Haploid and diploid generations alternate. A large number of individual genes were cloned and sequenced on the long and winding (and as yet unfinished) road towards the development of a malaria vaccine, and in the past few years the entire genome of several malaria parasites have been sequenced. *P. falciparum* has approximately 6000 genes in its 14 chromosomes and extrachromosomal elements compared with the 31 000 of its natural host. Codon composition is extremely biased to adenine and thymidine in *P. falciparum* but more evenly balanced in the other malaria parasite genomes. There appear to be some groupings of genes related to function. For example, the genes encoding the merozoite surface proteins are grouped. The many genes encoding the variant red cell surface antigens ('var' and 'rif' families), which contribute to the antigenic diversity necessary for the parasite to elude the host immune system, are also located close to each other near the telomeres.[15,63] The 'var' gene product, the variant surface

protein which mediates cytoadherence (PfEMP1) appears to be the main antigen determining the parasite population structure during chronic *falciparum* malaria infections.[64] Variation in surface antigenicity results from the activation of a different 'var' gene. This switching occurs at different rates, some of which exceed 2% per asexual cycle. It has been suggested that the diversity of these immunodominant variant repeat sequences interferes with the selection of high affinity antibody responses, and perpetuates low affinity responses in malaria. This 'confusion of the immune response' delays the development of effective immunity.[65] Immune selection also provides the selective pressure to maintain diversity in T- and B cell epitopes through a high frequency of non-synonymous base mutations during the asexual development of malaria parasites. On a larger scale, drug resistance has had a profound effect on the malaria parasite population structure. The progeny of single drug resistant parasites (first bearing chloroquine resistance and later sulfadoxine-pyrimethamine resistance) which originated in South-east Asia have swept across India and then spread across Southern and Eastern Africa.

The mechanisms maintaining genetic diversity within the parasite genome are many and complex.[66] Some of the polymorphic antigens identified are encoded by single gene copies in the haploid genome. These polypeptide antigens are characterized by tandem repeat sequences. Unequal crossing over during recombination can generate completely different sequences of these repeats. As these repeat sequences are also antibody targets, their variation provides antigenic diversity.

THE INFECTION

Genetic factors protecting against malaria

In 1949, J.B.S. Haldane suggested that people who were heterozygous for red cell abnormalities such as thalassaemia or sickle cell disease might be protected against malaria.[67] This, he said, would explain the high gene frequencies for the haemoglobinopathies in tropical areas and their rarity in colder climes. A state of 'balanced polymorphism' would exist, whereby the loss of the disadvantaged homozygotes would be offset by the survival advantage of heterozygotes. There is now good evidence from detailed epidemiological studies that this hypothesis is correct, although the mechanisms of protection vary considerably among the different erythrocyte abnormalities. The greatest protection is conferred by sickle cell trait, and Melanesian ovalocytosis.[68,69] These patients' red cells resist parasite invasion (in the case of sickle cell trait under low oxygen tensions), and once invaded the AS cells sickle readily, facilitating their clearance by the reticuloendothelial system. The protective effect conferred by the thalassaemias or glucose-6-phosphate dehydrogenase (G6PD) deficiency (which share a geographical distribution with malaria) is generally weaker.[70–72] In some studies, a protective effect has not been apparent, but recent large epidemiological studies on these genetic erythrocyte abnormalities do support the Haldane hypothesis. For example in two large African case-control studies, G6PD deficiency (both in female heterozygotes and male hemizygotes) was associated with 46–58% reduction in the risk of severe malaria.[71] The mechanism of protection in many of these haemoglobinopathies and how they interact with each other, is also less well understood.[72] The rate of decline of haemoglobin F in the first year of life is slower in α- and β-thalassaemia heterozygotes. Erythrocytes containing high haemoglobin F concentrations do not support parasite growth well. But studies from Vanuatu indicate that children with α-thalassaemia actually have more malaria (both *P. falciparum* and *P. vivax*) in the early years of life than their 'normal' counterparts, suggesting a complex interaction between malaria species and haemoglobin chain synthesis.[73] Melanesian ovalocytic erythrocytes both resist invasion by malaria parasites and provide a hostile intraerythrocytic ionic milieu for development. In the case of haemoglobin C, protection may be explained by abnormal presentation of the surface cytoadherence ligand PfEMP1 and consequent interference with sequestration.[74] Some haemoglobinopathies may protect against severe malaria but not uncomplicated malaria. For example, haemoglobin E heterozygotes (HbAE) are haematologically almost normal, and these individuals are susceptible to *falciparum* malaria but appear to be protected against severe malaria. Parasite multiplication at high densities is reduced.[75,76] Apart from the well established protection conferred by polymorphisms in the genes encoding haemoglobin, a large and confusing array of other polymorphisms associated with protection and susceptibility to malaria have been reported. For example, certain human leukocyte antigens (HLAs) are rare in Northern Europeans, but common in West Africans. Two of these, the class I antigen HLA-BW53 and the class II antigen HLA-DR B1* 1302, may also confer protection against severe malaria.[77] HLA molecules present processed antigenic peptides to cytotoxic T lymphocytes. HLA-B53-restricted cytotoxic T cells recognize a conserved nonamer peptide from a pre-erythrocytic (liver) stage-specific malaria antigen (LSA-1).[78] This suggests that cytotoxic T lymphocyte responses to the pre-erythrocytic stages of malaria may be important in immunity, and would explain how possession of HLA-B53 might confer a survival advantage.

In some cases, a polymorphism has been associated with protection in one study and susceptibility in another! Three different TNF promoter polymorphisms appear independently to be associated with severe malaria; Gambian children homozygous for the TNF-308A allele were at a seven-fold increased risk of dying or recovering with neurological sequelae.[79] Although this association was confirmed in East Africa, it was not found in two independent studies in Asia. TNF-238A was associated independently with severe anaemia,[80] and TNF-376A with susceptibility to cerebral malaria. A single nucleotide polymorphism in the inducible nitric oxide synthase gene promoter region was associated with severe anaemia in Gabon. Recent separate case–control studies on genetic polymorphisms in CD36 and ICAM-1, the two major receptors for *P. falciparum* cytoadherence, have given conflicting results. The CD36 polymorphism protected from severe malaria in one study but increased the risk in the other. An African ICAM-1 polymorphism predisposed to cerebral malaria in Kenya, was neutral in The Gambia, and protected in Gabon. In some of these associations, the possibility of linkage cannot be ruled out (i.e. the polymorphic gene lies close to another gene which is causally associated with the observed effect). For example the MHC III region, where the TNF promoter polymorphisms are located, contains a remarkably high density of genes with probable immune functions.[81] The contribution of epistasis, which is the interaction between genes, to malaria susceptibility and resistance has been underappreciated.[82] This makes interpretation of genetic associations very difficult, and probably explains many of the inconsistencies described above.

Expansion of the blood-stage infection

When the hepatic meronts (schizonts) rupture, they liberate approximately 10^5–10^6 merozoites into the circulation (i.e. the product of 5–100 successful sporozoites). These invade passing red cells immediately. In non-immune subjects the multiplication rate in *P. falciparum* often exceeds 10 per cycle (i.e. >50% efficiency)[59] and may reach 20-fold per cycle during the subsequent expanding phase of the infection (Figure 73.5).[83] For the first few cycles, the host is unaware of the brewing infection. On average, parasites are detectable in the blood by microscopy on the 11th day after sporozoite inoculation (the diligent microscopist can detect 20–50 parasites/μL reliably on thick films). At this stage, the host may still feel well, or may complain of vague non-specific symptoms of malaise, headache, myalgia, weakness or anorexia.[84,85] On average, the fever begins 2 days later, but in some cases, fever precedes detectable parasitaemia. The rise in parasite count is logarithmic initially, with a rising sine wave pattern of parasitaemia in *falciparum* malaria,[86,87] but in most cases the parasite expansion terminates abruptly to limit the infection at a parasite density of 10^4–10^5/μL (Figure 73.5). Only *P. falciparum* has the capacity for untrammelled multiplication. Parasitaemias may exceed 50% in some cases. Several factors converge to limit parasite multiplication. The host mobilizes specific and non-specific immune defences (particularly in the spleen). The parasite schizonts are damaged by high fevers.[88] The availability of suitable red cells is exhausted: *P. vivax* and *P. falciparum* prefer younger red cells and *P. malariae* prefers older cells. Interestingly, whereas *P. vivax* shows invasion restricted to only 13% of the red cell population, and *P. falciparum* causing uncomplicated malaria to 40%, *P. falciparum* parasites causing severe malaria in SE Asia show unrestricted invasion.[60]

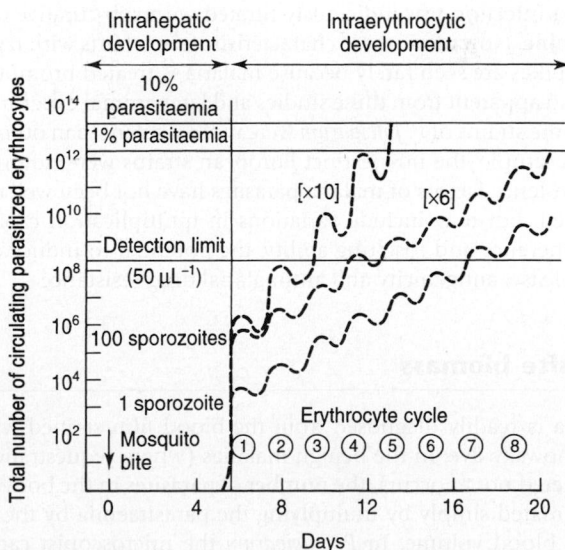

Figure 73.5 Logarithmic expansion of malaria infections in vivo. The vertical axis represents the total number of parasites circulating in the blood following infection of an adult of 50 kg. The infection rapidly reaches a lethal burden at high multiplication rates unless restrained. Maximum recorded multiplication rates are approximately ×20 per cycle in vivo. (From White and Krishna,[83] with permission.)

Thus, the untreated infection increases exponentially, then the rate of expansion decelerates rapidly, parasitaemia fluctuates, settles around a plateau, then declines and continues for several weeks or months at low levels before finally being eliminated. Although natural infections often contain two or more genetically different parasite strains, development tends to be relatively synchronous from the outset.[87] Further synchronization takes place in untreated infections in non-immune subjects, such that merogony ('sporulation') takes place within 1–2 h. This degree of synchronization is associated with fever spikes and rigors (the 'paroxysm'), and is more likely in *P. vivax*, *P. ovale* and *P. malariae* infections. Although one 'brood' predominates, in *P. falciparum* there is often at least one minor 'brood' or subpopulation cycling 24 h out of phase with the major brood.

The periodicity of malaria is enshrined in the terminology of the fever pattern. *P. malariae* has a 72-h life cycle, and so in untreated infections the paroxysm occurrs on the fourth day (using the Greek system of 'inclusive reckoning' the previous paroxysm is considered to occur on day one). This is termed 'quartan malaria'. The other human malarias are termed tertian (fever on the third day; 48-h asexual cycle). *P. knowlesi* has a 24-h cycle (quotidian). *P. falciparum* often synchronized to a daily fever spike (quotidian fever), presumably caused by two broods of approximately equal size oscillating 24 h out of phase, or failed to synchronize at all.[84–86] The classic descriptions of malaria symptomatology derive largely from detailed clinical observations made in the late nineteenth and early twentieth centuries, the experience with artificial infections in early chemotherapy trials, studies conducted by the military, and the extensive use of malaria therapy in the treatment of neurosyphilis. These observations were usually made on non-immune adults. In malaria therapy, patients with neurosyphilis were artificially infected by mosquito bites or transfusion, and the infections with *P. falciparum* or *P. vivax* were left untreated so that the patients experienced recurrent high fevers. If symptoms were severe then the malaria infection was judiciously titrated with sub-curative doses of quinine. Nowadays, these characteristic fever charts with regular fever spikes are seen rarely because malaria is treated promptly. It was also apparent from these studies and later animal experiments that some strains of *P. falciparum* were more virulent than others.[89–91] For example, the now extinct European strains were notorious. The virulence factors of malaria parasites have not been well characterized, but may include variations in multiplication capacity, cytoadherence and rosetting ability, the potential to induce cytokine release, antigenicity and antimalarial drug resistance.

Parasite biomass

Malaria is readily diagnosed from the blood film stained with a Romanowsky dye. In the benign malarias (where sequestration is considered not to occur), the number of parasites in the body may be estimated simply by multiplying the parasitaemia by the estimated blood volume. In *P. falciparum* the microscopist can see only the first third of the asexual life cycle. In the second two-thirds the parasitized cells are sequestered. As a consequence there may be large discrepancies between the number of parasites in the peripheral (circulating) blood and the number of parasites in the body (the parasite burden) (Figure 73.6).[83,92] This has often puzzled and misled clinicians; some patients appear to tolerate

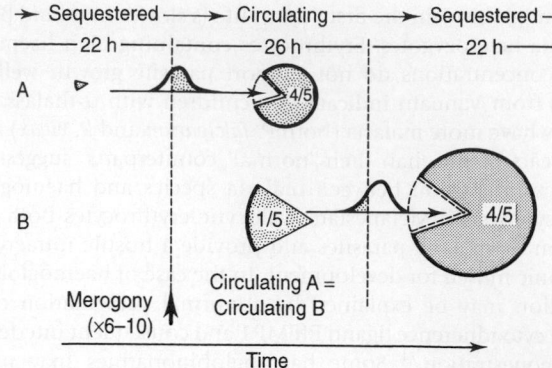

Figure 73.6 The problem of assessing the parasite burden from the peripheral parasitaemia in *P. falciparum* malaria. Sequestration hides the parasites causing harm. Two patients A and B have the same parasitaemia. In patient A, most of the parasites are circulating, and only a few from the previous cycle have yet to undergo merogony. In patient B, most of the parasites have already sequestered and only 20% of the biomass still circulates. There are over 60 times more parasites in patient B than in patient A. The clue to this difference lies in the stage distribution (shown crossing the hatched lines) of the circulating parasites which will be more mature in patient B. (From Silamut and White,[92] with permission.)

high parasitaemia with little adverse effect, whereas others die with low parasite counts. The clue to this apparent discrepancy lies both in the immune status of the host and in the stage of development of parasites on the peripheral blood smear.[92] A predominance of more mature parasites on the blood film suggests that the peripheral blood parasites are the trailing edge of a much greater sequestered parasite biomass, and it carries a worse prognosis for any parasitaemia than a predominance of younger forms. Two patients with the same peripheral parasitaemia may have as much as a one hundred-fold difference in the total number of parasites in the body. The presence of intraneutrophilic phagocytosed malaria pigment (in more than 5% of neutrophils) also reflects the degree of previous schizogony and is also a valuable prognostic index.[93,94] Measurement of proteins released by the parasite, such as Pf HRP2 in plasma, provides a good method of assessing this hidden pathogenic sequestered biomass.[95] In synchronous *P. falciparum* infections the peripheral blood parasite numbers fall at the time of sequestration, and rise abruptly at the time of merogony (when a predominance of tiny rings are seen) (Figure 73.5). The other explanation for the ability to tolerate high parasitaemias without apparent adverse effects relates to the development of 'anti-toxic' immunity.[96] The host adapts to repeated infection by producing fewer cytokines for a given quantum of parasites (see below).[97] Eventually a state is reached where infections are asymptomatic. This is called premunition.

Immunity

The precise mechanisms controlling malaria infections in the host are still incompletely understood. It was apparent from the era of malaria therapy for neurosyphilis, that a strain-specific immunity developed which protected against re-challenge with the same parasite strain, but did not protect from challenge with a different strain.[98] Effective immunity, as distinct from premunition, may be reached when there has been sufficient exposure to all local strains of malaria parasites. This is difficult to quantify as there is still no good in-vitro correlate of either antitoxic or strain-specific immunity to malaria. In controlling the acute infection, non-specific host defence mechanisms and the later development of more specific cell-mediated and humoral responses are both important.[99] Protective antibodies inhibit parasite expansion by agglutinating merozoites and by binding to parasitized erythrocytes. The opsonised parasitized red cells activate the Fc receptors of the monocyte-macrophage series resulting in splenic clearance.[100,101] The systemic and splenic monocyte-macrophage series appear to be the most important immune effector cells in the direct attack on parasitized erythrocytes and merozoites, although neutrophils may also play a role.[102,103] Non-specific effector mechanisms include non-opsonic phagocytosis via direct binding to monocyte-macrophage CD36, pro-inflammatory cytokine release, and the activation of phagocytic cells (including neutrophils) to release toxic oxygen species[104] and nitric oxide,[105] both of which are parasiticidal. The reaction of these oxygen intermediates with lipoproteins produces lipid peroxides. These are more stable cytotoxic molecules and are unaffected by antioxidants. There is also augmentation of splenic clearance function: the splenic thresholds for both filtration[106] and Fc receptor-mediated phagocytosis are lowered.[107,108] P. falciparum-infected erythrocytes are both more rigid[51,109] and more opsonized than uninfected red cells as they express both host- and parasite-derived neoantigens on the erythrocyte surface. However, the parasite proteins expressed on the red cell surface undergo antigenic variation[110,111] which prevents complete immune clearance and thereby sustains the untreated infection.

The immune response

Following natural infection there is a transient humoral response to sporozoite antigens; sporozoite antibodies decline then with a half-life of 3–4 weeks.[112] In areas of high transmission sporozoite antibody levels tend to plateau between 20 and 30 years of age, and do not correlate with premunition. Cytotoxic T cell immune responses cannot be directed against the blood stage parasite as red cells do not express human leukocyte (HLA) antigens, but the pre-erythrocytic liver stages of the parasite are vulnerable to T cell attack. Several lines of experimental evidence in animal malarias, and the observation that certain HLA types are relatively protected from severe malaria, indicate that class 1 restricted CD8(+) T cells play an important role in immunity. There is evidence supporting a role for both α–β and γ–δ CD4+ cells in the immune reponse to malaria.[113]

Strain-specific immunity to the asexual blood stage parasites develops slowly during natural untreated infections, but it then provides good protection against rechallenge. However, parasite populations are diverse, and cross-strain protection is initially weak or negligible. The development of immunity in endemic areas may represent the gradual acquisition of a repertoire of immunological memory for the range of local parasites. This involves strain-transcending immunity sufficient to ameliorate disease (antitoxic immunity) and a more strain-specific immunity, which protects from or attenuates the infection. The immune response to malaria is clearly very complex, and the relative importance of humoral and cellular immunity in man has not been defined clearly.[114] Infusions of hyperimmune serum to patients with acute malaria have reduced or eliminated parasitaemia[115,116] through opsonization and activation of phagocytic and cytotoxic effector functions by cytophilic IgG antibodies, augmentation of ring-form infected erythrocyte clearance,[117] and agglutination of merozoites. In addition to the role of cellular immunity in preventing pre-erythrocytic development, the increase in malaria severity in patients living in endemic areas with the acquired immune deficiency syndrome (HIV-AIDS) suggests that CD4+ cells play a significant role in modulating the severity of falciparum malaria.

PATHOPHYSIOLOGY

The pathophysiology of malaria results from destruction of erythrocytes, the liberation of parasite and erythrocyte material into the circulation, and the host reaction to these events. P. falciparum malaria-infected erythrocytes sequester in the microcirculation of vital organs, interfering with microcirculatory flow and host tissue metabolism.

Toxicity and cytokines

For many years malariologists hypothesized that parasites contained a toxin which was liberated at schizont rupture, and caused the symptoms of the paroxysm. No toxin in the strict sense of the word has ever been identified, but malaria parasites do induce release of cytokines in much the same way as bacterial endotoxin.[118,119] A glycolipid material with many of the properties of bacterial endotoxin is released on meront rupture.[120,121] This material is associated with the glycosylphosphatidylinositol anchor which covalently links proteins including the malaria parasite surface antigens to the cell membrane lipid bilayer.[122,123] This activates host inflammatory responses in macrophages by signalling through toll-like receptor (TLR) 2 and to a lesser extent TLR 4.[123,124] Malaria antigen-related IgE complexes also activate cytokine release. The limulus lysate assay, a test of endotoxin-like activity, is often positive in acute malaria. These products of malaria parasites, and the crude malaria pigment which is released at schizont rupture, induce activation of the cytokine cascade in a similar manner to the endotoxin of bacteria. But they are considerably less potent. For example an E.coli bacteraemia of 1 bacterium/mL carries an approximate mortality of 20% whereas in falciparum malaria only parasite densities of well over 10^9/mL produce such a lethal effect. Clearly, compared with bacteria, malaria parasites are notable for their lack of toxicity! Cells of the macrophage-monocyte series, γ/δ T cells, α/β T cells, CD14+ cells and endothelium are stimulated to release cytokines in a mutually amplifying chain reaction. Initially tumour necrosis factor (TNF), which plays a pivotal role, interleukin (IL)-1, and gamma interferon (γIFN) are produced and these in turn induce release of a cascade of other 'pro-inflammatory' cytokines including IL-6, IL-8, IL-12, IL-18.[125-127] These are balanced by production of the 'anti-inflammatory' cytokines, notably IL-10.[128] Cytokines are responsible for many of the symptoms and signs of the infection, particularly fever and malaise. Plasma concentrations of cytokines are elevated in both acute vivax and falciparum malaria.[125-127,129,130]

In established *vivax* malaria, which tends to synchronize earlier than *P. falciparum*, a pulse release of TNF occurs at the time of schizont rupture and this is followed by the characteristic symptoms and signs of the 'paroxysm', i.e. shivering, cool extremities, headache, chills, a spike of fever, and sometimes rigors followed by sweating, vasodilatation and defervescence.[129] For a given number of parasites *Plasmodium vivax* is a more potent inducer of TNF release than *P. falciparum*, which may explain its lower pyrogenic density.

It has been proposed that severe malaria and bacterial septicaemia may have a common cytokine-mediated pathology, despite considerable differences in their clinical, metabolic and haemodynamic manifestations. Cytokine concentrations in the blood fluctuate widely over a short period of time, and are high in both *P. vivax* and *P. falciparum*; indeed some of the highest TNF concentrations recorded in malaria occur during the paroxysms of synchronous *P. vivax* infections.[129] Nearly all the TNF measured in these assays is bound to soluble receptors; there is usually little or no bioactivity. Nevertheless, in most series there is a positive correlation between cytokine levels and prognosis in severe *falciparum* malaria. Acute malaria is associated with high levels of most cytokines but the balance differs in relation to severity. IL-12 and TGF-β 1, which may regulate the balance between pro-and antiinflammatory cytokines, are higher in uncomplicated than severe malaria.[130-132] IL-12 is inversely correlated with plasma lactate – a measure of disease severity.[133,134] IL-10, a potent antiinflammatory cytokine, increases markedly in severe malaria but, in fatal cases, does not increase sufficiently to restrain the production of TNF.[130] A reduced IL-10/TNF ratio has also been associated with childhood malarial anaemia in areas of high transmission.[133-135] All this points to a disturbed balance of cytokine production in severe malaria.

The first studies to associate elevations in plasma cytokine levels with disease severity focused on TNF and cerebral malaria, and led to the suggestion that TNF played a causal role in coma and cerebral dysfunction. Genetic studies from Africa indicated that children with the (308A) TNF2 allele, a polymorphism in the TNF promoter region, had a relative risk of 7 for death or neurological sequelae from cerebral malaria.[79] This finding was not confirmed in studies from South-east Asia. A separate polymorphism in this region which affects gene expression was associated with a four-fold increased risk of cerebral malaria.[81] On the other hand, the clinical studies in cerebral malaria with anti-TNF antibodies, and other strategies to reduce TNF production reported to date have shown no convincing effects other than reduction in fever.[136] In contrast to contradictory evidence in severe falciparum malaria, there is good evidence that cytokines do play a causal role in the pathogenesis of cerebral symptoms in murine models of severe malaria.[137] Numerous interventions have been beneficial in this model, but the clinical relevance of these observations is uncertain as Murine 'cerebral malaria' is clinically and pathologically unlike human cerebral malaria. There is no direct evidence that systemic release of TNF or other cytokines causes coma in humans (although mechanisms involving local release of nitric oxide and other medicators within the central nervous system and consequent inhibition of neurotransmission can be hypothesized). In a large prospective study in adults with severe malaria, elevated plasma TNF concentrations were associated specifically with renal dysfunction,[130] and TNF levels were actually lower in patients with pure cerebral malaria than those with other manifestations of severe disease. Severe malarial anaemia has been associated with yet another TNF promoter polymorphism (238A; odds ratio, OR 2.5).[80] Taken together, these various findings do not support a cytokine mediated pathology that is common to sepsis and malaria, although they do suggest some role for TNF and other cytokines in severe disease, (but not encephalopathy per se). The extent to which these cytokine abnormalities are a cause or an effect of severe disease remains to be determined.

Cytokines are probably involved in placental dysfunction, suppression of erythropoiesis and inhibition of gluconeogenesis, and certainly do cause fever in malaria. Tolerance to malaria, or premunition, reflects both immune regulation of the infection and also reduced production of cytokines in response to malaria ('antitoxic immunity'). Cytokines upregulate the endothelial expression of vascular ligands for *P. falciparum*-infected erythrocytes, notably ICAM-1, and thus promote cytoadherence. They may also be important mediators of parasite killing by activating leukocytes, and possibly other cells, to release toxic oxygen species,[138] nitric oxide, and by generating parasiticidal lipid peroxides, and causing fever. Thus, whereas high concentrations of cytokines appear to be harmful, lower levels probably benefit the host.

Sequestration

Erythrocytes containing mature forms of *P. falciparum* adhere to microvascular endothelium ('cytoadherence') and thus disappear from the circulation. This process is known as sequestration (Figure 73.7). The simian malaria parasites *P. coatneyi* and *P. fragile* infecting rhesus monkeys also sequester, but this does not occur to a significant extent with the other three human malaria parasites. Sequestration is thought to be central to the pathophysiology of *falciparum* malaria.[139-141]

The mechanics of cytoadherence are similar to leukocyte endothelial interactions. Tethering (the initial contact) is followed by rolling and then firm adherence (stasis). Once adherent, the parasitized cell remains stuck until schizogony and even afterwards the residual membranes (and often the attached pigment body) remain attached to the vascular endothelium. Rolling is probably the rate-limiting factor determining cytoadherence.[142]

Blood is a complex soup of deformable cells suspended in plasma proteins, electrolytes, and a variety of small organic molecules. Its effective viscosity changes non-linearly under the different shear rates encountered in the circulation (non-Newtonian behaviour). At haematocrits <12% (i.e. severe anaemia), red blood cell suspensions exhibit Newtonian behaviour. Under experimental conditions, changes in haematocrit over the range commonly encountered in severe malaria (venous haematocrit, 10–30%; capillary values are lower) have major effects on cytoadherence. Rolling increased five-fold as haematocrit rose from 10% to 20%, and cytoadhesion rose 12-fold between 10% and 30%. Over this range, the viscosity of blood approximately doubles, and so if shear stress is held constant, shear rates fall by approximately half allowing greater time for contact between cells and endothelium. The higher the haematocrit, the more that cells roll along the endothelial surface, and a higher proportion of these adhere to the vascular endothelium.[143]

Once infected red cells adhere, they do not enter the circulation again, remaining stuck until they rupture at merogony

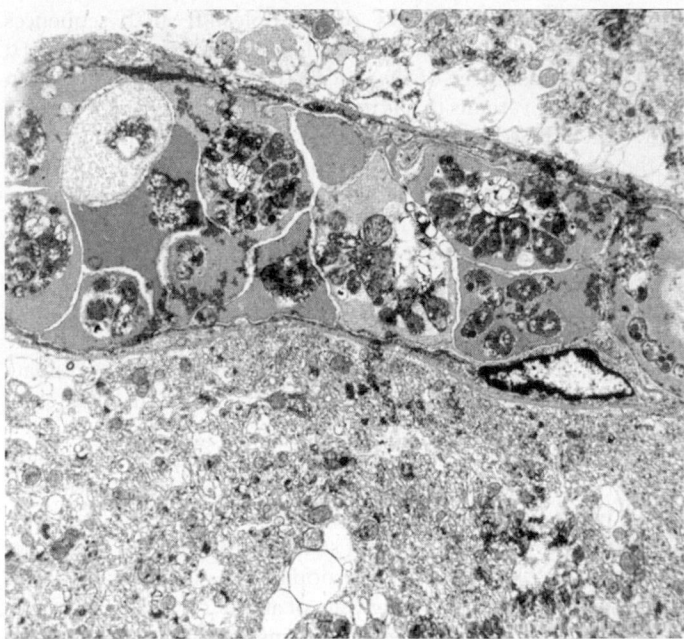

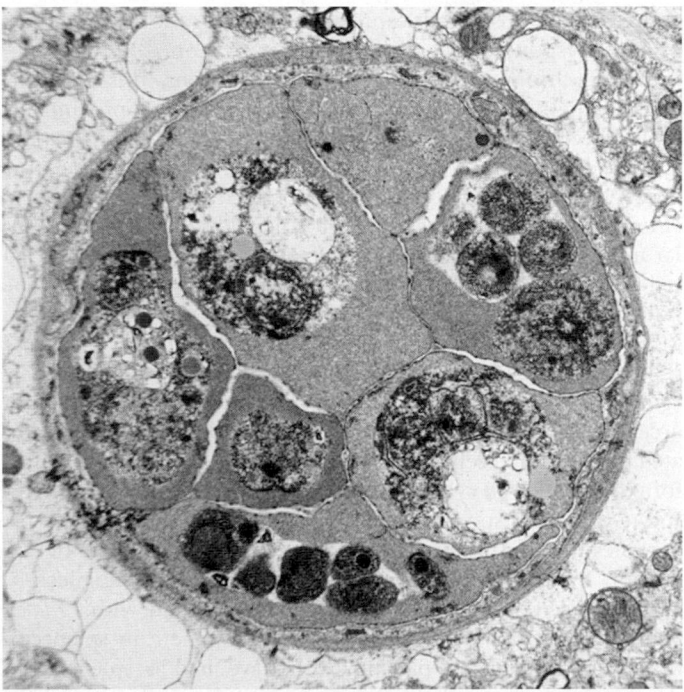

B

Figure 73.7 Two electron micrographs (×4320) showing densely packed parasitized erythrocytes sequestered in cerebral venules of a fatal case of cerebral malaria. Note that even when no intracellular parasite is seen, electron dense deposits are evident on the cell membranes indicating the red cell does contain a parasite, but that its body has been missed in the section. The packing of red cells is much tighter than in normal conditions. (Courtesy of Emsrii Pongponratn.)

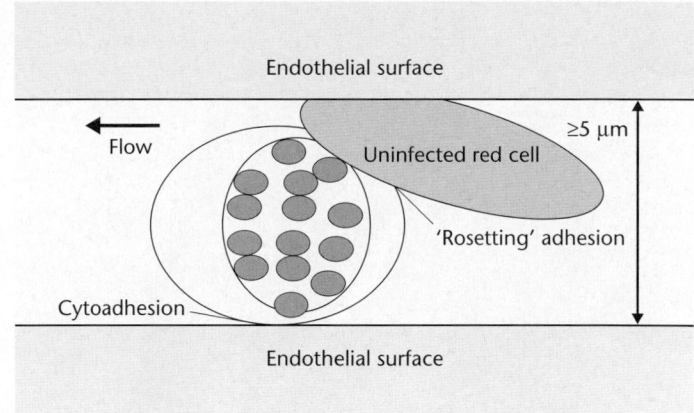

Figure 73.8 Uninfected red cells must squeeze past the static, rigid, spherical cytoadherent parasitized erythrocytes to maintain flow. This is compromised by the reduced deformability of uninfected red cells in severe malaria and the intererythrocytic adhesive forces that mediate rosetting.

(schizogony).[144] Under febrile conditions cytoadherence begins at approximately 12 h after merozoite invasion, and reaches 50% of maximum after 14–16 h. Adherence is essentially complete in the second half of the parasites' 48-h asexual life cycle. As a consequence, whereas in the other malarias of man mature parasites are commonly seen on blood smears, these forms are rare in *falciparum* malaria, and often indicate serious infection.[92] It was thought that ring stage-infected erythrocytes do not cytoadhere at all, but recent pathological and laboratory studies show that that they do, although much less so than more mature stages.[144,145] Ring form-infected parasites are also concentrated in the spleen and placenta, raising the intriguing possibility that the entire asexual cycle could take place away from the peripheral circulation. Sequestration occurs predominantly in the venules of vital organs (Figure 73.7). It is not distributed uniformly throughout the body, being greatest in the brain, particularly the white matter, prominent in the heart, eyes, liver, kidneys, intestines and adipose tissue, and least in the skin.[140,146] Even within the brain the distribution of sequestered erythrocytes varies markedly from vessel to vessel,[144] possibly reflecting differences in the expression of endothelial receptors (Figure 73.8). Cytoadherence and the related phenomena of rosetting and autoagglutination lead to microcirculatory obstruction in *falciparum* malaria (Figure 73.7).[147] The gross microcirculatory obstruction caused by cytoadherent erythrocytes has recently been clearly visualized in vivo using polarised light imaging (in the buccal and rectal microcirculation) and by high resolution fluoroscein angiography of the retinal circulation.[148,149]

The consequences of microcirculatory obstruction are activation of the vascular endothelium, endothelial dysfunction, together with reduced oxygen and substrate supply, which leads to anaerobic glycolysis, lactic acidosis and cellular dysfunction.

Cytoadherence

Cytoadherence is mediated by several different processes. The most important parasite ligands are a family of strain-specific,

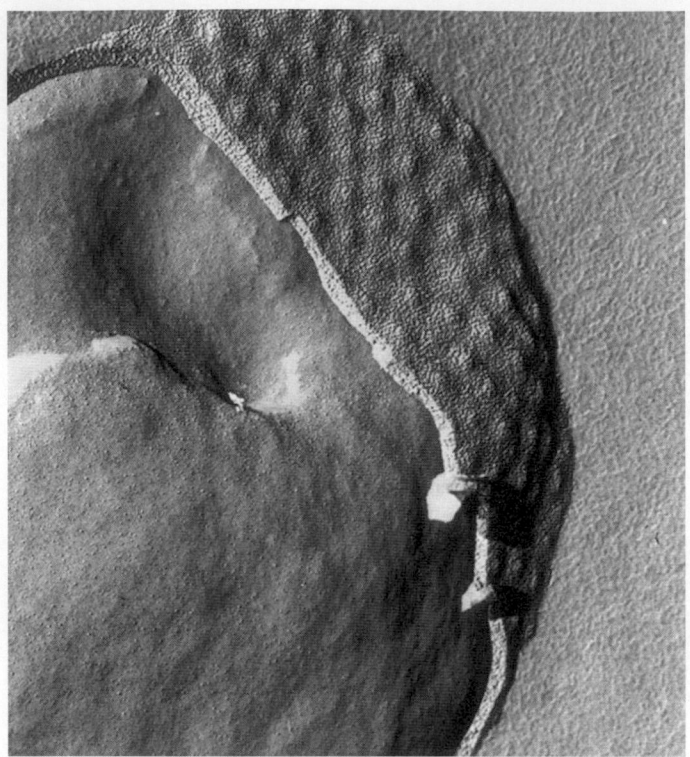

Figure 73.9 Freeze fracture electron micrograph of the membrane of a red cell containing mature *P. falciparum* showing regularly spaced surface knobs. (Courtesy of David Ferguson.)

high molecular weight parasite-derived proteins termed *P. falciparum* erythrocyte membrane protein 1 or PfEMP-1.[57,141,150] These variant surface antigen (VSA) proteins (molecular mass 240–260 kDa) are encoded by 'var' genes, a family of ~60 genes distributed in three general locations within the haploid genome: either immediately adjacent to the telomere, close to a telomeric 'var' gene, or in internal clusters.[151]

Each parasitized red cell expresses the product of a single gene, a process which is tightly controlled at the transcriptional level, and varies between different parasites and different PfEMP-1 genes.[152] PfEMP-1 is transcribed, synthesized, and stored within the parasite. Beginning at around 12 h of development, it is then exported to the surface of the infecting erythrocyte.[153] There it is apposed by an electrostatic interaction through the membrane to a submembranous accretion of parasite-derived knob-associated histidine-rich protein (KAHRP) which is in turn anchored to the red cell via the cytoskeleton protein ankryn.[154] These accretions cause humps or knobs on the surface of the red cell, which are the points of attachment to vascular endothelium (Figure 73.9). The protuberances are not essential for cytoadherence (Figure 73.10). A small subpopulation of naturally occurring parasites do not induce surface knobs, and parasites can be selected in culture which are knob negative (K−) but still cytoadhere. However, natural parasite isolates are nearly always knob positive (K+). PfEMP-1 protrudes from the red cell surface offering several Duffy binding-like (DBL) domains each capable of binding to particular

vascular 'receptors'. Analysis of multiple PfEMP-1 sequences has revealed common antigenic determinants in the DBL-1α domain, a constituent of the so-called 'head structure' common to all PfEMP-1 variants that is involved in the formation of rosettes and in cytoadherence. PfEMP-1 expression is greatest in the middle of the asexual cycle. PfEMP1 is an important adhesion molecule and as it is a parasite protein exposed to immune recognition, it is also a major antigenic determinant for the blood stage parasite. Two other variant surface antigens encoded by different gene families have been identified – the *Rifins* and the *Surfins*.[155,156] Their function is uncertain. Proteins expressed only on the younger ring stage infected red cells have also been identified in parasite lines which subsequently develop a chondroitin-sulphate A binding phenotype. These could play a role in ring stage cytoadherence.[157]

As in other protozoal parasites, the immunodominant surface antigen undergoes antigenic variation to 'change its coat' and avoid immune mediated attack. Each *P. falciparum* var gene appears to have different rates of switching on and off, with a net result that the infecting parasite population 'switches' to a new variant of PfEMP1 at an average rate of about 2% per asexual cycle in culture[158] although this may be considerably higher in vivo. Interestingly, the PfEMP-1 gene expressed shows some dependence on previous variant expression, reflecting the effects of host immune response on parasite antigenic variation.[159]

In the chronic phase of untreated infections, this antigenic variation results in small waves of parasitaemia approximately every three weeks. In addition to the 'var', 'rifin' and 'surfin' variant surface antigen gene superfamilies of *P. falciparum*, genome sequencing has revealed the 'vir' gene superfamily in *Plasmodium vivax*.[160] A protein similar to PfEMP-1 named sequestrin (molecular mass 270 kDa) has been identified on the surface of infected red cells using anti-idiotypic antibodies raised against one of the putative vascular receptors CD36 (see below).[161] The protein MESA may also be partially expressed on the surface of the red cell and has been suggested as a contributor to cytoadherence. The central role of parasite derived proteins in cytoadherence is not accepted by all. It has been suggested that cytoadherence is mediated by altered red cell membrane components such as a modified form of the red cell cytoskeleton protein band 3 (the major erythrocyte anion transporter, also called *Pfalhesin*).[162] In culture, most parasites lose the ability to cytoadhere after several cycles of replication. In vivo, cytoadherence may be modulated by the spleen.[163] This has been shown in *Saimiri* monkeys infected with *P. falciparum*. Parasitized erythrocytes do not cytoadhere in splenectomized monkeys. Rare patients who have had a splenectomy develop *falciparum* malaria and in some of these all stages of the parasite are seen in peripheral blood smears.[164]

Vascular endothelial ligands

A number of different cell adhesion molecules expressed on the surface of vascular endothelium have been shown to bind parasitized red cells (Figure 73.10). The interaction between these proteins and the variant surface adhesin of the parasitized red cell is complex. The property of cytoadherence can be studied in vitro with cells expressing the potential ligands on their surface (e.g. human umbilical vein/dermal microvascular or cerebral

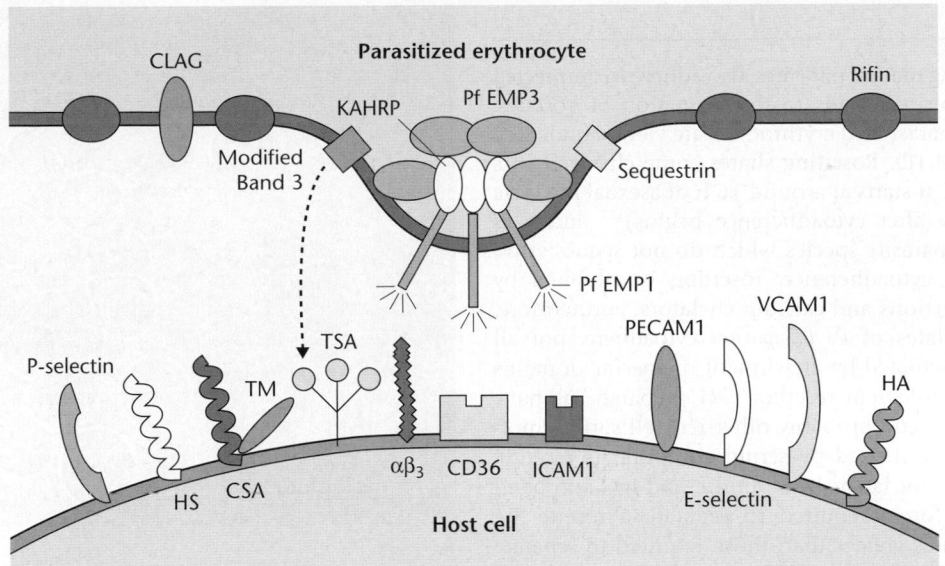

Figure 73.10 Schematic representation of cytoadherence in *falciparum* malaria. On the red cell side, the principal ligand is the variant antigen *Plasmodium falciparum* erythrocyte membrane protein 1 (PfEMP1). This is expressed on the surface of 'knobs' which protrude from the red cell surface. It is anchored beneath to the knob associated histidine rich protein (KAHRP), and stabilized by PfEMP3. The *rifin* and CLAG gene products are not directly involved in adhesion but CLAG does appear to be required for cytoadherence. Parasite modified band 3 (the major anion transporter) contributes to adhesion probably by binding to thrombospondin (TSA). Sequestrin is a distinct parasite derived protein also mediating adhesion. The ring stage adhesion[122] (not shown) is distinct from PfEMP1, and expressed in the first third of the asexual cycle. On the vascular endothelial side, many molecules facilitate adhesion by binding PfEMP1. The most important is the cellular differentiation antigen: CD36. Intercellular adhesion molecule 1 (ICAM 1) is important particularly in the brain, elsewhere it synergises with CD36. Chondroitin sulphate A (CSA) attached to thrombomodulin (TM) are very important for placental sequestration. Hyaluronic acid (HA) has also been implicated as a receptor for placental sequestration, but the evidence for this has weakened as it has emerged that HA is usually contaminated with CSA. The other identified adhesion molecules are vascular cell adhesion molecule 1 (VCAM1), E-selectin, platelet endothelial cell adhesion molecule 1 (PECAM1), $\alpha_v \beta_3$ integrin, heparan sulphate (HS) and P-selectin.

endothelial cells or transfected COS cells) or with the immobilized purified candidate ligand proteins. Probably the most important of these proteins is the leukocyte differentiation antigen CD36[165,166]; nearly all freshly obtained parasites bind to CD36.[167] Binding is increased at low pH (<7.0) and in the presence of high calcium concentrations.[168] CD36 is constitutionally expressed on vascular endothelium, platelets, and monocytes/macrophages but is usually not present on the surface of cerebral vessels,[169] although it has been suggested that parasitized erythrocytes could bind via CD36 to platelets adherent to cerebral vascular endothelium.[170]

The intercellular adhesion molecule (ICAM-1 or CD54), which is also the receptor for rhinovirus attachment, appears to be the major cytoadherence receptor in the brain.[169,171] ICAM-1, but not CD36, is upregulated by cytokines (notably TNFα), and provides a plausible pathological scenario whereby cytokine release enhances cytoadherence. At physiological shear rates (i.e. those likely to be encountered in the human microcirculation) the binding forces (c.10^{-10}N) are similar for CD36 and ICAM-1.[142,172,173] For both, the forces of attachment are lower than those required for detachment, which suggests post-attachment alterations to increase adhesion. Binding to the two ligands is synergistic.[174] Thrombospondin (a natural ligand for CD36) will also bind to some parasitized red cells (probably to modified band 3). Other proteins including VCAM-1, PECAM/CD31, E-selectin and the integrin alpha$_v$-beta$_3$ have also been shown to bind in some circumstances.[141] P-selectin has been shown to mediate rolling. The

relative importance of these molecules and their interactions in vivo is still not clear.

Chondroitin sulphate A (CSA) appears to be the major receptor for cytoadherence in the placenta.[175–177] Binding is mediated by a particular PfEMP1 (var2CSA) which gives hope for a specific vaccine against malaria in pregnancy.[178,179] Thus, the placenta selects a parasite subpopulation expressing this epitope. Antibodies which inhibit parasitized red cell cytoadherence by binding var2CSA are generally present in multigravidae in endemic areas, but not primigravidae.[180] This probably explains why the adverse effects of pregnancy on birth weight are greater in primigravidae.

Other as yet unidentified vascular receptors are also present, as sequestration also occurrs in vessels expressing none of the potential ligands identified so far. In summary ICAM-1 appears to be a major vascular ligand in the brain involved in cerebral sequestration, CSA is the major ligand in the placenta, and CD36 is probably the major ligand in the other organs. The relationship between cytoadherence, measured ex-vivo, and the severity of infection or clinical manifestations has been inconsistent between studies. This is not particularly surprising, as all parasitized erythrocytes cytoadhere. Severity is related to the number of parasites in the body and distribution of cytoadherence within the vital organs. The relative importance of parasite phenotype and the various potential vascular ligands in the pathophysiology of severe *falciparum* malaria and the precise role of the spleen as a modulator of cytoadherence still remains to be determined.

Rosetting

Erythrocytes containing mature parasites also adhere to uninfected erythrocytes.[181] This process leads to the formation of 'rosettes' when suspensions of parasitized erythrocytes are viewed under the microscope (Figure 73.11). Rosetting shares some characteristics of cytoadherence.[182,183] It starts at around 16 h of asexual life cycle development (slightly after cytoadherence begins)[184] and it is trypsin-sensitive. But parasite species which do not sequester do rosette[185] and unlike cytoadherence, rosetting is inhibited by certain heparin subfractions and calcium chelators. Furthermore, whereas all fresh isolates of *P. falciparum* cytoadhere, not all rosette. Rosetting is mediated by attachment of specific domains of PfEMP1 to the complement receptor CR1, heparan sulphate, blood group A antigen, and probably other red cell surface molecules. Attachment is facilitated by serum components recently identified as Complement factor D, albumin, and IgG anti-band 3 antibodies.[186] The forces required to separate a rosette are approximately five times greater than those required to separate cytoadherent cells, although shearing forces may still be effective in disrupting rosettes in vivo. When known rosetting parasite lines (K+R+) are perfused through the rat mesocaecum, an ex vivo model for the study of vascular perfusion, they cause significantly more microvascular obstruction than isolates which cytoadhere but do not rosette (K+R−).[139,187] Rosetting has been associated with severe malaria in some studies but not in others.[188–191] It has been suggested that rosetting might encourage cytoadherence by reducing flow (shear rate), which would enhance anaerobic glycolysis, reduce pH and facilitate adherence of infected erythrocytes to venular endothelium. Rosetting tends to start in venules, and this could certainly reduce flow. The adhesive forces involved in rosetting could impede forward flow of uninfected erythrocytes as they squeeze past sticky cytoadherent parasitized red cells in capillaries and venules (Figure 73.9).[192,193] The mechanical obstruction or 'static hindrance' would be compounded by the lack of deformability of the adherent, and circulating parasitized red cells.

Aggregation

Recently, a new adherence property of parasitized red cells has been characterized, and associated with disease severity.[194,195] This is the platelet mediated aggregation of parasitized erythrocytes and is mediated via platelet CD36. These cells clump together in ex vivo cultures. Aggregation could also contribute to vascular occlusion.

Red cell deformability

As *Plasmodium vivax* matures inside the erythrocyte, the cell enlarges and becomes more deformable.[52] *Plasmodium falciparum* does exactly the opposite; the normally flexible biconcave disc becomes progressively more spherical and rigid.[51,193] The reduction in deformability results from reduced membrane fluidity, increasing sphericity, and the enlarging and relatively rigid intraerythrocytic parasite. Infected red cells are less filterable than uninfected cells, and readily removed by the spleen. Indeed it has been argued that sequestration is an adaptive response to escape

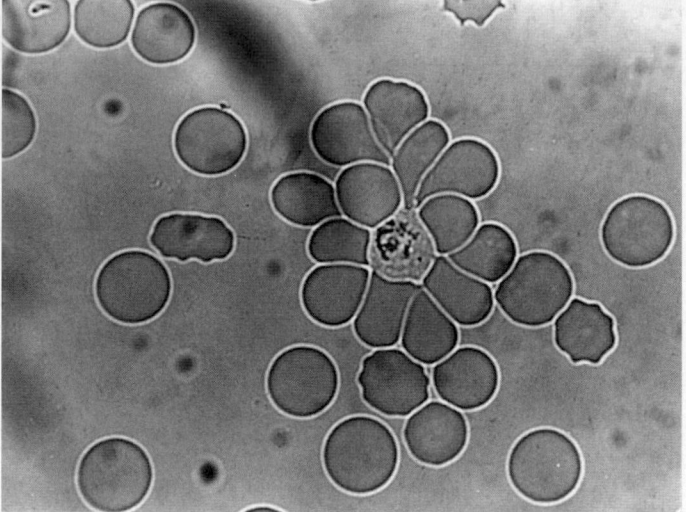

A

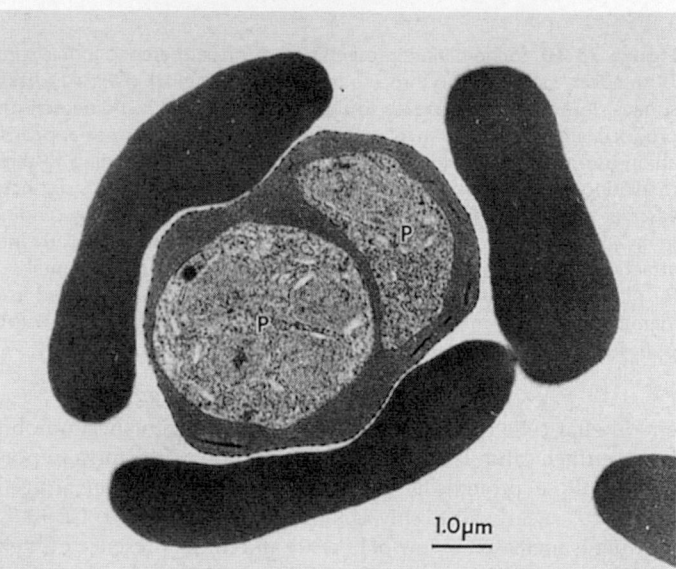

B

Figure 73.11 Rosetting. (A) Uninfected red blood cells bind to a *P. vivax*-infected erythrocyte. (Courtesy of R. Udomsangpetch.) (B) Transmission electron micrograph of a rosette around a *P. falciparum*-infected erythrocyte. (Courtesy of D. Ferguson.)

splenic filtration. However, reduced deformability alone cannot account for microvascular obstruction as it would lead to obstruction at the mid-capillary (i.e. the smallest internal diameter in the vasculature) and could not explain sequestration in venules.[193]

Even in severe malaria the majority of red cells are still uninfected. A reduction of uninfected red cell deformability has been recognized as a major contributor to disease severity and outcome. This phenomenon is specific to severe falciparum malaria; it is not found in sepsis.[147] Increased erythrocyte rigidity measured at the low shear stresses encountered in capillaries and venules is correlated closely with outcome in severe malaria.[193,196] When assessed at the higher shear rates encountered on the arterial side, and importantly in the spleen, reduced red cell deformability correlates with anaemia.[197]

Immunological processes

Given the very large amount of research conducted on the immunology of malaria it is remarkable how little we know of the contribution of immune processes to malaria pathology. It has been suggested that severe malaria, and in particular cerebral malaria, results from specific immune-mediated damage.[198] This is unlikely. Confusion arises when the term cerebral malaria is applied equally to human disease and to the neurological dysfunction in animal models infected with unusual parasites.[199] Neuropathology in rodent models does result from immune mediated damage, but human cerebral malaria has very different histopathological appearances. In relation to the degree of parasitized red cell sequestration, relatively few leukocytes are found in or around the cerebral vessels in fatal cases, although recent pathological studies have shown more host leukocyte and particularly platelet accumulation in the cerebral vasculature of African children who died from cerebral malaria compared to the findings in South-east Asian adults.[200] The degree of host leukocyte response depends on the stage of infection and is less than that seen in other organs, such as the kidney or lung, which may relate to the immunologically privileged state of the cerebral parenchyma. When excess intravascular leukocytes are seen in pathological specimens, they are often fulfilling their housekeeping role of clearing away residual cytoadherent membranes and pigment. There is little pathological evidence in man for cerebral vasculitis in cerebral malaria. There is evidence of systemic endothelial dysfunction, and recent neuropathological studies have shown evidence for intraparenchymal responses including widespread astroglial activation, evidence of blood–brain barrier leakage and axonal injury.[201,202]

Although some glomerular abnormalities have been noted in fatal malaria,[203] the clinical and pathological findings suggest that acute tubular necrosis, and not acute glomerulonephritis, is the cause of renal dysfunction. The pathogenesis of pulmonary oedema is uncertain – as it is for the adult respiratory distress syndrome in other conditions – but it is unlikely to involve a specific immune-mediated process. Thus despite the enormous intravascular antigenic load in malaria, with the formation and deposition of immune complexes and variable complement depletion,[204–207] there is little direct evidence of a specific immunopathological process in severe malaria.

While innate immune responses are very important in controlling malaria,[208] acute infections are associated with malaria antigen-specific unresponsiveness.[209–211] This selective paresis is one of the factors contributing to the slow development of an effective and specific immune response in malaria. Acute malaria is characterized by non-specific polyclonal B-cell activation. There is a reduction in circulating T cells with an increase in the γ/δ T-cell subset,[212] but other T-cell proportions are usually normal.[213] Although residents of hyperendemic or holoendemic malarious areas have hypergammaglobulinaemia, most of this antibody is not directed against malaria antigens.[214] In non-immune individuals, the acute antibody response to infection often comprises mostly IgM or IgG_2, isotypes which are unable to arm cytotoxic cells and thus kill asexual malaria parasites.[215] These observations have led to the suggestion that malaria induces an immunological 'smoke-screen' with broad-spectrum and non-specific activation that interferes with the orderly development of specific cellular immune responses and immune memory. In severe malaria there is evidence of a broader immune suppression,[216] with defects in monocyte and neutrophil chemotaxis, reduced monocytic phagocytic function, and a tendency to bacterial super-infection.[217,218] In the nephrotic syndrome associated with chronic *P. malariae* infections, malaria antigen and immune complexes can be eluted from the kidney, indicating an immunopathological progress in this condition.[219] But why some children are affected but the majority are not remains a mystery.

Permeability

There is evidence of a mild generalized increase in systemic vascular permeability in severe malaria.[220] Focal perivascular and intraparenchymal oedema is seen in the brain in 70% of fatal cases.[202] In the past, it was suggested that cerebral malaria resulted from a marked generalized increase in cerebral capillary permeability which led to brain swelling, coma and death,[221,222] but the imaging studies conducted to date indicate that, although there may be some increases in brain water, as would be expected given the widespread venular and capillary obstruction, the majority of adults and children with cerebral malaria do not have significant cerebral oedema (Figure 73.12).[223–226] However, the role of raised intracranial pressure in cerebral malaria still remains unclear. Whereas 80% of adults have opening pressures at lumbar puncture which are in the normal range (<200 mm CSF), 80% of children have elevated opening pressures (>100 mm CSF: the normal range is lower in children)[227,228] and intracranial pressure may rise transiently to very high levels. Uncontrolled epileptic seizure activity increases cerebral metabolism thereby increasing the imbalance between energy demand and limited supply (because of microvascular obstruction) and may cause brain swelling. Some patients with cerebral malaria die from acute respiratory arrest with neurological signs that are compatible with brain stem compression. But these signs are also common, and may persist for many hours, in survivors. The elevation in opening pressure is usually not great (in general, it is much lower than in bacterial or fungal meningitis), and there is no difference between these lumbar puncture opening pressures in surviving children and fatal cases.[229] Studies of computerized tomography (CT) or magnetic resonance imaging (MRI) have generally shown slight brain swelling in cerebral malaria (compatible with an increased intracerebral blood volume resulting from sequestration), sometimes discrete focal areas of oedema (particularly in white matter) or abnormal areas of signal attenuation in severe cases, but not severe generalized cerebral oedema.[223–226] Where generalized oedema has been reported it has been inferred from brain swelling on CT, and could have resulted from increased intracerebral blood volume.[230] Immunohistochemical studies on autopsy brain tissues indicate focal disruption of specialized endothelial cell tight junctions, and endothelial activation in areas of intense sequestration, but clinical investigations have also failed to detect major alterations in blood–brain barrier permeability.[231–234] In summary, raised intracranial pressure probably arises mainly from an increase in cerebral blood volume, which results from the addition of the circulating blood required to maintain cerebral perfusion and the considerable sequestered static biomass of intracerebral parasitized erythrocytes. Children may be particularly vulnerable

weeks following acute malaria and reticulocyte counts are usually low in the acute phase of the disease.[262-264] The cause of the dyserythropoiesis is thought to be related to intramedullary cytokine production. Severe malarial anaemia in African children has been associated with the 238A TNF promoter polymorphism and low levels of the anti-inflammatory cytokine IL-10.[80] Serum erythropoietin levels are usually elevated, although in some series it has been suggested that the degree of elevation was not sufficient for the degree of anaemia.[265-267] In *falciparum* malaria the entire red cell population (i.e. both infected and uninfected red cells) becomes more rigid. This loss of deformability correlates with disease severity and outcome,[147,196] and, when measured at the high shear rates encountered in the spleen, with the degree of resulting anaemia.[197] The mechanism responsible has not been identified, although there is evidence in acute malaria for increased oxidative damage which might compromise red cell membrane function and deformability.[268] In simian malarias there is evidence of an inversion of the erythrocyte membrane lipid bilayer in uninfected erythrocytes,[269] but this has not been studied in man. The role of antibody (i.e. Coombs'-positive haemolysis) in anaemia is unresolved.[270-272] The majority of studies to date do not show increased red cell immunoglobulin binding in malaria, but in the presence of a lowered recognition threshold for splenic clearance, this might be difficult to detect. The splenic threshold for the clearance of abnormal erythrocytes, whether because of antibody coating or reduced deformability, is lowered.[107,108] Thus, the spleen removes large numbers of relatively rigid cells causing shortened erythrocyte survival, particularly in severe malaria. This is unaffected by corticosteroids.[273] The spleen also fulfils its normative function of removing damaged intraerythrocytic parasites from red cells, (particularly following treatment with an artemisinin derivative), and returning the 'once parasitized' red cells back to the circulation by a process of 'pitting'.[274] These erythrocytes then have reduced survival.[275]

In the context of acute uncomplicated malaria, the anaemia is worse in younger children, and those with protracted infections. Loss of unparasitized erythrocytes accounts for approximately 90% of the acute anaemia resulting from a single uncomplicated infection.[276] Iron deficiency and malaria often coincide in the same patient, and in some areas routine iron supplementation following malaria promotes recovery from anaemia.

Coagulopathy and thrombocytopenia

In acute malaria, coagulation cascade activity is accelerated with accelerated fibrinogen turnover, consumption of antithrombin III, reduced factor XIII, and increased concentrations of fibrin degradation products.[277-282] In severe infections the antithrombin III, protein S and protein C are further reduced and prothrombin and partial thromboplastin times may be prolonged. In occasional patients (<5%) bleeding may be significant. The coagulation cascade is activated via the intrinsic pathway.[283] Intravascular thrombus formation is observed rarely at autopsy in fatal cases and on histopathological examination, fibrin deposition is sparse and platelets are unusual in adult cases,[140] in contrast to paediatric cases.[200]

Thrombocytopenia is common to all the four human malarias and is caused by increased splenic clearance.[284] Thrombocytopenia is associated with high levels of IL-10 and appropriately raised concentrations of thrombopoeitin (a key growth factor for platelet production).[285] Plasma concentrations of macrophage colony stimulating factor are high, which stimulate macrophage activity, and may increase platelet destruction.[286] Platelet turnover is increased. The role of platelet-bound antibody in malarial thrombocytopenia is controversial.[287-289] There has been evidence of platelet activation in some studies, but not others.[290] Erythrocytes containing mature parasites may activate the coagulation cascade directly,[291] and cytokine release is also procoagulant. The high plasma levels of P-selectin found in severe malaria may derive from platelets,[286] but could also come from vascular endothelium, as plasma concentrations of other endothelial derived proteins (thrombomodulin, E-selectin, ICAM-1, VCAM-1) are elevated as well.[292,293] It was suggested in the past that disseminated intravascular coagulation (DIC) is important in the pathogenesis of severe malaria,[294,295] but detailed prospective clinical and pathogenesis studies have refuted this. Coagulation cascade activity is directly proportional to disease severity,[281] but hypofibrinogenaemia resulting from DIC is significant in less than 5% of patients with severe malaria, and lethal haemorrhage (usually gastrointestinal) is very unusual.[296,297]

Blackwater fever

Blackwater fever (Figure 73.13) is a poorly understood condition in which there is massive intravascular haemolysis and the passage of 'Coca-Cola'-coloured urine.[297-299] Historically, this was linked to frequent quinine self-medication in expatriates living in

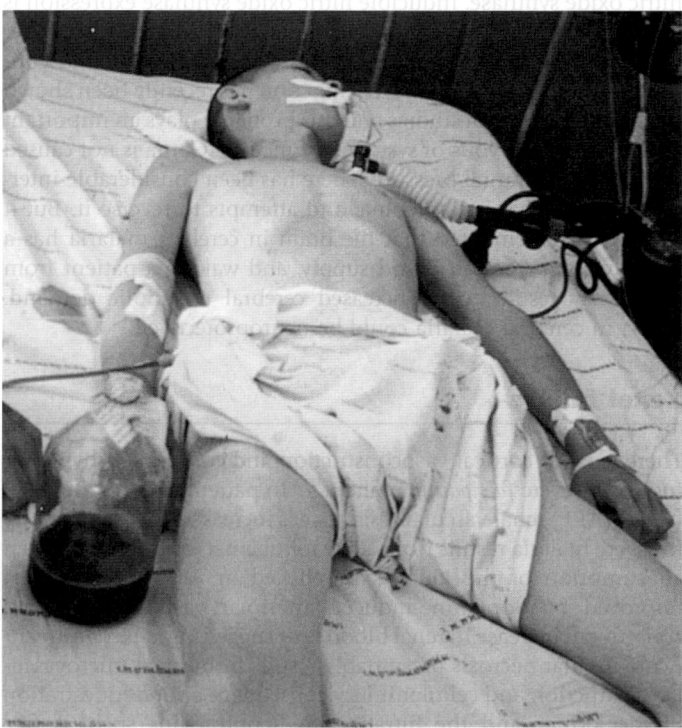

Figure 73.13 Blackwater fever. A 25-year-old male with severe malaria, pulmonary oedema, renal impairment and massive haemolysis.

malarious areas, and indeed blackwater fever almost disappeared from Africa during the 'chloroquine' era from 1950 to 1980. With the return of quinine blackwater fever has now reappeared.[300] Blackwater (black urine) occurs in four circumstances: (1) when patients with G6PD deficiency take oxidant drugs (e.g. primaquine, sulphones or sulphonamides) irrespective of whether they have malaria or not; (2) occasionally when patients with G6PD deficiency have malaria and receive quinine treatment; (3) in some patients with severe *falciparum* malaria who have normal erythrocyte G6PD levels irrespective of the treatment given and (4) when people who are exposed to malaria self-medicate frequently with quinine (or structurally related drugs).

In severe malaria, rates of blackwater in Asian patients are similar whether the patients receive quinine or an artemisinin derivative. How quinine causes blackwater in these last three situations is not known, as it is not an oxidant drug. G6PD-deficient red cells are particularly susceptible to oxidant stress as they are unable to synthesize adequate quantities of NADPH through the pentose shunt. This leads to low intraerythrocytic levels of reduced glutathione, and both alterations in the erythrocyte membrane and increased susceptibility to organic peroxides. Blackwater fever may be associated with acute renal failure, although in the majority of cases renal function remains normal.[298]

The spleen

There is considerable splenic enlargement in malaria, mainly as a result of cellular multiplication and structural change, and an increased capacity to clear red cells from the circulation both by Fc receptor-mediated (immune) mechanisms[107,108] and by recognition of reduced deformability (filtration).[106] There is considerable accumulation of parasitized erythrocytes.[301] The increased filtration of the spleen and the reduced deformability of the entire red cell population results in the rapid development of anaemia in severe malaria. The spleen may also modulate cytoadherence.[111] It plays a central role in limiting the acute expansion of the malaria infection by removing parasitized erythrocytes, and this has led to the suggestion that a failure to augment splenic clearance sufficiently rapidly may be a factor in the development of severe malaria. Characteristic changes to the immuno-architecture of the spleen are seen during infection which may reflect a central role for dendritic cells in orchestrating specific immune responses.[302]

The spleen is capable of removing damaged intraerythrocytic parasites and returning the once infected red cells to the circulation (a process known as 'pitting'),[274] where they have shortened survival.[275] This is an important contributor to parasite clearance following antimalarial drug treatment (particularly treatment with artemisinin derivatives).[303,304]

Gastrointestinal dysfunction

Abdominal pain may be prominent in acute malaria. Minor stress ulceration of the stomach and duodenum is common in severe malaria. The pattern of malabsorption of sugars, fats and amino acids suggests reduced splanchnic perfusion.[305–308] This results from both gut sequestration and visceral vasoconstriction. Gut permeability is increased,[309] and this may be associated with reduced local defences against bacterial toxins, or even whole bacteria in severe disease. Antimalarial drug absorption is remarkably unaffected in uncomplicated malaria, except for those drugs which have fat (i.e. food)-dependent absorption (halofantrine, atovaquone, lumefantrine).

Liver dysfunction

Jaundice is common in adults with severe malaria, and there is other evidence of hepatic dysfunction, with reduced clotting factor synthesis, reduced metabolic clearance of the antimalarial drugs, and a failure of gluconeogenesis which contributes to lactic acidosis and hypoglycaemia. Nevertheless, true liver failure (as in fulminant viral hepatitis) is very unusual. There is sequestration in the hepatic microvasculature and, although many patients with acute *falciparum* malaria have elevated liver blood flow values, in very severe infections liver blood flow is reduced.[308,310,311] In adults, liver blood flow values <15 mL/kg per min are associated with elevated venous lactate concentrations,[311] which suggests a flow limitation to lactate clearance and thus a contribution of liver dysfunction to lactic acidosis. Direct measurements of hepatic venous lactate concentrations in severe malaria confirm that the hepatosplanchnic extraction ratio is inversely correlated with mixed venous plasma lactate (i.e hyperlactataemia is associated with reduced liver clearance of lactate).[312] There is no relationship between liver blood flow and impairment of antimalarial drug clearance.[313] Jaundice in malaria appears to have haemolytic, hepatic, and cholestatic components. Cholestatic jaundice may persist well into the recovery period. There is no residual liver damage following malaria.

Acidosis

Acidosis is a major cause of death in severe *falciparum* malaria, both in adults and children. This has been considered to be mainly a lactic acidosis, although ketoacidosis (and sometimes salicylate intoxication) may predominate in children, and the acidosis of renal failure is common in adults.[312,314–317] In severe malaria, the arterial, capillary, venous and CSF concentrations of lactate rise in direct proportion to disease severity. Acid-base assessment or venous lactate concentrations on or 4 h after admission to hospital are very good indicators of prognosis in severe malaria.[315,318] In bacterial sepsis there is also hyperlactataemia, but, unless there is profound shock, the lactate-pyruvate ratio is usually <15. This indicates that hypermetabolism is the source of lactate accumulation in sepsis. In severe malaria, the pathogenesis is different; lactate-pyruvate ratios often exceed 30, reflecting tissue hypoxia and anaerobic glycolysis. Lactic acidosis results from several discrete processes: the tissue anaerobic glycolysis consequent upon microvascular obstruction; a failure of hepatic and renal lactate clearance; and the production of lactate by the parasite.[319,320] The role of hypovolaemia is controversial. Mature malaria parasites consume up to 70 times as much glucose as uninfected cells, and over 90% of this is converted to L+lactic acid (plasmodia do not have the complete set of enzymes necessary for the citric acid cycle). Interestingly, up to 6% of the lactic acid appears as D-lactate, but this does not contribute materially to the acidosis.[321] However, calculations based on glucose and lactate turnover in man indicate that the majority of the lactic acid produced in

Placenta

The placenta may be black from malaria pigment even if the mother is asymptomatic throughout pregnancy. Large numbers of mature parasites are seen on crush smears,[378] although the peripheral blood smear may be negative. There is often trophoblastic thickening, macrophage infiltration, pigment deposition and perivillous fibrin deposition. Active infection is associated with basement, membrane thickening, fibrinoid necrosis and syncitial knots.[379-383] Chronic infection is associated with marked mononuclear cell infiltration.

CLINICAL FEATURES IN RELATION TO TRANSMISSION INTENSITY

The clinical manifestations of malaria are dependent on the previous immune status of the host. In areas of intense *P. falciparum* malaria transmission, asymptomatic parasitaemia is usual in adults (premunition). Severe malaria never occurs in this age group: it is confined to the first years of life, and becomes progressively less frequent with increasing age. In Africa overall the average age of children admitted to hospital with severe malaria is 3 years, which corresponds with the peak mortality in the third year of life. The rate at which age-specific acquisition of premunition occurs is proportional to the intensity of malaria transmission. In areas with a constant high-level *P. falciparum* transmission (e.g. average infected anopheline biting frequencies of daily up to monthly), severe malaria occurs predominantly between 6 months and 3 years of age; milder symptoms are seen in older children, and adults are usually asymptomatic and have low parasitaemias. Malaria is common in pregnancy, but is oligosymptomatic or asymptomatic (although anaemia may be severe). The birth weight of babies born to primigravidae is reduced significantly. Spleen rates are high (>50%) in children between 2 and 9, corresponding with the epidemiological terms hyperendemic and holoendemic malaria. Severe anaemia in young children is the most common presentation of severe *falciparum* malaria in these circumstances. With lower or more seasonal or unstable transmission patterns the age distribution of severe malaria shifts upwards, severe malaria is seen in older children as well, and cerebral malaria becomes the most prominent manifestation (Figure 73.2). Spleen rates in children are lower than 50%. With even lower or more seasonal patterns of transmission, and when non-immunes travel to endemic areas, symptomatic disease is seen at all ages. Severe malaria does not occur commonly with *P. vivax*, *P. ovale*, or *P. malariae* but acute infection in a non-immune patient is still serious and debilitating. With more intense exposure, a state of premunition is also reached with these infections.

Incubation period

Precise data on the incubation period of malaria come from the detailed studies of malaria therapy for neurosyphilis, and also the many hundreds of volunteer experiments conducted between the turn of the century and 1965 (Table 73.1).[84-86,89,90] In the majority of mosquito-transmitted infections several heavily infected anophelines were allowed to bite. The sporozoite inocula were therefore probably larger than those received in most naturally acquired (autochthonous) infections. In most cases of *falciparum* or *vivax* malaria the incubation period is approximately 2 weeks. The shortest incubation period documented was reported by Shute[384] in a sailor who docked briefly in West Africa and somehow developed malaria 3 days later. Primary incubation periods can be long, particularly if the infection is suppressed by partially effective chemoprophylaxis. Most tropical strains of *P. vivax* had similar incubation periods to *P. falciparum*, but strains from cooler countries often had extremely long incubation periods. The primary infection began 9–12 months after sporozoite inoculation. This coincided with the short summer-time mosquito breeding season in these cold countries. These strains of *P. vivax* (e.g. *P. vivax* var *hibernans*) acquired in northern and Eastern Europe, Russia, central and northern China, are now nearly extinct but for a few areas of China, North Korea and South Korea near the demilitarized zone.

In the artificial infection experiments, the differences in recorded incubation periods between strains of the same *Plasmodia* species were small, although a negative correlation was apparent between the probable dose of sporozoites and the duration of the prepatent period (the time from sporozoite inoculation until the first positive blood film). The incubation period (time from sporozoite inoculation to fever) was prolonged by ineffective antimalarial treatment or prophylaxis – both of which reduce the effective multiplication rate.

The durations of the prepatent and incubation periods are also strongly influenced by previous exposure, i.e. 'immunity'. Effective immunity both reduces effective multiplication, which prolongs the prepatent period, and raises the threshold at which symptoms occur (premunition), which prolongs the incubation period. In *vivax* malaria the symptom threshold is raised disproportionately in immune individuals, i.e. the gap between the prepatent and incubation period widens.

Mixed species infections

The incidence of mixed species infections is always underestimated. Even with sensitive PCR detection methods, which reveal a higher rate than microscopy, mixed infections are underestimated. In simultaneous infection with *P. falciparum* and *P. vivax*, the former suppresses the latter, and the primary *vivax* malaria infection may not appear until several weeks later.[385-387] Sometimes the reverse occurs and *P. vivax* suppresses *P. falciparum*.[388] In sub-Saharan Africa *P. falciparum* commonly occurs together with *P. malariae* or *P. ovale*. In many areas outside Africa *P. falciparum* and *P. vivax* are both common and co-existent infections are frequent but, because of mutual suppression, the incidence is considerably underestimated.[385-391] For example, in Thailand approximately 30% of patients with *P. falciparum* malaria will have a subsequent symptomatic infection with *P. vivax* within 2 months of their primary *falciparum* malaria, without further exposure to malaria infection.[385] The converse (*P. vivax* malaria with undiagnosed coincident *P. falciparum* infection) occurs in approximately 8% of cases.[388] In low transmission settings coincident infection of *P. falciparum* with *P. vivax* reduces the risk of severe malaria four-fold,[392] reduces the degree of anaemia,[262] and reduces *P. falciparum* gametocyte carriage.[393] But in higher transmission settings the effect is opposite; mixed infections are associated with greater morbidity. Mixed infections with *P. malariae* and *P. ovale* are also underestimated.[390,391]

Pyrogenic density

The parasitaemia at which fever (>37.3°C) occurs is termed the 'pyrogenic density'. This varies widely: some non-immune patients will become febrile before parasites are visible on blood smears (i.e. the incubation period is shorter than the prepatent period), whereas immune adults or older children can on occasions tolerate up to 100 000 *P. falciparum* parasites/μL without fever. The pyrogenic density for *P. vivax* is generally lower than that of *P. falciparum*; in 76% of cases reported by Kitchen[394] the pyrogenic density was <100 parasites/μL. In *P. falciparum* infections average pyrogenic densities can be as high as 10 000/μL,[389] but it must be remembered that less than half the life cycle circulates in *falciparum* malaria.[356] The parasites in the blood smear are the circulating parasites in the generation subsequent to that which underwent pyrogenic merogony, and they are therefore an underestimate of the total parasite burden. The pyrogenic density is a marker of immunity. High pyrogenic densities indicate premunition, and a lower risk of severe disease. There are fewer data on pyrogenic densities in *P. malariae* infections, but it appears that they are higher than for *P. vivax*; values over 500/μL were found in 38% of Boyd's cases. There are limited data on *P. ovale*, but the available evidence suggests a pyrogenic density similar to *P. vivax*.

Uncomplicated malaria

The cardinal feature of malaria is fever. The clinical features of uncomplicated malaria are common to all four species, although there is a suggestion that *P. vivax*, which tends to synchronize rapidly, may cause more severe symptoms early in the course of the infection. *P. malariae* and possibly *P. ovale* both have a more gradual onset than *P. vivax*. *P. falciparum* is unpredictable: the onset ranges from gradual to fulminant. The first symptoms of malaria are non-specific and resemble influenza. They are similar for all four species of *Plasmodium*. Headache, muscular ache, vague abdominal discomfort, lethargy, lassitude and dysphoria often precede fever by up to 2 days. The temperature rises erratically at first, with shivering, mild chills, worsening headache and malaise, and loss of appetite. Children are irritable, lethargic and anorexic. If the infection is left untreated the fever in *P. vivax* and *P. ovale* regularizes to a 2-day cycle (tertian), and *P. malariae* fever spikes occur every 3 days (quartan pattern). *P. falciparum* remains erratic for longer, and may never regularize to a tertian pattern.[84] These terms derive from the Greek practice of inclusive reckoning, in which the beginning of the fever is considered day one. Thus, a tertian fever recurs every third day and a quartan fever every fourth day, with intervals of 2 and 3 days, respectively. Some infections consist of two broods cycling 24 h out of phase and in these there is a daily fever spike (quotidian fever). Even more complex fever patterns are described in detail in the early literature.

The classical malaria fever charts (which graced earlier editions of this textbook), and the teeth-chattering rigors and profuse sweats that characterized the 'paroxysm' (Figure 73.14), are relatively unusual today as malaria therapy of neurosyphilis is no longer practised (penicillin is more effective and more pleasant),

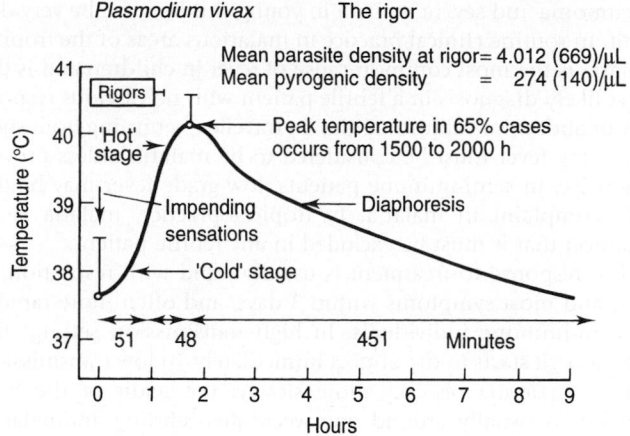

Figure 73.14 The rigor of *P. vivax* malaria. (The time course of signs and symptoms is taken from Kitchen SF, Puttnam P. Observations on the character of the paroxysm in vivax malaria. *J Natl Malaria Soc* 1946; 5:57–78.) True rigors are rare in *P. falciparum* malaria and occur with the other three human malarias only after the infections have synchronized sufficiently.

and symptomatic infections are treated as soon as they are diagnosed. In a true paroxysm, the temperature usually rises steeply from a normal or slightly elevated level to exceed 39°C. As the temperature begins to rise, there is intense headache and muscular discomfort. The patient feels cold, clutches at blankets, and curls up shivering and uncommunicative (the chill). There is peripheral vasoconstriction, and often 'goose-pimples'. Within minutes, the limbs begin to shake and the teeth chatter, and the temperature climbs rapidly to a peak (usually between 39 and 41.5°C). The rigor usually last 10–30 min, but can last up to 90 min (Figure 73.14). By the end of the rigor, there is peripheral vasodilatation and the skin feels hot. A profuse sweat then breaks out. The blood pressure is relatively low and there may be symptomatic orthostatic hypotension. The patient feels exhausted and may sleep. Defervescence usually takes 4–8 h. Paroxysms with rigors are more common in *P. vivax* and *P. ovale* than in *P. falciparum* or *P. malariae* malaria. They may begin a relapse, or occur after several days of more chaotic fever in primary infections with these two malaria species. True rigors are unusual in naturally acquired *falciparum* malaria. As the infection continues, the spleen and liver enlarge and anaemia develops. The patient loses weight. If no treatment is given, the natural infection stabilizes for several weeks or months and then gradually resolves. The duration of illness is proportional to the level of immunity and differs between the parasite species. Mild abdominal discomfort is common in malaria, and rarely patients may appear to have an 'acute abdomen'. Constipation or diarrhoea may occur. In some areas, watery diarrhoea is a prominent manifestation. However, there is usually no difficulty distinguishing malaria from gastroenteritis. A dry cough has been reported in some series, but this is not prominent. However, the respiratory rate may be raised, particularly in children, and this can give rise to diagnostic confusion in primary healthcare facilities where respiratory rate is used as the only criterion for the diagnosis of acute respiratory infection. On chest examination, there is no evidence of consolidation or effusion, but in an endemic area, the clinical distinction between early pneumonia and severe malaria in young children can be very difficult. In routine clinical practice in malarious areas of the tropics, malaria is the most common cause of fever in children and is the most likely diagnosis in a febrile patient with no obvious respiratory or abdominal abnormalities. In travellers returning from such areas, any fever must be considered to be malaria unless proved otherwise. In semi-immune patients, low-grade fever may be the only complaint in malaria. In tropical practice, malaria is so common that it must be excluded in any febrile patient.

The response to treatment is usually rapid with resolution of fever and most symptoms within 3 days, and often more rapidly in semi-immune individuals. In high transmission settings the haematocrit starts to rise almost immediately. In low transmission settings anaemia resolves more slowly; the nadir of the haematocrit is usually around one week after starting antimalarial treatment.

Relapse

Both *P. vivax* and *P. ovale* have a tendency to relapse after resolution of the primary infection. Relapse, which results from maturation of persistent hypnozoites in the liver, must be distinguished from recrudescence of the primary infection because of incomplete treatment. *P. falciparum* is the usual cause of recrudescent infections and these tend to arise 2–4 weeks following treatment (but this can be as long as 10 weeks following mefloquine treatment). Relapses occur weeks or months (or even years) after the primary infection. The proportion of cases relapsing and the intervals between relapses vary between strains. The pattern of relapse is determined largely by the geographical origin of the infection. For example, over 50% of *P. vivax* infections in Thailand relapse whereas in most of India the proportion is closer to 20%.[395] The rare subtropical *P. vivax* tends to have long gaps between relapses whereas tropical strains have short intervals (3–6 weeks). In Patrick Manson's famous experiment, conducted in September 1900, he infected his 23 year-old son with *P. vivax*, through mosquitoes sent by rail from Rome to London. His son became ill with 'double tertian fever', but was treated with quinine and recovered fully. In June 1901, he suddenly became ill again with *vivax* malaria; a relapse interval of 9 months.[396,397] In recent years, a relapse interval of 6 weeks has been quoted widely for tropical *Plasmodium vivax* infections but this is an artefact of the use of chloroquine for treatment, which suppresses the first relapse (at 3 weeks).[398] Blood chloroquine levels decline by the time of the second relapse at 6 weeks, and this is the first to manifest itself. The symptoms of a relapse start more abruptly than in the primary infection as the infection is more synchronous. They may begin with a sudden chill or rigor. Primaquine given for 14 days will eradicate hypnozoites and prevent relapse in over 80% of patients.

Malaria in pregnancy

In areas of intense transmission, the principal impact of *falciparum* malaria in pregnancy is an increased incidence of anaemia and a reduction in birth weight (approximately 170 g on average) of babies born to primigravidae.[345] Thus a greater proportion of babies have low birth weights (<2.5 kg). Low birth weight is a major risk factor for infantile death. Malaria reduces birth weight mainly by intrauterine growth retardation (IUGR). In high transmission areas, malaria may also cause prematurity.[399] In low transmission areas, prematurity is caused by symptomatic malaria close to term, not earlier in the pregnancy. The net result is an increased risk of neonatal death.[400] In high transmission settings, despite intense sequestration of parasites in the placenta, the mothers are usually asymptomatic, although they are more likely to be anaemic. In areas with lower levels of malaria transmission (mesoendemic or hypoendemic), symptomatic disease occurs and pregnant women are at an increased risk of severe *falciparum* malaria, particularly in the second and third trimesters. In low transmission areas, the adverse effects of malaria on birth weight extend to the first three pregnancies (and in non-immunes, to all pregnancies).[26] Anaemia is common and there is an increased risk of developing severe malaria. Anaemia itself is a risk factor for maternal mortality; moderate anaemia (Hb4-8 g/dL) carrying a relative risk of 1.35 and severe anaemia (Hb <4 g/dL), a risk of 3.5.[400] If a pregnant woman does develop severe malaria, fetal loss is common, and the maternal mortality is very high. The mortality of cerebral malaria in pregnancy is approximately 50%, compared with 15–20% in non-pregnant adults. Acute pulmonary oedema and hypoglycaemia are particular complications of severe malaria in pregnancy. The baby is commonly stillborn. The clinical features of uncomplicated *vivax*, *ovale* or *malariae* malaria are similar to those of uncomplicated *P. falciparum*. *P. vivax* infections also increase anaemia and they reduce birth weight by approximately 100 g. In contrast to *P. falciparum*, *vivax* malaria affects multigravidae more than primigravidae.[14] If a mother delivers with acute malaria, blood-borne transmission to the newborn is not uncommon, but this often resolves spontaneously. Nevertheless, babies must be observed closely for congenital malaria and malaria considered in the differential diagnosis of neonatal fever or anaemia.

Malaria in children

The majority of childhood malaria infections (Figure 73.15) present with fever and malaise, and respond rapidly to antimalarial treatment. Severe *falciparum* malaria is rare in the first six months of life, although when it does occur the mortality is high. In young children, the progression of *falciparum* malaria can be rapid. Generalized seizures are associated with fever, but they are more common in *P. falciparum* than *P. vivax* malaria, even in the absence of other signs of cerebral involvement. This suggests that cerebral sequestration causes significant pathology even in conscious patients. Coma, convulsions, acidosis, hypoglycaemia and severe anaemia are common presenting features of severe malaria in childhood.[401-404] At the bedside, the presence of respiratory distress (acidotic breathing) or deep coma defines children at high risk of dying.[36] These two overlapping clinical syndromes account for the majority of lethal infections. In areas of intense transmission, profound anaemia is the usual manifestation of severe malaria, and this occurs mainly in the 1–3 year age group. Severe malaria is rare in older children in high transmission settings. In areas of lower less stable transmission, cerebral malaria becomes a predominant manifestation of severe disease, and the age range shifts upwards. Jaundice and pulmonary oedema are unusual in

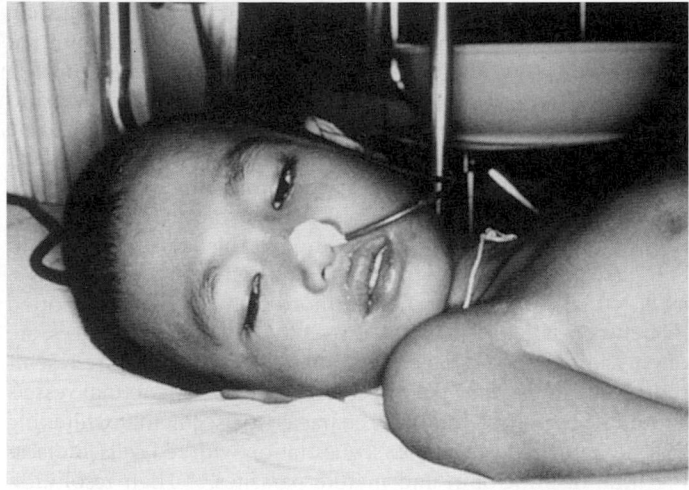

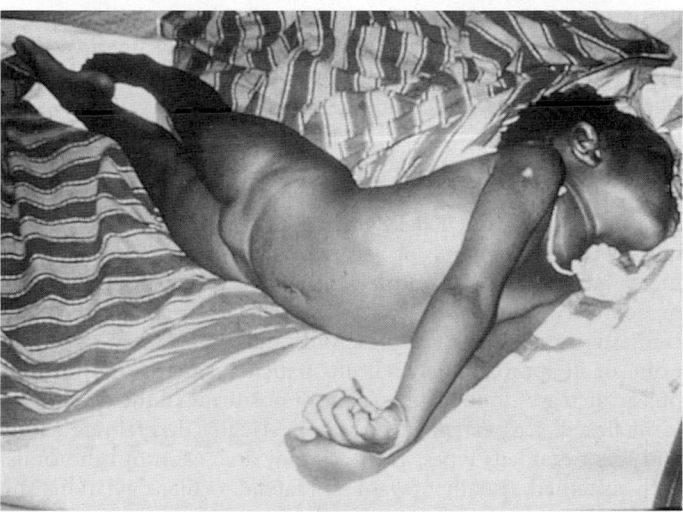

Figure 73.15 (A) A 6-year-old Thai boy with cerebral malaria. His father was admitted at the same time with cerebral malaria – both survived. (B) A 3-year-old Gambian girl with cerebral malaria and opisthotonos. (Courtesy of Jane Crawley.)

young children, and renal failure is very rare (a marked difference compared with adults). As a consequence, iatrogenic overhydration is less of a problem in children than in adults, although intravenous fluid administration must still be carefully supervised in small children. Dehydration is more common. In cerebral malaria seizures occurs frequently, particularly in the <3-year age group, and should be treated promptly. Hypoglycaemia is common, occurring in up to 30% of children with severe malaria, and is often accompanied by lactic acidosis. The blood glucose should be checked frequently and, where possible, continuous intravenous infusions of 5% or 10% dextrose given as a preventive measure.

In general, children tolerate the antimalarial drugs better than adults, and their symptoms resolve more quickly. The temptation to estimate body weight by 'eye' should be resisted, and all children should be weighed if possible so that the doses of anti-

malarial drugs can be given on a mg/kg basis. (Although administration of drugs adjusted to surface area is theoretically preferable, antimalarial doses have been devised on the basis of body weight). Children with acute malaria vomit readily, particularly if the temperature is high. Oral antimalarial treatment is more likely to be retained if it is palatable and the child is cool and calm before drug administration. In busy tropical clinics, only a minority of patients can be admitted to hospital, and many children with moderately severe malaria have to be treated on an out-patient basis. It is common practice to administer a single intramuscular dose of quinine and to send the patient home with the remainder of the oral regimen, and to give the parents advice to return if the child deteriorates further. In this situation, there is a danger of significant iatrogenic hypotension if the child is kept upright (e.g. on the mother's back). If possible the child should be observed for at least 2 h following parenteral drug administration and reassessed before discharge.

The diagnosis of severe malaria in children living in malaria endemic areas may be difficult. As a positive blood smear is common in apparently healthy children, finding malaria parasites in the blood of a sick child does not necessarily mean the child has severe malaria. Fever and rapid laboured breathing could be pneumonia even if the blood smear is positive. The obtunded child might have meningoencephalitis, and the shocked child might be septicaemic despite positive blood smears. The net result is that severe malaria in children tends to be overdiagnosed.

Malaria and HIV

When the enormity of the HIV epidemic in Africa was first recognized, it was thought that malaria and HIV infection did not interact significantly. This is not true. While asymptomatic HIV infection has little impact on malaria, with increasing immunosuppression in HIV-AIDS, immune control of malaria is impaired.[405–411] There is an increasing risk of parasitaemia, increasing risk of illness, and in low transmission settings an increased risk of severe malaria. HIV infection compounds malaria-associated reduction in birth weight. Therapeutic responses to antimalarial treatment are impaired so treatment failure rates are increased. Drug interactions between antiretrovirals and antimalarials have not yet been studied adequately. Where sulfadoxine-pyrimethamine is effective, then prophylaxis against opportunistic infections with trimethoprim-sulphamethoxazole will protect from malaria also.

Severe malaria

Death from acute *P. vivax*, *P. ovale* or *P. malariae* infections is rare. Occasionally already debilitated patients may succumb, and fatal haemorrhage may follow a ruptured spleen (either traumatic or spontaneous), but these events are very uncommon. There have been many case reports of 'cerebral *vivax* malaria'. Some of these may have been misdiagnoses, but there is increasing evidence, particularly from India and Indonesia, that *Plasmodium vivax* infections can be severe and life-threatening.[412,413]

Falciparum malaria is a major cause of death. The progression to severe disease can be rapid. In young children presenting with cerebral malaria a history of less than one day's illness is common. Although undernutrition is associated with an increased risk of clinical malaria and anaemia in high transmission settings,[414] cerebral malaria is rare in severe malnutrition and often seems to strike down the healthiest people. The great malariologist Ettore Marchiafava noted over 100 years ago how common severe malaria was in the 'hale and hearty' Italian shepherds who descended from the malaria-free mountains to the malarious valleys every autumn.[39] In adults, patients with severe malaria usually have a history of being ill for several days before admission to hospital.

Definitions of severe *falciparum* malaria are useful for clinical and epidemiological purposes. Definitions were proposed by working groups convened by the World Health Organization (WHO) in 1986, 1990[295] and 2000.[415] The widely used 1990 definition (Table 73.3[412]) was modified in a more recent series of recommendations, to make it more inclusive and practical, and to focus more on children (Table 73.4). Both are presented with comments.

In severe malaria, there is often evidence of multiple vital organ dysfunction, and more than one of the above criteria are fulfilled. Physicians should not worry unduly about definitions or semantics. They should treat *any patient about whom they are worried* as having severe malaria, even if they do not fall clearly into one of the above categories.

Cerebral malaria

This may be defined strictly as unrousable coma (i.e. there is a non-purposeful response or no response to a painful stimulus) in *falciparum* malaria. In practice, any patient with altered consciousness should be treated for severe malaria. Although cerebral malaria is the most prominent feature of severe *falciparum* malaria, some patients with ultimately lethal infections never lose consciousness until they die. In cerebral malaria, the onset of coma may be sudden, often following a generalized seizure, or gradual, with initial drowsiness, confusion, disorientation, delirium or agitation, followed by unconsciousness. Extreme agitation is a poor prognostic sign in *falciparum* malaria. The length of the prodromal history is usually several days in adults, but in children, can be as short as 6–12 h. A history of convulsions is common.

On examination, the patient is febrile and unrousable. There may be some passive resistance to neck flexion, but the board-like rigidity of meningitis is not found, and there are no other signs of meningeal irritation. There may be anaemia, which in some cases, particularly children, may be profound. Conversely, jaundice is relatively unusual in children but common in adults. Signs of bleeding are unusual and indicate a poor prognosis. The patient is usually warm, dry, and well perfused peripherally, with a low-normal blood pressure and a sinus tachycardia. Skin perfusion is variable. Poor capillary refill (refill time >2 s) is a serious prognostic sign in children. Intermittent 'goose-pimples' are common in association with cutaneous vasoconstriction. Sustained hyperventilation is a poor prognostic sign as it indicates metabolic acidosis if the chest is clear, or pneumonia or pulmonary oedema if it is not. The liver and spleen are commonly enlarged, but soft. Massive splenomegaly is not found. There is no lymphadenopathy and no rash. The clinical features are usually of a symmetrical encephalopathy. Focal signs are unusual. On examination of the nervous system, the gaze is usually normal or divergent (but there is no evidence of extraocular muscle paresis) (Figure 73.16). The pupils are usually mid-size and equally reactive. The fundus should be examined carefully. Five distinct fundoscopic abnormalities have been observed; retinal whitening, retinal haemorrhages, focal whitening of vessels, papilloedema and cotton wool spots.[416] These are more easily seen using indirect ophthalmoscopy, although this is usually unavailable. Papilloedema is unusual and is a sign of poor prognosis, as is retinal oedema. Retinal haemorrhages have been reported in between 6% and 37% of cases.[416–420] The haemorrhages are often flame or boat shaped, and may have a pale centre resembling Roth spots. They rarely affect the macula. The retinal vessels should be examined for a very characteristic segmental whitening that probably reflects intense sequestration with red cells containing little haemoglobin and mature parasites.[416] High resolution digital imaging retinal angiography shows irregular vascular lining in some vessels and obstruction reflecting cytoadherence.[420] In adult patients, the corneal reflexes are usually preserved but in children with deep coma they may be lost (a poor prognostic sign). It is important to examine the eyes carefully to exclude the rapid repetitive jerky movements that indicate covert seizure activity. There may be forced jaw closure with repetitive spontaneous teeth grinding (bruxism). The jaw jerk is sometimes brisk and there is often a pout reflex. Other frontal release signs are very unusual. Cranial nerve abnormalities are rare. Tone may be increased, decreased or normal. Likewise, the reflexes can be brisk or depressed. The abdominal reflexes are invariably absent, the cremasteric reflexes often preserved, and the plantar responses extensor in approximately half the patients. Patients may exhibit phasic increases in tone with extensor posturing of the decorticate (arm flexed, legs extended), or more usually decerebrate (arms and legs extended) types. The back may arch as in opisthotonus, with sustained, usually upward and lateral, ocular deviation. The posturing is commonly associated with noisy hyperventilation. Generalized or sometimes focal seizures may occur. The duration of coma varies considerably but overall is shorter in children (average 1 day) than in adults (average 2–3 days). Clinical evidence for seizure activity may be very subtle (e.g. tonic clonic eye movements without limb movement), and in some children there are no signs despite electroencephalographic evidence. Aspiration pneumonia is a potentially lethal sequel.

Untreated cerebral malaria is probably nearly always fatal. The overall mortality of treated cerebral malaria obviously depends on the referral practices and medical facilities available, but in reported studies with quinine treatment it averages 15% in children and 20% in adults (but up to 50% in pregnancy).[24–26,297,421] Some series have reported lower mortalities, but in these the definition of cerebral malaria has been more 'generous', i.e. they have included patients who were obtunded or delirious but not unrousable. Hospitals acting as secondary or tertiary referral centres often experience higher mortalities as they see a residue of more severe patients. The later the patient is referred, the higher the mortality. In the Vietnam War, the mortality of acute *falciparum* malaria was higher in soldiers who had returned to the USA than it was in Vietnam.[422] Obviously the diagnosis was made much more rapidly in Vietnam where physicians were well aware of malaria, than in the USA where they were not.

Table 73.3 1990 WHO Definition of severe malaria

1. Cerebral malaria – unrousable coma not attributable to any other cause in a patient with falciparum malaria. The coma should persist for at least 30 min (1 h in the 2000 definition) after a generalized convulsion to make the distinction from transient postictal coma. Coma should be assessed using the Blantyre coma scale in children or the Glasgow coma scale in adults (Table 73.12).

2. Severe anaemia – normocytic anaemia with haematocrit <15% or haemoglobin <5 g/dL in the presence of parasitaemia more than 10 000/μL. Note that finger prick samples may underestimate the haemoglobin concentration by up to 1 g if the finger is squeezed. If anaemia is hypochromic and/or microcytic, iron deficiency and thalassaemia/haemoglobinopathy must be excluded. (These criteria are rather generous; and would include many children in high transmission areas. A parasitaemia of >100 000/μL might be a more appropriate threshold.)

3. Renal failure – defined as a urine output of <400 mL in 24 h in adults, or 12 mL/kg in 24 h in children, failing to improve after rehydration, and a serum creatinine of more than 265 μmol/L (>3.0 mg/dL). (In practice for initial assessment, the serum creatinine alone is used.)

4. Pulmonary oedema or adult respiratory distress syndrome.

5. Hypoglycaemia – defined as a whole blood glucose concentration of less than 2.2 mmol/L (40 mg/dL).

6. Circulatory collapse or shock – hypotension (systolic blood pressure <50 mmHg in children aged 1–5 years or <70 mmHg in adults), with cold clammy skin or core-skin temperature difference >10°C. (The more recent review declined to give precise definitions, but noted the lack of sensitivity or specificity of core-peripheral measurements.) Capillary refill time is not mentioned but recent studies indicate this simple test provides a good assessment of severity.[449]

7. Spontaneous bleeding from gums, nose, gastrointestinal tract, etc. and/or substantial laboratory evidence of DIC. (This is relatively unusual.)

8. Repeated generalized convulsions – more than two observed within 24 h despite cooling. (In young children, these may be febrile convulsions, and the other clinical and parasitological features need to be taken into account.) Clinical evidence of seizure activity may be subtle (e.g. tonic clonic eye movements, profuse salivation, delayed coma recovery).

9. Acidaemia – defined as an arterial or capillary pH <7.35 (note temperature corrections are needed as most patients are hotter than 37°C; add 0.0147 pH unit per degree Celsius (°C) over 37°C), or acidosis defined as a plasma bicarbonate concentration <15 mmol/L or a base excess >10. (Operationally, the clinical presentation of 'respiratory distress' or 'acidotic breathing' is focused upon in the 2000 recommendations. Abnormal breathing patterns are a sign of severity indicating severe acidosis, pulmonary oedema or pneumonia.)

10. Macroscopic haemoglobinuria – if definitely associated with acute malaria infection and not merely the result of oxidant antimalarial drugs in patients with erythrocyte enzyme defects such as G6PD deficiency. (This is difficult to ascertain in practice: if the G6PD status is checked following massive haemolysis, the value in the remaining red cells may be normal even in mild G6PD deficiency. This part of the definition is not very useful.)

11. Postmortem confirmation of diagnosis. In fatal cases a diagnosis of severe falciparum malaria can be confirmed by histological examination of a postmortem needle necroscopy of the brain. The characteristic features, found especially in cerebral grey matter, are venules/capillaries packed with erythrocytes containing mature trophozoites and schizonts of *P. falciparum*. (These features may not be present in patients who die several days after the start of treatment, although there is usually some residual pigment in the cerebral vessels.)

The 2000 recommendations also include the following: (see Table 73.4)

12. Impairment of consciousness less marked than unrousable coma. (Any impairment of consciousness must be treated seriously. Assessment using the Glasgow Coma Scale is straightforward, but the Blantyre Scale needs careful local standardization particularly in younger children.)

13. Prostration: Inability to sit unassisted in a child who is normally able to do so. In a child not old enough to sit, this is defined as an inability to feed. This definition is based on examination not history.

14. Hyperparasitaemia – the relation of parasitaemia to severity of illness is different in different populations and age groups, but in general very high parasite densities are associated with increased risk of severe disease, e.g. >4% parasitaemia is dangerous in non-immunes, but may be well tolerated in semi-immune children. In non-immune children studied in Thailand a parasitaemia ≥4% carried a 3% mortality (30 times higher than in all uncomplicated malaria) but in areas of high transmission values much higher may be tolerated well. Many use a threshold definition of 10% parasitaemia in higher transmission settings.

The followings were not considered criteria of severe malaria:

Jaundice – detected clinically or defined by a serum bilirubin concentration >50 μmol/L (3.0 mg/dL). This is only a marker of severe malaria when combined with evidence of other vital organ dysfunction such as coma or renal failure.

Hyperpyrexia – a rectal temperature above 40°C in adults and children is no longer considered a sign of severity.

Table 73.4 Outline classification of severe malaria in children (WHO 2000)

GROUP 1
Children at immediately increased risk of dying who require parenteral antimalarial drugs and supportive therapy
Prostrated children (prostration is the inability to sit upright in a child normally able to do so, or to drink in the case of children too young to sit)
Prostrate but fully conscious
Prostrate with impaired consciousness but not in deep coma
Coma (the inability to localize a painful stimulus)
Respiratory distress (acidotic breathing)
Mild – sustained nasal flaring and/or mild intercostal indrawing (recession)
Severe – the presence of either marked indrawing (recession) of the bony structure of the lower chest wall or deep (acidotic) breathing

GROUP 2
Children who, though able to be treated with oral antimalarial drugs, require supervised management because of the risk of clinical deterioration, but who show none of the features of group 1 (above)
Children with a haemoglobin level <5 g/dL or a haematocrit <15%
Children with two or more convulsions within a 24 h period

GROUP 3
Children who require parenteral treatment because of persistent vomiting but who lack any specific clinical or laboratory features of groups 1 or 2 (above)

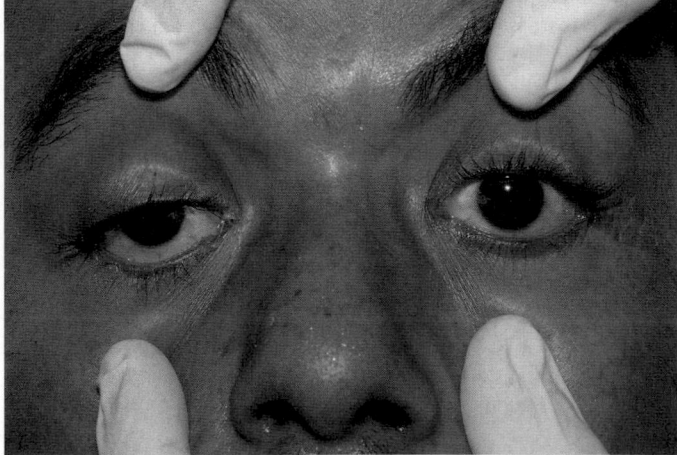

Figure 73.16 Divergent gaze in a 25-year-old Bangladeshi man with cerebral malaria.

Case history

A 2-year-old girl was brought to a large provincial African hospital by her mother in the late afternoon. She had had two generalized convulsions in the morning, and she was unrousable after the first of these. Her mother had noticed she was febrile, drowsy and apathetic and did not eat the previous evening, but before that, she had appeared to be well (although the mother had been working in the fields the previous day, and so could not be exact as to the time when symptoms began). After the first convulsion, the child was taken to a health centre where a presumptive diagnosis of malaria was made, and a single intramuscular injection was given into the buttock before the child was referred on to hospital. In the past, the child had received her immunizations, and had received treatment for malaria in the previous rainy season. She had also had several febrile episodes, which the mother had treated at home with antimalarial drugs and traditional medicines, and these had resolved without complications.

On examination, the child was unrousably comatose with only a non-localized motor response to a painful stimulus (Blantyre coma score 1). She was not anaemic or jaundiced, and she weighed 9 kg. The blood pressure was 85/65 mmHg, the pulse 138/min, and the rectal temperature 40.1°C. The child was not clinically dehydrated. The respiratory rate was 52/min. She was breathing deeply with the use of accessory muscles of respiration, intercostals indrawing, and flaring of the alar nasae. There were coarse breath sounds, particularly over the left lung field. The spleen tip was palpable and the liver 3 cm enlarged. There was some passive resistance to head flexion, but no other evidence of meningeal irritation. On fundoscopy a flame-shaped haemorrhage with a pale centre was visible adjacent to the superior nasal artery in the left eye. The optic discs were flat. The eyes were divergent. Positive findings on examination of the central and peripheral nervous systems were a pout reflex, a symmetrical increase in tone, and extensor plantar responses. Intermittent extensor posturing of the 'decerebrate' type, with extended arms and legs, sustained upward gaze and noisy hyperventilation lasting 10–15 s, occurred every 5 min. Blood was taken and an intravenous infusion of 5% dextrose water was started. A glucose oxidase stick test indicated the blood glucose was only 1.1.mmol/L; 8 mL (0.5 g/kg) of 50% dextrose was given by slow intravenous injection and the infusion was changed to 10% dextrose. There was no improvement in her clinical condition. The haematocrit was read as 36%, the white count was reported as 12 000/μL (no differential was available) and the parasitaemia on brief microscopic examination of the thin film was heavy; a subsequent count gave a value of 136/1000 red cells. In 25% of the parasites, pigment was evident indicating they were mature trophozoites, and 3% were schizonts. Phagocytosed pigment could be seen in 10% of the neutrophils. An infusion of quinine dihydrochloride was started. A loading dose of 160 mg (20 mg salt/kg) was drawn up (as close as possible to 0.53 mL of a 300 mg/mL solution in a 1 mL syringe) and injected into a 120 mL burette (infusion chamber) with 10% dextrose and set to run at 30 mL/h. (The hospital was fortunate to have a stock of paediatric infusion sets but if these had not been available, the quinine could have been given by split i.m. injections to the anterior thighs). A lumbar puncture was performed; the CSF was clear, there was clear CSF with free rise and fall with respiration, and the opening pressure was recorded as 140 mm CSF. The admitting physician was confident in a diagnosis of severe malaria, but was concerned there might also be pneumonia developing so she also started parenteral chloramphenicol succinate 25 mg/kg per 6-hourly, and requested a chest radiograph. Tepid sponging brought the rectal temperature down to 38.3°C. The posturing lessened in intensity and frequency. The vital signs remained stable over the next 4 h and the chest remained clear, but the respiratory rate increased to 60/min. The breathing was deep and noisy. The bed was wet, indicating that urine had been passed. A repeat blood glucose at 4 h was 3.2 mmol/L. At 5 h the blood pressure was 80/50, pulse 150/min, temperature 37.7°C and respiratory rate 62/min. The Blantyre coma score was still 1, and the neurological signs were unchanged. Some 20 minutes later the respiration became ataxic, and then stopped. She could not be resuscitated.

Comment

This child with cerebral malaria had several poor prognostic features on admission to hospital: deep coma, convulsions, extensor posturing, respiratory distress, hyperparasitaemia, a predominance of mature parasites on the peripheral blood smear, pigment in peripheral blood neutrophils and hypoglycaemia. The admitting physician was aware immediately that the outlook was bleak from the combination of coma and respiratory distress. The short history and absence of anaemia together with the high parasite count suggest a fulminant infection. The predominance of mature parasites suggests the possibility of a much greater sequestered parasite biomass than that evident from the peripheral parasitaemia. She was hypoglycaemic and almost certainly had lactic acidosis. Although the child had received an intramuscular injection before referral, the admitting physician could not be sure that it was quinine, and concluded correctly that the benefits of administering a quinine loading dose exceeded the risks of over treatment (note also that the injection had been given into the buttock, which is still sadly very common, despite the risks of significant sciatic nerve injury). Although the best available parenteral antimalarial treatment was started as soon as the diagnosis was made, irreversible pathological processes may already have taken place. As in many fatal cases in children, the exact cause of the final respiratory arrest was not known. The pragmatic decision to start antibiotics (chloramphenicol) as well as quinine illustrates the difficulties in excluding pneumonia or sepsis confidently in severely ill children, and under the circumstances was entirely reasonable. Could this child's life have been saved? If an effective treatment had been given earlier in the course of the illness the answer is almost certainly yes. Community pre-referral treatment with rectal artesunate has been shown to reduce the mortality of severe malaria in children under 5 years, by 25%. In very large studies conducted in Asia, parenteral artesunate reduced the mortality of severe malaria by 35%. Studies in African children comparing parenteral quinine and artesunate are in progress.

Convulsions

Seizures are common, particularly in young children. They are associated with *falciparum* malaria even in uncomplicated infections.[423] In the majority of cases, the child recovers uneventfully following one or two generalized convulsions, but some patients do not recover consciousness rapidly (<30 min) and may remain unrousable (cerebral malaria). In some cases, the cause of the protracted coma is status epilepticus. Focal seizures may also occur, but they are less common. Aspiration pneumonia is a common and preventable sequel to grand mal seizures. Repeated grand mal seizures in cerebral malaria are associated with residual neurological sequelae.

Post-malaria neurological syndromes and deficits

Residual neurological deficit

As severe malaria and seizures associated with malaria are so common in children, the possibility that these cause subtle but significant psychomotor impairment is of tremendous importance to tropical countries.[424] It is becoming increasingly clear that subtle but important neurocognitive deficits may follow recovery from cerebral malaria, particularly in children. The long-term prognosis of these has not yet been established. In approximately 3% of adults and 10–23% of children, there is a clinically obvious persistent neurological deficit following cerebral malaria (Figure 73.17).[425–429] In children, this is associated with profound and protracted coma, anaemia, and prolonged and repeated convulsions. In a retrospective study from Kenya, multiple seizures were associated with persistent motor deficits, malnutrition, hypoglycaemia and seizures with subsequent language deficits, and deep coma with cognitive impairment.[428] In The Gambia hypoglycaemia was not a risk factor for neurological deficit.[429] About 10% of children have demonstrable language deficit following cerebral malaria.[430,431] There is also an increased risk of epilepsy following severe malaria in childhood.[432]

In approximately 60% of severe cases with residual neurological deficit, there is a hemiparesis with variable hemisensory deficit and sometimes hemianopia.[427] Cortical blindness, diffuse cortical damage, tremor and occasionally isolated cranial nerve palsies may occur. Many of the deficits recover rapidly, and by 6 months, only 4% of survivors have obvious neurological abnormality.[427,429]

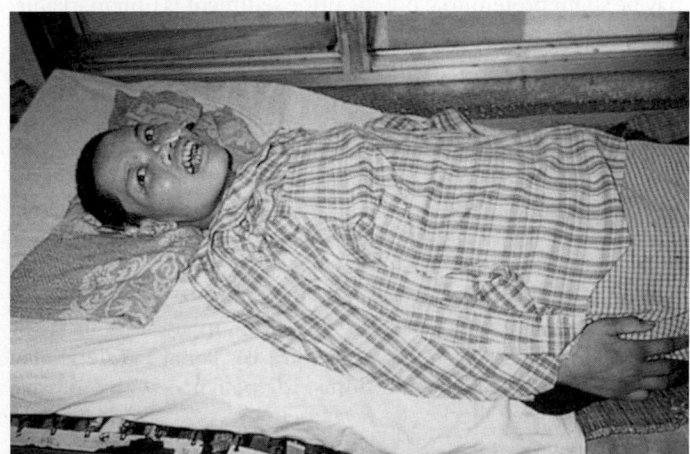

Figure 73.17 Permanent global residual neurological deficit following prolonged hypoglycaemia in a 33-year-old Vietnamese woman who had cerebral malaria in pregnancy. She had received intravenous quinine but, despite parenteral glucose administration, she was repeatedly severely hypoglycaemic.

Relapsing coma

Rarely, patients who recover from cerebral malaria may lapse into coma again, usually after a period of 1–2 days when they are rousable. In this condition, the CSF protein may be elevated (200–300 mg/dL) and there is sometimes an increase in CSF lymphocytes. There may be residual neurological deficit on recovery.

Post-malaria neurological syndromes

A variety of other late neurological complications may occur following recovery from cerebral malaria. These include psychosis, encephalopathy, Parkinsonian rigidity and tremor, a fine tremor and cerebellar dysfunction.[433–436] These post-malaria neurological syndromes (PMNS) may also rarely follow uncomplicated malaria, and could account for some of the cases previously attributed to mefloquine or chloroquine neurotoxicity. However, there appears to be a strong interaction between mefloquine and cerebral malaria, such that 5% of patients who receive mefloquine after severe malaria develop PMNS (a risk 10–50 times higher than following mefloquine treatment of uncomplicated malaria).[434] Mefloquine should not be used following cerebral malaria. The conditions are self-limiting, but very distressing, and usually resolve over several days, or sometimes 1–2 weeks. The syndrome of cerebellar ataxia occurring 2–3 weeks after acute uncomplicated malaria appears to be relatively common in Sri Lanka.[435] It too is usually self-limiting with recovery over a few weeks.

Acute renal failure

In some adult patients with severe malaria acute oliguric renal failure and other vital organ dysfunction is present on admission, whereas in others renal dysfunction becomes evident as the patient recovers from the acute phase of severe disease.[240,437,438] In the former fulminant presentation, there is a high incidence of associated hepatic dysfunction and metabolic acidosis, and pulmonary oedema is the usual terminal event. The blood pressure is normal. Jaundice is common and there may be a bleeding tendency. There may be slight proteinuria, but the urine sediment is unremarkable. The subacute presentation carries a better prognosis. The patient may be oliguric but is rarely anuric. The serum creatinine rises over a period of days until either dialysis is required because of hyperkalaemia or uraemic complications such as bleeding, pleural or pericardial effusions, encephalopathy or intractable vomiting, or there is gradual resolution with an increase in urine output. In the subacute presentation of acute renal failure parasitaemia may have cleared following antimalarial treatment before the patient is referred to hospital.[194] Although acute renal failure is a common complication of malaria in adults living in areas of low or unstable transmission, it is rare in children. Indeed, in high-transmission areas it is almost unheard of. Renal failure is also associated with haemoglobinuria in patients with massive haemolysis[439] (see Blackwater fever, below).

Metabolic acidosis

The main clinical indication of metabolic acidosis is laboured hyperventilation with increased inspiratory effort (often termed respiratory distress) and a clear chest initially on auscultation (Kussmaul's breathing). This usually results from accumulation of organic acids including lactic acid. Ketoacidosis may be present in children.[248,310–318,328] There is a wide anion gap.[328] Hypovolaemia is an important contributor and must be corrected. In areas where aspirin is still used widely salicylate intoxication should be considered.[440] Acidosis may be associated with renal failure in adults, but in the acute infection there is also a metabolic (lactic) acidosis. There may be a temporary worsening of lactic acidosis following grand-mal seizures, but the outlook in persistent acidosis is poor. Although blood pressure and tissue perfusion is usually adequate initially, hypotension commonly ensues.

Blackwater fever

The sinister reputation of blackwater fever derives from the high mortality (20–30%) documented in Europeans and Asians working in colonial Africa in the first half of the twentieth century.[298,439,441] Approximately half of these deaths were caused by renal failure. G.R. Ross,[441] writing from Southern Rhodesia (Zimbabwe), described blackwater fever as 'a disease to blanch the cheek of the bravest', and such was its reputation that magistrates considered it as an excuse for a felony! Today, the mortality is much lower. Indeed the passage of black (coca-cola coloured) or dark-brown-red urine is often not associated with significant renal impairment. Blackwater is usually transient and resolves without complications, but in severe cases renal failure may develop.[298,442] This behaves as acute tubular necrosis. Blackwater results from massive haemolysis. Some patients are G6PD deficient. In some patients, myoglobinuria may also be present. Transfused blood is also rapidly haemolysed. The mortality is highest when blackwater fever is associated with severe malaria and other evidence of vital organ dysfunction. Patients with blackwater fever and severe anaemia often have a slate-grey appearance, and their plasma may be red (haemoglobinaemia).

Acute pulmonary oedema

Hyperventilation or Kussmaul's breathing (respiratory distress) is a poor prognostic sign in malaria.[443] In the tachypnoea associated with high fever, breathing is shallow compared with the ominous laboured hyperventilation associated with metabolic acidosis, pulmonary oedema or bronchopneumonia. Acute pulmonary oedema may develop at any time in severe *falciparum* malaria. It is particularly common in pregnant women, but rare in children. This is one form of the adult respiratory distress syndrome,[246–248,444–446] and in some cases, may be difficult to distinguish clinically from pneumonia. The heart sounds are normal. The central venous pressure and pulmonary artery occlusion pressures are usually normal, the cardiac index is high, and systemic vascular resistance is low. This points to an increase in capillary permeability (unless the patient has been overhydrated). The chest radiograph shows increased interstitial shadowing and a normal heart size.

Hypotension

The majority of patients with severe malaria are febrile, with a high cardiac output, a low systemic vascular resistance, and a low-normal blood pressure. They are usually warm and well perfused. Patients with severe disease may develop sudden hypotension and become shocked. This was called 'algid malaria'.[447,448] In a proportion of cases, there is bacterial septicaemia, but in the majority blood cultures are subsequently negative. In children, poor capillary refill is a valuable prognostic sign.[449] Shock usually responds temporarily to saline infusion and inotropes, but pulmonary oedema may be provoked if too much salt is given and in adults if left-sided filling pressures (pulmonary artery wedge pressures) rise above 15 mmHg. The overall mortality is high. Orthostatic hypotension is common in acute uncomplicated malaria.[450,451] It is associated with impaired reflex cardioacceleration and is worsened by the quinolone antimalarial drugs.[452]

Rarely symmetrical peripheral gangrene can be associated with severe *falciparum* malaria. This does not appear to result from disseminated intravascular coagulation, but the roles of red cell and platelet agglutination and vascular obstruction have not been characterized.

Hypoglycaemia

Hypoglycaemia is either asymptomatic in severely ill patients, or presents as a further deterioration in the level of coma.[374–327,453] It is a sign of poor prognosis. In severe malaria, the usual signs of sweating and increased sympathetic nervous system activity are commonly absent or indistinguishable from the signs of malaria. Hypoglycaemia occurs in approximately 8% of adults and up to 30% of children with cerebral malaria. It is often recurrent. The clinical response to glucose is usually disappointing. In pregnant women with quinine-stimulated hyperinsulinaemic hypoglycaemia, the clinical features of hypoglycaemia are usually evident, and the patient responds dramatically to glucose. Hypoglycaemia can be often prevented by infusion of 10% dextrose but frequent monitoring is still necessary.

Anaemia

The degree of anaemia and the rate at which it develops vary enormously. The haemoglobin concentration may fall by up to 2 g/dL each day. Anaemia is a particular problem in children, where it may lead to sudden death. These complications are particularly likely with haemoglobin concentrations below 5 g/dL (15% haematocrit) and the risk rises steeply below 4 g/dL.[454] Some patients appear to tolerate severe malarial anaemia relatively well. These patients usually have an underlying chronic anaemia, and have adapted to chronic anaemia by right-shifting the oxygen dissociation curve which increases tissue unloading of oxygen. Thus, it is both the absolute haemoglobin concentration and the magnitude of the fall that determine the clinical consequences of anaemia. In the past, a syndrome of malaria-associated anaemic congestive heart failure was often diagnosed, and was managed by fluid restriction, and often very cautious blood transfusion. It is now clear that the majority of these children with severe anaemia, rapid deep breathing and low blood pressure are in fact hypovolaemic and acidotic and need quite the opposite treatment; intravenous rehydration and urgent blood transfusion.[455] Severe anaemia in high transmission settings has traditionally been ascribed to malaria but a recent detailed study from

Malawi (where the prevalence of HIV infection is high and iron deficiency is low) illustrates what a multifactorial problem this is usually. In children presenting with severe anaemia (Hb <5g/dL) bacteraemia, malaria, hookworm, HIV, G6PD deficiency, vitamin A deficiency and vitamin B12 deficiency were all associated with severe anemia whereas folate deficiency, sickle cell disease, and iron deficiency were not.[456]

Persistent fever

Patients with severe malaria may have persistent fever after parasite clearance. Although a proportion of cases have an identifiable chest or urinary tract infection, or in children blood cultures may grow *Salmonella* spp., the majority of cases have no clear explanation and the fever eventually resolves in a few days without further treatment.

LABORATORY FINDINGS

Haematology

There is a progressive normochromic normocytic anaemia. The white count is usually normal, but may be raised in very severe malaria, and very occasionally, there is a leucoerythroblastic picture. There is slight monocytosis, lymphopenia and eosinopenia, with reactive lymphocytosis and eosinophilia in the weeks following the acute infection.[457,458] The platelet count is reduced in all acute malarias, usually to around 100 000/µL, but thrombocytopenia is profound in some cases. Fibrinogen levels are usually elevated – a reduction indicates significant consumption (DIC). The fibrin degradation products are elevated. There is evidence of increased coagulation cascade activity through intrinsic pathway activation with antithrombin III depletion that is proportional to disease severity and there may be prolongation of the prothrombin and partial thromboplastin times. Polymorphonuclear leukocyte elastase levels are elevated in severe infection, suggesting neutrophil activation.[459]

Acute phase proteins

The C-reactive protein, orosomucoid (α_1-acid glycoprotein), procalcitonin and fibrinogen levels are raised, and immunoglobulin levels rise while albumin falls. Cytokine levels are raised in acute malaria; there are increased concentrations of circulating cytokine receptors, and there is an increase in urinary neopterin.

Biochemistry

There may be mild hyponatraemia[460] but the plasma potassium is remarkably normal, unless there is severe acidosis, although it may fall during the recovery phase from severe malaria.[461] The serum bicarbonate is often reduced and the anion gap widens in proportion to the acidosis. In adults, the serum creatinine and blood urea may be raised, with an increased urea to creatinine ratio. Total and conjugated bilirubin are often elevated in adults, the transaminase concentrations are often raised, and there may also be slight elevation of the hepatic alkaline phosphatase concentration. In children, the 5-nucleotidase is raised in proportion to disease severity. Creatinine phosphokinase, myoglobin and plasma urate levels are elevated in adults and children with severe malaria.[462] The serum calcium may be low and hypophosphataemia may be profound in severe infections.[332] Hypoglycaemia may occur, and in the absence of quinine treatment this is accompanied by elevated ketones, raised plasma lactate and alanine, and low insulin levels.[324–326] Lactate levels in arterial or venous blood, or CSF, are elevated and blood bicarbonate is reduced in proportion to disease severity.[463]

Cerebrospinal fluid

The pressures in adults and children are similar, averaging approximately 160 mm CSF. But because the normal range in children is lower (<100 mm) most values in children are elevated.[184] The CSF is usually normal in cerebral malaria, but moderately raised concentrations of protein are common (sometimes up to 200 mg/dL). There may be up to 10 cells/mL, and on occasions up to 50 are seen (usually all lymphocytes). The CSF lactate concentration is raised in cerebral malaria, and the glucose may be slightly low relative to blood. If the patient is deeply jaundiced the CSF may appear yellow.

Prognostic factors

The prognostic factors listed in Table 73.5 reflect vital organ dysfunction and the magnitude of the parasite burden. They are not absolute, and in fatal cases, several factors usually co-exist. Some of the apparently poor prognostic factors can have a benign explanation. Hyperventilation (respiratory distress) is usually a bad sign (indicating metabolic acidosis, pulmonary oedema, or pneumonia), but shallow tachypnoea can result from high fever alone (the tidal volume is lower). Upper gastrointestinal bleeding in cerebral malaria may also occur spontaneously. The prognostic implications of severe anaemia depend on the rate at which the haematocrit falls, the co-existing parasitaemia and metabolic abnormalities (particularly acidosis) and the stage of the infection. If anaemia develops gradually then even haemoglobin values less than 7 g/dL (packed cell volume <20%) can be surprisingly well tolerated as there is time for homeostatic adaptations such as the right shift in the oxygen dissociation curve, the increase in cardiac index and the fall in systemic vascular resistance. Hypotension is a poor prognostic sign only when associated with poor tissue perfusion, as evidenced by cool peripheries and poor capillary refill. Patients, particularly children, with acute malaria often have very low blood pressures but they are warm and well perfused. The biochemical measures are in general proportional to severity, but individual abnormalities can have other explanations. For example, hypoglycaemia carries a five-fold higher mortality in severe malaria, but in pregnant women treated with quinine hypoglycaemia may occur in uncomplicated infections because of quinine-stimulated hyperinsulinaemia. The concentration of lactate in venous or arterial blood or CSF is linearly proportional to the severity of disease. In terms of predictive prognostic value, the admission venous bicarbonate concentration has the best sensitivity and specificity, and it is available

Table 73.5 Laboratory indicators of a poor prognosis in severe malaria

BIOCHEMISTRY	
Hypoglycaemia	<2.2 mmol/L
Hyperlactataemia	>5 mmol/L[a]
Acidosis	Arterial pH < 7.3
	Venous plasma HCO₃ <15 mmol/L[a]
Serum creatinine	>265 µmol/L[b]
Total bilirubin	>50 µmol/L
Liver enzymes	sGOT (AST) >3 upper limit of normal
	sGPT (ALT) >3 upper limit of normal
	5-Nucleotidase ↑
Muscle enzymes	CPK ↑
	Myoglobin ↑
Urate	>600 µmol/L
HAEMATOLOGY	
Leukocytosis	>12 000/µL
	Severe anaemia (PCV <15%)
Coagulopathy	Platelets <50 000/µL[c]
	Prothrombin time prolonged >3 s
	Prolonged partial thromboplastin time
	Fibrinogen: <200 mg/dL
PARASITOLOGY	
Hyperparasitaemia	>100 000/µL – increased mortality[d]
	>500 000/µL – high mortality[d]
>20% of parasites are pigment-containing trophozoites and schizonts	
>5% of neutrophils contain visible malaria pigment	

PCV, packed cell volume; sGOT (AST), serum glutamic oxaloacetic transferase (aspartate aminotransferase); sGPT (ALT), serum glutamic pyruvic transaminase (alanine aminotransferase); CPK, creatine phosphokinase.
[a] Of all the laboratory indicators, measurements of acidosis have the best prognostic value.
[b] This is the criterion for adults. Less elevated values are found in children with severe malaria.
[c] Severe thrombocytopenia is only a poor prognostic sign if associated with other severity indicators.
[d] These refer to thresholds in non-immune adults. The thresholds are much higher in children in endemic areas; the most common threshold of 10% parasitaemia corresponds to approximately 300 000 parasites/µL at a haematocrit of 25%.

widely. Persistent acidosis with low plasma bicarbonate and elevated plasma lactate 4 h after admission indicates a poor prognosis. Although deep jaundice is often a bad sign, some adult patients develop a profound cholestatic jaundice without other evidence of vital organ dysfunction. Parasitaemia has traditionally been used as a measure of severity since the classic studies of Field and colleagues in Kuala Lumpur, Malaysia.[464,465] They observed that *P. falciparum* parasite counts over 100 000/µL were associated with an increased risk of dying, and that the mortality of a count over

Table 73.6 Severe manifestations of *P. falciparum* malaria in adults and children

PROGNOSTIC VALUE[a]			FREQUENCY[a]	
Children	Adults		Children	Adults
CLINICAL MANIFESTATIONS[b]				
+	(?)	Prostration	+++	+++
+++	++	Impaired consciousness	+++	++
+++	+++	Respiratory distress (acidotic breathing)	+++	++
+	++	Multiple convulsions	+++	+
+++	+++	Circulatory collapse	+	+
+++	+++	Pulmonary oedema (radiological)	+/–	+
+++	++	Abnormal bleeding	+/–	+
++	+	Jaundice	+	+++
+	+	Haemoglobinuria	+/–	+
LABORATORY FINDINGS				
+	+	Severe anaemia	+++	+
+++	+++	Hypoglycaemia	+++	++
+++	+++	Acidosis	+++	++
+++	+++	Hyperlactataemia	+++	++
+/–	++	Hyperparasitaemia	++	+
++	++	Renal impairment	+	+++

[a] On a scale from + to +++ ; +/– indicates borderline prognostic value of infrequent occurrence.
[b] Anuria and hypothermia (core temperature <36.5°C) are also poor prognostic signs.

500 000/μL was 50%. The distribution of parasite counts in severe malaria is shifted to higher parasitaemias in children living in areas of intense transmission, compared with non-immune adults. For example, parasite counts over 200 000/μL are not uncommon in ambulant semi-immune children who are mildly ill, whereas parasitaemias in this range are usually associated with severe disease in non-immune adults (Table 73.6). The sensitivity and specificity of parasitaemia alone as a prognostic indicator is limited, but can be improved by staging parasite development (more mature parasites – worse prognosis),[92] and counting the number of polymorphonuclear neutrophil leukocytes which contain pigment (>5% – poorer prognosis).[93,94] For any parasitaemia the prognosis is worse if >20% of parasites contain visible pigment, and better if >50% of parasites are at the tiny ring stage. Recent studies indicate that measurement of *Plasmodium falciparum* Histidine Rich protein2 (*Pf*HRP2) in plasma or serum can be used to estimate the sequestered parasite biomass in severe malaria.[95]

DIAGNOSIS

Malaria is diagnosed by microscopic examination of the blood. It is not a clinical diagnosis. In malaria endemic areas where malaria is the most common cause of fever (e.g. in children under 5 years in high transmission settings), then it is reasonable to treat for malaria if rapid tests or microscopy are not readily available.

Blood smears

Thick and thin blood films are made on clean, grease-free glass slides (Figure 73.18). Having written the patient's name, time and date, the glass slide can be cleaned by breathing on the surface and wiping with a clean cloth. The patient's finger should be cleaned with alcohol, allowed to dry, and then the side of the finger tip (or the dorsum below the nail-bed) should be pricked with a sharp sterile lancet or needle. Two drops of blood are placed at one end of the slide. The thin film is made immediately by placing the *smooth* leading edge of a second (spreader) slide in the central drop of blood, adjusting the angle (less blood – more acute) and, while holding the edges of the slide, smearing the blood with a swift and steady sweep along the surface. If the blood drop is too large, the spreader slide should be dunked in the drop, then 'jumped' to the slide surface carrying a smaller amount of blood – and then smeared. Making good thin films requires some practice. Anaemic blood smears poorly. The thick film should be stirred in a circular motion with the corner of the second slide until clotting takes place. The thick film must be of uneven thickness, but it should be possible to read the hands, but not the figures, of a watch face through the film.

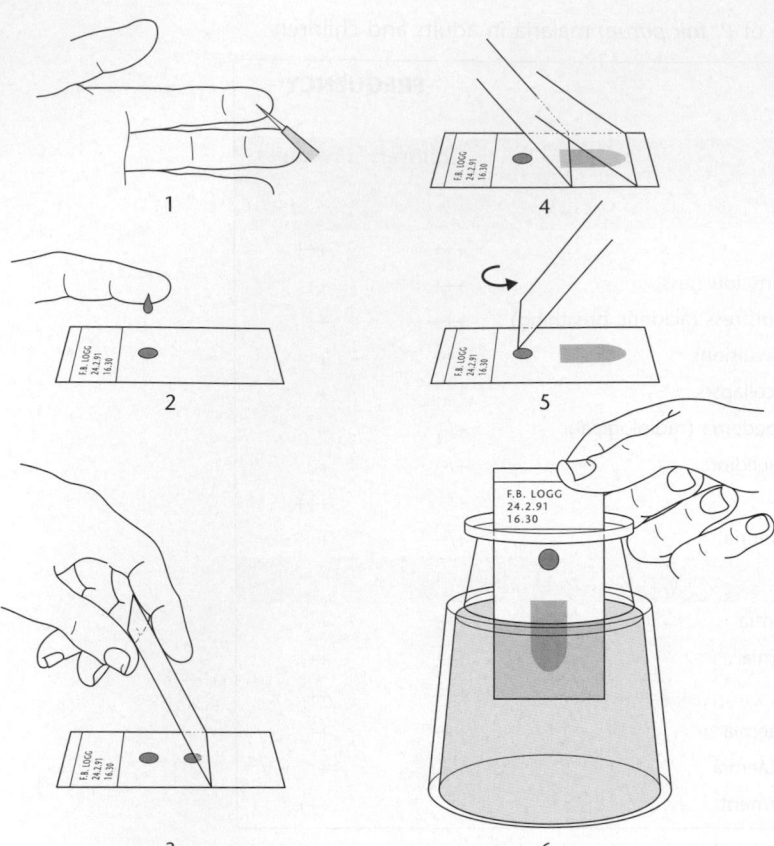

Figure 73.18 Making a peripheral blood smear.

Intradermal smears

Chinese researchers have shown that smears from intradermal blood may contain more mature forms of *P. falciparum* than the peripheral blood.[466] This is considered to allow a more complete assessment of severe malaria. The intradermal smears may also be positive or may show pigment containing leukocytes after the blood smear is negative. In terms of diagnostic sensitivity the intradermal smear is similar to the bone marrow (i.e. slightly more sensitive than peripheral blood). The smears are taken (Figure 73.19) from multiple intradermal punctures with a 25 G needle on the volar surface of the upper forearm. The punctures should not ooze blood spontaneously, but sero-sanguinous fluid can be expressed on to the slide by squeezing.

Staining and reading

The thick film should be dried thoroughly, otherwise it may wash away during staining. Drying may be accelerated by using a hair dryer. The thin film is then fixed by brief immersion in anhydrous methanol (taking care *not* to fix the thick film). Giemsa's stain buffered to a pH of 7.2 makes the best malaria slides, but for optimum results the stain should be left on the slide for 30 min. Field's stain is quicker and almost as good , but the thin and thick films are treated differently.[467] The thin film is immersed in the red stain (Field's B) for 6 s, then gently washed off for 5 s, then immersed in the blue stain (Field's A) for 3–4 s and then gently

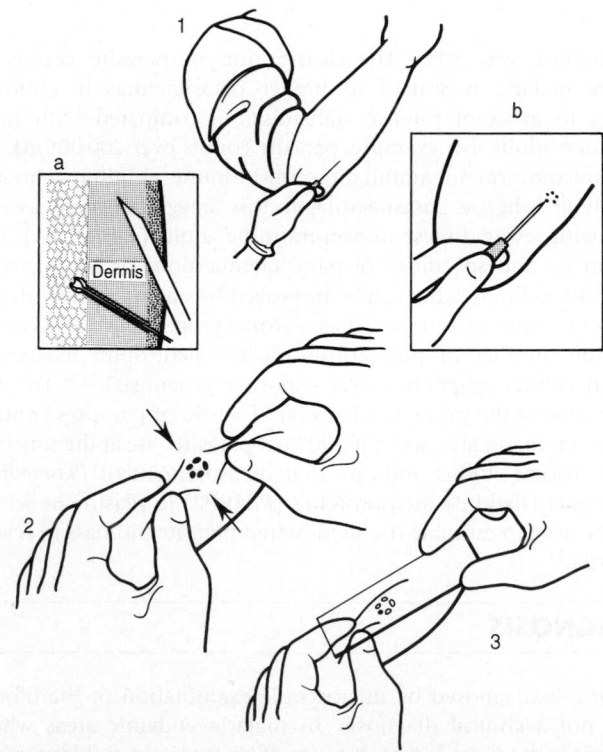

Figure 73.19 Making an intradermal smear.

washed off (5 s). The reverse order applies to the thick film: the slide is first immersed in the blue stain (Field's A) for 5 s, then gently washed off (5 s) then the red stain (Field's B) for 5 s, then gently washed off (5 s). Slides should be dried in a slide rack before examining under oil immersion at a magnification of ×1000.

Best results are obtained with fresh filtered stains and anhydrous methanol for fixing the thin film. Repeatedly reusing stains, which are full of precipitates, particles, and microorganisms, with methanol left in an open jar to absorb atmospheric water, and a poorly maintained fungus infected microscope (very familiar to all of us who work in the tropics) makes accurate parasite speciation and counting a lot more difficult.

Before going to oil immersion on the microsope (×1000 magnification), the slide should be scanned briefly under low magnification to identify the best area for detailed examination. For the thin film, the tail of the film should be examined; for the thick film, the area of optimum thickness and staining and least artefact is chosen. The thick film is approximately 30 times more sensitive than the thin film, although sensitivity and specificity depend to a great extent on the experience of the microscopist, the quality of the slides, stains and microscope, and the time spent examining the slide. Artefacts are common and often confusing. Speciation of malaria at the trophozoite stage is easier on the thin film, although gametocytes and schizonts are more likely to be seen on the thick film. The thin film is more accurate for parasite counting. The number of parasitized red cells per 1000 red cells should be counted. If there are two parasites in one red cell, this is counted

as one. At low parasitaemias (<5/1000 on the thin film) the thick film should be counted; the number of parasites per 200, or preferably 500 white cells is noted. These figures can then be corrected by the total red cell and white cell counts to give the number of parasites per unit blood volume (μL). If the white count is not available then the count is assumed to be 8000 μL. An alternative is to count all parasites in a fixed volume of blood. In severe malaria parasitaemias are usually high, and the stage of parasite development should be assessed on the thin film. The proportion of asexual parasites containing visible pigment (i.e. mature trophozoites and schizonts) should be counted. The presence of pigment in neutrophils and monocytes should also be noted and counted. In patients who have already received antimalarial treatment, pigment may still be present in leukocytes after clearance of parasitaemia, and this is an important clue to the diagnosis. Monocytes containing pigment are cleared more slowly than pigment containing neutrophils. The morphological characteristics of human malaria parasites are given in Table 73.7.

Rapid diagnostic tests

The introduction of simple, rapid, sensitive, highly specific, and increasingly affordable dipstick or card tests for the diagnosis of malaria has been a major advance in recent years. These are based on antibody detection of malaria specific antigens in blood samples; currently histidine rich protein 2 (*Pf*IRP2), parasite lactate dehydrogenase (which is antigenically distinct from the

Table 73.7 Morphological characteristics of human malaria parasites

	P. falciparum	*P. vivax*	*P. ovale*	*P. malariae*
Asexual parasites	Usually only ring forms seen. Fine blue cytoplasm oval, circular, comma-shaped or occasionally squeezed to the edge of the cell (appliqué form). One or two chromatin dots. Parasitaemia may exceed 2%	Irregular large fairly thick rings becoming very pleomorphic as the parasite matures. One chromatin dot	Regular dense ring enlarges to compact blue mature trophozoite. One chromatin dot	Dense thick rings, maturing to dense round trophozoites or rectangular or band-form trophozoites. Pigment associated with rings and trophozoites. Large red chromatin dot or band. Low parasitaemia usual
Meronts (Schizonts)	Rare in peripheral blood. 8–32 merozoites, dark brown-black pigment	Common. 12–18 merozoites, orange brown pigment	8–14 merozoites, brown pigment	8–10 merozoites, black pigment
Gametocytes	Banana-shaped. Male: light blue. Female: darker blue. Red-black nucleus with few scattered blue-black pigment granules in cytoplasm	Round or oval. Male: round, pale blue. Female: oval, dark blue. Triangular nucleus, few orange pigment granules	Large round dense blue like *P. malariae*, but prominent James' dots. Brown pigment	Large oval-shaped. Male: pale blue. Female: dense blue. Large black pigment granules
Red cell changes	Normal size. As parasite matures cytoplasm becomes pale, the cells become crenated, and a few small red dots appear over the cytoplasm (Maurer's clefts)	Enlarged. Pale red Schüffner's dots increase in number as parasite matures	Cells become oval with tufted ends. Prominent James' dots	Normal size and shape. No red dots

Note: Multiple invasion is often quoted as a feature of falciparum malaria. This is simply a function of higher parasite densities: at any given density, multiple invasion is over three times more frequent with *P. vivax* compared with *P. falciparum*. The simian parasite *P. knowlesi*, which is an important cause of human malaria in parts of South-east Asia, resembles *P. falciparum* at the ring stage, and *P. malariae* at the trophozoite stage.

host enzyme), and aldolase. Current *Pf*HRP2 and *Pf*LDH tests, based on colour reactions, provide a diagnostic sensitivity for *P. falciparum* similar to trained microscopists.[468–471] Recently, specific tests for *P. vivax* have been developed. Many tests also include 'pan-malaria' antibody which detects all malaria species. The cards or sticks then carry two band colour reactions plus a control (which should be positive). Thus a positive test with these two bands, with a negative in the *Plasmodium falciparum* test, signifies one of the other malaria species is causing the infection (and therefore, chloroquine rather than another antimalarial drug is required). This part of the test usually is less sensitive than good microscopy. The *P. falciparum* antigen detection tests may remain positive in patients with persistent gametocytaemia.[470] There are now many different tests from many different manufacturers, based on several different antibodies, and considerable variability between them in performance characteristics. Most available tests are based on *Pf*HRP2. These tests are the least expensive, simplest to perform, and the most robust under tropical conditions.[471,472] Variability in the diagnostic sensitivity of *Pf*HRP2 based tests also results from sequence diversity in the gene encoding *Pf*HRP2 and consequent variability in the number of antigenic repeats.

*Pf*HRP2 tests detect only *falciparum* malaria, and because *Pf*HRP2 is cleared very slowly from the blood, may remain positive for up to 1 month after the acute infection, particularly if the parasitaemia was high.[473] This is a disadvantage in areas where transmission is high, and infections frequent, but is very useful in the diagnosis of severely ill patients who have received previous antimalarial treatment. Their parasitaemia may have cleared but the *Pf*HRP2 test will remain strongly positive. In contrast, *Pf*LDH is cleared rapidly from blood, and so the test becomes negative within days of treatment. *Pf*HRP2 is present in parasitized erythrocytes but it is also secreted into plasma, and plasma concentrations (which can be assessed semi-quantitatively from the intensity of the colour reaction) are a guide to the parasite biomass and thus severity.[474] The *Pf*HRP2 test has proved useful in detecting mixed *P. falciparum* and *P. vivax* infections where the former was not evident microscopically.[388] False-positive tests may occur in patients with high concentrations of rheumatoid factor,[475] and false negatives have been reported in patients whose parasites have a rare antigenically variant form of *Pf*HRP2.

Other techniques

Unlike mature red cells, malaria parasites contain DNA and RNA. This can be stained with fluorescent dyes and visualized under ultraviolet light microscopy, or, with appropriate filters, seen under ordinary light. In the QBC™ technique blood samples are taken into a specialized capillary tube containing acridine orange stain and a float. Under high centrifugal forces (14 000 g) the infected erythrocytes, which have a higher buoyant density than uninfected cells, become concentrated around the float. Using a modified lens adaptor (Paralens™) with its own light source, the acridine orange fluorescence from malaria parasites can be visualized through an ordinary microscope.[476] In some series this system has proved more sensitive than conventional light microscopy, although it does not give parasite counts or speciation with accuracy, and it is relatively expensive. It is useful for screening large numbers of blood samples rapidly. DNA probes have also been developed for malaria diagnosis, but their utility outside epidemiological surveys is uncertain. Detection of malaria antibody can be useful in some circumstances, such as confirmation of earlier infection, but has no place in acute diagnosis.

Postmortem diagnosis

The diagnosis of cerebral malaria postmortem can be confirmed from a brain smear. A needle aspirate or biopsy is obtained through the superior orbital foramen or the foramen magnum. A smear of grey matter is examined after staining the slide in the same way as for a thin blood film.[174,477] Capillaries and venules are identified microscopically under low power, and examined under high power. If the patient died in the acute stage of cerebral malaria, the vessels are packed with erythrocytes containing mature parasites and a large amount of pigment.

THE ANTIMALARIAL DRUGS

History

Extracts of the plant huang hua hao (also often termed qinghao; *Artemesia annua*), known as qinghaosu, have been used in traditional medical practice in China for over two millenia. In 340AD, Ge Hong described use of qinghao infusions for the treatment of fever in the famous *Handbook of Emergency Treatments*. Thereafter qinghao is mentioned frequently in the Chinese materia medica as a treatment for agues. Antimalarial drug discovery has often been linked to war. With the growing conflict in Vietnam in the 1960s, Ho Chi Minh asked Zhou En Lai for assistance in combating malaria threatening his troops. Chinese scientists examined both synthetic and traditional medicine treatments. The antimalarial properties of qinghaosu were rediscovered in 1971 when low temperature ethyl-ether extracts of the plant were shown to have activity against experimental rodent malaria.[478] On the other side of the world, another medicinal plant came to medical attention during the reign of the Count of Cinchon as Viceroy of Peru between 1628 and 1629 (Figure 73.20). Legend has it that the Viceroy's wife, the Countess, was afflicted by ague in Lima. She was a well known and popular figure and news of her illness spread inland. It eventually reached Lloxa where a Spaniard was in governorship. He knew of a local remedy obtained from the bark of a tree and sent it to the ailing Countess. The therapeutic result was excellent; she improved rapidly, and was so impressed that she ordered the bark in quantity and dispensed it to the poor of Lima who commonly suffered from the dangerous tertian fevers. The pulverized bark became known as 'los polvos de la Condeca' or the Countess's powder, and Linnaeus subsequently named the tree from which the bark was obtained 'Cinchona' in honour of the Countess. Sadly, the detective work of one A.W. Haggis, reported in 1941,[479] has shown that 'the fabulous story of the Countess of Cinchon' is almost certainly a romantic fable. Nevertheless, it is likely that the bark was introduced to Europe by the Fathers of the Society of Jesus around the time of the story, or even earlier (c. 1630) and was widely promoted in Europe by the Jesuit Cardinal Juan de Hugo. For these reasons, it became known as Jesuit's bark.[480] Not everyone was convinced by the new remedy, and when in 1653 Archduke Leopold of Austria relapsed

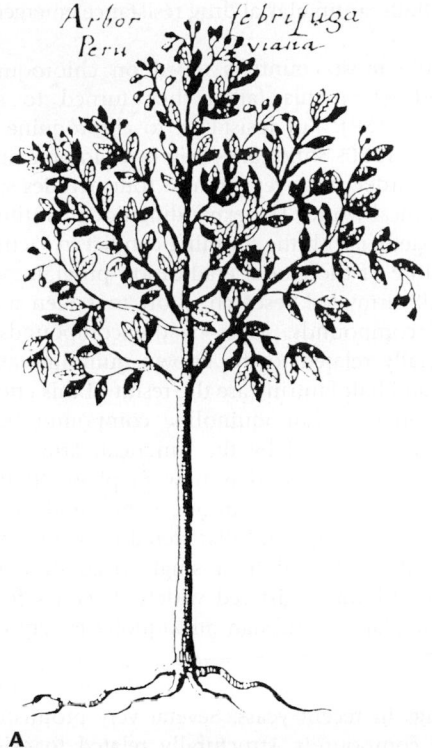

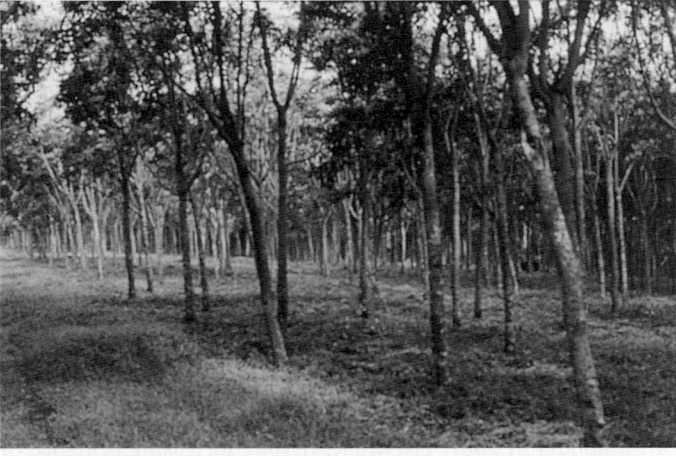

Figure 73.20 (A) The 'Arbor febrifuga Peruviana'. 'In the district of the city of Loja, diocese of Quito, grows a certain kind of large tree, which has a bark like cinnamon, a little more coarse and very bitter: which ground to powder is given to those who have fever, and with only this remedy, it leaves them' (Bernabé Cobo S. J. *Historia del Nuevo Mundo*; 1582–1657). (B) A cinchona plantation in Democratic Republic of Congo.

1 month after being cured of double quartan fever, his personal physician Jean-Jacques Chifflet began a bitter polemic on the merits of the bark which was to last for 200 years. Much of the dispute stemmed from the fact that many considered all fevers had the same cause, and clearly not all responded to Jesuit's bark. It was probably Torti in 1712 who first stated that the bark was 'specific solely for the ague'.

Another source of debate, and one that is still active today, was dosage. Sir Robert Talbor (Talbot) was one of the few physicians who was not afraid to give the bark in large and repeated doses, and when he cured the Dauphin (the son of Louis XIV) with his 'remede anglais' his fame spread far and wide. He subsequently treated Charles II of England successfully with the same medicament. Others were less enthusiastic. Many protestants believed the bark to be a poison disseminated by the Jesuits. The dose–response question was clarified in 1768 by Lind, who demonstrated clearly that in order to get best results the bark should be given in full doses as soon as the disease was diagnosed (advice that has stood the test of time).

In 1820, the French chemists Pierre Pelletier and Joseph Caventou isolated the alkaloid quinine from cinchona bark. Purification of the various cinchona alkaloids allowed standardization of dosage. Adequate doses could now be given in relatively small amounts of pure drug, but by the middle of the nineteenth century enormous doses (up to 100–150 grains over 2 days) were being prescribed. Toxicity was common and the popularity of the medicine declined. Gradually, however, the diagnosis of agues and the prescription of Cinchona alkaloids became more rational and logical. The new colonial powers recognized the importance of Cinchona, and improved methods of horticulture resulted in better yields of the alkaloids from the cultivated trees. The Dutch took the lead and vast plantations of high yielding *Cinchona ledgeriana* were started in the East Indies (principally in Java).[481]

Laveran, having identified haematozoa as the cause of paludism, later concluded that quinine cured the disease by killing the newly discovered parasites. This theory encountered considerable resistance in the years immediately following its publication. In 1880, Bacelli described the intravenous method of administering quinine (although there is evidence that this route had been used for 50 years before that). Laveran considered intravenous injection to be dangerous, giving rise to both local and general complications, and was only justified in 'the most grave and pernicious disease'. He also confirmed the earlier observations of Thomas Willis (1659) that cinchona cured the acute attacks of ague, but did not prevent relapses, and also appeared to have no effect on crescents (gametocytes of *P. falciparum*). The eminent Italian malariologists subsequently showed that quinine prevented asexual blood-stage development but could not stop sporulation of formed segmenters (meronts or schizonts).

In England in 1856, William Henry Perkin fortuitously discovered analine purple (mauve) while attempting to synthesize quinine from coal tar products. Thus began the synthetic dye industry. Later in Germany, the antimicrobial properties of those newly discovered aniline dyes were investigated. In 1890, Ehrlich showed that methylene blue had antimalarial activity against *P. cathemerium* in canaries, but the dye proved disappointing in clinical practice, and structural modifications did not lead to compounds with improved activity. During the Great War (1914–1918) whole armies were immobilized in the Balkans because of malaria, and there were heavy losses in Mesopotamia, East Africa and the Jordan Valley. The British and French armies used quinine extensively, and, despite frequent objections to the bitter medicament, many lives were saved. The military and strategic importance of antimalarial drugs stimulated much research immediately after the war.[482] In the early 1920s, the resurgent German chemical industry again focused its attention on new antimicrobial compounds. The first synthetic antimalarial was discovered in 1926. This was an aminoquinoline compound, pamaquine, also known as plasmoquine or plasmochin, a forerunner of the 8-aminoquinoline primaquine. Pamaquine was followed by the acridine compound mepacrine (quinacrine) in 1932, and the structurally related 4-aminoquinoline, chloroquine, in 1934. Initially chloroquine was rejected as being too toxic for human use, and the research team at Bayer were asked to produce a safer compound. They then produced 3-methylchloroquine (Sontoquine) but, despite clinical studies, these compounds were generally unavailable at the outbreak of World War II.

Armies fighting in tropical theatres of war usually lose more men to malaria than bullets.[482]At the outset of World War II, the Allies knew their position was precarious in the tropics, as most of the world's Cinchona was grown in Java,[483] and this was vulnerable to Japanese invasion. They embarked upon a tremendous combined research effort into the development and evaluation of new antimalarials. In the event, Java did fall to the Japanese, but widespread use of mepacrine (quinacrine) prophylaxis by the Allied soldiers proved highly effective (albeit somewhat toxic) and probably saved the day. Information on chloroquine was, in fact, available to the Allied Powers through pre-war reciprocal arrangements between the pharmaceutical companies, Bayer and Winthrop, but lay buried in documents until the defection of two French soldiers in North Africa in 1943. They brought with them a German antimalarial, later identified as Sontoquine. However, chloroquine was not fully evaluated until the end of the war.[484]

An entirely separate line of research in the UK led to the discovery in 1945 of the antimalarial biguanides, proguanil and subsequently chlorproguanil. These compounds were later shown to inhibit the plasmodial enzyme dihydrofolate reductase (DHFR). Researchers at the Wellcome Research Laboratories synthesizing purine analogues developed the antimitotic compound 6-mercaptopurine (and later azathioprine) and in 1952 discovered the antiprotozoal DHFR inhibitor pyrimethamine. This same line of Nobel Prize winning research later developed trimethoprim, which has considerably greater affinity for bacterial DHFR (but also inhibits the plasmodial enzyme), and also allopurinol, aciclovir and zidovudine (AZT).

By the early 1950s, the 4-aminoquinolines, chloroquine, and to a much lesser extent amodiaquine, had become the treatment of choice for all malaria throughout the world. Pyrimethamine was also used in treatment, and chloroquine, pyrimethamine and proguanil were used for prophylaxis. Primaquine was given to prevent relapses of P. vivax and P. ovale.[485] The Cinchona alkaloids were little used outside francophone Africa and, with the discontinuation of quinine, blackwater fever became a rarity. This was the heyday of the malaria eradication era,[486] and with the tremendous successes in Europe and North America and many urban areas of the tropics, interest in the development of new antimalarial drugs waned rapidly. But eradication in the tropics failed, and in the 1960s, antimalarial drug resistance emerged as a major threat.

Until 2005, most countries relied on chloroquine to treat malaria, and when this failed they turned to sulfadoxine-pyrimethamine (SP). But resistance to chloroquine emerged at the end of the 1950s simultaneously in Colombia and the Thai-Cambodian border and over the next four decades spread across the entire tropical world. The expanding tide of antimalarial drug resistance, together with the looming conflict in Vietnam and the manifest failure of the global eradication programme prompted a massive US army-led research effort to screen and test new antimalarial compounds. Most of the compounds developed were structurally related to the known quinoline antimalarials. Mefloquine and halofantrine are the result of this effort.[487] A new and more potent 8-aminoquinoline compound (tafenoquine) has also been developed by the American army research programme in recent years and is now in phase III trials. In the 1980s, the hydroxynaphthaquinone compound atovaquone (a modification of a compound discovered over 50 years ago) was combined with proguanil in a single fixed dose formulation (Malarone®) and was registered widely. It is a safe and highly effective antimalarial, although atovaquone is very expensive to manufacture.

It is the Chinese who have given us the most important antimalarial drugs in recent years. Several very promising synthetic antimalarial compounds, structurally related to existing drugs, have been produced, evaluated, and deployed. These are lumefantrine (formerly known as benflumetol), pyronaridine, piperaquine and naphthoquine. All are active against multi-drug resistant malaria. By far the most important development in malaria treatment in recent years has been the Chinese rediscovery and development of the drugs related to artemisinin (qinghaosu).[488–494] These drugs are structurally unrelated to existing antimalarials. They are rapidly and reliably effective and remarkably well tolerated and safe. But they were very slow to be adopted. The first countries outside China to deploy the artemisinin antimalarials were Vietnam, Thailand and Cambodia. In the 1990s in this part of South-east Asia, worsening multi-drug resistance in Plasmodium falciparum threatened the prospect of untreatable malaria, but treatment with artemisinin or its derivatives remained highly effective. Artemisinin combination treatments (initially artesunate-mefloquine) were introduced, and were first deployed nationally by Cambodia in 2001. Elsewhere, despite increasing evidence of efficacy and safety, there was initial reluctance to accept these drugs, which were significantly more expensive than the failing chloroquine and SP. Eventually worsening drug resistance in P. falciparum in Africa and the associated rising mortality finally created sufficient pressure on international agencies and donors to stop supporting the inexpensive but increasingly ineffective chloroquine and SP. The evidence in favour of these drugs is now overwhelming. There have been more clinical trials on artemisinin and its derivatives than any other antimalarial drugs. Artemisinin derivatives are used in parenteral or rectal formulations for severe disease and in combination with other antimalarial drugs for uncomplicated malaria. Artemisinin-based combination treatments (ACTs) are better than other antimalarials, and in 2006 were recommended by the World Health Organization antimalarial treatment guidelines as first-line treatment for all falciparum malaria in malaria endemic areas.

Between the 1960s and the 1990s, there was very little research on new antimalarial drugs by the international pharmaceutical industry. In recent years, increased international funding and the formation of public–private partnerships have led to a resurgence of research and development. There is now the 'healthiest' pipeline for developing antimalarials in living memory and over 15 new antimalarials are in various stages of development. The main concern is that most of these work on known targets and therefore may fall to common resistance mechanisms. New drugs for new parasite targets are needed.

Antimalarial drug resistance

In the last two decades of the twentieth century, the global death toll from malaria rose, while the mortality from other infectious diseases (with the notable exception of HIV-AIDS) generally fell. This was attributed directly to drug resistance. *Plasmodium falciparum* had developed resistance to all classes of antimalarial drugs with the general exception of the artemisinin derivatives.[495–500] Reduced in vitro susceptibility to artemether has been reported in French Guyana, but not elsewhere.[501]

The other human malarias are generally more sensitive to antimalarial drugs than *P. falciparum*, although resistance of *P. vivax* to antifols is widespread. Significant chloroquine resistance has now developed in *Plasmodium vivax* in Oceania, the island of New Guinea, parts of Indonesia, and to a lesser degree in several other diverse locations.[502–504] Quinine resistance in *P. falciparum* was first reported from Brazil in 1910,[505] but has never been high grade, and has not compromised use of the drug. Within years of the introduction of the antifols proguanil and pyrimethamine, resistance was noted in both *P. falciparum* and *P. vivax*, which certainly did compromise use of these drugs, but antimalarial resistance was not treated seriously until chloroquine resistance in *P. falciparum* developed almost simultaneously in South-east Asia and South America at the end of the 1950s. The selection of resistance may have resulted from the misguided use of chloroquine (and pyrimethamine) impregnated salt in an attempt to control malaria by mass prophylaxis.[506] During the 1970s chloroquine resistance in *P. falciparum* spread from South-east Asia and South America, and fuelled the resurgence of *falciparum* malaria in the tropics. By the early 1980s, chloroquine was no longer effective in many countries, and the first ominous reports of resistance from the east coast of Africa appeared. Since then chloroquine resistance spread remorselessly across Africa,[507] and today few countries in the tropics (such as those north of the Panama canal) are unaffected. Pyrimethamine resistance has also worsened rapidly, and the synergistic combination with sulphonamides (SP; sulphadoxine-pyrimethamine) is no longer effective in much of East Asia, Southern and Central Africa and South America. The importance of transcontinental spread of resistance in *P. falciparum* has been highlighted by recent molecular epidemiological studies which confirm that both the chloroquine resistance and the SP resistance that have wreaked such havoc in Africa, originated in South-east Asia.[508]

South-east Asia, and in particular the Thai-Cambodian border have traditionally had the world's most drug resistant malaria parasites and events there have acted as harbingers of the development of resistance elsewhere. Chloroquine resistance spread throughout the region in the 1960s and 1970s, and SP fell rapidly to resistance in the early 1980s. In 1984 mefloquine replaced quinine as the treatment of choice for *falciparum* malaria in Thailand. This was the first country in which mefloquine was used widely. It was introduced in combination with sulphadoxine and pyrimethamine in order to delay the onset of resistance. However, since 1988 mefloquine resistance developed rapidly in Thailand[120,508] and adjacent Cambodia and western Burma, and later in Vietnam, while sensitivity to quinine declined very gradually. By 1994, high level mefloquine resistance had developed in some areas with early treatment failures in 10% of cases. On the North-western border of Thailand, the combination of artesunate, given for 3 days, and high dose mefloquine (25 mg/kg) was introduced.[509] Despite the fact that *P. falciparum* there was already mefloquine resistant, this proved remarkably effective. In the subsequent 14 years cure rates have remained over 90%. Following deployment of the ACT there was an improvement of mefloquine sensitivity and[500,510–512] and a marked decline in the incidence of *falciparum* malaria. These results from the Thai-Burmese border, the dramatic declines in malaria mortality associated with artemisinin deployment in Vietnam,[513] and the combination of ACT deployment and improved vector control in KwaZulu Natal[514] led to a global initiative to evaluate antimalarial drug combinations based on the artemisinin derivatives. These combinations have proved safe and effective, and where they have been extensively deployed have usually resulted in a reduction in malaria. It is now widely accepted that ACTs should replace existing monotherapies for the treatment of malaria with the objective of ensuring sustained efficacy and preventing the emergence of resistance to the artemisinin derivatives. As ACTs are now central to all malaria control efforts, their loss to resistance would be a disaster. The recent observations of slow parasite clearance times following artemisinin treatment from the Thai-Cambodian border are therefore very worrying. This may reflect the development of tolerance to this essential class of antimalarial drugs. There is natural concern that antimalarial drug resistance could spread once again from this region.[478]

Antimalarial treatment

In general, the antimalarial drugs are more toxic than antibacterials, i.e. the therapeutic ratio is narrower, but serious adverse effects are rare. The available antimalarials fall into three broad groups: the aryl aminoalcohol (quinoline-related or quinoline-like) compounds (quinine, quinidine, chloroquine, amodiaquine, mefloquine, halofantrine, lumefantrine, piperaquine, pyronaridine, primaquine, tafenoquine); the antifols (pyrimethamine, proguanil, chlorproguanil, trimethoprim); and the artemisinin compounds (artemisinin, dihydroartemisinin, artemether, artemotil, artesunate). Of these, the artemisinin drugs have the broadest time window of action on the asexual malarial parasites, from young rings to early schizonts. This explains why they produce the most rapid therapeutic responses.[515,516] Rapid parasite clearance following artemisinin treatment reflects killing and removal of ring stage parasites. Several antibacterial drugs also have antiplasmodial activity, although in general their action is slow, and they are used in combination with the antimalarial drugs. Those used are the sulphonamides and sulphones, tetracyclines, clindamycin, macrolides, and inadvertently, chloramphenicol. Fosmidomycin is an

Table 73.9 Pharmacokinetic properties of the antimalarial drugs

Drug	ABSORPTION: TIME TO PEAK		Oral dose (mg/kg)	Plasma peak level (mg/L)	Binding (%)	V_d/f (L/kg)	Clearance/f (mL/kg/min)	$T_{1/2}\beta$ (h)	Comments
	p.o.	i.m.							
UNCOMPLICATED MALARIA									
Quinine	6	1–4	10	8	90	0.8	1.5	16	Protein binding increased. V_d and clearance further reduced in severe malaria. Rate of i.m. absorption (and pain!) proportional to concentration of injectate
Quinidine	1	–	10	5	85	1.3	1.7	10	
Chloroquine[a]	5	0.5	10	0.12	55	10–1000	2.0	30–60 days	Concentrated in red cells, white cells and platelets. Multiphasic elimination. Kinetics unaffected by disease severity
Amodiaquine			30					11 days DeAQ	Almost all antimalarial activity after oral administration is provided by the desethyl metabolite (DeAQ)
Piperaquine	6		55	0.15		728	23	28 days	Multiphasic elimination. Children have lower levels than adults at the beginning of the terminal elimination phase.
Mefloquine	17	–	25	–	>98	20	0.35	14 days	Multiphasic elimination. (+)RS enantiomer concentration higher, and (−)SR enantiomer lower, in whole blood than plasma. Interruption of enterohepatic cycling increases clearance
Halofantrine	15	–	8	0.9[b]	>98[c]	–	7.5	113	Metabolized to active desbutyl metabolite which is eliminated more slowly. Absorption increased by fats

Drug								Comments
Lumefantrine[a]	6	9	3.5[b]	>98[c]	2.7	3.0	86	Multiphasic elimination. Very variable bioavailability. Absorption markedly increased by fats
Pyrimethamine[b]	12	1.25	0.5	94	–	0.33	37	Concentrations in 2–5-year-old children significantly lower than in older children and adults
Chlorproguanil	4	–	0.1	75	30	20	35	Mainly a prodrug for active triazine metabolite chlorcycloguanil which is eliminated more rapidly
Atovaquone[a]	6	15	5[b]	99.5	6	2.5	30	Absorption increased by fats. Not metabolised
Artesunate[a]	1.5	4	0.5	–	0.15	50	0.75[a]	Rapidly hydrolysed in the stomach to dihydroartemisinin (DHA). Very little artesunate in blood after oral administration
Artemether[a]	2	3–18	1.5	95	2.7	54	1	Rapidly metabolized to DHA which predominates in plasma
Dihydroartemisinin	4	4	–	70	–	–	1	Absorption very formulation dependent.
HEALTHY SUBJECTS								
Primaquine	3	0.6	0.15	–	3	6	6	Active metabolites – still poorly characterized in relation to biological activity
Proguanil (Chloroguanide)[a]	3	3.5	0.17	75	24	19	16	Mainly a prodrug for active triazine metabolite cycloguanil which is eliminated more rapidly
Pyrimethamine[b]	4	0.3	0.35	–	2.9	0.4	85	–

[a] The pharmacokinetic properties of chloroquine, lumefantrine, sulphadoxine, artemether, artesunate, atovaquone, proguanil and presumably chlorproguanil in late pregnancy are significantly altered so that plasma concentrations are approximately half this in non-pregnant adults.

[b] Pyrimethamine and sulfadoxine plasma concentrations in young children aged 2–5 are approximately half those in older children and adults for the same administered dose.

phylaxis cumulative doses over 100 g (>5 years prophylaxis) are associated with an increased risk of retinopathy.[617] Retinal signs include a pale optic disc, arteriolar narrowing, peripheral retinal depigmentation, macular oedema, retinal granularity and oedema, and retinal pigmentary changes consisting of a circle of pigmentation and central pallor; the so called 'doughnut' or 'bull's eye' macula. Reversible corneal opacities can be seen in 30–70% of rheumatology patients within a few weeks of high dose treatment. Half are asymptomatic but others may complain of photophobia, visual halos around lights, and blurred vision. Residents on long-term chloroquine prophylaxis should probably have regular ophthalmological checks after taking the drug for 5 years, or if they experience any visual loss.[618] Myopathy is rare at the doses used in antimalarial prophylaxis. Less common cutaneous side-effects include lightening of skin colour, various rashes (photoallergic dermatitis, exacerbation of psoriasis, bullous pemphigoid, exfoliative dermatitis, pustular rash), skin depigmentation (with long-term use), and hair loss.[615] Parenteral chloroquine may cause hypotension if administered too rapidly or a large dose (>3.5 mg base/kg) is given by intramuscular or subcutaneous injection. In self-poisoning, chloroquine produces hypotension, arrhythmias, and coma, and is commonly lethal.[619] It has been suggested that diazepam is a specific antidote, but recent studies do not support a specific role for this drug above good haemodynamic and ventilatory support.[620]

Use

Chloroquine is still the drug of choice for sensitive malaria parasites. It is therefore used widely for *P. vivax*, *P. malariae* and *P. ovale*, and it is effective in *P.knowlesi* infections, but except in a very few areas, it has been replaced for *P. falciparum* treatment. The time-honoured oral chloroquine regimen of 25 mg base/kg spread over 3 days (10, 10, 5 or 10, 5, 5, 5 mg/kg at 24-h intervals) can be condensed into 36 h of drug administration.[621] The role of parental chloroquine has diminished considerably because of widespread resistance. Intravenous chloroquine should only be used if the infusion rate can be monitored carefully, otherwise intramuscular or subcutaneous administration is safer. Chloroquine is considered safe in pregnancy and in young children.

Amodiaquine

Amodiaquine is a 'Mannich base' 4-aminoquinoline with a similar mode of action to chloroquine. It is more active against resistant isolates of *P. falciparum*, and is combined with artesunate as an ACT. Amodiaquine is still effective against *falciparum* malaria in parts of South America, Western and Central Africa, and a few parts of Asia, but resistance is increasing. Despite being used for nearly 60 years, there is still little information on the pharmacology of amodiaquine. The newly developed fixed dose co-formulation is given as artesunate-amodiaquine 4/10 mg/kg daily for 3 days.

Pharmacokinetics

Oral amodiaquine undergoes extensive first-pass metabolism by intestinal and hepatic CYP 2C8 to the biologically active metabolite desethylamodiaquine.[622–624] This enzyme is polymorphic, and

is inhibited by several antiretroviral drugs, which suggests that there might be significant drug interactions.[625,626] The metabolite exerts the principal antimalarial activity. The parent compound has an elimination half-life of approximately 10 h[623] but, desethylamodiaquine, like chloroquine is extensively distributed, and eliminated slowly with an estimated terminal half-life of about 11 days.[627] There are no parenteral formulations commercially available, although a structurally similar compound, amopyraquine, is available for intramuscular administration in some countries.

Toxicity

Prophylactic use of amodiaquine is associated with an unacceptably high incidence of serious toxicity. Approximately 1 in 2000 people taking the drug regularly for prophylaxis develop agranulocytosis.[628] Serious hepatotoxicity also occurred at an estimated rate of 1 : 15 000. Agranulocytosis results from bioactivation to a reactive quinoneimine metabolite.[629] Simple modifications to the chemical structure prevent formation of this metabolite and, in theory, produce a much safer compound.[630] The incidence of these serious reactions is lower when amodiaquine is used in treatment, although precise estimates of the risk are still lacking.[630] Data on amodiaquine related side-effects are still few by comparison with other widely used antimalarials. Unusual fatigue has been prominent in some series. Case reports in the literature have documented rare neurological problems such as protruding tongue, intention tremor, excess salivation, and dysarthria in four African patients following amodiaquine treatment.[631] In two patients, these signs occurred on re-exposure to the drug. There is one case report of amodiaquine use over 1 year resulting in yellow pigmentation of skin and mucosae, the development of corneal and conjunctival inclusion bodies, and retinopathy. Minor adverse effects are similar to those of chloroquine, although pruritus is less of a problem, and although it still has an unpleasant taste, children find the drug more palatable. Upper gastrointestinal adverse effects are relatively commonly reported.

Mepacrine (quinacrine)

Mepacrine is structurally similar to chloroquine. It has the same side chain, but is an acridine instead of a quinoline. It is more toxic and less effective than chloroquine. It should not be used as an antimalarial.

Mefloquine

Mefloquine is a fluorinated 4-quinoline methanol compound used for the treatment of multi-drug resistant *falciparum* malaria. It has two asymmetric carbon atoms and is used clinically as a 50:50 racemic mixture of the erythroisomers. These have equal antimalarial activity but very different pharmacokinetic properties.[632–635] The parasiticidal action is similar to that of quinine. Mefloquine is very insoluble in water. It is available as tablets, which should be kept dry. There are no parenteral or paediatric liquid formulations. A fixed dose co-formulation with artesunate in a 2:1 ratio has just been developed.[632] Mefloquine has been combined with pyrimethamine and sulphadoxine, but this combination preparation offers no advantage over mefloquine alone, and carries the potential for severe sulphonamide toxicity.

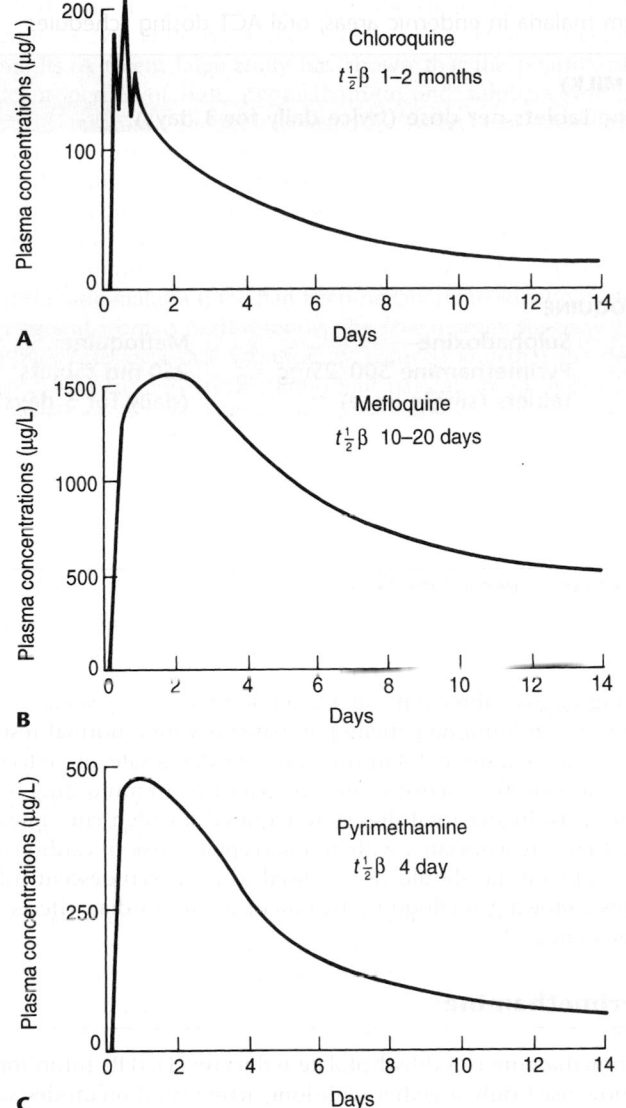

Figure 73.27 Plasma concentration time profiles following treatment doses of (A) chloroquine, (B) mefloquine, and (C) pyrimethamine.

Pharmacokinetics

Mefloquine is moderately well absorbed, extensively distributed, and slowly eliminated.[633–641] It is highly (>98%) bound to plasma proteins. Mefloquine is cleared principally by hepatic biotransformation to inactive metabolites. The apparent volume of distribution and clearance of the (+)RS enantiomer is four to six times higher than for the (−)SR enantiomer.[635,636] The overall terminal elimination half-life is approximately 3 weeks in healthy subjects and 2 weeks in malaria (Figure 73.27). The absorption of mefloquine is reduced in the acute phase of illness and bioavailability of the higher 25 mg/kg dose is improved by dividing it (e.g. giving 15 mg/kg initially and 10 mg/kg 8–24 h later, or 8 mg/kg per day for 3 days) or in combination with artesunate, by delaying mefloquine administration until the second day of treatment.[639,640] Splitting the dose also reduces the incidence of acute adverse effects.[632,641] Blood concentrations are higher in malaria than in healthy subjects and are reduced in diarrhoea (probably by interruption of enterohepatic recycling). Mefloquine clearance is increased in pregnancy.[642] The pharmacokinetics in adults and children are similar.[637] Co-administration with artesunate results in a more rapid recovery from malaria which enhances the oral bioavailability of the second (and third) doses. Although blood concentrations are higher with split dosing, early vomiting is reduced. The new fixed dose co-formulation is given as artesunate-mefloquine 4/8 mg/kg daily for 3 days (Table 73.11).

Toxicity

Nausea, vomiting, dizziness, weakness, sleep disturbances and dysphoria are relatively common with mefloquine.[615,643] Although children are more likely to vomit immediately after receiving mefloquine, and this was a significant problem when the drug was used alone, they otherwise tolerate the drug better than adults.[615,643–645] Women, in particular, commonly complain of dizziness and dysphoria for up to 4 days after receiving mefloquine treatment.[646] Mefloquine exacerbates malarial orthostatic hypotension. The main serious adverse effect of mefloquine is the development of acute but self-limiting neuropsychiatric reactions (convulsions, psychosis, encephalopathy).[647] The incidence of these is approximately 1:10000 when it is used as a prophylactic, but is higher with treatment (1:1000 in Asian patients, 1:200 in Caucasians or Africans) and 1:20 following severe malaria.[648–652] For these reasons, mefloquine should not be given following severe malaria. In one large study from Thailand, mefloquine treatment in pregnancy was associated with a four-fold increased risk of still-birth, although this effect was not seen in women exposed before conception (who would have had residual drug levels during early fetal organogenesis).[653] This effect was not seen in the other large study experience with mefloquine in pregnancy in Malawi.[654]

Use

Mefloquine is used for the oral treatment of uncomplicated multidrug resistant *falciparum* malaria. It is given in combination with artesunate 4 mg/kg per day for 3 days. The usual dose is 25 mg base/kg and should be split (15 mg/kg stat. followed by 10 mg/kg 8–24 h later, or preferably given in a fixed dose combination at 8 mg/kg per day for 3 days).[655] A single dose of 15 mg base/kg alone was widely used in semi-immune patients, but there is theoretical evidence that this leads more rapidly to resistance,[656] and it is no longer recommended.[657] If the patient vomits, the dose should be repeated (full dose if vomiting within 30 min, half dose 30–60 min, no further dose if after 1 h). Mefloquine is used for antimalarial prophylaxis at a dose of approximately 4 mg base/kg once weekly for both adults and children.

Halofantrine

Halofantrine is a 9-phenanthrene methanol. It has one asymmetric carbon atom and is used as a racemate. The enantiomers have equal antimalarial activity. Halofantrine is intrinsically more potent than quinine or mefloquine but, unfortunately, it is associated with rare but potentially lethal ventricular tachycardias which have rightly curtailed its use. It is available as tablets and a suspen-

concern is haemolysis and methaemoglobinaemia, and thus anaemia. Rare idiosyncratic reactions of sulphones (like sulphonamides) include leucopenia and agranulocytosis, cutaneous eruptions, peripheral neuropathy, psychosis, toxic hepatitis, cholestatic jaundice, nephrotic syndrome, renal papillary necrosis, severe hypoalbuminemia without proteinuria, an infectious mononucleosis-like syndrome, and minor neurological and gastrointestinal complaints.

Use

Proguanil has been used as a prophylactic taken once daily (3 mg/kg), often in combination with chloroquine. Chlorproguanil was available for many years for prophylactic use, but it is now available only in a fixed combination with dapsone as a treatment of uncomplicated chloroquine-resistant *falciparum* malaria.[686] The triple combination with artesunate was developed, but not deployed because of dapsone safety concerns (principally anaemia in G6PD deficient patients). Proguanil-dapsone and chlorproguanil-dapsone are both more active than SP against resistant *P. falciparum*, particularly the triple *DHFR* mutants currently prevalent in East Africa.[686–690] The treatment doses of proguanil used are 5–8 mg/kg per day (in combination with atovaquone), and for chlorproguanil 2 mg/kg per day is used in combination with dapsone 2.5 mg/kg. As both chlorproguanil and dapsone are eliminated more rapidly than pyrimethamine and sulphadoxine, use of this combination also provides less selective pressure for the emergence of resistance.[570,688]

Atovaquone-proguanil

This is a highly active antimalarial drug, a hydroxynaphthaquinone unlike other antimalarial drugs. Atovaquone is active even against multi-drug resistant *falciparum* malaria. The speed of therapeutic reponse is similar to that with mefloquine, and slower than that with artemisinin derivatives. Originally atovaquone alone was developed, but high level resistance developed in approximately 30% of treated patients.[691] This suggested that the point mutations in *cyt b*, which conferred resistance, emerged at an approximate frequency of 1 in 10^{12} parasites.[565,568] The fixed combination with proguanil proved much more effective, producing cure rates of nearly 100%, and emergence of resistance in less than 1:500 treated patients.[692–694] It is this combined formulation (Malarone®), which is now registered both for prophylaxis and treatment use in many countries. Nevertheless, it must be considered vulnerable, and for treatment use in endemic areas should be combined with an artemisinin derivative. This creates a highly effective and well tolerated artemisinin-based combination treatment.[694] Interestingly it is the parent compound proguanil which is the important contributor to antimalarial efficacy, as atovaquone-proguanil is equally effective against highly antifol resistant parasites, and also in individuals unable to convert proguanil to cycloguanil. Unfortunately, the very high cost of atovaquone synthesis makes this drug largely unaffordable in tropical countries.

Pharmacokinetics

Atovaquone is similar to halofantrine and lumefantrine in that oral absorption is augmented considerably by fats. Elimination is slower in patients of African origin ($T_{1/2}$ 70 h)[695] than in Oriental patients ($T_{1/2}$ 30 h). There are no significant interactions with proguanil or artesunate. Concentrations of both components were reduced by almost one half in late pregnancy (Table 73.9).[696]

Toxicity

The combination is really very well tolerated. Atovaquone-proguanil may cause vomiting in some patients. The adverse effects otherwise are similar to those of proguanil.

Use

Atovaquone-proguanil is becoming established as a safe, effective and expensive antimalarial prophylactic for travellers – as it is effective everywhere.[697] The adult prophylactic dose is 1 tablet (atovaquone 250 mg proguanil 100 mg) daily with food. It can be discontinued shortly after leaving the malaria transmission area. The treatment dose is 15–20/ 6–8 mg/kg per day for 3 days, which corresponds to an adult dose of 4 tablets/day. It is equally efficacious and well tolerated in young children.[698] The triple combination with artesunate is well tolerated and highly effective against multi-drug resistant *falciparum* malaria, and should be given if this drug is used in endemic areas. Artesunate-atovaquone-proguanil has been evaluated in pregnant women failing other treatments. It was well tolerated and effective, although plasma levels of all components were reduced, suggesting that a higher dose would be needed.[696,699,700] The high cost has been a major barrier to its use, and its use in treatment is confined almost exclusively to imported malaria in temperate countries.

Primaquine

Primaquine is an 8-aminoquinoline used mainly for its actions against the hypnozoites of *P. vivax* (to prevent relapse) and the gametocytes of *P. falciparum* (to prevent transmission).[701] Primaquine has significant liver stage activity against all the malarias (which accounts for its prophylactic efficacy) and it also has significant activity against asexual stage parasites of *P. vivax*, *P. malariae*, and *P. ovale*. Thus, the radical treatment of *vivax* and *ovale* in infections, where primaquine is combined usually with chloroquine, is a combination treatment which should provide mutual protection against resistance.

Pharmacokinetics

Primaquine is well absorbed after oral administration. It is cleared by hepatic biotransformation to the more polar metabolite carboxyprimaquine and several other metabolites with an elimination half-life of 8 h.[702–704] It is not known whether primaquine itself or one of its metabolites is responsible for the action against *P. vivax* hypnozoites (Table 73.9).

Toxicity

Nausea, headache, vomiting and abdominal pain or cramps are relatively common, particularly if higher doses (>30 mg) are taken on an empty stomach. Taking primaquine with food considerably improves tolerability. At an adult dose of 15 mg mild abdominal pain was reported in 3% of US Servicemen, and 22.5 mg produced abdominal symptoms in 12% which required treatment in 3%. Mild diarrhoea, chest pain, weakness, visual disturbances and pruritus occur occasionally. Significant methaemoglobinaemia (>10%), such that the patient appears cyanosed, occurs in less than 10% of adult patients receiving <22.5 mg day. The principal toxicity of primaquine is oxidant haemolysis.[705–707] This may result from oxidant species induced by the phenolic metabolite 5-hydroxyprimaquine. This is the most serious side-effect in individuals with glucose 6 phosphate dehydrogenasey (G6PD) deficiency, other enzyme deficiencies (e.g. glutathione synthetase) that counter oxidant stress, and several haemoglobinopathies (e.g. Hb Zurich, Hb Torino). Although first recognized in the 1920s with pamaquine, it was not until the early 1950s and the introduction of primaquine that haemolysis was noted as a significant problem among American soldiers of African descent. At that time, the cause of haemolysis was unknown and was labelled 'primaquine sensitivity'.[708] This led to the discovery of the sex-linked G6PD deficiency. The severity of haemolysis is related to the degree of G6PD deficiency and the primaquine dose. There are a large number of different G6PD genotypes. There is insufficient information on the relationship between genotype, red cell G6PD concentrations, and haemolytic tendency with primaquine. In general haemolysis is less severe in the common African (A⁻) form. In such patients, haemolysis tends to be self-limiting but in some of the Asian variants (e.g. Canton variant) and Mediterranean forms (B⁻) haemolysis may be severe. Haemolysis may be exacerbated by concurrent infections, liver disease (reduced primaquine metabolism), renal impairment (delayed excretion), and co-administration of other drugs with haemolytic potential, e.g. sulphonamides. Primaquine is contraindicated in pregnancy.

Use

Radical curative activity depends on the total dose administered and this is determined by adverse effects. Primaquine is given once daily in a dose of 0.25–0.5 mg/kg (adult doses 15–30 mg) together with food. The usual course of treatment for the radical treatment of vivax and ovale malaria is 14 days, and there is no good evidence to support shorter courses. In particular, there is no evidence that the commonly used 5-day regimen is effective.[709] There is no evidence for interactions with other antimalarial drugs. In patients with mild G6PD deficiency, a once-weekly dose of 0.6–0.8 mg/kg (adult dose 45 mg) is given for 6 weeks. For P. falciparum gametocytocidal activity a single dose of 0.5 mg/kg (30 mg) is given. For prophylaxis the adult dose evaluated has been 30 mg daily taken with food. This has been remarkably well tolerated.[710,711] In most vivax endemic areas, G6PD deficiency is prevalent but testing is not available, and there is no consensus on how primaquine should be used in these circumstances. If significant haemolysis occurs, primaquine should be stopped and the patient observed. Transfusion is rarely necessary except when there is severe deficiency.

Quinocide, Elubaquine and Tafenoquine

There are three other 8-aminoquinolines in use or development. Quinocide, a positional isomer of primaquine, was used predominantly in the USSR. It has very similar properties to primaquine and indeed is the main contaminant of primaquine drug substance.[712] Elubaquine (developed by CDRI, Lucknow) is an alternative to primaquine which is available in India. More data are needed on its pharmacokinetic properties in humans, and its relative safety and efficacy profiles.[713] Tafenoquine, formerly known as etaquine or WR 238605, is a slowly eliminated 8-aminoquinoline that was developed by the US army. It is currently undergoing phase III trials in antimalarial prophylaxis, and for the radical treatment of vivax malaria.[714,715] Tafenoquine has a terminal elimination half-life of approximately 2 weeks.[716] Tafenoquine is more efficacious and better tolerated than primaquine, although it still causes oxidant haemolysis in G6PD deficient subjects.

Qinghaosu (artemisinin)

Qinghaosu or artemisinin (Figure 73.28) is a sesquiterpene (15 carbon rings) lactone peroxide extracted from the leaves of the shrub Artemesia annua (variously termed huang hua hao or qinghao). Four derivatives are used widely: the oil-soluble methyl ethers artemether and artemotil (formerly known as arteether), the water-soluble hemisuccinate derivative artesunate, and dihydroartemisinin (DHA). A semisynthetic derivative artemisone, and a fully synthetic trioxalone compound (OZ 277) with similar modes of action are under development. Artesunate, artemether, and artemotil are all synthesized from DHA, and they are converted back to it within the body. Artemisinin itself is available in a few countries. It is 5–10 times less active than the derivatives, and is not metabolized to DHA. These drugs are the most rapidly acting of known antimalarials, and they have the broadest time window of antimalarial effect (from ring forms to early schizonts). They

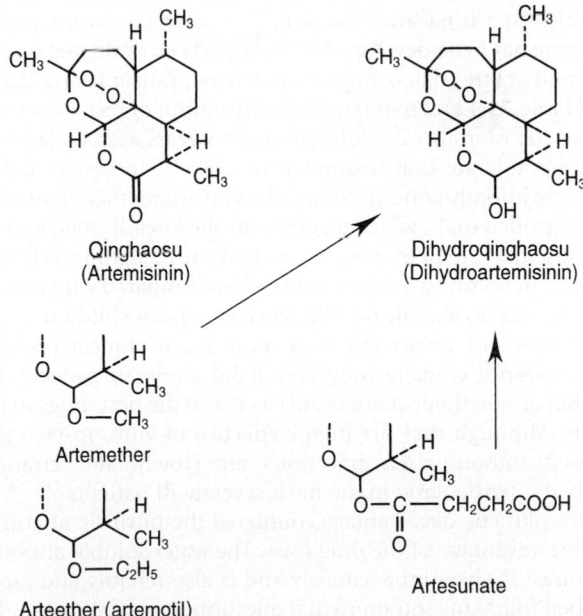

Figure 73.28 Qinghaosu: the parent compound artemisinin and the three derivatives. The oil-soluble ethers, artemether and arteether, and the water-soluble artesunate are all converted in vivo to a common biologically active metabolite dihydroartemisinin. The peroxide bridge in the sesquiterpene structure is essential for antimalarial activity. (From Hien and White,[494] with permission.)

Table 73.12 Dosage for rectal artesunate initial (pre-referral) treatment in children (aged 2–15 years and weighing at least 5 kg)

Weight (kg)	Age	Artesunate dose (mg)	Regimen (single dose)
5–8.9	0–12 months	50	One 50-mg suppository
9–19	13–42 months	100	One 100-mg suppository
20–29	43–71 months	200	Two 100-mg suppository
30–39	5–13 years	300	Three 100-mg suppositories
>40	≥14 years	400	One 400-mg suppository

Age ranges are a guide only–the target dose is 10 mg/kg

produce more rapid parasite clearance than other antimalarial drugs and they have proved to be very safe in clinical practice.[6,717–719] They are the best drugs for severe malaria.[720] In *falciparum* malaria, the artemisinin derivatives also effectively prevent progression to severe disease. For example in Western Thailand, a parasitaemia over 4% without vital organ dysfunction carries a 3% mortality (i.e. 30 times higher than uncomplicated malaria but less than one-fifth that of severe malaria). In this context, oral artesunate produces considerably superior therapeutic responses compared with an intravenous quinine loading dose.[721] This property of rapidly stopping parasite development and thereby arresting progression of the infection saves lives and also prevents development of severe malaria. Most deaths from severe malaria are in or near home and far from facilities capable of providing injections. Rectal formulations have been developed for community use as treatments for patients suspected of having severe malaria who are febrile and unable to take medications by mouth. Following the promising results with artemisinin suppositories in China and Vietnam,[722–724] a rectal formulation of artesunate has been developed.[725] This has been evaluated in a very large multicentre trial, conducted in Ghana, Tanzania and Bangladesh (Table 73.12). Pre-referral administration of rectal artesunate reduced the mortality of children under 5 years with malaria who could not tolerate oral treatment, by 25%.[726] In severe malaria, trials were initially conducted mainly with artemether. In randomized controlled trials, which together enrolled nearly 2000 patients, intramuscular artemether was associated with a significantly lower mortality in South-east Asian adults when compared with quinine, but there was no significant difference in African children.[719] Artemether was not associated with more rapid clinical responses (fever clearance, coma recovery) but it did accelerate parasite clearance. But artemether (or artemotil) were not the best drugs to have chosen. Although they are highly effective in vitro, in vivo these oil-based intramuscular injections are slowly and erratically absorbed – particularly in the most severely ill patients.[727,728] This pharmacokinetic disadvantage countered the intrinsic pharmacodynamic advantage of the drug class. The water soluble artesunate by contrast is given intravenously and is also reliably and rapidly absorbed following intramuscular injection. Recently, in a study of hospitalized severe malaria conducted in Bangladesh, Myanmar, Indonesia and India, which enrolled 1461 patients, parenteral artesunate reduced the mortality of severe malaria by 35% compared with quinine. This trial included 220 children in whom the beneficial effects were similar to adults.[720] The results were definitive and, combined with the results of smaller trials which gave

similar results, led to an immediate change in treatment recommendations for adults everywhere and for severe malaria in low transmission settings. But given the differences between African children and South-east Asian adults observed in the earlier artemether studies, uncertainty remained whether artesunate would be superior to quinine in children living in higher transmission areas. A large comparative study is therefore under way in Africa. In clinical studies in uncomplicated *falciparum* malaria the artemisinin derivatives provide both more rapid parasite and fever clearance than with other treatments, and also reduce gametocyte carriage, and thus transmission.[729,730] Concerns over their neurotoxic potential, revealed in animal studies, have not been confirmed in large and detailed clinical, neurophysiological and pathological studies.[731–733] Indeed their remarkable safety, efficacy, and lack of adverse effects[734] have led to widespread unregulated use and the manufacture of fake products.[735,736]

Artemisinin is available as capsules of powder or as suppositories. Artemether is formulated in peanut oil, and arteether in sesame seed oil, for intramuscular injection, and in capsules or tablets for oral use. Artesunate is formulated either as tablets, in a gel enclosed in gelatin for rectal administration, or as dry powder of artesunic acid for injection, supplied with an ampoule of 5% sodium bicarbonate. The powder is dissolved in the sodium bicarbonate, to form sodium artesunate, and then diluted in 5% dextrose or normal saline for intravenous or intramuscular injection. The majority of clinical data pertain to the most widely used derivative, artesunate.

Apart from the Thai-Cambodian border, there is no significant resistance to these drugs, which have become central to antimalarial treatment. Combinations of artemisinin derivatives with other antimalarial drugs (ACTs) provide high and sustained efficacy, and rapid therapeutic responses. This prevents the development of severe malaria and allows earlier return to school or work, mutual protection against resistance, and reduced gametocyte carriage which may reduce the incidence of malaria in low transmission settings. Community use of these drugs as monotherapies is strongly discouraged by the World Health Organization.

Pharmacokinetics

The artemisinin derivatives are rapidly absorbed and eliminated.[737] Artemisinin is cleared by metabolic conversion to inactive metabolites. It induces its own metabolism. Artesunate, artemether and artemotil are hydrolysed to the active metabolite dihydroartemisinin, which has an elimination half-life of approximately

45 min.[738,739] Although they are by far the most rapidly eliminated of the antimalarial drugs, because of their broad stage specificity of action they are highly effective when given once daily. Unlike some antibiotics, it is not necessary to exceed the MIC throughout the dosing interval for antimalarial drugs. After oral or parenteral administration, artesunate is hydrolysed rapidly (by stomach acid, and esterases in plasma and erythrocytes) and most of the antimalarial activity results from the DHA metabolite. Oral absorption is rapid and bioavailability is approximately 60%.[739,740] Rectal bioavailability is more variable;[741] following administration of the intrarectal formulation bioavailability averages 50% (although rates of absorption vary widely).[725] As for quinine, there is a contraction in the volume of distribution and reduced clearance in acute malaria, which increases blood concentrations. There may also be a malaria related inhibition of intestinal and hepatic first pass metabolism (by glucuronidation), which improves oral bioavailability. After oral administration, artemether is absorbed rapidly, but is converted more slowly (via CYP 3A4) to DHA, although the metabolite still accounts for the majority of antimalarial activity.[738] In contrast, after intramuscular administration absorption of artemether and artemotil (arteether) is slow and erratic.[728,732,738,742] Peak concentrations are often not reached for many hours. Following intramuscular administration concentrations of artemether exceed those of the active DHA metabolite. In some patients with severe malaria absorption may be inadequate.[727] Oral formulations of DHA contain excipients which promote absorption and give bioavailability comparable to that of artesunate. Elimination of DHA is largely by conversion to inactive glucuronides. No significant drug interactions have been identified with these compounds. Concentrations of artemisinin derivatives and DHA are similar in children and adults but are significantly reduced in late pregnancy (Table 73.9).[743]

Toxicity

The artemisinin-related compounds have been remarkably well tolerated in clinical evaluations. There has been no documented significant toxicity[734] other than rare type 1 hypersensitivity reactions (incidence approximately 1:3000 treatments).[744] In volunteer studies, a depression of reticulocyte counts has been noted, and haemoglobin recovery in the first week may be slightly slower than with other antimalarials but increased anaemia thereafter has not been observed in clinical studies. In animal studies, the artemisinin derivatives are much less toxic than the quinoline antimalarials. The principal toxicity in animals has been an unusual dose-related selective pattern of neuronal cell damage affecting certain brain stem nuclei.[745-747] This is a function of the pharmacokinetic properties of the drug. Neurotoxicity is related to protracted central nervous system exposure related to sustained blood concentrations, as follows intramuscular administration of the oil based artemether and artemotil. Much less neurotoxicity is seen in animal models following oral administration or intravenous artesunate because the drugs levels are not sustained.[748,749] Extensive clinical neurophysiological and smaller pathology studies have failed to show any evidence of neurotoxicity or cardiotoxicity in clinical use.[731,732,734] Initial animal studies also suggested effects on the electrocardiographic QT interval (ventricular repolarization) but this was probably secondary to neurotoxicity.[746] These drugs do not affect the heart in clinical use. The main concern over

their general use relates to early pregnancy.[750] In experimental animals, exposure during a critical time window in early pregnancy causes fetal loss as a result of inhibition of erythropoiesis.[751] Whether this effect could produce fetal developmental abnormalities in primates, and therefore in clinical use in the treatment of malaria has not been resolved. Detailed observations from prospective clinical studies in over 1000 exposed pregnancies are reassuring to date.[752,753] These drugs are therefore not recommended for the treatment of uncomplicated falciparum malaria in early pregnancy (first trimester) unless there are no effective alternatives. There is increasing confidence in their safety in the second and third trimesters. No adverse effects on the pregnancy or infant development have been seen in prospective studies.

Use

In severe malaria, artesunate is given by intravenous or intramuscular injection. The doses are 2.4 mg/kg given at 0, 12, 24 h then daily (earlier a lower maintenance dose of 1.2 mg/kg was recommended but this risked achieving inadequate blood concentrations).[754] Artemether and artemotil (arteether) are given by intramuscular injection to the anterior thigh. The dose of artemether is 3.2 mg/kg initially followed by 1.6 mg/kg daily (Table 73.10). Rectal artemisinin suppositories are very effective, but they are available only in Vietnam. The intrarectal artesunate formulation is used as a pre-referral treatment in a dose of 10 mg/kg per day until parenteral or oral treatment can be given (Table 73.12). For oral treatment, if used alone, the artemisinin derivatives should be given in a 7- (not 5) day course, but this should be combined with doxycycline or clindamycin where possible. The initial oral dose is 4 mg/kg followed by 2 mg/kg per day. The artemisinin derivatives should be used in fixed dose combinations with longer-acting drugs in order to accelerate the initial therapeutic response, to increase overall cure rates, and to protect them from resistance (Table 73.13).[558,565,568] Dose restrictions are not necessary in renal failure or with liver disease. The artemisinin derivatives are safe in children. They should not be used in the first trimester of pregnancy, but should be used in the second and third trimesters.[657] These drugs should be used for the treatment of severe malaria in pregnancy at any gestational age as they save lives and they are also safer than quinine.

Artemisinin combination treatments

The ACTs are rapidly effective and generally reliable treatments. They are now the treatment of choice for uncomplicated falciparum malaria in endemic areas. The artemisinin derivatives induce a rapid resolution of fever and illness. This may improve absorption of the combination partner (mefloquine, lumefantrine). While present in the blood (usually 3 days) they also protect the partner drug from the emergence of resistance and reduce gametocyte carriage. The partner drug then removes the relatively few parasites remaining after the 3-day course of treatment (a hundred million times less than when treatment started), and also protects the artemisinin derivative from resistance. But once the artemisinin derivative has been eliminated, the partner compound is no longer 'protected' and may then select for resistance. Thus, provided the partner is effective and full doses are absorbed, protection of the artemisinin component from resistance is complete, whereas protection of the partner drug is incomplete.

Table 73.13 Treatment of uncomplicated malaria (see also Table 73.11)

FIRST-LINE DRUGS IN ENDEMIC AREAS	
Malaria	**Drug treatment**
Known chloroquine sensitive *P. vivax, P. malariae, P. ovale, P. falciparum*[a]	Chloroquine 10 mg base/kg stat followed by 5 mg/kg at 12, 24 and 36 h; or 10 mg/kg at 24 h, 5 mg/kg at 48 h or Amodiaquine 10–12 mg base/kg/day – for 3 days or Any of the ACTs below[a]
Sensitive *P. falciparum* malaria[b]	Artesunate 4 mg/kg per day for 3 days + sulphadoxine 25 mg/kg + pyrimethamine 1.25 mg/kg (SP) single dose or Artesunate 4 mg/kg per day for 3 days + Amodiaquine 10 mg base/kg per day for 3 days
Multi-drug resistant *P. falciparum* malaria	Artemether–lumefantrine 1.5/9 mg/kg twice daily for three days with food. Adult dose 4 tablets b.d. for 3 days or Artesunate 4 mg/kg per day for 3 days + mefloquine 25 mg base/kg (either 8 mg/kg per day for 3 days or 15 mg/kg on day 2 then 10 mg/kg on day 3) or Dihydroartemisinin-piperaquine 3/16 mg/kg once daily for three days

SECOND-LINE TREATMENTS
Artesunate 2 mg/kg daily plus either (a) tetracycline 4 mg/kg 4 times daily or (b) doxycycline 3.5 mg/kg once daily or (c) clindamycin 10 mg/kg twice daily for 7 days. Several authorities recommend giving an initial dose of 4 mg/kg. Quinine 10 mg salt/kg 3 times daily plus either (a) tetracycline 4 mg/kg 4 times daily or (b) doxycycline 3 mg/kg once daily or (c) clindamycin 10 mg/kg twice daily for 7 days. Atovaquone–proguanil 20/8 mg/kg once daily for 3 days with food.

RADICAL TREATMENT
Patients with *P. vivax* and *P. ovale* infections should also be given primaquine 0.25 mg base/kg daily (0.375–0.5 mg base/kg in Oceania) with food for 14 days to prevent relapse. In mild G6PD deficiency 0.75 mg base/kg should be given once weekly for 6 weeks. Primaquine should not be given in severe G6PD deficiency.

GENERAL POINTS
In nearly all circumstances fixed dose combinations are preferable, and should replace use of separate tablets. Pregnancy: Mefloquine and artesunate should not be given in the first trimester. Halofantrine, primaquine, and tetracycline should not be used at any time in pregnancy, and sulphadoxine should not be used very near to term (if effective alternatives are readily available). Vomiting is less likely if the patient's temperature is lowered before oral drug administration. Short courses of artesunate or quinine (<7 days) alone are not recommended. In renal failure, the dose of quinine should be reduced by one-third to one-half after 48 h, and doxycycline (but not tetracycline) should be prescribed. The doses of all drugs (in mg/kg) are unchanged in children and pregnant women.[c] None of the tetracyclines or doxycycline should be given to pregnant women or children under 8 years of age. Mefloquine should not be given immediately following recovery from severe malaria, and treatment doses should not be used twice within one month.

[a] All ACTs are highly effective aginst *P. vivax, P. malariae,* and *P. ovale,* with the exception of combinations containing SP, as resistance to SP is widespread in *P. vivax.*

[b] If there is any doubt about the susceptibility of the infection, treat as if it was resistant.

[c] There is evidence that the mg/kg dose of sulfadoxin-pyrimethamine and dihydroartemisnin-piperaquine extrapolated from adults may be too low in children (5 years),[667,779] but higher dose regimens have not been evaluated.

Artemether-lumefantrine

Formerly called benflumetol, lumefantrine was developed by Chinese scientists. It is now available only in a fixed tablet combination with artemether. Each tablet contains artemether 20 mg and lumefantrine 120 mg. The combination is registered in many tropical countries and in Europe. Artemether-lumefantrine is very effective against multi-drug resistant *falciparum* malaria, and it is remarkably well tolerated. The price has fallen such that treatment courses for adults cost approximately US$1. After initial evaluations in Asia, it has become the most widely used of the ACTs.

Pharmacokinetics

Lumefantrine is lipophilic and hydrophobic. Its absorption is dose-limited and is considerably augmented by taking the drug together with food (a 16-fold increase with a fatty meal).[755,756] Only a small amount of fat is required. Dose finding studies with soya milk showed 36 mL (equivalent to 1.2 g fat) were required to produce 90% of maximum absorption.[757] The absorption of lumefantrine is reduced in the acute phase of malaria, but then increases considerably as symptoms resolve and the patient starts to eat.[755,756] Oral absorption is capacity limited, so increasing the current dose does not provide a corresponding increase in absorption.[758] This means the drug cannot be given once daily. Lumefantrine is metabolised to a desbutyl metabolite (principally via CYP 3 A4), which has antimalarial activity but contributes relatively little to overall antimalarial effect. The lumefantrine elimination half-life is 3–4 days.[756] As a result it provides a shorter duration of post-treatment prophylaxis compared with more slowly eliminated drugs such as mefloquine and piperaquine. The pharmacokinetic properties of lumefantrine are similar in adults and children. The principal pharmacokinetic variable which correlates with therapeutic response is the area under the plasma concentration curve (AUC).[756] The plasma level on day 7 after starting treatment is a good surrogate of the AUC.[759] On the Western border of Thailand when this drug was introduced, day 7 plasma levels of lumefantrine above 500 ng/mL were associated with a >90% cure rate.[760] Plasma concentrations of both drug components are reduced by approximately half in pregnancy[761] so the current dose regimen is insufficient for optimum cure rates in this important patient group (Table 73.11).

Toxicity

This combination is remarkably free of adverse effects. Concerns about possible cardiotoxicity, have been refuted by careful studies.[762] Lumefantrine is not cardiotoxic.

Use

There is now extensive experience with artemether-lumefantrine from all parts of the malaria affected world attesting to safety and efficacy. The treatment course initially recommended was 1.5/ 9 mg/kg (adult dose 4 tablets) given at 0, 8, 24, and 48 h. This was effective in patients with background immunity, but cure rates in non-immune patients with multi-drug resistant infections were approximately 80%[763] Increasing the regimen to six doses (i.e. twice daily for days) resulted in >95% cure rates[764,765] and this is now the recommended regimen.[766–769] Where it has

been assessed, adherence to this regimen has been relatively good.[770] The patient should be encouraged to take the drug with food or a small amount of milk. Recent studies suggest artemether-lumefantrine is safe in the second and third trimesters of pregnancy, although more information is needed and dose optimization is required. A paediatric formulation has been developed recently.

Pyronaridine

Structurally a relative of amodiaquine, pyronaridine was developed and used in China. It is active against multi-drug resistant *Plasmodium falciparum* malaria[771,772] and, like many drugs in this class, it is extensively distributed and slowly eliminated. Originally pyronaridine was deployed as an enteric-coated formulation for monotherapy (which had poor oral bioavailability), and was given in a 3-day course of 1200 mg or 1800 mg (adult dose) over 5 days. It is now being developed as a fixed co-formulation with artesunate. Clinical trials are in progress and preliminary results are excellent.

Piperaquine

Also developed in China, this bisquinoline compound and its hydroxy-derivative are active against multi-drug resistant *Plasmodium falciparum*.[773] Piperaquine replaced chloroquine as first-line treatment for *falciparum* malaria in China in 1978 and was used until 1994. Over 200 tonnes were dispensed. Resistance reportedly developed, but reversed after piperaquine was discontinued. In recent years, piperaquine has been available as a fixed combination with dihydroartemisinin (and also sometimes trimethoprim and primaquine). The currently available formulation contains 40 mg of dihydroartemisinin and 320 mg of piperaquine per tablet and in Asia is given in an adult dose of 3 tablets per day (equivalent to approximately 2.3/16 mg/kg, once daily for 3 days. It is relatively inexpensive (adult doses currently just over US$1). These combinations are registered and used in China, Vietnam and Cambodia. The combination is well tolerated, safe, and effective.

Pharmacokinetics

Oral dihydroartemisinin absorption is very dependent on the formulation and excipients. In current formulations, it is reliably and rapidly absorbed. Piperaquine is more slowly absorbed. It is extensively distributed and very slowly eliminated. The pharmacokinetic properties are generally similar to those of chloroquine.[774,775] Absorption may be increased by fats.[776] Latest estimates for the terminal elimination half-life exceed 1 month.[777,778] Children have an even slower terminal elimination half-life than adults but have lower plasma concentrations early in the terminal phase of elimination.[767,779,780] As with other slowly eliminated antimalarials, the day 7 plasma or blood concentration is a valuable predictor of efficacy.[759]

Toxicity

Piperaquine is safer than chloroquine. It is generally very well tolerated. Dosing is limited by abdominal discomfort. Apart from rare urticarial reactions to DHA, occasional abdominal discomfort and diarrhea have been reported in clinical trials which may have resulted from piperaquine. There is no evidence for cardiovascular toxicity with therapeutic doses. No serious adverse effects have been reported.

Use

Large trials in many countries attest to an excellent efficacy and safety profile. DHA-piperaquine has already established itself as an important antimalarial in the South-east Asian region.[778,781-783] It is effective against drug resistant *falciparum* and *vivax* malaria.[784,785] Dosing has been simplified to a once daily regimen.[786] When measured, adherence has been excellent.[787] Recent studies also indicate good efficacy and excellent tolerability in African children.[788] The long period of post-treatment prophylaxis conferred by the slowly eliminated piperaquine is both an advantage in preventing reinfections and suppressing *P. vivax* relapses, but also increases the selection pressure on resistance.

Antibacterials with antimalarial activity

The antibacterials which act on protein or nucleic acid synthesis often have significant antimalarial activity. But they are not sufficiently active to be used alone to treat malaria.[789] The sulphonamides and sulphones inhibit plasmodial folate synthesis by competing for the enzyme dihydropteroate synthetase. The sulphas are usually used in combination with pyrimethamine or the antimalarial biguanides with which they are synergistic. Trimethoprim is also an antifol; it has good antimalarial activity and shares resistance profiles with pyrimethamine. The tetracyclines are consistently active against all species of malaria. Doxycycline is the most widely used both for prophylaxis and treatment.[790] Clindamycin is as effective as the tetracyclines and has the advantage that it can be used in children and pregnant women.[791,792] The macrolides are active in vitro but are generally disappointing in vivo. Azithromycin is more active and has been evaluated both in prophylaxis and treatment. Rifampicin has a weak antimalarial effect in vivo. Chloramphenicol has antimalarial activity but this has not been well characterized. The fluoroquinolones have some activity but, despite one promising sentinel report, subsequent clinical experience has proved uniformly disappointing. Fosmidomycin has good antimalarial activity and is under investigation. These drugs all act relatively slowly, and they are therefore used in combination with more rapidly acting agents.

Manufacturing quality of antimalarial drugs

Several of the artemisinin derivatives and ACTs manufactured in Asia do not yet reach Internationally Accepted Good Manufacturing Practices or WHO pre-qualification standards. This does not mean that quality of the products has been poor – but that the manufacturing and quality assurance processes and documentation have not been sufficient to meet internationally accepted standards. This has been a major impediment to their acceptance and use outside the region, despite their evident efficacy and excellent safety profiles, as international donors will not purchase 'non GMP' products. (Hopefully by the next edition of this textbook, this section will no longer be necessary.)

Antimalarial drug interactions

Antimalarial drug interactions have not been well characterized. Mefloquine, halofantrine, quinidine and quinine are structurally similar and may compete for blood and tissue binding sites. Cardiotoxicity is assumed to be additive, and significant only for halofantrine, where there is a potentially dangerous interaction with mefloquine–probably because both act on potassium channels involved in cardiac repolarization.[592] It has been recommended that mefloquine should not be given to people also receiving quinine to avoid adverse cardiovascular effects, but no interaction has been demonstrated.[793] Inducers of CYP 3A4, such as rifampicin and anticonvulsant drugs, accelerate the clearance of quinine and mefloquine resulting in lower drug levels (and a greater chance of treatment failure).[794,795] When amodiaquine is coadministered with the antiretroviral efavirenz plasma concentrations of desethyamodiaquine are elevated and there is a significant risk of hepatotoxicity.[796] There is no evidence that the structurally dissimilar antimalarials interact with each other. Use of artesunate together with mefloquine improves the tolerance and absorption of mefloquine, presumably by curing malaria more rapidly. Similarly, the absorption of lumefantrine improves as the patient recovers.

There are many reports of synergy or antagonism between antimalarial drugs based on isobolograms drawn from in vitro observations. These are often used to justify a particular choice of antimalarial combination but, for the most part, the results are irrelevant to the clinical use of the drugs. Only when synergy or antagonism is extreme, such as the marked synergy between sulphadoxine and pyrimethamine, is this relevant clinically. There are no cases of marked antagonism between the available antimalarial drugs.

TREATING MALARIA

In severe malaria, rapidly acting rapidly bioavailable parenteral treatment should be given. Rectal formulations of artemisinin or its derivatives (particularly artesunate) offer the possibility of starting treatment in the home or village before referring to the hospital or health centre. Rectal artesunate should become much more widely available in the next few years parenteral artesunate has replaced quinine as the treatment of choice for severe malaria in low transmission settings. Quinine is still the mainstay of parenteral treatment in African children,[797] although studies are in progress to determine whether artesunate is more effective. It is certainly safer. Artemether occupies an intermediate position, having been shown to be more effective than quinine in Asian adults but not in African children. For uncomplicated *falciparum* malaria artemisinin-based combination treatments (ACTs) are now recommended as first-line treatment everywhere. WHO currently recommends one of four ACTs. The choice of partner drug depends on local patterns of sensitivity and cost. For the treatment of *P. vivax*, *P. malariae*, and *P. ovale* malaria chloroquine can still be relied upon in most areas although high-level resistance is now well established in Indonesia, Micronesia, and the island of New Guinea, and there are increasing reports of low-level resistance from many parts of Asia and South-America (Tables 73.9–73.12).

Table 73.14 WHO definitions of antimalarial treatment failure in uncomplicated falciparum malaria

Treatment outcome	Symptoms and signs
Early treatment failure	Development of danger signs or severe malaria on days 1–3 in the presence of parasitaemia
	Parasitaemia on day 2 higher than the day 0 count irrespective of axillary temperature
	Parasitaemia on day 3 with axillary temperature of ≥37.5°C
	Parasitaemia on day 3 of ≥25% of count on day 0.
Late treatment failure	Development of danger signs or severe malaria after day 3 in the presence of parasitaemia, without previously meeting any of the criteria of early treatment failure.
Late clinical failure	Presence of parasitaemia and axillary temperature of ≥37.5°C (or history of fever) on any day from day 4 to day 28, without previously meeting any of the criteria of early treatment failure.
Late parasitological failure	Presence of parasitaemia on any day from day 7 to day 28 and axillary temperature of <37.5°C, without previously meeting any of the criteria of early treatment failure or late clinical failure.
Adequate clinical and parasitological response	Absence of parasitaemia on day 28 irrespective of axillary temperature without previously meeting any of the criteria of early treatment failure, late clinical failure or late parasitological failure.

Assessment of the therapeutic response

Generally understood and standardized definitions of antimalarial drug treatment responses are important for epidemiological purposes, and helpful in therapeutic decision-making. The definitions of severe malaria and treatment failure and the methods of assessing the therapeutic response have all undergone changes in recent years.

In uncomplicated malaria, the immediate therapeutic response is usually assessed by the parasite and fever clearance times. Recent WHO definitions of treatment failure are shown in Table 73.14.[798]

Parasite clearance time (PCT)

This is the interval between beginning antimalarial treatment and the first negative blood slide. The accuracy of the measurement depends on the frequency with which blood slides are taken and the quality of microscopy. The PCT is directly proportional to the admission parasitaemia. The time, taken for parasitaemia to fall to half of the admission value (PCT_{50}) and to fall to 10% of the admission value (PCT_{90}) are also useful comparative measures unless initial parasitaemias are low.

Fever clearance time (FCT)

This is the interval from beginning antimalarial treatment until the patient is apyrexial. Fever does not come down linearly – it often fluctuates erratically. The method and site of measurements should be standardized and the use of antipyretics documented. One approach is to record when temperature first falls below 37.5°C (FCT_a), and then when the temperature falls and remains below 37.5°C for 24 h (FCT_b).

In vivo testing of antimalarial drug efficacy

The World Health Organization now recommends that antimalarial drug treatment policy should aim for cure rates of at least 95% and that there should be consideration of policy change if failure rates exceed 10%,[657] Continuous assessment of antimalarial drug efficacy is therefore needed to monitor antimalarial drug resistance and inform policy (Box 73.2). In comparative studies, the groups should reflect the population affected by malaria. Too many trials have been conducted in older children or adults in highly endemic areas. These groups have significant background immunity, few or no symptoms, and a high rate of self-cure.[398] Drug efficacy in the less immune younger children is therefore overestimated. The analysis should be age stratified if there is a wide age range included in the study. It is very important that patients, parents or guardians truly understand that participation in a drug trial is voluntary, and give informed consent. Ideally, pre-treatment with another antimalarial drug is an exclusion criterion, but in some areas this is very common. In which case, such patients should be included provided details are taken, and preferably a baseline blood level is taken.

In antimalarial drug trials, data should be entered on a case record form. Baseline clinical, and demographic details should be recorded and, at a minimum, the parasitaemia counted and haematocrit measured. In well-equipped sites, parasite culture to correlate the in vivo response with in vitro susceptibility can also be performed. A baseline whole blood sample (or blood spot on filter paper) should be stored for parasite genotyping. Molecular typing of *Plasmodium falciparum* (usually by assessment of size polymorphisms in fragments of the genes encoding MSP1, MSP2 and GLURP) has considerably improved the accuracy of drug trials conducted in endemic areas.[800–802] The genotype(s) of infections recurring within the follow-up period are compared to those in the initial isolate. If the same genotype is found the infection is considered a recrudescence (i.e. a treatment failure).[803] A different genotype indicates a newly acquired infection. The method is not foolproof; genotypes may be difficult to ascribe in mixed infections (which are usual in high transmission settings) and resistant infections might be subpatent on admission and therefore be considered erroneously as a new infection when they subsequently recrudesce.[804] But genotyping has been a considerable advance which allows large community-based drug assessments in *falci-*

Box 73.2 Design and conduct of antimalarial drug trials

An adequate sample size is required to assess the clinical efficacy of antimalarial drugs. For example, with a sample size of 60 studied patients and six treatment failures, the 95% confidence interval around the 90% cure rate is 82.4–97.6%. This study is too small for a definitive assessment as it leaves too much uncertainty as to the true cure rate in the population. In the past, antimalarial drug trials have been powered to detect differences between drugs – usually with 95% confidence and 80% power. This is a 'superiority' trial. But conducting such trials is increasingly difficult with cure rates over 90% because of the exponential increase in the sample size required.[799] The higher the standard treatment's cure rate, the more difficult it is to demonstrate conclusively a small difference in favour of a new treatment. An alternative approach is the non-inferiority trial, which aims to show that an experimental treatment is 'not worse' than the active control (i.e. current treatment) by more than a specified amount – the equivalence margin (often denoted δ). The null hypothesis being tested is that there *is* a difference between the two groups (i.e. it is the opposite to that in conventional superiority trials) and it is greater than the δ. The main limitation is that confounders introduced in a poorly conducted trial which affect both groups, and are unrelated to differences in the efficacy (or toxicity) of the trial regimens, can obscure significant differences. In a superiority trial this might lead to a failure to disprove the null hypothesis – i.e. failure to show difference – but in a non-inferiority trial the direction is opposite; a false rejection of the null hypothesis and conclusion of non-inferiority. This emphasizes the importance in antimalarial drug trials of avoiding errors in drug allocation and administration, poor adherence, errors in endpoint ascertainment (for antimalarial efficacy this refers particularly to identification of recrudescence), and loss to follow-up.

Blinding is often used to avoid bias in comparative trials although it is often difficult in antimalarial drug assessments because of differences in treatment regimens and the difficulties in masking the taste of the drugs. Compared with superiority trials, blinding does not protect against bias as well in non-inferiority trials because a biased investigator wishing to show non-inferiority can simply give all patients similar results. Analysis of non-inferiority trials requires a calculation of the difference between the failures rates in the treatment groups and a calculation of the confidence interval around this difference using appropriate methods and 'effective' sample sizes.[799]

parum malaria to be conducted in endemic areas. For studies of slowly eliminated drugs taking a blood level measurement at Day 7 in all patients helps to interpret treatment failures (i.e. whether they resulted from drug resistance or low blood concentrations).[805] For many drugs, simple filter paper whole antimalarial drug blood assays are now available.

Antimalarial treatment should be observed and adverse effects recorded. The patients should be followed daily until parasite clearance, then at weekly intervals. The rate of resolution of anaemia is a sensitive measure of the treatment response. The haemoglobin or haematocrit should be measured each time a parasite count is performed in therapeutic assessments. Four weeks is the minimum follow-up duration for rapidly eliminated drugs

and 6 weeks is the minimum for drugs with intermediate or long terminal elimination half-lives.[806] At least 90% follow-up at 4 weeks should be aimed for, and sample sizes adjusted for likely 'drop-out' rates. The appearance of *P. vivax*, *P. malariae* or *P. ovale* malaria requires chloroquine treatment. These patients' data are usually censored after treatment of *vivax* malaria.

Interpretation of trials

In antimalarial drug trials two or more groups of patients are followed for a pre-specified length of time after different antimalarial treatments. The cure rates, which means the proportions of patients who reach the end of this follow-up period without recrudescence of the infection, are compared. In the past, antimalarial treatment efficacy was usually assessed on a particular day (often day 14 or day 28 after starting treatment) so only patients followed to that day were included in the analysis. This is often referred as a '*per-protocol*' *(PP) analysis*. But in most trials, there are patients who do not complete the follow-up period, yet these patients do contribute useful information before they leave the trial, and their contribution can and should be used. If such a patient did not fail (i.e. remained aparasitaemic) when last observed, that patient's data are said to be 'censored' at the time they were last followed-up. The patient who has the appearance of *vivax* malaria following treatment of *falciparum* malaria is also usually censored at that time. The appropriate analysis for such data is *survival analysis*, which deals explicitly with censored values.[799] Patients with different follow-up periods cannot be treated the same way – someone who is followed up for longer has a greater chance of being recorded as treatment failure than another patient followed-up for a shorter time. Failure rates should be estimated using the Kaplan–Meier method. This is now endorsed by the current WHO recommendations for antimalarial resistance monitoring which suggest use of life tables (i.e. survival analysis) in analysing in vivo studies.[798] The '*intention to treat*' *(ITT) analysis*, which includes all missing patients or indeterminate values as treatment failures should be reported also, but it should not be the primary endpoint of an antimalarial drug study as it may overestimate the true failure rates.

Therapeutic assessments in *vivax* malaria

The design and conduct of studies in *vivax* malaria is similar to trials in *falciparum* malaria but the interpretation of results is more difficult. Unfortunately, genotyping does not distinguish reliably between recrudescence, relapse and new infection as approximately two-thirds of relapses are with a genotype different to that which caused the initial infection.[806,807] But in the assessment of chloroquine, any infection that recurs within 28 days can be regarded as resistant provided the whole blood chloroquine concentration is ≥100ng/mL. Assessment of anti-relapse activity is easiest if rapidly eliminated drugs are used (quinine, artesunate) as these do not suppress the first relapse.

Severe malaria trials

In addition to parasite and fever clearance, the rate of clinical recovery in survivors should be assessed. In unconscious children, the Blantyre Coma Scale (BCS) is most widely used and in adults the Glasgow Coma Score (GCS) should be measured. If possible, these should be assessed 4–6-hourly and the times to reach BCS scores of 3, 4 and 5 and GCS scores of 8, 11 and 15 recorded. The time to drink, sit, walk and leave hospital should also be documented. The changes in venous lactate, venous bicarbonate and, in adults, serum creatinine can also be followed and used as measures of the therapeutic response.

In vitro sensitivity testing

Both in vivo and in vitro assessments of antimalarial efficacy are needed to guide treatment recommendations and planning of policy. *P. falciparum* can be cultured relatively easily in vitro, whereas the other malaria parasites are more difficult to grow ex vivo. Short-term culture of *P. falciparum* over one cycle requires only simple sterile culture media, a candle jar and an incubator.[808,809] Short-term culture of *P. vivax* is also relatively easy with modifications to the conditions.[810,811] Antimalarial drug susceptibility can be tested by measuring the inhibition by different concentrations drugs of parasite maturation to the schizont stage, the degree of inhibition of radio-labelled (^{3}H) hypoxanthine uptake, or the synthesis of parasite specific lactate dehydrogenase or histidine rich protein 2.[812–814] The *Pf*LDH and *Pf*HRP2 tests require only an ELISA reader and have the additional advantage of being possible at low parasite densities. These are useful epidemiological tools, but they do not predict the clinical response to treatment in an individual because they do not reflect differences between people in antimalarial pharmacokinetics, immunity or stage of disease.

MANAGEMENT

In many tropical countries, 'malaria' is synonymous with 'fever'. Antimalarial drugs are self administered on a vast scale. Where possible, a definite species diagnosis should be obtained by microscopic examination of the blood smear or use of a suitable rapid antigen based diagnostic test (RDT). If there is any doubt, *Plasmodium falciparum* infection should be assumed. The management of malaria depends very much on the health facilities available and the endemicity of disease, i.e. the likely immune status of the patient. For example, in areas of intense transmission infants and young children are often parasitaemic. Distinguishing malaria from other infections as the cause of fever may be difficult or impossible, and so it is prudent to treat febrile children for malaria unless there is an evident alternative diagnosis. In these settings, asymptomatic parasitaemia is also common in older children and adults, but in these age groups, fever is more likely to be the result of some other infection. However, fever may precede detectable parasitaemia in non-immune adults or young children. The blood film should be re-checked in suspected cases. 'Blood smear-negative malaria' is a common diagnosis in the tropics – but one to be avoided. Other infections are more likely. If the patient has a sub-patent parasitaemia and no signs of severity it is safe to wait, seek other causes for the symptoms, and repeat the blood smears at 12–24 h intervals. In severely ill patients, antimalarial treatment should be started immediately in full doses, but other diagnoses sought. Patients may remain unconscious or develop renal failure after parasite clearance, but there is usually a clear history of previous treatment, and malaria pigment may still be found in monocytes in peripheral blood or intradermal smears,[473] and the *Pf*HRP2 dipstick will be positive.[518] If the temperature is high on admission (>38.5 °C) then symptomatic treatment with oral antipyretics (paracetamol, **not** aspirin) and tepid sponging bring symptomatic relief, and may also reduce the likelihood that the patient vomits the oral antimalarials. This is particularly important for young children who are less likely to have a seizure, and more likely to tolerate oral antimalarials when their temperature has been lowered and they are quiet and calm. Unfortunately, there are no paediatric formulations of mefloquine, or the artemisinin derivatives. For young children large pills should be crushed and given as a suspension in a small volume of sweet drink or milk when treating young children. A disposable syringe (*without* the needle!) may be used to draw up and give an accurate volume of the suspension into the child's mouth.

Benign malarias

Although *P. vivax*, *P. ovale* or *P. malariae* rarely kill, the disease can be moderately severe, requiring initial parenteral treatment. Occasional patients with *vivax* malaria do develop vital organ dysfunction, and these should be treated as for severe *falciparum* malaria. More usually, oral treatment with chloroquine (Table 73.13) leads to resolution of the fever within 2–3 days. The total dose is usually 25 mg base/kg. The initial dose is 10 mg base/kg and this is followed at 12-h intervals with subsequent doses of 5 mg/kg or the dose can be divided as 10, 10, 5 mg/kg on Days 0, 1 and 2, respectively. Resistance to SP is widespread and high level resistance to chloroquine in *P. vivax* is now a significant problem on the island of New Guinea and in parts of Indonesia. These infections respond to ACTs containing amodiaquine, piperaquine or mefloquine. *Plasmodium vivax* responds to antimalarial drugs similarly to *Plasmodium falciparum*.[815] The ACTs (with the exception of artesunate – SP) are highly effective against *vivax* malaria. Primaquine should be given to patients with *P. vivax* or *P. ovale* to prevent relapse. The incidence of relapse varies considerably by geographical region. The efficacy in preventing relapse is determined by the total dose of primaquine taken. The 5-day regimens widely used on the Indian subcontinent are insufficient. The usual adult dose has been 15 mg base/day (0.25 mg/kg) for 14 days although higher doses are needed for the relatively resistant 'Chesson-like' strains (found in East Asia and Oceania).[816] There is increasing use of 30 mg base/day for 14 days for infections from East Asia and Oceania. This is well tolerated if taken with food. Primaquine is often considered unnecessary if the patient is going to return immediately to a highly endemic area, although the risk-benefit assessment for use in children in Asia (where G6PD deficiency is common) has not been made. Primaquine should not be given to pregnant or lactating women or patients with known severe variants of G6PD deficiency. If mild variants of G6PD deficiency are known or likely then primaquine should be given in a dose of 0.75 mg/kg (45 mg) once weekly for 6 weeks. Primaquine does have significant activity against the asexual blood stages of *P. vivax* and this may mask chloroquine resistance in combined treatment, but may also protect against chloroquine resistance in areas with sensitive parasites.[817]

P. falciparum malaria

In endemic areas, uncomplicated *falciparum* malaria is treated on an out-patient basis in the same way as the other malarias. In temperate countries, imported cases should usually be hospitalized.

Table 73.15 Immediate clinical management of severe manifestations and complications of *falciparum* malaria

Manifestation/complication	Immediate management[a]
Coma (cerebral malaria)	Maintain airway, place patient on his or her side, exclude other treatable causes of coma (e.g. hypoglycaemia, bacterial meningitis); avoid harmful ancillary treatment such as corticosteroids, heparin and adrenaline; intubate if necessary.
Hyperpyrexia	Administer tepid sponging, fanning, cooling blanket and antipyretic drugs.
Convulsions	Maintain airways; treat promptly with intravenous or rectal benzodiazepine (lorazepam, midazolam or diazepam) or intramuscular paraldehyde.
Hypoglycaemia (blood glucose concentration of <2.2 mmol/L; <40 mg/100 mL)	Check blood glucose, correct hypoglycaemia and maintain with glucose-containing infusion.
Severe anaemia (haemoglobin <5 g/100 mL or packed cell volume <15%)	Transfuse with screened fresh whole blood.
Acute pulmonary oedema[b]	Prop patient up at an angle of 45°, give oxygen, give a diuretic, stop intravenous fluids, intubate and add positive end-expiratory pressure/continuous positive airway pressure in life-threatening hypoxaemia.
Acute renal failure	Exclude pre-renal causes, check fluid balance and urinary sodium; if in established renal failure add haemofiltration or haemodialysis, or if unavailable, peritoneal dialysis. The benefits of diuretics/dopamine in acute renal failure are not proven.
Spontaneous bleeding and coagulopathy	Transfuse with screened fresh whole blood (cryoprecipitate, fresh frozen plasma and platelets if available); give vitamin K injection.
Metabolic acidosis	Exclude or treat hypoglycaemia, hypovolaemia and septicaemia. If severe add haemofiltration or haemodialysis.
Shock	Suspect septicaemia, take blood for cultures; give parenteral antimicrobials, correct haemodynamic disturbances.
Hyperparasitaemia (e.g. >10% of circulating erythrocytes parasitized in non-immune patients with severe disease)	Treat with parenteral antimalarials initially

[a] It is assumed that appropriate antimalarial treatment will have been started in all cases.
[b] Prevent by avoiding excess hydration.

The choice of drugs will depend on the local pattern of resistance where the infection was acquired. Because of the propensity for *P. falciparum* infections to kill, careful assessment of severity is most important. There is obviously a distribution of severity from asymptomatic parasitaemia to fulminant lethal malaria. In practice, any patient who is unable to take oral medication will require parenteral treatment and careful observation, and any impairment of consciousness should be treated seriously. The progression to cerebral malaria can be rapid, particularly in young children.

Management of severe *P. falciparum* malaria (Table 73.15)

Severe malaria is a medical emergency. The airway should be secured in unconscious patients, an intravenous infusion should be started, and other resuscitation measures taken. A rapid clinical assessment of the degree of dehydration and the intravascular volume should be made. Vital signs and capillary refill time should be recorded. Particular attention should be paid to the respiratory pattern and any signs of respiratory distress (laboured deep breathing, flaring of the alar nasae, intercostal or substernal retraction) should be noted. The patient should be weighed if possible so that the antimalarials can be given on a body weight basis (for adults,

a simple method is for the stretcher-bearers to stand on bathroom scales with, and without, the patient). Immediate measurements of blood glucose (stick test), haematocrit, parasitaemia (parasite count, stage of development, and proportion of neutrophils containing malaria pigment) and, in adults, renal function (blood urea or creatinine) should be taken. The degree of acidosis is an important determinant of outcome; the plasma bicarbonate or venous lactate should be measured if possible (lactate rapid stick tests are now available). Arterial or capillary blood pH and gases should be measured in patients who are unconscious, hyperventilating, or shocked. Blood should be taken for cross-match, and later (if available) full blood count, platelet count, clotting studies, blood culture and full biochemistry. Parenteral antimalarial treatment should be given as soon as possible. Where there are adequate nursing facilities the antimalarial drugs should be given by intravenous infusion. There is no specific treatment for severe malaria other than antimalarial drugs. These are potentially life-saving and so it is very important that the dosing is correct (the first dose is by far the most important). Artesunate, which is the best treatment of severe malaria, should be given by intravenous or intramuscular injection, and artemether by intramuscular injection only. If quinine is used, a full loading dose (20 mg dihydrochloride salt/kg) should be given to all patients unless there is a clear history of adequate pre-treatment.[336,495,818,819] The quinoline antimalarials (chloroquine, quinine, quinidine) are compatible with saline or dextrose solutions. They should *never* be given by bolus intravenous injection. The assessment of fluid balance is critical in severe malaria. In children there is not a consensus as to optimum fluid management. Some children are clearly 'dry' on admission and need rehydration. Urgent blood transfusion is required for severely anaemic (haematocrit <15%) acidotic children, but the role of colloids otherwise remains controversial. In adults, there is a thinner dividing line between overhydration, which may precipitate pulmonary oedema, and underhydration which may contribute to shock or precipitate or worsen acidosis and renal impairment. Careful and frequent evaluations of the jugular venous pressure, peripheral perfusion, capillary refill, venous filling, skin turgor and urine output should be made. Where there is uncertainty over the jugular venous pressure, and if nursing facilities permit, a central venous catheter should be inserted and the pressure (CVP) measured directly. The CVP should be maintained between 0 and 5 cm. If the venous pressure is elevated (usually because of over-enthusiastic fluid administration), and the patient becomes breathless they should be nursed with the head at 45° and if necessary intravenous furosemide given. Acidotic breathing or respiratory distress, particularly in severely anaemic children, often indicates hypovolaemia and requires prompt rehydration and, if available, rapid blood transfusion.[318] Convulsions should be treated promptly with intravenous or rectal lorazepam (or midazolam or if unavailable, diazepam) or intramuscular paraldehyde. The role of prophylactic anticonvulsants is unresolved (see below).

When these immediate measures have been completed, a more detailed clinical examination should be conducted, with particular note of the level of consciousness and record of the coma score. Several coma scores have been advocated. The Glasgow coma scale (GCS)[820] is suitable for adults, and the simple Blantyre modification (BCS)[401] is readily performed in children (Table 73.16). Unconscious patients must have a diagnostic lumbar puncture to exclude bacterial meningitis. The opening pressure should be recorded and the rise and fall with respiration noted. The CSF should be sent for microscopic analysis, culture, and measurement of glucose, lactate and protein. Subsequent clinical observations should be as frequent as possible and should include vital signs, with an accurate assessment of respiratory rate and pattern, assessment of the coma score, and urine output. The blood glucose should be checked, using rapid stick tests every 4 h if possible, until recovery of consciousness. These stick tests may overestimate the frequency of hypoglycaemia so laboratory confirmation may be necessary. Important milestones on the road to recovery are the time to recover consciousness (GCS 15 or BCS 5), time to drink, and times to sit unaided and walk.

Cerebral malaria

When managing a patient who is unconscious with severe malaria, the physician must exclude, as far as possible, continuous seizure activity and hypoglycaemia as the cause. Both are more common in children than in adults. Many adjuvant therapies have been suggested, based on the prevailing pathophysiology hypothesis of

Table 73.16 Suitable coma scales to assess levels of consciousness in adults and children

The Blantyre coma scale for children	Score[a]	The modified Glasgow coma scale for adults	Score
BEST MOTOR RESPONSE		**BEST MOTOR RESPONSE**	
Localizes painful stimulus[b]	2	Obeys commands	6
Withdraws limb from pain[c]	1	Localizes pain	5
Non-specific or absent response	0	Withdraws limb from pain	4
		Flexion to pain	3
		Extension to pain	2
		None	1
VERBAL RESPONSE		**VERBAL RESPONSE**	
Appropriate cry	2	Oriented	5
Moan or inappropriate cry	1	Confused	4
None	0	Inappropriate words	3
		Incomprehensible sounds	2
		None	1
EYE MOVEMENTS		**EYE OPEN**	
Directed (e.g. follows mother's face)[d]	1	Spontaneously	4
Not directed	0	To speech	3
		To pain	2
		Never	1

[a] Total score can range from 0 to 5; 2 or less indicates 'unrousable coma'.
[b] Painful stimulus: rub knuckles on patient's sternum.
[c] Painful stimulus: firm pressure on thumbnail bed with horizontal pencil.
[d] Total score can range from 3 to 15; 'Unrousable coma' reflects a score of <9.

the time. These include heparin, low molecular weight dextran, urea, high-dose corticosteroids, aspirin, prostacyclin, pentoxifylline (oxpentifylline), desferrioxamine, anti-TNF antibody, ciclosporin and hyperimmune serum. Unfortunately, none has proved to be beneficial, and several have proved harmful.[821–827] None of these adjuvants should be used. The cornerstone of management is good intensive care and adequate appropriate antimalarial treatment.

Prophylactic phenobarbitone prevents seizures in cerebral malaria. But the role of prophylactic anticonvulsants is uncertain, since a large double-blind trial in Kenyan children with cerebral malaria showed a doubling of mortality in children receiving a single prophylactic intramuscular injection of phenobarbitone (20 mg/kg). Mortality was increased in children who received three or more doses of diazepam (i.e. had recurrent treated seizures), which suggests a possible interaction between these two drugs, and points to respiratory depression as the lethal effect.[827] Thus, the standard loading dose of phenobarbitone is contraindicated unless the patient can be ventilated. Some physicians give a smaller dose of phenobarbitone in unconscious patients, others do not give any seizure prophylaxis and rely on treatment. The safety and effectiveness of phenytoin, fosphenytoin and other anticonvulsants is not well characterized. The role of osmotic agents to treat raised intracranial pressure in cerebral malaria also remains uncertain. Although approximately 80% of children with cerebral malaria have moderately elevated pressures at lumbar puncture (whereas in adults 80% of pressures are in the normal range) and some children have very high pressures, there is no evidence that use of osmotic agents (such as mannitol) influences outcome. Those factors known to exacerbate raised intracranial pressure such as uncontrolled seizures and hypercapnoea should be treated promptly. Specific management includes care of the unconscious patient, careful fluid balance, rapid treatment of convulsions, treatment of hyperpyrexia, and early detection and treatment of other manifestations or complications of severe malaria. If there is any respiratory abnormality, or there are repeated seizures the patient should be ventilated, but great care should be taken to avoid hypercapnoea as the patient is intubated.

Hypoglycaemia should be suspected in any patient who deteriorates suddenly, and this should be treated empirically if glucose stick tests are unavailable. Supervening bacterial infections are common, particularly chest infections and catheter-related urinary tract infections, and spontaneous septicaemia may occur. Bacteraemia is more common in African children than in adults studied in South-east Asia. There is undoubtedly diagnostic overlap between severe malaria and bacterial septicaemia with incidental parasitaemia, but there is also a genuine predisposition to septicaemia in severe malaria. Empirical broad-spectrum antibiotics should certainly be given to any patient who deteriorates suddenly and in whom hypoglycaemia has been excluded, but many consider that all children with severe malaria in moderate and high transmission should receive antibiotics on admission. Aspiration pneumonia commonly follows generalized seizures. Patients should be nursed on their sides, and turned frequently. The role of prone positioning has not been studied. Most children will recover consciousness within 2 days, and most adults within 3 days. Rarely adults may remain unconscious for as long as 10 days. Obviously, with longer periods of coma complications such as pressure sores and secondary infections become increasingly likely, and parenteral nutrition is required.

Fluid balance

Children with severe malaria may be dehydrated, but renal failure and pulmonary oedema are extremely unusual in young children. A common mistake is to be too cautious in giving blood to an anaemic acidotic child for fear of precipitating 'congestive failure'. Recent studies indicate that anaemic congestive failure is uncommon, and that respiratory distress in these children represents metabolic acidosis not pulmonary oedema.[36,317,318] The acidosis is aggravated by anaemia and hypovolaemia.

In approximately 50% of adults admitted with severe malaria there is evidence of renal impairment. In the majority of these, there will be a transient period of oliguria, followed by uncomplicated recovery, but a minority will progress to established acute tubular necrosis. A polyuric phase is unusual. Adults with severe malaria are very vulnerable to fluid overload and the physician treads a narrow path between underhydration, and thus worsening renal impairment, and overhydration, with the risk of precipitating pulmonary oedema. Following admission, patients should be rehydrated carefully to a CVP of between 0 and 5 cm with 0.9% (normal) saline or other isotonic electrolyte solutions. Thereafter, the daily fluid requirements will depend on urine output (plus diarrhoea) and insensible losses, which can be considerable in febrile patients nursed in hot environments. Water and glucose are provided by 5% or 10% dextrose solutions. It is not possible to generalize on initial fluid requirements as these can vary from deficits of several litres to patients who are admitted oliguric and unconscious but well hydrated with a slightly elevated jugular venous pressure. Each patient's requirements should be assessed individually. It is well worth spending some time establishing clearly the level of the jugular venous pressure and if in doubt inserting a CVP line. If blood glucose is <4 mmol/L, then 10% glucose should be started following saline replacement; if it is <2.2 mmol/L, then hypoglycaemia should be treated immediately (0.3–0.5 g/kg of glucose). The fluid regimen must also be tailored around infusion of the antimalarial drugs. Artesunate and artemether are simple injections but quinine infusions must be rate controlled. Some physicians prefer to put the 24-h quinine maintenance dose in one 500 mL bottle of 0.9% saline or 5% dextrose water and infuse this at constant rate, whilst adjusting fluid balance as necessary through a separate piggy-backed line. Giving potassium or other electrolyte supplements can be guided by plasma concentration measurements. It is not usually necessary in the initial phase of management. Many patients will require blood transfusion. The exact criteria for transfusion will depend on blood availability, but in general, if the haematocrit falls below 20% then blood should be given, although in high transmission settings, this would necessitate too many transfusions. The lower threshold of 15% haematocrit is often used. In adults with severe malaria where there is a greater danger of precipitating pulmonary oedema, transmission of packed cells may be indicated. In practice, if blood is allowed to sediment in a bag or bottle, only the cells can be given. If the patient is volume overloaded the transfusion should be stopped, or continued very slowly adding furosemide (0.3 mg/kg) to each unit.

Acute renal failure

If the patient remains oliguric (<0.4 mL of urine/kg per hour), despite adequate rehydration, and the blood urea or creatinine are rising or already high, then fluids should be restricted to replace insensible losses only. Haemofiltration or dialysis should be started early particularly when there is evidence of multiple organ dysfunction. The role of dopamine and loop diuretics in preventing the progression of renal failure is controversial.[241] There is no evidence they are beneficial. Renal failure is hypercatabolic in the acute phase of the disease, and once conventional indications for dialysis have been reached (i.e. metabolic acidosis, uraemic complications, volume overload, or less commonly hyperkalaemia) the patient may deteriorate quickly or die suddenly. An electrocardiogram should be performed if acute renal failure is suspected and an immediate blood potassium measurement is unavailable. If there are signs of hyperkalaemia (peaked T waves, widening of the QRS complex) then calcium and glucose plus insulin should be given immediately. The tempo of disease is faster in patients with acute disease and multiple organ dysfunction, and dialysis should be started earlier than in those whose renal failure develops *after* other acute manifestations have resolved. Haemofiltration or haemodialysis are preferable to peritoneal dialysis. Haemofiltration is associated with a considerably more rapid resolution of biochemical abnormalities and a lower mortality than peritoneal dialysis. Despite the coagulopathy associated with severe malaria, bleeding problems are unusual. After the initial outlay for the pumps and balance, haemofiltration is also less expensive, although well-trained nursing care is essential. When there is no alternative to peritoneal dialysis the addition of hypertonic dextrose to the peritoneal dialysate can be used to remove excess fluid, and also to provide glucose in hypoglycaemic cases. The efficiency of peritoneal dialysis often improves after the first 24 h. Reduced peritoneal clearance is thought to be related to sequestration in the peritoneal microvasculature during the acute phase. Peritonitis (cloudy dialysis effluent) is relatively common if dialysis is continued for >72 h. The dose of quinine should be reduced by between one-third and one-half on the third day of treatment. Tetracycline is contraindicated, but doxycycline can still be given. The median time to recovery of urine flows (>20 mL/kg per 24 h) is 4 days. The overall prognosis and rate of recovery is better in oliguric than in anuric cases (Figure 73.29).

Patients with blackwater fever should be managed in the same way as other patients. Parenteral quinine should not be stopped unless an artemisinin derivative is available for substitution (both have been associated with blackwater). The preventative or therapeutic role of urinary alkalinization in blackwater fever has not been evaluated yet. Blood transfusion is often needed but the increase in haematocrit is often less than predicted because of the brisk haemolysis of the transfused cells. If the patient is volume overloaded, but needs blood, then dialysis or haemofiltration must be given first to create enough vascular 'space' for the blood. Packed cells should be given and the transfusion administered as slowly as possible.

Case history

A 46-year-old Brazilian forestry official was admitted to a large provincial hospital with a 5-day history of fever and malaise. Four

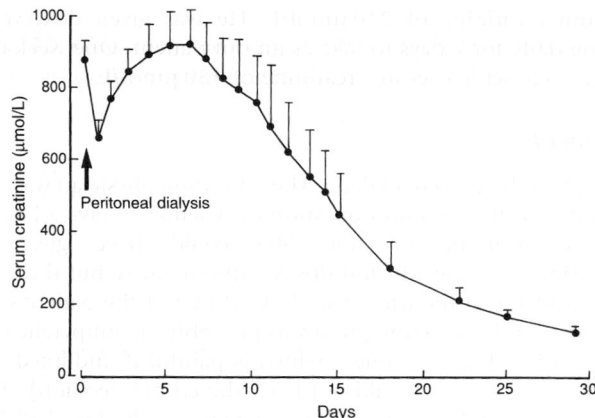

Figure 73.29 Recovery from malarial acute renal failure. This results from acute tubular necrosis. Many patients will not become oliguric, despite a rising serum creatinine in the first few days of hospitalization, and can be managed conservatively.

days previously, he had attended a health clinic and was told he had malaria. An intramuscular injection was given, and he was given three large white tablets to take immediately. A further 6 tablets were prescribed: two to be taken every 4–6 h. On direct questioning, he said that the injection was not painful (and looked like water), that the tablets were not particularly bitter, and that he did not have subsequent ringing in the ears or deafness. His symptoms did not improve, and so he left for the city. When he arrived, he was still febrile and felt ill so he consulted his private practitioner who gave him more white tablets (two to be taken three times daily) and red/yellow capsules (one to be taken four times daily). He found this medicine extremely bitter. By the time of admission he had taken four white tablets and two capsules, but had vomited twice the previous evening.

On examination, he was lucid, but slightly agitated, jaundiced and anaemic. His oral temperature was 38.7°C. He was slightly dehydrated; the blood pressure was 100/70 and the pulse 120/min. The cardiovascular and respiratory systems were normal, but the liver and spleen were both enlarged. The haematocrit was 24%, and the thick blood film showed a heavy P. falciparum parasitaemia with gametocytes. The thin film count was 58/1000 red cells (no mature parasites with pigment were seen). An urgent serum creatinine was 4.1 mg/dL (360 μmol/L) and blood glucose 72 mg/dL (4.0 mmol/L). The admitting physician put up an intravenous infusion and, after considering the history of previous treatment, gave a loading dose of quinine dihydrochloride (20 mg salt/kg) over 4 h. This was followed by further infusions of 10 mg/kg 8-hourly. The next day the serum creatinine had risen to 5.5 mg/dL (485 μmol/L), with a blood urea nitrogen of 120 mg/dL, but the serum potassium was 4.6 mmol/L and the urine output 1500 mL (positive balance 1200 mL). The parasite count was 22/1000 red cells. The following day, the serum creatinine was 6.3 mg/dL (554 μmol/L), the potassium 4.8 mmol/L and the urine output 1800 mL, but the fever had improved and the patient felt better. The quinine dose was reduced to 10 mg/kg 12-hourly. Thereafter, the patient improved steadily, and the serum creatinine fell. The fever clearance time was 74 h and parasite clearance time 82 h. The patient was discharged after 10 days with

molytic anaemia in Nigeria.[830] This often requires transfusion, in addition to antimalarial treatment and folate supplementation.

Uncomplicated malaria

Symptomatic malaria in pregnancy requires hospitalization where possible. Premature labour may occur and pregnant women receiving quinine are liable to develop hypoglycaemia. Chloroquine, pyrimethamine, proguanil, quinine and the sulphonamides are considered safe in pregnancy. Amodiaquine has been widely used but not well documented.[831] There is increasing evidence that the artemisinin derivatives are safe in the second and third trimesters,[752,753,830] but there is uncertainty in the first trimester, where they are not recommended. Mefloquine has been associated with a four-fold increased risk of stillbirth in Thailand,[654] but not in Malawi,[655] so there is some uncertainty over its safety. There is increasing confidence in the safety of artemether-lumefantrine and some preliminary experience with atovaquone-proguanil. Halofantrine and dihydroartemisinin-piperaquine, and have not been evaluated and should not be used. The tetracyclines and primaquine are contraindicated. As a consequence, the four established first-line artemisinin combination treatments are recommended for the treatment of *falciparum* malaria in the second and third trimesters. Quinine (10 mg salt/kg three times daily for 7 days) is still the treatment of choice for resistant *falciparum* malaria in the first trimester. The artemisinin derivatives and quinine should both be combined with clindamycin (10 mg/kg twice daily) to increase cure rates. Treatment failure rates are higher in pregnant women than in non-pregnant adults for any antimalarial regimen.[832] Pharmacokinetic studies indicate that blood concentrations of the artemisinin derivatives, lumefantrine, atovaquone, sulfadoxine, and proguanil are all significantly reduced in late pregnancy, so current dose recommendations may not be optimal.[696,743,761] Close follow-up of pregnant women is essential. Women in malarious areas should be encouraged to attend weekly antenatal clinics where blood smears and haematocrit can be checked, in addition to routine obstetric assessment.

Prophylaxis

If effective in the area and safe, antimalarial prophylaxis should be given during pregnancy.[833] Chloroquine (5 mg base/kg per week) is generally still very effective in preventing *P. vivax. P. ovale* and *P. malariae*. Unfortunately *P. falciparum* is usually present at the same time and usually resistant. In areas where *P. falciparum* is still sensitive to antifols daily proguanil (3.5 mg/kg per day) is safe and effective. There are some concerns over mefloquine in treatment use, although there is no significant evidence of an increased stillbirth risk when used as prophylaxis. Primaquine and doxycycline are contraindicated, and atovaquone-proguanil has not been evaluated yet.

Intermittent presumptive treatment (IPTp)

Studies conducted in high transmission areas of Africa have shown that administration of treatment doses of sulphadoxine-pyrimethamine (SP) two or three times during pregnancy was associated with reduced placental parasitization, reduced anaemia, and increased birth weight.[834] IPTp with SP has been increasingly adopted (although there have not yet been any pharmacokinetic studies of SP IPTp in pregnancy). More frequent administration is required in HIV-positive women. SP IPTp should not be given if co-trimoxazole is already being given. The beneficial effects of SP IPTp are still evident when failure rates with SP treatment in young children are high, which indicates that maternal immunity adds significantly to the pharmacological effect. SP IPTp is therefore still recommended by WHO. Since the original studies were conducted, resistance has worsened considerably in Africa.[835–840] It is not clear at what level of resistance SP IPTp is no longer cost-effective. Alternative drugs are under evaluation. There has been no consensus on whether IPTp should be used in low transmission settings nor on how IPTp works, although the simplest explanation is that it provides suppressive prophylaxis.

Breast-feeding

Nearly all the antimalarial drugs appear in breast milk, but where they have been measured the actual amounts excreted are small. Primaquine should be avoided, but otherwise there seems no reason to discourage breast-feeding in women receiving antimalarial drugs.

Case history

A 30-year-old female aid worker who was 28 weeks' pregnant returned to the UK from a project in rural western Cambodia. One week later, she developed headache, malaise and low-grade fever. She was found to have a *P. falciparum* infection; the peripheral blood parasite count was 48 000/µL, and she was referred to hospital. She had no relevant past medical history. In Cambodia, she had used repellents (DEET) and slept under an insecticide treated bed net but had not taken antimalarial prophylaxis. On examination, she was listless and febrile (oral temperature 38.9°C) but there were no other abnormal clinical or obstetric findings. As she was able to take fluids and there were no signs of severe malaria, she was given oral artemether-lumefantrine (4 tablets 80/480 mg) in a single dose on arrival at hospital, but 15 min later, she vomited. The dose was therefore repeated and this time the drug was retained. The next morning, her fever was higher (up to 40.4°C) but the parasite count had fallen risen to 5500/µL, and she remained lucid and able to sit and drink. Thereafter, the fever gradually subsided, the parasitaemia cleared (in 48 h), and she felt steadily better. She completed her 3-day six dose course of ACT, and was discharged after 5 days. But, 35 days after discharge, she was readmitted with fever and uterine contractions. There were no signs of fetal distress. A blood smear was again positive for *P. falciparum*; the count was 1800/µL. She was readmitted and treated with initially intravenous and then oral quinine (10 mg salt/kg three times daily). Her contractions stopped within 24 h but on the second day, she collapsed. She was found to be hypoglycaemic (plasma glucose 1.4 mmol/L) and this responded immediately to parenteral dextrose. The fever and parasitaemia resolved within 4 days and she was discharged with instructions to finish a 7-day course of treatment. Three weeks later (now 38 weeks' gestation), she returned to hospital in labour with a recurrence of symptoms. On examination, she was apyrexial but gave a history of fever, and she was clinically anaemic. The spleen tip was palpable. The blood smear was again positive (count 560/μL). She admitted having taken quinine for only 5 days in total because she was continually nauseated, had several episodes which she took to be hypoglycaemia, and felt the drug gave her a constant buzzing in the ears and made her dizzy. She was readmitted to hospital and 8 h later delivered a healthy 2.6 kg baby girl. She was treated with a supervised 3-day course of atovaquone-proguanil. Her haematocrit was 27% and the blood film was normochromic and normocytic. Iron and folic acid treatment was started. Thereafter she made an uncomplicated recovery, and had no further recrudescences of malaria.

Comment

Treating symptomatic malaria in late pregnancy is not easy! If possible these patients need hospitalization and careful monitoring. This case illustrates several points.

- Although infection risks are low in many parts of South-east Asia, there are still many forest fringe and forest areas where transmission occurs. The main vectors (*A.dirus* and *A.minimus*) in this area characteristically bite early in the evening before people go to sleep under their bed nets, and often before they apply insect repellents.
- Pregnant women are at increased risk from *falciparum* malaria and there is no suitable reliable prophylaxis; mefloquine resistance is prevalent, primaquine and doxycycline are contraindicated, and atovaquone-proguanil has not been sufficiently evaluated.[657]
- Vomiting after administration of oral antimalarials to patients with high fever is common. If vomiting occurs within 1 h the dose should be repeated, as was done in this case. If possible, the fever should have been brought down with antipyretics and tepid sponging and the patient made comfortable before being given the antimalarial treatment.
- Artemether-lumefantrine is generally a well tolerated and rapidly effective treatment for multi-drug resistant *falciparum* malaria. There are data now for artemisinin-derivatives in over 1000 prospectively studied women which attest to their safety in the second and third trimesters of pregnancy.
- This patient's infection was resistant. Both host and parasite factors may have contributed to treatment failure. Blood concentrations of artemether (and its active metabolite dihydroartemisinin) and lumefantrine in late pregnancy are approximately half those in non-pregnant adults.[761] The conventional 3-day, 6 dose, artemether-lumefantrine regimen may have been insufficient. In addition, resistant strains of *P. falciparum* are now prevalent in western Cambodia and eastern Thailand, and treatment responses following artemether-lumefantrine and artesunate-mefloquine are worse there than anywhere else in the world.[841–842]
- For parenteral treatment, artesunate is definitely preferable: it is simpler, safer and more effective (but for some reason not recommended for the treatment of severe malaria in the UK!). Quinine is poorly tolerated and is associated with a significant risk of hypoglycaemia in late pregnancy, particularly in patients with severe malaria (risk; 50%). Treatment failure rates with quinine alone are over 50% in non-immune pregnant women with *falciparum* malaria acquired in Cambodia and Thailand.

Poor adherence to the prescribed regimen is a major contributor to this poor therapeutic response, as in this case. If all doses had been taken then the addition of clindamycin to quinine would have increased the probability of cure to over 90%.
- By contrast atovaquone-proguanil is very well tolerated and has no adverse effects although published experience in pregnancy is confined to two pharmacokinetic studies which indicate that, as for artemether-lumefantrine, plasma levels are significantly reduced in late pregnancy.[696,700,761] This patient was fortunate then not to have had a further recrudescence.
- The suggested treatments for recrudescent infections are shown in Table 73.13.
- Anaemia is a common consequence of treatment failure in malaria, and a particular complication of malaria in later pregnancy.
- Malaria during pregnancy causes intrauterine growth retardation, and may have contributed to the relatively low birth weight. Symptomatic malaria near term often provokes labour, as in this case.

MALARIA IN CHILDREN

The greatest burden of malaria morbidity and mortality is in young children. Although maternal malaria is very common, congenital malaria is surprisingly rare given the high frequency with which placental smears are positive in endemic areas, and the not infrequent finding of parasites in cord blood smears.[843] Nevertheless, it may occur with any of the four human malarias. Congenital *falciparum* malaria is seldom severe. Congenital *P. vivax* or *P. ovale* infections do not require radical treatment as there are no pre-erythrocytic stages in the baby. Primaquine should not be given to neonates.

Severe malaria is relatively uncommon in the first 6 months of life, although when it does occur, the mortality is high. In young children, malaria presents as a febrile illness without focal signs. In *P. falciparum* infections, convulsions are an important complication in the first 3 years. They are twice as common as in *P. vivax* malaria, despite similar fever profiles. The progression to cerebral malaria in young children can be very rapid. Recovery is also rapid compared with adults. In areas of intense transmission, severe anaemia in the 1–3 year age group is the principal manifestation of severe *falciparum* malaria. A comparison of the relative frequencies of complications in adults and children is shown in Table 73.17.

Table 73.17 Relative incidence of severe *falciparum* malaria complications

	Non-pregnant adults	Pregnant women	Children
Anaemia	+	++	+++
Convulsions	+	+	+++
Hypoglycaemia	+	+++	+++
Jaundice	+++	+++	+
Renal failure	+++	+++	−
Pulmonary oedema	++	+++	+/−

Most of the deaths from malaria are in children and most of those are in Africa. Malaria is also an important cause of morbidity, failure to thrive, and probably increased susceptibility to other infections. Repeated attacks of fever and chronic anaemia are extremely common where malaria is not controlled. School attendance and performance are adversely affected. Whether cerebral malaria, malaria-associated convulsions, or the debilitating effects of repeated weakening febrile illnesses and anaemia cause developmental or intellectual retardation needs to be determined. There is now evidence for learning difficulties in children who have had seizures in malaria and in cerebral malaria survivors.[430-432] In general, children tolerate the antimalarial drugs better than adults. In severe malaria, fluid balance is also easier as renal failure is very unusual. However, the difficulties of providing adequate nursing in the tropics, of obtaining intravenous access, and the small volumes of intravenous fluid required often mean that antimalarial drugs are given by the intramuscular, subcutaneous or suppository routes. Children may deteriorate very rapidly in severe malaria. Sudden death is common in cerebral malaria but, if the child survives, recovery is more rapid than in adults. Iron deficiency is common in tropical countries and commonly co-exists with malaria. In general the benefits of iron supplementation in confirmed iron-deficiency, both on short-term anaemia and long-term neurocognitive development, outweigh the risks.[28] But a recent large carefully controlled study from Pemba, Tanzania shows clearly that the risks of death or severe illness of providing routine iron plus folic acid supplementation (in doses similar to those recommended by WHO) to young children exposed to high rates of malaria infection outweighed any immediate benefits.[29]

MALARIA WITH LIMITED RESOURCES

The majority of patients with malaria in the world are either untreated or treated inadequately by self-medication. In many countries, the private sector is the main source of antimalarial treatment. Fake or substandard drugs are common and incomplete treatment courses are often sold. Education of the public and the private commercial vendors is vitally important. Coherent and efficient schemes for the purchase and distribution of quality assured drugs are needed. In order to slow the pace of antimalarial resistance it is essential that whoever gives antimalarial treatment (parent, relative, village health worker, shop assistant) ensures a full course of treatment is administered. Most treatment regimens now are 3-day courses.

Most patients with severe malaria are not admitted to hospital; they are treated at home or at rural health clinics. Most deaths from malaria occur in or near home. Where intravenous infusions cannot be given, intramuscular administration is acceptable for quinine or the artemisinin derivatives. It is essential that sterile technique is adhered to fully. Artesunate intrarectal formulations are simple and effective alternatives to parenteral administration, and as a pre-referral treatment they have been shown to reduce the mortality of children (under 5 years) with malaria who cannot take oral medication by 25%. Where injections or suppositories are not possible then oral, or, if a tube is available, nasogastric instillation should be attempted, pending transfer of the patient.

The problem facing most tropical countries is serious. Their governments cannot afford to buy sufficient antimalarial drugs for

Table 73.18 Cost of antimalarial treatment for a 60 kg adult

Drug	US$[a]
Atovaquone-proguanil	30.0
Halofantrine	5.0
Artemether–lumefantrine	1.0[b]
Artesunate–mefloquine	2.5
Artesunate–amodiaquine	<1.0
Artesunate–sulphadoxine–pyrimethamine	<1.0
Artesunate	1.2
Quinine	1.5
Amodiaquine	0.30
Sulphadoxine–pyrimethamine	0.13
Chloroquine	0.10

[a] 2007 prices.
[b] Only through WHO approved sources.

their needs and most people cannot afford to purchase effective treatments.[842] The annual *per capita* expenditure on antimalarial drugs in most of sub-Saharan Africa is still <US$10. An adult (60 kg) course of chloroquine costs US$0.08, but the new artemisinin combinations cost more than five times this (Table 73.18). This is currently unaffordable to most patients. It is clear that if malaria is to be 'rolled back' then international financial support must be given to offset the costs of providing adequate treatment throughout the world.

PREVENTION

Insecticide treated bed nets

Insecticide spraying and insecticide-treated bed nets are the main methods of attacking the vector and controlling malaria. The chances of being bitten by a malaria-infected female anopheline mosquito can also be reduced considerably by simple measures. Covering exposed skin surfaces and remaining indoors or under a net at peak biting times will obviously reduce exposure. For example, most mosquitoes feed at night; sleeping indoors under insecticide (permethrin, deltamethrin)-treated bed nets reduces morbidity and mortality in malarious areas. A single impregnation of a cotton or nylon mosquito net will provide protection for 1 year.[845,846] Nylon tends to retain permethrin and deltamethrin better than cotton. The impregnated bed nets (ITN) can be washed and can tolerate small tears or holes without markedly reducing the protective effects. Recently, 'long lasting nets' have been developed which retain insecticidal activity for years. These are more expensive but may be cost-effective. At the time of writing, two types of long-lasting nets have received recommendations from the WHO Pesticide Evaluation Scheme (Olyset®, Sumitomo Chemical Co, Japan; and PermaNet® 1.0, Vestergaard-Frandsen, Denmark), although more are under development. The benefits conferred by bed nets depend greatly on the biting habits of the mosquito, the size and constitution of the nets, whether they are impregnated with insecticide, the number of nets being used in the village, and a variety of sociological factors that determine actual use of the nets in practice. The much lower protective efficacy of unimpregnated bed nets is variable and depends very much on the way in which they are used (Do they have holes? Are they tucked under the mattress?, etc.). These considerations are relatively unimportant for ITNs. In some studies, unimpregnated nets have not demonstrated protective efficacy. The use of ITNs has proved remarkably effective in some areas. In a pivotal study from The Gambia, use of ITNs reduced overall childhood mortality by 60%,[846] whereas earlier studies had shown malaria to account for approximately one-quarter of deaths in this age group, i.e. the reduction in mortality was over twice that expected.[847] This suggested either that malaria mortality had been seriously underestimated or that the debilitating effects of malaria may predispose to other infections, and consequent mortality. Many ITN studies have been conducted since and these give an overall estimated mortality reduction of 20%.[848–853] As a consequence, many countries have taken up ITN programmes as an important component of their antimalarial strategy. Unfortunately, even in areas where striking benefits have been demonstrated the proportion of people who have an ITN is still disappointingly low.[850] Despite subsidies, cost remains a significant barrier to their deployment. This emphasizes the importance of economic, educational, logistic and operational difficulties in limiting the success of proven effective antimalarial interventions. ITN deployment is a public good. Ideally ITN should be fully subsidised and donated free. Impregnation of household curtains, hammocks, clothing, or even cattle has been shown to reduce malaria.[854,855] It has been assumed that ITNs work mainly through personal protection, but their mass insecticidal effect may be more important in some contexts.[669] Thus, the protection afforded by sleeping without a net in a village where ITNs are used extensively, may be greater than sleeping under an ITN in a village where no-one else uses them!

Impregnated nets are effective throughout Africa but do not work in some other areas (notably parts of South-east Asia), because of different human and mosquito behaviour. If malaria is contracted by vectors which bite in the early evening or early morning away from human habitation then ITNs are not very effective.

Repellents

Other simple preventive measures, including the application of permethrin or deltamethrin to clothing or the use of insect repellents such as diethyltoluamide (DEET) on exposed skin surfaces, are also effective and need not be prohibitively expensive. DEET is generally very safe, including in pregnancy.[856] Coconut oil and DEET 'soap bar' preparations are available, which are cheap, stable and readily applied. Houses can be mosquito proofed by using wire-mesh grilles over windows, and designed in such a way as to discourage mosquito ingress. All these measures reduce the chances of an infection, but they do not eliminate it.

Chemoprophylaxis

Although the early colonists devised many ingenious methods of taking quinine regularly (including 'Indian tonic water'), they were generally neither pleasant nor fully effective. Quinine (a poor prophylactic) was relied upon by armies and colonists until after the Great War. The subsequent discovery of mepacrine (quinacrine, atebrine) in 1934 gave the Allied Powers an efficacious, albeit rather toxic, prophylactic, which prevented malaria effectively during World War II. However, it was the introduction of chloroquine, the antimalarial biguanides, and subsequently pyrimethamine after the war, that finally brought safe and effective antimalarial prophylaxis.[857] The DHFR inhibitors (pyrimethamine, proguanil, chlorproguanil) and atovaquone inhibit parasite development in the liver (pre-erythrocytic activity) and in the erythrocyte. They are sometimes called causal prophylactics. These drugs also inhibit development in the mosquito (sporontocidal activity). Chloroquine and mefloquine inhibit asexual blood-stage development but do not prevent development of the liver stages. Thus, the parasites emerge from the liver but cannot multiply in the red cells. Drugs with this action are called suppressive prophylactics. These drugs also have gametocytocidal activity against *P. vivax*, *P. malariae* and *P. ovale*, but not *P. falciparum*. Atovaquone-proguanil, doxycycline and primaquine have been added to the list of antimalarial prophylactics.[858] Each is active against resistant *P. falciparum* but each must be taken daily. Antimalarial prophylaxis must be taken regularly to ensure therapeutic (i.e. suppressive) antimalarial concentrations are maintained. Recommendations vary considerably, depending on risk, prevalence and drug resistance. Up-to-date recommendations are easily obtained on the internet (e.g. http://www.who.int) (Figure 73.30, for current World Health Organization recommendations for antimalarial prophylaxis by region). Increasing drug resistance in recent years has meant that many prophylactic drugs can no longer be relied upon, particularly in areas of multiple drug resistance such as South-east Asia and South America.[849–851]

The recommended prophylactic drug regimens are shown in Table 73.19. When prescribing antimalarial prophylaxis to travellers, it is important to emphasize that no antimalarial is completely effective, and that a febrile illness could still be malaria. It is essential that prophylaxis is taken regularly, and for most drugs continued for 4 weeks after leaving the transmission area. The need to take the drugs for a month after leaving the transmission area is to 'catch' any parasites acquired shortly before departure when they leave the liver. But drugs acting on the liver stages (atovaquone-proguanil, primaquine) can be stopped immediately (many advocate continuing for 1 week after exposure to ensure prevention). This is a particular advantage for travellers visiting a malarious area for a short time. It is prudent to begin prophylaxis 1 week before departing for a malarious area so that tolerance to the drug regimen can be assessed, and therapeutic concentrations are present on arrival. In some situations where the risks of acquiring *vivax* malaria are high (such as in military personnel), a full 2-week course of primaquine is given on leaving the endemic area. This is called 'terminal prophylaxis' and aims to eradicate hypnozoites. In anglophone countries, chloroquine is prescribed weekly, but in francophone countries it is given once daily (this is theoretically preferable). Mefloquine and pyrimethamine-dapsone are taken once a week and proguanil, atovaquone-proguanil, primaquine and doxycycline daily. Amodiaquine, quinine, sulphadoxine-pyrimethamine and the artemisinin drugs should not be used for prophylaxis.

In situations where the risk of infection is low, or there are no effective antimalarials available, or there is brief repeated exposure

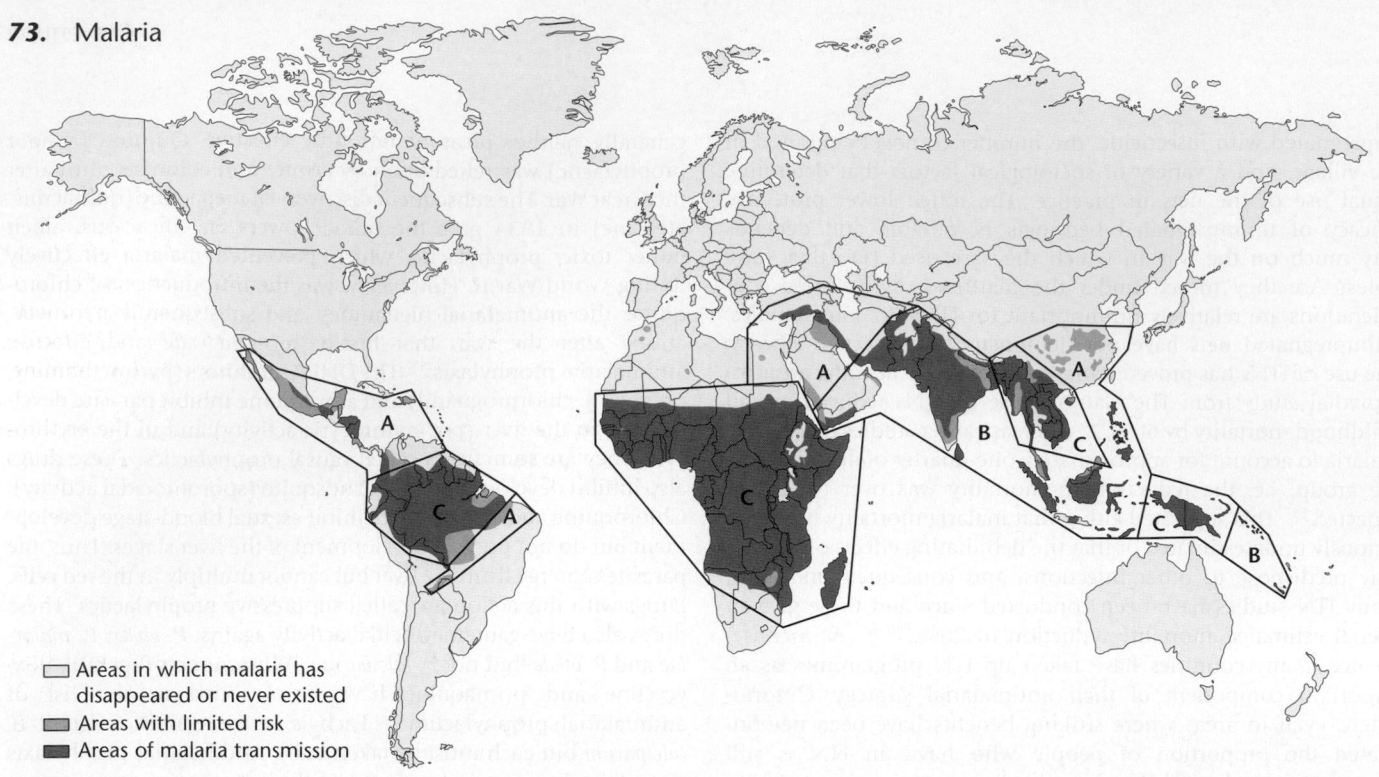

Figure 73.30 WHO recommendations for antimalarial prophylaxis.

Table 73.19 Antimalarial chemoprophylaxis

	Weight adjusted dose for children	Adult dose
CHLOROQUINE-SENSITIVE MALARIA		
Chloroquine[a]	5 mg base/kg weekly, or	300 mg base
	1.6 mg base/kg daily	100 mg base
and/or		
Proguanil	3.5 mg/kg daily	200 mg base
CHLOROQUINE-RESISTANT MALARIA		
Mefloquine[b]	5 base/kg weekly	250 mg base
or		
Doxycycline[c]	1.5 mg/kg daily	100 mg
or		
Primaquine	0.5 mg base/kg daily with food	30 mg base
or		
Atovaquone–proguanil	4/1.6 mg/kg daily	250/100 mg

Detailed local knowledge of *P. falciparum* antimalaria susceptibility and malaria risk should always be obtained.

[a] Chloroquine should not be taken by people with a history of seizures, generalized psoriasis or pruritus previously on chloroquine.

[b] Mefloquine is not recommended for babies <3 months of age. Mefloquine should not be taken by people with psychiatric disorders, epilepsy, or those driving heavy vehicles, trains, aeroplanes etc. or deep sea diving.

[c] Doxycycline may cause photosensitivity. Use of sunscreens is recommended.

For current World Health Organization recommendations see (http://www.who.int).

The WHO divides the world into three risk categories and makes the following recommendations:

A. Malaria risk low and seasonal, and *P. falciparum* is either absent or still sensitive to chloroquine.

This comprises Central America, north of the Panama Canal and northern Columbia, plus the southern and eastern ends of the malarious areas of Brazil, Turkey, Iraq, western Iran, and much of China (except for Yunnan, Hainan, and the areas adjoining Laos and Vietnam).

Prophylaxis: Chloroquine alone or no prophylaxis if very low risk.

B. Low malaria risk in most areas: chloroquine and proguanil still have significant efficacy.

This comprises Saudi Arabia, Yemen, the remainder of Iran, Afghanistan, Pakistan, India (except for the North East), Malaysia, Philippines, most of Indonesia, Micronesia.

Prophylaxis: Chloroquine + proguanil. 2nd choice: mefloquine.

C. Low malaria risk in Asia and most of South America, but high in most of Africa, lowland New Guinea, parts of Micronesia, and the Amazon basin. Drug resistance is more common.

Prophylaxis: 1st choice: mefloquine; 2nd choice: doxycycline. NB doxycycline is first choice for border areas of Cambodia, Myanmar and Thailand; 3rd choice: Chloroquine and proguanil.

to intermediate or high transmission (e.g. aircrews), travellers can be advised to carry a treatment course of antimalarial drugs with them. If they become ill, and there are no medical facilities for malaria diagnosis and treatment, the treatment course is self-administered.

The use of antimalarial prophylaxis by the inhabitants of malarious areas remains controversial.[833] It is generally agreed that pregnant women should take antimalarial prophylaxis if there is a significant risk of malaria, but that other adults should not. Chloroquine, pyrimethamine and proguanil are all considered safe in pregnancy, but are now largely ineffective against *P. falciparum*. Mefloquine is considered safe, although there are uncertainties as treatment use has been associated with stillbirth in one large series. Tetracyclines and primaquine are contraindicated in pregnancy (although some argue that they are safe in first trimester before the formation of fetal bones and dentition, and before the risk of acute fatty liver), and atovaquone-proguanil has not been evaluated. The use of antimalarial prophylaxis by children living in an endemic area has been shown to reduce mortality; in The Gambia administration of pyrimethamine and dapsone (Maloprim) in the 1–4 year age group reduced mortality by 25%.[847] Despite the reduction in mortality, a reduction in the incidence of clinical attacks of malaria and anaemia, improved nutrition and, in older children, a decrease in absenteeism from school, this practice has not been generally adopted, largely because of concerns that widespread deployment of chemoprophylaxis would encourage the spread of drug-resistant parasites and/or inhibit the development of naturally acquired immunity to malaria.

Intermittent preventive treatment in infancy (IPTi), childhood (IPTc) and in adults (IPTa)

Following the success of IPT in pregnancy (IPTp), the strategy of providing a treatment dose of antimalarials to all infants in high transmission settings at the time of EPI immunizations (usually given at 2, 3 and 9 months of age) has been developed. The two drugs evaluated mainly have been SP and, to a much lesser extent, amodiaquine. Although as for IPTp, there is no consensus how IPTi 'works' the most likely explanation is simply that of intermittent prophylaxis. The main benefit demonstrated has been a reduction in the incidence of clinical attacks of malaria and anaemia.[859–868] There has been no effect on mortality in the trials published to date. The initial description of IPTi claimed persistence of protection well into the second year of life, well after complete elimination of SP. Subsequent studies do not support this and indicate that protection following SP is for approximately 1 month only. This is important, as the majority of deaths occur after the first year of life. The benefits have been greatest in areas of high stable transmission. The World Health Organization recognizes the potential value of IPTi, but, because of uncertainty in the risk/benefit assessment and generally declining SP efficacy, does not recommend it currently. Predictably, the benefits of IPTi have been lower in areas of lower seasonal transmission where the major impact of malaria is after the first year of life, but studies in such areas (Senegal and Mali) showed that IPT given to older children during the malaria transmission season (IPTc) was very effective in preventing malaria.[861,862] IPT in older children can be delivered at school. Use of IPT in older children is likely to be

most effective in areas where a high level of malaria transmission is concentrated in a short period of the year. IPT has also been evaluated in parts of Asia where young men in inaccessible forested areas acquire malaria during the rainy season (IPTa). Widescale use of prophylaxis will encourage the selection of reasistance, although modelling studies to date are moderately reassuring. Another concern is that highly effective interventions such as prophylaxis together with ITN deployment might so reduce exposure to malaria that the acquisition of effective immunity was delayed, thereby increasing vulnerability to severe malaria at an older age. Again, the available evidence is reassuring, but more information is needed on these important issues. IPTi is still being evaluated. Several questions need to be addressed if IPTi is to be incorporated generally in malaria control programmes. Does IPTi add to the protection afforded by vector control measures, (ITN and residual spraying which, if applied intensively reduce transmission intensity and shift the distribution of the malaria burden to older children.)? Can an effective and sustainable delivery system be found (EPI is perfect but the ages targeted may be too young)? What drugs should be used (Should ACTs be used?)? What is the optimum timing of drug administration and the requisite interval between treatments? How should IPT be used in lower transmission settings? How much would this contribute to resistance?

Adverse effects of chemoprophylaxis

Adverse effects are a very important determinant of adherence to antimalarial prophylaxis regimens. As those taking the drugs prophylactically are healthy subjects, their tolerance of adverse effects is much lower than in treatment of malaria (where the patient often ascribes side-effects to the disease, and takes the drugs only for a brief period). About 20% of patients taking prophylactic antimalarial drugs report some adverse effects. These are usually minor and do not require a change in prophylaxis. Nausea is the most common side-effect. Chloroquine causes pruritus in subjects of African origin. Dizziness, dysphoria and sleep disturbances are particularly associated with mefloquine, visual disturbances with chloroquine, and photosensitivity and monilia with doxycycline. The risks of neuropsychiatric reactions or seizures are approximately 1 : 10 000, and appear similar for mefloquine and chloroquine.[651–653] There has been much televised publicity over the CNS adverse effects of mefloquine. Minor, but debilitating, CNS effects are reported more commonly in travellers taking mefloquine than in other groups of subjects.[653] Mefloquine prophylaxis should not be offered to subjects with epilepsy, psychiatric disorders, or to subjects in whom any CNS disturbances could have disastrous consequences such as pilots, coach drivers etc.

Primaquine (0.5 mg/kg per day) is well tolerated if taken with food. It should not be given to subjects who are G6PD deficient. Taken on an empty stomach, it causes abdominal discomfort. Atovaquone-proguanil is remarkably well tolerated (similar adverse effects to proguanil alone).

Mass treatment

Treatment of the entire at-risk population has been used in malaria elimination. Responses have been mixed, and this strategy is not generally recommended.[869]

management to flush out mosquito breeding areas, and to provide a hostile aquatic environment for mosquito egg and larval development, is an alternative to drainage. Changing water salinity or allowing organic matter pollution may also reduce vector populations. As always, major alterations to the environment should not be undertaken lightly: short-term benefits may be offset by long-term problems.

Human behaviour

Mosquitoes cannot fly far; most anophelines cannot fly more than 4 km, and in general, they remain within 2 km of their breeding sites. Of course they can be blown further, and occasionally they take plane journeys and deliver malaria around airports in other countries. If humans do not live near breeding sites, the chances of infection are reduced. Many vectors bite inside houses, and the design and protection offered by the dwelling are important determinants of malaria risk. Wire-mesh screens and other mosquito proofing measures are effective but expensive, and may also reduce ventilation. Where domestic species of anophelines exist (e.g. *A. stephensi* in India), water jars, tanks or containers should be closed to prevent mosquito access.[882]

Simple measures such as introducing polystyrene balls to float on top of well water may be remarkably effective. The use of mosquito-proof bed nets prevents human–vector contact, but they are considerably more effective in preventing malaria when impregnated with insect repellents or insecticides.[849] Pyrethroid insecticide (permethrin, deltamethrin)-impregnated nylon nets are best, and now long-lasting nets have been developed which retain activity for many years.[851]

Imagocides

Although chemical agents, such as the larvicide Paris green, and pyrethrum insecticides, had been widely used for vector control before World War II, the discovery of 2,2-bis-(*p*-chlorophenyl)-1,1,1-trichloroethane (DDT), with excellent activity against the adult mosquito (imagocidal activity), was a major advance in malaria control. DDT had residual imagocidal activity, which pyrethrum did not. It could be sprayed on the interior of houses, and would kill or deter mosquitoes for many months afterwards. DDT, along with two other chlorinated hydrocarbon residual insecticides, gamma benzene hexachloride (gamma HCH) and dieldrin were the principal weapons in the campaign to eradicate malaria and they had a tremendous beneficial impact on health and development in the tropics. Imagocides can be classified into three general categories.

Pyrethrins and pyrethroids

The naturally occurring compounds (derived from chrysanthemums) are light sensitive and unstable, but the synthetic pyrethroids (permethrin, deltamethrin) are both highly toxic to mosquitoes and stable, giving good residual activity. A single point mutation (resulting in phenyalanine or serine for leucine at position 1014) in the gene encoding a voltage-gated sodium channel protein is associated with pyrethroid and DDT resistance. Known as the pyrethroid knock down resistance (*kdr*) mutation, it has been found at several different locations, but predominantly in *A. gambiae* in West and South Africa.[884] Insecticide resistance is spreading and may represent a serious threat to the efficacy of impregnated bed nets and vector control.[885–889]

Chlorinated hydrocarbons

(DDT, gamma HCH, dieldrin) are widely used as water-dispersible powders which form an aqueous suspension suitable for spraying. Resistance, human toxicity and ecological concerns have restricted the use of DDT in recent years. This valuable insecticide was vastly overused in the agricultural sector. Use in disease control was relatively modest in comparison. But a global ban on DDT threw the baby out with the bathwater and threatened disease control in some areas where DDT was the only affordable and effective insecticide.[890] Fortunately, the ban has been relaxed for vector-borned disease control. Used appropriately DDT is still a very valuable malaria control tool (e.g. in Kwazulu Natal where *A. funestus* was pyrethroid resistant but DDT sensitive. Combined insecticide spraying and artemether-lumefantrine deployment terminated an epidemic of malaria in the late 1990s).[514] Dieldrin is now considered too toxic to humans and it is no longer used.

Anticholinesterases

These comprise the organophosphorous compounds (malathion, fenitrothion) and the carbamates (propoxur, trimethacarb, bendiocarb). Although resistance to the organophosphates has limited use in some areas, these compounds are still distributed widely. Malathion is the cheapest and most widely used. The anticholinesterases pose a potential health hazard to spraying teams, despite their wide therapeutic ratios.

General principles

Imagocides are also classified either by their portal of entry to the body of the mosquito, or to the method of application. Residual insecticides are applied as a deposit on to surfaces where the mosquitoes will rest (e.g. walls, ceilings). Space sprays fill the air with a mist or fog of insecticide. The choice of insecticide and application method will be determined by the sensitivity and behaviour of the local vectors and the nature of the environment. The anopheline mosquito vectors have countered these chemical assaults by changing their behaviour (resting and feeding preferences) and evolving resistance to the insecticides. This has had drastic consequences: reduced effectiveness; the necessity for more expensive replacements (to which resistance has also developed in some species); a disinclination of the chemical industry to invest further in a difficult and often unprofitable field; and as a consequence an inability of cash-strapped governments to pay for the new insecticides. Over 50 vector species are resistant to one or more of the organochlorine insecticides, over ten are resistant to the organophosphates, and pyrethroid resistance is spreading. Most important, *A. gambiae s.l.*, the dominant vector in Africa, has developed resistance to organochlorine insecticides in many areas. In Central America *A. albimanus* has developed multiple insecticide resistance. In India, the major vectors, *A. culicifacies* and *A. stephensi*, have become resistant to the organochlorines and malathion.

Larviciding

With the problems besetting use of residual imagocidal insecticides, there has been renewed interest in methods of larval control in recent years. These include environmental and water manipulation to prevent creation of mosquito breeding sites, the use of larvivorous fish and bacterial toxins, and the application of chemical agents. Mineral oils were the first larvicides to be employed, and diesel oil is still widely used today. Many of the imagocidal compounds described above are also used for larvicides. However, the organochlorines were highly effective but are no longer recommended because of their adverse environmental impact, and the development of resistance. The organophosphorous compounds are used widely and are relatively safe; for example, compounds such as temephos are safe to warm-blooded animals and fish and can be used to treat potable water.

Overall approach

The objectives of a malaria control programme will depend on the prevailing epidemiological situation, the availability of resources, and feasibility. One size definitely does not fit all! Local entomological knowledge and up-to-date knowledge on the patterns of antimalarial drug susceptibility are essential. Information on patterns of drug resistance is increasingly available through the World Health Organization and World Antimalarial Resistance Network (WARN). The first priority is the reduction of malaria mortality by making available facilities, personnel, diagnostics and drugs for diagnosis and effective treatment. Then activities should focus on reducing malaria morbidity (such programmes should focus on malaria in childhood and malaria in pregnancy), and rely on use of effective drugs and vector control. In low transmission settings, epidemics need to be anticipated. Having 'secured' the situation, it is also necessary to secure those areas free from malaria to prevent re-establishment of the infection. Finally, and in a carefully planned and multifaceted programme, work to eliminate the disease should begin. The Millenium Development Goals set a target of reducing the mortality of children under 5 years of age by two-thirds, and halting and reversing the spread of malaria, by the end of 2015. Now that greater resources are available to tropical countries for malaria control through the Global Fund for AIDS, TB and Malaria, and other national and international donor agencies, a more positive approach to global malaria control can become a reality. This has been given added impetus by Bill and Melinda Gates, who have effectively declared war on malaria, and committed their foundation to a programme of elimination. While increased support for national health structures and malaria control programmes are essential to sustain these initiatives, there is increasing support for a central subsidy for antimalarial drugs both to the public and private sectors such that they cost no more than chloroquine did, and therefore reach even the very remotest areas.[573] This is called the Affordable Medicines for Malaria facility (AMfM). This is a pragmatic approach to the sad reality that in most tropical countries access to affordable quality healthcare through the public sector is limited, so to reach everyone the private sector must also be involved. Similar arguments are made for insectcide-treated bed nets. Exactly how this will be operated remains a subject of considerable debate, but most are agreed that if everyone who needed an ITN and effective drugs actually received them, then malaria would indeed be rolled back, and that in economic terms this would be of tremendous humanitarian benefit and excellent value for the global economy. After decades of pessimism, there is increasing realization that we now have the necessary tools to control malaria.

REFERENCES

1. Bruce-Chwatt LJ. History of malaria from prehistory to eradication. In: Wernsdorfer WH, McGregor I, eds. *Malaria: Principles and Practice of Malariology*. Edinburgh: Churchill Livingstone; 1988:1–59.
2. Smith DC, Sanford LB. Laveran's germ: the reception and use of a medical discovery. *Am J Trop Med Hyg* 1988; 34:2–20.
3. Laveran CLA. Note sur un nouveau parasite trouvé dans le sang de plusieurs malades atteints de fievre palustre. *Bull Acad Med* 1880; 9:1235.
4. Ross R. On some peculiar pigmented cells found in two mosquitos fed on malarial blood. *BM J* 1897; 2:1786–1788.
5. Ross R. *The Prevention of Malaria*. 2nd edn. London: Murray.
6. Bignami A. Come si prendono le febbri malariche. *Boll R Acad Med Roma* 1899; 25:17–46.
7. Wagner-Jauregg J. *Lebenserinnerungen*. In: Schönbauer L. and Jantsch M., eds. Wien: Springer Verlag; 1950:157.8.
8. Cox-Singh J, DavisTM, Lee KS, et al. *Plasmodium* knowlesi malaria in humans is widely distributed and potentially life-threatening. *Clin Infect Dis* 2008; 46(2):165–171.
9. Mu J, Duan J, Makova KD, et al. Chromosome-wide SNPs reveal an ancient origin for *Plasmodium falciparum*. *Nature* 2002; 8; 418:323–326.
10. Joy DA, Feng X, Mu J, et al. Early origin and recent expansion of *Plasmodium falciparum*. *Science* 2003; 300:318–321.
11. Conway DJ, Fanello C, Lloyd JM, et al. Origin of Plasmodium falciparum malaria is traced by mitochondrial DNA. *Mol Biochem Parasitol* 2000; 111:163–171.
12. Price RN, Tjitra E, Guerra CA, et al. Vivax malaria: neglected and not benign. *Am J Trop Med Hyg* 2007; 77(Suppl 6):79–87.
13. Covell G. Spontaneous rupture of the spleen. *Trop Dis Bull* 1955; 52:705–723.
14. Nosten F, McGready R, Simpson JA, et al. The effects of *Plasmodium vivax* malaria in pregnancy. *Lancet* 1999; 354:546–549.
15. Gardner MJ, Hall N, Fung E, et al. Genome sequence of the human malaria parasite *Plasmodium falciparum*. *Nature* 2002; 419:498–511.
16. Gillies MT. Anopheline mosquitos: vector behaviour and bionomics. In: Wernsdorfer WH, McGregor I, eds. *Malaria: Principles and Practice of Malariology*. Edinburgh: Churchill Livingstone; 1988:453–485.
17. MacDonald G. *The Epidemiology and Control of Malaria*. London: Oxford University Press; 1957.
18. Snow RW, Guerra CA, Noor AM, et al. The global distribution of clinical episodes of *Plasmodium falciparum* malaria. *Nature* 2005; 434:214–217.
19. Smith DL, Dushoff J, Snow RW, et al. The entomological inoculation rate and *Plasmodium falciparum* infection in African children. *Nature* 2005; 438:492–495.
20. Greenwood BM, Bradley AK, Greenwood AM, et al. Mortality and morbidity from malaria among children in rural areas of The Gambia, West Africa. *Trans R Soc Trop Med Hyg* 1987; 81:478–486.
21. Smith DL, McKenzie FE. Statics and dynamics of malaria infection in Anopheles mosquitoes. *Malar J* 2004; 3:13.
22. Garnham PCC. *Malaria Parasites and Other Haemosporidia*. Oxford: Blackwell; 1966.
23. Baird JK, Jones TR, Danudirgo EW, et al. Age dependent acquired protection against *Plasmodium falciparum* in people having two years exposure to hyperendemic malaria. *Am J Trop Med Hyg* 1991; 45:65–76.

24. Desai M, ter Kuile FO, Nosten F, et al. Epidemiology and burden of malaria in pregnancy. *Lancet Infect Dis* 2007; 7:93–104.

25. Brabin BJ. Analysis of malaria in pregnancy in Africa. *Bull World Health Organ* 1983; 61:1005–1016.

26. Nosten F, ter Kuile F, Malankirri L, et al. Malaria in pregnancy in an area of unstable endemicity. *Trans R Soc Trop Med Hyg* 1991; 85:424–429.

27. Oppenheimer SJ, Gibson FD, Macfarland SB, et al. Iron supplementation increases prevalence and effects of malaria: report on clinical studies in Papua New Guinea. *Trans R Soc Trop Med Hyg* 1986; 80:603–612.

28. Iannotti LL, Tielsch JM, Black MM, et al. Iron supplementation in early childhood: health benefits and risks. *Am J Clin Nutr* 2006; 84:1261–1276.

29. Sazawal S, Black RE, Ramsan M, et al. Effects of routine prophylactic supplementation with iron and folic acid on admission to hospital and mortality in preschool children in a high malaria transmission setting: community-based, randomised, placebo-controlled trial. *Lancet* 2006; 367:133–143.

30. Breman JG, Mills A, Snow RW, et al. Conquering malaria. In: Jamison DT, Breman G, Measham AR, et al., eds. *Disease Control Prioritiew in Developing Countries.* 2nd edn. New York: Oxford University Press; 2006:413–422.

31. Jamison DT, Breman JG, Measham AR, et al. *Priorities in Health.* Washington DC: World Bank; 2006.

32. Mathers CDA, Lopez AD, Murray CJL. The burden of disease and mortality by condition; data, methods and results for 2001. In: Lopez AD, Mathers CD, Jamison DT, Murray CJL, eds. *Global Burden of Disease and Risk Factors.* New York: Oxford University Press; 2001 45–210.

33. McGregor IA. Epidemiology, malaria and pregnancy. *Am J Trop Med Hyg* 1984; 33:517–525.

34. Pasvol G, Weatherall DJ, Wilson RJM. Effects of fetal hemoglobin on susceptibility of red cells to *Plasmodium falciparum. Nature* 1977; 270:171–173.

35. Smith TA, Leuenberger R, Lengeler C. Child mortality and malaria transmission intensity in Africa. *Trends Parasitol* 2001; 17:145–149.

36. Marsh K, Forster D, Waruiru C, et al. Indicators of life-threatening malaria in African children. *N Engl J Med* 1995; 332:1399–1404.

37. Hendrickse RG, Hasan AH, Olumide LO, et al. Malaria in early childhood. An investigation of five hundred seriously ill children in whom a 'clinical' diagnosis of malaria was made on admission to the Children's Emergency Room at University College Hospital, Ibadan. *Ann Trop Med Parasitol* 1971; 65:1–20.

38. Lindsay SW, Wilkins HA, Zieler HA, et al. Ability of *Anopheles gambiae* mosquitos to transmit malaria during the dry and wet seasons in an area of irrigated rice cultivation in The Gambia. *J Trop Med Hyg* 1991; 94:313–324.

39. Marchiafava E. Pernicious malaria. *Am J Trop Med Hyg* 1932; 21:1–56.

40. McGregor IA. Consideration of some aspects of human malaria. *Trans R Soc Trop Med Hyg* 1965; 59:145–152.

41. Brewster DR, Greenwood BM. Seasonal variation of paediatric diseases in The Gambia, west Africa. *Ann Trop Paediatr* 1993; 13:133–146.

42. Luxemburger C, Kyaw Ley Thew, White NJ, et al. The epidemiology of malaria in a Karen population on the western border of Thailand. *Trans R Soc Trop Med Hyg* 1996; 90:105–111.

43. Garnham PCC. Malaria parasites of man: life cycles and morphology. In: Wernsdorfer WH, McGregor I, eds. *Malaria: Principles and Practice of Malariology.* Edinburgh: Churchill Livingstone; 1988:61–69.

44. Ponnudurai T, Lensen AHW, van-Gemart GJA, et al. Feeding behaviour and sporozoite ejection by infected Anopheles stephensi. *Trans R Soc Trop Med Hyg* 1991; 85:175–180.

45. Rosenburg R, Wirtz RA. An estimation of the number of sporozoites ejected by a feeding mosquito. *Trans R Soc Trop Med Hyg* 1990; 84:209–212.

46. Miller LH, Mason SJ, Clyde DF, et al. The resistance factor to *P. vivax* in Blacks: the Duffy blood group genotype. *N Engl J Med* 1976; 295:302–304.

47. Miller LH. Genetically determined human resistance factors. In: Wernsdorfer WH, McGregor I , eds. *Malaria: Principles and Practice of Malariology.* Edinburgh: Churchill Livingstone; 1988:487–500.

48. Cowman AF, Crabb BS. Invasion of red blood cells by malaria parasites. *Cell* 2006; 124: 755–766.

49. Mayer DC, Kaneko O, Hudson-Taylor DE, et al. Characterization of a *Plasmodium falciparum* erythrocyte-binding protein paralogous to EBA-175. *Proc Natl Acad Sci USA.* 2001; 24; 98:5222–5227.

50. Reed MB, Caruana SR, Batchelor AH, et al. Targeted disruption of an erythrocyte binding antigen in *Plasmodium falciparum* is associated with a switch toward a sialic acid-independent pathway of invasion. *Proc Natl Acad Sci USA* 2000; 97:7509–7514.

51. Cranston HA, Boylan CW, Carroll GL, et al. *Plasmodium falciparum* maturation abolishes physiologic red cell deformability. *Science* 1984; 223:400–402.

52. Suwanarusk R, Cooke BM, Dondorp AM, et al. The deformability of red blood cells parasitized by *Plasmodium falciparum* and *P. vivax. J Infect Dis* 2004; 189:190–194.

53. Pagola S, Stephens PW, Bohle DS, et al. The structure of malaria pigment beta-haematin. *Nature* 2000; 404:307–310.

54. Ginsburg H, Famin O, Zhang J, et al. Inhibition of glutathione-dependent degradation of heme by chloroquine and amodiaquine as a possible basis for their antimalarial mode of action. *Biochem Pharmacol* 1998; 56:1305–1313.

55. Kirk K, Saliba KJ. Targeting nutrient uptake mechanisms in Plasmodium. *Curr Drug Targets* 2007; 8:75–88.

56. Leech JH, Barnwell JW, Miller LH, et al. Identification of a strain-specific malarial antigen exposed on the surface of *Plasmodium falciparum* infected erythrocytes. *J Exp Med* 1984; 159:1567–1575.

57. Kraemer SM, Smith JD. A family affair: var genes, PfEMP1 binding, and malaria disease. *Curr Opin Microbiol* 2006; 9:374–380.

58. Singh B, Kim Sung L, Matusop A, et al. A large focus of naturally acquired *Plasmodium knowlesi* infections in human beings. *Lancet* 2004; 363:1017–1024.

59. Simpson JA, Aarons L, Collins WE, et al. Population dynamics of the *Plasmodium falciparum* parasite within the adult human host in the absence of antimalarial drugs. *Parasitology* 2002; 124:247–263.

60. Simpson JA, Silamut K, Chotivanich K, et al. Red cell selectivity in malaria: a study of multiple infected erythrocytes. *Trans R Soc Trop Med Hyg* 1999; 93:165–168.

61. Chotivanich K, Udomsangpetch R, Simpson JA, et al. Parasite multiplication potential and the severity of falciparum malaria. *J Infect Dis* 2000; 181:1206–1209.

62. Read AF, Nanara A, Nee S, et al. Gametocyte sex ratios as indirect measures of outcrossing rates in malaria. *Parasitology* 1992; 104:387–395.

63. Carlton J, Silva J, Hall N. The genome of model malaria parasites, and comparative genomics. *Curr Issues Mol Biol* 2005; 7:23–37.

64. Gupta S, Anderson RM. Population structure of pathogens: the role of immune selection. *Parasitol Today* 1999; 15:497–501.

65. Anders RF. Multiple cross reactivities amongst antigens of *Plasmodium falciparum* impair the development of protective immunity against malaria. *Parasite Immunol* 1986; 8:529–539.

66. Conway DJ. Molecular epidemiology of malaria. *Clin Microbiol Rev* 2007; 20:188–204.

67. Haldane JBS. Disease and evolution. *Ric Sci* 1949; 19(suppl):68–75.

68. Hill AVS. Malaria resistance genes: a natural selection. *Trans R Soc Trop Med Hyg* 1992; 86:225–226.

69. Allen SJ, O'Donnell A, Alexander ND, et al. Prevention of cerebral malaria in children in Papua New Guinea by South-east Asian ovalocytosis band 3. *Am J Trop Med Hyg* 1999; 60:1056–1060.

70. Weatherall DJ. Thalassaemia and malaria, revisited. *Ann Trop Med Parasitol* 1997; 91:885–890.

71. Ruwende C, Khoo SC, Snow RW, et al. Natural selection of hemi- and heterozygotes for G6P D deficiency in Africa by resistance to severe malaria. *Nature* 1995; 376:246–249.

72. Wambua S, Mwangi TW, Kortok M, et al. The effect of alpha+-thalassaemia on the incidence of malaria and other diseases in children living on the coast of Kenya. *PLoS Med* 2006; 3:e158.

73. Williams TN, Maitland K, Bennett S, et al. High incidence of malaria in alpha-thalassaemic children. *Nature* 1996; 383:522–525.

74. Fairhurst RM, Baruch DI, Brittain NJ, et al. Abnormal display of PfEMP-1 on erythrocytes carrying haemoglobin C may protect against malaria. *Nature* 2005; 435: 1117–1121.

75. Chotivanich K, Udomsangpetch R, Pattanapanyasat K, et al. Hemoglobin E; a balanced polymorphism protective against high parasitemias and thus severe falciparum malaria. *Blood* 2002; 100:1172–1176.

76. Hutagalung R, Wilairatana P, Looareesuwan S, et al. Influence of hemoglobin E trait on the severity of Falciparum malaria. *J Infect Dis* 1999; 179:283–286.

77. Hill AVS, Bennett S, Allsopp CEM, et al. Common West African HLA antigens are associated with protection from severe malaria. *Nature* 1991; 352:595–600.

78. Hill AVS, Elvin J, Willis AC, et al. Molecular analysis of an HLA-disease association: HLA-B53 and resistance to severe malaria. *Nature* 1992; 360:434–439.

79. McGuire W, Hill AV, Allsopp CE, et al. Variation in the TNF-alpha promoter region associated with susceptibility to cerebral malaria. *Nature* 1994; 371:508–510.

80. McGuire W, Knight JC, Hill AV, et al. Severe malarial anemia and cerebral malaria are associated with different tumor necrosis factor promoter alleles. *J Infect Dis* 1999; 179:287–290.

81. Kwiatkowski D. Genetic susceptibility to malaria getting complex. *Curr Opin Genet Dev* 2000; 10:320–324.

82. Williams TN, Mwangi TW, Wambua S, et al. Negative epistasis between the malaria-protective effects of alpha+-thalassemia and the sickle cell trait. *Nat Genet* 2005; 37:1253–1257.

83. White NJ, Krishna S. Treatment of malaria: some considerations and limitations of the current methods of assessment. *Trans R Soc Trop Med Hyg* 1989; 83:767–777.

84. Kitchen SF. Symptomatology: general considerations and falciparum malaria. In: Boyd MF, ed. *Malariology*. Vol. 2. Philadelphia: WB Saunders; 1949:996–1017.

85. James SP, Nichol WD, Shute PG. A study of induced malignant tertian malaria. *Proc R Soc Med* 1932; 25:1153–1186.

86. Fairley NH. Sidelights on malaria in man obtained by subinoculation experiments. *Trans R Soc Trop Med Hyg* 1947; 40:521–676.

87. White NJ, Chapman D, Watt G. The effects of multiplication and synchronicity on the vascular distribution of parasites in falciparum malaria. *Trans R Soc Trop Med Hyg* 1992; 86:590–597.

88. Kwiatkowski D, Nowak M. Periodic and chaotic host parasite interaction in human malaria. *Proc Natl Acad Sci USA* 1990; 88:5111–5113.

89. Wagner-Jauregg D. The treatment of general paresis by inoculation of malaria. *J Nerv Ment Dis* 1922; 55:369–375.

90. Jeffery GM. Epidemiological significance of repeated infections with homologous and heterologous strains and species of Plasmodium. *Bull World Health Organ* 1966; 35:873–882.

91. Schmidt LH. *Plasmodium falciparum* and *Plasmodium vivax* infections in the owl monkey (Aotus trivirgatus). 1. The course of untreated infections. *Am J Trop Med Hyg* 1978; 27:671–702.

92. Silamut K, White NJ. The relationship of stage of parasite development to prognosis in falciparum malaria. *Trans R Soc Trop Med Hyg* 1993; 87:436–443.

93. Phu NH, Day NPJ, Diep TS, et al. Intraleukocytic malaria pigment and prognosis in severe malaria. *Trans R Soc Trop Med Hyg* 1995; 89:197–199.

94. Lyke KE, Diallo DA, Dicko A, et al. Association of intraleukocytic *Plasmodium falciparum* malaria pigment with disease severity, clinical manifestations, and prognosis in severe malaria. *Am J Trop Med Hyg* 2003 Sep; 69(3):253–259.

95. Dondorp AM, Desakorn V, Pongtavornpinyo W, et al. Estimation of the total parasite biomass in acute falciparum malaria from plasma PfHRP2. *PLoS Medicine* 2005; 2:e204.

96. Playfair JHL, Taverne J, Bate CAW, et al. The malaria vaccine: anti-parasite or anti-disease immunity? *Immunol Today* 1990; 11:25–27.

97. Riley EM, Andersson L, Otoo N, et al. Cellular immune responses to *Plasmodium falciparum* antigens in Gambian children during and after an acute attack of falciparum malaria. *Clin Exp Immunol* 1988; 73:17–22.

98. Ciuca M, Baluf L, Chelarescu-Vierum. Immunity in malaria. *Trans R Soc Trop Med Hyg* 1934; 27:619–622.

99. Brown KN, Berzins K, Jarra W, et al. Immune responses to erythrocytic malaria. *Clin Immunol Allergy* 1986; 6:227–249.

100. Bouharoun-Tayoun H, Attanath P, Sabcharoen A, et al. Antibodies that protect humans against *P. falciparum* blood stages do not on their own inhibit parasite growth in vitro but act in co-operation with monocytes. *J Exp Med* 1990; 172:1633–1641.

101. McGilvray ID, Serghides L, Kapus A, et al. Nonopsonic monocyte/macrophage phagocytosis of Plasmodium falciparum-parasitized erythrocytes: a role for CD36 in malarial clearance. *Blood* 2000; 96:3231–3240.

102. Good MF, Doolan DL. Immune effector mechanisms in malaria. *Curr Opin Immunol* 1999; 11:412–419.

103. Yazdani SS, Mukherjee P, Chauhan VS, et al. Immune responses to asexual blood-stages of malaria parasites. *Curr Mol Med* 2006; 6:187–203.

104. Nnalue NA, Friedman MJ. Evidence for a neutrophil-mediated protective response in malaria. *Parasite Immunol* 1988; 10:47–58.

105. Rockett KA, Awburn MA, Aggarwal BB. In vivo induction of nitrite and nitrate by tumor necrosis factor, lymphotoxin and interleukin-1: possible role in malaria. *Infect Immun* 1992; 60:3725–3730.

106. Looareesuwan S, Ho M, Wattanagoon Y, et al. Dynamic alterations in splenic function in falciparum malaria. *N Engl J Med* 1987; 317:675–679.

107. Lee SH, Looareesuwan S, Wattanagoon Y, et al. Antibody dependent red cell removal during *P. falciparum* malaria: the clearance of red cells sensitised with IgG anti-D. *Br J Haematol* 1989; 73:396–402.

108. Ho M, White NJ, Looareesuwan S, et al. Splenic Fc receptor function in host defence and anaemia in acute falciparum malaria. *J Infect Dis* 1990; 161:555–561.

109. Lee MV, Ambrus JL, De Souza JM, et al. Diminished red blood cell deformability in uncomplicated human malaria. A preliminary report. *J Med* 1982; 13:479–485.

110. Marsh K, Howard R. Antigens induced on erythrocytes by *P. falciparum*. Expression of diverse and conserved determinants. *Science* 1986; 231:150–153.

111. Craig A, Scherf A. Molecules on the surface of the *Plasmodium falciparum* infected erythrocyte and their role in malaria pathogenesis and immune evasion. *Mol Biochem Parasitol* 2001; 115:129–143.

112. Webster HK, Brown AE, Chuenchitra C, et al. Characterisation of antibodies to sporozoites in *Plasmodium falciparum* malaria and correlation with protection. *J Clin Microbiol* 1988; 26:923–927.

113. Worku S, Bjorkman A, Troye-Blomberg M, et al. Lymphocyte activation and subset redistribution in the peripheral blood in acute malaria illness: distinct gammadelta+ T cell patterns in *Plasmodium falciparum* and *P. vivax* infections. *Clin Exp Immunol* 1997; 108:34–41.

114. Cohen S, McGregor IA, Carrington S. Gamma-globulin and acquired immunity to human malaria. *Nature* 1961; 192:735–737.

115. McGregor IA, Carrington S, Cohen S. Treatment of East African *P. falciparum* malaria with West African human gamma-globulin. *Trans R Soc Trop Med Hyg* 1963; 50:170–175.

116. Sabcharoen A, Burnouf T, Ouattara D, et al. Parasitologic and clinical response to immunoglobulin administration in falciparum malaria. *Am J Trop Med Hyg* 1991; 45:297–308.

117. Taliaferro WH, Mulligan MW. The histopathology of malaria with special reference to the function and origin of the macrophages in defence. *Indian Med Res Mem* 1937; 29:1–138.

118. Clark IA, Virelizier J-L, Carswell EA, et al. Possible importance of macrophage-derived mediators in acute malaria. *Infect Immun* 1981; 32:1058–1066.

119. Kwiatkowski D, Cannon J, Manogue K, et al. Tumour necrosis factor production in falciparum malaria and in association with schizont rupture. *Clin Exp Immunol* 1989; 77:361–366.

120. Bate CAW, Taverne J, Playfair JHL. Malaria parasites induce TNF production by macrophages. *Immunology* 1988; 64:227–231.

121. Bate CAW, Taverne J, Dave A, et al. Malaria exoantigens induce T-independent antibody that blocks their ability to induce TNF. *Immunology* 1990; 70:315–320.

122. Schofield L, Hackett F. Signal transduction in host cells by a glycosylphosphatidylinositol toxin of malaria parasites. *J Exp Med* 1993; 177:145–153.

123. Boutlis CS, Yeo TW, Anstey NM. Malaria tolerance – for whom the cell tolls? *Trends Parasitol* 2006; 22:371–377.

124. Krishnegowda G, Hajjar AM, Zhu J, et al. Induction of proinflammatory responses in macrophages by the glycosylphosphatidylinositols of *Plasmodium falciparum*: cell signaling receptors, glycosylphosphatidylinositol (GPI) structural requirement, and regulation of GPI activity. *J Biol Chem* 2005; 280:8606–8616.

125. Kern P, Hemmer CJ, Van Damme J, et al. Elevated tumor necrosis factor alpha and interleukin 6 serum levels as markers for complicated *Plasmodium falciparum* malaria. *Am J Med* 1989; 87:139–143.

126. Grau GE, Taylor TE, Molyneux ME, et al. Tumor necrosis factor and disease severity in children with falciparum malaria. *N Engl J Med* 1989; 320:1586–1591.

127. Kwiatkowski D, Hill AVS, Sambou I, et al. TNF concentrations in fatal cerebral, non-fatal cerebral, and uncomplicated *Plasmodium falciparum* malaria. *Lancet* 1990; 336:1201–1204.

128. Ho M, Schollaardt T, Snape S, et al. Endogenous IL-10 modulates proinflammatory response in *Plasmodium falciparum* malaria. *J Infect Dis* 1998; 178:520–525.

129. Karunaweera ND, Grau GE, Gamage P, et al. Dynamics of fever and serum levels of tumour necrosis factor are closely associated during clinical paroxysms in *Plasmodium vivax* malaria. *Proc Natl Acad Sci USA* 1992; 89:3200–3203.

130. Day NPJ, Hien TT, Schollaardt, et al. The pregnostic and pathophysiological role of pro- and anti-inflammatory cytokines in severe malaria. *J Infect Dis* 1999; 180:1288–1297.

131. Perkins DJ, Weinberg JB, Kremsner PG. Reduced interleukin-12 and transforming growth factor-beta1 in severe childhood malaria: relationship of cytokine balance with disease severity. *J Infect Dis* 2000; 182:988–992.

132. Luty AJ, Perkins DJ, Lell B, et al. Low interleukin-12 activity in severe Plasmodium falciparum malaria. *Infect Immun* 2000; 68:3909–3915.

133. Casals-Pascual C, Kai O, Lowe B, et al. Lactate levels in severe malarial anaemia are associated with haemozoin-containing neutrophils and low levels of IL-12. *Malar J* 2006; 5:101.

134. May J, Lell B, Luty AJ, et al. Plasma interleukin-10:Tumor necrosis factor (TNF)-alpha ratio is associated with TNF promoter variants and predicts malarial complications. *J Infect Dis* 2000; 182:1570–1573.

135. Clark IA, Chaudhri G. Tumour necrosis factor may contribute to the anaemia of malaria by causing dyserythropoiesis and erythrophagocytosis. *Br J Haematol* 1988; 70:99–103.

136. van Hensbroek MB, Palmer A, Onyiorah E, et al. The effect of a monoclonal antibody to tumor necrosis factor on survival from childhood cerebral malaria. *J Infect Dis* 1996; 174:1091–1097.

137. Lou J, Lucas R, Grau GE. Pathogenesis of cerebral malaria: recent experimental data and possible applications for humans. *Clin Microbiol Rev* 2001; 14:810–820.

138. Malhotra K, Salmon D, Le Bras J, et al. Susceptibility of *Plasmodium falciparum* to a peroxidase-mediated oxygen-dependent microbicidal system. *Infect Immun* 1988; 56:3305–3309.

139. Raventos-Suarez C, Kaul DK, Maculuso F, et al. Membrane knobs are required for the microcirculatory obstruction induced by *Plasmodium falciparum*-infected erythrocytes. *Proc Natl Acad Sci USA* 1985; 82:3829–3833.

140. MacPherson GG, Warrell MJ, White NJ, et al. Human cerebral malaria: a quantitative ultrastructural analysis of parasitized erythrocyte sequestration. *Am J Pathol* 1985; 119:385–401.

141. White NJ. Molecular mechanisms of cytoadherence in malaria. *Am J Physiol* 1999; 276:C1231–1242.

142. Yipp BG, Anand S, Schollaardt T, et al. Synergism of multiple adhesion molecules in mediating cytoadherence of Plasmodium falciparum-infected erythrocytes to microvascular endothelial cells under flow. *Blood* 2000; 96:2292–2298.

143. Flatt C, Mitchell S, Yipp B, et al. Attenuation of cytoadherence of Plasmodium falciparum to microvascular endothelium under flow by hemodilution. *Am J Trop Med Hyg* 2005; 72:660–665.

144. Silamut K, Phu NH, Whitty C, et al. A quantitative analysis of the microvascular sequestration of malaria parasites in the human brain. *Am J Path* 1999; 155:395–410.

145. Pouvelle B, Buffet PA, Lepolard C, et al. Cytoadhesion of Plasmodium falciparum ring-stage-infected erythrocytes. *Nat Med* 2000; 6:1264–1268.

146. Prommano O, Chaisri U, Turner GD, et al. A quantitative ultrastructural study of the liver and the spleen in fatal falciparum malaria. *South-east Asian J Trop Med Public Health* 2005; 36:1359–1370.

147. Dondorp AM, Pongponratn E, White NJ. Reduced microcirculatory flow in severe *falciparum* malaria: pathophysiology and electron-microscopic pathology. *Acta Trop* 2004; 89:309–317.

148. Beare NA, Taylor TE, Harding SP, et al. Malarial retinopathy: a newly established diagnostic sign in severe malaria. *Am J Trop Med Hyg* 2006; 75:790–797.

149. Dondorp A, Ince C, Charunwatthana P, et al. Direct in vivo assessment of microcirculatory disfunction in severe falciparum malaria. *J Infect Dis* 2008; 197:79–84.

150. Magowan C, Wollish W, Anderson L, et al. Cytoadherence by Plasmodium falciparum-infected erythrocytes is correlated with the expression of a family of variable proteins on infected erythrocytes. *J Exp Med* 1988; 168:1307–1320.

151. Su XZ, Heatwole VM, Wertheimer SP, et al. The large diverse gene family var encodes proteins involved in cytoadherence and antigenic variation of *Plasmodium falciparum*-infected erythrocytes. *Cell* 1995; 82:89–100.

152. Duffy MF, Reeder JC, Brown GV. Regulation of antigenic variation in *Plasmodium falciparum*: censoring freedom of expression? *Trends Parasitol* 2003; 19(3):121–124.

153. Treutiger CJ, Carlson J, Scholander C, et al. The time course of cytoadhesion, immunoglobulin binding, rosette formation, and serum-induced agglutination of *Plasmodium falciparum*-infected erythrocytes. *Am J Trop Med Hyg* 1998; 59:202–207.

154. Magowan C, Nunomura W, Waller KL, et al. *Plasmodium falciparum* histidine-rich protein 1 associates with the band 3 binding domain of ankyrin in the infected red cell membrane. *Biochim Biophys Acta* 2000; 1502:461–470.

155. Winter G, Kawai S, Haeggstrom M, et al. SURFIN is a polymorphic antigen expressed on *Plasmodium falciparum* merozoites and infected erythrocytes. *J Exp Med* 2005; 201:1853–1863.

156. Kyes SA, Rowe JA, Kriek N, et al. Rifins: a second family of clonally variant proteins expressed on the surface of red cells infected with Plasmodium falciparum. *Proc Natl Acad Sci USA* 96:9333–9338.

157. Pouvelle B, Buffet PA, Lepolard C, et al. Cytoadhesion of Plasmodium falciparum ring-stage-infected erythrocytes. *Nat Med* 2000; 6:1264–1268.

158. Roberts DJ, Craig AG, Berendt AR, et al. Rapid switching to multiple antigenic and adhesive phenotypes in malaria. *Nature* 1992; 357:689–692.

159. Horrocks P, Pinches R, Christodoulou Z, et al. Variable var transition rates underlie antigenic variation in malaria. *Proc Natl Acad Sci USA* 2004; 101(30):11129–11134.

160. del Portillo HA, Fernandez-Becerra C, Bowman S, et al. A superfamily of variant genes encoded in the subtelomeric region of *Plasmodium vivax*. *Nature* 2001; 410:839–842.

161. Ockenhouse CF, Klotz FW, Tandon NN, et al. Sequestrin, a CD36 recognition protein on *Plasmodium falciparum* malaria-infected erythrocytes identified by anti-idiotype antibodies. *Proc Natl Acad Sci USA* 1991; 88:3175–3179.

162. Sherman IW, Crandall I, Smith H. Membrane proteins involved in the adherence of *Plasmodium falciparum* infected erythrocytes to the endothelium. *Biol Cell* 1992; 74:161–178.

163. David PH, Hommel M, Miller LH, et al. Parasite sequestration in *Plasmodium falciparum* malaria: spleen and antibody modulation of

cytoadherence of infected erythrocytes. *Proc Natl Acad Sci USA* 1983; 80:5075–5079.

164. Bach O, Baier M, Pullwitt A, et al. Falciparum malaria after splenectomy: a prospective controlled study of 33 previously splenectomized Malawian adults. *Trans R Soc Trop Med Hyg* 2005; 99:861–867.

165. Barnwell JW, Asch AS, Nachman RL, et al. A human 88-kD membrane glycoprotein (CD36) functions in vitro as a receptor for a cytoadherence ligand on *Plasmodium falciparum* infected erythrocytes. *J Clin Invest* 1989; 84:765–772.

166. Ockenhouse CF, Ho M, Tandon NN, et al. Molecular basis of sequestration in severe and uncomplicated *Plasmodium falciparum* malaria. Differential adhesion of infected erythrocytes to CD36 and CD54 (ICAM-1). *J Infect Dis* 1991; 164:163–169.

167. Marsh K, Marsh VM, Brown J, et al. *Plasmodium falciparum*: the behavior of clinical isolates in an in vitro model of infected red blood cell sequestration. *Exp Parasitol* 1988; 65:202–208.

168. Crandall I, Smith H, Sherman IW. *Plasmodium falciparum*: the effect of pH and Ca^{2+} concentration on the in-vitro cytoadherence of infected erythrocytes to amelanotic melanoma cells. *Exp Parasitol* 1991; 73:362–368.

169. Turner GDH, Morrison H, Jones M, et al. An immunohistochemical study of the pathology of fatal malaria: Evidence for widespread endothelial activation and a potential role for intercellular adhesion molecule-1 in cerebral sequestration. *Am J Pathol* 1994; 145:1057–1069.

170. Wassmer SC, Combes V, Candal FJ, et al. Platelets potentiate brain endothelial alterations induced by *Plasmodium falciparum*. *Infect Immun* 2006; 74:645–653.

171. Berendt AR, Simmons DI, Tansey J, et al. Intercellular adhesion molecule-1 is an endothelial cell adhesion receptor for *Plasmodium falciparum*. *Nature* 1989; 341:57–59.

172. Wick TM, Louis V. Cytoadherence of *Plasmodium falciparum* infected erythrocytes to human umbilical vein and human dermal microvascular endothelial cells under shear conditions. *Am J Trop Med Hyg* 1991; 42:578–586.

173. Nash GB, Cooke BM, Marsh K, et al. Rheological analysis of the adhesive interactions of red blood cells parasitized by *Plasmodium falciparum*. *Blood* 1992; 79:798–807.

174. McCormick CJ, Craig A, Roberts D, et al. Intercellular adhesion molecule-1 and CD36 synergize to mediate adherence of *Plasmodium falciparum*-infected erythrocytes to cultured human microvascular endothelial cells. *J Clin Invest* 1997; 100:2521–2529.

175. Fried M, Duffy PE. Adherence of *Plasmodium falciparum* to chondroitin sulfate A in the human placenta. *Science* 1996; 272:1502–1504.

176. Reeder JC, Cowman AF, Davern KM, et al. The adhesion of *Plasmodium falciparum*-infected erythrocytes to chondroitin sulfate A is mediated by *P. falciparum* erythrocyte membrane protein 1. *Proc Natl Acad Sci USA* 1999; 96:5198–5202.

177. Fried M, Nosten F, Brockman A, et al. Maternal antibodies block malaria. *Nature* 1998; 395:851–852.

178. Fried M, Domingo GJ, Gowda CD, et al. *Plasmodium falciparum*: chondroitin sulfate A is the major receptor for adhesion of parasitized erythrocytes in the placenta. *Exp Parasitol* 2006; 113:36–42.

179. Costa FT, Fusai T, Parzy D, et al. Immunization with recombinant duffy binding-like-gamma3 induces pan-reactive and adhesion-blocking antibodies against placental chondroitin sulfate A-binding *Plasmodium falciparum* parasites. *J Infect Dis* 2003; 188:153–164.

180. Rogerson SJ, Hviid L, Duffy PE, et al. Malaria in pregnancy: pathogenesis and immunity. *Lancet Infect Dis* 2007; 7:105–117.

181. David PH, Handunnetti SM, Leech JH, et al. Rosetting: a new cytoadherence property of malaria-infected erythrocytes. *Am J Trop Med Hyg* 1988; 38:289–297.

182. Handunnetti SM, David PH, Perera KLR L, et al. Uninfected erythrocytes form 'rosettes' around *Plasmodium falciparum* infected erythrocytes. *Am J Trop Med Hyg* 1989; 40:115–118.

183. Udomsangpetch R, Wahlin B, Carlson J, et al. *Plasmodium falciparum*-infected erythrocytes form spontaneous erythrocyte rosettes. *J Exp Med* 1989; 169:1835–1840.

184. Angus BJ, Thanikkul K, Silamut K, et al. Rosette formation in *Plasmodium ovale* infection. *Am J Trop Med Hyg* 1996; 55: 560–561.

185. Udomsangpetch R, Thanikkul K, Pukrittayakamee S, et al. Rosette formation by *Plasmodium vivax*. *Trans R Soc Trop Med Hyg* 1995; 89:635–637.

186. Kaul DK, Roth EF, Nagel RL, et al. Rosetting of *Plasmodium falciparum* infected red blood cells with uninfected red blood cells enhances microvascular obstruction under flow conditions. *Blood* 1991; 78:812–819.

187. Luginbühl A, Nikolic M, Beck HP, et al. Complement factor D, albumin, and IgG anti-band 3 antibodies mimic serum in promoting rosetting of malaria-infected red cells. *Infect Immun* 2007; 75:1771–1777.

188. Carlson J, Helmby H, Hill AVS, et al. Human cerebral malaria: association with erythrocyte rosetting and lack of anti-rosetting antibodies. *Lancet* 1990; 336:1457–1460.

189. Ho M, Davis TME, Silamut K, et al. Rosette formation of P. falciparum infected erythrocytes from patients with acute malaria. *Infect Immun* 1991; 59:2135–2139.

190. Rowe A, Obeiro J, Newbold CI, et al. *Plasmodium falciparum* rosetting is associated with malaria severity in Kenya. *Infect Immun* 1995; 63:2323–2326.

191. al-Yaman F, Genton B, Mokela D, et al. Human cerebral malaria: lack of significant association between erythrocyte rosetting and disease severity. *Trans R Soc Trop Med Hyg* 1995; 89:55–58.

192. Nash GB, O'Brien E, Gordon-Smith EC, et al. Abnormalities in the mechanical properties of red blood cells caused by *Plasmodium falciparum*. *Blood* 1989; 74:855–861.

193. Dondorp AM, Kager PA, Vreeken J, et al. Abnormal blood flow and red blood cell deformability in severe malaria. *Parasitol Today* 2000; 16: 228–232.

194. Pain A, Ferguson DJ, Kai O, et al. Platelet-mediated clumping of *Plasmodium falciparum*-infected erythrocytes is a common adhesive phenotype and is associated with severe malaria. *Proc Natl Acad Sci USA* 2001; 98: 1805–1810.

195. Chotivanich K, Sritabal J, Uomsangpetch R, et al. Platelet-induced autoagglutination of P. falciparum infected red cells and disease severity in Thailand. *J Infect Dis* 2004; 189: 1052–1055.

196. Dondorp AM, Angus BJ, Hardeman MR, et al. Prognostic significance of reduced red cell deformability in severe falciparum malaria. *Am J Trop Med Hyg* 1997; 57:507–511.

197. Dondorp AM, Angus BJ, Chotivanich K, et al. Red cell deformability as a predictor of anemia in severe falciparum malaria. *Am J Trop Med Hyg* 1999; 60:733–737.

198. Schofield L, Grau GE. Immunological processes in malaria pathogenesis. *Nat Rev Immunol* 2005; 5:722–735.

199. Van der Heyde HC, Nolan J, Combes V, et al. A unified hypothesis for the genesis of cerebral malaria: sequestration, inflammation and hemostasis leading to microcirculatory dysfunction. *Trends Parasitol* 2006; 22:503–508.

200. Grau GE, Mackenzie CD, Carr RA, et al. Platelet accumulation in brain microvessels in fatal pediatric cerebral malaria. *J Infect Dis* 2003; 187:461–466.

201. Medana IM, Day NP, Hien TT, et al. Axonal injury in cerebral malaria. *Am J Pathol* 2002; 160:655–666.

202. Medana IM, Turner GD. Human cerebral malaria and the blood-brain barrier. *Int J Parasitol* 2006; 36:555–568.

203. Bhamarapravati N, Boonpucknavig S, Boonpucknavig V, et al. Glomerular changes in acute *Plasmodium falciparum* infection. *Arch Pathol* 1973; 96:298–293.

204. Adam C, Geniteau M, Gougerot-Pocidalo M, et al. Cryoglobulins, circulating immune complexes and complement activation in cerebral malaria. *Infect Immun* 1981; 31:530–535.

205. Neva FA, Howard WA, Glew RH, et al. Relationship of serum complement levels to events of the malarial paroxysm. *J Clin Invest* 1974; 54:451–460.

206. Petchclai B, Chutanondh R, Hiranras S, et al. Activation of classical and alternate complement pathways in acute falciparum malaria. *J Med Assoc Thai* 1977; 60:174–176.

207. Phanuphak P, Hanvanich M, Sakultamrung R, et al. Complement changes in falciparum malaria infection. *Clin Exp Immunol* 1985; 59:571–576.

208. Stevenson MM, Riley EM. Innate immunity to malaria. *Nat Rev Immunol* 2004; 4:169–180.

209. Ho M, Webster HK, Looareesuwan S, et al. Antigen-specific immuno-suppression in human malaria due to *Plasmodium falciparum*. *J Infect Dis* 1986; 153:763–771.

210. Ho M, Webster HK, Green B, et al. Defective production of and response to interleukin 2 in acute falciparum malaria. *J Immunol* 1988; 141:2755–2759.

211. Riley EM, MacLennan C, Kwiatkowski DK, et al. Suppression of in-vitro lymphoproliferative responses in acute malaria patients can be partially reversed by indomethacin. *Parasite Immunol* 1989; 11:509–517.

212. Ho M, Webster HK, Tongtawe P, et al. Increased gamma/delta T cells in acute falciparum malaria. *Immunol Lett* 1990; 25:139–142.

213. Ho M, Webster HK. T cell responses in acute falciparum malaria. *Immunol Lett* 1990; 25:135–138.

214. Hogh B. Clinical and parasitological studies on immunity to Plasmodium falciparum malaria in children. *Scand J Infect Dis* 1996; 102(suppl):1–53.

215. Bouharoun-Tayoun H, Druilhe P. *Plasmodium falciparum* malaria: evidence for an isotype imbalance which may be responsible for delayed acquisition of protective immunity. *J Clin Microbiol* 1992; 60:1473–1481.

216. Brasseur P, Agrapart M, Ballett JJ, et al. Impaired cell mediated immunity in *Plasmodium falciparum* infected patients with high parasitaemia and cerebral malaria. *Clin Immunol Immunopathol* 1983; 27:38–50.

217. Druilhe P, Brasseur P, Agrapart M, et al. T-cell responsiveness in severe *Plasmodium falciparum* malaria. *Trans R Soc Trop Med Hyg* 1983; 77:671–672.

218. Ward KN, Warrell MJ, Rhodes J, et al. Altered expression of human monocyte Fc receptor in *Plasmodium falciparum* malaria. *Infect Immun* 1984; 44:623–626.

219. Allison AC, Houba V, Hendrickse RG, et al. Immune complexes in the nephrotic syndrome of African children. *Lancet* 1969; ii:1232–1237.

220. Davis TME, Suputtamongkol Y, Spencer JL, et al. Measures of capillary permeability in acute falciparum malaria: relation to severity of infection and treatment. *Clin Infect Dis* 1992; 256–266.

221. Maegraith BG, Fletcher A. The pathogenesis of mammalian malaria. *Adv Parasitol* 1972; 10:49–75.

222. Migasena P, Areekul S. Capillary permeability function in malaria. *Ann Trop Med Parasitol* 1987; 81:549–560.

223. Looareesuwan S, Wilairatana P, Krishna S, et al. Magnetic resonance imaging of the brain in cerebral malaria. *Clin Infect Dis* 1995; 21:300–309.

224. Looareesuwan S, Warrell DA, White NJ, et al. Do patients with cerebral malaria have cerebral oedema? A computed tomography study. *Lancet* 1983; i:434–437.

225. Newton CR, Peshu N, Kendall B, et al. Brain swelling and ischaemia in Kenyans with cerebral malaria. *Arch Dis Child* 1994; 70:281–287.

226. Cordoliani YS, Sarrazin JL, Felten D, et al. MR of cerebral malaria. *AJNR Am J Neuroradiol* 1998; 19:871–874.

227. Newton CRJ C, Kirkham FJ, Winstanley PA, et al. Intracranial pressure in African children with cerebral malaria. *Lancet* 1991; 337:573–576.

228. Waller D, Crawley J, Nosten F, et al. Intracranial pressure in childhood cerebral malaria. *Trans R Soc Trop Med Hyg* 1991; 85:362–364.

229. White NJ. Lumbar puncture in cerebral malaria. *Lancet* 1991; 338:640–641.

230. Patankar TF, Karnad DR, Shetty PG, et al. Adult cerebral malaria: prognostic importance of imaging findings and correlation with postmortem findings. *Radiology* 2002; 224:811–816.

231. Warrell DA, Looareesuwan S, Phillips RE, et al. Function of the blood-cerebrospinal fluid barrier in human cerebral malaria: rejection of the permeability hypothesis. *Am J Trop Med Hyg* 1986; 35:882–889.

232. Badibanga B, Dayal R, Depierreux M, et al. Etude des principaux facteurs immunologiques et de la barriere hemato-meningee au cours de la malaria cerebrale chez l'enfant en pays d'endemie (Zaire). *Ann Soc Belg Med Trop* 1986; 66:23–27.

233. Brown HC, Chau TT, Mai NT, et al. Blood-brain barrier function in cerebral malaria and CNS infections in Vietnam. *Neurology* 2000; 55:104–111.

234. Brown H, Rogerson S, Taylor T, et al. Blood-brain barrier function in cerebral malaria in Malawian children. *Am J Trop Med Hyg* 2001; 64:207–213.

235. Newton CR, Hien TT, White NJ. Cerebral malaria. *J Neurol Neurosurg Psychiatry* 2000; 69:433–441.

236. Warrell DA, White NJ, Veall N, et al. Cerebral anaerobic glycolysis and reduced cerebral oxygen transport in human cerebral malaria. *Lancet* 1988; ii:534–538.

237. White NJ, Warrell DA, Looareesuwan S, et al. Pathophysiological and prognostic significance of cerebrospinal-fluid lactate in cerebral malaria. *Lancet* 1985; i:776–778.

238. Maneerat Y, Viriyavejakul P, Punpoowong B, et al. Inducible nitric oxide synthase expression is increased in the brain in fatal cerebral malaria. *Histopathology* 2000; 37:269–277.

239. Arthachinta S, Sitprija V, Kashemsant U. Selective renal angiography in renal failure due to infection. *Aust J Radiol* 1974; 18:446–452.

240. Trang TTM, Phu NH, Vinh H, et al. Acute renal failure in severe falciparum malaria. *Clin Infect Dis* 1992; 15:874–880.

241. Day NP, Phu NH, Mai NT, et al. Effects of dopamine and epinephrine infusions on renal hemodynamics in severe malaria and severe sepsis. *Crit Care Med* 2000; 28:1353–1362.

242. Boonpucknavig V, Sitprija V. Renal disease in acute *Plasmodium falciparum* infection in man. *Kidney Int* 1979; 16:44–52.

243. Hartenblower DL, Kantor GL, Rosen VJ. Renal failure due to acute glomerulonephritis during falciparum malaria. Case report. *Milit Med* 1972; 137:74–76.

244. Barratt JOW, Yorke W. An investigation into the mechanism of production of blackwater. *Ann Trop Med Parasitol* 1909–1910; 3:1–256.

245. Maegraith BG. *Pathological Processes in Malaria and Blackwater Fever*. Oxford: Blackwell; 1948:348–349.

246. James MFM. Pulmonary damage associated with falciparum malaria: a report of ten cases. *Ann Trop Med Parasitol* 1985; 79:123–138.

247. Charoenpan P, Indraprasit S, Kiatboonsri S, et al. Pulmonary edema in severe falciparum malaria. Hemodynamic study and clinicophysiologic correlation. *Chest* 1990; 9:1190–1197.

248. Day NP, Phu NH, Bethell DP, et al. The effects of dopamine and adrenaline infusions on acid-base balance and systemic haemodynamics in severe infection. *Lancet* 1996; 348:219–223.

249. Brooks MH, Malloy JP, Bartelloni PJ, et al. Pathophysiology of acute falciparum malaria. Correlation of clinical and biochemical abnormalities. *Am J Med* 1967; 43:735–744.

250. Chongsuphajaisiddhi T, Kasemuth R, Tajavanija S, et al. Changes in blood volume in falciparum malaria. *South-east Asian J Trop Med Public Health* 1971; 2:344–350.

251. Malloy JP, Brooks MH, Barry KG, et al. Pathophysiology of acute falciparum malaria. II. Fluid compartmentalization. *Am J Med* 1967; 43:745–750.

252. Sowunmi A, Newton CR, Waruiru C, et al. Arginine vasopressin secretion in Kenyan children with severe malaria. *J Trop Pediatr* 2000; 46:195–199.

253. Akech S, Gwer S, Idro R, et al. Volume expansion with albumin compared to gelofusine in children with severe malaria: results of a controlled trial. *PLoS Clin Trials* 2006; 1:e21.

254. Jarvis JN, Planche T, Bicanic T, et al. Lactic acidosis in Gabonese children with severe malaria is unrelated to dehydration. *Clin Infect Dis* 2006; 42:1719–1725.

255. Maitland K, Pamba A, English M, et al. Randomized trial of volume expansion with albumin or saline in children with severe malaria: preliminary evidence of albumin benefit. *Clin Infect Dis* 2005; 40:538–545.

256. Zuckerman A. Recent studies on factors involved in malarial anaemia. *Milit Med* 1966; 131(suppl):1201–1216.

257. Perrin LH, Mackey LJ, Miecher PA. The hematology of malaria in man. *Semin Hematol* 1982; 19:70–82.

258. Abdallah S, Weatherall DJ, Wickramasinghe SN, et al. The anaemia of P. falciparum malaria. *Br J Haematol* 1980; 46:171–183.

259. Looareesuwan S, Davis TME, Pukrittayakamee S, et al. Erythrocyte survival in severe falciparum malaria. *Acta Trop* 1991; 48:263–270.

260. Davis TME, Krishna S, Looareesuwan S, et al. Erythrocyte sequestration and anaemia in severe falciparum malaria. Analysis of acute changes in venous

haematocrit using a simple mathematical model. *J Clin Invest* 1990; 865:793–800.

261. Looareesuwan S, Merry AH, Phillips RE, et al. Reduced erythrocyte survival following clearance of malarial parasitaemia in Thai patients. *Br J Haematol* 1987; 67:473–478.

262. Price RN, Simpson J, Nosten F, et al. Factors contributing to anemia in uncomplicated falciparum malaria. *Am J Trop Med Hyg* 2001; 65(5):614–622.

263. Phillips RE, Looareesuwan S, Warrell DA, et al. The importance of anaemia in cerebral and uncomplicated falciparum malaria: role of complications, dyserythropoiesis and iron sequestration. *J Med* 1986; 58:305–323.

264. Knuttgen HJ. The bone marrow of non-immune Europeans in acute malaria infection: a topical review. *Ann Trop Med Parasitol* 1987; 81:567–576.

265. Vedovato M, De Paoli Vitali E, Dapporto M, et al. Defective erythropoietin production in the anaemia of malaria. *Nephrol Dial Transplant* 1999; 14:1043–1044.

266. Burgmann H, Looareesuwan S, Kapiotis S, et al. Serum levels of erythropoietin in acute *Plasmodium falciparum* malaria. *Am J Trop Med Hyg* 1996; 54:280–283.

267. Burchard GD, Radloff P, Philipps J, et al. Increased erythropoietin production in children with severe malarial anemia. *Am J Trop Med Hyg* 1995; 53:547–551.

268. Griffiths MJ, Ndungu F, Baird KL, et al. Oxidative stress and erythrocyte damage in Kenyan children with severe *Plasmodium falciparum* malaria. *Br J Haematol* 2001; 113:486–491.

269. Joshi P, Alam A, Chandra R, et al. Possible basis for membrane changes in non parasitized erythrocytes of malaria infected animals. *Biochim Biophys Acta* 1986; 862:220–222.

270. Facer CA, Bray RS, Brown J. Direct Coombs' antiglobulin reactions in Gambian children with *Plasmodium falciparum* malaria. I. Incidence and class specificity. *Clin Exp Immunol* 1979; 35:119–127.

271. Facer CA. Direct Coombs' antiglobulin reactions in Gambian children with *Plasmodium falciparum* malaria. II. Specificity of erythrocyte bound IgG. *Clin Exp Immunol* 1980; 39:279–288.

272. Merry AH, Looareesuwan S, Phillips RE, et al. Evidence against immune haemolysis in falciparum malaria in Thailand. *Br J Haematol* 1986; 64:187–194.

273. Charoenlarp P, Vanijanonta S, Chat-Panyaporn P. The effect of prednisolone on red cell survival in patients with falciparum malaria. *SE Asian J Trop Med Public Health* 1979; 10:127–131.

274. Angus B, Chotivanich K, Udomsangpetch R, et al. In-vivo removal of malaria parasites from red cells without their destruction in acute falciparum malaria. *Blood* 1997; 90:2037–2040.

275. Newton P, Chotivanich K, Chierakul W, et al. A comparison of the in vivo kinetics of Plasmodium falciparum ring – infected erythrocyte surface antigen (RESA) positive and negative erythrocytes. *Blood* 2001; 98:450–457.

276. Price RN, Simpson J, Nosten F, et al. Factors contributing to anemia in uncomplicated falciparum malaria. *Am J Trop Med Hyg* 2001; 65:614–612.

277. Jaroonvesama N. Intravascular coagulation in falciparum malaria. *Lancet* 1972; i:221–223.

278. Horstmann RD, Dietrich M. Haemostatic alterations in malaria correlate with parasitaemia. *Blut* 1975; 51:329–333.

279. Sucharit P, Chongsuphajaisiddhi T, Harinasuta T, et al. Studies on coagulation and fibrinolysis in cases of falciparum malaria. *SE Asian J Trop Med Public Health* 1975; 6:33–39.

280. Vogetseder A, Ospelt C, Reindl M, et al. Time course of coagulation parameters, cytokines and adhesion molecules in Plasmodium falciparum malaria. *Trop Med Int Health* 2004; 9:767–773.

281. Pukrittayakamee S, White NJ, Clemens R, et al. Activation of the coagulation cascade in falciparum malaria. *Trans R Soc Trop Med Hyg* 1989; 83:762–766.

282. Holst FG, Hemmer CJ, Foth C, et al. Low levels of fibrin-stabilizing factor (factor XIII) in human Plasmodium falciparum malaria: correlation with clinical severity. *Am J Trop Med Hyg* 1999; 60:99–104.

283. Clemens R, Pramoolsinsap C, Lorenz R, et al. Activation of the coagulation cascade in severe falciparum malaria through the intrinsic pathway. *Brit J Haematol* 1994; 87:100–105.

284. Skudowitz RB, Katz J, Lurie A, et al. Mechanisms of thrombocytopenia in malignant tertian malaria. *BMJ* 1973; ii:515–518.

285. Casals-Pascual C, Kai O, Newton CR, et al. Thrombocytopenia in falciparum malaria is associated with high concentrations of IL-10. *Am J Trop Med Hyg* 2006; 75:434–436.

286. Lee SH, Looareesuwan S, Chan J, et al. Plasma macrophage colony-stimulating factor and P-selectin levels in malaria-associated thrombocytopenia. *Thromb Haemost* 1997; 77:289–293.

287. Essien E. The circulating platelet in acute malaria infection. *Br J Haematol* 1989; 72:589–590.

288. Kelton JG, Keystone J, Moore J, et al. Immune-mediated thrombocytopenia of malaria. *J Clin Invest* 1983; 71:832–836.

289. Looareesuwan S, Davis JG, Allen DL, et al. Thrombocytopenia in malaria. *SE Asian J Trop Med Public Health* 1992; 23:44–50.

290. Supanaranond W, Davis TME, Dawes J, et al. In-vivo platelet activation and anomalous thrombospondin levels in severe falciparum malaria. *Platelets* 1992; 3:195–200.

291. Udeinya IJ, Miller LH. *Plasmodium falciparum*: effect of infected erythrocytes on clotting time of plasma. *Am J Trop Med Hyg* 1987; 37:246–249.

292. Ohnishi K. Serum levels of thrombomodulin, intercellular adhesion molecule-1, vascular cell adhesion molecule-1, and E-selectin in the acute phase of *Plasmodium vivax* malaria. *Am J Trop Med Hyg* 1999; 60:248–250.

293. Boehme MW, Werle E, Kommerell B, et al. Serum levels of adhesion molecules and thrombomodulin as indicators of vascular injury in severe *Plasmodium falciparum* malaria. *Clin Investig* 1994; 72:598–603.

294. Punyagupta S, Srichaikul T, Nitiyanant P, et al. Acute pulmonary insufficiency in falciparum malaria: summary of 12 cases with evidence of disseminated intravascular coagulation. *Am J Trop Med Hyg* 1974; 23:551–559.

295. Reid HA, Nkrumah FK. Fibrin-degradation products in cerebral malaria. *Lancet* 1972; i:218–221.

296. Borochovitz D, Crosley A, Metz J. Intravascular coagulation with fatal haemorrhage in cerebral malaria. *BMJ* 1970; ii:710.

297. World Health Organization, Control of Tropical Diseases. Severe and complicated malaria. 2nd edn. *Trans R Soc Trop Med Hyg* 1990; 84(suppl 2):1–65.

298. Chau TTH, Day NPJ, Chuong LV, et al. Blackwater fever in Southern Vietnam: a prospective descriptive study of 50 cases. *Clin Infect Dis* 1996; 23:1274–1281.

299. Rogier C, Imbert P, Tall A, et al. Epidemiological and clinical aspects of blackwater fever among African children suffering frequent malaria attacks. *Trans R Soc Trop Med Hyg* 2003; 97:193–197.

300. Bruneel F, Gachot B, Wolff M, et al. Resurgence of blackwater fever in long-term European expatriates in Africa: report of 21 cases and review. *Clin Infect Dis* 2001; 32:1133–1143.

301. Buffet PA, Milon G, Brousse V, et al. Ex vivo perfusion of human spleens maintains clearing and processing functions. *Blood* 2006; 107:3745–3752.

302. Urban BC, Hien TT, Day NP, et al. Fatal *Plasmodium falciparum* malaria causes specific patterns of splenic architectural disorganization. *Infect Immun* 2005; 73(4):1986–1994.

303. Chotivanich K, Udomsangpetch R, Dondorp A, et al. The mechanisms of parasite clearance after antimalarial treatment of *Plasmodium falciparum* malaria. *J Infect Dis* 2000; 182:629–633.

304. Buffet PA, Milon G, Brousse V, et al. Ex vivo perfusion of human spleens maintains clearing and processing functions. *Blood* 2006; 107:3745–3752.

305. Karney WW, Tong MJ. Malabsorption in *Plasmodium falciparum* malaria. *Am J Trop Med Hyg* 1972; 21:1–5.

306. Olsson RA, Johnston EH. Histopathologic changes and small bowel absorption in falciparum malaria. *Am J Trop Med Hyg* 1969; 18:355–359.

307. Segal HE, Hall AP, Jewell JS, et al. Gastrointestinal function, quinine absorption and parasite response in falciparum malaria. *SE Asian J Trop Med Public Health* 1974; 5:499–503.

308. Molyneux ME, Looareesuwan S. Menzies IS, et al. Reduced hepatic blood flow and intestinal malabsorption in severe falciparum malaria. *Am J Trop Med Hyg* 1989; 40:470–476.

309. Wilairatana P, Meddings JB, Ho M, et al. Increased gastrointestinal permeability in patients with *Plasmodium falciparum* malaria. *Clin Infect Dis* 1997; 24:430–435.

310. Pukrittayakamee S, White NJ, Davis TME, et al. Hepatic blood flow and metabolism in severe malaria: the clearance of intravenously administered galactose. *Clin Sci* 1992; 82:63–70.

311. Pukrittayakamee S, White NJ, Davis TME, et al. Glycerol metabolism in severe falciparum malaria. *Metabolism* 1994; 43:887–892.

312. Day NP, Phu NH, Mai NT, et al. The pathophysiologic and prognostic significance of acidosis in severe adult malaria. *Crit Care Med* 2000; 28:1833–1840.

313. Pukrittayakamee S, Looareesuwan S, Keeratithakul D, et al. A study of the factors affecting the metabolic clearance of quinine in malaria. *Eur J Clin Pharmacol* 1997; 52:487–493.

314. Taylor TE, Borgstein A, Molyneux ME. Acid-base status in paediatric Plasmodium falciparum malaria. *Q J Med* 1993; 86:99–109.

315. Krishna S, Waller DW, ter Kuile F, et al. Lactic acidosis and hypoglycaemia in children with severe malaria. *Trans R Soc Trop Med Hyg* 1994; 88:67–73.

316. English M, Sauerwein R, Waruiru C, et al. Acidosis in severe childhood malaria. *Q J Med* 1997; 90:263–270.

317. English M, Muambi B, Mithwani S, et al. Lactic acidosis and oxygen debt in African children with severe anaemia. *Q J Med* 1997; 90:563–569.

318. Newton CR, Valim C, Krishna S, et al. and Severe Malaria in African Children Network. The prognostic value of measures of acid/base balance in pediatric falciparum malaria, compared with other clinical and laboratory parameters. *Clin Infect Dis* 2005; 948–957.

319. Jensen MD, Conley M, Helstowski LD. Culture of *Plasmodium falciparum*: the role of pH glucose and lactate. *J Parasitol* 1983; 69:1060–1067.

320. Pfaller MA, Parquette AR, Krogstad DJ, et al. *Plasmodium falciparum*: stage-specific lactate production in synchronized cultures. *Exp Parasitol* 1982; 54:391–396.

321. Vander Jagt D, Hunsaker LA, Campos NM, et al. D-lactate production in erythrocytes infected with *Plasmodium falciparum*. *Mol Biochem Parasitol* 1990; 42:277–284.

322. Davis TME, Benn JJ, Suputtamongkol Y, et al. Lactate turnover and forearm lactate metabolism in severe falciparum malaria. *Endocrinol Metabol* 1996; 3:105–115.

323. Agbenyega T, Angus BJ, Bedu-Addo G, et al. Glucose and lactate kinetics in children with severe malaria. *J Clin Endocrinol Metab* 2000; 85:1569–1576.

324. White NJ, Warrell DA, Chanthavanich P, et al. Severe hypoglycaemia and hyperinsulinaemia in falciparum malaria. *N Engl J Med* 1983; 309:61–66.

325. White NJ, Miller KD, Marsh K, et al. Hypoglycaemia in African children with severe malaria. *Lancet* 1987; i:708–711.

326. Taylor TE, Molyneux ME, Wirima JJ, et al. Blood glucose levels in Malawian children before and during the administration of intravenous quinine in severe falciparum malaria. *N Engl J Med* 1988; 319:1040–1047.

327. English M, Wale S, Binns G, et al. Hypoglycaemia on and after admission in Kenyan children with severe malaria. *Q J Med* 1998; 91:191–197.

328. Dondorp AM, Chau TT, Phu NH, et al. Unidentified acids of strong prognostic significance in severe malaria. *Crit Care Med* 2004; 32:1683–1688.

329. Sasi P, English M, Berkley J, et al. Characterisation of metabolic acidosis in Kenyan children admitted to hospital for acute non-surgical conditions. *Trans R Soc Trop Med Hyg* 2006; 100:401–409.

330. Onongbu IC, Onyeneke EC. Plasma lipid changes in human malaria. *Tropenmed Parasitol* 1983; 34:193–196.

331. Davis TME, Supanaranond W, Pukrittayakamee S, et al. The pituitary-thyroid axis in severe falciparum malaria. *Trans R Soc Trop Med Hyg* 1990; 84:330–335.

332. Davis TME, Pukrittayakamee S, Woodhead JS, et al. Calcium and phosphate metabolism in acute falciparum malaria. *Clin Sci* 1991; 81:297–304.

333. Petithory JC, Lebeau G, Galeazzi G, et al. L'hypocalcemie palustre. Etudes des correlations avec d'autres parametres. *Bull Soc Pathol Exot Filiales* 1983; 76:455–462.

334. Brooks MH, Barry KG, Cirksen WJ, et al. Pituitary-adrenal function in acute falciparum malaria. *AMJ Trop Med Hyg* 1969; 18:872–877.

335. Davis TME, Looareesuwan S, Pukrittayakamee S, et al. Glucose turnover in severe falciparum malaria. *Metabolism* 1993; 42:334–340.

336. Dekker E, Romijn JA, Ekberg K, et al. Glucose production and gluconeogenesis in adults with uncomplicated falciparum malaria. *Am J Physiol* 1997; 272:E1059–1064.

337. Dekker E, Romijn JA, Waruiru C, et al. The relationship between glucose production and plasma glucose concentration in children with falciparum malaria. *Trans R Soc Trop Med Hyg* 1996; 90:654–657.

338. Okitolonda W, Delacollette C, Malengreau M, et al. High incidence of hypoglycaemia in African patients treated with intravenous quinine for severe malaria. *BMJ* 1987; 295:716–718.

339. Davis TME, Karbwang J, Looareesuwan S, et al. Comparative effects of quinine and quinidine on glucose metabolism in normal man. *Br J Clin Pharmacol* 1990; 30:397–403.

340. Davis TME, Pukrittayakamee S, Supanaranond W, et al. Glucose metabolism in quinine-treated patients with uncomplicated falciparum malaria. *Clin Endocrinol (Oxf)* 1990; 33:739–749.

341. Riley EM, Schneider G, Sambou I, et al. Suppression of cell-mediated immune responses to malaria antigens in pregnant Gambian women. *Am J Trop Med Hyg* 1989; 40:131–144.

342. Archibald HM. The influence of malaria infection of the placenta on the incidence of prematurity. *Bull World Health Organ* 1956; 15:842–845.

343. Jelliffe EFP. Low birth weight and malarial infection of the placenta. *Bull World Health Organ* 1968; 38:69–78.

344. Bray RS, Sinden RE. The sequestration of *Plasmodium falciparum* infected erythrocytes in the placenta. *Trans R Soc Trop Med Hyg* 1979; 73:716–719.

345. Brabin BJ. Analysis of malaria in pregnancy in Africa. *Bull World Health Organ* 1983; 61:1005–1016.

346. McGregor IA, Wilson ME, Billewicz WZ. Malaria infection of the placenta in The Gambia, West Africa: its incidence and relationship to stillbirth, birth weight and placental weight. *Trans R Soc Trop Med Hyg* 1983; 77:232–244.

347. Bray RS, Anderson MJ. Falciparum malaria and pregnancy. *Trans R Soc Trop Med Hyg* 1979; 73:427–431.

348. Nosten F, ter Kuile F, Malankirri L, et al. Malaria in pregnancy in an area of unstable endemicity. *Trans R Soc Trop Med Hyg* 1991; 85:424–429.

349. Looareesuwan S, Phillips RE, White NJ, et al. Quinine and severe falciparum malaria in late pregnancy. *Lancet* 1985; ii:4–8.

350. Bygbjerg IC, Lanng C. Septicaemia as a complication of falciparum malaria. *Trans R Soc Trop Med Hyg* 1982; 76:705.

351. Mabey DCW, Brown A, Greenwood BM. *Plasmodium falciparum* malaria and Salmonella infections in Gambian children. *J Infect Dis* 1987; 155:1319–1321.

352. Berkley J, Mwarumba S, Bramham K, et al. Bacteraemia complicating severe malaria in children. *Trans R Soc Trop Med Hyg* 1999; 93:283–286.

353. Walsh AL, Phiri AJ, Graham SM, et al. Bacteremia in febrile Malawian children: clinical and microbiologic features. *Pediatr Infect Dis J* 2000; 19:312–318.

354. Berkley JA, Lowe BS, Mwangi I, et al. Bacteremia among children admitted to a rural hospital in Kenya. *N Engl J Med* 2005; 352:39–47.

355. Bejon P, Berkley JA, Mwangi T, et al. Defining childhood severe falciparum malaria for intervention studies. *PLoS Med* 2007; 4:e251.

356. Marchiafava E, Bignami A. *On Summer–Autumnal Fever*. London: New Sydenham Society; 1894.

357. Dudgeon LS, Clarke C. A contribution to the microscopical histology of malaria. *Lancet* 1917; ii:153–156.

358. Dudgeon LS, Clarke C. An investigation on fatal cases of pernicious malaria caused by Plasmodium falciparum in Macedonia. *Q J Med* 1918; 12:372–390.

359. Gaskell JF, Millar WL. Studies on malignant malaria in Macedonia. *Q J Med* 1920; 13:381–426.

360. Kean BH, Smith JA. Death due to aestivo-autumnal malaria. A resume of one hundred autopsy cases 1925–1942. *Am J Trop Med Hyg* 1944; 24:317–322.

361. Edington GM. Pathology of malaria in West Africa. *BMJ* 1967; i:715–718.

362. Spitz S. Pathology of acute falciparum malaria. *Milit Med* 1946; 99: 555–572.

363. Pongponratn E, Riganti M, Punpoowong B, et al. Microvascular sequestration of parasitized erythrocytes in human falciparum malaria – a pathological study. *Am J Trop Med Hyg* 1991; 44:168–175.

364. Oo MM, Aikawa M, Than T. Human cerebral malaria: a pathological study. *J Neuropathol Exp Neurol* 1988; 46:223–231.

365. Igarashi I, Oo MM, Stanley H, et al. Knob antigen deposition in cerebral malaria. *Am J Trop Med Hyg* 1987; 37:511–515.

366. Boonpucknavig V, Boonpucknavig S, Udomsangpetch R, et al. An immunofluorescent study of cerebral malaria. *Arch Pathol Lab Med* 1990; 114:1028–1034.

367. Medana IM, Day NPJ, Hien TT, et al. Cellular stress and injury responses in the brains of adult Vietnamese patients with fatal Plasmodium falciparum malaria. *Neuropathol Appl Neurobiol* 2001; 27:421–433.

368. Duarte MIS, Corbett CEP, Boulos M, et al. Ultrastructure of the lung in falciparum malaria. *Am J Trop Med Hyg* 1985; 34:31–35.

369. Feldman RM, Singer V. Non-cardiogenic pulmonary edema and pulmonary fibrosis in falciparum malaria. *Rev Infect Dis* 1987; 9:134–139.

370. Anstey NM, Handojo T, Pain MC, et al. Lung injury in *vivax* malaria: pathophysiological evidence for pulmonary vascular sequestration and posttreatment alveolar-capillary inflammation. *J Infect Dis* 2007; 195:589–596.

371. Deller JJ, Cifarelli PS, Berque S, et al. Malaria hepatitis. *Milit Med* 1967; 132:614–620.

372. De Brito T, Barone AA, Faria RM. Human liver biopsy in *P. falciparum* and *P. vivax* malaria. A light and electron microscopy study. *Virchows Arch* 1969; 348:220–229.

373. Corcoran TE, Hegstrom GJ, Zoeckler SJ, et al. Liver structure in non fatal malaria. *Gastroenterology* 1953; 24:53–62.

374. Pongponratn E, Riganti M, Harinasuta T, et al. Electron microscopic study of phagocytosis in human spleen in falciparum malaria. *SE Asian J Trop Med Public Health* 1989; 20:31–39.

375. Weiss L. The spleen in malaria; the role of barrier cells. *Immunol Lett* 1990; 25:165–172.

376. Nguansangiam S, Day NP, Hien TT, et al. A quantitative ultrastructural study of renal pathology in fatal *Plasmodium falciparum* malaria. *Trop Med Int Health* 2007; 129(12):1037–1050.

377. Wickramasinghe SN, Looareesuwan S, Nagachinta B, et al. Dyserythropoiesis and ineffective erythropoiesis in *Plasmodium vivax* malaria. *Br J Haematol* 1989; 72:91–99.

378. Clark HC. The diagnostic value of the placental blood film in aestivo-autumnal malaria. *J Exp Med* 1915; 22:427–444.

379. Walter P, Gavin JF, Blot P. Placental pathologic changes in malaria. *Am J Pathol* 1982; 109:330–342.

380. Rogerson SJ, Pollina E, Getachew A, et al. Infiltrates in response to *Plasmodium falciparum* malaria infection and their association with adverse pregnancy outcomes. *Am J Trop Med Hyg* 2003; 68:115–119.

381. Galbraith RM, Fox H, Hsi B, et al. The human materno–fetal relationship in malaria. II. Histological, ultrastructural and immunopathological studies of the placenta. *Trans R Soc Trop Med Hyg* 1980; 74:61–72.

382. Ismail MR, Ordi J, Menendez C, et al. Placental pathology in malaria: a histological, immunohistochemical, and quantitative study. *Hum Pathol* 2000; 31:85–93.

383. Matteelli A, Caligaris S, Castelli F, et al. The placenta and malaria. *Ann Trop Med Parasitol* 1997; 91:803–810.

384. Shute PG. Malaria. *BMJ* 1951; 11:1280.

385. Looareesuwan S, White NJ, Chittamas S, et al. High rate of Plasmodium vivax relapse following treatment of falciparum malaria in Thailand. *Lancet* 1987; ii:1052–1055.

386. Mason DP, McKenzie FE. Blood-stage dynamics and clinical implications of mixed *Plasmodium vivax–Plasmodium falciparum* infections. *Am J Trop Med Hyg* 1999; 61:367–374.

387. Mayxay M, Newton PN, Pukrittayakamee S, et al. Mixed species malaria infections in humans. *Trends Parasitol* 2004; 20:233–240.

388. Mayxay M, Pukrittayakamee S, Chotivanich K, et al. Identification of cryptic co-infection with Plasmodium falciparum in patients presenting with *vivax* malaria. *Am J Trop Med* 2001; 65:588–592.

389. Luxemburger C, Kyaw Ley Thew, White NJ, et al. The epidemiology of malaria in a Karen population on the western border of Thailand. *Trans R Soc Trop Med Hyg* 1996; 90:105–111.

390. May J, Mockenhaupt FP, Ademowo OG, et al. High rate of mixed and subpatent malarial infections in southwest Nigeria. *Am J Trop Med Hyg* 1999; 61:339–343.

391. Zhou M, Liu Q, Wongsrichanalai C, et al. High prevalence of *Plasmodium malariae* and *Plasmodium ovale* in malaria patients along the Thai-Myanmar border, as revealed by acridine orange staining and PCR-based diagnoses. *Trop Med Int Health* 1998; 3:304–312.

392. Luxemburger C, Ricci F, Nosten F, et al. The epidemiology of severe malaria in an area of low transmission in Thailand. *Trans R Soc Trop Med Hyg* 1997; 91:256–262.

393. Price RN, Nosten F, Luxemburger C, et al. Risk factors for gametocyte carriage in uncomplicated falciparum malaria. *Am J Trop Med Hyg* 1999; 60:1019–1023.

394. Kitchen SF. Vivax malaria. In: Boyd, MF, ed. *Malariology*. Vol. 2. Philadephia: WB Saunders; 1949:1027–1045.

395. Rajgor DD, Gogtay NJ, Kadam VS, et al. Efficacy of a 14-day primaquine regimen in preventing relapses in patients with *Plasmodium vivax* malaria in Mumbai, India. *Trans R Soc Trop Med Hyg* 2003; 97:438–440.

396. Manson P. Experimental proof of the mosquito-malaria theory. *BMJ* 1900; ii:949–951.

397. Manson PT. Experimental malaria; recurrence after nine months. *BMJ* 1901; ii: 77.

398. White NJ. The assessment of antimalarial drug efficacy. *Trends Parasitol* 2002; 18:458–464.

399. Menendez C, Ordi J, Ismail MR, et al. The impact of placental malaria on gestational age and birth weight. *J Infect Dis* 2000; 181:1740–1745.

400. Brabin BJ, Hakimi M, Pelletier D. An analysis of anemia and pregnancy-related maternal mortality. *J Nutr* 2001; 131:604S–614S.

401. Molyneux ME, Taylor TE, Wirima JJ, et al. Clinical features and prognostic indicators in paediatric cerebral malaria: a study of 131 comatose Malawian children. *Q J Med* 1989; 71:441–459.

402. World Health Organization. Severe falciparum malaria. *Trans R Soc Trop Med Hyg* 2000; 94 Suppl 1:S1–90.

403. Waller D, Krishna S, Crawley J, et al. The clinical features and outcome of severe malaria in Gambian children. *Clin Infect Dis* 1995; 21:577–587.

404. Jaffar S, Van Hensbroek MB, Palmer A, et al. Predictors of a fatal outcome following childhood cerebral malaria. *Am J Trop Med Hyg* 1997; 57:20–24.

405. Whitworth J, Morgan D, Quigley M, et al. Effect of HIV-1 and increasing immunosuppression on malaria parasitaemia and clinical episodes in adults in rural Uganda: a cohort study. *Lancet* 2000; 356:1051–1056.

406. Cohen C, Karstaedt A, Frean J, et al. Increased prevalence of severe malaria in HIV-infected adults in South Africa. *Clin Infect Dis* 2005; 41:1631–1637.

407. Hewitt K, Steketee R, Mwapasa V, Whitworth J, French N. Interactions between HIV and malaria in non-pregnant adults: evidence and implications. *AIDS* 2006; 20:1993–2004.

408. Abu-Raddad LJ, Patnaik P, Kublin J. Dual infection with HIV and malaria fuels the spread of both diseases in sub-Saharan Africa. *Science* 2006; 314:1603–1606.

409. Shah SN, Smith EE, Obonyo CO, et al. HIV immunosuppression and antimalarial efficacy: sulfadoxine-pyrimethamine for the treatment of uncomplicated malaria in HIV-infected adults in Siaya, Kenya. *J Infect Dis* 2006; 194:1519–1528.

410. Laufer MK, van Oosterhout JJ, Thesing PC, et al. Impact of HIV-associated immunosuppression on malaria infection and disease in Malawi. *J Infect Dis* 2006; 193:872–878.

411. Van Geertruyden JP, Mulenga M, Mwananyanda L, et al. HIV-1 immune suppression and antimalarial treatment outcome in Zambian adults with uncomplicated malaria. *J Infect Dis* 2006; 194:917–925.

412. Kochar DK, Saxena V, Singh N, et al. *Plasmodium vivax* malaria. *Emerg Infect Dis* 2005; 11:132–134.

413. Anstey NM, Handojo T, Pain MC, et al. Lung injury in vivax malaria: pathophysiological evidence for pulmonary vascular sequestration and posttreatment alveolar-capillary inflammation. *J Infect Dis* 2007; 195:589–596.

414. Friedman JF, Kwena AM, Mirel LB, et al. Malaria and nutritional status among pre-school children: results from cross-sectional surveys in western Kenya. *Am J Trop Med Hyg* 2005; 73:698–704.

415. World Health Organization. Severe falciparum malaria. *Trans R Soc Trop Med Hyg* 2000; 94 Suppl 1:1–90.

416. Lewallen S, Harding SP, Ajewole J, et al. A review of the spectrum of clinical fundus findings in P. falciparum malaria in African children with a proposed classification and grading. *Trans R Soc Trop Med Hyg* 1999; 93:619–622.

417. Looareesuwan S, Warrell DA, White NJ, et al. Retinal haemorrhage, a common physical sign of prognostic significance in cerebral malaria. *Am J Trop Med Hyg* 1983; 32:911–915.

418. Lewallen S, Bakker H, Taylor TE, et al. Retinal findings predictive of outcome in cerebral malaria. *Trans R Soc Trop Med Hyg* 1996; 90:144–146.

419. Lewallen S, White VA, Whitten RO, et al. Clinical-histopathological correlation of the abnormal retinal vessels in cerebral malaria. *Arch Ophthalmol* 2000; 118:924–928.

420. Beare NA, Southern C, Chalira C, et al. Prognostic significance and course of retinopathy in children with severe malaria. *Arch Ophthalmol* 2004; 122:1141–1147.

421. Newton CR, Krishna S. Severe falciparum malaria in children: current understanding of pathophysiology and supportive treatment. *Pharmacol Ther* 1998; 79:1–53.

422. Dover AS, Western KA. Fatalities due to malaria in the United States, 1966–1969. *J Infect Dis* 1970; 121:573–575.

423. Wattanagoon Y, Srivilairit S, Looareesuwan S, et al. Convulsions in childhood malaria. *Trans R Soc Trop Med Hyg* 1994; 88: 426–428.

424. Holding PA, Snow RW. Impact of *Plasmodium falciparum* malaria on performance and learning: review of the evidence. *Am J Trop Med Hyg* 2001; 64(Suppl):68–75.

425. Omanga U, Nithinyurwa M, Shako D, et al. Les hemiplegies au cours de l'acces pernicieux a *Plasmodium falciparum* de l'enfant. *Ann Pediatr* 1983; 30:294–296.

426. Collomb H, Rey M, Dumas M, et al. Les hemiplegies au cours du paludisme aigue. *Bull Soc Med Afr Noire* 1967; 12:791–795.

427. Brewster DR, Kwiatkowski D, White NJ. Neurological sequelae of cerebral malaria in children. *Lancet* 1990; 336:1039–1043.

428. Holding PA, Stevenson J, Peshu N, et al. Cognitive sequelae of severe malaria with impaired consciousness. *Trans R Soc Trop Med Hyg* 1999; 93:529–534.

429. van Hensbroek MB, Palmer A, Jaffar S, et al. Residual neurologic sequelae after childhood cerebral malaria. *J Pediatr* 1997; 131:125–129.

430. Idro R, Carter JA, Fegan G, et al. Risk factors for persisting neurological and cognitive impairments following cerebral malaria. *Arch Dis Child* 2006; 91:142–148.

431. Carter JA, Lees JA, Gona JK, et al. Severe falciparum malaria and acquired childhood language disorder. *Dev Med Child Neurol* 2006; 48:51–57.

432. Carter JA, Neville BG, White S, et al. Increased prevalence of epilepsy associated with severe falciparum malaria in children. *Epilepsia* 2004; 45:978–981.

433. Newton CR, Hien TT, White N. Cerebral malaria. *J Neurol Neurosurg Psychiatry* 2000; 69:433–441.

434. Mai NTH, Day NPJ, Chuong LV, et al. Post-malaria neurological syndrome. *Lancet* 1996; 348:917–921.

435. De Silva HJ, Gamage R, Herath HKN, et al. A delayed onset cerebellar syndrome complicating falciparum malaria. *Ceylon Med J* 1986; 31:147–150.

436. Senanayake N. Delayed cerebellar ataxia: a new complication of falciparum malaria. *BMJ* 1987; 294:1253–1254.

437. Dukes DC, Sealey BJ, Forbes JL. Oliguric renal failure in blackwater fever. *Am J Med* 1948; 45:899–903.

438. Canfield CJ. Renal and hematologic complications of acute falciparum malaria in Vietnam. *Bull NY Acad Med* 1969; 45:1043–1057.

439. Blackie WK. Blackwater fever. *Clin Proc* 1944; 3:272–312.

440. English M, Marsh V, Amukoye E, et al. Chronic salicylate poisoning and severe malaria. *Lancet* 1996; 347:1736–1737.

441. Ross GR. Blackwater fever in Southern Rhodesia in retrospect. *Cent Afr Med J* 1962; 8:294–297.

442. Stone WJ, Hanchett JE, Knepshield JR. Acute renal insufficiency due to *falciparum* malaria. *Arch Intern Med* 1972; 129:620–628.

443. Taylor WR, Canon V, White NJ. Pulmonary manifestations of malaria: recognition and management. *Treat Respir Med* 2006; 5:419–428.

444. Brooks MH, Kiel FW, Sheehy TW, et al. Acute pulmonary edema in falciparum malaria. *N Engl J Med* 1968; 279:732–737.

445. Gurman G, Schlaeffer F, Alkan M, et al. Adult respiratory distress syndrome and pancreatitis as complications of falciparum malaria. *Crit Care Med* 1988; 16:205–206.

446. Fein LA, Rackow EC, Shapiro L. Acute pulmonary edema in *Plasmodium falciparum* malaria. *Am Rev Respir Dis* 1978; 118:425–429.

447. Sullivan J. Pernicious fever: febris algida and febris comatosa. *Med Times Gaz* 1876; 1:277–279.

448. Gage A. Algid malaria. *Ther Gaz* 1926; 50:77–81.

449. Evans JA, May J, Ansong D, et al. Capillary refill time as an independent prognostic indicator in severe and complicated malaria. *J Pediatr* 2006; 149:676–681.

450. Butler T, Weber DM. On the nature of orthostatic hypotension in acute malaria. *Trans R Soc Trop Med Hyg* 1973; 22:439–442.

451. Kofi-Ekue JM, Phiri DED, Mukunyandela M, et al. Severe orthostatic hypotension during treatment of malaria. *BMJ* 1988; 296:396.

452. Supanaranond W, Davis TME, Pukrittayakamee S, et al. Abnormal circulatory control in falciparum malaria: the effects of antimalarial drugs. *Eur J Clin Pharmacol* 1993; 44:325–329.

453. Das BA, Satpathy SK, Mohanty D, et al. Hypoglycaemia in severe falciparum malaria. *Trans R Soc Trop Med Hyg* 1988; 82:197–201.

454. Zucker JR, Lackritz EM, Ruebush TK 2nd, et al. Childhood mortality during and after hospitalization in western Kenya: effect of malaria treatment regimens. *Am J Trop Med Hyg* 1996; 55:655–660.

455. English M. Life-threatening severe malarial anaemia. *Trans R Soc Trop Med Hyg* 2000; 94:585–588.

456. Calis JC, Phiri KS, Faragher EB, et al. Severe anemia in Malawian children. *N Engl J Med* 2008; 358:888–899.

457. Davis TME, Ho M, Supanaranond W, et al. Changes in the peripheral blood eosinophil count in falciparum malaria. *Acta Trop* 1991; 48:243–245.

458. Hviid L, Kurtzhals JAL, Goka BQ Oliver-Commey JO, et al. Rapid reemergence of T cells into peripheral circulation following treatment of severe and uncomplicated *Plasmodium falciparum* malaria. *Infec. Immun* 1997; 65:1090–1093.

459. Pukrittayakamee S, Clemens R, Pramoolsinap C, et al. Polymorphonuclear leukocyte elastase in *Plasmodium falciparum* malaria. *Trans R Soc Trop Med Hyg* 1992; 86:598–601.

460. Miller LH, Makaranond P, Sitprija V, et al. Hyponatraemia in malaria. *Ann Trop Med Parasitol* 1967; 61:265–279.

461. Maitland K, Pamba A, Fegan G, et al. Perturbations in electrolyte levels in Kenyan children with severe malaria complicated by acidosis. *Clin Infect Dis* 2005; 40:9–16.

462. Miller KD, White NJ, Lott LA, et al. Biochemical evidence of muscle injury in African children with severe malaria. *J Infect Dis* 1989; 159:139–142.

463. White NJ, Miller KD, Brown J, et al. Prognostic value of CSF lactate in cerebral malaria. *Lancet* 1987; i:1261.

464. Field JW, Niven JC. A note on prognosis in relation to parasite counts in acute subtertian malaria. *Trans R Soc Trop Med Hyg* 1937; 30:569–574.

465. Field JW. Blood examination and prognosis in acute falciparum malaria. *Trans R Soc Trop Med Hyg* 1949; 43:33–68.

466. Li QQ, Guo X, Jian N, et al. Development state of *Plasmodium falciparum* in the intradermal, peripheral and medullary blood of patients with cerebral malaria. *Natl Med J Chin* 1983; 63:692–693.

467. White NJ, Silamut K. Rapid diagnosis of malaria. *Lancet* 1989; i:435.

468. Humar A, Ohrt C, Harrington MA, et al. Parasight F test compared with the polymerase chain reaction and microscopy for the diagnosis of *Plasmodium falciparum* malaria in travelers. *Am J Trop Med Hyg* 1997; 56:44–48.

469. Tjitra E, Suprianto S, Dyer M, et al. Field evaluation of the ICT malaria P. f/P. v immunochromatographic test for detection of *Plasmodium falciparum* and *Plasmodium vivax* in patients with a presumptive clinical diagnosis of malaria in eastern Indonesia. *J Clin Microbiol* 1999; 37:2412–2417.

470. Tjitra E, Suprianto S, McBroom J, et al. Persistent ICT malaria P. f/P. v panmalarial and HRP2 antigen reactivity after treatment of *Plasmodium falciparum* malaria is associated with gametocytemia and results in false-positive diagnoses of *Plasmodium vivax* in convalescence. *J Clin Microbiol* 2001; 39:1025–1031.

471. Proux S, Hkirijareon L, Ngamngonkiri C, et al. Paracheck-Pf: a new, inexpensive and reliable rapid test for *P. falciparum* malaria. *Trop Med Int Health* 2001; 6:99–101.

472. Chiodini PL, Bowers K, Jorgensen P, et al. The heat stability of Plasmodium lactate dehydrogenase-based and histidine-rich protein 2-based malaria rapid diagnostic tests. *Trans R Soc Trop Med Hyg* 2007; 101:331–337.

473. Mayxay M, Pukrittayakamee S, Chotivanich K, et al. Persistence of Plasmodium falciparum HRP-2 in successfully treated acute falciparum malaria. *Trans R Soc Trop Med Hyg* 2001; 95:179–182.

474. Desakorn V, Silamut K, Angus B, et al. Quantitative measurement of PfHRP2 antigen in blood and plasma; methods and applications. *Trans R Soc Trop Med Hyg* 1997; 91:479–483.

475. Iqbal J, Sher A, Rab A. *Plasmodium falciparum* histidine-rich protein 2-based immunocapture diagnostic assay for malaria: cross-reactivity with rheumatoid factors. *J Clin Microbiol.* 2000; 38:1184–1186.

476. Rickman LS, Long GW, Oberst R, et al. Rapid diagnosis of malaria by acridine orange staining of centrifuged parasites. *Lancet* 1989; i:68–71.

477. Raja RN. Post-mortem examination in cerebral malaria: a new simple method of demonstrating parasites in the capillaries of the brain. *Ind Med Gaz* 1922; 57:298–299.

478. White N. J Qinghaosu (artemisinin): the price of success. *Science* 2008; 320:330–334.

479. Haggis AW. Fundamental errors in the early history of Cinchona. *Bull Hist Med* 1941; 10:568–592.

480. Duran-Reynolds MG. *The Fever Bark Tree.* New York: Doubleday; 1946.

481. Dawson WT. Cinchona alkaloids and bark in malaria. *Int Clin* 1930; 2:121–149.

482. Melville CH. The prevention of malaria in war. In: Ross R, ed. *The Prevention of Malaria.* 2nd edn. London: Murray; 1911:577–599.

483. Taylor N. *Cinchona in Java.* New York: Greenberg; 1945.

484. Coatney GR. Pitfalls in a discovery: the chronicle of chloroquine. *Am J Trop Med Hyg* 1963; 12:121–128.

485. Covell G. Chemotherapy of malaria. *WHO Monograph Series* 1967: 27.

486. Pampana EJ. *A Textbook of Malaria Eradication.* 2nd edn. London: Oxford University Press; 1969.

487. Rozman RS, Canfield CJ. New experimental antimalarial drugs. *Adv Pharmacol Chemother* 1979; 16:1–43.

488. Ding GS. Recent studies on antimalarials in China: a review of literature since 1980. *Int J Exp Clin Chemother* 1988; 1:9–22.

489. Qinghaosu Antimalarial Coordinating Research Group. Antimalarial studies on qinghaosu. *Chin Med J* 1979; 92:811–816.

490. Klayman DL. Qinghaosu (artemisinin). An antimalarial drug from China. *Science* 1985; 228:1049–1055.

491. Jiang JB, Li GQ, Gao XB, et al. Antimalarial activity of mefloquine and qinghaosu. *Lancet* 1982; ii:285–288.

492. Lee IS, Hufford CD. Metabolism of antimalarial sequiterpene lactones. *Pharmacol Ther* 1990; 48:345–355.

493. Li GQ, Guo XB, Jiang R. Clinical studies on treatment of cerebral malaria with qinghaosu and its derivatives. *J Tradit Chin Med* 1982; 2:124–130.

494. Hien TT, White NJ. Qinghaosu. *Lancet* 1993; 341:603–608.

495. White NJ. Antimalarial drug resistance: the pace quickens. *J Antimicrob Chemother* 1992; 30:571–585.

496. Trape JF. The public health impact of chloroquine resistance in Africa. *Am J Trop Med Hyg* 2001; 64(suppl 1–2):12–17.

497. White NJ. Antimalarial drug resistance and mortality in falciparum malaria. *Trop Med Intl Hlth* 1999; 4:469–470.

498. Nosten F, ter Kuile F, Chongsuphajaisiddhi T, et al. Mefloquine-resistant falciparum malaria on the Thai–Burmese border. *Lancet* 1991; 337:1140–1143.

499. Simon F, Le-Bras J, Gaudebout C, et al. Reduced sensitivity of *Plasmodium falciparum* to mefloquine in West Africa. *Lancet* 1988; i:467–468.

500. Brockman A, Price RN, van Vugt M, et al. Plasmodium falciparum antimalarial drug susceptibility on the northwestern border of Thailand during five years of extensive use of artesunate-mefloquine. *Trans R Soc Trop Med Hyg* 2000; 94:537–544.

501. Jambou R, Legrand E, Niang M, et al. Resistance of *Plasmodium falciparum* field isolates to in-vitro artemether and point mutations of the SERCA-type PfATPase6. *Lancet* 2005; 366:1960–1963.

502. Rieckmann KH, Davis DR, Hutton DC. *Plasmodium vivax* resistance to chloroquine? *Lancet* 1989; ii:1183–1184.

503. Baird JK, Sustriayu Nalim MF, Basri H, et al. Survey of resistance to chloroquine by *Plasmodium vivax* in Indonesia. *Trans R Soc Trop Med Hyg* 1996; 90:409–411.

504. Baird JK. Chloroquine resistance in *Plasmodium vivax*. Antimicrob Agents Chemother 2004; 48:4075–4083.

505. Nocht B, Werner H. Beobachtungen uber relative Chininresistenz bei Malaria aus Brasilien. *Dtsch Med Wochenschr* 1910; 36:1557–1560.

506. Verdrager J. Epidemiology of emergence and spread of drug-resistant falciparum malaria in South-east Asia. *SE Asian J Trop Med Public Health* 1986; 17:111–118.

507. Trape JF, Pison G, Preziosi MP, et al. Impact of chloroquine resistance on malaria mortality. *C R Acad Sci III* 1998; 321:689–697.

508. Roper C, Pearce R, Nair S, et al. Intercontinental spread of pyrimethamine-resistant malaria. *Science* 2004; 305:1124.

509. Fontanet AL, Johnston DB, Walker AM, et al. High prevalence of mefloquine-resistant falciparum malaria in eastern Thailand. *Bull World Health Organ* 1993; 71:377–383.

510. Nosten F, Luxemburger C, ter Kuile FO, et al. Treatment of multi-drug resistant *Plasmodium falciparum* malaria with 3-day artesunate-mefloquine combination. *J Infect Dis* 1994; 170:971–977.

511. Nosten F, van Vugt M, Price R, et al. Effects of artesunate-mefloquine combination on incidence of *Plasmodium falciparum* malaria and mefloquine resistance in western Thailand; a prospective study. *Lancet* 2000; 356:297–302.

512. Carrara VI, Sirilak S, Thonglairuam J, et al. Deployment of early diagnosis and mefloquine-artesunate treatment of falciparum malaria in Thailand: the Tak Malaria Initiative. *PLoS Med* 2006; 3:e183.

513. Barat LM. Four malaria success stories: how malaria burden was successfully reduced in Brazil, Eritrea, India, and Vietnam. *Am J Trop Med Hyg* 2006; 74:12–16.

514. Barnes KI, Durrheim DN, Little F, et al. Effect of artemether-lumefantrine policy and improved vector control on malaria burden in KwaZulu-Natal, South Africa. *PLoS Med* 2005 2:e330.

515. Yayon a, Vande Waa JA, Yayon M, et al. Stage dependent effects of chloroquine on *Plasmodium falciparum* in vitro. *J Protozool* 1983; 30:642–647.

516. ter Kuile F, White NJ, Holloway P, et al. *Plasmodium falciparum*: in vitro studies of the pharmacodynamic properties of drugs used for the treatment of severe malaria. *Exp Parasitol* 1993; 76:85–95.

517. White NJ. Assessment of the pharmacodynamic properties of the antimalarial drugs in vivo. *Antimicrob Agents Chemother* 1997; 41:1413–1422.

518. Day NPJ, Diep PT, Ly PT, et al. Clearance kinetics of parasites and pigment-containing leukocytes in severe malaria. *Blood* 1996; 88:4696–4700.

519. White NJ. Why is it that antimalarial drugs do not always work? *Ann Trop Med Parasitol* 1998; 92:449–458.

520. York W, Macfie JWS. Observations on malaria made during treatment of general paralysis. *Trans R Soc Trop Med Hyg* 1924:12–44.

521. Watkins WM, Woodrow C, Marsh K. Falciparum malaria: differential effects of antimalarial drugs on ex vivo parasite viability during the critical early phase of therapy. *Am J Trop Med Hyg* 1993; 49:106–112.

522. Udomsangpetch R, Pipitaporn B, Krishna S, et al. Antimalarial drugs reduce cytoadherence and rosetting of *Plasmodium falciparum*. *J Infect Dis* 1996; 173:691–698.

523. Clyde DF, Shute GT. Resistance of East African varieties of Plasmodium falciparum to pyrimethamine. *Trans R Soc Trop Med Hyg* 1954; 48: 495–500.

524. Peters W. *Chemotherapy and Drug Resistance in Malaria*. 2nd edn. London: Academic Press; 1987.

525. Peterson DS, Walliker D, Wellems T. Evidence that a point mutation in dihydrofolate reductase-thymidylate synthase confers resistance to pyrimethamine in falciparum malaria. *Proc Natl Acad Sci USA* 1988; 85:9114–9118.

526. Imwong M, Pukrittakayamee S, Looareesuwan S, et al. Association of genetic mutations in *Plasmodium vivax* dhfr with resistance to sulfadoxine-pyrimethamine: geographical and clinical correlates. *Antimicrob Agents Chemother* 2001; 45:3122–3127.

527. Nzila A. The past, present and future of antifolates in the treatment of *Plasmodium falciparum* infection. *J Antimicrob Chemother* 2006; 57: 1043–1054.

528. Imwong M, Pukrittayakamee S, Renia L, et al. Novel point mutations in the dihydrofolate reductase gene of *Plasmodium vivax*: evidence for sequential selection by drug pressure. *Antimicrob Agents Chemother* 2003; 47:1514–1521.26, 527.

529. Biswas S, Escalante A, Chaiyaroj S, et al. Prevalence of point mutations in the dihydrofolate reductase and dihydropteroate synthetase genes of *Plasmodium falciparum* isolates from India and Thailand: a molecular epidemiologic study. *Trop Med Int Health* 2000; 5:737–743.

530. Anderson TJ, Nair S, Sudimack D, et al. Geographical distribution of selected and putatively neutral SNPs in South-east Asian malaria parasites. *Mol Biol Evol* 2005; 22:2362–2374.

531. Alker AP, Mwapasa V, Purfield A, et al. Mutations associated with sulfadoxine-pyrimethamine and chlorproguanil resistance in *Plasmodium falciparum* isolates from Blantyre, Malawi. *Antimicrob Agents Chemother* 2005; 49:3919–3921.

532. Peterson DA, Milhous WK, Wellems TE. Molecular basis of differential resistance to cycloguanil and pyrimethamine in *Plasmodium falciparum* malaria. *Proc Natl Acad Sci USA* 1990; 87:3018–3022.

533. Foote SJ, Galatis D, Cowman AF. Aminoacids in the dihydrofolate reductase-thymidylate synthase gene of *Plasmodium falciparum* involved in cycloguanil resistance differ from those involved in pyrimethamine resistance. *Proc Natl Acad Sci USA* 1990; 87:3014–3017.

534. Hyde JE. Drug-resistant malaria. *Trends Parasitol* 2005; 21:494–498.

535. Hyde JE, Sims PF. Sulfa-drug resistance in *Plasmodium falciparum*. *Trends Parasitol* 2001; 17:265–266.

536. Dokomajilar C, Lankoande ZM, Dorsey G, et al. Roles of specific *Plasmodium falciparum* mutations in resistance to amodiaquine and sulfadoxine-pyrimethamine in Burkina Faso. *Am J Trop Med Hyg* 2006; 75:162–165.

537. Marks F, Evans J, Meyer CG, et al. High prevalence of markers for sulfadoxine and pyrimethamine resistance in *Plasmodium falciparum* in the absence of drug pressure in the Ashanti region of Ghana. *Antimicrob Agents Chemother* 2005; 49:1101–1105.

538. Mugittu K, Ndejembi M, Malisa A, et al. Therapeutic efficacy of sulfadoxine-pyrimethamine and prevalence of resistance markers in Tanzania prior to revision of malaria treatment policy: *Plasmodium falciparum* dihydrofolate reductase and dihydropteroate synthase mutations in monitoring in vivo resistance. *Am J Trop Med Hyg* 2004; 71:696–697.

539. Krogstad D, Schlesinger PH. Acid vesicle function, intracellular pathogens and the action of chloroquine against *Plasmodium falciparum*. *N Engl J Med* 1987; 317:542–549.

540. Krugliak M, Ginsburg H. Studies on the antimalarial mode of action of quinoline-containing drugs: time dependence and irreversibility of drug

action, and interactions with compounds that alter the function of the parasite's food vacuole. *Life Sci* 1991; 49:1213–1219.

541. Chou AC, Chevli R, Fitch CD. Ferriprotoporphyrin IX fulfills the criteria for identification as the chloroquine receptor of malaria parasites. *Biochemistry* 1980; 19:1543–1549.

542. Bray PG, Ward SA, O'Neill PM. Quinolines and artemisinin: chemistry, biology and history. *Curr Top Microbiol Immunol* 2005; 295:3–38.

543. Foote SJ, Thompson JK, Cowman AF, et al. Amplification of the multidrug resistance gene in some chloroquine-resistant isolates of *Plasmodium falciparum*. *Cell* 1989; 57:921–930.

544. Price RN, Cassar C, Brockman A, et al. The pfmdr1 gene is associated with a multidrug resistance phenotype in *Plasmodium falciparum* from the western border of Thailand. *Antimicrob Agents Chemother* 1999; 43: 2943–2949.

545. Duraisingh MT, Jones P, Sambou I, et al. The tyrosine-86 allele of the pfmdr1 gene of *Plasmodium falciparum* is associated with increased sensitivity to the anti-malarials mefloquine and artemisinin. *Mol Biochem Parasitol* 2000; 108:13–23.

546. Reed MB, Saliba KJ, Caruana SR, et al. Pgh1 modulates sensitivity and resistance to multiple antimalarials in *Plasmodium falciparum*. *Nature* 2000; 403:906–909.

547. Valderramos SG, Fidock DA. Transporters involved in resistance to antimalarial drugs. *Trends Pharmacol Sci* 2006; 27:594–601.

548. Fidock DA, Nomura T, Talley AK, et al. Mutations in the *P. falciparum* digestive vacuole transmembrane protein PfCRT and evidence for their role in chloroquine resistance. *Mol Cell* 2000; 6:861–871.

549. Djimde A, Doumbo OK, Cortese JF, et al. A molecular marker for chloroquine-resistant falciparum malaria. *N Engl J Med* 2001; 344: 257–263.

550. Durand R, Jafari S, Vauzelle J, et al. Analysis of pfcrt point mutations and chloroquine susceptibility in isolates of *Plasmodium falciparum*. *Mol Biochem Parasitol* 2001; 114:95–102.

551. Laufer MK, Thesing PC, Eddington ND, et al. Return of chloroquine antimalarial efficacy in Malawi. *N Engl J Med* 2006; 355:1959–1966.

552. Suwanarusk R, Russell B, Chavchich M, et al. Chloroquine resistant *Plasmodium vivax*: In vitro characterisation and association with molecular polymorphisms. *PLoS ONE* 2007; 2:e1089.

553. Martin SK, Oduola AMJ, Milhous WK. Reversal of chloroquine resistance in *Plasmodium falciparum* by verapamil. *Science* 1987; 235:899–901.

554. Oduola AM, Omitowoju GO, Gerena L, et al. Reversal of mefloquine resistance with penfluridol in isolates of *Plasmodium falciparum* from south-west Nigeria. *Trans R Soc Trop Med Hyg* 1993; 87:81–83.

555. Sowunmi A, Oduola AM, Ogundahunsi OA, et al. Enhanced efficacy of chloroquine-chlorpheniramine combination in acute uncomplicated falciparum malaria in children. *Trans R Soc Trop Med Hyg* 1997; 91:63–67.

556. Brasseur P, Kouamouo J, Brandicourt O. Patterns of in-vitro resistance to chloroquine, quinine, and mefloquine of *Plasmodium falciparum* in Cameroon 1985–1986. *Am J Trop Med Hyg* 1988; 39:166–172.

557. Warsame M, Wernsdorfer WH, Payne D, et al. Susceptibility of *Plasmodium falciparum* in vitro to chloroquine, mefloquine, quinine and sulfadoxine/pyrimethamine in Somalia: relationship between the responses to different drugs. *Trans R Soc Trop Med Hyg* 1991; 85:565–569.

558. Srivastava IK, Rottenberg H, Vaidya AB. Atovaquone, a broad spectrum antiparasitic drug, collapses mitochondrial membrane potential in a malarial parasite. *J Biol Chem* 1997; 272:3961–3966.

559. Korsinczky M, Chen N, Kotecka B, et al. Mutations in *Plasmodium falciparum* cytochrome b that are associated with atovaquone resistance are located at a putative drug-binding site. *Antimicrob Agents Chemother* 2000; 44: 2100–2108.

560. Meshnick SR. Artemisinin antimalarials: mechanisms of action and resistance. *Med Trop* (Mars) 1998; 58(3 Suppl):13–17.

561. Olliaro PL, Haynes RK, Meunier B, et al. Possible modes of action of the artemisinin-type compounds. *Trends Parasitol* 2001; 17:122–126.

562. Eckstein-Ludwig U, Webb RJ, Van Goethem ID, et al. Artemisinins target the SERCA of *Plasmodium falciparum*. *Nature* 2003; 424:957–961.

563. Uhlemann AC, Cameron A, Eckstein-Ludwig U, et al. A single amino acid residue can determine the sensitivity of SERCAs to artemisinins. *Nat Struct Mol Biol* 2005; 12:628–629.

564. Uhlemann AC, Wittlin S, Matile H, et al. Mechanism of antimalarial action of the synthetic trioxolane RBX11160 (OZ277). *Antimicrob Agents Chemother* 2007; 51:667–672.

565. White NJ. Antimalarial drug resistance and combination chemotherapy. *Phil Trans R Soc Lond B* 1999; 354:739–749.

566. Curtis CF, Otoo LN. A simple model of the build up of resistance to mixtures of antimalarial drugs. *Trans R Soc Trop Med Hyg* 1986; 80: 889–892.

567. Hastings IM, D'Alessandro U. Modelling a predictable disaster: the rise and spread of drug-resistant malaria. *Parasitol Today* 2000; 16:340–347.

568. White NJ. Antimalarial drug resistance. *J Clin Invest* 2004; 113:1084–1092.

569. Watkins WM, Mosobo M. Treatment of *Plasmodium falciparum* malaria with pyrimethamine-sulphadoxine: selective pressure for resistance is a function of long elimination half-life. *Trans R Soc Trop Med Hyg* 1993; 87:75–78.

570. Hastings I, Watkins WM, White NJ. Pharmacokinetic parameters affecting the evolution of drug-resistance in malaria; The role of the terminal elimination half-life. *Philos Trans R Soc Lond B Biol Sci* 2002; 357:505–519.

571. Peters W. The prevention of antimalarial drug resistance. *Pharmacol Ther* 1990; 47:499–508.

572. White NJ, Nosten F, Looareesuwan S, et al. Averting a malaria disaster. *Lancet* 1999; 353:1965–1967.

573. Institute of Medicine. *Saving Lives, Buying Time, Economics of Antimalarial Drugs in an Age of Resistance*. Washington DC: National Academies Press; 2004.

574. Supanaranond W, Davis TME, Pukrittayakamee S, et al. Disposition of oral quinine in acute falciparum malaria. *Eur J Clin Pharmacol* 1991; 40:49–52.

575. Waller D, Krishna S, Craddock C, et al. The pharmacokinetic properties of intramuscular quinine in Gambian children with severe falciparum malaria. *Trans R Soc Trop Med Hyg* 1990; 84:488–491.

576. Mansor SM, Taylor TE, McGrath CS, et al. The safety and kinetics of intramuscular quinine in Malawian children with moderately severe falciparum malaria. *Trans R Soc Trop Med Hyg* 1990; 84:482–487.

577. Krishna S, Nagaraja NV, Planche T, et al. Population pharmacokinetics of intramuscular quinine in children with severe malaria. *Antimicrob Agents Chemother* 2001; 45:1803–1809.

578. Sabcharoen A, Chongsuphajaisiddhi T, Attanath P. Serum quinine concentrations following the initial dose in children with falciparum malaria. *SE Asian J Trop Med Public Health* 1989; 13:689–692.

579. White NJ, Looareesuwan S, Warrell DA, et al. Quinine pharmacokinetics and toxicity in cerebral and uncomplicated falciparum malaria. *Am J Med* 1982; 73:564–572.

580. White NJ, Chanthavanich P, Krishna S, et al. Quinine disposition kinetics. *Br J Clin Pharmacol* 1983; 16:399–404.

581. Krishna S, White NJ. Pharmacokinetics of quinine, chloroquine and amodiaquine. Clinical implications. *Clin Pharmacokinet* 1996; 30:263–299.

582. Phillips RE, Looareesuwan S, White NJ, et al. Quinine pharmacokinetics and toxicity in pregnant and lactating women with falciparum malaria. *Br J Clin Pharmacol* 1986; 21:677–683.

583. van Hensbroek MB, Kwiatkowski D, van den Berg B, et al. Quinine pharmacokinetics in young children with severe malaria. *Am J Trop Med Hyg* 1996; 54:237–242.

584. Pussard E, Barennes H, Daouda H, et al. Quinine disposition in globally malnourished children with cerebral malaria. *Clin Pharmacol Ther* 1999; 65:500–510.

585. Silamut K, Molunto P, Ho M, et al. Alpha-one acid glycoprotein (orosomucoid) and plasma protein binding of quinine in falciparum malaria. *Br J Clin Pharmacol* 1991; 32:311–315.

586. Silamut K, White NJ, Warrell DA, et al. Binding of quinine to plasma proteins in falciparum malaria. *Am J Trop Med Hyg* 1985; 34:681–686.

587. Mansor SM, Molyneux ME, Taylor TE, et al. Effect of *Plasmodium falciparum* malaria infection as the plasma concentration of alpha acid glycoprotein and the binding of quinine in Malawian children. *Br J Clin Pharmacol* 1991; 32:317–325.

588. White NJ, Looareesuwan S, Lavansiri K. Red cell quinine concentrations in falciparum malaria. *Am J Trop Med Hyg* 1983; 32:456–460.

589. Nontprasert A, Pukrittayakamee S, Kyle DE, et al. Antimalarial activity and interactions between quinine, dihydroquinine, and 3-hydroxyquinine against *P. falciparum* in vitro. *Trans R Soc Trop Med Hyg* 1996; 90: 553–555.

590. Newton P, Keeratithakul D, Teja-Isavadharm P, et al. Pharmacokinetics of quinine and 3-hydroxyquinine in severe falciparum malaria with acute renal failure. *Trans R Soc Trop Med Hyg* 1999; 93:69–72.

591. White NJ, Looareesuwan S, Warrell DA. Quinine and quinidine: a comparison of EKG effects during the treatment of malaria. *J Cardiovasc Pharmacol* 1983; 5:173–177.

592. White NJ. Cardiotoxicity of the antimalarial drugs. *Lancet Infect Dis* 2007; 7:549–558.

593. Dyson EH, Proudfoot AT, Prescott LF, et al. Death and blindness due to overdose of quinine. *BMJ* 1985; 291:31–33.

594. Boland ME, Brennand-Roper SM, Henry JA. Complications of quinine poisoning. *Lancet* 1985; i:384–385.

595. Henquin JC, Horeman B, Henquin M, et al. Quinine-induced modifications of insulin release and glucose metabolism by isolated pancreatic islets. *FEBS Lett* 1975; 57:280–284.

596. Bruce-Chwatt LJ. Quinine and the mystery of blackwater fever. *Acta Leiden* 1987; 55:181–196.

597. Yen LM, Dao LM, Day NPJ, et al. Role of quinine in the high mortality of intramuscular injection tetanus. *Lancet* 1994; 344: 786–787.

598. Hien TT, Day NPJ, Phu NH, et al. A controlled trial of artemether or quinine in Vietnamese adults with severe falciparum malaria. *N Engl J Med* 1996; 335:76–83.

599. van Hensbroek MB, Onyiorah E, Jaffar S, et al. A trial of artemether or quinine in children with cerebral malaria. *N Engl J Med* 1996; 335:69–75.

600. White NJ, Warrell DA, Looareesuwan S, et al. Quinine loading dose in cerebral malaria. *Am J Trop Med Hyg* 1983; 32:1–5.

601. Chongsuphajaisiddhi T, Sabcharoen A, Attanath P. In-vivo and in-vitro sensitivity to quinine in Thai children. *Ann Trop Paediatr* 1981; 1:21–26.

602. White NJ, Looareesuwan S, Warrell DA, et al. Quinidine in falciparum malaria. *Lancet* 1981; ii:1069–1072.

603. Phillips RE, Warrell DA, White NJ, et al. Intravenous quinidine for the treatment of severe falciparum malaria. Clinical and pharmacokinetic studies. *N Engl J Med* 1985; 312:1273–1278.

604. Karbwang J, Davis TME, Looareesuwan S, et al. A comparison of the pharmacokinetic and pharmacodynamic properties of quinine and quinidine in healthy Thai males. *Br J Clin Pharmacol* 1993; 35:265–271.

605. Miller KD, Greenberg AE, Campbell CC. Treatment of severe malaria in the United States with a continuous infusion of quinidine gluconate and exchange transfusion. *N Engl J Med* 1989; 321:65–70.

606. Kain KC, Gadd Ed, Gushulak B, et al. Errors in treatment recommendations for severe malaria. Committee to Advise on Tropical Medicine and Travel (CATMAT) *Lancet* 1996; 348:621–622.

607. Krogstad DJ, Pearson RD, Bennett JE, et al. Dosage for malaria treatment. *Lancet* 1996; 348:1311–1312.

608. White NJ, Warrell DA. Dosage for malaria treatment. *Lancet* 1996; 348: 1312.

609. Gustafsson LL, Walker O, Alvan G, et al. Disposition of chloroquine in man after single intravenous and oral doses. *Br J Clin Pharmacol* 1983; 15:471–479.

610. Frisk-Holmberg M, Bergqvist Y, Termond E, et al. The single dose kinetics of chloroquine and its major metabolite desethylchloroquine in healthy subjects. *Eur J Clin Pharmacol* 1984; 26:521–530.

611. White NJ, Watt G, Bergqvist Y, et al. Parenteral chloroquine in the treatment of falciparum malaria. *J Infect Dis* 1987; 155:192–201.

612. White NJ, Miller KD, Churchill FC, et al. Chloroquine treatment of severe malaria in children: pharmacokinetics, toxicity, and revised dosage recommendations. *N Engl J Med* 1988; 319:1493–1500.

73. Malaria

613. Walker O, Daurodu AH, Adeyokunnu AA, et al. Plasma chloroquine and desethylchloroquine concentrations in children during and after chloroquine treatment for malaria. *Br J Clin Pharmacol* 1983; 16:701–705.

614. Minker F, Iran J. Experimental and clinicopharmacological study of rectal absorption of chloroquine. *Acta Physiol Hung* 1991; 77:237–248.

615. Taylor WR, White NJ. Antimalarial drug toxicity: a review. *Drug Safety* 2004; 27:25–61.

616. Mnyika KS, Kihamia CM. Chloroquine-induced pruritus: its impact on chloroquine utilization in malaria control in Dar es Salaam. *J Trop Med Hyg* 1991; 94:27–31.

617. Easterbrook M. Ocular effects and safety of antimalarials. *Am J Med* 1988; 85(suppl 4a):23–29.

618. Peruval SPB, Meancock I. Chloroquine: ophthalmological safety and clinical assessment in rheumatoid arthritis. *BMJ* 1968; 3:579–584.

619. Riou B, Barriot P, Rimailho A, et al. Treatment of severe chloroquine poisoning. *N Engl J Med* 1988; 316:1–6.

620. Clemessy JL, Taboulet P, Hoffman JR, et al. Treatment of acute chloroquine poisoning: a 5-year experience. *Crit Care Med* 1996; 24:1189–1195.

621. Pussard E, Lepers JP, Clavier F, et al. Efficacy of a loading dose of oral chloroquine in a 36-hour treatment schedule for uncomplicated *Plasmodium falciparum* malaria. *Antimicrob Agents Chemother* 1991; 35: 406–409.

622. Li XQ, Bjorkman A, Andersson TB, et al. Amodiaquine clearance and its metabolism to N-desethylamodiaquine is mediated by CYP2C8: a new high affinity and turnover enzyme-specific probe substrate. *J Pharmacol Exp Ther* 2002; 300:399–407.

623. White NJ, Looareesuwan S, Edwards G, et al. Pharmacokinetics of intravenous amodiaquine. *Br J Clin Pharmacol* 1987; 23:127–135.

624. Hombhanje FW, Hwaihwanje I, Tsukahara T, et al. The disposition of oral amodiaquine in Papua New Guinean children with falciparum malaria. *Br J Clin Pharmacol* 2005; 59:298–301.

625. Hietala SF, Bhattarai A, Msellem M, et al. Population pharmacokinetics of amodiaquine and desethylamodiaquine in pediatric patients with uncomplicated falciparum malaria. *J Pharmacokinet Pharmacodyn* 2007; 34:669–686.

626. Parikh S, Ouedraogo JB, Goldstein JA, et al. Amodiaquine metabolism is impaired by common polymorphisms in CYP2C8: implications for malaria treatment in Africa. *Clin Pharmacol Ther* 2007; 82:197–203.

627. Pussard E, Verdier F, Faurisson F, et al. Disposition of monodesethylamodiaquine after a single oral dose of amodiaquine and three regimens for prophylaxis against *Plasmodium falciparum* malaria. *Eur J Clin Pharmacol* 1987; 33(4):409–414.

628. Hatton CS, Peto TEA, Bunch C, et al. Frequency of severe neutropenia associated with amodiaquine prophylaxis against malaria. *Lancet* 1986; i:411–414.

629. Harrison AC, Kitteringham NR, Clarke JB, et al. The mechanism of bioactivation and antigen formation of amodiaquine in the rat. *Biochem Pharmacol* 1992; 43:1421–1430.

630. O'Neill PM, Mukhtar A, Stocks PA, et al. Isoquine and related amodiaquine analogues: a new generation of improved 4-aminoquinoline antimalarials. *J Med Chem* 2003; 46:4933–4945.

631. Parikh S, Ouedraogo JB, Goldstein JA, et al. Amodiaquine metabolism is impaired by common polymorphisms in CYP2C8: implications for malaria treatment in Africa. *Clin Pharmacol Ther* 2007; 82:197–203.

632. Ashley EA, Lwin KM, McGready R, et al. An open label randomized comparison of mefloquine-artesunate as separate tablets vs. a new co-formulated combination for the treatment of uncomplicated multidrug-resistant falciparum malaria in Thailand. *Trop Med Int Health* 2006; 11:1653–1660.

633. Brocks DR, Mehvar R. Stereoselectivity in the pharmacodynamics and pharmacokinetics of the chiral antimalarial drugs. *Clin Pharmacokinet* 2003; 42:1359–1382.

634. Gimenez F, Pennie RA, Koren G, et al. Stereoselective pharmacokinetics of mefloquine in healthy Caucasians after multiple doses. *J Pharm Sci* 1994; 83:824–827.

635. Svensson US, Alin H, Karlsson MO, et al. Population pharmacokinetic and pharmacodynamic modelling of artemisinin and mefloquine enantiomers in patients with falciparum malaria. *Eur J Clin Pharmacol* 2002; 58:339–351.

636. Bourahla A, Martin C, Gimenez F, et al. Stereoselective pharmacokinetics of mefloquine in young children. *Eur J Clin Pharmacol* 1996; 50:241–244.

637. Karbwang J, White NJ. Clinical pharmacokinetics of mefloquine. *Clin Pharmacokinet* 1990; 19:264–279.

638. Looareesuwan S, White NJ, Warrell DA, et al. Studies of mefloquine bioavailability and kinetics using a stable isotope technique: a comparison of Thai patients with falciparum malaria and healthy Caucasian volunteers. *Br J Clin Pharmacol* 1987; 24:37–42.

639. Price RN, Simpson JA, Teja-Isavatharm P, et al. Pharmacokinetics of mefloquine combined with artesunate in children with acute falciparum malaria. *Antimicrob Agents Chemother* 1999; 43:341–346.

640. Simpson JA, Price RN, ter Kuile FO, et al. Population pharmacokinetics of mefloquine in patients with acute falciparum malaria. *Clin Pharmac Ther* 1999; 66:472–484.

641. Ashley EA, Stepniewska K, Lindegardh N, et al. Population pharmacokinetic assessment of a new regimen of mefloquine used in combination treatment of uncomplicated falciparum malaria. *Antimicrob Agents Chemother* 2006; 50:2281–2285.

642. Nosten F, Karbwang J, White NJ, et al. Mefloquine antimalarial prophylaxis in pregnancy: dose finding and pharmacokinetic study. *Br J Clin Pharmacol* 1990; 30:79–85.

643. Slutsker LM, Khoromana CD, Payne D, et al. Mefloquine therapy for *Plasmodium falciparum* malaria in children under 5 years of age in Malawi: in vivo/in vitro efficacy and correlation of drug concentration with parasitological outcome. *Bull World Health Organ* 1990; 68: 53–59.

644. Nosten F, ter Kuile F, Chongsuphajaisiddhi T, et al. Mefloquine pharmacokinetics and resistance in children with acute falciparum malaria. *Br J Clin Pharmacol* 1991; 31:556–559.

645. Luxemburger C, Price RN, Nosten F, et al. Mefloquine in infants and young children. *Ann Trop Paediatr* 1996; 16:281–286.

646. ter Kuile FO, Nosten F, Luxemburger C Kyle D, et al. Mefloquine treatment of acute falciparum malaria: A prospective study of non-serious adverse effects in 3673 patients. *Bull WHO* 1995; 73:631–642.

647. ter Kuile F, Nosten F, Thieren M, et al. High-dose mefloquine in the treatment of multidrug-resistant falciparum malaria. *J Infect Dis* 1992; 166:1393–1400.

648. Weinke T, Trautman M, Held T, et al. Neuropsychiatric side effects after the use of mefloquine. *Am J Trop Med Hyg* 1991; 45:86–91.

649. Luxemburger C, Nosten F, ter Kuiile F, et al. Mefloquine for multidrug-resistant malaria. *Lancet* 1991; 338:1268.

650. Bem JL, Kerr L, Stuerchler D. Mefloquine prophylaxis: an overview of spontaneous reports of severe psychiatric reactions and convulsions. *J Trop Med Hyg* 1992; 95:167–179.

651. Steffen R, Fuchs E, Schildknecht J, et al. Mefloquine compared with other malaria chemoprophylactic regimens in tourists visiting east Africa. *Lancet* 1993; 341:1299–1303.

652. Lobel HO, Miani M, Eng T, et al. Long-term malaria prophylaxis with weekly mefloquine. *Lancet* 1993; 34:848–851.

653. Schlagenhauf P. Mefloquine for malaria chemoprophylaxis 1992–1998: a review. *J Travel Med* 1999; 6:122–133.

654. Nosten F, Vincenti M, Simpson JA, et al. The effects of mefloquine treatment in pregnancy. *Clin Infect Dis* 1999; 28:808–815.

655. Steketee RW, Wirima JJ, Slutsker L, et al. Malaria treatment and prevention in pregnancy: indications for use and adverse events associated with use of chloroquine or mefloquine. *Am J Trop Med Hyg* 1996; 55(suppl 1):50–56.

656. Simpson JA, Watkins ER, Price RN, et al. Mefloquine pharmacokinetic-pharmacodynamic models: implications for dosing and resistance. *Antimicrob Agents Chemother*, 2000; 44:3414–3424.

657. World Health Organization. *Guidelines for the treatment of malaria.* Geneva: WHO; 2006.

658. Milton KA, Edwards G, Ward SA, et al. Pharmacokinetics of halofantrine in man: effects of food and dose size. *Br J Clin Pharmacol* 1989; 28:71–77.

659. Veenendaal JR, Parkinson AD, Kere N, et al. Pharmacokinetics of halofantrine and *n*-desbutylhalofantrine in patients with *falciparum* malaria following a multiple dose regimen of halofantrine. *Eur J Clin Pharmacol* 1991; 41:161–164.

660. Watkins WM, Oloo JA, Lury JD, et al. Efficacy of multiple dose halofantrine in treatment of chloroquine resistant falciparum malaria in children in Kenya. *Lancet* 1988; ii:247–250.

661. Nosten F, ter Kuile FO, Luxemburger C, et al. Cardiac effects of antimalarial treatment with halofantrine. *Lancet* 1993; 341:1054–1056.

662. Malvy D, Receveur MC, Ozon P, et al. Fatal cardiac incident after use of halofantrine. *J Travel Med* 2000; 7:215–216.

663. Akhtar T, Imran M. Sudden deaths while on halofantrine treatments – a report of two cases from Peshawar. *J Pak Med Assoc* 1994; 44:120–121.

664. Wesche DL, Schuster BG, Wang WX, et al. Mechanism of cardiotoxicity of halofantrine. *Clin Pharmacol Ther* 2000; 67:521–529.

665. ter Kuile FO, Dolan G, Nosten F, et al. Halofantrine versus mefloquine in the treatment of multi-drug resistant falciparum malaria. *Lancet* 1993; 341:1044–1049.

666. Winstanley P, Watkins WM, Newton CRJ C, et al. The disposition of oral and intramuscular Pyrimethamine/sulphadoxine in Kenyan children with high parasitaemia but clinically non-severe falciparum malaria. *Br J Clin Pharmacol* 1992; 33:143–148.

667. Barnes KI, Little F, Smith PJ, et al. Sulfadoxine-pyrimethamine pharmacokinetics in malaria: pediatric dosing implications. *Clin Pharmacol Ther* 2006; 80:582–596.

668. Miller KD, Lobel HO, Satriale RF, et al. Severe cutaneous reactions among American travellers using pyrimethamine-sulfadoxine (Fansidar™) for malaria prophylaxis. *Am J Trop Med Hyg* 1986; 35:451–458.

669. Bjorkman A, Phillips-Howard PA. Adverse reaction to sulfa drugs: implications for malaria chemotherapy. *Bull World Health Organ* 1991; 69:297–304.

670. von Seidlein L, Milligan P, Pinder M, et al. Efficacy of artesunate plus pyrimethamine-sulphadoxine for uncomplicated malaria in Gambian children: a double-blind, randomised, controlled trial. *Lancet* 2000; 355:352–357.

671. International Artemisinin Study Group. Artesunate combinations for treatment of malaria: meta analysis. *Lancet* 2004; 363:9–17.

672. Rogerson SJ, Chululuka E, Kanjala M, et al. Intermittent sulfadoxine-pyrimethamine in pregnancy: effectiveness against malaria morbidity in Blantyre, Malawi, in 1997–99. *Trans R Soc Trop Med Hyg* 2000; 94:549–553.

673. Wolfe EB, Parise ME, Haddix AC, et al. Cost-effectiveness of sulfadoxine-pyrimethamine for the prevention of malaria-associated low birth weight. *Am J Trop Med Hyg* 2001; 64:178–186.

674. Vallely A, Vallely L, Changalucha J, et al. Intermittent preventive treatment for malaria in pregnancy in Africa: what's new, what's needed? *Malar J* 2007; 6:16.

675. Schellenberg D, Menendez C, Kahigwa E, et al. Intermittent treatment for malaria and anaemia control at time of routine vaccinations in Tanzanian infants: a randomised, placebo-controlled trial. *Lancet* 2001; 357:1471–1477.

676. Greenwood B. Review: Intermittent preventive treatment – a new approach to the prevention of malaria in children in areas with seasonal malaria transmission. *Trop Med Int Health* 2006; 11:983–991.

677. Painter HJ, Morrisey JM, Mather MW, et al. Specific role of mitochondrial electron transport in blood-stage *Plasmodium falciparum*. *Nature* 2007; 446:88–91.

678. Wattanagoon Y, Taylor RB, Moody RR, et al. Single dose pharmacokinetics of proguanil and its metabolites in healthy adult volunteers. *Br J Clin Pharmacol* 1987; 24:775–780.

679. Winstanley P, Watkins W, Muhia D, et al. Chlorproguanil/dapsone for uncomplicated Plasmodium falciparum malaria in young children: pharmacokinetics and therapeutic range. *Trans R Soc Trop Med Hyg* 1997; 91:322–327.

680. Helsby NA, Ward SA, Edwards C, et al. The pharmacokinetics and activation of proguanil in man: consequences of variability in drug metabolism. *Br J Clin Pharmacol* 1990; 30:593–598.

681. Kaneko A, Kaneko O, Taleo G, et al. High frequencies of CYP2C19 mutations and poor metabolism of proguanil in Vanuatu. *Lancet* 1997; 349:921–922.

682. Wangboonskul J, White NJ, Nosten F, et al. Single dose pharmacokinetics of proguanil and its metabolites in pregnancy. *Eur J Clin Pharmacol* 1993; 44:247–251.

683. Simpson JA, Hughes D, Manyando C, et al. Population pharmacokinetic and pharmacodynamic modelling of the antimalarial chemotherapy chlorproguanil/dapsone. *Br J Clin Pharmacol* 2006; 61:289–300.

684. Harries AD, Forshaw AI, Friend HM. Malaria prophylaxis among British residents of Lilongwe and Kasungu districts, Malawi. *Trans R Soc Trop Med Hyg* 1988; 82:690–692.

685. Boots M, Phillips M, Curtis JR. Megaloblastic anaemia and pancytopenia due to proguanil in patients with chronic renal failure. *Clin Nephrol* 1982; 18:106–108.

686. Watkins WM, Brandling-Bennett Nevill CG, Carter JY, et al. Chlorproguanil/dapsone for the treatment of non-severe Plasmodium falciparum infection in Kenya. *Trans R Soc Trop Med Hyg* 1988; 82:398–403.

687. Amukoye E, Winstanley PA, Watkins WM, et al. Chlorproguanil-dapsone: effective treatment for uncomplicated falciparum malaria. *Antimicrob Agents Chemother* 1997; 41:2261–2264.

688. Nzila AM, Nduati E, Mberu EK, et al. Molecular evidence of greater selective pressure for drug resistance exerted by the long-acting antifolate Pyrimethamine/Sulfadoxine compared with the shorter-acting chlorproguanil/dapsone on Kenyan Plasmodium falciparum. *J Infect Dis* 2000; 181:2023–2028.

689. Krudsood S, Imwong M, Wilairatana P, et al. Artesunate-dapsone-proguanil treatment of falciparum malaria: genotypic determinants of therapeutic response. *Trans R Soc Trop Med Hyg* 2005, 99:142–149.

690. Bukirwa H, Garner P, Critchley J. Chlorproguanil-dapsone for treating uncomplicated malaria. *Cochrane Database Syst Rev* 2004; 18(4): CD004387.

691. Looareesuwan S, Viravan C, Webster HK, et al. Clinical studies of atovaquone, alone or in combination with other antimalarial drugs, for treatment of acute uncomplicated malaria in Thailand. *Am J Trop Med Hyg* 1996; 54:62–66.

692. Looareesuwan S, Wilairatana P, Chalermarut K, et al. Efficacy and safety of atovaquone/proguanil compared with mefloquine for treatment of acute *Plasmodium falciparum* malaria in Thailand. *Am J Trop Med Hyg* 1999; 60: 526–532.

693. Bustos DG, Canfield CJ, Canete-Miguel E, et al. Atovaquone-proguanil compared with chloroquine and chloroquine-sulfadoxine-pyrimethamine for treatment of acute *Plasmodium falciparum* malaria in the Philippines. *J Infect Dis* 1999; 179:1587–1590.

694. van Vugt M, Leonardi E, Phaipun L, et al. Treatment of uncomplicated multidrug-resistant falciparum malaria with artesunate-atovaquone-proguanil. *Clin Infect Dis* 2002; 35:1498–1504.

695. Hussein Z, Eaves J, Hutchinson DB, et al. Population pharmacokinetics of atovaquone in patients with acute malaria caused by *Plasmodium falciparum*. *Clin Pharmacol Ther* 1997; 61:518–530.

696. McGready R, Stepniewska K, Edstein MD, et al. The pharmacokinetics of atovaquone and proguanil in pregnant women with acute falciparum malaria. *Eur J Clin Pharm* 2003; 59:545–552.

697. Hogh B, Clarke PD, Camus D, et al. Atovaquone-proguanil versus chloroquine-proguanil for malaria prophylaxis in non-immune travellers: a randomised, double-blind study. Malarone International Study Team. *Lancet* 2000; 356:1888–1894.

698. Sabchareon A, Attanath P, Phanuaksook P, et al. Efficacy and pharmacokinetics of atovaquone and proguanil in children with multidrug-resistant *Plasmodium falciparum* malaria. *Trans R Soc Trop Med Hyg* 1998; 92:201–206.

699. McGready R, Ashley EA, Moo E, et al. A randomized comparison of artesunate-atovaquone-proguanil versus quinine in treatment for

uncomplicated falciparum malaria during pregnancy. *J Infect Dis* 2005; 192:846–853.

700. Na-Bangchang K, Manyando C, Ruengweerayut R, et al. The pharmacokinetics and pharmacodynamics of atovaquone and proguanil for the treatment of uncomplicated falciparum malaria in third-trimester pregnant women. *Eur J Clin Pharmacol* 2005; 61:573–582.

701. Baird JK, Hoffman SL. Primaquine therapy for malaria. *Clin Infect Dis* 2004; 39:1336–1345.

702. Mihaly GW, Ward SA, Edwards C, et al. Pharmacokinetics of primaquine in man: identification of the carboxylic acid derivative as a major plasma metabolite. *Br J Clin Pharmacol* 1984; 17:441–446.

703. Elmes NJ, Bennett SM, Abdalla H, et al. Lack of sex effect on the pharmacokinetics of primaquine. *Am J Trop Med Hyg* 2006; 74:951–952.

704. Kim YR, Kuh HJ, Kim MY, et al. Pharmacokinetics of primaquine and carboxyprimaquine in Korean patients with vivax malaria. *Arch Pharm Res* 2004; 27:576–580.

705. Carson PE, Flangan CL, Ickes CE, et al. Enzymatic deficiency in primaquine sensitive erythrocytes. *Science* 1956; 124:484–485.

706. Chan TK, Todd D, Tsao SC. Drug-induced haemolysis in glucose-6-phosphate dehydrogenase deficiency. *BMJ* 1976; ii:1227–1229.

707. Bowman ZS, Morrow JD, Jollow DJ, et al. Primaquine-induced hemolytic anemia: role of membrane lipid peroxidation and cytoskeletal protein alterations in the hemotoxicity of 5-hydroxyprimaquine. *J Pharmacol Exp Ther* 2005; 314:838–845.

708. Barrett EL. Glucose-6-phosphate dehydrogenase deficiency: a brief review. *Trans R Soc Trop Med Hyg* 1966; 60:267–275.

709. Galappaththy G, Omari A, Tharyan P. Primaquine for preventing relapses in people with *Plasmodium vivax* malaria. *Cochrane Database Syst Rev* 2007; 1: CD004389.

710. Fryauff DJ, Baird JK, Basri H, et al. Randomised placebo-controlled trial of primaquine for prophylaxis of falciparum and vivax malaria. *Lancet* 1995; 346:1190–1193.

711. Soto J, Toledo J, Rodriquez M, et al. Double-blind, randomized, placebo-controlled assessment of chloroquine/primaquine prophylaxis for malaria in nonimmune Colombian soldiers. *Clin Infect Dis* 1999; 29:199–201.

712. Brondz I, Mantzilas D, Klein U, et al. Nature of the main contaminant in the anti malaria drug primaquine diphosphate: a qualitative isomer analysis. *J Chromatogr B Analyt Technol Biomed Life Sci* 2004; 800:211–223.

713. Krudsood S, Wilairatana P, Tangpukdee N, et al. Safety and tolerability of elubaquine (bulaquine, CDRI 80/53) for treatment of *Plasmodium vivax* malaria in Thailand. *Korean J Parasitol* 2006; 44:221–228.

714. Lell B, Faucher JF, Missinou MA, et al. Malaria chemoprophylaxis with tafenoquine: a randomised study. *Lancet* 2000; 355:2041–2045.

715. Tafenoquine for the treatment of recurrent *Plasmodium vivax* malaria. *Am J Trop Med Hyg* 2007; 76:494–496.

716. Edstein MD, Nasveld PE, Kocisko DA, et al. Gender differences in gastrointestinal disturbances and plasma concentrations of tafenoquine in healthy volunteers after tafenoquine administration for post-exposure vivax malaria prophylaxis. *Trans R Soc Trop Med Hyg* 2007; 101:226–230.

717. Li GQ. Clinical studies on artemisinin suppository and on artesunate and artemether. In: Shen JX, ed. *Antimalarial Drug Development in China*. Beijing: National Institute of Pharmaceutical Research and Development; 1989:69–73.

718. Li GQ, Guo XB, Fu LC, et al. A summary of clinical studies on the treatment of malaria with qinghaosu suppositories. In: Li GQ, Guo XB, Yang F, eds. *Clinical Trials on Qinghaosu and its Derivatives*. Vol. 1. Guangzhou: College of Traditional Chinese Medicine, Sanya Tropical Medicine Institute; 1990:17–22.

719. The Artemether-Quinine Meta-analysis Study Group. A meta-analysis using individual patient data of trials comparing artemether with quinine in the treatment of severe falciparum malaria. *Trans R Soc Trop Med Hyg* 2001; 95:637–650.

720. Dondorp A, Nosten F, Stepniewska K, et al. Artesunate versus quinine for treatment of severe falciparum malaria: a randomised trial. *Lancet* 2005; 366:717–725.

721. Luxemburger C, Nosten F, Shotar RD, et al. Oral artesunate in the treatment of uncomplicated hyperparasitemic falciparum malaria. *Am J Trop Med Hyg* 1995; 53:522–525.

722. Hien TT, Arnold K, Vinh H, et al. Comparison of artemisinin suppositories with intravenous artesunate and intravenous quinine in the treatment of cerebral malaria. *Trans R Soc Trop Med Hyg* 1992; 86:582–583.

723. Phuong CXT, Bethell DB, Phuong PT, et al. Comparison of artemisinin suppositories, intramuscular artesunate, and intravenous quinine for the treatment of severe childhood malaria. *Trans R Soc Trop Med Hyg* 1997; 91:335–342.

724. Nosten F, van Vugt M, White NJ. Intrarectal artemisinin derivatives. *Med Trop* (Mars). 1998; 58(suppl 3):63–64.

725. Krishna S, Planche T, Agbenyega T, et al. Bioavailability and preliminary clinical efficacy of intrarectal artesunate in Ghanaian children with moderate malaria. *Antimicrob Agents Chemother* 2001; 45:509–516.

726. Gomes M. Rectocaps. *Lancet*.

727. Murphy SA, Mberu E, Muhia D, et al. The disposition of intramuscular artemether in children with cerebral malaria; a preliminary study. *Trans R Soc Trop Med Hyg* 1997; 91:3321–3334.

728. Hien TT, Davis TM, Chuong LV, et al. Comparative pharmacokinetics of intramuscular artesunate and artemether in patients with severe falciparum malaria. *Antimicrob Agents Chemother* 2004; 48:4234–4239.

729. Price RN, Nosten F, Luxemburger C, et al. The effects of artemisinin derivatives on malaria transmissability. *Lancet* 1996; 347:1654–1658.

730. Targett G, Drakeley C, Jawara M, et al. Artesunate reduces but does not prevent posttreatment transmission of *Plasmodium falciparum* to Anopheles gambiae. *J Infect Dis* 2001; 183:1254–1259.

731. van Vugt M, Angus BM, Price RN, et al. A case-control auditory evaluation of patients treated with artemisinin derivatives for multi-drug resistant *Plasmodium falciparum* malaria. *Am J Trop Med Hyg* 2000; 62:65–69.

732. Kissinger E, Hien TT, Hung NT, et al. Clinical and neurophysiological study of the effects of multiple doses of artemisinin on brain-stem function in Vietnamese patients. *Am J Trop Med Hyg* 2001; 63:48–55.

733. Hien TT, Turner GDH, Mai NTH, et al. Neuropathological assessment of artemether treated severe malaria. *Lancet* 2003; 362:295–296.

734. Price RN, van Vugt M, Phaipun L, et al. Adverse effects in patients with acute falciparum malaria treated with artemisinin derivatives. *Am J Trop Med Hyg* 1999; 60:547–555.

735. Newton P, Proux S, Green M, et al. Fake artesunate in SE Asia. *Lancet* 2001; 357:1948–1950.

736. Newton PN, Green MD, Fernandez FM, et al. Counterfeit anti-infective drugs. *Lancet Infect Dis* 2006; 6:602–613.

737. Navaratnam V, Mansor SM, Sit NW, et al. Pharmacokinetics of artemisinin-type compounds. *Clin Pharmacokinet* 2000; 39:255–270.

738. Teja-Isavadharm P, Nosten F, Kyle DE, et al. Comparative bio-availability of oral, rectal and intramuscular artemether in healthy subjects – use of simultaneous measurement by high performance liquid chromatography with electro-chemical detection and bioassay. *Brit J Clin Pharmacol* 1996; 42:599–604.

739. Batty KT, Thu LT, Davis TM, et al. A pharmacokinetic and pharmacodynamic study of intravenous vs oral artesunate in uncomplicated falciparum malaria. *Br J Clin Pharmacol* 1998; 45:123–129.

740. Newton P, Suputtamongkol Y, Teja-Isavadharm P, et al. Antimalarial bioavailability and disposition of artesunate in acute falciparum malaria. *Antimicrob Agents Chemother* 2000; 44:972–977.

741. Simpson JA, Agbenyega T, Barnes KI, et al. Population pharmacokinetics of artesunate and dihydroartemisinin following intra-rectal dosing of artesunate in malaria patients. *PLoS Med* 2006; 3: e444.

742. Mithwani S, Aarons L, Kokwaro GO, et al. Population pharmacokinetics of artemether and dihydroartemisinin following single intramuscular dosing of artemether in African children with severe falciparum malaria. *Br J Clin Pharmacol* 2004; 57:146–152.

743. McGready R, Stepniewska K, Ward SA, et al. Pharmacokinetics of dihydroartemisinin following oral artesunate treatment of pregnant women

with acute uncomplicated falciparum malaria. *Eur J Clin Pharmacol* 2006; 62:367–371.

744. Ribeiro IR, Olliaro P. Safety of artemisinin and its derivatives. A review of published and unpublished clinical trials. *Med Trop* (Mars) 1998; 58(suppl 3):50–53.

745. Leonardi-Nield E, Gilvary G, White NJ, et al. Severe allergic reactions to oral artesunate: a report of two cases. *Trans R Soc Trop Med Hyg* 2001; 95:182–183.

746. Brewer TG, Peggins JO, Grate SJ, et al. Neurotoxicity in animals due to arteether and artemether. *Trans R Soc Trop Med Hyg* 1994; 88(suppl 1):S33–S36.

747. Genovese RF, Newman DB, Petras JM, et al. Behavioral and neural toxicity of arteether in rats. *Pharmacol Biochem Behav* 1998; 60(2):449–458.

748. Nontprasert A, Nosten-Bertrand M, Pukrittayakamee S, et al. Assessment of the neurotoxicity of parenteral artemisinin derivatives in mice. *Am J Trop Med Hyg* 1998; 59:519–522.

749. Nontprasert A, Pukrittayakamee S, Nosten-Bertrand M, et al. Studies of the neurotoxicity of oral artemisinin derivatives in mice. *Am J Trop Med Hyg* 2000; 62:409–412.

750. Clark RL, White TE, A Clode S, et al. Developmental toxicity of artesunate and an artesunate combination in the rat and rabbit. *Birth Defects Res B Dev Reprod Toxicol* 2004; 71:380–394.

751. Longo M, Zanoncelli S, Torre PD, et al. In vivo and in vitro investigations of the effects of the antimalarial drug dihydroartemisinin (DHA) on rat embryos. *Reprod Toxicol* 2006; 22:797–810.

752. McGready R, Cho T, Keo, et al. Artemisinin antimalarials in pregnancy: a prospective treatment study of 539 multidrug resistant P. falciparum episodes *Clin Infect Dis* 2001; 33:2009–2016.

753. Dellicour S, Hall S, Chandramohan D, et al. The safety of artemisinins during pregnancy: a pressing question. *Malar J* 2007; 6:15.

754. Newton PN, Barnes KI, Smith PJ, et al. The pharmacokinetics of intravenous artesunate in adults with severe falciparum malaria *Eur J Clin Pharmacol* 2006; 62:1003–1009.

755. Ezzet F, van Vugt M, Nosten F, et al. The pharmacokinetics and pharmacodynamics of lumefantrine (benflumetol) in acute uncomplicated falciparum malaria. *Antimicrob Agents Chemother* 2000; 44:697–704.

756. White NJ, van Vugt M, Ezzet F. Clinical pharmacokinetics and pharmacodynamics of artemether-lumefantrine. *Clin Pharmacokinet* 1999; 37:105–125.

757. Ashley EA, Stepniewska K, Lindegardh N, et al. How much fat is necessary to optimize lumefantrine oral bioavailability? *Trop Med Int Health* 2007; 12:195–200.

758. Ashley EA, Stepniewska K, Lindegardh N, et al. Pharmacokinetic study of artemether-lumefantrine given once daily for the treatment of uncomplicated multidrug-resistant falciparum malaria. *Trop Med Int Health* 2007; 12:201–208.

759. White NJ, Stepniewska K, Barnes K, et al. Simplified antimalarial therapeutic monitoring: using the day-7 drug level? *Trends Parasitol* 2008; 24:159–163.

760. Price RN, Uhlemann AC, van Vugt M, et al. Molecular and pharmacological determinants of the therapeutic response to artemether-lumefantrine in multidrug-resistant Plasmodium falciparum malaria. *Clin Infect Dis* 2006; 42:1570–1577.

761. McGready R, Stepniewska K, Lindegardh N, et al. The pharmacokinetics of artemether and lumefantrine in pregnant women with uncomplicated falciparum malaria. *Eur J Clin Pharmacol* 2006; 62:1021–1031.

762. van Vugt M, Ezzet F, Nosten F, et al. No evidence of cardiotoxicity during antimalarial treatment with artemether-lumefantrine. *Am J Trop Med Hyg* 1999; 61:964–967.

763. van Vugt M, Brockman A, Gemperli B, et al. Randomised comparison of artemether-benflumetol and artesunate-mefloquine in the treatment of multi-drug resistant falciparum malaria. *Antimicrob Agents Chemother* 1998; 42:135–139.

764. van Vugt M, Wilairatana P, Gemperli B, et al. Efficacy of six doses of artemether-benflumetol in the treatment of multi-drug resistant falciparum malaria. *Am J Trop Med Hyg* 1999; 60:936–942.

765. van Vugt M, Looareesuwan S, Wilairatana P, et al. Artemether-lumefantrine for the treatment of multidrug resistant falciparum malaria. *Trans R Soc Trop Med Hyg* 2000; 94:545–548.

766. Zongo I, Dorsey G, Rouamba N, et al. Artemether-lumefantrine versus amodiaquine plus sulfadoxine-pyrimethamine for uncomplicated falciparum malaria in Burkina Faso: a randomised non-inferiority trial. *Lancet* 2007; 369:491–498.

767. Sagara I, Dicko A, Djimde A, et al. A randomized trial of artesunate-sulfamethoxypyrazine-pyrimethamine versus artemether-lumefantrine for the treatment of uncomplicated *Plasmodium falciparum* malaria in Mali. *Am J Trop Med Hyg* 2006; 75:630–636.

768. Bukirwa H, Yeka A, Kamya MR, et al. Artemisinin combination therapies for treatment of uncomplicated malaria in Uganda. *PLoS Clin Trials* 2006; 1:e7.

769. Martensson A, Stromberg J, Sisowath C, et al. Efficacy of artesunate plus amodiaquine versus that of artemether-lumefantrine for the treatment of uncomplicated childhood *Plasmodium falciparum* malaria in Zanzibar, Tanzania. *Clin Infect Dis* 2005; 41:1079–1086.

770. Piola P, Fogg C, Bajunirwe F, et al. Supervised versus unsupervised intake of six-dose artemether-lumefantrine for treatment of acute, uncomplicated *Plasmodium falciparum* malaria in Mbarara, Uganda: a randomised trial. *Lancet* 2005; 365:1467–1473.

771. Looareesuwan S, Kyle DE, Viravan C, et al. Clinical study of pyronaridine for the treatment of acute uncomplicated falciparum malaria in Thailand. *Am J Trop Med Hyg* 1996; 54:205–209.

772. Ringwald P, Bickii J, Basco LK. Efficacy of oral pyronaridine for the treatment of acute uncomplicated falciparum malaria in African children. *Clin Infect Dis* 1998; 26:946–953.

773. Chen L. Recent studies on antimalarial efficacy of piperaquine and hydroxypiperaquine. *Chin Med J* 1991; 104:161–163

774. Hung TY, Davis TM, Ilett KF, et al. Population pharmacokinetics of piperaquine in adults and children with uncomplicated falciparum or vivax malaria. *Br J Clin Pharmacol* 2004; 57:253–262.

775. Tarning J, Bergqvist Y, Day NP, et al.Characterization of human urinary metabolites of the antimalarial piperaquine. *Drug Metab Dispos* 2006; 34:2011–2019.

776. Sim IK, Davis TM, Ilett KF. Effects of a high-fat meal on the relative oral bioavailability of piperaquine. *Antimicrob Agents Chemother* 2005; 49:2407–2411.

777. Tarning J, Lindegardh N, Annerberg A, et al. *Antimicrob Agents Chemother* 2005; 49:5127–5128.

778. Hien TT, Mai PP, Phuong P, et al. Dihydroartemisinin-piperaquine against multidrug resistant falciparum malaria in Vietnam: randomized clinical trial. *Lancet* 2004; 363:18–22.

779. Tarning J, Ashley EA, Lindegardh N, et al. Population pharmacokinetics of piperaquine after two different treatment regimens with dihydroartemisinin-piperaquine in patients with *Plasmodium falciparum* malaria in Thailand. *Antimicrob Agents Chemother* 2008; 52:1052–1061.

780. Karunajeewa HA, Ilett KF, Mueller I, et al. Pharmacokinetics and efficacy of piperaquine and chloroquine in Melanesian children with uncomplicated malaria. *Antimicrob Agents Chemother* 2008; 52:237–243.

781. Denis MB, Davis TM, Hewitt S, et al. Efficacy and safety of dihydroartemisinin-piperaquine (Artekin) in Cambodian children and adults with uncomplicated falciparum malaria. *Clin Infect Dis* 2002; 35:1469–1476.

782. Ashley EA, Krudsood S, Phaiphun L, et al. Randomized, controlled dose-optimization studies of dihydroartemisinin-piperaquine for the treatment of uncomplicated multidrug-resistant falciparum malaria in Thailand. *J Infect Dis* 2004; 190:1773–1782.

783. Mayxay M, Thongpraseuth V, Khanthavong M, et al. An open, randomized comparison of artesunate plus mefloquine vs. dihydroartemisinin-piperaquine for the treatment of uncomplicated *Plasmodium falciparum* malaria in the Lao People's Democratic Republic (Laos). *Trop Med Int Health* 2006; 11:1157–1165.

784. Hasugian AR, Purba HL, Kenangalem E, et al. Dihydroartemisinin-piperaquine versus artesunate-amodiaquine: superior efficacy and

posttreatment prophylaxis against multidrug-resistant *Plasmodium falciparum* and *Plasmodium vivax* malaria. *Clin Infect Dis* 2007; 44: 1067–1074.

785. Ratcliff A, Siswantoro H, Kenangalem E, et al. Two fixed-dose artemisinin combinations for drug-resistant falciparum and vivax malaria in Papua, Indonesia: an open-label randomised comparison. *Lancet* 2007; 369:757–765.

786. Ashley EA, McGready R, Hutagalung R, et al. A randomized controlled study of a simple once daily regimen of dihydroartemisinin-piperaquine for the treatment of uncomplicated multi-drug resistant falciparum malaria. *Clin Infect Dis* 2005, 41:425–432.

787. Smithuis F, Kyaw MK, Phe O, et al. Efficacy and effectiveness of dihydroartemisinin-piperaquine versus artesunate-mefloquine in falciparum malaria: an open-label randomised comparison. *Lancet* 2006; 367:2075–2085.

788. Karema C, Fanello CI, van Overmeir C, et al. Safety and efficacy of dihydroartemisinin/piperaquine (Artekin) for the treatment of uncomplicated Plasmodium falciparum malaria in Rwandan children. *Trans R Soc Trop Med Hyg* 2006; 100:1105–1111.

789. Pukrittayakamee S, Clemens R, Chantra A, et al. Therapeutic responses to antibacterial drugs in vivax malaria. *Trans R Soc Trop Med Hyg* 2001; 95:524–528.

790. Taylor WR, Widjaja H, Richie TL, et al. Chloroquine/doxycycline combination versus chloroquine alone, and doxycycline alone for the treatment of *Plasmodium falciparum* and *Plasmodium vivax* malaria in northeastern Irian Jaya, Indonesia. *Am J Trop Med Hyg* 2001; 64:223–228.

791. Kremsner PG, Zotter GM, Feldmeier H, et al. A comparative trial of three regimens for treating uncomplicated falciparum malaria in Acre, Brazil. *J Infect Dis* 1988; 158:1368–1371.

792. Pukrittayakamee S, Chantra A, Vanijanonta S, et al. Therapeutic responses to quinine and clindamycin in multidrug-resistant falciparum malaria. *Antimicrob Agents Chemother* 2000; 44:2395–2398.

793. Supanaranond W, Suputamongkol Y, Davis TME, et al. Lack of a significant adverse cardiovascular effect of combined quinine and mefloquine therapy for uncomplicated malaria. *Trans R Soc Trop Med Hyg* 1997; 91:694–696.

794. Pukrittayakamee S, Prakongpan S, Wanwimolruk S, et al. Adverse effect of rifampin on quinine efficacy in uncomplicated falciparum malaria. *Antimicrob Agents Chemother* 2003; 47:1509–1513.

795. Ridtitid W, Wongnawa M, Mahatthanatrakul W, et al. Effect of rifampin on plasma concentrations of mefloquine in healthy volunteers. *J Pharm Pharmacol* 2000; 52:1265–1269.

796. German P, Greenhouse B, Coates C, et al. Hepatotoxicity due to a drug interaction between amodiaquine plus artesunate and efavirenz. *Clin Infect Dis* 2007; 44:889–891.

797. Zucker JR, Lackritz EM, Ruebush TK 2nd, et al. Childhood mortality during and after hospitalization in western Kenya: effect of malaria treatment regimens. *Am J Trop Med Hyg* 1996; 55:655–660.

798. WHO. Assessment and monitoring of antimalarial drug efficacy for the treatment of uncomplicated falciparum malaria WHO/HTM/RBM/2003.50. Geneva: World Health Organization 2003. Online. Available: http://www.who.int/malaria/resistance.

799. Stepniewska K, White NJ. Some considerations in the design and interpretation of antimalarial drug trials in uncomplicated falciparum malaria. *Malar J* 2006; 5:127.

800. Nosten F, Imvithaya S, Vincenti M, et al. Malaria on the Thai–Burmese border: treatment of 5182 patients with mefloquine-sulfadoxine-pyrimethamine combination. *Bull WHO* 1987; 65:891–896.

801. Farnert A, Arez AP, Babiker HA, et al. Genotyping of Plasmodium falciparum infections by PCR: a comparative multicentre study. *Trans R Soc Trop Med Hyg* 2001; 95:225–232.

802. WHO. Methods and techniques for clinical trials on antimalarial drug efficacy. Geneva: World Health Organization; 2008.

803. Looareesuwan S, Charoenpan P, Ho M, et al. Fatal *Plasmodium falciparum* malaria after an inadequate response to quinine treatment. *J Infect Dis* 1990; 161:577–580.

804. Brockman A, Paul REL, Anderson TJC, et al. Application of genetic markers to the identification of recrudescent *Plasmodium falciparum* infections on the northwestern border of Thailand. *Am J Trop Med Hyg,* 1999; 60:14–21.

805. Stepniewska K, Taylor WRJ, Mayxay M, et al. The in vivo assessment of antimalarial drug efficacy in falciparum malaria; the duration of follow-up. *Antimicrob Agents Chemother* 2004; 48:4271–4280.

806. Imwong M, Snounou G, Pukrittayakamee S, et al. Relapses of *Plasmodium vivax* infection usually result from activation of heterologous hypnozoites. *J infect Dis* 2007; 195:927–933.

807. Chen N, Auliff A, Rieckmann K, et al. Relapses of *Plasmodium vivax* infection result from clonal hypnozoites activated at predetermined intervals. *J infect Dis* 2007; 195:934–941.

808. Trager W, Jensen JB. Continuous culture of *Plasmodium falciparum*: its impact on malaria research. *Int J Parasitol* 1997; 27:989–1006.

809. Rieckmann KH. Visual in-vitro test for determining the drug sensitivity of *Plasmodium falciparum*. *Lancet* 1982; 1:1333–1335.

810. Chotivanich K, Silamut K, Stepniewska K, et al. Ex-vivo short term culture and developmental assessment of *Plasmodium vivax*. *Trans R Soc Trop Med Hyg* 2001; 95:677–680.

811. Russell BM, Udomsangpetch R, Rieckmann KH, et al. Simple in vitro assay for determining the sensitivity of *Plasmodium vivax* isolates from fresh human blood to antimalarials in areas where *P. vivax* is endemic. *Antimicrob Agents Chemother* 2003; 47:170–173.

812. Webster HK, Boudreau EF, Pavanand K, et al. Antimalarial drug susceptibility testing of *Plasmodium falciparum* in Thailand using a microdilution radioisotope method. *Am J Trop Med Hyg* 1985; 34:228–235.

813. Druilhe P, Moreno A, Blanc C, et al. A colorimetric in vitro drug sensitivity assay for *Plasmodium falciparum* based on a highly sensitive double-site lactate dehydrogenase antigen-capture enzyme-linked immunosorbent assay. *Am J Trop Med Hyg* 2001; 64:233–241.

814. Noedl H, Attlmayr B, Wernsdorfer WH, et al. A histidine-rich protein 2-based malaria drug sensitivity assay for field use. *Am J Trop Med Hyg* 2004; 71: 711–714.

815. Pukrittayakamee S, Chantra A, Simpson JA, et al. Therapeutic responses to different antimalarial drugs in vivax malaria. *Antimicrob Agents Chemother* 2000; 44:1680–1685.

816. Arnold J, Alving AS, Hockwald RS, et al. The effect of continuous and intermittent primaquine therapy on the relapse rate of Chesson strain vivax malaria. *J Lab Clin Med* 1954; 43:429–434.

817. Pukrittayakamee S, Vanijanonta S, Chantra A, et al. Blood stage antimalarial efficacy of primaquine in *Plasmodium vivax* malaria. *J Infect Dis* 1994; 169:932–935.

818. White NJ. Optimal regimens of parenteral quinine. *Trans R Soc Trop Med Hyg* 1995; 89:462–463.

819. van der Torn M, Thuma PE, Mabeza GF, et al. Loading dose of quinine in African children with cerebral malaria. *Trans R Soc Trop Med Hyg* 1998; 92:325–331.

820. Teasdale G, Jennett B. Assessment of coma and impaired consciousness. A practical scale. *Lancet* 1974; 2:81–84.

821. Punyagupta S, Srichaikul T, Nitiyanant P, et al. Acute pulmonary insufficiency in falciparum malaria: summary of 12 cases with evidence of disseminated intravascular coagulation. *Am J Trop Med Hyg* 1974; 23: 551–559.

822. Warrell DA, Looareesuwan S, Warrell MJ, et al. Dexamethasone proves deleterious in cerebral malaria. A double blind trial in 100 comatose patients. *N Engl J Med* 1982; 306:313–319.

823. Hoffman SL, Rustama D, Punjabi NH, et al. High-dose dexamethasone in quinine-treated patients with cerebral malaria: a double-blind, placebo-controlled trial. *J Infect Dis* 1988; 158:325–331.

824. Taylor TE, Molyneux ME, Wirima JJ, et al. Intravenous immunoglobulin in the treatment of paediatric cerebral malaria. *Clin Exp Immunol* 1992; 90:357–362.

825. van Hensbroek MB, Palmer A, Onyiorah E, et al. The effect of a monoclonal antibody to tumor necrosis factor on survival from childhood cerebral malaria. *J Infect Dis* 1996; 174:1091–1097.

826. Thuma PE, Mabeza GF, Biemba G, et al. Effect of iron chelation therapy on mortality in Zambian children with cerebral malaria. *Trans R Soc Trop Med Hyg* 1998; 92:214–218.

827. White NJ. Not much progress in treatment of cerebral malaria (editorial). *Lancet* 1998; 352: 594–595.

828. Crawley J, Waruiru C, Mithwani S, et al. Effect of phenobarbital on seizure frequency and mortality in childhood cerebral malaria: a randomised, controlled intervention study. *Lancet* 2000; 355:701–706.

829. Price RN, van Vugt M, Nosten F, et al. Artesunate versus artemether for the treatment of recrudescent multi-drug resistant falciparum malaria. *Am J Trop Med Hyg* 1998; 59:883–888.

830. McGready R, Brockman A, Cho T, et al. Randomized comparison of mefloquine-artesunate versus quinine in the treatment of multi-drug resistant falciparum malaria in pregnancy. *Trans R Soc Trop Med Hyg* 2000; 94:689–693.

831. Tagbor HK, Chandramohan D, Greenwood B. The safety of amodiaquine use in pregnant women. *Expert Opin Drug Saf* 2007; 6:631–635.

832. Barnes KI, Watkins WM, White NJ. Antimalarial dosing regimens and drug resistance. *Trends Parasitol* 2008; 24:127–134.

833. Greenwood BM. The use of anti-malarial drugs to prevent malaria in the population of malaria-endemic areas. *Am J Trop Med Hyg* 2004; 70:1–7.

834. Briand V, Cottrell G, Massougbodji A, et al. Intermittent preventive treatment for the prevention of malaria during pregnancy in high transmission areas. *Malar J* 2007; 6:160

835. White NJ. Intermittent presumptive treatment for malaria. A better understanding of the pharmacodynamics will guide more rational policymaking. *PLoS Medicine* 2005; 2:29–33.

836. Parise ME, Ayisi JG, Nahlen BL, et al. Efficacy of sulfadoxine-pyrimethamine for prevention of placental malaria in an area of Kenya with a high prevalence of malaria and human immunodeficiency virus infection. *Am J Trop Med Hyg* 1998; 59:813–822.

837. Vallely A, Vallely L, Changalucha J, et al. Intermittent preventive treatment for malaria in pregnancy in Africa: what's new, what's needed? *Malar J* 2007; 6:16.

838. Garner P, Gulmezoglu AM. Drugs for preventing malaria in pregnant women. *Cochrane Database Syst Rev* 2006; CD000169.

839. Kayentao K, Kodio M, Newman RD, et al. Comparison of intermittent preventive treatment with chemoprophylaxis for the prevention of malaria during pregnancy in Mali. *J Infect Dis* 2005; 191:109–116.

840. van Eijk AM, Ayisi JG, ter Kuile FO, et al. Effectiveness of intermittent preventive treatment with sulphadoxine-pyrimethamine for control of malaria in pregnancy in western Kenya: a hospital-based study. *Trop Med Int Health* 2004; 9:351–360.

841. Denis MB, Tsuyuoka R, Lim P, et al. Efficacy of artemether-lumefantrine for the treatment of uncomplicated falciparum malaria in northwest Cambodia. *Trop Med Int Health* 2006; 11:1800–1807.

842. Denis MB, Tsuyuoka R, Poravuth Y, et al. Surveillance of the efficacy of artesunate and mefloquine combination for the treatment of uncomplicated falciparum malaria in Cambodia. *Trop Med Int Health* 2006; 11:1360–1366.

843. Fischer PR. Congenital malaria: an African survey. *Clin Pediatr (Phila)* 1997; 36:411–413.

844. Foster SD. Pricing, distribution and use of antimalarial drugs. *Bull World Health Org* 1991; 69:349–363.

845. Lindsay SW, Gibson ME. Bed-nets revisited – old idea, new angle. *Parasitol Today* 1988; 4:270–272.

846. Alonso PL, Lindsay SW, Armstrong JRM, et al. The effect of insecticide-treated bed nets on mortality of Gambian children. *Lancet* 1991; 337:1499–1502.

847. Greenwood BM, Greenwood AM, Bradley AK, et al. Comparison of two strategies for control of malaria within a primary health care programme in the Gambia. *Lancet* 1988; 1:1121–1127.

848. Lengeler C. Comparison of malaria control interventions. *Bull World Health Org* 2001; 79:77.

849. Lengeler C. *Insecticide Treated Bed-nets and Curtains for Malaria Control (Cochrane Review)*. Oxford: The Cochrane Library; 2005.

850. WHO (2003) The Africa Malaria Report; 2003. (WHO/CDS/MAL/2003.1093). Available: http://whqlibdoc.who.int/hq/2003/WHO_CDS_MAL_2003.

851. Lindblade KA, Dotson E, Hawley WA, et al. Evaluation of long-lasting insecticidal nets after 2 years of household use. *Trop Med Int Health* 2005; 10:1141–1150.

852. Hawley WA, Phillips-Howard PA, ter Kuile FO, et al. Community-wide effects of permethrin-treated bed nets on child mortality and malaria morbidity in western Kenya. *Am J Trop Med Hyg* 2003; 68:121–127.

853. Phillips-Howard PA, Nahlen BL, Kolczak MS, et al. Efficacy of permethrin-treated bed nets in the prevention of mortality in young children in an area of high perennial malaria transmission in western Kenya. *Am J Trop Med Hyg* 2003; 68:23–29.

854. Rowland M, Durrani N, Kenward M, et al. Control of malaria in Pakistan by applying deltamethrin insecticide to cattle: a community-randomised trial. *Lancet* 2001; 357:1837–1841.

855. Curtis CF, Mnzava AE. Comparison of house spraying and insecticide-treated nets for malaria control. *Bull World Health Org* 2000; 78:1389–1400.

856. McGready R, Simpson JA, Htway M, et al. A double-blind randomized therapeutic trial of insect repellents for the prevention of malaria in pregnancy. *Trans R Soc Trop Med Hyg* 2001; 95:137–138.

857. Chen LH, Wilson ME, Schlagenhauf P. Prevention of malaria in long-term travelers. *JAMA* 2006; 296:2234–2244.

858. Shanks GD, Edstein MD. Modern malaria chemoprophylaxis. *Drugs* 2005; 65:2091–2110.

859. Rozendaal J. *Vector Control; Methods for Use by Individuals and Communities*. Geneva: World Health Organization; 1997.

860. Massaga JJ, Kitua AY, Lemnge MM, et al. Effect of intermittent treatment with amodiaquine on anaemia and malaria fevers in infants in Tanzania: a randomised, placebo-controlled trial. *Lancet* 2003; 361:1853–1860.

861. Chandramohan D, Owusu-Agyei S, Carneiro I, et al. Prevention of malaria in infants by intermittent preventive treatment in an area of high, seasonal transmission in Ghana. *BMJ* 2005; 331:727–733.

862. Cisse B, Sokhna C, Boulanger D, et al. Seasonal intermittent preventive treatment with artesunate and sulfadoxine pyrimethamine prevents malaria in Senegalese children. *Lancet* 2006; 367:659–667.

863. Dicko S, Sagara S, Sissoko MS, et al. Impact of intermittent preventive treatment with sulfadoxine-pyrimethamine targeting the transmission season on the incidence of clinical malaria in children aged 6 months to 10 years in Kambila, Mali. *Am J Trop Med Hyg* 2004; 71(suppl S4):6.

864. Clyde DF, McCarthy VC, Miller RM, et al. Specificity of protection of man immunized against sporozoite-induced malaria. *Am J Med Sci* 1973; 266:398–401.

865. Alonso PL, Sacarlal J, Aponte JJ, et al. Efficacy of the RTS,S/AS02A vaccine against *Plasmodium falciparum* infection and disease in young African children: randomised controlled trial. *Lancet* 2004; 364:1411–1420.

866. Graves P, Gelband H. Vaccines for preventing malaria (blood-stage). *Cochrane Database Syst Rev* 2006; 18(4):CD006199.

867. Gosling RD, Ghani AC, Deen JL, et al. Can changes in malaria transmission intensity explain prolonged protection and contribute to high protective efficacy of intermittent preventive treatment for malaria in infants? *Malar J* 2008; 3(7):54.

868. Mockenhaupt FP, Reither K, Zanger P, et al. Intermittent preventive treatment in infants as a means of malaria control: a randomized, double-blind, placebo-controlled trial in northern Ghana. *Antimicrob Agents Chemother* 2007; 51:3273–3281.

869. Kobbe R, Kreuzberg C, Adjei S, et al. A randomized controlled trial of extended intermittent preventive antimalarial treatment in infants. *Clin Infect Dis* 2007; 45:16–25.

870. von Seidlein L, Greenwood BM. Mass administrations of antimalarial drugs. *Trends Parasitol* 2003; 19:452–460.

871. Graves P, Gelband H. Vaccines for preventing malaria (pre-erythrocytic). *Cochrane Database Syst Rev*. 2006; 18(4):CD006198.

872. Epstein JE, Giersing B, Mullen G, et al. Malaria vaccines: are we getting closer? *Curr Opin Mol Ther* 2007; 9:12–24.

873. Hendrickse RG, Adeniyi A, Edington GM, et al. Quartan malarial nephrotic syndrome. Collaborative clinicopathological study in Nigerian children. *Lancet* 1977; i:1143–1149.

874. Gilles HM, Hendrickse RG. Nephrosis in Nigerian children: role of Plasmodium malariae and effect of antimalarial treatment. *BMJ* 1963; ii: 27–31.

875. Abdurrahman MB, Aikhionbare HA, Babaoye FA, et al. Clinicopathological features of childhood nephrotic syndrome in northern Nigeria. *Q J Med* 1990; 75:563–576.

876. Crane G. Tropical splenomegaly. Part II Oceania. *Clin Haematol* 1981; 10:976–982.

877. Martin-Peprah R, Bates I, Bedu-Addo G, et al. Investigation of familial segregation of hyperreactive malarial splenomegaly in Kumasi, Ghana. *Trans R Soc Trop Med Hyg* 2006; 100:68–73.

878. Piessens WF, Hoffman SL, Wadee AA, et al. Antibody mediated killing of T suppressor lymphocytes as a possible cause of macroglobulinaemia in the tropical splenomegaly syndrome. *J Clin Invest* 1985; 75: 1821–1827.

879. Hoffman SL, Piessens WF, Ratiwayanto S, et al. Reduction of suppressor T-lymphocytes in the tropical splenomegaly syndrome. *N Engl J Med* 1984; 310:337–341.

880. Bate I, Bedu-Addo G, Bevan DH, et al. Use of immunoglobulin gene rearrangements to show clonal lymphoproliferation in hyper-reactive malarial splenomegaly. *Lancet* 1991; 337:505–507.

881. Lam KMC, Syed N, Whittle H, et al. Circulating Epstein–Barr virus-carrying B cells in acute malaria. *Lancet* 1991; 337:876–879.

882. Nájera JA. Malaria control: achievements, problems and strategies. *Parasitologia* 2001; 43:1–89.

883. Molineaux L, Grammiccia G; *The Garki Project.* Geneva: World Health Organization; 1980.

884. Martinez-Torres D, Chandre F, Williamson MS, et al. Molecular characterization of pyrethroid knockdown resistance (kdr) in the major malaria vector *Anopheles gambiae* s.s. *Insect Mol Biol* 1998; 7:179–184.

885. Ranson H, Jensen B, Vulule JM, et al. Identification of a point mutation in the voltage-gated sodium channel gene of Kenyan *Anopheles gambiae* associated with resistance to DDT and pyrethroids. *Insect Mol Biol* 2000; 9:491–497.

886. Hargreaves K, Koekemoer LL, Brooke BD, et al. *Anopheles funestus* resistant to pyrethroid insecticides in South Africa. *Med Vet Entomol* 2000; 14: 181–189.

887. Hemingway J, Hawkes NJ, McCarroll L, et al. The molecular basis of insecticide resistance in mosquitoes. *Insect Biochem Mol Biol* 2004; 34:653–665.

888. Soderlund DM, Knipple DC. The molecular biology of knockdown resistance to pyrethroid insecticides. *Insect Biochem Mol Biol* 2003; 33: 563–577.

889. Chandre F, Darrier F, Manga L, et al. Status of pyrethroid resistance in *Anopheles gambiae* sensu lato. *Bull World Health Org* 1999; 77:230–234.

890. Attaran A, Roberts DR, Curtis CF, et al. Balancing risks on the backs of the poor. *Nat Med* 2000; 6:729–731.

Chapter 74

Peter L. Chiodini

Babesiosis

Babesia spp. are protozoan parasites of domestic and wild animals. They are members of the phylum Apicomplexa, order Piroplasmida, family Babesiidae.

Most human cases of babesiosis are due to *Babesia divergens* or *B. microti* species complex. *B. caucasica* has also been reported to infect humans, but Hoare[1] considered it to be synonymous with *B. bovis*. There is one case reportedly due to *B. canis*.[2] A new *Babesia*, WA1, now named *Babesia duncani* n.sp., was isolated from a patient in Washington State, USA.[3,4] Parasites isolated from cases of human babesiosis in California, USA, known as CA1-CA4, have been shown to be closely related to WA1 by molecular criteria.[3] A *Babesia divergens*-like parasite, MO1, has been isolated from a fatal case of babesiosis from Missouri, USA,[5] and another *B. divergens*-like parasite, unrelated to WA1, recorded from Washington state.[6] A previously uncharacterized *Babesia* distinct from *Babesia divergens* and closely related to *B. odocoilei*, a parasite of white-tailed deer has been described from Italy and Austria and named as EU1.[7] A *Babesia microti*-like organism has caused human infection in Taiwan.[8] Of considerable interest is the fact that *B. microti* can no longer be regarded as a single species, but exists as a worldwide species complex consisting of three clades, one containing zoonotic isolates.[9,10] As phylogenetic analysis based on molecular criteria develops further, there are likely to be more reports of new *Babesia* species and revision of the taxonomy of this genus.

LIFE CYCLE

Human babesiosis is a zoonosis acquired by tick bite when individuals accidentally interact with the natural life cycle of the parasite. Humans represent dead-end hosts for *Babesia* spp.

Bovine Babesias

Sporozoites are injected into the bloodstream by tick bite and penetrate erythrocytes. In contrast to the malaria life cycle, no tissue stage has ever been demonstrated for *B. bovis* or *B. divergens*. Within the erythrocyte the parasites vary in appearance, being oval, round or pear shaped.

Ring forms, especially, may be confused with malaria parasites, especially *Plasmodium falciparum*. However, *Babesia* does not form pigment and does not cause alterations in red cell morphology or staining, such as the Maurer clefts of *P. falciparum*, the Schüffner

dots of *P. vivax* or the James dots of *P. ovale*. *Babesia* multiplies in the red cell by budding (*Plasmodium* by schizogony). Release of daughter parasites is followed by reinvasion of fresh erythrocytes and further asexual multiplication.

Some of the sporozoites injected by the tick vector follow a different path of intraerythrocytic development, growing slowly and 'folding' to form accordion-like structures, thought to be gametocytes[11] that are destined to undergo further development in the tick vector.

Within the gut of the tick the accordion-like stage is able to resist digestion and eventually fuses with another, to form a zygote. Further development outside the intestine occurs in a variety of tissues, the salivary glands and ovaries being especially important for transmission.

Sporozoites in tick salivary glands are injected into the mammalian host at the next blood meal. Transovarial transmission of *B. bovis* also takes place so that newly hatched larvae are already infected. Trans-stadial transmission to nymph and then to adult stages can then take place.

Babesia microti

In the small mammal host of *B. microti*, sporozoites from the tick vector first enter lymphocytes and undergo merogony, the daughter parasites of which then enter erythrocytes.[11] There is no published report of this intralymphocytic stage in human *B. microti* infections. The presence of schizogony in lymphocytes of its vertebrate host is one of the factors which has led Uilenberg to conclude that *B. microti* is not a *Babesia* and could logically be called *Theileria microti*.[12] Until the taxonomic issue is further clarified, this chapter will continue to refer to *Babesia microti*.

B. microti does not undergo transovarial transmission,[11] but once a larva has become infected from a mammalian host it is able to pass on the infection trans-stadially to the nymph.

EPIDEMIOLOGY

Human infection follows tick bite or, rarely, blood transfusion or transplacental/perinatal infection. Each *Babesia*–vector–mammalian host system has its own characteristics, and the ecology and bionomics of the vector tick define the pattern of risk for the human population.

most of the anaemia is due to haemolysis. Total white blood cell counts are low or normal and there may be thrombocytopenia.[17]

Mean and differential lymphocyte counts and percentages of B lymphocytes and levels of T lymphocytes with the immunoglobulin (Ig) G Fc receptor were raised in acute infection. Polyclonal hypergammaglobulinaemia was found. Levels of serum IgG, IgM and C1q binding were significantly increased; C3 and C4 levels and haemolytic activity were reduced in acute-phase sera.[29]

There may be a mild increase in serum glutamic oxaloacetic transaminase (aspartate aminotransferase), alkaline phosphatase and bilirubin concentrations.[1]

Electron microscopy

This technique is not helpful for routine diagnosis of human babesiosis but may provide useful confirmation of the nature of the infection. Transmission electron microscopy of *B. microti* from a splenectomized patient also receiving systemic steroids showed considerable pleomorphism. All developmental stages were seen in both reticulocytes and mature erythrocytes. The same study identified convoluted cells with many free ribosomes, thought to represent an early gametocyte stage.[28]

Serodiagnosis

The indirect fluorescent antibody test (IFAT) is available for bovine *Babesia* and for *B. microti*. However, serology should not be seen as an alternative to blood film examination, especially in view of the fulminant nature of bovine *Babesia* infection in splenectomized patients. Demonstration of parasites in a blood film provides unequivocal proof of current infection. Some *B. microti* infections may have low level or transient parasitaemia,[32] and serology, with PCR testing of seropositive individuals,[27] has a useful part to play in establishing the diagnosis. Ruebush et al.[32] defined individuals with IFAT titres to *B. microti* of 64 or greater as seropositive. In patients with acute *B. microti* infection, IFAT titres were greater than or equal to 1 in 1024, and fell to 1 in 256 or 1 in 64 over 8–12 months. The possibility of cross-reaction with antimalarial antibody must be borne in mind when serological results are interpreted. The *B. microti* IFAT has a reported 88–96% sensitivity and 90–100% specificity.[33] A brief report describing an IgG ELISA for the detection of antibody to B.microti has been published. This assay has a reported sensitivity of 95.5% and specificity of 94.1% compared with the *B. microti* IFAT.[34]

Polymerase chain reaction

This technique has been applied to the diagnosis of *B. microti*, with a reported limit of detection of approximately three merozoites.[35] It is deployed increasingly to confirm infection in antibody-reactive individuals and to monitor the response to treatment.[27]

Animal inoculation

This is not used for routine diagnosis of individual cases, but *B. microti* from human cases can be isolated in hamsters,[17] and *B.*

divergens from a fatal human case was successfully passaged to gerbils and to a splenectomized calf.[25]

CLINICAL COURSE AND MANAGEMENT

Babesia bovis/divergens

If untreated, infection of splenectomized humans with bovine Babesias leads to fulminant illness and death. Specific treatment is based upon anecdotal case reports. Diminazene (Berenil) is active against *Babesia* in animals and was used in a case of human *B. divergens* infection, but the patient died.[36] Successful treatment of *B. divergens* (5% parasitaemia) in a splenectomized patient with pentamidine plus co-trimoxazole has been recorded.[36] The veterinary compound imidocarb was used successfully in the treatment of two cases of human infection with *B. divergens*[37] Quinine and chloroquine plus pyrimethamine have proven ineffective.[25]

Brasseur and Gorenflot[38] reported successful treatment of three cases with massive exchange blood transfusion (2–3 blood volumes) followed by intravenous clindamycin and oral quinine.

Atovaquone is effective against *B. divergens* in vitro.[39] In the absence of data from randomized controlled trials, current therapy should consist of exchange blood transfusion plus intravenous clindamycin and intravenous or oral quinine, depending upon the patient's condition.

Babesia microti

In most instances, patients suffer a mild illness from which they recover spontaneously. Recovery may be prolonged, with several months of fatigue and malaise.[17] Where treatment is required, oral quinine 650 mg every 8 h plus clindamycin 300–600 mg intravenously or intramuscularly every 6 h (adult doses) for 7–10 days has been regarded as the treatment of choice,[2,40] although it is not universally effective.[41] Paediatric dosage is oral quinine 25 mg/kg per day and intravenous or intramuscular clindamycin 20 mg/kg per day. Krause et al.[42] compared atovaquone 750 mg every 12 h plus azithromycin 500 mg on day 1 and 250 mg daily thereafter for 7 days with clindamycin 600 mg every 8 h and quinine 650 mg every 8 h for 7 days, all drugs being given orally. Atovaquone plus azithromycin proved to be as effective as clindamycin plus quinine and had fewer adverse reactions. The authors recommended that atovaquone plus azithromycin be considered for the treatment of non-life-threatening babesiosis in immunocompetent adult patients and in others who cannot tolerate clindamycin and quinine.[42] Weiss et al.[43] reported the successful use of azithromycin 12 mg/kg per day and atovaquone 40 mg/kg per day in neonates, without toxic effects, and had used a higher dose of azithromycin (600 mg per day) in combination with atovaquone (750 mg twice daily) in adults. They reported that the 600-mg daily dose of azithromycin led to earlier resolution of fever and rapid clearance of parasites from the blood.[43] The Infectious Diseases Society of America states that higher doses of azithromycin (600–1000 mg/day) may be used for immunocompromised patients with babesiosis.[44] Ranque[45] has suggested that a trial of atovaquone plus clindamycin should be performed.

Chloroquine is unhelpful. Diminazene was used in one case and the patient recovered but developed neurological complications resembling the Guillain-Barré syndrome.[46]

Whole blood or red cell exchange transfusion has produced a rapid and substantial fall in parasitaemia and its use as an adjunct to chemotherapy should be considered in severely ill patients with high parasitaemia.[47]

PREVENTION

There is no vaccine licensed for human use. Prevention of human babesiosis depends upon avoidance of tick bite: avoidance of tick habitats; wearing appropriate clothing to cover the lower part of the body; use of insect repellent (e.g. diethyltoluamide and permethrin-impregnated clothing); and prompt removal of ticks found on the person. In endemic areas, awareness of the possibility of transfusion-transmitted *Babesia* infection should be maintained so that those thought to be potentially infected with *Babesia* can be excluded from donation, although routine screening of donor blood is not yet established.[18]

REFERENCES

1. Hoare CA. Comparative aspects of human babesiosis. *Trans R Soc Trop Med Hyg* 1980; 74:143–148.
2. Telford SR III, Gorenflot A, Brasseur P, et al. Babesial infections in man and wildlife. In: Kreier JP, Baker JR, eds. *Parasitic Protozoa 5*. 2nd edn. San Diego: Academic Press; 1993:1–47.
3. Thomford JW, Conrad PA, Telford SR, et al. Cultivation and phylogenetic characterisation of a newly recognised human pathogenic protozoan. *J Infect Dis* 1994; 169:1050–1056.
4. Conrad PA, Kjemtrup AM, Carreno RA, et al. Description of Babesia duncani n.sp. (Apicomplexa: Babesiidae) from humans and its differentiation from other piroplasms. *Int J Parasitol* 2006; 36(7):779–789.
5. Herwaldt B, Persing DH, Precigout EA, et al. A fatal case of babesiosis in Missouri: identification of another piroplasm that infects humans. *Ann Intern Med* 1997; 124:643–650.
6. Herwaldt BL, de Bruyn G, Pieniazek NJ, et al. Babesia divergens-like infection, Washington State. *Emerg Infect Dis* 2004; 10(4): 622–629.
7. Herwaldt BL, Caccio S, Gherlinzoni F, et al. Molecular characterization of a non-Babesia divergens organism causing zoonotic babesiosis in Europe. *Emerg Infect Dis* 2003; 9(8):942–948.
8. Shih CM, Liu LP, Chung WC, et al. Human babesiosis in Taiwan: asymptomatic infection with a Babesia microti-like organism in a Taiwanese woman. *J Clin Microbiol* 1997; 35:450–454.
9. Gray JS. Identity of the causal agents of human babesiosis in Europe. *Int J Med Microbiol* 2006; 296(Suppl 40):131–136.
10. Sinski E, Bajer A, Welc R, et al. Babesia microti: prevalence in wild rodents and Ixodes ricinus ticks from the Mazury Lakes District of North-Eastern Poland. *Int J Med Microbiol* 2006; 296(Suppl 40):137–143.
11. Kakoma I, Mehlhorn H. Babesia of domestic animals. In: Kreier JP, ed. *Parasitic Protozoa*. 2nd edn. San Diego: Academic Press; 1993: 141–216.
12. Uilenberg G. Babesia – a historical overview. *Vet Parasitol* 2006; 138(1–2): 3–10.
13. Berry A, Morassin B, Kamar N, et al. Clinical picture: human babesiosis. *Lancet* 2001; 357:341.
14. Kjemtrup AM, Conrad PA. Human babesiosis: an emerging tick-borne disease. *Int J Parasitol* 2000; 30:1323–1337.
15. Meldrum SC, Birkhead GS, White DJ, et al. Human babesiosis in New York State: an epidemiological description of 136 cases. *Clin Infect Dis* 1992; 15:1019–1023.
16. Steketee RW, Eckman MR, Burgess EC, et al. Babesiosis in Wisconsin: a new focus of disease transmission. *JAMA* 1985; 253:2675–2678.
17. Ruebush TK II. Human babesiosis in North America. *Trans R Soc Trop Med Hyg* 1980; 74:149–152.
18. Leiby DA. Babesiosis and blood transfusion: flying under the radar. *Vox Sang* 2006; 90(3):157–165.
19. Leiby DA, Chung AP, Gill JE, et al. Demonstrable parasitemia among Connecticut blood donors with antibodies to Babesia microti. *Transfusion* 2005; 45(11):1804–1810.
20. Krause PJ, Telford SR III, Spielman A, et al. Concurrent Lyme disease and babesiosis. Evidence for increased severity and duration of illness. *JAMA* 1996; 275:1657–1660.
21. Swanson SJ, Neitzel D, Reed KD, et al. Coinfections acquired from ixodes ticks. *Clin Microbiol Rev* 2006; 19(4):708–727.
22. Benach JL, Habicht GS. Clinical characteristics of human babesiosis. *J Infect Dis* 1981; 144:481.
23. Ong KR, Stavropoulos C, Inada Y. Babesiosis, asplenia and AIDS. *Lancet* 1990; 336:112.
24. Falagas ME, Klempner MS. Babesiosis in patients with AIDS: a chronic infection presenting as fever of unknown origin. *Clin Infect Dis* 1996; 22:809–812.
25. Williams H. Human babesiosis. *Trans R Soc Trop Med Hyg* 1980; 74:157.
26. Uhnoo I, Cars O, Christensson D, et al. First documented case of human babesiosis in Sweden. *Scand J Infect Dis* 1992; 24:541–547.
27. Homer MJ, Aguilar-Delfin I, Telford SR III, et al. Babesiosis. *Clin Microbiol Rev* 2000; 13:451–469.
28. Sun T, Tenenbaum MJ, Greenspan J, et al. Morphologic and clinical observations in human infection with Babesia microti. *J Infect Dis* 1983; 148:239–248.
29. Benach JL, Habicht GS, Hamburger MI. Immunoresponsiveness in acute babesiosis in humans. *J Infect Dis* 1982; 146:369–380.
30. Hatcher JC, Greenberg PD, Antique J, et al. Severe babesiosis in Long Island: review of 34 cases and their complications. *Clin Infect Dis* 2001; 32: 1117–1125.
31. Clark IA, Budd AC, Hsue G, et al. Absence of erythrocyte sequestration in a case of babesiosis in a splenectomised human patient. *Malar J* 2006; 5:69.
32. Ruebush TK II, Juranek DD, Chisholm ES, et al. Human babesiosis on Nantucket Island. Evidence for self-limited and subclinical infections. *N Engl J Med* 1977; 297:825–827.
33. Krause PJ, Telford SR, Ryan R, et al. Diagnosis of babesiosis: evaluation of a serologic test for the detection of Babesia microti antibody. *J Infect Dis* 1994; 169:923–926.
34. Loa CC, Adelson ME, Mordechai E, et al. Serological diagnosis of human babesiosis by IgG enzyme-linked immunosorbent assay. *Curr Microbiol* 2004; 49(6):385–389.
35. Persing DH, Mathiesen D, Marshall WF, et al. Detection of Babesia microti by polymerase chain reaction. *J Clin Microbiol* 1992; 30:2097–2103.
36. Raoult D, Soulayrol L, Toga B, et al. Babesiosis, pentamidine and cotrimaxozole. *Ann Intern Med* 1987; 107:944.
37. Vial HJ, Gorenflot A. Chemotherapy against babesiosis. *Vet Parasitol* 2006; 138(1–2):147–160.
38. Brasseur P, Gorenflot A. Human babesiosis in Europe. *Mem Inst Oswaldo Cruz* 1992; 87:131–132.
39. Pudney M, Gray JS. Therapeutic efficacy of atovaquone against the bovine intraerythrocytic parasite, Babesia divergens. *J Parasitol* 1997; 83:307–310.
40. Gelfand JA, Poutsiaka D. Babesia. In: Mandell GL, Bennett JE, Dolin R, eds. *Principles and Practice of Infectious Diseases*. 5th edn. Philadelphia: Churchill Livingstone; 2000:2899–2902.
41. Anonymous. Clindamycin and quinine treatment for Babesia microti infections. *MMWR Morb Mortal Wkly Rep* 1983; 32:65–71.

42. Krause PJ, Lepore T, Sikand VK, et al. Atovaquone and azithromycin for the treatment of babesiosis. *N Engl J Med* 2000; 343:1454–1458.

43. Weiss LM, Wittner M, Tanowitz HB. The treatment of babesiosis. *N Engl J Med* 2001; 344:773.

44. Wormser GP, Dattwyler RJ, Shapiro ED, et al. Single-dose prophylaxis against Lyme disease. *Lancet Infect Dis* 2007; 7(6):371–373.

45. Ranque S. The treatment of babesiosis. *N Engl J Med* 2001; 344:773–774.

46. Ruebush TK II, Rubin RH, Wolpow ER, et al. Neurologic complications following the treatment of human Babesia microti infection with diminazene aceturate. *Am J Trop Med Hyg* 1979; 28:184–189.

47. Evenson DA, Perry E, Kloster B, et al. Therapeutic apheresis for babesiosis. *J Clin Apheresis* 1998; 13:32–36.

Chapter 75 Christian Burri and Reto Brun

Human African Trypanosomiasis

HISTORICAL BACKGROUND

David Livingstone (1813–1873) had been convinced in the mid-nineteenth century that the tsetse fly was responsible for the transmission of 'nagana', a disease that affected cattle in central Africa. This is clearly recorded in his classic *Missionary Travels*, first published in 1857. It seems probable that Livingstone had in fact associated the bite of *Glossina palpalis* with 'nagana' as early as 1847. It was not until 1894, however, that the causative role of *Trypanosoma* (later designated *T. brucei*) was delineated in nagana, and this resulted from the brilliant work of David Bruce (Figure 75.1) in Zululand, where he had been posted from military duty in Natal. Shortly before this, animal trypanosomes had been visualized, and in 1878 Timothy Lewis had first indicated that trypanosomes could cause infection in mammals.

A febrile illness associated with cervical lymphadenopathy and lethargy had been clearly recorded in Sierra Leone by T. M. Winterbottom (1765–1859) in 1803. In 1902, Joseph Dutton (1874–1905) and John Todd (1876–1949) demonstrated that *Trypanosoma* spp. were responsible for this condition, then named 'trypanosome fever' in West Africa; their observations were made on an Englishman who had been infected in The Gambia.

Early in the twentieth century an outbreak that was described at the time as 'negro lethargy' swept central Africa; this involved the northern shores of Lake Victoria in Nyanza. No one, it seems, equated the disease with 'trypanosome fever'. In 1902, the Royal Society sent a Sleeping Sickness Expedition, consisting of Low, Castellani (1877–1971) and Christy (1864–1932), in an attempt to determine the aetiological agent responsible for this disease. Manson was of the opinion that *Filaria perstans* was responsible; he had visualized this parasite in three cases of sleeping sickness investigated in London. After a great deal of painstaking work, Castellani concluded that the disease was caused by a streptococcus. He also visualized *Trypanosoma* spp. in the cerebrospinal fluid (CSF) of a single patient with 'negro lethargy'; however, he disregarded this organism, and favoured the streptococcal theory. The Royal Society proceeded to send a second team to Uganda in 1903, consisting of Bruce (Figure 75.1) and David Nabarro (1874–1958). They demonstrated *Trypanosoma* spp. in numerous cases of sleeping sickness (in both CSF and blood) and, furthermore, were able to transmit *T. gambiense* to monkeys via the bite of infected *Glossina palpalis* (the local species of tsetse fly); this work clinched the aetiological agent responsible for this disease.

Several years were to pass before the animal reservoirs of African trypanosomiasis were delineated. Was the causative organism of nagana identical with that which caused African trypanosomiasis? It was not until 1910 that J. W. W. Stephens (1865–1946) and H. B. Fantham (1875–1937) discovered *T. rhodesiense* in Nyasaland (now Malawi) and northern Rhodesia (now Zimbabwe). In 1911, Allan Kinghorn (?–1955) and Warrington Yorke (1883–1943) demonstrated the transmission of *T. rhodesiense* to humans by *Glossina morsitans*.

It is now known that human African trypanosomiasis ('sleeping sickness') is caused by the protozoan parasites *Trypanosoma brucei gambiense* in west and central Africa, and by *Trypanosoma brucei rhodesiense* in eastern Africa. By the end of the 1960s, the disease had been almost eliminated by means of large-scale control and intervention programmes. However, the situation has deteriorated since and by the year 2000, the number of cases was estimated at 300 000 to 500 000 with about 60 million people at risk, but fewer than 4 million under appropriate surveillance. Major outbreaks have been reported from the Democratic Republic of Congo, Angola, Sudan and Uganda. Today, the number of cases is again decreasing due to improved surveillance and vector control.

GEOGRAPHICAL DISTRIBUTION AND EPIDEMIOLOGY

Sleeping sickness is endemic only in areas where *Glossina* species are found. The ecological limit of Glossina distribution is approximately a line from 14°N from Senegal in the west to 10°N in southern Somalia in the east, and 20°S corresponding to the northern fringes of the Kalahari and Namibian Deserts. The distribution of Glossina is determined by climatic factors (temperature and humidity) through its effects on vegetation. It is anticipated that satellite technology will be of increasing use in defining fly distribution in relation to habitats.[1] Comparison of such images over time will, in association with geographical information system (GIS) techniques, be of value in predicting tsetse distribution in relation to changes in environment. Rogers and Williams[2] examined how GIS can contribute to studies of human and animal trypanosomiasis and how data from meteorological

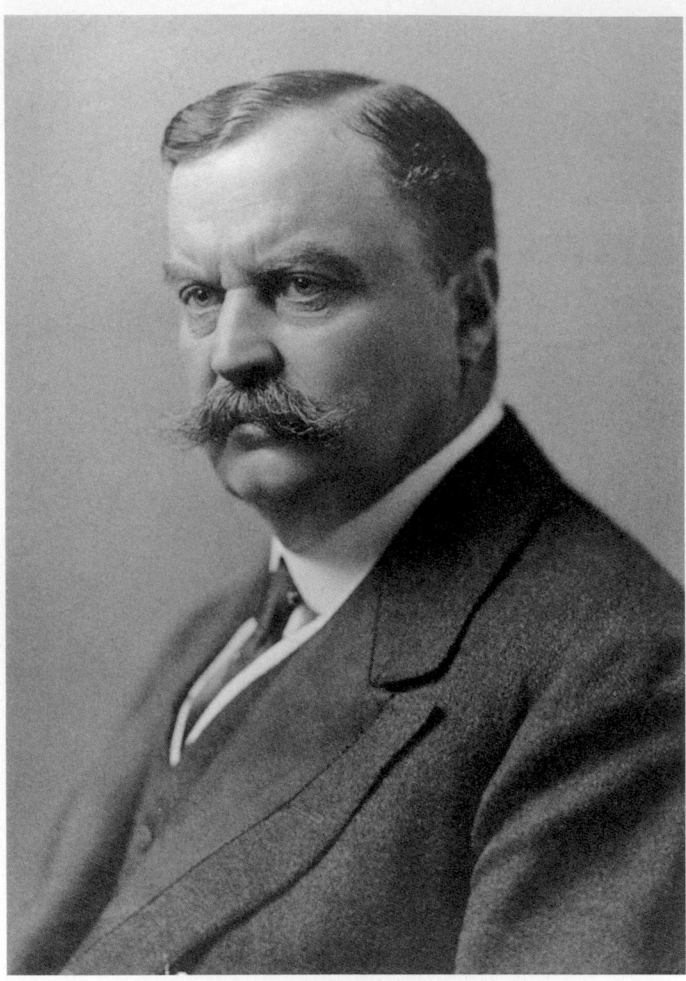

Figure 75.1 David Bruce (1855–1931) established the causes of nagana in Zululand and of 'negro lethargy' in Uganda. (From Gillespie SH et al., eds. *Principles and Practice of Clinical Parasitology.* Chichester: Wiley; 2001.)

Table 75.1 Major vectors of *T.b. gambiense* and *T.b. rhodesiense* and geographical distribution

T.b. gambiense

  G. palpalis palpalis, G. palpalis gambiensis

    Angola, Benin, Burkina Faso, Cameroon, Central African Republic, Congo, Democratic Republic of Congo, Gabon, Gambia, Ghana, Guinea, Guinea-Bissau, Ivory Coast, Liberia, Mali, Nigeria, Senegal, Sierra Leone, Togo

  G. tachinodes

    Benin, Burkina Faso, Cameroon, Central African Republic, Chad, Ethiopia, Ghana, Guinea, Ivory Coast, Mali, Niger, Nigeria, Sudan, Togo

  G. fuscipes quanzensis, G. fuscipes martinii

    Angola, Congo, Democratic Republic of Congo

  G. fuscipes fuscipes

    Cameroon, Central African Republic, Chad, Congo, Democratic Republic of Congo, Sudan, Uganda

T.b. rhodesiense

  G. morsitans morsitans, G. morsitans centralis

    Angola, Botswana, Burundi, Malawi, Mozambique, Rwanda, Tanzania, Zambia, Zimbabwe

  G. pallidipes

    Burundi, Ethiopia, Kenya, Malawi, Mozambique, Rwanda, Sudan, Tanzania, Uganda, Zambia, Zimbabwe

  G. swynnertoni

    Kenya, Tanzania

  G. fuscipes fuscipes

    Ethiopia, Kenya, Tanzania, Uganda

satellites help to understand the spatial distribution of vectors and disease.

There are over 20 species of *Glossina* and a number of subspecies, most of which are capable of acting as vectors of trypanosomes that cause human sleeping sickness (as well as animal disease). The tsetse flies are separated into three groups, of which two groups are mainly responsible for the transmission of sleeping sickness: the *palpalis* group transmits *T.b. gambiense*, which is responsible for the chronic form of the disease; and the *morsitans* group transmits *T.b. rhodesiense*, which causes a more acute disease. In Uganda, epidemic *T.b. rhodesiense* is transmitted by the riverine tsetse fly *G. fuscipes*. The major vectors and their geographical distribution are listed in Table 75.1. The current distribution of sleeping sickness in Africa is shown in Figure 75.2. Jordan[3] provides an up-to-date summary of *Glossina* biology and control.

Sleeping sickness is endemic in over 200 known foci in 36 countries and *Glossina* spp. infest approximately 10 million km² or about one-third of the African continent.

In the late 1990s, WHO had not only emphasized the recrudescence of the disease, with major flare-ups in many endemic countries, but also the dramatic lack of awareness about the disease situation. The resulting under-surveillance had led to reporting of approximately 25 000 new cases per year and estimates of the infection level reaching over 300 000 new cases.[4] In the meantime, major events have impacted control of the disease, such as the interruption of war and civil conflicts in several affected countries; the commitment of several non-governmental organizations to combat the disease under extremely difficult circumstances; and the investments of several governments in large scale bilateral projects. The WHO played a crucial role through reinforcing networks and advocacy, and particularly through a partnership with two major pharmaceutical companies, which not only secured the continued production of the trypanocidal drugs, but also allowed the provision of the treatments for free and created additional financial means to promote capacity building of national programmes and to implement active case-finding using appropriate tools. As a consequence, during the past 5 years, surveillance activities have increased, raising the total number of people screened through surveys of active case-finding, leading to a substantial and regular decline in the number of new cases.[5–10] The reported number of cases per year is now 17 500 and the new estimated cumulative rate 50 000–70 000 cases. In view of this significant progress, the International Scientific Council for Trypanosomiasis Research and Control at its 28th conference in Addis Ababa in September 2005 recommended that WHO should launch an elimination programme for sleeping sickness.[11] To reach this goal, the continued efforts in the development of safer drugs and simpler and more reliable diagnostic tests will also be key, as this will allow the treatment to be implemented also in primary healthcare facilities. The main challenge will be to maintain awareness, strengthen surveillance and sustain efforts to achieve the goal of elimination. It must not be forgotten that neglecting the disease will inevitably lead to a new resurgence. In this light the situation in Uganda merits special attention: the area affected by *T.b. rhodesiense* has increased 2.5-fold since 1985, and the active disease focus is now only 150 km from areas currently affected by *T.b. gambiense*.

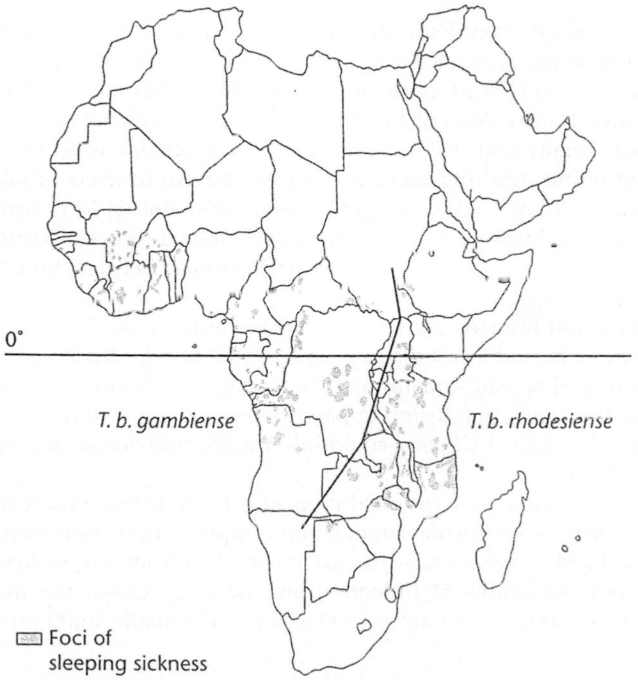

BIOLOGY

T. brucei subspecies trypanosomes of the subgenus Trypanozoon are morphologically indistinguishable. However, since the 1970s, much research has been undertaken to find biochemical and molecular markers that might define clinical disease and epidemiology. The problems that these extensive studies have addressed are the identity and potential infectivity to humans of trypanosomes circulating in domestic and game animals, and those isolated from *Glossina*.

The morphology of *T. brucei* is described by Hoare[12] (Figure 75.3). Parasites are pleomorphic, extracellular in the blood and tissues, and vary in length from 12 to 42 μm; they have a small subterminal kinetoplast and a free flagellum. Parasite multiplication is impaired by specific antibodies produced by the host, resulting in a decrease in the parasitaemia. However, some parasites escape the immune response by the mechanism of antigenic variation, a mechanism that enables the trypanosomes to produce a surface coat composed of a different glycoprotein.[13] The result is a fluctuating parasitaemia with multiple progressive pathological changes, which vary in pattern and intensity with the different parasite strains and host.

T. brucei organisms are infective to laboratory animals: inoculation of infective material from human, animal reservoir and *Glossina* produces infection in a range of laboratory animals. *T.b. rhodesiense* can be propagated in mice, rats, rabbits and guinea pigs. However, *T.b. gambiense* infections are much less virulent and can be propagated only in the multimammate rat (*Mastomys natalensis*), *Grammomys* spp.[14] or in mice with severe combined immune deficiency (SCID).[15] The development of a kit for in vitro isolation of trypanosomes, known as KIVI,[16] enables the isolation of procyclic (insect gut) forms and the characterization of such isolates using polymerase chain reaction (PCR). However, to study drug

Figure 75.2 Distribution of human African trypanosomiasis. (Reproduced with permission from the World Health Organization.[4])

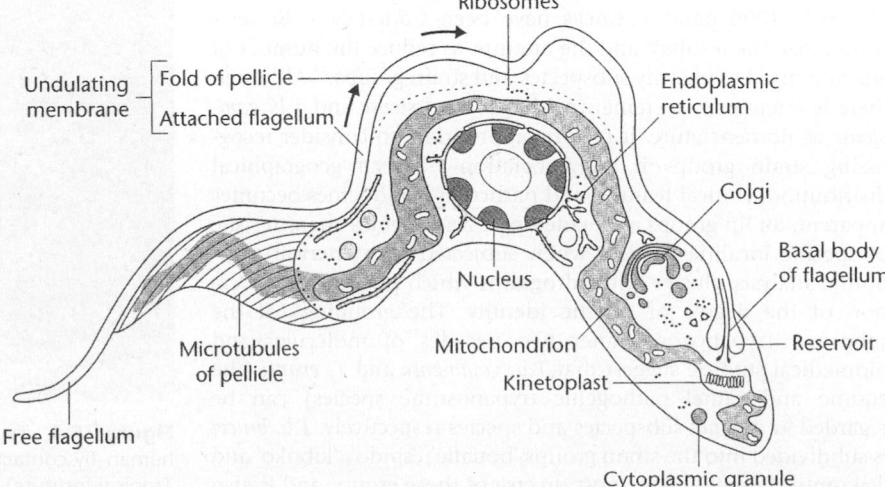

Figure 75.3 Morphology of *Trypanosoma brucei*. (Reproduced with permission from Allen and Unwin.)

resistance, bloodstream forms are required. Those can be obtained from procyclic forms after a full passage through the tsetse vector.[17] Alternatively, infected patients' blood can be cryopreserved in the field using, e.g. the cryomedium Triladyl® and liquid nitrogen.[18] In the laboratory, the frozen blood sample can be thawed and injected into a susceptible rodent for propagation.[19]

It is generally recognized that *T.b. brucei* is the animal infective form of the subgenus Trypanozoon, which is not infective to humans because of its sensitivity to human serum. *T.b. brucei* is lysed by human serum; this is associated with high-density lipoprotein molecules, which are trypanocidal.[20,21] The lytic effect of human serum was the basis for the development of the blood incubation infectivity test (BIIT).[22] This test involved incubation of trypanosomes in human serum before inoculation into rats. Jenni and Brun[23] developed an in vitro test in which the viability of the test organisms is compared in parallel cultures containing 20% human serum or 20% heat-inactivated horse serum as control. The method can detect single serum-resistant forms in a population of sensitive forms. Today PCR methods are available which make use of the *T.b. rhodesiense* specific SRA (serum resistance associated) gene[24] or the *T.b. gambiense* specific TgsGP gene.[25]

The analysis of parasite populations using modern technologies revealed the diversity and complexity of the trypanosomes infective to humans. The problem of understanding the relationships between different populations has been compounded by the demonstration that *T. brucei* can hybridize in *Glossina* in the laboratory.[26] It could also be shown that human serum resistance can be passed on from a parent to the offspring of a cross *T.b. rhodesiense × T.b. brucei*.[27] Neither the frequency of hybridization in the wild nor its significance in terms of epidemiology and patterns of drug resistance is yet known. PCR analysis of mobile genetic elements[28] and the use of microsatellite markers[29] are new technologies which will help to distinguish different strains of *T. brucei* across all three subspecies and notably among *T.b. gambiense* which is the least genetically variable *T.b. brucei* subspecies.

These studies have provoked extensive discussion on the genetics of wild populations of parasites and the relative importance of clonality[30] and sexuality in such populations. The application and use of modern techniques in the epidemiology of trypanosomiasis are described by Gibson and Miles.[31] Extensive studies of nearly 1000 parasite stocks have been undertaken. Reviews summarize the results[32] and the attempt to reduce the number of enzymes used to identify subspecies and strain groups.[33] Although there is a tendency to remain with *T.b. rhodesiense* and *T.b. gambiense* as nomenclature, it may be appropriate to consider recognizing strain groups if an association between geographical distribution, clinical features and particular zymodemes becomes apparent. Strain groups are made up of zymodemes characteristic of specific localities which, when subjected to numerical taxonomic analysis, cluster in dendrograms which provide an indication of the degree of genetic identity. The groupings of the subgenus Trypanozoon, after two decades of molecular and biomedical studies, suggest that *T.b. gambiense* and *T. evansi* (the equine and camel pathogenic trypanosome species) can be regarded as distinct subspecies and species respectively. *T.b. brucei* is subdivided into the strain groups 'bouaflé', 'sindo', 'kiboko' and 'kakumbi'. Bouaflé is the most diverse of these groups and is also

found in West African animals. Some of the stocks of bouaflé are infective to humans; some isolates of bouaflé are also found in East Africa. The relationship between *T.b. rhodesiense* and *T.b. brucei* is complex. *T.b. rhodesiense* in the classical sense is divided into Zambezi and Busoga strain groups with characteristic isoenzyme profiles and DNA banding.[33] The Zambezi group of isolates from humans in Zambia is of relatively low virulence; Busoga stocks are from people in northern and central areas of the *T.b. rhodesiense* distribution.

EPIDEMIOLOGY

T.b. gambiense

T.b. gambiense is endemic throughout West and Central Africa, and is frequently associated with foci of infection, which historically were recognized as areas where prevalence was often 10-fold higher. Transmission of *T.b. gambiense* is associated with particular sites, usually near riverine vegetation, river crossings, water collection points, washing sites and villages adjacent to rivers or lakes (Figures 75.4, 75.5). *T.b. gambiense* transmission is 'site associated', and intense transmission was considered to occur particularly at the end of the dry season when contact between humans and *G. palpalis* was most frequent. Flies require regular blood meals and humans are always available at these particular sites. In more humid forest regions, however, *G. palpalis* distribution is more widespread and human–fly contact is less intense. Once infected, a fly can transmit trypanosomes each time it bites; hence a single infected *Glossina* could infect many individuals at a particular site.

The most recent categorization of *T.b. gambiense* places this organism in a particular strain group comprised of six zymodemes (stocks with characteristic isoenzyme profiles). There are, however, chronic infections of humans from the Ivory Coast, the most sampled area, which are now placed in the bouaflé strain group

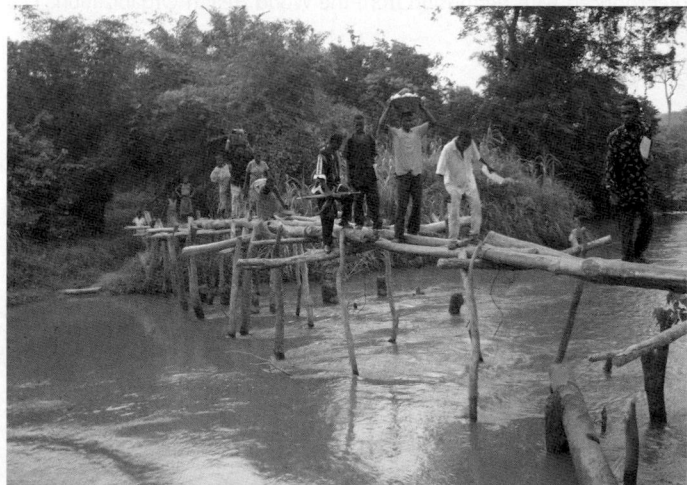

Figure 75.4 Typical site of transmission of *T.b. gambiense* where human–fly contact is high; habitat of *G. palpalis*. (From C. Burri (Swiss Tropical Institute), Kikongotanga, Democratic Republic of Congo.)

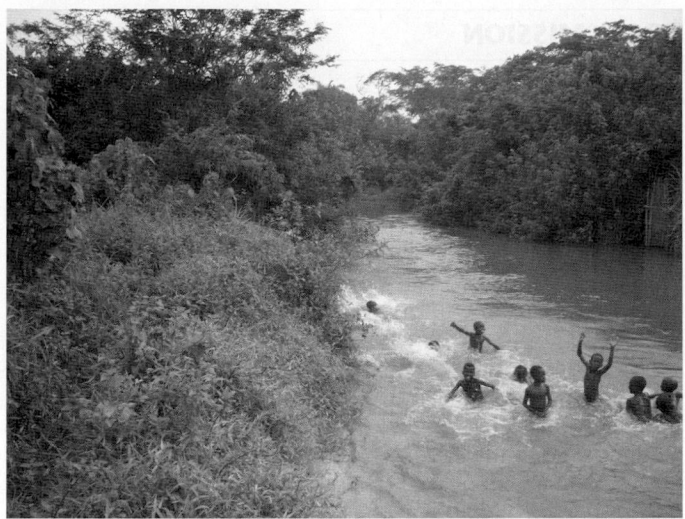

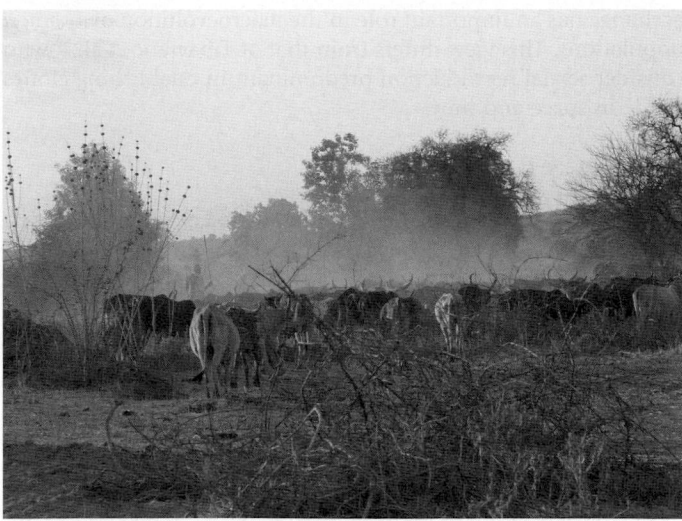

Figure 75.5 Typical site of transmission of *T.b. gambiense* where human–fly contact is high; habitat of *G. palpalis*. (From C. Burri (Swiss Tropical Institute), Kikongotanga, Democratic Republic of Congo.)

Figure 75.6 Typical site of transmission of *T.b. rhodesiense;* habitat of *G. morsitans*. (From I. Küpfer (Swiss Tropical Institute), Urambo District, Tanzania.)

and which belong to the same zymodeme as stocks isolated from a range of wild and domestic animals.[34] Classical *T.b. gambiense* strains (termed type 1) cannot be propagated in laboratory rodents nor be transmitted by *morsitans* group tsetse flies. There is also a second type of *T.b. gambiense* circulating in Central and West Africa (termed type 2) which shares characteristics with *T.b. rhodesiense*, such as developing high parasitaemias in laboratory rodents and being transmitted by *morsitans* group tsetse flies. Information on the animal reservoir of *T.b. gambiense* is scarce and consists of the examination of a few animals; epidemiological studies are missing. Pigs, dogs and cattle but also the game animal species kob (*Kobus kob*) and hartebeest (*Alcelaphus buselaphus*) have been found infected with *T.b. gambiense*. A study in Cameroon examined 164 wild animals by PCR and found 8% (rodents, antelopes, monkeys and carnivores) infected with *T.b. gambiense*.[35] Early experimental studies demonstrated that a range of domestic and wild animals was capable of being infected with isolates of *T.b. gambiense* from humans.

Recent decades have seen a considerable increase in our understanding of the complex interrelationships of the subgenus *Trypanozoon*. Earlier studies were handicapped by a lack of methods for parasite isolation and identification. Isoenzyme analysis and molecular methods have provided a strong base for future detailed epidemiological studies, particularly using PCR, to identify precisely the strain group from small amounts of parasite material from humans, mammals or *Glossina*.

T.b. rhodesiense

The endemic situation

T.b. rhodesiense is the causative agent of the acute form of sleeping sickness. It is distributed from Uganda in the northern part of East Africa to Botswana in the south. Recent biochemical and molecular studies have identified two main strain groups associated with

acute sleeping sickness, Zambezi and Busoga, the strain groups representing the southern and northern limits of distribution, respectively. Zambezi strains from Zambia and Malawi are often less virulent than the Busoga strain group.[36,37]

Sleeping sickness is endemic throughout eastern and southeastern Africa, and humans are infected by the bite of *Glossina* spp. associated with woodland savannah habitats (Figure 75.6). The *morsitans* group, particularly *G. pallidipes* and *G. swynnertoni*, as well as *G. morsitans* itself, are the vectors; these species are preferentially bovid feeders and are not attracted to humans. Savannah *Glossina* spp. therefore feed on humans only when other hosts are not available. In Uganda also the *palpalis* group species *G. fuscipes* is a main vector for *T.b. rhodesiense*. The classical view of the epidemiology of *T.b. rhodesiense* trypanosomiasis is that specific groups of people are more at risk of becoming infected – usually those whose activities or occupations bring them into more frequent contact with *Glossina*. Examples of such groups are honey gatherers, fishermen, game wardens, poachers and firewood collectors. *T.b. rhodesiense* is a zoonosis; the known reservoir hosts are domestic animals such as cattle, sheep and goat, and a variety of game animals including carnivores.[38] The difference between *T.b. brucei* and *T.b. rhodesiense* is the sensitivity or resistance to human serum. Responsibility lies with the serum resistance associated gene, which is coexpressed with the variant surface antigen in *T.b. rhodesiense* stocks.[24,39,40]

Analysis of the zymodemes of *T. brucei* from the Lambwe Valley, Kenya, by Cibulskis,[41] using a contingency table approach, has suggested that particular zymodemes are associated with particular mammalian hosts and that such relationships are stable, at least over a 32-month period. Earlier studies in this locality showed that the *T. brucei* population changed during the sleeping sickness outbreak in 1980,[42,43] showing that outbreaks arose from within the locality rather than through the introduction of strains from outside. In the context of the experimental finding of sexual recombination in *T. brucei*, Cibulskis[41] suggested that genetic exchange has an important role in the macroevolution of *T. brucei* populations. This view differs from that of Tibayrenc et al.,[30] who consider sexual reproduction predominant in establishing clones stable in space and time.

Epidemic *T.b. rhodesiense*

Epidemics of acute disease have been observed over many decades, but most recently in Busoga, Uganda. This epidemic involved around 8000 cases per year in the mid-1980s but could be brought under control through a combination of interventions: intense surveillance, diagnosis and treatment, and vector control. The epidemic in Busoga was believed to be caused by a change in the agriculture of the area when cotton and coffee production ceased and the land was not cultivated, allowing the weed *Lantana camara* to become abundant. This shrub provided a suitable habitat for *G. f. fuscipes* to invade Busoga from the lakeside. A similar invasion of *G. f. fuscipes* occurred in Alego, Kenya,[43] and was associated with an earlier epidemic. In both of these epidemics, cattle have been implicated as reservoir hosts.[42-44] Detailed analysis of zymodemes has allowed the characterization of these parasites into the strain group Busoga, with a smaller number of isolates belonging to the Zambezi strain group which is more characteristic of Zambia. *G. f. fuscipes* flies can be found in peridomestic situations in East Africa, associated with cattle and pigs as a reservoir. This situation parallels peridomestic populations of West African riverine flies where, in humid areas, peridomestic *G. palpalis* group flies are associated with domestic pig populations living close to or within villages.[45]

TRANSMISSION

T. brucei subspecies are transmitted to mammalian hosts by the bite of tsetse flies (*Glossina* spp.). A tsetse fly gets infected when taking a bloodmeal on an infected mammalian host. A complex developmental cycle in the fly ends with the infective metacyclic stage in the lumen of the salivary glands (Figure 75.7). This process may take 3–4 weeks. Metacyclic trypanosomes are injected into the skin of the mammalian host during the probing and feeding process. Development in the tsetse fly involves a complex series of changes in the morphology and biochemistry of the parasite. Several factors play key roles in these changes: lectins present in *Glossina* midgut and haemolymph, the presence of Rickettsia-like organisms, and molecular signals that influence parasite transformation, establishment and maturation.[46] Lectins in the tsetse midgut kill incoming trypanosomes. Feeding lectin-inhibitory sugars or procyclin to flies significantly increased the midgut infection rates. While lectins are detrimental for the establishment of a midgut infection, the same lectins are required for maturation to the infective metacyclic stage. Knowledge of the parasite–vector interactions could eventually lead to novel control strategies to interrupt transmission.

The possibility of mechanical (non-cyclical) transmission by biting insects or *Glossina* has been suggested, although there is only circumstantial evidence to support the idea. Mechanical transmission has been suggested as the reason for the clustering of cases in a household or where cases are found outside the normal range of *Glossina*.

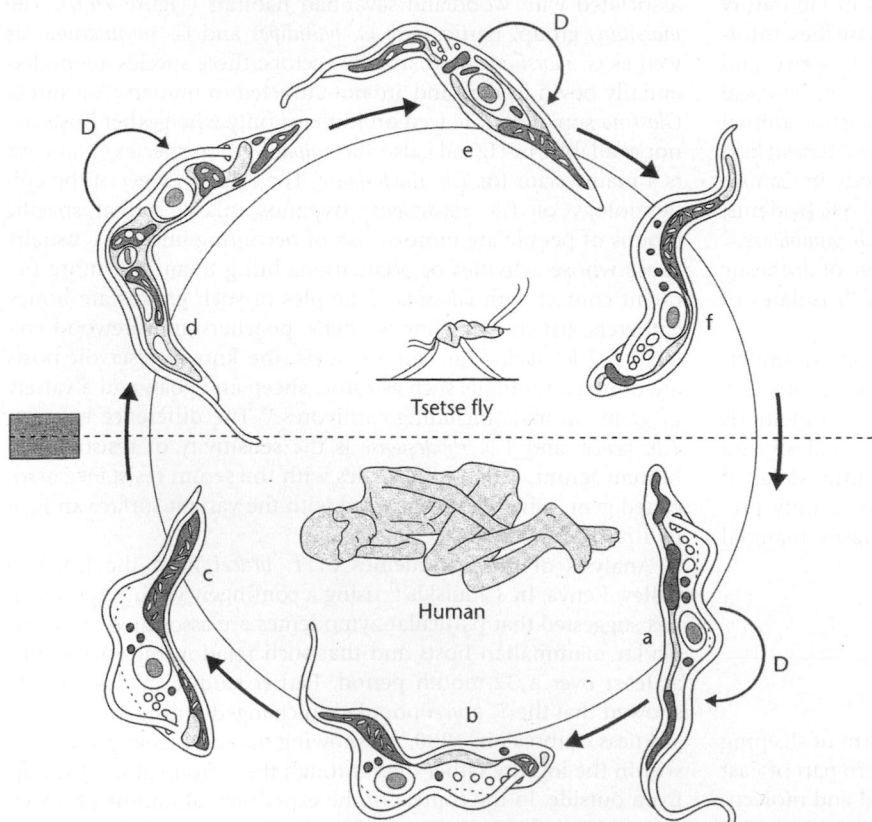

Figure 75.7 Cycle of *T. brucei* spp. showing the different morphological forms in the human and in the tsetse fly. In the blood and lymphatic system of humans (a) slender, (b) intermediate and (c) short stumpy forms are present. Stumpy forms differentiate in the fly midgut to (d) procyclic forms, then to (e) epimastigote forms and finally in the salivary glands to (f) infective metacyclic forms. Bloodstream forms (a–c) and metacyclic forms are covered by the variable surface glycoprotein (VSG) coat. 'D' indicates the capability to undergo cell division. (From Brun R. Sleeping sickness in Africa; on the rise again. *Karger Gazette* 1999; 63:5–7, with permission from Karger, Basel.)

DIAGNOSIS

The diagnosis of *T.b. gambiense* human African trypanosomiasis (HAT usually follows a three-step pathway: screening, diagnostic confirmation, and staging. Suspected cases detected by serological methods (usually the card agglutination test for trypanosomiasis; CATT) undergo parasitological diagnosis by investigation of the blood and/or lymph (Figure 75.8) and in case of a positive result, examination of the CSF follows for stage determination.[47] *T.b. rhodesiense* is usually directly detected in the blood.

Immunodiagnostic methods

Field diagnosis of infections with *Trypanosoma brucei gambiense* relies on the initial screening with the card agglutination trypanosomiasis test (CATT/*T.b. gambiense*) in most endemical areas. The test is a cheap, quick, and practical serological test that has been widely used since it was developed in 1978.[48] The basis is a reagent composed of stained freeze-dried trypanosomes of selected variable antigen types (VATs), which can be obtained from the Institute of Tropical Medicine, Antwerp, Belgium. The CATT is an agglutination test of high sensitivity and specificity, and is easy to perform in the field. A drop of heparinized whole blood is mixed with a drop of the reagent on a card and, in the presence of specific antibodies, the trypanosomes in the reagent will agglutinate. It is inexpensive and results are obtained within 5 min.[4] Use of the CATT has considerably increased the detection rate in active surveys compared with the sole use of parasitological assays. No such test exists presently for *T.b. rhodesiense*, but parasite detection in the blood is much easier in this form of the disease. The specificity of the CATT can be further improved when performed on diluted plasma (CATT-P) or serum or when the biological fluid is titrated. However, until today there has been no consensus about the cut-off. Still, confirmatory diagnosis by parasitological methods is the gold standard. If the treatment decision is based on the CATT dilution the epidemiological situation has to be considered and a stage determination must be performed to prevent patients being unnecessarily exposed to drugs with a high risk for severe adverse drug reactions.[49–51]

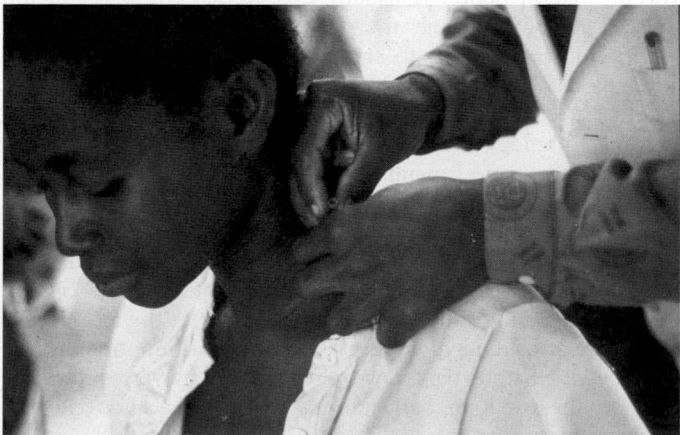

Figure 75.8 Lymph node aspiration for diagnosis. (From J. Blum (Swiss Tropical Institute), Vanga, Democratic Republic of Congo.)

Alternative tests, such as the card indirect antigen test for trypanosomiasis (CIATT), in which specific antibodies are coupled to latex beads and used to trap antigens in serum or whole blood,[37] or The LATEX/*T.b. gambiense* which has been developed as a field alternative to the CATT.[52] The test is based on the combination of three purified variable surface antigens, LiTat 1.3, 1.5, and 1.6, coupled with suspended latex particles. The test procedure is similar to the CATT, including the use of a similar rotator. Compared to the CATT, the LATEX/*T.b. gambiense* showed a higher specificity (96–99%) but a lower or similar sensitivity (71–100%) in recent field studies conducted in several Western and Central African countries. Further evaluations are needed before it can be recommended for routine field use.[47]

Different PCR assays have been developed; but none of them has been validated for diagnostic purposes. The methods are summarized in Chappuis et al.[47] For laboratory use, other methods, such as immunofluorescence (IF), indirect haemagglutination (IHA), enzyme-linked immunosorbent assay (ELISA) and different PCR methods, have been described.

Simple and inexpensive methods will be required to allow the future diagnosis of sleeping sickness in primary healthcare facilities. Several methods are currently under investigation, and one of them, a simple molecular dipstick for visualization of PCR products underwent Phase I evaluation.[53]

Parasitological methods

Serological indication of a trypanosome infection alone does not justify treatment because of the relative toxicity of all drugs in use. Therefore, the detection of the parasite is of great importance.

The body fluids that are most commonly examined for the presence of trypanosomes are blood, lymph node aspirates and CSF. Trypanosomes may also be detected in bone marrow aspirates and ascites fluid.

Different techniques are used for diagnosis in blood:

- Blood films (thin, thick or wet) can be used for direct detection of trypanosomes. Wet blood films are used for the detection of motile trypanosomes, whereas thin and thick blood films are fixed in methanol and Giemsa stained
- Concentration methods increase the chances for detection of the parasite because the parasitaemia, especially in *T.b. gambiense* infections, is usually very low
- The microhaematocrit centrifugation technique (m-HCT)[54] is based on microscopic examination of the buffy coat zone of blood cells using a long working distance objective following centrifugation in microhaematocrit capillaries. This method is used widely in the field
- The miniature anion-exchange centrifugation technique (m-AECT)[55] is based on the detection of trypanosomes in the eluate after the passage of infected blood through an anion-exchange (diethylaminoethyl cellulose) column followed by centrifugation in microhaematocrit capillaries. This method has proven to be more sensitive under field conditions than other methods
- For analysis of the lymph, a wet preparation[4] of the aspirate from enlarged lymph nodes is examined at a magnification of 400×

- In vivo inoculation of biological material from humans, animal hosts or vectors into susceptible animals has been used to detect trypanosomes. Mice and rats are used for detecting *T.b. rhodesiense*, whereas immunosuppressed *Mastomys natalensis*, suckling rats or SCID (severe combined immunodeficient) mice should preferably be used for *T.b. gambiense*.

DETERMINATION OF THE STAGE OF THE DISEASE

Chemotherapy, especially the use of melarsoprol for second-stage disease, bears a significant risk. Today the treatment decision follows the staging and therefore a correct determination of the stage is crucial before commencing treatment.

Examination of the CSF is used to determine the stage of the disease. Parasites can sometimes be seen during white cell counting, but detection after concentration by single or, better, double centrifugation is substantially more sensitive.

The criteria for second-stage infection are: either trypanosomes detected in the CSF and/or a raised leukocyte count of more than 5 cells/mm³. This cut-off is similar to that currently used in neurology.[4] A small-scale investigation had indicated that infections of up to 20 cells/mm³ may be treated with the first-stage drug pentamidine with only a minor increase in the relapse rate.[56] Based on these results, Angola has changed the national criteria for second-stage treatment accordingly. Unfortunately, results of this large-scale application are still outstanding. However, in the meantime, other investigations have indicated that the cut-off should rather be maintained at 5 cells/mm³. In one study, the risk of treatment failure in patients with a CSF leukocyte count of 6–10 cells/mm³ was more than three times higher than in those with a count of 0–5 cells/mm³.[10] In another investigation, patients with cell counts of 11–20 cells/mm³ had 7.1 times higher odds to relapse than patients with a lower cell count (95% confidence interval 1.4–36).[57]

An increased protein content of the CSF was formerly used as an additional criterion for staging, but due to the frequent lack of materials, variability of the results and the lesser predictive value compared with white blood cell counting, this method is only rarely used today.[58]

The CSF of second-stage HAT patients contains high levels of immunoglobulins, especially IgM, and an increased CSF IgM concentration has thus been considered by some as a strong potential marker of second-stage HAT for a long time. A latex agglutination test for IgM in CSF (LATEX/IgM) designed for field use has recently been developed. Following initial promising results,[59] the LATEX/IgM was evaluated with CSF samples from patients from several countries where infection is endemic.[60] CSF end titres obtained by the LATEX/IgM paralleled the IgM concentrations determined by nephelometry and ELISA. At a cut-off value of = 1:8, the sensitivity and specificity of LATEX/IgM for intrathecal IgM synthesis were 89% and 93%, respectively. Future prospective studies with large numbers of patients are needed for LATEX/IgM validation.

Sleep–wake recordings may become another useful tool to detect the CNS involvement and second-stage disease. In a small scale investigation, the 24-h distribution of sleep–wake, the altered sleep structure, sleep onset REM sleep periods (SOREMP) and the EEG morphological alterations were recorded in first and second-stage patients. The sleep–wake cycle and sleep structure were totally disrupted in second-stage patients, these alterations being alleviated by treatment with melarsoprol. However, similar alterations were also observed in some Stage I or 'intermediate' patients (5–20 cells/mm³) and more work will be necessary.[61]

DIFFERENTIAL DIAGNOSIS

Owing to the many clinical variations of sleeping sickness, it is difficult to describe a 'typical' case of the disease; differential diagnosis might therefore be of unusual importance. In first-stage human African trypanosomiasis, other causes of protracted febrile illness such as drug-resistant malaria, typhoid fever and viral hepatitis should be considered. The prominent lymphadenopathy can be suggestive of mononucleosis or tuberculous lymphadenitis. In second-stage disease, syphilitic meningomyelitis, cerebral tumour, cerebral tuberculosis, HIV-associated cryptococcal meningitis and chronic viral encephalitis must be considered.

CLINICAL SYMPTOMS AND SIGNS

T.b. gambiense and *T.b. rhodesiense* differ in many respects, such as biology, transmission and epidemiology, as well as the clinical picture and treatment of their respective infections (Table 75.2).

T.b. gambiense

T.b. gambiense infections run a chronic course of years from infection to extensive nervous system involvement and the classical picture of sleeping sickness. The symptoms and signs described in the literature, especially for second-stage disease, vary considerably. This is in part explained by the largely varying status of the patient at hospital admission, which depends on the social status of the local population, nutrition and transport facilities, and the virulence of the trypanosome strain. A typical list of second-stage signs and symptoms observed is given in Table 75.3.[62]

First-stage illness

The incubation period is usually 2–3 weeks. The onset of the disease is very unspecific; the only sign may be irregular fever, varying in cycles of one to several days and not responding to antimalarials. This scheme reflects the stimulation of the immune system by changing variant surface glycoproteins (VSGs; see Immunopathology below). Lymphadenopathy, headache, myalgia, fatigue and general malaise may accompany this phase. The initial phase may be followed by a relatively asymptomatic phase lasting for several months to, sometimes, a few years.

The posterior cervical lymph nodes are enlarged in as many as 85% of hospitalized patients (classic Winterbottom's sign) (Figure 75.9). Pruritus and transient oedema (mostly of the face, Figure 75.10) are also frequently observed. Cutaneous eruptions of the papuloerythematous type may be found, but are very difficult to spot on the trunk of dark-skinned individuals, and generally resolve spontaneously.

With progress of the disease, the symptoms associated with the waves of parasitaemia become less frequent, and parasites become

Table 75.2 Differences between *T.b. gambiense* and *T.b. rhodesiense* sleeping sickness

	West African (Gambian)	East African (Rhodesian)
Parasite	*T.b. gambiense*	*T.b. rhodesiense*
Main vectors	*Palpalis* group	*Morsitans* group
Main habitat	Near water	Savannah, cleared bush
Highest incidence	Congo (DRC), Angola, South Sudan, North Uganda	South-east Uganda, Tanzania
Main reservoir	Humans	Antelope and cattle
	Pig, dog	
Disease type	Chronic (years)	Acute (months)
Parasitaemia	Low	Moderate
Diagnosis	Lymph node aspiration	Blood
	CSF (lumbar puncture)	CSF (lumbar puncture)
Serology	CATT	None
TREATMENT		
First-stage	Pentamidine	Suramin
Second-stage	Melarsoprol	Melarsoprol
Alternative treatment	Eflornithine and Nifurtimox	(Melarsoprol and Nifurtimox)
Disease control	Active case search and tsetse trapping	Tsetse trapping

Adapted from Pepin (2000).[64]

Table 75.3 Typical symptoms and signs of second-stage *T.b. gambiense* sleeping sickness

Symptoms and signs	(%)
Headache	78.7
Sleeping disorder	74.4
Adenopathy	56.1
Pruritus	51.1
Splenomegaly[a]	42.5
Motor weakness	34.8
Hepatomegaly[a]	25.5
Malnutrition	25.2
Unusual behaviour	24.7
Disturbed appetite	22.9
Walking difficulties	21.7
Tremor	21.0
Fever	16.1
Speech disorder	13.4
Abnormal movements	10.5

Compiled data from 2541 second-stage sleeping sickness patients from different countries and settings who were treated in a multinational drug utilization study on an abridged treatment with melarsoprol (Impamel II).
[a] Information only available on 504 patients. Adapted from Blum et al. (2006).[62]

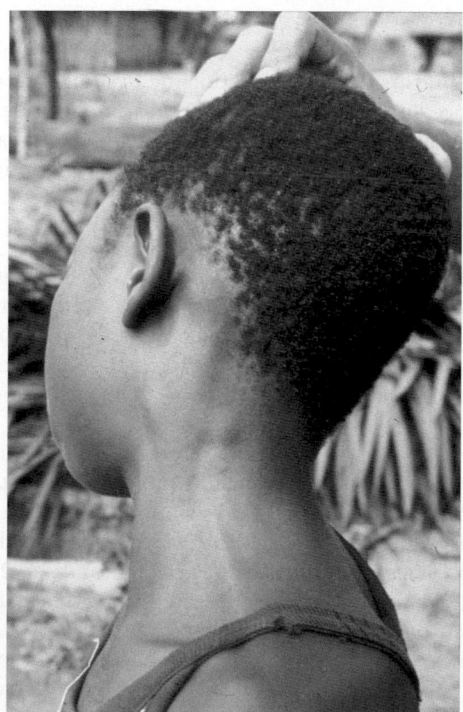

Figure 75.9 Winterbottom's sign; enlarged cervical lymph nodes in a patient with *T.b. gambiense* infection. (From J. Blum (Swiss Tropical Institute), Vanga, Democratic Republic of Congo.)

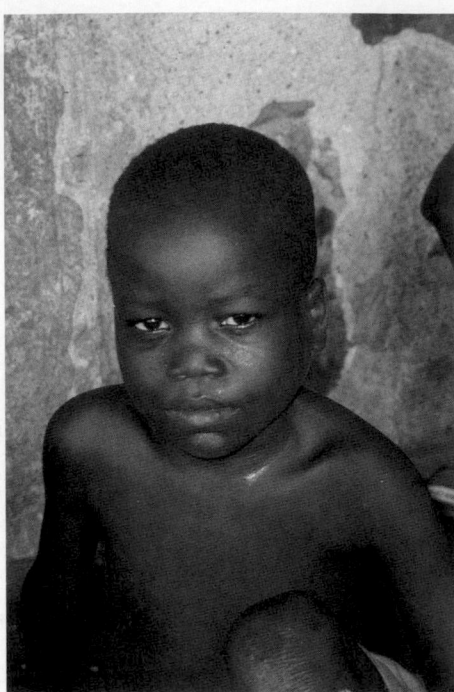

Figure 75.10 Facial oedema in a patient with first-stage *T.b. gambiense* infection. (From C. Burri (Swiss Tropical Institute), Dondo, Angola.

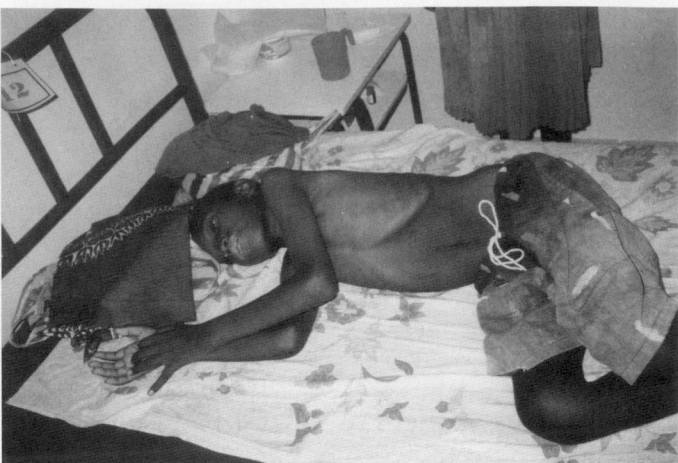

Figure 75.11 Patient with advanced second stage *T.b. gambiense* infection. (From C. Burri (Swiss Tropical Institute), Viana, Angola.)

difficult to find in the blood. Endocrine dysfunctions occur at a more advanced phase and may manifest as amenorrhoea, reduced libido, impotence and a high abortion rate. Profound anaemia is another feature that may be observed at this stage of infection.

Second-stage illness

Invasion of the trypanosomes into the CNS marks the onset of the second stage of the infection. It occurs first in the least protected areas such as the choroid plexus, thalamus, area postrema, median eminence, and pineal and hypophyseal regions.[63] This localization may explain in part the principal clinical and neurological signs observed.

The second stage is the result of a chronic meningoencephalitis, with characteristic symptoms such as progressive mental deterioration proceeding to coma.

The interval between the start of the infection and the second, encephalitic, stage is in the order of several months to 2 years, but much longer periods have been observed. The average duration of this stage is from 4 months to 1 year.

Headaches become constant and may be unresponsive to analgesics. Motor functions become seriously impaired, and the patient may only be able to walk aided. Speech becomes slurred and abnormal movements and tremor occur; the picture may resemble Parkinsonism. At this stage mental changes of considerable variation may become obvious. The pattern ranges from basic lethargy with bouts of mania, to delirium, paranoia, aggressive behaviour and schizoid attacks. Involvement of sleep-regulating regions such as the thalamus, area postrema, median eminence

and the pineal region cause sleep derangements characteristic for *T.b. gambiense* infection. Patients are often indifferent to activities going on around them (Figure 75.11). Two major disturbances of the sleep pattern were identified in second-stage patients: First, the nychthemeral (night and day) alternation of sleep and wakefulness is altered proportionally to the severity of the disease. Short sleep episodes occur equally by day and night. Second, the structure of sleep episodes is altered, with frequent sleep onset REM sleep periods (SOREMP), REM sleep episodes occurring soon after long wakefulness transitions with a latency shorter than 15 min (International Classification of Sleep Disorders, 1990). The sleep–wake cycle alteration as well as the SOREMPs recede or disappear after melarsoprol treatment.[61]

General pruritus and bedsores are a frequent feature at this stage, as well as weight loss and substantial wasting. It is generally accepted that sleeping sickness is ultimately fatal in all patients, if left untreated. The patient finally becomes comatose and will die, often from bacterial superinfections such as aspiration pneumonia. Most of the neurological signs described above remain reversible with treatment for a long time, confirming the predominance of potentially reversible inflammatory processes over destructive lesions.

T.b. rhodesiense

The East African form of the disease is a much more acute infection: the incubation period, the first stage, and the second stage with CNS involvement develop over a few weeks.

First-stage illness

An inoculation chancre, which often remains invisible in Africans, develops 5–15 days after the bite. It is a painful, circumscribed, indurated dusky-red papule 2–5 cm in diameter, which disappears after 2–3 weeks. Regional lymphadenopathy or adjacent cellulitis occurs. Fever and parasitaemia appear hours to days later or, in the absence of a chancre, within 1–3 weeks of the infective bite.[64]

Generally, the parasites are more numerous in the blood than in the gambiense form of the disease. Cervical lymphadenopathy (Winterbottom's sign) is less common than in Gambian human African trypanosomiasis, but submandibular, axillary or inguinal lymph nodes may be enlarged. Keratitis and conjunctivitis have been observed.

Second-stage illness

The disease progresses much more rapidly than for *T.b. gambiense*, causing the death of the patient within 6–9 months. Symptoms and signs of CNS involvement may be absent, except for drowsiness and tremors. Pericardial effusion and congestive heart failure have been described in *T.b. rhodesiense* infection, and in one-third of patients, abnormal electrocardiograms were found.[65]

PATHOLOGY AND PATHOGENESIS

Sleeping sickness produces multiple pathological changes that involve most organs and systems. The changes are progressive and their anatomy, histology, physiology, biochemistry and immunology have been described extensively. The damage results from a complex interplay of factors between the different systems.

Pathology

A local inflammatory response with oedema and mononuclear infiltration occurs at the site of infection. The trypanosomes then spread to the lymphatic system and glands, and to the bloodstream. The lymph glands become enlarged and trypanosomes can be found in lymph gland aspirates. Microscopically the follicles are enlarged with prominent reactive centres and many plasma cells in the sinuses. The main feature of the pathological change is a vasculitis.

The spleen is slightly enlarged. The malpighian follicles are few and inconspicuous. There is a general proliferation of the reticuloendothelium, congestion at the periphery of the splenic sinuses, often focal necrosis with endothelial macrophages and ingested red corpuscles.

The liver may be slightly enlarged in some cases; there is infiltration with mononuclear cells in the periportal tracts and microscopical mononuclear cell granulomas.

In *T.b. rhodesiense* infections there is a pancarditis involving all layers of the heart including mural and valvular endocardium. In experimental infections in monkeys, myocarditis with trypanosomes in the interstitial tissues, especially the endocardium, was observed. Histologically there is a marked interstitial infiltration with plasma and morular cells, with disappearance of muscle fibres and fibrosis.

- Proliferative glomerulonephritis leading to fibrosis has been observed
- The bone marrow is hypercellular with areas of gelatinous degeneration
- The lesions in the lungs are characterized by intravascular proliferation of the reticuloendothelium, which may block the capillaries with fibrosis, and collapse of the alveoli
- Localized oedema due to collections of lymphocytes may be observed in the eyelids, perineum and the skin of the back.

Typical pathological lesions of the CNS are seen only after invasion of the trypanosomes. No gross lesions of the nerve centres are present, but there is progressive chronic leptomeningitis, especially in the Virchow-Robin spaces (where the pia sheathes the blood vessels and the fluid acts as lymph) and also on the vertex (Dürck's nodes).

The dura may be adherent to the skull and to the arachnoid. The brain itself is congested and oedematous, the surface smooth, with convolutions flattened by increased pressure. The consistency of the brain tissues is unaltered except for softening around any haemorrhages that may occur. The ventricles are distended with fluid. In all cases there is perivascular round-cell infiltration (perivascular cuffing) throughout the brain tissue and meninges, varying in amount and in different anatomical regions. The invading cells are glia cells, lymphocytes, the morular (Mott) and Marhalko cells. The two latter types are degenerative plasmocytes. Trypanosomes have been found in the brain, mainly in frontal lobe, pons and medulla. Demyelination and neuronal damage have been described. The organisms also invade the CSF, which they enter by the canal from the choroidal plexus.[65]

Patients have markedly altered plasma albumin : globulin ratios; the macroglobulinaemia is characteristic of both the Gambian and Rhodesian forms. The increases are highest for IgM with the first parasitaemia, whereas IgG responses are not so marked. This is followed by a progressive suppression, which is selective for the IgG production, with IgM levels remaining high. Another obvious change in plasma is the increase in total lipid content, which in rabbits may be up to four times that of uninfected animals. Large amounts of cholesterol and β-lipoprotein(s) are present, together with increased amounts of free fatty acids (e.g. linoleic, oleic, palmitic and stearic). Disturbances of other plasma constituents (e.g. decrease of calcium and bicarbonate, increase of phosphate, urea and creatinine levels) indicate renal damage. Gross pathological changes to the kidney are not a usual feature of patients with sleeping sickness, but glomerulonephritis has been observed in experimental animals.

The aetiology of the anaemia in sleeping sickness is multifactorial, with haemolysis, haemodilution and disordered and/or non-compensatory erythropoiesis having continued with variable contributions during the infection. Haemolysis is largely responsible, with phagocytosis of red cells that have become coated with immune complexes in the spleen sinusoids and by the Kupffer cells of the liver. The haemolysis may also result in part from haemolytic factors liberated by trypanosomes. As infection progresses the blood and plasma volumes become progressively enlarged, thus causing a haemodilution effect. Red cell production by the bone marrow is significantly reduced. The defect here is associated with a failure of iron incorporation into the red cell precursors, with a large excess of storage iron not employed for haemoglobin synthesis.

Patients may also have a moderate leukocytosis; differential counts regularly show monocytosis, lymphocytosis and plasmacytosis, and large Mott morular cells may also be found.

Blood homeostasis becomes seriously disturbed. The disease is commonly associated with minor haemorrhages and multiple petechiae, although these are rarely sufficiently severe to be life threatening. The pathogenesis is associated with vascular injury, coagulopathy with increased fibrinolysis, and thrombocytopenia. The coagulopathy is most common in acute *T.b. rhodesiense* disease

thrombocytopenia. Pruritus is more frequent with concomitant filariasis.

About 99.7% of the drug is bound to plasma proteins (e.g. albumin, globulins, fibrinogen), which places suramin in the class of the most extensively bound drugs. Suramin has one of the longest half-lives of all drugs given to humans. In patients with HIV/AIDS who were given suramin once weekly for 5 weeks, the drug accumulated during the time of administration and then diminished, with a half-life of 44–54 days;[85] in patients with onchocerciasis the terminal half-life was 92 days.[86] Total plasma levels remained above 100 mg/mL for several weeks. The volume of distribution was 38–46 L, and total clearance was less than 0.5 mL/min.[85] The renal clearance contributed essentially to the removal of the drug from the body.

Suramin inhibits, rather non-specifically, numerous enzymes including L-α-glycerophosphate oxidase, glycerol-3-phosphate dehydrogenase, RNA polymerase and kinases, thymidine kinase, dihydrofolate reductase, hyaluronidase, urease, hexokinase, fumarase, trypsin, reverse transcriptase and the receptor-mediated uptake of low-density lipoprotein by trypanosomes. Suramin is taken up by trypanosomes by pinocytosis, as a plasma protein-bound complex.[87] The accumulation of suramin in the trypanosomes was hypothesized to be one of the reasons for the differential toxicity between the host and the parasite.

Treatment of second stage

Melarsoprol

The organo-arsenical drug melarsoprol (Arsobal®, Aventis), was developed in 1949 by the addition of the heavy metal chelator dimercaptopropanol (British Anti-Lewisite; BAL) to the trivalent arsenic of melarsen oxide.[88] Despite the high frequency of severe adverse drug reactions and a significant increase of the number of the patients refractory to treatment in certain areas,[89] the drug is still the most frequently used for treatment of second-stage sleeping sickness owing to a lack of good alternatives.

An abridged schedule for treatment of second-stage *T.b. gambiense* sleeping sickness with melarsoprol has been extensively evaluated and was recently recommended as the standard schedule.[90-92] The new schedule supersedes a wide range of different empirically derived treatment regimens used in the past. These schedules with various dosages shared the application of the drug in repeated series of three to four injections every 24 h, spaced by 7–10 days.

Owing to irritating properties of the solvent propylene glycol, melarsoprol has to be given strictly as an intravenous injection; a paravasal deposition of the drug has to be avoided.

Adverse drug reactions of melarsoprol may be severe and life-threatening. The most important is an encephalopathic syndrome, which occurs in 5–10% of all treated cases, and which is fatal for about 10–70% of those patients. Clinically, the syndrome has been defined either as convulsions, the rapid deterioration of neurological symptoms and progressive coma, or psychotic reactions/abnormal behaviour.[4,93]

The cause of the reaction to melarsoprol and the influence of the treatment schedule on its frequency have been discussed exten-

sively during the past decade. An immune reaction is generally thought to underlie the syndrome, but the detailed mechanisms remain unknown.[93] Trypanosome antigens can be excluded as a unique trigger, because identical encephalopathic syndromes were also observed in patients treated experimentally with melarsoprol for advanced leukaemia.[94] The temporal distribution of the occurrence of the syndrome was virtually identical under standard treatment interrupted with breaks compared with the continuous daily application for 10 days in a large-scale controlled clinical trial.[90] As the drug pressure in the CSF during the continuous new treatment schedule is uninterrupted and constantly increasing until the end of treatment, another postulated reason, namely non-curative treatment leading to a reaction against recurrent trypanosomes in the CSF, can also be excluded. Another possible target for stimulating a delayed immune reaction not yet investigated is the hapten consisting of one of the melarsoprol metabolites and plasma proteins.[95] The immunological nature of the encephalopathic syndromes was corroborated by the preliminary finding that patients with two human leukocyte antigen haplotypes (C*14/B*15 and A*23/C*14) were at a significantly higher risk to develop an encephalopathic syndrome (J. Seixas, pers comm).

In a large-scale clinical trial the concomitant application of prednisolone at 1 mg/kg body weight has been shown to reduce the incidence of encephalopathic syndromes by two-thirds (i.e. 11.4–4.1%; difference in percentage −7.3% (CI$_{95}$ −11.7% to −2.7%) and the mortality rate by one-third (i.e. 7.5–5.2%; difference in percentage −2.3% (CI$_{95}$ −6.3% to +1.7%)).[96] It is possible that two different reactions lead to the syndrome: the prognosis of patients with a single convulsion is reasonably good, whereas 50–70% of those rapidly developing coma die within 3 days.[93]

Management of encephalopathic syndromes is attempted by the application of anticonvulsants (diazepam, phenobarbital, phenytoin) and high-dose parenteral steroids (dexamethasone, hydrocortisone) to reduce cerebral oedema. Adrenaline (epinephrine) is often given, but its beneficial use has not been proven, and dimercaprol is contraindicated.

Other frequent adverse drug reactions to melarsoprol are pyrexia, headache, general malaise and thrombophlebitis at the sites of injection. Skin reactions, such as pruritus and maculopapular eruptions are quite common, but severe complications such as bullous eruptions occur only in less than 1% of cases.[4] Other occasional adverse reactions are peripheral motoric or sensorial (paraesthesia) neuropathy, cardiac failure, renal dysfunction (proteinuria and hypertension) as well as hepatotoxicity (raised levels of liver enzymes, bilirubinaemia).[97]

Serum concentrations of melarsoprol determined by biological assay and atomic absorption spectrometry were, respectively, in the range of 2.5–6 μg/mL at 5 min and 220 (±80) ng/mL at 120 h after the fourth injection of the therapy courses. Melarsoprol is rapidly metabolized to melarsen oxide with a half-life of 0.5 h; melarsen oxide decays with a half-life of 3.9 h, not solely due to a rapid elimination but also because of irreversible binding to plasma proteins of more than 20 kDa in size.[95] The mean terminal elimination half-life of melarsoprol determined as total trypanocidal activity by bioassay is approximately 35 h, the volume of distribution is about 2 L/kg and total clearance is 1 mL/min per kg.[98] CSF samples are obtained by spinal tap, and therefore only marginal information about this compartment is available from humans. The CSF drug levels are generally very low, in the range of 2% of those in the serum in humans and monkeys, and the half-life of activity in this compartment was about 5 days in a monkey model.

The mechanisms of action of melarsoprol are not completely understood. Trypanothione (N^1,N^8-bis(glutathionyl)-spermidine), which plays a major role in the dithioldisulfide redox balance in trypanosomes and forms an adduct with melarsen oxide (MelT), was proposed as the primary target of melarsoprol. However, this idea was contested based on the high K_i value required for this target, and a modest decrease in intracellular levels of reduced trypanothione and glutathione.[84] Additionally, melarsen oxide was found inside treated trypanosomes and inhibited pyruvate kinase, phosphofructokinase and fructose-2, 6-biphosphatase. In summary, melarsoprol appears to be a highly non-discriminating inhibitor of a large number of mammalian and trypanosomal enzymes that contain dithiols.

Eflornithine

In 1990, the US Food and Drug Administration (FDA) approved eflornithine (α-difluoromethylornithine; DFMO, Ornidyl® Aventis) for the treatment of *gambiense* sleeping sickness. The most commonly used dosage regimen consists of 100 mg of eflornithine/kg body weight at 6-h intervals for 14 days (150 mg/kg body weight in children) by short infusions over a period of at least 30 min.

A recent retrospective analysis of a large patient number corroborated the impression that 14 days of therapy with intravenous eflornithine resulted in significantly fewer deaths and severe adverse events than did 10 days of therapy with intravenous melarsoprol. No evidence of increased death or relapse rates within 12 months after the end of eflornithine treatment was found. However, the lack of trained medical staff in many remote healthcare centres and the insufficient financial and technical logistic capacities in most endemic countries still hamper the universal use of eflornithine. Local phlebitis, bacterial abscesses and septicaemia, which were earlier reported to be a major obstacle, can efficiently be avoided with adequate nursing care.[99]

Adverse drug reactions are frequent and the characteristics are similar to those of other cytotoxic drugs. Their occurrence and intensity increases with the duration of treatment and the severity of the general condition of the patient. The most frequent adverse effects are bone marrow toxicity (anaemia, leucopenia, thrombocytopenia) in 25–50% of treated patients. Gastrointestinal symptoms such as nausea, vomiting and diarrhoea can be observed in about 10%, alopecia, usually towards the end of the treatment, is seen in about 5–10%, and neurological symptoms such as convulsions in 7% of treated patients. Generally, adverse drug reactions of eflornithine are reversible after the end of the treatment course. The drug arrests embryonic development in mice, rats and rabbits; the excretion into breast milk is unknown.[100]

After low oral doses (5–10 mg/kg), peak plasma concentrations were reached 1.5–6 h later. The mean half-life was 3.3 h and the volume of distribution in the range of 0.35 L/kg. Renal clearance was about 2 mL/min per kg (after intravenous application) and accounted for more than 80% of drug elimination. Bioavailability of an orally administered 10 mg/kg dose was estimated at 54%. Eflornithine produces CSF:plasma ratios of between 0.13 and 0.51.[101]

Eflornithine acts by inhibiting the trypanosomal enzyme ornithine decarboxylase (ODC), which catalyses the conversion of ornithine to putrescine, the first and rate-limiting step in the synthesis of putrescine and of the polyamines spermidine and spermine.[102] Polyamines are involved in nucleic acid synthesis, contribute to the regulation of protein synthesis and are essential for the growth and multiplication of all eukaryotic cells.[103] Trypanosomes are more susceptible to the drug than human cells, possibly because of the slow turnover of this enzyme in *T.b. gambiense*.[102] The rapid turnover is also responsible for the innate resistance of *T.b. rhodesiense* to eflornithine.[89]

Nifurtimox

Nifurtimox (Lampit®; Bayer) is a drug that was introduced in the late 1960s for use in patients with Chagas' disease.[104] The drug is not registered for use in sleeping sickness, and its use is currently restricted to compassionate treatment in combination with other trypanocidal drugs of patients not responding to melarsoprol. Nifurtimox was tested empirically in HAT case series during the 1970s and 1980s with conflicting results.[105] These evaluations differed in treatment regimens and evaluation criteria, making them difficult to compare. For treatment schedules, refer to the section 'combination treatment' and Table 75.4.

Nifurtimox is generally not well tolerated, and only about one-third of the patients remain free from adverse drug reactions[106] but generally adverse effects are not severe, very rarely fatal, and dose related.[96] Gastrointestinal disturbances with nausea, abdominal pains and vomiting are very frequent, and neurological adverse reactions with general convulsions, tremor or agitation may occur. The development of peripheral polyneuropathy and generalized skin reactions were seen as occasional events. All adverse reactions were rapidly reversible after discontinuation of the drug.

In healthy human volunteers given a single oral dose of 15 mg/kg nifurtimox average peak plasma levels of 751 (range 356–1093) ng/mL were reached within 2–3 h. The drug has an apparent volume of distribution of about 755 L (approximately 15 L/kg) and a high apparent clearance of 193 L/h (about 64 mL/min per kg). Nifurtimox is quickly eliminated, with an average plasma elimination half-life of 3 (range 2–6) h.[107]

The mechanism of action of nifurtimox is not completely elucidated. Its trypanocidal action may be related to its ability to undergo partial reduction to form chemically reactive radicals causing the production of superoxide anions, hydrogen peroxide and hydroxyl radicals. These free radicals may react with cellular macromolecules and cause membrane injury, enzyme inactivation, damage to DNA and mutagenesis.[108]

Therapy for treatment failures and relapses and combination treatment

Background

The relapse rate after melarsoprol treatment was generally in the range of 3–10% for both forms of human African trypanosomiasis. Only during the last decade has this proportion increased in some areas with epidemic *T.b. gambiense*, to 30% in north-west Uganda,[109] 21% in south Sudan and 25% in north Angola.[110]

Reasons for these treatment failures might be: (1) the parasite (drug-resistant trypanosomes, pronounced tissue tropism that allows the trypanosomes to escape to niches inaccessible to the drug) or (2) the host (altered drug metabolism resulting in changed pharmacokinetics). The use of incremental doses of melarsoprol was discussed to support the increase of relapse rates.[111] A Ugandan *T.b. rhodesiense* isolate from 1960–1961 was recently re-analysed and found to have a 10-fold decreased melarsoprol sensitivity in vitro and to be resistant in the mouse model at 20 mg/kg for four consecutive days.[89] However, no drug-resistant *T.b. gambiense* isolates have yet been described, although trypanosome populations from relapse patients were examined.[89] Studies in north Angola[112] and north-west Uganda[113] indicated that melarsoprol levels were identical in relapsing patients and those who could be cured.

Molecular investigations have shown that the genes *TbAT1* cooling for the purine transporter P2 which also mediates the uptake of melarsoprol and diamidines, and *TbMRPA* which encodes a putative trypanothione-conjugate efflux pump, are potentially involved in a reduced drug susceptibility. Overexpression of *TbMRPA* can cause melarsoprol resistance and disruption of *TbAT1* in *Trypanosoma brucei* reduced sensitivity to these trypanocides. A major challenge is to determine the contribution of *TbAT1* and *TbMRPA* to drug resistance in the field, in particular to melarsoprol treatment failures in *T.b. gambiense* patients. TbAT1r alleles were shown to be significantly more prevalent in melarsoprol relapses than in newly infected *T.b. gambiense* patients.[113,114] However, polymorphisms were also detected among *TbAT1* genes from different drug-sensitive trypanosomes (Mäser and Kaminsky, unpublished data).

Combination treatment

To overcome the precarious situation, combination of the existing drugs was envisaged. A preliminary clinical trial combining melarsoprol and nifurtimox indicated the potential usefulness of the approach.[115] A further trial conducted in Omugo, Uganda was designed to compare three different combination treatment regimens: melarsoprol-nifurtimox (M + N), melarsoprol-eflornithine (M + E), and nifurtimox-eflornithine (N + E). The dosages of the drugs were equal in each arm: melarsoprol 1.8 mg/kg per day i.v., once daily for 10 days; eflornithine 100 mg/kg in slow i.v. infusion, every 6 h for 7 days; and nifurtimox 5 mg/kg (adults) or 6.5 mg/kg (children, <15 years) orally, every 8 h for 10 days. The sample size had originally had been set at 145 patients per arm (435 in total) to test equivalence in cure rates after 24 months of follow-up. However, the enrolment was suspended after only 54 patients for ethical reasons due to the high fatality observed in the M + N arm and the strong contrast of overall toxicity per arm. An intention-to-treat analysis was performed and yielded cure rates of 44.4% for M + N, 78.9% for M + E, and 94.1% for N + E. There was also a strong difference in the case fatality of M + N (n = 4) and M + E (n = 1) and N + E (n = 0) and the major adverse events (grades 3 and 4) between M + N (n = 18) and M + E (n = 9) and N + E (n = 5), although the small number of observations did not allow a demonstration of significance.[105] Despite the clear sample size limitations of this study it was recommended to follow-up this approach, and to this end a multicentre study of a shorter course of intravenous eflornithine

administered twice per day with a course of oral nifurtimox is now underway.[99]

New developments

The development of orally applicable drug pafuramidine maleate (DB289) for treatment of first stage human African trypanosomiasis caused by *Trypanosoma brucei gambiense* was pursued up to phase III clinical trials which were conducted in DRC, Angola and Sudan. Pafuramidine would have become the first oral therapy for this disease, however, the development programme had to be cancelled by the Consortium for Parasitic Drug Devlopment due to unexpected liver and renal toxicity observed during a last safety run in parallel with the Phase III trail.[115,116] Research on novel oral diamidines is continuing by a consortium under the leadership of the University of North Carolina, USA, to find a clinical candidate for the second stage of the disease (personal communication R. Brun).

Treatment follow-up

Because of the increasing frequency of treatment-refractory infections, the policy of performing a confirmatory lumbar puncture 1 day after the last drug application of each second-stage case should be recommended. The CSF should be analysed with a sensitive method for parasite detection (any concentration technique). The white cell count is not a helpful criterion at this point, because it may remain raised for several weeks. All patients should be monitored for 2 years, with lumbar punctures performed every 6 months. First-stage patients should be considered to have relapsed if they present at any examination with a white cell count >20 cells/mm^3 and should be retreated with melarsoprol. In case of equivocal results the patient should be seen again after 1–2 months. A relapse is confirmed if trypanosomes can be found in the CSF at any follow-up examination. There is no analytical method for distinguishing between relapse and reinfection. A relapse is suspected if the CSF white cell count is 50 cells/mm^3 or more, and has doubled since the previous examination, or 20–49 cells/mm^3 with recurrence of symptoms. Retreatment with melarsoprol may be attempted once in regions with a low relapse rate, but drug combinations are recommended in regions where treatment failure is common.

DISEASE CONTROL

Infected persons may remain almost asymptomatic for long periods before they develop signs of sleeping sickness but they always represent a reservoir. Therefore, the most important control measure for *gambiense* trypanosomiasis is active case-finding followed by treatment of the identified infected subjects. Populations of endemic areas (foci) with a prevalence of over 1% should be examined once a year by mobile teams. In areas with a prevalence below 1%, active case detection may be maintained with a reduced periodicity.[4] The use of the CATT has become a routine tool, and its increased sensitivity over lymph node aspiration has partially made up for the lower participation of the population today compared with that in colonial times. CATT-positive patients should be subjected to the diagnostic path described in the section on diagnosis. However, the parasitological methods have a limited sensitivity and therefore do not allow all HAT patients with a positive screening result to be confirmed parasitologically and receive treatment. One option is to examine these serologically suspect individuals at regular intervals (e.g. every 3 months) for 1 to 2 years, but compliance with this procedure is usually low. A more promising option is to determine a subgroup of serologically suspected individuals at high risk of being infected with *T.b. gambiense* and to treat them. It was suggested to treat all serologically suspect individuals with a CATT end titre of = 1:16, when the prevalence of HAT in the investigated population is sufficiently high. It remains an open question which prevalence threshold should be chosen for this approach, but it should probably be no less than 1%.[47] However, the risk of unnecessary treatment has also to be considered, and thus other factors like poor access to care and the absence of concentration methods for the parasitological diagnosis may positively influence the decision to perform titration of serum and treat individuals with a CATT end titre of = 1:16.

In highly endemic areas, the additional use of tsetse fly traps placed in spots of high risk of transmission supports the control of the disease.

For *T.b. rhodesiense* generally, a fixed post-surveillance approach is chosen because the symptoms are severe and patients tend to volunteer for treatment.[4]

Chemoprophylaxis is no longer in use because of the poor risk–benefit ratio owing to the adverse effects of the drugs in use.

Indicators for monitoring the efficacy of national control programmes have been suggested and may assist in improvement of the activities.[118]

REFERENCES

1. PAAT (Program Against African Trypanosomiasis). Information System. 2006. Online. Available: http://wwwfaoorg/paat/html/gishtm

2. Rogers DJ, Williams BG. Monitoring trypanosomiasis in space and time. *Parasitology* 1993; 106(suppl):S77–S92.

3. Jordan AM. *Trypanosomiasis Control and African Rural Development.* London: Longman; 1986.

4. WHO. *Control and surveillance of African trypanosomiasis.* Geneva: World Health Organization; 1998.

5. Abel PM, Kiala G, Loa V, et al. Retaking sleeping sickness control in Angola. *Trop Med Int Health* 2004; 9(1):141–148.

6. Lutumba P. Trypanosomiasis control, democratic republic of Congo, 1993–2003. *Emerg Infect Dis* 2005; 11(9):1382–1389.

7. Robays J, Bilengue MM, Stuyft PV, et al. The effectiveness of active population screening and treatment for sleeping sickness control in the Democratic Republic of Congo. *Trop Med Int Health* 2004; 9(5):542–550.

8. Ruiz JA, Simarro PP, Josenando T. Control of human African trypanosomiasis in the Quicama focus, Angola. *Bull World Health Organ* 2002; 80(9):738–745.

9. Simarro PP, Franco JR, Ndongo P, et al. The elimination of Trypanosoma brucei gambiense sleeping sickness in the focus of Luba, Bioko Island, Equatorial Guinea. *Trop Med Int Health* 2006; 11(5):636–646.

10. Balasegaram M, Harris S, Checchi F, et al. Treatment outcomes and risk factors for relapse in patients with early-stage human African trypanosomiasis (HAT) in the Republic of the Congo. *Bull WHO* 2006; 84:777–782.

11. Anonymous. *Weekly Epidemiological Record* 2006; 8:71–80.

12. Hoare CA. *The Trypanosomes of Mammals (A Zoological Monograph).* Oxford: Blackwell Scientific; 1972.

13. Vickerman K. Antigenic variation in trypanosomes. *Nature* 1978; 273(5664):613–617.

14. Buscher P, Bin Shamamba SK, Ngoyi DM, et al. Susceptibility of Grammomys surdaster thicket rats to Trypanosoma brucei gambiense infection. *Trop Med Int Health* 2005; 10(9):850–855.

15. Inoue N, Narumi D, Mbati PA, et al. Susceptibility of severe combined immuno-deficient (SCID) mice to Trypanosoma brucei gambiense and T. b. rhodesiense. *Trop Med Int Health* 1998; 3(5):408–412.

16. Truc P, Aerts D, McNamara JJ, et al. Direct isolation in vitro of Trypanosoma brucei from man and other animals, and its potential value for the diagnosis of Gambian trypanosomiasis. *Trans R Soc Trop Med Hyg* 1992; 86(6):627–629.

17. Dukes P, Kaukas A, Hudson KM, et al. A new method for isolating Trypanosoma brucei gambiense from sleeping sickness patients. *Trans R Soc Trop Med Hyg* 1989; 83(5):636–639.

18. Maina NW, Kunz C, Brun R. Cryopreservation of Trypanosoma brucei gambiense in a commercial cryomedium developed for bull semen. *Acta Trop* 2006; 98(3):207–211.

19. Maina NWN, Oberle M, Otieno C, et al. Isolation and propagation of Trypanosoma brucei gambiense from sleeping sickness patients in South Sudan. *Trans R Soc Trop Med Hyg* 2007; 101(6):540–546.

20. Tomlinson S, Raper J. Natural human immunity to trypanosomes. *Parasitol Today* 1998; 14(9):354–359.

21. Pays E, Vanhollebeke B, Vanhamme L, et al. The trypanolytic factor of human serum. *Nat Rev Microbiol* 2006; 4(6):477–486.

22. Rickman LR, Robson J. The blood incubation infectivity test: A simple test which may serve to distinguish Trypanosoma brucei from T. rhodesienses. *Bull WHO* 1970; 42(4):650–651.

23. Jenni L, Brun R. A new in vitro test for human serum resistance of Trypanosoma (T.) brucei. *Acta Trop* 1982; 39(3):281–284.

24. Radwanska M, Chamekh M, Vanhamme L, et al. The serum resistance-associated gene as a diagnostic tool for the detection of Trypanosoma brucei rhodesiense. *Am J Trop Med Hyg* 2002; 67(6):684–690.

25. Berberof M, Perez-Morga D, Pays E. A receptor-like flagellar pocket glycoprotein specific to Trypanosoma brucei gambiense. *Mol Biochem Parasitol* 2001; 113(1):127–138.

26. Jenni L, Marti S, Schweizer J, et al. Hybrid formation between African trypanosomes during cyclical transmission. *Nature* 1986; 322(6075): 173–175.

27. Gibson WC, Mizen VH. Heritability of the trait for human infectivity in genetic crosses of Trypanosoma brucei ssp. *Trans R Soc Trop Med Hyg* 1997; 91(2):236–237.

28. Simo G, Herder S, Njiokou F, et al. Trypanosoma brucei s.l.: characterisation of stocks from Central Africa by PCR analysis of mobile genetic elements. *Exp Parasitol* 2005; 110(4):353–362.

29. Balmer O, Palma C, MacLeod A, et al. Characterization of di-, tri- and tetranucleotide microsatellite markers with perfect repeats for Trypanosoma brucei and related species. *Molecular Ecology Notes* 2006; 6:508–510.

30. Tibayrenc M, Kjellberg F, Ayala FJ. A clonal theory of parasitic protozoa: the population structures of Entamoeba, Giardia, Leishmania, Naegleria, Plasmodium, Trichomonas, and Trypanosoma and their medical and taxonomical consequences. *Proc Natl Acad Sci USA* 1990; 87(7): 2414–2418.

31. Gibson W, Miles MA. Application of new technologies to epidemiology. *Brit Med Bull* 1985; 41(2):115–121.

32. Godfrey DG, Baker RD, Rickman LR, et al. The distribution, relationships and identification of enzymic variants within the subgenus Trypanozoon. *Adv Parasitol* 1990; 29:1–39.

33. Stevens JR, Godfrey DG. Numerical taxonomy of Trypanozoon based on polymorphisms in a reduced range of enzymes. *Parasitology* 1992; 104:75–86.

34. Stevens JR, Lanham SM, Allingham R, et al. A simplified method for identifying subspecies and strain groups in Trypanozoon by isoenzymes. *Ann Trop Med Parasitol* 1992; 86(1):9–28.

35. Herder S, Simo G, Nkinin S, et al. Identification of trypanosomes in wild animals from southern Cameroon using the polymerase chain reaction (PCR). *Parasite* 2002; 9(4):345–349.

36. Buyst H. The epidemiology of sleeping sickness in the historical Luangwa valley. *Ann Soc Belge Med Trop* 1977; 57(4–5):349–359.

37. MacLean L, Chisi JE, Odiit M, et al. Severity of human African trypanosomiasis in East Africa is associated with geographic location, parasite genotype, and host inflammatory cytokine response profile. *Infect Immun* 2004; 72(12):7040–7044.

38. Geigy R, Mwambu PM, Kauffmann M. Sleeping sickness survey in Musoma district, Tanzania. IV. Examination of wild mammals as a potential reservoir for T. rhodesiense. *Acta Trop* 1971; 28(3):211–220.

39. De Greef C, Imberechts H, Matthyssens G, et al. A gene expressed only in serum-resistant variants of Trypanosoma brucei rhodesiense. *Mol Biochem Parasitol* 1989; 36(2):169–176.

40. Xong HV, Vanhamme L, Chamekh M, et al. A VSG expression site-associated gene confers resistance to human serum in Trypanosoma rhodesiense. *Cell* 1998; 95(6):839–846.

41. Cibulskis RE. Genetic variation in Trypanosoma brucei and the epidemiology of sleeping sickness in the Lambwe Valley, Kenya. *Parasitology* 1992; 104(Part 1):99–109.

42. Gibson WC, Wellde BT. Characterization of Trypanozoon stocks from the South Nyanza sleeping sickness focus in Western Kenya. *Trans R Soc Trop Med Hyg* 1985; 79(5):671–676.

43. Onyango RJ, van Hoeve K, de Raadt P. The epidemiology of T. rhodesiense sleeping sickness in Alego location, central Nyanza, Kenya. I. Evidence that cattle may act as reservoir hosts of trypanosomes infective to man. *Trans R Soc Trop Med Hyg* 1966; 60:175.

44. Gibson WC, Gashumba JK. Isoenzyme characterization of some Trypanozoon stocks from a recent trypanosomiasis epidemic in Uganda. *Trans R Soc Trop Med Hyg* 1983; 77(1):114–118.

45. Baldry DAT, Chaudhuri MFB. Epidemiology of African trypanosomiasis. *Insect Sci Appl* 1980; 1(1):85–93.

46. Welburn SC, Maudlin I. Tsetse-trypanosome interactions: rites of passage. *Parasitol Today* 1999; 15(10):399–403.

47. Chappuis F, Loutan L, Simarro P, et al. Options for field diagnosis of human African trypanosomiasis. *Clin Microbiol Rev* 2005; 18(1): 133–146.

48. Magnus E, Vervoort T, Van Meirvenne N. A card agglutination test with stained trypanosomes (CATT) for the serological diagnosis of T.b. gambiense trypanosomiasis. *Ann Soc Belge Med Trop* 1978; 58:169–176.

49. Chappuis F, Stivalello E, Adams K, et al. Card agglutination test for trypanosomiasis (CATT) end-dilution titer and cerebrospinal fluid cell count as predictors of human African trypanosomiasis (Trypanosoma brucei gambiense) among serologically suspected individuals in Southern Sudan. *Am J Trop Med Hyg* 2004; 71:313–317.

50. Inojosa WO, Augusto I, Bisoffi Z, et al. Diagnosing human African trypanosomiasis in Angola using a card agglutination test: observational study of active and passive case finding strategies. *BMJ* 2006; 332(7556):1479.

51. Simarro PP, Ruiz JA, Franco JR, et al. Attitude towards CATT-positive individuals without parasitological confirmation in the African Trypanosomiasis (T.b. gambiense) focus of Quicama (Angola). *Trop Med Int Health* 1999 Dec.; 4(12):858–861.

52. Buscher P, Lejon V, Magnus E, et al. Improved latex agglutination test for detection of antibodies in serum and cerebrospinal fluid of Trypanosoma brucei gambiense infected patients. *Acta Trop* 1999; 73(1):11–20.

53. Deborggraeve S, Claes F, Laurent T, et al. Molecular dipstick test for diagnosis of sleeping sickness. *J Clin Microbiol* 2006; 44(8):2884–2889.

54. Woo PT. The haematocrit centrifuge for the detection of trypanosomes in blood. *Can J Zool* 1969; 47(5):921–923.

55. Lumsden WGR, Kimber CD, Evans DA, et al. Trypanosoma brucei: Miniature anion exchange centrifugation for detection of low parasitemias: Adaptation for field use. *Trans R Soc Trop Med Hyg* 1979; 73:313–317.

56. Doua F, Miezan TW, Sanon Singaro JR, et al. The efficacy of pentamidine in the treatment of early-late stage Trypanosoma brucei gambiense trypanosomiasis. *Am J Trop Med Hyg* 1996; 55(6):586–588.

57. Lejon V, Legros D, Savignoni A, et al. Neuro-inflammatory risk factors for treatment failure in 'early second stage' sleeping sickness patients treated with Pentamidine. *J Neuroimmunol* 2003; 144(1–2):132–138.

58. Lejon V, Buscher P. Cerebrospinal fluid in human African trypanosomiasis: a key to diagnosis, therapeutic decision and post-treatment follow-up [Review Article]. *Trop Med Int Health* 2005; 10(5):395–403.

59. Lejon V, Buscher P, Sema NH, et al. Human African trypanosomiasis: A latex agglutination field test for quantifying IgM in cerebrospinal fluid. *Bull WHO* 1998; 76(6):553–558.

60. Lejon V, Legros D, Richer M, et al. IgM quantification in the cerebrospinal fluid of sleeping sickness patients by a latex card agglutination test. *Trop Med Int Health* 2002; 7(8):685–692.

61. Buguet A, Bisser S, Josenando T, et al. Sleep structure: a new diagnostic tool for stage determination in sleeping sickness. *Acta Trop* 2005; 93(1): 107–117.

62. Blum J, Schmid C, Burri C. Clinical aspects of 2541 patients with second stage human African trypanosomiasis. *Acta Trop* 2006; 97(1):55–64.

63. Schultzberg M, Ambatsis M, Samuelsson EB, et al. Spread of Trypanosoma brucei to the nervous system: early attack on circumventricular organs and sensory ganglia. *J Neurosci Res* 1988; 21(1):56–61.

64. Pepin J. African trypanosomiasis. In: Strickland GT, ed. *Hunter's Tropical Medicine and Emerging Infectious Diseases*. 8th edn. Philadelphia: Saunders; 2000:643–654.

65. Manson-Bahr PEC, Bell DR. *African Trypanosomiasis. Manson's Tropical Diseases*. 19th edn. London: Baillière and Tindall; 1987:54–73.

66. Molyneux DH, Pentreath V, Doua F. African trypanosomiasis in man. In: Cook GC, ed. *Manson's Tropical Diseases*. 20th edn. London: Saunders; 1996:1171–1196.

67. Kristensson K, Bentivoglio M. Pathology of African trypanosomiasis. In: Dumas M, Bouteille B, Buguet A, eds. *Progress in Human African Trypanosomiasis, Sleeping Sickness*. Paris: Springer; 1999:157–182.

68. Mansfield JM, Paulnock DM. Regulation of innate and acquired immunity in African trypanosomiasis. *Parasite Immunol* 2005; 27(10–11):361–371.

69. MacLean L, Odiit M, Sternberg JM. Nitric oxide and cytokine synthesis in human African trypanosomiasis. *J Infect Dis* 2001; 184(8):1086–1090.

70. Baetselier PD, Namangala B, Noel W, et al. Alternative versus classical macrophage activation during experimental African trypanosomosis. *Int J Parasitol* 2001; 31(5–6):575–587.

71. Lejon V, Reiber H, Legros D, et al. Intrathecal immune response pattern for improved diagnosis of central nervous system involvement in trypanosomiasis. *J Infect Dis* 2003; 187(9):1475–1483.

72. Sternberg J. Human African trypanosomiasis: clinical presentation and immune response. *Parasite Immunol* 2004; 26(11–12):469–476.

73. Bisser S, Ouwe-Missi-Oukem-Boyer ON, Toure FS, et al. Harbouring in the brain: A focus on immune evasion mechanisms and their deleterious effects in malaria and human African trypanosomiasis. *Int J Parasitol* 2006; 36(5):529–540.

74. Vincendeau P, Bouteille B. Immunology and immunopathology of African trypanosomiasis. *An Acad Bras Cienc* 2006; 78(4):645–665.

75. Berriman M, Ghedin E, Hertz-Fowler C, et al. The genome of the African trypanosome Trypanosoma brucei. *Science* 2005; 309(5733): 416–422.

76. El-Sayed NM, Myler PJ, Blandin G, et al. Comparative genomics of trypanosomatid parasitic protozoa. *Science* 2005; 309(5733): 404–409.

77. Hutchinson OC, Webb H, Picozzi K, et al. Candidate protein selection for diagnostic markers of African trypanosomiasis. *Trends Parasitol* 2004; 20(11):519–523.

78. Agranoff D, Stich A, Abel P, et al. Proteomic fingerprinting for the diagnosis of human African trypanosomiasis. *Trends Parasitol* 2005; 21(4):154–157.

79. Apted FIC. Treatment of human trypanosomiasis. In: Mulligan HW, ed. *The African Trypanosomiasis*. London: Allen & Unwin; 1970:684–710.

80. Sands M, Kron MA, Brown RB. Pentamidine: A review. *Review in Infectious Diseases* 1985; 7:625–634.

81. Doua F, Yapo FB. Human trypanosomiasis in the Ivory Coast – therapy and problems. *Acta Trop* 1993; 54(3–4):163–168.

82. Bronner U, Doua F, Ericsson O, et al. Pentamidine concentrations in plasma, whole blood and cerebrospinal fluid during treatment of Trypanosoma gambiense infection in Côte d'Ivoire. *Trans R Soc Trop Med Hyg* 1991; 85(5):608–611.

83. Berger BJ, Lombardy RJ, Marbury GD, et al. Metabolic N-hydroxylation of pentamidine in vitro. *Antimicrob Agents Chemother* 1990; 34(9):1678–1684.

84. Wang CC. Molecular mechanisms and therapeutic approaches to the treatment of African trypanosomiasis. *Annu Rev Pharmacol Toxicol* 1995; 35:93–127.

85. Collins JM, Klecker RWJ, Yarchoan R, et al. Clinical pharmacokinetics of suramin in patients with HTLV-III/LAV infection. *J Clin Pharmacol* 1986; 26:22–26.

86. Chijioke CP, Umeh RE, Mbah AU, et al. Clinical pharmacokinetics of suramin in patients with onchocerciasis. *Eur J Clin Pharmacol* 1998; 54(3):249–251.

87. Fairlamb AH, Bowman BR. Uptake of the trypanocidal drug suramin by bloodstream forms of Trypanosoma brucei and its effect in respiration and growth rate in vivo. *J Biochem Pathol* 1980; 1:315–333.

88. Friedheim EAH. Mel B in the treatment of human trypanosomiasis. *Am J Trop Med Hyg* 1949; 29:173–180.

89. Brun R, Schumacher R, Schmid C, et al. The phenomenon of treatment failures in human African trypanosomiasis. *Trop Med Int Health* 2001; 6(11):906–914.

90. Burri C, Nkunku S, Merolle A, et al. Efficacy of new, concise treatment schedule for melarsoprol in treatment of sleeping sickness caused by *Trypanosoma brucei gambiense*: a randomised trial. *Lancet* 2000; 355: 1419–1425.

91. Schmid C, Richer M, Bilenge CM, et al. Effectiveness of a 10-day melarsoprol schedule for the treatment of late-stage human African trypanosomiasis: Confirmation from a multinational study (Impamel II). *J Infect Dis* 2005; 191(11):1922–1931.

92. Jannin J, Cattand P. Treatment and control of human African trypanosomiasis. *Curr Opin Infect Dis* 2004; 17(6):565–571.

93. Blum J, Nkunku S, Burri C. Clinical description of encephalopathic syndromes and risk factors for their occurrence and outcome during melarsoprol treatment of human African trypanosomiasis. *Trop Med Int Health* 2001; 6(5):390–400.

94. Soignet SL, Tong WP, Hirschfeld S, et al. Clinical study of an organic arsenical, melarsoprol, in patients with advanced leukemia. *Cancer Chemother Pharmacol* 1999; 44(5):417–421.

95. Keiser J, Ericsson O, Burri C. Investigations of the metabolites of the trypanocidal drug melarsoprol. *Clin Pharmacol Therapeutics* 2000; 67(5): 478–488.

96. Pepin J, Milord F, Mpia B, et al. An open clinical trial of nifurtimox for arseno-resistant Trypanosoma brucei gambiense sleeping sickness in central Zaire. *Trans R Soc Trop Med Hyg* 1989; 83(4):514–517.

97. Van Nieuwenhove S. Present strategies in the treatment of human African trypanosomiasis. In: Dumas M, Bouteille B, Buguet A, eds. *Progress in Human African Trypanosomiasis, Sleeping Sickness*. Paris: Springer; 1999:253–280.

98. Burri C, Baltz T, Giroud C, et al. Pharmacokinetic properties of the trypanocidal drug melarsoprol. *Chemotherapy* 1993; 39(4):225–234.

99. Chappuis F, Udayraj N, Stietenroth K, et al. Eflornithine is safer than melarsoprol for the treatment of second-stage Trypanosoma brucei gambiense human African trypanosomiasis. *Clin Infect Dis* 2005; 41(5): 748–751.

100. Burri C, Brun R. Eflornithine for treatment of human African trypanosomiasis. *Parasitol Res* 2003; 90(suppl 1):S49–S52.

101. Dow MM. Ornidyl label. *Ornidyl Patient Information*; 1991.

102. Bacchi CJ, Nathan HC, Hutner SH, et al. Polyamine metabolism: a potential therapeutic target in trypanosomes. *Science* 1980; 210(4467): 332–334.

103. Pegg AE, McCann PP. Polyamine metabolism and function. *Am J Physiol* 1982; 243(5):C212–C221.

104. Gonnert R. Nifurtimox: causal treatment of Chagas' disease. *Drug Res* 1972; 22(9):1563.

105. Priotto G, Fogg C, Balasegaram M, et al. Three drug combinations for late-stage Trypanosoma brucei gambiense sleeping sickness: A randomized clinical trial in Uganda. *PLoS Clin Trials* 2006; 1(8):e39:1–8.

106. Wegner DH, Rohwedder RW. Experience with nifurtimox in chronic Chagas' infection. Preliminary report. *Drug Res* 1972; 22(9):1635–1641.

107. Paulos C, Paredes J, Vasquez I, et al. Pharmacokinetics of a nitrofuran compound, nifurtimox, in healthy volunteers. *Int J Clin Pharmacol Ther Toxicol* 1989; 27(9):454–457.

108. Docampo R, Moreno SN. Free radical metabolism of antiparasitic agents. *Fed Proc* 1986; 45(10):2471–2476.

109. Legros D, Evans S, Maiso F, et al. Risk factors for treatment failure after melarsoprol for *Trypanosoma brucei gambiense* trypanosomiasis in Uganda. *Trans R Soc Trop Med Hyg* 1999; 93:439–442.

110. Stanghellini A, Josenando T. The situation of sleeping sickness in Angola: a calamity. *Trop Med Int Health* 2001; 6(5):330–334.

111. Pepin J, Mpia B. Trypanosomiasis relapse after melarsoprol therapy, Democratic Republic of Congo, 1982–2001. *Emerg Infect Dis* 2005; 11(6):921–927.

112. Burri C, Keiser J. Pharmacokinetic investigations in patients from northern Angola refractory to melarsoprol treatment. *Trop Med Int Health* 2001; 6(5):412–420.

113. Matovu E, Enyaru JC, Legros D, et al. Melarsoprol refractory T.b. gambiense from Omugo, north-western Uganda. *Trop Med Int Health* 2001; 6(5): 407–411.

114. Matovu E, Geiser F, Schneider V, et al. Genetic variants of the TbAT1 adenosine transporter from African trypanosomes in relapse infections following melarsoprol therapy. *Mol Biochem Parasitol* 2001; 117(1):73–81.

115. Bisser S, Van Nieuwenhove S, Lejon V, et al. New therapeutic regimen for sleeping sickness. Description, results and lessons from the clinical trial established in Bwamanda (Equateur, RDC). Bruges: COST B9 Meeting; 2000.

116. Immtech. Immtech Report Fiscal Year End 2008 Results. Online. Available: http://www.immtechpharma.com/documents/news_061808a.pdf.

117. Anonymous. *$22.6 Million Gates Foundation Grant Targets New Treatment for African Sleeping Sickness*. 2006. Online. Available: http://wwwuncedu/news/archives/may06/may06shtml

118. Bouchet B, Legros D, Lee E. Key indicators for the monitoring and evaluation of control programmes of human African trypanosomiasis due to Trypanosoma brucei gambiense. *Trop Med Int Health* 1998; 3(6):474–481.

Chapter 76   Michael A. Miles

American Trypanosomiasis (Chagas' Disease)

HISTORY

American trypanosomiasis, which results from infection with the protozoan parasite *Trypanosoma cruzi*, is justly referred to as Chagas' disease in homage to the great discoveries of the Brazilian scientist, Carlos Chagas. In 1907, Carlos Chagas left the beautiful city of Rio de Janeiro to work at Lassance in the state of Minas Gerais as a malaria control officer. The local inhabitants who lived in poor-quality housing complained that they were attacked at night by a large blood-sucking insect, the triatomine bug (Hemiptera, Reduviidae). Carlos Chagas immediately suspected that such blood-sucking insects might transmit a human infectious disease. He collected examples of the bug (*Panstrongylus megistus*; Figure 76.1) and found abundant protozoan flagellates in the bug faeces. He sent specimens of the insect back to Rio de Janeiro, to his mentor, Oswaldo Cruz. Marmosets exposed to infected bugs developed a circulating trypanosome which Chagas named *Trypanosoma cruzi*. Back in Lassance, he began to look for human infections and found the same organisms circulating in the blood of children with an acute febrile illness (Figure 76.2). As far as I am aware, this discovery is unique as the disease agent was first found in the insect vector and only subsequently in patients.

Carlos Chagas went on to describe all the major features of the *T. cruzi* life cycle in experimental animals and to discover natural reservoir hosts, such as the armadillo. The mechanism of transmission from the vector was hotly debated but was finally proven in 1912, by Emile Brumpt, to be by contamination with infected bug faeces, rather than directly through the bite of the triatomine bug.

The clinical and public health significance of Chagas' disease remained controversial for several years, until its widespread distribution in Latin America became recognized. There are several historical and political accounts of the extraordinary discovery of Chagas' disease.[1]

Serological surveys throughout Latin America eventually revealed that up to 18 million people might carry *T. cruzi*. At its peak, it was estimated that up to 90 million people might be exposed to infection. Of those infected, 5–10%, especially children, might be expected to die in the initial acute phase of infection. In some regions, up to 30% of those surviving the acute phase might suffer the chronic consequences: chagasic heart disease and, more rarely, enlargement and dysfunction of the oesophagus and colon.[2]

Vector-borne Chagas' disease is essentially a disease of poverty and poor housing. As we shall see, in the last decade, enormous progress has been made through national and international control programmes, in reducing the incidence of infection. *T. cruzi* can also be transmitted by blood transfusion, and screening of donor blood is thus an essential part of prevention. Congenital transmission and oral transmission, usually via food contaminated with infected bug faeces, are also known. An infected individual usually retains low-level infection for life. An immunocompromised state, as in human immunodeficiency virus (HIV) infection or in organ recipients, can reactivate the acute infection.

Like other trypanosomatids (trypanosomes and leishmanias), *T. cruzi* has generated intense research interest because of its molecular biology and the uncertain pathogenesis of Chagas' disease. Epidemiologically, the disease is enigmatic because the prognosis is unpredictable and many of those infected remain healthy for life. Fundamental to the understanding of Chagas' disease has been the demonstration that *T. cruzi* has remarkable heterogeneity, with at least two major subspecific divisions, which have distinct geographical distributions, ecologies and epidemiologies.[3,4]

A second human trypanosomiasis can be found in the New World, resulting from *Trypanosoma rangeli* infection. *T. rangeli* is, however, considered to be non-pathogenic, although it may complicate the diagnosis of Chagas' disease (see below).

A recent volume gives a detailed review of many aspects of the South American and African trypanosomiases.[5]

GEOGRAPHICAL DISTRIBUTION

Human *T. cruzi* infection is confined to the Americas. It extends from approximately 40°45′ South in Argentina into the southern states of the USA. Human infection is rare in the USA and still relatively uncommon in the vast Amazon basin of South America, for reasons that will be explained (see Epidemiology). Natural cycles of *T. cruzi* infection, involving many different triatomine bug species and mammal hosts, are much more widespread than the human infection, from southern Argentina and Chile (46° South) to northern California (42° North). Rarely, sporadic cases of transmission are detected outside the normal geographical distribution

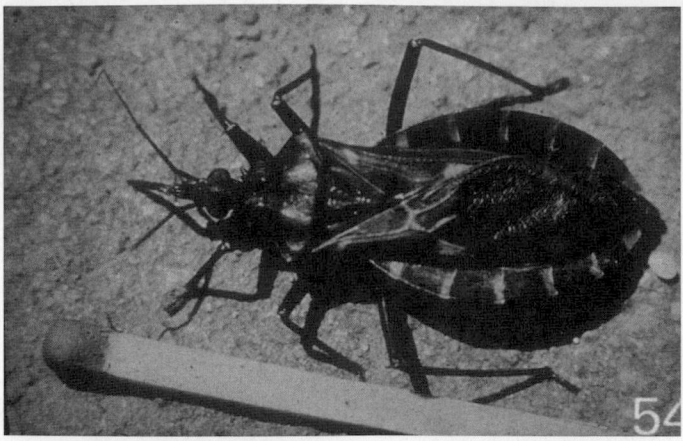

Figure 76.1 The triatomine bug *Panstrongylus megistus*, female with egg. (Courtesy of T. V. Barrett.)

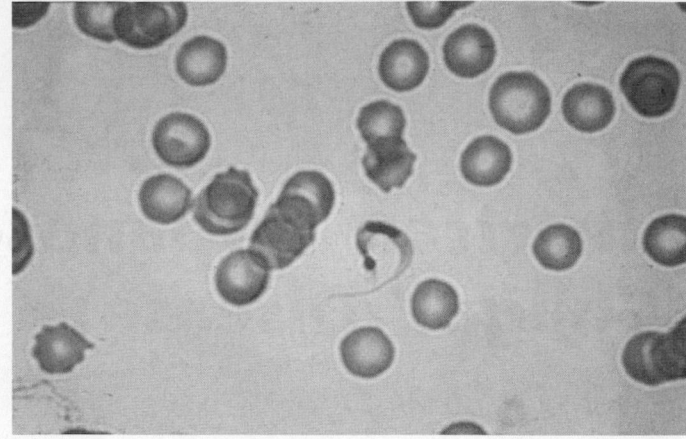

Figure 76.3 Typical trypomastigote of *Trypanosoma cruzi* in blood, showing C shape and large posterior kinetoplast.

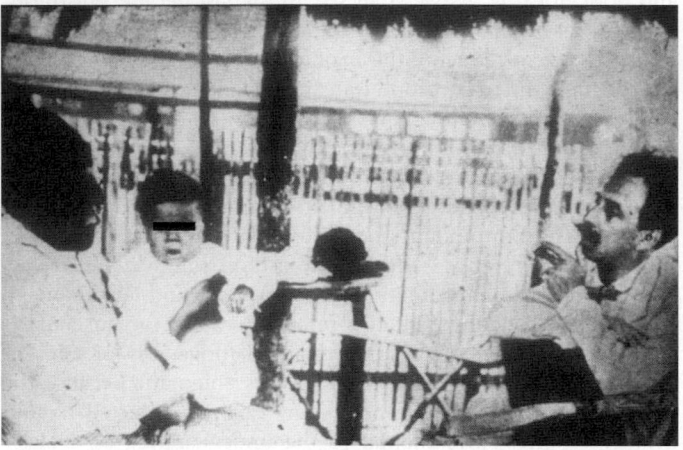

Figure 76.2 Carlos Chagas in Lassance, Minas Gerais State, Brazil, with one of the first infants with diagnosed Chagas' disease.

if infected donor blood is transfused into a naive recipient, or due to congenital transfer of infection across the placenta.[6] Further details of the geographical distribution are given in conjunction with the description of the epidemiology (see below).

AETIOLOGY

T. cruzi is a eukaryotic, single-celled, protozoan parasite of the order Kinetoplastida and the family Trypanosomatidae. Like other kinetoplastid organisms, *T. cruzi* has mitochondrial DNA in the form of a discrete organelle, the kinetoplast. The kinetoplast can be seen by light microscopy in stained blood films or tissue sections and is an important diagnostic feature, together with the infected cell type as *T. cruzi* can be found in non-phagocytic cells (Figure 76.3).

The morphological stages in the life cycle of *T. cruzi* are defined by the position of the kinetoplast relative to the nucleus and by the presence and extent of the free flagellum (Figure 76.4).[7] Unlike the African trypanosome, *Trypanosoma brucei*, *T. cruzi* does not

divide in the blood of the mammalian host, but divides intracellularly in non-phagocytic and phagocytic cells. Thus *T. cruzi* is predominantly an intracellular parasite in mammals, and this influences the pathogenesis of the disease and the nature of the immune response to infection. In the triatomine bug vector, *T. cruzi* divides solely within the intestinal tract and does not escape into the haemocoel. Division is by binary fission in the lumen of the gut, largely as epimastigotes, which have the kinetoplast adjacent to the nucleus. In the rectum of the triatomine bug, epimastigotes attach by the flagellum to the epithelium of the rectum wall and transform to infective (metacyclic) trypomastigotes. When the bug takes a blood meal, metacyclic trypomastigotes are released with the faeces and urine, and can establish infection in the mammalian host either by crossing mucous membranes, such as the conjunctiva, nasal or oral mucosae, or through abraded skin such as the wound made by the bite of the bug. Trypomastigotes cannot cross the barrier of intact skin, however, and once the bug faeces is dry it is no longer infective. Bugs acquire infection by feeding on the blood of an infected mammal or, rarely, by piercing the intestinal tract of another recently fed, infected bug, or by probing freshly deposited faeces of an infected bug (coprophagy). There is no transmission of *T. cruzi* infection from the bug through its egg stage to its offspring (transovarial transmission).

The infective metacyclic trypomastigotes in bug faeces are slender and highly motile. Inside the mammal they can penetrate non-phagocytic cells, particularly muscle cells, but also phagocytic cells and a wide variety of cell types. Inside the cell, *T. cruzi* escapes from the cell vacuole (phagolysosome) to lie free in the cytoplasm. There it loses its flagellum and transforms to a small oval amastigote stage which multiplies by binary fission, forming a false cyst or pseudocyst. After about 5 days, the amastigotes in the mature pseudocyst transform to small C-shaped trypomastigotes which are released when the pseudocyst ruptures. Multiplication may occur locally at the initial site of infection, causing a cutaneous or ocular lesion, before systemic spread of the organism (see Clinical features, below). Trypomastigotes released from pseudocysts are of two types: a slender, highly active trypomastigote, which can be found in the blood only in severe acute infections, and a smaller, broader, less motile trypomastigote, which is the

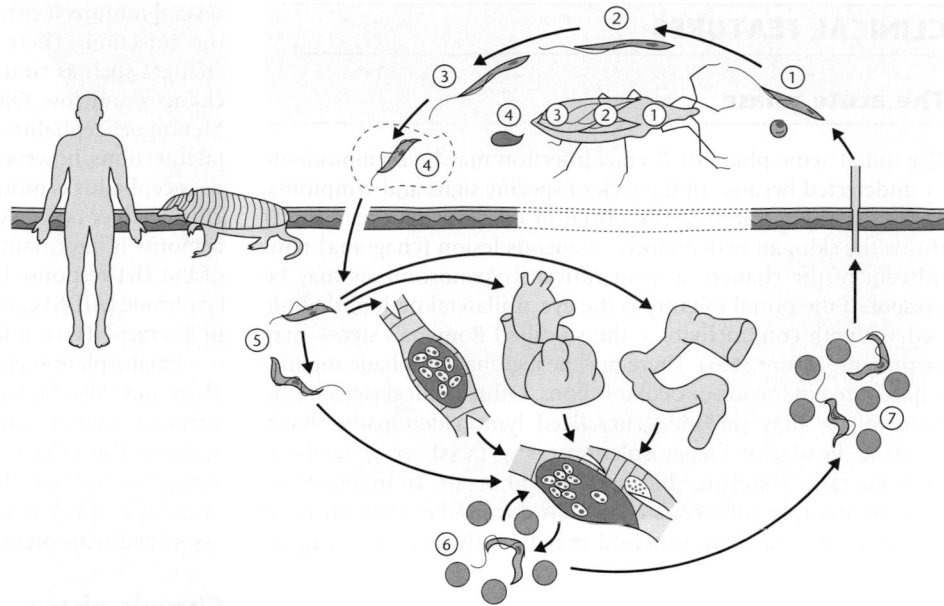

Figure 76.4 Summary of the life cycle of *Trypanosoma cruzi*, in the vector (1–4) and mammalian host (5–7). (Courtesy of Meddia.)

most common form found circulating in the blood. It is thought that these two forms have distinct functions. The slender form may be designed to re-establish the next intracellular cycle, whereas the short broad forms are more usually taken up by the insect vector. Pseudocysts may be very widely distributed among tissues of an infected mammal but they are frequently abundant in heart muscle, skeletal muscle or smooth muscle of the alimentary tract, in accord with the pathology of chronic Chagas' disease. Microscopically patent blood parasitaemia, if present, is usually transient in the acute phase of infection. Nevertheless, low numbers of circulating trypomastigotes usually remain for life and the host is a lifelong potential source of infection to triatomine bugs. If the host is attacked by bugs, trypomastigotes transform in the bug foregut to amastigotes and sphaeromastigotes (with a free flagellum) and begin to multiply by binary fission, which continues in the midgut as the epimastigote stage, thus completing the cycle. Bugs become infective 10–15 days after taking the infected blood meal.

All stages of the life cycle can be readily reproduced in tissue culture. Thus epimastigotes can be grown in liquid media or in liquid overlay above blood agar base. Transformation to metacyclic trypomastigotes may occur in older cultures but is not guaranteed with all strains; 2% sterile human urine has been shown to supplement growth. Intracellular amastigotes can be grown in many different mammalian cell lines: small, motile trypomastigotes can be seen in vitro in infected mammalian cells ('boiling cells') just before rupture, which releases trypomastigotes into the liquid overlay.

As already noted, there are important secondary methods of transmission in addition to vector-borne transmission. Of these, blood transfusion transmission has been particularly important epidemiologically (see below). Congenital transmission is also well documented (Figure 76.5). Reported congenital transmission rates vary but around 1% of infants born to seropositive mothers may acquire infection in utero. Strain specific congenital transmis-

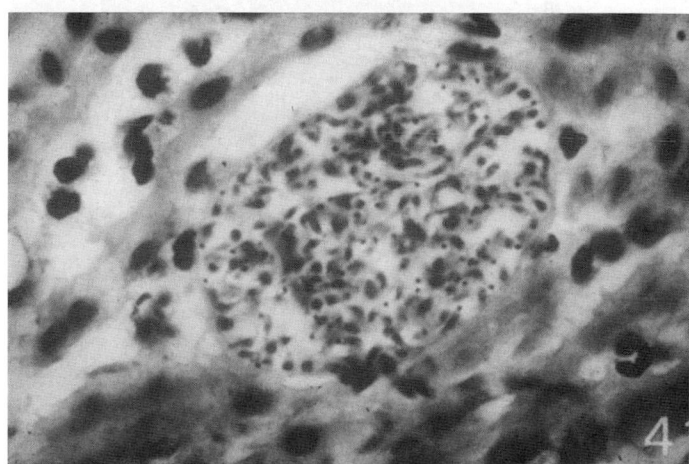

Figure 76.5 Mature pseudocyst of *Trypanosoma cruzi* in umbilical cord, from a congenital case of Chagas' disease. (Courtesy of Hipolito de Almeida.)

sion of *T. cruzi* has not been demonstrated; it has been suggested that exposure of the mother to multiple re-infection predisposes to congenital transmission.[8] Oral outbreaks may occur from food, particularly sugar cane and palm juices, contaminated by triatomine faeces, or through consumption of raw infected meat of a reservoir host. Sexual transmission is not known but may rarely occur. Milk transmission from mother to child occurs rarely. Oral transmission may be important in sustaining zoonotic *T. cruzi* infection among reservoir hosts, many of which eat insects. Anal gland infections occur in the opossum (*Didelphis*) with the glands containing life cycle stages typical of those found in the insect vector. It is not known whether this represents a primitive or a secondary stage of the life cycle, but anal gland secretions are presumably highly infective.

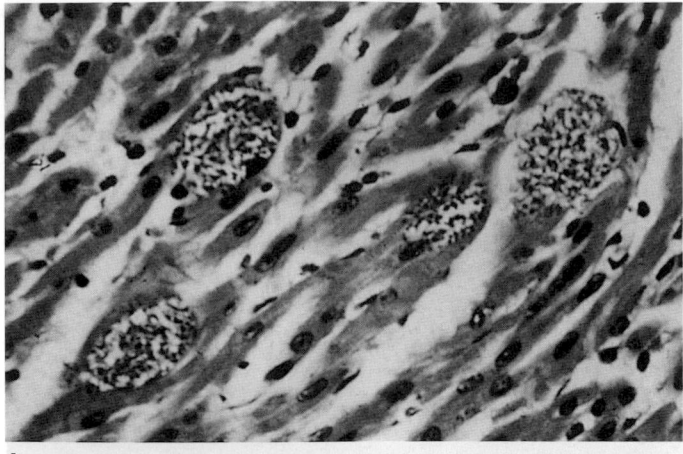

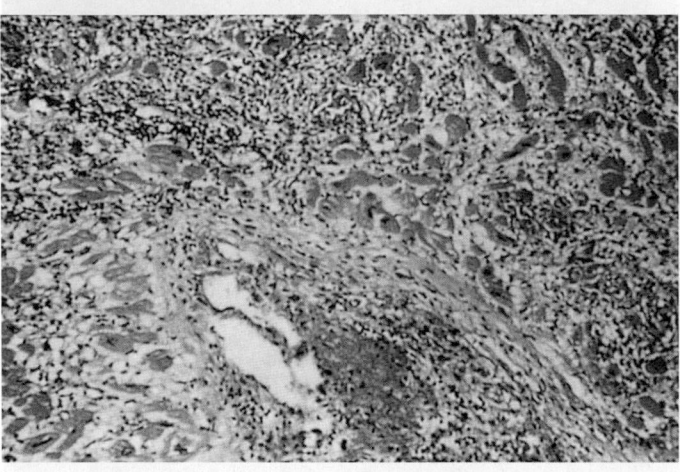

Figure 76.10 (A) Early acute-phase *Trypanosoma cruzi* infection: myocardium showing unruptured pseudocysts with no inflammatory reaction. (B) Later infection showing destruction of myocardium and inflammatory response.

similar correlations between ECG abnormalities and the distribution of lesions. Furthermore, it is quite clear that there is a marked loss of ganglion cells in megacardia, megaoesophagus and megacolon. This appears primarily to affect the parasympathetic innervation, leading to a sympathetic overload. The frequency of right bundle branch block (RBBB) in chronic Chagas' disease is thought to be due to the fact that the right conducting system of the heart is less diffuse and more vulnerable to focal lesions than the bifascicular left conducting system. The pathogenesis of 'neurogenic' Chagas' disease is thus partially explained in terms of: (1) pseudocyst rupture which deposits antigens on uninfected cells around the site of the pseudocyst; (2) focal immunological destruction of uninfected cells carrying adsorbed *T. cruzi* antigens, including ganglion cells; (3) further loss of ganglion cells with age; and (4) dysfunction and enlargement of the affected organs when the loss of ganglion of cells crosses a critical threshold. The latter may occur at any time after the acute phase, or not at all during the life of the infected individual. The majority of neurological damage is

thought to occur in the acute phase of the infection and to be related to the level of parasitaemia. The sympathetic overload can be mimicked in experimental rats by the inoculation of catecholamines, and this alone may induce apical aneurysm.[11]

The inflammatory response in the tissues normally subsides after the acute phase of the infection. In some patients this inflammatory response appears to be renewed, leading to a progressive myocarditis and a slow decline in cardiac function. This 'myogenic' picture is thought to have an autoimmune component. Cross-reactive antibodies between *T. cruzi* and normal host tissues can be generated experimentally, and tissue cross-reactive antibodies have been reported in patients with chronic Chagas' disease. Some reports show that heart transplants from normal mice into syngeneic chagasic mice suffer autoimmune rejection. In contrast, conflicting reports show the survival of such syngeneic transplants without autoimmune rejection unless the heart is parasitized.[12] Hence, the influence of residual small numbers of parasites on the prognosis of chronic Chagas' disease is unpredictable, and it is not straightforward to eliminate them by chemotherapy (see below).

Much of the pathogenesis of Chagas' disease has been worked out by studies in Brazil.[5] It is notable that megasyndromes are said to be less common in the north of South America and in Central America, although fewer studies have been undertaken. It has been suggested that regional differences in the pathology of Chagas' disease may be related to radically distinct subspecific strains of *T. cruzi* (see Epidemiology).

DIAGNOSIS

In a known endemic area of Chagas' disease, Romana's sign is suggestive of acute infection, although there are other potential causes of unilateral conjunctivitis such as insect bite or injury. Many of the systemic signs of early Chagas' disease are not specific and could be confused with other febrile illnesses. In chronic disease, particular ECG abnormalities (e.g. RBBB) are highly indicative if associated with positive serological findings. Hirschsprung's megacolon can be distinguished from chagasic megacolon because the former is rare in adults; if necessary, radiography or electromanometry can be used for differential diagnosis.[2] For immigrants or travellers returning from Latin America who have symptoms that might be attributable to Chagas' disease, it is essential to investigate thoroughly for the presence of a supporting history, such as exposure to triatomine bugs or blood transfusion. Rarely, infection in endemic areas might be acquired by food contaminated with infected material from triatomine bugs or reservoir hosts. In all such cases serology, correctly performed, should be positive if Chagas' disease is present. Exhaustive investigation for Chagas' disease is pointless if serology is consistently negative.

Parasitological examination may reveal the presence of trypanosomes in peripheral blood during the acute phase of infection. In some acute cases direct microscopy of unstained wet blood films may be positive. Methods for detecting scanty trypomastigotes include:[13] (a) microscopy of thick blood films; (b) microscopy of the buffy coat layer after haematocrit centrifugation (be careful to avoid exposure to infection if tubes are inadequately sealed); (c) searching for trypomastigotes in centrifuged serum after blood coagulation (Strout's method); and (d) centrifugation of blood after lysis of red cells with 0.87% ammonium chloride.

Note that *T. cruzi* is a relatively fragile organism and if thin films are prepared a high angle between the lower slide and smearing slide is required or the organisms disintegrate.

All of these concentration methods may fail to detect trypomastigotes in some acute cases. After the acute-phase infection, the parasitaemia subsides to very low levels that are usually subpatent to all these direct techniques. However, patent parasitaemia may re-occur in immunocompromised patients.

The only parasitological techniques that may be effective in the chronic phase are xenodiagnosis or blood culture.[14] In xenodiagnosis, triatomine bugs from laboratory colonies reared by feeding on birds (which are insusceptible to *T. cruzi* infection) are fed on the patient. Some 20–25 days later the intestinal tract of each triatomine bug is removed, mixed with sterile physiological saline (using a blunt spatula) and observed microscopically for the presence of epimastigotes. Care must be taken to avoid exposure to infective metacyclic trypomastigotes in bug faeces. Bugs are usually fed on the underside of the patient's forearm, enclosed in plastic pots within black bags. Xenodiagnosis is quite sensitive, with up to 50% of seropositive patients yielding a positive xenodiagnosis when 10 or 20 bugs are used. It is essential to use sterile saline for the dissection or contaminanting free living protozoa may confuse diagnosis, if *Triatoma infestans* is used for xenodiagnosis, examination for colonies must be carried out beforehand to detect the presence of *Blastocrithidia triatomae*, which is a natural invertebrate parasite of this species. Local triatomine bug species should be used for xenodiagnosis because susceptibility to different strains of *T. cruzi* may vary. Delayed hypersensitivity reactions following xenodiagnosis may require treatment. Anaphylactic reactions are extremely rare, but two cases are known. Multiple cultures using a sensitive blood agar base with physiological saline overlay may, under ideal conditions, be as sensitive as xenodiagnosis. However, contamination of cultures, particularly in the field, may interfere. Through-the-cap inoculation of cultures reduces contamination. Xenodiagnosis is generally the preferred method rather than blood culture because it is so robust. Adult bugs are not recommended because they are less resistant to starvation. Normally, starved fourth or fifth instars are used as they can be kept unfed for weeks and transported easily, as long as they are protected from high temperatures.

Theoretically, detection of parasite DNA by the polymerase chain reaction (PCR) is a reliable alternative to detect intact trypomastigotes. PCR methods are available but are not yet sufficiently practical, routine or low cost to replace parasitological diagnosis.

In the absence of effective treatment, *T. cruzi* infection and antibodies are almost always retained for life. Many serological tests have been described since the development of the complement fixation test in 1913. The most reliable and frequently applied are the indirect immunofluorescent antibody test (IFAT) and the enzyme-linked immunosorbent assay (ELISA). The IFAT requires a fluorescent microscope; results must be interpreted with care, positive and negative controls should be run on each slide, and serum dilutions of less than 1 : 80 may give false-positive results. The ELISA requires careful standardization and the inclusion of positive and negative controls on every plate but, once established, has the advantages that very large numbers of samples may be screened simultaneously and positives and negatives may be distinguished by eye, as well as by measurement of light absorp-tion in a spectrophotometer. Commercial kits are available but are expensive and may be somewhat less sensitive than IFAT or ELISA. Blood spots, stored dry, can be used in place of serum, but serum samples give accurate measurement of antibody titre. Note that IgM in bloodspots deteriorates quickly unless they are maintained at −20°C. Cross-reactions may occur, for example with visceral or cutaneous leishmaniasis. Ideally a proportion of serum samples should be referred to reference centres for checking. Children born of seropositive mothers may be antibody positive for up to 9 months because IgG crosses the placenta. The presence of IgM antibodies to *T. cruzi* in a newborn child is usually indicative of congenital infection. Such antibodies may be detected with an IgM-specific conjugate.

MANAGEMENT

Only two effective drugs have been developed for the treatment of *T. cruzi* infection. Nifurtimox (Lampit®) is an orally administered synthetic nitrofuran, which has not always been readily available. However, the manufacturer, Bayer, has recently safeguarded supply by restarting production in El Salvador. Nifurtimox is given in three divided daily doses at 8–10 mg/kg for 90 days. Double doses are recommended for infected children. There are significant potential side-effects, which may lead to interruption of treatment. These include anorexia, loss of weight, psychological disturbances, excitability, drowsiness, nausea and vomiting.[15] Hospitalization is usually recommended to monitor the side-effects and to ensure compliance. The second, more frequently used drug is benznidazole (Rochagan®) which is a nitroimidazole, also orally administered. The dosage is 5–7 mg/kg in two divided daily doses for 60 days, or 10 mg/kg for children. As with nifurtimox there are many potential side-effects that may cause interruption of treatment; prominent among these are cutaneous changes such as hypersensitivity and dermatitis but there may also be oedema, lymphadenopathy, myalgia and depression of bone marrow.[15] The mode of action of these drugs is not clear but the two proposed mechanisms are increase of oxidative stress on *T. cruzi* and damage to DNA.

Acute cases should always be treated with benznidazole, as this may be life saving and may drastically reduce the parasite load or eliminate the infection. As there are fewer side-effects in children, recent recommendations are that children in the chronic phase should also be treated.[16] The value of treatment for the chronic phase in adults is debated because of side-effects and treatment failure, and also because the role of continued low-level infection in the pathogenesis of the disease is still somewhat controversial. Case-by-case decision to treat adults may depend, for example, on the presence of symptoms, the possible impact of side-effects and whether a female patient is of child-bearing age, with a slight risk of congenital transmission of infection. High doses are used to treat congenital cases: up to 25 mg/kg nifurtimox daily for 30 days or up to 10 mg/kg benznidazole daily for 30–60 days. Immunocompromised patients must be treated. Double or even higher doses are recommended for treatment if meningoencephalitis is present. An indicator of cure for acute cases is serological reversion within 1 year but for chronic cases reversion may take several years. Persistently negative xenodiagnosis may be an encouraging sign but is not an unequivocal indicator.

Supportive chemotherapy is vital for treatment of acute symptoms and for heart failure in patients with chronic Chagas' disease. Chagasic heart disease may be treated by restricted sodium intake, diuretics, vasodilatation (angiotensin-converting enzyme inhibitors) and maintenance of serum potassium concentration. Digitalis may be recommended in acute Chagas' disease with heart involvement, but is a last resort in those with chronic heart disease because it can make arrhythmias worse by causing premature ventricular beats or impeding AV conduction. Acute meningoencephalitis may be managed with anticonvulsants, sedatives and intravenous mannitol. Pacemakers may be fitted if bradycardia does not respond to atropine, or for complete AV block or for atrial fibrillation with a slow ventricular response that does not improve with vagolytic drugs. Lidocaine (lignocaine), mexiletine, propafenone, flecainide, β-adrenoreceptor antagonists and amiodarone are effective for the treatment of ventricular extrasystoles; the most effective drug in the management of arrhythmias is amiodarone. Treatment of arrhythmias may prolong the life expectancy of patients but may also aggravate symptoms. In emergencies, lidocaine may be used intravenously. Experienced physicians and expert reports, for example from the World Health Organization,[9] should be consulted to ensure optimal case management.

Surgery is a vital part of the treatment of chronic Chagas' disease, particularly for megaoesophagus and megacolon. Mild megaoesophagus can be treated by control of diet or balloon dilatation of the cardiac sphincter. In more severe megaoesopha-

gus, a section of muscle is removed surgically from the junction of the oesophagus and stomach, which alleviates the condition and retains muscle control of the stomach (the Heller–Vasconcelos procedure).[17] As a last resort, partial surgical removal of the distal oesophagus may be required, followed by replacement with a section from elsewhere in the alimentary tract, such as the jejunun. Less severe megacolon can be treated with laxatives, colonic lavage or manual evacuation, if necessary with laparotomy. Decompressing intubation before surgery can release sigmoid volvulus. Surgery may be simplified by initial sigmoidostomy as subsequently more of the colon may be retained. Severe megacolon may be corrected effectively by the modified Duhamel–Haddad operation which consists of resection of the sigmoid loop, closing the rectal stump, and bringing the descending colon into the rear wall of the rectum (Figure 76.11).[17] The operation is performed in two stages, the first of which leaves a perineal colostomy, and the second in which a wide join is made between the colon and the rectal stump, with peridural anaesthesia. Surgical resection may also be part of treatment of chagasic heart disease to remove aneurysms or arrhythmic regions.

EPIDEMIOLOGY

The natural habitats of triatomine bugs are the nests and resting sites of mammals and birds, particularly palm trees, hollow trees,

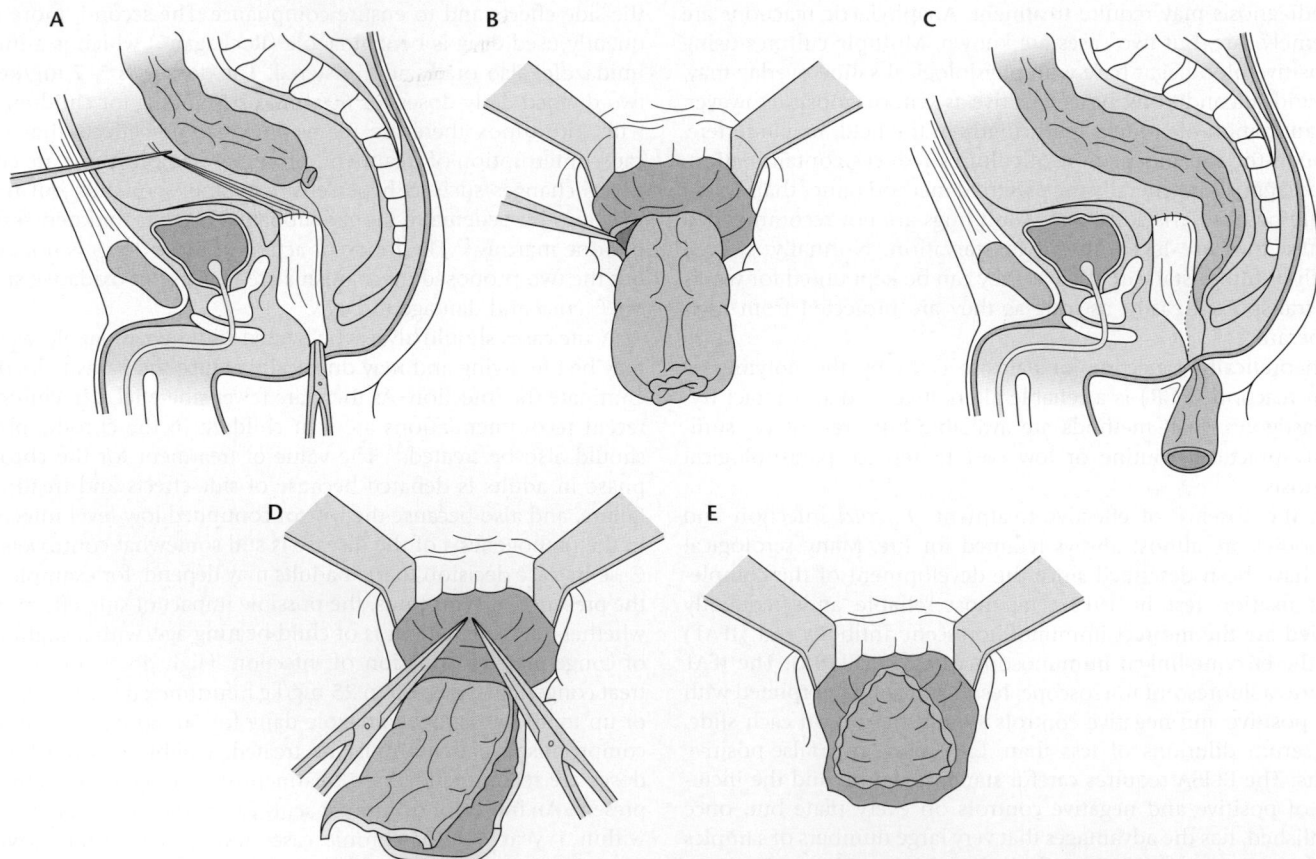

Figure 76.11 Modified Duhamel–Haddad procedure for surgical correction of megacolon in chronic Chagas' disease.

tree cavities, burrows and rock crevices. The vast majority of approximately 137 species are confined to the New World.[18,19] Seven of 13 Old World species are closely related to *Triatoma rubrofasciata*, which has been disseminated around the world by shipping, in association with the rat (*Rattus rattus*). *T. rubrofasciata* transmits *Trypanosoma conorhini* to rats by the contaminative route. The strange Old World genus *Linshcosteus* has six species. An unidentified trypanosome species similar to *T. conorhini* has recently been isolated from *Linshcosteus* in India.

Five species of triatomine bug have become notorious vectors of Chagas' disease because they have adapted so well to colonize human dwellings. *T. infestans* is the main vector in the southern cone countries of South America (Argentina, Bolivia, Brazil, Chile, Paraguay and Uruguay). *Rhodnius prolixus* and *T. dimidiata* are the principal vectors in northern South America and Central America. *Panstrongylus megistus* is an important vector in central and eastern Brazil, and *Triatoma brasiliensis* in north-east Brazil. There are several other domestic vector species of secondary importance in different geographical areas, such as *Rhodnius ecuadoriensis* in Peru. Some silvatic species also rarely form domestic colonies or invade houses as flying adults, causing sporadic cases of Chagas' disease. Male and female bugs are obligatory blood-feeders and they require at least one blood meal before moulting to the next of their five instars. Fifth-stage nymphs have rudimentary wing lappets; only adults are fully winged. One species, *Triatoma spinolai*, has wingless females and winged or wingless males. While virtually all species feed on mammal, bird or reptilian blood, a few species, such as *Eratyrus mucronatus*, have also been reported to take invertebrate blood, particularly during early stages.

All mammal species are considered to be susceptible to *T. cruzi*, and more than 150 species of 24 families have been reported as infected. Birds and reptiles are not susceptible to *T. cruzi* infection, but chickens are nevertheless particularly important epidemiologically as they may sustain large triatomine colonies in chicken houses. Guinea pigs that are bred within or adjacent to houses, dogs, cats, rats and mice may carry *T. cruzi* and be attacked by triatomine bugs. Cats probably acquire infection by the oral route through eating mice and infected bugs. *T. cruzi* prevalence rates in pigs, goats, cattle and horses are usually very low. The mammal reservoir host first described by Carlos Chagas was the armadillo, *Dasypus novemcinctus*; the most commonly infected silvatic mammal is the common opossum, *Didelphis* species.

Serological surveys have been used to establish the prevalence of Chagas' disease in South America. The prevalence of human infection in endemic areas rises with age, as is to be expected because the contamination route of transmission is precarious. Locally acquired Chagas' disease is very rare in North America as the local bug species rarely colonize houses, although adult bugs occasionally fly into campsites, attracted to light. Similarly in the vast Amazon basin no triatomine bug species has yet adapted well to colonize houses. Most of the 300 or so cases of Chagas' disease known from the Amazon basin are due to adult bugs flying into houses, to oral outbreaks through contaminated food or to *Rhodnius brethesi*, a silvatic species that attacks gatherers of piassaba palm fronds. *Panstrongylus geniculatus* has been found in peridomestic pigs in the Amazon basin.[20] Silvatic *T. cruzi* infection where human Chagas' disease is rare, such as in the Amazon basin or the USA, is referred to as enzootic transmission. The regional distribution of chronic Chagas' disease does not correspond with the prevalence of *T. cruzi* infection. Thus mega-syndromes are reported as common in the southern cone countries but much less so in northern South America and Central America, although studies there have been less intense.

The disparate distribution of chronic Chagas' disease and many other factors relating to the biology of *T. cruzi* led to the suggestion that *T. cruzi* was not a single entity but a diverse species. Thus response to chemotherapy, infectivity to triatomine bug species, behaviour in experimental animals, morphology, antigenic profiles and biochemical characteristics suggested heterogeneity within the species. This was proven in the 1970s by phenotyping *T. cruzi* strains using multi locus enzyme electrophoresis (MLEE). In particular, the first of these studies noted that strains of *T. cruzi* from domestic and silvatic transmission cycles in eastern Brazil were radically distinct (more so than recognized species of *Leishmania*) and involved different triatomine vector species, *Panstrongylus megistus* inside houses, and *Triatoma tibiamaculata* outside houses in opossum refuges. This approach strengthened the concept that in some localities domestic and silvatic transmission cycles are separate, or overlapping (Figure 76.12), as is now known to be the case in certain regions of Venezuela where the domestic vector is *R. prolixus* and where *R. prolixus* also infests palm trees. The distinction between transmission cycle types is vital for planning control programmes.[1] In the Amazon basin (and the USA), transmission cycles are 'enzootic',[4] without domiciliated triatomines in houses but with sporadic cases due to adult infected vectors flying into houses or contaminating food, such as palm or sugar cane presses, giving rise to oral outbreaks of acute Chagas' disease (Figure 76.12).

The heterogeneity of *T. cruzi* has been reaffirmed many times by many methods, including profiles of randomly amplified polymorphic DNA (RAPD), microsatellites and diversity of 24S alpha, miniexon, 18S RNA genes, and many other target genes, including those encoding enzyme genes used in MLEE. Isoenzyme electrophoresis originally classified *T. cruzi* into principal zymodemes Z1, Z2 and Z3.[21] Many different studies over several decades have shown that there are at least two major subspecific divisions within the species. These are named by international consensus simply as *T. cruzi* I and *T. cruzi* II (*T. cruzi* I corresponding with Z1 and *T. cruzi* II encompassing Z2). By DNA sequence analysis, TCI consists of a single less heterogeneous clade, whereas TCII emerges as three phylogenetic clades (IIa, b, c), with two relatively recent aneuploid hybrid lineages (IId, IIe), which have haplotypes split across the IIb and IIc clades.[22,23] In contrast, TCIIb and TCI appear to be less complex lineages. This present concept of *T. cruzi* divisions may change as more *T. cruzi* isolates are examined with a wider range of methods. Phylogenetic analyses and production of hybrids in the laboratory have shown that *T. cruzi* has both an ancient and active capacity for genetic exchange.[23] This capacity may have profound epidemiological implications for the origin and spread of virulent or drug resistant strains, and for adaptation to new hosts and niches.

We have proposed that TCI has an evolutionary history associated with *Didelphis*, and possibly the triatomine tribe Rhodniini and the palm tree ecotope. Forms similar to infective stages in the triatomine vector are isolated from anal gland secretions of *Didelphis*, suggesting a supplementary non-vectorial route of transmission in this particular host. In contrast, the natural hosts of TCII have not been clearly resolved. However, we recently isolated

A. Separate

B. Overlapping

C. Enzootic

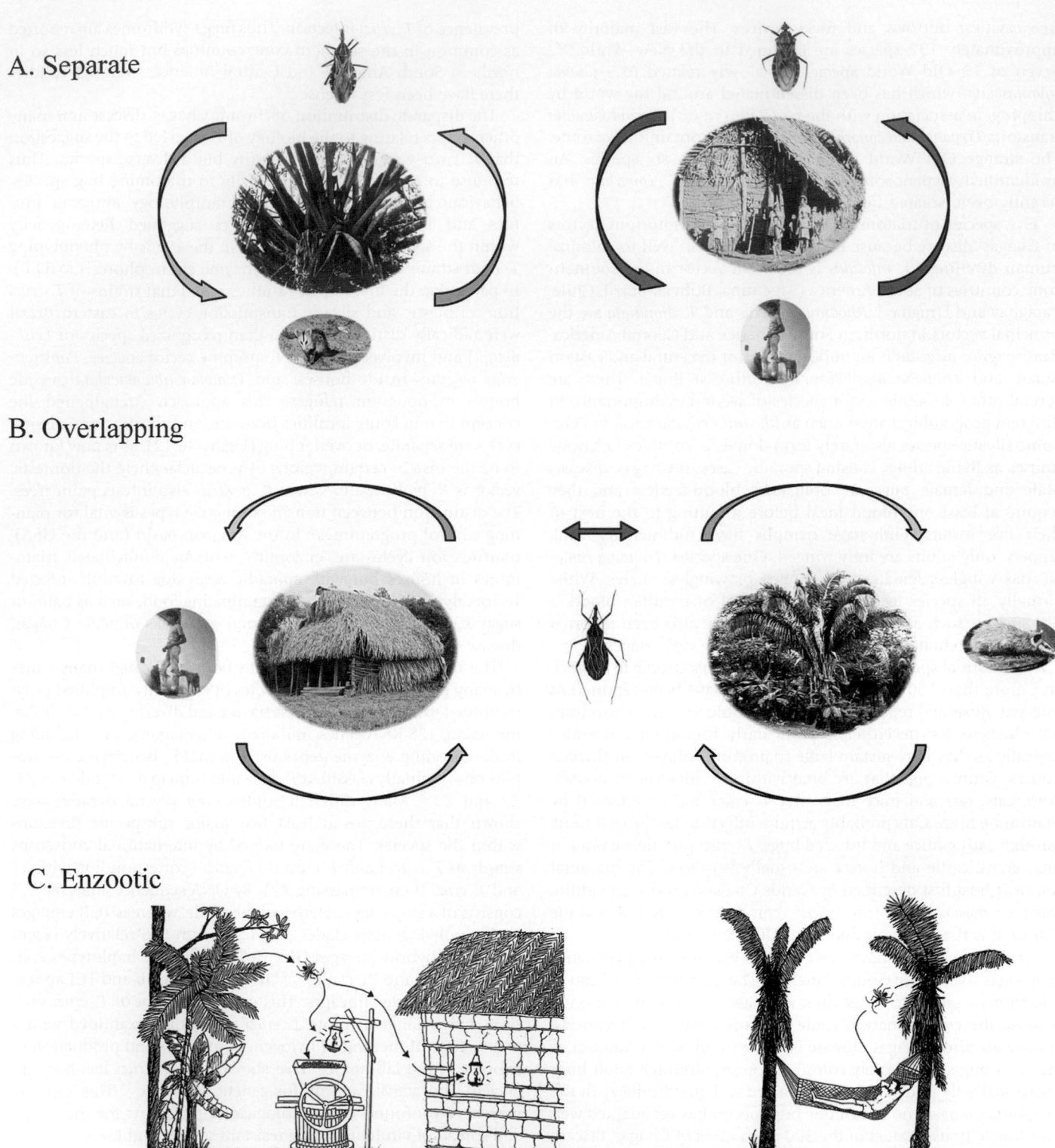

Figure 76.12 Transmission cycles of *Trypanosoma cruzi*. (A) An example of separate silvatic and domestic transmission cycles, in Bahia State, Brazil: *T. cruzi* I in the silvatic cycle (principal silvatic host the opossum, *Didelphis albiventris*, vector *Triatoma tibiamaculata*, and *T. cruzi* II in the domestic transmission cycle (vector *Panstrongylus megistus*). (B) An example of overlapping silvatic and domestic transmission cycles, in parts of Venezuela: *T. cruzi* I in both the domestic and silvatic transmission cycles (vector *Rhodnius prolixus* in houses and in palm trees). (C) Enzootic transmission in the Amazon basin: sporadic cases of Chagas' disease occur due to adult bugs flying to palm presses (orally transmitted outbreaks) or houses but not forming domestic colonies; also forest workers harvesting the piassaba palm may be attacked by *Rhodnius brethesi*. (Courtesy of J. S. Patterson.)

several *T. cruzi* II subgroups from armadillos.[24] The ancient South American ancestry of opossums and armadillos, and their respective arboreal and terrestrial niches, suggests that they may have long-standing evolutionary associations with different *T. cruzi* lineages.

Trypanosoma cruzi I was originally described from the silvatic cycle in Brazil. This has led to the misconception that TCI is always associated with silvatic transmission cycles, which is certainly not the case. TCI predominates from the Amazon basin northwards, where it is also the main cause of Chagas' disease in endemic areas such as Venezuela. In contrast, TCII predominates in domestic transmission cycles in southern cone countries of South America (Argentina, Brazil, Bolivia, Chile, Paraguay and Uruguay). Differences in pathology associated with TCI and TCII infections remain enigmatic. In the southern cone region (TCII) chagasic mega syndromes are common, whereas they are considered virtually absent north of the Amazon (TCI). The implication is that TCII, although not the exclusive agent of Chagas' disease, is more pathogenic than TCI.[25] Virtually nothing is known of the comparative pathogenesis of TCIIa–e. Strikingly, the hybrid genotypes predominate among human infections in Paraguay, Chile, Argentina, Bolivia and Southern Brazil, despite the abundance of other genotypes in silvatic cycles in these regions, suggesting that the hybrids may indeed have an enhanced propensity to thrive in the human host.[24]

PREVENTION AND CONTROL

Transmission by blood transfusion contributes significantly to the public health problem of Chagas' disease.[26] Congenital transmission and oral transmission are important for the unfortunate few infected by these routes. Nevertheless the overwhelming majority of cases of Chagas' disease are disseminated by triatomine bugs. When I first set foot in South America in 1971, I was dismayed to see the way in which triatomine bugs multiplied unimpeded in poor-quality housing. Chagas' disease is thus largely a disease of poverty. There is no chemoprophylaxis. There is no vaccine. It is unlikely that there will ever be a vaccine as induction of autoimmunity[27] must be reliably excluded from any candidate vaccine preparation, and vaccine trials are difficult to envisage when chronic side-effects might be revealed decades later. Fortunately there are proven, highly effective, methods for controlling both triatomine bugs and blood transfusion transmission of Chagas' disease.

Many attempts have been made to devise strategies for controlling triatomine bugs. Most, such as juvenile hormone mimics to prevent development, household traps and release of parasitic wasps that grow in triatomine eggs, have been abandoned. Effective control depends on insecticide spraying (Figure 76.13), supported by health education, community participation and house improvement (Figure 76.14).[28] The insecticides of choice are synthetic pyrethroids. Effective control campaigns have three phases: preparatory, attack and vigilance. In the preparatory phase, the distribution of all dwellings is mapped, the abundance of triatomine infestation assessed, and the attack and vigilance phases are planned and costed. In the attack phase, all houses and peridomestic buildings are sprayed irrespective of whether bugs have been found. Chicken houses or other peridomestic infestations

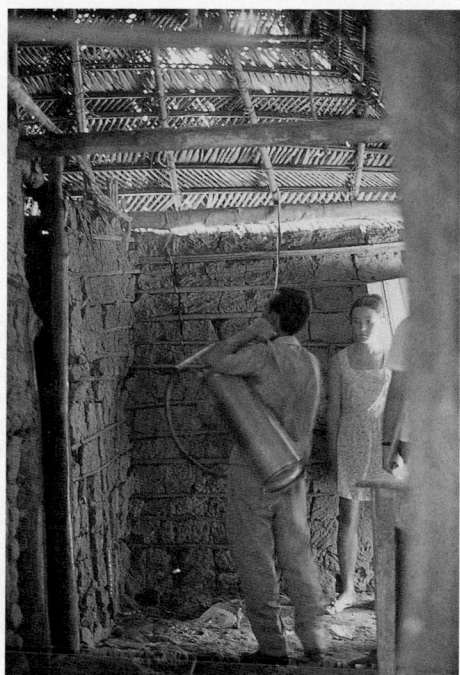

Figure 76.13 Spraying a triatomine-infested house.

that are missed may lead to rapid reinvasion. In the vigilance phase, appropriate sections of the community report residual infestations, which brings in a rapid response team to spray such dwellings and surrounding sites.[28]

Serological testing is an essential part of monitoring the success of vector control. All children born after the beginning of a vector control campaign should be seronegative except for those <9 months of age and born of seropositive mothers, who will have acquired IgG transplacentally, and except for occasional congenital cases. Thus, tracing seropositive children will reveal residual triatomine infestations. Low-cost assays, such as the ELISA, allow entire endemic regions to be screened. In addition, serological testing provides a means of screening blood donors, organ donors and organ recipients. In highly endemic areas contaminated blood can be treated with crystal violet (250 mg/L) and stored at 4°C for at least 24 h to kill *T. cruzi*. Prophylactic benznidazole should be given to immunosuppressed organ recipients.

The enormous economic burden of chronic Chagas' disease is much greater than the cost of prevention and control. This has stimulated national and international campaigns. In the southern cone countries of South America, virtually the only important domestic triatomine vector is *T. infestans*. This species is thought to have spread from silvatic habitats in Bolivia and/or the Chaco region as elsewhere it has been found only in domestic and peridomestic sites.[29] The realization that reinvasion should not be a significant problem in southern cone countries led to the launch of the southern cone programme, to eliminate *T. infestans* from Argentina, Bolivia, Brazil, Chile, Paraguay, Uruguay and southern Peru.[30] Although not yet complete or uniformly adopted, the programme has been a resounding success. It is reported that 85% of domestic transmission has been eliminated from Brazil. Chile and Uruguay are essentially free of domestic transmission, which is

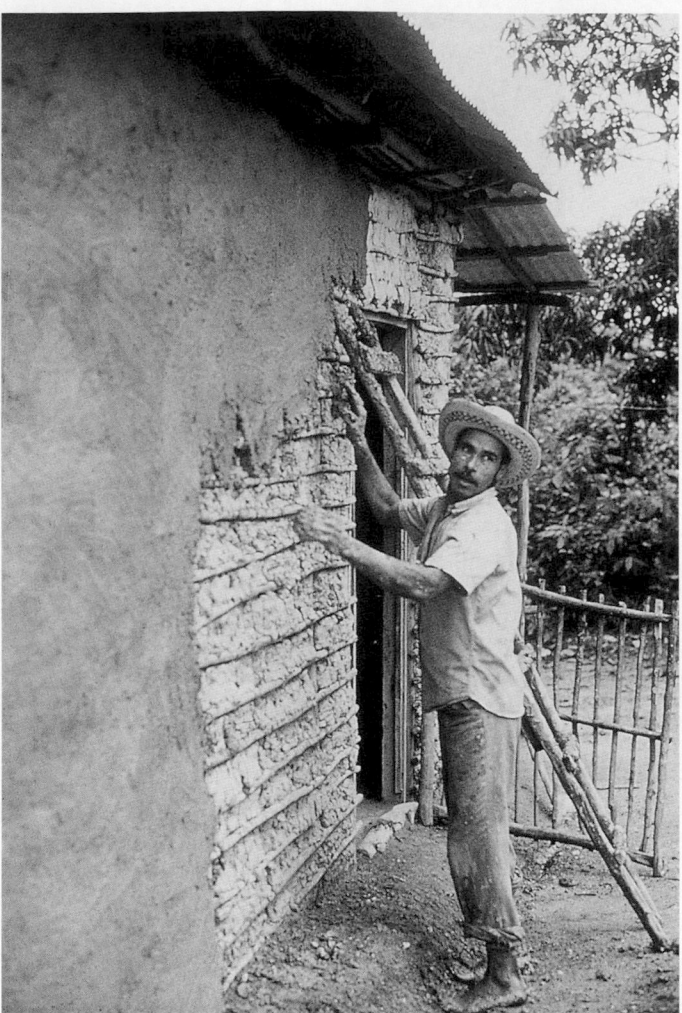

Figure 76.14 A new roof and plastered walls to combat *Rhodnius prolixus* infestation in Venezuela.

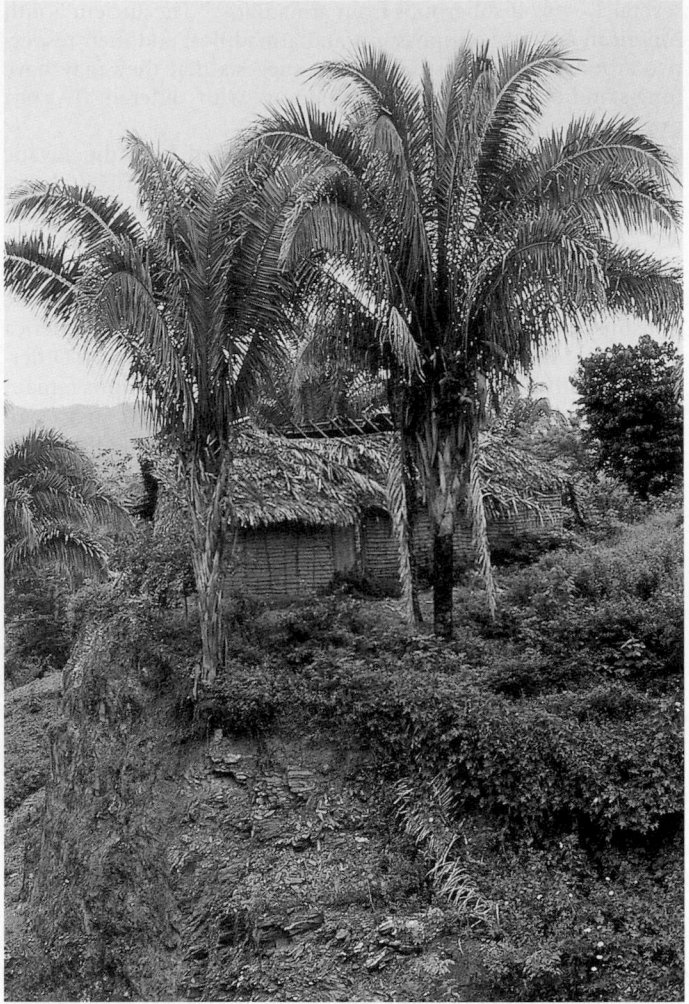

Figure 76.15 Palms adjacent to a house in Venezuela: *Rhodnius prolixus* may replenish the domestic cycle from the sylvatic habitat.

also much reduced in the remaining countries. The southern cone programme provides a model for international collaboration in disease control.

New international control initiatives are now in progress for the Andean Pact countries and for Central America.[31] Here control may be less straightforward because the geographical distribution of *R. prolixus* in palm trees is not fully known, and it is clear that in some regions reinvasion of houses from the silvatic habitat occurs (Figures 76.12, 76.15). Palm trees around dwellings may now be surveyed by a new triatomine bug trap, the Noireau trap, in which bugs are trapped on adhesive tape around a plastic vessel containing a sentinel mouse.[29] Effective methods for insecticide treatment of infested palms need to be devised. Secondary domestic species may also emerge as complications for vector control. In the Amazon basin a surveillance programme has been proposed to respond rapidly to any domestic bug species brought in from outside endemic areas.[31] Furthermore some Amazonian species, such as *P. geniculatus*, reported from peridomestic pigsties, may adapt to live in human dwellings. In addition, food prepara-

tion plants such as palm or sugar-cane presses should be protected from contamination by triatomine bugs attracted to artificial light. Although eradication of *T. cruzi* as a zoonotic infection is neither required nor feasible, there is reason for optimism that Chagas' disease in future may be largely eliminated as a public health problem.[31]

The molecular biology of *T. cruzi* and other trypanosomatids is of immense research interest. The availability of the full genome sequence of *T. cruzi* may help to identify new drug targets.[32] A low-cost, non-toxic, oral drug is needed to eliminate the reservoir of human infection. Further research is also required to elucidate the epidemiological significance of subspecific diversity.[4]

TRYPANOSOMA RANGELI

The primary importance of *T. rangeli* is that it may confuse the diagnosis of Chagas' disease. Thus, if *R. prolixus* is used for xenodiagnosis of a suspect case, positive xenodiagnosis bugs may be

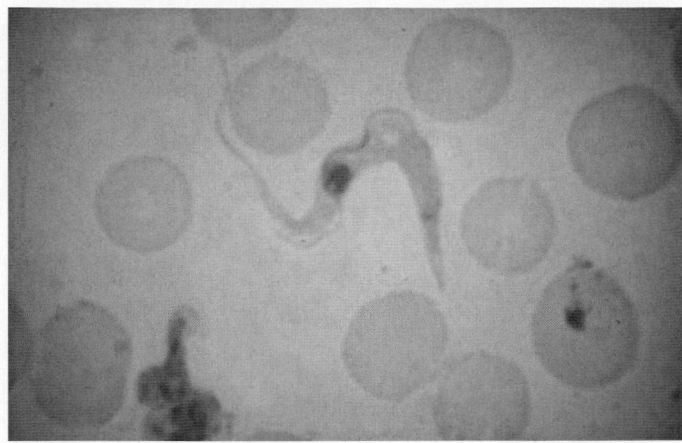

Figure 76.16 Trypomastigote of *Trypanosoma rangeli* in blood.

due to the acquisition of *T. rangeli* infection and not *T. cruzi*, or to both organisms. With appropriate training, *T. rangeli* in triatomine bugs can be distinguished from *T. cruzi* by the presence of epimastigotes of up to 80 μm in length, by the smaller kinetoplast, or by the fact that *T. rangeli* escapes from the lumen of the intestinal tract to reach the haemocoel and infect the salivary glands in some infected bugs. A drop of haemolymph may be removed for microscopic examination by severing one of the bug legs and extruding the haemolymph under a coverslip placed on a microscope slide. *T. rangeli* may be pathogenic to *Rhodnius*, causing malformation and defects in moulting.

T. rangeli is not considered to be pathogenic in humans; it is very rarely seen in human blood (Figure 76.16). Trypomastigotes of *T. rangeli* in blood are much larger than those of *T. cruzi*, and they also have a smaller subterminal kinetoplast. The main natural host of this appears to be the common opossum (*Didelphis*). The species *T. rangeli* is heterogeneous, with at least two genetic lineages that appear to be associated with different vector species and geographical distributions.[33] *T. rangeli* is thought to divide in peripheral blood, but the full life cycle in the mammalian host is uncertain. Transmission is by triatomine bite, with heavy metacyclic trypomastigote infections occurring in the salivary glands of *Rhodnius*. Antibodies to *T. rangeli* may be fairly prevalent where *R. prolixus* is the domestic triatomine vector. Theoretically, such antibodies may cross-react with *T. cruzi*, although the extent of such cross-reactions in *T. rangeli* infections is not clear. It is certain that antibodies to *T. cruzi* in chronic Chagas' disease, which may have titres in excess of 1 in 10^6, do cross-react with *T. rangeli*.

REFERENCES

1. Miles MA. The discovery of Chagas disease: progress and prejudice. *Infect Dis Clin North Am* 2004; 18:247–260.
2. Miles MA. Chagas disease and chagasic megacolon. In: Kamm MA, Lennard-Jones JE, eds. *Constipation*. Petersfield: Wrightson Biomedical; 1994:205–210.
3. Gaunt M, Miles MA. The ecotopes and evolution of triatomine bugs (Triatominae) and their associated trypanosomes. *Mem Inst Oswaldo Cruz* 2000; 95:557–565.
4. Miles MA, Feliciangeli MD, Arias AR. American trypanosomiasis (Chagas disease) and the role of molecular epidemiology in guiding control strategies. *BMJ* 2003; 326:1444–1448.
5. Maudlin I, Holmes P, Miles MA, eds. *The Trypanosomiases*. London: CABI; 2004.
6. Riera C, Guarro A, Kassab HE, et al. Congenital transmission of *Trypanosoma cruzi* in Europe (Spain): a case report. *Am J Trop Med Hyg* 2006; 75:1078–1081.
7. Hoare CA. *The Trypanosomes of Mammals*. Oxford: Blackwell; 1972.
8. Torrico F, Vega CA, Suarez E, et al. Are maternal re-infections with *Trypanosoma cruzi* associated with high morbidity and mortality of congenital Chagas disease? *Trop Med Int Health* 2006; 11:628–635.
9. WHO. *Control of Chagas Disease*. WHO Technical Report Series 905. Geneva: World Health Organization; 2002.
10. Pan American Health Organization. *Chagas Disease and the Nervous System*. Scientific Publication No. 547. Washington, DC: PAHO; 1994.
11. Miles MA. New World trypanosomiasis. In: Cox FEG, Kreier JP, Wakelin D, eds. Topley, Wilson's *Microbiology and Microbial Infections: Parasitology*. London: Arnold, 2005:376–398.
12. Tarleton RL, Zhang L, Downs MO. 'Autoimmune' rejection of neonatal heart transplants in experimental Chagas disease is a parasite-specific response to infected host tissue. *Proc Natl Acad Sci USA* 1997; 94:3932–3937.
13. Cheesborough M. *District Laboratory Practice in Tropical Countries*, Part 1. Cambridge: Cambridge University Press; 1999.
14. Miles MA. Culturing and biological cloning of *Trypanosoma cruzi*. In: Hyde JE, ed. *Protocols in Molecular Parasitology*. Totowa: Humana Press; 1993:15–28.
15. Castro JA, de Mecca MM, Bartel LC. Toxic side-effects of drugs used to treat Chagas disease (American trypanosomiasis). *Hum Exp Toxicol* 2006; 25:471–479.
16. Estani SS, Segura EL, Ruiz AM, et al. Efficacy of chemotherapy with benznidazole in children in the indeterminate phase Chagas disease. *Am J Trop Med Hyg* 1998; 59:526–529.
17. Raia AA. *Manifestaçoes Digestivas da Moléstia de Chagas*. São Paulo: Sarvier Brasil, 1983.
18. Lent H, Wygodzinsky P. Revision of the Triatominae (Hemiptera, Reduviidae), and their significance as vectors of Chagas disease. *Bull Am Mus Nat Hist* 1979; 163:123–520.
19. Dujardin JP, Schofield CJ. Triatominae: Systematics, morphology and population Biology. In: Maudlin I, Holmes P, Miles MA, eds. *The Trypanosomiases*. London: CABI; 2004:181–201.
20. Valente VC, Valente SAS, Noireau F, et al. Chagas disease in the Amazon Basin: association of *Panstrongylus geniculatus* (Hemiptera: Reduviidae) with domestic pigs. *J Med Entomol* 1998; 35:99–103.
21. Miles MA, Souza A, Povoa M, et al. Isozymic heterogeneity of *Trypanosoma cruzi* in the first autochthonous patients with Chagas disease in Amazonian Brazil. *Nature* 1978; 272:819–821.
22. Machado CA, Ayala FJ. Nucleotide sequences provide evidence of genetic exchange among distantly related lineages of *Trypanosoma cruzi*. *Proc Natl Acad Sci USA* 2001; 98:7396–7401.
23. Gaunt MW, Yeo M, Frame IA, et al. Mechanism of genetic exchange in American trypanosomes. *Nature* 2003; 421:936–939.
24. Yeo M, Acosta N, Llewellyn M, et al. Origins of Chagas disease: Didelphis species are natural hosts of *Trypanosoma cruzi* I and armadillos hosts of *Trypanosoma cruzi* II, including hybrids. *Int J Parasitol* 2005; 35:225–233.
25. Freitas JM, Lages-Silva E, Crema E, et al. Real time PCR strategy for the identification of major lineages of *Trypanosoma cruzi* directly in chronically infected human tissues. *Int J Parasit* 2005; 35:411–417.
26. Moraes-Souza H, Bordin JO, Langhi D. Control of blood transfusion transmission of American Trypanosomiasis. In: Maudlin I, Holmes P, Miles MA, eds. *The Trypanosomiases*. London: CABI; 2004:479–490.
27. Kali J, Cunha-Neto E. Autoimmunity in Chagas disease cardiomyopathy: fulfilling the criteria at last. *Parasitol Today* 1996; 12:396–399.
28. Dias JCP. Control of Chagas disease in Brazil. *Parasitol Today* 1987; 3:336–341.
29. Noireau F, Cortez MG, Monteiro FA, et al. Can wild *Triatoma infestans* foci in Bolivia jeopardize Chagas disease control efforts? *Trends Parasitol* 2005; 21:7–10.
30. Schofield CJ, Dias JCP. The southern cone initiative against Chagas disease. *Adv Parasitol* 1998; 2:2–22.

31. Schofield CJ, Jannin J, Salvatella R. The future of Chagas disease control. *Trends Parasitol* 2006; 22:583–588.

32. El-Sayed, Myler NM, Bartolomeu DC, et al. The genome sequence of *Trypanosoma cruzi*, etiologic agent of Chagas disease. *Science* 2005; 309:409–415.

33. Urrea DA, Carranza JC, Cuba CA, et al. Molecular characterization of *Trypanosoma rangeli* strains isolated from *Rhodnius ecuadoriensis* in Peru, *R. colombiensis* in Colombia and *R. pallescens* in Panama supports a co-evolutionary association between parasites and vectors. *Infect Genet Evol* 2005; 5:123–129.

Chapter 77

Jean-Pierre Dedet and Francine Pratlong

Leishmaniasis

Leishmaniases are parasitic diseases caused by protozoan flagellates of the genus *Leishmania*, parasites infecting numerous mammal species, including humans, and transmitted through the infective bite of an insect vector, the phlebotomine sandfly.

The Leishmaniases threaten 350 million people in 88 countries of four continents. The annual incidence of new cases is estimated between 1.5 and 2 million.[1] In numerous underdeveloped countries, they remain a major public health problem.

The genus *Leishmania* includes around 30 different taxa, the majority of which commonly infect humans, in whom they are responsible for various types of disease: visceral, cutaneous (of localized or diffuse type) and mucocutaneous leishmaniases. This variability of the clinical features results from both the diversity of the *Leishmania* species and the immune response of the hosts.

PARASITE

Leishmania are protozoa belonging to the order Kinetoplastida and the family Trypanosomatidae, which includes other parasites of mammals, including humans (genus *Trypanosoma*), of plants (*Phytomonas*) and of insects (*Leptomonas*, *Crithidia*, etc.).

Description

Leishmania are dimorphic parasites, which present as two principal morphological stages: the intracellular amastigote, within the mononuclear phagocytic system of the mammalian host, and the flagellated promastigote within the intestinal tract of the insect vector and in culture medium.

The amastigote stage is a round or oval body about 2–6 μm in diameter, containing a nucleus, a kinetoplast and an internal flagellum seen clearly in electron micrographs. The amastigotes multiply within the parasitophorous vacuoles of macrophages.

The promastigote stage has a long and slender body (about 15–30 μm by 2–3 μm), with a central nucleus, a kinetoplast and a long free anterior flagellum.

Identification

Since the origin of the genus *Leishmania* by Ross,[2] the number of species described has significantly increased. As the different species are indistinguishable by their morphology, other criteria have been used for their identification. Lumsden distinguished between extrinsic characters (such as clinical features, geographical distribution, behaviour in culture, laboratory animals or vectors) and intrinsic ones (such as immunological, biochemical or molecular criteria).[3] Among them, isoenzyme electrophoresis remains the current gold standard technique. DNA-based techniques are being used increasingly for identification. They are used to generate phylogenetic trees, so far limited to taxonomic groups of epidemiological importance, such as for the complexes *L. donovani*,[4] *L. tropica*,[5] and *L. braziliensis*.[6]

Applied to *Leishmania* initially by Gardener et al.,[7] isoenzyme analysis has been widely developed for the study of these parasites. Its success principally results from the existence of a high degree of polymorphism, expressed as stable and relatively specific electromorphs. These have permitted characterization of the strains by their enzymatic profiles and their grouping in homogeneous electrophoretic taxonomic units termed zymodemes. Recently, a sequencing approach of isoenzyme genes was developed for studying their genetic diversity and for further use for typing by an MLST (multilocus sequence typing) approach.[8,9]

Isoenzyme characterization is currently the reference technique for *Leishmania* identification at specific and infra-specific levels, and for classification of the genus.[10]

Classification

Various types of classification have been successively applied to the genus. Those proposed between 1916 and 1987 were monothetic Linnean classifications based on few hierarchical characters. Lainson and Shaw are the authors who worked the most on these types of classification and who made them evolutive. Their last classification[11] divided the genus *Leishmania* into two subgenera: *Leishmania* sensu stricto, present in both Old and New Worlds, and *Viannia*, restricted to the New World. Within these two subgenera various species complexes were individualized.

Since the 1980s, Adansonian phenetic classifications have been employed. They are based on a number of similarly weighted characters (absence of hierarchy) used simultaneously (polythetic classification) without a prior hypothesis. They were at first phe-

also extracellular) amastigotes are ingested by the insect. Inside the blood meal, amastigotes transform into motile promastigotes, which escape through the peritrophic membrane enveloping the blood meal. The promastigotes multiply intensively inside the intestinal tract of the sandfly, successively as free elongated promastigotes (nectomonads) or as attached pro- and paramastigotes (haptomonads).[18] This intraluminal development occurs in the midgut (*Leishmania* subgenus, previously section Suprapylaria according to Lainson and Shaw[19]), or in the hindgut and the midgut (*Viannia* subgenus, previously section Peripylaria). Whatever the multiplication site, the parasites subsequently migrate to the anterior part of the sandfly midgut, where they change into free-swimming metacyclic promastigotes, the stage infective for the vertebrate host.

The bite of an infected sandfly deposits infective metacyclic promastigotes in the mammal's skin, which are rapidly phagocytosed by cells of the mononuclear phagocyte system. The intracellular parasites change into amastigotes, which multiply by simple mitosis. The molecular aspects of the parasite–cell interaction in the mammalian host are briefly summarized below (see Pathology, below).

Transmission

The inoculation of metacyclic promastigotes through the sandfly bite is the usual method of Leishmaniasis transmission. Other routes remain exceptional.

In visceral leishmaniasis (VL), a few cases of congenital and of blood transfusion transmission have been reported. A case of direct transmission by sexual contact has been reported.[20] Exchange of syringes has been incriminated to explain the high prevalence of *L. infantum*/HIV co-infection in intravenous drug-users in southern Europe.[21]

In cutaneous leishmaniasis (CL), contact with the active lesion is innocuous; infection should require inoculation of material from active sores, as was carried out in ancient times by various populations of endemic areas as a crude form of vaccination.

Geographical distribution

Leishmaniases are widely distributed around the world. They range over the intertropical zones of America and Africa, and extend into temperate regions of South America, southern Europe and Asia. Their extension limits are latitude 45° north and 32° south. Geographical distribution of the diseases is related to that of the sandfly species acting as vectors, their ecology and the conditions of internal development of the parasite.

Leishmaniases are present in 88 countries in four continents, of which 16 are industrialized and 72 developing countries, 13 of them among the poorest in the world. There are an estimated 12 million cases in a worldwide population of exposed at risk estimated at 350 million people. One-and-a-half to 2 million new cases occur each year.[1]

VL is found in 47 countries and its mean annual incidence is estimated at around 500000 new cases. The main historical foci of endemic VL are located, east to west, in China, India, Central Asia, East Africa, the Mediterranean basin and Brazil (Figure 77.2). The anthroponotic species *L. donovani* is restricted to China, India and East Africa, while the zoonotic species *L. infantum* extends from China to Brazil. India is certainly the biggest focus of VL in the world. Between 1875 and 1950, the disease there took on an epidemic feature, with three severe outbreaks in Assam and a subsequent extension to other Indian states.[22]

At the present time, 90% of the VL cases in the world are in Bangladesh, India and Nepal, Sudan and Brazil. Bihar State in India experienced a dramatic epidemic, with more than 300000 cases reported between 1977 and 1990 and a mortality rate over 2%.[23] In southern Sudan, an outbreak was responsible for 100000 deaths from 1989 to 1994, in a population of Upper Nile Province of less than 1 million.[24] Population movements, such as rural to suburban migration in north-eastern Brazil,[25] are factors for VL extension, by exposing thousands of non-immune individuals to the risk of infection.

The large majority of Old World CL (Figure 77.3) is due to the two species *L. major* and *L. tropica* and proceeds from countries of the Near and Middle East: Afghanistan, Iran, Saudi Arabia and Syria. *L. major*, the species responsible for zoonotic CL, has a large distribution area, including West, North and East Africa, the Near and Middle East and Central Asia. Economic developments have been accompanied by movements of populations which have caused dramatic epidemic outbreaks of this species in several countries of the Middle East, but also in Algeria and Tunisia. The anthroponotic species *L. tropica* is present in various cities of the Near and Middle East, but extends also to Tunisia and Morocco, where an animal reservoir is suspected in some foci. Other species have restricted distribution areas: *L. aethiopica* to Ethiopia and Kenya, *L. arabica* to Saudi Arabia and *L. killicki* to Tunisia and Algeria. *L. turanica* and *L. gerbilli* are Central Asian species restricted to rodents.

In the New World (Figure 77.4), *L. braziliensis* is the species with the widest distribution area. It extends from south of Mexico to north of Argentina. *L. amazonensis* has a large distribution in South America, but human cases of this rodent enzootic species are unusual. Other species have more restricted areas: *L. guyanensis* (north of the Amazonian basin), *L. panamensis* (Colombia and Central America), *L. mexicana* (Mexico and Central America), and lastly *L. peruviana*, which is restricted to the Andean valleys of Peru. With the exception of this latter species, all other American dermotropic species are responsible for wild zoonoses of the rainforest.

PATHOLOGY

The bite of an infected sandfly results in the intradermal inoculation of metacyclic promastigotes. Their establishment in the mammalian host is facilitated in a remarkable way by the sandfly saliva delivered at the same time, which enhances *Leishmania* infectivity.[26] Sandfly saliva contains various pharmacologically active substances, which globally prevent haemostatic mechanisms of the host, and cause vasodilatation and local immunosuppression.[27]

Within the dermis of mammalian skin, the metacyclic promastigotes escape complement activation, thanks to their surface com-

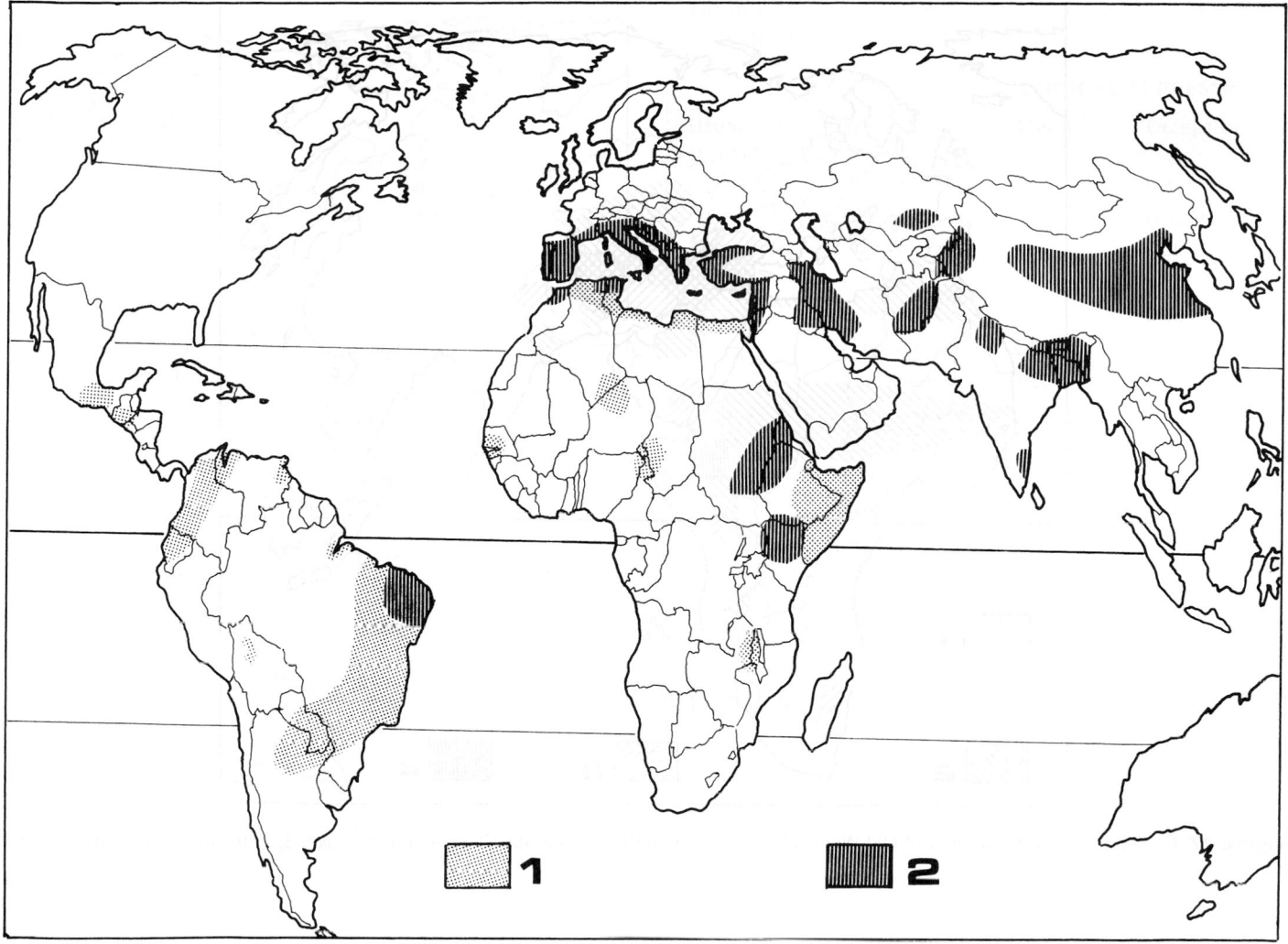

Figure 77.2 Geographical distribution of visceral leishmaniasis. 1, Low-endemicity areas; 2, High-endemicity areas.

ponents, mainly lipophosphoglycan and glycoprotein (63 kDa). They are then phagocytosed by macrophages within which they transform into amastigotes, and have the capacity to resist intracellular digestion. Their survival in these cells is the result of several factors related to the cell itself (decrease in the production of oxidative and nitrogenic derivatives triggered by the presence of the parasite) and to the amastigote's ability to resist lysosomal hydrolases, a property probably related to surface glyco-inositol-phospholipids.[28]

When the intracellular development of the amastigotes remains localized at the inoculation site, various cytokines are released and cell reactions are generated, resulting in the development of a localized lesion of CL.[29] In other instances, the parasites spread to the organs of the mononuclear phagocytic system, giving rise to VL. Amastigotes may also spread to other cutaneous sites, as in diffuse cutaneous leishmaniasis (DCL), or to mucosae in the case of mucocutaneous leishmaniasis (MCL).

The localization of the parasite to the various organs of the patient results in the clinical expression of the disease. It is directly related to the tropism of the parasite species (Table 77.2). In that sense, the genus *Leishmania* can be divided broadly into viscerotropic (*L. donovani*, *L. infantum*) and dermotropic species (roughly all other species). *L. braziliensis*, and more rarely *L. panamensis*, are known for their secondary mucosal spread.

In spite of this general tropism of the species, some exceptions occur, which are independent of the clinical status of the patient harbouring the parasite. Thus, well-established viscerotropic species can occasionally be responsible for limited cutaneous lesions without signs or symptoms of any visceral involvement. One of the best examples is the dermotropic enzymatic variant of the normally visceralizing species *L. infantum* in the Mediterranean basin.[30] This unusual tropism of certain populations of a species may be explained by intraspecific variation of the parasite genome, the markers of which remain unknown.

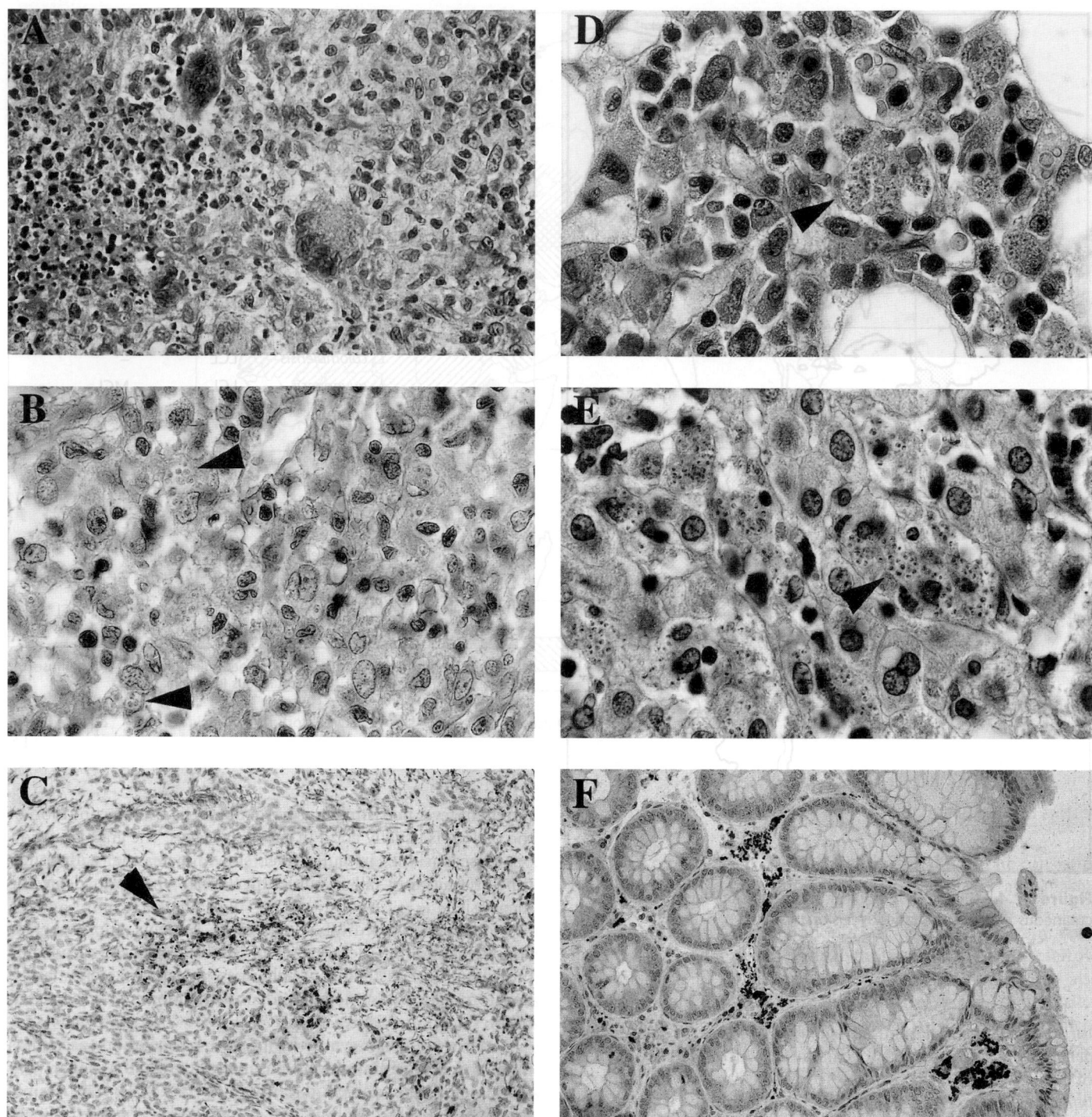

Figure 77.5 Cutaneous and visceral leishmaniasis: histopathology. (A) Skin: CL due to *L. major*. Mature granuloma and giant cells; no parasite detected (H&E staining, ×250). (B) Skin: CL. Infiltrate by histiocytes, lymphocytes and plasma cells; numerous amastigotes in histiocytes (H&E staining, ×400). (C) Skin: CL. Amastigotes of *L. major* detected by immunohistochemistry using a mouse anti-*L. amazonensis* immune serum (streptavidin peroxidase method and amino-ethyl carbazole (AEC) as chromogen, ×250). (D) Bone marrow. VL due to *L. infantum* (H&E staining, ×400). (E) Liver. VL due to *L. infantum*. Numerous parasitized histiocytes (H&E staining, ×400). (F) Colon. HIV/*Leishmania* co-infection. Amastigotes in the submucosae (immunohistochemistry: streptavidin peroxidase and AEC, ×400). Arrowheads indicate the presence of parasites. (From M. Huerre and J. C. Antoine, Institut Pasteur, Paris, France, reproduced with permission.)

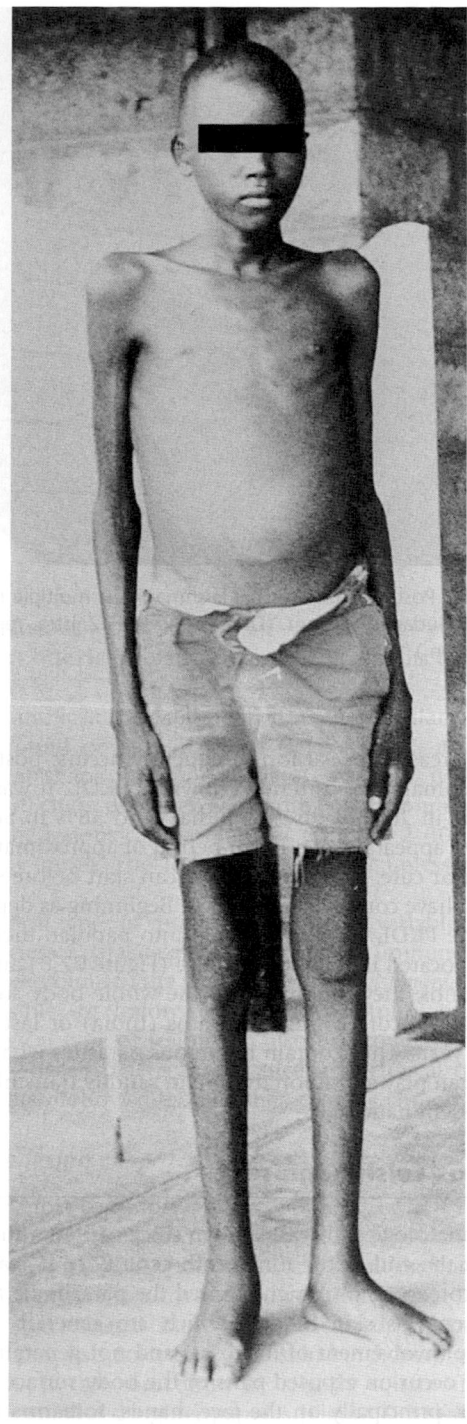

Figure 77.6 General presentation of visceral leishmaniasis: weight loss and splenomegaly in an East African patient (J. P. Dedet).

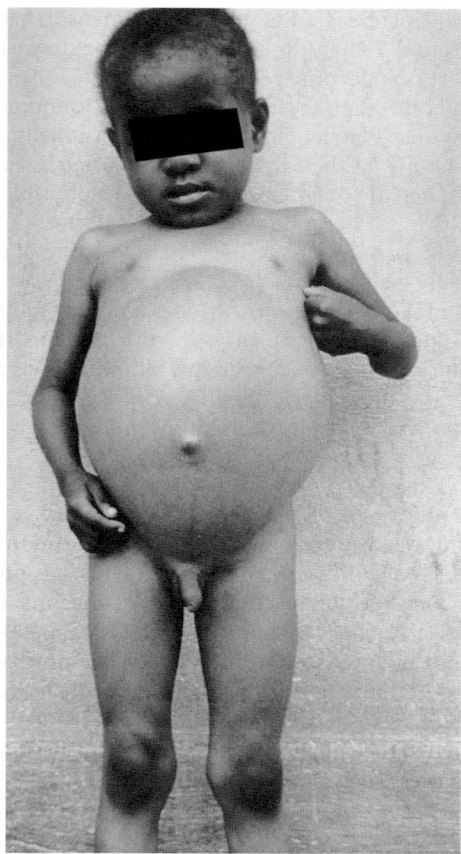

Figure 77.7 Visceral leishmaniasis: protuberant abdomen caused by massive enlargement of spleen and liver. (From IRD, INSERM and P. Desjeux, reproduced with permission from LePont et al. Leishmaniases et phlebotomes en Bolivie. Editions ORSTOM et INSERM, ©1992.)

during evolution. The nodes are small, firm painless and mobile.

Anaemia is responsible for an extreme paleness of skin and mucosa. In India, patient skin has a greyish pigmentation, which gives rise to the local name of the disease (kala-azar). Other symp-

toms can be found, such as digestive, pulmonary and bleeding manifestations.

Diarrhoea is frequently reported and is related to ulcerations of the digestive mucosa. Pulmonary involvement can occur, with a dry, non productive cough. Episodes of bleeding are principally epistaxis, and more rarely bleeding from the gums, purpura, petechiae and menorrhagia.

During evolution, the clinical presentation progressively worsens, with amplification of the above-described symptoms. Ascites is considered as a late sign of bad prognosis, sometimes associated with oedema and pleural effusion. These unusual signs are more common in Indian kala-azar. As a result of albuminuria and immune complex deposition, renal involvement may occur as a late complication.

Biological parameters

VL is characterized by haematological as well as plasmatic protein alterations.

Anaemia is the major and most frequent haematological sign. Generally of normochromic and normocytic type, it progressively

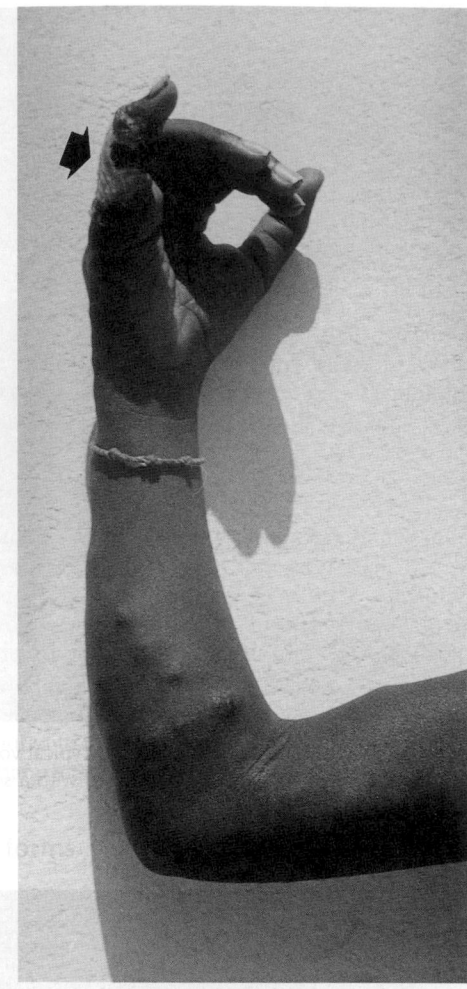

Figure 77.12 Lymphangitic extension along the forearm and the arm, from a finger-localized cutaneous lesion (arrow). (From Société de Pathologie Exotique, reproduced with permission.)

Other types of lesions

More rarely, other clinical types of lesions are encountered: closed nodular type, infiltrative plaques, eczematoid, warty and pseudo-tumoural. This clinical polymorphism of the lesions is unrelated to species.

Lymphangitic dissemination

Solitary or multiple subcutaneous nodules in the draining territory are sometimes associated with a cutaneous lesion (Figure 77.12). Palpation easily detects a lymphangitic cord, regularly enlarged in small round and painless nodules, containing parasites. They can occasionally become open to the skin and transform into secondary lesions. This type of dissemination ('sporotrichoid spread') is mainly reported with *L. major*, *L. braziliensis*, *L. guyanensis* and *L. panamensis*.

Evolution

Whatever the clinical type of lesion, the evolution is chronic and leads most often to spontaneous cure, after a time varying accord-ing to the *Leishmania* species from a few months (about 6 months for *L. major*, *L. mexicana* or *L. peruviana*) to a few years (more than 1 year for *L. aethiopica*, *L. infantum*, *L. tropica* or *L. guyanensis*). The cure, either spontaneous or following treatment, results in an indelible scar, pinkish or whitish on pale skin and hyperpigmented on dark skin. Depending on the clinical feature of the lesion, the scar is generally depressed (ulcerative lesion). The evolution of CL does not generally lead to mutilations, with the exception of chiclero's ulcer, which is occasionally responsible for partial amputation of the ear auricle.

Clinical cure does not always lead to a complete disappearance of the parasites. In about 10% of cases it is followed by the resurgence of an active lesion on the scar. This reactivation can occur between a few months to a few years following the initial cure. This secondary lesion will also spontaneously cure.

Diffuse cutaneous Leishmaniasis

This particularly severe form of CL was described from Venezu-ela.[49] It is a peculiar and scarce clinical form, resulting from the parasitism of particular *Leishmania* species, *L. amazonensis* and occasionally *L. mexicana*[50] in the New World, and *L. aethiopica* in the Old World, in patients with an antileishmanial specific defect in cell-mediated immunity.[51] Since HIV infection has spread to Leishmaniasis endemic areas, DCL cases have been occasionally reported due to unusual species, such as *L. braziliensis* in the New World[52] and *L. infantum*[53] and *L. major*[54] in the Old World.

A non-ulcerated nodule rich in parasites represents the basic cutaneous lesion of this form of disease. The nodules are numer-ous, at first isolated, then joining to form large patches, dissemi-nated to the whole of the body, to the face, as well as to the trunk and limbs. The general appearance of the patient mimics the pre-sentation of lepromatous leprosy, with 'leonine' facies. The pathol-ogy of the lesion is characteristic, with a homogeneous epidermal and dermal infiltrate of vacuolized macrophages full of *Leishmania* amastigotes. The leishmanin skin test is consistently negative.

During the development of this condition, there is no ulcer-ation, nor mucosal or visceral involvement, but a slow constant aggravation by successive relapses, interrupted with phases of remission. This form is resistant to therapy by classical antileish-manial drugs, and especially to pentavalent antimonials, and never cures spontaneously.

Leishmaniasis recidivans

This is a chronic form of Leishmaniasis, due essentially to *L. tropica* in the Old World and occasionally to *L. braziliensis* in the New World.[55] The lesion is located on the face and follows an acute lesion, after numerous months of evolution. The lesion shows a peripheral active zone, constantly enlarging, around a central healing part (Figure 77.13). The presentation mimics that of lupus vulgaris. The lesion contains a small number of parasites and cor-responds to an exaggerated cell-mediated immune response on the part of the host.

Mucocutaneous Leishmaniasis

MCL, also named 'espundia' since its early description,[56] is a par-ticular nosological entity mainly due to the species *L. braziliensis*,

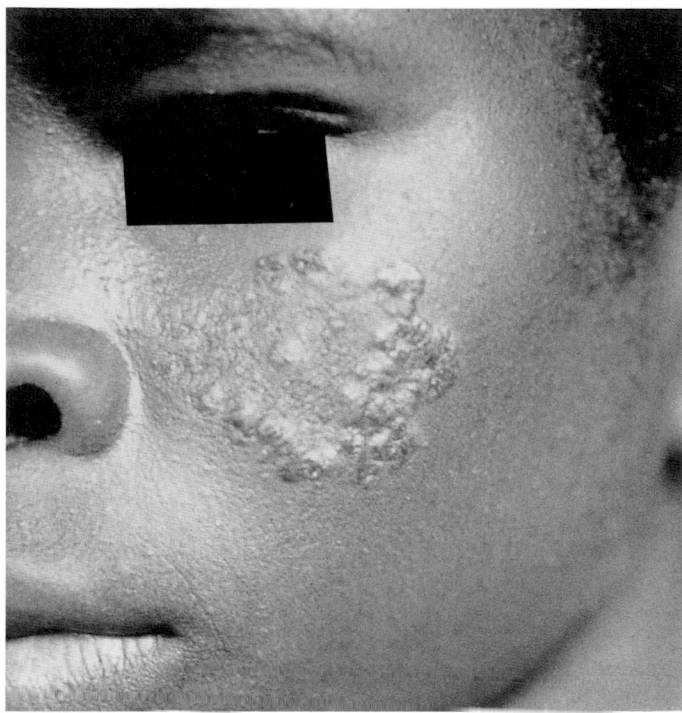

Figure 77.13 Leishmaniasis recidivans. (From P. Desjeux, reproduced with permission.)

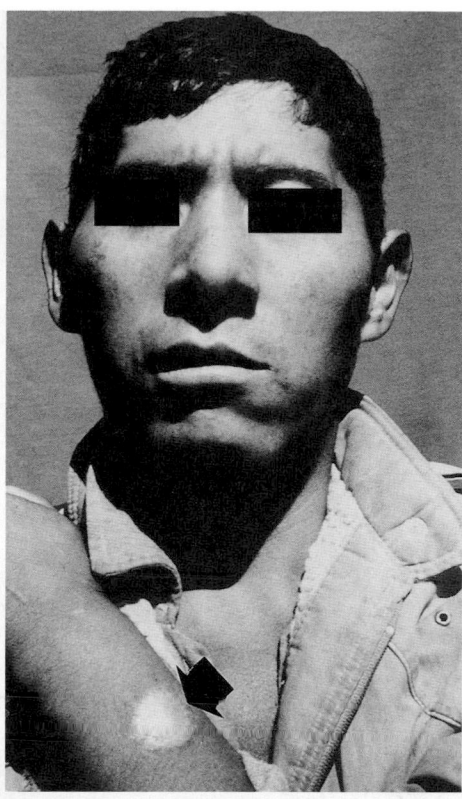

Figure 77.14 Mucocutaneous leishmaniasis. Classical presentation of the patient harbouring the scar of the initial cutaneous lesion (arrow), and consulting for congestion and oedema of the nasal pyramid. (From L. Valda Rodriguez, reproduced with permission.)

and occasionally to *L. panamensis*. It is a wild zoonosis, of which the natural reservoirs remain unknown. It occurs from southern Mexico to the north of Argentina.

This form of leishmaniasis evolves in two stages: a primary cutaneous lesion, eventually followed, after a variable time of latency, by secondary mucosal involvement.

The initial cutaneous lesion does not fundamentally differ from the localized lesions occurring during infection by other *Leishmania* dermotropic species (see above), and its evolution generally leads to spontaneous cure. Once the primary cutaneous lesion(s) cure, the *Leishmanial* infection remains for a variable period of time, which can be very long, sometimes indefinite. The frequency of occurrence of secondary mucosal involvement appears variable, according to foci considered and authors. The period of time between cutaneous lesion and subsequent appearance of the mucosal involvement extends from several weeks to many years. Very long time intervals have been occasionally observed by several authors.[57]

If it occurs, the mucosal involvement starts on the nasal mucosa. The patient suffers with nasal congestion (Figure 77.14), which causes nocturnal discomfort. Epistaxis can also be the initial symptom.[57] The initial nasal lesion is generally localized to the anterior, cartilaginous part of the nasal septum. It appears as a small-sized hyperaemic inflammatory granuloma, rapidly evolving to an ulcer.[58] The septum is rapidly invaded and destroyed, which leads to the perforation of the nasal septum in its anterior part, which is generally considered a symptom pathognomonic of MCL (Figure 77.15).[57] The involvement of nasal mucosa can be apparent from the exterior, even as early as the initial inflammatory stage, and manifests as congestion and oedema of the nasal

pyramid (Figure 77.14). At the stage of septum destruction, the nose shape is flattened and weighed down, and is classically described as 'tapir nose' (Figure 77.16).

The buccal mucosa is commonly affected at a later stage of the disease, with or without contiguous spread from the nasal lesions. The mucosae of the palate and of the interior lips are the most frequently involved, while the tongue generally remains uninjured. The palatal lesions are granulomatous and extensive, and reach the velum (Figure 77.17). They produce the classical 'Escomel cross'. The lip lesions are inflamed and ulcerated, sometimes extending to the external part, with frequent tissue destruction. A palatal perforation can occur in the later stages and results in the nasal fossae and mouth cavity becoming interconnected.

Laryngeal extension follows the rhino-buccal-pharyngeal localization of the parasite. The lesion is firstly infiltrative and manifests as dysphonia and metallic cough. When granulomatous, the laryngeal lesion can cause obstruction of the respiratory tract, with possible fatal consequences due to acute respiratory distress. Dysphagia and the resulting undernutrition have serious consequences for the physical condition of the patient.

Tissue necrosis and disfigurement appear in the advanced stage of the condition and can be extremely severe. They result in disfiguring mutilations: the nose and lips can totally disappear, at which time the mouth and nasal cavity become connected by a single hole. Socio-psychological consequences are considerable for the patient, often leading to suicide.

infection; it is a relatively non-invasive method and, as such, much appreciated by HIV co-infected as well as immunocompetent patients, and its sensitivity seems comparable in both groups.

Parasites have been found in a variety of unusual sites, such as cerebrospinal fluid, normal skin, digestive mucosa, bronchiolo-alveolar fluid and pleural liquid. These sites of parasite research are not included in the current diagnosis route, but have been fortuitously used in immunocompromised HIV patients.

Cutaneous and mucocutaneous leishmaniasis

The circumstances in which parasites are found in the skin are: CL of Old and New Worlds, PKDL in India and East Africa, and even in healthy skin during *Leishmania*/ HIV co-infection. Skin material is obtained by superficial scraping with a scarifier or a Brock curette, by needle aspiration, or by tissue collection made with a dental broach or biopsy punch. The site from which diagnostic material is collected is the determining factor in the discovery of the parasite and depends on the clinical type of the lesion. For example, the inflammatory edge of an ulcerative cutaneous lesion is the elected place for parasite detection. In the particular case of mucosal lesions, material is collected with biopsy forceps.

Detection methods

Collected material can be smeared on to a microscope slide, cultured, fixed for pathological examination or more recently, submitted to the polymerase chain reaction (PCR) technique. Inoculation into laboratory animals is rarely performed.

The staining method most appropriate for *Leishmania* detection is one employing panoptic May Grünwald-Giemsa stain. Amastigotes are typically intramonocytic, but frequently extracellular in smears, the nucleus and kinetoplast staining characteristically purple (Figure 77.19). Direct examination of smears may give a rapid diagnosis if carefully practised, but has a limited sensitivity, inferior to that of culture and particularly that of new PCR techniques. Specific staining of biopsy material using mouse anti-*Leishmania* immune serum and peroxidase conjugate can be used for an easy detection of the parasites, the immune serum cross-reacting with various taxa of *Leishmania* (Figure 77.5C, F).

Culture has a higher sensitivity than direct detection of parasites on smears, and is a useful complement to parasitological

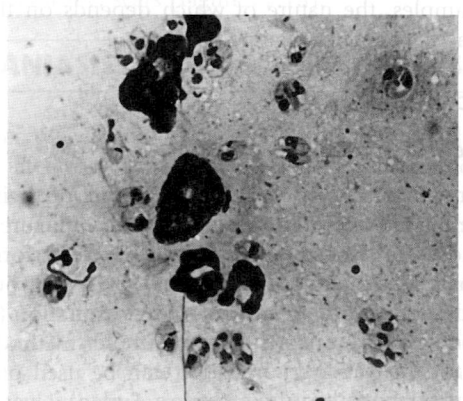

Figure 77.19 *Leishmania* amastigotes stained by May Grünwald-Giemsa technique on smears prepared from a cutaneous lesion.

diagnosis. In addition, isolation of the parasite strain allows parasite drug sensitivity testing and parasite identification, by isoenzyme electrophoresis, monoclonal antibodies or specific probes hybridization. The classical blood agar NNN medium is the most currently used, but numerous diphasic and liquid media are presently available. The ease with which parasites may be established in culture varies according to species, and even to strains, some being difficult to cultivate in vitro (*L. venezuelensis*, *L. braziliensis*). Guidelines for *Leishmania* culture and isolation can be found in Evans et al.[65] *Leishmania* cultures are incubated at 24–26°C. The parasite develops as a mobile promastigote stage, and grows slowly with a doubling time of about 48–72 h.

Animal inoculation into the golden hamster, one of the most susceptible laboratory animals, is an alternative to in vitro cultivation, but is not really practical in current diagnosis.

Molecular diagnosis has been increasingly used in the last decade, and can be applied to any type of tissue sample, hence to any form of leishmaniasis.[66] The detection of the parasite DNA is essentially achieved through PCR amplification. The advantages of this method are its high sensitivity coupled to a theoretically quasi absolute specificity. Other advantages include the possibility of detecting the parasite on contaminated samples or cultures, and the relative promptness of the result as compared with in vitro cultivation, as well as the possibility to carry out species identification simultaneously or at least using the same DNA extract. In real life, PCR assays are not standardized and a huge number of in-house methods are in use, leading to wide variations in performances among laboratories.

Molecular diagnosis has been successfully applied to the diagnosis of VL[67–70] and of CL.[71–73] In both conditions, it has been found to be more sensitive than classical diagnostic procedures, including cultivation. In VL, a PCR assay has proved almost 100% sensitive using peripheral blood, avoiding bone marrow sampling and making it particularly applicable in immunosuppressed patients as a relatively non-invasive diagnostic method.[67] This also allows the therapeutic follow-up of patients over relatively long periods of time. Molecular diagnosis has been applied to canine leishmaniasis with variable success, but the use of an 'ultrasensitive' PCR assay allowed the detection of a very high rate of asymptomatic carriage.[74] Recent developments rely upon the use of quantitative real-time PCR. In VL, the use of an 'ultrasensitive' method again allowed the detection of asymptomatic carriage also in man, including during immunosuppression, and allowed the definition of a parasitaemia threshold above which symptoms are likely to appear.[75]

Immunological diagnosis

During VL and DCL, the immune response of the patient is of humoral type, with the development of high levels of specific circulating antibodies in serum which, however, can be absent in immunocompromised patients. During CL and MCL, the preponderant immune response is of cell-mediated type, which can be explored by a delayed hypersensitivity test.

Various serological tests have been developed to detect circulating specific antibodies for the diagnosis of VL. The techniques proposed are numerous and differ in their sensitivity and specificity, and their use depends on their cost and reagent availability:

indirect fluorescent antibody technique (IFAT, the most commonly used), immuno-enzymatic techniques, counter-current immuno-electrophoresis, indirect haemagglutination test and immunoblot. There are a few which are relatively easy to practise in field conditions: direct agglutination test (DAT), rK39 immunochromatography dipstick, latex particle agglutination, dot-ELISA and fast-ELISA. According to the antigen used, cross-reactions may occur with other infectious diseases, such as malaria, trypanosomiasis, mycobacteriosis and schistosomiasis. Immunological diagnosis is a relatively non-invasive approach, and useful to combine with direct demonstration of the parasite, which, of course, remains the reference technique. The presence of specific antibodies is not necessarily correlated to an active disease and can reveal a subclinical infection. The immunological diagnosis has some limits, particularly for post-treatment follow-up (specific antibodies remain present for a long time after treatment) and in immunocompromised patients, in whom the immune response can be weak or even negative.

The immunoblot analysis is a more sensitive technique than IFAT or ELISA, which detect antibodies against specific antigens according to Leishmania species. It is a method useful not only for diagnosis confirmation, but also for patient follow-up during treatment.[76] Moreover, it is of epidemiological interest, being able to detect asymptomatic infections in patients living in endemic areas.[63]

A latex agglutination test for the detection of Leishmania antigens in urine has been developed[77] and evaluated in various countries, including India and Nepal, Sudan, Brazil and Spain. It appears efficient for initial diagnosis of VL before treatment.

The leishmanin skin test[78] measures delayed-type hypersensitivity. It consists of an intradermal injection of a suspension of promastigotes killed by heat and phenol; the test is read 48–72 h later; only an induration of at least 5 mm is considered positive. It is usually positive during LCL and MCL. It is always negative during DCL. It is negative during acute VL, in which it usually turns positive several months after clinical cure. The leishmanin skin test is useful for epidemiological studies, during which it reveals asymptomatic infections.

TREATMENT

Treatment of leishmaniases remains difficult, due to the multiplicity of the existing Leishmania species, and their often variable susceptibility to available drugs, which are old, toxic and expensive products. Resistance to the existing products is developing in some foci, such as India.

There have been no significant changes in the treatment of leishmaniases for many years. Since the 1920s, treatment has been based on pentavalent antimonial compounds. Following the increasing incidence of VL cases in immunocompromised patients and the rise of acquired resistance to antimonials, amphotericin B, mainly in its liposomal form, has joined the antimonials as a first-line drug for Leishmaniasis. Miltefosine, a new oral compound, has shown promising results and appears to be an efficient alternative for the treatment of Indian kala-azar. Other products, such as aminosidine or imidazoles, could find new applications, but there is no really new product in development at present time. Alternative drugs are investigated for many years without passing the step of clinical trials.

We first consider the available products, and will then discuss their indications according to the different clinical forms of Leishmaniasis.

Products

Antimonials

Two closely related pentavalent antimonials are currently used: meglumine antimoniate (Glucantime®, Aventis), available in France, Latin America and Francophone countries, and sodium stibogluconate (Pentostam®, Glaxo-SmithKline), available in English-speaking countries. For a few years, a generic formulation of sodium stibogluconate has been manufactured in India (Albert David Ltd). These two chemically close antimonial salts have distinct antimony content of respectively 85 and 100 mg Sb/mL. When properly manufactured and stored, they have comparable efficacy and toxicity.

Antimonials have proven to be efficient in Leishmaniasis treatment through a century of use and about 15 randomized trials. However, the mechanism of action as antileishmanial agents remains unclear.

It may involve inhibition of ATP synthesis. It might be possible that antimonial salts have to be concentrated within the macrophage or parasite and transformed into active trivalent metabolites to be efficient. Antimonials have poor oral absorption and therefore are administered by the parenteral route. They are rapidly excreted by the kidneys.

In spite of numerous side-effects attributed to antimonials, the scarcity of documented accidents allows their continued use. Their side-effects on the fetus remaining unknown, their use during pregnancy is not recommended. Some of the side-effects of pentavalent antimonials are related to intolerance action and are of anaphylactic type, including shivers, fever, arthralgias, myalgias, skin rashes, abdominal symptoms and headache. Other side-effects seem to be linked to accumulation of product. They include reversible elevation of hepatocellular enzymes, subclinical pancreatitis, and decrease in haemoglobin level and platelet count. Cardiac side-effects are the most worrisome. Several electrocardiogram (ECG) changes occur, of which flattening and/or inversion of T waves is the most common. Patients can develop prolongation of the corrected QT interval, concave ST abnormality and prolongation of the PR interval. These ECG changes are transient; they gradually approach normal in a 1–3-week period after patients complete therapy. Exceptional sudden deaths have been reported for a few patients who received more than the recommended dose of Sb^V.

Sodium stibogluconate is supplied in multi-dose 100 mL bottles (100 mg Sb^V/mL), while meglumine antimoniate is supplied as 5 mL ampoules (85 mg Sb^V/mL). They are administered on the basis of their Sb^V content. The recommended dosage of Sb^V is 20 mg/kg per day, for 20 days in CL and 28 days in VL and MCL.[79,80] They are currently injected by the intravenous (i.v.) or intramuscular (i.m.) route. The i.v. route is preferred when the volume of drug is high, as it is for most adults. The appropriate volume of drug is mixed with 50 mL of 5% dextrose in sterile water and infused over at least a 10-min interval. In the case of a few localized cutaneous lesions, intralesional injections are used.

Where resources permit, an ECG, serum chemistries and a complete blood count should be obtained for all patients before

Localized cutaneous leishmaniasis

Management of patients with LCL depends on the type and characters of the lesion(s), the *Leishmania* species involved, the risk of extension and the opinion of the patient. Briefly, three options are possible: therapeutic abstention, or local or general treatment.

Mild, rapidly self-healing forms of CL, such as those due to *L. major* or *L. peruviana*, can ultimately remain untreated, if the patient wishes. Belazzoug and Neal[87] showed that, out of two groups of patients with *L. major* CL, the group receiving distilled water as placebo was more rapidly cured than that receiving pentavalent antomonial.

Various local treatments have been proposed, including diverse physical means (diathermy, cryotherapy, radiotherapy, laser), surgical excision or local applications of ointments. They were all limited trials, made without control groups, the results of which were inconclusive. These procedures cannot be generalized.

Local infiltrations of pentavalent antomonials are recommended for the treatment of small numbers of lesions. Various protocols have been proposed consisting of a course of 5–10 infiltrations of 1–5 mL of antimonial, often accompanied by a local anaesthetic in order to avoid pain, associated or not with cryotherapy. Infiltrations are done two or three times a week.

Systemic treatment is recommended for CL with large and/or multiple lesions, with lymphangitic dissemination, those of recidivans type or with a risk of mucosal involvement. CL of immuno-compromised patients should also be treated by systemic treatment. The currently used systemic treatment is that of a course of 20 days of pentavalent antimonial, at a dose of 20 mg Sb^V/kg per day. Oral imidazoles can occasionally be used as alternatives to antimonials in the case of *L. major* CL (fluconazole) or of *L. mexicana* CL (ketoconazole). A course of four to five i.m. injections of pentamidine (4 mg/kg per injection) on alternate days is the first-line treatment for CL due to *L. guyanensis* and *L. panamensis*. Miltefosine has been proposed as an alternative treatment for *L. panamensis* CL.[88]

Diffuse cutaneous Leishmaniasis

Once established, DCL is resistant to treatment. Systematic pentavalent antimonials can improve the clinical evolution temporarily. Pentamidine showed some efficacy, but with high doses close to toxicity. A combination of paromomycin and antimonial gave good results in two Ethiopian patients.[89] There is an urgent need for testing various new molecules or formulations (liposomal amphotericin B, IFNγ). But the scarcity of cases does not allow randomized clinical trials with control groups.

Mucocutaneous Leishmaniasis

Systemic treatment of the primary cutaneous lesion is recommended, with the hope of avoiding parasite extension to facial mucosae. The treatment currently used in endemic areas is pentavalent antimonial, a 20-day course of i.m. injections, 20 mg Sb^V/kg per day. A recent publication reports the cure of a single patient by liposomal amphotericin B,[90] an observation which needs to be repeated. However, it has been shown that a correct treatment does not consistently prevent the development of secondary mucosal lesions.

The treatment of mucosal lesions should be as early as possible, in order to avoid the extension of lesions and subsequent mutilations. The antimonials, at standard doses, are injected daily over 28 days. The level of cure is variable according to country and the evolution grade of the lesions. Amphotericin B has been currently used for cases with long evolution or poorly responding to antimonials. Cure was sometimes obtained from 1 g, but superior doses (2–3 g) were often necessary. Amphotericin B was used as first-line drug during a mass campaign in Bolivia.[91] Cases of resistance seem to exist, but few documented observations are available. Liposomal amphotericin B and association of IFNγ or paromomycin to antimonials can be an alternative solution.

PROPHYLAXIS

Intervention strategies for prevention or control are hampered by the variety of the structure of Leishmaniasis foci, with many different animals able to act as reservoir hosts of zoonotic forms and a multiplicity of sandfly vectors, each with a different pattern of behaviour. In 1990, a WHO Expert Committee described no less than 11 distinct eco-epidemiological entities and defined control strategies for each of them.[92]

The aim of prevention is avoiding host infection (human or canine) and its subsequent disease. It includes means to prevent intrusion of people into natural zoonotic foci and ways to protect against infective bites of sandflies. Prevention can be at an individual or collective level.

Control programmes are intended to interrupt the life cycle of the parasite, to limit or, ideally, to eradicate, the disease. The two main targets in control programmes are the vector and the reservoir, which are not mutually exclusive. As the majority of the Leishmaniases are zoonoses, control programmes are generally limited and rarely pass beyond the experimental stage. In the New World, almost all the Leishmaniases are sylvatic, and control is not usually feasible. Even removal of the forest itself may not reach the objective, as various *Leishmania* species have proved to be remarkably adaptable to environment degradation. For example, *L. braziliensis* survived the great deforestation of eastern Brazil.

Whatever type of intervention strategy is selected, an active participation of the population is essential to success. Public information on the natural history of the parasite, transmission and the disease is a prerequisite for any prevention measure or development of a control programme.

Prevention

Prevention includes all individual or collective measures aimed at preventing infection of the human or canine population.

Individual prevention

Numerous individual protective means are available but are not equally feasible. The simplest measure is avoiding exposure to risk. Other means include mechanical, chemical or therapeutic measures.

Avoiding risk exposure

The risk of infection is geographically and temporally localized. A simple preventive measure is, therefore, to avoid the vicinity of sandfly development or resting sites in endemic areas during critical periods (seasons and activity cycles of the vector). This is less feasible in tropical than temperate regions where transmission seasons are limited, but occasionally it can be applicable elsewhere. However, this way of avoiding risk is not applicable to the general situation of many developing countries where regular migration leads to human settlements inside the heart of natural foci. This results in a high exposure to risk by non-immune, uninformed populations.

Mechanical means

Mechanical means have the objective of protection from sandfly bites. They include wearing clothes that cover as much skin as possible and using bed nets.

Sandflies bite uncovered skin and do not have the ability to bite through clothes, even thin material like cotton. Wearing full clothes during the hours of sandfly activity is a good preventive measure which can decrease the number of cutaneous lesions, even if it does not avoid all contamination.

Sandflies can generally pass through the mesh of mosquito bed nets, and therefore it is generally recommended to use fine bed nets of terylene. A disadvantage of these nets is that they impede air circulation, and are thus uncomfortable in hot weather. The present trend is to use conventional mosquito bed nets impregnated with various insecticides, including the pyrethroids permethrin ($300 mg/m^2$), deltamethrin ($15–25 mg/m^2$) and lambda cyhalothrin ($10 mg/m^2$). They have been found to be efficient because of both their repellent and residual killing effects. But the intrinsic limitation of bed nets is related to the behaviour of the people who tend to be at greatest risk between sunset and bedtime. This method therefore provides more protection for women and children than for male adults.[93] Pilot control programmes with impregnated bed nets are ongoing in Bolivia, Afghanistan, Iran, Sudan and Syria.

Chemical means

Sandflies are sensitive to various repellents used against mosquitoes. They are sprayed or spread on uncovered skin before the hours of sandfly activity (dusk and night). The duration of efficacy depends not only on the product but also on the climatic conditions, mainly heat and humidity. It is generally considered that protection is limited to 2–6 h.

For dogs, two products are available for specific protection against sandflies:deltamethrin-impregnated collar, Scalibor® (Intervet) and a permethrin-based ectoparasiticide, Adventix® Spot-on (Bayer Health Care).

Self-protection insecticides can reduce man–vector contact. Mosquito coils containing pyrethroid insecticides provide good protection during the time of combustion (6–8 h). Electrically heated fumigation mats are also efficient, but need electricity, which is often unavailable in rural areas of developing countries. Insecticide spraying has a good but temporary efficacy.

Chemoprophylaxis and vaccine

Neither chemoprophylaxis nor vaccines are available against Leishmaniasis.

Various vaccines have been made and experimentally tested in different animal models, but none has prevented human or canine Leishmaniasis. Putative vaccines include live, irradiated or killed parasites, parasitic crude fractions and recombinant parasitic antigens.[94]

The first vaccines contained live *L. major* promastigotes and were empirically used in the past in Central Asian republics of the former USSR, Israel and later intensively in Iran during the war against Iraq. Similar vaccines were developed in Brazil for American CL. Vaccines containing killed promastigotes, with or without BCG as an adjuvant, were then used in field trials in several countries including Brazil, Venezuela and Iran.

A variety of second-generation vaccines are at different developmental stages and include recombinant *Leishmania*, bacteria or viruses expressing *Leishmania* antigens, and defined recombinant subunits and synthetic peptides. But none of them is presently available for human or canine use.

Collective measures

Independently of an established control programme, the human population can be collectively protected through a few measures to keep sandflies away from people. To reduce peridomestic transmission, environmental changes have been proposed in particular situations, such as forest clearings around human settlements. Insecticide application inside houses is also occasionally recommended.

Forest clearance

The establishment of human settlements in South American primary forest results in outbreaks of CL. In such situations, a high level of human infection is related to domestic or peridomestic transmission by sandflies flying from the neighbouring forest. Establishment of a forest-free zone of about 400 m around a human settlement in French Guiana resulted in a dramatic decrease in human cases during the following years.[95] Such changes in the environment must, however, be maintained, as secondary forest appeared to favour an increase in *Lutzomyia flaviscutellata* and rodent populations, leading to an increase in enzootic rodent Leishmaniasis.[96]

Indoor residual spraying

This is a simple, cost-effective method for controlling endophilic vectors which can have a long-lasting effect, depending on the insecticide. Sandflies are sensitive to all classes of insecticides: organochlorines, organophosphates, carbamates or pyrethroids. Vectors of VL remain sensitive to DDT even in places where *P. papatasi* shows some level of resistance.[97] It is therefore the first-line insecticide for indoor spraying owing to its low cost and long residual action.

Control

The structure and dynamics of natural foci of Leishmaniasis are so diverse that a standard control programme cannot be defined

56. Escomel E. La Espundia. *Bull Soc Pathol Exot* 1911; 4:489–492.

57. Walton BC. American cutaneous and mucocutaneous Leishmaniasis. In: Peters W, Killick-Kendrick R, eds. *The Leishmaniases in Biology and Medicine.* Vol. 2. London: Academic Press; 1987:637–664.

58. Marsden PD, Nonata RR. Mucocutaneous Leishmaniasis: a review of clinical aspects. *Rev Soc Bras Med Trop* 1975; 9:309–326.

59. Desjeux P, Alvar J. *Leishmania*/HIV co-infections: epidemiology in Europe. *Ann Trop Med Parasitol* 2003; 97:S3–S15.

60. Alvar J. Leishmaniasis and AIDS co-infection: the Spanish example. *Parasitol Today* 1994; 10:160–163.

61. Dereure J, Pratlong F, Reynes J, et al. Haemoculture as a tool for diagnosing visceral Leishmaniasis in HIV-negative and HIV-positive patients: interest for parasite identification. *Bull World Health Organ* 1998; 76:203–206.

62. Campino L, Santos-Gomes G, Pratlong F, et al. The isolation of *Leishmania donovani* MON-18 from an AIDS patient in Portugal: possible needle transmission. *Parasite* 1994; 1:391–392.

63. Mary C, Lamouroux D, Dunan S, et al. Western-blot analysis of antibodies to *Leishmania infantum* antigens: potential of the 14-kD and 16-kD antigens for diagnosis and epidemiologic purposes. *Am J Trop Med Hyg* 1992; 47:764–771.

64. Basset D, Faraut F, Marty P, et al. Visceral Leishmaniasis in organ transplant recipients: 11 new cases and a review of the literature. *Microbes Infect* 2005; 7:1370–1375.

65. Evans DA, Godfrey D, Lanham S, et al. *Handbook on Isolation, Characterization and Cryopreservation of Leishmania.* Geneva: World Health Organization; 1989.

66. Reithinger R, Dujardin JC. Molecular diagnosis of Leishmaniasis: current status and future applications. *J Clin Microbiol* 2007; 45:21–25.

67. Lachaud L, Dereure J, Chabbert E, et al. Optimized PCR using patient blood samples for diagnosis and follow-up of visceral Leishmaniasis, with special reference to AIDS patients. *J Clin Microbiol* 2000; 38:236–240.

68. Costa JM, Durand R, Deniau M, et al. PCR enzyme-linked immunosorbent assay for diagnosis of Leishmaniasis in human immunodeficiency virus-infected patients. *J Clin Microbiol* 1996; 34:1831–1833.

69. Riera C, Fisa R, Ribera E, et al. Value of culture and nested polymerase chain reaction of blood in the prediction of relapses in patients co-infected with *Leishmania* and human immunodeficiency virus. *Am J Trop Med Hyg* 2005; 73:1012–1015.

70. Cruz I, Chicharro C, Nieto J, et al. Comparison of new diagnostic tools for management of pediatric Mediterranean visceral Leishmaniasis. *J Clin Microbiol* 2006; 44:2343–2347.

71. Lopez M, Inga R, Cangalaya M, et al. Diagnosis of *Leishmania* using the polymerase chain reaction: a simplified procedure for field work. *Am J Trop Med Hyg* 1993; 49:348–356.

72. Pirmez C, Silva Trajano V, Paes-Oliveira Neto M, et al. Use of PCR in diagnosis of human American tegumentary Leishmaniasis in Rio de Janeiro, Brazil. *J Clin Microbiol* 1999; 37:1819–1823.

73. Vega-Lopez F. Diagnosis of cutaneous Leishmaniasis. *Curr Opin Infect Dis.* 2003; 16:97–101.

74. Lachaud L, Chabbert E, Dubessay P, et al. Value of two PCR methods for the diagnosis of canine visceral Leishmaniasis and the detection of asymptomatic carriers. *Parasitol* 2002; 125:197–207.

75. Mary C, Faraut F, Drogoul MP, et al. Reference values for *Leishmania infantum* parasitemia in different clinical presentations: quantitative polymerase chain reaction for therapeutic monitoring and patient follow-up. *Am J Trop Med Hyg* 2006; 75:858–863.

76. Kumar P, Pai K, Tripathi K, et al. Immunoblot analysis of the humoral immune response to *Leishmania donovani* polypeptides in cases of human visceral Leishmaniasis : its usefulness in prognosis. *Clin Diagn Lab Immunol* 2002; 9:1119–1123.

77. Attar ZJ, Chance ML, El-Safi S, et al. Latex agglutination test for the detection of urinary antigens in visceral Leishmaniasis. *Acta Trop* 2001; 78:11–16.

78. Montenegro J. A cutis reaçao na leishmaniose. *Ann Fac Med Sao Paulo* 1926; 1:323–330.

79. Herwaldt BL, Berman JD. Recommendations for treating Leishmaniasis with sodium stibogluconate (Pentostam®) and review of pertinent clinical studies. *Am J Trop Med Hyg* 1992; 46:296–306.

80. World Health Organization. *WHO Model Prescribing Information, Drugs Used in Parasitic Diseases.* Geneva: WHO; 1997.

81. Bern C, Adler-Moore J, Berenguer J, et al. Liposomal amphotericin B for the treatment of visceral Leishmaniasis. *Clin Infect Dis* 2006; 43:917–924.

82. Davidson RN, Di Martino L, Gradoni L, et al. Short-course treatment of visceral Leishmaniasis with liposomal amphotericin B (AmBisome). *Clin Infect Dis* 1996; 22:938–943.

83. Olliaro PL, Guerin PJ, Gerst S, et al. Treatment options for visceral Leishmaniasis: a systematic review of clinical studies done in India, 1980–2004. *Lancet Infect Dis* 2005; 5:763–774.

84. Sundar S, Jha TK, Thakur CP, et al. Single-dose liposomal amphotericin B in the treatment of visceral Leishmaniasis in India: a multicentric study. *Clin Infect Dis* 2003; 37:800–804.

85. Sundar S. Drug resistance in Indian visceral Leishmaniasis. *Trop Med Int Health* 2001; 6:849–854.

86. Davidson RN. Practical guide for the treatment of the Leishmaniases. *Drugs* 1998; 56:1009–1018.

87. Belazzoug S, Neal RA. Failure of meglumine antimoniate to cure cutaneous lesions due to *Leishmania major* in Algeria. *Trans R Soc Trop Med Hyg* 1986; 80:670–671.

88. Soto J, Arana BA, Toledo J, et al. Miltefosine for New World cutaneous Leishmaniasis. *Clin Infect Dis* 2004; 38:1266–1272.

89. Teklemariam S, Hiwot AG, Frommel D, et al. Aminosidine and its combination with sodium stibogluconate in the treatment of diffuse cutaneous Leishmaniasis caused by *Leishmania aethiopica*. *Trans R Soc Trop Med Hyg* 1994; 88:334–339.

90. Brown M, Noursadeghi M, Boyle J, et al. Successful liposomal amphotericin B treatment of *Leishmania braziliensis* cutaneous Leishmaniasis. *Br J Dermatol* 2005; 153:203–205.

91. Dedet JP, Melogno R, Cardenas F, et al. Rural campaign to diagnose and treat mucocutaneous Leishmaniasis in Bolivia. *Bull World Health Organ* 1995; 73:339–345.

92. World Health Organization. *Control of the* Leishmaniases. Report of a WHO Expert Committee. 1990 Technical Report Series 793.

93. Elnaiem DA, Elnahas AM, Aboud MA. Protective efficacy of lambdacyhalothrin-impregnated bednets against *Phlebotomus orientalis*, the vector of visceral Leishmaniasis in Sudan. *Med Vet Entomol* 1999; 13:310–314.

94. Modabber F. Vaccines against Leishmaniasis. *Ann Trop Med Parasitol* 1995; 89:83–88.

95. Esterre P, Chippaux JP, Lefait JF, et al. Evaluation d'un programme de lutte contre la leishmaniose cutanée dans un village forestier de Guyane française. *Bull World Health Organ* 1986; 64:559–565.

96. Ready PD, Lainson R, Shaw JJ. Leishmaniasis in Brazil. XX. Prevalence of 'enzootic rodent Leishmaniasis' (*Leishmania mexicana amazonensis*), and apparent absence of 'pian bois' (*Le. braziliensis guyanensis*), in plantations of introduced tree species and other non-climax forests in eastern Amazonia. *Trans R Soc Trop Med Hyg* 1983; 77:775–785.

97. Mukhopadhyay AK, Hati AK, Chakraborty S, et al. Effect of DDT on *Phlebotomus* sandflies in Kala-azar endemic foci in West Bengal. *J Commun Dis* 1996; 28:171–175.

98. Sanyal RK, Alam SN, Kaul SN, et al. Some observations of epidemic of current outbreaks of kala-azar in Bihar. *J Commun Dis* 1979; 11:170–182.

99. Guan LR. Current status of kala-azar and vector control in China. *Bull World Health Organ* 1991; 69:595–601.

100. Lacerda MM. The Brazilian Leishmaniasis control programme. *Mem Inst Oswaldo Cruz* 1994; 89:489–495.

101. Dye C. The logic of visceral Leishmaniasis control. *Am J Trop Med Hyg* 1996; 55:125–130.

102. Saf'janova V M. Leishmaniasis control. *Bull World Health Organ* 1971; 44:561–566.

103. Sanyal RK, Banjerjeeb DP, Ghosh TK, et al. A longitudinal review of kala-azar in Bihar. *J Commun Dis* 1979; 11:149–169.

104. Davies CR, Llanos-Cuentas A, Canales J, et al. The fall and rise of Andean cutaneous Leishmaniasis: transient impact of the DDT campaign in Peru. *Trans R Soc Trop Med Hyg* 1994; 88:389–393.

105. Alencar JE de. Profilaxia do calazar no Ceara, Brasil. *Rev Inst Med Trop Sao Paulo* 1961; 3:175–180.

106. Hertig M, Fairchild GB. The control of Phlebotomus in Peru with DDT. *Am J Med* 1947; 28:207–230.

107. Ready PD, Arias JR, Freitas RA. A pilot study to control *Lutzomyia umbratilis* (Diptera, Psychodidae), the major vector of *Leishmania braziliensis guyanensis*, in a peri-urban rainforest of Manaus, Amazonas State, Brazil. *Mem Inst Oswaldo Cruz* 1985; 80:27–36.

108. Joshi GC, Kaul SM, Wattal BL. Susceptibility of sandflies to organochlorine insecticides in Bihar, India: further report. *J Commun Dis* 1979; 11: 209–213.

Transmission of Toxoplasmosis

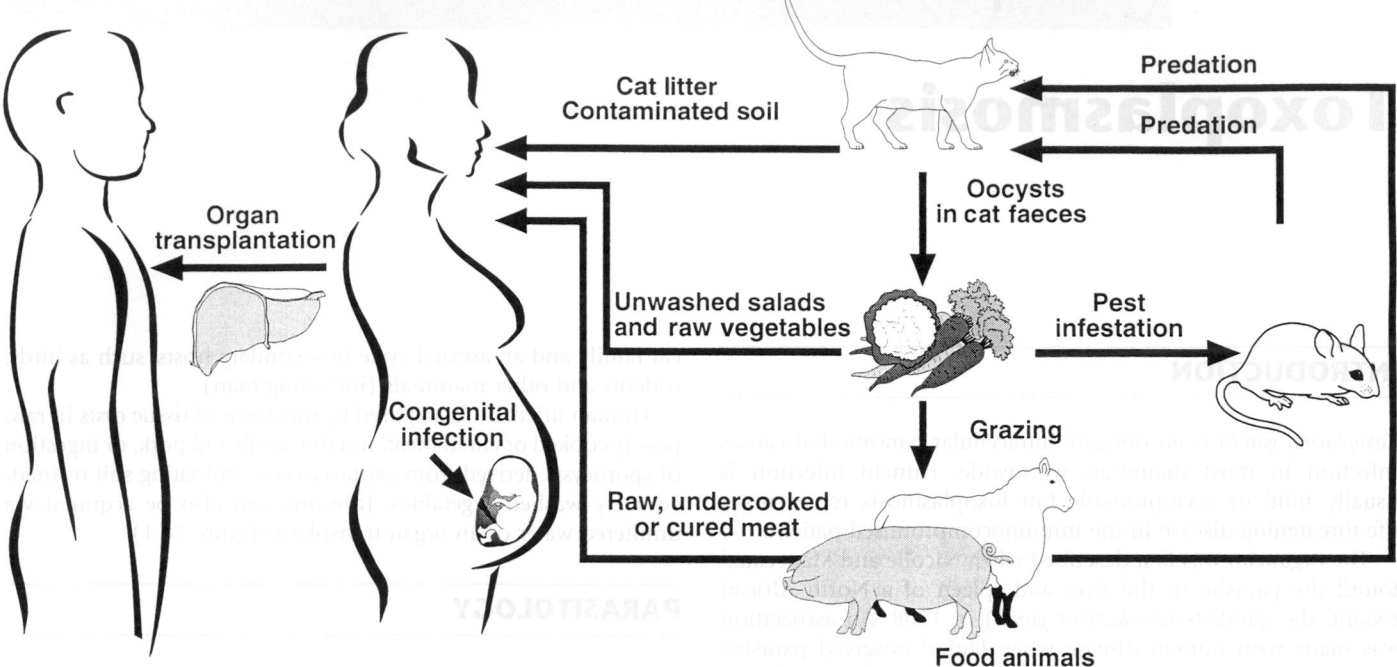

Figure 78.1 Transmission of toxoplasmosis.

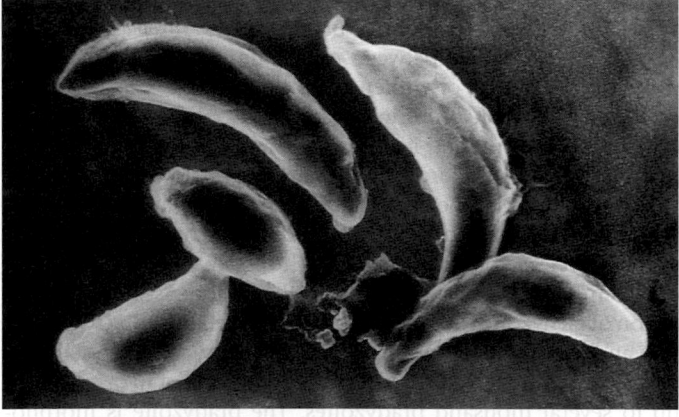

Figure 78.2 Trophozoites of *T. gondii* (scanning electron micrograph).

Eventually tissue cysts form, containing quiescent bradyzoites. Periodic excystation occurs, controlled by mechanisms which are not established. Release of toxoplasma results in cellular destruction due to invasion and disruption by tachyzoites as well as damage associated with the host immune response.

Immunity is predominantly cell mediated. Activated macrophages and T cells play a central role, while interferon-γ and other cytokines induce an effective immune response.[10] Specific antibody in the presence of complement eliminates extracellular parasites.

PATHOLOGY

Lesions observed at histopathological examination result from the dissemination of the parasite in the circulation, cytolytic action of the organism and the immune response of the host. Tissue necrosis is associated with thrombosis of small vessels.

Lymphadenopathy in the immunocompetent individual shows follicular hyperplasia and collections of mononuclear cells, usually at the periphery of the node. The normal tissue architecture is preserved and the parasites are rarely identified unless immunohistochemical stains are used.[11] The immunosuppressed patient, by contrast, may have abundant toxoplasma in the tissues. In cases of toxoplasmic encephalitis with the acquired immune deficiency syndrome (AIDS), cerebral tissues show central necrosis with surrounding astrocytosis. Pseudocysts are seen at the necrotic margins.[12] Necrosis, thrombosis and pseudocysts are present in the heart, liver, lung and brain of immunosuppressed patients with disseminated toxoplasmosis.

Congenital toxoplasmosis can be generalized or predominantly localized in the CNS. Brain tissue shows encephalitis with multiple infarcts and necrosis, particularly in the cortex, basal ganglia and periventricular areas. Characteristic glial nodules are formed. Focal calcification with zones of necrosis is present in severe disease of prolonged duration. Hydrocephalus results from obstruction of the aqueduct of *Sylvius* or cerebral tissue destruction.[13] The infected placenta has chronic inflammation in the decidua and focal reaction within the villi.[14] Infected ocular tissue shows destruction of areas of the retina, with proliferation of pigment at the borders of lesions during healing. Occasionally parasites may be seen at the margins.[15]

CLINICAL MANIFESTATIONS

The immunocompetent patient

In most cases of toxoplasmosis, the source of infection cannot be identified but the usual incubation period is between 1 and 3 weeks. The majority of individuals suffer no discernible illness and the acute infection passes unnoticed. The most common presentation of symptomatic toxoplasmosis is painless cervical lymphadenopathy, which may be accompanied by fever. Fewer persons experience generalized lymphadenopathy with malaise and myalgia which follows a course of relapse and remission over several weeks or months. The differential diagnosis includes lymphoma and infectious mononucleosis. Rarely, cutaneous rash, arthralgia, pericarditis or acute chorioretinitis may be associated with postnatal toxoplasma infection.[16] Some studies have suggested a link between hepatitis and toxoplasmosis but this remains contentious.[17]

Congenital infection

The incidence and presentation of acute toxoplasmosis in the pregnant woman does not differ from that in the population as a whole. Consequently, most infections pass unrecognized unless systematic screening is undertaken. The primary risk of congenital toxoplasmosis is associated with maternal parasitaemia and subsequent placentitis. As parasitaemia is normally limited to <20 days' duration, the greatest risk of fetal infection is associated with maternal infection acquired during pregnancy. A number of cases of congenital toxoplasmosis have been reported where the mother acquired the infection well before conception, but this is likely to be a rare event.[18] The rate of maternal–fetal transmission of infection rises as the gestational age at the time of maternal infection progresses. If left untreated, the risk of fetal infection is <15% when the mother acquires her infection during the first trimester, but over 60% if maternal infection is acquired in the third trimester. Conversely, the risk of severe fetal damage is highest if the infection crosses the placenta in early pregnancy.[19]

The features of congenital toxoplasmosis range from a severely damaged infant, with death in the perinatal period, to an infected but clinically unaffected child. Severe congenital toxoplasmosis presents with hydrocephalus, mental retardation, cerebral calcification and retinochoroiditis. Skin rash, hepatitis, pneumonia, myocarditis and myositis may be present.[20] Only 10% of all congenitally infected infants suffer such severe disease. Studies suggest some children born with congenital infection will develop ocular disease in later life, regardless of the clinical status at birth.[21]

Ocular toxoplasmosis

Most cases of ocular toxoplasmosis are thought to result from periodic reactivation of infection established in the prenatal period. However, some studies have proposed that most cases of ocular toxoplasmosis are associated with postnatal rather than congenital infection.[22] Excystation of the parasite is associated with acute inflammatory episodes and progressive retinal damage occurs. Retinal lesions may be apparent at birth but most often present as late sequelae in the second and third decades of life. Severe congenital disease is associated with microphthalmia, cataract, strabismus and nystagmus. The characteristic lesion is that of necrotizing retinitis, which appears as yellow-white 'cotton-wool' patches in the fundus during acute episodes. The lesions appear 'punched out' and pigmented when quiescent. The degree of visual disturbance depends on the location of the lesions within the retina. In the adult, acute ocular toxoplasmosis presents with sudden onset blurring of vision. An indistinct retinal lesion may be seen through a vitreous haze, the 'headlight in the fog' sign. The differential diagnosis of ocular toxoplasmosis includes: colobomatous defect, intraocular haemorrhage, defects of retinal blood vessels, retinoblastoma and glioma.[23]

Toxoplasmosis and AIDS

In the absence of effective antiviral therapy, toxoplasmosis is the most common cause of focal brain lesions and one of the most frequent opportunistic infections in patients with AIDS. Most cases result from secondary reactivation of a chronic, previously quiescent infection associated with impairment of the individual's immune function. Features of cerebral infection predominate and the characteristic presentation is that of fever, persistent headache, deterioration of mental status and focal neurological signs. Retinochoroiditis, following extension of CNS infection, and pulmonary disease (presenting with cough and dyspnoea) are also described. Disseminated infection involving the heart, liver, CNS and lungs may be found at postmortem.[24,25] The differential diagnosis of cerebral toxoplasmosis with AIDS includes lymphoma, cryptococcal infection and bacterial brain abscess. Human immunodeficiency virus (HIV)-infected patients with residual cell-mediated immune function (pre-AIDS) may present with an indolent illness comprising malaise, chronic headache and lymphadenopathy, usually associated with primary toxoplasma infection.

Toxoplasmosis and organ transplantation

Toxoplasmosis represents a life-threatening complication to organ graft recipients. Severe toxoplasma infection in association with solid organ transplantation (heart, heart–lung, liver and kidney) is restricted to the recipient without pre-existing immunity to toxoplasma (seronegative) who is given an organ containing viable cysts of the parasite (seropositive donor). The frequency of infection in such 'mismatches' reflects the likelihood of the organ transplant containing cysts. Consequently, infection is most frequent after cardiac transplant and least common in association with renal transplantation. The infected recipient develops fever, deterioration of consciousness and signs of respiratory failure, reflecting disseminated disease, usually 3–6 weeks after the operation.[26] Such complications are effectively prevented by routine co-trimoxazole prophylaxis for solid organ graft recipients.

As the duration of parasitaemia following acute infection is limited, blood transfusion will rarely transmit toxoplasmosis. The risk is greater after granulocyte transfusion. Toxoplasmosis associated with bone marrow transplant is a rare event and is usually due to reactivation of the recipient's previously quiescent, chronic infection. Fever, CNS signs and pulmonary dysfunction are characteristic findings 15–150 days after transplantation. Overall mortality is 80%.[27]

Other associations

A number of studies have shown an association between human behaviour,[28] schizophrenia[29] and toxoplasma infection. It is not established if these represent a causal effect or if parasite specific therapy is of benefit.

DIAGNOSIS

In most instances, the non-specific nature of the signs and symptoms of toxoplasmosis does not permit reliable diagnosis based solely on the clinical findings. Due to the diversity of toxoplasma infection, investigations must be selected which are appropriate to that patient group.[30] Suitable test selections are given in Table 78.1.

Isolation

T. gondii can be isolated from infected tissues by animal inoculation or tissue culture. Intraperitoneal injection into mice is a highly sensitive diagnostic method but results are only available 3–6 weeks after inoculation. Tissue culture is less sensitive but produces a result within 10 days.

Parasite detection

Histological examination can be helpful, particularly following excision of enlarged lymph nodes or biopsy of a cerebral lesion in AIDS. The sensitivity of these investigations is improved if immunohistochemical studies are employed. A number of antigen detection methods have been developed utilizing enzyme-linked immunosorbent assay (ELISA) and agglutination systems. Antigen detection is most valuable when investigating the immunocompromised where the serological response is altered. The limitation of antigen detection has been the relative lack of sensitivity of the assay. Methods based on the detection of toxoplasma DNA by hybridization with specific probes or amplification using the polymerase chain reaction represent a considerable advance,[31] particularly when applied to testing amniotic fluid in suspected toxoplasmosis during pregnancy.[32]

Serology

A wide range of antibody detection methods are available and serology is often the investigation of choice. T. gondii contains a large number of membranous and cytoplasmic antigens which are incorporated into the different serological assays in variable proportions. It is not possible to compare antibody levels recorded by different tests. Whole organisms are used as the antigen source in the dye test, direct agglutination test and fluorescent antibody assay. Disrupted organisms are fixed to carrier particles in the indirect haemagglutination test and latex agglutination test and provide the antigen source for ELISA-based systems.[30]

Table 78.1 Investigation of toxoplasmosis

	Parasite isolation	Histology	Parasite detection	Serology	Other
IMMUNOCOMPETENT PATIENT					
Lymphadenopathy	–	Excision biopsy	–	IgG, IgM	–
Pregnancy	–	–	Amniotic fluid	IgG, IgM, IgA, avidity tests	–
Ocular disease	–	–	Ocular fluid	IgG, local antibody production	–
IMMUNOSUPPRESSED PATIENT					
Fetus	Amniotic fluid, blood cells	–	Amniotic fluid, blood cells	IgM, IgA	Total IgM, liver function tests
Neonate	Placenta, blood cells	–	Blood cells	Sequential IgG assessment, Western blot, IgM, IgA	Radiology of brain, ocular examination
AIDS	Brain biopsy	Brain biopsy	Brain biopsy	IgG	Radiology of brain, therapeutic trial
ORGAN TRANSPLANT					
Heart, lung, liver, kidney	Tissue biopsy, bone marrow	Tissue biopsy	–	IgG, IgM	–
Bone marrow	Bone marrow, blood cells	–	Bone marrow	–	Therapeutic trial

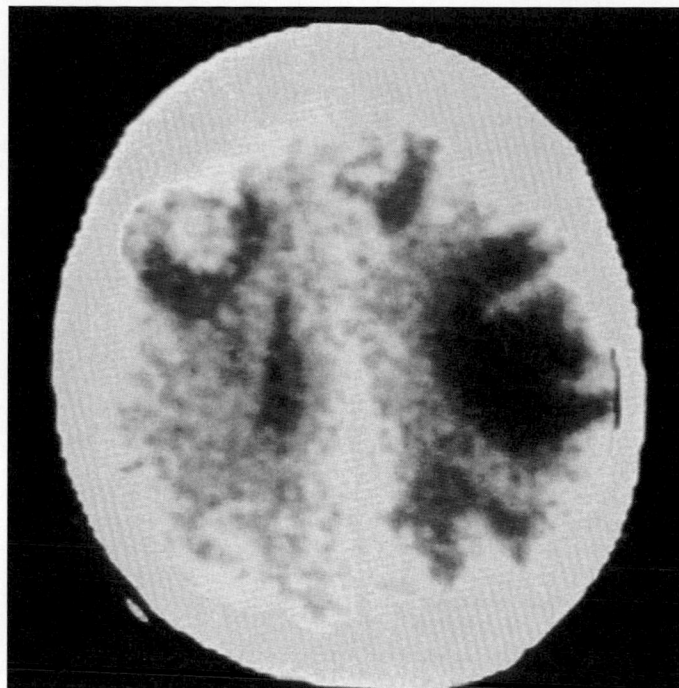

Figure 78.3 Computed tomography of the brain in cerebral toxoplasmosis associated with AIDS.

The presence of specific IgG indicates prior exposure to the parasite and the potential for reactivation in the immunocompromised. Specific IgM, IgA or low-avidity IgG is associated with more recent infection of the immunocompetent individual. The dye test remains the 'gold standard' test and the availability of this bioassay has been increased by the production of tachyzoites in tissue culture.

Other methods

Cell-mediated immunity can be measured by a skin test or in vitro assays but has limited clinical applications. Computed tomography of the brain is useful in the investigation of patients with congenital toxoplasmosis and AIDS (Figure 78.3). Therapeutic trials of antiparasite drugs may be required to confirm the diagnosis of toxoplasmosis in the profoundly immunosuppressed.[24]

MANAGEMENT

None of the agents currently available for clinical use shows activity against the encysted form of the parasite. Consequently, treatment is directed against the active tachyzoite form and complete eradication of the parasite is not attempted.[6,33]

Immunocompetent patients

Specific therapy has not been shown to be effective in otherwise healthy individuals and is rarely indicated in view of the potential toxicity of antitoxoplasma agents. Therapy may be considered when the illness is protracted or unusually severe. Sulfadiazine (2 g/day) with pyrimethamine (25 mg/day) is given by the oral route. Sulfadimidine may be substituted for sulfadiazine. Vitamin supplementation consisting of folinic acid (15 mg twice weekly) or yeast tablets BPC (8 tablets twice weekly) is given to prevent bone marrow toxicity.[34] Increasingly, azithromycin (3 g/day for 10 days) is used to avoid sulfonamide toxicity.

The pregnant woman

The macrolide antibiotic spiramycin should be given at a dose of 3 g/day throughout the confinement in an attempt to reduce the risk of transplacental passage of the parasite. If fetal infection is confirmed by amniocentesis or ultrasound investigation, antiparasite therapy is given to reduce the severity of congenital disease. Sulfadiazine (50–100 mg/kg per day)–pyrimethamine (0.5–1.0 mg/kg per day) with vitamin supplement is given for 3 weeks, followed by a further 3 weeks' therapy consisting of spiramycin (3 g/day). Alternating 3 weeks' drug courses are given until delivery.[6] However, the clinical benefits of this approach are uncertain.[35]

Congenital infection

All infected infants are given specific therapy until the age of 1 year, irrespective of the severity of the disease. Rotating 3-week courses of sulfadiazine with pyrimethamine and folinic acid (doses as for the pregnant woman) followed by spiramycin (100 mg/kg per day) are given.[6,36] The role of corticosteroids is not fully established but these are often given when ventricular dilatation is noted.

Ocular disease

Quiescent lesions recognized beyond the age of 1 year require observation only. When active inflammation is noted sulfadiazine (2 g/day) or clindamycin (1.2 g/day) given with pyrimethamine (25 mg/day) and vitamin supplementation is advised. Treatment is continued for 10 days after inflammation subsides. Systemic corticosteroids are usually administered during the antiparasite therapy. However, clinical practice varies widely and there is no consensus of optimal management.[37] Laser or cryotherapy was previously used in an attempt to limit the spread of a lesion across the retina but this approach has been shown to be ineffective.[38]

Toxoplasmosis with AIDS

Acute therapy comprises sulfadiazine (4–8 g/day)–pyrimethamine 50–75 g/day) with vitamin supplements continued for 6 weeks. Clindamycin (2.4–4.8 g/day) can be substituted if severe sulfonamide toxicity is experienced. Reduced dose maintenance therapy may be given after an acute episode to prevent relapse while the CD4 count remains low.[25]

Organ transplant recipients

Seronegative recipients of a seropositive heart, heart–lung or liver donor should be given pyrimethamine (25 mg/day) prophylaxis for 6 weeks after the operation to prevent primary infection.[39]

When significant disease is established in any organ graft recipient high-dose therapy, similar to that given in AIDS, is indicated. Maintenance therapy is not required unless the period of immunosuppression is likely to be prolonged.

PREVENTION AND CONTROL

Health education

Women contemplating pregnancy or shown to be seronegative after conception should be offered guidance to reduce the risk of acquiring toxoplasmosis during pregnancy. Foods eaten without further preparation, such as vegetables and fruit, should be washed to remove contaminating soil and sporocysts. Gloves should be worn when gardening or emptying cat litter trays. Meats that might contain tissue cysts should be cooked until 'well done' and handwashing after preparing raw meat should be emphasized.[40] Similar advice can be given to HIV-infected individuals.

Previously, deliberate exposure to the parasite prior to puberty was encouraged in some areas by the habit of eating raw meat. This practice is no longer considered ethical due to the risk of reactivated infection should the individual later become immunosuppressed.

Vaccination

Short-lived immunity can be induced when using non-viable toxoplasma, while viable organisms of reduced pathogenicity are associated with chronic infection and potential reactivation.[41] A non-cyst-forming strain of *T. gondii* is available for sheep[42] but there is presently no vaccine suitable for humans.

Antenatal screening

Any screening programme should be evaluated in four main areas: frequency and severity of the disease; sensitivity, specificity, performance and cost of diagnosis; effectiveness of management; administrative structure.[43] In France, a programme based on IgG seroconversion is in operation and similar schemes have been promoted in other countries.[44] Further research is required to establish the harm : benefit ratio of screening for toxoplasmosis in pregnancy before the diversion of scarce funds from other health projects can be justified.

REFERENCES

1. Nicolle C, Manceaux L. Sur une infection à corps de leishman (où organisme voisins) du gondii. *CR Acad Sci* 1908; 147: 763–766.
2. Janků J. Pathogensa a pathologiká anatomie tak nazvaného vrozeného kolobomu zluté skurny v oku normálne velikém a mikrophthalmickém s nálezem parazitu v sítnici. *Cas Lék Ces* 1923; 62:1021–1027.
3. Wolf A, Cowen D. Granulomatous encephalomyelitis due to an encephalitozoan (encephalitozoic encephalomyelitis): a new protozoan disease of man. *Bull Neurol Inst NY* 1937; 6:306–371.
4. Pinkerton H, Weinman D. Toxoplasma infection in man. *Arch Pathol* 1940; 30:374–392.
5. Sabin AB, Feldman HA. Dyes as microchemical indicators of a new immunity phenomenon affecting a protozoan parasite. *Science* 1948; 108: 660–663.
6. Montoya JG, Liesenfeld O. Toxoplasmosis. *Lancet* 2004; 363:1965–1976.
7. Cook AJ, Gilbert RE, Buffolano W, et al. Sources of toxoplasma infection in pregnant women: European multicentre case-control study. *BMJ* 2000; 321:142–147.
8. Grigg ME, Bonnefoy S, Hehl AB, et al. Success and virulence in toxoplasma as the result of sexual recombination between two distinct ancestries. *Science* 2001; 294:161–165.
9. Joiner K. Cell attachment and entry by Toxoplasma gondii. *Behring Inst Mitt* 1991; 88:20–26.
10. Suzuki Y, Orellana MA, Schreiber RD, et al. Interferon gamma, the major mediator of resistance against Toxoplasma gondii. *Science* 1988; 240: 516–518.
11. Eapen M, Mathyew CF, Aravindan KP. Evidence based criteria for the histopathological diagnosis of toxoplasmic lymphadenopathy. *J Clin Pathol* 2005; 58:1143–1146.
12. Falangola MF, Reichler BD, Petito CK. Histopathology of cerebral toxoplasmosis in human immunodeficiency virus infection: a comparison between patients with early-onset and late-onset acquired immunodeficiency syndrome. *Hum Pathol* 1994; 25:1091–1097.
13. Frenkel JK. Toxoplasma: mechanisms of infection, laboratory diagnosis and management. *Curr Top Pathol* 1971; 54:27–75.
14. Elliot WG. Placental toxoplasmosis: report of a case. *Am J Clin Pathol* 1970; 53:413–417.
15. Roberts F, Mets MB, Ferguson DJ, et al. Histopathological features of ocular toxoplasmosis in the fetus and infant. *Arch Ophthalmol* 2001; 119:51–58.
16. Kean BH. Clinical toxoplasmosis – 50 years. *Trans R Soc Trop Med Hyg* 1972; 66:549–571.
17. Dogan N, Kabukcuoglu S, Vardareli E. Toxoplasmic hepatitis in an immunocompetent patient. *Turkiye Parazitoloji Dergisi* 2007; 31:260–263.
18. Holliman RE. Clinical sequelae of chronic maternal toxoplasmosis. *Rev Med Microbiol* 1994; 5:47–55.
19. Dunn D, Wallon M, Peyron F, et al. Mother-to-child transmission of toxoplasmosis: risk estimates for clinical counselling. *Lancet* 1999; 353: 1829–1833.
20. Safadi MA, Berezin EN, Farhat CK, et al. Clinical presentation and follow up of children with congenital toxoplasmosis in Brazil. *Braz J infect Dis* 2003; 7:325–331.
21. Koppe JG, Loewer-Sieger DH, de Roever-Bonnet H. Results of 20 year follow-up of congenital toxoplasmosis. *Lancet* 1986; 1:254–255.
22. Gilbert RE, Stranford M. Is ocular toxoplasmosis caused by prenatal or postnatal infection? *Br J Ophthalmol* 2000; 84:224–226.
23. de Jong PT. Ocular toxoplasmosis: common and rare symptoms and signs. *Int Ophthalmol* 1989; 13:391–397.
24. Holliman RE. Toxoplasmosis and the acquired immune deficiency syndrome. *J Infect* 1988; 16:121–128.
25. Nissapatorn V, Quek KF, Leong CL, et al. Toxoplasmosis in HIV/AIDS patients: a current situation. *Jpn J Infect Dis* 2004; 57:160–165.
26. Wreghitt TG, Hakim M, Gray JJ, et al. Toxoplasmosis in heart and heart and lung transplant recipients. *J Clin Pathol* 1989; 42:194–199.
27. Mele A, Paterson PJ, Prentice HG, et al. Toxoplasmosis in bone marrow transplantation: A report of two cases and systematic review of the literature. *Bone Marrow Transplant* 2002; 29:691–698.
28. Flegr J, Zitkova S, Kodym P, et al. Introduction of changes in human behaviour by the parasitic protozoan Toxoplasma gondii. *Parasitol* 1996; 113:49–54.
29. Torrey EF, Yolken RH. Toxoplasma gondii and schizophrenia. *Emerg Infect Dis* 2003; 9:1375–1379.
30. Holliman RE. The diagnosis of toxoplasmosis. *Serodiagn Immunother Infect Dis* 1990; 4:83–93.

31. Savva D, Morris JC, Johnson JD, et al. Polymerase chain reaction for detection of Toxoplasma gondii. *J Med Microbiol* 1990; 32:25–31.

32. Filisetti D, Gorcii M, Pernot-Marino E, et al. Diagnosis of congenital toxoplasmosis: comparison of targets for detection of toxoplasma gondii by PCR. *J Clin Microbiol* 2003; 41:4826–4828.

33. McCabe RE, Oster S. Current recommendations and future prospects in the treatment of toxoplasmosis. *Drugs* 1989; 38:973–987.

34. Krick JA, Remington JS. Toxoplasmosis in the adult: an overview. *N Engl J Med* 1978; 298:550–553.

35. Gilbert R, Gras L. Effect of timing and type of treatment on the risk of mother to child transmission of Toxoplasma gondii. *Br J Obstet Gynaecol* 2003; 110:112–120.

36. Holliman RE. Uncommon infections: toxoplasmosis, toxocariasis and cryptosporidiosis. *Prescribers J* 1992; 32:127–132.

37. Holland GN, Lewis KG. An update on current practices in the management of ocular toxoplasmosis. *Am J Ophthalmol* 2002; 134:102–114.

38. Desmettre T, Labalette P, Fortier B, et al. Laser photocoagulation around the foci of toxoplasma retinochoroiditis: a descriptive statistical analysis of 35 patients with long-term follow-up. *Ophthalmologia* 1996; 210:90–94.

39. Holliman RE, Johnson JD, Adams S, et al. Toxoplasmosis and heart transplantation. *J Heart Lung Transplant* 1991; 10:608–610.

40. Carter AO, Gelmon SB, Wells GA, et al. The effectiveness of a prenatal education programme for the prevention of congenital toxoplasmosis. *Epidemiol Infect* 1989; 103:539–545.

41. Bhopale GM. Development of a vaccine for toxoplasmosis: current status. *Microbes Infect* 2003; 5:457–462.

42. Buxton D, Innes EA. A commercial vaccine for ovine toxoplasmosis. *Parasitology* 1995; 110:S11–S16.

43. Wilson JM, Junger G. Principles and practice of screening for disease. *Public Health Papers No. 34*. WHO: Geneva; 1968.

44. McCabe RE, Remington JS. Toxoplasmosis: the time has come. *N Engl J Med* 1988; 318:313–315.

E. dysenteriae for the pathogenic amoeba and *E. dispar* for the non-pathogenic amoeba. Because Brumpt was unable to distinguish morphologically between the two proposed species and because there was growing evidence that cysts obtained from asymptomatic carriers could produce experimental infection, his explanation gained little support. It regained favour only after Sargeaunt and associates[8,9] were able to distinguish pathogenic strains of *E. histolytica* from non-pathogenic strains on the basis of isoenzyme typing. Since then, many other markers that allow the discrimination between both groups have been identified. In 1993, Diamond and Clark,[10] using all the biochemical, immunological and genetic evidence for distinguishing pathogenic from non-pathogenic strains of *E. histolytica*, redescribed *E. histolytica* Schaudinn, 1903, formally separating it from *E. dispar* Brumpt, 1925. In 1997, a World Health Organization (WHO) expert committee met in Mexico City and endorsed the separation of pathogenic and non-pathogenic strains into two separate species.[11,12]

The organism

Taxonomy

The systematics of amoeboid eukaryotes is in a state of flux. *E. histolytica* was considered by some authors to be an early branching of the eukaryotic lineage, as it appeared to lack mitochondria, peroxisomes, rough endoplasmic reticulum and Golgi system, and has an unusual glycolytic metabolism. Many of these features are shared with other amitochondriate protists known as Archezoa.[13] However, small-subunit ribosomal RNA-based phylogenetic trees placed *E. histolytica* in a branch that arises more recently than several lineages with typical eukaryotic organelles and metabolism.[13,14] The demonstration that *E. histolytica* has a cryptic organelle that corresponds to a rudimentary mitochondrion[15,16] and the identification of genes involved in vesicular transport[17] have seriously undermined the hypothesis that Entamoeba represent early branching eukaryotes. In 1998, Cavalier-Smith revised the position of *E. histolytica* and placed it in the kingdom Protozoa, sub-kingdom Neozoa, infra-kingdom Sarcomastigota, phylum Amoebozoa, sub-phylum Conosa.[18] The species formerly termed *Entamoeba histolytica* should now be broken down into *E. histolytica* and *E. dispar*, the latter being non-pathogenic.

Structure

The trophozoite is distinguished from other intestinal amoebae by morphological characteristics of diagnostic importance. It ranges in size from 20 to 40 mm. Two zones can be recognized within the cytoplasm: an outer zone, or ectoplasm, and an inner zone, or endoplasm. The ectoplasm is clear, refractive and sharply separated from the endoplasm. The endoplasm contains abundant vesicles embedded in a cytoplasmic matrix, which gives them the appearance of ground glass. The cytoplasmic vesicles sometimes contain ingested red blood cells in various stage of disintegration. Using DNA-specific stains it is possible to identify a small spherical DNA-containing body 1–2 μm in size that corresponds to rudimentary mitochondria.[19] Ribosomes appear to be ordered in helical arrays. The cytoskeleton is characterized by microfilaments, generally found immediately below the plasma membrane at the sites of attachment of the amoeba to the substrate and where phagocytic channels are formed. The nucleus is not usually visible, although it may be faintly discerned as a finely granular ring in the unstained amoeba. When stained with haematoxylin, trichrome or Lawless stain, details of nuclear structure may be observed. The nucleus is spherical and 4–7 mm in diameter. The nuclear membrane is clearly defined; its inner surface is lined with uniform and closely packed fine granules of chromatin. In the centre of the nucleus is a small mass of chromatin, the karyosome. A clear halo surrounding the karyosome and a 'linin' network giving a 'cartwheel' appearance has been described, but these probably represent fixation artefacts. The presence of a rough endoplasmic reticulum or Golgi system has not been demonstrated. However, the presence of genes encoding proteins involved in vesicular transport and translational machinery suggest that functional equivalents may exist.[17]

In fresh isolates, *E. histolytica* can move as fast as 5 mm/s. Trophozoites move by means of pseudopodia, cytoplasmic protrusions that may be formed at any point on the surface of the organism. Actively moving trophozoites have a well-defined morphological polarity. The clear glass-like ectoplasm flows out to form the pseudopodium, slowly followed by the more granular endoplasm as the amoeba moves in the direction in which it was extruded. The pseudopodial extension is accompanied by recycling of the cytoplasm and the formation of a posterior appendix, commonly referred to as the uroid. The uroid accumulates capped ligands as bacteria, lectins or antibodies and, by an unknown mechanism, is detached from the amoeba without damaging the parasite.

The precyst amoebae are colourless, round or oval cells that are smaller than the trophozoite but larger than the cyst. They may be distinguished by a rounded single nucleus, absence of ingested material and lack of a cyst wall. The cytoplasm usually contains deposits of diffuse glycogen and, occasionally, chromatoid bodies are seen. The nuclear morphology is often confusing at this stage and it is best to rely upon either trophozoites or cysts for specific identification.

The cysts are round or oval, slightly asymmetrical hyaline bodies, 10–16 mm in diameter, with a smooth, refractive, non-staining wall about 0.5 mm thick. The immature cyst has a single nucleus, about one-third of its diameter, whereas the mature infective cyst contains four smaller nuclei, rarely more. The nuclei may at times appear as small refractive spheres within the cytoplasm of the unstained cyst, but more often they are not visible. The cytoplasm of the young cysts contains vacuoles with glycogen and chromatoid bodies. These chromatoid bodies, so named because they stain with haematoxylin like the chromatin of the nucleus, are reported to contain ribonucleic and deoxyribonucleic acids and phosphates, and tend to disappear as the cyst matures, so that they may be absent in about half of the cysts. When stained with iodine, the cytoplasm of the cyst will be yellow-green to yellow-brown in colour; the nuclear membrane and karyosome are distinct and light brown. Chromatoidal bars do not stain and appear as clear spaces in the cytoplasm. If glycogen is present in the cytoplasm, it will stain a dark yellow-brown.

Microbiology

The main reservoir of *E. histolytica* is the human, although morphologically similar amoebae may be found in primates, dogs and cats. The complete life cycle of *E. histolytica* consists of four consecutive stages: the trophozoite, precyst, cyst and metacyst. The cyst is resistant to gastric acid, and on ingestion it passes into the small intestine. The amoeba within the cyst becomes active in the neutral or alkaline environment of the small intestine. The cyst wall is digested, probably by the digestive enzymes within the lumen of the gut. The encysted amoeba becomes very active and each of the four nuclei in the emerging E. histolytica undergoes one round of division, thus forming eight amoebae, smaller than the trophozoites seen in the colon, from a single cyst. They are carried into the caecum where they complete their maturation. They multiply by binary fission, the nucleus dividing by modified mitosis. As the amoebae pass down the colon they become dehydrated and assume a spherical shape known as a precyst. A thin cyst wall is secreted, forming an unripe cyst. Two mitotic divisions occur, resulting in a cyst that contains four nuclei. They are evacuated in the stool and discharged into the environment. Cysts remain viable and infective for several days in faeces and water, but are easily killed by desiccation.

Diamond's[20] medium allows the cultivation of E. histolytica without bacteria or other living organisms (i.e. axenically). Optimal growth occurs at 35–37°C, at pH 7.0, and under reduced oxygen tension.

Metabolism

Carbohydrates are the main source of energy for the parasite. The uptake of glucose involves a specific transport system that provides approximately 100 times the amount incorporated by endocytosis. Glucose is degraded to pyruvate via the Embden–Meyerhof pathway. The principal end-products of the anaerobic carbohydrate metabolism are ethanol and carbon dioxide; lactate is not produced and lactate dehydrogenase has not been reported. In many of the glycolytic reactions inorganic pyrophosphate, rather

than adenosine triphosphate (ATP), is used as an energy source. Amoeba are obligate fermenters that lack pyruvate dehydrogenase and the enzymes for oxidative phosphorylation and Krebs cycle.[21] The fermentation enzymes include the pyruvate: ferredoxin oxidoreductase, ferredoxin and alcohol dehydrogenase, which are most similar to the equivalent enzymes in anaerobic bacteria.[22] Alcohol dehydrogenase and ferredoxin are found throughout the cytosol.[15] In contrast, pyruvate:ferredoxin oxidoreductase is located in the plasma membrane and in a cytoplasmic structure that most likely corresponds to the rudimentary mitochondria.[23]

Synthesis of nucleic acids depends on the salvage of preformed purines as E. histolytica lacks a de novo purine pathway. It is also able to salvage pyrimidine bases, although it is able to synthesize them de novo.

Genetics

E. histolytica has been sequenced to completion (http://pathema. tigr.org). The genome is 20.6 Mb in size, 51% coding, and it includes 8197 genes. The total genome G + C content is low (about 24%), with a G + C content of coding regions approximately 33% higher. Several copies of ribosomal DNA (rDNA) are present as extrachromosomal circular elements, but their functional significance is unknown.

The first widely used system to characterize E. histolytica strains was based on the migration of six isoenzymes (hexokinase, phosphoglucomutase, aldolase, acetylglucosaminidase, peptidase and nicotinamide-adenine dinucleotide (NAD) diaphorase). It allowed workers to divide E. histolytica into two distinct groups: pathogenic and non-pathogenic (Figure 79.1).[8] Since then other typing systems have been introduced, including a polymerase chain reaction (PCR)-based system based on repeats in the tRNA genes.[24]

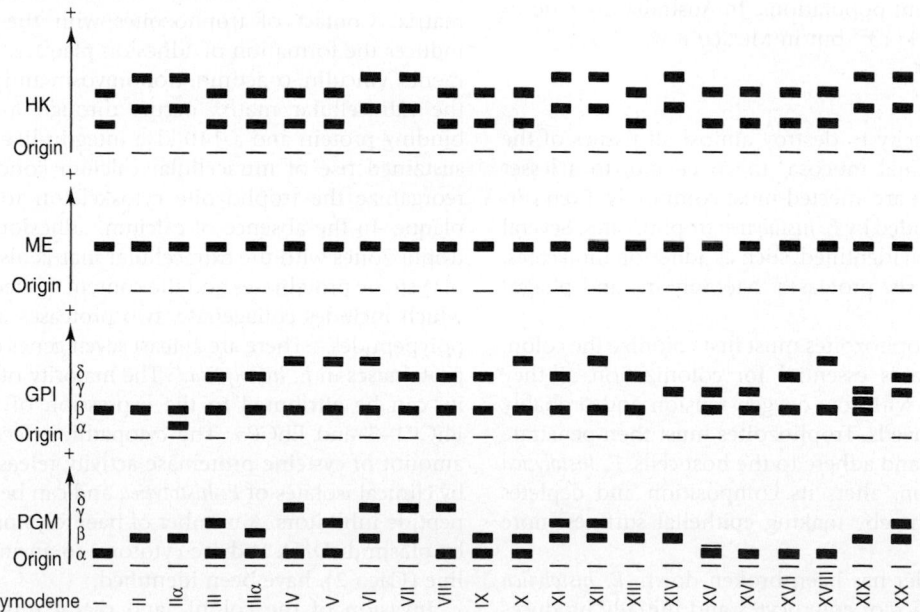

Figure 79.1 Zymodemes of E. histolytica identified by using GPI (EC 5.3.1.9), L-malate:NADP⁺ oxidoreductase (ME; oxaloacetate decarboxylating) (EC 1.1.1.4.0), PGM (EC 2.7.5.1) and HK (EC 2.7.1.1). Pathogenic zymodemes include II, IIa, VI,VII, XI, XII, XIII, XIV, XIX and XX. Non-pathogenic zymodemes include I, III, IIIa, IV, V, VIII, IX, X, XV, XVI, XVII, XVIII and (not shown) XXI. (From Bruckner D. A. Amebiasis. Clin Microbiol Rev 1992; 5:356–369.)

Epidemiology

E. histolytica has a worldwide distribution and is endemic in most countries with low socioeconomic conditions. Before the separation of the 'non-pathogenic strains' into a different species, it was estimated that approximately 480 million people, or 12% of the world's population, were infected and 40 000–110 000 persons died anually.[25] In endemic areas, it is now clear that *E. dispar* is the more prevalent species, by a ratio of up to 10 : 1. The risk of asymptomatic carriers of *E. histolytica* developing invasive disease is estimated at about 10%.[26] In Europe and North America, where invasive amoebiasis is rare, almost all infections previously ascribed to *E. histolytica* were in fact due to *E. dispar*. When these data are taken into account, it is more likely that only 10% of the 480 million infections (approximately 48 million people) are infected with *E. histolytica*, whereas the rest have infections with *E. dispar*.

Infection occurs via the faecal–oral route, food and drink becoming contaminated through exposure to human faeces. Food-borne outbreaks of disease are due to insanitary handling of food and its preparation by infected individuals. Therefore, it is not surprising that prevalence is high in places where human faeces are used for fertilizer. Cyst carriers are the main reservoir of infection. Epidemics occur when raw sewage contaminates water supplies. Sexual transmission also occurs. Recognized high-risk groups include travellers, immigrants, migrant workers, immunocompromised individuals, individuals in mental institutions, prisons and, possibly, children in day-care centres. Severe infections occur in very young children, pregnant women, the malnourished and individuals taking corticosteroids. Patients with AIDS do not have an increased risk of severe infection. Recent attempts to re-write the epidemiology of amoebiasis, using molecular tools to distinguish *E. histolytica* from *E. dispar*, suggest that generalizations will be difficult and the relative frequency of these two amoebic infections will differ in different populations. In Australia the ratio of histolytica to dispar was 1 : 13[27] but in Mexico it was 1.5 : 1.[28]

Pathogenesis

E. histolytica has the capacity to destroy almost all tissues of the human body. The intestinal mucosa, the liver and, to a lesser extent, the brain and skin are affected most commonly. Even cartilage and bone can be eroded by *E. histolytica* trophozoites. Several virulence factors have been identified, such as adhesion molecules, contact-dependent cytolysis, proteases, haemolysins and phagocytic activity.

To produce damage, trophozoites must first colonize the colon. The presence of bacteria is essential for colonization as they provide an environment with low oxygen tension and probably supply other metabolic needs. Trophozoites must then penetrate through the mucus layer and adhere to the host cells. *E. histolytica* enhances mucus secretion, alters its composition and depletes goblet cells of mucin, thereby making epithelial surfaces more vulnerable to invasion.

Once the mucus barrier has been broken down, *E. histolytica* reaches the luminal surface of enterocytes and initially produces a contact-dependent focal and superficial epithelial erosion. Trophozoites adhere to colonic mucins and host cells through the N-acetyl-D-galactosamine-inhibitable lectin, a 260-kDa protein also known as the Gal/GalNAc adherence lectin, composed of a

170-kDa and a 35/31-kDa subunit. The 170-kDa subunit is immunologically similar to the integrins.[29] Other molecules are involved in adhesion including a 220-kDa lectin, a 112-kDa adhesin and a surface lipophosphoglycan.

Although there is evidence to suggest that *E. histolytica* can induce apoptosis of host cells,[30] cell damage is primarily contact dependent. The Gal/GalNAc adherence lectin is not directly cytotoxic but it is required for cytolysis as target cell lysis is reduced in the presence of galactose. Furthermore, a monoclonal antibody against the heavy subunit is capable of partially inhibiting cytolysis without blocking adherence. It has been suggested that cell lysis is produced through the channel-forming peptides of *E. histolytica* (amoebapores). Three isoforms have been identified, amoebapores A, B and C, which are present in a ratio of 35 : 10 : 1, with the genes showing 35–57% deduced amino acid sequence identity. Their structure is now known.[31] Like other pore-forming peptides, amoebapores are readily soluble but are capable of changing rapidly into a membrane-inserted stage. Oligomerization occurs by formation of a channel through the plasma membrane, allowing the passage of water, ions and other small molecules, and thus lysing the target cell. Amoebapore C seems to be the most effective, while amoebapore A is not efficient in lysing erythrocytes. Amoebapores are found in cytoplasmic vesicles and show maximum activity in acidic pH, which is consistent with previous observations that lysis of target cells by *E. histolytica* required a pH of 5.0 within amoebic vesicles. In spite of all the advances in the characterization of amoebapores, their participation in the cytolytic event produced by *E. histolytica* has not yet been demonstrated. Amoebapores are not spontaneously secreted from viable trophozoites. The presence of pore-forming activity in the non-pathogenic *E. dispar*, although 60% less potent, suggests that the primary function of amoebapores is to destroy phagocytosed bacteria.

During the invasion to deeper layers of the mucosa, trophozoites must lyse surrounding cells and degrade the extracellular matrix. Contact of trophozoites with the extracellular matrix induces the formation of adhesion plaques, containing actin filaments, vinculin, α-actinin, tropomyosin and myosin I. Binding to the extracellular matrix occurs through a 37-kDa fibronectin-binding protein and a 140-kDa integrin-like receptor, inducing a sustained rise of intracellular calcium concentration needed to reorganize the trophozoite cytoskeleton to form the adhesion plaque. In the absence of calcium, adhesion is poor. Contact of trophozoites with the extracellular matrix also induces the release of cysteine proteinases and the content of electron-dense granules, which includes collagenase, two proteases and at least 25 other polypeptides.[32] There are at least seven genes encoding for cysteine proteinases in *E. histolytica*.[33] The majority of the proteinase activity can be attributed to the expression of four of these genes, EhCP1–3 and EhCP5. The cytopathic effect correlates with the amount of cysteine proteinase activity released into the medium by clinical isolates of *E. histolytica* and can be inhibited by specific peptide inhibitors. A number of haemolysins, which are encoded by plasmid rDNA and are cytotoxic to an intestinal mucosal cell line (Caco 2), have been identified.

Invasion of the colonic and caecal mucosa by *E. histolytica* begins in the interglandular epithelium. This is a site of low resistance where intestinal cells are normally shed as the final stage in the renewal of the epithelium. Cell infiltration around invading amoebae leads to rapid lysis of inflammatory cells and tissue necrosis; thus, acute inflammatory cells are seldom found in biopsy samples or in scrapings of rectal mucosal lesions. Ulceration may deepen and progress under the mucosa. Further progression of the lesion may produce loss of the mucosa and submucosa, and eventually perforation of the colon.

Amoebae probably spread from the intestine to the liver through the portal circulation. The presence and extent of liver involvement bears no relationship to the degree of intestinal amoebiasis, and these conditions do not necessarily coincide. The early stages of hepatic amoebic invasion have not been studied in humans. In experimental animals, inoculation of E. histolytica trophozoites into the portal vein produces multiple foci of neutrophil accumulation around parasites, followed by focal necrosis and granulomatous infiltration. As the lesions extend in size, the granulomas are gradually substituted by necrosis, until the lesions coalesce and necrotic tissue occupies progressively greater portions of the liver. Hepatocytes close to the early lesions show degenerative changes that lead to necrosis, but direct contact of liver cells with amoebae is rarely observed. It is thought that liver damage is not caused directly by the amoebae but rather by the lysosomal enzymes of lysed polymorphonuclear neutrophils (PMNs) and monocytes that accumulate around the parasite. During experimental infection, hypocomplementaemic and leucopenic animals demonstrate reduced amoebic-induced liver damage when compared with normal animals.

In severe cases, especially in patients treated with corticosteroids, amoebic trophozoites can be found in virtually every organ of the body, including the brain, lungs and eyes.

Immunity

The first contact of the trophozoite with the immune system is through the epithelial intestinal cells. E. histolytica stimulates human intestinal epithelial cells to secrete interleukin (IL) 8 and tumour necrosis factor (TNF)α.[34,35] Neutrophils are rapidly recruited and activated in response to the proinflammatory cytokine IL-8. Cell infiltration around invading amoebae leads to rapid lysis of inflammatory cells followed by tissue necrosis.

E. histolytica in axenic culture is susceptible to complement lysis, whereas when grown in the presence of human serum or after passage through animals they become resistant. Complement resistance is mediated in part by the Gal/GalNAc adherence lectin. The adhesin binds to C8 and C9, inhibiting their assembly and therefore C5b-9-mediated lysis. The immune complex disappears from the amoebic surface, probably by capping, as the biochemical analysis of the uroid reveals the presence of complement components. The resistance to complement-mediated lysis decreases after incubation of the trophozoite with either cytochalasin B or trypsin, and after glutaraldehyde fixation. This suggests that intact membrane mobility and a trypsin-sensitive surface component are necessary to inhibit the activation of the alternative complement pathway. Inactivation of the anaphylotoxins C3a and C5a by secreted cysteine proteases of E. histolytica may also play a role in mediating resistance to complement lysis.[36]

Invasive infection with E. histolytica produces a marked immune response which results in the development of protective immunity, though immunity to intestinal infection is incomplete.[37] Recurrence of amoebic colitis or abscess is unusual. De Leon[38] monitored more than 1000 patients with amoebic liver abscess for

5 years and found a recurrence rate of 0.29%. Patients with AIDS, surprisingly, do not appear to be more susceptible to amoebic disease than those without AIDS, even though asymptomatic carriage is common.[39] Intestinal invasion by E. histolytica results in a prompt local secretory antibody response followed by a systemic antibody response. Circulating antibodies can be demonstrated as early as 1 week after the onset of invasive amoebiasis in humans and experimental animals. All immunoglobulin classes are involved, but there seems to be a predominance of IgG$_2$ antibodies. However, it has been demonstrated that the cysteine proteinases of E. histolytica can degrade both IgA[40] and IgG[41] antibody, which may limit the effectiveness of the host humoral response.

Clinical features

The clinical spectrum (see also Chapter 10) of intestinal E. histolytica infection ranges from asymptomatic carrier state or acute colitis, to fulminant colitis with perforation.

Asymptomatic infection

Asymptomatic cyst carriage of E. histolytica is well documented. The majority will clear the infection spontaneously. An epidemiological study in a semirural area in South Africa showed that 90% of asymptomatic carriers of E. histolytica cleared the infection within a year; the remaining 10% developed amoebic colitis.[26]

Intestinal amoebiasis (Table 79.1)

The onset is insidious, except in fulminating cases, with abdominal discomfort, loose motions or frank diarrhoea, not necessarily with blood or excessive mucus. In more severe cases the stools rapidly become bloodstained with mucus. Tenesmus occurs in half of the patients and is always associated with rectosigmoid involvement. Constitutional symptoms are not prominent. On physical examination tenderness may be localized anywhere in the lower abdomen but is usually over the caecum, transverse colon

Table 79.1 Symptoms and findings in acute colitis

	(%)
Symptoms	
Duration of symptoms (weeks)	
0–1	48
2–4	37
>4	15
Diarrhoea	100
Dysentery	99
Abdominal pain	85
Low back pain	66
Physical findings	
Fever	38
Abdominal tenderness	83

Source: Adams EB, MacLeod IN. Invasive amebiasis. I. Amebic dysentery and its complications. Medicine 1977; 56:315–323.

or sigmoid. The liver may be slightly enlarged and tender. Recto-sigmoidoscopy and colonoscopy of mild or moderate cases usually reveals the presence of small ulcers (3–5 mm in diameter) which most frequently involve the caecum and rectum but may be scattered throughout the colon and are especially numerous in the region of the flexures. Rarely, the disease may involve the terminal ileum. The ulcers are initially superficial with hyperaemic borders and a necrotic base covered with a yellowish exudate. There is normal mucosa between sites of invasion. However, diffuse inflammation has also been described, making firm diagnosis on gross appearance difficult. On rare occasions involvement of the blood vessels at the base of the ulcer may produce brisk bleeding. More rarely, an ulcer may perforate and the patient may die from peritonitis. Extensive inflammatory polyposis has been demonstrated as a complication of amoebic colitis and this may be a source of confusion with idiopathic inflammatory bowel disease. Acute amoebic dysentery must be differentiated from bacterial colitis caused by *Shigella* spp., *Salmonella* spp., *Campylobacter jejuni*, enteroinvasive and enterohaemorrhagic *Escherichia coli*, and *Yersinia enterocolitica*.

In surgical specimens ulcers look flat and oval in shape, without induration of the underlying bowel wall. Histologically, there is non-specific diffuse inflammation around the superficial ulcerations. As the disease advances, the classically described flask-shaped ulcers with undermined edges are formed. The lamina propria is infiltrated by plasma cells, lymphocytes, neutrophils and eosinophils. There is oedema and focal haemorrhage. The infiltrate also involves the surface epithelium, and frequently there is an overlying exudate within which trophozoites may be found (Figure 79.2).

Fulminant colitis is the result of confluent ulceration and necrosis of the colon. The clinical picture is virtually indistinguishable from that of fulminant ulcerative colitis. The bowel is dilated, particularly in its transverse portion. The patient is extremely febrile and toxic, and shows signs of hypovolaemia and electrolyte imbalance. Despite the severity of the illness, amoebae may not be readily recovered from the stools of these patients. Surgical

specimens reveal extensive areas of necrosis within which some patches of intact hyperaemic mucosa are found.

An amoeboma, or amoebic granuloma, may result from repeated invasion of the colon by *E. histolytica*, complicated by pyogenic infection. Amoebomas may be found anywhere in the colon but are more frequent at the caecum (40%) and rectosigmoid junction (20%). Lesions are usually single and involve a short segment of the colon. These mass lesions are often mistaken for malignancy and may occasionally be palpable. Histologically the amoeboma is non-fibrotic and contains granulation tissue with lymphocytes, plasma cells, eosinophils and giant cells. There is remarkably little inflammation and most of the swelling is due to oedema. Amoebae are scanty and difficult to demonstrate. Fibrous tissue is formed later.

Amoebic liver abscess

This is the most common extraintestinal form of invasive amoebiasis. Amoebic abscesses (Table 79.2) may be found in all age groups, but are 10 times more frequent in adults than in children,

Table 79.2 Symptoms and findings in amoebic liver abscess

	(%)
Symptoms	
Duration of symptoms (weeks)	
<2	37–66
2–4	20–40
4–12	16–42
>12	5–11
Pain	90
Diarrhoea and/or dysentery	14–66
Weight loss	33–53
Cough	10–32
Dyspnoea	4
Physical findings	
Localized tenderness	80–95
Enlarged liver	43–93
Fever	75–98
Rales, rhonchi	8–47
Localized intercostal tenderness	40
Epigastric tenderness	22
Swelling over the liver	10
Jaundice	10–25
Laboratory findings	
Increased bilirubin	10–25
White blood cell count >10 × 10⁹/L	63–94
Raised transaminases	26–50
Raised alkaline phosphatase	38–84
Increased erythrocyte sedimentation rate	81

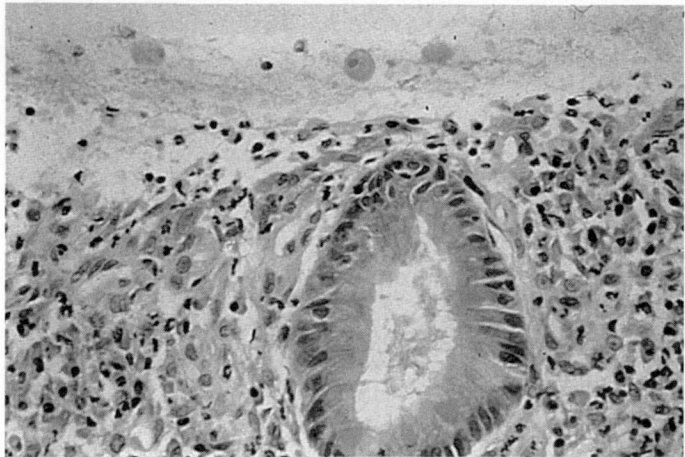

Figure 79.2 Colonic mucosa showing superficial ulceration with amoebic invasion. (H&E stain; magnification ×400.) (Courtesy of Paola Domizio, Department of Morbid Anatomy, St Bartholomew's Hospital, London.)

Source: Martinez-Palomo A. *The Biology of Entamoeba histolytica*. Chichester: University Research Press/Wiley; 1982.

and are more frequent in males than in females. They are more common in the poorest sectors or urban populations. Approximately 20% of patients have a past history of dysentery. About 10% of patients have diarrhoea or dysentery at the time of diagnosis of amoebic liver abscess. The parasite can be detected in faeces in less than 50% of cases if standard microscopy is used; the prevalence rises to 75% if culture is used. The onset of symptoms is usually abrupt, with pain in the upper abdomen and high fever. The pain is intense and constant, radiating to the scapular region and right shoulder; it increases with deep breathing or coughing, or when the patient rests on the right side. When the abscess is localized on the left lobe, pain occurs on the left side of the abdomen and may radiate to the left shoulder. Localized tenderness in the region of the abscess, most commonly at the lower right intercostal spaces, is frequent even in the absence of diffuse liver pain. Fever is present in most cases; it varies between 38° and 40°C, frequently in spikes but sometimes constant over several days, with rigors and profuse sweating. Anorexia, weight loss, nausea, vomiting and fatigue may all be present. On physical examination the cardinal sign of amoebic liver abscess is painful hepatomegaly. Digital pressure and fist percussion will often produce intense pain in the liver region. On palpation the liver is soft and smooth. Hepatomegaly may not be detected in patients with amoebic abscess of the dome of the liver because the enlargement is upward. Mild jaundice is quite common, but severe obstructive jaundice is rare. Amoebic abscess and cirrhosis may coexist, so a hard liver does not exclude the diagnosis. Movement of the right side of the chest and diaphragm is restricted and there is hypoventilation of the right lower lobe of the lung. This is frequently associated with atelectasis or effusion in the right chest. The presentation may be so abrupt that it can be confused with an acute surgical abdomen. The usual clinical diagnosis in such a case is acute cholecystitis or appendicitis. Differential diagnosis with pyogenic liver abscess should be established, particularly in non-endemic areas.

Lesions are usually single and most are found in the right lobe of the liver in the posterior, external and superior portions. The incidence of amoebic abscess of the left lobe ranges from 5% to 21%. The liver abscess has a thin capsular wall with a necrotic centre composed of a thick fluid, an intermediate zone of coarse stroma and an outer zone of nearly normal tissue. Typically, abscess fluid is odourless, resembling 'chocolate syrup' or 'anchovy paste', and bacteriologically sterile, although secondary bacterial invasion may occur. Microscopic examination of the abscess fluid reveals granular eosinophilic debris with no or few cells; amoebae tend to be located at the periphery of the abscess. Liver abscesses may heal, rupture or disseminate. The mortality rate has been estimated to be around 0.2–2.0% in adults and up to 26% in children.[42]

Invasive amoebic lesions in humans, whether localized in the large intestine, liver or skin, almost invariably heal without the formation of scar tissue, if treated properly. The absence of fibrotic tissue following necrosis is particularly striking in the liver.

Peritoneal amoebiasis

This is caused by the rupture of a hepatic liver abscess or, less frequently, by perforation of the caecum. It is characterized by a sudden increase in abdominal pain, frequently generalized, which resembles that of septic peritonitis. A plain abdominal radiograph will reveal the presence of free air in the peritoneal cavity. In some instances the perforation may be smaller and the abdominal signs are more localized.

Pericardial amoebiasis

Pericardial involvement is the most serious complication of an amoebic liver abscess. It occurs in less than 1% of all amoebic liver abscesses, especially of the left lobe. Although there may be a presuppurative stage that is associated with a sterile effusion, perforation of the abscess into the pericardium is usually followed by progressive tamponade or the sudden development of shock. Although the mortality rate from pericardial involvement has decreased from >90% to <40%, it is still frequently necessary to perform open drainage because of the development of loculations and thickened pericardium.

Pleuropulmonary amoebiasis

Invasion of the pleural cavity or the lung parenchyma is most commonly due to extension from a liver abscess and occurs in <1% of those with amoebic dysentery, in 3% of all autopsies on people dying from amoebiasis and in 15% of patients with liver abscess. Haematogenous spread is rare. The first clinical symptoms are those of the liver abscess, followed by severe pain in the lower chest, often radiating to the right shoulder. There may be dyspnoea and non-productive cough. Bronchohepatic fistulas are characterized by expectoration of large amounts of dark brown material. Superimposed bacterial infections are common.

Cerebral amoebiasis

Cerebral involvement has been documented in 1.2–2.5% of patients who have amoebiasis at autopsy, but in <0.1% of patients whose cases are reported in studies of large clinical series. Although the symptoms of cerebral amoebiasis depend on the site and size of the lesion, as many as 50% of patients may have abrupt onset of symptoms and die from cerebellar involvement or rupture within 12–72 h. The availability of metronidazole, which penetrates the blood–brain barrier, should greatly improve the prognosis of this unusual complication.

Genitourinary amoebiasis

Renal amoebiasis, a rare complication of amoebic liver abscess, is thought to occur by rupture of a hepatic abscess, haematogenous spread from lesions in the liver or lungs, or extension through the lymphatics. Patients who have renal amoebiasis usually respond well to aspiration and medical therapy. Genital lesions also occur infrequently and are usually caused by fistulas from a liver abscess or rectocolitis. Typically, lesions are painful punched-out ulcers with profuse discharge. Medical treatment is usually sufficient for resolution of the lesions.

Cutaneous amoebiasis

This results from perforation of an abscess or intestine into the skin. It may also develop from surgical wounds infected secondarily with an internal amoebic lesion or in the perineal-genital area. Histologically, there is ulceration with extensive necrosis in the base, pseudoepitheliomatous hyperplasia at the margins, and a non-specific inflammatory infiltrate extending into the deep dermis and subcutaneous tissues beneath the ulcer base. Sometimes there is extensive pseudoepitheliomatous hyperplasia involving much of the lesion with only small punctate areas of ulceration. This may resemble verrucous carcinoma. *E. histolytica* may be found in the overlying exudate.

Diagnosis and differential diagnosis

Detection of the parasite

Amoebiasis, although often suspected clinically, requires confirmation in the laboratory by finding cysts and trophozoites in the stools (which need to be differentiated by special tests from those of *E. dispar*) or trophozoites in the various tissues (see also Appendix II). The detection of the organism depends on appropriate specimen collection, processing and examination by trained personnel (Table 79.3). Molecular diagnosis of amoebiasis can now include the polymerase chain reaction.[24]

Stools

The diagnosis of invasive intestinal amoebiasis is based on the identification of *E. histolytica* trophozoites in rectal smears or recently evacuated stools and on the results of rectosigmoidoscopy. Fresh samples should be examined for detection of trophozoites containing erythrocytes. However, the test is useful only if the sample is examined within 30 min of the passage of the specimen. Three types of wet mount preparation should be made from each specimen: mounts in saline solution (to observe amoebic motility in a warm specimen); mounts in saline plus iodine (to differentiate *E. histolytica* cysts from other amoebic species and helminth ova); and mounts in saline plus methylene blue (to distinguish cysts from leukocytes, which stain blue). It is advisable always to confirm the diagnosis by using a permanent-stained slide (iron haematoxylin or trichrome). The presence of trophozoites containing ingested red blood cells is strongly suggestive of *E. histolytica* and invasive disease.

Examination of material scraped or aspirated from mucosal surfaces during sigmoidoscopy may reveal the presence of trophozoites. Microscopic examination of wet preparations may be difficult because of the need for low light intensity and difficulties in

differentiating the unstained *E. histolytica* from other amoebae and from inflammatory cells (Table 79.4). The mucosal material may also be smeared, fixed and stained with trichrome stain. Fixation of stool smears can be achieved by immersion of the slide in Schaudinn's solution or by adding two or three drops of polyvinyl alcohol to the mucosal material directly on the slide, mixing it, and allowing the slide to air dry.

Examination for ova and parasites in a minimum of three stool specimens, using concentration and permanent stain techniques, is the standard method of detection and identification of cysts of the organism. If possible, the stools should be examined before the administration of antimicrobial, antidiarrhoeal and antacid preparations or barium because all these agents may interfere with the recovery of amoebae. However, the cysts of *E. dispar* are indistinguishable from those of *E. histolytica* and, therefore, positive stools should be reported as containing *E. histolytica/E. dispar*.[11] Many research techniques have been used to differentiate between these species but only one of them has achieved commercialization. The *Entamoeba histolytica* II kit (TechLab, Blacksburg, Virginia, USA) is based on the detection of epitopes of the 170-kDa adhesin, present only in *E. histolytica*. The specificity and sensitivity of the assay for detection of *E. histolytica* in stool was estimated at 93% and 95%, respectively.[43] However, its high cost limits its use, particularly in the developing world where *E. histolytica* is endemic. A differential diagnosis should also be made with *E. hartmanni*, which is morphologically identical to *E. histolytica* and can be positively identified only by measuring its size.

Sigmoidoscopy

This is of value in symptomatic cases. The mucosal lesions should be aspirated and the material examined for trophozoites. Biopsies may be taken from the edge of the ulcers and stained with periodic acid-Schiff solution.

Liver aspirate

This should be collected in a number of different containers as it is obtained from the abscess. The amoebae are sparse in necrotic material from the centre of the abscess, but they are more abundant on the marginal walls and are therefore more commonly

Table 79.3 Microscopic diagnosis of *E. histolytica*

Sample	Fixative	Examination	Stain
Stool	PVA, 10% formalin, Schaudinn's fixative, sodium acetate-acetic acid formalin	Concentrate, permanently stained slide	Gomori trichrome, iron haematoxylin
Sigmoid colon Aspirate	PVA, Schaudinn's fixative	Permanently stained slide	Gomori trichrome, iron haematoxylin
Direct	None	Wet mount with or without enzyme digest	
Fixed	PVA, Schaudinn's fixative	Permanently stained slide	Gomori trichrome, iron haematoxylin, periodic acid
Biopsy	Formalin	Routine histology	Schiff, haematoxylin and eosin

PVA, polyvinyl alcohol with either $HgCl_2$ or $CuSO_4$; with periodic acid-Schiff organism stains intensely pink and has a distinct outline, but cytoplasmic and nuclear details are obscured. H&E stain cytoplasm pink and nucleus blue; in sections the nucleolus may not always be present.
Source: Bruckner DA. Amebiasis. *Clin Microbiol Rev* 1992; 5:356–369.

Table 79.4 Differential characteristics of host cells, *E. coli* and *E. hartmanni*, commonly mistaken for *E. histolytica*, in wet preparations

Cell	Diameter or length (µm)	Motility	NUCLEUS		Cytoplasm	
			No.	Visibility nucleus: cytoplasm ratio	Appearance (stained)	Inclusions
E. HISTOLYTICA/E. DISPAR						
Trophozoites	20–40	Progressive with hyaline finger-like pseudopodia; may be rapid	1	Hard to see in unstained preparations (1:10–1:12)	Ground glass appearance. Clear differentiation of ectoplasm and endoplasm; vacuoles usually small	Presence of erythrocytes diagnostic
Cysts	10–20	None	1–4	1:2–1:3	Clear	Chromidial bodies (stained) may be present; usually elongate with blunt, smooth rounded edges; round or oval
E. COLI						
Trophozoites	15 50	Sluggish. non-directional; blunt, granular pseudopodia	1	Often visible in unstained preparation	Granular, little differentiation into ectoplasm and endoplasm; usually vacuolated	Bacteria, yeast cells other debris
Cysts	10–35	None	1–8	≥16 nuclei seen occasionally	Clear	Chromidial bodies (stained) may be present, less frequently than in *E. histolytica/E. dispar*; splinter shape with rough pointed ends
E. HARTMANNI						
Trophozoites	6–10	Progressive, with hyaline finger-like pseudopodia; may be rapid	1	Hard to see in unstained preparations 1:10–1:12	Ground glass appearance. Clear differentiation of ectoplasm and endoplasm; vacuoles usually small	Can only be differentiated from *E. histolytica* by direct measurement of either trophozoite or cyst
Cysts	5–8	None	1–4	1:2–1:3	Clear	–
HOST CELLS						
PMNs	Average 16	None	1	2–4 segments; if lobed, nucleus fragments may mimic the four nuclei found in *E. histolytica* cyst (1:1).	Granular	None
Macrophages	20–60; may be 5–10	Sluggish	1	Large, may be irregular in shape (like monocyte); may mimic *E. histolytica* trophozoite; can also ingest erythrocytes	Coarse; may be highly vacuolated	Usually contain ingested debris, PMNs and erythrocytes

Source: Bruckner DA. Amebiasis. *Clin Microbiol Rev* 1992; 5:356–369.

found in the last portions of aspirated material. Demonstration of the organism is often extremely difficult because trophozoites may be trapped in viscous pus or debris and will not exhibit typical motility.

Laboratory investigations

In mild cases of colitis laboratory tests are normal (see also Appendix I). With severe disease, leukocytosis is present. About 75% of patients with amoebic liver abscesses have a white blood cell count >10 000/mm³. The occasional patient with leucopenia will usually have long-standing disease and may have underlying alcoholism or folate deficiency. Eosinophilia is not associated with extraintestinal amoebiasis. Anaemia is common, particularly in patients who have chronic amoebic liver abscesses. The level of alkaline phosphatase is raised in >75% of patients, particularly in those with long-standing disease. Levels of transaminases may be increased in 50% of cases, especially in patients with acute disease or complications. The levels of transaminases usually return to normal soon after therapy is initiated, although alkaline phosphatase concentration may remain raised for several months. In extraintestinal amoebiasis, organisms may or may not be found in the stool; therefore, the presence of antibodies against *E. histolytica* may be useful. Serology can be useful in the diagnosis of amoebiasis, particularly in non-endemic areas. Antibody response is present in 85–95% of patients with invasive disease. Virtually all known serological tests have been employed to detect anti-amoebic antibody, including immunofluorescent antibody tests, indirect haemagglutination assays (IHAs), radio-immunoassay, countercurrent immunoelectrophoresis and enzyme-linked immunosorbent assays (ELISAs). ELISAs are the most sensitive and do not give false-negative results in patients with amoebic liver abscesses. ELISA is also specific, giving only 3.6% false-positive results in controls living in endemic areas. The results of serological tests may be negative in patients who present acutely and should be repeated in 5–7 days. Serological responses measured by agar gel diffusion, countercurrent immunoelectrophoresis and ELISA usually become negative within 6–12 months, although they may persist for more than 3 years. However, results of IHAs may remain positive for more than 10 years after clinical and parasitological cure, even in the absence of reinfection. Therefore these tests should be interpreted with caution as antibody may be present for prolonged periods, and in areas of high endemicity a high prevalence of seropositivity already exists. Clinical laboratories should check with their local health authorities for guidelines for use and interpretation of serological tests.

Radiology

Radiological changes in the colon consist of mucosal oedema, haustral blunting and ulceration, usually localized to one part of the colon. Ulcers are initially shallow but may deepen and assume a 'collar-button' or flasked-shaped appearance. There may be toxic dilatation of the colon. Amoebomas manifest as an intraluminal mass, an annular lesion or irregularity of the bowel wall with lack of normal distensibility. Differential diagnosis with carcinoma may be difficult; rapid disappearance of the lesion after treatment favours the diagnosis.

In patients with hepatic involvement, plain radiography of the thorax may reveal elevation of the right hemidiaphragm, pleural reaction obscuring the right costophrenic angle. Radiologically, unruptured abscesses do not show a fluid level, and calcification of the liver parenchyma is rare. Non-invasive radiographic studies have dramatically increased early diagnosis of amoebic liver abscesses and their potential complications. The isotope liver scan is very useful as it becomes positive within the first days of illness, often before other imaging techniques. Presumably these early changes reflect either a focal decrease in blood supply or injury to the Kupffer cells rather than liquefaction necrosis. Ultrasonography of an amoebic liver abscess typically reveals a round or oval hypoechoic area that is contiguous to the liver capsule and without significant wall echoes (Figure 79.3). Computed tomography and magnetic resonance imaging are also sensitive studies for demonstrating amoebic liver abscesses (Figure 79.4). More than 80% of patients who have symptoms of an abscess for more than 10 days have a single lesion of the right lobe of the liver, while 50% of patients who present acutely may have multiple lesions. Abscesses resolve slowly and may increase in size during the first few weeks after therapy, even with successful treatment. The ultrasonographic abnormalities resolve within 6 months in two-thirds of the patients with amoebic liver abscess; however, 10% remain abnormal for more than 1 year after treatment. The differential diagnosis includes pyogenic liver abscess, gallbladder disease and sepsis.

MANAGEMENT

Two classes of drugs are used in the treatment of amoebic infections. Luminal amoebicides, such as diloxanide furoate and iodoquinol, act on organisms in the intestinal lumen and are not effective against organisms in tissue. Tissue amoebicides, such as metronidazole, dehydroemetine and chloroquine, are effective in the treatment of invasive amoebiasis but less effective in the treatment of organisms in the bowel lumen (Table 79.5).

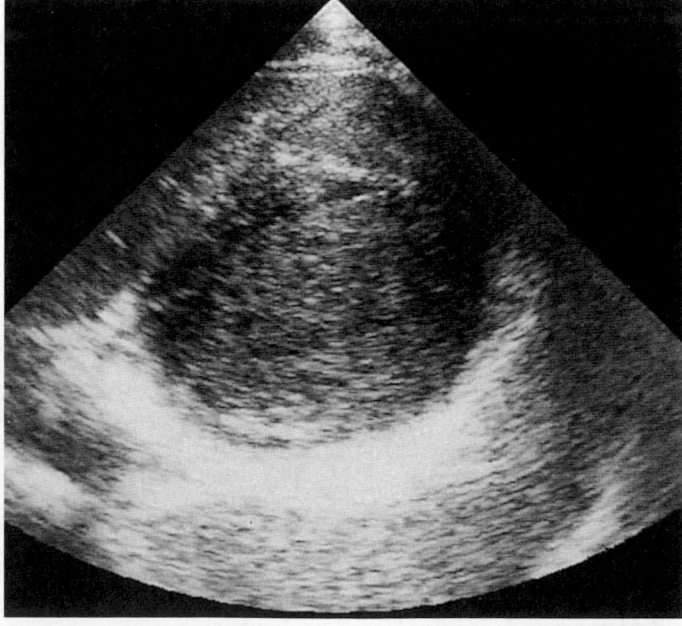

Figure 79.3 Liver ultrasonogram demonstrating an amoebic hepatic abscess. (Courtesy of Alison McLean.)

Table 79.5 Treatment of amoebiasis

		Adult dosage	Paediatric dosage (mg/kg daily)
ASYMPTOMATIC INTESTINAL CARRIER			
1st choice	Diloxanide furoate	500 mg t.i.d. × 10 days	20 (divided in 3 doses for 10 days)
2nd choice	Paromomycin	25–30 mg/kg daily in 3 doses for 7–10 days	25–30 (divided in 3 doses for 7–10 days)
or	Iodoquinol	650 mg t.i.d. for 20 days	20–40 (divided in 3 doses for 20 days)
INTESTINAL INFECTION			
1st choice	Metronidazole followed by diloxanide furoate[a]	750–800 mg t.i.d. for 10 days 500 mg t.i.d. for 10 days	35–50 (divided in 3 doses for 10 days) 20 (divided in 3 doses for 10 days)
or	Tinidazole followed by diloxanide furoate[a]	2 g/day for 2–3 days 500 mg t.i.d. for 10 days	50–60 (for 3 days) 20 (divided in 3 doses for 10 days)
2nd choice	Paromomycin	25–30 mg/kg daily in 3 doses for 7–10 days	25–30 (divided in 3 doses for 7–10 days)
or	Nitazoxanide	500 mg b.d. for 3 days	100–200 mg b.d. for 3 days depending on body size
AMOEBIC LIVER ABSCESS			
1st choice	Metronidazole followed by diloxanide furoate[a]	750–800 mg t.i.d. for 10 days 500 mg t.i.d. for 10 days	35–50 (divided in 3 doses for 7–10 days 20 (divided in 3 doses for 10 days)
or	Tinidazole followed by diloxanide furoate[a]	2 g/day for 3–5 days 500 mg t.i.d. for 10 days	20 (divided in 3 doses for 10 days) 50–60 (for 5 days)
2nd choice	Dehydroemetine followed by diloxanide furoate[a]	1–1.5 mg/kg daily (max. 90 mg/day) i.v. for 5 days 500 mg t.i.d. for 10 days	1 (for 10 days maximum) 20 (divided in 3 doses for 10 days)

[a] Paromomycin or iodoquinol may be used as an alternative to diloxanide furoate.

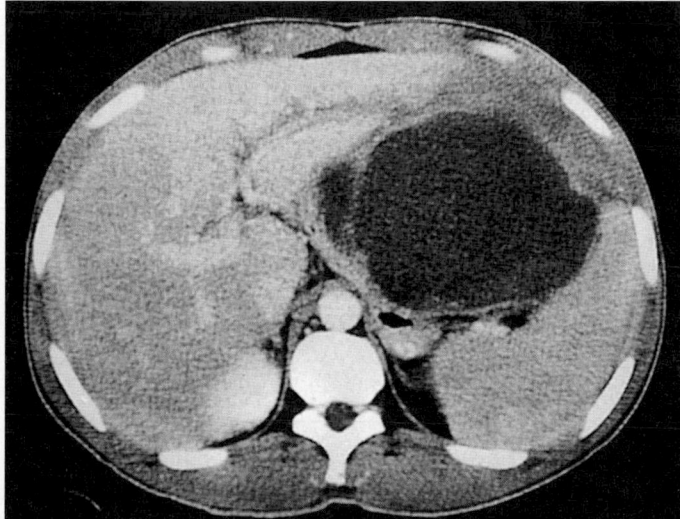

Figure 79.4 Computed tomogram of the liver demonstrating a left lobe amoebic abscess. (Courtesy of Alison McLean.)

Asymptomatic patients

The WHO has suggested that, in asymptomatic individuals, treatment is not appropriate when *E. histolytica*/*E. dispar* has been detected but *E. histolytica* has not been identified with specific tests, unless there are reasons to suspect infection with *E. histolytica*, including high specific antibody titres, a history of close contact with a case of invasive amoebiasis, or an outbreak of amoebiasis.[11] Patients with demonstrated *E. histolytica* infection can be treated with diloxanide furoate, paromomycin or iodoquinol. Iodoquinol and its analogue iodochlorhydroxyquin are effective against intraluminal amoebae but have been reported to cause myelo-optic neuropathy after long-term use.

Intestinal infection

Metronidazole or tinidazole are the drugs of choice for amoebic colitis as they are very effective against the trophozoite; however, they have little effect on the cyst and therefore treatment should be followed by a luminal agent such as diloxanide furoate. Other imidazole compounds such as ornidazole may be used.

Liver abscess

Metronidazole or tinidazole followed by diloxanide furoate is the treatment of choice. The potential cardiovascular and gastrointestinal adverse effects of dehydroemetine and emetine limit their use, and they are used only as second-line treatment. Higher relapse rates are associated with chloroquine than with other therapeutic agents.

Aspiration of the abscess may be necessary in some cases (Table 79.6).[44] However, the need for open surgical drainage has decreased

Table 79.6 Indications for aspiration of amoebic liver abscess

FORMAL INDICATIONS
To rule out a pyogenic abscess, particularly with multiple lesions
As adjunct to medical therapy (no response after 72 h)
If rupture is believed to be imminent
Abscess in the left lobe where the risk of rupture is increased
POSSIBLE INDICATIONS
To reduce the period of disability[47] (further trials are necessary to confirm this indication)

since the success of percutaneous drainage. Surgery should be reserved for patients with rupture of the abscess, with bacterial superinfection, or when an abscess that needs drainage cannot be approached.

Prevention

The control of invasive amoebiasis could be achieved through improvement of living standards and the establishment of adequate sanitary conditions in countries where the disease is prevalent. Methods of attack should aim at: (1) the community, through the improvement of environmental sanitation including water supply, adequate disposal of faeces, food safety and health education to prevent faecal–oral transmission; and (2) the individual, through early detection and treatment in cases of infection and disease.

Cysts remain viable and infective for several days in faeces and may survive in soil for at least 8 days at 34–38°C, and for 1 month at 10°C. They also remain infective in fresh water, sea water, sewage and wet soil. Cysts survive for up to 45 min in faecal material lodged under the fingernails but are killed within 1 min by desiccation on the surface of the hands. Amoebic cysts are destroyed by exposure to 200 parts/10^6 of iodine, 5–10% acetic acid, and heating at a temperature above 68°C. They can be removed from water by sand filtration but are not killed by the quantity of chlorine ordinarily used to purify water; therefore chlorination alone cannot prevent epidemics originating from faecal contamination of water. In places where purification of water supplies is inadequate, boiling for 10 min will kill all cysts.

There is no vaccine available against amoebiasis. Several antigens of E. histolytica have been developed as possible immunogens. These have different degrees of purity and are used in conjunction with a variety of adjuvants. As yet these have been tried only in animal models. Individual chemoprophylaxis for travellers is not indicated because the possibility of acquiring the infection has been shown to be very low (0.3%).[45]

Entamoeba dispar (formerly known as non-pathogenic E. histolytica)

E. dispar is the most frequently found Entamoeba both in humans and primates. It is morphologically identical to E. histolytica and is its closest genetic relative in the genus Entamoeba. Unlike E. histolytica, E. dispar does not cause disease in humans. However, there is some evidence to suggest that E. dispar is capable of inducing focal surface erosion of the colonic mucosa without invading the submucosa or causing ulcers.[46] Although up to 20% of E. dispar infections may lead to seropositivity for standard immunodiagnosis of E. histolytica, the antibody levels during E. dispar infection never approach those seen with E. histolytica. Infection is asymptomatic and does not require treatment.[11]

Several biological differences have been described between E. dispar and E. histolytica, but none of them fully explains why E. dispar is unable to produce invasive disease. E. dispar produces less protease,[47] does not bind to target cells as strongly and is less cytotoxic, has a thinner glycocalyx, higher surface charge and has less phagocytic activity than E. histolytica.[48] In vitro, E. dispar is less likely to be lysed by complement.[49]

Entamoeba moshkovskii ('E. histolytica-like' amoebae)

E. moshkovskii was originally isolated from sewage in Moscow and subsequently reported in many parts of the world. E. moshkovskii is described as morphologically indistinguishable from E. histolytica but is isolated from free-living sources, usually in the sediment of sewage-polluted waters. Similar amoebae have been isolated from humans and were grouped under the name of 'E. histolytica-like amoebae'. The best known of these is the 'Laredo' strain. Initially, they were thought to represent atypical E. histolytica. Numerous studies revealed differences between these strains and true E. histolytica, including a lack of serological cross-reactivity, dissimilar DNA base composition and distinctive isoenzyme profiles. Recently, analysis of the small subunit rRNA gene has suggested that these amoebae are strains of E. moshkovskii and are not closely related to E. histolytica. This amoeba has a wide temperature tolerance, multiplying at 10–37°C. It produces contractile vacuoles in hypotonic media and is highly resistant to amoebicidal drugs.

Entamoeba chattoni

This amoeba frequently infects apes and monkeys, in which it causes no clinical symptoms. Asymptomatic infection in individuals who are in close contact with monkeys has been reported.[50]

Endolimax nana

Endolimax nana is a cosmopolitan and common intestinal amoeba of humans, primates and pigs which can be confused with E. histolytica. Endolimax nana is non-pathogenic. The trophozoites are small (6–15 mm in diameter). Movement is by pseudopodia but this fails to produce directional locomotion. The cysts are 8–10 mm in diameter and have a refractile cyst wall. The details of nuclear structure and the appearance of the cytoplasm closely resemble those of Iodamoeba bütschlii. Usually there is only one nucleus in trophozoites, but there are four nuclei in immature cysts. Endolimax nana has no chromidial body in stained samples, and the nuclear membrane appears to be devoid of peripheral chromatin.

Iodamoeba bütschlii

Iodamoeba bütschlii is the most common amoeba of swine, and the pig was probably its original host. It is also frequently found in humans and monkeys. Trophozoites vary greatly in size, ranging from 6 to 20 mm in diameter. The cytoplasm contains one or more glycogen mass(es) that may be seen after iodine staining, as well as bacteria, yeasts and debris; red blood cells are never ingested. The nucleus is usually not visible but permanent stains will reveal a characteristic appearance with a large central karyosome surrounded by a ring of small chromatin granules. Cysts of *I. bütschlii* are 8–15 mm in diameter, commonly ovoidal or irregularly pyriform in shape. The cysts are distinctive in preparations stained with iodine because of the constant presence of the large, sharply outlined and dense glycogen-containing vacuole. Only one nucleus is found in most cysts.

I. bütschlii is non-pathogenic; only exceptionally has the presence of this parasite been linked to symptomatic infection in humans. As is the case with other amoebae commonly found in the human colon, *I. bütschlii* has a distinct isoenzyme profile.

Dientamoeba fragilis

According to morphological and molecular evidence, *Dientamoeba fragilis* is now considered to be an aberrant trichomonad flagellate, not an amoeba. Infection with this organism may be associated with gastrointestinal symptoms, such as diarrhoea and abdominal pain, but most cases are asymptomatic.[51] *D. fragilis* is a small (6–12 mm) cosmopolitan parasite. Only trophozoites are known; they can be differentiated from other intestinal amoebae by the presence of two nuclei in the majority of them. However, around 30–40% of organisms are mononucleate and may be confused with *Blastocystis hominis*, which is more common. Trichrome stains should always be performed. Culture is possible and the parasite can be differentiated by its distinct isoenzyme profile. Polymerase chain reaction (PCR)-restriction fragment length polymorphism analysis of its ribosomal genes suggests the presence of two genetically distinct forms.[52] Further studies are needed to determine whether there is a correlation between these genetic groups and virulence.

THE MASTIGOPHORA (FLAGELLATES)

Giardia intestinalis

Giardia intestinalis (syn. *lamblia*, *duodenalis*) is the most common human protozoan enteropathogen and there is now compelling evidence to indicate that infection with this parasite can cause both acute and chronic diarrhoea.[53] Intestinal malabsorption may be severe, such that chronic infection in children may be associated with retardation of growth and development. Molecular and genetic analysis of the parasite has shown that *Giardia* has a unique place in evolution as it is probably the first organism to emerge from the prokaryotic to the eukaryotic state.[54] Our knowledge of this parasite has expanded rapidly since it was first cultured in the 1970s, but many aspects of its biology and interactions with its mammalian hosts remain unanswered. There is no unifying explanation for the diverse clinical spectrum seen in giardiasis, which ranges from asymptomatic carriage to persistent diarrhoea

with malabsorption. As yet, no classical virulence factors have been identified and thus a clear explanation of pathogenesis is lacking. In addition, despite extensive investigation in animal models and to some extent during human infection, the key immunological determinants for clearance of acute infection and the development of protective immunity remain only partially defined. There is now good evidence that this infection is a zoonosis that can be transmitted through domestic water supplies; control within the environment is therefore an important public health issue.

The organism

Taxonomy

Giardia is in the kingdom Protozoa, sub-kingdom Archezoa, phylum Metamonada, subphylum Mastigophora.[55] Members of the genus *Giardia* have an adhesive disc on the ventral surface, unlike other members of the family Hexamitidae. There are three major morphological subtypes of *Giardia*: *G. agilis* from amphibians, *G. muris* from mice and *G. intestinalis* from humans and some other vertebrates (Figure 79.5). These different types can be distinguished by the overall shape and dimensions of the trophozoite body and also by the distinctive shapes of the median bodies. Two other *Giardia* isolates have been described: *G. psittaci* isolated from a budgerigar and *G. ardeae* from the great blue heron. Again, these can be distinguished from the other subtypes by an absence of the ventrolateral flange in the former and a single (rather than a double) caudal flagellum in the latter.

The chemotaxonomy of *Giardia* has been explored using a variety of techniques, including antigen, isoenzyme and DNA analysis. These approaches have clearly shown that *Giardia* isolates differ from one to another, although the sensitivity of the techniques varies. Molecular genetic approaches have shown that human *Giardia* isolates may be subdivided into two major genotypes, which are now often referred to as assemblages A and

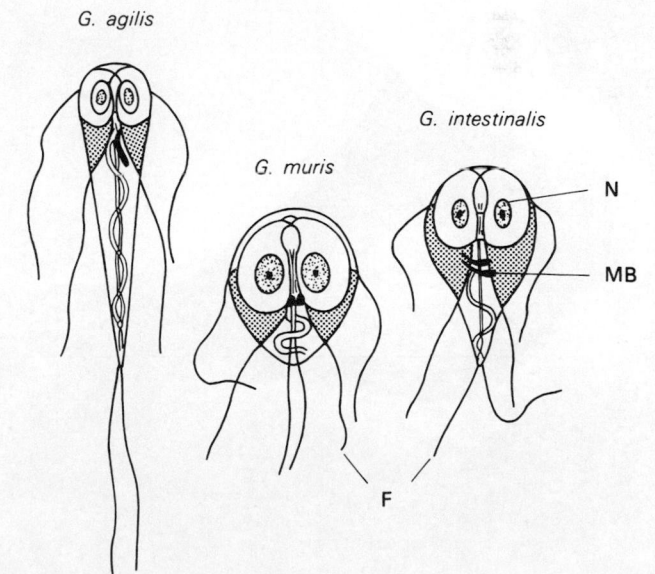

Figure 79.5 *G. agilis*, *G. muris* and *G. intestinalis*. N, nucleus; MB, median body; F, flagellum.

B, though there are many subtypes within these assemblages. There is evidence that giardiasis is a zoonosis, but evidence of anthroponotic transmission (i.e. from human to human) also exists.

Structure

Giardia exists as a trophozoite, which colonizes the proximal small intestine and is responsible for the production of diarrhoea and malabsorption, and as a cyst, which is able to exist outside the host in a suitable environment and is the form of the parasite by which giardiasis is usually transmitted.

The trophozoite, when fixed for light microscopy, is 12–15 mm long and 5–9 mm wide (Figure 79.6). It has two nuclei and four symmetrically placed flagella originating from basal bodies at the anterior pole of the nuclei. The median body is found posteriorly and varies in shape according to subtype (see Figure 79.5). A median body contains cytoskeletal proteins, including the giardins, actin and α-actinin. The trophozoite has a convex dorsal surface and a concave ventral surface containing the ventral disc. This organelle is unique to *Giardia* and is a rigid structure consisting of microtubules, cross-bridges attached to microtubules and microribbons which run perpendicularly to both the microtubules and the cross-bridges. The disc contains a variety of cytoskeletal

proteins, including the family of giardins, actin, α-actinin, myosin and tropomyosin. α₁-*Giardin* has been identified structurally and functionally to be an annexin with a typical calcium-binding domain.[56] These proteins give the disc flexibility and allow it to change shape, a process that is thought to be important for attachment. The flagella have the usual eukaryotic structure consisting of nine pairs of microtubules with two central single microtubules.

Giardia trophozoites are largely devoid of cytoplasmic organelles, the major structure being multiple ovoid vacuoles which appear to resemble lysosomes, containing a variety of hydrolases, including acid phosphatase, proteinases and DNases and RNases. Other structures include what may be a primitive Golgi apparatus that is involved in protein sorting, bacterial endosymbionts and a 35-nm double-stranded RNA virus. The role of these organisms in the life cycle of *Giardia* has not been established.

Cysts are ovoid or elliptical, approximately 7–10 mm in length. The cyst wall is composed of a layer of fibrils arranged as a felt-like web. There is controversy as to whether N-acetylglucosamine or galactosamine is the major cyst wall sugar. The cyst contains two or four nuclei; a median body and cytoskeletal components can usually be identified. The cyst is able to survive in a cool, moist environment for weeks or even months.

Microbiology

The life cycle of *Giardia* is simple, involving the ingestion of cysts in contaminated water or food or through direct person-to-person contact, infection being initiated with as few as 10–100 cysts. Excystation occurs in the proximal small intestine where the trophozoite multiplies. The cycle is completed when encystation occurs in the distal small intestine and colon, and cysts are excreted again into the environment in faeces at a concentration of approximately 150 000–200 000 cysts per gram of faeces.

Colonization involves three processes: excystation, attachment to the intestinal epithelium and multiplication. Excystation is thought to be triggered by low pH and duodenal and pancreatic secretions. The intracellular vacuoles have been observed to discharge their contents during excystation, suggesting that hydrolases are required to complete the process.[57]

Giardia attaches to the intestinal epithelium, probably by a variety of mechanisms, although it seems likely that the ventral disc plays a major part, either by flagella-generated hydrodynamic forces beneath the disc or by direct disc movement mediated by its contractile proteins, particularly those in the peripheral regions of the disc. Pharmacological disruption of microfilament function inhibits attachment, supporting a central role for the ventral disc. In addition, like many microorganisms, *Giardia* possesses a mannose-binding surface lectin that appears to exist as a prolectin in the cytoplasm and is activated by trypsin. This lectin has been purified and shown to have a molecular weight of 28–30 kDa. Experiments in attachment models using mammalian intestinal epithelial cells or culture cell lines suggest that both disc and lectin-mediated mechanisms are important, at least in vitro.

Giardia trophozoites divide by binary fission but the mechanisms by which growth is controlled and the factors that are essential for growth remain poorly defined. Bile has been shown to promote growth of *Giardia* both in vivo and in vitro.[58] This probably relates to *Giardia*'s absolute requirement for preformed phospholipid, uptake being facilitated by the presence of conju-

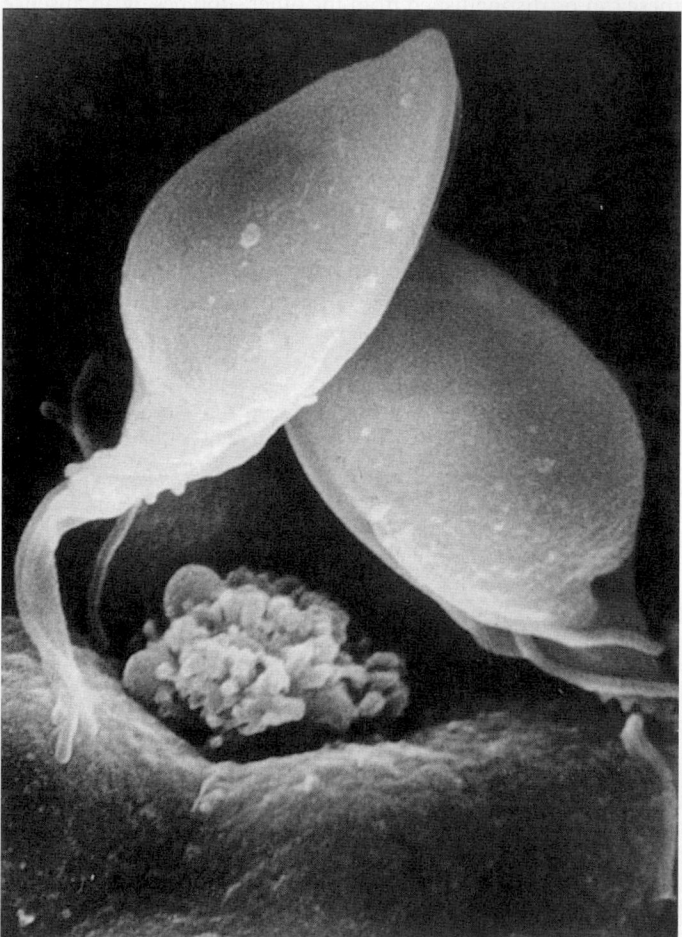

Figure 79.6 Scanning electron micrograph showing two *G. intestinalis* trophozoites.

gated bile salts. Bile salt uptake has been shown to occur by an active transport process, suggesting that a specific carrier may be present in the surface membrane. Other factors that are known to be essential for growth include a carbohydrate source, usually glucose, and a low partial pressure of oxygen.

The final stage of the life cycle, encystation, can also be completed in vitro following exposure of trophozoites to high concentrations of conjugated bile salts and myristic acid at neutral pH. Thus, bile and bile salts may have a dual role in the parasite life cycle, on one hand promoting growth and multiplication, while at the same time ensuring that the parasite completes its life cycle by encystation. An encystation-specific promoter for glucosamine-6-phosphate isomerase directs synthesis of the first enzyme required for N-acetylgalactosamine synthesis during encystation.[59]

Metabolism

Following the development of methods for axenic cultivation of *Giardia*, knowledge of the parasite's biochemistry and metabolism expanded rapidly. *Giardia* lacks mitochondria and mitochondrial enzymes, and respires in the presence of oxygen by a flavin, iron-sulphur protein-mediated electron transport system. Glucose is the major energy source, and is converted to pyruvate by Embden–Meyerhof and hexose monophosphate shunt pathways. Glucose is metabolized incompletely to carbon dioxide, ethanol and acetate. In strictly anaerobic environments, alanine is produced from pyruvate and ketoglutarate, whereas in the presence of low oxygen concentrations ethanol production increases and alanine production is reduced.

Giardia predominantly acquires membrane and other lipids from the culture medium and has little or no capacity for in vivo synthesis. Phosphatidylglycerol has been identified as a major phospholipid of *Giardia* and is probably esterified by parasite phospholipases. Trophozoites can use exogenous arachidonic acid for phosphatidylinositol synthesis.

Giardia is unable to synthesize purines and pyrimidines, which distinguishes it from most other eukaryotes. *Giardia* relies therefore on salvage pathways for both of the nucleic acids which must be synthesized exogenously. Pyrimidines are taken up by active transport processes, one for uridine and cytosine and another for thymidine.

The calcium-binding protein calmodulin has been detected in *Giardia* trophozoites and probably has a similar function in maintaining intracellular calcium homeostasis as it does in other eukaryotes.

Genetics

Sequencing of the *Giardia* genome is approaching completion (http://gmod.mbl.edu/perl/site/giardia/). The genome is 12 Mb on 5 chromosomes, with 4746 putative genes.

Giardia has five chromosomes with four or as many as eight copies in each nucleus.[60] Chromosome size varies between 1 and 4×10^6 base pairs (bp), giving a total of 1.2×10^7 bp for the five chromosomes. Densitometric scanning of restriction endonuclease digests of *Giardia* DNA produces a similar genome size. *Giardia* nuclei appear to be haploid, and thus genetic diversity is explained on the basis of clonal divergence.

The G + C content of the *G. intestinalis* genome has been estimated to be 42–48%, that of the protein-coding gene sequences

to be from 49% to >60%, and that of the rDNA gene to be 75%.[60] The non-coding regions are relatively A + T rich. *Giardia* rRNAs are smaller than other eukaryotes and eubacteria. The rDNA gene is only 5566 bp in *G. intestinalis* and slightly larger in *G. muris* and *G. ardeae*. Sequence analysis of the 16S-like RNA has demonstrated *Giardia*'s intermediate position between prokaryotes and eukaryotes.

Epidemiology

Giardiasis is found worldwide but in high prevalence in the developing world, where prevalence rates can reach 20–30%. Prevalence rates can often underestimate the overall impact of a pathogen. In rural Guatemala, 45 children were followed from birth through the first 3 years of life; all were found to have giardiasis during this period and many had recurrent and prolonged infections with the parasite. Prevalence in Peruvian children reached 40% by the age of 6 months, and stool examination confirmed prevalence rates of about 20% in children in Zimbabwe and Bangladesh. Age-specific prevalence rises throughout infancy and childhood, declining only in adolescence. In the industrialized world, prevalence varies between 2% and 5%, although within these low prevalence areas there may be localized regions of higher prevalence.

Age appears to be a risk factor for susceptibility to giardiasis, infection being more common in infants and young children, although giardiasis is rare during the first 6 months of life, particularly where breast-feeding is practised. Undernutrition may increase the susceptibility to infection, as indicated by a study in Gambian children with chronic diarrhoea and malnutrition of whom 45% had giardiasis compared with only 12% of healthy age- and sex-matched controls.[61]

Giardiasis is well recognized to occur in travellers, although overall it accounts for no more than 5% of cases of traveller's diarrhoea. However, 30% of travellers to the former Soviet Union were positive for *Giardia* in one study and >40% of Scandinavian visitors to St Petersburg acquired the infection.[62] Travelling within the USA may be hazardous, particularly for skiers in Colorado and visitors to National Parks, if they drink the apparently clean surface water.

Individuals with hypogammaglobulinaemia or agammaglobulinaemia are at risk of chronic giardiasis, but individuals with HIV and AIDS do not seem to be at particularly increased risk of developing symptomatic disease, although carriage rates are generally higher than in the general population. These observations are consistent with the view that secretory immunity in the intestinal lumen is more important for clearance than cell-mediated responses within the intestinal mucosa.

A key factor in transmission of giardiasis is the ability of the cyst to survive for long periods in a suitable environment outside the host. Surface water in many parts of the world, including North America and Europe, is contaminated with *Giardia* cysts, which are not inactivated by chlorination alone. Interruption of the ancillary water purification procedures can lead to contamination of municipal water supplies and has been shown to account for many of the reported epidemics of water-borne giardiasis.[63] A survey in the USA suggested that there may be as many as 2.5 million cases of giardiasis each year.[64] Water-borne transmission has also been shown to occur in swimming pools. Despite these epidemics, water-borne transmission probably represents a relatively small proportion of the total infections worldwide. Food has also been shown to be a vehicle for transmission of giardiasis, although again this is probably a relatively uncommon route of transmission.

Direct person-to-person spread by faecal–oral transmission certainly accounts for the high prevalence of giardiasis in day-care centres, schools and residential institutions, where prevalence may be as high as 35%. Person-to-person spread is also known to occur as a result of sexual contact.

The major reservoirs of *Giardia* cysts are the human host and contaminated surface water. There is increasing evidence that a variety of domestic and wild animals carry *Giardia* spp. that are genotypically indistinguishable from human isolates. Although there is as yet no direct evidence that transmission has occurred from animals to humans, the higher prevalence of *Giardia* in companion animals that are in close contact with humans, particularly children in the home, makes this a strong possibility.

Pathogenesis

As yet, no specific virulence factors have been identified in *Giardia* and thus no unifying hypothesis for pathogenesis has yet emerged. Current evidence suggests that *Giardia* is able to perturb mucosal structure and function; at the same time there may be additional factors operating in the intestinal lumen, which may also contribute to diarrhoea and malabsorption (Table 79.7).[65,66]

Mucosal factors

Disruption of intestinal structure

In human giardiasis, the full spectrum of abnormalities of villous architecture has been described, ranging from normal to subtotal villous atrophy (Figure 79.7). A majority of infected individuals have relatively mild abnormalities of villous architecture, with associated crypt hyperplasia. Infections in experimental models produce similar changes but, as in human infection, the abnor-

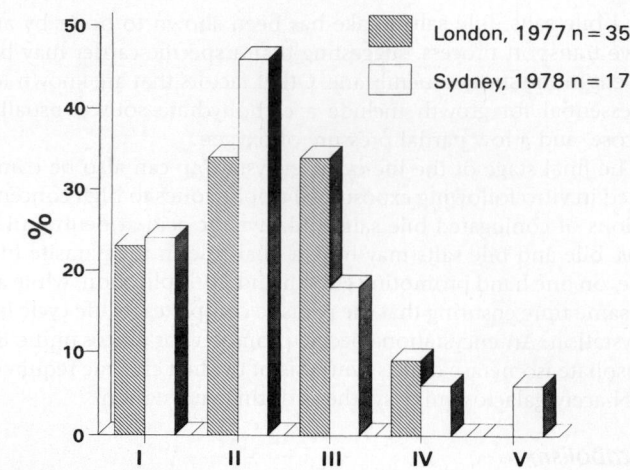

Figure 79.7 Percentage of patients with giardiasis with normal (I), mild (II), moderate (III) and severe (IV) partial villous atrophy, and subtotal villous atrophy (V).

malities are generally mild. The gerbil provides a good model for studying small intestinal structure and function as weanling gerbils develop diarrhoea and by the 6th day of infection have villous shortening in the duodenum and crypt hyperplasia throughout the small intestine. However, as with murine giardiasis there is no associated mucosal inflammation.

Even in the absence of gross changes in villous architecture, ultrastructural abnormalities, such as shortening and disruption of microvilli have been described in both humans and the gerbil model. Recent work in a neonatal rat model of giardiasis confirmed the reduction in villous height and an increase in crypt depth.

These morphological abnormalities are associated with reduction in disaccharidase activity. In animal models, diarrhoea is at its peak when disaccharide activities are most profoundly reduced.

Intestinal dysfunction

Intestinal solute and electrolyte absorption is impaired in gerbil and neonatal rat models of infection. Perfusion of a lactose-containing solution in neonatal rats exaggerated the abnormalities of water and electrolyte absorption and also showed impaired glucose absorption compared with non-infected controls. In vitro studies in Ussing chambers and brush-border membrane vesicles from infected mice provide further support for an impairment of glucose and amino acid transport.

Mechanisms of mucosal injury

A variety of mechanisms has been proposed to explain these structural and functional abnormalities of the intestinal mucosa. Attachment of *Giardia* trophozoites to the epithelium can disrupt and distort microvilli, particularly in murine giardiasis. It seems unlikely that this degree of disruption can account for the widespread changes of microvillous membrane surface area and other abnormalities of villous architecture observed in the small intestine. However, work in tissue culture cell lines has shown that *Giardia* trophozoites induce localized condensation of F-actin and

Table 79.7 Pathogenesis of giardiasis: possible mechanisms

MUCOSAL FACTORS
Direct damage by trophozoites
Microvilli
Disaccharidases
Transport proteins
Parasite products
Proteases
Lectin
Immune mediated
T cell activation
LUMINAL FACTORS
Bacterial overgrowth
Inhibition of digestive enzymes
Bile salt deconjugation
Bile salt uptake by trophozoites

loss of perijunctional α-actinin, and tight junction changes have been associated with alterations in claudin.[66,67] These cytoskeletal rearrangements could account for early changes in epithelial cell function.[68]

There is some evidence to suggest that *Giardia* trophozoites produce cytopathic substances that might be responsible for this disruption of epithelial structure and function. *Giardia* is known to produce a variety of proteinases that could find cleavage sites in proteins of the microvillous membrane. *Giardia* also has a mannose-binding surface lectin, which could interact with mannose residues on relatively immature enterocytes and again contribute to epithelial damage. Other dietary plant lectins are known to be able to produce substantial abnormalities of villous architecture.

There is increasing evidence to suggest that T cell activation within the intestinal mucosa can produce villous atrophy.[69] This mechanism is thought to operate in graft-versus-host disease and in coeliac disease. T cell activation in normal human fetal small intestinal explants with pokeweed mitogen or with an anti-CD3 antibody results in villous atrophy, crypt hyperplasia and increased IL-2 production, confirming T cell activation. Further support for this hypothesis has been obtained from studies of experimental *G. muris* infection in athymic nu/nu mice. Recent evidence implicates neuronal nitric oxide (NO) as an important contributor to clearance of infection (Li), though excess NO also causes epithelial damage.

Luminal factors

Bacterial overgrowth

Giardiasis has been associated with increased numbers of aerobic and/or anaerobic bacteria in the upper small intestine of the indigenous Indian population or in travellers to the Indian subcontinent. Bacterial overgrowth can produce architectural abnormalities in the small intestine similar to those seen in giardiasis and thus may have a role in the pathogenesis of mucosal damage.

Bile salt deconjugation

Conjugated bile salts have an important role in dietary fat absorption, but if deconjugated by luminal bacteria, they lose their detergent properties and may damage cell membranes. One study in Indian patients with giardiasis showed evidence of bile salt deconjugation, although this was not confirmed by a further study of patients in the UK. *Giardia* itself does not have the ability to deconjugate bile salts.

Bile salt uptake

As discussed above, bile salts have an important role in the life cycle of *Giardia*. There is evidence to suggest that the organism takes up bile salts during growth by an energy-requiring active transport process, possibly involving a membrane carrier.[70] Although the precise metabolic advantages to the parasite have not been defined, a secondary effect of this process could be the depletion of intraluminal bile salt, thus impairing micellar solubilization of dietary fats and at the same time inhibition of pancreatic lipase, which is dependent on bile salts for full expression of hydrolytic activity.

Pancreatic enzyme inhibition

Several studies have suggested that concentrations of pancreatic enzymes in the duodenum are reduced in patients with giardiasis. Although there is no evidence of primary pancreatic failure in giardiasis, *Giardia* trophozoites are able to inhibit trypsin and lipase activity in vitro.[71] The precise mechanisms by which the organism achieves this have not been established, although it seems likely that this may relate to a direct effect of *Giardia* proteinases on the secreted pancreatic proteins.

Until specific virulence factors have been identified, it is unlikely that the relative importance of these mucosal and luminal mechanisms in pathogenesis will be established. At present it seems reasonable to assume that the process is multifactorial, involving a combination of varying degrees of mucosal injury combined with disruption of the luminal phases of digestion and absorption.

Immunity

Studies in experimental models and limited studies in human giardiasis have made it possible to attribute essential roles to the immune system in the eradication of acute infection and to determine, at least in part, the determinants of persistent infection in an otherwise immunocompetent host.[72] There is increasing evidence to suggest that immunological factors are important in protecting mammalian hosts from reinfection, and thus the development of protective immunity. It seems unlikely that a single infection provides long-lasting protective immunity because age-specific prevalence increases throughout childhood and into early adolescence, suggesting that multiple exposures to the parasite are required before protection is achieved.

Giardia *antibodies*

Serum antibody

Anti-*Giardia* IgG can be detected in >80% of patients with symptomatic infection; antibody titres may remain raised for months or even years after primary infection. In endemic areas anti-*Giardia* IgG titres are increased in individuals without infection, suggesting widespread previous exposure to the parasite. Anti-*Giardia* IgM titres increase early in infection and then decline rapidly. Studies in India and The Gambia indicate that only 30% of patients with infection have detectable anti-*Giardia* IgA. *Giardia*sis has also been associated with raised total serum IgE, although in one case where this was investigated in depth this was not directed towards *Giardia* but possibly to food antigens as a result of increased intestinal permeability following acute giardiasis.[73] Similar patterns in antibody responses have been demonstrated in murine and neonatal rat models of giardiasis.

Secretory antibody

The secretory(s) IgA response in giardiasis is likely to be the most important aspect of immune response for parasite clearance. This is probably the reason why individuals with immunoglobulin deficiency have persistent giardiasis, which is often refractory to treatment. Specific sIgA has been detected on the surface of *G. lamblia* trophozoites in human jejunal biopsies and in human jejunal fluid. Anti-*Giardia* sIgA has also been detected in human milk and saliva, and epidemiological evidence suggests that the presence of these antibodies may contribute to protection from giardiasis in breast-fed infants.

Experimental infections in mice and neonatal rats support a role for sIgA and IgG antibodies in parasite clearance. Administration of anti-IgM to mice produces a profound reduction in sIgA and results in chronic giardiasis. Protective effects of immune milk have also been demonstrated experimentally in mice. However, anti-*Giardia* sIgA is clearly not the only determinant of chronic infection, as C3H/He mice develop persistent infection despite normal concentrations of anti-*Giardia* sIgA. The human secretory response is directed to a range of *Giardia* membrane antigens.

Giardia *antigens*

The surface antigen profile varies between *Giardia* isolates and this may be one contributory factor to the delay in achieving protective immunity to this parasite. Thus, ideally all studies seeking to identify immunodominant antigens should relate to the serum or secretory antibody responses to the particular isolate in each given infection. This is extremely difficult and probably impossible to achieve on a wide scale. A variety of antigens (24–225 kDa) has been detected by immunoprecipitation and immunoblotting techniques using polyclonal antisera, monospecific antisera and monoclonal antibodies. Some antigens have been studied in more depth, particularly a 170-kDa surface antigen which has been partly cloned and sequenced. This is one of a series of cysteine-rich proteins that appear to be immunogenic, although their role in the parasite clearance of protective immunity has not been established.

An 82–88-kDa surface antigen has also been studied by several groups and is known to be a target for the immune response in human giardiasis. Recently a *Giardia* heat shock antigen has also been shown to be important in human giardiasis, and failure to produce an antibody response to this antigen may be an important factor leading to persistent infection. Expression of this antigen is now known to occur not only following a temperature shift but also on exposure to the physical and chemical environment found in duodenal fluid. This antigen has homology with hsp70, a highly conserved family of heat shock proteins found throughout the animal kingdom and shown to be important determinants of the host immune response in other bacterial and parasitic infections.

Giardia has also been shown to be able to vary expression of certain of its surface antigens in both experimental and human infection, and this may be a way in which the parasite evades immune clearance. These variant-specific surface proteins (VSPs) constitute a family of related proteins, the expression of which is regulated by the organism.

Cell-mediated immunity

Cellular immune responses are thought to be important in the immune response to this parasite, although evidence stems largely from work in animal models. Increased numbers of lamina propria and intraepithelial lymphocytes have been reported in both experimental giardiasis and in human infection, although an increase in absolute lymphocyte numbers does not appear to be a prerequisite for parasite clearance. There have, however, been no detailed studies on lymphocyte phenotype in human giardiasis.

T lymphocytes

The most compelling evidence of a role for T lymphocytes in parasite clearance has been obtained from the natural history of murine giardiasis in the athymic nu/nu T cell-deficient mouse. Infection is prolonged in this strain but can be eradicated by reconstitution with lymphocytes from syngeneic mice with normal immune function. These experiments have suggested that CD4 cells are critically important for the ability of mice to clear *G. muris* infection and may be involved in switching B cell IgM to IgA production during infection. Recent work in B cell-deficient mice has clearly shown the importance of T cells in controlling acute *Giardia* infection.[74] Genetic factors are also important because immunocompetent mice with different genetic backgrounds vary in their susceptibility to infection with G. muris and in their ability to eradicate infection.

B lymphocytes

Total B cell numbers increase in human small intestinal mucosa infected with G. intestinalis, IgM-bearing cells being the predominant subtype. IgM cells are prominent early in infection and in nodular lymphoid hyperplasia of the small intestine, which occurs in some patients with giardiasis. A further study found only IgA and IgG cells, although this may reflect differences in sampling time because it would be expected that, during the later stages of infection, IgM-producing cells would switch to IgA production.

Mast cells, macrophages and polymorphonuclear leukocytes

Mast cell deficiency prolongs experimental infection in mice but the role of mast cells in human infection has not been established. Macrophages may also act as effector cells, their phagocytic activity for *Giardia* trophozoites being increased in the presence of specific antibodies. Neutrophils from patients with giardiasis also exhibit antibody-dependent cell-mediated cytotoxicity (ADCC) against *Giardia* trophozoites in vitro.

Integrated immune response in giardiasis

The immune system, particularly T cells, has a major role in parasite clearance during acute infection, the control of mucosal invasion and ultimately the development of protective immunity. Current evidence suggests that anti-*Giardia* sIgA also has a role in clearing *Giardia* from the gut lumen, possibly by trophozoite agglutination and/or inhibition of flagella motility.[75] Monoclonal antibodies have been shown to be directly cytotoxic to *Giardia* trophozoites and it is likely that ADCC may occur within the intestinal lumen.

Invasion of the intestinal epithelium by *Giardia* trophozoites is a rare event but a variety of mechanisms is available within the mucosa to inhibit this process; these include cytotoxic intraepithelial lymphocytes, ADCC and the complement system.

The immunological determinants of long-term protective immunity remain to be discovered. Clinical and experimental evidence suggests that secretory antibody in the intestinal lumen is likely to be important, although the antigenic determinants are as yet not defined. Preliminary evidence suggests that *Giardia* heat shock antigen, one of the family of hsp70 proteins, may be involved.

Clinical features

The most common form of giardiasis is asymptomatic carriage. This is common in highly endemic areas in the developing world, although it also occurs in Europe and North America. Such individuals appear to suffer no ill effects from the parasite, although there have been no systematic studies of the subclinical impact of such an infection. It is unclear whether asymptomatic infections relate to carriage of 'non-pathogenic' strains or whether the host is able to maintain parasite numbers at a level below expression of clinical disease without complete clearance of the infection (see also Chapter 10).

Acute giardiasis has been well characterized in individuals travelling from areas of low to high endemicity. Symptoms usually begin within 3–20 (mean 7) days of arrival within a high-risk area and in the vast majority recovery occurs within 2–4 weeks. In up to 25% of travellers with giardiasis, symptoms may persist for 7 weeks or more. Diarrhoea is the major symptom and is usually watery initially but subsequently develops the features of steatorrhoea, often associated with nausea, abdominal discomfort, bloating and weight loss (Table 79.8).

Although giardiasis is self-limiting in the majority of healthy immunocompetent individuals, a proportion, possibly 30–50%, goes on to have persistent diarrhoea, usually with features of steatorrhoea. Weight loss can be profound, with losses of 10–20% of the usual or ideal body weight. In symptomatic patients with persistent diarrhoea, 50% will have biochemical evidence of fat malabsorption and possibly of other nutrients, including vitamin A and vitamin B_{12} (Table 79.9). Secondary lactase deficiency is well recognized to occur in human giardiasis and in experimental models, and patients may take many weeks to recover even after clearance of the parasite.

Clinical complications of giardiasis

Retardation of growth and development

A series of hospital-based studies has clearly shown the potential of giardiasis to impair growth and development in infants and young children. This is a highly selected population, biased towards more severely affected children, and thus gives no indication as to the impact of giardiasis in the community. Several studies from Central America and West Africa suggest that giardiasis does have an independent inhibitory effect on child growth, but it is difficult to arrive at firm conclusions because within these populations many other factors contribute to undernutrition and impaired development.

Allergic and inflammatory conditions

Lymphoid nodular hyperplasia has been associated with chronic giardiasis and immune deficiency. There is no clear indication as to the precise pathogenetic relationship between these phenom-

Table 79.8 Symptoms of acute giardiasis in travellers

Clinical features	Patients (%)
Diarrhoea	95
Weakness	76
Weight loss	68
Abdominal pain	69
Nausea	60
Steatorrhoea	56
Flatulence	35
Vomiting	29
Fever	17

Table 79.9 Intestinal malabsorption in giardiasis

SUBJECTS WITH NORMAL RESULTS (%)							
Study	Location	No. of subjects	D-xylose	Lactose	Fat	Vitamin B_{12}	Vitamin A
Veghelyi 1939	Hungary	14	–	–	71	–	–
Katsampes 1944	USA	15	–	–	–	–	100
Cantor 1967	Argentina	20	–	–	25	–	–
Hoskins 1967	USA	6	50	100	40	100	–
Alp 1969	Australia	5	20	20	100	–	–
Barbieri 1970	Brazil	11[a]	27	–	82	–	–
Ament 1972	USA	77	–	–	66	100	–
Cowen 1973	USA	3	100	–	60	100	–
Tewari 1974	India	30	23	–	50	6	–
Rabassa 1975	Cuba	50	62	27	34	–	–
Wright 1977	UK	40	45	–	35	–	–
Tandon 1977	India	63	4	–	27	0	–
Hartong 1979	USA	12	55	–	64	60	–
Mahalanabis 1979	India	4	79	–	50	–	100
Mean (%)			47	49	55	61	100

[a] Asymptomatic children.

ena, although there is some evidence to suggest that a common feature may be a predominance of IgM-producing B cells, possibly as a result of the failure to switch from IgM to IgA production within the intestine. IgE-mediated allergic phenomena are uncommon in giardiasis, unlike many helminth infections, although occasional cases have been described.

Protein-losing enteropathy

This is a rare occurrence in giardiasis but has been described in children in West Africa and may contribute to undernutrition.[76]

Diagnosis

Clinically, giardiasis is often suggested by a typical history which often includes a period of recent foreign travel. The main differential diagnoses include other causes of intestinal malabsorption such as tropical sprue and coeliac disease. Other infective causes of persistent diarrhoea include strongyloidiasis, cryptosporidiosis, microsporidiosis and cyclosporiasis. Many clinicians treat giardiasis empirically with a nitroimidazole derivative, even without achieving a firm microscopic diagnosis.

Microscopy

Giardia cysts and occasionally *Giardia* trophozoites are detected in faecal specimens by light microscopy, which continues to be the gold standard for the diagnosis of giardiasis. Faecal specimens are examined, either fresh or fixed with polyvinyl alcohol formalin, and then stained with trichrome or iron haematoxylin. Cyst detection can be improved by concentration techniques using formalin-ethyl acetate or zinc sulphate. Immunofluorescent anticyst antibodies have been used to assist the detection of cysts in faecal specimens. Examination of multiple faecal specimens increases the chances of making a positive diagnosis, with up to 70% of positive stools detected following examination of a single faecal specimen, rising to 85% when at least three separate stool specimens are examined. Trophozoites are usually found only in freshly passed watery diarrhoea. Trophozoites can also be detected microscopically in duodenal fluid and, although overall this technique has a lower sensitivity than faecal microscopy, it does complement the latter, in that some patients with negative stool microscopy will have a positive duodenal aspirate.[77] Trophozoites may also be detected by endoscopic brush cytology or in mucosal impression smears of small intestinal biopsies.

Faecal antigen ELISA

Antigen tests come in two main formats: ELISAs and rapid strip tests. Generally, these tests offer simplicity and they save time in the lab, but their sensitivity is not much higher than microscopy, anywhere between 44% and 82%.[78,79] Specificity is generally high, over 95%. False positives, however, are almost always reported in these assays and the interpretation of these findings is difficult. Enthusiasts for the test will regard this as 'microscopy-negative' giardiasis, but the pessimist will merely regard this as a true false positive, possibly due to the presence of cross-reacting faecal antigens. It seems likely, however, that microscopy-negative cases of giardiasis do exist and the more sensitive methods of detection such as ELISA or DNA-based diagnostic techniques will eventually prove the case.

Serology

Anti-*Giardia* IgG titres are not helpful in diagnosis because they are commonly found to be increased in non-infected individuals in endemic areas. Anti-*Giardia* IgM titres are usually increased only in infected individuals and have been shown to be useful in a research setting for detecting individuals with acute giardiasis in endemic areas such as India and The Gambia. Sensitivity and specificity decrease, however, in children with persistent diarrhoea, in some of whom anti-*Giardia* IgM titres persist for several months.

DNA-based techniques

Specific DNA probes for *Giardia* are now available, although preliminary studies suggest that there may be difficulties in liberating DNA from *Giardia* cysts. Much more importantly, PCR-based assays have come into use both for detection and for genotyping that amplifies the intergenic spacer region of multicopy rRNA gene followed by nested PCR appears to be a rapid and reliable technique for detecting *Giardia* in stool.[80]

Management

In many healthy immunocompetent individuals, giardiasis is a self-limiting illness, with the parasite being eradicated by host defence mechanisms without specific treatment. Administration of an antigiardial drug will generally reduce the severity of symptoms and the duration of the illness. Although symptomatic patients with giardiasis are generally offered antimicrobial chemotherapy, the question as to whether asymptomatic patients, particularly those in an endemic area, should be treated continues to be discussed. Since the development of in vitro culture techniques for *Giardia* isolates, methods have been developed to assess drug sensitivity in vitro. However, the precise relationship between indices of drug susceptibility in vitro and the subsequent behaviour of the drug in vivo has not been clearly established. Treatment failures do occur and it is thought that at least some of these episodes are related to drug resistance.

Three classes of drugs are commonly used to treat giardiasis: the nitroimidazole derivatives, the acridine dyes, such as mepacrine, and the nitrofurans such as furazolidone. Some commonly used treatment regimens for adults and children are shown in Table 79.10. Nitroimidazole derivatives are probably the drugs of choice, particularly when used as short-course regimens. Mepacrine has a similar efficacy but is generally less well tolerated. Furazolidone has a lower efficacy but is popular for the treatment of giardiasis in childhood as it has relatively few adverse effects and is available as a suspension. The adverse effects of these agents are summarized in Table 79.11.

A variety of other chemotherapeutic agents has been assessed in vitro and some have also been used in the clinical setting. The benzimidazole drugs appear to have some antigiardial activity, which almost certainly relates to their ability to inhibit cytoskeletal function. Albendazole has been shown to have antigiardial activity in vitro[81] and recent clinical trial data support its value in human infection. Other drugs such as sodium fusidate, D- and DL-propranolol, mefloquine, doxycycline and rifampicin have all been shown to have antigiardial activity,[82] although the majority have not been subjected to rigorous evaluation in

Table 79.10 Drug treatment of giardiasis

Drug	Adults	Children	Efficacy (%)
Metronidazole	2 g (single dose) daily for 3 days or 400 mg three times daily for 5 days	15 mg/kg per day (max. 750 mg) for 10 days	>90
Tinidazole	2 g single dose	50–75 mg/kg single dose	>90
Mepacrine (quinacrine)	100 mg three times daily for 5–7 days	2 mg/kg three times daily for 5–7 days	>90
Furazolidone	100 mg four times daily for 7–10 days	2 mg/kg three times daily for 7–10 days	>80
Nitazoxanide	500 mg b.d. for 3 days	100–200 mg b.d. for 3 days depending on body size	

Table 79.11 Adverse effects of antigiardial drugs

Drugs	Adverse effects
Metronidazole and tinidazole	Nausea, vomiting, metallic taste, gastrointestinal disturbances, rashes, urticaria and angio-oedema Rarely drowsiness, headache, dizziness, ataxia Prolonged use, peripheral neuropathy Disulfiram-like reaction with alcohol Avoid in pregnancy and breast-feeding
Mepacrine (quinacrine)	Gastrointestinal disturbances, dizziness, headache, nausea and vomiting Occasionally toxic psychosis Prolonged use, yellow discolouration of skin, sclerae and urine, chronic dermatoses, hepatitis and aplastic anaemia Avoid in pregnancy, hepatic impairment, psoriasis, the elderly and history of psychosis
Furazolidone	Nausea, vomiting Haemolysis in glucose-6-phosphate dehydrogenase deficiency
Nitazoxanide	Lemon-yellow discolouring of sclerae during treatment of over 5 days; this can mislead practitioners into thinking jaundice is developing but serum bilirubin remains normal

clinical practice. Nitazoxanide is a promising drug for treatment of giardiasis.[83]

Prevention

It seems highly unlikely that *Giardia* spp. will ever be eliminated from the environment, as they can survive for weeks or months outside the host in water or a moist environment and it is now well established that surface water in many parts of the world is contaminated with *Giardia* cysts. This reservoir could potentially maintain the animal reservoir of *Giardia*, which is increasingly thought to be another potential source of human infection. Despite vigilance about water quality, it is vital to ensure that contaminated surface water collecting grounds are appropriately treated before water enters the public water supply. Attention to personal hygiene in order to break the faecal–oral cycle is also important, particularly in residential institutions and day-care centres.

There is compelling evidence that breast-feeding protects against giardiasis; this can be partly attributed to passive immunization. Whether active immunization in the form of a vaccine is feasible, or even appropriate, continues to be evaluated. Parenteral immunization with adjuvants can protect experimental animals from challenge with *G. intestinalis*, and the epidemiological evidence in humans that protective immunity does eventually develop, probably over a number of years, suggests that

immunological approaches to prevention are feasible. However, it is unclear as to why the development of protective immunity following natural infection appears to require repeated exposure to the organism. It is possible that this is related, at least in part, to the variable antigenic profiles of different *Giardia* isolates. In addition, it is known that the expression of certain *Giardia* antigens can vary during both experimental and human infection, thus providing a way in which the organism may evade the host immune response. Failure to mount an antibody response to *Giardia* heat shock antigen in children with chronic diarrhoea in The Gambia suggests that impaired response may also be a factor. Clearly all of these issues need to be taken into account in planning a vaccine development strategy.

Non-pathogenic flagellates

There are a number of other flagellates found in humans that do not appear to cause disease. *Trichomonas hominis* is commonly found in faeces of individuals living in the developing world. Only the trophozoite form is recognized; it varies from 5 to 14 mm in length. There is a single nucleus, anterior to which are basal bodies from which arise three to four flagella.

Chilomastix mesnili occurs as both cysts and trophozoite and is larger than *Trichomonas hominis*, being usually 10–15 mm in length, although it may occasionally be as large as 20 mm. The trophozoite has a large spiral longitudinal cleft anteriorly and an anterior single nucleus. Basal bodies at the anterior pole of the nucleus give rise to three anterior flagella, two fibrils that support the margins of the longitudinal cleft (the mouth), and a fourth flagellum, which moves within the longitudinal cleft. There are no cytoskeletal elements, the parasite maintaining its shape by a pellicle. The cyst is pear-shaped and approximately 18 mm in length. Internal structures are apparent in the stained cyst in which one or two nuclei may be observed.

Rare non-pathogenic flagellates include *Embadomonas intestinalis* and *Enteromonas hominis*.

THE CILIOPHORA

Members of this class are all relatively large in size and covered by short hair-like organelles called cilia, which give the organism its motility. They have two nuclei, one somatic and one germinal. Reproduction is by binary fission, although conjugation does occur when nuclear material is exchanged between parasites. The only ciliate that is pathogenic to humans is *Balantidium coli*.

Balantidium coli

Balantidium coli is the largest and probably least common protozoan pathogen of humans.[84] It can cause a severe life-threatening colitis, which is potentially avoidable by appropriate antibiotic therapy. Fatalities are almost invariably due to diagnostic imprecision.

The organism

B. coli exists as a trophozoite (usually found in stools of acute infection) and cysts, which become more apparent in chronic infection or asymptomatic carriers. The trophozoite is oval in shape, about 17 µm long and 15 µm wide. In its favoured host, the pig, trophozoites may reach 200 µm in length, when they can be seen with the aid of a hand lens or in some cases with the naked eye. The trophozoite is covered with cilia which propel the organism through the fluid contents of the intestinal lumen. At the anterior end of the trophozoite there is a cytostome (a mouth) leading into the cytopharynx, which extends approximately one-third of the body length. Posteriorly there is a cytopyge (anus).

There are two nuclei, a larger macronucleus and a smaller micronucleus which lies in the concavity of the macronucleus. There are two contractile vacuoles connected by a canal. Intracellular organelles are limited, the major features being food vacuoles which circulate through the endoplasm. The trophozoite multiplies by lateral transverse fission, which may be preceded by conjugation, in which nuclear material is exchanged between trophozoites.

B. coli forms a large spherical cyst which may reach 60 mm in diameter. Cysts can survive outside the mammalian host for several weeks in moist conditions but are rapidly destroyed in hot, dry conditions. Infection is usually transmitted by the cyst.

Epidemiology

The parasite is found in northern and southern hemispheres, although it is most commonly reported in tropical and subtropical regions, particularly Central and South America, Iran, Papua New Guinea and the Philippines. Prevalence is usually <1%, although higher rates are reported in hyperendemic areas and some residential institutions. *B. coli* is found in many mammals other than humans, particularly pigs and monkeys. Swine appear to be the most important animal reservoir for human disease, although enteric disease does not seem to occur in this host. The largest reported endemic of balantidiasis, involving 110 persons, resulted from gross contamination of ground and surface water supplies by pig faeces after a severe typhoon.[85] Communities that live in close association with swine tend to have increased prevalence of the disease because carriage by pigs has been estimated to be 40–90%.

Pathogenesis

The trophozoite is able to invade the distal ileal and colonic mucosa to produce intense mucosal inflammation and ulceration. The mechanisms involved are not clearly understood, although it is considered that the motile trophozoite is able to penetrate the mucosa and submucosa, and even in some instances, the muscle layers of the colon. Invasion is thought to be facilitated by the enzyme hyaluronidase, produced by the parasite. The resulting inflammation may be mediated partly by other products liberated by the parasite and possibly by recruitment of mucosal inflammatory cells, particularly neutrophils.

Clinical features

In many respects, the illness produced by infection with *B. coli* closely resembles amoebic colitis. Clinical presentation occurs in three forms: (1) the asymptomatic carrier state, most commonly seen in persons in institutional care and possibly accounting for up to 80% of all infections; (2) acute and acute fulminant colitis; and (3) chronic infection. In the acute form, diarrhoea with blood and mucus begins abruptly and may be associated with nausea, abdominal discomfort and marked weight loss. Proctosigmoidoscopy reveals inflammatory changes, including discrete ulceration, although the rectum is not invariably involved. The illness can progress rapidly, accompanied by fever and prostration, and lead to death, usually due to peritonitis from colonic perforation. A protracted course with intermittent diarrhoea but only occasional blood in the stools is typical of the chronic form of the disease. A few cases of balantidial appendicitis have been reported.

Diagnosis and differential diagnosis

The large motile trophozoites are the predominant form of the parasite excreted in faeces and these can often be seen with the aid of a hand lens. Trophozoites may also be obtained from material from the margins of ulcers seen in the rectum at proctosigmoidoscopy. The macroscopic appearances at sigmoidoscopy do not, however, distinguish balantidiasis from other forms of infective or non-specific inflammatory bowel disease. Specific antibody responses to the parasite can be detected in serum but the value of serological tests in clinical diagnosis has not been clearly determined.

Management

The most commonly used treatment is tetracycline 500 mg four times daily for 10 days. The parasite is also sensitive to bacitracin, ampicillin, metronidazole and paromomycin. Surgery may be required in fulminant disease, as in amoebiasis, although a conservative approach should be taken wherever possible.

THE COCCIDIA

Cryptosporidium parvum

Tyzzer,[86] in 1907, was the first to describe an organism of this genus with a short account of *Cryptosporidium muris* in the gastric mucosa of laboratory mice. He identified the mode of transmission as faecal–oral, and provisionally classified the organism with the *coccidia*. A further report in 1912 by the same author demonstrated a similar parasite in the small intestine; as he was unable to cross-infect from one site to the other with the two organisms, he recognized that they were different species. This latter organism is probably *C. parvum*. For many years only these two species were recognized, but recently, there has been an explosion of understanding of the genus *Cryptosporidium*, and now 13 species are recognized, with the possibility that many more will be named. Current valid species are: *C. muris*, *C. parvum*, *C. hominis*, *C. andersoni*, *C. wrairi*, *C. felis*, *C. canis*, *C. meleagridis*, *C. baileyi*, *C. galli*, *C. serpentis*, *C. saurophilum*, and *C. molnari*.[87] Of these, only *C. parvum* and *C. hominis* infect humans. Cryptosporidiosis (the infection due to *Cryptosporidium* spp.) is now recognized to represent a substantial threat to HIV-infected individuals, with a lifetime risk of infection of around 10%, but it is also responsible for substantial outbreaks of water-borne diarrhoea in the immunocompetent, and for diarrhoea in travellers and in children.

The organism

Taxonomy

C. parvum is a protozoan, of the phylum Apicomplexa, class Sporozoasida, subclass Coccidiasina, order Eucoccidiorida.

Structure and ultrastructure

It is characteristic of these *coccidia* that the life cycle (Figure 79.8) includes merogony, gametogony and sporogony, and takes place within a vertebrate host. The ingested form is the oocyst, which has probably already sporulated before shedding. Excystation takes place in the small intestine, with four sporozoites being released from each oocyst. These are actively motile and penetrate the enterocyte. Electron micrographs show that the trophozoite takes up an intracellular but extracytoplasmic position (Figure 79.9). Merogony or schizogony leads to the liberation of eight merozoites from the cell in the first cycle and four in the second, and direct invasion of neighbouring enterocytes takes place, magnifying the infection. Sexual multiplication takes place, leading to the formation of the zygote, and subsequently to the development of thin-walled oocysts (20%) and thick-walled oocysts (80%). Thick-walled oocysts are excreted in the faeces, but it is thought that thin-walled oocysts may lead to autoinfection.

Genetics

In the past 5 years, enormous progress has been made in establishing the genome sequences of three Cryptosporidium species:

C. parvum, *C. muris* and *C. hominis*. Preliminary assemblies are available at: http://cryptodb.org/. There are eight chromosomes. As yet, there are no data on genes responsible for pathogenicity or virulence.

Epidemiology

Immunocompetent individuals

Substantial evidence has accumulated implicating *C. parvum* in outbreaks of water-borne diarrhoea[88] and in stable endemic childhood diarrhoea among the poor of the developing world. Travellers' diarrhoea may result from infection with this parasite. The evidence for the water-borne nature of the infection comes from epidemics that have occurred along water distribution patterns and the finding that oocysts can be detected in the water supply by filtration of large volumes through 1-mm pores. As cryptosporidiosis is a common pathogen in calf and lamb diarrhoea, it is probably a zoonosis, transmitted in surface run-off water contaminated by calf faeces. Chlorination of water at usual levels fails to inactivate oocysts. It is probably this resistance to chlorination that allowed transmission of 70 cases following contamination of a swimming pool in the UK, and in a similar outbreak reported from California.

Data from the Public Health Laboratory Service in north Wales,[89] based on diagnostic laboratory returns, show an age distribution of infection, with a peak between 1 and 5 years, and a marked reduction over the age of 35 years. The incidence is seasonal and varies with rainfall. Cryptosporidial infection is a common cause of diarrhoea outbreaks in children, and these may cluster in nurseries. The spring peak in incidence in the UK closely parallels that observed for lambs, according to reports from the Central Veterinary Laboratories. Cases have been identified in which the only apparent transmission opportunity has been exposure to horse manure used as garden fertilizer. Veterinary students have an increased risk of infection, as do dairy farmers compared with other farming groups. Indirect transmission has occurred to young urban children from the clothing of mechanical digger operators returning home with boots and clothes soiled by farm manure.

Cryptosporidiosis is an important contributor to childhood diarrhoea, with a prevalence among children with diarrhoea of 1–3% in the industrialized world and 4–17% in developing countries. Values of 1–13% have been reported in several studies from China.[90] In the developed world, cryptosporidiosis is found in outbreaks clustered around day-care nurseries. In a careful prospective study in Guinea-Bissau, cryptosporidia were found in 6.1% of patients with acute (<2 weeks) diarrhoea and in 15% of those with chronic diarrhoea, with a relative mortality in children with cryptosporidial diarrhoea in the first year of life of 2.9.[91]

Insight into the transmission and pathobiology of the infection arises from the report of an outbreak of cryptosporidiosis in Denmark in 1990.[92] The setting was an infectious disease ward with a mixed population of HIV-seropositive and -seronegative patients; the index case was a demented seropositive man with cryptosporidial diarrhoea who contaminated an ice machine with faeces. None of the 73 HIV-seronegative inpatients became infected, but 18 (32%) of 57 HIV-positive patients developed infection, 17 of whom had AIDS. The mean incubation time was at least 13 days.

series of Zairean patients, 89% had intermittent diarrhoea and the mean duration was 9 months; no difference was demonstrated between patients with cryptosporidiosis and those with other forms of HIV-related diarrhoea.

Patients in all areas of the globe show considerable wasting as AIDS progresses, but it is difficult to discern how much can be attributed to any particular infection. There is certainly anorexia in AIDS, and oral and oesophageal candidiasis exacerbate the problem. There is no evidence that cryptosporidiosis is associated with a greater degree of nutritional impairment than any other enteric manifestation of AIDS. Phillips et al.,[94] however, showed an association between cryptosporidial infection and nutritional impairment in immunocompetent children. Children in Guinea-Bissau who were undernourished were not more likely to develop the infection, but did suffer adverse nutritional consequences afterwards.[91]

Some patients develop small bowel disease alone, while others may also have involvement of the biliary tract. The first large study of biliary disease in AIDS[104] described a syndrome of sclerosing cholangitis, sometimes associated with cholecystitis. This may be associated with cryptosporidial infection of the biliary tract, with microsporidiosis (see below) or with cytomegalovirus, or it may be impossible to identify a cause. The disorder usually occurs in patients with chronic diarrhoea and is associated with progressive right upper quadrant abdominal pain. The patients tend to have had other opportunistic infections by this stage of the HIV infection. Biochemical tests of hepatic damage usually show raised serum levels of alkaline phosphatase and γ-glutamyltransferase in the absence of jaundice. Transaminase concentrations may or may not be increased. Ultrasonographic examination of the liver may show irregularly dilated intrahepatic bile ducts. The definitive test is endoscopic retrograde cholangiopancreatography, which shows this distortion of the biliary anatomy, with or without papillary stenosis. Forbes et al.[105] found cryptosporidia in 13 of 20 cases, and estimated that up to one in six of all cases of AIDS-related cryptosporidiosis may also have sclerosing cholangitis. In the last decade, the introduction of antiretroviral therapy has had a dramatic and positive impact on HIV-infected individuals, but although the number of patients with severe, chronic cryptosporidiosis has fallen where these drugs are available, cases still do occur, especially in Africa.

Cryptosporidiosis is associated with malnutrition and increased mortality in children in developing countries.[106] Longitudinal studies in Guinea-Bissau have demonstrated that cryptosporidiosis precedes the development of growth failure. In malnourished children with persistent diarrhoea in Zambia, cryptosporidiosis was associated with higher mortality independently of HIV infection.[107]

Diagnosis

Current diagnostic methods rely heavily on the identification of the oocysts in faeces. Three staining methods are in common use: auramine staining, modified Ziehl–Neelsen staining and immunofluorescence using monoclonal antibodies to oocysts. These techniques are relatively insensitive. The threshold of reliable (100%) detection was found to be 10 000 cysts/g in watery stool, but in formed stool thresholds were 50 000/g by immunofluorescence and 500 000/g by acid-fast staining.[108]

ELISAs that incorporate anti-oocyst antibodies to detect cryptosporidial antigen in faeces have been developed, and rapid strip tests are also available. Several different assays using PCR have been published for detection of DNA in stool or biopsies.[80] Serological tests have been described, but have not reached the stage of routine use.

Management

There is no effective treatment that will eradicate cryptosporidial infection in all cases; over 100 drugs have been tested. Several controlled trials have now confirmed that nitazoxanide is effective against *C. parvum* in well-nourished and malnourished HIV-uninfected children.[109] A 3-day course is effective: children under 4 years receive 100 mg twice daily and those over 4 years 200 mg twice daily, orally. A Cochrane review suggests that none of the treatments evaluated was consistently effective in immunocompromised adults or children, but the number of trials available for inclusion in the meta-analysis was small.[110] The most important aspect of treatment is fluid and electrolyte replacement with oral rehydration solutions, although intravenous therapy may be necessary. Symptomatic treatment with codeine phosphate or powerful opiates should be given readily, according to resources, and nutritional support is probably beneficial.

Prevention

When dealing with a disease affecting mainly the immunocompromised, it is difficult to evaluate measures directed at reduction of incidence. On the basis of what little we know about transmission, it would seem prudent to advise those at risk, including HIV-infected individuals, to boil all drinking water and to avoid swimming in public water. There is no immediate prospect of effective immunization against the infection.

Prevention of nosocomial or laboratory-acquired infection requires strict attention to containment and generous washing of any contaminated areas. Disposables should be used where possible. The oocysts are resistant to many disinfectants, but are reliably inactivated by boiling, freezing, drying and 3% hydrogen peroxide.[111]

Isospora belli

This coccidian was first described in 1915 but has received much less attention in the world literature than cryptosporidia, probably because of its comparative rarity in the developed world. It has recently attracted interest because of its identification in patients with AIDS. The infective form of the parasite is the oocyst, which releases sporozoites, leading to a small bowel infection. The parasite there takes up an intracellular location and undergoes merogony and sporogony.

Epidemiology

The route of transmission of the parasite is not established but faecal-oral spread seems likely. Infection is uncommon in the developed world, as reflected by the prevalence in European and North American patients with AIDS (compared with Africans) shown in Table 79.12. In Paris, in a series of 3500 patients from the tropics studied before the HIV pandemic, only five (0.1%)

cases of isosporiasis were found. A survey of 55 421 stool specimens in Chile over a 10-year period revealed only 452 (0.8%) positives.[112]

Pathogenesis

Isosporiasis is associated with mild to a subtotal villous atrophy. This is seen in patients with AIDS, but was also reported before the HIV pandemic.[113] Inflammatory cells and eosinophils are seen in the lamina propria.

Clinical features

As with cryptosporidiosis, isosporiasis leads to a self-limiting diarrhoea in the immunocompetent, and to chronic diarrhoea in the immunocompromised. The illness in the apparently immunocompetent may be prolonged, extending to 20 years in one report.[114] There is little evidence regarding the frequency with which isosporiasis spontaneously remits in patients with AIDS. In AIDS, isosporiasis is associated with wasting and dehydration. The most thorough analysis remains that of De Hovitz et al.,[115] in which 15 patients with *Isospora belli* were identified among 131 Haitian patients with AIDS; their main complaints were watery diarrhoea, cramping abdominal pain and nausea.

Diagnosis

Diagnosis rests on stool examination using wet preparations and modified Ziehl–Neelsen acid-fast stained smears. The oocysts appear oval, larger than cryptosporidial oocysts (20–30 × 11–19 mm); some oocysts are sporulated before leaving the host and have two easily identified sporoblasts. The oocysts fluoresce with the phenol auramine stain under ultraviolet light. The parasites may also be recognized in small bowel biopsies, visible within enterocyte cytoplasmic vacuoles under electron microscopy and light microscopy.[113]

Management

Treatment with oral co-trimoxazole (sulfamethoxazole 800 mg and trimethoprim 160 mg) four times daily for 10 days eliminated the parasite from stool in most cases, with an interruption in diarrhoea.[116] Unfortunately, this was followed by relapse in 50%, usually within 12 weeks. Retreatment was usually effective. Prophylactic co-trimoxazole may be necessary. Pyrimethamine-sulphonamide combinations are also effective.[116] There is little information on the regimen of choice for those who are intolerant of sulphonamides.

Sarcocystis species

Infection with this coccidian, formerly known as *Isospora hominis*, is uncommonly recognized. The parasite is similar to *I. belli* in its biology,[112] but the life cycle requires alternating infection of intermediate hosts, such as cattle and pigs, and definitive hosts, such as humans. In Strasbourg, the infection was present in 286 patients over a 5-year period, representing 0.4–1.5% of all stool specimens. The infection has not so far been recognized in AIDS. In the Strasbourg series, 30% of patients had peripheral eosinophilia. Biopsy specimens may show an eosinophilic infiltrate. Sporocysts are recognized in stool with the same stains as are used for isosporiasis, but the cysts are smaller (15 × 10 mm).

Cyclospora cayetanensis

During the mid-1980s, a new intestinal pathogen was identified in the stools of individuals with persistent diarrhoea; these were initially known as cyanobacterium-like bodies. It has subsequently become evident that this organism is a member of the *coccidia*, of the genus *Cyclospora*. The organism was tentatively named *Cyclospora cayetanensis*,[117] which now appears to have been formally adopted.

The organism

Until the recent reports in humans, organisms of the genus *Cyclospora* have been identified only in reptiles, myriapods, insectivores and rodents. Oocysts of the human parasite differ morphologically from oocysts in these animal species, and it thus appears that the human isolate is a new species. Each oocyst has two sporocysts. Sporulation has been effected in vitro after 7–13 days in culture. Excystation results in the liberation of two sporozoites which are crescent shaped, approximately 9 mm in length and 1.2 mm in width.[117] The ultrastructural characteristics of the oocysts are entirely consistent with those of other members of the *coccidia*. The parasite life cycle would appear to have both sexual and asexual components. The asexual stages of sporozoite, trophozoite, schizont and merozoite have been identified by electron microscopy in human duodenal biopsies.[118] However, it was assumed that the sexual cycle had also taken place because oocysts were also detected in the patient's stool. It was concluded, therefore, that *Cyclospora* requires only a single host to complete its entire life cycle in humans. Recent molecular phylogenetic analysis indicates that *Cyclospora* is closely related to Eimeria species.[119]

Epidemiology

Cyclospora spp. were first identified in individuals with a history of foreign travel and those infected with HIV. Seasonal outbreaks were described in Nepal among foreign residents and travellers, and a small outbreak has been reported in medical staff in a Chicago hospital. Since these initial observations a more detailed study in Nepal has revealed new information about the infection. As yet the global prevalence of the infection is unknown, although a prevalence of 4–7% has been reported in foreign residents in Nepal, with peak prevalence rates occurring during the warmer months with higher rainfall.[120] *Cyclospora* diarrhoea has now been described in the Americas, the Caribbean, Africa, Bangladesh, South-east Asia, Australia, England and Eastern Europe. The incubation period is quite short, ranging from 1 to 7 days. Transmission appears to be by the faecal–oral route, with water being the most important vehicle. The first water-borne outbreak in the USA was reported in 1995.[121] However, in 1996, a major outbreak of cyclosporiasis was investigated in the USA, which was found to be due to the ingestion of Guatemalan raspberries.[122] Several further outbreaks have been documented in the USA and Canada, which again were thought to be associated with the consumption of berries.

which is septated. For this reason, it was originally given the name *Septata intestinalis*. Most series report that it is less common in patients with AIDS and persistent diarrhoea than *E. bieneusi*, but it is more sensitive to albendazole.[135]

REFERENCES

1. World Health Organization. *The World Health Report 1998. Life in the 21st Century: A Vision for All*. Geneva: WHO; 1998.
2. Löch FD. Massive development of amebas in the large intestine. Translated and reprinted in *Am J Trop Med Hyg* 1875; 24:383–392.
3. Osler W. On the *Amoeba coli* in dysentery and in dysenteric liver abscess. *Johns Hopkins Hosp Bull* 1890; 1:53–54.
4. Councilman WT, Lafleur HA. Amoebic dysentery. *Johns Hopkins Hosp Rep* 1891; 2:395–548.
5. Schaudinn F. Untersuchungen über die Fortpflanzung einiger Rhizopoden (Vorläufige Mittheilung). *Arb Kaiserlichen Gesundheitsamte* 1903; 19: 547–576.
6. Walker EL, Sellards AW. Experimental entamoebic dysentery. *Philippine J Sci B Trop Med* 1913; 8:253–330.
7. Brumpt E. Etude sommaire de l' '*Entamoeba dispar*' n. sp. Amibe à kystes quandrinuclées, parasite de l'homme. *Bull Acad Med (Paris)* 1925; 94: 943–952.
8. Sargeaunt PG, Williams JE, Grene JD. The differentiation of invasive and non-invasive *Entamoeba histolytica* by isoenzyme electrophoresis. *Trans R Soc Trop Med Hyg* 1978; 72:519–521.
9. Sargeaunt PG, Williams JE. Electrophoretic isoenzyme patterns of the pathogenic and non-pathogenic intestinal amoebae of man. *Trans R Soc Trop Med Hyg* 1979; 73:225–227.
10. Diamond LS, Clark CG. A redescription of *Entamoeba histolytica* Schaudinn, 1903 (Amended Walker, 1911) separating it from *Entamoeba dispar* Brumpt, 1925. *J Eukaryot Microbiol* 1993; 40:340–344.
11. WHO/PAHO/UNESCO. A consultation with experts on amoebiasis. Mexico City, Mexico 28–29 January, 1997. *Epidemiol Bull* 1997; 18:13–14.
12. WHO. Amoebiasis. *Wkly Epidemiol Rec* 1997; 72:97–99.
13. Cavalier-Smith T. Kingdom protozoa and its 18 phyla. *Microbiol Rev* 1993; 57:953–994.
14. Silberman JD, Clark CG, Diamond LS, et al. Phylogeny of the genera Entamoeba and Endolimax as deduced from small-subunit ribosomal RNA sequences. *Mol Biol Evol* 1999; 16:1740–1751.
15. Mai Z, Ghosh S, Frisardi M, et al. Hsp60 is targeted to a cryptic mitochondrion-derived organelle ('crypton') in the microaerophilic protozoan parasite *Entamoeba histolytica*. *Mol Cell Biol* 1999; 19: 2198–2205.
16. Tovar J, Fischer A, Clark CG. The mitosome, a novel organelle related to mitochondria in the amitochondrial parasite *Entamoeba histolytica*. *Mol Microbiol* 1999; 32:1013–1021.
17. Azam A, Paul J, Sehgal D, et al. Identification of novel genes from *Entamoeba histolytica* by expressed sequence tag analysis. *Gene* 1996; 181:113–116.
18. Cavalier-Smith T. A revised six-kingdom system of life. *Biol Rev Camb Philos Soc* 1998; 73:203–266.
19. Ghosh S, Field J, Rogers R, et al. The *Entamoeba histolytica* mitochondrion-derived organelle (crypton) contains double-stranded DNA and appears to be bound by a double membrane. *Infect Immun* 2000; 68:4319–4322.
20. Diamond LS. Techniques of axenic cultivation of *Entamoeba histolytica* Schaudinn, 1903 and *E. histolytica*-like amebae. *J Parasitol* 1968; 54: 1047–1056.
21. Reeves RE. Metabolism of *Entamoeba histolytica* Schaudinn, 1903. *Adv Parasitol* 1984; 23:105–142.
22. Rosenthal B, Mai Z, Caplivski D, et al. Evidence for the bacterial origin of genes encoding fermentation enzymes of the amitochondriate protozoan parasite *Entamoeba histolytica*. *J Bacteriol* 1997; 179:3736–3745.
23. Rodriguez MA, Garcia-Perez RM, Mendoza L, et al. The pyruvate: ferredoxin oxidoreductase enzyme is located in the plasma membrane and in a cytoplasmic structure in Entamoeba. *Microb Pathog* 1998; 25:1–10.
24. Ali IK, Zaki M, Clark CG. Use of PCR amplification of tRNA gene-linked short tandem repeats for genotyping *Entamoeba histolytica*. *J Clin Microbiol* 2005; 43: 842–847.
25. Walsh JA. Problems in recognition and diagnosis of amebiasis: estimation of the global magnitude of morbidity and mortality. *Rev Infect Dis* 1986; 8:228–238.
26. Gathiram V, Jackson TF. A longitudinal study of asymptomatic carriers of pathogenic zymodemes of *Entamoeba histolytica*. *S Afr Med J* 1987; 72:669–672.
27. Fotedar R, Stark D, Beebe N, et al. PCR detection of *Entamoeba histolytica, Entamoeba dispar*, and *Entamoeba moshkovskii* in stool samples from Sydney, Australia. *J Clin Microbiol* 2007; 45:1035–1037.
28. Ramos F, Moran P, Gonzalez E, et al. *Entamoeba histolytica* and *Entamoeba dispar*: prevalence of infection in a rural Mexican community. *Exp Parasitol* 2005; 110:327–330.
29. Adams SA, Robson SC, Gathiram V, et al. Immunological similarity between the 170 kD amoebic adherence glycoprotein and human beta 2 integrins. *Lancet* 1993; 341:17–19.
30. Huston CD, Houpt ER, Mann BJ, et al. Caspase 3-dependent killing of host cells by the parasite *Entamoeba histolytica*. *Cell Microbiol* 2000; 2: 617–625.
31. Leippe M, Bruhn H, Hecht O, et al. Ancient weapons: the three-dimensional structure of amoebapore A. *Trends Parasitol* 2005; 21:5–7.
32. Leon G, Fiori C, Das P, et al. Electron probe analysis and biochemical characterization of electron-dense granules secreted by *Entamoeba histolytica*. *Mol Biochem Parasitol* 1997; 85:233–242.
33. Que X, Reed SL. Cysteine proteinases and the pathogenesis of amebiasis. *Clin Microbiol Rev* 2000; 13:196–206.
34. Yu Y, Chadee K. *Entamoeba histolytica* stimulates interleukin 8 from human colonic epithelial cells without parasite-enterocyte contact. *Gastroenterology* 1997; 112:1536–1547.
35. Seydel KB, Li E, Swanson PE, et al. Human intestinal epithelial cells produce proinflammatory cytokines in response to infection in a SCID mouse-human intestinal xenograft model of amebiasis. *Infect Immun* 1997; 65:1631–1639.
36. Reed SL, Ember JA, Herdman DS, et al. The extracellular neutral cysteine proteinase of *Entamoeba histolytica* degrades anaphylatoxins C3a and C5a. *J Immunol* 1995; 155:266–274.
37. Haque R, Mondal D, Duggal P, et al. *Entamoeba histolytica* infection in children and protection from subsequent amoebiasis. *Infect Immun* 2006; 74:904–909.
38. De Leon A. Pronóstico tardío en el absceso hepático amibiano. *Arch Invest Med* 1970; 1:205–206.
39. Moran P, Ramos F, Ramiro M, et al. Infection by HIV-1 is not a risk for amebiasis. *Am J Trop Med Hyg* 2005; 73:296–300.
40. Kelsall BL, Ravdin JI. Degradation of human IgA by *Entamoeba histolytica*. *J Infect Dis* 1993; 168:1319–1322.
41. Tran VQ, Herdman DS, Torian BE, et al. The neutral cysteine proteinase of *Entamoeba histolytica* degrades IgG and prevents its binding. *J Infect Dis* 1998; 177:508–511.
42. Carrada-Bravo T. Invasive amebiasis as a public health problem. *Biol Med Hosp Infant Mex* 1989; 46:139–148.
43. Haque R, Neville LM, Hahn P, et al. Rapid diagnosis of Entamoeba infection by using Entamoeba and *Entamoeba histolytica* stool antigen detection kits. *J Clin Microbiol* 1995; 33:2558–2561.
44. Freeman O, Akamaguna A, Jarikre LN. Amoebic liver abscess: the effect of aspiration on the resolution or healing time. *Ann Trop Med Parasitol* 1990; 84:281–287.
45. Weinke T, Friedrich-Janicke B, Hopp P, et al. Prevalence and clinical importance of *Entamoeba histolytica* in two high-risk groups: travelers returning from the tropics and male homosexuals. *J Infect Dis* 1990; 161:1029–1031.

46. Vohra H, Bhatti HS, Ganguly NK, et al. Virulence of pathogenic and non-pathogenic zymodemes of *Entamoeba histolytica* (Indian strains) in guinea-pigs. *Trans R Soc Trop Med Hyg* 1989; 83:648–650.

47. Bruchhaus I, Jacobs T, Leippe M, et al. *Entamoeba histolytica* and *Entamoeba dispar*: differences in numbers and expression of cysteine proteinase genes. *Mol Microbiol* 1996; 22:255–263.

48. Espinosa-Cantellano M, Gonzales-Robles A, Chavez B, et al. *Entamoeba dispar*: ultrastructure, surface properties and cytopathic effect. *J Eukaryot Microbiol* 1998; 45:265–272.

49. Walderich B, Weber A, Knobloch J. Sensitivity of *Entamoeba histolytica* and *Entamoeba dispar* patient isolates to human complement. *Parasite Immunol* 1997; 19:265–271.

50. Sargeaunt PG, Patrick S, O'Keeffe D. Human infections of *Entamoeba chattoni* masquerade as *Entamoeba histolytica*. *Trans R Soc Trop Med Hyg* 1992; 86:633–634.

51. Stark DJ, Beebe N, Marriott D, et al. Dientamoebiasis: clinical importance and recent advances. *Trends Parasitol* 2006; 22:92–96.

52. Johnson JA, Clark CG. Cryptic genetic diversity in *Dientamoeba fragilis*. *J Clin Microbiol* 2000; 38:4653–4654.

53. Farthing MJG. Giardiasis as a disease. In: Reynoldson JA, Thompson RCA, Lymbery AJ, eds. *Giardia: From Molecules to Disease and Beyond*. London: CAB International; 1993:15–37.

54. Kabnick KS, Peattie DA. *Giardia*: a missing link between prokaryotes and eukaryotes. *Am Sci* 1991; 79:34–43.

55. Cox FEG. Classification and introduction to the parasitic protozoa. In: Cox FEG, Wakelin D, Gillespie SH, Despommier DD, eds. *Topley, Wilson's Parasitology*. 10th edn. London: Edward Arnold; 2007:186–199.

56. Bauer B, Engelbrecht S, Bakker-Grunwald T, et al. Functional identification of alpha 1-giardin as an annexin of *Giardia lamblia*. *FEMS Microbiol Lett* 1999; 173:147–153.

57. Hetsko ML, McCaffery JM, Svard SG, et al. Cellular and transcriptional changes during excystation of *Giardia lamblia* in vitro. *Exp Parasitol* 1998; 88:172–183.

58. Farthing MJG, Keusch GT, Carey MC. Effects of bile and bile salts on growth and membrane lipid uptake by *Giardia lamblia*: possible implication for pathogenesis of intestinal disease. *J Clin Invest* 1985; 76:1727–1732.

59. Knodler LA, Svard SG, Silberman JD, et al. Developmental gene regulation in *Giardia lamblia*: first evidence for an encystation-specific promoter and differential 5′ mRNA processing. *Mol Microbiol* 1999; 34:327–340.

60. Adam RD. The *Giardia lamblia* genome. *Int J Parasitol* 2000; 30:475–484.

61. Sullivan PB, Marsh MN, Phillips MB, et al. Prevalence and treatment of giardiasis in chronic diarrhoea and malnutrition. *Arch Dis Child* 1991; 66:304–306.

62. Jokipii L, Jokipii AM. Giardiasis in travelers: a prospective study. *J Infect Dis* 1974; 30:295–299.

63. Karanis P, Kourenti C, Smith H. Waterborne transmission of protozoan parasites: a worldwide review of outbreaks and lessons learnt. *J Water Health* 2007; 5:1–38.

64. Furness BW, Beach MJ, Roberts JM. Giardiasis surveillance – United States, 1992–1997. *Morbid Mortal Weekly* 2000; 49:1–13.

65. Katelaris PH, Farthing MJG. Diarrhoea and malabsorption in giardiasis: a multifactorial process. *Gut* 1992; 33:295–297.

66. Buret AG. Mechanisms of epithelial dysfunction in giardiasis. *Gut* 2007; 56:316–317.

67. Troeger H, Epple H-J, Schneider T, et al. Effect of chronic *Giardia lamblia* infection on epithelial transport and barrier function in human duodenum. *Gut* 2007; 56:328–335.

68. Teoh DA, Kamieniecki D, Pang G, et al. *Giardia lamblia* rearranges F-actin and alpha-actinin in human colonic and duodenal monolayers and reduces transepithelial electrical resistance. *J Parasitol* 2000; 86:800–806.

69. Scott KG, Logan MR, Klammer GM, et al. Jejunal brush border microvillous alterations in *Giardia muris*-infected mice: role of T lymphocytes and interleukin-6. *Infect Immun* 2000; 68:3412–3418.

70. Das S, Schteingart CD, Hofmann AF, et al. *Giardia lamblia*: evidence for carrier-mediated uptake and release of conjugated bile acids. *Exp Parasitol* 1997; 87:133–141.

71. Seow F, Katelaris PH, Ngu M. The effect of *Giardia lamblia* trophozoites on trypsin, chymotrypsin and amylase in vitro. *Parasitology* 1993; 106:233–238.

72. Faubert G. Immune response to *Giardia duodenalis*. *Clin Microbiol Rev* 2000; 13:35–54.

73. Farthing MJG, Chong S, Walker-Smith JA. Acute allergic phenomena in giardiasis. *Lancet* 1984; ii:1428.

74. Singer SM, Nash TE. T-cell-dependent control of acute *Giardia lamblia* infections in mice. *Infect Immun* 2000; 68:170–175.

75. Char S, Cevallos AM, Yamson P, et al. Impaired IgA response to *Giardia* heat shock antigen in children with persistent diarrhoea and giardiasis. *Gut* 1992; 34:38–40.

76. Sullivan PB, Lunn PG, Northrop-Clewes CA, et al. Parasitic infection of the gut and protein-losing enteropathy. *J Pediatr Gastroenterol Nutr* 1992; 15:404–407.

77. Goka AKJ, Rolston DDK, Mathan VI, et al. The relative merits of faecal and duodenal juice microscopy in the diagnosis of giardiasis. *Trans R Soc Trop Med Hyg* 1990; 84:66–67.

78. Oster N, Gehrig-Feistel H, Jung H, et al. Evaluation of the immunochromatographic CORIS *Giardia* strip test for rapid diagnosis of *Giardia lamblia*. *Eur* 2006; 25:112–115.

79. Weitzel T, Dittrich S, Mohl I, et al. Evaluation of seven commercial antigen detection tests for *Giardia* and *Cryptosporidium* in stool samples. *Clin Microbiol Infect* 2006; 12:656–659.

80. Amar CF, East CL, Gray J, et al. Detection by PCR of eight groups of enteric pathogens in 4,627 faecal samples. *J Clin Microbiol Infect Dis* 2007; 26:311–323.

81. Meloni BP, Thompson RCA, Reynoldson JA, et al. Albendazole: a more effective antiGiardial agent in vitro than metronidazole or tinidazole. *Trans R Soc Trop Med Hyg* 1990; 84:375–379.

82. Crouch AA, Seow WK, Whitman LM, et al. Sensitivity in vitro of *Giardia intestinalis* to dyadic combinations of azithromycin, doxycycline, mefloquine, tinidazole and furazolidone. *Trans R Soc Trop Med Hyg* 1990; 84:246–248.

83. Rossignol JF, Ayoub A, Ayers MS. Treatment of diarrhea caused by *Giardia intestinalis* and *Entamoeba histolytica* or *E. dispar*: a randomized, double-blind, placebo-controlled study of nitazoxanide. *J Infect Dis* 2001; 184:381–384.

84. Arean VM, Koppisch E. Balantidiasis: a review and report of cases. *Am J Pathol* 1956; 32:1089–1115.

85. Walzer PD, Judson FN, Murphy KB, et al. Balantidiasis outbreak in Truk. *Am J Trop Med Hyg* 1973; 22:33–41.

86. Tyzzer EE. A sporozoan found in the peptic glands of the common mouse. *Proc Soc Exp Biol Med* 1907; 5:12–13.

87. Xiao L, Fayer R, Ryan U, et al. Cryptosporidium taxonomy: recent advances and implications for public health. *Clin Microbiol Rev* 2004; 17:72–97.

88. Smith HV, Rose JB. Waterborne cryptosporidiosis. *Parasitol Today* 1990; 6:8–12.

89. Casemore DP. Epidemiological aspects of human cryptosporidiosis. *Epidemiol Infect* 1990; 104:1–28.

90. Zu SX, Zhu SY, Li JF. Human cryptosporidiosis in China. *Trans R Soc Trop Med Hyg* 1992; 86:639–640.

91. Molbak K, Hojlyng N, Gottschau A, et al. Cryptosporidiosis in infancy and childhood mortality in Guinea-Bissau, West Africa. *BMJ* 1993; 307:417–420.

92. Ravn P, Lungren JD, Kjaeldgaard P, et al. Nosocomial outbreak of cryptosporidiosis in AIDS patients. *BMJ* 1991; 302:277–280.

93. Blanshard C, Jackson AM, Shanson DC, et al. Cryptosporidiosis in HIV seropositive patients. *Q J Med* 1992; 85:813–823.

94. Phillips AD, Thomas AG, Walker-Smith JA. Cryptosporidium, chronic diarrhoea and the proximal small intestinal mucosa. *Gut* 1992; 33:1057–1061.

95. Kelly P, Makumbi FA, Carnaby S, et al. Variable distribution of *Cryptosporidium parvum* in small and large intestine in AIDS revealed by polymerase chain reaction. *Eur J Gastro Hepatol* 1998; 10:855–858.

96. Kelly P, Thillainayagam AV, Smithson J, et al. Jejunal water and electrolyte transport in human cryptosporidiosis. *Dig Dis Sci* 1996; 41:2095–2099.

97. O'Hara SP, Small AJ, Nelson JB, et al. The HIV-1 tat protein enhances *Cryptosporidium parvum*-induced apoptosis in cholangiocytes via a Fas ligand-dependent mechanism. *Infect Immun* 2007; 75:684–696.

98. MacDonald V, Kelly P. Intestinal *coccidia*: cryptosporidiosis, isosporiasis, cyclosporiasis. In: Cox FEG, Wakelin D, Gillespie SH, Despommier DD, eds. *Topley, Wilson's Parasitology*, 10th edn. London: Edward Arnold; 2007:399–421.

99. Jacyna MR, Parkin J, Goldin R, et al. Protracted enteric cryptosporidial infection in selective immunoglobulin A and saccharomyces opsonin deficiencies. *Gut* 1990; 31:714–716.

100. Kelly P, Jack D, Naeem A, et al. Mannose binding lectin is a contributor to mucosal defence against *Cryptosporidium parvum* in AIDS patients. *Gastroenterology* 2000; 119:1236–1242.

101. Connolly GM, Dryden MS, Shanson DC, et al. Cryptosporidial diarrhoea in AIDS and its treatment. *Gut* 1988; 29:593–597.

102. McGowan I, Hawkins A, Weller I. The natural history of cryptosporidial diarrhoea in HIV infected patients. *AIDS* 1993; 7:349–354.

103. Colebunders R, Francis H, Mann JM, et al. Persistent diarrhea, strongly associated with HIV infection in Kinshasa, Zaire. *Am J Gastroenterol* 1987; 82:859–864.

104. Teixidor HS, Godwin TA, Ramirez EA. Cryptosporidiosis of the biliary tract in AIDS. *Radiology* 1991; 180:51–56.

105. Forbes A, Blanshard C, Gazzard B. Natural history of AIDS related sclerosing cholangitis: a study of 20 cases. *Gut* 1993; 34:116–121.

106. Molbak K, Andersen M, Aaby P, et al. Cryptosporidium infection in infancy as a cause of malnutrition: a community study from Guinea-Bissau, West Africa. *Am J Clin Nutr* 1997; 65:149–152.

107. Amadi BC, Kelly P, Mwiya M, et al. Intestinal and systemic infection, HIV and mortality in Zambian children with persistent diarrhoea and malnutrition. *J Pediatr Gastroenterol Nutr* 2001; 32:550–554.

108. Weber R, Bryan RT, Bishop HS, et al. Threshold of detection of Cryptosporidium oocysts in human stool specimens: evidence for low sensitivity of current diagnostic methods. *J Clin Microbiol* 1991; 29:1323–1327.

109. Amadi BC, Mwiya M, Musuku J, et al. Effect of nitazoxanide on morbidity and mortality in Zambian children with cryptosporidiosis: a randomised controlled trial. *Lancet* 2002; 360:1375–1380.

110. Abubakar I, Aliyu SH, Arumugam C, et al. Prevention and treatment of cryptosporidiosis in immunocompromised patients. *Cochrane Database of Systematic Reviews* 2007, Issue 1. Art No. CD004932. DOI:10.1002/14651858.CD004932.pub2.

111. Casemore DP, Blewett DA, Wright SE. Cleaning and disinfection of equipment for gastrointestinal flexible endoscopy: interim recommendations of a working party of the British Society of Gastroenterology. *Gut* 1990; 31:1156–1157 (letter).

112. Stürchler D. Parasitic diseases of the small intestinal tract. *Baillières Clin Gastroenterol* 1987; 1:397–424.

113. Brandborg LL, Goldberg SB, Breidenbach WC. Human coccidiosis – a possible cause of malabsorption. *N Engl J Med* 1970; 283:1306–1313.

114. Trier JS, Moxey PC, Schimmel EM, et al. Chronic intestinal coccidiosis in man: intestinal pathology and response to treatment. *Gastroenterology* 1974; 66:923–935.

115. De Hovitz JA, Pape JW, Boncy M, et al. Clinical manifestations and therapy of Isospora belli infection in patients with AIDS. *N Engl J Med* 1986; 315:87–90.

116. Pape JW, Verdier RI, Johnson WD. Treatment and prophylaxis of *Isospora belli* infections in patients with AIDS. *N Engl J Med* 1989; 320:1044–1047.

117. Ortega YR, Sterling CR, Gilman RH, et al. Cyclospora species – a new protozoan pathogen of humans. *N Engl J Med* 1993; 328:1308–1312.

118. Sun T, Hardi CF, Asnis D, et al. Light and electron microscopic identification of *Cyclospora* species in the small intestine: evidence of the presence of asexual life cycle in human host. *Am J Clin Pathol* 1996; 105:215–220.

119. Relman DA, Schmidt TM, Gajadhar A, et al. Molecular phylogenetic analysis of *Cyclospora*, the human intestinal pathogen, suggests that it is closely related to Eimeria species. *J Infect Dis* 1996; 173:440–445.

120. Hoge CW, Shlim DR, Rajah R, et al. Epidemiology of diarrhoeal illness associated with coccidian-like organism among travellers and foreign residents in Nepal. *Lancet* 1993; 341:1175–1179.

121. Huang P, Weber JT, Sosin DM, et al. The first reported outbreak of diarrheal illness associated with *Cyclospora* in the United States. *Ann Intern Med* 1995; 123:409–414.

122. Herwaldt BI, Ackers M-L, Farrar J, et al. An outbreak in 1996 of cyclosporiasis associated with imported raspberries. *N Engl J Med* 1997; 336:1548–1556.

123. Bendall RP, Lucas S, Moody A, et al. Diarrhoea associated with cyanobacterium-like bodies: a new coccidian enteritis of man. *Lancet* 1993; 341:590–592.

124. Hoge CW, Shlim DR, Ghimire M, et al. Placebo-controlled trial of co-trimoxatole for *Cyclospora* infections among travellers and foreign residents in Nepal. *Lancet* 1995; 345:667–668, 691–693.

125. Verdier R-I, Fitzgerald DW, Johnson WD Jr, et al. Trimethoprim-sulfamethoxazole compared with ciprofloxacin for treatment and prophylaxis of *Isospora belli* and *Cyclospora cayetanensis* infection in HIV-infected patients. A randomized, controlled trial. *Ann Intern Med* 2000; 132:885–888.

126. Desportes-Livage I. Biology of microsporidia. In: Petry F, ed. *Cryptosporidiosis and Microsporidiosis. Contributions to Microbiology.* Vol. 6. Basel: Karger; 2000:116–139.

127. Modigliani R, Bories C, le Charpentier Y, et al. Diarrhoea and malabsorption in AIDS: a study of four cases with special emphasis on opportunistic protozoan infections. *Gut* 1985; 26:179–187.

128. Cali A, Owen RL. Intracellular development of *Enterocytozoon*, a unique microsporidian found in the intestine of AIDS patients. *J Protozool* 1990; 37:145–155.

129. Orenstein JM, Tenner M, Kotler DP. Localization of infection by the microsporidian *Enterocytozoon bieneusi* in the gastrointestinal tract of AIDS patients with diarrhoea. *AIDS* 1992; 6:195–197.

130. Field AS, Hing MC, Millikan ST, et al. Microsporidia in the small intestine of HIV-infected patients. A new diagnostic technique and a new species. *Med J Aust* 1993; 158:390–394.

131. Pol S, Romana CA, Richard S, et al. Microsporidia infection in patients with HIV and unexplained cholangitis. *N Engl J Med* 1993; 328:95–99.

132. Weber R, Bryan RT, Owen RL, et al. Improved light microscopical detection of microsporidia spores in stool and duodenal aspirates. *N Engl J Med* 1992; 326:161–166.

133. Blanshard C, Ellis DS, Tovey DG, et al. Treatment of intestinal microsporidiosis with albendazole in patients with AIDS. *AIDS* 1992; 6:311.

134. Molina JM, Tourneur M, Sarfati C, et al. Fumagillin treatment of intestinal microsporidiosis. *New Engl J Med* 2002; 346:1963–1969.

135. Molina JM, Oksenhendler E, Beauvais B, et al. Disseminated microsporidiosis due to *Septata intestinalis* in patients with AIDS: clinical features and response to albendazole therapy. *J Infect Dis* 1995; 171:245–249.

Chapter 80

David C. Warhurst

Potentially Pathogenic Free-living Amoebae

Facultatively parasitic free-living amoebae, normally found in soil and water, cause three important diseases in man: primary amoebic meningoencephalitis (PAM), granulomatous amoebic encephalitis (GAE) with invasion of other tissues, and chronic amoebic keratitis (CAK). Both PAM and CAK occur in healthy individuals, while GAE and related diseases are generally associated with immunodeficient states.[1]

The free-living amoebae concerned belong to two main groups of small free-living amoebae: the amoeboflagellates and the Acanthamoebidae. One case of a brain abscess caused by the larger free-living amoeba *Sappinia diploidea* has been reported in an immunocompetent farmer.[2,3]

Amoeboflagellates

Naegleria fowleri, which causes PAM, is found worldwide in warm fresh water, normally feeding on bacteria. Its life cycle has three stages: the feeding, growing, multiplying form or trophozoite found on surfaces of vegetation and mud, the rapidly motile biflagellate form (Figure 80.1) often found in the surface layers of water and the dormant cyst form found in the same locations as the trophozoite. Experimental and epidemiological evidence supports the infectivity to man of the trophozoite and flagellate. Infection takes place through the olfactory epithelium of the nose when the organisms are inhaled in contaminated water, usually during swimming, penetrate the epithelium and pass along the olfactory nerve branches in the cribriform plate to enter the meninges, where they multiply in the CSF of the perivascular Virchow–Robin spaces. Trophozoites penetrate the dura mater and enter the substance of the brain, ingesting cerebral tissue (Figure 80.2). The symptoms and features of the CSF are characteristic of a purulent bacterial meningitis, but there is no response to antibacterials. Coma culminates in death. The application of specific therapy after early diagnosis of the condition has led to recovery in only three authentic instances among about 300 recorded cases (Table 80.1). Although relatively few cases of PAM are recorded, the disease is significant among those associated with recreational water use because of its almost invariably fatal outcome. In the 10 years from 1989, 22 cases of PAM caused by *N. fowleri* were reported in the USA, all fatal.[4] In the latest report from MMWR (2006), the only death in 2003–2004 from infection associated with recreational water was caused by *N. fowleri*.[5]

Acanthamoebidae

Acanthamoeba species

Acanthamoeba spp. which cause GAE and CAK, are found worldwide and also feed on bacteria (In some earlier studies the organism was referred to as *Hartmannella* but the genera are now recognized to be distinct). *Acanthamoeba* spp., unlike *Naegleria*, can multiply in fresh or brackish water. The life cycle consists only of the trophozoite and cyst forms, and either of these can be a source of infection for man. Several species have been isolated from human tissue, and the ubiquitous distribution of these organisms means that human exposure is widespread. For example, it is estimated that humans inhale one of the resistant cysts every day.[6] As a corollary of this wide exposure, the organism finds it difficult to colonize man, and infections are generally restricted to the immunodeficient, or to immunoprivileged sites, the most common of which is the cornea (Figures 80.3, 80.4). Infections are generally of a chronic type and there is a marked granulomatous reaction. Treatment by medical or surgical means is usually successful in ocular infection, but a few successes have been reported in systemic infection.

Acanthamoeba and upper respiratory infection

Association of *Acanthamoeba* with upper respiratory infections was suspected in the 1960s,[7] and the organism has been regularly isolated from oronasal swabs. Several strains isolated from room and outside air using a slit sampler were found to be cytopathic to mammalian cell cultures.[6] Although there is a suggestive link between the isolation of *Acanthamoeba* from the upper respiratory tract and nose bleeding, rhinitis and upper respiratory infections, the connection has not yet been convincingly drawn. It may be argued that, in some cases at least, isolations from the nose represent trapped air-borne cysts, and not active infections.

Balamuthia mandrillaris

Among case reports of GAE, mainly due to infection with *Acanthamoeba* spp., an increasing number of systemic infections with the acanthamoebid free-living amoeba *Balamuthia mandrillaris* are being reported.[1,8,9] This organism has not yet been shown to cause CAK. The life cycle resembles that of *Acanthamoeba*, but the

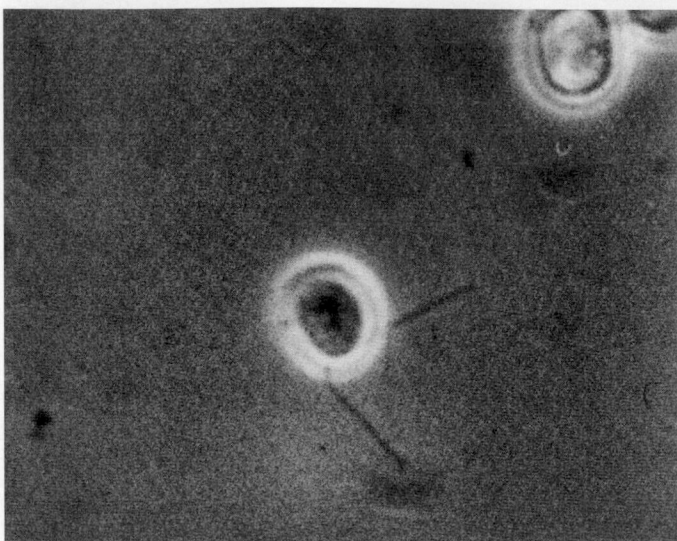

Figure 80.1 Flagellate stage of *Naegleria fowleri*. (Environmental isolate; organism fixed with osmic acid vapour and examined under phase contrast.)

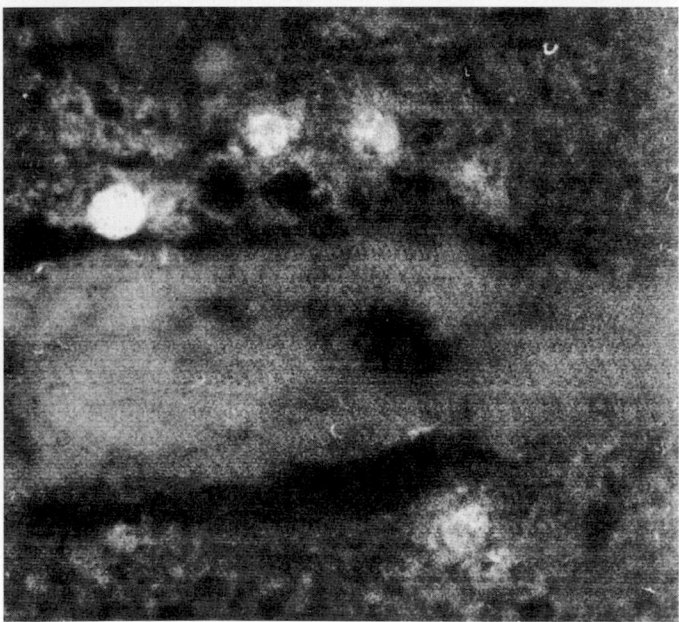

Figure 80.2 *Naegleria fowleri* in human brain section. (Stained by specific fluorescent antibody test.) This shows a cerebral vessel, and *Naegleria* trophozoites invading the brain tissue from the perivascular CSF.

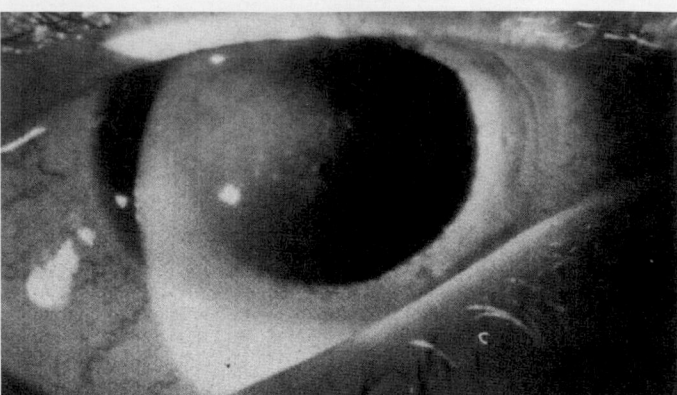

Figure 80.3 *Acanthamoeba* species keratitis. Corneal ulceration, hypopyon, conjunctival hyperaemia and radial neuritis are visible in this photograph of an infected eye.

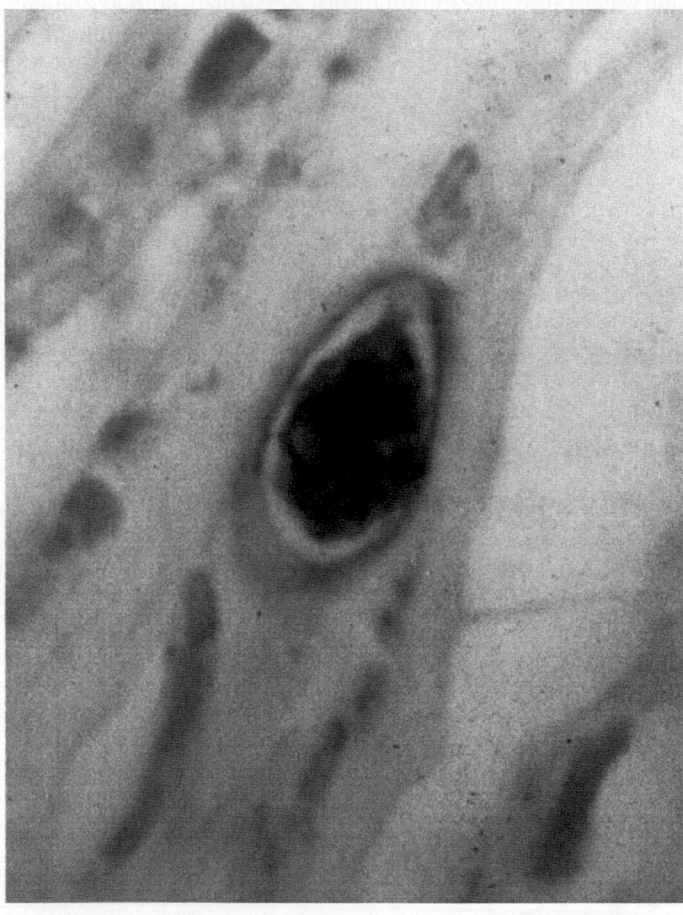

Figure 80.4 Encysting trophozoite of *Acanthamoeba* species in corneal laminae. (Stained with immunoperoxidase using rabbit anti-*Acanthamoeba* serum. Note cellular infiltration and the heavily stained amoebic trophozoite.)

organism infects apparently immunocompetent as well as immunosuppressed adults and children. There are reports of successful treatment of early diagnosed cases.[10,11] Isolation and diagnosis by culture is difficult, serum IFAT titres can be helpful[12,13] and PCR is now a preferred diagnostic approach.[1] Study of DNA homologies has confirmed a close relationship with *Acanthamoeba* spp., but ruled out inclusion in the genus.[14]

Environmental isolation[15,16] is possible using cell cultures or other free-living amoebae as food.

Association of free-living amoebae with *Legionella* and other bacteria

Acanthamoeba and *Naegleria* spp. can harbour pathogenic microorganisms, such as *Legionella*[17,18] and the *cholera vibrio*[19] and have

Table 80.1 Successful treatments of culture- or PCR-proved *Naegleria fowleri* meningoencephalitis

Location	Culture or PCR proof of *N. fowleri*	Delay in diagnosis (cerebral oedema, coma etc.)	Antiamoebic drug treatment
CASE 1			
S. Australia 1972[a]	Yes. Culture	>3 days (coma, but responding to painful stimuli)	AmB:1.0 mg/kg per day i.v. ×5, then 0.5 mg intrathecally and a ventricular reservoir fitted to allow 10 doses of 0.1 mg on alternate days, with stemetil premedication. The intraventricular amphotericin dose was mixed with CSF prior to administration
CASE 2			
California 1982[42]	Yes. Culture and, later, PCR	3 days (mild coma, responding to painful stimuli)	AmB: 1.5 mg/kg per day i.v. in 2 divided doses for 3 days with 1.5 mg AmB/day intrathecally. Then 1 mg AmB every other day for 8 days: miconazole i.v. at 350 mg/m² per day in 3 divided doses for 9 days: miconazole intrathecally, 10 mg/day and then 10 mg every other day for 8 days, and rifampicin orally at 10 mg/kg per day in 3 divided doses for 9 days. Dexamethasone and phenytoin were given respectively for increased intracranial pressure and for seizures
CASE 3			
Mexico 2005[41]	Yes. Culture, later PCR and antigen confirmation	On admission, severe headache, vomiting and fever. After 9 h ataxic gait, mild confusion, seizures and coma	Dexamethasone 0.6 mg/kg 6-hourly i.v., ceftriaxone 100 mg/kg per day i.v. initially; after 9 h, AmB 0.25 mg/kg daily i.v. rising to 1 mg/kg, for 14 days, fluconazole 10 mg/kg daily i.v. first, followed by oral for 1 month, and oral rifampicin 10 mg/kg oral daily for 1 month. Recovery began within a few hours and on the 3rd day afebrile and awake

AmB, amphotericin B deoxycholate.
[a] K. Anderson, pers comm; Anderson K, Jamieson A. Primary amoebic meningoencephalitis. *Lancet* 1972; ii:379.

the potential to act as chlorine-resistant infection reservoirs for these organisms in water supply networks.

PRIMARY AMOEBIC MENINGOENCEPHALITIS

Clinical features[20]

Naegleria fowleri is normally restricted to the central nervous system but in one severely malnourished case, the organism was found disseminated in many tissues.[21,22] The illness attacks healthy persons, 3–7 days after exposure to contaminated water. It starts with headache and slight pyrexia, in some cases associated with sore throat and rhinitis. Over the next 3 days the disease progresses, with rising fever and increasing headache, vomiting and stiff neck. The severely disoriented or comatose patient is admitted to hospital with a diagnosis of acute pyogenic meningitis. Lumbar puncture reveals a purulent cerebrospinal fluid (CSF) but no bacteria are demonstrated. The CSF pressure is generally raised. No response is noted to antibacterials. Deep coma is followed by cardiorespiratory failure and death ensues.[23] Haemorrhagic pulmonary oedema may develop during the course of the disease and this is thought to be neurogenic.[24] In addition, myocarditis may be detected at postmortem.[25] Although involvement with water

sports antecedes most cases, some fatal infections reported from Australia were acquired from the mains water supply.[24] In one US case,[26] the patient, a narcotic addict, who had recently had teeth extracted, had no history of water contact other than with public water supplies; and a Nigerian farmer is thought to have become infected after ritual nose rinsing with water from a local pond.[27]

Diagnosis

The major problem in diagnosis of PAM is to distinguish between it and other encephalitides of rapid onset such as meningococcal, acute tubercular and viral meningitis. Distinction from all but non-tubercular bacterial meningitis is relatively straightforward because on CSF examination there is a markedly raised cell count, mainly polymorphonuclear cells. In tubercular or viral meningitis the cellular increase, when present, is composed mainly of mononuclear cells. The presence of erythrocytes in CSF has been suggested as characteristic of PAM, but evidence so far does not confirm its specificity and erythrocytes may contaminate CSF during the lumbar puncture procedure. CSF protein is generally raised around 1 g/L and may reach 10 g/L, and this contrasts with viral meningitis where low values are usually found. Glucose may be lower than normal, as in bacterial meningitis, but this is not a useful diagnostic feature.

It is recommended that in investigation of CSF from meningitis cases a fraction of the CSF should be put on one side while the film is being stained for bacteria, so that if bacteria are not seen the CSF can be examined in wet film in more detail. Observation of fresh CSF under a coverslip is a procedure which may give much information. First, in the case of bacterial meningitis, the presence of bacteria may be observed directly, before cultures have grown. If no bacteria are seen, amoebic trophozoites may be discovered. Here there is scope for error. Highly active mononuclear or other white cells may be found in the CSF, and unless careful observation is made to detect the large granular nucleus (amoebae have a small to invisible nucleus) and the non-progressive movement of the mammalian cells, the cells may be mistaken for amoebae. In CSF at 37°C, *Naegleria* moves actively at a rate of one to three body lengths per minute. The movement is progressive and the body is elongated like a slug during movement, with characteristic explosive protrusion of a clear pseudopodium on alternate sides of the anterior. Warming the wet preparation may be a useful method of stimulating movement.

As well as wet microscopy, examination of cytospin films stained by a Romanovsky stain should be carried out. An acridine orange stain with examination under the fluorescent microscope may also be useful to differentiate the amoebae from leukocytes, the small nucleus and large area of reddish foamy cytoplasm of the amoebae being particularly noteworthy.[28]

To confirm the diagnosis after treatment has been instituted, cultures of the CSF sample upon 1.5% non-nutrient agar coated with washed *E. coli* bacteria and maintained in a moist box at 37°C overnight should be examined. The agar may be made up in distilled water or ideally in the dilute amoeba saline solution of Page[29]:

NaCl	0.12 g
$MgSO_4 \cdot 7H_2O$	0.004 g
$CaCl_2 \cdot 2H_2O$	0.004 g
Na_2HPO_4	0.14 g
KH_2PO_4	0.136 g

in 1 L distilled water, autoclaved in 100 mL aliquots and stored at room temperature.

N. fowleri will grow in cell cultures used in the usual virus isolation techniques, and these may be used as an isolation method. It is important to ensure that antifungals such as amphotericin (Fungizone) are not included in the cultures.

N. fowleri-specific monoclonal antibodies have been developed which are likely to prove valuable in diagnosis,[30] and isoenzyme,[31] restriction digestion and polymerase chain reaction (PCR) techniques for identification of *N. fowleri* and other pathogenic free living amoebae from environmental and pathological material have been described.[32] Nevertheless, the urgency of diagnosis makes direct examination of the CSF the primary basis for going ahead with treatment. Confirmation by other means should be available within 24 h, but delay is undesirable.

Management

There is a shortage of successful treatments on which to base recommendations. Schuster and Visvesvara give five case reports of successful treatment[33] in Table 3 of their recent review, but I have excluded four from this Table 80.1, since available evidence indicates *N. fowleri* was not involved.[34,35,36,37,38,39,40]

There remain in the literature then, only three convincing successfully-treated cases. In all three, success followed early diagnosis of the infection and the institution (gradual in case 3[41]) of a high-dose regimen of amphotericin B deoxycholate (AmB), with, in the two most recent, a concomitant azole drug i.v. and/or intrathecally and oral rifampicin (Table 80.1). The choice of intravenous azole drug appears to lie between miconazole and fluconazole, with miconazole more active in vitro. It is informative to contrast successful and unsuccessful treatments in female children of 9 (case 2, Table 80.1)[42] and 11 years of age.[43] A mild headache was the first indication of the disease, with no upper respiratory symptoms noted. Treatment in the former case was successful. The patient had been swimming in a hot spring where a fatal case of PAM had been acquired in 1971.[44] Before admission the patient had a 3-day history of symptoms, initially headache, followed by nausea, vomiting and increasing lethargy. On the morning of admission she was comatose but responsive to painful stimuli. A diagnosis of bacterial meningitis was made on the cell count and chemical features of the CSF. Because of the previous case from the same hot spring, a wet preparation of CSF was examined. Cells with amoeboid movement were observed in the CSF and in stained preparations[45] in the County Hospital to which she was transferred, and a diagnosis of PAM was made. The treatment was begun while the patient was responsive to pain and to tactile stimulation. Although nuchal rigidity and diffuse papilloedema were present, muscle tone and deep tendon reflexes were normal. Serum electrolytes, blood urea nitrogen and glucose were within normal limits and, significantly, computed tomography showed cerebral oedema was mild. Combination drug treatment was successful in achieving removal of detectable amoebae from the CSF and stabilization of the patient's condition after 3 days. During the remainder of her stay in hospital the patient's condition continued to improve, although after discharge some decrease in pain sensation in the left leg was noted, which resolved within 2 months, while the CSF remained abnormal for several months. Subsequent cases in the USA treated with a similar though not identical regimen have not survived.[46]

The contrasting patient, at Bath Spa, UK, was also admitted to hospital with a 3-day history of headache and a 1-day history of pyrexia, vomiting and blurred vision. She had swum in a warm mineral water pool 6 days previously. The patient was drowsy, with slight neck stiffness. Eye movements and fundi were normal. Thus the clinical condition on admission to hospital was apparently no worse than in the first case. On the basis of purulent CSF and other characteristic features a diagnosis of pyogenic meningitis was made, and treatment with antibacterial antibiotics was instituted. The condition of the patient deteriorated during the next few hours, and convulsions began to occur, which were controlled with phenytoin, diazepam and intramuscular paraldehyde. The optic fundi remained normal, but cerebral oedema was assumed to be present, and mannitol was given intravenously. Respiratory arrest occurred 20 h after admission, and at 36 h identification of amoebae was made in the CSF, organisms were successfully cultured, and antiamoebic therapy (amphotericin B 0.5 mg/kg per day by single 6-hourly intravenous infusion, concurrently with sulfadimidine and rectal metronidazole) was begun. Amphotericin B (0.15 mg) was administered through a ventricular catheter. Although it had been planned to increase the intravenous amphotericin dose to 1 mg/kg per day, poor urinary output and rising blood urea led to only 0.6 mg/kg being achieved. On day 3, 0.05 mg amphotericin was given, and on day 4, 0.1 mg intraventricularly. Although amoebae were then visually and culturally absent from the CSF, the patient did not wake from her coma and died on day 5 after cardiac arrest.

A significant difference between the two cases is that the clinicians and laboratory staff in the first were aware of the possibility of PAM, having seen an earlier fatal case acquired from the same stream, and identification of amoebae in the CSF was made soon after the patient was admitted to hospital. Differences in the treatment may also have been significant, in particular the initial lower intravenous dose of amphotericin in the fatal case, but early diagnosis is clearly to be aimed at. It is, however, important to note that studies on DNA from the isolate from the Californian case indicate that the N. fowleri involved was an unusual variety which had a restriction pattern that diverges most from all other strains tested.[47]

Recommendations for treatment were made by Duma.[48] The administration of high dose amphotericin B should not be unduly delayed once diagnosis of the condition has been made. The approach that is normally made to intravenous amphotericin treatment for other conditions, that is, to start at a lower dose (0.25–0.5 mg/kg per day) and increase it cautiously to detect idiosyncrasy and delay kidney damage, is inappropriate (although this presupposes the diagnosis is reliable). After a low trial dose, the maximum dose possible should be given immediately, by slow intravenous infusion. Judging by the intrathecal dose of amphotericin B used in case 1, it appears that there is some scope for increase. It is recognized that children can tolerate higher doses of amphotericin B than adults.[49,50] An argument advanced by Ferrante[51] is that too high a dose of the drug leads to lysis of amoebae and an adverse immunological reaction to the released foreign protein. Ferrante's point is probably best addressed by the judicious use of corticosteroids to moderate the inflammatory reaction, as in cases 2 and 3 (Table 80.1).

It is important to monitor the blood urea nitrogen value daily during amphotericin treatment, and the manufacturers recommend that if this rises above 17.8 mmol/L (50 mg/dL), or the creatinine above 310 μmol/L (3.5 mg/dL), 1 day of therapy should be omitted and the next dose lowered. Amphotericin B methyl ester, a less toxic modification of the drug, though active in vitro, has not been found effective in protecting experimental mice.[52] Findings have been reported for liposomal amphotericin B.[53]

The use of drug combinations

In in vitro and animal studies a potentiative synergism of amphotericin with tetracycline,[54,55] miconazole[56] and rifampicin[57] has been reported. The rationale for using combination drug treatment with miconazole is supported by in vitro studies carried out on the strain of N. fowleri isolated from the CSF in the Californian case, since synergism was seen with amphotericin. Synergism was not demonstrated between rifampicin and amphotericin, but there was clearly an additive effect, while the effects of rifampicin and miconazole were apparently mildly antagonistic. Although there is not enough evidence from human studies to support

combination drug treatments, there seems no reason not to try them. It is worth noting that for Candida albicans miconazole is antagonistic to amphotericin B,[58] but this was not seen for N. fowleri. Ketoconazole appears to be an alternative to miconazole and potentially less toxic. However, it is less effective than miconazole in vitro. Recent work in vitro and in the mouse model indicates that the azole voriconazole may be worth trying[59] and that azithromycin may be useful in synergy with AmB.[60]

Pathology and pathogenesis

N. fowleri injures nerve cells by two alternate mechanisms: trogocytosis (ingestion of the cytoplasm through a feeding cup), and contact-dependent lysis due to alteration of the permeability of the target cell by lytic proteins. Cell death is due to the release of ions, followed later by the loss of large macromolecules.[61]

The pathogenic process in the brain is probably similar to that in bacterial meningitis. An inflammatory reaction develops in the meninges and the cellular influx leads to damage of the cellular functions of the blood–brain barrier. In addition there is damage to the integrity of the barrier due to direct invasion of amoebae into the brain tissue, which occurs without obvious cellular reaction.

Although it probably has no relevance to the pathogenesis of PAM, it is interesting to note that even non-pathogenic species of Naegleria harbour an agent capable of causing cytopathic changes in cultured vertebrate cells. The agent is termed NACM (Naegleria amoeba cytopathic agent) and is a protein of 35 kDa. NACM shows the features of an infectious agent, with some similarity to a prion.[62]

Immunology

Reciprocal titres in the indirect fluorescent antibody test of 5–20 were found in a survey of normal human sera in New Zealand.[63] It will probably be concluded that for such low titres to be found in such a sensitive test indicates little exposure and probable cross-reactivity with antigens from related or unrelated species. The disease course is too rapid in the majority of clinical cases for humoral antibody to be stimulated, but it has been demonstrated in a recovered case. Although a low total serum IgA level has been postulated to be a predisposing factor in infection,[64] this has not been confirmed.[65] Evidence has been obtained experimentally in BALB/c mice that immunity can be transferred by immune spleen cells but not by immune serum.[66] However, an earlier study did show transfer by immune serum.[67] There is experimental evidence that immunity is manifested at the nasal mucosa by polymorphonuclear leukocytes, which kill the amoebae, and also by the shedding of necrotic epithelium.[68]

Although the amoebae are unaffected by recombinant human interleukin 1 or tumour necrosis factor,[69] the latter stimulates the adherence of neutrophils to N. fowleri, with destruction of the amoeba. This is independent of complement or specific immunoglobulin. Ingestion of neutrophils by trophozoites was observed following more prolonged incubation, particularly in the absence of tumour necrosis factor. Ability of trophozoites to ingest host neutrophils may represent a virulence factor.[70] The trophozoites are killed by complement[71] in the bloodstream, and this probably explains the usual restriction to the CNS.

In recent immunization studies in mice, intranasal adjuvants which increase amoeba-specific mucosal IgA levels in nasal fluids have been shown to enhance protection.[72]

Epidemiology

N. fowleri has been isolated from thermally elevated aquatic environments worldwide, but temperature factors associated with occurrence of the amoeba remain relatively undefined. It is interesting that, although N. fowleri will grow well at temperatures up to 45°C, cysts are not readily produced at high temperatures, in contrast to the non-pathogenic species N. lovaniensis,[73] which also grows at 45°C. This may perhaps explain the persistence of N. fowleri in areas of fluctuating temperature or exposure to a temperature gradient. At Bath Spa[74] N. fowleri was isolated from water in an area where warm water mixed with cool, and only N. lovaniensis in a site where the water was uniformly at a high temperature. In a study of a newly created cooling reservoir (Clinton Lake, Illinois) before and after thermal additions from a nuclear power plant, N. fowleri was isolated from the thermally elevated arm but not from the ambient-temperature arm of the reservoir. The probability of isolating thermophilic Naegleria and pathogenic N. fowleri increased significantly with temperature. Repetitive DNA restriction fragment profiles of the N. fowleri Clinton Lake isolates and a known N. fowleri strain of human origin were homologous.[75] This suggests that even in temperate areas we can expect N. fowleri colonization of any newly introduced heated freshwater habitats, such as warm pools. Isolation of the amoebae from environmental sources is difficult since overgrowth of non-pathogenic species, such as N. lovaniensis, readily takes place. To avoid this, it is recommended that multiple small water samples of 10 mL should be collected, concentrated by gentle centrifugation, and each sediment cultured on a different culture plate.[76] The use of swab samples from surfaces has also been reported to increase success in isolating pathogenic free-living amoebae.[77]

Prevention

In the North Island of New Zealand, the bathing places fed by hot springs are generally lined with earth, and the only preventive measures which are applicable are warnings not to immerse the head. These are presented to the public in graphic notices around the pools. In the UK, the contaminated pools associated with the Bath Spa mineral spring have been closed for bathing, for several years. A borehole has been drilled into the aquifer, allowing hot water to reach the surface uncontaminated, further measures have been taken on the other pools and the complex has reopened.

Water treatment

Filtration

Treatment of raw water to be used for drinking purposes by coagulation and filtration is generally effective for removal of organisms which do not multiply in the environment, such as bacterial pathogens, Entamoeba histolytica and Giardia. In the case of the potentially pathogenic free-living amoebae, even one organism which passes through the filter is significant, since unlimited multiplication is possible in the 'purified' water provided a suitable bacterial food source is present. Chemical or physical disinfection is therefore **always** indicated in addition to other measures.

Physical treatment

N. fowleri is not usually isolated from waters at temperatures below 25°C. The cysts and trophozoites are killed by temperatures above 60°C. Attractive recreational waters generally exceed 25°C and are at well below amoebicidal temperatures. The amoebae will grow at a wide range of pH in culture, although growth halts below pH 4.6 and above pH 9.5. Ultraviolet radiation appears ineffective in preventing Naegleria or bacterial contamination of swimming pools.[78] It has been shown that post-UV treatment repair processes in the related species N. gruberi are highly effective.[79] However, a combination of intensive UV treatment and chlorination, together with regular bacteriological and amoebic monitoring, has been applied at the newly opened Bath Spa Complex.

Chemical treatment

N. fowleri will not grow in brackish water. Concentrations of sodium chloride of more than 0.75% will inhibit growth. It has also been shown experimentally that high concentrations of calcium (40–60 mmol/L) are inhibitory.[80] The cysts of N. fowleri, like those of E. histolytica and Giardia, need a free chlorine residual concentration (mg/L) × time (min) factor (CT factor) in the region of 40 for 99.9% inactivation,[81] i.e. 4 mg/L for 10 min or 2 mg/L for 20 min. Depending on the amount of organic material capable of reacting with chlorine present in the water, an initial quantity of chlorine added will produce different residual concentrations of chlorine available for microbial inactivation. In any experimental study it is therefore important to determine the concentration of chlorine (or residual) which remains after the experiment. Only this level is relevant in determination of microbial sensitivity. The pH of the water affects activity, since the active chemical species HOCl, hypochlorous acid, decreases in concentration as pH is raised. However, in contrast to the cysts, the trophozoites are killed by lower chlorine residuals in the antibacterial region of 0.5–1 mg/L. Since disinfection efficiency of chlorine is inversely related to pH, these values are valid up to pH 7.5, but not higher. It is also important to note that chlorination is less efficient at lower temperatures. If bacterial growth is prevented, and this can be confirmed in water masses by a low or nil total plate count, growth of the amoebae should not be possible in the mass of water. However it is still possible that bacteria and amoebae may be growing on and in surfaces not adequately in contact with the disinfectant or in surface films. For example, in the Czechoslovakian series of infections associated with a chlorinated swimming pool at Usti nad Labem, the amoebae were being harboured in unchlorinated water behind a false wall at one end of the pool.[82] In the Bath Spa episode (1978), there was a channel of communication between contaminated unchlorinated warm spring water flowing under the swimming pool and the chlorinated contents. The South Australian series of PAM cases were apparently infected from the public water supply, which was piped over desert after chlorination and thus lost its chlorine content and allowed amoebae to grow. The problem was solved by introducing supplementary chlorination points along the desert pipeline.[83] In addition, the disinfectant monochloramine has been used because it is more persistent than chlorine itself.[84] Ozonation has been tested with some success.[85]

Although the problem of eliminating *Naegleria* from swimming pools seems immense, this is a much more serious problem for natural waters than for artificial pools, where careful design and proper maintenance should be able to achieve effective control.[86]

GRANULOMATOUS AMOEBIC ENCEPHALITIS

The first evidence for involvement of *Acanthamoeba* in human cerebral granulomatous disease was reported in the early 1970s. For *Acanthamoeba*, Kenney[87] examined 1000 sera collected on a routine basis from patients in a New York hospital and found two which reacted at a high titre with *A. culbertsoni* antigen in a complement fixation test. One of the patients had suffered from gastrointestinal problems, and there was little other evidence to incriminate amoebae. (It is interesting to note that we have seen *A. culbertsoni* infection in the small intestinal wall of a Malaysian patient.) The other died of a cerebrovascular accident, and amoebae similar to *Acanthamoeba* were demonstrated at postmortem histological examination of the brain in the case described by Jager and Stamm.[88] Several species of the genus have now been identified in human pathological material. The organism produces infections in various tissues in the immunocompromised or debilitated, including those with the acquired immune deficiency syndrome (AIDS).

Clinical features

The incubation period is generally prolonged. The signs and symptoms are typical of a variety of conditions resulting from space-occupying lesions in the brain and include hemiparesis, seizures and, in about 70%, altered mental ability (stupor or lethargy, and later disorientation, irritability and combativeness). The predisposing factors include use of corticosteroids (42%), antibiotics, chemotherapy, alcoholism, AIDS, diabetes and pregnancy. Although the disease is generally found in immunocompromised states and is prolonged and chronic, acute *Acanthamoeba* meningoencephalitis has been seen associated with *Acanthamoeba* keratitis and uveitis in a child.[89] The relationship of amoebic proteases from an isolate from GAE to cytopathology has been examined recently, and degradation of extracellular matrix by a serine protease has been pinpointed as of importance for blood–brain barrier penetration.[90]

Martinez[91] reviewed 15 cases of GAE known or assumed to be due to *Acanthamoeba*. The patients, six female and nine male, were aged from 5 to 58 years, 11 were white and four black, and their illnesses lasted from 7 to 120 days. In six cases, there was a history of chronic skin ulceration or other visceral or superficial lesion. The symptoms were those of a focal or diffuse encephalopathy, with meningeal irritation. Fever, mental abnormalities, seizures, headache and hemiparesis were predominant. On admission to hospital none of these patients was in coma, in contrast to the situation often found with PAM. Cirrhosis or other liver disease was also present in three of the 15 patients; pneumonitis, diabetes, Hodgkin's disease and glucose-6-phosphate dehydrogenase defi-

ciency were also seen. Apart from antibiotic treatment, eight (53%) had been given corticosteroids. Six had been given cancer chemotherapy, three radiation therapy, three were alcoholic and two of the four females of child-bearing age were pregnant. More than 65 cases have now been reported as due either to *Acanthamoeba* or some other free-living amoeba causing GAE and there have been cases following bone marrow transplantation.[92]

No patient in this series had any recent history of swimming or water sports.

Acanthamoebidae: *Balamuthia mandrillaris*

The involvement of this soil amoeba in disease was not discovered until 1989, when Visvesvara was able to detect and culture an unusual amoeba[93] in the brain of a baboon showing symptoms similar to those of meningoencephalitis and GAE, and it soon became clear that several human GAE cases which had been thought to be caused by *Acanthamoeba*, but where the amoebae in sections did not stain with *Acanthamoeba*- or *Naegleria*-specific serum, were caused by a similar organism. Subsequently, an infection was seen in an AIDS case.[94]

Clinical features and diagnosis of GAE

The disease can mimic a deep mycosis with systemic dissemination. In five cases reviewed by Jager and Stamm[88] there was frontal headache, fluctuating coma, with or without significant history of a predisposing disease. The route of infection of the brain in the Hodgkin's lymphoma case they reviewed is thought to have been intranasal, since there were basal cortical changes in the brain, with the olfactory lobes affected. Presence of amoebae in the vessel walls gives rise to a vasculitis of an allergic type. Dead and dying organisms and cysts are found, and there is evidence of a foreign body giant cell reaction. It is noteworthy that amoebic cysts are seen in the tissues in GAE and CAK, unlike the situation in Naegleria PAM.

The CSF cell count was raised in all patients, lymphocytes being markedly elevated, composing 19–100% of the cells present. Glucose concentrations, where measured, were not appreciably lowered, as would be found in bacterial meningitis or PAM.

Although amoebic trophozoites have been reported in CSF in a few cases of GAE, there is no doubt that this is an extremely unusual finding, which may, however, be more frequent in AIDS.[95]

Further clarification on the clinical features of *B. mandrillaris* infection is developing. An initial lesion of the skin is often seen, sometimes in the nasal pyramid, which may be compact, firm and well delineated. This may or may not ulcerate, and can persist for several months before cerebral symptoms develop.[96] The cerebral lesions are characterized by angiitis/vasculitis, which leads to thrombosis and infarct, when the brain tissue is then locally infiltrated by amoebae to give granulomatous lesions (Figure 80.5).[97] In Peru, the disease has been diagnosed in cases of stroke in immunocompetent children. Headaches, lethargy and coma may supervene. In one patient with neutropenia, CSF glucose was extremely low or unmeasurable.[98] Survival after development of cerebral symptoms is generally a matter of days or weeks.

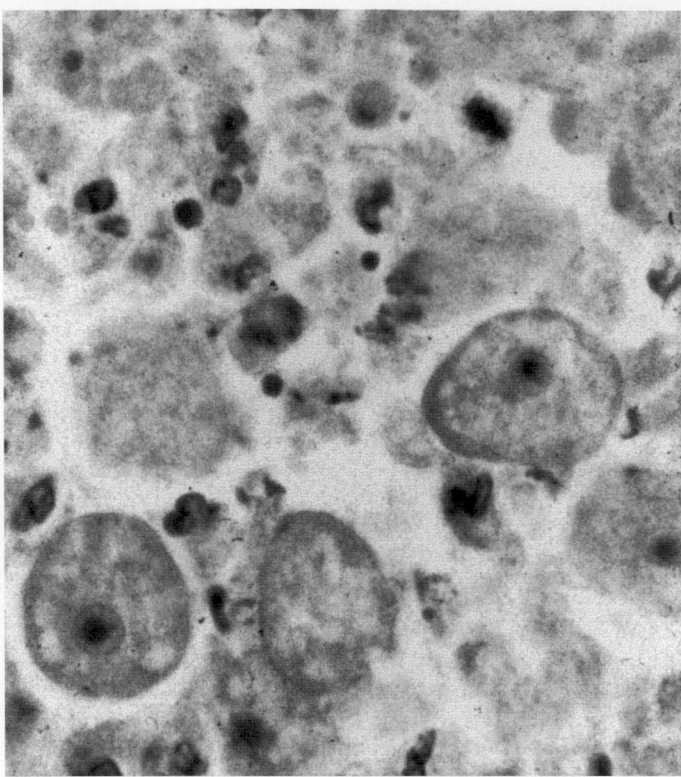

Figure 80.5 Section of brain from AIDS patient showing necrotic granuloma containing trophozoites of *Balamuthia mandrillaris*, showing typical nuclear features of free-living amoebae (H&E).

Importance of serology in diagnosis of chronic systemic and/or cerebral infections by *Acanthamoeba* and *Balamuthia*

In view of the chronic nature of the infection with *Acanthamoeba* and *Balamuthia* and the invasive character of attempts to obtain biopsy specimens, the ideal initial investigation would seem to be serological. The case reported by Kenney[87] illustrates this.

Cerebral biopsy is not an uncommon procedure, and specific polyclonal antibody has been used on wax-embedded sections in immunofluorescence[99] or immunoperoxidase techniques.

Plate cultures (as above for *Naegleria*) may be made from fresh biopsy material and incubated at 37°C for up to a week under humid conditions. *Balamuthia* does not grow well under these conditions, but as with *Naegleria* and *Acanthamoeba*, can be isolated in cell cultures. Attempts at culture from CSF can also be made.

PCR techniques for the identification of axenic *Acanthamoeba* isolates at the generic and specific level have been described[100] but these are not currently suitable for detection of low numbers of the organism in clinical material. However, rhodamine- and fluorescein-labelled probes have been developed, the former reacting with RNA and DNA of the genus *Acanthamoeba* and the latter with type T4 (most often associated with amoebic keratitis) of 12 ssu-rRNA subgeneric sequences.[101,102] Because samples containing only cysts may be difficult to grow, and amoebae may be very scanty

and need culture amplification before detection, the best system for diagnosis would be to divide the sample, to probe one portion, and to culture the other, repeating the probing on the culture. The multiplex real time PCR[32] appears now the PCR method of choice for both genera and for confirmation of *Naegleria* infection.

Management

There are reports of the successful use of rifampicin, paromomycin in treatment of *Acanthamoeba* infections in mice.[103] Experience is being gained in the treatment of *Acanthamoeba* GAE in humans.[104] Successful treatment of a solitary *Acanthamoeba* brain lesion in AIDS by excision and fluconazole/sulfadiazine has been reported.[105]

Pathology and pathogenesis

Acanthamoeba probably injures cells by two mechanisms: trogocytosis (ingestion of the cytoplasm through a feeding cup), and contact-mediated lysis of cellular components due to secreted enzymes. Much of the pathology is probably related to attraction of a granulomatous cellular response. It has been shown that collagenase, for example, is effective in attracting cells into the cornea (see Chronic *Acanthamoeba* keratitis, below).

Immunology

More than 90% of adult sera have reciprocal titres of up to 80 in the indirect fluorescent antibody test.

CHRONIC *ACANTHAMOEBA* KERATITIS

Acanthamoeba is present in all types of environments throughout the world. Since its cysts are resistant to drying, the chance of cyst inoculation into a mucous surface is high. The cornea is an immunoprivileged site, because there is no direct contact with the blood, and it is possible for cysts or trophozoites of this organism to infect corneal stroma.

Acanthamoeba keratitis or keratouveitis presents a serious diagnostic and treatment problem to ophthalmologists. Since the first reports from the UK and the USA in the early 1970s, many further cases have been seen in Europe, the USA and other countries. The major part of the increase in developed countries is probably related to contact lens use and is related to direct inoculation of amoebic trophozoites or cysts into the cornea during insertion of the contaminated lens.

Clinical features

The first ocular infections[106,107] were thought to be associated with trauma to the cornea, leading to invasion of the amoebae, and were not linked to contact lens use. However, 85% of *Acanthamoeba* eye infections in a US survey were in hard or soft contact lens wearers.[108]

Symptoms characteristically mimic those of herpes keratitis, although the condition is generally more painful than the viral disease.

Retrospective studies of keratitis material in London prior to 1973 failed to reveal any earlier cases.[109]

Lang and von Heimburg-Elliger[110] in 1991 reviewed 108 literature case reports: eight (7%) patients were wearing hard contact lenses; 19 (17%) remembered trauma; four (4%) had visited a hot tub; 61 (56%) needed penetrating keratoplasty, 11 (10%) rekeratoplasty; five (5%) eyes were enucleated; in 21 (19%) of the patients the diagnosis was made on histological grounds.

Acanthamoeba keratitis has occurred in both male and female patients from the early 20s to the elderly. Inflammation of the cornea (keratitis) is seen, generally with a larger or smaller epithelial defect. Accumulation of pus in the anterior chamber (hypopyon) is a common feature, together with a ring infiltrate. Following erosion of the cornea the posterior membrane (Descemet's membrane) may bulge forwards (descemetocele) and may perforate, releasing the aqueous humour. There may also be secondary infection with bacteria, graft rejection, swelling of the conjunctiva (chemosis) or accumulation of blood in the anterior chamber (hyphema). Secondary glaucoma (increased intraocular tension related to inflammation of the ciliary body) may complicate the disease.[111] Radial neuritis is reported to be a pathognomonic sign.[112] The disease runs a slow relapsing course; often a ring abscess is persistent, epithelial breakdown is recurrent, and the hypopyon waxes and wanes.

Diagnosis

Clinical signs[113] have been confused not only with those of other infective entities but also with those due to topical anaesthetic abuse.[114]

Diagnosis may be made by observation of characteristic cysts in wet mounts (10% KOH wet mount is reported to be satisfactory[115]) of corneal ulcer scrapings, and subsequent culture. Cultures made from superficial scrapings of the cornea, or from punch biopsies[116] are valuable. Suggestive but not conclusive evidence for the infection is obtained when the amoeba is isolated from the contact lenses themselves, the cases or washing fluid. The fluorescent dye Calcofluor has been used to stain the cysts in smears, but it does not detect the trophozoites well.

The temperature of the eye is lower than that of the rest of the human body; therefore *Acanthamoeba* strains that grow at lower temperatures may also contribute to infection. This should be taken into account in cultivation, and a sample should always be cultured at 30°C and at 37°C if there is sufficient material. Further comments on the value of nucleic acid-based diagnosis and cultures will be seen above in the section on diagnosis of GAE.

Epidemiology

Acanthamoeba is ubiquitous in air, soil and water. In a study of the moist areas in physiotherapy departments of 10 hospitals, 61% of the swabs taken in those areas were positive for one or several species of amoebae cultivated on non-nutrient agar according to Page. A total of 47 strains of *Acanthamoeba* and only two non-pathogenic strains of *Naegleria* were isolated. Six of the 47 strains of *Acanthamoeba* isolated revealed pathogenic characters in mice.[117]

Management

The most effective therapeutic drugs so far examined have been the diamidines: propamidine and dibromopropamidine.[118] It is important to remember that *Acanthamoeba*, unlike *Naegleria*, encysts in infected tissues. Clinical cure often utilizes medication in combination with surgical procedures, such as keratoplasty or, sometimes, debridement.[119] Antiinflammatory corticosteroids are thought to increase the susceptibility of the eye to *Acanthamoeba* infection, but their judicious use in conjunction with drug treatment has been valuable in many cases. This problem is discussed with respect to several eye infections by Stern and Buttross.[120]

The first patient treated successfully at Moorfields Eye Hospital had a 4-month history of suppurative keratitis, associated with an epithelial defect, hypopyon and secondary glaucoma. *Acanthamoeba* was isolated from the eye on three occasions. Intensive therapy with propamidine isethionate (0.1%) drops hourly by day and night, with dibromopropamidine ointment (0.15%) 4-hourly, was instituted. After 9 days, although corneal improvement was noted, signs of toxicity, including reddening of the eye and swelling of the lids, were seen. The intensive propamidine treatment was discontinued, neomycin drops were instilled 4-hourly day and night, and the 4-hourly dibromopropamidine treatment was continued. After 1 month the epithelium had healed and 4-hourly prednisolone drops were added, with steady improvement in the corneal inflammation. The treatment was tapered off over a further month, leaving only the neomycin drops, which were continued for 1 year, when some toxic signs developed (limbal follicles, with some increased palpebral conjunctival hyperaemia and cellularity, but no signs of skin irritation). Following cessation of all topical therapy, 4 months elapsed, with disappearance of limbal and conjunctival signs and no recurrence of the disease. Some 22 months after initial presentation, a penetrating keratoplasty (corneal graft) was carried out. The excised corneal disc showed no special changes and no morphologically identifiable *Acanthamoeba* on light and electron microscopical examination. Using the indirect fluorescent antibody technique and rabbit anti-*Acanthamoeba* serum it was possible to see small curved arcs, which probably represented fragments of cyst wall.

Propamidine isethionate drops were instilled four times a day for 2 months, in addition to the usual postoperative topical steroids and antibiotics. There was no evidence of adverse effect(s) on the graft or the remainder of the eye. The graft remained clear for a further 9 months, when a rejection episode developed which was readily controlled with topical corticosteroids. Because of persisting secondary glaucoma, the intraocular pressure needed to be controlled using timolol maleate (0.25%) drops twice daily.

The initial intensive treatment probably need not be continued for more than 1 week because intensive therapy with propamidine may give rise to corneal toxicity.[121] More recent observations confirm the effectiveness of propamidine (or dibromopropamidine) and neomycin.[122] However, one case was successfully treated with propamidine isethionate and 'Neosporin' (neomycin/polymyxin/gramicidin) at 30-min intervals for 11 and 9 days,[123] whereas in seven other cases 1% miconazole topically was used successfully in triple therapy with a less intensive course of the other two agents.[124] Earlier studies at Moorfields and in the author's laboratory showed that the gramicidin component of 'Neosporin' was irritating and relatively non-toxic to amoebae. A successful regimen used neomycin, polymyxin and dibromopropamidine together with gentamicin.[125]

An early report of the efficacy of oral ketoconazole (200 mg twice a day) and topical miconazole[111] encouraged the use of these antifungals, which have shown some success. Miconazole or ketoconazole drops have been used, with or without 'Neosporin' drops.[126] In a more recent study, the new antifungal itraconazole was used orally with topical 0.1% miconazole hourly during the day. The therapy was successful after 5, 8 and 9 weeks in three patients.[127]

Resistance to topical dibromopropamidine was observed in a case of bilateral keratitis. Eradication of amoebae was finally achieved following prolonged topical therapy and two corneal grafts in each eye. Paromomycin, benzethonium chloride, clotrimazole and R 11/29 (a phenanthridinium compound) were continued topically for 3 months postoperatively. There were no further recurrences during a 14-month follow-up. Drug sensitivities were performed for three isolates of *Acanthamoeba* species, which demonstrated the development of resistance to dibromopropamidine. In addition, the resistant isolates were temperature-sensitive mutants which would not grow at temperatures above 30°C.[128]

A novel treatment with a polyhexamethylene biguanide (PHMB) biocide, first shown to be active on free-living amoebae in the early 1970s,[129] 'Baquacil' or 'ReNu', has shown promise in the elimination of *Acanthamoeba* from the human eye. It is active at low concentrations against the cysts,[130] unlike most other agents, and this means that it attacks one of the main sources of treatment failure because drug treatment may stimulate encystment.[131,132] Chlorhexidine, another biguanide, is now regularly used with success, alone or in combination with other agents.[133]

Animal models of *Acanthamoeba* keratitis have been developed and are important in understanding the pathogenic mechanisms involved in the disease and in testing new drug treatments. It may be that improvements will be possible when the host response is better understood.[134,135]

Pathology and pathogenesis

In acanthamoebic keratitis, the organisms apparently depend on the cellular components of the cornea as substrates for growth.[136] Parasite-conditioned medium contains both collagenase and lower concentrations of other proteolytic enzymes. However, most of the collagenolytic and pathogenic activity is directly attributable to specific collagenase. Intrastromal injection of sterile, *Acanthamoeba*-conditioned culture medium into naive Lewis rats produces corneal lesions clinically similar to and closely resembling those found in biopsy specimens of human patients diagnosed with acanthamoebic keratitis. There is moderate to severe neutrophil infiltration, disruption of stromal lamellae and oedema. Identical pathological sequelae have been produced by intrastromal injection of purified collagenase (25 units/mL).[137]

Commensal bacteria on the eyelids, conjunctiva and tear film may have a role in pathogenesis.[138] This may also be the case for viruses. Many cases of human keratitis due to *Acanthamoeba* species have a pseudoherpetic appearance and the infection is known to have followed diagnosed herpes infection in some cases. After herpetic and amoebic co-infection rabbits show severe corneal lesions, and when the viral infection is treated the amoebic

co-infection progresses unchecked with severe lesions until day 37 post-infection, with numerous trophozoites and cysts.[139] This may have significant implications in human disease. However, experimental infections have also been established in the rabbit without co-infection with herpes,[140] and several rat models have now been described.[141] In the Wistar rat model, the inflammatory cell profile was observed to change at intervals. In tissue sections the cellular response consisted of neutrophils on the first day but predominantly macrophages on the following days. Some T lymphocytes but no B lymphocytes were observed.[142]

Immunology

Immunity against these amoebae involves a combination of complement, antibody and cell-mediated immunity. Evidence suggests that the major mechanism is activation of phagocytic cells, especially neutrophils, by lymphokines and opsonization of the amoebae by antibody, which promotes an antibody-dependent cellular destruction of the organism.[143] Oral immunization of hamsters with amoebic mannose binding protein gave partial protection against experimental keratitis.[144]

Prevention of contact lens-related *Acanthamoeba* eye infection

There can be little doubt that the reason for the increase in case numbers of *Acanthamoeba* keratitis in the developed world since the 1970s has been the introduction of contact lenses, and of soft contact lenses in particular.[145] The type of lens and the way the lenses are handled by the patient may be crucial in raising the risk of infection. Adequate means for lens cleaning, disinfection, rinsing and storage need to be available. In addition, for patients who are careless or persist in using non-sterile rinsing solutions, user-friendly and foolproof adequate methods of disinfection will be of great help in prevention.[146]

When storage cases for contact lenses of 102 asymptomatic lens wearers were tested for contamination by bacteria and free-living amoebae, 43 had significant counts of viable bacteria. Seven had contamination by *Acanthamoebae*.[147] In a recent study, infection of the eye by *Acanthamoeba* has been conclusively linked to the contact lens storage container, the home-made saline solution and the kitchen cold water tap. The authors recommend that the use of home-made saline solutions and the rinsing of contact lenses in tap water be strongly discouraged.[148]

Unfortunately, many contact lens users receive poor lens care instructions or cannot be relied on to follow appropriate routines. Finding a foolproof means of lens disinfection for them is critical. Recently, several disinfection systems were tested against *A. castellanii* and *A. polyphaga* cysts and trophozoites to see which might prove most effective. Effective systems included heat disinfection at 70–80°C for 10 min, 3% hydrogen peroxide for 2–3 h, 0.001% thimerosal with edetate for 4 h, 0.005% benzalkonium chloride with edetate for 4 h, and either 0.001% chlorhexidine for 4 h or 0.004% chlorhexidine for 1 h.

Problems associated with chemical disinfection (with, e.g. 3% hydrogen peroxide) of plastic contact lenses include lens fit alterations, which may lead to epithelial trauma. In addition, antimicrobial chemicals need to be rinsed, neutralized or degraded after use, as they can injure the corneal and conjunctival epithelium.[149] In a study of contamination of lenses in 101 users,[150] 81% of cases were found to be microbiologically contaminated. While 75% used hydrogen peroxide solution for decontamination, all contaminating organisms were catalase positive. Where the lens material will resist it, heat disinfection at 70–80°C for 10 min, or 3% hydrogen peroxide for 2–3 h, is recommended. A neutralization step should follow exposure to the peroxide.

Adherence of cysts and trophozoites to the contact lens is probably important in mediation of infection. Trophozoites of *A. polyphaga* adhered in vitro to low and high water content nonionic soft contact lenses. Adherence was greater to high water content soft lenses. Cyst attachment occurred only to the soft lenses, and was higher for the high water content lenses. Attachment of cysts to each lens tested was significantly lower than that of trophozoites. Recommended cleaning procedures using two commercial solutions (10% sodium tridecyl ether sulphate for rigid gas-permeable lenses; EDTA and sorbic acid for soft contact lenses) removed all adherent trophozoites and cysts from lenses. Correctly applied lens cleaning agents which remove adherent trophozoites, cysts and epithelial cells from the lenses and cases may reduce the risk of infection.[151]

The use of disposable hydrogel contact lenses, which are worn continuously and then discarded, is thought to protect against lens-related infection. But if lenses are removed during the period of use, or rinsed or stored in tap water or well water, this protective effect may be lost.[152]

REFERENCES

1. Schuster FL, Visvesvara GS. Free-living amoebae as opportunistic and non-opportunistic pathogens of humans and animals. *Int J Parasitol* 2004; 34:1001–1027.

2. Gelman BB, Rauf SJ, Nader R, et al. Amoebic encephalitis due to *Sappinia diploidea*. *JAMA* 2001; 285(19):2450–2451.

3. Gelman BB, Popov V, Chaljub G, et al. Neuropathological and ultrastructural features of amebic encephalitis caused by *Sappinia diploidea*. *J Neuropathol Exp Neurol* 2003; 62:990–998.

4. Barwick RS, Levy DA, Craun GF, et al. Surveillance for waterborne-disease outbreaks – United States, 1997–1998. *MMWR CDC Surveill Summ* 2000; 49(4):1–21. [The figure stated in the text includes MMWR reports from 1989 onwards].

5. Dziuban EJ, Liang JL, Craun GF, et al. Surveillance for waterborne disease and outbreaks associated with recreational water – United States, 2003–2004. *MMWR Surveill Summ* 2006; 55:1–30.

6. Kingston D, Warhurst DC. Isolation of amoebae from the air. *J Med Microbiol* 1969; 2:27–36.

7. Warhurst DC. Ryan virus and the lipovirus: examples of *Acanthamoeba* (Hartmannella) contamination of cell cultures. *Parasitol Today* 1989; 5:161–162

8. Intalapaporn P, Suankratay C, Shuangshoti S, et al. *Balamuthia Mandrillaris* Meningoencephalitis: The First Case In Southeast Asia. *Am J Trop Med Hyg* 2004; 70:666–669.

9. Bakardjiev A, Azimi PH, Ashouri N, et al. Amebic encephalitis caused by *Balamuthia mandrillaris*: report of four cases. *Pediatr Infect Dis J* 2003; 22: 447–452.

10. Deetz TR, Sawyer MH, Billman G, et al. Successful Treatment of *Balamuthia* Amoebic Encephalitis: Presentation of 2 Cases. *CID* 2003; 37:1304–1312.

11. Sungmi Jung S, Schelper RL, Visvesvara GS, et al. *Balamuthia mandrillaris* meningoencephalitis in an immunocompetent patient an unusual clinical

12. White JML, Barker RD, Salisbury JR, et al. Granulomatous amoebic encephalitis. *Lancet* 2004; 364:220

13. Jayasekera S, Sissons J, Tucker J, et al. Post-mortem culture of *Balamuthia mandrillaris* from the brain and cerebrospinal fluid of a case of granulomatous amoebic meningoencephalitis, using human brain microvascular endothelial cells. *J Med Microbiol* 2004; 53:1007–1012.

14. Booton GC, Carmichael JR, Visvesvara GS, et al. Genotyping of *Balamuthia Mandrillaris* based on nuclear 18s and mitochondrial 16s Rrna genes *Am J Trop Med Hyg* 2003; 68:65–69.

15. Schuster FL, Dunnebacke TH, Booton GC, et al. Environmental isolation of *Balamuthia mandrillaris* associated with a case of amebic encephalitis. *J Clin Microbiol* 2003; 41:3175–3180.

16. Dunnebacke TH, Schuster FL, Yagi S, et al. *Balamuthia mandrillaris* from soil samples. *Microbiology* 2004; 150:2837–2842.

17. Rowbotham TJ. Preliminary report of the pathogenicity of *Legionella pneumophila* for freshwater and soil amoebae. *J Clin Pathol* 1980; 33:1179–1183.

18. Kilvington S, Price J. Survival of Legionella pneumophila within cysts of *Acanthamoeba* polyphaga following chlorine exposure. *J Appl Bacteriol* 1990; 68:519–525.

19. Thom S, Warhurst DC, Drasar BS. Association of *Vibrio cholerae* with fresh water amoebae. *J Med Microbiol* 1992; 36:303–306.

20. Martinez AJ. Clinical manifestations of free-living amoeba infections. In: Rondanelli EG, ed. *Amphizoic Amoebae: Human Pathology*. Padua: Piccin Press; 1987:161–177.

21. Derrick EH. A fatal case of generalized amoebiasis due to a protozoon closely resembling if not identical to *Iodamoeba buetschlii*. *Trans R Soc Trop Med Hyg* 1948; 42:191–198.

22. Stamm WP. The staining of free-living amoebae by indirect immunofluorescence. *Ann Soc Belg Med Trop* 1974; 54:321–325.

23. Carter RF. Primary amoebic meningoencephalitis: an appraisal of present knowledge. *Trans R Soc Trop Med Hyg* 1972; 66:193–213.

24. Miller G, Cullity G, Walpole I, et al. Primary amoebic meningoencephalitis in Western Australia. *Med J Aust* 1982; 1:352–357.

25. Markowitz SM, Martinez AJ, Duma RJ, et al. Myocarditis associated with primary amoebic meningoencephalitis. *Am J Clin Pathol* 1974; 62:619–628.

26. Patras D, Andujar J. Meningoencephalitis due to Hartmannella (*Acanthamoeba*). *Am J Clin Pathol* 1966; 46:226–233.

27. Lawande RV, MacFarlane JT, Weir WC, et al. A case of primary amebic meningoencephalitis in a Nigerian farmer. *Am J Trop Med Hyg* 1980; 29:21–25.

28. Medley S. Acridine orange: method for diagnosis of amoebic meningitis? *Med J Aust* 1980; 2:635.

29. Page FC. Taxonomic criteria for *limax amoebae*, with descriptions of 3 new species of *Hartmannella* and 3 of *Vahlkampfia*. *J Protozool* 1967; 14: 499–521.

30. Flores BM, Garcia CA, Stamm WE, et al. Differentiation of *Naegleria fowleri* from *Acanthamoeba* species by using monoclonal antibodies and flow cytometry. *J Clin Microbiol* 1990; 28:1999–2005.

31. Kilvington S, Mann PG, Warhurst DC. Differentiation between *Naegleria fowleri* and *N. lovaniensis* using isoenzyme electrophoresis of aspartate aminotransferase. *Trans R Soc Trop Med Hyg* 1984; 78:562–563.

32. Qvarnstrom Y, Visvesvara GS, Sriram R, et al. Multiplex real-time pcr assay for simultaneous detection of *Acanthamoeba* spp., *Balamuthia mandrillaris*, and *Naegleria fowleri*. *J Clin Microbiol* 2006; 3589–3595.

33. Schuster FL, Visvesvara GS. Opportunistic amoebae: challenges in prophylaxis and treatment. *Drug Resist Update* 2004; 7:41–51.

34. Apley J, Clarke SK, Roome AP, et al. Primary amoebic meningoencephalitis in Britain. *BMJ* 1970; 1:596–599.

35. Saygi G, Warhurst DC, Roome AP. A study of amoebae isolated from the Bristol cases of primary amoebic encephalitis. *Proc R Soc Med* 1973; 66(3):277–282.

course and a favorable outcome. *Arch Pathol Lab Med* 2004; 128: 466–468.

36. Warhurst DC, Thomas SC. An isozyme difference between a smooth and a rough (R) strain of *Naegleria gruberi*. *Protistologica* 1978; XIV:87–89.

37. Brown RL. Successful treatment of primary amebic meningoencephalitis. *Arch Intern Med* 1991; 151(6):1201–1202.

38. Martinez AJ. Comment on: *Arch Intern Med* 1991; 151:1201–1202. Amebic encephalitis unlikely. *Arch Intern Med* 1992; 152: 1330–1331.

39. Jain R, Prabhakar S, Modi M, et al. Naegleria meningitis: a rare survival. *Neurol India* 2002; 50:470–472.

40. Wang A, Kay R, Poon WS, et al. Successful treatment of amoebic meningoencephalitis in a Chinese living in Hong Kong. *Clin Neurol Neurosurg* 1993; 95(3):249–252.

41. Vargas-Zepeda J, Gomez-Alcala AV, Vasquez-Morales JA, et al. Successful treatment of *Naegleria fowleri* meningoencephalitis by using intravenous amphotericin B, fluconazole and rifampicin. *Arch Med Res* 2005; 3 6:83–86.

42. Seidel JS, Harmatz P, Visvesvara GS, et al. Successful treatment of primary amebic meningoencephalitis. *N Engl J Med* 1982; 306:346–348.

43. Cain ARR, Wiley PE, Brownell B, et al. Primary amoebic meningoencephalitis. *Arch Dis Child* 1981; 56:140–143.

44. Hecht RH, Cohen AH, Stoner J, et al. Primary amebic meningoencephalitis in California. *Calif Med* 1972; 117:69–73.

45. Boyle AL, Friedman TA, Braustein H, et al. Rapid diagnosis of primary amoebic meningoencephalitis due to *Naegleria*: detection of organisms with bacterial stains. *J Clin Pathol* 1979; 32:306–307.

46. Stevens AR, Shulman ST, Lansen TA, et al. Primary amebic meningoencephalitis: a report of two cases and antibiotic and immunologic studies. *J Infect Dis* 1981; 143:193–199.

47. De Jonckheere JF. Characterization of *Naegleria* species by restriction endonuclease digestion of whole-cell DNA. *Mol Biochem Parasitol* 1987; 24:55–66.

48. Duma RJ. Disease caused by free-living amoebae. *Infect Dis Newslett* 1989; 8:25–32.

49. Drutz DJ. Rapid infusion of amphotericin B: is it safe, effective and wise? *Am J Med* 1992; 93:119–121.

50. Cruz JM, Peacock JE, Loomer L, et al. Rapid intravenous infusion of amphotericin B: a pilot study. *Am J Med* 1992; 93:123–130.

51. Ferrante A. Free living amoebae: pathogenicity and immunity. *Parasite Immunol* 1991; 13:31–47.

52. Ferrante A. Comparative sensitivity of *Naegleria fowleri* to amphotericin B and amphotericin B methyl ester. *Trans R Soc Trop Med Hyg* 1982; 76: 476–478.

53. Goswick SM, Brenner GM. Activities of therapeutic agents against *Naegleria fowleri* in vitro and in a mouse model of primary amebic meningoencephalitis. *J Parasitol* 2003; 89(4):837–842.

54. Thong YH, Rowan-Kelly B, Ferrante A, et al. Synergism between tetracycline and amphotericin B in experimental amoebic meningoencephalitis. *Med J Aust* 1978; 1:663–664.

55. Thong YH. Delayed treatment of primary amoebic meningoencephalitis with amphotericin B and tetracycline. *Trans R Soc Trop Med Hyg* 1979; 73:806–808.

56. Thong YH. Chemotherapy for primary amebic meningoencephalitis. *N Engl J Med* 1982; 306:1295–1296.

57. Thong YH, Rowan-Kelly B, Ferrante A. Treatment of experimental *Naegleria* meningoencephalitis with a combination of amphotericin B and rifamycin. *Scand J Infect Dis* 1979; 11:151–153.

58. Schachter LP, Owellen RJ, Rathbun HK, et al. Antagonism between miconazole and amphotericin-B. *Lancet* 1976; ii:318.

59. Schuster FL, Guglielmo BJ, Visvesvara GS. In-vitro activity of miltefosine and voriconazole on clinical isolates of free-living amebas: *Balamuthia mandrillaris, Acanthamoeba* spp., and *Naegleria fowleri*. *J Eukaryot Microbiol* 2006; 53:121–126.

60. Soltow SM, Brenner GM. Synergistic activities of azithromycin and amphotericin B against *Naegleria fowleri* in vitro and in a mouse model of primary amebic meningoencephalitis. *Antimicrob Agents Chemother* 2007; 51:23–27.

61. Marciano-Cabral R, Zoghby KL, Bradley SG. Cytopathic action of *Naegleria fowleri* amoebae on rat neuroblastoma target cells. *J Protozool* 1990; 37:138–144.

62. Dunnebacke TH, Dixon JS. NACM, a cytopathogenic protein from *Naegleria gruberi*, EGs: purification, production of monoclonal antibody, and the immunoidentification of a product that develops in NACM-treated vertebrate cell cultures. *J Protozool* 1990; 37:11S–16S.

63. Cursons RTM, Brown TJ, Keys EA, et al. Immunity to pathogenic free living amoebae: role of humoral antibody. *Infect Immun* 1980; 29:401–407.

64. Cursons RM, Keys EA, Brown TM, et al. IgA and primary amoebic meningoencephalitis. *Lancet* 1979; i:223–224.

65. Cain ARR, Mann PG, Warhurst DC. IgA and primary amoebic meningoencephalitis. *Lancet* 1979; i:441.

66. Ahn MH, Min DY. Resistance to *Naegleria fowleri* infection passively acquired from immunized splenocyte, serum or milk. *Kisaengchunghak Chapchi* 1989; 27:79–86.

67. Thong YH, Ferrante A, Shepherd C, et al. Resistance of mice to *Naegleria* meningoencephalitis transferred by immune serum. *Trans R Soc Trop Med Hyg* 1978; 72:650–652.

68. Thong YH, Carter RF, Ferrante A, et al. Site of expression of immunity to *Naegleria fowleri* in immunized mice. *Parasite Immunol* 1983; 5:67–76.

69. Fischer-Stenger K, Cabral GA, Marciano-Cabral F. The interaction of *Naegleria fowleri* amoebae with murine macrophage cell lines. *J Protozool* 1990; 37:168–173.

70. Michelson MK, Henderson WR Jr, Chi EY, et al. Ultrastructural studies on the effect of tumor necrosis factor on the interaction of neutrophils and *Naegleria fowleri*. *Am J Trop Med Hyg* 1990; 42:225–233.

71. Rowan-Kelly B, Ferrante A, Thong YH. Activation of complement by *Naegleria*. *Trans R Soc Trop Med Hyg* 1980; 74:333–336.

72. Rojas-Hernandez S, Rodriguez-Monroy MA, Lopez-Revilla R, et al. Intranasal coadministration of the Cry1Ac protoxin with amoebal lysates increases protection against *Naegleria fowleri* meningoencephalitis. *Infect Immun* 2004; 72(8):4368–4375.

73. Aufy S, Kilvington S, Mann PG, et al. Improved selective isolation of *Naegleria fowleri* from the environment. *Trans R Soc Trop Med Hyg* 1986; 80:350–351.

74. Kilvington S, Mann PG, Warhurst DC. Pathogenic Naegleria amoebae in the waters of Bath: A fatality and its consequences. *Bath: Bath City Council* 1991; 89–96.

75. Huizinga HW, McLaughlin GL. Thermal ecology of *Naegleria fowleri* from a power plant cooling reservoir. *Appl Environ Microbiol* 1990; 56:2200–2205.

76. Pernin P, Pelandakis M, Rouby Y, et al. Comparative recoveries of *Naegleria fowleri* amoebae from seeded river water by filtration and centrifugation. *Appl Environ Microbiol* 1998; 64: 955–959.

77. John DT, Howard MJ. Techniques for isolating thermotolerant and pathogenic freeliving amebae. *Folia Parasitol (Praha)* 1996; 43:267–271.

78. De Jonckheere JF. Hospital hydrotherapy pools treated with ultraviolet light: bad bacterial quality and presence of thermophilic Naegleria. *J Hyg (Camb)* 1982; 88:205–214.

79. Hillebrandt S, Muller I. Repair of damage caused by UV- and X-irradiation in the amoeboflagellate *Naegleria gruberi*. *Radiat Environ Biophys* 1991; 30:123–130.

80. Brown TM, Cursons RTM. Prophylaxis. In: Rondanelli EG, ed. *Amphizoic Amoebae: Human Pathology*. Padua: Piccin Press; 1987:217–236.

81. Chang SL. Resistance of pathogenic Naegleria to some common physical and chemical agents. *Appl Environ Microbiol* 1978; 35:368–375.

82. Kadlec V, Cerva L, Skvarova J. Virulent *Naegleria fowleri* in an indoor swimming pool. *Science* 1978; 201:1025.

83. Dorsch MM, Cameron AS, Robinson BS. The epidemiology and control of primary amoebic meningoencephalitis with particular reference to South Australia. *Trans R Soc Trop Med Hyg* 1983; 77:372–377.

84. Esterman A, Roder DM, Cameron AS, et al. Determinants of the microbiological quality of South Australian swimming pools. *Appl Env Microbiol* 1984; 47:325–328.

85. Cursons RTM, Brown TJ, Keys EA. Effect of disinfectants on pathogenic free-living amoebae: in axenic conditions. *Appl Environ Microbiol* 1980; 40:401–407.

86. Lyons TB, Kapur R. Limax amoebae in public swimming pools of Albany, Schenectady and Rensselaer counties, New York: their concentration, correlations and significance. *Appl Environ Microbiol* 1977; 33:551–555.

87. Kenney M. The Micro-Kolmer complement fixation test in routine screening for soil ameba infection. *Health Lab Sci* 1971; 8:5–10.

88. Jager BV, Stamm WP. Brain abscesses caused by free living amoeba probably of the genus *Hartmannella* in a patient with Hodgkin's disease. *Lancet* 1972; ii:1343–1345.

89. Jones DB, Visvesvara GS , Robinson NM. *Acanthamoeba* polyphaga keratitis and *Acanthamoeba* uveitis associated with fatal meningoencephalitis. *Trans Ophthalmol Soc UK* 1975; 95:221–232.

90. Sissons J, Alsam S, Goldsworthy G, et al. Identification and properties of proteases from an *Acanthamoeba* isolate capable of producing granulomatous encephalitis. *BMC Microbiology* 2006; 6:42.

91. Martinez AJ. Is *Acanthamoeba* encephalitis an opportunistic infection? *Neurology* 1980; 30:567–574.

92. Anderlini P, Przepiorka D, Luna M, et al. *Acanthamoeba* meningoencephalitis after bone-marrow transplantation. *Bone Marrow Transplant* 1994; 14:459–461.

93. Visvesvara GS, Martinez AJ, Schuster FL, et al. *Leptomyxid ameba,* a new agent of amebic meningoencephalitis in humans and animals. *J Clin Microbiol* 1990; 28:2750–2756.

94. Anzil AP, Rao C, Wrzolek MA, et al. Amebic meningoencephalitis in a patient with AIDS caused by a newly recognized opportunistic pathogen, leptomyxid ameba. *Arch Pathol Lab Med* 1991; 115:21–22.

95. Hawley HB, Czachor JS, Malhotra V, et al. *Acanthamoeba* encephalitis in patients with AIDS. *AIDS Reader* 1997; 7:137–144.

96. Deol I, Robledo L, Meza A, et al. Encephalitis due to a free-living amoeba (*Balamuthia mandrillaris*): case report with literature review. *Surg Neurol* 2000; 53:611–616.

97. Recavarren-Arce S, Velarde C, Gotuzzo E, et al. Amoeba angiitic lesions of the central nervous system in *Balamuthia mandrillaris* amoebiasis. *Hum Pathol* 1999; 30:269–273.

98. Katz JD, Ropper AH, Adelman L, et al. A case of *Balamuthia mandrillaris* meningoencephalitis. *Arch Neurol* 2000; 57:1210–1212.

99. Warhurst DC. Naegleria and *Acanthamoeba* in tissue sections. In: Edwards J, Taylor, C, Tomlinson A, eds. *Immunofluorescence techniques in Diagnostic Microbiology.* London: HMSO; 1982:46–48.

100. Vodkin M, Howe DK, Visvesvara GS, et al. Identification of *Acanthamoeba* at the generic and specific levels using the polymerase chain reaction. *J Protozool* 1992; 39:378–385.

101. Stothard DR, Hay J, Schroeder-Diedrich JM, et al. Fluorescent oligonucleotide probes for clinical and environmental detection of *Acanthamoeba* and the T4 18S rRNA gene sequence type. *J Clin Microbiol* 1999; 37:2687–2693.

102. Stothard DR, Schroeder-Diedrich JM, Awwad MH, et al. The evolutionary history of the genus *Acanthamoeba* and the identification of eight new 18S rRNA gene sequence types. *J Eukaryotic Microbiol* 1998; 45:45–54.

103. Mazur T, Kasprzak W, Zagarska-Nowak G. Sensitivity of limax amoebae to some antiparasitic drugs II activity in vivo. *Wiadomosci Parazitologiczne* 1983; 29:271–272.

104. Slater CA, Sickel JZ, Visvesvara GS, et al. Brief report: successful treatment of disseminated *Acanthamoeba* infection in an immunocompromised patient. *N Engl J Med* 1994; 331:85–87.

105. Seijo-Martinez M, Gonzalez-Medeiro G, Santiago P, et al. Granulomatous amebic encephalitis in a patient with AIDS: isolation of *Acanthamoeba* sp. group II from brain tissue and successful treatment with sulfadiazine and fluconazole. *J Clin Microbiol* 2000; 38:3892–3895.

106. Nagington J, Watson PG, Playfair TJ, et al. Amoebic infection of the eye. *Lancet* 1974; ii:1537–1540.

107. Visvesvara GS, Jones DB, Robinson NM. Isolation, identification, and biological characterization of *Acanthamoeba* polyphaga from a human eye. *Am J Trop Med Hyg* 1975; 24:784–790.

108. Stehr-Green JK, Bailey TM, Visvesvara GS. The epidemiology of *Acanthamoeba* keratitis in the United States. *Am J Ophthalmol* 1989; 107:331–336.

109. Ashton N, Stamm WP. Amoebic infection of the eye: a pathological report. *Trans Ophthalmol Soc UK* 1975; 95:214–220.

110. Lang GE, von Heimburg-Elliger A. *Acanthamoeba* keratitis in hard contact lens wearers. Case report and review of the literature of 108 cases. *Klin Monatsbl Augenheilkd* 1991; 198:290–294.

111. Hirst LW, Green WR, Merz W, et al. Management of *Acanthamoeba* keratitis: a case report and review of the literature. *Ophthalmology* 1984; 91:1105–1111.

112. McCulley JP, Alizadeh H, Niederkorn JY. *Acanthamoeba* keratitis. *CLAO J* 1995; 21:73–76.

113. Visvesvara GS. Acanthamoebiasis and naegleriasis. In: Balows A, Hausler WJ, Ohashi M, Turano A, eds. *Laboratory Diagnosis of Infectious Disease.* New York: Springer; 1988:723–730.

114. Rosenwasser GO, Holland S, Pflugfelder SC, et al. Topical anesthetic abuse. *Ophthalmology* 1990; 97:967–972.

115. Sharma S, Srinivasan M, George C. Diagnosis of *Acanthamoeba* keratitis: a report of four cases and review of literature. *Indian J Ophthalmol* 1990; 38:50–56.

116. Lee P, Green WR. Corneal biopsy: indications, techniques, and a report of a series of 87 cases. *Ophthalmology* 1990; 97:718–721.

117. Michel R, Menn T. *Acanthamoeba,* Naegleria and invertebrates in wet areas of physiotherapy equipment in hospitals. *Zentralbl Hyg Umweltmed* 1991; 191:423–437.

118. Wright P, Warhurst DC, Jones BR. *Acanthamoeba* keratitis successfully treated medically. *Br J Ophthalmol* 1985; 69:778–782.

119. Osato MS, Robinson NM, Wilhelmus KR, et al. In vitro evaluation of antimicrobial compounds for cysticidal activity against *Acanthamoeba. Rev Infect Dis* 1991; 13(suppl):S431–S435.

120. Stern GA, Buttross M. Use of corticosteroids in combination with antimicrobial drugs in the treatment of infectious corneal disease. *Ophthalmology* 1991; 98:847–853.

121. Johns KJ, Head WS, O'Day DM. Corneal toxicity of propamidine. *Arch Ophthalmol* 1988; 106:68–69.

122. Maudgal PC. *Acanthamoeba* keratitis: report of three cases. *Bull Soc Belg Ophthalmol* 1989; 231:135–148.

123. John T, Lin J, Sahm DF. *Acanthamoeba* keratitis successfully treated with prolonged propamidine isethionate and neomycin-polymyxin-gramicidin. *Ann Ophthalmol* 1990; 22:20–23.

124. Berger ST, Mondino BJ, Hoft RH, et al. Successful medical management of *Acanthamoeba* keratitis. *Am J Ophthalmol* 1990; 110:395–403.

125. Beattie AM, Slomovic AR, Rootman DS, et al. *Acanthamoeba* keratitis with two species of *Acanthamoeba. Can J Ophthalmol* 1990; 25:260–262.

126. Sharma S, Srinivasan M, George C. *Acanthamoeba* keratitis in non-contact lens wearers. *Arch Ophthalmol* 1990; 108:676–678.

127. Ishibashi Y, Matsumoto Y, Kabata T, et al. Oral itraconazole and topical miconazole with debridement for *Acanthamoeba* keratitis. *Am J Ophthalmol* 1990; 109:121–126.

128. Ficker L, Seal D, Warhurst D, et al. *Acanthamoeba* keratitis: resistance to medical therapy. *Eye* 1990; 4:835–838.

129. Warhurst DC, Singer M. Inhibition of growth of *Naegleria* by a swimming pool additive. *Trans R Soc Trop Med Hyg* 1975; 69:7.

130. Kilvington S. Activity of water biocide chemicals and contact lens disinfectants on pathogenic free-living amoebae. *Int Biodeterioration* 1990; 26:127–138.

131. Kim BG, McCann PP, Byers TJ. Inhibition of multiplication of *Acanthamoeba castellanii* by specific inhibitors of ornithine decarboxylase. *J Protozool* 1987; 34:264–266.

132. Byers TJ, Kim BG, King LE, et al. Molecular aspects of the cell cycle and encystment in *Acanthamoeba. Rev Infect Dis* 1991; 13:S378–S384.

133. Hay J, Kirkness CM, Seal DV, et al. Drug resistance and *Acanthamoeba* keratitis: the quest for alternative antiprotozoal chemotherapy. *Eye* 1994; 8:555–563.

134. Badenoch PR. The pathogenesis of *Acanthamoeba* keratitis. *Aust NZJ Ophthalmol* 1991; 19:9–20.

135. He Y G, Niederkorn JY, Alizadeh H, et al. A pig model of *Acanthamoeba* keratitis: transmission via contaminated contact lenses. *Invest Ophthalmol Vis Sci* 1992; 33:126–133.

136. Stopak SS, Roat MI, Nauheim RC, et al. Growth of *Acanthamoeba* on human corneal epithelial cells and keratocytes in vitro. *Invest Ophthalmol Vis Sci* 1991; 32:354–359.

137. He YG, Niederkorn JY, McCulley JP, et al. In vivo and in vitro collagenolytic activity of *Acanthamoeba* castellanii. *Invest Ophthalmol Vis Sci* 1990; 31:2235–2240.

138. Larkin DF, Easty DL. External eye flora as a nutrient source for *Acanthamoeba*. *Graefes Arch Clin Exp Ophthalmol* 1990; 228:458–460.

139. Paniagua-Crespo E, Tsouria-Belaid A, Bellon C, et al. Amoebic keratitis caused by *Acanthamoeba* sp. May HSV1 infection play a role? *J Fr Ophthalmol* 1991; 14:25–31.

140. Cote MA, Irvine JA, Rao NA, et al. Evaluation of the rabbit as a model of *Acanthamoeba* keratitis. *Rev Infect Dis* 1991; 13(suppl):S443–S444.

141. Larkin DF, Easty DL. Experimental *Acanthamoeba* keratitis: I. Preliminary findings. *Br J Ophthalmol* 1990; 74:551–555.

142. Larkin DF, Easty DL. Experimental *Acanthamoeba* keratitis: II. Immunohistochemical evaluation. *Br J Ophthalmol* 1991; 75:421–424.

143. Ferrante A. Free living amoebae: pathogenicity and immunity. *Parasite Immunol* 1991; 13:31–47.

144. Garate M, Alizadeh H, Neelam S, et al. Oral immunization with *Acanthamoeba castellanii* Mannose-binding protein ameliorates amoebic keratitis. *Infect Immun* 2006; 74:7032–7034

145. Meisler DM, Rutherford I. *Acanthamoeba* and disinfection of soft contact lenses. *Rev Infect Dis* 1991; 13(suppl):S410–S412.

146. Moore MB. *Acanthamoeba* keratitis and contact lens wear: the patient is at fault. *Cornea* 1990; 9(suppl):S33–S35.

147. Larkin DF, Kilvington S, Easty DL. Contamination of contact lens storage cases by *Acanthamoeba* and bacteria. *Br J Ophthalmol* 1990; 74: 133–135.

148. Kilvington S, Larkin DF, White DG, et al. Laboratory investigation of *Acanthamoeba* keratitis. *J Clin Microbiol* 1990; 28:2722–2725.

149. Chandler JW. Biocompatibility of hydrogen peroxide in soft contact lens disinfection: antimicrobial activity vs. biocompatibility – the balance. *CLAO J* 1990; 16(suppl):S43–S45.

150. Gray TB, Cursons RTM, Sherwan JF, et al. *Acanthamoeba*, bacterial and fungal contamination of contact lens storage cases. *Br J Ophthalmol* 1995; 79:601–605.

151. Kilvington S, Larkin DF. *Acanthamoeba* adherence to contact lenses and removal by cleaning agents. *Eye* 1990; 4:589–593.

152. Heidemann DG, Verdier DD, Dunn SP, et al. *Acanthamoeba* keratitis associated with disposable contact lenses. *Am J Ophthalmol* 1990; 110:630–634.

Chapter 81

Gordon C. Cook

Trichomonal Infection

Trichomonas vaginalis is a pathogenic protozoan with a high degree of site specificity – affecting predominantly the lower female genitourinary tract.[1] Infection may or may not be symptomatic; it can be sexually transmitted. In women, <10^4, and in men, 4×10^6, organisms produce an infection. Related organisms are: *T. tenax* and *Pentatrichonomas hominis*; while these colonize the gums and colon, respectively, neither is of proven pathogenicity.

First visualized by Donné in 1836, *T. vaginalis* was first shown in the early twentieth century, as a result of inoculation studies, to be pathogenic. It is an ovoid organism, 10–20 μm wide; 'twitching' motility is brought about by four anterior flagella and a recurrent flagellum (embedded in an undulating membrane, which runs along two-thirds of the cell). It is actively phagocytic, optimal growth occurring under moderately anaerobic conditions. Reproduction is by binary fission; unlike many pathogenic protozoa, cysts are not formed. When subjected to either in vitro or in vivo study, a strain variation in virulence is apparent.

DISTRIBUTION AND EPIDEMIOLOGY

Infection occurs worldwide – in both urban and rural settings.[1] In the 1970s, the World Health Organization (WHO) estimated an annual world incidence of 180 million cases; however, *T. vaginalis* infection is not notifiable, and data on prevalence tend therefore to be highly unreliable. In sexually transmitted disease (STD) clinics, overall figures varying from 7% to 32% have been recorded. Highest prevalence rates are in groups with a high level of sexual activity. In female prostitutes, figures of up to 80% have been noted. In tropical populations, recorded prevalence has varied from 3% in Manila university students, to 15–20% in clinic populations studied in Asia and Africa. Three studies from Nigeria give an insight into the prevalence of infection in West Africa.[2–4] Infection was detected in 505 (24.7%) out of 2048 urine specimens submitted by students at a 'higher institution'; 374 (74%) occurred in women, and 131 (26%) in men.[2] At Jos, infection rates of 37.6% and 24.8% were recorded in groups (250 were examined in each group) of urban and rural women, respectively.[3] Specimens from 2224 adult women examined at the cytology clinic at University College Hospital, Ibadan, revealed an infection rate of 9.8%.[4] In Turkish women with a vaginal discharge, a 13% incidence has been recorded.[5] Other studies have shown significant prevalence rates in Tanzania,[6] Iran,[7] Korea,[8] and Ghana.[9] Infection tends to be high in HIV-infected individuals.[10–16] At Dar-es-Salaam, Tanzania, an investigation of 359 gynaecological in-patients revealed that those infected with *T. vaginalis* had an almost three-fold higher risk of being infected with HIV.[17] A high rate of infection has also been demonstrated in pregnant women in a rural community in north-eastern Nigeria.[18] In men (in whom the disease is usually asymptomatic and self-limiting [see below]), meaningful prevalence figures are virtually non-existent. The organism is frequently co-existent with another infection, e.g. candidiasis, gonorrhoea, syphilis or HIV infection; it is therefore important to screen an infected woman for another STD(s), which often has a greater medical significance. Although non-venereal transmission of *T. vaginalis* is rare, the organism can survive for several hours in a moist environment. Perinatal infection in about 5% of female babies born (vaginally) to infected mothers has been recorded.

PATHOGENESIS AND PATHOLOGY

The organism involves squamous (rather than columnar) epithelium; only rarely can it be isolated from the endocervix, but the urethra is involved in 90% of infected cases. Rarely, it has been demonstrated in the epididymis and prostate, and occasionally causes non-gonococcal (tetracycline-resistant) urethritis (NGU). *T. vaginalis* infection is accompanied by large numbers of polymorphonuclear neutrophils (PMNs) (which, together with macrophages, kill the organism) and a consequent vaginal discharge. The organism is not invasive, existing either free in the vaginal cavity or adherent to epithelium; in about 50% of cases, microscopic haemorrhage is apparent using an appropriate technique. Local IgA is usually detectable (see below); however, serum antibody concentration remains low, and is of no use diagnostically (see below).

CLINICAL ASPECTS

Classical presentation consists of vulvo-vaginitis.[19–22] In an experimentally induced infection, the incubation period ranges from 3 to 28 days. Although 50–90% of infected women are symptomatic, it is frequently difficult to attribute symptoms directly to *T. vaginalis*, because another organism(s) is co-existent. In 50–75%

of those infected, a vaginal discharge (often frothy and greenish-yellow,[3,5] and sometimes odorous) is present; 25–50% of women infected suffer from vulval irritation,[2,3] while 50% experience dyspareunia; mild dysuria is sometimes present. Lower abdominal discomfort is described by 10% of infected women; it may be accompanied by salpingitis, although this may have a different aetiology – possibly another STD. A yellowish vaginal discharge is present in 50–75% of those infected, while vulval erythema is present in less than one-third. It is probably a cause of female infertility.[23]

In men, NGU may be present,[24–29] but the majority of cases are asymptomatic. When symptomatic, infection may resemble NGU of another aetiology;[26,27] it is usually recognized following failure of response to standard chemotherapeutic regimens.[28,29] *T. vaginalis* can be detected in 70% of men who have experienced sexual intercourse with an infected woman within the previous 48 hours. It is one of several STDs to affect male homosexuals.[30] Involvement of the epididymis and prostate are rare events.

A small percentage of female infants born to infected mothers may be infected (see above), but a *T. vaginalis* infection in older children may indicate sexual abuse.

In the long term, *T. vaginalis* infection is benign. There is no evidence that it directly predisposes to cervical carcinoma; an associated organism(s), e.g. a papillomavirus,[21] may, however, be implicated in this pathology.

DIAGNOSIS

Definitive diagnosis depends on demonstration of the parasite in a specimen from a symptomatic woman (see above) – who in many cases has recently had sexual intercourse with a 'new' partner. Recent use of an antibiotic(s) suggests the possibility of a *Candida* spp. infection. Presence of another STD should be sought by careful examination of the vulva using a speculum; further examination after trichomoniasis has been treated may also reveal an associated (co-existent) infection. Vaginal inflammation is present with both *T. vaginalis* and *Candida* spp. infection, but not usually in bacterial vaginosis.[19,21,31,32] The cervix should be examined for evidence of cervicitis and a purulent or mucopurulent discharge.

T. vaginalis can be demonstrated using a vaginal swab. The specimen can either be transferred directly to a microscope slide, or the swab agitated in a tube containing about 1 mL saline.[33] The organism can be cultured using a variety of media.

Normal vaginal pH is <4.5; this is maintained in most women suffering from vulvovaginal candidiasis. However, more than 75% of women with a *T. vaginalis* infection, accompanied by bacterial vaginosis,[1] have a pH > 4.5. Cervical discharge has an elevated pH; therefore, that in vaginal material may be artificially elevated; recent coitus also significantly elevates pH (semen is significantly more alkaline than vaginal secretion). Following determination of pH, several drops of 10–20% potassium hydroxide can be added to the discharge obtained during speculum examination; a pungent, fishy, amine-like odour is present in 75% of women with a *T. vaginalis* infection,[5] and most of those with bacterial vaginosis;[31] this test is negative in vulvovaginal candidiasis.

For a definitive diagnosis, microscopic examination of vaginal discharge is mandatory; a drop of wet-mount preparation should be examined under a coverslip.[33,34] In a *T. vaginalis* infection, the flora consists of rods or coccobacilli, while epithelial cells are unaltered and PMNs plentiful; motile *T. vaginalis* (decreasing in older, cooled preparations) can be visualized in 40–80% of those infected. Gram staining is virtually useless for recognition of *T. vaginalis*; Giemsa staining is 50% sensitive, and an acridine-orange technique about 60% sensitive. Use of a routine Papanicolaou technique[34] on a cervical specimen detects *T. vaginalis* in 60–70% of cases. Newer fluorescent antibody techniques[33] possess a sensitivity of 80–90% when compared with culture. In bacterial vaginosis, the normal flora consisting of rods is replaced by coccobacilli (which encrust the epithelial cells); few PMNs are present.

In men, diagnosis is usually more difficult;[35] occasionally, a wet-mount preparation of urethral discharge will reveal motile organisms. The most effective means of diagnosis is by culture (see below) of a urethral specimen or sample of urine sediment following prostatic massage.[25]

Culture techniques (with a sensitivity of >95%) are not widely used, but these increase the detection rate.[36,37] *T. vaginalis* grows best on a suitable medium in an anaerobic environment at 37°C; selective growth can be achieved by addition of an appropriate antibiotic(s). Recently, an enzyme-linked immunosorbent assay has been compared with wet-mount and culture techniques for detecting *T. vaginalis*;[37–40] culture proved to be more sensitive. Other recently developed techniques include: employment of monoclonal antibodies;[33] a molecular probe for identification of *T. vaginalis* DNA;[38] a PCR;[32] and detection of anti-*T. vaginalis* antibodies in cervical secretions and serum samples.[40–46]

Local IgA is detectable in most infected women (see above);[37,40,41] however, there is not a significant elevation of the serum concentration.

TREATMENT

T. vaginalis is usually highly sensitive (minimal inhibitory concentration <1 µg/mL) to the 5-nitroimidazole compounds,[47] but not to most other antimicrobial agents. A study carried out in Basra, Iraq, for example, failed to demonstrate any therapeutic effect from doxycycline or praziquantel.[48] Recently, however, relative resistance to metronidazole in some strains has been demonstrated.[22,33,49,50]

In women, metronidazole is thus most widely used[19,22,30,31,51–53] with a recommended dose regimen of 2.0 g as a single dose; this cures 85% of cases, and, when the sexual partner is treated simultaneously, the success rate rises to 95%. Another regimen utilizes a single-day divided dose of 1.6 g. A regimen using 250 mg three times a day for 7 days probably gives a comparable result. In men, a 7-day course is of proven efficacy, while the single-dose regimen has not been adequately assessed. Metronidazole possesses significant side-effects (Chapter 79), including the development of a *Candida* spp. infection. Although there is no evidence of teratogenicity in *Homo sapiens*, metronidazole should, if possible, be avoided during the first trimester of pregnancy.[33] Experience with tinidazole is limited,[33,47,54,55] but results using a single-dose regimen are encouraging; it has the advantage of being significantly less expensive, and possesses minimal side-effects. A 100% cure rate has been recorded using nimorazole (4 g in two equally divided doses 24 hours apart).[47] Clotrimazole 100 mg intravaginally at night usually relieves symptoms, but a 7-day course cures only about 20%. Clindamycin is also an alternative.[31] Mebendazole, furazolidone and anisomycin may all be effective in 5-nitroimidazole-resistant *T. vaginalis*;[55] however, 'prospective, randomized, double-blind, active-control comparative studies' are required.[56] More recently, paromomycin has proved effective in metronidazole-resistant infection.[57] A study recently carried out in Botswana concluded that 'management guidelines' for infection with *T. vaginalis* in antenatal care should be revised.[58]

Use of condoms is effective in prevention of infection.[2] A spermatocide, nonoxinol 9 – which is present in many vaginal preparations – possesses significant trichomonacidal properties.[55]

REFERENCES

1. Hook EW. Trichomonas vaginalis – no longer a minor STD. *Sex Transm Dis* 1999; 26:388–389.

2. Anosike JC, Onwuliri D, Inyang RE, et al. Trichomoniasis amongst students of a higher institution in Nigeria. *Appl Parasitol* 1993; 34:19–25.

3. Ogbonna CI, Ogbonna IB, Ogbonna AA, et al. Studies on the incidence of *Trichonomas vaginalis* amongst pregnant women in Jos area of Plateau State, Nigeria. *Angew Parasitol* 1991; 32:198–204.

4. Konje JC, Otolorin ED, Ogunniyi JD, et al. The prevalence of *Gardnerella vaginalis*, *Trichomonas vaginalis* and *Candida albicans* in the cytology clinic at Ibadan, Nigeria. *Afr J Med Sci* 1991; 20:29–34.

5. Yereli K, Balcioglu IC, Degerli K, et al. Incidence of *Trichomonas vaginalis* among women having vaginal discharge, in Manisa, Turkey. *J Egypt Soc Parasitol* 1997; 27:905–911.

6. Klinger EV, Kapiga SH, Sam NE, et al. A community-based study of risk factors for *Trichomonas vaginalis* infection among women and their male partners in Moshi urban district, northern Tanzania. *Sex Transm Dis* 2006; 33:712–718.

7. Shobeiri F, Nazari M. A prospective study of genital infections in Hamedan, Iran. *Southeast Asian J Trop Med Publ Hlth* 2006; 37(suppl 3):174–177

8. Ryu JS, Min DY. *Trichomonas vaginalis* and trichomoniasis in the Republic of Korea. *Korean J Parasitol* 2006; 44:101–116.

9. Adu-Sarkodie Y, Opoku BK, Crucitti T, et al. Lack of evidence for the involvement of rectal and oral trichomonads in the aetiology of vaginal trichomoniasis in Ghana. *Sex Transm Dis* 2007; 83:130–132.

10. Jackson DJ, Rakwar JP, Bwayo JJ, et al. Urethral *Trichomonas vaginalis* infection and HIV-1 transmission. *Lancet* 1997; 350:1076.

11. Press N, Chavez VM, Ticona E, et al. Screening for sexually transmitted diseases in human immunodeficiency virus-positive patients in Peru reveals an absence of *Chlamydia trachomatis* and identifies *Trichomonas vaginalis* in pharyngeal specimens. *Clin Infect Dis* 2001; 32:808–814.

12. Niccolai LM, Kopicko JJ, Kassie A, et al. Incidence and predictors of reinfection with *Trichomonas vaginalis* in HIV-infected women. *Sex Transm Dis* 2000; 27:284–288.

13. Price MA, Stewart SR, Miller WC, et al. The cost-effectiveness of treating male trichomoniasis to avert HIV transmission in men seeking sexually transmitted disease care in Malawi. *J Acquir Immune Defic Syndr* 2006; 43:202–209.

14. Råssjö EB, Mirembe FM, Darj E. Vulnerability and risk factors for sexually transmitted infections and HIV among adolescents in Kampala, Uganda. *AIDS Care* 2006; 18:710–716.

15. Hagan JE, Dulmaa N. Risk factors and prevalence of HIV and sexually transmitted infections among low-income female commercial sex workers in Mongolia. *Sex Transm Dis* 2007; 34:83–87.

16. McClelland RS, Sangare L, Hassan WM, et al. Infection with *Trichomonas vaginalis* increases the risk of HIV-1 acquisition. *J Infect Dis* 2007; 195:698–702.

17. ter Meulen J, Mgaya HN, Chang-Claude J, et al. Risk factors for HIV infection in gynaecological inpatients in Dar es Salaam, Tanzania, 1988–1990. *East Afr Med J* 1992; 69:688–692.

18. Nwosu CO, Djieyep NA. Candidiasis and trichomoniasis among pregnant women in a rural community in the semi-arid zone, north-eastern Nigeria. *West Afr J Med* 2007; 26:17–19.

19. Kent HL. Epidemiology of vaginitis. *Am J Obstet Gynecol* 1991; 165:1168–1176.

20. Sobel JD. Vulvovaginitis. *Dermatol Clin* 1992; 10:339–359.

21. Hatch KD. Vulvar and vaginal disorders. *Curr Opin Obstet Gynecol* 1992; 4:904–906.

22. Heine P, McGregor JA. *Trichomonas vaginalis*: a reemerging pathogen. *Clin Obstet Gynecol* 1993; 36:137–144.

23. el-Sharkawy IM, Hamza SM, el-Sayed MK. Correlation between *Trichomonas vaginalis* and female infertility. *J Egypt Soc Parasitol* 2000; 30:287–294.

24. Fowler JE Jr. Urethritis in men. *Semin Urol* 1991; 9:15–27.

25. Saxena SB, Jenkins RR. Prevalence of *Trichomonas vaginalis* in men at high risk for sexually transmitted diseases. *Sex Transm Dis* 1991; 18:138–142.

26. Krieger JN, Jenny C, Verdon M, et al. Clinical manifestations of trichomoniasis in men. *Ann Intern Med* 1993; 118:844–849.

27. Krieger JN, Verdon M, Siegel N, et al. Natural history of urogenital trichomoniasis in men. *J Urol* 1993; 149:1455–1458.

28. Bakare RA, Ashiru JO, Adeyemi-Doro FA, et al. Non-gonococcal urethritis (NGU) due to *Trichomonas vaginalis* in Ibadan. *West Afr J Med* 1999; 18:64–68.

29. el-Seoud SF, Abbas MM, Habib FS. Study of trichomoniasis among Egyptian male patients. *J Egypt Soc Parasitol* 1998; 28:263–270.

30. Levine GI. Sexually transmitted parasitic diseases. *Prim Care* 1991; 18:101–128.

31. Majeroni BA. New concepts in bacterial vaginosis. *Am Fam Physician* 1991; 44:1215–1218.

32. Hart G. Factors associated with trichomoniasis, candidiasis and bacterial vaginosis. *Int J STD AIDS* 1993; 4:21–25.

33. Lossick JG, Kent HL. Trichomoniasis: trends in diagnosis and management. *Am J Obstet Gynecol* 1991; 165:1217–1222.

34. Weinberger MW, Harger JH. Accuracy of the Papanicolaou smear in the diagnosis of asymptomatic infection with *Trichomonas vaginalis*. *Obstet Gynecol* 1993; 82:425–429.

35. Krieger JN, Verdon M, Siegel N, et al. Risk assessment and laboratory diagnosis of trichomoniasis in men. *J Infect Dis* 1992; 166:1362–1366.

36. Boeke AJ, Dekker JH, Peerbooms PG. A comparison of yield from cervix versus vagina for culturing *Candida albicans* and *Trichomonas vaginalis*. *Genitourin Med* 1993; 69:41–43.

37. Sharma P, Malla N, Gupta I, et al. A comparison of wet mount, culture and enzyme linked immunosorbent assay for the diagnosis of trichomoniasis in women. *Trop Geogr Med* 1991; 43:257–260.

38. Rubino S, Muresu R, Rappelli P, et al. Molecular probe for identification of *Trichomonas vaginalis* DNA. *J Clin Microbiol* 1991; 29:702–706.

39. Riley DE, Roberts MC, Takayama T, et al. Development of polymerase chain reaction-based diagnosis of *Trichomonas vaginalis*. *J Clin Microbiol* 1992; 30:465–472.

40. Romia SA, Othman TA. Detection of antitrichomonal antibodies in sera and cervical secretions in trichomoniasis. *J Egypt Soc Parasitol* 1991; 21:373–381.

41. Bhatt R, Pandit D, Deadhar L. Detection of serum antitrichomonal antibodies in urogenital trichomoniasis by immunofluorescence. *J Postgrad Med* 1992; 38:72–74.

42. Okuyama T, Takahashi R, Mori M, et al. Polymerase chain reaction amplification of *Trichomonas vaginalis* DNA from Papanicolaou-stained smears. *Diagn Cytopathol* 1998; 19:437–440.

43. Madico G, Quinn TC, Rompalo A, et al. Diagnosis of *Trichomonas vaginalis* infection by PCR using vaginal swab samples. *J Clin Microbiol* 1998; 36:3205–3210.

44. van Der Schee C, van Belkum A, Zwijgers L, et al. Improved diagnosis of *Trichomonas vaginalis* infection by PCR using vaginal swabs and urine specimens compared to diagnosis by wet mount microscopy, culture, and fluorescent staining. *J Clin Microbiol* 1999; 37:4127–4130.

45. Ryu JS, Chung HL, Min DY, et al. Diagnosis of trichomoniasis by polymerase chain reaction. *Yonsei Med J* 1999; 40:56–60.

46. Mayta H, Gilman RH, Calderon MM, et al. 18S ribosomal DNA-based PCR for diagnosis of *Trichomonas vaginalis*. *J Clin Microbiol* 2000; 38:2683–2687.

47. Chunge CN, Kangethe S, Pamba HD, et al. Treatment of symptomatic trichomoniasis among adult women using oral nitroimidazoles. *East Afr Med J* 1992; 69:398–401.

48. Mahdi NK, Gany ZH, Sharief M. Alternative drugs against *Trichomonas vaginalis*. *East Mediterr Health J* 2006; 12:679–684.

49. Sobel JD, Nagappan V, Nyirjesy P. Metronidazole-resistant vaginal trichomoniasis – an emerging problem. *N Engl J Med* 1999; 341:292–293.

50. Snipes LJ, Gamard PM, Narcisi EM, et al. Molecular epidemiology of metronidazole resistance in a population of *Trichomonas vaginalis* clinical isolates. *J Clin Microbiol* 2000; 38:3004–3009.

51. Hager WD, Rapp RP. Metronizadole. *Obstet Gynecol Clin North Am* 1992; 19:497–510.

52. Anonymous. Drug-resistant *Trichomonas vaginalis*. *Commun Dis Rep CDR Weekly* 1993; 3:141.

53. Ikeh EI, Bello CS, Ajayi JA. In vitro susceptibility of *Trichomonas vaginalis* strains to metronizadole – a Nigerian experience. *Genitourin Med* 1993; 69:241–242.

54. Hamed KA, Studemeister AE. Successful response of metronizadole-resistant trichomonal vaginitis to tinidazole. A case report. *Sex Transm Dis* 1992; 19:339–340.

55. O-Prasertsawat P, Jetsawangsri T. Split-dose metronizadole or single-dose tinidazole for the treatment of vaginal trichomoniasis. *Sex Transm Dis* 1992; 19:295–297.

56. Livengod CH, Lossick JG. Resolution of resistant vaginal trichomoniasis associated with the use of intravaginal nonoxynol-9. *Obstet Gynecol* 1991; 78:954–956.

57. McCutchan JA, Ronald AR, Corey L, et al. Evaluation of new anti-infective drugs for the treatment of vaginal infections. Infectious Diseases Society of America and the Food and Drug Administration. *Clin Infect Dis* 1992; 15(suppl 1):S115–S122.

58. Romoren M, Velauthapillai M, Rahman M, et al. Trichomoniasis and bacterial vaginosis in pregnancy: inadequately managed with the syndromic approach. *Bull World Health Organ* 2007; 85:297–304.

Chapter 82 Andrew Davis

Schistosomiasis

The term human schistosomiasis includes a complex group of acute and chronic parasitic infections caused by mammalian blood flukes (*Schistosoma*). These infections are transmitted by specific aquatic or amphibious snails in a wide variety of freshwater habitats.

The various species of the genus *Schistosoma* are members of the family Schistosomatidae-dioecious digenean parasites whose habitat is the blood–vascular system of vertebrates. The family is divided into three, the Schistosomatinae, Bilharziellinae and Gigantobilharziinae, and contains 12 genera, of which several are confined to birds and five to mammals; only *Schistosoma* is associated with humans.

A general feature of the family is that the female is longer and more slender than the male and is normally carried in a ventral groove, the gynaecophoric canal, formed by ventrally flexed lateral outgrowths of the male body. Of all the mammalian blood flukes, the genus *Schistosoma* has achieved the greatest geographical distribution and diversification.[1]

Of the 16 species of schistosome known to infect humans or animals, only five are responsible for the overwhelming proportion of human infections: *Schistosoma haematobium, S. intercalatum, S. mansoni, S. japonicum* and *S. mekongi*. Rarely, other zoophilic species or hybrids may be found in humans.[2] The five principal species infecting humans are subdivided into three groups characterized by the size and appearance of the eggs produced by the female schistosome:

- Eggs with a terminal spine: *S. haematobium, S. intercalatum*
- Eggs with a lateral spine: *S. mansoni*
- Rounded or ovoid minutely spined eggs: *S. japonicum* and *S. mekongi*.

HISTORY

S. haematobium

Chronic haematuria and various bladder disorders occurred in Egypt and Mesopotamia from the earliest times in association with the agricultural civilizations of the great river valleys. Haematuria was described in the *Gynaecological Papyrus of Kahun*, written in the mid-XIIth dynasty period, about 1900BC. Many remedies for haematuria were recorded from the time of the Ebers Papyrus and it can be assumed that the condition was widespread.[3] Calcified ova of the parasite were demonstrated in the kidneys of two Egyptian mummies of the XXth dynasty (1250–1000BC).[4]

During the Napoleonic invasion of Egypt (1799–1801), symptoms of the disease in troops were rife,[5] yet it was not until 1851 that the causal agent (*Distoma haematobium*, now *Schistosoma haematobium*), a blood fluke, was found by Theodor Bilharz in a mesenteric vein during a postmortem examination at the Kasr el Aini Hospital in Cairo.[6]

S. mansoni

In 1902, Manson found lateral spined eggs in the faeces of a West Indian patient in London and postulated the existence of a second species of blood fluke.[7] Subsequent controversy between A. Looss and L. W. Sambon, eminent scientists of the day, was resolved by the work of Leiper at El Marg, a village in the present Qualyubia Governorate, just north of Cairo, in 1915; Leiper established beyond doubt the existence of two distinct species of schistosome and the presence of snail intermediate hosts belonging not only to two different genera but also to two different subfamilies.[8] In the New World, eggs with a lateral spine were found in Bahia (Brazil) in 1904 and described in 1908[9] and in Venezuela in 1906.[10]

S. japonicum

In 1847, the clinical entities 'Kabure itch' and 'Katayama syndrome' were described in a village in the Hiroshima Prefecture in Japan,[11] while in 1904 Katsurada[12] recovered worms from the portal system of a cat and named the species *Schistosomum japonicum*. From 1909 to 1915, the biology of this parasite, its life cycle and the pathology it caused were elucidated and described by Japanese and other investigators.[13–16]

The investigation was recognized clinically in both China[17] and the Philippines in the early years of the twentieth century[18] and in Sulawesi, Celebes, in the 1930s.[19]

In China, the Oncomelania intermediate hosts were discovered in 1924[20] and in the Philippines in 1932.[21]

S. intercalatum

Suspicion arose in 1923 that, because some cases of human 'intestinal' schistosomiasis in the Yakusu area near Kisangani in present-day Zaire showed an atypical clinical picture and possessed an unusual egg morphology, a species distinct from *S. haematobium* was involved.[22] Follow-up of this work led to a description in 1934 of a new species, *S. intercalatum*, of which the snail intermediate host was a member of the *Bulinus africanus* group.[23] The recent description of a new species of human schistosome, *Schistosoma guineensis* led to a call for more phylogenetic studies of the genus *Schistosoma*; this is ongoing but seems to treat *S. intercalatum* and *S. guineenisis* as separate taxa closely related to *S. haematobium*.[24,25]

S. mekongi

Described initially in 1978,[26] the parasite causes human schistosomiasis in an, as yet, restricted area in Laos and Kampuchea (Cambodia). The intermediate host, *Tricula aperta*, is aquatic and is not susceptible to strains of *S. japonicum*.[27] A monograph provides the most authoritative account of the species to date.[28]

GEOGRAPHICAL ASPECTS

Schistosomiasis is now endemic in 76 countries and territories;[29] *S. mansoni* is found in 55 countries, ranging from the Arabian Peninsula, numerous countries in the African continent and, of the Indian Ocean islands, solely in Madagascar. High-prevalence endemicity exists in the Nile valley, particularly the neighbours Sudan and Egypt. In the New World, the infection exists in Brazil, Surinam, Venezuela and several islands in the Caribbean. Brazil stands out, with 25 million people resident in endemic areas and 3 million infected (Figures 82.1, 82.2).

S. haematobium is now endemic in 53 countries in the Middle East, most of the African continent and some islands in the Indian Ocean: Mauritius (although now near to extinction), Madagascar, Zanzibar and Pemba. In India, a focus of urinary schistosomiasis was described at Gimvi, in the Ratnagiri district, Maharashtra State.[30] Re-examination in 1981 was confirmatory,[31] but a combined Indian government/World Health Organization (WHO)/World Bank mission in 1985 found only two persons infected of 352 examined by Nuclepore filtration of urine. The presumed intermediate host, a freshwater limpet, *Ferrissia tenuis*, was found in all water bodies of major human water contact.[32] This ill-defined focus still excites scientific interest but should soon be controlled absolutely. In 40 countries, double infections with *S. mansoni* and *S. haematobium* are endemic.[33]

S. japonicum infection in humans is found only in mainland China, Indonesia (Lindu Lake valley and the Napu valley in central Sulawesi) and the Philippines. There is no evidence of recent transmission in Thailand, and schistosomiasis was eradicated in Japan some three decades ago.

A parasite resembling *S. japonicum* (*S. malayensis*), transmitted by *Robertsiella kaporensis*, has been found in humans in Pahang State, Malaysia.[34] Wild rats are the only known natural hosts and it is thought that the human is not an important host for this parasite.

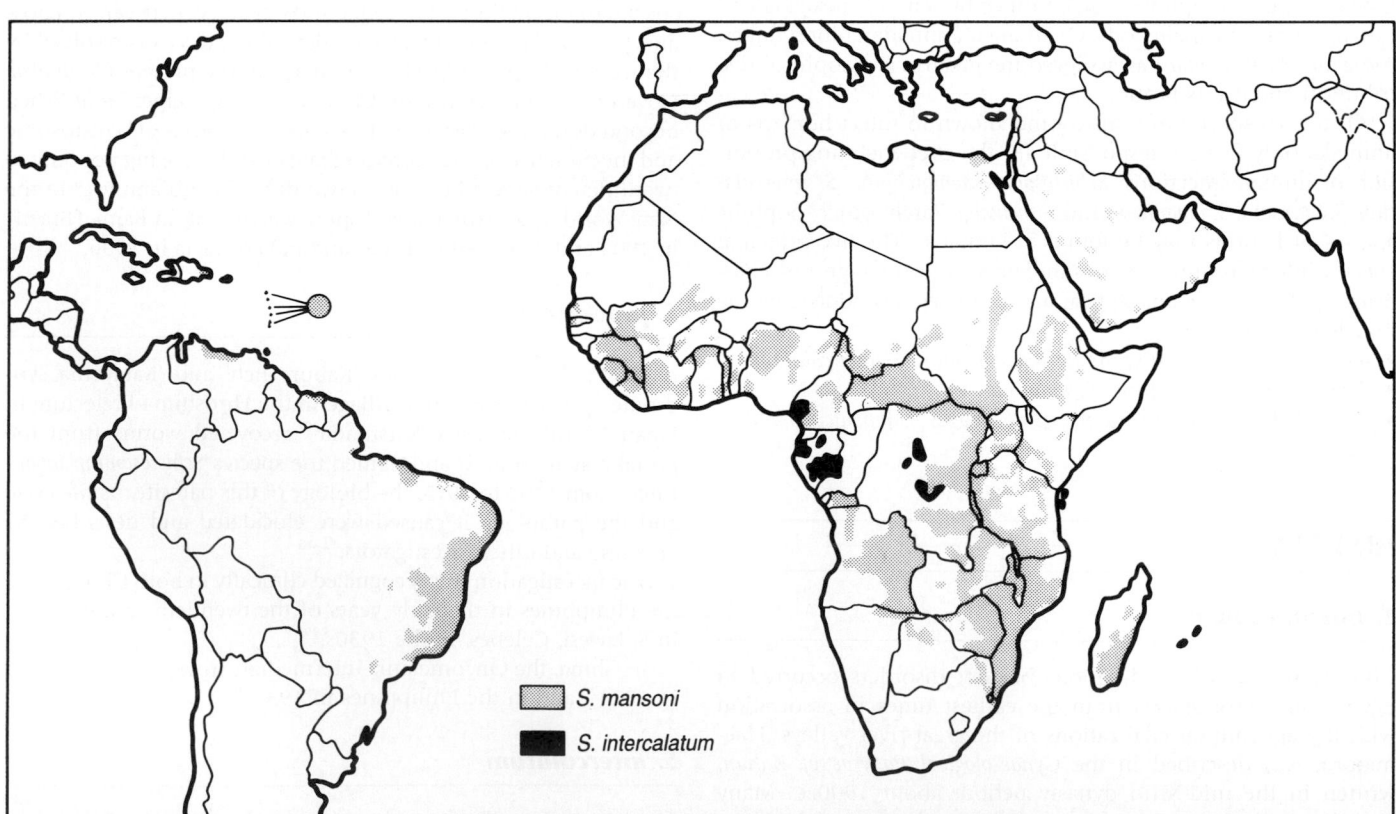

Figure 82.1 Global distribution of schistosomiasis due to *Schistosoma mansoni* and *S. intercalatum*, 1985.

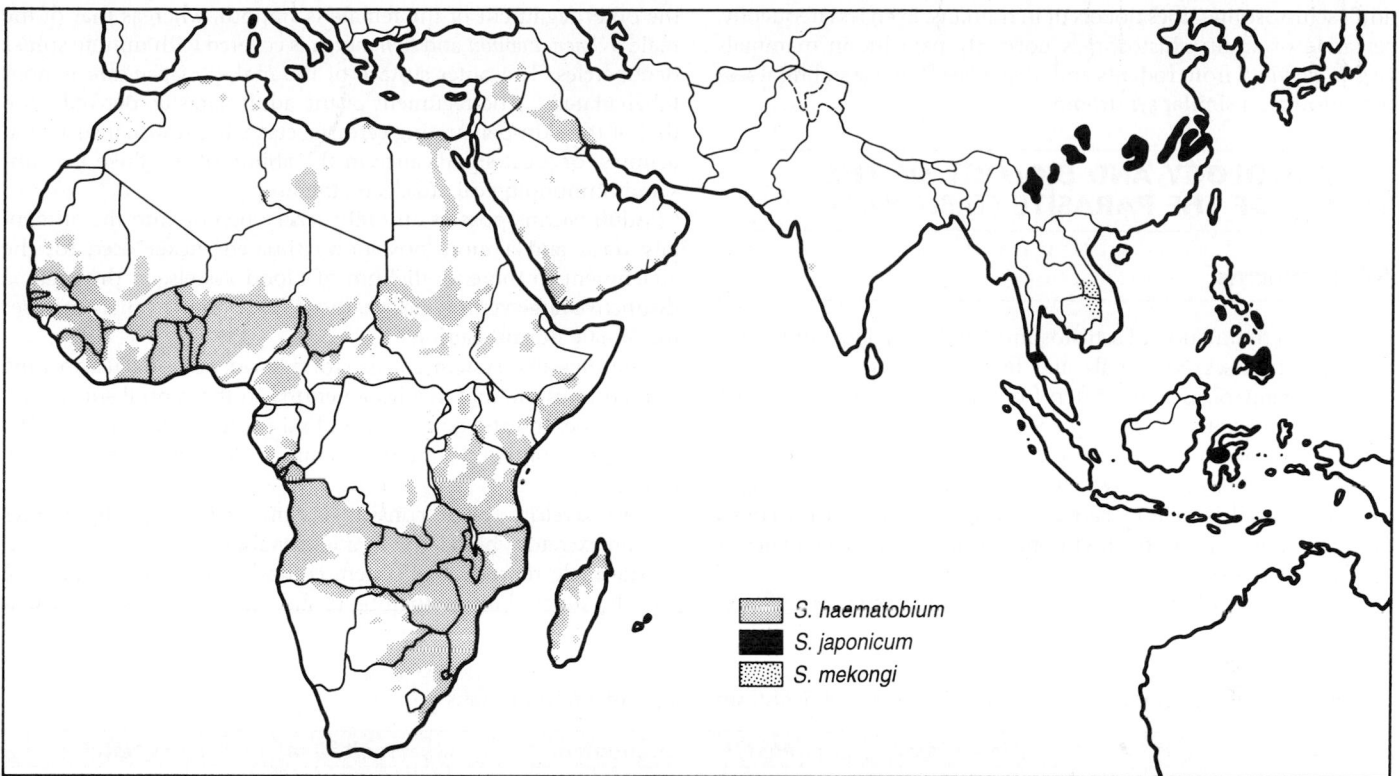

S. haematobium
S. japonicum
S. mekongi

Figure 82.2 Global distribution of schistosomiasis due to *Schistosomiasis haematobium*, *S. japonicum* and *S. mekongi* 1985.

S. intercalatum is endemic in 10 countries in central and west Africa.[35]

S. mekongi is endemic on Khong Island, Lao People's Democratic Republic, and in some areas of Democratic Kampuchea.[36]

AETIOLOGY

Of the five species of the genus, *Schistosoma* is responsible for most human infections; *S. mansoni*, *S. japonicum* and *S. mekongi* inhabit the pericolonic venules within the distribution of the portal venous system. The eggs of *S. mansoni* are characterized by a laterally placed spine; those of *S. japonicum* and *S. mekongi* are smaller and are round or ovoid with a rudimentary spine. All of these species produce 'intestinal' or 'rectal' schistosomiasis.

S. haematobium inhabits the terminal venules in the wall of the bladder, the genitourinary system and the pelvic plexus within the distribution of the inferior vena cava; its eggs have a terminal spine and it causes 'urinary' or 'vesical' schistosomiasis.

Neither *S. haematobium* nor *S. mansoni* is restricted exclusively in their anatomical vascular habitats within the respective distributions of the inferior vena caval or the portal venous systems. *S. haematobium* can exist in the perirectal venules and its eggs may be found in the stools, although almost invariably they are dead. *S. mansoni* may live in the pelvic plexus and its eggs can be detected in urine ('mansonuria'), although this is an uncommon finding during epidemiological surveys.

Much less is known on human infection with *S. intercalatum* than is the case with the other species. Two geographical strains

('Cameroon' and 'Zaire') have been described,[37,38] each with distinct and different intermediate snail hosts and patterns of egg distribution within the host. *S. intercalatum* appears to be a species distinct from *S. haematobium*; it produces terminal-spined eggs of characteristic morphology and the clinical syndrome of infection is that of a lower bowel colitis, i.e. lower abdominal discomfort or pain with either dysentery or diarrhoea. This should be qualified with the reminder that many cases are asymptomatic. Its geographical distribution is restricted to central and west Africa. Natural hybridization has been described.[39–41] Experimentally, hybridization between *S. mansoni* and *S. intercalatum* in a monkey (*Erythrocebus patas*) from Nigeria has been reported.[42] *S. mekongi* is, as yet, confined to Laos and Kampuchea (Cambodia), is transmitted by an aquatic intermediate host, *Tricula aperta*, and is also found in dogs.

Infrequently, humans are infected by schistosomes that normally live in other mammalian hosts, for example *S. bovis*, a member of the *S. haematobium* complex and a common parasite in cattle and sheep; *S. mattheei*, which has multiple hosts in both domestic and wild animals in southern Africa, and *S. margrebowiei*, a parasite frequent in antelopes in central Africa. Such infections in humans are seldom of pathological significance but suggestions have been advanced that they may confer a relative type of immunity (heterologous immunity) against *S. mansoni* and *S. haematobium* infections in areas where all species co-exist.[43,44] The cercariae of certain avian blood flukes, *Trichobilharzia*, *Gigantobilharzia* and *Ornithobilharzia*, may penetrate human skin producing cercarial dermatitis or 'swimmer's itch'. Outbreaks may occur in either tropical or temperate climates but development of cercariae into adult schistosomes does not occur in humans. Even less frequently, cercariae of adult schistosomes normally parasitic in mammals (e.g. *S. douthitti* from rodents and *S. spindale* from water buffaloes) may produce a similar syndrome.

PARASITOLOGY AND BIOLOGY OF THE STAGES OF THE PARASITE (TABLE 82.1)

Adult worms

In nature, a population of schistosomes in the final definitive host usually comprises both male and female worms (Figure 82.3). Since the genus *Schistosoma* differs from most digenetic trematodes in being dioecious, a consequence of heteromorphic chromosomes in the ovum,[45] a population could conceivably be unisexual (male or female worms only). Under laboratory conditions, single miracidial snail infections carried through to cercarial infections of the final host result in either populations of unisexual males or unisexual females.[46]

Adult worms, of separate sex, are small, with a species variation in length of 6–28 mm and in breadth of 0.25–1 mm. In all species,

the outer tegument of the female is smooth, whereas that of the male *S. haematobium* and *S. mansoni* is covered with minute spines or tubercles. The outer surface of the male *S. japonicum* is non-tuberculated.[47] The tegument of the adult parasite, derived from that of the skin-penetrating cercarial stage, has unusual structural features, of great significance in the ability of the fluke to withstand immunological attacks by the host.

Adult worms possess an oral sucker opening into the alimentary tract, and a more posteriorly situated sucker used for the attachment to the endothelium of blood vessels. In the male, a distinctive large ventral groove, the gynaecophoric canal, encloses the female during pairing.

The digestive system consists of a short oesophagus opening into an intestine that divides anteriorly to the ventral sucker and reunites behind the gonads as a blind posterior gut caecum. The black gut contents contain haematin derived from ingested blood.

The excretory system consists of flame cells, collecting tubules and an excretory bladder with a terminal pore.

The male reproductive system comprises four or five pairs of dorsally situated testes opening to the exterior through a vas deferens and seminal vesicle through an infolded cirrus.

Table 82.1 Comparison of principal features of *Schistosoma* spp. infecting humans

	S. japonicum	*S. mekongi*[a]	*S. mansoni*	*S. haematobium*	*S. intercalatum*
ADULT WORMS					
Location of adult in host	Mesenteric veins	Mesenteric veins	Mesenteric veins	Vesical plexus	Mesenteric veins
Length of posterior gut caecum	Medium	Medium	Very long	Short	Short
MALE					
Length (mm)	10–20	115	6–13	10–15	11–14
Width (mm)	0.55	0.41	1.10	0.90	0.3–0.4
No. of testes	6–7	6–7	4–13 (6–9)[b]	4–5	2–7 (4–5)[b]
Tubercles	Absent	Absent?	Coarse	Fine	Fine
FEMALE					
Length (mm)	20–30	112	10–20	16–26	10–14
Width (mm)	0.30	0.23	0.16	0.25	0.15–0.18
Ovary: position in body	Middle	Rear half	Front third	Rear third	Rear half
Uterus: position in body	Front half	Front half	Front half	Front two-thirds	Front two-thirds
Length	Short	Short	Very short	Long	Long
No. of eggs	50–200	10+	1–2	10–50	5–60
MATURE EGG					
Shape	Round	Round	Ovoid	Ovoid	Ovoid
Size (μm)	6 × 100	57 × 66	61 × 140	62 × 150	61 × 176
Spine	Lateral (reduced)	Lateral (reduced)	Lateral (prominent)	Terminal (prominent)	Terminal (prominent)
Normally passed in	Faeces	Faeces	Faeces	Urine	Faeces (and urine)
Eggs/female per day	3500	?	100–300	20–300	150–400
Reaction of egg shell to Ziehl–Neelsen stain[c]	+ve	?	+ve	−ve	+ve
INTERMEDIATE HOST SNAIL	*Oncomelania*	*Tricula*	*Biomphalaria*	*Bulinus*	*Bulinus*

[a]From experimental animal infections. [b]Usual range. [c]In histological sections. (Courtesy of R. F. Sturrock, Department of Medical Parasitology, London School of Hygiene and Tropical Medicine. Reproduced with permission from Jordan P. Webbe G., Sturrock, eds. *Human Schistosomaniasis*. Wallingford: CAB International; 1993.)

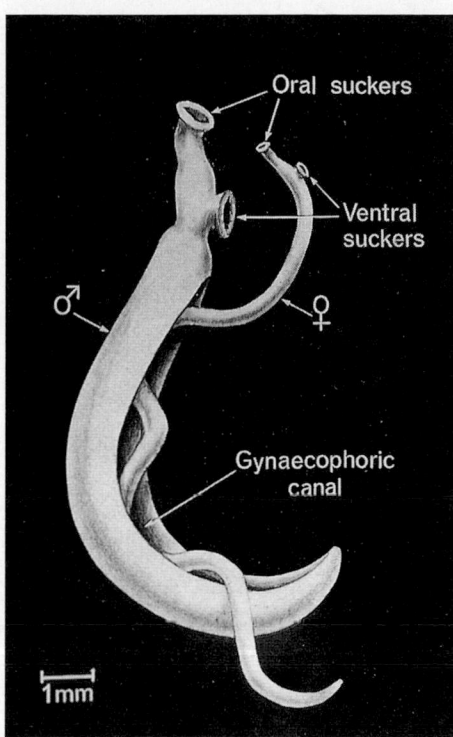

Figure 82.3 Male and female schistosomes. (Courtesy of Tropical Resources Unit.)

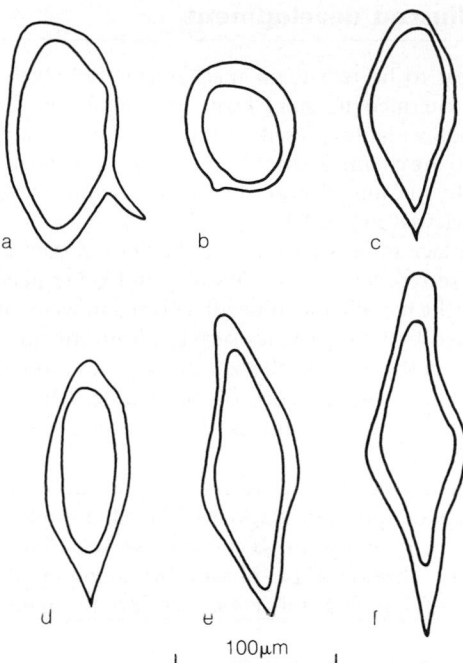

Figure 82.4 Eggs of *Schistosoma* spp. (A) *S. mansoni*, (B) *S. japonicum*, (C) *S. haematobium*, (D) *S. intercalatum*, (E) *S. mattheei*, (F) *S. bovis*.

In females, the reproductive system consists of a pear-shaped ovary in the mid-body line from which the oviduct runs anteriorly to join the common reproductive duct formed after fusion with a vitelline duct. The common duct enters the ootype, which in turn opens into the uterus which eventually opens to the exterior just below the ventral sucker.

The lifespan of the adult worm in humans is not known accurately. In the past, stress was laid on evidence of longevity with periods quoted ranging from 18 to 28 years,[48] to >30 years.[49] Since the 1970s, epidemiological studies of the excretal egg outputs of groups of infected people, in the absence of treatment or in the absence of reinfection after successful treatment, have suggested that a proportion of children, in particular, cease to pass eggs in the excreta within a relatively short time. This has been interpreted as indicative of the mortality of established worm burdens and has led to the popular (but not necessarily correct) current concept of the mean length of life of the female schistosome being of the order of 3–8 years.[50]

Detailed reviews of the somewhat fragmentary knowledge of the physiology, biochemistry and genetic constitution are given in specialist publications.[51,52] A later – most useful – review of advances in cell biology and mechanisms of protective immunity together with prospects for the advancement of vaccine studies is available.[53]

Eggs

A general description of egg morphology is given in the section on Aetiology, above; the microscopic appearance is diagnostic of the parent schistosome species (Figure 82.4) and the eggs are laid by fertilized female schistosomes intravascularly towards the periphery of the capillary venules. Eggs are non-operculate, possess a spine and contain an embryo, the miracidium, which develops inside the egg within a period of some 16 days. As a rough generalization it is supposed that approximately 50% of eggs pass through the walls of the bladder, the genitourinary apparatus or the colon, to be excreted in urine or faeces and the remainder are retained within the tissues.[52–54] The latter die about 21 days after oviposition. Excreted eggs usually contain embryos seen to be viable by observation of flame cell, ciliary or whole-body movement on microscopy. In a suitable environment of fresh water and warmth (10–30°C), the embryos (miracidia) hatch and leave the egg through slits induced partly by their own activity and partly by osmotic effects.

An adult *S. haematobium* female produces 20–200 terminal-spined eggs/day, *S. mansoni* produces 100–300 or more lateral-spined eggs/female per day and *S. japonicum* produces 500–3500 ovoid eggs with a rudimentary lateral 'knob'/female per day. The fecundity of *S. intercalatum* (another terminal-spined species and *S. mekongi* (ovoid eggs with a rudimentary lateral spine) is unknown.

Miracidia

Although miracidia of different species differ in size, they have similar morphological features and behavioural patterns. Details are given in specialist texts.[54]

On hatching from an egg in appropriate conditions, miracidia swim actively (at 2 mm/s), have behavioural patterns similar to those of the molluscan intermediate hosts and are infective to snails for 8–12 h.

1429

Intramolluscan development

There appear to be two main mechanisms by which miracidia locate the intermediate snail host: miracidial responses to the main physical variables present in the environment and also their responses to the chemical stimuli originating from snail hosts. The considerable amount of published experimental work on these topics is reviewed in specialist texts.[55,56]

After contact, miracidia penetrate the body surface of the snail through a secretion from the apical gland cells; penetration is initiated by the papilla, the miracidial boring movement probably being assisted by lytic enzymes secreted from the gut.[57] Penetration occurs via the foot of the snail in 70%, other points of entry being the tentacle or the edge of the mantle.[58] In *S. japonicum* infections, penetration points are found over the whole of the cephalopedal area.[59]

After penetration, the ciliated surface of the miracidium disappears and, in an appropriate species of snail, a mother sporocyst develops near the entry site. If the snail is not a potential host, miracidia are destroyed by phagocytic action. Only a small proportion of entering miracidia develop to mature mother sporocysts.

At 96 h, the mother sporocyst is an elongated sac filled with germinal cells and small, centrally located, vacuoles; at 8 days it has undergone further considerable growth. Germ cells are budded off from the epithelial lining; these develop into daughter sporocysts which migrate to other parts of the body of the snail, mainly through the loose connective tissue, to the digestive gland. Further germ ball production ensues, resulting in the final form of the larvae, the cercariae.

As a result of this asexual multiplication process within mother and daughter sporocysts, thousands of cercariae are formed, all of the same sex, and all originating from a single miracidium.

A proportion of infected snails have a shortened lifespan or become sterile. Some exhibit self-cure and their egg-laying returns to normal; some die.

From the time of miracidial penetration, production of mature cercariae occurs after 4–5 weeks in *S. mansoni* infection, 5–6 weeks in *S. haematobium* and 7 weeks or longer in *S. japonicum*. Numerous physical, environmental and biological factors account for these variations in time.

Cercariae

All cercariae originating from one miracidium are of the same sex; when mature, they emerge from the snail as a free-swimming stage adaptable to invasion of the definitive host (Figure 82.5).

Cercariae are furcocercous (brevifurcate), have no eye spots or pharynx, are <1 cm in length, have an oral muscular sucker occupying about one-third of the body, and a small ventral sucker or acetabulum. Their trilaminar tegument is covered with minute spines and hairs; the digestive system has a mouth in the centre of the oral sucker, an oesophagus and a pair of dorsally placed caeca; behind the oral sucker is a mass of nerve fibres from which three pairs of nerves emerge; the excretory system consists of flame cells, collecting tubules, an excretory bladder and one pair of protonephridia in the tail. Six pairs of cephalic glands subserve the emergence from the snail and penetration of the host skin,

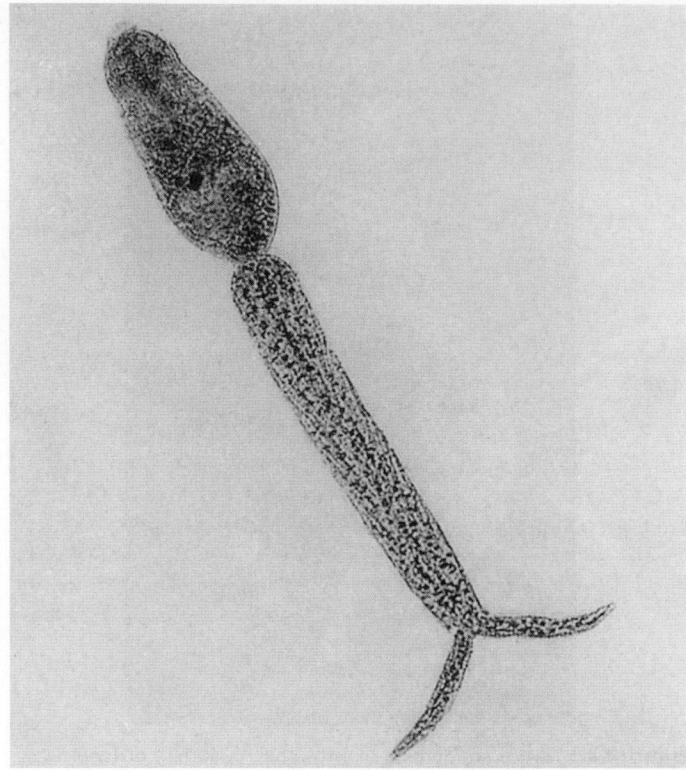

Figure 82.5 Schistosome cercaria. (Courtesy of O. D. Standen.)

aided by enzymatic secretions which have an adhesive function as the cercariae move over the skin in host location.

Cercarial production

In *S. haematobium* and *S. mansoni* the main stimulus for the release of cercariae is light, usually at temperatures between 10 and 30°C. Cercariae can, however, be shed in small numbers in the dark. In the laboratory, marked differences in shedding patterns are seen between the two species. Patterns of shedding in the field are, as might be anticipated, variable and reference should be made to biology texts.[60,61]

In *S. japonicum* infections in the field, cercarial numbers are maximal during the early night; minimal concentrations were recorded at 15:00 h and maxima at 23:00 h. Prolonged exposure to light seems to be essential in this species.

Cercarial production varies daily. Correlated with the susceptibility of a snail to infection, a small number excreted initially rises to a peak and then falls to a relatively constant level throughout the life of the snail or until spontaneous cure occurs. The size of the intermediate snail host is probably the most important variable determining cercarial output; other things being equal, large snails shed more than small snails; high cercarial outputs from *Biomphalaria glabrata* are common: 1000–3000 cercariae/day; African *Biomphalaria* spp. shed some 500 cercariae daily and rarely exceed 1500; among the larger Bulinids, similar numerical shedding occurs but rarely is 2000 cercariae per day exceeded. In *S. japonicum* infections, the snail hosts are much smaller and estimates of natural shedding in *Ocomelania hupensis* quadrasi were as low as 15/day, although, under particular conditions, 160/day were obtained. In Japan,[61] *O. h. nosophora* is thought to produce many more cercariae than *O. h. Quadrasi*. Cercarial lifespan is short: 36–48 h. As they are non-feeding organisms dependent on their large glycogen reserves, adverse environmental variables that stimulate glycogen usage reduce cercarial viability. Water velocity studies relating cercarial penetration and infection rates have produced anomalous results; patently, most cercariae are infective to vertebrate hosts under field conditions.

Schistosomula

After cercariae have penetrated human skin (or pharyngeal mucosa), a rapid process aided by lytic substances from the penetration glands, they lose their tails and become schistosomula. A remarkable additional transition is from a 'freshwater environment' to a 'saltwater environment' within the body.

Schistosomula are thus tail-less and worm-like in appearance, shed the glycocalyx, and the skin becomes the seven-layered of the adult worm, consisting of two closely opposed lipid bilayers. They then traverse the subcutaneous tissues within 48 h, penetrate the peripheral or venous channels, and are transported to the right side of the heart and lungs, where the peak concentration is attained in 5–7 days. Further developments in length and surface area occur. While controversy on the route of migration of schistosomula from the lungs to the hepatic portal system has existed for 60 years,[62] more recent evidence suggests that lung development adapts schistosomula for intravascular migration and the parasites exit the lungs in the direction of blood flow, pass to the left side of the heart, and are then distributed to system

organs in proportion to cardiac output – a totally intravascular route.

Those parasites entering splanchnic organs penetrate capillary networks rapidly, enter the hepatic portal venous system and most are trapped in the liver. The parasites distributed to organs supplied by the systemic circulation eventually return to the lungs in venous blood.[62] This implies that individual organisms may make repeated circuits of the pulmonary-systemic circulation before entering a blood vessel leading to the hepatic portal system. On arrival in the hepatic portal system, the majority of schistosomula begin to feed on blood, increase in mass and, from a primary location in the smallest hepatic portal distributaries, grow and move upstream into larger vessels.[62] The parasites shorten in dimension, experience a marked loss in motility and undergo various metabolic changes, and, once schistosomula have transformed to adult worms in the liver, lose their ability to undertake intravascular migration.

In experiments with *S. mansoni* pairing occurred 28–35 days after infection. This was succeeded by migration of paired adults to egg-laying sites in the distribution of the mesenteric superior and inferior veins, or the veins of the vesical and pelvic plexus.

LIFE CYCLE

The life cycle of all species of schistosome that infect humans has a common pathway from a sexual generation of adult schistosomes within the vascular system of the definitive host, an asexual phase in the freshwater intermediate snail host and a return to the human via cercarial invasion of the skin or mucosa on a host's exposure to cercaria-infested water (Figure 82.6).

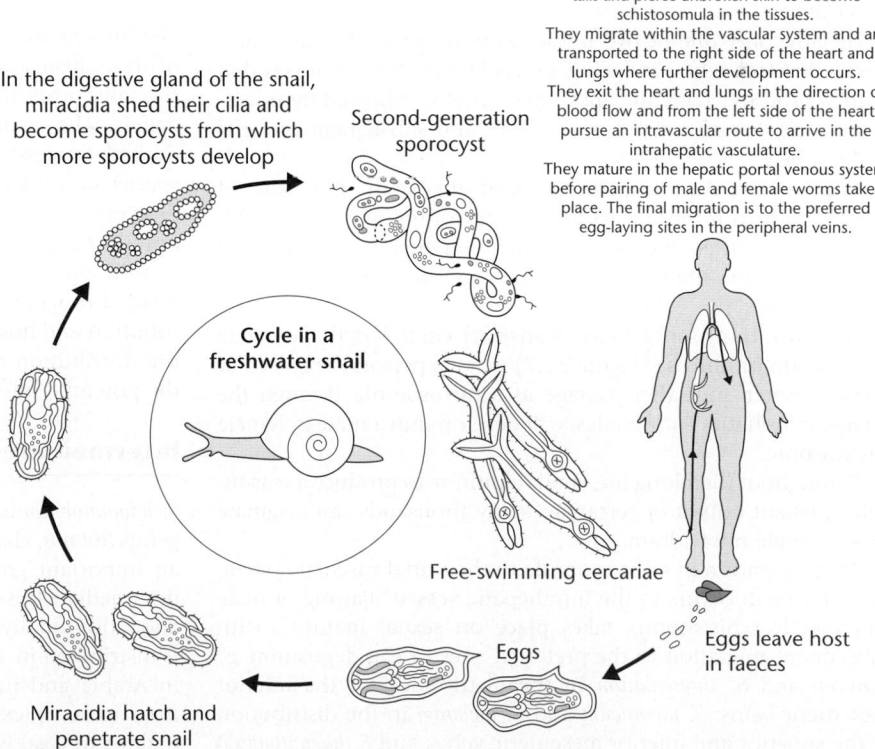

In the digestive gland of the snail, miracidia shed their cilia and become sporocysts from which more sporocysts develop

Second-generation sporocyst

Cycle in a freshwater snail

Free-swimming cercariae

Eggs

Miracidia hatch and penetrate snail

Eggs leave host in faeces

Person infested by cercariae which shed their tails and pierce unbroken skin to become schistosomula in the tissues.
They migrate within the vascular system and are transported to the right side of the heart and lungs where further development occurs.
They exit the heart and lungs in the direction of blood flow and from the left side of the heart pursue an intravascular route to arrive in the intrahepatic vasculature.
They mature in the hepatic portal venous system before pairing of male and female worms takes place. The final migration is to the preferred egg-laying sites in the peripheral veins.

Figure 82.6 Life cycle of *S. mansoni*. (Courtesy of Tropical Resources Unit.)

Adult schistosomes, living as pairs within capillary blood vessels, the slender females held in the gynaecophoric canal of the male, copulate and the females produce eggs daily throughout their life, the numbers varying with the species (see section on Eggs, above).

Eggs, the microscopic appearance of which is diagnostic of the parent schistosome species, are laid intravascularly toward the peripheral branches of the capillary venules. Partly mature at oviposition, some eggs pass through the vessel wall, aided by their spine and cytolytic secretions, into the lumen of the genitourinary tract (*S. haematobium*) or the bowel (*S. mansoni*, *S. japonicum*, *S. mekongi*, *S. intercalatum*) and reach the external world in the excreta (urine and/or faeces). Other eggs, which are the immune-stimulating and pathogenic agents in the tissues, embolize from their intravascular origin to liver, lung and many other sites.

When viable schistosome eggs are excreted and reach fresh water, either by direct deposition or by being washed in from a neighbouring site, in a suitable environment of warmth and light, the larvum within each egg becomes active and, aided by osmosis, the egg ruptures or 'hatches'; the larvum, now termed a miracidium, emerges. Miracidia are mobile organisms swimming actively by means of ciliary movements. Miracidial behaviour is related in a general way to the ecology of the snail intermediate host, and adaptive behavioural patterns have been described. During a short lifespan, miracidia are infective to snail intermediate hosts for some 8–12 h, and must find a suitable freshwater snail for continuance of their life cycle; such snails (intermediate hosts) are specific for each species of schistosome.

Miracidia then penetrate the soft tissues of the snail, influenced by numerous variables, including chemotaxis, the relative number of larvae and snails within a water body, length of contact time and physical characteristics of the surrounding medium, i.e. water temperature, velocity of flow, turbulence and the presence of ultraviolet light.

Usually, only one or two miracidia undergo further intramolluscan development, producing a sacculate mother sporocyst that in turn produces daughter sporocysts. This is followed by migration to the digestive gland of the snail and subsequent cercarial development.

After an incubation period within the snail, the time of which varies with the species and the surrounding physical environment, cercariae escape from the daughter sporocysts and emerge from the snail under suitable conditions of temperature, light and pH.

Free-swimming fork-tailed cercariae, <1 cm in length, penetrate human skin or mucosa (Figure 82.7) when a person is exposed to infested water and, after passage as schistosomula through the tissues, lymphatics and venules, will develop into a male or female schistosome.

Throughout their long life, snails continue to produce a reasonably constant output of cercariae; many thousands can originate from a single miracidium.

After migration of schistosomula to the portal vascular system, further growth occurs in the intrahepatic vessels. Pairing of male and female schistosomes takes place on sexual maturity, with subsequent migration to the preferred sites of egg deposition: *S. mansoni* and *S. intercalatum* in the distribution of the inferior mesenteric veins; *S. japonicum* and *S. mekongi* in the distribution of the superior and inferior mesenteric veins; and *S. haematobium*

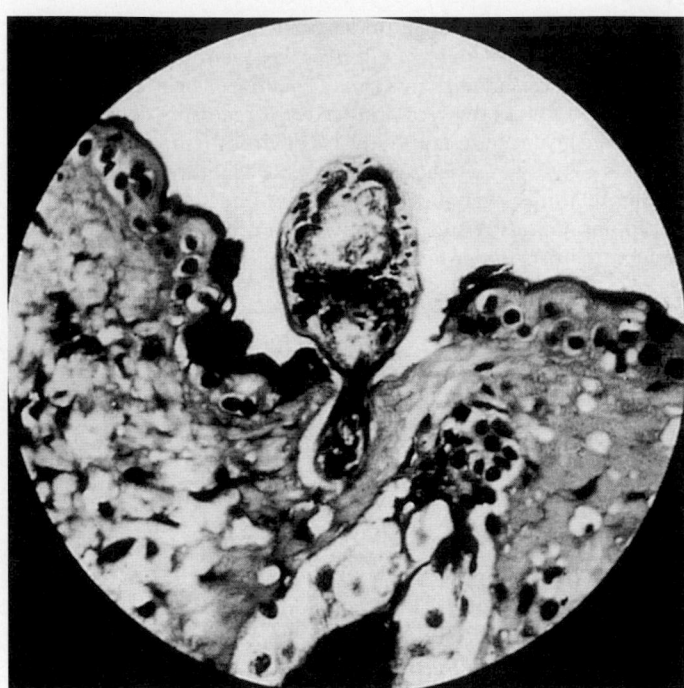

Figure 82.7 Cercarial penetration in schistosomiasis. (Courtesy of O. D. Standen.)

in the distribution of the vesical veins and the pelvic plexus. Egg deposition and excretal egg excretion begins.

INTERMEDIATE HOSTS

The biology of the intermediate snail hosts (Figures 82.8–82.10) of the schistosomes is a complex subject covered in numerous specialist texts to which reference should be made for specific details. The snail host range of schistosomes is comparatively limited. Successful parasitism of the approximately 18 recognized species of schistosome depends on the ability of the parasite to develop in a small number of species of intermediate hosts within only 10 genera.[64]

Although the schistosomes and their intermediate hosts can be divided roughly into groups reflecting their zoogeographical distribution and host specificity, the situation is complicated because the distribution of schistosomes does not exactly match that of the potential intermediate hosts.[66]

Intermediate hosts of *S. haematobium*

S. haematobium is transmitted by some 30 nominal species of the genus *Bulinus*, classified into four species-groups: *Bulinus africanus*, an important group medically as species within the group are intermediate hosts of *S. haematobium* in Africa south of the Sahara and, additionally, some cattle schistosomes; the *B. forskalli* group is distributed in a pan-African fashion with representatives found in Arabia and in some Indian Ocean islands; the *B. truncatus/tropicus* complex, again of pan-African distribution, extends from Malawi to east, west and north Africa and the Middle East as far

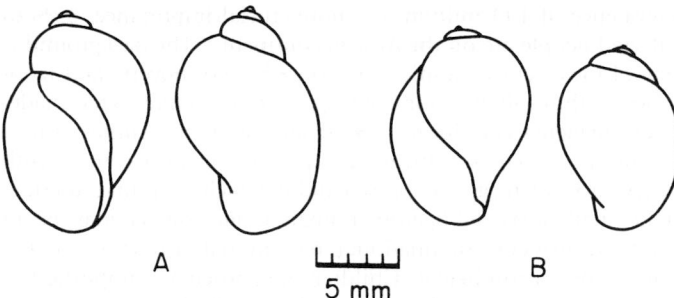

Figure 82.8 Snails of the *Bulinus* genus hosts of *S. haematobium*. (A) *Bulinus truncatus* group. (B) *B. africanus* group.

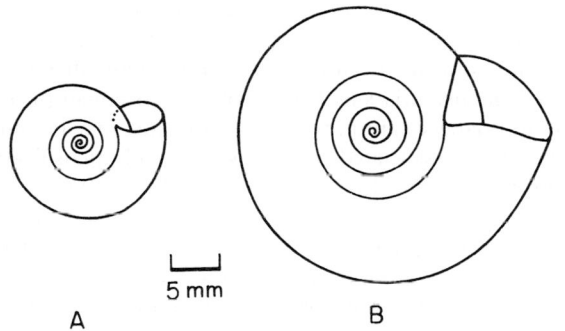

Figure 82.9 Snails of the *Biomphalaria* genus hosts of *S. mansoni*. (A) *Biomphalaria alexandrina*. (B) *B. glabrata*.

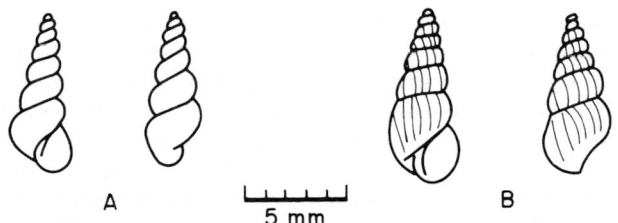

Figure 82.10 Snails of the *Oncomelania* genus host of *S. japonicum*. (A) *Oncomelania hupensis nosophora*. (B) *O. h. hupensis*.

as Iran; a small group, *B. reticulatus* is found patchily in Africa (e.g. in Ethiopia) and in isolated habitats in the Arabian peninsula.

Intermediate hosts of *S. intercalatum*

Of the two biologically distinct strains of *S. intercalatum* known to exist, one is transmitted by snails of the *Bulinus africanus* group and occurs in a restricted area of north-east Zaire; the other is transmitted by *B. forskalli* and occurs in Cameroon and Gabon. Each strain is unable to develop in a snail with which the other is compatible and, additionally, there are differences in prepatent periods and in certain enzyme patterns of the parasite.

Intermediate hosts of *S. mansoni*

S. mansoni is transmitted by species of the genus *Biomphalaria*, widely distributed in the Old World throughout Africa, the Nile

valley and the Arabian peninsula but not in Iraq or Iran. In the New World the genus is found in the southern USA, several Caribbean islands (notably Puerto Rico, St Lucia, Guadeloupe and the Dominican Republic) and on the South American continent in Brazil, Surinam and Venezuela.

The framework for the taxonomic status was described in 1978;[62] and four species-groups are still recognized. In the Old World the *Biomphalaria pfeifferi* group has several forms and is found in all parts of Africa south of the Sahara, the Malagasy Republic, in Aden, Yemen and Saudi Arabia; the *choanomphala* group has only a few forms restricted to certain of the great natural African lakes; the *alexandrina* group has a scattered distribution in Africa and is common in the Sudan and Egypt. *B. sudanica* has both east and west African species components.

In the New World, the genus *Biomphalaria* is represented by some 20 species but, of these, only *B. glabrata* (*Say*), *B. straminea* (*Dunker*) and *B. tenagophila* (*Orbigny*) have been found to be naturally infected with *S. mansoni*.

Parasite-intermediate host relationships

There are many complex and complicated variations in the relationships between schistosomes and their intermediate hosts; parasite infectivity is as important as intermediate host susceptibility and differences in relationships occur even within limited geographical areas. Both environmental and genetic factors play a part in influencing the transmission of a schistosome through a particular species of snail.

The genera *Bulinus* and *Biomphalaria* are aquatic snails and are identified on a basis of various conchological, anatomical and biological characteristics. This is a highly specialized field and requires biological expertise. The snails are found in many different habitats including permanent or semipermanent small ponds, marshes, swamps, rivers and streams, and large permanent water bodies such as lakes, dams, irrigation channels and rice fields. Their biology varies with their environment and lengthy studies are required to elucidate the details.

Cross-fertilization is usual in aquatic snail intermediate hosts but they are in fact hermaphrodites and capable of self-fertilization. Ova are laid in water as egg masses some 5–10 mm in diameter. Hatching of free-living snails occurs in 1–2 weeks; a steady growth ensues, and maximal size and maturity is seen in 3–6 months. Snail intermediate hosts have an enormous reproductive potential because egg-laying continues throughout life and lifespans have wide variations in the different species; e.g. *Bulinus globosus* infected with *S. haematobium* lived for 400 days and *Biomphalaria pfeifferi* infected with *S. mansoni* survived for 213 days.[63,64]

Intermediate hosts of *S. japonicum*

S. japonicum is transmitted by amphibious snails, populations of polytypic *Oncomelania hupensis*, of which there are six subspecies: *O. h. hupensis* in mainland China; *O. h. quadrasi* in the Philippines; *O. h. nosophora* in Japan; *O. h. lindoensis* in Sulawesi, Indonesia; and *O. h. formosana* and *O. h. chiui* in Taiwan, where schistosomiasis is confined to animals and does not exist in humans. A

Concomitant immunity, in experimental terms, describes the resistance, partial or total, of an actively infected host to a subsequent challenge infection by the same type of organism. Adult worms evade the immune responses by adding a layer of host-specific antigens to their tegmental membranes. Adult worms of a primary infection are unharmed by cercarial challenge but the invading forms of the challenge infection tend to be destroyed. Concomitant immunity occurs in schistosome infections and challenges in many experimental hosts and in humans.[80]

Further exploratory progress was made through longitudinal field studies involving detailed quantitation of egg outputs and water contact in children, allied to the technique of reinfection studies. Chemotherapy is given to remove existing infections; the levels of newly acquired infections (reinfections) are observed, quantitated and related to water contact and degree of exposure. These techniques produced strong evidence that age-dependent resistance to reinfection is distinct from age-dependent exposural change, in two areas, The Gambia and Kenya, for both *S. haematobium* and *S. mansoni* infection. For example, in The Gambia, changes in intensity of infection with time were compared in two communities, in one of which transmission had been interrupted by mollusciciding. In this area, the mean lifespan of the worms was 3–4 years, allowing comparison with the untreated area (control) of the numbers of eggs deposited by worms over the same 3-year period. The acquisition of new infections by adults over 25 years of age was 1000-fold less than that of 5–8-year-old children. This difference could not be attributed to a 1000-fold reduction of water contact in the adults, thus suggesting age-dependent acquisition of immunity to superinfection.[81–83] Thus the role of immunity in limited schistosome infections in communities in two areas endemic for *S. haematobium* and *S. mansoni* was placed on a firmer footing. However, the immunity is probably not absolute, is evident only after years of exposure to infection, and some data suggest that it occurs earlier in areas of high prevalence and intensity.

The balance of the immune response in the early years of exposure to infection is directed towards production of blocking antibodies, which may be of IgM, IgG or IgG4. Protective antibodies, IgE or other immunoglobulin isotypes, are detected in both older children and adults who appear to be resistant to infection.[84] Later data led to a surmise that 'resistance' to acquired infection, or reinfection after successful chemotherapy, is multifactorial and compartmentalized. It may involve both humoral and cellular responses at different stages of parasitic invasion. Known influencing variables are an IgE response, high levels of interferon γ (IFNγ) and tumour necrosis factor α (TNFα) and peripheral blood mononuclear cell (PBMC) responses involving different groups of cells and various cytokines, allied to a possible genetic factor on chromosome 5q31–q33. Further molecular exploration is ongoing.[85]

PATHOGENESIS

The lesions that occur during this long-lived infection are caused largely by schistosome eggs. Adult worms are impervious to the immune system of the host and by themselves cause little or no pathology, although they excrete antigens, such as the gut-associated soluble antigens found in the sera of patients with schistosomiasis and which are now used both as a marker for infection and as an indicator of therapeutic success through estimation of the cathode- and anode-associated antigens.[86]

Schistosome eggs cannot traverse capillary beds unaided because they measure up to 70 μm in width. Slightly less than half of the eggs are laid into the lumen of the gut or urinary tract. The remainder are laid in the walls of the organ or embolize into the portal radicles or lung arterioles. Collateral vascular bypasses enable eggs to reach many other organs in the body.

At oviposition, eggs are immature but miracidial maturation takes place within a few days. Soluble egg antigens (SEAs) originating from the secretory glands of miracidia enclosed within eggs diffuse out through submicroscopic pores in the eggshell and induce a host hypersensitivity response. The immunopathology of schistosomiasis is considered to be due to granuloma formation around tissue-deposited eggs and is a manifestation of delayed hypersensitivity through a T cell-mediated immune response.

During an active infection, a range of early, mature and involuting granulomas is present.[87] Granulomas vary with the immune status of the host: in primary infections with marked reactions to soluble egg antigens, large florid granulomas occur with some central necrosis. The florid granuloma is composed of the schistosome egg surrounded by cellular aggregates of eosinophils, mononuclear phagocytes, lymphocytes, neutrophils, plasma and fibroblasts. Activated macrophages cluster close to the eggshell, while lymphocytes and plasma cells are peripherally placed. Fibroblasts appear early and throughout the lengthy involution process replace other cell types. Many granulomas are of sizes much greater than those of schistosome eggs.

After the acute phase of some 3 months, modulation of host immune responses to SEAs results in relatively small granulomas which have fewer surrounding cells.

There are consistent and strong correlations of high organ and tissue egg loads and severe pathology in quantitative autopsy studies in *S. haematobium* and *S. mansoni*;[88,89] clinico-epidemiological findings are in agreement. Other factors may operate, such as direct and indirect fibroblastic proliferation and induced abnormalities of types I and III collagen.

Thus the pathology of schistosomiasis results from collections of granulomas, from fibroblastic lesions obstructing vessels and fibroinflammatory swellings containing millions of eggs. Unlike early granulomas, these late and obstructive and fibrous lesions respond poorly to antischistosomal chemotherapy.

There is a plethora of systemic host responses to schistosome infection, as cercariae, schistosomula, adult worms and eggs all generate multiple antigens to which the host immune system responds through immunocompetent cells. Antibodies specific to each stage are long lived and persist after successful chemotherapy. Several defined schistosome antigens have been detected; the most useful in clinical work is the cathode-associated antigen. Other antigens are complexed to immunoglobulins and can be found at various sites, e.g. Schistosomal nephropathy.[90]

Von Lichtenber[87] has strikingly contrasted the pathogenetic variables and prognosis in the hepatosplenomegaly of the early infection resulting from cell proliferation with florid granulomas, reticuloendothelial hyperplasia and diffuse inflammatory infiltrates, all reversible by specific chemotherapy, with the hepatosplenomegaly of the advanced disease induced by fibrovascular pathology with periportal fibrosis, portal hypertension and its associated effects on the spleen in which the prognosis is far less dependent on chemotherapy but more on surgical alleviation of a mechanical obstructive condition.

The influence of genetic factors on immunopathology and on protective immunity remains unclear. While two studies in Egypt[92] and the Philippines[92] suggested a relationship between severe disease and specific human leukocyte antigen (HLA) haplotypes, the association was not found in Brazil.[93] However, a more recent Brazilian study demonstrated that host genetic factors were implicated in human resistance to *S. mansoni* in one specific focus. No firm generalizations can yet be made.[94]

PATHOLOGY

It is useful to consider the pathology and pathophysiology of the various schistosome infections within the stages of the life cycle and their timeframes:

- cercarial invasion and schistosomular migration
- maturation of schistosomes, pairing and commencement of egg-laying
- established infection with continuous egg-laying
- late stages and complications.

Attempts to link discrete clinical entities with these stages should be made only with the realization that the apparently endless series of epidemiological, immunological and physiological interactions encountered, particularly in endemic areas, make resultant associations and correlations less than clearcut.

Frequently, much clearer relationships between clinical expressions and pathophysiological derangements are seen in non-immune visitors, transients or immigrants who become infected in endemic areas. In parallel, infected travellers or holidaymakers returning to temperate locations may present clear pictures of infections acquired in endemic zones.

Cercarial invasion of the skin or mucosal penetration on exposure to infested water, particularly when the quantum of infection is high, can occur in <15 min; the clinical complement of cercarial dermal invasion is a schistosome (cercarial or allergic) dermatitis lasting for some 24–48 h.

The pathophysiological response is the initiation of the first mechanisms of the immune response with marked eosinophilia and an antibody-dependent cell-mediated cytotoxic response involving IgG.

At widely different times, ranging from 2 to 16 weeks after cercarial invasion, during the migration of schistosomula, their maturation, pairing and initiation of egg-laying, the clinical manifestations of acute toxaemic schistosomiasis or Katayama syndrome may arise. Worm and/or egg antigens produce a marked antigenic stimulus with rapidly rising antibody levels and an increase in serum IgG, IgA and IgM levels. Circulating antigen-antibody complexes are found and may be deposited in glomeruli, producing immune complex glomerulopathy. The whole clinical picture is one resembling the acute serum sickness syndrome.

At variable times after infection, from some 2 months onwards, the stage of established infection occurs, with continuous egg-laying associated with the 'classical' symptoms and signs of established schistosomiasis. SEAs from miracidia in the eggs provoke a T lymphocyte-mediated host response which, in time, results in the characteristic granuloma with eosinophils prominent in the destruction of the eggs.

After some years, changes in clinical symptoms and physical signs appear, and there is superimposition of late-stage complications such as obstructive uropathy, hydronephrosis and pyelonephritic renal failure in *S. haematobium* infection, or portal hypertension which may be 'compensated' or 'decompensated' with ascites, and hepatosplenomegaly with or without gastrointestinal bleeding in *S. mansoni*, *S. japonicum* and *S. mekongi* infections. Modulation by T suppressor lymphocytes and antibody blockade diminish the host immune response over time; fibroblasts stimulate collagen production and fibrotic complications involving a variety of anatomical sites (e.g. periportal hepatic fibrosis and obstructive uropathy) ensue.

Pathology of established infection

S. haematobium

Urinary bladder

The urinary bladder is the most frequently affected organ. Cystoscopy, surgery or autopsy reveal the gross lesions, which are often multiple. A hyperaemic mucosa on cystoscopy is universal. 'Sandy patches' occur in one-third; these are raised greyish-yellow mucosal irregularities associated with heavy egg deposition and surrounded by dense fibrous tissue. Calcification may occur. They are sited most commonly at the trigone and near the ureteric orifices.

Other raised lesions are granulomas, nodules and polyps, which may be sessile or pedunculated and are related to local heavy tissue egg loads. Focal granulomas are of pin-head size with the customary histological appearances.

Vesical ulcers are less common and can vary in size from a small irregular defect to an irregular deep transverse fissure. They occur mainly on the posterior wall of the bladder.

Many degrees of bladder muscle hypertrophy are found at autopsy but specific associations with tissue egg loads or local lesions are lacking; muscle hypertrophy appears to be more frequent in cases with obstructive uropathy. Obstructive lesions from fibrosis of the neck of the bladder in periurethral granulomatous reactions are a common complication, as are bladder calculi.

Bladder calcification is common and is often encountered both in clinical practice and in radiological surveys. Calcification is linear, occurring along lines of deposited eggs. Calcified bladders usually retain normal elasticity.

Ureters

Although the ureters are less frequently affected than the bladder, their involvement is important for it leads to morbidity and is the forerunner of obstructive uropathy. Tissue egg loads in the ureters are greater in cases with obstructive uropathy than in those without.[95] Arguments on whether unilateral disease predominates more on the left than on the right side have continued for at least a decade. In a quantitative analysis, tissue egg burdens were much higher in the right lower ureter than in the left, but unilateral obstructive uropathy occurred equally on both sides.[96] Bilateral ureteric involvement is the rule.

The histopathological appearance of the ureteric lesions resembles that of bladder lesions. Granulomatous lesions resolve and lead to ureteral fibrotic stenosis. Rising back pressure leads to hydroureter, with or without hydronephrosis, the collective title of which is obstructive uropathy. This condition predisposes to *Escherichia coli* or *Salmonella* urinary tract infection, which can lead to chronic pyelonephritis and Gram-negative septicaemia.[97–99]

Genital organs

Because *S. haematobium* parasitizes the vesical plexus, eggs are not uncommonly found in both male and female genital organs, but the long-running debate of their functional significance has not yet been concluded.

In males, the mean *S. haematobium* egg count/g of seminal vesicle tissue was 20 000 in one investigation.[100] The resultant enlargement, muscular hypertrophy and fibrosis produced an increase in weight of the seminal vesicles that correlated with the presence of obstructive uropathy. Much less commonly affected were the prostate, testes, epididymis and penis. A causal role for these lesions in the production of male infertility has not been substantiated.

In females, the finding of eggs in the female genital organs is similarly frequent; eggs may be found in the vulva, vagina and cervix, where ulcerating polypoid or nodular lesions may be seen. Nodules in the perianal skin are not rare. The internal female genital organs – ovaries, Fallopian tubes and uterus – are much less commonly affected. In Malawi, gynaecological complications of schistosomiasis were considered a significant cause of female morbidity, particularly when the lower genital tract was involved; ovarian, uterine and tubal pathologies were not major causes of morbidity, but diagnosis was difficult.[99a] There is a dearth of recent reports associating ectopic pregnancy or infertility and *S. haematobium* infection.[100]

Schistosomiasis has little impact on female infertility and rarely renders a woman anovulatory, despite the proximity of eggs to the gonads, tubes and uterus. A recent well-conducted study in rural Zimbabwe confirmed that sandy patches, neovascularization and vessel pathology were strongly associated with schistosome ova. There was however, no association of *S. haematobium* ova with ulcers, leukoplakia, papillomatous tumours and polypoid. Disappointingly, praziquantel treatment was not associated with a significant reduction in genital lesions or contact bleeding over a 12-month period and the findings were independent of HIV status.[101]

Gastrointestinal tract

S. haematobium eggs are found frequently in the gastrointestinal tract, their density being highest in the appendix with a gradual decrease in density down to the distal tract. Polyps have been recorded in the rectosigmoid colon in an autopsy study of *S. haematobium* cases; the polyps were inflammatory and were often ulcerated.[100]

S. haematobium eggs are often seen in rectal biopsy material but are usually dead.

Kidney

Although Schistosomal granulomas are rare in the parenchyma, renal lesions occur as a sequel of obstructive uropathy and are manifest as pyelonephritis.

Schistosomal antigens in mesangial areas of the glomeruli in uncomplicated cases of *S. haematobium* infection have been observed by immunofluorescent microscopy as well as granular deposits of IgG, IgM and C3, yet there was a lack of basement membrane changes, an absence of clinical renal disease and normal renal function.[102] There remains doubt about whether *S. haematobium* causes a specific nephropathy in the face of other mechanisms of renal failure.[103] A reversible nephrotic syndrome in *S. haematobium* complicated by *Salmonella* infection has been described.[104]

Lung

Pulmonary arteritis and cor pulmonale are rare in pure *S. haematobium* infection, yet egg granulomas are frequently encountered at autopsy.

Ectopic lesions

Migration of *S. haematobium* within the vascular system and subsequent egg-laying may produce a variety of ectopic lesions.

It was formerly considered that *S. haematobium* in Egypt was not a cause of Symmer's periportal hepatic fibrosis (despite the common finding of *S. haematobium* granulomas in the liver).[105,106] More recent studies, and in particular those using ultrasonography, have shown that *S. haematobium* in Egypt does indeed cause schistosomal hepatic fibrosis, hepatic granulomas, cellular infiltration of the portal tracts, and obstruction and substitution of portal radicles by granulomas.

Cutaneous deposition of *S. haematobium* eggs is not uncommon and has been recognized for decades.[107] Papular or nodular lesions occur in many sites, most frequently in the genital and perigenital areas but also in the neck, chest and abdominal wall.[108–112]

Other sites of ectopic lesions are in the central nervous system (CNS), an occurrence less frequent than in infections due to *S. japonicum* or *S. mansoni*.

The finding of eggs of *S. haematobium* in the CNS without clinical sequelae is not rare; eggs appear to produce minimal or no histological reaction, in contrast to the production of inflammatory responses when laid elsewhere.[113] The spinal cord is affected more often than the brain.[113]

Rare and curious lesions have been described, such as multiple *S. haematobium* egg deposition in the pericardium, causing a fibrous pericarditis,[114] and the demonstration of an adult *S. haematobium* worm in the choroid plexus.[115]

Bladder cancer and S. haematobium *infection*

Despite at least 14 reviews of the relationship between bladder cancer and *S. haematobium* infection published since the early 1980s, the aetiological significance of the parasite in the causation of this cancer remains a topic for argument.[116]

In Egypt, where *S. haematobium* has been hyperendemic for centuries and despite the fact that the prevalence and intensity of infection has decreased rapidly and substantially since the 1960s, cancer in a bladder infected with schistosomiasis occupies the primary rank among all recorded cancers.[117]

In certain other countries, for instance Iraq, coastal Kenya, Ghana, Malawi, Mozambique, Zambia and Zimbabwe, a consistent association between the presence of *S. haematobium* and bladder carcinoma seems to exist. However, in Nigeria, South

Africa and Saudi Arabia, all countries with a moderate or high prevalence of *S. haematobium*, the association is not present: bladder cancer is no more frequent than in non-endemic countries.

When cancer is associated with urinary schistosomiasis, the tumour may occur at any site in the bladder, yet it rarely originates in the trigone, a frequent site of origin in non-Schistosomal cancers and the commonest site of 'sandy patches' and heavy egg deposition.

Schistosomal bladder cancer occurs in an age group significantly younger than that in which cancer occurs in non-Schistosomal areas. In the Nile delta, where men do most of the agricultural work, which involves repeated exposure to cercaria-infested waters, the ratio of male : female bladder cancer with histological evidence of past Schistosomal infection is as high as 12 : 1, whereas the sex ratio among those with no such evidence approximates the 4 : 1 ratio seen in the UK.[118]

The histopathology of cancer in association with schistosomiasis is dominated by squamous cell tumours, in contrast to the commoner transitional cell carcinoma encountered in non-Schistosomal areas.[118,119]

Most squamous cell cancers in Schistosomal bladders are fairly well differentiated, largely indolent and localized, spreading directly through the bladder wall with late and infrequent lymphatic spread. Bloodstream metastasis is rare. This picture contrasts sharply with that of transitional cell carcinoma.

Bladder cancer has been produced experimentally in monkeys and baboons infected with *S. haematobium*,[120,121] species not known for the common occurrence of bladder tumours. However, two large consecutive autopsy studies conducted in Cairo showed no differences of significance in the frequency or type of urothelial malignancies in patients with or without urinary schistosomiasis.[95,96] Several mechanisms have been suggested to explain the suspected role of *S. haematobium* in bladder cancer, none of which is proven; for example, fibrosis induced by schistosome eggs may induce proliferation, abnormal hyperplasia and metaplasia, all possible precancerous changes, in epithelial cells; chronic urinary bacterial infection and the production of nitrosamines (well-known bladder carcinogens) from their precursors in urine; urinary stasis allowing concentration of endogenous carcinogens leading to their absorption from urine and exposure of the bladder epithelium; raised urinary β-glucuronidase levels originating from miracidia and adult schistosomes liberating carcinogenic amines in urine.[122]

In summary, carcinogenic change associated with *S. haematobium* occurs only after many years of infection. The Schistosomal infection is considered to be a tumour promoter, potentiating carcinogenesis, rather than a direct inducer. The various co-factors necessary for malignant neoplasia are not known with certainty.[123]

However, arguments against an association between urinary schistosomiasis and bladder cancer still remain.[124] Possibly, the next few decades will provide clarification of the relationship. Large-scale population-based chemotherapy directed at the control of morbidity would be expected to lower cancer incidence rates in the most badly affected endemic countries, and studies to this end are in place in Egypt. The critical problem will be the acquisition of accurate and acceptable population-based incidence estimates of bladder cancer.

Should this prove to be the case, it will validate the most penetrating report to date on the relationship between *S. haematobium* and bladder cancer from the International Agency for Research on Cancer[125] (IARC), which concluded that there is sufficient evidence in humans for the carcinogenicity of infection with *Schistosoma haematobium* and arrived at the overall evaluation that infection with *Schistosoma haematobium* is carcinogenic to humans.

S. mansoni

A range of chronic lesions is found, from scattered granulomas of the intestinal tract to gross hepatic periportal fibrosis (Symmer's pipe-stem fibrosis; bilharzial clay-pipe stem fibrosis).

Focal granulomas and fibrosis may occur in any part of the intestinal tract, most frequently in the rectosigmoid colon because the preferred habitat of adult *S. mansoni* is in the tributaries of the inferior mesenteric vein. These lesions rarely lead to gross clinical symptoms. Pathology in the small bowel is not as severe as that in the large gut, even though in late-stage infections, particularly in Egypt and Brazil, there was a shift in egg deposition from the colon to the small intestine at autopsy.[126]

Colonic polyposis, a syndrome peculiar but not exclusive to Egypt, occurs in young patients and is related directly to the intensity of infection. The colon and rectum are the sites of multiple pedunculated polyps with associated mucosal swelling, hyperaemia and oedema. The concentration of eggs within the polyps is much higher than at other sites in the intestine. The clinical accompaniments are significant blood and protein losses producing anaemia, chronic diarrhoea, tenesmus and a protein-losing enteropathy.

Occasionally pseudotumours of Schistosomal eggs surrounded by extensive fibrous tissue occur in *S. mansoni* infection and are termed 'bilharziomas'. Sites of predilection are the omentum, mesenteric lymph nodes, paracaecal region and infrequently the wall of the gut. Occasional and rare reports appear in the literature relating intestinal obstruction caused by chronic Schistosomal infection.[126]

Schistosomal granulomas in bowel and liver are illustrated in Figures 82.11 and 82.12.

Hepatosplenic schistosomiasis

The major, and undoubtedly the most important, complication of chronic *S. mansoni* infection is periportal hepatic fibrosis; because the basic pathology is sited in and around the portal tracts and the hepatic parenchyma is normal in uncomplicated cases, the term cirrhosis is inappropriate. A cut section of the liver, which may or may not be enlarged, shows macroscopic wide bands of fibrosis around portal tracts, resembling the stems of a number of clay pipes (see Figure 82.19). The surface of the liver may be smooth, granular or nodular. Between portal fields, the hepatic parenchyma does not exhibit the nodularity of Laënnec's cirrhosis.

Deposited eggs produce granulomas with surrounding inflammatory infiltrates in the connective tissue that surrounds the hepatic veins, proximal to presinusoidal vessels. Affected portal tracts become blocked with granulomas and disorganized by inflammation, fibrosis and pyelophlebitis.[127] Eggs, an eosinophilic

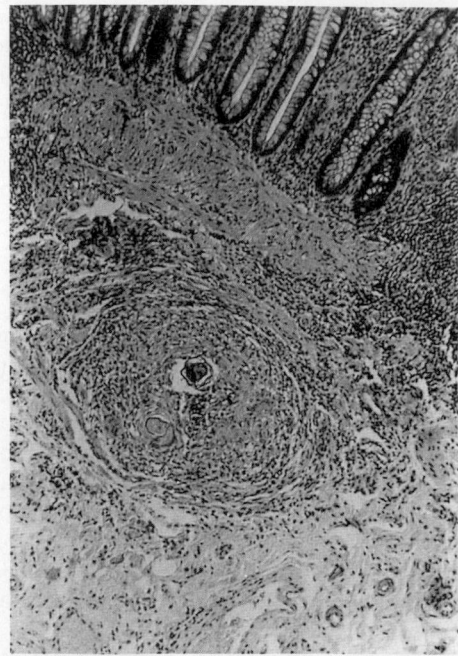

Figure 82.11 Schistosomal granuloma (*S. mansoni*) of bowel. The structureless mass at the centre is an egg.

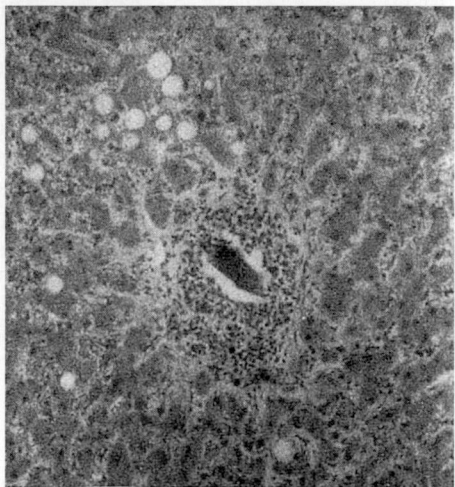

Figure 82.12 Schistosomal granuloma (*S. mansoni*) in liver. The structureless mass at the centre is an egg. (Courtesy of B. H. Kean.)

infiltrate, schistosomal pigment and/or organizing thrombi are found. The accumulation of egg granulomas around sites of blockage leads to further portal enlargement, and simultaneously the hepatic arteries enlarge and push out new branching capillaries. Thus the presinusoidal portal hypertension produces a compensatory arterial flow. Total intrahepatic blood flow remains within normal limits, with maintenance of hepatocellular integrity.

The diminished portal blood flow from portal hypertension is compensated for by the increase in hepatic arterial supply and the rich capillary arterial network around the portal branches which communicates with the portal vein[127] there remain unexplained

discrepancies between clinical and pathological interpretations of the arterial origin of the hepatic capillary network.[128] Hepatic fibrosis results from the accumulation of collagen[129,130] and may originate in the proliferation of collagen-synthesizing cells, increased synthesis by existing cells or deficiency in collagen degradation. In experimental animals, the amount of collagen in the liver increases in parallel with egg granuloma formation. In human hepatic schistosomiasis, there is increased collagen content and marked collagen synthesis in wedge liver biopsy material when compared with control tissue. The natural course of pure periportal fibrosis is slow and is termed 'compensated' because liver cell function tests show only slight abnormalities, if any. Over time, the consequences of portal hypertension with splenomegaly and/ or variceal haemorrhage, with or without ascites, appear, although hepatic decompensation does not develop until an advanced stage of the process. In countries where there is a high prevalence of viral hepatitis (hepatitis B, C, D or E), these may co-exist with hepatosplenic schistosomiasis, and the clinical progression of decompensated hepatic fibrosis presents a much more rapid progress because hepatocellular pathology is much more severe than in the 'pure' state of Schistosomal hepatic fibrosis.

Spleen

Splenomegaly is the usual accompaniment of hepatic schistosomiasis and is due to portal venous hypertension, chronic passive congestion and reticuloendothelial hyperplasia. Focal infarcts and trabecular haemorrhages may occur and the spleen is tough and fibrotic. Hypersplenism may produce pancytopenia or leucoerythroblastic anaemia. The spleen may become enormously enlarged (Egyptian splenomegaly or Banti's syndrome in the older literature), as in kala-azar (visceral leishmaniasis) or the myeloproliferative syndromes. Lymphomas have been reported occasionally.[131]

Lungs and heart

Pulmonary hypertension caused by granulomatous pulmonary arteritis originating from large-scale embolization of eggs is commonly the result of hepatic pipe-stem fibrosis with extensive portocaval shunts occurring in *S. mansoni* or *S. japonicum* infections. This may produce Schistosomal cor pulmonale. Strangely, and despite a direct access to the lungs via the inferior vena cava, cor pulmonale occurs less frequently in pure or mixed *S. haematobium* infection than would be anticipated. There are fewer reports of cor pulmonale in *S. japonicum* than in *S. mansoni* infection despite the similar pathogenetic mechanisms.[132]

Granulomatous inflammation occludes distal pulmonary arterial branches and eventually produces a rise in pulmonary arterial pressure with right ventricular hypertrophy and strain; the smaller arterioles show fibrointimal sclerosis; fibrinoid necrosis and angiomatoid formation is widespread in alveolar tissue. This complication arises in long-standing cases of heavy infection and presents clinically as congestive heart failure arising in chronic cor pulmonale.

Kidney

Renal lesions (Schistosomal nephropathy; glomerulonephritis), consisting of deposition of immune complexes of host immunoglobulins with adult worm or egg antigens in the glomerular mesangium and basement membrane, occur in *S. mansoni* infection. A variety of glomerular lesions has been found at autopsy in hepatosplenic patients.[132] Mild proteinuria is common in *S. mansoni* infection, and in hepatosplenic cases progressive nephropathy leading to renal failure occurs in a small proportion, although the clinical course is slow and the greater risks are from the hepatic complications.[132]

Amyloidosis has been demonstrated in renal biopsy material from patients with the nephrotic syndrome and schistosomiasis in Egypt.[133]

Egg deposition in the kidney is rare and is not thought to be responsible for serious renal pathology.

Central nervous system

Various forms of 'neurological schistosomiasis' occur in infections due to *S. mansoni*, *S. japonicum* and *S. haematobium*. Yet, in view of the global total of infected people, CNS localization is rare. Eggs of all three species have been found in the brain and spinal cord, and adult worms have been demonstrated at various sites.

'Cerebral' schistosomiasis has traditionally been associated with *S. japonicum* infection, but eggs of *S. mansoni* and *S. haematobium* have also been found in the brain, rather more frequently with *S. mansoni*. The route of infection is thought to be via Batson's valveless intervertebral plexus or by arterial egg embolism.[134] Eggs may be present in the CNS with little or no histological reaction and, in a randomly selected series of hepatosplenic cases of schistosomiasis coming to autopsy, one-quarter had *S. mansoni* eggs in the brain;[134] these cases may be symptom free.

Myelopathy with various motor and/or sensory presentations occurs, more commonly in *S. mansoni* than in *S. haematobium* infection, and cord transection with paraparesis is well known. Not infrequently, spinal cord schistosomiasis is recognized in the acute toxaemic stages that occur in tourists and transient visitors to endemic areas on their return to temperate climates after a short tropical stay.

Other ectopic lesions

Cutaneous lesions due to *S. mansoni* are rare, although papular or nodular lesions at different sites are known.

In Egypt, genital lesions are commonly found at autopsy. Placental schistosomiasis has been reported from Brazil.[135]

S. japonicum

The intestinal and hepatic lesions of *S. japonicum* are in general similar to those occurring in *S. mansoni* infection but with several specific differences. The primary lesion is a T cell-mediated granuloma formation around the eggs, but modulation of the granuloma size is largely antibody mediated, whereas in *S. mansoni* infection cell mediation is the dominant mechanism.

The adult worms are located in the branches of the inferior mesenteric vein and in the superior haemorrhoidal vein[136] and an adult female deposits 1000–3500 eggs/day in highest density in the large intestine and, in descending order, in the rectum, sigmoid and descending colon. The small intestine is relatively lightly infected.

Knowledge of the pathological anatomy (gross and microscopic) of *S. japonicum* lags behind that of *S. mansoni* infection because autopsy studies are fewer; are currently seldom performed in the countries endemic for *S. japonicum*; and, in the broad public health sense, schistosomiasis has been declining progressively as a cause of death for some decades.[132,137,138]

Gastrointestinal lesions in experimental animals are focal and isolated, and are interspersed with normal bowel. Segmental lesions occur in humans and multiple lesions are common, including mucosal hyperplasia, pseudopolyposis, ulceration and thickening of the intestinal wall.

Gastric schistosomiasis is seen frequently in surgical or biopsy specimens. Subclinical cases are probably common but unrecognized, owing to non-diagnostic symptoms and insensitive diagnostic techniques.

Macroscopic hepatic changes in the chronic phase parallel those in *S. mansoni* infection. The liver is frequently enlarged with an irregular surface. On cross-section, the characteristic wide bands of fibrous tissue surrounding the larger portal tracts are seen and Symmer's periportal (clay-pipe stem) fibrosis is found at autopsy. Microscopically, the picture is one of chronic pseudotubercles with chronic inflammation, cellular infiltrates around eggs, extensive fibrosis and neovascularization in the portal tracts. The accompanying manifestations of portal hypertension (i.e. splenomegaly with or without gastrointestinal varices, with or without bleeding) are to be anticipated.

Although *S. japonicum* eggs are often found in the lung and obliterative pulmonary arteritis is similar to that seen in *S. mansoni*, clinical cor pulmonale has not been reported as in *S. mansoni* infection.

In contrast to *S. mansoni* and *S. haematobium*, the brain is more commonly affected in *S. japonicum* infection, although spinal cord involvement appears to be less frequent. The cerebral lesions are held to be caused by intracranial egg deposition or embolism via a vascular route.

In the first half of the twentieth century, Schistosomal dwarfism with retardation of growth and sexual development was recognized as a not uncommon occurrence in China. This syndrome is rare in modern times.

Cancer and S. japonicum infection

Epidemiological studies have not demonstrated any direct relationships between gastric cancer and *S. japonicum* infection.[132]

The situation regarding a relationship between colonic or rectal cancer and *S. japonicum* is much more complex. Case-control studies in China and the Philippines, and an epidemiological cross-sectional survey in China, have suggested both positive and negative associations. One case-control study in China showed a strong association between *S. japonicum* infection and rectal cancer but no association between colonic cancer and a history of *S. japonicum* infection.[132] No definitive conclusions can be reached from the studies to date. Improved designs of further studies are essential for clarification.

A similar position exists regarding the presence or absence of a relationship between primary liver cell cancer and schistosomiasis. The ubiquity of hepatitis B infection, a known precancerous condition, in areas endemic for *S. japonicum*, has complicated study designs. Again, the correlation is speculative. The authorita tive IARC monograph[125] concluded that there is limited evidence in humans and experimental animals for the carcinogenicity of infection with *S. japonicum*, although the overall evaluation was that infection with *S. japonicum* is possibly carcinogenic to humans. Simultaneously the evaluation concluded that infection with *S. mansoni* is not classifiable with regard to its carcinogenicity to humans.

S. mekongi

Although the clinical manifestations of *S. mekongi* infection are similar to those of *S. japonicum*, the morbidity and pathology resulting from the former is compounded by the presence of *Opisthorcis viverrini* in areas endemic for *S. mekongi*. Objective descriptions of detailed pathology in humans are lacking.

S. intercalatum

The distribution of *S. intercalatum* is restricted in 10 countries in central and west Africa, and more information exists on experimental infection than does pathological description.[139]

The disease is mild, and in proctoscopy in hospital inpatients, the rectal and colonic mucosa was considered abnormal in 47 out of 85 patients. Non-specific lesions predominated: mucosal congestion, oedema, bleeding and/or ulceration. In liver biopsies, granulomatous lesions, of a size smaller than those seen in *S. mansoni* infection, were seen in the portal tracts. Tissue reaction to eggs was slight or absent in some patients. No portal hypertension was seen.[139,140–148]

The newly described *S. guineensis*, the only schistosome species on the island of Sao Tome, has been shown to produce 'pipe stem type' hepatic portal septal fibrosis and genital involvement. Other pathological sequelae are currently under investigation. It is suspected that hybridization with *S. intercalatum* occurs. The parasite is susceptible to treatment with praziquantel but may require increased dosage or courses of chemotherapy.[25]

A Global Burden of Disease Study attributed a low disability weight, based on disability adjusted life years (DALY). Yet a penetrating meta-analysis produced evidence of significant associations between human Schistosomal infections and diarrhoea, abdominal pain, fatigue in addition to having total deficit, undernutrition and reduced exercise tolerance. Many of these presumed indirect effects of schistosomiasis cannot be directly compared with the classical well-known sequelae of chronic infections but led the authors to conclude that the ranking of schistosomiasis in the Global Burden of Disease study should be up-graded to a surprising extent. Proof of indirect disease association is not yet forthcoming but general expert opinion remains that the infection is underrated, in addition to the well-known direct pathological sequelae.

CLINICAL FEATURES

General

To the clinician, particularly in the tropics, schistosomiasis can be a frustrating infection. With the exception of haematuria in urinary schistosomiasis, there is no one diagnostic symptom or sign; even the commonly described various symptoms and signs are rarely pathognomic. Schistosomiasis is a collection of infections of protean manifestations.

Whereas clinical medicine is taught in the context of classical descriptions of symptoms and signs, these were, in the past, culled from classical and advanced cases. This is rarely the rule in practice, for classical and advanced cases represent only a small proportion of an extensive frequency distribution of clinical syndromes. 'Classical' cases of schistosomiasis are in a minority: many patients have non-specific symptoms and many are symptom free or ignore their symptoms, and infection is discovered only on purposive surveys or during investigation for some unrelated complaint. This is due to the biological phenomenon of the overdispersed distribution of parasites within hosts; this aggregated distribution means that, in any population of hosts, there exists only a small proportion of 'heavy' infections with 'typical' symptoms, and the majority of cases are moderate or light infections with a corresponding freedom from symptoms – or even a complete lack of symptoms.

While it is useful to consider schistosomiasis within the 'classical' stages of the life history – i.e. cercarial invasion, transformation of schistosomula and maturation of adults, established infection, late stages and complications – in an attempt to link clinical pointers to these stages, it should be realized that the stages merge into one another and are rarely clearcut, especially in endemic areas in those who are semi-immune. Non-immune visitors to endemic areas or transients who become infected often provide a clearer clinical description than residents of endemic zones.

Syndromes common to all schistosome infections

Cercarial dermatitis

Seldom, if ever, described in indigenous inhabitants of endemic areas, especially in Africa, and only rarely in non-immune visitors, cercarial dermatitis occurs more commonly on exposure to avian cercariae where symptoms are more intense than in cases exposed to human Schistosomal cercaria-infested waters.

Arising within a few minutes of exposure and receding within 24–72 h, itching (pruritus) of the skin is the prime symptom, accompanied in some cases by erythema and/or a papular eruption. The condition can occur after exposure to any of the five common schistosomes infecting humans.

Acute Schistosomiasis

Also termed acute toxaemic schistosomiasis, Katayama syndrome or Katayama fever, after the Katayama region in Hiroshima prefecture, Japan, where it was originally described, this acute illness can be found after exposure to any of the schistosomes infecting humans but is most marked in primary infections in non-immune individuals.

Recent reports from China indicate that this acute syndrome due to *S. japonicum* is not limited to uninfected individuals living in an endemic area at the time of first exposure, but may occur even in those with an active chronic infection or in persons with a recent history of infection and documented treatment and cure.[132]

In the acute syndrome due to *S. mansoni* infection, a diminution in transmission produced by control measures has led to a relative increase in reports of acute cases, and this phenomenon has been observed in Puerto Rico and Venezuela.

Acute schistosomiasis is much less commonly reported for *S. haematobium* infection and there are no data on its occurrence with *S. intercalatum* or *S. mekongi*.

As the incubation periods of the different schistosome infections are not known accurately and have been the subject of numerous estimates, only broad descriptions of the time phases of the occurrence of the syndrome after initial cercarial exposure can be given.

In *S. japonicum* infection, the mean period between exposure and the onset of fever in 105 people with no previous history of infection and with only a single day's exposure to cercaria-infested water was 41.5 (range 14–84) days.[132] For *S. mansoni*, the incubation period of the Katayama syndrome ranges from 4 to 87 days, but is generally between 3 and 7 weeks.[126]

Surprisingly short incubation periods may be encountered in non-immunes who became infected in endemic areas. For example, within 35 days of returning from Botswana, symptoms occurred in 12 of 13 US travellers with a history of water contact; symptoms lasted for 1–30 (mean 8) days, and 9 of 11 had eggs of *S. mansoni* in the stools during the symptomatic period.[142] Three Dutch non-immunes infected in Mali developed illness within 1–4 weeks of exposure and all had eggs of both *S. mansoni* and *S. haematobium* in the stools at 12 weeks.

The clinical picture is one of an acute pyrexial illness; continuing fever is a prime characteristic; the patient feels ill and may have rigors, sweating, general myalgia and headache. An urticarial skin rash may appear and lymphadenopathy or other non-specific signs may occur. Anorexia, nausea, abdominal discomfort and loose stools or diarrhoea, sometimes with blood and mucus, are not rare. The liver is frequently slightly enlarged and tender, and a slightly enlarged spleen occurs in about one-third of patients.

A cough with, on physical examination, dry or moist rales, is frequent, and an intense eosinophilia is almost invariably present.

Cerebral symptoms may appear and the occurrence of spinal cord syndromes or suggestive initial symptoms is an indication for urgent investigative measures.

Established infections

S. haematobium (urinary schistosomiasis)

With the proviso that many patients will have minimal symptoms, the cardinal complaint is recurrent painless haematuria. Other urinary tract symptoms may precede or be associated, for instance burning on micturition, frequency, suprapubic discomfort or pain. Bladder involvement may lead to precipitancy, dribbling or incontinence. In fact, in an endemic area, any urinary tract symptom is an indication to explore for the presence of *S. haematobium*. However, in many countries in Africa, in the young age groups and early teenagers, macroscopic haematuria may be virtually universal; in boys it provokes little comment and is regarded as a natural sign of puberty and an approach to manhood.

In the phase of established infection it is common practice to recognize two stages: (1) an active stage in children, adolescents and young patients, with egg deposition in many organs and egg excretion in the urine with proteinuria and haematuria, macroscopic or microscopic; and (2) in older patients, urinary egg excretion is sparse or absent but extensive pathology has developed. Even in the later stages of obstructive uropathy, symptoms may be absent or minimal. Chronic bladder lesions may produce persistent urinary dribbling and occasionally multiple fistulas in the perineum, with the picture of the 'watering-can scrotum'; this is also seen in areas of heavy transmission in children and young teenagers where exposure is maximal, but the phenomenon is much rarer nowadays than in the past, coincidental with the widespread use of chemotherapy at the peripheral and school level of healthcare.

Surveys have shown wide regional variation in co-existent bacteriuria; when present, the predominant organisms are *E. coli*, *Klebsiella* spp., *Pseudomonas* spp. and *Salmonella* spp.

In Egypt, recurrent *Salmonella* bacteraemia is a well recognized complication of *S. haematobium* infection. Patients with urinary schistosomiasis presenting with a recurrence of salmonellosis should first be treated for the *S. haematobium* infection.[143] In the later stages of obstructive uropathy, hydronephrosis may develop and cause renal parenchymal dysfunction which, added to urinary tract infection, leads to impaired kidney function.[143] The ominous relationship between bilateral Schistosomal uropathy, bacteriuria with impairment of hydrogen ion excretion, non-functioning kidneys and death has been well described.[144]

S. intercalatum (intestinal or urinary schistosomiasis)

In comparison with *S. haematobium* or *S. mansoni* infection, clinical symptoms of disease are commonly mild or absent in *S. intercalatum* infection and it is not regarded as a serious public health problem.[145] Active infection is seen in children and adolescents, and pathology is detected only in those with egg excretion in excess of 400 eggs/g of faeces.

The usual clinical presentation is one of diarrhoea, often with blood in the faeces, and lower abdominal pain or discomfort. However, some patients may present with haematuria and, in a report from Nigeria, *S. intercalatum* eggs were found in the urine, but not in faeces, in 6% of the 1709 people surveyed.[146] The known existence of natural hybridization between *S. intercalatum* and *S. haematobium* can produce atypical clinical pictures with ectopic localization of worms.[147,148]

S. mansoni, *S. japonicum* and *S. mekongi* (intestinal schistosomiasis)

The wide spectrum of clinical presentations has been emphasized in recent decades by the increasing use of community-based surveys as a tool of investigation, in contrast with the customary descriptions of infection and disease rooted in hospital patients. Many, if not the majority, of persons infected with *S. mansoni* or *S. japonicum* are symptom free or have minimal and non-specific symptoms, findings again in agreement with the known epidemiological and biological distribution of the parasite within the human host.

Clinical features are encountered in only a small proportion of patients with persistent or heavy infections. Intestinal disease is shown by a chronic or intermittent diarrhoea with blood in the stools, abdominal discomfort or pain and colicky cramps. Severe dysentery is rare but certainly does occur. Secondary symptoms of fever, weakness, fatigue, anorexia and weight loss are frequent.

In epidemiological surveys, there are significant correlations between visible or occult blood in the stools, abdominal pain and diarrhoea.

Hepatomegaly, often of the left lobe, and splenomegaly are frequent accompaniments. In the later stages of infection, there occurs a chronic catarrhal state of the intestine with a swollen, granular mucosa and loose stools with blood and/or mucus or an intermittent dysenteric syndrome.

The primary complications of polyposis and hepatosplenic schistosomiasis have their own symptomatology; polyposis produces what is in effect a severe chronic dysentery with blood and protein loss. Intussusception and/or rectal prolapse may occur.

Hepatosplenic schistosomiasis, often remarkably symptom free, presents as upper abdominal discomfort, left upper abdominal pain or a swelling of the abdomen. Physical signs include a firm enlargement of the liver, often with splenomegaly. The spleen may become greatly enlarged, sometimes extending downwards past the umbilicus into the left iliac fossa, and may even at times fill most of the abdomen. Ascites may be present, but the classical signs of hepatocellular disease, spider-web angiomata, gynaecomastia, palmar erythema, jaundice and alterations in hair distribution are not present in 'pure' Schistosomal disease. They may, however, be found where hepatitis B, C, D or E co-exist with Schistosomal periportal fibrosis and lead to post-hepatitic hepatocellular damage. In advanced cases, endocrine changes can be found: growth retardation, infantilism, retarded bone age, all probably due to hypopituitarism. Amenorrhoea, early menopause, infertility and loss of libido have been attributed to a similar cause.[132]

A not uncommon primary presenting sign of hepatosplenic disease in schistosomiasis is haematemesis from gastrooesophageal varices. This may occur without warning or may be preceded by a feeling of weakness or upper abdominal discomfort; patients have classical signs of acute blood loss with sweating, pallor, thirst, somnolence and a lowered blood and pulse pressure. In many cases, melaena follows, and this acute episode may precipitate ascites and/or peripheral oedema. Fatalities may occur with the primary haemorrhage if treatment is not available; recurrent multiple haemorrhagic episodes are usual. Unless complicated by hepatitis B, C, D or E, liver function and hepatic encephalopathy does not develop. Where mixed infections of S. mansoni or S. japonicum and the various hepatitis viruses co-exist, the downhill clinical course is correspondingly rapid and the typical signs of hepatocellular failure appear with, in parallel, a poor prognosis.

S. japonicum and S. mekongi

While infections with the oriental schistosomes follow a broadly similar clinical course to that of S. mansoni, several distinct differences emerge. In general, infection with S. mekongi is milder than that with S. japonicum. Hepatosplenomegaly is common but cerebral and cardiopulmonary complications are not reported.

In the past there have been more hospital-based clinical studies of S. japonicum than community-based investigations. Hence the clinical descriptions have been slanted towards advanced cases. In fact, at least half of patients infected with S. japonicum are asymptomatic. General symptoms, fatigue, weakness, nonspecific abdominal discomfort, and irregular bowel movements or intermittent diarrhoea are frequent. Chronic diarrhoea is said to be a common complaint and lower abdominal pain is a frequent symptom.[132]

The later signs of hepatosplenic schistosomiasis evolve as do those of S. mansoni infection. Although Schistosomal dwarfism was not uncommon in China in the first half of the twentieth century, it has become a rarity nowadays. Cardiopulmonary and renal complications are well known.

The main difference clinically is the occurrence of cerebral schistosomiasis in S. japonicum infection. Spinal cord involvement appears less frequently than with S. mansoni, but such generalizations are difficult, if not impossible, to confirm scientifically.

In the acute phase of cerebral schistosomiasis, the presenting symptoms and signs are those of a meningoencephalitis, with pyrexia, headache, vomiting, blurred vision and disturbed consciousness. In the established or chronic phase of the infection, several distinct neurological presentations are recognized; most common is epilepsy which may be generalized but is more frequently Jacksonian in type; signs suggestive of a space occupying lesion or a stroke are also described. Advances in neuroradiology, with or without operational biopsy, are diagnostic.

DIFFERENTIAL DIAGNOSIS

In an infection of such diverse clinical manifestations it is scarcely surprising that schistosomiasis in any of its forms can be confused with many other disease processes. Acute schistosomiasis (Katayama syndrome) must be differentiated from typhoid (leucopenia, no eosinophilia), brucellosis, malaria, leptospirosis and numerous other causes of pyrexia of uncertain origin (PUO). Pyrexia and eosinophilia occur in trichinosis, tropical eosinophilia, visceral larva migrans and infections with Opisthorcis, Paragonimiasis and Clonorchis spp.

In the established stage, S. haematobium must be distinguished from haemoglobinurias, cancer of the urogenital tract, other infections such as acute nephritides, and rarer conditions such as renal tuberculosis with haematuria.

S. mansoni, with its common presentation of non-specific abdominal symptoms, may suggest peptic ulcer, biliary disease or pancreatitis; in such cases, symptoms disappear after specific antiSchistosomal treatment.

Lower abdominal conditions to be excluded are the various forms of dysentery, particularly amoebic dysentery, ulcerative colitis and non-Schistosomal polyposis.

The differential diagnosis of hepatosplenic schistosomiasis is wide and embraces all causes of hepatomegaly and splenomegaly, separately and combined. The marked splenic enlargement of portal hypertension due to periportal fibrosis must be distinguished from kala-azar (visceral leishmaniasis), certain of the chronic leukaemias or myeloproliferative syndromes, some of the haemoglobinopathies (e.g. thalassaemias) and the tropical splenomegaly syndrome.

In endemic areas, schistosomiasis must always be considered as one of the causes of cor pulmonale and virtually any neurological presentation, but particularly the various forms of epilepsy and the different types of myelopathy or spinal cord compression syndromes.

A sound knowledge of local or regional epidemiological patterns of parasitic and other infectious diseases and a high index of diagnostic suspicion contribute greatly to the avoidance of diagnostic error.

DIAGNOSIS

A definitive diagnosis is made by the direct visual demonstration of the eggs of the parasite in body excretions or secretions, overwhelmingly stool and urine (Figures 82.13–82.16); or alternatively in material from rectal biopsy or biopsies from liver or surgically removed tissue. A sensitive direct diagnosis can also be made by hatching tests in which swimming miracidia originating from excreted eggs can be seen with the naked eye. This is an indication beyond doubt that the eggs are viable and have originated from living fertilized female schistosomes.

A recent addition to direct diagnostic techniques is the detection of schistosome antigens in serum or urine: circulating anodic antigen (CAA) and circulating cathodic antigen (CCA). These two glycoprotein circulating antigens associated with the gut of the adult worm are well characterized, are genus specific and their presence indicates active infection in persons by *S. mansoni*, *S. haematobium* or *S. intercalatum*. They are detected by enzyme immunoassay and have virtually 100% specificity and very high sensitivity. Patently they offer new possibilities for epidemiological and post-chemotherapeutic monitoring, but are expensive, are 'high technology', need complex reagents and require standardization and controlled trials before operational use in control programmes. At present, they are used at the research level in

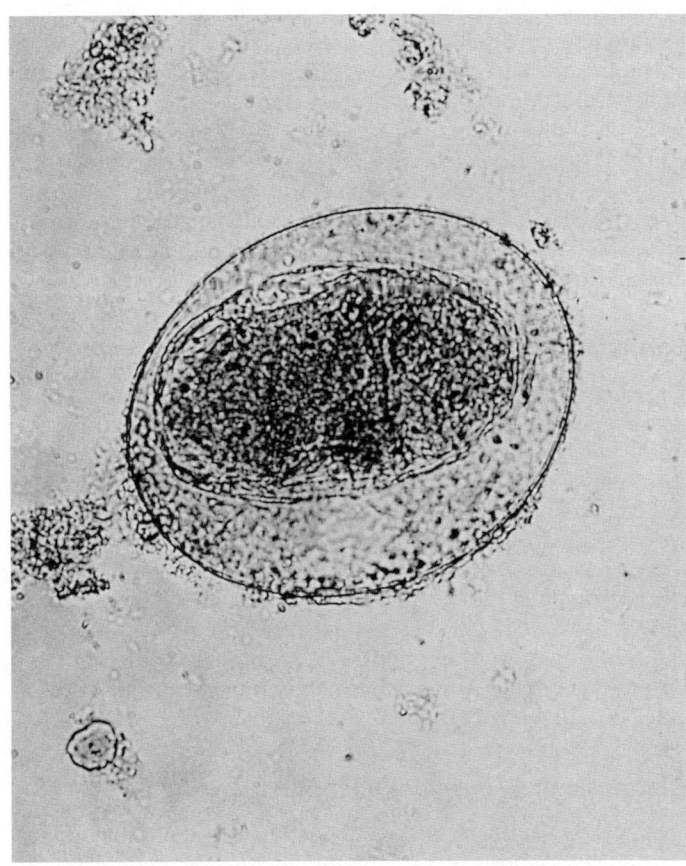

Figure 82.15 Egg of *S. japonicum*. (Courtesy of Tropical Resources Unit.)

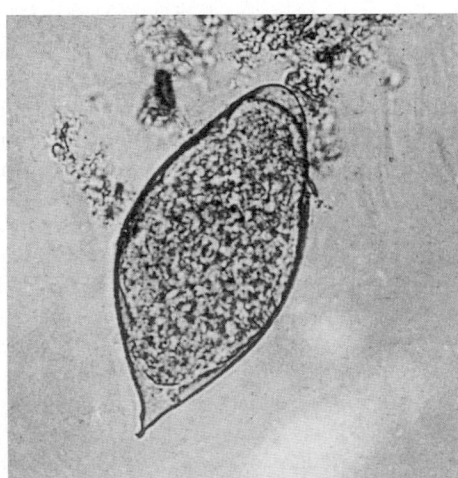

Figure 82.13 Egg of *S. haematobium*. (Courtesy of Tropical Resources Unit.)

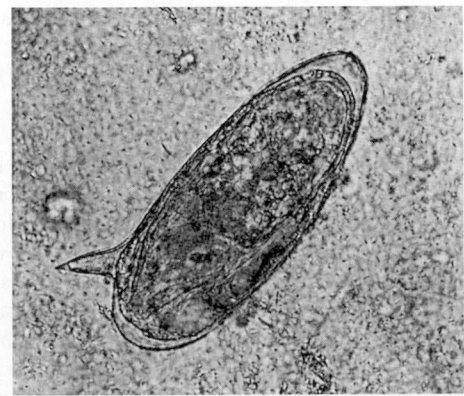

Figure 82.14 Egg of *S. mansoni*. (Courtesy of O. D. Standen.)

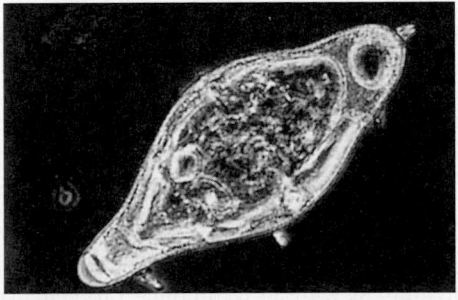

Figure 82.16 Egg of *S. intercalatum*. (Courtesy of V. R. Southgate.)

individual patients or in small groups[149–153] (see Immunodiagnosis, below).

All other methods of diagnosis, whether clinical, immunological, radiological (see Figures 82.17, 82.18), ultrasonographic (see Figures 82.19, 82.20) or endoscopic without biopsy, are essentially indirect.

Direct diagnostic techniques

Parasitological diagnosis

No single optimal technique applicable to all situations exists. Most of the current techniques can be interpreted qualitatively or quantitatively depending on the diagnostic setting. Quantitative techniques are virtually always used in research, in experimental chemotherapy and clinical trials, in epidemiological surveys and in the evaluation of intervention measures.

In an individual clinical setting, it is customary to examine repeated specimens of excreta parasitologically (in practice, three specimens) before declaring a patient to be 'negative'. Confirmation of a diagnosis by hatching tests demonstrates that the eggs are viable and an active infection exists; the finding of dead eggs only in the excreta is not an indication for chemotherapy.

Egg counting

The direct demonstration of eggs represents an enormous advantage over all other diagnostic measures because specificity is obviously maximal, yet a slavish belief in the absolute virtues of quantitative diagnosis is scarcely justified. Egg counts are merely indirect estimates of worm loads; they vary in time and place and with technicians, and the assumed Poisson distribution of eggs in the excreta may not hold.[154] Conclusions on chemotherapeutic efficacy of drugs based on single post-treatment examinations should be viewed with cynicism; coefficients of variation of daily egg output are very high and in *S. haematobium* infections egg output is subject to a circadian rhythm: it peaks and is least variable from 10:00 to 14:00 h.

Diagnosis of *S. haematobium* infection

Ova of *S. haematobium* are usually detected easily in the urine. A qualitative diagnosis is made by the microscopic examination of a sedimented or centrifuged urine specimen. Exercise before specimen collection is unnecessary. Eggs of *S. mansoni* or *S. intercalatum* are found not infrequently in the urine. In one series, 15% of patients with a sole *S. mansoni* infection had 'mansonuria', but this is an unusually high rate.[155]

Nowadays, filtration techniques, giving a quantitative estimation of egg excretion, have tended to replace simple sedimentation and/or centrifugation and are certainly the 'norm' in epidemiological studies. Currently, urine samples are passed through filter paper,[156] polycarbonate[157,158] or a polyamide material[159–162] by a variety of syringes or pumps. The principle common to all is that eggs are retained on the filter and can be counted with or without staining. Many different stains are in use and preferences are largely personal; eggs may be 'stored' in preservative or a preservative-stain mixture. As with all techniques, problems arise during field usage. False epidemiological results may occur from loss of eggs during bulk transport of dried filter papers,[162] and, in a small but significant proportion, eggs are retained on polyamide filters (Nytrel) even after careful attempts to reuse them. As a general rule, any filter should be used once only and then discarded.

Diagnosis of intestinal dwelling schistosomes

In infections with *S. mansoni*, *S. japonicum*, *S. mekongi* and *S. intercalatum*, where eggs are excreted in the faeces, simple comminution of the stool and sedimentation before microscopy is a reliable diagnostic technique. Direct saline microscopy of stool has a very low diagnostic sensitivity owing to the small amount of the faecal sample examined.

Many concentration techniques have been described.[163–167] All involve removal of fat, faecal debris and mucus, and of necessity require more sophisticated laboratory facilities. They find their optimal use in the detection of 'light' infections where egg excretion is of a low intensity or is intermittent.

In South Africa, a popular and efficient technique for egg recovery from stools in both medical and veterinary practice is based on twin nylon gauze filters and the use of water pressure to break up faecal material. Claims of high sensitivity have been advanced.[168]

Nowadays, the cellophane thick faecal smear, the Kato technique or one of its numerous modifications has become a standard diagnostic tool[169,170] in both clinical and epidemiological studies. Essentially a semi-concentration-clearing-staining process, it is a simple microscopic method examining 20–50 mg of stool, depending on the template used, and is quantitative, thus permitting the comparisons of internationally acquired data. It can be performed in the field and may be used at the primary healthcare level. The prepared slide takes some time to clear; this varies with ambient temperature and humidity. Slides can be stored for at least 1 week, often longer, the time again being variable, so that assessments of technicians' counts can be incorporated into a system of quality control. A further advantage lies in its use in the diagnosis and counting of eggs of many intestinal nematodes or cestodes (e.g. *Ascaris lumbricoides*, *Trichuris trichuria*, *Taenia* spp. and hookworms), although to assess hookworm egg excretion, counts must be made 15–30 min after slide preparation because hookworm eggs disappear after this period owing to solution from the Kato slides, and assessment is useless after 1 h. A historical fact of interest is that the original Kato technique was invented and adopted during the major national ascariasis control campaigns conducted in Japan after World War II, directed against the public health problems existing in the country at that time. The exact details of the procedure must be calibrated for each working location, taking into account environmental variables, resources and locally available material and human skills. Disadvantages of the Kato technique are that watery or diarrhoeal stools cannot be processed and dietary habits may result in hard fibrous stools that are difficult to process. Additionally, there is a definite lower limit of sensitivity of 50–100 eggs/g of stool detectable by a single smear. Numerous variants of the technique exist and it is common practice to examine two or three subsamples of single faecal specimen. Whichever technique is used, it is vital that the amount of stool examined, whether in a single examination or by a number of subsample examinations, should be reported so that valid comparisons can be made between areas.

A variant of the thick smear technique for S. mansoni infections is the glass sandwich technique[171,172] which has been used widely in the Sudan and Malawi. The technique requires no reagents and it has been suggested that it is more cost-effective than other similar quantitative methods. A small-scale experiment showed no significant differences in egg recovery or in methods, readers or slides prepared from the same stool specimens and processed by either the Kato or glass sandwich technique.[173] Further comparisons on a larger scale are needed, and a major disadvantage of this technique is that it is limited to use in restricted endemic areas; hence comparison of findings with other endemic areas is, at present, invalid.

Miracidial hatching

Described originally by Fulleborn in 1921[174] and in routine use in biological and chemotherapeutic studies for decades, it is surprising that more attention has not been given to this technique in clinical medicine because hatching is generally accepted as the most sensitive of all parasitological methods in all forms of schistosomiasis. The method remains essential for adequate post-treatment evaluation in clinical trials. However, adaptation to field studies has been uncommon because standardization and quantification are more difficult than in techniques where eggs can simply be counted. Nevertheless, it is salutary to recall that diagnosis and follow-up of treated patients in the huge Chinese control programmes of the 1960s and 1970s were based on a 'nylon network running water sedimentation technique', essentially a field-adapted miracidial hatching process.[175,176]

The relative ease of isolation of eggs from urine led to many more attempts to quantify hatching procedures in S. haematobium than in S. mansoni infections. As a rough estimate of the numbers of hatchable eggs, the miradiascope was used as a macroscopic technique routinely for surveys in southern Africa.[177,178] More sensitive and accurate hatching techniques have followed[179,180] and further refinements are appearing;[181–184] undoubtedly the use of 'wet' preparations has complicated field standardization, but hatching retains its primacy as the most sensitive diagnostic tool in S. haematobium infections.

In S. mansoni infections, many variants of hatching techniques exist, some semiquantitative and all possessing high sensitivity.[185,186] In S. japonicum endemic areas in China, miracidial hatching is widely and routinely used for both epidemiological surveys and as an indicator of parasitological cure after chemotherapy.[132]

Rectal biopsy

Used for decades as a simple direct diagnostic technique at the individual clinical level, rectal biopsy may be employed in addition to faecal examination and provides an effective way of visualizing eggs. Small biopsy specimens of mucosa are soaked in water and examined microscopically as a crush preparation. In the intestinal dwelling species, egg viability can often be determined by observation of flame cell or miracidial movement within the eggshell. Biopsies may be taken from rectal valves via a crocodile forceps or with a curette and proctoscope, a much simpler procedure; the mucosa is pulled over the end of the proctoscope and cut off with the curette.[187]

Ova of S. haematobium in rectal snips are usually non-viable and black.

In Brazil, the oogram technique (a quantitative rectal biopsy with division of eggs into developmental stages) is commonly used. If an oogram is used in addition to faecal examination in an assessment of the effects of anti-Schistosomal drugs, it can be confidently predicted that estimates of 'cure rates' based solely on excretal examination will be considerably reduced.[187]

Other biopsy sites

As expected, schistosome ova are frequently found in other biopsy locations, such as the liver, bladder, cervix, vagina, perineum and skin, and indications for a biopsy of such sites lie at the individual clinical level.

Indirect diagnostic techniques

A high index of epidemiological suspicion with appropriate physical or radiological signs, seroimmunological assessment of antibody levels by a variety of assays and, in S. haematobium infections, the detection of red blood cells and protein in the urine in subjects in endemic areas all remain indirect diagnostic techniques.

Chemical reagent strips

Indirect diagnostic techniques are used most frequently in S. haematobium infections. The application of chemical reagent strips (CRSs) in a semiquantitative fashion is highly useful as a diagnostic surrogate in endemic areas of the disease; a positive result is interpreted as indicating active infection.

Reagent strips in current use have ranges of sensibility of 5–15 red blood cells/mL and 0.015–0.03 mg of haemoglobin per 100 mL urine. They use a peroxide compound and orthotolidine as a chromogen. The colour distinction between negative and the first level of reactivity on the strips is well defined, and in the presence of blood, the colour indicators show distinct changes from yellow or pale orange to green or blue.[188] False-positive reactions occur in myoglobinuria and in the presence of bacterial peroxidases resulting from heavy bacteriuria, and inhibition of the reactions may occur if urinary ascorbic acid levels exceed 10 mg/100 mL urine.

CRSs that measure levels of proteinuria semiquantitatively use tetrabromophthalein ethylester with a buffer. The colour discrimination between negative and the first level of proteinuria is, however, not well defined. Precise assessment of colour change from yellow-green to green-blue is difficult. False positives occur in alkaline urines or when quinine or a quinine derivative is present. False negatives have occurred in strongly acid urine with Bence Jones proteinuria and in urine containing predominantly γ-globulin.

Many experiences of the use of CRSs in areas endemic for S. haematobium[189–192] have confirmed the consistent and significant correlation between reagent strip reactions indicating haematuria and/or proteinuria and increasing intensity of egg output.

Good predictive values resulting from high sensitivity and specificity emphasize the limitations of conventional single microscopic examinations at very low egg output levels and confirm the validity of CRSs in detecting those with a 'high' egg output (i.e.

over 50 eggs/10 mL urine in this case).[192] CRSs can be used in areas of both high and low transmission patterns and find an optimal use in the detection of those with 'heavy' infections who are a priority for chemotherapy. The use of CRSs can be expected to increase at primary healthcare levels in programmes of morbidity control in *S. haematobium* infection.

Immunodiagnosis

Serodiagnostic techniques are used for the detection of either specific antibodies or genus-specific antigens.

Antibodies to adult worm, schistosomular, cercarial or egg antigens are detected by a multiplicity of procedures, including the various forms of enzyme-linked immunosorbent assay (ELISA), radioimmunoassay (RIA), indirect immunofluorescence tests (IFAT), gel precipitation techniques (GPT), indirect haemagglutination (IHA), latex agglutination (LAT) and circumoval precipitin tests (COPT) that have superseded the older Cercarienhüllen reactions (CHR) and complement fixation tests (CFT).

In general, antibody detection techniques have been less useful to the practising physician and epidemiologist than the techniques of direct parasitological diagnosis. Their basic disadvantage is that they all point to past exposure to mammalian or, in rare instances, avian schistosomes without indicating the duration, activity or quantum of infection. Further disadvantages are an absence of globally agreed criteria of performance and standards; the necessity for expensive equipment, costly or labile reagents; the need for skilled technical personnel; and the slow diminution of specific antibody level after treatment, thus reducing their value as a marker of chemotherapeutic success. Each laboratory in endemic or non-endemic areas has tended to use its own particular antigen and assay procedure. The WHO has conducted several collaborative studies[193,194] in attempts to improve the technology and to standardize both antigens and procedures. Agreement is not yet in sight. A most useful review of the present position has been produced.[195]

In striking contrast, very real advances have been made in antigen detection. Improvements in the production of monoclonal antibodies have led to new diagnostic tests of CAA and CCA in serum and urine.

A recent review details the technological advances made in one leading research centre,[196] compares the efficacy of antigen detection with both parasitological and antibody determinations in a range of clinico-epidemiological situations, and summarizes the 'pros' and 'cons' of these techniques. It appears that no single method can be optimal in all circumstances and the availability of laboratory facilities, the need for a rapid diagnosis and the local logistical frame, plus, of course, the overall costs, will determine whether antigen detection, antibody detection or parasitological examination will be dominant in practical usage. This seems to point to a north–south divide in the provision of laboratory facilities.

Radiology

As a form of indirect diagnosis, various radiological procedures (Figures 80.17, 80.18) for detecting morbidity from Schistosomal infection have long been in use in hospital practice and have included plain abdominal radiography to detect calcification,

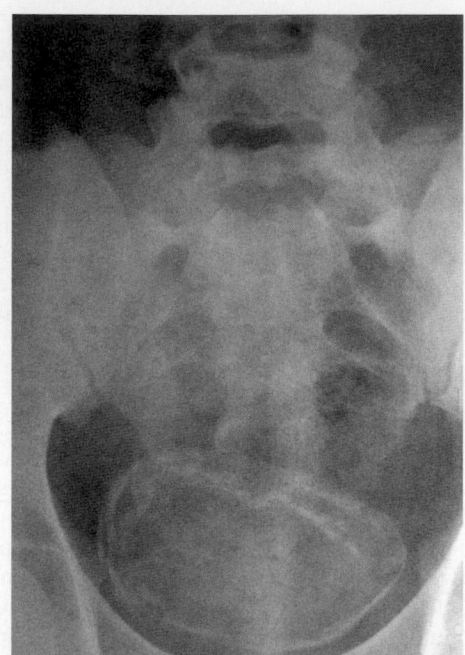

Figure 82.17 Calcification of the bladder in late *S. haematobium* infection.

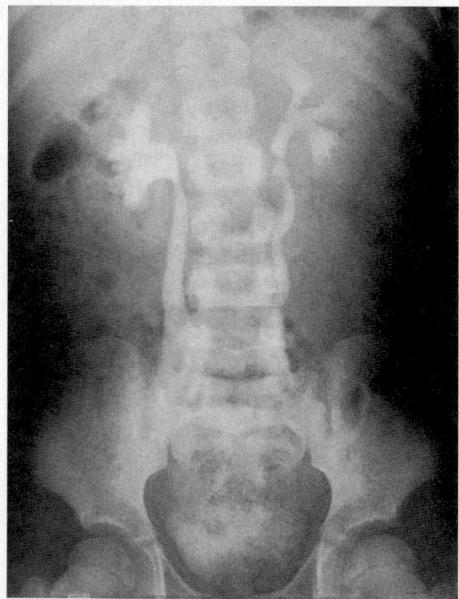

Figure 82.18 Dilated ureters, calcified bladder and hydronephrosis caused by *Schistosoma* infection. (Courtesy of D. M. Forsyth.)

intravenous pyelography to detect bladder and ureteral changes or obstructive uropathy, isotope renography, computed tomography for cerebral schistosomiasis, myelography for suspected cord damage, and portal venography for hepatosplenic schistosomiasis with portal venous hypertensive changes. Complications, such as gastrointestinal bleeding, may require the use of specialized techniques, such as abdominal ultrasonography, splenoportography

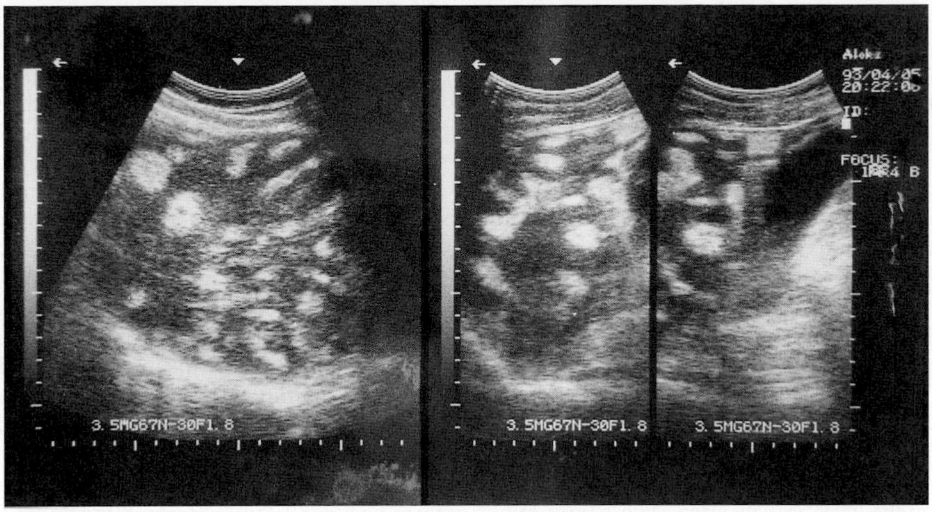

Figure 82.19 Symmer's periportal fibrosis in *S. mansoni* infection (Courtesy of Dr Ashraf Omar, Department of Tropical Medicine, Cairo University.)

and nuclear isotopic studies of hepatic blood flow. The rapidly advancing techniques in radiology make this an area which is becoming a specialist zone.

The indications for a particular investigation lie at the individual patient level and are the joint responsibilities of the physician and the radiologist.

Ultrasonography

Major changes in the diagnostic approach in individual patients and in the epidemiological assessment of morbidity in communities have occurred in parallel with the introduction and expanded use of ultrasonography (Figures 80.19, 80.20). The technique is non-invasive, simple, portable, has no biological hazard to the patient or the operator and either complements or is an alternative diagnostic method to many invasive techniques. With the exception of hydroureter, ureteral calculi and bladder calcification, it has, in comparison with other diagnostic procedures, high specificity and sensitivity, is superior to physical examination in measuring liver and spleen size, and is the best technique for grading Schistosomal periportal fibrosis, portal hypertension, hydronephrosis, urinary bladder wall lesions and renal and bladder stones.[197] An extensive review of technical and clinical experience is available.[198]

Following field use of portable ultrasonography, particularly in Egypt, where it is widely used, an agreed protocol for standardized investigations and methods of reporting was produced by the WHO.[199]

It has been demonstrated in community studies that sonographic lesions of periportal fibrosis in *S. mansoni* infection, with thickening of portal tracts and portal vein walls, correlated with the number of eggs in the stool.[200] Fine measurements of hepatic pathology are possible and are superior to clinical examination.[201] Where available, ultrasonography should replace clinical grading and physical examination as a preferred method of assessing liver and spleen enlargement.[202]

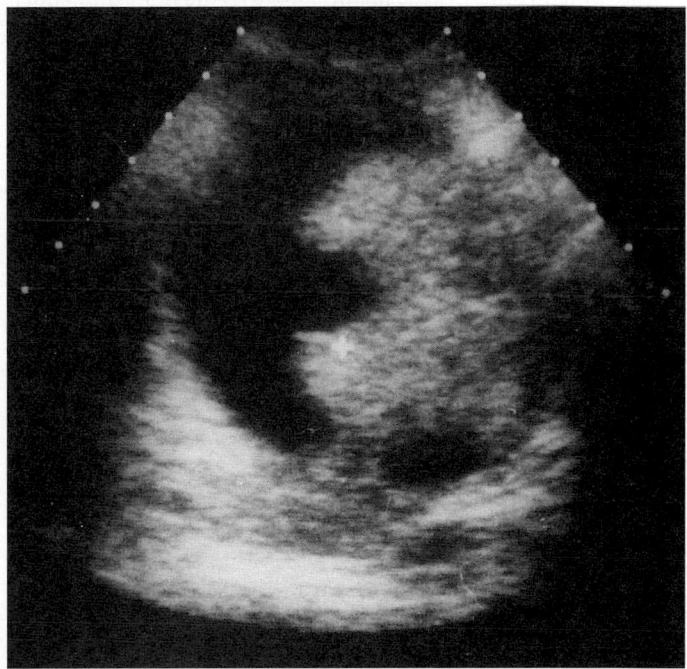

Figure 82.20 Carcinoma of the bladder in *S. haematobium* infection. (Courtesy of Dr Ashraf Omar, Department of Tropical Medicine, Cairo University.)

The sonographic patterns of Schistosomal hepatic fibrosis are characteristic and are distinct from those of other hepatic diseases. Schistosomiasis can now be distinguished from cirrhosis with confidence.

Additionally, an ultrasonographic scoring system is of clinical use in the prediction of both oesophageal varices and the likelihood of bleeding from them.[203]

An interesting outcome of ultrasonographic studies has been the demonstration that *S. haematobium* can cause mild degrees of Schistosomal periportal fibrosis in an area where *S. mansoni* does not exist;[105] this confirms an observation, first made in 1974 in Upper Egypt, that hepatosplenic disease caused by *S. haematobium* is a distinct entity.[106]

The use of abdominal ultrasonography to determine the decrease in morbidity following population-based chemotherapy programmes can be expected to grow dramatically.

MANAGEMENT

For no other parasitic diseases have there been such major advances in chemotherapy as have occurred since the 1960s, in the treatment of schistosomiasis. The introduction and widespread use, at both the individual patient level and in large-scale community-based operations, of the current highly effective, orally administered, well tolerated, anti-Schistosomal drugs have provided physicians, epidemiologists and public health practitioners with therapeutic opportunities not in existence at the end of the 1960s.

The primary objective of chemotherapy is cure of the individual patient by eradication of the infection (or the infection with two species) from which he or she suffers. Cure leads to cessation of egg deposition, the pathogenic agent in the tissues, and this prevents additional organ damage; existing lesions will, in the vast majority of cases, regress. In large-scale community-based chemotherapy programmes, where compromises on dosage may have to be made to ensure a viable delivery system and optimal population coverage, the main aim is to reduce the community egg load and excretion by the greatest amount possible. Individual 'cure' may or may not occur; the community benefits as a whole by the blocking of the egg–miracidium–snail stage of the biological cycle, which reduces transmission by minimizing excretal pollution of water supplies and thus diminishes cercarial contamination of human water contact sites. Of even greater importance is the reduction of community morbidity caused by schistosomiasis; nowadays this can be measured and the success of interventions can be evaluated with some accuracy and precision.

Since the last edition of this book, major changes in the outlook for anti-Schistosomal chemotherapy have taken place.[204] Whereas three anti-Schistosomal compounds were used globally and were all on the 'WHO List of Essential Drugs', the position now is totally different. Metrifonate has been withdrawn from the market and pursues, under a different nomenclature and with pharmacological refinements, a role in the treatment of dementia.

Oxamniquine is available currently in only very few countries, but its manufacturer has assured the WHO that production will continue for the foreseeable future.

Praziquantel

Praziquantel is the drug of choice, and is effective against all schistosome species that occur in humans. It is also effective in the other snail-borne trematode infections – clonorchiasis, paragonimiasis and opisthorchiasis – and in infections due to the adult cestodes, *Taenia solium*, *T. saginata*, *Hymenolepis nana* and *Diphyllobothrium* spp. It is active against the secondary larval stages of *T. solium* in humans, dermal cysticercosis and neurocysticercosis, but has little or no effect in ocular cysticercosis. Praziquantel is not active in the human secondary larval stages of *Echinococcus* spp. and is generally ineffective in *Fasciola hepatica* infections. There is no therapeutic activity in protozoan or nematode infections including the filariae.

Although dosage is standardized in large-scale epidemiologically based morbidity control programmes, there is frequently a variation in dose in the treatment of the individual patient. In field programmes, a single oral dose of 40 mg/kg is effective in *S. haematobium*, *S. mansoni* and *S. intercalatum* infections. For *S. japonicum* infection, the dosages employed originally were a total dose of 60 mg/kg, given at 4-hourly intervals as three 20-mg/kg doses or two 30-mg/kg doses, but present field practice, since the mid-1980s, has been to use a single oral dose of 40 mg/kg.

The usual total dose for *S. mekongi* is 60 mg/kg, although there is evidence that repeated treatment at this dosage may be necessary for cure of this species.[205–208]

For treatment of individual patients with heavy infections with *S. mansoni* (over 800 eggs/g of stool), a total dose of 50 or 60 mg/kg, given in two equally divided doses 4–6 h apart, may be needed; single doses are best given after food and, if possible, in the evening.

Patient tolerance is extremely good and virtually all trials have confirmed the absence of toxicity in the liver, kidney, haematopoietic system, or other body organs and functions. However, minor side-effects do occur; those related to the gastrointestinal tract are epigastric or generalized abdominal pain or discomfort, nausea, rarely vomiting, anorexia and loose stools. These side-effects are mild, transient and, even if their incidence is high, rarely if ever require medication. A rare event in patients heavily infected with *S. mansoni* or *S. japonicum* is the passage of blood in the stools after praziquantel treatment. The explanation is unknown; it occurs a few hours after dosage but recovery is rapid and without clinical sequelae.

Headache and dizziness may be encountered, as may fever, pruritus or a transient skin eruption, none of which is serious or lasting. Side-effects that occur in field treatments tend to be more frequent in foci of intense transmission, and should not be used as an argument for reduction of the dose.

'Cure rates' are high; it can be expected that with the appropriate dosage they will be around 80% in small groups. In large-scale field operations, where supervision is of necessity less stringent and where total compliance may be difficult to ensure, rates of 50–60% will be found when a single oral dose of 40 mg/kg is used; egg output reduction in those not 'cured' should exceed 90% of pretreatment output.

A disturbing trend has appeared in field programmes of control in recent years. 'Resistance' or 'tolerance' to praziquantel has been claimed and documented on several occasions in the treatment and control of *S. mansoni*,[209,210] and resistance can be induced in laboratory studies.[211]

Cure rates after praziquantel treatment in a new highly endemic focus of intense transmission of *S. mansoni* in northern Senegal in the early 1990s were alarmingly low.[212–214] However, a WHO consultation decided that the intensity of transmission in this focus was such as to cause the initially observed low cure rates, because praziquantel is ineffective or at least less effective against maturing worms. In a new focus in non-immunes with a high intensity of transmission, these would be present in the majority of infections.

There is good evidence from Egypt that in the delta some 2–3% of patients were still excreting eggs after two or three praziquantel treatments. Some 20% of field isolates showed a normal susceptibility to praziquantel, but some of the remaining sampled isolates required two to six times the normal dose to achieve a 50% reduction in worm numbers in laboratory studies. However, this reduced susceptibility was not increased upon repeated passages under drug pressure. Thus evidence exists that certain schistosome isolates or strains of the parasite are inherently less susceptible to praziquantel. Persistent monitoring and surveillance is obviously essential to detect the emergence of true drug resistance. The picture is not clear, and the story unfolds.[209] In Egypt, follow-up of isolates in areas where praziquantel was used intensively in man indicated that the use of the drug has not resulted in a dramatic change in its curative efficacy.[210] These findings confirm the vital importance of a monitoring system – essential to detect the emergence of true resistance/tolerance. The recent introduction of a simple new technique for assessing praziquantel effect on miracidia hatched from eggs may, if confirmed in different species, offer an affordable surveillance device to predict praziquantel 'resistance' or 'tolerance'.[215]

Although this 'resistance-tolerance' phenomenon has been reported in human S. mansoni infections, no evidence exists at present of 'resistance' in S. japonicum or S. haematobium infections. Field trials of praziquantel treatment monitored over many years in China[216] and in Kenya[217] have produced consistent 'cure rates' year on year during annual treatments of both S. japonicum and S. haematobium infections. In the latter case, theoretical mathematical modelling suggested that the emergence of resistance might take some 7 years on an annual treatment coverage of 100% of an infected population. As this coverage is rarely, if ever, obtained in field practice, where a range of 25–75% compliance is more usual, emergence of resistance may take 10–15 years.

Oxamniquine

A tetrahydroquinolone compound distantly related to hycanthone, oxamniquine is effective only against S. mansoni. In animal models, it proved inactive against S. japonicum and early trials in humans showed virtually no activity against S. haematobium or S. matthei.

In the animal studies, one peculiarity was that male worms proved more susceptible than female worms. Egg-laying by surviving females ceased in the absence of males after successful treatment, thus removing the basic pathogenetic mechanism in S. mansoni infection.[218,219]

Oxamniquine is available as capsules of 250 mg or as a syrup containing 50 mg/mL, and is marketed as Mansil® in South America and as Vansil® in Africa. In the USA, capsules have a yellow body marked PFIZER 641 with a dark green cap marked VANSIL. The shelf life is 5 years for capsules and 3 years for the syrup.

Oxamniquine is used at all stages, from acute toxaemic to chronic and complicated S. mansoni infections, with good results.

Advanced S. mansoni infection with hepatosplenomegaly, portal hypertension and/or ascites responds well, and in Schistosomal polyposis there are great improvements in both the associated anaemia and protein-losing enteropathy.[220–222]

High cure rates (60–90% in different samples) are seen after oxamniquine treatment of uncomplicated S. mansoni infections.

From 1975 to 1979 oxamniquine was used in a major control campaign in Brazil, when some 5 million doses were given in the field programmes with high cure rates and very good tolerance.[223]

The dose of oxamniquine varies with the geographical origin of the S. mansoni infection, the age and hence the surface area of the patient. In South America, adults are given 15 mg/kg of body weight as a single oral dose; in children 20 mg/kg is preferred, given in two divided portions each of 10 mg/kg with an interval of 4–6 h between doses. If practicable, the drug should be given after food or just before sleep.

With S. mansoni occurring on the African continent, only those with strains of West African origin are given the same doses as in South America. In Egypt, Sudan and southern Africa, a total dose of 60 mg/kg body weight is used, either as 15 mg/kg for 2 days or as 20 mg/kg once daily for 3 days. In East Africa, a total dose of 30–40 mg/kg is given in a split regimen over 1 or 2 days.

In general, oxamniquine is well tolerated. There are virtually no contraindications but classes of patients exist who require close monitoring. Patients with a history of any form of epilepsy must be supervised for 48 h after treatment because a small number of epileptiform convulsions have been reported, as have generalized seizures after the drug, fortunately without sequelae and with clinical and electroencephalographic recovery.[224]

As with many other drugs, treatment should not be given during the first 4 months of pregnancy.

Any patient whose occupation involves care of heavy machinery or who is employed in the transport industry (e.g. pilots, truckers, dockers, crane drivers) should be placed off work for 48 h after treatment.

Side-effects are uncommon; dizziness, drowsiness and headache are most frequent but last for some 4–6 h only. Hallucinations and a state of excitement are very rare events. Although abdominal discomfort, vomiting and diarrhoea do occur, there is no constant statistical correlation and, in practice, adverse effects have had no influence on compliance in field programmes.

A harmless orange–red discolouration of the urine may occur but is transitory, and a syndrome of peripheral blood eosinophilia, scattered pulmonary infiltrates and increased immune complexes in serum with urinary excretion of Schistosomal antigens is known in Egypt but has not been described in other locations.[225]

An eosinophilia after treatment occurs commonly and is maximal in 7–10 days; it represents a reaction to dead or dying schistosomes. Changes in hepatic enzyme levels may be seen but no constant pattern exists.

In summary, oxamniquine is a highly useful drug for treatment of all forms of S. mansoni infection, including many advanced and complicated syndromes. Resistance to oxamniquine is known in South America but is not yet a public health problem, as such patients are treated successfully with praziquantel.[226]

The future of chemotherapy

Regrettably, for economic reasons, there appears to be little possibility of major pharmaceutical industry investment in exploration of new anti-Schistosomal compounds. Cost recovery in Third World endemic countries is highly questionable even disregarding the profit motive. Thus the importance of monitoring control programmes for true 'drug resistance' cannot be overemphasized, although at present there are lamentably few such efforts.

The recent introduction of a simple new technique for assessing the effects of praziquantel on miracidia hatched from eggs may, if confirmed in different species, offer an affordable surveillance device to predict praziquantel 'resistance' or 'tolerance'.[215]

Myrrh

In Egypt, Mirazid, prepared from myrrh (Arabian or Somali), an oleo-gum resin from the stem of thorny trees (*Commiphora motiviol* Engier), containing 23–40% resin myrrhia was reported to possess anti-Schistosomal activity and has been used widely in rural practice. However, a multicentre trial of its effects in mice and hamsters with strains of *S. mansoni* of Egyptian, Puerto Rican and Brazilian origin failed to provide any worthwhile anti-Schistosomal effects in contrast with praziquantel-treated animals which produced the usual effects.[227] Furthermore, a well-conducted clinical trial in the Egyptian Delta produced only a very low 'cure rate' when compared with praziquantel treatment in a randomized study.[228] These results raised serious doubts on the anti-Schistosomal properties of myrrh and it cannot currently be considered as an addition to therapy.

Artemisinin derivatives (artemether, artesunate)

It is known that artemisinin derivatives, by killing immature worms, have preventive effects in *S. japonicum* infections in animal models.[229,230] This action was confirmed in humans in randomized double-blind placebo-controlled trials in China during recent floods, where the incidence and intensity of infection in endemic areas was reduced significantly.[231]

Artemisinin, the active ingredient of the herb *Artemesia annua*, is a sesquiterpene lactone containing a peroxide bridge and was isolated in the 1970s. Several semi-synthetic derivatives have been generated and they are the most potent antimalarials currently available.

Activity against *S. japonicum* was discovered later in animals with highest efficacy against schistosomula. Since artemether and praziquantel showed maximal activities against juvenile and adult worms, respectively, combinations of the two compounds were naturally suggested. Many randomized controlled trials of artemether against *S. japonicum* were pursued in China and high protective efficacy was observed.[232,233] (Further details of schistosomiasis in China can be found in *Acta Tropica*, Volume 96, Issue 2–3,[234] a resource highly recommended for those studying this subject)

However, because artemisinin derivatives are one of the current mainstays in antimalarial chemotherapy and because endemic malaria and endemic schistosomiasis co-exist in numerous areas, especially in Africa, wider use of these derivatives must await the clarification of several epidemiological and public health issues. There may be a risk of selecting schistosome strains less sensitive to praziquantel if artemether is given at an early stage after infection when maturing schistosomes are known to be insensitive to praziquantel. Furthermore, the effects of repeated doses of artemether (or other derivatives) on the biology and local epidemiology of malaria are as yet unknown. Further work remains to be done before these problems are clarified in many areas of Africa.

Assessment of chemotherapy

Assessment of patients treated for schistosomiasis is conducted by repeated clinical observation, evaluation of symptomatic improvement, and diminution or disappearance of physical, radiological, particularly ultrasonographic and endoscopic signs.

Direct parasitological examination of urine, stool or rectal biopsy is essential and should be performed on repeated (three) specimens of excreta at about 6–8 weeks and 4–6 months after treatment, by a selection of appropriate techniques detailed above.

Follow-up is simple if no reinfection risk is present; the explanation of viable eggs in the excreta at 4–6 months is less clear in endemic areas where transmission persists. It may be due to a maturing prepatent infection unaffected by chemotherapy, a true reinfection or a therapeutic failure. It is not always easy to decide which event, or even combination of events, is responsible. Increased use of antigen detection techniques (e.g. CAA, CCA) offers real possibilities for clarification of these problems.

Special clinical syndromes and management

Neurological schistosomiasis

The efficacy and safety of modern anti-Schistosomal drugs has led to early treatment of encephalopathies, myelopathies or other spinal cord syndromes, reasonably suspected, even if not proven, to be due to schistosomiasis. This improves prognosis as cord damage in myelopathy is closely related to time of diagnosis.

An ELISA using keyhole limpet haemocyanin is said to distinguish between antibody responses in acute and chronic Schistosomal infection,[235] and CAA can be diagnostic where eggs are not yet excreted. These two diagnostic techniques should be used when available; unfortunately they are, as yet, restricted to certain high-technology centres.

The use of corticosteroids remains controversial. Laminectomy is an important technique in acute paraplegia with spinal compression or block, or in deteriorating clinical circumstances during conservative treatment.

In *S. japonicum*, suspected cerebral schistosomiasis should be localized with modern imaging techniques and treated with praziquantel, which is safe and effective. Computed tomography demonstrates resolution of intracerebral masses, regression of cerebral oedema and the subsequent disappearance of epilepsy.[236] Appropriate neurosurgical supervision should be on hand.

Acute toxaemic schistosomiasis (Katayama syndrome)

Early diagnosis of a suspicious clinical presentation can now be made with the keyhole limpet haemocyanin antibody assay and CAA antigen detection techniques. Disputes remain whether steroids should be added to specific drug treatment with praziquantel or oxamniquine, and the position has not yet been resolved. As a general principle, patients should be treated with praziquantel, which is effective against all species.

Associated salmonellosis

The chronic bacteraemia due to *Salmonella typhi* or *S. paratyphi* is due to the attachment of the bacteria to the integument or in the gut of the adult schistosome. Although clinical response to antibiotics is good, bacteraemia will recur unless the underlying schistosomiasis is treated. The therapeutic response to anti-Schistosomal drugs is good.

Associated hepatitis

Even if, in hepatosplenic schistosomiasis, there is serological or other evidence of an associated hepatitis B infection (or C, D or E), and activity of schistosomiasis is still present, it is worthwhile treating the latter with praziquantel.

Portal hypertension

Chemotherapy is but one part of patient care, as complications are mainly due to the mechanical obstructive pathology resulting from periportal fibrosis. Where eggs are still found in the excreta, treatment with praziquantel or oxamniquine is indicated and gives the usual response.

Gastrointestinal bleeding

Admission to a specialized centre is essential because that is where skills in assessment, immediate resuscitation, fibreoptic endoscopy, balloon tamponade and/or endoscopic sclerotherapy are present. The treatment of this complication is beyond the scope of the general physician and is preferably a matter for specialists in this area of intensive care. Emergency portocaval shunts have fallen into disrepute as a high proportion of operative deaths may occur and, in the survivors, there is frequently a loss of shunt patency and/or encephalopathy. A selective distal splenorenal shunt has been claimed to offer a lower haemorrhage recurrence rate and an improved survival rate.[237]

The clinical application of β-adrenergic blockade using non-selective β-blockers (e.g. propranolol) for the prevention of an initial gastrointestinal haemorrhage in either cirrhosis or portal hypertension from Schistosomal periportal fibrosis is ambiguous. It is not yet clear which clinical variables are the best predictors of response to β-blockers.

In endemic rural areas, the major difficulty is diagnosing the presence of oesophageal varices in the absence of a history or an actual bleed, for the necessary diagnostic facilities are not there. Thus referral to a specialized centre possessing the essential facilities is the optimal, if Elysian, form of management.

Schistosomiasis without eggs

This title describes cases where no ova can be found on investigation but there exists a high index of clinical suspicion of Schistosomal infection, usually based upon an epidemiological history of exposure, existing cases in fellow members of a group, an unexplained eosinophilia in a presenting suspect and/or a suggestive or suspicious seroimmunodiagnostic test result.

In areas endemic for *S. haematobium*, the presence of a positive test for microhaematuria on CRS examination is taken as indicative of infection.

Again, the simplicity of use of modern drugs has clarified many difficult diagnostic situations and frequently treatment is undertaken on 'suspicion alone', a practice justifiable only when exhaustive efforts to reach a parasitological or serological diagnosis have failed.

Detailed monographs on the properties of anti-Schistosomal drugs and their use in clinical and field practice have been produced.[238–241]

PREVENTION AND CONTROL

Both prevention and control depend on an area-specific, species-specific and epidemiologically-specific mixture of intervention methods. The characteristics of endemic areas, the transmission patterns, the infecting parasite species and strains, the intermediate snail host(s), the availability or otherwise of water supplies and sanitary facilities, the behavioural customs of the human communities, especially their water contact patterns and above all the socioeconomic background, all contribute to a multiplicity of interactions to produce a vast mosaic of transmission and epidemiological pictures. An accurate diagnosis of all of these variables, quantitative when possible, is necessary before entering into prevention and control programmes. The aims of both prevention and control are:

1. The reduction in the number of eggs excreted from infected people reaching waters harbouring the intermediate snail host(s); this is dependent on health education, the provision and use of adequate sanitary facilities, and specific anti-Schistosomal chemotherapy for infected communities and individuals.
2. The reduction in the probability of miracidial/snail contact; this relies on all factors in (1.), appropriate modifications of the aquatic environment and reduction of intermediate snail host numbers by application of chemical molluscicides or the use of suitable biological control means.
3. The reduction of cercarial densities, which will occur as a result of all of the preceding actions but overwhelmingly from the employment of molluscicides.
4. The reduction of the probability of cercariae locating a definitive host, again due to the cumulative effects of all of the preceding factors plus the reduction of human water contact with infected water bodies by the provision of adequate domestic or peridomestic water supplies and the substitution of safe recreational water sites.
5. The reduction of the longevity of the adult worms in the human host, a function of chemotherapy.

1453

Multiple overlaps are obvious in these processes and, conventionally, stress in 'prevention' is directed towards health education and the provision of adequate water supplies and sanitation supplemented by environmental improvements. 'Control' is dominated by chemotherapy and molluscicides, yet integration of these interventions is essential for success and each endemic focus or region requires an individual clinico-epidemiological, zoogeographical, sociological and environmental approach based on the common principles listed above.

In the past, emphasis was given to 'transmission control', largely through repetitive mollusciciding. This was expensive; molluscicides did not achieve total kills of snails and their eggs in operationally difficult terrains, and the techniques require skilled biologists and technical personnel. Epidemiological extrapolation of the successes of modern chemotherapy and the employment of simple low-cost diagnostic techniques led inevitably to a reappraisal of the strategy and tactics of control. Many schistosomiasis control operations operated through a single disease control mechanism are simply beyond the financial and human resources of the great majority of endemic countries in Africa, where 85% of the global prevalence exists. A strategy of control has now evolved that stresses repetitive population-based chemotherapy, aimed at 'morbidity control' rather than 'transmission control'. It is implemented through the peripheral healthcare workers in the primary healthcare system adopted by all countries, and many successes have been documented that have been evaluated by epidemiological, parasitological and ultrasonographic tools.

Advances in control using population-based chemotherapy have been numerous. The philosophical and economic benefits of vertically based programmes have been laid out by Canning.[242] New initiatives are listed in a recent article.[243] Two major programmes, the Schistosomiasis Control Initiative, funded by the Bill and Melinda Gates Foundation, currently operating in Uganda, Burkina Faso, Mali, Niger, Tanzania and Zambia, and the formation by WHO of a 'Great Neglected Diseases Programme' will stimulate further national control programmes. The basic foundation of these programmes will use the spearhead of mass chemotherapy and will be applied, not only to schistosomiasis, but to soil transmitted helminths, lymphatic filariasis, onchocerciasis, and trachoma, all using appropriate chemotherapeutic agents. When prevalence and intensity of infection has been lowered to a satisfactory level, then it is hoped that residual disease will be dealt with through the Primary Health system – this has yet to be proven. Patently, integration of the attack phases of these operations is essential and a recent example from Nigeria, the largest sub-Saharan country, has pointed the way.[244] The latest example of successful control using a chemotherapeutic spearhead is of an 8-year programme in Cambodia where *S. mekongi* was attacked with mass chemotherapy with praziquantel and followed with mebendazole for soil-transmitted helminths. The success was attributed to political commitment even in a country with minimal resources.[245] However, the naive supposition that chemotherapy alone will provide the definitive answer to schistosomiasis control is not substantiated. In such a multi-faceted socioeconomic, biological, human behavioural and clinical syndrome, 'control' certainly needs chemotherapy as a spearhead but also needs to be reinforced by such snail control measures as required by epidemiological criteria. Reinfection after chemotherapy is a risk that is ever present against a background of unchanging socioeconomic conditions, because the constraints of achieving total population coverage with drugs and the less than absolute cure rates mean that egg deposition continues, albeit at a much lower level, and therefore transmission continues.

Add to this the difficulties in environmental improvement, the provision of sanitation and water supplies and the deployment of continuing health education, and the 'control' of schistosomiasis implying a permanent cessation of transmission is clearly a Herculean task. Patently, the constraining factors are political and economic, not technical.

A summary of the current rationale for control and data on its employment are provided in the last two reports of the WHO Expert Committee.[246]

Mollusciciding

The use of molluscicides in the control of schistosomiasis is a highly specialized field. Synthetic chemical molluscicides are virtually restricted nowadays to one compound, niclosamide (Bayluscide; Bayer) and, although other chemicals lethal to snails exist, their practical use is minimal. Although many molluscicides of plant origin are known,[247] the eventual outlook for the isolation, characterization, toxicological screening, large-scale production and distribution of their active ingredients for use in endemic countries is blurred.

A useful specialist text on indications, technical use, application in different habitats and evaluation of molluscicides has been produced by the WHO.[248]

Molluscicides will continue in use as one of the integral specific control tools, but techniques have changed markedly from the old 'blanket application' to a much more focused approach guided by the epidemiological criteria of high prevalence, high intensity and rapidity of reinfection rates in any particular focus or area of infection.

Vaccines and vaccination

The limitations of current control measures have changed the old aims of 'transmission control', with implied eradication after cessation of transmission, to the current strategy of 'morbidity control', with an uncertain diminution of transmission but recognition that some residual infection will continue.

These factors, added to the virtually unchanging socioeconomic circumstances in many countries, especially in Africa where 85% of current prevalence is found, and added to the recent explosion of new techniques in biotechnology, led to a huge rise in research aimed at the production of vaccines against the invasive stages of schistosomiasis or the pathology produced. While advances in molecular biology have led to the identification and characterization of an impressive number of schistosome antigens, progress in human vaccination studies has lagged behind those in animal models. One view emerging is that a vaccine, even with a long-term protective effect, would probably be insufficient as a sole control mechanism but would need to be given in conjunction with chemotherapy and other control methods.[249,250] The antigenic identities of the biologically active molecules selected as candidates for Schistosomal vaccine development are: a variant of the isoenzyme glutathione S-transferase (Sm28GST); paramyosin

(Sm97); an irradiation-associated vaccine antigen (IrV-5); the glycolytic enzyme triose-phosphate isomerase (TPI); and the membrane antigen Sm23 and a fatty acid-binding protein (FABP) 14 (Sm14).[252] However, further testing of these six antigens in mice by two independent laboratories experienced in experimental schistosomiasis research showed that a stated modest goal of consistent induction of 40% protection or better was not reached with any of the molecules tested.[250]

Currently, the only vaccine candidate molecule with what appeared to be satisfactory antigenic properties is a glutathione S-transferase (Sh28GST) in *S. haematobium* infections. Preliminary phase 1a safety trials in humans have been conducted in France and Senegal, and are leading to efficacy studies. Results might be anticipated in 1–2 years' time.[251]

The case for the sceptics of the feasibility or even utility of a vaccine in schistosomiasis has been argued recently and persuasively by Gryseels.[252] It was pointed out that, apart from the complex technical problems to be met and solved, there were marked differences from the campaigns with vaccines against the childhood viral and bacterial diseases, and there were fundamental differences in the public health concepts involved.

While a vaccine programme of sequential steps of preclinical development, independent testing of antigens at all stages, human correlate studies, scale-up, subsequent field trials and large-scale production has been initiated by the UNDP/World Bank/WHO Tropical Diseases Research Programme (TDR), many problems exist. There remain many unanswered questions on the immunology of schistosomiasis and on the mechanisms of protection when it exists, and formidable challenges lie ahead regarding large-scale antigen production and the improvement of the current modest levels of protection achieved to date in animal models. A view of vaccine-linked chemotherapy is emerging from scientists in the field and the arguments are laid out by Bergquist et al.[250] but as yet they do not negate the necessity of a multi-faceted approach to control.

It has been estimated that a vaccine development and scale-up programme leading to market availability will take some 10 years – not dissimilar to a drug development schedule.[253] It will be some years before vaccines in humans evolve from the present enthusiastic hopes to realistic practical usage in the field, and the methodological difficulties in assessing their possible application in the numerous epidemiological mosaics of schistosomiasis transmission foci will be profound.

REFERENCES

1. Rollinson D, Southgate VR. The genus Schistosoma: a taxonomic appraisal. In: Rollinson D, Simpson AJG, eds. *The Biology of Schistosomes. From Genes to Latrines.* London: Academic Press; 1987:1–4.

2. World Health Organization. The control of schistosomiasis. *World Health Organ Tech Rep Ser* 1985; 728:1–49.

3. Farooq M. Historical development. In: *Epidemiology and Control of Schistosomiasis (Bilharziasis)*. Basle: Karger; 1973:1–16.

4. Ruffer MA. Note on the presence of Bilharzia haematobia in Egyptian mummies of the 20th dynasty 1220–1000 BC. *BMJ* 1910; I:16.

5. Larrey DJ. *(Haematurie) Mémoires de Chirurgie Militaire et Campagnes.* Paris: Smith; 1812–1817.

6. Bilharz TM. Fernere Beobachtungun uber das die Pfortader des Menschen bewohnende Distomum haematobium und sein verhaltniss zu gewissen pathologischen Bildungen aus brieflichen Mitheilungen an Professor v. Siebold vom 29 Marz 1852. *Acta Tropica* 1852; 4:72–76.

7. Manson P. Report of a case of bilharzia from the West Indies. *BMJ* 1902; ii:1894–1895.

8. Leiper RT. *Researches on Egyptian Bilharziosis.* (A report to the War Office on the results of the Bilharzia Mission in Egypt, 1915). London: John Bale Sons and Danielson; 1918:1–140. Reprinted from JR Army Medical Corps 1915; XXV:1, 147, 253; 1916; XXVII:171; 1918; XXX:235.

9. da Silva M. La schistosomose à Bahia. *Arch Parasitol* 1908; 13:231–302. Contribution to the study of schistosomiasis in Bahia, Brazil (English translation of original paper). *J Trop Med Hyg* 1909; 12:159–164.

10. Soto VR. Naturaleza de la disenteria en Caracas. Doctoral thesis, No. 63 1906.

11. Fujii Y. *Chugai Iji Shimpo* 1847; 691:55 [in Japanese].

12. Katsurada F. Schistosomum japonicum, a new parasite of man by which an endemic disease in various areas of Japan is caused. *Annot Zool Japan* 1904; 5:146–160.

13. Miyagaawa Y. *Mitte Med Fak Univ Tokyo* 1913; 1383:1–3 [in Japanese].

14. Miyairi K, Suzuki M. *Tokyo Iji Shinshi* 1913; 1386:1 [in Japanese].

15. Miyairi K, Suzuki M. *Mitte Med Fak Kais Univ Kyushu (Fukuoka)* 1914; 1:187.

16. Leiper RT, Atkinson EL. Observations of the spread of Asiatic schistosomiasis. *Chin Med J* 1915; 29:143–149.

17. Logan OT. Three cases of infection with Schistosoma japonicum in Chinese subjects. *J Trop Med Hyg* 1906; 9:294–296.

18. Woolley PG. The occurrence of schistosomiasis japonicum vel cattoi in the Philippine islands. *Phillipine J Sci* 1906; 1:83–90.

19. Brug SL, Tesch JW. Parasitic worm infestations in inhabitants around Lake Lindoe, Celebes. *Geneeskd T Ned Ind* 1937; 77:2151–2158.

20. Faust EC, Meleney HE. Studies on schistosomiasis japonica. With a supplement on the molluscan hosts of the human blood fluke in China and Japan, and species liable to be confused with them, by Nelson Anandale. *Am J Hyg (Monogr Ser)* 1924; 3:1–139.

21. Tubangui MA. The molluscan intermediate host in the Phillipines of the oriental blood fluke Schistosoma japonicum. *Philippine J Sci* 1932; 49:295–304.

22. Chesterman CC. Note sur la bilharziose dans la region de Stanleyville (Congo Belge). *Ann Soc Belg Méd Trop* 1923; 3:73.

23. Fisher AC. A study of the schistosomiasis of the Stanleyville district of the Belgian Congo. *Trans R Soc Trop Med Hyg* 1934; 28:277–306.

24. Pages JR, Jourdane J, Southgate, VR, et al. Reconnaissance deux especes jumelles au sein du taxon Schistosoma intercalatum Fisher 1934, agent de la schistosome humaine rectale en Afrique. N. sp. In: Coombes C, Jourdane J, eds. *Taxonomy, Ecology and Evolution of Metazoan Parasites.* Vol. 11. Perpignan: Presses Universitaires de Perpignan; 2003.

25. Webster BL, Southgate VR, Littlewood DT. A revision of the interrelationships of Schistosoma including the recently described Schistosoma guineensis. *Int J Parasitol* 2006; 36:974–955.

26. Voge M, Bruckner D, Bruce JI. Schistosoma melongi sp.n. from man and animals compared with four strains of Schistosoma japonicum. *J Parasitol* 1978; 64:577–584.

27. LiangYS, Kitikoon V. Susceptibility of Lithoglyphopsis aperta to Schistosoma mekongi and Schistosoma japonicum. In: Bruce JI, Sornmani S, Asch HL et al., eds. The Mekong Schistosome. *Malacol Rev* 1980; (suppl 2):53–60.

28. Bruce JI, Sornmani S, Asch HL, et al., eds. The Mekong Schistosome. *Malacol Rev* 1980; (suppl 2):1–282.

29. World Health Organization. Report of the WHO Informal Consultation on Schistosomiasis Control, Geneva, 2–4 December 1998. WHO/CDS/CPC/SIP/99.2. Geneva: WHO; 1999.

30. Gadgie RK, Shah SN. Human schistosomiasis in India. Discovery of an endemic focus in the Bombay state. *Indian J Med Sci* 1952; 6:760–763.

31. Sathe BD, Mukerji S, Gaitonde BB, et al. Reinvestigation of an old focus of schistosomiasis in Gimvi village, District Ratnagiri, in Maharashtra State, India. *Bull Haffkine Inst* 1981; 9:34–37.

32. World Health Organization. Assessment of the risk of introduction of schistosomiasis in water resources development projects and a survey of schistosomiasis in Gimvi, Ratnagiri District, Mararashtra State, India. A report of a joint mission. British Museum (Natural History), Haffkine Institute, Maharashtra State Directorate of Health, National Institute of Communicable Diseases, World Bank, World Health Organization, 13–22 November 1985. *Wkly Epidemiol Rec* 1985; 60:43.

33. Doumenge JP, Mott KE, Cheung C, et al. Atlas de la Répartition Mondiale des Schistosomiases. Talence, CEGET-CRNS. Geneva: WHO; 1987:400.

34. Davis GM, Greer GJ. A new genus and two new species of Triculinae (Gastropoda Prosobranchia) and the transmission of a Malaysian mammalian Schistosoma sp. *Proc Acad Nat Sci Philadelphia* 1980; 132:245–276.

35. Chitsulo L, Engles D, Montresor A, et al. The global status of schistosomiasis and its control. *Acta Tropica* 2000; 77(1):41–51.

36. Davis A. Schistosomiasis. In: Robinson D, ed. *Epidemiology and the Community Control of Disease in Warm Climate Countries*, 2nd edn. Edinburgh: Churchill Livingstone; 1985:389–412.

37. Browne DS, Sarfati C, Southgate VR, et al. Observations on Schistosoma intercalatum in southeast Gabon. *Z Parasitenkd* 1984; 70:243–253.

38. Wolfe MS. Schistosoma intercalatum infection in an American family. *Am J Trop Med Hyg* 1974; 23:45–50.

39. Wright CA, Southgate VR, van Wijk HB, et al. Hybrids between Schistosoma intercalatum and *S. haematobium* in Cameroon. *Trans R Soc Trop Med Hyg* 1974; 68:413–414.

40. Burchard GD, Kern P. Probable hybridization between S. intercalatum and S. haematobium in Western Gabon. *Trop Geogr Med* 1985; 37:119–123.

41. Southgate VR, van Wijk HB, Wright CA. Schistosomiasis at Loum, Cameroon: Schistosoma haematobium, S. intercalatum and their natural hybrid. *Z Parasitenk* 1976; 49:145–159.

42. Kuntz RE, McCullough B, Huang TC et al. Schistosoma intercalatum, Fisher 1934 (Cameroon) infection in the patas monkey. (Erythrocebus patas, Schreber, 1775). *Int J Parasitol* 1978; 8:65–68.

43. Nelson GS, Amin MA, Saoud MFA, et al. Studies on heterologous immunity in schistosomiasis. 1. Heterologous schistosome immunity in mice. *Bull World Health Organ* 1968; 38:9–17.

44. Amin MA, Nelson GS, Saoud MFA. Studies on heterologous immunity in mice. 2. Heterologous schistosome immunity in rhesus monkeys. *Bull World Health Organ* 1968; 38:19–27.

45. Short RB. Sex and the single chromosome. *J Parasitol* 1983; 69:3–22.

46. Erasmus DA. The adult schistosome; structure and reproductive biology. In: Rollinson D, Simpson AJG, eds. *The Biology of Schistosomes. From Genes to Latrines*. London: Academic Press; 1987:51–82.

47. Webbe G. The life cycle of the parasites. In: Jordan P, Webbe G, eds. *Schistosomiasis, Epidemiology, Treatment and Control*. London: Heinemann; 1982:50–78.

48. Christopherson JB. Longevity of parasitic worms. The term of living existence of Schistosoma haematobium in the human body. *Lancet* 1924; i:742–743.

49. Chabasse D, Bertrand G, Leroux JP, et al. Bilharziose à Schistosoma mansoni evolutive découverte 37 ans après l'infection. *Bull Soc Pathol Exot Filiales* 1985; 78:643–647.

50. World Health Organization. Immunology of schistosomiasis. *Bull World Health Organ* 1974; 51:553–595.

51. Simpson AJG. Schistosome molecular biology. In: Rollinson D, Simpson AJG, eds. *The Biology of Schistosomes. From Genes to Latrines*. London: Academic Press; 1987:147–161.

52. Rumjanek FD. Biochemistry and physiology. In: Rollinson D, Simpson AJG, eds. *The Biology of Schistosomes. From Genes to Latrines*. London: Academic Press; 1987:163–183.

53. Capron A. Schistosomiasis. Forty years war on the worm. *Parasitol Today* 1998; 14:379–384.

54. Jourdane J, Théron A. Larval development; eggs to cercariae. In: Rollinson D, Simpson AJG, eds. *The Biology of Schistosomes. From Genes to Latrines*. London: Academic Press; 1987:83–113.

55. Pesigan TP, Farooq M, Hairston N, et al. Studies on Schistosoma japonicum in the Philippines. 1. General considerations and epidemiology. *Bull World Health Organ* 1958; 18:345–455.

56. Wilson RA. Cercariae to liver worms: development and migration in the mammalian host. In: Rollinson D, Simpson AJG, eds. *The Biology of Schistosomes. From Genes to Latrines*. London: Academic Press; 1987:115–146.

57. Miller P, Wilson RA. Migration of the schistosomula of Schistosoma mansoni from the lungs to the hepatic portal system. *Parasitology* 1980; 80:267–288.

58. Wright WH. Geographical distribution of schistosomes and their intermediate hosts. In: Ansari N, ed. *Epidemiology and Control of Schistosomiasis (Bilharziasis)*. Basle: Karger; 1973:32–249.

59. Hairston NG. The dynamics of transmission. In: Ansari N, ed. *Epidemiology and Control of Schistosomiasis (Bilharziasis)*. Basle: Karger; 1973:250–336.

60. Browne DS. *Freshwater Snails of Africa and their Medical Importance*. London: Taylor & Francis; 1980:1–488.

61. Webbe G. The intermediate hosts and host-parasite relationships. In: Jordan P, Webbe G, eds. *Schistosomiasis, Epidemiology, Treatment and Control*. London: Heinemann; 1982:16–49.

62. Southgate VR, Rollinson D. Natural history of transmission and interactions. In: Rollinson D, Simpson AJG, eds. *The Biology of Schistosomes. From Genes to Latrines*. London: Academic Press; 1987:347–378.

63. Fryer SE. Studies on the epidemiology of a Nigerian strain of Schistosoma haematobium with particular reference to the molluscan hosts. PhD thesis, University of Wales; 1986.

64. Meulemann EA. Host-parasite relationships between the freshwater pulmonate Biomphalaria pfeifferi and the trematode Schistosoma mansoni. *Neth J Zool* 1972; 22:355–427.

65. Jordan P, Webbe G. Epidemiology. In: Jordan P, Webbe G, eds. *Schistosomiasis: Epidemiology, Treatment and Control*. London: Heinemann; 1982:227–292.

66. Wilkins HA. Epidemiology of schistosome infections in man. In: Rollinson D, Simpson AJG, eds. *The Biology of Schistosomes. From Genes to Latrines*. London: Academic Press; 1987:379–397.

67. Rollinson D, Simpson AJG, eds. *The Biology of Schistosomes. From Genes to Latrines*. London: Academic Press; 1987.

68. Cheng TH. Schistosomiasis in mainland China. A review of research and control programs since 1949. *Am J Trop Med Hyg* 1971; 20:26–53.

69. Fenwick A. Baboons as reservoir hosts of Schistosoma mansoni. *Trans R Soc Trop Med Hyg* 1969; 66:557–567.

70. Combes C, Delattre P. Principaux paramétrès de l'infestation des rats (Rattus rattus et Rattus norvegicus) par Schistosoma mansoni dans un foyer de schistosomiase intestinale de la region caraibe. *Oecol Appl* 1981; 2:63–79.

71. Dounge JP, Mott KE, Rollinson D, et al. Schistosoma mansoni from naturally infected Rattus rattus in Guadeloupe: identification, prevalence and enzyme polymorphism. *Parasitology* 1986; 93:39–53.

72. WHO. Consultation Bergqvist R. Prospects of vaccination against schistosomiasis. *Scand J Infect Dis* 1990; 76:60–71.

73. Davis A, Butterworth AE. Immunity in human schistosomiasis. In: Prospects for immunological intervention in human schistosomiasis. Proceedings of a Meeting of the Scientific Working Group on Schistosomiasis 26–28 May 1986, Geneva. *Acta Tropica* 1987; (suppl 12):31–40.

74. Khalife J, Capron M, Grzych J-M, et al. Immunity in human schistosomiasis. Regulation of protective immune mechanisms by IgM blocking antibodies. *J Exp Med* 1986; 164:1626–1640.

75. Cheng TH. Schistosomiasis in mainland China. In: Butterworth AE, Bensted-Smith R, Capron A, et al., eds. Immunity in human schistosomiasis mansoni: prevention by blocking antibodies of the expression of immunity in young children. *Parasitology* 1987; 94:281–300.

76. Butterworth AE, Fulford AJC, Dunne DW, et al. Longitudinal studies on human schistosomiasis. *Philos Trans R Soc Lond [Biol]* 1988; 321:495–511.

77. Capron A, Dessaint JP, Capron M, et al. Immunity to schistosomes: progress toward vaccine. *Science* 1987; 238:1065–1072.

78. Dalton PR. A sociological approach to the control of Schistosoma mansoni in St Lucia. *Bull World Health Organ* 1976; 54:587–595.

79. Colley DG, Colley MD. Protective immunity and vaccines to schistosomiasis. *Parasitol Today* 1989; 5:350–354.

80. Corrêa-Oliveira R, Caldas IR, Gazzinelli G. Natural versus drug-induced resistance in Schistosoma mansoni infection. *Parasitol Today* 2000; 16:397–399.

81. Wilkins HA, Goll PH, Marshall TF, et al. Dynamics of Schistosoma haematobium infection in a Gambian community. I. The patterns of human infection in the study area. *Trans R Soc Trop Med Hyg* 1984; 78:216–221.

82. Goll PH, Wilkins HA, Marshall TF, et al. Dynamics of Schistosoma haematobium infection in a Gambian community. II. The effect on transmission of control of Bulinus senegalensis by the use of niclosamide. *Trans R Soc Trop Med Hyg* 1984; 78:222–226.

83. Wilkins HA, Goll PH, Marshall TF, et al. Dynamics of Schistosoma haematobium infection in a Gambian community. III. Acquisition and loss of infection. *Trans R Soc Trop Med Hyg* 1984; 78:227–232.

84. Butterworth AE, Hagan P. Immunity in human schistosomiasis. *Parasitol Today* 1987; 3:11–16.

85. Hagan P. Reinfection, exposure and immunity in human schistosomiasis. *Parasitol Today* 1992; 8:12–16.

86. De Jonge N, Gryseel B, Hilberath GW, et al. Detection of circulating anodic antigen by ELISA for seroepidemiology of schistosomiasis mansoni. *Trans R Soc Trop Med Hyg* 1988; 82:591–594.

87. von Lichtenberg F. Consequences of infections with schistosomes. In: Rollinson D, Simpson AJG, eds. *The Biology of Schistosomes: From Genes to Latrines*. London: Academic Press; 1987:185–232.

88. Smith JH, Christie JD. The pathobiology of Schistosoma haematobium in humans. *Hum Pathol* 1986; 17:333–345.

89. Cheever AW, Kamel IA, Elwi AM, et al. Schistosoma mansoni and S. haematobium infections in Egypt. II. Quantitative parasitological findings at necropsy. *Am J Trop Med Hyg* 1977; 26:702–716.

90. Hoshino-Shimizu B, Brito T, Kanamura HY. Human schistosomiasis. Schistosoma mansoni antigen detection in renal glomeruli. *Trans R Soc Trop Med Hyg* 1976; 70:492–496.

91. Abdel-Salam E, Ishaak S, Mahmoud AAF. Histocompatibility linked susceptibility for hepatosplenomegaly in human schistosomiasis mansoni. *J Immunol* 1979; 123:1829–1851.

92. Sazazuki T, Ohuta N, Kanoeoka R, et al. Association between an HLA haplotype and low responsiveness to Schistosomal worm antigen in man. *J Exp Med* 1979; 152:314–318.

93. Pereira DM da SM. Sistemas HLA, ABO e Rhe caracteristicas racais em patientes com hepatosplomegalia equistossomitca. Thesis, University of Brazilia; 1979.

94. Abel L, Demenais F, Prata A, et al. Evidence for the segregation of a major gene on human susceptibility/resistance to infection by Schistosoma mansoni. *Am J Hum Genet* 1991; 48:959–970.

95. Smith JH, Kamel IA, Elwi A, et al. A quantitative post mortem analysis of urinary schistosomiasis in Egypt. I. Pathology and pathogenesis. *Am J Trop Med Hyg* 1974; 23:1054–1071.

96. Smith JH, Elwi A, Kamel IA, et al. A quantitative post mortem analysis of urinary schistosomiasis in Egypt. II. Evolution and epidemiology. *Am J Trop Med Hyg* 1975; 24:806–822.

97. Farid Z. Chronic urinary Salmonella carriers with intermittent bacteraemia. *J Egypt Public Health Assoc* 1970; 45:157–160.

98. Farid Z, Trabolsi B, Hafez A. Escherichia coli bacteraemia in chronic schistosomiasis. *Ann Trop Med Parasitol* 1984; 78:661–662.

99. Wright ED, Chiphangi J, Hutt MSR. Schistosomiasis of the female genital tract. A histopathological study of 176 cases from Malawi. *Trans R Soc Trop Med Hyg* 1982; 76:822–829.

100. Chen MG, Mott KE. Progress in the assessment of morbidity due to Schistosoma haematobium. A review of recent literature. In: Progress in assessment of morbidity due to Schistosomiasis. *Trop Dis Bull* 1989; 86:R1–R36.

101. Kjetland EF, Mudaluza T, Ndhiovu PD, et al. Genital schistosomiasis in women: a clinical 12-month study in vivo study following treatment with praziquantel. *Trans Roy Soc Trop Med Hyg* 2006; 100:740–752.

102. Higashi GI, Abdel-Salam E, Soliman M, et al. Immunofluorescent analysis of renal biopsies in uncomplicated Schistosoma haematobium infections in children. *J Trop Med Hyg* 1984; 87:123–129.

103. Sadigursky M, Andrade ZA, Danner R et al. Absence of Schistosomal glomerulopathy in Schistosoma haematobium infection in man. *Trans R Soc Trop Med Hyg* 1976; 70:322–323.

104. Farid Z, Higashi GI, Bassily S, et al. Chronic salmonellosis, urinary schistosomiasis and massive proteinuria. *Am J Trop Med Hyg* 1972; 21:578–581.

105. Nafeh MA, Medhat A, Swifae Y, et al. Ultrasonographic changes of the liver in Schistosoma haematobium infection. *Am J Trop Med Hyg* 1992; 47:225–230.

106. Nooman ZM, Nafeh MA, El-Kateb H, et al. Hepatosplenic disease caused by Bilharzia haematobium in Upper Egypt. *J Trop Med Hyg* 1974; 77:42–48.

107. Girges R. *Schistosomiasis (Bilhariasis)*. London: John Bale Sons and Danielson; 1934.

108. Adeyemi-Doro FAB, Osoba AO, Junaid TA. Perigenital cutaneous schistosomiasis. *Br J Vener Dis* 1979; 55:446–449.

109. Develoux M, Blanc L, Veller JM, et al. Bilharziose cutanée thoracique. *Ann Dermatol Vener* 1987; 114:695–697.

110. Hull PR, Hay IT. Peri-umbilical cutaneous schistosomiasis. *S Afr Med J* 1979; 53:654.

111. Macdonald DM, Morrison JGL. Cutaneous ectopic schistosomiasis. *BMJ* 1976; ii:619–620.

112. Obasi OE. Cutaneous schistosomiasis in Nigeria. An update. *Br J Dermatol* 1986; 114:597–602.

113. Scrimgeour EM, Gajdusek DC. Involvement of the central nervous system in Schistosoma mansoni and S. haematobium infection, a review. *Brain* 1985; 108:1023–1038.

114. van der Horst R. Schistosomiasis of the pericardium. *Trans R Soc Trop Med Hyg* 1979; 73:243–244.

115. Chitiyo ME. Schistosomal involvement of the choroid plexus. *Centr Afr J Med* 1972; 18:45–47.

116. Isebai I. Parasites in the aetiology of cancer: bilharziasis and bladder cancer. *CA Cancer J Clin* 1977; 27:100–106.

117. Makhyoun NA, El-Kashlan KM, Al-Ghorab MM, et al. Aetiological factors in bilharzial bladder cancer. *J Trop Med Hyg* 1971; 74:73–78.

118. Prates MD, Gillman J. Carcinoma of the urinary bladder in the Portuguese East Africa with special reference to bilharzial cystitis and preneoplastic reactions. *S Afr Med Sci* 1959; 24:13–40.

119. Lucas SB. Squamous cell carcinoma of the bladder and schistosomiasis. *East Afr Med J* 1982; 59:345–351.

120. Kuntz RE, Cheevers AW, Myers BJ. Proliferative epithelial lesions of the urinary bladder of nonhuman primates infected with Schistosoma haematobium. *J Natl Cancer Inst* 1972; 48:223–235.

121. Hicks RM, James C, Webbe G. Effect of S. haematobium and N-butyl-N-(4-hydroxy butyl)nitrosamine on the development of urothelial neoplasia in the baboon. *Br J Cancer* 1980; 42:730–755.

122. Hicks RM, Ismael MM, Walters CL, et al. Association of bacteriuria and urinary nitrosamine formation with Schistosoma haematobium infection in the Qualyub area of Egypt. *Trans R Soc Trop Med Hyg* 1982; 76:519–528.

123. Cheever AW. Schistosomiasis and neoplasia. *J Natl Cancer Inst* 1978; 61:13–18.

124. Attah EB, Nkposong EO. Schistosomiasis and carcinoma of the bladder: a critical review of causal relationship. *Trop Geogr Med* 1976; 28:268–272.

125. World Health Organization. Schistosomes, liver flukes and Helicobacter pylori. *IARC Monographs on the Evaluation of Carcinogenic Risks to Humans.* Vol. 61. Geneva: WHO; 1994.

126. Chen MG, Mott KE. Progress in assessment of morbidity due to Schistosoma mansoni infection. In: Progress in assessment of morbidity due to schistosomiasis. Reviews of recent literature. *Trop Dis Bull* 1988; 85:R1–R56.

127. Warren KS. The kinetics of hepatosplenic schistosomiasis. *Semin Liver Dis* 1984; 4:293–300.

128. Dunn MA, Kamel R. Hepatic schistosomiasis. *Hepatology* 1981; 1:653–661.

129. Warren KS. The relevance of schistosomiasis. *N Engl J Med* 1980; 303:203–206.

130. Dunn MA, Kamel R, Kamel IA, et al. Liver collagen synthesis in schistosomiasis mansoni. *Gastroenterology* 1979; 76:978–982.

131. Andrade ZA, Abreu WN. Follicular lymphoma of the spleen in patients with hepatosplenic schistosomiasis mansoni. *Am J Trop Med Hyg* 1971; 20:237–243.

132. Chen MG, Mott KE. Progress in assessment of morbidity due to Schistosoma japonicum. A review of recent literature. In: Progress in assessment of morbidity due to Schistosomiasis. *Trop Dis Bull* 1988; 85:R1–R45.

133. Barsoum RS, Bassily S, Soliman MM, et al. Renal amyloidosis and schistosomiasis. *Trans R Soc Trop Med Hyg* 1979; 73:367–374.

134. Pitella JEH, Lana-Peixoto M. Brain involvement in hepatosplenic schistosomiasis mansoni. *Brain* 1981; 104:621–632.

135. Bittencourt AL, Almeida MAC, Inues MAF, et al. Placental involvement in schistosomiasis mansoni; report of four cases. *Am J Trop Med Hyg* 1980; 29:571–575.

136. Chen MG. Relative distribution of Schistosoma japonicum eggs in the intestine of man: a subject of inconsistency. *Acta Trop* 1990; 48:163–171.

137. Mao SP, He YX, Yang YQ, et al. Schistosoma japonicum and schistosomiasis japonica. In: Wu ZJ, Mao SP, Wang JW, eds. *Chinese Medical Encyclopaedia, Parasitology and Parasitic Diseases.* Shanghai: Shanghai Publishing House for Sciences and Technology; 1984:44–55 [in Chinese].

138. Santos AT. The present status of schistosomiasis in the Philippines. *Southeast Asian J Trop Med Public Health* 1984; 15:439–445.

139. Garin D, Chapalain JC, Thierry J, et al. Le point sur Schistosoma intercalatum. *Med Trop* 1990; 50:433–440.

140. van Wijk HB, Elias EA. Hepatic and rectal pathology in Schistosoma intercalatum infection. *Trop Geogr Med* 1975; 27:237–248.

141. Stuiver PC. Acute schistosomiasis (Katayama fever). *BMJ* 1984; 288:221–222.

142. Centers for Disease Control. Acute schistosomiasis in US travelers returning from Africa. *MMWR* 1990; 39:141–148.

143. Farid Z, Bassily S, Kent DC, et al. Chronic urinary salmonella carriers with intermittent bacteraemia. *Am J Trop Med Hyg* 1970; 73:153–156.

144. Farid Z, Kilpatrick ME, Ishak EA. S. Haematobium and S. Intercalatum. Clinical and pathological aspects. In: Jordan P, Webbe G, Sturrock RF, eds. *Human Schistosomiasis*, 3rd edn. Wallingford: CAB International; 1993:159–193.

145. Simarro PP, Sima FO, Mir M. African trypanosomiasis and Schistosoma intercalatum infection in Equatorial Guinea: comparative epidemiology and feasibility of integrated control. *Trop Med Parasitol* 1989; 40:159–162.

146. Simarro PP, Sima FO, Mir M. Urban epidemiology of Schistosoma intercalatum in the city of Bata, Equatorial Guinea. *Trop Med Parasitol* 1990; 41:254–256.

147. Arene FO, Ukpeibo ET, Nwanze EA. Studies on schistosomiasis in the Niger Delta; Schistosoma intercalatum in the urban city of Port Harcourt, Nigeria. *Public Health* 1989; 103:295–301.

148. Corachan M, Escosa R, Mass J, et al. Clinical presentations of Schistosoma intercalatum infestation. *Lancet* 1987; I:1139.

149. Deelder AM, De Jonge N, Boerman OC, et al. Sensitive determination of circulating anodic antigen in Schistosoma mansoni infected individuals by an enzyme-linked immunosorbent assay using monoclonal antibodies. *Am J Trop Med Hyg* 1989; 40:268–272.

150. De Jonge J, Fillié YE, Hilberath GW, et al. Presence of the schistosome circulating anodic antigen (CAA) in urine of patients with Schistosoma mansoni or S. haematobium infections. *Am J Trop Med Hyg* 1989; 41:563–569.

151. De Jonge N, Schommer G, Krikger FW, et al. Presence of circulating anodic antigen in serum of Schistosoma intercalatum-infected patients from Gabon. *Acta Trop* 1989; 46:115–120.

152. De Jonge N, Rabello ALT, Krijger FW, et al. Levels of the schistosome circulating anodic and cathodic antigens in serum of schistosomiasis patients from Brazil. *Trans R Soc Trop Med Hyg* 1991; 85:756–759.

153. Kremsner PG, De Jonge N, Simarro PP, et al. Quantitative determination of circulating anodic and cathodic antigens in serum and urine of individuals infected with Schistosoma intercalatum. *Trans R Soc Trop Med Hyg* 1993; 87:167–169.

154. Braun-Munzinger RA, Southgate BA. Repeatability and reproducibility of egg counts of Schistosoma haematobium in urine. *Trop Med Parasitol* 1992; 43:149–154.

155. Cook JA, Jordan P. Excretion of Schistosoma mansoni eggs in the urine. *Trans R Soc Trop Med Hyg* 1970; 64:793–794.

156. Bell DR. In East African Institute for Medical Research: Annual Report 1961–1962. Kenya: Government Printer; 1962:24.

157. Dazo BC, Biles JE. Two new field techniques for detection and counting of Schistosoma haematobium eggs in urine samples. *Bull World Health Organ* 1974; 51:399–408.

158. Peters PA, Warren KS, Mahmoud AAF. Rapid accurate quantification of schistosome eggs via nuclepore filters. *J Parasitol* 1976; 62:154–155.

159. Peters PA, Mahmoud AAF, Warren KS, et al. Field studies of rapid accurate means of quantifying Schistosoma haematobium eggs in urine samples. *Bull World Health Organ* 1976; 54:159–162.

160. Mott KE, Baltes R, Bambahga J, et al. Field studies of a reusable polyamide filter for detection of Schistosoma haematobium eggs by urine filtration. *Trop Med Parasitol* 1981; 33:227–228.

161. Mott KE. A reusable polyamide filter for diagnosis of S. haematobium infection by urine filtration. *Bull Soc Pathol Exot* 1983; 76:101–104.

162. Braun-Munzinger RA, Rohde R. False epidemiological results from the bulk transport of dried filter paper in urinary schistosomiasis. *Trop Med Parasitol* 1986; 37:286–289.

163. Ritchie LS. An ether sedimentation technique for routine stool examination. *Bull US Army Med Dept* 1948; 8:326.

164. Hunter GW III, Hodges EP, Jahnes WG, et al. Studies on schistosomiasis. II. Summary of further studies on methods of recovering eggs of S. japonicum. *Bull US Army Med Dept* 1948; 8:128–131.

165. Blagg W, Schaegel EL, Mansour NS. A new concentration technique for the demonstration of protozoa and helminthic eggs in the faeces. *Am J Trop Med Hyg* 1955; 4:23–28.

166. Knight WB, Hiatt RA, Cline BL, et al. A modification of the formol-ether concentration technique for increased sensitivity in detecting Schistosoma mansoni eggs. *Am J Trop Med Hyg* 1970; 25:818–823.

167. Allen AVH, Ridley DS. Further observations on the formol-ether concentration technique for faecal parasites. *J Clin Pathol* 1970; 23:545–546.

168. Visser PS, Pitchford RJ. A simple apparatus for rapid recovery of helminthic eggs from excreta with special reference to Schistosoma mansoni. *S Afr Med J* 1972; 46:1344–1346.

169. Komiya Y, Kobayashi A. Evaluation of Kato's thick smear with a cellophane cover for helminth eggs in faeces. *Jpn J Med Sci Biol* 1966; 19:59–64.

170. Katz N, Chaves A, Pellegrino J. A simple device for quantitative thick smear technique in schistosomiasis mansoni. *Rev Inst Med Trop Sâo Paulo* 1972; 14:397–400.

171. Teesdale CH, Amin MA. Comparison of the Bell technique, a modified Kato thick smear technique and a digestion method for the field diagnosis of schistosomiasis mansoni. *J Helminthol* 1976; 59:17–20.

172. Teesdale CH, Amin MA. A simple thick smear technique for the diagnosis of Schistosoma mansoni infection. *Bull World Health Organ* 1976; 54:703–705.

173. Chitsulo L, Teesdale CH, Dixon H. Comparison of the Teesdale glass sandwich and Kato-Katz techniques for the diagnosis of Schistosoma mansoni; a double-blind study. *Trop Med Parasitol* 1990; 41:447–449.

174. Fulleborn F. Über den Nachweis der Schistosomum mansoni: Eir in Stuhle. *Arch Schiffs Tropenkr Hamburg* 1921; 25:334–340.

175. Fun-Zhi. Schistosomiasis Shou Chai, 2nd edn. (Prevention and control of schistosomiasis handbook compiled by the Revolutionary Committee of Shanghai Schistosomiasis Research Institute.) Shanghai: People's Press; 1971 [in Chinese].

176. Shanghai Municipal Institute for Prevention and Treatment of Schistosomiasis. Handbook on the Prevention and Treatment of

Schistosomiasis (translated by the US Department of Health, Education and Welfare, Public Health Service, National Institutes of Health). DHEW publication No. NIH77-1290. 1977:61-69.

177. Gorman S, Ross WF, Blair DM. The macroscopic diagnosis of urinary schistosomiasis. *S Afr Med J* 1947; 21:853-854.

178. Meeser SV, Ross WF, Blair DM. Further observations on the macroscopic diagnosis of urinary schistosomiasis. *J Trop Med Hyg* 1948; 51:54-59.

179. Weber MC. Miracidial hatching. *Centr Afr J Med* 1973; 19(suppl 9):11-14.

180. Davis A. Field trials of 'Ambilhar' in the treatment of urinary bilharziasis in schoolchildren. *Bull World Health Organ* 1966; 35:827-835.

181. Davis A. Comparative trials of antimonial drugs in urinary schistosomiasis. *Bull World Health Organ* 1968; 38:197-227.

182. Braun-Munzinger RA, Southgate BA. Egg viability in urinary schistosomiasis. I. New methods compared with available methods. *J Trop Med Hyg* 1993; 96:22-27.

183. Braun-Munzinger RA, Southgate BA. Egg viability in urinary schistosomiasis. II. Simplifying modifications and standardization of new methods. *J Trop Med Hyg* 1993; 96:71-75.

184. Braun-Munzinger RA, Southgate BA. Egg viability in urinary schistosomiasis. III. Repeatability and reproducibility of new methods. *J Trop Med Hyg* 1993; 96:179-185.

185. Upatham ES, Sturrock RF, Cook JA. Studies on the hatchability of Schistosoma mansoni from a naturally infected human community on St Lucia, West Indies. *Parasitology* 1976; 73:253-264.

186. Zicker F, Katz N, Wolf J. Availaçao do teste de ecloso de miracidios na equistossoma mansonica. *Rev Bras Malariol Doencas Trop* 1977; 30:65-75.

187. Da Cunha AS. A availiaçao terapéutica da oxamniquine na equistossomose mansoni humana pelo metodo do oograma per biopsia de mucosa rectal. *Rev Inst Med Trop Sâo Paulo* 1982; 24:88-94.

188. Briggs M, Chatfield M, Mummery D, et al. Screening with reagent strips. *BMJ* 1971; iii:433-434.

189. Wilkins HA, Goll P, Marshall TF, et al. The significance of proteinuria and haematuria in Schistosoma haematobium infection. *Trans R Soc Trop Hyg* 1979; 73:74-80.

190. Pugh RNH, Bell DR, Gilles HM. Malumfashi endemic diseases research project. XV. The potential medical importance of bilharzia in northern Nigeria: a suggested rapid cheap and effective solution for control of Schistosoma haematobium infection. *Ann Trop Med Parasitol* 1980; 74:597-613.

191. Feldmeir H, Doehring E, Dafallah AA. Simultaneous use of a sensitive filtration technique and reagent strips in urinary schistosomiasis. *Trans R Soc Trop Med Hyg* 1982; 76:416-421.

192. Savioli L, Hatz C, Dixon H, et al. Control of morbidity due to Schistosoma haematobium on Pemba Island: egg excretion and haematuria as indicators of infection. *Am J Trop Med Hyg* 1990; 43:289-295.

193. Mott KE, Dixon H. Collaborative study on antigens for immunodiagnosis of schistosomiasis. *Bull World Health Organ* 1981; 60:729-753.

194. Mott KE, Dixon H, Carter CE, et al. Collaborative study on antigens for immunodiagnosis of Schistosoma japonicum infections. *Bull World Health Organ* 1987; 65:233-244.

195. Bergquist R. In: Bergquist R, ed. *Immunodiagnostic Approaches in Schistosomiasis.* Chichester: Wiley; 1992:1-8.

196. van Lieshout L, Polderman AM, Deelder AM. Immunodiagnosis of schistosomiasis by determination of the circulating antigens CAA and CCA, in particular in individuals with recent or light infection. *Acta Tropica* 2000; 77:69-80.

197. Abdel-Waheb MF, Strickland GT. Abdominal ultrasonography for assessing morbidity from schistosomiasis. 2. Hospital studies. *Trans R Soc Trop Med Hyg* 1993; 87:135-137.

198. Hatz C, Jenkins JM, Tanner M. Ultrasound in schistosomiasis. *Acta Tropica* 1992; 51:1-97.

199. World Health Organization. Meeting on ultrasonography in Schistosomiasis. UNDP/World Bank/WHO Special Programme for Research and Training in Tropical Diseases. TDR/SCH/ULTRASON/91.3, CTD/91.3. Geneva: WHO; 1991:1-32 (unpublished document).

200. Abdel-Wahab MF, Esmat G, Narooz SI, et al. Sonographic studies of schoolchildren in a village endemic for Schistosoma haematobium. *Trans R Soc Trop Med Hyg* 1990; 84:69-73.

201. Abdel-Waheb MF, Esmat G, Farrag A, et al. Grading of hepatic schistosomiasis by the use of ultrasonography. *Am J Trop Med Hyg* 1992; 46:403-408.

202. Abdel-Wahab MF, Esmat G, Milad M, et al. Characteristic sonographic patterns of Schistosomal hepatic fibrosis. *Am J Trop Med Hyg* 1989; 40:72-76.

203. Abdel-Waheb MF, Esmat G, Farrag A, et al. Ultrasonographic prediction of esophageal varices in schistosomiasis mansoni. *Am J Gastroenterol* 1993; 88:560-563.

204. Davis A. The Professor Gerald Webbe Memorial Lecture. Global control of schistosomiasis. *Trans R Soc Trop Med Hyg* 2000; 94:609-615.

205. Ajana F, Dei-Cas E, Colin JJ, et al. La bilharziose humaine à Schistosoma mekongi; problèmes diagnostiques et thérapeutiques. *Méd Mal Infect* 1986 3:141-146.

206. Chidiac C, Beaucaire G, Mouton Y, et al. Echecs au praziquantel dans le traitement des bilharzioses; intérêt de la biopsie de muqueuse rectale et du suivi prolonge. *Méd Mal Infect* 1986; 5:380-384.

207. Duong TH, Furet Y, Lorett G, et al. Traitement de la bilharziose à Schistosoma mekongi par le praziquantel. *Méd Trop* 1988; 48:39-43.

208. Manoury V, Guillemot F, Mathieu-Chandelier C, et al. Bilharzioses à Schistosoma mekongi diagnostiquées par biopsie rectale et traitées par praziquantel; à propos de 5 cases. *Gastroenterol Clin Biol* 1990; 14:1032-1033.

209. Ismael M, Metwally A, Farghaly A, et al. Characterization of isolates of Schistosoma mansoni from Egyptian villagers that tolerate high doses of praziquantel. Am J Trop Med Hyg 1996; 55:212-218.

210. Ismael M, Botros S, Metwally A, et al. Resistance to praziquantel. Direct evidence from Schistosoma mansoni isolated from Egyptian villagers. Am J Trop Med Hyg 1999; 60:932-935.

211. Fallon PG, Doenhoff MJ. Drug resistant schistosomiasis: resistance to praziquantel and oxamniquine induced in Schistosoma mansoni in mice is drug specific. *Am J Trop Med Hyg* 1994; 51:83-89.

212. Gryseels B, Stelma FF, Talla I, et al. Epidemiology, immunology and chemotherapy of Schistosoma mansoni infections in a recently expressed community in Senegal. *Trop Geogr Med* 1994; 46:209-219.

213. Stelma FF, Talma I, Sow S, et al. Efficacy and side-effects of praziquantel in an epidemic focus of Schistosoma mansoni. *Am J Trop Med Hyg* 1995; 53:167-170.

214. Guissé F, Polman K, Stelma FF, et al. Therapeutic evaluation of two different dose regimens of praziquantel in a recent Schistosoma mansoni focus in northern Senegal. *Am J Trop Med Hyg* 1997; 56:511-514.

215. Liang YS, Coles GC, Doenhoff MJ. Detection of praziquantel resistance in schistosomes. *Trop Med Int Health* 2000; 5:72.

216. Liang YS, Dai JR, Ning A, et al. Susceptibility of Schistosoma japonicum to praziquantel in China. *Trop Med Int Health* 2001; 6(9):707-714.

217. King CH, Muchiri EM, Ouma JH. Evidence against rapid emergence of praziquantel resistance in Schistosoma haematobium, Kenya. *Emerg Infect Dis* 2000; 6(6):585-593.

218. Foster R, Cheetham BL. Studies with the schistosomicide oxamniquine (UK-4721). I. Activities in rodents and in vitro. *Trans R Soc Trop Med Hyg* 1973; 67:674-684.

219. Foster R, Cheetham BL, King DF. Studies with the schistosomicide oxamniquine (UK-4271). II. Activity in primates. *Trans R Soc Trop Med Hyg* 1973; 67:685-693.

220. Bassily S, Farid Z, Higashi GI, et al. Treatment of complicated schistosomiasis mansoni with oxamniquine. *Am J Trop Med Hyg* 1978; 27:1284-1286.

221. Farid Z, Higashi GI, Bassily S. Treatment of advanced hepatosplenic with oxamniquine. *Trans R Soc Trop Med Hyg* 1980; 74:400-401.

222. Abaza HH, Hammouda N, Abd Rabbo H, et al. Chemotherapy of Schistosomal polyposis with oxamniquine. *Trans R Soc Trop Med Hyg* 1978; 72:602-604.

223. Machado PA. The Brazilian control programme for schistosomiasis control 1975–1979. *Am J Trop Med Hyg* 1982; 31:76–86.

224. Stokvis H, Bauer AGC, Stuiver PC, et al. Seizures associated with oxamniquine therapy. *Am J Trop Med Hyg* 1986; 35:330–331.

225. Higashi GI, Farid Z. Oxamniquine fever: drug induced or immune complex reaction. *BMJ* 1979; 2:830.

226. Katz N, Rocha RS, De Souza CP, et al. Efficacy of alternating therapy with oxamniquine and praziquantel to treat Schistosoma mansoni in children following failure of first treatment. *Am J Trop Med Hyg* 1991; 44:509–512.

227. Botros S, William S, Ebeid F, et al. Lack of evidence for an antischistosomal activity of myrrh in experimental animals. *Am J Trop Med Hyg* 2004; 71(2):206–210.

228. Barakat R, Elmorshedy H, Fenwick A. Efficacy of myrrh in the treatment of human Schistosomiasis mansoni. *Am J Trop Med Hyg* 2005; 73(2): 365–367.

229. Xiao SH, You JQ, Yang YQ, et al. Experimental studies on early treatment of Schistosomal infection with artemether. Southeast Asian. *J Trop Med Public Health* 1995; 26:306–318.

230. Xiao SH, You JQ, Mei JY, et al. Preventive effect of artemether in rabbits infected with Schistosoma japonicum cerariae. *Acta Pharmacol Sin* 1998; 19:63–66.

231. Xiao SH, Booth M, Tanner M. The prophylactic effect of artemether against Schistosoma japonicum infections. *Parasitol Today* 2000; 16:122–126.

232. Xiao SH, Catto BA. In vitro and in vivo studies of the effect of artemether on Schistosoma mansoni. *Antimicrob Agents Chemother* 1989; 33:1557–1562.

233. Xiao SH, Chollet J, Weiss NA, et al. Preventive effect of artemether in experimental animals infected with Schistosoma mansoni. *Parasitol Int* 2000; 49:19–24.

234. Bergquist R, Ming-Gang C, Xiao-Nong Z, et al, (eds.). Control of schistosomiasis in China. *Acta Tropica* 2005; 96:67–328.

235. Mansour NM, Omer Ali P, Farid Z, et al. Serological differentiation of acute and chronic schistosomiasis mansoni by antibody responses to keyhole limpet haemocyanin. *Am J Trop Med Hyg* 1989; 41:338–344.

236. Watt G, Adapon B, Long GW, et al. Praziquantel in treatment of cerebral schistosomiasis. *Lancet* 1986; ii:529–532.

237. Ezzat FA, Abu-Elmagd KM, Aly MA, et al. Selective shunt versus nonshunt surgery for management of both Schistosomal and nonSchistosomal variceal bleeders. *Ann Surg* 1990; 212:97–108.

238. Davis A. Metriphonate. In: Dollery C, ed. *Therapeutic Drugs*. Vol. 2. Edinburgh: Churchill Livingstone; 1991:M164–M170.

239. Davis A. Oxamniquine. In: Dollery C, ed. *Therapeutic Drugs*. Vol. 2. Edinburgh: Churchill Livingstone; 1991:O42–O45.

240. Wegner DHG. Praziquantel. In Dollery C (ed.) *Therapeutic Drugs*. Vol. 2. Edinburgh: Churchill Livingstone; 1991:P189–P195.

241. Davis A. AntiSchistosomal drugs and clinical practice. In: Jordan P, Webbe G, Sturrock RF, eds. *Human Schistosomiasis*. 3rd edn. Wallingford: CAB International; 1993:367–404.

242. Canning D. Priority setting and the 'neglected' tropical diseases. *Trans R Soc Trop Med Hyg* 2006; 100(6):499–504.

243. Fenwick A. New initiatives against Africa's worms. *Trans R Soc Trop Med Hyg* 2006; 100(3):200–207.

244. Richards FO Jr, Eigege A, Miri ES, et al. Integration of mass drug administration programmes in Nigeria: The challenge of schistosomiasis. *Bull World Health Org* 2006; 84(8):673–676.

245. Sinuon M, Tsuyuoka R, Socheat D, et al. Control of Schistosoma mekongi in Cambodia: results of eight years of control activities in the two endemic provinces. *Trans R Soc Trop Med Hyg* 2007; 101(1):34–39.

246. World Health Organization. The control of schistosomiasis. Second Report of the WHO Expert Committee. *WHO Tech Rep Ser* 1993; 830: 1–86.

247. Mott KE, ed. *Plant Molluscicides*. Published on behalf of the UNDP/World Bank/WHO Special Programme for Research and Training in Tropical Diseases. Chichester: Wiley; 1987.

248. McCullough FS. The use of mollusciciding in Schistosomiasis control. WHO/SCHISTO/92.107 Geneva: WHO; 1992 (unpublished document).

249. Bergquist NR. Controlling schistosomiasis by vaccination: a realistic option? *Parasitol Today* 1995; 11:191–194.

250. Bergquist NR, Colley DG. Schistosomiasis vaccines: research to development. *Parasitol Today* 1998; 14(3):99–104.

251. Capron A, Rriveau G, Capron M. Vaccine strategies against schistosomiasis: from concepts to clinical trials. In: *Conference and Abstract Book: New Challenges in Tropical Medicine and Parasitology*, 18–22 September, Oxford, 2000:58–59 (Abstract PL10.2).

252. Gryseels B. Schistosomiasis vaccines: a devil's advocate view. *Parasitol Today* 2000; 16(2):46–47.

253. Stuck M-M. Chances and risks of developing vaccines. *Vaccine* 1996; 14(14):1301–1302.

Chapter 83   Paiboon Sithithaworn, Banchob Sripa, Sasithorn Kaewkes and Melissa Haswell-Elkins

Food-borne Trematodes

The liver flukes (*Fasciola, Opisthorchis, Clonorchis*), lung flukes (*Paragonimus*) and intestinal flukes (*Fasciolopsis, Echinostoma, Heterophyes*) are important causes of human disease. Although these are commonly thought of as 'tropical' parasites, some species are not limited to hot climates. An extreme example is *Opisthorchis felineus* which is commonly acquired through the consumption of raw frozen fish in Siberia. The availability of freshwater flora and fauna and a preference for eating them raw or incompletely cooked are the most important factors determining their distribution in man.

All food-borne trematodes belong to the subclass Digenea. Digenean trematodes undergo sexual reproduction in their definitive hosts (e.g. human or mammals) and asexual reproduction in their intermediate hosts (snail) (Table 83.1). Their life cycles are complex and involve one or more intermediate hosts (the first always being a snail) and several morphological stages. Eggs pass out of the definitive host in faeces (in some cases sputum) and those which reach freshwater can infect susceptible snails. Development in the snail results in the release of numerous cercariae which swim about until they contact a suitable plant or animal where encystment occurs to form metacercariae. The life cycle is completed and continues when viable metacercariae are ingested by susceptible definitive hosts.

Among the thousands of food-borne trematodes, hundreds may infect man, and new species are still being discovered.[1-3] Because most species also parasitize other animals and are of veterinary importance, the term 'accidental' is sometimes used to describe human infections. The term is appropriate for some representatives, such as *Fasciola*, which in most endemic areas occurs in isolated cases or outbreaks, or for flukes rarely reported in humans, e.g. *Watsoni, Dicrocoelium, Eurytrema, Metorchis*. However, estimates that 40 million people harbour food-borne trematodes[4,5] argue against a major role of chance in most infections.

The endemic areas of these parasites often overlap, since people often enjoy many kinds of raw food. For example, adult worms of 13 food-borne trematode species (plus *Taenia saginata*) were found among 224 residents of a single village in north-east Thailand.[2] Up to seven species have been reported in a single individual.[6] Some authors have reported an association between 'tastiness' of fish and the season or species with the highest intensity of infective stages.[7] This may reflect an influence of human taste preference on parasite life cycles.

Food-borne trematodes have received less attention than other helminth infections, perhaps because of their focal distribution and lack of acute symptoms. However, some authors have mistak-enly reported them as comparatively benign, which is certainly not the case for the liver flukes and *Paragonimus*, as reviewed here. Severity of disease is associated with the number of worms present, except perhaps in the case of ectopic infections, where a single worm can cause serious pathology.

Due to growing tourism, migration and international trade of fishery products, infections previously confined to endemic areas are increasingly being reported in non-endemic countries.[4,5] There is also evidence that some endemic areas are expanding due to domestic migration, environmental changes that favour snail proliferation, declining economic conditions and sanitation, and increasing availability of contaminated foods through wider distribution networks in the absence of food inspections.[1,8-11] On the other hand, as newly industrialized countries alter their natural environment and pollute their river systems, native snail, crustacean and fish fauna decline. Night-soil and manure, potentially containing fluke eggs, are being replaced by chemical fertilizer. Thus risk of infection by eating raw 'wild' foods might be gradually replaced by risk of exposure to potentially hazardous chemicals.

Efforts to control food-borne parasites are largely dependent on chemotherapy. The drug of choice for treatment of most food-borne trematodes is praziquantel, which is now inexpensive and widely available. In the case of *Fasciola*, an effective drug for treatment is triclabendazole.[12] However, in addition to anthelmintic treatment to cure current infection, improvements in sanitation and health promotion to encourage the cooking of foods involved in transmission are important components of control to prevent reinfection. Although eating habits have cultural and social significance and often are difficult to change, finding ways to reduce exposure to parasites through food is essential.[13,14] Introduction of good aquaculture practices for fish farmers in accordance with the requirements for the production of safe and quality fish, particularly on a commercial sector for food processing for safe consumption of fish, should be encouraged.[5]

LIVER FLUKES

Opisthorchiasis and clonorchiasis

Aetiology

The human liver flukes, *Clonorchis sinensis, Opisthorchis viverrini* and *O. felineus*, remain important public health problems in many

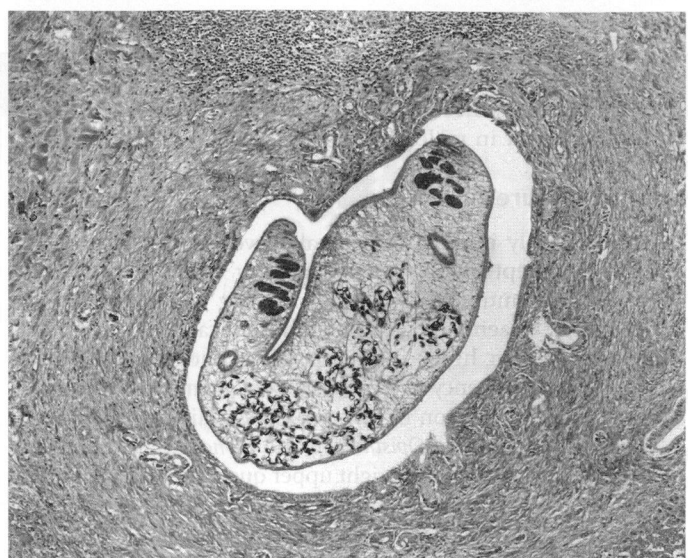

Figure 83.3 Histopathology of chronic *Opisthorchis viverrini* infection in human. An adult fluke is seen in the bile duct lumen. Adenomatous hyperplasia and inflammation with prominent periductal fibrosis are noted.

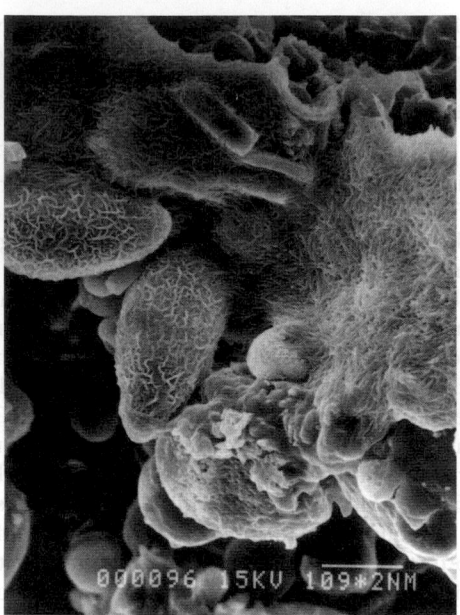

Figure 83.4 Scanning electron micrograph of gallstone showing liver fluke eggs with typical mush-melon-eggshell surface in the nidus of the stone.

(odds ratio = 8.6).[52] A history of raw fish consumption, positive serological test for clonorchiasis[52] and area of residence[53] were also linked to increased risk of CCA.

A special feature of *O. felineus* infection, not often reported for the other species, is acute opisthorchiasis.[36] This is characterized by hepatosplenomegaly and tenderness, eosinophilia up to 40%, and chills and fever. It occurs early in infection and may be associated with primary exposure to a large dose of metacercariae. However, there appear to be no recent reports of this phenomena.

Pathology and pathogenesis

Liver enlargement and dilated subcapsular bile ducts with thick fibrotic walls can be seen grossly in heavily infected cases.[17,18,20,28,34,54] Microscopically, bile duct pathology is characterized by desquamation of epithelial cells of secondary and tertiary ducts and chronic inflammation with infiltration of lymphocytes, monocytes, eosinophils and plasma cells (Figure 83.3). Granulomatous inflammation around the eggs is occasionally observed along the bile ducts. Epithelial hyperplasia may occur at early stage of infection. In severe cases, adenomatous hyperplasia, and goblet cell metaplasia may be seen. Periductal fibrosis is the most prominent histological feature of chronic infection.[32,54] This corresponds to periportal echoes detected by ultrasonography. Inflammation, necrosis and atrophy of hepatic cells have also been reported.

The pathology of fluke-associated cholecystitis consists of fibrosis, infiltration of mast cells and eosinophils and mucosal hyperplasia of the gallbladder wall.[54,55] Perforation of the gallbladder wall is uncommon in liver fluke infection. Parasites and eggs have been observed in the nidus of gallbladder and intrahepatic stones (Figure 83.4).[34,56]

The pathogenesis of liver fluke-mediated tissue damage may be directly via mechanical or chemical irritation and/or immune-mediated.[32,54,57,58] Mechanical injury from the activities of feeding, movement and migration of flukes contributes to biliary ulceration through its suckers. Chemical irritation results as the liver fluke secretes or excretes metabolic products from the tegument and excretory openings into the bile. Some of these products are highly mitogenic to fibroblast or biliary cell lines when co-cultured in vitro with the flukes.[54,59] This suggests that excreted or secreted fluke products may cause the long observed hyperplasia of biliary epithelial cells typical of opisthorchiasis. Moreover, the fluke excretory–secretory products are also highly immunogenic and stimulate marked inflammatory infiltration in the intrahepatic and extrahepatic bile ducts in animals experimentally infected with *Opisthorchis*.[58] Nitric oxide and other reactive oxygen intermediates produced by inflammatory cells during infection might exert direct cytotoxic and mutagenic effects and increased cell proliferation.[60] Increased formation of 8-nitroguanine (8-NO_2-G) and 8-oxo-7,8-dihydro-2'-deoxyguanosine (8-oxodG) has been observed in experimentally infected animals, a response that is enhanced with repeated infection and considered to be mutagenic.[61,62] Increased endogenous production of *N*-nitroso compounds and enhanced hepatic activation of carcinogens in these areas of fibrosis may create highly mutagenic conditions for the chronically proliferating bile duct epithelium. All together these form an ideal environment for cancer development.[19,63–65]

Diagnosis and investigation

Egg detection in faeces or bile content is the traditional diagnostic method for liver fluke infection. The most frequently used methods to detect eggs in the faeces are the Kato thick smear, Stoll's dilution and the quantitative formalin ethyl acetate concentration technique. All three techniques effectively detect moderate and heavy infections. However, comparative studies in low-intensity areas have shown that a single reading of the concentration and dilution techniques detect about 70% of infections, while the sensitivity of Kato is considerably lower (45%). Worm burden and egg count correlate closely, with an estimated egg output of 53/g of faeces per worm (using Stoll's dilution technique).[66] Stoll's egg counts tend to be higher than those derived using the concentration technique.

Although egg detection is almost always used in surveys and treatment programmes, several immunodiagnostic tests have been described for *Opisthorchis* and *Clonorchis* infections.[34,67,68] While most antigens of these flukes are non-specific and antibodies persist long after treatment, good results have been gained from new serological tests using individual antigens and those detecting isotype-specific antibodies. Faecal antigen detection by enzyme-linked immunosorbent assays (ELISAs) using monoclonal antibodies against secretory antigens and DNA probes also shows promise.[69,70] However, more recent attention has been focused on the detection of egg DNA in faecal specimen by polymerase chain reaction (PCR) which is effective in the diagnosis of liver fluke infection in experimental animals as well as in humans.[71-73]

Management

Treatment with praziquantel at 40 mg/kg body weight in a single dose is effective against opisthorchiasis and clonorchiasis.[12,32,74] This regimen has been used most commonly in large-scale treatment programmes. The most effective recommended regimen particularly for clonorchiasis is 25 mg/kg three times over 1 day (total dose 75 mg/kg).[32] Side-effects, such as dizziness, vomiting and abdominal pain, occur frequently but are transient and rarely severe. Most abnormalities of the gallbladder are also eliminated by elimination of the parasite.[46] Concerns have been raised that praziquantel treatment could possibly be dangerous for people with early cholangiocarcinoma, since the sudden expulsion of many worms might aggravate obstruction caused by the tumour. The drug hexachloroparaxylol (Chloxyle) has also been used extensively for the treatment of *O. felineus*, but it may be less effective than praziquantel.

Prevention and control

Prevention of human liver fluke infection can be facilitated by treatment (to reduce the excretion of eggs), sanitation (to prevent eggs from reaching water sources) and health education (to discourage the eating of raw fish).[10,13,32] The application of Hazard Analysis Critical Control Point principles and procedures during fish farming can reduce metacercarial contamination of fish.[75] Control of snail vectors by molluscicides is not considered feasible because of their widespread distribution and resistance to adverse conditions. To be most effective, health education should be designed and delivered in a culturally sensitive manner with the aim of stimulating behaviour change as well as simply providing information. Targeting young age groups, for example, school children, may be an attractive choice for long-term control. Large-scale efforts in endemic areas by public health ministries have probably had a major impact on the intensity of all three infections.

Fascioliasis

There are an estimated 2.4 million people infected with the two larger human liver flukes, *Fasciola hepatica* and *Fasciola gigantica*, often causing serious acute and chronic morbidity.[4,76,77] These parasites commonly infect domestic ruminants and wildlife throughout the world and indirectly impact on human well-being through massive economic loss in the livestock industry. Humans usually become infected by eating aquatic plants grown in water that is contaminated with faeces from animals harbouring *Fasciola*.

History and seminal discoveries

Fasciola hepatica was the first trematode to be described – 500 years before most others (de Brie, 1379; cited in Beaver et al. 1984[28]). Its complete life cycle was identified by Leuckart (1882) and Thomas (1883); this greatly facilitated the elucidation of other trematode life cycles. The successful search for effective veterinary vaccines through elegant immunological and molecular biochemistry studies has increased our understanding of host and trematode parasite relationship.

Aetiology and life cycle

F. hepatica (the sheep liver fluke) and *F. gigantica* (mainly of cattle) cause human fascioliasis. The parasites vary in adult and egg size and shape (Figure 83.5) and species of the snail host of the family Lymnaeidae. *F. hepatica* is common in temperate and subtropical areas, especially in sheep-raising areas. Human infections are relatively common in Europe (especially France, Spain, UK and Portugal), the Middle East (particularly Egypt and Iran), Central and South America (Cuba, Peru, Ecuador and Bolivia) and Africa.[76,77] *F. gigantica* occurs in South and South-east Asia and Africa. The two co-exist in some countries, and differentiation is difficult.

The adult worm lives in the bile duct of the final host, which may be sheep (*F. hepatica*), cattle/buffalo (*F. gigantica*) or humans. Eggs are excreted in the faeces. The eggs undergo further development upon reaching a water body; miracidia then hatch and penetrate a suitable snail host. After multiplication as sporocysts and rediae, free-swimming mature cercariae exit the snail, attach to aquatic vegetation and become metacercarial cysts. These cysts establish infection upon ingestion by man and other mammals. They excyst in the duodenum, then migrate through the intestinal wall, into the body cavity, through Glisson's capsule across the liver parenchyma and into the bile ducts, where they may live for many years. Eggs are excreted 3–4 months after ingestion, and the entire cycle is completed in 4–6 months. High humidity, moderate temperatures and rainfall favour transmission.[11,78]

Epidemiology

Human infection with *Fasciola* is most common in villages and larger towns within rural areas, especially sheep- and cattle-grazing areas.[79] Levels of infection depend on the frequency of humans eating plants (mainly watercress in Europe, morning glory in Asia) from water bodies contaminated with animal faeces. In most endemic areas, human infection is relatively rare, even where prevalence among domestic animals is high. Outbreaks of *F. hepatica* occur in households and communities and are often traced to

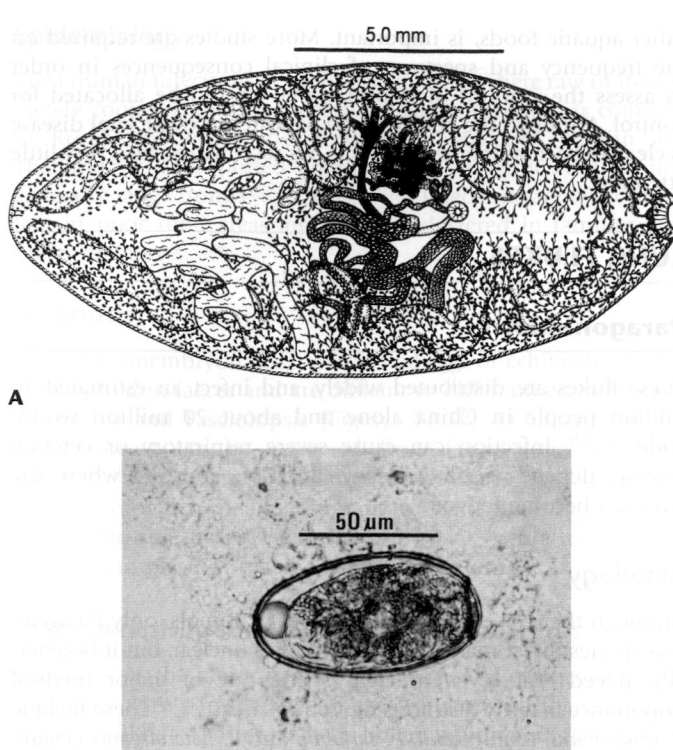

Figure 83.9 (A) Adult worm of *Paragonimus heterotremus*. (B) Egg of *P. heterotremus*.

Epidemiology

Human infection most often results from consumption of raw or incompletely cooked pickled, wine- or brine-soaked crabs, crayfish and shrimps harbouring metacercariae.[121,122,126,129] Alternatively, transmission may occur via eating wild boar, pigs, or small animals harbouring pre-adult worms. Metacercariae may also be ingested during preparation of these foods via contamination of hands or utensils. In addition to dietary preferences, raw crab meat and juice are thought to have medicinal properties for enhancing fertility, reducing fever and treating measles.[129] This last practice once caused high levels of infection in Korean children, while Philippine children enjoy eating incompletely roasted crabs.[130]

Although endemic pockets are still being discovered in Korea, the number infected has dropped dramatically in recent years.[129] High prevalences of infection (up to 45%) were observed during a skin test survey in endemic communities in Korea in 1959. Infection levels have also significantly dropped in Japan in the past 50 years. However, changing dietary practices and reluctance to stop eating raw crabs are leading to increased infection levels in some areas.[123,127] The infection is endemic throughout China, although again, vigorous control efforts have successfully reduced prevalences in some areas.[122] Surveys in the Philippines found prevalences of 0.5–12% in human communities, while 50–100% of crabs in endemic areas harbour *Paragonimus*.[130] Although eating raw food is not a widespread habit in India, 39 cases of Paragonimus were reported from Manipur State.[125]

Pathogenesis and pathology

The site of pathology of paragonimiasis depends upon the migratory route of the larvae and the tissue in which they lodge.[28,84,121] Inflammatory responses to the adult worms, immature worms and eggs are similar, regardless of location. Resulting lesions are granulomatous, beginning with leukocyte (mainly eosinophil) infiltration and finally resulting in thick cysts or abscesses and ultimately calcification. The parasites live within these fibrotic, greyish-white capsules (1.5–5 cm in diameter) in pairs or triplets, surrounded by thick, blood-streaked fluid and numerous eggs. Later, the capsules may be empty or fluid filled. Eggs trapped in the tissue may also provoke granulomas at the periphery of the necrotic area. The capsules occur most frequently in the upper right quadrant of the lungs and, in the fewer cases of cerebral involvement, the posterior portion of the brain is usually affected.

In both human and experimental infections there appears to be a subsidence of inflammation in later periods. This may be due to modulation of the immune response.

Clinical features

Pulmonary infection is accompanied by a chronic productive cough, with brownish purulent sputum containing streaks of blood and parasite eggs in *P. westermani*, *P. heterotremus* and African and American paragonimiasis. Chest pain and night sweats may also occur. The signs mimic bronchiectasis, bronchopneumonia, or tuberculosis not responding to antibiotics. Eosinophilia of 20–25% is common.

Pleural effusion and pneumothorax with marked eosinophilia in the exudate and peripheral blood occur particularly frequently in *P. miyazakii* infections in Japan. Although there may be a persistent cough, neither brownish sputum nor eggs are expelled in *P. skrjabini* and *P. miyazakii* infections.

Cerebral paragonimus may cause eosinophilic meningitis, which is characterized by headache, convulsions of the focal Jacksonian type, hemiplegia and visual impairment with insidious onset.[84,131] Most cases involve males under 10 years of age. Flukes in the spinal cord may cause spastic paraplegia. Pulmonary symptoms (cough with brownish sputum) usually accompany cerebral disease. Cutaneous paragonimiasis occurs when the parasites lodge in subcutaneous tissue, forming painless, mobile swellings which may contain immature worms. The patient may also exhibit mild pulmonary abnormalities. This manifestation occurs frequently in *P. skrjabini* infection, which does not localize to the lungs.

Sometimes the flukes migrate through the peritoneal cavity eliciting the formation of multiple nodules (abdominal paragonimiasis) which often appear similar to malignant tumours.

Mortality has been reported, either due to parasites and resulting abscesses in the heart or to fulminating infection in the abdominal cavity.

Diagnosis and investigations

The clinical signs are fairly pathognomonic, particularly when diet history and residence in an endemic area are known, but misdiagnosis is commonly due to unfamiliarity with the disease.[125] Tests to rule out tuberculosis, skin tests and sputum smear and culture are helpful in differentiation. Eggs of *Paragonimus* may be found in the faeces, sputum, gastric washings, plural effusion or tissue.

Blood in the sputum contains sufficient eggs to be visualized by direct smear. Sputum without blood should be collected over 24 h, centrifuged and the sediment dissolved in 3% sodium hydroxide for examination for eggs. Eggs may not be present in the sputum of infected children or elderly people, but faecal examination using a concentration technique may reveal eggs. Adult worms might be expectorated after treatment or found in skin lesions.

Skin and immunodiagnostic tests using parasite antigens are highly sensitive and useful for surveys and in diagnosing the infection(s).[125,132,133] Complement fixation tests and ELISA detect early as well as chronic infection and titres decline rapidly (becoming negative in 1–2 months) after cure. These tests therefore assist in assessing cure following treatment.

Radiological investigations, particularly plain radiography and computed tomography, are useful in diagnosing pulmonary disease. Lesions typically show a nodular or ring shadow, patchy infiltration and cavities.[125,134] In eosinophilic meningitis, computed tomography reveals a 'soap bubble appearance' of dilated ventricles and multiple dense calcification and calcified cystic lesions.[131] Magnetic resonance images of the brain reveal conglomerates of multiple ring-like enhancements in the cerebral hemisphere of the brain in cerebral paragonimiasis.[135]

Management

Long regimens of bithionol, totalling 10–15 doses of 30 mg/kg body weight on alternate days, and niclofan (2 mg/kg, single dose) are effective and have been used widely. Praziquantel has been the drug of choice, with a course of 3×25 mg/kg body weight for 3 days being nearly 100% effective against all species.[122,136] Side-effects are usually mild and pulmonary abnormalities decrease within 4 months. Cutaneous paragonimiasis with flare-up may occur after praziquantel treatment for pulmonary disease. Caution is required in the treatment of cerebral disease; one such patient became comatose for 48 h, while others showed no severe effects. Some studies have also shown triclabendazole to be effective.[126,137] Doses ranging from 5 mg/kg body weight once daily for 3 days, 10 mg/kg twice on 1 day, to 10 mg/kg in a single dose have been found to be better tolerated and as effective as praziquantel in eliminating infection of *P. mexicanus*.[137]

Prevention and control

In addition to drug treatment, health education to discourage the consumption of raw crustaceans is recommended, particularly addressing the special danger of infection to children. Increased recognition of the problem by health workers and the population may facilitate earlier treatment and dietary change. Folk beliefs regarding medicinal properties of raw crabs, plus the inability of rapid dry cooking or soaking in brine, soy sauce or alcohol to kill the parasites, may require special attention in health promotion messages.

REFERENCES

1. Chai JY, Park JH, Han ET, et al. Mixed infections with *Opisthorchis viverrini* and intestinal flukes in residents of Vientiane Municipality and Saravane Province in Laos. *J Helminthol* 2005; 79:283–289.

2. Kaewkes S. *The epidemiology and taxonomy of minute intestinal flukes in Northeast Thailand*, PhD thesis. University of Queensland; 1993.

3. Radomyos B, Wongsaroj T, Wilairatana P, et al. Opisthorchiasis and intestinal fluke infections in northern Thailand. *Southeast Asian J Trop Med Public Health* 1998; 29:123–127.

4. WHO. Control of food-borne trematode infections. *WHO Tech Rev Serv*; 1995.

5. WHO. *Report of Joint WHO/FAO workshop on food-borne trematode infections in Asia*. Hanoi; 2004.

6. Radomyos P, Radomyos B, Tungtrongchitr A. Multi-infection with helminths in adults from northeast Thailand as determined by post-treatment fecal examination of adult worms. *Trop Med Parasitol* 1994; 45:133–135.

7. Cho SY, Kang SY, Lee, et al. B. Metagonimiasis in Korea. *Drug Res* 1984; 34:1211–1213.

8. Cross JH. Changing patterns of some trematode infections in Asia. *Drug Res* 1984; 34:1224–1126.

9. Graczyk TK, Fried B. Echinostomiasis: a common but forgotten food-borne disease. *Am J Trop Med Hyg* 1998; 58:501–504.

10. Jongsuksuntigul P, Imsomboon T. Opisthorchiasis control in Thailand. *Acta Trop* 2003; 88:229–232.

11. Mas-Coma S, Angles R, Esteban JG, et al. The Northern Bolivian Altiplano: a region highly endemic for human fascioliasis. *Trop Med Int Health* 1999; 4:454–467.

12. Keiser J, Utzinger J. Chemotherapy for major food-borne trematodes: a review. *Expert Opin Pharmacother* 2004; 5:1711–1726.

13. Seo BS. Socio-economic and cultural aspects of human trematode infections in Korea. *Drug Res* 1984; 34:1116–1118.

14. Eckert J. Workshop summary: food safety: meat- and fish-borne zoonoses. *Vet Parasitol* 1996; 64:143–147.

15. Lun ZR, Gasser RB, Lai DH, et al. Clonorchiasis: a key foodborne zoonosis in China. *Lancet Infect Dis* 2005; 5:31–41.

16. IARC. *IARC Monographs on the Evaluation of Carcinogenic Risks to Humans*. 1994; 61:121–175.

17. Haswell-Elkins MR, Satarug S, Elkins DB. *Opisthorchis viverrini* infection in northeast Thailand and its relationship to cholangiocarcinoma. *J Gastroenterol Hepatol* 1992; 7:538–548.

18. Hoeppli R. Histological changes in the liver of sixty-six Chinese infected with *Clonorchis sinensis*. *Chin Med* 1933; 47:1125–1141.

19. Thamavit W, Bhamarapravati N, Sahaphong S, et al. Effects of dimethylnitrosamine on induction of cholangiocarcinoma in *Opisthorchis viverrini*-infected Syrian golden hamsters. *Cancer Res* 1978; 38:4634–4639.

20. Vatanasapt V, Tangvoraphonkchai V, Titapant V, et al. A high incidence of liver cancer in Khon Kaen Province, Thailand. *Southeast Asian J Trop Med Public Health* 1990; 21:489–494.

21. Kaewkes S. Taxonomy and biology of liver flukes. *Acta Trop* 2003; 88:177–186.

22. Lee SU, Huh S. Variation of nuclear and mitochondrial DNAs in Korean and Chinese isolates of *Clonorchis sinensis*. *Korean J Parasitol* 2004; 42:145–148.

23. Park GM. Genetic comparison of liver flukes, *Clonorchis sinensis* and *Opisthorchis viverrini*, based on rDNA and mtDNA gene sequences. *Parasitol Res* 2007; 100:351–357.

24. Park GM, Yong TS. Geographical variation of the liver fluke, *Clonorchis sinensis*, from Korea and China based on the karyotypes, zymodeme and DNA sequences. *Southeast Asian J Trop Med Public Health* 2001; 32(suppl 2):12–16.

25. Sithithaworn P, Nuchjungreed C, Srisawangwong T, et al. Genetic variation in *Opisthorchis viverrini* (Trematoda: Opisthorchiidae) from northeast Thailand and Laos PDR based on random amplified polymorphic DNA analyses. *Parasitol Res* 2007; 100:613–617.

26. Saijuntha W, Sithithaworn P, Wongkham S, et al. Genetic markers for the identification and characterization of *Opisthorchis viverrini*, a medically important food borne trematode in Southeast Asia. *Acta Trop* 2006; 100:246–251.

116. Velasquez CC. Heterophyidiasis. In: Hillyer GV, Hopla CE, section eds. *Section C: Parasitic Zoonoses*, Vol. III. Boca Raton: CRC Press; 1982: 99–107.

117. Sukontason K, Unpunyo P, Sukontason KL, et al. Evidence of *Haplorchis taichui* infection as pathogenic parasite: three case reports. *Scand J Infect Dis* 2005; 37:388–390.

118. Africa C, Leon WD E, Garcia EY. Intestinal heterophyidiasis with cardiac involvement: a contribution to etiology of heart failure. *J Philippine Islands Med Assoc* 1935; 15:358–361.

119. Lee SH, Hwang SW, Chai JY, et al. Comparative morphology of eggs of *Heterophyids* and *Clonorchis sinensis* causing human infections in Korea. *Kisaengchunghak Chapchi* 1984; 22:171–180.

120. Ditrich O, Giboda M, Scholz T, et al. Comparative morphology of eggs of the Haplorchiinae (Trematoda: Heterophyidae) and some other medically important *heterophyid* and *opisthorchid* flukes. *Folia Parasitol* 1992; 39:123–132.

121. Miyazaki I. Paragonimiasis. In: Hillyer GV, Hopla CE, section eds. *Section C: Parasitic Zoonoses*, Vol. III. Boca Raton: CRC Press; 1982:143–164.

122. Zhi-Biao X. Studies on clinical manifestations, diagnosis and control of paragonimiasis in China. In: Cross JH, ed. *Emerging Problems in Food-Borne Parasitic Zoonosis: Impact on Agriculture and Public Health*. Bangkok: Thai Watana Panich Press; 1991:345–348.

123. Gyoten J. Changes of living habits related to the infection in human paragonimiasis in Japan, based on the epidemiological data. *Japan J Parasitol* 1994; 43:462–470.

124. Pozio E. Current status of food-borne parasitic zoonoses in Mediterranean and African regions. In: Cross JH, ed. *Emerging Problems in Food-Borne Parasitic Zoonosis: Impact on Agriculture and Public Health*. Bangkok: Thai Watana Panich Press; 1991:85–87.

125. Singh TS, Mutum SS, Razaque MA. Pulmonary paragonimiasis: clinical features, diagnosis and treatment of 39 cases in Manipur. *Trans R Soc Trop Med Hyg* 1986; 80:967–971.

126. Blair D, Xu Z B, Agatsuma T. Paragonimiasis and the genus *Paragonimus*. *Adv Parasitol* 1998; 42:113–222.

127. Uchiyama F, Morimoto Y, Nawa Y. Re-emergence of paragonimiasis in Kyushu, Japan. *Southeast Asian J Trop Med Public Health* 1999; 30: 686–691.

128. Nishimura K, Hung T. Current views on geographic distribution and modes of infection of neurohelminthic diseases. *J Neurol Sci* 1997; 145:5–14.

129. Choi DW. *Paragonimus* and paragonimiasis in Korea. *Korean J Parasitol* 1990; 28:79–102.

130. Belizario V, Guan M, Borja L, et al. Pulmonary paragonimiasis and tuberculosis in Sorsogon, Philippines. *Southeast Asian J Trop Med Public Health* 1997; 28(suppl 1):37–45.

131. Jaroonvesama N. Differential diagnosis of eosinophilic meningitis. *Parasitol Today* 1988; 4:262–266.

132. Lee JS, Lee J, Kim SH, et al. Molecular cloning and characterization of a major egg antigen in *Paragonimus westermani* and its use in ELISA for the immunodiagnosis of paragonimiasis. *Parasitol Res* 2007; 100:677–681.

133. Zhang R, Gao S, Geng Y, et al. Epidemiological study on *Clonorchis sinensis* infection in Shenzhen area of Zhujiang delta in China. *Parasitol Res* 2007; 101:179–183.

134. Devi KR, Narain K, Bhattacharya S, et al. Pleuropulmonary paragonimiasis due to *Paragonimus heterotremus*: molecular diagnosis, prevalence of infection and clinicoradiological features in an endemic area of northeastern India. *Trans R Soc Trop Med Hyg* 2007; 101:786–792.

135. Kang SY, Kim TK, Kim TY, et al. A case of chronic cerebral *paragonimiasis westermani*. *Korean J Parasitol* 2000; 38:167–171.

136. Udonsi JK. Clinical field trials of praziquantel in pulmonary paragonimiasis due to Paragonimus uterobilateralis in endemic populations of the Igwun Basin, Nigeria. *Trop Med Parasitol* 1989; 40:65–68.

137. Calvopina M, Guderian RH, Paredes W, et al. Treatment of human pulmonary paragonimiasis with triclabendazole: clinical tolerance and drug efficacy. *Trans R Soc Trop Med Hyg* 1998; 92:566–569.

Chapter 84   Paul E. Simonsen

Filariases

The filariases result from infection with vector-borne tissue-dwelling nematodes called filariae. Depending on the species, adult filariae may live in the lymphatics, blood vessels, skin, connective tissues or serous membranes. The females produce larvae (microfilariae) which live in the bloodstream or skin. All true filariae that infect humans (superfamily Filarioidea; family Onchocercidae) are transmitted by dipteran vectors. The guinea worm (superfamily Dracunculoidea) is not a true filaria, but is included in this section as a related nematode transmitted by arthropod vectors. A summary of the common filarial worms infecting humans and the common disease symptoms is shown in Table 84.1. A few species of animal filariae may accidentally infect humans. The transmission of human filariae is confined to warm climates, a high temperature being necessary for the parasites to develop in the vectors.

The pattern of the life cycle of all species of filariae is shown in Figure 84.1. Detailed life cycles of the species infecting humans are given in Appendix III. The infective form is the third-stage larva which is transmitted by the vector. The rate of growth and differentiation of worms and longevity of both microfilariae and adult worms differ markedly between different species. Some adult worms may live as long as 20 years. A high specificity of the filaria-vector and the filaria-host relationships has evolved over a long period of time.

From the public health point of view, onchocerciasis and lymphatic filariasis are the most important filarial infections. Dracunculiasis (guinea worm infection) results in severe ulceration, and Calabar swellings and other clinical manifestations of loiasis may have severe consequences for the patient.

LYMPHATIC FILARIASIS

Three species of lymphatic dwelling filarial worms, *Wuchereria bancrofti*, *Brugia malayi* and *B. timori*, cause lymphatic filariasis in humans. The vectors are species of mosquitoes (*Anopheles*, *Culex*, *Aedes* and *Mansonia* spp). Infection with *W. bancrofti* is sometimes called bancroftian filariasis, while brugian filariasis refers to infection by the other two species. *W. bancrofti* is geographically much more widespread than the *Brugia* spp. Lymphatic filariasis is a major cause of debilitating and disfiguring chronic disease manifestations (especially lymphoedema, elephantiasis and hydrocele) in endemic areas.[1]

Historical background

Our present knowledge of filariasis owes much to investigations carried out towards the end of the nineteenth and the beginning of the twentieth centuries. Microfilariae, recovered in hydrocele fluid from a Cuban patient, were first described by Jean-Nicolas Demarquay in Paris in 1863.[2] Three years later, microfilariae were found in chylous urine in a patient in Brazil by Otto Wucherer, who was unaware of the earlier French report.[3] Timothy Lewis, working in India, first reported the finding of microfilariae in human blood in 1872.[4] Adult worms were recovered by Joseph Bancroft in Australia in 1876 and named *Filaria bancrofti*.[5] In 1921 this species was included in the genus *Wuchereria*.

The distinguished pioneer of tropical medicine, Sir Patrick Manson, while working in Amoy in China, made several contributions to the understanding of the biology of *W. bancrofti*.[6] Thus, in 1877 he observed the development of the parasite in mosquitoes fed on the blood of his microfilaraemic gardener, and he speculated that it was transmitted by mosquitoes. He also noticed that microfilariae could not always be found in the blood of infected patients. By serial blood examinations every few hours, he then revealed the nocturnal periodicity of the microfilariae.

Examination of specimens of adult worms revealed two new species, subsequently called *Brugia malayi* (1960) and *B. timori* (1977). A detailed history of lymphatic filariasis has been written.[7]

Geographical distribution

The distribution of the three causal parasites of lymphatic filariasis, *W. bancrofti*, *B. malayi* and *B. timori*, is shown in Figure 84.2. *W. bancrofti* is distributed throughout the tropical regions of Asia, Africa, the Americas and the Pacific, and is particularly prevalent in areas with hot and humid climates. *B. malayi* is found in Southeast Asia and in areas of south-west India, whereas *B. timori* occurs only on some islands in Indonesia.

In 1997, it was estimated that at least 128 million individuals were infected, 115 million with *W. bancrofti* and 13 million with the *Brugia* spp.[8] India (48 million cases) and sub-Saharan Africa (51 million cases) accounted for most of this burden. Results from many recent surveys indicate that the true figures could be much higher. Lymphatic filariasis has disappeared from North America,

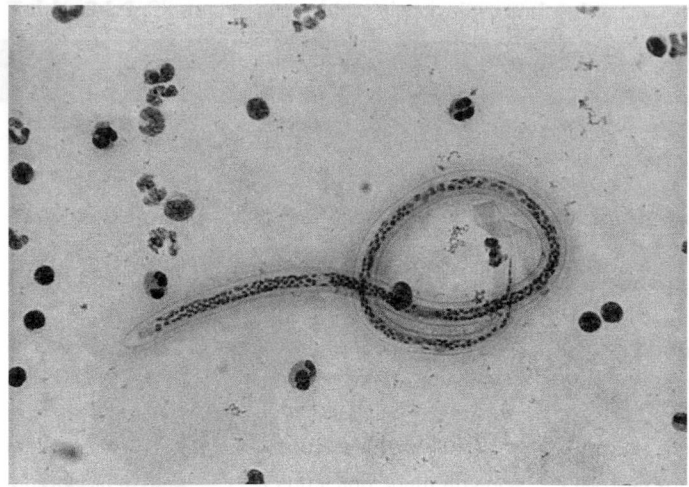

Figure 84.3 Microfilaria of *W. bancrofti* in thick blood film.

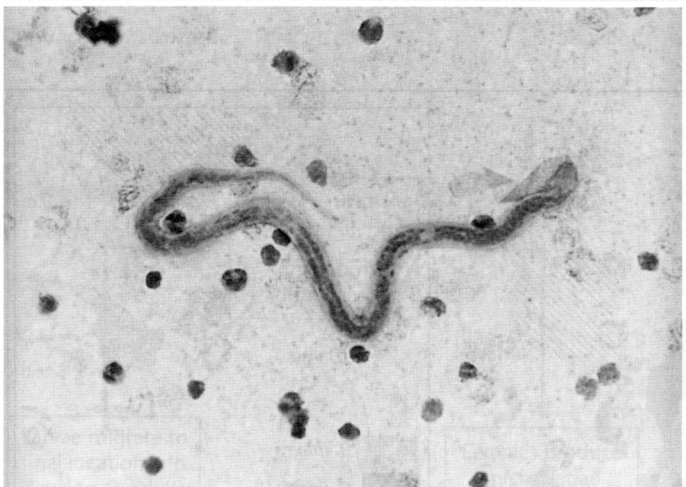

Figure 84.4 Microfilaria of *B. malayi* in thick blood film.

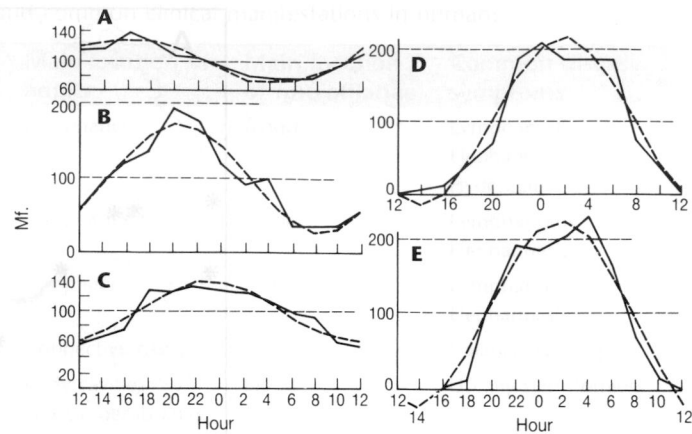

Figure 84.5 Observed (—) and theoretical (- - -) periodicity of microfilariae in peripheral blood. (A) Diurnally subperiodic *W. bancrofti* in the South Pacific. (B) Nocturnally subperiodic *W. bancrofti* from west Thailand. (C) Nocturnally subperiodic *B. malayi* in the Philippines. (D) Nocturnally periodic *B. malayi* in Malaysia. (E) Nocturnally periodic *W. bancrofti* in Malaysia. (Reproduced from *Control of Lymphatic Filariasis. A Manual for Health Personnel.* Geneva: WHO; ©1987.)

respectively. A strain of *B. malayi* also exhibits nocturnal sub-periodicity (Figure 84.5).

The periodicity is due to a biological rhythm inherent in the microfilariae but influenced by the circadian rhythm of the host. Microfilaraemia of nocturnally periodic *W. bancrofti* ceases to be periodic in persons who start work at night and sleep during the day, and in patients who have been hospitalized for long periods.

Clinical features

Lymphatic filariasis is characterized by a wide range of clinical presentations.

One group of individuals in the endemic community shows no clinical manifestations or microfilariae. This includes individuals who have not been sufficiently exposed to be infected, individuals with prepatent infection or adult worm infection without micro-

filaraemia, and individuals who have cleared the infection. Another group of individuals in the endemic community shows microfilariae in their blood but no obvious clinical manifestations. Some of these may remain microfilaraemic and asymptomatic for years or even for the rest of their lives.

Recent surveys employing diagnostic tests that detect circulating antigens from adult *W. bancrofti* worms have demonstrated that many of the amicrofilaraemic individuals in endemic areas actually harbour adult worms.[10] Through the use of ultrasonography and lymphoscintigraphy it has been recognized that most infected but apparently asymptomatic individuals (with or without microfilaraemia) suffer from subclinical lymphatic abnormalities, especially dilatation of the vessels (lymphangiectasis).[11,12]

Obvious symptomatic filarial disease manifests itself in both acute and chronic forms, and may be with or without infection.

Bancroftian filariasis

Common clinical manifestations of bancroftian filariasis are acute adenolymphangitis, hydrocele, lymphoedema and elephantiasis. Chyluria and tropical pulmonary eosinophilia are more rarely seen manifestations. Although frequent in males, genital manifestations do not appear to be a substantial problem in females.[13]

Acute manifestations

Manifestations of acute filarial disease ('filarial fever'), often described as adenolymphangitis (ADL), are characterized by episodic attacks of malaise, fever and chills, and by the appearance of enlarged painful lymph nodes draining the affected part, usually the lower limb, followed by an acute, warm and tender swelling. The episodes usually resolve spontaneously after about a week, and may recur several times within a year. Regression of the swelling after an ADL attack of the leg is commonly followed by excessive skin exfoliation.[14] In males the genitals are frequently affected and attacks may present as acute funiculitis or epididymo-orchitis. Acute attacks may be unilateral or bilateral, and commonly occur also in individuals with chronic manifestatons.[15]

Two distinct syndromes of acute filarial attacks in the extremities have recently been recognized.[16] One, called acute filarial lymphangitis (AFL), is caused by the death of adult worms, either spontaneously or after treatment. It presents as a circumscribed inflammatory nodule or cord centred around degenerating adult worms, with lymphangitis spreading in a descending (centrifugal) fashion. It usually has a mild clinical course and rarely causes residual lymphoedema. The other syndrome, acute dermato-lymphangioadenitis (ADLA) is not caused by filarial worms per se, but probably results from secondary bacterial infections in the legs with compromised lymphatics. It is characterized by diffuse subcutaneous inflammation with or without ascending lymphangitis, and is often accompanied by oedema in the affected leg. It is believed to be the common cause of chronic lymphoedema and elephantiasis.

Hydrocele

Hydrocele is the most common chronic manifestation in bancroftian filariasis. It results from the accumulation of clear straw-coloured fluid in the sac surrounding the testicles. The onset may be silent, i.e., without accompanying acute episodes, or it may be preceded by one or more attacks of funiculitis or epididymo-orchitis. Following early acute episodes, the swelling around the testis usually disappears completely, but over the years the tunica vaginalis becomes thickened and there is progressive enlargement of the hydrocele (Figure 84.6). Most cases are unilateral, but bilateral hydrocele, often with different sizes on the two sides, is not uncommon. Rarely, the fluid may have a milky appearance if lymph from a ruptured lymphatic vessel pours into the hydrocele to form a chylocele.

In clinical surveys, hydrocele is graded according to developmental stage and size. A commonly used scale records swelling of the spermatic cord as hydrocele grade I, and true hydroceles are classified from their length as grade II (6.0–8.0 cm), III (8.1–11.0 cm), IV (11.1–15.0 cm) and V (>15 cm).[17,18]

Lymphoedema and elephantiasis

Chronic lymphoedema progressing to elephantiasis most commonly affects the legs (Figure 84.7). The arms (Figure 84.8), scrotum, penis, vulva and breasts may also more rarely be affected. Following recurrent episodes of acute attacks, first pitting oedema and then chronic non-pitting oedema with loss of skin elasticity and fibrosis develops. The development of elephantiasis may be arrested at any stage. It commences on one side but often becomes bilateral.

In the leg, loss of contour is first observed around the ankles. Following initial attacks the limb returns to normal. Over several years the oedema becomes non-pitting with thickening and loss of skin elasticity. Further progression leads to evident elephantiasis with skin folds, dermatosclerosis and papillomatous lesions. Secondary bacterial and fungal infections are common in the lymphoedematous skin, and probably exacerbate the progression of elephantiasis. In severe cases pus may ooze from chronic ulcerations in the affected part, which may also emanate a foul smell.

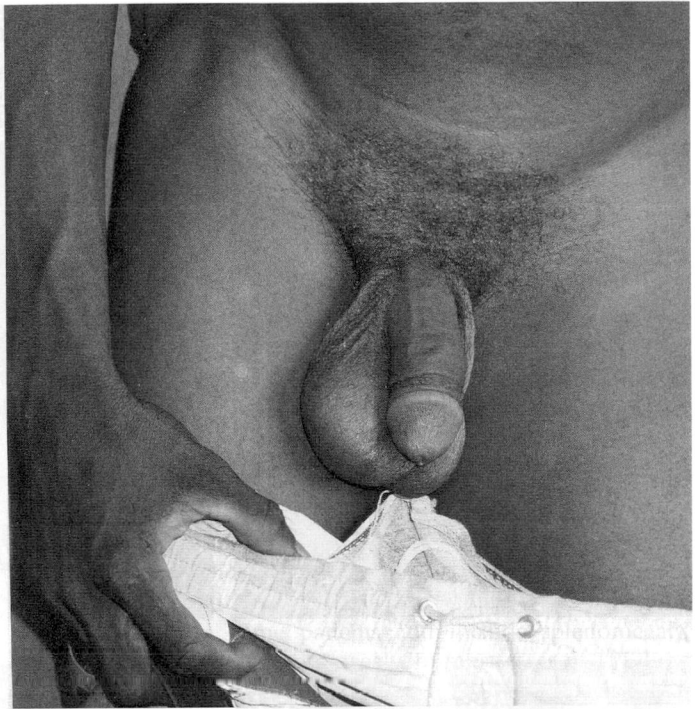

A

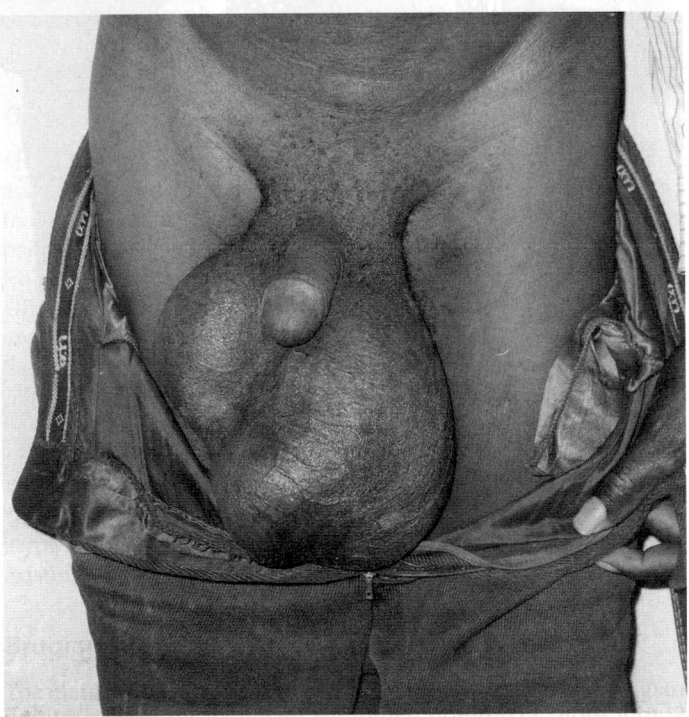

B

Figure 84.6 Lymphatic filariasis: hydrocele. (A) Early; (B) advanced.

Geographical variation in clinical picture

Clinical manifestations of lymphatic filariasis have been reported in the past to differ considerably between geographical zones. However, as examination and grading procedures become more standardized, differences appear to be less marked.

Most cases of TPE and chyluria have been reported from south and South-east Asian countries. In Africa, the prevalence of both chyluria and TPE is low. A recent search for TPE cases in a highly endemic lymphatic filariasis area of Tanzania confirmed the rarity of this syndrome in the population.[24]

In *W. bancrofti* endemic areas of Papua New Guinea, microfilarial prevalences can be exceedingly high, reaching 60–80% for the overall population, whereas clinical sign rates for hydrocele and elephantiasis tend to be similar or even lower than those seen in highly endemic areas (overall 15–30% microfilarial prevalence) elsewhere in the world.[25]

Diagnosis

Clinical diagnosis

Acute or chronic manifestations resembling those described above in individuals who live in or who have visited areas endemic for transmission of *W. bancrofti*, *B. malayi* or *B. timori* are indicative of lymphatic filariasis.

A sudden onset of fever, accompanied by acute groin pain with swollen tender lymph glands and/or oedematous swelling of the leg distinguishes an acute attack of filarial ADL from the many other causes of fever and adenitis that occur in tropical countries. Filarial funiculitis needs to be differentiated from funiculitis due to bacterial infection.

Inguinal hernia is the most common scrotal swelling that needs to be distinguished from hydrocele. If the hernia is irreducible then the translucency test and the inability of the examiner to get above the swelling distinguish it from hydrocele. Both irreducible hernias and hydroceles often exist in the same patient. Obstructed hernias, tumours of the testis, tuberculosis and other bacterial infections of the epididymis, *Schistosoma haematobium* of the cord and acute lymphadenitis of the groin glands need to be distinguished from genital lesions of filarial origin.

Common conditions that need to be distinguished from filarial lymphoedema are swollen limbs due to congestive cardiac failure, subacute nephritis or blockage of venous (thrombosis) or lymphatic (tuberculosis, leprosy) systems, and Kaposi's sarcoma. In all these conditions the patient's history greatly assists in differentiating them from filarial elephantiasis. The oedema of cardiac failure and subacute nephritis has a painless onset and is bilateral. Secondary carcinoma of lymph glands and surgical ablation may also result in elephantiasis of the limbs.

An endemic form of leg elephantiasis occurs in many parts of Africa at altitudes that preclude a filarial aetiology.[26] Mineral particles from volcanic soils, absorbed through the plantar skin of bare-footed peoples, are believed to be the causative agents (see Chapter 33). Such non-filarial tropical elephantiasis has also been reported from South and Central America.

Early stages of scrotal elephantiasis need to be distinguished from other conditions that affect the scrotal skin, such as fungal infections, scrotal oedema due to onchocerciasis and the thickened skin that results from the intense itching and scratching in scabies infections.

TPE should be differentiated from bronchial asthma and other allergic conditions, tuberculosis and eosinophilic leukaemia. TPE must also be distinguished from helminth infections that have a stage of the life cycle that involves lung tissue: *Ascaris*, *Strongyloides*, *Schistosoma* spp. and trichinosis. Confusion may also arise with visceral larva migrans caused by *Toxocara*. A rapid beneficial response to DEC therapy distinguishes TPE from the above-mentioned conditions.

Parasitological diagnosis

Adult worms are recovered only rarely from the tissues, and parasitological diagnosis is usually based on recovery of microfilariae from the patient's blood. Amicrofilaraemia does not exclude filarial disease, nor does microfilaraemia denote it. Blood samples taken from patients with clinical manifestations, whether acute or chronic, are often negative for microfilariae. In individuals there is no relationship between microfilarial density and severity of disease. Microfilariae frequently occur in hydrocele fluid and may occasionally be seen in urine or other body fluids.

For parasitological diagnosis of lymphatic filariasis, a blood specimen should be obtained at the time of the day when the peak concentration of microfilariae is expected (e.g. between 21:00 and 03:00 hours for nocturnally periodic forms).[9]

Many techniques have been described for demonstrating microfilariae in blood samples (see also Appendix I). The counting chamber technique is fast, quantitative and cheap.[27] An aliquot of 100 mL of finger-prick blood is added to a tube containing 0.9 mL of 3% acetic acid. Microfilariae are counted in a counting chamber under the low power of a compound microscope. If only one species of filaria is present in the area, this technique is the most suitable for routine hospital diagnosis as well as for field surveys. Species identification of the microfilariae may be difficult with the counting chamber technique.

In areas where more than one species of blood microfilaria exists, staining techniques are recommended. These are simple to perform but sensitivity is rather low owing to the small amount of blood examined and loss of microfilariae during the staining procedure. Microfilariae of *W. bancrofti*, *B. malayi* and *B. timori* have sheaths (see Figures 84.3 and 84.4). Microfilariae of *W. bancrofti* measure on average 260×8 μm, whereas those of *B. malayi* are slightly shorter and can be distinguished from microfilariae of *W. bancrofti* by the two isolated nuclei at the tip of the tail and the absence of nuclei in the cephalic space (see Appendix III). Microfilariae of *B. timori* are longer than those of *B. malayi*. Apart from microfilariae of *W. bancrofti*, two other species of microfilariae found in the blood in parts of Africa are those of *Loa loa* and *Mansonella perstans*. Staining with Giemsa or haematoxylin enables microfilariae of these species to be differentiated morphologically. *M. perstans* and *M. ozzardi* microfilariae also occur in the blood in South America and the West Indies.

The membrane (Nuclepore) filtration techniques are sensitive and excellent if the high cost of filters can be afforded. Staining of filters enables identification of the microfilariae. The techniques are impractical for field surveys because venous blood is needed. If filters are not available for examination of large quantities of blood, the Knott concentration technique may be used as an alternative, highly sensitive test (see Appendix I).

Diethylcarbamazine provocative day test

Nocturnally periodic microfilariae of *W. bancrofti* and *B. malayi* may be provoked, by the administration of DEC, to enter the peripheral blood in the daytime. Between 30 and 60 min is the optimum time for blood examination after the administration of a dose of 2 mg/kg of DEC (usually 100 mg of DEC is given to adults and 50 mg to children below 12 years of age).[28] The DEC provocative day test results in a significant long-term reduction of microfilaraemia, and therefore should not be used for diagnosis in follow-up studies on microfilaraemia.[29]

In contrast to its daytime action on nocturnally periodic *W. bancrofti*, the administration of DEC at night reduces the microfilaraemia. A similar reduction occurs following the daytime administration of the drug to diurnally subperiodic *W. bancrofti*. In hospitalized patients and others whose sleep rhythms have been altered, the test is of little use. Because of the risk of a severe Mazzotti reaction, the test is contraindicated in onchocerciasis endemic regions. A similar provocative effect is not exerted by daytime administration of ivermectin or albendazole.[30]

Immunological and polymerase chain reaction (PCR)-based diagnosis

Filarial worms induce a wide range of immune responses in the host, and several immunodiagnostic techniques for lymphatic filariasis, based on the detection of specific antibodies in the patient's serum, have been devised in the past. These have generally been of limited value in endemic areas, because most individuals are positive for antibodies to crude filarial antigens as a result of constant exposure. They have furthermore suffered from cross-reactions to other nematode infections and from being unable to distinguish past and present infection. The tests can be of some value in diagnosing visitors to endemic areas who develop symptoms of lymphatic filariasis but have no microfilaraemia.

The development of new, specific and sensitive immunodiagnostic tests has been a priority in lymphatic filariasis research. Cross-reactions have been reduced through detection for specific IgG4 antibodies, and specific IgG4 has been reported to be a good marker of active infection. Such tests may be of particular value in brugian filariasis, for which progress in development of circulating antigen detection-based diagnosis has been limited. A rapid format dipstick test (Brugia Rapid) detecting IgG4 to a *B. malayi* recombinant antigen in whole blood is currently undergoing field evaluation.[31] Other recombinant antigen based antibody assays are being developed and tested for their usefulness in monitoring human exposure and infection in control programs.[32] Specific IgG4 can also be detected in the urine of patients infected with *W. bancrofti*.[33]

Highly sensitive and specific tests for detection of specific circulating filarial antigens (CFAs) have been produced for bancroftian filariasis. These tests rely on the capture of filarial antigens in serum, plasma or blood specimens by use of specific monoclonal antibodies. Two different test principles have been utilized by two companies in the manufacture of test kits, which are now commercially available.[34,35] The TropBio-test (TropBio Pty Ltd, Austra-

lia) is a semiquantitative sandwich ELISA for detection of CFA in serum or plasma specimens. A sub-version of this test is adapted for analysis of finger-prick blood collected on filter paper discs. The NOW® Filariasis Test (Binax Inc., USA) is an immunochromatographic card test that in a few minutes can provide a yes/no answer for serum or fresh finger-prick blood specimens. In contrast to the parasitological tests, the CFA-based tests diagnose adult worm infection and not just microfilaraemia. Their sensitivity and specificity appear to be close to 100%. As the tests are not dependent on the microfilarial periodicity, blood specimens can be collected and examined at any time of the day. No such test is currently available for brugian filariasis.

Polymerase chain reaction (PCR) assays for the detection of microfilarial infections in humans have been developed for both *W. bancrofti* and *B. malayi*.[36,37] The techniques need at least one microfilaria in the volume of blood used for DNA extraction, and therefore are not more sensitive than microscopic blood examination for microfilariae. In contrast, these tests appear to be powerful tools for detection of infection in vectors.

Ultrasonography

Adult *W. bancrofti* can be detected by ultrasonography in lymphatic vessels of the scrotal area of infected males.[38,39] They are more dispersed and more difficult to detect within the lymphatic system of infected females.[40] The live worms wriggle continuously inside the dilated vessel ('filaria dance sign'). There are often several worms clumped together, and they show a remarkable long-term stability in location. Attempts to detect adult *B. malayi* by ultrasonography in the scrotal lymphatics of infected males have failed, but they were recently detected in the breast, the thigh, the calf and in an inguinal lymph node of infected individuals.[41]

Pathology and immunology

Most of the pathology in lymphatic filariasis is associated with the adult worms and their location in the lymphatics. A wide range of manifestations is seen in endemic regions. On the one hand are people with no obvious signs of infection or disease and asymptomatic microfilaria carriers, and on the other are those who develop signs of lymphatic responsiveness to adult worms, with fever, and who later develop chronic lymphatic pathology. In the case of TPE there is a vigorous immune response directed against the microfilariae, with consequent pathology. The pathogenesis of lymphatic filariasis has long been a matter of debate.

The majority of individuals in endemic areas mount an immunological response to filarial antigens as a result of the constant exposure. Polarization of the antibody and T cell responses towards a T helper cell (Th) type 2 response in microfilaraemic individuals, as opposed to a Th1-type response in patients with chronic disease, has been recognized.[42] A relative Th1-type hyporesponsiveness in infected individuals appears to be limited to filarial antigens, and its existence is presumably important for the successful persistence of the parasites within the host.

When examining patients with filariasis in studies on pathogenesis, a common approach has been to compare and contrast two poles in the clinical spectrum, namely individuals with detectable microfilaraemia but with no evident clinical manifestations, and individuals with chronic lymphatic disease who have generally been assumed to be amicrofilaraemic.[42] A hypothesis claiming a developmental sequence from the first to the second of these categories has been supported by the observation of more vivid immunological sensitization to filarial antigen in patients with chronic disease than in those with asymptomatic microfilaraemia. According to this hypothesis, microfilaraemic individuals are in a state of immunological tolerance. Breakdown of tolerance (for whatever reason) and activation of host protective responses would lead to clearing of the parasites but would at the same time have detrimental immunopathological effects.

This hypothesis of a basically immune-mediated pathogenesis of lymphatic disease has recently been challenged by observations from several lines of research. Analysis of epidemiological data has shown that in most endemic communities microfilaraemia is equally likely to occur in individuals with or without chronic pathology.[10,18,43] Use of strict classification criteria based on circulating antigenaemia, microfilaraemia and clinical status has furthermore indicated that host immune responses are more related to infection status than to disease status in the endemic population.[44-46] Further evidence for a different pathway of disease development in lymphatic filariasis comes from studies applying the imaging techniques of ultrasonography and lymphoscintigraphy in the assessment of lymphatic damage, and from detailed clinical, microbiological and histological observations.[44,47] According to these, two different pathological syndromes may lead to lymphatic filarial disease (Figure 84.10).

Dilatation of the lymphatics (lymphangiectasia) appears to be the basic lesion in the more common and more severe of these syndromes. Lymphangiectasia is present in virtually all individuals with adult worms whether or not they are microfilaraemic or have obvious signs of clinical disease. Apparently, the adult worms themselves are capable of inducing endothelial cell proliferation and lymphatic dilatation via mechanisms that do not involve lymphatic obstruction or involvement of the host's immune responses. Toxins released from endosymbiotic *Wolbachia* bacteria, which are found in abundance within the *W. bancrofti* and *B. malayi* worms, have been suspected to play a role.[48] The lymphangiectasia impairs lymphatic function and predisposes to microbial infection that may result in acute dermatolymphangioadenitis (ADLA). This is frequently accompanied by oedema in the affected part, and repeated attacks of ADLA might lead the way to chronic lymphoedema.[16] Recurrent secondary bacterial and fungal infections gaining access via entry lesions in the skin thus become important co-factors in the development of filarial lymphoedema and elephantiasis.[49,50]

The second syndrome is caused by the death of adult worms, either naturally or drug induced. The subsequent activation of host inflammatory reactions may result in formation of granulomatous nodules and episodes of acute filarial lymphangitis (AFL). These usually have a mild clinical course, and rarely cause residual lymphoedema in the extremities. Acute hydrocele appears to result from an AFL attack in the intrascrotal lymphatics, with granuloma formation and temporary obstruction of the lymphatic flow from the tunica vaginalis.[51] Most acute hydroceles disappear within a short time. The risk factors for progression to chronic hydrocele are still unclear, but probably include worm burden and granuloma location.

In the case of TPE there is a vigorous immune response directed against the microfilariae, with consequent pathology. Patients with TPE are immunologically hyperresponsive to filarial antigens.[21] Laboratory studies demonstrate high serum levels of filaria-specific IgG and IgE, and marked peripheral blood eosinophilia. The manifestations of TPE are most marked in the lungs. Lung biopsies have shown inflammatory foci around degenerating microfilariae. These findings, together with the absence of circulating microfilariae, suggest that an antibody-mediated mechanism of microfilaria destruction occurs in the lungs of these patients.

Protective immunity has not been proved in lymphatic filariasis. Epidemiological analyses of observed age-infection patterns in endemic communities do not generally suggest that infection prevalence is systematically reduced in older age groups, which would be expected as a consequence of acquired immunity.[52,53]

Visitors to endemic from non-endemic areas only rarely develop microfilaraemia, but they may acquire adult worms. Expatriates, exposed to intense transmission, may develop symptoms faster than is the case with resident natives of the endemic area. During World War II, 40 000 American service personnel were exposed to infection with *W. bancrofti*. More than 10 000 cases of disease were diagnosed, but microfilaraemia developed in fewer than ten of these. In a study of expatriate mineworkers with a length of exposure ranging from 1 to 8 years, some were positive for specific IgG1 and IgG4 antibody responses to the parasite but none was positive for specific circulating antigens.[54]

The effects of human immunodeficiency virus (HIV) infection on concurrent lymphatic filariasis, and vice versa, are largely unknown, but a positive cross-sectional relation between HIV and lymphatic filariasis has been observed among adults in an endemic area of Tanzania.[55]

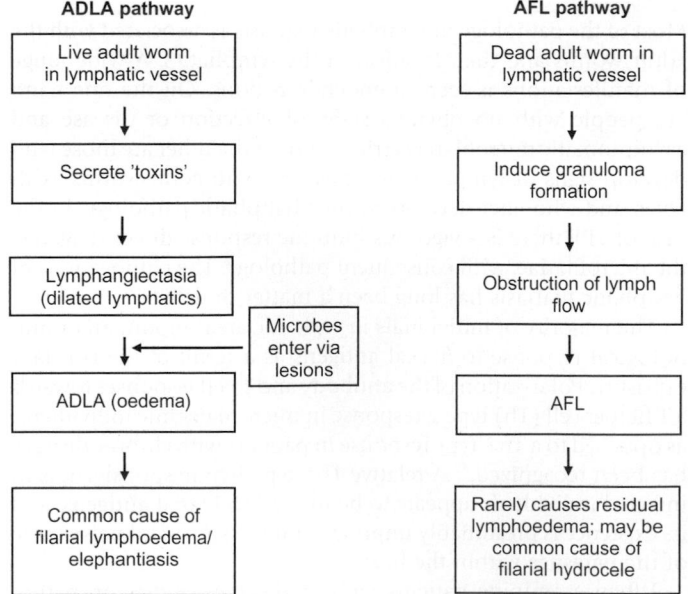

Figure 84.10 Sequence of development of the two types of acute filarial syndromes, acute dermatolymphangioadenitis (ADLA) and acute filarial lymphangitis (AFL), and their possible relationship to chronic filarial disease.

Table 84.2 Effect of diethylcarbamazine and ivermectin on microfilariae and adults of human filarial parasites

Drug	Stage	*Wuchereria bancrofti* and *Brugia* spp.	*Loa loa*	*Mansonella perstans*	*Mansonella streptocerca*	*Mansonella ozzardi*	*Onchocerca volvulus*
Diethylcarbamazine	Microfilaria	++	++[a]	+	++	–	++[a]
	Adult	+	+	–	++	–	–
Ivermectin	Microfilaria	++	++[a]	–	++	++	++
	Adult	–	?	?	?	?	–?

–, No effect; +, few/some are eliminated; ++, most are eliminated; ?, unknown. [a] Severe side-effects may occur.

Management

Individual treatment of filariasis aims to prevent or reverse progression of disease. Detailed accounts of current knowledge and experience on the treatment and management of lymphatic filariasis in its different clinical forms have been given.[19,56]

Antifilarial drugs

For almost half a century, the drug most commonly used has been diethylcarbamazine citrate (DEC). DEC is a microfilaricidal agent also capable of killing a proportion of the adult *W. bancrofti*, *B. malayi* and *B. timori* (Table 84.2). Ivermectin (Mectizan®) is a potent microfilaricide, but has no macrofilaricidal effect. A promising area of research is the use of antibiotics to deplete the filarial worms of endosymbiontic *Wolbachia* bacteria. Trials with a 6–8 week course of doxycycline have shown significant activity against adult worms and microfilariae as well as improvement of pathology.[57,58]

Diethylcarbamazine

DEC exerts no direct lethal action on the microfilariae but apparently modifies them so that they are removed by the host's immune system. The lethal effect of DEC on adult worms in vivo can be directly monitored by ultrasonography.[59]

DEC treatment of microfilaraemic patients (and amicrofilaraemic circulating antigen-positive patients) may prevent development of lymphatic damage by eliminating adult worms. It apparently has little or no effect on already induced lymphatic damage, or on chronic obstructive disease.[60] Dying adult worms following DEC treatment may trigger transient attacks of acute filarial lymphangitis.[16] DEC treatment is not recommended during acute episodes because it may provoke additional adult worm death and exacerbate the inflammatory response.

DEC is administered orally. The recommended therapeutic dose is 6 mg/kg body weight daily, in three divided doses after food, for 12 days. The number of microfilariae in the blood usually decreases rapidly after the start of treatment and then increases, usually at reduced intensity, after some months. Clearance of circulating filarial antigen is highly variable, probably because some living adult worms persist after treatment.[59,61] Drug reactions, due to dying parasites, may commence a few hours after the start of treatment. They are less severe in bancroftian filariasis than in brugian filariasis. There are two groups of reactions: systemic and local.[62] Systemic reactions include headache, joint and body pain, dizziness, anorexia, malaise and vomiting. Fever and sys-

temic reactions tend to be related to the intensity of infection. Localized reactions include lymphadenitis, abscess formation and transient lymphoedema. In bancroftian filariasis funiculitis, epididymitis and hydrocele formation also occur. These local reactions tend to occur later and last longer than the systemic effects. Interruption of treatment is not usually necessary. Side-effects of DEC therapy are reduced, and efficacy increased, when treatment is spaced, for example when single doses (6 mg/kg) are given weekly or monthly. The passing of *Ascaris* worms is often a beneficial side-effect of DEC therapy.

Treatment may be repeated every 6 months for as long as the person remains microfilaraemic or has symptoms. There may be severe reactions to DEC in persons infected with *Onchocerca volvulus* or *Loa loa*. Therefore, special care must be taken in areas where these two parasites occur.

The recommended treatment for TPE is a 3-week course of DEC. Following DEC therapy most patients show rapid improvement. Repeat treatment may be necessary.

Ivermectin

Owing to its efficacy in killing microfilariae of *O. volvulus*, studies were initiated to test the efficiency of ivermectin against *W. bancrofti* and *B. malayi* (Table 84.2). Results indicated that a single oral dose of ivermectin (150 µg/kg body weight) effectively removes microfilariae of *W. bancrofti*,[63] but microfilariae reappear in the blood faster than after treatment with a dose of DEC and there is no evidence of a macrofilaricidal effect. In brugian filariasis the fall in microfilaraemia is more gradual than is the case in bancroftian filariasis. Side-effects of ivermectin therapy are generally similar to those mentioned above for DEC. Ivermectin should not be used in pregnant women or in children below 5 years of age.

The major role of ivermectin in lymphatic filariasis is for treatment and control of infection in areas that are co-endemic for onchocerciasis and/or loiasis (i.e. many parts of Africa). Since it has no macrofilaricidal effect, repeated half-yearly or yearly treatments are needed to keep the microfilaraemia at a low level. Ivermectin also has an effect against *Ascaris*, hookworm and scabies infection.

Symptomatic treatment

It has increasingly been recognized that microbial co-infections play an important role in the aetiology of most ADL attacks, and that foot care combined with antibiotic and antifungal therapy can play an important role in their prevention and cure.[20,64,65]

Chronic lymphoedema and elephantiasis can also benefit greatly from prevention and treatment of superficial bacterial and fungal infections. Patient education should emphasize the importance of hygiene and skin care to reduce the number of acute attacks and thereby to prevent progression of the disease.[20] Wearing of shoes, made to fit the often deformed feet, is an important way to limit the risk of skin lesions. Physiotherapy and bandaging are more professional approaches which can be very helpful to alleviate and reduce the lymphoedema. Elevation of the affected limb during rest and sleep may also be beneficial.

Surgical management

Before any surgical procedure, a course of DEC is recommended. Chronic hydroceles require excision and eversion of the sac. In scrotal elephantiasis the surgical removal of the grossly elephantoid skin and scrotal tissues with preservation of the penis and testicles has proved worthwhile. Surgical treatment of limb elephantiasis has generally proved unsuccessful. Earlier techniques involving the excision of redundant tissue from severely affected limbs generally led to long-term results that were unsatisfactory. More beneficial responses have been obtained recently with lymphovenous procedures, followed by removal of excess subcutaneous and fatty tissue from the affected extremities and adequate postural drainage and physiotherapy. In chyluria, if conservative approaches using DEC therapy and restriction of dietary fats are not helpful, then surgery is indicated.

Epidemiology

Humans are infected by mosquitoes carrying infective larvae. There is no evidence for animals being infected with *W. bancrofti* under natural conditions. The nocturnally periodic form of *B. malayi* has been reported only in humans, but the subperiodic form is found also in a wide variety of domestic and wild animals (monkeys, cats). There appears to be no animal reservoir of *B. timori*.

Microfilariae of all species can be transmitted in blood transfusions and will circulate in the recipient's blood for weeks. Congenital transmission of microfilariae has been reported but seems to be of little significance, and these microfilariae do not undergo further development.

Infection and disease in the endemic community

Characteristic patterns of microfilaraemia, circulating antigenaemia and disease are seen in affected populations in endemic areas.[10,17,18] An example of this pattern in a highly *W. bancrofti* endemic East African village is seen in Figure 84.11. Usually, microfilaraemia starts to appear in children of about 5 years of age. The prevalence then rises with increasing age and commences to level out above the age of 30 years. The prevalence rarely goes above 40–50% in any age group. It may decrease slightly in older persons. The prevalence of specific circulating antigenaemia is higher than that of microfilaraemia in all age groups. Signs of disease begin to develop around the onset of puberty or in early adult life, with recurrent ADL attacks. Hydroceles also begin to appear around this age. The prevalence of signs rises steadily, and in highly endemic areas the majority of elderly males may have

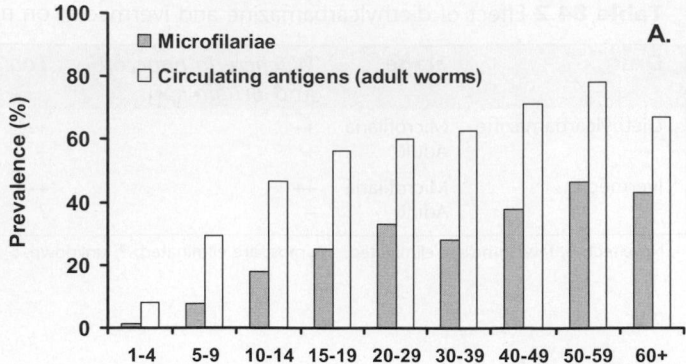

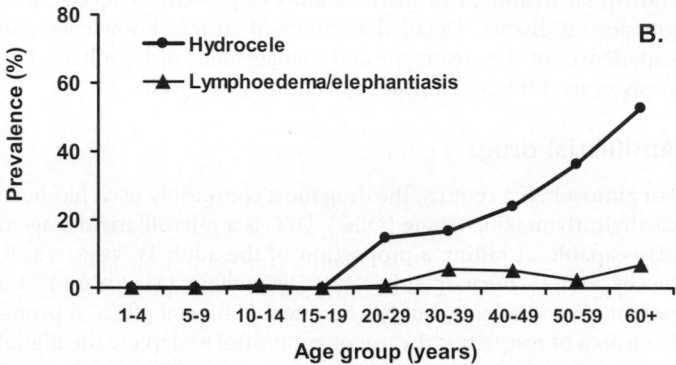

Figure 84.11 The pattern of *W. bancrofti* infection and chronic disease as seen in an endemic village on the coast of north-east Tanzania. Prevalence of (A) microfilaraemia and circulating filarial antigenaemia among all, and (B) prevalence of hydrocele grade 2 and above among males and lymphoedema/elephantiasis among all. (Based on Simonsen et al.[10])

hydroceles. In stable endemic communities elephantiasis is seen mainly in older people, but younger persons may also be affected. The overall burden of infection and disease in the endemic community is proportional to the intensity of transmission.

Cross-sectional surveys, although providing important information on the distribution of infection and disease in the affected population, give only a static view of the situation. In reality there is a dynamic sequel in development of infection and disease. Some of the people who are uninfected during the survey may have been positive for microfilariae or adult worms previously, or will become so later. Also, clinical manifestations often develop late in the course of infection, when some people have reached an uninfected stage. However, a recent 26-year follow-up survey indicated that once infection has been acquired, the chance of ever becoming naturally free of infection is small.[66] In many surveys the prevalence and intensity of microfilaraemia has been slightly higher in males than in females, and this appears to be especially significant for those aged 15–40 years. It has been suggested that hormonal factors in females of reproductive age make them more resistant to infection than males of the same age group.[67]

Exposure to intense transmission over long periods is necessary before a patent infection with microfilariae is acquired, and visitors to endemic areas rarely acquire microfilaraemia. Prenatal exposure to parasite antigens may explain why children born to microfilaraemic mothers appear to have a higher chance of developing microfilaraemia later, than do those born to amicrofilaraemic mothers,[18,68] but increased household exposure may also be a contributing factor.[69]

Geographical variation in transmission

The epidemiology of *W. bancrofti* and *B. malayi* infections varies in different geographical areas, especially with respect to the prevalence and intensity of infection, the transmission pattern and the clinical manifestations. Differences in vectorial capacity and density are important factors influencing these epidemiological parameters in different endemic areas.[70] Even within the endemic community there can be considerable variation in vector abundance and transmission between different sections and from one household to the next.[71]

There are also inherent differences in the parasite; for example, three strains of *W. bancrofti* and two strains of *B. malayi* have been recognized on the basis of differences in periodicity of the microfilariae. In most areas the microfilariae of *W. bancrofti* are nocturnally periodic, being adapted to transmission by night-biting *Culex* and *Anopheles* mosquitoes. A diurnal subperiodic form is found in the South Pacific and in the Andaman and Nicobar Islands (India), whereas a nocturnally subperiodic form is found in Thailand. *B. malayi* occurs both in a nocturnal periodic and a nocturnal subperiodic form, whereas *B. timori* is nocturnally periodic. The subperiodic forms are transmitted by vectors that bite mainly during the daytime. It is possible that variation in worm habitat preferences within the host's lymphatic system may contribute to differences in clinical manifestations.

For details of the vector species and their bionomics, see Appendix IV. Different geographical vector zones have been recognized on the basis of the predominant vector species responsible for transmission in the areas.[72] *Culex quinquefasciatus* is the principal vector of *W. bancrofti* in urban and semiurban areas of southern and South-east Asia, East Africa and America. Increased pollution of freshwater bodies and the introduction of pit latrines, which favour breeding of this mosquito, has led to increased transmission in many areas. *C. quinquefasciatus* is an endophilic night-biter. There is no evidence that it is transmitting filariasis in West Africa. In rural areas of Asia and Africa, *Anopheles* spp. are the main vectors, with the *A. gambiae* complex and *A. funestus* being the most important vectors in Africa. The main vectors of the *Anopheles* spp. bite indoors at night and breed in open, rather clean, water.

In the South Pacific islands the predominant vectors of *W. bancrofti* belong to day-biting *Aedes* spp., especially *A. polynesiensis*. The majority of these mosquitoes bite outdoors and breed in small temporary water collections: tree holes, empty cans and bottles, coconut shells, plant axils and crab holes. In Papua New Guinea night-biting *Anopheles* spp. are the principal vectors.

The nocturnally subperiodic form of *B. malayi* is transmitted by *Mansonia* mosquitoes in dense swamp forest areas. This form is commonly found also in wild monkeys. Nocturnally periodic *B. malayi* has been reported only from humans. It is transmitted in open plains and agricultural areas, mainly by *Mansonia* spp. mosquitoes, although in some areas species of *Anopheles* and *Aedes* also play a role. The larvae and pupae of *Mansonia* mosquitoes

obtain their oxygen directly from the cells of certain species of aquatic plants present in clean water-bodies. Survival of the *Mansonia* spp. is dependent on the association with the plants. Increased pollution has in some places led to a decrease in breeding of *Mansonia*, with a subsequent drop in transmission of *B. malayi*. *Mansonia* spp. prefer to feed outside and biting usually commences shortly after dusk. *A. barbirostris* is the only mosquito to date to have been identified as a vector of *B. timori*.

Control

In communities endemic for lymphatic filariasis, the disfiguring and debilitating clinical manifestations result in much suffering and have severe socioeconomic and psychological consequences for those affected.[73,74] The objective of control is to reduce transmission and morbidity, thereby eliminating lymphatic filariasis as a public health problem. Successful programmes for the control of lymphatic filariasis must be based on a thorough understanding of the distribution and dynamics of the disease in the targeted population. The diverse characteristics of communities in endemic foci, as well as differences in vector, parasite and disease parameters, emphasize the importance of having multiple measures and approaches for control.

The main method used in the control of lymphatic filariasis is mass chemotherapy.[75] It may be supplemented by mosquito control.[72] Morbidity control through patient management (hygiene, antimicrobial treatment, physiotherapy) and establishment of self-help groups is recommended.[20] To achieve success in a control programme it is necessary for the community to be actively involved. Community leaders and motivated persons should be identified and approached for the purpose of obtaining their cooperation. Adequate health education should be given regarding the nature of the disease and on the methods used for its control.[76,77]

Before starting a control programme, knowledge of the geographical delimitation of the disease is essential. Rapid assessment procedures are based on examination of specific age-sex groups in selected populations to determine the prevalence of easily recognizable signs such as hydrocele or circulating antigenaemia. Geographical information system (GIS) has been utilized for large-scale mapping of the disease.[78,79] All areas with indigenously acquired infections are considered to be endemic. Criteria for distinguishing different levels of endemicity have so far not been established.

Mathematical models of lymphatic filariasis transmission, infection and disease within the endemic community have been developed. It is envisaged that such models can be used to predict the outcome of control based on different measures, and thus can provide guidance towards the most cost-effective control strategies in specific settings.[80,81]

Chemotherapeutic control

Chemotherapeutic control of lymphatic filariasis is generally based on mass treatment, i.e. the drug is administered to the total population in the community (except individuals in whom it is contraindicated). In mass treatment campaigns there is no need to conduct parasitological or other diagnoses before treatment. Thus cost is reduced. The amicrofilaraemic infections and persons

More than 99% of all cases are in Africa in a zone that spreads from west to east. This band extends between 15°N and 15°S in the west, and widens slightly towards the east. As a result of recent mapping surveys, the estimate for numbers infected in Africa is likely to be revised upwards.[91]

Foci in Guatemala and Mexico of about 90 000 infected individuals exist mainly on the Pacific slope of the Sierra Madra between altitudes of 500 and 1500 m. Northern Venezuela has a focus with about 40 000 infected individuals. Smaller foci have been found in southern Venezuela, Columbia, Brazil, Ecuador and Yemen.[90]

Life cycle and transmission

The general filarial life cycle is shown in Figure 84.1. For details of the life cycle of *O. volvulus*, see also Appendix III.

Adult worms live mainly in subcutaneous nodules or are free in the skin. The ratio of adult females : males in nodules is about 3 : 1. The adults are slender white worms, the male being 2–5 cm × 0.2 mm and the females 35–70 cm × 0.4 mm. The female produces sheathless microfilariae measuring 300 × 8 µm with an expanded head free of nuclei and a sharply pointed tail (Figure 84.14).

Microfilariae are found mainly in the upper dermis and in nodules but may also appear in blood, urine or any body fluid, particularly in heavy infections. They are common in the eye, with direct spread from adjacent skin appearing to be their main mode of entry. Microfilarial loads can be as high as 2000/mg of skin, and heavily infected individuals may harbour >100 000 000 microfilariae. The microfilariae have a lifespan of 1–2 years.

Microfilariae present in the skin are ingested by the *Simulium* vector when feeding. Some of the ingested microfilariae migrate from the gut of the blackfly into the thoracic muscles and develop via two moults into infective larvae over a period of 6–12 days (for a description of the development in the fly see Appendix III, and for the life history of *Simulium* see Appendix IV). Transmission of infective larvae to humans occurs when the fly takes its next blood meal. The larvae migrate to the subcutaneous tissues, moult twice, and then develop over several months to adult worms. The gravid female releases microfilariae, which may appear in the skin after a prepatent period of 10–15 months after the introduction of infective larvae. Some 500–1500 microfilariae are released per female per day, and the mean duration of female reproductive life has been estimated at 9–11 years.

Simulium flies can breed only in well oxygenated water. The gravid female oviposits into free-flowing rivers and streams, particularly in rapids, and transmission takes place mainly near these locations, hence the name 'river blindness'.

Transmission in utero of microfilariae of *O. volvulus* has been reported. These microfilariae do not undergo further development.

Clinical features

The main clinical manifestations of onchocerciasis are skin lesions, eye lesions and nodule formation. In general, clinical manifestations develop after long exposure to infection, and their severity depends on the intensity of infection. Many individuals who have

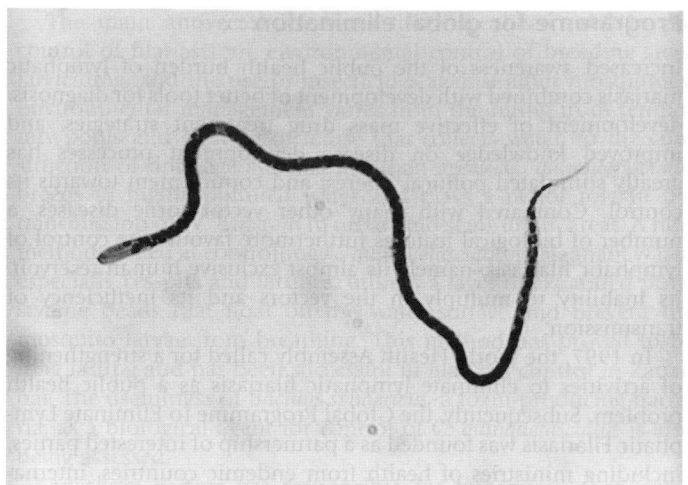

Figure 84.14 Skin microfilaria of *O. volvulus*.

microfilariae in the skin, especially those with light infections, have no symptoms or signs.

Skin lesions

Dermal changes occur when the microfilariae undergo destruction in the skin and vary from a few papules to the extensive pigmentary and chronic atrophic changes.[92] A clinical classification and grading system of the cutaneous changes in onchocerciasis has been developed, with the main recognized categories being acute papular onchodermatitis, chronic papular onchodermatitis, lichenified onchodermatitis, skin atrophy, and skin depigmentation.[93] Frequently a combination of these categories exists in the same person. In Africa, the skin lesions are most common over the legs but may cover the whole body. A range of skin lesions is shown in Figure 84.15.

Itching and rash are the most important early manifestations of onchocercal dermatitis. The rash consists of many raised papules, which are due to microabscess formation, and may disappear within a few days or may spread. Often the rash is confined to one anatomical quarter of the body. The resulting pruritus can be very intense (filarial itch), and the skin often becomes secondarily infected following scratching. In the later stages there may be heavy lichenification and thickening of the skin (lizard skin).

The more chronic changes are probably related to the repeated occurrence of local pathology around dying parasites. There is skin atrophy with loss of elasticity, giving a prematurely aged appearance (presbyderma). Loss of elastic fibres in the skin of the groin may lead to hernia, and to the classical 'hanging groin' with inguinal and/or femoral glands contained in pendulous folds.

A condition called leopard skin (Figure 84.15B) may occur. This results from loss of pigment, degeneration of the dermal collagen and thinning of the epidermis. Leopard skin particularly affects the pretibial regions, where trauma or scratching following the bites of *Simulium* flies may exacerbate, or even cause, the depigmentation of this condition.

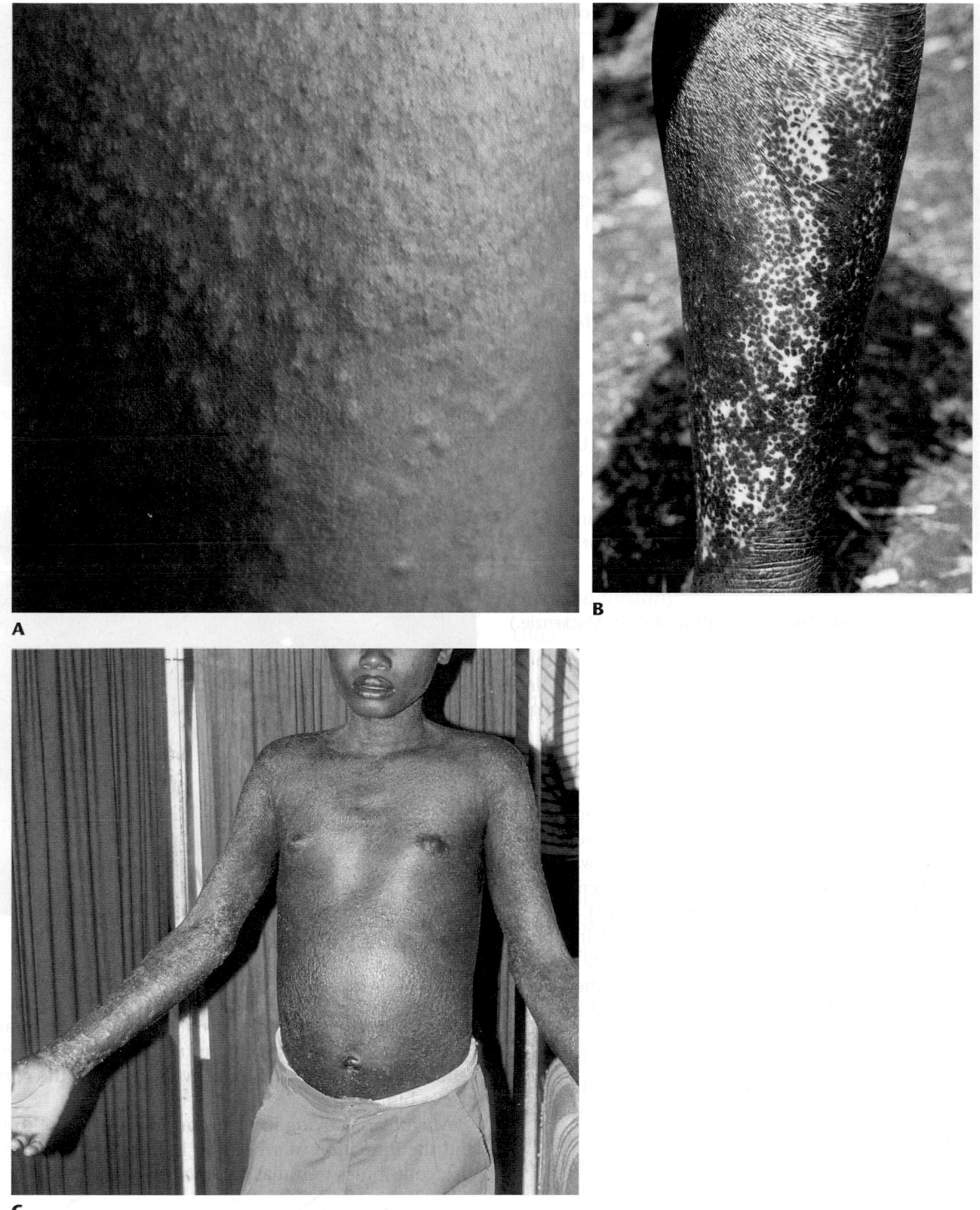

Figure 84.15 Onchocerciasis: skin lesions. (A) Papules on skin (courtesy of C. D. Mackenzie); (B) depigmentation and leopard skin (courtesy of C. D. Mackenzie); (C) lichenified eczematoid dermatitis of the body and arms (courtesy of E. M. Pedersen).

Sowda

Sowda (Figure 84.16), from the Arabic for black or dark, is a localized form of onchodermatitis. It is common in the Yemen, but is also found elsewhere.

Sowda is the result of a strong immune response on the part of the host. The condition is usually localized to one limb but both legs and/or arms or the trunk may be involved. It is characterized by intense itching. The involved skin becomes swollen and darkened, and covered with scaly papules. Local

Snips are immersed in isotonic saline, for instance in wells of a microtitration plate. Microfilariae that have emerged after 0.5–24 h are counted under the low power of a compound microscope. Teasing of the skin is unnecessary. The sensitivity of skin snips to diagnose infection depends upon the number of skin snips taken and on the intensity of infection. Microfilariae of *O. volvulus* are 270–320 μm long, unsheathed, and have a characteristic head and a pointed tail (see Figure 84.14). They must be differentiated from the smaller skin-dwelling microfilariae of *M. streptocerca* in Africa and *M. ozzardi* in South America. Blood microfilariae – *W. bancrofti*, *Loa loa* and *M. perstans* – occasionally appear in skin snips contaminated by blood.

Immunological and PCR-based diagnosis

Several immunodiagnostic tests have been devised for onchocerciasis.[102] Adult *O. volvulus* isolated from nodules, or adult worms or microfilariae of *O. gibsoni* or *O. gutturosa* from cattle, have frequently been used as the source of antigen. Generally, immunodiagnosis based on detection of antibodies to crude antigens is of limited practical use owing to the low specificity and sensitivity of the tests. Cross-reactions to other nematode infections are common and the tests cannot distinguish between past and present infections. In endemic areas, where the population is continuously exposed to infection, most people are positive to the tests. Such tests may be of value in the diagnosis of onchocerciasis in persons from non-endemic areas who have visited an endemic area.

The development of specific and sensitive immunodiagnostic tests has been a priority in onchocerciasis research. The specificity of tests has been improved by the detection of specific IgG4 antibodies and by the identification and use of specific antigens. Tests utilizing specific recombinant antigens have been developed, and an ELISA with a cocktail made from three of these antigens has shown a high sensitivity and specificity.[103] A field applicable rapid-format card test that detects IgG4 to a recombinant antigen in serum or blood specimens has also proved to be sensitive and specific,[104] but is not yet commercially available. Tests for detection of specific circulating antigens in onchocerciasis have given mixed results, and in general have not been as successful as in lymphatic filariasis. However, a highly sensitive and specific dipstick assay for the detection of *O. volvulus* antigens in urine was recently described.[105]

A PCR technique with high specificity for *O. volvulus* DNA has been developed. In addition to identifying worm DNA in skin snips from infected humans, this technique is capable of distinguishing between various strains of the parasite and of detecting *O. volvulus* larvae in extracts of blackfly vectors.[101]

Pathology and immunology

Large numbers of live microfilariae may be present in the skin without inducing any tissue reaction (Figure 84.20). Pathology in the skin and in the anterior segment of the eye is caused mainly by dying and dead microfilariae. Like many other filarial parasites, *O. volvulus* contains endosymbiontic bacteria of the genus *Wolbachia*. Recent studies have implicated products from these endosymbionts in the pathogenesis of onchocerciasis, especially the ocular manifestations.[48,106]

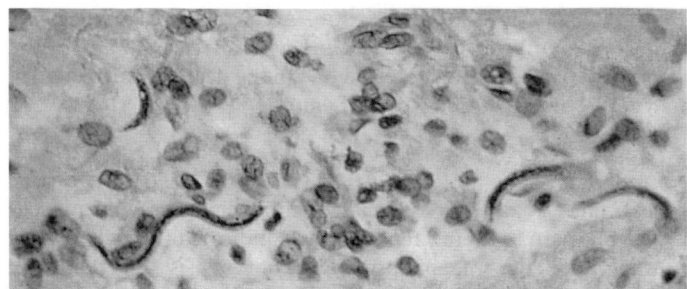

Figure 84.20 Onchocerciasis: microfilariae of *O. volvulus* in subcutaneous tissue.

The initial lesions comprise foci of inflammatory reactions around degenerating microfilariae, composed mainly of eosinophils, neutrophils and macrophages.[107,108] Antibodies, immune complex formation and complement activation on the surface of the microfilariae may be involved in attracting the immunocompetent cells.[109] The dermal tissue between the early focal lesions shows no changes. Later, dermal fibroblasts increase in numbers, leading to fibrosis, and the normal collagen and elastic fibres of the dermis are gradually replaced by hyalinized scar tissue. There may also be loss of pigment in the skin. The histological appearance of the skin in advanced cases closely resembles the skin of very old subjects (i.e. presbyderma). Some of the skin damage observed in onchocerciasis patients may also be caused by the mechanical effects of scratching, by toxins inoculated when blackflies take a blood meal or by secondary infections.

In the skin condition Sowda, there is immunological hyperactivity, and the most striking histopathological feature is the presence of an extensive inflammatory cell infiltrate of the upper dermis. Identification of *O. volvulus* collagen as a principal antigen recognized by antibodies in patients with Sowda raises the possibility that this condition might arise through cross-reactivity between these antibodies and human collagen.[110]

Using a slit lamp, live microfilariae can be seen in the cornea of the eye. There is no visible tissue response to their presence. Dead microfilariae give rise to foci of inflammation which cause the characteristic punctate ('snowflake') keratitis, with opacities around each microfilaria. The major pathology of the anterior segment is due to sclerosing keratitis. Chronic inflammation and vascularization leading to scarring eventually result in complete opacification of the cornea. This process normally starts from each side and from below, and resembles an inflammatory immune response. The aetiology of the posterior segment lesions is less clear.[111]

Some adult worms are found free in the subcutaneous tissues but most are contained in nodules. Nodules are essentially granulomatous reactions around adult worms. They often have separate chambers containing several worms. Nodules have thick fibrous walls and a variable degree of cellular infiltration (Figure 84.21) with macrophages being the predominant cell type.[108] Calcification may occur in older nodules and in dead worms.

Specific humoral immune responses of individuals living in areas endemic for onchocerciasis are usually marked. Most infected individuals have a diminished cellular responsiveness to *O. volvulus* antigens in comparison to apparently uninfected persons from

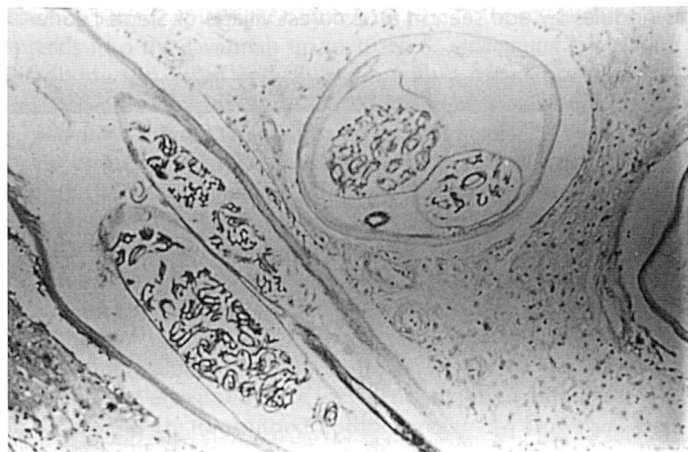

Figure 84.21 Onchocerciasis: adult *O. volvulus* in nodule. (Courtesy of H. Zaiman.)

the same endemic areas and to patients with the more localized Sowda.[108] A major role of immune responses appears to be to contain or limit inflammation around dying or dead microfilariae. Antibodies mediating cellular killing of microfilariae and infective larvae in vitro have been observed in sera from some persons living in endemic areas.[109] The presence of such antibodies may indicate that immune elimination of larval stages occurs in some infected individuals, although protective immunity has not been proved in onchocerciasis. In utero exposure to *O. volvulus* antigens may affect the child's immune responses and perhaps his or her susceptibility to *O. volvulus* infection later in life.[112]

In individuals from non-endemic areas who become infected during visits to endemic areas, infections are usually mild and the most common clinical presentation is dermatitis.[113] Microfilaraemia may be of low density or absent. Nodules or eye lesions are rare. The patients usually have specific antibody responses to *O. volvulus* and raised eosinophil levels.

Immune responses to mycobacterial infections[114] and to tetanus vaccination[115] are downregulated in *O. volvulus*-infected individuals. HIV-infected onchocerciasis patients exhibit significantly impaired antibody responses to *O. volvulus* antigens and tend to lose their reactivity to these antigens over time.[116]

Management

Drug treatment

DEC is no longer recommended for the treatment of onchocerciasis. It can induce severe adverse reactions, especially in heavily infected individuals, and may precipitate or aggravate ocular lesions. It has now been replaced by ivermectin (Mectizan®) as the drug of choice.[90] Both of these drugs have a strong microfilaricidal effect, whereas adult worms remain essentially unaffected (see Table 84.2).

Suramin, although largely used as a macrofilaricide, also has some microfilaricidal effects. Fatalities due to drug toxicity may occur and its use is not recommended. The macrofilaricidal effects of benzimidazoles are being investigated. Endosymbiontic bacteria (*Wolbachia* spp.), recently discovered in *O. volvulus*, are potential new targets for chemotherapy with antibiotics.[117]

Ivermectin

Ivermectin in a single oral dose of 150 µg/kg body weight causes a rapid elimination of microfilariae from the skin.[118] More than 80% of skin microfilariae are eliminated in the first 48 h and this then slowly increases to 97%. The low level of microfilaraemia is maintained over a period of several months, after which there is a gradual increase. Retreatment may be necessary and follow-up skin snips should be examined 6–12 months after the initial treatment. Treatment is contraindicated in pregnant women, breast-feeding women with infants below 1 week old, children below 5 years of age, or individuals with serious acute or chronic illnesses.

Adverse reactions resemble, but appear to be much less severe than, those associated with DEC therapy. In a study in Sierra Leone[119] the most common side-effect of ivermectin was the passing of *Ascaris* worms! Other effects in descending order of frequency were itching and/or rash, muscle and/or joint pains, fever, headache, swelling of the limbs, joint or face, dizziness, tender lymphadenopathy, conjunctivitis and tender nodules. Other investigators have noted severe postural hypotension and bronchoconstriction to be side-effects of ivermectin therapy. These conditions are reported to be transient and to respond to symptomatic management. The single-dose ivermectin regimens have no known long-lasting effect on mature worms, but the drug causes intrauterine degeneration and temporary sequestration of unborn microfilariae. Recent studies suggest that the drug may have a macrofilaricidal effect if more frequent (3-monthly) treatments are given.[120]

The disappearance of microfilariae from the eye is much more gradual than microfilarial reduction in the skin. Available data on the impact of repeated doses of ivermectin on ocular onchocercal disease indicate regression of early lesions of the anterior segment, including iridocyclitis and sclerosing keratitis. It also appears to have a beneficial effect on optic nerve disease and visual field loss, but not on chorioretinitis.[121]

Nodulectomy

Nodulectomy has only limited use because many worms are present outside the nodules and some nodules are not palpable. Head nodules should be excised because their presence increases the risk of eye disease and blindness.

Epidemiology

O. volvulus is transmitted between humans and the vectors. The infection is not a zoonosis. Many species and subspecies of *Simulium* flies can act as vectors. Despite geographical variation in pathogenicity, *O. volvulus* parasites are morphologically indistinguishable throughout their range of distribution.

Infection and disease in the endemic community

The epidemiology of onchocerciasis varies throughout its distribution. Different patterns of infection and disease are associated with differences in the abundance, vector competence and feeding characteristics of the local blackfly populations, differences in parasite strains and differences in the human host response to the

treatment with ivermectin became the principal strategy for onchocerciasis control. It reduces the microfilarial burden and thus transmission in the community.[139] Since ivermectin is only microfilaricidal, treatments should continue for a period equivalent to the reproductive lifespan of the adult female worms, in order to halt transmission. Currently a dose of 150 mg/kg body weight once yearly is being encouraged for most endemic areas. Children under the age of 5 years should not be treated.

The manufacturer of Mectizan® (Merck) has made this product available free of charge through the Mectizan® Donation Program to governmental and non-governmental healthcare organizations involved in onchocerciasis control programmes.[140]

Repeated treatments with ivermectin result in significant improvement of itching and severe onchocercal skin disease[141] and in regression of both early and advanced lesions of the anterior segment of the eye.[94,121] As an additional benefit ivermectin reduces the prevalence and intensity of *Ascaris* infections.

Following the initial field testing of ivermectin, the OCP started large-scale distribution for transmission and morbidity control in the programme area.[91,135] Numerous smaller control programmes utilizing mass treatment were also started in other endemic areas. Partnerships of non-governmental organizations involved in blindness prevention, international organizations (including the WHO and the World Bank) and governments of endemic countries subsequently established the African Programme for Onchocerciasis Control (APOC) and the Onchocerciasis Elimination Program in the Americas (OEPA) for the promotion and coordination of control activities on the African and American continents, respectively. APOC took over as the leading coordinating body of onchocerciasis control in Africa when the OCP ended its activities in 2002.

Serious reactions, including death, after mass ivermectin treatment for onchocerciasis have recently been reported in individuals with high-intensity *Loa loa* microfilaraemia,[142] and call for caution when using ivermectin in loiasis endemic areas. Most of these reactions have been observed in Cameroon.

To date, resistance of *O. volvulus* to ivermectin has not been observed.[143] However, there is an urgent need for development of new backup drugs should this occur. In particular it would be beneficial with a safe and easily administered macrofilaricidal drug, which could reduce the time needed to eliminate the adult worms from endemic areas.[91,144]

Nodulectomy

Nodulectomy campaigns have been encouraged in some countries, especially in those where head nodules are common. The impact of such campaigns on ocular disease can be difficult to assess. In Guatemala, for example, where systematic campaigns have been associated with decreased blindness, other factors, particularly changes in socioeconomic conditions, may have decreased human–vector contact.

OTHER FILARIAL INFECTIONS

In addition to the filarial worms resulting in human lymphatic filariasis and onchocerciasis, four other species of filariae commonly infect humans. These are *Loa loa*, *Mansonella perstans*, *M.*

streptocerca and *M. ozzardi* (see Table 84.1). A few species of animal filariae cause rare zoonotic infections in humans.

Loa loa

Loa loa is a filarial parasite of humans in parts of West and Central Africa.[145] It is commonly known as the 'eye-worm', because adult worms are occasionally seen to move across the eye of the patient.

Life cycle and transmission

Adult *L. loa* live and move around in the connective tissues of humans. They frequently wander through the subcutaneous tissues and may sometimes pass beneath the conjunctiva of the eye. The females measure 50–70 × 0.5 mm and the males 30–35 × 0.4 mm. More detailed morphology is given in Appendix III. The sheathed microfilariae circulate in the blood and measure 230–300 × 6–8 μm (Figure 84.22).

Human *L. loa* is transmitted by tabanid flies of the genus *Chrysops*. The microfilarial periodicity is adapted to the day-biting habits of the vectors. It is diurnal, with peak concentration in the peripheral blood around noon (Figure 84.23). Microfilariae ingested by the vectors during feeding penetrate the stomach wall of the flies and migrate to the fat body where they develop in 8–12 days. Infective larvae (2 mm × 25 μm) then move via the thorax to the proboscis. The larvae burrow into the skin of the human host when the vector feeds. The minimum prepatent period (until appearance of microfilariae) is 5–6 months, but it can be much longer, and adult worms may live for 17 years or more.

Clinical features

The most common clinical manifestations of loiasis are recurrent angio-oedema (Calabar swellings) and pruritus. Adult worms may be noticed when they pass under the conjunctiva of the eye (Figure 84.24) or under the skin (Figure 84.25).[146–148] They usually appear and then disappear within 10–15 min, leaving no trace behind.

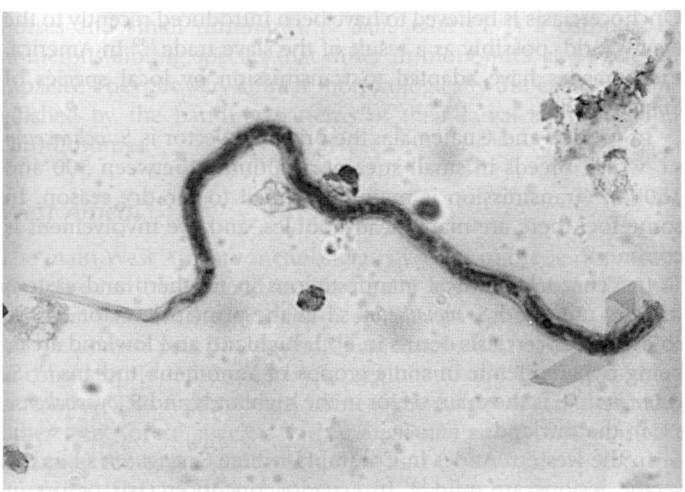

Figure 84.22 Microfilaria of *L. loa*.

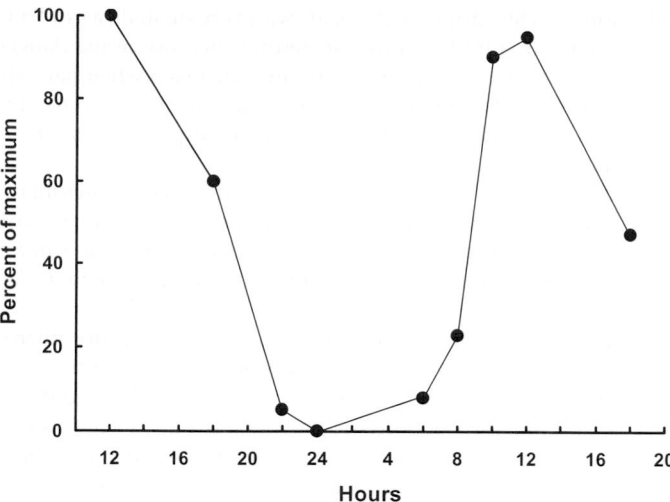

Figure 84.23 Periodicity of *L. loa* microfilariae in the peripheral blood.

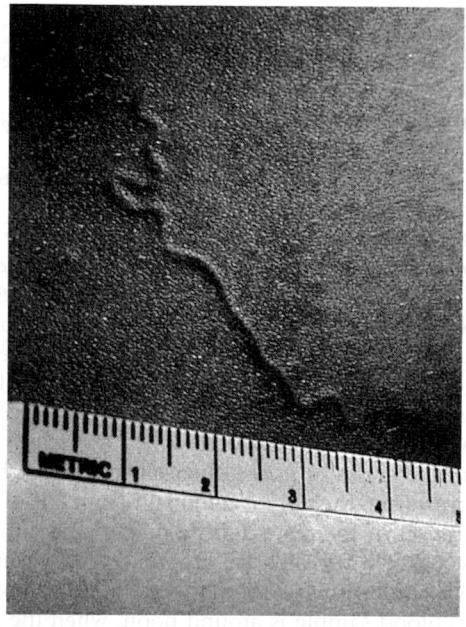

Figure 84.25 *L. loa* migrating under the skin. (Courtesy of P. G. P. Manson-Bahr.)

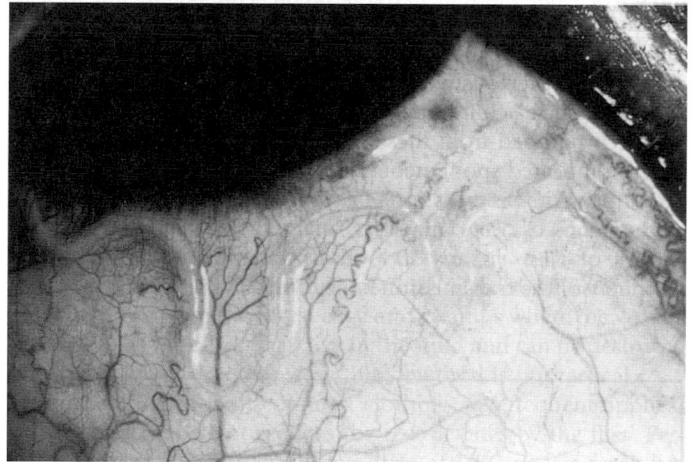

Figure 84.24 Transocular migration of adult *L. loa*. (Courtesy of J. Anderson.)

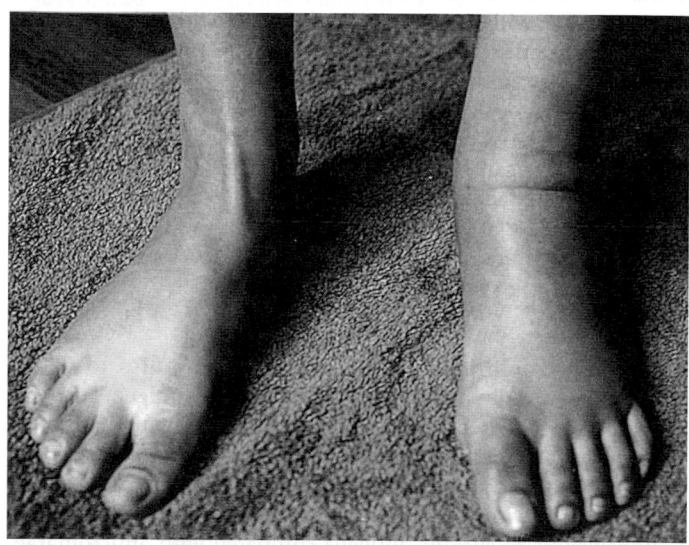

Figure 84.26 Calabar swelling.

Hypereosinophilia, especially in expatriates, is common. Calabar swellings (Figure 84.26) are most commonly observed on the hands, wrists and forearms, but they may appear anywhere on the body. The swellings are painless, and do not pit on pressure. They may last from a few hours to several days. Usually one swelling occurs at a time, and may recur at irregular intervals for years after the patient has left the endemic area. Calabar swellings probably reflect the host's response to parasite antigens at the site of the swellings. Other common symptoms include generalized pruritus, fatigue and arthralgia. The death of an adult worm may occasionally cause a localized abscess. Dead worms sometimes calcify and are then easily seen on radiography.

More serious complications can occur when *L. loa* invade the central nervous system and other vital organs. An epidemiological correlation has been observed between loiasis and the occurrence of endomyocardial fibrosis, and it is possible that hypereosinophilia induced by the infection may lead to the cardiac damage.[149]

Nephropathy and encephalopathy are less common pathological changes. Nodules in the conjunctiva, swelling of the eyelids and proptosis were previously reported from Uganda as complications of loiasis. However, histological evidence has shown that these lesions are due to *M. perstans*.[150] (For Ocular loiasis, see Chapter 18.)

As in other filarial infections, expatriates entering an endemic area are more troubled by clinical manifestations than are the indigenous inhabitants. However, the prevalence of microfilaraemia is apparently lower in expatriates than in the local inhabitants.[148,151]

Diagnosis is by recovering the microfilariae (Figure 84.29) from the blood. Blood samples may be obtained at any time of the day, and techniques similar to those used for concentration and examination of blood samples for the diagnosis of lymphatic filariasis are utilized. For morphological features of the microfilariae, see Appendix III.

Ivermectin has no effect on *M. perstans* (see Table 84.2). DEC (200 mg twice daily for 21 days with a gradual dosage increase the first 3 days) reduces the microfilaraemias, but mebendazole (100 mg twice daily for 28 days) appears to be more effective in eliminating the infection. A combination of mebendazole and DEC resulted in a significantly higher activity than each of these drugs alone.[165] Albendazole (400 mg twice daily) given for 10 days resulted in a slow but significant decrease in *M. perstans* of microfilaraemia after 1–3 months.[166]

Few studies have been carried out on the epidemiology of *M. perstans* infections. The microfilarial prevalence is generally higher in adults than in children, and males are usually more frequently infected than females.[167] In some localities very high prevalences of microfilaraemia are found.[168]

The main vectors in Africa are *C. grahami* and *C. inornatipennis*, but other species of *Culicoides* also play a role. The species of *Culicoides* transmitting *M. perstans* in the Americas have not been identified. *M. perstans* is found commonly in chimpanzees and gorillas, but it is also widespread in areas where there are no large apes.

Mansonella streptocerca

M. streptocerca is a filarial parasite of humans, having a limited distribution in Central and West Africa (Figure 84.30). A new focus in Uganda was described recently.[169] The adult worms inhabit the dermis of the upper thorax and shoulders, but they have rarely been recovered and very few have been examined in detail. The adult female measures 27×0.08 mm and the male 17×0.05 mm. The microfilariae (Figure 84.31) also inhabit the dermis. They are unsheathed, measure $180–240 \times 3–5$ μm and exhibit no periodicity.

M. streptocerca is transmitted by tiny biting midges of the genus *Culicoides*, the most common vector probably being *C. grahami*. Complete development in the vector has been observed experimentally to take 9 days. Information on the development of *M. streptocerca* in the human host is lacking, and the prepatent period is unknown.

The infection generally causes few clinical manifestations. Dermatitis is the most common sign and is most marked over the thorax and shoulders.[169] It is characterized by pruritus, hypopigmented macules and papules. Microscopically, infected skin shows dilated dermal lymphatics, and it has been suggested that *M. streptocerca* might be a cause of lymphoedema and elephantiasis. Clinically the infection must be distinguished from onchocerciasis and leprosy.

Diagnosis is made by finding the unsheathed microfilariae of *M. streptocerca* in skin snips (for the technique, see Onchocerciasis). The microfilariae have a characteristic 'shepherd's crook' tail. Other distinguishing features of the microfilariae are shown in Figure 84.31 and mentioned in Appendix III. A sensitive and specific PCR assay for specific detection of *M. streptocerca* DNA in skin biopsies has been developed.[170]

DEC eliminates both microfilariae and adults (see Table 84.2) of *M. streptocerca* when given in a dosage of 2–6 mg/kg body weight for 21 days. In most patients, the DEC treatment causes intense pruritus and development of cutaneous papules in which degenerating adult worms may be found. Other side reactions similar to the Mazzotti reaction during DEC treatment of onchocerciasis may occur but are not common. Ivermectin in a single dose of 150 μg/kg body weight leads to sustained suppression of microfilaraemia in the skin.[171] Common short-term adverse reactions are increased pruritus and dermatitis.

Adults and microfilariae of *M. streptocerca* are found in the skin of chimpanzees, but whether the infection is a zoonosis is not known.

Mansonella ozzardi

M. ozzardi is a human filarial parasite found only in the New World. Foci exist in Central America, in northern South America and in some Caribbean islands (Figure 84.32). A new focus in Bolivia was described recently.[172] Adult worms have been recov-

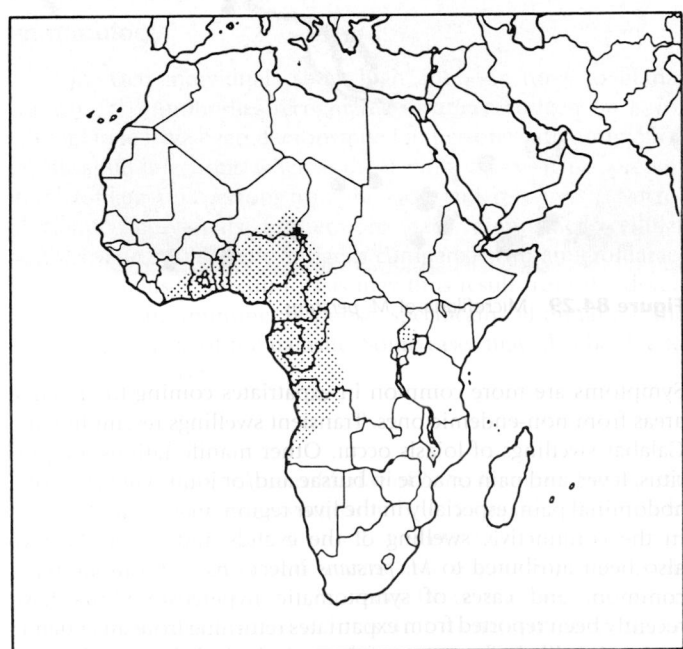

Figure 84.30 Geographical distribution of *M. streptocerca*.

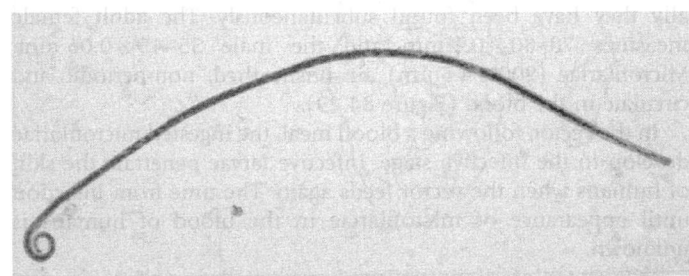

Figure 84.31 Microfilaria of *M. streptocerca*. (Courtesy of P. Fischer.)

on the importa
Special monofil
ing water, but ef
polyester cloth[
cloth. To preven
health educatio
guinea worm u
control can be a
ticide temephos
veillance on the
is being adop
sible control r
containment).

REFERENCE:

1. World Health
   Fifth report of
   1992; 821.
2. Demarquay JN
   laiteux (galact
   l'on peut cons
   Gaz Méd Paris
3. Wucherer OE.
   descripta, enc
   Brazil. *Gaz Me*
4. Lewis TR. On
   chyluria and o
5. Cobbold TS. I
   Lancet 1877; ii
6. McGregor IA.
   birth of the sc
   89:1–8.
7. Grove DI. *A H*
   1990.
8. Michael E, Bu
   Today 1997; 1:
9. Simonsen PE,
   Tanzania: mic
   microfilarial ir
10. Simonsen PE,
    infection, dise
    low endemicit
    550–559.
11. Dreyer G, Add
    dilatation in tl
    Trop Med Hyg
12. Freedman DO
    lymphatic abn
    J Infect Dis 19:
13. Bernhard P, M
    reproductive h
    area in Tanzan
14. Dunyo SK, Nk
    in acute lympl
    539–540.
15. Gasarasi DB, I
    to bancroftian
    75:19–28.
16. Dreyer G, Mec
    persons living
    two syndrome

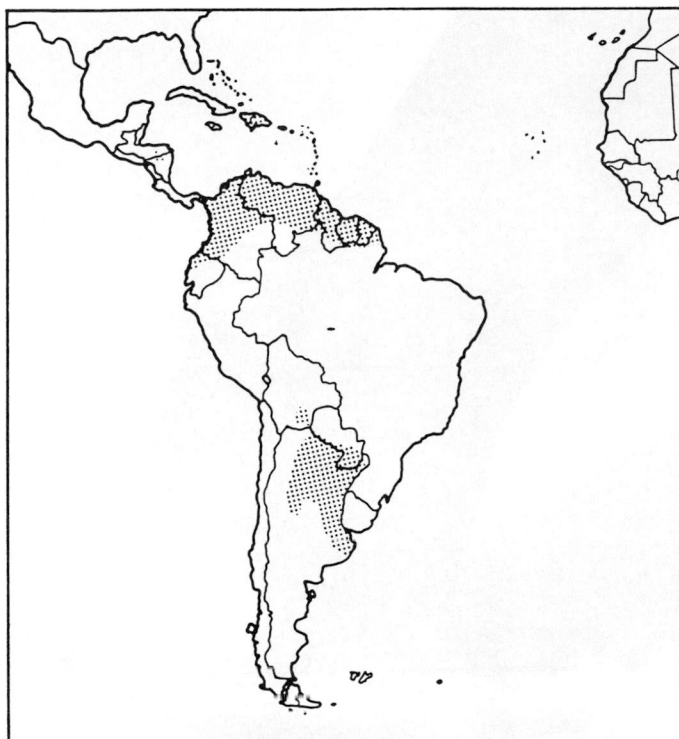

Figure 84.32 Geographical distribution of *M. ozzardi*.

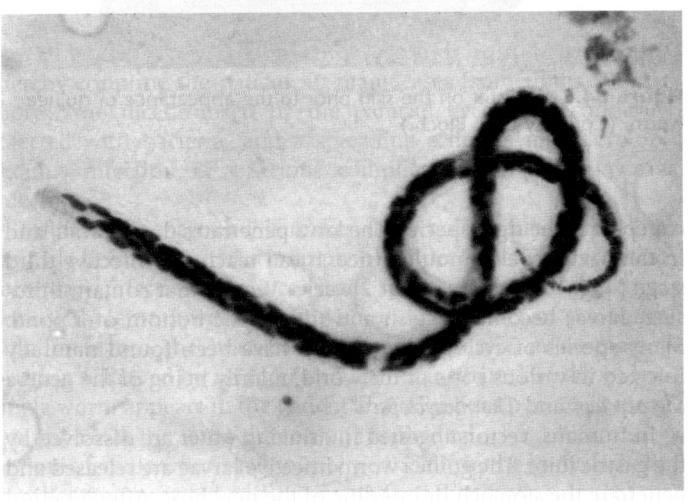

Figure 84.33 Microfilaria of *M. ozzardi*. (Courtesy of M. Eberhard.)

ered from the peritoneal cavity of humans. Females measure 50×0.15 mm and males 26×0.07 mm. The microfilariae (220×3–4 μm, see Figure 84.33) are unsheathed, non-periodic and are found in both blood and skin.

Two groups of vectors have been shown to transmit *M. ozzardi* infections. In the Caribbean islands the vectors are biting midges of the genera *Culicoides*, whereas in the Amazon basin *Simulium* blackflies have been incriminated. The development of the parasite has been studied in the vectors and in experimental infections in patas monkeys. In the monkeys the prepatent period was 5–6

months. Natural *M. ozzardi* infections have not been reported from animals. In endemic foci, human infections tend to be highly prevalent, with the microfilarial infection rates increasing with age.[172,173]

Most people infected with *M. ozzardi* are symptomless. Symptoms of severe articular pain, headache, fever and pruritus have been reported, but these have generally not been closely associated to infection.[172,173] Eosinophilia is common. Individuals in endemic areas have high titres of antibodies against filarial antigens.

The infection is diagnosed by finding the microfilariae in blood or in skin biopsies.[174] The techniques described under Lymphatic filariasis and Onchocerciasis can be used. For characteristics of the microfilariae, see Figure 84.33 and Appendix III. DEC has little or no effect on *M. ozzardi* infections (see Table 84.2), but a single dose of 6 mg ivermectin has been reported to provide significant long-term reduction in microfilaraemia.[175]

Rare filarial infections

Humans occasionally become infected with species of filariae normally found in animals.[150] Among these zoonotic infections, those due to *Dirofilaria* spp. are the most frequently reported and the most widespread.

Dirofilariasis

Dirofilaria spp. are natural parasites of various species of carnivores. In these hosts, the microfilariae circulate in the blood. Transmission is by mosquitoes. In human infections, parasite development is impaired and no microfilariae are produced.[176,177]

Pulmonary dirofilariasis

D. immitis is a filarial parasite of dogs. It is transmitted worldwide, except in cold climates. In the dog, adult *D. immitis* inhabit the pulmonary arteries and right ventricle of the heart, where they may occur in large coiled masses. Pulmonary dirofilariasis in humans results from infection with *D. immitis*. In humans, the parasite may develop partially in the pulmonary arterial tree, where it ultimately dies, perhaps as a result of an inflammatory response. Typically a spherical nodule 1–3 cm in diameter is discovered in the lungs on routine radiography (a 'coin lesion') or at autopsy. A single worm, usually necrotic and sometimes calcified, is present in the lumen of the artery. Most patients are asymptomatic. When present, symptoms include cough, chest pain, eosinophilia, haemoptysis and fever. Diagnosis is usually based on biopsy. Serological diagnosis has not been very successful. The only treatment is surgical excision.

Subcutaneous dirofilariasis

D. repens is a natural parasite of dogs and cats in warmer climates of the Old World. It has not been reported from America. In the normal hosts, adult worms are located in the subcutaneous tissues. In humans, occasional infections may result in the formation of subcutaneous nodules consisting of a degenerating immature worm surrounded by granulomatous tissue.[178] Nodules occur in

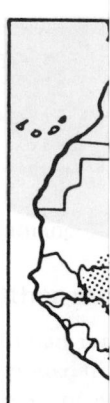

Figure 84.

A techn
eruption t
gical remo
in guinea
No ant
niridazole
been repo
allowing
infections

Epidem

Human gu
spread, bu
distributic
Africa (Fig
The oc
use of sm
contract tl
cyclopoid
immersin
release of
mission o
lecting dri
The tra
the major
within a f

129. Makunde WH, Salum FM, Massaga JJ, et al. Clinical and parasitological aspects of itching caused by onchocerciasis in Morogoro, Tanzania. *Ann Trop Med Parasitol* 2000; 94:793–799.

130. Zimmerman PA, Katholi CR, Wooten MC, et al. Recent evolutionary history of American *Onchocerca volvulus*, based on analysis of a tandemly repeated DNA sequence family. *Mol Biol Evol* 1994; 11:384–392.

131. Botto C, Gillespie AJ, Vivas-Martinez S, et al. Onchocerciasis hyperendemic in the Unturán Mountains: the value of recombinant antigens in describing a new transmission area in southern Venezuela. *Trans R Soc Trop Med Hyg* 1999; 93:25–30.

132. Corredor A, Nicholls RS, Duque S, et al. Current status of onchocerciasis in Columbia. *Am J Trop Med Hyg* 1998; 58:594–598.

133. Guderian RH, Shelley AJ. Onchocerciasis in Ecuador: the situation in 1989. *Mem Inst Oswaldo Cruz* 1992; 87:405–415.

134. Evans TG. Socioeconomic consequences of blinding onchocerciasis in West Africa. *Bull World Health Organ* 1995; 73:495–506.

135. Vlassoff C, Weiss M, Ovuga EB L, et al. Gender and the stigma of onchocercal skin disease in Africa. *Soc Sci Med* 2000; 50:1353–1368.

136. Boatin B, Molyneux DH, Hougard JM, et al. Patterns of epidemiology and control of onchocerciasis in West Africa. *J Helminthol* 1997; 71:91–101.

137. Hougard J-M, Yaméogo L, Sékétéli A, et al. Twenty-two years of blackfly control in the Onchocerciasis Control Programme in West Africa. *Parasitol Today* 1997; 13:425–431.

138. De Sole G, Awadzi K, Remme J, et al. A community trial of ivermectin in the onchocerciasis focus of Asubende, Ghana. II. Adverse reactions. *Trop Med Parasitol* 1989; 40:375–382.

139. Boatin BA, Hougard J-M, Alley ES, et al. The impact of Mectizan on the transmission of onchocerciasis. *Ann Trop Med Parasitol* 1998; 92:S47–S60.

140. Alleman MM, Twum-Danso NA Y, Thylefors BI. The Mectizan® Donation Program – highlights from 2005. *Filaria J* 2006; 5:11.

141. Brieger WR, Awedoba AK, Eneanya CI, et al. The effects of ivermectin on onchocercal skin disease and severe itching: results of a multicentre trial. *Trop Med Int Hlth* 1998; 3:951–961.

142. Gardon J, Gardon-Wendel N, Demanga-Ngangue, et al. Serious reactions after mass treatment of onchocerciasis with ivermectin in an area endemic for *Loa loa* infection. *Lancet* 1997; 350:18–22.

143. Awadzi K, Boakye DA, Edwards G, et al. An investigation of persistent microfilaridermia despite multiple treatments with ivermectin in two onchocerciasis endemic foci in Ghana. *Ann Trop Med Parasitol* 2004; 98: 231–249.

144. Hopkins AD. Ivermectin and onchocerciasis: is it all solved? *Eye* 2005; 19:1057–1066.

145. Boussinesq M. Loiasis. *Ann Trop Med Parasitol* 2006; 100:715–731.

146. Noireau F, Apembet JD, Nzoulani A, et al. Clinical manifestations of loiasis in an endemic area in the Congo. *Trop Med Parasitol* 1990; 41:37–39.

147. Klion AD, Massougbodji M, Sadeler B-C, et al. Loiasis in endemic and non-endemic populations: immunologically mediated differences in clinical presentation. *J Infect Dis* 1991; 163:1318–1325.

148. Andy JJ, Bishara FF, Soyinka OO. Relation of severe eosinophilia and microfilariasis to chronic African endomyocardial fibrosis. *Br Heart J* 1981; 45:672–680.

149. Lukiana T, Mandina M, Situakibanza NH, et al. A possible case of spontaneous *Loa loa* encephalopathy associated with a glomerulopathy. *Filaria J* 2006; 5:6.

150. Orihel TC, Eberhard ML. Zoonotic filariasis. *Clin Microbiol Rev* 1998; 11: 366–381.

151. Churchill DR, Morris C, Kakoya A, et al. Clinical and laboratory features of patients with loiasis (*Loa loa* filariasis) in the UK. *J Infect* 1996; 33: 103–109.

152. Dupont A, Zue-N'dong J, Pinder M. Common occurrence of amicrofilaraemic *Loa loa* filariasis within the endemic region. *Trans R Soc Trop Med Hyg* 1988; 82:730.

153. Klion AD, Vijaykumar A, Oei T, et al. Serum immunoglobulin G4 antibodies to the recombinant antigen, Ll-SXP-1, are highly specific for *Loa loa* infection. *J Infect Dis* 2003; 187:128–133.

154. Touré FS, Mavoungou E, Kassambara L, et al. Human occult loiasis: field evaluation of a nested polymerase chain reaction assay for the detection of occult infection. *Trop Med Int Hlth* 1998; 3:505–511.

155. Pinder M, Dupont A, Egwang TG. Identification of a surface antigen on *Loa loa* microfilariae the recognition of which correlates with the amicrofilaraemic state in man. *J Immunol* 1988; 141:2480–2486.

156. Baize S, Wahl G, Soboslay PT, et al. T helper responsiveness in human *Loa loa* infection; defective specific proliferation and cytokine production by CD4⁺ T cells from microfilaraemic subjects compared with amicrofilaraemics. *Clin Exp Immunol* 1997; 108:272–278.

157. Klion AD, Ottesen EA, Nutman TB. Effectiveness of diethylcarbamazine in treating loiasis acquired by expatriate visitors to endemic regions: long-term follow-up. *J Infect Dis* 1994; 169:604–610.

158. Duong TH, Kombila M, Ferrer A, et al. Reduced *Loa loa* microfilaria count ten to twelve months after a single dose of ivermectin. *Trans R Soc Trop Med Hyg* 1997; 91:592–593.

159. Hoegaerden MV, Ivanoff B, Flocard F, et al. The use of mebendazole in the treatment of filariases due to *Loa loa* and *Mansonella perstans*. *Ann Trop Med Parasitol* 1987; 81:275–282.

160. Tabi T-E, Befidi-Mengue R, Nutman TB, et al. Human loiasis in a Cameroonian village: A double-blind, placebo-controlled, crossover clinical trial of a three-day albendazole regimen. *Am J Trop Med Hyg* 2004; 71:211–215.

161. Klion AD, Horton J, Nutman TB. Albendazole therapy for loiasis refractory to diethylcarbamazine treatment. *Clin Infect Dis* 1999; 29:680–682.

162. Wanji S, Tendongfor N, Esum M, et al. Heterogeneity in the prevalence and intensity of loiasis in five contrasting bioecological zones in Cameroon. *Trans R Soc Trop Med Hyg* 2003; 97:182–187.

163. Nutman TB, Miller KD, Mulligan M, et al. Diethylcarbamazine provides effective prophylaxis for human loiasis. *N Engl J Med* 1988; 319:752–756.

164. Fux CA, Chappuis B, Holzer B, et al. *Mansonella perstans* causing symptomatic hypereosinophilia in a missionary family. *Travel Med Infect Dis* 2006; 4: 275–280.

165. Bregani ER, Rovellini A, Mbaïdoum M, et al. Comparison of different anthelminthic drug regimens against *Mansonella perstans* filariasis. *Trans R Soc Trop Med Hyg* 2006; 100:458–463.

166. Duong TH, Kombila M, Ferrer A, et al. Decrease in *Mansonella perstans* microfilaraemia after albendazole treatment. *Trans R Soc Trop Med Hyg* 1998; 92:459.

167. Fischer P, Kilian AH D, Bamuhiiga J, et al. Prevalence of *Mansonella perstans* in western Uganda and its detection using the QBC-fluorescence method. *Appl Parasitol* 1996; 37:32–37.

168. Onapa AW, Simonsen PE, Baehr I, et al. Rapid assessment of the geographical distribution of *Mansonella perstans* infections in Uganda, by screening schoolchildren for microfilariae. *Ann Trop Med Parasitol* 2005; 99:383–393.

169. Fischer P, Bamuhiiga J, Büttner DW. Occurrence and diagnosis of *Mansonella streptocerca* in Uganda. *Acta Trop* 1997; 63:43–55.

170. Fischer P, Büttner DW, Bamuhiiga J, et al. Detection of the filarial parasite *Mansonella streptocerca* in skin biopsies by a nested polymerase chain reaction-based assay. *Am J Trop Med Hyg* 1998; 58:816–820.

171. Fischer P, Tukesiga E, Büttner DW. Long-term suppression of *Mansonella streptocerca* microfilariae after treatment with ivermectin. *J Infect Dis* 1999; 180:1403–1405.

172. Bartoloni A, Cancrini G, Bartalesi F, et al. *Mansonella ozzardi* infection in Bolivia: prevalence and clinical association in the Chaco Region. *Am J Trop Med Hyg* 1999; 61:830–833.

173. McNeeley DF, Raccurt CP, Boncy J, et al. Clinical evaluation of *Mansonella ozzardi* in Haiti. *Trop Med Parasitol* 1988; 40:107–110.

174. Post RJ, Adams Z, Shelley AJ, et al. The morphological discrimination of microfilariae of *Onchocerca volvulus* from *Mansonella ozzardi*. *Parasitology* 2003; 127:21–27.

175. González AA, Chadee DD, Rawlins SC. Single dose of ivermectin to control mansonellosis in Trinidad: a four-year follow-up study. *Trans R Soc Trop Med Hyg* 1998; 92:570–571.

176. Simón F, López-Belmonte J, Marcos-Atxutegi C, et al. What is happening outside North America regarding human dirofilariasis. *Vet Parasitol* 2005; 133:181–189.

177. Theis JH. Public health aspects of dirofilariasis in the United States. *Vet Parasitol* 2005; 133:157–180.

178. Pampiglione S, Trotti GC, Rivasi F. Human dirofilariasis due to *Dirofilaria (Nochtiella) repens*: a review of world literature. *Parassitologia* 1995, 37: 149–193.

179. Yelifari L, Frempong E, Olsen A. The intermediate hosts of *Dracunculus medinensis* in Northern Region, Ghana. *Ann Trop Med Parasitol* 1997; 91: 403–409.

180. Bloch P, Simonsen PE. Immunoepidemiology of *Dracunculus medinensis* infections. I. Antibody responses in relation to infection status. *Am J Trop Med Hyg* 1998; 59:978–984.

181. Bloch P, Simonsen PE. Immunoepidemiology of *Dracunculus medinensis* infections. II. Variation in antibody responses in relation to transmission season and patency. *Am J Trop Med Hyg* 1998; 59:985–990.

182. Rohde JE, Sharma BL, Patton H, et al. Surgical extraction of guinea worm: disability reduction and contribution to disease control. *Am J Trop Med Hyg* 1993; 48:71–76.

183. Issaka-Tinorgah A, Magnussen P, Bloch P, et al. Lack of effect of ivermectin on prepatent guinea-worm: a single-blind, placebo-controlled trial. *Trans R Soc Trop Med Hyg* 1994; 88:346–348.

184. Bimi L, Freeman AR, Eberhard ML, et al. Differentiating *Dracunculus medinensis* from *D. insignis*, by the sequence analysis of the rRNA gene. *Ann Trop Med Parasitol* 2005; 99:511–517.

185. Ruiz-Tiben E, Hopkins DR. Dracunculiasis (Guinea worm disease) eradication. *Adv Parasitol* 2006; 61:275–309.

186. Hunter JM. Bore holes and the vanishing of guinea worm disease in Ghana's Upper Region. *Soc Sci Med* 1997; 45:71–89.

187. Olsen A, Magnussen P, Anemana S. The acceptability and effectiveness of a polyester drinking-water filter in a dracunculiasis-endemic village in Northern Region, Ghana. *Bull World Health Organ* 1997; 75: 449–452.

immune reaction is humoral, associated with a polarized T helper 2 (Th2)-type profile,[43] and is directed against the migrating larval stage. The reaction to adult worms in unusual locations is cellular.

The antigens which elicit antibodies are released at the moulting period between the second and third larval stages, when there are markedly elevated levels of IgE and a peripheral eosinophilia.[44,45] A further response is elicited in the bowel between the fourth and fifth stages, at which time there may be a marked loss of worm burden; this may be a regulatory mechanism in natural infections. However, whether this humoral response confers protection from reinfection remains unresolved.[14]

Adult worms in the bowel elicit no response, but when they wander into tissues the reaction is cellular and results in a granuloma. Immediate hypersensitivity to adult *A. lumbricoides* antigens develops in some people.

Clinical features

Natural history

Most *A. lumbricoides* infections are symptomless, but heavy infections in childhood give rise to symptoms. These heavy infections are controlled by immunity, or by diminished exposure, so that adults have much lighter infections, although reinfection can occur throughout life.

Incubation period

The incubation period from infection after swallowing eggs to the first appearance of eggs in the stools is 60–70 days. In larval ascariasis, pulmonary symptoms occur 4–6 days after infection.

Symptoms and signs

Light infections do not usually cause symptoms, though a single adult worm can cause a liver abscess or block the common bile duct. Acute manifestations are roughly proportional to the number of worms harboured and serious disease may be caused when the burden amounts to 100 worms or more.

Ascariasis

During the migratory stages the larvae cause a pneumonitis 4–16 days after infection, with fever, cough, sputum and radiological infiltration of the lungs. There is a high eosinophilia and larvae can be found in the sputum or gastric juice, especially if a quantity is collected, digested with trypsin and centrifuged. It seems that Löffler's syndrome occurs with seasonal ascariasis, rather than with continued transmission throughout the year.[46,47] The pneumonitis is of short duration – about 3 weeks (in contrast to tropical pulmonary eosinophilia (TPE), which lasts for many months). There may be asthma, which can be so intense as to cause status asthmaticus, and the liver may be affected, becoming enlarged and tender.

On reaching the general circulation, larvae may cause symptoms similar to those of *Toxocara* spp. Neurological disorders including convulsions, meningism and epilepsy, palpebral oedema, insomnia and tooth grinding during the night may occur. When the larvae wander into the brain they cause granulomas, presenting as small tumours in the eye, retina or brain.

The commonest complication of ascariasis is small-bowel obstruction (Figure 85.10).[48] The incidence of *Ascaris*-induced intestinal obstruction (AI-IO) is non-linearly related to the prevalence of infection and estimated to be in the range of 0–0.25 cases per year per 1000 in endemic areas. The case fatality rate is up to 5%.[48] AI-IO is most common among children below the age of 10 years, possibly because of their narrower intestinal lumen diameter and high worm burden, and as many as 1000 worms have been removed from one patient. Gastrointestinal discomfort, colic and vomiting are quite common. Plain abdominal radiography and abdominal ultrasonography featuring the characteristic 'railway track' sign and 'bull's eye' appearance help to confirm the diagnosis.[49]

Adult worms tend to migrate when their environment is disturbed. In the presence of tetrachloroethylene, anaesthetics or fever, they migrate and wander into the bile ducts, ampulla of Vater, appendix, perineal sinuses and Eustachian tubes. They can cause volvulus and gangrene of the bowel, intestinal perforation and peritonitis, acute pancreatitis, suppurative cholangitis, liver abscess, acute cholecystitis and obstructive jaundice.

For these reasons it is important not to give tetrachloroethylene when there is a possibility of *A. lumbricoides* infection and to deworm children when they are ill and febrile or before giving an anaesthetic. With the advent of the imidazoles and other anthelmintics, the use of tetrachloroethylene is virtually extinct.

Differential diagnosis

The syndrome of pulmonary symptoms, radiological lung infiltration and hypereosinophilia is common to a number of helminthic and other infections. Larval ascariasis must be distinguished from toxocariasis, hookworm, *Strongyloides stercoralis*, schistosomiasis and TPE. Essentially, larval ascariasis is a short-term illness lasting 2–3 weeks with a rapidly falling eosinophilia.

Often associated with *A. lumbricoides*, *Toxocara* spp. cause the visceral larva migrans (VLM) syndrome, which persists for many months with a persistently high eosinophilia, and lung symptoms are not prominent. Wandering *Toxocara* larvae cause almost identical lesions of the brain and eye as *A. lumbricoides* and can be diagnosed by specific serological tests.

The invasive stage of hookworm lasts 2–3 months, subsiding gradually, ova being found in the stool from 42 days onwards. It may be preceded by a localized eruption on the legs (ground itch).

The invasive stage of schistosomiasis (Katayama syndrome) can last 2–3 months. There is usually splenomegaly and specific serology is available for diagnosis.

TPE may closely resemble *Ascaris* pneumonia. It occurs mainly in adults, has a much longer duration, and specific filarial serological tests will be positive (older tests using less specific antigens cross-reacted with *Ascaris*). It responds rapidly to diethylcarbamazine.

Pulmonary aspergillosis, drug reactions and eosinophilic leukaemia are all more chronic.

Diagnosis

A diagnosis can be made from passage of worms in the stool or by finding eggs in faeces. Fertile eggs are oval and measure about

60×45 μm. The shell is transparent, is surrounded by an outer mamillated shell stained by bile pigments, and contains an unsegmented embryo (see Figure 85.9A). Non-fertile eggs are longer and narrower (90×40 μm), have a thinner shell and more irregular outer covering, and are found in about two-thirds of infections, due either to a shortage or absence of males. Intensity of infection can be assessed by quantitative egg count methods such as the Kato–Katz method. The WHO definition of a heavy infection is ≥50 000 eggs/g of faeces (see Table 85.1).

Decorticated eggs are usually found in ectopic sites where they have had the outer shell removed and present as smooth oval objects (see Figure 85.9B).

Eosinophilia

In larval ascariasis there is a high eosinophilia, but in adult infections there is little or none. If a marked eosinophilia occurs in adult infections, then an associated *Toxocara* spp. or *S. stercoralis* infection must be suspected.

Adult worms

Sometimes the passage of an adult worm from the nose, mouth or anus will be reported and causes distress. The size and shape will distinguish it from other worms, especially tapeworms, which may be noticed by patients.

Radiography

Radiographic examination 4–6 hours after an opaque meal displays the worms as cylindrical filling defects or as string-like shadows produced by the opaque substance which the worms have ingested. Modern imaging techniques are now increasingly available.[33]

Serological diagnosis

Since there is much cross-reactivity with other helminthic antigens, immunodiagnosis is of little help in *Ascaris* infection, either adult or larval.

Management

Both albendazole and mebendazole are highly effective against *A. lumbricoides*[23] and are the drugs of choice (see Table 85.2). Levamisole and pyrantel pamoate are also effective. Treatment is best given between meals.

Treatment of complications

Treatment of complications responds dramatically to prednisolone therapy. Anthelmintics should be given 2 weeks after lung involvement.

Conservative treatment – antispasmodics, analgesics, gastric decompression via a nasogastric tube, administration of intravenous fluids – is usually successful. An anthelmintic, preferably in soluble form and quick-acting (levamisole, pyrantel), is given when the acute phase of the illness is over and intestinal function restored. If this fails, surgical removal is needed.[35]

Conservative treatment is the first choice for dealing with complication – antispasmodics, gastric decompression, intravenous fluids, liquid paraffin and anthelmintics – and is usually successful.

If surgical intervention is decreed necessary because of fever, tachycardia, visible peristalsis, severe pain or lack of remission within 48 hours of conservative treatment, this should be as conservative as possible, e.g. careful unknotting of the worm bolus and milking of the worms into the colon. Rarely is enterotomy required.

Epidemiology and control

Biological similarities between *A. lumbricoides* and *T. trichiura* mean they share similar climatic envelopes,[24] which explains in part the close correspondence of *A. lumbricoides* and *T. trichiura* prevalence in different regions of the world.[50]

Many of the epidemiological features of *A. lumbricoides* are also similar to those for *T. trichiura* (see p. 1517): marked age-dependency in infection patterns, highly aggregated distributions within communities,[51] household clustering of heavy infection,[26,52] and evidence of predisposition (for a review, see Crompton[53]).

As with *T. trichiura*, control of *A. lumbricoides* is based on a combination of personal hygiene, proper disposal of faeces, health education and chemotherapy (see pp. 1536–1539).

Toxocariasis

Toxocariasis in man is the result of infection with the dog ascarid *Toxocara canis* or the cat ascarid *Toxocara cati*. These geohelminths do not undergo normal development in humans but are arrested at the larval stage, causing toxocariasis, visceral larva migrans (VLM), ocular toxocariasis or covert toxocariasis.

Geographical distribution

T. canis has a worldwide distribution: rates in humans vary from 2% to 50% in developed countries and up to 86% in developing countries, where environmental conditions favour geohelminth transmission.[54,55] The importance of *T. cati* in humans remains under-appreciated.[56]

VLM, which was first described in the southern USA has been recognized mainly in the southern and eastern USA but also in Europe, the Caribbean, Central and South America, the Philippines, Australia, and north, west and southern Africa.

Ocular toxocariasis (granulomatous ophthalmitis), also first described in the USA,[57] has been recognized in many parts of the world and serological surveys report numerous cases of ocular toxocariasis in Europe.[58]

Aetiology

T. canis and *T. cati* are roundworm infections in dogs and cats, respectively. The morphology resembles that of *A. lumbricoides* (see p. 1519), the males being 4–6 cm long and the females 6.5–10 cm long. Eggs, which are pitted superficially, measure 85×75 μm, being larger than those of *A. lumbricoides*. They are not found in humans, only in dog and cat faeces and contaminated soil.

Life cycle

In both dogs and cats the life cycle is similar to that of *A. lumbricoides* in humans except that transplacental infection is common and the offspring born with a patent infection shed numerous

day-to-day variation in egg output, diagnostic sensitivity is increased by examining multiple stool samples over consecutive days.[96] Heavy infections are defined as intensities of ≥4000 eggs/g of faeces (see Table 85.1).

Adult worms

The eggs of *A. duodenale* and *N. americanus* are morphologically almost identical. Species differentiation is achieved by morphological examination of the buccal apparatus of adult worms obtained by explusion techniques or of larval stages cultured from eggs by the Harada–Mori method.

Serological diagnosis

Multiplex real-time PCR methods have been used to detect and quantify *A. duodenale* and *N. americanus* in faecal samples, and distinguish infections from *Oesophagostomum biurcum*, whose eggs are morphologically indistinguishable from hookworm.[97]

Management

Treatment consists of elimination of the parasites and treatment of the anaemia, if present. Treatment of the anaemia is the first priority but there is no reason why both objectives should not be proceeded with concurrently. Treatment is usually directed against the adult stages but there is evidence that albendazole in a single dose of 400 mg is active against the pre-intestinal larval stages of *N. americanus*.[98]

Albendazole is highly effective against both *A. duodenale* and *N. americanus* (see Table 85.2). A single dose of 400 mg will produce an 80% cure rate and 200 mg daily for 3 days will give 100% cure.[23] It is also highly effective against *Ascaris lumbricoides* and *Trichuris trichiura* and is therefore especially suitable for mass treatment. Mebendazole is only partially effective against *A. duodenale* and *N. americanus*,[23] and treatment over several days may be required for heavy infections. Levamisole and pyrantel pamoate may also be used, although in some areas, e.g. north-western Australia, pyrantel pamoate is ineffective.[99]

Treatment of anaemia

The anaemia is treated by the administration of iron by mouth, in the form of ferrous sulphate or gluconate, 200 mg three times daily, which should be continued for 3 months after a normal haemoglobin level has been achieved. This will restore the iron reserves to normal.

After starting iron therapy, a reticulocyte response may be seen in about 1 week. In most cases the haemoglobin will rise by 1.0 g per week. Folic acid, 5 mg daily, should be given for at least 1 month to cover the erythopoeitic response. Many patients in the tropics fail to correct the haemoglobin fully and develop macrocytosis if this is not done.

Parenteral iron – iron–dextran complex or iron–poly (sorbitol gluconic acid) complex – may be used in patients who cannot tolerate oral iron, in patients where compliance is in doubt, and in patients in whom regular follow-up is difficult or unlikely.

Epidemiology and control

The main reservoir of infection is man, although *N. americanus* has been recovered on occasion from non-human primates.[100] In general, however, the transmission of hookworm infection depends upon an adequate source of infection in the human population, the deposition of eggs in a favourable environment for extrinsic development of the parasite, appropriate conditions of the soil (moisture and warmth) to allow larvae to develop, and suitable conditions for the infective larvae to penetrate the skin.

Recent analysis employing GIS and remote sensing shows that hookworm is able to thrive more in hotter environments and has a more cosmopolitan distribution than *T. trichiura* and *A. lumbricoides*.[24] This is suggested to be due in part to the ability of larvae to migrate downward into the soil, thereby avoiding desiccation. In addition, hookworms have a longer adult lifespan and can find refuge from external temperatures for longer than the other geohelminth species, increasing the chances of hookworm transmission stages being deposited and developing in suitable thermal conditions. In some temperate climates local environmental conditions may allow transmission, as in the Cornish tin mines and Swiss railway tunnels in the past[101] and in the Rand in South Africa today. Cultural and agricultural practices such as the use of human faeces for fertilizer provide good opportunities for infection.[102]

Epidemiological studies show that children can be infected with hookworm as young as 6 months. Subsequently, infection prevalence typically rises monotonically with increasing age to a plateau in adulthood.[103] Increases in prevalence among the eldery have been observed in some populations.[104,105] Because of logistic and social difficulties, estimates of worm numbers by chemotherapeutic expulsion in an age-stratified host population have been very few,[103] with most studies having relied on an indirect measure of intensity: quantitative egg counts. The few age-stratified estimates of hookworm burden using anthelmintic expulsion indicate that *N. americanus* worm burdens tend to increase in hosts up to age 15–25 years and remain constant thereafter.[73,103]

As with other geohelminths, the distribution of hookworms per host is highly aggregated within populations.[106] There is also evidence of household clustering and small-scale spatial variation, determined in part by local variation in socioeconomic status and environmental factors.[52,107]

The basis of hookworm control is described on pp. 1536–1539.

Cutaneous larva migrans (creeping eruption, sandworm, plumber's itch, duckhunter's itch)

Cutaneous larva migrans (CLM) is a cutaneous eruption resulting from exposure of the skin to the infective filariform larvae of non-human hookworm (*Ancylostoma braziliense*, *A. caninum*) and *Strongyloides* of the nutria and racoon. The infective larvae cannot complete their normal life cycle in the human host but persist under the skin, without developing further, where they cause CLM.

Geographical distribution

CLM occurs in most warm, humid, tropical and subtropical areas, being especially common in the southern USA, along the coast of the Gulf of Mexico and Florida.[108] It is also common on the coast of sub-Saharan Africa, South and South-east Asia, and Latin America.

Aetiology

Ancyclostoma

A. braziliense is the hookworm of dogs and cats. It is smaller than *A. duodenale* (female 1 cm and male 8.5 mm long), the internal pair of ventral teeth are smaller, and the dorsal rays in the copulatory bursa are distinctive (Figure III.62). The eggs are indistinguishable from those of human hookworms. The life cycle is similar to that of *A. duodenale* but man is an unsuitable host and the third-stage larva does not enter the bloodstream but wanders under the skin, causing CLM.

A. caninum is the dog hookworm. Its life history is similar to that of *A. braziliense*.

Strongyloides

Filariform larvae of *S. stercoralis* can re-enter the skin as part of autoinfection around the anus and buttocks, where they cause 'larva currens', a rash rather like that of CLM.

S. myopotami (nutria) and *S. procyonis* (racoon) both produce similar lesions in the human host, in which they cannot complete their normal life cycle. The lesions are more persistent.

Transmission

Infection is acquired from damp contaminated soil through the skin of that part of the body in contact with the soil (foot, abdomen, buttock).

Pathology

The filariform larvae are unable to penetrate below the stratum germinativum of human skin, where they form a tunnel with the corium as a floor and the stratum granulosum as a roof. Local eosinophilia and round cell infiltration occur round the tunnel and may persist for months. Rarely the larvae reach the lungs, where they cause transitory pulmonary symptoms and eosinophilia and may be recovered from bronchial washings. They do not mature in the intestine.

Immunity

Little is known about immunity. There is no protective immunity and people can be infected more than once.

Clinical features

Natural history

The larvae wander under the skin and can persist for months before they eventually die.

Incubation period

Symptoms start immediately after penetration of the skin, a matter of a few hours only.

Symptoms and signs

There is a red itchy papule at the site of entry, which becomes elevated and vesicular. The larvae move several millimetres to a few centimetres each day and leave tunnels which become dry and crusted. The track is linear and twists and turns (Figure 85.13). It causes an intense pruritus and the skin is scratched and becomes secondarily infected.[109] The lesions may be single or multiple. The most common sites are the hands and buttocks with *A. braziliense*[110] but the abdomen is often infested in plumber's itch and the lesions may be very numerous indeed (Figure 85.14). A second form of CLM associated with folliculitis has also been reported.[111]

The lesions produced by non-human hookworms (CLM) are well defined, move very slowly and persist for months. There is little surrounding flare and the track is indurated. In contrast, the lesions produced by *Strongyloides* (larva currens) are less well defined, have a red flare on the outside, move much more rapidly and persist for a few hours only.

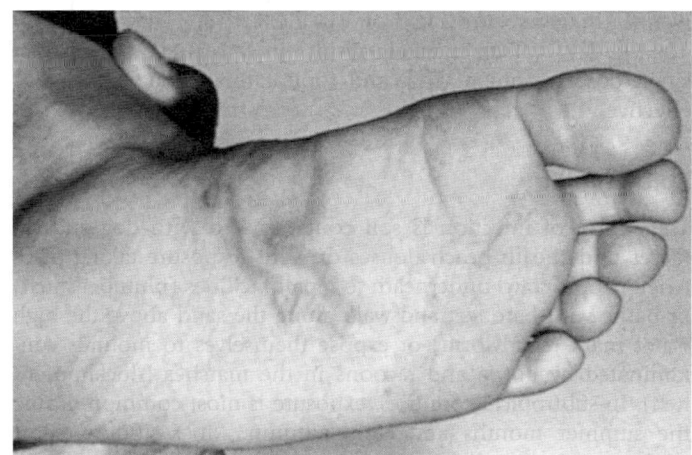

Figure 85.13 Cutaneous larva migrans (*A. braziliense*).

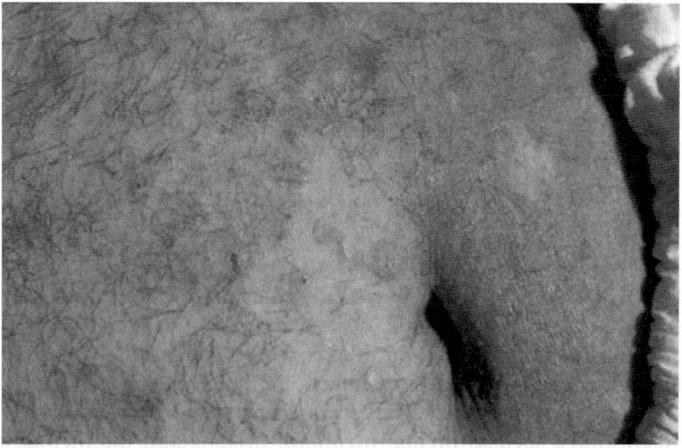

Figure 85.14 Multiple burrows of cutaneous larva migrans (creeping eruption).

pinpoint larval granulomas. The larvae may carry microorganisms, and an overwhelming septicaemia caused by *E. coli* has been caused in this way. In light infections, jejunal biopsy has shown oedema, cellular infiltration and eosinophilic infiltration of the mucosa with partial villous atrophy. At postmortem, ulceration and atrophy of the mucosa are seen, with numerous adult worms in the wall of the duodedum and jejunum. At times, filariform larvae fail to break out of the alveoli, gain access to the general circulation and can invade the brain, intestine, lymph glands, liver, lungs and, rarely, myocardium.

Transmission

Infection is acquired originally from contaminated soil via free-living filariform infective larvae. Once established, further infection may be acquired from the colon or anal skin from parasitic infective larvae. The transmission of *S. stercoralis* through the milk has been demonstrated in several animal species and it is possible that this occurs in man.

Immunity

Immunity to reinfection develops in most individuals after a primary infection and the *Strongyloides* adults and larvae are confined to the small intestine and the worm burden is controlled. Immunity is both antibody and cell mediated.

Humoral antibody-mediated immunity is elicited by the secretions of infective larvae with a type I response, an eosinophilic tissue response, and a peripheral eosinophilia – often with urticarial rashes. Antibodies are produced which cross-react with many other helminths, including filariae.

Cell-mediated immunity is elicited by adult and larval worms in the tissues, which are localized and destroyed by a cell-mediated granulomatous reaction. If cell-mediated immunity is depressed for any reason, such as immunosuppressive states of drugs, then a generalized hyperinfection results, causing massive strongyloidiasis.

Among persons co-infected with human T cell lymphotropic virus type 1 (HTLV-1), production of IFNγ may decrease the production of antibodies that participate in the host immune response against infection.[115]

Clinical features

Natural history

In the majority of cases, a small population of adult worms maintains itself in the small intestine for many years (30 or more) in the absence of any further infection from the outside, causing recurrent symptoms when filariform larvae enter the perianal skin, and cause a recurrent rash – 'larva currens' – associated with urticaria. In a small minority of cases, the defences of the body break down and a generalized severe infection ensues.

Incubation period

The pre-patent period from infection to the appearance of rhabditiform larvae in the stools is 1 month.

Symptoms and signs

The vast majority of infections in endemic areas are symptomless. When, for various reasons, the number of *Strongyloides* present in the intestine increases, then symptoms develop.

Primary infection

This is rarely seen in endemic areas and descriptions are based on self-induced experimental infections. A pruritic erythematous eruption, which lasts about 3 weeks, occurs at the site of entry of the larvae. A dry cough or sore throat appears on the 6th–9th day together with abdominal fullness, aching in the right lower quadrant of the abdomen and a watery diarrhoea alternating with constipation. Larvae are first detected in the stools 27 days after infection.

Chronic uncomplicated strongyloidiasis

This is characterized by epigastric and right upper quadrant pain together with nausea, chronic diarrhoea and weight loss.

Skin rashes

There are two types of skin rashes. One, occurring around the anus and anywhere on the trunk, is a linear eruption – 'larva currens' – in which the larvae migrate under the skin causing an itching rash with a larval track which is not indurated and has a red flare at the edge which moves quite rapidly (2–10 cm per hour), disappearing in a few hours (Figure 85.17), in contrast to the more indurated and persistent track of non-human hookworm (cutaneous larva migrans). The second form is urticaria caused by allergy to the larvae penetrating the skin in an individual who has already been sensitized. It occurs predominantly in the buttocks, with pruritus ani, and around the waist, lasts 1–2 days and recurs at regular intervals. The creeping type of eruption, which is seen mainly in infections from Indo-China and was common in prisoners of war in the Far East in the Second World War, can last for 30 years or more.[116] A strongyloides-related glomerulonephritis has been reported.[117]

Severe complicated strongyloidiasis

In persons debilitated by disease, malnutrition or serious illness, severe and potentially fatal complications may result from massive invasion of the tissues by *S. stercoralis* (i.e. when *S. stercoralis* disseminate). The same results can occur in immunocompromised individuals, for example, as a result of treatment with immunosuppressive drugs for lymphoma and organ transplantation and/or immunosuppression due to the effects of co-infection with HTLV-1.[115] It has recently been suggested that host immunosup-

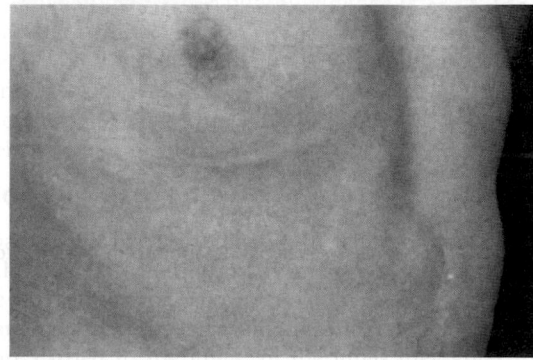

Figure 85.17 Skin rash (larva currens) of *Strongyloides stercoralis*.

pression favours the direct development of infective larvae, thereby promoting hyperinfection. Interestingly, it seems that in HIV-positive persons with poor immune function, indirect development – rather than direct development – of infective larvae in the gut is favoured.[118] This observation may explain the notable absence of disseminated strongyloidiasis in late-stage HIV disease.

First-stage larvae develop in the duodenum and jejunum, bore into the bowel wall, become adult and produce ova. In this way the number of *Strongyloides* is immensely increased and infective larvae invade the tissues and circulate, causing massive strongyloidiasis. Severe abdominal pain, vomiting and diarrhoea together with a sprue-like syndrome may develop: a protein-losing enteropathy, hypoalbuminaemia and generalized oedema occur. Fever, hypertension, abdominal tenderness and distension, reduced bowel sounds, paralytic ileus and a necrotizing jejunitis have been reported.

In the lungs, pulmonary symptoms resembling tropical pulmonary eosinophilia with hypereosinophilia, pneumonitis, diffuse crepitations, scattered bronchi, pleural effusion and pulmonary abscess, and gross respiratory failure may occur.[119]

Neurological complications with headache, convulsions, confusion, stupor, meningitis and focal neurological signs occur. In 30% of immunocompromised patients, a Gram-negative (*E. coli*) meningitis is found.

Other complications include a septicaemia with enteric organisms, shock, multiple petechiae on the chest and abdomen, and periumbilical purpura.

Laboratory findings

Raised serum IgE levels are found. Towards the end of the early stage of infection there is a high leukocytosis of up to 25×10^9/L; an eosinophilia of $10-12 \times 10^9$/L is characteristic. Later, when the infection is chronic, there is a moderate eosinophilia which may persist for years. In severe complicated strongyloidiasis, the eosinophilia disappears and is an indication of poor prognosis.

Differential diagnosis

Strongyloidiasis must be differentiated from other tissue-invading helminths: *A. lumbricoides*, hookworm and liver flukes. Disseminated strongyloidiasis may closely resemble tropical pulmonary eosinophilia, especially since serology cross-reacts. 'Larva currens' resembles cutaneous larva migrans, but, in distinction from it, in 'larva currens' the rash is situated mainly round the buttocks and on the trunk, lasts only a few hours and may occur intermittently for many years.

Diagnosis

Only adults or rhabditiform larvae (Figure 85.16) appear in the stools, duodenal aspirate or by the Entero test capsule. They can be demonstrated by the faecal examination methods or cultured in charcoal at 26°C for a week (see Appendix III).

The Kato–Katz method, the most commonly used diagnostic method in geohelminth epidemiology, does not detect *S. stercoralis*, and this feature probably explains why the global prevalence of *S. stercoralis* is likely to be underestimated. More sensitive coprological methods include a modified agar plate[120] and the Baermann technique. However, because of low larval densities, multiple examinations are often necessary.[121] Serological methods using ELISA, which detect serum IgG against a crude extract of infective larvae,[122] are more sensitive than coprology, but are labour-intensive and prone to cross-reactions with other helminths and filariae. A gelatin particle indirect agglutination test is considered to be more practical than the ELISA for mass screening for strongyloidiasis.[123]

Management

S. stercoralis should usually be treated whether or not the infection is giving rise to symptoms. It should be looked for and treated especially in immunosuppressed patients – for example, those on corticosteroid therapy or immunosuppressive drugs, persons infected with HIV, or persons from endemic areas in whom transplantation is being contemplated. Ivermectin is highly efficacious and the drug of choice (see Table 85.2). Albendazole, mebendazole and thiabendazole can also be used but are generally less efficacious.[124] There is often a decrease in the efficacy of treatment in persons coinfected with HTLV-1.

Epidemiology

Man is the most important host of *S. stercoralis* but dogs and chimpanzees have been found infected with strains indistinguishable from those of man. Larvae are unable to survive temperatures below 8°C or above 40°C or desiccation. Strongyloidiasis thrives in conditions of overcrowding on damp soil in tropical conditions such as in rural villages in South-east Asia and the Amazon. Due to difficulties in diagnosis, few detailed epidemiological studies exist; however, infection is normally more prevalent among males than females and increases with age.[125,126] Household clustering also occurs.[127] It was very common among prisoners of war in Burma and Indo-China in the Second World War[116] and Vietnam veterans.

Control

Control methods are the same as for other geohelminths (see pp. 1536–1539).

Strongyloides fülleborni

This is widely distributed in tropical forest regions of Central and East Africa. The main source of infection is monkey faeces, although human-to-human transmission may occur. In most cases there are no symptoms; 24% of pygmies in Zaire were found to be passing ova and very heavy infections were found without any evidence of disease.

Aetiology

S. fülleborni can be distinguished from *S. stercoralis* by the prominent vulvar lips, narrowing behind the vulva and a prominent oesophagus. Eggs are passed in the stool in contrast to *S. stercoralis* and resemble those of hookworm, for which they are commonly mistaken. Treatment is as for *S. stercoralis*.

age-specificity of infection with the different species: the peak intensities of *A. lumbricoides* and *T. trichiura* occur in children under 10 years of age; and of hookworms and *S. stercoralis* in adults over 20 years of age. Whether programmes targeted at individual differences are cost-effective has yet to be determined, but seems improbable.

Three chemotherapeutic strategies can be used: mass chemotherapy, i.e. treatment of all persons if the prevalence of infection is 50% or over; selective population chemotherapy, i.e. treatment of all infected persons at the time of a survey; targeted chemotherapy, i.e. treatment of specific groups likely to suffer the greatest morbidity.

WHO has identifed three key groups which are given priority for treatment: a) school-age children, b) pre-school children and c) pregnant women. The 2001 World Health assembly established regular treatment of 75% of schoolchildren by 2010 as the key target.[133,134]

a) School-age children

School-based programmes have been shown to be a cost-effective approach for controlling the intensity of intestinal helminth infection even in environments where transmission is high.[135]

The effectiveness of these programs reflects the epidemiological observation that treatment of an intensely infected age group or subpopulation reduces transmission overall,[136] and the economic observation that this results in externalities that greatly increase the cost-effectiveness of the approach.[137-140] The increase in school participation worldwide as one of the key Millennium Development Goals, as well as the specific promotion of school health programmes as part of these efforts, provides an additional strong policy incentive to deliver deworming through school systems.[141,142] The sustainability of at-scale, school-based national programmes has been demonstrated in several erstwhile low-income countries that have now transitioned to middle-income status or above – including Japan, Korea, Brazil and Sri Lanka.[143,144] In all of these cases the transition was from a school-based chemotherapy programme as part of a national school health system approach to management through the established health services as infection declined.

School-based deworming can reduce rates of anaemia[145,146] and improve growth, particularly in weight.[145] Antenatal anthelmintic treatment improves haemoglobin levels,[147] birth weight and infant survival.[148]

Meta-analyses of randomized trials have given equivocal results[149] but more recent analyses demonstrate increases in growth, especially ponderal weight gain.[150] Quantifying the impact on educational measures remains a challenge, with stronger evidence for impacts on cognition than on educational outcomes, probably because the latter depends on education quality.[20,21]

The demonstrated cost-effectiveness of deworming as a school-based intervention has encouraged more interest by development agencies in this intervention. The increased availabilty of development aid for deworming, as well as the availability of free anthelmintics through large-scale donations by the pharmaceutical industry, has resulted in a growth in community-wide progammes. Whether these are sustainable or cost-effective has yet to be determined, and efforts to enhance sustainability and cost-savings by integrating programmes are being evaluated.

b) Pre-school children

Progammes for pre-school children have been developed as part of micronutrient or other health campaigns, as part of health programmes delivered through pre-schools, and as an addition to 'child health days' that provide a range of health interventions to young children on a demand basis. There is evidence that all these approaches are effective in improving the growth and nutrition of pre-school children and, where they build on existing systems, are cost-effective.[151,152]

c) Pregnant women

Infection during pregnancy is widespread and affects the health of the mother, fetal development, and the survival and subsequent development of the child.[147,148,153] Previous advice was that anthelmintic treatment should be avoided in pregnancy, but it is now recommended that infected pregnant mothers should be treated, ideally after the first trimester.[154]

In recent years, there have been significant advances in the design of chemotherapy control strategies,[155] one of the most important of which are the improvements in methods for identifying populations for treatment using geographical information systems (GIS).[156] Practical, low-cost methods of using GIS for planning and targeting national progammes have now been developed and implemented at national scale.[24]

Resistance to anthelmintic drugs

Resistance is now widespread in the gastrointestinal nematodes of ruminants, particularly sheep and goats.[157] Although resistance by human nematodes has rarely been reported, managers of control programmes should be alerted to the possibility, particularly since the current biological assays do not detect resistance until the resistance genotype is already common and fixed in the worm population. A possible genetic marker for resistance to treatment of *S. stercoralis* has been identified,[158] and the genotypic markers of resistance in veterinary nematodes have been identified in the common nematodes of humans, but not yet developed into assays appropriate for surveillance.

Mebendazole drug failure against *N. americanus* in Mali[159] and pyrantel drug failure against *A. duodenale* in Western Australia have been reported,[99] but in the absence of any definitions of resistance for these species it is difficult to interpret these findings. Careful monitoring of mass treatment programmes is therefore essential,[160] and it is very important that the available anthelmintics are used in ways that will delay or prevent drug resistance, such as ensuring the existence of refuge populations (e.g. by targeting specific age groups), by maintaining low treatment pressure through infrequent cycles of treatment, and possibly by the use of combination therapies as is advocated for malaria. A 2007 WHO/World Bank meeting on drug resistance has developed a way forward for more structured surveillance.

Sanitation

Marked improvements in environmental hygiene are the ultimate answer to the control and elimination of geohelminth infections, but for many low-income countries and for poor and disenfranchised communities in middle-income countries these are expensive and long-term objectives.

In the medium term, however, many varieties of affordable latrines are available, e.g. ventilated improved pit latrines and double-vault latrines.[161] These have proved to be culturally acceptable in many countries; they are easy to install, operate and maintain. Further, they allow adequate composting of human excretion as fertilizer.

It must be appreciated that the effect of sanitation is slow to develop, and that therefore periodic anthelmintic treatments should be maintained until sanitation has had an impact on transmission.

Investment in sanitation is justified in terms of a broad range of returns to health and social outcomes, and avoidance of worm infection alone could not justify the substantial investment required. However, improvements in hygiene have been achieved at very much lower cost than improvements in sanitation, with programmes to encourage hand-washing with soap achieving important health benefits with existing technologies and at low cost.[161]

Health education

Human behaviour is of great importance in the transmission of geohelminths, and the success or failure of control programmes often hinges on the modification of behavioural patterns. Health education must target its activities on this crucial criterion, aiming to determine which local cultures and practices are conducive to the transmission of infection and need to be modified to reduce the risk. If beneficial cultural practices are identified, these should be reinforced to enhance compliance. As many stakeholders as possible should be involved in the planning process, paying particular attention to cultural diversity, gender and the specific needs of the target group. Improvements in personal hygiene, especially hand-washing, should be actively encouraged, and where programmes are linked to school health activities, the health and hygiene message should be part of the curriculum and reinforced by IEC messages in the community. Modern audiovisual technology may be used when appropriate.

Community participation

This is crucial for the success of any control programme. Active participation of the community in the planning and execution of any intervention is mandatory. The schedule should suit the convenience of the community and be discussed and agreed by them. As with all the diseases of poverty, economic development is mandatory for effective community involvement.

Monitoring and evaluation

Monitoring and evaluation are essential and should be used to review or revise any control programme, demonstrate health benefits, but also to assess cost-effectiveness.[162] Since the main aim underlying geohelminth control is the prevention of disease rather than to reduce or eradicate transmission, it is important that evaluation focuses on both intensity of infection and morbidity measures where possible, and not the sole use of infection prevalence.

Targeted chemotherapy implemented within an existing health infrastructure has been shown to achieve an overall reduction in the prevalence and intensity of *A. lumbricoides* and *T. trichiura* infection in children aged 2–15 years at one-fifth of the drug purchase cost of mass chemotherapy, and with few of the attendant costs of drug delivery.[135,136]

CLINICAL PHARMACOLOGY OF ANTHELMINTIC DRUGS

A number of single-dose, orally administered drugs are available for the treatment and control of STH infections. These include albendazole, mebendazole, pyrantel and levamisole. Each of these drugs is recommended by WHO for use in large-scale control programmes.[132] They are all broad-spectrum benzimidazole anthelmintics, although their efficacy against individual STH species varies (Table 85.3). Because benzimidazoles are poorly

Table 85.3 Effectiveness* of single anthelmintic drugs.

	Albendazole	Mebendazole	Pyrantel	Levamisole
Ascaris lumbricoides	CR[†] = 88% (79–83%) ERR = >99%	CR = 95% (91–97%) ERR = >99%	CR = 88% (79–93%) ERR = >95%	CR = >87% ERR = >92%
Trichuris trichiura	CR = 28% (13–39%) ERR = 80% (28–100%)	CR = 36% (16–51%) ERR = >80% (50–80%)	CR = 28% ERR = ~40%	CR = 9% ERR = ~40%
Hookworm	CR = 72 (59–81%) ERR = 80% (62–100%)	CR = 15% (1–27%) ERR = >80% (38–100%)	CR = 31% (19–42%) ERR = >99%	CR = 38% ERR = ~60%
Strongyloides stercoralis	CR[‡] = 40–60% ERR = NA	Low effectiveness	Low effectiveness	Low effectiveness

* Effectiveness measures the effect of a drug against a parasite in a field setting, whereas efficacy measures the effect of a drug in ideal settings
† CR = cure rate, the percentage of individuals among whom parasites are cleared; ERR = egg reduction rate, changes in mean egg count before and after treatment. NA = not available. Median of estimates (for CR, 95% confidence interval and for ERR, range in parenthensis) based on reviews by Bennett & Guyatt,[23] Horton [182] and a recent systematic review and meta analysis by Keiser & Utzinger.[165]
‡ 400mg daily for 3 days.

absorbed, they reach and kill the parasites in the intestinal tract, causing few side-effects. Since their development in the 1970s, these broad-spectrum benzimidazoles have revolutionized the community control of the geohelminths and, to date, millions of individuals have been treated, with minimal side-effects.[165]

Albendazole

This is the most widely used anthelmintic for the community control of multiple STH infections. Albendazole is poorly absorbed from the gastrointestinal tract and is rapidly and extensively metabolized by the liver to sulphoxide and sulphone metabolites. The sulphoxide metabolite is an active anthelmintic and may be responsible for most of the drug effects in vivo. The drug binds to intracellular tubulin, impairing essential absorptive functions in the parasite.

It is known to be teratogenic and embryotoxic in some animals, but only after doses considerably higher than used in clinical practice. Given the fact that STH-related morbidity can develop rapidly in pregnant women and treatment confers health benefits, WHO now recommends treatment of lactating women and of pregnant women after the first trimester.[166] It has also recently been recommended that children as young as 12 months can be safely treated, with the recommended dose for children aged 1–2 years being 200 mg.

Adverse effects are mild and transient, and include epigastric pain, diarrhoea, headache, nausea, vomiting, dizziness, constipation, pruritus and dry mouth.

Mebendazole

Mebendazole is effective against adult worms and larval stages. It binds to nematode tubulin, preventing the formation of microtubules, and selectively inhibits cell division and glucose uptake in nematodes; this latter effect results in increased utilization of helminth glycogen and deprivation for the worms of their main source of energy. Oral absorption is limited by its poor solubility. The small amount absorbed is metabolized extensively by the liver to inactive compounds. As with albendazole, mebendazole is now recommended for lactating and pregnant women and young children living in endemic areas.[166]

Adverse effects are mild and transient, including gastrointestinal discomfort, headache and dizziness.

Rarely, mebendazole stimulates *Ascaris* worms to emerge from the mouth and nostrils, which alarms the patients unless they are forewarned.

Pyrantel

Pyrantel binds to acetylcholine receptors of parasites and owes its activity to its action on the neuromuscular system of the worms. It paralyses the worms, which are then expelled in the faeces. It is poorly absorbed from the gastrointestinal tract, with less than 15% excreted in the urine as unchanged drug and metabolites and 70% excreted unchanged in the faeces. Safe use in pregnancy has not been established.

Adverse effects include mild and transient gastrointestinal discomfort, headache, dizziness, drowsiness, insomnia and skin rash.

Pyrantel and piperazine are antagonistic and should not be administered concurrently.

Levamisole

Levamisole has a similar mode of action to pyrantel and causes spastic paralysis followed by passive elimination of parasites. It is rapidly absorbed from the gastrointestinal tract, achieving peak plasma levels within 2 hours, and is eliminated within 3 days. Much of the absorbed drug is metabolized in the liver. There is no evidence of teratogenicity, although it should not be given in the first trimester.

Adverse effects include abdominal pain, nausea, vomiting, dizziness and headache.

Piperazine

Piperazine is used in the treatment of *A. lumbricoides*, especially in the presence of intestinal or biliary obstruction, with reported cure rates of 60% and above.[164] Recommended dosage is 75 mg/kg. It is also used for the treatment of *E. vermicularis*, at a dosage of 50 mg/kg daily for seven successive days. Safe use in pregnancy has not been established.

Nitazoxanide

Nitazoxanide is a antiparasitic drug noted for its treatment of protozoan infections but has also been shown to be effective against STH infections.[167,168] Pharmaceutical compositions of nitazoxanide include both nitazoxanide and its derivative, tizoxanide, as active ingredients, with particle sizes of the active drug substance ranging from 5 to 200 μm. Adverse effects are mild and transient and include abdominal pain, nausea, vomiting and diarrhoea. Two daily doses (100 mg to 400 mg) are required for three or more days.

Tribendimidine

Tribendimidine is a new class of anthelmintic, which was first synthesized in China in the 1980s.[169] Preliminary trials in humans demonstrate that single-dose tribendimidine is effective against *A. lumbricoides*, both species of hookworm and *E. vermicularis*, and has efficacy superior to that of albendazole for the treatment of hookworm when used as a single dose of 400 mg.[169] Further efficacy trials are underway.

Side-effects are minimal and transient, and include abdominal pain, nausea, vomiting and diarrhoea.

OTHER NEMATODES FOR WHICH MAN IS NOT THE NORMAL HOST

Trichinosis (*Trichinella spiralis*)

Geographical distribution

Trichinosis has a worldwide distribution and as many as 11 million people are infected globally (Figure 85.18).[170] The incidence of human trichinosis has declined markedly in North America and

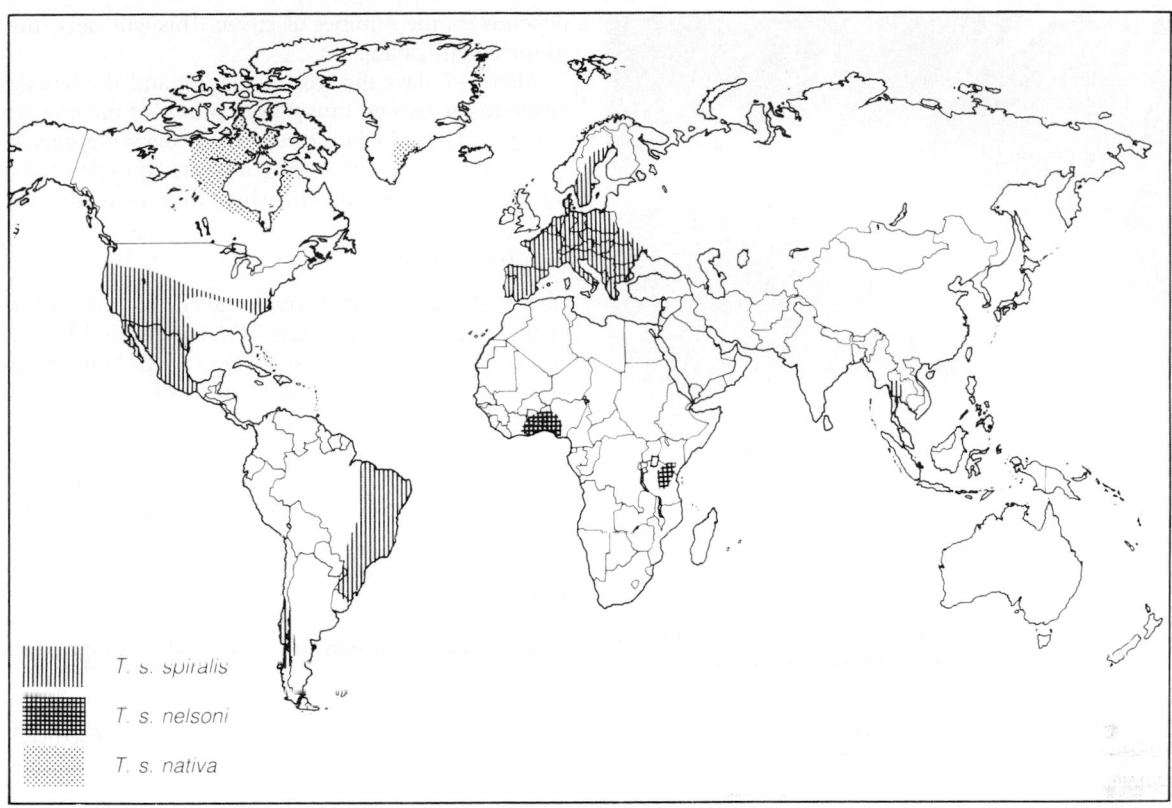

Figure 85.18   Geographical distribution of trichinosis.

Europe; however, sporadic outbreaks still occur. Large outbreaks also occur in China, Mexico, Argentina, Chile, the Balkans, Russia and the Baltic States.[171] It is also an important cause of disease and death in the Arctic, where polar explorers have died as a result of trichinosis; it is less important in the tropics but occurs in both East and West Africa. It is not a soil-transmitted helminth infection.

Aetiology

Trichinella spiralis occurs in two forms: adult and cystic. The adult *T. spiralis* (see Appendix III) is a white worm just visible to the naked eye and inhabits the small intestine. The male (1.6 × 0.04 mm) has a cloaca situated posteriorly between two caudal papillae. The female (3–4 × 0.06 mm) has a vulva in the anterior fifth, an ovary in the posterior half of the body, and a coiled uterine tube in the anterior portion.

Life cycle (see Appendix III)

The female lives for 30 days and is viviparous. The eggs (20 μm) live in the upper uterus and the larvae (100 × 6 μm) break out, living free in the uterine cavity. One female produces more than 1500 larvae. The larvae, which emerge as early as 4–7 days after infection, continue to be produced for 4–16 weeks. They make their way via the lymphatics and blood circulation to the right heart and lungs, enter the arterial circulation and reach striated muscle, where they encyst.

Cystic stage

The cyst is formed by the larva encapsulated by the host tissue. The capsule is an adventitious ellipsoidal sheath [s1] with blunt ends, resulting from cellular reaction around the tightly coiled larva (Figure 85.19). The long axis parallels that of the muscle fibres, and host amino acids nourish it so that it can remain alive for many years. In man, calcification may take place after 6 months and lead to death of the larva. When consumed by a carnivorous host, the cysts are digested in the stomach, and, after encysting, the larvae, which are resistant to gastric juice, invade the duodenal and jejunal mucosa, where they penetrate the columnar epithelium and develop into adults after 36 hours. The period between infection and the encysting stage in the muscles is 17–21 days.

Species and strains of *Trichinella*

T. spiralis contains three subspecies which can infect man. They are indistinguishable morphologically but vary in their host specificity and can be distinguished enzymatically:[172]

- *T. spiralis spiralis* of temperate regions, with domestic pigs the main source of human infection. The parasite can also persist in sylvatic reservoir hosts (e.g. foxes) independent of whether or not infection among domestic animals or humans occurs.[173]
- *T. spiralis nativa* of the Arctic regions; a parasite of carrion-feeding carnivores; polar bears and walruses are the main sources of human infection.

1541

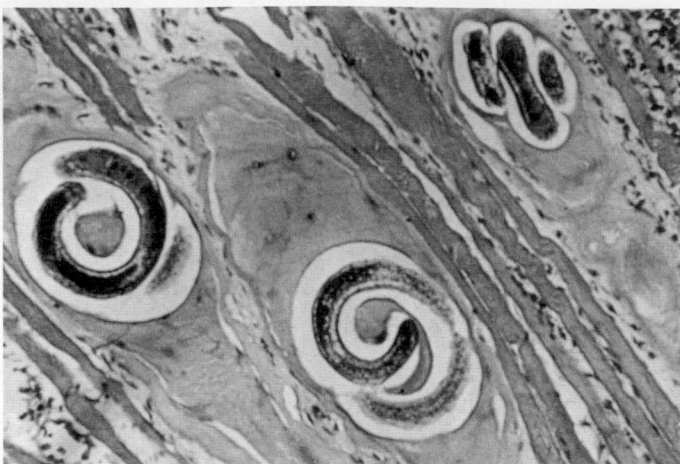

Figure 85.19 Larvae of *Trichinella spiralis* in muscle.

- *T. spiralis nelsoni* in Africa and southern Europe in wild carnivores, with wild pigs the source of human infection.

T. s. nativa is very resistant to freezing and *T. s. nelsoni* and *T. s. nativa* have a low infectivity for domestic pigs and rats.

Transmission

Transmission is by mouth from eating undercooked meat.

T. s. spiralis

Human infection is acquired from eating undercooked pork from infected pigs. The pigs are infected from eating raw garbage or perhaps from eating synanthropic rats which themselves become infected from garbage. Horse meat consumption was implicated in *T. spiralis* outbreaks in France and Italy.[174] An epidemic due to *T. pseudospiralis* was reported from Thailand, affecting 59 individuals, all of whom ate raw pork from a wild pig that was distributed to villagers by a local hunter.[175] Raptorial migrating birds from Asia are thought to have recently introduced *T. pseudospiralis* into Eastern Europe.[176]

T. s. nativa

Human infection is acquired from eating bear meat (the top predator), polar bear in the Arctic and brown bears in sub-Arctic regions of the former USSR and North America. Walrus meat can also be infective. Polar explorers have died as a result of eating polar bear meat.

T. s. nelsoni

Human infection results from eating meat of the bush pig or warthog which are themselves infected from carrion.

Pathology

The capsule of the infective larva is digested in the intestine since it is resistant to the gastric juice and penetrates the duodenal and jejunal mucosa, where the amount of trauma and irritation depends on the number of larvae. This will cause the symptoms of the enteric phase.

After 5–7 days the worms mature and the females discharge larvae to the tissues, causing symptoms of the migratory or invasive stage. Later, the larvae encyst, causing symptoms of the encystment stage. Larvae only encyst in striated muscle but travel through the brain and heart muscle, where they are unable to encyst.

Striated muscle

Larvae, after travelling through the circulation, encyst in muscles of the diaphragm, masseters, intercostals, and laryngeal, tongue and ocular muscles. At first there is a basophilic degeneration of the muscle fibres followed by formation of a hyaline capsule around the larva with an inflammatory infiltrate of lymphocytes and a few eosinophils (Figure 85.19). Foreign body giant cells may be present. The infiltrate subsides and fat is deposited at the poles and after 6 months calcification takes place, eventually leading to death of the larva.

Brain

Larvae migrate through the brain and meninges, causing leptomeningitis, granulomatous nodules in the basal ganglia, medulla and cerebellum, and perivascular cuffing in the cortex. They can be found in the cerebrospinal fluid with a raised cell count and increased protein.

Heart

The larvae cause considerable damage on passage through the myocardium, cellular infiltration and necrosis with subsequent fibrosis of the myocardial bundles.

Immunity

Natural immunity

Natural immunity is confined to cold-blooded animals with a temperature below 37°C.

Acquired immunity

A well-marked immunity to reinfection develops after the first infection but it is necessary for the infective larvae to develop through to the adult stage before immunity is produced, which is both anti-adult and anti-larval. Cell-mediated immunity is largely responsible but humoral antibodies develop. Immunized mice respond rapidly to challenge infections, with an inflammatory reaction in the bowel and the elimination of adult worms. Cellular immunity can be transferred by cellular elements and diminished by corticosteroids, adrenalectomy and whole body irradiation.

Clinical features

Natural history

Trichinosis is a self-limiting infection lasting in light infections 2–3 weeks and in heavy ones at the most 2–3 months. Except in heavy infections, mortality is low. Light infections are often asymptomatic and routine examinations of diaphragms at autopsy have shown a significant number containing calcified cysts in endemic areas.

Incubation period

From eating infected meat, the development of symptoms during the enteric phase is up to 7 days after infection, and for the migratory phase, from 7 to 21 days.

Symptoms and signs

The symptomatology depends on the level of infection and can be related to the number of larvae per gram of muscle: light infections (subclinical), up to 10 larvae; moderate, 50 to 500 larvae; and severe and possibly fatal infections, more than 1000. In symptomatic cases, symptoms develop in three stages: enteric (invasion of the intestine) phase, migration of the larvae (invasive phase) and a period of encystation in the muscles.

Enteric phase

Irritation and inflammation of the duodenum and jejunum where the larvae penetrate cause nausea, vomiting, colic and sweating, resembling an attack of acute food poisoning. There may be a maculopapular skin rash, and in a third of cases symptoms of a pneumonitis occur between the 2nd and 6th day, lasting about 5 days.

Migratory (invasion) phase

The cardinal symptoms and signs of this phase are severe myalgia, periorbital oedema and eosinophilia. There is difficulty in mastication, breathing and swallowing, due to the involvement of the muscles, and there may be some muscular paralysis of the extremities. There is a high remittent fever with typhoidal symptoms, splinter haemorrhages under the nails and in the conjunctivae, and blood and albumin in the urine. Characteristically there is a hypereosinophilia from the 14th day, which decreases after a week and persists at a lower level. An absence of eosinophilia denotes a poor prognosis. The lymph glands may be enlarged, as well as the parotid and submental glands. Occasionally there is splenomegaly. In severe cases there may be subpleural, gastric and intestinal haemorrhages.

Rarely, myocardial complications can occur[177] and in 10–20% of patients neurological complications when larvae pass through the central nervous system.[178]

Encystment phase

This is the third stage and may be severe. There may be cachexia, oedema and extreme dehydration. During the second month after infection there is a decrease in muscle tenderness, fever and itching subside, and congestive heart failure may appear. Damage to the brain may persist, with protean neurological signs which may clear up later or persist. Gram-negative septicaemia from organisms introduced by the larvae, permanent hemiplegia and Jacksonian epilepsy 10 years after an attack of trichinosis have been described.

Differential diagnosis

Trichinosis resembles many conditions: typhoid, encephalitis, myositis and tetanus; due to the association with a high eosinophilia it closely resembles the tissue stages of schistosomiasis (Katayama syndrome), hookworm, *Strongyloides* and other helminthic infections. Trichinosis may also resemble collagen disorders such as periarteritis nodosa and acute rheumatoid arthritis.

Diagnosis

Diagnosis is made by demonstrating larvae, by immunological and molecular methods.[179]

Demonstration of larvae

Larvae have been isolated from peripheral blood in the early stages of the migration phase by mixing blood with dilute acetic acid and centrifuging. Larvae may be demonstrated in muscle by trichinoscopy.

Trichinoscopy

This can only be used when the encystment phase has started, from 7 days after infection onwards. Samples of deltoid, biceps, gastrocnemius or pectoralis major are digested with 1% pepsin and 1% hydrochloric acid for several hours at 37°C, filtered or centrifuged, and the number of larvae per gram of muscle estimated. Larvae can also be seen on muscle pressed between two slides, which is more useful in the first 3 weeks of the disease.

Xenodiagnosis can be performed by feeding diaphragmatic tissue to uninfected albino white rats and examining them 1 month later.

The following immunological and antigen detection tests have been used: indirect immunofluoresence; an enzymatic immunohistochemical technique; colorimetric sandwich ELISA; microfluorescence; enhanced chemiluminescence; dissociated enhanced lanthemide fluoroimmunoassay (DELFIA); Western blot test. DELFIA is the most sensitive for detecting antigen.[179]

Management

Treatment is directed against the larvae and the immune reaction they invoke. Ten days of oral mebendazole (200 mg twice a day) or thiabendazole (25 m/kg twice a day) are both effective, although the former is better tolerated by patients.[180] In severe life-threatening infections the immulone response must be controlled, and prednisolone 20 mg three times daily is given initially, reducing and finally discontinuing over a period of 2–3 weeks. Some cases are resistant to prednisolone.

Epidemiology (Figure 85.20)

Man is not the normal host of *T. spiralis* and becomes infected only after eating raw or undercooked flesh. The usual type, *T. s. spiralis*, found in Europe and North America, is an infection of synanthropic rats, by which it is propagated. These rats are cannibalistic and may be eaten by domestic pigs, which infect man when raw or undercooked pork is eaten. Pigs can also become infected after eating carcasses of sylvatic reservoir hosts, such as foxes.

Clinical illness is most likely to occur when meat prepared from a single heavily infected pig is eaten by a family or community. Where the meat has been diluted by uninfected meat, the disease is mild or subclinical. Garbage that contains unsterilized pig scraps and other trimmings is the most common source of infection in pigs. Another possible source is the ingestion of faeces of other infected animals, mice, rats, foxes and other pigs, at a

Temperate zone: *T.s. spiralis*

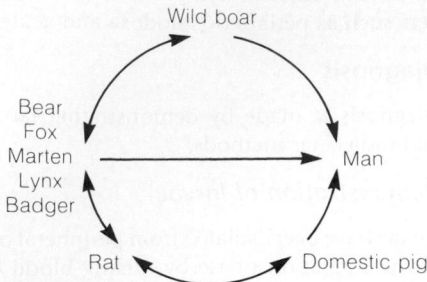

Africa: *T.s. nelsoni*

Arctic: *T.s. nativa*

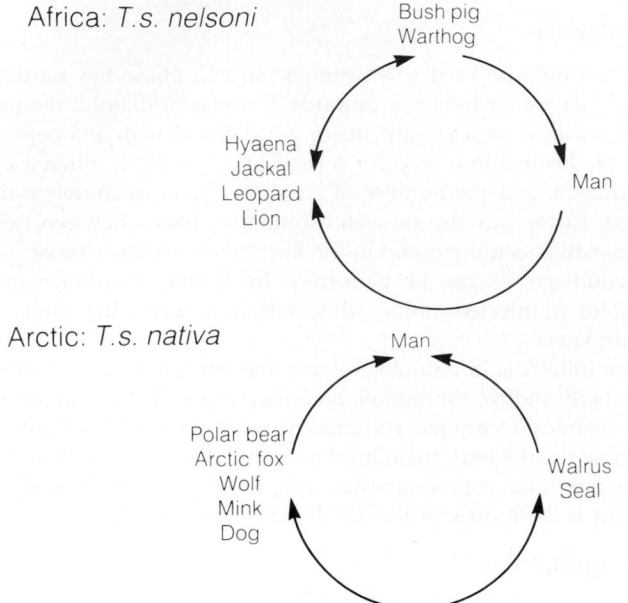

Figure 85.20 Epidemiology of *Trichinella spiralis*.

time when mature larvae are becoming established in the intestinal wall. The majority of infections are symptomless.

T. s. nativa is found mainly in Alaska and the northern regions of the world. Here, trichinosis is found in the white whale, walrus, hair seal, tree squirrel, black and white polar bear, dog, wolf, fox and wolverine. The polar bear, which is at the top of the Arctic food pyramid, is usually heavily infected and is the usual source, along with black and brown bear, of human infections.

T. s. nelsoni is found in sub-Saharan Africa, where it has been described from East Africa and Senegal. The infection is found in bush pigs (*Potamochoerus porcus*) and in the lion, leopard, cheetah and hyena. Man is infected by eating bush pig; domestic pigs are not infected.

One of the most extensive, single-source outbreaks ever recorded in China, involving more than 600 infections and over 300 clinical cases, was reported in 1997. The entire episode was attributed to the infection of undercooked pork dumplings at one restaurant.[181] An exhaustive review on trichinellosis has been published.[182]

Prevention

The main method of prevention is thorough cooking of all meat and regular meat inspection by means of trichinoscopy of all pork. Effective treatment of pork may be instituted by means of refrigeration. Storage of pork in deep-freeze units at −18°C to −15°C is effective. The cysts are destroyed by storage at −15°C for 20 days, −20°C for 10 days, −25°C for 6 days, and immediately by quick freezing at −37°C.

Cooking of all garbage will prevent the infection in pigs, and dressed pork may be irradiated by cobalt-60 or caesium-137, which kills the cysts.

REFERENCES

1. Jardine M, Kokai GK, Dalzell A M. *Enterobius vermicularis* and colitis in children. *J Pediatr Gastroenterol Nutr* 2006; 43:610–612.
2. Macedo T, MacCarty RL. Eosinophilic ileocolitis secondary to *Enterobius vermicularis*: case report. *Abdom Imaging* 2000; 25:530–532.
3. Zahariou A, Karamouti M, Papaioannou P. *Enterobius vermicularis* in the male urinary tract: a case report. *J Med Case Reports* 2007; 1:137.
4. Arca MJ, Gates RL, Groner JI, et al. Clinical manifestations of appendiceal pinworms in children: an institutional experience and a review of the literature. *Pediatr Surg Int* 2004; 20:372–375.
5. Bundy DA, Cooper ES. *Trichuris* and trichuriasis in humans. *Adv Parasitol* 1989; 28:107–173.
6. de Silva NR, Brooker S, Hotez PJ, et al. Soil-transmitted helminth infections: updating the global picture. *Trends Parasitol* 2003; 19:547–551.
7. Bethony J, Brooker S, Albonico M, et al. Soil-transmitted helminth infections: ascariasis, trichuriasis, and hookworm. *Lancet* 2006; 367:1521–1532.
8. Bundy DAP, Chan MS, Medley GF, et al. Intestinal nematode infections. In: Murray CJL, Lopez AD, Mathers CD, eds. *Global Epidemiology of Infectious Disease – Global Burden of Disease (IV)*. Geneva: World Health Organization; 2004:243–300.
9. Geissler PW, Mwaniki D, Thiong F, et al. Geophagy as a risk factor for geohelminth infections: a longitudinal study of Kenyan primary schoolchildren. *Trans R Soc Trop Med Hyg* 1998; 92:7–11.
10. Jung RC, Beaver PC. Clinical observations on *Trichocephalus trichiurus* (whipworm) infestation in children. *Pediatrics* 1951; 8:548–557.
11. Cooper ES, Ramdath DD, Whyte-Alleng C, et al. Plasma proteins in children with trichuris dysentery syndrome. *J Clin Pathol* 1997; 50:236–240.
12. Duff EM, Anderson NM, Cooper ES. Plasma insulin-like growth factor-1, type 1 procollagen, and serum tumour necrosis factor alpha in children recovering from Trichuris dysentery syndrome. *Paediatrics* 1999; 103:69.
13. Shin JL, Gardiner GW, Deitel W, et al. Does whipworm increase the pathogenicity of *Campylobacter jejuni*? A clinical correlate of an experimental observation. *Can J Gastroenterol* 2004; 18:175–177.
14. Bradley JE, Jackson JA. Immunity, immunoregulation and the ecology of trichuriasis and ascariasis. *Parasite Immunol* 2004; 26:429–441.
15. Jackson JA, Turner JD, Rentoul L, et al. T helper cell type 2 responsiveness predicts future susceptibility to gastrointestinal nematodes in humans. *J Infect Dis* 2004; 190:1804–1811.
16. Bundy DA, Cooper ES, Thompson DE, et al. Predisposition to *Trichuris trichiura* infection in humans. *Epidemiol Infect* 1987; 98:65–71.
17. Cooper ES, Bundy DA, MacDonald TT, et al. Growth suppression in the Trichuris dysentery syndrome. *Eur J Clin Nutr* 1990; 44:285–291.
18. Stephenson LS, Holland CV, Cooper ES. The public health significance of *Trichuris trichiura*. *Parasitology* 2000; 121(suppl):S73–S95.
19. Cooper ES, Bundy DA, Henry FJ. Chronic dysentery, stunting, and whipworm infestation. *Lancet* 1986; 2:280–281.
20. Watkins WE, Pollitt E. 'Stupidity or worms': do intestinal worms impair mental performance? *Psychol Bull* 1997; 121:171–191.

21. Jukes MCH, Drake LJ, Bundy DAP. *Health, Nutrition and Education for All: Levelling the Playing Field*. Wallingford: CABI Publishing; 2008.

22. Ismail MM, Jayakody RL. Efficacy of albendazole and its combinations with ivermectin or diethylcarbamazine (DEC) in the treatment of *Trichuris trichiura* infections in Sri Lanka. *Ann Trop Med Parasitol* 1999; 93: 501–504.

23. Bennett A, Guyatt H. Reducing intestinal nematode infection: efficacy of albendazole and mebendazole. *Parasitol Today* 2000; 16:71–74.

24. Brooker S, Clements ACA, Bundy DAP. Global epidemiology, ecology and control of soil-transmitted helminth infections. *Adv Parasitol* 2006; 62: 221–261.

25. Kightlinger LK, Seed JR, Kightlinger MB. *Ascaris lumbricoides* intensity in relation to environmental, socioeconomic, and behavioral determinants of exposure to infection in children from southeast Madagascar. *J Parasitol* 1998; 84:480–484.

26. Forrester JE, Scott ME, Bundy DA, et al. Clustering of *Ascaris lumbricoides* and *Trichuris trichiura* infections within households. *Trans R Soc Trop Med Hyg* 1988; 82:282–288.

27. Bundy DA, Medley GF. Immuno-epidemiology of human geohelminthiasis: ecological and immunological determinants of worm burden. *Parasitol* 1992; 104(suppl):S105–S119.

28. Quinnell RJ. Genetics of susceptibility to human helminth infection. *Int J Parasitol* 2003; 33:1219–1231.

29. de Silva NR, Chan MS, Bundy DA. Morbidity and mortality due to ascariasis: re-estimation and sensitivity analysis of global numbers at risk. *Trop Med Int Health* 1997; 2:519–528.

30. Khuroo MS, Zargar SA, Mahajan R. Hepatobiliary and pancreatic ascariasis in India. *Lancet* 1990; 335:1503–1506.

31. Shah OJ, Zargar SA, Robbani I. Biliary ascariasis: a review. *World J Surg* 2006; 30:1500–1506.

32. Shah OJ, Robbani I, Khan F, et al. Management of biliary ascariasis in pregnancy. *World J Surg* 2005; 29:1294–1298.

33. Ng KK, Wong HF, Kong MS, et al. Biliary ascariasis: CT, MR cholangiopancreatography, and navigator endoscopic appearance – report of a case of acute biliary obstruction. *Abdom Imaging* 1999; 24:470–472.

34. Pilankar KS, Amarapurkar AD, Joshi RM, et al. Hepatolithiasis with biliary ascariasis – a case report. *BMC Gastroenterol* 2003; 3:35.

35. Beckingham IJ, Cullis SN, Krige JE, et al. Management of hepatobiliary and pancreatic *Ascaris* infestation in adults after failed medical treatment. *Br J Surg* 1998; 85:907–910.

36. Cooper PJ, Barreto ML, Rodrigues LC. Human allergy and geohelminth infections: a review of the literature and a proposed conceptual model to guide the investigation of possible causal associations. *Br Med Bull* 2006; 79–80:203–218.

37. Cooper PJ, Chico ME, Vaca MG, et al. Effect of albendazole treatments on the prevalence of atopy in children living in communities endemic for geohelminth parasites: a cluster-randomised trial. *Lancet* 2006; 367:1598–1603.

38. Tripathy K, Duque E, Bolanos O, et al. Malabsorption syndrome in ascariasis. *Am J Clin Nutr* 1972; 25:1276–1281.

39. Hlaing T. Ascariasis and childhood malnutrition. *Parasitology* 1993; 107(suppl):S125–S136.

40. Jalal F, Nesheim MC, Agus Z, et al. Serum retinol concentrations in children are affected by food sources of beta-carotene, fat intake, and anthelmintic drug treatment. *Am J Clin Nutr* 1998; 68:623–629.

41. O'Lorcain P, Holland CV. The public health importance of *Ascaris lumbricoides*. *Parasitology* 2000; 121(suppl):S51–S71.

42. Crompton DW, Nesheim MC. Nutritional impact of intestinal helminthiasis during the human life cycle. *Annu Rev Nutr* 2002; 22:35–59.

43. Cooper PJ, Chico ME, Sandoval C, et al. Human infection with *Ascaris lumbricoides* is associated with a polarized cytokine response. *J Infect Dis* 2000; 182:1207–1213.

44. Palmer DR, Hall A, Haque R, et al. Antibody isotype responses to antigens of *Ascaris lumbricoides* in a case-control study of persistently heavily infected Bangladeshi children. *Parasitology* 1995; 111:385–393.

45. King EM, Kim HT, Dang NT, et al. Immuno-epidemiology of *Ascaris lumbricoides* infection in a high transmission community: antibody responses and their impact on current and future infection intensity. *Parasite Immunol* 2005; 27:89–96.

46. Gelpi AP, Mustafa A. Seasonal pneumonitis with eosinophilia. A study of larval ascariasis in Saudi Arabs. *Am J Trop Med Hyg* 1967; 16:646–657.

47. Spillman RK. Pulmonary ascariasis in tropical communities. *Am J Trop Med Hyg* 1975; 24:791–800.

48. de Silva NR, Guyatt HL, Bundy DA. Morbidity and mortality due to Ascaris-induced intestinal obstruction. *Trans R Soc Trop Med Hyg* 1997; 91:31–36.

49. Wasadikar PP, Kulkarni AB. Intestinal obstruction due to ascariasis. *Br J Surg* 1997; 84:410–412.

50. Booth M, Bundy D A. Comparative prevalences of *Ascaris lumbricoides*, *Trichuris trichiura* and hookworm infections and the prospects for combined control. *Parasitology* 1992; 105:151–157.

51. Anderson RM. The population dynamics and epidemiology of intestinal nematode infections. *Trans R Soc Trop Med Hyg* 1986; 80:686–696.

52. Brooker S, Alexander N, Geiger S, et al. Contrasting patterns in the small-scale heterogeneity of human helminth infections in urban and rural environments in Brazil. *Int J Parasitol* 2006; 36:1143–1151.

53. Crompton DW. Ascaris and ascariasis. *Adv Parasitol* 2001; 48:285–375.

54. Thompson DE, Bundy DA, Cooper ES, et al. Epidemiological characteristics of *Toxocara canis* zoonotic infection of children in a Caribbean community. *Bull World Health Organ* 1986; 64:283–290.

55. Despommier D. Toxocariasis: clinical aspects, epidemiology, medical ecology, and molecular aspects. *Clin Microbiol Rev* 2003; 16:265–272.

56. Fisher M. *Toxocara cati*: an underestimated zoonotic agent. *Trends Parasitol* 2003; 19:167–170.

57. Wilder HC. Nematode endophthalmitis. *Trans Am Acad Ophthalmol Otolaryngol* 1950; 55:99–109.

58. Good B, Holland CV, Taylor MR, et al. Ocular toxocariasis in schoolchildren. *Clin Infect Dis* 2004; 39:173–178.

59. Wolfe A, Wright IP. Human toxocariasis and direct contact with dogs. *Vet Rec* 2003; 152:419–422.

60. Overgaauw PA. Aspects of Toxocara epidemiology: human toxocarosis. *Crit Rev Microbiol* 1997; 23:215–231.

61. Nicoletti A, Bartoloni A, Sofia V, et al. Epilepsy and toxocariasis: a case-control study in Burundi. *Epilepsia* 2007; 48:894–899.

62. Stewart JM, Cubillan LD & Cunningham ET Jr. Prevalence, clinical features, and causes of vision loss among patients with ocular toxocariasis. *Retina* 2005; 25:1005–1013.

63. Maetz HM, Kleinstein RN, Federico D, et al. Estimated prevalence of ocular toxoplasmosis and toxocariasis in Alabama. *J Infect Dis* 1987; 156:414.

64. Sharghi N, Schantz PM, Caramico L, et al. Environmental exposure to Toxocara as a possible risk factor for asthma: a clinic-based case-control study. *Clin Infect Dis* 2001; 32:E111–E116.

65. Gonzalez MT, Ibanez O, Balcarce N, et al. Toxocariasis with liver involvement. *Acta Gastroenterol Latinoam* 2000; 30:187–190.

66. de Savigny DH, Voller A, Woodruff AW. Toxocariasis: serological diagnosis by enzyme immunoassay. *J Clin Pathol* 1979; 32:284–288.

67. Glickman L, Schantz P, Dombroske R, et al. Evaluation of serodiagnostic tests for visceral larva migrans. *Am J Trop Med Hyg* 1978; 27:492–498.

68. Nunes CM, Tundisi RN, Heinemann MB, et al. Toxocariasis: serological diagnosis by indirect antibody competition ELISA. *Rev Inst Med Trop Sao Paulo* 1999; 41:95–100.

69. Noordin R, Smith HV, Mohamad S, et al. Comparison of IgG-ELISA and IgG4-ELISA for Toxocara serodiagnosis. *Acta Trop* 2005; 93:57–62.

70. Yamasaki H, Araki K, Lim PK, et al. Development of a highly specific recombinant *Toxocara canis* second-stage larva excretory-secretory antigen for immunodiagnosis of human toxocariasis. *J Clin Microbiol* 2000; 38: 1409–1413.

71. Paco JM, Campos DM, Oliveira JA. Wild rodents as experimental intermediate hosts of *Lagochilascaris minor* Leiper, 1909. *Mem Inst Oswaldo Cruz* 1999; 94:441–449.

72. Calvopina M, Guevara AG, Herrera M, et al. Treatment of human lagochilascariasis with ivermectin: first case report from Ecuador. *Trans R Soc Trop Med Hyg* 1998; 92:223–224.

73. Brooker S, Bethony J, Hotez PJ. Human hookworm infection in the 21st century. *Adv Parasitol* 2004; 58:197–288.

74. Hawdon JM, Hotez PJ. Hookworm: developmental biology of the infectious process. *Curr Opin Genet Dev* 1996; 6:618–623.

75. Schad GA, Chowdhury AB, Dean CG, et al. Arrested development in human hookworm infections: an adaptation to a seasonally unfavorable external environment. *Science* 1973; 180:52–54.

76. Yu SH, Jiang ZX, Xu LQ. Infantile hookworm disease in China. A review. *Acta Trop* 1995; 59:265–270.

77. Del Valle A, Jones BF, Harrison LM, et al. Isolation and molecular cloning of a secreted hookworm platelet inhibitor from adult *Ancylostoma caninum*. *Mol Biochem Parasitol* 2003; 129:167–177.

78. Roche M, Layrisse M. The nature and causes of 'hookworm anemia.' *Am J Trop Med Hyg* 1966; 15:1029–1102.

79. Stoltzfus RJ, Albonico M, Chwaya HM, et al. Hemoquant determination of hookworm-related blood loss and its role in iron deficiency in African children. *Am J Trop Med Hyg* 1996; 55:399–404.

80. Stoltzfus RJ, Chwaya HM, Tielsch JM, et al. Epidemiology of iron deficiency anemia in Zanzibari schoolchildren: the importance of hookworms. *Am J Clin Nutr* 1997; 65:153–159.

81. Pritchard DI, Quinnell RJ, Moustafa M, et al. Hookworm (*Necator americanus*) infection and storage iron depletion. *Trans R Soc Trop Med Hyg* 1991; 85:235–238.

82. Gilles HM, Watson-Williams EJ, Ball PAJ. Hookworm infection and anaemia: an epidemiological, clinical and laboratory study. *Q J Med* 1964; 331:1–24.

83. Brooker S, Peshu N, Warn PA, et al. The epidemiology of hookworm infection and its contribution to anaemia among pre-school children on the Kenyan coast. *Trans R Soc Trop Med Hyg* 1999; 93:240–246.

84. Stoltzfus RJ, Chwaya HM, Montresor A, et al. Malaria, hookworms and recent fever are related to anemia and iron status indicators in 0- to 5-y old Zanzibari children and these relationships change with age. *J Nutr* 2000; 130:1724–1733.

85. Quinnell RJ, Pritchard DI, Raiko A, et al. Immune responses in human necatoriasis: association between interleukin-5 responses and resistance to reinfection. *J Infect Dis* 2004; 190:430–438.

86. Geiger S, Caldas IR, McGlone BE, et al. Stage-specific immune responses in human *Necator americanus* infection. *Parasite Immunol* 2007; 29:347–358.

87. Quinnell RJ, Bethony J, Pritchard DI. The immunoepidemiology of human hookworm infection. *Parasite Immunol* 2004; 26:443–454.

88. Fujiwara RT, Geiger SM, Bethony J, et al. Comparative immunology of human and animal models of hookworm infection. *Parasite Immunol* 2006; 28:285–293.

89. Bethony J, Loukas A, Smout M, et al. Antibodies against a secreted protein from hookworm larvae reduce the intensity of hookworm infection in humans and vaccinated laboratory animals. *FASEB J* 2005; 19:1743–1745.

90. Lwambo NJ, Bundy DA, Medley GF. A new approach to morbidity risk assessment in hookworm endemic communities. *Epidemiol Infect* 1992; 108:469–481.

91. Anyaeze CM. Reducing burden of hookworm disease in the management of upper abdominal pain in the tropics. *Trop Doct* 2003; 33:174–175.

92. Maxwell C, Hussain R, Nutman TB, et al. The clinical and immunologic responses of normal human volunteers to low dose hookworm (*Necator americanus*) infection. *Am J Trop Med Hyg* 1987; 37:126–134.

93. Wright V, Bickle Q. Immune responses following experimental human hookworm infection. *Clin Exp Immunol* 2005; 142:398–403.

94. Brooker S, Hotez PJ, Bundy DAP. Hookworm-related anemia among pregnant women: a systematic review. PLoS Negl Trop.

95. Sakti H, Nokes C, Hertanto WS, et al. Evidence for an association between hookworm infection and cognitive function in Indonesian school children. *Trop Med Int Health* 1999; 4:322–334.

96. Booth M, Vounatsou P, N'Goran EK, et al. The influence of sampling effort and the performance of the Kato-Katz technique in diagnosing *Schistosoma mansoni* and hookworm co-infections in rural Cote d'Ivoire. *Parasitology* 2003; 127:525–531.

97. Verweij JJ, Brienen EA, Ziem J, et al. Simultaneous detection and quantification of *Ancylostoma duodenale*, *Necator americanus*, and *Oesophagostomum bifurcum* in fecal samples using multiplex real-time PCR. *Am J Trop Med Hyg* 2007; 77:685–690.

98. Cline BL, Little MD, Bartholomew RK, et al. Larvicidal activity of albendazole against *Necator americanus* in human volunteers. *Am J Trop Med Hyg* 1984; 33:387–394.

99. Reynoldson JA, Behnke JM, Pallant LJ, et al. Failure of pyrantel in treatment of human hookworm infections (*Ancylostoma duodenale*) in the Kimberley region of north west Australia. *Acta Trop* 1997; 68:301–312.

100. Michaud C, Tantalean M, Ique C, et al. A survey for helminth parasites in feral New World non-human primate populations and its comparison with parasitological data from man in the region. *J Med Primatol* 2003; 32:341–345.

101. Peduzzi R, Piffaretti JC. *Ancylostoma duodenale* and the Saint Gothard anaemia. *Br Med J* 1983; 287:1942–1945.

102. Humphries DL, Stephenson LS, Pearce EJ, et al. The use of human faeces for fertilizer is associated with increased intensity of hookworm infection in Vietnamese women. *Trans R Soc Trop Med Hyg* 1997; 91:518–520.

103. Bundy DAP. Is the hookworm just another geohelminth? In: Schad GA, Warren KS, eds. *Hookworm Disease: Current Status and New Directions*. London: Taylor and Francis; 1990:147–164.

104. Bethony J, Chen J, Lin S, et al. Emerging patterns of hookworm infection: influence of aging on the intensity of *Necator* infection in Hainan Province, People's Republic of China. *Clin Infect Dis* 2002; 35:1336–1344.

105. Brooker S, Jardim-Botelho A, Quinnell RJ, et al. Age-related changes in hookworm infection, anaemia and iron deficiency in an area of high *Necator americanus* hookworm transmission in south-eastern Brazil. *Trans R Soc Trop Med Hyg* 2007; 101:146–154.

106. Schad GA, Anderson RM. Predisposition to hookworm infection in humans. *Science* 1985; 228:1537–1540.

107. Raso G, Vounatsou P, Gosoniu L, et al. Risk factors and spatial patterns of hookworm infection among schoolchildren in a rural area of western Cote d'Ivoire. *Int J Parasitol* 2006; 36:201–210.

108. Yosipovitch G, Sugeng MW, Seow CS, et al. Widespread and unusual presentations of cutaneous larva migrans acquired in tropical sandy beach resorts. *J Eur Acad Dermatol Venereol* 2002; 16:284–285.

109. Heukelbach J, Wilcke T, Feldmeier H. Cutaneous larva migrans (creeping eruption) in an urban slum in Brazil. *Int J Dermatol* 2004; 43:511–515.

110. Jackson A, Heukelbach J, Calheiros CM, et al. A study in a community in Brazil in which cutaneous larva migrans is endemic. *Clin Infect Dis* 2006; 43:e13–18.

111. Caumes E, Ly F, Bricaire F. Cutaneous larva migrans with folliculitis: report of seven cases and review of the literature. *Br J Dermatol* 2002; 146:314–316.

112. Veraldi S, Rizzitelli G. Effectiveness of a new therapeutic regimen with albendazole in cutaneous larva migrans. *Eur J Dermatol* 1999; 9:352–353.

113. Caumes E. Treatment of cutaneous larva migrans. *Clin Infect Dis* 2000; 30:811–814.

114. Tremblay A, MacLean JD, Gyorkos T, et al. Outbreak of cutaneous larva migrans in a group of travellers. *Trop Med Int Health* 2000; 5:330–334.

115. Carvalho EM, Da Fonseca Porto A. Epidemiological and clinical interaction between HTLV-1 and *Strongyloides stercoralis*. *Parasite Immunol* 2004; 26:487–497.

116. Gill GV, Welch E, Bailey JW, et al. Chronic *Strongyloides stercoralis* infection in former British Far East prisoners of war. *Q J Med* 2004; 97:789–795.

117. Wong TY, Szeto CC, Lai FF, et al. Nephrotic syndrome in strongyloidiasis: remission after eradication with anthelmintic agents. *Nephron* 1998; 79:333–336.

118. Viney ME, Brown M, Omoding NE, et al. Why does HIV infection not lead to disseminated strongyloidiasis? *J Infect Dis* 2004; 190:2175–2180.

119. Wehner JH, Kirsch CM. Pulmonary manifestations of strongyloidiasis. *Semin Respir Infect* 1997; 12:122–129.

120. Koga K, Kasuya S, Khamboonruang C, et al. A modified agar plate method for detection of *Strongyloides stercoralis. Am J Trop Med Hyg* 1991; 45:518–521.

121. Sato Y, Kobayashi J, Toma H, et al. Efficacy of stool examination for detection of Strongyloides infection. *Am J Trop Med Hyg* 1995; 53:248–250.

122. Conway DJ, Bailey JW, Lindo JF, et al. Serum IgG reactivity with 41-, 31-, and 28-kDa larval proteins of *Strongyloides stercoralis* in individuals with strongyloidiasis. *J Infect Dis* 1993; 168:784–787.

123. Sithithaworn J, Sithithaworn P, Janrungsopa T, et al. Comparative assessment of the gelatin particle agglutination test and an enzyme-linked immunosorbent assay for diagnosis of strongyloidiasis. *J Clin Microbiol* 2005; 43:3278–3282.

124. Igual-Adell R, Oltra-Alcaraz C, Soler-Company E, et al. Efficacy and safety of ivermectin and thiabendazole in the treatment of strongyloidiasis. *Expert Opin Pharmacother* 2004; 5:2615–2619.

125. Yori PP, Kosek M, Gilman RH, et al. Seroepidemiology of strongyloidiasis in the Peruvian Amazon. *Am J Trop Med Hyg* 2006; 74:97–102.

126. Steinmann P, Zhou XN, Du ZW, et al. Occurrence of *Strongyloides stercoralis* in Yunnan Province, China, and comparison of siagnostic methods. *PLoS Negl Trop Dis* 2007; 1:e75.

127. Lindo JF, Robinson RD, Terry SI, et al. Age-prevalence and household clustering of *Strongyloides stercoralis* infection in Jamaica. *Parasitology* 1995; 110:97–102.

128. Ashford RW, Barnish G, Viney ME. *Strongyloides fuelleborni kellyi*: infection and disease in Papua New Guinea. *Parasitol Today* 1992; 8:314–318.

129. Yong TS, Lee JH, Shin S, et al. Differential diagnosis of *Trichostrongylus* and hookworm eggs via PCR using ITS-1 sequence. *Korean J Parasitol* 2007; 45:69–74.

130. Ralph A, O'Sullivan MV, Sangster NC, et al. Abdominal pain and eosinophilia in suburban goat keepers–trichostrongylosis [corrected]. *Med J Aust* 2006; 184:467–469.

131. Loukas A, Bethony J, Brooker S, et al. Hookworm vaccines: past, present, and future. *Lancet Infect Dis* 2006; 6:733–741.

132. WHO. *WHO Model Prescribing Information: Drugs Used in Parasitic Diseases.* 2nd edn. Geneva: World Health Organization; 1995.

133. WHO. *107th Session of WHO's Executive Board.* Geneva: World Health Organization; 2001.

134. WHO. *Prevention and Control of Schistosomiasis and Soil-transmitted Helminthiasis. Report of a WHO Expert Committee.* Geneva: World Health Organization; 2002.

135. Warren KS, Bundy DAP, Anderson RM, et al. Helminth infection. In: Jamison DT, Mosley WH, Measham AR, et al., eds. *Disease Control Priorities in Developing Countries.* New York: Oxford University Press; 1993.

136. Bundy DA, Wong MS, Lewis LL, et al. Control of geohelminths by delivery of targeted chemotherapy through schools. *Trans R Soc Trop Med Hyg* 1990; 84:115–120.

137. Miguel E, Kremer M. Worms: identifying impacts on education and health in the presence of treatment externalities. *Econometrica* 2004; 72:159–217.

138. The Partnership for Child Development. The cost of large-scale school health programmes which deliver anthelmintics to children in Ghana and Tanzania. *Acta Trop* 1999; 73:183–204.

139. Bleakley H. Disease and development: evidence from hookworm eradication in the American South. *J Eur Econ Assoc* 2003; 1:376–386.

140. Guyatt H. The cost of delivering and sustaining a control programme for schistosomiasis and soil-transmitted helminthiasis. *Acta Trop* 2003; 86:267–274.

141. UNESCO. *The Dakar Framework for Action: Education for All – Meeting our Collective Commitments.* UNESCO: World Education Forum, Dakar; 2000.

142. The World Bank. *The FRESH Framework: A Toolkit for Task Managers. Human Development Network.* Washington, DC: The World Bank; 2000.

143. Hotez PJ, Bundy DAP, Beegle K, et al. Helminth infections: soil-transmitted helminth infections and schistosomiasis. In: Jamison DT, Breman JG, Measham AR, et al., eds. *Disease Control Priorities in Developing Countries.* 2nd edn. New York: The World Bank and Oxford University Press; 2006:467–497.

144. Bundy DAP, Shaeffer S, Jukes M, et al. School based health and nutrition programs. In: Jamison DT, Breman JG, Measham AR, et al., eds. *Disease Control Priorities in Developing Countries.* 2nd edn. New York: The World Bank and Oxford University Press; 2006:1091–1108.

145. Stoltzfus RJ, Albonico M, Tielsch JM, et al. School-based deworming program yields small improvement in growth of Zanzibari school children after one year. *J Nutr* 1997; 127:2187–2193.

146. Guyatt HL, Brooker S, Kihamia CM, et al. Evaluation of efficacy of school-based anthelmintic treatments against anaemia in children in the United Republic of Tanzania. *Bull World Health Organ* 2001; 79:695–703.

147. Torlesse H, Hodges M. Anthelminthic treatment and haemoglobin concentrations during pregnancy. *Lancet* 2000; 356:1083.

148. Christian P, Khatry S, West K. Antenatal anthelmintic treatment, birthweight, and infant survival in rural Nepal. *Lancet* 2004; 364:981–983.

149. Dickson R, Awasthi S, Williamson P, et al. Effects of treatment for intestinal helminth infection on growth and cognitive performance in children: systematic review of randomised trials. *BMJ* 2000; 320:1697–1701.

150. Taylor-Robinson DC, Jones AP, Garner P. Deworming drugs for treating soil-transmitted intestinal worms in children: effects on growth and school performance. *Cochrane Database Syst Rev* 2007; (4):CD000371.

151. Stoltzfus RJ, Chway HM, Montresor A, et al. Low dose daily iron supplementation improves iron status and appetite but not anemia, whereas quarterly anthelminthic treatment improves growth, appetite and anemia in Zanzibari preschool children. *J Nutr* 2004; 134:348–356.

152. Alderman H, Konde-Lule J, Sebuliba I, et al. Effect on weight gain of routinely giving albendazole to preschool children during child health days in Uganda: cluster randomised controlled trial. *BMJ* 2006; 333:122.

153. Bundy DA, Chan MS, Savioli L. Hookworm infection in pregnancy. *Trans R Soc Trop Med Hyg* 1995; 89:521–522.

154. Allen HE, Crompton DW, de Silva N, et al. New policies for using anthelmintics in high risk groups. *Trends Parasitol* 2002; 18:381–382.

155. Albonico M, Montresor A, Crompton DW, et al. Intervention for the control of soil-transmitted helminthiasis in the community. *Adv Parasitol* 2006; 61:311–348.

156. Brooker S, Beasley M, Ndinaromtan M, et al. Use of remote sensing and a geographical information system in a national helminth control programme in Chad. *Bull World Health Organ* 2002; 80:783–789.

157. Geerts S, Gryseels B. Drug resistance in human helminths: current situation and lessons from livestock. *Clin Microbiol Rev* 2000; 13:207–222.

158. Satoh M, Toma H, Sato Y, et al. Production of a high level of specific IgG4 antibody associated with resistance to albendazole treatment in HLA-DRB1*0901-positive patients with strongyloidiasis. *Am J Trop Med Hyg* 1999; 61:668–671.

159. De Clercq D, Sacko M, Behnke J, et al. Failure of mebendazole in treatment of human hookworm infections in the southern region of Mali. *Am J Trop Med Hyg* 1997; 57:25–30.

160. Albonico M, Engels D, Savioli L. Monitoring drug efficacy and early detection of drug resistance in human soil-transmitted nematodes: a pressing public health agenda for helminth control. *Int J Parasitol* 2004; 34:1205–1210.

161. Mooijman A, van den Berg C, Jensen LO, et al. *Toolkit on Hygiene, Sanitation, and Water in Schools.* Washington, DC: World Bank, WSP & UNICEF; 2005.

162. Brooker S, Whawell S, Kabatereine NB, et al. Evaluating the epidemiological impact of national control programmes for helminths. *Trends Parasitol* 2004; 20:537–545.

163. Horton J. Albendazole: a review of anthelmintic efficacy and safety in humans. *Parasitology* 2000; 121(suppl):S113–S132.

164. Keiser J, Utzinger J. Efficacy of current drugs against soil-transmitted helminth infections. Systematic review and meta-analysis. *JAMA* 2008; 299:1937–1948.

165. Urbani C, Albonico M. Anthelmintic drug safety and drug administration in the control of soil-transmitted helminthiasis in community campaigns. *Acta Tropica* 2003; 86:215–221.

Box 86.1 Recommendations for the laboratory diagnosis and follow-up of human CE

Primary diagnostic approach (screening and confirmation)
Serum antibody detection[a] and/or imaging procedure

Seronegative samples AND negative imaging findings	Seronegative samples AND 'positive' imaging findings	Seropositive samples AND 'positive' or negative imaging findings
Persons with documented infection risk only: Serological and imaging follow-up every 6 months for 2 years. Differential diagnosis[b]	Differential diagnosis[b] *Asymptomatic cases* Extended/advanced imaging procedures; Repeat serodiagnosis with a new serum sample and immunoblotting; FNAB[38] or biopsy for PCR (tissue) or antigen detection (fluid), if appropriate; If lesions are fully calcified: Serological and imaging follow-up after 6 months to confirm parasite inactivity *Symptomatic cases* Consideration of percutaneous drainage or surgical intervention and/or chemotherapy without serodiagnostic confirmation	*Asymptomatic AND symptomatic cases* Species-specific (secondary) serology with: – ELISA using appropriate (purified) antigens – Immunoblot for the detection of Antigen B subunits or other specific bands

Post-surgical and/or chemotherapeutical follow-up

Post-surgical follow-up	Chemotherapeutical follow-up (assessing viability)
– CT and/or MRI and/or ultrasound – Serum antibody detection by ELISA – Serum antigen detection by ELISA[c]	– CT and/or MRI and/or ultrasound – Serum antibody detection by ELISA – Serum antigen detection by ELISA[c]

[a] ELISA for IgG detection, IHAT and latex agglutination test (LAT) with crude parasite antigen, alone or in combination, are commonly used.
[b] Clinical differential diagnosis for AHD (in some cases for cysticercosis) or neoplasias may be required.[30,31,33]
[c] Only in those patients with initially detectable circulating antigens.[37]

Whatever surgical procedure is chosen, care has to be taken to avoid spillage of cyst content or, more specifically, protoscolices, which is the main predictor of recurrent disease. To achieve this, the peritoneal cavity should be carefully protected, and the cyst evacuated and sterilized with scolicidal agents. The use of formalin and hypertonic saline should be abandoned since they can induce caustic injury to the biliary tree.[49,50] Formalin and hypertonic saline have also been associated with severe acidosis and hypernatraemia, respectively.[51] Currently used scolicidal agents include chlorhexidine, hydrogen peroxide, cetrizamide and, most preferably, ethanol.[43,51] Pretreatment with benzimidazole compounds (affecting the germinal layer) – optionally complemented with praziquantel (affecting protoscolices) – has been proposed to avoid the use of dangerous scolicidal agents and to decrease the rate of recurrence.[52–54]

Radical surgery – hepatectomy or pericystectomy – has relatively low relapse rates, ranging from 8.5% to 22%,[43,44,51,55,56] whereas relapse occurs in up to 75% after non-radical surgery (Table 86.1).[46,57,58] Recently, minimally invasive approaches have

been successfully used.[59–61] Local recurrence has been ascribed to the formation of exogenous daughter cysts which are left behind in the case of non-radical surgery.

Rupture into the biliary tree has been successfully treated with choledochojejunostomy or T-tube drainage;[62,63] in a comparative series, choledochojejunostomy was found to result in fewer instances of recurrent jaundice than T-tube drainage.[63] Endoscopic sphincterotomy with or without nasobiliary drainage has been successfully used in the treatment of obstructive jaundice due to biliary rupture.[64,65] Sphincterotomy is also useful in cases of post-operative biliary leaks.[65] In selected cases, cyst removal and lavage with hypertonic saline by ERCP can lead to cure.[66]

In rare cases, in particular where radical surgery has not been possible, liver transplantation may have to be considered and has been successfully carried out.[11]

Pulmonary cysts can be of primary origin, but are also often the result of infected or ruptured hepatic cysts. About 40% of patients present with complications, mainly infection but also pneumothorax.[67] In these cases, surgical treatment is mandatory.

Table 86.1 Selection of recurrence rates (as a percentage of the total series) after surgery for CE

Authors	*n*	Radical (%)[a]	Non-radical (%)[b]	PAIR (%)[c]
Akhan et al.[57]	31	–	–	3.2
Behrns and van Heerden[46]	23	0	50.0	–
Magistrelli et al.[58]	119	16.9	4.2	–
Morel et al.[44]	42	2.4	27.3	–

[a] Includes formal hepatic resections and total pericystectomy.
[b] Includes different procedures such as capitonnage or partial pericystectomy.
[c] PAIR: Puncture, aspiration, inoculation and reaspiration (see text).

Treatment consists of wedge resection or lobectomy,[68] a two-stage procedure sometimes being necessary.[67] Recently, minimally invasive approaches for concurrent hepatic and pulmonary disease have been reported.[69] Recurrence of pulmonary disease appears to be rare.[56,67,68] A placebo controlled trial of albendazole in pulmonary hydatid disease showed cure in 45% in the verum group as opposed to 0 in the placebo group; thus, primary pharmacotherapy can be considered in uncomplicated cases.[70] Cardiac involvement necessitates surgery using bypass.[71]

Surgery is also the treatment of choice for renal involvement, nephrectomy being necessary only in about 15%, the others being able to be treated with pericystectomy alone.[58,72] For the treatment of hydatid cysts of the central nervous system recovery can be expected if the whole cyst can be extracted[16]; results of pharmacological treatment are uncertain.[16]

PAIR, once a rather controversial procedure, is now widely used in selected cases but requires experienced specialists. In a randomized trial comparing pericystectomy with PAIR plus albendazole, hospital stay was shorter and complications fewer in the patients treated with PAIR compared to the surgical group.[73] PAIR is indicated for:[2] patients refusing surgery; infected cysts not communicating with the biliary vessel system; inoperable patients (see contraindications for surgery); pregnant patients; children >3 years; anechoic lesion = 5 cm in diameter; cysts with a regular double laminated layer; cysts with multiple septal divisions of more than five; multiple cysts (= 5 cm in diameter) in different liver segments; relapse after surgery; and failure to respond to chemotherapy. Relative contraindications for PAIR are inaccessible or risky location of the cyst in the liver; multiple septal divisions; cysts with echogenic lesions; inactive cysts or calcified lesions; communicating cysts; cysts located in the lung and bones and some others. It should not be performed when exophytic cysts or dilated bile ducts are observed on preoperative imaging.[74] A multicentric study, based on the use of 95% ethanol as a scolicidal agent, reported the successful treatment of 231 cysts in 163 Italian and Kenyan patients with abdominal, mainly hepatic CE.[75] Other experiences with PAIR were obtained in 61 patients with 84 hepatic hydatid cysts.[76] In this study, hydatid cysts were sterilized by the injection of one of two scolicidal agents: 20% hypertonic saline solution (38 patients) or 0.5% silver nitrate (23 patients), respectively. All patients underwent follow-up examinations for 1 month to 6 years after PAIR: serial sonographic examinations revealed a heterogeneous echo pattern in 78 cysts (93%); a progressive decrease in diameter in 76 cysts (90%); calcification of the cyst wall, cystic contents or both in 10 cysts (12%); and complete disappearance of one cyst (1%) in a patient who had been monitored for over 6 years. Similar results were reported by Men and colleagues.[77] However, complications are not infrequent after PAIR. No recurrence of CE after PAIR was observed in Odev's series[76] over the follow-up period of 72 months, while there were three local recurrences and one rupture into the biliary tree in the series by Men et al.[77] and 2.8% in another Turkish series.[78] Recently, a percutaneous approach employing radiofrequency ablation has been described with good immediate results[79] but long-term results are not yet available.

Pharmacotherapy

Two benzimidazole compounds – mebendazole and albendazole – and praziquantel have activity against *E. granulosus* in vitro and in animal models.[80,81] No controlled studies have ever been performed in man but large series with the benzimidazoles have been published (Table 86.2).[82–90] Albendazole appears preferable to mebendazole because of its better bioavailability.[91,92] Both drugs penetrate into the cysts,[93,94] but sometimes heroic doses are needed to achieve a therapeutic plasma concentration of mebendazole.[95] Mebendazole should be given after a fat-rich meal and levels monitored 4 hours after the morning dose.[93] Plasma levels of mebendazole are unrelated to dose;[94,95] the generally accepted therapeutic levels are around 250 nmol/L. The therapeutic level of albendazole sulphoxide, the major active metabolite in serum,[96] has not been defined in vivo yet. Better absorption of albendazole when given with a fatty meal has also been reported.[97] Cholestasis increases the blood levels of both drugs.[98] The former use of albendazole in cycles of 4 weeks, followed by a drug-free interval of 2 weeks, has been increasingly replaced by continuous treatment.[2,99] The initial idea for the cyclic treatment had been to diminish toxicity and to avoid autoinduction of its metabolism.[96] However, more recently continuous administration was found to be more efficacious in a small comparative study than administration in cycles: 6/6 patients on continuous therapy showed cyst involution, while relapse occurred in the cycling group.[100]

Side-effects of the two drugs appear to be similar and include mainly leucopenia, hair loss and hepatotoxicity.[82,98] For both benzimidazoles it appears likely that they act not truly parasiticidally in vivo but rather parasitostatically. Thus, in those treated with

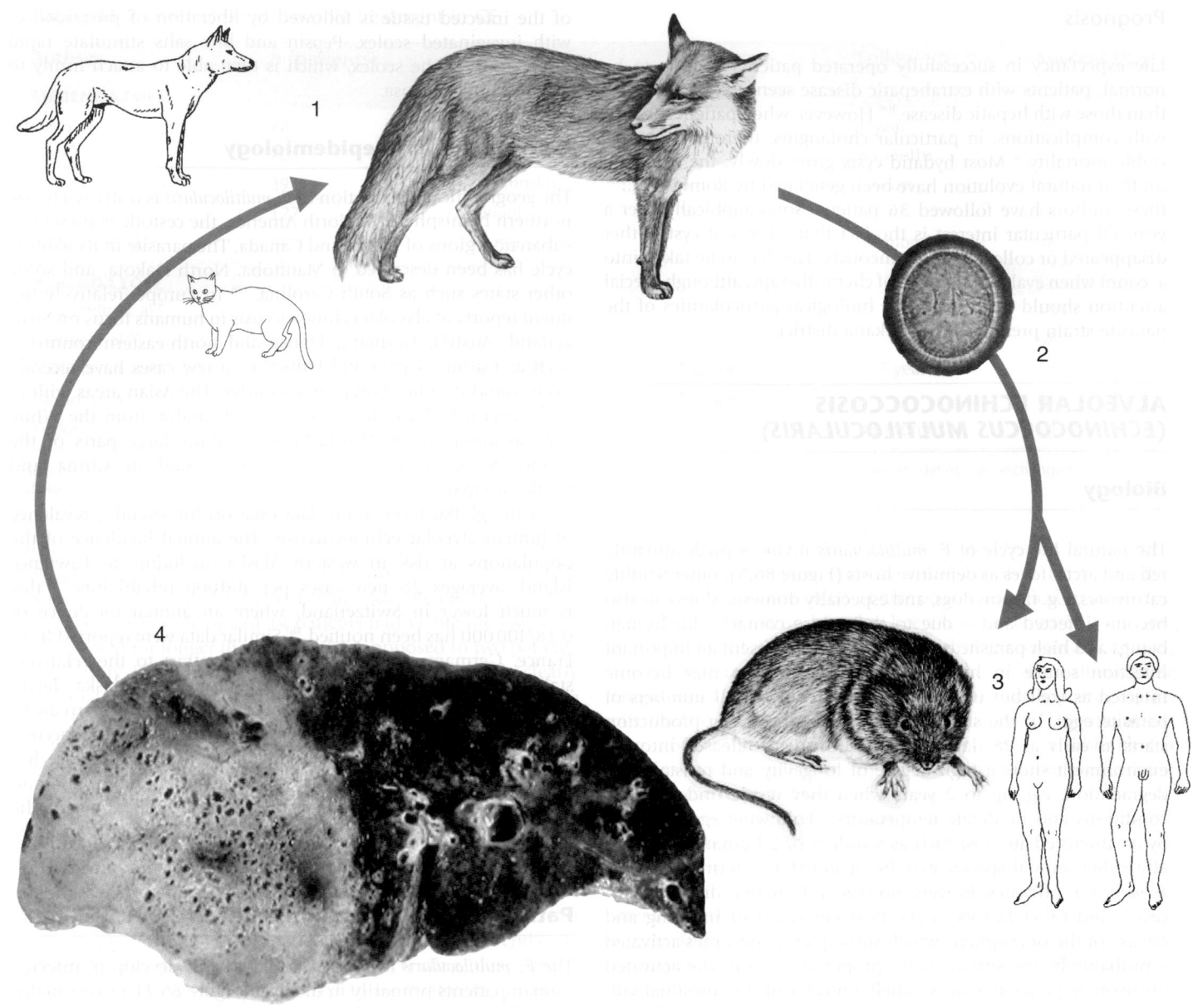

Figure 86.5 The life cycle of *E. multilocularis* involves predominantly foxes as definitive hosts (1), occasionally other carnivores such as domestic dogs or house cats. When parasite eggs (2) are ingested by a suitable intermediate host (3) including man and various rodents, the parasite metacestode will primarily become established in the liver (4). Macroscopically, the typical lesion is characterized by a dispersed mass of fibrous tissue with a multitude of interconnected vesicles ranging from a few millimetres to centimetres in size. The peroral uptake of protoscoleces-containing metacestodes by definitive hosts, e.g. when eating infected mice, terminates the life cycle.

exhibiting an early 'dying out' or 'abortion' of the metacestode (Figure 86.6).[114] Thus, after infection with *E. multilocularis*, not every person appears susceptible to unlimited metacestode proliferation and will become actual patients within 5–15 years following infection.[115] The host mechanisms modulating the course of infection are most likely of immunological nature, including primarily T cell interactions. Thus, the periparasitic granuloma, mainly composed of macrophages, myofibroblasts and T cells,

contains a large number of CD4+ T cells in patients with abortive or died-out lesions, whereas in patients with active metacestodes the number of CD8+ T cells is increased;[116] and an immunosuppressive process is assumed to downregulate the lymphoid macrophage system. Conversely, the status of cured AE is generally reflected by a high parasite antigen-specific in vitro lymphoproliferative response. The cytokine mRNA levels following *E. multilocularis* antigen stimulation of lymphocytes shows a rather

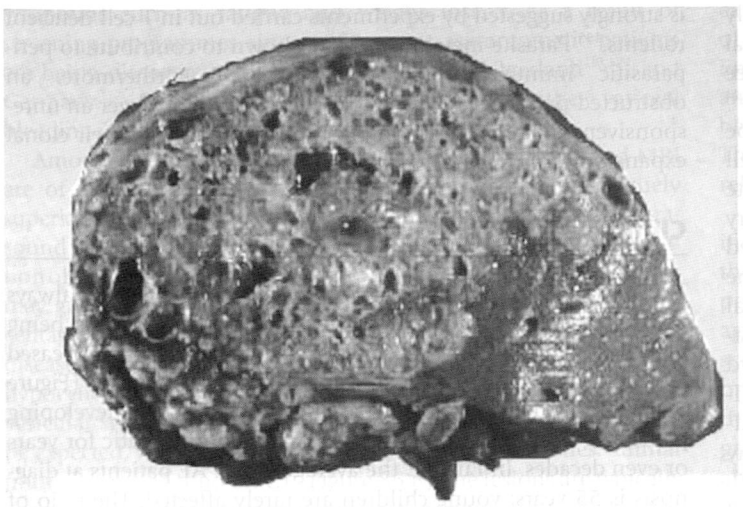
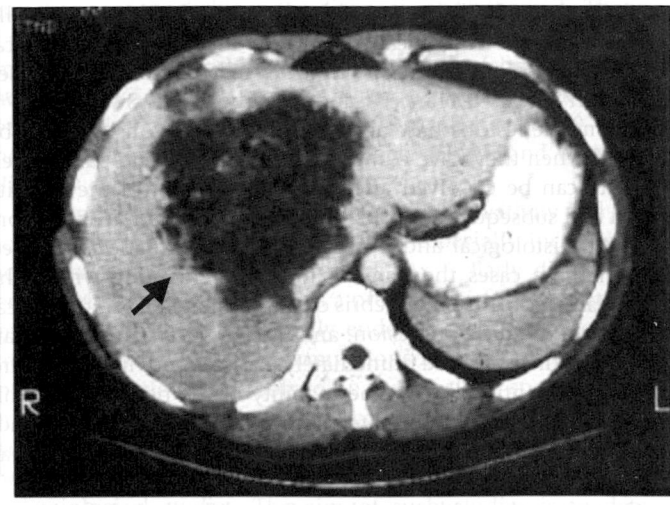
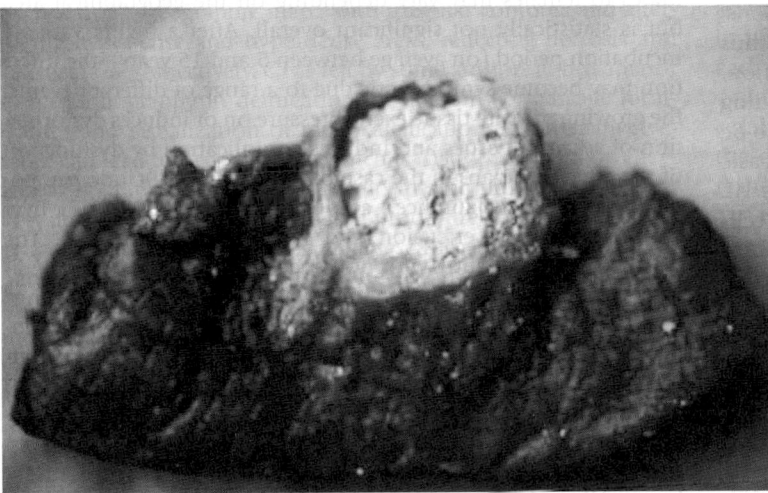
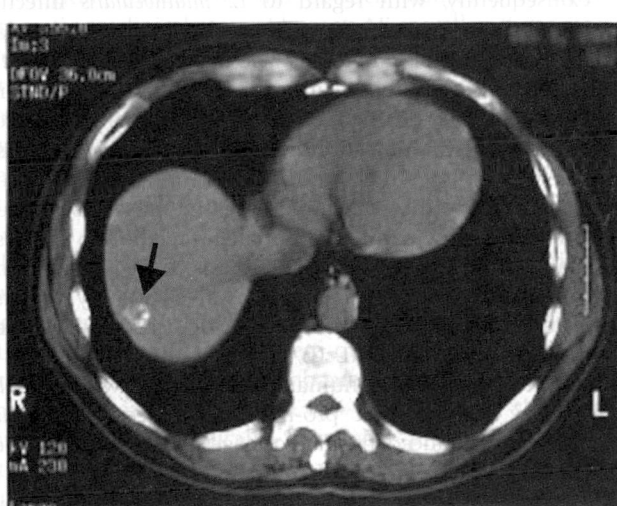

Figure 86.6 In the first row, an *E. multilocularis* active liver AE lesion is shown, while the second row presents a 'died-out' lesion. Left column: macroscopic presentation of resected and cross-sected liver lesion; right column: CT visualization of similar lesion type, parasitic mass denoted by arrow. Note in the CTs the hypodensity of the large lesions (arrow) in active AE, while the 'died-out' lesion (second row) will appear as a small fully calcified white mass (arrow).

Th2-oriented production of cell cytokine transcripts including IL-3, IL-4 and IL-10.[117] The phenomenon of immunological or constitutional resistance may be dependent upon a potential immunogenetic predisposition with the potential of an HLA-DR type association.[118,119] Conversely, lack of Th cell activity such as in advanced AIDS is associated with a rapid and unlimited growth and dissemination of the parasite in AE, as exemplified by a young AIDS patient who died from AE at the age of 6 years.[120] Chemotherapeutic restorage of CD4+ cell numbers in an AIDS patient regained control of the progression of AE by benzimidazole treatment.[121] As for *E. granulosus*, the primary site of interaction between *E. multilocularis* and its host is the mucosa of the gastrointestinal tract. Scarce information is available on the immune response against migrating and subsequently established oncospheres and their development into larvae of *E. multilocularis* in humans. Therefore, the following considerations will focus on the immune response to fully developed and progressively proliferating metacestodes. Many patients with AE respond with a marked synthesis of parasite-specific antibodies, including all isotypes of immunoglobulins. There is no evidence that specific antibodies have a direct restricting role on the growth of the metacestode. However, protoscolices and oncospheres of *E. multilocularis* can be lysed by antibody mediated complement inactivation. Antibodies appear to be involved in the rare chronic granulomatous course of the disease. In contrast to antibodies, T lymphocyte interactions appear to be of immunopathophysiological significance. The concept that T lymphocytes are the main determinant of host response is supported by different findings in animal models of alveolar echinococcosis. Thus, depletion of T cells enhances metastasis formation in mice, and in congenitally athymic nude mice. Peritoneal macrophages also contribute significantly to NO-mediated periparasitic immunosuppression.[122,123]

In 'resistant' human AE patients – as mentioned above – mass proliferation of the intrahepatic metacestode is putatively inhibited by an appropriate host immune response. The process finally

observed in 8 of 11 untreated patients; however, duration of treatment of at least 2 years is needed to observe such favourable effects, and viable material was found in patients treated for up to 48 months.[188] In contrast, in two patients treated for a short time with albendazole no growth could be observed,[180] which is in contrast to some other experience.[183] Finally, benzimidazole treatment has been found to render some patients – initially judged to be unresectable – fit for radical surgery.[191]

OTHER *ECHINOCOCCUS* SPECIES

Echinococcus vogeli

E. vogeli is maintained primarily in a silvatic predator–prey cycle which includes the bush dog and occasionally domestic dogs as definitive host and pacas as intermediate hosts. Humans are rarely infected. The metacestode of *E. vogeli* is polycystic and fluid filled, with a tendency to form multi-chambered conglomerates; the predilection site in the intermediate host is the liver. Endogenous proliferation and convolution of both germinal and laminated layers lead to the formation of secondary subdivisions of the primary vesicle, including production of brood capsules and protoscolices.[192] The geographical distribution of *E. vogeli* includes the northern half of South America.

Polycystic hydatid disease due to *E. vogeli* in humans has been reported from Argentina, Brazil, Colombia, Ecuador, Panama and Venezuela. While the most frequent primary site is the liver, primary polycystic infections have also occurred elsewhere in the abdominal cavity, in the lungs and in other thoracic organs.[193,194] Patients with polycystic echinococcosis usually present with a painful right hypochondrial mass, jaundice or an hepatic abscess, rarely with signs and symptoms of pulmonary disease – in particular cough and haemoptysis.[194] Commonly, the evolution of the disease is rather benign; recovery was reported following surgical resection, and sometimes spontaneously. Diagnostic imaging is hampered especially with regard to the differentiation from CE and AE. Laboratory tests rarely reveal eosinophilia; antibodies against homologous antigens, determined by ELISA and immunoblot, help in diagnosis.[195] In inoperable cases, albendazole yields much the same result(s) as in *E. granulosus*, with cure or improvement observed in four of six patients in a recent small series.[196]

Echinococcus oligarthrus

E. oligarthrus infects only felids (mainly the cougar, the jaguar, the ocelot, the jaguarundi and Geoffroyi's cat) as definitive hosts, with the larval stage occurring in subcutaneous muscles of large South American rodents such as agoutis and pacas. The metacestode is, like *E. vogeli*, polycystic and fluid filled. There is less subdivision into secondary chambers and the laminated layer is significantly thinner than that of *E. vogeli*. So far very few infections with larval *E. oligarthrus* have been reported in humans, e.g. in Venezuela,[197] Brazil,[198] Surinam[199] and India.[200]

Other Echinococcus species

E. equinus and *E. ortleppi* have previously been attributed to *E. granulosus* as a species, but more recent phylogenetic analyses provided evidence for an own speciation.[1] Due to their practical absence of infectivity to humans, these species will not be further presented and discussed in this chapter.

In the Qinghai-Tibet plateau, both *E. multilocularis* and *E. granulosus* are sympatrically distributed. A new species was recently isolated from the Tibetan fox, *Vulpes ferrilata*, and also found in pika, *Ochotona curzoniae*, as intermediate host.[201] Morphological, genetic and ecological features of the cestode led to designation of a new species, *Echinococcus shiquicus*. However, no infections in humans caused by *E. shiquicus* have yet been identified.

REFERENCES

1. Nakao M, McManus DP, Schantz PM, et al. A molecular phylogeny of the genus *Echinococcus* inferred from complete mitochondrial genomes. *Parasitology* 2007; 134(Pt 5):713–722.
2. Eckert J, Gemmell MA, Meslin FX, et al. *WHO/OIE Manual on Echinococcosis in Humans and Animals: a Public Health Problem of Global Concern*. Paris: WHO/OIE; 2001.
3. Campos-Bueno A, Lopez-Abente G, Andres-Cercadillo AM. Risk factors for *Echinococcus granulosus* infection: a case-control study. *Am J Trop Med Hyg* 2000; 62:329–334.
4. Attanasio E, Ferretti G, Palmas C. Hydatidosis in Sardinia: review and recommendations. *Trans R Soc Trop Med Hyg* 1985; 79:154–158.
5. Yalin R, Aktan AO, Yegen C, et al. Significance of intracystic pressure in abdominal hydatid disease. *Br J Surg* 1992; 79:1182–1183.
6. Siles-Lucas S, Gottstein B: Review: Molecular tools for the diagnosis of cystic and alveolar echinococcosis. *Trop Med Int Health* 2001; 6:463–475.
7. Ferreira AM, Irigoin F, Breijo M, et al. How *Echinococcus granulosus* deals with complement. *Parasitol Today* 2000; 16:168–172.
8. Dixon JB. Echinococcosis. *Comp Immunol Microbiol Infect Dis* 1997; 20: 87–94.
9. Ellis ME, Sinner W, Asraf AM, et al. Echinococcal disease and mycobacterial infection. *Ann Trop Med Parasitol* 1991; 85:243–251.
10. Zhang W, McManus DP. Recent advances in the immunology and diagnosis of echinococcosis. *FEMS Immunol Med Microbiol* 2006; 47:24–41.
11. Moreno-Gonzalez E, Segurola CL, et al. Liver transplantation for *Echinococcus granulosus* hydatid disease. *Transplantation* 1994; 58:797–800.
12. Gottstein B, Reichen J. Hydatid lung disease. In: Sharma OP, ed. *Tropical Lung Disease*. 2nd edn. New York: Taylor and Francis; 2006:327–350.
13. Yagmur O, Demircan O, Atilla E, et al. Cardiac tamponade due to rupture of hydatid cyst into the pericardium. *Dig Surg* 1992; 9:329–331.
14. Agarwal DK, Agarwal R, Barthwal SP. Interventricular septal hydatid cyst presenting as complete heart block. *Br Heart J* 1996; 75:266.
15. Sinha PR, Jaipuria N, Avasthey P. Intracardiac hydatid cyst and sudden death in a child. *Int J Cardiol* 1995; 51:293–295.
16. Khaldi M, Mohamed S, Kallel J, et al. Brain hydatosis: report on 117 cases. *Childs Nerv Syst* 2000; 16:765–769.
17. Benomar A, Yahyaoui M, Birouk N, et al. Middle cerebral artery occlusion due to hydatid cysts of myocardial and intraventricular cavity cardiac origin: 2 cases. *Stroke* 1994; 25:886–888.
18. Salinas JC, Torcal J, Lozano R, et al. Intracystic infection of liver hydatidosis. *Hepatogastroenterology* 2000; 47:1052–1055.
19. Kervancioglu R, Bayram M, Elbeyli L. CT findings in pulmonary hydatid disease. *Acta Radiol* 1999; 40:510–514.
20. Harris KM, Morrisl DL, Tudor R, et al. Clinical and radiographic features of simple and hydatid cysts of the liver. *Br J Surg* 1986; 73:835–838.
21. Doyle DJ, Hanbidge AE, O'Malley ME. Imaging of hepatic infections. *Clin Radiol* 2006; 61:737–748.
22. Taori K, Sanyal R, Mahajan S, et al. *Australasian Radiol* 2006; 50:298–305.
23. Bezzi M, Teggi A, De Rosa F, et al. Abdominal hydatid disease: US findings during medical treatment. *Radiology* 1987; 162:91–95.

24. Hira PR, Lindberg LG, Francis I, et al. Diagnosis of cystic hydatid disease: role of aspiration cytology. *Lancet* 1988; ii:655–657.

25. Horchani A, Nouira Y, Kbaier I, et al. Hydatid cyst of the kidney: a report of 147 controlled cases. *Eur Urol* 2000; 38:461–467.

26. Khabiri AR, Begheri F, Assmar M, et al. Analysis of specific IgE and IgG subclass antibodies for diagnosis of *Echinococcus granulosus*. *Parasite Immunol* 2006; 28:357–362.

27. Mamuti W, Sako Y, Nakao M, et al. Recent advances in characterization of Echinococcus antigen B. *Parasit Int* 2005; 55 Suppl:S57–S62.

28. Wattal C, Mohan C, Agarwal SC. Evaluation of specific immunoglobulin E by enzyme-linked immunosorbent assay in hydatid disease. *Int Arch Allergy Appl Immunol* 1987; 87:98–100.

29. Pinon JM, Poirriez J, Lepan J, et al. Value of isotypic characterization of antibodies of *Echinococcus granulosus* by enzyme-linked immuno-filtration assay. *Eur J Clin Microbiol* 1987; 6:291–295.

30. Poretti D, Felleisen E, Grimm F, et al. Differential immunodiagnosis between cystic hydatid disease and other cross-reactive pathologies. *Am J Trop Med Hyg* 1999; 60:193–198.

31. Dar FK, Buhidma MA, Kidwai SA. Hydatid false positive serological test results in malignancy. *BMJ* 1984; 288:1197.

32. Ben-Ismail R, Rouger P, Carme B, et al. Comparative automated assay of anti-P1 antibodies in acute hepatic distomiasis (fascioliasis) and in hydatidosis. *Vox Sang* 1980; 38:156–168.

33. Pfister M, Gottstein B, Cerny T, et al. Immunodiagnosis of echinococcosis in cancer patients. *Clin Microbiol Infect* 1999; 5:693–697.

34. Iacona A, Pini C, Vicari G. Enzyme-linked immunosorbent assay (ELISA) in the serodiagnosis of hydatid disease. *Am J Trop Med Hyg* 1980; 29:95–99.

35. Rigano R, Profumo E, Ioppolo S, et al. Cytokine patterns in seropositive and seronegative patients with *Echinococcus granulosus* infection. *Immunol Lett* 1998; 64:5–8.

36. Lightowlers MW, Liu D, Haralambous A, et al. Subunit composition and specificity of the major cyst fluid antigens of *Echinococcus granulosus*. *Mol Biochem Parasitol* 1989; 37:171–182.

37. Ferragut G, Ljungstrom I, Nieto A. Relevance of circulating antigen detection to follow-up experimental and human cystic hydatid infections. *Parasite Immunol* 1998; 20:541–549.

38. Stefaniak J. Fine needle aspiration biopsy in the differential diagnosis of the liver cystic echinococcosis. *Acta Trop* 1997; 67:107–111.

39. MacPherson CNL, Romig T, Zehyle E, et al. Portable ultrasound scanner versus serology in screening for hydatid cysts in a Nomadic population. *Lancet* 1987; ii:259–261.

40. Shambesh MA, Craig PS, Macpherson CN, et al. An extensive ultrasound and serologic study to investigate the prevalence of human cystic echinococcosis in northern Libya. *Am J Trop Med Hyg* 1999; 60:462–468.

41. Frider B, Larrieu E, Odriozola M. Long-term outcome of asymptomatic liver hydatidosis. *J Hepatol* 1999; 30:228–231.

42. Dziri C, Haouet K, Fingerhut A. Treatment of hydatid cyst of the liver: Where is the evidence? *World J Surg* 2004; 28:731–736.

43. Langer JC, Rose DB, Keystone JS, et al. Diagnosis and management of hydatid disease of the liver: a 15-year North American experience. *Ann Surg* 1984; 119:412–417.

44. Morel P, Robert J, Rohner A. Surgical treatment of hydatid disease of the liver: a survey of 69 patients. *Surgery* 1988; 104:859–862.

45. Elhamel A. Pericystectomy for the treatment of hepatic hydatid cysts. *Surgery* 1990; 107:316–320.

46. Behrns KE, van Heerden JA. Surgical management of hepatic hydatid disease. *Mayo Clin Proc* 1991; 66:1193–1197.

47. Khoury G, Abiad F, Geagea T, et al. Laparoscopic treatment of hydatid cysts of the liver and spleen. *Surg Endosc* 2000; 14:243–245.

48. Seven R, Berber E, Mercan S, et al. Laparoscopic treatment of hepatic hydatid cysts. *Surgery* 2000; 128:36–40.

49. Kehila M, Korbi S, Tlili K, et al. Les cholangites sclérosantes secondaires et les séquelles biliaires fibrosantes du kyste hydatique du foie. *Med Chir Dig* 1989; 18:467–476.

50. Belghiti J, Benhamou JP, Houry S, et al. Caustic sclerosing cholangitis: a complication of the surgical treatment of hydatid disease of the liver. *Arch Surg* 1986; 121:1162–1165.

51. Schaefer JW, Khan MY. Echinococcosis (hydatid disease): lessons from experience with 59 patients. *Rev Infect Dis* 1991; 13:243–247.

52. Morris DL. Pre-operative albendazole therapy for hydatid cyst. *Br J Surg* 1987; 74:805–806.

53. French CM. Mebendazole and surgery for human hydatid disease in Turkana. *East Afr Med J* 1984; 61:113–119.

54. Cobo F, Yarnoz C, Sesma B, et al. Albendazole plus praziquantel versus albendazole alone as a pre-operative treatment in intra-abdominal hydatidosis caused by Echinococcus granulosus. *Trop Med Int Health* 1998; 3:462–466.

55. Little JM, Hollands MJ, Ekberg H. Recurrence of hydatid disease. *World J Surg* 1988; 12:700–704.

56. Cangiotti L, Giulini SM, Muiesan P, et al. Hydatid disease of the liver: long-term results of surgical treatment. *J Chir* 1991; 12:501–504.

57. Akhan O, Özmen MN, Dincer A, et al. Liver hydatid disease: long-term results of percutaneous treatment. *Radiology* 1996; 198:259–265.

58. Magistrelli P, Masetti R, Coppola R, et al. Surgical treatment of hydatid disease of the liver. *Arch Surg* 1991; 126:518–523.

59. Khoury G, Abiad F, Geagea T, et al. Laparoscopic treatment of hydatid cysts of the liver and spleen. *Surg Endosc* 2000; 14:243–245.

60. Ertem M, Karahasanoglu T, Yavuz N, et al. *Arch Surg* 2002; 137:1170–1173.

61. Kayaalp C. Evacuation of hydatid liver cysts using laparoscopic trocar. *World J Surg* 2002; 26:1324–1327.

62. Alper A, Ariogul O, Emre A, et al. Choledocho-duodenostomy for intrabiliary rupture of hydatid cysts of liver. *Br J Surg* 1987; 74:243–245.

63. Xynos E, Zoras O-J L, Pechlivanidis G, et al. Intrabiliary rupture of hydatid cyst of the liver. *Dig Surg* 1990; 7:148–152.

64. Leong S, Kim YI, Gray R, et al. Endoscopic and surgical management of intrabiliary rupture of hydatid liver cyst. *Can J Gastroenterol* 1992; 6:135–139.

65. Iscan M, Duren M. Endoscopic sphincterotomy in the management of postoperative complications of hepatic hydatid disease. *Endoscopy* 1991; 23:282–283.

66. Singh V, Reddy DC, Verma GR, et al. *Liver Int* 2006; 26:621–624.

67. Safioleas M, Misiakos EP, Dosios T, et al. Surgical treatment for lung hydatid disease. *World J Surg* 1999; 23:1181–1185.

68. Novick RJ, Tchervenkov CI, Wilson JA, et al. Surgery for thoracic hydatid disease: a North American experience. *Ann Thorac Surg* 1987; 43:681–686.

69. Lone GN, Bhat MA, Ali N, et al. Minimally invasive transthoracotomy-transphrenotomy for concurrent hepatic and pulmonary hydatid disease. *Br J Surg* 2005; 92:729–733.

70. Keshmiri M, Baharvahdat H, Fattahi SH, et al. A placebo controlled study of albendazole in the treatment of pulmonary echinococcosis. *Eur Respir J* 1999; 14:503–507.

71. Miralles A, Bracamonte L, Pavie A, et al. Cardiac echinococcosis: surgical treatment and results. *J Thorac Cardiovasc Surg* 1994; 107:184–190.

72. Horchani A, Nouira Y, Kbaier I, et al. Hydatid cyst of the kidney: a report of 147 controlled cases. *Eur Urol* 2000; 38:461–467.

73. Khuroo MS, Wani NA, Javid G, et al. Percutaneous drainage compared with surgery for hepatic hydatid cysts. *N Engl J Med* 1997; 337:881–887.

74. Lewall DB, Nyak P. Hydatid cysts of the liver: two cautionary signs. *Br J Radiol* 1998; 71:37–41.

75. Filice C, Brunetti E. Use of PAIR in human cystic echinococcosis. *Acta Trop* 1997; 64:95–107.

76. Odev K, Paksoy Y, Arslan A, et al. Sonographically guided percutaneous treatment of hepatic hydatid cysts: long-term results. *J Clin Ultrasound* 2000; 28:469–478.

77. Men S, Hekimoglu B, Yucesoy C, et al. Percutaneous treatment of hepatic hydatid cysts: an alternative to surgery. *AJR* 1999; 172:83–89.

78. Ustunsoz B, Akhan O, Kamiloglu MA, et al. Percutaneous treatment of hydatid cysts of the liver: long-term results. *AJR* 1999; 172:91–96.

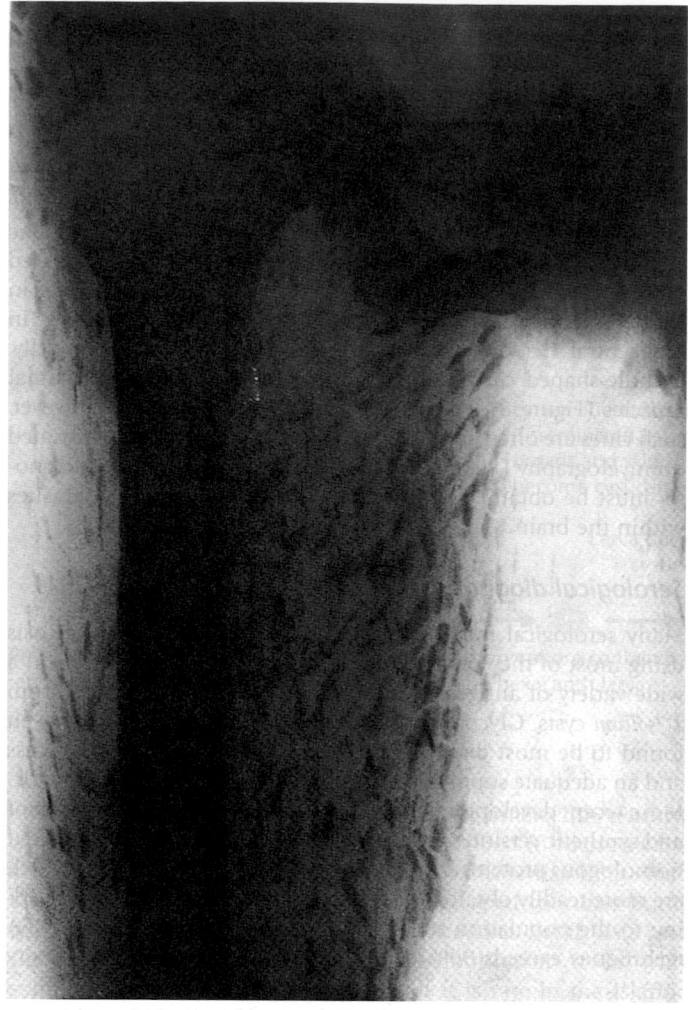

Figure 87.3 Very large numbers of calcified cysticerci in thigh muscle.

with other helminthic infections, particularly hydatidosis and taeniasis, remains a problem but has been reduced with the use of more refined antigens.[14] The detection of antibodies or antigen in the CSF in combination with conventional serology marginally improves overall sensitivity. Antigen can also be detected in the blood and declining serum levels have been associated with successful treatment.[16]

Even the simpler serological tests are a valuable clinical tool. In endemic areas, they can be used to screen epileptic and other neurological patients. Positive cases can be confirmed by imaging and may then benefit from specific treatment. In a series of 630 patients seen at neurology clinics in Zimbabwe, 12% had antibodies detected by ELISA, using a crude cyst fluid antigen. The test had a positive predictive value of 87% and a negative predictive value of 85% for active neurocysticercosis potentially amenable to treatment.[17]

Imaging

Modern imaging techniques have proved very powerful in demonstrating the presence of cysticerci in the brain and have also taught us a good deal about the natural history of the disease. A

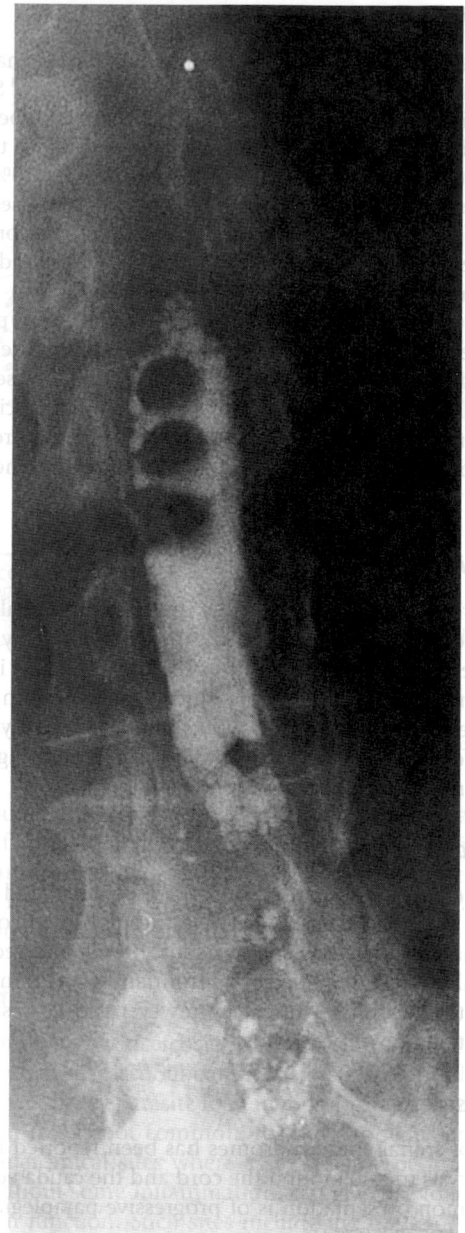

Figure 87.4 Cysticerci around the cauda equina on myelography.

number of appearances have been described on CT (Figure 87.5).

- Calcified lesions
- Small (<2 cm) hypodense lesions
- Similar hypodense lesions with a bright central spot representing the protoscolex within the cyst. This is visible in a little under half of such lesions
- Similar-sized lesions showing ring or disc enhancement. The natural history of these enhancing lesions is that they are likely to disappear from the CT image within 12 months
- Occasionally there may be much larger cysts, up to 6 cm across, in which case other cestode larvae such as hydatid and coenurosis as well as racemose cysticercosis (see below) should be considered.

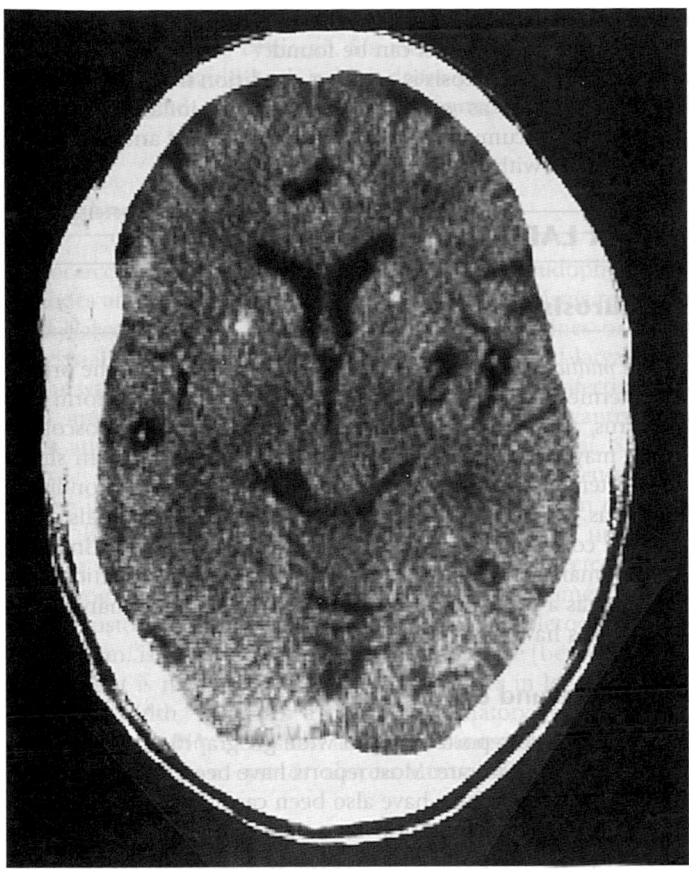

Figure 87.5 CT image of the head showing calcified and viable cerebral cysticerci, some with the protoscolex visible as a central opacity.

Similar appearances are seen with magnetic resonance imaging,[18] which is particularly valuable, as with other pathologies, in demonstrating posterior fossa and spinal lesions. It is also superior for imaging ventricular cysts which, having a similar radiodensity to CSF, are less easily visualized on CT.

Management

Until the 1980s there was no drug therapy that was known to be effective against cysticercosis. Treatment was therefore mostly symptomatic, although surgical intervention to remove cysts or to deal with their consequences, such as hydrocephalus, was sometimes appropriate. Since that time it has been shown that anthelmintics can be effective in reducing the number of cysts present on CT.[19] The extent to which this leads to clinical benefit is more problematical and the exact role of anthelmintics remains the subject of debate. In adults with parenchymal cysts demonstrated by CT which do not show significant enhancement, there is evidence of both radiographical and clinical improvement after anthelmintic treatment.[19] In almost all other groups of patients, however, information is either contradictory or lacking. Patients with calcified cysts on CT, even though they may persist in having epilepsy, are unlikely to gain any benefit from anthelmintic treatment. Markedly enhancing parenchymal lesions, which constitute

the most common appearance in children, have been shown to disappear spontaneously from the CT image within a year.[20] From this observation it has been suggested that such cases can generally be managed with symptomatic treatment and corticosteroids to reduce the local inflammatory response and that anthelmintics are unnecessary. This very benign view of childhood cysticercosis reflects experience with imported disease in North America. In contrast, reports from tropical countries have shown that a proportion of children have chronic disease and frequently relapsing symptoms; some of these develop severe neurological consequences such as hydrocephalus.[21] There is a consensus that single enhancing lesions do not require anticysticercotic treatment and that when the inflammatory response dominates the clinical picture, as in cysticercotic encephalitis, anticysticercotics are likely to exacerbate the condition in the short term and should be avoided.[22] Some recent controlled studies have shown more rapid resolution of enhancing cysts with anticysticercotics[23] but clinical benefit is more difficult to demonstrate and there remains no general agreement on the management of multiple enhancing lesions. Each case must be evaluated on its merits, but symptomatic treatment and close observation may sometimes be a reasonable approach.

The first drug to be shown to be effective was praziquantel, given at 50 mg/kg daily for 15 days.[19] Albendazole has also been studied extensively. In substantial doses (15 mg/kg daily for 30 days), it appears to have at least an equivalent effect on reducing cysts present on CT[24] and has come to be the drug of first choice. The ideal dose of both drugs remains uncertain. Eight days of albendazole appears to be of equivalent efficacy to the original 30 days[24] and has been widely adopted. Much shorter courses of praziquantel, e.g. 50 mg/kg daily for 8 days or even 3 doses of 25 mg/kg at 2-hourly intervals on a single day,[25] have been shown to be effective in small numbers of cases. These shorter courses of anthelmintics, repeated after a period of months if necessary, offer the promise of a less expensive regimen for developing countries.

The significant adverse effects of anticysticercal therapy are similar for the two drugs. They appear to be directly related to the damage inflicted on *cysticerci* and the consequent acute inflammatory response. This may result in cerebral oedema and raised intracranial pressure, particularly if there are many cysts. Typically, a severe headache arises – sometimes within a few hours of commencing therapy but more often after 2–4 days. If treated symptomatically most of these will resolve without sequelae but a minority will develop a severe acute illness with cerebral infarction, and deaths have been reported. Concomitant use of corticosteroids in substantial doses is effective in suppressing this in most (though not all) cases and is almost always appropriate. Steroids have the unwanted effect of decreasing levels of praziquantel, though not albendazole.

Surgical excision is still conventionally recommended for intraventricular cysts. Neuroendoscopic removal is now the preferred technique. Meningeal disease may require protracted steroid therapy to control arachnoiditis, as well as anticysticercotics.[22]

Control

Control of the parasite has been achieved in developed countries by the interruption of its life cycle at two points. The systematic

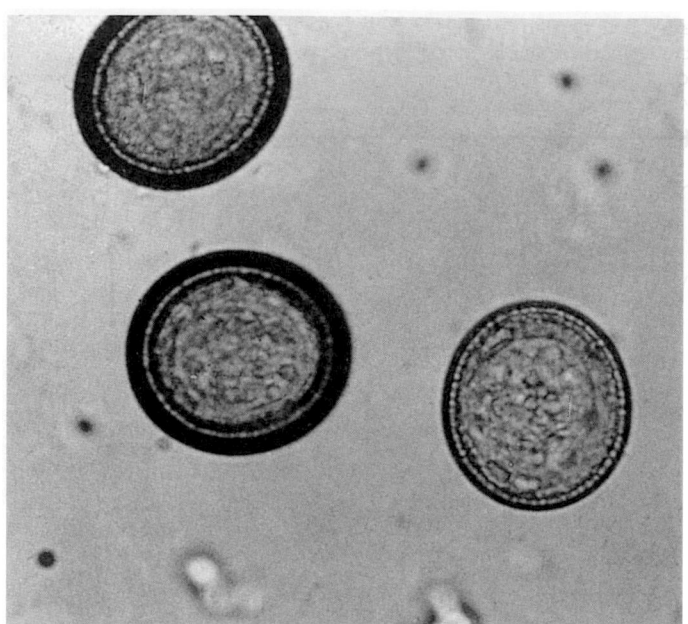

Figure 87.11 *Taenia* ova. (Courtesy of Tropical Resources Unit, Wellcome Trust.)

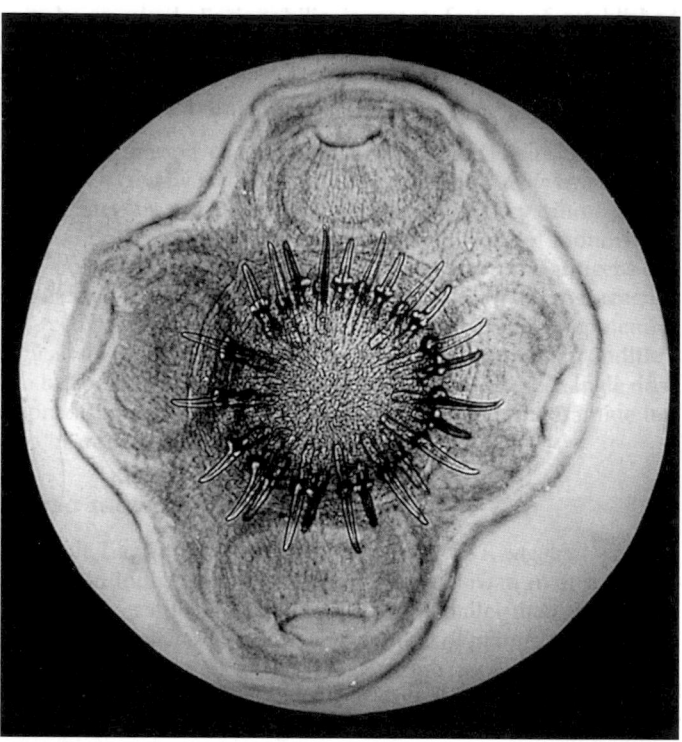

A

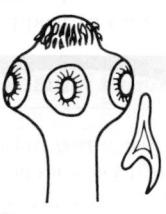

B

Figure 87.12 (A) *T. solium* (pig tapeworm) (armed tapeworm) scolex showing hooklets. (Courtesy of Tropical Resources Unit, Wellcome Trust.) (B) *T. solium* head, showing suckers and the arrangement of the hooklet.

dying worm were believed to constitute a risk of cysticercosis through internal autoinfection. No evidence has ever emerged to support this hypothesis and purgation is no longer regarded as necessary.

Hymenolepis nana

The dwarf tapeworm *H. nana* (Figure 87.13) is unique among cestodes in that the life cycle is maintained between humans without the necessity for any other host species; indeed, the same individual acts as intermediate and definitive host. Ingested ova (Figure 87.14) are activated by the gut and invade the small intestinal mucosa where they encyst within a villus. Within 3–4 days the protoscolex of this cercocyst evaginates to become the scolex of an adult worm. This attaches to the intestinal wall, the remainder of the worm developing to a mature length of 3–4 cm over about a month, after which egg production begins. Detached proglottids degenerate during passage through the intestine, releasing their cargo of ova, and are not seen in the faeces. Infections involving several hundred worms are common. Spread is by faecal–oral transmission with autoinfection, particularly amongst children, amplifying the intensity of infection. Rodents may act as an alternative definitive host and insects are capable of infection with the larval stage but neither of these appear to be important in parasite transmission.

Prevalence and distribution

H. nana is a very common parasite in warm climates where sanitation is poor, particularly in children, amongst whom the prevalence is often in the region of 2–3%.

Clinical features

A variety of symptoms have been attributed to *H. nana* infection, including abdominal pain and anorexia as well as systemic complaints such as irritability and headache. Eosinophilia is common. Several reports have associated infection with growth retardation.[40] It is difficult to be certain whether these features are truly a direct result of the parasite or whether it is acting as a marker of faecal–oral infection, insanitation and poverty, but heavy infections probably do have significant clinical consequences.

Diagnosis and treatment

Diagnosis is by detecting the characteristic ova on faecal microscopy. The cercocyst stage is in contact with the host immune system and consequently, unlike other tapeworm infections, there is a sufficiently predictable humoral response for serology to be of some diagnostic value. An enzyme linked immunosorbent assay (ELISA) has been developed with sensitivity of about 80%.[41]

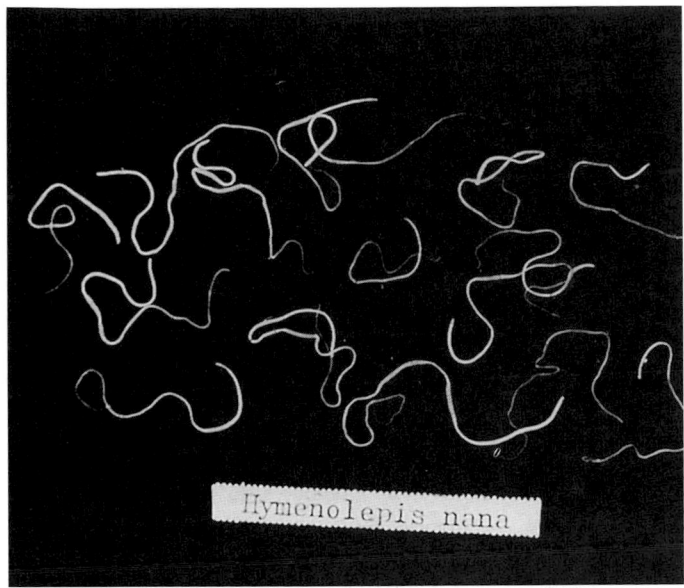

Figure 87.13 *H. nana* (dwarf tapeworm). (Courtesy of Tropical Resources Unit, Wellcome Trust.)

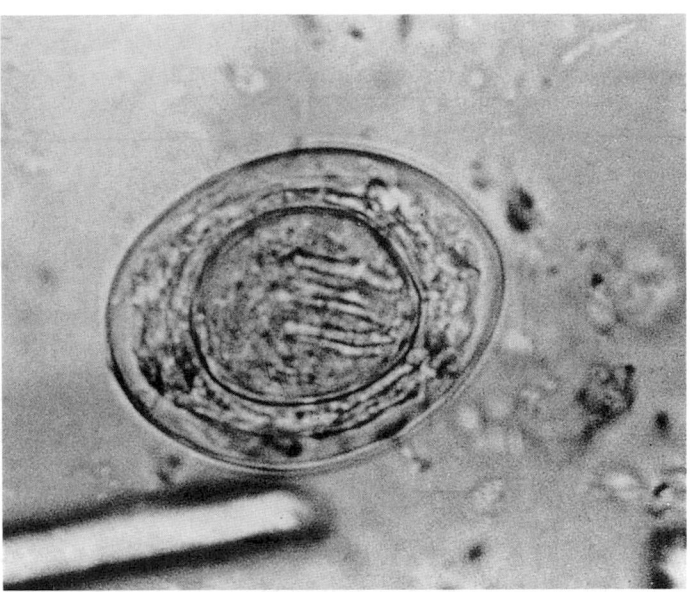

Figure 87.14 *H. nana* (dwarf tapeworm). Ovum. (Courtesy of Tropical Resources Unit.)

Table 87.1 Species of *Diphyllobothrium* infecting humans

Species	Second intermediate host	Principal definitive host	Geographical range
D. latum	Pike, perch, etc.	Man	Widespread
D. cordatum	?	Bearded seals	Greenland, Alaska
D. dalliae	Blackfish	Canines?	Alaska, Eastern Siberia
D. dendriticum	Char, salmon, trout	Gulls	Throughout sub-Arctic
D. klebanovskii	Pacific salmon	Marine mammals	Eastern Siberia
D. nihonkaiense	Pacific salmon	Marine mammals?	Japan
D. pacificum	Var. marine fish	Sea lions	Pacific South America
D. ursi	Pacific salmon	Bears	Alaska, Canada

There is extensive cross-reaction with other cestode infections. A single dose of praziquantel is effective therapy. At least 20 mg/kg is recommended. Niclosamide has also been widely used. Mebendazole only gives cure rates around 50%.

Control

As with other faecal–oral infections, control depends on sanitation and education.

Diphyllobothrium latum

Man can act as definitive host for a variety of pseudophyllidean tapeworms of the genus *Diphyllobothrium* (Table 87.1). Various tiny aquatic invertebrates, especially *Cyclops* water fleas, are the first intermediate host for these parasites (Figure 87.15). The plerocercoid larvae ascend to the apex of the aquatic food chain, with species specificity in their adaptation to particular larger fish. Definitive hosts include birds and marine and terrestrial mammals.

D. latum, the fish tapeworm, is the species adapted to humans; bears and other terrestrial carnivores may act as paratenic hosts but man is generally the host that is significant in transmission. It is a large (up to 10 m), slightly translucent tapeworm (Figure 87.16) inhabiting the small intestine where it attaches by means of two longitudinal slit-like suckers or bothria. Infections are commonly multiple and occasionally there may be more than a hundred individual worms. The largest recorded total length of *D. latum* tapeworm(s) expelled from one patient is 330 m.[42] The preferred second intermediate hosts are temperate freshwater fish, especially pike, perch and burbot.[43] Human infection is acquired by eating undercooked fish. Both freezing and cooking effectively destroy the parasite.

Prevalence and distribution

Although the disease is reported from many parts of the world, most transmission occurs in Russia. The original heartland of *D. latum* infection extended from eastern Scandinavia across

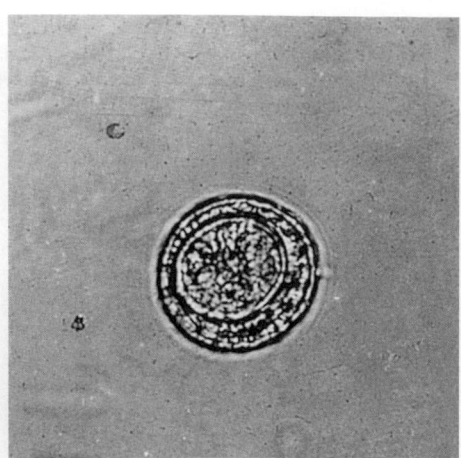

Figure 87.20 Egg of Dipylidium caninum.

proglottids the size of rice grains are passed intact in the stool; free ova (Figure 87.20) are difficult to detect. Infection is most often asymptomatic and there are no known serious consequences. Treatment is with praziquantel.

Diphyllobothrium spp

A number of species of *Diphyllobothrium* other than *D. latum* have been reported as infecting man (Table 87.1). *D. dendriticum* is the cause of human diphyllobothriasis among the indigenous people of the subarctic region where it infects salmonid fish, especially Arctic char.[43] Gulls are the most significant definitive hosts. Prevalences of 30% and more have been recorded in Canadian Inuit communities. Several other parasites infect humans around the northern Pacific, through Pacific salmon, including *D. klebanovskii* which is the principal parasite in the Russian Far East and *D. nihonkaiense* in Japan. *D. pacificum* occurs in Chile and Peru and is acquired through the consumption of the traditional dishes of marinated raw fish known as 'ceviche'. The clinical consequences of all these infections have not been well studied but are considered to be minor.

REFERENCES

1. Henneberg R. Die tierischen Parasiten des Zentralnervensystem. In: Lewandowsky M, ed. *Handbuch der Neurologie*. Berlin: Springer; 1912.
2. Mahajan RC. Geographical distribution of human cysticercosis. In: Flisser A, Willms K, Laclette JP, et al., eds. *Cysticercosis. Present State of Knowledge and Perspectives*. New York: Academic Press; 1982.
3. Gajdusek DC. Introduction of Taenia solium into west New Guinea with a note on an epidemic of burns from cysticercus epilepsy in the Ekari people of the Wissel Lakes area. *Papua New Guinea Med J* 1978; 21(4):329–342.
4. Rabiela-Cervantes MT, Rivas-Hernandez A, Rodriguez-Ibarra J, et al. Anatomopathological aspects of human brain cysticercosis. In: Flisser A, Willms K, Laclette JP, et al., eds. *Cysticercosis. Present State of Knowledge and Perspectives*. New York: Academic Press; 1982.
5. McGill RJ. Cysticercosis resembling myopathy. *Lancet* 1948; ii:728–730.
6. Medina MT, Rosas E, Rubio-Donnadieu F, et al. Neurocysticercosis as the main cause of late-onset epilepsy in Mexico. *Arch Int Med* 1990; 150(2):325–327.
7. Chopra JS, Kaur U, Mahajan RC. Cysticerciasis and epilepsy: a clinical and serological study. *Trans Roy Soc Trop Med Hyg* 1981; 75(4):518–520.
8. van As A D, Joubert J. Neurocysticercosis in 578 black epileptic patients. *S Afr Med J* 1991; 80(7):327–328.
9. Forlenza OV, Filho AH, Nobrega JP, et al. Psychiatric manifestations of neurocysticercosis: a study of 38 patients from a neurology clinic in Brazil. *J Neurol Neurosurg Psychia* 1997; 62(6):612–616.
10. Chandramuki A, Nayak P. Sub acute and chronic meningitis in children – an immunological study of cerebrospinal fluid. *Indian J Pediatr* 1990; 57(5):685–691.
11. Rangel R, Torres B, Del Bruto O, et al. Cysticercotic encephalitis: a severe form in young females. *Am J Trop Med Hyg* 1987; 36(2):387–392.
12. Chandy MJ, Rajshekhar V, Ghosh S, et al. Single small enhancing CT lesions in Indian patients with epilepsy: clinical, radiological and pathological considerations. *J Neurol Neurosurg Psychiat* 1991; 54(8):702–705.
13. Restrepo BI, Obregón-Henao A, Mesa M, et al. Characterization of the carbohydrate components of *Taenia solium* metacestode glycoprotein antigens. *Int J Parasitol* 2000; 30:689–696.
14. Bueno EC, Scheel CM, Vaz AJ, et al. Application of synthetic 8-kD and recombinant GP50 antigens in the diagnosis of neurocysticercosis by enzyme-linked immunosorbent assay. *Am J Trop Med Hyg* 2005; 72(3):278–283.
15. Espindola NM, Iha AH, Fernandes I, et al. Cysticercosis immunodiagnosis using 18- and 14-kilodalton proteins from Taenia crassiceps cysticercus antigens obtained by immunoaffinity chromatography. *J Clin Microbiol* 2005; 43(7):3178–3184.
16. Garcia HH, Parkhouse RM, Gilman RH, et al. Serum antigen detection in the diagnosis, treatment, and follow-up of neurocysticercosis patients. *Trans Roy Soc Trop Med Hyg* 2000; 94(6):673–676.
17. Mason P, Houston S, Gwanzura L. Neurocysticercosis: experience with diagnosis by ELISA serology and computerised tomography in Zimbabwe. *Cent Afr J Med* 1992; 38(4):149–154.
18. do Amaral LL, Ferreira RM, da Rocha AJ, et al. Neurocysticercosis: evaluation with advanced magnetic resonance techniques and atypical forms. *Top Magn Reson Imaging* 2005; 16(2):127–144.
19. Sotelo J, Escobedo F, Rodriguez-Carbajal J, et al. Therapy of parenchymal brain cysticercosis with praziquantel. *N Engl J Med* 1984; 310(16):1001–1007.
20. Mitchell WG, Crawford TO. Intraparenchymal cerebral cysticercosis in children: diagnosis and treatment. *Pediatrics* 1988; 82(1):76–82.
21. Lopez-Hernandez A, Garaizar C. Analysis of 89 cases of infantile cerebral cysticercosis. In: Flisser A, Willms K, Laclette JP, et al., eds. *Cysticercosis. Present state of knowledge and perspectives*. New York: Academic Press; 1982.
22. Garcia HH, Evans CA, Nash TE, et al. Current consensus guidelines for treatment of neurocysticercosis. *Clin Microbiol Rev* 2002; 15(4):747–756.
23. Del Brutto OH, Roos KL, Coffey CS, et al. Meta-analysis: Cysticidal drugs for neurocysticercosis: albendazole and praziquantel. *Ann Intern Med* 2006; 145(1):43–51.
24. Sotelo J, Del Brutto OH, Penagos P, et al. Comparison of therapeutic regimen of anticysticercal drugs for parenchymal brain cysticercosis. *J Neurol* 1990; 237(2):69–72.
25. Corona T, Lugo R, Medina R, et al. Single-day praziquantel therapy for neurocysticercosis. *N Engl J Med* 1996; 334(2):125.
26. Allan JC, Velasquez-Tohom M, Fletes C, et al. Mass chemotherapy for intestinal Taenia solium infection: effect on prevalence in humans and pigs. *Trans Roy Soc Trop Med Hyg* 1997; 91(5):595–598.
27. Sciutto E, Morales J, Martinez JJ, et al. Further evaluation of the synthetic peptide vaccine S3Pvac against Taenia solium cysticercosis in pigs in an endemic town of Mexico. *Parasitology* 2007; 134(Pt 1):129–133.
28. Jung RC, Rodriguez MA, Beaver PC, et al. Racemose cysticercus in human brain. A case report. *Am J Trop Med Hyg* 1981; 30(3):620–624.
29. Lachberg S, Thompson RC, Lymbery AJ. A contribution to the etiology of racemose cysticercosis. *J Parasitol* 1990; 76(4):592–594.
30. Templeton AC. Anatomical and geographical location of human coenurus infection. *Trop Geogr Med* 1971; 23(1):105–108.
31. Ing MB, Schantz PM, Turner JA. Human coenurosis in North America: case reports and review. *CID* 1998; 27(3):519–523.

32. Maillard H, Marionneau J, Prophette B, et al. Taenia crassiceps cysticercosis and AIDS. *AIDS* 1998; 12(12):1551–1552.

33. Holodniy M, Almenoff J, Loutit J, et al. Cerebral sparganosis: case report and review. *Rev Infect Dis* 1991; 13(1):155–159.

34. Torres JR, Noya OO, Noya BA, et al. Treatment of proliferative sparganosis with mebendazole and praziquantel. *Trans Roy Soc Trop Med Hyg* 1981; 75(6):846–847.

35. Montenegro TC, Miranda EA, Gilman R. Production of monoclonal antibodies for the identification of the eggs of Taenia solium. *Ann Trop Med Parasitol* 1996; 90(2):145–155.

36. Allan JC, Velasquez-Tohom M, Torres-Alvarez R, et al. Field trial of the coproantigen-based diagnosis of Taenia solium taeniasis by enzyme-linked immunosorbent assay. *Am J Trop Med Hyg* 1996; 54(4):352–356.

37. Fan PC, Chung WC. Taenia saginata asiatica: epidemiology, infection, immunological and molecular studies. *J Microbiol Immunol Infect* 1998; 31(2):84–89.

38. Zarlenga DS, McManus DP, Fan PC, et al. Characterization and detection of a newly described Asian taeniid using cloned ribosomal DNA fragments and sequence amplification by the polymerase chain reaction. *Experimental Parasitology* 1991; 72(2):174–183.

39. Diaz CS, Candil RA, Uribe, et al. Serology as an indicator of Taenia solium tapeworm infections in a rural community in Mexico. *Trans Roy Soc Trop Med Hyg* 1990; 84(4):563–566.

40. Khalil HM, el Shimi S, Sarwat MA, et al. Recent study of Hymenolepis nana infection in Egyptian children. *J Egypt Soc Parasitol* 1991; 21(1):293–300.

41. Castillo RM, Grados P, Carcamo C, et al. Effect of treatment on serum antibody to Hymenolepis nana detected by enzyme-linked immunosorbent assay. *J Clin Microbiol* 1991; 29(2):413–414.

42. Ostling G. Treatment of tapeworm infection with desaspidin, a new phloroglucinol derivative isolated from Finnish fern. *Am J Trop Med Hyg* 1961; 10:855–858.

43. Curtis MA, Bylund G. Diphyllobothriasis: fish tapeworm disease in the circumpolar north. *Arctic Med Res* 1991; 50(1):18–24.

44. von Bonsdorff B. *Diphyllobothriasis in man*. London: Academic Press, 1977.

45. Dupouy-Camet J, Peduzzi R. Current situation of human diphyllobothriasis in Europe. *Euro Surveill* 2004; (5):31–35.

Chapter 88

Graham B. White

Ectoparasites: Leeches and Leech Infestation, Myiasis, Jigger Fleas, Scabies, Louse Infestation

LEECHES AND LEECH INFESTATION

Geographical distribution

Land leeches are common in South-east Asia, the Pacific islands, the Indian subcontinent and South America. Aquatic leeches have a worldwide distribution.

Aetiology

Leeches that attack humans have the following position in the animal kingdom:

Phylum   Annelida
Class   Hirudinea
Order   Gnathobdellida
Family   Hirudinidae

Gnathobdellida leeches are invertebrates, having a smooth cuticle, a mouth lacking a proboscis but with three jaws, two suckers (one surrounding the mouth, the other at the posterior end) and powerful muscles, circular and longitudinal. They attach themselves by the posterior sucker, the anterior end moving about freely. When unfed, they are usually about 2.5 cm long and 5 mm thick; some are bigger. When full of blood they are dark, bloated objects.

The muscular jaws are covered with chitin and produce a characteristic triradiate wound in the skin of the victim. The mouth leads to a pharynx, with salivary glands that secrete the anticoagulant hirudin, a crop in which ingested blood can be stored, a stomach, intestine, rectum and anal pore near the posterior sucker. The excretory system consists of 17 pairs of nephridia. There is a vascular system and a nervous system.

Leeches are hermaphrodites, each one possessing testes and ovaries. The spermatozoa of one individual are deposited during copulation on the cuticle (to migrate through the tissues to reach the ovary) or into the vagina of the other member of the copulating pair. Some leeches deposit egg masses on objects submerged in water; others form a cocoon to be deposited in water or mud, from which the young hatch and attach themselves to water plants. Others carry their young until they are able to suck.

Leeches that attack humans may be divided into two classes: land leeches, which have powerful jaws that can penetrate the skin so that they can attach anywhere on the external surface of the body, and aquatic leeches, which have weak jaws and require soft tissues to feed on. They gain entrance to orifices such as the pharynx and vagina.

Land leeches

Land leeches live in the vegetation of tropical rainforests and tend to breed near springs, streams and wells frequented by cattle, horses and other vertebrates. The species noted for attacks on humans include Haemadipsa zelanica, H. sylvestris and H. picta. Land leeches attach themselves to the skin and feed; when fed, they fall off on to the ground, having remained attached for a comparatively short time.

Clinical features

The punctures made in the skin by land leeches are painless, and remain open and bleeding after the leech has gone; healing is slow. Leeches take much more blood than they need and if they remain attached, or are numerous, they can take so much that the person becomes seriously anaemic and may die from loss of blood.

Management

Leeches that attach themselves to the skin must be induced to detach; however, they must not be simply pulled off because they may then leave behind their jaws, which could become the starting point of destructive ulceration. Drops of strong salt solution, alcohol or strong vinegar applied around the mouth, or heat from a lighted match or cigarette applied to the body, will cause the leech to release its hold. The wound can then be treated with a styptic and an antiseptic agent.

Prevention

People in countries where land leeches are common should, when travelling in infested country, wear boots and trousers thick enough to prevent access by the leeches to the skin. Additional protection is afforded if the garments or the skin are treated with repellents, such as diethyl toluamide (DEET), dimethyl or dibutyl phthalate (DMP, DBP) or indalone. DEET and DBP last longer on clothing and, if applied about once every 2 weeks at the rate of 28 mL/set

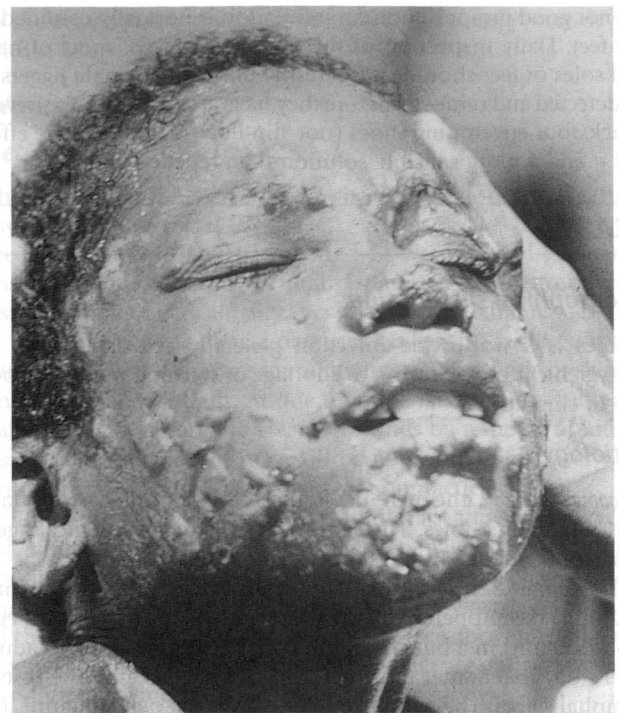

Figure 88.4 Crusted scabies. (Courtesy of P. Rotmil.)

the mote and convert the papule into a pustule. Local sensitization is followed by the appearance of a rash.

The generalized rash of scabies is an itchy erythematous rash, the distribution of which does not correspond to the site of the mites. It is a phenomenon of hypersensitivity in which it may be impossible to demonstrate mites. The eruption occurs most commonly in the axillae, around the waist, at the inner aspect of the thighs and at the back of the legs, from which it may spread all over the body. It commonly occurs in reinfection, and the number of mites present may be small.

Immunosuppression and crusted scabies

Evidence for acquired immunity to scabies comes from the finding that, in immunosuppressed persons, the mites escape control and multiply considerably, leading to encrustation of the skin, a condition known as crusted or Norwegian scabies. Steroid therapy to control undiagnosed itching may change ordinary into crusted scabies.

This is a severe type of scabies accompanied by profuse crusting and hyperkeratotic plaques (Figure 88.4). It is common in the tropics and used to be common in leprosy. Burrows are not formed and a large number of scabies mites may be present on the surface of the skin.

Scabies in children

Scabies in children is atypical. During the first year of life the lesions are general and resemble pemphigus, the buttocks and perineum being most often severely affected. Burrows are often impossible to find, and secondarily infected excoriations and scattered pustules are the most characteristic lesion (Figure 88.5).

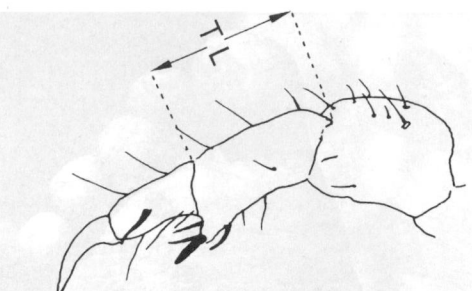

Figure 88.5 The second leg of *Pediculus*, showing the length of the tibia (TL). In *P. capitis* TL = approximately 0.3 mm, and in *P. humanus* TL = approximately 0.4 mm.

Sarcoptic mange (animal scabies)

This is sometimes contracted by people following contact with dogs, cats and cattle infested with zoonotic races of *Sarcoptes*. It may be distinguished from human scabies by the distribution of papules and vesicles on the arms, shoulders, trunks and thighs, and by the absence of burrows on the hands. Sarcoptic mange responds rapidly to treatment with ivermectin or sulphur.

Important complication: nephritis

Secondary infection of scabies lesions is very common, especially in children. Scabies infected with nephritogenic strains of β-haemolytic streptococci is an important cause of glomerulonephritis, and in some parts of the world may be a more frequent cause of nephritis than streptococcal throat infection. Secondarily infected scabies should always be treated with a course of antibiotics at the same time as antiscabetic treatment.

Differential diagnosis

Scabies in the tropics is atypical in appearance, especially in children, in whom crusted scabies may be difficult to distinguish from eczema and pyoderma. Itching is severe in scabies, in which it may be possible to identify burrows. In adults, onchocerciasis (also intensely pruritic) and lepromatous leprosy (with which scabies may co-exist) must be thought of.

Diagnosis

Scabies burrows between the fingers may be seen with a magnifying glass. After opening a burrow, the mite at the end can be extracted with a needle and examined under mineral oil. Scrapings from ulcers may reveal mites or eggs.

Management (see also Chapter 19)

All members of the family in contact with the patient should be treated at the same time. In addition to affected areas of the head, it is important to treat the whole body from the neck down. Mites are found only above the neck in infants.

Benzyl benzoate 20% emulsion should be applied from the neck down after a bath and allowed to dry, when the clothes may be put on again. After 24 h a second bath should be taken, and the clothes and bedclothes washed in the meantime. A second treatment should be given 1 week later. Crusted lesions should first be removed with a mixture of sulphur and salicylic acid. Secondary infection is treated with a 5-day course of penicillin.

NBIN emulsion concentrate consists of 68% benzyl benzoate, 6% DDT, 12% benzocaine and 14% polysorbate 80. This requires a dilution of 1:15 in water before use.

Tetmosol (tetraethylthiuram monosulphide) in a 5% solution can be used as benzyl benzoate. In soap form, it is of little value.

Crotamiton (Eurax) is applied daily for 5 days and is suitable for infants. It is more expensive but has powerful antipruritic properties.

Lotions of 0.5% malathion or 1% BHC are also effective, and sting less than benzyl benzoate.

Epidemiology and control

Human scabies waxes and wanes in incidence over 15–20-year cycles, probably as a result of changing immunity patterns. Scabies is widespread in the tropics, especially among children. Infection is associated with poor hygiene – the result of inadequate water supply.

Good personal hygiene, plus the search for and treatment of infected families, is the best form of control in the community.

Prevention is by avoidance of skin contact with infected persons and clothing. People able to wash themselves frequently do not suffer much from scabies.

LOUSE INFESTATION

Three species of louse are parasitic to humans:
- *Pediculus humanus* (body louse)
- *Pediculus capitis* (head louse)
- *Phthirus pubis* (crab louse).

Pediculus humanus and *P. capitis* are morphologically similar but have different habits. Although experimental interbreeding is possible, this does not happen in nature. The majority of lice are host specific, and although lice from domestic animals may be found on humans they do not persist. Most lice do not survive for long when removed from the host.

Pediculus humanus (body louse)

Aetiology

P. humanus is larger (0.4 mm) than *P. capitis* (0.3 mm) and there are minor morphological differences (Figures 88.5, 88.6). The female *P. humanus* sometimes attaches her eggs (nits) to body hair, but more often cements them to clothing fibres, usually along seams and folds in garments. The female lice produce an average of four to five eggs per day during their life of up to 1 month. The

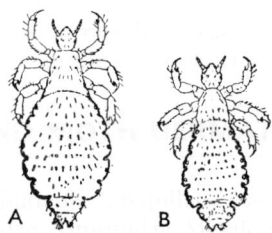

Figure 88.6 (A) Female *Pediculus humanus*. (B) Female *Pediculus capitis*.

nymphs hatch in 8 days, becoming adult after three moults in 18 days. Nymphs and adults take blood meals two to five times a day throughout life.

Transmission

Pediculus infestation is usually acquired through close contact with lousy persons, shared clothes and bedding. Lice tend to leave patients with fever and sweating, thus promoting the spread of disease. They avoid light and leave a corpse as it becomes cold.

Clinical features

Body lice cause itching and a generalized red maculopapular rash. Scratching may cause secondary infection and impetigo may result. *P. humanus* is the sole transmitter of louse-borne typhus (*Rickettsia prowazeki*), trench fever (*Bartonella quintana*) (see Chapter 49) and louse-borne relapsing fever (*Borrelia recurrentis*) (see Chapter 69).

Diagnosis

Eggs (nits) should be searched for on body hair. Adults, nymphs and eggs should be looked for in the seams and folds of clothing.

Pediculus capitis (head louse)

P. capitis females cement their eggs (nits) to the base of head hairs, and growth of the hair eventually brings the empty egg cases into view after the eggs have hatched. They are confined to the scalp.

Transmission

This is by close contact, usually head-to-head transfer.

Clinical features

Head lice seldom cause noticeable signs or symptoms, and infestation is principally a hygienic and aesthetic nuisance. In heavy infections, some dermatitis of the scalp can result from scratching. *P. capitis* is not known to be a vector for any disease.

Diagnosis

Diagnosis is by searching for the presence of 'nits' in the hair or observing the lice themselves.

Phthirus pubis (crab louse)

Crab lice occur worldwide, and are found exclusively on humans.

Aetiology

Phthirus is shorter and broader then *Pediculus* and has massive claws on the second and third legs by which it clings to hair (Figure 88.7). It is found most commonly in the genital and inguinal regions, but may be found on any of the body hair except that of the scalp, including the beard, chest hair and eyelashes. It cannot survive off the host for more than 24 h.

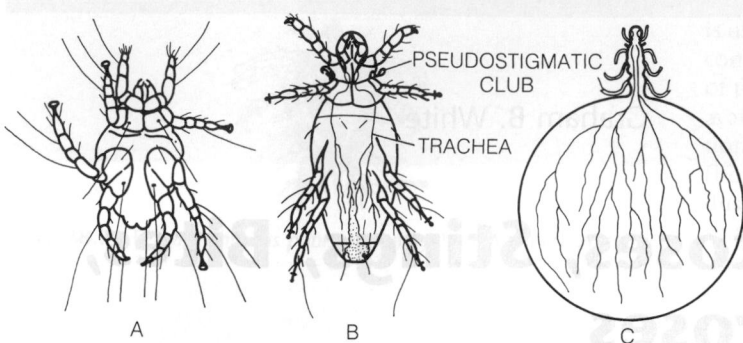

Figure 89.1 *Pyemotes tritici*. (A) Male. (B) Female. (C) Pregnant female with brood sac (×80).

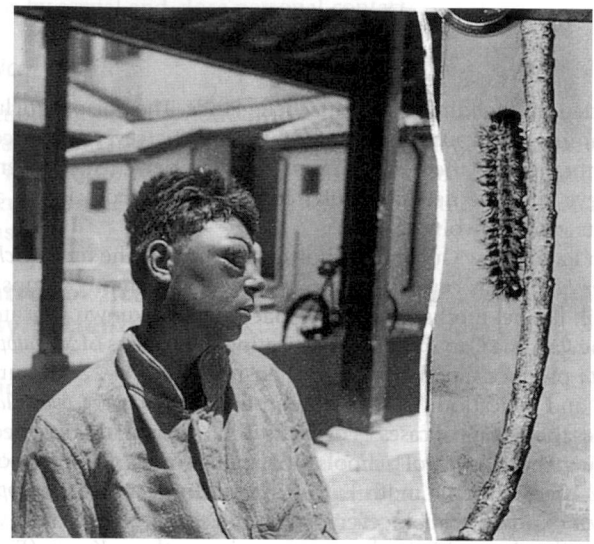

Figure 89.2 Urticating dermatitis caused by contact with a processionary caterpillar of the moth *Thaumetopoea wilkinsoni*.

dockers unloading ships' cargoes have developed dyspnoea and erucic stomatitis from the inhalation and ingestion of detached hairs.

The family Meloidae contains some species known as blister beetles because their body fluids contain cantharidin, a cytotoxic principle that causes vesicular dermatitis when applied to the skin. The best known species is the so-called Spanish fly *Lytta vesicatoria*, and in India *Mylabris cichorii* and *Epicauta hirticornis* are troublesome. In the Gilbert Islands, severe blistering is caused by the coconut beetles *Sessinia collaris* and *Ananca decolor* of the family Oedemeridae. The bushmen of South Africa use body fluids from the larvae of the *chrysomelid* beetle *Diamphidia nigroornata* as a lethal arrow poison, which causes death from a general paralysis. *Staphylinid* beetles of the genus *Paederus* cause urticaria and blistering, and minute species of the genera *Atheta* and *Oxytelus* fly in numbers and may enter the eye, causing a burning sensation.

OTHER INSECTS

Other insects that cause dermatitis are *ceratopogonid* flies (biting midges) of the genus *Culicoides*. In Brazil *C. paraensis* is a public health problem in this way, and in El Salvador an increase in biting *Culicoides* was correlated with decreasing standards of sanitation and the cessation of a control campaign against the breeding sites of the mosquito *Aedes aegypti*. In Japan there are records of eczema following the bites of *C. erairai*, and long-lasting sores (3–4 months) following bites by *C. obsoletus*. Mosquito bites in persons sensitized to their saliva can cause troublesome chronic ulcers which will respond dramatically to topical steroids. Sandflies and black flies can similarly cause quite severe reactions in sensitized persons which will respond fairly readily to steroid ointment such as betamethasone valerate. An irritant vesicular rash, superficially resembling scabies, can be caused by *Thysanoptera* (see also Appendix IV).

BEE AND WASP STINGS

The stings of bees, wasps and hornets may produce a mild reaction that is easily soothed with an ice-pack, diluted vinegar or antihistamine ointment. They may be very serious in the case of multiple stinging or stings in the mouth. Some people react violently to bee stings and may become increasingly hypersensitive with each successive sting. In such cases anaphylaxis may result, which can be fatal. Massive anaphylaxis causes muscular paralysis and suggests a curare-like action on synapses of muscle end-plates. The antidote is an injection of adrenaline (epinephrine).

People who are extremely sensitive to bee stings should always have access to a pressurized bronchodilator spray and use two puffs while breathing in; this procedure can be repeated in 15 min. Such patients, however, may quickly become faint and lose consciousness, and should be taken immediately into medical care.[4,5]

Bee and wasp venoms contain histamine, acetylcholine and enzymes (phospholipase A and hyaluronidase); the more superficial aspects of a sting are due to the histamine. The Africa honey bee *Apis mellifica adansonii* is abundant in equatorial and warm temperate southern Africa, and is a fairly aggressive species. In 1956 this species was introduced into South America and hybridization with local bees has produced an extremely aggressive race of Brazilian honey bees. The spread of these bees has been very rapid from South America to the USA. A number of fatalities has resulted from the abundance and special behavioural characteristics of the bee. The slightest disturbance near the hive can cause hundreds of bees to become air-borne; they may then sting any animal or human within 100 m of the apiary and may pursue fleeing victims for over 1 km.[6,7]

In the honey bee, the sting is torn out by the act of stinging, but the poison gland (which is attached to the sting) continues to inject venom into the wound. For this reason, the sting should be carefully removed as soon as possible and the remaining venom expressed from the gland with forceps.

Sometimes, stingless social bees (*Melipona*, etc.) are prone to aggressive mass biting, and some neotropical species squirt caustic fluid, but these insects are rarely more than a nuisance. Some tiny stingless sweat bees (*Trigona*) can be annoying in the African savannah regions and, because of their numbers and persistence, are sometimes mistaken for *Simulium* (black flies).

Wasps (*Vespula*) and hornets (*Vespa*) can sting repeatedly because, unlike the honey bee, the sting is not torn out by the action of stinging. Wasp venom contains a higher proportion of histamine and 5-hydroxytryptamine (serotonin), which is distinctly more active than that of the honey bee. *Scleroderma nipponensis* (Bethylidae), in one incident in Japan, attacked 340 people, who were left with reddish swellings and injuries leading to suppuration and lymphangitis. Some parasitic wasps of the family Ichneumonidae, such as *Ophion*, *Netelia* and *Ichneumon*, can inflict painful stings. Sensitive patients may be ill for some weeks following these stings.

Paper-wasps of the genus *Polistes* also cause many fatalities in the New World. These wasps build their nests under the eaves of houses or in ornamental shrubs and trees where people are likely to be exposed to their stings.

Arthropod venoms are considered in Chapter 31, and by Beard[8] and Bucherl and Buckley.[9]

POISONOUS HONEY

Occasionally, the honey produced by hive bees, wild honey bees, bumble-bees and stingless bees may be toxic if particular plants are foraged or if polluted liquid resources are used in the absence of clean drinking water (which should be provided in the case of honey bees).

ANTS

Ants can bite, sting and squirt formic acid. Mostly, the attacks of ants produce only mild effects, but, as in wasps, the stinging apparatus is a modified ovipositor that can be extracted after each sting and used repeatedly; multiple stinging may induce an anaphylactic response. Some ants may also be mechanical transmitters of disease; for example, Pharaoh's ants (*Monomorium pharaonis*) have been found to carry *Salmonella*, *Pseudomonas*, *Staphylococcus*, *Streptococcus* and *Clostridium* spp.[10]

The venom of ants is largely proteinaceous but in the southeastern USA, *Solenopsis richteri* is a dangerous fire ant in which the venom is non-proteinaceous and exhibits necrotic activity resembling the bites of *Loxosceles* spiders. When a colony is disturbed, the ants erupt in thousands and 3000–5000 stings may be administered in a matter of seconds. Allergic reactions to such stings, and anaphylactic shock, may sometimes result in the death of sensitive individual. This subject is reviewed elsewhere, by Gurney.[11]

OTHER BITES AND ALLERGIES

Skin reactions of both immediate and delayed hypersensitivity type were common following the bite of *Triatoma infestans* and *T. maxima* in Brazil, where the former was the major human-biting triatomid (*Hemiptera*). The reactions were sufficiently severe to prevent the use of these bugs for xenodiagnosis.[12]

Other orders that contain insects capable of inflicting bites or stings include other *Hemiptera* (plant bugs) and some *Orthoptera*. Chicken bugs in Mexico (*Haematosiphon inodorus*) and Brazil (*Ornithocoris toledo*) attack poultry, but may incidentally bite humans and may produce a polymorphous dermatitis with pustules, scabs and linear scars. The bite of the giant water-bugs (*Belostomatidae*) may be nearly as severe as a bee sting. Many other bugs will bite if handled incautiously. The larger coreid and pentatomid bugs can squirt a jet of irritant fluid from the metathoracic glands into the eye of the beholder, which may cause a very painful reaction for a day or two.

The bites of several insects not mentioned above may also produce allergic reactions. Recorded cases involve adult flies of the rhagionid genus *Symphoromyia* and larvae of *Therevidae*[13] and *Tabanidae*[14] (*Diptera*), and the possibility of such reactions following the bite of almost any insect must be considered; if possible, suspected specimens should be collected and identified by a specialist.

In addition to bites, other allergic reactions are not uncommon. Inhalant allergens may be acquired from acarine sources in house dust (especially from *Dermatophagoides pteronyssinus*) or among stored products from the grain weevil *Sitophilus granarius* or the Mexican bean weevil *Zabrotes subfasciatus*.

Some aquatic insects such as *Ephemeroptera* and *Trichoptera* emerge in vast numbers, and their cast exuviae are fragmented and wind-borne and become inhalant allergens. Chironomidae ('green nimitti') have also been associated with asthma and other allergic symptoms along the Nile.[15] Terrestrial counterparts that cause similar allergies are the prolific aphids.

Allergic reactions to the bites and stings of insects and other arthropods have been considered by Frazier[16] and Frazier and Brown.[17] Tu[18] has surveyed the whole field of arthropod poisons, allergens and venoms.

For the identification of arthropods of medical importance, Lane and Crosskey[19] should be consulted.

NEUROSES

Many people have a morbid fear of insects. The extreme manifestation of this is in delusory parasitosis (Ekbom's syndrome), also loosely referred to as parasitophobia, acarophobia or entomophobia. In these cases, patients suffering from dermatitis artefacta, usually of emotional origin, believe that they are infested with insects or other parasites which cause the itching. They then scratch the affected parts until the skin breaks down. Further skin damage may be caused by the overuse of disinfectants or insecticides. Such cases are difficult, and best treated by a psychiatrist, but every effort should be made to establish that there are in fact no minute biting insects such as *Culicoides* or allergen-producing mites or insects, particularly of the type bearing or shedding